DATE DUE

CASARETT AND DOULL'S
TOXICOLOGY
THE BASIC SCIENCE OF POISONS

What is there that is not poison?
All things are poison and nothing (is)
without poison. Solely the dose
determines that a thing is not a poison.

Paracelsus
(1493–1541)

NOTICE

Medicine is an ever-changing science. As new research and clinical experience broaden our knowledge, changes in treatment and drug therapy are required. The authors and the publisher of this work have checked with sources believed to be reliable in their efforts to provide information that is complete and generally in accord with the standards accepted at the time of publication. However, in view of the possibility of human error or changes in medical sciences, neither the authors nor the publisher nor any other party who has been involved in the preparation or publication of this work warrants that the information contained herein is in every respect accurate or complete, and they disclaim all responsibility for any errors or omissions or for the results obtained from use of the information contained in this work. Readers are encouraged to confirm the information contained herein with other sources. For example and in particular, readers are advised to check the product information sheet included in the package of each drug they plan to administer to be certain that the information contained in this work is accurate and that changes have not been made in the recommended dose or in the contraindications for administration. This recommendation is of particular importance in connection with new or infrequently used drugs.

CASARETT AND DOULL'S
TOXICOLOGY
THE BASIC SCIENCE OF POISONS

Seventh Edition

EDITOR

Curtis D. Klaassen, Ph.D.

University Distinguished Professor and Chair
Department of Pharmacology, Toxicology, and Therapeutics
University of Kansas Medical Center
Kansas City, Kansas

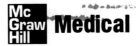
McGraw Hill Medical

New York   Chicago   San Francisco   Lisbon   London   Madrid   Mexico City
New Delhi   San Juan   Seoul   Singapore   Sydney   Toronto

Casarett and Doull's Toxicology: The Basic Science of Poisons

3   4   5   6   7   8   9   0   CCI/CCI   12   11   10

ISBN 978-0-07-147051-3
MHID 0-07-147051-4

This book was set in Times Roman by Aptara, Inc.
The editors were James F. Shanahan and Christie Naglieri.
The production supervisor was Sherri Souffrance.
Project management was provided by Aptara, Inc.
The cover designer was Janice Bielawa.
Cover photo: Macrophage and asbestos. Credit: VEM/Photo Researchers, Inc.
Courier Kendalville was printer and binder.

This book is printed on acid-free paper.

Library of Congress Cataloging-in-Publication Data

Casarett and Doull's toxicology: the basic science of poisons/editor, Curtis D. Klaassen. – 7th ed.
    p. ; cm.
Includes bibliographical references and index.
ISBN-13: 978-0-07-147051-3 (hardcover : alk. paper)
ISBN-10: 0-07-147051-4 (hardcover : alk. paper)
1. Toxicology. I. Casarett, Louis J. II. Klaassen, Curtis D. III. Title: Toxicology : the basic science of poisons.
[DNLM: 1. Poisoning. 2. Poisons. QV 600 C335 2007]
RA1211.C296 2007
615.9–dc22   2007015656

CONTENTS

See color insert between pages 760 and 761

CONTRIBUTORS

Michael Aschner, Ph.D.
Gray E.B. Stahlman Chair in Neuroscience
Professor of Pediatrics and Pharmacology
and Senior Investigator of the Kennedy Center
Vanderbilt University
Nashville, Tennessee
Chapter 16

S. Satheesh Anand, Ph.D.
Research Toxicologist
DuPont Haskell Laboratory for Health and Environmental Sciences
Newark, Delaware
Chapter 24

John C. Bloom, V.M.D., Ph.D.
Executive Director
Distinguished Medical Fellow, Diagnostic
  and Experimental Medicine
Eli Lilly and Company
Indianapolis, Indiana
Chapter 11

William K. Boyes, Ph.D.
Neurotoxicology Division
National Health and Environmental Effects Research Laboratory
Office of Research and Development
U.S. Environmental Protection Agency
Durham, North Carolina
Chapter 17

John T. Brandt, M.D.
Medical Fellow II
Diagnostic and Experimental Medicine
Eli Lilly and Company
Indianapolis, Indiana
Chapter 11

James V. Bruckner, Ph.D.
Department of Pharmaceutical and Biomedical Sciences
College of Pharmacy
University of Georgia
Athens, Georgia
Chapter 24

George A. Burdock, Ph.D., D.A.B.T., F.A.C.N.
President, Burdock Group
Vero Beach, Florida
Chapter 30

Louis R. Cantilena Jr.
Professor of Medicine and Pharmacology
Director, Division of Clinical Pharmacology and Medical Toxicology
Uniformed Services University
Bethesda, Maryland
Chapter 32

Charles C. Capen, D.V.M., M.Sc., Ph.D.
Distinguished University Professor
The Ohio State University
Department of Veterinary Biosciences
Columbus, Ohio
Chapter 21

Luis G. Costa, Ph.D.
Professor, Department of Environmental
and Occupational Health Sciences
University of Washington
Seattle, Washington
Chapter 22

Daniel L. Costa, Sc.D.
National Program Director for Air Research
Office of Research and Development
Environmental Protection Agency
Research Triangle Park,
North Carolina
Chapter 28

Robert T. Di Giulio, Ph.D.
Professor, Nicholas School of the Environment and Earth Sciences
Duke University
Durham, North Carolina
Chapter 29

David L. Eaton, Ph.D.
Professor of Environmental and Occupational Health Sciences
  and Public Health Genetics
School of Public Health and Community Medicine
and Associate Vice Provost for Research
University of Washington
Seattle, Washington
Chapter 2

Elaine M. Faustman
Professor and Director
Institute for Risk Analysis and Risk Communication
Department of Environmental and Occupational Health Sciences
University of Washington
Seattle, Washington
Chapter 4

Paul M. D. Foster, Ph.D.
National Toxicology Program
National Institute of Environmental Health Sciences
Research Triangle Park, North Carolina
Chapter 20

Donald A. Fox, Ph.D.
Professor of Vision Sciences, Biology and
   Biochemistry, and Pharmacology
University of Houston
Houston, Texas
Chapter 17

Michael A. Gallo, Ph.D.
UMDNJ-Robert Wood Johnson Medical School
Piscataway, New Jersey
Chapter 1

Steven G. Gilbert, Ph.D., D.A.B.T.
Director, Institute of Neurotoxicology and Neurological Discoders
   (INND)
Affilate Associate Professor
Department of Environmental and Occupational Health Sciences
University of Washington
Seattle, Washington
Chapter 2

Robert A. Goyer, M.D.
Professor Emeritus Department of Pathology
University of Western Ontario
London, Ontario, Canada
Chapter 23

L. Earl Gray, Jr. Ph.D.
NHEERL Reprotoxicology Division Endocrinology Branch
U.S. Environmental Protection Agency
Research Triangle Park, North Carolina
Chapter 20

Zoltán Gregus, M.D., Ph.D., D.Sc., D.A.B.T.
Department of Pharmacology and Therapeutics
Toxicology Section
University of Pécs, Medical School
Pécs, Hungary
Chapter 3

Naomi H. Harley, Ph.D.
New York University School of Medicine
Department of Environmental Medicine
New York, New York
Chapter 25

George R. Hoffman, Ph.D.
Professor, Department of Biology
College of Holy Cross
Worcester, Massachusetts
Chapter 9

Michael P. Holsapple, Ph.D., F.A.T.S.
Executive Director
ILSI Health and Environmental Sciences Institute (HESI)
Washington DC
Chapter 12

Hartmut Jaeschke, Ph.D.
Professor, Department of Pharmacology, Toxicology and Therapeutics
University of Kansas Medical Center
Kansas City, Kansas
Chapter 13

Lisa M. Kamendulis, Ph.D.
Assistant Professor
Department of Pharmacology and Toxicology
Indiana University School of Medicine
Indianapolis, Indiana
Chapter 8

Norbert E. Kaminski, Ph.D.
Professor, Pharmacology & Toxicology
Director, Center for Integrative Toxicology
Michigan State University
East Lansing, Michigan
Chapter 12

Y. James Kang, D.V.M., Ph.D., F.A.T.S.
Professor, Departments of Medicine, and Pharmacology and Toxicolgy
University of Louisville School of Medicine
Louisville, Kentucky
Chapter 18

Barbara L. Faubert Kaplan, Ph.D.
Assistant Professor
Center for Integrative Toxicology
Michigan State University
East Lansing, Michigan
Chapter 12

Robert J. Kavlock, Ph.D.
National Health and Environmental Effects Research Laboratory
United States Environmental Protection Agency
Research Triangle Park, North Carolina
Chapter 10

James E. Klaunig, Ph.D.
Robert B. Forney Professor of Toxicology;
Director, Center for Environmental Health;
Associate Director, IU Cancer Center,
School of Medicine, Indiana University
Indianapolis, Indiana
Chapter 8

Frank N. Kostonis, Ph.D.
Department of Food Microbiology and Toxicology
Food Research Institute, University of Wisconsin
Madison, Wisconsin
Chapter 30

Jerold A. Last, Ph.D.
Professor, Department of Pulmonary and Critical Care Medicine
University of California
Davis, California
Chapter 15

Lois D. Lehman-McKeeman, Ph.D.
Distinguished Research Fellow
Discovery Toxicology
Bristol-Myers Squibb Company
Princeton, New Jersey
Chapter 5

Jie Liu, Ph.D.

Staff Scientist, Inorganic Carcinogenesis
Laboratory of Comparative Carcinogenesis
National Cancer Institute at NIEHS
Research Triangle Park, North Carolina
Chapter 23

Theodora M. Mauro, M.D.

Associate Professor in Residence and Vice Chairman
Department of Dermatology
University of California, San Francisco; and
    Service Chief, Department of Dermatology
VA Medical Center San Francisco
San Francisco, California
Chapter 19

Virginia C. Moser, Ph.D., D.A.B.T.

Toxicologist, Neurotoxicology Division
National Health and Environmental Effects Research Laboratory
US Enviromental Protection Agency
Research Triangle Park, North Carolina
Chapter 16

Michael D. Newman, Ph.D.

Professor of Marine Science
School of Marine Science
College of William and Mary
Gloucester Point, Virginia
Chapter 29

Stata Norton, Ph.D.

Emeritus Professor
Department of Pharmacology, Toxicology and Therapeutics
University of Kansas Medical Center
Kansas City, Kansas
Chapter 27

Brian W. Ogilvie, B.A.

Director of Drug Interactions
XenoTech, LLC
Lenexa, Kansas
Chapter 6

Gilbert S. Omenn, M.D., Ph.D.

Professor of Internal Medicine
Human Genetics, Public Health and Computational Biology
University of Michigan
Ann Arbor, Michigan
Chapter 4

Andrew Parkinson, Ph.D.

Chief Executive Officer
XenoTech, LLC
Lenexa, Kansas
Chapter 6

Martin A. Philbert, Ph.D.

Professor and Senior Associate Dean for Research
University of Michigan School of Public Health
Ann Arbor, Michigan
Chapter 16

Kent E. Pinkerton, Ph.D.

Professor, Center for Health and the Environment
University of California
Davis, California
Chapter 15

Alphonse Poklis, Ph.D.

Professor of Pathology
Director of Toxicology
Department of Pathology
Virginia Commonwealth University
Chapter 31

R. Julian Preston, Ph.D.

Associate Director for Health, National Health and
    Environmental Effects Laboratory
U.S. Environmental Protection Agency
Research Triangle Park
North Carolina
Chapter 9

Rudy J. Richardson, S.D., D.A.B.T.

Professor of Toxicology
Department of Environmental Health Sciences
School of Public Health
University of Michigan
Ann Arbor, Michigan
Chapter 16

Robert H. Rice, Ph.D.

Professor, Department of Environmental Toxicology
University of California, Davis
Davis, California
Chapter 19

John M. Rogers, Ph.D.

Chief
Developmental Biology Branch
Reproductive Toxicology Division
National Health and Environmental Effects Research Laboratory
Office of Research and Development
U.S. Environmental Protection Agency
Research Triangle Park, North Carolina
Chapter 10

Rick G. Schnellmann, Ph.D.

Professor and Chair
Department of Pharmaceutical Sciences
Medical University of South Carolina
Charleston, South Carolina
Chapter 14

Danny D. Shen, Ph.D.

Professor, Department of Pharmacy and Pharmaceutics
School of Pharmacy
University of Washington
Seattle, Washington
Chapter 7

Peter S. Thorne, Ph.D.

Professor and Director Environmental Health Sciences Research Center
The University of Iowa
Iowa City, Iowa
Chapter 33

Laura S. Van Winkle, Ph.D.

Associate Adjunct Professor
Department of Anatomy
Physiology and Cell Biology, School of Veterinary Medicine; and
    Center for Health and the Environment
University of California at Davis
Davis, California
Chapter 15

Michael P. Waalkes, Ph.D.
Chief Inorganic Carcinogenesis Section
Laboratory of Comparative Carcinogenesis
National Cancer Institute at the National Institue of Environmental
    Health Sciences
Research Triangle Park, North Carolina
Chapter 23

D. Alan Warren, M.P.H., Ph.D.
Program Director
Environmental Health Science
University of South Carolina Beaufort
Beaufort, South Carolina
Chapter 24

John B. Watkins III, Ph.D., D.A.B.T.
Assistant Dean and Director
Professor of Pharmacology and Toxicology
Medical Sciences Program
Indiana University School of Medicine
Bloomington, Indiana
Chapter 26

Hanspeter R. Witschi, M.D., D.A.B.T., F.A.T.S.
Professor of Toxicology
Institute of Toxicology and Environmental Health and Department of
    Molecular Biosciences
School of Veterinary Medicine
University of California
Davis, California
Chapter 15

PREFACE

The seventh edition of *Casarett and Doull's Toxicology: The Basic Science of Poisons*, as the previous six, is meant to serve primarily as a text for, or an adjunct to, graduate courses in toxicology. Because the six previous editions have been widely used in courses in environmental health and related areas, an attempt has been made to maintain those characteristics that make it useful to scientists from other disciplines. This edition will again provide information on the many facets of toxicology, especially the principles, concepts, and modes of thoughts that are the foundation of the discipline. Mechanisms of toxicity are emphasized. Research toxicologists will find this book an excellent reference source to find updated material in areas of their special or peripheral interests.

The overall framework of the seventh edition is similar to the sixth edition. The seven units are "General Principles of Toxicology" (Unit 1), "Disposition of Toxicants" (Unit 2), "Non-Organ-Directed Toxicity" (carcinogenicity, mutagenicity, and teratogenicity) (Unit 3), "Target Organ Toxicity" (Unit 4), "Toxic Agents" (Unit 5), "Environmental Toxicology" (Unit 6), and "Applications of Toxicology" (Unit 7).

This edition reflects the marked progress made in toxicology during the last few years. For example, the importance of apoptosis, cytokines, growth factors, oncogenes, cell cycling, receptors, gene regulation, transcription factors, signaling pathways, transgenic animals, "knock-out" animals, polymorphisms, microarray technology, genomics, proteonomics, etc., in understanding the mechanisms of toxicity are included in this edition. More information on environmental hormones is also included. References in this edition include not only traditional journal and review articles, but, internet sites also. (Readers who would like a Power-Point version of the figures and tables can obtain the same from the publisher.)

The editor is grateful to his colleagues in academia, industry, and government who have made useful suggestions for improving this edition, both as a book and as a reference source. The editor is especially thankful to all the contributors, whose combined expertise has made possible a volume of this breadth. I especially recognize John Doull, the original editor of this book, for his continued support.

PREFACE TO THE FIRST EDITION

This volume has been designed primarily as a textbook for, or adjunct to, courses in toxicology. However, it should also be of interest to those not directly involved in toxicologic education. For example, the research scientist in toxicology will find sections containing current reports on the status of circumscribed areas of special interest. Those concerned with community health, agriculture, food technology, pharmacy, veterinary medicine, and related disciplines will discover the contents to be most useful as a source of concepts and modes of thought that are applicable to other types of investigative and applied sciences. For those further removed from the field of toxicology or for those who have not entered a specific field of endeavor, this book attempts to present a selectively representative view of the many facets of the subject.

Toxicology: The Basic Science of Poisons has been organized to facilitate its use by these different types of users. The first section (Unit I) describes the elements of method and approach that identify toxicology. It includes those principles most frequently invoked in a full understanding of toxicologic events, such as dose-response, and is primarily mechanistically oriented. Mechanisms arc also stressed in the subsequent sections of the book, particularly when these are well identified and extend across classic forms of chemicals and systems. However, the major focus in the second section (Unit II) is on the systemic site of action of toxins. The intent therein is to provide answers to two questions: What kinds of injury are produced in specific organs or systems by toxic agents? What are the agents that produce these effects?

A more conventional approach to toxicology has been utilized in the third section (Unit III), in which the toxic agents are grouped by chemical or use characteristics. In the final section (Unit IV) an attempt has been made to illustrate the ramifications of toxicology into all areas of the health sciences and even beyond. This unit is intended to provide perspective for the nontoxicologist in the application of the results of toxicologic studies and a better understanding of the activities of those engaged in the various aspects of the discipline of toxicology.

It will be obvious to the reader that the contents of this book represent a compromise between the basic, fundamental, mechanistic approach to toxicology and the desire to give a view of the broad horizons presented by the subject. While it is certain that the editors' selectivity might have been more severe, it is equally certain that it could have been less so, and we hope that the balance struck will prove to be appropriate for both toxicologic training and the scientific interest of our colleague.

L.J.C.
J.D.

Although the philosophy and design of this book evolved over a long period of friendship and mutual respect between the editors, the effort needed to convert ideas into reality was undertaken primarily by Louis J. Casarett. Thus, his death at a time when completion of the manuscript was in sight was particularly tragic. With the help and encouragement of his wife, Margaret G. Casarett, and the other contributors, we have finished Lou's task. This volume is a fitting embodiment of Louis J. Casarett's dedication to toxicology and to toxicologic education.

J.D.

CASARETT AND DOULL'S
TOXICOLOGY
THE BASIC SCIENCE OF POISONS

What is there that is not poison?
All things are poison and nothing (is)
without poison. Solely the dose
determines that a thing is not a poison.
Paracelsus
(1493–1541)

UNIT 1

GENERAL PRINCIPLES
OF TOXICOLOGY

HISTORY AND SCOPE
OF TOXICOLOGY

Michael A. Gallo

HISTORY OF TOXICOLOGY

    Antiquity
    Middle Ages
    Age of Enlightenment

MODERN TOXICOLOGY

AFTER WORLD WAR II

Toxicology has been defined as the study of the adverse effects of xenobiotics and thus is a borrowing science that has evolved from ancient poisoners. Modern toxicology goes beyond the study of the adverse effects of exogenous agents to the study of molecular biology, using toxicants as tools. Currently, many toxicologists are studying the mechanisms of endogenous compounds such as oxygen radicals and other reactive intermediates generated from xenobiotics and endobiotics. Historically, toxicology formed the basis of therapeutics and experimental medicine. Toxicology in this and last century (1900 to the present) continues to develop and expand by assimilating knowledge and techniques from most branches of biology, chemistry, mathematics, and physics. A recent addition to the field of toxicology (1975 to the present) is the application of this discipline to safety evaluation and risk assessment.

The contributions and activities of toxicologists are diverse and widespread. In this biomedical area, toxicologists are concerned with mechanisms of action and exposure to chemicals as a cause of acute and chronic illness. Toxicologists contribute to physiology and pharmacology by using toxic chemicals to understand physiological phenomena. They are involved in the recognition, identification, and quantification of hazards resulting from occupational exposure to chemicals and the public health aspects of chemicals in air, water, other parts of the environment, food, and drugs. Traditionally, toxicologists have been intimately involved in the discovery and development of new drugs, food additives, and pesticides. Toxicologists also participate in the development of standards and regulations designed to protect human health and the environment from the adverse effects of chemicals. Environmental toxicologists (a relatively new subset of the discipline) have expanded toxicology to study the effects of chemicals on flora and fauna. Molecular toxicologists are studying the mechanisms by which toxicants modulate cell growth and differentiation and how cells respond to toxicants at the level of the gene. In all branches of toxicology, scientists explore the mechanisms and modes of action by which chemicals produce adverse effects in biological systems. Clinical toxicologists develop antidotes and treatment regimens to ameliorate poisonings from xenobiotic injury. Toxicologists carry out some or all of these activities as members of academic, industrial, and governmental organizations. In fact, these activities help them to share methodologies for obtaining data for toxicity of materials and to make reasonable predictions regarding the hazards of the material to people and the environment using this data. Although different, these complementary activities characterize the discipline of toxicology.

Toxicology, like medicine, is both a science and an art. The science of toxicology is defined as the observational and data-gathering phase, whereas the art of toxicology consists of utilization of data to predict outcomes of exposure in human and animal populations. In most cases, these phases are linked because the facts generated by the science of toxicology are used to develop extrapolations and hypotheses to explain the adverse effects of chemical agents in situations where there is little or no information. For example, the observation that the administration of TCDD (2,3,7,8-tetrachlorodibenzo-*p*-dioxin) to female Sprague Dawley rats induces hepatocellular carcinoma is a fact. However, the conclusion that it will also have a similar affect in humans is unclear whether it is a prediction or hypothesis. Therefore, it is important to distinguish facts from predictions. When we fail to distinguish the science from the art, we confuse facts with predictions and argue that they have equal validity, which they clearly do not suggest. In toxicology, as in all sciences, theories have a higher level of certainty than do hypotheses, which in turn are more certain than speculations, opinions, conjectures, and guesses. An insight into modern toxicology and the roles, points of view, and activities of toxicologists can be obtained by examining the evolution of this discipline.

HISTORY OF TOXICOLOGY

Antiquity

Toxicology dates back to the earliest humans, who used animal venom and plant extracts for hunting, warfare, and assassination. The knowledge of these poisons must have predated recorded history. It is safe to assume that prehistoric humans categorized some plants as harmful and others as safe. The same is probably true for the classification of snakes and other animals. The Ebers papyrus (circa 1500 BC) contains information pertaining to many recognized poisons, including hemlock (the state poison of the Greeks), aconite (a Chinese arrow poison), opium (used as both a poison and an antidote), and metals such as lead, copper, and antimony. There is also an indication that plants containing substances similar to digitalis and belladonna alkaloids were known. Hippocrates (circa 400 BC) added a number of poisons and clinical toxicology principles pertaining to bioavailability in therapy and overdosage, while the Book of Job (circa 400 BC) speaks of poison arrows (Job 6:4). In the literature of ancient Greece, there are several references to poisons and their use. Some interpretations of Homer have Odysseus obtaining poisons for his arrows (Homer, circa 600 BC). Theophrastus (370–286 BC), a student of Aristotle, included numerous references to poisonous plants in *De Historia Plantarum*. Dioscorides, a Greek physician in the court of the Roman emperor Nero, made the first attempt to classify poisons, which was accompanied by descriptions and drawings. His classification into plant, animal, and mineral poisons not only remained a standard for 16 centuries but is still a convenient classification (Gunther, 1934). Dioscorides also dabbled in therapy, recognizing the use of emetics in poisoning and the use of caustic agents and cupping glasses in snakebite. Poisoning with plant and animal toxins was quite common. Perhaps the best-known recipient of poison used as a state method of execution was Socrates (470–399 BC), whose cup of hemlock extract was apparently estimated to be the proper dose. Expeditious suicide on a voluntary basis also made use of toxicologic knowledge. Demosthenes (385–322 BC), who took poison hidden in his pen, was one of many examples. The mode of suicide calling for one to fall on his sword, although manly and noble, carried little appeal and less significance for the women of the day. Cleopatra's (69–30 BC) knowledge of natural primitive toxicology permitted her to use the more genteel method of falling on her asp.

The Romans too made considerable use of poisons in politics. One legend tells of King Mithridates VI of Pontus, whose numerous acute toxicity experiments on unfortunate criminals led to his eventual claim that he had discovered an antidote for every venomous reptile and poisonous substance (Guthrie, 1946). Mithridates was so fearful of poisons that he regularly ingested a mixture of 36 ingredients (Galen reports 54) as protection against assassination. On the occasion of his imminent capture by enemies, his attempts to kill himself with poison failed because of his successful antidote concoction, and he was forced to use a sword held by a servant. From this tale comes the term "mithridatic," referring to an antidotal or protective mixture. The term "theriac" has also become synonymous with "antidote," although the word comes from the poetic treatise *Theriaca* by Nicander of Colophon (204–135 BC), which dealt with poisonous animals; his poem "Alexipharmaca" was about antidotes.

Poisonings in Rome reached epidemic proportions during the fourth century BC (Livy). It was during this period that a conspiracy of women to remove men from whose death they might profit was uncovered. Similar large-scale poisoning continued until Sulla issued the *Lex Cornelia* (circa 82 BC). This appears to be the first law against poisoning, and it later became a regulatory statute directed at careless dispensers of drugs. Nero (AD 37–68) used poisons to do away with his stepbrother Brittanicus and employed his slaves as food tasters to differentiate edible mushrooms from their more poisonous kin.

Middle Ages

Come bitter pilot, now at once run on
The dashing rocks thy seasick weary bark!
Here's to my love! O true apothecary!
Thy drugs are quick. Thus with a kiss I die.
                    (Romeo and Juliet, act 5, scene 3)

Before the Renaissance, the writings of Maimonides (Moses ben Maimon, AD 1135–1204) included a treatise on the treatment of poisonings from insects, snakes, and mad dogs (*Poisons and Their Antidotes*, 1198). Maimonides, like Hippocrates before him, wrote on the subject of bioavailability, noting that milk, butter, and cream could delay intestinal absorption. Malmonides also refuted many of the popular remedies of the day and stated his doubts about others. It is rumored that alchemists of this period (circa AD 1200), in search

of the universal antidote, learned to distill fermented products and made a 60% ethanol beverage that had many interesting powers.

In the early Renaissance, the Italians, with characteristic pragmatism, brought the art of poisoning to its zenith. The poisoner became an integral part of the political scene. The records of the city councils of Florence, particularly those of the infamous Council of Ten of Venice, contain ample testimony about the political use of poisons. Victims were named, prices set, and contracts recorded; when the deed was accomplished, payment was made.

An infamous figure of the time was a lady named Toffana who peddled specially prepared arsenic-containing cosmetics (*Agua Toffana*). Accompanying the product were appropriate instructions for its use. Toffana was succeeded by an imitator with organizational genius, Hieronyma Spara, who provided a new fillip by directing her activities toward specific marital and monetary objectives. A local club was formed of young, wealthy, married women, which soon became a club of eligible young wealthy widows, reminiscent of the matronly conspiracy of Rome centuries earlier. Incidentally, arsenic-containing cosmetics were reported to be responsible for deaths well into the twentieth century (Kallett and Schlink, 1933).

Among the prominent families engaged in poisoning, the Borgias were the most notorious. However, many deaths that were attributed to poisoning are now recognized as having resulted from infectious diseases such as malaria. It appears true, however, that Alexander VI, his son Cesare, and Lucrezia Borgia were quite active. The deft application of poisons to men of stature in the Catholic Church swelled the holdings of the papacy, which was their prime heir.

In this period Catherine de Medici exported her skills from Italy to France, where the prime targets of women were their husbands. However, unlike poisoners of an earlier period, the circle represented by Catherine and epitomized by the notorious Marchioness de Brinvillers depended on developing direct evidence to arrive at the most effective compounds for their purposes. Under the guise of delivering provender to the sick and the poor, Catherine tested toxic concoctions, carefully noting the rapidity of the toxic response (onset of action), the effectiveness of the compound (potency), the degree of response of the parts of the body (specificity, site of action), and the complaints of the victim (clinical signs and symptoms).

The culmination of the practice in France is represented by the commercialization of the service by Catherine Deshayes, who earned the title "La Voisine." Her business was dissolved by her execution. Her trial was one of the most famous of those held by the Chambre Ardente, a special judicial commission established by Louis XIV to try such cases without regard to age, sex, or national origin. La Voisine was convicted of many poisonings, with over 2000 infants among her victims.

Age of Enlightenment

All substances are poisons; there is none which is not a poison. The right dose differentiates poison from a remedy.

                                        Paracelsus

A significant figure in the history of science and medicine in the late Middle Ages was the renaissance man Philippus Aureolus Theophrastus Bombastus von Hohenheim-Paracelsus (1493–1541). Between the time of Aristotle and the age of Paracelsus, there was little substantial change in the biomedical sciences. In the sixteenth century, the revolt against the authority of the Catholic Church was accompanied by a parallel attack on the godlike authority exercised by the followers of Hippocrates and Galen. Paracelsus personally and professionally embodied the qualities that forced numerous changes in this period. He and his age were pivotal, standing between the philosophy and magic of classical antiquity and the philosophy and science willed to us by figures of the seventeenth and eighteenth centuries. Clearly, one can identify in Paracelsus's approach, point of view, and breadth of interest numerous similarities to the discipline that is now called toxicology.

Paracelsus, a physician-alchemist and the son of a physician, formulated many revolutionary views that remain an integral part of the structure of toxicology, pharmacology, and therapeutics today (Pagel, 1958). He promoted a focus on the "toxicon," the primary toxic agent, as a chemical entity, as opposed to the Grecian concept of the mixture or blend. A view initiated by Paracelsus that became a lasting contribution held as corollaries that (1) experimentation is essential in the examination of responses to chemicals, (2) one should make a distinction between the therapeutic and toxic properties of chemicals, (3) these properties are sometimes but not always indistinguishable except by dose, and (4) one can ascertain a degree of specificity of chemicals and their therapeutic or toxic effects. These principles led Paracelsus to introduce mercury as the drug of choice for the treatment of syphilis, a practice that survived 300 years but led to his famous trial. This viewpoint presaged the "magic bullet" (arsphenamine) of Paul Ehrlich and the introduction of the therapeutic index. Further, in a very real sense, this was the first sound articulation of the dose–response relation, a bulwark of toxicology (Pachter, 1961).

The tradition of the poisoners spread throughout Europe, and their deeds played a major role in the distribution of political power throughout the Middle Ages. Pharmacology as it is known today had its beginnings during the Middle Ages and early Renaissance. Concurrently, the study of the toxicity and the dose–response relationship of therapeutic agents was commencing.

The occupational hazards associated with metalworking were recognized during the fifteenth century. Early publications by Ellenbog (circa 1480) warned of the toxicity of the mercury and lead exposures involved in goldsmithing. Agricola published a short treatise on mining diseases in 1556. However, the major work on the subject, *On the Miners' Sickness and Other Diseases of Miners* (1567), was published by Paracelsus. This treatise addressed the etiology of miners' disease, along with treatment and prevention strategies. Occupational toxicology was further advanced by the work of Bernardino Ramazzini. His classic, published in 1700 and entitled *Discourse on the Diseases of Workers,* set the standard for occupational medicine well into the nineteenth century. Ramazzini's work broadened the field by discussing occupations ranging from miners to midwives and including printers, weavers, and potters.

The developments of the Industrial Revolution stimulated a rise in many occupational diseases. Percival Pott's (1775) recognition of the role of soot in scrotal cancer among chimney sweepers was the first reported example of polyaromatic hydrocarbon carcinogenicity, a problem that still plagues toxicologists today. These findings led to improved medical practices, particularly in prevention. It should be noted that Paracelsus and Ramazzini also pointed out the toxicity of smoke and soot.

The nineteenth century dawned in a climate of industrial and political revolution. Organic chemistry was in its infancy in 1800, but by 1825 phosgene ($COCl_2$) and mustard gas (bis[B-chloroethyl]sulfide) had been synthesized. These two chemicals were used in World War I as war gases, and as late as the Iraq–Iran War in the late twentieth century. By 1880 over 10,000 organic compounds had been synthesized including chloroform, carbon tetrachloride, diethyl ether, and carbonic acid, and petroleum and coal gasification by-products were used in trade (Zapp, 1982). The toxicity of benzene was established at the turn of the twentieth century. Determination of the toxicologic potential of these newly created chemicals became the underpinning of the science of toxicology as it is practiced today. However, there was little interest during the mid-nineteenth century in hampering industrial development. Hence, the impact of industrial toxicology discoveries was not felt until the passage of worker's insurance laws, first in Germany (1883), then in England (1897), and later in the United States (1910).

Experimental toxicology accompanied the growth of organic chemistry and developed rapidly during the nineteenth century. Magendie (1783–1885), Orfila (1787–1853), and Bernard (1813–1878) carried out truly seminal research in experimental toxicology and laid the groundwork for pharmacology and experimental therapeutics as well as occupational toxicology.

Orfila, a Spanish physician in the French court, was the first toxicologist to use autopsy material and chemical analysis systematically as legal proof of poisoning. His introduction of this detailed type of analysis survives as the underpinning of forensic toxicology (Orfila, 1818). Orfila published the first major work devoted expressly to the toxicity of natural agents (1815). Magendie, a physician and experimental physiologist, studied the mechanisms of action of emetine, strychnine, and "arrow poisons" (Olmsted, 1944). His research into the absorption and distribution of these compounds in the body remains a classic in toxicology and pharmacology. One of Magendie's more famous students, Claude Bernard, continued the study of arrow poisons (Bernard, 1850) but also added works on the mechanism of action of carbon monoxide. Bernard's treatise, *An Introduction to the Study of Experimental Medicine* (translated by Greene in 1949), is a classic in the development of toxicology.

Many German scientists contributed greatly to the growth of toxicology in the late nineteenth and early twentieth centuries. Among the giants of the field are Oswald Schmiedeberg (1838–1921) and Louis Lewin (1850–1929). Schmiedeberg made many contributions to the science of toxicology, not the least of which was the training of approximately 120 students who later populated the most important laboratories of pharmacology and toxicology throughout the world. Many of today's toxicologists and pharmacologists can trace their scientific heritage back to Schmiedeberg. His research focused on the synthesis of hippuric acid in the liver and the detoxification mechanisms of the liver in several animal species (Schmiedeberg and Koppe, 1869). Lewin, who was educated originally in medicine and the natural sciences, trained in toxicology under Liebreich at the Pharmacological Institute of Berlin (1881). His contributions on the chronic toxicity of narcotics and other alkaloids remain a classic. Lewin also published much of the early work on the toxicity of methanol, glycerol, acrolein, and chloroform (Lewin, 1920, 1929).

MODERN TOXICOLOGY

Toxicology has evolved rapidly during the 1900s. The exponential growth of the discipline can be traced to the World War II era with its marked increase in the production of drugs, pesticides, munitions, synthetic fibers, and industrial chemicals. The history of many sciences represents an orderly transition based on theory, hypothesis testing, and synthesis of new ideas. Toxicology, as a gathering and an applied science, has, by contrast, developed in fits and starts. Toxicology calls on almost all the basic sciences to test its hypotheses. This fact, coupled with the health and occupational regulations that have driven toxicology research since 1900, has made this discipline exceptional in the history of science. The differentiation of toxicology as an art and a science, though arbitrary, permits the presentation of historical highlights along two major lines.

Modern toxicology can be viewed as a continuation of the development of the biological and physical sciences in the late nineteenth and twentieth centuries (Table 1-1). During the second half of the nineteenth century, the world witnessed an explosion in science that produced the beginning of the modern era of genetics, medicine, synthetic chemistry, physics, and biology. Toxicology has drawn its strength and diversity from its proclivity to borrowing. With the advent of anesthetics and disinfectants and the advancement of experimental pharmacology in the late 1850s, toxicology as it is currently understood got its start. The introduction of ether, chloroform, and carbonic acid led to several iatrogenic deaths. These unfortunate outcomes spurred research into the causes of the deaths and early experiments on the physiological mechanisms by which these compounds caused both beneficial and adverse effects. By the late nineteenth century the use of organic chemicals was becoming more widespread, and benzene, toluene, and the xylenes went into larger-scale commercial production. Interestingly, benzene was used as a drug to treat leukemia in the early 1900s.

During this period, the use of "patent" medicines was prevalent, and there were several incidents of poisonings from these medicaments. The adverse reactions to patent medicines, coupled with the response to Upton Sinclair's exposé of the meat-packing industry in *The Jungle,* culminated in the passage of the Wiley Bill (1906), the first of many U.S. pure food and drug laws (see Hutt and Hutt, 1984, for regulatory history).

A working hypothesis about the development of toxicology is that the discipline expands in response to legislation, which itself is a response to a real or perceived tragedy. The Wiley bill was the first such reaction in the area of food and drugs, and the worker's compensation laws cited above were a response to occupational toxicities. In addition, the National Safety Council was established in 1911, and the Division of Industrial Hygiene was established by the U.S. Public Health Service in 1914. A corollary to this hypothesis might be that the founding of scientific journals and/or societies is sparked by the development of a new field. The *Journal of Industrial Hygiene* began in 1918. The major chemical manufacturers in

Table 1.1
Selection of Developments in Toxicology

Development of early advances in analytic methods
  Marsh, 1836: development of method for arsenic analysis
  Reinsch, 1841: combined method for separation and analysis of As and Hg
  Fresenius, 1845, and von Babo, 1847: development of screening method for general poisons
  Stas-Otto, 1851: detection and identification of phosphorus
Early mechanistic studies
  F. Magendie, 1809: study of "arrow poisons," mechanism of action of emetine and strychnine
  C. Bernard, 1850: carbon monoxide combination with hemoglobin, study of mechanism of action of strychnine, site of action of curare
  R. Bohm, ca. 1890: active anthelmintics from fern, action of croton oil catharsis, poisonous mushrooms
Introduction of new toxicants and antidotes
  R. A. Peters, L. A. Stocken, and R. H. S. Thompson, 1945: development of British Anti Lewisite BAL) as a relatively specific antidote for arsenic, toxicity of monofluorocarbon compounds
  K. K. Chen, 1934: introduction of modern antidotes (nitrite and thiosulfate) for cyanide toxicity
  C. Voegtlin, 1923: mechanism of action of As and other metals on the SH groups
  P. Müller, 1944–1946: introduction and study of DDT (dichlorodiphenyltrichloroethane) and related insecticide compounds
  G. Schrader, 1952: introduction and study of organophosphorus compounds
  R. N. Chopra, 1933: indigenous drugs of India
Miscellaneous toxicologic studies
  R. T. Williams: study of detoxication mechanisms and species variation
  A. Rothstein: effects of uranium ion on cell membrane transport
  R. A. Kehoe: investigation of acute and chronic effects of lead
  A. Vorwald: studies of chronic respiratory disease (beryllium)
  H. Hardy: community and industrial poisoning (beryllium)
  A. Hamilton: introduction of modern industrial toxicology
  H. C. Hodge: toxicology of uranium, fluorides; standards of toxicity
  A. Hoffman: introduction of lysergic acid and derivatives; pscyhotomimetics
  R. A. Peters: biochemical lesions, lethal synthesis
  A. E. Garrod: inborn errors of metabolism
  T. T. Litchfield and F. Wilcoxon: simplified dose-response evaluation
  C. J. Bliss: method of probits, calculation of dosage-mortality curves

the United States (Dow, Union Carbide, and DuPont) established internal toxicology research laboratories to help guide decisions on worker health and product safety.

During the 1890s and early 1900s, the French scientists Becquerel and the Curies reported the discovery of "radioactivity." This opened up for exploration a very large area in physics, biology, and medicine, but it would not affect the science of toxicology for another 40 years. However, another discovery, that of vitamins, or "vital amines," was to lead to the use of the first large-scale bioassays (multiple animal studies) to determine whether these "new" chemicals were beneficial or harmful to laboratory animals. The initial work in this area took place at around the time of World War I in several laboratories, including the laboratory of Philip B. Hawk in Philadelphia. Hawk and a young associate, Bernard L. Oser, were responsible for the development and verification of many early toxicologic assays that are still used in a slightly amended form. Oser's contributions to food and regulatory toxicology were extraordinary. These early bioassays were made possible by two major advances in toxicology: the availability of developed and refined strains of inbred laboratory rodents (Donaldson, 1912), and the analytical chemical capability to assay urine and blood for residues.

The 1920s saw many events that began to mold the fledgling field of toxicology. The use of arsenicals for the treatment of diseases such as syphilis (arsenicals had been used in agriculture since the mid-nineteenth century) resulted in acute and chronic toxicity. Prohibition of alcoholic beverages in the United States opened the door for early studies of neurotoxicology, with the discovery that triorthocresyl phosphate (TOCP), methanol, and lead (all products of "bootleg" liquor) are neurotoxicants. TOCP, which until recently was a gasoline additive, caused a syndrome that became known as "ginger-jake" walk, a spastic gait resulting from drinking adulterated ginger beer. Mueller's discovery of DDT (dichlorodiphenyl-trichloroethane) and several other organohalides, such as hexachlorobenzene and hexachlorocyclohexane, during the late 1920s resulted in wider use of insecticidal agents. Other scientists were hard at work attempting to elucidate the structures and activity of the estrogens and androgens. Work on the steroid hormones led to the use of several assays for the determination of the biological activity of organ extracts and synthetic compounds. Efforts to synthesize steroid-like chemicals were spearheaded by E. C. Dodds and his co-workers, one of whom was Leon Golberg, a young organic chemist. Dodds's work on the bioactivity of the estrogenic compounds resulted in the synthesis of diethylstilbestrol (DES), hexestrol, and other stilbenes and the discovery of the strong estrogenic activity of substituted stilbenes; eventually leading to the Nobel Prize in Medicine. Golberg's intimate involvement in this work stimulated his interest in biology, leading to degrees in biochemistry and medicine and a career in toxicology in which he oversaw the creation of the laboratories of the British Industrial Biological Research Association (BIBRA) and the Chemical Industry Institute of Toxicology (CIIT). Interestingly, the initial observations that led to the discovery of DES were the findings of feminization of animals treated with the experimental carcinogen 7,12-dimethylbenz[a]anthracene (DMBA).

The 1930s saw the world preparing for World War II and a major effort by the pharmaceutical and chemical industries in Germany and the United States to manufacture the first mass-produced antibiotics, and warfare agents. One of the first journals expressly dedicated to experimental toxicology, *Archiv für Toxikologie,* began publication in Europe in 1930, the same year that Herbert Hoover signed the act that established the National Institutes of Health (NIH) in the United States.

The discovery of sulfanilamide was heralded as a major event in combating bacterial diseases. However, for a drug to be effective, there must be a reasonable delivery system, and sulfanilamide is highly insoluble in an aqueous medium. Therefore, it was originally prepared in ethanol (elixir). However, it was soon discovered that the drug was more soluble in diethylene glycol, which is a dihydroxy rather than a monohydroxy ethane. The drug was sold in the diethylene glycol solution but was labeled as an elixir, and several patients died of acute renal failure resulting from the metabolism of the glycol to oxalic acid and glycolic acid, with the acids, along with the active drug, crystallizing in the kidney tubules. This tragic event led to the passage of the Copeland bill in 1938, the second major bill involving the formation of the U.S. Food and Drug Administration (FDA). The sulfanilamide disaster played a critical role in the further development of toxicology, resulting in work by Eugene Maximillian Geiling (a direct scientific offspring of John Jacob Abel and Schmiedeberg) in the Pharmacology Department of the University of Chicago that elucidated the mechanism of toxicity of both sulfanilamide and ethylene glycol. Studies of the glycols were simultaneously carried out at the U.S. FDA by a group led by Arnold Lehman. The scientists associated with Lehman and Geiling were to become the leaders of toxicology over the next 40 years. With few exceptions, toxicology in the United States owes its heritage to Geiling's innovativeness and ability to stimulate and direct young scientists and Lehman's vision of the use of experimental toxicology in public health decision making. Because of Geiling's reputation, the U.S. government turned to this group for help in the war effort. There were three main areas in which the Chicago group took part during World War II: the toxicology and pharmacology of organophosphate chemicals, antimalarial drugs, and radionuclides. Each of these areas produced teams of toxicologists who became academic, governmental, and industrial leaders in the field.

It was also during this time that DDT and the phenoxy herbicides were developed for increased food production and, in the case of DDT, control of insect-borne diseases. These efforts between 1940 and 1946 led to an explosion in toxicology. Thus, in line with the hypothesis advanced above, the crisis of World War II caused the next major leap in the development of toxicology.

If one traces the history of the toxicology of metals over the past 45 years, the role of the Chicago group, and Rochester, is quite apparent. This story commences with the use of uranium for the "bomb" and continues today with research on the role of metals in their interactions with DNA, RNA, and growth factors. Indeed, the Manhattan Project created a fertile environment that resulted in the initiation of quantitative biology, drug metabolism and structure activity relationships (with antimalarials), radiotracer technology, and inhalation toxicology. These innovations have revolutionized modern biology, chemistry, therapeutics, and toxicology.

Inhalation toxicology began at the University of Rochester under the direction of Stafford Warren, who headed the Department of Radiology. He developed a program with colleagues such as Harold Hodge (pharmacologist), Herb Stokinger (chemist), Sid Laskin (inhalation toxicologist), and Lou and George Casarett (toxicologists). These young scientists were to go on to become giants in the field. The other sites for the study of radionuclides were Chicago for the "internal" effects of radioactivity and Oak Ridge, Tennessee, for the effects of "external" radiation. The work of the scientists on these teams gave the scientific community data that contributed to the early understanding of macromolecular binding of xenobiotics, cellular mutational events, methods for inhalation toxicology and therapy, and toxicological properties of trace metals, along with a better appreciation of the complexities of the dose–response curve.

Another seminal event in toxicology that occurred during the World War II era was the discovery of organophosphate cholinesterase inhibitors. This class of chemicals, which was discovered by Willy Lange and Gerhard Schrader, was destined to become a driving force in the study of neurophysiology and toxicology for several decades. Again, the scientists in Chicago played major roles in elucidating the mechanisms of action of this new class of compounds. Geiling's group, Kenneth Dubois in particular, were leaders in this area of toxicology and pharmacology. Dubois's students, particularly Sheldon Murphy (and his students), continued to be in the forefront of this special area. The importance of the early research on the organophosphates has taken on special meaning in the years since 1960, when these non-bioaccumulating insecticides were destined to replace DDT and other organochlorine insectides.

Early in the twentieth century, it was demonstrated experimentally that quinine has a marked effect on the malaria parasite [it had been known for centuries that chincona bark extract is efficacious for "Jesuit fever" (malaria)]. This discovery led to the development of quinine derivatives for the treatment of the disease and the formulation of the early principles of chemotherapy. The pharmacology department at Chicago was charged with the development of antimalarials for the war effort. The original protocols called for testing of efficacy and toxicity in rodents and perhaps dogs and then the testing of efficacy in human volunteers. One of the investigators charged with generating the data needed to move a candidate drug from animals to humans was Fredrick Coulston. This young parasitologist and his colleagues, working under Geiling, were to evaluate potential drugs in animal models and then establish human clinical trials. It was during these experiments that the use of nonhuman primates came into vogue for toxicology testing. It had been noted by Russian scientists that some antimalarial compounds caused retinopathies in humans but did not apparently have the same adverse effect in rodents and dogs. This finding led the Chicago team to add one more step in the development process: toxicity testing in rhesus monkeys just before efficacy studies in people. This resulted in the prevension of blindness in untold numbers of volunteers and perhaps some of the troops in the field. It also led to the school of thought that nonhuman primates may be one of the better models for humans and the establishment of primate colonies for the study of toxicity. Coulston pioneered this area of toxicology and remained committed to it until his death in 2003.

Another area not traditionally thought of as toxicology but one that evolved during the 1940s as an exciting and innovative field is experimental pathology. This branch of experimental biology developed from bioassays of estrogens and early experiments in chemical- and radiation-induced carcinogenesis. It is from these early studies that hypotheses on tumor promotion and cancer progression have evolved.

Toxicologists today owe a great deal to the researchers of chemical carcinogenesis of the 1940s. Much of today's work can be traced to Elizabeth and James Miller at Wisconsin. This husband and wife team started under the mentorship of Professor Rusch, the director of the newly formed McArdle Laboratory for Cancer Research, and Professor Baumann. The seminal research of the Millers, and a young Allen Conney, led to the discovery of the role of reactive intermediates in carcinogenicity and that of mixed-function oxidases in the endoplasmic reticulum. Conney's discovery of benzo(a)pyrene hydroxylase induction in the 1950s opened the field of chemical

metabolism that has resulted in the elucidation of the arylhydrocarbon receptor in the 1970s and 1980s. These findings, which initiated the great works on the cytochrome-P450 family of proteins, were aided by two other major discoveries for which toxicologists (and all other biological scientists) are deeply indebted: paper chromatography in 1944 and the use of radiolabeled dibenzanthracene in 1948. Other major events of note in drug metabolism included the work of Bernard Brodie on the metabolism of methyl orange in 1947. This piece of seminal research led to the examination of blood and urine for chemical and drug metabolites. It became the tool with which one could study the relationship between blood levels and biological action. The classic treatise of R. T. Williams, *Detoxication Mechanisms,* was published in 1947. This text described the many pathways and possible mechanisms of detoxication and opened the field to several new areas of study.

The decade after World War II was not as boisterous as the period from 1935 to 1945. The first major U.S. Pesticide Act was signed into law in 1947. The significance of the initial Federal Insecticide, Fungicide, and Rodenticide Act was that for the first time in U.S. history a substance that was neither a drug nor a food had to be shown to be safe and efficacious. This decade, which coincided with the Eisenhower years, saw the dispersion of the groups from Chicago, Rochester, and Oak Ridge and the establishment of new centers of research. Adrian Albert's classic *Selective Toxicity* was published in 1951. This treatise, which has appeared in several editions, presented a concise documentation of the principles of the site-specific action of chemicals.

AFTER WORLD WAR II

You too can be a toxicologist in two easy lessons, each of ten years.
Arnold Lehman (circa 1955)

The mid-1950s witnessed the strengthening of the U.S. Food and Drug Administration's commitment to toxicology under the guidance of Arnold Lehman. Lehman's tutelage and influence are still felt today. The adage "*You too can be a toxicologist...*" is as important a summation of toxicology as the often-quoted statement of Paracelsus: "*The dose makes the poison.*" The period from 1955 to 1958 produced two major events that would have a long-lasting impact on toxicology as a science and a professional discipline. Lehman, Fitzhugh, and their co-workers formalized the experimental program for the appraisal of food, drug, and cosmetic safety in 1955, updated by the U.S. FDA in 1982, and the Gordon Research Conferences established a conference on toxicology and safety evaluation, with Bernard L. Oser as its initial chairman. These two events led to close relationships among toxicologists from several groups and brought toxicology into a new phase. At about the same time, the U.S. Congress passed and the President of the United States signed the additives amendments to the Food, Drug, and Cosmetic Act. The Delaney clause (1958) of these amendments stated broadly that any chemical found to be carcinogenic in laboratory animals or humans could not be added to the U.S. food supply. The impact of this food additive legislation cannot be overstated. Delaney became a battle cry for many groups and resulted in the inclusion at a new level of biostatisticians and mathematical modelers in the field of toxicology. It fostered the expansion of quantitative methods in toxicology and led to innumerable arguments about the "one-hit" theory of carcinogenesis. Regardless of one's view of Delaney, it has served as an excellent starting point for understanding the complexity of the biological phenomenon of carcinogenicity and the development of risk assessment models. One must remember that at the time of Delaney, the analytic detection level for most chemicals was 20 to 100 ppm (today, parts per quadrillion). Interestingly, the Delaney clause has been invoked only on a few occasions, and it has been stated that Congress added little to the food and drug law with this clause (Hutt and Hutt, 1984).

Shortly after the Delaney Amendment and after three successful Gordon Conferences, the first American journal *Toxicology and Applied Pharmacology* dedicated to toxicology was launched by Coulston, Lehman, and Hayes. Since 1960, over 50 journals and innumerable societies have been launched to disseminate toxicological information. The founding of the Society of Toxicology followed shortly afterward, and became its official publication. The Society's founding members were Fredrick Coulston, William Deichmann, Kenneth DuBois, Victor Drill, Harry Hayes, Harold Hodge, Paul Larson, Arnold Lehman, and C. Boyd Shaffer. These researchers deserve a great deal of credit for the growth of toxicology. DuBois and Geiling published their *Textbook of Toxicology* in 1959. The text you are reading is a continuum of the DuBois and Geiling classic.

The 1960s were a tumultuous time for society, and toxicology was swept up in the tide. Starting with the tragic thalidomide incident, in which several thousand children were born with serious birth defects, and the publication of Rachel Carson's *Silent Spring* (1962), the field of toxicology developed at a feverish pitch. Attempts to understand the effects of chemicals on the embryo and fetus and on the environment as a whole gained momentum. New legislation was passed, and new journals were founded. The education of toxicologists spread from the deep traditions at Chicago and Rochester to Harvard, Miami, Albany, Iowa, Jefferson, and beyond. Geiling's fledglings spread as Schmiedeberg's had a half century before. Many new fields were influencing and being assimilated into the broad scope of toxicology, including environmental sciences, aquatic and avian biology, biostatistics, risk modeling, cell biology, analytic chemistry, and molecular genetics.

During the 1960s, particularly the latter half of the decade, the analytic tools used in toxicology were developed to a level of sophistication that allowed the detection of chemicals in tissues and other substrates at part per billion concentrations (today, parts per quadrillion may be detected). Pioneering work in the development of point mutation assays that were replicable, quick, and inexpensive led to a better understanding of the genetic mechanisms of carcinogenicity (Ames, 1983). The combined work of Ames, the Millers (Elizabeth C. and James A.) at McArdle Laboratory, Cooney, and others allowed the toxicology community to make major contributions to the understanding of the carcinogenic process.

The low levels of detection of chemicals and the ability to detect point mutations rapidly created several problems and opportunities for toxicologists and risk assessors that stemmed from interpretation of the Delaney amendment. Cellular and molecular toxicology developed as a subdiscipline, and risk assessment became a major product of toxicological investigations.

The establishment of the National Center for Toxicologic Research (NCTR), the expansion of the role of the U.S. FDA, and the establishment of the U.S. Environmental Protection Agency (EPA) and the National Institute of Environmental Health Sciences (NIEHS) were considered clear messages that the government had taken a strong interest in toxicology. Several new journals appeared during the 1960s, and new legislation was written quickly after *Silent Spring* and the thalidomide disaster.

The end of the 1960s witnessed the "discovery" of TCDD as a contaminant in the herbicide Agent Orange (the original discovery

of TCDD toxicity, as the "Chick Edema Factor," was reported in 1957). The research on the toxicity of this compound has produced seminal findings regarding signal transduction, and some very poor research in the field of toxicology. The discovery of a high-affinity cellular binding protein designated the "Ah" receptor (see Poland and Knutsen, 1982, for a review) at the McArdle Laboratory and work on the genetics of the receptor at NIH (Nebert and Gonzalez, 1987; Thomas *et al.*, 1972) have revolutionized the field of toxicology. The importance of TCDD to toxicology lies in the fact that it forced researchers, regulators, and the legal community to look at the role of mechanisms of toxic action in a different fashion. The compound is a potent carcinogen in several species but is not a mutagen.

At least two other events precipitated a great deal of legislation during the 1970s: Love Canal and Kepone in the James River. The "discovery" of Love Canal led to major concerns regarding hazardous wastes, chemical dump sites, and disclosure of information about those sites. Soon after Love Canal, the EPA listed several equally contaminated sites in the United States. The agency was given the responsibility to develop risk assessment methodology to determine health risks from exposure to effluents and to attempt to remediate these sites. These combined efforts led to broad-based support for research into the mechanisms of action of individual chemicals and complex mixtures. Love Canal and similar issues created the legislative environment that led to the Toxic Substances Control Act and eventually to the Superfund bill. These omnibus bills were created to cover the toxicology of chemicals from initial synthesis to disposal (cradle to grave).

The expansion of legislation, journals, and new societies involved with toxicology was exponential during the 1970s and 1980s and shows no signs of slowing down. Currently, in the United States there are dozens of professional, governmental, and other scientific organizations with thousands of members and over 120 journals dedicated to toxicology and related disciplines.

In addition, toxicology continues to expand in stature and in the number of programs worldwide. The International Congress of Toxicology is made up of toxicology societies from Europe, South America, Asia, Africa, and Australia and brings together the broadest representation of toxicologists.

The original Gordon Conference series has changed to Mechanisms of Toxicity, and several other conferences related to special areas of toxicology are now in existence. The Society of Toxicology in the United States has formed specialty sections and regional chapters to accommodate the over 5000 scientists involved in toxicology today. The American College of Toxicology has developed into an excellent venue for regulatory and industrial toxicology, and two boards have been established to accredit and certify toxicologists (The Academy of Toxicological Sciences and the American Board of Toxicology). Texts and reference books for toxicology students and scientists abound. Toxicology has evolved from a borrowing science to a seminal discipline seeding the growth and development of several related fields of science and science policy.

The history of toxicology has been interesting and varied but never dull. Perhaps as a science that has grown and prospered by borrowing from many disciplines, it has suffered from the absence of a single goal, but its diversification has allowed for the interspersion of ideas and concepts from higher education, industry, and government. As an example of this diversification, one now finds toxicology graduate programs in medical schools, schools of public health, and schools of pharmacy as well as programs in environmental science and engineering, as well as undergraduate programs in toxicology at several institutions. Surprisingly, courses in toxicology are now being offered in several liberal arts undergraduate schools as part of their biology and chemistry curricula. This has resulted in an exciting, innovative, and diversified field that is serving science and the community at large.

Few disciplines can point to both basic sciences and direct applications at the same time. Toxicology—the study of the adverse effects of xenobiotics (and more recently endobiotics)—may be unique in this regard.

REFERENCES

Albert A: *Selective Toxicity.* London: Methuen, 1951.

Ames BN: Dietary carcinogens and anticarcinogens. *Science* 221:1249–1264, 1983.

Bernard C: Action du curare et de la nicotine sur le systeme nerveux et sur le systme musculaire. *CR Soc Biol* 2:195, 1850.

Bernard C: *Introduction to the Study of Experimental Medicine,* trans., in Greene HC, Schuman H (eds.) New York: Dover, 1949.

Carson R: *Silent Spring.* Boston: Houghton Mifflin, 1962.

Christison R: *A Treatise on Poisons,* 4th ed. Philadelphia: Barrington & Howell, 1845.

Doll R, Peto R: *The Causes of Cancer.* New York: Oxford University Press, 1981.

Donaldson HH: The history and zoological position of the albino rat. *Natl Acad Sci* 15:365–369, 1912.

DuBois K, Geiling EMK: *Textbook of Toxicology.* New York: Oxford University Press, 1959.

Gunther RT: *The Greek Herbal of Dioscorides.* New York: Oxford University Press, 1934.

Guthrie DA: *A History of Medicine.* Philadelphia: Lippincott, 1946.

Handler P: Some comments on risk assessment, in *The National Research Council in 1979: Current Issues and Studies.* Washington, DC: NAS, 1979.

Hutt PB, Hutt PB II: A history of government regulation of adulteration and misbranding of food. *Food Drug Cosmet J* 39:2–73, 1984.

Kallet A, Schlink FJ: *100,000,000 Guinea Pigs: Dangers in Everyday Foods, Drugs and Cosmetics.* New York: Vanguard, 1933.

Levey M: Medieval arabic toxicology: The book on poisons of Ibn Wahshiya and its relation to early Indian and Greek texts. *Trans Am Philos Soc* 56(7): 1966.

Lewin L: *Die Gifte in der Weltgeschichte: Toxikologische, allgemeinverstandliche Untersuchungen der historischen Quellen.* Berlin: Springer, 1920.

Lewin L: *Gifte und Vergiftungen.* Berlin: Stilke, 1929.

Loomis TA: *Essentials of Toxicology,* 3rd ed. Philadelphia: Lea & Febiger, 1978.

Macht DJ: Louis Lewin: Pharmacologist, toxicologist, medical historian. *Ann Med Hist* 3:179–194, 1931.

Meek WJ: *The Gentle Art of Poisoning.* Medico-Historical Papers. Madision: University of Wisconsin, 1954; reprinted from *Phi Beta Pi Quarterly,* May 1928.

Muller P: Uber zusammenhange zwischen Konstitution und insektizider Wirkung I. *Helv Chim Acta* 29:1560–1580, 1946.

Munter S (ed.): *Treatise on Poisons and Their Antidotes. Vol. II of the Medical Writings of Moses Maimonides.* Philadelphia: Lippincott, 1966.

Nebert D, Gonzalez FJ: P450 genes: Structure, evolution and regulation. *Annu Rev Biochem* 56:945–993, 1987.

Olmsted JMD: *François Magendie: Pioneer in Experimental Physiology and Scientific Medicine in XIX Century France.* New York: Schuman, 1944.

Orfila MJB: *Secours a Donner aux Personnes Empoisonees et Asphyxiees.* Paris: Feugeroy, 1818.

Orfila MJB: *Traite des Poisons Tires des Regnes Mineral, Vegetal et Animal, ou, Toxicologie Generale Consideree sous les Rapports de la Physiologie, de la Pathologie et de la Medecine Legale.* Paris: Crochard, 1814–1815.

Pachter HM: *Paracelsus: Magic into Science.* New York: Collier, 1961.

Pagel W: *Paracelsus: An Introduction to Philosophical Medicine in the Era of the Renaissance.* New York: Karger, 1958.

Paracelsus (Theophrastus ex Hohenheim Eremita): *Von der Besucht.* Dillingen, 1567.

Poland A, Knutson JC: 2,3,7,8-Tetrachlorodibenzo-*p*-dioxin and related halogenated aromatic hydrocarbons, examination of the mechanism of toxicity. *Annu Rev Pharmacol Toxicol* 22:517–554, 1982.

Ramazzini B: *De Morbis Artificum Diatriba.* Modena: Typis Antonii Capponi, 1700.

Robert R: *Lehrbuch der Intoxikationen.* Stuttgart: Enke, 1893.

Schmiedeberg O, Koppe R: *Das Muscarin das giftige Alkaloid des Fliegenpilzes.* Leipzig: Vogel, 1869.

Thomas PE, Kouri RE, Hutton JJ.The genetics of AHH induction in mice: a single gene difference between C57/6J and DBA/2J. *Biochem Genet.* 6:157–168,1972.

Thompson CJS: *Poisons and Poisoners: With Historical Accounts of Some Famous Mysteries in Ancient and Modern Times.* London: Shaylor, 1931.

U.S. FDA: *Toxicologic Principles for the Safety Assessment of Direct Food Additives and Color Additives Used in Food.* Washington, DC: U.S. Food and Drug Administration, Bureau of Foods, 1982.

Voegtlin C, Dyer HA, Leonard CS: On the mechanism of the action of arsenic upon protoplasm. *Public Health Rep* 38:1882–1912, 1923.

Williams RT: *Detoxication Mechanisms,* 2nd ed. New York: Wiley, 1959.

Zapp JA Jr, Doull J: Industrial toxicology: Retrospect and prospect, in Clayton GD, Clayton FE (eds.): *Patty's Industrial Hygiene and Toxicology,* 4th ed. New York: Wiley Interscience, 1993, pp. 1–23.

SUPPLEMENTAL READING

Adams F (trans.): *The Genuine Works of Hippocrates.* Baltimore: Williams & Wilkins, 1939.

Beeson BB: Orfila—pioneer toxicologist. *Ann Med Hist* 2:68–70, 1930.

Bernard C: Analyse physiologique des proprietes des systemes musculaire et nerveux au moyen du curare. *CR Acad Sci (Paris)* 43:325–329, 1856.

Bryan CP: *The Papyrus Ebers.* London: Geoffrey Bales, 1930.

Clendening L: *Source Book of Medical History.* New York: Dover, 1942.

Gaddum JH: *Pharmacology,* 5th ed. New York: Oxford University Press, 1959.

Garrison FH: *An Introduction to the History of Medicine,* 4th ed. Philadelphia: Saunders, 1929.

Hamilton A: *Exploring the Dangerous Trades.* Boston: Little, Brown, 1943. (Reprinted by Northeastern University Press, Boston, 1985.)

Hays HW: *Society of Toxicology History, 1961–1986.* Washington, DC: Society of Toxicology, 1986.

Holmstedt B, Liljestrand G: *Readings in Pharmacology.* New York: Raven Press, 1981.

PRINCIPLES OF TOXICOLOGY

David L. Eaton and Steven G. Gilbert

INTRODUCTION TO TOXICOLOGY

Toxicology is the study of the adverse effects of chemical or physical agents on living organisms. A *toxicologist* is trained to examine and communicate the nature of those effects on human, animal, and environmental health. Toxicological research examines the cellular, biochemical, and molecular mechanisms of action as well as functional effects such as neurobehavioral and immunological, and assesses the probability of their occurrence. Fundamental to this process is characterizing the relation of exposure (or dose) to the response. *Risk assessment* is the quantitative estimate of the potential effects on human health and environmental significance of various types of chemical exposures (e.g., pesticide residues on food, contaminants in drinking water). The variety of potential adverse effects and the diversity of chemicals in the environment make toxicology a broad science, which often demands specialization in one area of toxicology. Our society's dependence on chemicals and the need to assess potential hazards have made toxicologists an increasingly important part of the decision-making processes.

Different Areas of Toxicology

The professional activities of toxicologists fall into three main categories: descriptive, mechanistic, and regulatory (Fig. 2-1). Although each has distinctive characteristics, each contributes to the other, and all are vitally important to chemical risk assessment (see Chap. 4).

A *mechanistic toxicologist* is concerned with identifying and understanding the cellular, biochemical, and molecular mechanisms by which chemicals exert toxic effects on living organisms (see Chap. 3 for a detailed discussion of mechanisms of toxicity). The results of mechanistic studies are very important in many areas of applied toxicology. In risk assessment, mechanistic data may be very useful in demonstrating that an adverse outcome (e.g., cancer, birth defects) observed in laboratory animals is directly relevant to humans. For example, the relative toxic potential of organophosphate insecticides in humans, rodents, and insects can be accurately predicted on the basis of an understanding of common mechanisms (inhibition of acetylcholinesterase) and differences in biotransformation for these insecticides among the different species. Similarly, mechanistic data may be very useful in identifying adverse

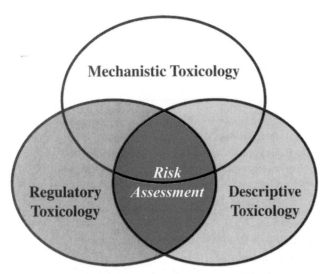

Figure 2-1. Graphical representation of the interconnections between different areas of toxicology.

responses in experimental animals that may not be relevant to humans. For example, the propensity of the widely used artificial sweetener saccharin to cause bladder cancer in rats may not be relevant to humans at normal dietary intake rates. This is because mechanistic studies have demonstrated that bladder cancer is induced only under conditions where saccharin is at such a high concentration in the urine that it forms a crystalline precipitate (Cohen, 1998). Dose–response studies suggest that such high concentrations would not be achieved in the human bladder even after extensive dietary consumption.

Mechanistic data are also useful in the design and production of safer alternative chemicals and in rational therapy for chemical poisoning and treatment of disease. For example, the drug thalidomide was originally marketed in Europe and Australia as a sedative agent for pregnant women. However, it was banned for clinical use in 1962 because of devastating birth defects that occurred if the drug was ingested during a critical period in pregnancy. But mechanistic studies over the past several decades have demonstrated that this drug may have a unique molecular mechanism of action that interferes with the expression of certain genes responsible for blood vessel formation (angiogenesis). With an understanding of this mechanism, thalidomide has been "rediscovered" as a valuable therapeutic agent that may be highly effective in the treatment of certain infectious diseases (e.g., leprosy and AIDS), a variety of inflammatory diseases, and some types of cancer. This provides an interesting example of how a highly toxic drug with selectivity toward a specific population (pregnant women) can be used safely with proper precautions. Following its approval for therapeutic use in 1998, a program was established that required all clinicians, pharmacists, and patients that receive thalidomide to enroll in a specific program (System for Thalidomide Education and Prescribing Safety, STEPS). The population at risk for the potential teratogenic effects of thalidomide (all women of childbearing age) were required to use two forms of birth control, and also have a negative pregnancy test within 24 hours of beginning therapy, and periodically the patients registered with the STEPS program, 6000 were females of childbearing age. Remarkably, after 6 years of use, only one patient actually received thalidomide during her pregnancy. She initially tested negative at the beginning of therapy; on a subsequent test she was identified

as positive, and the drug was stopped. The pregnancy ended up as a miscarriage (Uhl *et al.*, 2006). Thus, a clear understanding of mechanism of action led to the development of strict prescribing guidelines and patient monitoring, thereby allowing a potentially dangerous drug to be used safely and effectively to treat disease in tens of thousands of patients who would otherwise not have benefited from the therapeutic actions of the drug (Lary *et al.*, 1999).

In addition to aiding directly in the identification, treatment, and prevention of chemical toxicity, an understanding of the mechanisms of toxic action contributes to the knowledge of basic physiology, pharmacology, cell biology, and biochemistry. The advent of new technologies in molecular biology and genomics now provide mechanistic toxicologists with the tools to explore exactly how humans may differ from laboratory animals in their response to toxic substances. These same tools are also being utilized to identify individuals who are genetically susceptible to factors in the environment or respond differently to a chemical exposure. For example, it is now recognized that a small percentage of the population genetically lacks the ability to detoxify the chemotherapeutic drug, 6-mercaptopurine, used in the treatment of some forms of leukemia. Young children with leukemia who are homozygous for this genetic trait (about one in 300) may experience serious toxic effects from a standard therapeutic dose of this drug. Numerous genetic tests for polymorphisms in drug metabolizing enzymes and transporters are now available that can identify genetically susceptible individuals in advance of pharmacological treatment (Eichelbaum *et al.*, 2006).

These new areas of "pharmacogenomics" and "toxicogenomics" provides an exciting opportunity in the future for mechanistic toxicologists to identify and protect genetically susceptible individuals from harmful environmental exposures, and to customize drug therapies that enhance efficacy and minimize toxicity, based on an individual's genetic makeup.

A *descriptive toxicologist* is concerned directly with toxicity testing, which provides information for safety evaluation and regulatory requirements. The appropriate toxicity tests (as described later in this chapter and other chapters) in cell culture systems or experimental animals are designed to yield information to evaluate risks posed to humans and the environment from exposure to specific chemicals. The concern may be limited to effects on humans, as in the case of drugs and food additives. Toxicologists in the chemical industry, however, must be concerned not only with the risk posed by a company's chemicals (insecticides, herbicides, solvents, etc.) to humans but also with potential effects on fish, birds, and plants, as well as other factors that might disturb the balance of the ecosystem. Descriptive toxicology is of course not divorced from mechanistic studies, as such studies provide important clues to a chemical's mechanism of action, and thus contribute to the development of mechanistic toxicology through hypothesis generation. Such studies are also a key component of risk assessments that are used by regulatory toxicologists. The recent advent of so-called "omics" technologies (genomics, transcriptomics, proteomics, metabonomics, etc.) form the basis of the emerging subdiscipline of toxicogenomics. The application of these new technologies to toxicity testing is in many ways "descriptive" in nature, yet affords great mechanistic insights into how chemicals produce their toxic effects. This exciting new area of toxicology is discussed in more detail later in the chapter.

A *regulatory toxicologist* has the responsibility for deciding, on the basis of data provided by descriptive and mechanistic toxicologists, whether a drug or other chemical poses a sufficiently low risk to be marketed for a stated purpose or subsequent human or environmental exposure resulting from its use. The Food and Drug Administration (FDA) is responsible for allowing drugs, cosmetics, and food additives to be sold in the market according to the Federal Food, Drug and Cosmetic Act (FFDCA). The U.S. Environmental Protection Agency (EPA) is responsible for regulating most other chemicals according to the Federal Insecticide, Fungicide and Rodenticide Act (FIFRA), the Toxic Substances Control Act (TSCA), the Resource Conservation and Recovery Act (RCRA), the Safe Drinking Water Act, and the Clean Air Act. In 1996, the U.S. Congress passed the Food Quality Protection Act (FQPA) which fundamentally changed the pesticide and food safety laws under FIFRA and FFDCA requiring stricter safety standards particularly for infants and children, who were recognized as more susceptible to health effects of pesticides. The EPA is also responsible for enforcing the Comprehensive Environmental Response, Compensation and Liability Act [CERCLA, later revised as the Superfund Amendments Reauthorization Act (SARA)], more commonly called the Superfund Act. This regulation provides direction and financial support for the cleanup of waste sites that contain toxic chemicals that may present a risk to human health or the environment. The Occupational Safety and Health Administration (OSHA) of the Department of Labor was established to ensure that safe and healthful conditions exist in the workplace. The National Institute for Occupational Safety and Health (NIOSH) as part of the Centers for Disease Control and Prevention (CDC) in the Department of Health and Human Services is responsible for conducting research and making recommendations for the prevention of work-related injury and illness. The Consumer Product Safety Commission is responsible for protecting consumers from hazardous household substances, whereas the Department of Transportation (DOT) ensures that materials shipped in interstate commerce are labeled and packaged in a manner consistent with the degree of hazard they present. Regulatory toxicologists are also involved in the establishment of standards for the amount of chemicals permitted in ambient air, industrial atmospheres, and drinking water, often integrating scientific information from basic descriptive and mechanistic toxicology studies with the principles and approaches used for risk assessment (see Chap. 4).

In addition to the above categories, there are other specialized areas of toxicology such as forensic, clinical, and environmental toxicology. *Forensic toxicology* is a hybrid of analytic chemistry and fundamental toxicological principles. It is concerned primarily with the medicolegal aspects of the harmful effects of chemicals on humans and animals. The expertise of forensic toxicologists is invoked primarily to aid in establishing the cause of death and determining its circumstances in a postmortem investigation (see Chap. 31). *Clinical toxicology* designates an area of professional emphasis in the realm of medical science that is concerned with disease caused by or uniquely associated with toxic substances (see Chap. 32). Generally, clinical toxicologists are physicians who receive specialized training in emergency medicine and poison management. Efforts are directed at treating patients poisoned with drugs or other chemicals and at the development of new techniques to treat those intoxications. Public contact about treatment and prevention is often through the national network of poison control centers. *Environmental toxicology* focuses on the impacts of chemical pollutants in the environment on biological organisms. Although toxicologists concerned with the effects of environmental pollutants on human health fit into this definition, it is most commonly associated with studies on the impacts of chemicals on nonhuman organisms such as fish, birds, terrestrial animals, and plants. *Ecotoxicology* is a specialized area within environmental toxicology that focuses more specifically

on the impacts of toxic substances on population dynamics in an ecosystem. The transport, fate, and interactions of chemicals in the environment constitute a critical component of both environmental toxicology and ecotoxicology.

Toxicology and Society

Information from the toxicological sciences, gained by experience or research, has a growing influence on our personal lives as well as for human and environmental health across the globe. Knowledge about the toxicological effects of a compound affects consumer products, drugs, manufacturing processes, waste clean up, regulatory action, civil disputes, and broad policy decisions. The expanding influence of toxicology on societal issues is accompanied by the responsibility to be increasingly sensitive to the ethical, legal, and social implications of toxicological research and testing.

The convergence of multiple elements has highlighted the evolving ethical dynamics of toxicology. First, experience and new discoveries in the biological sciences have emphasized our interconnectedness with nature and the need for well-articulated visions of human, animal, and environmental health. One vision is that we have "condition(s) that ensure that all living things have the best opportunity to reach and maintain their full genetic potential" (Gilbert, 2005a). Second, we have experience with the health consequences of exposure to such things as lead, asbestos, and tobacco, along with the detailed mechanistic research to understand the long-term risks to individuals and society. This has precipitated many regulatory and legal actions and public policy decisions, not to mention costly and time-consuming lawsuits. Third, we have an increasingly well-defined framework for discussing our social and ethical responsibilities. There is growing recognition that ethics play a crucial role in public health decision-making that involve conflicts between individual, corporate, and social justice goals (Callahan and Jennings, 2002; Kass, 2001; Lee, 2002). Fourth, is the appreciation that all research involving humans or animals must be conducted in a responsible and ethical manner. Fifth, is managing both the uncertainty and biological variability inherent in the biological sciences. Decision-making often includes making judgments with limited or uncertain information, which often includes an overlay of individual values and ethics. Finally, individuals involved in toxicological research must be aware of and accountable to their own individual biases and possible conflicts of interest and adhere to the highest ethical standards of the profession (Maurissen *et al.*, 2005).

Ethical reasoning and philosophy has a long and deep history, but more pragmatic bioethical reasoning can be traced to Aldo Leopold, who is arguably, America's first bioethicist: "A thing is right when it tends to preserve the integrity, stability, and beauty of the biotic community. It is wrong when it tends otherwise." (Leopold, 1949). The essence of toxicology is to understand the effects of chemicals on the biotic community. This broader definition of an ethic became more focused with examples such as the mercury poisoning in Minamata Bay, Japan, thalidomide, and the effects of pesticides as brought to public awareness by Rachel Carson's "Silent Spring" (Carson, 1962). In the United States, these events supported the public and political will to establish the EPA, strengthening of the FDA and other regulations designed to protect human and environmental health. The appreciation that some segments of our society were deferentially at risk from chemical exposures evolved into an appreciation of environmental justice (Coburn, 2002; EPA, 2005; Lee, 2002; Morello-Frosch *et al.*, 2002). The EPA defines environmental justice as "the fair treatment and meaningful involvement of all people regardless of race, color, national origin, or income with respect to the development, implementation, and enforcement of environmental laws, regulations, and policies..." (EPA, 2005). Environmental justice is now an important component of numerous community-based programs of interest, and is relevant to the field of toxicology. There is growing recognition of the direct financial and indirect costs to individuals and society from environmental exposures that are not equally distributed across society (Landrigan et al., 2002).

On a parallel track, biomedical ethics developed out of the lessons of World War II and related abuses of human subjects. The four principle of biomedical ethics—respect for autonomy, beneficence (do good), non-maleficence (do no harm), and justice (be fair)—became well established as a basis for decision-making in health care settings (Beauchamp and Childress, 1994). These principles formed the basis of rules and regulations regarding the conduct of human research. The demands of ethics and science made it clear that the highest standards of care produced the best results in both human and animal research. Rules and regulations regarding the housing and conduct of animal studies evolved similarly. Professional toxicology societies now require their members to adhere to the highest ethical standards when conducting research with humans or animals. A further refinement and expansion of biomedical ethical principles is the development of community-based participatory research that takes into consideration community needs to ensure the best results and benefit to the community (Arcury et al., 2001; Gilbert, 2006; O'Fallon and Dearry, 2002).

A glance at the daily newspaper confirms the number of current, sometimes controversial issues that are relevant to the field of toxicology. Decisions and action are often demanded or required even when there is a certain level of uncertainty in the toxicological data. The classic example of this challenge is establishing causation of the health effects of tobacco products. In part to address issues related to the health effects of tobacco products, Bradford Hill defined criteria for determining causation (Hill, 1965). These criteria are briefly summarized below.

1. Strength of association (relationship between independent and dependent variables)
2. Consistency of findings (replication of results by different studies)
3. Biological gradient (strength of the dose-response relationship)
4. Temporal sequence ("cause" before effect)
5. Biologic or theoretical plausibility (mechanism of action)
6. Coherence with established knowledge (no competing hypotheses)
7. Specificity of association (cause is tightly linked to an outcome)

Quantitative risk assessment was developed in part to address issues of uncertainty related to potential harm. The risk assessment process summarized data for risk managers and other decision makers, who must take into consideration to some degree the qualitative elements of ethical, social and political issues. Whereas risk management clearly has an ethical and values based aspect, risk assessment is not immune from the influence of one's values, bias or perspective. Ultimately action is required and as Bradford Hill (1965) noted: "All scientific work is incomplete—whether it be observational or experimental. All scientific work is liable to be upset or modified by advancing knowledge. That does not confer upon us a freedom to ignore the knowledge we already have or postpone the action that it appears to demand at a given time." These so-called "Bradford Hill criteria" were developed largely as a "weight of evidence" approach for interpreting a body of epidemiology data, yet are relevant as well to toxicology. Guzelian et al. (2005) provide a more detailed, evidence-based approach for determining causation in toxicology, primarily for application in the legal arena.

Although the scientific data may be the same, there are substantial differences in how toxicological data are used in a regulatory framework to protect public health versus establishing individual causation in the courtroom (Eaton, 2003). The approach to regulatory decision-making is in part directed by policy. For example, the experience with thalidomide and other drugs motivated the U.S. Congress to give the FDA broad power to ensure the efficacy and safety of new medicines or medical procedures. In this situation the pharmaceutical company or proponents of an activity must invest in the appropriate animal and human studies to demonstrate safety of the product. We have instituted a very precautionary approach with regard to drugs and medical devices. The approach to industrial chemicals is defined by the Toxic Substance Control Act and does not stipulate such a rigorous approach when introducing a new chemical.

Building on the work of Hill and others particularly from Europe, the Precautionary Principle was defined at the Wingspread Conference, in 1998: "When an activity raises threats of harm to human health or the environment, precautionary measures should be taken even if some cause and effect relationships are not fully established scientifically." (Gilbert, 2005b; Myers and Raffensperger, 2006; Raffensperger and Tickner, 1999). The precautionary principle incorporates elements of science and ethical philosophy into a single statement, acknowledging that ethics and values are part of the decision making process. Although the conceptual value of the precautionary principle to public health protection is obvious, the actual implementation of it in toxicological risk assessment is not straightforward, and remains a point of considerable debate (Marchant, 2003; Goldstein, 2006; Peterson, 2006).

With the increased relevance of toxicological data and evaluation in issues fundamental to society there has been increased awareness of the possibility of conflicts of interest influencing the decision-making process (Maurissen et al., 2005). The disclosure of conflicts of interest as well as the development of appropriate guidelines continues to be a challenge (NAS, 2003; Goozner, 2004; Krimsky and Rothenberg, 2001). These issues go to the core of one's individual values and integrity in the interpretation and communication of research results. Many professional societies, including the Society of Toxicology (http://www.toxicology.org/ai/asot/ethics.asp), have developed codes of ethics for their members.

As the field of toxicology has matured and its influence on societal issues has increased so has the need for the profession to make a commitment to examine the ethical, legal, and social implications of research and practice of toxicology.

General Characteristics of the Toxic Response

One could define a *poison* as any agent capable of producing a deleterious response in a biological system, seriously injuring function or producing death. This is not, however, a useful working definition for the very simple reason that virtually every known chemical has the potential to produce injury or death if it is present in a sufficient amount. Paracelsus (1493–1541), a Swiss/German/Austrian physician, scientist, and philosopher, phrased this well when he noted, "What is there that is not poison? All things are poison and nothing

Table 2.1

Approximate Acute LD$_{50}$s of Some Representative Chemical Agents

AGENT	LD$_{50}$, MG/KG*
Ethyl alcohol	10000
Sodium chloride	4000
Ferrous sulfate	1500
Morphine sulfate	900
Phenobarbital sodium	150
Picrotoxin	5
Strychnine sulfate	2
Nicotine	1
d–Tubocurarine	0.5
Hemicholinium-3	0.2
Tetrodotoxin	0.10
Dioxin (TCDD)	0.001
Botulinum toxin	0.00001

*LD$_{50}$ is the dosage (mg/kg body weight) causing death in 50% of exposed animals.

[is] without poison. Solely the dose determines that a thing is not a poison."

Among chemicals there is a wide spectrum of doses needed to produce deleterious effects, serious injury, or death. This is demonstrated in Table 2-1, which shows the dosage of chemicals needed to produce death in 50% of treated animals (LD$_{50}$). Some chemicals produce death in microgram doses and are commonly thought of as being extremely poisonous. Other chemicals may be relatively harmless after doses in excess of several grams. It should be noted, however, that measures of acute lethality such as LD$_{50}$ may not accurately reflect the full spectrum of toxicity, or hazard, associated with exposure to a chemical. For example, some chemicals with low acute toxicity may have carcinogenic, teratogenic, or neurobehavioral effects at doses that produce no evidence of acute toxicity. In addition, there is growing recognition that genetic factors can account for individual susceptibility to a range of responses.

CLASSIFICATION OF TOXIC AGENTS

Toxic agents are classified in a variety of ways, depending on the interests and needs of the classifier. In this textbook, for example, toxic agents are discussed in terms of their target organs (liver, kidney, hematopoietic system, etc.), use (pesticide, solvent, food additive, etc.), source (animal and plant toxins), and effects (cancer, mutation, liver injury, etc.). The term *toxin* generally refers to toxic substances that are produced by biological systems such as plants, animals, fungi, or bacteria. The term *toxicant* is used in speaking of toxic substances that are produced by or are a by-product of anthropogenic (human-made) activities. Thus, zeralanone, produced by a mold, is a toxin, whereas "dioxin" [2,3,7,8-tetrachlorodibenzo-*p*-dioxin (TCDD)], produced during the production and/or combustion of certain chlorinated organic chemicals, is a toxicant. Some toxicants can be produced by both natural and anthropogenic activities. For example, polyaromatic hydrocarbons are produced by the combustion of organic matter, which may occur both through natural processes (e.g., forest fires) and through anthropogenic activities (e.g., combustion of coal for energy production; cigarette smoking). Arsenic, a toxic metalloid, may occur as a natural contaminant of groundwater or may contaminate groundwater secondary to indus-

trial activities. Generally, such toxic substances are referred to as toxicants, rather than toxins, because, although they are naturally produced, they are not produced by biological systems.

Toxic agents may also be classified in terms of their physical state (gas, dust, liquid), their chemical stability or reactivity (explosive, flammable, oxidizer), general chemical structure (aromatic amine, halogenated hydrocarbon, etc.), or poisoning potential (extremely toxic, very toxic, slightly toxic, etc.). Classification of toxic agents on the basis of their biochemical mechanisms of action (e.g., alkylating agent, cholinesterase inhibitor, methemoglobin producer) is usually more informative than classification by general terms such as irritants and corrosives. But more general classifications such as air pollutants, occupation-related agents, and acute and chronic poisons can provide a useful focus on a specific problem. It is evident from this discussion that no single classification is applicable to the entire spectrum of toxic agents and that combinations of classification systems or a classification based on other factors may be needed to provide the best rating system for a special purpose. Nevertheless, classification systems that take into consideration both the chemical and the biological properties of an agent and the exposure characteristics are most likely to be useful for regulatory or control purposes and for toxicology in general.

SPECTRUM OF UNDESIRED EFFECTS

The spectrum of undesired effects of chemicals is broad. Some effects are deleterious and others are not. In therapeutics, for example, each drug produces a number of effects, but usually only one effect is associated with the primary objective of the therapy; all the other effects are referred to as *undesirable* or *side effects* of that drug for that therapeutic indication. However, some of these side effects may be desired for another therapeutic indication. For example, the "first-generation" antihistamine diphenhydramine (Benadryl) is effective in reducing histamine responses associated with allergies, but it readily enters the brain and causes mild central nervous system (CNS) depression (drowsiness, delayed reaction time). With the advent of newer and selective histamine receptor antagonists that do not cross the blood–brain barrier and thus do not have this CNS-depressant side effect, diphenhydramine is used less commonly today as an antihistamine. However, it is widely used as an "over the counter" sleep remedy, often in combination with analgesics (e.g., Tylenol PM, Excedrin PM, etc), taking advantage of the CNS-depressant effects. Some side effects of drugs are never desirable and are always deleterious to the well-being of humans. These are referred to as the *adverse, deleterious,* or *toxic* effects of the drug.

Allergic Reactions

Chemical allergy is an immunologically mediated adverse reaction to a chemical resulting from previous sensitization to that chemical or to a structurally similar one. The term *hypersensitivity* is most often used to describe this allergic state, but *allergic reaction* and *sensitization reaction* are also used to describe this situation when pre-exposure of the chemical is required to produce the toxic effect (see Chap. 12). Once sensitization has occurred, allergic reactions may result from exposure to relatively very low doses of chemicals; therefore population-based dose–response curves for allergic reactions have seldom been obtained. Because of this omission, some people assumed that allergic reactions are not dose-related. Thus, they do not consider the allergic reaction to be a true toxic response. However, for a given allergic individual, allergic reactions are dose-related. For example, it is well known that the allergic response to pollen in sensitized individuals is related to the concentration of pollen in the air. In addition, because the allergic response is an undesirable, adverse, deleterious effect, it obviously is also a toxic response. Sensitization reactions are sometimes very severe and may be fatal.

Most chemicals and their metabolic products are not sufficiently large to be recognized by the immune system as a foreign substance and thus must first combine with an endogenous protein to form an antigen (or immunogen). A molecule that must combine with an endogenous protein to elicit an allergic reaction is called a *hapten.* The hapten–protein complex (antigen) is then capable of eliciting the formation of antibodies, and usually at least 1 or 2 weeks is required for the synthesis of significant amounts of antibodies. Subsequent exposure to the chemical results in an antigen–antibody interaction, which provokes the typical manifestations of allergy. The manifestations of allergy are numerous. They may involve various organ systems and range in severity from minor skin disturbance to fatal anaphylactic shock. The pattern of allergic response differs in various species. In humans, involvement of the skin (e.g., dermatitis, urticaria, and itching) and involvement of the eyes (e.g., conjunctivitis) are most common, whereas in guinea pigs, bronchiolar constriction leading to asphyxia is the most common. However, chemically induced asthma (characterized by bronchiolar constriction) certainly does occur in some humans, and the incidence of allergic asthma has increased substantially in recent years. Hypersensitivity reactions are discussed in more detail in Chap. 12.

Idiosyncratic Reactions

Chemical idiosyncrasy refers to a genetically determined abnormal reactivity to a chemical (Goldstein *et al.*, 1974; Levine, 1978). The response observed is usually qualitatively similar to that observed in all individuals but may take the form of extreme sensitivity to low doses or extreme insensitivity to high doses of the chemical. However, while some people use the term *idiosyncratic* as a catchall to refer to all reactions that occur with low frequency, it should not be used in that manner (Goldstein *et al.*, 1974). A classic example of an idiosyncratic reaction is provided by patients who exhibit prolonged muscular relaxation and apnea (inability to breathe) lasting several hours after a standard dose of succinylcholine. Succinylcholine usually produces skeletal muscle relaxation of only short duration because of its very rapid metabolic degradation by an enzyme that is present normally in the bloodstream called plasma butyrylcholinesterase (also referred to as pseudocholinesterase). Patients exhibiting this idiosyncratic reaction have a genetic polymorphism in the gene for the enzyme butyrylcholinesterase, which is less active in breaking down succinylcholine. Family pedigree and molecular genetic analyses have demonstrated that the presence of low plasma butyrylcholinesterase activity is due to the presence of one or more single nucleotide polymorphisms in this gene (Bartels *et al.*, 1992). Similarly, there is a group of people who are abnormally sensitive to nitrites and certain other chemicals that have in common the ability to oxidize the iron in hemoglobin to produce *methemoglobin,* which is incapable of carrying oxygen to the tissues. The unusual phenotype is inherited as an autosomal recessive trait and is characterized by a deficiency in NADH-cytochrome b5 reductase activity. The genetic basis for this idiosyncratic response has been identified as a single nucleotide change in codon 127, which results in replacement of serine with proline (Kobayashi *et al.*, 1990). The consequence of this genetic deficiency is that these individuals may suffer from a serious lack of oxygen delivery to tissues after exposure to doses of methemoglobin-producing chemicals that would be harmless to individuals with normal NADH-cytochrome b5 reductase activity.

Immediate versus Delayed Toxicity

Immediate toxic effects can be defined as those that occur or develop rapidly after a single administration of a substance, whereas delayed toxic effects are those that occur after the lapse of some time. Carcinogenic effects of chemicals usually have a long latency period, often 20 to 30 years after the initial exposure, before tumors are observed in humans. For example, daughters of mothers who took diethylstilbestrol (DES) during pregnancy have a greatly increased risk of developing vaginal cancer, but not other types of cancer, in young adulthood, some 20 to 30 years after their in utero exposure to DES (Hatch *et al.*, 1998). Also, delayed neurotoxicity is observed after exposure to some organophosphorus insecticides that act by covalent modification of an enzyme referred to as *neuropathy target esterase* (NTE), a neuronal protein with serine esterase activity (Glynn *et al.*, 1999). Binding of certain organophosphates (OP) to this protein initiates degeneration of long axons in the peripheral and central nervous system. The most notorious of the compounds that produce this type of neurotoxic effect is triorthocresylphosphate (TOCP). The effect is not observed until at least several days after exposure to the toxic compound. In contrast, most substances produce immediate toxic effects but do not produce delayed effects.

Reversible versus Irreversible Toxic Effects

Some toxic effects of chemicals are reversible, and others are irreversible. If a chemical produces pathological injury to a tissue, the ability of that tissue to regenerate largely determines whether the effect is reversible or irreversible. Thus, for a tissue such as liver, which has a high ability to regenerate, most injuries are reversible, whereas injury to the CNS is largely irreversible because differentiated cells of the CNS cannot divide and be replaced. Carcinogenic and teratogenic effects of chemicals, once they occur, are usually considered irreversible toxic effects.

Local versus Systemic Toxicity

Another distinction between types of effects is made on the basis of the general site of action. Local effects are those that occur at the site of first contact between the biological system and the toxicant. Such effects are produced by the ingestion of caustic substances or the inhalation of irritant materials. For example, chlorine gas reacts with lung tissue at the site of contact, causing damage and swelling of the tissue, with possibly fatal consequences, even though very little of the chemical is absorbed into the bloodstream. The alternative to local effects is systemic effects. Systemic effects require absorption and distribution of a toxicant from its entry point to a distant site, at which deleterious effects are produced. Most substances except highly reactive materials produce systemic effects. For some materials, both effects can be demonstrated. For example, tetraethyl lead produces effects on skin at the site of absorption and then is transported systemically to produce its typical effects on the CNS and other organs. If the local effect is marked, there may also be indirect systemic effects. For example, kidney damage after a severe acid burn is an indirect systemic effect because the toxicant does not reach the kidney.

Most chemicals that produce systemic toxicity do not cause a similar degree of toxicity in all organs; instead, they usually elicit their major toxicity in only one or two organs. These sites are referred to as the *target organs* of toxicity of a particular chemical. The target organ of toxicity is often not the site of the highest concentration of the chemical. For example, lead is concentrated in bone, but its toxicity is due to its effects in soft tissues, particularly the brain. DDT is concentrated in adipose tissue but produces no known toxic effects in that tissue.

The target organ of toxicity most frequently involved in systemic toxicity is the CNS (brain and spinal cord). Even with many compounds having a prominent effect elsewhere, damage to the CNS can be demonstrated by the use of appropriate and sensitive methods. Next in order of frequency of involvement in systemic toxicity are the circulatory system; the blood and hematopoietic system; visceral organs such as the liver, kidney, and lung; and the skin. Muscle and bone are least often the target tissues for systemic effects. With substances that have a predominantly local effect, the frequency with which tissues react depends largely on the portal of entry (skin, gastrointestinal tract, or respiratory tract).

Interaction of Chemicals

Because of the large number of different chemicals an individual may come in contact with at any given time (workplace, drugs, diet, hobbies, etc.), it is necessary, in assessing the spectrum of responses, to consider how different chemicals may interact with each other. Interactions can occur in a variety of ways. Chemical interactions are known to occur by a number of mechanisms, such as alterations in absorption, protein binding, and the biotransformation and excretion of one or both of the interacting toxicants. In addition to these modes of interaction, the response of the organism to combinations of toxicants may be increased or decreased because of toxicologic responses at the site of action.

The effects of two chemicals given simultaneously produce a response that may simply be additive of their individual responses or may be greater or less than that expected by addition of their individual responses. The study of these interactions often leads to a better understanding of the mechanism of toxicity of the chemicals involved. A number of terms have been used to describe pharmacologic and toxicologic interactions. An *additive* effect occurs when the combined effect of two chemicals is equal to the sum of the effects of each agent given alone (example: $2 + 3 = 5$). The effect most commonly observed when two chemicals are given together is an additive effect. For example, when two organophosphate insecticides are given together, the cholinesterase inhibition is usually additive. A *synergistic* effect occurs when the combined effects of two chemicals are much greater than the sum of the effects of each agent given alone (example: $2 + 2 = 20$). For example, both carbon tetrachloride and ethanol are hepatotoxic compounds, but together they produce much more liver injury than the mathematical sum of their individual effects on liver at a given dose would suggest. *Potentiation* occurs when one substance does not have a toxic effect on a certain organ or system but when added to another chemical makes that chemical much more toxic (example: $0 + 2 = 10$). Isopropanol, for example, is not hepatotoxic, but when it is administered in addition to carbon tetrachloride, the hepatotoxicity of carbon tetrachloride is much greater than when it is given alone. *Antagonism* occurs when two chemicals administered together interfere with each other's actions or one interferes with the action of the other (example: $4 + 6 = 8$; $4 + (-4) = 0$; $4 + 0 = 1$). Antag-

onistic effects of chemicals are often very desirable in toxicology and are the basis of many antidotes. There are four major types of antagonism: functional, chemical, dispositional, and receptor. *Functional antagonism* occurs when two chemicals counterbalance each other by producing opposite effects on the same physiologic function. Advantage is taken of this principle in that the blood pressure can markedly fall during severe barbiturate intoxication, which can be effectively antagonized by the intravenous administration of a vasopressor agent such as norepinephrine or metaraminol. Similarly, many chemicals, when given at toxic dose levels, produce convulsions, and the convulsions often can be controlled by giving anticonvulsants such as the benzodiazepines (e.g., diazepam). *Chemical antagonism* or *inactivation* is simply a chemical reaction between two compounds that produces a less toxic product. For example, dimercaprol (British antilewisite, or BAL) chelates with metal ions such as arsenic, mercury, and lead and decreases their toxicity. The use of antitoxins in the treatment of various animal toxins is also an example of chemical antagonism. The use of the strongly basic low-molecular-weight protein protamine sulfate to form a stable complex with heparin, which abolishes its anticoagulant activity, is another example. *Dispositional antagonism* occurs when the disposition—that is, the absorption, distribution, biotransformation, or excretion of a chemical—is altered so that the concentration and/or duration of the chemical at the target organ are diminished. Thus, the prevention of absorption of a toxicant by ipecac or charcoal and the increased excretion of a chemical by administration of an osmotic diuretic or alteration of the pH of the urine are examples of dispositional antagonism. If the parent compound is responsible for the toxicity of the chemical (such as the anticoagulant warfarin) and its metabolic breakdown products are less toxic than the parent compound, increasing the compound's metabolism (biotransformation) by administering a drug that increases the activity of the metabolizing enzymes (e.g., a "microsomal enzyme inducer" such as phenobarbital) will decrease its toxicity. However, if the chemical's toxicity is largely due to a metabolic product (as in the case of the organophosphate insecticide parathion), inhibiting its biotransformation by an inhibitor of microsomal enzyme activity (SKF-525A or piperonyl butoxide) will decrease its toxicity. *Receptor antagonism* occurs when two chemicals that bind to the same receptor produce less of an effect when given together than the addition of their separate effects (example: $4 + 6 = 8$) or when one chemical antagonizes the effect of the second chemical (example: $0 + 4 = 1$). Receptor antagonists are often termed *blockers*. This concept is used to advantage in the clinical treatment of poisoning. For example, the receptor antagonist naloxone is used to treat the respiratory depressive effects of morphine and other morphine-like narcotics by competitive binding to the same receptor. Another example of receptor antagonism is the use of the antiestrogen drug tamoxifen to lower breast cancer risk among women at high risk for this estrogen-related cancer. Tamoxifen competitively block estradiol from binding to its receptor. Treatment of organophosphate insecticide poisoning with atropine is an example not of the antidote competing with the poison for the receptor (cholinesterase) but involves blocking the receptor (cholinergic receptor) for the excess acetylcholine that accumulates by poisoning of the cholinesterase by the organophosphate (see Chap. 22).

Tolerance

Tolerance is a state of decreased responsiveness to a toxic effect of a chemical resulting from prior exposure to that chemical or to a structurally related chemical. Two major mechanisms are responsible for tolerance: one is due to a decreased amount of toxicant reaching the site where the toxic effect is produced (*dispositional tolerance*), and the other is due to a reduced responsiveness of a tissue to the chemical. Comparatively less is known about the cellular mechanisms responsible for altering the responsiveness of a tissue to a toxic chemical than is known about dispositional tolerance. Two chemicals known to produce dispositional tolerance are carbon tetrachloride and cadmium. Carbon tetrachloride produces tolerance to itself by decreasing the formation of the reactive metabolite (trichloromethyl radical) that produces liver injury (see Chap. 13). The mechanism of cadmium tolerance is explained by induction of metallothionein, a metal-binding protein. Subsequent binding of cadmium to metallothionein rather than to critical macromolecules decreases its toxicity.

CHARACTERISTICS OF EXPOSURE

Toxic effects in a biological system are not produced by a chemical agent unless that agent or its metabolic breakdown (biotransformation) products reach appropriate sites in the body at a concentration and for a length of time sufficient to produce a toxic manifestation. Many chemicals are of relatively low toxicity in the "native" form but, when acted on by enzymes in the body, are converted to intermediate forms that interfere with normal cellular biochemistry and physiology. Thus, whether a toxic response occurs is dependent on the chemical and physical properties of the agent, the exposure situation, how the agent is metabolized by the system, the concentration of the active form at the particular target site(s), and the overall susceptibility of the biological system or subject. Thus, to characterize fully the potential hazard of a specific chemical agent, we need to know not only what type of effect it produces and the dose required to produce that effect but also information about the agent, the exposure, and its disposition by the subject. Two major factors that influence toxicity as it relates to the exposure situation for a specific chemical are the route of exposure, and the duration, and frequency of exposure.

Route and Site of Exposure

The major routes (pathways) by which toxic agents gain access to the body are the gastrointestinal tract (ingestion), lungs (inhalation), skin (topical, percutaneous, or dermal), and other parenteral (other than intestinal canal) routes. Toxic agents generally produce the greatest effect and the most rapid response when given directly into the bloodstream (the intravenous route). An approximate descending order of effectiveness for the other routes would be inhalation, intraperitoneal, subcutaneous, intramuscular, intradermal, oral, and dermal. The "vehicle" (the material in which the chemical is dissolved) and other formulation factors can markedly alter absorption after ingestion, inhalation, or topical exposure. In addition, the route of administration can influence the toxicity of agents. For example, an agent that acts on the CNS, but is efficiently detoxified in the liver, would be expected to be less toxic when given orally than when given via inhalation, because the oral route requires that nearly all of the dose pass through the liver before reaching the systemic circulation and then the CNS.

Occupational exposure to toxic agents most frequently results from breathing contaminated air (inhalation) and/or direct and prolonged contact of the skin with the substance (dermal exposure), whereas accidental and suicidal poisoning occurs most frequently by oral ingestion. Comparison of the lethal dose of a toxic substance by different routes of exposure often provides useful information about its extent of absorption. In instances when the toxic dose after oral or dermal administration is similar to the toxic dose after intravenous administration, the assumption is that the toxic agent is absorbed readily and rapidly. Conversely, in cases where the toxic dose by the dermal route is several orders of magnitude higher than the oral toxic dose, it is likely that the skin provides an effective barrier to absorption of the agent. Toxic effects by any route of exposure can also be influenced by the concentration of the agent in its vehicle, the total volume of the vehicle and the properties of the vehicle to which the biological system is exposed, and the rate at which exposure occurs. Studies in which the concentration of a chemical in the blood is determined at various times after exposure are often needed to clarify the role of these and other factors in the toxicity of a compound. For more details on the absorption of toxicants, see Chap. 5.

Duration and Frequency of Exposure

Toxicologists usually divide the exposure of experimental animals to chemicals into four categories: acute, subacute, subchronic, and chronic. Acute exposure is defined as exposure to a chemical for less than 24 hours, and examples of exposure routes are intraperitoneal, intravenous, and subcutaneous injection; oral intubation; and dermal application. Whereas acute exposure usually refers to a single administration, repeated exposures may be given within a 24-hours period for some slightly toxic or practically nontoxic chemicals. Acute exposure by inhalation refers to continuous exposure for less than 24 hours, most frequently for 4 hours. Repeated exposure is divided into three categories: subacute, subchronic, and chronic. *Subacute exposure* refers to repeated exposure to a chemical for 1 month or less, *subchronic* for 1 to 3 months, and *chronic* for more than 3 months, although usually this refers to studies with at least 1 year of repeated dosing. These three categories of repeated exposure can be by any route, but most often they occur by the oral route, with the chemical added directly to the diet.

In human exposure situations, the frequency and duration of exposure are usually not as clearly defined as in controlled animal studies, but many of the same terms are used to describe general exposure situations. Thus, workplace or environmental exposures may be described as *acute* (occurring from a single incident or episode), *subchronic* (occurring repeatedly over several weeks or months), or *chronic* (occurring repeatedly for many months or years).

For many chemicals, the toxic effects that follow a single exposure are quite different from those produced by repeated exposure. For example, the primary acute toxic manifestation of benzene is central nervous system (CNS) depression, but repeated exposures can result in bone marrow toxicity and an increased risk for leukemia. Acute exposure to chemicals that are rapidly absorbed is likely to produce immediate toxic effects but also can produce delayed toxicity that may or may not be similar to the toxic effects of chronic exposure. Conversely, chronic exposure to a toxic chemical may produce some immediate (acute) effects after each administration in addition to the long-term, low-level, or chronic effects of the toxic substance. In characterizing the toxicity of a specific chemical, it is evident that information is needed not only for the single-dose (acute) and long-term (chronic) effects but also for exposures of intermediate duration. The other time-related factor that is important in the temporal characterization of repeated

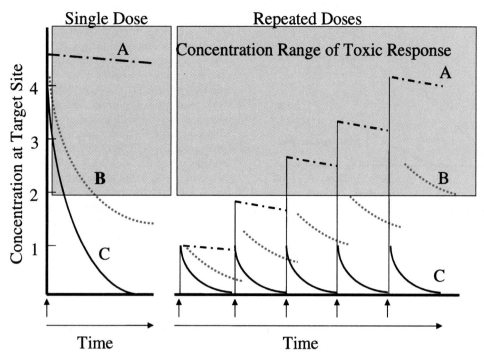

Figure 2-2. Diagrammatic view of the relationship between dose and concentration at the target site under different conditions of dose frequency and elimination rate.

Line A. A chemical with very slow elimination (e.g., half-life of 1 year). *Line B.* A chemical with a rate of elimination equal to frequency of dosing (e.g., 1 day). *Line C.* Rate of elimination faster than the dosing frequency (e.g., 5 h). Blue-shaded area is representative of the concentration of chemical at the target site necessary to elicit a toxic response.

exposures is the frequency of exposure. The relationship between elimination rate and frequency of exposure is shown in Fig. 2-2. A chemical that produces severe effects with a single dose may have no effect if the same total dose is given in several intervals. For the chemical depicted by line B in Fig. 2-2, in which the half-life for elimination (time necessary for 50% of the chemical to be removed from the bloodstream) is approximately equal to the dosing frequency, a theoretical toxic concentration (shown conceptually as two Concentration Units in Fig. 2-2) is not reached until the fourth dose, whereas that concentration is reached with only two doses for chemical A, which has an elimination rate much slower than the dosing interval (time between each repeated dose). Conversely, for chemical C, where the elimination rate is much shorter than the dosing interval, a toxic concentration at the site of toxic effect will never be reached regardless of how many doses are administered. Of course, it is possible that residual cell or tissue damage occurs with each dose even though the chemical itself is not accumulating. The important consideration, then, is whether the interval between doses is sufficient to allow for complete repair of tissue damage. It is evident that with any type of repeated exposure, the production of a toxic effect is influenced not only by the frequency of exposure but may, in fact, be totally dependent on the frequency rather than the duration of exposure. Chronic toxic effects may occur, therefore, if the chemical accumulates in the biological system (rate of absorption exceeds the rate of biotransformation and/or excretion), if it produces irreversible toxic effects, or if there is insufficient time for the system to recover from the toxic damage within the exposure frequency interval. For additional discussion of these relationships, see Chaps. 5 and 7.

DOSE–RESPONSE RELATIONSHIP

The characteristics of exposure and the spectrum of toxic effects come together in a correlative relationship customarily referred to as the *dose–response relationship*. Whatever response is selected for measurement, the relationship between the degree of response of the biological system and the amount of toxicant administered assumes a form that occurs so consistently as to be considered the most fundamental and pervasive concept in toxicology.

From a practical perspective, there are two types of dose–response relationships: (1) the individual dose–response relationship, which describes the response of an *individual* organism to varying doses of a chemical, often referred to as a "graded" response because the measured effect is continuous over a range of doses, and (2) a quantal dose–response relationship, which characterizes the distribution of individual responses to different doses in a *population* of individual organisms.

Individual, or Graded, Dose–Response Relationships

Individual dose–response relationships are characterized by a dose-related increase in the severity of the response. The dose relatedness of the response often results from an alteration of a specific biochemical process. For example, Fig. 2-3 shows the dose–response relationship between different dietary doses of the organophosphate insecticide chlorpyrifos and the extent of inhibition of two

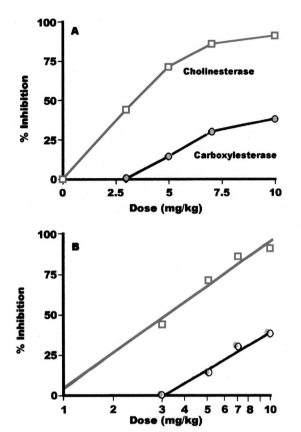

Figure 2-3. *Dose–response relationship between different doses of the organophosphate insecticide chlorpyrifos and esterase enzyme inhibition in the brain.*

Open circles and blue lines represent acetylcholinesterase activity and closed circles represent carboxylesterase activity in the brains of pregnant female Long-Evans rats given 5 daily doses of chlorpyrifos. *A.* Dose–response curve plotted on an arithmetic scale. *B.* Same data plotted on a semi-log scale. (Data derived from Lassiter *et al.*, Gestational exposure to chloryprifos: Dose response profiles for cholinesterase and carboxylesterase activity. *Toxicol Sci* 52:92–100, 1999, with permission from Oxford University Press.)

different enzymes in the brain and liver: acetylcholinesterase and carboxylesterase. In the brain, the degree of inhibition of both enzymes is clearly dose-related and spans a wide range, although the amount of inhibition per unit dose is different for the two enzymes. From the shapes of these two dose–response curves it is evident that, in the brain, cholinesterase is more easily inhibited than carboxylesterase. The toxicologic response that results is directly related to the degree of cholinesterase enzyme inhibition in the brain. Thus, clinical signs and symptoms for chlorpyrifos would follow a dose–response relationship similar to that for brain cholinesterase. However, for many chemicals, more than one effect may result because of multiple different target sites in different tissues. Thus, the observed response to varying doses of a chemical in the whole organism is often complicated by the fact that most toxic substances have multiple sites or mechanisms of toxicity, each with its own "dose–response" relationship and subsequent adverse effect. Note that when these dose–response data are plotted using the base 10 log of the dose on the abscissa (Fig. 2.3*B*), a better "fit" of the data to a straight line usually occurs. This is typical of many graded as well as quantal dose–response relationships.

Quantal Dose–Response Relationships

In contrast to the "graded" or continuous-scale dose–response relationship that occurs in individuals, the dose–response relationships in a *population* are by definition quantal—or "all or none"—in nature; that is, at any given dose, an individual in the population is classified as either a "responder" or a "nonresponder." Although these distinctions of "quantal population" and "graded individual" dose–response relationships are useful, the two types of responses are conceptually identical. The ordinate in both cases is simply labeled *the response,* which may be the degree of response in an individual or system or the fraction of a population responding, and the abscissa is the range in administered doses.

A widely used statistical approach for estimating the response of a population to a toxic exposure is the "Effective Dose" or ED. Generally, the mid-point, or 50%, response level is used, giving rise to the "ED_{50}" value. However, any response level, such as an ED_{01}, ED_{10} or ED_{30} could be chosen. A graphical representation of an approximate ED_{50} is shown in Fig. 2-4. Note that these data are

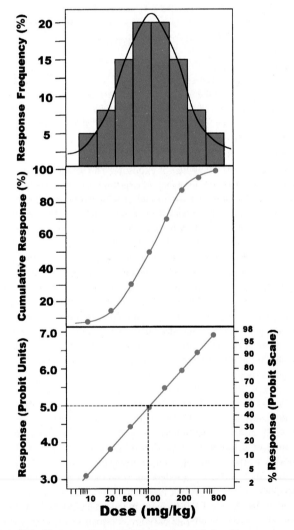

Figure 2-4. *Diagram of quantal dose–response relationship.*

The abscissa is a log dosage of the chemical. In the top panel the ordinate is response frequency, in the middle panel the ordinate is percent response, and in the bottom panel the response is in probit units (see text).

"quantal". Where death is the measured end-point, the ED_{50} would be referred to as the Lethal Dose 50 (LD_{50}). Historically, determination of the LD_{50} was often the first experiment performed with a new chemical. Today, it is widely recognized that the LD_{50} is of marginal value as a measure of hazard, although it does provide a useful "ball park" indication of the relative hazard of a compound to cause serious, life-threatening poisoning from a single exposure. Although death is an obvious quantal end-point to measure, it should be noted that any quantal response could be used. For example, the LD_{50} of lead or DDT is not a relevant endpoint when characterizing hazards of the agents to children or wildlife, respectively. Even continuous variables can be converted to quantal responses if desired. For example, an antihypertensive drug that lowers blood pressure might be evaluated in a population by assigning a "responder" as an individual who's blood pressure was lowered by 10 mm Hg or more. Note that, in this example, an individual that responded to a change in blood pressure of 50 mm Hg would classified the same as an individual with a change in only 10 mm Hg, yet an individual with a change in 8 mm Hg would be classified as a "non-responder". The top panel of Fig. 2-4 shows that quantal dose responses typically exhibit a normal or Gaussian distribution. The frequency histogram in this panel also shows the relationship between dose and effect. The bars represent the percentage of animals that responded at each dose minus the percentage that responded at the immediately lower dose. One can clearly see that only a few animals responded to the lowest dose and the highest dose. Larger numbers of animals responded to doses intermediate between these two extremes, and the maximum frequency of response occurred in the middle portion of the dose range. Thus, we have a bell-shaped curve known as a *normal frequency distribution.* The reason for this normal distribution is that there are differences in susceptibility to chemicals among individuals; this is known as biological variation. Animals responding at the left end of the curve are referred to as *hypersusceptible,* and those at the right end of the curve are called *resistant.* If the numbers of individuals responding at each consecutive dose are added together, a cumulative, quantal dose–response relationship is obtained. When a sufficiently large number of doses is used with a large number of animals per dose, a sigmoid dose–response curve is observed, as depicted in the middle panel of Fig. 2-4. With the lowest dose (6 mg/kg), 1% of the animals respond. A normally distributed sigmoid curve such as this one approaches a response of 0% as the dose is decreased and approaches 100% as the dose is increased; but—theoretically—it never passes through 0 and 100%. However, the minimally effective dose of any chemical that evokes a stated all-or-none response is called the *threshold dose* even though it cannot be determined experimentally.

For a normally distributed population response, the sigmoid curve has a relatively linear portion between 16 and 84%. These values represent the limits of 1 standard deviation (SD) of the mean (and the median) in a population with truly normal or Gaussian distribution. However, it is usually not practical to describe the dose–response curve from this type of plot because one does not usually have large enough sample sizes to define the sigmoid curve adequately. In a normally distributed population, the mean ±1 SD represents 68.3% of the population, the mean ±2 SD represents 95.5% of the population, and the mean ±3 SD equals 99.7% of the population. Because quantal dose–response phenomena are usually normally distributed, one can convert the percent response to units of deviation from the mean or normal equivalent deviations (NEDs). Thus, the NED for a 50% response is 0; an NED of +1 is equated

with an 84.1% response. Traditionally, units of NED are converted by the addition of 5 to the value to avoid negative numbers; these converted units are called *probit units* (Bliss, 1957). The probit (from the contraction of *prob*ability un*it*), then, is an NED plus 5. In this transformation, a 50% response becomes a probit of 5, a +1 deviation becomes a probit of 6, and a −1 deviation is a probit of 4.

The data given in the top two panels of Fig. 2-4 are replotted in the bottom panel with the response plotted in probit units. The data in the middle panel (which was in the form of a sigmoid curve) and the top panel (a bell-shaped curve) form a straight line when transformed into probit units. In essence, what is accomplished in a probit transformation is an adjustment of quantal data to an assumed normal population distribution, resulting in a straight line. The ED_{50} is obtained by drawing a horizontal line from the probit unit 5, which is the 50% response point, to the dose–effect line. At the point of intersection, a vertical line is drawn, and this line intersects the abscissa at the ED_{50} point. It is evident from the line that information with respect to the effective dose for 90% or for 10% of the population also may be derived by a similar procedure. Mathematically, it can be demonstrated that the range of values encompassed by the confidence limits is narrowest at the midpoint of the line (ED_{50}) and widest at both extremes (ED_{10} and ED_{90}) of the dose–response curve (dotted lines in Fig. 2-5). In addition to the ED_{50}, the slope of the dose–response curve can also be obtained. Figure 2-5 demonstrates the dose–response curves for the response of two compounds. Compound A exhibits a "flat" dose–response curve, showing that a large change in dosage is required before a significant change in response will be observed. However, compound B exhibits a "steep" dose–response curve, where a relatively small change in dosage will cause a large change in response. It is evident that the ED_{50} for both compounds is the same (8 mg/kg). However, the slopes of the dose–response curves are quite different. At one-half of ED_{50} of the compounds (4 mg/kg), less than 1% of the animals exposed to compound B would respond but 20% of the animals given compound A would respond.

In Figs. 2-4 and 2-5 the dosage has been given on a log basis. Although the use of the log of the dosage is empiric, log-dosage plots for normally distributed quantal data provide a more nearly linear representation of the data. It must be remembered, however,

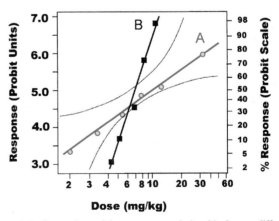

Figure 2-5. Comparison of dose–response relationship for two different chemicals, plotted on a log dose-probit scale.

Note that the slope of the dose–response is steeper for chemical *B* than chemical *A*. Dotted lines represents the confidence limits for chemical *A*.

Table 2.2
Allometric Scaling of Dose Across Different Species

SPECIES	WEIGHT (kg)	SURFACE AREA (cm²)*	FOLD DIFFERENCE, RELATIVE TO HUMANS, NORMALIZED BY BODY WEIGHT		
			mg/kg	(BW)$^{2/3}$	(BW)$^{3/4}$
Mouse	0.30	103	1	13.0	7.0
Rat	0.2	365	1	6.9	4.3
Guinea pig	0.4	582	1	5.5	3.6
Rabbit	1.5	1410	1	3.5	2.6
Cat	2	1710	1	3.2	2.4
Monkey	4	2720	1	2.6	2.0
Dog	12	5680	1	1.8	1.5
Human	70	18500	1	1.0	1.0

*Surface area of animals is closely approximated by the formula: SA = 10.5 × (Body wt, in grams)$^{2/3}$.

that this is not universally the case. Some radiation effects, for example, give a better probit fit when the dose is expressed arithmetically rather than logarithmically. There are other situations in which other functions (e.g., exponentials) of dosage provide a better fit to the data than does the log function. It is also conventional to express the dosage in milligrams per kilogram. It might be argued that expression of dosage on a mole-per-kilogram basis would be better, particularly for making comparisons among a series of compounds. Although such an argument has considerable merit, dosage is usually expressed in milligrams per kilogram.

One might also view dosage on the basis of body weight as being less appropriate than other bases, such as surface area. The term *Allometry* refers to the field of study that examines the relationships between body weight and other biological and physical parameters such as rate of basal metabolism (caloric consumption), heart rate, blood flow, etc. Allometric studies revealed that the relationship between body weight and various other physiological parameters can be closely estimated by the formula, $Y = aW^b$, where Y is the biological parameter of interest, a and b are constants that relate Y to body weight (Rodricks *et al.*, 2001). In general, organ sizes between species seem to scale best when b is equal to 1, whereas metabolically derived parameters scale better when b is 0.67–0.75. The relationship between body surface area and body weight across most mammalian species is closely described by the formula SA = $10.5 \times$ (body weight, in grams)$^{0.67}$ (Harkness and Wagner, 1995). Empirical comparisons of toxicity data across species confirm that this relationship is appropriate for toxicological scaling. For example, Travis and White (1988) analyzed a number of toxicity testing data sets for 27 different chemotherapeutic drugs for which toxicity data were available in mouse, rat, hamster, dog, monkey, and human. They found that the exponent of body weight that gave the best correlation with toxicity was 0.73, with 95% confidence bounds of 0.69–0.77 (Rodricks *et al.*, 2001). Table 2-2 illustrates the differences in comparative doses when scaling is done by body weight (mg/kg) versus an allometric approach that uses an exponent of either 0.67 or 0.75. Thus, if a scaling factor of (BW)$^{2/3}$ is used, a mouse would need to receive a dose 13 times greater than humans for an equivalent toxic response, where as a it would be seven times greater if a scaling factor of (BW)$^{3/4}$ was used. However, not all toxic responses will necessarily scale across species in the same way. For example, acute lethality seemed to correlate better across species when body weight, rather than body surface area, was used (Rhomberg and Wolf, 1998).

Shape of the Dose–Response Curve

Essential Nutrients   The shape of the dose–response relationship has many important implications in toxicity assessment. For example, for substances that are required for normal physiologic function and survival (e.g., vitamins and essential trace elements such as chromium, cobalt, and selenium), the shape of the "graded" dose–response relationship in an individual over the entire dose range is actually U-shaped (Fig. 2-6). That is, at very low doses, there is a high level of adverse effect, which decreases with an increasing dose. This region of the dose–response relationship for essential nutrients is commonly referred to as a *deficiency*. As the dose is increased to a point where the deficiency no longer exists, no adverse response is detected and the organism is in a state of homeostasis. However, as the dose is increased to abnormally high levels, an adverse response (usually qualitatively different from that observed at deficient doses) appears and increases in magnitude with increasing dose, just as with other toxic substances. Thus, it is recognized that high doses of vitamin A can cause liver toxicity and birth defects,

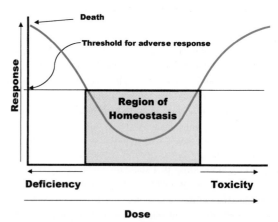

Figure 2-6. Individual dose–response relationship for an essential substance such as a vitamin or trace element.

It is generally recognized that, for most types of toxic responses, a threshold exists such that at doses below the threshold, no toxicity is evident. For essential substances, doses below the minimum daily requirement, as well as those above the threshold for safety, may be associated with toxic effects. The blue-shaded region represents the "region of homeostasis"—the dose range that results in neither deficiency or toxicity.

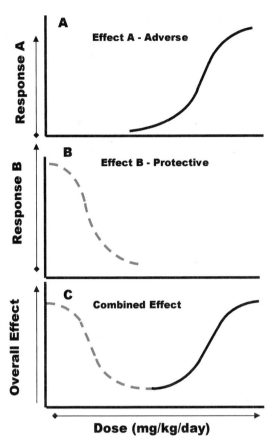

Figure 2-7. Hypothetical dose–response relationship depicting characteristics of hormesis.

Hormetic effects of a substance are hypothesized to occur when relatively low doses result in the stimulation of a beneficial or protective response (*B*), such as induction of enzymatic pathways that protect against oxidative stress. Although low doses provide a potential beneficial effect, a threshold is exceeded as the dose increases and the net effects will be detrimental (*A*), resulting in a typical dose-related increase in toxicity. The complete dose–response curve (*C*) is conceptually similar to the individual dose–response relationship for essential nutrients shown in Fig. 2-6.

high doses of selenium can affect the brain, and high doses of estrogens may increase the risk of breast cancer, even though low doses of all these substances are essential for life.

Hormesis   There is considerable evidence to suggest that some nonnutritional toxic substances may also impart beneficial or stimulatory effects at low doses but that, at higher doses, they produce adverse effects. This concept of "hormesis" was first described for radiation effects but may also pertain to most chemical responses (Calabrese and Blaine, 2005). Thus, in plotting dose versus response over a wide range of doses, the effects of hormesis may also result in a "U-shaped" dose–response curve. In its original development, the concept of hormesis pertained to the ability of substances to stimulate biological systems at low doses but to inhibit them at high doses. The application of the concept of hormesis to whole-animal toxicologic dose–response relationships may also be relevant but requires that the "response" on the ordinate be variant with dose. For example, chronic alcohol consumption is well recognized to increase the risk of esophageal cancer, liver cancer, and cirrhosis of the liver at relatively high doses, and this response is dose-related

(curve A, Fig. 2-7). However, there is also substantial clinical and epidemiologic evidence that low to moderate consumption of alcohol reduces the incidence of coronary heart disease and stroke (curve B, Fig. 2-7) (Hanna *et al.*, 1997). Thus, when all responses are plotted on the ordinate, a "U-shaped" dose–response curve is obtained (curve C, Fig. 2-7). U-shaped dose–response relationships have obvious implications for the process of low dose extrapolation in risk assessment.

Threshold   Another important aspect of the dose–response relationship at low doses is the concept of the threshold. It has long been recognized that acute toxicologic responses are associated with thresholds; that is, there is some dose below which the probability of an individual responding is zero. Obviously, the identification of a threshold depends on the particular response that is measured, the sensitivity of the measurement, and the number of subjects studied. For the individual dose–response relationship, thresholds for most toxic effects certainly exist, although interindividual variability in response and qualitative changes in response pattern with dose make it difficult to establish a true "no effects" threshold for any chemical. The biological basis of thresholds for acute responses is well established and frequently can be demonstrated on the basis of mechanistic information (Aldridge, 1986). The traditional approaches to establishing acceptable levels of exposure to chemicals are inherently different for threshold versus nonthreshold responses. The existence of thresholds for chronic responses is less well defined, especially in the area of chemical carcinogenesis. It is, of course, impossible to scientifically prove the absence of a threshold, as one can never prove a negative. Nevertheless, for the identification of "safe" levels of exposure to a substance, the absence or presence of a threshold is important for practical reasons (see Chap. 4). A classic example of the difficulty of establishing thresholds experimentally is provided by the "ED01" study, where over 24,000 mice and 81 different treatment groups were used to determine the shape of the dose–response relationship for the prototypical carcinogen 2-acetylaminofluorene (2-AAF). The study was designed to identify a statistically significant response of 1% (0.01 probability). The mice were exposed to 2-AAF at one of seven different doses in the dose range of 30 to 150 ppm (plus 0 dose control) (Littlefield *et al.*, 1979). Eight "sacrifice intervals" were used to determine how quickly tumors developed. The dose–response relationship between 2-AAF exposure and liver and bladder cancer at 24 and 33 months of exposure are shown in Fig. 2-8. Both types of tumors demonstrated increasing incidence with increasing dose, but the shapes of the two curves are dramatically different. For liver tumors, no clear threshold was evident, whereas for bladder tumors, an apparent threshold was evident. However, the apparent threshold, or "no observable adverse effect level" (NOAEL), for bladder cancer was lower at 33 months (45 ppm) than at 24 months (75 ppm). Of course, the ability to detect a low incidence of tumors depends on the number of animals used in the study. Thus, although a threshold (a dose below which no response occurs) appears evident for bladder tumors in Fig. 2-8, one cannot say for certain that tumors would not occur if more animals had been included in the lower-dose groups. (See Chap. 4 for more discussion on statistical issues related to extrapolation of dose–response curves and the determination of NOAELs.)

In evaluating the shape of the dose–response relationship in populations, it is realistic to consider inflections in the shape of the dose–response curve rather than absolute thresholds. That is, the slope of the dose–response relationship at high doses may be

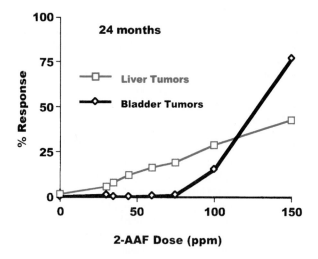

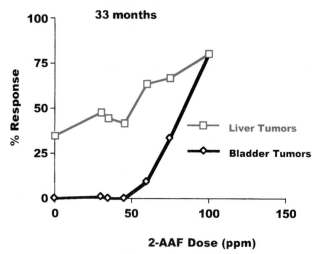

Figure 2-8.   Dose–response relationship for carcinogens.

Eight groups of male mice were administered 2-acetylaminofluorine (2-AAF) in the diet from weaning. The percent of animals with liver (*blue line*) or bladder (*black line*) tumors at 24 months (*A*) or 33 months (*B*) are shown. Most of the animals in the high-dose group (150 ppm) did not survive to 33 months; thus, those data are not shown in *B*.

substantially different from the slope at low doses, usually because of dispositional differences in the chemical. Saturation of biotransformation pathways, protein-binding sites or receptors, and depletion of intracellular cofactors represent some reasons why sharp inflections in the dose–response relationship may occur. For example, the widely used analgesic acetaminophen has a very low rate of liver toxicity at normal therapeutic doses. Even though a toxic metabolite [*N*-acetyl-*p*-benzoquinoneimine (NAPQI)] is produced in the liver at therapeutic doses, it is rapidly detoxified through conjugation with the intracellular antioxidant glutathione. However, at very high doses, the level of intracellular glutathione in the liver is depleted and NAPQI accumulates, causing serious and potentially fatal liver toxicity. This effect is analogous to the rapid change in pH of a buffered solution that occurs when the buffer capacity is exceeded. Some toxic responses, most notably the development of cancer after the administration of genotoxic carcinogens, are often considered to be linear at low doses and thus do not exhibit a threshold. In such circumstances, there is no dose with "zero" risk,

although the risk decreases proportionately with a decrease in the dose. The existence or lack of existence of a threshold dose for carcinogens has many regulatory implications and is a point of considerable controversy and research in the field of quantitative risk assessment for chemical carcinogens (see Chap. 4).

Assumptions in Deriving the Dose–Response Relationship

A number of assumptions must be considered before dose–response relationships can be used appropriately. The first is that the response is due to the chemical administered. To describe the relationship between a toxic material and an observed effect or response, one must know with reasonable certainty that the relationship is indeed a causal one. For some data, it is not always apparent that the response is a result of chemical exposure. For example, an epidemiologic study might result in the discovery of an "association" between a response (e.g., disease) and one or more variables. Frequently, the data are presented similarly to the presentation of "dose response" in pharmacology and toxicology. Use of the dose response in this context is suspect unless other convincing evidence supports a causal connection between the estimated dose and the measured endpoint (response). Unfortunately, in nearly all retrospective and case-control studies and even in many prospective studies, the dose, duration, frequency, and routes of exposure are seldom quantified, and other potential etiologic factors are frequently present. In its most strict usage, then, the dose–response relationship is based on the knowledge that the effect is a result of a known toxic agent or agents.

A second assumption seems simple and obvious: The magnitude of the response is in fact related to the dose. Perhaps because of its apparent simplicity, this assumption is often a source of misunderstanding. It is really a composite of three other assumptions that recur frequently:

1. There is a molecular target site (or sites) with which the chemical interacts to initiate the response.
2. The production of a response and the degree of response are related to the concentration of the chemical at the target site.
3. The concentration at the site is, in turn, related to the dose administered.

The third assumption in using the dose–response relationship is that there exists both a quantifiable method of measuring and a precise means of expressing the toxicity. For any given dose–response relationship, a great variety of criteria or endpoints of toxicity could be used. The ideal criterion would be one closely associated with the molecular events resulting from exposure to the toxicant. It follows from this that a given chemical may have a family of dose–response relationships, one for each toxic endpoint. For example, a chemical that produces cancer through genotoxic effects, liver damage through inhibition of a specific enzyme, and CNS effects via a different mechanism may have three distinct dose–response relationships, one for each endpoint. Early in the assessment of toxicity, little mechanistic information is usually available; thus establishing a dose–response relationship based on the molecular mechanism of action is usually impossible. Indeed, it might not be approachable even for well-known toxicants. In the absence of a mechanistic, molecular ideal criterion of toxicity, one looks to a measure of toxicity that is unequivocal and clearly relevant to the toxic effect. Such measures are often referred to as "effects-related biomarkers." For example, with a new compound chemically related to the class of organophosphate insecticides, one might approach the measurement of toxicity by measuring the inhibition of cholinesterase in blood. In this way, one would be measuring, in a readily accessible system and using a technique that is convenient and reasonably precise, a prominent effect of the chemical and one that is usually pertinent to the mechanism by which toxicity is produced.

The selection of a toxic endpoint for measurement is not always so straightforward. Even the example cited above may be misleading, as an organophosphate may produce a decrease in blood cholinesterase, but this change may not be directly related to its toxicity. As additional data are gathered to suggest a mechanism of toxicity for any substance, other measures of toxicity may be selected. Although many endpoints are quantitative and precise, they are often indirect measures of toxicity. Changes in enzyme levels in blood can be indicative of tissue damage. For example, alanine aminotransferase (ALT) and aspartate aminotransferase (AST) are used to detect liver damage. Use of these enzymes in serum is yet another example of an effects-related biomarker because the change in enzyme activity in the blood is directly related to damage to liver cells. Much of clinical diagnostic medicine relies on effects-related biomarkers, but to be useful the relationship between the biomarker and the disease must be carefully established. Patterns of isozymes and their alteration may provide insight into the organ or system that is the site of toxic effects. As discussed later in this chapter, the new tools of toxicogenomics provide an unprecedented opportunity to discover new "effects-related biomarkers" in toxicology.

Many direct measures of effects are also not necessarily related to the mechanism by which a substance produces harm to an organism but have the advantage of permitting a causal relation to be drawn between the chemical and its action. For example, measurement of the alteration of the tone of smooth or skeletal muscle for substances acting on muscles represents a fundamental approach to toxicological assessment. Similarly, measures of heart rate, blood pressure, and electrical activity of heart muscle, nerve, and brain are examples of the use of physiologic functions as indices of toxicity. Measurement can also take the form of a still higher level of integration, such as the degree of motor activity or behavioral change.

The measurements used as examples in the preceding discussion all assume prior information about the toxicant, such as its target organ or site of action or a fundamental effect. However, such information is usually available only after toxicological screening and testing based on other measures of toxicity. With a new substance, the customary starting point is a single dose acute toxicity test designed to provide preliminary identification of target organ toxicity. Studies specifically designed with lethality as an end-point are no longer recommended by United States or international agencies. Data from acute studies provides essential information for choosing doses for repeated dosing studies as well as choosing specific toxicological endpoints for further study. Key elements of the study design must be a careful, disciplined, detailed observation of the intact animal extending from the time of administration of the toxicant to any clinical signs of distress, which may include detailed behavioral observations or physiological measures. It is recommended that these observations be taken over a 14-day period. From properly conducted observations, immensely informative data can be gathered by a trained toxicologist. Second, an acute toxicity study ordinarily is supported by histological examination of major tissues and organs for abnormalities. From these observations, one can usually obtain more specific information about the events leading to the various

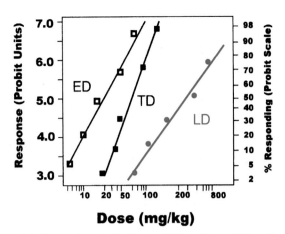

Figure 2-9. Comparison of effective dose (ED), toxic dose (TD), and lethal dose (LD).

The plot is of log dosage versus percentage of population responding in probit units.

endpoints, the target organs involved, and often a suggestion about the possible mechanism of toxicity at a relatively fundamental level.

Evaluating the Dose–Response Relationship

Comparison of Dose Responses Figure 2-9 illustrates a hypothetical quantal dose–response curve for a desirable effect of a chemical effective dose (ED) such as anesthesia, a toxic dose (TD) effect such as liver injury, and the lethal dose (LD). As depicted in Fig. 2-9, a parallelism is apparent between the ED curve and the curve depicting mortality (LD). It is tempting to view the parallel dose–response curves as indicative of identity of mechanism—that is, to conclude that the lethality is a simple extension of the therapeutic effect. Whereas this conclusion may ultimately prove to be correct in any particular case, it is not warranted solely on the basis of the two parallel lines. The same admonition applies to any pair of parallel "effect" curves or any other pair of toxicity or lethality curves.

Therapeutic Index The hypothetical curves in Fig. 2-9 illustrate two other interrelated points: the importance of the selection of the toxic criterion and the interpretation of comparative effect. The concept of the "therapeutic index," which was introduced by Paul Ehrlich in 1913, can be used to illustrate this relationship. Although the therapeutic index is directed toward a comparison of the therapeutically effective dose to the toxic dose of a chemical, it is equally applicable to considerations of comparative toxicity. The *therapeutic index* (TI) in its broadest sense is defined as the ratio of the dose required to produce a toxic effect and the dose needed to elicit the desired therapeutic response. Similarly, an index of comparative toxicity is obtained by the ratio of doses of two different materials to produce an identical response or the ratio of doses of the same material necessary to yield different toxic effects.

The most commonly used index of effect, whether beneficial or toxic, is the median effect dose (ED_{50}). The therapeutic index of a drug is an approximate statement about the relative safety of a drug expressed as the ratio of the adverse endpoint or toxic dose (historically the lethal dose) to the therapeutic dose:

$$\text{Therapeutic Index} = TD_{50}/ED_{50}$$

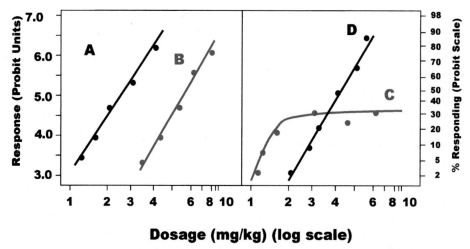

Figure 2-10. Schematic representation of the difference in the dose–response curves for four chemicals (A–D), illustrating the difference between potency and efficacy (see text).

From Fig. 2-9 one can approximate a therapeutic index by using these median doses. The larger the ratio, the greater the relative safety. The ED_{50} is approximately 20, and the TD_{50} is about 60; thus, the therapeutic index is 3, a number indicating that reasonable care in exposure to the drug is necessary to avoid toxicity. However, the use of the median effective and median toxic doses is not without disadvantages, because median doses tell nothing about the slopes of the dose–response curves for therapeutic and toxic effects.

Margins of Safety and Exposure One way to overcome this deficiency is to use the ED_{99} for the desired effect and the TD_1 for the undesired effect. These parameters are used in the calculation of the margin of safety (MOS):

$$\text{Margin of safety} = TD_1/ED_{99}$$

The quantitative comparisons described above have been used mainly after a single administration of chemicals. However, for chemicals for which there is no beneficial or effective dose and exposures are likely to occur repeatedly, the ratio of TD_1 to ED_{99} has little relevance. Thus, for non-drug chemicals, the term *margin of safety* has found use in risk-assessment procedures as an indicator of the magnitude of the difference between an estimated "exposed dose" to a human population and the NOAEL or other benchmark dose determined in experimental animals.

A measure of the degree of accumulation of a chemical and/or its toxic effects can also be estimated from quantal toxicity data. The *chronicity index* of a chemical is a unitless value obtained by dividing its 1-dose TD_{50} by its 90-dose (90-day) TD_{50}, with both expressed in milligrams per kilogram per day. Theoretically, if no cumulative effect occurs over the doses, the chronicity index will be 1. If a compound were absolutely cumulative, the chronicity index would be 90.

Historically, statistical procedures similar to those used to calculate the LD_{50} can also be used to determine the lethal time 50 (LT_{50}), or the time required for half the animals to die (Litchfield, 1949). The LT_{50} value for a chemical indicates the time course of the toxic effects but does not indicate whether one chemical is more toxic than another.

Frequently, dose–response curves from repeated-dose experimental animal studies (subacute, subchronic, or chronic) are used to estimate the NOAEL, or some other "benchmark" measure of minimal toxic response, such as the dose estimated to produce toxic effects in 10% of the population (TD_{10}) (see also Chap. 4). These estimates of minimal toxic dose, derived from quantal dose–response curves, can be used in risk assessment to derive a "margin of exposure" (MOE) index. This index compares the estimated daily exposure, in milligrams per kilogram per day, that might occur under a given set of circumstances to some estimated value from the quantal dose–response relationship (e.g., NOAEL or TD_{10}). Like the MOS, the MOE is often expressed as a ratio of these two values. Thus, for example, if an estimate of human exposure to a pesticide residue yielded a value of 0.001 mg/kg/day, and a TD_{10} of 1 mg/kg/day was determined for that same pesticide, the MOE would be 1000. This value indicates that the estimate of daily exposure under the described set of conditions is 1/1000 the estimated daily dose that would cause evident toxicity in 10% of exposed animals. (See Chap. 4 for a more complete discussion of benchmark doses, NOAELs, and MOE.)

Potency versus Efficacy To compare the toxic effects of two or more chemicals, the dose response to the toxic effects of each chemical must be established. One can then compare the potency and maximal efficacy of the two chemicals to produce a toxic effect. These two important terms can be explained by reference to Fig. 2-10, which depicts dose–response curves to four different chemicals for the frequency of a particular toxic effect, such as the production of tumors. Chemical A is said to be more potent than chemical B because of their relative positions along the dosage axis. Potency thus refers to the range of doses over which a chemical produces increasing responses. Thus, A is more potent than B and C is more potent than D. Maximal efficacy reflects the limit of the dose–response relationship on the response axis to a certain chemical. Chemicals A and B have equal maximal efficacy, whereas the maximal efficacy of C is less than that of D.

VARIATION IN TOXIC RESPONSES

Selective Toxicity

Selective toxicity means that a chemical produces injury to one kind of living matter without harming another form of life even though the two may exist in intimate contact (Albert, 1965, 1973). The living matter that is injured is termed the *uneconomic form* (or undesirable), and the matter protected is called the *economic form* (or desirable). They may be related to each other as parasite and host or may be two tissues in one organism. This biological diversity interferes with the ability of ecotoxicologists to predict the toxic effects of a chemical in one species (humans) from experiments performed in another species (laboratory animals). However, by taking advantage of the biological diversity, it is possible to develop chemicals that are lethal for an undesired species and harmless for other species. In agriculture, for example, there are fungi, insects, and even competitive plants that injure the crop, and thus selective pesticides are needed. Similarly, animal husbandry and human medicine require chemicals, such as antibiotics, that are selectively toxic to the undesirable form but do not produce damage to the desirable form.

Drugs and other chemicals used for selective toxic purposes are selective for one of two reasons. Either (1) the chemical is equally toxic to both economic and uneconomic cells but is accumulated mainly by uneconomic cells or (2) it reacts fairly specifically with a cytological or a biochemical feature that is absent from or does not play an important role in the economic form (Albert, 1965, 1973). Selectivity resulting from differences in distribution usually is caused by differences in the absorption, biotransformation, or excretion of the toxicant. The selective toxicity of an insecticide spray may be partly due to a larger surface area per unit weight that causes the insect to absorb a proportionally larger dose than does the mammal being sprayed. The effectiveness of radioactive iodine in the treatment of hyperthyroidism (as well as its thyroid carcinogenicity) is due to the selective ability of the thyroid gland to accumulate iodine. A major reason why chemicals are toxic to one, but not to another, type of tissue is that there are differences in accumulation of the ultimate toxic compound in various tissues. This, in turn, may be due to differences in the ability of various tissues to transport or biotransform the chemical into the ultimate toxic product.

Selective toxicity caused by differences in comparative cytology is exemplified by a comparison of plant and animal cells. Plants differ from animals in many ways—for example, absence of a nervous system, an efficient circulatory system, and muscles as well as the presence of a photosynthetic mechanism and cell walls. The fact that bacteria contain cell walls and humans do not has been utilized in developing selective toxic chemotherapeutic agents, such as penicillin and cephalosporins, that kill bacteria but are relatively nontoxic to mammalian cells.

Selective toxicity can also be a result of a difference in biochemistry in the two types of cells. For example, bacteria do not absorb folic acid but synthesize it from *p*-aminobenzoic acid, glutamic acid, and pteridine, whereas mammals cannot synthesize folic acid but have to absorb it from the diet. Thus, sulfonamide drugs are selectively toxic to bacteria because the sulfonamides, which resemble *p*-aminobenzoic acid in both charge and dimensions, antagonize the incorporation of *p*-aminobenzoic acid into the folic acid molecule—a reaction that humans do not carry out.

Species Differences

Although a basic tenet of toxicology is that "experimental results in animals, when properly qualified, are applicable to humans," it is important to recognize that both quantitative and qualitative differences in response to toxic substances may occur among different species. As discussed above, there are many reasons for selective

toxicity among different species. Even among phylogenetically similar species (e.g., rats, mice, guinea pigs, and hamsters), large differences in response may occur. For example, the LD_{50} for the highly toxic dioxin, 2,3,7,8-tetrachlorodibenzo-*p*-dioxin (TCDD), differs by more than 1000-fold between guinea pigs and hamsters. Not only does the lethal dose for TCDD vary widely among species, so do the particular target organs affected. Species differences in response to carcinogenic chemicals represent an important issue in regulatory risk assessment. As discussed in Chap. 4, extrapolation of laboratory animal data to infer human cancer risk is currently a key component of regulatory decision making. The validity of this approach of course depends on the relevance of the experimental animal model to humans. Large differences in carcinogenic response between experimental animal species are not unusual. For example, mice are highly resistant to the hepatocarcinogenic effects of the fungal toxin aflatoxin B_1. Dietary doses as high as 10,000 parts per billion (ppb) failed to produce liver cancer in mice, whereas in rats dietary doses as low as 15 ppb produced a significant increase in liver tumors (Wogan *et al.*, 1974). The mechanistic basis for this dramatic difference in response appears to be entirely related to species differences in the expression of a particular form of glutathione *S*-transferase (mGSTA3-3) that has unusually high catalytic activity toward the carcinogenic epoxide of aflatoxin (Eaton and Gallagher, 1994). Mice express this enzyme constitutively, whereas rats normally express a closely related form with much less detoxifying activity toward aflatoxin epoxide. Interestingly, rats do possess the gene for a form of glutathione *S*-transferase with high catalytic activity toward aflatoxin epoxide (rGSTA5-5) that is inducible by certain dietary antioxidants and drugs. Thus, dietary treatment can dramatically change the sensitivity of a species to a carcinogen.

Other examples in which large species differences in response to carcinogens have been observed include the development of renal tumors from 2,3,5-trimethylpentane and *d*-limonene in male rats (Lehman-McKeeman and Caudill, 1992), the production of liver tumors from "peroxisomal proliferators" such as the antilipidemic drug clofibrate and the common solvent trichloroethylene (Roberts, 1999), and the induction of nasal carcinomas in rats after inhalation exposure to formaldehyde (Monticello and Morgan, 1997).

Identifying the mechanistic basis for species differences in response to chemicals is an important part of toxicology because only through a thorough understanding of these differences can the relevance of animal data to human response be verified.

Individual Differences in Response

Even within a species, large interindividual differences in response to a chemical can occur because of subtle genetic differences. Hereditary differences in a single gene that occur in more than 1% of the population are referred to as *genetic polymorphism* and may be responsible for idiosyncratic reactions to chemicals, as discussed earlier in this chapter. However, genetic polymorphism may have other important but less dramatic effects than those described for acute idiosyncratic responses (such as that occurring in pseudocholinesterase-deficient individuals after succinylcholine exposure). For example, it is recognized that approximately 50% of the Caucasian population has a gene deletion for the enzyme glutathione S-transferase M1. This enzyme has no apparent significant physiologic function, and thus homozygotes for the gene deletion (e.g., those who lack both copies of the normal gene) are functionally and physiologically normal. However, epidemiologic studies have indicated that smokers who are homozygous for the null allele may be at slightly increased risk of developing lung cancer compared with smokers who have one or both copies of the normal gene (Mohr *et al.*, 2003). Chapter 6 provides additional examples of genetic differences in biotransformation enzymes that may be important determinants of variability in individual susceptibility to chemical exposures.

Genetic polymorphism in physiologically important genes may also be responsible for interindividual differences in toxic responses. For example, studies in transgenic mice have shown that mice possessing one copy of a mutated *p53* gene (a so-called tumor suppressor gene; see Chap. 8) are much more susceptible to some chemical carcinogens than are mice with two normal copies of the gene (Tennant *et al.*, 1999). In humans, there is evidence that possessing one mutated copy of a tumor suppressor gene greatly increases the risk of developing certain cancers. For example, retinoblastoma is a largely inherited form of cancer that arises because of the presence of two copies of a defective tumor suppressor gene (the Rb gene) (Wiman, 1993). Individuals with one mutated copy of the Rb gene and one normal copy are not destined to acquire the disease (as are those with two copies of the mutated gene), although their chance of acquiring it is much greater than that of persons with two normal Rb genes. This is the case because both copies of the gene must be nonfunctional for the disease to develop. With one mutated copy present genetically, the probability of acquiring a mutation of the second gene (potentially from exposure to environmental mutagens) is much greater than the probability of acquiring independent mutations in both copies of the gene as would be necessary in people with two normal Rb alleles. (See Chap. 8 for additional discussion of tumor suppressor genes.)

As our understanding of the human genome increases, more "susceptibility" genes will be discovered, and it is likely that the etiology of many chronic diseases will be shown to be related to a combination of genetics and environment. Simple blood tests may ultimately be developed that allow an individual to learn whether he or she may be particularly susceptible to specific drugs or environmental pollutants. Although the public health significance of this type of information could be immense, the disclosure of such information raises many important ethical and legal issues that must be addressed before wide use of such tests.

The study of "gene-environment" interactions, or "Ecogenetics" (Costa and Eaton, 2006) is a rapidly developing field of substantial relevance to toxicology. It is likely that the majority of chronic diseases develop as a result of the complex interplay between multiple genes and the myriad of environmental factors, including diet, lifestyle, and occupational and/or environmental exposures to toxic substances.

DESCRIPTIVE ANIMAL TOXICITY TESTS

Two main principles underlie all descriptive animal toxicity testing. The first is that the effects produced by a compound in laboratory animals, when properly qualified, are applicable to humans. This premise applies to all of experimental biology and medicine. On the basis of dose per unit of body surface, toxic effects in humans are usually in the same range as those in experimental animals. On a body weight basis, humans are generally more vulnerable than are experimental animals. When one has an awareness of these quantitative differences, appropriate safety factors can be applied to calculate relatively safe doses for humans. All known chemical carcinogens in humans, with the possible exception of arsenic, are carcinogenic in some species but not in all laboratory animals. It has become increas-

ingly evident that the converse—that all chemicals carcinogenic in animals are also carcinogenic in humans—is not true (Dybing and Sanner, 1999; Grisham, 1997; Hengstler *et al.*, 1999). However, for regulatory and risk assessment purposes, positive carcinogenicity tests in animals are usually interpreted as indicative of potential human carcinogenicity. If a clear understanding of the mechanism of action of the carcinogen indicates that a positive response in animals is not relevant to humans, a positive animal bioassay may be considered irrelevant for human risk assessment (see Chap. 4). This species variation in carcinogenic response appears to be due in many instances to differences in biotransformation of the procarcinogen to the ultimate carcinogen (see Chap. 6).

The second principle is that exposure of experimental animals to chemicals in high doses is a necessary and valid method of discovering possible hazards in humans. This principle is based on the quantal dose–response concept that the incidence of an effect in a population is greater as the dose or exposure increases. Practical considerations in the design of experimental model systems require that the number of animals used in toxicology experiments always be small compared with the size of human populations at risk. Obtaining statistically valid results from such small groups of animals requires the use of relatively large doses so that the effect will occur frequently enough to be detected. However, the use of high doses can create problems in interpretation if the response(s) obtained at high doses does not occur at low doses. Thus, for example, it has been shown that bladder tumors observed in rats fed very high doses of saccharin will not occur at the much lower doses of saccharin encountered in the human diet. At the high concentrations fed to rats, saccharin forms an insoluble precipitate in the bladder that subsequently results in chronic irritation of bladder epithelium, enhanced cell proliferation, and ultimately bladder tumors (Cohen, 1998, 1999). In vitro studies have shown that precipitation of saccharin in human urine will not occur at the concentrations that could be obtained from even extraordinary consumption of this artificial sweetener. Examples such as this illustrate the importance of considering the molecular, biochemical, and cellular mechanisms responsible for toxicological responses when extrapolating from high to low dose and across species.

Toxicity tests are not designed to demonstrate that a chemical is safe but to characterize the toxic effects a chemical can produce. Although there are no set toxicology tests that have to be performed on every chemical intended for commerce, a tiered approach typical of many hazard assessment programs is shown illustrated in Fig. 2-11. Depending on the eventual use of the chemical, the toxic effects produced by structural analogs of the chemical, as well as the toxic effects produced by the chemical itself, contribute to the determination of the toxicology tests that should be performed. The FDA, EPA, and Organization for Economic Cooperation and Development (OECD) have written good laboratory practice (GLP) standards that stipulate that procedure must be defined and accountability documented. These guidelines are expected to be followed when toxicity tests are conducted in support of the introduction of a chemical to the market.

The following sections provide an overview of basic toxicity testing procedures in use today. For a detailed description of these tests, the reader is referred to several authoritative texts on this subject (Williams and Hottendorf, 1999; Hayes, 2001; Jacobson-Kram and Keller, 2001).

Although different countries have often had different testing requirements for toxicity testing/product safety evaluation, efforts to "harmonize" such testing protocols have resulted in more

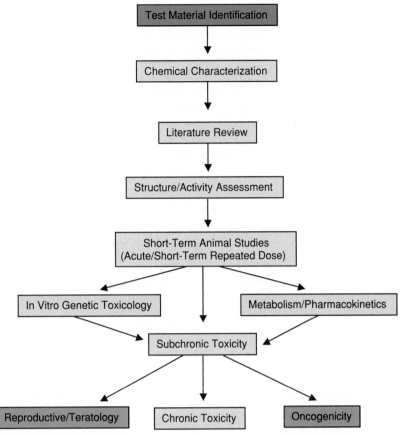

Figure 2-11. Typical Tiered Testing Scheme for the Toxicological Evaluation of New Chemicals

(Adapted from: Wilson *et al.*, 2001. In: Hayes, 2001; *Principles and Methods in Toxicology*, 4th ed, Fig. 19-1, p. 918.)

standardized approaches. The International Conference on Harmonization of Technical Requirements for Registration of Pharmaceuticals for Human Use (ICH) includes regulatory authorities from Europe, Japan, and the United States (primarily the FDA), as well as experts from the pharmaceutical industry in the three regions, who worked together to develop internationally recognized scientific and technical approaches to pharmaceutical product registration. ICH has adopted guidelines for most areas of toxicity testing (Table 2-3). In addition to safety assessment (ICH Guidelines designated with an "S"), ICH has also established guidelines on Quality (Q), Efficacy (E) and Multidisciplinary (M) topics. [see: http://www.ich.org/cache/compo/276-254-1.html for a description of current ICH guidelines and (Pugsley and Curtiss, 2006) for a detailed discussion of in vitro and in vivo pharmacological methods development that has been informed by the ICH regulatory guidance document for pre-clinical safety testing of drugs].

Typically, a tiered approach is used, with subsequent tests dependent on results of initial studies. A general framework for how new chemicals are evaluated for toxicity is shown in Fig 2-11. Early studies require careful chemical evaluation of the compound or mixture to assess purity, stability, solubility, and other physicochemical factors that could impact the ability of the test compound to be delivered effectively to animals. Once this information is obtained, the chemical structure of the test compound is compared with similar chemicals for which toxicological information is already available. Structure-activity relationships may be derived from a

review of existing toxicological literature, and can provide additional guidance on design of acute and repeated dose experiments, and what specialized tests need to be completed. Once such basic information has been compiled and evaluated, the test compound is then administered to animals in acute and repeated dose studies.

Acute Toxicity Testing

Generally, the first toxicity test performed on a new chemical is acute toxicity, determined from the administration of a single exposure. The objectives of acute toxicity testing are to: (1) provide an estimate of the intrinsic toxicity of the substance, often times expressed as an approximate lethal dose (e.g., LD_{50}), (2) provide information on target organs and other clinical manifestations of toxicity, (3) identify species differences and susceptible species, (4) establish the reversibility of the toxic response, and (5) provide information that will assist in the design and dose selection for longer term (sub-chronic, chronic) studies. It should be noted that the ICH recommended in 1991 (D'Arcy and Harron, 1992) the elimination of LD_{50} determinations for pharmaceuticals, although other regulatory requirements, e.g., pesticide registration, may still require determinations of LD_{50}s.

The LD_{50} and other acute toxic effects are determined after one or more routes of administration (one route being oral or the intended route of exposure) in one or more species. The species most often used are the mouse and rat. Studies are performed in both adult

Table 2.3

International Conference on Harmonization (ICH) Codification of "Safety" Protocols. Titles and abbreviations adopted November, 2005

Carcinogenicity studies	
S1A	Need for Carcinogenicity Studies of Pharmaceuticals
S1B	Testing for Carcinogenicity of Pharmaceuticals
S1C(R1)	Dose Selection for Carcinogenicity Studies of Pharmaceuticals & Limit Dose
Genotoxicity studies	
S2A	Guidance on Specific Aspects of Regulatory Genotoxicity Tests for Pharmaceuticals
S2B	Genotoxicity: A Standard Battery for Genotoxicity Testing of Pharmaceuticals
Toxicokinetics and pharmacokinetics	
S3A	Note for Guidance on Toxicokinetics: The Assessment of Systemic Exposure in Toxicity Studies
S3B	Pharmacokinetics: Guidance for Repeated Dose Tissue Distribution Studies
Toxicity testing	
	Single Dose Toxicity Tests
S4	Duration of Chronic Toxicity Testing in Animals (Rodent and Non Rodent Toxicity Testing)
Reproductive toxicology	
S5(R2)	Detection of Toxicity to Reproduction for Medicinal Products & Toxicity to Male Fertility
Biotechnological products	
S6	Preclinical Safety Evaluation of Biotechnology-Derived Pharmaceuticals
Pharmacology studies	
S7A	Safety Pharmacology Studies for Human Pharmaceuticals
S7B	The Non-Clinical Evaluation of the Potential for Delayed Ventricular Repolarization (QT Interval Prolongation) by Human Pharmaceuticals
Immunotoxicology studies	
S8	Immunotoxicity Studies for Human Pharmaceuticals
Joint safety/efficacy (multidisciplinary) topic	
M3(R1)	Non-Clinical Safety Studies for the Conduct of Human Clinical Trials for Pharmaceuticals

Data from: http://www.ich.org/cache/compo/276-254-1.html.

male and female animals. Food is often withheld the night before dosing. The number of animals that die in a 14-day period after a single dosage is tabulated. In addition to mortality and weight, daily examination of test animals should be conducted for signs of intoxication, lethargy, behavioral modifications, morbidity, food consumption, and so on.

Determination of the LD_{50} has become a public issue because of increasing concern for the welfare and protection of laboratory animals. The LD_{50} is not a biological constant. Many factors influence toxicity and thus may alter the estimation of the LD_{50} in any particular study. Factors such as animal strain, age, and weight, type of feed, caging, pretrial fasting time, method of administration, volume and type of suspension medium, and duration of observation have all been shown to influence adverse responses to toxic substances. These and other factors have been discussed in detail in earlier editions of this textbook (Doull, 1980). Because of this inherent variability in LD_{50} estimates, it is now recognized that for most purposes it is only necessary to characterize the LD_{50} within an order of magnitude range such as 5–50 mg/kg, 50–500 mg/kg, and so on.

There are several traditional approaches to determining the LD_{50} and its 95% confidence limit as well as the slope of the probit line. The reader is referred to the classic works of Litchfield and Wilcoxon (1949), Bliss (1957), and Finney (1971) for a description of the mechanics of these procedures. Other statistical tech-

niques that require fewer animals, such as the "moving averages" method of Thompson and Weill (Weil, 1952), are available but do not provide confidence limits for the LD_{50} and the slope of the probit line. Finney (1985) has succinctly summarized the advantages and deficiencies of many of the traditional methods. For most circumstances, an adequate estimate of the LD_{50} and an approximation of the 95% confidence intervals can be obtained with as few as 6 to 9 animals, using the "up-and-down" method as modified by Bruce (1985). When this method was compared with traditional methods that typically utilize 40 to 50 animals, excellent agreement was obtained for all 10 compounds tested (Bruce, 1987). In mice and rats the LD_{50} is usually determined as described above, but in the larger species only an approximation of the LD_{50} is obtained by increasing the dose in the same animal until serious toxic effects are evident.

If there is a reasonable likelihood of substantial exposure to the material by dermal or inhalation exposure, acute dermal and acute inhalation studies are performed. When animals are exposed acutely to chemicals in the air they breathe or the water they (fish) live in, the dose the animals receive is usually not known. For these situations, the lethal concentration 50 (LC_{50}) is usually determined; that is, the concentration of chemical in the air or water that causes death to 50% of the animals. In reporting an LC_{50}, it is imperative that the time of exposure be indicated. The acute dermal toxicity test is usually performed in rabbits. The site of application is shaved. The test substance is kept in contact with the skin for 24 hours by wrapping the skin with an impervious plastic material. At the end of the exposure period, the wrapping is removed and the skin is wiped to remove any test substance still remaining. Animals are observed at various intervals for 14 days, and the LD_{50} is calculated. If no toxicity is evident at 2 g/kg, further acute dermal toxicity testing is usually not performed. Acute inhalation studies are performed that are similar to other acute toxicity studies except that the route of exposure is inhalation. Most often, the length of exposure is 4 hours.

Although by themselves LD_{50} and LC_{50} values are of limited significance given the growing sophistication of target organ toxicity endpoints and mechanistic analysis. The most meaningful scientific information derived from acute toxicity tests comes from clinical observations and postmortem examination of animals rather than from the specific LD_{50} value.

Skin and Eye Irritations

The ability of a chemical to irritate the skin and eye after an acute exposure is usually determined in rabbits. For the dermal irritation test (Draize test), rabbits are prepared by removal of fur on a section of the back by electric clippers. The chemical is applied to the skin (0.5 mL of liquid or 0.5 g of solid) under four covered gauze patches (1 in. square; one intact and two abraded skin sites on each animal) and usually kept in contact for 4 hours. The nature of the covering patches depends on whether occlusive, semiocclusive, or nonocclusive tests are desired. For occlusive testing, the test material is covered with an impervious plastic sheet; for semiocclusive tests, a gauze dressing may be used. Occasionally, studies may require that the material be applied to abraded skin. The degree of skin irritation is scored for erythema (redness), eschar (scab), and edema (swelling) formation, and corrosive action. These dermal irritation observations are repeated at various intervals after the covered patch has been removed. To determine the degree of ocular irritation, the chemical is instilled into one eye (0.1 mL of liquid or 100 mg of solid) of each test rabbit. The contralateral eye is used as the control. The eyes of the rabbits are then examined at various times after application.

Controversy over this test has led to the development of alternative in vitro models for evaluating cutaneous and ocular toxicity of substances. The various in vitro methods that have been evaluated for this purpose include epidermal keratinocyte and corneal epithelial cell culture models. These and other in vitro tests have been reviewed recently (Davila et al., 1998).

Sensitization

Information about the potential of a chemical to sensitize skin is needed in addition to irritation testing for all materials that may repeatedly come into contact with the skin. Numerous procedures have been developed to determine the potential of substances to induce a sensitization reaction in humans (delayed hypersensitivity reaction), including the Draize test, the open epicutaneous test, the Buehler test, Freund's complete adjuvant test, the optimization test, the split adjuvant test, and the guinea pig maximization test (Maibach and Patrick, 2001; Rush et al., 1995). Although they differ in regard to route and frequency of duration, they all utilize the guinea pig as the preferred test species. In general, the test chemical is administered to the shaved skin topically, intradermally, or both and may include the use of adjuvant to enhance the sensitivity of the assay. Multiple administrations of the test substance are generally given over a period of 2 to 4 weeks. Depending on the specific protocol, the treated

area may be occluded. Some 2 to 3 weeks after the last treatment, the animals are challenged with a nonirritating concentration of the test substance and the development of erythema is evaluated.

Subacute (Repeated-Dose Study)

Subacute toxicity tests are performed to obtain information on the toxicity of a chemical after repeated administration and as an aid to establish doses for subchronic studies. A typical protocol is to give three to four different dosages of the chemicals to the animals by mixing it in their feed. For rats, 10 animals per sex per dose are often used; for dogs, three dosages and 3 to 4 animals per sex are used. Clinical chemistry and histopathology are performed after 14 days of exposure, as described below in the section on subchronic toxicity testing.

Subchronic

The toxicity of a chemical after subchronic exposure is then determined. Subchronic exposure can last for different periods of time, but 90 days is the most common test duration. The principal goals of the subchronic study are to establish a NOAEL and to further identify and characterize the specific organ or organs affected by the test compound after repeated administration. One may also obtain a "lowest observed adverse effect level" (LOAEL) as well as the NOAEL for the species tested. The numbers obtained for NOAEL and LOAEL will depend on how closely the dosages are spaced and the number of animals examined. Determinations of NOAELs and LOAELs have numerous regulatory implications. For example, the EPA utilizes the NOAEL to calculate the *reference dose* (RfD), which may be used to establish regulatory values for "acceptable" pollutant levels (Barnes and Dourson, 1988) (see Chap. 4). An alternative to the NOAEL approach referred to as the *benchmark dose* uses all the experimental data to fit one or more dose–response curves (Crump, 1984). These curves are then used to estimate a benchmark dose that is defined as "the statistical lower bound on a dose corresponding to a specified level of risk" (Allen et al., 1994a). Although subchronic studies are frequently the primary or sole source of experimental data to determine both the NOAEL and the benchmark dose, these concepts can be applied to other types of toxicity testing protocols, such as that for chronic toxicity or developmental toxicity (Allen et al., 1994a, 1994b; Faustman et al., 1994) (see also Chap. 4 for a complete discussion of the derivation and use of NOAELs, RfDs, and benchmark doses). If chronic studies have been completed, these data are generally used for NOAEL and LOAEL estimates in preference to data from subchronic studies.

A subchronic study is usually conducted in two species (usually rat and dog for FDA; and mouse for EPA) by the route of intended exposure (usually oral). At least three doses are employed (a high dose that produces toxicity but does not cause more than 10% fatalities, a low dose that produces no apparent toxic effects, and an intermediate dose) with 10 to 20 rodents and 4 to 6 dogs of each sex per dose. Each animal should be uniquely identified with permanent markings such as ear tags, tattoos, or electronically coded microchip implants. Only healthy animals should be used, and each animal should be housed individually in an adequately controlled environment. When the test compound is administered in the diet over a prolonged period of time (sub-chronic and chronic studies), the concentration in the diet should be adjusted periodically (weekly for the first 12–14 weeks) to maintain a constant intake of material based on food consumption and rate of change in body weight (Wilson et al., 2001). Animals should be observed once or twice daily for signs of toxicity, including changes in body weight, diet consumption, changes in fur color or texture, respiratory or cardiovascular distress, motor and behavioral abnormalities, and palpable masses. All premature deaths should be recorded and necropsied as soon as possible. Severely moribund animals should be terminated immediately to preserve tissues and reduce unnecessary suffering. At the end of the 90-day study, all the remaining animals should be terminated and blood and tissues should be collected for further analysis. The gross and microscopic condition of the organs and tissues (about 15 to 20) and the weight of the major organs (about 12) are recorded and evaluated. Hematology and blood chemistry measurements are usually done before, in the middle of, and at the termination of exposure. Hematology measurements usually include hemoglobin concentration, hematocrit, erythrocyte counts, total and differential leukocyte counts, platelet count, clotting time, and prothrombin time. Clinical chemistry determinations commonly made include glucose, calcium, potassium, urea nitrogen, alanine aminotransferase (ALT), serum aspartate aminotransferase (AST), gamma-glutamyltranspeptidase (GGT), sorbitol dehydrogenase, lactic dehydrogenase, alkaline phosphatase, creatinine, bilirubin, triglycerides, cholesterol, albumin, globulin, and total protein. Urinalysis is usually performed in the middle of and at the termination of the testing period and often includes determination of specific gravity or osmolarity, pH, proteins, glucose, ketones, bilirubin, and urobilinogen as well as microscopic examination of formed elements. If humans are likely to have significant exposure to the chemical by dermal contact or inhalation, subchronic dermal and/or inhalation experiments may also be required. Subchronic toxicity studies not only characterize the dose–response relationship of a test substance after repeated administration but also provide data for a more reasonable prediction of appropriate doses for chronic exposure studies.

For chemicals that are to be registered as drugs, acute and subchronic studies (and potentially additional special tests if a chemical has unusual toxic effects or therapeutic purposes) must be completed before the company can file an Investigational New Drug (IND) application with the FDA. If the application is approved, clinical trials can commence. At the same time phase I, phase II, and phase III clinical trials are performed, chronic exposure of the animals to the test compound can be carried out in laboratory animals, along with additional specialized tests.

Chronic

Long-term or chronic exposure studies are performed similarly to subchronic studies except that the period of exposure is longer than 3 months. In rodents, chronic exposures are usually for 6 months to 2 years. Chronic studies in nonrodent species are usually for 1 year but may be longer. The length of exposure is somewhat dependent on the intended period of exposure in humans. For example, for pharmaceuticals, the ICH S4 guidance calls for studies of 6 months in duration in rodents, and 9 months in non-rodents. However, if the chemical is a food additive with the potential for lifetime exposure in humans, a chronic study up to 2 years in duration is likely to be required.

Dose selection is critical in these studies to ensure that premature mortality from chronic toxicity does not limit the number of animals that survive to a normal life expectancy. Most regulatory guidelines require that the highest dose administered be the estimated maximum tolerable dose (MTD). This is generally derived from subchronic studies, but additional longer studies (e.g.,

6 months) may be necessary if delayed effects or extensive cumulative toxicity are indicated in the 90-day subchronic study. The MTD has had various definitions (Haseman, 1985). The MTD has been defined by some regulatory agencies as the dose that suppresses body weight gain slightly (i.e., 10%) in a 90-day subchronic study (Reno, 1997). However, regulatory agencies may also consider the use of parameters other than weight gain, such as physiological and pharmacokinetic considerations and urinary metabolite profiles, as indicators of an appropriate MTD (Reno, 1997). Generally, one or two additional doses, usually fractions of the MTD (e.g., one-half and one-quarter MTD), and a control group are tested.

Chronic toxicity tests may include a consideration of the carcinogenic potential of chemicals so that a separate lifetime feeding study that addresses carcinogenicity does not have to be performed. However, specific chronic studies designed to assess the carcinogenic potential of a substance may be required (see below).

Developmental and Reproductive Toxicity

The effects of chemicals on reproduction and development also need to be determined. *Developmental toxicology* is the study of adverse effects on the developing organism occurring anytime during the life span of the organism that may result from exposure to chemical or physical agents before conception (either parent), during prenatal development, or postnatally until the time of puberty. *Teratology* is the study of defects induced during development between conception and birth (see Chap. 10). *Reproductive toxicology* is the study of the occurrence of adverse effects on the male or female reproductive system that may result from exposure to chemical or physical agents (see Chap. 20).

Several types of animal tests are utilized to examine the potential of an agent to alter development and reproduction. General fertility and reproductive performance (segment I) tests are usually performed in rats with two or three doses (20 rats per sex per dose) of the test chemical (neither produces maternal toxicity). Males are given the chemical 60 days and females 14 days before mating. The animals are given the chemical throughout gestation and lactation. Typical observations made include the percentage of females that become pregnant, the number of stillborn and live offspring, and the weight, growth, survival, and general condition of the offspring during the first 3 weeks of life.

The potential of chemicals to disrupt normal embryonic and/or fetal development (teratogenic effects) is also determined in laboratory animals. Current guidelines for these segment II studies call for the use of two species, including one nonrodent species (usually rabbits). Teratogens are most effective when administered during the first trimester, the period of organogenesis. Thus, the animals (usually 12 rabbits and 24 rats or mice per group) are usually exposed to one of three dosages during organogenesis (day 7 to 17 in rodents and days 7 to 19 in rabbits), and the fetuses are removed by cesarean section a day before the estimated time of delivery (gestational days 29 for rabbit, 20 for rat, and 18 for mouse). The uterus is excised and weighed and then examined for the number of live, dead, and resorbed fetuses. Live fetuses are weighed; half of each litter is examined for skeletal abnormalities and the remaining half for soft tissue anomalies.

The perinatal and postnatal toxicities of chemicals also are often examined (segment III). This test is performed by administering the test compound to rats from the 15th day of gestation throughout delivery and lactation and determining its effect on the birthweight, survival, and growth of the offspring during the first 3 weeks of life.

In some instances a multigenerational study may be chosen, often in place of segment III studies, to determine the effects of chemicals on the reproductive system. At least three dosage levels are given to groups of 25 female and 25 male rats shortly after weaning (30 to 40 days of age). These rats are referred to as the F_0 generation. Dosing continues throughout breeding (about 140 days of age), gestation, and lactation. The offspring (F_1 generation) have thus been exposed to the chemical in utero, via lactation, and in the feed thereafter. When the F_1 generation is about 140 days old, about 25 females and 25 males are bred to produce the F_2 generation, and administration of the chemical is continued. The F_2 generation is thus also exposed to the chemical in utero and via lactation. The F_1 and F_2 litters are examined as soon as possible after delivery. The percentage of F_0 and F_1 females that get pregnant, the number of pregnancies that go to full term, the litter size, the number of stillborn, and the number of live births are recorded. Viability counts and pup weights are recorded at birth and at 4, 7, 14, and 21 days of age. The fertility index (percentage of mating resulting in pregnancy), gestation index (percentage of pregnancies resulting in live litters), viability index (percentage of animals that survive 4 days or longer), and lactation index (percentage of animals alive at 4 days that survived the 21-day lactation period) are then calculated. Gross necropsy and histopathology are performed on some of the parents (F_0 and F_1), with the greatest attention being paid to the reproductive organs, and gross necropsy is performed on all weanlings.

The International Commission on Harmonization (ICH) guidelines provide for flexible guidelines that address six "ICH stages" of development: premating and conception (stage A), conception to implantation (stage B), implantation to closure of the hard palate (stage C), closure of the hard palate to end of pregnancy (stage D), birth and weaning (stage E), and weaning to sexual maturity (stage F). All of these stages are covered in the segment I to segment III studies described above (Christian, 1997).

Numerous short-term tests for teratogenicity have been developed (Faustman, 1988). These tests utilize whole-embryo culture, organ culture, and primary and established cell cultures to examine developmental processes and estimate the potential teratogenic risks of chemicals. Many of these in utero test systems are under evaluation for use in screening new chemicals for teratogenic effects. These systems vary in their ability to identify specific teratogenic events and alterations in cell growth and differentiation. In general, the available assays cannot identify functional or behavioral teratogens (Faustman, 1988).

Mutagenicity

Mutagenesis is the ability of chemicals to cause changes in the genetic material in the nucleus of cells in ways that allow the changes to be transmitted during cell division. Mutations can occur in either of two cell types, with substantially different consequences. Germinal mutations damage DNA in sperm and ova, which can undergo meiotic division and therefore have the potential for transmission of the mutations to future generations. If mutations are present at the time of fertilization in either the egg or the sperm, the resulting combination of genetic material may not be viable, and the death may occur in the early stages of embryonic cell division. Alternatively, the mutation in the genetic material may not affect early embryogenesis but may result in the death of the fetus at a later developmental period, resulting in abortion. Congenital abnormalities may also result from mutations. Somatic mutations refer to mutations in all

other cell types and are not heritable but may result in cell death or transmission of a genetic defect to other cells in the same tissue through mitotic division. Because the initiating event of chemical carcinogenesis is thought to be a mutagenic one, mutagenic tests are often used to screen for potential carcinogens.

Numerous in vivo and in vitro procedures have been devised to test chemicals for their ability to cause mutations. Some genetic alterations are visible with the light microscope. In this case, cytogenetic analysis of bone marrow smears is used after the animals have been exposed to the test agent. Because some mutations are incompatible with normal development, the mutagenic potential of a chemical can also be evaluated by the dominant lethal test. This test is usually performed in rodents. The male is exposed to a single dose of the test compound and then is mated with two untreated females weekly for 8 weeks. The females are killed before term, and the number of live embryos and the number of corpora lutea are determined.

The test for mutagens that has received the widest attention is the *Salmonella*/microsome test developed by Ames and colleagues (Ames *et al.*, 1975). This test uses several mutant strains of *Salmonella typhimurium* that lack the enzyme phosphoribosyl ATP synthetase, which is required for histidine synthesis. These strains are unable to grow in a histidine-deficient medium unless a reverse or back-mutation to the wild type has occurred. Other mutations in these bacteria have been introduced to enhance the sensitivity of the strains to mutagenesis. The two most significant additional mutations enhance penetration of substances into the bacteria and decrease the ability of the bacteria to repair DNA damage. Because many chemicals are not mutagenic or carcinogenic unless they are biotransformed to a toxic product by enzymes in the endoplasmic reticulum (microsomes), rat liver microsomes are usually added to the medium containing the mutant strain and the test chemical. The number of reverse mutations is then quantified by the number of bacterial colonies that grow in a histidine-deficient medium.

Strains of yeast have recently been developed that detect genetic alterations arising during cell division after exposure to nongenotoxic carcinogens as well as mutations that arise directly from genotoxic carcinogens. This test identifies deletions of genetic material that occur during recombination events in cell division that may result from oxidative damage to DNA, direct mutagenic effects, alterations in fidelity of DNA repair, and/or changes in cell cycle regulation (Galli and Schiestl, 1999). Mutagenicity is discussed in detail in Chap. 9.

With the advent of techniques that readily allow manipulation of the mouse genome, transgenic animals have been developed that allow for in vivo assessment of mutagenicity of compounds. For example, two commercially available mouse strains, the "MutaMouse", and "BigBlue" contain the *lac* operon of *E. coli* that has been inserted into genomic DNA using a lambda phage to DNA to produce a recoverable shuttle vector. Stable, homozygous strains of these transgenic animals (both mice and rats have been engineered) can be exposed to potential mutagenic agents. Following in vivo exposure, the target *lac* genes can be recovered from virtually any cell type or organ and analyzed for mutations (Brusick, 2001).

Oncogenicity Bioassays

Oncogenicity studies are both time consuming and expensive, and are usually only done when there is reason to suspect that a chemcial may be carcinogenic, or when there may be wide spread, long term exposures to humans (e.g., widely used food additives, drinking water contaminants, or pharmaceuticals that are likely to be administered repeatedly for long periods of time). Chemicals that test positive in several mutagenicity assays are likely to be carcinogenic, and thus are frequent candidates for oncogenicity bioassay assessment. In the United States, the National Toxicology Program (NTP) has the primary responsibility for evaluating non-drug chemicals for carcinogenic potential. For pharmaceuticals, the FDA may require the manufacturer to conduct oncogenicity studies as part of the preclinical assessment, depending on the intended use of the drug, and the results of mutagenicity assays and other toxicological data.

Studies to evaluate the oncogenic (carcinogenic) potential of chemicals are usually performed in rats and mice and extend over the average lifetime of the species (18 months to 2 years for mice; 2 to 2.5 years for rats). To ensure that 30 rats per dose survive the 2-year study, 60 rats per group per sex are often started in the study. Both gross and microscopic pathological examinations are made not only on animals that survive the chronic exposure but also on those that die prematurely. The use of the MTD in carcinogenicity has been the subject of controversy. The premise that high doses are necessary for testing the carcinogenic potential of chemicals is derived from the statistical and experimental design limitations of chronic bioassays. Consider that a 0.5% increase in cancer incidence in the United States would result in over 1 million additional cancer deaths each year—clearly an unacceptably high risk. However, identifying with statistical confidence a 0.5% incidence of cancer in a group of experimental animals would require a minimum of 1000 test animals, and this assumes that no tumors were present in the absence of exposure (zero background incidence).

Figure 2-12 shows the statistical relationship between minimum detectable tumor incidence and the number of test animals per group. This curve shows that in a chronic bioassay with 50 animals per test group, a tumor incidence of about 8% could exist even though no animals in the test group had tumors. This example assumes that there are no tumors in the control group. These statistical considerations illustrate why animals are tested at doses higher than those that occur in human exposure. Because it is impractical to use the large number of animals that would be required to test the potential carcinogenicity of a chemical at the doses usually encountered by people, the alternative is to assume that there is a relationship between the administered dose and the tumorigenic response and give animals doses of the chemical that are high enough to produce a measurable tumor response in a reasonable size test group, such as 40 to 50 animals per dose. The limitations of this approach are discussed in Chap. 4. For non-mutagenic pharmaceutical agents, ICH S1C provides the following guidance on dose selection for oncogenicity studies: "The doses selected for rodent bioassays for non-genotoxic pharmaceuticals should provide an exposure to the agent that (1) allow an adequate margin of safety over the human therapeutic exposure, (2) are tolerated without significant chronic physiological dysfunction and are compatible with good survival, (3) are guided by a comprehensive set of animal and human data that focus broadly on the properties of the agent and the suitability of the animal (4) and permit data interpretation in the context of clinical use."

Another approach for establishing maximum doses for use in chronic animal toxicity testing of drugs is often used for substances for which basic human pharmacokinetic data are available (for example, new pharmaceutical agents which have completed phase I clinical trials). For chronic animal studies performed on drugs where single-dose human pharmacokinetic data are available, a daily dose that would provide an area under the curve (AUC) in laboratory animals equivalent to 25 times the AUC in humans given the highest (single) daily dose to be used therapeutically may be used, rather than the MTD. Based on a series of assumptions regarding allometric scaling between rodents and humans (Table 2-2), the ICH noted that it may not be necessary to exceed a dose of 1500 mg/kg/day where there is no evidence of genotoxicity, and where the maximum recommended human dose does not exceed 500 mg/day.

Most regulatory guidelines require that both benign and malignant tumors be reported in oncogenicity bioassays. Statistical increases above the control incidence of tumors (either all tumors or specific tumor types) in the treatment groups are considered indicative of carcinogenic potential of the chemical unless there are qualifying factors that suggest otherwise (lack of a dose response, unusually low incidence of tumors in the control group compared with "historic" controls, etc.; Huff, 1999). Thus, the conclusion as to whether a given chronic bioassay is positive or negative for carcinogenic potential of the test substance requires careful consideration of background tumor incidence. Properly designed chronic oncogenicity studies require that a concurrent control group matched for variables such as age, diet, housing conditions be used. For some tumor types, the "background" incidence of tumors is surprisingly high. Figure 2-13 shows the background tumor incidence for various tumors in male and female F-344 rats used in 27 National Toxicology Program 2-year rodent carcinogenicity studies. The data shown represent the percent of animals in control (nonexposed) groups that developed the specified tumor type by the end of the 2-year study. These studies involved more than 1300 rats of each sex. Figure 2-14 shows similar data for control (nonexposed) male and female B6C3F1 mice from 30 recent NTP 2-year carcinogenicity studies and includes data from over 1400 mice of each sex. There are several key points that can be derived from these summary data:

1. Tumors, both benign and malignant, are not uncommon events in animals even in the absence of exposure to any known carcinogen.
2. There are numerous different tumor types that develop "spontaneously" in both sexes of both rats and mice, but at different rates.

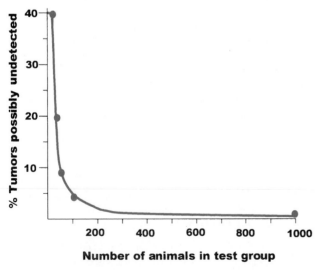

Figure 2-12. *Statistical limitations in the power of experimental animal studies to detect tumorigenic effects.*

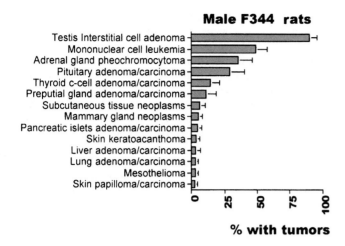

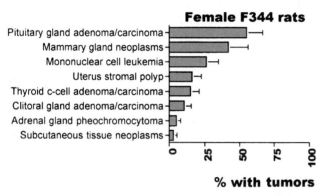

Figure 2-13. Most frequently occurring tumors in untreated control rats from recent NTP 2-year rodent carcinogenicity studies.

The values shown represent the mean ±SD of the percentage of animals developing the specified tumor type at the end of the 2-year study. The values were obtained from 27 different studies involving a combined total of between 1319 and 1353 animals per tumor type.

3. Background tumors that are common in one species may be uncommon in another (for example, testicular interstitial cell adenomas are very common in male rats but rare in male mice; liver adenomas/carcinomas are about 10 times more prevalent in male mice than in male rats).

4. Even within the same species and strain, large gender differences in background tumor incidence are sometimes observed (for example, adrenal gland pheochromocytomas are about seven times more prevalent in male F344 rats than in female F344 rats; lung and liver tumors are twice as prevalent in male B6C3F1 mice as in female B6C3F1 mice).

5. Even when the general protocols, diets, environment, strain and source of animals, and other variables are relatively constant, background tumor incidence can vary widely, as shown by the relatively large standard deviations for some tumor types in the NTP bioassay program. For example, the range in liver adenoma/carcinoma incidence in 30 different groups of unexposed (control) male B6C3F1 mice went from a low of 10% to a high of 68%. Pituitary gland adenomas/carcinomas ranged from 12 to 60% and 30 to 76% in unexposed male and female F344 rats, respectively, and from 0 to 36% in unexposed female B6C3F1 mice.

Taken together, these data demonstrate the importance of including concurrent control animals in such studies. In addition, comparisons of the concurrent control results to "historic" controls accumulated over years of study may be important in identifying potentially spurious "false-positive" results. The relatively high variability in background tumor incidence among groups of healthy, highly inbred strains of animals maintained on nutritionally balanced and consistent diets in rather sterile environments highlights the dilemma in interpreting the significance of both positive and negative results in regard to the human population, which is genetically diverse, has tremendous variability in diet, nutritional status, and overall health; and lives in an environment full of potentially carcinogenic substances, both natural and human-made.

Finally, it should be noted that both inbred and outbred strains have distinct background tumor patterns and the NTP and most other testing programs select strains based on the particular needs of the agent under study. For example, the NTP used the Wistar rat for chemicals that may have the testis as a target organ, based on acute, sub-chronic or other bioassay results. Similarly, the NTP used the Sprague-Dawley strain of rat in studies of estrogenic agents such as genistein because its mammary tumors are responsive to estrogenic stimulation, as are humans.

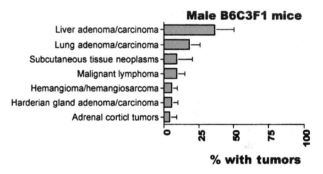

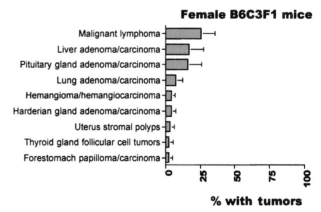

Figure 2-14. Most frequently occurring tumors in untreated control mice from recent NTP 2-year rodent carcinogenicity studies.

The values shown represent the mean ±SD of the percentage of animals developing the specified tumor type at the end of the 2-year study. The values were obtained from 30 different studies involving a total of between 1447 and 1474 animals per tumor type.

Neurotoxicity Assessment

Neurotoxicity or a neurotoxic effect is defined as an adverse change in the chemistry, structure or function of the nervous system following exposure to a chemical or physical agent. The structure, function, and development of the nervous system and its vulnerability to chemicals, is examined in Chap. 16. When evaluating the potential neurological effects of a compound, effects may be on the central or peripheral nervous system or related to exposure that occurred during development or as an adult. The developing nervous system is particularly sensitive to chemical exposures (see Chap. 10).

In vitro systems often using cell culture techniques is a rapidly developing area of neurotoxicity assessment. Specific cell lines are available to examine effects on neuron or glial cells such as proliferation, migration, apoptosis, synpatogenesis and other endpoints. In vitro assays have a number of potential advantages including minimizing the use of animal, lower costs, and adaptable to high through put screening. It is also possible to use an in vitro model to examine the interaction of chemicals, such as food additives, on neuronal cells (Lau *et al.*, 2006). The principle and challenges on in vitro neurotoxicity testing are well described (Tiffany-Castiglioni, 2004).

Procedures for the neurobehavioral evaluation of animals were initially developed as part of the scientific investigation of behavioral motivation. Some of these procedures were then used to evaluate the neuropharmacological properties of new drugs. Now animals are commonly used to evaluate the neurotoxic properties of chemicals. A wide range of adult and developmental animal tests are used to access neurobehavioral function. In addition, neuropathological assessment is an important part of the neurotoxicity evaluation and best practices have been developed for developmental neurotoxicity (Bolon *et al.*, 2006). Irwin developed a basic screen for behavioral function in mice (Irwin, 1968), which was subsequently refined to the functional observational battery (FOB) (Moser, 2000). The FOB can also be used in the evaluation of drug safety (Redfern *et al.*, 2005).

The U.S. EPA established a protocol for the evaluation of developmental neurotoxicity (DNT) in laboratory animals (U.S. EPA 870.6300 and OECD 426) (EPA, 1998; OECD 2004). These protocols include tests of neurobehavioral function, such as auditory startle, learning and memory function, changes in motor activity, and neuropathologic examination and morphometric analysis. Methods and procedures for developmental neurotoxicity evaluation are well established (Claudio *et al.*, 2000; Cory-Slechta *et al.*, 2001; Dorman *et al.*, 2001; Garman *et al.*, 2001; Mileson and Ferenc, 2001). Recent studies examine the neurotoxicity of multiple chemical exposures in animals (Moser *et al.* 2006). Methods are also available to examine cognitive measures on weanling rodents in DNT studies (Ehman and Moser 2006). Non-human primates have been invaluable in evaluating the effects of neurotoxoicants and the risk assessment process (Burbacher and Grant 2000). Sophisticated assessment of operant behavior, and learning and memory assessment of rodents has been used to evaluate the effects of lead (Cory-Slechta, 1995, 1996, 2003). Monkeys can also be used to evaluate the low level effects of neurotoxicants such as mercury on vision, auditory function and vibration sensitivity (Burbacher *et al.*, 2005; Rice and Gilbert, 1982, 1992, 1995). There is remarkable concordance between human and animal neurotoxicity assessment, for example, in lead, mercury, and PCBs (Rice, 1995).

Human testing for the neurological effects of occupational exposures to chemicals is advancing rapidly (Anger, 2003; Farahat *et al.*, 2003; Kamel *et al.*, 2003; McCauley *et al.*, 2006) and even the neurotoxic effects of war (Binder *et al.*, 1999, 2001). These methods have also been applied to Hispanic workers (Rohlman *et al.*, 2001b) and populations with limited education or literacy (Rohlman *et al.*, 2003). The WHO has also recommended a test battery for humans (Anger *et al.*, 2000). There are also neurobehavioral test batteries for assessing children (Rohlman *et al.*, 2001a). Evaluation of the childhood neurological effects of lead (Lanphear *et al.*, 2005; Needleman and Bellinger, 1991) and mercury (Myers *et al.*, 2000) have added enormously to our understanding of the health effects of these chemicals and to the methodology of human neurobehavioral testing.

In summary, the neurontoxicological evaluation is an important aspect of developing a hazard and risk assessment of environmental chemicals and drugs.

Immunotoxicity Assessment

Under normal conditions, the immune system is responsible for host defense against pathogenic infections and certain cancers. However, environmental exposures can alter immune system development and/or function and lead to hypersensitivity, autoimmunity, or immunosuppression, the outcome of which may be expressed as a pathology in most any organ or tissue (see Chap. 12). Our understanding of the biological processes underlying immune system dysfunction remains incomplete. However, advances in molecular biology (including use of transgenic/knockout mice), analytical methods (including gene expression arrays and multiparameter flow cytometry), animal models (including adoptive transfers in immunocompromised mice and host resistance to viral, bacterial, or tumor cell challenge), and other methods are greatly advancing our knowledge.

From a toxicologist's perspective, evaluation of immune system toxicity represents special challenges. Development of hypersensitivity can take various forms, depending on the mechanism underlying the associated immune response, and standard assumptions regarding dose-response relationships may not necessarily apply. For example, a single or incidental exposure to beryllium has been associated with chronic beryllium disease in some individuals. We are only just beginning to understand the biological basis underlying such individual susceptibility. In the case of chronic beryllium disease, a genetic polymorphism in a gene involved in antigen recognition may be associated with increased susceptibility (see Bartell *et al.*, 2000). Although our ability to predict immunogenicity remains poor, research efforts are continuing to identify aspects of the chemical and the individual that confer immunogenicity and underlie hypersensitivity. For example, the increasing incidence of allergic asthma among preschool-age children in the United States since the 1980s, may be associated with exposure to allergens (e.g., dust mites, molds, and animal dander), genetic factors, and other factors in the *in utero* and post-natal environment (see Donovan and Finn, 1999; Armstrong *et al.*, 2005).

Immunosuppression is another form of immune system toxicity, which can result in a failure to respond to pathogenic infection, a prolonged infection period, or expression of a latent infection or cancer. Various chemicals have been associated with immunosuppression. Broad spectrum and targeted immunosuppressive chemicals are designed and used therapeutically to reduce organ transplant rejection or suppress inflammation. However, a large number of chemicals have been associated with immunosuppression, including organochlorine pesticides, diethylstilbesterol, lead, and halogenated aromatic hydrocarbons (including TCDD), and exposures that occur during critical stages may present special risk to development (Holladay, 2005).

Autoimmunity is a specific immune system disorder in which components of the immune system attack normal (self) tissues. Cases of autoimmunity have been reported for a wide range of chemicals including therapeutic drugs, metals, pesticides, and solvents. As with other forms of immune system toxicity, autoimmunity can present in most any tissue.

Finally, new forms of immunotoxicity are appearing based on novel forms of clinical therapy and immunomodulation. These include the variously classified "tumor lysis syndromes" and "cytokine storms" that arise from massive cytokine dysregulation. A recent example involved six healthy volunteers who had enrolled in a Phase 1 clinical trial in the UK who developed a severe cytokine response to an anti-CD28 monoclonal antibody leading to systemic organ failures (Bhogal and Combes, 2006). Such cases are stark reminders of the challenges we face in understanding how the immune system is regulated, developing reliable test systems for identifying such risks prior to human use, and safe means for testing these agents in humans.

As described in Chapter 12, current practice for evaluating potential toxic effects of xenobiotic exposures on the immune system involves a tiered approach to immunotoxicity screening (Luster *et al.*, 2003). This tiered approach is generally accepted world-wide in the registration of novel chemical and therapeutic products. Most recently, final guidance to the pharmaceutical industry was published in April, 2006 by the International Conference on Harmonization of Technical Requirements for Registration of Pharmaceuticals for Human Use (Table 2-3). This guidance, which applies to the nonclinical (animal) testing of human pharmaceuticals is the accepted standard in the U.S., EU, and Japan, and demonstrates the continued commitment by these regulatory bodies to understand the potential risks posed by novel therapeutics.

Tiered testing relies on the concept that standard toxicity studies can provide good evidence for immunotoxicity when considered with known biological properties of the chemical, including structural similarities to known immunomodulators, disposition, and other clinical information, such as increased occurrence of infections or tumors. Evaluation of hematological changes, including differential effects on white blood cells and immunoglobulin changes, and alterations in lymphoid organ weights or histology, can provide strong evidence of potential effects to the immune system. Should such evaluations indicate a potential effect on immune system function, more detailed evaluations may be considered, including the evaluation of functional effects (e.g., T-cell dependent antibody response or Natural Killer cell activity), flow cytometric immunophenotyping, or host resistance studies. Thus, as with other areas of toxicology, the evaluation of immune system toxicity requires the toxicologist to be vigilant in observing early indications from a variety of sources in developing a weight-of-evidence assessment regarding potential injury/dysfunction.

Other Descriptive Toxicity Tests

Most of the tests described above will be included in a "standard" toxicity testing protocol because they are required by the various regulatory agencies. Additional tests may be required or included in the protocol to provide information relating a special route of exposure, such as inhalation. Inhalation toxicity tests in animals usually are carried out in a dynamic (flowing) chamber rather than in static chambers to avoid particulate settling and exhaled gas complications. Such studies usually require special dispersing and analytic methodologies, depending on whether the agent to be tested is a gas, vapor, or aerosol; additional information on methods, concepts,

and problems associated with inhalation toxicology is provided in Chaps. 15 and 28. The duration of exposure for inhalation toxicity tests can be acute, subchronic, or chronic, but acute studies are more common with inhalation toxicology. Other special types of animal toxicity tests include toxicokinetics (absorption, distribution, biotransformation, and excretion), the development of appropriate antidotes and treatment regimens for poisoning, and the development of analytic techniques to detect residues of chemicals in tissues and other biological materials.

TOXICOGENOMICS

In the past decade, numerous new genome-based technologies have become available that allow for the large-scale analysis of biological responses to external stimuli. Traditional scientific approaches to elucidate the biochemical and molecular effects of toxic substances focused largely on examining biochemical pathways that were logically connected to observed responses identified through gross pathology, histology, blood chemistry, or behavioral observations. Such "hypothesis driven" research into understanding mechanism of action remains a mainstay of current scientific investigations in toxicology. However, technologies now available allow one to examine the entire "universe" of biological responses to a toxic substance (Fig. 2-15). These new "hypothesis generating" technologies include: genomics (characterization of much or all of the genome of an organism), transcriptomics (characterization of most or all of the mRNAs, or transcriptome, expressed in a given cell/tissue), proteomics (characterization of most or all of the proteins expressed in a given cell/tissue), and metabonomics (characterization of most or all of the small molecules in a cell or tissue, including substrates, products, and co-factors of enzyme reactions). Other "omics" approaches (e.g., "lipidomics", "nutrigenomics") are being devised to look broadly at the biological response of an organism to change. The integration of all of these levels of molecular function (genomics, transcriptomics, proteomics, metabonomics, etc.) to the understanding of how a living organism functions at the cellular level is sometimes referred to as "Systems Biology" (Weston and Hood, 2004). Because each level of analysis generates a very large quantity of data, the collection, organization, evaluation and statistical analysis is in itself an enormous undertaking. The field of "Bioinformatics" has been developed to address the many computational and statistical challenges of "omics" data. In the field of toxicology, the term "toxicogenomics" is used to define the area of research that "combines transcript, protein and metabolite profiling with conventional toxicology to investigate the interaction between genes and environmental stress in disease causation" (Waters and Fostel, 2004). A conceptual model for how the various new "omics" technologies can be incorporated into toxicological evaluation is shown in Fig. 2-15.

Genomics: The genome of an organism represents the full complement of genes that are determined at fertilization by the combination of the parental DNA. Thus, each cell of an organism has the same genome, characterized by the nucleotide sequences inherited from its parents. The human genome consists of approximately 3 billion base pairs of deoxyribonucleotides. Within the human genome, there is, on average, about 0.1% variability in DNA sequence between any two individuals, and it is these differences that contribute to the uniqueness of each person. Most of this variability exists as "single nucleotide polymorphism", or SNPs, although larger segments of DNA may be variable between individuals, including the duplication or loss of entire genes. The identification of particular genetic variants, such as the GSTM1 polymorphism, that might

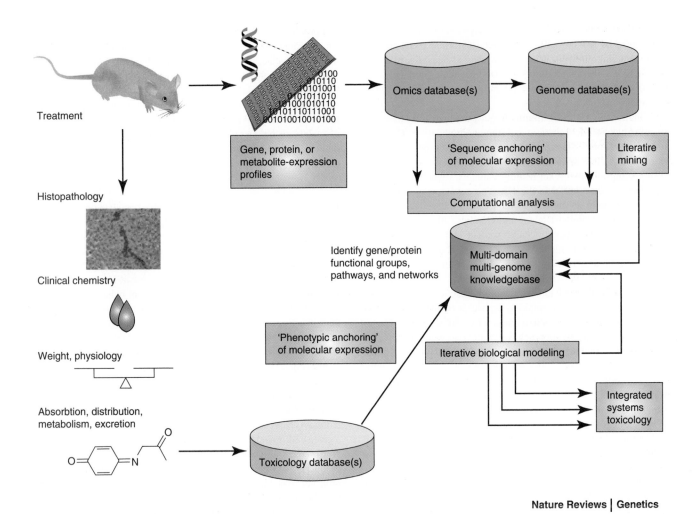

Figure 2-15. Conceptual approach for incorporating "omics" technologies and resulting large databases into toxicological evaluation.

Data from experiments that evaluate the effects of a chemical on global patterns of gene expression (transcriptomics), protein content (proteomics), and small molecules/metabolites (metabonomics/metabolomics), combined with genomic information from both the test species (e.g. rats, mice) and the target species of interest (e.g., humans), are analyzed by computational tools (bioinformatics) for unique or potentially predictive patterns of toxicity. Essential to the use of omics data for predictive toxicology/safety assessment is the ability to reliably tie observed omics patterns to traditional measures of toxicity, such as histopathology and clinical chemistry (phenotypic anchoring).
(From: Waters MD, Fostel JM: Toxicogenomics and systems toxicology: Aims and prospects. *Nat Rev Genet* 5(12):936–948, 2004, with permission from Nature Publishing Group.)

contribute to interindividual differences in susceptibility to chemicals or other environmental factors discussed previously, represents a relatively new and growing area of study that aims to understand the complex interactions between the human genome and the environment (Costa and Eaton, 2006).

Although the genome provides the blueprint for biological function, in order for the genomic information to be utilized in a cell, it must be expressed. Expression of the genome occurs when the coding sequence of DNA is converted to messenger RNA (mRNA). For any given cell, transcription of the genomic information contained in that cell is only partial. It is the differential expression of genes in a given cell that is largely responsible for the diverse function of the thousands of different cells, tissues, and organs that constitute an individual organism. Thus, understanding which genes are expressed

in a given tissue, at what level, and how toxicants perturb the "transcriptome" is of great relevance to toxicology. In addition to coding for mRNAs that provide the blueprint for protein synthesis, genomic DNA also generates small interfering RNAs (siRNA, microRNAs) which are biologically active and can participate in the regulation of gene expression. Furthermore, methylation of DNA is an important determinant of gene expression in cells and tissues, and exogenous chemicals can interfere with transcriptional function via altering DNA methylation (Watson and Goodman, 2002). Importantly, although such epigenetic changes do not result in the alteration of the genomic sequence, they can result in heritable phenotypic changes. Thus, genomic analyses in toxicology may also include techniques to identify toxicant-induced changes in DNA methylation patterns (Watson and Goodman, 2002).

Transcriptomics: Among the first changes that a cell will exhibit following exposure to a toxic substance is a change in gene expression. The transcriptome (all of the mature mRNA species present in a cell at a given point in time) is dynamic, and represents the steady-state between the rate of synthesis (transcription) and degradation of mRNAs in a cell. Toxicologists have utilized the so-called "Northern blot" analysis to assess the level of expression of individual genes in cells or tissues for decades. The "Reverse Transcriptase Polymerase Chain Reaction" (RT-PCR) allows one to quantitatively measure the relative number of mRNA species in a sample for specific genes. Using general primers, it is also possible to amplify the entire transcriptome quantitatively to make many complete copies of the transcriptome in a test tube. Thus, large amounts of material for analysis can be obtained from a relatively small number of cells. Finally, using microarray technologies, where tens of thousands of unique oligonucleotides (or cDNAs) are anchored on a solid matrix, toxicologists can now quantitatively assess the expression of thousands of unique mRNAs in a single sample, thus capturing an "expression profile" of the entire transcriptome in one analysis.

There is great promise that gene expression profiles may be used to provide signatures of specific types of toxic responses, such as a cellular response to DNA damage or oxidative stress. There is also hope that such signature changes in gene expression could be used to facilitate more accurate cross-species extrapolation, allowing comparison of, for example, toxicant-induced changes in gene expression in rat hepatocytes with that of human hepatocytes under identical experimental conditions. However, one of the major challenges in toxicogenomics is the recognition that transcriptional regulation is highly dynamic, and that gene expression profiles can change dramatically with both dose and time. Because microarray experiments are relatively expensive and highly data intensive, it becomes both costly and challenging to conduct and analyze experiments with extensive dose and time course data (although costs are declining). Although changes in gene expression often contribute to, or are reflective of, phenotypic changes that occur in response to a toxic substance, the transcriptome is still somewhat far removed from the ultimate biochemical functions that dictate the actual biological function of the cell. Because the functional expression of a gene generally requires the translation of the mRNA to a protein, there is also great interest in looking at the "proteome"–the entire compliment of *proteins* that are present in a cell or tissue at a given point in time.

Proteomics: Analysis of the proteome of a cell or tissue is much more difficult than analysis of the transcriptome, primarily because it is not yet possible to "amplify" the number of copies of proteins in a cell. Furthermore, unambiguous identification of specific proteins is much more difficult than that for individual mRNAs. Identification of specific proteins is generally done using a combination of separation techniques (e.g., 2D-gel electrophoresis, high performance liquid chromatography), followed by tandem mass spectrometry for identification (Aebersold and Mann, 2003). Because of size limitations for accurate mass spectrometry, protein mixtures are usually digested to smaller peptide fragments. The mixture of peptide fragments is resolved into individual components, and the identity of the specific peptides is determined based on high resolution mass analysis and sequential degradation (sequential loss of single amino acids) of the peptides by various means (Aebersold and Mann, 2003). The large and complex set of peptide mass fragments is then analyzed by computers and compared with a large database of mass fragments of known peptides/proteins. Because as few as 5 amino acid

sequences may provide unique identification of a specific protein, the presence and relative abundance of specific proteins in a sample can then be reconstructed through bioinformatic analyses. As with transcriptomics, it is hoped that changes in protein expression can be used as specific biomarkers for particular types of toxic responses. Of course, such conceptual approaches have been used for years, e.g., use of serum transaminase proteins as indicators of liver damage, or the presence of prostate specific antigen (PSA) in serum as a potential biomarker of early stage prostate hyperplasia or cancer. The potential power of proteomics lies in the ability to identify unique patterns of protein expression, or identification of unique proteins or peptides, that are predictive of early toxic response or later development of disease.

Metabonomics/metabolomics: These two terms are often used interchangeably to describe the analysis of the "universe" of small molecules that serve as substrates, products, and co-factors of the milieu of enzymatic reactions and other metabolic processes that define living cells, and thus the organism. Metabonomics has been defined as "the comprehensive and simultaneous systematic profiling of metabolite levels and their systematic and temporal change through such effects on diet, lifestyle, environment, genetic and pharmaceuticals, both beneficial and adverse, in whole organisms" (Lindon *et al.*, 2003, 2006). The term "metabolomics" has been used principally in studies in plants and in vitro or single cell systems (Fiehn, 2002). Regardless of the specific term used (metabonomics will be used here), the concept of quantitatively analyzing toxicant-induced changes in the "metabolic profile" (the "metabonome") of a cell, tissue or body fluid in some ways represents the "Holy Grail" of toxicogenomics, because the changes in these small molecules must represent a biologically relevant integration of all of the molecular, biochemical and cellular perturbations that lead to the development of toxicity (Fig. 2-15). In other words, changes in the metabonome should reflect the biologically relevant changes in gene transcription, translation, protein function, and other cellular processes, including temporal and adaptive responses, while ignoring biologically irrelevant changes in these factors. Although conceptually superior to either transcriptomics or proteomics for predictive toxicology, metabonomics lags significantly in technological development of readily accessible tools for thorough analysis of the metabonome.

Two approaches for identifying and measuring hundreds, or even thousands, of small molecules in biological samples have emerged – Nuclear Magnetic Resonance (NMR), and mass spectrometry (Lindon *et al.*, 2003, 2006). Both have their advantages and limitations, and it is likely that the most successful approaches to applying metabonomics to toxicological problems will utilize both techniques.

Bioinformatics: One feature in common among all of the various "omics" technologies is the ability to generate very large volumes of data (literally millions of data points from a single experiment). Both the data management and statistical evaluation of toxicogenomics studies represents an enormous challenge. The emerging field of bioinformatics has developed to address these challenges. Numerous commercial platforms for conducting microarray analysis of the transcriptome are available, and sophisticated software is available for both data management and analysis. One of the major challenges in statistical analysis of large data sets is the large number of "false positives" that will result from multiple comparisons. In a typical gene array experiment, it is not uncommon for an investigator to make >20,000 different comparisons. At the typical "95%" statistical confidence limit, one would expect more than 1000 of the noted differences to occur just by chance alone. Thus, more rigorous statistical methods have been developed to reduce the so-called "false discovery rate" in such experiments (Storey *et al.*, 2005; Gao, 2006).

Challenges in using "omics" technologies for predictive toxicology and risk assessment: A conceptual framework for incorporating these new technologies into toxicology, sometimes referred to as "Systems Toxicology" is shown in Fig. 2-15. Several key components of such an approach include: (1) large databases of treatment-specific information, such as results of transcriptomic, proteomic and metabonomic analyses from target tissues and/or body fluids derived from toxicant-treated animals, (2) genomic databases that describe the DNA sequence information from the species of interest, (3) computational tools that extract information from these and other databases and the published literature to identify critical pathways and networks that are altered by the toxicant treatment, and (4) comparison with traditional toxicological endpoints to ensure that the observed "omics responses are closely aligned with the toxicant-related pathophysiology in the animal (histopathology, clinical chemistry, etc) – a process called "phenotypic anchoring" (Waters and Fostel, 2004).

Toxicogenomics tools are becoming indespensible for research aimed at identifying the mechanisms and mode of action of toxic substances. However, the incorporation of such approaches into routine toxicity assessment presents numerous challenges. Numerous working group reports and publications have addressed the challenges of incorporating toxicogenomics data into predictive toxicology and risk assessment (Bammler, 2006; Maggioli *et al.*, 2006; Boverhof and Zacharewski, 2006).

One of the major challenges to incorporating toxicogenomic data into risk assessment is related to the highly dynamic processes that preceded an observed toxic response. Traditional measure of toxicity, such as histopathological changes in a tissue, tend to be stable or even irreversible, whereas the myriad of molecular, biochemical, and cellular changes that give rise to the toxic response(s) are highly dynamic, frequently changing by the hour. Thus, the profiles of mRNAs, proteins and/or metabolites captured at a single point in time may be dramatically different, depending on the specific point in time the sample was collected. Many of the observed changes may be the result of direct effects of the toxicant on specific targets, whereas others will be compensatory or feedback mechanisms invoked in response to the initial damage. Nevertheless, patterns of change in transcript, protein and/or metabolite profiles are likely to provide informative "signatures" of toxic response that will be of great value in predictive toxicology. Such approaches may be particularly useful in pharmaceutical development, where toxicogenomic profiles may help to accelerate preclinical evaluation of drug candidates by identifying "class prediction" profiles indicative of certain types of desirable (pharmacological efficacy) as well as adverse (e.g., DNA damage, oxidative stress) responses.

Finally, it is likely that the introduction of omics technologies to toxicity testing will eventually contribute to the reduction, refinement and replacement (the "3Rs") of animals in toxicity testing and product safety evaluations (Kroeger, 2006).

REFERENCES

Aebersold R, Mann M: Mass spectrometry-based proteomics. *Nature* 422:198–207, 2003.

Albert A: Fundamental aspects of selective toxicity. *Ann NY Acad Sci* 123:5–18, 1965.

Albert A: *Selective Toxicity.* London: Chapman and Hall, 1973.

Aldridge WN: The biological basis and measurement of thresholds. *Annu Rev Pharmacol Toxicol* 26:39–58, 1986.

Allen BC, Kavlock RJ, Kimmel CA, *et al.*: Dose–response assessment for developmental toxicity: II. Comparison of generic benchmark dose estimates with no observed adverse effect levels. *Fundam Appl Toxicol* 23:487–495, 1994a.

Allen BC, Kavlock RJ, Kimmel CA, *et al.*: Dose–response assessment for developmental toxicity: III. Statistical models. *Fundam Appl Toxicol* 23:496–509, 1994b.

Ames BN, McCann J, Yamasaki E: Methods for detecting carcinogens and mutagens with the *Salmonella*/mammalian-microsome mutagenicity test. *Mutat Res* 31:347–364, 1975.

Anger WK, Liang YX, Nell V, *et al.*: Lessons learned—15 years of the WHO-NCTB: A review. *Neurotoxicology* 21(5):837–846, 2000.

Anger WK: Neurobehavioural tests and systems to assess neurotoxic exposures in the workplace and community. *Occup Environ Med* 60:531–538, 474, 2003.

Arcury TA, Quandt SA, Dearry A: Farmworker pesticide exposure and community-based participatory research: Rationale and practical applications. *Environ Health Perspect* 109(Suppl 3):429–434, 2001.

Armstrong JM, Loer-Martin D, Leibnitz R: Developmental immunotoxicant exposure and exacerbated postnatal immune responses: Asthma, in Holladay SD (ed): *Developmental Immunotoxicology.* Boca Raton: CRC Press, pp. 229–281, 2005.

Bammler T, Beyer RP, Bhattacharya S, *et al.*: Standardizing global gene expression analysis between laboratories and across platforms. *Nat Methods* 2:351–356, 2005.

Barnes DG, Dourson M: Reference dose (RfD): Description and use in health risk assessments. *Regul Toxicol Pharmacol* 8:471–486, 1988.

Bartell SM, Takaro TK, Ponce RA, *et al.*: Risk assessment and screening strategies for beryllium exposure. *Technology* 7:241–249, 2000.

Bartels CF, James K, La Du BN: DNA mutations associated with the human butyrylcholinesterase J-variant. *Am J Hum Genet* 50:1104–1114, 1992.

Beauchamp TL, Childress JF: *Principles of Biomedical Ethics*, 4th ed. New York: Oxford University Press, 1994.

Bhogal N, Combes R: TGN1412: Time to change the paradigm for the testing of new pharmaceuticals. *Altern Lab Anim* 34:225–239, 2006.

Binder LM, Storzbach D, Anger WK, *et al.*: Subjective cognitive complaints, affective distress, and objective cognitive performance in Persian Gulf War veterans. *Arch Clin Neuropsychol* 14:531–536, 1999.

Binder LM, Storzbach D, Campbell KA, *et al.*: Neurobehavioral deficits associated with chronic fatigue syndrome in veterans with Gulf War unexplained illnesses. *J Int Neuropsychol Soc* 7:835–839, 2001.

Bliss CL: Some principles of bioassay. *Am Sci* 45:449–466, 1957.

Bolon B, Garman R, Jensen K, Krinke G, Stuart B: A "best practices" approach to neuropathologic assessment in developmental neurotoxicity testing—for today. *Toxicol Pathol* 34(3):296–313, 2006.

Boverhof DR, Zacharewski TR: Toxicogenomics in risk assessment: Applications and needs. *Toxicol Sci* 89:352–360, 2006.

Bruce RD: A confirmatory study of the up-and-down method for acute oral toxicity testing. *Fundam Appl Toxicol* 8:97–100, 1987.

Bruce RD: An up-and-down procedure for acute toxicity testing. *Fundam Appl Toxicol* 5:151–157, 1985.

Brusick D: Genetic toxicology, in Hayes AW (ed): *Principles and Methods of Toxicology*, 4th ed, London: Taylor and Francis, 2001, Chapter 17, pp. 819–852.

Burbacher TM, Grant KS, Mayfield DB, *et al.*: Prenatal methylmercury exposure affects spatial vision in adult monkeys. *Toxicol Appl Pharmacol* 208:21–28, 2005.

Burbacher TM, Grant KS: Methods for studying nonhuman primates in neurobehavioral toxicology and teratology. *Neurotoxicol Teratol* 22:475–486, 2000.

Calabrese EJ, Blain R: The occurrence of hormetic dose responses in the toxicological literature, the hormesis database: An overview. *Toxicol Appl Pharmacol* 202:289–301, 2005.

Callahan D, Jennings B: Ethics and public health: Forging a strong relationship. *Am J Public Health* 92:169–176, 2002.

Carson R: Silent spring. Boston: Houghton Mifflin, 2002, c 1962.

Christian M: Reproductive and developmental toxicity studies, in Sipes IG, McQueen CA, Gandolfi AJ (eds): *Comprehensive Toxicology*; Williams PD, Hottendorf GH (eds): Vol 2. *Toxicological Testing and Evaluation*. New York: Pergamon Press, 1997, pp. 145–154.

Claudio L, Kwa WC, Russell AL, Wallinga D: Testing methods for developmental neurotoxicity of environmental chemicals. *Toxicol Appl Pharmacol* 164(1):1–14, 2000.

Claudio L: An analysis of the U.S. Environmental Protection Agency neurotoxicity testing guidelines. *Regul Toxicol Pharmacol* 16(2):202–212, 1992.

Cohen SM: Calcium phosphate–containing urinary precipitate in rat urinary bladder carcinogenesis. *IARC Sci Publ* 147:175–189, 1999.

Cohen SM: Cell proliferation and carcinogenesis. *Drug Metab Rev* 30:339–357, 1998.

Corburn J: Environmental justice, local knowledge, and risk: The discourse of a community-based cumulative exposure assessment. *Environ Manage* 29:451–466, 2002.

Cory-Slechta DA, Crofton KM, Foran JA, *et al.*: Methods to identify and characterize developmental neurotoxicity for human health risk assessment. I: behavioral effects. *Environ Health Perspect* 109(Suppl 1):79–91, 2001.

Cory-Slechta DA: Lead-induced impairments in complex cognitive function: Offerings from experimental studies. *Child Neuropsychol* 9:54–75, 2003.

Cory-Slechta DA: Legacy of lead exposure: Consequences for the central nervous system. *Otolaryngol Head Neck Surg* 114:224–226, 1996.

Cory-Slechta DA: Relationships between lead-induced learning impairments and changes in dopaminergic, cholinergic, and glutamatergic neurotransmitter system functions. *Annu Rev Pharmacol Toxicol* 35:391–415, 1995.

Costa LG, Eaton DL: *Gene-Environment Interactions: Fundamentals of Ecogenetics*. New York: Wiley Press, 2006, 557 pp.

Crump KS: An improved procedure for low-dose carcinogenic risk assessment from animal data. *J Environ Pathol Toxicol Oncol* 5:339–348, 1984.

D'Arcy PF, Harron DWG (eds). *Proceedings of the First International Conference on Harmonisation*. Queen's University of Belfast, 1992.

Davila JC, Rodriguez RJ, Melchert RB, *et al.*: Predictive value of in vitro model systems in toxicology. *Annu Rev Pharmacol Toxicol* 38:63–96, 1998.

Donovan CE, Finn PW: Immune mechanisms of childhood asthma. *Thorax* 54: 938–946, 1999.

Dorman DC, Allen SL, Byczkowski JZ, *et al.*: Methods to identify and characterize developmental neurotoxicity for human health risk assessment. III: Pharmacokinetic and pharmacodynamic considerations. *Environ Health Perspect* 109(Suppl 1):101–111, 2001.

Doull J: Factors influencing toxicity, in Doull J, Klaassen CD, Amdur MO (eds): *Casarett and Doull's Toxicology: The Basic Science of Poisons*, 2nd ed, New York: Macmillan, 1980, pp. 70–83.

Dybing E, Sanner T: Species differences in chemical carcinogenesis of the thyroid gland, kidney and urinary bladder. *IARC Sci Publ* 147:15–32, 1999.

Eaton DL. Scientific judgment and toxic torts: A primer in toxicology for judges and lawyers. *J Law and Policy* 12:5–42, 2003.

Eaton DL, Gallagher EP: Mechanisms of aflatoxin carcinogenesis. *Annu Rev Pharmacol Toxicol* 34:135–172, 1994.

Ehman KD, Moser VC: Evaluation of cognitive function in weanling rats: A review of methods suitable for chemical screening. *Neurotoxicol Teratol* 28(1):144–161, 2006.

Eichelbaum M, Ingelman-Sundberg M, Evans WE: Pharmacogenomics and individualized drug therapy. *Annu Rev Med* 57:119–137, 2006.

EPA: Environmental Justice. Environmental Protection Agency. Available: http://www.epa.gov/compliance/environmentaljustice/, 2005.

EPA: Health Effects Test Guidlines. OPPTS 870.6300 Developmental Neurotoxicidy Toxicity Study, U.S. Environmental Protection Agency, 1998.

Farahat TM, Abdelrasoul GM, Amr MM, *et al.*: Neurobehavioural effects among workers occupationally exposed to organophosphorous pesticides. *Occup Environ Med* 60:279–286, 2003.

Faustman EM, Allen BC, Kavlock RJ, *et al.*: Dose–response assessment for developmental toxicity: I. Characterization of database and determination of no observed adverse effect levels. *Fundam Appl Toxicol* 23:478–486, 1994.

Faustman EM: Short-term tests for teratogens. *Mutat Res* 205:355–384, 1988.

Fiehn O: Metabolomics—the link between genotypes and phenotypes. *Plant Mol Biol* 48:155–171, 2002.

Finney DJ: *Probit Analysis*. Cambridge: Cambridge University Press, 1971.

Finney DJ: The median lethal dose and its estimation. *Arch Toxicol* 56:215–218, 1985.

Galli A, Schiestl RH: Cell division transforms mutagenic lesions into deletion-recombinagenic lesions in yeast cells. *Mutat Res* 429:13–26, 1999.

Gao X: Construction of null statistics in permutation-based multiple testing for multi-factorial microarray experiments. *Bioinformatics* 22:1486–1494, 2006.

Garman RH, Fix AS, Jortner BS, *et al.*: Methods to identify and characterize developmental neurotoxicity for human health risk assessment. II: Neuropathology. *Environ Health Perspect* 109(Suppl 1):93–100, 2001.

Gilbert G: Ethical, Legal, and Social Issues: Our Children's Future. *Neurotoxicology* 26:521–530, 2005a.

Gilbert SG: Public health and the precautionary principle. *Northwest Public Health Spring/Summer*: 4, 2005b.

Gilbert SG: Supplementing the traditional institutional review board with an environmental health and community review board. *Environ Health Perspect* 114:1626–1629, 2006.

Glynn P, Read DJ, Lush MJ, *et al.*: Molecular cloning of neuropathy target esterase (NTE). *Chem Biol Interact* 119(120):513–517, 1999.

Goldstein BD: The precautionary principle: Is it a threat to toxicological science? *Int J Toxicol* 25:3–7, 2006.

Goldstein A, Aronow L, Kalman SM: *Principles of Drug Action*. New York: Wiley, 1974.

Goozner M: Unrevealed: Non-disclosure of conflicts of interest in four leading medical and scientific journals: Center for Science in the Public Interest, 2004.

Grisham JW: Interspecies comparison of liver carcinogenesis: Implications for cancer risk assessment. *Carcinogenesis* 18:59–81, 1997.

Guzelian PS, Victoroff MS, Halmes NC, *et al.*: Evidence-based toxicology: A comprehensive framework for causation. *Hum Exp Toxicol* 24:161–201, 2005.

Hanna EZ, Chou SP, Grant BF: The relationship between drinking and heart disease morbidity in the United States: Results from the National Health Interview Survey. *Alcohol Clin Exp Res* 21:111–118, 1997.

Harkness JE, Wagner JE: *The Biology and Medicine of Rabbits and Rodents*, 4th ed, New York: Williams and Wilkens, 1995.

Haseman JK: Issues in carcinogenicity testing: Dose selection. *Fundam Appl Toxicol* 5:66–78, 1985.

Hatch EE, Palmer JR, Titus-Ernstoff L, *et al.*: Cancer risk in women exposed to diethylstilbestrol in utero. *JAMA* 280:630–634, 1998.

Hayes AW, (ed). *Principles and Methods of Toxicology*, 4th ed, New York: Taylor and Francis, 2001.

Hengstler JG, Van der Burg B, Steinberg P, *et al.*: Interspecies differences in cancer susceptibility and toxicity. *Drug Metab Rev* 31:917–970, 1999.

Hill AB: The environment and disease: Association or causation? *Proc Royal Soc Med* 58:295–300, 1965.

Holladay SD (ed): *Developmental immunotoxicology*. Boca Raton: CRC Press, 2005, p 364.

Huff JE: Value, validity, and historical development of carcinogenesis studies for predicting and confirming carcinogenic risk to humans, in Kitchin KT (ed): *Carcinogenicity Testing: Predicting & Interpreting Chemical Effects*. New York: Marcel Dekker, 1999, pp. 21–123.

Irwin S: Comprehensive observational assessment: Ia. A systematic, quantitative procedure for assessing the behavioral and physiologic state of the mouse. *Psychopharmacologia* 13(3):222–257, 1968.

Jacobson-Kram D, Keller KA: *Toxicology Testing Handbook: Principles, Applications and Data Interpretation*, New York: Marcel Dekker, 2001.

Kamel F, Rowland AS, Park LP, *et al.*: Neurobehavioral performance and work experience in Florida farmworkers. *Environ Health Perspect* 111:1765–1772, 2003.

Kass NE: An ethics framework for public health. *Am J Public Health* 91:1776–1782, 2001.

Kobayashi Y, Fukumaki Y, Yubisui T, *et al.*: Serine-proline replacement at residue 127 of NADH-cytochrome b5 reductase causes hereditary methemoglobinemia, generalized type. *Blood* 75:1408–1413, 1990.

Krimsky S, Rothenberg LS: Conflict of interest policies in science and medical journals: Editorial practices and author disclosures. *Sci Eng Ethics* 7:205–218, 2001.

Kroeger M: How omics technologies can contribute to the "3R" principles by introducing new strategies in animal testing. *Trends Biotech* 24:343–346, 2006.

Landrigan PJ, Schechter CB, Lipton JM, *et al.*: Environmental pollutants and disease in American children: Estimates of morbidity, mortality, and costs for lead poisoning, asthma, cancer, and developmental disabilities. *Environ Health Perspect* 110:721–728, 2002.

Lanphear BP, Hornung R, Khoury J, *et al.*: Low-level environmental lead exposure and children's intellectual function: An international pooled analysis. *Environ Health Perspect* 113:894–899, 2005.

Lary JM, Daniel KL, Erickson JD, *et al.*: The return of thalidomide: Can birth defects be prevented? *Drug Saf* 21:161–169, 1999.

Lau K, McLean WG, Williams DP, Howard CV: Synergistic interactions between commonly used food additives in a developmental neurotoxicity test. *Toxicol Sci* 90:178–187, 2006.

Lee C: Environmental justice: Building a unified vision of health and the environment. *Environ Health Perspect* 110(Suppl 2):141–144, 2002.

Lehman-McKeeman LD, Caudill D: Biochemical basis for mouse resistance to hyaline droplet nephropathy: Lack of relevance of the alpha 2u-globulin protein superfamily in this male rat-specific syndrome. *Toxicol Appl Pharmacol* 112:214–221, 1992.

Leopold A: A Sand County Almanac, 1949; Reprinted by Ballantine Books, 1991.

Levine RR: *Pharmacology: Drug Actions and Reactions*. Boston: Little, Brown, and Company, 1978.

Lindon JC, Nicholson JK, Holmes E, *et al.*: Contemporary issues in toxicology the role of metabonomics in toxicology and its evaluation by the COMET project. *Toxicol Appl Pharmacol* 187:137–146, 2003.

Lindon JC, Holmes E, Nicholson JK: Metabonomics techniques and applications to pharmaceutical research & development. *Pharm Res* 23:1075–1088, 2006.

Litchfield J, Wilcoxon F: Simplified method of evaluating dose-effect experiments. *J Pharmacol Exp Ther* 96:99–113, 1949.

Litchfield JT: A method for rapid graphic solution of time-percent effective curve. *J Pharmacol Exp Ther* 97:399–408, 1949.

Littlefield NA, Farmer JH, Gaylor DW, *et al.*: Effects of dose and time in a long-term, low-dose carcinogenicity study, in Staffa JA, Mehlman MA (eds): *Innovations in Cancer Risk Assessment (ED01 Study)*. Park Forest South, IL: Pathotox Publishers, 1979.

Luster MI, Dean JH, Germolec DR: Consensus workshop on methods to evaluate developmental immunotoxicity. *Environ Health Perspect* 111:579–583, 2003.

Maggioli J, Hoover A, Weng L: Toxicogenomic analysis methods for predictive toxicology. *J Pharmacol Toxicol Methods* 53:31–37, 2006.

Maibach HI, Patrick E: Dermatotoxicology, in Hayes AW (ed): *Principles and Methods of Toxicology*. New York: Taylor and Francis, 2001, pp. 1039–1084.

Maurissen JP, Gilbert SG, Sander M, *et al.*: Workshop proceedings: Managing conflict of interest in science. A little consensus and a lot of controversy. *Toxicol Sci* 87:11–14, 2005.

Marchant, G: From general policy to legal rule: aspirations and limitations of the precautionary principle. *Environ Health Perspect* 111:1799–1803, 2003.

McCauley LA, Anger WK, Keifer M, *et al.*: Studying health outcomes in farmworker populations exposed to pesticides. *Environ Health Perspect* 114:953–960, 2006.

Mileson BE, Ferenc SA: Methods to identify and characterize developmental neurotoxicity for human health risk assessment: Overview. *Environ Health Perspect* 109(Suppl 1):77–78, 2001.

Mohr LC, Rodgers JK, Silvestri GA. Glutathione S-transferase M1 polymorphism and the risk of lung cancer. *Anticancer Res* 23:2111–2124, 2003.

Monticello TM, Morgan KT: Chemically-induced nasal carcinogenesis and epithelial cell proliferation: A brief review. *Mutat Res* 380:33–41, 1997.

Morello-Frosch R, Pastor M, Jr, Porras C, Sadd J: Environmental justice and regional inequality in southern California: Implications for future research. *Environ Health Perspect* 110(Suppl 2):149–154, 2002.

Moser VC, Simmons JE, Gennings C: Neurotoxicological interactions of a five-pesticide mixture in preweanling rats. *Toxicol Sci* 92:235–245, 2006.

Moser VC: The functional observational battery in adult and developing rats. *Neurotoxicology* 21(6):989–996, 2000.

Myers GJ, Davidson PW, Cox C, *et al.*: Twenty-seven years studying the human neurotoxicity of methylmercury exposure. *Environ Res* 83:275–285, 2000.

Myers NJ, Raffensperger C (eds): Precautionary Tools for Reshaping Environmental Policy. Cambridge: MIT Press, 2006.

NAS: Policy on Committee Composition and Balance and Conflicts of Interest for Committees Used in the Development of Reports, National Academies Press, 2003.

Needleman HL, Bellinger D: The health effects of low level exposure to lead. *Annu Rev Public Health* 12:111–140, 1991.

OECD: Draft Guidance Document on Reproductive Toxicity Testing and Assessment, Series on Testing and Assessment No. 43. Environment Directorate, Organisation for Economic Cooperation and Development, 2004.

O'Fallon LR, Dearry A: Community-based participatory research as a tool to advance environmental health sciences. *Environ Health Perspect* 110(Suppl 2):155–159, 2002.

Peterson M: The precautionary principle is incoherent. *Risk Anal* 26:595–601, 2006.

Pugsley MK, Curtis MJ: Safety pharmacology in focus: New methods developed in the light of the ICH S7B guidance document. *J Pharmacol Toxicol Methods*, 54:94–98, 2006.

Raffensperger C, Tickner J (ed): *Protecting Public Health & the Environment: Implementing the Precautionary Principle*. Washington, DC: Island Press, 1999.

Redfern WS, Strang I, Storey S, *et al.*: Spectrum of effects detected in the rat functional observational battery following oral administration of non-CNS targeted compounds. *J Pharmacol Toxicol Methods* 52:77–82, 2005.

Reno FE: Carcinogenicity studies, in Sipes IG, McQueen CA, Gandolfi AJ (eds): *Comprehensive Toxicology.* Williams PD, Hottendorf GH (eds): Vol 2. *Toxicological Testing and Evaluation.* New York: Pergamon Press, 1997, pp. 121–131.

Rhomberg LR, Wolff SK: Empirical scaling of single oral lethal doses across mammalian species based on a large database. *Risk Anal* 18:741–753, 1998.

Rice DC, Gilbert SG: Early chronic low-level methylmercury poisoning in monkeys impairs spatial vision. *Science* 216(4547):759–761, 1982.

Rice DC, Gilbert SG: Effects of developmental methylmercury exposure or lifetime lead exposure on vibration sensitivity function in monkeys. *Toxicol Appl Pharmacol* 134:161–169, 1995.

Rice DC, Gilbert SG: Exposure to methyl mercury from birth to adulthood impairs high-frequency hearing in monkeys. *Toxicol Appl Pharmacol* 115:6–10, 1992.

Rice DC: Neurotoxicity of lead, methylmercury, and PCBs in relation to the Great Lakes. *Environ Health Perspect* 103(Suppl 9):71–87, 1995.

Roberts RA: Peroxisome proliferators: Mechanisms of adverse effects in rodents and molecular basis for species differences. *Arch Toxicol* 73:413–418, 1999.

Rodricks JV, Gaylor DW, Turnbull D: Quantitative Extrapolations in Toxicology, in Hayes AW (ed): *Principles and Methods in Toxicology*, 4th ed, Philadelphia: Taylor & Francis, 2001, Chapter 8, pp. 365–386.

Rohlman DS, Anger WK, Tamulinas A, *et al.*: Development of a neurobehavioral battery for children exposed to neurotoxic chemicals. *Neurotoxicology* 22:657–665, 2001a.

Rohlman DS, Bailey SR, Anger WK, McCauley L: Assessment of neurobehavioral function with computerized tests in a population of hispanic adolescents working in agriculture. *Environ Res* 85:14–24, 2001b.

Rohlman DS, Gimenes LS, Eckerman DA, *et al.*: Development of the Behavioral Assessment and Research System (BARS) to detect and characterize neurotoxicity in humans. *Neurotoxicology* 24:523–531, 2003.

Rush RE, Bonnette KL, Douds DA, *et al.*: Dermal irritation and sensitization, in Derelanko MJ, Hollinger MA (eds): *CRC Handook of Toxicology.* New York: CRC Press, 1995, pp. 105–162.

Storey JD, Xiao W, Leek JT, *et al.*: Significance analysis of time course microarray experiments. *Proc Natl Acad Sci U S A* 102:12837–12842, 2005.

Tennant RW, Stasiewicz S, Mennear J, *et al.*: Genetically altered mouse models for identifying carcinogens. *IARC Sci Publ* 146:123–150, 1999.

Tiffany-Castiglioni E (ed): In Vitro Neurotoxicology: Principles and Challenges (Methods in Pharmacology and Toxicology): Humana Press, 2004.

Travis CC, White RK: Interspecific scaling of toxicity data. *Risk Anal* 8:119–125, 1988.

Uhl K, Cox E, Rogan R, *et al.*: Thalidomide use in the US: Experience with pregnancy testing in the S.T.E.P.S. programme. *Drug Safety* 29:321–329, 2006.

Waters MD, Fostel JM: Toxicogenomics and systems toxicology: Aims and prospects. *Nat Rev Genet* 5:936–948, 2004.

Watson RE, Goodman JI: Epigenetics and DNA methylation come of age in toxicology. *Toxicol Sci* 67:11–16, 2002.

Weil C: Tables for convenient calculation of median-effective dose (LD50 or ED50) and instruction in their use. *Biometrics* 8:249–263, 1952.

Weinshilboum RM, Otterness DM, Szumlanski CL: Methylation pharmacogenetics: Catechol O-methyltransferase, thiopurine methyltransferase, and histamine N-methyltransferase. *Annu Rev Pharmacol Toxicol* 39:19–52, 1999.

Weston AD, Hood L: Systems biology, proteomics, and the future of health care: Toward predictive, preventative, and personalized medicine. *J Proteome Res* 3:179–196, 2004.

Williams PD, Hottendorf GH: Toxicological tesing and evaluation, in IG Sipes, CA McQueen, AJ Gandolfi(eds): *Comprehensive Toxicology*, Vol. 2, New York: Pergamon Press, 1997.

Wiman KG: The retinoblastoma gene: Role in cell cycle control and cell differentiation. *FASEB J* 7:841–845, 1993.

Wilson NH, Hardisty JF, Hayes JR: Short-term, subchronic and chronic toxicology studies, in Hayes AW (ed): *Principles and Methods of Toxicology*, Philadelphia: Taylor & Francis, 2001, Chapter 19, pp. 917–958.

Wogan GN, Paglialunga S, Newberne PM: Carcinogenic effects of low dietary levels of aflatoxin B1 in rats. *Food Cosmet Toxicol* 12:681–685, 1974.

CHAPTER 3

MECHANISMS OF TOXICITY

Zoltán Gregus

STEP 1—DELIVERY: FROM THE SITE OF EXPOSURE TO THE TARGET

    Absorption versus Presystemic Elimination

        Absorption

        Presystemic Elimination

    Distribution to and Away from the Target

        Mechanisms Facilitating Distribution to a Target

        Mechanisms Opposing Distribution to a Target

    Excretion versus Reabsorption

        Excretion

        Reabsorption

    Toxication versus Detoxication

        Toxication

        Detoxication

STEP 2—REACTION OF THE ULTIMATE TOXICANT WITH THE TARGET MOLECULE

    Attributes of Target Molecules

    Types of Reactions

        Noncovalent Binding

        Covalent Binding

        Hydrogen Abstraction

        Electron Transfer

        Enzymatic Reactions

    Effects of Toxicants on Target Molecules

        Dysfunction of Target Molecules

        Destruction of Target Molecules

        Neoantigen Formation

    Toxicity Not Initiated by Reaction with Target Molecules

STEP 3—CELLULAR DYSFUNCTION AND RESULTANT TOXICITIES

    Toxicant-Induced Cellular Dysregulation

        Dysregulation of Gene Expression

        Dysregulation of Ongoing Cellular Activity

    Toxic Alteration of Cellular Maintenance

        Impairment of Internal Cellular Maintenance: Mechanisms of Toxic Cell Death

        Impairment of External Cellular Maintenance

STEP 4—INAPPROPRIATE REPAIR AND ADAPTATION

    Mechanisms of Repair

        Molecular Repair

        Cellular Repair: A Strategy in Peripheral Neurons

        Tissue Repair

    Mechanisms of Adaptation

        Adaptation by Decreasing Delivery to the Target

        Adaptation by Decreasing the Target Density or Responsiveness

        Adaptation by Increasing Repair

        Adaptation by Compensating Dysfunction

    When Repair and Adaptation Fail

        When Repair Fails

        When Adaptation Fails

    Toxicity Resulting from Inappropriate Repair and Adaptation

        Tissue Necrosis

        Fibrosis

        Carcinogenesis

CONCLUSIONS

Depending primarily on the degree and route of exposure, chemicals may adversely affect the function and/or structure of living organisms. The qualitative and quantitative characterization of these harmful or toxic effects is essential for an evaluation of the potential hazard posed by a particular chemical. It is also valuable to understand the mechanisms responsible for the manifestation of toxicity—that is, how a toxicant enters an organism, how it interacts with target molecules, and how the organism deals with the insult.

An understanding of the mechanisms of toxicity is of both practical and theoretical importance. Such information provides a rational basis for interpreting descriptive toxicity data, estimating the probability that a chemical will cause harmful effects, establishing procedures to prevent or antagonize the toxic effects, designing drugs and industrial chemicals that are less hazardous, and developing pesticides that are more selectively toxic for their target organisms. Elucidation of the mechanisms of chemical toxicity has led to

a better understanding of fundamental physiologic and biochemical processes ranging from neurotransmission (e.g., curare-type arrow poisons) through deoxyribonucleic acid (DNA) repair (e.g., alkylating agents) to transcription, translation, and signal transduction pathways (e.g., chemicals acting through transcription factors, such as the aryl hydrocarbon receptor). Pathologic conditions such as cancer and Parkinson's disease are better understood because of studies on the mechanism of toxicity of chemical carcinogens and 1,2,3,6-tetrahydro-1-methyl-4-phenylpyridine (MPTP), respectively. Continued research on mechanisms of toxicity will undoubtedly continue to provide such insights.

This chapter reviews the cellular mechanisms that contribute to the manifestation of toxicities. Although such mechanisms are dealt with elsewhere in this volume, they are discussed in detail in this chapter in an integrated and comprehensive manner. We provide an overview of the mechanisms of chemical toxicity by relating a

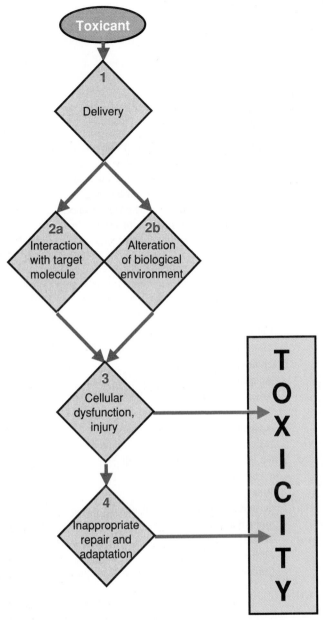

Figure 3-1. Potential stages in the development of toxicity after chemical exposure.

series of events that begins with exposure, involves a multitude of interactions between the invading toxicant and the organism, and culminates in a toxic effect. This chapter focuses on mechanisms that have been identified definitively or tentatively in humans or animals.

As a result of the huge number of potential toxicants and the multitude of biological structures and processes that can be impaired, there are a tremendous number of possible toxic effects. Correspondingly, there are various pathways that may lead to toxicity (Fig. 3-1). A common course is when a toxicant delivered to its target reacts with it, and the resultant cellular dysfunction manifests itself in toxicity. An example of this route to toxicity is that taken by the puffer fish poison, tetrodotoxin. After ingestion, this poison reaches the voltage-gated Na^+ channels of motoneurons (step 1). Interaction of tetrodotoxin with this target (step 2a) results in blockade

of Na^+ channels, inhibition of the activity of motor neurons (step 3), and ultimately skeletal muscle paralysis. No repair mechanisms can prevent the onset of such toxicity.

Sometimes a xenobiotic does not react with a specific target molecule but rather adversely influences the biological (micro) environment, causing molecular, organellar, cellular, or organ dysfunction leading to deleterious effects. For example, 2,4-dinitrophenol, after entering the mitochondrial matrix space (step 1), collapses the outwardly directed proton gradient across the inner membrane by its mere presence there (step 2b), causing mitochondrial dysfunction (step 3), which is manifest in toxic effects such as hyperthermia and seizures. Chemicals that precipitate in renal tubules and block urine formation represent another example for such a course (step 2b).

The most complex path to toxicity involves more steps (Fig. 3-1). First, the toxicant is delivered to its target or targets (step 1), after which the ultimate toxicant interacts with endogenous target molecules (step 2a), triggering perturbations in cell function and/or structure (step 3), which initiate repair mechanisms at the molecular, cellular, and/or tissue levels as well as adaptive mechanisms to diminish delivery, boost repair capacity and/or compensate for dysfunction (step 4). When the perturbations induced by the toxicant exceed repair and adaptive capacity or when repair and adaptation becomes malfunctional, toxicity occurs. Tissue necrosis, cancer, and fibrosis are examples of chemically induced toxicities whose development follow this four-step course.

STEP 1—DELIVERY: FROM THE SITE OF EXPOSURE TO THE TARGET

Theoretically, the intensity of a toxic effect depends primarily on the concentration and persistence of the ultimate toxicant at its site of action. The ultimate toxicant is the chemical species that reacts with the endogenous target molecule (e.g., receptor, enzyme, DNA, microfilamental protein, lipid) or critically alters the biological (micro) environment, initiating structural and/or functional alterations that result is toxicity. Often the ultimate toxicant is the original chemical to which the organism is exposed (parent compound). In other cases, the ultimate toxicant is a metabolite of the parent compound or a reactive oxygen or nitrogen species (ROS or RNS) generated during the biotransformation of the toxicant. Occasionally, the ultimate toxicant is an unchanged or altered endogenous molecule (Table 3-1).

The concentration of the ultimate toxicant at the target molecule depends on the relative effectiveness of the processes that increase or decrease it's concentration at the target site (Fig. 3-2). The accumulation of the ultimate toxicant at its target is facilitated by its absorption, distribution to the site of action, reabsorption, and toxication (metabolic activation). Conversely, presystemic elimination, distribution away from the site of action, excretion, and detoxication oppose these processes and work against the accumulation of the ultimate toxicant at the target molecule.

Absorption versus Presystemic Elimination

Absorption Absorption is the transfer of a chemical from the site of exposure, usually an external or internal body surface (e.g., skin, mucosa of the alimentary and respiratory tracts), into the systemic circulation. Whereas transporters may contribute to the gastrointestinal absorption of some chemicals (e.g., salicylate and valproate by monocarboxylate transporters, some β-lactam antibiotics and ACE inhibitor drugs by peptide transporters, Fe^{2+}, Cd^{2+}, as well

Table 3.1
Types of Ultimate Toxicants and Their Sources

Parent xenobiotics as ultimate toxicants		
Pb ions		
Tetrodotoxin		
TCDD		
Methylisocyanate		
HCN		
CO		
Xenobiotic metabolites as ultimate toxicants		
Amygdalin	$\rightarrow$	HCN
Arsenate	$\rightarrow$	Arsenite
Fluoroacetate	$\rightarrow$	Fluorocitrate
Ethylene glycol	$\rightarrow$	Oxalic acid
Hexane	$\rightarrow$	2,5-Hexanedione
Acetaminophen	$\rightarrow$	N-Acetyl-p-benzoquinoneimine
CCl_4	$\rightarrow$	$CCl_3OO^\bullet$
Benzo[a]pyrene (BP)	$\rightarrow$	BP-7,8-diol-9,10-epoxide
Benzo[a]pyrene (BP)	$\rightarrow$	BP-Radical cation
Reactive oxygen or nitrogen species as ultimate toxicants		
Hydrogen peroxide		
Diquat, doxorubicin, nitrofurantoin	$\rightarrow$	Hydroxyl radical ($HO^\bullet$)
Cr(V), Fe(II), Mn(II), Ni(II)		
Paraquat $\rightarrow O_2^{\bullet-} + NO^\bullet$	$\rightarrow$	Peroxynitrite ($ONOO^-$)
Endogenous compounds as ultimate toxicants		
Sulfonamides $\rightarrow$ albumin-bound bilirubin	$\rightarrow$	Bilirubin
$CCl_3OO^\bullet \rightarrow$ unsaturated fatty acids	$\rightarrow$	Lipid peroxyl radicals
$CCl_3OO^\bullet \rightarrow$ unsaturated fatty acids	$\rightarrow$	Lipid alkoxyl radicals
$CCl_3OO^\bullet \rightarrow$ unsaturated fatty acids	$\rightarrow$	4-Hydroxynon-2-enal
$HO^\bullet \rightarrow$ proteins	$\rightarrow$	Protein carbonyls

as some other divalent metal ions by the divalent metal-ion transporter, and arsenate by phosphate transporters), the vast majority of toxicants traverse epithelial barriers and reach the blood capillaries by diffusing through cells. The rate of absorption is related to the concentration of the chemical at the absorbing surface, which depends on the rate of exposure and the dissolution of the chemical. It is also related to the area of the exposed site, the characteristics of the epithelial layer through which absorption takes place (e.g., the thickness of the stratum corneum in the skin), the intensity of the subepithelial microcirculation, and the physicochemical properties of the toxicant. Lipid solubility is usually the most important property influencing absorption. In general, lipid-soluble chemicals are absorbed more readily than are water-soluble substances.

Presystemic Elimination During transfer from the site of exposure to the systemic circulation, toxicants may be eliminated. This is not unusual for chemicals absorbed from the gastrointestinal (GI) tract because they must first pass through the GI mucosal cells, liver, and lung before being distributed to the rest of the body by the systemic circulation. The GI mucosa and the liver may eliminate a significant fraction of a toxicant during its passage through these tissues, decreasing its systemic availability. For example, ethanol is oxidized by alcohol dehydrogenase in the gastric mucosa (Lim *et al.*, 1993), cyclosporine is returned from the enterocyte into the intestinal lumen by P-glycoprotein (an ATP-dependent xenobiotic transporter) and is also hydroxylated by cytochrome P450 (CYP3A4) in these cells (Lin *et al.*, 1999), morphine is glucuronidated in intestinal mu-

cosa and liver, and manganese is taken up from the portal blood into liver and excreted into bile. Such processes may prevent a considerable quantity of chemicals from reaching the systemic blood. Thus, presystemic or first-pass elimination reduces the toxic effects of chemicals that reach their target sites by way of the systemic circulation. In contrast, the processes involved in presystemic elimination may contribute to injury of the digestive mucosa, liver, and lungs by chemicals such as ethanol, iron salts, α-amanitin, and paraquat because these processes promote their delivery to those sites.

Distribution to and Away from the Target

Toxicants exit the blood during the distribution phase, enter the extracellular space, and may penetrate into cells. Chemicals dissolved in plasma water may diffuse through the capillary endothelium via aqueous intercellular spaces and transcellular pores called fenestrae and/or across the cell membrane. Lipid-soluble compounds move readily into cells by diffusion. In contrast, highly ionized and hydrophilic xenobiotics (e.g., tubocurarine and aminoglycosides) are largely restricted to the extracellular space unless specialized membrane carrier systems are available to transport them.

During distribution, toxicants reach their site or sites of action, usually a macromolecule on either the surface or the interior of a particular type of cell. Chemicals also may be distributed to the site or sites of toxication, usually an intracellular enzyme, where the ultimate toxicant is formed. Some mechanisms facilitate whereas others delay the distribution of toxicants to their targets.

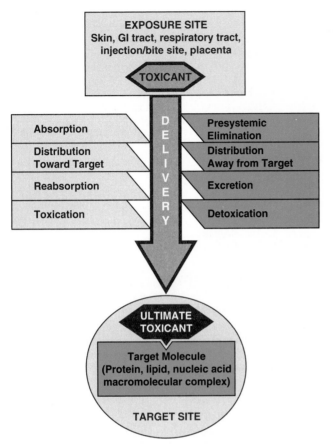

Figure 3-2. *The process of toxicant delivery is the first step in the development of toxicity.*

Mechanisms Facilitating Distribution to a Target   Distribution of toxicants to specific target sites may be enhanced by (1) the porosity of the capillary endothelium, (2) specialized membrane transport, (3) accumulation in cell organelles, and (4) reversible intracellular binding.

Porosity of the Capillary Endothelium   Endothelial cells in the hepatic sinusoids and in the renal peritubular capillaries have larger fenestrae (50 to 150 nm in diameter) that permit passage of even protein-bound xenobiotics. This favors the accumulation of chemicals in the liver and kidneys.

Specialized Transport Across the Plasma Membrane   Specialized ion channels and membrane transporters can contribute to the delivery of toxicants to intracellular targets. For example, aquaglyceroporin channels may mediate influx of arsenite, which is present at physiological pH as uncharged $As(OH)_3$, voltage-gated Ca^{2+} channels permit the entry of cations such as lead or barium ions into excitable cells, and Na^+, K^+-ATPase promotes intracellular accumulation of thallous ion. Paraquat enters into pneumocytes via hitherto unspecified transporters, hepatocellular uptake of α-amanitin is mediated by the Na-dependent bile acid transporter (NTCP) and an organic anion transporting polypeptide (OATP1B3) and that of microcystin by OATP1B1 and OATP1B3, organic anion transporters such as human OAT1 and OAT3 mediate renal tubular uptake of ochratoxin and mercuric ion (the latter as the di-cysteine conjugate Cys-Hg-Cys), whereas both OAT1 and amino acid transporters can carry methylmercury as its cysteine conjugate CH_3-Hg-Cys, and an MPTP metabolite (MPP^+) enters into extrapyramidal dopamin-

ergic neurons by means of the dopamine transporter. Endocytosis of some toxicant-protein complexes, such as Cd-metallothionein or hydrocarbons bound to the male rat-specific α_{2u}-globulin, by renal proximal tubular cells can also occur. In addition, lipoprotein receptor–mediated endocytosis contributes to entry of lipoprotein-bound toxicants into cells equipped with such transporters. Membrane recycling can internalize cationic aminoglycosides associated with anionic phospholipids in the brush border membrane of renal tubular cells (Laurent *et al.*, 1990). This process may also contribute to cellular uptake of heavy metal ions. Such uptake mechanisms facilitate the entry of toxicants into specific cells, rendering those cells targets. Thus, carrier-mediated uptake of paraquat by pneumocytes and internalization of aminoglycosides by renal proximal tubular cells expose those cells to toxic concentrations of those chemicals.

Accumulation in Cell Organelles   Amphipathic xenobiotics with a protonable amine group and lipophilic character accumulate in lysosomes as well as mitochondria and cause adverse effects there. Lysosomal accumulation occurs by pH trapping, i.e., diffusion of the amine (e.g., amiodarone, amitriptyline, fluoxetine) in unprotonated form into the acidic interior of the organelle, where the amine is protonated, preventing its efflux. The entrapped amine inhibits lysosomal phospholipases, impairing degradation of lysosomal phospholipids, and causing phospholipidosis. Mitochondrial accumulation takes place electrophoretically. The amine is protonated in the intermembrane space (to where the mitochondria eject protons). The cation thus formed will then be sucked into the matrix space by the strong negative potential there ($-220\,mV$), where it may impair β-oxidation and oxidative phosphorylation. By such mechanisms, the valued antiarrhytmic drug amiodarone is entrapped in the hepatic lysosomes and mitochondria, causing phospholipidosis (Kodavanti and Mehendale, 1990) and microvesiculas steatosis with other liver lesions (Fromenty and Pessayre, 1997), respectively. The cationic metabolite of MPTP (MPP^+) also electrophoretically accumulates in the mitochondria of dopaminergic neurons, causing mitochondrial dysfunction and cell death, whereas highly lipophilic local anesthetics (e.g., tetracaine, bupivacaine), when overdosed or inadvertently injected into a blood vessel, accumulate in cardiac mitochondria, compromising mitochondrial energy production and causing cardiac failure. Human equilibrative nucleoside transporter 1 (ENT1) in the mitochondrial inner membrane appears responsible for targeting fialuridine (an already withdrawn thymidine nucleoside analogue antiviral drug) into human mitochondria, where it inhibits mitochondrial DNA synthesis, thereby inducing hepatotoxicity. The fact that ENT1 is not localized in rodent mitochondria may account for the dramatic difference in mitochondrial toxicity of fialuridine between humans and rodents (Lee *et al.*, 2006).

Reversible Intracellular Binding   Binding to the pigment melanin, an intracellular polyanionic aromatic polymer, is a mechanism by which chemicals such as organic and inorganic cations and polycyclic aromatic hydrocarbons can accumulate in melanin-containing cells in the retina, the substantia nigra, and the skin (Larsson, 1993). The release of melanin-bound toxicants is thought to contribute to the retinal toxicity associated with chlorpromazine and chloroquine, injury to substantia nigra neurons by MPTP and manganese, and the induction of melanoma by polycyclic aromatics. Keratins are the major structural proteins in the epidermis and its appendages (nail and hair), constituting up to 85% of fully differentiated keratinocytes (skin cells). As keratins are abundant in cysteine residues, they can sequester thiol-reactive metal ions and metalloid compounds, whose nail and hair contents are indicative of exposure. Release of keratin-bound arsenic in keratinocytes may adversely affect these cells, leading to dermal lesions common in arsenicism.

Mechanisms Opposing Distribution to a Target Distribution of toxicants to specific sites may be hindered by several processes. The processes include (1) binding to plasma proteins, (2) specialized barriers, (3) distribution to storage sites such as adipose tissue, (4) association with intracellular binding proteins, and (5) export from cells.

Binding to Plasma Proteins As long as xenobiotics such as DDT and TCDD are bound to high-molecular-weight proteins or lipoproteins in plasma, they cannot leave the capillaries by diffusion. Even if they exit the bloodstream through fenestrae, they have difficulty permeating cell membranes. Dissociation from proteins is required for most xenobiotics to leave the blood and enter cells. Therefore, strong binding to plasma proteins delays and prolongs the effects and elimination of toxicants.

Specialized Barriers Brain capillaries have very low aqueous porosity because their endothelial cells lack fenestrae and are joined by extremely tight junctions. This blood–brain barrier prevents the access of hydrophilic chemicals to the brain except for those that can be actively transported. In the choroid plexus, where the capillaries are fenestrated, the choroidal epithelial cells are sealed together by tight junctions, forming the blood-cerebrospinal fluid barrier. Water-soluble toxicants also have restricted access to reproductive cells, which are separated from capillaries by other cells. The oocyte in the ovary is surrounded by multiple layers of granulosa cells, and the spermatogenic cells are supported by Sertoli cells that are tightly joined in the seminiferous tubules to form the blood-testis barrier (see Chap. 20). Transfer of hydrophilic toxicants across the placenta is also restricted. However, none of these barriers are effective against lipophilic substances.

Distribution to Storage Sites Some chemicals accumulate in tissues (i.e., storage sites) where they do not exert significant effects. For example, highly lipophilic substances such as chlorinated hydrocarbon insecticides concentrate in adipocytes, whereas lead is deposited in bone by substituting for Ca^{2+} in hydroxyapatite. Such storage decreases the availability of these toxicants for their target sites and acts as a temporary protective mechanism. However, insecticides may return to the circulation and be distributed to their target site, the nervous tissue, when there is a rapid lipid loss as a result of fasting. This contributes to the lethality of pesticide-exposed birds during migration or during the winter months, when food is restricted. The possibility that lead is mobilized from the bone during pregnancy is of concern.

Association with Intracellular Binding Proteins Binding to non-target intracellular sites also reduces the concentration of toxicants at the target site, at least temporarily. Metallothionein, a cysteine-rich cytoplasmic protein, serves such a function in acute cadmium intoxication (Klaassen et al., 1999).

Export from Cells Intracellular toxicants may be transported back into the extracellular space. This occurs in brain capillary endothelial cells. In their luminal membrane, these cells contain ATP-dependent membrane transporters (ATP-binding cassette or ABC transporters) such as the multidrug-resistance protein (MDR1), or P-glycoprotein, which extrudes chemicals and contributes to the blood-brain barrier (Schinkel, 1999). Compared to normal mice, mice with disrupted *mdr1a* gene exhibit 100-fold higher brain levels of and sensitivity to ivermectin, a neurotoxic pesticide and human antihelmintic drug

that is one of many P-glycoprotein substrates (Schinkel, 1999). The ocyte is also equipped with the P-glycoprotein that provides protection against chemicals that are substrates for this efflux pump (Elbling et al., 1993). Hematopoietic stem cells (and perhaps other stem cells) are also protected by ABC transporters, such as MDR1, MRP1 and BCRP (breast cancer resistance protein), of which the latter confers these cells resistance to mitoxantrone. ABC transporters that export drugs were first identified in tumor cells which often overexpress them, thereby making these cells resistant to antitumor drugs these transporters pump out.

Excretion versus Reabsorption

Excretion Excretion is the removal of xenobiotics from the blood and their return to the external environment. Excretion is a physical mechanism whereas biotransformation is a chemical mechanism for eliminating the toxicant.

For nonvolatile chemicals, the major excretory structures in the body are the renal glomeruli, which hydrostatically filter small molecules (<60 kDa) through their pores, and the proximal renal tubular cells and hepatocytes, which actively transport chemicals from the blood into the renal tubules and bile canaliculi, respectively. These cells are readily exposed to blood-borne chemicals through the large endothelial fenestrae; they have transporters of the solute carrier (SLC) family (e.g., OAT, OCT, and OATP type) that mediate the basolateral uptake of particular chemicals and transporters of the ATP-binding cassette (ABC) carrier family (e.g., MRP and MDR type) that mediate the luminal export of certain chemicals (see Chap. 5). Renal transporters have a preferential affinity for smaller (<300-Da), and hepatic transporters for larger (>400-Da), amphiphilic molecules. A less common "excretory" mechanism consists of diffusion and partition into the excreta on the basis of their lipid content (see below) or acidity. For example, morphine is transferred into milk and amphetamine is transferred into gastric juice by nonionic diffusion. This is facilitated by pH-trapping of those organic bases in those fluids, which are acidic relative to plasma (see Chap. 5).

The route and speed of excretion depend largely on the physicochemical properties of the toxicant. The major excretory organs—kidney and liver—can efficiently remove only highly hydrophilic, usually ionized chemicals such as organic acids and bases. The reasons for this are as follows: (1) in the renal glomeruli, only compounds dissolved in plasma water can be filtered; (2) transporters in hepatocytes and renal proximal tubular cells are specialized for secretion of highly hydrophilic organic acids and bases; (3) only hydrophilic chemicals are freely soluble in the aqueous urine and bile; and (4) lipid-soluble compounds are readily reabsorbed by transcellular diffusion.

There are no efficient elimination mechanisms for nonvolatile, highly lipophilic chemicals such as polyhalogenated biphenyls and chlorinated hydrocarbon insecticides. If they are resistant to biotransformation, such chemicals are eliminated very slowly and tend to accumulate in the body upon repeated exposure. Three rather inefficient processes are available for the elimination of such chemicals: (1) excretion by the mammary gland after the chemical is dissolved in the milk lipids; (2) excretion in bile in association with biliary micelles and/or phospholipid vesicles; and (3) intestinal excretion, an incompletely understood transport from blood into the intestinal lumen. Volatile, nonreactive toxicants such as gases and volatile liquids diffuse from pulmonary capillaries into the alveoli and are exhaled.

Reabsorption Toxicants delivered into the renal tubules may diffuse back across the tubular cells into the peritubular capillaries. This process is facilitated by tubular fluid reabsorption, which increases the intratubular concentration as well as the residence time of the chemical by slowing urine flow. Reabsorption by diffusion is dependent on the lipid solubility of the chemical. For organic acids and bases, diffusion is inversely related to the extent of ionization, because the nonionized molecule is more lipid-soluble. The ionization of weak organic acids, such as salicylic acid and phenobarbital, and bases, such as amphetamine, procainamide, and quinidine, is strongly pH-dependent in the physiologic range. Therefore their reabsorption is influenced significantly by the pH of the tubular fluid. Acidification of urine favors the excretion of weak organic bases, whereas alkalinization favors the elimination of weak organic acids. Some organic compounds may be reabsorbed from the renal tubules by transporters. For example, peptide transporters (PEPT) can move some β-lactam antibiotics and angiotensin converting enzyme inhibitor drugs across the brush border membrane. Carriers for the physiologic oxyanions mediate the reabsorption of some toxic metal oxyanions in the kidney. Chromate and molybdate are reabsorbed by the sulfate transporter, whereas arsenate is reabsorbed by the phosphate transporter.

Toxicants delivered to the GI tract by biliary, gastric, and intestinal excretion and secretion by salivary glands and the exocrine pancreas may be reabsorbed by diffusion across the intestinal mucosa. Because compounds secreted into bile are usually organic acids, their reabsorption is possible only if they are sufficiently lipophilic or are converted to more lipid-soluble forms in the intestinal lumen. For example, glucuronides of toxicants such as diethylstilbestrol, and glucuronides of the hydroxylated metabolites of polycyclic aromatic hydrocarbons, chlordecone, and halogenated biphenyls are hydrolyzed by the β-glucuronidase of intestinal microorganisms, and the released aglycones are reabsorbed (Gregus and Klaassen, 1986). Glutathione conjugates of hexachlorobutadiene and trichloroethylene are hydrolyzed by intestinal and pancreatic peptidases, yielding the cysteine conjugates, which are reabsorbed and serve as precursors of some nephrotoxic metabolites (Anders, 2004).

Toxication versus Detoxication

Toxication A number of xenobiotics (e.g., strong acids and bases, nicotine, aminoglycosides, ethylene oxide, methylisocyanate, heavy-metal ions, HCN, CO) are directly toxic, whereas the toxicity of others is due largely to metabolites. Biotransformation to harmful products is called *toxication* or *metabolic activation.* With some xenobiotics, toxication confers physicochemical properties that adversely alter the microenvironment of biological processes or structures. For example, oxalic acid formed from ethylene glycol may cause acidosis and hypocalcaemia as well as obstruction of renal tubules by precipitation as calcium oxalate. Occasionally, chemicals acquire structural features and reactivity by biotransformation that allows for a more efficient interaction with specific receptors or enzymes. For example, the organophosphate insecticide parathion is biotransformed to paraoxon, an active cholinesterase inhibitor; the rodenticide fluoroacetate is converted in the citric acid cycle to fluorocitrate, a false substrate that inhibits aconitase; as a result of its CYP2E1-catalyzed oxidation, the general anesthetic methoxyflurane releases fluoride ion which inhibits several enzymes (including enolase in the glycolytic pathway) and which contributes to renal injury after prolonged anesthesia; some cephalosporin antibiotics (e.g., cephoperazone) may cause hemorrhage because they undergo biotransformation with release of 1-methyltetrazole-5-thiol that inhibits vitamin K epoxide reductase and thus impairs activation clotting factors; and fialuridine, an antiviral drug withdrawn from development because it produced lethal hepatotoxicity in patients involved in the clinical trial, is phosphorylated to the triphosphate, which inhibits DNA polymerase-γ and thus impairs synthesis of mitochondrial DNA (Lewis *et al.*, 1996). Most often, however, toxication renders xenobiotics and occasionally other molecules in the body, such as oxygen and nitric oxide ($^{\bullet}$NO), indiscriminately reactive toward endogenous molecules with susceptible functional groups. This increased reactivity may be due to conversion into (1) electrophiles, (2) free radicals, (3) nucleophiles, or (4) redox-active reactants.

Formation of Electrophiles Electrophiles are molecules containing an electron-deficient atom with a partial or full positive charge that allows it to react by sharing electron pairs with electron-rich atoms in nucleophiles. The formation of electrophiles is involved in the toxication of numerous chemicals (Table 3-2) (see Chap. 6). Such reactants are often produced by insertion of an oxygen atom, which withdraws electrons from the atom it is attached to, making that electrophilic. This is the case when aldehydes, ketones, epoxides, arene oxides, sulfoxides, nitroso compounds, phosphonates, and acyl halides are formed (Table 3-2). In other instances, conjugated double bonds are formed, which become polarized by the electron-withdrawing effect of an oxygen, making one of the double-bonded carbons electron-deficient (that is, electrophilic). This occurs when α, β-unsaturated aldehydes and ketones as well as quinones, quinoneimines, and quinonemethides are produced (Table 3-2). Formation of many of these electrophilic metabolites is catalyzed by cytochrome P450s.

Cationic electrophiles may be produced as a result of heterolytic bond cleavage. For example, methyl-substituted aromatics such as 7,12-dimethylbenzanthracene and aromatic amines (amides), such as 2-acetylaminofluorene, are hydroxylated to form benzylic alcohols and N-hydroxy arylamines (amides), respectively (Miller and Surh, 1994). These metabolites are then esterified, typically by sulfotransferases. Heterolytic cleavage of the C—O or N—O bonds of these esters results in a hydrosulfate anion and the concomitant formation of a benzylic carbonium ion or arylnitrenium ion, respectively (see Chap. 6). The antiestrogen tamoxifen undergoes similar activation by hydroxylation and sulfation to form a carbocationic metabolite (Kim *et al.*, 2004). After being C-hydroxylated by CYP2E1, the hepatocarcinogen dimethylnitrosamine undergoes spontaneous decomposition, finally a heterolytic cleavage of the C—N bond to form methyl carbonium cation ($^{+}CH_3$) (see Chap. 6). In a similar process, the tobacco-specific nicotine-derived nitrosamine ketone (NNK), the most potent carcinogen in tobacco, may generate either methyl carbonium cation or piridyloxobutyl carbonium cation, depending on the site of C-hydroxylation that initiates its decomposition. Formally, spontaneous heterolytic cleavage of the C—Cl bond results in formation of reactive epi- sulfonium ion from the vesicant chemical warfare agent sulfur mustard (2,2'-bis-chloroethylsulfide). An episulfonium ion metabolite is also the ultimate toxicant produced from the fumigant 1,2-dibromoethane following its conjugation with glutathione to form S-(2-bromoethyl)glutathione conjugate, a so called half-sulfur mustard (Anders, 2004). The oxidation of mercury (Hg^0) to Hg^{2+} by catalase, reduction of CrO_4^{2-} to DNA-reactive Cr^{3+} by ascorbate (Quievryn *et al.*, 2002) and reduction of the phosphate-mimicking AsO_4^{3-} to thiol-reactive AsO_3^{2-}/As^{3+} by enzymes catalyzing

Table 3.2
Toxication by Formation of Electrophilic Metabolites

ELECTROPHILIC METABOLITE	PARENT TOXICANT	ENZYMES CATALYZING TOXICATION	TOXIC EFFECT
Nonionic electrophiles			
Aldehydes, ketones			
Acetaldehyde	Ethanol	ADH	Hepatic fibrosis(?)
Zomepirac glucuronide	Zomepirac	GT→isomerization	Immune reaction(?)
2,5-Hexanedione	Hexane	CYP	Axonopathy
α, β-Unsaturated aldehydes, ketones			
Acrolein	Allyl alcohol	ADH	Hepatic necrosis
Acrolein	Allyl amine	MAO	Vascular injury
Muconic aldehyde	Benzene	Multiple	Bone marrow injury
4-Hydroxynon-2-enal	Fatty acids	Lipid peroxidation	Cellular injury(?)
Quinones, quinoneimines			
DES-4,4'-quinone	DES	Peroxidases	Carcinogenesis(?)
N-Acetyl-p-benzoquinoneimine	Acetaminophen	CYP, peroxidases	Hepatic necrosis
Epoxides, arene oxides			
Aflatoxin B$_1$ 8,9-epoxide	Aflatoxin B$_1$	CYP	Carcinogenesis
2-Chlorooxirane	Vinyl chloride	CYP	Carcinogenesis
Bromobenzene 3,4-oxide	Bromobenzene	CYP	Hepatic necrosis
Benzo[a]pyrene 7,8-diol 9,10-oxide	Benzo[a]pyrene	CYP	Carcinogenesis
Sulfoxides			
Thioacetamide S-oxide	Thioacetamide	FMO	Hepatic necrosis
Nitroso compounds			
Nitroso-sulfamethoxazole	Sulfamethoxazole	CYP	Immune reaction
Phosphonates			
Paraoxon	Parathion	CYP	ChE inhibition
Acyl halides			
Phosgene	Chloroform	CYP	Hepatic necrosis
Trifluoroacetyl chloride	Halothane	CYP	Immune hepatitis
Thionoacyl halides			
2,3,4,4-Tetrachlorothiobut-3-enoic acid chloride	HCBD	GST→GGT →DP→CβCL	Renal tubular necrosis
Thioketenes			
Chloro-1,2,2-trichlorovinyl-thioketene	HCBD	GST→GGT →DP→CCβL	Renal tubular necrosis
Cationic electrophiles			
Carbonium ions			
Benzylic carbocation	7,12-DMBA	CYP→ST	Carcinogenesis
Carbonium cation	DENA	CYP→s.r.	
Nitrenium ions			
Arylnitrenium ion	AAF, DMAB, HAPP	CYP→ST	Carcinogenesis
Sulfonium ions			
Episulfonium ion	1,2-dibromoethane	GST	Carcinogenesis
Metal ions			
Mercury(II) ion	Elemental Hg	Catalase	Brain injury
Diaquo-diamino platinate(II)	Cisplatinum	s.r.	Renal tubular necrosis

KEY: AAF = 2-acetylaminofluorene, ADH = alcohol dehydrogenase, CCβL = cysteine conjugate β-lyase; ChE = cholinesterase; CYP = cytochrome P450; DENA = diethylnitrosamine; DMAB N,N-dimethyl-4-aminoazobenzene; 7,12-DMBA = 7,12-dimethylbenzanthracene; DES = diethylstilbestrol; DP = dipeptidase; FMO = flavin-containing monooxygenase; GT = UDP-glucuronosyltransferase; GGT = gamma-glutamyltransferase; GST = glutathione S-transferase; HAPP = heterocyclic arylamine pyrolysis products; HCBD = hexachlorobutadiene; ST = sulfotransferase; s.r. = spontaneous rearrangement.

phosphorolytic reactions, such as glyceraldehyde-3-phosphate dehydrogenase (Gregus and Németi, 2005), are examples for formation of electrophilic toxicants from inorganic chemicals.

Formation of Free Radicals   A free radical is a molecule or molecular fragment that contains one or more unpaired electrons in its outer orbital. Radicals are formed by (1) accepting an electron or (2) losing an electron, or by (3) homolytic fission of a covalent bond.

1. Xenobiotics such as paraquat, doxorubicin, and nitrofurantoin can accept an electron from reductases to give rise to radicals

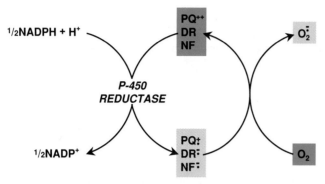

Figure 3-3. *Production of superoxide anion radical ($O_2^{\bullet-}$) by paraquat (PQ^{++}), doxorubicin (DR), and nitrofurantoin (NF).*

Note that formation of ($O_2^{\bullet-}$) is not the final step in the toxication of these xenobiotics, because $O_2^{\bullet-}$ can yield the much more reactive hydroxyl radical, as depicted in Fig. 3-4.

(Fig. 3-3). These radicals typically transfer the extra electron to molecular oxygen, forming a superoxide anion radical ($O_2^{\bullet-}$) and regenerating the parent xenobiotic, which is ready to gain a new electron (Kappus, 1986). Through this "redox cycling," one electron acceptor xenobiotic molecule can generate many $O_2^{\bullet-}$ molecules. There are also endogenous sources of $O_2^{\bullet-}$. This radical is generated in large quantities by NADPH oxidase (Nox) in activated macrophages and granulocytes during "respiratory burst," and in smaller quantities by many other cells, such as endothelial cells and vascular smooth muscle cells, which also express Nox in the plasma membrane (Bokoch and Knaus, 2003). Growth factor receptor stimulation in these non-phagocytotic cells is coupled to Nox activation. $O_2^{\bullet-}$ is also produced by the mitochondrial electron transport chain, especially

by complexes I and III. The significance of $O_2^{\bullet-}$ stems to a large extent from the fact that $O_2^{\bullet-}$ is a starting compound in two toxication pathways (Fig. 3-4); one leading to formation of hydrogen peroxide (HOOH) and then hydroxyl radical (HO$^{\bullet}$), whereas the other produces peroxynitrite (ONOO$^-$) and ultimately nitrogen dioxide ($^{\bullet}$NO$_2$), and carbonate anion radical ($CO_3^{\bullet-}$).

2. Nucleophilic xenobiotics such as phenols, hydroquinones, aminophenols, aromatic amines (e.g., benzidine), hydrazines, phenothiazines (e.g., chlorpromazine; see Fig. 3-6), and thiols are prone to lose an electron and form free radicals in a reaction catalyzed by peroxidases (Aust *et al.*, 1993). Some of these chemicals, such as catechols and hydroquinones, may undergo two sequential one-electron oxidations, producing first semiquinone radicals and then quinones. Quinones are not only reactive electrophiles (Table 3-2) but also electron acceptors with the capacity to initiate redox cycling or oxidation of thiols and NAD(P)H. Polycyclic aromatic hydrocarbons with sufficiently low ionization potential, such as benzo[a]pyrene and 7,12-dimethylbenzanthracene, can be converted via one-electron oxidation by peroxidases or cytochrome P450 to radical cations, which may be the ultimate toxicants for these carcinogens (Cavalieri and Rogan, 1992). Like peroxidases, oxyhemoglobin (Hb-FeII-O$_2$) can catalyze the oxidation of aminophenols to semiquinone radicals and quinoneimines. This is another example of toxication, because these products, in turn, oxidize ferrohemoglobin (Hb-FeII) to methemoglobin (Hb-FeIII), which cannot carry oxygen.

3. Free radicals are also formed by homolytic bond fission, which can be induced by electron transfer to the molecule (reductive fission). This mechanism is involved in the conversion of CCl$_4$ to the trichloromethyl free radical (Cl$_3$C$^{\bullet}$) by an electron transfer from cytochrome P450 or the mitochondrial electron

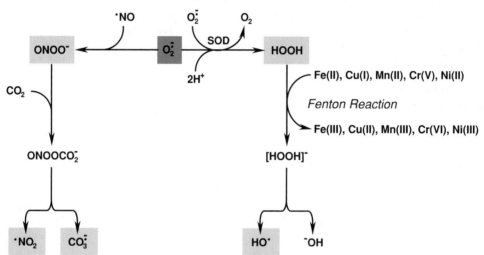

Figure 3-4. *Two pathways for toxication of superoxide anion radical ($O_2^{\bullet-}$) via nonradical products (ONOO$^-$ and HOOH) to radical products ($^{\bullet}$NO$_2$, $CO_3^{\bullet-}$ and HO$^{\bullet}$).*

In one pathway, conversion of ($O_2^{\bullet-}$) to HOOH is spontaneous or is catalyzed by superoxide dismutase (SOD). Homolytic cleavage of HOOH to hydroxyl radical and hydroxyl ion is called the Fenton reaction and is catalyzed by the transition metal ions shown. Hydroxyl radical formation is the ultimate toxication for xenobiotics that form $O_2^{\bullet-}$ (see Fig. 3-3) or for HOOH, the transition metal ions listed, and some chemicals that form complexes with these transiton metal ions. In the other pathway, $O_2^{\bullet-}$ reacts avidly with nitric oxide ($^{\bullet}$NO), the product of $^{\bullet}$NO synthase (NOS), forming peroxynitrite (ONOO$^-$). Spontaneous reaction of ONOO$^-$ with carbon dioxide (CO$_2$) yields nitrosoperoxy carbonate (ONOOCO$_2^-$) that is homolytically cleaved to nitrogen dioxide ($^{\bullet}$NO$_2$) and carbonate anion radical ($CO_3^{\bullet-}$). All three radical products indicated in this figure are oxidants, whereas $^{\bullet}$NO$_2$ is also a nitrating agent.

transport chain (reductive dehalogenation) (Recknagel *et al.*, 1989). The $Cl_3C^\bullet$ reacts with O_2 to form the even more reactive trichloromethylperoxy radical ($Cl_3COO^\bullet$) (Hippeli and Elstner, 1999).

The hydroxyl radical ($HO^\bullet$), a free radical of paramount toxicological significance, is also generated by homolytic fission. Such a process yields large amounts of $HO^\bullet$ from water upon ionizing radiation. Reductive homolytic fission of hydrogen peroxide (HOOH) to $HO^\bullet$ and HO^- is called the *Fenton reaction* (Fig. 3-4). This is catalyzed by transition metal ions, typically Fe(II) or, Cu(I), Cr(V), Ni(II), or Mn(II), and is a major toxication mechanism for HOOH and its precursor $O_2^{\bullet-}$ as well as for transition metals. Moreover, the toxicity of chemicals, such as nitrilotriacetic acid, bleomycin, and orellanin (Hippeli and Elstner, 1999), which chelate transition metal ions is also based on Fenton chemistry because chelation increases the catalytic efficiency of some transition metal ions. Complexation with some endogenous oligopeptides also increases the catalytic efficiency of weakly Fenton-active metal ions, such as Ni(II). The pulmonary toxicity of inhaled mineral particles such as asbestos and silica is caused, at least in part, by the formation of $HO^\bullet$ triggered by Fe ions on the particle surface (Vallyathan *et al.*, 1998; Castranova, 2004). Hydrogen peroxide is a direct or indirect by-product of several enzymatic reactions, including monoamine oxidase, acyl-coenzyme A oxidase, xanthine oxidoreductase (Harrison, 2002) and CYP2E1 (Caro and Cederbaun, 2004). It is produced in large quantities by spontaneous or superoxide dismutase-catalyzed dismutation of $O_2^{\bullet-}$.

Homolytic cleavage is also involved in free radical generation from $ONOO^-$ (Squadrito and Pryor, 1998) (Fig. 3-4). The facile reaction of $ONOO^-$ with the ubiquitous CO_2 yields nitrosoperoxycarbonate ($ONOOCO_2^-$), which can spontaneously homolyze into two radicals, the oxidant and nitrating agent nitrogen dioxide ($^\bullet NO_2$) and the oxidant carbonate anion radical ($CO_3^{\bullet-}$). Thus, formation of $ONOO^-$ and the latter radicals represent a toxication mechanism for $O_2^{\bullet-}$ and $^\bullet NO$. As $^\bullet NO$ is the product of nitric oxide synthase (NOS), this mechanism is especially relevant in and around cells that express NOS constitutively (i.e., neurons and endothelial cells) as well as in and around cells that express the inducible form of NOS in response to cytokines. Inside the cell, a predominant site for formation of $ONOO^-$ as well as its products $CO_3^{\bullet-}$ and $^\bullet NO_2$ are the mitochondria, wherein the lipophilic $^\bullet NO$ can readily diffuse and where the electron transport chain and the citric acid cycle produces $O_2^{\bullet-}$ and CO_2, respectively (Denicola and Radi, 2005).

Formation of Nucleophiles The formation of nucleophiles is a relatively uncommon mechanism for activating toxicants. Examples include the formation of cyanide from amygdalin, which is catalyzed by bacterial β-glucosidase in the intestine; from acrylonitrile after epoxidation and subsequent glutathione conjugation; and from sodium mitroprusside by thiol-induced decomposition. Carbon monoxide is a toxic metabolite of dihalomethanes that undergo oxidative dehalogenation. Hydrogen selenide, a strong nucleophile and reductant, is formed from selenite by reaction with glutathione or other thiols.

Formation of Redox-Active Reactants There are specific mechanisms for the creation of redox-active reactants other than those already mentioned. Examples include the formation of the methemoglobin-producing nitrite from nitrate by bacterial reduction in the intestine or from esters of nitrous or nitric acids in reaction with

glutathione. Dapsone hydroxylamine and 5-hydroxyprimaquine, hydroxylated metabolites of the respective drugs, produce methemoglobin by cooxidation (Fletcher *et al.*, 1988). Reductants such as ascorbic acid and reductases such as NADPH-dependent flavoenzymes reduce Cr(VI) to Cr(V) (Shi and Dalal, 1990). Xenobiotic radicals formed in redox cycling (e.g., those depicted in Fig. 3-3) as well as $O_2^{\bullet-}$ can reduce Fe(III) bound to ferritin and consequently release it as Fe(II). Cr(V) and Fe(II) thus formed catalyze $HO^\bullet$ formation (Fig. 3-4).

In summary, the most reactive metabolites are electron-deficient molecules and molecular fragments such as electrophiles and neutral or cationic free radicals. Although some nucleophiles are reactive (e.g., HCN, CO), many (e.g., hydroquinones) are activated by conversion to electrophiles. Similarly, free radicals with an extra electron (e.g., those shown in Fig. 3-3) cause damage by giving rise to the neutral $HO^\bullet$ radical after the formation and subsequent homolytic cleavage of HOOH.

Detoxication Biotransformation that eliminates an ultimate toxicant or prevents its formation is called *detoxication*. In some cases, detoxication may compete with toxication for a chemical. Detoxication can take several pathways, depending on the chemical nature of the toxic substance.

Detoxication of Toxicants with No Functional Groups In general, chemicals without functional groups, such as benzene and toluene, are detoxicated in two phases. Initially, a functional group such as hydroxyl or carboxyl is introduced into the molecule, most often by cytochrome-P450 enzymes. Subsequently, an endogenous acid, such as glucuronic acid, sulfuric acid, or an amino acid, is added to the functional group by a transferase. With some exceptions, the final products are inactive, highly hydrophilic organic acids that are readily excreted. Carbonyl reduction catalyzed by at least five enzymes (e.g., 11-β-hydroxysteroid dehydrogenase-1, carbonyl reductase and three members of aldo-keto reductase superfamily) initiates detoxication of the potent carcinogen nicotine-derived nitrosamine ketone [NNK; 4-(methylnitrosamino)-1-(3-pyridyl)-1-butanone]. The formed nicotine-derived nitrosamine alcohol is then readily glucuronidated at its hydroxyl moiety and is excreted into urine (Maser, 2004).

Detoxication of Nucleophiles Nucleophiles are generally detoxicated by conjugation at the nucleophilic functional group. Hydroxylated compounds are conjugated by sulfation, glucuronidation, or rarely by methylation, whereas thiols are methylated or glucuronidated and amines and hydrazines are acetylated. These reactions prevent peroxidase-catalyzed conversion of the nucleophiles to free radicals and biotransformation of phenols, aminophenols, catechols, and hydroquinones to electrophilic quinones and quinoneimines. An alternative mechanism for the elimination of thiols, amines, and hydrazines is oxidation by flavin-containing monooxygenases (Krueger and Williams, 2005). Some alcohols, such as ethanol, are detoxicated by oxidation to carboxylic acids by alcohol and aldehyde dehydrogenases. A specific detoxication mechanism is the biotransformation of cyanide to thiocyanate by rhodanese or mercaptopyruvate sulfurtransferase.

Detoxication of Electrophiles A general mechanism for the detoxication of electrophilic toxicants is conjugation with the thiol nucleophile glutathione (Ketterer, 1988). This reaction may occur spontaneously or can be facilitated by glutathione S-transferases. Metal ions—such as Ag^+, Cd^{2+}, Hg^{2+}, and CH_3Hg^+ ions—readily react with and are detoxicated by glutathione. Specific mechanisms

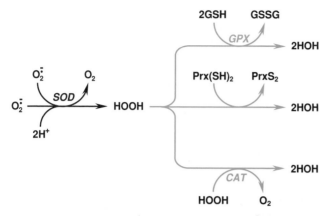

Figure 3-5. Detoxication of superoxide anion radical ($O_2^{\bullet-}$) by superoxide dismutase (SOD), and of HOOH by glutathione peroxidase (GPX), peroxiredoxin (Prx-(SH)$_2$), and catalase (CAT).

The byproducts are glutathione disulfide (GSSG) and peroxiredoxin disulfide (PrxS$_2$), from which glutathione (GSH) and Prx-(SH)$_2$ are regenerated by glutathione reductase and thioredoxin-reductase, respectively.

for the detoxication of electrophilic chemicals include epoxide hydrolase-catalyzed biotransformation of epoxides and arene oxides to diols and dihydrodiols, respectively, and carboxylesterase-catalyzed hydrolysis of organophosphate ester pesticides. Others are two-electron reduction of quinones to hydroquinones by NAD(P)H:quinone oxidoreductase (NQO1) and NRH:quinone oxidoreductase (NQO2), reduction of α, β-unsaturated aldehydes (e.g., the lipidperoxidation product 4-oxonon-2-enal) to alcohols or to their saturated derivative by carbonyl reductase (Maser, 2006), or oxidation of α, β-unsaturated aldehydes to acids by aldehyde dehydrogenases. Complex formation of thiol-reactive metal ions by metallothionein and the redox-active ferrous iron by ferritin are special types of detoxications. Covalent binding of electrophiles to proteins can also be regarded as detoxification provided that the protein has no critical function and does not become a neoantigen or otherwise harmful. Carboxylesterases, for example, inactivate organophosphates not only by hydrolysis but also by covalent binding.

Detoxication of Free Radicals   Because $O_2^{\bullet-}$ can be converted into much more reactive compounds (Fig. 3-4), its elimination is an important detoxication mechanism. This is carried out by superoxide dismutases (SOD), high-capacity enzymes located in the cytosol (Cu, Zn-SOD) and the mitochondria (Mn-SOD), which convert $O_2^{\bullet-}$ to HOOH (Fig. 3-5). Subsequently, HOOH is reduced to water by

catalase in the peroxisomes (also in the mitochondria in cardiac muscle), by the selenocysteine-containing glutathione peroxidases in the cytosol and mitochondria, and by peroxiredoxins in the cytosol, mitochondria and endoplasmic reticulum (Fig. 3-5) (Rhee et al., 2005).

No enzyme eliminates HO$^\bullet$. Whereas some relatively stable radicals, such as peroxyl radicals (see Fig. 3-9), can readily abstract a hydrogen atom from glutathione, α-tocopherol (vitamin E), or ascorbic acid (vitamin C), thus becoming nonradicals, these antioxidants are generally ineffective in detoxifying HO$^\bullet$ (Sies, 1993). This is due to its extreme reactivity and thus short half-life (10^{-9}s), which provides little time for the HO$^\bullet$ to reach and react with antioxidants. Therefore the only effective protection against HO$^\bullet$ is to prevent its formation by elimination of its precursor, HOOH, via conversion to water (Fig. 3-5).

ONOO$^-$ (which is not a free radical oxidant) is significantly more stable than HO$^\bullet$ (half-life of about 1 second). Nevertheless, the small biological antioxidant molecules (glutathione, uric acid, ascorbic acid, α-tocopherol) are relatively inefficient in intercepting it, because ONOO$^-$ rapidly reacts with CO_2 (Squadrito and Pryor, 1998) to form reactive free radicals (Fig. 3-4). More efficient are the selenocysteine-containing glutathione peroxidase and peroxiredoxins, which can reduce ONOO$^-$ to nitrite (ONO$^-$) the same way they reduce HOOH to water (Fig. 3-5). Selenoprotein P, which contains 10 selenocysteine residues and coats the surface of endothelial cells, also reduces ONOO$^-$ and may serve as a protectant against this oxidant in blood. In addition, ONOO$^-$ reacts with oxyhemoglobin, heme-containing peroxidases and albumin, all of which could be important sinks for ONOO$^-$. Furthermore, elimination of the two ONOO$^-$ precursors—i.e., $^\bullet$NO by reaction with oxyhemoglobin (to yield methemoglobin and nitrate) and $O_2^{\bullet-}$ by SODs (see above)—is a significant mechanism in preventing ONOO$^-$ buildup (Squadrito and Pryor, 1998).

Peroxidase-generated free radicals are eliminated by electron transfer from glutathione. This results in the oxidation of glutathione, which is reversed by NADPH-dependent glutathione reductase (Fig. 3-6). Thus, glutathione plays an important role in the detoxication of both electrophiles and free radicals.

Detoxication of Protein Toxins   Presumably, extra- and intracellular proteases are involved in the inactivation of toxic polypeptides. Several toxins found in venoms, such as α- and β-bungaratoxin, erabutoxin, and phospholipase, contain intramolecular disulfide bonds that are required for their activity. These proteins are inactivated by thioredoxin, an endogenous dithiol protein that reduces the essential disulfide bond (Lozano et al., 1994).

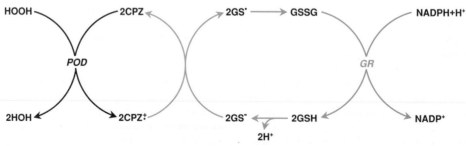

Figure 3-6. Detoxication of peroxidase (POD)–generated free radicals such as chlorpromazine free radical (CPZ$_\bullet^+$) by glutathione (GSH).

The by-products are glutathione thiyl radical (GS$^\bullet$) and glutathione disulfide (GSSG), from which GSH is regenerated by glutathione reductase (GR).

When Detoxication Fails   Detoxication may be insufficient for several reasons:

1. Toxicants may overwhelm detoxication processes, leading to saturation of the detoxication enzymes, consumption of the cosubtrates, or depletion of cellular antioxidants such as glutathione, ascorbic acid, and α-tocopherol. This results in the accumulation of the ultimate toxicant.

2. Occasionally, a reactive toxicant inactivates a detoxicating enzyme. For example, $ONOO^-$ incapacitates Mn-SOD, which normally would counteract $ONOO^-$ formation (Murphy, 1999) (see Fig. 3-4).

3. Some conjugation reactions can be reversed. For example, 2-naphthylamine, a bladder carcinogen, is N-hydroxylated and glucuronidated in liver, with the glucuronide excreted into urine. While in the bladder, the glucuronide is hydrolyzed, and the released arylhydroxylamine is converted by protonation and dehydration to the reactive electrophilic arylnitrenium ion (Bock and Lilienblum, 1994). Isocyanates and isothiocyanates form labile glutathione conjugates from which they can be released. Thus, methylisocyanate readily forms a glutathione conjugate in the lung after inhalation. From there, the conjugate is distributed to other tissues, where the reactive electrophilic parent compound may be regenerated (Baillie and Kassahun, 1994). Such conjugates are considered transport forms of toxicants.

4. Sometimes detoxication generates potentially harmful by-products, such as the glutathione thiyl radical and glutathione disulfide, which are produced during the detoxication of free radicals (Fig. 3-6). Glutathione disulfide can form mixed disulfides with protein thiols, whereas the thiyl radical ($GS^\bullet$), after reacting with thiolate (GS^-), forms a glutathione disulfide radical anion ($GSSG^{\bullet -}$), which can reduce O_2 to $O_2^{\bullet -}$. Conjugation with glutathione may lead to HCN generation in the course of acrylonitrile biotransformation, the first step of which is epoxidation of acrylonitrile ($H_2C{=}CH{-}CN$). Whereas glutathione conjugation detoxifies this epoxide if it takes place at the carbon adjacent to the nitrile group (-CN), it causes release of this group as HCN if glutathione conjugates with the epoxide at the carbon not linked to the nitrile moiety.

STEP 2—REACTION OF THE ULTIMATE TOXICANT WITH THE TARGET MOLECULE

Toxicity is typically mediated by a reaction of the ultimate toxicant with a target molecule (step 2a in Fig. 3-1). Subsequently, a series of secondary biochemical events occur, leading to dysfunction or injury that is manifest at various levels of biological organization, such as at the target molecule itself, cell organelles, cells, tissues and organs, and even the whole organism. Because interaction of the ultimate toxicant with the target molecule triggers the toxic effect, consideration is given to (1) the attributes of target molecules, (2) the types of reactions between ultimate toxicants and target molecules, and (3) the effects of toxicants on the target molecules (Fig. 3-7). Finally, consideration is given to toxicities that are initiated not by reaction of the ultimate toxicant with target molecules, but rather by alteration of the biological (micro)environment (step 2b in Fig. 3-1) in which critical endogenous molecules, cell organelles, cells, and organs operate.

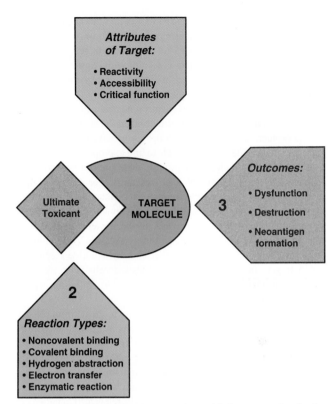

Figure 3-7. Reaction of the ultimate toxicant with the target molecule: the second step in the development of toxicity.

Attributes of Target Molecules

Practically all endogenous compounds are potential targets for toxicants. The identification and characteristics of the target molecules involved in toxicity constitute a major research priority, but a comprehensive inventory of potential target molecules is impossible. Nevertheless, the most prevalent and toxicologically relevant targets are macromolecules such as nucleic acids (especially DNA) and proteins. Among the small molecules, membrane lipids are frequently involved, whereas cofactors such as coenzyme A and pyridoxal rarely are involved.

To be a target, an endogenous molecule must possess the appropriate reactivity and/or steric configuration to allow the ultimate toxicant to enter into covalent or noncovalent reactions. For these reactions to occur, the target molecule must be accessible to a sufficiently high concentration of the ultimate toxicant. Thus, endogenous molecules that are exposed to reactive chemicals or are adjacent to sites where reactive metabolites are formed are frequently targets. Technical advances in the field of proteonomics make it increasingly possible to identify potential protein targets of reactive chemicals as chemical-protein adducts. A compendium of proteins adducted by reactive toxicant metabolites has been established at the University of Kansas (http://tpdb.medchem.ku.edu:8080/ protein_database/search.jsp). The first target for reactive metabolites is often the enzyme that catalyzes their production or the adjacent intracellular structures. For example, thyroperoxidase, the enzyme involved in thyroid hormone synthesis, converts some nucleophilic xenobiotics (such as methimazole, amitrole, and resorcinol) into reactive free radicals that inactivate thyroperoxidase (Engler *et al.*, 1982). This is the basis for the antithyroid as well as the thyroid tumor–inducing effect of these chemicals. Carbon tetrachloride, which is activated by cytochrome P450, destroys this enzyme as well as the neighboring microsomal membranes (Osawa *et al.*, 1995). Several mitochondrial enzymes are convenient targets for nephrotoxic cysteine conjugates such as dichlorovinyl cysteine, because these conjugates are converted to electrophiles by mitochondrial enzymes with cysteine conjugate β-lyase activity (e.g., aspartate aminotransferase and branched chain amino acid aminotransferase) that can readily channel their reactive products to neighboring enzymes such as α-ketoglutarate dehydrogenase (Anders, 2004). Reactive metabolites that are unable to find appropriate endogenous reaction partners in close proximity to their site of formation may diffuse until they encounter such reactants. For example, hard electrophiles such as the arylnitrenium ion metabolite of *N*-methyl-4-aminoazobenzene react readily with hard nucleophilic atoms in nucleic acids, and thus target DNA in the nucleus, even though the electrophiles are produced in the cytoplasm. Vinyl chloride epoxide formed in the hepatocytes from vinyl chloride reaches its DNA targets in the neighboring endothelial cells (that are more sensitive to this genotoxin than the liver cells), initiating hepatic hemangiosarcoma.

Not all targets for chemicals contribute to the harmful effects. Thus, while carbon monoxide causes toxicity by binding to ferrohemoglobin, it also associates with the iron in cytochrome P450 with little or no consequence. Covalent binding of toxicants to various intracellular proteins, including enzymes and structural proteins, has been demonstrated, yet it is often uncertain which protein(s) is/are involved in binding that is toxicologically relevant (Cohen *et al.*, 1997; Pumford and Halmes, 1997; Rombach and Hanzlik, 1999). Arylation of some hepatic mitochondrial proteins by acetaminophen (4'-hydroxyacetanilide) is thought to be causally related to the liver injury induced by this drug because the nonhepatotoxic regioisomer of acetaminophen (3'-hydroxyacetanilide) does not readily bind covalently to these proteins (Cohen *et al.*, 1997; Jaeschke and Bajt, 2006). In contrast, arylation of a number of hepatic cytoplasmic proteins by acetaminophen is likely to be inconsequential because the nonhepatotoxic regioisomer of this drug also arylates those proteins (Nelson and Pearson, 1990). Covalent binding to proteins without adverse consequences may even represent a form of detoxication by sparing toxicologically relevant targets. This principle is best exemplified by covalent binding of organophosphate insecticides to plasma cholinesterase, which is a significant protective mechanism, as it counteracts phosphorylation of acetylcholinesterase, the target

molecule. Thus, to conclusively identify a target molecule as being responsible for toxicity, it should be demonstrated that the ultimate toxicant (1) reacts with the target and adversely affects its function, (2) reaches an effective concentration at the target site, and (3) alters the target in a way that is mechanistically related to the observed toxicity.

Types of Reactions

The ultimate toxicant may bind to the target molecules noncovalently or covalently and may alter it by hydrogen abstraction, electron transfer, or enzymatically.

Noncovalent Binding This type of binding can be due to apolar interactions or the formation of hydrogen and ionic bonds and is typically involved in the interaction of toxicants with targets such as membrane receptors, intracellular receptors, ion channels, and some enzymes. For example, such interactions are responsible for the binding of strychnine to the glycine receptor on motor neurons in the spinal cord, TCDD to the aryl hydrocarbon receptor, saxitoxin to sodium channels, phorbol esters to protein kinase C, and warfarin to vitamin K 2,3-epoxide reductase. Such forces also are responsible for the intercalation of chemicals such as acridine yellow and doxorubicin into the double helix of DNA. These chemicals are toxic because the steric arrangement of their atoms allows them to combine with complementary sites on the endogenous molecule more or less as a key fits into a lock. Noncovalent binding usually is reversible because of the comparatively low bonding energy.

Covalent Binding Being practically irreversible, covalent binding is of great toxicologic importance because it permanently alters endogenous molecules (Boelsterli, 1993). Covalent adduct formation is common with electrophilic toxicants such as nonionic and cationic electrophiles and radical cations. These toxicants react with nucleophilic atoms that are abundant in biological macromolecules, such as proteins and nucleic acids. Electrophilic atoms exhibit some selectivity toward nucleophilic atoms, depending on their charge-to-radius ratio. In general, soft electrophiles prefer to react with soft nucleophiles (low charge-to-radius ratio in both), whereas hard electrophiles react more readily with hard nucleophiles (high charge-to-radius ratio in both). Examples are presented in Table 3-3. Metal ions such as silver and mercury are also classified as soft

Table 3.3

Examples of Soft and Hard Electrophiles and Nucleophiles

ELECTROPHILES		NUCLEOPHILES
Carbon in polarized double bonds (e.g., quinones, α,β-unsaturated ketones)	Soft	Sulfur in thiols (e.g., cysteinyl residues in proteins and glutathione)
Carbon in epoxides, strained-ring lactones, aryl halides	↑	Sulfur in methionine
Aryl carbonium ions		Nitrogen in primary and secondary amino groups of proteins (e.g., lysine ε-amino group)
Benzylic carbonium ions, nitrenium ions		Nitrogen in amino groups in purine bases in nucleic acids
Alkyl carbonium ions	↓	Oxygen of purines and pyrimidines in nucleic acids
	Hard	Phosphate oxygen in nucleic acids

SOURCE: Based on Coles (1984).

electrophiles. These prefer to react covalently with soft nucleophiles (especially thiol groups). Conversely, hard electrophiles such as lithium, calcium, and barium, react preferentially as cations with hard nucleophiles (e.g., carboxylate and phosphate anions). Metals falling between these two extremes, such as chromium, zinc, and lead, exhibit universal reactivity with nucleophiles. The reactivity of an electrophile determines which endogenous nucleophiles can react with it and become a target.

A covalent reaction of special biological significance can take place between HOOH (a soft electrophile) and protein thiol groups, preferentially those with low pK_a value, i.e., with a propensity of being in the strongly nucleophilic thiolate anion form (Prot-S$^-$) at physiological pH. This reaction produces protein sulfenic acid (Prot-S-OH):

$$\text{Prot-SH} + \text{HOOH} \rightarrow \text{Prot-S-OH} + \text{HOH}$$

The S atom in a sulfenic acid is electrophilic as it is made electron deficient by the electron withdrawing effect of O. Therefore, a protein-sulfenic acid can react with another thiol group of the same or a different protein or of glutathione (GSH), resulting in, respectively, formation of an intramolecular disulfide, intermolecular disulfide or a mixed disulfide of the protein and glutathione (i.e., glutathionylation of the protein):

$$\text{Prot}_1\text{-S-OH} + \text{Prot}_2\text{-SH} \rightarrow \text{Prot}_1\text{-S-S-Prot}_2 + \text{HOH}$$

$$\text{Prot-S-OH} + \text{GSH} \rightarrow \text{Prot-S-SG} + \text{HOH}$$

Not only HOOH, but also hydroperoxides (e.g., lipid hydroperoxides, LOOH; see Fig. 3-9) may enter into such reactions, producing protein-sulfenic acids, protein-disulfides and glutathionylated proteins, which can be considered as posttranslational modifications with a role in redox signaling (Forman *et al.*, 2004).

Neutral free radicals such as HO$^\bullet$, $^\bullet$NO$_2$, and Cl$_3$C$^\bullet$ can also bind covalently to biomolecules. The addition of Cl$_3$C$^\bullet$ to double-bonded carbons in lipids or to lipid radicals yields lipids containing chloromethylated fatty acids. The addition of hydroxyl radicals to DNA bases results in the formation of numerous products, including 8-hydroxypurines, 5-hydroxymethylpyrimidines, and thymine and cytosine glycols (Breen and Murphy, 1995).

Nucleophilic toxicants are in principle reactive toward electrophilic endogenous compounds. Such reactions occur infrequently because electrophiles are rare among biomolecules. Examples include the covalent reactions of amines and hydrazides with the aldehyde pyridoxal, a cosubstrate for several enzymes, including glutamate decarboxylase. Carbon monoxide, cyanide, hydrogen sulfide, and azide form coordinate covalent bonds with iron in various hemeproteins. Other nucleophiles react with hemoglobin in an electron-transfer reaction (see below).

Hydrogen Abstraction   Neutral free radicals, such as those generated in reactions depicted in Fig. 3-4, can readily abstract H atoms from endogenous compounds, converting those compounds into radicals. Abstraction of hydrogen from thiols (R—SH) creates thiyl radicals (R—S$^\bullet$), which upon radical recombination with HO$^\bullet$ form sulfenic acids (R—S—OH) that are precursors of disulfides (R—S—S—R) (see above). Radicals can remove hydrogen from CH$_2$ groups of free amino acids or from amino acid residues in proteins and convert them to carbonyls. These carbonyls react covalently with amines, forming cross-links with DNA or other proteins. Hydrogen

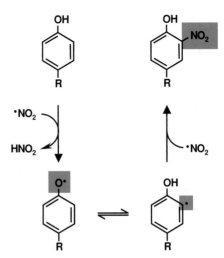

Figure 3-8. *Formation of 3-nitrotyrosine residues in proteins by reaction with nitrogen dioxide ($^\bullet$NO$_2$).*

$^\bullet$NO$_2$ is an oxidizing and nitrating species generated from ONOO$^-$ (Fig. 3-4). In addition, $^\bullet$NO$_2$ is a contaminant in cigarette smoke, exhaust of gas engines and stoves, as well as the causative agent of "silo-filler's disease."

abstraction from deoxyribose in DNA yields the C-4'-radical, the first step to DNA cleavage (Breen and Murphy, 1995). Abstraction of hydrogen from fatty acids produces lipid radicals and initiates lipid peroxidation. As depicted in Fig. 3-8, nitration of tyrosine residues in proteins purportedly involves H abstraction followed by radical recombination, i.e., covalent binding between the resultant tyrosyl radical and $^\bullet$NO$_2$ (Squadrito and Pryor, 1998).

Electron Transfer   Chemicals can oxidize Fe(II) in hemoglobin to Fe(III), producing methemoglobinemia. Nitrite can oxidize hemoglobin, whereas N-hydroxyl arylamines (such as dapsone hydroxylamine), phenolic compounds (such as 5-hydroxy primaquine), and hydrazines (such as phenylhydrazine) are cooxidized with oxyhemoglobin, forming methemoglobin and hydrogen peroxide (Coleman and Jacobus, 1993).

Enzymatic Reactions   A few toxins act enzymatically on specific target proteins. For example, the plant toxins ricin and abrin are N-glycosidases; they hydrolyse a specific glycosidic bond in ribosomal RNS, blocking protein synthesis. Botulinum toxin acts as a Zn-protease; it hydrolyses the fusion proteins that assist in exocytosis of the neurotransmitter acetylcholine in cholinergic neurons, most importantly motoneurons, causing paralysis. The lethal factor component of anthrax toxin is also a Zn-protease, which inactivates mitogen-activated protein kinase kinase (MAPKK), inducing cell death. Other bacterial toxins catalyze the transfer for ADP-ribose from NAD$^+$ to specific proteins. Through such a mechanism, diphtheria toxin blocks the function of elongation factor 2 in protein synthesis and cholera toxin activates a G protein. Snake venoms contain hydrolytic enzymes that destroy biomolecules.

In summary, most ultimate toxicants act on endogenous molecules on the basis of their chemical reactivity. Those with more than one type of reactivity may react by different mechanisms with various target molecules. For example, quinones may act as electron acceptors and initiate thiol oxidation or free radical reactions that lead to lipid peroxidation, but they may also act as soft electrophiles and bind covalently to protein thiols. The lead ion acts as a soft electrophile when it forms coordinate covalent bonds with critical thiol groups in δ-aminolevulinic acid dehydratase, its major target enzyme in heme synthesis (Goering, 1993). However, it behaves like a hard electrophile or an ion when it binds to protein kinase C or blocks calcium channels, substituting for the natural ligand Ca^{2+} at those target sites.

Effects of Toxicants on Target Molecules

Reaction of the ultimate toxicant with endogenous molecules may cause dysfunction or destruction; in the case of proteins, it may render them foreign (i.e., an antigen) to the immune system.

Dysfunction of Target Molecules   Some toxicants activate protein target molecules, mimicking endogenous ligands. For example, morphine activates opioid receptors, clofibrate is an agonist on the peroxisome proliferator–activated receptor, and phorbol esters and lead ions stimulate protein kinase C.

More commonly, chemicals inhibit the function of target molecules. Several xenobiotics—such as atropine, curare, and strychnine—block neurotransmitter receptors by attaching to the ligand-binding sites or by interfering with the function of ion channels. Tetrodotoxin and saxitoxin, for example, inhibit opening of the voltage-activated sodium channels in the neuronal membrane, whereas DDT and the pyrethroid insecticides inhibit their closure. Some toxicants block ion transporters, others inhibit mitochondrial electron transport complexes, and many inhibit enzymes. Chemicals that bind to tubulin (e.g., vinblastine, colchicine, paclitaxel, trivalent arsenic) or actin (e.g., cytochalasin B, phalloidin) impair the assembly (polymerization) and/or disassembly (depolymerization) of these cytoskeletal proteins.

Protein function is impaired when conformation or structure is altered by interaction with the toxicant. Many proteins possess critical moieties, especially thiol groups, which are essential for catalytic activity or assembly to macromolecular complexes. Proteins that are sensitive to covalent and/or oxidative modification of their thiol groups include the enzymes glyceraldehyde 3-phosphate dehydrogenase (see Table 3-6), and pyruvate dehydrogenase (see Fig. 3-13), the Ca^{2+} pumps (see Fig. 3-14, Table 3-7), the DNA repair enzyme O^6-methylguanine-DNA-methyltransferase, the DNA-methylating enzyme C^5-cytosine-DNA-methyltransferase, ubiquitin-conjugating enzymes, peroxiredoxins, protein tyrosine phosphatases (e.g., cdc25) the lipid phosphatase PTEN (phosphatase and tensin homologue) (Rhee et al., 2005), caspases (see Fig. 3-16), the transcription factor AP-1, and the electrophile-sensor protein Keap1 (see Fig. 3-23), just to name a few. These and many other proteins are inactivated by thiol-reactive chemicals, causing impaired maintenance of the cell's energy and metabolic homeostasis and/or altered signal transduction. As to the latter outcome, covalent and/or oxidative modification of thiol groups in Keap1 triggers the adaptive electrophile stress response, which is cytoprotective (see Fig. 3-23). Conversion of the catalytic thiol group (-SH) in protein tyrosine phosphatases (PTP) to sulfenic acid group (-S-OH) upon reaction with HOOH or lipid hydroperoxides (see reaction scheme above) inactivates these enzymes. As PTPs keep protein kinase-mediated signal transduction pathways under control (see Fig. 3-11), PTP inactivation permit such signaling to surge, thereby launching, for example, a mitogenic response. Formation of protein sulfenic acids by the oxidative stress product HOOH is thus considered as an initiating event of

redox signaling (Forman et al., 2004). It is important to note that protein sulfenic acid formation is readily reversed by reaction of the sulfenic acid with a thiol (e.g., glutathione), resulting in a protein disulfide (e.g., protein-S-SG; see the scheme above) which in turn is reduced by thioredoxin or glutaredoxin as shown in Fig. 3-19, thereby regenerating the active PTP in thiol form and terminating the signaling. Protein tyrosine nitration (see Fig. 3-8) may also alter protein function or may interfere with signaling pathways that involve tyrosine kinases and phosphatases.

Toxicants may interfere with the template function of DNA. The covalent binding of chemicals to DNA causes nucleotide mispairing during replication. For example, covalent binding of aflatoxin 8,9-oxide to N-7 of guanine results in pairing of the adduct-bearing guanine with adenine rather than cytosine, leading to the formation of an incorrect codon and the insertion of an incorrect amino acid into the protein. Such events are involved in the aflatoxin-induced mutation of the Ras proto-oncogene and the p53 tumor suppressor gene (Eaton and Gallagher, 1994). 8-Hydroxyguanine and 8-hydroxyadenine are mutagenic bases produced by $HO^\bullet$ that can cause mispairing with themselves as well as with neighboring pyrimidines, producing multiple amino acid substitutions (Breen and Murphy, 1995). Cr(III) produced from chromate (Cr(VI)) via reduction by ascorbate, alone or complexed to ascorbate, forms coordinate covalent bond with phosphate in DNA, thereby inducing a mutation (Quievryn et al., 2002). Chemicals such as doxorubicin, that intercalate between stacked bases in the double-helical DNA, push adjacent base pairs apart, causing an even greater error in the template function of DNA by shifting the reading frame.

Destruction of Target Molecules   In addition to adduct formation, toxicants alter the primary structure of endogenous molecules by means of cross-linking and fragmentation. Bifunctional electrophiles, such as 2,5-hexanedione, carbon disulfide, acrolein, 4-oxonon-2-enal, 4-hydroxynon-2-enal, and nitrogen mustard alkylating agents, cross-link cytoskeletal proteins, DNA, or DNA with proteins. HOOH and hydroxyl radicals can also induce cross-linking by converting proteins into either reactive electrophiles (e.g., protein sulfenic acids and protein carbonyls, respectively), which react with a nucleophilic group (e.g., thiol, amine) in another macromolecule. Radicals (e.g., those shown in Fig. 3-4) may induce cross-linking of macromolecules by converting them into radicals, which react with each other by radical recombination. Cross-linking imposes both structural and functional constraints on the linked molecules.

Some target molecules are susceptible to spontaneous degradation after chemical attack. Free radicals such as $Cl_3COO^\bullet$ and $HO^\bullet$ can initiate peroxidative degradation of lipids by hydrogen abstraction from fatty acids (Recknagel et al., 1989). The lipid radical ($L^\bullet$) formed is converted successively to lipid peroxyl radical ($LOO^\bullet$) by oxygen fixation, lipid hydroperoxide (LOOH) by hydrogen abstraction, and lipid alkoxyl radical ($LO^\bullet$) by the Fe(II)-catalyzed Fenton reaction. Subsequent fragmentation gives rise to hydrocarbons such as ethane and reactive aldehydes such as 4-hydroxynon-2-enal and malondialdehyde (Fig. 3-9). Thus, lipid peroxidation not only destroys lipids in cellular membranes but also generates endogenous toxicants, both free radicals (e.g., $LOO^\bullet$, $LO^\bullet$) and electrophiles (e.g., 4-oxonon-2-enal, 4-hydroxynon-2-enal). These substances can readily react with adjacent molecules, such as membrane proteins, or diffuse to more distant molecules such as DNA. F_2-isoprostanes are stable peroxidation products of arachidonic acid; these are not only sensitive markers of lipid

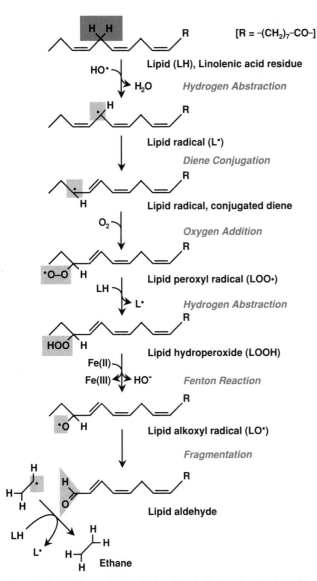

[R = –(CH₂)₇–CO–]

Lipid (LH), Linolenic acid residue

HO•

H₂O

Hydrogen Abstraction

Lipid radical (L•)

Diene Conjugation

Lipid radical, conjugated diene

O₂

Oxygen Addition

Lipid peroxyl radical (LOO•)

LH

L•

Hydrogen Abstraction

Lipid hydroperoxide (LOOH)

Fe(II)

Fe(III) HO⁻

Fenton Reaction

Lipid alkoxyl radical (LO•)

Fragmentation

Lipid aldehyde

LH

L•

Ethane

Figure 3-9. Lipid peroxidation initiated by the hydroxyl radical (HO•).

Many of the products, such as the radicals and the α,β-unsaturated aldehydes, are reactive, whereas others, such as ethane, are nonreactive but are indicators of lipid peroxidation.

peroxidation, but also potent pulmonary and renal vasoconstrictors (Basu, 2004).

Apart from hydrolytic degradation by toxins and radiolysis, toxicant-induced fragmentation of proteins is not well documented. There are, however, examples for destruction of the prosthetic group in enzymes. For instance, cytochrome P450 converts allyl isopropyl acetamide into a reactive metabolite, which alkylates the heme moiety of the enzyme. This leads to loss of the altered heme and to porphyria (De Matteis, 1987). Arsine (AsH₃) acutely induces heme release from oxyhemoglobin, which may underlie its hemolytic effect. Aconitase is attacked by ONOO⁻ at its $[4Fe-4S]^{2+}$ cluster, whose one Fe atom is genuinely labile (as is complexed to inorganic sulfur and not to enzyme-bound cysteines like the others). As a result of the oxidant action of ONOO⁻, the labile Fe is lost, inactivating the enzyme (Castro *et al.*, 1994) and compromising the citric acid cycle where aconitase functions.

Several forms of DNA fragmentation are caused by toxicants. For instance, attack of DNA bases by HO• can result in the formation of imidazole ring–opened purines or ring–contracted pyrimidines, which block DNA replication. Formation of a bulky adduct at guanine *N*-7 destabilizes the *N*-glycosylic bond, inducing depurination. Depurination results in apurinic sites that are mutagenic. Single-strand breaks typically are caused by hydroxyl radicals via abstraction of H from desoxyribose in DNA yielding the C-4′ radical, followed by $O_2^{\bullet-}$ addition, Criegee rearrangement, and cleavage of the phosphodiester bond (Breen and Murphy, 1995). Multiple hydroxyl radical attacks on a short length of DNA, which occur after ionizing radiation, cause double-strand breaks that are typically lethal to the affected cell.

Neoantigen Formation Whereas the covalent binding of xenobiotics or their metabolites is often inconsequential with respect to the function of the immune system, in some individuals these altered proteins, which carry the xenobiotic adduct as a hapten, evoke an immune response. Some chemicals (e.g., dinitrochlorobenzene, penicillin, and nickel-ion) are sufficiently reactive to bind to proteins spontaneously. Others may obtain reactivity by autooxidation to quinones (e.g., urushiols, the allergens in poison ivy) or by enzymatic biotransformation (Park *et al.*, 2005). For example, cytochrome P450 biotransforms halothane to an electrophile, trifluoroacetyl chloride, which binds as a hapten to microsomal and cell surface proteins in the liver, inducing a hepatitis-like immune reaction in sensitive patients.

Haptenized proteins released from cells may evoke antibody-mediated (humoral) and/or T-cell-mediated (cellular) immune response. In the humoral response, B-cells play the leading role: they bind the complete antigen through their B-cell receptors and associate with T-helper cells (CD4⁺). Antigen binding (as signal 1) and cell surface co-stimulatory molecules on T-helper cells (as signal 2) induce differentiation of B-cells into plasma B-cells that manufacture and secrete antibody. By binding to the antigen, the antibody assists in destruction of the antigen by phagocytosis, however, harmful consequences may also result. For example, when penicillin-bound proteins as antigens react with IgE-type antibodies on the surface of mast cells, the reaction triggers release of mast cell mediators (e.g., histamine, leukotrienes), which in turn may cause bronchoconstriction (asthma), vasodilatation, and plasma exudation (wheal, anaphylactic shock).

In cellular immune response, T-cells are the main mediators. T-helper cells become activated by two signals coming from antigen-presenting cells (APC), such as macrophages in internal tissues and dendritic cells in tissues that are in contact with external environment (i.e., skin and mucosal lining of the respiratory and gastrointestinal tract). The APC phagocytoses the haptenized protein and migrates to the lymph nodes where most T-cells are located. Meanwhile, the APC processes the antigen into appropriate peptides, externalizes and transfers the processed antigen to the MHC (major histocompatibility complex) on its surface. On reaching the lymph node, the APC presents the MHC-bound peptide to the T-cell receptor (TCR) of T-helper cells (signal 1). In addition, cell surface co-activator molecules (e.g., CD80 and CD86) on APC bind to their counterparts (e.g., CD28) on T-cells (signal 2). Without signal 2 (which verifies that the antigen detected is foreign) the T-cell becomes functionally inert (anergic). On receiving both signals, the helper T-cell becomes specific to one particular antigen, expresses the T-cell growth factor IL-2 and its receptor, proliferate and differentiate. Using IL-2 and other cytokines, helper T-cells can activate cytotoxic T-cells (CD8[+]) and induce expression of adhesion molecules at the site of allergen contact. Whereas this response is protective against virus-infected cells and tumor cells, it causes inflammation and cell injury in cells containing xenobiotic neoantigens. This model describes the response to contact allergens, such as nickel and urushiols, and is the basis of detecting contact allergens in mice with the local lymph node assay.

Besides the above-described classical mechanism of neoantigen-initiated APC-mediated T-cell activation, xenobiotics may cause T-cell activation by more direct ways. For example, Ni-ions may not only form co-ordinate covalent bonds with proteins, making them neoantigens, but apparently crosslink MHC of APC with the TCR of T-cells, activating the latter. Moreover, some drugs (e.g., sulfamethoxazole), which can be biotransformed into adduct forming metabolites (e.g., nitroso-sulfamethoxazole) that triggers T-cell activation by the classical mechanism, purportedly may also stimulate the TCR of T-cells directly, without involvement of APC. Furthermore, the immune response may be facilitated by toxic and inflammatory cell injury because these "danger signals" upregulate the co-stimulatory molecules on T-cells.

Drug-induced lupus and possibly many cases of drug-induced agranulocytosis are thought to be mediated by immune reactions triggered by drug-protein adducts. The causative chemicals are typically nucleophiles, such as aromatic amines (e.g., aminopyrine, clozapine, procainamide, and sulfonamides), hydrazines (e.g., hydralazine and isoniazid), and thiols (e.g., propylthiouracil, methimazole, and captopril). These substances can be oxidized by myeloperoxidase of granulocytes and monocytes (the precursors of APC) or by the ROS/RNS such cells produce (HO[•], ONOO[−], HOCl, see Fig. 3-22) to reactive metabolites that bind to the surface proteins of these cells, making them antigens (Uetrecht, 1992). The reactive metabolites may also activate monocytes and thus promote the immune reaction. Activation of CD4[+] T-cells by inhibition of promoter methylation of specific genes by procainamide and hydralazine as a possible lupus-inducing mechanism is discussed under dysregulation of transcription.

Toxicity Not Initiated by Reaction with Target Molecules

Some xenobiotics do not only interact with a specific endogenous target molecule to induce toxicity, but instead alter the biological microenvironment (see step 2b in Fig. 3-1). Included here are (1) chemicals that alter H^+ ion concentrations in the aqueous biophase, such as acids and substances biotransformed to acids, such as methanol and ethylene glycol, as well as protonophoric uncouplers such as 2,4-dinitrophenol and pentachlorophenol, which dissociate their phenolic protons in the mitochondrial matrix, thus dissipating the proton gradient that drives ATP synthesis; (2) solvents and detergents that physicochemically alter the lipid phase of cell membranes and destroy transmembrane solute gradients that are essential to cell functions; and (3) other xenobiotics that cause harm merely by occupying a site or space. For example, some chemicals (e.g., ethylene glycol, methotrexate, acyclovir) form water-insoluble precipitates in the renal tubules. By occupying bilirubin binding sites on albumin, compounds such as the sulfonamides induce bilirubin toxicity (kernicterus) in neonates. Carbon dioxide displaces oxygen in the pulmonary alveolar space and causes asphyxiation.

STEP 3—CELLULAR DYSFUNCTION AND RESULTANT TOXICITIES

The reaction of toxicants with a target molecule may result in impaired cellular function as the third step in the development of toxicity (Fig. 3-1). Each cell in a multicellular organism carries out defined programs. Certain programs determine the destiny of cells—that is, whether they undergo division, differentiation (i.e., express proteins for specialized functions), or apoptosis. Other programs control the ongoing (momentary) activity of differentiated cells, determining whether they secrete more or less of a substance, whether they contract or relax, and whether they transport and metabolize nutrients at higher or lower rates. For regulations of these cellular programs, cells possess signaling networks (such as those shown in Figs. 3-11 and 3-12) that can be activated and inactivated by external signaling molecules. To execute the programs, cells are equipped with synthetic, metabolic, kinetic, transport, and energy-producing systems as well as structural elements, organized into macromolecular complexes, cell membranes, and organelles, by which they maintain their own integrity (internal functions) and support the maintenance of other cells (external functions).

As outlined in Fig. 3-10, the nature of the primary cellular dysfunction caused by toxicants, but not necessarily the ultimate outcome, depends on the role of the target molecule affected. If the target molecule is involved in cellular regulation (signaling), dysregulation of gene expression, and/or dysregulation of momentary cellular function occurs primarily. However, if the target molecule is involved predominantly in the cell's internal maintenance, the resultant dysfunction can ultimately compromise the survival of the cell. The reaction of a toxicant with targets serving external functions can influence the operation of other cells and integrated organ systems. The following discussion deals with these consequences.

Toxicant-Induced Cellular Dysregulation

Cells are regulated by signaling molecules that activate specific cellular receptors linked to signal transducing networks that transmit the signals to the regulatory regions of genes and/or to functional proteins. Receptor activation may ultimately lead to (1) altered gene expression that increases or decreases the quantity of specific proteins and/or (2) a chemical modification of specific proteins, typically by phosphorylation, which activates or inhibits proteins. Programs controlling the destiny of cells primarily affect gene expression, whereas those regulating the ongoing activities primarily influence the activity of functional proteins; however, one signal often evokes both responses because of branching and interconnection of signaling networks.

Dysregulation of Gene Expression   Dysregulation of gene expression may occur at elements that are directly responsible for transcription, at components of the intracellular signal transduction pathway, and at the synthesis, storage, or release of the extracellular signaling molecules.

Dysregulation of Transcription   Transcription of genetic information from DNA to mRNA is controlled largely by interplay between transcription factors (TFs) and the regulatory or promoter region of genes. By binding to nucleotide sequences in this region, activated TFs facilitate the formation of the preinitiation complex, promoting transcription of the adjacent gene. Xenobiotics may interact with the

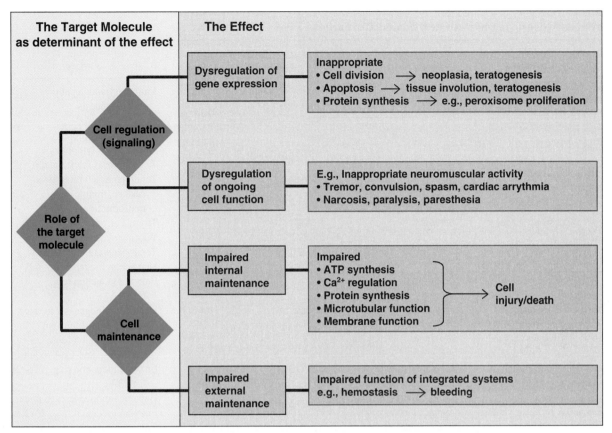

Figure 3-10. The third step in the development of toxicity: alteration of the regulatory or maintenance function of the cell.

TFs (or other components of the preinitiation complex) and with the promoter region of the gene.

Dysregulation of Transcription by Chemicals Acting Through Ligand-Activated Transcription Factors   Several endogenous compounds, such as hormones (e.g., steroids, thyroid hormones) and vitamins (retinoids and vitamin D), influence gene expression by binding to and activating TFs (Table 3-4). Xenobiotics may mimic the natural ligands. For example, fibric acid–type lipid-lowering drugs and phthalate esters substitute for polyunsaturated fatty acids as ligands for the peroxisome proliferator-activated receptor (PPARα) (Poellinger *et al.*, 1992), and xenoestrogens (e.g., diethylstilbestrol, DDT, methoxychlor) substitute estradiol, an endogenous ligand for estrogen receptors.

Acting through ligand-activated TFs, natural or xenobiotic ligands when administered at extreme doses or at critical periods during ontogenesis may cause toxicity by inappropriately influencing the fate of cells and inducing cell death or mitosis (Table 3-4). Glucocorticoids induce apoptosis of lymphoid cells. Whereas desirable in the treatment of lymphoid malignancies, this is an unwanted response in many other conditions. TCDD, a ligand of the aryl hydrocarbon receptor (AHR), produces thymic atrophy by causing apoptosis of thymocytes. Estrogens exert mitogenic effects in cells that express estrogen receptors (ER), such as those found in the female reproductive organs, the mammary gland, and the liver. ER-mediated proliferation appears to be responsible, at least in part, for formation of tumors in these organs during prolonged estrogen exposure (Green, 1992), as well as for induction of the rare vaginal adenocarcinoma in late puberty after transplacental exposure to the synthetic estrogen diethylstilbestrol (DES). Stimulation of these receptors during

a critical prenatal period of differentiation reprograms the estrogen target tissue (i.e., Mullerian duct), resulting in benign and malignant abnormalities in the reproductive tract later in life (Newbold, 2004). Mice exposed neonatally with DES served to model DES-induced late carcinogenesis in the reproductive tract. Compared to the wild-type animals, mice overexpressing ERα were exceedingly sensitive to DES-induced uterine adenocarcinoma, whereas ERα-knockout mice were resistant, indicating the role of ERα in tumorigenesis. It has been speculated that environmental xenoestrogens such as DDT, polychlorinated biphenyls, bisphenol A, and atrazine contribute to an increased incidence of breast cancer. Zearalenone, a mycoestrogen feed contaminant, causes vulval prolapse in swine, an example of an ER-mediated proliferative lesion. The mitogenic and hepatic tumor-promoting effects of peroxisome proliferators in rodents are also receptor-mediated, because it is not observed in PPARα-null mice (Peters *et al.*, 1998). Humans do not respond with hepatocellular and peroxisomal proliferation to fibrates and express PPARα at low levels and often in nonfunctional forms. Humanized mice (i.e., PPARα-null mice transfected with human PPARα) also fail to exhibit hepatocellular and peroxisomal proliferation after fibrate treatment (Gonzalez and Yu, 2006). Nevertheless, transfection of rat PPARα into human hepatocytes does not convey inducibility of peroxisomes by PPARα ligands, implying additional species differences in this signaling. Chemicals that act on ligand-activated TFs, such as glucocorticoids, TCDD, and retinoids, induce fetal malformations that may be regarded as inappropriate gene expression. Candidate target genes are the homeobox genes that determine the body plan during early ontogenesis.

Table 3.4
Toxicants Acting on Ligand-Activated Transcription Factors

LIGAND-ACTIVATED TRANSCRIPTION FACTOR	ENDOGENOUS LIGAND	EXOGENOUS LIGAND	EFFECT
Estrogen receptor (ER)	Estradiol	Ethynylestradiol Diethylstilbestrol DDT, Methoxychlor Zeralenone	Mammary and hepatic carcinogenesis Porcine vulval prolapse
Glucocorticoid receptor (GR)	Cortisol	Dexamethasone	Apoptosis of lymphocytes Teratogenesis (cleft palate)
Retinoic acid receptor (RAR, RXR)	All-*trans*-retinoic acid	13-*cis* retinoic acid	Teratogenesis (craniofacial, cardiac, thymic malformations)
Aryl hydrocarbon receptor (AHR)	Unknown	TCDD PCBs PAHs	Thymic atrophy Wasting syndrome Teratogenesis (cleft palate) Hepatocarcinogenesis in rats Enzyme induction (e.g., CYP1A1)
Peroxisome proliferator–activated receptor (PPARα)	Fatty acids	Fibrate esters (e.g., clofibrate) Phthalate esters (e.g., DEHP)	Hepatocarcinogenesis in mice Peroxisome proliferation Enzyme induction (e.g., CYP4A1, acyl-CoA oxidase)
Constitutive androstane receptor (CAR)	3α,5α-androstenol 3α,5α-androstanol (inhibitors)	TCPOBOP, Phenobarbital* DDT, PCP Chlorpromazine	Enzyme induction (e.g., CYP2B, CYP3A) Hepatocarcinogenesis in mice
Pregnane X receptor (PXR)	Pregnenolone Progesterone	PCN, Dexamethasone Spironolactone, Cyproterone Rifampicin, Zearalenone Litocholic acid	Enzyme induction (e.g., CYP3A) Transporter induction (e.g., Oatp2, Mdr1, Mrp1, Mrp2, Mrp3)

TCPOBP = 1,2-bis[2-(3,5-dichloropyridyloxy)benzene, *Phenobarbital indirectly activates CAR not as a ligand.

Compounds that act on ligand-activated TFs can also change the pattern of cell differentiation by overexpressing various genes. For example, the PPARα-ligand fibric acid derivatives stimulate genes that encode peroxisomal enzymes and induce proliferation of peroxisomes in rodent liver (Green, 1992). TCDD, phenobarbital, and pregnenolone 16α-carbonitrile (PCN) activate AHR, the constitutive androstane receptor (CAR), and the pregnane X receptor (PXR), respectively (Table 3-4), thereby exerting their well known cytochrome P450–inducing effects. However, rodent, rabbit and human PXRs and CARs exhibit low degree of sequence conservation in their ligand-binding domains. This accounts for marked species differences in the induction potential of their ligands, such as PCN, rifampicin, and TCPOBOP (Gonzalez and Yu, 2006). Genes of several xenobiotic metabolizing enzymes may be activated by these chemicals. For example, TCDD increases the expression of cytochrome-P450 1A1, UDP-glucuronosyltransferase-1, and several subunits of mouse and rat glutathione *S*-transferase because the promoter region of their genes contains a dioxin (or xenobiotic) response element that is recognized by the TCDD-activated AHR complexed with its nuclear translocator protein ARNT (also called HIF-1β). In AHR-null mice, TCDD induces neither these enzymes nor the adverse effects listed in Table 3-4 (Gonzalez and Fernandez-Salguero, 1998).

Dysregulation of Transcription by Chemicals Altering the Regulatory Region of Genes   Xenobiotics may dysregulate transcription by also altering the regulatory gene regions through direct chemical interaction or by changing their methylation pattern. It has been hypothesized that thalidomide (or its hydrolysis product) exerts teratogenic effect in the embryo by intercalating to GGGCGG sequences (also called GC boxes) that are binding sites for Sp1, a transcription activator for RNA polymerase II (Stephens *et al.*, 2000). Thalidomide would thus impair insulin-like growth factor-1 (IGF-2) and fibroblast growth factor-2 (FGF-2) signaling pathways necessary for angiogenesis and limb formation, because both pathways encompass multiple proteins whose genes contain GC boxes in the regulatory region (but lack TATA and CCAAT boxes). Another chemical feature of thalidomide that may account for impaired Sp1-mediated transcriptional activation is that the hydrolysis product of this drug is a glutamine analogue and thus mimics the glutamine-rich activation domain of Sp1 protein.

As described in more detail in this chapter under carcinogenesis, methylation of cytosines in CpG islands located in the promoter of genes is a major epigenetic mechanism, which together with coupled histone modifications (e.g., acetylation, methylation) influences the transcriptional activity of the adjacent gene. Promoter methylation silences genes, whereas demethylation permits their activation. Importantly, when DNA replication occurs, the methylation pattern is copied from the parent strand to the daughter strand by DNA methyltransferase-1 (Dnmt1), making the pattern heritable. Nevertheless, promoter methylation is subject to environmental influences, which can thus cause heritable changes in gene regulation. Altered promoter methylation has been implicated in chemically induced systemic lupus erythemathosus (SLE), in developmental deficiencies manifested postnatally or even in subsequent generations, and in cancer. The antiarrhytmic drug procainamide and the antihypertensive hydralazine often induce SLE, an autoimmune inflammatory disease. Both drugs inhibit DNA methylation and induce global DNA hypomethylation in CD4$^+$ T lymphocytes with concomitant overexpression of proteins important in inflammation, such as CD11a (an integrin subunit), CD70 (a B cell costimulatory molecule), and perforin (a cell killing molecule) (Ballestar *et al.*, 2006). Idiopathic lupus also involves global DNA hypomethylation in T cells with overexpression of these proinflammatory proteins. Therefore, promoter hypomethylation and overexpression of critical genes that convert T cells into aggressive inflammatory cells appears fundamental in the pathogenesis of both idiopathic and drug-induced SLE.

The so-called genomically imprinted genes are especially susceptible for epigenetic dysregulation. Normally, we carry equally expressed two copies (i.e., maternal and paternal alleles) of the vast majority of genes. However, for the relatively few (100–200) genomically imprinted genes, either the paternal or maternal copy is silenced by methylation, whereas the other allele is expressed. Dysregulation of imprinting can range from loss of imprinting, which results in bi-allelic expression and double amounts of the gene product, to silencing of both alleles. Dysregulation of the genomically imprinted insulin-like growth factor-2 gene (*Igf2*) has been implicated in the growth deficit observed in mouse embryos in response to TCDD exposure in the preimplantation stage (Wu *et al.*, 2004). The retarded growth is purportedly caused by decreased expression of *Igf2*, whose imprint control region becomes hypermethylated. TCDD also increased DNA methyltransferase activity in the embryos probably because *Dnmt1* gene expression is controlled by the transcription activator Sp1, which in turn is Ah-receptor inducible.

The genome is especially susceptible to epigenetic alterations during early development, as in the preimplantation mammalian embryo the genome (except for the imprinted genes) undergoes extensive demethylation, and appropriate patterns of cytosine methylation are reestablished after implantation. Developing mammalian germ cells are also subject to such changes: primordial germ cells undergo genomic demethylation while they migrate into the early gonad, and then they undergo remethylation during sex determination in the gonad, e.g., testis development. During this period (embryonic 11–15 day in the rat), the androgen receptor and estrogen receptor-β are expressed in the developing testis, and ligands of these nuclear receptors can influence the methylation process. Indeed, transient exposure of gestating female rats during the period of gonadal sex determination to vinclozolin (an agricultural fungicide with antiandrogenic activity) or methoxychlor (a DDT type insecticide with estrogenic activity) decreased the spermatogenic capacity (with reduced spermium number and viability) in the adult male offspring and increased the incidence of male infertility (Anway *et al.*, 2005). Importantly, these effects were transferred through the male germ line to nearly all males of the subsequent three generations. These adverse transgenerational effects on reproduction correlate with altered DNA methylation patterns in the germ line. Thus endocrine disruptors have the potency to epigenetically reprogram the germ line and promote transgenerational disease state, although the relevance of these findings under human exposure conditions is still uncertain.

Transcription is also severely dysregulated in cancer cells by altered promoter methylation (i.e., global DNA hypomethylation and tumor suppressor gene hypermethylation). DNA methylation, including its biochemistry, its influence on histone modifications (acetylation and methylation) and its role in chemical carcinogenesis, is discussed in this chapter under mechanisms of action of epigenetic carcinogens.

Dysregulation of Signal Transduction Extracellular signaling molecules, such as growth factors, cytokines, hormones, and neurotransmitters, can ultimately activate TFs utilizing cell surface receptors and intracellular signal transducing networks. Figure 3-11 depicts a simplified scheme for such networks and identifies some of the most important signal-activated TFs that control transcriptional activity of genes that influence cell cycle progression and thus determine the fate of cells. Among these TFs are the c-Fos and c-Jun proteins, which bind in dimeric combinations (called AP-1) to the tetradecanoylphorbol acetate (TPA) response element (TRE), for example, in the promoter of cyclin D gene whose product promotes the cell division cycle (see Figs. 3-21 and 3-27). Other signal-activated TFs that up regulate the transcription of cyclin D gene by binding to their cognate nucleotide sequences include c-Myc, E2F, NF-κB, CREB and STAT. Mitogenic signaling molecules thus induce cell proliferation. In contrast, TGF-β induces the expression of cyclin-dependent kinase inhibitor proteins (e.g., p15, p57) that mediates its antimitotic effect (Johnson and Walker, 1999) (see Fig. 3-27).

The signal from the cell surface receptors to the TFs is relayed mainly by successive protein-protein interactions and protein phosphorylations at specific serine, threonine, or tyrosine hydroxyl groups. Cell surface growth factor receptors (item 4 in Fig. 3-11) are in fact phosphorylating enzymes (i.e., receptor protein tyrosine kinases). Their ligands induce them to phosphorylate themselves, which, in turn, enable these receptors to bind adapter proteins. Through these, the growth factor receptors can initiate proliferative signaling via two important pathways: (1) by activating Ras, they set in motion the mitogen-activated kinase (MAPK) cascade (Qi and Elion, 2005), and (2) by activating phosphatidilinositol-3-kinase (PI3K), they start the PI3K-Akt pathway. A crucial step in the latter is the PI3K-catalyzed phosphorylation of a plasma membrane lipid to generate phosphatidylinositol-3,4,5-triphosphate (PIP$_3$) that recruits protein kinase Akt to the membrane for activation. Because Akt (also called protein kinase B) has numerous substrates, the PI3K-Akt pathway branches (Morgensztern and McLeod, 2005). For example, branches lead toward the transcription factor NF-κB and the protein kinase mTOR, whose phosphorylated products facilitate ribosomal translation of proteins (for the branch leading from Akt to mTOR, see Fig. 3-25).

The intracellular signal transducer proteins are typically but not always activated by phosphorylation—that is catalyzed by protein kinases—and are usually inactivated by dephosphorylation, which is carried out by protein phosphatases. Interestingly, growth factor receptors can amplify their signals by inducing formation of HOOH. As discussed earlier, by attacking protein thiolate groups and converting them into sulfenic acid groups, HOOH reversibly inactivates protein tyrosine phosphatases and PTEN, a lipid phosphatase that eliminates PIP$_3$ (Rhee *et al.*, 2005). The source of HOOH is O$_2^{\bullet-}$ produced by the enzyme complex NADPH oxidase (Nox), which is activated by growth factor receptors via the PI3K → PIP$_3$ → Rac (a

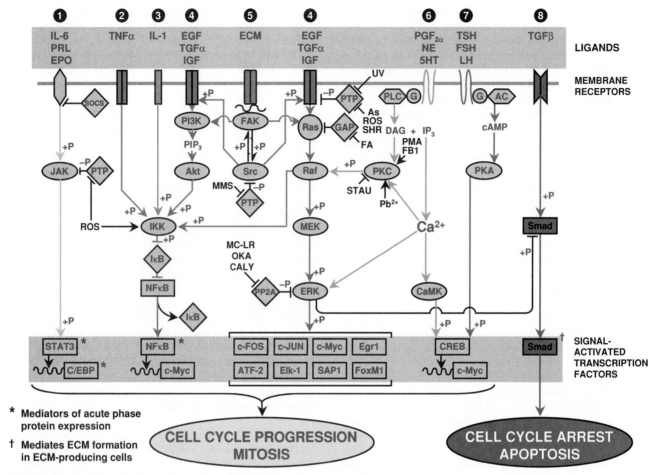

Figure 3-11. Signal transduction pathways from cell membrane receptors to signal-activated nuclear transcription factors that influence transcription of genes involved in cell-cycle regulation.

The symbols of cell membrane receptors are numbered 1–8 and some of their activating ligands are indicated. Circles represent G proteins, oval symbols protein kinases, rectangles transcription factors, wavy lines genes, and diamond symbols inhibitory proteins, such as protein phosphatases (PTP, PP2A), the GTPase-activating protein GAP, and inhibitory binding proteins, such as IκB and SOCS (suppressor of cytokine signaling). Arrowheads indicate stimulation or formation of second messengers (e.g., DAG, IP$_3$, PIP$_3$, cAMP, Ca^{2+}), whereas blunt arrows indicate inhibition. Phosphorylation and dephosphorylation are indicated by +P and –P, respectively. Abbreviations for interfering chemicals are printed in black (As = arsenite; CALY = calyculin A; FA = fatty acids; FB1 = fumonisin B; MC-LR = microcystin-LR; OKA = okadaic acid; MMS = methylmethane sulfonate; PMA = phorbol miristate acetate; ROS = reactive oxygen species; SHR = SH-reactive chemicals, such as iodoacetamide; STAU = staurosporin).

Two important proliferative signaling can be evoked by growth factors, such as EGF, acting on their tyrosine kinase receptors (#4), which are duplicated in the figure for clarity. These receptors use adaptor proteins (Shc, Grb2, and SOS; not shown) to activate Ras by converting it from inactive GDP-bound form to active GTP-bound state, which in turn activates the MAP-kinase phosphorylation cascade built up from specific forms of MAPKKK, MAPKK and MAPK proteins (here Raf, MEK, and ERK, respectively). The phosphorylated MAPK (e.g., ERK) moves into the nucleus and phosphorylates transcription factors (e.g., c-FOS) thereby enabling them to bind to cognate sequences in the promoter regions of genes (e.g., cyclin genes) to facilitate transcription. The same growth factor receptors (#4) can signal through the phosphatidilinositol-3-kinase (PI3K) – Akt – IκB-kinase (IKK) – IκB – NF-κB pathway (see the text for more details). There are numerous interconnections between the signal transduction pathways. For example, the G-protein-coupled receptor (#6) can relay signal into the MAPK pathway via phospholipase C (PLC)-catalyzed formation of second messengers that activate protein-kinase C (PKC), whereas signals from TNFα and IL-1 receptors (#2 and 3) are channeled into the (PI3K) – Akt – NF-κB pathway by phosphorylating IKK. The integrin receptor (#5) whose ligands are constituents of the extracellular matrix (ECM), can also engage the growth factor receptors and Ras as well as PI3K via focal adhesion kinase (FAK) and the tyrosine kinase Src. The cell cycle acceleration induced by these and other signal transduction pathways is further enhanced by the ERK-catalyzed inhibitory phosphorylation of Smad that blocks the cell-cycle arrest signal from the TGF-β receptor (#9). Activation of protein kinases (PKC, CaMK, MAPK) by Ca^{2+} can also trigger mitogenic signaling. Several xenobiotics that are indicated in the figure may dysregulate the signaling network. Some may induce cell proliferation either by activating mitogenic protein kinases (e.g., PKC), or inhibiting inactivating proteins, such

G-protein that associates with Nox) pathway. Although once thought to be restricted to phagocytes, Nox occurs in the plasma membrane of many other cells, such as endothelial cells and vascular smooth muscle cells (Bokoch and Knaus, 2003). Although, Nox in these cells is much less efficient to produce $O_2^{\bullet-}$ than Nox in the phagocytes, the non-phagocytotic Nox releases $O_2^{\bullet-}$ into the cytoplasm, whereas the phagocytotic Nox delivers it to the external face of the plasma membrane (El-Benna et al., 2005).

Chemicals may cause aberrant signal transduction in a number of ways, most often by altering protein phosphorylation, occasionally by interfering with the GTPase activity of G proteins (e.g., Ras), by disrupting normal protein-protein interactions or by establishing abnormal ones, or by altering the synthesis or degradation of signaling proteins. Such interventions may ultimately influence cell cycle progression.

Chemically Altered Signal Transduction with Proliferative Effect Xenobiotics that facilitate phosphorylation of signal transducers often promote mitosis and tumor formation. Such are the phorbol esters and fumonisin B that activate protein kinase C (PKC). These chemicals mimic diacylglycerol (DAG), one of the physiologic activators of PKC (Fig. 3-11). The other physiologic PKC activator Ca^{2+} is mimicked by Pb^{2+}, whose effect on $PKC\alpha$ is concentration-dependent: stimulatory at picomolar concentration, when Pb^{2+} occupies only high-affinity binding sites on PKC, and inhibitory at micromolar concentration, where the low affinity sites are also occupied (Sun et al., 1999). Lead acetate does induce marked hepatocellular proliferation in rats. The activated PKC promotes mitogenic signaling at least in two ways: (1) by phosphorylating Raf, the first protein kinase in the MAPK pathway (Fig. 3-11), and (2) by phosphorylating a protein phosphatase that dephosphorylates the transcription factor c-Jun at specific sites (Thr 231, Ser 234, and Ser 249), thereby permitting its binding to DNA. Protein kinases may also be activated by interacting proteins that had been altered by a xenobiotic. For example, the TCDD-liganded AhR binds to MAPK. This may contribute to the TCDD-induced overexpression of cyclins and cyclin-dependent kinases in guinea pig liver (Ma and Babish, 1999).

Aberrant phosphorylation of proteins may result not only from increased phosphorylation by kinases, but also from decreased dephosphorylation by phosphatases. Inhibition of phosphatases, including the lipid phosphatase PTEN, appears to be the underlying mechanism of the mitogenic effect of various chemicals, oxidative stress, and ultraviolet (UV) irradiation (Herrlich et al., 1999). Protein tyrosine phosphatases and dual-specificity phosphatases (i.e., enzymes that remove phosphate from phosphorylated tyrosine as well as serine and threonine residues) as well as PTEN contain a catalytically active cysteine, and are susceptible to inactivation by HOOH via sulfenic acid formation and by covalent reaction with other SH-reactive chemicals (Forman et al., 2004; Rhee et al., 2005). Indeed, xenobiotics such as the SH-reactive iodoacetamide, the organometal compound tributyltin, arsenite, as well as HOOH cause phosphorylation of the epidermal growth factor (EGF) receptor (item 4 in Fig. 3-11) by interfering with the protein tyrosine phosphatase that would dephosphorylate and thus "silence" this receptor (Herrlich et al., 1999; Chen et al., 1998). Arsenite activates NADPH oxidase (Nox) in various cells, producing oxidative stress (Lynn et al., 2000; Smith et al., 2001). This may result from the arsenite-activated growth factor receptors that send an activating signal through the $PI3K \rightarrow PIP_3 \rightarrow Rac$ path to the neighboring Nox, also localized in the plasma membrane. It is tempting to speculate that Nox activation and related $O_2^{\bullet-}$ production in endothelial cells and vascular smooth muscle cells contributes to the vasculotoxic effects of arsenic. Arsenite may also inactivate the dual-specificity phosphatase that dephosphorylates and "silences" certain MAPKs (JNK, p38), whereas methylmethane sulfonate (MMS) appears to inhibit a protein phosphatase that inactivates Src, a protein tyrosine kinase (Herrlich et al., 1999). The thiol oxidizing agent diamide (which increases phosphorylation of MAPKs) and phenolic antioxidants (which form phenoxyl radicals and increase c-Fos and c-Jun expression) (Dalton et al., 1999) may also act by incapacitating protein tyrosine phosphatases. Protein phosphatase 2A (PP2A) is the major soluble ser/thr phosphatase in cells and is likely responsible, at least in part, for reversing the growth factor-induced stimulation of MAPK, thereby keeping the extent and duration of MAPK activity under control (Goldberg, 1999). PP2A also removes an activating phosphate from a mitosis-triggering protein kinase (p34[cdc2]). Several natural toxins are extremely potent inhibitors of PP2A; including the blue–green algae poison microcystin-LR and the dinoflagellate-derived okadaic acid (Toivola and Eriksson, 1999), which are tumor promoters in experimental animals subjected to prolonged low-dose exposure. It is to be noted, however, that acute high-dose exposure to microcystin induces severe liver injury, whereas such exposure to okadaic acid is the underlying cause of the diarrhetic shellfish poisoning. In these conditions, hyperphosphorylation of proteins other than those involved in proliferative signaling (e.g., hepatocellular microfilaments in microcystin poisoning) may be primarily responsible for the pathogenesis.

Apart from phosphatases, there are also inhibitory binding proteins that can keep signaling under control. Such is IκB, which binds to NF-κB, preventing its transfer into the nucleus and its function as a TF. Upon phosphorylation by its designated IκB kinase (IKK), IκB is degraded by the proteosome and NF-κB is set free. IKK can be phosphorylated (activated) by other protein kinases, such as Raf, a member of the MAPK cascade, and by Akt a member of the PI3K-Akt pathway (Fig. 3-11). NF-κB is an important contributor to proliferative and pro-life signaling, because via the above pathways, growth factor receptor stimulation can cause IκB phosphorylation and thus the release of NF-κB, and because the released NF-κB transactivates genes whose products accelerate the cell division cycle (e.g., cyclin D1 and c-Myc) and inhibit apoptosis (e.g., antiapoptotic Bcl proteins and the caspase inhibitor IAP proteins) (Karin, 2006). NF-κB activation, via the Akt-mediated IKK phosphorylation, is involved in the proliferative (and possibly carcinogenic) effect of arsenite, nicotine, and the nicotine-derived

---

as protein phosphatases (PTP, PP2A), GAP or IκB. Others, e.g., inhibitors of PKC, oppose mitosis and facilitate apoptosis.

This scheme is oversimplified and tentative in several details. Virtually all components of the signaling network (e.g., G proteins, PKCs, MAPKs) are present in multiple, functionally different forms whose distribution may be cell specific. The pathways depicted are not equally relevant for all cells. In addition, these pathways regulating gene expression determine not only the fate of cells, but also control certain aspects of the ongoing cellular activity. For example, NF-κB induces synthesis of acute phase proteins.

nitrosamine ketone (NNK). In addition, because NF-κB also targets the genes of several cytokines (e.g., TNF-α, IL-1β) and acute phase proteins (e.g., C-reactive protein, α1-acid glycoprotein), and because such cytokines acting on their receptors (items 2 and 3 in Fig. 3-11) activate NF-κB, this TF plays a leading role also in inflammatory and acute phase reactions, as well as in cancer caused by chronic inflammation (Karin, 2006; Waddick and Uckun, 1999).

Another site from which aberrant mitogenic signals may originate is the GTP/GDP binding protein Ras, which is active in GTP-bound form but inactive in GDP-bound form. The activity of Ras is normally terminated via stimulation of its own GTPase activity by a GTPase-activating protein (GAP) (Fig. 3-11) that returns Ras into its inactive GDP-bound state. Fatty acids, which may accumulate, for example, in response to phospholipase A activation and exposure to peroxysome proliferators (Rose *et al.*, 1999), inhibit GAP and can delay the turning off of Ras. As discussed in more detail later in the chapter, genotoxic carcinogens may mutate Ras, and if the mutation leads to a loss of its GTPase activity, this would result in a permanent signaling for the MAPK pathway—a condition that contributes to malignant transformation of the affected cell population.

Chemically Altered Signal Transduction with Antiproliferative Effect   Downturning of increased proliferative signaling after cell injury may compromise replacement of injured cells. This prediction has been made from a study on cultured Hepa 1-6 cells that exhibited the following, seemingly consequential alterations upon exposure to acetaminophen (follow the path in Fig. 3-11): inhibition of Raf $\rightarrow$ diminished degradation of IκB $\rightarrow$ diminished binding of NF-κB to DNA $\rightarrow$ diminished expression of c-Myc mRNA (Boulares *et al.*, 1999). Down regulation of a normal mitogenic signal is a step away from survival and toward apoptosis. Indeed, inhibitors of PKC (staurosporin), PI3K (wortmannin), and of IκB degradation (gliotoxin) (Waddick and Uckun, 1999) are apoptosis inducers. TGF-β and glucocorticoids increase IκB synthesis and, in turn, decrease NF-κB activation and c-Myc expression (Waddick and Uckun, 1999). These mechanisms may contribute to the apoptotic effect of TGF-β and glucocorticoids, the latter in lymphoid cells.

Dysregulation of Extracellular Signal Production   Hormones of the anterior pituitary exert mitogenic effects on endocrine glands in the periphery by acting on cell surface receptors. Pituitary hormone production is under negative feedback control by hormones of the peripheral glands. Perturbation of this circuit adversely affects pituitary hormone secretion and, in turn, the peripheral gland. For example, xenobiotics that inhibit thyroid hormone production (e.g., the herbicide amitrole and the fungicide metabolite ethylenethiourea) or enhance thyroid hormone elimination (e.g., phenobarbital) reduce thyroid hormone levels and increase the secretion of thyroid-stimulating hormone (TSH) because of the reduced feedback inhibition. The increased TSH secretion stimulates cell division in the thyroid gland, which is responsible for the goiters or thyroid tumors caused by such toxicants (see Chap. 21). Decreased secretion of pituitary hormone produces the opposite adverse affect, with apoptosis followed by involution of the peripheral target gland. For example, estrogens produce testicular atrophy in males by means of feedback inhibition of gonadotropin secretion. The low sperm count in workers intoxicated with the xenoestrogen chlordecone probably results from such a mechanism.

Dysregulation of Ongoing Cellular Activity   Ongoing control of specialized cells is exerted by signaling molecules acting on membrane receptors that transduce the signal by regulating Ca^{2+} entry into the cytoplasm or stimulating the enzymatic formation of intracellular second messengers. The Ca^{2+} or other second messengers ultimately alter the phosphorylation of functional proteins, changing their activity and, in turn, cellular functions almost instantly. Toxicants can adversely affect ongoing cellular activity by disrupting any step in signal coupling.

Dysregulation of Electrically Excitable Cells   Many xenobiotics influence cellular activity in excitable cells, such as neurons, skeletal, cardiac, and smooth muscle cells. Cellular functions such as the release of neurotransmitters and muscle contraction are controlled by transmitters and modulators synthesized and released by adjacent neurons. The major mechanisms that control such cells are shown schematically in Fig. 3-12, and chemicals that interfere with these mechanisms are listed in Table 3-5.

Altered regulation of neural and/or muscle activity is the basic mechanism of action of many drugs and is responsible for toxicities associated with drug overdosage, pesticides, and microbial, plant, and animal toxins (Herken and Hucho, 1992). As neurons are signal-transducing cells, the influence of chemicals on neurons is seen not only on the neuron affected by the toxicant but also on downstream cells influenced by the primary target. Thus, tetrodotoxin, which blocks voltage-gated Na^+ channels (item 7 in Fig. 3-12) in motor neurons, causes skeletal muscle paralysis. In contrast, cyclodiene insecticides, which block GABA receptors (item 3 in Fig. 3-12) in the central nervous system, induce neuronal excitation and convulsions (Narahashi, 1991).

Perturbation of ongoing cellular activity by chemicals may be due to an alteration in (1) the concentration of neurotransmitters, (2) receptor function, (3) intracellular signal transduction, or (4) the signal-terminating processes.

Alteration in Neurotransmitter Levels   Chemicals may alter synaptic levels of neurotransmitters by interfering with their synthesis, storage, release, or removal from the vicinity of the receptor. The convulsive effect of hydrazine and hydrazides (e.g., isoniazid) is due to their ability to decrease the synthesis of the inhibitory neurotransmitter GABA (Gale, 1992). Reserpine causes its several adverse effects by inhibiting the neuronal storage of norepinephrine, 5-hydroxytryptamine, and dopamine, thereby depleting these transmitters. Skeletal muscle paralysis caused by botulinum toxin is due to inhibition of acetylcholine release from motor neurons and the lacking stimulation of the acetylcholine receptors at the neuromuscular junction (receptor 1 in Fig. 3-12). In contrast, inhibition of acetylcholinesterase by organophosphate or carbamate insecticides or chemical warfare agents (e.g., soman) prevents the hydrolysis of acetylcholine, resulting in massive stimulation of cholinergic receptors (receptors 1, 5, and 11 in Fig. 3-12) and a cholinergic crisis (Table 3-5). Inhibition of the neuronal reuptake of norepinephrine by cocaine or tricyclic antidepressants is responsible for overexcitation of alpha$_1$-adrenergic receptors on vascular smooth muscles, resulting in nasal mucosal ulceration and myocardial infarction in heavy cocaine abusers, whereas overstimulation of beta$_1$-adrenergic receptors contributes to life-threatening arrhythmias. Similar cardiac complications may result from amphetamine abuse, because amphetamine enhances the release of norepinephrine from adrenergic neurons and competitively inhibits neuronal reuptake of this transmitter. A hypertensive crisis can occur with the combined use of tricyclic antidepressants and monoamine oxidase inhibitors, drugs that block different mechanisms of norepinephrine elimination (Hardman *et al.*, 1995). Concomitant use of drugs that increase the

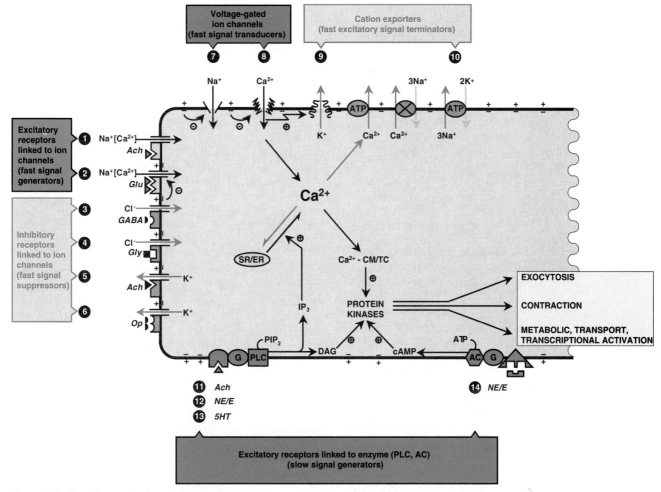

Figure 3-12. Signaling mechanisms for neurotransmitters.

This simplified scheme depicts major cellular signaling mechanisms that are operational in many neurons and muscle and exocrine cells. Chemicals acting on the numbered elements are listed in Table 3-5. Fast signaling is initiated by the opening of ligand-gated Na^+/Ca^{2+} channels (1,2). The resultant cation influx decreases the inside negative potential (i.e., evokes depolarization) and thus triggers the opening of the voltage-gated Na^+ and Ca^{2+} channels (7,8). As a second messenger, the influxed Ca^{2+} activates intracellular Ca^{2+}-binding proteins such as calmodulin (CM) and troponin C (TC), which, in turn, enhance the phosphorylation of specific proteins, causing activation of specific cellular functions. The signal is terminated by channels and transporters (e.g., 9,10) that remove cations from the cells and thus reestablish the inside negative resting potential (i.e., cause repolarization) and restore the resting Ca^{2+} level. Fast signaling can be suppressed by opening the ligand-activated Cl^- or K^+ channels (3-6), which increases the inside negativity (i.e., induces hyperpolarization) and thus counteracts opening of the voltage-gated Na^+ and Ca^{2+} channels (7,8). Signal transduction from other receptors (11–14) that are coupled to G_s proteins involves enzymatic generation of second messengers: inositol 1,4,5-trisphosphate (IP_3) and diacylglycerol (DAG) by phospholipase C (PLC) and cyclic AMP (cAMP) by adenylyl cyclase (AC). These messengers influence cellular activities by activating protein kinases directly or by mobilizing Ca^{2+} from the sarcoplasmic or endoplasmic reticulum (SR and ER), as IP_3 does. For clarity, this figure does not depict that inhibitory receptors 5 and 6 are G_i protein-coupled and that besides opening K^+ channels, they also inhibit AC. Ach = acetylcholine; Glu = glutamate; GABA = γ-aminobutyric acid; Gly = glycine; Op = opioid peptides; NE = norepinephrine; E = epinephrine; 5HT = 5-hydroxytryptamine; G = G protein; PIP_2 = phosphatidylinositol 4,5-bisphosphate. Encircled positive and negative signs indicate activation and inhibition, respectively.

level of serotonin (5-HT) by enhancing its neuronal release, decreasing its neuronal reuptake (e.g., fluoxetine) or its biotransformation (e.g., monoamine oxidase inhibitors) induce the serotonin syndrome with cognitive and behavioral changes, autonomic dysfunction, and neuromuscular abnormalities. It is thought that cytotoxic antineoplastic drugs (e.g., cisplatin) and radiation cause nausea and emesis, a disturbing reaction to chemo- and radiotherapy, by inducing re-

lease of 5-HT from enterochromaffin cells of the intestinal mucosa, which stimulates the 5-HT$_3$-receptors (5-HT-gated cation channel, functionally similar to item 1 in Fig. 3-12) on the adjacent vagal afferent neurons, thereby evoking the vomiting reflex (Endo *et al.*, 2000). Intestinal release of 5-HT and stimulation of vagal affarent neurons are also involved in the emetic effect of ipecac syrup and its alkaloids (cephaelin and emetine). The alpha$_2$-adrenergic receptor

Table 3.5

Agents Acting on Signaling Systems for Neurotransmitters and Causing Dysregulation of the Momentary Activity of Electrically Excitable Cells Such as Neurons and Muscle Cells*

Receptor/Channel/Pump		Agonist/Activator		Antagonist/Inhibitor	
NAME	LOCATION	AGENT	EFFECT	AGENT	EFFECT
1. Acetylcholine nicotinic receptor	Skeletal muscle	Nicotine Anatoxin-a Cytisine *Ind:* ChE inhibitors	Muscle fibrillation, then paralysis	Tubocurarine, lophotoxin α-Bungarotoxin α-Cobrotoxin α-Conotoxin Erabutoxin b *Ind:* botulinum toxin	Muscle paralysis
	Neurons	See above	Neuronal activation	Pb^{2+}, general anesthetics	Neuronal inhibition
2. Glutamate receptor	CNS neurons	*N*-Methyl-*D*-aspartate Kainate, domoate Quinolinate Quisqualate *Ind:* hypoxia, HCN → glutamate release	Neuronal activation → convulsion, neuronal injury ("excitotoxicity")	Phencyclidine Ketamine General anesthetics	Neuronal inhibition →anesthesia Protection against "excitotoxicity"
3. GABA$_A$ receptor	CNS neurons	Muscimol, avermectins sedatives (barbiturates, benzodiazepines) General anaesthetics (halothane) Alcohols (ethanol)	Neuronal inhibition → sedation, general anaesthesia, coma, depression of vital centers	Bicuculline Picrotoxin Pentylenetetrazole Cyclodiene insecticides Lindane, TCAD *Ind:* isoniazid	Neuronal activation → tremor, convulsion
4. Glycine receptor	CNS neurons, motor neurons	Avermectins (?) General anesthetics	Inhibition of motor neurons → paralysis	Strychnine *Ind:* tetanus toxin	Disinhibition of motor neurons → tetanic convulsion
5. Acetylcholine M$_2$ muscarinic receptor	Cardiac muscle	*Ind:* ChE inhibitors	Decreased heart rate and contractility	Belladonna alkaloids (e.g., atropine) atropinelike drugs (e.g., TCAD)	Increased heart rate
6. Opioid receptor	CNS neurons, visceral neurons	Morphine and congeners (e.g., heroin, meperidine) *Ind:* clonidine	Neuronal inhibition → analgesia, central respiratory depression, constipation, urine retention	Naloxone	Antidotal effects in opiate intoxication
7. Voltage-gated Na$^+$ channel	Neurons, muscle cells, etc.	Aconitine, veratridine Grayanotoxin Batrachotoxin Scorpion toxins Ciguatoxin DDT, pyrethroids	Neuronal activation → convulsion	Tetrodotoxin, saxitoxin μ-Conotoxin Local anaesthetics Phenytoin Quinidine	Neuronal inhibition → paralysis, anesthesia Anticonvulsive action
8. Voltage-gated Ca^{2+} channel	Neurons, muscle cell, etc.	Maitotoxin (?) Atrotoxin (?) Latrotoxin (?)	Neuronal/muscular activation, cell injury	ω-Conotoxin Pb^{2+}	Neuronal inhibition → paralysis

(continued)

Table 3.5
(Continued)

Receptor/Channel/Pump		Agonist/Activator		Antagonist/Inhibitor	
NAME	LOCATION	AGENT	EFFECT	AGENT	EFFECT
9. Voltage/Ca^{2+}-activated K^+ Channel	Neurons, smooth and skeletal muscle cardiac muscle	Pb^{2+}	Neuronal/muscular inhibition	Ba^{2+} Apamin (bee venom) Dendrotoxin 20-HETE hERG inhibitors (e.g., cisapride, terfenadine)	Neuronal/muscular activation → convulsion/spasm vasoconstriction PMV tachycardia (torsade de pointes)
10. Na^+,K^+-ATPase	Universal			Digitalis glycosides Oleandrin Chlordecone	Increased cardiac contractility, excitability Increased neuronal excitability → tremor
11. Acetylcholine M_3 muscarinic receptor	Smooth muscle, glands	*Ind:* ChE inhibitors	Smooth muscle spasm Salivation, lacrimation	Belladonna alkaloids (e.g., atropine) Atropinelike drugs (e.g., TCAD)	Smooth muscle relaxation → intestinal paralysis, decreased salivation, decreased perspiration
Acetylcholine M_1 muscarinic receptor	CNS neurons	Oxotremorine *Ind:* ChE inhibitors	Neuronal activation → convulsion	See above	
12. Adrenergic $alpha_1$ receptor	Vascular smooth muscle	(Nor)epinephrine *Ind:* cocaine, tyramine amphetamine, TCAD	Vasoconstriction → ischemia, hypertension	Prazosin	Antidotal effects in intoxication with $alpha_1$-receptor agonists
13. $5-HT_2$ receptor	Smooth muscle	Ergot alkaloids (ergotamine, ergonovine)	Vasoconstriction → ischemia, hypertension	Ketanserine	Antidotal effects in ergot intoxication
14. Adrenergic $beta_1$ receptor	Cardiac muscle	(Nor)epinephrine *Ind:* cocaine, tyramine amphetamine, TCAD	Increased cardiac contractility and excitability	Atenolol, metoprolol	Antidotal effects in intoxication with $beta_1$-receptor agonists

*Numbering of the signaling elements in this table corresponds to the numbering of their symbols in Fig. 3-12. This tabulation is simplified and incomplete. Virtually all receptors and channels listed occur in multiple forms with different sensitivity to the agents. The reader should consult the pertinent literature for more detailed information. CNS = central nervous system; ChE = cholinesterase; *Ind* = indirectly acting (i.e., by altering neurotransmitter level); 20-HETE = 20-hydroxy 5,8,11,14-eicosatetraenoic acid; PMV = polymorphic ventricular; TCAD = tricyclic antidepressant.

agonist clonidine induces release in the brain of beta-endorphin, an endogenous peptide that stimulates opioid receptors (item 6 in Fig. 3-12). This explains why clonidine intoxication mimics several symptoms of morphine poisoning, including depressed respiration and pin-point pupils.

Toxicant–Neurotransmitter Receptor Interactions Some chemicals interact directly with neurotransmitter receptors, including (1) agonists that associate with the ligand-binding site on the receptor and mimic the natural ligand, (2) antagonists that occupy the ligand-binding site but cannot activate the receptor, (3) activators, and (4) inhibitors that bind to a site on the receptor that is not directly involved in ligand binding. In the absence of other actions, agonists and activators mimic, whereas antagonists and inhibitors block, the physiologic responses characteristic of endogenous ligands. For example, muscimol, a mushroom poison, is an agonist at the inhibitory $GABA_A$ receptor (item 3 in Fig. 3-12), whereas barbiturates, benzodiazepines, general anesthetics, and alcohols are activators (Narahashi, 1991). Thus, all these chemicals cause inhibition of central nervous system activity, resulting in sedation, general anesthesia, coma, and ultimately blockade of the medullary respiratory center, depending on the dose administered. There are also similarities in the responses evoked by agonist/activators on excitatory receptors and those elicited by antagonists/inhibitors on inhibitory sites. Thus, glutamate receptor agonists and muscarinic receptor agonists cause neuronal hyperactivity in the brain and ultimately convulsions, as do inhibitors of $GABA_A$ receptor. It is also apparent that chemicals acting as agonists/activators on inhibitory receptors and those acting as antagonists/inhibitors on excitatory receptors may exert similar effects. Moreover, general anesthetic solvents induce general anesthesia not only by activating the inhibitory ligand-gated chloride-ion channels (i.e., $GABA_A$ and glycine receptors; see items 3 and 4, respectively, in Fig. 3-12) but also by inhibiting the excitatory ligand-gated cation channels (i.e., neuronal nicotinic acetylcholine receptor and glutamate receptors; see items 1 and 2, respectively, in Fig. 3-12) (Franks and Lieb, 1998; Perouansky et al., 1998). Because there are multiple types of receptors for each neurotransmitter, these receptors may be affected differentially by toxicants. For example, the neuronal nicotinic acetylcholine receptor is extremely sensitive to inhibition by lead ions, whereas the muscular nicotine receptor subtype is not (Oortgiesen et al., 1993). Other chemicals that produce neurotransmitter receptor–mediated toxicity are listed in Table 3-5.

Some sensory neurons have receptors that are stimulated by chemicals, such as the capsaicin receptor, which is a ligand-gated cation channel (Herken and Hucho, 1992). This receptor mediates the burning sensation of the tongue and reflex stimulation of the lacrimal gland associated with exposure to red pepper and other irritants. Lacrimators in tear gas, which are typically thiol-reactive chemicals, also stimulate these neurons, though their precise mode of action is unclear.

Toxicant–Signal Transducer Interactions   Many chemicals alter neuronal and/or muscle activity by acting on signal-transduction processes. Voltage-gated Na^+ channels (item 7 in Fig. 3-12), which transduce and amplify excitatory signals generated by ligand-gated cation channels (receptors 1 and 2 in Fig. 3-12), are activated by a number of toxins derived from plants and animals (Table 3-5) as well as by synthetic chemicals such as DDT, resulting in overexcitation (Narahashi, 1992). In contrast, chemicals that block voltage-gated Na^+ channels (such as tetrodotoxin and saxitoxin) cause paralysis. The Na^+ channels are also important in signal transduction in sensory neurons; therefore, Na^+-channel activators evoke sensations and reflexes, whereas Na^+-channel inhibitors induce anesthesia. This explains the reflex bradycardia and burning sensation in the mouth that follow the ingestion of monkshood, which contains the Na^+-channel activator aconitine, as well as the use of Na^+-channel inhibitors such as procaine and lidocaine for local anesthesia.

Toxicant–Signal Terminator Interactions   The cellular signal generated by cation influx is terminated by removal of the cations through channels or by transporters (Fig. 3-12). Inhibition of cation efflux may prolong excitation, as occurs with the blockade of Ca^{2+}-activated K^+ channels (item 9 in Fig. 3-12) by Ba^{2+}, which is accompanied by potentially lethal neuroexcitatory and spasmogenic effects. The arachidonic acid metabolite 20-hydroxy 5,8,11,14-eicosatetraenoic acid (20-HETE) also blocks Ca^{2+}-activated K^+ channels, causing vasoconstriction. Induction by cyclosporine of 20-HETE production in renal proximal tubular cells and the resultant decrease in renal cortical blood flow may underlie the nephrotoxic effect of cyclosporine (Seki et al., 2005). Blockade of specific voltage-gated K^+ channels (called hERG channels; item 9 in Fig. 3-12) in the heart delays cardiac repolarization (as indicated by prolonged QT time in ECG) and may evoke polymorphic ventricular tachycardia (termed torsade de pointes), which may cause sudden death if degenerates into ventricular fibrillation (Sanguinetti and Mitcheson, 2005). Several drugs with such an effect (e.g., astemizole, cisapride, grepafloxacin, terfenadine) have been withdrawn from clinical use. Glycosides from digitalis and other plants inhibit Na^+,K^+-ATPase (item 10 in Fig. 3-12) and thus increase the intracellular Na^+ concentration, which, in turn, decreases Ca^{2+} export by Ca^{2+}/Na^+ exchange (Fig. 3-12). The resultant rise in the intracellular concentration of Ca^{2+} enhances the contractility and excitability of cardiac muscle. Inhibition of brain Na^+,K^+-ATPase by chlordecone may be responsible for the tremor observed in chlordecone-exposed workers (Desaiah, 1982). Lithium salts, although used therapeutically, have the potential to produce hyperreflexia, tremor, convulsions, diarrhea, and cardiac arrhythmias (Hardman et al., 1995). Lithium also markedly potentiates cholinergically mediated seizures. Besides inhibition of Li^+-sensitive enzymes (e.g., inositol monophosphatase, bisphosphate 3′-nucleotidase), another possible reason for these toxic effects is inefficient repolarization of neurons and muscle cells in the presence of Li^+. Whereas Li^+ readily enters these cells through Na^+ channels, contributing to the signal-induced depolarization, it is not a substrate for the Na^+,K^+ pump. Therefore, the cells fail to repolarize properly if a fraction of intracellular Na^+ is replaced by Li^+.

Failure of the Na^+,K^+ pump is also believed to contribute to the neuronal damage resulting from hypoxia, hypoglycemia, and cyanide intoxication. Inasmuch as 70% of the ATP produced in neurons is used to drive the Na^+,K^+ pump; cessation of ATP synthesis causes a cell to become or remain depolarized. The depolarization-induced release of neurotransmitters such as glutamate from such neurons is thought to be responsible for the hypoxic seizures and further amplification of neuronal injury by the neurotoxic actions of glutamate (Patel et al., 1993).

Dysregulation of the Activity of Other Cells   While many signaling mechanisms also operate in nonexcitable cells, disturbance of these processes is usually less consequential. For example, rat liver cells possess alpha$_1$-adrenergic receptors (item 12 in Fig. 3-12) whose activation evokes metabolic changes, such as increased glycogenolysis and glutathione export, through elevation of intracellular Ca^{2+}, which may have toxicologic significance.

Many exocrine secretory cells are controlled by muscarinic acetylcholine receptors (item 11 in Fig. 3-12). Salivation, lacrimation, and bronchial hypersecretion after organophosphate insecticide poisoning are due to stimulation of these receptors. In contrast, blockade of these receptors contributes to the hyperthermia characteristic of atropine poisoning. Kupffer cells, resident macrophages in the liver, secrete inflammatory mediators (see Fig. 3-22) that can harm the neighboring cells. Because Kupffer cells possess glycine receptors, i.e., glycine-gated Cl^- channels (item 4 in Fig. 3-12), the secretory function of these macrophages (e.g., secretion of inflammatory mediators) can be blocked by administration of glycine, which induces hyperpolarization via influx of Cl^-. Such intervention alleviates ethanol-induced liver injury (Yin et al., 1998).

The discovery that some sulfonamides produce hypoglycemia in experimental animals led to the development of oral hypoglycemic agents for diabetic patients. These drugs inhibit K^+ channels in pancreatic beta cells, inducing sequentially depolarization, Ca^{2+} influx through voltage-gated Ca^{2+} channels, and exocytosis of insulin (Hardman et al., 1995). The antihypertensive diazoxide acts in the opposite fashion on K^+ channels and impairs insulin secretion. Whereas this effect is generally undesirable, it is exploited in the treatment of inoperable insulin-secreting pancreatic tumors.

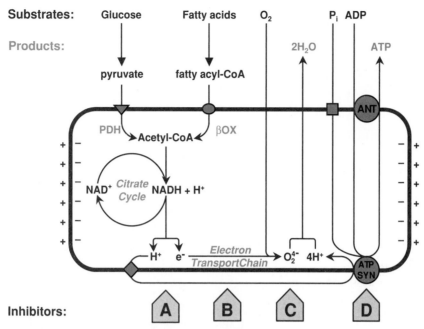

Figure 3-13. ATP synthesis (oxidative phosphorylation) in mitochondria.

Arrows with letters A to D point to the ultimate sites of action of four categories of agents that interfere with oxidative phosphorylation (Table 3-6). For simplicity, this scheme does not indicate the outer mitochondrial membrane and that protons are extruded from the matrix space along the electron transport chain at three sites. βOX = beta-oxidation of fatty acids; e^- = electron; P_i = inorganic phosphate; ANT = adenine nucleotide translocator; ATP SYN = ATP synthase (F_oF_1ATPase).

Toxic Alteration of Cellular Maintenance

Numerous toxicants interfere with cellular maintenance functions. In a multicellular organism, cells must maintain their own structural and functional integrity as well as provide supportive functions for other cells. Execution of these functions may be disrupted by chemicals, resulting in a toxic response.

Impairment of Internal Cellular Maintenance: Mechanisms of Toxic Cell Death   For survival, all cells must synthesize endogenous molecules; assemble macromolecular complexes, membranes, and cell organelles; maintain the intracellular environment; and produce energy for operation. Chemicals that disrupt these functions, especially the energy-producing function of mitochondria and protein synthesis controlling function of the genome, jeopardize survival and may cause toxic cell death.

There are three critical biochemical disorders that chemicals inflicting cell death may initiate, namely, ATP depletion, sustained rise in intracellular Ca^{2+}, and overproduction of ROS and RNS. In the following discussion, these events and the chemicals that may cause them are individually characterized. Then it is pointed out how their concerted action may induce a bioenergetic catastrophe, culminating in necrosis. Finally, there follows a discussion of the circumstances under which the cell can avoid this disordered decay and how it can execute death by activating catabolic processes that bring about an ordered disassembly and removal of the cell, called apoptosis.

Primary Metabolic Disorders Jeopardizing Cell Survival: ATP Depletion, Ca^{2+} Accumulation, ROS/RNS Generation Depletion of ATP   ATP plays a central role in cellular maintenance both as a chemical for biosynthesis and as the major source of energy. It is utilized in numerous biosynthetic reactions, activating endogenous compounds by phosphorylation and adenylation, and is incorporated into cofactors as well as nucleic acids. It is required for muscle contraction and polymerization of the cytoskeleton, fueling cellular motility, cell division, vesicular transport, and the maintenance of cell morphology. ATP drives ion transporters, such as the Na^+,K^+-ATPase in the plasma membrane, the Ca^{2+}-ATPase in the plasma and the endoplasmic reticulum membranes, and H^+-ATPase in the membrane of lysosomes and neurotransmitter-containing vesicles. These pumps maintain conditions essential for various cell functions. For example, the Na^+ concentration gradient across the plasma membrane generated by the Na^+,K^+ pump drives Na^+-glucose and Na^+-amino acid cotransporters as well as the Na^+/Ca^{2+} antiporter, facilitating the entry of these nutrients and the removal of Ca^{2+}.

Chemical energy is released by hydrolysis of ATP to ADP or AMP. The ADP is rephosphorylated in the mitochondria by ATP synthase (Fig. 3-13). Coupled to oxidation of hydrogen to water, this process is termed *oxidative phosphorylation*. In addition to ATP synthase, oxidative phosphorylation requires the (1) delivery of hydrogen in the form of NADH to the initial electron transport complex; (2) delivery of oxygen to the terminal electron transport complex; (3) delivery of ADP and inorganic phosphate to ATP synthase; (4) flux of electrons along the electron transport chain to O_2, accompanied by ejection of protons from the matrix space across the inner membrane; and (5) return of protons across the inner membrane into the matrix space down an electrochemical gradient to drive ATP synthase (Fig. 3-13).

Several chemicals impede these processes, interfering with mitochondrial ATP synthesis (Commandeur and Vermeuien, 1990; Wallace and Starkow, 2000). These chemicals are divided into five groups (Table 3-6). Substances in class A interfere with the delivery of hydrogen to the electron transport chain. For example, fluoroacetate inhibits the citric acid cycle and the production of reduced cofactors. Class B chemicals such as rotenone and cyanide

Table 3.6
Agents Impairing Mitochondrial ATP Synthesis*

A. Inhibitors of hydrogen delivery to the electron transport chain acting on/as
  1. Glycolysis (critical in neurons): hypoglycemia; iodoacetate and NO^+ at GAPDH
  2. Gluconeogenesis (critical in renal tubular cells): coenzyme A depletors (see below)
  3. Fatty acid oxidation (critical in cardiac muscle): hypoglycin, 4-pentenoic acid
  4. Pyruvate dehydrogenase: arsenite, DCVC, p-benzoquinone
  5. Citrate cycle
      (a) Aconitase: fluoroacetate, $ONOO^-$
      (b) Isocitrate dehydrogenase: DCVC
      (c) Succinate dehydrogenase: malonate, DCVC, PCBD-cys, 2-bromohydroquinone, 3-nitropropionic acid, cis-crotonalide fungicides
  6. Depletors of TPP (inhibit TPP-dependent PDH and α-KGDH): ethanol
  7. Depletors of coenzyme A: 4-(dimethylamino)phenol, p-benzoquinone
  8. Depletors of NADH
      (a) See group A.V.1. in Table 3-7
      (b) Activators of poly(ADP-ribose) polymerase: agents causing DNA damage (e.g., MNNG, hydrogen peroxide, $ONOO^-$)
B. Inhibitors of electron transport acting on/as
  1. Inhibitors of electron transport complexes
      (a) NADH–coenzyme Q reductase (complex I): rotenone, amytal, MPP^+, paraquat
      (b) Cycotochrome Q–cytochrome c reductase (complex III): antimycin-A, myxothiazole
      (c) Cytochrome oxidase (complex IV): cyanide, hydrogen sulfide, azide, formate, $^\bullet NO$, phosphine (PH_3)
      (d) Multisite inhibitors: dinitroaniline and diphenylether herbicides, $ONOO^-$
  2. Electron acceptors: CCl_4, doxorubicin, menadione, MPP^+
C. Inhibitors of oxygen delivery to the electron transport chain
  1. Chemicals causing respiratory paralysis: CNS depressants (e.g., opioids), convulsants
  2. Chemicals impairing pulmonary gas exchange: CO_2, "deep pulmonary irritants" (e.g., NO_2, phosgene, perfluoroisobutene)
  3. Chemicals inhibiting oxygenation of Hb: carbon monoxide, methemoglobin-forming chemicals
  4. Chemicals causing ischemia: ergot alkaloids, cocaine
D. Inhibitors of ADP phosphorylation acting on/as
  1. ATP synthase: oligomycin, cyhexatin, DDT, chlordecone
  2. Adenine nucleotide translocator: atractyloside, DDT, free fatty acids, lysophospholipids
  3. Phosphate transporter: N-ethylmaleimide, mersalyl, p-benzoquinone
  4. Chemicals dissipating the mitochondrial membrane potential (uncouplers)
      (a) Cationophores: pentachlorophenol, dinitrophenol-, benzonitrile-, thiadiazole herbicides, salicylate, cationic amphiphilic drugs (amiodarone, perhexiline), valinomycin, gramicidin, calcimycin (A23187)
      (b) Chemicals permeabilizing the mitochondrial inner membrane: PCBD-cys, chlordecone
E. Chemicals causing mitochondrial DNA damage and/or impaired transcription of key mitochondrial proteins
  1. Antiviral drugs: zidovudine, zalcitabine, didanosine, fialuridine
  2. Chloramphenicol (when overdosed)
  3. Ethanol (when chronically consumed)

---

*The ultimate sites of action of these agents are indicated in Fig. 3-13. DCVC = dichlorovinyl-cysteine; GAPDH = glyceraldehyde 3-phosphate dehydrogenase; α-KGDH = α-ketoglutarate dehydrogenase; MNNG = N-methyl-N'-nitro-N-nitrosoguanidine; MPP^+ = 1-methyl-4-phenylpyridinium; PCBD-cys = pentachlorobutadienyl-cysteine; PDH = pyruvate dehydrogenase; TPP = thyamine pyrophosphate

inhibit the transfer of electrons along the electron transport chain to oxygen. Class C agents interfere with oxygen delivery to the terminal electron transporter, cytochrome oxidase. All chemicals that cause hypoxia ultimately act at this site. Chemicals in class D inhibit the activity of ATP synthase, the key enzyme for oxidative phosphorylation. At this site, the synthesis of ATP may be inhibited in one of four ways: (1) direct inhibition of ATP synthase, (2) interference with ADP delivery, (3) interference with inorganic phosphate delivery, and (4) deprivation of ATP synthase from its driving force, the controlled influx of protons into the matrix space. Protonophoric chemicals (uncouplers) such as 2,4-dinitrophenol and pentachlorophenol import protons into the mitochondrial matrix, dissipating the proton gradient that drives the controlled influx of protons into the matrix, which, in turn, drives ATP synthase. Finally, chemicals causing mi-

tochondrial DNA injury, and thereby impairing synthesis of specific proteins encoded by the mitochondrial genome (e.g., subunits of complex I and ATP synthase), are listed in group E. These include the dideoxynucleoside antiviral drugs used against AIDS, such as zidovudine. Table 3-6 lists other chemicals that impair ATP synthesis.

Impairment of oxidative phosphorylation is detrimental to cells because failure of ADP rephosphorylation results in the accumulation of ADP and its breakdown products as well as depletion of ATP. Accordingly, hepatocytes exposed to KCN and iodoacetate exhibit a rapid rise in cytosolic H^+ and Mg^{2+} as a result of the hydrolysis of adenosine di- and triphosphates (existing as Mg salts) and the release of phosphoric acid and Mg^{2+} (Herman *et al.*, 1990). The increased conversion of pyruvate to lactate also may contribute to the acidosis. The lack of ATP compromises the operation of ATP-requiring ion

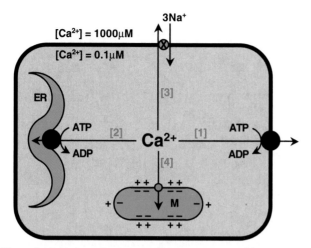

Figure 3-14. Four mechanisms for the elimination of Ca^{2+} from the cytoplasm: Ca^{2+}-ATPase-mediated pumping into (1) the extracellular space as well as (2) the endoplasmic reticulum (ER) and ion-gradient–driven transport into (3) the extracellular space (by the Ca^{2+}/Na^+ exchanger) as well as (4) the mitochondria (M; by the Ca^{2+} uniporter).

Some chemicals that inhibit these mechanisms are listed in Table 3-7, group B.

pumps, leading to the loss of ionic and volume-regulatory controls (Buja *et al.*, 1993). Shortly after intracellular acidosis and hypermagnesemia, liver cells exposed to KCN and iodoacetate exhibit a rise in intracellular Na^+, probably as a result of failure of the Na^+ pump, after which plasma membrane blebs appear. The intracellular phosphoric acidosis is beneficial for the cells presumably because the released phosphoric acid forms insoluble calcium phosphate, preventing the rise of cytosolic Ca^{2+}, with its deleterious conse-

quences (see below). In addition, a low pH also directly decreases the activity of phospholipases and inhibits mitochondrial permeability transition (see later). Terminally, the intracellular pH rises, increasing phospholipase activity, and this contributes to irreversible membrane damage (i.e., rupture of the blebs) not only by degrading phospholipids but also by generating endogenous detergents such as lysophospholipids and free fatty acids. The lack of ATP aggravates this condition because the reacylation of lysophospholipids with fatty acids is impaired.

Sustained Rise of Intracellular Ca^{2+} Intracellular Ca^{2+} levels are highly regulated (Fig. 3-14). The 10,000-fold difference between extracellular and cytosolic Ca^{2+} concentration is maintained by the impermeability of the plasma membrane to Ca^{2+} and by transport mechanisms that remove Ca^{2+} from the cytoplasm (Richter and Kass, 1991). Ca^{2+} is actively pumped from the cytosol across the plasma membrane and is sequestered in the endoplasmic reticulum and mitochondria (Fig. 3-14). Because mitochondria are equipped with a low-affinity Ca^{2+} transporter, they play a significant role in Ca^{2+} sequestration only when the cytoplasmic levels rise into the micromolar range. Under such conditions, a large amount of Ca^{2+} accumulates in the mitochondria, where it is deposited as calcium phosphate.

Toxicants induce elevation of cytoplasmic Ca^{2+} levels by promoting Ca^{2+} influx into or inhibiting Ca^{2+} efflux from the cytoplasm (Table 3-7). Opening of the ligand- or voltage-gated Ca^{2+} channels or damage to the plasma membrane causes Ca^{2+} to move down its concentration gradient from extracellular fluid to the cytoplasm. Toxicants also may increase cytosolic Ca^{2+} by inducing its leakage from the mitochondria or the endoplasmic reticulum. They also may diminish Ca^{2+} efflux through inhibition of Ca^{2+} transporters or depletion of their driving forces. Several chemicals that can cause a sustained rise in cytoplasmic Ca^{2+} levels are listed in Table 3-7.

Table 3.7
Agents Causing Sustained Elevation of Cytosolic Ca^{2+}

A. Chemicals inducing Ca^{2+} influx into the cytoplasm
I.   Via ligand-gated channels in neurons:
   1. Glutamate receptor agonists ("excitotoxins"): glutamate, kainate, domoate
   2. TRPV1 receptor (capsaicin receptor) agonists: capsaicin, resiniferatoxin
II. Via voltage-gated channels: maitotoxin (?), $HO^\bullet$
III. Via "newly formed pores": maitotoxin, amphotericin B, chlordecone, methylmercury, alkyltins
IV. Across disrupted cell membrane:
   1. Detergents: exogenous detergents, lysophospholipids, free fatty acids
   2. Hydrolytic enzymes: phospholipases in snake venoms, endogenous phospholipase A_2
   3. Lipid peroxidants: carbon tetrachloride
   4. Cytoskeletal toxins (by inducing membrane blebbing): cytochalasins, phalloidin
V.   From mitochondria:
   1. Oxidants of intramitochondrial NADH: alloxan, *t*-BHP, NAPBQI, divicine, fatty acid hydroperoxides, menadione, MPP^+
   2. Others: phenylarsine oxide, gliotoxin, $^\bullet NO$, $ONOO^-$
VI. From the endoplasmic reticulum:
   1. IP_3 receptor activators: γ-HCH (lindan), IP_3 formed during "excitotoxicity"
   2. Ryanodine receptor activators: δ-HCH

B. Chemicals inhibiting Ca^{2+} export from the cytoplasm (inhibitors of Ca^{2+}-ATPase in cell membrane and/or endoplasmic reticulum)
I.   Covalent binders: acetaminophen, bromobenzene, CCl_4, chloroform, DCE
II. Thiol oxidants: cystamine (mixed disulfide formation), diamide, *t*-BHP, $O_2^{\bullet-}$ and HOOH generators (e.g., menadione, diquat)
III. Others: vanadate, Cd^{2+}
IV. Chemicals impairing mitochondrial ATP synthesis (see Table 3-6)

KEY: DCE = 1,1-dichloroethylene; *t*-BHP = *t*-butyl hydroperoxide; HCH = hexachlorocyclohexane; MPP^+ = 1-methyl-4-phenylpyridinium; NAPBQI = *N*-acetyl-*p*-benzoquinoneimine.

Sustained elevation of intracellular Ca^{2+} is harmful because it can result in (1) depletion of energy reserves, (2) dysfunction of microfilaments, (3) activation of hydrolytic enzymes, and (4) generation of ROS and RNS. There are at least three mechanisms by which sustained elevations in intracellular Ca^{2+} unfavorably influence the cellular energy balance. First, high cytoplasmic Ca^{2+} concentrations cause increased mitochondrial Ca^{2+} uptake by the Ca^{2+} "uniporter," which, like ATP synthase, utilizes the inside negative mitochondrial membrane potential ($\Delta\Psi m$) as the driving force. Consequently, mitochondrial Ca^{2+} uptake dissipates $\Delta\Psi m$ and inhibits the synthesis of ATP. Moreover, chemicals that oxidize mitochondrial NADH activate a transporter that extrudes Ca^{2+} from the matrix space (Richter and Kass, 1991). The ensuing continuous Ca^{2+} uptake and export ("Ca^{2+} cycling") by the mitochondria further compromise oxidative phosphorylation. Second, Ca^{2+} may also impair ATP synthesis by causing oxidative injury to the inner membrane by mechanisms described later. Third, a sustained rise in cytoplasmic Ca^{2+} not only impairs ATP synthesis but also increases ATP consumption by the Ca^{2+}-ATPases working to eliminate the excess Ca^{2+}.

A second mechanism by which an uncontrolled rise in cytoplasmic Ca^{2+} causes cell injury is microfilamental dissociation (Nicotera *et al.*, 1992; Leist and Nicotera, 1997). The cellwide network of actin filaments maintains cellular morphology by attachment of the filaments to actin-binding proteins in the plasma membrane. An increase of cytoplasmic Ca^{2+} causes dissociation of actin filaments from α-actinin and fodrin, proteins that promote anchoring of the filament to the plasma membrane. This represents a mechanism leading to plasma membrane blebbing, a condition that predisposes the membrane to rupture.

A third event whereby high Ca^{2+} concentrations are deleterious to cells is activation of hydrolytic enzymes that degrade proteins, phospholipids, and nucleic acids (Nicotera *et al.*, 1992; Leist and Nicotera, 1997). Many integral membrane proteins are targets for Ca^{2+}-activated neutral proteases, or calpains (Liu *et al.*, 2004). Calpain-mediated hydrolysis of actin-binding proteins also may cause membrane blebbing. Indiscriminate activation of phospholipases by Ca^{2+} causes membrane breakdown directly and by the generation of detergents. Activation of a Ca^{2+}-Mg^{2+}-dependent endonuclease causes fragmentation of chromatin. Elevated levels of Ca^{2+} can lock topoisomerase II in a form that cleaves but does not religate DNA. In summary, intracellular hypercalcaemia activates several processes that interfere with the ability of cells to maintain their structural and functional integrity. The relative importance of these processes in vivo requires further definition.

Overproduction of ROS and RNS   There are a number of xenobiotics that can directly generate ROS and RNS, such as the redox cyclers (Fig. 3-3) and the transition metals (Fig. 3-4). In addition, overproduction of ROS and RNS can be secondary to the intracellular hypercalcaemia, as Ca^{2+} activates enzymes that generate ROS and/or RNS in the following ways:

1. Activation of the dehydrogenases in the citric acid cycle by Ca^{2+} accelerates the hydrogen output from the citrate cycle and, in turn, the flux of electrons along the electron transport chain (see Fig. 3-13). This, together with the suppressed ATP-synthase activity (owing to the Ca^{2+}-induced uncoupling), increases the formation of $O_2^{\bullet-}$ by the mitochondrial electron transport chain.

2. Ca^{2+}-activated proteases proteolytically convert xanthine dehydrogenase into xanthine oxidase, whose byproducts are $O_2^{\bullet-}$ and HOOH (Harrison, 2002).

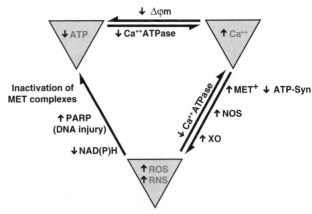

Figure 3-15. Interrelationship between the primary metabolic disorders (ATP depletion, intracellular hypercalcemia, and overproduction of ROS/RNS) that ultimately cause necrosis or apoptosis.

See text for details. ATP-Syn = ATP synthase, MET = mitochondrial electron transport; NOS = nitric oxide synthase; PARP = poly(ADP-ribose) polymerase; ROS = reactive oxygen species; RNS = reactive nitrogen species; XO = xanthine oxidase; $\Delta\psi m$ = mitochondrial membrane potential.

3. Neurons and endothelial cells constitutively express NOS that is activated by Ca^{2+}. Given the extremely high reactivity of $^{\bullet}NO$ with $O_2^{\bullet-}$, co-production of these radicals will inevitably lead to formation of $ONOO^-$, a highly reactive oxidant (Murphy, 1999) (Fig. 3-4). Moreover, $ONOO^-$ can increase its own formation by incapacitating the highly sensitive Mn-SOD, which would eliminate $O_2^{\bullet-}$, a precursor of $ONOO^-$.

Interplay between the Primary Metabolic Disorders Spells Cellular Disaster   The primary derailments in cellular biochemistry discussed above do not remain isolated but interact and amplify each other in a number of ways (Fig. 3-15):

1. Depletion of cellular ATP reserves deprives the endoplasmic and plasma membrane Ca^{2+} pumps of fuel, causing elevation of Ca^{2+} in the cytoplasm. With the influx of Ca^{2+} into the mitochondria, $\Delta\Psi m$ declines, hindering ATP synthase.

2. As stated above, intracellular hypercalcaemia facilitates formation of ROS and RNS, which oxidatively inactivate the thiol-dependent Ca^{2+} pump, which in turn, aggravates the hypercalcaemia.

3. The ROS and RNS can also drain the ATP reserves. $^{\bullet}NO$ is a reversible inhibitor of cytochrome oxidase, NO^+ (nitrosonium cation, a product of $^{\bullet}NO$) S-nitrosylates and thus inactivates glyceraldehyde 3-phosphate dehydrogenase, impairing glycolysis, whereas $ONOO^-$ irreversibly inactivates respiratory chain complexes I, II, III, and aconitase (by reacting with their Fe-S center) (Murphy, 1999). Therefore, $^{\bullet}NO$ and $ONOO^-$ inhibit cellular ATP synthesis.

4. Furthermore, $ONOO^-$ can induce DNA single-strand breaks, which activate poly(ADP-ribose) polymerase (PARP) (Szabó, 1996). As part of the repair strategy, activated PARP transfers multiple ADP-ribose moieties from NAD^+ to nuclear proteins and PARP itself (D'Amours *et al.*, 1999). Consumption of NAD^+ severely compromises ATP synthesis (see Fig. 3-13), whereas resynthesis of NAD^+ consumes ATP. Hence a major

consequence of DNA damage by $ONOO^-$ is a cellular energy deficit (Murphy, 1999).

The chain of events and their contribution to the worsening metabolic conditions are somewhat cell- and toxicant-specific. For example, cyanide toxicity in neurons is associated with depolarization and glutamate release (Patel *et al.*, 1993), followed by Ca^{2+} influx through voltage-gated as well as glutamate-gated channels (see items 8 and 12, respectively, in Fig. 3-12). As they express Ca^{2+}-activated NOS, neurons are also prone to generate "nitrosative stress," which affects not only themselves but perhaps more significantly the neighboring astrocytes (Szabó, 1996). In contrast, in cyanide- and iodoacetate-poisoned liver cells, the increase in cytoplasmic Ca^{2+} is not an early event (Herman *et al.*, 1990). A nitrosative stress critically contributes to propagation of acetaminophen-induced hepatocellular injury, in which the initiating event is covalent binding of N-acetyl-p-benzoquinoneimine (NAPBQI) to mitochondrial proteins (Jaeschke and Bajt, 2006). This purportedly causes a surge in mitochondrial $O_2^{\bullet-}$ generation, followed by in situ formation of $ONOO^-$. Owing to depletion of the protective glutathione by NAPBQI, $ONOO^-$ readily nitrates mitochondrial proteins. Concomitantly, covalent binding incapacitates the plasma membrane Ca^{2+} pump and the resultant hypercalcemia further deteriorates mitochondrial function and ATP production. It appears that in this and many other cytotoxicities the interplay of ATP depletion, intracellular hypercalcemia, and overproduction of ROS and RNS, involving multiple vicious cycles (Fig. 3-15), can progressively aggravate the biochemical disorder until it becomes a disaster.

Mitochondrial Permeability Transition (MPT) and the Worst Outcome: Necrosis   Mitochondrial Ca^{2+} uptake, decreased $\Delta\Psi m$, generation of ROS and RNS, depletion of ATP, and consequences of the primary metabolic disorders (e.g., accumulation of inorganic phosphate, free fatty acids, and lysophosphatides) are all considered as causative factors of an abrupt increase in the mitochondrial inner-membrane permeability, termed MPT. This is thought to be caused by misfolded proteins from the inner and outer membrane, which aggregate and open a proteinaceous pore ("megachannel") that spans both mitochondrial membranes (Kroemer *et al.*, 1998; Kim *et al.*, 2003; Rodriguez-Enriquez *et al.*, 2004). As this pore is permeable to solutes of size <1500 Da, its opening permits free influx into the matrix space of protons, causing rapid and complete dissipation of $\Delta\Psi m$ and cessation of ATP synthesis as well as osmotic influx of water, resulting in mitochondrial swelling. Ca^{2+} that accumulates in the matrix space effluxes through the pore, flooding the cytoplasm. Such mitochondria are not only incapable of synthesizing ATP but even waste the remaining resources because depolarization of the inner membrane forces the ATP synthase to operate in the reverse mode, as an ATPase, hydrolyzing ATP. Then even glycolysis may become compromised by the insufficient ATP supply to the ATP-requiring glycolytic enzymes (hexokinase, phosphofructokinase). A complete bioenergetic catastrophe ensues in the cell if the metabolic disorders evoked by the toxic chemical (such as one listed in Tables 3-6 and 3-7) is so extensive that most or all mitochondria in the cell undergo MPT, causing depletion of cellular ATP (see Fig. 3-17). Degradative processes already outlined (e.g., oxidative and hydrolytic degradation of macromolecules and membranes as well as disintegration of intracellular solute and volume homeostasis) will go to completion, causing a complete failure in maintenance of cellular structure and functions and culminating in cell lysis or necrosis.

An Alternative Outcome of MPT: Apoptosis   Chemicals that adversely affect cellular energy metabolism, Ca^{2+} homeostasis, and redox state and ultimately cause necrosis, may also induce apoptosis, another form of cell demise. Whereas the necrotic cell swells and lyses, the apoptotic cell shrinks; its nuclear and cytoplasmic materials condense, and then it breaks into membrane-bound fragments (apoptotic bodies) that are phagocytosed (Wyllie, 1997).

As discussed above, the multiple metabolic defects that a cell suffers in its way to necrosis are causal yet rather random in sequence. In contrast, the routes to apoptosis are ordered, involving cascade-like activation of catabolic processes that finally disassemble the cell. A scheme of the apoptotic pathways is presented in Fig. 3-16.

It appears that most if not all chemical-induced cell deaths will involve the mitochondria, and the resulting mitochondrial dysfunction (such as Ca^{2+} accumulation, dissipation of $\Delta\Psi m$, and overproduction of ROS/RNS) may ultimately trigger either necrosis or apoptosis, and that MPT can be a crucial event in both. A related event is release into the cytoplasm of cytochrome *c* (cyt *c*), a small positively charged hemeprotein that normally resides in the mitochondrial intermembrane space attached electrostatically to cardiolipin, a specific inner membrane phospholipid with excess negative charge. Peroxidation of cardiolipin results in detachment of cyt *c* from the lipid, which may be a critical first step of cyt *c* release into the cytoplasm (Orrenius, 2004).

The significance of cyt *c* release is twofold (Cai *et al.*, 1998): (1) As cyt *c* is the penultimate link in the mitochondrial electron transport chain, its loss will block ATP synthesis, increase formation of $O_2^{\bullet-}$ (instead of O_2^{4-} as shown in Fig. 3-13), and potentially thrust the cell toward necrosis. (2) Simultaneously, the unleashed cyt *c* (and some other proteins set free from the mitochondria) represents a signal or an initial link in the chain of events directing the cell to the apoptotic path (Cain, 2003) (Fig. 3-16). Cyt *c* together with dATP/ATP induces the cytoplasmic adapter protein Apaf-1 to oligomerize and bind the latent procaspase-9 (forming a complex called apoptosome), facilitating its conversion to active caspase-9.

Caspases are cysteine proteases (that is, they possess a catalytically active cysteine) that cleave proteins after specific aspartate residues. They reside mostly in the cytoplasm in inactive forms, as procaspases, which are activated either by dimerization (initiators) or proteolytic cleavage (effectors) (Boatright *et al.*, 2003). Perhaps in order to guarantee that inadvertent activation of caspases should not occur, inhibitor of apoptosis proteins (IAP), such as XIAP and cIAP, reside in the cytoplasm and physically capture caspases that might have become activated (Cain, 2003). Therefore, cyt *c* alone probably could not induce sufficiently strong caspase activation if it were not for a gang of proteins that physically remove the IAPs from the caspases just being activated. These proteins, named Smac and Omi (or Diablo and HtrA2, respectively), are not only the helpers of cyt *c*, but also residents of the mitochondrial intermembrane space, from where they are jointly mobilized to promote the caspase cascade. Some caspases on the "top" of the cascade, (e.g., 8 and 9) cleave and activate procaspases. Thereby these initiator caspases carry the activation wave to the so-called effector caspases (e.g., 3, 6, and 7), which cleave specific cellular proteins, activating or inactivating them. It is the hydrolysis of these specific proteins that accounts directly or indirectly for the morphologic and biochemical alterations in apoptotic cells. For example, proteolytic inactivation of PARP prevents futile DNA repair and wasting of ATP; hydrolysis of the inhibitor of caspase-activated DNase (ICAD) permits caspase-activated DNase (CAD) to translocate to the nucleus and

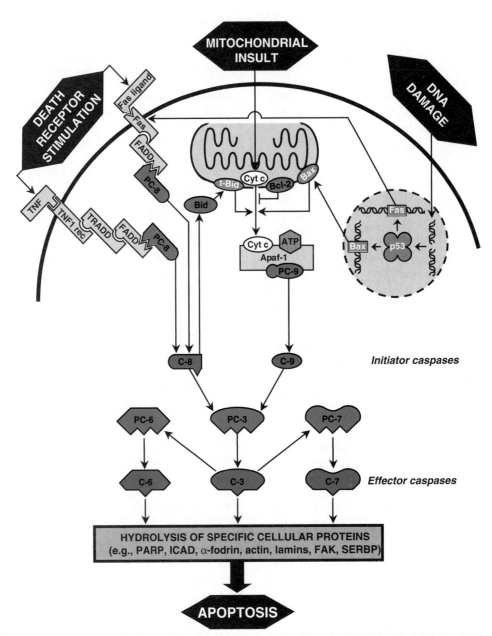

Figure 3-16. Apoptotic pathways initiated by mitochondrial insult, nuclear DNA insult, and Fas or TNF receptor-1 stimulation.

The figure is a simplified scheme of three pathways to apoptosis. (1) Mitochondrial insult (see text) ultimately opens the permeability transition pore spanning both mitochondrial membranes and/or causes release of cytochrome c (Cyt c) and other pro- and antiapoptotic proteins (not shown) from the mitochondria. Cyt c release is facilitated by Bax or truncated Bid (tBid) proteins and opposed by Bcl-2 protein. (2) DNA insult, especially double-strand breaks, activates p53 protein which increases the expression of Bax (that mediates Cyt c release) and the membrane receptor protein Fas. (3) Fas ligand or tumor necrosis factor (TNF) binds to and activates their respective receptor, Fas and TNF1 receptor. These ligand-bound receptors and the released Cyt c interact with specific adapter proteins (i.e., FADD, TRADD and Apaf-1) through which they activate initiator procaspases (PC; e.g., PC-8 and PC-9) to active caspases (C). The latter in turn cleave and activate other proteins e.g., Bid and the main effector procaspase PC-3. The active effector caspase-3 activates other effector procaspases (PC-6, PC-7). Finally, C-3, C-6, and C-7 cleave specific cellular proteins, leading to morphological and biochemical features of apoptosis. These pathways are not equally relevant in all types of cells and other pathways, such as those employing TGF-β as an extracellular signaling molecule, and ceramide as an intracellular signaling molecule, also exist. FAK = focal adhesion kinase; ICAD = inhibitor of caspase-activated DNase; PARP = poly(ADP-ribose) polymerase; SREBP = sterol regulatory element binding protein.

cleave internucleosomal DNA; cleavage of structural proteins (α-fodrin, actin, lamins) aids in disassembly of the cell; incapacitation of focal adhesion kinase (see Fig. 3-11) permits detachment of the cell from the extracellular matrix; and hydrolytic activation of sterol regulatory element-binding proteins may contribute to accumulation of sterols and externalization of phosphatidylserine in the plasma membrane that identify the apoptotic cell to phagocytes. Besides caspases, DNA fragmentation can be induced by apoptosis-inducing factor (AIF) and endonuclease G that are also released from the mitochondrial intermembrane space and may contribute to DNA fragmentation during apoptosis and acetaminophen-induced caspase-independent hepatocellular necrosis (Jaeschke and Bajt, 2006).

The decisive mitochondrial event of cell death, i.e., release of cyt c and other pro-apoptotic proteins (e.g., Smac, AIF), are controlled by the Bcl-2 family of proteins, which includes members that facilitate (e.g., Bax, Bak, Bad, Bid, Puma, Noxa) and those that inhibit (e.g., Bcl-2, Bcl-XL) these processes. The death-promoting members can oligomerize and form pores in the mitochondrial outer membrane. By doing so, they may facilitate release of cyt c and other intermembrane proapoptotic proteins via MPT induced by toxic insult of the mitochondria; however, mitochondrial outer membrane permeabilization (MOMP) alone by Bax and its congeners is sufficient to evoke egress of cyt c from the mitochondria. MOMP induced by Bax, Bak, and/or Bid is responsible for cyt c release in apoptosis initiated at extramitochondrial targets, including death receptors and the nuclear DNA (see below). The death-suppressor Bcl-2 and Bcl-XL can dimerize with the death-inducing counterparts and neutralize them. Thus, the relative amount of these antagonistic proteins functions as a regulatory switch between cell survival and death (Reed et al., 1998).

The proapoptotic Bax and Bid proteins, which can induce MOMP, represent links whereby death programs initiated extramitochondrially, e.g., by DNA damage in the nucleus or by stimulation of the so-called death receptors (Fas receptor and TNF receptor-1) at the cell surface, can engage the mitochondria into the apoptotic process (Green, 1998) (Fig. 3-16). DNA damage (evoked by ionizing and UV radiations, alkylating chemicals, and topoisomerase II inhibitors, such as doxorubicin (Adriamycin)) induces stabilization and activation of p53 protein, a transcription factor, which increases expression of proapoptotic members of the Bcl-family of proteins, such as Bax, Puma and Noxa (Liu and Chen, 2006) (see also Fig. 3-28). As discussed further on, DNA damage is potentially mutagenic and carcinogenic; therefore, apoptosis of cells with damaged DNA is an important self-defense of the body against oncogenesis. Furthermore, the antitumor drugs targeting the nuclear DNA exert their desirable toxic effects against tumor cells (and also their undesirable cytotoxic effects against rapidly dividing normal cells such as hematopoietic cells and small intestinal mucosal cells) by inducing apoptosis primarily via a p53-dependent mechanism.

Stimulation of TNF receptor-1 or Fas receptor by their ligands induces receptor oligomerization and recruitment of adapter proteins to activate the caspase cascade through their initiator procaspase, caspase-8 (Fig. 3-16). Nevertheless, death receptor activation can also engage the mitochondria into the apoptosis program via caspase-8-mediated cleavage of Bid. The Fas system is involved in cell-mediated cytotoxicity, as cytotoxic T lymphocytes express the Fas ligand that activates the Fas receptor in the membrane of potential target cells, such as those of the liver, heart, and lung. Cholestatic liver injury involves apoptosis induced by the retained hydrophobic bile acids mediated partly through their mitochondrial effect (i.e., MPT) and through the death receptors

(Higuchi and Gores, 2003). By activating PKC, toxic bile acids promote trafficking of Fas receptor and TRAIL-receptor-2 (another death receptor) from the Golgi complex into the plasma membrane of liver cells, where the increased receptor density induces spontaneous (i.e., ligand-independent) receptor oligomerization and caspase activation. Increased expression of soluble FasL and Fas receptor is thought to play a causative role in the apoptosis of pulmonary alveolar epithelial cells underlying acute lung injury (or acute respiratory distress syndrome) (Martin et al., 2005), a potentially lethal outcome of various pathologies and heroin intoxication. The Fas system also mediates germ cell apoptosis in the testes of rodents exposed to mono-(2-ethylhexyl)phthalate or 2,5-hexanedione, the ultimate toxicant formed from hexane. These chemicals damage the microtubules in the Sertoli cells that normally nurse the germ cells. Unable to support the germ cells, Sertoli cells overexpress the Fas ligand to limit the number of germ cells (which up-regulate their Fas receptor) by deleting them via apoptosis (Cohen et al., 1997; Lee et al., 1997).

Thus, apoptosis can be executed via multiple pathways, most involving caspase activation. The route preferred will depend, among others, on the initial insult (Fig. 3-16) as well as on the type and state of the cell. For example, T lymphocytes lacking the *Bax* gene can still undergo p53-dependent death in response to ionizing radiation, probably by increasing Fas expression (Fig. 3-16), whereas *Bax*-null fibroblasts cannot.

What Determines the Form of Cell Death? For reasons discussed later, it is not inconsequential for the surrounding tissue whether a cell dies by apoptosis or necrosis. Therefore considerable research has focused on what determines the form of cell death. Interestingly, there are some common features in the process of apoptosis and necrosis. Both forms of cell death caused by cytotoxic agents may involve similar metabolic disturbances and MPT (Kim et al., 2003; Kroemer et al., 1998; Quian et al., 1999), and blockers of the latter (e.g., cyclosporin A, Bcl-2 overexpression) prevent both apoptosis and necrosis in different settings. Furthermore, many xenobiotics—such as the hepatotoxicant 1,1-dichloroethylene, thioacetamide, and cadmium as well as the nephrotoxicant ochratoxin—can cause both apoptosis and necrosis (Corcoran et al., 1994). However, toxicants tend to induce apoptosis at low exposure levels or early after exposure at high levels, whereas they cause necrosis later at high exposure levels. This indicates that the severity of the insult determines the mode of cell death. Based on experimental evidence it appears that larger toxic insults cause necrotic cell death rather than apoptosis because it incapacitates the cell to undergo apoptosis. This incapacitation may result from three causatively related cellular events, i.e., increasing number of mitochondria undergoing MPT, depletion of ATP, and failed activation of caspases or their inactivation.

Lemasters and coworkers (Kim et al., 2003; Rodriguez-Enriquez et al., 2004) used confocal microscopy to visualize mitochondria in cells exposed to an apoptogenic stimulus and found that MPT does not occur uniformly in all mitochondria. They proposed a model in which the number of mitochondria undergoing MPT (which probably depends on the degree of chemical exposure) determines the fate of the cell. According to this model, when only a few mitochondria develop MPT, they are removed by lysosomal autophagy and the cell survives. When more mitochondria suffer MPT, the autophagic mechanism becomes overwhelmed, and the released proapoptotic factors (e.g., cyt c, Smac, AIF) initiate caspase activation and apoptosis (Fig. 3-16). When MPT involves virtually all mitochondria, cytolysis occurs. Figure 3-17 illustrates an expanded version of this model.

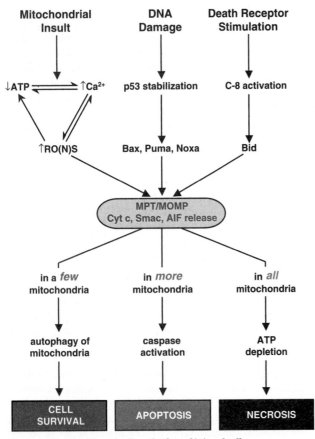

Figure 3-17. "Decision plan" on the fate of injured cell.

See the text for details. MOMP = mitochondrial outer membrane permeabilization; MPT = mitochondrial permeability transition; Puma = p53-up-
regulated modulator of apoptosis; RO(N)S = reactive oxygen or nitrogen
species.

For reasons discussed above, ATP is bound to become severely
depleted in cells in which most mitochondria suffer MPT. The degree of ATP depletion may decide the fate of the cell. In experimental
models as distinct as Ca^{2+}-exposed hepatocytes, Fas-stimulated T
lymphocytes, and HOOH-exposed endothelial cells, necrosis occurs
instead of apoptosis when cells are depleted of ATP, whereas apoptosis takes place rather than necrosis when ATP depletion is alleviated
by providing substrates for ATP generation (Leist *et al.*, 1997; Kim
et al., 2003; Lelli *et al.*, 1998). Lack of ATP can prevent execution
of the apoptotic program, because apoptosis involves ATP-requiring
steps, such as activation of procaspase-9 in the apoptosome complex
(Fig. 3-16).

Failure of caspase activation can also result from direct action
of reactive toxicants on these enzymes. The active site of caspases
is composed of a pentapeptide (QACXG) with a reactive cysteine
in it. At high concentrations, soft electrophiles, disulfides (e.g., glutathione disulfide) and oxidants (e.g., ROS), can react with this
cysteine, causing caspase inactivation and ablation of the apoptotic program, with necrosis rather than apoptosis as the final outcome. Such a scenario has been demonstrated for cell death evoked
by tributyltin, pyrrolidine dithiocarbamate, and arsenic trioxide
(Orrenius, 2004) and might also underlie the acetaminophen-
induced hepatocellular necrosis, which involves cyt *c* release with
no caspase activation or apoptosis (Jaeschke and Bajt, 2006).

Induction of Cell Death by Unknown Mechanisms   In addition to
chemicals that ultimately injure mitochondria by disrupting oxidative phosphorylation and/or control of intracellular Ca^{2+}, there are
toxicants that cause cell death by affecting other functions or structures primarily. Included here are (1) chemicals that directly damage the plasma membrane, such as lipid solvents, detergents, and
venom-derived hydrolytic enzymes; (2) xenobiotics that damage the
lysosomal membrane, such as aminoglycoside antibiotics and hydrocarbons binding to α_{2u}-globulin; (3) toxins that destroy the
cytoskeleton, such as the microfilamental toxins phalloidin and
cytochalasins, and the microtubular toxins colchicine and 2,5-
hexanedione; (4) the protein phosphatase inhibitor hepatotoxicant
microcystin, which causes hyperphosphorylation of microfilaments
and other cellular proteins (Toivola and Eriksson, 1999); (5) toxins
that disrupt protein synthesis, such as α-amanitin and ricin; and (6)
cholesterol lowering drugs (statins) that inhibit HMG-coenzyme A
reductase, the rate limiting enzyme in the mevalonate pathway, and
rarely cause myotoxicity.

The events leading to cell death after exposure to these chemicals are generally unknown. It is likely that cell death caused by
these chemicals is ultimately mediated by impairment of oxidative
phosphorylation, sustained elevation of intracellular Ca^{2+}, and/or
overproduction of ROS/RNS, and that it takes the form of necrosis
if these processes are abrupt, but apoptosis if they are protracted.
For example, direct injury of the plasma membrane would lead
rapidly to increased intracellular Ca^{2+} levels. Neurofilamental toxins that block axonal transport cause energy depletion in the distal
axonal segment. HMG-coenzyme A reductase inhibitors diminish
not only the synthesis of cholesterol, but may also compromise formation of other products of the mevalonate pathway. Such are the
mitochondrial electron transporting molecule ubiquinone (also
called coenzyme Q) and isopentenyl pyrophosphate, which is utilized for isopentenylation of selenocysteinyl-tRNA, an obligatory
step for synthesis of selenoproteins, including the antioxidant glutathione peroxidase (see Fig. 3-5) and thioredoxin reductase (see
Fig. 3-19). These alterations may contribute to statin-induced myopathy and rhabdomyolysis.

Impairment of External Cellular Maintenance   Toxicants also
may interfere with cells that are specialized to provide support to
other cells, tissues, or the whole organism. Chemicals acting on the
liver illustrate this type of toxicity. Hepatocytes produce and release
into the circulation a number of proteins and nutrients. They remove
cholesterol and bilirubin from the circulation, converting them into
bile acids and bilirubin glucuronides, respectively, for subsequent
excretion into bile. Interruption of these processes may be harmful
to the organism, the liver, or both. For example, inhibition of hepatic synthesis of coagulation factors by coumarins does not harm the
liver, but may cause death by hemorrhage (Hardman *et al.*, 1995).
This is the mechanism of the rodenticidal action of warfarin. In the
fasting state, inhibitors of hepatic gluconeogenesis, such as hypoglycin, may be lethal by limiting the supply of glucose to the brain.
Similarly, Reye's syndrome, which is viewed as a hepatic mitochondrial injury caused by a combination of a viral disease (which may
induce hepatic NOS) and intake of salicylate (which provokes MPT)
(Fromenty and Pessayre, 1997; Kim *et al.*, 2003), causes not only
hepatocellular injury but also severe metabolic disturbances (hypoglycemia, hyperammonemia) that affect other organs as well. Chemical interference with the β-oxidation of fatty acids or the synthesis,
assembly, and secretion of lipoproteins overloads the hepatocytes

with lipids, causing hepatic dysfunction (Fromenty and Pessayre, 1997). α-Naphthylisothiocyanate causes separation of the intercellular tight junctions that seal bile canaliculi (Krell *et al.*, 1987), impairing biliary secretion and leading to the retention of bile acids and bilirubin; this adversely affects the liver as well as the entire organism.

STEP 4—INAPPROPRIATE REPAIR AND ADAPTATION

The fourth step in the development of toxicity is inappropriate repair and adaptation (Fig. 3-1). As noted previously, many toxicants alter macromolecules, which eventually cause damage at higher levels of the biological hierarchy in the organism. Progression of toxic lesions can be intercepted by repair mechanisms operating at molecular, cellular, and tissue levels (Fig. 3-18). Another strategy whereby the organism can resist the noxious chemical is by increasing its own readiness to cope with it and with its harmful effects. This phenomenon is called adaptation. Because the capacity of the organism to repair itself and adapt to the toxic exposure and effects is so important in determining the outcome of chemical exposure, the mechanisms of repair and adaptation will be discussed below.

Mechanisms of Repair

Molecular Repair Damaged molecules may be repaired in different ways. Some chemical alterations, such as oxidation of protein thiols and methylation of DNA, are simply reversed. Hydrolytic removal of the molecule's damaged unit or units and insertion of a newly synthesized unit or units often occur with chemically altered DNA and peroxidized lipids. In some instances, the damaged molecule is totally degraded and resynthesized. This process is time-consuming but unavoidable in cases such as the regeneration of cholinesterase after organophosphate intoxication.

Repair of Proteins Thiol groups are essential for the function of numerous proteins, such as receptors, enzymes, cytoskeletal proteins, and TFs. Oxidation of protein thiols (Prot-SHs) to protein disulfides (Prot-SS, $Prot_1$-SS-$Prot_2$), protein-glutathione mixed disulfides (Prot-SSG), and protein sulfenic acids (Prot-SOH) as well

as oxidation of methionine in proteins to methionine sulfoxide can be reversed by enzymatic reduction (Watson *et al.*, 2004; Gravina and Mieyal, 1993; Moskovitz, 2005) (Fig. 3-19). The endogenous reductants are thioredoxins and glutaredoxins, small, ubiquitous proteins with two redox-active cysteines in their active centers (Holmgren *et al.*, 2006). These proteins as well as thioredoxin-reductase have two isoenzymes; those labeled 1 are located in the cytosol, whereas 2 are mitochondrial. Because the catalytic thiol groups in these proteins become oxidized, they are reduced by NADPH, which is generated by $NADP^+$-dependent isocitrate dehydrogenase localized in various cell compartments (cytosol, mitochondria, peroxysomes), as well as by the cytosolic glucose-6-phosphate dehydrogenase and 6-phosphogluconate dehydrogenase in the pentose phosphate pathway. Repair of oxidized hemoglobin (methemoglobin) occurs by means of electron transfer from cytochrome b_5, which is then regenerated by a NADH-dependent cytochrome b_5 reductase (also called methemoglobin reductase).

Soluble intracellular proteins are susceptible to denaturation (misfolding) and aggregation by physical or chemical insults. Molecular chaperones such as the heat-shock proteins can rescue denatured proteins by ATP-dependent disaggregation and refolding, or by engaging the chaperone-dependent ubiquitin ligase CHIP, assist in their degradation by proteasomes (Lee and Tsai, 2005). Proteasomes are large ATP-consuming protease complexes in the cytosol that not only control the level of regulatory proteins (e.g., p53, IκB, Nrf2, cyclins), but also have a predominant role in eliminating oxidized, misfolded, or otherwise damaged intracellular proteins (Poppek and Grune, 2006). For example, CYP2E1, in which the heme becomes cross-linked to the protein as a consequence of reductive dechlorination of CCl_4 to the trichloromethyl free radical by this enzyme, is eliminated by proteosomal degradation. Damaged proteins are first conjugated with ubiquitin in an ATP-dependent manner, allowing their recognition by the proteosome that degrades them. Damaged proteins can be eliminated also by proteolysis in lysosomes. For example, lysosomal proteases degrade the immunogenic trifluoroacylated proteins that are formed in the liver during halothane anesthesia (Cohen *et al.*, 1997). Damaged proteins enter lysosomes by autophagy, i.e., ATP-demanding enclosure into membrane vesicles (autophagosomes) that fuse with lysosomes (Meijer and Codogno, 2004). Erythrocytes have

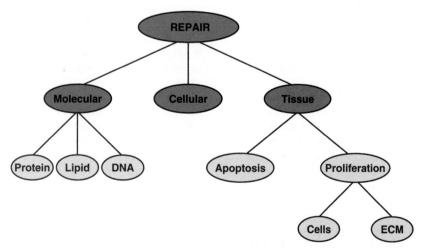

Figure 3-18. Repair mechanisms.

Dysfunction of these mechanisms results in dysrepair, the fourth step in the development of numerous toxic injuries. ECM = extracellular matrix.

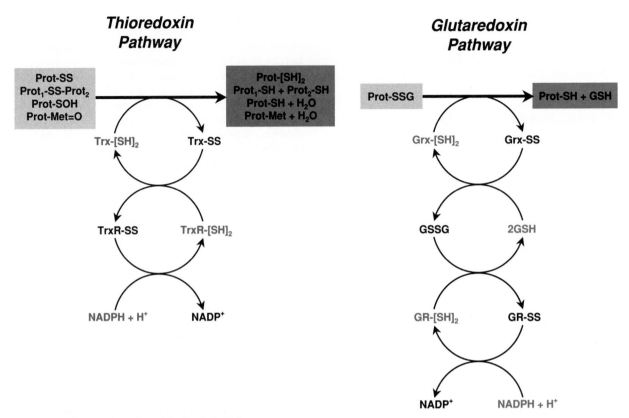

Figure 3-19. Repair of proteins oxidized at their thiol groups.

Protein disulfides (Prot-SS, $Prot_1$-SS-$Prot_2$), protein sulfenic acids (Prot-SOH) and protein methionine sulfoxides (Prot-Met=O) are reduced by thioredoxin (Trx-[SH]$_2$) with methionine sulfoxide reductases catalyzing the latter process. Protein-glutathione mixed disulfides (Prot-SSG) are reduced by glutaredoxin (Grx-[SH]$_2$), which is also called thioltransferase. The figure also indicates how Trx-[SH]$_2$ and Grx-[SH]$_2$ are regenerated from their disulfides (Trx-SS and Grx-SS, respectively). In the mitochondria, Trx-SS also can be regenerated by the dithiol dihydrolipoic acid, a component of the pyruvate- and α-ketoglutarate dehydrogenase complexes. GSH = glutathione; GSSG = glutathione disulfide; GR-[SH]$_2$ and GR-SS = glutathione reductase (dithiol and disulfide forms, respectively); TrxR-[SH]$_2$ and Trx-SS = thioredoxin-reductase (dithiol and disulfide forms, respectively).

ATP-independent, nonlysosomal proteolytic enzymes that rapidly and selectively degrade proteins denatured by HO$^\bullet$ (Davies, 1987). Removal of damaged and aggregated proteins is especially critical in the eye lens for maintenance of its transparency.

Repair of Lipids   Peroxidized lipids are repaired by a complex process that operates in concert with a series of reductants as well as with glutathione peroxidase and reductase (Fig. 3-20). Phospholipids containing fatty acid hydroperoxides are preferentially hydrolyzed by phospholipase A2, with the peroxidized fatty acids replaced by normal fatty acids (van Kuijk *et al.*, 1987). Again, NADPH is needed to "repair" the reductants that are oxidized in the process.

Repair of DNA   Despite its high reactivity with electrophiles and free radicals, nuclear DNA is remarkably stable, in part because it is packaged in chromatin and because several repair mechanisms are available to correct alterations. The mitochondrial DNA, however, lacks histones and efficient repair mechanisms and therefore is more prone to damage. Different types of damages are corrected by specialized mechanisms, each employing a different set of repair proteins (Christmann *et al.*, 2003).

Direct Repair   Certain covalent DNA modifications are directly reversed by enzymes such as DNA photolyase, which cleaves adjacent pyrimidines dimerized by UV light. Inasmuch as this chromophore-equipped enzyme uses the energy of visible light to correct damage, its use is restricted to light-exposed cells.

Minor adducts, such as methyl groups, attached to DNA bases by alkylating agents (e.g., methylmethane sulfonate) may be removed by special enzymes (Christmann *et al.*, 2003). Such groups attached to the O^6 position of guanine are cleaved off by O^6-methyguanine-DNA-methyltransferase (MGMT). While repairing the DNA, this alkyltransferase sacrifices itself, transferring the adduct onto one of its cysteine residues. This results in its inactivation, ubiquitination, and proteosomal degradation. Thus, like glutathione, which is depleted during detoxication of electrophiles, MGMT is consumed during the repair of DNA. Methyl groups attached to N^1 of adenine and guanine, and N^3 of thymine and cytosine are removed by oxidative demethylation catalyzed by DNA dioxygenases (ABH2 and ABH3). These peculiar O_2, Fe^{2+}, ascorbate, and 2-oxoglutarate dependent enzymes oxygenate the methyl group adduct, which in turn leaves as formaldehyde, while 2-oxoglutarate is oxidatively decarboxylated to succinate.

Excision Repair   Base excision and nucleotide excision are two mechanisms for removing damaged bases from DNA (see

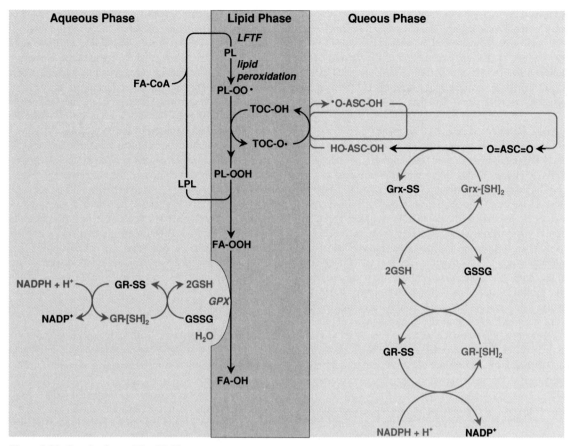

Figure 3-20. Repair of peroxidized lipids.

Phospholipid peroxyl radicals (PL-OO$^\bullet$) formed as a result of lipid peroxidation (Fig. 3-9) may abstract hydrogen from alpha-tocopherol (TOC-OH) and yield phospholipid hydroperoxide (PL-OOH). From the latter, the fatty acid carrying the hydroperoxide group is eliminated via hydrolysis catalyzed by phospholipase (PLase), yielding a fatty acid hydroperoxide (FA-OOH) and a lysophospholipid (LPL). The former is reduced to a hydroxy-fatty acid (FA-OH) by glutathione peroxidase (GPX), utilizing glutathione (GSH), or by peroxiredoxins (not shown), whereas the latter is reacylated to phospholipid (PL) by lysophosphatide fatty acyl-coenzyme A transferase (LFTF), utilizing long-chain fatty acid-coenzyme A (FA-CoA). The figure also indicates regeneration of TOC-OH by ascorbic acid (HO-ASC-OH), regeneration of ascorbic acid from dehydroascorbic acid (O=ASC=O) by glutaredoxin (Grx-[SH]$_2$), and reduction of the oxidized glutaredoxin (Grx-SS) by GSH. Oxidized glutathione (GSSG) is reduced by glutathione reductase (GR-[SH]$_2$), which is regenerated from its oxidized form (GR-SS) by NADPH, the ultimate reductant. NADPH is produced by NADP$^+$-dependent isocitrate dehydrogenases and during metabolism of glucose via the pentose phosphate shunt. TOC-O$^\bullet$ = tocopheroxyl radical; $^\bullet$O-ASC-OH = ascorbyl radical.

Chaps. 8 and 9). Lesions that do not cause major distortion of the helix typically are removed by base excision, in which the altered base is recognized by a relatively substrate-specific DNA-glycosylase that hydrolyzes the N-glycosidic bond, releasing the modified base and creating an apurinic or apyrimidinic (AP) site in the DNA. For example, 8-hydroxyguanine (8-OH-Gua), a major mutagenic product of oxidative stress, is removed from the DNA by specific 8-OH-Gua DNA glycosylase. The AP site is recognized by the AP endonuclease, which hydrolyzes the phosphodiester bond adjacent to the abasic site. After its removal, the abasic sugar is replaced with the correct nucleotide by a DNA polymerase and is sealed in place by a DNA ligase. Interestingly, AP endonuclease is a bifunctional protein and is also called redox factor-1 (Ref-1). In concert with thioredoxin and thioredoxin-reductase, it maintains transcription factors with sensitive thiol groups in their DNA-binding domain (Fos, Jun, NF-κB) in an active reduced state (Hansen *et al.*, 2006).

Bulky lesions such as adducts produced by aflatoxins or aminofluorene derivatives and dimers caused by UV radiation are removed by nucleotide-excision repair, which employs approximately 30 proteins (Christmann *et al.*, 2003). Lesions in the non-transcribed strands or the non-transcribed regions of the genome are corrected by the global genomic repair system. This involves proteins that recognize the distorted double helix at the lesion, unwind the DNA, excise a number of intact nucleotides on both sides of the lesion together with the one containing the adduct. The excised section of the strand is restored by insertion of nucleotides into the gap by DNA polymerase and ligase, using the complementary strand as a template. Lesions in the transcribed DNA strand blocking the RNA polymerase in the actively transcribed genes are removed by another variation of nucleotide excision repair, the transcription-coupled repair system. This involves assembly of repair proteins to remove the stalled RNA polymerase before excision of the damage and filling the gap. Resynthesis of the removed section of the strand is designated "unscheduled DNA synthesis" and can be detected by the appearance of altered deoxynucleosides in urine. Excision repair has a remarkably low error rate of less than 1 mistake in 10^9 bases repaired.

Poly(ADP-ribose)polymerase (PARP) appears to be an important contributor in excision repair. Upon base damage or single-strand break, PARP binds to the injured DNA and becomes activated. The active PARP cleaves NAD^+ to use the ADP-ribose moiety of this cofactor for attaching long chains of polymeric ADP-ribose to nuclear proteins, such as histones. Because one ADP-ribose unit contains two negative charges, the poly(ADPribosyl)ated proteins accrue negativity and the resultant electrorepulsive force between the negatively charged proteins and DNA causes decondensation of the chromatin structure. It is hypothesized that PARP-mediated opening of the tightly packed chromatin allows the repair enzymes to access the broken DNA and fix it. Thereafter, poly(ADP-ribose) glycohydrolase gains access to the nucleus from its perinuclear localization and reverses the PARP-mediated modification of nuclear proteins (D'Amours *et al.*, 1999). Other features of PARP that are relevant in toxicity—such as destruction of PARP by caspases during apoptosis as well as the significance of NAD^+ (and consequently ATP) wasting by PARP in necrosis—have been discussed earlier in this chapter.

Recombinational (or Postreplication) Repair   Recombinational repair occurs when the excision of a bulky adduct or an intrastrand pyrimidine dimer fails to occur before DNA replication begins. At replication, such a lesion prevents DNA polymerase from polymerizing a daughter strand along a sizable stretch of the parent strand that carries the damage. The replication results in two homologous ("sister") yet dissimilar DNA duplexes; one has a large postreplication gap in its daughter strand and an intact duplex synthesized at the opposite leg of the replication fork. This intact sister duplex is utilized to complete the postreplication gap in the damaged sister duplex. This is accomplished by recombination ("crossover") of the appropriate strands of the two homologous duplexes. After separation, the sister duplex that originally contained the gap carries in its daughter strand a section originating from the parent strand of the intact sister, which in turn carries in its parent strand a section originating from the daughter strand of the damaged sister. This strand recombination explains the phenomenon of "sister chromatid exchange," which is indicative of DNA damage corrected by recombinational repair. This process also repairs double breaks, which can also be repaired by the so-called DNA nonhomologous end-joining system that ligates DNA ends and employs several proteins including DNA-dependent protein kinase. A combination of excision and recombinational repairs occurs in restoration of DNA with interstrand cross-links.

Cellular Repair: A Strategy in Peripheral Neurons   Repair of damaged cells is not a widely applied strategy in overcoming cellular injuries. In most tissues, injured cells die, with the survivors dividing to replace the lost cells. A notable exception is nerve tissue, because mature neurons have lost their ability to multiply. In peripheral neurons with axonal damage, repair does occur and requires macrophages and Schwann cells. Macrophages remove debris by phagocytosis and produce cytokines and growth factors, which activate Schwann cells to proliferate and transdifferentiate from myelinating operation mode into a growth-supporting mode. Schwann cells play an indispensable role in promoting axonal regeneration by increasing their synthesis of cell adhesion molecules (e.g., N-CAM), by elaborating extracellular matrix proteins for base membrane construction, and by producing an array of neurotrophic factors (e.g., nerve growth factor, glial–cell line–derived growth factor) and their receptors (Fu and Gordon, 1997). While comigrating with the regrowing axon, Schwann cells physically guide as well as chemically lure the axon to reinnervate the target cell.

In the mammalian central nervous system, axonal regrowth is prevented by growth inhibitory glycoproteins (e.g., NI 35, myelin-associated glycoprotein) and chondroitin sulfate proteoglycans produced by the oligodendrocytes and by the scar produced by astrocytes (Johnson, 1993). Thus, damage to central neurons is irreversible but is compensated for in part by the large number of reserve nerve cells that can take over the functions of lost neurons. For example, in Parkinson's disease, symptoms are not observed until there is at least an 80% loss of nigrostriatal neurons.

Tissue Repair   In tissues with cells capable of multiplying, damage is reversed by deletion of the injured cells and regeneration of the tissue by proliferation. The damaged cells are eliminated by apoptosis or necrosis.

Apoptosis: An Active Deletion of Damaged Cells   Apoptosis initiated by cell injury can be regarded as tissue repair for two reasons, the first of which is that it may intercept the process leading to necrosis, as discussed earlier (see Fig. 3-17). Necrosis is a more harmful sequel than apoptosis for the tissue in which the injured cell resides. A cell destined for apoptosis shrinks; its nuclear and cytoplasmic materials condense, and then it breaks into membrane-bound fragments (apoptotic bodies) that are phagocytosed (Bursch *et al.*, 1992). During necrosis, cells and intracellular organelles swell and disintegrate with membrane lysis. Whereas apoptosis is orderly, necrosis is a disorderly process that ends with cell debris in the extracellular environment. The constituents of the necrotic cells attract aggressive inflammatory cells, and the ensuing inflammation amplifies cell injury (see further on). With apoptosis, dead cells are removed without inflammation. Second, apoptosis may intercept the process leading to neoplasia by eliminating the cells with potentially mutagenic DNA damage. This function of apoptosis is discussed in more detail in the final section of this chapter.

It must be emphasized, however, that apoptosis of damaged cells has a full value as a tissue repair process only for tissues that are made up of constantly renewing cells (e.g., the bone marrow, the respiratory and gastrointestinal epithelium, and the epidermis of the skin), or of conditionally dividing cells (e.g., hepatic and renal parenchymal cells), because in these tissues the apoptotic cells are readily replaced. The value of apoptosis as a tissue repair strategy is markedly lessened in organs containing nonreplicating and nonreplaceable cells, such as the neurons, cardiac muscle cells, and female germ cells, because deletion of such cells, if extensive, can cause a deficit in the organ's function. Apoptosis in the pulmonary alveolar epithelium, an extremely tight barrier, could cause flooding of the alveolar space with interstitial fluid, a potentially lethal outcome.

Proliferation: Regeneration of Tissue   Tissues are composed of various cells and the extracellular matrix. Tissue elements are anchored to each other by transmembrane proteins. Cadherins allow adjacent cells to adhere to one another, whereas connexins connect neighboring cells internally by associating these proteins into tubular structures (gap junctions). Integrins link cells to the extracellular matrix. Therefore, repair of injured tissues involves not only regeneration of lost cells and the extracellular matrix but also reintegration of the newly formed elements. In parenchymal organs such as liver, kidney, and lung, various types of cells are involved in the process of tissue restoration. Nonparenchymal cells of mesenchymal origin residing in the tissue, such as resident macrophages and endothelial cells, and those migrating to the site of injury, such as blood monocytes, produce factors that stimulate parenchymal cells to divide and stimulate some specialized cells (e.g., the stellate cells in the liver) to synthesize extracellular matrix molecules.

Replacement of Lost Cells by Mitosis   Soon after injury, cells adjacent to the damaged area enter the cell division cycle (Fig. 3-21). Enhanced DNA synthesis is detected experimentally as an increase in the labeling index, which is the proportion of cells that incorporate administered ^{3}H-thymidine or bromodeoxyuridine into their nuclear DNA during the S phase of the cycle. Also, mitotic cells can be observed microscopically. As early as 2 to 4 hours after administration of a low dose of carbon tetrachloride to rats, the mitotic index in the liver increases dramatically, indicating that cells already in the G_2 phase progress rapidly to the M phase. The mitotic activity of the hepatocytes culminates at 36 to 48 hours, after a full transit through the cycle, indicating that quiescent cells residing in G_0 enter and progress to mitosis (M). Peak mitosis of nonparenchymal cells occurs later, after activation and replication of parenchymal cells. In some tissues, such as intestinal mucosa and bone marrow, stem cells first divide to provide self-renewal and then differentiate to replace more mature cells lost through injury. Stem cell-derived cells, called oval cells, are also located in the liver, in the bile ductules. In severe toxic liver injury, when hepatocyte replication is impaired (e.g., in rats dosed with galactosamine or acetylaminofluorene, and in humans intoxicated with acetaminophen), the oval cells proliferate and differentiate into both hepatocytes and biliary epithelial cells (Fausto *et al.*, 2006; Vessey and Hall, 2001). As these cells produce α-fetoprotein, the level of serum α-fetoprotein correlates with improved outcome of acetaminophen-induced injury. In an ozone-exposed lung, the nonciliated Clara cells and type II pneumocytes undergo mitosis and terminal differentiation to replace, respectively, the damaged ciliated bronchial epithelial cells and type I pneumocytes (Mustafa, 1990).

Sequential changes in gene expression occur in the cells that are destined to divide. In rats subjected to partial hepatectomy to study the regeneration of the liver, oligonucleotide microarray analysis revealed that more than 150 genes involved in the early gene response with up or down-regulation (Su *et al.*, 2002). The overexpressed genes include those that code for transcription factors important in proliferative signaling, such as c-*fos*, c-*jun*, *Egr1*, and c-*myc* (see Fig. 3-11), the genes of the antiapoptotic protein Bcl-X_L (see Fig. 3-16), and that of the cell cycle accelerator protein mdm2 (see Fig. 3-27). Interestingly, some genes whose products decelerate the cell cycle also become temporarily overexpressed (e.g., the cyclin dependent kinase inhibitor p21 and gadd45; see Fig. 3-27), suggesting that this duality keeps tissue regeneration precisely regulated. Nevertheless, the genetic expression is apparently reprogrammed so that DNA synthesis and mitosis gain priority over specialized cellular activities. For example, as a result of dedifferentiation, regenerating hepatocytes underexpress cytochrome P450, N-acetyltransferase-2 as well as PPARα, and hepatic stellate cells cease to accumulate fat and vitamin A.

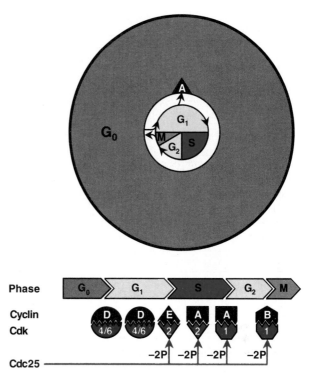

Figure 3-21. The cell division cycle and the participating cyclins and cyclin-dependent protein kinases.

Areas representing phases of the cycle are meant to be proportional to the number of cells in each phase. Normally, most cells are in G_0 phase, a differentiated and quiescent state. After receiving signals to divide, they progress into the G_1 phase of the cell division cycle. G_0/G_1 transition involves activation of immediate early genes so that cells acquire replicative competence. Now increasingly responsive to growth factors, these cells progress to the phase of DNA synthesis (S). If this progression is blocked (e.g., by the accumulated p53 protein), the cells may undergo apoptosis (A). After DNA replication, the cells prepare further for mitosis in the G_2 phase. Mitosis (M) is the shortest phase of the cell cycle (approximately 40 min out of the 40-h-long cycle of hepatocytes) and most likely requires the largest energy expenditure per unit of time. The daughter cells produced may differentiate and enter into the pool of quiescent cells (G_0), substituting for those which had been lost. During the cycle, the levels of various cyclins temporarily surge by synthesis and degradation (see figure). These proteins bind to and activate specific cyclin-dependent protein kinases (Cdk, see figure), which, in turn, phosphorylate and thus activate enzymes and other proteins required for DNA replication and cell division (Johnson and Walker, 1999) (see Fig. 3-27). In addition to cyclines, phosphorylation also regulate the activity of Cdks: phosphorylation by Wee1 protein kinase inactivates Cdk 1 and Cdk 2, whereas dephosphorylation by cdc25 phosphatases activates them. After tissue necrosis, the number of cells entering the cell division cycle markedly increases at areas adjacent to the injury. The proportion of cells that are in S phase in a given period is reflected by the labeling index, whereas the percentage of cells under going mitosis is the mitotic index (see text).

It has been speculated that the regenerative process is initiated by the release of chemical mediators from damaged cells. The nonparenchymal cells, such as resident macrophages and endothelial cells, are receptive to these chemical signals and produce a host of secondary signaling molecules, cytokines, and growth factors that promote and propagate the regenerative process (Fig. 3-22). In rodents subjected to partial hepatectomy the initial or priming phase of liver regeneration is controlled by the cytokines TNF-α and IL-6, whose hepatic mRNA and serum levels increase. TNF-α originates

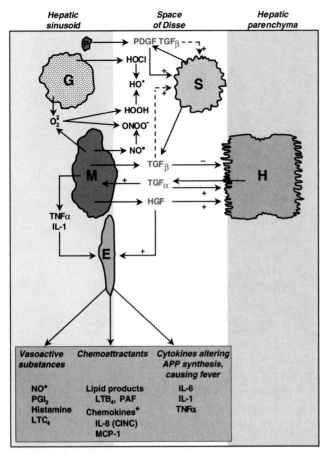

Figure 3-22. Mediators of tissue repair and side reactions to tissue injury in liver: (1) growth factors promoting replacement of cells and the extracellular matrix; (2) mediators of inflammation, acute-phase protein AAP synthesis, and fever; and (3) cytotoxic mediators of inflammatory cells.

HGF = hepatocyte growth factor; PDGR = platelet-derived growth factor; TGF-α = transforming growth factor-alpha, TGF-β = transforming growth factor-beta; NO$^\bullet$ = nitric oxide; PGI$_2$ = prostacyclin; LTC$_4$ = leukotriene C$_4$; IL = interleukin; LTB$_4$ = leukotriene B$_4$; PAF = platelet-activating factor; CINC (the rat homolog of IL-8) = cytokine-induced neutrophil chemoattractant; MCP-1 = monocyte chemotactic protein; TNF = tumor necrosis factor. Cells presented are E = endothelial cells; G = granulocyte; H = hepatocyte; M = macrophage (Kupffer cell); S = stellate cell (also called perisinusoidal, Ito or fat-storing cell). *Rather than the endothelial cells, other stromal cells are the main sources of chemokines (e.g., stellate cells for MCP-1). Solid arrows represent effects of growth factors on cell division, whereas the dashed arrow shows the effect on extracellular matrix formation. Positive and negative signs indicate stimulation and inhibition, respectively. See text for further details.

from the Kupffer cells. This cytokine acts on these macrophages in an autocrine manner, activating its receptor (item 2 in Fig. 3-11) and the coupled signal transducing network. This in turn causes activation of NF-κB, which increases IL-6 expression. The secreted IL-6 then acts on the hepatocytes and through its receptor (item 1 in Fig. 3-11) activates JAK (Janus kinase) and induces transcription factors (e.g., Stat3, C/EBPβ), which activate several target genes. This cytokine network promotes transition of the quiescent liver cells (G$_0$) into cell cycle (G$_1$) and makes them receptive to growth factors ("priming"). Growth factors, especially the hepatocyte growth factor (HGF), transforming growth factor-α (TGF-α), and heparin-binding epidermal growth factor-like growth factor

(HB-EGF), initiate the progression of the "primed" cells in the cycle toward mitosis (Costa *et al.*, 2003; Fausto *et al.*, 2006). Despite its name, neither the formation nor the action of HGF is restricted to the liver. It is produced by resident macrophages and endothelial cells of various organs—including liver, lung, and kidney—and in a paracrine manner activates receptors on neighboring parenchymal cells (Fig. 3-22). In rats intoxicated with carbon tetrachloride, the synthesis of HGF in hepatic and renal nonparenchymal cells increases markedly (Noji *et al.*, 1990) and HGF levels in blood rise rapidly (Lindroos *et al.*, 1991). The communication between parenchymal and nonparenchymal cells during tissue repair is mutual. For example, TGF-α, a potent mitogen produced by regenerating hepatocytes, acts both as an autocrine and a paracrine mediator on liver cells as well as on adjacent nonparenchymal cells (Fig. 3-22). By activating their receptors (item 4 in Fig. 3-11), these growth factors initiate signaling through the MAPK pathway and the PI3K – Akt pathway (Fig. 3-11), thereby mediate activation of transcription factors (c-Jun, c-Fos, c-Myc, FoxM1B, NF-κB, Stat3). These among others, induce cyclins and the protein phosphatase cdc25, two groups of short-lived regulatory proteins. Then cyclins activate Cdks by associating with them (Figs. 3-21), whereas cdc25 activates Cdk1 and Cdk2 by dephosphorylating their two amino-acid residues (Thr14 and Tyr15). The activated Cdks accelerate the cell cycle mainly by phosphorylation of pRb. This in turn releases the transcription factor E2F, which induces enzymes and regulatory proteins needed for cell cycle progression (Fig. 3-27). The growth factor signaling also activates mTOR (mammalian target of rapamycin) which up-regulates mRNA translation, thereby meeting the demand for increased protein synthesis (see Fig. 3-25). Similar signaling appears to mediate regeneration of the *S*-(1,2-dichlorovinyl)-L-cysteine-injured kidney that exhibits increased expression of the cytokine IL-6, the growth factors TGF-α and HB-EGF, the growth factor receptors EGFR (also receptor for TGF-α) and IGF-1R, and the MAP kinase isoform Erk1 (Vaidya *et al.*, 2003).

Although the cytokine- and growth factor-controlled mitotic cell replacement is likely an essential part in the repair of most tissues built up of cells with proliferative capacity, there are also tissue specific features of tissue repair. For example in the liver, bile acids also stimulate hepatocyte proliferation through their nuclear receptor, FXR (Huang *et al.*, 2006). In mice subjected to partial hepatectomy, liver regrowth is hastened by bile acid feeding, but is markedly delayed when FXR is deleted or recirculation of bile acids from the intestine to the liver is prevented. Epithelia composed of a single cell layer form important barriers; therefore replacement of mortally injured epithelial cells, which become detached from the basement membrane, is an urgent need. This can be achieved more rapidly by cell migration than by mitotic cell replacement. For example, in the damaged mucosa of the gastrointestinal tract, cells of the residual epithelium rapidly migrate to the site of injury as well as elongate and thin to reestablish the continuity of the surface even before this could be achieved by cell replication. Cell movement involves orderly dissociation of cadherin-mediated cell-cell contacts (involving β-catenin phosphorylation) and integrin-mediated cell-ECM contacts at focal adhesions (involving FAK phosphorylation), assembly of actin stress fibers, and formation of lamellopodia (cell projection filled with F-actin meshwork). Mucosal repair is dictated not only by growth factors and cytokines operative in tissue repair elsewhere but also by trefoil factors (TFF). TFFs are small (7–12 kDa) protease-resistant proteins that are abundantly secreted from specific mucosal cells (e.g., intestinal goblet cells) and are associated with the mucous layer of the gastrointestinal tract (Taupin and Podolsky, 2003). TFF expression is rapidly up-regulated at the margins of mucosal injury by cytokine and growth factor signaling. Whereas growth factors (e.g., HGF and EGF) exert both motogenic (motility-increasing) and mitogenic effects on enterocytes, TFFs are potent motogens, but are not mitogens. Although TFFs do not act alone, they are the only peptides shown to be essential for restitution of the injured intestinal mucosa. Normal mice exposed to dextran sodium sulfate in the drinking water develop diffuse colonic mucosal injury some exhibiting bloody diarrhea. In contrast, the majority of TFF3-null mice develop frank bloody diarrhea and die in response to dextran sodium sulfate. The immediate target molecule (e.g., receptor) for TFFs remains unknown. Migration of the surviving cells also precedes mitotic cell replacement in the tubular epithelium of the injured kidney. It appears that extracellular matrix components, such as collagen IV, beneath the tubular epithelial cells aid in the restitution of the injured epithelium and reestablishment of its polarity (Nony and Schnellmann, 2003).

Replacement of the Extracellular Matrix   The extracellular matrix is composed of proteins, glycosaminoglycans, and the glycoprotein and proteoglycan glycoconjugates (Gressner, 1992). In liver, these molecules are synthesized by stellate or fat storing cells located in the space of Disse, between the hepatic sinusoid and the hepatocytes (Fig. 3-22). The stellate cells become activated during liver regeneration, undergoing mitosis and major phenotypic changes. The latter changes include not only increased synthesis and secretion of extracellular matrix constituents, but also expression of α-smooth muscle actin and loss of fat, vitamin A and PPARγ content. Thus, resting stellate cells become transdifferentiated into myofibroblast-like contractile and secretory cells. Activation of stellate cells is mediated chiefly by two growth factors—platelet-derived growth factor (PDGF) and transforming growth factor-β (TGF-β) (Fig. 3-22). Both may be released from platelets (that accumulate and degranulate at sites of injury) and later from the activated stellate cells themselves. The main sources of TGF-β, however, are the neighboring tissue macrophages residing in the hepatic sinusoids (Gressner, 1992). A dramatic increase in TGF-β mRNA levels in Kupffer cells is observed with in situ hybridization after carbon tetrachloride-induced hepatic necrosis. Proliferation of stellate cells is induced by the potent mitogen PDGF, whereas TGF-β acts on the stellate cells to induce their transdifferentiation and to stimulate the synthesis of extracellular matrix components, including collagens, fibronectin, tenascin, and proteoglycans. TGF-β acts through its Ser/Thr kinase receptor (item 8 in Fig. 3-11), which phosphorylates the transcription factors Smad2 and 3 (Flanders, 2004). TGF-β also plays a central role in extracellular matrix formation in other tissues. In kidney and lung, for example, TGF-β targets the mesangial cells and the septal fibroblasts, respectively. Remodeling of the extracellular matrix is aided by matrix metalloproteinases, which hydrolyse specific components of the matrix, as well as by tissue inhibitors of matrix metalloproteinases. The former group of these proteins originates from various types of nonparenchymal cells, including inflammatory cells; however, their inhibitors are mainly produced by stellate cells (Arthur *et al.*, 1999).

The way in which tissue regeneration is terminated after repair is unclear, but the gradual dominance of TGF-β, which is a potent antimitogen and apoptogen, over mitogens is a contributing factor in the termination of cell proliferation. Extracellular matrix production may be halted by an intracellular negative feedback mechanism in the ECM producing cells, i.e., by induction of Smad7 (an inhibitory Smad), which competitively inhibits phosphorylation of the receptor-activated Smads (Smad2 and 3). In addition, extracel-

lular products of the proliferative response, such as the proteoglycan decorin and the positive acute phase protein alpha$_2$-macroglobulin, can bind and inactivate TGF-β, thereby they may contribute to its silencing (Gressner, 1992).

Side Reactions to Tissue Injury   In addition to mediators that aid in the replacement of lost cells and the extracellular matrix, resident macrophages and endothelial cells activated by cell injury also produce other mediators that induce ancillary reactions with uncertain benefit or harm to tissues (Fig. 3-22). Such reactions include inflammation, altered production of acute-phase proteins, and generalized reactions such as fever.

Inflammation-Leukocyte Invasion   Alteration of the microcirculation and accumulation of inflammatory cells are the hallmarks of inflammation. These processes are largely initiated by resident macrophages secreting cytokines, such as TNF-α and interleukin-1 (IL-1), in response to tissue damage (Baumann and Gauldie, 1994) (Fig. 3-22). These cytokines, in turn, stimulate neighboring stromal cells, such as the endothelial cells and fibroblasts, to release mediators that induce dilation of the local microvasculature and cause permeabilization of capillaries. Activated endothelial cells also facilitate the egress of circulating leukocytes into the injured tissue by releasing chemoattractants and expressing cell-adhesion molecules, which are cell surface glycoproteins (Jaeschke, 1997). One group of cell-adhesion molecules, called selectins, located on the membrane of endothelial cells, interact with their ligands on the surface of leukocytes, thereby slowing down the flow of these cells and causing them to "roll" on the capillary surface. Subsequently a stronger interaction (adhesion) is established between the endothelial cells and leukocytes with participation of intercellular adhesion molecules (e.g., ICAM-1) expressed on the endothelial cell membrane and integrins expressed on the membrane of leukocytes. This interaction is also essential for the subsequent transendothelial migration of leukocytes. This is facilitated by gradients of chemoattractants that induce expression of leukocyte integrins. Chemoattractants originate from various stromal cells and include chemotactic cytokines (or chemokines), such as the monocyte chemotactic protein-1 (MCP-1) and IL-8 (whose rat homolog is the cytokine-induced neutrophil chemoattractant or CINC), as well as lipid-derived compounds, such as platelet-activating factor (PAF) and leukotriene B$_4$ (LTB$_4$). Ultimately all types of cells in the vicinity of injury express ICAM-1, thus promoting leukocyte invasion; the invading leukocytes also synthesize mediators, thus propagating the inflammatory response. Production of most inflammatory mediators is induced by signaling, turned on by TNF-α and IL-1, which results in activation of transcription factors, notably NF-κB and C/EBP (Poli, 1998) (see Fig. 3-11). Genes of many of the proteins mentioned above (e.g., selectins, ICAM-1, MCP-1, IL-8) and below (e.g., inducible nitric oxide synthase, acute phase proteins) as well as the genes of TNF-α and IL-1 themselves contain binding sites for the NF-κB (Lee and Burckart, 1998).

Inflammation-ROS and RNS Production   Macrophages, as well as leukocytes, recruited to the site of injury undergo a respiratory burst, discharging free radicals and enzymes (Weiss and LoBuglio, 1982) (Fig. 3-22). Free radicals are produced in the inflamed tissue in three ways, each of which involves a specific enzyme: NADPH oxidase (Nox), nitric oxide synthase, or myeloperoxidase.

Nox is an electron-transporting protein complex composed of two transmembrane proteins (one of them the FAD- and heme-containing catalytic subunit) and four cytoplasmic proteins (including the G-protein Rac) (El-Benna *et al.*, 2005). In resting cells Nox is dormant, however, in activated cells the cytoplasmic subunits become extensively phosphorylated and move to the membrane to assemble the Nox complex. Constituents of microorganisms, such as the bacterial lipopolysaccharide (LPS; the active endotoxin component of Gram negative bacteria), acting through the cell surface Toll-like receptors (TLR), and PKC activators, such phorbol miristate acetate (PMA), may evoke Nox activation. Unlike in nonphagocytic cells, in macrophages and granulocytes activation causes a sudden and rapid electron transfer from NADPH through the FAD and heme in Nox to the molecular oxygen, releasing the thus formed superoxide anion radical ($O_2^{\bullet-}$) in a burst ("respiratory burst") at the external membrane surface into the phagocytic vacuole:

$$NADPH + 2O_2 \rightarrow NADP^+ + H^+ + 2O_2^{\bullet-}$$

The $O_2^{\bullet-}$ can give rise to the hydroxyl radical ($HO^{\bullet}$) in two sequential steps: The first is spontaneous or is catalyzed by superoxide dismutase, and the second, the Fenton reaction, is catalyzed by transition metal ions (see also Fig. 3-4):

$$2O_2^{\bullet-} + 2H^+ \rightarrow O_2 + HOOH$$

$$HOOH + Fe^{2+} \rightarrow Fe^{3+} + HO^- + HO^{\bullet}$$

Macrophages, but not granulocytes, generate another cytotoxic free radical, nitric oxide ($^{\bullet}NO$). This radical is produced from arginine by nitric oxide synthase (Wang *et al.*, 1993), which is inducible in macrophages by bacterial endotoxin and the cytokines IL-1 and TNF:

$$\text{L-arginine} + O_2 \rightarrow \text{L-citrulline} + {}^{\bullet}NO$$

Subsequently, $O_2^{\bullet-}$ and $^{\bullet}NO$, both of which are products of activated macrophages, can react with each other, yielding peroxynitrite anion; upon reaction with carbon dioxide, this decays into two radicals, nitrogen dioxide and carbonate anion radical (Fig. 3-4):

$$O_2^{\bullet-} + {}^{\bullet}NO \rightarrow ONOO^-$$

$$ONOO^- + CO_2 \rightarrow ONOOCO_2^-$$

$$ONOOCO_2^- \rightarrow {}^{\bullet}NO_2 + CO_3^{\bullet-}$$

Granulocytes, but not macrophages, discharge the lysosomal enzyme myeloperoxidase into engulfed extracellular spaces, the phagocytic vacuoles (Wang *et al.*, 1993). Myeloperoxidase catalyzes the formation of hypochlorous acid (HOCl), a powerful oxidizing agent, from hydrogen peroxide (HOOH) and chloride ion:

$$HOOH + H^+ + Cl^- \rightarrow HOH + HOCl$$

Like HOOH, HOCl can form $HO^{\bullet}$ as a result of electron transfer from Fe^{2+} or from $O_2^{\bullet-}$ to HOCl:

$$HOCl + O_2^{\bullet-} \rightarrow O_2 + Cl^- + HO^{\bullet}$$

All these reactive chemicals, as well as the discharged lysosomal proteases, are destructive products of inflammatory cells. Although these chemicals exert antimicrobial activity at the site of microbial invasion, at the site of toxic injury they can damage the adjacent healthy tissues and thus contribute to propagation of tissue injury (see "Tissue Necrosis," below). Moreover, in some chemically induced injuries, inflammation plays the leading role. For example, α-naphthyl-isothiocyanate (ANIT), a cholestatic chemical, causes neutrophil-dependent hepatocellular damage. ANIT apparently acts on bile duct epithelial cells, causing them to release chemoattractants for neutrophil cells, which upon invading the liver, injure hepatocytes (Hill *et al.*, 1999). Kupffer cell activation, TNF-α release, and subsequent inflammation are also prominent and causative events in galactosamine-induced liver injury in rats (Stachlewitz *et al.*, 1999).

Whereas it is well recognized that chemical-inflicted tissue injury can induce inflammation as a side reaction of tissue repair, it is becoming clear that inflammation (even if harmless alone) can precipitate an overt tissue injury upon chemical exposure that is noninjurious alone. For example, a small harmless dose of the macrophage activator LPS converts nontoxic doses of monocrotaline, aflatoxin B$_1$ and allyl alcohol into ones that are markedly hepatotoxic (Roth *et al.*, 2003). Moreover, in rats pretreated with LPS, unlike in untreated animals, chlorpromazine, ranitidine and trovafloxacin caused liver injury. These drugs (and many others) when given to patients can induce rare, unexpected and not obviously dose-related liver injury. Therefore, it is hypothesized that such idiosyncratic drug reactions develop when some endotoxin exposure decreases the threshold for drug toxicity by priming the Kupffer cells that produce ROS and inflammatory mediators discussed above. Manifest or subclinical infection, gastrointestinal disturbance or alcohol consumption (which greatly increases the intestinal permeability for endotoxin) may be the source of endotoxin. It is not surprising that most idiosyncratic drug reactions affect the liver, because this organ contains 80–90% of the body's fixed macrophages (i.e., Kupffer cells), because the liver is the first organ to be exposed to LPS translocating from the intestinal lumen, and because the Kupffer cells are not only activated by LPS but also remove it from the circulation, thereby protecting other organs from its inflammatory effects (Roth *et al.*, 2003). However, the causative relationship between inflammation and idiosyncrasy needs further substantiation.

Altered Protein Synthesis: Acute-Phase Proteins Cytokines released from macrophages and endothelial cells of injured tissues also alter protein synthesis, predominantly in the liver (Baumann and Gauldie, 1994) (Fig. 3-18). Mainly IL-6 but also IL-1 and TNF act on cell surface receptors and increase or decrease the transcriptional activity of genes encoding certain proteins called positive and negative acute-phase proteins, respectively, utilizing primarily the transcription factors NF-κB, C/EBP, and STAT (Poli, 1998; see Fig. 3-12). Many of the hepatic acute-phase proteins, such as C-reactive protein, are secreted into the circulation, and their elevated levels in serum are diagnostic of tissue injury, inflammation, or neoplasm. Increased sedimentation of red blood cells, which is also indicative of these conditions, is due to enrichment of blood plasma with positive acute-phase proteins such as fibrinogen.

Apart from their diagnostic value, positive acute-phase proteins may play roles in minimizing tissue injury and facilitating repair. For example, many of them, such as alpha$_2$-macroglobulin and alpha$_1$-antiprotease, inhibit lysosomal proteases released from the injured cells and recruited leukocytes. Haptoglobin binds hemoglobin in blood, metallothionein complexes metals in the cells, heme oxygenase oxidizes heme to biliverdin, and opsonins facilitate phagocytosis. Thus, these positive acute-phase proteins may be involved in the clearance of substances released upon tissue injury.

Negative acute-phase proteins include some plasma proteins, such as albumin, transthyretin, and transferrin, as well as hepatic enzymes (e.g., several forms cytochrome P450 and glutathione *S*-transferase), ligand-activated transcription factors (e.g., PPARα and the bile acid receptor FXR), and transporters, such as bile acid transporters at the sinusoidal and canalicular membrane of hepatocytes (Ntcp and Bsep, respectively) and the bile canalicular export pump Mrp2. Because the latter enzymes and transporters play important roles in the toxication, detoxication and excretion of endo- and xenobiotics, the disposition and toxicity of bile acids and toxicants may be altered markedly during the acute phase of tissue injury.

Although the acute-phase response is phylogenetically preserved, some of the acute-phase proteins are somewhat species-specific. For example, during the acute phase of tissue injury or inflammation, C-reactive protein and serum amyloid A levels dramatically increase in humans but not in rats, whereas the concentrations of alpha$_1$-acid glycoprotein and alpha$_2$-macroglobulin increase markedly in rats but only moderately in humans.

Generalized Reactions Cytokines released from activated macrophages and endothelial cells at the site of injury also may evoke neurohumoral responses. Thus IL-1, TNF, and IL-6 alter the temperature set point of the hypothalamus, triggering fever. IL-1 possibly also mediates other generalized reactions to tissue injury, such as hypophagia, sleep, and "sickness behavior" (Rothwell, 1991). In addition, IL-1 and IL-6 act on the pituitary to induce the release of ACTH, which in turn stimulates the secretion of cortisol from the adrenals. This represents a negative feedback loop because corticosteroids inhibit cytokine gene expression.

Mechanisms of Adaptation

Adaptation may be defined as a noxa-induced capability of the organism for increased tolerance to the noxa itself. It involves responses acting to preserve or regain the biological homeostasis in the face of increased harm. Theoretically, adaptation to toxicity may result from biological changes causing (1) diminished delivery of the causative chemical(s) to the target, (2) decreased size or susceptibility of the target, (3) increased capacity of the organism to repair itself, and (4) strengthened mechanisms to compensate the toxicant-inflicted dysfunction. Mechanistically, adaptation involves sensing the noxious chemical and/or the initial damage or dysfunction, and a response that typically occurs through altered gene expression. Such mechanisms will be briefly overviewed below.

Adaptation by Decreasing Delivery to the Target The first step in the development of toxicity is delivery of the ultimate toxicant (a xenobiotic, its metabolite or xenobiotic-generated ROS and RNS) to the target (Fig. 3-2). Certain chemicals induce adaptive changes that lessen their delivery by diminishing the absorption, increasing their sequestration by intracellular binding proteins, enhancing their detoxication, or promoting their cellular export.

Repression of Iron Absorption An adaptive mechanism affecting absorption is induced by iron whose uptake from the intestinal lumen into the enterocyte is mediated by the divalent metal transporter 1 (DMT1). High iron intake diminishes the expression of DMT1 in the apical membrane of enterocytes, whereas low intake has the opposite effect. This regulation occurs at the translational level by the intracellular iron-regulatory proteins (IRP). IRP1 contains a [4Fe-4S] cluster that, when in this form, prevents its binding to mRNA. Iron deficiency causes loss of Fe from the cluster, allowing the thus formed IRP1 apoprotein to bind to the DMT1 mRNA. This protects the mRNA from enzymatic degradation, thereby increasing its level and allowing more DMT1 protein to be translated. Conversely, iron overload saturates IRP1 with Fe, making it incapable of binding to and stabilizing the DMT1 mRNA. The conse-

quential loss of DMT1 mRNA and protein then markedly limits Fe^{2+} absorption. This adaptive mechanism has utmost physiological importance in maintenance of iron homeostasis. Its toxicological relevance is that DMT1 also mediates the transport of Cd^{2+}, therefore DMT1 overexpression in iron deficiency increases intestinal absorption of this highly toxic metal ion (Park *et al.*, 2002).

Induction of Ferritin and Metallothionein Adaptive cellular accumulation of the binding proteins ferritin and metallothionein (MT) is protective against their respective ligands, iron and cadmium ions. Interestingly, up-regulation of ferritin by iron overload, like down-regulation of DMT1, is also translationally mediated by IRP1. However, the apoIRP1 (that is formed in iron deficiency) acts oppositely on ferritin mRNA and blocks its translation. Iron overload relieves this blockade, as it yields IPR1 with the [4Fe-4S] cluster, which does not bind to the ferritin mRNA, thus causing a surge in ferritin translation. Ferritin is protective as it removes iron from the Fenton reaction (Fig. 3-4).

MT is greatly induced by cadmium and elevated levels of MT protect the liver by restricting distribution of this toxic metal ion to sensitive intracellular targets (Klaassen *et al.*, 1999). Induction of MT by Cd^{2+} is likely indirect; mediated by Zn (displaced from intracellular binding sites), which activates the metal-responsive transcription factor 1 (MTF-1) that in turn augments transcription of the MT gene by binding to the metal-responsive elements in its promoter (Lichtlen and Schaffner, 2001).

Induction of Detoxication—The Electrophile Response, Part 1 Adaptive increases in detoxication (i.e., elimination of xenobiotics, their reactive metabolites, harmful endobiotics, or ROS and RNS by biotransformation) and cellular export have a major role in limiting toxicity. Such adaptation is typically induced by compounds with thiol reactivity (i.e., soft electrophiles, oxidants and those generating oxidative stress), which are sensed by the cytosolic Keap1-Nrf2 protein complex. The response is initiated by the transcription factor Nrf2, which activates genes with electrophile-response element (EpRE) in their regulatory region (Fig. 3-23; Dinkova-Kostova *et al.*, 2005). Normally Nrf2 is retained in the cytoplasm by Keap1, a homodimeric protein with ubiquitin ligase activity. Keap1 keeps Nrf2 inactive and at low intracellular levels by targeting it for proteosomal degradation by ubiquitination. Upon disruption of the Keap1-Nrf2 complex, the active Nrf2 escapes rapid degradation and accumulates in the cell. Electrophiles, such as quinones (e.g., *t*-butylquinone), qinoneimines (e.g., derived from acetaminophen), quinone methides (e.g., metabolite of butylated hydroxytoluene), α, β-unsaturated aldehydes and ketones (e.g., the lipid peroxidation products 4-oxonon-2-enal, 4-hydroxynon-2-enal and 15-A_{2t}-isoprostane), isothiocyanates (e.g., α-naphthylisothiocyanate), thiol-reactive metal ions (e.g., Cd^{2+}), and trivalent arsenicals, as well as direct and indirect oxidants (e.g., HOOH, diquat, quinones) may attack Keap1 at its reactive cysteine thiol groups by binding to them covalently or oxidizing them, thereby forcing Keap1 to release Nrf2. Alternatively, Nrf2 release may be induced via phosphorylation of Keap1 by kinases, such as PKC and those in the MAPK and the PI3K-Akt signaling pathways (Fig. 3-11) that may be turned on by chemical stresses (Jaiswal, 2004). After being released from Keap1, Nrf2 translocates into the nucleus, forms a heterodimer with small Maf proteins, and activates genes through binding to EpREs.

There are many genes with EpRE motifs that encode proteins known to be important in detoxication and export (Fig. 3-23). These include genes that code for (1) enzymes that detoxify xenobiotics (e.g., NQO1, NQO2, AR, GST, UGT), (2) enzymes that eliminate $O_2^{\bullet-}$ and HOOH (e.g., SOD1, GPX2, catalase), (3) proteins that detoxify

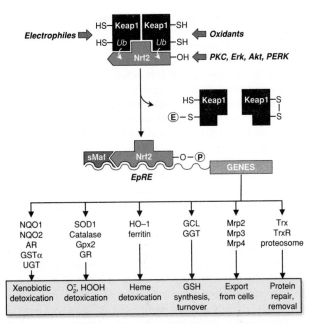

Figure 3-23. Signaling by Keap1/Nrf2 mediates the electrophile response.

Normally Nrf2 (NF-E2-related factor 2) is kept inactive and at a low intracellular level by interacting with Keap1 which promotes its proteosomal degradation by ubiquitination. Electrophiles covalently bind to, whereas oxidants oxidize the reactive thiol groups of Keap1, causing Keap1 to release Nrf2. Alternatively, Nrf2 release may follow phosphorylation of Keap1 by protein kinases. After being released from Keap1, the active Nrf2 accumulates in the cell, translocates into the nucleus and forms a heterodimer with small Maf proteins to activate genes that contain electrophile response element (EpRE) in their promoter region. These include enzymes, binding proteins, and transporters functioning in detoxication and elimination of xenobiotics, ROS, and endogenous reactive chemicals, as well as some proteins that can repair or eliminate oxidized proteins. Induction of such proteins represents an electrophile-stress response that provides protection against a wide range of toxicants. Abbreviations: AR, aldose reductase; G6PDH, glucose 6-phosphate dehydrogenase; GCL, glutamate-cysteine ligase; GGT, gamma-glutamyl transpeptidase; GPX2, glutathione peroxidase 2; GR, glutathione reductase; GSTα, glutathione S-transferase α subunit; HO-1, heme oxygenase 1; NQO1, NAD(P)H:quinone oxidoreductase; NQO2, NRH:quinone oxidoreductase; 2; Mrp2, Mrp3 and Mrp4, multidrug-resistance protein 2, 3 and 4; SOD1, superoxide dismutase 1; UGT, UDP-glucuronosyltransferase; SOD1, superoxide dismutase 1; Trx, thioredoxin; TrxR, thioredoxin reductase.

heme (e.g., HO-1, ferritin), (4) enzymes involved in the synthesis and regeneration of GSH (e.g., GCL and the NADPH-forming G6PDH), and (5) transporters (e.g., Mrp2, 3 and 4) that pump xenobiotics and their metabolites out of cells. Other Nrf2-induced proteins of known toxicological relevance will be mentioned later.

As demonstrated in Fig. 3-24, these Nrf2-mediated adaptive changes facilitate elimination and detoxication of electrophilic chemicals, as well as ROS that may be generated by them, and assist in repairing or removing damaged proteins (to be discussed later); therefore Nrf2 conveys protection against a wide range of toxicants. Indeed, Nrf2 knockout mice are more sensitive to the hepatotoxicity of acetaminophen, the pulmonary toxicity of butylated hydroxytoluene, hyperoxia, or cigarette smoke, the neurotoxicity of 3-nitropropionic acid, and the carcinogenicity of benzo[a]pyrene (Dinkova-Kostova et al., 2005). Conversely, liver specific deletion of Keap1 constitutively activates Nrf2 in hepatocytes, causing

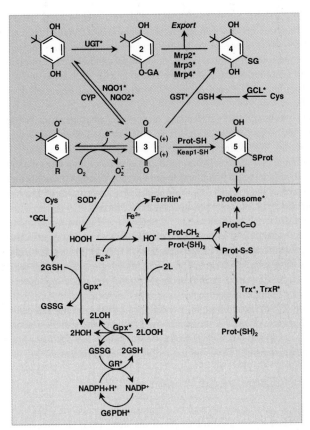

Figure 3-24. Adaptive changes in response to the t-butylhydroquinone (tBHQ)-induced electrophile stress that influence the metabolic fate and some effects of (tBHQ) and of superoxide anion radical generated in the course of tBHQ biotransformation.

This figure illustrates the numerous proteins (i.e., enzymes, exporters, repair proteins), which when induced in response to the tBHQ-induced electrophile stress, facilitates the detoxication and export of tBHQ and/or its metabolites, the detoxication of ROS formed during the biotransformation of tBHQ, and repair or removal of proteins damaged by the reactive metabolites. Proteins induced by Nrf2 as a result of adaptation to the electrophile stress are marked with an asterisk.

tBHQ (1) can be detoxified by UDP-glucuronosyltransferase to form tBHQ-glucuronide (2) and toxified by cytochrome P450-catalyzed dehydrogenation to t-butylquinone (tBQ; 3), which contains electrophilic carbon atoms (+), and is believed to be the actual inducer of electrophile stress response. tBQ can undergo three biotransformations. First, it can be detoxified by conjugation with glutathione (GSH) to form tBHQ-SG (4), which together with tBHQ-glucuronide, are exported from the cell by Mrp 2, 3 and 4. Secondly, tBQ can covalently bind to SH groups in proteins (5), including Keap1. Thirdly, by accepting an electron (e), tBQ can form t-butylsemiquinone radical (6), which can pass the electron to molecular oxygen to form superoxide anion radical ($O_2^{\bullet}$), completing a redox cycle. In a process catalyzed by superoxide dismutase (SOD), $O_2^{\bullet}$ can form HOOH, which is detoxified by GSH-peroxidase (GPX), using GSH (whose synthesis is rate-limited by GCL), or toxified by Fe^{2+}-catalyzed Fenton reaction to form hydroxyl radical ($HO^{\bullet}$). $HO^{\bullet}$ can react with proteins to form oxidized proteins (Prot-C=O, Prot-S-S), which can be degraded in the proteosome, or Prot-S-S can also be repaired through reduction by the thioredoxin (Trx) – thioredoxin reductase (TrxR) system. $HO^{\bullet}$ can also react with lipid (L) and form lipid hydroperoxide (LOOH), which can be reduced to lipid alcohol (LOH) by GPX at the expense of GSH. This results in formation of glutathione disulfide (GSSG), which can be reduced back to GSH by glutathione reductase (GR) at the expense of NADPH generated by glucose-6-phosphate dehydrogenase (G6PDH). Virtually all of these processes become more effective after the electrophile stress response.

them to overexpress many detoxifying enzymes and become resistant to acetaminophen-induced hepatotoxicity. Nrf2 can be activated by treatment with several chemicals of low toxicity, such as t-butyl hydroquinone (tBHQ), butylated hydroxyanisole (BHA), sulforaphane (an isothiocyanate in broccoli) and oltipraz (a dithiolenethione compound whose metabolites can form mixed disulfides with thiols, probably also with those on Keap1). These chemicals induce Nrf2 target genes and protect from toxicant-induced tissue injury and cancer. Of these chemopreventive agents, some (e.g., tBHQ and BHA) are antioxidants. Hence the inappropriate names "antioxidant response" and "antioxidant-response element" or ARE for the Nrf2-mediated adaptive alterations and the cognate DNA-binding site for Nrf2, respectively. It became apparent only later that the electrophilic quinone metabolites of these chemicals are the inducers and not the antioxidants.

Adaptation by Decreasing the Target Density or Responsiveness
Decreasing the density and sensitivity of the xenobiotic target is an adaptation mechanism for several cell surface receptors. Such alterations underlie the tolerance induced by opioids, abused drugs of considerable clinical toxicological interests.

Induction of Opioid Tolerance The main target of opioids (e.g., morphine, heroine, methadone) is the μ-opioid receptor. Stimulation of this G_i-protein-coupled inhibitory receptor by an agonist results in adenyl-cyclase inhibition (causing decline in cyclic AMP levels and PKA activity) and K^+ channel opening (causing hyperpolarization) (Fig. 3-12) in neurons with opioid receptors, such as those in the midbrain periaqueductal gray. Even brief stimulation induces adaptive alterations: the receptor is desensitized by G-protein receptor kinase-mediated phosphorylation and β-arrestin binding, then becomes uncoupled from the G protein and internalized via a clathrin-dependent pathway. Whereas some receptors are recycled to the cell membrane, others are degraded in the lysosomes, causing receptor down regulation (Bailey and Connor, 2005). Upon prolonged stimulation, adenyl-cyclase signaling undergoes a compensatory increase. Tolerance to opioids, though far from being clarified mechanistically, may result from down-regulation of the receptors and up-regulation of adenyl-cyclase signaling. These changes would require increasing doses of agonist to produce an effect (i.e., inhibition of adenyl-cyclase signaling) as intensive as after its first application. These adaptive changes could also explain the withdrawal reaction, i.e., appearance of clinical symptoms (dysphoria, excitement, pain sensation), contrasting with the pharmacologic effects of opioids (euphoria, sedation, analgesia), upon abrupt termination of drug treatment, because withdrawal of the opioid would disinhibit the reinforced signaling it had inhibited. Nevertheless, mechanistic relationships between tolerance and the withdrawal reaction remain controversial (Bailey and Connor, 2005). An important clinical feature of opioid tolerance is that the tolerance to the respiratory depressive effect is short-lived and sensitivity returns after some abstinence. Therefore abusers then often kill themselves with a dose tolerated earlier.

Adaptation by Increasing Repair There are several repair mechanisms that can be induced after toxicant exposure. Some of these may aid in repairing damaged molecules, proteins and DNA, others in regenerating the injured tissue.

Induction of Enzymes Repairing Oxidized Proteins—The Electrophile Response, Part 2 After sublethal exposure to chemicals, such as tBHQ, 4-hydroxynon-2-enal, and Cd^{2+}, not only

enzymes functioning in xenobiotic detoxication, but also some of those mediating protein repair become overexpressed as part of the above-described electrophile response. The induced proteins include thioredoxin 1 (Trx1) and thioredoxin-reductase 1 (TR1), which can reduce oxidized proteins (protein disulfides, -sulfenic acids, and -methionine sulfoxides) (Fig. 3-19), and several subunits of the proteosome complex, which hydrolyses damaged proteins. These repair proteins are transcribed from genes containing EpRE, and their transcription is controlled by Nrf2 (Fig. 3-23). As Trx1 and TR1 are reduction partners for ribonucleotide reductase, they support this enzyme in forming deoxyribonucleotides for DNA synthesis. Thus induction of Trx1 and TR1 also assists DNA repair.

Induction of Chaperones Repairing Misfolded Proteins—The Heat-shock Response The cellular abundance of many molecular chaperones, which can disaggregate and refold denatured proteins, also increases after physical and chemical stresses (e.g., heat, ionizing radiation, oxidants, metal ions). Two adaptive reactions involving overexpression of chaperones are known; they are the heat-shock response and the endoplasmic reticulum (ER) stress response.

Although first observed as a result of hyperthermia, the heat-shock response is an adaptive mechanism also triggered by various pathologic conditions (e.g., trauma, tissue ischemia) and by virtually all reactive chemicals and/or their metabolites (e.g., electrophiles, oxidants, lipid peroxidation products, metal ions, arsenite) that denature proteins. Thus it takes place simultaneously with the electrophile response discussed above. This reaction, however, is governed by heat-shock transcription factors (HSF), mainly HSF1, which transactivate genes that encode heat-shock proteins (Hsp) through heat-shock response elements (HSE) within the promoter region. HSF1, like Nrf2, normally resides in the cytoplasm, where it associates with Hsp90, Hsp70, and Hsp40. Upon heat- or chemical-induced protein damage, these Hsps are purportedly sequestered by damaged proteins, allowing HSF1 to be released. HSF1 then migrates into the nucleus, trimerizes, undergoes phosphorylation and stimulates the transcription of Hsp genes. The chaperones Hsp90 and Hsp70, together with co-chaperone proteins, are especially important in maintaining the integrity of hundreds of proteins. The client proteins include not only those carrying out house-keeping functions, but also those involved in signaling and apoptosis. Therefore, induction of Hsps has pleiotropic effects besides increased protection from cytotoxity.

Induction of Chaperones Repairing Misfolded Proteins—The Endoplasmic-Reticulum Stress Response All proteins that are destined for export or insertion into cellular membranes pass through the ER where disulfide bonds are formed and the proteins are correctly folded. This process is catalyzed by ER-resident chaperones, such as glucose-regulated proteins Grp78, Grp94, and protein disulfide isomerase. Damage of proteins being processed in the ER by reactive intermediates (e.g., free radicals formed from CCl_4) or depletion of Ca^{2+} in the ER lumen (e.g., by inactivation of the ER Ca^{2+}-ATPase; see Fig. 3-14) causes accumulation of unfolded proteins in the ER that evokes the ER stress response (also called unfolded protein response) (Cribb *et al.*, 2005). This is initiated by removal of Grp78 by the damaged proteins from IRE1-α, an endoribonuclease. This in turn splices the mRNA for XBP1 into mature XBP1, allowing its translation into XBP1 protein, a transcription factor activating transcription of the ER-resident chaperones, such as Grp78 and Grp94, whose genes contain unfolded protein response elements (UPRE) in their promoter. Concomitantly, another transcription factor, ATF6 (activating transcription factor 6), becomes activated by proteolytic cleavage of its precursor in the

Golgi complex. Through binding to the ER stress response element (ERSE), ATF6 also promotes the transcription of the chaperones Grp78 and Grp94, as well as that of XBP1. Indeed, cells exposed to CCl_4, exhibit rapid induction of Grp78. This response fails to occur in cells that lack CYP2E1, indicating that the ER stress response is mediated by $Cl_3C^\bullet$ and $Cl_3COO^\bullet$ formed by CYP2E1 and/or by the CYP2E1-generated ROS (Lewis and Roberts, 2005). In addition to enrolling new ER-associated molecular chaperones to cope with the increase in damaged proteins, other measures are also taken by this complex adaptive program, such as temporary attenuation of mRNA translation (by engaging the ER-resident kinase PERK which catalyzes inactivating phosphorylation of eIF2α, a translation initiation factor) and increased removal of unfolded and misfolded proteins from the ER through translocon pores and their delivery to the cytoplasmic proteosome.

Induction of Enzymes Repairing DNA—The DNA Damage Response Upon DNA damage an adaptive response is initiated in which the protagonist is p53, a protein that can play the role of a transcription factor regulating gene expression and the role of an associate protein affecting the function of its interacting protein partner. Normally, p53 is kept inactive and at low levels by its binding protein mdm2 (see Fig. 3-28), which ubiquitinates p53, facilitating its proteosomal degradation. DNA damage activates kinases, such as ATM (ataxia telangiectasia mutated), ATR (ataxia telangiectasia related) and DNA-PK (DNA-dependent protein kinase), which through checkpoint kinases (Chk1, Chk2) phosphorylate p53 (Christmann *et al.*, 2003; McGowan and Russel, 2004). Upon phosphorylation, p53 escapes from mdm2, allowing its activation and stabilization. Indeed, the levels of p53 protein in cells increase dramatically in response to DNA damage caused by UV or gamma irradiation or genotoxic chemicals. p53 then facilitates DNA repair by a number of mechanisms. For example, mainly by transcriptionally up-regulating the cyclin-dependent kinase inhibitor protein p21, p53 arrests cells in G1 phase of the cell cycle (see Fig. 3-28), allowing more time for DNA repair. As a transcription factor, p53 also increases expression of proteins directly involved in DNA repair (Harms *et al.*, 2004). Such proteins include (a) GADD45 (growth arrest and DNA damage inducible), that interacts with histones and facilitates access of proteins (e.g., topoisomerase) to DNA, (b) XPE and XPC, members of the xeroderma pigmentosum group of proteins important in UV-induced DNA damage recognition before nucleotide excision repair, (c) MSH2 and PCNA (proliferating cell nuclear antigen) operating in mismatch repair, and (d) a form of ribonucleotide reductase that provides deoxyribonucleotides for filling in DNA gaps. As a partner protein, p53 supports the function of several proteins of the nucleotide excision machinery (e.g., TFIH, XPB, XPD). Other roles p53 plays in apoptosis and in carcinogenesis as a tumor suppressor protein are illustrated in Figs. 3-16 and 3-28 and discussed elsewhere in this chapter.

Adaptive Increase in Tissue Repair—A Proliferative Response Many toxicants potentially injurious to cells, e.g., electrophiles, oxidants and those inducing oxidative stress, can initiate a mitogenic signaling as a prelude to tissue repair via cell replacement. It appears that the need for mitogenesis is sensed by protein tyrosine phosphatases (PTP, e.g., PTP1B) and the lipid phosphatase PTEN, which contain reactive cysteine-thiols at their active site (Rhee *et al.*, 2005). These phosphatases serve as brakes on the growth factor receptor-initiated mitogenic signaling, as PTPs dephosphorylate (and inactivate) the receptors themselves (e.g., EGFR, PDGFR, IGFR) as well as some protein kinases (e.g., Src and JAK), whereas PTEN dephosphorylates PIP_3, an important second messenger in the PI3K–Akt–IKK–NF-κB pathway (Fig. 3-11). Electrophiles covalently bind to essential cysteine-SH groups in these phosphatases. HOOH can oxidize the critical –SH group in PTEN to an intramolecular disulfide, whereas it oxidizes the -SH group of PTP1B, through sulfenic acid (-S-OH), to a five-membered cyclic sulfenyl amide species in which the sulfur atom is covalently linked to the nitrogen of the neighboring serine (Rhee *et al.*, 2005). Inactivation of PTPs and PTEN, which decrease the proliferative signal transduction, amplifies intracellular signaling for mitosis and survival.

It has been known for some time that oxidative stress, if not severe, activates the transcription factor NF-κB (Dalton *et al.*, 1999). For example, silica, which can produce ROS on its surface, activates NF-κB as well as PI3K when added to various cells (Castranova, 2004). In light of new information discussed above, NF-κB activation is now attributed to the fact that this transcription factor is situated downstream of growth factor receptors (which are negatively controlled by the ROS-sensitive PTP) and PIP_3 (which is eliminated by ROS-sensitive PTEN) (Fig. 3-11). Furthermore, NF-κB is at the focal point of proliferative and pro-life signaling, as it transactivates genes producing cell cycle accelerators (e.g., cyclin D1 and c-Myc) and apoptosis inhibitors (e.g., antiapoptotic Bcl proteins and the caspase inhibitor IAP proteins) (Karin, 2006). In addition, NF-κB also transactivates the genes of ferritin, GST, SOD1, HO-1, a proteosome subunit, and GADD45, facilitating detoxication and molecular repair. All these roles of NF-κB explain its involvement in tolerance to chemically induced tissue injury, resistance against cholestatic liver injury caused by bile acids, in adaptation to ionizing radiation, as well as in the phenomenon termed preconditioning. This is a tolerance to ischemic tissue injury (e.g., myocardial infarction); a tolerance induced by temporarily enhanced ROS formation evoked by hyperoxia or brief periods of ischemia-reperfusion.

In addition to signaling for cell replacement in damaged tissue–in which NF-κB plays a leading role–the growing cells need to boost protein synthesis. This is done under the control of the protein kinase mTOR (mammalian target of rapamycin). As shown in Fig. 3-25, mTOR activation results from signaling through both pathways coupled to growth factor receptors, i.e., the MAPK-pathway leading to phosphorylation of the MAPK isoform Erk, and the PI3K-pathway leading to phosphorylation of Akt (see Fig. 3-11). Importantly, these pathways are subject to activation in response to oxidant or electrophile exposure as they are controlled by PTPs and PTEN. Erk and Akt protein kinases activate mTOR through a complex mechanism (Fig. 3-25), and mTOR in turn phosphorylates and regulates effectors of protein synthesis, such as the translation repressor protein 4EBP1 and the protein kinase S6K, which modifies ribosomes increasing their translational efficiency (Shaw and Cantley, 2006). As described under hypoxia response and energy stress response, mTOR signaling is switched off in the cell to save energy as a measure to adapt to the energy shortage caused by hypoxia or toxic impairment of ATP synthesis.

Adaptation by Compensating Dysfunction Dysfunctions caused by toxicants or drug overdose manifested at the level of organism (e.g., hypoxia), organ system (e.g., hypo- and hypertension), or organ (e.g., renal tubular dysfunction) may evoke compensatory mechanisms.

Adaptation to Hypoxia—The Hypoxia Response When O_2 delivery is impaired and hypoxia persists for more than a few minutes, a response involving gene expression alteration is initiated.

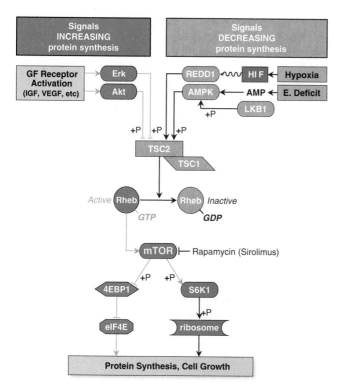

Figure 3-25. Modulation of protein synthesis at translational level by signaling through the mTOR pathway as a means for cellular adaptation – increased signaling via mTOR supports cell growth and proliferation, whereas attenuated signaling permits energy conservation when hypoxia or toxic injury cause energy deficit.

Growth factor receptors signaling via either the MAPK-pathway, leading to phosphorylation of Erk, or via the PI3K-pathway, leading to phosphorylation of Akt (see Fig. 3-11), activate the serine/threonine kinase, mTOR (mammalian target of rapamycin; rapamycin is also called sirolimus), by an indirect mechanism. The protein kinases Erk and Akt catalyze inactivating phosphorylation of TSC2, a member of TSC1/2 complex. TSC2 is a GTPase-activating protein whose substrate is Rheb, a small G protein (ras homologue), which is active in the GTP-bound form and inactive in the GDP-bound form. With its GTPase activity inactivated by Erk or Akt, TSC2 cannot convert Rheb-GTP into inactive Rheb-GDP, and thus Rheb-GTP activates mTOR. In turn, mTOR phosphorylates two substrates which are necessary to initiate translation of mRNA into proteins, i.e., (1) 4EBP1 (eukaryotic initiation factor 4E-binding protein-1), which thus releases the translational initiation factor eIF4E, and (2) S6K1 (ribosomal protein S6 kinase-1), which phosphorylates ribosomal protein S6, thereby increasing translational efficiency of mRNAs that encode ribosomal proteins ("ribosomal biogenesis"). Regulation of protein synthesis by mTOR controls cell size and proliferation.

Protein synthesis for cell growth and proliferation, however, is halted in times of energy deficit resulting from hypoxia or toxic impairment of ATP production. Then AMP levels increase and AMP binds to the AMP-activated protein kinase (AMPK), facilitating its phosphorylation by protein kinase LKB1. Activated AMPK phosphorylates TSC2 (at a site different from that targeted by Akt and Erk), thereby increasing the GTPase-activating capacity of TSC2. This in turn switches Rheb off, making mTOR inactive and bringing mRNA translation to a halt. Hypoxia can initiate this process in a more specific way as well, i.e., via stabilization of the hypoxia inducible factor (HIF). This transcription factor induces the synthesis of REDD1, by a mechanism that is not completely understood, activates TSC2. See text for further details on cellular responses to hypoxia and energy deficit.

This reaction is mainly orchestrated by hypoxia inducible factor-1α (HIF-1α), a ubiquitous transcription factor whose activity and cellular abundance is greatly increased in response to hypoxia (Maxwell and Salnikow, 2004; Pouyssegur *et al.*, 2006). HIF-1α is maintained at very low intracellular levels because of its continuous hydroxylation of two proline residues by HIF-prolyl hydroxylases. This permits a ubiquitin ligase subunit (called von Hippel Lindau protein or VHL) to capture HIF-1α and initiate its destruction by proteosomal degradation. Indeed, HIF-1α is one of the shortest lived proteins with a half-life of less than 5 minutes. In addition, HIF-1α is kept transcriptionally inactive by hydroxylation at one of its asparagine residues by HIF-asparagine hydroxylases, which prevents interaction of HIF-1α with transcriptional co-activators, such as p300 and CBP. These two types of HIF hydroxylases are O_2 sensors: they use O_2 as a substrate to carry out proline/asparagine hydroxylations with concomitant oxidative decarboxylation of 2-oxoglutarate to succinate, with the K_M of O_2 being close to the ambient O_2 concentration. As the O_2 concentration falls, decreases in the hydroxylation rate of HIF-1α as well as its VHL-mediated ubiquitination and proteosomal degradation occur, and this increases its abundance and transcriptional activity. HIF hydroxylases belong to the Fe^{2+} and ascorbate-dependent dioxygenases (the largest group of non-heme oxidases), therefore not only hypoxia, but also Fe^{2+} deficiency impairs their activity. This latter feature explains why iron chelators (e.g., deferoxamine) or Fe^{2+}-mimicking metal ions (e.g., Co^{2+} and Ni^{2+}) also induce and activate HIF-1α (Maxwell and Salnikow, 2004). When induced after hypoxic conditions, HIF-1α dimerizes with HIF-1β (also called Arnt, which coincidentally, is the dimerization partner for the Ah receptor as well). The HIF complex transactivates a vast array of genes with hypoxia response element (HRE) in their promoter. Many of the gene products assist in acclimatization to hypoxia (Pouyssegur *et al.*, 2006). These include (1) erythropoietin (EPO) that is produced largely in kidney and activates erythropoiesis in bone marrow, (2) vascular endothelial growth factor (VEGF) and angiopoietin-2 that stimulate blood vessel growth (i.e., angiogenesis), (3) proteins facilitating anaerobic ATP synthesis from glucose (i.e., glycolysis), such as the glucose transporter GLUT1 and some glycolytic enzymes, (4) proteins that correct acidosis caused by glycolytic overproduction of lactate (e.g., a monocarboxylate transporter and a Na^+/H^+ exchanger for export of lactate and H^+, respectively), (5) the REDD1 signal transducer protein that initiates a complex signaling pathway that leads to suspension of the ATP-consuming protein synthesis via inactivation of the protein kinase mTOR (Fig. 3-25), and (6) many other proteins, such as those that promote extracellular matrix remodeling (e.g., matrix metalloproteinase-2) and cell migration (perhaps to facilitate access of the cells to the blood vessel), as well as BNIP3, a pro-apoptotic member of Bcl-2 family (perhaps to induce apoptosis upon extreme hypoxia). Experiments on mice kept in low O_2 environment (hypoxic preconditioning) demonstrated that HIF-1α became stabilized in the retina of these animals, hypoxia-responsive genes (EPO, VEGF) were induced, and the retina became resistant to light toxicity (Grimm *et al.*, 2005). Adaptation to hypoxia also occurs, for example, in response to high altitude hypoxia, chronic cardiorespiratory dysfunction, ischemic preconditioning, along with other adaptive responses discussed above. The hypoxia response is also expected to develop as a result of toxicities causing hypoxia acutely or subacutely (e.g., respiratory muscle weakness after organophosphate intoxication, diquat-induced pulmonary injury) or as a delayed sequel (e.g., respiratory surface restriction in hard metal disease).

Adaptation to Energy Depletion—The Energy Stress Response
Cells try to maintain their adenosine nucleotide pool in triphosphorylated, energized state, which is in the form of ATP. When the re-phosphorylation rate of AMP and ADP to ATP does not keep up with the rate of ATP use, because, for example, oxidative phosphorylation is impaired or ATP use for muscle contraction or ion pumping is excessive, the ratio of AMP to ATP increases. A cellular mechanism has evolved to sense this menacing energy deficit and, in order to compensate, boosts ATP production and curtails ATP consumption (Hardie *et al.*, 2006). The sensor is a ubiquitous heterotrimeric intracellular protein complex called AMP-activated protein kinase (AMPK). AMP strongly activates AMPK allosterically, and also by making it susceptible for phosphorylation by protein kinase LKB1 (or by the calmodulin dependent protein kinase kinase, CaMKK, in neurons). The phosphorylated, and thus activated AMPK, targets two sets of proteins. One set includes those whose activation facilitates ATP production from catabolism of glucose and fatty acids as well as by promoting the biogenesis of mitochondria. For example, AMPK activation increases (a) glucose uptake (via recruiting to the cell membrane or activating glucose transporters GLUT4 and GLUT1), (b) glycolysis (via phosphorylation and activation of 6-phosphofructo-2-kinase (PFK-2) whose product, fructose-2,6-bisphosphate is a glycolytic activator), and (c) fatty acid oxidation in mitochondria (via phosphorylation and inactivation of acetyl-CoA-carboxylase, whose product, malonyl-CoA, is an allosteric inhibitor of carnitine palmitoyltransferase-1, or CPT-1, which mediates uptake of long-chain fatty acid CoA esters into mitochondria). Another set of proteins, which are inactivated by AMPK (directly or indirectly), include those that are involved in biosynthetic ATP consuming reactions. Thus, AMPK inhibits (a) glycogen synthesis via phosphorylation and inactivation of glycogen synthase, (b) lipid synthesis by phosphorylating and inactivating acetyl-CoA-carboxylase, whose product, malonyl-CoA, is an essential substrate for fatty acid synthesis, (c) cholesterol synthesis by phosphorylating and inactivating HMG-CoA reductase, (d) glucose synthesis via inactivating phosphorylation of a transcriptional coactivator, TORC2, which then decreases expression of key gluconeogenetic enzymes, such as phosphoenolpyruvate carboxykinase (PEPCK) and glucose-6-phosphatase, and (e) protein synthesis, and thus cell growth, by inhibiting the protein kinase mTOR (Fig. 3-25). AMPK-mediated modulation of cellular energy supply and consumption involves mainly kinase reactions rather than new protein synthesis. Therefore, this adaptation is a rapid process. It can be a response to any harmful condition that compromises oxidative phosphorylation, such as hypoxia, hypoglycemia (especially in neurons) and chemically induced mitochondrial toxicity. For example, cells exposed to arsenite exhibit rapid increases in the AMP/ATP ratio and AMPK activity, with concomitant declines in HMG-CoA reductase activity as well as fatty acid and cholesterol synthesis (Corton *et al.*, 1994).

After surveying the major cellular adaptation mechanisms to toxicants, it is easy to recognize that one noxa may initiate several adaptive responses. For example, cells exposed to a hypoxic environment can rapidly respond with both AMPK-mediated program of energy stabilization, and HIF-1α-directed adaptation to oxygen shortage. Theoretically, an electrophile toxicant that can bind covalently to cellular macromolecules and can also generate oxidative stress, such as a redox cycling quinone, would be expected to induce a number of adaptive processes, including the electrophile response, the heat-shock response, the endoplasmic-reticulum stress response, the DNA-damage response, and the proliferative response, and if it compromises ATP synthesis as well, it even induces the energy-stress response.

Adaptation by Neurohumoral Mechanisms   There are numerous adaptive responses to dysfunctions of organs or organ systems that are mediated by humoral or neuronal signals between cells located in the same or different organs. For example, the rapid hyperventilation evoked by acute hypoxia or HCN inhalation, mediated by a neural reflex initiated by glomus cells in the carotid body. These chemosensitive cells generate a Ca^{2+} signal via the above-described AMP-sensor, AMPK, which becomes activated by hypoxia or CN^- through impairment of oxidative phosphorylation in these cells, causing rise in the AMP/ATP ratio (Evans *et al.*, 2005). Besides CN^-, mitochondrial electron transport inhibitors (e.g., rotenone, antimycin A, myxothiazole), uncouplers (e.g., 2,4-dinitrophenol) or ATP-synthase inhibitors (e.g., oligomycin) (see Table 3-6 and Fig. 3-13) as well as AMPK activators mimic the response to hypoxia in these cells. There are numerous other neurohumoral adaptive mechanisms in the body, such as the sympathetic reflex as well as activation of the renin-angiotensin-aldosterone system in response to hypotension, and the feedback systems between endocrine glands and the hypothalamus-hypophysis, which correct abnormal hormone levels. For information on these and other mechanisms, the reader is referred to textbooks of physiology.

When Repair and Adaptation Fail

When Repair Fails   Although repair mechanisms operate at molecular, cellular, and tissue levels, for various reasons they often fail to provide protection against injury. First, the fidelity of the repair mechanisms is not absolute, making it possible for some lesions to be overlooked. However, repair fails most typically when the damage overwhelms the repair mechanisms, as when protein thiols are oxidized faster than they can be reduced. In other instances, the capacity of repair may become exhausted when necessary enzymes or cofactors are consumed. For example, alkylation of DNA may lead to consumption of O^6-methguanine-DNA-methyltransferase, and lipid peroxidation can deplete alpha-tocopherol. Sometimes the toxicant-induced injury adversely affects the repair process itself. For example, ethanol generates ROS via CYP2E1 which impairs proteosomal removal of damaged proteins. After exposure to necrogenic chemicals, mitosis of surviving cells may be blocked and restoration of the tissue becomes impossible (Mehendale, 2005). Finally, some types of toxic injuries cannot be repaired effectively, as occurs when xenobiotics are covalently bound to proteins. Thus, toxicity is manifested when repair of the initial injury fails because the repair mechanisms become overwhelmed, exhausted, or impaired or are genuinely inefficient.

It is also possible that repair contributes to toxicity. This may occur in a passive manner, for example, if excessive amounts of NAD^+ are cleaved by PARP when this enzyme assists in repairing broken DNA strands, or when too much NAD(P)H is consumed for the repair of oxidized proteins and endogenous reductants. Either event can compromise oxidative phosphorylation, which is also dependent on the supply of reduced cofactors (see Fig. 3-13), thus causing or aggravating ATP depletion that contributes to cell injury. Excision repair of DNA and reacylation of lipids also contribute to cellular deenergization and injury by consuming significant amounts of ATP. However, repair also may play an active role in toxicity. This is observed after chronic tissue injury, when the repair process goes astray and leads to uncontrolled proliferation instead of tissue remodeling. Such proliferation of cells may yield neoplasia whereas overproduction of extracellular matrix results in fibrosis.

When Adaptation Fails   Although adaptation mechanisms, such as the Nrf2-mediated electrophile response and the NF-κB-induced proliferative reaction, boost the capacity of the organism to withstand toxicant exposure and damage, excessive exposure can overwhelm this protective response. Moreover, toxicants may impair the adaptive process. For example, moderate oxidative stress activates NF-κB, AP-1, and Nrf2 to initiate adaptive protection. However, extensive oxidant exposure, aborts this program because it leads to oxidation of thiol groups in the DNA-binding domain of these transcription factors (Hansen *et al.*, 2006). Similarly, Hg^{2+} can incapacitate NF-κB, thus inhibiting the pro-life program activated by this transcription factor. This promotes Hg^{2+}-induced renal tubular cell injury (Dieguez-Acuna *et al.*, 2004).

Some adaptive mechanisms may be harmful under extreme conditions. For example, acute tubular injury, which impairs tubular reabsorption and causes polyuria, triggers a tubuloglomerular feedback mechanism that reduces glomerular blood flow and filtration. Ultimately, this may precipitate anuric renal failure. It is possible that an adaptive mechanism that is beneficial in the short term, may become harmful when forced to operate for a prolonged period of time. As discussed earlier, NF-κB activation is indispensable for repair via proliferation of the acutely injured tissue. However, NF-κB also targets cytokine genes, and the cytokines (e.g., TNF-α, IL-1β) in turn activate NF-κB through their receptors (see Fig. 3-11). This vicious cycle may lead to chronic inflammation and cancer when repetitive tissue injury maintains NF-κB signaling (Karin, 2006). This occurs after occupational exposure to silica (Castranova, 2004). Sustained activation of HIF-1α in tumors facilitates invasiveness, in part by increasing VEGF expression and angiogenesis. In the kidney HIF-1α may be involved in fibrogenesis, as it targets critical genes, like tissue inhibitor of metalloproteinase-1.

Toxicity Resulting from Inappropriate Repair and Adaptation

Like repair, dysrepair occurs at the molecular, cellular, and tissue levels. Some toxicities involve dysrepair at an isolated level. For example, hypoxemia develops after exposure to methemoglobin-forming chemicals if the amount of methemoglobin produced overwhelms the capacity of methemoglobin reductase. Because this repair enzyme is deficient at early ages, neonates are especially sensitive to chemicals that cause methemoglobinemia. Formation of cataracts purportedly involves inefficiency or impairment of lenticular repair enzymes, such as the endo- and exopeptidases, which normally reduce oxidized crystalline and hydrolyze damaged proteins to their constituent amino acids. Dysrepair also is thought to contribute to the formation of Heinz bodies, which are protein aggregates formed in oxidatively stressed and aged red blood cells. Defective proteolytic degradation of the immunogenic trifluoroacetylated proteins may make halothane-anesthetized patients victims of halothane hepatitis.

Several types of toxicity involve failed and/or derailed repairs at different levels before they become apparent. This is true for the most severe toxic injuries, such as tissue necrosis, fibrosis, and chemical carcinogenesis.

Tissue Necrosis   As discussed above, several mechanisms may lead to cell death. Most or all involve molecular damage that is potentially reversible by repair mechanisms. If repair mechanisms operate effectively, they may prevent cell injury or at least retard its progression. For example, prooxidant toxicants cause no lipid fragmentation in microsomal membranes until alpha-tocopherol is depleted in those membranes. Membrane damage ensues when this endogenous antioxidant, which can repair lipids containing peroxyl radical groups (Fig. 3-20), becomes unavailable (Scheschonka *et al.*, 1990). This suggests that cell injury progresses toward cell necrosis if molecular repair mechanisms are inefficient or the molecular damage is not readily reversible.

Progression of cell injury to tissue necrosis can be intercepted by two repair mechanisms working in concert: apoptosis and cell proliferation. As discussed above, injured cells can initiate apoptosis, which counteracts the progression of the toxic injury. Apoptosis does this by preventing necrosis of injured cells and the consequent inflammatory response, which may cause injury by releasing cytotoxic mediators. Indeed, the activation of Kupffer cells, the source of such mediators in the liver, by the administration of bacterial lipopolysaccharide (endotoxin) greatly aggravates the hepatotoxicity of galactosamine. In contrast, when the Kupffer cells are selectively eliminated by pretreatment of rats with gadolinium chloride, the necrotic effect of carbon tetrachloride is markedly alleviated (Edwards *et al.*, 1993). Blockade of Kupffer cell function with glycine (via the inhibitory glycine receptor; see item 4 in Fig. 3-12) also protects the liver from alcohol-induced injury (Yin *et al.*, 1998).

Another important repair process that can halt the propagation of toxic injury is proliferation of cells adjacent to the injured cells. This response is initiated soon after cellular injury. A surge in mitosis in the liver of rats administered a low (nonnecrogenic) dose of carbon tetrachloride is detectable within a few hours. This early cell division is thought to be instrumental in the rapid and complete restoration of the injured tissue and the prevention of necrosis. This hypothesis is corroborated by the finding that in rats pretreated with chlordecone, which blocks the early cell proliferation in response to carbon tetrachloride, a normally nonnecrogenic dose of carbon tetrachloride causes hepatic necrosis (Mehendale, 2005). The sensitivity of a tissue to injury and the capacity of the tissue for repair are apparently two independent variables, both influencing the final outcome of the effect of injurious chemical—that is, whether tissue restitution ensues with survival or tissue necrosis occurs with death. For example, variations in tissue repair capacity among species and strains of animals appear to be responsible for certain variations in the lethality of hepatotoxicants (Soni and Mehandale, 1998).

It appears that the efficiency of repair is an important determinant of the dose-response relationship for toxicants that cause tissue necrosis. Following chemically induced liver or kidney injury, the intensity of tissue repair increases up to a threshold dose, restraining injury, whereupon it is inhibited, allowing unrestrained progression of injury (Mehendale, 2005). Impaired signaling to mitosis (see Fig. 3-11), caused by high tissue concentrations of toxicants (e.g., acetaminophen in the liver or *S*-(1,2-dichlorovinyl)-L-cysteine in the kidney) and their reactive metabolites may account for lagging tissue repair (Boulares *et al.*, 1999; Vaidya *et al.*, 2003), but maintenance of DNA and protein synthesis, mitotic machinery, and energy supply may also be impaired at high-dose chemical exposures. That is, tissue necrosis is caused by a certain dose of a toxicant not only because that dose ensures sufficient concentration of the ultimate toxicant at the target site to initiate injury but also because that quantity of toxicant causes a degree of damage sufficient to compromise repair, allowing for progression of the injury. Experimental observations with hepatotoxicants indicate that apoptosis and cell proliferation are operative with latent tissue injury caused by low (nonnecrogenic) doses of toxicants, but are inhibited with severe injury induced by high (necrogenic) doses. For example, 1,1-dichloroethylene, carbon tetrachloride, and thioacetamide all induce apoptosis in the liver at low doses, but cause hepatic necrosis after high-dose exposure (Corcoran *et al.*, 1994). Similarly, there is an early mitotic response in the liver to low-dose carbon tetrachloride, but this response is absent after administration of the solvent at necrogenic doses (Mehendale, 2005). This suggests that tissue necrosis occurs because the injury overwhelms and disables the repair mechanisms, including (1) repair of damaged molecules, (2) elimination of damaged cells by apoptosis, and (3) replacement of lost cells by cell division.

Fibrosis Fibrosis is a pathologic condition characterized by excessive deposition of an extracellular matrix of abnormal composition. Hepatic fibrosis, or cirrhosis, results from chronic consumption of ethanol or high dose retinol (vitamin A), treatment with methotrexate, and intoxication with hepatic necrogens such as carbon tetrachloride and iron. Pulmonary fibrosis is induced by drugs such as bleomycin and amiodarone and prolonged inhalation of oxygen or mineral particles. Doxorubicin may cause cardiac fibrosis, whereas exposure to ionizing radiation induces fibrosis in many organs. Most of these agents generate free radicals and cause chronic cell injury.

Fibrosis is a specific manifestation of dysrepair of the chronically injured tissue. As discussed above, cellular injury initiates a surge in cellular proliferation and extracellular matrix production, which normally ceases when the injured tissue is remodeled. If increased production of extracellular matrix is not halted, fibrosis develops.

The cells that manufacture the extracellular matrix during tissue repair (e.g., stellate cells and myofibroblasts in liver, mesangial cells in the kidney, fibroblasts-like cells in lungs and skin) are the ones that overproduce the matrix in fibrosis. These cells are controlled and phenotypically altered ("activated") by cytokines and growth factors secreted by nonparenchymal cells, including themselves (see Fig. 3-22). TGF-β appears to be the major mediator of fibrogenesis, although other factors are also involved. These include growth factors, such as connective tissue growth factor (CTGF; a TGF-β-induced growth factor) and platelet-derived growth factor, vasoactive peptides, such as endothelin-1 and angiotensin-II, and the adipocyte-derived hormone leptin (Lotersztajn *et al.*, 2005). The evidence is compelling to indicate that TGF-β, acting through its receptor (item 8 in Fig. 3-11), and receptor activated transcription factors (Smad2 and 3), is a highly relevant causative factor of fibrosis. For example, subcutaneous injection of TGF-β induces local fibrosis, whereas overexpression of TGF-β in transgenic mice produces hepatic fibrosis. Smad3-null mice are relatively resistant to radiation-nduced cutaneous fibrosis, bleomycin-induced pulmonary fibrosis and CCl$_4$-induced hepatic fibrosis. TGF-β antagonists, such as anti-TGF-β immunoglobulin and decorin, as well as Smad3 antagonists, such as halofuginone and overexpressed Smad7 protein (that is antagonistic to Smad 2 and 3), ameliorate chemically induced fibrogenesis (Flanders, 2004). In several types of experimental fibrosis and in patients with active liver cirrhosis, overexpression of TGF-β in affected tissues has been demonstrated.

The increased expression of TGF-β is a common response mediating regeneration of the extracellular matrix after an acute injury. However, whereas TGF-β production ceases when repair is complete, this does not occur when tissue injury leads to fibrosis. Failure to halt TGF-β overproduction could be caused by continuous injury or a defect in the regulation of TGF-β. Indeed, after acute CCL$_4$-induced liver injury hepatic stellate cells exhibit a TGF-β-mediated induction of Smad7 (which purportedly terminates the fibrotic signal by inhibiting activation of Smad2 and Smad3 by TGF-β receptor), however, after chronic injury, Smad7 induction fails to occur (Flanders, 2004).

The fibrotic action of TGF-β is due to (1) stimulation of the synthesis of individual matrix components by specific target cells and (2) inhibition of matrix degradation by decreasing expression of matrix metalloproteinase-1 and increasing the expression of matrix degrading enzyme inhibitors, such as tissue inhibitor of metalloproteinase-1 (TIMP-1) and plasminogen activator inhibitor-1 (PAI-1) (Arthur *et al.*, 1999; Flanders, 2004). Interestingly, TGF-β induces transcription of its own gene in target cells (Flanders, 2004), suggesting that the TGF-β produced by these cells can amplify in an autocrine manner the production of the extracellular matrix. This positive feedback (autoinduction) may facilitate fibrogenesis.

Fibrosis involves not only excessive accumulation of the extracellular matrix but also changes in its composition. The basement membrane components, such as collagen IV and laminin, as well as the fibrillar type collagens (collagen I and III), which confer rigidity to tissues, increase disproportionately, during fibrogenesis (Gressner, 1992).

Fibrosis is detrimental in a number of ways:

1. The scar compresses and may ultimately obliterate the parenchymal cells and blood vessels.
2. Deposition of basement membrane components between the capillary endothelial cells and the parenchymal cells presents a diffusional barrier which contributes to malnutrition of the tissue cells.
3. An increased amount and rigidity of the extracellular matrix unfavorably affect the elasticity and flexibility of the whole tissue, compromising the mechanical function of organs such as the heart and lungs.
4. Furthermore, the altered extracellular environment is sensed by integrins. Through these transmembrane proteins and the coupled intracellular signal transducing networks (see Fig. 3-11), fibrosis may modulate several aspects of cell behavior, including polarity, motility, and gene expression (Raghow, 1994).

Carcinogenesis Chemical carcinogenesis involves inappropriate function of various repair and adaptive mechanisms, including (1a) insufficient adaptive response to DNA damage with failure of DNA repair that leads to mutation of critical genes, (1b) inappropriate control at regulatory gene regions over expression of critical genes, (2) failure to induce apoptosis, and (3) failure to terminate cell proliferation.

As to be described in more detail later, carcinogenesis entails gene expression alterations initiated by two fundamentally distinct types of mechanisms that often work simultaneously and in concert, i.e., genetic and epigenetic mechanisms. Genetic mechanisms bring about *qualitative* change in gene expression, i.e., expression of an altered gene product, a mutant protein, with gain or loss in activity. In contrast, epigenetic mechanisms cause *quantitative* change in

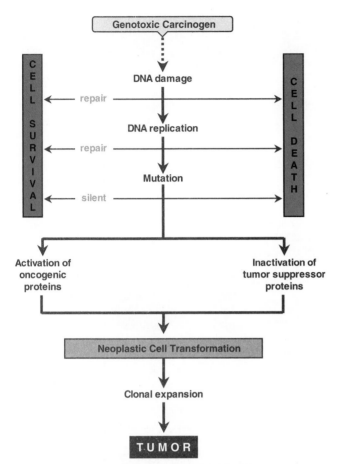

Figure 3-26. The process of carcinogenesis initiated by genotoxic carcinogens.

The figure indicates that activating mutation of proto-oncogenes that encode permanently active oncoproteins and inactivating mutation of tumor suppressor genes that encode permanently inactive tumor suppressor proteins can cooperate in neoplastic transformation of cells. It is important to realize that overexpression of normal proto-oncogenes (e.g., by hypomethylation of their promoter) and under-expression (silencing) of normal tumor suppressor genes (e.g., by hypermethylation of their promoter) may also contribute to such transformation (see text for explanation).

gene expression resulting in more or less protein product. Whereas genetic mechanisms affect the coding sequences of critical genes, causing DNA damage, epigenetic mechanisms influence the regulatory (promoter) region of genes, causing increased or decreased transcriptional activity of the gene. Thus, chemical and physical insults may induce neoplastic transformation of cells by affecting critical genes through genotoxic and nongenotoxic (i.e., epigenetic) mechanisms. However, either mechanism ultimately induces cancer by causing cellular failures in initiating apoptosis and/or terminating cell proliferation.

Inappropriate Repair of the Coding Region of Critical Genes: Mutation, an Initiating Event in Carcinogenesis   Chemicals that react with DNA may cause damage such as adduct formation, oxidative alteration, and strand breakage (Fig. 3-26). In most cases, these lesions are repaired or injured cells are eliminated. If neither event occurs, a lesion in the parental DNA strand may induce a heritable alteration, or mutation, in the daughter strand during replication. The mutation may remain silent if it does not alter the protein encoded

by the mutant gene or if the mutation causes an amino acid substitution that does not affect the function of the protein. Alternatively, the genetic alteration may be incompatible with cell survival. The most unfortunate scenario for the organism occurs when the altered genes express mutant proteins that reprogram cells for multiplication and avoidance of apoptosis (i.e., immortalization). When such cells undergo mitosis, their descendants also have a similar propensity for proliferation. Moreover, because enhanced DNA replication and cell division increases the likelihood of mutations, these cells eventually acquire additional mutations that may further increase their growth advantage over their normal counterparts. The final outcome of this process is a nodule, followed by a tumor consisting of transformed, rapidly proliferating cells (Fig. 3-26).

The critical role of DNA repair in preventing carcinogenesis is attested by the human heritable disease xeroderma pigmentosum. Affected individuals lack excision repair proteins of the XP series and exhibit a greatly increased incidence of sunlight-induced skin cancers. Cells from these patients are also hypersensitive to DNA-reactive chemicals, including aflatoxin B_l, aromatic amines, polycyclic hydrocarbons, and 4-nitroquinoline-1-oxide (Lehmann and Dean, 1990). Also, mice with ablated PARP gene are extremely sensitive to γ-rays and N-methylnitrosourea and show genomic instability, as indicated by increases in the levels of both sister chromatid exchanges and chromatid breaks following genotoxic insult (D'Amours *et al.*, 1999).

A small set of cellular genes are the targets for genetic alterations that initiate neoplastic transformations. Included are proto-oncogenes and tumor-suppressor genes (Barrett, 1992).

Mutation of Proto-oncogenes   Proto-oncogenes are highly conserved genes encoding proteins that stimulate the progression of cells through the cell cycle (Smith *et al.*, 1993). The products of proto-oncogenes include (1) growth factors; (2) growth factor receptors; (3) intracellular signal transducers such as G proteins, protein kinases, cyclins, and cyclin-dependent protein kinases; and (4) nuclear transcription factors. Figure 3-27 depicts several proto-oncogene products that are closely involved in initiating the cell-division cycle. The legend of that figure outlines some important details on the function of these proteins and their interaction with tumor suppressor proteins (to be discussed below). Transient increases in the production or activity of proto-oncogene proteins are required for regulated growth, as during embryogenesis, tissue regeneration, and stimulation of cells by growth factors or hormones. In contrast, permanent activation and/or overexpression of these proteins favor neoplastic transformation. One mechanism whereby genotoxic carcinogens induce neoplastic cell transformation is by producing an activating mutation of a proto-oncogene. Such a mutation is so named because the altered gene (then called an *oncogene*) encodes a permanently active protein that forces the cell into the division cycle. An example of mutational activation of an oncogene protein is that of the Ras proteins.

Ras proteins are G-proteins with GTP/GDP binding capacity as well as GTPase activity (Anderson *et al.*, 1992). They are localized on the inner surface of the plasma membrane and function as crucial mediators in responses initiated by growth factors (see Figs. 3-11 and 3-27). Ras is located downstream from growth factor receptors and nonreceptor protein tyrosine kinases and upstream from mitogen-activated protein kinase (MAPK) cascade whose activation finally up-regulates the expression of cyclin D and initiates the mitotic cycle (Fig. 3-27). In this pathway, Ras serves as a molecular switch, being active in the GTP-bound form and inactive in the GDP-bound form. Some mutations of the *Ras* gene (e.g., a

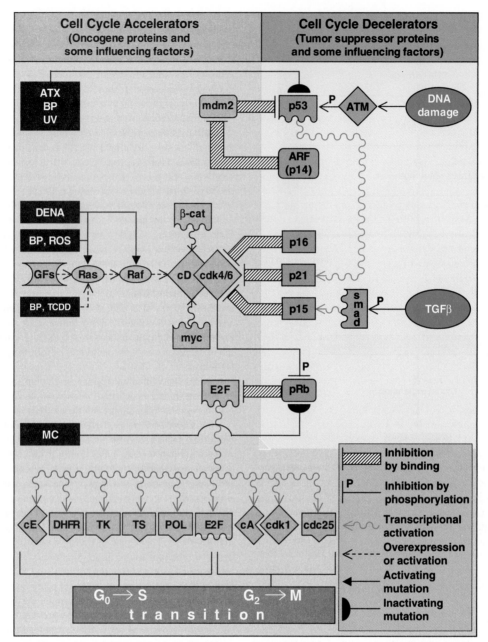

Figure 3-27. Key regulatory proteins controlling the cell division cycle with some signaling pathways and xenobiotics affecting them.

Proteins on the left, represented by gray symbols, accelerate the cell cycle and are oncogenic if permanently active or expressed at high level. In contrast, proteins on the right, represented by blue symbols, decelerate or arrest the cell cycle and thus suppress oncogenesis, unless they are inactivated (e.g., by mutation).

Accumulation of cyclin D (cD) is a crucial event in initiating the cell division cycle. cD activates cyclin-dependent protein kinases 4 and 6 (cdk4/6), which in turn phosphorylate the retinoblastoma protein (pRb) causing dissociation of pRb from transcription factor E2F (Johnson and Walker, 1999). Then the unleashed E2F is able to bind to and transactivate genes whose products are essential for DNA synthesis, such as dihydrofolate reductase (DHFR), thymidine kinase (TK), thymidylate synthetase (TS), and DNA polymerase (POL), or are regulatory proteins, such as cyclin E (cE), cyclin A (cA) and cyclin-dependent protein kinase 1 (cdk1), that promote further progression of the cell cycle. Expression of cD is increased, for example, by signals evoked by growth factors (GFs) via Ras proteins and by transcription factors, such as myc and β-catenin (β-cat). Some carcinogens, e.g., benzpyrene (BP) and reactive oxygen species (ROS), and diethylnitrosamine (DENA) may cause mutation of the *Ras* or *Raf* gene that results in permanently active mutant Ras protein, but BP as well as TCDD may also induce simple overexpression of normal Ras protein.

Cell cycle progression is counteracted, for example, by pRb (which inhibits the function of E2F), by cyclin-dependent protein kinase inhibitors (such as p15, p16, and p21), by p53 (that transactivates the *p21* gene), and by ARF (also called p14 that binds to mdm2, thereby neutralizing the antagonistic effect of mdm2 on p53). Signals point mutation in codon 12) dramatically lower the GTPase activity of the protein. This in turn locks Ras in the permanently active GTP-bound form. Continual rather than signal-dependent activation of Ras can lead eventually to uncontrolled proliferation and transformation. Indeed, microinjection of Ras-neutralizing monoclonal antibodies into cells blocks the mitogenic action of growth factors as well as cell transformation by several oncogenes. Numerous carcinogenic chemicals induce mutations of Ras proto-oncogenes that lead to constitutive activation of Ras proteins (Anderson *et al.*, 1992). These include *N*-methyl-*N*-nitrosourea, polycyclic aromatic hydrocarbons, benzidine, aflatoxin B$_l$, and ionizing radiation. Most of these chemicals induce point mutations by transversion of G$_{35}$ to T in codon 12.

Another example for activating mutation of a proto-oncogene is *B-Raf* mutation, although *Ras* and *Raf* mutations are mutually exclusive (Shaw and Cantley, 2006). Raf proteins are protein kinases; lying just downstream from Ras and being the first signal transducers in the MAP kinase pathway (see Fig. 3-11). After recruitment by Ras to the cell membrane, Raf is activated by the growth factor receptor (see item 4 in Fig. 3-11) through phosphorylation in its activating segment. B-Raf mutations occur in mouse liver tumors induced by diethylnitrosamine (Jaworski *et al.*, 2005) in 66% of malignant melanomas and a wide range of human cancers. All mutations are within the activation segment of B-Raf, with a single amino acid substitution (V599E) accounting for the majority. The mutant B-Raf protein has elevated kinase activity probably because substitution of the non-polar valine with the negatively charged glutamate mimics an activating phosphorylation. Thus, the constitutively active B-Raf continually sends Ras-independent proliferative signal down the MAPK pathway. Indeed, transfection of the mutant *B-Raf* gene into cells induced neoplastic transformation even in the absence of Ras proteins (Davies *et al.*, 2002). Another proto-oncogene product that often undergoes activating mutation in breast and colon tumors is p110α, the catalytic subunit of PI3K (Shaw and Cantley, 2006). This can cause permanent proliferative signaling via the GF receptor–PI3K–Akt pathway (see Fig. 3-11).

Whereas constitutive activation of oncogene proteins, as a result of point-mutation, is a common initiator of chemical carcinogenesis, permanent overexpression of such proteins also can contribute to neoplastic cell transformation. Overexpression of proto-oncogene proteins may result from amplification of the proto-oncogene (i.e., the formation more than one copy) (Anderson *et al.*, 1992). Such event may be initiated by DNA strand breaks, and therefore often observed after exposure to ionizing radiation; however, proto-oncogene amplification also occurs in spontaneous human cancer. Overexpression of proto-oncogene proteins as a result of nongenotoxic, epigenetic mechanisms will be discussed later.

Mutation of Tumor-Suppressor Genes   Tumor-suppressor genes encode proteins that inhibit the progression of cells in the division cycle, or promote apoptosis upon DNA damage. Figure 3-27 depicts such proteins, which include, for example, cyclin-dependent protein kinase inhibitors (e.g., p15, p16, and p21), transcription factors (e.g., p53 and Smad) that activate genes encoding cyclin-dependent protein kinase inhibitors, proteins (e.g., pRb) that block transcription factors involved in DNA synthesis and cell division, and proteins (e.g., ARF) that block inhibitors of tumor suppressor proteins. Other notable tumor suppressor gene products include, for example, the protein kinases (e.g., ATM, ATR) that sense the DNA damage and signal for the p53-controlled response shown in Fig. 3-28, proapotic proteins (e.g., Bax, Puma, Noxa) induced after DNA damage (Fig. 3-28), the phosphatase PTEN (that dephosphorylates the membrane lipid phosphatidylinositol-3,4,5-triphosphate, an essential intermediate in the PI3K-Akt pathway) that turns off the PI3K-Akt pathway-mediated proliferative signaling (Fig. 3-11), and the GTPase activating protein TSC2 (tuberous sclerosis complex-2) that prevents activation of mTOR (Fig. 3-25). Uncontrolled proliferation can occur when the mutant tumor-suppressor gene encodes a protein that cannot suppress cell division. Inactivating mutations of specific tumor suppressor genes in germ cells are responsible for the inherited predisposition to cancer, as in familial retinoblastoma (pRb), Wilms' tumor (WT1), familial polyposis (Smad4), and Li-Fraumeni syndrome (p53). Mutations of tumor-suppressor genes in somatic cells contribute to nonhereditary cancers. The genes of p16, PTEN, pRb are frequently mutated in human cancer. The best-known tumor suppressor gene involved in both spontaneous and chemically induced carcinogenesis is p53.

The p53 tumor suppressor gene encodes a 53 kDa protein with multiple functions (Fig. 3-28). Acting as a transcriptional modulator, the p53 protein (1) transactivates genes whose products arrest the cell cycle (e.g., p21 and gadd45), repair damaged DNA (e.g., XPE, MSH2), or promote apoptosis (e.g., Bax, Puma, and Fas receptor) and (2) represses genes that encode cell cycle accelerators (e.g., cyclin B1, Cdk1), or antiapoptotic proteins (e.g., bcl-2 and IGF-1 receptor) (Bennett *et al.*, 1999; Liu and Chen, 2006). DNA damage activates protein kinases to phosphorylate and stabilize the p53 protein, causing its accumulation (Fig. 3-28). The accumulated p53 may induce cell cycle arrest, DNA repair and apoptosis of the affected cells. Thus, p53 eliminates cancer-prone cells from the replicative pool, counteracting neoplastic transformation (Fig. 3-26); therefore it is commonly designated as guardian of the genome.

Indeed, cells that have no p53 are a million times more likely to permit DNA amplification than are cells with a normal level of the suppressor gene. Furthermore, mice with the p53 gene deleted develop cancer by 6 to 9 months of age, attesting to the crucial role of the p53 tumor-suppressor gene in preventing carcinogenesis.

Mutations in the p53 gene are found in 50 percent of human tumors and in a variety of induced cancers. The majority are "missense mutations" that change an amino acid and result in a faulty or altered protein (Bennett *et al.*, 1999). The faulty p53 protein forms a complex with endogenous wild-type p53 protein and inactivates it. Thus, the mutant p53 not only is unable to function as a tumor suppressor protein but also prevents tumor suppression by the wild-type p53.

Carcinogens may cause characteristic pattern of mutations in the p53 tumor-suppressor gene. An example is the point mutation in codon 249 from AGG to AGT, which changes amino acid 249 in the p53 protein from arginine to serine. This mutation predominates

---

evoked by DNA damage and TGF-β will ultimately result in accumulation of p53 and p15 proteins, respectively, and deceleration of the cell cycle. In contrast, mutations that disable the tumor suppressor proteins facilitate cell cycle progression and neoplastic conversion and are common in human tumors. Aflatoxin B$_1$ (ATX), BP and UV light cause such mutations of the *p53* gene (Bennet *et al.*, 1999), whereas *pRb* mutations occur invariably in methylcholanthrene (MC)-induced transplacental lung tumors in mice (Miller, 1999).

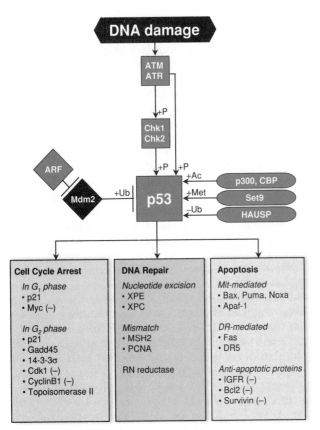

Figure 3-28. The guardian of the genome: p53 tumor suppressor protein—its role and regulation.

When activated upon DNA damage, the p53 protein may mediate cell cycle arrest, DNA repair and apoptosis. p53 can induce these effects by acting chiefly as a transcription factor that can activate the transcription of most target genes, while repressing some of others, such as those marked with (-) in the figure (Liu and Chen, 2006). For example, p53 transactivates *p21* and *gadd45* genes (whose products are inhibitors of cyclin–cyclin-dependent protein kinase complexes) and arrest the cell cycle in G_1 and G_2 phases, respectively, but p53 represses the *Cdk1* and *cyclin B1* genes (whose products are indispensable for the cells to transit from G_2 phase to M) (see Fig. 3-21). p53 also transactivates the genes of some DNA repair proteins and pro-apoptotic proteins (e.g., bax and fas; see Fig. 3-16) and represses the genes of anti-apoptotic proteins (e.g., bcl-2 and insulin-like growth factor-1 [IGF-1] receptor), whereby it promotes apoptosis. These (and other) p53-induced pro-apoptotic mechanisms may be cell specific, i.e., all are not necessarily occurring in the same cell at the same time.

The intracellular level and activity of p53 depends primarily on the presence of mdm2 protein, which inactivates p53 by ubiquitinating it; monoubiquitination causes export of p53 from the nucleus, whereas polyubiquitination promotes its proteosomal degradation. The influence of mdm2 on p53 may be disrupted by overexpression of the ARF (or p14) protein (which binds to mdm2 and removes it from p53) or by posttranslational modification of p53 through phosphorylation by protein kinases (see below), acetylation by acetyltransferases (e.g., p300 and CBP), and methylation by methyltransferases (e.g., Set9) (Liu and Chen, 2006). These mechanisms release p53 from mdm2, stabilize the p53 protein, thereby greatly increasing its abundance and activity. Phosphorylation of p53 is induced by DNA damage. This is sensed by kinases, such as ATM (ataxia telangiectasia mutated) and ATR (ataxia telangiectasia related), which directly or through checkpoint kinases (Chk1, Chk2) phosphorylate p53 to induce cell cycle arrest, DNA repair or apoptosis (McGowan and Russel, 2004).

It is important to emphasize that there is also a p53-independent mechanism to arrest the cells suffering DNA damage before mitosis. Like induction of p53, this is also initiated by the activated Chk1, which phosphorylates and

in hepatocellular carcinomas in individuals living where food is contaminated with aflatoxin B_1 (Bennett *et al.*, 1999). Because aflatoxin B_1 induces the transversion of G to T in codon 249 of the p53 tumor-suppressor gene in human hepatocytes (Aguilar *et al.*, 1993), it appears likely that this mutation is indeed induced by this mycotoxin. Although the detected mutation in patients presumably contributes to the hepatocarcinogenicity of aflatoxin B_1 in humans, it is not required for aflatoxin B_1–induced hepatocarcinogenesis in rats, as rats do not show this aberration in the transformed liver cells.

Inappropriate Activation or Responsiveness of the Regulatory Region of Critical Genes: Epigenetic Mechanisms in Carcinogenesis
Whereas some chemicals cause cancer by reacting with DNA and inducing a mutation, others do not damage DNA, yet induce cancer after prolonged exposure (Barrett, 1992). These chemicals are designated *nongenotoxic* or *epigenetic carcinogens* and include (1) xenobiotic mitogens, such as the PKC activator phorbol esters and fumonisin B_1, as well as some other chemicals that promote mitogenic signaling, such as the protein phosphatase inhibitor okadaic acid (see Fig. 3-11); (2) endogenous mitogens, such as growth factors (e.g., TGF-α) and hormones with mitogenic action on specific cells [e.g., estrogens on mammary gland or liver cells, TSH on the follicular cells of the thyroid gland, and luteinizing hormone (LH) on Leydig cells in testes]; (3) toxicants that, when given chronically, cause sustained cell injury (such as chloroform and *d*-limonene); (4) xenobiotics that are nongenotoxic carcinogens in rodents but not in humans, such as phenobarbital, DDT, TCDD and peroxisomal proliferators (e.g., fibrates, WI-14643, di- and trihalogenated acetic acids); and (5) ethionine and diethanolamine, which interfere with formation of endogenous methyl donors (Poirier, 1994). Because several of the listed chemicals promote the development of tumors after neoplastic transformation has been initiated by a genotoxic carcinogen, they are referred to as *tumor promoters*. Despite the initial belief that promoters are unable to induce tumors by themselves, studies suggest that they can do so after prolonged exposure.

It is apparent that nongenotoxic chemicals, like the genotoxic ones, ultimately also influence proto-oncogenes and/or tumor suppressor genes, but in a different manner: they increase the transcriptional activity of proto-oncogenes and/or decrease the transcription rate of tumor suppressor genes. Therefore, nongenotoxic carcinogens, when continuously present, can permanently induce the synthesis of normal proto-oncogene proteins and/or repress the synthesis of normal tumor suppressor proteins, rather than inducing the synthesis of permanently active mutant proto-oncogene proteins or permanently inactive mutant tumor suppressor proteins, as the mutagenic genotoxic carcinogens do.

---

inactivates cdc25A, a protein phosphatase, which normally would dephosphorylate Cdk1 and activate the Cdk1-cyclin B complex (see Fig. 3-21). Thus when cdc25A is inactivated Cdk1 stalls and mitosis is delayed. Interestingly, p53 assists in keeping Cdk1, this mitosis-driving molecular motor, off track as it induces 14-3-3σ, a cytoplasmic binding protein, which associates with both cdc25A and the Cdk1-cyclin B complex and sequesters them in the cytoplasm.

By arresting division of cells with potentially mutagenic DNA damage, facilitating the DNA repair or eliminating such cells, p53 protein counteracts neoplastic development. *p53*-null mice, like *ARF*-null mice, develop tumors with high incidence. Mutational inactivation of the p53 protein is thought to contribute to the carcinogenic effect of aflatoxin B_1, sunlight and cigarette smoke in humans. Overexpression of mdm2 can lead to constitutive inhibition of p53 and thereby promotes oncogenesis even if the *p53* gene is unaltered. See the text for more details.

The ultimate target of epigenetic carcinogens is the promoter region of critical genes where they can act via two distinct modes. First, they may alter the abundance and/or activity of transcription factors, typically by influencing upstream signaling elements ranging from extracellular signaling molecules (e.g., TSH) to intracellular transducer proteins (e.g., PKC). Obviously both xenobiotic and endogenous mitogens mentioned above can thus activate proliferative pathways (see Fig. 3-11) that descend to transcription factors (e.g., Myc) that act on the promoter of proto-oncogenes (e.g., cyclins). It is easy to recognize that even epigenetic carcinogens of the cytotoxic type act in this manner. As discussed under tissue repair, cell injury evokes the release of mitogenic growth factors such as HGF and TGF-α from tissue macrophages and endothelial cells. Thus, cells in chronically injured tissues are exposed continuously to endogenous mitogens. Although these growth factors are instrumental in tissue repair after acute cell injury, their continuous presence is potentially harmful because they may ultimately transform the affected cells into neoplastic cells. Indeed, transgenic mice that overexpress TGF-α develop hepatomegaly at a young age and tumors by 12 months (Fausto *et al.*, 2006). Mitogenic cytokines secreted by Kupffer cells are apparently involved in hepatocyte proliferation and, possibly, tumor formation induced by peroxysome proliferators in rats (Rose *et al.*, 1999) and in the formation of the endothelial cell-derived hepatic hemangiosarcoma in mice exposed to 2-butoxyethanol (Corthals *et al.*, 2006).

Epigenetic carcinogens can alter expression of critical genes also by a second major mechanism, i.e., by altering the responsiveness of the promoter region of these genes to transcription factors. Promoter responsiveness is typically controlled by methylation at C_5 of specific cytosine residues located in CpG islands (i.e., clusters of CpG dinucleotides) in the promoter. It is well known that promoter methylation decreases the transcriptional activity of genes. For example, tissue specific genes (e.g., the genes of gastrointestinal trefoil factors) are fully methylated in tissues where they are not expressed, but are typically demethylated in tissues where they are expressed.

Promoter methylation by DNA cytosine methyltransferases (e.g., DNMT1, DNMT3a, and DNMT3b) can silence genes because it weakens binding of transcription factors to the promoter and because it can reduce accessibility of the promoter for transcription factors (Esteller, 2005). This latter mechanism involves modification of core histone proteins at their protruding amino-terminal tails by deacetylation and methylation of lysine residues. This makes the histone more compact, thereby diminishing access to the gene promoter of transcription factors and other proteins involved in transcription initiation. Histone deacetylases that remove the acetyl group from histone tails may be recruited by DNMTs directly, or through proteins that recognize and bind to the methylated CpG dinucleotides (e.g., MeCP1, MeCP2, MBD2, MBD3). Some of these methyl-CpG binding domain containing proteins (e.g., MBD2, MBD3) also have histone deacetylase activity. Finally, both DNMTs and MBDs can recruit histone methyltransferases (HMT) to methylate histone tail lysines.

While methylation of CpG dinucleotides codes for gene silencing via histone deacetylation and methylation ("histone code"), unmethylated genes are alert. In fact, CpG islands in the 5'-end region (promoter, untranslated region, exon 1) of genes are relatively unmethylated in normal tissues, except for tissue-specific or germline-specific genes, and genomically imprinted genes (see earlier). Thus, if the appropriate transcription factors are available for a particular gene, and if the CpG island remains unmethylated, the histones acetylated and unmethylated, then the gene will be transcribed

(Esteller, 2005). Histones are acetylated by histone acetyltransferases, such as p300 and CBP, which also acetylate other proteins, including p53 (see Fig. 3-28), and are also transcriptional coactivators.

It is well documented that the normal methylation pattern of DNA is disrupted in cancer cells. Such cells are characterized by global (average) hypomethylation, i.e., decreased content of genomic 5'-methylcytosine. Paradoxically, DNA hypomethylation occurs in the face of hypermethylation of the CpG islands in the promoter region tumor suppressor genes, which are normally demethylated (Esteller, 2005). Among the frequently hypermethylated tumor suppressor genes in human cancers are, for example, the Cdk inhibitor p15 and p16, the mdm2-binding protein ARF, pRb that tethers E2F (see Fig. 3-30), the DNA repair enzyme O^6-methyguanine-DNA-methyltransferase (MGMT) and the lipid phosphatase PTEN. Importantly, both the global hypomethylation and tumor suppressor gene hypermethylation intensify with increased malignancy of the tumor. Relevance of hypermethylation-induced silencing of tumor suppressor genes in carcinogenesis is supported by the finding that inhibitors of DNMTs (such as 5-aza-2'-deoxycytidine) can stop the growth of cancer cells and induce their differentiation by demethylating the dormant tumor suppressor genes, thereby restoring their expression (Esteller, 2005). The consequence of global hypomethylation of DNA is less clear. Nevertheless, demethylation of proto-oncogenes and increased expression of their products is a plausible mechanism (Goodman and Watson, 2002), although others have also been proposed (e.g., chromosomal instability, reactivation of transposable DNA elements and loss of genomic imprinting). On comparing mouse strains, it has been suggested that their sensitivity to chemical carcinogens may be related inversely to their capacity to maintain normal patterns of DNA methylation. It is worth noting that DNA methylation is more stable in human cells than in rodent cells (Goodman and Watson, 2002).

It appears that some of the epigenetic carcinogens alter DNA methylation. Inhibition of DNA methylation is a plausible mechanism that underlies tumorigenesis induced by ethionine, which depletes S-adenosyl-methionine (the methyl donor for DNMTs), and diethanolamine, which inhibits cellular uptake of choline, a dietary methyl group source for methylation of homocysteine to methionine. Upon prolonged administration, virtually all nongenotoxic rodent liver carcinogens listed above decrease DNA methylation. In addition to global DNA hypomethylation, promoter hypomethylation of the following proto-oncogenes have been observed in mouse or rat liver: *Ras* or *Raf,* following phenobarbital treatment, *c-Jun, c-Myc,* and *IGF-2,* after treatment with dichloro-, dibromo-, or trichloroacetic acid, and *c-Myc* after WY-14643 dosing. Long-term arsenic exposure of mice also induces hypomethylation of hepatic DNA globally and in the promoter of estrogen receptor-α (ERα), a hormone-activated transcription factor. This is associated with an increase of cyclin D, a potentially ERα-linked gene (Chen *et al.*, 2004). In contrast, in human keratinocytes TCDD induces promoter hypermethylation in the tumor suppressor genes p16 and p53 as well as immortalization of these cells (Ray and Swanson, 2004). Although the mechanisms that initiate altered promoter methylation are currently unknown, it is possible that that altered promoter methylation plays a role in tumor promotion by these nongenotoxic carcinogens.

Cooperation of Genotoxic and Epigenetic Mechanisms in Carcinogenesis   Genotoxic and epigenetic mechanisms most likely complement and amplify each other in chemical carcinogenesis. For example, tumor suppressor genes are often silenced by promoter methylation in tumors induced by genotoxic carcinogens (like in spontaneous human tumors). In aflatoxin B$_1$-induced mouse lung tumor and in skin tumor induced by 7,12-dimethylbenzanthracene, tumor suppressor genes such as *p16*, *ARF* and *MGMT* exhibit increased methylation. Conversely, global DNA hypomethylation and tumor suppressor gene hypermethylation may increase the occurrence of mutations in cells exposed to epigenetic carcinogens. In this sense, epigenetic mechanisms may also initiate carcinogenesis (Goodman and Watson, 2002). Furthermore, one chemical may exert both genotoxic and epigenetic effects. This has been proposed for estrogens that may produce mutagenic free radicals via redox cycling of their quinone and hydroquinone metabolites and also induce receptor-mediated proliferative effect (Newbold, 2004). The antiestrogen tamoxifen, a hepatocarcinogen in rats (but not in humans), exerts genotoxic effect and induces global hypomethylation of DNA and histones in rat liver (Tryndyak *et al.*, 2006).

Cooperation of Proto-oncogenes and Tumor-Suppressor Genes in Carcinogenesis   The accumulation of genetic damage in the form of mutant proto-oncogenes (which encode activated proteins) and mutant tumor-suppressor genes (which encode inactivated proteins) as well as increased activation of normal proto-oncogenes (causing expression of more cell cycle accelerator proteins) and silencing of normal tumor suppressor genes (causing expression of less cell cycle decelerator proteins) are the forces that drive transformation of normal cells with controlled proliferative activity to malignant cells with uncontrolled proliferative activity. Because the number of cells in a tissue is regulated by a balance between mitosis and apoptosis, the uncontrolled proliferation results from perturbation of this balance (Fig. 3-29).

Failure of Apoptosis: Promotion of Mutation and Clonal Growth

As discussed earlier, in cells suffering DNA damage, the stabilized p53 protein may induce cell death by apoptosis (Fig. 3-28). Apoptosis thus eliminates cells with DNA damage, preventing mutations to initiate carcinogenesis. Initiated preneoplastic cells have much higher apoptotic activity than do normal cells (Bursch *et al.*, 1992) and this can counteract their clonal expansion. In fact, facilitation of apoptosis can induce tumor regression. This occurs when hormone dependent tumors are deprived of the hormone that promotes growth and suppresses apoptosis. This is the rationale for the use of tamoxifen, an antiestrogen, and gonadotropin-releasing hormone analogs to combat hormone-dependent tumors of the mammary gland and the prostate gland, respectively (Bursch *et al.*, 1992).

Thus, the inhibition of apoptosis is detrimental because it facilitates both mutations and clonal expansion of preneoplastic cells. Indeed, apoptosis inhibition plays a role in the pathogenesis of human B-cell lymphomas, in which a chromosomal translocation, results in aberrantly increased expression of Bcl-2 protein, which overrides programmed cell death after binding to and inactivating the proapoptotic Bax protein (see Fig. 3-16). Increased levels of Bcl-2 are also detected in other types of cancer, and a high Bcl-2/Bax ratio in a tumor is a marker for poor prognosis (Jäättelä, 1999). Other antiapoptotic proteins, such as Hsp 27, 70, and 90 (Sreedhar and Csermely, 2004) and IAP family members, may also contribute to progression of neoplasia. Survivin, a member of the IAP family, is expressed in all cancer cells but not in adult differentiated cells (Jäättelä, 1999).

Inhibition of apoptosis is one mechanism by which the rodent tumor promoter phenobarbital promotes clonal expansion of preneoplastic cells. This has been demonstrated in rats given a single dose of *N*-nitrosomorpholine followed by daily treatments with phenobarbital for 12 months to initiate and promote, respectively,

neoplastic transformation in liver (Schulte-Hermann *et al.*, 1990). From 6 months onward, phenobarbital did not increase DNA synthesis and cell division in the preneoplastic foci, yet it accelerated foci enlargement. The foci grow because phenobarbital lowers apoptotic activity, allowing the high cell replicative activity to manifest itself. The peroxisome proliferator nafenopin, a nongenotoxic hepatocarcinogen, also suppresses apoptosis in primary rat hepatocyte cultures (Bayly *et al.*, 1994), supporting the hypothesis that this mechanism may play a role in the hepatocarcinogenicity of peroxisome proliferators in rodents.

Failure to Terminate Proliferation: Promotion of Mutation, Proto-Oncogene Expression, and Clonal Growth

Enhanced mitotic activity, whether it is induced by oncogenes inside the cell or by external factors such as xenobiotic or endogenous mitogens, promotes carcinogenesis for a number of reasons.

1. First, the enhanced mitotic activity increases the probability of mutations. This is due to activation of the cell-division cycle, which invokes a substantial shortening of the G$_l$ phase. Thus, less time is available for the repair of injured DNA before replication, increasing the chance that the damage will yield a mutation. Although repair still may be feasible after replication, postreplication repair is error-prone. In addition, activation of the cell-division cycle increases the proportion of cells that replicate their DNA at any given time. During replication, the amount of DNA doubles and the DNA becomes unpacked, greatly increasing the effective target size for DNA-reactive mutagenic chemicals, including ROS.

2. Enhanced mitotic activity may compromise DNA methylation, which occurs in the early postreplication period and carried out by DNMTs that copy the methylation pattern of the parental DNA strand to the daughter strand (maintenance methylation). Limitation of DNMTs by shortened G$_2$ phase or by presence of other transacting factors might impair methylation and may contribute to overexpression of proto-oncogens, starting a vicious cycle.

3. Another mechanism by which proliferation promotes the carcinogenic process is through clonal expansion of the initiated cells to form nodules (foci) and tumors.

4. Finally, cell-to-cell communication through gap junctions (constructed from connexins) and intercellular adhesion through cadherins are temporarily disrupted during proliferation. Lack of these junctions contributes to the invasiveness of tumor cells. Several tumor promoters, such as phenobarbital, phorbol esters, and peroxisome proliferators, decrease gap junctional intercellular communication. It has been hypothesized that this contributes to neoplastic transformation. Increased susceptibility of connexin-knockout mice to spontaneous and chemically induced liver tumors supports this hypothesis (Chipman *et al.*, 2003).

It appears that genotoxic carcinogens induce cancer *primarily* by causing mutations in critical genes whose aberrant products promote mitosis and inhibit apoptosis, and *secondarily* by causing aberrant methylation of critical genes whose normal products produced in abnormal quantities, there by further tilting the balance of mitosis and apoptosis to the favor of the former. In contrast, nongenotoxic carcinogens cause cancer by promoting carcinogenesis initiated by genotoxic agents or spontaneous DNA damage (Fig. 3-30). Spontaneous DNA damage, which occasionally gives rise to mutation, commonly occurs in normal cells (Barrett, 1992). It is estimated

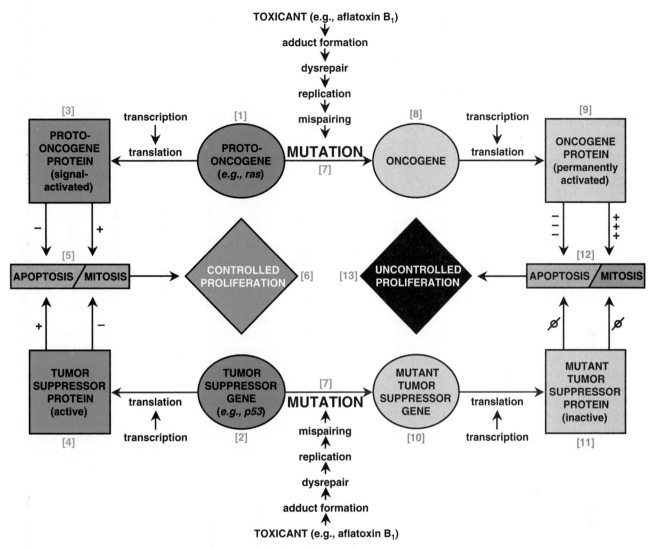

Figure 3-29. A model of cooperation between a proto-oncogene (1) and a tumor suppressor gene (2) before and after mutation.

The model shows that the normal proteins encoded by the cellular proto-oncogenes and the tumor suppressor genes [(3) and (4), respectively] reciprocally influence mitosis and apoptosis (5) and thus ensure controlled cell proliferation (6). However, the balance between the effects of these two types of proteins is offset by a toxicant-induced mutation of their genes (7) if the mutant proto-oncogene (oncogene) (8) encodes a constitutively (i.e., permanently) active oncogene protein (9) and the mutant tumor suppressor gene (10) encodes an inactive tumor suppressor protein (11). Under this condition, the effect of the oncogene protein on mitosis and apoptosis is unopposed (12), resulting in uncontrolled proliferation. Such a scenario may underlie the carcinogenicity of aflatoxin B₁, which can induce mutations in *Ras* proto-oncogene and the *p53* tumor suppressor gene (see text for details). Positive and negative signs represent stimulation and inhibition, respectively; Ø means "no effect." It is important to realize that in addition to activating mutation of proto-oncogenes and inactivating mutation of tumor suppressor genes overexpression of normal proto-oncogenes (e.g., by hypomethylation of their promoter) and under-expression (silencing) of normal tumor suppressor genes (e.g., by hypermethylation of their promoter) may also contribute to and cooperate in neoplastic transformation of cells (see text for explanation).

that in human cells, 1 out of 10^8 to 10^{10} base pairs suffers spontaneous mutation. Genotoxic carcinogens increase the frequency 10- to 1000-fold. Nongenotoxic carcinogens also increase the frequency of spontaneous mutations through a mitogenic effect and by the mechanisms discussed earlier. In addition, nongenotoxic carcinogens, by inhibiting apoptosis, increase the number of cells with DNA damage and mutations. Both enhanced mitotic activity and decreased apoptotic activity brought about by nongenotoxic carcino-

gens expand the population of transformed cells, promoting cancer development. In summary, nongenotoxic carcinogens appear to act by enhancing cell division and/or inhibiting apoptosis.

CONCLUSIONS

This overview systematically surveys the mechanisms of the potential events that follow toxicant exposure and contribute to toxicity.

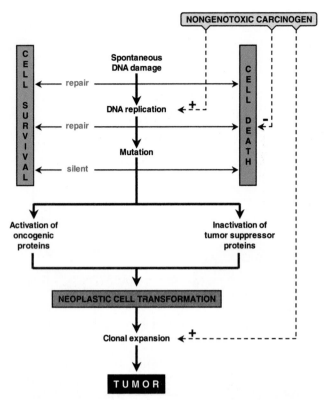

Figure 3-30. The process of carcinogenesis promoted by nongenotoxic carcinogens.

Positive and negative signs represent stimulation and inhibition, respectively. See text for explanation.

This approach is also useful in the search for mechanisms responsible for (1) selective toxicity, that is, differences in the sensitivity to toxicants of various organisms, such as different species and strains of animals, organs, and cells, and (2) alteration of toxicity by exogenous factors such as chemicals and food and physiologic or pathologic conditions such as aging and disease. To identify the mechanisms that underlie selective toxicity or alterations in toxicity, all steps where variations might occur must be considered systematically. Selective or altered toxicity may be due to different or altered (1) exposure; (2) delivery, thus resulting in a different concentration of the ultimate toxicant at the target site; (3) target molecules; (4) biochemical processes triggered by the reaction of the chemical with the target molecules; (5) repair at the molecular, cellular, or tissue level; or (6) altered gene expression-based stress responses as well as circulatory and thermoregulatory reflexes by which the affected organism can adapt to some of the toxic effects.

In this chapter, a simplified scheme has been used to give an overview of the development of toxicity (Fig. 3-1). In reality, the route to toxicity can be considerably more diverse and complicated. For example, one chemical may yield several ultimate toxicants, one ultimate toxicant may react with several types of target molecules, and reaction with one type of target molecule may have a number of consequences. Thus, the toxicity of one chemical may involve several mechanisms which can interact with and influence each other in an intricate manner.

This chapter has emphasized the significance of the chemistry of a toxicant in governing its delivery to and reaction with the target molecule as well as the importance of the biochemistry, molecular and cell biology, immunology, and physiology of the affected organism in its response to the action of the toxicant. An organism has mechanisms that (1) counteract the delivery of toxicants, such as detoxication; (2) reverse the toxic injury, such as repair mechanisms; and (3) offset some dysfunctions, such as adaptive responses. Thus, toxicity is not an inevitable consequence of toxicant exposure because it may be prevented, reversed, or compensated for by such mechanisms. Toxicity develops if the toxicant exhausts or impairs the protective mechanisms and/or overrides the adaptability of biological systems.

REFERENCES

Aguilar F, Hussain SP, Cerutti P: Aflatoxin Bl induces the transversion of G → T in codon 249 of the p53 tumor suppressor gene in human hepatocytes. *Proc Natl Acad Sci U S A* 90:8586–8590, 1993.

Anders MW: Glutathione-dependent bioactivation of haloalkanes and haloalkenes. *Drug Metab Rev* 36:583–594, 2004.

Anderson MW, Reynolds SH, You M, Maronpot RM: Role of proto-oncogene activation in carcinogenesis. *Environ Health Perspect* 98:13–24, 1992.

Anway MD, Cupp AS, Uzumcu M, Skinner MK: Epigenetic transgenerational actions of endocrine disruptors and male fertility. *Science* 308:1466–1469, 2005.

Arthur MJP, Iredale JP, Mann DA: Tissue inhibitors of metalloproteinases: Role in liver fibrosis and alcoholic liver disease. *Alcohol Clin Exp Res* 23:940–943, 1999.

Aust SD, Chignell CF, Bray TM, et al: Free radicals in toxicology. *Toxicol Appl Pharmacol* 120:168–178, 1993.

Bailey CP, Connor M: Opioids: Cellular mechanisms of tolerance and physical dependence. *Curr Opin Pharmacol* 5:60–68, 2005.

Baillie TA, Kassahun K: Reversibility in glutathione-conjugate formation. *Adv Pharmacol* 27:163–181, 1994.

Ballestar E, Esteller M, Richardson BC: The epigenetic face of systemic lupus erythematosus. *J Immunol* 176:7143–7147, 2006.

Barrett JC: Mechanisms of action of known human carcinogens, in Vainio H, Magee PN, McGregor DB, McMichael AJ (eds): *Mechanisms of Carcinogenesis in Risk Identification.* Lyons, France: International Agency for Research on Cancer, 1992, pp 115–134.

Basu S: Isoprostanes: Novel bioactive products of lipid peroxidation. *Free Radic Res* 38:105–22, 2004.

Baumann H, Gauldie J: The acute phase response. *Immunol Today* 15:74–80, 1994.

Bayly AC, Roberts RA, Dive C: Suppression of liver cell apoptosis in vitro by the nongenotoxic hepatocarcinogen and peroxisome proliferator nafenopin. *J Cell Biol* 125:197–203, 1994.

Bennett WP, Hussain SP, Vahakangas KH, et al: Molecular epidemiology of human cancer risk: Gene-environment interactions and *p53* mutation spectrum in human lung cancer. *J Pathol* 187:8–18, 1999.

Boatright KM, Salvesen GS: Mechanisms of caspase activation. *Curr Opin Cell Biol* 15:725–731, 2003.

Bock KW, Lilienblum W: Roles of uridine diphosphate glucuronosyltransferases in chemical carcinogenesis, in Kauffman FC (ed). *Conjugation-Deconjugation Reactions in Drug Metabolism and Toxicity.* Berlin: Springer-Verlag, 1994, pp 391–428.

Boelsterli UA: Specific targets of covalent drug-protein interactions in hepatocytes and their toxicological significance in drug-induced liver injury. *Drug Metab Rev* 25:395–451, 1993.

Bokoch GM, Knaus UG: NADPH oxidases: Not just for leukocytes anymore! *Trends Biochem Sci* 28:502–508, 2003.

Boulares HA, Giardina C, Navarro CL, et al: Modulation of serum growth factor signal transduction in Hepa 1-6 cells by acetaminophen: An inhibition of c-*myc* expression, NF-κB activation, and Raf-1 kinase activity. *Tox Sci* 48:264–274, 1999.

Breen AP, Murphy JA: Reactions of oxyl radicals with DNA. *Free Rad Biol Med* 18:1033–1077, 1995.

Buja LM, Eigenbrodt ML, Eigenbrodt EH: Apoptosis and necrosis: Basic types and mechanisms of cell death. *Arch Pathol Lab Med* 117:1208–1214, 1993.

Bursch W, Oberhammer F, Schulte-Hermann R: Cell death by apoptosis and its protective role against disease. *Trends Pharmacol Sci* 13:245–251, 1992.

Cai J, Yang J, Jones DP: Mitochondrial control of apoptosis: The role of cytochrome *c*. *Biochim Biophys Acta* 1366:139–149, 1998.

Cain K: Chemical-induced apoptosis: Formation of the Apaf-1 apoptosome. *Drug Metab Rev* 35:337–363, 2003.

Caro AA, Cederbaum AI: Oxidative stress, toxicology, and pharmacology of CYP2E1. *Annu Rev Pharmacol Toxicol* 44:27–42, 2004.

Castro L, Rodriguez M, Radi R: Aconitase is readily inactivated by peroxynitrite, but not by its precursor, nitric oxide. *J Biol Chem* 269:29409–29415, 1994.

Castranova V: Signaling pathways controlling the production of inflammatory mediators in response to crystalline silica exposure: Role of reactive oxygen/nitrogen species. *Free Radic Biol Med* 37:916–925, 2004.

Cavalieri EL, Rogan EG: The approach to understanding aromatic hydrocarbon carcinogenesis: The central role of radical cations in metabolic activation. *Pharmacol Ther* 55:183–199, 1992.

Chen H, Li S, Liu J, et al: Chronic inorganic arsenic exposure induces hepatic global and individual gene hypomethylation: implications for arsenic hepatocarcinogenesis. *Carcinogenesis* 25:1779–1786, 2004.

Chen W, Martindale L, Holbrook NJ, Liu Y: Tumor promoter arsenite activates extracellular signal-regulated kinase through a signaling pathway mediated by epidermal growth factor receptor and Shc. *Mol Cell Biol* 18:5178–5188, 1998.

Chipman JK, Mally A, Edwards GO: Disruption of gap junctions in toxicity and carcinogenicity. *Toxicol Sci* 71:146–153, 2003.

Christmann M, Tomicic MJ, Roos W, Kaina B: Mechanism of human DNA repair: An update. *Toxicology* 193:3–34, 2003.

Cohen SD, Pumford NR, Khairallah EA, et al: Contemporary issues in toxicology: Selective protein covalent binding and target organ toxicity. *Toxicol Appl Pharmacol* 143:1–2, 1997.

Coleman MD, Jacobus DP: Reduction of dapsone hydroxylamine to dapsone during methaemoglobin formation in human erythrocytes in vitro. *Biochem Pharmacol* 45:1027–1033, 1993.

Coles B: Effects of modifying structure on electrophilic reactions with biological nucleophiles. *Drug Metab Rev* 15:1307–1334, 1984.

Commandeur JNM, Vermeulen NPE: Molecular and biochemical mechanisms of chemically induced nephrotoxicity: A review. *Chem Res Toxicol* 3:171–194, 1990.

Corcoran GB, Fix L, Jones DP, et al: Apoptosis: Molecular control point in toxicity. *Toxicol Appl Pharmacol* 128:169–181, 1994.

Corthals SM, Kamendulis LM, Klaunig JE: Mechanisms of 2-butoxyethanol-induced hemangiosarcomas. *Toxicol Sci* 92:378–386, 2006.

Corton JM, Gillespie JG, Hardie DG: Role of the AMP-activated protein kinase in the cellular stress response. *Curr Biol* 4:315–324, 1994.

Costa RH, Kalinichenko VV, Holterman AX, Wang X: Transcription factors in liver development, differentiation, and regeneration. *Hepatology* 38:1331–1347, 2003.

Cribb AE, Peyrou M, Muruganandan S, Schneider L: The endoplasmic reticulum in xenobiotic toxicity. *Drug Metab Rev* 37:405–442, 2005.

Dalton TP, Shertzer HG, Puga A: Regulation of gene expression by reactive oxygen. *Annu Rev Pharmacol Toxicol* 39:67–101, 1999.

D'Amours D, Desnoyers S, D'Silva I, Poirier GG: Poly(ADP-ribosyl)ation reactions in the regulation of nuclear functions. *Biochem J* 342:249–268, 1999.

Davies H, Bignell GR, Cox C, et al: Mutations of the BRAF gene in human cancer. *Nature* 417:949–954, 2002.

Davies KJ: Protein damage and degradation by oxygen radicals: I. General aspects. *J Biol Chem* 262:9895–9901, 1987.

De Matteis F: Drugs as suicide substrates of cytochrome P450, in De Matteis F, Lock EA (eds): *Selectivity and Molecular Mechanisms of Toxicity*. Houndmills, England: Macmillan, 1987, pp 183–210.

Denicola A, Radi R: Peroxynitrite and drug-dependent toxicity. *Toxicology* 208:273–288, 2005.

Desaiah D: Biochemical mechanisms of chlordecone neurotoxicity: A review. *Neurotoxicology* 3:103–110, 1982.

Dieguez-Acuna FJ, Polk WW, Ellis ME, et al: Nuclear factor κB activity determines the sensitivity of kidney epithelial cells to apoptosis: Implications for mercury-induced renal failure. *Toxicol Sci* 82:114–123, 2004.

Dinkova-Kostova AT, Holtzclaw WD, Kensler TW: The role of Keap1 in cellular protective responses. *Chem Res Toxicol* 18:1779–1791, 2005.

Eaton DL, Gallagher EP: Mechanisms of aflatoxin carcinogenesis. *Annu Rev Pharmacol Toxicol* 34:135–172, 1994.

Edwards MJ, Keller BJ, Kauffman FC, Thurman RG: The involvement of Kupffer cells in carbon tetrachloride toxicity. *Toxicol Appl Pharmacol* 119:275–279, 1993.

El-Benna J, Dang PM, Gougerot-Pocidalo MA, Elbim C: Phagocyte NADPH oxidase: A multicomponent enzyme essential for host defenses. *Arch Immunol Ther Exp* 53:199–206, 2005.

Elbling L, Berger W, Rehberger A, et al: P-Glycoprotein regulates chemosensitivity in early developmental stages of the mouse. *FASEB J* 7:1499–1506, 1993.

Endo T, Minami M, Hirafuji M, et al: Neurochemistry and neuropharmacology of emesis—the role of serotonin. *Toxicology* 153:189–201, 2000.

Engler H, Taurog A, Nakashima T: Mechanism of inactivation of thyroid peroxidase by thioureylene drugs. *Biochem Pharmacol* 31:3801–3806, 1982.

Esteller M: Aberrant DNA methylation as a cancer-inducing mechanism. *Annu Rev Pharmacol Toxicol* 45:629–656, 2005.

Evans AM, Mustard KJ, Wyatt CN, et al: Does AMP-activated protein kinase couple inhibition of mitochondrial oxidative phosphorylation by hypoxia to calcium signaling in O_2-sensing cells? *J Biol Chem* 280:41504–41511, 2005.

Fausto N, Campbell JS, Riehle KJ: Liver regeneration. *Hepatology* 43:S45–S53, 2006.

Flanders KC: Smad3 as a mediator of the fibrotic response. *Int J Exp Pathol* 85:47–64, 2004.

Fletcher KA, Barton PF, Kelly JA: Studies on the mechanisms of oxidation in the erythrocyte by metabolites of primaquine. *Biochem Pharmacol* 37:2683–2690, 1988.

Forman HJ, Fukuto JM, Torres M: Redox signaling: Thiol chemistry defines which reactive oxygen and nitrogen species can act as second messengers. *Am J Physiol Cell Physiol* 287:C246–C256, 2004.

Franks NP, Lieb WR: Which molecular targets are most relevant to general anaesthesia? *Toxicol Lett* 100–101:1–8, 1998.

Fromenty B, Pessayre D: Impaired mitochondrial function in microvesicular steatosis. Effects of drugs, ethanol, hormones and cytokines. *J Hepatol* 26:43–53, 1997.

Fu SY, Gordon T: The cellular and molecular basis of peripheral nerve regeneration. *Mol Neurobiol* 14:67–116, 1997.

Gale K: Role of GABA in the genesis of chemoconvulsant seizures. *Toxicol Lett* 64–65:417–428, 1992.

Goering PL: Lead-protein interactions as a basis for lead toxicity. *Neurotoxicology* 14:45–60, 1993.

Goldberg Y: Protein phosphatase 2A: Who shall regulate the regulator? *Biochem Pharmacol* 4:321–328, 1999.

Gonzalez FJ, Yu AM: Cytochrome P450 and xenobiotic receptor humanized mice. *Annu Rev Pharmacol Toxicol* 46:41–64, 2006.

Gonzalez FJ, Fernandez-Salguero P: The aryl hydrocarbon receptor. Studies using the AHR-null mice. *Drug Metab Dispos* 26:1194–1198, 1998.

Goodman JI, Watson RE: Altered DNA methylation: A secondary mechanism involved in carcinogenesis. *Annu Rev Pharmacol Toxicol* 42:501–525, 2002.

Gravina SA, Mieyal JJ: Thioltransferase is a specific glutathionyl mixed disulfide oxidoreductase. *Biochemistry* 32:3368–3376, 1993.

Green DR: Apoptotic pathways: The roads to ruin. *Cell* 94:695–698, 1998.

Green S: Nuclear receptors and chemical carcinogenesis. *Trends Pharmacol Sci* 13:251–255, 1992.

Gregus Z, Klaassen CD: Enterohepatic circulation of toxicants, in Rozman K, Hanninien O (eds): *Gastrointestinal Toxicology.* Amsterdam: Elsevier/North Holland, 1986, pp 57–118.

Gregus Z, Németi B, The glycolytic enzyme glyceraldehyde-3-phosphate dehydrogenase works as an arsenate reductase in human red blood cells and rat liver cytosol. *Toxicol Sci* 85:859–869, 2005.

Gressner AM: Hepatic fibrogenesis: The puzzle of interacting cells, fibrogenic cytokines, regulatory loops, and extracellular matrix molecules. *Z Gastroenterol* 30(Suppl 1):5–16, 1992.

Grimm C, Hermann DM, Bogdanova A, et al: Neuroprotection by hypoxic preconditioning: HIF-1 and erythropoietin protect from retinal degeneration. *Semin Cell Dev Biol* 16:531–538, 2005.

Hansen JM, Go Y-M, Jones DP: Nuclear and mitochondrial compartmentation of oxidative stress and redox signaling. *Ann Rev Pharmacol Toxicol* 46:215–234, 2006.

Hardie DG, Hawley SA, Scott JW: AMP-activated protein kinase—development of the energy sensor concept. *J Physiol* 574:7–15, 2006.

Hardman JG, Gilman AG, Limbird LL (eds): *Goodman & Gilman's The Pharmacological Basis of Therapeutics,* 9th ed. New York, McGraw-Hill: 1995.

Harms K, Nozell S, Chen X: The common and distinct target genes of the p53 family transcription factors. *Cell Mol Life Sci* 61:822–842, 2004.

Harrison R.: Structure and function of xanthine oxidoreductase: Where are we now? *Free Radic Biol Med* 33:774–797, 2002.

Herken H, Hucho F (eds): *Selective Neurotoxicity.* Berlin: Springer-Verlag, 1992.

Herman B, Gores GJ, Nieminen AL, et al: Calcium and pH in anoxic and toxic injury. *Crit Rev Toxicol* 21:127–148, 1990.

Herrlich P, Rahmsdorf HJ, Bender K: Signal transduction induced by adverse agents: "Activation by inhibition." The UV response 1997, in Puga A, Wallace KB (eds): *Molecular Biology of the Toxic Response.* Philadelphia: Taylor & Francis, 1999, pp 479–492.

Higuchi H, Gores GJ: Bile acid regulation of hepatic physiology: IV. Bile acids and death receptors. *Am J Physiol* 284:G734–G738, 2003.

Hill DA, Jean PA, Roth RA: Bile duct epithelial cells exposed to alpha-naphthylisothiocyanate produce a factor that causes neutrophildependent hepatocellular injury in vitro. *Toxcol Sci* 47:118–125, 1999.

Holmgren A, Johansson C, Berndt C, Lonn ME, Hudemann C, Lillig CH: Thiol redox control via the thioredoxin and glutaredoxin systems. *Biochem Soc Trans* 33:1375–1377, 2005.

Hippeli S, Elstner EF: Transition metal ion-catalyzed oxygen activation during pathogenic processes. *FEBS Lett* 443:1–7, 1999.

Huang W, Ma K, Zhang J, et al: Nuclear receptor-dependent bile acid signaling is required for normal liver regeneration. *Science* 312:233–236, 2006.

Jäättelä M: Escaping cell death: Survival proteins in cancer. *Exp Cell Res* 248:30–43, 1999.

Jaeschke H: Cellular adhesion molecules: Regulation and functional significance in the pathogenesis of liver diseases. *Am J Physiol* 273:G602–G611, 1997.

Jaeschke H, Bajt ML: Intracellular signaling mechanisms of acetaminophen-induced liver cell death. *Toxicol Sci* 89:31–41, 2006.

Jaiswal AK: Nrf2 signaling in coordinated activation of antioxidant gene expression. *Free Rad Biol Med* 36:1199–1207, 2004.

Jaworski M, Buchmann A, Bauer P, Riess O, Schwarz M: B-raf and Ha-ras mutations in chemically induced mouse liver tumors. *Oncogene* 24:1290–1295, 2005.

Johnson AR: Contact inhibition in the failure of mammalian CNS axonal regeneration. *Bioessays* 15:807–813, 1993.

Johnson DG, Walker CL: Cyclins and cell cycle checkpoints. *Annu Rev Pharmacol Toxicol* 39:295–312, 1999.

Kappus H: Overview of enzyme systems involved in bio-reduction of drugs and in redox cycling. *Biochem Pharmacol* 35:1–6, 1986.

Karin M: Nuclear factor-κB in cancer development and progression. *Nature* 441:431–436, 2006.

Ketterer B: Protective role of glutathione and glutathione transferases in mutagenesis and carcinogenesis. *Mutat Res* 202:343–361, 1988.

Kim JS, He L, Lemasters JJ: Mitochondrial permeability transition: A common pathway to necrosis and apoptosis. *Biochem Biophys Res Commun* 304:463–470, 2003.

Kim SY, Suzuki N, Laxmi YR, Shibutani S: Genotoxic mechanism of tamoxifen in developing endometrial cancer. *Drug Metab Rev* 36:199–218, 2004.

Klaassen CD, Liu J, Choudhuri S: Metallothionein: An intracellular protein to protect against cadmium toxicity. *Annu Rev Pharmacol Toxicol* 39:267–294, 1999.

Kodavanti UP, Mehendale HM: Cationic amphiphilic drugs and phospholipid storage disorder. *Pharmacol Rev* 42:327–353, 1990.

Krell H, Metz J, Jaeschke H, et al: Drug-induced intrahepatic cholestasis: Characterization of different pathomechanisms. *Arch Toxicol* 60:124–130, 1987.

Kroemer G, Dallaporta B, Resche-Rigon M: The mitochondrial death/life regulator in apoptosis and necrosis. *Annu Rev Physiol* 60:619–642, 1998.

Krueger SK, Williams DE: Mammalian flavin-containing monooxygenases: Structure/function, genetic polymorphisms and role in drug metabolism. *Pharmacol Ther* 106:357–387, 2005.

Larsson BS: Interaction between chemicals and melanin. *Pigment Cell Res* 6:127–133, 1993.

Laurent G, Kishore BK, Tulkens PM: Aminoglycoside-induced renal phospholipidosis and nephrotoxicity. *Biochem Pharmacol* 40:2383–2392, 1990.

Lee J, Richburg JH, Younkin SC, Boekelheide K: The Fas system is a key regulator of germ cell apoptosis in the testis. *Endocrinology* 138:2081–2088, 1997.

Lee JI, Burckart GJ: Nuclear factor kappa B: Important transcription factor and therapeutic target. *J Clin Pharmacol.* 38:981–993, 1998.

Lee EW, Lai Y, Zhang H, Unadkat JD. Identification of the mitochondrial targeting signal of the human equilibrative nucleoside transporter 1 (hENT1): Implications for interspecies differences in mitochondrial toxicity of fialuridine. *J Biol Chem* 281:16700–16706, 2006.

Lee S, Tsai FTF: Molecular chaperones in protein quality control. *J Biochem Mol Biol* 38:259–265, 2005.

Lehmann AR, Dean SW: Cancer-prone human disorders with defects in DNA repair, in Cooper CS, Grover PL (eds): *Chemical Carcinogenesis and Mutagenesis II.* Berlin: Springer-Verlag, 1990, pp 71–101.

Leist M, Nicotera P: Calcium and neuronal death. *Rev Physiol Biochem Pharmacol* 132:79–125, 1997.

Leist M, Single B, Castoldi AF, et al: Intracellular adenosine triphosphate (ATP) concentration: A switch in the decision between apoptosis and necrosis. *J Exp Med* 185:1481–1486, 1997.

Lelli JL, Becks LL, Dabrowska MI, Hinshaw DB: ATP converts necrosis to apoptosis in oxidant-injured endothelial cells. *Free Rad Biol Med* 25:694–702, 1998.

Lewis MD, Roberts BJ: Role of CYP2E1 activity in endoplasmic reticulum ubiquitination, proteasome association, and the unfolded protein response. *Arch Biochem Biophys* 436:237–245, 2005.

Lewis W, Levine ES, Griniuviene B, et al: Fialuridine and its metabolites inhibit DNA polymerase γ at sites of multiple adjacent analog incorporation, decrease mtDNA abundance, and cause mitochondrial structural defects in cultured hepatoblasts. *Proc Natl Acad Sci* 93:3592–3597, 1996.

Lichtlen P, Schaffner W: The "metal transcription factor" MTF-1: Biological facts and medical applications. *Swiss Med Wkly* 131:647–652, 2001.

Lim RT Jr, Gentry RT, Ito D, et al: First-pass metabolism of ethanol is predominantly gastric. *Alcohol Clin Exp Res* 17:1337–1344, 1993.

Lin JH, Chiba M, Baillie TA: Is the role of the small intestine in first-pass metabolism overemphasized? *Pharmacol Rev* 51:135–137, 1999.

Lindroos PM, Zarnegar R, Michalopoulos GK: Hepatocyte growth factor (hepatopoietin A) rapidly increases in plasma before DNA synthesis and liver regeneration stimulated by partial hepatectomy and carbon tetrachloride administration. *Hepatology* 13:743–750, 1991.

Liu G, Chen X: Regulation of the p53 transcriptional activity. *J Cell Biochem* 97:448–458, 2006.

Liu X, Van Vleet T, Schnellmann RG: The role of calpain in oncotic cell death. *Annu Rev Pharmacol Toxicol* 44:349–370, 2004.

Lotersztajn S, Julien B, Teixeira-Clerc F, et al: Hepatic fibrosis: Molecular mechanisms and drug targets. *Annu Rev Pharmacol Toxicol* 45:605–628, 2005.

Lozano RM, Yee BC, Buchanan BB: Thioredoxin-linked reductive inactivation of venom neurotoxins. *Arch Biochem Biophys* 309:356–362, 1994.

Lynn S, Gurr JR, Lai HT, Jan KY: NADH oxidase activation is involved in arsenite-induced oxidative DNA damage in human vascular smooth muscle cells. *Circ Res* 86:514–519, 2000.

Ma X, Babish JG: Activation of signal transduction pathways by dioxins. "Activation by inhibition." The UV response 1997. Puga A, Wallace KB (eds): *Molecular Biology of the Toxic Response.* Philadelphia: Taylor & Francis, 1999, pp 493–516.

Martin TR, Hagimoto N, Nakamura M, Matute-Bello G: Apoptosis and epithelial injury in the lungs. *Proc Am Thorac Soc* 2:214–220, 2005.

Maser E: Significance of reductases in the detoxification of the tobacco-specific carcinogen NNK. *Trends Pharmacol Sci* 25:235–237, 2004.

Maser E: Neuroprotective role for carbonyl reductase? *Biochem Biophys Res Commun* 340:1019–1022, 2006.

Maxwell P, Salnikow K: HIF-1, an oxygen and metal responsive transcription factor. *Cancer Biol Ther* 3:29–35, 2004.

McGowan CH, Russell P: The DNA damage response: Sensing and signaling. *Curr Opin Cell Biol* 16:629–633, 2004.

Mehendale HM: Tissue repair: An important determinant of final outcome of toxicant-induced injury. *Toxicol Pathol* 33:41–51, 2005.

Meijer AJ, Codogno P: Regulation and role of autophagy in mammalian cells. *Int J Biochem Cell Biol* 36:2445–2462, 2004.

Miller JA, Surh Y-J: Sulfonation in chemical carcinogenesis, in Kauffman FC (ed): *Conjugation-Deconjugation Reactions in Drug Metabolism and Toxicity.* Berlin: Springer-Verlag, 1994, pp 429–457.

Miller MS: Tumor suppressor genes in rodent lung carcinogenesis. Mutation of *p53* does not appear to be an early lesion in lung tumor pathogenesis. *Toxicol Appl Pharmacol* 156:70–77, 1999.

Morgensztern D, McLeod HL: PI3K/Akt/mTOR pathway as target for cancer therapy. *Anti-Cancer Drugs* 16:797–803, 2005.

Moskovitz J: Methionine sulfoxide reductases: Ubiquitous enzymes involved in antioxidant defense, protein regulation, and prevention of aging-associated diseases. *Biochim Biophys Acta* 1703:213–219, 2005.

Murphy MP: Nitric oxide and cell death. *Biochim Biophys Acta* 1411:401–414, 1999.

Mustafa MG: Biochemical basis of ozone toxicity. *Free Radic Biol Med* 9:245–265, 1990.

Narahashi T: Nerve membrane Na^+ channels as targets of insecticides. *Trends Pharmacol Sci* 13:236–241, 1992.

Narahashi T: Transmitter-activated ion channels as the target of chemical agents, in Kito S, Segawa T, Olsen R (eds): *Neuroreceptor Mechanisms in the Brain.* New York: Plenum Press, 1991, pp 61–73.

Nelson SD, Pearson PG: Covalent and noncovalent interactions in acute lethal cell injury caused by chemicals. *Annu Rev Pharmacol Toxicol* 30:169–195, 1990.

Newbold RR: Lessons learned from perinatal exposure to diethylstilbestrol. *Toxicol Appl Pharmacol* 199:142–150, 2004.

Nicotera P, Bellomo G, Orrenius S: Calcium-mediated mechanisms in chemically induced cell death. *Annu Rev Pharmacol Toxicol* 32:449–470, 1992.

Noji S, Tashiro K, Koyama E, et al: Expression of hepatocyte growth factor gene in endothelial and Kupffer cells of damaged rat livers, as revealed by in situ hybridization. *Biochem Biophys Res Commun* 173:42–47, 1990.

Nony PA, Schnellmann RG: Mechanisms of renal cell repair and regeneration after acute renal failure. *J Pharmacol Exp Ther* 304:905–912, 2003.

Oortgiesen M, Leinders T, van Kleef RG, Vijverberg HP: Differential neurotoxicological effects of lead on voltage-dependent and receptor-operated ion channels. *Neurotoxicology* 14:87–96, 1993.

Orrenius S: Mitochondrial regulation of apoptotic cell death. *Toxicol Lett* 149:19–23, 2004.

Osawa Y, Davila JC, Nakatsuka M, et al: Inhibition of P450 cytochromes by reactive intermediates. *Drug Metab Rev* 27:61–72, 1995.

Park BK, Kitteringham NR, Maggs JL, Pirmohamed M, Williams DP. The role of metabolic activation in drug-induced hepatotoxicity. *Annu Rev Pharmacol Toxicol* 45:177–202, 2005.

Park JD, Cherrington NJ, Klaassen CD: Intestinal absorption of cadmium is associated with divalent metal transporter 1 in rats. *Toxicol Sci* 68:288–294, 2002.

Patel MN, Yim GK, Isom GE: *N*-methyl-*D*-aspartate receptors mediate cyanide-induced cytotoxicity in hippocampal cultures. *Neurotoxicology* 14:35–40, 1993.

Perouansky M, Kirson ED, Yaari Y: Mechanism of action of volatile anesthetics: Effects of halothane on glutamate receptors in vitro. *Toxicol Lett* 100–101:65–69, 1998.

Peters JM, Aoyama T, Cattley RC, et al: Role of peroxisome proliferator-activated receptor α in altered cell cycle regulation in mouse liver. *Carcinogenesis* 19:1989–1994, 1998.

Poellinger L, Göttlicher M, Gustafsson JA: The dioxin and peroxisome proliferator-activated receptors: Nuclear receptors in search of endogenous ligands. *Trends Pharmacol Sci* 13:241–245, 1992.

Poirier LA: Methyl group deficiency in hepatocarcinogenesis. *Drug Metab Rev* 26:185–199, 1994.

Poli V: The role of C/EBP isoforms in the control of inflammatory and native immunity functions. *J Biol Chem* 273:29279–29282, 1998.

Poppek D, Grune T: Proteasomal defense of oxidative protein modifications. *Antioxid Redox Signal* 8:173–184, 2006.

Pouyssegur J, Dayan F, Mazure NM: Hypoxia signaling in cancer and approaches to enforce tumor regression. *Nature* 441:437–443, 2006.

Pumford NR, Halmes NC: Protein targets of xenobiotic reactive intermediates. *Annu Rev Pharmacol Toxicol* 37:91–117, 1997.

Qi M, Elion EA: MAP kinase pathways. *J Cell Sci* 118: 3569–3572, 2005.

Qian T, Herman B, Lemasters JJ: The mitochondrial permeability transition mediates both necrotic and apoptotic death of hepatocytes exposed to Br-A23187. *Toxicol Appl Pharmacol* 154:117–125, 1999.

Quievryn G, Messer J, Zhitkovich A, Carcinogenic chromium(VI) induces cross-linking of vitamin C to DNA in vitro and in human lung A549 cells. *Biochemistry* 41:3156–3167, 2002.

Raghow R: The role of extracellular matrix in postinflammatory wound healing and fibrosis. *FASEB J* 8:823–831, 1994.

Ray SS, Swanson HI: Dioxin-induced immortalization of normal human keratinocytes and silencing of p53 and p16INK4a. *J Biol Chem* 279:27187–27193, 2004.

Recknagel RO, Glende EA Jr, Dolak JA, Waller RL: Mechanisms of carbon tetrachloride toxicity. *Pharmacol Ther* 43:139–154, 1989.

Reed JC, Jurgensmeier JM, Matsuyama S: Bcl-2 family proteins and mitochondria. *Biochim Biophys Acta* 1366:127–137, 1998.

Rhee SG, Kang SW, Jeong W: Intracellular messenger function of hydrogen peroxide and its regulation by peroxiredoxins. *Curr Opin Cell Biol* 17:183–189, 2005.

Richter C, Kass GE: Oxidative stress in mitochondria: Its relationship to cellular Ca^{2+} homeostasis, cell death, proliferation, and differentiation. *Chem Biol Interact* 77:1–23, 1991.

Rodriguez-Enriquez S, He L, Lemasters JJ: Role of mitochondrial permeability transition pores in mitochondrial autophagy. *Int J Biochem Cell Biol* 36:2463–2472, 2004.

Rombach EM, Hanzlik RP: Detection of adducts of bromobenzene 3,4-oxide with rat liver microsomal protein sulfhydryl groups using specific antibodies. *Chem Res Toxicol* 12:159–163, 1999.

Rose ML, Rusyn I, Bojes HK, et al: Role of Kupffer cells in peroxisome proliferator-induced hepatocyte proliferation. *Drug Metab Rev* 31:87–116, 1999.

Roth RA, Luyendyk JP, Maddox JF, Ganey PE: Inflammation and drug idiosyncrasy—is there a connection? *J Pharmacol Exp Ther* 307:1–8, 2003.

Rothwell NJ: Functions and mechanisms of interleukin 1 in the brain. *Trends Pharmacol Sci* 12:430–436, 1991.

Sanguinetti MC, Mitcheson JS: Predicting drug-hERG channel interactions that cause acquired long QT syndrome. *Trends Pharmacol Sci* 26:119–124, 2005.

Scheschonka A, Murphy ME, Sies H: Temporal relationships between the loss of vitamin E, protein sulfhydryls and lipid peroxidation in microsomes challenged with different prooxidants. *Chem Biol Interact* 74:233–252, 1990.

Schinkel AH: P-glycoprotein, a gatekeeper in the blood-brain barrier. *Adv Drug Delivery Rev* 36:179–194, 1999.

Schulte-Hermann R, Timmermann-Trosiener I, Barthel G, Bursch W: DNA synthesis, apoptosis, and phenotypic expression as determinants of growth of altered foci in rat liver during phenobarbital promotion. *Cancer Res* 50:5127–5135, 1990.

Seki T, Ishimoto T, Sakurai T, et al: Increased excretion of urinary 20-HETE in rats with cyclosporine-induced nephrotoxicity. *J Pharmacol Sci* 97:132–137, 2005.

Shaw RJ, Cantley LC: Ras, PI(3)K and mTOR signalling controls tumour cell growth. *Nature* 441:424–430, 2006.

Shi X, Dalal NS: NADPH-dependent flavoenzymes catalyze one electron reduction of metal ions and molecular oxygen and generate hydroxyl radicals. *FEBS Lett* 276:189–191, 1990.

Sies H: Strategies of antioxidant defense. *Eur J Biochem* 215:213–219, 1993.

Smith KR, Klei LR, Barchowsky A: Arsenite stimulates plasma membrane NADPH oxidase in vascular endothelial cells. *Am J Physiol* 280:L442–L449, 2001.

Smith MR, Matthews NT, Jones KA, Kung HE: Biological actions of oncogenes. *Pharmacol Ther* 58:211–236, 1993.

Soni MG, Mehendale HM: Role of tissue repair in toxicologic interactions among hepatotoxic organics. *Environ Health Perspect* 106:1307–1317, 1998.

Squadrito GL, Pryor WA: Oxidative chemistry of nitric oxide: The roles of superoxide, peroxynitrite, and carbon dioxide. *Free Rad Biol Med* 25:392–403, 1998.

Sreedhar AS, Csermely P: Heat-shock proteins in the regulation of apoptosis: New strategies in tumor therapy: A comprehensive review. *Pharmacol Ther* 101:227–257, 2004.

Stachlewitz RF, Seabra V, Bradford B, et al: Glycine and uridine prevent D-galactosamine hepatoxicity in the rat: Role of the Kupffer cells. *Hepatology* 29:737–145, 1999.

Stephens TD, Bunde CJ, Fillmore BJ: Mechanism of action in thalidomide teratogenesis. *Biochem Pharmacol* 59:1489–1499, 2000.

Su AI, Guidotti LG, Pezacki JP, et al: Gene expression during the priming phase of liver regeneration after partial hepatectomy in mice. *Proc Natl Acad Sci USA* 99:11181–11186, 2002.

Sun X, Tian X, Tomsig JL, Suszkiw JB: Analysis of differential effects of Pb^{2+} on protein kinase C isozymes. *Toxicol Appl Pharmacol* 156:40–45, 1999.

Szabó C: DNA strand breakage and activation of poly-ADP ribosyltransferase: A cytotoxic pathway triggered by peroxynitrite. *Free Rad Biol Med* 21:855–869, 1996.

Taupin D, Podolsky DK: Trefoil factors: Initiators of mucosal healing. *Nat Rev Mol Cell Biol* 4:721–732, 2003.

Toivola DM, Eriksson JE: Toxins affecting cell signalling and alteration of cytoskeletal structure. *Toxicol In Vitro* 13:521–530, 1999.

Tryndyak VP, Muskhelishvili L, Kovalchuk O, et al: Effect of long-term tamoxifen exposure on genotoxic and epigenetic changes in rat liver: Implications for tamoxifen-induced hepatocarcinogenesis. *Carcinogenesis* 27:1713–1720, 2006.

Uetrecht JP: The role of leukocyte-generated reactive metabolites in the pathogenesis of idiosyncratic drug reactions. *Drug Metab Rev* 24:299–366, 1992.

Vaidya VS, Shankar K, Lock EA, et al: Molecular mechanisms of renal tissue repair in survival from acute renal tubule necrosis: Role of ERK1/2 pathway. *Toxicol Pathol* 31:604–618, 2003.

Vallyathan V, Shi X, Castranova V: Reactive oxygen species: Their relation to pneumoconiosis and carcinogenesis. *Environ Health Perspect* 106:1151–1155, 1998.

Van Kuijk FJGM, Sevanian A, Handelman GJ, Dratz EA: A new role for phospholipase A2: Protection of membranes from lipid peroxidation damage. *TIBS* 12:31–34, 1987.

Vessey CJ, Hall PM: Hepatic stem cells: A review. *Pathology* 33:130–141, 2001.

Waddick KG, Uckun FM: Innovative treatment programs against cancer: II. Nuclear factor-κB (NF-κB) as a molecular target. *Biochem Pharmacol* 57:9–17, 1999.

Wallace KB, Starkov AA: Mitochondrial targets of drug toxicity. *Annu Rev Pharmacol Toxicol* 40:353–388, 2000.

Wang JF, Komarov P, de Groot H: Luminol chemiluminescence in rat macrophages and granulocytes: The role of NO, O_2^-/H_2O_2, and HOCl. *Arch Biochem Biophys* 304:189–196, 1993.

Watson WH, Yang X, Choi YE, Jones DP, Kehrer JP: Thioredoxin and its role in toxicology. *Toxicol Sci* 78:3–14, 2004.

Weiss SJ, LoBuglio AF: Phagocyte-generated oxygen metabolites and cellular injury. *Lab Invest* 47:5–18, 1982.

Wu Q, Ohsako S, Ishimura R, Suzuki JS, Tohyama C: Exposure of mouse preimplantation embryos to 2,3,7,8-tetrachlorodibenzo-p-dioxin (TCDD) alters the methylation status of imprinted genes H19 and Igf2. *Biol Reprod* 70:1790–1797, 2004.

Wyllie AH: Apoptosis: An overview. *Brit Med Bull* 53:451–465, 1997.

Yin M, Ikejima K, Arteel GE, et al: Glycine accelerates recovery from alcohol-induced liver injury. *J Pharmacol Exp Therap* 286:1014–1019, 1998.

RISK ASSESSMENT

Elaine M. Faustman and Gilbert S. Omenn

INTRODUCTION AND HISTORICAL CONTEXT

Toxicologic research and toxicity testing constitute the scientific core of an important activity known as risk assessment, which is used for the evaluation of potential adverse health impacts from chemical exposures. Risk evaluation is not new since for decades the American Conference of Governmental Industrial Hygienists (ACGIH) has set threshold limit values for occupational exposures and the U.S. Food and Drug Administration (FDA) has established acceptable daily intakes for pesticide residues and food additives. In 1958, the U.S. Congress instructed the FDA in the Delaney Clause to prohibit the addition to the food supply of all substances found to cause cancer in animals or humans. Pragmatically, this policy allowed food sources that had nondetectable levels of these additives to be declared "safe." As advances in analytic chemistry revealed that "nondetects" were not equivalent to "not present," regulatory agencies were forced to develop "tolerance levels" and "acceptable risk levels." Risk assessment methodologies blossomed in the 1970s with the rising need to address these issues and statues (Albert, 1994).

In *Risk Assessment in the Federal Government: Managing the Process* (The Red Book), the National Research Council (NRC) detailed steps for hazard identification, dose–response assessment, exposure analysis, and characterization of risks (NRC, 1983). This framework has evolved into the scheme shown in Fig. 4-1, and provides a consistent risk assessment framework across agencies. The figure illustrates a framework with bidirectional arrows demonstrating an ideal situation where mechanistic research feeds directly into risk assessments and critical data uncertainty drives research. Initially, attention was focused on cancer risks; in subsequent years, noncancer endpoints were examined with similar methods. Continuing advances in toxicology, epidemiology, exposure assessment, biologically-based modeling of adverse responses, the modeling of variability and uncertainty, and the rapidly growing area of genomics have contributed to improvements in risk assessment. Nevertheless, public policy objectives often require extrapolations that go far beyond the observation of actual effects and reflect different approaches for addressing risks, generating controversy.

The National Academy of Sciences (NAS) 1994 report entitled *Science and Judgment in Risk Assessment* captured in its title the combination of qualitative and quantitative approaches essential for effective assessment of risks (NRC, 1994). The report discussed in detail the challenges and provided approaches for incorporating new scientific findings into the risk assessment process. It also highlighted approaches to deal with uncertainty when insufficient scientific information was available. To address these challenges, the Presidential/Congressional Commission on Risk Assessment and Risk Management (Risk Commission, 1997) formulated a comprehensive framework that (1) put each environmental problem or issue into public health and/or ecological context and (2) proactively called for engaging relevant stakeholders, often affected or potentially affected community groups, from the very beginning of the six-stage process shown in Fig. 4-2. This report emphasized that particular exposures and potential health effects must be evaluated across sources and exposure pathways and in light of multiple endpoints, not just one chemical, in one environmental medium (air, water, soil, food, products), for one health effect at a time. This has been the general approach up to the present. The importance of defining the risk problem is critical to risk assessment, a process that has been outlined by the U.S. Environmental Protection Agency (EPA) (www.epa.gov/pesticides/ecosystem/ecorisk.htm). Similar frameworks have been used by the Health and Safety Executive Risk Assessment Policy Unit of the United Kingdom (Health and Safety Executive, 2000) and by the World Health Organization (WHO).

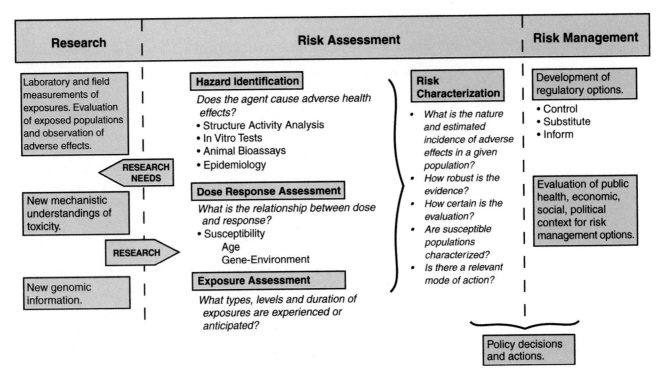

Figure 4-1. Risk assessment/risk management framework.

This framework shows in blue the four key steps of risk assessment: hazard identification, dose–response assessment, exposure assessment, and risk characterization. It shows an interactive, two-way process where research needs from the risk assessment process drive new research, and new research findings modify risk assessment outcomes. (Adapted from NRC, 1983, 1994; Calkins, 1980; Faustman, 1996; Gargas, 1999, reprinted with permission from the National Academic Press, National Academy of Sciences.)

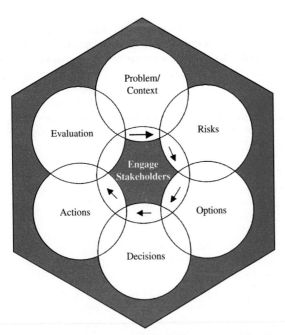

Figure 4-2. Risk management framework for environmental health from the U.S. Commission on Risk Assessment and Risk Management.

The framework comprises six stages: (1) formulating the problem in a broad public health context; (2) analyzing the risks; (3) defining the options; (4) making risk-reduction decisions; (5) implementing those actions; and (6) evaluating the effectiveness of the actions taken. Interactions with stakeholders are critical and thus have been put at the center of the framework. (Charnley and Omenn, 1997; Risk Commission, 1997).

DEFINITIONS

Risk assessment is the systematic scientific evaluation of potential adverse health effects resulting from human exposures to hazardous agents or situations (NRC, 1983, 1994; Omenn, 2000). *Risk* is defined as the probability of an adverse outcome based upon the exposure and potency of the hazardous agent(s). Although historically there have been differences in how the term *hazard* has been used, international risk harmonization activities have allowed for current consensus on hazard as reference to intrinsic toxic properties. Risk assessment requires an integration of both qualitative as well as quantitative scientific information. For example, qualitative information about the overall evidence and nature of the endpoints and hazards are integrated with quantitative assessment of the exposures, host susceptibility factors, and the magnitude of the hazard. A description of the uncertainties and variability in the estimates is a significant part of risk characterization and an essential component of risk assessment. Analogous approaches are applied to ecologic risks, as demonstrated by EPA's ecological risk assessment guidelines (http://www.epa.gov/pesticides/ecosystem/ecorisk.htm). The objectives of risk assessment are outlined in Table 4-1.

The phrase *characterization of risk* reflects the combination of qualitative and quantitative analysis. Increasingly, the use of the term "hazard characterization" versus "hazard identification" has been seen in both the EPA (2005a) and WHO (World Health Organization, 2004) documents. This shift recognizes the difficulties in evaluating only hazard information without dose–response information. Unfortunately, many users equate risk assessment with quantitative risk assessment, generating a number for an overly precise risk estimate, while ignoring crucial information about the

Table 4.1

Objectives of Risk Assessment

1. Balance risks and benefits.
   Drugs
   Pesticides
2. Set target levels of risk.
   Food contaminants
   Water pollutants
3. Set priorities for program activities.
   Regulatory agencies
   Manufacturers
   Environmental/consumer organizations
4. Estimate residual risks and extent of risk reduction after steps are taken to reduce risks.

uncertainties of the risk assessment, mechanism, and type of effect across species. In January 2006, the Office of Management and Budget (OMB) in collaboration with the Office of Science and Technology Policy (OSTP) proposed standards and guidelines for agency risk assessments with the aim of improving the technical quality and transparency of information used in risk assessment and subsequent public policy and regulation. In part, the draft guidelines have emphasized the need to provide uncertainty and variability characterization in the estimate of risk. The NAS reviewed the OMB proposal in 2007.

Risk management refers to the process by which policy actions are chosen to control hazards identified in the risk assessment stage of the framework (Fig. 4-2). Risk managers consider scientific evidence and risk estimates—along with statutory, engineering, economic, social, and political factors—in evaluating alternative options and choosing among those options (Risk Commission, 1997).

Risk communication is the challenging process of making risk assessment and risk management information comprehensible to community groups, lawyers, local elected officials, judges, business people, labor, and environmentalists (Morgan, 1993; Sandman, 1993; Fischhoff *et al.*, 1996; NRC, 1996). Part of this analytic-deliberative process is the crucial, too-often neglected requirement of considering the fears, perceptions, priorities, and proposed remedies of these "stakeholders" (Risk Commission, 1997; Drew *et al.*, 2003; Judd *et al.*, 2005). Sometimes the decision makers and stakeholders simply want to know the "bottom line": is a substance or a situation "safe" or not? Others will be keenly interested in knowing why the risk estimates are uncertain and may be well prepared to challenge underlying assumptions about context and methodology. The *perception of risk* is further discussed at the end of this chapter.

DECISION MAKING

Risk management decisions are reached under diverse statutes in the United States. Table 4-2 lists examples of major environmental statutes and the year of initial enactment. Some statutes specify reliance on risk alone, whereas others require a balancing of risks and benefits of the product or activity. Risk assessments provide a valuable framework for priority setting within regulatory and health agencies, in the chemical development process within companies, and in resource allocation by environmental organizations. Similar approaches for risk assessment have been developed in many other countries and through such international organizations as the International Programme for Chemical Safety (IPCS) within the WHO. Currently within the IPCS, there are significant efforts toward a global harmonization of risk assessment methodology. The goal is to develop confidence and acceptance of different assessment approaches through a common understanding and agreement on basic principles of testing and assessment.

A major challenge for risk assessment, risk communication, and risk management is to work across disciplines to demonstrate the biological plausibility and clinical significance of the conclusions from epidemiologic, lifetime animal, short-term in vitro and in vivo, and structure–activity studies of chemicals thought to have

Table 4.2

Examples of Major Toxic Chemical Laws in the United States by Responsible Agency and Year of Initial Enactment

EPA	Air pollutants	Clean Air Act 1970
	Water pollutants	Federal Water Pollution Control Act 1948
	Drinking water	Safe Drinking Water Act 1974
	Pesticides	Fungicides, Insecticides & Rodenticides Act (FIFRA) 1947 Food Quality Protection Act (FQPA) 1996
	Ocean dumping	Marine Protection, Research and Sanctuaries Act (MPRSA) or Ocean Dumping Act (1972)
	Toxic chemicals	Toxic Substances Control Act (TSCA) 1976
	Hazardous wastes	Resource Conservation and Recovery Act (RCRA) 1976
	Abandoned hazardous wastes	Superfund (CERCLA) 1980
CEQ	Environmental impacts	National Environmental Policy Act (NEPA) 1969
OSHA	Workplace	Occupational Safety and Health (OSH) Act 1970
FDA	Foods, drugs and cosmetics	Food and Drugs Act 1906 Food, Drugs and Cosmetics Act (FDC) 1938 FDA Modernization Act 1997
CPSC	Dangerous consumer products	Consumer Product Safety Act (CPSA) 1972
DOT	Transport of hazardous materials	Hazardous Materials Transportation Act (HMTA) 1975

EPA, Environmental Protection Agency; CEQ, Council for Environmental Quality (now Office of Environmental Policy); OSHA, Occupational Safety and Health Administration; FDA, Food and Drug Administration; CPSC, Consumer Product Safety Commission; DOT, Department of Transportation.

potential adverse effects. Biomarkers of exposure, effect, or individual susceptibility can link the presence of a chemical in various environmental compartments to specific sites of action in target organs and to host responses (NRC, 1989a,b, 1992a,b). Mechanistic investigations of the actions of specific chemicals can help us penetrate the "black box" approach of simply counting tumors, for example, in exposed animals in routine bioassays. Greater appreciation of the mechanisms and extent of individual variation in susceptibility among humans can improve protection of subgroups of susceptible populations and better relate findings in animals to the characterization of risk for humans. Individual behavioral and social risk factors may be critically important both to the risk and to the reduction of risk. Finally, public and media attitudes toward local polluters, other responsible parties, and relevant government agencies may lead to what has been labeled "the outrage factor" (Sandman, 1993), greatly influencing the communication process and the choices for risk management.

HAZARD IDENTIFICATION

Assessing Toxicity of Chemicals—Introduction

In order to assess the toxicity of chemicals, information from four types of studies is used: structure–activity relationships (SAR), in vitro or short-term studies, in vivo animal bioassays, and information from human epidemiological studies. In many cases, toxicity information for chemicals is limited. For example, in 1998, the EPA evaluated high production volume (HPV) chemicals (those produced in excess of 1 million lb/y) to ascertain the availability of chemical hazard data. Their study found that for 43% of these HPV chemicals, there were no publicly available studies for any of the basic toxicity endpoints (EPA, 1998a). In response, EPA established a voluntary program called the HPV Challenge Program (www.epa.gov/hpv/). Industry participants in this program committed to filling the data gaps for HPV chemicals. Since its inception, there have been over 2,200 chemicals sponsored for additional testing. International efforts such as the Organization for Economic Cooperation and Development's screening information data set (OECD/SIDS) program are also addressing data needs related to HPV, highlighted by the publication of their Manual for Investigation of HPV Chemicals (www.oecd.org).

Data requirements for specific chemicals can vary greatly by compound type and applicable regulatory statutes. Introduced in 2003 and approved in 2006, the European Union released a regulatory framework for Registration, Evaluation and Authorisation of Chemicals (REACH) (http://ec.europa.eu/environment/chemicals/reach/reach_intro.htm). Under the REACH framework, starting in 2007, all stakeholders must submit physical, chemical, and toxicological data as well as risk assessment studies for all chemicals in use. Table 4-3 shows requirements and costs during 1997 for one example class of agents, pesticides (Stevens, 1997); 40 CFR 158.340 (EPA, 1998b, 2000a). It also illustrates current international efforts to harmonize these testing guidelines by listing examples of the new harmonized 870 test guidelines (EPA, 2000b).

Assessing Toxicity of Chemicals—Methods

Structure–Activity Relationships Given the cost of $2 to $4 million and the 3–5 years required for testing a single chemical in a lifetime rodent carcinogenicity bioassay, initial decisions on whether to continue development of a chemical, to submit pre-manufacturing

notice (PMN), or to require additional testing may be based largely on results from structure–activity relationships (SARs) and limited short-term assays.

A chemical's structure, solubility, stability, pH sensitivity, electrophilicity, volatility, and chemical reactivity can be important information for hazard identification. Historically, certain key molecular structures have provided regulators with some of the most readily available information on the basis of which to assess hazard potential. For example, 8 of the first 14 occupational carcinogens were regulated together by the Occupational Safety and Health Administration (OSHA) as belonging to the aromatic amine chemical class. The EPA Office of Toxic Substances relies on SARs to meet deadlines to respond to pre-manufacturing notice for new chemical manufacture under the Toxic Substances Control Act (TSCA). Structural alerts such as N-nitroso or aromatic amine groups, amino azo dye structures, or phenanthrene nuclei are clues to prioritize chemicals for additional evaluation as potential carcinogens. The database of known developmental toxicants limits SARs to a few chemical classes, including chemicals with structures related to those of valproic acid, retinoic acid, phthalate esters, and glycol ethers (NRC, 2000). More recently, omic technologies have been used to supplement SAR relationship databases, as seen with the creation of the National Cancer Institute's (NCI) gene expression database (http://dtp.nci.nih.gov/).

SARs have been used for assessment of complex mixtures of structurally related compounds. A prominent application has been the assessment of risks associated with 2,3,7,8-tetrachlorodibenzo-p-dioxin (TCDD), related chlorinated and brominated dibenzo-p-dioxins, dibenzofurans, and planar biphenyls, and chemicals generally present as mixtures in the environment. The use of toxicity equivalence factors (TEFs) is used to evaluate health risks associated with closely related chemicals. For the TCDD class, this is based on a common mechanism of aryl-hydrocarbon (Ah) receptor induction (EPA, 1994b). The estimated toxicity of environmental mixtures containing these chemicals is calculated as the sum of the product of the concentration of each chemical multiplied by its TEF value. The World Health Organization has organized efforts to reach international consensus on the TEFs used for polychlorinated biphenyls (PCBs), polychlorinated dibenzo-p-dioxins (PCDDs), and polychlorinated dibenzofurans (PCDFs) for both humans and wildlife, and has recently updated its values and published the supporting database (Van den Berg et al., 1998, 2006; Haws et al., 2006). Under the auspices of WHO, the dioxin-like PCB congeners have been assigned TEFs reflecting their toxicity relative to TCDD, which itself has been assigned a TEF of 1.0.

Computerized SAR methods have, in general, given disappointing results in the National Toxicology Program (NTP) 44-chemical rodent carcinogenicity prediction challenge (Ashby and Tennant, 1994; Omenn et al., 1995; Benigni and Zito, 2004). More focused efforts are those of pharmaceutical companies successfully using combinatorial chemistry and three-dimensional (3D) molecular modeling approaches to design ligands (new drugs) that can sterically fit into the "receptors of interest." However, for environmental pollutants where selective binding to specific receptors is rare, these applications of SAR has had limited applications within risk assessment.

In Vitro and Short-Term Tests The next level of biological information obtained within the hazard identification process includes assessment of the test chemical in in vitro or short-term tests, ranging from bacterial mutation assays performed entirely in vitro to more elaborate short-term tests, such as skin-painting studies in mice or

Table 4.3

EPA/FIFRA Requirement for Hazard Evaluation of Pesticides

GUIDE-ELINE NO.	REVISED 870 GUIDELINE	TYPE OF TOXICITY STUDY	TEST SYSTEM	OBJECTIVE	APPROXIMATE COST/STUDY (US$)
81-1	1100	Acute oral	Rats	Define toxic dose by ingestion	2000
81-2	1200	Acute dermal	Rabbits	Define toxic dose by absorption through skin	1500
81-3	1300	Acute inhalation	Rats	Define toxic dose by inhalation	5000
81-4	2400	Ocular	Rabbits	Assess eye irritation/injury	1500
81-5	2500	Skin irritation	Rabbits	Assess skin irritation/injury	100
81-6	2600	Sensitization	Guinea pigs	Assess allergic potential	3000
81-7	6100–6855	Neurotoxicity*[†]	Hens/rats	Assess nervous system injury	25,000[†]
84-2	5100–5915	Mutagenicity[‡]	In vivo/in vitro	Determine genotoxic potential; screen for carcinogenicity	5,000[§]
82-1	3050–3465	Range-finding[‡] Subacute (28- to 90-day§)	Rats	Determine effects following repeated doses; set dose level	70,000
			Mice		70,000
			Dogs	for longer studies	100,000
			Rabbits		75,000
			Tats	Identify target organs; set dose	190,000
			Mice levels for chronic studies		190,000
83-5	4200–4300	Carcinogenicity/ Chronic toxicity	Rats	Determine potential to induce	1,400,000
83-2			Mice	tumors; define dose-response relationships (lifetime)	800,000
83-1			Dogs	Determine long-term toxic effects (1 year)	400,000
83-3	3550–3800	Reproduction and teratogenicity	Rats	Determine potential to cause fetal	505,000
83-4			Rabbits	abnormalities and effects on development, fertility, pregnancy, and development of offspring over at least two generations	
85-1	7485	Toxicokineties	Rats Mice	Determine and quantitate the metabolic fate of a pesticide	100,000

*Required for organophosphate insecticides only.

[†]Additional neurotoxicity tests 81-7, 81-8, 82-6, 82-7, and 83-6 have been added to requirements for certain materials and can include tests such as functional observational battery, motor activity, developmental landmarks, and learning and memory assessments (Sette, 1991). Costs listed for this type of study are only those for the initial study, not additional testing.

[‡]Range-finding studies are not required, but provide justification for setting dose levels in required studies. EPA-required studies can include reverse mutation assays in *Salmonella*, forward mutation assays in mammalian cells—e.g., Chinese hamster ovary cells, mouse lymphoma L5178Y (the locus cells)—and in vivo cytogenetics (Dearfield, 1990).

[§]Indicates per assay cost and represent 1997 estimates using guideline 81 series.

SOURCE: Adapted from Stevens, (1997), and updated with newly revised EPA 870 guideline information (EPA, 2000b). For details on changes in the Health Effects test guidelines reflective of the harmonization of the toxicology guidelines between the Office of Pollution Prevention and Toxics (OPPT) and the Office of Pesticide Programs (OPP), within the EPA and with the Organization for Economic Cooperation and Development (OECD) guidelines, see EPA (2000b) (http://www.epa.gov/OPPTS_Harmonized/870_Health_Effects_Test_Guidelines).

altered rat liver–foci assays conducted in vivo. For example, EPA mutagenicity guidelines call for assessment of reverse mutations using the Ames *Salmonella typhimurium* assay; forward mutations using mammalian cells, mouse lymphoma L5178Y, Chinese hamster ovary, or Chinese hamster lung fibroblasts; and in vivo cytogenetics assessment (bone marrow metaphase analysis or micronucleus tests). Chapter 8 discusses uses of these assays for identifying chemical carcinogens and Chap. 9 describes in detail various assays

of genetic and mutagenic endpoints. Other assays evaluate developmental toxicity (Faustman, 1988; Schwetz, 1993; Whittaker and Faustman, 1994; Brown *et al.*, 1995; Lewandowski *et al.*, 2000; NRC, 2000), reproductive toxicity (Gray, 1988; Harris *et al.*, 1992; Shelby *et al.*, 1993), neurotoxicity (Atterwill *et al.*, 1992; Costa, 2000), and immunotoxicity (Chap. 12). Less information is available on the extrapolation of these test results for noncancer risk assessment than for the mutagenicity or carcinogenicity endpoints;

however, mechanistic information obtained in these systems has been applied to risk assessment (Abbott *et al.*, 1992; EPA, 1994a; Leroux *et al.*, 1996; NRC, 2000).

Overall, progress in developing new in vitro assays has been slow and frustrating. The 2005 EPA guidelines for carcinogen risk assessment lists standard tests for gene mutations in bacteria and mammalian cells and for structural chromosomal aberrations as relevant in vitro methods. In addition, they highlight the option of newer methods including mouse mutations and cancer transgenic models.

The Interagency Coordinating Committee on the Validation of Alternative Methods (ICCVAM) of NTP has reinvigorated the validation process in the United States as a result of Public Law 103-43 and coordinates cross-agency issues relating to development, validation, acceptance, and national/international harmonization of toxicological test methods for use in risk assessments. The committee has put forth recommendations for various short-term/in vitro assays, such as the cell-free corrosivity test, and for the mouse local lymph node assay for assessing chemical potential to elicit allergic contact dermatitis (NIEHS, 1999a,b). In addition, in 2006 the committee released a draft document that extensively reviews in vitro acute toxicity methods (http://ntp-apps.niehs.nih.gov/iccvampb/SearchDoc.cfm). The European Centre on the Validation of Alternative Methods (ECVAM) was also formed to "support the development, validation, and acceptance of methods that could reduce, refine, or replace the use of laboratory animals" (http://ecvam.jrc.cec.eu.int/index.htm). Recent successes of ECVAM are described in Hartung *et al.* (2003).

The validation and application of short-term assays is particularly important to risk assessment because such assays can be designed to provide information about mechanisms of effects, moreover, they are fast and inexpensive compared with lifetime bioassays (McGregor *et al.*, 1999). Validation of in vitro assays, like other kinds of tests, requires determination of their sensitivity (ability to identify true carcinogens), specificity (ability to recognize noncarcinogens as noncarcinogens), and predictive value for the toxic endpoint under evaluation. The societal costs of relying on such tests, with false positives (noncarcinogens classified as carcinogens) and false negatives (true carcinogens not detected) are the subject of a value-of-information model for testing in risk assessment and risk management (Lave and Omenn, 1986; Omenn and Lampen, 1988).

Efforts to improve our ability to utilize short-term tests for carcinogenicity prediction include increased attention to improving the mechanistic basis of short-term testing. Examples of this approach include the development and application of several knockout transgenic mouse models as shorter-term in vivo assays to identify carcinogens and currently under evaluation by NTP (Nebert and Duffy, 1997; Tennant *et al.*, 1999). The primary use of short-term tests continues to be for mechanistic evaluations. In that context, results from short-term assays have impacted risk assessments. For example, evidence of nonmutagenicity in both in vitro and in vivo short-term assays play an essential role, allowing regulators to consider nonlinear cancer risk assessment paradigms for nongenotoxic carcinogens (EPA, 1999b). Mechanistic information from short-term in vitro assays can also be used to extend the range of biological observations available for dose–response assessment. In addition, assay methods building on new knowledge from molecular and developmental biology for developmental toxicity risk assessment that acknowledge the highly conserved nature of developmental pathways across species should accelerate use of a broader range of model organisms and assay approaches for noncancer risk assessments (NRC, 2000).

Animal Bioassays Animal bioassays are a key component of the hazard identification process. A basic premise of risk assessment is that chemicals that cause tumors in animals can cause tumors in humans. All human carcinogens that have been adequately tested in animals produce positive results in at least one animal model. Thus, "although this association cannot establish that all agents and mixtures that cause cancer in experimental animals also cause cancer in humans, nevertheless, in the absence of adequate data on humans, it is biologically plausible and prudent to regard agents and mixtures for which there is sufficient evidence of carcinogenicity in experimental animals as if they presented a carcinogenic risk to humans" (IARC, 2000)—a reflection of the "precautionary principle." The USEPA Cancer Guidelines (EPA, 2005b) also assume relevance of animal bioassays unless lack of relevance for human assessment is specifically determined. In general, the most appropriate rodent bioassays are those that test exposure pathways of most relevance to predicted or known human exposure pathways. Bioassays for reproductive and developmental toxicity and other noncancer endpoints have a similar rationale. The National Toxicology Program Center for the Evaluation of Risks to Human Reproduction (CERHR) serves as a resource to the public and regulatory agencies regarding the interpretation and assessment of adverse effects of chemicals on reproduction and development (http://cerhr.niehs.nih.gov/).

Consistent features in the design of standard cancer bioassays include testing in two species and both sexes, with 50 animals per dose group and near lifetime exposure. Important choices include the strains of rats and mice, the number of doses, and dose levels [typically 90, 50, and 10–25% of the maximally tolerated dose (MTD)], and the details of the required histopathology (number of organs to be examined, choice of interim sacrifice pathology, etc.). The NTP website lists details on study designs and protocols (http://ntp-server.niehs.nih.gov/). Positive evidence of chemical carcinogenicity can include increases in number of tumors at a particular organ site, induction of rare tumors, earlier induction (shorter latency) of commonly observed tumors, and/or increases in the total number of observed tumors.

The cancer bioassay, designed for hazard identification, is frequently used to evaluate dose–response. The relatively limited number of evaluated doses and the use of high doses have caused issues for low-dose extrapolations and has limited the use of cancer bioassays as a "gold standard" for prediction of human carcinogenicity risk (McClain, 1994; Cohen, 1995; Risk Commission, 1997; Rodericks *et al.*, 1997; Capen *et al.*, 1999; Rice *et al.*, 1999). Tumors may be increased only at the highest dose tested, which is usually at or near a dose that causes systemic toxicity (Ames and Gold, 1990). Second, even without toxicity, the high dose may trigger different events than do low-dose exposures.

Rats and mice give concordant positive or negative results in only 70% of bioassays, so it is unlikely that rodent/human concordance would be higher (Lave *et al.*, 1988). Haseman and Lockhart (1993) concluded that most target sites in cancer bioassays showed a strong correlation (65%) between males and females—especially for forestomach, liver, and thyroid tumors—so they suggested, for efficiency, that bioassays could rely on a combination of male rats and female mice. Even when concordant, positive results are observed, there can still be large differences in potency, as observed in aflatoxin-induced tumors in rats and mice. In this example, an almost 100,000-fold difference in susceptibility to aflatoxin B_1 (AFB$_1$)-induced liver tumors is seen between the sensitive rat and trout species versus the more resistant mouse strains. Genetic differences in the expression of cytochrome P450 and glutathione-*S*-transferases explain most of these species differences and suggest that humans may be as sensitive to AFB_1-induced liver tumors as rats (Eaton and Gallagher, 1994; Eaton *et al.*, 1995, 2001). These species differences have been supported by research results (Groopman and Kensler, 1999) and have been extended within epidemiological studies to demonstrate the interaction of hepatitis C infection with AFB_1 exposure to fully explain elevated human liver cancer risks.

Lifetime bioassays have been enhanced with the collection of additional mechanistic data and with the assessment of multiple noncancer endpoints. It is feasible and desirable to integrate such information together with data from mechanistically oriented short-term tests and biomarker and genetic studies in epidemiology (Perera and Weinstein, 2000). In the example of AFB_1 induced liver tumors, AFB_1-DNA adducts have proved to be an extremely useful biomarker. A highly linear relationship was observed between liver tumor incidence (in rats, mice, and trout) and AFB_1-DNA adduct formation over a dose range of five orders of magnitude (Eaton and Gallagher, 1994). Such approaches may allow for an extension of biologically observable phenomena to doses lower than those leading to frank tumor development and help to address the issues of extrapolation over multiple orders of magnitude to predict response at environmentally relevant doses.

Table 4-4 presents some mechanistic details about rodent tumor responses that are no longer thought to be directly predictive of cancer risk for humans. This table lists examples of both qualitative and quantitative considerations useful for determining relevance of rodent tumor responses for human risk evaluations. An example of qualitative considerations is the male rat kidney tumor observed following exposure to chemicals that bind to a_{2u}-globulin (e.g., unleaded gasoline, 1,4-dichlorobenzene, D-limonene). The a_{2u}-globulin is a male-rat-specific low-molecular-weight protein not found in female rats, humans, or other species, including mice and monkeys (McClain, 1994; Neumann and Olinn, 1995; Oberdorster, 1995; Omenn *et al.*, 1995; Risk Commission, 1997; Rodericks *et al.*, 1997).

Table 4-4 also illustrates quantitative considerations important for determining human relevance of animal bioassay information. For example, doses of compounds so high as to exceed solubility in the urinary tract outflow lead to tumors of the urinary bladder in male rats following crystal precipitation and local irritation leading to hyperplasia. Such precipitates are known to occur following saccharin or nitriloacetic acid exposure (Cohen *et al.*, 2000). The decision to exclude saccharin from the NTP list of suspected human carcinogens reaffirms the nonrelevance of such high-dose responses for likely human exposure considerations (Neumann and Olinn, 1995; National Toxicology Program, 2005). A gross overloading of the particle clearance mechanism of rat lungs via directly administered particles, as was seen in titanium dioxide (TDO) exposures, resulted in EPA's delisting TDO as a reportable toxicant for the Clean Air Act Toxic Release Inventory (EPA, 1988c; Oberdorster, 1995).

Table 4.4

Examples of Mechanistic Considerations for Carcinogens: Explanation for Special Cases of Rodent Bioassay Data Lacking Relevance for Human Risk Evaluation

SYSTEM	TARGET ORGAN	MECHANISM FOR SUSCEPTIBLE SPECIES	SPECIES DIFFERENCES	ILLUSTRATIVE CHEMICAL AGENTS
Urinary tract	Renal tumors in male rats	Chemicals bind to a_{2U}-globulin Accumulation in target kidney cells Increased necrosis Increased regenerative hyperplasia Renal tubular calcification neoplasia	a_{2U}-globulin male rat specific low-molecular weight protein not found in female rats, humans, mice, monkeys	Unleaded gasoline 1,4-Dichlorobenzene D-limonene Isophorons Dimethyl-methylphosphonate Perchloroethylene Pentachloroethane Hexachloroethane
	Bladder	Reactive hyperplasia from cytotoxic precipitated chemicals	Rodent exposure levels exceed solubility, not relevant for human exposure	Saccharin, melamine, nitrilotriacetic acid, fosetyl-A2
Gastric	Forestomach	Direct oral gavage Local cytotoxicity Hyperplasia	Rodent gavage treatment, exposure conditions not relevant for human exposure	BHA, propionic acid, ethyl acrylate
Endocrine	Thyroid gland tumors	Alteration in thyroid homeostasis Decreased thyroid hormone production Sustained increase in thyroid stimulating hormone (TSH) Thyroid tumors	Lack of thyroid-binding protein in rodents versus humans Decreased $t_{1/2}$ for T_4; increased TSH levels in rodents	Ethylene bisdithio-carbamate, fungicides, amitrol, goitrogens, sulfamethazine
Respiratory	Rat lung	Overwhelming clearance mechanisms	High dose effects seen with rodent models	Various particles, titanium dioxide

SOURCE: Neumann, 1995; Oberdörster, 1995; Omenn, 1995; McClain, 1994; Risk Commission, 1997; Rodericks, 1997.

Table 4.5

Example of Three Types of Epidemiological Study Designs

METHODOLOGICAL ATTRIBUTES	TYPE OF STUDY		
	COHORT	CASE-CONTROL	CROSS-SECTIONAL
Initial classification	Exposure–nonexposure	Disease–nondisease	Either one
Time sequence	Prospective	Retrospective	Present time
Sample composition	Nondiseased individuals	Cases and controls	Survivors
Comparison	Proportion of exposed with disease	Proportion of cases with exposure	Either one
Rates	Incidence	Fractional (%)	Prevalence
Risk index	Relative risk-attributable risk	Relative odds	Prevalence
Advantages	Lack of bias in exposure; yields incidence and risk rates	Inexpensive, small number of subjects, rapid results, suitable for rare diseases, no attrition	Quick results
Disadvantages	Large number of subjects required, long follow-up, attrition, change in time of criteria and methods, costly, inadequate for rare diseases	Incomplete information, biased recall, problem in selecting control and matching, yields only relative risk—cannot establish causation, population of survivors	Cannot establish establish causation (antecedent consequence); population of survivors; inadequate for rare diseases

SOURCES: Gamble and Battigelli, 1978, 1991.

Other rodent responses not likely to be predictive for humans include localized forestomach tumors after gavage. Ethyl acrylate, which produces such tumors, was delisted on the basis of extensive mechanistic studies (National Toxicology Program, 2005). In general, for risk assessment, it is desirable to use the same route of administration as the likely exposure pathway in humans to avoid such extrapolation issues. Despite the example of forestomach tumors, tumors in unusual sites—like the pituitary gland, the eighth cranial nerve, or the Zymbal gland—should not be immediately dismissed as irrelevant, since organ-to-organ correlation is often lacking (NRC, 1994). The EPA cancer guidelines provide a good list of considerations for evaluating relevance in the sections on evaluating weight of evidence (EPA, 2005b).

In an attempt to improve the prediction of cancer risk to humans, transgenic mouse models have been developed as possible alternative to the standard two-year cancer bioassay. Transgenic models use knockout or transgenic mice that incorporate or eliminate a gene that has been linked to human cancer. NTP evaluated some of these models and found the p53 deficient (p53+/− heterozygous) and Tg.AC (v-Ha-ras transgene) models to be particularly useful in identifying carcinogens and mechanisms of action (Bucher, 1998; Chhabra et al., 2003). The use of transgenic models has the power to improve the characterization of key cellular and mode of action of toxicological responses (Mendoza et al., 2002; Gribble et al., 2005). However, these studies have been used primarily for mechanistic characterization than for hazard identification. Transgenic models have been shown to reduce cost and time as compared to the standard 2-year assay but also have been shown to be somewhat limited in their sensitivity (Cohen, 2001). As stated in the current EPA Cancer Guidelines, transgenic models should not be used to replace the standard 2-year assay, but should be used in conjunction with other types of data to assist in the interpretation of additional toxicological and mechanistic evidence (EPA, 2005b).

Use of Epidemiologic Data in Risk Assessment The most convincing line of evidence for human risk is a well-conducted epidemiologic study in which a positive association between exposure and disease has been observed (NRC, 1983). Epidemiologic studies are essentially opportunistic. Studies begin with known or presumed exposures, comparing exposed versus nonexposed individuals, or with known cases, compared with persons lacking the particular diagnosis.

Table 4-5 shows examples of epidemiologic study designs and provides clues on types of outcomes and exposures evaluated. Although convincing, there are important limitations inherent in epidemiologic studies. When the study is exploratory, hypotheses are often weak. Robust exposure estimates are often difficult to obtain as they are frequently done retrospectively and have a long latency before clinical manifestations appear. Another challenge for interpretation is that there are often exposures to multiple chemicals, especially when a lifetime exposure period is considered. There is always a trade-off between detailed information on relatively few persons and very limited information on large numbers of persons. Contributions from lifestyle factors, such as smoking and diet, are important to assess as they can have a significant impact on cancer development. Human epidemiology studies provide very useful information for hazard assessment and can provide quantitative information for data characterization. Several good illustrations of epidemiological studies and their interpretation for toxicological evaluation are available (Gamble and Battigelli, 1991; Checkoway, 1997; Lippmann and Schlesinger, 2000).

There are three major types of epidemiology study designs: cross-sectional studies, cohort studies, and case-control studies, as detailed in Table 4-5. Cross-sectional studies survey groups of humans to identify risk factors (exposure) and disease but are not useful for establishing cause and effect. Cohort studies evaluate individuals selected on the basis of their exposure to a chemical under study. Thus, based on exposure status, these individuals are monitored for development of disease. These prospective studies monitor over time individuals who initially are disease-free to determine the rates at which they develop disease. In case-control studies subjects are selected on the basis of disease status: disease cases and matched cases of disease-free individuals. Exposure histories of the two groups are compared to determine key consistent features in their exposure histories. All case-control studies are retrospective studies.

In risk assessment, epidemiologic findings are judged by the following criteria: strength of association, consistency of observations (reproducibility in time and space), specificity (uniqueness in quality or quantity of response), appropriateness of temporal relationship (did the exposure precede responses?), dose–responsiveness, biological plausibility and coherence, verification, and analogy (biological extrapolation) (Hill, 1965). In addition, epidemiologic study designs should be evaluated for their power of detection, appropriateness of outcomes, verification of exposure assessments, completeness of assessing confounding factors, and general applicability of the outcomes to other populations at risk. Power of detection is calculated using study size, variability, accepted detection limits for endpoints under study, and a specified significance level (Healey, 1987; Dean, 1995; EGRET, 1994).

Recent advances from the human genome project, increased sophistication and molecular biomarkers, and improved mechanistic bases for epidemiologic hypotheses, have allowed epidemiologists to get within the "black box" of statistical associations and move forward our understanding of biological plausibility and clinical relevance. "Molecular epidemiology," the integration of molecular biology into traditional epidemiologic research, is a new focus of human studies where improved molecular biomarkers of exposure, effect, and susceptibility have allowed investigators to more effectively link molecular events in the causative disease pathway. Epidemiologists can now include the contribution of potential genetic factors with environmental risk factors to the determination of the etiology, distribution, and prevention of disease. Highlighting the potential power of genetic information to epidemiological studies, the Human Genome Epidemiology Network (HuGE) was launched in 2001, providing a literature database of published, population-based epidemiologic studies of human genes (Lin et al., 2006).

With the advance of genomics, the range of biomarkers has grown dramatically and includes identification of single nucleotide polymorphisms (SNPs), genomic profiling, transcriptome analysis, and proteomic analysis (Simon and Wang, 2006). Implications of these improvements for risk assessment are tremendous, as they provide an improved biological basis for extrapolation across the diversity of human populations and allow for improved cross-species comparisons with rodent bioassay information. In addition, genomics allows for "systems-based" understanding of disease and response, moving risk assessment away from a linear, single-event-based concept and improving the biological plausibility of epidemiologic associations (Toscano and Oehlke, 2005).

Integrating Qualitative Aspects of Risk Assessment

Qualitative assessment of hazard information should include a consideration of the consistency and concordance of findings, including a determination of the consistency of the toxicological findings across species and target organs, an evaluation of consistency across duplicate experimental conditions, and a determination of the adequacy of the experiments to detect the adverse endpoints of interest.

NTP uses several categories to classify bioassay results, with the category *clear evidence of carcinogenicity* describing bioassays where dose-related increases in malignant or combined malignant and benign neoplasms are seen across doses including at least a significant increase in two of the four species/sex test groups. NTP's evaluation guidelines specify the additional categories of *some, equivocal, no evidence,* and *inadequate study.*

Qualitative assessment of animal or human evidence is done by many agencies, including the EPA and International Agency for Research on Cancer (IARC). Similar evidence classifications have been used for both the animal and human evidence categories by both agencies. These evidence classifications have included levels of sufficient, limited, inadequate, and no evidence (EPA, 1994a, 2005b) or *evidence suggesting lack of carcinogenicity* (IARC, 2000). For both agencies, these classifications are used for overall weight-of-evidence approach for carcinogenicity classification.

Weight-of-evidence is an integrative step used by the EPA to "characterize the extent to which the available data support the hypothesis that an agent causes cancer in humans" (EPA, 2005b). It is the process of "weighing" all of the evidence to reach a conclusion about carcinogenicity. With this method, the likelihood of human carcinogenic effect is evaluated in addition to an understanding of the conditions under which such effects may be expressed. Weight of evidence can consider both the quality and quantity of data as well as any underlying assumptions. The evidence includes data from all of the hazard assessment and characterization studies such as SAR data, in vivo and/or in vitro studies and epidemiological data. Using this type of information and weight-of-evidence approach, the EPA includes hazard descriptors to define carcinogenic potential and to provide a measure of clarity and consistency in the characterization narrative: "carcinogenic to humans," "likely to be carcinogenic to humans," "suggestive evidence of carcinogenic potential," "inadequate information to assess carcinogenic potential," and "not likely to be carcinogenic to humans." In this section, approaches for evaluating cancer endpoints are discussed. Similar weight-of-evidence approaches have been proposed for reproductive risk assessment (refer to *sufficient* and *insufficient evidence* categories in EPA's guidelines for reproductive risk (EPA, 1996b)).

The Institute for Evaluating Health Risks defined an "evaluation process" by which reproductive and developmental toxicity data can be consistently evaluated and integrated to ascertain their relevance for human health risk assessment (Moore et al., 1995). This evaluation process now serves as the basis for NTP's Center for the Evaluation of Risks to Human Reproduction (CERHR) (http://cerhr.niehs.nih.gov/). Application of such carefully deliberated approaches for assessing noncancer endpoints should help avoid the tendency to list chemicals as yes or no (positive or negative) without human relevancy information.

Mode of Action   The EPA has emphasized in their revised cancer guidelines, the importance of using "weight of evidence" to arrive at insights to possible "mode(s) of action" (MOA) (EPA, 2005b). MOA information describes key events and processes leading to molecular and functional effects that would in general explain the overall process of cancer development. In many cases these could be plausible hypothesized MOAs for both specific toxicity endpoints, but the detailed mechanistic nuances of the pathway might not yet be fully known. EPA has proposed using such MOA information to suggest nondefault approaches for cancer risk assessments and for evaluating toxicity of compounds with common MOAs in cumulative risk assessments (EPA, 1996b, 1998a).

Within the EPA's new Carcinogenic Risk Assessment Guidelines, the MOA framework considers evidence from animal studies, relevance to humans, and life stage or population susceptibility (EPA, 2005b). Chemical-specific adjustment factors for interspecies differences and human variability have been proposed and build upon guidance developed by the WHO's International Programme on Chemical Safety Harmonization Project (World Health Organization, 2000). Critical to the MOA development is the use of "criteria of causality" considerations, which build on Hill criteria used in epidemiology (Hill, 1965; Faustman et al., 1996; EPA, 1999b; Klaunig et al., 2003), and consider dose–response relationships and temporal associations, as well as the biological plausibility, coherence, strength, consistency, and specificity of the postulated MOA.

DOSE–RESPONSE ASSESSMENT

Integrating Quantitative Aspects of Risk Assessment

Quantitative considerations in risk assessment include dose–response assessment, exposure assessment, variation in susceptibility, and characterization of uncertainty. For dose–response assessment, varying approaches have been proposed for threshold versus nonthreshold endpoints. Traditionally, in the United States, threshold approaches have been applied for assessment of noncancer endpoints, and nonthreshold approaches have been used for cancer endpoints. As we have learned more about nongenotoxic mechanisms of carcinogenicity, these processes have been evaluated using threshold approaches. Each approach and its inherent assumptions are discussed below, as are recent efforts to include more detailed mechanistic considerations to harmonize these approaches (Bogdanffy et al., 2001).

In general, human exposure data for prediction of human response to environmental chemicals are quite limited; thus, animal bioassay data have primarily served as the basis for most quantitative risk assessments and have required extrapolation for human health evaluation. The risk assessor, however, is normally interested in low environmental exposures when considering human risk, exposures which are well below the experimentally observable range of responses in most animal assays. Thus, methods for extrapolating from high dose to low dose as well as extrapolating from animal risk to human risk are required and comprise a major portion of dose–response assessment.

The fundamental basis of the quantitative relationships between exposure to a chemical and the incidence of an adverse response is the dose–response assessment. Analysis of dose–response relationships must start with the determination of the critical effects to be quantitatively evaluated. It is usual practice to choose the most robust data sets with adverse effects occurring at the lowest levels of exposure from studies using the most relevant exposure routes. The "critical" adverse effect is defined as the significant adverse biological effect that occurs at the lowest exposure level (Barnes and Dourson, 1988). EPA has issued toxicity-specific guidelines that are useful in identifying such critical effects (for developmental toxicity (EPA, 1991b); reproductive toxicity (EPA, 1996b); neurotoxicity (EPA, 1995); cancer (EPA, 1994a, 1996a, 1999b, 2005b)). IPCS has recently compiled a document cited as the Principles for Modeling Dose–Responses for the Risk Assessments of Chemicals (World Health Organization, 2004). It outlines key concepts and considerations for dose–response evaluations within the context of a risk assessment.

Threshold Approaches Approaches for characterizing threshold dose–response relationships include identification of "no observed adverse effect level" (NOAELs) or "lowest observed adverse effect levels" (LOAELs). On the dose–response curve illustrated in Fig. 4-3, the doses tested in the bioassay are given as E, F, G, H, and I. The statistical significance of points G, H, and I is indicated using an asterisk (*). The threshold (T) represents the dose below which no additional increase in response is observed. The NOAEL (F) is identified as the highest nonstatistically significant dose tested; in this example the NOAEL occurs at approximately 2 mg/kg body weight. Point G is the LOAEL (~2.3 mg/kg body weight), as it is the lowest dose tested with a statistically significant effect. Lines A–D represent possible extrapolations below the point of departure (POD), which is represented on this figure as an (*) and is labeled as point E. The POD is used to specify the estimated dose near the lower end of the observed dose range, below which, extrapolation to lower exposures is necessary (EPA, 2005b). In Fig. 4-3, the POD occurs at 10% effective dose or ED_{10}. The type of extrapolation below the POD is depending on the type of data available. The importance of choosing an appropriate POD and extrapolation type is discussed further in the following sections of the chapter.

In general, most animal bioassays are constructed with sufficient numbers of test animals to detect biological responses at the 10% response range; however, this is dependent upon endpoint and

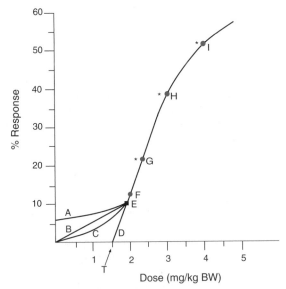

Figure 4-3. Dose–response curve.

This figure is designed to illustrate a typical dose–response curve with points E to I indicating the biologically determined responses. Statistical significance of these responses is indicated with a "*" symbol. The threshold dose is shown by T, a dose below which no change in biological response occurs. Point E represents the point of departure (POD), the dose near the lower end of the observed dose–response range, below which, extrapolation to lower doses is necessary (EPA, 2005b). Point F is the highest nonstatistically significant response point, hence it is the "no observed adverse effect level" (NOAEL) for this example. Point G is the "lowest observed adverse response level" (LOAEL). Curves A–D show some options for extrapolating the dose–response relationship below the range of biologically observed data points, POD, point E.

the background rate of the endpoint in control animals. The risk assessor should always understand the biological significance of the responses being evaluated in order to put statistical observations in context. *Significance* thus usually refers to both biological and statistical criteria (Faustman *et al.*, 1994) and is dependent upon the number of dose levels tested, the number of animals tested at each dose, and background incidence of the adverse response in the nonexposed control groups. The NOAEL should not be perceived as risk-free, as several reports have shown that the response of NOAELs for continuous endpoints averages 5% risk, and NOAELs based on quantal endpoints can be associated with risk of greater than 10% (Allen *et al.*, 1994; Faustman *et al.*, 1994).

As described in Chap. 2, approaches for characterizing dose–response relationships include identification of effect levels such as LD_{50} (dose producing 50% lethality), LC_{50} (concentration producing 50% lethality), ED_{10} (dose producing 10% response), as well as NOAELs.

NOAELs have traditionally served as the basis for risk assessment calculations, such as reference doses or acceptable daily intake (ADI) values. Reference doses (RfDs) or concentrations (RfCs) are estimates of a daily exposure to an agent that is assumed to be without adverse health impact in humans. The ADIs are used by WHO for pesticides and food additives to define "the daily intake of chemical, which during an entire lifetime appears to be without appreciable risk on the basis of all known facts at that time" (World Health Organization, 1962; Dourson *et al.*, 1985). Reference doses (first introduced in Chap. 2) and ADI values typically are calculated from NOAEL values by dividing by uncertainty (UF) and/or modifying factors (MF) (Dourson and Stara, 1983; Dourson and DeRosa, 1991; EPA, 1991b).

$$RfD = NOAEL/(UF * MF)$$
$$ADI = NOAEL/(UF * MF)$$

Tolerable daily intakes (TDI) can be used to describe intakes for chemicals that are not "acceptable" but are "tolerable" as they are below levels thought to cause adverse health effects. These are calculated in a manner similar to ADI. In principle, dividing by the uncertainty factors allows for interspecies (animal-to-human) and intraspecies (human-to-human) variability with default values of 10

each. An additional uncertainty factor is used to account for experimental inadequacies—for example, to extrapolate from short-exposure-duration studies to a situation more relevant for chronic study or to account for inadequate numbers of animals or other experimental limitations. If only a LOAEL value is available, then an additional 10-fold factor commonly is used to arrive at a value more comparable to a NOAEL. For developmental toxicity endpoints, it has been demonstrated that the application of the 10-fold factor for LOAEL-to-NOAEL conversion is too large (Allen *et al.*, 1994). Traditionally, a safety factor of 100 would be used for RfD calculations to extrapolate from a well-conducted animal bioassay (10-fold factor animal to human) and to account for human variability in response (10-fold factor human-to-human variability).

Modifying factors can be used to adjust the uncertainty factors if data on mechanisms, pharmacokinetics, or relevance of the animal response to human risk is available. For example, if there is kinetic information suggesting that rat and human metabolism are very similar for a particular compound, producing the same active target metabolite, then—rather than using a 10-fold uncertainty factor to divide the NOAEL from the animal toxicity study to obtain a human relevant RfD—a factor of 3 for that uncertainty factor might be used. Of particular interest is the recent addition of an extra 10-fold factor through the Food Quality and Protection Act (FQPA) to ensure protection of infants and children (EPA, 1996a). Under this law an additional uncertainty factor is added to ensure protection of children's health; it is currently being used for determining allowable pesticide chemical residues. This factor is designed to take into account potential pre- and postnatal toxicity and to overcome the incompleteness of toxicity and exposure data (FQPA; PL 104-170). Illustrative discussions on how such a legislatively mandated uncertainty factor might be applied are available for chlorpyrifos (EPA, 1999a; Schardein and Scialli, 1999). In this case, this factor was reduced due to the availability of specific animal experiments assessing developmental toxicity at sensitive life stages (Zhao *et al.*, 2006) (www.epa.gov/iris/subst/0026.htm).

To reduce uncertainty in calculating RfDs and ADIs, there has been a transition from the use of traditional 10-fold uncertainty factors to the use of data-derived and chemical-specific adjustment factors. Such efforts have included reviewing the human pharmacologic literature from published clinical trials (Silverman

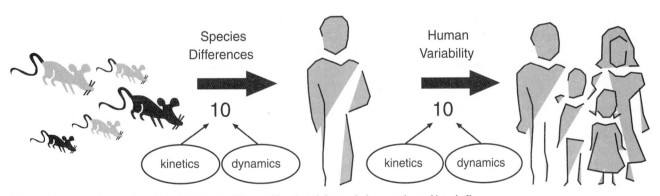

Figure 4-4. Toxicokinetic (TK) and toxicodynamic (TD) considerations inherent in interspecies and interindividual extrapolations.

Toxicokinetics refers to the processes of absorption, distribution, elimination, and metabolism of a toxicant. *Toxicodynamics* refers to the actions and interactions of the toxicant within the organism and describes processes at organ, tissue, cellular, and molecular levels. This figure shows how uncertainty in extrapolation both across and within species can be considered as being due to two key factors: a kinetic component and a dynamic component. Refer to the text for detailed explanations.

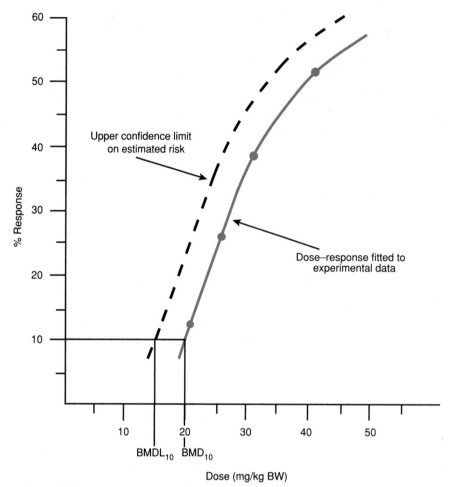

Figure 4-5. Illustration of benchmark dose (BMD) approach.

This figure shows the $BMDL_{10}$ and BMD_{10}, the lower confidence limit and dose (ED_{10}) associated with a 10% incidence of adverse response, respectively.

et al., 1999) and developing human variability databases for a large range of exposures and clinical conditions (Renwick, 1991, 1999; Johnson *et al.*, 1997). Toward this goal, Renwick has separated the intra- and interspecies uncertainty factors into two components: toxicokinetic (TK) and toxicodynamic (TD) aspects (Renwick, 1991, 1999; Johnson *et al.*, 1997). Figure 4-4 shows these distinctions. A key advantage of this approach is that it provides a structure for incorporating scientific information on specific aspects of the overall toxicologic process into the reference dose calculations; thus, relevant data can replace a portion of the overall "uncertainty" surrounding these extrapolations. Current WHO guidance uses a 4.0- and 2.5-fold factor for the TK and TD interspecies components, respectively (World Health Organization, 2005), and inter-individual TK and TD factors of 3.16 (Renwick and Lazarus, 1998).

NOAEL values have also been utilized for risk assessment by evaluating a "margin of exposure" (MOE), where the ratio of the NOAEL determined in animals and expressed as mg/kg/day is compared with the level to which a human may be exposed. For example, human exposures to a specific chemical are calculated to be solely via drinking water, and the total daily intake of the compound is 0.04 mg/kg/day. If the NOAEL for neurotoxicity is 100 mg/kg/day, then the MOE would be 2,500 for the oral exposure route for neurotoxicity. Such a large value is reassuring to public health officials. Low values of MOE indicate that the human levels

of exposure are close to levels for the NOAEL in animals. There is usually no factor included in this calculation for differences in human or animal susceptibility or animal-to-human extrapolation; thus, MOE values of less than 100 have been used by regulatory agencies as flags for requiring further evaluation.

The NOAEL approach has been criticized on several points, including that (1) the NOAEL must, by definition, be one of the experimental doses tested and (2) once this is identified, the rest of the dose–response curve is ignored. Because of these limitations, an alternative to the NOAEL approach, the benchmark dose (BMD) method, was proposed (Crump, 1984). In this approach, the dose–response is modeled and the lower confidence bound for a dose at a specified response level [benchmark response (BMR)] is calculated. The BMR is usually specified at 1, 5, or 10%. Figure 4-5 shows the BMD using a 10% benchmark response (BMD_{10}) and a 95% lower confidence bound on dose ($BMDL_{10}$). The $BMDx$ (with *x* representing the percent benchmark response) is used as an alternative to the NOAEL value for reference dose calculations. Thus, the RfD would be

$$RfD = BMDx/UF\,{}^{*}\,MF$$

EPA has developed software for the application of benchmark dose methods and developed a technical guidance document to provide guidelines for application of BMDs for both cancer and noncancer endpoints (EPA, 2000a). The 2004 WHO guidelines for dose–response modeling for risk assessment also discuss BMD approaches (World Health Organization, 2004). Both the EPA and WHO guidelines distinguish NOAEL versus BMD based approaches. Harmonization of approaches available for assessments is discussed in these documents.

The benchmark dose approach has been applied to study several noncancer endpoints, including developmental (Allen *et al.*, 1994) and reproductive toxicity (Auton, 1994). The most extensive studies with developmental toxicity have shown that BMD_{05} values were similar to a statistically derived NOAEL for a wide range of developmental toxicity endpoints and that results from using generalized dose–response models were similar to statistical models designed specifically to represent unique features of developmental toxicity testing.

Advantages of the benchmark dose approach can include (1) the ability to take into account the dose–response curve; (2) the inclusion of a measure of variability (confidence limit); and (3) the use of a consistent benchmark response level for RfD calculations across studies. Obviously, limitations in the animal bioassays in regard to minimal test doses for evaluation, shallow dose responses, and use of study designs with widely spaced test doses will limit the utility of these assays for any type of quantitative assessments, whether NOAEL- or BMD-based approaches.

Nonthreshold Approaches As Fig. 4-3 shows, numerous dose–response curves can be proposed in the low-dose region of the dose–response curve if a threshold assumption is not made. Because the risk assessor generally needs to extrapolate beyond the region of the dose–response curve for which experimentally observed data are available; the choice of models to generate curves in this region has received lots of attention. For nonthreshold responses, methods for dose–response assessments have also utilized models for extrapolation to de minimus (10^{-4} to 10^{-6}) risk levels at very low doses, far below the biologically observed response range and far below the effect levels evaluated for threshold responses.

EPA guidelines define the dose–response methods as requiring two steps: (1) defining the "point of departure" (POD) or the lowest dose associated with adverse effects within the range of the experimental data and (2) the extrapolation from the POD to low environmentally relevant exposure levels based on experimental data. The extrapolation can be done with a linear model or a nonlinear model with this choice dependent on the amount and type of experimental data available. Risk estimates using the linear model (biological response increases proportionally with level of exposure) are higher that nonlinear models where the biological response does not vary proportionally with the dose. For example, in 2003, the EPA released a Dioxin Reassessment and used the BMD dose–response method. The reassessment used a POD based on a 1% response with a linear extrapolation model based on the position that the scientific data were inadequate to rule out the EPA's standard default linear assumption. The EPA dioxin reassessment was evaluated in a National Academies Report in 2006 (NAS, 2006) and this review discusses remaining extrapolation issues.

Two general types of dose–response models exist for extrapolation: statistical (or probability distribution models) and mechanistic models (Krewski and Van Ryzin, 1981). The distribution models are based on the assumption that each individual has a tolerance level for a test chemical and that this response level is a variable following a specific probability distribution function. These responses can be modeled using a cumulative dose–response function. Chapter 2 discusses the common normal distribution pattern (see Fig. 2-3). A log probit model estimates the probability of response at a specified dose (d); thus, $P(d) = \phi[a + \beta\log d]$, where ϕ is the cumulative function for a standard normal distribution of the log tolerances with standard deviations σ and mean μ, a equals μ/σ, and β equals the slope of the probit line ($-1/\sigma$). The probit curve at low doses usually assumes an S-shape. Chapter 2 discusses determination of the LD_{50} value from such a curve. However, extrapolation of the experimental data from 50% response levels to a "safe," "acceptable," or "de minimus" level of exposure—e.g., one in a million risk above background—illustrates the huge gap between scientific observations and highly protective risk limits (sometimes called *virtually safe doses* or those corresponding to a 95% upper confidence limit on adverse response rates).

The log logistic model was derived from chemical kinetic theory. The probability of response at dose d is defined as $P(d) = [1 - \exp(a + \beta\log d)]^{-1}$. Like the probit model, this model defines sigmoidal curves that are symmetrical around the 50% response level; however, the log logistic curves approach the 0 and 100% response levels with a shallow curve shape. The logit and probit curves are indistinguishable in fitting the data in the region of the response curve where experimentally derived data are present (Brown, 1984; Hartung, 1987).

Models Derived from Mechanistic Assumptions This modeling approach designs a mathematical equation to describe dose–response relationships that are consistent with postulated biological mechanisms of response. These models are based on the idea that a response (toxic effect) in a particular biological unit (animal, human, pup, etc.) is the result of the random occurrence of one or more biological events (stochastic events).

Radiation research has spawned a series of such "hit models" for cancer modeling, where a hit is defined as a critical cellular event that must occur before a toxic effect is produced. The simplest mechanistic model is the one-hit (one-stage) linear model in which only one hit or critical cellular interaction is required for a cell to be altered. For example, based on somatic mutation theory, a single mutational change would be sufficient for a cell to become cancerous through a transformational event and dose-independent clonal expansion. The probability statement for these models is $P(d) = 1 - \exp^{(-\lambda d)}$, where λd equals the number of hits occurring during a time period. A single molecule of a genotoxic carcinogen would have a minute but finite chance of causing a mutational event.

As theories of cancer have grown in complexity, so too have these hit-based mechanistic models. Multihit models have been developed that can describe hypothesized single-target multihit events, as well as multitarget, multihit events in carcinogenesis. The probability statements for these models is $P(d) = \int^{\lambda d} \chi^{k-1} \exp(-x)/\Gamma(k)dx$, where $\Gamma(k)$ denotes the gamma function with k = critical number of hits for the adverse response. The Weibull model has a dose–response function with characteristics similar to those of the multihit models, where the response equation is $P(d) = 1 - \exp[-\lambda d^k]$. Here again, k = critical number of hits for the toxic cellular response.

Armitage and Doll (1957) developed a multistage model for carcinogenesis that was based on these equations and on the hypothesis that a series of ordered stages was required before a cell could undergo mutation, initiation, transformation, and progression to form a tumor. This relationship was generalized by Crump (1980) by maximizing the likelihood function over polynomials, so that the

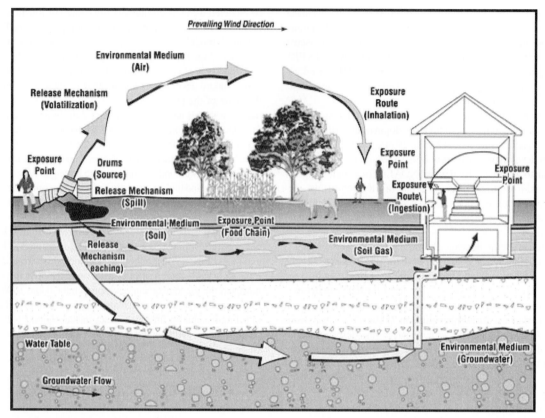

Figure 4-6. Exposure pathway schematic.

Within the risk assessment process, a critical early step is the identification of the exposure pathway(s). To fully characterize exposure, the site-specific and chemical-specific exposure pathways must be identified. This hypothetical exposure pathway schematic illustrated the various ways in which contaminants can move from the source through media to points of exposure. (http://www.atsdr.cdc.gov/HAC/PHAManual/images/figure6_2.jpg).

probability statement is:

$$P(d) = 1 - \exp\left[- \left(\lambda_0 + \lambda_1 d^1 + \lambda_2 d^2 + \cdots \lambda_k d^k \right) \right]$$

If the true value of λ_1 is replaced with λ_1^* (the upper confidence limit of λ_1), then a linearized multistage model can be derived where the expression is dominated by $(\lambda d^*)d$ at low doses. The slope on this confidence interval, q_1^*, has been used by EPA for quantitative cancer assessment. To obtain an upper 95% confidence interval on risk, the q_1^* value (risk/Δ dose in mg/kg/day) is multiplied by the amount of exposure (mg/kg/day). Thus, the upper-bound estimate on risk (R) is calculated as:

$$R = q_1^* [\text{risk}(\text{mg/kg/day})^{-1}] \times \text{exposure (mg/kg/day)}$$

This relationship has been used to calculate a "virtually safe dose" (VSD), which represents the lower 95% confidence limit on a dose that gives an "acceptable level" of risk (e.g., upper confidence limit for 10^{-6} excess risk). The integrated risk information system (IRIS) (www.epa.gov/iriswebp/iris) developed by EPA gives q^* values for many environmental carcinogens (EPA, 2000c). Because both the q_1^* and VSD values are calculated using 95% confidence intervals, the values are believed to represent conservative, protective estimates.

The EPA has utilized the LMS model to calculate "unit risk estimates" in which the upper confidence limit on increased individual lifetime risk of cancer for a 70-kg human breathing 1 μg/m^3 of contaminated air or drinking 2 L/day of water containing 1 ppm (1 mg/L) is estimated over a 70-year life span. The example given in Fig. 4-7 shows the calculation of incremental lifetime cancer risk (ILCR) of skin cancer using soil exposure and q^* values for inorganic arsenic. If a POD-based approach is used for low dose extrapolation, the model would be used to extrapolate from the POD or upper confidence limit and these slopes would be considered for the q^* values.

Toxicologic Enhancements of the Models   Three exemplary areas of research that have improved the models used in risk extrapolation are time to tumor information, physiologically based toxicokinetic modeling, and biologically based dose–response modeling (Albert, 1994). Chapter 7 discusses in detail improvements in our estimation of exposure and offers approaches on how to model "target internal effective dose" in risk assessment rather than just using single-value "external exposure doses." In this chapter we discuss the biologically based dose–response (BBDR) modeling.

BBDR modeling aims to make the generalized mechanistic models discussed in the previous section more clearly reflect specific biological processes. Measured rates are incorporated into the mechanistic equations to replace default or computer-generated values. For example, the Moolgavkar–Venson–Knudson (MVK) model

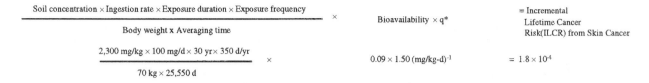

A. Ingestion of Arsenic from Soil—Point Estimation Method

$$\frac{\text{Soil concentration} \times \text{Ingestion rate} \times \text{Exposure duration} \times \text{Exposure frequency}}{\text{Body weight} \times \text{Averaging time}} \times \quad \text{Bioavailability} \times q^* \qquad \begin{array}{l}= \text{Incremental}\\ \text{Lifetime Cancer}\\ \text{Risk(ILCR) from Skin Cancer}\end{array}$$

$$\frac{2{,}300 \text{ mg/kg} \times 100 \text{ mg/d} \times 30 \text{ yr} \times 350 \text{ d/yr}}{70 \text{ kg} \times 25{,}550 \text{ d}} \times \quad 0.09 \times 1.50 \text{ (mg/kg-d)}^{-1} \qquad = 1.8 \times 10^{-4}$$

B. Ingestion of Arsenic from Soil—Probabilistic Methods

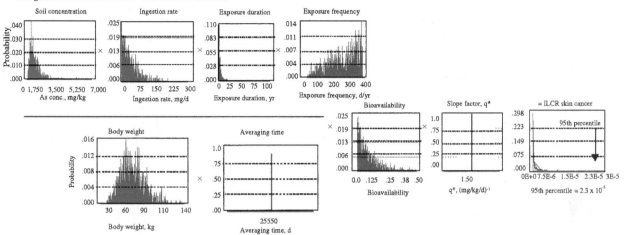

Figure 4-7. Example of risk calculations for incremental lifetime cancer risk (ILCR) of skin cancer due to ingestion of arsenic in soil.

A. Point exposure estimation method for calculation of ILCR. Point estimates for arsenic exposure input parameters are used in this example to calculate the ILCR. This exposure estimate is multiplied by the bioavailability of arsenic in soil to calculate the dose. Multiplication of the dose by the slope factor (q^*) yields the lifetime risk. **B.** Probabilistic exposure methods for calculating the incremental lifetime cancer risk (ILCR) from arsenic ingestion. In this example, the soil concentration, ingestion rate, exposure duration and frequency, body weight, and bioavailability are modeled as distributions. Note that q^* and averaging time (years) are given as single-point estimations. This method yields a distribution of ILCR, with a 95th percentile upper confidence interval of 2.3×10^{-5}. (Data from Calabrese, 1989; Davis, 1990; EPA, 1989a,b, 1992, 1999b; Israeli, 1992; Brorby, 1993; ATSDR, 1998.)

is based on a two-stage model for carcinogenesis, where two mutations are required for carcinogenesis and birth and death rates of cells are modeled through clonal expansion and tumor formation. This model has been applied effectively to human epidemiologic data on retinoblastoma. In animal studies, kidney and liver tumors in the 2-acetylaminofluorene (2-AAF) "mega mouse" study, rat lung tumors following radiation exposure, rat liver tumors following N-nitrosomorpholine exposure, respiratory tract tumors following benzo[a]pyrene exposure, and mouse liver tumors following chlordane exposure have been modeled (Cohen and Ellwein, 1990; Moolgavkar and Luebeck, 1990). EPA relied primarily on the receptor binding theory in its dioxin risk reassessments (EPA, 1994a, 2003). Kohn *et al.* (1993) and Anderson *et al.* (1993) have used physiologically based toxicokinetics (PBTK) and BBDR information to improve dioxin risk assessment.

Development of biologically based dose–response models for endpoints other than cancer are limited; however, several approaches have been explored in developmental toxicity, utilizing mode of action information on cell cycle kinetics, enzyme activity, and cytotoxicity as critical endpoints (Faustman *et al.*, 1989, 2005; Shuey *et al.*, 1994; Leroux *et al.*, 1996; Gohlke *et al.*, 2002, 2004, 2005, 2007). Approaches have been proposed that link pregnancy-specific toxicokinetic models with temporally sensitive toxicodynamic models

for developmental impacts (Faustman *et al.*, 1999, 2006). Unfortunately, there is a lack of specific, quantitative biological information on kinetics and dynamics for most toxicants and endpoints (NRC, 2000; EPA, 2004).

RISK CHARACTERIZATION

Risk characterization is a summary of the risk assessment components and serves to outline the key findings and inform the risk manager in public health decisions. It is an analysis and integration of the conclusions from the hazard assessment, the dose–response, and the exposure assessment. EPA outlines the science policy and elements for completing a risk characterization in their *Risk Characterization Handbook* (EPA, 2000d).

For many years there has been an information-sharing process aimed at harmonization of chemical testing regimes and clinical trials methodologies, so that data might be accepted in multiple countries. Recent efforts by WHO and IPCS have included the Harmonization of Approaches to the Assessment of Risk from Exposure to Chemicals Project (www.who.int/ipcs/methods/harmonization/en/). This project has the goal of globally harmonizing but not standardizing the approaches to risk assessment by increasing understanding and developing basic principles and guidance on specific chemical risk assessment issues. The WHO has worked to harmonize dose–response methodologies (DRM) and released a report providing a descriptive guidance for risk assessors in using DRM in hazard characterization (World Health Organization, 2004).

Variation in Susceptibility

Risk assessment methodologies incorporating human variability have been slow to develop. Generally, assay results utilize means and standard deviations to measure variation, or even standard errors of the mean. This ignores variability in response due to differences in age, sex, health status, and genetics. Default factors of 10X are overutilized to describe cross- and between-species differences and toxicokinetic and dynamic data are rare. Nevertheless, EPA and OSHA are expected under the Clean Air Act and the Occupational Safety and Health Act to promulgate standards that protect the most susceptible subgroups or individuals in the population (Omenn et al., 1990; Faustman and Omenn, 2006; Kramer et al., 2006; Cullen et al., in revision).

Ecogenetics has been defined as the study of critical genetic determinants that define susceptibility to environmentally influenced adverse health effects (Costa and Eaton, 2006). Ecogenetic variation can affect biotransformation systems that activate and detoxify chemicals or alter the response in target tissues. With the completion of the Human Genome Project in April 2003, the identification of human polymorphisms has greatly expanded our potential for understanding how genetic variability can impact biological response and susceptibility. There have been numerous activities initiated with the goal of understanding the linkage between genes and the environment and the following databases and initiatives are designed to identify polymorphisms, including single-nucleotide polymorphisms (SNP). These include the SNP consortium (http://snp.cshl.org/), the DNA Polymorphism Discovery Resource (www.genome.gov/10001552), the National Center for Biotechnology Information (NCBI) SNP databases (www.ncbi.nlm.nih.gov/SNP/) (www.ncbi.nlm.nih.gov/-entrez/?db=snp), and the NIH GAIN program (www.genome.gov/19518664). Using the information from such databases, researchers hope to identify genetic similarities and differences in human beings with the goal of identifying genes that affect health, disease, and individual responses to medications and environmental factors. It should be noted that this type of information raises ethical, social, and legal concerns regarding protections of individual donors (Hsieh, 2004).

One of the key challenges for toxicologists doing risk assessments will be the interpretation and linking of observations from highly sensitive molecular and genome-based methods with the overall process of toxicity (Eisen et al., 1998; Limbird and Taylor, 1998; Andersen and Barton, 1999; NRC, 2000). The basic need for linkage of observations was highlighted in early biomarker work. NRC reports on biomarkers (NRC, 1989a,b, 1992a,b) drew distinctions for biomarkers of effect, exposure, and susceptibility across a continuum of exposure, effect, and disease/toxicity. Biomarkers of early effects, like frank clinical pathology, arise as a function of exposure, response, and time. Early, subtle, and possibly reversible effects can generally be distinguished from irreversible disease states. Chemical-specific biomarkers have the potential to provide critical information, but there is an inherent complexity in pulling the information together. If biomarkers are considered a reflection of exposure or disease state, then considerations have to be made regarding the interactions between genes and the environment and the difference between a population-based assessment and individual assessment (Groopman and Kensler, 1999).

Nowhere is the challenge for interpretation of early and highly sensitive response biomarkers clearer than in the complicated data from gene expression arrays (toxicogenomics). Because our relatively routine ability to monitor gene responses—up to tens of thousands of them simultaneously—has grown exponentially in the last decade, the need for toxicologists to interpret such observations for risk assessment and for the overall process of toxicity has been magnified with equal or greater intensity. Recent papers from several toxicogenomics projects have confirmed the repeatability and cross-platform concordance of microarray data (Bammler et al., 2005; Guo et al., 2006; Nature Biotechnology Editorial, 2006; Patterson et al., 2006).

Microarray analysis for risk assessment requires sophisticated analyses beyond the basic cluster analysis (Eisen et al., 1998b) to arrive at a functional interpretation and linkage to conventional toxicological endpoints. Because of the vast number of measured responses with gene expression arrays, pattern analysis techniques are being used through pathway mapping platforms such as MAPPfinder and GenMAPP (Moggs et al., 2004; Currie et al., 2005). The Gene Ontology Consortium has developed a controlled vocabulary (ontology) for sharing biological information. Database users can then annotate their gene products with gene ontology (GO) terms, establishing a consistent description and definition across databases and studies. Through the power of GO terms, new analysis methods are being developed to allow for a quantitative time- and dose-dependent interpretation of genomic response at the biological and cellular level (Yu et al., 2006).

Both the EPA and FDA have formally recognized the power of genomic information as well as its potential limitations. Both agencies have issued interim policies guiding how to include genomic information into risk assessments and state to use genomic information in conjunction with standard risk assessment data (www.epa.gov/osa/genomics.htm, www.fda.gov/oc/initiatives/criticalpath/whitepaper.html).

EXPOSURE ASSESSMENT

The primary objectives of exposure assessment are to determine source, type, magnitude, and duration of contact with the chemical of interest. Obviously, this is a key element of the risk assessment process, as hazard does not occur in the absence of exposure. However, it is also frequently identified as the key area of uncertainty in the overall risk determination. Here, the primary focus is on uses of exposure information in quantitative risk assessment.

Obviously, the primary goal of such calculations is to determine not only the type and amount of total exposure, but also to find out specifically how much may be reaching target tissues. A key step in making an exposure assessment is determining what exposure pathways are relevant for the risk scenario under development. Figure 4-6 shows an example exposure diagram used to illustrate possible exposure pathways from a hazardous waste site release. The subsequent steps entail quantitation of each pathway identified as a potentially relevant exposure and then summarizing these pathway-specific exposures for calculation of overall exposure. Such calculations can include an estimation of total exposures for a specified population as well as calculation of exposure for highly exposed individuals. The EPA has published numerous documents which provide guidelines for determining such exposures (EPA, 1989a, 1992, 1997), with the recognition that special considerations need to be adopted when assessing childhood exposures (EPA, 2006).

Conceptually, calculations are designed to represent "a plausible estimate" of exposure of individuals in the upper 90th percentile of the exposure distribution. Upper-bound estimations would be "bounding calculations" designed to represent exposures at levels that exceed the exposures experienced by all individuals in the exposure distribution and are calculated by assuming limits for all exposure variables. A calculation for individuals exposed at levels near the middle of the exposure distribution is a central estimate. Figure 4-7 gives example risk calculations using two types of exposure estimation procedures (EPA, 1989a,b, 1992). Part A shows a point estimation method for the calculation of arsenic (As) exposure via a soil ingestion route. In this hypothetical scenario, As exposure is calculated using point estimates, and a lifetime average daily dose (LADD) is calculated as follows:

$$\text{LADD} = \frac{\begin{array}{c}\text{Concentration of} \times \text{Contact} \times \text{Contact} \times \text{Exposure} \\ \text{the toxicant in the} \quad \text{rate} \quad \text{fraction} \quad \text{duration} \\ \text{exposure media}\end{array}}{\text{(body weight) (lifetime)}}$$

Many exposures are now estimated using exposure factors probability distributions rather than single-point estimates for the factors within the LADD equation (Finley et al., 1994; Cullen and Frey, 1999). Such approaches can provide a reality check and can be useful for generating more realistic exposure profiles. Part B of Fig. 4-7 shows how this is done using an example arsenic risk scenario with soil As concentration, ingestion rate, exposure duration, frequency, body weight, and bioavailability modeled as distributed variables. Using Monte Carlo simulation techniques, an overall incremental lifetime cancer risk (ILCR) distribution can be generated and a 95th percentile for population risk obtained. The *EPA Exposure Factors Handbook,* which is online (www.epa.gov/ncea/efh/pdfs/efh-chapter01.pdf), provides useful information about exposure distributions (EPA, 1997). In 2006, the EPA released a supplemental document with child-specific exposure factors to address the special considerations necessary when evaluating childhood exposures (EPA, 2006).

Additional considerations for exposure assessments include how time and duration of exposure are evaluated in risk assessments. In general, estimates for cancer risk use average exposure over a lifetime (see LADD example above). In a few cases, short-term exposure limits (STELs) are required (e.g., ethylene oxide) and characterization of brief but high levels of exposure is required. In these cases exposures are not averaged over the lifetime and the effects of high, short-term doses are estimated. With developmental

toxicity, a single exposure can be sufficient to produce an adverse developmental effect; thus, daily doses are used, rather than lifetime weighted averages (EPA, 1991b; Weller et al., 1999).

The Food Quality Protection Act of 1996 has highlighted the need for several additional exposure and risk considerations (EPA, 1996c). These include the need to evaluate total exposures by determining aggregate exposure measures for all exposures to a single substance. Cross-media exposure analyses, such as those conducted for lead and mercury, are good examples of the value of looking at such total exposures in evaluating human risks and complex models are available [see EPA's integrated exposure uptake biokinetic model for lead in children (IEUBK)]. *Cumulative exposures* and *cumulative risk* refer to the total exposure to a group of compounds with similar modes of toxicity. For example, EPA is identifying and categorizing pesticides that act by a common mode of action, and such discussions of cumulative exposures to classes of organophosphates with similar modes of toxic action have been used as examples of classes of pesticides for which cumulative exposure and cumulative risk estimates are needed (ILSI, 1999).

INFORMATION RESOURCES

There are numerous information resources available for toxicology including the Toxicology Data Network (http://toxnet.nlm.nih.gov/) from the U.S. National Library of Medicine, the U.S. National Toxicology Program (http://ntp-server.niehs.nih.gov/), the WHO International Programme on Chemical Safety (www.who.int/pcs/IPCS/index.htm), and the International Agency for Research on Cancer (www.iarc.fr/).

RISK PERCEPTION AND COMPARATIVE ANALYSES OF RISK

Individuals respond differently to information about hazardous situations and products, as do communities and whole societies (Fischhoff, 1981; Fischhoff et al., 1993, 1996; Sandman, 1993; NRC, 1996; Risk Commission, 1997; Institute of Medicine, 1999). Understanding these behavioral responses is critical in stimulating constructive risk communication and evaluating potential risk management options. In a classic study, students, League of Women Voters members, active club members, and scientific experts were asked to rank 30 activities or agents in order of their annual contribution to deaths (Slovic et al., 1979, 2005). Club members ranked pesticides, spray cans, and nuclear power as safer than did other lay persons. Students ranked contraceptives and food preservatives as riskier and mountain climbing as safer than did others. Experts ranked electric power, surgery, swimming, and X-rays as

Table 4.6

Example Exposure Factor Handbook Information: Drinking Water Intake

AGE GROUP	MEAN	INTAKE (mL/day) 10th–90th PERCENTILES	MEAN	INTAKE (mL/day) 10th–90th PERCENTILES
Infants (<1 year)	302	0–649	43.5	0–101.8
Children (1–10 years)	736	286–1,294	35.5	12.5–64.4
Teens (11–19 years)	965	353–1,701	18.2	6.5–32.3
Adults (20–64 years)	1,366	559–2,268	19.9	8.0–33.7
Adults (64+ years)	1,459	751–2,287	21.8	10.9–34.7
All ages	1,193	423–2,092	22.6	8.2–39.8

SOURCE: US EPA, 1997; Ershow and Cantor, 1989.

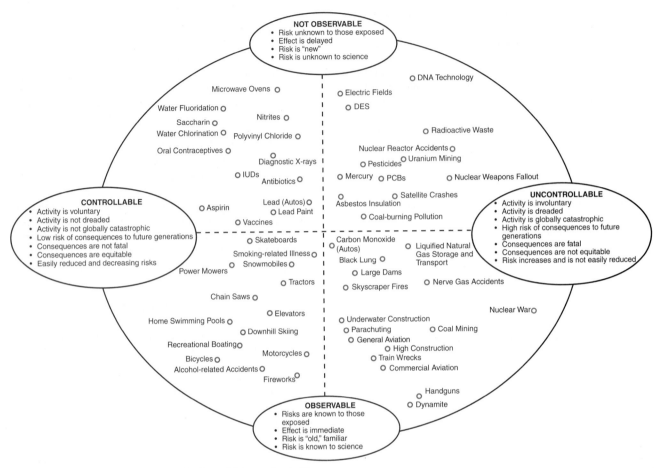

Figure 4-8. Perceptions of risk illustrated using a "risk space" axis diagram.

Risk space has axes that correspond roughly to a hazard's perceived "dreadedness" and to the degree to which it is familiar or observable. Risks in the upper right quadrant of this space are most likely to provoke calls for government regulation.

more risky, but nuclear power and police work as less risky than did lay persons. There are also group differences in perceptions of risk from chemicals among toxicologists, correlated with their employment in industry, academia, or government (Neal *et al.*, 1994).

Psychological factors such as dread, perceived uncontrollability, and involuntary exposure interact with factors that represent the extent to which a hazard is familiar, observable, and "essential" for daily living (Lowrance, 1976; Morgan, 1993). Figure 4-8 presents a grid on the parameters controllable/uncontrollable and observable/not observable for a large number of risky activities; for each of the two-paired main factors, highly correlated factors are described in the boxes.

Public demand for government regulations often focuses on involuntary exposures (especially in the food supply, drinking water, and air) and unfamiliar hazards, such as radioactive waste, electromagnetic fields, asbestos insulation, and genetically modified crops and foods. The public can respond negatively when they perceive that information about hazards or new technologies has been withheld or underrated. This can explain some of the very strong responses to genetically modified foods, HIV-contaminated blood transfusions in the 1980s, or hazardous chemical and radioactive wastes.

Perceptions of risk led to the addition of an extra safety factor (default value 10) for children in the Food Quality Protection Act of 1996. Engineering based "as low as reasonably achievable"

(ALARA) approaches also reflect the general "precautionary principle," which is strongly favored by those who, justifiably, believe we are far from knowing all risks given the limited toxicity testing (Roe *et al.*, 1997).

SUMMARY

The NRC and Risk Commission frameworks for risk assessment and risk management provide a consistent framework-based approach for evaluating risks and taking action to reduce risks. The objectives of risk assessments vary with the issues, risk management needs, and statutory requirements. Hence, setting the context and problem formation for risk evaluation is essential. The frameworks are sufficiently flexible to address various objectives and to accommodate new knowledge while also providing guidance for priority setting in industry, environmental organizations, and government regulatory and public health agencies. Toxicology, epidemiology, exposure assessment, and clinical observations can be linked with biomarkers, cross-species investigations of mechanisms of effects, and systematic approaches to risk assessment, risk communication, and risk management. Advances in toxicology are certain to improve the quality of risk assessments for a broad array of health endpoints as scientific findings substitute data for assumptions and help to describe and model uncertainty more credibly.

REFERENCES

Abbott BD, Harris MW, Birnbaum LS: Comparisons of the effects of TCDD and hydrocortisone on growth factor expression provide insight into their interaction in the embryonic mouse palate. *Teratology* 45(1):35–53, 1992.

Albert RE: Carcinogen risk assessment in the US Environmental Protection Agency. *Crit Rev Toxicol* 24:75–85, 1994.

Allen BC, Kavlock RJ, Kimmel CA, Faustman EM: Dose response assessments for developmental toxicity: II. Comparison of generic benchmark dose estimates with no observed adverse effect levels. *Fundam Appl Toxicol* 23:487–495, 1994.

Ames BN, Gold LS: Too many rodent carcinogens: Mitogenesis increases mutagenesis. *Science* 247:970–971, 1990.

Andersen ME, Barton HA: Biological regulatoin of receptor-hormone complex C in relation to dose–response assessments of endocrine-active compounds. *Toxicol Sci* 48:38–50, 1999.

Anderson ME, Mills JJ, Gargas ML: Modeling receptor-mediated processes with dioxin: Implications for pharmacokinetics and risk assessment. *Risk Anal* 13:25–36, 1993.

Armitage P, Doll R: A two-stage theory of carcinogenesis in relation to the age distribution of human cancer. *Br J Cancer* 11:161–169, 1957.

Ashby J, Tennant RW: Prediction of rodent carcinogenicity of 44 chemicals: Results. *Mutagenesis* 9:7–15, 1994.

ATSDR: Toxicological Profile for Arsenic (draft). Atlanta, US: Department of Health and Human Services, 1998.

Atterwill CK, Johnston H, Thomas SM: Models for the in vitro assessment of neurotoxicity in the nervous system in relation to xenobiotic and neurotrophic factor-mediated events. *Neurotoxicology* 13:39–54, 1992.

Auton TR: Calculation of benchmark doses from teratology data. *Regul Toxicol Pharmacol* 19:152–167, 1994.

Bammler T, Beyer RP, Bhattacharya S, *et al.*: Standardizing global gene expression analysis between laboratories and across platforms. *Nat Meth.* 2(5):351–356, 2005.

Barnes DG, Dourson MJ: Reference dose (RfD): Description and use in health risk assessment. *Regul Toxicol Pharmacol* 8:471–486, 1988.

Benigni R, Zito R: The second National Toxicology Program comparative exercise on the prediction of rodent carcinogenicity: definitive results. *Mutat Res* 566(1):49–63, 2004.

Bogdanffy MS, Daston G, Faustman EM, *et al.*: Harmonization of cancer and noncancer risk assessment: Proceedings of a consensus-building workshop. *Toxicol Sci* 61(1):18–31, 2001.

Brorby G, Finley G: Standard probability density functions for routine use in environmental health risk assessment, *Society for Risk Analysis Annual Meeting*. Savannah, GA, 1993.

Brown CC: High-to-low-dose extrapolation in animals, in Rodricks JV, Tardiff RG (eds.): *Assessment and Management of Chemical Risks*. Washington, DC, American Chemical Society, 1984, pp. 57–79.

Brown NA, Spielmann H, Bechter R: Screening chemicals for reproductive toxicity: The current alternatives: The report and recommendations of an ECVAM/ETS workshop. *Alt Lab Anim* 23:868–882, 1995.

Bucher JR: Update on national toxicology program (NTP) assays with genetically altered or "transgenic" mice. *Environ Health Perspect* 106(10):619–621, 1998.

Calabrese EJ, Pastides H, Barnes R: How much soil do young children ingest: An epidemiologic study, in Kostecki, PT, Calabrese, EJ (eds.): *Petroleum Contaminated Soils*. Chelsea, MI: Lewis Publishers, 1989, pp. 363–397.

Calkins DR, Dixon RI, Gerber CR: Identification, characterization, and control of potential human carcinogens: A framework for federal decision-making. *J Natl Cancer Inst* 61:167–175, 1980.

Capen CC, Dybing E, Rice JM, Wilbourn JD: Species differences in thyroid, kidney and urinary bladder carcinogenesis. IARC Scientific Publication (147).

Charnley G, Omenn GS: A summary of the findings and recommendations of the commission on risk assessment and risk management (and accompanying papers prepared for the commission). *Hum Ecol Risk Assess* 3:701–711, 1997.

Checkoway H: Epidemiology, in Rosenstock L, Cullen M (eds.): *Textbook of Clinical Occupational and Environmental Medicine*. Philadelphia, Saunders, 1997, pp. 150–168.

Chhabra RS, Bucher JR, Wolfe M, Portier C: Toxicity characterization of environmental chemicals by the US National Toxicology Program: an overview. *Int J Hyg Environ Health* 206(4–5):437–445, 2003.

Cohen SM: Human relevance of animal carcinogenicity studies. *Regul Toxicol Pharmacol* 21(1):75–80, 1995; discussion 81–86.

Cohen SM: Alternative models for carcinogenicity testing: Weight of evidence evaluations across models. *Toxicol Pathol* 29 Suppl:183–190, 2001.

Cohen SM, Arnold LL, Cano M, Ito M, Garland EM, Shaw RA: Calcium phosphate-containing precipitate and the carcinogenicity of sodium salts in rats. *Carcinogenesis* 21(4):783–792, 2000.

Cohen SM, Ellwein LB: Proliferative and genotoxic cellular effects in 2-acetylaminofluorene bladder and liver carcinogenesis: Biological modeling of the EDO1 study. *Toxicol Appl Pharmacol* 104:79–93, 1990.

Costa L, Eaton D: Introduction, in Costa L, Eaton. Hoboken D (eds.): *Gene-Environment Interactions: Fundamentals Of Ecogenetics*. Hoboken, NJ: Wiley, 2006.

Costa LG: *Biochemical and Molecular Neurotoxicology*. New York: Wiley, 2000.

Crump KS: An improved procedure for low-dose carcinogenic risk assessment from animal data. *J Environ Pathol Toxicol* 5:349–358, 1980.

Crump KS: A new method for determining allowable daily intakes. *Fundam Appl Toxicol* 4:854–871, 1984.

Cullen A, KramerCB, Faustman EM: The Application of genetic information for regulatory standard setting under the clean air act: a decision analytic approach. *Risk Analysis* (in revision).

Cullen AC, Frey HC: Probabilistic techniques in exposure assessment, *A Handbook for Dealing with Variability and Uncertainty in Models and Inputs*. New York: Plenum Press, 1999.

Currie RA, Bombail V, Oliver JD, Moore DJ, Lim FL, Gwilliam V, Kimber I, Chipman K, Moggs JG Orphanides G: Gene ontology mapping as an unbiased method for identifying molecular pathways and processes affected by toxicant exposure: application to acute effects caused by the rodent non-genotoxic carcinogen diethylhexylphthalate. *Toxicol Sci* 86(2):453–469, 2005.

Davis S, Waller P, Buschborn R: Quantitative estimates of soil ingestion in normal children between the ages of 2 and 7 years: Population-based estimates using aluminum, silicon, and titanium as soil tracer elements. *Arch Environ Health* 45:112–122, 1990.

Dean AG, Dean JA, Coulombier D: Epi info, Version 6: A word processing, database, and statistics program for public health on IBM-compatible microcomputers. Atlanta: Centers for Disease Control and Prevention (CDC), 1995.

Dearfield KL: Pesticide assessment guidelines, Subdivision F, Hazard evaluation. Series 84, 1990.

Dourson MJ, Hertzberg RC, Hartung R, Blackburn K: Novel methods for the estimation of acceptable daily intake. *Toxicol Ind. Health* 1:23–41, 1985.

Dourson ML, DeRosa CT: The use of uncertainty factors in establishing safe levels of exposure, in Krewski D, Franklin C (eds.): *Statistics in Toxicology*. New York: Gordon & Breach, 1991, pp. 613–627.

Dourson ML, Stara JF: Regulatory history and experimental support of uncertainty (safety factors). *Regul Toxicol Pharmacol* 3:224–238, 1983.

Drew CH, Grace DA, Silbernagel SM, Hemmings ES, Smith A, Griffith WC, Takaro TK, Faustman EM: Nuclear waste transportation: Case studies of identifying stakeholder risk information needs. *Environ Health Perspect* 111(3):263–272, 2003.

Eaton DL, Bammler TK, Kelly EJ: Interindividual differences in response to chemoprotection against aflatoxin-induced hepatocarcinogenesis: Implications for human biotransformation enzyme polymorphisms. *Adv Exp Med Biol* 500:559–576, 2001.

Eaton DL, Gallagher EP: Mechanisms of aflatoxin carcinogenesis. *Annu Rev Pharmacol Toxicol* 34:135–172, 1994.

Eaton DL, Gallagher EP, Bammler TK Kunze KL: Role of cytochrome P4501A2 in chemical carcinogenesis: implications for human variability in expression and enzyme activity. *Pharmacogenetics* 5(5):259–274, 1995.

EGRET: Statistics and Epidemiology Research Corporation (SERC). Seattle: Statistics and Epidemiology Research Corporation, 1994.

Eisen MB, Spellman PT, Brown PO, Botstein D: Cluster analysis and display of genome-wide expression patterns. *Proc Natl Acad Sci USA* 95:14863–14868, 1998.

EPA: Proposed guidelines for assessing female reproductive risk. *Fedl Reg* 53:24834–24847, 1988.

EPA: Exposure factors handbook, *Final report: EPA*. Washington, DX: Office of Health and Environmental Assessment, 1989a. http://www.epa.gov/nceawww1/exposure.htm

EPA: Risk assessment guidance for Superfund, *Human Health Evaluation Manual*. Washington, DC: Office of Policy Analysis and Office of Emergency and Remedial Response, 1989b, Part A, Vol. 1.

EPA: *Alpha2u-Globulin*. Washington, DC: EPA, 1991a.

EPA: Guidelines for developmental toxicity risk assessment. *Fed Reg* 56:63798–63826, 1991b.

EPA: Guidelines for exposure assessment. *Fed Reg* 57:22888–22938, 1991b.

EPA: Guidelines for Carcinogen Risk Assessment (Draft Revisions). Washington, DC: Office of Health and Environmental Assessment, 1994a.

EPA: Health Assessment Document for 2,3,7,8-Tetrachlorodibenzo-p-Diosin (TCDD) and Related Compounds. Washington, DC: Office of Research and Development, 1994b.

EPA: Proposed guideline for neurotoxicity risk assessment. 60:52032–52056, 1995.

EPA: *Food quality Protection Act (FQPA)*. Washington, DC: Office of Pesticide Programs, 1996a.

EPA: Guidelines for reproductive toxicity risk assessment. *Fed Reg* 61:56278–56322, 1996b.

EPA: Proposed guidelines for ecological risk assessment. Fed Reg 61, 1996c.

EPA: The EPA Exposure factors handbook. 1997.

EPA: *Chemical Hazard Avilability Study*. Washington, DC: Office of Pollution Prevention and Toxics, 1998a.

EPA: Guidance for identifying pesticides that have a common mechanism of toxicity: Notice of avilability and solicitation of public comments. *Fed Reg* 63:42031–42032, 1998b.

EPA: Health effects test guidelines. Developmental neurotoxicity study. Washington, DC, 1998c.

EPA: Chlorpyrifos-report of the FQPA safety factor committee. HED Doc No. 013296. Washington, DC, 1999a.

EPA: Guidelines for carcinogen risk assessment, draft. NCEA-F-0644. Washington, DC, 1999b.

EPA: Benchmark Dose Technical Guidance Document. Washington, DC, United States Environmental Protection Agency, 2000a.

EPA: Health effects test guidelines. 870 Series final guidelines. Washington, DC, Office of prevention, Pesticides and toxic substances, 2000b. http://www.epa.gov/opptsfrs/publications/OPPTS_Harmonized/870_Health_Effects_Test_Guidelines/index.html

EPA: Integrated risk information system. Washington, DC, Office of research and development, National center for environmental assessment, 2000c.

EPA: Risk Characterization, Science Policy Council Handbook. Office of Science Policy. Washington, DC, U.S. Environmental Protection Agency, 2000d.

EPA: Exposure and human health reassessment of 2,3,7,8-tetrachlorodibenzo-*p*-dioxin (TCDD) and related compounds. National Center for Environmental Assessment, 2003.

EPA: Modeling developmental processes in animals: Applications in neurodevelopmental toxicology, 2004.

EPA: Glossary of IRIS terms, 2005a. http://www.epa.gov/iris/gloss8.htm#w, 6/20/2006

EPA: Guidelines for Carcinogen Risk Assessment (Cancer Guidelines). Federal Register Notice, 2005b. http://cfpub.epa.gov/ncea/cfm/recordisplay.cfm?deid=116283,

EPA: Child-Specific Exposure Factors Handbook, 2006.

Ershow AG, Cantor KP: Total water and tapwater intake in the United States, in Bethesda MD (ed.): *Populations-Based Estimates of Quantities and Sources*, Life Sciences Research Office, Federation of American Societies for Experimental Biology, 1989, pp. 328–334.

Faustman E, Gohlke J, Lewandowski T, Bartell S, Judd N, Vigoren E, Griffith W: Modeling Developmental Processes in Animals: Applications in Neurodevelopmental Toxicology. EPA/600/P-04/110A, 2006.

Faustman E, Gohlke JM, Judd NL, Lewandowski TA, Bartell SM, Griffith, WC: Modeling developmental processes in animals: Applications in neurodevelopmental toxicology. *Environ Toxicol Pharmacol* May 19(3): 615–624, 2005.

Faustman E, Omenn G: Risk assessment and the impact of ecogenetics, in Costa L, Eaton D (eds.): *Gene–Environment Interactions: Fundamentals of Ecogenetics*., Huboken, NJ, Wiley and Sons.

Faustman EM: Short-term test for teratogens. *Mutat Res* 205:355–384, 1988.

Faustman EM, Allen BC, Kavlock RJ, Kimmel CA: Dose–response assessment for developmental toxicity: I. Characterization of data base and determination of no observed adverse effect levels. *Fundam Appl Toxicol* 23:478–486, 1994.

Faustman EM, Lewandowski TA, Ponce RA, Bartell SM: Biologically based dose–response models for developmental toxicants: Lessons from methylmercury. *Inhal Toxicol* 11:101–114, 1999.

Faustman EM, Ponce RA, Seeley MR, Whittaker SG: Experimental approaches to evaluate mechanisms of developmental toxicity, in Hood R (ed.): *Handbook of Developmental Toxicology*. Boca Raton, FL, CRC Press, 1996, pp. 13–41.

Faustman EM, Wellington DG, Smith WP, Kimmel CS: Characterization of a developmental toxicity dose response model. *Environ Health Perspect* 79:229–241, 1989.

Finley G, Proctor D, Scott P: Recommended distributions for exposure factors frequently used in health risk assessment. *Risk Anal* 14:533–553, 1994.

Fischhoff B: Cost–benefit analysis: An uncertain guide to public policy. *Am NY Acad Sci* 363:173–188, 1981.

Fischhoff B, Bostrom A, Quandrel MJ: Risk perception and communication. *Annu Rev Public Health* 14:183–203, 1993.

Fischhoff B, Bostrom A, Quandrel MJ: Risk perception and communication, in Detels R, Holland W, McEwen J, Omenn GS (eds.): *Oxford Textbook of Public Health*. New York, Oxford University Press, 1996, pp. 987–1002.

Gamble JF, Battigelli MC: Epidemiology, in Clayton GD, Clayton FE (eds.): *Patty's Industrial Hygiene and Toxicology*. New York, Wiley, 1978, pp. 113–127.

Gamble JF, Battigelli MC: Occupational epidemiology: Some guideposts, in Clayton GD, Clayton FE (eds.): *Patty's Industrial Hygiene and Toxicology*. New York, Wiley, 1991.

Gargas ML, Finley BL, Paustenback DJ, Long TF: Environmental health risk assessment: theory and practice, in Ballantyne B, Marrs T and Syversen T (eds.): *General and Applied Toxicology*. New York, Grove's Dictionaries, 1999, pp. 1749–1809.

Gohlke JM, Griffith WC, Bartell SM, Lewandowski TA, Faustman EM: A computational model for neocortical neuronogenesis predicts ethanol-induced neocortical neuron number deficits. *Dev Neurosci* 24(6):467–477, 2002.

Gohlke JM, Griffith WC, Faustman E: Computational Models of Neocortical Neuronogenesis and Programmed Cell Death in the Developing Mouse, Monkey and Human. Cerebral Cortex. (in press)

Gohlke JM, Griffith WC, Faustman EM: The role of cell death during neo-cortical neurogenesis and synaptogenesis: Implications from a computational model for the rat and mouse. *Brain Res Dev Brain Res* 151(1–2):43–54, 2004.

Gohlke JM, Griffith WC, Faustman EM: A systems-based computational model for dose–response comparisons of two mode of action hypotheses for ethanol-induced neurodevelopmental toxicity. *Toxicol Sci* 86(2):470–484, 2005.

Gray TJB: *Application of in Vitro Systems in Male Reproductive Toxicology.* San Diego, CA, Academic Press, 1988.

Gribble EJ, Hong SW, Faustman EM: The magnitude of methylmercury-induced cytotoxicity and cell cycle arrest is p53-dependent. *Birth Defects Res A Clin Mol Teratol* 73(1):29–38, 2005.

Groopman JD, Kensler TW: The light at the end of the tunnel for chemical-specific biomarkers: Daylight or headlight? *Carcinogenesis* 20(1):1–11, 1999.

Guo L, Lobenhofer EK, Wang C, et al.: Rat toxicogenomic study reveals analytical consistency across microarray platforms. *Nat Biotechnol* 24(9):1162–1169, 2006.

Harris MW, Chapin RE, Lockhart AC: Assessment of a short-term reproductive and developmental toxicity screen. *Fundam Appl Toxicol* 19:186–196, 1992.

Hartung R: Dose–response relationships, in Tardiff RG, Rodricks JV (eds.): *Toxic Substances and Human Risk: Principles of Data Interpretation.* New York, Plenum Press, 1987, pp. 29–46.

Hartung T, Bremer S, Casati S, et al.: ECVAM's response to the changing political environment for alternatives: Consequences of the European Union chemicals and cosmetics policies. *Altern Lab Anim* 31(5):473–481, 2003.

Haseman JK, Lockhart AM: Correlations between chemically related site-specific carcinogenic effects in long-term studies in rats and mice. *Environ Health Perspect* 101:50–54, 1993.

Haws LC, Su SH, Harris M, et al.: Development of a refined database of mammalian relative potency estimates for dioxin-like compounds. *Toxicol Sci* 89(1):4–30, 2006.

Healey GF: Power calculations in toxicology, 1987.

Health and Safety Executive: *Reducing Risks, Protecting People.* Suffolk, UK, HSE Books, 2000.

Hill AB: The environment and disease: Association or causation. *Proc R Soc Med* 58:295–300, 1965.

Hsieh A: A nation's genes for a cure to cancer: Evolving ethical, social and legal issues regarding population genetic databases. *Columbia J Law Soc Probl* 37(3):359–411, 2004.

IARC: *IARC Monographs on the Evaluation of Carcinogenic Risks to Humans.* Lyon, France, World Health Organization, 2000.

ILSI: *A Framework for Cumulative Risk Assessment.* Washington, DC, International Life Science Institute, 1999.

Institute of Medicine: *Toward Environmental Justice.* Washington, DC, National Academy Press, 1999.

Israeli M, Nelson CB: Distribution and expected time of residence for United States households. *Risk Anal* 12:65–72, 1992.

Johnson DE, Wolfgang GHI, Gledin MA, Braeckman RA: Toxicokinetics and toxicodynamics, in Sipes I, McQueen C, Gandolfi A (eds.): *Comprehensive Toxicology.* Oxford, UK, Pregamon, Elsevier Sciences, 1997, pp. 169–181.

Judd NL, Drew CH, Acharya C, et al.: Framing scientific analyses for risk management of environmental hazards by communities: Case studies with seafood safety issues. *Environ Health Perspect* 113(11):1502–1508, 2005.

Kavlock RJ, Allen BC, Faustman EM, Kimmel CA: Dose response assessments for developmental toxicity: IV. Bencgmark doses for fetal weight changes. *Fundam Appl Toxicol* 26:211–222, 1995.

Klaunig JE, Babich M, Baetcke K, Cook J, et al.: PPARα agonist-induced rodent tumors: Modes of action and human relevance. *Crit Rev Toxicol* 33(6):655–780, 2003.

Kohn MC, Lucier GW, Clark GC: A mechanistic model of effects of dioxin on gene expression in the rat liver. *Toxicol Appl Pharmacol* 120:138–154, 1993.

Kramer CB, Cullen AC, Faustman EM: Policy implications of genetic information on regulation under the Clean Air Act: The case of particulate matter and asthmatics. *Environ Health Perspect* 114(3):313–319, 2006.

Krewski D, Van Ryzin J: Dose response models for quantal response toxicity data, in Csorgo M, Dawson D, Rao J, Seleh A (eds.): *Statistics and Related Topics.* North-Holland, Amsterdam, 1981, pp. 201–229.

Lave LB, Ennever F, Rosenkranz HS, Omenn GS: Information value of the rodent bioassay. *Nature* 336:631–633, 1988.

Lave LB, Omenn GS: Cost-effectiveness of short-term tests for carcinogenicity. *Nature* 334:29–34, 1986.

Leroux BG, Leisenring WM, Moolgavkar SH, Faustman EM: A biologically based dose-response model for development. *Risk Anal* 16:449–458, 1996.

Lewandowski TA, Ponce RA, Whittaker SG, Faustman EM: In vitro models for evaluating developmental toxicity, in Gad S (ed.): *Vitro Toxicology.* New York, Taylor & Francis, 2000, pp. 139–187.

Limbird LE, Taylor P: Endocrine disruptors signal the need for receptor models and mechanisms to inform policy. *Cell Press* 93:157–163, 1998.

Lin BK, Clyne M, Walsh M, et al.: Tracking the epidemiology of human genes in the literature: The HuGE Published Literature database. *Am J Epidemiol* 164(1):1–4, 2006.

Lippmann M, Schlesinger RB: Toxicological bases for the setting of health-related air pollution standards. *Annu Rev Public Health* 21:309–333, 2000.

Lowrance WW: *Of Acceptable Risk.* Los Altos, CA, William Kaufmann, 1976.

McClain RM: Mechanistic considerations in the regulation and classification of chemical carcinogens, in Kotsonis F, Mackey M, Hjelle J (eds.): *Nutritional Toxicology.* New York, Raven Press, 1994, pp. 278–304.

McGregor DB, Rice JM, Venitt S: The use of short- and medium-term tests for carcinogens and data on genetic effects in carcinogenic hazard evaluation. Lyon, France, IARC, 1999.

Mendoza MA, Ponce RA, Ou YC, Faustman EM: p21(WAF1/CIP1) inhibits cell cycle progression but not G2/M-phase transition following methylmercury exposure. *Toxicol Appl Pharmacol* 178(2):117–125, 2002.

Moggs JG, Tinwell H, Spurway T, et al.: Phenotypic anchoring of gene expression changes during estrogen-induced uterine growth. *Environ Health Perspect* 112(16):1589–1606, 2004.

Moolgavkar SH, Luebeck G: Two-event model for carcinogenesis: Biological, mathematical, and statistical considerations. *Risk Anal* 10:323–341, 1990.

Moore JA, Daston GP, Faustman EM: An evaluative process for assessing human reproductive and developmental toxicity of agents. *Reprod Toxicol* 9:61–95, 1995.

Morgan GM: Risk analysis and management. *Sci Am* 269:32–41, 1993.

NAS: *Health Risks from Dioxin and Related Compounds: Evaluation of the EPA Reassessment.* Washington, DC, National Academies Press, 2006.

National Toxicology Program: 11th Report on Carcinogens. US Department of Human and Health Services, 2005. http://ntp.niehs.nih.gov/index.cfm?objectid=32BA9724-F1F6-975E-7FCE50709CB4C932

Nature Biotechnology Editorial: Making the most of microarrays. *Nat Biotechnol* 24(10 Suppl):1039, 2006.

Neal N, Malmfors T, Slovic P: Intuitive toxicology: Expert and lay judgments of chemical risks. *Toxicol Pathol* 22:198–201, 1994.

Nebert DW, Duffy JJ: How knockout mouse lines will be used to study the role of drug-metabolizing enzymes and their receptors during reproduction, development, and environmental toxicity, cancer and oxidative stress. *Biochem Pharmacol* 53:249–254, 1997.

Neumann DA, Olinn SS: Urinary bladder carcinogenesis: A working group approach to risk assessment. *Food Chem Toxicol* 33:701–704, 1995.

NIEHS: *Corrositex: An in Vitro Test Method for Assessing Dermal Corrosivity Potential of Chemicals.* Washington, DC, ICCVAM: 33109–33111, 1999a.

NIEHS: *The Murine Local Lymph Node Assay: A Test Method for Assessing the Allergic Contact Dermatitis Potential of Chemicals/Compounds.* Washington, DC, ICCVAM: 14006–14007, 1999b.

NRC: *Risk Assessment in the Federal Government: Managing the Process.* Washington, DC: National Academy Press, 1983.

NRC: *Biological Markers in Pulmonary Toxicology.* Washington, DC: National Academy Press, 1989a.

NRC: *Biological Markers in Reproductive Toxicology.* Washington, DC: National Academy Press, 1989b.

NRC: *Biological Markers in Immunotoxicology.* Washington, DC: National Academy Press, 1992a.

NRC: *Environmental Neurotoxicology.* Washington, DC: National Academy Press, 1992b.

NRC: *Science and Judgement in Risk Assessment.* Washington, DC: National Academy Press, 1994.

NRC: *Understanding Risk.* Washington, DC: National Academy Press, 1996.

NRC: *Scientific Frontiers in Developmental Toxicology and Risk Assessment.* Washington, DC: National Research Council, 2000.

Oberdorster G: Lung particle overload: Implications for occupational exposure to particles. *Regul Toxicol Pharmacol* 12:123–135, 1995.

Omenn GS: The genomic era: a crucial role for the public health sciences. *Environ Health Perspect* 108(5):A204–A205, 2000.

Omenn GS, Lampen A: Scientific and cost-effectiveness criteria in selecting batteries of short-term tests. *Mutat Res* 205:41–49, 1988.

Omenn GS, Omiecinski CJ, Eaton DE: Eco-genetics of chemical carcinogens, in Cantor C, Caskey C, Hood L (eds.): *Biotechnology and Human Genetic Predisposition to Disease.* New York: Wiley-Liss, 1990, pp. 81–93.

Omenn GS, Stuebbe S, Lave LB: Predictions of rodent carcinogenicity testing results: Interpretation in light of the Lave-Omenn value-of-information model. *Mol Carcinogen* 14:37–45, 1995.

Patterson TA, Lobenhofer EK, Fulmer-Smentek SB, *et al.*: Performance comparison of one-color and two-color platforms within the MicroArray Quality Control (MAQC) project. *Nat Biotechnol* 24(9):1140–1150, 2006.

Perera F, Weinstein IB: Molecular epidimiology: recent advances and future directions (review). *Carcinogenesis* 21:517–524, 2000.

Renwick AG: Safety factors and the establishment of acceptable daily intakes. *Food Addit Contam* 8:135–150, 1991.

Renwick AG: Toxicokinetics, in Ballantyne B, Marrs T, Syversen T (eds.): *General And Applied Toxicology.* New York: Grove's Dictionaries, 1999, pp. 67–95.

Renwick AG, Lazarus NR: Human variability and noncancer risk assessment—An analysis of the default uncertainty factor. *Regul Toxicol Pharmacol* 27:3–20, 1998.

Rice JM, Baan RA, Blettner M: Rodent tumors of urinary bladder, renal cortex, and thyroid gland. IARC Monographs: Evaluations of carcinogenic risk to humans. *Toxicol Sci* 49(166–171), 1999.

Risk Commission: *The Presidential/Congressional Commission on Risk Assessment and Risk Management.* Washington, DC: Government Printing Office, 1997.

Rodericks JV, Rudenko I, Starr TB, Turnbull D: Risk Assessment, in Sipes I, McQueen C, Gandolfi A (eds.): *Comprehensive Toxicology.* Oxford, UK: Pergamon, Elsevier Sciences, 1997, pp. 315–338.

Roe D, Pease W, Florini K, Silbergeld E: *Toxic Ignorance.* Washington, DC: Environmental Defense Fund, 1997.

Sandman PM: *Responding to Community Outrage: Strategies for Effective Risk Communication.* Fairfax, VA: American industrial Hygiene Association, 1993.

Schardein JL, Scialli AR: The legislation of toxicologic safety factors: the food quality protection act with chlorpyrifos as a test case. *Reprod Toxicol Rev* 13:1–14, 1999.

Schwetz BA: in vitro approaches in developmental toxicity. *Reprod Toxicol* 7:125–127, 1993.

Sette WF: Pesticide assessment guidelines, Subdivision D, Hazard evaluation, Human and Domestic Animals, Addendum 10 Neurotoxicity Series 81, 82 and 83 PB91-154617. Washington, DC: National technical information services, 1991.

Shelby MD, Bishop JB, Mason JM, Tindall KR: Fertility, reproduction and genetic disease: Studies on the mutagenic effects of environmental agents on mammalian germ cells. *Environ Health Perspect* 200:283–291, 1993.

Shuey DL, Lau C, Logsdon TR: Biologically based dose–response modeling in developmental toxicology: Biochemical and cellular sequelae of 5-fluorouracil exposure in the developing rat. *Toxicol Appl Pharmacol* 126:129–144, 1994.

Silverman KC, Naumann BD, Holder DJ: Establishing data-derived adjustment factors from published pharmaceutical clinical trial data. *Hum Ecol Risk Assess* 5:1059–1089, 1999.

Simon R, Wang SJ: Use of genomic signatures in therapeutics development in oncology and other diseases. *Pharmacogenomics J* 6(3):166–173, 2006.

Slovic P, Baruch F, Lichtenstein S: Rating the risks. *Environ* 21:1–20, 36–39, 1979.

Slovic P: Risk perception, in Travis C (ed.): *Carcinogen Risk Assessment.* New York, Plenum Press, 1988, pp. 171–192.

Slovic P, Peters E, Finucane ML, Macgregor DG: Affect, risk, and decision making. *Health Psychol* 24(4 Suppl):S35–S40, 2005.

Stevens JT: Risk assessment of pesticides, in Williams P, Hottendorf G (eds.): *Comprehensive Toxicology.* Oxford, UK: Pergamon, Elsevier Sciences, 1997, pp. 17–26.

Tennant RW, Stasiewicz S, Mennear J: Genetically altered mouse models for identifying carcinogens, in McGregor DB, Rice JM, Venitt S (eds.): *The Use of Short- and Medium-Term Tests for Carcinogens and Data on Genetic Effects in Carcinogenic Hazard Evaluation.* Lyon, France: IARC Scientific Publications, 1999, Vol. 146, pp. 123–150.

Toscano WA, Oehlke KP: Systems biology: New approaches to old environmental health problems. *Int J Environ Res Public Health* 2(1):4–9, 2005.

Van den Berg M, Birnbaum L, Bosveld ATC: Toxic equivalency factors (TEFs) for PCBs, PCDDs, PCDFs for humans and wildlife. *Environ Health Perspect* 106:775–792, 1998.

Van den Berg M, Birnbaum LS, Denison M, *et al.*: The 2005 World Health Organization reevaluation of human and mammalian toxic equivalency factors for dioxins and dioxin-like compounds. *Toxicol Sci* 93(2):223–241, 2006.

Weller E, Long N, Smith A: Dose–rate effects of ethylene oxide exposure on developmental toxicity. *Toxicol Sci* 50:259–270, 1999.

Whittaker SG, Faustman EM: *In Vitro Assays for Developmental Toxicity.* New York: Raven Press, 1994.

World Health Organization: Principles in governing consumer safety in relation to pesticide residues. WHO tech rep ser 240, 1962.

World Health Organization: IPCS/OECD Joint Project on Harmonization of Chemical Hazards, 2000.

World Health Organization: Principles for modeling dose–response for the risk assessment of chemicals, 2004.

World Health Organization: Chemical-specific adjustment factors for interspecies differences and human variability: Guidance document for use of data in dose/concentration-response assess, 2005. http://whqlibdoc.who.int/publications/2005/9241546786_eng.pdf, 6/19/06

Yu X, Griffith WC, Hanspers K, *et al.*: A system based approach to interpret dose and time-dependent microarray data: Quantitative integration of GO ontology analysis for risk assessment. *Toxicol Sci*, 92(2): 560–77, 2006.

Zhao Q, Dourson M, Gadagbui B: A review of the reference dose for chlorpyrifos. *Regul Toxicol Pharmacol* 44(2):111–124, 2006.

UNIT 2

DISPOSITION OF TOXICANTS

CHAPTER 5

ABSORPTION, DISTRIBUTION, AND EXCRETION OF TOXICANTS

Lois D. Lehman-McKeeman

INTRODUCTION

The disposition of a chemical or *xenobiotic* is defined as the composite actions of its *absorption*, *distribution*, *biotransformation*, and *elimination*. This chapter will focus on the contribution of absorption, distribution, and elimination to xenobiotic toxicity, whereas Chap. 6 is dedicated to biotransformation. The quantitative characterization of xenobiotic disposition is termed *pharmacokinetics* or *toxicokinetics* and is reviewed in Chap. 7.

The various factors and organs involved in affecting disposition of a toxicant are depicted in Fig. 5-1. The complexity of this diagram is intended to illustrate that, although they will be discussed separately, all processes related to disposition are likely to occur simultaneously. Fundamentally, the disposition of any compound is a major contributor to its potential for toxicity. Specifically, as discussed previously (see Chaps. 2 and 3), the toxicity of a substance is directly dependent on the dose, where "dose" is defined as the amount that ultimately reaches the site or sites of action (tissue, cell, or molecular target). Therefore, because the disposition of a chemical determines its concentration at the site of action, the concerted action of absorption, distribution, and elimination dictates the potential for adverse events to occur.

The skin, lungs, and alimentary canal are the main barriers that separate higher organisms from an environment containing a large number of chemicals. Toxicants must cross one or several of these incomplete barriers to exert deleterious effects, and only chemicals that are caustic and corrosive (acids, bases, salts, oxidizers), which act directly at the point of contact, are exceptions to this generalization. A chemical absorbed into the bloodstream or lymphatics through any of the major barriers is distributed, at least to some extent, throughout the body, including the site where it produces damage. This site is called the *target organ* or *target tissue*. A chemical may have one or several target organs, and, in turn, several chemicals may have the same target organ or organs. However, target organ concentration is not the only factor that can influence the susceptibility of organs to toxicants, and the organ or tissue with the highest concentration of a toxicant is not necessarily the site where toxicity is observed. A classical example of this distinction is dichlorodiphenyltrichloroethane (DDT), a chlorinated hydrocarbon insecticide that achieves high concentrations in fat depots but is not toxic to that tissue.

Poor absorption of a toxicant, resulting from a low amount absorbed or a low rate of absorption, limits or prevents toxicity because a chemical may never attain a sufficiently high concentration at a potential site of action to cause toxicity. Similarly, if a chemical is well absorbed but rapidly biotransformed or eliminated from an organism, it is less likely to be toxic because the rapid excretion prevents it from reaching a sufficiently high concentration at a potential site of action to cause toxicity. These are examples of how the disposition of toxicants contributes to the fundamental concept (see Chap. 1) that the "dose makes the poison."

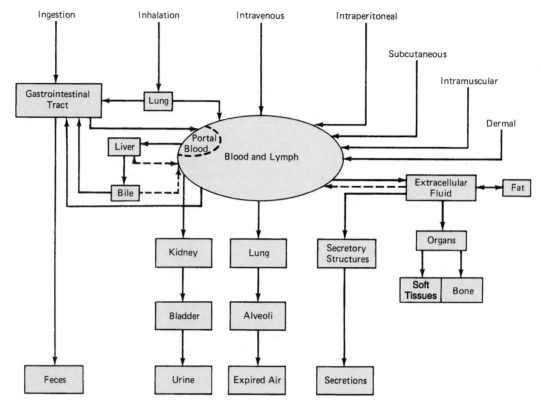

Figure 5-1. *Summary of the disposition of toxicants as determined by absorption, distribution, and excretion in the body.*

Collectively, all the processes comprising xenobiotic disposition are interrelated and influence each other. The integrated relationship of these processes is illustrated in Fig. 5-1. In this chapter, the qualitative aspects of absorption, distribution, and excretion are presented with emphasis on the functional features and molecular determinants of these processes. As all these processes involve passage across biological membranes, we begin with a discussion of this important and ubiquitous barrier.

CELL MEMBRANES

Toxicants usually pass through a number of cells, such as the stratified epithelium of the skin, the thin cell layers of the lungs or the gastrointestinal (GI) tract, capillary endothelium, and ultimately the cells of the target organ. The plasma membranes surrounding all these cells are remarkably similar. The basic unit of the cell membrane is a phospholipid bilayer composed primarily of phosphatidylcholine and phosphatidylethanolamine. Phospholipids are amphiphilic, consisting of a hydrophilic polar head and a hydrophobic lipid tail. In membranes, polar head groups are oriented toward the outer and inner surfaces of the membrane, whereas the hydrophobic tails are oriented inward and face each other to form a continuous hydrophobic inner space. The thickness of the cell membrane is about 7–9 nm. Numerous proteins are inserted or embedded in the bilayer, and some *transmembrane* proteins traverse the entire lipid bilayer, functioning as important biological receptors or allowing the formation of aqueous pores and ion channels (Fig. 5-2). Some cell membranes (eukaryotic) have an outer coat or glycocalyx consisting of glycoproteins and glycolipids. The fatty acids of the membrane do not have a rigid crystalline structure but are semifluid

at physiologic temperatures. The fluid character of membranes is determined largely by the structure and relative abundance of unsaturated fatty acids. The more unsaturated fatty acids the membranes contain, the more fluid-like they are, facilitating more rapid active or passive transport.

Toxicants cross membranes either by passive processes in which the cell expends no energy or by mechanisms in which the cell provides energy to translocate the toxicant across its membrane.

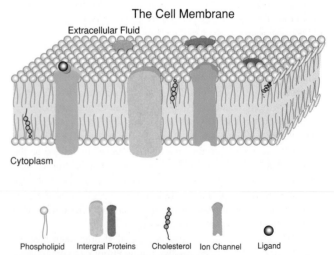

Figure 5-2. *Schematic model of a biological membrane. (www.bioeng. auckland.ac.nz/images/database/bioinformatics/cell_membrane/gif; with permission).*

Passive Transport

Simple Diffusion   Most toxicants cross membranes by simple diffusion, following the principles of Fick's law which establishes that chemicals traverse from regions of higher concentration to regions of lower concentration without any energy expenditure. Small hydrophilic molecules (up to about 600 Da) permeate membranes through aqueous pores (Benz *et al.*, 1980), in a process termed paracellular diffusion, whereas hydrophobic molecules diffuse across the lipid domain of membranes (transcellular diffusion). The smaller a hydrophilic molecule is, the more readily it traverses membranes by simple diffusion through aqueous pores. Consequently, a small, water-soluble compound such as ethanol is rapidly absorbed into the blood from the GI tract and is distributed just as rapidly throughout the body by simple diffusion from blood into all tissues.

Many toxicants are larger organic molecules with differing degrees of lipid solubility. For such compounds, the rate of transport across membranes correlates with lipid solubility, which is frequently expressed as octanol/water partition coefficients of the uncharged molecules, or log *P* as listed in Table 5-1. The log *P* is an extremely informative physicochemical parameter relative to assessing potential membrane permeability, with positive values associated with high lipid solubility. Thus, the amino acids such as glycine are water soluble and have a negative log *P*, whereas the environmental contaminants DDT and TCDD are very lipid soluble and have a high, positive log *P*.

Many chemicals are weak organic acids or bases which in solution are ionized according to Arrhenius' theory. The ionized form usually has low lipid solubility and thus does not permeate readily through the lipid domain of a membrane. There may be some transport of organic anions and cations (depending on their molecular weight) through the aqueous pores, but this is a slow and inefficient process. In contrast, the nonionized form of weak organic acids and bases is to some extent lipid soluble, resulting in diffusion across the lipid domain of a membrane. The rate of transport of the nonionized form is proportional to its lipid solubility. The molar ratio of ionized to nonionized molecules of a weak organic acid or base in solution depends on the ionization constant. The ionization constant provides a measure for the weakness of organic acids and bases. The pH at which a weak organic acid or base is 50% ionized is called its pK_a or pK_b. Like pH, both pK_a and pK_b are defined as the negative logarithm of the ionization constant of a weak organic acid or base. With the equation $pK_a = 14 - pK_b$, pK_a can also be calculated for weak organic bases. An organic acid with a low pK_a is relatively a strong acid, and one with a high pK_a is a weak acid. The opposite is true for bases. The numerical value of pK_a does not indicate whether a chemical is an organic acid or a base. Knowledge of the chemical structure is required to distinguish between organic acids and bases.

The degree of ionization of a chemical depends on its pK_a and on the pH of the solution. The relationship between pK_a and pH is described by the Henderson–Hasselbalch equations.

$$\text{For acids: } pK_a - pH = \log \frac{[\text{nonionized}]}{[\text{ionized}]}$$

$$\text{For bases: } pK_a - pH = \log \frac{[\text{ionized}]}{[\text{nonionized}]}$$

The effect of pH on the degree of ionization of an organic acid (benzoic acid) and an organic base (aniline) is shown in Fig. 5-3. According to the Brönsted–Lowry acid–base theory, an acid is a proton (H^+) donor and a base is a proton acceptor. Thus, the ionized and nonionized forms of an organic acid represent an acid–base pair, with the nonionized moiety being the acid and the ionized moiety being the base. At a low pH, a weak organic acid such as benzoic acid is largely nonionized. At pH 4, exactly 50% of benzoic acid is ionized and 50% is nonionized because this is the pK_a of the compound. As the pH increases, more and more protons are neutralized by hydroxyl groups, and benzoic acid continues to dissociate until almost all of it is in the ionized form. For an organic

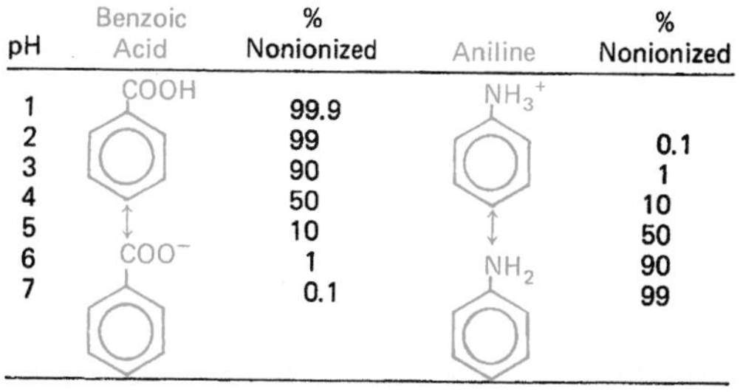

Table 5-1
Octanol/Water Partition Coefficients (*P*) of Different Molecules Expressed as log P

COMPOUND	LOG *P*
Paraquat	Charged molecule
Sulfobromophthalein	Charged molecule
Cephalosporin C	−4.72
Cystine	−4.45
Glycine	−3.21
Glutathione	−3.05
Gluconic acid	−2.89
Cysteine	−2.35
Glucose	−2.21
Edetic acid	−1.93
Ethylene glycol	−1.37
Lead acetate	−0.63
Ouabain	−0.35
p-Aminohippuric acid	−0.25
Dimercaprol	0.18
Scopolamine	0.30
Sarin	0.45
Aspirin	1.02
Colchicine	1.19
Atropine	1.32
Benzoic acid	1.88
Benzene	2.14
Salicylic acid	2.19
Digoxin	2.27
Methyl salicylate	2.34
2,4-D	2.73
Warfarin	2.89
Digitoxin	3.05
Parathion	3.47
DDT	6.76
TCDD	7.05

pH	Benzoic Acid	% Nonionized	Aniline	% Nonionized
1	COOH	99.9	NH₃⁺	
2		99		0.1
3		90		1
4		50		10
5		10		50
6	COO⁻	1	NH₂	90
7		0.1		99

Figure 5-3. Effect of pH on the ionization of benzoic acid (pK_a 4) and aniline ($pK_a = 5$).

base such as aniline, the inverse is true. At a low pH, when protons are abundant, almost all of aniline is protonated, i.e., ionized. This form of aniline is an acid because it can donate protons. As the pH increases, ions from aniline continue to dissociate until almost all the aniline is in the nonionized form, which is the aniline base. As transmembrane passage is largely restricted to the nonionized form, benzoic acid is more readily translocated through a membrane from an acidic environment, whereas more aniline is transferred from an alkaline environment.

Filtration   When water flows in bulk across a porous membrane, any solute small enough to pass through the pores flows with it. Passage through these channels is called *filtration*, as it involves bulk flow of water caused by hydrostatic or osmotic force. One of the main differences between various membranes is the size of these channels. In renal glomeruli, a primary site of filtration, these pores are relatively large (about 70 nm) allowing molecules smaller than albumin (approximately 60 kDa) to pass through. In contrast, there are no aqueous pores at cellular tight junctions, and channels in most cells are much smaller (3–6 Å), thereby only permitting substantial passage of molecules with molecular weights of no more than a few hundred daltons (Schanker, 1962; Lin, 2006).

Special Transport

There are numerous compounds whose movement across membranes cannot be explained by simple diffusion or filtration. Some compounds are too large to pass through aqueous pores or too insoluble in lipids to diffuse across the lipid domains of membranes. Nevertheless, they are often transported very rapidly across membranes, even against concentration gradients. To explain these phenomena, specialized transport systems have been identified. These systems are responsible for the transport (both influx and efflux) across cell membranes of many nutrients, such as sugars and amino and nucleic acids, along with some foreign compounds. Based on the sequencing of the human genome, there are at least 500 genes whose putative function involves membrane transport (Venter *et al.*, 2001). However, not all of these genes contribute to the disposition of toxicants. Throughout this chapter, transporters known to contribute to the disposition and subsequent effects of xenobiotics will be emphasized. Importantly, the role of xenobiotic transporters in chemical disposition is an emerging research field, and new information regarding their function, molecular regulation, and genetic polymorphisms is likely to modify traditional concepts in toxicology.

Active Transport   Active transport is characterized by: (1) movement of chemicals against electrochemical or concentration gradients, (2) saturability at high substrate concentrations, (3) selectivity for certain structural features of chemicals, (4) competitive inhibition by chemical cogeners or compounds that are carried by the same transporter, and (5) requirement for expenditure of energy, so that metabolic inhibitors block the transport process.

Substances actively transported across cell membranes presumably form a complex with a membrane-bound macromolecular carrier on one side of the membrane. The complex subsequently traverses to the other side of the membrane, where the substance is released. Afterward, the carrier returns to the original surface to repeat the transport cycle.

Xenobiotic Transporters   Significant advances in identifying and understanding the carrier-mediated transport systems for xenobiotics have been made in the recent years. In total, it is estimated that at least 5% of all human genes are transporter related, indicative of the importance of the transport function in normal biological and toxicological outcomes (Hediger *et al.*, 2004). Transporters mediate the influx (uptake) or efflux of xenobiotics and can be divided into two categories, determined by whether they mediate active or facilitated transfer of compounds. The first active, energy-dependent xenobiotic transporter identified was a phosphoglycoprotein overexpressed in tumor cells that showed resistance to anticancer drugs. The gene conferred multidrug resistance (MDR) to the cells, and was also called P-glycoprotein (P-gp). This transporter functions as an efflux pump, which in cancerous cells, exudes cytotoxic drugs out of the tumor cells, and thus contributes to their resistance (Ambudkar *et al.*, 1999). In humans, the major form of P-gp involved in xenobiotic transport is a single protein (MDR1), whereas in rodents there are two drug-transporting P-gp homologs identified as Mdr1a and Mdr1b. There is an additional member of the MDR family (Mdr2) that is involved in phospholipid transport but does not play an important role in xenobiotic disposition. Similarly, the bile salt export pump (BSEP) functions specifically to transport bile acids.

P-gp was the first member of a large superfamily of transport proteins known as ATP-binding cassette (ABC) transporters. There are now seven subfamilies of ABC transporters identified, with 48 genes in humans (Dean *et al.*, 2001). The second important ABC transport subfamily is the multiresistant drug protein (MRP) family for which MRP1 was also originally isolated from multidrug resistant cells (see Box 5-1). Members of this family excrete chemicals from cells, and MRP2 and MRP3 are particularly important in the efflux of xenobiotic metabolites, particularly those conjugated with UDP-glucuronic acid or glutathione. Breast cancer resistance protein (BCRP), which was originally isolated from a breast cancer cell line, is expressed in normal and malignant tissue and appears to play a role in the efflux transport of numerous endogenous and xenobiotic sulfate conjugates (Mao and Unadkat, 2005).

ABC transporters exhibit all the characteristics of the active transport outlined above, and most notably, they require the expenditure of energy to function. For most ABC transporters, the binding and hydrolysis of ATP provides the energy required to move their substrates across membranes. The typical structure of most ABC transporters consists of two types of structural domains including hydrophobic membrane spanning domain (MSD) and the hydrophilic, intracellular nucleotide binding domain (NBD) where ATP binds and is hydrolyzed (Fig. 5-4). The typical structural organization of the ABC transporter, as exemplified by P-gp, is a tandem repeat of two domains (1 MSD followed by 1 NBD). The two repeated halves are joined by a polypeptide linker sequence. MRPs are distinguished from P-gp in that they comprise five domains, with an extra MSD that comprises five transmembrane segments and an extracytosolic amino terminus, whereas BCRP is a "half-transporter" that comprises a single MSD with six transmembrane segments preceded by a single NBD. Recent evidence suggests that BCRP forms a homodimer or a homotetramer to function as an efflux pump (Leslie *et al.*, 2005). These differences in structure account for differences in molecular weight (approximately 170, 190, and 70 kDa for P-gp, MRP1, and BCRP, respectively), but there remains considerable overlap in many of the xenobiotics that are transported by these proteins.

Box 5-1
Major ABC Transporters Involved in Xenobiotic Disposition

ABBREVIATION	NAME	GENE SYMBOL	FUNCTION
MDR1/P-gp	Multidrug resistant protein/P-glycoprotein	*ABCB1*	Efflux from gut, brain, and placenta; biliary excretion
MDR2	Multidrug resistant protein 2	*ABCB4*	Phospholipid transport
BSEP	Bile salt export pump	*ABCB11*	Bile salt transport
MRP1	Multidrug resistance associated protein 1	*ABCC1*	Multidrug resistance in many tissues
MRP2	Multidrug resistance associated protein 2	*ABCC2*	Organic anion efflux, glucuronide, and glutathione conjugates
MRP3	Multidrug resistance associated protein 3	*ABCC3*	Organic anion efflux, glucuronide, and glutathione conjugates
MRP4	Multidrug resistance associated protein 4	*ABCC4*	Nucleoside transport
MRP5	Multidrug resistance associated protein 5	*ABCC5*	Nucleoside transport
MRP6	Multidrug resistance associated protein 6	*ABCC6*	Unknown
BCRP	Breast cancer resistance protein	*ABCG2*	Organic anion efflux, mainly sulfate conjugates

NOTE: Gene nomenclature denotes those genes identified in humans.

Members of the ABC transport family are expressed constitutively in many cells, and collectively they play important roles in absorption from the GI tract and elimination into bile or into urine for a diverse array of xenobiotics. They are also critical to maintaining the barrier function of numerous tissues sites including the blood–brain barrier, the blood–testis barrier, and the maternal–fetal barrier or placenta. Hence, they play a central role in the disposition and toxicity of xenobiotics. Their function in absorption, distribution, and excretion will be discussed throughout the remaining sections of this chapter.

The second major type of xenobiotic transporters is that which function predominantly as facilitative transporters. A major family of such transporters is known as solute carriers (SLCs), for which there are now 43 gene families known. Many of the nearly 300 genes comprising the 43 distinct SLC families play important roles in the disposition of endogenous compounds, including glucose, neurotransmitters, nucleotides, essential metals, and peptides. Additionally, there are several families that are vital to xenobiotic disposition, regulating the movement of many diverse organic anions and cations across cell membranes (Hediger *et al.*, 2004).

Genes in families SLC21 and SLC22 are extremely important in xenobiotic disposition (see Box 5-2). The organic-anion transporting peptides (OATP, SLCO family) are important membrane transport proteins that mediate the sodium-independent transport of a wide range of compounds, including organic acids, bases, and neutral compounds. Although they are largely regarded as influx pumps, solutes can move bidirectionally, and these proteins appear to be especially important in the hepatic uptake of xenobiotics. In human liver, three OATPs (OATP1B1, OATP1B3, and OATP2B1) have been identified, whereas the major Oatps in rat liver are Oatp1a1, Oatp1a4, and Oatp1b2. For Oatps, the mechanism of transport is anion exchange such that the cellular influx of an organic compound is thought to be coupled to the efflux of bicarbonate, glutathione, or glutathione conjugates.

The organic-anion transporter (OAT; SLC22) family is particularly important in the renal uptake of anions, and four human proteins (OAT1, 2, 3, and 4) have been identified in the kidney, whereas Oat1 and Oat3 are the major transporters identified in the rat kidney. The organic-cation transporter (OCT; also SLC22) family is important in both the renal and hepatic uptake of xenobiotics. In this family, OCT1 is expressed in human liver, whereas only OCT2 has been detected in human kidney. In rats, Oct1 is found in liver, whereas both Oct1 and Oct2 are expressed in rat kidney. Novel organic-cation transporters (OCTNs; also SLC22) have also been identified which transport exogenous cations along with important endogenous compounds such as carnitine. OATs transport substrates against an electrochemical gradient in exchange for intracellular dicarboxylates, such as α-ketoglutarate, whereas the driving force for Oct-mediated transport is the electrochemical gradient of the transported cation, typical of faciliated diffusion (described below). Peptide transporters (PEPT1 and PEPT2) are responsible for the transport of di- and tri-peptides as well as drugs and toxicants such as the β-lactam antibiotics.

Facilitated Diffusion Facilitated diffusion applies to carrier-mediated transport that exhibits the properties of active transport except that the substrate is not moved against an electrochemical or concentration gradient, and the transport process does not require the input of energy; that is, metabolic poisons do not interfere with this transport. The transport of glucose from the GI tract across the basolateral membrane of the intestinal epithelium, from plasma into red blood cells, and from blood into the central nervous system (CNS) occurs by facilitated diffusion. As noted earlier, OCTs, which function in the uptake of organic cations particularly

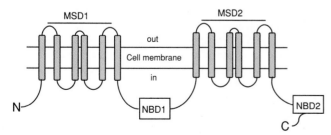

Figure 5-4. Diagrammatic representation of the structure of p-glycoprotein, illustrating the membrane spanning domains (MSD) and ATP-binding domains (NBD).

Box 5-2

Major Members of the Solute Carrier Transporters Involved in Xenobiotic Disposition

ABBREVIATION	NAME	GENE FAMILY	HUMAN PROTEINS	FUNCTION
OATP	Organic anion transporting polypeptide	*SLCO*	OATP1A2 OATP1B1 OATP1B3 OATP1C1 OATP2A1 OATP2B1 OATP3A1 OATP4A1 OATP4C1 OATP5A1 OATP6A1	Transport of organic anions, cations, and neutral compounds
OAT	Organic-anion transporter	*SLC22*	OAT1 OAT2 OAT3 OAT4 OAT5	Transport of organic anions, predominantly in kidney
OCT and OCTN	Organic-cation transporter	*SLC22*	OCT1 OCT2 OCT3 OCTN1 OCTN2	Transport of organic cations, predominantly in kidney OCTN2 specifically involved in carnitine transport
PepT	Peptide transporter	*SLC15*	PEPT1 PEPT2	Transport of di- and tripeptides, some xenobiotics

NOTE: Gene and protein members of the solute carrier families are compiled from Mizuno *et al.* (2003), Hagenbuch and Meier (2004), Sahi (2005), and Lin (2006).

in the liver and kidney, mediate cation movement by faciliated diffusion.

Additional Transport Processes Other forms of specialized transport have been proposed, but their overall importance is not as well established as that of active transport and facilitated diffusion. Phagocytosis and pinocytosis are proposed mechanisms for cell membranes flowing around and engulfing particles. This type of transfer has been shown to be important for the removal of particulate matter from the alveoli by phagocytes and from blood by the reticuloendothelial system of the liver and spleen.

ABSORPTION

The process by which toxicants cross body membranes and enter the bloodstream is referred to as *absorption*. There are no specific systems or pathways for the sole purpose of absorbing toxicants. Xenobiotics penetrate membranes during absorption by the same processes as do biologically essential substances such as oxygen, foodstuffs, and other nutrients. The main sites of absorption are the GI tract, lungs, and skin. However, absorption may also occur from other sites, such as the subcutis, peritoneum, or muscle, if a chemical is administered by special routes. Experimentalists and medical professionals often distinguish between parenteral and enteral administration of drugs and other xenobiotics. Enteral administration includes all routes pertaining to the alimentary canal (sublingual, oral, and rectal), whereas parenteral administration involves all other routes (intravenous, intraperitoneal, intramuscular, subcutaneous, etc.).

Absorption of Toxicants by the Gastrointestinal Tract

The GI tract is one of the most important sites where toxicants are absorbed. Many environmental toxicants enter the food chain and are absorbed together with food from the GI tract. This site of absorption is also particularly relevant to toxicologists because accidental ingestion is the most common route of unintentional exposure to a toxicant (especially for children) and intentional overdoses most frequently occur via the oral route.

The GI tract may be viewed as a tube traversing the body. Although it is within the body, its contents can be considered exterior to the body. Therefore, unless a noxious agent has caustic or irritating properties, poisons in the GI tract usually do not produce systemic injury to an individual until they are absorbed.

Absorption of toxicants can take place along the entire GI tract, even in the mouth and the rectum. Therefore, although the majority of drugs are given orally, drugs such as nitroglycerin are administered sublingually whereas others are administered as rectal suppositories. If a toxicant is an organic acid or base, it tends to be absorbed by simple diffusion in the part of the GI tract where it exists in its most lipid-soluble (nonionized) form. Because gastric juice is acidic (pH about 2) and the intestinal contents are nearly neutral, the lipid solubility of weak organic acids or bases can differ markedly in these two areas of the GI tract. One can determine by the Henderson–Hasselbalch equations the fraction of a toxicant that is in the nonionized (lipid-soluble) form and estimate the rate of absorption from the stomach or intestine. According to this equation, a weak organic acid is present mainly in the nonionized (lipid-soluble) form in the stomach and predominantly in the ionized form in the intestine. Therefore, weak organic acids are absorbed more readily from the stomach than from the intestine. In contrast, organic bases (except very weak organic bases) are likely to be ionized and not lipid soluble in the stomach, but are more likely to be in the nonionized form in the intestine, suggesting that the absorption of such compounds occurs predominantly in the intestine rather than in the stomach. However, the Henderson–Hasselbalch equations have to be interpreted with some qualifications because other factors—including the mass action law, surface area, and blood flow rate—have to be taken into consideration in examining the absorption of weak organic acids or bases. For example, only 1% of benzoic acid is present in the lipid-soluble form in the intestine. Therefore, one might conclude that the intestine has little capacity to absorb this organic acid. However, absorption is a dynamic process. The

blood keeps removing benzoic acid from the lamina propria of the intestine, and according to the mass action law, the equilibrium will always be maintained at 1% in the nonionized form, providing continuous availability of benzoic acid for absorption. Moreover, absorption by simple diffusion is also proportional to the surface area. The small intestine has a very large surface because the villi and microvilli increase the surface area approximately 600-fold, such that the overall capacity of the intestine for absorption of benzoic acid is quite large. Similar considerations are valid for the absorption of all weak organic acids from the intestine (Box 5-3).

The mammalian GI tract has numerous specialized transport systems (carrier-mediated) for the absorption of nutrients and electrolytes (Table 5-2). The absorption of some of these substances is complex and depends on a number of factors. The absorption of iron, for example, depends on the need for iron and takes place in two steps: Iron first enters the mucosal cells and then moves into the blood. The first step is relatively rapid, whereas the second is slow. Consequently, iron accumulates within the mucosal cells as a protein–iron complex termed *ferritin*. When the concentration of iron in blood drops below normal values, some iron is liberated from the mucosal stores of ferritin and transported into the blood. As a consequence, the absorption of more iron from the intestine is triggered to replenish these stores. Calcium is also absorbed by a two-step process: absorption from the lumen followed by exudation into the interstitial fluid. The first step is faster than the second, and therefore intracellular calcium rises in mucosal cells during absorption. Vitamin D is required for both steps of calcium transport.

Some xenobiotics are absorbed by the same specialized transport systems, thereby leading to potential competition or interaction. For example, 5-fluorouracil is absorbed by the pyrimidine transport system (Yuasa *et al.*, 1996), thallium utilizes the system that normally absorbs iron (Leopold *et al.*, 1969), lead can be absorbed by the calcium transporter (Fullmer *et al.*, 1992), and cobalt and manganese compete for the iron transport system (Flanagan *et al.*, 1980).

Numerous xenobiotic transporters are expressed in the GI tract where they function to increase or decrease absorption of xenobiotics (Fig. 5-5). Several proteins in the SLC families are expressed in the intestine where they are predominantly localized on the apical brush border membranes of the enterocytes and increase uptake from the lumen into the enterocytes. In humans OATP2B1, 3A1, and 4A1 have been identified, whereas in rodents Oatp1a5 is the predominant uptake transporter. OCTs, particularly OCT1 and 2, have also been identified in the human intestine. There are also peptide transporters (PEPT1) in the GI tract that mediate the transport of peptide-like drugs such as antibiotics, particularly those containing a β-lactam structure (Tsuji *et al.*, 1993; Dantzig *et al.*, 1994). Transepithelial absorption of dipeptides (e.g., glycylsarcosine) and β-lactam antibiotics at low concentrations occurs predominantly by active carrier-mediated mechanisms at both apical and basolateral membranes (Thwaites *et al.*, 1993).

The primary active efflux transporters such as P-gp, MRP2, and BCRP are also expressed on enterocyte brush border membranes where they function to excrete their subsrates into the lumen, thereby decreasing the net absorption of xenobiotics. MRP3 is also found in the intestine, but is localized to the basolateral membrane. P-gp expression in the intestine increases from the duodenum to colon, whereas MRP2 expression is highest in the duodenum and decreases to undetectable levels in the terminal ileum and colon, and BCRP is found throughout the small intestine and colon. There will be a net reduction in the absorption of chemicals that are substrates for these transporters, and this is a desirable outcome for toxic chemicals. For example, the dietary

Box 5-3

FOR WEAK ACIDS

$$pK_a - pH = \log \frac{[\text{nonionized}]}{[\text{ionized}]}$$

Benzoic acid $pK_a \approx 4$

Stomach pH ≈ 2

$$4 - 2 = \log \frac{[\text{nonionized}]}{[\text{ionized}]}$$

$$2 = \log \frac{[\text{nonionized}]}{[\text{ionized}]}$$

$$10^2 = \log \frac{[\text{nonionized}]}{[\text{ionized}]}$$

$$100 = \log \frac{[\text{nonionized}]}{[\text{ionized}]}$$

Ratio favors absorption

Intestine pH ≈ 6

$$4 - 6 = \log \frac{[\text{nonionized}]}{[\text{ionized}]}$$

$$-2 = \log \frac{[\text{nonionized}]}{[\text{ionized}]}$$

$$10^{-2} = \frac{[\text{nonionized}]}{[\text{ionized}]}$$

$$\frac{1}{100} = \frac{[\text{nonionized}]}{[\text{ionized}]}$$

FOR WEAK BASES

$$pK_a - pH = \log \frac{[\text{ionized}]}{[\text{nonionized}]}$$

Aniline $pK_a \approx 5$

Stomach pH ≈ 2

$$5 - 2 = \log \frac{[\text{ionized}]}{[\text{nonionized}]}$$

$$3 = \log \frac{[\text{ionized}]}{[\text{nonionized}]}$$

$$10^3 = \log \frac{[\text{ionized}]}{[\text{nonionized}]}$$

$$1000 = \log \frac{[\text{ionized}]}{[\text{nonionized}]}$$

Intestine pH ≈ 6

$$5 - 6 = \log \frac{[\text{ionized}]}{[\text{nonionized}]}$$

$$-1 = \log \frac{[\text{ionized}]}{[\text{nonionized}]}$$

$$10^{-1} = \frac{[\text{ionized}]}{[\text{nonionized}]}$$

$$\frac{1}{10} = \frac{[\text{ionized}]}{[\text{nonionized}]}$$

Ratio favors absorption

Table 5-2

Site Distribution of Specialized Transport Systems in the Small Intestine of Man and Animals

SUBSTRATES	UPPER	MIDDLE	LOWER	COLON
Sugar (glucose, galactose, etc.)	+ +	+ + +	+ +	0
Neutral amino acids	+ +	+ + +	+ +	0
Basic amino acids	+ +	+ +	+ +	?
Gamma globulin (newborn animals)	+	+ +	+ + +	?
Pyrimidines (thymine and uracil)	+	+	?	?
Triglycerides	+ +	+ +	+	?
Fatty acid absorption and conversion to triglyceride	+ + +	+ +	+	0
Bile salts	0	+	+ + +	
Vitamin B_{12}	0	+	+ + +	0
Na^+	+ + +	+ +	+ + +	+ + +
H^+ (and/or HCO_3^- secretion)	0	+	+ +	+ +
Ca^{2+}	+ + +	+ +	+	?
Fe^{2+}	+ + +	+ +	+	?
Cl^-	+ + +	+ +	+	0

SOURCE: Adapted from Wilson TH: *Mechanisms of Absorption.* Philadelphia: WB Saunders, 1962, pp. 40–68.

carcinogen, 2-amino-1-methyl-6-phenylimidazo(4,5-b)pyridine (PhIP), a heterocyclic amine produced during the cooking of meat, is a substrate for MRP2. Studies comparing the disposition of PhIP in wild-type and Mrp2-deficient rats showed that MRP is very important in limiting the oral absorption of this harmful compound (Dietrich *et al.*, 2001). However, whereas limiting absorption of toxicants and carcinogens is beneficial, these transporters can also function to limit the oral absorption of drugs. For example, the immunosuppressive drug cyclosporine and the chemotherapeutic anticancer drugs paclitaxel (taxol), colchicine, and vincristine are not readily absorbed from the GI tract because they are good substrates for P-gp.

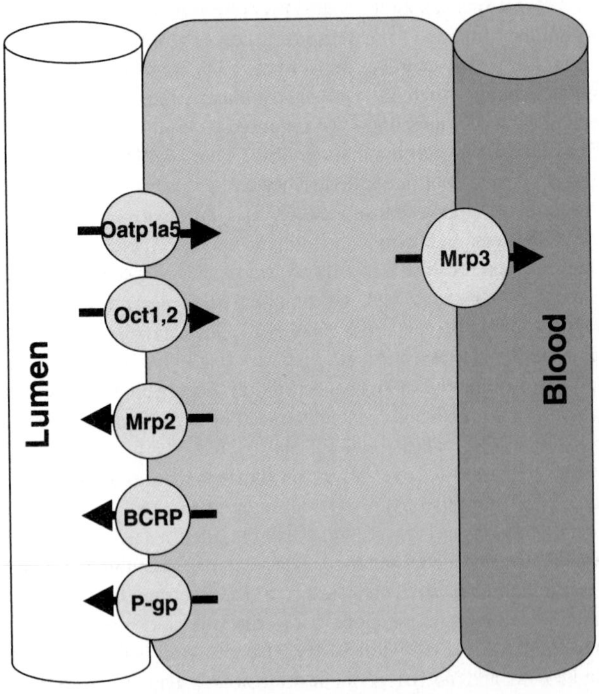

The number of toxicants actively absorbed by the GI tract is low; most enter the body by simple diffusion. Although lipid-soluble substances are absorbed by this process more rapidly and extensively than are water-soluble substances, the latter may also be absorbed to some degree. After oral ingestion, about 10% of lead, 4% of manganese, 1.5% of cadmium, and 1% of chromium salts are absorbed. If a compound is very toxic, even small amounts of absorbed material produce serious systemic effects. An organic compound that would not be expected to be absorbed on the basis of the pH-partition hypothesis is the fully ionized quaternary ammonium compound pralidoxime chloride (2-PAM; molecular weight 137), yet it is absorbed almost entirely from the GI tract. The mechanism by which some lipid-insoluble compounds are absorbed is not entirely clear. It appears that organic ions of low molecular weight (<200) can be transported across the mucosal barrier by paracellular transport, that is, passive penetration through aqueous pores at the tight junctions (Aungst and Shen, 1986), or by active transport as discussed above.

Particles and particulate matter can also be absorbed by the GI epithelium. In this case, particle size determines absorption and factors such as the lipid solubility or ionization characteristics are less important. For particles, size is inversely related to absorption such that absorption increases with decreasing particle diameter (Florence *et al.*, 1995). This explains why metallic mercury is relatively nontoxic when ingested orally and why powdered arsenic was found to be significantly more toxic than its coarse granular form (Schwartze, 1923). Emulsions of polystyrene latex particles 22 μm in diameter enter intestinal cells by pinocytosis, a process that is much more prominent in newborns than in adults (Williams and Beck, 1969), after which they are carried through the intestinal epithelium in intact vesicles and discharged into the interstices of the lamina propria. Absorption into gut-associated lymphoid tissue (such as Peyer's patches) and the mesenteric lymph supply play a key role in systemic absorption of particles (Jani *et al.*, 1990; Florence *et al.*, 1995).

There is recent interest in particles of very small diameter that may be used in a variety of chemical and biological processes. *Nanoparticles* or nanomaterials are typically less than 100 nm in

Figure 5-5. Schematic model showing the important xenobiotic transport systems present in the gastrointestinal tract. Oatp1a5 is expressed in rat intestine whereas in humans, OATP2B1, 3A1, 4A1 are found.

size, and numerous issues have been raised regarding the toxic potential of these entities. Although the absorption of large particles is typically limited, absorption of nanoparticles by the GI tract in rats is as high as 30% for particles that are 50 nm in diameter (Jani *et al.*, 1990), and nonionized particles showed higher absorption than those modified to possess an ionized surface (Florence *et al.*, 1995).

It is clear that the absorption of a toxicant from the GI tract depends on its physical properties, including lipid solubility and its dissolution rate. Although it is often generalized that an increase in lipid solubility increases the absorption of chemicals, an extremely lipid-soluble chemical is unlikely to dissolve in the aqueous fluids within the GI tract, and thus, absorption of a highly lipid soluble compound from the GI tract is likely to be very low (Houston *et al.*, 1974). Similarly, if the toxicant is a solid and is relatively insoluble in GI fluids, it will again have limited contact with the GI mucosa and its rate of absorption will be low.

In addition to the characteristics of the compounds themselves, there are numerous additional factors relating to the GI tract itself that influence the absorption of xenobiotics. These factors include pH, the presence of food, digestive enzymes, bile acids, and bacterial microflora in the GI tract, and the motility and permeability of the GI tract. Chemical resistance or lack of resistance to alteration by the acidic pH of the stomach, enzymes of the stomach or intestine, or the intestinal flora are extremely important. A toxicant may be hydrolyzed by stomach acid or biotransformed by enzymes in the GI tract or the microflora to new compounds with a toxicity greatly different from that of the parent compound. For example, snake venoms, which are proteinaceous, are much less toxic by the oral route relative to intravenous exposure because they are broken down by digestive enzymes of the GI tract. In direct contrast, a variety of nitroaromatic compounds are reduced by intestinal microflora to potentially toxic and carcinogenic aromatic amines. For example, 2,6-dinitrotoluene requires nitroreduction to 2,6-diaminotoluene in the GI tract to produce long-term adverse effects, and these effects including mutagenicity and carcinogenicity, are not seen in germ-free animals (Rickert *et al.*, 1984). Similarly, the nitroaromatic perfume, musk xylene, can inhibit the activity of cytochrome P450 enzymes in the liver only after it is reduced to an amine derivative by resident microflora in the GI tract and subsequently absorbed (Lehman-McKeeman *et al.*, 1997). It has also been shown that ingestion of well water with a high nitrate content produces methemoglobinemia much more frequently in infants than in adults. In this case, bacteria in the GI tract convert nitrate to nitrite, increasing the likelihood of methemoglobinemia (Mensinga *et al.*, 2003). Infants are more susceptible to methemoglobinemia because the higher pH of the neonatal GI tract is permissive for the growth of bacteria (such as *Escherichia coli*) that convert nitrate to nitrite. The contribution of bacteria in the GI tract to other aspects of xenobiotic disposition, particularly enterohepatic circulation, is discussed in greater detail later in this chapter.

Agents such as the chelator, ethylenediaminetetraacetic acid (EDTA), increase absorption of some toxicants by increasing intestinal permeability. An increase in permeability is thought to result from the chelation of calcium that is involved in the formation and maintenance of tight intercellular junctions (Ballard *et al.*, 1995) such that binding of calcium reduces the integrity of the cell junctions, allowing more paracellular absorption. Furthermore, simple diffusion is proportional not only to the surface area and the permeability but also to the residency time within various segments of the GI tract. Therefore, the rate of absorption of a toxicant remaining for longer periods in the intestine increases, whereas that with a shorter residency time decreases. Experiments have shown that the oral toxicity of some chemicals is increased by diluting the dose (Borowitz *et al.*, 1971). This phenomenon may be explained by more rapid stomach emptying induced by increased dosage volume, which in turn leads to greater absorption in the duodenum because of the larger surface area there. Furthermore, some agents used as laxatives alter absorption of xenobiotics by increasing intestinal motility (Levine, 1970), whereas agents used as antidiarrheals may increase absorption by slowing intestinal motility.

The amount of a chemical that enters the systemic circulation after oral administration depends on several factors. The amount absorbed into the cells of the GI tract is important, and transporters can influence this amount by affecting the uptake or efflux from the cells. Further, before a chemical enters the systemic circulation, it can be biotransformed by the cells in the GI tract or extracted by the liver and excreted into bile with or without prior biotransformation. This phenomenon of the removal of chemicals before entrance into the systemic circulation is referred to as *presystemic elimination* or *first-pass effect*. The lung can also contribute to the biotransformation or elimination of chemicals before their entrance into the systemic circulation, although its role is less well-defined than that of the intestine and the liver. Chemicals that have a high first-pass effect will appear to have a lower absorption because they are eliminated as quickly as they are absorbed. For toxicants, a high first-pass effect will serve to limit exposure and typically minimizes toxic potential.

A number of other factors have been shown to alter absorption. For example, although lead and many other heavy metal ions are not absorbed readily from the GI tract, EDTA and other chelators increase the lipid solubility and thus the absorption of complexed ions. Thus, it is important not to give a chelator orally when excess metal is still present in the GI tract after oral ingestion. Furthermore, metal ions can affect absorption of other ions. For example, cadmium decreases the absorption of zinc and copper, calcium decreases cadmium absorption, and magnesium decreases absorption of fluoride (Pfeiffer, 1977). Consumption of grapefruit juice can also influence GI absorption through the actions of naringin, a flavonoid, that inhibits intestinal cytochrome P450 3A activity (see Chap. 6) and alters the function of P-gp (Evans, 2000). Grapefruit juice increases the GI absorption of numerous pharmaceutical agents (such as calcium-channel blockers and cholesterol-lowering agents) and in some cases, this effect leads to toxic or adverse reactions resulting from increased exposure to the drugs.

Species differences in absorption across the GI tract are widely recognized. As one example, absorption of nadolol after intraperitoneal and oral dosing was compared across species by calculating the plasma area-under-the-curve (AUC) and was found to be essentially complete in dogs, substantially less in humans, and quite limited in rats (Table 5-3). Urinary and fecal excretion of nadolol support the bioavailability data, as the low oral absorption of nadolol in rats is consistent with the large amount of drug recovered in feces. However, excretory data further indicate that in addition to the nonabsorbed portion of this compound, biliary and possibly nonbiliary sources also contribute to the fecal excretion of this compound. Similar comparisons across species provide further evidence for species differences in the absorption of numerous compounds, indicating that nadolol is not an exceptional case (Calabrese, 1984).

The factors that contribute to species differences in absorption are not fully understood. Anatomical considerations are likely to contribute to species differences in intestinal absorption, and substantial functional differences exist between species. Because most

Table 5-3

Absorption and Excretion of Radioactivity in Rats, Dogs, and Man after Nadolol Dosages*

SPECIES	DOSE (mg/kg)	PERCENT OF DOSE EXCRETED			PERCENT OF DOSE ABSORBED
		ROUTE	URINE	FECES	
Rat	20	Po	11	84	18
	20	Ip	62	31	(100)
Dog	25	Po	76	28	102
	25	Ip	75	12	(100)
Man	2	Po	25	77	34
	2	Ip	73	23	(100)

*SOURCE: Modified from Dreyfus *et al.* (1978).

Table 5-4

pH of the Gastrointestinal Contents of Various Species*

SPECIES	pH				
	STOMACH	JEJUNUM	CECUM	COLON	FECES
Monkey	2.8	6.0	5.0	5.1	5.5
Dog	3.4	6.6	6.4	6.5	6.2
Rat	3.8	6.8	6.8	6.6	6.9
Rabbit	1.9	7.5	6.6	7.2	7.2

*SOURCE: Modified from Smith (1965).

xenobiotics are transported across the GI mucosa by passive diffusion, and because this transport is surface area- and site-dependent, it can be expected that these factors will be responsible for species differences in some instances. Furthermore, species differences in the pH along the GI tract exist (Table 5-4), varying by as much as 2 pH units. The magnitude of this diversity can translate into differences up to two orders of magnitude in the concentration of the nonionized versus ionized moiety of a weak organic acid or base available for absorption. In addition, the GI absorption is often higher in dogs compared to other species because paracellular absorption is thought to occur to a greater extent in dogs.

Another factor that may result in species-dependent absorption of xenobiotics is the presence and function of the GI microflora. Bacteria in the GI tract are highly abundant, with strict anaerobes (oxygen intolerant) being the most prevalant. More than 400 species of bacteria have been found in the GI tract. In general, the intestinal

Table 5-5

Number of Microbes and their Distribution along the Gastrointestinal Tract of Various Species*

SPECIES	STOMACH	JEJUNUM	COLON	FECES
Monkey	23	24	41	38
Dog	19	20	40	43
Rat	18	23	37	38
Rabbit	4	5	13	13
Man	2	4	10	—

*Expressed as $\log_{10}$ of viable counts.
SOURCE: Modified from Smith (1965) and Rowland *et al.* (1985).

microflora in animals is remarkably similar, although qualitative and quantitative differences have been reported (Rowland *et al.*, 1985). For example, rabbit and humans are distinguished from other species in that the number of microbes found in the upper regions of the GI tract is relatively low (Table 5-5). The lower pH of the stomach in rabbits and humans contributes to the lower number of microbes found in this region. Importantly, bacterial metabolism is a prerequisite for absorption of some xenobiotics, and species differences in absorption may result from differences in the type and number of microbes in the GI tract.

Absorption of Toxicants by the Lungs

Toxic responses to chemicals can occur from absorption following inhalation exposure. A frequent cause of death from poisoning—carbon monoxide—and an important occupational disease—silicosis—both result from absorption or deposition of airborne poisons in the lungs.

A major group of toxicants that are absorbed by the lungs are gases (e.g., carbon monoxide, nitrogen dioxide, and sulfur dioxide), vapors of volatile or volatilizable liquids (e.g., benzene and carbon tetrachloride), and aerosols. Because the absorption of inhaled gases and vapor differs from that of aerosols, aerosols are discussed separately below. However, the absorption of gases and vapors is governed by the same principles, and therefore the word *gas* is used to represent both in this section.

Gases and Vapors   The absorption of inhaled gases takes place mainly in the lungs. However, when inhaled, gases first pass through the nose, filtering through delicately scrolled, simple epithelial-lined turbinates, which serve to increase the surface area of exposure. Because the mucosa of the nose is covered by a film of fluid, gas molecules can be retained by the nose and not reach the lungs if they are very water soluble or react with cell surface components. Therefore, the nose acts as a "scrubber" for water-soluble gases and highly reactive gases, partially protecting the lungs from potentially injurious insults. Although these actions may serve to reduce systemic exposure or to protect the lungs, they also increase the risk that the nose could be adversely affected. Such is the case with formaldehyde (Kerns *et al.*, 1983) and vinyl acetate (Bogdanffy *et al.*, 1999), which cause tumors of the nasal turbinates in rats.

Absorption of gases in the lungs differs from intestinal and percutaneous absorption of compounds in that the dissociation of acids and bases and the lipid solubility of molecules are less important factors in pulmonary absorption because diffusion through cell membranes is not rate-limiting in the pulmonary absorption of gases. There are at least three reasons for this. First, ionized molecules are of very low volatility, so that they do not achieve significant concentrations in normal ambient air. Second, the epithelial cells lining the alveoli—that is, type I pneumocytes—are very thin and the capillaries are in close contact with the pneumocytes, so that the distance for a chemical to diffuse is very short. Third, chemicals absorbed by the lungs are removed rapidly by the blood, and blood moves very quickly through the extensive capillary network in the lungs.

When a gas is inhaled into the lungs, gas molecules diffuse from the alveolar space into the blood and then dissolve. Except for some gases with a special affinity for certain body components (e.g., the binding of carbon monoxide to hemoglobin), the uptake of a gas by a tissue usually involves the simple physical process of dissolving. The end result is that gas molecules partition between the two media: air and blood during the absorptive phase and blood and other tissues during the distributive phase. As the contact of the inspired gas with blood continues in the alveoli, more molecules dissolve in blood until gas molecules in blood are in equilibrium with gas molecules in the alveolar space. At equilibrium, the ratio of the concentration of chemical in the blood and chemical in the gas phase is constant. This solubility ratio is called the *blood-to-gas partition coefficient*, and it is unique for each gas. Note that whereas the ratio is constant, the concentrations achieved vary in accordance with Henry's law, which dictates that the amount of gas dissolved in a liquid is proportional to the partial pressure of the gas in the gas phase at any given concentration before or at saturation. Thus, the higher the inhaled concentration of a gas (i.e., the higher the partial pressure), the higher the gas concentration in blood, but the blood:gas ratio does not change unless saturation has occurred. When equilibrium is reached, the rate of transfer of gas molecules from the alveolar space to blood equals the rate of removal by blood from the alveolar space. For example, chloroform has a relatively high blood-to-gas partition coefficient (approximately 20), whereas ethylene has a low coefficient (0.14). By comparison, a smaller percentage of the total ethylene in the lungs is removed into the blood during each circulation because the low blood-to-gas partition coefficient dictates that blood is quickly saturated with this gas. Therefore, an increase in the respiratory rate or minute volume does not change the transfer of such a gas to blood. In contrast, an increase in the rate of blood flow increases the rate of uptake of a compound with a low solubility ratio because of more rapid removal from the site of equilibrium, that is, the alveolar membranes. It has been calculated that the time to equilibrate between the blood and the gas phase for a relatively insoluble gas is about 10–20 minutes.

A gas with a high blood-to-gas partition coefficient, such as chloroform, is readily transferred to blood during each respiratory cycle so that little if any remains in the alveoli just before the next inhalation. The more soluble a toxic agent is in blood, the more of it will be dissolved in blood by the time equilibrium is reached. Consequently, the time required to equilibrate with blood is much longer for a gas with a high blood-to-gas partition coefficient than for a gas with a low ratio. This has been calculated to take a minimum of 1 hour for compounds with a high solubility ratio, although it may take even longer if the gas also has high tissue affinity (i.e., high fat solubility). With highly soluble gases, the principal factor limiting the rate of absorption is respiration. Because the blood is already removing virtually all gases with a high solubility ratio from the lungs, increasing the blood flow rate does not substantially increase the rate of absorption. However, the rate can be accelerated greatly by increasing the rate of respiration.

The blood carries the dissolved gas molecules to the rest of the body. In each tissue, the gas molecules are transferred from the blood to the tissue until equilibrium is reached at a tissue concentration dictated by the tissue-to-blood partition coefficient. After releasing part of the gas to tissues, blood returns to the lungs to take up more of the gas. The process continues until a gas reaches equilibrium between blood and each tissue according to the tissue-to-blood partition coefficients characteristic of each tissue. This equilibrium is referred to as *steady state*, and at this time, no net absorption of gas takes place as long as the exposure concentration remains constant.

Aerosols and Particles   Absorption of aerosol and particles is distinguished from gases and vapors by the factors that determine absorption from the inhalation route of exposure. The absorption of gases and vapors by inhalation is determined by the partitioning of the compound between the blood and the gas phase along with its solubility and tissue reactivity. In contrast, the important characteristics that affect absorption after exposure to aerosols are the aerosol size and water solubility of any chemical present in the aerosol.

The site of deposition of aerosols and particulates depends largely on the size of the particles. This relationship is discussed in detail in Chap. 15. In general, the smaller the particle, the further into the respiratory tree the particle will deposit (Fig. 5-6). Particles ranging from 5 μm or larger, described as "course particles" usually are deposited in the nasopharyngeal region. Those deposited on the unciliated anterior or rostral portion of the nose tend to remain at the site of deposition until they are removed by nose wiping, blowing, or sneezing. The mucous blanket of the ciliated nasal surface propels insoluble particles by the movement of the cilia. These particles and particles inhaled through the mouth are swallowed within minutes. Soluble particles may dissolve in the mucus and be carried to the pharynx or may be absorbed through the nasal epithelium into the blood.

Particulate matter with diameters of approximately 2.5 μm, referred to as "fine particles" are deposited mainly in the tracheobronchiolar regions of the lungs, from which they may be cleared by retrograde movement of the mucus layer in the ciliated portions of the respiratory tract (also known as the mucociliary escalator). The rate of cilia-propelled movement of mucus varies in different parts of the respiratory tract, although in general it is a rapid and efficient transport mechanism. Toxicants or viral infections that damage cilia may impair the efficiency of this process. Measurements have shown transport rates between 0.1 and 1 mm per minute, resulting in removal half-lives between 30 and 300 minutes. Coughing and sneezing greatly increase the movement of mucus and particulate matter toward the mouth. Particles eventually may be swallowed and absorbed from the GI tract or expectorated.

Particles 1 μm and smaller penetrate to the alveolar sacs of the lungs. Ultrafine or nanoparticles are those that are less than 0.1 μm (100 nM) in diameter. Those particles that are approximately 10–20 nm in size have the greatest likelihood of depositing in the alveolar region. These extremely small particles may be absorbed into blood or cleared through the lymphatics after being scavenged by alveolar macrophages (Oberdorster *et al.*, 2005).

In addition to being a major determinant of lung deposition, as particle size decreases, the number of particles in a unit of space increases along with the total surface area of the particles. This relationship, illustrated in Table 5-6, indicates that nanoparticles have the propensity to deliver high amounts of particulates to the lung. The contribution of nanoparticles to toxic responses, with special emphasis on their disposition (and factors that influence disposition including size, composition, surface structure, surface group modification, solubility, and aggregation) are major areas of toxicological and human health effects research (Nel *et al.*, 2006).

The mechanisms responsible for the removal or absorption of particulate matter from the alveoli are less clear than those responsible for the removal of particles deposited in the tracheobronchial tree. Removal appears to occur by three major mechanisms. First, particles may be removed from the alveoli by a physical process. As described earlier, it is thought that particles deposited on the fluid layer of the alveoli are aspirated onto the mucociliary escalator of the tracheobronchial region. From there, they are transported to the mouth and may be swallowed. The origin of the thin fluid layer in the alveoli is probably a transudation of lymph and secretions of lipids and other components by the alveolar epithelium. The alveolar fluid flows by an unknown mechanism to the terminal

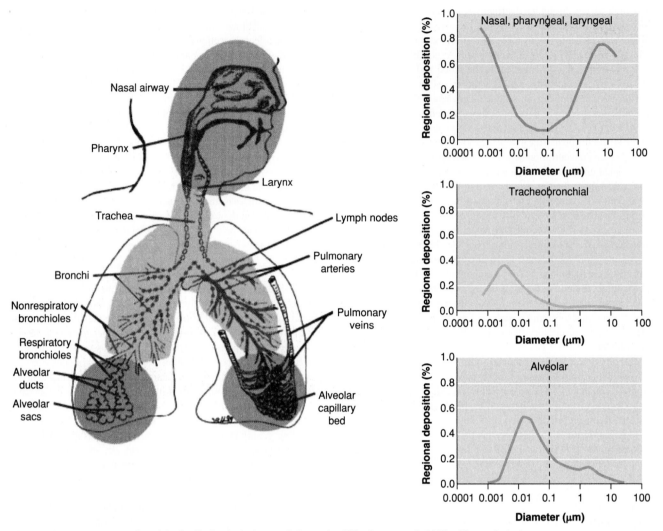

Figure 5-6. Representation of particle distribution in the lungs relative to size. (Oberdorster et al., 2005, with permission).

bronchioles. This flow seems to depend on lymph flow, capillary action, the respiratory motion of the alveolar walls, the cohesive nature of the respiratory tract's fluid blanket, the propelling power of the ciliated bronchioles, and the surface tension within the fluid layer. Second, particles from the alveoli may be removed by phagocytosis. The principal cells responsible for engulfing alveolar debris are the resident alveolar macrophages. These phagocytic cells are found in large numbers in normal lungs and contain many phago-

Table 5-6
Particle Number and Surface Area for 10 μg/m^3 Airborne Particles

PARTICLE DIAMETER (μm)	PARTICLES/mL AIR	PARTICLE SURFACE AREA (μm^2/mL AIR)
5	0.15	12
2	2	30
0.5	153	120
0.02	2,400,000	3016
0.05	153,000,000	12,000

SOURCE: Modified from Oberdorster *et al.* (2005) and Nel *et al.* (2006).

cytized particles of both exogenous and endogenous origin. They apparently migrate to the distal end of the mucociliary escalator and are cleared and eventually swallowed. Third, removal may occur via the lymphatics. The endothelial cells lining lymphatic capillaries are permeable to very large molecules (molecular weight $>10^6$) and for particles, although the rate of penetration is low above a molecular weight of 10,000. Nevertheless, the lymphatic system plays a prominent role in collecting high-molecular-weight proteins leaked from cells or blood capillaries and particulate matter from the interstitium and the alveolar spaces. Particulate matter may remain in lymphatic tissue for long periods, and this explains the phenomenon of "dust store of the lungs."

In general, the overall removal of particles from the alveoli is relatively inefficient. The rate of clearance by the lungs can be predicted by a compound's solubility in lung fluids. The lower the solubility, the lower the removal rate. Thus, it appears that removal of particles that enter the alveoli is largely due to the dissolution and vascular transport. Some particles may remain in the alveoli indefinitely. This may occur when long-lived alveolar macrophages phagocytose indigestible dust particles and secrete cytokines that stimulate the development of a local network of type I and III collagen fibers to form an alveolar dust plaque or nodule.

Absorption of Toxicants Through the Skin

Skin is the largest body organ and provides a relatively good barrier for separating organisms from their environment. Overall, human skin comes into contact with many toxic chemicals, but exposure is usually limited by its relatively impermeable nature. However, some chemicals can be absorbed by the skin in sufficient quantities to produce systemic effects. For example, there are several insecticides for which fatal exposures have occurred in agricultural workers after absorption through intact skin (see Chap. 22). In addition, there are numerous chemicals that increase tumor development in other organs after dermal application.

The skin comprises two major layers, the epidermis and dermis (Fig. 5-7). The epidermis is the outermost layer and comprises keratinocytes that are metabolically competent and able to divide. Dividing keratinocytes in the stratum germinativum displace maturing keratinocyte layers upward until they reach the outermost layer, the stratum corneum. The stratum corneum comprises densely packed keratinized cells that have lost their nuclei and are biologically inactive. The stratum corneum is replaced approximately every 3 to 4 weeks in human adults. This complex process involves dehydration and polymerization of intracellular matrix forming keratin-filled dried cell layers. During the process, the cell walls apparently double in thickness and transform to a dry, keratinous semisolid state with much lower permeability for diffusion of toxicants. The stratum corneum is unique anatomically and represents the single most important barrier to preventing fluid loss from the body while also serving as the major barrier to prevent the absorption of xenobiotics into the body.

The dermis is situated beneath the epidermis and comprises primarily of fibroblasts. This region also contains the vascular network that provides the dermis and epidermis with blood supply and serves to carry absorbed compounds into the body. Although the major anatomical area that controls absorption across the skin is the stratum corneum, compounds may also be absorbed through dermal appendages, including sweat and sebaceous glands and hair follicles found in the dermis. Sweat glands and hair follicles are scattered in varying densities on skin. These appendages account for no more than 1% of the total cross-sectional area of the total skin surface, and in general, passage through these areas is much more rapid than

passage through the stratum corneum. Ultimately, to be absorbed a chemical must pass the barrier of the stratum corneum and then traverse the other six layers of the skin (Dugard, 1983; Poet and McDougal, 2002).

In contrast to the complexity of the GI tract, the skin is a simpler penetration barrier for chemicals because passage through the stratum corneum is the rate-determining step. All toxicants move across the stratum corneum by passive diffusion. In general, lipophilic (fat-soluble) compounds are absorbed more readily across the stratum corneum, whereas the penetration of hydrophilic (water-soluble) compounds is more limited. Nonpolar toxicants diffuse through the skin in a manner that is proportional to their lipid solubility and inversely related to molecular weight. However, although lipophilic compounds may pass more readily through the stratum corneum, their passage through the dermis may become rate-limiting. Hydrophilic compounds are more likely to penetrate the skin through appendages such as hair follicles.

Human stratum corneum displays significant differences in structure and chemistry from one region of the body to another, and these differences affect the permeability of the skin to chemicals. Skin from the plantar and palmar regions is much different from skin from other areas of the body in that the stratum corneum of the palms and soles is adapted for weight bearing and friction and there are no hair follicles present. The stratum corneum of the rest of the body surface is adapted for flexibility and fine sensory discrimination. The permeability of the skin also depends on both the diffusivity and the thickness of the stratum corneum. Whereas the stratum corneum is much thicker on the palms and soles (400–600 μm in callous areas) than on the arms, back, legs, and abdomen (8–15 μm), it has much higher diffusivity per unit thickness. In contrast, the skin of the scrotum is characterized by a thin stratum corneum and a high diffusivity. Consequently, as illustrated by the comparative absorption of malathion across different human skin sites (Table 5-7), toxicants are likely to readily cross scrotal skin, whereas absorption across forehead skin is less extensive, and penetration across the palm is lowest because of the thickness of the stratum corneum and the lack of dermal appendages.

The second phase of percutaneous absorption consists of diffusion of the toxicant through the lower layers of the epidermis (stratum granulosum, spinosum, and germinativum) and the dermis. Despite possessing tight intercellular junctions, these cell layers are far inferior to the stratum corneum as diffusion barriers. In contrast to the stratum corneum, they contain a porous, nonselective, aqueous diffusion medium. Toxicants pass through this area by diffusion and enter the systemic circulation through the numerous venous and lymphatic capillaries in the dermis. The rate of diffusion depends on

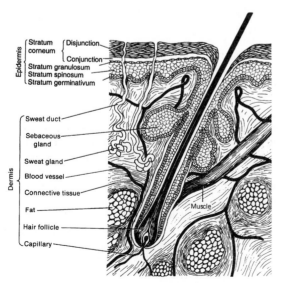

Figure 5-7. Diagram of a cross section of human skin.

Table 5-7

Absorption of Malathion Across Different Human Skin Regions

ANATOMICAL REGION	ABSORPTION (%)	STRATUM CORNEUM THICKNESS (μm)	HAIR FOLLICLES/cm^2
Scrotum	101.6	5	60
Forehead	23.2	13	770
Hand (back)	12.5	49	18
Palm	5.8	400	—

SOURCE: Adapted from Poet and McDougal (2002).

blood flow, interstitial fluid movement, and perhaps other factors, including interactions with dermal constituents.

There are several factors that can influence the absorption of toxicants through the skin, including: (1) the integrity of the stratum corneum, (2) the hydration state of the stratum corneum, (3) temperature, (4) solvents as carriers, and (5) molecular size. Because the stratum corneum plays a critical role in determining cutaneous permeability, removal of this layer causes a dramatic increase in the permeability of the epidermis for a variety of large or small molecules, both lipid-soluble and water-soluble (Poet and McDougal, 2002). Caustic agents such as acids and alkalis that damage the stratum corneum increase its permeability. The most frequently encountered penetration-enhancing damage to the skin results from burns and various skin diseases. Water also plays an extremely important role in skin permeability. Under normal conditions, the stratum corneum is partially hydrated, containing about 7% water by weight. This amount of water increases the permeability of the stratum corneum approximately 10-fold over the permeability that exists when it is completely dry. On contact with water, the stratum corneum can increase its weight of tightly bound water up to fivefold, and this can increase permeability an additional two- to threefold. In many studies, the site of application will be covered with plastic wrap (occlusive application), as originally described by Draize *et al.* (1944), which hydrates the stratum corneum and enhances the absorption of some toxicants. Similarly, an increase in temperature will increase dermal penetration by increasing dermal blood flow. This is particularly important for occupational exposures to agents such as insecticides in which agricultural workers are likely to be working strenuously at relatively high temperatures. Such environmental conditions increase dermal penetration and may increase the risk of systemic toxicity.

Solvents used to dissolve compounds of interest can also influence dermal penetration. In general, lower absorption will be observed if a toxicant is highly soluble in the vehicle, whereas low solubility of the toxicant in the vehicle will tend to increase dermal penetration. In addition, solvents such as dimethyl sulfoxide (DMSO) facilitate the penetration of toxicants through the skin by increasing the permeability of the stratum corneum. Although the mechanism by which DMSO enhances skin permeability is not fully understood, it has been suggested that DMSO: (1) removes much of the lipid matrix of the stratum corneum, making holes on artificial shunts in the penetration barrier; (2) produces reversible configurational changes in protein structure brought about by the substitution of integral water molecules; and (3) functions as a swelling agent (Dugard and Embery, 1969). Finally, it is generally recognized that compounds with molecular weights greater than 400 Da will exhibit poor dermal penetration. As described earlier, nanomaterials represent a unique new area in which the small size of the particles is likely to increase penetration and systemic exposures to these small molecules.

Dermal absorption has been studied in most laboratory animals including rats, mice, rabbits, guinea pigs, primates, and pig, and dermal absorption varies widely across these species. As a general rule, dermal absorption across rodent skin is much greater than human skin, whereas the cutaneous permeability characteristics of guinea pigs, pigs, and monkeys are often similar to those observed in humans (Wester and Maibach, 1993). Species differences in percutaneous absorption account for the differential toxicity of insecticides in insects and humans. For example, the LD_{50} of injected DDT is approximately equal in insects and mammals, but DDT is much less toxic to mammals than to insects when it is applied to the skin. This appears to be due to the fact that DDT is poorly absorbed through the skin of mammals but passes readily through the chitinous exoskeleton of insects. Furthermore, insects have a much greater body surface area relative to weight than do mammals.

Species differences in dermal absorption of xenobiotics result from several anatomic, physiologic, and biochemical factors (Dugard, 1983; Poet and McDougal, 2002). First, the composition and thickness of the stratum corneum along with the nature of the the the dermal appendages are highly variable across species. The stratum corneum is much thicker in humans than in most laboratory animals, making human skin typically less permeable than animal skin. However, the thinner stratum corneum in animals is often compensated for by a relatively thick hair cover, diminishing direct contact of the skin with a xenobiotic. Sweat and pilosebaceous ducts also reveal great species variability. Eccrine sweat glands are located in the pads of the extremities of all mammals. However, the general body surface of humans contains 100 to $600/m^2$ of coiled tubular sweat glands, whereas rodents, rabbits, cats, and dogs have none. The number of pilosebaceous ducts in humans and pigs is similar (about $40/cm^2$), but rodents may have up to 100 times more. Another important potential rate-limiting step in the dermal absorption of chemicals is the cutaneous blood flow. Owing to an important thermoregulatory function of the skin in humans as opposed to furred animals, there is a much more extensive vasculature in humans than in most mammals (Calabrese, 1984). Biotransformation reactions in skin can also facilitate absorption, and the presence of metabolizing enzymes is highly variable across species. Xenobiotic transporters, including Mrp1, 3, 4, 5, and 6, have been identifed in skin keratinocytes and may also contribute to species differences in dermal absorption of toxicants (Kao *et al.*, 1985; Baron *et al.*, 2001).

Overall, commonly-used laboratory animals are typically not good models of human absorption of toxicants. An example of the species differences and lack of concordance with human data for dermal absorption of the herbicide 2,4-dichlorophenoxyacetic acid (2,4-D) is illustrated in Table 5-8. In general, absorption through primate or pig skin is considered to most closely predict human dermal absorption (Wester and Maibach, 1993). Additionally, in vitro methods using human skin may provide reasonable alternatives to the use of laboratory animals for evaluating dermal absorption of toxicants (Bronaugh *et al.*, 1982).

Absorption of Toxicants after Special Routes of Administration

Toxicants usually enter the bloodstream after absorption through the skin, lungs, or GI tract. However, in studying the effects of chemicals in laboratory animals, other routes of administration may also be used. The most common routes are: (1) intravenous, (2) intraperitoneal, (3) subcutaneous, and (4) intramuscular. The intravenous route introduces the toxicant directly into the bloodstream, eliminating the process of absorption. Intraperitoneal injection results in rapid absorption of xenobiotics because of the rich peritoneal and mesenteric blood supply and the relatively large surface area of the peritoneal cavity. In addition, this route of administration circumvents the delay and variability of gastric emptying. Intraperitoneally administered compounds are absorbed primarily through the portal circulation and therefore must pass through the liver before reaching other organ. Subcutaneously and intramuscularly administered toxicants are usually absorbed at slower rates but enter directly into the general circulation. The rate of absorption by these two routes can be altered by changing the blood flow to the injection site. For

Table 5-8

Comparison of Dermal Absorption of 2,4-D Across Species

SPECIES	WASH TIME (hour)	COLLECTION TIME (hour)	% ABSORBED
Rat	24	336	20
Rabbit	24	336	12
Monkey	24	336	6
Human	4	120	3.7

NOTE: Data modified from Ross *et al.* (2005) and represent application of the dimethyl-lamine salt of 2,4-D. In all cases, the dose applied was 4 μg/cm^2. For rats, rabbits, and monkeys, the application site was washed after 24 hours, whereas human skin was washed after 4 hours. The collection time denotes the interval over which data were collected to determine absorption.

example, epinephrine causes vasoconstriction and will decrease the rate of absorption if it is coinjected intramuscularly with a toxicant. The formulation of a xenobiotic may also affect the rate of absorption, as toxicants are typically absorbed more slowly from suspensions than from solutions.

The toxicity of a chemical may or may not depend on the route of administration. If a toxicant is injected intraperitoneally, most of the chemical enters the liver via the portal circulation before reaching the general circulation. Therefore, an intraperitoneally administered compound may be completely extracted and biotransformed by the liver with subsequent excretion into bile without gaining access to the systemic circulation. Propranolol (Shand and Rangno, 1972) and lidocaine (Boyes *et al.*, 1970) are two drugs with efficient extraction during the first pass through the liver. A chemical with a high first-pass effect that is toxic in an organ other than the liver and GI tract is likely to be less toxic when administered intraperitoneally than when administered by other routes (intravenously, intramuscularly, or subcutaneously) because the intraperitoneal route favors extraction in the liver to reduce what is available systemically. In contrast, compounds with no appreciable biotransformation in the liver are likely to show similar toxicity independent of the route of administration if the rates of absorption are equal. Therefore, preliminary information on the contribution of biotransformation and excretion of xenobiotics to toxic outcome can be derived by comparing toxic responses after administration by different routes.

DISTRIBUTION

After entering the blood by absorption or intravenous administration, a toxicant is distributed to tissues throughout the body. Distribution usually occurs rapidly. The rate of distribution to organs or tissues is determined primarily by blood flow and the rate of diffusion out of the capillary bed into the cells of a particular organ or tissue. The final distribution depends largely on the affinity of a xenobiotic for various tissues. In general, the initial phase of distribution is dominated by blood flow, whereas the eventual distribution is determined largely by affinity. The penetration of toxicants into cells occurs by passive diffusion or special transport processes, as was discussed previously. Small water-soluble molecules and ions apparently diffuse through aqueous channels or pores in the cell membrane. Lipid-soluble molecules readily permeate the membrane itself. Very polar molecules and ions of even moderate size (molecular weight of 50 or more) cannot enter cells easily except by special transport mechanisms because they are surrounded by a hydration shell, making their actual size much larger.

Volume of Distribution

Total body water is derived from that which is either extracellular or intracellular and represents three distinct compartments: plasma water and interstitial water comprise the extracellular compartment and are distinguished from intracellular water. The concentration of a toxicant in blood depends largely on its volume of distribution. The volume of distribution (Vd) is used to quantify the distribution of a xenobiotic throughout the body. It is defined as *the volume in which the amount of drug would need to be uniformly dissolved in order to produce the observed blood concentration.* Illustrated below are examples of observed plasma concentrations after absorption of 1 g of a compound in a 70-kg human, which are determined by the Vd. For example, a high concentration would be observed in the plasma if the chemical were distributed into plasma water only (a low Vd), and a much lower concentration would be reached if it were distributed into a large pool, such as total body water (a high Vd). However, the distribution of toxicants is complex and under most circumstances cannot be equated with distribution into one of the water compartments of the body. Binding to and/or dissolution in various storage sites of the body, such as fat, liver, and bone, are usually more important factors in determining the distribution of chemicals (Box 5-4).

Some toxicants do not readily cross cell membranes and therefore have restricted distribution, whereas other toxicants rapidly pass through cell membranes and are distributed throughout the body. Some toxicants selectively accumulate in certain parts of the body as a result of protein binding, active transport, or high solubility in fat. The target organ for toxicity may be the site of accumulation, but this is not always the case. If a toxicant accumulates at a site other than the target organ or tissue, the accumulation is likely to be protective because plasma levels and consequently its concentration at the site of action is reduced. In this case, it is assumed that the chemical in the storage depot is toxicologically inactive. However, a chemical in a storage depot is also in equilibrium with the free fraction of the toxicant in plasma, so that it is released into the circulation as the unbound fraction of toxicant is eliminated.

Box 5-4

COMPARTMENT	% OF TOTAL	LITERS IN 70-kg HUMAN	PLASMA CONCENTRATION AFTER 1 g OF CHEMICAL
Plasma water	4.5	3	333 mg/L
Total extracellular water	20	14	71 mg/L
Total body water	55	38	26 mg/L
Tissue binding	—	—	0–25 mg/L

Storage of Toxicants in Tissues

Because only the free fraction of a chemical is in equilibrium throughout the body, binding to or dissolving in certain body constituents greatly alters the distribution of a xenobiotic. Some xenobiotics attain their highest concentrations at the site of toxic action, such as carbon monoxide, which has a very high affinity for hemoglobin, and paraquat, which accumulates in the lungs. Other chemicals concentrate at sites other than the target organ. For example, lead is stored in bone, but manifestations of lead poisoning appear in soft tissues. The compartment where a toxicant is concentrated is described as a storage depot. Toxicants in these depots are always in equilibrium with the free fraction in plasma, so that as a chemical is biotransformed or excreted from the body, more is released from the storage site. As a result, the biological half-life of stored compounds can be very long. The following discussion deals with the major storage sites for xenobiotics in the body.

Plasma Proteins as Storage Depot Binding to plasma proteins is the major site of protein binding, and several different plasma proteins bind xenobiotics and some endogenous constituents of the body. As depicted in Fig. 5-8, albumin is the major protein in plasma and it binds many different compounds. α_1-Acid glycoprotein, although present at a much lower concentration than albumin, is also an important protein in plasma, and compounds with basic characteristics tend to bind to it. Transferrin, a beta globulin, is important for the transport of iron in the body. The other major metal-binding protein in plasma is ceruloplasmin, which carries copper. The alpha- and beta-lipoproteins are very important in the transport of lipid-soluble compounds such as vitamins, cholesterol, and steroid hormones as well as xenobiotics. Plasma gamma globulins are antibodies that function specifically in immunological reactions. (Wilkinson, 1983). Overall, plasma proteins bind acidic compounds such as phenylbutazone, basic compounds such as imipramine, and neutral compounds such as digitoxin.

Albumin, present in the plasma at a concentration of 500–600 μM, is the most abundant protein in plasma and serves as both a depot and multivalent transport protein for many endogenous and exogenous compounds. Protein–ligand interactions occur primarily as a result of hydrophobic forces, hydrogen bonding, and Van der Waals forces. Because of their high molecular weight, plasma proteins and the toxicants bound to them cannot cross capillary walls.

Consequently, the fraction of a toxicant bound to plasma proteins is not immediately available for distribution into the extravascular space or filtration by the kidneys. However, the interaction of a chemical with plasma proteins is a reversible process, and as unbound chemical diffuses out of capillaries, bound chemical dissociates from the protein until the free fraction reaches equilibrium between the vascular space and the extravascular space. In turn, diffusion in the extravascular space to sites more distant from the capillaries continues, and the resulting concentration gradient provides the thermodynamic force for continued dissociation of the bound fraction in plasma. Active transport processes are not limited by the binding of chemicals to plasma proteins.

The binding of toxicants to plasma proteins is usually determined by equilibrium dialysis or ultrafiltration. The total amount in plasma is determined prior to these separation methods, and the fraction that passes through a dialysis membrane or appears in the ultrafiltrate is the unbound (or free) fraction. The bound fraction is determined as the difference between the total and unbound fractions. Binding of toxicants to plasma proteins can be assessed through the use of Scatchard analysis (Scatchard, 1949) in which the ratio of bound to free ligand (toxicant) is plotted on the ordinate and the concentration of bound ligand is plotted on the abscissa, depicted in Fig. 5-9. From this analysis, the number of ligand binding sites (N) per molecule of protein and the affinity constant of the protein–ligand complex can be determined. Although Fig. 5-9 shows a linear relationship, Scatchard plots frequently exhibits nonlinearity, indicating the presence of two or more classes of binding sites with different affinities and capacity characteristics. The extent of plasma protein binding varies considerably among xenobiotics. Some, such as antipyrine, are not bound; others, such as secobarbital, are bound to about 50%; and some, like warfarin, are 99% bound.

The binding of chemicals to plasma proteins is an important concept in toxicology for two reasons. Toxicity is typically manifested by the amount of a xenobiotic that is unbound. Therefore, a compound with a high degree of plasma protein binding may not show toxicity when compared to one that is less extensively bound to plasma proteins. Ironically, a high degree of protein binding also tends to increase the risk of adverse effects resulting from

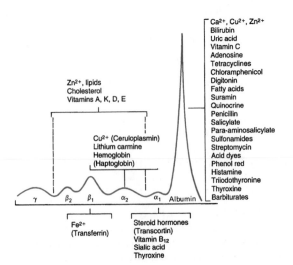

Figure 5-8. Ligand interactions with plasma proteins.

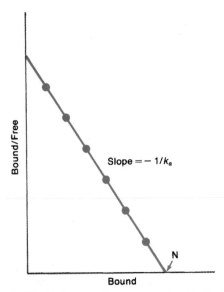

Figure 5-9. Schematic representation of the Scatchard plot for the analysis of the binding of toxicants to proteins.

Table 5-9

Plasma Protein Binding and Half-life of Clofibric Acid in the Mouse, Rat, and Man

SPECIES	PLASMA PROTEIN BINDING (%)	HALF-LIFE (hour)
Man	97	21
Rat	75	6
Mouse	45	2

SOURCE: Modified from Cayen (1980).

interactions with other highly bound compounds. In particular, severe toxic reactions can occur if a toxicant with a high degree of protein binding is displaced from plasma proteins by another agent, increasing the free fraction of the toxicant in plasma. This interaction increases the equilibrium concentration of the toxicant in a target organ, thereby increasing the potential for toxicity. Most research on the adverse interactions associated with binding of xenobiotics to plasma proteins has been conducted with drugs. For example, if a strongly bound sulfonamide is given concurrently with an antidiabetic drug, the sulfonamide may displace the antidiabetic drug and induce a hypoglycemic coma. Similarly, interactions resulting from displacement of warfarin can lead to inappropriate blood clotting and possible deleterious effects. Xenobiotics can also compete with and displace endogenous compounds that are bound to plasma proteins. The importance of this phenomenon was demonstrated in a clinical trial comparing the efficacy of tetracycline with that of a penicillin–sulfonamide mixture in the management of bacterial infections in premature infants (Silverman *et al.*, 1956). The penicillin–sulfonamide mixture led to much higher mortality than did the tetracycline, because the sulfonamide displaced a considerable amount of bilirubin from albumin. Free bilirubin then diffused into the brain of the newborns (because the blood–brain barrier is not fully developed), causing a severe form of brain damage termed *kernicterus*. In addition to drugs, some chemicals, such as the insecticide dieldrin, also bind avidly to plasma proteins (99%). Therefore, it is to be expected that chemical–chemical interactions that alter plasma protein binding occur with many different xenobiotics.

Plasma protein binding can also give rise to species differences in the disposition of xenobiotics. For example, plasma protein binding of clofibric acid is considerably different between mice, rats, and humans and correlates with the half-lives of this compound in these species (Table 5-9). Because clofibric acid is primarily eliminated in all three species by glomerular filtration without tubular reabsorption, differences in the free fraction of this compound in plasma across the species contribute to the observed species differences in drug half-life. Additional factors that influence plasma protein binding across species include differences in the concentration of albumin, in binding affinity, and/or in competitive binding of endogenous substances.

Liver and Kidney as Storage Depots The liver and kidney have a high capacity for binding many chemicals. These two organs probably concentrate more toxicants than do all the other organs combined, and in most cases, active transport or binding to tissue components are likely to be involved.

Hepatic uptake of lead illustrates how rapidly liver binds foreign compounds: just 30 minutes after a single dose, the concentration of lead in liver is 50 times higher than the concentration in plasma (Klaassen and Shoeman, 1974). In addition, some proteins serve to sequester xenobiotics in the liver or kidney. For example, metallothionein (MT), a specialized metal-binding protein, sequesters both essential and toxic metals including zinc and cadmium (Cd) with high affinities in the kidney and liver. In liver, Cd bound to MT serves to concentrate and sequester the heavy metal while preventing its excretion into bile. In the kidney, however, the Cd–MT complex is very toxic and is mechanistically involved in the chronic toxicity of Cd (Klaassen and Liu, 1997). Another protein that sequesters certain toxicants in the kidney is α2u-globulin. This protein, which is synthesized in large quantities only in male rats, binds to a diverse array of xenobiotics including metabolites of D-limonene (a major constituent of orange juice and 2,4,4-trimethylpentane (found in unleaded gasoline). The chemical-α2u-globulin complex is taken up by the kidney, where it accumulates within the lysosomal compartment and damages the proximal tubule cells. Ultimately, the accumulation of this complex in the kidney is responsible for male-rat-specific nephrotoxicity and carcinogenicity (Lehman-McKeeman, 1997).

Fat as Storage Depot There are many organic compounds that are highly stable and lipophilic, leading to their accumulation in the environment. The lipophilic nature of these compounds also permits rapid penetration of cell membranes and uptake by tissues, and it is not surprising that highly lipophilic toxicants are distributed and concentrated in body fat. The environmental accumulation and potential toxicological significance of long-term storage of numerous compounds including the pesticides aldrin, chlordane, DDT, dieldrin, endrin, heptachlor, mirex, and toxaphene, along with polychlorinated and polybrominated biphenyls, dioxins, and furans has led to international treaties controlling the use of these persistent organic pollutants. The potential for these compounds to produce toxicity, including carcinogenic, developmental, and endocrine effects is related to their accumulation and storage in body fat (Jandacek and Tso, 2001).

Toxicants appear to accumulate in fat by dissolution in neutral fats, which constitute about 50% and 20% of the body weight of obese individuals and lean athletic individuals, respectively. Thus, toxicants with a high lipid/water partition coefficient may be stored in body fat, and higher amounts are likely to be retained in obese individuals. Storage lowers the concentration of the toxicant in the target organ such that toxicity is likely to be less severe in an obese person than in a lean individual. However, of more practical toxicological concern is the possibility that a sudden increase in the concentration of a chemical in blood and the target organ of toxicity may occur if rapid mobilization from fat occurs. Several studies have shown that signs of intoxication can be produced by short-term starvation of experimental animals that were previously exposed to persistent organochlorine insecticides.

There have been numerous attempts to alter storage of lipophilic toxins in adipose tissues in animal models and humans. Changes in body fat composition appear to be the most effective in reducing body burdens, and interventions designed to reduce the absorption of these compounds from the GI tract appear to be somewhat helpful in reducing storage depots of persistent organic pollutants in fat (Jandacek and Tso, 2001).

Bone as Storage Depot Compounds such as fluoride, lead, and strontium may be incorporated and stored in the bone matrix. For example, 90% of the lead in the body is eventually found in the skeleton. Skeletal uptake of xenobiotics is essentially a surface chemistry phenomenon, with exchange taking place between the bone surface and the fluid in contact with it. The fluid is the extracellular fluid, and the surface is that of the hydroxyapatite crystals of bone mineral. Many of those crystals are very small, resulting in a large surface area relative to the mass of the bone. The extracellular fluid brings the toxicant into contact with the hydration shell of the hydroxyapatite, allowing diffusion through it and penetration of the crystal surface. As a result of similarities in size and charge, F^- may readily displace OH^-, whereas lead or strontium may substitute for calcium in the hydroxyapatite lattice matrix through an exchange–absorption reaction.

Foreign compounds deposited in bone are not sequestered irreversibly by that tissue. Toxicants can be released from the bone by ionic exchange at the crystal surface and dissolution of bone crystals through osteoclastic activity. An increase in osteolytic activity such as that seen after parathyroid hormone administration leads to enhanced mobilization of hydroxyapatite lattice, which can be reflected in an increased plasma concentration of toxicants. Ultimately, deposition and storage of toxicants in bone may or may not be detrimental. Lead is not toxic to bone, but the chronic effects of fluoride deposition (skeletal fluorosis) and radioactive strontium (osteosarcoma and other neoplasms) are well documented.

Blood–Brain Barrier

Access to the brain is restricted by the presence of two barriers: the blood–brain barrier (BBB) and the blood–cerebral spinal fluid barrier (BCSFB). Although neither represents an absolute barrier to the passage of toxic agents into the CNS, many toxicants do not enter the brain in appreciable quantities because of these barriers.

The BBB is formed primarily by the endothelial cells of blood capillaries in the brain (Fig. 5-10). Each endothelial cell forms a tight junction with adjacent cells, essentially forming a tight seal between the cells and preventing diffusion of polar compounds through paracellular pathways. Diffusion of more lipophilic compounds through endothelial cell membranes is counteracted by xenobiotic efflux transporters present in the endothelial cells. Glial cells, particularly astrocytes, contribute to the BBB by secreting chemical factors that modulate endothelial cell permeability, and astrocytes and perivascular microglial cells extend processes that support the integrity of the BBB. For small- to medium-sized water-soluble molecules, the tighter junctions of the capillary endothelium and the lipid membranes of the glial cell processes represent the major barrier. Although the absorption of lipid-soluble compounds is favored in the brain, such compounds must traverse the membranes of the endothelial cells, not be substrates for xenobiotic transporters, and then traverse the glial cell processes to enter the brain.

The BCSFB is found between the circulating blood and the circulating cerebral spinal fluid in the brain (Fig. 5-11). It comprises

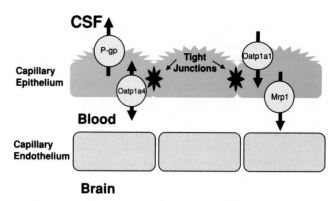

Figure 5-11. Schematic model showing the xenobiotic transporting systems that contribute to the blood–cerebral spinal fluid barrier.

elements of the choroid plexus, the arachnoid membrane, and certain periventricular locations (including the area postrema). The choroid plexus has highly permeable endothelial cells on the blood side but is lined by epithelial cells on the CSF side that form the barrier. Xenobiotic transporters also contribute to removing compounds that may enter the endothelial cells. Furthermore, the protein concentration in CSF is much lower than that in other body fluids. The low protein content of the CSF also limits the movement of water-insoluble compounds by paracellular transport, which is possible in a largely aqueous medium only when such compounds are bound to proteins. Furthermore, in most cases, toxicants achieve concentrations in the CSF that are no higher than the concentration of the unbound toxicant in the plasma. The BCSFB is more of an anatomical entity than a true barrier, but it does provide some protection against the distribution of toxicants to the CNS, thereby affording some protection against toxicity.

Active transport processes represent a key mechanism that decreases the concentration of xenobiotics in the brain. Four ATP-dependent transporters have been identified as part of the BBB including P-gp, Mrp2, Mrp4, and BCRP (deLange, 2004; Leslie et al., 2005). These transporters are located on the luminal (blood side) plasma membrane and function to move xenobiotics absorbed into the capillary endothelial cells out into the blood (Fig. 5-10). Oatp1a4 is also found on the luminal side and could drive a concentrative efflux if coupled energetically to the electrical potential difference across the endothelial cell membrane. Collectively, these transporters can efficiently efflux a wide range of anionic (Mrp2, Mrp4), cationic (P-gp, BCRP), uncharged (all four), and numerous drug conjugates (Oatp1a4, Mrp2) from the brain.

Xenobiotic transporters are also expressed in the choroid plexus, but within the BSCFB, P-gp and Mrp1 are thought to play the most important roles (Fig. 5-10). In this barrier, P-gp is expressed on the luminal side, with efflux from the choroidal epithelial cells into the CSF. In contrast, Mrp1 is expressed on the basolateral side of the choroidal epithelium, catalyzing the transport of xenobiotics out of the cells and into the vascular compartment (deLange, 2004). Members of the Oatp, Oat, Oct, and peptide transporters are also expressed at the choriod plexus. Oatp3, Oat3, and Pept2 are particularly important in regulating xenobiotic concentrations in the CSF (deLange, 2004).

The importance of transport processes to the maintenance of the BBB has been demonstrated in genetically modified mouse models. Compounds that are substrates for P-gp achieve much higher brain levels in P-gp null ($Mdr1a^{-/-}/Mdr1b^{-/-}$) mice relative to wild-type

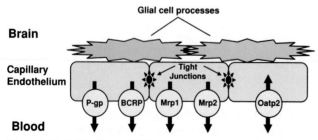

Figure 5-10. Schematic model showing the xenobiotic transporting systems that contribute to the blood–brain barrier.

mice, and are likely to show increased toxicity as well. Seminal studies demonstrated that P-gp null mice were far more sensitive to the insecticide, ivermectin, and the anticancer agent, vinblastine. The brain uptake of these compounds was increased 26- and 80-fold, respectively, and the sensitivity to neurotoxicity or lethality was increased up to 100-fold (Schinkel *et al.*, 1994; Lankas *et al.*, 1997). Expression of Mrp1 in the choroid plexus has been shown to modulate the concentrations of toxicants in the cerebral spinal fluid, but no studies have yet shown a correlation to neurotoxic potential relative to Mrp1 function.

The effectiveness of the blood–brain barrier varies from one area of the brain to another. For example, the cortex, the lateral nuclei of the hypothalamus, the area postrema, the pineal body, and the posterior lobe of the hypophysis are more permeable than are other areas of the brain. It is not clear whether this is due to the increased blood supply to those areas, or because the BSCFB represents a more permeable barrier, or both. In general, the entrance of toxicants into the brain follows the same principle that applies to transfer across other cells in the body. Only the free fraction of a toxicant (i.e., not bound to plasma proteins) equilibrates rapidly with the brain. Lipid solubility plays an important role in determining the rate of entry of a compound into the CNS, as does the degree of ionization, as discussed earlier. Lipid solubility enhances the rate of penetration of toxicants into the CNS, whereas ionization greatly diminishes it. Pralidoxime (2-PAM), a quaternary nitrogen derivative, does not readily penetrate the brain and is ineffective in reversing the inhibition of brain cholinesterase caused by organophosphate insecticides. Some very lipophilic compounds may enter the brain but are so efficiently removed by xenobiotic transporters that they do not reach appreciable concentrations. This is particularly true for agents like cyclosporin. TCDD, which is highly lipophilic, is also not readily distributed into the brain, but it is not known whether transporters influence its distribution to the brain or not. It is likely that strong binding to plasma proteins or lipoproteins, as well as the composition of the brain (mainly phospholipids), limits the entry of very lipophilic compounds into the brain. Some xenobiotics, although very few, appear to enter the brain by carrier-mediated processes. For example, methylmercury combines with cysteine, forming a structure similar to methionine (see Box 5-5), and the complex is then accepted by the large neutral amino acid carrier of the capillary endothelial cells (Clarkson, 1987).

The blood–brain barrier is not fully developed at birth, and this is one reason why some chemicals are more toxic in newborns than adults. The example of kernicterus resulting from increased brain levels of bilirubin in infants was noted earlier. In addition, morphine is 3–10 times more toxic to newborn than to adult rats because of the higher permeability of the brain of a newborn to morphine. Similarly, lead produces encephalomyelopathy in newborn rats but not in adults, apparently because of differences in the stages of development of the blood–brain barrier.

Passage of Toxicants Across the Placenta

The term *placental barrier* has been associated with the concept that the main function of the placenta is to protect the fetus against the passage of noxious substances from the mother. However, the placenta is a multifunctional organ that also provides nutrition for the conceptus, exchanges maternal and fetal blood gases, disposes of fetal excretory material, and maintains pregnancy through complex hormonal regulation. Placental structure and function show more species differences than any other mammalian organ. Anatomically, the placental barrier consists of a number of cell layers interposed between the fetal and maternal circulations, but the number of cell layers varies across species and with the stage of gestation. Placentas in which the maximum number of cell layers are present (all six layers) are called *epitheliochorial* (Table 5-10). Those in which the maternal epithelium is absent are referred to as *syndesmochorial*. When only the endothelial layer of the maternal tissue remains, the tissue is termed *endotheliochorial*; when even the endothelium is gone (as in humans), the chorionic villi bathe in the maternal blood, and the tissue is called *hemochorial*. In some species, some of the fetal layers are absent and are called *hemoendothelial*. Within the same species, the placenta may also change its histologic classification during gestation. For example, at the beginning of gestation, the placenta of a rabbit has six major layers (epitheliochorial), and at the end it has only one (hemoendothelial). Overall, there are marked species differences in placental structure. The animal models that are most similar to the organization of the human placenta based on its hemochorial histological organization are rodents and primates, but the decidual nature of the rodent placenta still differs markedly from that of humans (Myllynen *et al.*, 2005; Leiser and Kauffman, 1994).

Most of the vital nutrients necessary for the development of the fetus are transported by active transport systems. For example, vitamins, amino acids, essential sugars, and ions such as calcium and iron are transported from mother to fetus against a concentration gradient (Ganapathy *et al.*, 2000; Ginsburg, 1971). In contrast, most toxic chemicals pass the placenta by simple diffusion. The only exceptions are a few antimetabolites that are structurally similar to endogenous purines and pyrimidines, which are the physiologic substrates for active transport from the maternal to the fetal circulation. The placenta also has biotransformation capabilities that may prevent some toxic substances from reaching the fetus (Syme *et al.*, 2004). Among the substances that cross the placenta by passive diffusion, more lipid-soluble substances rapidly attain a maternal-fetal equilibrium. Under steady-state conditions, the concentrations of a toxic compound in the plasma of the mother and fetus are usually the same.

Many foreign substances can cross the placenta, and the same factors that dictate the passage of xenobiotics across biological membranes are important determinants of the placental transfer. In addition to chemicals, viruses (e.g., rubella virus), cellular pathogens (e.g., syphilis spirochetes), and globulin antibodies can traverse the placenta. In this regard, the placental barrier is not as precise an anatomical unit like the BBB. The human placenta

Box 5-5

$$CH_3Hg^+ + {}^-S-CH_2-CH-COO^-$$
$$\overset{|}{NH_3^+}$$
Cysteine

$$CH_3-Hg-S-CH_2-CH-COO^-$$
$$\overset{|}{NH_3^+}$$
Methylmercury–Cysteine (complex)

$$CH_3-S-CH_2-CH_2-CH-COO^-$$
$$\overset{|}{NH_3^+}$$
Methionine

Table 5-10
Tissues Separating Fetal and Maternal Blood

| | MATERNAL TISSUE | | | FETAL TISSUE | | | |
	ENDOTHELIUM	CONNECTIVE TISSUE	EPITHELIUM	TROPHOBLAST	CONNECTIVE TISSUE	ENDOTHELIUM	SPECIES
Epitheliochorial	+	+	+	+	+	+	Pig, horse, donkey
Syndesmochorial	+	+	—	+	+	+	Sheep, goat, cow
Endotheliochorial	+	—	—	+	+	+	Cat, dog
Hemochorial	—	—	—	+	+	+	Human, monkey
Hemoendothelial	—	—	—	—	—	+	Rat, rabbit, guinea pig

SOURCE: Modified from Morris *et al.* (1994).

comprises the syncytiotrophoblast and cytotrophoblast layers. The apical membrane of the syncytiotrophoblast, which forms a continuous epithelial layer, is bathed in maternal blood and the basolateral surface is in contact with either the discontinuous cytotrophoblast layer, the stromal tissue or the fetal vasculature (Fig. 5-12). To reach the fetus, toxins must traverse the apical and basolateral membranes of the syncytiotrophoblast as well as the endothelium of the fetal capillaries. Xenobiotic transporters are differentially expressed in these various cells and contribute to the barrier function that restricts distribution of toxicants to the fetus. In particular, P-gp, Mrp2, and BCRP are expressed on the apical border of the syncytiotrophoblast, whereas Mrp1 is localized to the basolateral membranes of syncytiotrophoblasts and the fetal capillary endothelial cells. These transporters play important roles in protecting the fetus while regulating the movement of essential nutrients. There are numerous other transporters in the placenta, many of which are critical to the transfer of nutrients to or the removal of waste products from the fetus. In addition, transporters from the OAT, OCT, and OCTN families have been identified in the placenta, but the precise function and/or membrane location has not been fully established (Ganapathy *et al.*, 2000). For example, the homozygous offspring of female P-gp null mice (*Mdr1a⁻/⁻/Mdr1b⁻/⁻*) develop cleft palate when treated with a photoisomer of avermectin, whereas heterozygous littermates showed intermediate susceptibility and wild-type mice were resistant to this adverse effect (Lankas *et al.*, 1998).

BCRP, whose expression is highest in the human placenta relative to any other organ, has also been shown to protect the fetus from exposure to toxicants, and Mrp2 is likely to be particularly important for preventing the passage of conjugated metabolites of toxicants from the maternal to fetal circulation. Finally, Mrp1, lo-

cated on the fetal capillary endothelium is proposed to prevent or limit the entry of organic anions into the fetal circulation.

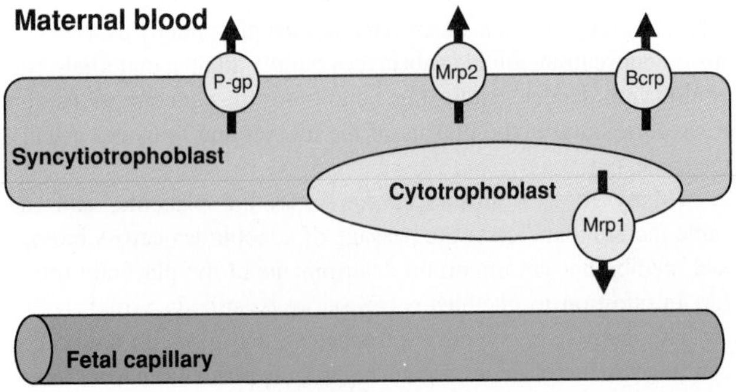

Despite the presence of biotransformation systems and xenobiotic transporters designed to nourish and protect the fetus, the transfer of xenobiotics across the placenta can still occur. One important consequence of placental transfer is that of transplacental carcinogenesis. In this case exposing the mother during gestation increases the likelihood of tumor development in the offspring later in life (see Chap. 8). The most well-known transplacental carcinogen in humans is diethylstilbestrol (Newbold and McLachlan, 1996), but other compounds such as the anti-viral drug zidovudine (Diwan *et al.*, 1999) and inorganic arsenic (Waalkes *et al.*, 2003) induce tumors in mice when exposed to these chemicals only during gestation.

Redistribution of Toxicants

The most critical factors that affect the distribution of xenobiotics are the organ blood flow and its affinity for a xenobiotic. The initial phase of distribution is determined primarily by blood flow to the various parts of the body. Therefore, a well-perfused organ such as the liver may attain high initial concentrations of a xenobiotic. However, chemicals may have a high affinity for a binding site (e.g., intracellular protein or bone matrix) or to a cellular constituent (e.g., fat), and with time, will redistribute to these high affinity sites. For example, although 50% of a dose of lead is found in the liver 2 hours after administration, 1 month later, 90% of the lead remaining in the body is associated with the crystal lattice of bone. Similarly, persistent organic pollutants do not distribute rapidly to fat, but accumulate selectively in adipose tissue over time.

EXCRETION

Toxicants are eliminated from the body by several routes. The kidney is perhaps the most important organ for the excretion of xenobiotics because more chemicals are eliminated from the body by this route than by any other (see Chap. 14). Biotransformation to more water-soluble products is usually a prerequisite to the excretion of xenobiotics through urine (see Chap. 6). The second important route of elimination of many xenobiotics is through feces, and the third, primarily for gases, is through the lungs. Biliary excretion of xenobiotics and/or their metabolites is most often the major source of fecal excretion, but a number of other sources can be significant for some compounds. All body secretions appear to have the ability to excrete chemicals; toxicants have been found in sweat, saliva, tears, and milk.

Figure 5-12. Schematic model showing the transport systems that contribute to the barrier function of the placenta.

Urinary Excretion

The kidney is a very efficient organ for the elimination of toxicants from the body. The functional unit of the kidney is the nephron, comprising the glomerulus, a capillary tuft that initiates the process of filtration of the blood, and tubular elements within the renal cortex and medulla that function to produce and concentrate urine. Toxic compounds are excreted in urine by the same mechanisms the kidney uses to remove the endproducts of intermediary metabolism from the body including glomerular filtration, tubular excretion by passive diffusion, and active tubular secretion. In general, the excretion of small molecular weight (<350 Da), water-soluble compounds is favored in urine.

The kidney receives about 25% of the cardiac output, about 20% of which is filtered at the glomeruli. The glomerular capillaries have large pores (approximately 70 nm) which filter compounds up to a molecular weight of about 60 kDa (smaller than albumin). The degree of plasma protein binding affects the rate of filtration because protein-xenobiotic complexes, particularly those bound to albumin, will not be filtered by the glomerulus. Glomerular filtration rates vary considerably across species, ranging from a high of approximately 10 mL/min/kg in mice to about 1.8 mL/min/kg in humans. This difference appears to be determined by the relative number of nephrons per kilogram of body weight, with mice being the highest (Lin, 1995).

A toxicant filtered at the glomerulus may remain in the tubular lumen and be excreted with urine. Depending on the physicochemical properties of a compound, it may be reabsorbed across the tubular cells of the nephron back into the bloodstream. The principles governing the reabsorption of toxicants across the kidney tubules are the same as those discussed earlier in this chapter for passive diffusion across cell membranes. Thus, toxicants with a high lipid/water partition coefficient are reabsorbed efficiently, whereas polar compounds and ions are excreted with urine. The pH of urine may vary but it is usually slightly acidic (approximately 6–6.5). Just as the Henderson–Hasselbach calculations determine the absorption of nonionized compounds from the GI tract, they also determine urinary excretion. In this case, urinary excretion (i.e., not reabsorbed) of the ionized moiety is favored, such that bases are excreted to a greater extent at lower pH whereas

excretion of acids predominates at higher urinary pH. A practical application of this knowledge is illustrated by the treatment of phenobarbital poisoning with sodium bicarbonate. The percentage of ionization can be increased markedly within physiologically attainable pH ranges for a weak organic acid such as phenobarbital (pK_a 7.2). Consequently, alkalinization of urine by the administration of sodium bicarbonate results in a significant increase in the excretion of phenobarbital. Acceleration of salicylate loss via the kidney can be achieved through the administration of sodium bicarbonate. In a similar manner, urinary acidification can be used to increase the excretion of a weak base like phencyclidine (PCP) in drug abusers.

Toxic agents can also be excreted from plasma into urine by passive diffusion through the tubule. This process is probably of minor significance because filtration is much faster than excretion by passive diffusion through the tubules, providing a favorable concentration gradient for reabsorption rather than excretion. Exceptions to this generalization may be some organic acids ($pK_a \approx 3$–5) and bases ($pK_a \approx 7 - 9$) that would be largely ionized and thus trapped at the pH of urine (pH $\approx$ 6). For renal excretion of such compounds, the flow of urine is likely to be important for the maintenance of a concentration gradient, favoring excretion. Thus, diuretics can hasten the elimination of weak organic acids and bases.

Xenobiotics can also be excreted into urine by active secretion. This process involves the uptake of toxicants from the blood into the cells of the renal proximal tubule, with subsequent efflux from the cell into the tubular fluid from which urine is formed. Figure 5-13 illustrates the various families of transporters expressed in the rodent kidney that are directly involved in xenobiotic disposition. There are numerous other transporters such as specific glucose transporters or nucleotide transporters that play a role predominantly in the flux of endogenous substances which are not presented here. Transporters may be expressed on the lumenal side of the cell where they contribute to tubular secretion and reabsorption, whereas other transporters are localized to the basolateral membranes, serving to transport xenobiotics to and from the circulation and the renal tubular cells. Renal functional activity, as may be altered by toxicant exposure, can also be evaluated by determining the renal clearance of transporter substrates such as the widely used organic anion, p-aminohippurate (PAH).

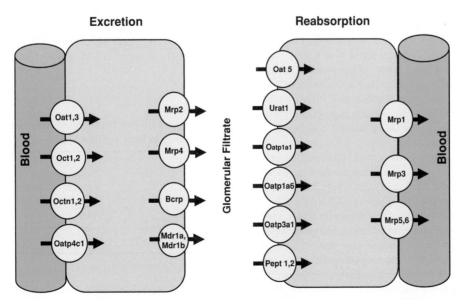

Figure 5-13. Schematic model showing the transport systems in the proximal tubule of the kidney.

Transporters expressed on the basolateral side of the renal tubules include OATs, OCTs, and selected members of the organic anion transporting polypeptides (OATP). The OAT family mediates the renal uptake of organic acids such as PAH and is important in the renal exchange of dicarboxylates. In humans, OAT1, 2, 3 are expressed on the basolateral membrane, whereas OAT4 is localized to the brush border membrane. In rodents, Oat1 and 3 are localized to the basolateral membranes. Although the OATs play an important role in the physiological exchange of metabolites in the kidney, they can also contribute to the development of renal toxicity. In particular, the clinical use of antiviral drugs cidofovir and adefovir is limited by nephrotoxicity that is mediated by the accumulation of these drugs in the proximal tubule by OAT1 (Ho et al., 2000). Oat5 is reported to transport ochratoxin A, and may play a role in the nephrotoxicity associated with exposure to this naturally occurring mycotoxin.

The OCT family is responsible for the renal uptake of some cations, particularly those of low molecular weight. Substrates for OCTs include endogenous compounds such as choline, tetraethylammonium (TEA), and certain cationic drugs including cimetidine and acyclovir. OCT2 is highly expressed in human kidney, whereas Oct1 and 2 are expressed on the basolateral membranes of the rodent kidney (Shitara et al., 2005). A second cation transporter is OCTN, and two isoforms, OCTN1 and 2 are localized to the brush border membranes in human and rodent kidney. Substrates include cations like TEA, and OCTN2 is particularly important in the renal reabsorption of carnitine, which is an essential cofactor for fatty acid β-oxidation.

In kidney, peptide transporters, localized to the brush border membrane of the proximal tubule are important for the reuptake of di- and tripeptides. Two transporters, Pept1 and 2 have been identified in the human and rodent kidney, with Pept1 localized in the upper region of the proximal tubule (pars convoluta) and Pept2 expressed in the lower region (pars recta) of the convoluted tubule.

P-gp, MRP2, and MRP4 are also found on the luminal brush border of the proximal tubule, where they contribute to the efflux of xenobiotics out of the cells and into the tubular fluid, thereby enhancing excretion. Mrp1 is also expressed in the rodent kidney, but it is primarily found in the epithelial cells of the loop of Henle and the collecting ducts, whereas in humans, MRP1 has been detected in the glomerulus. In Mrp1$^{(-/-)}$ null mice, the anticancer drug VP-16 causes polyuria indicative of damage to the collecting duct, suggesting that Mrp1 is likely to be involved in the clearance of the compound from the kidney (Wijnholds et al., 1998). Finally, Bcrp is expressed at high levels in the rat and mouse kidney, where it is localized to the apical brush border of the proximal tubule epithelium. This transporter appears to play an important role in the efflux of certain sulfate conjugates of xenobiotics. In contrast, BCRP has not been detected in the human kidney, suggesting that species differences in the urinary excretion of sulfated compounds could occur.

As in all active transport systems, there is competition for renal secretion of xenobiotics. This fact was taken advantage of during World War II, when penicillin was in short supply. Penicillin is actively secreted by the organic acid systems (OATs) of the kidney. To lengthen its half-life and duration of action, another acid was sought to compete with penicillin for renal secretion, and probenecid was successfully introduced for this purpose. Uric acid is also secreted actively by renal tubules, and a unique member of the OAT family, the urate transporter (URAT1) is expressed only in the kidney where it functions specifically as a mechanism for reabsorption of urate.

Various uricosuric agents, including probenecid and phenylbutazone inhibit URAT1 to facilitate the excretion of uric acid from the body.

Because many functions of the kidney are incompletely developed at birth, some xenobiotics are eliminated more slowly in newborns than in adults, and therefore may be more toxic to newborns. For example, the clearance of penicillin by premature infants is only about 20% of that observed in older children. In general, the OATs is not fully developed at birth, but its development can be stimulated by the administration of substances normally excreted by this system (Hirsch and Hook, 1970). Some compounds, such as cephaloridine, are known to be nephrotoxic in adult animals but not in newborns. Because active uptake of cephaloridine by the kidneys is not well developed in newborns, this chemical is not concentrated in the tubules and consequently is not nephrotoxic. If the development of active transport in newborns is stimulated, the kidneys take up cephaloridine more readily and nephrotoxicity is observed (Wold et al., 1977).

The renal proximal tubule reabsorbs small plasma proteins that are filtered at the glomerulus. This largely occurs by pinocytosis at the brush border membrane of the proximal tubule epithelium. If a toxicant binds to those small proteins, it can be carried into the proximal tubule cells and exert toxicity. As discussed previously, cadmium bound to metallothionein is readily taken up by the kidney and is the major cause of Cd-induced nephrotoxicity (Klaassen and Liu, 1997). Similarly, chemicals such as limonene and 2,4,4-trimethyl pentane bind to the male-rat-specific protein, α_{2u}-globulin, and are taken up by the proximal tubule to produce hyaline droplet nephropathy and eventually renal tumors in male rats (Lehman-McKeeman, 1997).

Species differences in regard to the urinary excretion of weak organic acids and bases are observed frequently, as the pH of urine varies widely among species. Differences in renal clearance also can occur for compounds filtered at the glomeruli because of differences in plasma protein binding. Similarly, differences in xenobiotic transporter expression, regulation, and function can contribute to differences in the renal excretion of toxicants.

Additional factors affecting the excretion of xenobiotics are exemplified by the disposition of griseofulvin in rats and rabbits (Table 5-11). Rabbits metabolize griseofulvin to 6-demethylgriseofulvin (a phase-I metabolite), a low-molecular weight species that is predominantly excreted in urine. In contrast, rats metabolize griseofulvin to many conjugates (phase-II metabolites) which are higher molecular weight species (>350) that are preferentially excreted in bile. In this example, species differences

Table 5-11

Urinary and Biliary Excretion of Griseofulvin and/or Metabolites in Rats and Rabbits

	RATS*		RABBITS*	
	URINE	BILE	URINE	BILE
Total	12	77	78	11
Phase I metabolites	ND†	23	70	3
Phase II metabolites	ND	54	8	8

*Expressed as percent of dose.
†ND, not determined.
SOURCE: Modified from Symchowicz et al. (1967), with permission.

in biotransformation ultimately determine the route of excretion of griseofulvin.

Fecal Excretion

Fecal excretion is the other major pathway for the elimination of xenobiotics from the body. Fecal excretion of chemicals is a complex process that is not as well understood as urinary excretion. Several important sources and many more minor sources contribute to the excretion of toxicants via the feces.

Nonabsorbed Ingesta In addition to undigested material, varying proportions of nutrients and xenobiotics that are present in food or are ingested voluntarily (drugs) pass through the alimentary canal unabsorbed, contributing to fecal excretion. The physicochemical properties of xenobiotics and the biological characteristics that facilitate absorption were discussed earlier in this chapter. Although most chemicals are lipophilic to some extent and thereby available for absorption, it is rare for 100% of a compound to be absorbed. At the same time, some macromolecules and some essentially completely ionized compounds of higher molecular weight are not absorbed at all. For example, the absorption of polymers or quaternary ammonium bases is quite limited in the intestine. Consequently, most of a dose of orally administered sucrose polyester, cholestyramine, or paraquat can be found in feces. Therefore, the nonabsorbed portion of xenobiotics contributes to the fecal excretion of most chemicals to some extent. One other factor contributing to fecal excretion is intestinal secretion, which likely occurs by passive diffusion out of enterocytes or via exfoliation of intestinal cells during the normal turnover of this epithelium.

Biliary Excretion The biliary route of elimination is perhaps the most significant source contributing to the fecal excretion of xenobiotics and is even more important for the excretion of metabolites. The liver plays an important role in removing toxic chemicals from blood after absorption from the GI tract, because blood from the GI tract passes via the portal circulation through the liver before reaching the general circulation. A compound can be extracted by the liver, thereby preventing its distribution to other parts of the body. The liver is also the main site for biotransformation of toxicants, and metabolites may be excreted directly into bile. In this manner, the liver can remove xenobiotics and their metabolites before entering the general circulation (Fig. 5-14). Furthermore, xenobiotics and/or their metabolites excreted into bile enter the intestine and may be excreted with feces. However, if the physicochemical properties favor reabsorption, an enterohepatic circulation may ensue (discussed below).

The biliary excretion of two organic acids, sulfobromophthalein (BSP) and indocyanine green (ICG), is used to evaluate liver function. This diagnostic test is performed by injecting either BSP or ICG intravenously and determining its disappearance from plasma. A lack of proper plasma clearance of BSP or ICG indicates reduced biliary excretion, suggesting liver dysfunction or injury.

Toxic chemicals bound to plasma proteins are fully available for active biliary excretion. The factors that determine whether a chemical will be excreted into bile or into urine are not fully understood. However, as a general rule, low-molecular-weight compounds (<325) are poorly excreted into bile whereas compounds or their conjugates with molecular weights exceeding about 325 can be excreted in appreciable quantities. Glutathione and glucuronide conjugates have a high predilection for excretion into bile, but there are marked species differences in the biliary excretion of foreign compounds with consequences for the biological half-life of a compound and its toxicity (Klaassen *et al.*, 1981). Table 5-12 provides examples of species differences in biliary excretion, and demonstrates that species variation in biliary excretion is also compound specific. It is therefore difficult to categorize species into "good" or "poor" biliary excretors but, in general, rats and mice tend to be better biliary excretors than are other species (Klaassen and Watkins, 1984).

Foreign compounds excreted into bile are often divided into three classes on the basis of the ratio of their concentration in bile versus that in plasma. Class A substances have a ratio of nearly 1

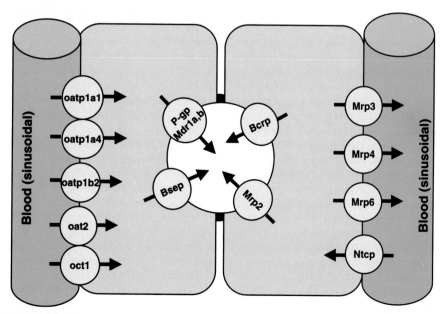

Figure 5-14. Schematic model showing the xenobiotic transporting systems present in the liver.

Table 5-12
Biliary Excretion of Xenobiotic Conjugates Across Species

	INDOCYANINE GREEN	PHENOLPHTHALEIN GLUCURONIDE	SULFADIMETHYOXINE n-GLUCURONIDE	STILBESTROL GLUCURONIDE
Molecular Wt	775	495	487	445
% EXCRETED IN BILE				
Rat	82	54	43	95
Dog	97	81	43	65
Rabbit	97	13	10	32
Guinea pig	Not done	6	12	20

SOURCE: Data modified from Lin (1995).

and include sodium, potassium, glucose, mercury, thallium, cesium, and cobalt. Class B substances have a ratio of bile to plasma greater than 1 (usually between 10 and 1000). Class B substances include bile acids, bilirubin, SBP, lead, arsenic, manganese, and many other xenobiotics. Class C substances have a ratio below 1 (e.g., inulin, albumin, zinc, iron, gold, and chromium). Compounds rapidly excreted into bile are usually class B substances. However, a compound does not have to be highly concentrated in bile for biliary excretion to be of quantitative importance. For example, mercury is not concentrated in bile, yet bile is the main route of excretion for this slowly eliminated substance.

Biliary excretion is regulated predominantly by xenobiotic transporters present on the canalicular membrane. Transporters present on the sinusoidal membranes of hepatocytes also contribute to hepatic uptake and efflux, and thereby contribute to hepatobiliary clearance of xenobiotics. There are four known transporters expressed on the canalicular membrane that are directly involved in biliary excretion. These include P-gp, Mrp2, BCRp, and BSEP. P-gp, Mrp2, and Bcrp are important in the biliary excretion of many xenobiotics, whereas BS is critical for the secretion of bile and the regulation of bile flow. Mrp2 is extremely important in biliary excretion because it is largely responsible for the transport of organic anions including the glucuronide and glutathione conjugates of many xenobiotics. BCRP has particular affinity for sulfated conjugates of toxicants, whereas P-gp primarily transports cationic substrates into bile.

The important contribution of Mrp2 to biliary excretion of toxicants was established in part by the characterization of two naturally occurring mutant strains of rat, the Groningen/Yellow transport deficient (TR^-) and the Eisai hyperbilirubinemic rat (EHBR), both of which lack functional Mrp2 protein. These rats are phenotypically similar to humans suffering from Dubin–Johnson syndrome, a rare inherited disorder associated with mutations in MRP2 and characterized by chronic conjugated hyperbilirubinemia. The mutant rats also present with conjugated hyperbilirubinemia, show reduced biliary excretion of glutathione, and are defective in the normal biliary excretion of glucuronide and glutathione conjugates of many xenobiotics. An $Mrp2^{-/-}$ null mouse has been developed, and like its mutant rat counterparts, shows marked reductions in bile flow, biliary glutathione concentrations, and reduced ability to eliminate xenobiotics. For example, plasma levels of the food-derived carcinogen, PhIp, was increased 1.9-fold in $Mrp2^{-/-}$ null mice compared to wild-type controls, demonstrating that functional Mrp2 plays a role in reducing exposure to toxic chemicals (Vlaming et al., 2006). Finally, species differences in Mrp2 function may contribute to the qualitative differences observed across species in biliary excretion. In a direct comparison of the transport of 2,4-dinitrophenyl-S-glutathione (DNP-SG) across canalicular membrane vesicles from various species, clearance (μL/min/mg protein) ranged from a high rate of 64.2 in rats to a low of 3.8 in humans, with intermediate values for other species including mouse, guinea pig, rabbit, and dog (Ishizuka et al., 1999). Such differences are likely to contribute to the observed species differences in biliary excretion illustrated in Table 5-12.

Although the highest levels of Bcrp are found in the placenta, the transporter is expressed on the bile canalicular membrane of hepatocytes where it preferentially transports sulfate conjugates of xenobiotics. Known substrates for BCRP include estrone 3-sulfate and 4-methylembelliferone sulfate and methotrexate. P-gp is important in the biliary elimination of compounds such as doxorubicin and vinblastine.

The biliary excretion of xenobiotics mediated by Mrp2, Bcrp, and P-gp usually results in increased excretion of toxicants out of hepatocytes and into bile. In doing so, these transporters increase excretion of xenobiotics and generally limit the likelihood of toxicity in the liver. However, adverse reactions can occur if the function of these transporters is inhibited, as evidenced by the examples illustrated above for the genetic mutant or knockout models. Furthermore, although BSEP does not appear to play a major role in the excretion of xenobiotics, some compounds can inhibit the function of this transporter, thereby decreasing the biliary excretion of bile acids and leading to cholestasis (defined as a decrease in bile flow with increased serum bilirubin) and cholestatic liver injury (Arrese and Ananthanarayanan, 2004). For example, inhibition of BSEP by the pharmaceutical agent, troglitazone, and to a much greater extent, troglitazone sulfate, competitively inhibits BSEP function, leading to intrahepatic cholestasis, which may contribute to the hepatotoxicity of troglitazone. Furthermore, inhibition of BSEP contributes to the cholestasis observed with steroids such as estradiol.

Although the transporters located on the canalicular membrane are directly responsible for biliary excretion of xenobiotics, other xenobiotic transporters localized to the sinusoidal membranes are also important in determining hepatic concentrations of toxicants and thereby contribute to hepatic disposition and biliary elimination. Transporters present on rat sinusoidal membranes include the ABC transport family members, Mrp3, Mrp4, and Mrp6, along with Oatps, Oats, and Oct. The Na^+/taurocholate cotransporting polypeptide (NCTP) is also found on the sinusoidal membrane where it functions in the uptake of bile acids into the liver.

Mrp3 transports many of the same organic anions that are substrates for Mrp2 from the liver into the blood circulation. It has recently been shown to be important in the excretion of acetaminophen- and morphine glucuronide conjugates from liver into blood (Borst *et al.*, 2006). In humans, it is upregulated during cholestasis and in patients with Dubin–Johnson syndrome, and in a similar manner, it is increased in TR⁻ and EHBR rats. The increase in Mrp3 is recognized as a compensatory response that helps to protect hepatocytes from toxic chemicals for cells deficient in Mrp2. Mrp4 is specifically involved in the cellular efflux of purine analogs, nucleoside antiviral drugs, and cyclic nucleotides, including cAMP and cGMP. It has also been shown to be a carrier for some xenobiotics including conjugated and unconjugated compounds (Borst *et al.*, 2006). A major role for Mrp6 in xenobiotic disposition has not been established, but mutations in human MRP6 are associated with pseudoxanthoma elasticum, a hereditary disease affecting the elasticity of connective tissues (Bergen *et al.*, 2007).

Several Oatps are located on the basolateral membrane of hepatocytes where they contribute to the uptake of many organic anions. The Oatps exhibit broad substrate specificity and play an important role in the hepatic uptake of numerous drugs and xenobiotics along with a variety of hormones, including thyroxin, and hormone conjugates. Oat2 is expressed in liver and transports small organic anions such as indomethacin and salicylate along with prostaglandins (Anzai *et al.*, 2006). Oct1 is also expressed in human and rodent liver, and contributes to the uptake of organic cations. This includes numerous endogenous compounds such as choline and dopamine as well as cationic xenobiotics. It has recently been shown that the biguanide compound, metformin, which is used to treat type 2 diabetes, is a substrate for OCT1. Metformin can cause lactic acidosis through alterations in mitochondrial function, and Oct1$^{-/-}$ knockout mice are generally resistant to lactic acidosis compared to wild-type mice (Wang *et al.*, 2003), suggesting an important role for this transporter in the elimination and toxic potential of this compound. In concert, the Oatps, OAT, and OCT family of transporters are important in the uptake of toxicants into the liver, a step that can contribute to metabolism in the liver or efflux into the bile, or back into the circulation. Overall, these uptake transporters are important in determining the distribution to and excretion from the liver.

An important concept relating to biliary excretion is the phenomenon of enterohepatic circulation. After a compound is excreted into bile, it enters the intestine where it can be reabsorbed or eliminated with feces. Many organic compounds are conjugated with UDP-glucuronic acid, sulfate, or glutathione (see Chap. 6) before excretion into bile, and these polar metabolites are not sufficiently lipid-soluble to be reabsorbed. However, enzymes found in the intestinal microflora may hydrolyze glucuronide and sulfate conjugates, liberating a more lipophilic moiety and increasing the likelihood of reabsorption. Reabsorption of the liberated xenobiotic completes a cycle in which the compound can return to the liver, where it can again be metabolized and excreted back into bile. Repeated enterohepatic cycling may lead to very long half-lives of xenobiotics in the body. Therefore, it is often desirable to interrupt this cycle to hasten the elimination of a toxicant from the body. This principle has been utilized in the treatment of dimethylmercury poisoning; ingestion of a polythiol resin binds the mercury and thus prevents its reabsorption (Magos and Clarkson, 1976).

An increase in hepatic excretory function also has been observed after pretreatment with some drugs (Klaassen and Watkins, 1984). For example, it has been demonstrated that phenobarbital increases plasma disappearance of BSP by enhancing its biliary excretion. The increase in bile flow caused by phenobarbital is an important factor in increasing the biliary excretion of BSP. However, other factors, including induction of phase-II enzymes (see Chap. 6) and xenobiotic transporters may also enhance biliary elimination. Induction of metabolizing enzymes and transporters work in concert to increase the clearance of a toxicant from the plasma. In particular, induction of these processes increases the capacity for a xenobiotic to be: (1) taken up into the liver; (2) metabolized to conjugates that are likely to be excreted into bile; and (3) excreted into bile and removed from the general circulation. However, not all microsomal enzyme inducers increase bile flow and excretion, as agents such as 3-methylcholanthrene and benzo[a]pyrene are relatively ineffective in this regard.

An increase in biliary excretion often decreases the toxicity of xenobiotics. For example, in laboratory animals, phenobarbital treatment enhances the biliary excretion and elimination of methylmercury from the body (Magos and Clarkson, 1976). Two steroidal agents, spironolactone and pregnenolone-16α-carbonitrile, which also increase bile production and enhance biliary excretion of BSP, decrease the toxicity of cardiac glycosides at least in part by increasing their biliary excretion. This in turn decreases the concentration of cardiac glycosides in the heart, their target organ of toxicity (Castle and Lage, 1973; Klaassen, 1974).

The toxicity of some compounds can also be directly related to their biliary excretion. For example, the intestinal toxicity of several xenobiotics and drugs is increased by their excretion into bile. This is the case for nonsteroidal anti-inflammatory drugs which cause intestinal ulcerations that can be abolished by bile-duct ligation (Duggan *et al.*, 1975). More recently, irinotecan, an anticancer drug, was found to induce severe GI toxicity (severe diarrhea) in humans and rats. The mechanism for the effect of this drug involved metabolism to an active metabolite that was a good substrate for Mrp2. The excretion into bile mediated by Mrp2 results in high concentrations of the toxic metabolite in the intestinal lumen and

Table 5-13

Urinary, Biliary, and Fecal Excretion of Indomethacin and/or its Metabolites in Dogs and Monkeys after Intravenous Dosage

	URINE		BILE		FECES	
COMPOUND	DOG	MONKEY	DOG	MONKEY	DOG	MONKEY
Indomethacin	0.6*	10.5	3.8	33.6	68.7	4
Phase I metabolites	4.1	24.2	NI†	NI	2.7	6
Phase II metabolites	3.3	17.9	52.1	8.1	3.1	NI
Total dose excreted	7.9	52.7	55.9	51.7	76.3	10

*Values represent % of dose excreted.

†NI, not identified or very small amounts.

SOURCE: Modified from Hucker *et al.* (1966) and Yesair *et al.* (1970), with permission.

toxicity ensues. The toxicity of irinotecan can be modulated by inhibiting Mrp2 function (Chu *et al.*, 1997).

Many xenobiotic transporters are not expressed early in development, and the hepatic excretory system is not fully developed in newborns. As a result, there are numerous examples of compounds that are more toxic to newborns than to adults (Klaassen and Slitt, 2005). For example, ouabain is about 40 times more toxic in newborn than in adult rats. This is due to an almost complete inability of the newborn rat liver to remove ouabain from plasma. The development of hepatic excretory function can be promoted in newborns by administering microsomal enzyme inducers.

Often the elimination of a compound occurs by different routes in different species, as shown in the case of indomethacin in the dog and the rhesus monkey (Table 5-13). Dogs excrete most of a dose in feces, whereas monkeys excrete the majority of a dose in urine. Both species excrete similarly large quantities of a dose in bile. Because dogs excrete most of a dose in bile as conjugates (MW > 500 Da), it is to be expected that these hydrophilic indomethacin derivatives will not be reabsorbed unless they are hydrolyzed by intestinal bacteria to the reabsorbable parent compound, or to phase-I metabolites (which do have good bioavailability). Based on available experimental data, it is not possible to determine whether this occurs in dogs. It appears that indomethacin undergoes enterohepatic circulation with repeated conjugation in the liver and deconjugation in the small intestine, with a gradual "loss" of conjugates into the large intestine. However, because almost all of fecal excretion consists of indomethacin, it is apparent that the large intestinal flora hydrolyzes the indomethacin conjugates. Limited reabsorption of indomethacin is not surprising ($pK_a \approx 4.5$, colon pH ≈ 8), because more than 99.7% of indomethacin is ionized in the large intestine, which has a small surface area (compared to the small intestine). This does not allow for a sufficiently rapid shift in the mass balance to result in substantial reabsorption.

Monkeys also have extensive enterohepatic recycling of indomethacin (51.7% of dose excreted in bile within 2 hours). However, most of the biliary excretion consists of parent compound, which is readily reabsorbed in the small intestine, as indicated by the small amount lost into feces (about 10% of dose). In contrast to dogs, monkeys excrete most of a dose as phase-I metabolites (24.2% of dose) and indomethacin (10.5% of dose). Because indomethacin has a molecular weight of 358 and phase-I metabolites have molecular weights of 220–345, these compounds are more readily excreted in urine.

Exhalation

Substances that exist predominantly in the gas phase at body temperature are eliminated mainly by the lungs. Because volatile liquids are in equilibrium with their gas phase in the alveoli, they may also be excreted via the lungs. The amount of a liquid eliminated via the lungs is proportional to its vapor pressure. A practical application of this principle is seen in the breath analyzer test for determining the amount of ethanol in the body. Highly volatile liquids such as diethyl ether and certain volatile anesthetics (nitrous oxide) are excreted almost exclusively by the lungs.

No specialized transport systems have been described for the excretion of toxic substances by the lungs. Some xenobiotic transporters, including Mrp1 and P-gp, have been identified in the lung, but overall, compounds excreted via exhalation in the lung are most likely to be eliminated by simple diffusion. Elimination of gases is roughly inversely proportional to the rate of their absorption. Therefore, gases with low solubility in blood, such as ethy-lene, are rapidly excreted, whereas chloroform, which has a much higher solubility in blood, is eliminated very slowly by the lungs. Trace concentrations of highly lipid-soluble anesthetic gases such as halothane and methoxyflurane may be present in expired air for as long as 2–3 weeks after a few hours of anesthesia. Undoubtedly, this prolonged retention is due to deposition in and slow mobilization from adipose tissue of these very lipid-soluble agents. The rate of elimination of a gas with low solubility in blood is perfusion-limited, whereas that of a gas with high solubility in blood is ventilation-limited.

Other Routes of Elimination

Cerebrospinal Fluid A specialized route of removal of toxic agents from a specific organ is represented by the cerebrospinal fluid (CSF). All compounds can leave the CNS with the bulk flow of CSF through the arachnoid villi. In addition, lipid-soluble toxicants also can exit at the site of the blood–brain barrier. As discussed earlier, toxicants also can be removed from the CSF by active transport, using the transport systems present in the BCSFB.

Milk The secretion of toxic compounds into milk is extremely important because (1) a toxic material may be passed with milk from the mother to the nursing offspring and (2) compounds can be passed from cows to people via dairy products. Toxic agents are excreted into milk by simple diffusion. Because milk has an acidic pH (about 6.5), basic compounds may be concentrated in milk, whereas acidic compounds may attain lower concentrations in milk than in plasma (Findlay, 1983; Wilson, 1983). More important, about 3–4% of milk consists of lipids, and the lipid content of colostrum after parturition is even higher. Lipid-soluble xenobiotics diffuse along with fats from plasma into the mammary glands and are excreted with milk during lactation. Many of the same compounds that can accumulate in fat such as aldrin, chlordane, DDT, and polychlorinated and polybrominated biphenyls, dibenzo-*p*-dioxins, and furans (Van den Berg *et al.*, 1987; Li *et al.*, 1995) have been found in human breast milk, and milk can be a major route of their excretion. More recently, other persistent compounds such as nitromusk perfume ingredients have been identified in milk, but it is unclear as to whether the presence of these compounds is directly responsible for possible adverse effects (Leibl *et al.*, 2000). Species differences in the excretion of xenobiotics with milk are to be expected, as the proportion of milk fat derived from the circulation versus that synthesized de novo in the mammary gland differs widely among species. Metals chemically similar to calcium, such as lead, and chelating agents that form complexes with calcium also can be excreted into milk to a considerable extent.

Sweat and Saliva The excretion of toxic agents in sweat and saliva is quantitatively of minor importance. Again, excretion depends on the diffusion of the nonionized, lipid-soluble form of an agent. Toxic compounds excreted into sweat may produce dermatitis. Substances excreted in saliva enter the mouth, where they are usually swallowed to become available for GI absorption.

CONCLUSION

Humans are in continuous contact with toxic chemicals. Toxicants are in the food we eat, the water we drink, and the air we breathe. Depending on their physical and chemical properties, toxic chemicals may be absorbed by the GI tract, the lungs, and/or the skin. Fortunately, the body has the ability to biotransform and excrete these

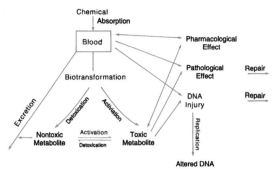

Figure 5-15. Schematic representation of the disposition and toxic effects of chemicals.

compounds into urine, feces, and air. However, when the rate of absorption exceeds the rate of elimination, toxic compounds may accumulate and reach a critical concentration at a certain target site, and toxicity may ensue (Fig. 5-15). Whether a chemical elicits toxicity depends not only on its inherent potency and site specificity but also on whether, and if so how, it is absorbed, distributed, and eliminated.

Therefore, knowledge of the disposition of chemicals is of great importance in judging the toxicity of xenobiotics. For example, for a potent CNS suppressant that displays a strong hepatic first-pass effect, oral exposure is of less concern than is exposure by inhalation. Also, two equipotent gases, with the absorption of one being perfusion rate-limited and that of the other being ventilation rate-limited, will exhibit completely different toxicity profiles at a distant site because of differences in the concentrations attained in the target organ.

Many chemicals have very low inherent toxicity but can be metabolically activated into toxic metabolites, and toxicity may be determined by the rate of formation of toxic metabolites. Alternatively, a very potent toxicant may be detoxified rapidly by biotransformation. The fundamental and overarching concept is that adverse effects are related to the unbound concentration of the "toxic chemical" at the site of action (in the target organ), whether a chemical is administered or generated by biotransformation in the target tissue or at a distant site. Accordingly, the toxic response exerted by chemicals is critically influenced by the rates of absorption, distribution, biotransformation, and excretion.

REFERENCES

Ambudkar SV, Dey S, Hrycyna CA, Ramachandra M, Pastan I, Gottesman MM: Biochemical, cellular and pharmacological aspects of the multidrug transporter. *Annu Rev Pharmacol Toxicol* 39:361–398, 1999.

Anzai N, Kanai Y, Endou H: Organic anion transporter family: Current knowledge. *J Pharmacol Sci* 100:411–426, 2006.

Arrese M, Ananthanarayanan M: The bile salt export pump: Molecular properties, function and regulation. *Pflugers Arch* 449:123–131, 2004.

Aungst B, Shen DD: Gastrointestinal absorption of toxic agents, in Rozman K, Hanninen O (eds.): *Gastrointestinal Toxicology.* Amsterdam/New York/Oxford: Elsevier, 1986, pp. 29–56.

Ballard ST, Hunter JH, Taylor AE: Regulation of tight-junction permeability during nutrient absorption across the intestinal epithelium. *Annu Rev Nutr* 15:35–55, 1995.

Baron JM, Holler D, Schiffer R, *et al.*: Expression of multiple cytochrome P450 enzymes and multidrug resistance-associated transport proteins in human skin keratinocytes. *J Invest Dermatol* 116:541–548, 2001.

Benz R, Janko K, Länger P: Pore formation by the matrix protein (porin) to *Escherichia coli* in planar bilayer membranes. *Ann NY Acad Sci* 358:13–24, 1980.

Bergen AA, Plomp AS, Hu X, deJong PT, Gorgels TG: ABCC6 and pseudoxanthoma elasticum. *Pflugers Arch* 453:685–691, 2007.

Bogdanffy MS, Manning LA, Sarangapani R: High-affinity nasal extraction of vinyl acetate vapor is carboxylesterase dependent. *Inhal Toxicol* 11:927–941, 1999.

Borowitz JL, Moore PF, Him GKW, Miya TS: Mechanism of enhanced drug effects produced by dilution of the oral dose. *Toxicol Appl Pharmacol* 19:164–168, 1971.

Borst P, Zelcer N, van de Wetering K: MRP2 and 3 in health and disease. *Cancer Lett* 234:51–61, 2006.

Boyes RN, Adams HJ, Duce BR: Oral absorption and disposition kinetics of lidocaine hydrochloride in dogs. *J Pharmacol Exp Ther* 174:1–8, 1970.

Bronaugh RL, Stewart RF, Congdon ER, Giles AL, Jr: Methods for in vitro percutaneous absorption studies. I. Comparison with in vivo results. *Toxicol Appl Pharmacol* 62:474–480, 1982.

Calabrese EJ: Gastrointestinal and dermal absorption: Interspecies differences. *Drug Metab Rev* 15:1013–1032, 1984.

Castle MC, Lage GL: Enhanced biliary excretion of digitoxin following spironolactone as it relates to the prevention of digitoxin toxicity. *Res Commun Chem Pathol Pharmacol* 5:99–108, 1973.

Cayen MN: Metabolic disposition of antihyperlipidemic agents in man and laboratory animals. *Drug Metab Rev* 11:291–323, 1980.

Chu XY, Kato Y, Niinuma K, Sudo KI, Hakusui H, Sugiyama Y: Multispecific organic anion transporter (cMOAT) is responsible for the biliary excretion of the camptothecin derivative irinotecan, CPT-11 and its metabolites in rats. *J Pharmacol Exp Ther* 281:304–314, 1997.

Clarkson TW: Metal toxicity in the central nervous system. *Environ Health Perspect* 75:59–64, 1987.

Dantzig AH, Duckworth DC, Tabas LB: Transport mechanisms responsible for the absorption of loracarbef, cefixime, and cefuroxime axetil into human intestinal Caco-2 cells. *Biochem Biophys Acta* 1191:7–13, 1994.

Dean M, Rzhetsy A, Allikmets R: The human ATP-binding cassette (ABC) transporter superfamily. *Genome Res* 11:1156–1166, 2001.

deLange ECM: Potential role of ABC transporter as a detoxification system at the blood–CSF barrier. *Ad Drug Delivery Rev* 56:1793–1809, 2004.

Dietrich CG, Rudi de Waart D, Ottenhoff R, Schoots IG, Oude Elferink RPJ: Increased bioavailability of the food-derived carcinoge 2-amino-1-methyl-6-phenylimidazo[4,5]pyridine in MRP2-deficient rats. *Mol Pharmacol* 59:974–980, 2001.

Diwan BA, Riggs CW, Logsdon D, *et al.*: Multiorgan transplacental and neonatal carcinogenicity of 3′-axido-3′-deoxythymidine in mice. *Toxicol Appl Pharmacol* 161:82–99, 1999.

Dowling RH: Compensatory changes in intestinal absorption. *Br Med Bull* 23:275–278, 1967.

Draize JH, Woodard G, Calvery HO: Methods for the study of irritation and toxicity of substances applied topically to the skin and mucous membranes. *J Pharmacol Exp Ther* 82:377–390, 1944.

Dreyfuss J, Shaw JM, Ross JJ: Absorption of the adrenergic-blocking agent, nadol, by mice, rats, hamsters, rabbits, dogs, monkeys and man: Unusual species differences. *Xenobiotica* 8:503–510, 1978.

Dugard PH: Skin permeability theory in relation to measurements of percutaneous absorption in toxicology, in Marzulli FN, Maibach HI (eds.): *Dermatotoxicology,* 2nd ed. Washington/New York/London: Hemisphere, 1983, pp. 91–116.

Dugard PH, Embery G: The influence of dimethylsulphoxide on the percutaneous migration of potassium butyl [^{35}S]sulphate, potassium methyl [^{35}S]sulphate and sodium [^{35}S]sulphate. *Br J Dermtol* 81(Suppl 4):69–74, 1969.

Duggan DE, Hooke KF, Noll RM, Kwan KC: Enterohepatic circulation of indomethacin and its role in intestinal irritation. *Biochem Pharmacol* 24:1749–1754, 1975.

Evans AM: Influence of dietary components on the gastrointestinal metabolism and transport of drug. *Ther Drug Monit* 22:131–136, 2000.

Findlay JWA: The distribution of some commonly used drugs in human breast milk. *Drug Metab Rev* 14:653–686, 1983.

Flanagan PR, Haist J, Valberg LS: Comparative effects of iron deficiency induced by bleeding and low-iron diet on the intestinal absorptive interactions of iron, cobalt, manganese, zinc, lead and calcium. *J Nutr* 110:1754–1763, 1980.

Florence AT, Hillery AM, Hussain N, Jani PU: Factors affecting the oral uptake and translocation of polystyrene nanoparticles: Histological and analytical evidence. *J Drug Target* 3:65–70, 1995.

Fullmer CS: Intestinal interactions of lead and calcium. *Neurotoxicology* 13:799–807, 1992.

Ganapathy V, Prasad PD, Ganapathy ME, Leibach FH: Placental transporters relevant to drug disposition across the maternal-fetal interface. *J Pharmacol Exp Ther* 294:413–420, 2000.

Ginsburg J: Placental drug transfer. *Annu Rev Pharmacol* 11:387–408, 1971.

Hagenbuch B, Meier PJ: Organic anion transporting polypeptides of the OATP/SLC21 family: Phylogenetic classification as OATP/SLCO superfamily, new nomenclature and molecular/functional properties. *Pflugers Arch* 447:653–665, 2004.

Hediger MA, Romero MF, Peng J-B, Rolfs A, Takanaga H, Bruford EA: The ABCs of solute carriers: Physiological, pathological and therapeutic implications of human membrane transport proteins. *Pflugers Arch* 447:465–468, 2004.

Hirsch GH, Hook JB: Maturation of renal organic acid transport substrate stimulation by penicillin and *p*-aminohippurate (PAH). *J Pharmacol Exp Ther* 171:103–108, 1970.

Ho ES, Lin DC, Mendel DB, Cihlar T: Cytotoxicity of antiviral nucleotides adefovir and cidofovir induced by the expression of the human renal organic anion transporter I. *J Am Soc Nephrol* 11:383–393, 2000.

Houston JB, Upshall DG, Bridges JW: A re-evaluation of the importance of partition coefficients in the gastrointestinal absorption of nutrients. *J Pharmacol Exp Ther* 189:244–254, 1974.

Hucker HB, Hutt JE, White SD, et al.: Studies on the absorption, distribution and excretion of indomethacin in various species. *J Pharmacol Exp Ther* 153:237–249, 1966.

Ishizuka H, Donno K, Shiina T, et al.: Species differences in the transport activity for organic anions across the bile canalicular membrane. *J Pharmacol Exp Ther* 290:1324–1330, 1999.

Jandacek RJ, Tso P: Factors affecting the storage and excretion of toxic lipophilic xenobiotics. *Lipids* 36:1289–1305, 2001.

Jani P, Halbert GW, Langridge J, Florence AT: Nanoparticle uptake by the rat gastrointestinal mucosa: Quantitation and particle size dependency. *J Pharm Pharmacol* 42:821–826, 1990.

Kao J, Patterson FU, Hall J: Skin penetration and metabolism of topically applied chemicals in six mammalian species, including man: An *in vitro* study with benzo(a)pyrene and testosterone. *Toxicol Appl Pharmacol* 81:502–516, 1985.

Kerns WD, Pavkov KL, Donofrio DJ, Gralla EJ, Swenberg JA: Carcinogenicity of formaldehyde in rats and mice after long-term inhalation exposure. *Cancer Res* 43:4382–4392, 1983.

Klaassen CD: Effect of microsomal enzyme inducers on the biliary excretion of cardiac glycosides. *J Pharmacol Exp Ther* 191:201–211, 1974.

Klaassen CD, Eaton DL, Cagen SZ: Hepatobiliary disposition of xenobiotics, in Bridges JW, Chasseaud LF (eds.): *Progress in Drug Metabolism*. New York: Wiley, 1981, pp. 1–75.

Klaassen CD, Liu J: Role of metallothionein in cadmium-induced hepatotoxicity and nephrotoxicity. *Drug Metab Rev* 29:79–102, 1997.

Klaassen CD, Shoeman DW: Biliary excretion of lead in rats, rabbits and dogs. *Toxicol Appl Pharmacol* 29:434–446, 1974.

Klaassen CD, Watkins JB: Mechanisms of bile formation, hepatic uptake, and biliary excretion. *Pharmacol Rev* 36:1–67, 1984.

Klaassen CD, Slitt AL: Regulation of hepatic transporters by xenobiotic receptors. *Curr Drug Metab* 6: 309–328, 2005.

Lankas GR, Cartwright ME, Umbenhauer D: P-glycoprotein deficiency in a subpopulation of CF-1 mice enhances avermectin-induced neurotoxicity. *Toxicol Appl Pharmacol* 143:357–365, 1997.

Lankas GR, Wise LD, Cartwright ME, et al.: Placental p-glycoprotein deficiency enhances susceptibility to chemically induced birth defects in mice. *Reprod Toxicol* 12:457–463, 1998.

Lehman-McKeeman LDL: α2u-globulin nephropathy, in Sipes IG, McQueen CA, Gandolfi AJ (eds.): *Comprehensive Toxicology*. New York: Elsevier, 1997, pp. 693–692.

Lehman-McKeeman LD, Johnson DR, Caudill D: Induction and inhibition of mouse cytochrome P450 2B enzymes by musk xylene. *Toxicol Appl Pharmacol* 142:169–177, 1997.

Leibl B, Mayer R, Ommer S, Sonnichsen C, Koletzko B: Transition of nitro musks and polycyclic musks into human milk. *Adv Exp Med Biol* 478:289–305, 2000.

Leiser P, Kaufmann R: Placental structure: In a comparative aspect. *Exp Clin Endocrinol* 102:122–134, 1994.

Leopold G, Furukawa E, Forth W, Rummel W: Comparative studies of absorption of heavy metals in vivo and in vitro. *Arch Pharmacol Exp Pathol* 263:275–276, 1969.

Leslie EM, Deeley RG, Cole SPC: Multidurg resistance proteins: Role of P-glycoprotein, MRP1, MRP2, and BCRP (ABCG2) in tissue defense. *Toxicol Appl Pharmacol* 204:216–237, 2005.

Levine RR: Factors affecting gastrointestinal absorption of drugs. *Am J Dig Dis* 15:171–188, 1970.

Li X, Weber LWD, Rozman KK: Toxicokinetics of 2,3,7,8-tetrachlorodibenzo-*p*-dioxin (TCDD) in female Sprague-Dawley rats including placental and lactational transfer to fetuses and neonates. *Fundam Appl Toxicol* 27:70–76, 1995.

Lin JH: Species similarities and differences in pharmacokinetics. *Drug Metab Dispo* 23:1008–1021, 1995.

Lin JH: Tissue distribution and pharmacodynamics: A complicated relationship. *Curr Drug Metab* 7:39–65, 2006.

Mao Q, Unadkat JD: Role of the breast cancer resistance protein (ABCG2) in drug transport. *The AAPS Journal* 7:E118–E133, 2005.

Magos L, Clarkson TW: The effect of oral doses of a polythiol resin on the excretion of methylmercury in mice treated with cystein, D-penicillamine or phenobarbitone. *Chem Biol Interact* 14:325–335, 1976.

Mensinga TT, Speijers GJ, Meulenbelt J: Health implications of exposure to environmental nitrogenous compounds. *Toxicol Rev* 22:41–51, 2003.

Morris Jr, FH, Boyd DH, Mahendran D: Placental transport, in Knobel E, Neill JD (eds.): *The Physiology of Reproduction*. New York, NY: Raven Press Ltd, 1994, pp. 813–861.

Myllynen P, Pasanen M, Pelkonen O: Human placenta: A human organ for developmental toxicology research and biomonitoring. *Placenta* 26:361–371, 2005.

Mizuno N, Niwa T, Yotsumoto Y, Sugiyama Y: Impact of drug transporter studies on drug discovery and development. *Pharmacol Rev* 55:425–461, 2003.

Nel A, Xia T, Madler L, Li N: Toxic potential of materials at the nanolevel. *Science* 311:622–627, 2006.

Newbold RR, McLachlan JA: Transplacental hormonal carcinogenesis: Diethylstilbestrol as an example. *Prog Clin Biol Res* 394:131–147, 1996.

Oberdorster G, Oberdorster E, Oberdorster J: Nanotoxicology: An emerging discipline evolving from studies of ultrafine particles. *Environ Health Perspect* 113:823–539, 2005.

Pfeiffer CJ: Gastroenterologic response to environmental agents—absorption and interactions, in Lee DHK (ed.): *Handbook of Physiology. Section 9: Reactions to Environmental Agents*. Bethesda, MD: American Physiological Society, 1977, pp. 349–374.

Poet TS, McDougal JN: Skin absorption and human risk assessment. *Chem Biol Interact* 140:19–34, 2002.

Rickert DE, Butterworth BE, Popp JA: Dinitrotoluene: Acute toxicity, oncogenicity, genotoxicity and metabolism. *CRC Crit Rev Toxicol* 13:217–234, 1984.

Ross JH, Driver JH, Harris SA, Maibach HI: Dermal absorption of 2,4-D: A review of species differences. *Reg Toxicol Pharmacol* 41:82–91, 2005.

Rowland IR, Mallet AK, Wise A: The effect of diet on mammalian gut flora and its metabolic activities. *CRC Crit Rev Toxicol* 16:31–103, 1985.

Sahi J: Use of in vitro transporter assays to understand hepatic and renal disposition of new drug candidates. *Expert Opin Drug Metab Toxicol* 1:409–427, 2005.

Scatchard G: The attraction of proteins for small molecules and ions. *Ann NY Acad Sci* 51:660–672, 1949.

Schanker LS: Passage of drugs across body membranes. *Pharmcol Rev* 74:501–530, 1962.

Schinkel A, Smith JJM, van Tellingen O, *et al.*: Disruption of the mouse mdr1a p-glycoprotein gene leads to a deficiency in the blood–brain barrier and to increased sensitivity to drugs. *Cell* 47:491–502, 1994.

Schwartze EW: The so-called habituation to arsenic: Variation in the toxicity of arsenious oxide. *J Pharmacol Exp Ther* 20:181–203, 1923.

Shand DG, Rangno RE: The deposition of propranolol: I. Elimination during oral absorption in man. *Pharmacology* 7:159–168, 1972.

Shitara Y, Sato H, Sugiyama Y: Evaluation of drug–drug interaction in the hepatobiliary and renal transport of drugs. *Annu Rev Pharmacol Toxicol* 45:689–723, 2005.

Silverman WA, Andersen DH, Blanc WA, Crozier DN: A difference in mortality rate and incidence of kernicterus among premature infants allotted to two prophylactic antibacterial regimens. *Pediatrics* 18:614–625, 1956.

Smith HW: Observations on the flora of the alimentary tract of animals and factors affecting its composition. *J Pathol Bacteriol* 89:95–107, 1965.

Symchowicz S, Staub MS, Wong KKA: Comparative study of griseofulvin-^{14}C metabolism in the rat and rabbit. *Biochem Pharmacol* 16:2405–2411, 1967.

Syme MR, Paxton JW, Keelan JA: Drug transfer and metabolism by the human placenta. *Clin Pharmacokinet* 43:487–514, 2004.

Thwaites DT, Brown CD, Hirst BH, Simmons NL: H+-coupled dipeptide (glycylsarcosine) transport across apical and basal borders of human intestinal Caco-2 cell monolayers display distinctive characteristics. *Biochem Biophys Acta* 1151:237–245, 1993.

Tsuji A, Tamai 1, Nakanishi M, *et al.*: Intestinal brush-border transport of the oral cephalosporin antibiotic, cefdinir, mediated by dipeptide and monocarboxylic acid transport systems in rabbits. *J Pharm Pharmacol* 45:996–998, 1993.

Van den Berg M, Heeremans C, Veerhoven E, Olie K: Transfer of polychlorinated dibenzo-*p*-dioxins and dibenzofurans to fetal and neonatal rats. *Fundam Appl Toxicol* 9:635–644, 1987.

Venter JC, Adams MD, Myers EW, *et al.*: The sequence of the human genome. *Science* 291:1304–1351, 2001.

Vlaming MLH, Morhmann K, Wagenaar E, *et al.*: Carcinogen and anticancer drug transport by Mrp2 in vivo: Studies using Mrp2 (Abcc2) knockout mice. *J Pharmacol Exp Ther* 318:319–327, 2006.

Wang DS, Kusuhara H, Kato Y, Jonker JW, Schinkel AH, Sugiyama Y: Involvement of organic cation transporter 1 in the lactic acidosis caused by metformin. *Mol Pharmacol* 63:844–848, 2003.

Waalkes MP, Ward JM, Liu J, Diwan BA: Transplacental carcinogenesis of inorganic arsenic in drinking water: Induction of hepatic, ovarian, pulmonary and adrenal tumors in mice. *Toxicol Appl Pharmacol* 186:7–17, 2003.

Wester RC, Maibach HI: Animal models for percutaneous absorption, in Wang RGM, Knaak JB, Maibach HI (eds.): *Health Risk Assessment—Dermal and Inhalation Exposure and Absorption of Toxicants.* Boca Raton: CRC Press, 1993, pp. 89–103.

Wihnholds J, Scheffer GL, van der Valk M, *et al.*: Multidrug resistance protien 1 protects the oropharyngeal mucosal layer and the testicular tubules against drug-induced damage. *J Exp Med* 188:797–808, 1998.

Wilkinson GR: Plasma and tissue binding considerations in drug disposition. *Drug Metab Rev* 14:427–465, 1983.

Williams RM, Beck F: A histochemical study of gut maturation. *J Anat* 105:487–501, 1969.

Wilson JT: Determinants and consequences of drug excretion in breast milk. *Drug Metab Rev* 14:619–652, 1983.

Wold JS, Joust RR, Owen NV: Nephrotoxicity of cephaloridine in newborn rabbits: Role of the renal anionic transport system. *J Pharmacol Exp Ther* 201:778–785, 1977.

Yesair DW, Callahan M, Remington L, Kensler CJ: Role of the enterohepatic cycle of indomethacin on its metabolism, distribution in tissues and its excretion by rats, dogs, and monkeys. *Biochem Pharmacol* 19:1579–1590, 1970.

Yuasa H, Matsuhisa E, Watanabe J: Intestinal brush border transport mechanism of 5-fluorocuracil in rats. *Biol Pharm Bull* 19:94–99, 1996.

CHAPTER 6

BIOTRANSFORMATION OF XENOBIOTICS

Andrew Parkinson and Brian W. Ogilvie

INTRODUCTION

PRINCIPLES OF XENOBIOTIC BIOTRANSFORMATION

HYDROLYSIS, REDUCTION, AND OXIDATION

  Hydrolysis
    Carboxylesterases
    Cholinesterase (AChE and BChE)
    Paraoxonases (Lactonases)
    Prodrugs and Alkaline Phosphatase
    Peptidases
    Epoxide Hydrolases
  Reduction
    Azo- and Nitro-Reduction
    Carbonyl Reduction—SDRs and AKRs
    Disulfide Reduction
    Sulfoxide and *N*-Oxide Reduction
    Quinone Reduction—NQO1 and NQO2
    Dihydropyrimidine Dehydrogenase (DPD)
    Dehalogenation
    Dehydroxylation—Cytochrome b_5 and Aldehyde Oxidase
    Aldehyde Oxidase—Reductive Reactions
  Oxidation
    Alcohol, Aldehyde, Ketone Oxidation–Reduction Systems

Alcohol Dehydrogenase
Aldehyde Dehydrogenase
Dihydrodiol Dehydrogenase
Molybdenum Hydroxylases (Molybdozymes)
Xanthine Oxidoreductase
Aldehyde Oxidase
Monoamine Oxidase, Diamine Oxidase, and Polyamine Oxidase
Semicarbazide-Sensitive Amine Oxidase (SSAO)
Aromatization
Peroxidase-Dependent Cooxidation
Flavin Monooxygenases
Cytochrome P450
Activation of Xenobiotics by Cytochrome P450
Inhibition of Cytochrome P450
Induction of Cytochrome P450—Xenosensors

CONJUGATION

  Glucuronidation
  Sulfonation
  Methylation
  Acetylation
  Amino Acid Conjugation
  Glutathione Conjugation
  Thiosulfate Sulfurtransferase (Rhodanese)
  Phosphorylation—The Dog That Did Not Bark

INTRODUCTION

In 2003, my father, Edward William Parkinson, died of Lou Gehrig disease, otherwise known as ALS in America and as MND in Britain. He died beeping. The beeping came from a portable, electronic syringe that periodically injected my father with glycopyrrolate, an anticholinergic drug that blocks the production of saliva that many ALS patients have difficulty swallowing. Glycopyrrolate is a quaternary ammonium salt, hence, it is positively charged at physiological pH. As such, glycopyrrolate does not readily cross lipid bilayers, which is why it is injected intravenously or intramuscularly, it has fewer CNS effects (it does not readily cross the blood–brain barrier), and a relatively small volume of distribution at steady state ($V_{ss} = 0.42$ L/kg). Glycopyrrolate is rapidly eliminated in the urine. The mean elimination half-life increases from 19 minutes in patients with normal kidney function to 47 minutes in patients with severe kidney impairment, indicating that renal disease impairs the elimination of glycopyrrolate. Although it is excreted in the urine largely as unchanged drug, glycopyrrolate reinforces a number of principles about xenobiotic biotransformation, the most important of which is: xenobiotic biotransformation is the process—actually a series of enzyme-catalyzed processes—that alters the physiochemical properties of foreign chemicals (xenobiotics) from those that favor absorption across biological membranes (namely, lipophilicity) to those favoring elimination in urine or bile (namely, hydrophilicity). Without xenobiotic biotransformation, the numerous foreign chemicals to which we are exposed (which includes both man-made and natural chemicals such as drugs, industrial chemicals, pesticides, pollutants, pyrolysis products in cooked food, alkaloids, secondary plant metabolites, and toxins produced by molds, plants, etc.) either unintentionally or, in the case of drugs, intentionally would—if they are sufficiently lipophilic to be absorbed from the gastrointestinal tract and other sites of exposure—eventually accumulate to toxic levels. Furthermore, absent xenobiotic biotransformation, many of the drugs in use today would have an unacceptably long duration of action. In contrast, drugs that are not lipophilic, like glycopyrrolate, are not absorbed from the gastrointestinal tract (hence they are not orally active), and if they are administered parenterally they are not biotransformed (because they are already hydrophilic), and they are rapidly eliminated from the body.

The enzymes that catalyze xenobiotic biotransformation are often called drug-metabolizing enzymes. The acronym ADME stands for **a**bsorption, **d**istribution, **m**etabolism, and **e**limination. This acronym is used widely in the pharmaceutical industry to describe the four main processes governing drug disposition. This chapter describes some fundamental principles of xenobiotic biotransformation, and describes the major enzyme systems involved in the biotransformation (or metabolism) of drugs and other xenobiotics. The examples given are biased toward drugs and human enzyme systems for two reasons. First, many of the fundamental principles of xenobiotic biotransformation stem from such studies. This is especially true of drugs with a narrow therapeutic index (where the toxic dose is not much greater than the therapeutic dose), which have revealed a large number of genetic and environmental factors that affect xenobiotic biotransformation and, hence, drug toxicity. Second, adverse drug reactions are one of the leading causes of death in the United States. Lazarou *et al.* (1998) estimated that in 1994 over 2 million hospitalized patients had serious adverse drug events (ADEs) and 106,000 had fatal outcomes, placing ADEs only behind heart disease, cancer, stroke, and pulmonary disease as a leading cause of death. Furthermore, of the 548 new chemical entities approved by the FDA between 1974 and 1999, ~10% (56 drugs) required black box warnings or were withdrawn from the market because of ADEs that included hepatotoxicity, cardiotoxicity (several as a result of drug–drug interactions), myelotoxicity, immunotoxicity, and warnings to pregnant women (Lasser *et al.*, 2002; Thomas, 2002). In many cases, xenobiotic biotransformation is central to understanding these ADEs.

PRINCIPLES OF XENOBIOTIC BIOTRANSFORMATION

It is difficult to make categorical statements about xenobiotic biotransformation because there is an exception to every rule. Nevertheless, the following points, which might be considered principles or rules, apply in the majority of cases:

Point 1 Xenobiotic biotransformation or drug metabolism is the process of converting lipophilic (fat soluble) chemicals, which are readily absorbed from the gastrointestinal tract and other sites, into hydrophilic (water soluble) chemicals, which are readily excreted in urine or bile. There are exceptions even to this most basic rule. For example, acetylation and methylation are biotransformation reactions that can actually decrease the water solubility of certain xenobiotics. As a general rule, xenobiotics with a log $D_{7.4} > 0$ require biotransformation to facilitate their elimination (Williams *et al.*, 2003b).

Point 2 The biotransformation of xenobiotics is catalyzed by various enzyme systems that can be divided into four categories based on the reaction they catalyze:

1. Hydrolysis (e.g., carboxylesterase)
2. Reduction (e.g., carbonyl reductase)
3. Oxidation (e.g., cytochrome P450)
4. Conjugation (e.g., UDP-glucuronosyltransferase)

The mammalian enzymes involved in the hydrolysis, reduction, oxidation, and conjugation of xenobiotics are listed in Table 6-1, together with their principal subcellular location. The conjugation reactions include glucuronidation, sulfonation (often called sulfation), acetylation, methylation, conjugation with glutathione (mercapturic acid synthesis) and conjugation with amino acids (such as glycine, taurine, and glutamic acid). Examples of the major chemical groups that undergo biotransformation together with the enzymes that commonly mediate their biotransformation are given in Table 6-2 (Williams *et al.*, 2003b).

Xenobiotic biotransformation is generally catalyzed by enzymes, but there are exceptions. For example, hydrolysis of certain carboxylic and phosphoric acid esters, reduction of sulfoxides to sulfides (e.g., rabeprazole), isomerization involving enol–keto tautomerization (e.g., thalidomide), and the conjugation of certain xenobiotics with glutathione can occur nonenzymatically at an appreciable rate. Certain reactions are catalyzed by gastric acid, such as the hydrolysis of esters and the conversion of indole-3-carbinol to a dimer that is a potent agonist of the aryl hydrocarbon receptor (AhR) and, consequently, an inducer of various enzymes including certain cytochrome P450 enzymes (CYP1A1, 1A2, 1B1, and 2S1).

Point 3 In general, individual xenobiotic-biotransforming enzymes are located in a single organelle. In Table 6-1, some enzymes are listed with two or more subcellular locations. However, in such cases, the enzyme name generally refers to two or more enzymes, each with its own distinct subcellular location. For example, the epoxide hydrolase located in microsomes is a different enzyme from the epoxide hydrolase located in cytosol (i.e., they are distinct gene products). From a practical perspective, it is noteworthy that during the homogenization of tissue and the preparation of subcellular fractions, a certain degree of cross-contamination of organelles occurs. For example, microsomes contain detectable levels of monoamine oxidase due to their contamination with the outer mitochondrial membrane.

Point 4 In general, xenobiotic biotransformation is accomplished by a limited number of enzymes with broad substrate specificities. In humans, for example, two cytochrome P450 enzymes—namely, CYP2D6 and CYP3A4—metabolize over half the orally effective drugs in current use (Gonzalez and Tukey, 2006). The broad and sometimes overlapping substrate specificities of xenobiotic-biotransforming enzymes preclude the possibility of naming the individual enzymes after the reactions they catalyze (which is how most other enzymes are named). Many of the enzymes involved in xenobiotic biotransformation are named according to nomenclature systems based on the primary amino acid sequence of the individual enzymes. Some enzymes are given the same name across all mammalian species, whereas others are named in a species-specific manner. For example, some cytochrome P450 enzymes, such as CYP1A1, CYP1A2, and CYP1B1, are so named in all mammalian species, whereas cytochrome P450 enzymes in the CYP2, CYP3, and CYP4 families (with certain exceptions such as CYP2E1) are named in a species-specific manner. The convention of using italic and normal letters to distinguish between the gene and gene products (mRNA and protein), respectively, and the convention of using lower case letters to designate mouse genes and gene products will not be followed in this chapter.

The structure (i.e., amino acid sequence) of a given xenobiotic-biotransforming enzyme may differ among individuals, which can give rise to differences in rates of drug metabolism. In general, a variant form of a xenobiotic-biotransforming enzyme (known as an *allelic variant* or an *allelozyme*) has diminished enzymatic activity compared with that of the wild-type enzyme, although this is not always the case (see section "Alcohol Dehydrogenase"). The impact of amino acid substitution(s) on the catalytic activity of a xenobiotic-biotransforming enzyme may be substrate dependent, such that an allelic variant may interact normally with some substrates (and inhibitors) but interact atypically with others.

Point 5 Hydrolysis, reduction, and oxidation expose or introduce a functional group (such as –OH, –NH$_2$, –SH, or –COOH) that can be converted to a water-soluble conjugate (see Table 6-2).

Table 6-1

General Pathways of Xenobiotic Biotransformation and Their Major Subcellular Location

REACTION	ENZYME OR SPECIFIC REACTION	LOCALIZATION
Hydrolysis	Carboxylesterase	Microsomes, cytosol, lysosomes, blood
	Alkaline phosphatase	Plasma membrane
	Peptidase	Blood, lysosomes
	Epoxide hydrolase	Microsomes, cytosol
Reduction	Azo- and nitro-reduction	Microflora
	Carbonyl (aldo-keto) reduction	Cytosol, microsomes, blood
	Disulfide reduction	Cytosol
	Sulfoxide reduction	Cytosol
	Quinone reduction	Cytosol, microsomes
	Dihydropyrimidine dehydrogenase	Cytosol
	Reductive dehalogenation	Microsomes
	Dehydroxylation (cytochrome b_5)	Microsomes
	Dehydroxylation (aldehyde oxidase)	Cytosol
Oxidation	Alcohol dehydrogenase	Cytosol
	Aldehyde dehydrogenase	Mitochondria, cytosol
	Aldehyde oxidase	Cytosol
	Xanthine oxidase	Cytosol
	Monoamine oxidase	Mitochondria
	Diamine oxidase	Cytosol
	Peroxidase	Microsomes, lysosomes, saliva
	Flavin-monooxygenases	Microsomes
	Cytochrome P450	Microsomes
Conjugation	UDP-Glucuronosyltransferase	Microsomes
	Sulfotransferase	Cytosol
	Glutathione transferase	Cytosol, microsomes, mitochondria
	Amino acid transferase	Mitochondria, microsomes
	N-Acetytransferase	Mitochondria, cytosol
	Methytransferase	Cytosol, microsomes, blood

The first three reactions (hydrolysis, reduction, and oxidation) are often called Phase 1 reactions, and the conjugation reactions are often called Phase 2 reactions. The classification of xenobiotic-biotransforming enzymes into Phase 1 and Phase 2 (and the extension of this system to classify xenobiotic transporters as Phase 3) has been criticized lately by Josephy *et al.* (2005), as being both misleading and contrary to the original principles of Williams (1959), the drug metabolism pioneer who coined the phrases to distinguish reactions that resulted in either a decrease or increase in xenobiotic toxicity (Phase 1) from reactions that resulted in only a decrease in toxicity (Phase 2). The arguments against the Phase 1–Phase 2 classification are as follows.

First, although the conjugation of many xenobiotics is preceded by hydrolysis, reduction, or oxidation (such that xenobiotics can be said to undergo Phase 1 before Phase 2 metabolism), there are several cases where a xenobiotic undergoes oxidation after it has been conjugated (such that Phase 2 precedes Phase 1 metabolism). For example, gemfibrozil is conjugated with glucuronic acid before it undergoes oxidation by cytochrome P450 (Ogilvie *et al.*, 2006). Second, there are numerous xenobiotics that are conjugated directly. For example, the majority of acetaminophen (Tylenol) is conjugated directly with glucuronic acid and, to a lesser extent, sulfonic acid. Third, the original idea that Phase 2 metabolism results in only detoxication is incorrect. Indeed, all xenobiotic-metabolizing enzymes are capable of increasing the toxicity of one or more xenobiotics, including the conjugating enzymes that R.T. Williams classified as Phase 2 (detoxifying) enzymes. For example, conjugation of carboxylic acid-containing drugs with glucuronic acid to form acyl glucuronides is thought to be responsible for the hepatotoxicity observed with numerous NSAIDs (nonsteroidal anti-inflammatory drugs). In fact, in the United States, NSAIDs and other carboxylic acid-containing drugs represent the largest category of drugs whose clinical development was halted or whose regulatory approval was subsequently withdrawn because of liver toxicity in humans (Fung *et al.*, 2001). Finally, some enzymes do not fit neatly into the Phase 1 or Phase 2 category. Epoxide hydrolase, for example, might be considered a Phase 1 enzyme because it introduces a functional group (-OH) for subsequent conjugation reactions, but it might also be considered a Phase 2 enzyme because it catalyzes the addition of water to aliphatic epoxides and arene oxides that are often formed by cytochrome P450. In this chapter, the terms Phase 1 and Phase 2 metabolism will not be used; instead the pathways of xenobiotic biotransformation will be divided into four categories: hydrolysis, reduction, oxidation, and conjugation.

Point 6 Not all biotransformation reactions are catalyzed by the mammalian enzymes listed in Table 6-1. Some biotransformation reactions are catalyzed by enzymes in the gut microflora (largely anaerobic bacteria in the colon), whereas the biotransformation of still other xenobiotics is catalyzed by enzymes that participate in intermediary (endobiotic) metabolism. This principle is illustrated in Fig. 6-1 for three xenobiotics that are all converted to benzoic acid and then hippuric acid. The conversion of toluene to hippuric acid

Table 6-2

Common Chemical Groups and Enzymes Possibly Involved in Their Metabolism

CHEMICAL GROUP	ENZYME(S)	REACTION(S)
Alkane R—CH₂—R	CYP	Hydroxylation, dehydrogenation
Alkene R₂C=CR₂	CYP, GST	Epoxidation, glutathione adduct formation
Alkyne R—C≡C—R	CYP	Oxidation to carboxylic acid
Aliphatic alcohol R—CH₂—OH	CYP, ADH, catalase, UGT, SULT	Oxidation, glucuronidation, sulfonation
Aliphatic amine R—NH₂	CYP, FMO, MAO, UGT, SULT, MT, NAT, peroxidase	N-Dealkylation, N-oxidation, deamination, N-glucuronidation, N-carbamoyl glucuronidation, N-sulfonation, N-methylation, N-acetylation
Amidine HN=CR—NH₂	CYP	N-Oxidation
Arene (R-substituted benzene)	CYP	Hydroxylation and epoxidation
Carboxylic acid R—COOH	UGT, amino acid transferases	Glucuronidation, amino acylation
Epoxide (oxirane ring)	Epoxide hydrolase, GST	Hydrolysis, glutathione adduct formation
Lactone (cyclic ester)	Lactonase (paraoxonase)	Hydrolysis (ring opening)
Aldehyde R—CH=O	CYP, ALDH	Oxidative de-formylation, oxidation to carboxylic acid
Amide R—C(=O)—NH—R	Amidase (esterase)	Hydrolysis
Aniline (phenyl-NH₂)	CYP, NAT, UGT, peroxidase, SULT	N-Hydroxylation, N-acetylation, N-glucuronidation, N-oxidation, N-sulfonation
Aromatic azaheterocycles (quinoline ring)	UGT, CYP, aldehyde oxidase	N-Glucuronidation, hydroxylation, N-oxidation, ring cleavage, oxidation
Carbamate R—NH—C(=O)—O—R	CYP, esterase	Oxidative cleavage, hydrolysis
Ester R—CH₂—O—C(=O)—R	CYP, esterase	Oxidative cleavage, hydrolysis
Ether R—CH₂—O—CH₂—R	CYP	O-Dealkylation
Ketone R—CH₂—C(=O)—R	CYP, SDR, AKR	Baeyer–Villiger oxidation, reduction
Phenol (phenyl-OH)	CYP, UGT, SULT, MT	Ipso-substitution, glucuronidation, sulfonation, methylation
Thioether R—CH₂—S—CH₂—R	CYP, FMO	S-Dealkylation, S-oxidation

ADH, alcohol dehydrogenase; ALDH, aldehyde dehydrogenase; AKR, aldo-keto reductases; FMO, flavin monoxygenase; GST, glutathione transferase; MAO, monoamine oxidase; MT, methyltransferase; SDR, short-chain dehydrogenases/reductases; NAT, N-acetyltransferase; SULT, sulfotransferase; UGT, UDP-glucuronosyltransferase.

SOURCE: Data adapted from Williams JA, Hurst SI, Bauman J, *et al.*: Reaction phenotyping in drug discovery: moving forward with confidence? *Curr Drug Metab* 4:527–534, 2003b.

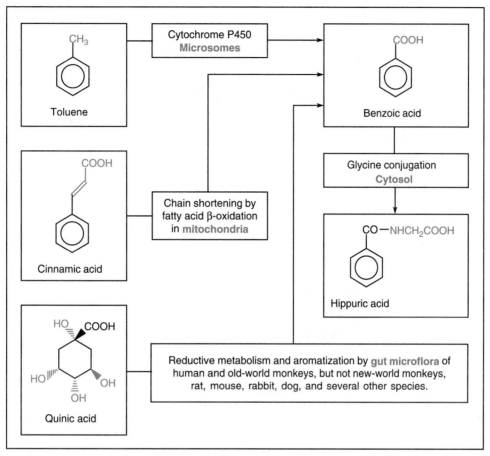

Figure 6-1. Examples of xenobiotic biotransformation by different enzyme systems: a xenobiotic-biotransforming enzyme (cytochrome P450), an endobiotic-metabolizing enzyme, and gut microflora.

is catalyzed by some of the xenobiotic biotransforming enzymes listed in Table 6-1: Microsomal cytochrome P450 converts toluene to benzoic acid in three oxidative steps (R-CH$_3$ → R-CH$_2$OH → RCHO → RCOOH), which introduces a functional group (namely, –COOH) that is conjugated with glycine to produce hippuric acid, which is excreted in urine. Cinnamic acid is also converted to benzoic acid but, in this case, the reaction is catalyzed by the mitochondrial enzymes involved in the β-oxidation of fatty acids. Quinic acid is also converted to benzoic acid, but this reductive, multistep reaction is catalyzed by gut microflora. Incidentally, the conversion of benzoic acid to hippuric acid is of historical interest because it is generally recognized as the first xenobiotic biotransformation reaction to be discovered (in dogs by Woehler in 1828, and in humans by Ure in 1841).

Some drugs are intentionally designed to be biotransformed by endobiotic-metabolizing enzymes. For example, the anti-HIV drug zidovudine (AZT) is converted to a triphosphate nucleoside by enzymes in the salvage pathway (nucleoside kinase, nucleoside monophosphate kinase or NMK, and nucleoside diphosphate kinase or NDK). HIV reverse transcriptase inhibitors, like zidovudine, are administered as nonphosphorylated analogs to facilitate their absorption and cellular uptake. Conversely, some drugs are administered as a phosphorylated prodrug (e.g., fosamprenavir) to promote their water solubility and rate of dissolution. The luminal surface of the small intestine contains high levels of alkaline phosphatase, which hydrolyzes prodrugs like fosamprenavir and thereby releases

the active drug at the surface of the enterocyte, where it is readily absorbed. Generally speaking, kinase and alkaline phosphatase are not usually considered to be xenobiotic-biotransforming enzymes.

Point 7   Just as some xenobiotics are biotransformed by the so-called endobiotic-metabolizing enzymes (Point 6), certain endobiotics are biotransformed by the so-called xenobiotic-metabolizing enzymes. For example, the same cytochrome P450 enzymes implicated in xenobiotic biotransformation also contribute to the hepatic catabolism of steroid hormones, and the same UDP-glucuronosyltransferases that conjugate xenobiotics also glucuronidate bilirubin, thyroid hormones, and steroid hormones. Benzoic acid, a xenobiotic, is conjugated with glycine (as shown in Fig. 6-1), and so are bile acids (endobiotics). Certain leukotrienes are glutathione conjugates. From the few examples in Points 6 and 7, it is apparent that, on a case-by-case basis, there is no clear-cut distinction between endobiotic- and xenobiotic-biotransforming enzymes.

The human genome project has helped to establish that what were once thought to be two distinct enzymes, one involved in the metabolism of endobiotics and one involved in the metabolism of xenobiotics, are in fact one and the same enzyme. For example, the microsomal enzyme known as 11β-hydroxysteroid dehydrogenase is identical to the xenobiotic-metabolizing enzyme known as microsomal carbonyl reductase.

Point 8   Several xenobiotic-biotransforming enzymes are inducible, meaning their expression can be increased (upregulated) usually in response to exposure to high concentrations of xenobiotics. Induction is mediated by ligand-activated receptors (so-called xenosensors) that are activated by xenobiotics (ligands) to DNA-binding proteins that upregulate the transcription of various genes encoding xenobiotic-biotransforming enzymes, especially cytochrome P450 (CYP) enzymes, which are usually induced to the greatest extent (in terms of fold increase). The major xenosensors are the aryl hydrocarbon receptor (AhR), which induces CYP1 enzymes, the constitutive androstane receptor (CAR), which induces CYP2B, 2C, and 3A enzymes, the pregnane X receptor (PXR), which also induces CYP2B, 2C, and 3A enzymes, and the peroxisome proliferator activated receptor alpha (PPARα), which induces CYP4 enzymes. CAR and PXR are closely related, and they tend to be activated by the same ligands and bind to the same DNA-response elements (i.e., the same discrete regions of DNA that control gene expression), for which reason there is said to be considerable *cross-talk* between these two xenosensors. There is also considerable cross-talk between xenosensors and several other nuclear receptors including nuclear factor kappa-B (NF-κB), the receptor activated during infectious and inflammatory diseases, which suppress CYP expression and induction because NF-κB represses all four xenosensors (and several other nuclear receptors). Certain xenosensors are activated by endogenous ligands (e.g. bilirubin, bile acids, and fatty acids activate CAR, PXR, and PPARα, respectively), and certain nuclear receptors, such as the vitamin D receptor (VDR) can mimic PXR and induce CYP3A4, which inactivates the active metabolite of vitamin D. These examples illustrate how xenosensors are not just involved in xenobiotic disposition but also play a role in endobiotic homeostasis. Two proteins called KEAP-1 (Kelch-like ECH-related protein) and Nrf2 (nuclear factor E2 p45-related factor-2) function as xenosensors in as much as they induce enzymes in response to oxidative stress, which is often associated with xenobiotic biotransformation. Binding of the transcription factor Nrf2 to the region of DNA known as the antioxidant response element (also known as the electrophilic response element) induces enzymes that detoxify electrophiles and metabolites that generate reactive oxygen species (ROS), including glutathione transferase (GSTA1), microsomal epoxide hydrolase, aldo-keto reductase (AKR7A, also known as aflatoxin aldehyde reductase), NAD(P)H-quinone oxidoreductase (NQO1, also known as DT-diaphorase), and glutamate-cysteine ligase (GCL), which catalyzes the rate-limiting step in glutathione synthesis. Induction of GCL increases the rate of glutathione synthesis under conditions of oxidative stress and a decrease in glutathione concentration (Lee and Johnson, 2004).

Induction is a reversible, adaptive response to xenobiotic exposure. The induced enzymes (and transporters) usually accelerate the elimination of the xenobiotic that triggered the induction process, in which case the xenobiotic is said to be an auto-inducer (one that induces its own metabolism). However, xenobiotics often induce enzymes that are not capable of metabolizing them, in which case the induction is said to be gratuitous. Induction is a pleiotropic response: Activation of AhR, CAR, PXR, PPARα, and Nrf2 all result in alterations in the expression of numerous genes, some of which are upregulated (or induced) and some of which are downregulated (or suppressed).

Point 9   The ability of certain xenobiotic-biotransforming enzymes to metabolize hormones and other endobiotics (Point 7) and the ability of certain xenobiotics to induce xenobiotic-biotransforming enzymes (Point 8) have implications for understanding an important mechanism by which certain xenobiotics can alter homeostasis or cause toxicity. Persistent exposure to xenobiotics that are enzyme inducers can increase the rate of steroid hor-

mone oxidation by cytochrome P450 and increase the rate of thyroid hormone glucuronidation and sulfonation which, in rodents, can lead to the development of Leydig cell tumors (due to elevated levels of LH and FSH) and thyroid follicular tumors (due to elevated levels of TSH), respectively (Grasso *et al.*, 1991). Persistent exposure to enzyme inducers can also cause liver tumors, although the mechanism is not fully understood. Activation of certain xenosensors is critical to liver tumor development, although upregulation of xenobiotic-biotransforming enzymes appears to be less important than other xenosensor-dependent events, such as the down-regulation of gap junctional proteins, which diminishes cell–cell communication.

Phenobarbital, Wy-14,643, methapyrilene, and Ponceau S are representatives of four classes of nongenotoxic rodent tumorigens (epigenetic tumor promoters) that cause hepatocellular hyperplasia and hypertrophy in association with proliferation of the endoplasmic reticulum, peroxisomes, mitochondria, and lysosomes, respectively (Grasso *et al.*, 1991). In the first two cases, the hepatocellular changes depend on activation of CAR (in the case of phenobarbital) and PPARα (in the case of Wy-14,643). Prolonged activation of these receptors in rodents results in the development of liver and/or thyroid tumors. However, this is thought to be a rodent-specific phenomenon because, in the case of phenobarbital and other enzyme-inducing antiepileptic drugs (EIAEDs), there is compelling epidemiological evidence that these chemicals do not cause liver tumors in humans even after 30+ years of treatment (Parkinson *et al.*, 2006).

The major UDP–glucuronosyltransferase responsible for conjugating bilirubin is UGT1A1, which is inducible by CAR agonists such as phenobarbital and scoparone (6,7-dimethylesculetin). At one time, the management of neonatal jaundice included treatment with phenobarbital to induce bilirubin conjugation, but this practice has been discontinued. However, the Chinese herbal Yin Zhi Wuang (active ingredient scoparone) is still used to treat neonatal jaundice. Bilirubin is also a CAR agonist, and high levels of bilirubin induce UGT1A1 and bilirubin/bilirubin glucuronide transporters to increase the rate of bilirubin elimination when bilirubin levels are elevated (e.g., during hemolytic anemia).

Point 10   Xenobiotic biotransformation can alter the biological properties of a xenobiotic. It can make the xenobiotic less toxic (detoxication), but in some cases it can make it more toxic (activation). The oxidation of ethanol (alcohol) to acetaldehyde is an example of xenobiotic activation, and the subsequent oxidation of acetaldehyde to acetic acid is an example of detoxication. The biotransformation of drugs can result in (1) a loss of pharmacological activity (e.g., the conversion of acetaminophen to acetaminophen glucuronide and the conversion of morphine to morphine 3-glucuronide), (2) no change in pharmacological activity (e.g., the conversion of fluoxetine to its N-demethylated metabolite norfluoxetine), or (3) an increase in pharmacological activity (e.g., the conversion of codeine to morphine, as well as the conversion of morphine to morphine 6-glucuronide).

Point 11   In many cases, the toxicity of a xenobiotic is due to the parent compound (the compound that was absorbed), in which case xenobiotic biotransformation serves as a detoxication mechanism. This is illustrated by the clinical observation that the incidence of adverse drug events is often higher in individuals with a poor metabolizer phenotype (discussed later in Point 23). However, xenobiotic-biotransforming enzymes can convert certain xenobiotics to reactive (electrophilic) metabolites, and this activation process plays an important role in chemical toxicity and chemical mutagenicity/carcinogenicity; the former often involves the covalent binding of electrophilic metabolites to critical cellular nucleophiles like proteins, whereas the latter involves covalent binding to one or more purine or pyrimidine bases in DNA. Cytochrome P450 is particularly effective at converting proximate carcinogens to ultimate carcinogens by converting the former to electrophilic metabolites that bind to and mutate DNA, thereby leading to mutations and tumor initiation. The Ames' bacterial mutagenicity assay, which is representative of several mutagenicity tests, is performed in the absence and presence of cytochrome P450 (i.e., liver microsomes) to evaluate the mutagenic potential of both the parent compound and any electrophilic metabolites, respectively. Polycyclic aromatic hydrocarbons (combustion pollutants and components of tobacco smoke), aromatic amines (industrial chemicals), aflatoxin (a mycotoxin), cooked-food pyrolysis products, and tobacco-specific nitrosamines are all examples of proximate carcinogens that require metabolic activation to form electrophilic, DNA-binding metabolites (ultimate carcinogens).

Certain anticancer drugs require activation by xenobiotic-metabolizing enzymes in order to exert their antineoplastic effects. For example, cyclophosphamide is activated by CYP2B6 and several other cytochrome P450 enzymes, and TLK286 is activated by glutathione transferase, which is often over-expressed in tumors thereby conferring resistance against certain anticancer drugs (see section "Glutathione Conjugation") (Gonzalez and Tukey, 2006).

Point 12   The toxicity and potential carcinogenicity of electrophilic metabolites produced by cytochrome P450 and other xenobiotic-biotransforming enzymes is reduced and often altogether eliminated by their conjugation with glutathione, which is often described as a noncritical cellular nucleophile. In the majority of cases, conjugation with glutathione represents a detoxication reaction; one that protects critical cellular nucleophiles, such as protein and DNA, from covalent modification. However, there are cases (e.g., dibromoethane) where conjugation with glutathione actually produces a DNA-reactive (mutagenic) metabolite. Conjugation with glutathione can occur both enzymatically (by glutathione S-transferase) and nonenzymatically.

Point 13   The biotransformation of some xenobiotics results in the production of reactive oxygen species (ROS), which can cause cell toxicity (including DNA damage) through oxidative stress and lipid peroxidation. Glutathione, glutathione transferases, and glutathione peroxidases all limit the toxic effects of ROS just as they limit the toxicity of reactive metabolites formed directly from xenobiotics. Oxidative stress and the formation of electrophilic metabolites reduce glutathione levels and thus result in the concurrent oxidation of KEAP-1, which then releases Nrf2, which in turn upregulates the expression of enzymes that detoxify electrophilic metabolites (e.g., epoxides) and those metabolites that generate ROS (e.g., quinones) (see Point 8).

Point 14   The balance between activation and detoxication by xenobiotic-biotransforming enzymes is often a key determinant of chemical toxicity, and is often the basis for organ or species differences in toxicity. For example, aflatoxin is converted by liver microsomal cytochrome P450 to a reactive epoxide that is thought to be responsible for the hepatotoxic and hepatocarcinogenic effect of this mycotoxin. The fact that this reaction occurs in the liver explains why aflatoxin causes liver toxicity and liver tumors. On this basis, mice would be expected to be more sensitive than rats to the hepatotoxic effects of aflatoxin because mice catalyze the epoxidation of aflatoxin faster than rats. However, through glutathione conjugation, mice also detoxify aflatoxin epoxide faster than rats. Consequently, despite their slower rate of activation, rats are more

susceptible than mice to the toxic effects of aflatoxin. Coumarin is hepatotoxic to rats, but not to humans. This species difference is attributable to differences in the metabolites formed by cytochrome P450. Rats convert coumarin to a reactive epoxide that rearranges to a reactive aldehyde, whereas humans convert coumarin to the relatively nontoxic metabolite 7-hydroxycoumarin (umbelliferone).

The enzymes involved in xenobiotic activation and detoxication play important roles in determining the susceptibility of mammals to the hepatotoxic effects of acetaminophen, which is the leading cause of acute liver failure in humans (Kaplowitz, 2005). Acetaminophen is activated to a reactive metabolite by cytochrome P450, including CYP2E1, which is detoxified by conjugation with glutathione (see section "Glutathione Conjugation"). Experiments with so-called knockout mice have established that gene deletion of CYP2E1 protects mice from acetaminophen hepatotoxicity, whereas depletion of glutathione (by chemical, not genetic means) potentiates it. However, gene deletion experiments have identified a host of factors that increase the susceptibility of mice to acetaminophen hepatotoxicity, including deletion of CAR, glutathione transferase-Pi, Jun Kinase-2 (JNK2), DNAse 1, interferon-γ (IFN-γ), lipopolysaccharide-binding protein (LPS-BP), Toll-like receptor-4 (TRL4), and osteopontin, as well as depletion of neutrophil and NK/NKT cells. Conversely, other gene deletions have been shown to protect mice from the hepatotoxic effects of acetaminophen, including Nrf2, interleukin-6 (IL-6), interleukin-10 (IL-10), cyclooxygenase-2 (Cox-2), chemokine receptor-2 (CCR2), and chemokine receptor-5 (CCR5), as well as depletion of Kupffer cells (Kaplowitz, 2005). The important point here is that the factors that determine whether a xenobiotic will or will not cause cellular toxicity go far beyond the enzymes involved in xenobiotic activation and detoxication, and these additional factors can also play a role in determining organ and species differences in xenobiotic toxicity. This principle is illustrated by the anti-HIV drug abacavir, hypersensitivity to which is determined not by an individual's enzymatic capacity to activate or detoxify the drug but by an individual's human leukocyte antigen (HLA) subtype (Mallal et al., 2002).

Point 15   Exposure to xenobiotics (especially drugs) is largely through oral ingestion, and the small intestine and liver are highly developed to limit systemic exposure to orally ingested xenobiotics, a process known as *first-pass elimination* (or *presystemic elimination*). The enterocytes at the tips of the small intestinal villi express the efflux transporter *P*-glycoprotein (also known as MDR1 or ABCB1), which serves to limit xenobiotic absorption. The enterocytes express high levels of certain cytochrome P450 and UDP-glucuronosyltransferase enzymes, which biotransform a wide variety of xenobiotics. The liver expresses a number of uptake transporters that actively remove xenobiotics from the blood. They also express a number of efflux transporters that actively discharge xenobiotics or their metabolites (especially conjugates) into the bile canaliculus for biliary excretion, or that actively discharge xenobiotic metabolites (especially conjugates) across the sinusoidal membrane back into the blood for urinary excretion. The liver expresses the largest number and, with few exceptions, the highest concentrations of xenobiotic-biotransforming enzymes.

Although the liver contains higher concentrations of most xenobiotic-biotransforming enzymes, and because the number of hepatocytes in the liver exceeds the number of enterocytes in the small intestine, it might be assumed that, compared with the liver, the small intestine would make only a small contribution to first-pass metabolism, but this is not the case. Furanocoumarins in grapefruit juice inhibit intestinal but not hepatic CYP3A4 and yet grapefruit juice increases systemic exposure to felodipine and other drugs that undergo first-pass metabolism by CYP3A4 (Paine *et al.*, 2006). The impact of the CYP3A4 inhibitor ketoconazole on the disposition of the CYP3A4 substrate midazolam depends on whether midazolam is given orally or intravenously. When midazolam is given intravenously, such that its clearance is dependent only on hepatic metabolism, ketoconazole causes a three- to fivefold increase in the area-under-the-plasma-concentration-time curve (AUC). However, when midazolam is given orally, ketoconazole causes a 10- to 15-fold increase in AUC, the difference reflecting the significant role of intestinal metabolism to the presystemic clearance of midazolam. In rats, administration of the general cytochrome P450 inhibitor 1-aminobenzotriazole (ABT) by the intravenous route (which inhibits only hepatic CYP enzymes) and the oral route (which inhibits both intestinal and hepatic CYP enzymes) can be used to assess the relative role of the intestine and liver to the first-pass metabolism of a drug or other xenobiotic (Strelevitz *et al.*, 2006).

The small intestine and liver are exposed to high concentrations of xenobiotics, and they possess high levels of the enzymes that potentially convert xenobiotics to reactive or toxic metabolites. It is perhaps not surprising, therefore, that both tissues possess protective mechanisms to minimize the risk of xenobiotic toxicity and carcinogenicity. As already mentioned, both tissues have enzymes and transporters that facilitate the elimination of xenobiotics and their metabolites. In both tissues, several of the xenobiotic-biotransforming enzymes and transporters are inducible, enabling the liver and the small intestine to respond to high levels of xenobiotics by enhancing the rate of xenobiotic biotransformation and elimination. In the small intestine, the enterocytes at the villus tips undergo extensive turnover, such that the mature cells that are exposed to high levels of xenobiotics and/or reactive metabolites are quickly lost (exfoliated) and replaced in a matter of days. In liver, high levels of glutathione (5–10 mM), a large proportion of diploid (binucleated) cells, and a high regenerative capacity all protect the liver from xenobiotic toxicity or help the liver to repair chemical-mediated toxicity. In addition, severely damaged hepatocytes can undergo apoptosis (cell-programmed death) to eliminate precancerous cells (i.e., cells with extensive DNA damage).

Point 16   Some of the same mechanisms that protect the small intestine and liver from xenobiotic toxicity also protect certain organs such as the brain and reproductive organs. Xenobiotics that enter the systemic circulation are often excluded from the brain by the blood–brain barrier, which poses a physical barrier to xenobiotic transport (in the form of tight junctions) and a biochemical barrier notably in the form of the efflux transporter *P*-glycoprotein (MDR1 or ABCB1). Germ cells in the testis are protected in part by a blood–testis barrier, by high levels of glutathione (and glutathione transferase and glutathione peroxidase), and by high cell turnover (as in the case of enterocytes). The ovum, with virtually no cell turnover, possesses high levels of glutathione (8 mM and more), which protects it from DNA-reactive electrophiles and from the oxidative stress that accompanies both xenobiotic exposure and fertilization. Efflux transporters and glutathione transferases are often over-expressed in tumor cells as a result of chromosomal rearrangements that place the genes encoding these proteins under the control of a strong promoter. The over-expression of a transporter and/or glutathione transferase can confer resistance to certain cancer chemotherapeutic agents (many of which are intended to be converted to reactive metabolites that damage DNA and kill tumor cells).

Point 17   In view of the important role of cytochrome P450 in the metabolic activation of proximate carcinogens to ultimate carcinogens, it may seem paradoxical to list cytochrome P450 induction among the defense mechanisms that protect organisms from the carcinogenic effects of xenobiotics. Activation by cytochrome P450 is definitely required for certain xenobiotics to exert their carcinogenic effects, and induction of cytochrome P450 is associated with an increase in the toxicity of certain xenobiotics. However, contrary to expectation, treatment of rodents with a cytochrome P450 inducer prior to treatment with a known proximate carcinogen (such as aflatoxin, various nitrosamines, or polycyclic aromatic hydrocarbons) is generally associated with a decrease, not an increase, in tumor incidence (Parkinson and Hurwitz, 1991). The route of exposure to the carcinogen can affect the impact of enzyme induction; it protects against orally administered drugs but may increase the tumorigenicity of carcinogens applied directly to their site of action (Nebert *et al.*, 2004), and prolonged treatment of rodents with an enzyme inducer *after* application of the initiating carcinogen can lead to an increase in tumor incidence because many enzyme inducers act as tumor promoters (see Point 9). Nevertheless, enzyme induction appears, for the most part, to provide protection against chemical carcinogenesis.

Point 18   Although the small intestine and liver contain the highest concentrations, xenobiotic-biotransforming enzymes are nevertheless widely distributed throughout the body. In terms of specific content (i.e., the amount of enzyme on a per-mg-protein basis), some of the highest concentrations of xenobiotic-metabolizing enzymes are to be found in nasal epithelium, a portal of entry for many volatile xenobiotics. Xenobiotic-biotransforming enzymes in the lung, eye, and skin can be especially important for the metabolism of drugs delivered by inhalation, eye drop, or topical application, respectively. The kidney expresses several xenobiotic-biotransforming enzymes, in addition to numerous transporters that actively secrete xenobiotics (especially acidic metabolites) into urine. The kidney also metabolizes glutathione conjugates formed in the liver.

Point 19   Species differences in xenobiotic-biotransforming enzymes are often the basis for species differences in both the qualitative and quantitative aspects of xenobiotic biotransformation and toxicity. As mentioned in Point 14, species difference in coumarin metabolism and toxicity (activation by epoxidation in rats, detoxication by aromatic hydroxylation in humans) reflects a species difference in hepatic microsomal cytochrome P450, whereas species differences in glutathione transferase activity account for the difference between rats and mice in terms of their susceptibility to aflatoxin-induced liver toxicity. Species differences in the fetal expression of xenobiotic-biotransforming enzymes have raised questions about the suitability of laboratory animals to assess the risk of human teratogenicity because human fetal liver expresses CYP3A7, an enzyme capable of activating aflatoxin to reactive metabolites, whereas no such enzyme is expressed in the fetus of rodents (Li *et al.*, 1997).

Biotransformation, inhibition, and induction can occur in a species-specific manner. For example, furafylline and omeprazole are inhibitors and inducers of human CYP1A2, respectively, but they do not inhibit or induce CYP1A2 in rodents. Such species differences are the impetus for the development of so-called humanized mice, which involves substituting the murine genes that encode xenobiotic-metabolizing enzymes (and the receptors that regulate their expression) with their human counterparts (Gonzalez, 2003; Gonzalez and Yu, 2006).

In some species, entire pathways of xenobiotic biotransformation are low or absent. For example, cats and dogs are considered poor glucuronidators and poor acetylators of xenobiotics, respectively. Metabolism by gut microflora can occur in a species-dependent manner. For example, as shown in Fig. 6-1, quinic acid is converted to benzoic acid in humans and old-world monkeys but not in new-world monkeys, mice, rats, and most other laboratory animals (Adamson *et al.*, 1970).

Point 20   In sexually mature rats and, to a lesser extent, mice there are marked gender differences in the expression of certain xenobiotic-biotransforming enzymes (both oxidative and conjugating enzymes). In other species, including humans, gender differences either do not exist or they generally represent less than a twofold difference, whereas the differences in rodents can be an order of magnitude or greater. Against a large background of interindividual variation in each gender, it is often difficult to discern gender differences in xenobiotic biotransformation in humans although, in general, women appear to have lower CYP1A2 and higher CYP3A4 activity than men (reviewed in Parkinson *et al.*, 2004). It is particularly interesting that, compared with men, women appear to have a higher incidence of idiosyncratic drug toxicity (Walgren *et al.*, 2005), which has been the cause of a number of drug withdrawals and black box warnings (see Point 21).

Point 21   Idiosyncratic drug reactions (IDRs) are rare adverse events ($<0.1\%$) that do not involve an exaggerated pharmacological response, do not occur in most patients at any dose, and typically do not occur immediately after exposure but do so after weeks or months of repeated administration (Walgren *et al.*, 2005). IDRs are also known as Type B reactions, and they can be divided into allergic and nonallergic IDRs. The former tend to develop relatively quickly (in days or weeks) and, after the drug is discontinued, patients respond robustly when rechallenged with the same or a closely related drug, whereas the latter tend to develop relatively slowly (with symptoms sometimes appearing after 6 months or more of drug treatment) and patients may or may not respond to rechallenge with the drug. Evidence for an immune component to allergic IDRs is often circumstantial or lacking, as is the evidence for the lack of an immune component to nonallergic IDRs. Hepatotoxicity is a prevalent IDR. Drugs that were withdrawn from the U.S. market or carry a black box warning for idiosyncratic hepatotoxicity are listed in Table 6-3. The drugs are structurally diverse and fall into numerous therapeutic classes. In many cases there is evidence implicating a reactive metabolite in the idiosyncratic hepatotoxicity, although such metabolites tend to be formed in all individuals, leaving unanswered the critical question of what factor or factors predispose a small proportion of the population to the hepatotoxic effects of certain drugs, many of which cause little or no discernible liver toxicity in laboratory animals. In several cases, the drugs listed in Table 6-3 have closely related structures that do not cause idiosyncratic hepatotoxicity. For example, rosiglitazone and pioglitazone contain the same thiazolidinedione ring that in troglitazone is converted to a reactive metabolite, and yet only troglitazone has been withdrawn from the market because of idiosyncratic hepatotoxicity. This difference may be due to the much larger daily dose of troglitazone (300 mg) compared with rosiglitazone (4–8 mg) and pioglitazone (15–45 mg). Uetrecht (2001) has proposed the general rule that drugs administered at a daily dose of 10 mg or less do not cause idiosyncratic toxicity, and this rule is consistent with the dosing information shown in Table 6-3. Other examples of closely related drugs where one does and one does not cause hepatotoxicity include tolcapone/entacapone, ticlopidine/clopidogrel, amineptine/tianeptine,

tamoxifen/toremifene, ibufenac/ibuprofen, ebrotidine/famotidine, and niperotidine/ranitidine (Walgren *et al.*, 2005). Labetrol has two chiral centers and is a racemic mixture of four enantiomers, one of which is dilevalol. Although labetrol carries a black box warning for hepatotoxicity, dilevalol was not approved by the FDA because it caused a high incidence of liver toxicity during clinical trials. In some cases the difference is thought to be due to differences in dose (which is invariably higher for the drug partner that causes hepatotoxicity), but in other cases the basis for the difference is not known.

Point 22   The same dose of drug (or any other xenobiotic) administered to humans often results in large interindividual differences in exposure to the parent compound (typically measured as the area under the plasma concentration–time curve or AUC). This variation can reflect genetically determined differences in the activity of xenobiotic-biotransforming enzymes or transporters (genetic polymorphisms) or environmental differences, such as drug–drug interactions.

Point 23   The study of the causes, prevalence, and impact of heritable differences in xenobiotic-biotransforming enzymes is known as *pharmacogenetics*. It is the basis for the concept of individualized medicine, whereby the dosage of drugs with a narrow therapeutic index (such as anticancer drugs) is adjusted in accordance with an individual's genotype (i.e., drug-metabolizing potential).

Genetic variation in a xenobiotic-metabolizing enzyme produces four discernable phenotypes: poor metabolizers (PMs), intermediate metabolizers (IMs), extensive metabolizers (EMs), and ultrarapid metabolizers (UM), which arise from the expression of no functional alleles ($-/-$) for PMs, one nonfunctional allele and one partially functional allele or two partially active alleles ($-/^*$ or $^*/^*$) for IMs, one or two functional alleles ($+/-$, $+/^*$, or $+/+$) for EMs, and gene duplication ($[+/+]n$) for UMs. This traditional classification scheme has been revised recently on the basis of an activity score, which assigns to each allelic variant a functional activity value from 1 (for the wild type or ^{*1} allele) to zero (for any completely nonfunctional allele), as shown in Table 6-4 (Zineh *et al.*, 2004).

For those enzymes that are polymorphically expressed, such as CYP2D6, the incidence of the PM (and UM) genotype can vary widely from one ethnic group to the next. For example, the CYP2D6 PM genotype is common among Caucasians but not Asians, whereas the converse is true of the CYP2C19 PM genotype.

When the clearance of a drug is largely determined by a polymorphically expressed enzyme, such as CYP2D6, exposure follows the rank order: poor metabolizers (PMs) > intermediate metabolizers (IMs) > extensive metabolizers (EMs) > ultrarapid metabolizers (UMs). Exposure to metabolites (especially the maximum concentration, C_{max}) follows the opposite rank order. The difference in exposure between PMs and EMs (i.e., the fold increase in AUC associated with the PM phenotype versus the EM phenotype) depends on fractional metabolism (*fm*), a measure of how much of the drug's clearance is determined by CYP2D6 (or whatever enzyme is responsible for metabolizing the drug in question). The fold increase in AUC (AUC_{PM}/AUC_{EM}) is equal to $1/(1 - fm)$; hence, the impact of the polymorphism increases dramatically as *fm* approaches unity. If CYP2D6 accounted for half of a drug's clearance ($fm = 0.5$), exposure to that drug would increase twofold in CYP2D6 PMs. However, if CYP2D6 accounted for 90% of a drug's clearance ($fm = 0.9$), then exposure to that drug would increase tenfold in CYP2D6 PMs. This is why PMs are often at increased risk of adverse drug events either due to an exaggerated

Table 6-3

Drugs That Have Been Withdrawn or Carry a Black Box Warning for Idiosyncratic Hepatotoxicity[a]

DRUG NAME	TYPICAL DOSE (mg)	INDICATION	REACTIVE METABOLITE AND EVIDENCE OF MECHANISM-BASED ENZYME INHIBITION	INDUCTION[b], IMMUNOLOGICAL AND OTHER MECHANISTIC ASPECTS
Drugs withdrawn				
Benoxaprofen	300–600	NSAID	Acyl glucuronide	Inducer (rat AhR and PPARα agonist)
Bromfenac	25–50	NSAID	Acyl glucuronide	
Iproniazid	25–150	Depression	Multiple. MBI of MAO-B	Anti-MAO-B and antimitochondria
Nefazodone	200	Depression	Quinoneimine. MBI of CYP3A4	
Tienilic acid	250–500	Diuretic	Thiophene epoxide, sulfoxide. MBI of CYP2C9	Anti-LKM$_2$ (anti-CYP2C9)
Troglitazone	400	Diabetes	Quinone methide, sulfenic acid, α-ketoisocyanate	Inducer (CAR/PXR agonist)
Black box warnings				
Acitretin	25–50	Psoriasis	No. Acitretin, a retinoid, is esterified to etretinate	Etretinate was withdrawn in 2002
Bosentan	125–250	PAH	No	Inhibits BSEP. Inducer (PXR agonist)
Dacarbazine	140–315	Melanoma, lymphoma	Methyl diazohydroxide and methyl cation (CH$_3^+$)	Hepatotoxic to laboratory animals
Dantrolene	300–400	Muscle relaxant	Nitro-reduction intermediates bind to GSH	Inducer (AhR agonist)
Felbamate	1200	Epilepsy	2-Phenylpropenal (atropaldehyde)	Inducer (PXR agonist)
Flutamide	750	Prostate cancer	Unknown metabolites bind to protein and GSH	Inhibits mitochondrial respiration
Gemtuzumab	9 mg/m^2	AML	Reductive activation to a di-radical	Designed to intercalate and bind DNA
Isoniazid	300	Tuberculosis	Multiple. MBI of CYP1A1, 2A6, 2C19, and 3A4.	Radicals formed by myeloperoxidase
Ketoconazole	200	Fungal infections	Di-aldehyde	Auto-inhibitor (inhibits CYP3A4)
Naltrexone	50	Alcoholism, addiction	No	
Nevirapine	200–400	AIDS	No	Inducer (PXR agonist)
Pemoline	37.5–112.5	Hyperactivity	No	
Tolcapone	300	Parkinsonism	Nitro reduction and then quinoneimine formation	Uncouples mitochondrial respiration
Trovafloxacin	100–500	Antibiotic	No, but it has a lipophilic difluorinated side chain present in a toxic fluoroquinolone—now withdrawn	Eosinophilia suggests an immune-mediated hepatitis
Valproic acid (VPA)	1000–4200	Epilepsy	CoA esterification and epoxidation of 4-ene-VPA	Disrupts mitochondrial β-oxidation

[a] Data Adapted from Walgren JL, Mitchell MD, Thompson DC: Role of metabolism in drug-induced idiosyncratic hepatotoxicity. *Crit Rev Toxicol* 35:325–361, 2005.

[b]The receptor agonist assignment is based on the CYP-induced enzyme (CYP1A for AhR; CYP2B, CYP2C, and/or CYP3A for CAR/PXR; CYP4A for PPARα).
AhR, aryl hydrocarbon receptor; AIDS, acquired immunodeficiency syndrome; AML, acute myeloid leukemia; anti-LKM$_2$, auto-antibodies against liver and kidney microsomes
(anti-LKM$_1$ contains antibodies against CYP2D6, whereas anti-LKM$_2$ contains antibodies against CYP2C9); BSEP, bile salt export pump (a bile canalicular transporter);
CYP, cytochrome P450; GSH, glutathione; MAO, monoamine oxidase; MBI, mechanism-based inhibitor (a.k.a. suicide inactivator); NSAID, nonsteroidal anti-inflammatory
drug; PAH, pulmonary arterial hypertension; PPARα, peroxisome proliferator activated receptor-alpha; PXR, pregnane X receptor; VPA, valproic acid.

Table 6-4

The Relationship Between Genotype and Phenotype for a Polymorphically Expressed Enzyme with Active (wt), Partially Active (*x), and Inactive (*y) Alleles

GENOTYPE	ALLELES	CONVENTIONAL PHENOTYPE[a]	ACTIVITY SCORE[b]	ACTIVITY SCORE PHENOTYPE[c]
Duplication of active alleles ($n = 2$ or more)	(wt/wt)n	UM	$2 \times n$	UM
Two fully active wild-type (wt) alleles	wt/wt	EM	$1 + 1 = 2$	High EM
One fully active + one partially active allele	wt/*x	EM	$1 + 0.5 = 1.5$	Medium EM
One fully active + one inactive allele	wt/*y	EM	$1 + 0 = 1$	Low EM
Two partially active alleles	*x/*x	EM or IM	$0.5 + 0.5 = 1$	Low EM
One partially active + one inactive allele	*x/*y	IM	$0.5 + 0 = 0.5$	IM
Two inactive alleles	*y/*y	PM	$0 + 0 =$ zero	PM

[a]The phenotypes are ultrarapid metabolizer (UM), extensive metabolizer (EM), intermediate metabolizer (IM), and poor metabolizer (PM), based on the particular combination of alleles that are fully active (wt), partially active (*x), or inactive (*y).

[b]In the case of CYP2D6 (Data from Zineh *et al.*, 2004), various activity scores have been determined experimentally as follows:

Activity score = 1.0 for each *1 (wt), *2, *35, and *41 [2988G].
Activity score = 0.75 for each *9, *29, *45, and *46.
Activity score = 0.5 for each *10, *17, and *41 [2988A].
Activity score = 0 for each *3, *4, *5, *6, *7, *8, *11, *12, *15, *36, *40, and *42.

[c]Activity scores are classified as follows (from Zineh *et al.*, 2004):

UM activity score => 2.0 (e.g., [*1/*1]n where n is 2 or more gene duplications).
High EM activity score = 1.75 to 2.0 (e.g., *1/*1).
Medium EM activity score = 1.5 (e.g., *1/*17 or *9/*9).
Low EM activity score = 1.0 to 1.25 (e.g., *1/*4, *17/*17, or *9/*17).
IM activity score = 0.5 to 0.75 (e.g., *4/*9 or *4/*17).
PM activity score = 0 (e.g., *4/*4).

pharmacological response to the drug or due to its toxic side effects. An exception is omeprazole and other proton pump inhibitors, which actually provide improved control over gastroesophageal reflux disease (GERD) in CYP2C19 PMs compared with EMs (Furuta *et al.*, 2005).

There are a minority of cases where the UMs, not the PMs, are at increased risk, especially in cases where the polymorphic enzyme catalyzes the formation of a pharmacologically active or toxic metabolite. For example, CYP2D6 converts the prodrug codeine into the active metabolite morphine, and there are reports of morphine intoxication in CYP2D6 UMs; one case being the death of a baby being breast fed by a CYP2D6 UM mother who was prescribed codeine (Gasche *et al.*, 2004; Koren *et al.*, 2006).

Many cases have now been described where the PM phenotype requires dosage adjustment to prevent drug toxicity or an exaggerated pharmacological response. For example, CYP2D6 PMs are at increased risk for perhexiline hepatotoxicity and at increased risk for an exaggerated pharmacological response to debrisoquine and sparteine, three drugs that were not approved in the USA because of the high incidence of adverse events in the PMs. On the other hand, when drugs are converted to active metabolites by CYP2D6, then PMs derive inadequate therapeutic effect. For example, CYP2D6 converts codeine to morphine; hence, codeine is a less-effective analgesic in PMs. Similarly, CYP2D6 converts the breast cancer drug tamoxifen to endoxifen (which is 30- to 100-fold more potent than tamoxifen in suppressing estrogen-dependent cell proliferation), hence, CYP2D6 PMs are at increased risk for breast cancer recurrence following tamoxifen adjuvant therapy (Goetz *et al.*, 2005). Other examples of genetic polymorphisms that affect drug disposition in humans include CYP2C9 (warfarin), CYP2C19 (omeprazole), CYP3A4 (clopidogrel, irinotecan, thioridazine), CYP3A5 (tacrolimus), UGT1A1 (irinotecan), UGT2B7 (morphine), TPMT (6-mercaptopurine), NAT2 (isoniazid), COMT (levodopa), DPD (5-

fluorouracil), and the efflux transporter P-glycoprotein (digoxin) (Robert *et al.*, 2005; Relling and Giacomini, 2006). Most of these drugs identified in parentheses all have a narrow therapeutic target. Details of these genetic polymorphisms are given later in the chapter.

Genetic polymorphisms in xenobiotic-biotransforming enzymes have an impact on the incidence of certain environmental diseases. For example, ethnic differences in the incidence of polymorphisms in alcohol dehydrogenase and aldehdye dehydrogenase impact the incidence of alcoholism (Li, 2000). Genetic polymorphisms in CYP2A6 impact the incidence of cigarette-smoking-induced lung cancer. Individuals lacking CYP2A6 are PMs of nicotine (so they tend to smoke less than CYP2A6 EMs) and are poor activators of tobacco-specific mutagens (so they form fewer DNA-reactive metabolites than do CYP2A6 EMs) (Kamataki *et al.*, 2005).

Genetic polymorphisms can be the underlying cause of a disease. For example, the severe and mild hyperbilirubinemia associated with Crigler–Najjar syndrome and Gilbert's syndrome, respectively, reflect a complete and partial loss of the UDP-glucuronosyltransferase responsible for conjugating bilirubin, namely, UGT1A1. The hyperbilirubinemic Gunn rat is the rodent equivalent of Crigler–Najjar syndrome.

Genetic polymorphisms have been described in laboratory animals. For example, laboratory-bred rabbits have about 50:50 chance of being a poor or rapid acetylator of certain drugs a (such as isoniazid) because *N*-acetyltransferase 2 (NAT2) is polymorphically expressed in rabbits.

Point 24 Environmental factors can introduce as much variation in drug metabolism as can genetic factors, and this is especially true of drug–drug interactions. To take CYP3A4 as an example, PMs can be created pharmacologically with inhibitors (such as ketoconazole and erythromycin), whereas UMs can be created pharmacologically with inducers (such as rifampin and the herbal agent

St. John's wort). Whereas the impact of genetic polymorphisms on drug disposition and safety is often identified during clinical trials, the impact of drug–drug interactions may not be identified until after the drug has been approved and is under postmarketing surveillance.

Drugs (and other xenobiotics) can be viewed from a *victim* and *perpetrator* perspective. A drug whose clearance is largely determined by a single route of elimination, such as metabolism by a single CYP enzyme, is considered a victim drug (also known as a sensitive or object drug). Such drugs have a high victim potential because a diminution or loss of that elimination pathway, either due to a genetic deficiency in the relevant CYP enzyme or due to its inhibition by another, concomitantly administered drug, will result in a large decrease in victim drug clearance and a correspondingly large increase in exposure (the magnitude of which will depend on fractional metabolism, as indicated in Point 23). Some victim drugs have a high therapeutic index, hence, they are therapeutically effective in PMs to UMs and cause roughly the same incidence of adverse effects regardless of genotype. However, in the case of victim drugs with a narrow therapeutic index, dosage must be increased in UMs to achieve a therapeutic effect and/or it must be decreased in PMs to prevent adverse drug events.

Perpetrators are those drugs (or other environmental factors) that inhibit or induce the enzyme that is otherwise responsible for clearing a victim drug. In other words, perpetrators are drugs that cause drug–drug interactions. Perpetrators are also known as precipitants. Genetic polymorphisms that result in the partial or complete loss of enzyme activity can also be viewed as perpetrators inasmuch they cause a decrease in the clearance of—and an increase in exposure to—victim drugs.

Terfenadine (Seldane), cisapride (Propulsid), astemizole (Hismanal), and cerivastatin (Baycol) are all victim drugs, so much so that they have all been withdrawn from the market (Fung *et al.*, 2001). The first three are all victim drugs because they are extensively metabolized by CYP3A4. Inhibition of CYP3A4 by various antimycotic drugs, such as ketoconazole, and antibiotic drugs, such as erythromycin, decrease the clearance of terfenadine, cisapride, and astemizole and increase their plasma concentrations to levels that, in some individuals, cause ventricular arrhythmias (QT prolongation) which can result in fatal heart attacks. Cerivastatin is extensively metabolized by CYP2C8. Its metabolism is inhibited by gemfibrozil (actually by gemfibrozil glucuronide), and the combination of cerivastatin (Baycol) and gemfibrozil (Lopid) was associated with a high incidence of fatal, cerivastatin-induced rhabdomyolysis (Ogilvie *et al.*, 2006).

Mibefradil (Posicor) is the only drug withdrawn from the U.S. market largely because of its perpetrator potential. This calcium channel blocker not only causes extensive inhibition of CYP3A4, it causes prolonged inhibition of the enzyme by virtue of being a metabolism-dependent inhibitor of CYP3A4. By inactivating CYP3A4 in an irreversible manner—such that restoration of normal CYP3A4 activity required the synthesis of new enzyme—mibefradil inhibits CYP3A4 long after treatment with the drug is discontinued.

The in vitro technique of reaction phenotyping (also known as enzyme mapping) is the process of identifying which enzyme or enzymes are largely responsible for metabolizing a drug candidate (Williams *et al.*, 2003b; Ogilvie *et al.*, 2007). Reaction phenotyping allows an assessment of the victim potential of a drug candidate or other xenobiotic. Drug candidates can also be evaluated in vitro for their potential to inhibit or induce cytochrome P450, which allows

an assessment of their perpetrator potential (Tucker *et al.*, 2001; Bjornsson *et al.*, 2003; U.S. Food and Drug Administration, 2006).

Herbal remedies can also interact with drugs. For example, St. John's wort contains hyperforin, which is a potent PXR agonist and, as such, is an inducer of CYP3A4 (along with several other xenobiotic-metabolizing enzymes) and *P*-glycoprotein (MDR1 or ABCB1). To prevent a loss of therapeutic efficacy, the use of St. John's wort is not recommended for patients on antirejection drugs (such as cyclosporine and tacrolimus), anti-HIV drugs (such as indinavir and nevirapine), anticoagulants (such as warfarin and phenprocoumon), or oral contraceptive steroids (Pal and Mitra, 2006). Food can affect drug disposition in a number of ways. It can affect absorption, which is why some drugs are taken with meals and others are taken between meals. Large quantities of cruciferous vegetables (e.g., broccoli and Brussels sprouts) can induce hepatic CYP1A2 (Conney, 1982), whereas grapefruit juice can inhibit intestinal CYP3A4 (Paine *et al.*, 2006).

Point 25   Although drug–drug interactions can cause an increase in the incidence of adverse events or, in the case of induction, a loss of therapeutic efficacy, not all drug–drug interactions are undesirable. For example, some anti-HIV drugs, like ritonavir, inhibit CYP3A4 and thereby improve the pharmacokinetic profile of other anti-HIV drugs, like saquinavir and lopinavir. Tumors often over-express various transporters and glutathione transferases, which limit the effectiveness of several anticancer drugs. Drugs that inhibit transporters and glutathione transferase are being developed to enhance the efficacy of anticancer drugs.

Point 26   Although the amount of functional enzyme determines whether an individual is a poor or rapid metabolizer, there are other factors that can impact the rate of xenobiotic metabolism. Not surprisingly, severe liver disease decreases the rate of metabolism of a large number of drugs whose clearance is determined by hepatic metabolism. For certain xenobiotic-metabolizing enzymes, particularly the conjugating enzymes, cofactor availability can impact the rate of xenobiotic biotransformation. The liver usually has sufficient NADPH to saturate reactions catalyzed by cytochrome P450, but it does not have sufficient levels of UDP-glucuronic acid (UDPGA) or 3′-phosphoadenosine-5′-phosphosulfate (PAPS) to saturate the enzymes responsible for glucuronidating or sulfonating xenobiotics. Consequently, alterations in the levels of these cofactors can impact the rate or extent of glucuronidation and sulfonation. For example, fasting lowers hepatic levels of these cofactors, and fasting decreases the extent to which acetaminophen is conjugated. Consequently, fasting increases the extent to which acetaminophen is metabolized to a toxic metabolite by cytochrome P450 (including CYP2E1, which is induced by fasting), for which reason fasting is suspected of being one of the risk factors for acetaminophen hepatotoxicity (Whitcomb, 1994).

Point 27   Stereochemical aspects can play an important role in the interaction between a xenobiotic and its biotransforming enzyme (both from a substrate and inhibitor perspective), and xenobiotic-biotransforming enzymes can play a key role in converting one stereoisomer to another, a process known as *mutarotation* or *inversion of configuration*.

A xenobiotic that contains a chiral center can exist in two mirror-image forms called stereoisomers or enantiomers. The biotransformation of some chiral xenobiotics occurs stereoselectively; meaning that one enantiomer (stereoisomer) is biotransformed faster than its antipode. For example, the antiepileptic drug Mesantoin®, which is a racemic mixture of *R*- and *S*-mephenytoin, is biotransformed stereoselectively in humans, such that the *S*-enantiomer is rapidly hydroxylated (by CYP2C19) and eliminated faster than the R-enantiomer. The ability of some chiral xenobiotics to inhibit xenobiotic-biotransforming enzymes can also occur stereoselectively. For example, quinidine is a potent inhibitor of CYP2D6, where as quinine, its antipode, has relatively little inhibitory effect on this enzyme. In some cases, achiral molecules (or achiral centers) are converted to a mixture of enantiomeric metabolites, and this conversion may proceed stereoselectively such that one enantiomer is formed preferentially over its antipode. For example, several cytochrome P450 enzymes catalyze the 6-hydroxylation of steroid hormones. Some P450 enzymes (such as the rat enzyme CYP2A1) preferentially catalyze the 6α-hydroxylation reaction, whereas other P450 enzymes (such as the CYP3A enzymes in all mammalian species) preferentially catalyze the 6β-hydroxylation reaction (which is a major route of hepatic steroid biotransformation).

Inversion of configuration is the process whereby one enantiomer is converted to its antipode via an achiral intermediate. This interconversion can occur nonenzymatically, as in the case of thalidomide, or it can be catalyzed by a xenobiotic-metabolizing enzyme, as in the case of lisofylline, or by an endobiotic-metabolizing enzyme, as in the case of simvastatin (Fig. 6-2).

In the case of thalidomide, inversion of configuration (as shown in Fig. 6-2) occurs spontaneously, although the process is facilitated by albumin (Eriksson *et al.*, 1998). In the mid-to-late 1950s, mainly in Europe, thalidomide was prescribed to pregnant women in the first trimester to treat morning sickness. Unfortunately, whereas (R)-thalidomide is an effective sedative, the (S)-enantiomer is a teratogen that produces phocomelia (limb shortening) and other congenital defects in the offspring largely as a result of its ability to inhibit angiogenesis (vasculogenesis). The teratogenic effect of thalidomide cannot be circumvented by administering only the (R)-enantiomer because spontaneous or albumin-facilitated racemization quickly produces the teratogenic (S)-enantiomer. Thalidomide blocks the release of tissue necrosis factor alpha (TNFα) and it has been approved for the treatment of erythema nodosum leprosum (an acute inflammatory reaction associated with lepromatous leprosy), and is useful in the treatment of several other inflammatory conditions and immune-mediated diseases. Because of its ability to inhibit angiogenesis (the process that supplies tumors with new blood vessels), thalidomide is also under investigation as an anticancer drug. It is ironic that a drug with antivascular side effects that was originally prescribed as a sedative is now in clinical trials for vascular diseases with sedation as a side effect (Franks *et al.*, 2004).

Ketones can be reduced by carbonyl reductases to a mixture of enantiomeric secondary alcohols, and this can occur with a high degree of stereoselectivity. For example, pentoxifylline is reduced by carbonyl reductases in blood and liver to a mixture of secondary alcohols with the major metabolite having an S-configuration, as shown in Fig. 6-2. Interestingly, the minor metabolite, a secondary alcohol with the R-configuration, has pharmacological properties distinct from those of its S-antipode and its ketone precursor, pentoxifylline. This minor metabolite is known as lisofylline, which is under clinical investigation for the treatment of various diseases. Through the action of carbonyl reductase, lisofylline is oxidized to pentoxifylline and then reduced to its antipode (i.e., R-alcohol $\rightarrow$ ketone $\rightarrow$ S-alcohol), the net result being an inversion of configuration (Lillibridge *et al.*, 1996). The same type of interconversion explains why the administration of pure R-albuterol to human volunteers results in the formation of S-albuterol, just as the admin-

istration of pure S-albuterol leads to the formation of R-albuterol (Boulton and Fawcett, 1997).

In the case of simvastatin (which contains a β-hydroxy-lactone), the interconversion of two secondary alcohols (β-hydroxy-lactone $\leftrightarrow$ α-hydroxy-lactone) involves hydrolysis of the lactone ring (by paraoxonase 3 [hPON3] in humans) followed by formation of a thioether with coenzyme A, the first step in the β-oxidation of fatty acids, followed by dehydration to an achiral intermediate. Reversal of the steps by a combination of hydrolysis and lactonization (condensation) restores the lactone ring with the hydroxyl group in the original β-configuration or in the opposing α-configuration. In humans, the initial hydrolysis of the lactone ring and the final lactonization (condensation) reaction are both catalyzed by paraoxonase-3 (hPON3) (Draganov and La Du, 2004).

Point 28   Mass spectrometry is widely used to characterize the structure of metabolites, and many instruments now come equipped with software to assist in this process, based on the fact that certain xenobiotic reactions are associated with discrete changes in mass. For example, the loss of 2 atomic mass units (amu) signifies dehydrogenation, whereas the loss of 14 amu usually signifies demethylation ($-CH_2$). Several reactions result in an increase in mass, including reduction (+2 amu = 2H), methylation (+14 amu = CH_2), oxidation (+16 amu = O), hydration (+18 amu = H_2O), acetylation (+42 amu = C_2H_2O), glucosylation (+162 = $C_6H_{10}O_5$), sulfonation (+80 amu = SO_3), glucuronidation (+176 amu = $C_6H_8O_6$), and conjugation with glutathione (+305 amu = $C_{10}H_{15}N_3O_6S$), glycine (+74 amu = $C_2H_4NO_2$), and taurine (+42 amu = $C_2H_6NO_3S$).

Occasionally, routine changes in mass can arise from unexpected reactions. For example, ziprasidone is converted to two metabolites, each of which involves an increase of 16 amu, which normally indicates addition of oxygen (e.g., hydroxylation, sulfoxidation, N-oxygenation). One of the metabolites is indeed formed by addition of oxygen to ziprasidone (sulfoxidation), as shown in Fig. 6-3 (Beedham *et al.*, 2003). However, the other metabolite is formed by a combination of reduction (+2 amu) and methylation (+14). Therefore, care must be exercised in interpreting routes of metabolism based on changes in mass.

Mass spectrometry can typically provide information on which region of a molecule has undergone biotransformation, but it can seldom distinguish between several closely related possibilities. For example, based on mass spectrometry alone, it might be possible to ascertain that a certain phenyl group has been hydroxylated. However, analysis by nuclear magnetic resonance (NMR) is required to ascertain whether the hydroxylation occurred at the ortho, meta, or para position.

Point 29   As mentioned in Point 18, xenobiotic-biotransforming enzymes are widely distributed throughout the body. The advent of high-throughput assays based on quantitative real-time reverse-transcription polymerase chain reaction (QPCR) has facilitated comprehensive measurements of the levels of mRNA encoding numerous xenobiotic-biotransforming enzymes, transporters, and xenosensors in a wide range of human tissues (Nishimura *et al.*, 2003, 2004; Furukawa *et al.*, 2004; Nishimura and Naito, 2005, 2006). These data are very informative as far as mRNA expression is concerned, but it can be difficult to draw conclusions about the activity of a given enzyme in a given tissue based on mRNA levels alone. For instance, based on mRNA levels in human liver, the levels of the top-ten CYP enzymes follow the rank order: CYP2E1 $\gg$ 2A6 > 2C8 > 2C18 $\approx$ 1A2 $\approx$ 4A11 $\approx$ 8B1 $\approx$ 2C9 $\approx$ 3A4 > CYP51A1 (Nishimura *et al.*, 2003). This contrasts substantially from the levels of CYP

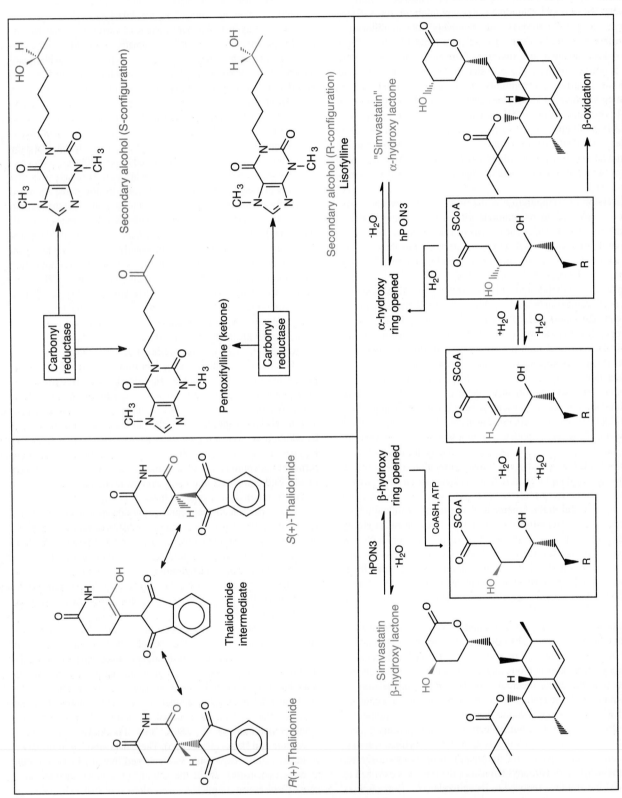

Figure 6-2. *Stereochemical aspects of xenobiotic biotransformation: Inversion of configuration by nonenzymatic means (thalidomide), by carbonyl reductase (liso-fylline), and by hydrolysis and condensation (lactonization) of a lactone ring (simvastatin).*

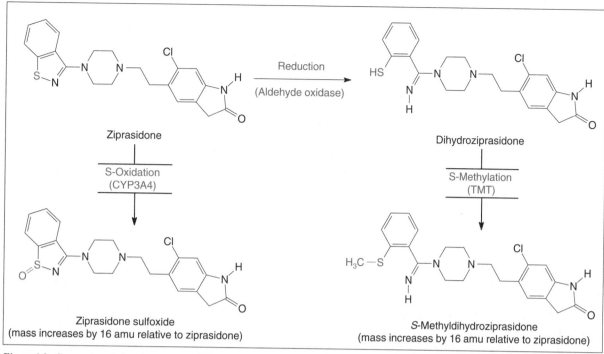

Figure 6-3. *Conversion of ziprasidone to two different metabolites both involving a mass increase of 16 amu (relative to ziprasidone).*

protein, which follow the rank order: CYP3A4 > 2C9 ≈ 3A5 ≈ 2E1 > 1A2 > 2A6 > 2C8 > 2C19 > 2B6 > 2D6 (Rowland-Yeo *et al.*, 2004; Howgate *et al.*, 2006). In the case of CYP2E1, hepatic mRNA levels are more than 17 times higher than the levels of CYP3A4 mRNA, but CYP2E1 protein levels are less than half those of CYP3A4. This discrepancy is due to the fact that, under normal conditions, most of the mRNA encoding CYP2E1 is sequestered in the cytoplasm and is not available for translation (Gonzalez, 2007). The mRNA for FMO2 is present at very high levels in human lung, but is not translated into functional enzyme due to the presence of a truncation mutation in Caucasians and Asians. However, about 26% of African Americans, 7% of Puerto Ricans, and 2% of Mexicans have one normal allele and express a functional protein (Cashman and Zhang, 2006).

HYDROLYSIS, REDUCTION, AND OXIDATION

Hydrolysis

Mammals contain a variety of enzymes that hydrolyze xenobiotics containing such functional groups as a carboxylic acid ester (delapril and procaine), amide (procainamide), thioester (spironolactone), phosphoric acid ester (paraoxon), acid anhydride (diisopropyl-fluorophosphate [DFP]), and lactone (spironolactone), as shown in Fig. 6-4. The major hydrolytic enzymes are the carboxylesterases, cholinesterases, and paraoxonases (for which lactonase is a more encompassing name), but they are by no means the only hydrolytic enzymes involved in xenobiotic biotransformation. The first two classes of hydrolytic enzymes, the carboxylesterases and cholinesterases, are known as serine esterases because their catalytic site contains a nucleophilic serine residue that participates in the hydrolysis of various xenobiotic and endobiotic substrates. This serine residue becomes phosphorylated by organophosphorus (OP) compounds, such as those used as insecticides, herbicides, fungi-

cides, nematicides, and plant growth regulators. However, following completion of the human genome project, it was determined that, of the estimated 22,500 human genes, about 5% (1227 genes) can be classified as serine hydrolases based on structural features (motifs) predicted from their DNA sequence, of which about 150 can be classified as serine proteases (Casida and Quistad, 2005).

Based on the large number of potential serine hydrolases, it is not surprising that enzymes other than those described in this chapter (namely, the carboxylesterases, cholinesterases, and paraoxonases) may participate in xenobiotic metabolism. Aldehyde dehydrogenases, carbonic anhydrases, carboxypeptidases, lipases, proteases, and even albumin have all been shown to have hydrolytic (esteratic) activity toward various xenobiotics. Cytochrome P450 can catalyze the cleavage of certain xenobiotics containing a carboxylic acid ester (see section "Cytochrome P450" for examples).

Based on the large number of potential serine hydrolases, it is not surprising that enzymes other than carboxylesterases and cholinesterases represent additional targets for phosphorylation and inactivation by OP compounds. Some of these OP targets have been identified; they include enzymes involved in the hydrolysis of endobiotics and certain receptors (reviewed in Casida and Quistad, 2005). Differential binding to these numerous sites may account for some of the differences observed among OP compounds. However, in insects, nematodes, and mammals, the critical site is acetylcholinesterase, the cholinesterase that hydrolyzes acetylcholine and thereby terminates its neurotransmitter activity. Phosphorylation of acetylcholinesterase is the principal mechanism of OP toxicity, with 70–90% inhibition usually proving lethal, and reversal of this phosphorylation event is one of the strategies to treat OP poisoning (e.g., with pralidoxime).

In the presence of an alcohol, carboxylesterases and certain other hydrolytic enzymes can catalyze the transesterification of xenobiotics, which accounts for the conversion of cocaine (a methyl ester) to ethylcocaine (the corresponding ethyl ester) (Fig. 6-4).

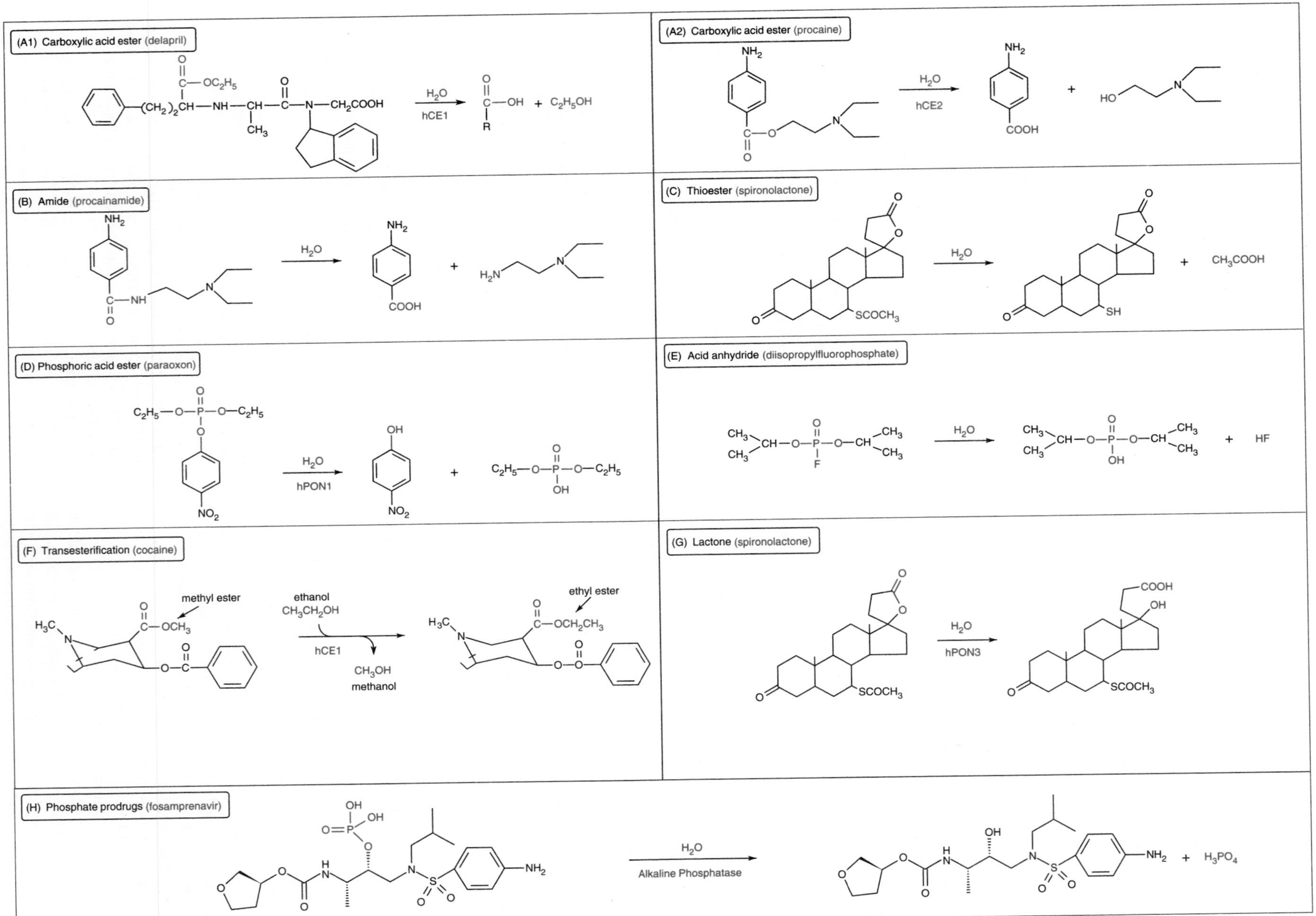

Figure 6-4. *Examples of reactions catalyzed by carboxylesterases, cholinesterases, organophosphatases, and alkaline phosphatase. hCE1 and hCE2, human carboxylesterases 1 and 2; hPON1 and hPON3 (human) paraoxonase 1 and 3.*

Transesterification occurs when ethanol, not water, cleaves the catalytic transition state, i.e., the esteratic bond between the active serine residue on the enzyme and the carbonyl group on the xenobiotic:

$$\text{Enzyme}-\text{O}-\text{CO}-\text{R} + \text{CH}_3\text{CH}_2\text{OH}$$
$$\rightarrow \text{Enzyme}-\text{OH} + \text{CH}_3\text{CH}_2-\text{O}-\text{CO}-\text{R}$$

Carboxylesterases in serum, liver, intestine, and other tissues and the cholinesterases in blood (and muscles depending on the route of xenobiotic exposure) collectively determine the duration and site of action of certain drugs. For example, procaine—a carboxylic acid ester—is rapidly hydrolyzed, which is why this drug is used mainly as a local anesthetic. In contrast, procainamide, the amide analog of procaine, is hydrolyzed much more slowly; hence, this drug reaches the systematic circulation, where it is useful in the treatment of cardiac arrhythmia. In general, enzymatic hydrolysis of amides occurs more slowly than esters, although electronic factors can influence the rate of hydrolysis. The presence of electron-withdrawing substituents weakens an amide bond, making it more susceptible to enzymatic hydrolysis.

The hydrolysis of xenobiotics by carboxylesterases and other hydrolytic enzymes is not always a detoxication process. Figure 6-5 shows some examples in which carboxylesterases convert xenobiotics to toxic and tumorigenic metabolites.

In 1953, Aldridge classified hydrolytic enzymes on the basis of their interaction with OP compounds, classifying those that hydrolyze OP compounds as A-esterases, those that are inhibited by OP compounds as B-esterases, and those that do not interact with OP compounds as C-esterases. Although the terms are still widely used, the classification system of Aldridge can be somewhat confusing because it divides the paraoxonases into the A- and C-esterase class (the human paraoxonase hPNO1 hydrolyzes OP compounds and so can be classified as an A-esterase, whereas hPON2 and hPON3 can be classified as C-esterases because they do not hydrolyze OP compounds, nor are they inhibited by them). Furthermore, carboxylesterases and cholinesterases, two distinct classes of hydrolytic enzymes, are both B-esterases according to Aldridge because both are inhibited by OP compounds.

Carboxylesterases Carboxylesterases are ~60 kDa glycoproteins that are present in a wide variety of tissues, including serum. Most of the carboxylesterase activity in liver is associated with the endoplasmic reticulum, although considerable carboxylesterase activity is present in lysosomes and cytosol. Although by some estimates human liver and brain may express 5 and 30 carboxylesterases, respectively (Liederer and Borchardt, 2006), the hydrolysis of xenobiotic esters and amides in humans is largely catalyzed by just two carboxylesterases called hCE1 and hCE2. hCE1 mRNA is detected at very high levels in the liver, followed by the trachea and lung (at less than 10% of the level detected in the liver) (Nishimura and Naito, 2006). It is encoded by two genes, namely, CES1A1 and CES1A2, that differ only in the amino acid sequence of the encoded signal peptide, for which reason both genes are considered to encode the same enzyme, hCE1. The second human carboxylesterase, hCE2, is encoded by CES2A1, and is expressed to approximately the same extent in the liver and small intestine, followed by the colon and kidney (at less than half of the level detected in the liver) (Nishimura and Naito, 2006). In various mammalian species, carboxylesterases are found in the plasma, whereas human plasma does not contain carboxylesterases, meaning that

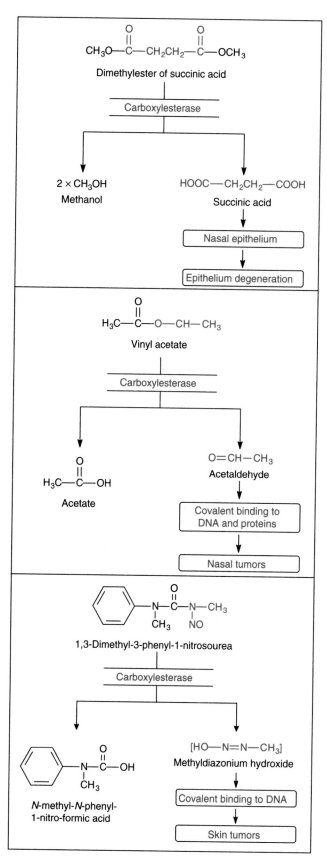

Figure 6-5. Activation of xenobiotics to toxic and tumorigenic metabolites by carboxylesterases.

butyrylcholinesterases and paraoxonases, not carboxylesterases, are responsible for the hydrolysis of amide and ester-containing compounds in the plasma (Satoh and Hosokawa, 2006). In rats, hydrolases A and B appear to be the counterparts of hCE1 and hCE2, respectively. The HUGO Gene Nomenclature Committee has officially approved gene names for CES1, 2, 3, 4, and 7 (http://www.gene.ucl.ac.uk/nomenclature/index.html), with CES1 and CES2 corresponding to hCE1 and hCE2. However, Satoh and Hosokawa (2006) have proposed that in all mammalian species, the carboxylesterases can be assigned to one of five gene families (designated CES 1–5) with three human genes in the first gene family (namely, CES1A1, 1A2, and 1A3), and a single member of the remaining families (i.e., CES2A1, 3A1, 4C1, and 5A1).

As illustrated in Fig. 6-4, hCE1 generally catalyzes the hydrolysis of xenobiotics with a small alcoholic leaving group (such as ethanol, as in the case of delapril) whereas hCE2 generally catalyzes the hydrolysis of xenobiotics with a small acidic or large alcoholic leaving group (as in the case of procaine), although there are xenobiotics that are hydrolyzed by both enzymes. hCE1 is more active than hCE2 at catalyzing the hydrolysis of numerous xenobiotics such as oseltamivir, benazepril, cilazepril, quinapril, temocapril, imidapril, meperidine, delapril, and clopidogrel, as well as the transesterification of the methyl esters of cocaine (Fig. 6-4), whereas hCE2 is more active than hCE1 at hydrolyzing aspirin, heroin, cocaine benzoyl ester, 6-acetylmorphine, oxybutynin, and the anticancer drug irinotecan (7-ethyl-10-[4-(1-piperidino)-1-piperidino]carbonyoxycamptothecin, also known as CPT-11) (Satoh and Hosokawa, 2006; Shi et al., 2006; Tang et al., 2006). The hydrolysis of irinotecan by hCE2 (and, to a much lesser extent, by hCE1) produces SN-38, a topoisomerase inhibitor that is responsible for both the anticancer effects of irinotecan and many of its side effects, especially diarrhea, which can be understood, at least in part, by the high levels of hCE2 in the intestine (Satoh et al., 2002).

Genetic polymorphisms (single nucleotide polymorphisms or SNPs) have been described for hCE2, some of which appear to lower the rate of hydrolysis of irinotecan to SN-38 (Kubo et al., 2005). Genetic polymorphisms have also been described for hCE1, but these are less likely to impair overall hCE1 because the enzyme is encoded by two genes. Therefore, a true hCE1 PM would only arise if genetic polymorphisms affected both alleles of both hCES1A1 and hCES1A2. A phenotype for hCE1 that might be classified as high extensive metabolizer has been described. It arises from a single nucleotide polymorphism in the promoter region of hCES1A2 (but not hCES1A1) that increases the expression of hCE1 and thereby increases the rate of hydrolysis of imidapril to its active metabolite imidaprilat, an angiotensin-converting enzyme (ACE) inhibitor, which increases its antihypertensive effect (Geshi et al., 2005).

In addition to hydrolyzing xenobiotics, carboxylesterases hydrolyze numerous endogenous compounds, such as palmitoyl-CoA, monoacylglycerol, diacylglycerol, retinyl ester, platelet-activating factor, and other esterified lipids. Carboxylesterases can also catalyze the synthesis of fatty acid ethyl esters, which represents a nonoxidative pathway of ethanol metabolism in adipose and certain other tissues. In the case of platelet-activating factor, carboxylesterases catalyze both the deacetylation of PAF and its subsequent esterification with fatty acids to form phosphatidylcholine (Satoh and Hosokawa, 1998).

Certain carboxylesterases also have a physiologic function in anchoring other proteins to the endoplasmic reticulum. For example, the lysosomal enzyme β-glucuronidase is also present in the endoplasmic reticulum, where it is anchored in the lumen by egasyn, a microsomal carboxylesterase related to hCE1. Egasyn binds to β-glucuronidase at its active site serine residue, which effectively abolishes the carboxylesterase activity of egasyn, although there is no corresponding loss of β-glucuronidase activity. Binding of OP compounds to egasyn causes the release of β-glucuronidase into plasma, which serves as the basis for a test for OP exposure (Fujikawa et al., 2005). The retention of β-glucuronidase in the lumen of the ER is thought to be physiologically significant. Glucuronidation by microsomal UGTs is a major pathway in the clearance of many of the endogenous aglycones (such as bilirubin) and xenobiotics (such as drugs). However, hydrolysis of glucuronides by β-glucuronidase complexed with egasyn in the lumen of the ER appears to be an important mechanism for recycling endogenous compounds, such as steroid hormones (Dwivedi et al., 1987). The acute-phase response protein, C-reactive protein, is similarly anchored in the endoplasmic reticulum by egasyn.

The mechanism of catalysis by carboxylesterases is analogous to the mechanism of catalysis by serine-proteases. In the case of carboxylesterases, it involves charge relay among a catalytic triad comprising an acidic amino acid residue (glutamate [Glu_{335}]), a basic residue (histidine [His_{448}]), and a nucleophilic residue (serine [Ser_{203}]) (Yan et al., 1994; Satoh and Hosokawa, 1998). (These amino acid residues, numbered for a rat carboxylesterase, differ slightly in other species, but the overall location and function of these residues are the same in all mammalian carboxylesterases.) The mechanism of catalysis of carboxylesterases is shown in Fig. 6-6, and is discussed in more detail in the section on *Epoxide Hydrolase*. Organophosphorus compounds bind to the nucleophilic OH-group on the active site serine residue to form a phosphorus–oxygen bond, which is not readily cleaved by water. Therefore, OP compounds bind stoichiometrically to carboxylesterases and inhibit their enzymatic activity, for which reason they are also classified as B-esterases (Aldridge, 1953). Surprisingly, the stoichiometric binding of OP compounds to carboxylesterases is an important determinant of OP toxicity, as outlined in the following section on cholinesterases.

Cholinesterases (AChE and BChE)   Acetylcholinesterase (AChE) and butyrylcholinesterase (BChE, also known as pseudocholinesterase) are related enzymes. As the names imply, AChE and BChE have high activity toward acetylcholine and butyrylcholine (and propionylcholine), respectively. BChE can also hydrolyze bambuterol, chlorpropaine, cocaine, methylprednisolone acetate, heroin, isosorbide diaspirinate, mivacurium, procaine, succinylcholine, tetracaine, and other drugs. Eserine is an inhibitor of both enzymes, whereas BW284C51 is a selective inhibitor of AChE, and iso-OMPA is a selective inhibitor of BChE (Liederer and Borchardt, 2006). Drugs that selectively inhibit brain AChE and BChE activity, such as rivastigmine (Exelon®), have been used to treat Alzheimer's disease. Other drugs that inhibit AChE and are used to treat Alzheimer's disease include tacrine (Cognex®), gelantamine (Reminyl®), and donepezil (Aricept®).

Both enzymes exist in six different forms with differing solubility: monomer (G1), dimer (G2), tetramer (G4), tailed tetramers (A4), double tetramers (A8), and triple tetramers (A12). G1, G2, and G4 contain 1, 2, and 4 subunits, each with a catalytic site. These various forms can each exist in three states: soluble (hydrophilic), immobilized (asymmetric), and amphiphilic globular (membrane-bound through trachment to the phospholipid bilayer) (Nigg and Knaak, 2000). All forms are expressed in muscle. In the case of AChE, the

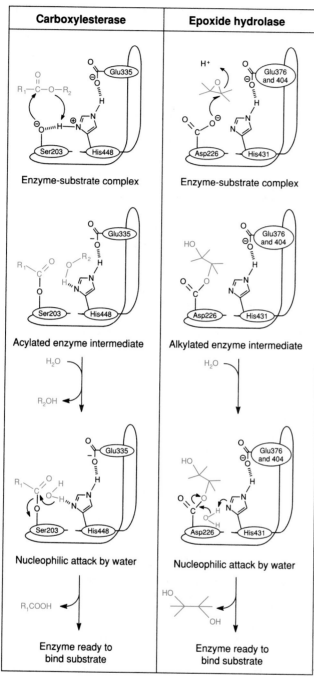

Figure 6-6. *Catalytic cycle of microsomal carboxylesterase (left) and microsomal epoxide hydrolase (right), two α/β-hydrolase fold enzymes.*

Based on measurements of erythrocyte AChE activity, familial reductions of 30% have been reported, and a reduction of 50% has been linked to paroxysmal nocturnal hemoglobinuria (Nigg and Knaak, 2000).

At least 10 genetic variants of BChE have been described following the discovery of PMs of succinylcholine. Succinylcholine is a muscle relaxant whose duration of action is determined by serum BChE. In some individuals ($\sim$2% of Caucasians), succinylcholine causes prolonged muscular relaxation and apnea, which led to the discovery of a genetic variant of BChE ($Asp_{70} \rightarrow Gly_{70}$) (La Du, 1992; Lockridge, 1992). Although this allelozyme has markedly diminished activity toward succinylcholine (which is the genetic basis for the exaggerated response to this muscle relaxant in affected individuals), it nevertheless has appreciable activity toward other substrates, such as acetylcholine and benzoylcholine. The wild type and variant form of BChE are equally sensitive to the inhibitory effect of OP compounds, but the allelic variant is relatively resistant to the inhibitory effect of dibucaine, a local anesthetic, which forms the basis of a diagnostic test for its presence (frequently called a test for atypical pseudocholinesterase). The discovery of the BChE allelozyme (the so-called atypical pseudocholinesterase) is of historical interest because it ushered in the new field of pharmacogenetics. Since its initial discovery in the late 1950s, several allelic variants of BChE and many other xenobiotic-biotransforming enzymes have been identified (see Point 23).

Carboxylesterases and cholinesterases in the blood and tissues play an important role in limiting the amount of OP compounds that reaches AChE in the brain, inhibition of which is the mechanism of toxicity of OP pesticides (and carbamate insecticides), such that a 70–90% loss of AChE activity is lethal to mammals, insects, and nematodes. The symptoms of OP toxicity resemble those caused by excessive stimulation of cholinergic nerves. The covalent interaction between OP compounds and brain AChE is analogous to their binding to the active site serine residue in all serine esterases (B-esterases). As previously mentioned, certain OP compounds are hydrolyzed by A-esterases (the paraoxonases) but bind stoichiometrically and, for the most part, irreversibly to B-esterases (carboxylesterases and cholinesterases). Surprisingly, stoichiometric binding of OP compounds to carboxylesterase and cholinesterase (and perhaps to numerous other enzymes and receptors that have structural features common to serine esterases) plays an important role in limiting the toxicity of OP compounds. Numerous studies have shown an inverse relationship between serine esterase activity and susceptibility to the toxic effect of OP compounds. Factors that decrease serine esterase activity potentiate the toxic effects of OP compounds, whereas factors that increase serine esterase activity have a protective effect. For example, the susceptibility of animals to the toxicity of parathion, malathion, and diisopropylfluorophosphate (DFP) is inversely related to the level of serum esterase activity (which reflects both carboxylesterase and BChE activity). Differences in the susceptibility of several mammalian species to OP toxicity can be abolished by pretreatment with selective serine esterase inhibitors such as cresylbenzodioxaphosphorin oxide, the active metabolite of tri-*ortho*-tolylphosphate (which is also known as tri-*ortho*-cresylphosphate or TOCP). Esterases are not the only enzymes involved in the detoxication of OP pesticides. Certain OP compounds are detoxified by cytochrome P450, flavin monooxygenases, and glutathione transferases. However, paraoxonases, enzymes that catalyze the hydrolysis of certain OP compounds, appear to play only a minor role in determining susceptibility to OP toxicity, as outlined in the following section.

major form in brain is the tetramer G4 (anchored with a 20-kDa side chain containing fatty acids), but the major form in erythrocytes is the dimer G2 (anchored with a glycolipid-phosphatidylinositol side chain). In the case of BChE, the major form in serum is the tetramer G4 (a glycoprotein with Mr 342 kDa). In both AChE and BChE, the esteratic site (containing the active site serine residue) is adjacent to an anionic (negatively charged) site that interacts with the positively charged nitrogen on acetylcholine and butyrylcholine.

Genetic variants of AChE that severely impair its activity have not been described, which is not surprising given the key role that AChE plays in terminating neurotransmission by acetylcholine.

Paraoxonases (Lactonases) Paraoxonases catalyze the hydrolysis of a broad range of organophosphates, organophosphinites, aromatic carboxylic acid esters, cyclic carbonates, and lactones. They are calcium-dependent enzymes containing a critical sulfhydryl (-SH) group; as such they are inhibited by EDTA, metal ions (Cu and Ba), and various mercurials such as phenylmercuric acetate (PMA) and *para*-chloromercuribenzoate (PCMB). Based on the observation that A-esterases are inhibited by PCMB but not OP compounds, Augustinsson (1966) postulated that, in the case of paraoxonases, OP compounds bind to a nucleophilic SH-group on an active site cysteine residue and form a phosphorus–sulfur bond, which is readily cleaved by water. A strong argument against this postulate is the fact that there is no loss of activity when the only potential active site cysteine residue in human paraoxonase (Cys283) is substituted with serine or alanine (Sorenson *et al.*, 1995). Paraoxonase requires Ca^{2+}, both for stability and catalytic activity, which raises the possibility that the hydrolysis of OP compounds by paraoxonase involves metal-catalyzed hydrolysis, analogous to that proposed for calcium-dependent phospholipase A2 or zinc-dependent phosphotriesterase activity (Sorenson *et al.*, 1995).

Humans express three paraoxonases designated hPON1, hPON2, and hPON3. hPON1 is present in liver microsomes and plasma, where it is associated exclusively with high-density lipoprotein (HDL). hPON2 is not present in plasma but it is expressed in several tissues. hPON3 is expressed in serum and liver and kidney microsomes. In addition to differences in tissue distribution, the three paraoxonases in mice respond differently to oxidative stress, which decreases PON1, increases PON3, and has no effect on PON2.

Only hPON1 has appreciable arylesterase activity and the ability to hydrolyze the toxic oxon metabolites of OP insecticides such as parathion, diazinon, and chlorpyrifos (Draganov and La Du, 2004). However, all three enzymes can catalyze the hydrolysis of various lactones, for which reason the name "lactonase" is more encompassing. They also catalyze the reverse reaction, i.e., the lactonization of hydroxy-carboxylic acids, as illustrated in Fig. 6-2. Hydrolysis and lactonization of statins, such a lovastatin and simvastatin, is catalyzed only by hPON3. Reports of the same reaction being catalyzed by hPON1 appear to be attributable to trace contamination with hPON3 (Draganov and La Du, 2004). The lactone dihydrocoumarin is the only substrate reported for hPON2.

There is evidence to suggest that hPON1 protects against atherosclerosis by hydrolyzing specific derivatives of oxidized cholesterol and/or phospholipids in atherosclerotic lesions and in oxidized low-density lipoprotein (LDL). For example, mice lacking PON1 (knockout mice or PON1 null mice) are predisposed to atherogenesis (Draganov and La Du, 2004). It has been suggested that PON1 has two active sites, one involved in hydrolytic reactions and the other involved in protecting LDL against oxidation. The ability of PON1 to protect LDL from copper-induced oxidation requires a cysteine residue at position 284 (which is *not* required for esteratic activity) but which does not require calcium (which *is* required for catalytic activity).

Based on its ability to hydrolyze OP compounds, it seems reasonable to assume that PON1 would play an important role in determining susceptibility to OP toxicity, but this may not be the case. PON1 knockout mice are no more susceptible than wild-type mice to the toxic effects of paraoxon (the active metabolite of parathion). However, it is possible that PON1 plays a larger role in limiting the toxicity of other OP compounds such as diazoxon and chlorpyrifos oxon because it hydrolyzes these oxons 10–20

times faster than it hydrolyzes paraoxon (Draganov and La Du, 2004).

hPON1 hydrolyzes the unsaturated cyclic carbonate prodrug prulifloxacin to its active metabolite NM394, and the rate of hydrolysis is influenced by a genetic polymorphism at amino acid 192. Whether this position is a glutamine or arginine residue affects the hydrolytic activity of hPON1 in a substrate-dependent manner, with some substrates being hydrolyzed faster by hPON1$_{192R}$, such as paraoxon, and others being hydrolyzed faster by hPON1$_{192Q}$, such as certain lactones. There is clinical evidence supporting—but also some excluding—a link between the hPON1$_{192R}$ genetic polymorphism and the development of cardiovascular disease, which is consistent with the decreased ability of this allelozyme to metabolize oxidized lipids (Draganov and La Du, 2004).

Diisopropylfluorophosphatase (DFPase), which catalyzes the release of fluoride from DFP, is a hydrolytic enzyme related to the paraoxonases. It hydrolyzes the nerve gas agents sarin and soman (Liederer and Borchardt, 2006).

Prodrugs and Alkaline Phosphatase Many prodrugs are designed to be hydrolyzed by hydrolytic enzymes (reviewed by Liederer and Borchardt, 2006). Some prodrugs, such as propranolol ester, are hydrolyzed by both carboxylesterases and cholinesterases (both AChE and BChE), whereas others are preferentially or specifically hydrolyzed by carboxylesterases (capecitabine, irinotecan), BChE (bambuterol, methylprednisolone acetate), hPNO1 (prulifloxacin) or hPON3 (lovastatin, simvastatin). In some cases the prodrug is hydrolyzed by an enzyme that has yet to be fully characterized. For example, the hydrolysis of valacyclovir to the antiviral drug acyclovir is catalyzed by a human enzyme named valacyclovirase (genesymbol: BPHL). Some prodrugs are hydrolyzed with a high degree of stereoselectivity. For example, in the case of prodrugs of ibuprofen and flurbiprofen, the *R*-enantiomer is hydrolyzed about 50 times faster than the *S*-enantiomer.

Some prodrugs, such as fosphenytoin (Cerebyx®) and fosamprenavir (Lexiva®), are designed to be hydrolyzed by alkaline phosphatase, high concentrations of which are present on the luminal surface of the enterocytes lining the wall of the small intestine. Hydrolysis of these prodrugs by alkaline phosphatase releases the active drug at the surface of the enterocytes, where it can be readily absorbed.

As a result of their ability to hydrolyze prodrugs, hydrolytic enzymes may have clinical applications in the treatment of certain cancers. They might be used, for example, to activate prodrugs in vivo and thereby generate potent anticancer agents in highly selected target sites (e.g., at the surface of tumor cells, or inside the tumor cells themselves). For example, carboxylesterases might be targeted to tumor sites with hybrid monoclonal antibodies (i.e., bifunctional antibodies that recognize the carboxylesterase and the tumor cell), or the cDNA encoding a carboxylesterase might be targeted to the tumor cells via a viral vector. In the case of irinotecan, this therapeutic strategy would release the anticancer drug SN-38 in the vicinity of the tumor cells, which would reduce the systemic levels and side effects of this otherwise highly toxic drug (Senter *et al.*, 1996). Some prodrugs, such as capecitabine, are activated by hydrolytic enzymes in the tumors themselves. There is evidence to suggest that, by hydrolyzing SN-38-glucuronide (a metabolite of the anticancer drug irinotecan), β-glucuronidase in colonic tumor cells may play a role in exposing such tumors to the topoisomerase inhibitor SN-38 (Tobin *et al.*, 2006).

Peptidases With the advent of recombinant DNA technology, numerous human peptides have been mass-produced for use as therapeutic agents, and several recombinant peptide hormones, growth factors, cytokines, soluble receptors, and humanized monoclonal antibodies currently are used clinically. To avoid acid-precipitation and proteolytic degradation in the gastrointestinal tract, peptides are administered parenterally. Nevertheless, peptides are hydrolyzed in the blood and tissues by a variety of peptidases, including aminopeptidases and carboxypeptidases, which hydrolyze amino acids at the *N*- and C-terminus, respectively, and endopeptidases, which cleave peptides at specific internal sites (trypsin, for example, cleaves peptides on the C-terminal side of arginine or lysine residues) (Humphrey and Ringrose, 1986). Peptidases cleave the amide linkage between adjacent amino acids, hence, they function as amidases. As in the case of carboxylesterases, the active site of peptidases contains either a serine or cysteine residue, which initiates a nucleophilic attack on the carbonyl moiety of the amide bond. As previously noted, the mechanism of catalysis by serine proteases, such as chymotrypsin, is similar to that by serine esterases (B-esterases).

Epoxide Hydrolases Epoxide hydrolases catalyze the *trans*-addition of water to alkene epoxides and arene oxides (oxiranes), which can form during the cytochrome P450-dependent oxidation of aliphatic alkenes and aromatic hydrocarbons, respectively. As shown in Fig. 6-7, the products of this hydrolysis are vicinal diols with a *trans*-configuration (i.e., *trans*-1,2-dihydrodiols); a notable exception being the conversion of leukotriene A₄ (LTA4) to leukotriene B₄(LTB4), in which case the two hydroxyl groups that result from epoxide hydrolysis appear on nonadjacent carbon atoms. Epoxide hydrolases play an important role in detoxifying electrophilic epoxides that might otherwise bind to proteins and nucleic acids and cause cellular toxicity and genetic mutations. Although the levels vary from one tissue to the next, epoxide hydrolase has been found in the microsomal fraction of virtually all tissues, including the liver, testis, ovary, lung, kidney, skin, intestine, colon, spleen, thymus, brain, and heart.

There are five distinct forms of epoxide hydrolase in mammals: microsomal epoxide hydrolase (mEH, which is the product of the gene EPHX1), soluble epoxide hydrolase (the gene product of EPHX2), cholesterol epoxide hydrolase, leukotriene A₄ (LTA₄, the gene product of LTA4H) hydrolase, and hepoxilin hydrolase (Fretland and Omiecinski, 2000; Morisseau and Hammock, 2005).

As their names imply, the latter three enzymes appear to hydrolyze endogenous epoxides exclusively, and have virtually no capacity to detoxify xenobiotic oxides. LTA₄ hydrolase is distinct from the other epoxide hydrolases because it is a bifunctional zinc metalloenzyme that has both epoxide hydrolase and peptidase activity, and because the two hydroxyl groups introduced during the conversion of LTA₄ to LTB₄ are eight carbon atoms apart.

In contrast to the high degree of substrate specificity displayed by the cholesterol, LTA₄ and hepoxilin epoxide hydrolases, mEH hydrolyzes a wide variety of xenobiotics with an alkene epoxide or arene oxide. sEH hydrolyzes some xenobiotic epoxides and oxides, such a *trans*-stilbene oxide, but it also plays an important role in the hydrolysis of endogenous fatty acid epoxides, such as the epoxyeicosatrienoic acids (EETs) that are formed by epoxidation of arachidonic acid by cytochrome P450 and the leukotoxins that are formed by the epoxidation of linoleic acid by leukocytes (Fretland and Omiecinski, 2000; Morisseau and Hammock, 2005).

In the case of EETs, hydrolysis by sEH terminates their vasodilatory effects. Male sEH knockout mice (sEH null mice) have significantly lower blood pressure than wild-type mice, supporting the important role of sEH in EET hydrolysis (and the important vasodilatory effects of EETs), and supporting the notion that inhibitors of sEH might be useful in the treatment of hypertension. In the case of leukotoxins, hydrolysis by sEH can be considered an activation process because it produces diols that perturb membrane permeability and calcium homeostasis, which results in vascular inflammation and cardio-pulmonary toxicity, including acute respiratory distress syndrome (ARDS) and multiple organ failure (Morisseau and Hammock, 2005).

In general, mEH prefers mono-substituted epoxides and di-substituted epoxides with a *cis* configuration, such as *cis*-stilbene oxide, whereas sEH prefers tetra- and tri-substituted epoxides and di-substituted epoxides with a *gem* configuration (both substituents on the same carbon atom) or the *trans* configuration, such as *trans*-stilbene oxide, as shown in Fig. 6-8. In rodents, sEH and mEH are both inducible enzymes; sEH is under the control of PPARα, so it is induced following treatment of rats and mice with peroxisome

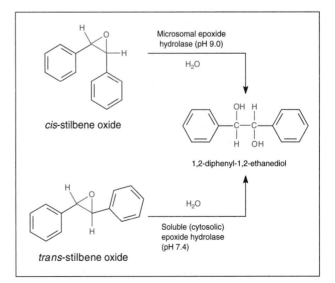

Figure 6-8. Stereoselective hydrolation of stilbene oxide by microsomal and soluble epoxide hydrolase.

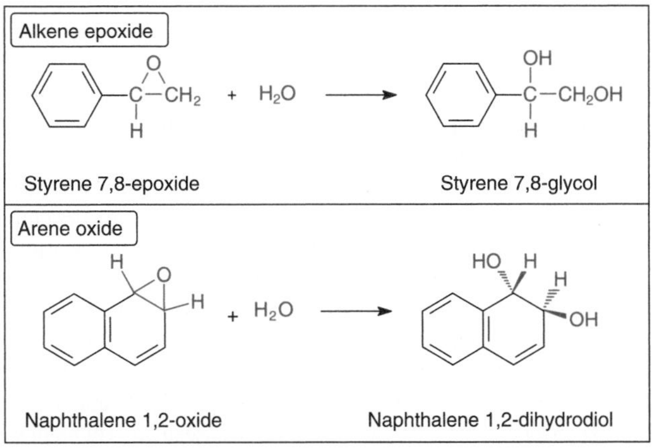

Figure 6-7. Examples of the hydrolation of an alkene epoxide (top) and an arene oxide (bottom) by epoxide hydrolase.

proliferators, whereas mEH is under the control of Nrf2, so it is induced in response to oxidative stress or exposure to electrophiles and glutathione depletors (see section "Quinone Reduction—NQO1 and NQO2"). Treatment of mice with the CAR agonist phenobarbital induces mEH about two- to threefold, whereas treatment with Nrf2 activators such as butylated hydroxytoluene (BHT), butylated hydroxyanisole (BHA), and ethoxyquin induces mEH by an order of magnitude or more.

Many epoxides and oxides are intermediary metabolites formed during the cytochrome P450-dependent oxidation of unsaturated aliphatic and aromatic xenobiotics. These electrophilic metabolites might otherwise bind to proteins and nucleic acids and cause cellular toxicity and genetic mutations. In general, sEH and mEH are found in the same tissues and cell types that contain cytochrome P450. For example, the distribution of epoxide hydrolase parallels that of cytochrome P450 in liver, lung, and testis. In other words, both enzymes are located in the centrilobular region of the liver (zone 3), in Clara and type II cells in the lung, and in Leydig cells in the testis. The co-localization of epoxide hydrolase and cytochrome P450 presumably ensures the rapid detoxication of alkene epoxides and arene oxides generated during the oxidative metabolism of xenobiotics.

Electrophilic epoxides and arene oxides are constantly produced during the cytochrome P450-dependent oxidation of unsaturated aliphatic and aromatic xenobiotics, and are highly reactive to cellular macromolecules such as DNA and protein. Epoxide hydrolase can rapidly convert these potentially toxic metabolites to the corresponding dihydrodiols, which are less reactive and easier to excrete. Thus, epoxide hydrolases are widely considered as a group of detoxication enzymes. In some cases, however, further oxidation of a dihydrodiol can lead to the formation of diol epoxide derivatives that are no longer substrates for epoxide hydrolase because the oxirane ring is protected by bulky substituents that sterically hinder interaction with the enzyme. This point proved to be extremely important in elucidating the mechanism by which polycyclic aromatic hydrocarbons cause tumors in laboratory animals (Conney, 1982). Tumorigenic polycyclic aromatic hydrocarbons, such as benzo[a]pyrene, are converted by cytochrome P450 to a variety of arene oxides that bind covalently to DNA, making them highly mutagenic to bacteria. One of the major arene oxides formed from benzo[a]pyrene, namely, the 4,5-oxide, is highly mutagenic to bacteria but weakly mutagenic to mammalian cells. This discrepancy reflects the rapid inactivation of benzo[a]pyrene 4,5-oxide by epoxide hydrolase in mammalian cells. However, one of the arene oxides formed from benzo[a]pyrene, namely, benzo[a]pyrene 7,8-dihydrodiol-9,10-oxide, is not a substrate for epoxide hydrolase and is highly mutagenic to mammalian cells and considerably more potent than benzo[a]pyrene as a lung tumorigen in mice.

Benzo[a]pyrene 7,8-dihydrodiol-9,10-oxide is known as a bay-region diolepoxide, and analogous bay-region diolepoxides are now recognized as tumorigenic metabolites of numerous polycyclic aromatic hydrocarbons. A feature common to all bay-region epoxides is their resistance to hydrolyation by epoxide hydrolase, which results from steric hindrance from the nearby dihydrodiol group. As shown in Fig. 6-9, benzo[a]pyrene 7,8-dihydrodiol-9,10-oxide is formed in three steps: Benzo[a]pyrene is converted to the 7,8-oxide, which is converted to the 7,8-dihydrodiol, which is converted to the corresponding 9,10-epoxide. The first and third steps are epoxidation reactions catalyzed by cytochrome P450 or prostaglandin H synthase, but the second step is catalyzed by epoxide hydrolase. Consequently, even though epoxide hydrolase plays a major role in detoxifying sev-

eral benzo[a]pyrene oxides, such as the 4,5-oxide, it nevertheless plays a role in converting benzo[a]pyrene to its ultimate tumorigenic metabolite, benzo[a]pyrene 7,8-dihydrodiol-9,10-oxide.

The importance of mEH in the conversion of polycyclic aromatic hydrocarbons to their ultimate carcinogenic metabolites, namely, diol-epoxides, is illustrated by the observation that mEH knockout mice (mEH-null mice) are less sensitive than wild-type mice to the tumorigenic effects of 7,12-dimethylbenz[a]anthracene (DMBA) (Fretland and Omiecinski, 2000; Morisseau and Hammock, 2005).

Not all epoxides are highly reactive and toxic to the cells that produce them. The major metabolite of carbamazepine is an epoxide, which is so stable that carbamazepine 10,11-epoxide is a major circulating metabolite in patients treated with this antiepileptic drug. (Carbamazepine is converted to a second epoxide, which is less stable and more cytotoxic, as shown in the section on *Cytochrome P450*.) Vitamin K epoxide is also a nontoxic epoxide, which is formed and consumed during the vitamin K-dependent γ-carboxylation of prothrombin and other clotting factors in the liver. Vitamin K epoxide is not hydrated by epoxide hydrolase but is reduced by vitamin K epoxide reductase. This enzyme is inhibited by warfarin and related coumarin anticoagulants, which interrupts the synthesis of several clotting factors. Some drugs actually contain an epoxide, such as scopolamine and tiotropium.

Epoxide hydrolase is one of several proteins (so-called preneoplastic antigens) that are overexpressed in chemically induced foci and nodules that eventually develop into liver tumors. Several alcohols, ketones, and imidazoles stimulate microsomal epoxide hydrolase activity in vitro. Epoxide hydrolase cannot be inhibited by antibodies raised against the purified enzyme, but it can be inhibited by certain epoxides, such as 1,1,1-trichloropropene oxide and cyclohexene oxide, and certain drugs, such as valpromide (the amide analog of valproic acid) and progabide, a γ-aminobutyric acid (GABA) agonist. These latter two drugs potentiate the neurotoxicity of carbamazepine by inhibiting epoxide hydrolase, leading to increased plasma levels of carbamazepine 10,11-epoxide and presumably the more toxic 2,3-epoxide (Kroetz et al., 1993). Several genetic polymorphisms have been identified in the coding region and the 5' region (i.e., the regulatory region) of the gene encoding human mEH (Daly, 1999). Two variants involve substitutions at amino acid 113 (Tyr → His) or amino acid 139 (His → Arg), which are encoded by exons 3 and 4, respectively. Although these allelic variant forms of mEH have near-normal enzymatic activity (at least 65% of normal), they appear to be less stable than the wild-type enzyme. The possibility that these amino acid substitutions might predispose individuals to the adverse effects of antiepileptic drugs has been examined, but no such association was found (Daly, 1999). More recently, a case was reported of a man who had a defect in mEH expression and suffered acute and severe phenytoin toxicity (Morisseau and Hammock, 2005).

The microsomal and soluble forms of epoxide hydrolase show no evident sequence identity and, accordingly, are immunochemically distinct proteins (Beetham et al., 1995). Nevertheless, mEH and sEH catalyze reactions by the same mechanism, and similar amino acids are involved in catalysis, namely, a nucleophilic acid (Asp_{226} in mEH and Asp_{334} in sEH), a basic histidine (His_{431} in mEH and His_{523} in sEH), an orienting acid (Glu_{404} in mEH and Asp_{495} in sEH) and polarizing tyrosine residues (Tyr_{299} and Tyr_{374} in mEH and Tyr_{382} and Tyr_{465} in mEH) (Morisseau and Hammock, 2005). The mechanism of catalysis by epoxide hydrolase is similar to that of carboxylesterase, in that the catalytic site comprises

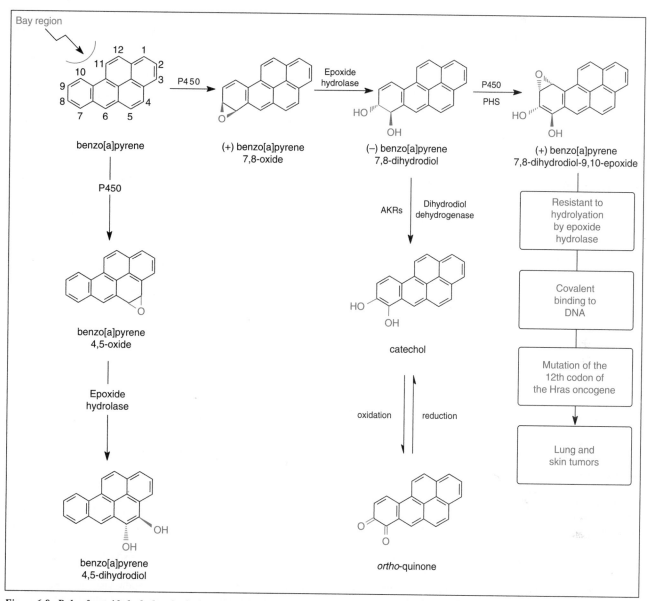

Figure 6-9. Role of epoxide hydrolase in the inactivation of benzo[a]pyrene 4,5-oxide and in the conversion of benzo[a]pyrene to its tumorigenic bay-region diolepoxide. Also shown is the role of dihydrodiol dehydrogenase, a member of the aldo–keto reductase (AKR) superfamily, in the formation of reactive catechol and ortho-quinone metabolites of benzo[a]pyrene.

three amino acid residues that form a catalytic triad, as shown in Fig. 6-6. The attack of the nucleophile Asp$_{226}$ on the carbon of the oxirane ring initiates enzymatic activity, leading to the formation of an α-hydroxyester–enzyme intermediate, with the negative charge developing on the oxygen atom stabilized by a putative oxyanion hole. The His$_{431}$ residue (which is activated by Glu$_{376}$ and Glu$_{404}$) activates a water molecule by abstracting a proton (H^{+}). The activated (nucleophilic) water then attacks the Cγ atom of Asp$_{226}$, resulting in the hydrolysis of the ester bond in the acyl–enzyme intermediate, which restores the active enzyme and results in formation of a vicinal diol with a trans-configuration (Armstrong, 1999). The second step, namely, cleavage of the ester bond in the acyl–enzyme intermediate, resembles the cleavage of the ester or amide bond in substrates for serine esterases and proteases.

Although epoxide hydrolase and carboxylesterase both have a catalytic triad comprising a nucleophilic, basic, and acidic amino

acid residue, there are striking differences in their catalytic machinery, which account for the fact that carboxylesterases primarily hydrolyze esters and amides, whereas epoxide hydrolases primarily hydrolyze epoxides and oxides. In the triad, both enzymes have histidine as the base and either glutamate or aspartate as the acid, but they differ in the type of amino acids for the nucleophile. Even during catalysis, there is a major difference. In carboxylesterases, the same carbonyl carbon atom of the substrate is attacked initially by the nucleophile Ser$_{203}$ to form an α-hydroxyester-enzyme ester that is subsequently attacked by the activated water to release the alcohol product. In contrast, two different atoms in epoxide hydrolase are targets of nucleophilic attacks. First the less hindered carbon atom of the oxirane ring is attacked by the nucleophile Asp$_{226}$ to form a covalently bound ester, and next this ester is hydrolyzed by an activated water molecule that attacks the Cγ atom of the Asp$_{226}$ residue, as illustrated in Fig. 6-6. Therefore, in carboxylesterase,

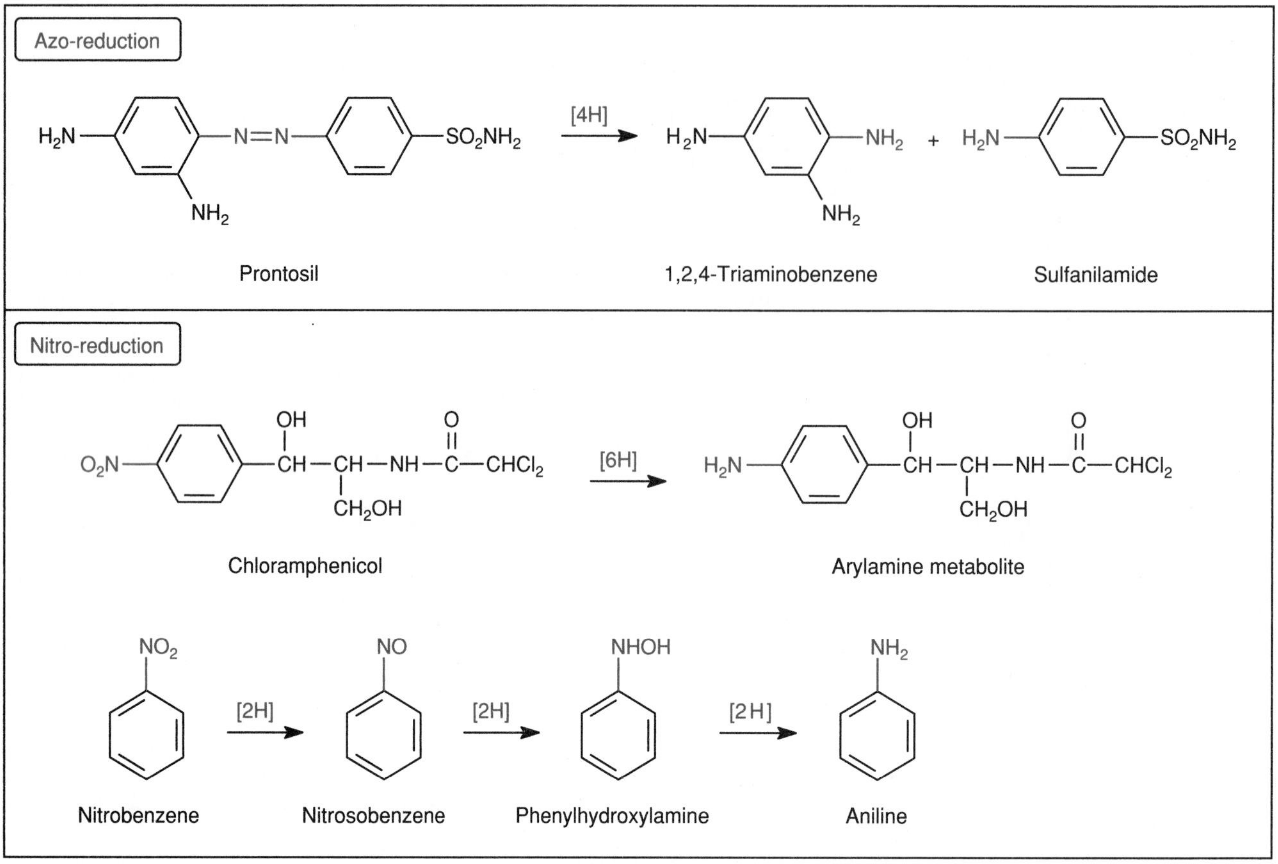

Figure 6-10. Examples of drugs that undergo azo reduction (prontosil) and nitro reduction (chloramphenicol and nitrobenzene).

the oxygen introduced to the product is derived from the activated water molecule. In contrast, in epoxide hydrolase, the oxygen introduced to the product is derived from the nucleophile Asp_{226} (Fig. 6-6).

Carboxylesterases and epoxide hydrolases exhibit no primary sequence identity, but they share surprising similarities in the topology of the structure and sequential arrangement of the catalytic triad. Both are members of the α/β-hydrolase fold enzymes, a superfamily of proteins that include lipases, esterases, and haloalkane dehydrogenases (Beetham *et al.*, 1995). Functionally, proteins in this superfamily all catalyze hydrolytic reactions; structurally, they all contain a similar core segment that is composed of eight β-sheets connected by α-helices. They all have a catalytic triad and the arrangement of the amino acid residues in the triad (i.e., the order of the nucleophile, the acid, and the base in the primary sequence) is the mirror image of the arrangement in other hydrolytic enzymes such as trypsin. All three active-site residues are located on loops that are the best conserved structural features in the fold, which likely provides catalysis with certain flexibility to hydrolyze numerous structurally distinct substrates.

Reduction

Certain metals (e.g., pentavalent arsenic) and xenobiotics containing an aldehyde, ketone, alkene, disulfide, sulfoxide, quinone, *N*-oxide, hydroxamic acid, amidoxime, isoxazole, isothiazole, azo, or nitro group are often reduced in vivo, although it is sometimes difficult to ascertain whether the reaction proceeds enzymatically or

nonenzymatically by interaction with reducing agents (such as the reduced forms of glutathione, FAD, FMN, and NAD[P]). Some of these functional groups can be either reduced or oxidized. For example, aldehydes (R–CHO) can be reduced to an alcohol (R–CH$_2$OH) or oxidized to a carboxylic acid (R–COOH), whereas sulfoxides (R_1–SO–R_2) can be reduced to a sulfide (R_1–S–R_2) or oxidized to a sulfone (R_1–SO$_2$–R_2). Likewise, some enzymes, such as alcohol dehydrogenase, aldehyde oxidase, and cytochrome P450, can catalyze both reductive and oxidative reactions depending on the substrate or conditions. In the case of halogenated hydrocarbons, such as halothane, dehalogenation can proceed by an oxidative or reductive pathway, both of which are catalyzed by the same enzyme (namely, cytochrome P450). In some cases, such as azo-reduction, nitro-reduction, and the reduction of certain alkenes, the reaction is largely catalyzed by intestinal microflora.

Azo- and Nitro-Reduction Prontosil and chloramphenicol are examples of drugs that undergo azo- and nitro-reduction, respectively, as shown in Fig. 6-10. Reduction of prontosil is of historical interest. Treatment of streptococcal and pneumococcal infections with prontosil marked the beginning of specific antibacterial chemotherapy. Subsequently, it was discovered that the active drug was not prontosil but its metabolite, sulfanilamide (*para*-aminobenzene sulfonamide), a product of azo-reduction. During azo-reduction, the nitrogen–nitrogen double bond is sequentially reduced and cleaved to produce two primary amines, a reaction requiring four reducing equivalents. Nitro-reduction requires six reducing equivalents,

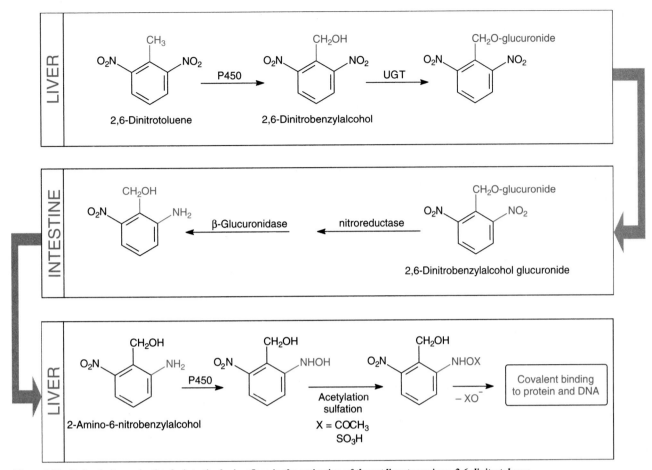

Figure 6-11. Role of nitro reduction by intestinal microflora in the activation of the rat liver tumorigen, 2,6-dinitrotoluene.

which are consumed in three sequential reactions, as shown in Fig. 6-10 for the conversion of nitrobenzene to aniline.

Azo- and nitro-reduction reactions are generally catalyzed by intestinal microflora. However, under certain conditions, such as low oxygen tension, the reactions can be catalyzed by liver microsomal cytochrome P450 and NAD(P)H-quinone oxidoreductase (NQO1, a cytosolic flavoprotein that is also known as DT-diaphorase) and, in the case of nitroaromatics, by cytosolic aldehyde oxidase. The anaerobic environment of the lower gastrointestinal tract is well suited for azo- and nitro-reduction, which is why intestinal microflora contribute significantly to these reactions. The reduction of quinic acid to benzoic acid is another example of a reductive reaction catalyzed by gut microflora, as shown in Fig. 6-1.

Nitro-reduction by intestinal microflora is thought to play an important role in the toxicity of several nitroaromatic compounds including 2,6-dinitrotoluene, which is hepatotumorigenic to male rats. The role of nitro-reduction in the metabolic activation of 2,6-dinitrotoluene is shown in Fig. 6-11 (Long and Rickert, 1982; Mirsalis and Butterworth, 1982). The biotransformation of 2,6-dinitrotoluene begins in the liver, where it is oxidized by cytochrome P450 and conjugated with glucuronic acid. This glucuronide is excreted in bile and undergoes biotransformation by intestinal microflora. One or both of the nitro groups are reduced to amines by nitroreductase, and the glucuronide is hydrolyzed by β-glucuronidase. The deconjugated metabolites are absorbed and transported to the liver, where the newly formed amine group is

N-hydroxylated by cytochrome P450 and conjugated with acetate or sulfonate. These conjugates form good leaving groups, which renders the nitrogen highly susceptible to nucleophilic attack from proteins and DNA; this ostensibly leads to mutations and the formation of liver tumors. The complexity of the metabolic scheme shown in Fig. 6-11 underscores an important principle, namely, that the activation of some chemical tumorigens to DNA-reactive metabolites involves several different biotransforming enzymes and may take place in more than one tissue. Consequently, the ability of 2,6-dinitrotoluene to bind to DNA and cause mutations is not revealed in most of the short-term assays for assessing the genotoxic potential of chemical agents. These in vitro assays for genotoxicity do not make allowance for biotransformation by intestinal microflora or, in some cases, the conjugating enzymes.

Nitro-reduction by intestinal microflora also plays an important role in the biotransformation of musk xylene (1,3,5-trinitro-2-*t*butyl-4,6-dimethylbenzene). Reduction of one or both of the nitro groups is required for musk xylene to induce (as well as markedly inhibit) liver microsomal cytochrome P450 (namely, CYP2B) in rodents (Lehman-McKeeman *et al.*, 1999).

Carbonyl Reduction—SDRs and AKRs   A variety of xenobiotics contain a carbonyl function (R–CHO and R_1–CO–R_2) that undergoes reduction in vivo. The reduction of aldehydes to primary alcohols and of ketones to secondary alcohols is generally

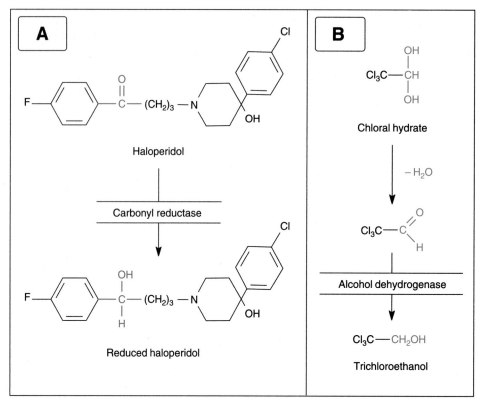

Figure 6-12. Reduction of xenobiotics by carbonyl reductase (A) and alcohol dehydrogenase (B).

catalyzed in mammals by NAD(P)H-dependent reductases belonging to one of two superfamilies, the aldo–keto reductases (AKRs), and the short-chain dehydrogenases/reductases (SDRs), as shown in Table 6-5 (Jez and Penning, 2001; Oppermann *et al.*, 2001; Matsunaga *et al.*, 2006). Humans contain 39 SDR members, two of which, namely, cytosolic and microsomal carbonyl reductase, play a role in the reduction of a wide variety of carbonyl-containing xenobiotics (other species express more than two carbonyl reductases). Erythrocytes also contain carbonyl reductase, which contributes significantly to the reduction of haloperidol, as shown in Fig. 6-12. From the alternative names given in Table 6-5, it is apparent that the cytosolic and microsomal carbonyl reductases have both been studied for their role in endobiotic metabolism, namely, the reduction of prostaglandin derivatives and 11β-hydroxysteroids, respectively. The AKRs are members of a superfamily of cytosolic enzymes that reduce both xenobiotic and endobiotic compounds, as their alternative names imply (Table 6-5). Various members of the AKR superfamily can function as dihydrodiol dehydrogenases and oxidize the *trans*-dihydrodiols of various polycyclic aromatic hydrocarbon oxiranes (formed by epoxide hydrolase) to the corresponding *ortho*-quinones, as shown previously in Fig. 6-9. The role of AKR as an oxidizing enzyme is discussed in the section on oxidative enzymes (see section "Dihydrodiol Dehydrogenase"). As mentioned earlier (see Point 8), one of the AKRs, namely, AKR7A (also known as aflatoxin aldehyde reductase) is one of the many enzymes induced following activation of Nrf2 by oxidative stress, exposure to electrophiles, or depletion of glutathione.

In certain cases, the reduction of aldehydes to alcohols can be catalyzed by alcohol dehydrogenase, as shown in Fig. 6-12

for the conversion of the sedative-hypnotic, chloral hydrate, to trichloroethanol. As shown in Table 6-5, alcohol dehydrogenases belong to the medium chain dehydrogenases/reductases (MDRs). They typically convert alcohols to aldehydes, for which reason they are discussed later in the section on oxidative reactions (see section "Alcohol Dehydrogenases"). In the case of chloral hydrate, the reverse reaction is favored by the presence of the trichloromethyl group, which is a strong electron-withdrawing group.

The SDR carbonyl reductases are monomeric, NADPH-dependent enzymes present in erythrocytes and both the cytosolic and microsomal fraction of the liver, kidney, brain, and many other tissues. The major circulating metabolite of the antipsychotic drug, haloperidol, is a secondary alcohol formed by carbonyl reductases in the blood and liver, as shown in Fig. 6-12. Other xenobiotics that are reduced by carbonyl reductases include pentoxifylline (see Fig. 6-2), acetohexamide, daunorubicin, doxorubicin, loxoprofen, menadione, 4-nitroacetophenone, timiperone, and *R*-warfarin (Rosemond and Walsh, 2004). As shown in Fig. 6-2, the reduction of ketones to secondary alcohols by carbonyl reductases may proceed with a high degree of stereoselectivity, as in the case of pentoxifylline (Lillibridge *et al.*, 1996).

Liver cytosol and microsomes contain different forms of carbonyl reductase, and these can differ in the degree to which they stereoselectively reduce ketones to secondary alcohols. For example, keto-reduction of pentoxifylline produces two enantiomeric secondary alcohols: one with the *R*-configuration (which is known as lisofylline) and one with the *S*-configuration, as shown in Fig. 6-2. Reduction of pentoxifylline by cytosolic carbonyl reductase results in the stereospecific formation of the optical antipode of lisofylline, whereas the same reaction catalyzed by microsomal

Table 6-5

Human Aldo–Keto Reductases (AKRs), Short-Chain Dehydrogenases/Reductases (SDRs), Medium-Chain Dehydrogenases/Reductases (MDRs), and Quinone Reductases (NQOs)

ENZYME SUPERFAMILY	EXAMPLE ENZYMES	ALTERNATIVE NAMES	SUBCELLULAR LOCALIZATION
Aldo–keto reductase (AKR) 13 enzymes	AKR1A1	Aldehyde reductase	Cytosol
	AKR1B1	Aldose reductase	Cytosol
	AKR1B10	Small intestine reductase	Cytosol
	AKR1C1	20α-Hydroxysteroid dehydrogenase	Cytosol
	AKR1C1, 1C2, 1C4	Dihydrodiol dehydrogenases (DD1, DD2, DD4)	Cytosol
	AKR1C1, 1C2, 1C3, 1C4	3α-Hydroxysteroid dehydrogenase	Cytosol
	AKR1C3	17β-Hydroxysteroid dehydrogenase type V	Cytosol
	AKR1C4	Chlordecone reductase	Cytosol
	AKR1D1	Δ^4-3-Ketosteroid-5β-reductase	Cytosol
	AKR6A3, 6A5, 6A9	Shaker-channel subunit Kvb1, Kvb2, Kvb3	Cytosol
	AKR7A2	Aflatoxin B$_1$ aldehyde reductase 2	Golgi
	AKR7A3	Aflatoxin B$_1$ aldehyde reductase 3	Cytosol
Short chain dehydrogenase/ reductases (SDR) 39 enzymes	Cytosolic carbonyl reductase	Xenobiotic ketone reductase with pH 6.0 activity; Prostaglandin 9-ketoreductase; Human placental NADP-linked 15-hydroprostaglandin dehydrogenase	Cytosol
	Microsomal carbonyl reductase	11β-Hydroxysteroid dehydrogenase; 11β-reductase, 11-oxidoreductase	Microsomes
Medium chain dehydrogenase/ reductases (MDR) 7 ADH enzymes	ADH1A	Class I ADH; ADH1, α, β, γ; hADH1,2,3	Cytosol
	ADH1B	Class I ADH; ADH2, β, γ; ADHII; hADH4	Cytosol
	ADH1C	Class I ADH; ADH3, γ	Cytosol
	ADH4	Class II ADH; π, hADH7	Cytosol
	ADH5	Class III ADH; χ	Cytosol
	ADH6	Class V ADH	Cytosol
	ADH7	Class IV ADH; μ or σ	Cytosol
NQO 2 enzymes	NQO1	DT diaphorase, menadione reductase	Cytosol
	NQO2	N-Ribosyldihydronicotinamide dehydrogenase	Cytosol

NQO, NADPH-Quinone oxidoreducta2e.

carbonyl reductase produces both lisofylline and its optical antipode in a ratio of about 1 to 5 (Lillibridge *et al.*, 1996).

In rat liver cytosol, the reduction of quinones is primarily catalyzed by NQO1 and NQO2 (see section "Quinone Reduction—NQO1 and NQO2"), whereas in human liver cytosol, quinone reduction is catalyzed by both NQO and carbonyl reductases.

Various members of the AKR superfamily have been implicated in the reduction of such carbonyl-containing xenobiotics as the tobacco-specific nitrosamine NNK, acetohexamide, daunorubicin, naloxone, naltrexone, befunolol, ethacrynic acid, ketoprofen, ketotifen, haloperidol, loxoprofen, metyrapone, oxo-nortyptyline, and numerous aromatic and aliphatic aldehydes (Rosemond and Walsh, 2004). Many of the xenobiotics reduced by AKRs and also reduced by SDRs, and in most cases the relative contribution of individual carbonyl-reducing enzymes is not known. Genetic polymorphisms of AKRs or SDRs have not been shown to impact the disposition or safety of carbonyl-containing drugs, and there appear to be no reports of drug–drug interactions involving the inhibition or induction of AKRs or SDRs (Rosemond and Walsh, 2004).

Disulfide Reduction Some disulfides are reduced and cleaved to their sulfhydryl components, as shown in Fig. 6-13 for the alcohol deterrent, disulfiram (Antabuse). As shown in Fig. 6-13, disulfide reduction by glutathione is a three-step process, the last of which is catalyzed by glutathione reductase. The first steps can be catalyzed by glutathione transferase, or they can occur nonenzymatically.

Sulfoxide and N-Oxide Reduction Thioredoxin-dependent enzymes in liver and kidney cytosol have been reported to reduce sulfoxides, which themselves may be formed by cytochrome P450 or flavin monooxygenases (Anders *et al.*, 1981). It has been suggested that recycling through these counteracting enzyme systems may prolong the half-life of certain xenobiotics. Sulindac is a sulfoxide that undergoes reduction to a sulfide, which is excreted in bile and reabsorbed from the intestine (Ratnayake *et al.*, 1981). This enterohepatic cycling prolongs the duration of action of the drug such that this nonsteroidal anti-inflammatory drug (NSAID) need only be taken twice daily.

Sulfoxide reduction may also occur nonenzymatically at an appreciable rate, as in the case of the proton pump inhibitor rabeprazole (Miura *et al.*, 2006). Diethyldithiocarbamate methyl ester, a metabolite of disulfiram, is oxidized to a sulfine, which is reduced to the parent methyl ester by glutathione. In the latter reaction, two molecules of glutathione (GSH) are oxidized with reduction

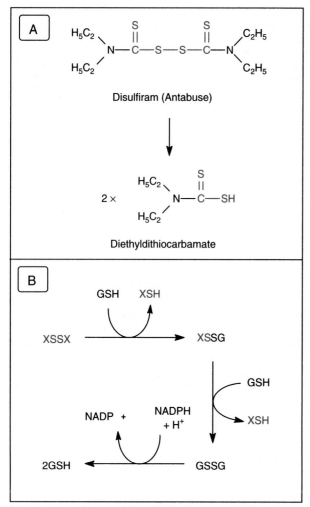

Figure 6-13. Biotransformation of disulfiram by disulfide reduction (A) and the general mechanism of glutathione-dependent disulfide reduction of xenobiotics (B).

GSH, glutathione; XSSX, xenobiotic disulfide; GSSG, reduced glutathione. The last reaction in (B) is catalyzed by glutathione reductase.

of the sulfine oxygen to water (Madan *et al.*, 1994), as shown below:

$$R_1R_2C = S^+ \!-\! O^- + 2GSH \rightarrow R_1R_2C = S + GSSG + H_2O$$

Just as sulfoxide reduction can reverse the effect of sulfoxidation, so the reduction of *N*-oxides can reverse the *N*-oxygenation of amines, which is catalyzed by flavin monooxygenases and cytochrome P450. Under reduced oxygen tension, reduction of the *N*-oxides of imipramine, tiaramide, indicine, and *N*,*N*-dimethylaniline can be catalyzed by mitochondrial and/or microsomal enzymes in the presence of NADH or NADPH (Sugiura and Kato, 1977). The NADPH-dependent reduction of *N*-oxides in liver microsomes appears to be catalyzed by cytochrome P450 (Sugiura *et al.*, 1976), although in some cases NADPH-cytochrome P450 reductase may play an important role.

As a class, *N*-oxides are not inherently toxic compounds. However, certain aromatic and aliphatic *N*-oxides have been exploited as bioreductive drugs (also known as DNA affinic drugs) for the treatment of certain cancers and infectious diseases (Wardman *et al.*, 1995). In these cases, *N*-oxides have been used as prodrugs that are converted to cytotoxic or DNA-binding drugs under hypoxic conditions. The fact that *N*-oxides of certain drugs are converted to toxic metabolites under hypoxic conditions is the basis for their selective toxicity to certain solid tumors (namely, those that are hypoxic and, hence, resistant to radiotherapy) and anaerobic bacteria. For example, tirapazamine (SR 4233) is a benzotriazine di-*N*-oxide that is preferentially toxic to hypoxic cells, such as those present in solid tumors, apparently due to its rapid activation by one-electron reduction of the *N*-oxide to an oxidizing nitroxide radical, as shown in Fig. 6-14 (Walton *et al.*, 1992). This reaction is catalyzed by cytochrome P450 and NADPH-cytochrome P450 reductase (Saunders *et al.*, 2000). Two-electron reduction of the di-*N*-oxide, SR 4233, produces a mono-*N*-oxide, SR 4317, which undergoes a second *N*-oxide reduction to SR 4330. Like SR 4233, the antibacterial agent, quindoxin, is a di-*N*-oxide whose cytotoxicity is dependent on reductive activation, which is favored by anaerobic conditions.

Bioreductive alkylating agents, which include such drugs as mitomycins, anthracyclins, and aziridinylbenzoquinones represent another class of anticancer agents that require activation by reduction. However, for this class of agents, bioactivation also involves a two-electron reduction reaction, which is largely catalyzed by NQO, which is described in the next section.

Quinone Reduction—NQO1 and NQO2 Quinones can be reduced to hydroquinones by two closely related, cytosolic flavoproteins, namely, NQO1 and NQO2. The former enzyme, NAD(P)H-quinone oxidoreductase-1, is also known as DT-diaphorase. The latter enzyme, NAD(P)H-quinone oxidoreductase-2, is also known as NRH-quinone oxidoreductase because it prefers the unusual electron donor dihydronicotinamide riboside (NMR) over NAD(P)H. Although they are closely related enzymes (both contain two 27-kDa subunits each with an FAD prosthetic group), NQO1 and NQO2 have different substrate specificities, and they can be distinguished on the basis of their differential inhibition by dicoumarol and quercetin (which are selective inhibitors of NQO1 and NQO2, respectively). NQO2 may have a physiological role in the metabolism of vitamin K hydroquinone (Chen *et al.*, 2000).

An example of the type of reaction catalyzed by NQO is shown in Fig. 6-15. Formation of the hydroquinone involves a two-electron reduction of the quinone with stoichiometric oxidation of NAD[P]H *without* oxygen consumption. (The two-electron reduction of certain quinones can also be catalyzed by carbonyl reductase, especially in humans.) In contrast, NADPH-cytochrome P450 reductase, a microsomal flavoprotein, catalyzes the one-electron reduction of quinones to semiquinone radicals that, in addition to being reactive metabolites themselves, cause oxidative stress by reacting with oxygen to form reactive oxygen species (ROS), which leads to nonstoichiometric oxidation of NADPH and oxygen consumption, as shown in Fig. 6-15. The two-electron reduction of quinones is a nontoxic reaction—one that is not associated with semiquinone formation and oxidative stress—provided the resultant hydroquinone is sufficiently stable to undergo glucuronidation or sulfonation. However, there are quinone-containing xenobiotics that, despite undergoing two-electron reduction by NQO, produce semiquinone free radicals, oxidative stress, DNA damage, and cytotoxicity. Many of these xenobiotics are being developed as anticancer drugs because NQO1 is often overexpressed in tumor cells. The properties of the hydroquinone determine whether, during the metabolism of quinone-containing xenobiotics, NQO functions as a protective antioxidant

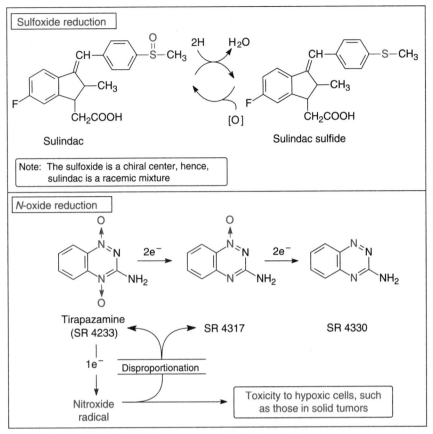

Figure 6-14. *Examples of sulfoxide and N-oxide reduction.*

Note that tirapazamine (3-amino-1,2,4-benzotriazine-1,4-dioxide) is a representative of a class of agents
that are activated by reduction, which may be clinically useful in the treatment of certain tumors.

or a pro-oxidant activator leading to the formation of reactive oxy-gen species and reactive semiquinone free radicals. The latter are thought to form not from the one-electron reduction of the quinone but from the two-electron reduction of the quinone (Q) to the hy-droquinone (QH$_2$), which then undergoes one-electron oxidation or perhaps disproportionation to form the reactive semiquinone (QH):

$$QH_2 + Q \leftrightarrow 2QH$$

Drugs or drug candidates that are activated by NQO to anti-cancer agents include the aziridinylbenzoquinone diaziquone, the anthraquinone mitoxantrone, the indolquinones mitomycin C and EO9 (an analog of mitomycin C that is more rapidly reduced by NQO1), and the anthracycline antibiotics daunorubicin and dox-orubicin (Gutierrez, 2000). These so-called bioreductive alkylating agents are reduced by NQO1 to generate semiquinone free radicals and other reactive intermediates that undergo nucleophilic additions with DNA, resulting in single-strand DNA breaks. The reason such drugs are preferentially toxic to tumor cells is that tumor cells, es-pecially those in solid tumors, are hypoxic, and hypoxia induces the synthesis of NQO1 (by a mechanism that involves the Acti-vator Protein 1 [AP-1] and Nuclear Factor-κB [NF-κB] response elements in the 5′-promoter region of the NQO1 gene). There-fore, tumor cells often express high levels of NQO1, which pre-disposes them to the toxic effects of quinone-reductive anticancer drugs like mitomycin C. Interestingly, mitomycin C also upregu-lates the expression of NQO1, which may enable this anticancer

drug to stimulate its own metabolic activation in tumor cells (Yao *et al.*, 1997). Some cancer chemotherapeutic agents, such as the *N*-oxide SR 4233, are inactivated, not activated, by NQO, as shown in Fig. 6-14.

NQO can activate certain nitroaromatic compounds (R–NO$_2$) to the corresponding hydroxylamine (R–NHOH), which can be acti-vated by acetylation or sulfonation (by pathways analogous to those shown in Fig. 6-11). Dinitropyrenes and the nitroaromatic com-pound CB 1954 are activated by NQO. The latter compound was under consideration as an anticancer agent. However, although it is activated by reduction by rat NQO, the nitroaromatic compound CB 1954 is not activated by human NQO.

Oxidative stress appears to be an important component to the mechanism of toxicity of several xenobiotics that either contain a quinone or can be biotransformed to a quinone (Anders, 1985). The production of superoxide anion radicals and oxidative stress are responsible, at least in part, for the cardiotoxic effects of dox-orubicin (adriamycin) and daunorubicin (daunomycin), the pul-monary toxicity of paraquat and nitrofurantoin, and the neurotoxic effects of 6-hydroxydopamine. Oxidative stress also plays an im-portant role in the destruction of pancreatic beta cells by alloxan and dialuric acid. Tissues low in superoxide dismutase activity, such as the heart, are especially susceptible to the oxidative stress associated with the redox cycling of quinones. This accounts, at least in part, for the cardiotoxic effects of adriamycin and related anticancer agents, although other susceptibility factors have been proposed (Mordente *et al.*, 2001).

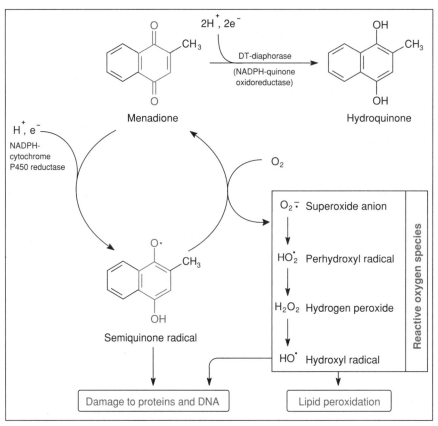

Figure 6-15. Two-electron reduction of menadione to a hydroquinone, and production of reactive oxygen species during its one-electron reduction to a semiquinone radical.

As already mentioned in this section, it is now apparent that the structure of the hydroquinones produced by NQO determines whether the two-electron reduction of quinones results in xenobiotic detoxication or activation. Hydroquinones formed by two-electron reduction of unsubstituted or methyl-substituted 1,4-naphthoquinones (such as menadione) or the corresponding quinone epoxides are relatively stable to autoxidation, whereas the methoxyl, glutathionyl, and hydroxyl derivatives of these compounds undergo autoxidation with production of semiquinones and reactive oxygen species. The ability of glutathionyl derivatives to undergo redox cycling indicates that conjugation with glutathione does not prevent quinones from serving as substrates for NQO. The glutathione conjugates of quinones can also be reduced to hydroquinones by carbonyl reductases, which actually have a binding site for glutathione. In human carbonyl reductase, this binding site is Cys_{227}, which is involved in binding both substrate and glutathione (Tinguely and Wermuth, 1999). Although oxidative stress is an important mechanism by which quinones cause cellular damage (through the intermediacy of semiquinone radicals and the generation of reactive oxygen species), it should be noted that quinones are Michael acceptors, and cellular damage can occur through direct alkylation of critical cellular proteins and/or DNA (Bolton *et al.*, 2000).

NQO1 is inducible up to tenfold by two classes of inducers, which have been categorized as *bifunctional* and *monofunctional* inducers (Prochaska and Talalay, 1988). The bifunctional inducers include compounds like β-naphthoflavone, benzo[a]pyrene, 3-methylcholanthrene and 2,3,7,8-tetrachlorodibenzo-p-dioxin (TCDD or dioxin), which induce both oxidative enzymes (such as the cytochrome P450 enzyme CYP1A1) and conjugating enzymes (such as glutathione transferase and UDP-glucuronosyltransferase). The monofunctional inducers tend to induce conjugating and other non-CYP enzymes (although in mice, monofunctional inducers can induce CYP2C55 and 2U1, as well as aldehyde oxidase). These inducers signal through two distinct mechanisms, one involving the XRE (xenobiotic-response element) and one involving the ARE (antioxidant response element), which is also known as the EpRE (electrophilic response element). (Response elements are short sequences of DNA, often located in the 5′-promoter region of a gene, that bind the transcription factors that control gene expression.) Some enzymes, such as CYP1A1, are largely regulated by the XRE, whereas others are largely regulated by ARE, such as glutathione transferase (see Point 8). Some enzymes, such as NQO1, are regulated by both. The monofunctional inducers can be subdivided into two chemical classes: those that cause oxidative stress through redox cycling (e.g., the quinone, menadione, and the phenolic antioxidants *tert*-butylhydroquinone and 3,5-di-*tert*-butylcatechol), and those that cause oxidative stress by depleting glutathione (e.g., fumarates, maleates, acrylates, isothiocyanates, and other Michael acceptors that react with glutathione).

The flavonoid β-naphthoflavone and the polycyclic aromatic hydrocarbon benzo[a]pyrene induce NQO1 by both mechanisms; the parent compound binds to the *Ah* receptor and is responsible for inducing CYP1A1, as well as NQO1, via the XRE, whereas electrophilic and/or redox active metabolites of β-naphthoflavone and benzo[a]pyrene are responsible for inducing glutathione

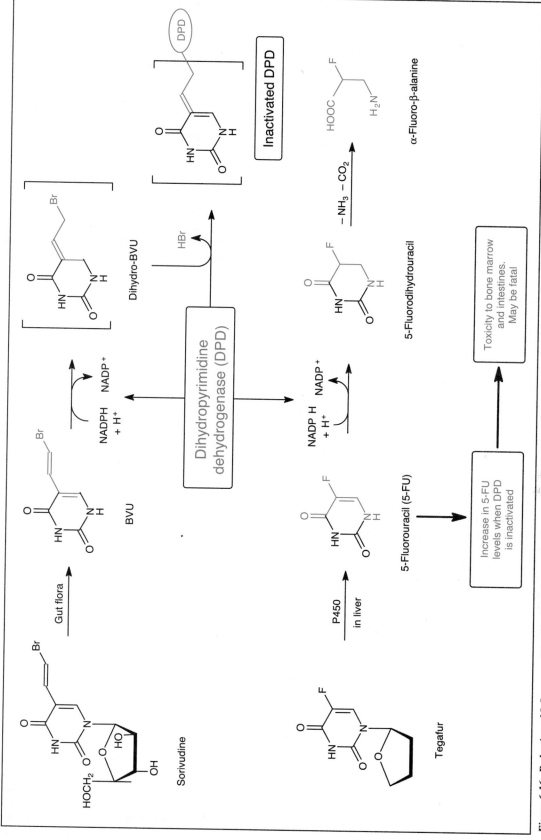

Figure 6-16. Reduction of 5-fluorouracil by dihydropyrimidine dehydrogenase and its inhibition (suicide inactivation) by Sorivudine.
Note: Inhibition of dihydropyrimidine dehydrogenase is the mechanism of fatal interactions between Sorivudine and the 5-fluorouracil prodrug, tegafur.

transferase, as well as NQO1, via the ARE. The situation with benzo[*a*]pyrene is quite intriguing. This polycyclic aromatic hydrocarbon binds directly to the *Ah* receptor, which binds to the XRE and induces the synthesis of CYP1A1, which in turn converts benzo[*a*]pyrene to electrophilic metabolites (such as arene oxides and diolepoxides) and redox active metabolites (such as catechols), as shown in Fig. 6-9. These electrophilic and redox active metabolites then induce enzymes that are regulated by the ARE. However, the catechol metabolites of benzo[*a*]pyrene are further converted by dihydrodiol dehydrogenase to *ortho*-quinones (Fig. 6-9), and are thereby converted back into planar, hydrophobic compounds that are highly effective ligands for the *Ah* receptor (Burczynski and Penning, 2000). This may be toxicologically important, because the *Ah* receptor may translocate *ortho*-quinone metabolites of benzo[*a*]pyrene into the nucleus, where they might damage DNA (Bolton *et al.*, 2000).

Among the monofunctional inducers that apparently increase NQO1 via ARE is sulforaphane, an ingredient of broccoli that may be responsible for the anticarcinogenic effects of this cruciferous vegetable (Zhang *et al.*, 1992). Isothiocyanates (which are also present at high levels in cruciferous vegetables) likely exert their chemopreventive effects largely through induction of the detoxifying enzymes under the control of ARE, namely, glutathione transferase (GSTA1), microsomal epoxide hydrolase, aldo–keto reductase (AKR7A, also known as aflatoxin aldehyde reductase), NAD(P)H-quinone oxidoreductase (NQO1, also known as DT-diaphorase), glutamate-cysteine ligase (GCL), as well as genes involved in apoptosis. One isothiocyanate in particular, phenethyl isothiocyanate, has been found to activate Nrf2 and activate numerous genes in addition to those encoding xenobiotic-biotransforming enzymes and oxidant defense systems. Microarray studies carried out in wild-type and Nrf2 knockout mice treated with phenethylisothiocyanate showed that the most highly inducible genes include the very low density lipoprotein (VLDL) receptor, G-protein signaling modulator 2, early growth response 1, pancreatic lipase-related protein 2, histocompatibility 2 (K region), general transcription factor IIB, myoglobin, potassium voltage-gated channel Q2, and SLC39A10 (Hu *et al.*, 2006). As with other xenosensors, activation of Nrf2 results in a pleiotypic response in which a large number of genes are activated (or repressed). As mentioned above (this section), hypoxia and the anticancer agent mitomycin C are also inducers of NQO1, which has implications for cancer chemotherapy.

NQO1 and NQO2 are polymorphically expressed enzymes, and several lines of evidence suggest that NQO1 and/or NQO2 plays a key role in protecting bone marrow from the hematotoxic effects of benzene or other environmental factors (Iskander and Jaiswal, 2005). In humans, a high percentage of individuals with myeloid and other types of leukemia are homo- or heterozygous for a null mutant allele of NQO1. This polymorphism, NQO1*2, is a SNP ($C_{609}T$) that changes Pro_{187} to Ser_{187}, which destabilizes the protein and targets it for rapid degradation by the ubiquitin proteasomal pathway (Ross, 2005). Mice lacking NQO1 or NQO2 (knockout or null mice) have no developmental abnormalities but have increased granulocytes in the blood and myelogenous hyperplasia of the bone marrow (due to decreased apoptosis). Mice lacking NQO1 are substantially more susceptible than wild-type mice to benzene-induced hematotoxicity (Iskander and Jaiswal, 2005; Ross, 2005). The hematotoxicity of benzene is thought to involve its conversion to hydroquinone in the liver and its subsequent oxidation to benzo-quinone by myeloperoxidase in the bone marrow (discussed later in

the section on *Peroxidase-dependent cooxidation*). NQO would be expected to play a role in detoxifying benzoquinone, and the loss of this protective mechanism may be the mechanism by which loss of NQO potentiates benzene hematotoxicity. However, loss of NQO also impairs apoptosis, which also represents a plausible explanation for the association between loss of NQO and increased susceptibility to benzene hematotoxicity. This latter mechanism (i.e., impaired apoptosis) likely accounts for the observation that NQO1 and NQO2 null mice are more susceptible than wild-type mice to skin carcinogenesis by benzo[*a*]pyrene and 7,12-dimethylbenz[*a*]anthracene, an effect attributable to the diol-epoxides, not the quinone metabolites, of these polycyclic aromatic hydrocarbons (Iskander and Jaiswal, 2005).

Dihydropyrimidine Dehydrogenase (DPD)   In 1993, 15 Japanese patients died as a result of an interaction between two oral medications: Sorivudine—a new antiviral drug for herpes zoster—and Tegafur—a prodrug that is converted in the liver to the anticancer agent, 5-fluorouracil. The deaths occurred within 40 days of the Japanese government's approval of Sorivudine for clinical

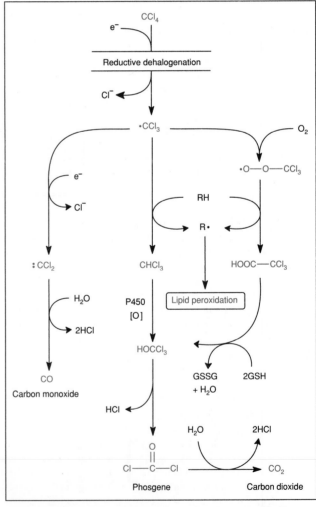

Figure 6-17. Reductive dehalogenation of carbon tetrachloride to a trichloromethyl free radical that initiates lipid peroxidation.

RH, unsaturated lipid; R·, lipid dienyl radical; GSH, reduced glutathione; GSSG, oxidized glutathione.

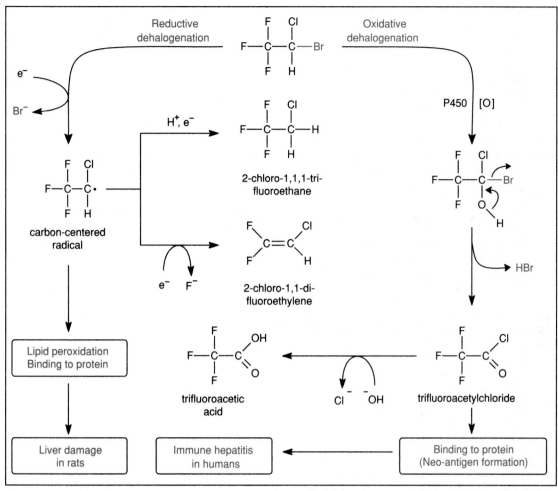

Figure 6-18. *Activation of halothane by reductive and oxidative dehalogenation and their role in liver toxicity in rats and humans.*

use. The mechanism of the lethal interaction between Sorivudine and Tegafur is illustrated in Fig. 6-16, and involves inhibition of dihydropyrimidine dehydrogenase (DPD), an NADPH-requiring, homodimeric protein (Mr ~210 kDa) containing FMN/FAD and an iron–sulfur cluster in each subunit. The enzyme is located mainly in liver cytosol, where it catalyzes the reduction of 5-fluorouracil and related pyrimidines. Sorivudine is converted in part by gut flora to (*E*)-5-(2-bromovinyl) uracil (BVU), which lacks antiviral activity but which is converted by DPD to a metabolite that binds covalently to the enzyme. The irreversible inactivation (a.k.a. suicidal inactivation) of DPD by Sorivudine causes a marked inhibition of 5-fluorouracil metabolism, which increases blood levels of 5-fluorouracil to toxic and, in some cases, lethal levels (Ogura *et al.*, 1998; Kanamitsu *et al.*, 2000).

Several genetic polymorphisms that result in a partial or complete loss of DPD activity have been described (van Kuilenburg *et al.*, 2004; Robert *et al.*, 2005). Severe 5-fluorouracil toxicity has also been documented in individuals who are heterozygous for allelic variants of DPD, and 5-fluorouracil lethality has been documented in rare individuals who are completely deficient in DPD (one individual in about 10,000). 5-Fluorouracil is one of the most frequently prescribed anticancer drugs, for which reason assessing an individual's DPD genotype (by analyzing DNA for allelic variants) or phenotyping (by measuring DPD activity in peripheral blood

mononuclear cells or PBMCs) is advocated prior to 5-fluorouracil therapy so that the dosage of this anticancer drug can be adjusted on an individual basis.

Dehalogenation   There are three major mechanisms for removing halogens (F, Cl, Br, and I) from aliphatic xenobiotics (Anders, 1985). The first, known as *reductive dehalogenation*, involves replacement of a halogen with hydrogen, as shown below:

$$X-\underset{\underset{X}{|}}{\overset{\overset{X}{|}}{C}}-\underset{\underset{H}{|}}{\overset{\overset{X}{|}}{C}}-X \quad \xrightarrow[-HX]{+2H} \quad X-\underset{\underset{X}{|}}{\overset{\overset{X}{|}}{C}}-\underset{\underset{H}{|}}{\overset{\overset{X}{|}}{C}}-H$$

Pentahaloethane   Tetrahaloethane

In the second mechanism, known as *oxidative dehalogenation*, a halogen and hydrogen on the same carbon atom are replaced with oxygen. Depending on the structure of the haloalkane, oxidative dehalogenation leads to the formation of an acylhalide or aldehyde, as shown below:

$$X-\underset{\underset{X}{|}}{\overset{\overset{X}{|}}{C}}-\underset{\underset{H}{|}}{\overset{\overset{X}{|}}{C}}-X \quad \xrightarrow[-HX]{+[O]} \quad X-\underset{\underset{X}{|}}{\overset{\overset{X}{|}}{C}}-\overset{\overset{X}{|}}{C}=O$$

Pentahaloethane   Tetrahaloacetylhalide

A third mechanism of dehalogenation involves the elimination of two halogens on adjacent carbon atoms to form a carbon–carbon double bond, as shown below:

$$X-\overset{\overset{\textstyle X}{|}}{\underset{\underset{\textstyle X}{|}}{C}}-\overset{\overset{\textstyle X}{|}}{\underset{\underset{\textstyle H}{|}}{C}}-X \quad \xrightarrow[-2HX]{+2H} \quad \overset{\overset{\textstyle X}{}}{\underset{\underset{\textstyle X}{}}{C}}=\overset{\overset{\textstyle X}{}}{\underset{\underset{\textstyle H}{}}{C}}$$

Pentahaloethane   Trihaloethylene

A variation on this third mechanism is *dehydrohalogenation*, in which a halogen and hydrogen on adjacent carbon atoms are eliminated to form a carbon–carbon double bond.

Reductive and oxidative dehalogenation are both catalyzed by cytochrome P450. (The ability of cytochrome P450 to catalyze both reductive and oxidative reactions is explained later in the section on *Cytochrome P450*.) Dehalogenation reactions leading to double bond formation are catalyzed by cytochrome P450 and glutathione transferase. These reactions play an important role in the biotransformation and metabolic activation of several halogenated alkanes, as the following examples illustrate.

The hepatotoxicity of carbon tetrachloride (CCl_4) and several related halogenated alkanes is dependent on their biotransformation by reductive dehalogenation (Plaa, 2000). The first step in reductive dehalogenation is a one-electron reduction catalyzed by cytochrome P450, which produces a potentially toxic, carbon-centered radical and inorganic halide. In the case of CCl_4, reductive dechlorination produces a trichloromethyl radical ($\bullet CCl_3$), which initiates lipid peroxidation and produces a variety of other metabolites, as shown in Fig. 6-17.

Halothane can also be converted by reductive dehalogenation to a carbon-centered radical, as shown in Fig. 6-18. The mechanism is identical to that described for carbon tetrachloride, although in the case of halothane the radical is generated through loss of bromine, which is a better leaving group than chlorine. Figure 6-18 also shows that halothane can undergo oxidative dehalogenation, which involves oxygen insertion at the C–H bond to generate an unstable halohydrin ($CF_3COHClBr$) that decomposes to a reactive acylhalide (CF_3COCl), which can bind to cellular proteins (particularly to amine groups) or further decompose to trifluoroacetic acid (CF_3COOH).

Both the oxidative and reductive pathways of halothane metabolism generate reactive intermediates capable of binding to proteins and other cellular macromolecules. The relative importance of these two pathways to halothane-induced hepatotoxicity appears to be species dependent. In rats, halothane-induced hepatotoxicity is promoted by those conditions favoring the reductive dehalogenation of halothane, such as moderate hypoxia (10–14% oxygen) plus treatment with the cytochrome P450 inducers, phenobarbital, and pregnenolone-16α-carbonitrile. In contrast to the situation in rats, halothane-induced hepatotoxicity in guinea pigs is largely the result of oxidative dehalogenation of halothane (Lunam *et al.*, 1989). In guinea pigs, halothane hepatotoxicity is not enhanced by moderate hypoxia and is diminished by the use of deuterated halothane, which impedes the oxidative dehalogenation of halothane because the P450-dependent insertion of oxygen into a carbon–deuterium bond is energetically less favorable (and therefore slower) than inserting oxygen into a carbon–hydrogen bond.

Halothane hepatitis in humans is a rare but severe form of liver necrosis associated with repeated exposure to this volatile anesthetic. In humans, as in guinea pigs, halothane hepatotoxicity

appears to result from the oxidative dehalogenation of halothane, as shown in Fig. 6-18. Serum samples from patients suffering from halothane hepatitis contain antibodies directed against neoantigens formed by the trifluoroacetylation of proteins. These antibodies have been used to identify which specific proteins in the endoplasmic reticulum are targets for trifluoroacetylation during the oxidative dehalogenation of halothane (Pohl *et al.*, 1989).

The concept that halothane is activated by cytochrome P450 to trifluoroacetylhalide, which binds covalently to proteins and elicits an immune response, has been extended to other volatile anesthetics, such as enflurane, methoxyflurane, and isoflurane. In other words, these halogenated aliphatic hydrocarbons, like halothane, may be converted to acylhalides that form immunogens by binding covalently to proteins. In addition to accounting for rare instances of enflurane hepatitis, this mechanism of hepatotoxicity can also account for reports of a *cross-sensitization* between enflurane and halothane, in which enflurane causes liver damage in patients previously exposed to halothane.

One of the metabolites generated from the reductive dehalogenation of halothane is 2-chloro-1,1-difluoroethylene (Fig. 6-18). The formation of this metabolite involves the loss of two halogens

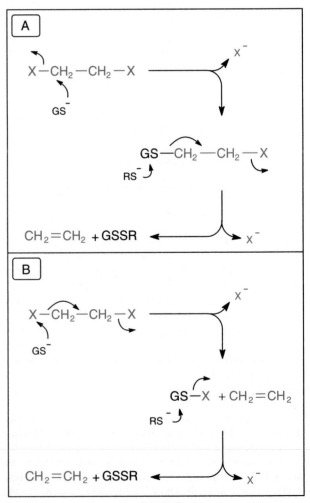

Figure 6-19. Glutathione-dependent dehalogenation of 1,2-dihaloethane to ethylene. (A) Nucleophilic attack on carbon and (B) nucleophilic attack on halide.

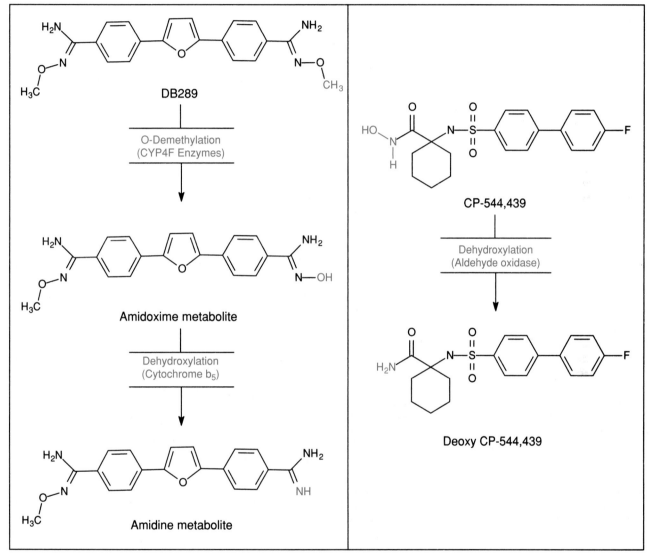

Figure 6-20. *Dehydrochlorination of the pesticide DDT to DDE, a glutathione-dependent reaction.*

Figure 6-21. *Dehydroxylation by cytochrome b₅ and aldehyde oxidase.*

from adjacent carbon atoms with formation of a carbon–carbon double bond. This type of dehalogenation reaction can also be catalyzed by glutathione transferases. Glutathione initiates the reaction with a nucleophilic attack either on the electrophilic carbon to which the halogen is attached (mechanism A) or on the halide itself (mechanism B), as shown in Fig. 6-19 for the dehalogenation of 1,2-dihaloethane to ethylene. The insecticide DDT is detoxified by dehydrochlorination to DDE by DDT-dehydrochlorinase, as shown in

Fig. 6-20. The activity of this glutathione-dependent reaction correlates well with resistance to DDT in houseflies.

Dehydroxylation—Cytochrome b₅ and Aldehyde Oxidase
In the presence of NADH and NADH-cytochrome b₅ reductase (CYB5R3), the microsomal hemoprotein cytochrome b₅ (CYB5A) can catalyze the N-dehydroxylation of various amidoximes, as shown in Fig. 6-21 for the amidoxime metabolite of

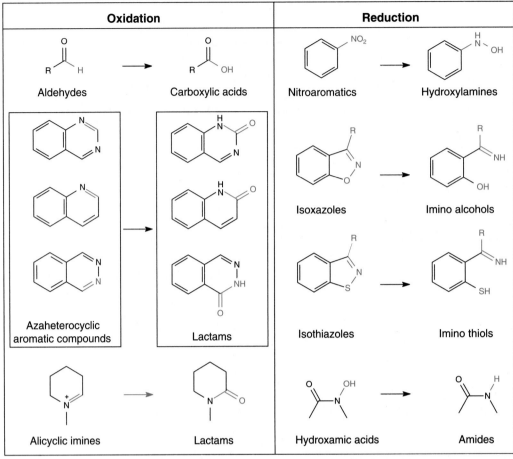

Figure 6-22. Examples of oxidation and reduction catalyzed by aldehyde oxidase.

the antimicrobial prodrug DB289 (Saulter *et al.*, 2005). The complex of NADH-cytochrome b$_5$ reductase and cytochrome b$_5$, in the presence of NADH, can also efficiently reduce arylhydroxylamine metabolites of drugs such as sulfamethoxazole and dapsone, as well as carcinogens that are generated through the oxidation of compounds such as 4-aminobiphenyl and PhIP by CYP1A1, 1A2, 1B1, lactoperoxidase, and myeloperoxidase (see sections "Cytochrome P450" and "Peroxidase-Dependent Cooxidation") (Kurian *et al.*, 2006). Because these carcinogenic arylhydroxylamines can be further activated by glucuronidation, sulfonation, or acetylation in various tissues (see sections "Glucuronidation," "Sulfonation," and "Acetylation"), reduction by NADH-cytochrome b$_5$ reductase and cytochrome b$_5$ represents a competing detoxication pathway. Figure 6-21 also shows a similar dehydroxylation reaction catalyzed by aldehyde oxidase, an enzyme that can catalyze both reductive and oxidative reaction, as discussed in the next section.

Aldehyde Oxidase—Reductive Reactions Aldehyde oxidase is a cytosolic molybdozyme that catalyzes the oxidation of some xenobiotics and the reduction of others. The types of oxidative and reductive reactions catalyzed by aldehyde oxidase are shown in Fig. 6-22. In contrast to the large number of drugs that are known to be (or suspected of being) oxidized by aldehyde oxidase in vivo, only a few drugs are known to be (or suspected of being) reduced by aldehyde oxidase in vivo, including nitrofurazone, zonisamide, and ziprasidone. The reductive metabolism of ziprasidone by aldehyde

oxidase is shown in Fig. 6-3, and the reductive dehydroxylation of CP-544,439 is shown in Fig. 6-21. The features of aldehyde oxidase and the oxidative reactions it catalyzes are discussed later in the section on "Aldehyde Oxidase."

Oxidation

Alcohol, Aldehyde, Ketone Oxidation–Reduction Systems Alcohols, aldehydes, and ketones are oxidized by a number of enzymes, including alcohol dehydrogenase, aldehyde dehydrogenase, AKRs (such as those with dihydrodiol dehydrogenase activity), the molybdenum-containing enzymes, aldehyde oxidase, and xanthine dehydrogenase/oxidase, and cytochrome P450. For example, simple alcohols (such as methanol and ethanol) are oxidized to aldehydes (namely, formaldehyde and acetaldehyde) by alcohol dehydrogenase. These aldehydes are further oxidized to carboxylic acids (formic acid and acetic acid) by aldehyde dehydrogenase, as shown in Fig. 6-23. Many of the aforementioned enzymes can also catalyze the reduction of xenobiotics, as discussed in the previous section on "Reduction."

Alcohol Dehydrogenase Alcohol dehydrogenases (ADHs) belong to the medium-chain dehydrogenases/reductases (MDRs), as shown in Table 6-5. ADHs are zinc-containing, cytosolic enzymes present in several tissues including liver, which has the highest levels, kidney, lung, and gastric mucosa (Agarwal, 1992). Human ADHs are dimeric proteins consisting of two 40-kDa subunits designated

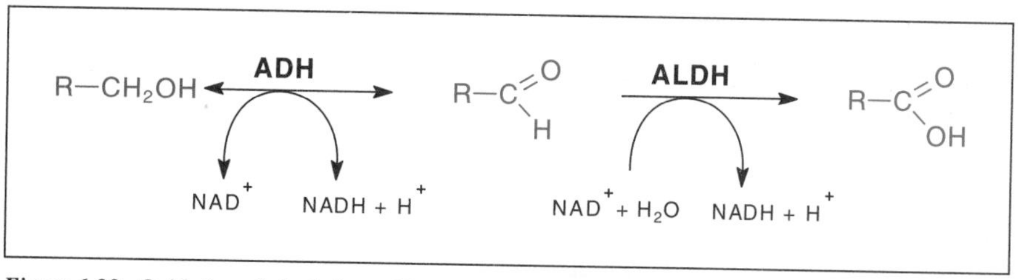

Figure 6-23. *Oxidation of alcohols to aldehydes and carboxylic acids by alcohol dehydrogenase (ADH) and aldehyde dehydrogenase (ALDH).*

α, β, γ, π, χ, and either σ or μ. As shown in Table 6-5, there are seven human ADHs, and these are categorized into five classes (I–V). Class I comprises three enzymes: ADH1A, which contains at least one alpha subunit ($\alpha\alpha$, $\alpha\beta$, or $\alpha\gamma$), ADH1B, which contains at least one beta subunit ($\beta\beta$ or $\beta\gamma$), and ADH1C, which contains two gamma subunits ($\gamma\gamma$). ADH1A, -1B, and 1C were formerly known as ADH1, -2, and -3. Class II contains ADH4, which is composed of two pi subunits ($\pi\pi$). Class III contains ADH5, which is composed of two chi subunits ($\chi\chi$). Class IV contains ADH7, which is composed of two subunits designated mu ($\mu\mu$) or sigma ($\sigma\sigma$). Class V contains ADH6 (for which there is no subunit designation) (Brennan *et al.*, 2004); see also www.gene.ucl.ac.uk/ nomenclature/genefamily/ADH.shtml.

Of the seven ADHs, only ADH1B and ADH1C are polymorphic. There are three allelic variants of the beta subunit (β_1, β_2, and β_3), which differ by a single amino acid, and two allelic variants of the gamma subunit (γ_1 and γ_2), which differ by two amino acids. Consequently, the human ADH enzymes comprise nine subunits, all of which can combine as homodimers. In addition, the α, β, and γ subunits (and their allelic variants) can form heterodimers with each other (but not with the π, χ, or σ/μ subunits, which only form homodimers). ADH1B enzymes that differ in the type of β subunits are known as allelozymes, as are ADH1C enzymes that differ in the type of γ subunit.

The class I ADH isozymes (ADH1A or α-ADH, ADH1B or β-ADH, and ADH1C or γ-ADH) are responsible for the oxidation of ethanol and other small, aliphatic alcohols, and they are strongly inhibited by pyrazole and its 4-alkyl derivatives (e.g., 4-methylpyrazole). High levels of class I ADH isozymes are expressed in liver and adrenals, with lower levels in kidney, lung, blood vessels (in the case of ADH1B) and other tissues, but not brain.

The class II enzyme ADH4 (π-ADH) is primarily expressed in liver (with lower levels in stomach), where it preferentially oxidizes larger aliphatic and aromatic alcohols. ADH4 differs from the ADH1 isozymes in that it plays little or no role in ethanol and methanol oxidation, and it is not inhibited by pyrazole.

The class III enzyme ADH5 (χ-ADH) preferentially oxidizes long-chain alcohols (pentanol and larger) and aromatic alcohols (such as cinnamyl alcohol). Like ADH4, ADH5 is not inhibited by pyrazole. However, in contrast to ADH4, which is largely confined to the liver, ADH5 is ubiquitous, being present in virtually all tissues (including brain), where it appears to play an important role in detoxifying formaldehyde. In fact, ADH5 and formaldehyde dehydrogenase are identical enzymes (Koivusalo *et al.*, 1989).

The class IV enzyme ADH7 (μ- or σ-ADH) is a low-affinity (high K_m), high-capacity (high V_{max}) enzyme, and is the most active of the medium-chain ADHs in oxidizing retinol. It is the major ADH expressed in human stomach and other areas of the gas-

trointestinal tract (esophagus, gingiva, mouth, and tongue). In contrast the other ADHs, ADH7 is not expressed in adult human liver. Inasmuch as ADH7 is expressed in the upper gastrointestinal tract, where chronic alcohol consumption leads to cancer development, there is considerable interest in the role of ADH7 in the conversion of ethanol to acetaldehyde (a suspected upper GI tract carcinogen or co-carcinogen) and in its role in the metabolism of retinol (a vitamin required for epithelial cell growth and differentiation), which might be inhibited by alcohol consumption (Seitz and Oneta, 1998).

The class I ADH isozymes differ in their capacity to oxidize ethanol. Even the allelozymes, which differ in a single amino acid, differ markedly in the affinity (K_m) and/or capacity (V_{max}) for oxidizing ethanol to acetaldehyde. The homodimer, $\beta_2\beta_2$ and heterodimers containing at least one β_2 subunit (i.e., the ADH1B*2 allelozymes) are especially active in oxidizing ethanol at physiological pH. ADH1B*2 (formerly known as ADH2*2) is known as *atypical* ADH, and is responsible for the unusually rapid conversion of ethanol to acetaldehyde in 90% of the Pacific Rim Asian population (Japanese, Chinese, Korean). The atypical ADH is expressed to a much lesser degree in Caucasians (<5% of Americans, ~8% of English, ~12% of Germans, and ~20% of Swiss), African Americans (<10%), Native Americans (0%), and Asian Indians (0%) (Agarwal, 1992). The three ADH1B alleles, ADH1B*1 (β_1-ADH), ADH1B*2 (β_2-ADH), and ADH1B*3 (β_3-ADH) are mainly expressed in Caucasians (up to 95%), Pacific Rim Asians (~90%), and Africans/African Americans (~24%), respectively. These population differences in ADH1B allelozyme expression contribute to ethnic differences in alcohol consumption and toxicity, as discussed in the next section on *Aldehyde Dehydrogenase.*

Unlike the allelic variants of ADH1B, the allelic variants of ADH1C do not differ markedly in their ability to oxidize ethanol. However, as in the case of the ADH1B allelozymes, the expression of the ADH1C allelozymes also varies from one ethnic group to the next. The two allelozymes of ADH1C, namely, ADH1C*1 (γ_1-ADH) and ADH1C*2 (γ_2-ADH), are respectively expressed 50:50 in Caucasians, but 90:10 in Pacific Rim Asians (Li, 2000).

The various class I ADH isozymes and allelozymes in human liver oxidize ethanol with a K_m of 50 μM to 4 mM. For comparison, legal intoxication in the United States is defined as a blood alcohol level of 0.08%, which corresponds to 18 mM (Edenberg, 2000). Therefore, during intoxication, the hepatic metabolism of ethanol by ADH becomes saturated, and the kinetics of ethanol disappearance conform to zero-order kinetics, meaning that a constant *amount* of ethanol is metabolized per unit time. When the concentration of ethanol falls within the range of K_m, the kinetics of ethanol disappearance conform to a first-order process, meaning that a constant *percentage* of the remaining ethanol is metabolized per unit time.

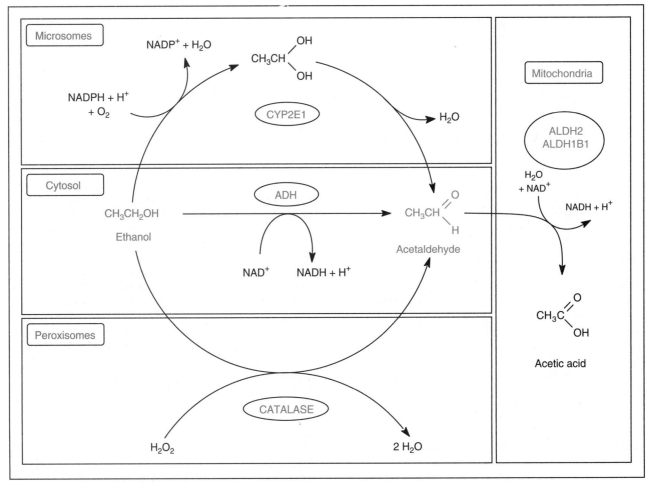

Figure 6-24. Oxidation of alcohol to acetaldehyde by alcohol dehydrogenase (ADH), cytochrome P450 (CYP2E1), and catalase.

Note: The oxidation of alcohol to acetic acid involves multiple organelles.

The metabolism of alcohol is usually thought of as a linear progression from ethanol to acetaldehyde to acetic acid. However, ADH1 not only oxidizes ethanol to acetaldehyde, it also reduces acetaldehyde back to ethanol. Umulis *et al.* (2005) estimated that, if the reverse reaction did not occur, levels of acetaldehyde would be 10 times higher than those actually observed in vivo. Acetaldehyde is considerably more toxic than ethanol or acetic acid; hence, blood levels of acetaldehyde are an important determinant of alcohol tolerability, as discussed in the next section on Aldehyde Dehydrogenases.

Compared with hepatic ADH, gastric ADH has a lower affinity (higher K_m) but higher capacity (larger V_{max}) for oxidizing ethanol; the former being dominated by the class I ADH isozymes (ADH1A, -1B, and 1C), the latter by the class IV enzyme ADH7. Although ethanol is largely biotransformed by hepatic ADH1, gastric ADH7 nevertheless can limit the systemic bioavailability of alcohol. This first-pass elimination of alcohol by gastric ADH7 can be significant depending on the manner in which the alcohol is consumed; large doses over a short time produce high ethanol concentrations in the stomach, which compensate for the low affinity (high K_m) of gastric ADH7. Young women have lower gastric ADH7 activity than do men, and gastric ADH7 activity tends to be lower in alcoholics (Frezza *et al.*, 1990). Some alcoholic women have no detectable gastric ADH7, and blood levels of ethanol after oral consumption of alcohol are the same as those that are obtained after intravenous administration. Gastric ADH7 activity decreases during fasting, which is one reason alcohol is more intoxicating when consumed on an empty stomach. Several commonly used drugs (e.g., cimetidine, ranitidine, aspirin) are noncompetitive inhibitors of gastric ADH7. Under certain circumstances these drugs increase the systemic availability of alcohol, although the effect is too small to have serious medical, social, or legal consequences (Levitt, 1993). About 30% of Asians appear to be genetically deficient in class IV ADH7, the main gastric ADH. In addition to biotransforming ethanol and retinol, class IV ADH7 also detoxifies the dietary carcinogen, nitrobenzaldehyde. It has been suggested that a lack of class IV ADH7 in Japanese subjects may impair their ability to detoxify nitrobenzaldehyde and may possibly be linked to the high rate of gastric cancer observed in the Japanese population (Seitz and Oneta, 1998).

Alcohols can be oxidized to aldehydes by non-ADH enzymes in microsomes and peroxisomes, although these are quantitatively less important than ADH for ethanol oxidation (Lieber, 2004). The microsomal ethanol oxidizing system (formerly known as MEOS) is the cytochrome P450 enzyme, CYP2E1. The corresponding peroxisomal enzyme is catalase. The oxidation of ethanol to acetaldehyde by these three enzyme systems is shown in Fig. 6-24.

Table 6-6
Properties of the Human Aldehyde Dehydrogenases (ALDHs)

ALDH	ALTERNATIVE NAMES	TISSUE	SUBCELLULAR LOCALIZATION	MAJOR SUBSTRATE
1A1	ALDH1	Liver, stomach, etc.	Cytosol	Retinal
1A2	ALDH11	Testis, liver, kidney, etc.	Cytosol	Retinal
1A3	ALDH6	Prostate, salivary gland, stomach, kidney	Cytosol	Aliphatic aldehyde, retinal
1B1	ALDH5	Muscle, liver, kidney, etc.	Mitochondria	Acetaldehyde
1L1	FDH	Liver, kidney, pancreas, muscle	Cytosol	10-Formyltetrahydrofolate
1L2	FLJ38508	Cervix, uterus	Cytosol	Unknown
2	ALDM	Liver, stomach, muscle, etc.	Mitochondria	Acetaldehyde
3A1	ALDH3	Trachea, stomach, lung, etc.	Cytosol	Aromatic aldehydes
3A2	FALDH	Adrenal, liver, heart, muscle, etc.	Microsomes	Fatty and aromatic aldehydes
3B1	ALDH7	Kidney, lung	Microsomes	Aliphatic and aromatic aldehydes
3B2	ALDH8	Parotid	Microsomes	Unknown
4A1	ALDH4	Liver, kidney	Mitochondria	Glutamate, γ-semialdehyde
5A1	SSDH	Brain, liver, heart	Mitochondria	Succinic semialdehyde
6A1	MMSDH	Kidney, liver, heart	Mitochondria	Methylmalonate semialdehyde
7A1	ATQ1	Kidney, heart, ovary, etc.	Cytosol	Unknown
8A1	ALDH12	Liver, kidney, etc.	Cytosol	Unknown
9A1	γABHD, ALDH9	Liver, kidney, muscle	Cytosol	Amine aldehyde
16A1	MGC10204	Uterus, placenta	Unknown	Unknown
18A1	Δ^1–P5CS[a]	Kidney, heart, muscle, etc.	Mitochondria	Glutamate

[a] Δ^1-Pyrroline-5-carboxylate synthase, P5CS.

γABHD, 4-aminobutyraldehyde; FALDH, fatty aldehyde dehydrogenase; SSDH, succinic dehydrogenase; MMSDH, methylmalonate semialdehyde dehydrogenase.

Data adapted from Sládek NE: Human aldehyde dehydrogenases: Potential pathological, pharmacological, and toxicological impact. *J Biochem Mol Toxicol* 17:7–23, 2003; Vasiliou V, Pappa A, Estey T: Role of human aldehyde dehydrogenases in endobiotic and xenobiotic metabolism. *Drug Metab Rev* 36:279–299, 2004.

Aldehyde Dehydrogenase   Aldehyde dehydrogenase (ALDH) oxidizes aldehydes to carboxylic acids with NAD$^+$ as the cofactor. Several ALDH enzymes are involved in the oxidation of xenobiotic aldehydes. The enzymes also have esterase activity (Yoshida *et al.*, 1998). Formaldehyde dehydrogenase, which specifically oxidizes formaldehyde that is complexed with glutathione, is not a member of the ALDH family but is a class III ADH (ADH5) (Koivusalo *et al.*, 1989). At least 19 ALDH genes have been identified in humans, and a correspondingly large number of ALDH genes appear to be present in other mammalian species (Sládek, 2003; Vasiliou *et al.*, 2004). The name, tissue distribution, subcellular location, and major substrate for the human ALDHs are summarized in Table 6-6. The ALDHs differ in their primary amino acid sequences. They may also differ in the quaternary structure. For example, ALDH3A1 appears to be a dimer of two 85-kDa subunits, whereas ALDH1A1 and ALDH2 appear to be homotetramers of 54-kDa subunits (Goedde and Agarwal, 1992). In contrast to ALDH1A1 and ALDH2, which specifically reduce NAD$^+$, ALDH3A1 reduces both NAD$^+$ and NADP$^+$ due to its low affinity for these cofactors.

As shown in Fig. 6-24, ALDH2 is a mitochondrial enzyme that, by virtue of its high affinity, is primarily responsible for oxi-

dizing simple aldehydes, such as acetaldehyde (K_m for acetaldehyde <5 μM at pH 7.4). A genetic polymorphism for ALDH2 has been documented in humans. A high percentage (45–53%) of Japanese, Chinese, Koreans, Taiwanese, and Vietnamese populations are deficient in ALDH2 activity due to a point mutation (Glu$_{487}$ $\rightarrow$ Lys$_{487}$). This inactive allelic variant of ALDH2 is known as ALDH2*2, to distinguish it from the active, wild-type enzyme, ALDH2*1. This same population (i.e., Pacific Rim Asians) also have a high incidence of the atypical form of ADH (i.e., ADH2*2), which means that they rapidly convert ethanol to acetaldehyde but only slowly convert acetaldehyde to acetic acid. (They also have a relatively high prevalence of a deficiency of class IV ADH activity, which impairs gastric metabolism of ethanol.) As a result, many Asian subjects experience a flushing syndrome after consuming alcohol due to a rapid build-up of acetaldehyde, which triggers the dilation of facial blood vessels through the release of catecholamines. Native Americans also experience a flushing syndrome after consuming alcohol, apparently because they express another allelic variant of ALDH2 and/or because acetaldehyde oxidation in blood erythrocytes is impaired in these individuals, possibly due to the expression of a variant form of ALDH1A1. The functional genetic variants of

ADH that rapidly convert ethanol to acetaldehyde (i.e., ADH2*2), and the genetic variants of ALDH that slowly detoxify acetaldehyde both protect against heavy drinking and alcoholism. Inhibition of ALDH by disulfiram (Antabuse) causes an accumulation of acetaldehyde in alcoholics. The nauseating effect of acetaldehyde serves to deter continued ethanol consumption (Goedde and Agarwal, 1992). However, it is important to note that a predisposition toward alcoholism is not simply determined by factors that affect the pharmacokinetics of ethanol and its metabolites. Studies in humans and rodents implicate serotonin 1b receptor, dopamine D2 receptor, tryptophan hydroxylase, and neuropeptide Y as candidate targets of genetic susceptibility in the pharmacodynamic actions of ethanol (Li, 2000). Monoamine oxidase may also be a risk factor for alcoholism, as discussed later (see section "Monoamine Oxidase").

Genetic deficiencies in other ALDHs impair the metabolism of other aldehydes, which is the underlying basis of certain diseases. For example, ALDH4A1 deficiency disturbs proline metabolism and causes type II hyperprolinemia, symptoms of which include mental retardation and convulsions. Various missense and other mutations in the ALDH3A2 gene (formerly ALDH10 or FALDH) cause a deficiency of the active enzyme that detoxifies fatty aldehydes, which disturbs the metabolism of membrane lipids, and is the underlying basis of Sjögren–Larsson syndrome, symptoms of which include ichthyosis, neurological problems, and oligophrenia. Treatment of Sjögren–Larsson syndrome consists of inhibition of 5-lipoxygenase (ALOX5) with zileuton and stimulation of ALDH3A2 transcription with the PPAR agonist bezafibrate in patients with certain missense mutations (Rizzo, 2007).

The toxicological consequences of an inherited (i.e., genetic) or acquired (e.g., drug-induced) deficiency of ALDH illustrate that aldehydes are more cytotoxic than the corresponding alcohol. This is especially true of allyl alcohol (CH_2=CHCH$_2$OH), which is converted by ADH to the highly hepatotoxic aldehyde, acrolein (CH_2=CHCHO).

The oxidation of ethanol by ADH and ALDH leads to the formation of acetic acid, which is rapidly oxidized to carbon dioxide and water. However, in certain cases, alcohols are converted to toxic carboxylic acids, as in the case of methanol and ethylene glycol, which are converted via aldehyde intermediates to formic acid and oxalic acid, respectively. Formic and oxalic acids are considerably more toxic than acetic acid. For this reason, methanol and ethylene glycol poisoning are commonly treated with ethanol, which competitively inhibits the oxidation of methanol and ethylene glycol by ADH and ALDH. The potent inhibitor of ADH, 4-methylpyrazole (fomepizole), is also used to treat methanol and ethylene glycol poisoning.

The reduction of aldehydes and ketones to primary and secondary alcohols by carbonyl reductases has already been discussed (see section "Carbonyl Reduction—SDRs and AKRs"). In contrast to ADH and ALDH, carbonyl reductases typically use NADPH as the source of reducing equivalents. Aldehydes, especially aromatic aldehydes, can also be oxidized by aldehyde oxidase and xanthine oxidase, which are discussed in the section "Molybdenum Hydroxylases."

Dihydrodiol Dehydrogenase As mentioned in the section on "Carbonyl Reduction—SDRs and AKRs", several members of the aldo–keto reductase (AKR) superfamily are dihydrodiol dehydrogenases that oxidize the *trans*-dihydrodiols of various polycyclic aromatic hydrocarbons to the corresponding *ortho*-quinones, as shown in

Fig. 6-9 (Penning, 1997; Burczynski and Penning, 2000). There is also a gene, DHDH, that is unrelated to AKRs and encodes a dimeric enzyme that is only expressed in the intestine (Arimitsu *et al.*, 1999). Polycyclic aromatic hydrocarbons can be oxidized by cytochrome P450 to an arene oxide, an electrophilic and potentially toxic metabolite that is detoxified by its conversion to a *trans*-dihydrodiol by epoxide hydrolase. By oxidizing the *trans*-dihydrodiol to an *ortho*-quinone, AKRs generate yet another potentially toxic metabolite. In terms of their ability to cause oxidative stress and cellular toxicity, *ortho*-quinones can be considered equivalent to *para*-quinones, which were discussed earlier in the section "Quinone Reduction—NQO1 and NQO2."

Molybdenum Hydroxylases (Molybdozymes) There are two major molybdenum hydroxylases or molybdozymes that participate in the biotransformation of xenobiotics: aldehyde oxidase and xanthine oxidoreductase (XOR, also known as xanthine oxidase) (Rettie and Fisher, 1999; Beedham, 2002). Sulfite oxidase is a third molybdozyme; it will not be described here except to say sulfite oxidase, as the name implies, oxidizes sulfite, an irritating air pollutant, to sulfate, which is relatively innocuous. Genetic deficiencies in the synthesis of molybdenum cofactor results in the loss of xanthine oxidoreductase, aldehyde oxidase, and sulfite oxidase, but it is loss of the latter enzyme that gives rise to the progressive neurological damage that leads to death in early childhood (Reiss and Johnson, 2003).

All three molybdozymes are flavoprotein enzymes consisting of two identical ~150 kDa subunits, each of which contains FAD, molybdenum, in the form of a pterin molybdenum cofactor ([Mo^{VI} (=S) (=O)]$^{2+}$) and two iron–sulfur (Fe$_2$S$_2$) centers (known as FeSI and FeSII). The catalytic cycle involves an interaction between the molybdenum center with a reducing substrate, which results in the reduction of the molybdenum cofactor, after which reducing equivalents are transferred intramolecularly to the flavin and iron–sulfur centers, with reoxidation occurring via the flavin moiety by molecular oxygen (in the case of aldehyde oxidase and xanthine oxidase) or NAD$^+$ (in the case of xanthine dehydrogenase). During substrate oxidation, aldehyde oxidase and xanthine oxidase are reduced and then reoxidized by molecular oxygen; hence, they function as true oxidases. The oxygen incorporated into the xenobiotic is derived from water rather than oxygen, which distinguishes the oxidases from oxygenases. The overall reaction is as follows:

$$RH \xrightarrow[-2H^+, -2e^-]{+H_2O} ROH$$

Additional details of the catalytic cycle are described in the next section "Xanthine Oxidoreductase." Xanthine oxidase and aldehyde oxidase catalyze the oxidation of electron-deficient sp^2-hybridized (i.e., double-bonded) carbon atoms found, more often than not, in nitrogen heterocycles, such as purines, pyrimidines, pteridines, and iminium ions. This contrasts with oxidation by cytochrome P450, which generally catalyzes the oxidation of carbon atoms with a high electron density. For this reason, xenobiotics that are good substrates for molybdozymes tend to be poor substrates for cytochrome P450, and vice versa (Rettie and Fisher, 1999). In nitrogen heterocycles, the carbon atom with lowest electron density is adjacent to the nitrogen atom, for which reason xanthine oxidase and aldehyde oxidase tend to hydroxylate the α-carbon atom to form a hydroximine that rapidly tautomerizes to the corresponding α-aminoketone. As the name implies, aldehyde oxidase can convert certain aldehydes to the

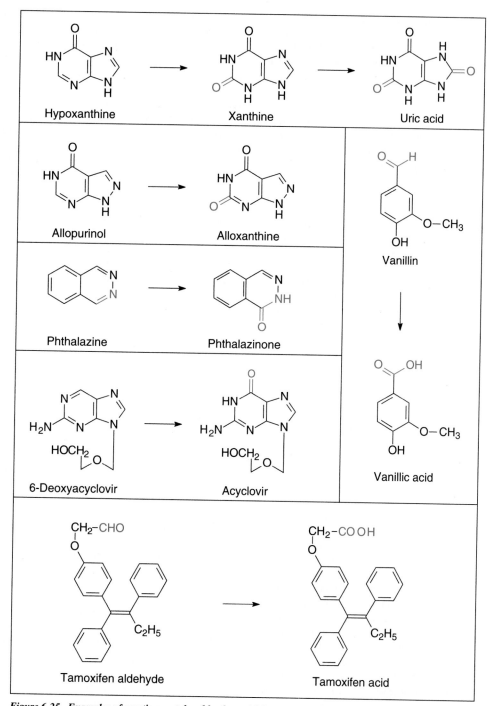

Figure 6-25. Examples of reactions catalyzed by the molybdozymes, xanthine oxidase, and aldehyde oxidase.

corresponding carboxylic acid; a property that is also shared by xanthine oxidase, albeit with lower activity. Certain aromatic aldehydes, such as tamoxifen aldehyde and benzaldehyde, are good substrates for aldehyde oxidase and xanthine oxidase, whereas aliphatic aldehydes tend to be poor substrates. Consequently, aldehyde oxidase and xanthine oxidase contribute negligibly to the metabolism of acetaldehyde. Some reactions catalyzed by aldehyde oxidase and xanthine oxidase are shown in Fig. 6-25. Under certain conditions, both enzymes can also catalyze the reduction of xenobiotics. Examples of reductive reactions catalyzed by aldehyde oxidase are shown in Fig. 6-22.

Xanthine Oxidoreductase Xanthine dehydrogenase (XD) and xanthine oxidase (XO) are two forms of the same enzyme that differ in the electron acceptor used in the final step of catalysis. In the case of XD, the final electron acceptor is NAD$^+$ (dehydrogenase activity), whereas in the case of XO the final electron acceptor is oxygen (oxidase activity). XD is converted to XO by oxidation of cysteine residues (Cys$_{993}$ and Cys$_{1326}$ of the human enzyme) and/or proteolytic cleavage. The conversion of XD to XO by cysteine oxidation appears to be reversible. Under normal physiologic conditions, XD is the predominant form of the enzyme found in vivo. However, during tissue processing, the dehydrogenase form tends to be converted to the oxidase form; hence, most in vitro studies are conducted with XO or a combination of XO and XD. The induction (upregulation) of XD and/or the conversion of XD to XO in vivo is thought to play an important role in ischemia-reperfusion injury, lipopolysaccharide (LPS)-mediated tissue injury, and alcohol-induced hepatotoxicity (Pacher et al., 2006). During ischemia, XO levels increase because hypoxia induces XOR gene transcription, and because XD is converted to XO. During reperfusion, XO contributes to oxidative stress and lipid peroxidation because the oxidase activity of XO involves the reduction of molecular oxygen, which can lead to the formation of reactive oxygen species of the type shown in Fig. 6-15. Similarly, treatment with LPS, a bacterial endotoxin that triggers an acute inflammatory response, increases XO activity both by inducing XOR transcription and by converting XD to XO. The associated increase in oxidative stress has been implicated in LPS-induced cytotoxicity. Ethanol facilitates the conversion of XD to XO, and the conversion of ethanol to acetaldehyde provides a substrate and, hence, a source of electrons for the reduction of oxygen. Hereafter, the two forms of the enzyme will be referred to as xanthine oxidoreductase (XOR).

Typical reactions catalyzed by XOR are shown in Fig. 6-25. XOR contributes significantly to the first-pass elimination of several purine derivatives (e.g., 6-mercaptopurine and 2,6-dithiopurine), and limits the therapeutic effects of these cancer chemotherapeutic agents. In contrast, certain prodrugs are activated by xanthine oxidase. For example, the antiviral prodrugs 6-deoxyacyclovir and 2′-fluoroarabino-dideoxypurine, which are relatively well absorbed after oral dosing, are oxidized by xanthine oxidase to their respective active forms, acyclovir and 2′-fluoroarabino-dideoxyinosine, which are otherwise poorly absorbed (see Fig. 6-25). Furthermore, XOR has been implicated in the bioactivation of mitomycin C and related antineoplastic drugs, although this bioactivation reaction is thought to be largely catalyzed by NQO1 (DT-diaphorase), as discussed previously in the section "Quinone Reduction–NQO1 and NQO2."

XOR catalyzes an important physiological reaction, namely, the sequential oxidation of hypoxanthine to xanthine and uric acid, as shown in Fig. 6-25 (Rajagopalan, 1980). By competing with hypoxanthine and xanthine for oxidation by XD/XO, allopurinol inhibits the formation of uric acid, making allopurinol a useful drug in the treatment of gout (a complication of hyperuricemia). Allopurinol can also be used to evaluate the contribution of XOR to xenobiotic biotransformation in vivo. Like allopurinol, hydroxylated coumarin derivatives, such as umbelliferone (7-hydroxycoumarin) and esculetin (7,8-dihydroxycoumarin), are potent inhibitors of XD/XO. Allopurinol and other XOR inhibitors are being evaluated for the treatment of various types of ischemia-reperfusion and vascular injury that appear to be mediated, at least in part, by XOR (Pacher et al., 2006).

Monomethylated xanthines are preferentially oxidized to the corresponding uric acid derivatives by XD/XO. In contrast, dimethylated and trimethylated xanthines, such as theophylline (1,3-dimethylxanthine) and caffeine (1,3,7-trimethylxanthine), are oxidized to the corresponding uric acid derivatives primarily by cytochrome P450. Through two sequential N-demethylation reactions, cytochrome P450 converts caffeine to 1-methylxanthine, which is converted by XOR to 1-methyluric acid. The urinary ratio of 1-methylxanthine to 1-methyluric acid provides an in vivo marker of XOR activity.

The mechanism of catalysis by molybdozymes depicted in Fig. 6-26 is based on studies xanthine oxidase by Okamoto et al. (2004) and Amano et al. (2007). The molybdopterin active center

of the enzyme consists of molybdenum (Mo) bound to the following groups: pterin cofactor, thioxo (=S), oxo (=O) and hydroxyl (−OH). The hydroxyl group (Mo-OH) is activated by a nearby glutamic acid residue in the enzyme to Mo-O-, which initiates a nucleophilic attack on the substrate. This oxygen is incorporated into the substrate (e.g., xanthine) to form product (e.g., uric acid) and is replaced by oxygen from water. The resting enzyme is restored by the removal of two reducing equivalents, which may be transferred to NAD (in the case of XD) or oxygen (in the case of XO), as shown in Fig. 6-26.

In humans, XOR is a cytosolic enzyme that is widely distributed throughout the body, with the highest levels in heart, brain, liver, skeletal muscle, pancreas, small intestine, colon, and placenta. In humans, XOR appears to be encoded by a single gene (i.e., XDH). Although the sequences of two enzymes have been reported in the literature, the first report is now known to describe the sequence of human aldehyde oxidase. A complete deficiency of XOR (which may also involve a deficiency of aldehyde oxidase) gives rise to the rare genetic disorder, xanthinuria.

Aldehyde Oxidase Aldehyde oxidase is the second of two molybdozymes that play an important role in xenobiotic biotransformation; the other being xanthine oxidase (discussed in the preceding section). Whereas xanthine oxidase exists in two forms, a dehydrogenase form (XD) that relays electrons to NAD$^+$ and an oxidase form (XO) that relays electrons to molecular oxygen, aldehyde oxidase exists only in the oxidase form apparently because it lacks an NAD$^+$ binding site (Terao et al., 1998). Another significant difference between these two molybdozymes is that high levels of xanthine oxidase appear to be widely distributed throughout the body, whereas high levels of aldehyde oxidase are found in the liver, with considerably less activity in other tissues, at least in humans. Apart from these differences, many of the features of xanthine oxidase apply to aldehyde oxidase, including subcellular location (cytosol), enzyme structure and cofactor composition, mechanism of catalysis, preference for oxidizing carbon atoms adjacent to the nitrogen atoms in nitrogen heterocycles, and its preference for oxidizing aromatic aldehydes over aliphatic aldehydes. Furthermore, aldehyde oxidase also transfers electrons to molecular oxygen, which can generate reactive oxygen species and lead to oxidative stress and lipid peroxidation. Therefore, the pathophysiologic features described for xanthine oxidase may similarly apply to aldehyde oxidase, especially in the case of ethanol-induced liver damage.

As shown in Figs. 6-22 and 6-25, aldehyde oxidase can oxidize a number of substituted pyrroles, pyridines, pyrimidines, purines, pteridines, and iminium ions by a mechanism that is presumably similar to that described for xanthine oxidase in the previous section. Aldehyde oxidase can oxidize aldehydes to their corresponding carboxylic acids, but the enzyme shows a marked preference for aromatic aldehydes (e.g., benzaldehyde, tamoxifen aldehyde). Consequently, aldehyde oxidase contributes negligibly to the oxidation of aliphatic aldehydes, such as acetaldehyde. Rodrigues (1994) found that, in a bank of human liver samples, aldehyde oxidase activity toward N^1-methylnicotinamide varied more than 40-fold, whereas activity toward 6-methylpurine varied less than threefold. Although this suggests human liver cytosol contains two or more forms of aldehyde oxidase, subsequent Southern blot analysis has provided evidence for only a single copy of the aldehyde oxidase gene in humans (Terao et al., 1998), although genomic analysis of chromosome 2 has revealed the presence of 3 nearby pseudogenes

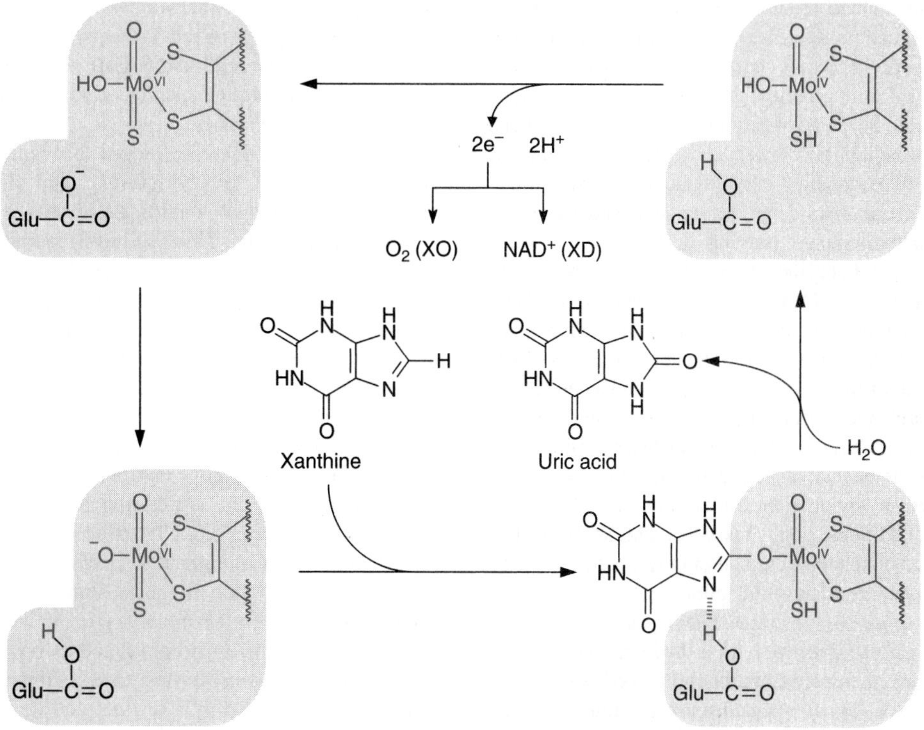

Figure 6-26. Catalytic cycle of the molybdozyme xanthine oxidoreductase.

Xanthine oxidoreductase is a molybdozyme with xanthine dehydrogenase (XD) and xanthine oxidase (XO) activities. During the final step of the catalytic cycle, the enzyme is re-oxidized by transferring electrons to NAD$^+$ (in the case of XD) or oxygen (in the case of XO). The same mechanism of catalysis likely applies to aldehyde oxidase, although there is no dehydrogenase form of this molybdozyme.

(Dupl. 1-3) (Garrattini *et al.*, 2003). On the other hand, the mouse likely expresses multiple aldehyde oxidase enzymes because the mouse AOX1 gene (on chromosome 1) is followed by three homologous genes (AOH1-3) that, in contrast to human Dupl. 1-3, appear to encode functional enzymes.

A number of physiologically important aldehydes are substrates for aldehyde oxidase, including homovanillyl aldehyde (formed from dopamine), 5-hydroxy-3-indoleacetaldehyde (formed from serotonin), and retinal, which is converted by aldehyde oxidase to retinoic acid, an important regulator of cell growth, differentiation, and morphogenesis. The catabolism of catecholamines by monoamine oxidase produces dihydromandelaldehyde, which is oxidized by aldehyde oxidase to dihydromandelic acid. Therefore, aldehyde oxidase plays an important role in the catabolism of biogenic amines and catecholamines. In humans, the gene for aldehyde oxidase has been mapped to chromosome 2q33, placing it near a genetic marker that co-segregates with the recessive familial form of amyotrophic lateral sclerosis (Lou Gehrig disease). In mouse brain, aldehyde oxidase is localized in the choroid plexus and motor neurons, which lends further support to the proposal that aldehyde oxidase is a candidate gene for this particular motor neuron disease (Bendotti *et al.*, 1997).

In general, xenobiotics that are good substrates for aldehyde oxidase are poor substrates for cytochrome P450, and vice versa (Rettie and Fisher, 1999). Naphthalene (with no nitrogen atoms) is oxidized by cytochrome P450, but not by aldehyde oxidase, whereas the opposite is true of pteridine (1,3,5,8-tetraazanaphthalene), which contains four nitrogen atoms. The intermediate structure, quinazolone (1,3-diazanaphthalene) is a substrate for both enzymes. This complementarity in substrate specificity reflects the opposing preference of the two enzymes for oxidizing carbon atoms; cytochrome P450 prefers to oxidize carbon atoms with high electron density, whereas aldehyde oxidase (and XD/XO) prefers to oxidize carbon atoms with low electron density. The substrate specificity of aldehyde oxidase differs among mammalian species, with substrate size being the main differentiating factor. The active site of human aldehyde oxidase accommodates much smaller substrates than rabbit or guinea pig aldehyde oxidase. Substituents on a substrate that increase electronegativity tend to enhance V_{max}, whereas substituents that increase lipophilicity tend to increase affinity (decrease K_m). Another interesting species difference is that dogs possess little or no aldehyde oxidase activity. However, aldehyde oxidase in human liver has proven to be rather unstable, which complicates an in vitro assessment of species differences in aldehyde oxidase activity (Rodrigues, 1994; Rettie and Fisher, 1999). A further complication is the observation of species differences in the relative roles of aldehyde oxidase and XOR in xenobiotic biotransformation. For example, the 6-oxidation of antiviral deoxyguanine prodrugs is catalyzed exclusively in rats by XD/XO, but by aldehyde oxidase in humans (Rettie and Fisher, 1999).

Aldehyde oxidase is the second of two enzymes involved in the formation of cotinine, a major metabolite of nicotine excreted in the urine of cigarette smokers. The initial step in this reaction is the formation of a double bond (C=N) in the pyrrole ring, which produces nicotine $\Delta^{1',5'}$-iminium ion. Like nicotine, several other drugs are oxidized either sequentially or concomitantly by cytochrome P450 and aldehyde oxidase, including quinidine, azapetine, cyclophosphamide, carbazeran, and prolintane. Other drugs that are oxidized by aldehyde oxidase include bromonidine, citalopram, proprion-aldehyde, O^6-benzylguanine, 6-mercaptopurine, metyrapone, quinine, pyrazinamide, methotrexate, vanillin, isovanillin, zaleplon, and famciclovir (an antiviral prodrug that is converted by aldehyde oxidase to penciclovir). Several pyrimidine derivatives are oxidized by aldehyde oxidase, including 5-ethyl-2($1H$)-pyrimidone, which is converted by aldehyde oxidase to 5-ethynyluracil. Like Sorivudine, 5-ethynyluracil is a metabolism-dependent (suicide) inactivator of dihydropyrimidine dehydrogenase (see Fig. 6-16).

Raloxifene and perphenazine are extraordinarily potent inhibitors of aldehyde oxidase (Obach, 2004). Menadione is also a potent inhibitor of aldehyde oxidase ($K_i \sim 0.1$ μM) and is often used together with allopurinol to discriminate between aldehyde oxidase- and XOR-catalyzed reactions. Hydralazine has been used to assess the role of aldehyde oxidase in human drug metabolism in vivo. The ability of proadifen to inhibit aldehyde oxidase is noteworthy because this methadone analog, commonly known as SKF 525A, is widely used as a cytochrome P450 inhibitor.

Under certain conditions, aldehyde oxidase and XOR can also catalyze the reduction of xenobiotics, including azo-reduction (e.g., 4-dimethylaminoazobenzene), nitro-reduction (e.g., 1-nitropyrene), N-oxide reduction (e.g., S-(-)-nicotine-1′-N-oxide), nitrosamine reduction (e.g., N-nitrosodiphenylamine), hydroxamic acid reduction (e.g., N-hydroxy-2-acetylaminofluorene), sulfoxide reduction (e.g., sulindac; see Fig. 6-14), and epoxide reduction (e.g., benzo[a]pyrene 4,5-oxide). Oximes (C=NOH) can also be reduced by aldehyde oxidase to the corresponding ketimines (C=NH), which may react nonenzymatically with water to produce the corresponding ketone or aldehyde (C=O) and ammonia. An analogous reaction allows aldehyde oxidase to catalyze the reductive ring opening of zonisamide and 1,2-benzisoxazole, which results in the formation of an oxo-containing metabolite and ammonia (Sugihara et al., 1996). The reduction of ziprasidone by aldehyde oxidase is shown in Fig. 6-3, and examples of other reductive reactions catalyzed by aldehyde oxidase are shown in Fig. 6-22. Xenobiotic reduction by aldehyde oxidase in vitro requires anaerobic conditions or the presence of a reducing substrate, such as N^1-methylnicotinamide, 2-hydroxypyrimidine, or benzaldehyde. These "co-substrates" reduce the enzyme, which in turn catalyzes azo-reduction, nitro-reduction, etc. by relaying electrons to xenobiotics (rather than molecular oxygen). These unusual requirements make it difficult to assess the degree to which aldehyde oxidase functions as a reductive enzyme in vivo.

Monoamine Oxidase, Diamine Oxidase, and Polyamine Oxidase

Monoamine oxidase (MAO; gene symbols MAOA and MAOB), diamine oxidase (DAO; gene symbol ABP1), and polyamine oxidase (PAO; gene symbol PAOX) are all involved in the oxidative deamination of primary, secondary, and tertiary amines (Benedetti, 2001; Agostinelli et al., 2004; Edmondson et al., 2004). Substrates for these enzymes include several naturally occurring amines, such as the monoamine serotonin (5-hydroxytryptamine), the diamine putrescine, and monoacetylated derivatives of the polyamines spermine and spermidine. A number of xenobiotics are substrates for these enzymes, particularly MAO. Oxidative deamination of a primary amine produces ammonia and an aldehyde, whereas oxidative deamination of a secondary amine produces a primary amine and an aldehyde. (The products of the former reaction—i.e., an aldehyde and ammonia—are those produced during the reductive biotransformation of certain oximes by aldehyde oxidase, as described in the

preceding section on "Aldehyde Oxidase"). The aldehydes formed by MAO are usually oxidized further by other enzymes to the corresponding carboxylic acids, although in some cases they are reduced to alcohols. Examples of reactions catalyzed by MAO, DAO, and PAO are shown in Fig. 6-27.

Monoamine oxidase is located throughout the brain, and is present in the liver, kidney, intestine, and blood platelets in the outer membrane of mitochondria. Its substrates include milacemide (Fig. 6-27), a dealkylated metabolite of propranolol (Fig. 6-27), primaquine, haloperidol, doxylamine, β-phenylethylamine, tyramine, catecholamines (dopamine, norepinephrine, epinephrine), tryptophan derivatives (tryptamine, serotonin), and tryptophan analogs known as triptans, which include the antimigraine drugs sumatriptan, zolmitriptan, and rizatriptan.

There are two forms of monoamine oxidase, called MAO-A and MAO-B. MAO-A preferentially oxidizes serotonin (5-hydroxytryptamine), norepinephrine, and the dealkylated metabolite of propranolol, and is preferentially inhibited by clorgyline, whereas MAO-B preferentially oxidizes β-phenylethylamine and benzylamine, and is preferentially inhibited by L-deprenyl (selegiline). Species differences in the substrate specificity of MAO have been documented. For example, dopamine is oxidized by MAO-B in humans, but by MAO-A in rats, and by both enzymes in several other mammalian species. Most tissues contain both forms of the enzyme, each encoded by a distinct gene, although some tissues express only one MAO. In humans, for example, only MAO-A is expressed in the placenta, whereas only MAO-B is expressed in blood platelets and lymphocytes. The distribution of MAO in the brain shows little species variation, with the highest concentration of MAO-A in the locus coeruleus, and the highest concentration of MAO-B in the raphe nuclei. MAO-A is expressed predominantly in catecholaminergic neurons, whereas MAO-B is expressed largely in serotonergic and histaminergic neurons and glial cells. The distribution of MAO throughout the brain does not always parallel that of its substrates. For example, serotonin is preferentially oxidized by MAO-A, but MAO-A is not found in serotonergic neurons.

MAO-A and -B are encoded by two distinct genes, both localized on the X-chromosome (Xp11.4-p11.3) and both comprise 15 exons with an identical intron–exon organization, which suggests they are derived from a common ancestral gene (Shih et al., 1999). The amino acid sequence of MAO-A (Mr 59.7 kDa) is 70% identical to that of MAO-B (Mr 58.0 kDa). The deletion of both MAO-A and -B gives rise to Norrie disease, an X-linked recessive neurologic disorder characterized by blindness, hearing loss, and mental retardation (Shih et al., 1999). Selective loss of MAO-A (due to a point mutation) gives rise to abnormal aggressiveness, whereas alterations in MAO-B have been implicated in Parkinson's disease (discussed later in this section).

The mechanism of catalysis by monoamine oxidase is illustrated below:

$$RCH_2NH_2 + FAD \rightarrow RCH=NH + FADH_2$$
$$RCH=NH + H_2O \rightarrow RCHO + NH_3$$
$$FADH_2 + O_2 \rightarrow FAD + H_2O_2$$

The substrate is oxidized by the enzyme, which itself is reduced (FAD $\rightarrow$ FADH$_2$). The oxygen incorporated into the substrate is derived from water, not molecular oxygen; hence, the enzyme functions as a true oxidase. The catalytic cycle is completed by reoxidation of the reduced enzyme (FADH$_2$ $\rightarrow$ FAD) by oxygen, which generates hydrogen peroxide (which may be a cause of oxidative

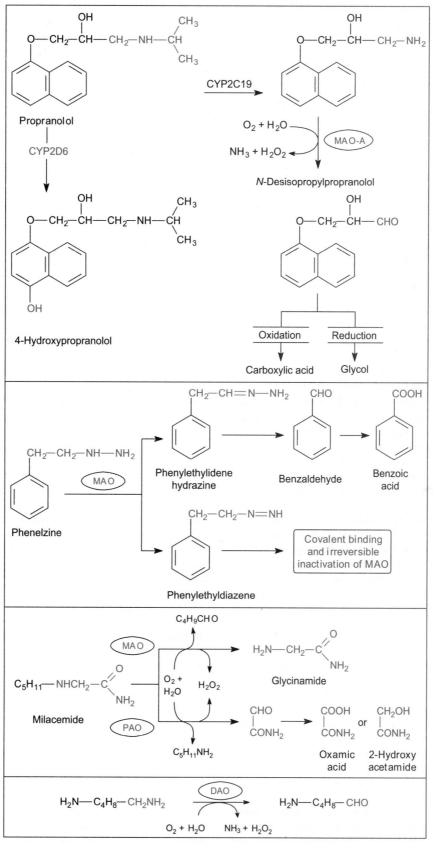

Figure 6-27. Examples of reactions catalyzed by monoamine oxidase (MAO), diamine oxidase (DAO), and polyamine oxidase (PAO).

Note that phenelzine is a metabolism-dependent (mechanism-based) inhibitor of MAO-A and MAO-B.

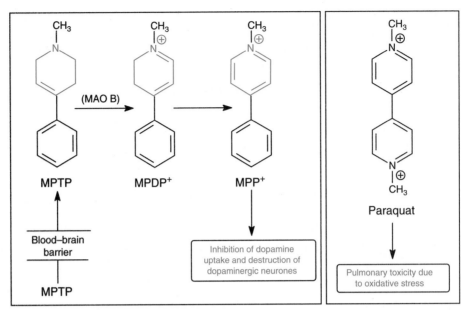

Figure 6-28. *Activation of MPTP (1-methyl-4-phenyl-1,2,5,6-tetrahydropyridine) to the neurotoxic metabolite, MPP$^+$ (1-methyl-4-phenylpyridine), by monoamine oxidase B.*

The toxic pyridinium metabolite, MPP$^+$, is structurally similar to the herbicide paraquat MPDP$^+$, 1-methyl-4-phenyl-2,3-dihydropyridine.

stress). The initial step in the catalytic cycle appears to be abstraction of hydrogen from the α-carbon adjacent to the nitrogen atom, hence, the oxidative deamination of xenobiotics by MAO is generally blocked by substitution of the α-carbon. For example, amphetamine and other phenylethylamine derivatives carrying a methyl group on the α-carbon atom are not oxidized well by MAO. (Amphetamines can undergo oxidative deamination, but the reaction is catalyzed by cytochrome P450.) The abstraction of hydrogen from the α-carbon adjacent to the nitrogen atom can occur stereospecifically; therefore, only one enantiomer of an α-substituted compound may be oxidized by MAO. For example, whereas MAO-B catalyzes the oxidative deamination of both *R*- and *S*-β-phenylethylamine, only the *R*-enantiomer is a substrate for MAO-A. The oxidative deamination of the dealkylated metabolite of propranolol is catalyzed stereoselectively by MAO-A, although in this case the preferred substrate is the *S*-enantiomer (which has the same absolute configuration as the *R*-enantiomer of β-phenylethylamine) (Benedetti and Dostert, 1994).

Clorgyline and L-deprenyl (selegiline) are metabolism-dependent inhibitors (i.e., mechanism-based or suicide inactivators) of MAO-A and MAO-B, respectively. Both enzymes are irreversibly inhibited by phenelzine, a hydrazine that can be oxidized either by abstraction of hydrogen from the α-carbon atom, which leads to oxidative deamination with formation of benzaldehyde and benzoic acid, or by abstraction of hydrogen from the terminal nitrogen atom, which leads to formation of phenylethyldiazene and covalent modification of the enzyme, as shown in Fig. 6-27.

Monoamine oxidase has received considerable attention for its role in the activation of MPTP (1-methyl-4-phenyl-1,2,5,6-tetrahydropyridine) to a neurotoxin that causes symptoms characteristic of Parkinson's disease in humans and monkeys but not rodents (Gerlach *et al.*, 1991). In 1983, Parkinsonism was observed in young individuals who, in attempting to synthesize and use a narcotic drug related to meperidine (Demerol®), instead synthesized and self-administered MPTP, which causes selective destruc-

tion of dopaminergic neurons in the substantia nigra. MPTP crosses the blood–brain barrier, where it is oxidized by MAO in the astrocytes (a type of glial cell) to 1-methyl-4-phenyl-2,3-dihydropyridine (MPDP$^+$), which in turn autoxidizes to the neurotoxic metabolite, 1-methyl-4-phenylpyridine MPP$^+$, as shown in Fig. 6-28. Because it is transported by the dopamine transporter, MPP$^+$ concentrates in dopaminergic neurons, where it impairs mitochondrial respiration. The neurotoxic effects of MPTP can be blocked with pargyline (an inhibitor of both MAO-A and MAO-B), by L-deprenyl (a selective inhibitor of MAO-B) but not by clorgyline (a selective inhibitor of MAO-A). This suggests that the activation of MPTP to its neurotoxic metabolite is catalyzed predominantly by MAO-B. This interpretation is consistent with the finding that MAO-B knockout mice (i.e., transgenic mice that lack MAO-B) do not sustain damage to the dopaminergic terminals of nigrostriatal neurons after MPTP treatment (Shih *et al.*, 1999; Quinn *et al.*, 2007).

Genetic and environmental factors both appear to play important roles in the etiology of Parkinson's disease. Apart from MPTP, Parkinsongenic neurotoxins to which humans are exposed have not been identified unequivocally; hence, the environmental factors that cause Parkinson's disease remain to be identified. It is interesting that the bipyridyl herbicide, paraquat, is similar in structure to the toxic metabolite of MPTP, as shown in Fig. 6-28. Some epidemiological studies have shown a positive correlation between herbicide exposure and the incidence of Parkinsonism in some but not all rural communities. Haloperidol can also be converted to a potentially neurotoxic pyridinium metabolite (Subramanyam *et al.*, 1991).

MAO-B may be among the genetic factors that affect susceptibility to Parkinson's disease. MAO-B activity in the human brain increases with aging, perhaps due to a proliferation of glial cells. It has been proposed that increased oxidation of dopamine by MAO-B in the elderly may lead to a loss of dopaminergic neurons in the substantia nigra, which underlies Parkinson's disease. Such damage may be caused by the oxidative stress associated with the oxidative deamination of dopamine by MAO-B. In support of this proposal,

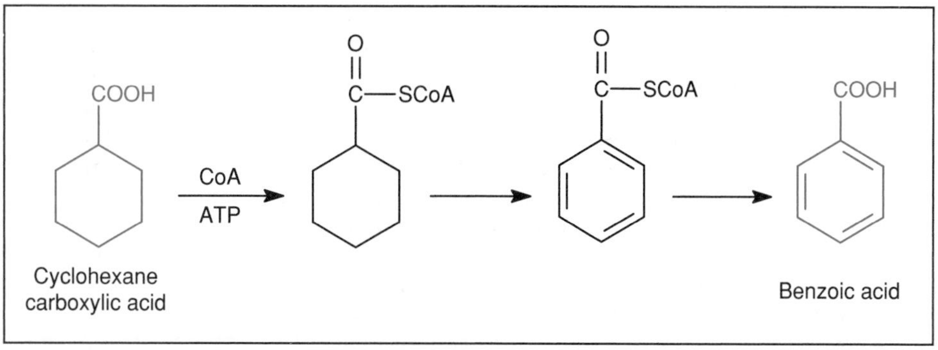

Figure 6-29. Aromatization of cyclohexane carboxylic acid, a reaction catalyzed by rabbit and guinea pig liver mitochondria.

patients with Parkinson's disease have elevated MAO-B activity in the substantia nigra, and the MAO-B inhibitor L-deprenyl (selegiline) delays the progression of symptoms (Sano *et al.*, 1997). Furthermore, there are allelic variants of MAO-B, some of which (such as allele 1 and allele B4) appear to be associated with an increased risk of developing Parkinson's disease (Shih *et al.*, 1999). No such association has been found between Parkinson's disease and MAO-A gene polymorphisms. Cigarette smoking, which carries a number of health risks, has been shown nevertheless to provide some protection against Parkinson's disease (Gorell *et al.*, 1999). Although the mechanism of protection remains to be determined, it is interesting to note that cigarette smokers are known to have decreased levels of MAO-B (and MAO-A) (Shih *et al.*, 1999), the degree of which is proportional to cigarette usage (i.e., it is dose related) (Whitfield *et al.*, 2000).

MAO-A knockout mice have elevated brain levels of serotonin and a distinct behavioral syndrome, including enhanced aggression in adult males. The enhanced aggressive behavior exhibited by MAO-A knockout mice is consistent with the abnormal aggressive behavior in individuals who lack MAO-A activity due to a point mutation in the MAO-A gene (Shih *et al.*, 1999). Other polymorphisms in the MAO-A gene appear to be risk factors for alcoholism among Euro-Americans and Han Chinese (Shih *et al.*, 1999). MAO-B may also be a factor in alcoholism inasmuch as alcoholics (especially male Type 2 alcoholics) tend to have lower MAO activity in platelets, which only contain MAO-B. However, MAO-B activity is not lower in alcoholics when cigarette smoking status is taken into account, which suggests that MAO-B activity tends to be lower in alcoholics because smoking and alcohol dependence are strongly associated with each other (Whitfield *et al.*, 2000).

Although not present in mitochondria, PAO resembles MAO in its cofactor requirement and basic mechanism of action. Both enzymes use oxygen as an electron acceptor, which results in the production of hydrogen peroxide. The MAO inhibitor pargyline also inhibits PAO. The anticonvulsant milacemide is one of the few xenobiotic substrates for PAO, although it is also a substrate for MAO (Fig. 6-27). By converting milacemide to glycine (via glycinamide), MAO plays an important role in the anticonvulsant therapy with milacemide (Benedetti and Dostert, 1994).

Diamine oxidase is a cytosolic, copper-containing, pyridoxal phosphate-dependent enzyme present in liver, kidney, intestine, and placenta. Its preferred substrates include histamine and simple alkyl diamines with a chain length of 4 (putrescine) or 5 (cadaverine) carbon atoms. Diamines with carbon chains longer than 9 are not substrates for DAO, although they can be oxidized by MAO. DAO

or a similar enzyme is present in cardiovascular tissue and appears to be responsible for the cardiotoxic effects of allylamine, which is converted by oxidative deamination to acrolein. Although histamine is a substrate for DAO, there is little or no DAO in brain (nor is there a receptor-mediated uptake system for histamine, in contrast to other neurotransmitters). For this reason, the major pathway of histamine metabolism in the brain is by methylation (see section "Methylation").

Semicarbazide-Sensitive Amine Oxidase (SSAO)   Semicarbazide-sensitive amine oxidase (SSAO; gene symbol AOC3) is a copper-containing enzyme that catalyzes fundamentally the same reaction catalyzed by monoamine oxidase:

$$RCH_2NH_2 + H_2O + O_2 \rightarrow RCHO + H_2O_2 + NH_3$$

SSAO can be distinguished from MAO by its sensitivity to inhibitors (it is inhibited by semicarbazide but not by clorgyline, deprenyl, or pargyline, whereas the opposite is true for MAO), and it is found on various cell surfaces and in plasma, whereas MAO is found in mitochondria. SSAO has been cloned and shown to be identical to vascular adhesion protin-1 (VAP-1). Plasma SSAO is a soluble, proteolytic cleavage product of membrane-bound SSAO. SSAO levels are increased in diabetic patients and decreased in individuals with major depression. Although SSAO activity in vitro is measured with benzylamine, there is little evidence to suggest that SSAO plays a major role in the metabolism of drugs or other xenobiotics in vivo (Obata, 2006; Roessner *et al.*, 2006; Wang *et al.*, 2006a).

Aromatization   The conversion of MPTP to MPP$^+$ (Fig. 6-28) is an example of a xenobiotic whose oxidation involves the introduction of multiple double bonds to achieve some semblance of aromaticity (in this case, formation of a pyridinium ion). Aromatization of xenobiotics is an unusual reaction, but some examples have been documented. A mitochondrial enzyme in guinea pig and rabbit liver can oxidize several cyclohexane derivatives to the corresponding aromatic hydrocarbon, as shown in Fig. 6-29 for the aromatization of cyclohexane carboxylic acid (hexahydrobenzoic acid) to benzoic acid. Mitochondria from rat liver are less active, and those from cat, mouse, dog, monkey, and human are completely inactive. The reaction requires magnesium, coenzyme A, oxygen, and ATP. The first step appears to be the formation of hexahydrobenzoyl-CoA, which is then dehydrogenated to the aromatic product. Glycine

Table 6-7

Characteristics of Some Human Peroxidases

PEROXIDASES	CELLULAR LOCATION	SUBCELLULAR LOCATION	HOMOLOGY WITH MPO
Myeloperoxidase (MPO)	Neutrophils, leukocytes	Lysosomes (human milk)	100%
Eosinophil peroxidase (EPO)	Eosinophils	Lysosomes	70%
Lactoperoxidase (LPO)	Mammary duct epithelial cells	Saliva, tears (bovine milk)	61%
Thyroid peroxidase (TPO)	Thyroid follicular cells	Microsomes, Golgi	47%
Prostaglandin-H synthase			
PHS1	Numerous extrahepatic tissues	Microsomes	
PHS2	Inflammatory cells	Microsomes	

Data adapted from O'Brien PJ: Peroxidases. *Chem Biol Interact* 129:113–139, 2000.

stimulates the reaction, probably by removing benzoic acid through conjugation to form hippuric acid. The conversion of androgens to estrogens involves aromatization of the A-ring of the steroid nucleus. This reaction is catalyzed by CYP19A1, one of the cytochrome P450 enzymes involved in steroidogenesis. Gut microflora can catalyze aromatization reactions, as shown in Fig. 6-1 for the conversion of quinic acid to benzoic acid.

Peroxidase-Dependent Cooxidation   The oxidative biotransformation of xenobiotics generally requires the reduced pyridine nucleotide cofactors, NADPH and NADH. An exception is xenobiotic biotransformation by peroxidases, heme-containing enzymes that couple the reduction of hydrogen peroxide (or a lipid hydroperoxide) to the oxidation of other substrates (O'Brien, 2000; Tafazoli and O'Brien, 2005). Several different peroxidases catalyze the biotransformation of xenobiotics (in addition to performing important physiological functions), and these enzymes occur in a variety of tissues and cell types. Peroxidases do not play an important role in the first-pass metabolism or clearance of drugs and most other xenobiotics because their contribution is usually negligible compared with cytochrome P450 and other oxidative enzymes. However, peroxidases do play an important role in xenobiotic toxicity, especially the activation of drugs associated with idiosyncratic hepatotoxicity, blood dyscrasias (e.g., agranulocytosis, aplastic anemia) and skin rashes, and the activation of xenobiotics (including the activation of proximate carcinogens to ultimate carcinogens) in skin, bladder, bone marrow, and various other extrahepatic tissues.

In humans, the family of peroxidases includes myeloperoxidase (MPO), eosinophil peroxidase (EPO; gene symbol EPX), lactoperoxidase (LPO), thyroid peroxidase (TPO), and two forms of prostaglandin H synthase (PHS1 and PHS2; gene symbols PTGS1 and 2). Some basic features of these peroxidases are summarized in Table 6-7. These peroxidases all have physiological functions: MPO, EPO, and LPO are lysosomal enzymes present in neutrophils, eosinophils, and secretory cells of exocrine glands, respectively. During infection, MPO and EPO are released into phagocytic vacuoles (granules) and into the plasma, whereas LPO is released into saliva and tears, where they kill microorganisms and thereby provide protection against infectious agents such as bacteria and parasites. (Peroxidases are also present in milk: LPO is the predominant peroxidase in cow's milk, whereas MPO is the predominant peroxidase in human milk.) The hydrogen peroxide required by MPO and EPO is produced by a membrane-bound NADPH oxidase that is activated by the presence of infectious agents. Unlike MPO, EPO, and LPO, which are soluble enzymes, TPO is a membrane-bound peroxidase located on the apical membrane of thyroid follicular cells; it

catalyzes the iodination of tyrosine residues and the oxidative coupling of di- and mono-iodinated tyrosine residues in thyroglobulin to form triiodothyronine- and thyroxine-bound thyroglobulin, from which thyroid hormones are released. An NAD(P)H-oxidase known as p138 TOX (gene symbol DUOX2), which is also localized on the apical plasma membrane, produces the hydrogen peroxide required by TPO to synthesize thyroid hormones. PHS1 and PHS2 are the peroxidase component of cyclooxygenase 1 and 2 (COX1 and COX2); they are enzymes that convert arachidonic acid (and closely related fatty acids) to a variety of eicosanoids (prostaglandins, leukotrienes, thromboxane, and prostacyclin). In contrast to the other peroxidases, PHS1 and PHS2 do not require a source of hydrogen peroxide (although they can use it); hence, their activity is not dependent on an H_2O_2-generating NAD(P)H-oxidase. Catalase is also a peroxidase. This peroxisomal enzyme catalyzes the disproportionation of hydrogen peroxide to water and oxygen ($2H_2O_2 \rightarrow 2H_2O + O_2$). At low concentrations of hydrogen peroxide, catalase can catalyze the oxidation of ethanol (see Fig. 6-24) and various other small molecules. Glutathione peroxidases (GPXs) are a family of selenium-containing enzymes that also detoxify hydrogen peroxide (and lipid hydroperoxides) by reducing it to water, which is associated with the formation of oxidized glutathione as follows:

$$2GSH + HOOH \rightarrow GS.SG + H_2O + H_2O$$

In mammalian peroxidases (in contrast to plant peroxidases), the heme prosthetic group is covalently attached to the enzyme. Iron is bound to four pyrrole nitrogens with the nitrogen on the imidazole ring of histidine serving as the usual fifth ligand. The sixth coordination position is vacant so that peroxidases can interact with hydrogen peroxide (or other hydroperoxides), just as the sixth coordinate position of hemoglobin and myoglobin (both of which have low peroxidase activity) is available to bind molecular oxygen. The oxidation of a xenobiotic ($X \rightarrow XO$ or $2XH \rightarrow 2X\bullet + H_2O$) by peroxidase involves the conversion of hydrogen peroxide to water or the conversion of a hydroperoxide to the corresponding alcohol ($ROOH \rightarrow ROH$), during which the peroxidase (Fe^{III}) is converted to spectrophotometrically distinct states known as Compound I and Compound II, as shown below for the conversion of a xenobiotic phenol (X–OH) to the corresponding phenoxyl radical (R–O):

$$Peroxidase + ROOH \rightarrow Compound\ I + ROH$$
$$Compound\ I + XOH \rightarrow Compound\ II + XO\bullet + H^+$$
$$Compound\ II + XOH \rightarrow Peroxidase + XO\bullet + H_2O$$

In this example, the hydroperoxide is converted to the corresponding alcohol ($ROOH \rightarrow ROH$), and the peroxyl oxygen atom is reduced to water (H_2O) by the one-electron oxidation of two molecules of xenobiotic (XOH) to produce two xenobiotic radicals (XO•). In some cases, the oxygen from the hydroperoxide is incorporated into the xenobiotic itself (XH → XOH). Examples of each reaction are given later in this section. The conversion of ROOH to ROH involves the release of an oxygen atom that coordinates with the heme iron (initially in the ferric or Fe^{III} state). This iron-bound oxygen formally contains only six (instead of eight) valence electrons, making it a powerful oxidizing species. One electron is removed from the iron to produce Fe^{IV}=O, and a second electron is removed from the tetrapyrrole ring to produce a π-porphyrin–cation radical (Por•$^+$), which corresponds to Compound I (Fe^{IV}=O–Por•$^+$). The transfer of an electron from a xenobiotic (XOH → XO• + H$^+$) to the porphyrin cation radical produces Compound II (Fe^{IV}=O–Por). In some cases, such as PHS, the electron donated to the initial Fe=O complex comes directly or indirectly from an amino acid rather than the tetrapyrrole ring, and this accounts in part for some of the differences among the various peroxidases (such as the ability of TPO to catalyze the iodination of tyrosine residues and the subsequent formation of thyroid hormones).

Although peroxidases are renowned for catalyzing one-electron oxidation reactions, they can catalyze the two-electron oxidation of iodide (I$^-$) to hypoiodous acid (HOI) and iodine which, in the case of TPO, is important for the synthesis of thyroid hormones:

Peroxidase Compound I(O) + I$^-$ + H$^+$ → HOI (hypoiodous acid)
Peroxidase Compound I(O) + 2 × I$^-$ + H$^+$ → I$_2$ (iodine) + OH$^-$

MPO, EPO, and LPO can all oxidize the pseudo-halide thiocyanate (SCN$^-$) faster than iodide, which in turn is oxidized faster than bromide, which is oxidized much faster than chloride. In fact, MPO is the only peroxidase with appreciable ability to oxidize chloride to hypochlorous acid. There is an inverse relationship between the rate of conversion of halides to hypohalous acids and their physiological plasma concentrations: chloride = 100–140 mM, bromide = 20–100 μM, and iodide = 0.1–0.5 μM. Consequently, the relatively low rate of chloride oxidation is offset by the high levels of chloride such that about half (20–70%) of the hydrogen peroxide produced by activated neutrophils is converted to hypochlorous acid, which reacts with glutathione, proteins, thiols, and amines, unsaturated fatty acids and cholesterol, all of which disrupt cell membranes and lead to cell lysis and death (of both infectious organisms and host cells). Formation of hypochlorous acid by MPO is not only important from a physiological perspective but also from a drug metabolism and toxicity perspective, as discussed later in this section. The preferred "halide" substrate for MPO is thiocyanate, which is present in plasma at concentrations ranging from 20 to 120 μM, which is sufficiently high that oxidation of thiocyanate consumes the other half of the hydrogen peroxide produced by activated neutrophils. Whereas MPO oxidizes chloride to hypochlorous acid, which is cytotoxic, it oxidizes thiocyanate to thiocyanogen [(SCN$_2$)], which rapidly hydrolyzes to hypothiocyanic acid (HOSCN). Hypothiocyanic acid is much less reactive and cytotoxic than hypochlorous acid, such that the oxidation of thiocyanate by peroxidases is a mechanism to remove hydrogen peroxide without forming hypochlorous acid. This appears to represent an important mechanism of hydrogen peroxide detoxication in saliva, which contains low levels of catalase but high levels (1–5 mM) of thiocyanate, and in the stomach, where the levels of thiocyanate in parietal cells are three times greater than plasma levels, which allows gastric peroxidase to inactivate hydrogen peroxide that

otherwise stimulates gastric acid secretion by stimulating histamine release from mast cells. Inactivation of gastric peroxidase by aspirin, dexamethasone, indomethacin, or methimazole can result in gastric ulceration due to impaired detoxication of hydrogen peroxide and impaired synthesis of cytoprotective prostaglandins.

MPO and EPO can be distinguished by (1) their cellular distribution (neutrophils/leukocytes versus eosinophils); (2) their ability to oxidize halides (MPO is better than EPO at converting chloride to hypochlorous acid whereas EPO is better than MPO at converting bromide to hypobromous acid), and (3) their sensitivity to inhibitors (MPO is more sensitive to the inhibitory effect of cyanide over azide, whereas the opposite is true of EPO).

The level of EPO (or a related peroxidase) in uterine epithelial cells is regulated by estrogen; uterine peroxidase activity is inducible several hundred fold by estrogenic steroids, including the synthetic estrogens diethylstilbestrol and tamoxifen. The level of TPO in thyroid follicular cells is regulated by TSH. The enzyme is inactivated by a variety of ethylenethiourea drugs, such as propylthiouracil and methimazole (which is used as an antithyroid drug in patients with Grave's disease), as well as a number of naturally occurring flavonoid/resorcinol compounds that also have antithyroid effects. By inactivating TPO and impairing thyroid hormone synthesis, these chemicals trigger a large and prolonged increase in TSH that in rodents (but apparently not in humans) can result in thyroid follicular cell tumor formation.

MPO is an abundant enzyme is granulocytes, where it accounts for 5% of the dry weight. MPO can be used as a diagnostic marker to differentiate myeloid leukemia from lymphoid leukemia.

MPO has been implicated in the formation of reactive metabolites of drugs that cause idiosyncratic agranulocytosis, including clozapine, aminopyrine, vesnarinone, propylthiouracil, dapsone, sulfonamides, procainamide, amodiaquine, and ticlopidine (Liu and Uetrecht, 2000; O'Brien, 2000; Tafazoli and O'Brien, 2005). Many of these drugs are aromatic amines, and both MPO and PHS have also been implicated in the activation of several carcinogenic aromatic amines, such as benzidine, methylaminoazobenzene, and aminofluorene. Furthermore, inactivating polymorphisms in MPO (such as MPO-463A) appear to afford protection against both the activation of aromatic amines and PAH in tobacco smoke and the tumor-promoting effects of hydrogen peroxide formed by tobacco smoke-activated neutrophils (O'Brien, 2000).

In the presence of hydrogen peroxide and chloride (which are converted to hypochlorous acid by MPO), activated neutrophils and monocytes oxidize the aforementioned drugs to reactive intermediates (such as nitrogen-centered radicals, hydroxylamines, N-chloramines and, in the case of aromatic amines with a hydroxyl group in the para-position, quinoneimines or the corresponding semiquinoneimine radicals). In the case of ticlopidine, MPO converts the thiophene ring of this antiplatelet drug to a thiophene-S-chloride, a reactive metabolite that rearranges to 2-chloroticlopidine (minor) and dehydro-ticlopidine (major), or reacts with glutathione, as shown in Fig. 6-30. When catalyzed by activated neutrophils, ticlopidine oxidation is inhibited by low concentrations of azide and catalase. When catalyzed by purified myeloperoxidase, ticlopidine oxidation requires hydrogen peroxide and chloride, although all components of this purified system can be replaced with hypochlorous acid (HOCl). It is not known whether drugs that cause agranulocytosis are activated in the bone marrow by neutrophils or their precursors that contain myeloperoxidase, or are activated in neutrophils in the general circulation. In the latter case, agranulocytosis would presumably involve an immune response triggered by neoantigens

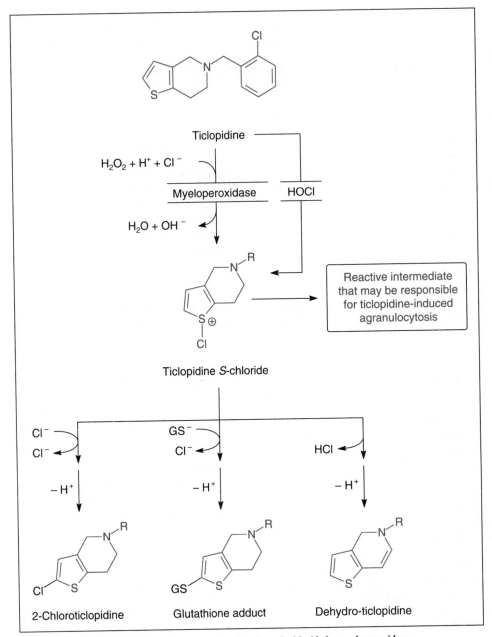

Figure 6-30. Activation of ticlopidine to a reactive thiophene S-chloride by myeloperoxidase.

formed in neutrophils by the covalent modification of cellular component by one or more of the reactive metabolites formed by MPO.

MPO has also been implicated in the formation of pro-oxidant phenoxyl radicals of etoposide, a topoisomerase inhibitor that causes myelogenous leukemia, and both MPO and PHS have been implicated in the formation of phenoxyl radicals of benzene, an industrial solvent linked to bone marrow suppression and leukemia. MPO and PHS cannot oxidize benzene itself. Liver cytochrome P450 converts benzene to phenol, which in turn is oxidized to hydroquinone, which can be converted to DNA-reactive metabolites by MPO in bone marrow leukocytes and by PHS in bone marrow. The myelosuppressive effect of benzene can be blocked by the PHS inhibitor, indomethacin, which suggests an important role for PHS-dependent activation in the myelotoxicity of benzene. The formation of phenol and hydroquinone in the liver is also impor-

tant for myelosuppression by benzene. However, such bone marrow suppression cannot be achieved simply by administering phenol or hydroquinone to mice, although it can be achieved by coadministering hydroquinone with phenol. Phenol stimulates the MPO- and PHS-dependent activation of hydroquinone. Therefore, bone marrow suppression by benzene involves the cytochrome P450-dependent oxidation of benzene to phenol and hydroquinone in the liver, followed by the phenol-enhanced, MPO- and PHS-catalyzed peroxidative oxidation of hydroquinone to reactive intermediates that bind to protein and DNA in the bone marrow (Fig. 6-31). It is noteworthy that the cytochrome CYP enzyme responsible for hydroxylating benzene has been identified as CYP2E1 (see section "Cytochrome P450"). Although CYP2E1 was first identified in liver, this same enzyme has been identified in bone marrow where it can presumably convert benzene to phenol and possibly hydroquinone.

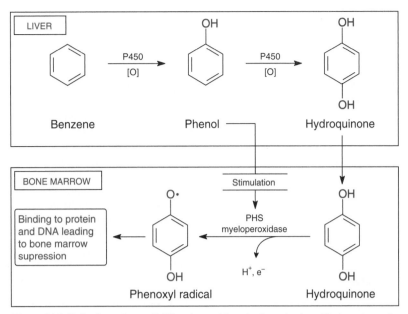

Figure 6-31. Role of cytochrome P450 and peroxidases in the activation of benzene to myelotoxic metabolites.

The importance of CYP2E1 in the metabolic activation of benzene was confirmed by the demonstration that CYP2E1 knockout mice are relatively resistant to the myelosuppressive effects of benzene (Gonzalez, 2003; Gonzalez and Yu, 2006).

Prostaglandin H synthase (PHS) is one of the most extensively studied peroxidases involved in xenobiotic biotransformation. As shown in Fig. 6-32, PHS is a dual-function enzyme composed of a *cyclooxygenase*, which converts arachidonic acid to PGG$_2$, a 15-hydroperoxide-endoperoxide (which involves the addition of two molecules of oxygen to each molecule of arachidonic acid), and a *peroxidase* that converts the 15-hydroperoxide to the corresponding 15-alcohol PGH$_2$, which can be accompanied by the oxidation of xenobiotics. The two forms of PHS, namely, PHS1 and PHS2, are better known as two forms of cyclooxygenase, namely, COX1 and COX2. A third cyclooxygenase, namely, COX3, has also been described, and is expressed predominantly in the cerebral cortex and heart. This enzyme is a splice variant of PHS1; one that retains the first intron in its mRNA (Chandrasekharan *et al.*, 2002). PHS1 is a microsomal enzyme expressed in a wide variety of tissues that synthesize and release eicosanoids (prostaglandins, leukotrienes, thromboxane, prostacyclin), which generally bind to G-coupled cell surface receptors and regulate cellular function, largely in a paracrine (local) fashion. In contrast, PHS2 is expressed on the nuclear membrane of cells that respond to inflammatory cytokines, mitogens, tumor promoters, and AhR agonists (i.e., agents such as TNF-α, lipopolysaccharide, phorbol esters, TPA, dioxin). PGH2 appears to produce prostaglandins that activate receptors on the nuclear membrane, and high levels of the enzyme are expressed in colorectal and other tumors, which appear to be important for tumor promotion and angiogenesis (the process of stimulating the blood vessel supply). Both enzymes play an important role in the activation of xenobiotics to toxic or tumorigenic metabolites, particularly in extrahepatic tissues that contain low levels of cytochrome P450. PHS2 (COX2) also appears to play an important role in the subsequent response of tissues to cell damage and tumor initiation, and is a possible target for the treatment or prevention of certain types of cancer.

In certain cases, the oxidation of xenobiotics by peroxidases involves direct transfer of the peroxide oxygen to the xenobiotic, as shown in Fig. 6-32 for the conversion of substrate X to product XO. An example of this type of reaction is the PHS-catalyzed epoxidation of benzo[*a*]pyrene 7,8-dihydrodiol to the corresponding 9,10-epoxide (see Fig. 6-9). Although PHS can catalyze the final step (i.e., 9,10-epoxidation) in the formation of this tumorigenic metabolite of benzo[*a*]pyrene, it cannot catalyze the initial step (i.e., 7,8-epoxidation), which is catalyzed by cytochrome P450. Several lines of evidence suggest that both PHS1 and PHS2 play an important role in PAH-induced skin carcinogenesis. First, PHS1 knockout and PHS2 knockout mice are both resistant to PAH-induced skin cancer. (It is noteworthy that PHS1 knockout mice appear normal despite having only 1% of the prostaglandin levels of wild-type mice, whereas only 60% of PHS2 knockout mice survive until weaning, and the 40% that survive past weaning usually die within the year of kidney disease.) Resveratrol (an inhibitor of PHS1 and CYP1A1) and SC-58125 (an inhibitor of PHS2) both block PAH-induced skin cancer in mice.

PHS can also catalyze the 8,9-epoxidation of aflatoxin B$_1$, which is one of the most potent hepatotumorigens known. Epoxidation by cytochrome P450 is thought to be primarily responsible for the hepatotumorigenic effects of aflatoxin B$_1$. However, aflatoxin B$_1$ also causes neoplasia of rat renal papilla. This tissue has very low levels of cytochrome P450, but contains relatively high levels of PHS, which is suspected, therefore, of mediating the nephrotumorigenic effects of aflatoxin (Fig. 6-33).

The direct transfer of the peroxide oxygen from a hydroperoxide to a xenobiotic is not the only mechanism of xenobiotic oxidation by peroxidases, nor is it the most common. Xenobiotics that can serve as electron donors, such as amines and phenols, can be oxidized to free radicals during the reduction of a hydroperoxide. In this case, the hydroperoxide is still converted to the corresponding alcohol, but the peroxide oxygen is reduced to water instead of being incorporated into the xenobiotic. For each molecule of hydroperoxide reduced (which is a two-electron process), two molecules of xenobiotic can be oxidized (each by a one-electron process). Important

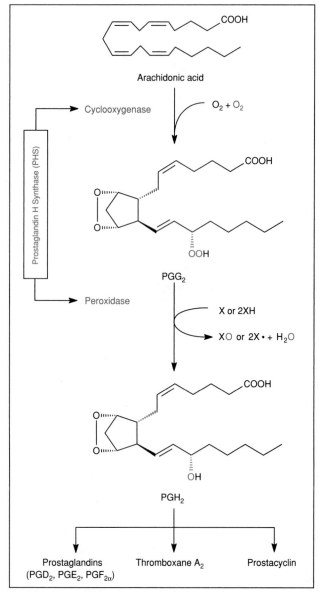

Figure 6-32. Cooxidation of xenobiotics (X) during the conversion of arachidonic acid to PGH₂ by prostaglandin H synthase.

classes of compounds that undergo one-electron oxidation reactions by peroxidase include aromatic amines, phenols, hydroquinones, and polycyclic hydrocarbons. Many of the metabolites produced are reactive electrophiles. For example, polycyclic aromatic hydrocarbons, phenols, and hydroquinones are oxidized to electrophilic quinones. Acetaminophen is similarly converted to a quinoneimine, namely, *N*-acetyl-benzoquinoneimine, a cytotoxic electrophile that binds to cellular proteins, as shown in Fig. 6-34. The formation of this toxic metabolite by cytochrome P450 causes centrilobular necrosis of the liver. However, acetaminophen can also damage the kidney medulla, which contains low levels of cytochrome P450 but relatively high levels of PHS; hence, PHS may play a significant role in the nephrotoxicity of acetaminophen. The two-electron oxidation of acetaminophen to *N*-acetyl-benzoquinoneimine by PHS likely involves the formation of a one-electron oxidation product, namely, *N*-acetyl-benzosemiquinoneimine radical. Formation of this semiquinoneimine radical by PHS likely contributes to the

nephrotoxicity of acetaminophen and related compounds, such as phenacetin and 4-aminophenol.

Like the kidney medulla, urinary bladder epithelium also contains low levels of cytochrome P450 but relatively high levels of PHS. Just as PHS in kidney medulla can activate aflatoxin and acetaminophen to nephrotoxic metabolites, so PHS in urinary bladder epithelium can activate certain aromatic amines, such as benzidine, 4-aminobiphenyl, and 2-aminonaphthalene, to DNA-reactive metabolites that cause bladder cancer in certain species, including humans and dogs. PHS can convert aromatic amines to reactive radicals, which can undergo nitrogen–nitrogen or nitrogen–carbon coupling reactions, or they can undergo a second one-electron oxidation to reactive diimines. Binding of these reactive metabolites to DNA is presumed to be the underlying mechanism by which several aromatic amines cause bladder cancer in humans and dogs. In some cases the one-electron oxidation of an amine leads to N-dealkylation. For example, PHS catalyzes the N-demethylation of aminopyrine, although in vivo this reaction is mainly catalyzed by cytochrome P450. In contrast to cytochrome P450, PHS does not

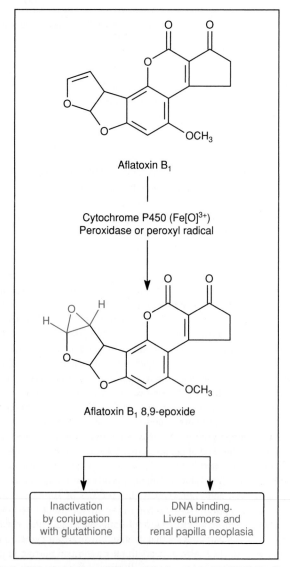

Figure 6-33. Activation of aflatoxin B₁ by cytochrome P450, leading to liver tumor formation, and by peroxidases, leading to renal papilla neoplasia.

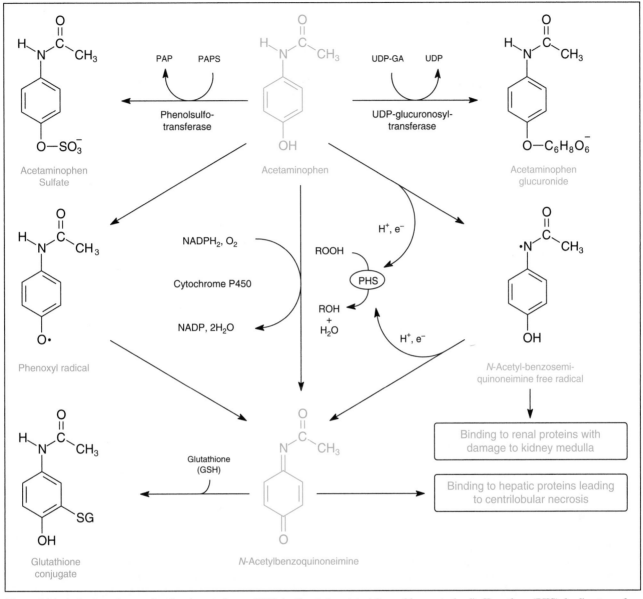

Figure 6-34. *Activation of acetaminophen by cytochrome P450, leading to hepatotoxicity, and by prostaglandin H synthase (PHS), leading to nephrotoxicity.*

Conjugation with sulfonate, glucuronic acid, or glutathione represents detoxication reactions.

appear to catalyze the N-hydroxylation of carcinogenic aromatic amines (an important step in their metabolic activation), although MPO and LPO have been shown to catalyze this reaction. In liver, activation of aromatic amines by N-hydroxylation appears to be catalyzed predominantly by CYP1A2, whereas this same reaction in the bladder epithelium appears to be catalyzed by another enzyme, possibly a CYP enzyme other than CYP1A2, such as CYP2A13, CYP4B1, or CYP2S1 (Nakajima *et al.*, 2006), or a peroxidase other than PHS.

Many of the aromatic amines known or suspected of causing bladder cancer in humans have been shown to cause bladder tumors in dogs. In rats, however, aromatic amines cause liver tumors by a process that involves N-hydroxylation by cytochrome P450, followed by conjugation with acetate or sulfonate, as shown in Fig. 6-11. This species difference has complicated an assessment of the role of PHS in aromatic amine-induced bladder cancer,

because such experiments must be carried out in dogs. However, another class of compounds, the 5-nitrofurans, such as *N*-[4-(5-nitro-2-furyl)-2-thiazole]formamide (FANFT) and its deformylated analog 2-amino-4-(5-nitro-2-furyl)thiazole (ANFT), are substrates for PHS and are potent bladder tumorigens in rats. The tumorigenicity of FANFT is thought to involve deformylation to ANFT, which is oxidized to DNA-reactive metabolites by PHS. The ability of FANFT to cause bladder tumors in rats is blocked by the COX inhibitor, aspirin, which suggests that PHS plays an important role in the metabolic activation and tumorigenicity of this nitrofuran. Unexpectedly, combined treatment of rats with FANFT and aspirin causes forestomach tumors, which are not observed when either compound is administered alone.

Increased expression of PHS2 (COX2) has been documented in a number of tumors, including human colorectal, gastric, esophageal, pulmonary, and pancreatic carcinomas (Gupta and

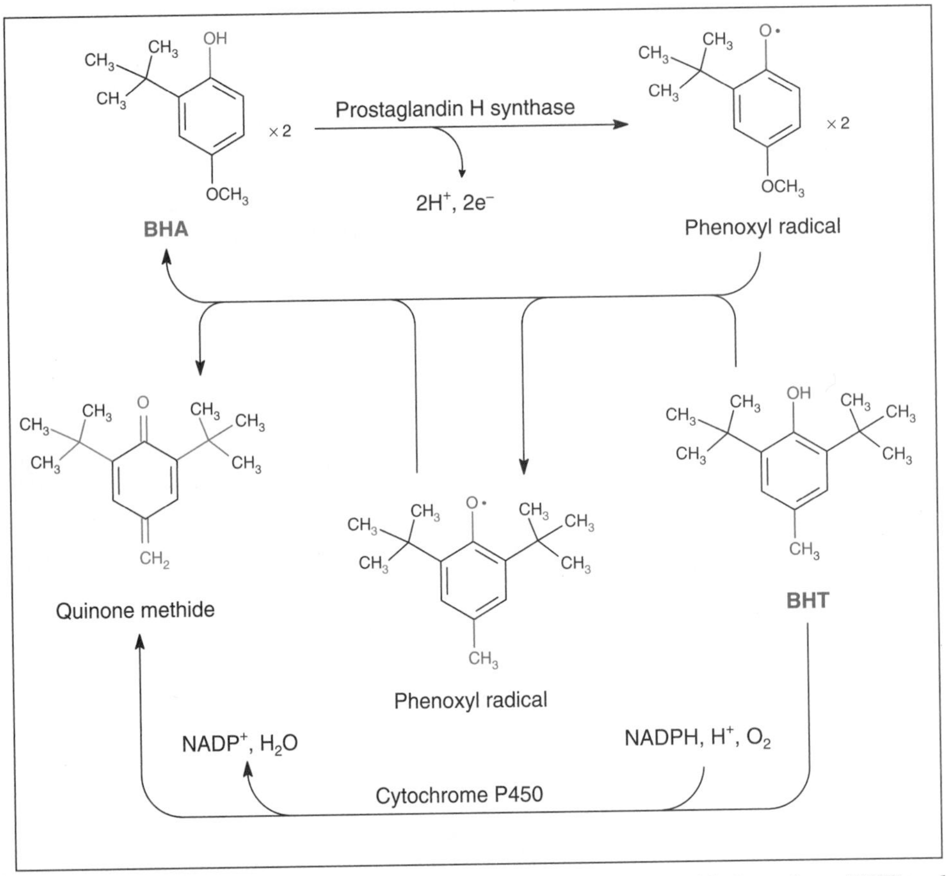

Figure 6-35. *Metabolite interaction between the phenolic antioxidants, butylated hydroxytoluene (BHT), and butylated hydroxyanisole (BHA).*

Note that activation of BHT to a toxic quinone methide can be catalyzed by cytochrome P450 or, in the presence of BHA, by prostaglandin H synthase.

DuBois, 1998; Molina *et al.*, 1999). Aspirin and other nonsteroidal anti-inflammatory drugs (NSAIDs) block the formation of colon cancer in experimental animals, and there is epidemiological evidence that long-term use of certain NSAIDs (aspirin and sulindac), but not acetaminophen (which does not inhibit COX2), decreases the incidence of colorectal polyps and cancer in humans, and also decreases the number of deaths from esophageal, gastric, and rectal cancers. The incidence of intestinal neoplasms in Apc$^{\Delta 716}$ knockout mice is dramatically suppressed by crossing these transgenic animals with PHS2 (COX-2) knockout mice (Oshima *et al.*, 1996). From these few examples it is apparent that PHS2 may play at least two distinct roles in tumor formation; it may convert certain xenobiotics to DNA-reactive metabolites (and thereby *initiate* tumor formation), and it may somehow *promote* subsequent tumor growth, perhaps through formation of growth-promoting eicosanoids.

Many phenolic compounds can serve as reducing substrates for PHS peroxidase. The phenoxyl radicals produced by one-electron oxidation reactions can undergo a variety of reactions, including binding to critical nucleophiles, such as protein and DNA, reduction by antioxidants such as glutathione, and self-coupling. The reactions of phenoxyl radicals are analogous to those of the nitrogen-centered free radicals produced during the one-electron oxidation of aromatic amines by PHS.

It was previously mentioned in this section that phenol can enhance the peroxidative metabolism of hydroquinone, which is an important component to benzene myelotoxicity. An analogous interaction has been described between the phenolic antioxidants, butylated hydroxytoluene (BHT), and butylated hydroxyanisole (BHA). In mice, the pulmonary toxicity of BHT, which is a relatively poor substrate for PHS, is enhanced by BHA, which is a relatively good substrate for PHS. The mechanism by which BHA enhances the pulmonary toxicity of BHT appears to involve the peroxidase-dependent conversion of BHA to a phenoxyl radical that interacts with BHT, converting it to a phenoxyl radical (by one-electron oxidation) or a quinone methide (by two-electron oxidation), as shown in Fig. 6-35. Formation of the toxic quinone methide of BHT can also be catalyzed by cytochrome P450, which is largely responsible for activating BHT in the absence of BHA.

Several reducing substrates, such as phenylbutazone, retinoic acid, 3-methylindole, sulfite, and bisulfite, are oxidized by PHS to carbon- or sulfur-centered free radicals that can trap oxygen to form a peroxyl radical, as shown in Fig. 6-36 for phenylbutazone. The peroxyl radical can oxidize xenobiotics in a peroxidative manner. For example, the peroxyl radical of phenylbutazone can convert benzo[*a*]pyrene 7,8-dihydrodiol to the corresponding 9,10-epoxide.

PHS is unique among peroxidases because it can both generate hydroperoxides and catalyze peroxidase-dependent reactions, as shown in Fig. 6-32. Xenobiotic biotransformation by PHS is controlled by the availability of arachidonic acid. The biotransformation of xenobiotics by other peroxidases is controlled by the availability

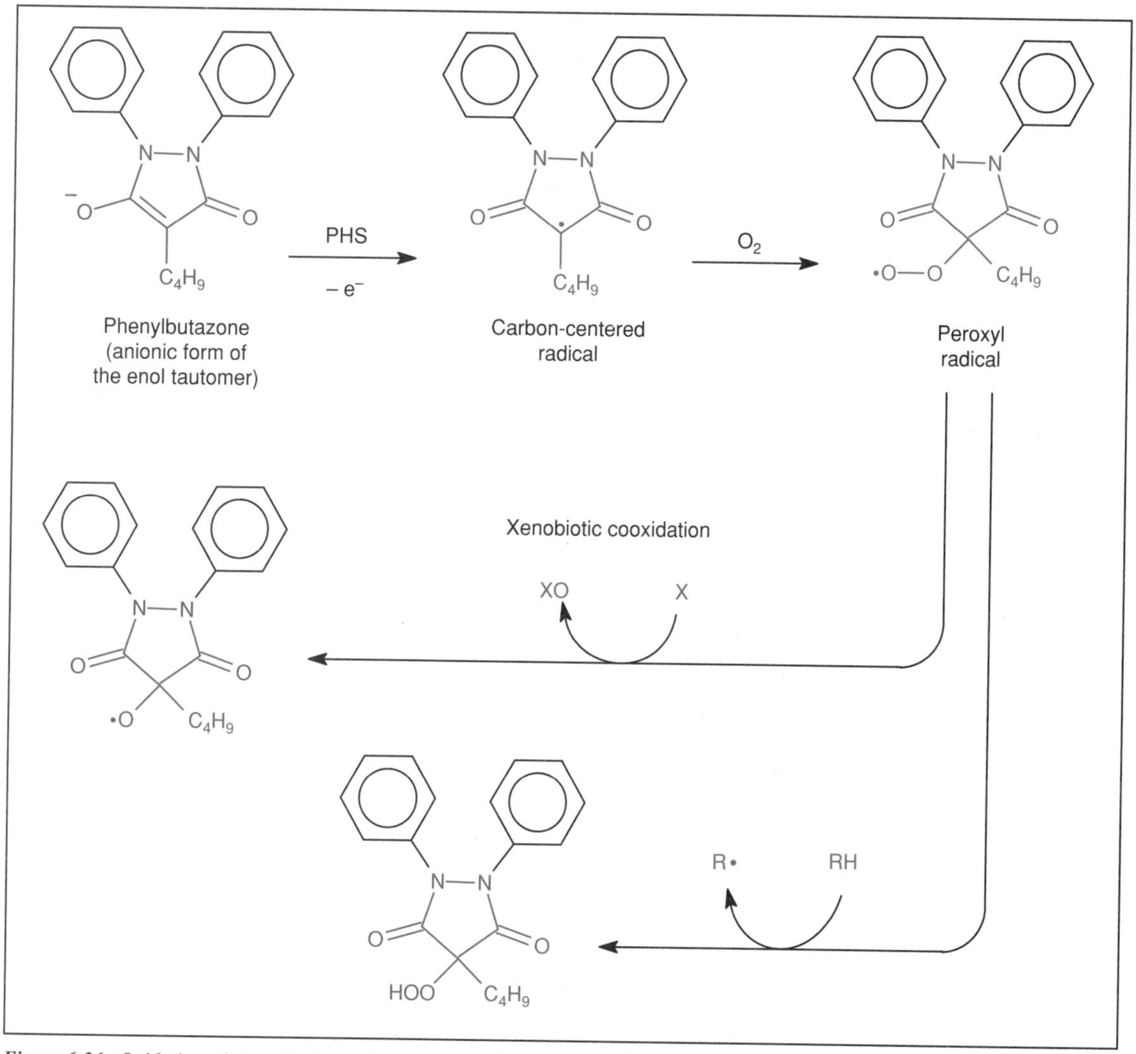

Figure 6-36. Oxidation of phenylbutazone by prostaglandin H synthase (PHS) to a carbon-centered radical and peroxyl radical.

Note that the peroxyl radical can oxidize xenobiotics (X) in a peroxidative manner.

of hydroperoxide substrates. Hydrogen peroxide is a normal product of cellular respiration, and lipid peroxides can form during lipid peroxidation. The level of these peroxides and their availability for peroxidase reactions depends on the efficiency of hydroperoxide scavenging by glutathione peroxidase and catalase.

Flavin Monooxygenases   Liver, kidney, intestine, brain, and lung contain one or more FAD-containing monooxygenases (FMO) that oxidize the nucleophilic nitrogen, sulfur, and phosphorus heteroatom of a variety of xenobiotics (Ziegler, 1993; Lawton *et al.*, 1994; Cashman, 1995, 1999; Rettie and Fisher, 1999; Cashman and Zhang, 2006). The mammalian FMO gene family comprises five enzymes (designated FMO1–FMO5) that contain 532–558 amino acid residues each and are 48–60% identical in amino acid sequence within a species, whereas orthologous forms are 82–86% identical across species (Hines *et al.*, 2002). Up to six FMO pseudogenes have also been observed, including one that shares 71% sequence identity with FMO3, namely, FMO6, for which nine distinct transcripts were identified in liver, but not kidney. All of these variant FMO6 transcripts arise by alternative splicing and lead to truncated,

and therefore nonfunctional, enzymes. The possibility remains that rare SNPs in the FMO6 pseudogene would lead to normal expression in some rare individuals, but this has not yet been documented (Hines *et al.*, 2002). The tertiary structure of human FMO has not yet been determined, but each FMO enzyme contains a highly conserved glycine-rich region (residues 4-32) that binds one mole of FAD (noncovalently) near the active site, which is adjacent to a second highly conserved glycine-rich region (residues 186–213) that binds NADPH. Other structural motifs have been reviewed in detail by Ziegler (2002).

Like CYP, the FMOs are microsomal enzymes that require NADPH and O_2, and many of the reactions catalyzed by FMO also can be catalyzed by CYP. Several in vitro techniques have been developed to distinguish reactions catalyzed by FMO from those catalyzed by CYP. In general, and in contrast to CYP, FMO is heat labile and can be inactivated in the absence of NADPH by warming microsomes to 50°C for 1 minute. By comparison, CYP can be inactivated with nonionic detergent, such as 1% Emulgen 911, which has a minimal effect on FMO activity. The pH optimum for FMO-catalyzed reactions (pH 8–10) tends to be higher than that for most (but not all) CYP reactions (pH 7–8). Antibodies raised against

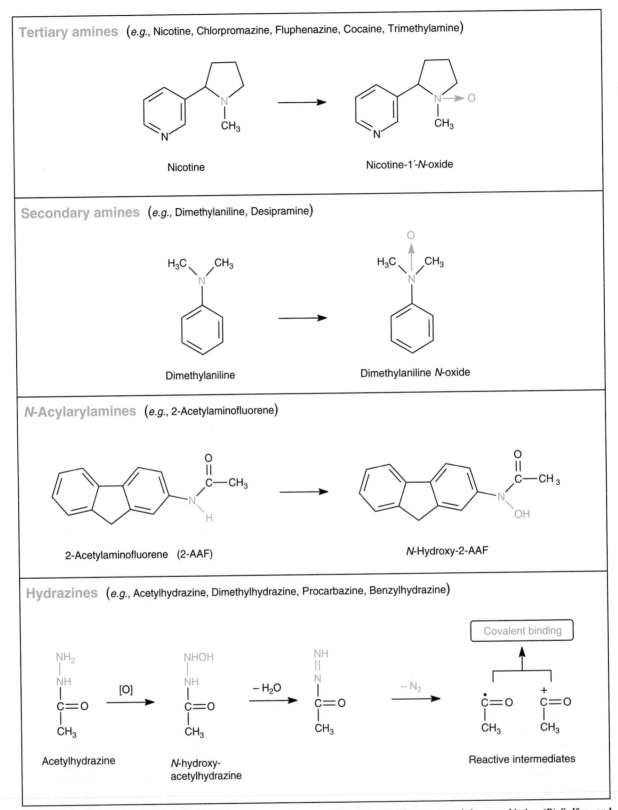

Figure 6-37. Examples of reactions catalyzed by flavin monooxygenases (FMO). (A) Nitrogen-containing xenobiotics. (B) Sulfur- and phosphorus-containing xenobiotics.

Thiols (*e.g.*, Cysteamine)

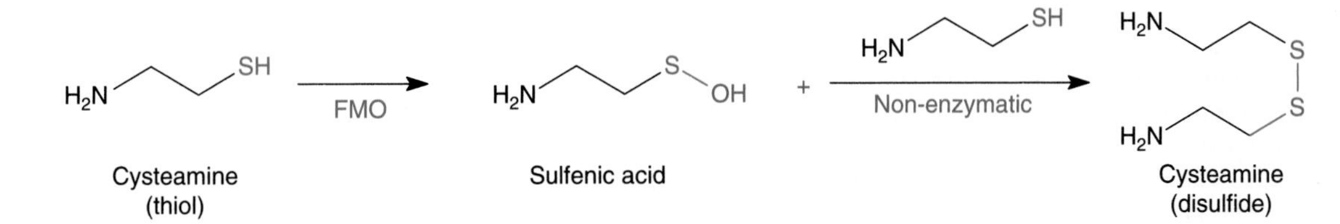

Cysteamine
(thiol)

FMO

Sulfenic acid

+

Non-enzymatic

Cysteamine
(disulfide)

Sulfide (*e.g.*, Cimetidine, Aldicarb, Phorate)

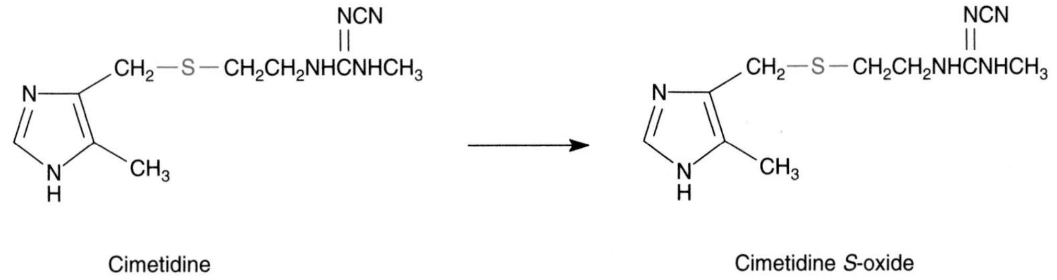

Cimetidine

Cimetidine *S*-oxide

Thioamides (*e.g.*, Thiobenzamide, Thioacetamide, Methimazole, Propylthiouracil)

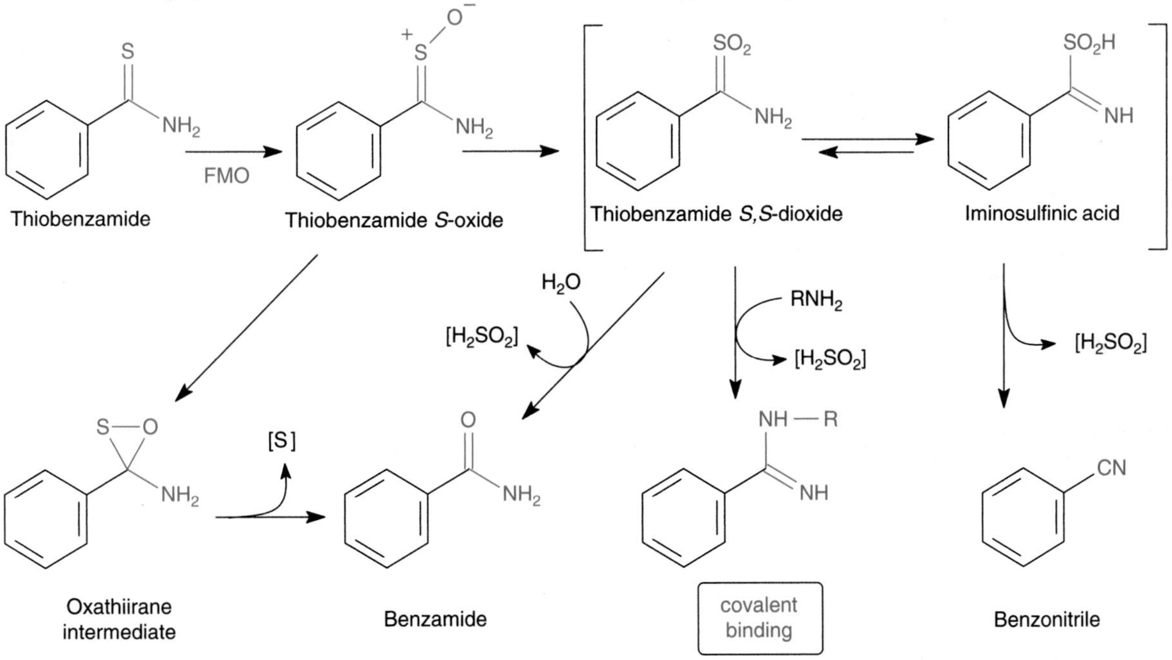

Thiobenzamide

FMO

Thiobenzamide *S*-oxide

Thiobenzamide *S,S*-dioxide

Iminosulfinic acid

H_2O

$[H_2SO_2]$

RNH_2

$[H_2SO_2]$

$[H_2SO_2]$

[S]

Oxathiirane
intermediate

Benzamide

covalent
binding

Benzonitrile

Phosphines (*e.g.*, Diphenylmethylphosphine)

Diphenylmethylphosphine

Diphenylmethylphosphine oxide

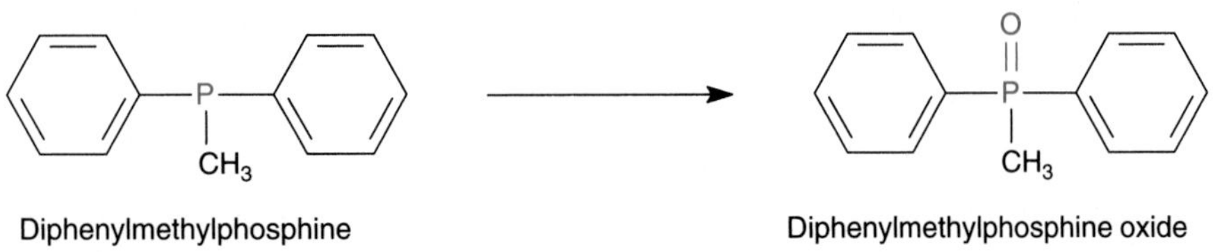

(*Continued.*)

purified CYP enzymes can be used not only to establish the role of CYP in a microsomal reaction but also to identify which particular CYP enzyme catalyzes the reaction. In contrast, antibodies raised against purified FMO do not inhibit the enzyme. The use of chemical inhibitors to ascertain the relative contribution of FMO and CYP to microsomal reactions is often complicated by a lack of specificity. For example, cimetidine and SKF 525A, which are well-recognized CYP inhibitors, are both substrates for FMO. Conversely, the FMO inhibitor methimazole is known to inhibit several of the CYP enzymes in human liver microsomes (namely, CYP2B6, CYP2C9, and CYP3A4). The situation is further complicated by the observation that the various forms of FMO differ in their thermal stability and sensitivity to detergents and other chemical modulators (examples of which are described later in this section).

FMO catalyzes the oxidation of nucleophilic tertiary amines to N-oxides, secondary amines to hydroxylamines and nitrones, and primary amines to hydroxylamines and oximes. Amphetamine, benzydamine, chlorpromazine, clozapine, guanethidine, imipramine, methamphetamine, olanzapine, and tamoxifen are examples of nitrogen-containing drugs that are N-oxygenated by FMO (and by CYP in most cases). FMO also oxidizes several sulfur-containing xenobiotics (such as thiols, thioethers, thiones, and thiocarbamates) and phosphines to S- and P-oxides, respectively. Cimetidine and sulindac sulfide are examples of sulfur-containing drugs that are converted to sulfoxides by FMO. Figure 6-14 shows how sulindac is reduced to sulindac sulfide, only to be oxidized by FMO back to the parent drug in what is often called a futile cycle. Hydrazines, iodides, selenides, and boron-containing compounds are also substrates for FMO. Examples of FMO-catalyzed reactions are shown in Fig. 6-37a and b. Zwitterions, positively-multiple charged compounds, and diamines such as cadaverine are generally not substrates (Krueger *et al.*, 2006).

In general, the metabolites produced by FMO are the products of a chemical reaction between a xenobiotic and a peracid or peroxide, which is consistent with the mechanism of catalysis of FMO (discussed later in this section). The reactions catalyzed by FMO are generally detoxication reactions, although there are exceptions to this rule, which are described below (this section). Inasmuch as FMO attacks nucleophilic heteroatoms, it might be assumed that substrates for FMO could be predicted simply from their pKa values (i.e., from a measure of their basicity). Although there is some truth to this—for example, xenobiotics containing an sp^3-hybridized nitrogen atom with a pK of 5–10 are generally good substrates for FMO—predictions of substrate specificity based on pKa alone are not very reliable presumably because steric effects influence access of substrates to the FMO active site, which is consistent with the reported lack of rabbit FMO2 activity toward imipramine and chlorpromazine (Rettie and Fisher, 1999; Krueger *et al.*, 2006).

With few exceptions, FMO acts as an electrophilic oxygenating catalyst, which distinguishes it from most other flavoprotein oxidases and monooxygenases (which will be discussed further in the section "Cytochrome P450"). The mechanism of catalysis by FMO is depicted in Fig. 6-38. After the FAD moiety is reduced to FADH$_2$ by NADPH, the oxidized cofactor, NADP$^+$, remains bound to the enzyme. FADH$_2$ then binds oxygen to produce a peroxide (i.e., the 4a-hydroperoxyflavin of FAD). The peroxide is relatively stable, probably because the active site of FMO comprises nonnucleophilic, lipophilic amino acid residues, and this is thought to be the form in which FMO exists in vivo. During the oxygenation of xenobiotics, the 4a-hydroperoxyflavin is converted to 4a-hydroxyflavin with transfer of the flavin peroxide oxygen to the substrate (depicted

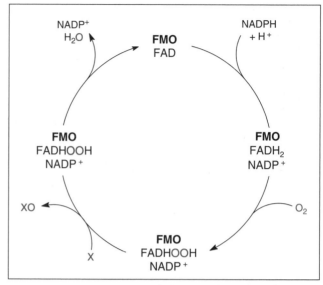

Figure 6-38. Catalytic cycle of flavin monooxygenase (FMO).

X and XO are the xenobiotic substrate and oxygenated product, respectively. The 4a-hydroperoxyflavin and 4a-hydroxyflavin of FAD are depicted as FADHOOH and FADHOH, respectively.

as X → XO in Fig. 6-38). From this latter step, it is understandable why the metabolites produced by FMO are generally the products of a chemical reaction between a xenobiotic and a peroxide or peracid. The final step in the catalytic cycle involves dehydration of 4a-hydroxyflavin (which restores FAD to its resting, oxidized state) and release of NADP$^+$. This final step is important because it is rate limiting, and it occurs after substrate oxygenation. Consequently, this step determines the upper limit of the rate of substrate oxidation. Therefore all good substrates for FMO are converted to products at the same maximum rate (i.e., V_{max} is determined by the final step in the catalytic cycle). Binding of NADP$^+$ to FMO during catalysis is important because it prevents the reduction of oxygen to H$_2$O$_2$. In the absence of bound NADP$^+$, FMO would function as an NADPH-oxidase that would consume NADPH and cause oxidative stress through excessive production of H$_2$O$_2$.

The oxygenation of substrates by FMO does not lead to inactivation of the enzyme, even though some of the products are strong electrophiles capable of binding covalently to critical and noncritical nucleophiles such as protein and glutathione, respectively. The products of the oxygenation reactions catalyzed by FMO and/or the oxygenation of the same substrates by CYP can inactivate CYP. For example, the FMO-dependent S-oxygenation of spironolactone thiol (which is formed by the deacetylation of spironolactone by carboxylesterases, as shown in Fig. 6-4) leads to the formation of an electrophilic sulfenic acid (R–SH → R–SOH) that can undergo redox cycling, or be further converted to the reactive sulfinic acid that inactivates CYP and binds covalently to other proteins (Krueger *et al.*, 2006).

In humans, FMO plays an important role in the biotransformation of several drugs (e.g., benzydamine, cimetidine, clozapine, guanethidine, methimazole, olanzapine, ranitidine, sulindac sulfide, tamoxifen, hydrazines such as procarbazine, and various dimethylaminoalkyl phenothiazine derivatives such as chlorpromazine and imipramine), xenobiotics (e.g., aldicarb, cocaine, disulfoton, fenthion, methamphetamine, nicotine, tyramine), and endogenous substrates (e.g., trimethylamine, cysteamine, and lipoic acid). The major flavin monooxygenase in human liver microsomes, FMO3, is predominantly if not solely responsible for converting (S)-nicotine to (S)-nicotine N-1′-oxide (which is one of the reactions shown in Fig. 6-37a). The reaction proceeds stereospecifically; only the trans isomer is produced by FMO3, and this is the only isomer of (S)-nicotine N-1′-oxide excreted in the urine of cigarette smokers or individuals wearing a nicotine patch (Cashman and Zhang, 2006). Therefore, the urinary excretion of trans-(S)-nicotine N-1′-oxide can be used as an in vivo probe of FMO3 activity in humans. FMO3 is also the principal enzyme involved in the S-oxygenation of cimetidine, an H_2-antagonist widely used in the treatment of gastric ulcers and other acid-related disorders (this reaction is shown in Fig. 6-37b). Cimetidine is stereoselectively sulfoxidated by FMO3 to an 84:16 mixture of (+) and (−) enantiomers, which closely matches the 75:25 enantiomeric composition of cimetidine S-oxide in human urine. Therefore, the urinary excretion of cimetidine S-oxide, like that of (S)-nicotine N-1′-oxide, is an in vivo indicator of FMO3 activity in humans.

Sulindac is a sulfoxide that exists in two stereochemical forms (as do most sulfoxides), and a racemic mixture of R- and S-sulindac is used therapeutically as a nonsteroidal anti-inflammatory drug (NSAID). As shown in Fig. 6-14, the sulfoxide group in sulindac is reduced to the corresponding sulfide (which is achiral), which is then oxidized back to sulindac (a process often described as futile cycling). In human liver, the sulfoxidation of sulindac sulfide is catalyzed by FMO3 with little or no contribution from CYP. At low substrate concentrations (30 μM), FMO3 converts sulindac sulfide to R- and S-sulindac in an 87:13 ratio (Hamman et al., 2000). Consequently, although sulindac is administered as a racemic mixture (i.e., a 1:1 mixture of R- and S-enantiomers), the reduction of this drug to the corresponding sulfide and its preferential sulfoxidation by FMO3 to R-sulindac results in stereoselective enrichment of R-sulindac in serum and urine.

In the case of sulindac sulfide, stereoselective sulfoxidation occurs not only with human FMO3 (the major drug-metabolizing FMO in human liver), but also with porcine FMO1 (the major form expressed in pig liver) and rabbit FMO2 (the major form expressed in rabbit lung) (Hamman et al., 2000). However, this conformity is the exception, rather than the rule. For example, in contrast to the stereoselective oxygenation of (S)-nicotine and cimetidine by human FMO3 (see above), FMO1 (which is the major FMO expressed in pig, rat, and rabbit liver) converts (S)-nicotine to a 1:1 mixture of cis- and trans-(S)-nicotine N-1′-oxide, and similarly converts cimetidine to a 1:1 mixture of (+) and (−) cimetidine S-oxide, respectively. Therefore, statements concerning the role of FMO in the disposition of xenobiotics in humans may not apply to other species, or vice versa.

Several sulfur-containing xenobiotics are oxygenated by FMO to electrophilic reactive intermediates. Such xenobiotics include various thiols, thioamides, 2-mercaptoimidazoles, thiocarbamates, and thiocarbamides. The electrophilic metabolites of these xenobiotics do not inactivate FMO, but they can covalently modify and inactivate neighboring proteins, including CYP. Some of these same xenobiotics are substrates for CYP, and their oxygenation to electrophilic metabolites leads to inactivation of CYP, a process known variously as metabolism-dependent inhibition, mechanism-based inhibition, and suicide inactivation. 2-Mercaptoimidazoles undergo sequential S-oxygenation reactions by FMO, first to sulfenic acids and then to sulfinic acids (R–SH → R–SOH → R–SO_2H). These electrophilic metabolites, like the sulfenic acid metabolite produced from spironolactone thiol (see above), bind to critical nucleophiles

(such as proteins) or interact with glutathione to form disulfides. The thiocarbamate functionality present in numerous agricultural chemicals is converted by FMO to S-oxides (sulfoxides), which can be further oxygenated to sulfones. These reactions involve S-oxygenation adjacent to a ketone, which produces strong electrophilic acylating agents, which may be responsible for the toxicity of many thiocarbamate herbicides and fungicides. The hepatotoxicity of thiobenzamide is dependent on S-oxidation by FMO and/or CYP. As shown in Fig. 6-37b, the S-oxidation of thiobenzamide produces an S-oxide, which can rearrange to an oxathiirane (a three-membered ring of carbon, sulfur, and oxygen) upon photolysis or thermolysis. However, such oxathiiranes are readily reduced back to the S-oxide. In vivo, the S,S-dioxide is more likely to form, which readily tautomerizes to iminosulfinic acid, binds covalently to protein (which leads to hepatocellular necrosis) or rearranges to benzamide, a reaction known as oxidative group transfer.

Endogenous FMO substrates include cysteamine, which is oxidized to the disulfide, cystamine, and trimethylamine (TMA), which is converted to TMA N-oxide (Fig. 6-37b). By converting cysteamine to cystamine, FMO may serve to produce a low-molecular weight disulfide-exchange agent, which may participate in the formation of disulfide bridges during peptide synthesis or the renaturation of proteins. By converting TMA to TMA N-oxide, FMO converts a malodorous and volatile dietary product of choline, lecithin, and carnitine catabolism to an inoffensive metabolite. TMA smells of rotting fish, and people who are genetically deficient in FMO3 suffer from trimethylaminuria or fish-odor syndrome, which is caused by the excretion of TMA in urine, sweat, and breath (Ayesh and Smith, 1992). The underlying genetic basis of trimethylaminuria is a mutation ($Pro_{153} \rightarrow Leu_{153}$) in exon 4 of the FMO3 gene (Dolphin et al., 1997). Although this mutation (and hence trimethylaminuria) occurs only rarely, it is now known to be just one of several mutations that decrease or eliminate FMO3 activity; these other mutations include missense mutations ($Glu_{32} \rightarrow Lys_{32}$, $Ala_{52} \rightarrow Thr_{52}$, $Met_{66} \rightarrow Ile_{66}$, $Met_{82} \rightarrow Thr_{82}$, $Glu_{314} \rightarrow X_{314}$, $Arg_{387} \rightarrow Leu_{387}$, $Arg_{492} \rightarrow Trp_{492}$, etc.) and the nonsense mutation $Glu_{305} \rightarrow X_{305}$ (Cashman et al., 2000; Cashman and Zhang, 2006). As might be expected, trimethylaminuria is associated with an impairment of nicotine N-oxidation and other pathways of drug biotransformation that are primarily catalyzed by FMO3 (Rettie and Fisher, 1999). For instance, benzydamine N-oxygenation has been correlated with FMO3 genotype in trimethylaminurics (Cashman and Zhang, 2006).

Humans and other mammals express five different flavin monooxygenases (FMO1, FMO2, FMO3, FMO4, and FMO5) in a species- and tissue-specific manner, as shown in Table 6-8 (adapted from Cashman, 1995; Cashman and Zhang, 2006; Zhang and Cashman, 2006). For example, the major hepatic FMOs expressed in humans are FMO3 and FMO5, whereas FMO1 is the major FMO expressed in rat, rabbit, and pig liver. Previously, FMO3 has been considered to be the dominant FMO in human liver, but FMO5 expression is higher, but has activity toward fewer xenobiotic substrates, and likely plays only a minor role in xenobiotic metabolism (Cashman and Zhang, 2006). FMO5 is also the most highly expressed FMO in the small intestine. In humans, high levels of FMO1 are expressed in the kidney, and low levels of FMO2 are expressed in the lungs of Caucasians and Asians. However, lung microsomes from other species, particularly rabbit, mouse, and monkey, contain high levels of expressed FMO2, and of the FMO transcripts detected in human lung, the FMO2 transcript is found at the highest levels by far (Zhang and Cashman, 2006). The uncharacteristically low levels of active FMO2 in human lung is caused by a mutation (a C → T

Table 6-8
Putative Tissue Levels of Flavin Monooxygenase (FMO) Enzymes Present in Animals and Humans

	FMO1	FMO2	FMO3	FMO4	FMO5
Liver					
Mouse	Low	None	High	Unknown	Low
Rat	High	Unknown	Low	Unknown	Low
Rabbit	High	None	Low	Unknown	Low
Human[a]	Trace	Low	Very high	High	Very high
Kidney					
Mouse	High	Unknown	High	Unknown	Low
Rat	High	Unknown	High	High	Low
Rabbit	Low	Low	Trace	High	Low
Human[a]	High	High	Low	Medium	Medium
Lung					
Mouse	Unknown	High	Trace	None	Low
Rat	Unknown	Unknown	Unknown	None	Low
Rabbit	Unknown	Very high	Unknown	None	None
Human[a]	Low	Variable[b]	Medium	Low	Medium
Small intestine					
Human[a]	Low	Low	Trace	Trace	Medium

[a] Human levels are based on tissue expression of FMO as reported in Cashman and Zhang (2006) and are based on mRNA levels.

[b] FMO2 mRNA levels in human lung are high, but this mRNA is not translated into functional enzyme due to the presence of a truncation mutation in Caucasians and Asians. About 26% of African Americans, 7% of Puerto Ricans, and 2% of Mexicans have one normal allele and express a functional protein.

SOURCE: Data adapted from Cashman JR, Zhang J: Human flavin-containing monooxygenases. *Annu Rev Pharmacol Toxicol* 46:65–100, 2006; Zhang J, Cashman JR: Quantitative analysis of FMO gene mRNA levels in human tissues. *Drug Metab Dispos* 34:19–26, 2006; Cashman JR: Structural and catalytic properties of the mammalian flavin-containing monooxygenase. *Chem Res Toxicol* 8:166–181, 1995.

transition at codon 472) in the major human FMO2*2 allele found in Caucasians and Asians, which results in the synthesis of a nonfunctional, truncated protein (one lacking the last 64 amino acid residues from the C-terminus) (Dolphin *et al.*, 1998). In contrast, 26% of African Americans, 7% of Puerto Ricans, and 2% of Mexicans have one normal allele and express a functional protein (Cashman and Zhang, 2006). In pulmonary microsomes from individuals who express one or more functional FMO2 alleles, the protein level is equal to or greater than that of CYPs. Functional FMO2 appears to have high S-oxygenation activity toward thioureas and thioamides, which implies that individuals who express a functional FMO2 may be more susceptible to the toxic effects of sulfenic acids, whereas Caucasians and Asians may be protected from thioether-containing pesticides (Cashman and Zhang, 2006). FMO4 appears to be expressed at low levels in the brain of several mammalian species, where it might terminate the action of several centrally active drugs and other xenobiotics. FMO4 is unstable, however, which makes its characterization somewhat difficult (Cashman and Zhang, 2006).

The various forms of FMO are distinct gene products with different physical properties and substrate specificities. For example, FMO2 N-oxygenates n-octylamine, whereas such long aliphatic primary amines are not substrates for FMO1, although they stimulate its activity toward other substrates (in some cases causing a change in stereospecificity). Conversely, short-chain tertiary amines, such as chlorpromazine, orphenadrine, and imipramine, are substrates for FMO1 but not FMO2. FMO2 exhibits no activity toward phenothiazine derivatives with only a 3-carbon side chain or 1,3-diphenylthiourea (Krueger *et al.*, 2006). FMO3 is highly selective in the N-oxygenation of trimethylamine, whereas FMO5 is selective for the N-oxygenation of short-chain aliphatic primary amines such as *N*-octylamine, but has little activity toward other typical

FMO substrates (Krueger *et al.*, 2006). The substrate specificity of FMO4 also appears to be somewhat restricted. Certain substrates are oxygenated stereospecifically by one FMO enzyme but not another. For example, FMO2 and FMO3 convert (*S*)-nicotine exclusively to *trans*-(*S*)-nicotine N-1′-oxide, whereas the N-oxides of (*S*)-nicotine produced by FMO1 are a 1:1 mixture of *cis* and *trans* isomers. FMO2 is heat stable under conditions that completely inactivate FMO1, and FMO2 is resistant to anionic detergents that inactivate FMO1. Low concentrations of bile acids, such as cholate, stimulate FMO activity in rat and mouse liver microsomes but inhibit FMO activity in rabbit and pig liver.

The FMO enzymes expressed in liver microsomes are not under the same regulatory control as CYP enzymes. In rats, the expression of FMO1 is suppressed rather than induced by treatment with phenobarbital or 3-methylcholanthrene (although some studies point to a modest [∼3 fold] induction of rat FMO1 by 3-methylcholanthrene). Indole-3-carbinol, which induces the same CYP enzymes as 3-methylcholanthrene, causes a marked decrease in FMO activity in rat liver and intestine. A similar decrease in FMO3 activity occurs in human volunteers following the consumption of large amounts of Brussels sprouts, which contain high levels of indole-3-carbinol and related indoles. The decrease in FMO3 activity may result from direct inhibition of FMO3 by indole-3-carbinol and its derivatives rather than from an actual decrease in enzyme levels (Cashman *et al.*, 1999). However, the AHR-agonist, TCDD was found to induce FMO2 and FMO3 mRNA levels in mice by 30- and 80-fold, respectively (Tijet *et al.*, 2006).

The levels of FMO3 and, to a lesser extent, the levels of FMO1 in mouse liver microsomes are sexually differentiated (female > male) due to suppression of expression by testosterone. The opposite is true of FMO1 levels in rat liver microsomes, the expression of which is positively regulated by testosterone and negatively regulated by estradiol. In pregnant rabbits, lung FMO2 is positively regulated by progesterone and/or corticosteroids.

Species differences in the relative expression of FMO and CYP appear to determine species differences in the toxicity of the pyrrolizidine alkaloids, senecionine, retrorsine, and monocrotaline. These compounds are detoxified by FMO, which catalyzes the formation of tertiary amine N-oxides, but are activated by CYP, which oxidizes these alkaloids to pyrroles that generate toxic electrophiles through the loss of substituents on the pyrrolizidine nucleus (details of which appear in the section "Cytochrome P450"). Rats have a high pyrrole-forming CYP activity and a low N-oxide forming FMO activity, whereas the opposite is true of guinea pigs. This likely explains why pyrrolizidine alkaloids are highly toxic to rats but not to guinea pigs. Many of the reactions catalyzed by FMO are also catalyzed by CYP, but differences in the oxidation of pyrrolizidine alkaloids by FMO and CYP illustrate that this is not always the case.

Cytochrome P450   Of all the xenobiotic-biotransforming enzymes, the cytochrome P450 (CYP) enzyme system ranks first in terms of catalytic versatility and the sheer number of xenobiotics it detoxifies or activates to reactive intermediates. The highest levels of CYP enzymes involved in xenobiotic biotransformation are found in liver endoplasmic reticulum (microsomes), but CYP enzymes are present in virtually all tissues. The liver microsomal CYP enzymes play a very important role in determining the intensity and duration of action of drugs, and they also play a key role in the detoxication of xenobiotics. CYP enzymes in liver and extrahepatic tissues play important roles in the activation of xenobiotics to toxic and/or tumorigenic metabolites. The catalytic versatility of CYP enzymes is apparent from Table 6-2, which shows some of the many chemical groups that can be metabolized by cytochrome P450.

Microsomal and mitochondrial CYP enzymes play key roles in the biosynthesis or catabolism of steroid hormones, bile acids, fat-soluble vitamins such as vitamins A and D, fatty acids, and eicosanoids such as prostaglandins, thromboxane, prostacyclin, and leukotrienes, which underscores the catalytic versatility of cytochrome P450. In humans, the metabolism of the aforementioned endobiotics and the biotransformation of innumerable xenobiotics are catalyzed by 57 CYP enzymes, as shown in Table 6-9. In several cases, there is no clear functional distinction in terms of endobiotic and xenobiotic metabolism because there are many examples of CYP enzymes playing an important role in the metabolism of both an endobiotic and a drug or other xenobiotic.

All CYP enzymes are heme-containing proteins. The heme iron in cytochrome P450 is usually in the ferric (Fe^{3+}) state. When reduced to the ferrous (Fe^{2+}) state, cytochrome P450 can bind ligands such as O_2 and carbon monoxide (CO). The complex between ferrous cytochrome P450 and CO absorbs light maximally at 450 nm, from which cytochrome P450 derives its name. The absorbance maximum of the CO complex differs slightly among different CYP enzymes and ranges from 447 nm to 452 nm. All other hemoproteins that bind CO absorb light maximally at ~420 nm. The unusual absorbance maximum of cytochrome P450 is due to an unusual fifth ligand to the heme (a cysteine-thiolate). The amino acid sequence around the cysteine residue that forms the thiolate bond with the heme moiety is highly conserved in all CYP enzymes. When this thiolate bond is disrupted, cytochrome P450 is converted to a catalytically inactive form called cytochrome P420.

Table 6-9

Classification of the 57 Human CYP Enzymes

XENOBIOTICS	STEROIDOGENIC	FATTY ACIDS/ EICOSANOIDS	UNKNOWN
CYP1A1	CYP11A1	CYP4A11	CYP2A7
CYP1A2	CYP11B1	CYP4B1	CYP2S1
CYP1B1	CYP11B2	CYP4F2	CYP2U1
CYP2A6	CYP17A1	CYP4F8	CYP2W1
CYP2A13	CYP19A1	CYP4F12	CYP3A43
CYP2B6	CYP21A2	CYP5A1[a]	CYP4A22
CYP2C8[b]		CYP8A1[c]	CYP4F11
CYP2C9[b]	BILE ACID		CYP4F22
CYP2C18	CYP7A1	VITAMIN D	CYP4V2
CYP2C19	CYP7B1	CYP24A1	CYP4X1
CYP2D6	CYP8B1	CYP26C1[d]	CYP4Z1
CYP2E1	CYP27A1[e]	CYP27B1	CYP20A1
CYP2F1	CYP39A1	CYP2R1	CYP27C1
CYP2J2[b]	CYP46A1		
CYP3A4[f]	CYP51A1[g]	RETINOIC ACID	
CYP3A5		CYP26A1	
CYP3A7		CYP26B1	
CYP4F3[b]			

[a] Thromboxane A synthase (TBXAS1).
[b] Also involved in fatty acid and eicosanoid metabolism.
[c] Prostaglandin I_2 (prostacyclin) synthase (PTGIS).
[d] Also involved in retinoic acid metabolism.
[e] Also involved in vitamin D metabolism.
[f] Also involved in bile acid synthesis.
[g] Also involved in cholesterol biosynthesis.

By competing with oxygen, CO inhibits cytochrome P450. The inhibitory effect of carbon monoxide can be reversed by irradiation with light at 450 nm, which photodissociates the cytochrome P450–CO complex. These properties of cytochrome P450 are of historical importance. The observation that treatment of rats with certain chemicals, such as 3-methylcholanthrene, causes a shift in the peak absorbance of cytochrome P450 (from 450 nm to 448 nm) provided some of the earliest evidence for the existence of multiple forms of cytochrome P450 in liver microsomes. The conversion of cytochrome P450 to cytochrome P420 by detergents and phospholipases helped to establish the hemoprotein nature of cytochrome P450. The inhibition of cytochrome P450 by CO and the reversal of this inhibition by photodissociation of the cytochrome P450–CO complex established cytochrome P450 as the microsomal and mitochondrial enzyme involved in drug biotransformation and steroid biosynthesis.

The basic reaction catalyzed by CYP enzymes is monooxygenation in which one atom of oxygen is incorporated into a substrate, designated RH, and the other is reduced to water with reducing equivalents derived from NADPH, as follows:

$$\text{Substrate (RH)} + O_2 + \text{NADPH} + H^+ \rightarrow$$
$$\text{Product (ROH)} + H_2O + \text{NADP}^+$$

Although cytochrome P450 functions as a monooxygenase, the products are not limited to alcohols and phenols due to rearrangement reactions (Guengerich, 1991, 2001b; Isin and Guengerich, 2007). During catalysis, cytochrome P450 binds directly to the substrate and molecular oxygen, but it does not interact directly with NADPH or NADH. The mechanism by which cytochrome

P450 receives electrons from NAD(P)H depends on the subcellular localization of cytochrome P450. In the endoplasmic reticulum, which is where most of the CYP enzymes involved in xenobiotic biotransformation are localized, electrons are relayed from NADPH to cytochrome P450 via a flavoprotein called NADPH-cytochrome P450 reductase (also known as an oxidoreductase or OR; gene symbol POR). Within this flavoprotein, electrons are transferred from NADPH to cytochrome P450 via FMN and FAD. In mitochondria, which house many of the CYP enzymes involved in steroid hormone biosynthesis and vitamin D metabolism, electrons are transferred from NAD(P)H to cytochrome P450 via two proteins; an iron–sulfur protein called ferredoxin (gene symbol FDX1), and an FMN-containing flavoprotein called ferredoxin reductase (gene symbol FDXR). These proteins are also known as adrenodoxin and adrenodoxin reductase. In bacteria such as *Pseudomonas putida* electron flow is similar to that in mitochondria (NADH → flavoprotein → putidaredoxin → P450).

There are some notable exceptions to the general rule that cytochrome P450 requires a second enzyme (i.e., a flavoprotein) for catalytic activity. One exception applies to two CYP enzymes involved in the conversion of arachidonic acid to eicosanoids, namely, thromboxane A synthase (CYP5A1) and prostaglandin I_2 synthase, which is also known as prostacyclin synthase (CYP8A1). These two CYP enzymes convert the endoperoxide, PGH_2, to thromboxane (TXA_2) and prostacyclin (PGI_2) in platelets and the endothelial lining of blood vessels, respectively. In both cases, cytochrome P450 functions as an isomerase and catalyzes a rearrangement of the oxygen atoms introduced into arachidonic acid by cyclooxygenase (see Fig. 6-32). The plant cytochrome P450, allene oxide synthase (CYP74A1), and certain invertebrate CYP enzymes also catalyze the rearrangement of oxidized chemicals.

The second exception is represented by two CYP enzymes expressed in the bacterium *Bacillus megaterium*, which are known as BM-1 (CYP106A1) and BM-3 (CYP102A1). These CYP enzymes are considerably larger than most CYP enzymes because they are linked directly to a flavoprotein. In other words, the cytochrome P450 moiety and oxidoreductase flavoprotein are expressed in a single protein encoded by a single gene. Through recombinant DNA techniques, mammalian CYP enzymes have been linked directly to NADPH-cytochrome P450 reductase and, like the bacterial enzyme, the resultant fusion protein is catalytically active. Most mammalian CYP enzymes are not synthesized as a single enzyme containing both the hemoprotein and flavoprotein moieties, but this arrangement is found in the nitric oxide (NO) synthases. In addition to its atypical structure, the CYP enzyme expressed in *Bacillus megaterium*, CYP102A1, is unusual for another reason: It is inducible by phenobarbital, which has provided insight into the mechanism of cytochrome P450 induction.

Phospholipids and cytochrome b_5 also play an important role in cytochrome P450 reactions. Cytochrome P450 and NADPH-cytochrome P450 reductase are embedded in the phospholipid bilayer of the endoplasmic reticulum, which facilitates their interaction. When the C-terminal region that anchors NADPH-cytochrome P450 reductase in the membrane is cleaved with trypsin, the truncated flavoprotein can no longer support cytochrome P450 reactions, although it is still capable of reducing cytochrome c and other soluble electron acceptors. The ability of phospholipids to facilitate the interaction between NADPH-cytochrome P450 reductase and cytochrome P450 does not appear to depend on the nature of the polar head group (serine, choline, inositol, ethanolamine), although certain CYP enzymes (those in the CYP3A subfamily)

have a requirement for phospholipids containing unsaturated fatty acids.

Cytochrome b_5 can donate the second of two electrons required by cytochrome P450. Although this would be expected simply to increase the rate of catalysis of cytochrome P450, cytochrome b_5 can also increase the apparent affinity with which certain CYP enzymes bind their substrates, hence, cytochrome b_5 can increase V_{max} and/or decrease the apparent K_m of cytochrome P450 reactions. Liver microsomes contain numerous forms of cytochrome P450 but contain a single form of NADPH-cytochrome P450 reductase (POR) and cytochrome b_5 (CYB5A). For each molecule of NADPH-cytochrome P450 reductase in rat liver microsomes, there are 5–10 molecules of cytochrome b_5 and 10–20 molecules of cytochrome P450. NADPH-cytochrome P450 reductase will reduce electron acceptors other than cytochrome P450, which enables this enzyme to be measured based on its ability to reduce cytochrome c (which is why NADPH-cytochrome P450 reductase is often called NADPH-cytochrome c reductase). NADPH-cytochrome P450 reductase can transfer electrons much faster than cytochrome P450 can use them, which more than likely accounts for the low ratio of NADPH-cytochrome P450 reductase to cytochrome P450 in liver microsomes. Low levels of NADPH-cytochrome P450 reductase may also be a safeguard to protect cells from the often deleterious one-electron reduction reactions catalyzed by this flavoprotein (see Fig. 6-15). In addition to supporting certain CYP-catalyzed reactions, cytochrome b_5 and NADH-cytochrome b_5 reductase can catalyze the dehydroxylation of certain amidoximes and arylhydroxylamines (formed by N-hydroxylation of aromatic amines), which can reverse their formation by CYP enzymes (see Fig. 6-21).

The catalytic cycle of cytochrome P450 is shown in Fig. 6-39 (Dawson, 1988). The first part of the cycle involves the activation of oxygen, and the final part of the cycle involves substrate oxidation, which entails the abstraction of a hydrogen atom or an electron from the substrate followed by oxygen rebound (radical recombination). Following the binding of substrate to the CYP enzyme, the heme iron is reduced from the ferric (Fe^{3+}) to the ferrous (Fe^{2+}) state by the addition of a single electron from NADPH-cytochrome P450 reductase. The reduction of cytochrome P450 is facilitated by substrate binding, possibly because binding of the substrate in the vicinity of the heme moiety converts the heme iron from a low-spin to a high-spin state. Oxygen binds to cytochrome P450 in its ferrous state, and the $Fe^{2+}O_2$ complex is converted to an $Fe^{2+}OOH$ complex by the addition of a proton (H^+) and a second electron, which is derived from NADPH-cytochrome P450 reductase or cytochrome b_5. Introduction of a second proton cleaves the $Fe^{2+}OOH$ complex to produce water and an $(FeO)^{3+}$ complex, which transfers its oxygen atom to the substrate. Release of the oxidized substrate returns cytochrome P450 to its initial state. If the catalytic cycle is interrupted (uncoupled) following introduction of the first electron, oxygen is released as superoxide anion (see "Other Reactions" in Fig. 6-39). If the cycle is interrupted after introduction of the second electron, oxygen is released as hydrogen peroxide (H_2O_2). The final oxygenating species $(FeO)^{3+}$ can be generated directly by the transfer of an oxygen atom from hydrogen peroxide and certain other hydroperoxides, a process known as the peroxide shunt. For this reason certain P450 reactions can be supported by hydroperoxides in the absence of NADPH-cytochrome P450 reductase and NADPH.

Cytochrome P450 catalyzes several types of oxidation reactions, including:

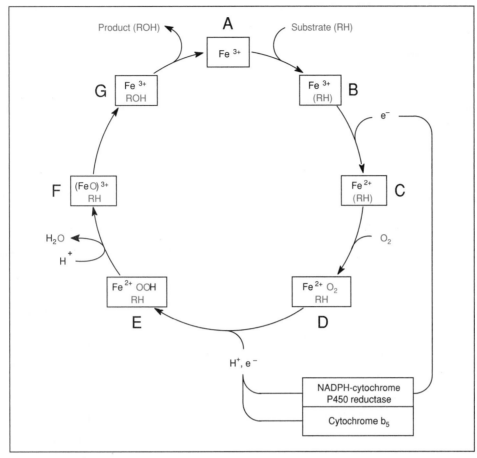

Other reactions

One-electron reduction	**C** $(Fe^{2+}\,RH)$	$\longrightarrow$	**A** $(Fe^{3+}) + RH\dot{}^{-}$
Superoxide anion production	**D** $(Fe^{2+}\,O_2\,RH)$	$\longrightarrow$	**B** $(Fe^{3+}\,RH) + O_2\dot{}^{-}$
Hydrogen peroxide production	**E** $(Fe^{2+}OOH\,RH) + H^{+}$	$\longrightarrow$	**B** $(Fe^{3+}RH) + H_2O_2$
Peroxide shunt	**B** $(Fe^{3+}\,RH) + XOOH$	$\longrightarrow$	**F** $(FeO)^{3+}\,RH + XOH$

Figure 6-39. Catalytic cycle of cytochrome P450.

1. Hydroxylation of an aliphatic or aromatic carbon;
2. Epoxidation of a double bond;
3. Heteroatom (S-, N-, and I-) oxygenation and N-hydroxylation;
4. Heteroatom (O-, S-, and N-) dealkylation;
5. Oxidative group transfer;
6. Cleavage of esters;
7. Dehydrogenation.

In the first three cases, oxygen from the $(FeO)^{3+}$ complex is incorporated into the substrate, which otherwise remains intact. In the fourth case, oxygenation of the substrate is followed by a rearrangement reaction leading to cleavage of an amine (N-dealkylation) or an ether (O- and S-dealkylation). Oxygen from the $(FeO)^{3+}$ complex is incorporated into the alkyl-leaving group, producing an aldehyde or ketone. In the fifth case, oxygenation of the substrate is followed by a rearrangement reaction leading to loss of a heteroatom (oxidative group transfer). The sixth case, the cleavage of esters, resembles

heteroatom dealkylation in that the functional group is cleaved with incorporation of oxygen from the $(FeO)^{3+}$ complex into the leaving group, producing an aldehyde. In the seventh case, two hydrogens are abstracted from the substrate with the formation of a double bond (C=C, C=O, or C=N), with the reduction of oxygen from the $(FeO)^{3+}$ complex to water. It should be noted that this long list of reactions does not encompass all the reactions catalyzed by cytochrome P450. Cytochrome P450 can catalyze reductive reactions (such as azo reduction, nitro reduction, and reductive dehalogenation) and isomerization reactions (such as the conversion of PGH_2 to thromboxane and prostacyclin). During the synthesis of steroid hormones, cytochrome P450 catalyzes the cleavage of carbon–carbon bonds, which occurs during the conversion of cholesterol to pregnenolone by side-chain cleavage enzyme (CYP11A1, which is also known as P450$_{scc}$) and the aromatization of a substituted cyclohexane, which occurs during the conversion of androgens to estrogens by aromatase (CYP19A1, also known as CYP19 and P450$_{arom}$).

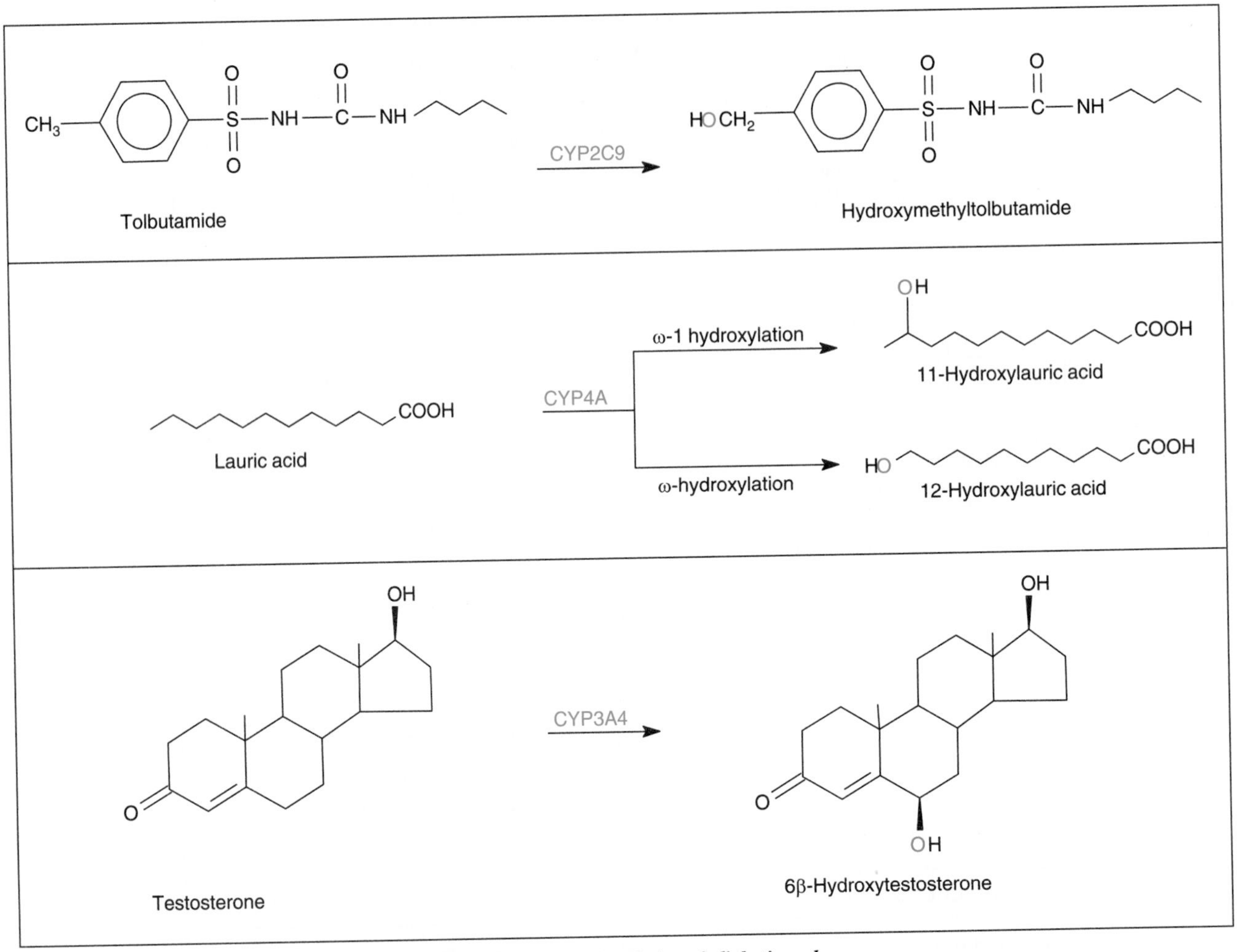

Figure 6-40. *Examples of reactions catalyzed by cytochrome P450: Hydroxylation of aliphatic carbon.*

Examples of aliphatic and aromatic hydroxylation reactions catalyzed by cytochrome P450 are shown in Figs. 6-40 and 6-41, respectively. The hydroxylation of aromatic hydrocarbons may proceed via an oxirane intermediate (i.e., an arene oxide) that isomerizes to the corresponding phenol. Alternatively, aromatic hydroxylation can proceed by a mechanism known as direct insertion. The *ortho*-hydroxylation and *para*-hydroxylation of chlorobenzene proceed via 2,3- and 3,4-epoxidation, whereas *meta*-hydroxylation proceeds by direct insertion, as shown in Fig. 6-42. When aromatic hydroxylation involves direct insertion, hydrogen abstraction (i.e., cleavage of the C–H bond) is the rate-limiting step, so that substitution of hydrogen with deuterium or tritium considerably slows the hydroxylation reaction. This *isotope effect* is less marked when aromatic hydroxylation proceeds via an arene oxide intermediate. Arene oxides are electrophilic and, therefore, potentially toxic metabolites that are detoxified by such enzymes as epoxide hydrolase (see Figs. 6-7 to 6-9) and glutathione transferase (see section "Glutathione Conjugation"). Depending on the ring substituents, the rearrangement of arene oxides to the corresponding phenol can lead to an intramolecular migration of a substituent (such as hydrogen or a halogen) from one carbon to the next. This intramolecular migration occurs at the site of oxidation and is known as the NIH shift; so named for its discovery at the National Institutes of Health.

Aliphatic hydroxylation involves insertion of oxygen into a C–H bond. As in the case of aromatic hydroxylation by direct insertion, cleavage of the C–H bond by hydrogen abstraction is the rate-limiting step, as shown below:

$$(FeO)^{3+} \quad HC{-} \longrightarrow Fe(OH)^{3+} \quad {\cdot}C{-} \longrightarrow Fe^{3+} \quad HO{-}C{-}$$

In the case of simple, straight-chain hydrocarbons, such as *n*-hexane, aliphatic hydroxylation occurs at both the terminal methyl groups and the internal methylene groups. In the case of fatty acids and their derivatives (i.e., eicosanoids such as prostaglandins and leukotrienes), aliphatic hydroxylation occurs at the ω-carbon (terminal methyl group) and the ω-1 carbon (penultimate carbon), as shown for lauric acid in Fig. 6-40. Most CYP enzymes preferentially catalyze the ω-1 hydroxylation of fatty acids and their derivatives, but one group of CYP enzymes (those encoded by the CYP4A genes) preferentially catalyzes the ω-hydroxylation of fatty acids, which can be further oxidized to dicarboxylic acids.

Xenobiotics containing a carbon–carbon double bond (i.e., alkenes) can be epoxidated (i.e., converted to an oxirane) in an analogous manner to the oxidation of aromatic compounds to arene oxides. Just as arene oxides can isomerize to phenols, so aliphatic epoxides can isomerize to the corresponding ene-ol, the formation of which may involve an intramolecular migration (NIH shift) of a substituent at the site of oxidation. Like arene oxides, aliphatic epoxides are also potentially toxic metabolites that are inactivated by other xenobiotic-metabolizing enzymes. Oxidation

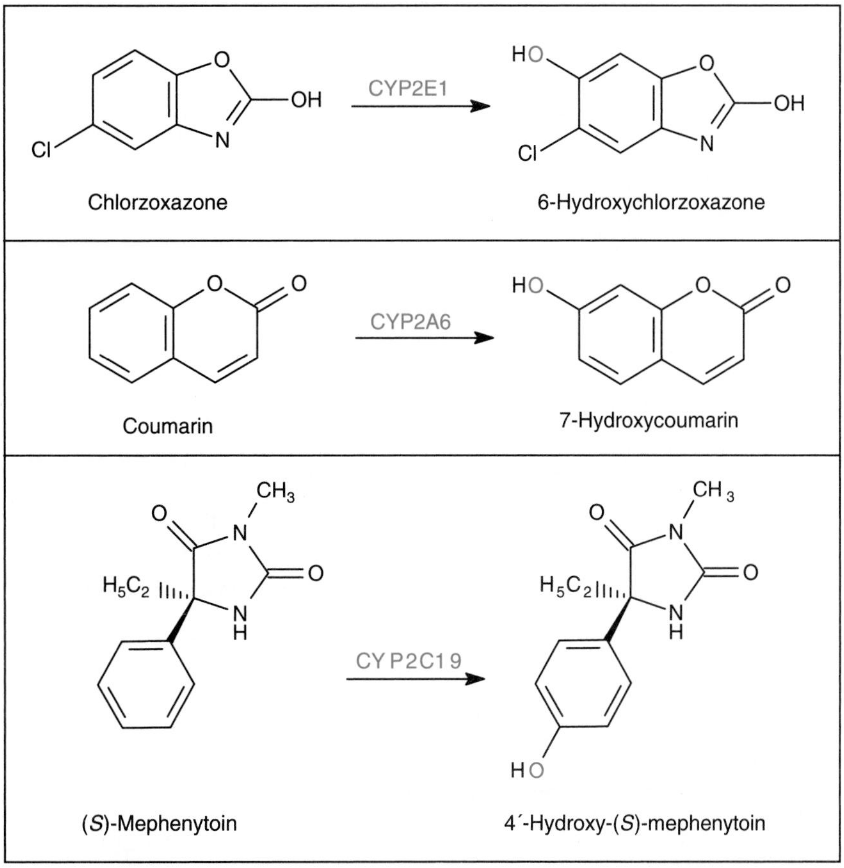

Figure 6-41. Examples of reactions catalyzed by cytochrome P450: Hydroxylation of aromatic carbon.

of some aliphatic alkenes and alkynes produces metabolites that are sufficiently reactive to bind covalently to the heme moiety of cytochrome P450, a process known as suicide inactivation or mechanism-based inhibition (discussed later in section "Inhibition of Cytochrome P450"). As previously discussed in the section on epoxide hydrolase, not all epoxides are highly reactive electrophiles. Although the 3,4-epoxidation of coumarin produces an hepatotoxic metabolite, the 10,11-epoxidation of carbamazepine produces a stable, relatively nontoxic metabolite (Fig. 6-42).

In the presence of NADPH and O_2, liver microsomes catalyze the oxygenation of several sulfur-containing xenobiotics, including chlorpromazine, cimetidine, lansoprazole, and omeprazole. Sulfur-containing xenobiotics can potentially undergo two consecutive sulfoxidation reactions: one that converts the sulfide (S) to the sulfoxide (SO), which occurs during the sulfoxidation of chlorpromazine and cimetidine, and one that converts the sulfoxide (SO) to the sulfone (SO_2), which occurs during the sulfoxidation of omeprazole and lansoprazole, as shown in Fig. 6-43. Albendazole is converted first to a sulfoxide and then to a sulfone. All of these reactions are catalyzed by FMO (as shown in Fig. 6-37b) and/or cytochrome P450 (as shown in Fig. 6-43). Both enzymes are efficient catalysts of S-oxygenation, and both contribute significantly to the sulfoxidation of various xenobiotics. For example, the sulfoxidation of omeprazole, lansoprazole, chlorpromazine, and phenothiazine by human liver microsomes is primarily catalyzed by a CYP enzyme (namely, CYP3A4), whereas the sulfoxidation of cimetidine is primarily catalyzed by FMO (namely, FMO3).

In the presence of NADPH and O_2, liver microsomes catalyze the oxygenation of several nitrogen-containing xenobiotics, including chlorpromazine, doxylamine, oflaxacin, morphine, nicotine, MPTP, methapyrilene, methaqualone, metronidazole, pargyline, pyridine, senecionine, strychnine, trimethylamine, trimipramine, and verapamil, all of which are converted to stable N-oxides. Whereas S-oxygenation might be catalyzed by both cytochrome P450 and FMO, N-oxygenation is more likely to be catalyzed by just one of these enzymes. For example, the conversion of (S)-nicotine to trans-(S)-nicotine N-1'-oxide by human liver microsomes is catalyzed by FMO3, with little or no contribution from cytochrome P450. Conversely, the conversion of pyridine to its N-oxide is primarily catalyzed by cytochrome P450. Both enzymes can participate in the N-oxygenation of certain xenobiotics. For example, the N-oxygenation of chlorpromazine is catalyzed by FMO3 and, to a lesser extent, by two CYP enzymes (CYP2D6 and CYP1A2). In general, FMO catalyzes the N-oxygenation of xenobiotics containing electron-deficient nitrogen atoms, whereas cytochrome P450 catalyzes the N-oxygenation of xenobiotics containing electron-rich nitrogen atoms. Therefore, substrates primarily N-oxygenated by cytochrome P450 are somewhat limited to pyridine-containing xenobiotics, such as the tobacco-specific nitrosamine NNK and the antihistamine temelastine, and to xenobiotics containing a quinoline or isoquinoline group, such as the muscle relaxant 6,7-dimethoxy-4-(4'-chlorobenzyl)isoquinoline.

The initial step in heteroatom oxygenation by cytochrome P450 involves the abstraction of an electron from the heteroatom (N, S,

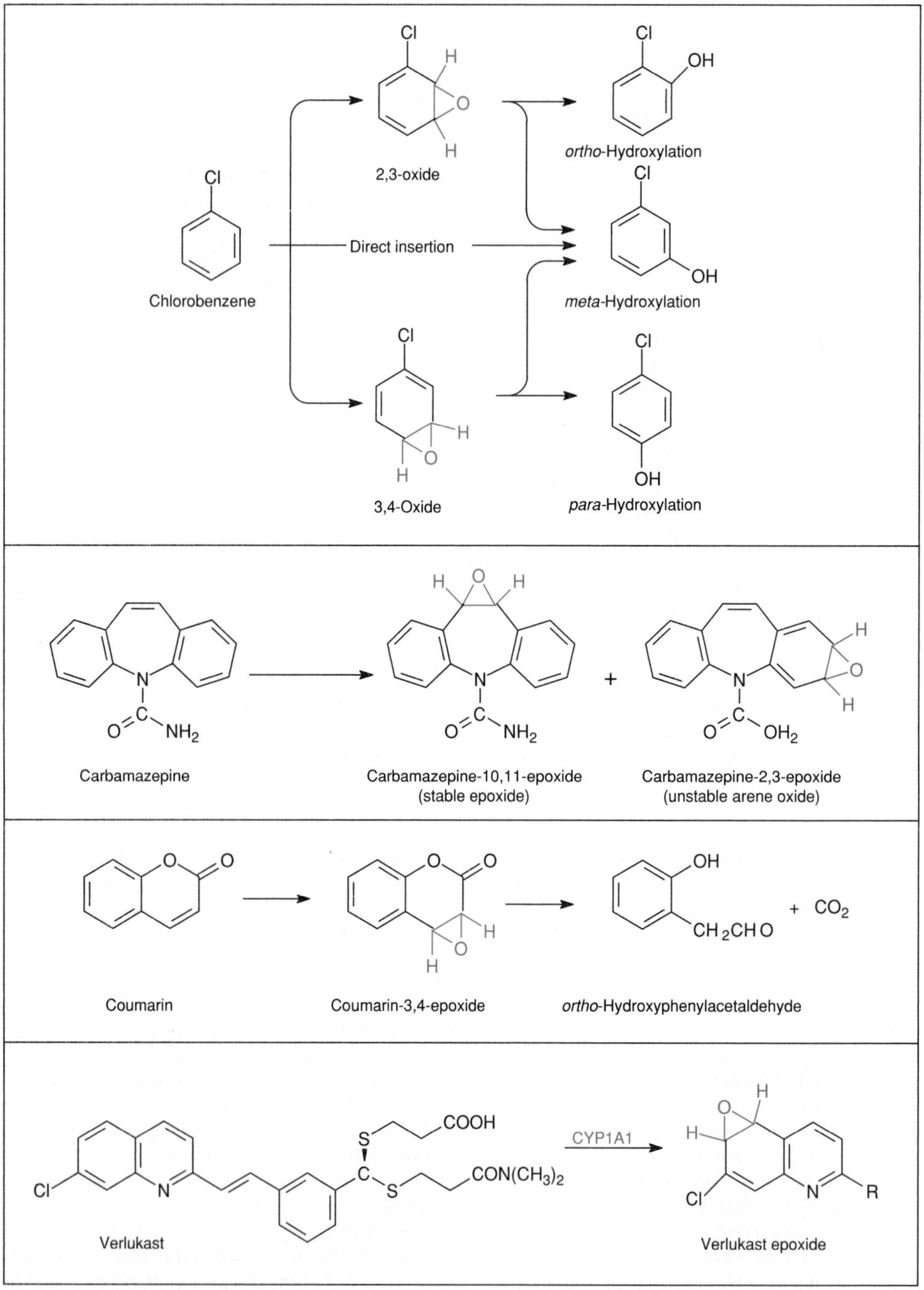

Figure 6-42. *Examples of reactions catalyzed by cytochrome P450: Epoxidation.*

or *I*) by the (FeO)$^{3+}$ complex, as shown below for sulfoxidation.

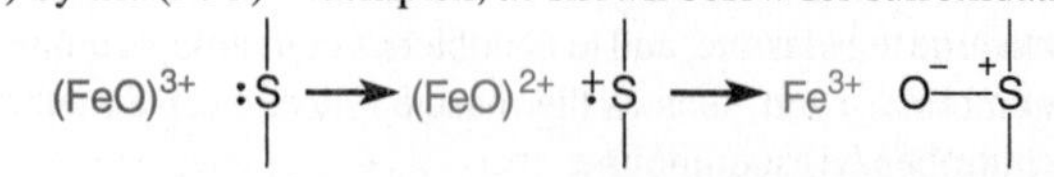

$$(FeO)^{3+} \ :\!\overset{|}{\underset{|}{S}} \ \longrightarrow \ (FeO)^{2+} \ \ddagger\overset{|}{\underset{|}{S}} \ \longrightarrow \ Fe^{3+} \ \ O^{-}\!\!-\!\!\overset{+}{\underset{|}{S}}$$

Abstraction of an electron from *N*, *O*, or *S* by the (FeO)$^{3+}$ complex is also the initial step in heteroatom dealkylation, but in

this case abstraction of the electron from the heteroatom is quickly followed by abstraction of a proton (H$^+$) from the α-carbon atom (the carbon atom attached to the heteroatom). Oxygen rebound leads to hydroxylation of the α-carbon, which then rearranges to form the corresponding aldehyde or ketone with cleavage of the α-carbon from the heteroatom, as shown below for the N-dealkylation of an

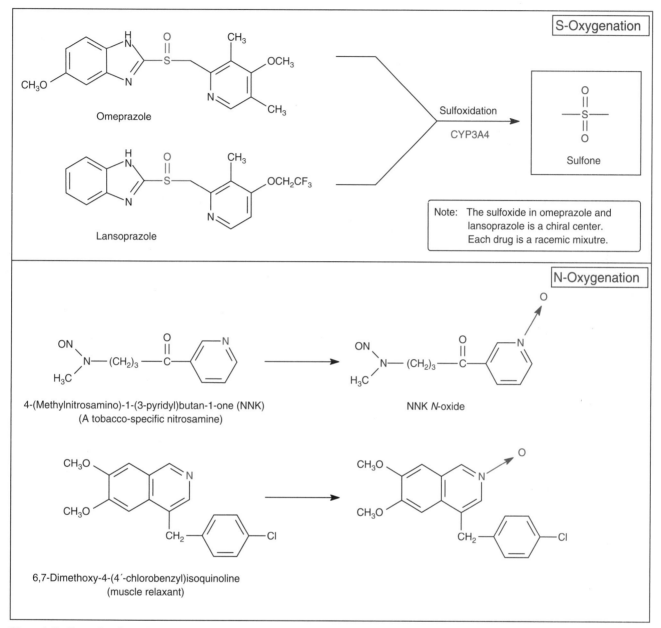

Figure 6-43. *Examples of reactions catalyzed by cytochrome P450: Heteroatom oxygenation.*

N-alkylamine:

$(FeO)^{3+}$:N— $\longrightarrow$ $(FeO)^{2+}$ $\overset{+}{\cdot}$N— $\longrightarrow$ $Fe(OH)^{3+}$:N— $\longrightarrow$
CH₂R ... CH₂R ... ·CHR

Fe^{3+} :N— $\longrightarrow$:N— + O=CHR
HOCHR ... H

Although the initial steps in heteroatom oxygenation and heteroatom dealkylation are the same (abstraction of an electron from the heteroatom to produce a radical cation), the nature of the radical cation determines whether the xenobiotic will undergo oxygenation or dealkylation. The sulfur radical cations of numerous xenobiotics are sufficiently stable to allow oxygen rebound with the heteroatom itself, which results in S-oxygenation. However, this is not generally the case with nitrogen radical cations, which undergo rapid deprotonation at the α-carbon, which in turn results in N-dealkylation. In general, therefore, cytochrome P450 catalyzes the N-dealkylation, not the N-oxygenation, of amines. N-Oxygenation by cytochrome P450 can occur if the nitrogen radical cation is stabilized by a nearby electron-donating group (making the nitrogen electron rich) or if α-protons are either absent (e.g., aromatic amines) or inaccessible (e.g., quinidine). In the case of primary and secondary aromatic amines, N-oxygenation by cytochrome P450 usually results in the formation of arylhydroxylamines, as illustrated in Fig. 6-11. N-Hydroxylation of aromatic amines with subsequent O-acetylation or O-sulfonation is one mechanism by which tumorigenic aromatic amines, such as 2-acetylaminofluorene and 4-aminobiphenyl, are converted to electrophilic reactive intermediates that bind covalently to DNA.

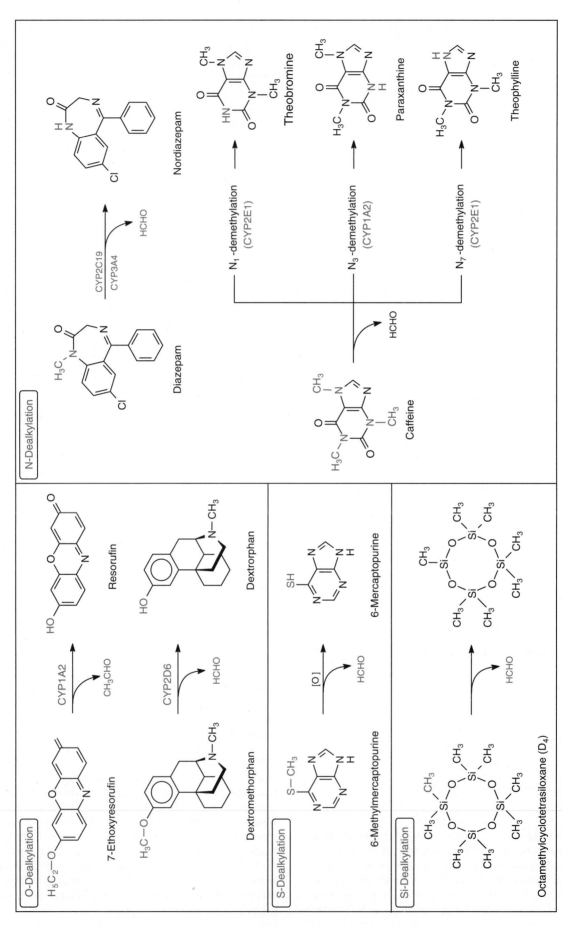

Figure 6-44. Examples of reactions catalyzed by cytochrome P450: Heteroatom dealkylation.

In contrast to cytochrome P450, which oxidizes nitrogen-containing xenobiotics by a radicaloid mechanism involving an initial one-electron oxidation of the heteroatom, FMO oxidizes nitrogen-containing xenobiotics by a heterolytic mechanism involving a two-electron oxidation by the 4a-hydroperoxide of FAD (see Fig. 6-38). These different mechanisms explain why the N-oxygenation of xenobiotics by cytochrome P450 generally results in N-dealkylation, whereas N-oxygenation by the FMO results in *N*-oxide formation. In contrast to cytochrome P450, FMO does not catalyze N-, O-, or S-dealkylation reactions.

Numerous xenobiotics are N-, O-, or S-dealkylated by cytochrome P450, and some examples of these heteroatom dealkylation reactions are shown in Fig. 6-44. The dealkylation of xenobiotics containing an N-, O-, or S-methyl group results in the formation of formaldehyde, which can easily be measured by a simple colorimetric assay to monitor the demethylation of substrates in vitro. The expiration of ^{13}C- or ^{14}C-labelled carbon dioxide following the demethylation of drugs containing a ^{13}C- or ^{14}C-labelled methyl group has been used to probe cytochrome P450 activity in vivo (Watkins, 1994). The activity of the human CYP enzymes involved in the N-demethylation of aminopyrine, erythromycin, and caffeine can be assessed by this technique. Although caffeine has three *N*-methyl groups, all of which can be removed by cytochrome P450, the major pathway in humans involves N3-demethylation of caffeine to paraxanthine (see Fig. 6-44).

Whereas the metabolism of *N*-methyl amines by cytochrome P450 generally results in N-demethylation, with the hydroxylation of the methyl group leading to the release of formaldehyde, the metabolism of *N*-methyl amides and carbamates by cytochrome P450 often results in the formation of a stable methyl-hydroxylated metabolite; one that does not release formaldehyde (which would otherwise complete an N-demethylation reaction) possibly because of the hydroxymethyl metabolite formation of a six-membered configuration that is stabilized by hydrogen bonding, as illustrated below:

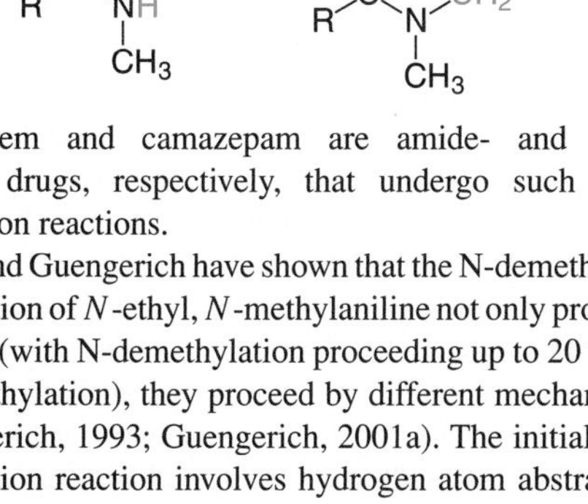

Zolpidem and camazepam are amide- and carbamate-containing drugs, respectively, that undergo such *N*-methyl-hydroxylation reactions.

Seto and Guengerich have shown that the N-demethylation and N-deethylation of *N*-ethyl, *N*-methylaniline not only proceed at different rates (with N-demethylation proceeding up to 20 times faster than N-deethylation), they proceed by different mechanisms (Seto and Guengerich, 1993; Guengerich, 2001a). The initial step in the N-deethylation reaction involves hydrogen atom abstraction from the α-carbon atom (i.e., the carbon atom attached to the nitrogen) whereas the initial step in the N-demethylation reaction involves a much faster reaction, namely, a one-electron transfer from the nitrogen atom, which is transferred to the FeO^{3+} complex in cytochrome

P450. Although the N-demethylation of *N*,*N*-substituted *amines* proceeds by the relatively rapid process of one-electron transfer, the *N*-demethylation of *N*,*N*-substituted *amides*, where the adjacent carbonyl causes electrons to be withdrawn from the nitrogen atom, proceeds by the relatively slow process of hydrogen atom abstraction, for which reason the latter reactions, in contrast to the former, show a large intrinsic isotope effect when the hydrogen atoms are replaced with deuterium (because it requires more energy to break a C–D bond than a C–H bond).

In addition to N-dealkylation, primary amines can also undergo oxidative deamination by cytochrome P450, which is an example of oxidative group transfer. The mechanism is similar to that of N-dealkylation: The α-carbon adjacent to the primary amine is hydroxylated, which produces an unstable intermediate that rearranges to eliminate ammonia with the formation of an aldehyde or ketone. The conversion of amphetamine to phenylacetone is an example of oxidative deamination, as shown in Fig. 6-45. Oxidative deamination is also catalyzed by monoamine oxidase (MAO). In the example given above, however, the substrate, amphetamine, contains an α-methyl group which renders it a poor substrate for MAO (as described in the section "Monoamine Oxidase, Diamine Oxidase, and Polyamine Oxidase", above).

In addition to oxidative deamination, cytochrome P450 catalyzes two other types of oxidative group transfer, namely, oxidative desulfuration and oxidative dehalogenation. In all cases the heteroatom (*N*, *S*, or halogen) is replaced with oxygen. As shown in Fig. 6-46, oxidative desulfuration converts parathion, which has little insecticidal activity, to paraoxon, which is a potent insecticide. The same reaction converts thiopental to pentobarbital. Diethyldithiocarbamate methyl ester, a metabolite of disulfiram, also undergoes oxidative desulfuration. The initial reaction involves S-oxidation by cytochrome P450 or FMO to a sulfine (R$_1$R$_2$C = S → R$_1$R$_2$C = S$^+$–O$^-$). In the presence of glutathione (GSH) and glutathione transferase, this sulfine is either converted back to the parent compound (R$_1$R$_2$C = S$^+$–O$^-$ + 2 GSH → R$_1$R$_2$C = S + GSSG + H$_2$O) or it undergoes desulfuration (R$_1$R$_2$C = S$^+$–O$^-$ + 2 GSH → R$_1$R$_2$C = O + GSSG + H$_2$S) (Madan *et al.*, 1994).

Cytochrome P450 catalyzes both reductive and oxidative dehalogenation reactions (Guengerich, 1991). During oxidative dehalogenation, a halogen and hydrogen from the same carbon atom are replaced with oxygen (R$_1$R$_2$CHX → R$_1$R$_2$CO) to produce an aldehyde or acylhalide, as shown in Fig. 6-18 for the conversion of halothane (CF$_3$CHClBr) to trifluoroacetylchloride (CF$_3$COCl). Oxidative dehalogenation does not involve a direct attack on the carbon–halogen bond, but it involves the formation of an unstable halohydrin by oxidation of the carbon atom bearing the halogen substituent. The carbon–halogen bond is broken during the rearrangement of the unstable halohydrin. When the carbon atom contains a single halogen, the resulting product is an aldehyde, which can be further oxidized to a carboxylic acid or reduced to a primary alcohol. When the carbon atom contains two halogens, the dihalohydrin intermediate rearranges to an acylhalide, which can be converted to the corresponding carboxylic acid (see Fig. 6-18). As discussed previously, aldehydes and, in particular, acylhalides are reactive compounds that can bind covalently to protein and other critical cellular molecules. The immune hepatitis caused by repeated exposure of humans to halothane and related volatile anesthetics is dependent on oxidative dehalogenation by cytochrome P450, with neoantigens produced by the trifluoroacetylation of proteins, as shown in Fig. 6-18.

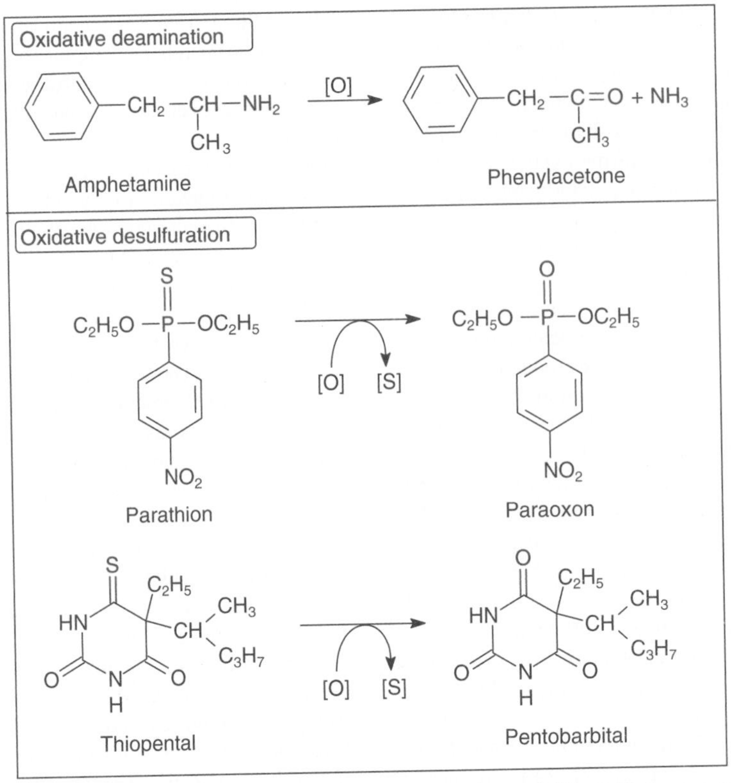

Figure 6-45. Examples of reactions catalyzed by cytochrome P450: Oxidative group transfer.

Cytochrome P450 can catalyze the reductive dehalogenation of halogenated alkanes (see Figs. 6-17 and 6-18) and the reduction of certain azo- and nitro-containing xenobiotics, although these latter reactions are largely catalyzed by gut microflora (see Fig. 6-10). The ability of cytochrome P450 to reduce xenobiotics can be understood from the catalytic cycle shown in Fig. 6-39. Binding of a substrate to cytochrome P450 is followed by a one-electron reduction by NADPH–cytochrome P450 reductase. Under aerobic conditions, reduction of the heme iron to the ferrous state permits binding of oxygen. Anaerobic conditions, in contrast, interrupt the cycle at this point, which allows cytochrome P450 to reduce those substrates capable of accepting an electron. Therefore, cytochrome P450 can catalyze reduction reactions, such as azo-reduction, nitro-reduction, and reductive dehalogenation, particularly under conditions of low oxygen tension. In effect, the substrate rather than molecular oxygen accepts electrons and is reduced. In fact, oxygen acts as an inhibitor of these reactions because it competes with the substrate for the reducing equivalents. The toxicity of many halogenated alkanes is dependent on their biotransformation by reductive dehalogenation. The first step in reductive dehalogenation is a one-electron reduction catalyzed by cytochrome P450, which produces a potentially toxic, carbon-centered radical and inorganic halide. The conversion of CCl_4 to a trichloromethyl radical and other toxic metabolites is shown in Fig. 6-17.

The oxidative desulfuration of parathion (see Fig. 6-45) involves the production of an intermediate that rearranges to paraoxon (as shown in Fig. 6-46). This same intermediate can decompose to 4-nitrophenol and diethylphosphorothioic acid, which are the same products formed by the hydrolysis of parathion (Fig. 6-46). In addition to facilitating the hydrolysis of phosphoric acid esters, cy-

tochrome P450 also catalyzes the cleavage of carboxylic acid esters, as shown in Fig. 6-46. Carboxylic acid esters typically are cleaved by carboxylesterases, which results in the formation of an acid and an alcohol ($R_1COOCH_2R_2 + H_2O \rightarrow R_1COOH + R_2CH_2OH$). In contrast, cytochrome P450 converts carboxylic acid esters to an acid plus aldehyde ($R_1COOCH_2 R_2 + [O] \rightarrow R_1COOH + R_2CHO$), as shown in Fig. 6-46. The deacylation of loratadine is the major route of biotransformation of this nonsedating antihistamine. The reaction is catalyzed predominantly by cytochrome P450 (namely, CYP3A4 with a minor contribution from CYP2D6), with little contribution from carboxylesterases.

Cytochrome P450 can also catalyze the dehydrogenation of a number of compounds, including acetaminophen, nifedipine, and related dihydropyridine calcium-channel blockers, sparteine, nicotine, and testosterone, as shown in Fig. 6-47. Dehydrogenation by cytochrome P450 converts acetaminophen to its hepatotoxic metabolite, N-acetylbenzoquinoneimine, as shown in Fig. 6-34. The formation of a double bond during the conversion of digitoxin (dt_3) to 15′-dehydro-dt_3 leads to cleavage of the terminal sugar residue to produce digitoxigenin bisdigitoxoside (dt_2) (Fig. 6-47), which can similarly be converted to 9′-dehydro-dt_2, which undergoes digitoxosyl cleavage to digitoxigenin monodigitoxoside (dt_1). In contrast to digitoxin, this latter metabolite is an excellent substrate for glucuronidation. In rats, the CYP enzymes responsible for converting digitoxin to dt_1 (namely, the CYP3A enzymes) and the UGT responsible for glucuronidating dt_1 are inducible by dexamethasone, pregnenolone-16α-carbonitrile and spironolactone, all of which protect rats from the toxic effects of digitoxin. The dehydrogenation of nicotine produces nicotine $\Delta^{1',5'}$-iminium ion, which is oxidized by cytosolic aldehyde oxidase to cotinine, a major metabolite of nicotine excreted in the urine of cigarette smokers (see Fig. 6-47).

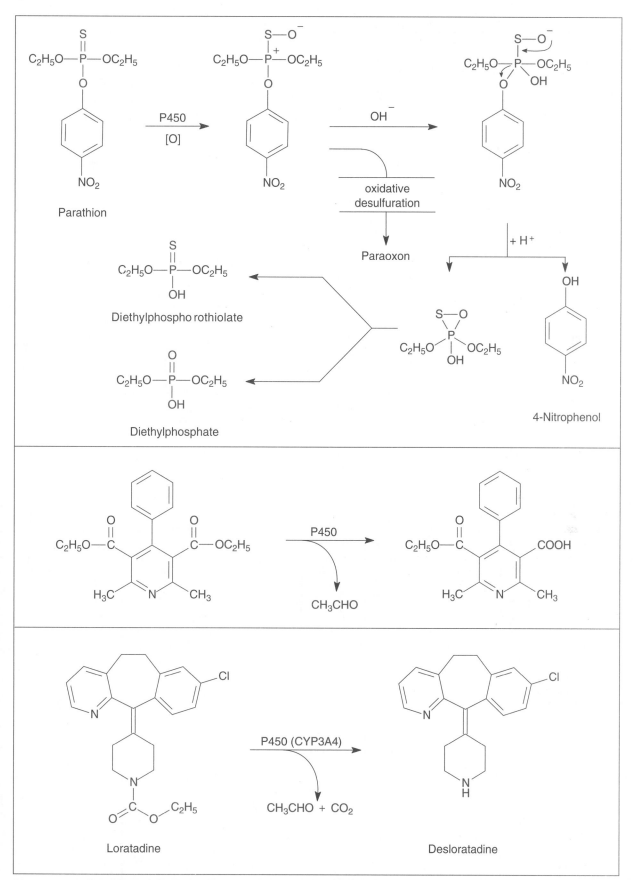

Figure 6-46. Examples of reactions catalyzed by cytochrome P450: Cleavage of esters.

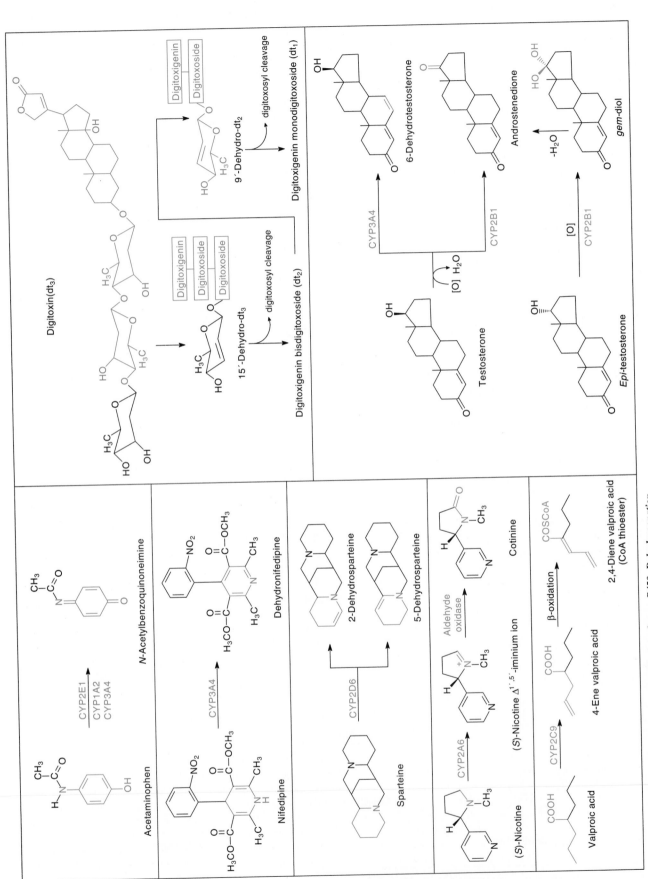

Figure 6-47. *Examples of reactions catalyzed by cytochrome P450: Dehydrogenation.*

Testosterone is dehydrogenated by cytochrome P450 to two metabolites: 6-dehydrotestosterone, which involves formation of a carbon–carbon double bond, and androstenedione, which involves formation of a carbon–oxygen double bond, as shown in Fig. 6-47. The conversion of testosterone to androstenedione is one of several cases where cytochrome P450 converts a primary or secondary alcohol to an aldehyde or ketone, respectively. The reaction can proceed by formation of a *gem*-diol (two hydroxyl groups on the same carbon atom), with subsequent dehydration to a keto group, as shown in Fig. 6-24 for the conversion of ethanol to acetaldehyde. However, *gem*-diols are not obligatory intermediates in the oxidation of alcohols by cytochrome P450, and in fact the conversion of testosterone to androstenedione by CYP2B1 (the major phenobarbital-inducible CYP enzyme in rats) does not involve the intermediacy of a *gem*-diol but proceeds by direct dehydrogenation (Fig. 6-47). In contrast, a *gem*-diol is involved in the formation of androstenedione from *epi*-testosterone (which is identical to testosterone except the hydroxyl group at C17 is in the α-configuration, not the β-configuration). The fact that formation of androstenedione from *epi*-testosterone involves formation of a *gem*-diol, whereas its formation from testosterone does not, makes it difficult to generalize the mechanism by which cytochrome P450 converts alcohols to aldehydes and ketones.

Liver microsomes from all mammalian species contain numerous CYP enzymes, each with the potential to catalyze the various types of reactions shown in Figs. 6-40 through 6-47. In other words, all of the CYP enzymes expressed in liver microsomes have the potential to catalyze xenobiotic hydroxylation, epoxidation, dealkylation, oxygenation, dehydrogenation, and so forth. The broad and often overlapping substrate specificity of liver microsomal CYP enzymes precludes the possibility of naming these enzymes for the reactions they catalyze, which are now categorized into families and subfamilies and named individually on the basis of their amino acid sequence. As shown in Table 6-9, the CYP enzymes involved in xenobiotic biotransformation belong mainly to the CYP1, 2, and 3 gene families. The CYP enzymes involved in endobiotic metabolism generally have the same name in all mammalian species. Some of the xenobiotic-biotransforming CYP enzymes have the same name in all mammalian species, whereas others are named in a species-specific manner. For example, all mammalian species contain two CYP enzymes belonging to the CYP1A subfamily, and in all cases these are known as CYP1A1 and CYP1A2 because the function and regulation of these enzymes are highly conserved among mammalian species. The same is true of CYP1B1, 2E1, 2R1, 2S1, 2U1, and 2W1, all of which are highly conserved orthologs that can be given the same name across mammalian species. In most other cases, functional or evolutionary relationships are not immediately apparent; hence, the CYP enzymes are named in a species-specific manner, and the names are assigned in chronological order regardless of the species of origin. For example, human liver microsomes express CYP2D6, but this is the only functional member of the CYP2D subfamily found in human liver. CYP2D7 and 2D8 are human pseudogenes. The other members of this subfamily (i.e., CYP2D1–CYP2D5 and CYP2D5 onward) are the names given to CYP2D enzymes in other species.

Without exception, the levels and activity of each CYP enzyme have been shown to vary from one individual to the next, due to environmental and/or genetic factors. Decreased CYP enzyme activity can result from (1) a genetic mutation that either blocks the synthesis of a CYP enzyme or leads to the synthesis of a catalytically compromised, inactive, or unstable enzyme, which give rise to the poor and intermediate metabolizer (PM and IM) genotypes; (2) exposure to an environmental factor (such as an infectious disease or an inflammatory process) that suppresses CYP enzyme expression, or (3) exposure to a xenobiotic that inhibits or inactivates a preexisting CYP enzyme. By inhibiting cytochrome P450, one drug can impair the biotransformation of another, which may lead to an exaggerated pharmacological or toxicological response to the second drug. In this regard, inhibition of cytochrome P450 by a drug (and suppression of cytochrome P450 by infection, vaccination, or inflammation) essentially mimics the effects of a genetic deficiency in CYP enzyme expression (i.e., these environmental factors mimic the IM or PM genotype depending on the degree to which they decrease CYP activity). Genetic deficiencies in CYP expression, CYP inhibition and, to a lesser extent, CYP suppression all contribute significantly to inter-individual variability in drug metabolism and toxicity, and inhibition of CYP activity is a major cause of drug–drug interactions. Examples of the impact of these genetic and environmental factors on drug metabolism and toxicity are given later in this section in the overviews of individual CYP enzymes and in the section "Inhibition of Cytochrome P450."

Increased CYP enzyme activity can result from (1) gene duplication leading to overexpression of a CYP enzyme, which gives rise to the ultra-rapid metabolizer (UM) genotype; (2) exposure to drugs and other xenobiotics that induce the synthesis of cytochrome P450, or (3) exposure to drugs and other xenobiotics that stimulate the activity of a preexisting enzyme (a process known as homotropic or heterotropic activation depending on whether the drug stimulates its own metabolism or the metabolism of other drugs, respectively). Activation of cytochrome P450 has been documented in vitro and in some in situ situations, such as the pronounced (up to 25-fold) activation of *R*-warfarin 10-hydroxylation by quinidine in rabbit liver microsomes and perfused rabbit liver (Chen *et al.*, 2004a). However, in general, activation does not appear to be a major cause of drug–drug interactions. Although duplication of functional CYP2D6 genes has been documented (and shown to be relevant to drug metabolism and safety [see section "CYP2D6"]), induction of cytochrome P450 by xenobiotics is the most common mechanism by which CYP enzyme activity is increased to a pharmacologically relevant extent. By inducing cytochrome P450, one drug can stimulate the metabolism of a second drug and thereby decrease or ameliorate its therapeutic effect. Enzyme induction is a particular concern when it compromises the therapeutic effectiveness of drugs that have a narrow therapeutic index and are being used to treat a life-threatening illness, such as anti-HIV drugs, antirejection drugs (like cyclosporine and tacrolimus), and oral anticoagulants (like warfarin), or when it is used with drugs that exhibit a quantal (all-or-nothing) dose–response relationship, such as oral contraceptive steroids (which either block or don't block ovulation and thereby provide or don't provide protection against unwanted pregnancy).

The environmental factors known to affect P450 levels include medications (e.g., prescription drugs as well as herbal remedies), foods (e.g., cruciferous vegetables, charcoal-broiled beef), social habits (e.g., alcohol consumption, cigarette smoking), and disease status (diabetes, infection, inflammation, vaccination, liver and kidney disease, and both hyper- and hypothyroidism). When environmental factors influence CYP enzyme levels, considerable variation may be observed during repeated measures of xenobiotic biotransformation (e.g., drug metabolism) in the same individual. Such variation is not observed when alterations in CYP activity are determined genetically.

Due to their broad substrate specificity, it is possible that two or more CYP enzymes can contribute to the metabolism of a single compound. For example, two CYP enzymes, designated CYP2D6 and CYP2C19, both contribute significantly to the metabolism of propranolol in humans: CYP2D6 oxidizes the aromatic ring to give 4-hydroxypropranolol, whereas CYP2C19 oxidizes the isopropanolamine side chain to give naphthoxylactic acid (see Fig. 6-27). Consequently, changes in either CYP2D6 or CYP2C19 alone do not markedly affect the disposition of propranolol, but a rare combined genetic deficiency of both enzymes severely impairs propranolol metabolism. Three human CYP enzymes, CYP1A2, CYP2E1, and CYP3A4, can convert the commonly used analgesic, acetaminophen, to its hepatotoxic metabolite, N-acetylbenzoquinoneimine (Figs. 6-34 and 6-47). It is also possible for a single CYP enzyme to catalyze two or more metabolic pathways for the same drug. For example, CYP2D6 catalyzes both the O-demethylation and 5-hydroxylation (aromatic ring hydroxylation) of methoxyphenamine, and CYP3A4 catalyzes the 3-hydroxylation and N-oxygenation of quinidine, the 1′- and 4-hydroxylation of midazolam, the *tert*-butyl-hydroxylation and N-dealkylation of terfenadine, and several pathways of testosterone oxidation, including 1β-, 2β-, 6β-, and 15β-hydroxylation and dehydrogenation to 6-dehydrotestosterone (Figs. 6-40 and 6-47).

The pharmacological or toxic effects of certain drugs are exaggerated in a significant percentage of the population due to a heritable deficiency in a CYP enzyme (Meyer, 1994; Tucker, 1994). The observation that individuals who are genetically deficient in a particular CYP enzyme are poor metabolizers of one or more drugs illustrates a very important principle, namely, that the rate of elimination of drugs can be largely determined by a single CYP enzyme. This observation seems to contradict the fact that CYP enzymes have broad and overlapping substrate specificities. The resolution to this apparent paradox lies in the fact that although more than one human CYP enzyme can catalyze the biotransformation of a xenobiotic, they may do so with markedly different affinities. Consequently, xenobiotic biotransformation in vivo, where only low substrate concentrations are usually achieved, is often determined by the CYP enzyme with the highest affinity (lowest apparent K_m) for the xenobiotic. For example, the N-demethylation of diazepam (shown in Fig. 6-44) and the 5-hydroxylation of omeprazole are both catalyzed by two human CYP enzymes, namely, CYP2C19 and CYP3A4. However, these reactions are catalyzed by CYP3A4 with such low affinity that the N-demethylation of diazepam and the 5-hydroxylation of omeprazole in vivo are largely determined by CYP2C19. When several CYP enzymes catalyze the same reaction, their relative contribution to xenobiotic biotransformation is determined by the kinetic parameter, V_{max}/K_m, which is a measure of in vitro intrinsic clearance at low substrate concentrations ($<10\%$ of K_m).

A drug whose clearance is largely determined by a single CYP enzyme (or any single route of elimination) is said to have high *victim* or *object* potential, meaning its rate of clearance will be decreased by genetic polymorphisms and inhibitory drugs that result in a loss of that particular CYP activity and increased by drugs and other xenobiotics that induce that particular CYP enzyme. For example, a drug that is largely cleared by CYP2D6 will be slowly metabolized in CYP2D6 PMs and rapidly metabolized in CYP2D6 UMs, whereas a drug whose clearance is largely determined by CYP3A4 will be slowly metabolized in the presence of ketoconazole (and other CYP3A4 inhibitors) and rapidly metabolized in the presence of rifampin or St. John's wort (and other CYP3A4 in-

ducers). Accordingly, for drugs under development, considerable attention is paid to identifying which CYP enzyme or enzymes are involved in eliminating the drug, a process known as *reaction phenotyping* or *enzyme mapping*. Four in vitro approaches have been developed for reaction phenotyping. Each has its advantages and disadvantages, and a combination of approaches is usually required to identify which human CYP enzyme is responsible for metabolizing a xenobiotic. The four approaches to reaction phenotyping are as follows:

1. Correlation analysis, which involves measuring the rate of xenobiotic metabolism by several samples of human liver microsomes and correlating reaction rates with the variation in the level or activity of the individual CYP enzymes in the same microsomal samples. This approach is successful because the levels of the CYP enzymes in human liver microsomes vary enormously from sample to sample (up to 100-fold) but vary independently from each other.

2. Chemical inhibition, which involves an evaluation of the effects of known CYP enzyme inhibitors on the metabolism of a xenobiotic by human liver microsomes. Chemical inhibitors of cytochrome P450, which are discussed later, must be used cautiously because most of them can inhibit more than one CYP enzyme. Some chemical inhibitors are mechanism-based inhibitors that require biotransformation to a metabolite that inactivates or noncompetitively inhibits cytochrome P450.

3. Antibody inhibition, which involves an evaluation of the effects of inhibitory antibodies against selected CYP enzymes on the biotransformation of a xenobiotic by human liver microsomes. Due to the ability of antibodies to inhibit selectively and noncompetitively, this method alone can potentially establish which human CYP enzyme is responsible for biotransforming a xenobiotic. Unfortunately, the utility of this method is limited by the availability of specific inhibitory antibodies.

4. Biotransformation by purified or recombinant (cDNA-expressed) human CYP enzymes, which can establish whether a particular CYP enzyme can or cannot biotransform a xenobiotic, but it does not address whether that CYP enzyme contributes substantially to reactions catalyzed by human liver microsomes. The information obtained with purified or recombinant human CYP enzymes can be improved by taking into account large differences in the extent to which the individual CYP enzymes are expressed in human liver microsomes, which is summarized in Table 6-10.

Some CYP enzymes, such as CYP1A1 and CYP1B1, are expressed at such low levels in human liver microsomes that they do not contribute significantly to the hepatic biotransformation of xenobiotics that are excellent substrates for these enzymes. Other CYP enzymes are expressed in some but not all livers. For example, CYP3A5 is expressed in ~25% of human livers. It should be emphasized that reaction phenotyping in vitro is not always carried out with pharmacologically or toxicologically relevant substrate concentrations. As a result, the CYP enzyme that appears responsible for biotransforming the drug in vitro may not be the CYP enzyme responsible for biotransforming the drug in vivo. This may be particularly true of CYP3A4, which metabolizes several drugs with high capacity but low affinity.

Reaction phenotyping (often in conjunction with clinical observation) has been used to characterize the substrate specificity of many of the CYP enzymes expressed in human liver microsomes.

Table 6-10

Concentration of Individual P450 Enzymes in Human Liver and Intestinal Microsomes

	LIVER				INTESTINE
P450 ENZYME	SPECIFIC CONTENT (PMOL/MG PROTEIN)				
	SOURCE 1[a]	SOURCE 2[b]	SOURCE 3[b]	SOURCE 4[b]	SOURCE 5[c]
CYP1A2	52	45	42	15	
CYP2A6	36	68	42	12	
CYP2B6	11	39	1.0	3.0	
CYP2C8	24	64			
CYP2C9	73	96			11
CYP2C18	1	<2.5			
CYP2C19	14	19			2.1
CYP2D6	8	10	5.0	15	0.7
CYP2E1	61	49	22		
CYP3A4	155	108	98	40	58
CYP3A5	68	1.0			16
TOTAL	503	534	344		

[a]Data from Howgate EM, Rowland YK, Proctor NJ, Tucker GT, Rostami-Hodjegan A: Prediction of in vivo drug clearance from in vitro data. I: Impact of inter-individual variability. *Xenobiotica* 36:473–497, 2006; Rowland-Yeo K, Rostami-Hodjean A, Tucker GT: Abundance of cytochromes P450 in human liver: A meta-analysis. *Br J Clin Pharmacol* 57:687, 2004.

[b]Data from Rodrigues A: Integrated cytochrome P450 reaction phenotyping. *Biochem Pharmacol* 57:465–480, 1999.

[c]Data from Paine MF, Widmer WW, Hart HL, *et al.*: A furanocoumarin-free grapefruit juice establishes furanocoumarins as the mediators of the grapefruit juice-felodipine interaction. *Am J Clin Nutr* 83:1097–1105, 2006.

Examples of reactions catalyzed by individual human CYP enzymes are shown in Figs. 6-40 through 6-47, and lists of substrates, inhibitors, and inducers for each CYP enzyme are given in Table 6-11. The examples listed in Table 6-11 are largely based on examples cited by the U.S. Food and Drug Administration (FDA), which has provided, where possible, the following lists to guide the conduct of in vitro and in vivo pharmacokinetic drug–drug interaction studies: (1) preferred and acceptable CYP substrates and chemical inhibitors for reaction phenotyping in vitro; (2) sensitive probe substrates to monitor CYP activity in vivo (a sensitive substrate is one whose clearance is largely [>80%] determined by a single CYP enzyme such that loss of that CYP enzyme causes a fivefold or higher increase in exposure); (3) drugs that are strong or weak inhibitors of CYP enzymes in vivo; (4) preferred and acceptable inhibitors and inducers for use as positive controls for CYP inhibition and induction studies in vitro, and (5) drugs that are effective inducers of CYP enzymes in vivo (U.S. Food and Drug Administration, 2006).

The global features of the major xenobiotic-biotransforming human CYP enzymes are as follows:

1. Two CYP enzymes, namely, CYP2D6 and CYP3A4, metabolize the majority of orally effective drugs, but they often metabolize different drugs and they do not metabolize all drugs; consequently there are many drugs whose clearance is largely determined by CYP enzymes other than CYP2D6 or CYP3A4. Inter-individual variation in CYP2D6, which is largely confined to the liver, is largely determined by genetic factors whereas inter-individual variation in CYP3A4, which is expressed in liver and small intestine, is largely determined by environmental factors (such as inhibitory and inducing drugs).

2. CYP2D6, CYP2C9, CYP2C19, and CYP3A5 are four xenobiotic-biotransforming CYP enzymes whose expression is significantly influenced by genetic polymorphisms that give rise to poor metabolizer (PM) and extensive metabolizer (EM) phenotypes, the incidence of which varies from one ethnic group to

the next. Genetic polymorphisms do affect other CYP enzymes, but not to the same extent as these four CYP enzymes.

3. The induction of CYP3A4 is often associated with induction of CYP2A6, 2B6, 2C8, 2C9, and 2C19. CYP1A2, and CYP2E1 are also inducible enzymes, but they are induced by different mechanisms and xenobiotics. Consequently, CYP1A2, 2E1, and 3A4 represent three distinct classes of inducible human CYP enzymes. CYP2D6 is considered a noninducible enzyme.

The salient features of each of the major xenobiotic-biotransforming CYP enzymes, with emphasis on the CYP enzymes in human liver microsomes, are summarized below:

CYP1A1/2   All mammalian species possess two inducible CYP1A enzymes, namely, CYP1A1 and CYP1A2. Human liver microsomes contain relatively high levels of CYP1A2, but not CYP1A1, even though this enzyme is readily detectable in the human lung, intestine, skin, lymphocytes, and placenta, particularly from cigarette smokers. In contrast to CYP1A1, CYP1A2 is not expressed in extrahepatic tissues; therefore, in humans, CYP1A2 and CYP1A1 can be considered hepatic and extrahepatic enzymes, respectively. In addition to cigarette smoke, inducers of the CYP1A enzymes include charcoal-broiled meat (a source of polycyclic aromatic hydrocarbons), cruciferous vegetables (a source of various indoles), and omeprazole and lansoprazole, two proton-pump inhibitors used to suppress gastric acid secretion. In contrast, oral contraceptive drugs suppress the expression of CYP1A2.

CYP1A1 and CYP1A2 both catalyze the O-dealkylation of 7-methoxyresorufin and 7-ethoxyresorufin (see Fig. 6-44). Reactions preferentially catalyzed by CYP1A1 include the hydroxylation and epoxidation of polycyclic aromatic hydrocarbons (PAHs) like benzo[a]pyrene (B[a]P) (see Fig. 6-9) and the epoxidation of the leukotriene D_4 receptor antagonist, verlukast (Fig. 6-42). CYP1A2 catalyzes the N-hydroxylation of aromatic amines, such as 4-aminobiphenyl, 2-aminonaphthalene, and several carcinogenic

Table 6-11

Examples of Clinically Relevant Substrates, Inhibitors, and Inducers of the Major Human Liver Microsomal P450 Enzymes Involved in Xenobiotic Biotransformation

	CYP1A2	CYP2A6	CYP2B6	CYP2C8	CYP2C9	CYP2C19	CYP2E1
Substrates	Alosetron[a]	Coumarin[d]	Bupropion[d]	Amodiaquine[b]	Diclofenac[d]	Fluoxetine[b]	Aniline[b]
	Caffeine[b,c]	Nicotine[d]	Efavirenz[c,d]	Cerivastatin	Fluoxetine[b]	S-Mephenytoin[d,e]	Chlorzoxazone[d]
	Duloxetine[a]		Propofol[b]	Paclitaxel[d,e]	Flurbiprofen[b]	Lansoprazole[c]	Lauric acid[b]
	7-Ethoxyresorufin[b]		S-Mephenytoin[b]	Rosiglitazone[b,c]	Phenytoin[e]	Moclobemide	4-Nitrophenol[b]
	Phenacetin[d]		Cyclophosphamide	Repaglinide[a,c]	Tolbutamide[c,d]	Omeprazole[a–c]	
	Tacrine[b]		Ketamine		S-Warfarin[c–e]	Pantoprazole[c]	
	Tizanidine[e]		Meperidine				
	Theophylline[b,c,e]		Nevirapine				
Inhibitors	Acyclovir[f]	Methoxsalen[d]	Clopidogrel[b]	Gemfibrozil[b,c,h]	Amiodarone[c,g]	Fluvoxamine[c]	Clomethiazole[b]
	Cimetidine[f]	Pilocarpine[b]	3-Isopropenyl-3-methyl	Montelukast[d]	Capecitabine	Moclobemide[c]	Diallyldisulfide[b]
	Ciprofloxacin[g]	Tranylcypromine[d]	diamantane[b]	Pioglitazone[b]	Fluconazole[b,c,g]	Nootkatone[b]	Diethyldithiocarbamate[b]
	Famotidine[f]	Tryptamine[b]	2-Isopropenyl-2-	Quercetin[d]	Fluoxetine[b]	Omeprazole[c,h]	Disulfiram[c]
	Fluvoxamine[c,h]		methyladamantane[b]	Rosiglitazone[b]	Fluvoxamine[b]	Ticlopidine[b]	
	Furafylline[d]		Phencyclidine[b]	Rosuvastatin	Oxandrolone[g]		
	Mexiletene[g]		Sertraline[b]	Trimethoprim[b,f]	Sulfaphenazole[d]		
	α-Naphthoflavone[b]		Thio-TEPA[b]		Sulfinpyrazone[f]		
	Norfloxacin[f]		Ticlopidine[b]		Tienilic acid		
	Propafenone[g]		Phenylethylpiperidine				
	Verapamil[f]						
	Zileuton[g]						
Inducers	3-Methylcholanthrene[d]	Dexamethasone[d]	Phenobarbital[d]	Phenobarbital[b]	Phenobarbital	Phenobarbital	Ethanol[c]
	β-Naphthoflavone[d]	Pyrazole[b]	Phenytoin[b]	Rifampin[c,d]	Rifampin	Rifampin[c,d]	Isoniazid
	Omeprazole[d]		Rifampin				
	Lansoprazole[b]						
	TCDD						

[a] Classified by the FDA as a "sensitive substrate" (i.e., drugs whose plasma AUC values have been shown to increase by ≥fivefold when coadministered with a known CYP inhibitor).

[b] FDA-acceptable in vitro substrate, inhibitor, or inducer.

[c] FDA-provided examples of in vivo substrates, inhibitors, or inducers for oral administration. Substrates in this category have plasma AUCs that are increased by at least twofold (fivefold for CYP3A4 substrates) when co-administered with inhibitors of the enzyme. Inhibitors in this category increase the AUC of substrates for that enzyme by at least twofold (fivefold for CYP3A4). Inducers in this category decrease the plasma AUC of substrates for that enzyme by at least 30%.

[d] FDA-preferred in vitro substrate, inhibitor, or inducer.

[e] Classified by the FDA as a "substrate with narrow therapeutic range" (i.e., drugs whose exposure-response indicates that increases in their exposure levels by concomitant use of CYP inhibitors may lead to serious safety concerns such as Torsades de Pointes).

[f] Classified by the FDA as a "weak inhibitor" (i.e., caused a ≥1.25-fold but <twofold increase in plasma AUC or 20–50% decrease in the clearance of sensitive CYP substrates when the inhibitor was given at the highest approved dose and the shortest dosing interval in clinical evaluations).

[g] Classified by the FDA as a "moderate inhibitor" (i.e., caused a ≥ twofold but < fivefold increase in plasma AUC or 50–80% decrease in the clearance of sensitive CYP substrates when the inhibitor was given at the highest approved dose and the shortest dosing interval in clinical evaluations).

[h] Classified by the FDA as a "strong inhibitor" (i.e., caused a ≥ fivefold increase in plasma AUC or ≥ 80% decrease in the clearance of CYP substrates in clinical evaluations).

Note: All FDA classifications are based on information available as of May 1, 2006 at the following URL: http://www.fda.gov/cder/drug/drugInteractions/tableSubstrates.htm#classInhibit

Substrates

CYP2D6		CYP3A4				
Atomoxetine[c]	(R)-Metoprolol	Alfentanil[e]	Clopidogrel	Fentanyl[e]	Midazolam[a,c,d]	Saquinavir[a]
Amitriptyline	Methylphenidate	Alfuzosin	Cyclosporine[e]	Fluticasone[a]	Mifepristone	Sildenafil[a,c]
Aripiprazole	Mexiletine	Alprazolam	Depsipeptide	Gallopamil	Mosapride	Sibutramine
Brofaromine	Morphine	Amlodipine	Dexamethasone	Gefitinib	Nicardipine	Simvastatin[a,c]
(±)-Bufuralol[d]	Nortriptyline	Amprenavir	Dextromethorphan[b]	Gepirone	Nifedipine[b]	Sirolimus[e]
(S)-Chlorpheniramine	Ondansetron	Aprepitant	Diergotamine[e]	Granisetron	Nimodipine	Sunitinib
Chlorpromazine	Paroxetine	Artemether	α-Dihydroergocriptine	Gestodene	Nisoldipine	Tacrolimus[e]
Clomipramine	Perhexiline	Astemizole[e]	Disopyramide	Halofantrine	Nitrendipine	Tadalafil
Codeine	Pimozide	Atazanavir	Docetaxel	Laquinimod	Norethindrone	Telithromycin
Debrisoquine[b]	Propafenone	Atorvastatin	Domperidone	Imatinib	Oxatomide	Terfenadine[b,e]
Desipramine[a,c]	(+)-Propranolol	Azithromycin	Dutasteride	Indinavir	Oxybutynin	Testosterone[d]
Dextromethorphan[c,d]	Sparteine	Barnidipine	Ebastine	Isradipine	Perospirone	Tiagabine
Dolasetron	Tamoxifen	Bexarotene	Eletriptan[a,c]	Itraconazole	Pimozide[e]	Tipranavir
Duloxetine	Thioridazine[e]	Bortezomib	Eplerenone[a]	Karenitecin	Pranidipine	Tirilazad
Fentanyl	Timolol	Brotizolam	Ergotamine[e]	Ketamine	Praziquantel	Tofisopam
Haloperidol (reduced)	Tramadol	Budesonide[a]	Erlotinib	Levomethadyl	Quetiapine	Triazolam[a-c]
Imipramine	(R)-Venlafaxine	Buspirone[a,c]	Erythromycin[b]	Lonafarnib	Quinidine[e]	Trimetrexate
Loperamide		Capravirine	Eplerenone	Lopinavir	Quinine	Vardenafil[a]
		Carbamazepine	Ethosuximide	Loperamide	Reboxetine	Vinblastine
		Cibenzoline	Etoperidone	Lovastatin[a,c]	Rifabutin	Vincristine
		Cilastazol	Everolimus	Medroxyprogesterone	Ritonavir	Vinorelbine
		Cisapride[e]	Ethinyl estradiol	Methylprednisolone	Rosuvastatin	Ziprasidone
		Clarithromycin	Etoricoxib	Mexazolam	Ruboxistaurin	Zonisamide
		Clindamycin	Felodipine[a,c]		Salmetrol	

Inhibitors

CYP2D6		CYP3A4				
Amiodarone[f]	Fluoxetine[c,h]	Amiodarone	Cimetidine[f]	Fluvoxamine	Itraconazole[c,d,h]	Saquinavir[c,h]
Buproprion	Methadone	Amprenavir[g]	Clarithromycin[c,h]	Fosamprenavir[g]	Mibefradil	St. John's wort
Chlorpheniramine	Mibefradil	Aprepitant[g]	Diltiazem[g]	Gestodene	Nefazodone[c,h]	Telithromycin[c,h]
Cimetidine	Paroxetine[c,h]	Atazanavir[c,h]	Erythromycin[g]	Grapefruit Juice	Nelfinavir[c,h]	Troleandomycin[b]
Clomipramine	Quinidine[c,d]	Azamulin[b]	Felbamate	Ketoconazole[c,d,h]	Ritonavir[c,h]	Verapamil[b,g]
Duloxetine[g]	Sertraline[f]	Bosentan	Fluconazole[g]	Indinavir[c,h]	Roxithromycin	
Haloperidol	Terbinafine[g]					

Inducers

CYP2D6		CYP3A4				
NA		Amprenavir	Efavirenz	Nifedipine	Rifampin[c,d]	Troglitazone[b]
		Avasimibe	Etoposide	Omeprazole	Rifapentine[b]	Troleandomycin
		Bosentan	Guggulsterone	Paclitaxel[b]	Ritonavir	Vitamin E
		Carbamazepine[c]	Hyperforin	PCBs	Simvastatin	Vitamin K2
		Clotrimazole	Lovastatin	Phenobarbital[b]	Spironolactone	Yin zhi wuang
		Cyproterone acetate	Mifepristone	Phenytoin[b]	Sulfinpyrazole	
		Dexamethasone[b]	Nelfinavir	Rifabutin	Topotecan	

aromatic amines in tobacco smoke or cooked food, which in many cases represents the initial step in the conversion of aromatic amines to tumorigenic metabolites (see Fig. 6-11). Compared with their wild-type littermates, CYP1A1 knockout mice and CYP1A2 knockout mice would be expected to be resistant to the tumorigenic effects of PAHs like B[a]P and aromatic amines like 4-aminobiphenyl and the cooked-food mutagens IQ and PhIP, but they are not: Deletion of CYP1A2 has a potentiating effect on adduct and tumor formation (and methemoglobinemia) by aromatic amines, whereas deletion of CYP1A1 has a potentiating effect on the acute toxicity of oral B[a]P and the levels of adduct formation in extrahepatic tissues, presumably because CYP1A1 in the liver and small intestine of mice plays an important role in the presystemic clearance of B[a]P (which does not cause tumors in these tissues). These results suggest that, at least in mice, enzymes other than CYP1A1 (such as peroxidases and other CYP enzymes like CYP1B1) play important roles in the activation of PAH to reactive metabolites that induce skin and lung tumors, whereas enzymes other than CYP1A2 (such as peroxidases and other CYP enzymes, possibly members of the CYP2-4 families) play important roles in the activation of aromatic amines to reactive metabolites that cause liver and bladder tumors (Nebert and Dalton, 2006).

Drugs and other xenobiotics that are substrates, inhibitors, or inducers of human CYP1A2 are shown in Table 6-11. CYP1A2 catalyzes the O-dealkylation of phenacetin and the 4-hydroxylation of acetanilide, both of which produce acetaminophen, which can be converted by CYP1A2 and other CYP enzymes to a toxic benzoquinoneimine (Fig. 6-34). As shown in Fig. 6-44, CYP1A2 catalyzes the N3-demethylation of caffeine to paraxanthine. By measuring rates of formation of paraxanthine in blood, urine, or saliva or by measuring the exhalation of isotopically labeled CO_2 from ^{13}C- or ^{14}C-labeled caffeine, the N3-demethylation of caffeine can be used as an in vivo probe of CYP1A2 activity, which varies enormously from one individual to the next.

Although CYP1A1 and CYP1A2 are expressed in all mammals, there are species differences in their function and regulation.

For example, although CYP1A1 is not expressed in human liver (or in the liver of most other mammalian species), it appears to be constitutively expressed in Rhesus monkey and guinea pig liver. Conversely, although CYP1A2 is expressed in human liver (and in most other mammalian species), it does not appear to be constitutively expressed in Cynomolgus monkey liver. Polycyclic and polyhalogenated aromatic hydrocarbons appear to induce CYP1A enzymes in all mammalian species. In contrast, omeprazole is an inducer of CYP1A enzymes in humans, but not in mice or rabbits (Diaz *et al.*, 1990). The function of the CYP1A enzymes is fairly well conserved across species, although there are subtle differences. For example, in some species, such as the rat, CYP1A1 is considerably more effective than CYP1A2 as a catalyst of 7-ethoxyresorufin O-dealkylation, whereas the opposite is true in other species, such as rabbit. In mice, CYP1A1 and CYP1A2 catalyze the O-dealkylation of 7-ethoxyresorufin at comparable rates. In the rat, CYP1A1 preferentially catalyzes the O-dealkylation of 7-ethoxyresorufin whereas CYP1A2 preferentially catalyzes the O-dealkylation of 7-methoxyresorufin. However, in other species, such as the mouse and the human, CYP1A2 catalyzes the O-dealkylation of 7-ethoxyresorufin and 7-methoxyresorufin at about the same rate. In addition to differences in tissue distribution and substrate specificity, CYP1A1 and 1A2 can be distinguished by differences in their affinity for various inhibitors. Ellipticine and resveratrol preferentially inhibit CYP1A1, whereas the mechanism-based inhibitor furafylline is a specific inhibitor of CYP1A2 (in humans, but not in other species). CYP1A1 and CYP1A2 are both inhibited by α-naphthoflavone.

Although the levels of CYP1A2 vary enormously from one individual to the next, genetic defects in CYP1A2 (i.e., CYP1A2 poor metabolizers) are extremely rare. Several clinical studies have reported gender differences in CYP1A2, with most—but not all—studies reporting slightly higher CYP1A2 in males compared with females (with wide variation in both genders). Rasmussen *et al.* (2002) reported that, based on a clinical study of caffeine metabolism in 378 individuals, males have higher CYP1A2 activity than females. Although oral contraceptive treatment reduces CYP1A2 activity, the gender difference reported by Rasmussen *et al.* was significant even when women on oral contraceptive steroids were excluded from the analysis. Rasmussen *et al.* (2002) also demonstrated a strong correlation in CYP1A2 activity between identical (monozygous) twins and concluded that, despite the large number of environmental factors that can potentially influence CYP1A2 expression, genetic factors account for 70–75% of the observed variation in CYP1A2 activity.

CYP1B1 Human CYP1B1 shares many properties with CYP1A1: Both can activate polycyclic aromatic hydrocarbons (PAHs) to DNA-reactive (mutagenic) metabolites; both are expressed in extrahepatic tissues but not liver, and both are inducible by TCDD and other Ah receptor agonists, such that the levels of CYP1B1 in the aerodigestive tract, like those of CYP1A1, are elevated in cigarette smokers (Port *et al.*, 2004). In addition to being expressed in the respiratory and gastrointestinal tract, CYP1B1 is expressed in several estrogen-responsive tissues, such as mammary gland, ovary, and uterus. CYP1B1 is expressed in the eye, and genetic polymorphisms in CYP1B1 are associated with primary congenital glaucoma. CYP1B1 knockout mice also have structural eye defects, which suggest that CYP1B1 has an important physiological role in eye development. In addition to metabolizing PAHs, CYP1B1 also catalyzes the 4-hydroxylation of 17β-estradiol, which produces a catechol that can potentially oxidize to a toxic *ortho*-quinone.

Methylation of 4-hydroxyestradiol acts as a detoxication pathway in some tissues, as discussed in the section entitled *Methylation*. A role for CYP1B1 in chemical carcinogenesis is suggested by the observation that, compared with their wild-type littermates, CYP1B1 knockout mice are relatively resistant to PAH-induced tumor and lymphoma formation.

In addition to being under the transcriptional control of the Ah receptor, the expression of human CYP1B1 is controlled post-transcriptionally by the microRNA known as miR-27b, a small noncoding RNA that blocks the synthesis of CYP1B1 by binding to near-perfect matching sequences in the 3′-untranslated region of CYP1B1. The level of miR-27b is decreased and the level of CYP1B1 is correspondingly increased (overexpressed) in breast cancerous cells (and other cancerous tissues) (Tsuchiya *et al.*, 2006). The overexpression of CYP1B1 in malignant cells (coupled with and its ability to activate xenobiotics to reactive metabolites) is being exploited to activate a prodrug to a cytotoxic metabolite as a possible cancer treatment. A related approach is the development of CYP1B1 DNA vaccine, which has been shown in clinical trials to kill CYP1B1-expressing cancer cells (Maecker *et al.*, 2003).

CYP2A6 and 2A13 Enzymes belonging to the *CYP2A* gene family show marked species differences in catalytic function. For example, the two CYP2A enzymes expressed in rat liver, namely, CYP2A1 and CYP2A2, primarily catalyze the 7α- and 15α-hydroxylation of testosterone, respectively. In contrast, the CYP2A enzyme expressed in human liver, namely, CYP2A6, catalyzes the 7-hydroxylation of coumarin, as shown in Fig. 6-41. Just as rat CYP2A1 and CYP2A2 have little or no capacity to 7-hydroxylate coumarin, human CYP2A6 has little or no capacity to hydroxylate testosterone. Mouse liver microsomes contain three CYP2A enzymes; a testosterone 7α-hydroxylase (CYP2A12), a testosterone 15α-hydroxylase (CYP2A4), and a coumarin 7-hydroxylase (CYP2A5). Functionally, CYP2A5 can be converted to CYP2A4 by a single amino acid substitution (Phe$_{209}$ → Leu$_{209}$). In other words, this single amino substitution converts CYP2A5 from a coumarin 7-hydroxylating to a testosterone 15α-hydroxylating enzyme (Lindberg and Negishi, 1989). The fact that a small change in primary structure can have a dramatic effect on substrate specificity makes it difficult to predict whether orthologous proteins in different species (which are structurally similar but never identical) will catalyze the same reactions.

Differences in CYP2A function have important implications for the adverse effects of coumarin, which is hepatotoxic to rats but not humans. Whereas coumarin is detoxified in humans by conversion to 7-hydroxycoumarin, which is subsequently conjugated with glucuronic acid and excreted, a major pathway of coumarin biotransformation in rats involves formation of the hepatotoxic metabolite, coumarin 3,4-epoxide, as shown in Fig. 6-42. In addition to catalyzing the 7-hydroxylation of coumarin, CYP2A6 converts 1,3-butadiene to butadiene monoxide and nicotine to nicotine $\Delta^{1',5'}$-iminium ion, which is further oxidized by aldehyde oxidase to cotinine, as shown in Fig. 6-47.

Humans possess two functional CYP2A genes, namely, CYP2A6 and 2A13, and one nonfunctional CYP2A gene, namely, CYP2A7. CYP2A6 and the nonfunctional CYP2A7 are expressed in the liver but few extrahepatic tissues (with the notable exception of mammary gland), whereas CYP2A13 is expressed mainly in the lung (bronchus and trachea) and bladder, with lower levels in reproductive organs such as testis, ovary, uterus, and mammary gland. Hepatic CYP2A6 plays a major role in the metabolism of coumarin and nicotine, and plays a role in the metabolism of tegafur, fadrozole, methoxyflurane, and valproic acid. 8-Methoxypsoralen, a structural analog of coumarin, is a potent, mechanism-based inhibitor of CYP2A6. Other inhibitors of CYP2A6 are listed in Table 6-11. CYP2A13 does not appear to contribute to drug clearance, but it may play an important role in the activation of xenobiotics to toxic and carcinogenic metabolites in lung and bladder. CYP2A6 and CYP2A13 both activate nitrosamines to DNA-reactive (mutagenic) metabolites, especially those nitrosamines with bulky alkyl substituents such as NNK, N'-nitrosonorcotinine, and related nitrosomines found in tobacco smoke. (CYP2E1 also activates nitrosamines, but it preferentially activates nitrosamines with small alkyl substituents such as N-nitrosodimethylamine.)

The identification of three Japanese individuals who were poor metabolizers of SM-12502, an antiplatelet drug whose clearance is largely determined by CYP2A6, led to the identification of a genetic polymorphism that, in homozygous individuals, leads to the complete loss of CYP2A6 (CYP2A6*4C/*4C). The incidence of the CYP2A6 PM genotype is relatively high in Asians (up to 5% of Japanese, 3% of Chinese, 1.9% of Koreans, and 1.5% of Thais), but no such CYP2A6 PMs have been identified in Caucasians. Individuals who are genetically deficient in CYP2A6 have a considerably lower risk of cigarette-smoking-induced lung cancer presumably because these individuals have a reduced capacity for activating tobacco-smoke nitrosamines to carcinogenic metabolites (Kamataki et al., 2005). In support of this interpretation, the CYP2A inhibitor 8-methoxypsoralen protects mice from NNK-induced lung adenomas. CYP2A6 PMs are not only poor metabolizers of nitrosamines but they also are poor metabolizers of nicotine. Therefore, decreased cigarette consumption may also contribute to the lowered risk of lung cancer in CYP2A6 PMs. CYP2A6 is detectable in human lung, but the levels are considerably less than those of CYP2A13, which can activate the same carcinogens as CYP2A6. Therefore, it is not immediately obvious why a genetic deficiency in CYP2A6 protects against lung cancer. A similar situation occurs with CYP2D6 inasmuch as individuals lacking this hepatic enzyme (i.e., CYP2D6 PMs) also have a decreased risk of cigarette-smoking-induced lung cancer.

It seems somewhat paradoxical but just as CYP2A6 PMs have a decreased risk of lung cancer, so they have an increased risk of nasopharyngeal cancer, which is rare in Caucasians (Western countries) but endemic in Southern China and Southeast Asia. It has been postulated that, in the absence of CYP2A6, higher levels of nitrosamines and other carcinogens reach the nasal epithelium where they can be activated to carcinogenic metabolites by CYP2E1 and CYP2A13, both of which are expressed in nasal epithelium (Tiwawech et al., 2006).

Like CYP2A6, CYP2A13 can activate several carcinogens including many of the nitrosamines (e.g., NNK) and aromatic amines (e.g., 4-aminobiphenyl) that are present in cigarette smoke, and the mycotoxin aflatoxin B1. CYP2A13 is suspected of playing a role in the activation of carcinogens in tobacco smoke because it is localized in the two sites where cigarette smoking causes cancer, namely, the lung bronchus and bladder (Nakajima et al., 2006).

CYP2B6 CYP2B6 is expressed in human liver and, to a lesser extent, in kidney, intestine, and lung. It plays a major role in the metabolism of bupropion, efavirenz, and propofol, and the metabolism of these substrates (in addition to the N-demethylation, but not the 4'-hydroxylation, of S-mephenytoin) can be used in vitro or in vivo to assess CYP2B6 activity, as shown in Table 6-11. Other substrates for CYP2B6 include the anticancer drugs cyclophosphamide and tamoxifen. As shown in Table 6-11, several drugs have been shown to inhibit CYP2B6, and many of them do

so in a metabolism-dependent manner, such as clopidogrel, ticlopidine, and thio-TEPA. CYP2B6 is an inducible enzyme; it is generally co-induced with CYP3A4 and several CYP2C enzymes by xenobiotics that activate CAR and/or PXR, such as rifampin, the enzyme-inducing antiepileptic drugs (EIAEDs) such as phenobarbital, phenytoin, carbamazepine, and felbamate, and the herbal preparation of St. John's wort, which is the topic of a subsequent section (see the section "Induction of Cytochrome P450—Xenosensors").

CYP2C Enzymes Humans express four CYP2C enzymes, namely, CYP2C8, CYP2C9, 2C18, and 2C19. With the exception of CYP2C18, these CYP2C enzymes play a significant role in drug metabolism, and their inhibition or induction is the basis of a number of clinically important drug interactions. In the case of CYP2C9 and 2C19, genetic polymorphisms give rise to a PM phenotype, which also impacts the metabolism and safety or efficacy of certain drugs. As a general rule (to which there are many exceptions), CYP2C8 metabolizes large, acidic drugs, including several glucuronide conjugates; CYP2C9 metabolizes (or is inhibited by) smaller acid- or sulfonamide-containing drugs, and CYP2C19 metabolizes drugs often with a high degree of stereoselectivity (i.e., it preferentially metabolizes one enantiomer over the other). All four enzymes appear to be inducible by CAR/PXR agonists; hence, they tend to be co-induced together with CYP2B6 and CYP3A4. Substrates, inhibitors, and inducers of CYP2C8, 2C9, and 2C19 are listed in Table 6-11.

CYP2C8 CYP2C8 has been implicated in the metabolism of the following drugs and endobiotics: all-*trans* retinoic acid, arachidonic acid, amiodarone, amodiaquine, carbamazepine, cerivastatin (withdrawn), chloroquine, cilostazol, *R*-ibuprofen, lovastatin, morphine, pioglitazone, paclitaxel (Taxol®), repaglinide, rosiglitazone, rosuvastatin, simvastatin, tazarotene, torsemide, troglitazone (withdrawn), verapamil and zopiclone. However, with the exception of the antidiabetic drug, repaglinide, all of the above drugs are metabolized to a significant extent by enzymes other than CYP2C8. Repaglinide is classified by the FDA as a sensitive CYP2C8 substrate. In the presence of the CYP2C8 inhibitor gemfibrozil, exposure to repaglinide (based on plasma AUC) increases about eightfold (from 5.5 to 15-fold).

Substrates for CYP2C8 tend to be large and acidic as evidenced by the observation that CYP2C8 metabolizes several glucuronides. For example, whereas 17β-estradiol and diclofenac are metabolized by CYP2C9, the glucuronide metabolites of these compounds (namely, estradiol-17β-glucuronide and diclofenac acyl glucuronide) are metabolized by CYP2C8 (at the same site as that metabolized by CYP2C9, which is distal to the glucuronide moiety).

The ability of CYP2C8 to metabolize glucuronide conjugates appears to play an important role in the mechanism by which the hypolipidemic drug gemfibrozil inhibits the metabolism, and thereby increases in the toxicity (a sometimes fatal muscle disorder known as rhabdomyolysis) of cerivastatin (Baycol), a member of the statin class of cholesterol synthesis inhibitors that was withdrawn from the market (Ogilvie et al., 2006). Gemfibrozil glucuronide, but not gemfibrozil itself, is a potent mechanism-based inhibitor of CYP2C8. In other words, CYP2C8 metabolizes gemfibrozil glucuronide to a metabolite that inactivates the enzyme. The sometimes fatal interaction between gemfibrozil (the perpetrator drug) and cerivastatin (the victim drug) was a significant factor in the decision to withdraw cerivastatin from the U.S., European, and Japanese markets.

CYP2C9 CYP2C9 plays a major role in the metabolism of a wide variety of therapeutic agents including NSAIDs (e.g., diclofenac, celecoxib, ibuprofen, flurbiprofen, naproxen, piroxicam, mefenamic acid, and suprofen), oral hypoglycemics (e.g., glyburide, glipizide, glimepiride, tolbutamide), oral anticoagulants (e.g., S-warfarin, S-acenocoumarol, and phenprocoumon), diuretics and uricosurics (e.g., sulfinpyrazone sulfide, torsemide, tienilic acid [ticrynafen]), angiotensin II blockers (e.g., candesartan, irbesartan, losartan), anticonvulsants (e.g., phenytoin), and many others. It also metabolizes Δ^9-tetrahydrocannabinol and certain endobiotics such as arachidonic acid, linoleic acid, and serotonin (5-hydroxytryptamine). Substrates for—and inhibitors of—CYP2C9 tend to be acid- or sulfonamide-containing compounds, but there are exceptions to this general rule. In fact, the most potent CYP2C9 inhibitors known, namely, benzbromarone and 2-methyl-3-(3',5'-diiodo-4'-hydroxybenzoyl)benzofluran, are neither acid- nor sulfonamide-containing compounds (Rettie and Jones, 2005).

CYP2C9 is a polymorphically expressed enzyme. Two allelic variants, CYP2C9*2 and CYP2C9*3, are each present in about 10% of Northern European populations such that about 40% of Caucasians possess one or two allelic variants of CYP2C9. CYP2C9*2 is generally associated with no more than a small decrease in catalytic activity, whereas CYP2C*3 is associated with a marked decrease in catalytic activity. Individuals who are homozygous for the *3 allele are considered CYP2C9 PMs (i.e., poor metabolizers of drugs that are otherwise cleared by CYP2C9). Estimates of the CYP2C9 PM genotype are in the range of 1–10% in Caucasians, 1–4% in Africans, and 0–2% in Asians. The PM genotype is particularly important for S-warfarin, tolbutamide, and phenytoin. These three drugs have a low therapeutic index, and their dose must be reduced in CYP2C9 PMs to prevent adverse drugs events. Dosage adjustment is also required when these drugs are combined with a CYP2C9 inhibitor or inducer, examples of which are given in Table 6-11.

Tienilic acid is also metabolized by CYP2C9, but with potentially deleterious effects. CYP2C9 converts tienilic acid to an electrophilic thiophene sulfoxide that can react either with water to give 5-hydroxytienilic acid or with a nucleophilic amino acid in CYP2C9 to form a covalent adduct, which inactivates the enzyme (Lecoeur et al., 1994). Antibodies directed against the adduct between CYP2C9 and tienilic acid are thought to be responsible for the immunoallergic hepatitis that develops in about 1 out of every 10,000 patients treated with this uricosuric diuretic drug. As shown in Table 6-3, these auto-antibodies against CYP2C9 are known as anti-LKM$_2$ because they are directed against **L**iver and **K**idney **M**icrosomes. The subscript number 2 distinguishes these antibodies against CYP2C9 from those against CYP2D6, which are known as anti-LKM$_1$.

CYP2C18   In contrast to the other three CYP2C enzymes expressed in human liver, CYP2C18 appears to play little or no role in drug metabolism. CYP2C18 is the most abundant CYP2C enzyme in skin and lung, and it also appears to be expressed in brain, uterus, mammary gland, kidney, and duodenum. CYP2C18 is more than an order of magnitude more active than either CYP2C9 or CYP2C19 at catalyzing the *para*-hydroxylation of phenytoin to HPPH, and CYP2C18 can further hydroxylate HPPH to a catechol (Kinobe et al., 2005). Autoxidation of this catechol to an *ortho*-quinone is thought to be responsible, at least in part, for rare incidences of hypersensitivity reactions to phenytoin. Therefore, although hepatic CYP2C9 and CYP2C19 are largely responsible for determining the systemic clearance of phenytoin, it is possible that CYP2C18 is responsible for activating phenytoin by the catechol/quinone pathway

in the skin, the tissue where the first signs of hypersensitivity to phenytoin are observed.

CYP2C19   CYP2C19 is a polymorphically expressed enzyme that metabolizes several drugs with a high degree of stereospecificity such that, in the case of drugs administered as a racemic mixture, it metabolizes one enantiomer faster than the other, as in the case of mephenytoin (Mesantoin®), which is of historical interest with respect to CYP2C19. A genetic polymorphism for the metabolism of S-mephenytoin was first described in 1984 (reviewed in Wilkinson et al., 1989). The deficiency affects the 4'-hydroxylation (aromatic ring hydroxylation) of this anticonvulsant drug (see Fig. 6-41). The other major pathway of S-mephenytoin metabolism, namely, N-demethylation to S-nirvanol, is not affected. (This pathway was subsequently shown to be catalyzed by CYP2B6.) Consequently, poor metabolizers excrete little or no 4'-hydroxymephenytoin in their urine, but they do excrete increased amounts of the N-demethylated metabolite, S-nirvanol (S-phenylethylhydantoin). The enzyme responsible for this genetic polymorphism is CYP2C19, and it is highly stereoselective for the S-enantiomer of mephenytoin. In contrast to the S-enantiomer, the R-enantiomer is not converted to 4'-hydroxymephenytoin, but it is N-demethylated to R-nirvanol (R-phenylethylhydantoin). Individuals who are genetically deficient in CYP2C19 are at increased risk of adverse events from Mesantoin® (a racemic mixture of the S- and R-enantiomers of mephenytoin). An exaggerated central response has been observed in CYP2C19 PMs administered Mesantoin® at doses that were without effect in CYP2C19 EMs.

CYP2C19 plays an important role in the metabolism of several proton pump inhibitors including omeprazole and lansoprazole, the structures of which are shown in Fig. 6-43. The sulfoxide group in omeprazole and lansoprazole (and other proton pump inhibitors) is a chiral center, and CYP2C19 preferentially metabolizes one enantiomer over the other: it preferentially hydroxylates the R-enantiomer in the case of omeprazole, and it preferentially hydroxylates the S-enantiomer in the case of lansoprazole. These reactions are equivalent inasmuch as these two proton pump inhibitors are hydroxylated on opposite ends of the molecule (on the pyridine ring in the case of omeprazole and on the benzimidazole ring in the case of lansoprazole), meaning the sulfoxide in each case binds to the active site of CYP2C19 in the same orientation (Kim et al., 2003). CYP2C19 PMs are poor metabolizers of omeprazole and lansoprazole. However, CYP2C19 PMs are not at increased risk for adverse drug events but actually derive greater therapeutic benefit (better control of gastroesophageal reflux disease or GERD) from standard doses of proton pump inhibitors (Furuta et al., 2005). Esomeprazole, the S-enantiomer of omeprazole, was approved for the treatment of GERD and related gastric acid disorders. Compared with the R-enantiomer, esomeprazole is not rapidly metabolized by CYP2C19, and its improved pharmacokinetic behavior provides CYP2C19 EMs with the same therapeutic benefit as CYP2C19 PMs administered omeprazole. Other substrates, inhibitors, and inducers of CYP2C19 are listed in Table 6-11.

The incidence of the CYP2C19 PM genotype varies considerably from one ethnic group to the next: It ranges from 13 to 23% in Japanese, Chinese, Korean, Turkish, and Saudi Arabian subjects, but the incidence is considerably lower (1–5%) in Caucasians and Africans. No CYP2C19 UMs (individuals with functional CYP2C19 gene duplications) have been identified, although CYP2C19 is an inducible enzyme whose activity can be increased by CAR/PXR agonists (see Table 6-11).

CYP2D6   In the late 1950s, clinical trials in the United States established that sparteine was as potent as oxytocin for inducing labor at term. However, the duration and intensity of action of sparteine was dramatically increased in ~7% of all patients tested. The exaggerated response to sparteine included prolonged (tetanic) uterine contraction and abnormally rapid labor. In some cases, sparteine caused the death of the fetus. The drug was not recommended for clinical use because these side effects were unpredictable and occurred at doses of 100–200 mg, which were well tolerated by other patients. The antihypertensive drug, debrisoquine, was subsequently found to cause a marked and prolonged hypotension in 5–10% of patients, and a genetic polymorphism for the metabolism of debrisoquine and sparteine was discovered in 1977–1979. Poor metabolizers lack CYP2D6, which catalyzes the 4-hydroxylation of debrisoquine and the dehydrogenation (Δ^2- and Δ^5-oxidation) of sparteine (see Fig. 6-47).

In addition to debrisoquine and sparteine, CYP2D6 biotransforms an extraordinarily large number of drugs, as shown in Table 6-11. Individuals lacking CYP2D6 have an exaggerated response to some but not all these drugs. For example, even though debrisoquine and propranolol are both biotransformed by CYP2D6, the effects of propranolol are not exaggerated in poor metabolizers of debrisoquine, for two reasons. First, 4-hydroxypropranolol is a β-adrenoceptor antagonist, so the 4-hydroxylation of propranolol by CYP2D6 does not terminate the pharmacological effects of the drug. Second, CYP2D6 is not the only CYP enzyme to biotransform propranolol. As mentioned above, CYP2C19 catalyzes the side-chain oxidation of propranolol to naphthoxylactic acid (see Fig. 6-27). Because CYP2D6 and CYP2C19 both contribute significantly to the biotransformation of propranolol, a deficiency in either one of these enzymes does not markedly alter the pharmacokinetics of this beta blocker. However, in one individual who lacked both enzymes, the total oral clearance of propranolol was markedly reduced (Wilkinson *et al.*, 1989). The biotransformation of substrates for CYP2D6 occurs 5–7.5Å from a basic nitrogen, which interacts with an anionic residue (Glu[301]) in the enzyme's substrate-binding site. Quinidine is a potent inhibitor of CYP2D6 because it interacts favorably with the anionic site on CYP2D6 but it cannot be oxidized at a site 5–7.5Å from its basic nitrogen atoms. Quinidine, paroxetine, and fluoxetine (and especially norfluoxetine, its *N*-demethylated metabolite) are strong CYP2D6 inhibitors in vivo, and a PM phenotype can be induced pharmacologically with these particular inhibitors. Quinine, the levorotatory diastereomer of quinidine, is not a potent inhibitor of CYP2D6, and neither drug is a potent inhibitor of the CYP2D enzymes expressed in rats.

As shown in Fig. 6-44, CYP2D6 catalyzes the O-demethylation of dextromethorphan to dextrorphan, which is glucuronidated and excreted in urine. Dextromethorphan can also be N-demethylated, a reaction catalyzed predominantly by CYP3A4 and CYP2B6, but this metabolite is not glucuronidated and excreted in urine. Because the urinary excretion of dextromethorphan is dependent on O-demethylation, this over-the-counter antitussive drug can be used to identify individuals lacking CYP2D6, and it can be used as an in vivo probe to identify drugs capable of causing clinically significant inhibition of CYP2D6. Other FDA-acceptable in vivo probes of CYP2D6 include desipramine and atomoxetine (see Table 6-11).

Genetic polymorphisms of CYP2D6 have been so extensively studied that it is possible not only to categorize individuals into four genotypes, namely, poor metabolizers (PMs), intermediate metabolizers (IMs), extensive metabolizers (EMs), and ultra-rapid metabolizers (UMs), but it is also possible to subdivide the extensive metabolizers into three categories, namely, High Activity EM, Medium Activity EM, and Low Activity EM, as summarized in Table 6-4. The incidence of the CYP2D6 PM genotype varies considerably from one ethnic group to the next: It is 5–7% in Caucasians, 2–4% in Africans and African Americans, and 1–2% in Turkish and Asian (Thai, Chinese, and Japanese) subjects. Similarly, the incidence of the CYP2D6 gene duplication, which gives rise to the CYP2D6 UM genotype, varies among ethnic groups: It is up to 29% in Ethiopians, 20% in Saudi Arabians, 5–10% in Southern European Caucasians, but only 1–2% of Northern European Caucasians, 5–10% of Turkish subjects, and up to 2% in African, African-American, and Asian subjects. CYP2D6 PMs are often at increased risk of an exaggerated pharmacological response, such as the prolonged uterine contractions caused by sparteine or the prolonged hypotension caused by debrisoquine, or a toxicological response, such as the hepatotoxic effects of perhexiline (three drugs that, because of the adverse events in CYP2D6 PMs, were not approved by the FDA). Some drugs, such as the analgesic codeine (which is O-demethylated to morphine) and the anticancer drug tamoxifen (which is hydroxylated and N-demethylated to endoxifen), are converted to pharmacologically active metabolites by CYP2D6. Consequently, CYP2D6 PMs derive less therapeutic benefit than CYP2D6 EMs. In contrast, in the case of codeine, CYP2D6 UMs are at increased risk from morphine toxicity. The death of an elderly man administered a recommended dose of codeine and the death of baby who was breast-fed by a woman on codeine have been attributed to the CYP2D6 UM genotype that causes rapid conversion of codeine to morphine (which causes respiratory suppression) (Gasche *et al.*, 2004; Koren *et al.*, 2006).

Individuals lacking CYP2D6 have an unusually low incidence of some chemically induced neoplastic diseases (Idle, 1991). For example, CYP2D6 PMs appear to be relatively resistant to lung cancer whereas CYP2D6 UMs appear to be at increased risk (Agundez *et al.*, 2001). It has been hypothesized that CYP2D6 may play a role in the metabolic activation of chemical carcinogens, such as those present in the environment, in the diet, and/or in cigarette smoke. According to this hypothesis, CYP2D6 PMs have a low incidence of cancer because they fail to activate chemical carcinogens, whereas CYP2D6 UMs have an increased risk because they rapidly and/or extensively activate pro-carcinogens. However, CYP2D6 appears to play little or no role in the activation of known chemical carcinogens to DNA-reactive or mutagenic metabolites, with the notable exception of the tobacco-smoke-specific nitrosamine, 4-(methylnitrosamino)-1-(3-pyridyl)-1-butanone (NNK), which is also activated by numerous other CYP enzymes (see the previous section on "CYP2A6 and 2A13"). Although the association between CYP2D6 status and lung cancer incidence was first described in 1984, the mechanism underlying this association remains to be determined.

CYP2E1   As shown in Fig. 6-24, CYP2E1 was first identified as the microsomal ethanol oxidizing system (MEOS, Lieber, 1999). In addition to ethanol, CYP2E1 catalyzes the biotransformation—and in many cases the metabolic activation—of a large number of halogenated alkanes and nitrosamines, as shown in Table 6-12 (Guengerich *et al.*, 1991). CYP2E1 is expressed constitutively in human liver and several extrahepatic tissues, such as the kidney, lung, bone marrow, and lymphocytes. As illustrated in Fig. 6-31, CYP2E1 in the liver and possibly the bone marrow itself plays an important role in activating benzene to myelotoxic metabolites, as evidenced by the protective effect of CYP2E1 gene deletion in mice (Gonzalez, 2003).

Table 6-12

Examples of Xenobiotics Activated by Human P450

CYP1A2	**CYP2E1**
Acetaminophen	Acetaminophen
2-Acetylaminofluorene	Acrylonitrile
4-Aminobiphenyl	Benzene
2-Aminofluorene	Carbon tetrachloride
2-Naphthylamine	Chloroform
NNK	Dichloromethane
Amino acid pyrolysis products	1,2-Dichloropropane
(DiMeQx, MeIQ, MeIQx, Glu P-1,	Ethylene dibromide
Glu P-2, IQ, PhIP, Trp P-1, Trp P-2)	Ethylene dichloride
Tacrine	Ethyl carbamate
CYP2A6 and 2A13	Halothane
NNK and bulky nitrosamines	N-Nitrosodimethylamine
N-Nitrosodiethylamine	Styrene
Aflatoxin B1	Trichloroethylene
CYP2B6	Vinyl chloride
6-Aminochrysene	**CYP3A4**
Cyclophosphamide	Acetaminophen
Ifosfamide	Aflatoxin B_1 and G_1
CYP2C8, 9, 18, 19	6-Aminochrysene
Tienilic acid	Benzo[a]pyrene 7,8-dihydrodiol
Phenytoin	Cyclophosphamide
Valproic acid	Ifosfamide
CYP2D6	1-Nitropyrene
NNK	Sterigmatocystin
CYP2F1	Senecionine
3-Methylindole	$Tris$(2,3-dibromopropyl) phosphate
Acetaminophen	**CYP4B1**
Valproic acid	Ipomeanol
CYP1A1 and 1B1	3-Methylindole
Benzo[a]pyrene and	2-Aminofluorene
other polycyclic	
aromatic hydrocarbons	

NNK, 4-(methylnitrosamino)-1-(3-pyridyl)-1-butanone, a tobacco-specific nitrosamine.
Data adapted from Guengerich FP, Shimada T: Oxidation of toxic and carcinogenic chemicals by human cytochrome
    P-450 enzymes. *Chem Res Toxicol* 4:391–407, 1991.

The function and regulation of CYP2E1 are relatively well conserved among mammalian species. In humans and most other mammalian species, CYP2E1 is inducible by ethanol, isoniazid, and ketone bodies (which form during uncontrolled diabetes). In contrast to the induction of most other CYP enzymes, the induction of CYP2E1 often involves increased translation of preexisting mRNA and/or protein stabilization rather than transcriptional activation of the CYP2E1 gene; hence, induction of CYP2E1 often occurs in the absence of an increase in mRNA levels.

CYP2E1 can activate acetaminophen to the hepatotoxic metabolite, N-acetylbenzoquinoneimine, as shown in Figs. 6-34 and 6-47. Compared with their wild-type littermates, CYP2E1 knockout mice are relatively resistant to acetaminophen hepatotoxicity (Gonzalez, 2003). The mechanism by which alcohol potentiates the hepatotoxic effects of acetaminophen (Tylenol®) is thought to involve increased activation of acetaminophen, due to the induction of CYP2E1, and decreased inactivation, due to a lowering of glutathione levels. Induction of CYP2E1 by isoniazid stimulates the dehalogenation of the volatile anesthetics, enflurane and isoflurane. In human liver microsomes, CYP2E1 activity can be conveniently measured by the 6-hydroxylation of chlorzoxazone and the hydroxylation of 4-nitrophenol (Table 6-11). The 6-hydroxylation of chlorzoxazone can also be catalyzed by CYP1A1, but this enzyme is rarely expressed in human liver. Chlorzoxazone is an FDA-approved muscle relaxant (Paraflex®), and the urinary excretion of 6-hydroxychlorzoxazone and the plasma ratio of 6-hydroxychlorzoxazone to chlorzoxazone have been used as noninvasive in vivo probes of CYP2E1. The levels of CYP2E1 are by no means constant among individuals, but they do not exhibit the marked interindividual variation characteristic of other CYP enzymes. CYP2E1 is one of the CYP enzymes that require cytochrome b_5, which lowers the K_m for several substrates biotransformed by CYP2E1.

CYP2F1 and 2J2   CYP2F1 is expressed in the lung and plays an important role in activating the pulmonary toxin 3-methylindole to a reactive metabolite (formed by a dehydrogenation reaction analogous to those shown in Fig. 6-47 (Nichols *et al.*, 2003).

CYP2J2 is expressed in liver, small intestine, heart, and kidney. Although it has been shown to contribute significantly to the biotransformation of ebastine and, to a lesser extent, astemizole, CYP2J2 is better known for its ability to epoxygenate arachidonic acid to vasoactive metabolites, such as *cis*-11,12-epoxyeicosatrienoic acid (11,12-EET), which is one of four EETs formed by the CYP-dependent epoxygenation of arachidonic acid (Liu *et al*., 2006a; Spiecker and Liao, 2006). As such, CYP2J2 is one of several CYP enzymes involved in EET formation, including other members of the CYP2 family (see "CYP2C8" and "CYP2C9" above) and several members of the CYP4 family (see "CYP4 Enzymes" below).

CYP2R1, 2S1, 2U1, and 2W1   CYP2R1, 2S1, 2U1, and 2W1 are four of the eight members of the CYP1 and 2 families that are so well conserved from an evolutionary perspective that they have been given the same names across all mammalian species (the other members are CYP1A1, 1A2, 1B1, and 2E1). These enzymes have been conserved during evolution presumably because they perform an important physiological function. In support of this possibility, CYP2R1, 2S1, 2U1, and 2W1 have been shown to metabolize vitamin D, all-*trans* retinoic acid, fatty acids, and arachidonic acid, respectively, although the ability of CYP2W1 to metabolize arachidonic acid (or any of several other fatty acids) is not supported by recent studies (Yoshioka *et al*., 2006). Notwithstanding their ability to metabolize all-*trans* retinoic acid or fatty acids, CYP2S1, 2U1, and 2W1 are suspected of performing an as-yet unidentified physiologic function, for which reason they are classified as orphan enzymes of unknown function (Table 6-9).

Like CYP1A1, CYP1A2, and CYP1B1, the recently identified CYP enzyme known as CYP2S1 is inducible by TCDD and other Ah receptor agonists. Like CYP1A1 and CYP1B1, CYP2S1 is expressed mainly in extrahepatic tissues such as lung, trachea, stomach, small intestine, colon, spleen, bladder, and skin. CYP2S1 metabolizes all-*trans* retinoic acid, which is a physiologic substrate. In view of its structural similarities to—and co-localization with—CYP2A13, and in view of its inducibility by Ah receptor agonists, CYP2S1 has been conjectured to play a role in the metabolic activation of xenobiotics in extrahepatic tissues. However, in bacterial mutagenicity assays, CYP2S1 has been shown NOT to activate the pro-carcinogens NNK, PhIP, aflatoxin B1, and a series of polycyclic aromatic hydrocarbons and their diol-epoxides (Wang *et al*., 2005b; Wu *et al*., 2006).

CYP2W1 is expressed in a large number of tumors, and yet it does not appear to be expressed to a significant extent in normal (i.e., noncancerous) hepatic or extrahepatic tissues (Karlgren *et al*., 2006). Like CYP1B1, which is also overexpressed in malignant cells (see "CYP1B1" above), CYP2W1 can activate a wide variety of polycyclic aromatic hydrocarbons and their diol-epoxides to mutagenic metabolites (Wang *et al*., 2005b; Wu *et al*., 2006). Whether expression of CYP2W1 contributes to tumor formation or is expressed only as a result of malignancy remains to be determined.

CYP3A Enzymes   The most abundant CYP enzymes in human liver microsomes belong to the CYP3A gene subfamily, which includes CYP3A4, 3A5, 3A7, and 3A43. CYP3A43 is considered an orphan enzyme of unknown function (see Table 6-9). CYP3A7 is considered a fetal enzyme that may play a role in the activation of drugs to teratogenic metabolites (Li *et al*., 1997). This is a concern because laboratory animals do not express a fetal CYP3A enzyme, raising the possibility that teratogenic metabolites formed

by CYP3A7 may go undetected during reproductive toxicity testing in animals. Whereas CYP3A7 is considered to be a fetal enzyme, CYP3A4 and 3A5 are considered to be adult enzymes, although livers from some adults contain CYP3A7 and some fetal livers contain CYP3A5.

CYP3A4   CYP3A4 is abundantly expressed in liver and small intestine, where it biotransforms an extraordinary array of steroid hormones and xenobiotics, including drugs from numerous therapeutic classes (Table 6-11). By some estimates, CYP3A4 metabolizes about 70% of all drugs. A large number of clinically significant drug–drug, drug–herbal, and drug–food interactions involve the inhibition or induction of hepatic and/or intestinal CYP3A4. Three victim drugs whose clearance is mainly determined by CYP3A4, namely, terfenadine (Seldane), cisapride (Propulsid), and astemizole (Hismanal), have been withdrawn from the market because of their potential to cause ventricular arrhythmias (and on rare occasions heart attacks) when their metabolism by CYP3A4 was inhibited by drugs like ketoconazole and erythromycin. One perpetrator drug, namely, mibefradil (Posicor) has been withdrawn from the market because of its ability to cause marked and prolonged inhibition of CYP3A4 by virtue of its ability to cause mechanism-based inhibition of CYP3A4 (which persists after the inhibitory drug is withdrawn and until new enzyme is synthesized).

CYP3A4 is abundantly expressed in the small intestine where it contributes substantially to the first-pass metabolism (presystemic clearance) of numerous drugs. The inhibition of intestinal CYP3A4 by furanocoumarins in grapefruit juice, which can cause large increases in exposure to drugs that otherwise undergo first-pass elimination, is an important mechanism of drug–food interaction. The induction of intestinal and hepatic CYP3A4 by St. John's wort, which can result in a loss of therapeutic efficacy of oral contraceptive steroids, anti-HIV, and antiorgan rejection drugs, is an important mechanism of drug–herbal interactions.

The induction of CYP3A4 is mediated by CAR and PXR, agonists for which include several antibiotics, such as rifampin and rifabutin, and several enzyme-inducing antiepileptic drugs (EIAEDs), such as phenobarbital, phenytoin, carbamazepine, and felbamate, as shown in Table 6-11 (a more complete list of CYP3A4 inducers is given in the later section "Cytochrome P450 Induction - Xenosensors)."

The function and regulation of the CYP3A enzymes is fairly well conserved among mammalian species, with some notable exceptions. For example, rifampin is an inducer of the CYP3A enzymes in humans and rabbits but not rats or mice, whereas the opposite appears to be true of pregnenolone-16α-carbonitrile (PCN). In adult rats, the levels of CYP3A2 in males are much greater (>tenfold) than in females. In humans, men do not have higher levels of CYP3A4 than women; in fact there is evidence to suggest that the reverse is true; that women have slightly higher levels of CYP3A4 than men, although it should be noted that CYP3A4 levels vary widely in both men and women.

CYP3A4 metabolizes more drugs than any other xenobiotic-biotransforming enzyme, which is apparent from the large list of CYP3A4 substrates listed in Table 6-11. Like CYP2C8, CYP3A4 can metabolize large substrates, such as paclitaxel (Taxol®), which is a substrate for both enzymes. The active site of CYP3A4 is sufficiently large to bind two drugs simultaneously, and individual drugs tend to bind to discrete regions, which has several consequences. First, the binding of two substrates to CYP3A4 allows for homotropic activation (where a substrate stimulates its own metabolism, as in the case of testosterone and diazepam) and heterotropic activation (where one compound, such as α-naphthoflavone, stimulates the metabolism of another). These effects give rise to non-Michaelis–Menten or atypical enzyme kinetics, which is characteristic of the metabolism of several drugs by CYP3A4. The binding of one ligand (substrate, inhibitor, or activator) to CYP3A4 can cause conformational changes that increase the size of the active site by 80% or more, which allows additional ligands to bind, possibly in a stacked or side-by-side configuration (Ekroos and Sjögren, 2006). Second, substrates can bind to relatively discrete sites within the active site. Testosterone and midazolam appear to bind to distinct sites (called the steroid and benzodiazepine binding site, respectively); consequently these two prototypical substrates only weakly inhibit each other's metabolism by CYP3A4. As a result of these different substrate-binding sites or orientations, it is possible for a drug to inhibit CYP3A4 in a substrate-dependent manner. However, inhibitors that coordinate directly with the heme moiety of CYP3A4 will inhibit the metabolism of all CYP3A4 substrates, as will most mechanism-based inhibitors of CYP3A4 (see the later section "Inhibition of Cytochrome P450"). Although the active site of CYP3A4 is sufficiently large to bind substrates in apparently discrete sites and to bind two molecules simultaneously, it nevertheless often catalyzes reactions with a high degree of regio- and stereoselectivity. In the case of testosterone, for example, CYP3A4 catalyzes hydroxylation at several sites on the β-face of the molecule (e.g., 1β-, 2β-, 6β-, and 15β-hydroxylation) but none on the α-face.

CYP3A5 CYP3A5 is a polymorphically expressed enzyme. Functional enzyme (encoded by the CYP3A5*1 or wild-type allele) is expressed in the liver of only 10–30% of Caucasians, ~50% of Chinese, ~60% of African Americans, and 60–70% of Japanese. No CYP3A5 UMs (individuals with functional CYP3A5 gene duplications) have been identified. There are conflicting reports on the relative levels of CYP3A5 and CYP3A4 in liver. Some reports indicate that the levels of CYP3A5 are uniformly low (Patki *et al.*, 2003; Westlind-Johnsson *et al.*, 2003) whereas others indicate that, in some liver samples, the levels of CYP3A5 can approach those of CYP3A4 (Lin *et al.*, 2002). There are also conflicting reports on the relative rate of drug and steroid metabolism by CYP3A5 and CYP3A4. Studies with recombinant enzymes generally show that CYP3A4 is considerably more active than CYP3A5 in the metabolism of a wide range of substrates. Many of these studies were recently criticized (Huang *et al.*, 2004) on the basis that few of them were conducted with recombinant enzymes in the presence of both NADPH-cytochrome P450 reductase and cytochrome b_5. Under such conditions, the catalytic activity of CYP3A5 can rival or even surpass that of CYP3A4. Of the eight substrates examined, midazolam represented the extreme case. In the presence of both NADPH-cytochrome P450 reductase and cytochrome b_5, recombinant CYP3A5 was three times more active than CYP3A4 at catalyzing the 1'-hydroxylation of midazolam, based on estimates of in vitro intrinsic clearance (i.e., V_{max}/K_m) (Huang *et al.*, 2004). However, when this same group evaluated the metabolism of the same eight substrates in two pools ($n = 10$) of human liver microsomes each with the same levels of CYP3A4 but with markedly different levels of CYP3A5 (to mimic the CYP3A5 polymorphism), it was found that CYP3A5 contributed nothing to the metabolism of testosterone, carbamazepine, lidocaine, terfenadine, dextromethorphan, or itraconazole, but contributed 27, 26, and 35% to the metabolism of midazolam, erythromycin, and flunitrazepam, respectively.

The recent study by Huang *et al.* (2004) demonstrated that, under certain in vitro conditions, the catalytic activity of CYP3A5 can surpass that of CYP3A4 (in a substrate-dependent manner) and predicted that CYP3A5 could potentially contribute to the metabolism of midazolam, a drug whose disposition is known to be highly dependent on CYP3A-catalyzed metabolism in the liver and small intestine. The studies by (Huang *et al.*, 2004) predict a role, albeit not a major role, for CYP3A5 in the metabolism of midazolam. However, two in vivo studies have shown that CYP3A5 genotype has no influence on the disposition of midazolam in vivo (Goh *et al.*, 2002; Shih and Huang, 2002). Possible reasons for the discrepancy between the in vitro prediction of the contribution of CYP3A5 to drug metabolism and the in vivo observation have been reviewed by Williams *et al.* (2003a).

Other studies have evaluated the influence of CYP3A5 genotype on the disposition of cyclosporine and tacrolimus, two immunosuppressive (antirejection) drugs that are substrates for both *P*-glycoprotein and CYP3A4. The results with cyclosporine were unexpected: In individuals identified by genotyping analysis to be CYP3A5 poor metabolizers, the oral clearance of cyclosporine was 31% higher compared with CYP3A5 extensive metabolizers, suggesting that not only did CYP3A5 fail to contribute to the metabolism of cyclosporine, but that the expression of functional CYP3A5 somehow impaired the metabolism of cyclosporine by CYP3A4 (Yates *et al.*, 2002). In contrast to the unexpected findings with cyclosporine, two clinical studies provide evidence that CYP3A5 genotype significantly influences the disposition of tacrolimus, such that patients who expressed high levels of CYP3A5 required higher doses of tacrolimus to achieve desired blood levels of this calcineurin inhibitor (Macphee *et al.*, 2002; Zheng *et al.*, 2003).

Finally, it is noteworthy that, when evaluated as inhibitors of recombinant human CYP3A enzymes, 14 out of 14 compounds inhibited CYP3A4 more potently than they inhibited CYP3A5 (by a factor of 3.9- to 142-fold) (Ekins *et al.*, 2003).

CYP4 Enzymes Humans express 12 members of the CYP4 family, namely, CYP4A11, 4A22, 4B1, 4F2, 4F3, 4F8, 4F11, 4F12, 4F22, 4V2, 4X1, and 4Z1. For the most part, these enzymes can be divided into two groups: a group that is known to metabolize fatty acids and/or eicosanoids and a group that has no known function (so-called orphan enzymes), as shown in Table 6-9. The first group (CYP4A11, 4B1, 4F2, 4F3, 4F8, and 4F12) is part of a larger group of fatty acid- and eicosanoid-metabolizing enzymes, which includes CYP2C8, 2C9, and 2J2. These enzymes are collectively involved in the formation or further metabolism of numerous vasoactive agents, such as the various epoxidation products of arachidonic acid (EETs), leukotoxins (formed by the epoxidation of C_{18} unsaturated fatty acids) and mediators of inflammation, such as prostaglandins and leukotrienes (notably LTB_4) (Baer and Rettie, 2006; Kalsotra and Strobel, 2006). In many cases, these enzymes hydroxylate the terminal methyl group (ω-hydroxylation) distal to the carboxylic group, which is thermodynamically unfavorable compared with hydroxylation of a methylene group (e.g., ω-1 hydroxylation). Following ω-hydroxylation, the terminal hydroxymethyl group can be further oxidized to convert the original fatty acid/eicosanoid to a dicarboxylic acid.

Several CYP4 enzymes have been shown to metabolize drugs and other xenobiotics, but in nearly all cases the drugs that are metabolized by the CYP4 enzymes are also metabolized more extensively by CYP1, 2, or 3 family members. A notable exception is the antiparasitic prodrug DB-287, which is O-demethylated in human liver microsomes by CYP4F2 and CYP4F3 with negligible contribution from CYP enzymes in the 1, 2, or 3 family, as shown in Fig. 6-21 (Wang *et al.*, 2006b). Another notable exception is CYP4B1, which is expressed in a wide range of extrahepatic tissues and which activates several protoxicants including the pneumotoxins ipomeanol and 3-methylindole, and the bladder carcinogen 2-aminofluorene (Baer and Rettie, 2006).

Activation of Xenobiotics by Cytochrome P450 Biotransformation by cytochrome P450 does not always lead to detoxication, and several examples have been given previously where the toxicity or tumorigenicity of a chemical depends on its activation by cytochrome P450. The role of individual human CYP enzymes in the activation of selected procarcinogens and protoxicants is summarized in Table 6-12 (adapted from Guengerich and Shimada, 1991). A variety of cytochrome P450-dependent reactions are involved in the activation of the chemicals listed in Table 6-12. The conversion of polycyclic aromatic hydrocarbons to tumor-forming metabolites involves the formation of bay-region diolepoxides, as shown in Fig. 6-9, for the conversion of benzo[*a*]pyrene to benzo[*a*]pyrene 7,8-dihydrodiol-9,10, epoxide. Epoxidation generates hepatotoxic metabolites of chlorobenzene and coumarin (Fig. 6-42), and generates an hepatotumorigenic metabolite of aflatoxin B_1 (Fig. 6-33).

The initial step in the conversion of aromatic amines to tumor-forming metabolites involves N-hydroxylation, as shown for 2-amino-6-nitrobenzylalcohol (Fig. 6-11) and 2-acetylaminofluorene (Fig. 6-37a). In the case of acetaminophen, activation to hepatotoxic metabolite involves dehydrogenation to *N*-acetylbenzoquinoneimine, as shown in Fig. 6-34. A similar reaction converts butylated hydroxytoluene to a toxic quinone methide, as shown in Fig. 6-35. The myelotoxicity of benzene depends on its conversion to phenol and hydroquinone (Fig. 6-31). The toxicity of several organophosphorus insecticides involves oxidative group transfer to the corresponding organophosphate, as shown for the conversion of parathion to paraoxon in Figs. 6-45 and 6-46. The hepatotoxicity of carbon tetrachloride involves reductive dechlorination to a trichloromethyl free radical, which binds to protein and initiates lipid peroxidation, as shown in Fig. 6-17. The hepatotoxicity and nephrotoxicity of chloroform involves oxidative dechlorination to phosgene (Fig. 6-17). Oxidative and reductive dehalogenation both play a role in the activation of halothane, although hepatotoxicity in rats is more dependent on reductive dehalogenation, whereas the immune hepatitis in humans is largely a consequence of oxidative dehalogenation, which leads to the formation of neoantigens (Pohl *et al.*, 1989). Formation of neoantigens (by covalent binding to CYP2C9) is also the mechanism by which the uricosuric diuretic drug, tienilic acid, causes immune hepatitis (Lecoeur *et al.*, 1994).

Some of the chemicals listed in Table 6-12 are activated to toxic or tumorigenic metabolites by mechanisms not mentioned previously. For example, *N*-nitrosodimethylamine, which is representative of a large class of tumorigenic nitrosamines, is activated to an alkylating electrophile by *N*-demethylation, as shown in Fig. 6-48. The activation of ethyl carbamate (urethane) involves two sequential reactions catalyzed by cytochrome P450 (CYP2E1): dehydrogenation to vinyl carbamate followed by epoxidation, as shown in Fig. 6-48. CYP2E1 is one of several CYP enzymes that can catalyze the epoxidation of tetrachloroethylene. The rearrangement of this epoxide to a carbonyl is accompanied by migration of chlorine,

which produces the highly reactive metabolite, trichloroacetyl chloride, as shown in Fig. 6-48. The toxic pyrrolizidine alkaloids, such as senecionine, are cyclic arylamines that are dehydrogenated by cytochrome P450 (CYP3A4) to the corresponding pyrroles. Pyrroles themselves are nucleophiles, but electrophiles are generated through the loss of substituents on the pyrrolizidine nucleus, as shown in Fig. 6-48. Cyclophosphamide and ifosfamide are examples of chemicals designed to be activated to toxic electrophiles for the treatment of malignant tumors and other proliferative diseases. These drugs are nitrogen mustards, which have a tendency to undergo intramolecular nucleophilic displacement to form an electrophilic aziridinium species. In the case of cyclophosphamide and ifosfamide, the nitrogen mustard is stabilized by the presence of a phosphoryl oxygen, which delocalizes the lone pair of nitrogen electrons required for intramolecular nucleophilic displacement. For this reason, formation of an electrophilic aziridinium species requires hydroxylation by cytochrome P450, as shown in Fig. 6-48 for cyclophosphamide. Hydroxylation of the carbon atom next to the ring nitrogen leads spontaneously to ring opening and elimination of acrolein. In the resultant phosphoramide mustard, delocalization of the lone pair of nitrogen electrons to the phosphoryl oxygen is now disfavored by the presence of the lone pair of electrons on the oxygen anion; hence, the phosphoramide undergoes an intramolecular nucleophilic elimination to generate an electrophilic aziridinium species. This reaction is catalyzed by CYP3A4 and CYP2B6. Activation of cyclophosphamide by CYP enzymes in the skin would generate a cytotoxic metabolite at the base of hair follicles, which may be the reason why hair loss is one of the side effects of cyclophosphamide treatment.

Many of the chemicals listed in Table 6-12 are also detoxified by cytochrome P450 by biotransformation to less toxic metabolites. In some cases, the same CYP enzyme catalyzes both activation and detoxication reactions. For example, CYP3A4 activates aflatoxin B_1 to the hepatotoxic and tumorigenic 8,9-epoxide, but it also detoxifies aflatoxin B_1 by 3-hydroxylation to aflatoxin Q_1. Similarly, CYP3A4 activates senecionine by converting this pyrrolizidine alkaloid to the corresponding pyrrole, but it also detoxifies senecionine through formation of an *N*-oxide (a reaction mainly catalyzed by FMO3). Epoxidation of trichloroethylene by CYP2E1 appears to be both an activation and detoxication pathway, as shown in Fig. 6-48. Rearrangement of trichloroethylene epoxide can be accompanied by migration of chlorine, which produces chloral (trichloroacetaldehyde), or hydrogen, which produces dichloroacetylchloride. Chloral is much less toxic than dichloroacetylchloride; hence, migration of the chlorine during epoxide rearrangement is a detoxication reaction, whereas migration of the hydrogen is an activation reaction. These few examples serve to underscore the complexity of factors that determine the balance between xenobiotic activation and detoxication.

Inhibition of Cytochrome P450 Inhibition of cytochrome P450 is a major cause of drug–drug interactions (and occasionally the withdrawal of regulatory approval), as illustrated by the examples cited earlier (terfenadine, cisapride, astemizole, cerivastatin, and mibefradil) in the sections "CYP3A4" and "CYP2C8".

Inhibitory drug interactions generally fall into two categories: direct and metabolism-dependent inhibition. Direct inhibition can be subdivided into two types. The first involves competition between two drugs that are metabolized by the same CYP enzyme. For example, omeprazole and diazepam are both metabolized by

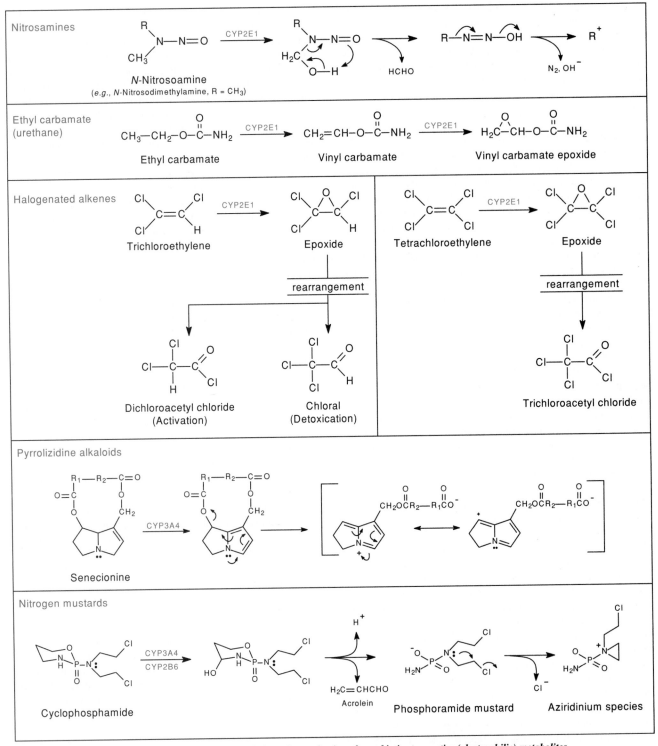

Figure 6-48. Additional mechanisms of cytochrome P450-dependent activation of xenobiotics to reactive (electrophilic) metabolites.

CYP2C19. When the two drugs are administered simultaneously, omeprazole decreases the plasma clearance of diazepam and prolongs its plasma half-life. The inhibition of diazepam metabolism by omeprazole is presumed to involve competition for metabolism by CYP2C19 because no such inhibition occurs in CYP2C19 PMs (individuals who lack CYP2C19). The second type of direct inhibition is when the inhibitor is not a substrate for the affected CYP enzyme. The inhibition of dextromethorphan biotransformation by

quinidine is a good example of this type of drug interaction. Dextromethorphan is O-demethylated by CYP2D6, and the clearance of dextromethorphan is impaired in individuals lacking this polymorphically expressed enzyme. The clearance of dextromethorphan is similarly impaired when this antitussive drug is taken with quinidine, a potent inhibitor of CYP2D6. However, quinidine is not biotransformed by CYP2D6, even though it binds to this enzyme with high affinity ($K_i \sim 100$ nM). Quinidine is actually biotransformed by CYP3A4, and is a weak competitive inhibitor of this enzyme ($K_i > 100$ μM), although its effects are highly dependent on the CYP3A4 substrate employed.

Although there are many exceptions, certain structural motifs are often associated with the inhibition of certain xenobiotic-metabolizing CYP enzymes some of which were discussed in the sections on individual CYPs (e.g., sections "CYP1A1/2," "CYP2C Enzymes," "CYP2D6," and "CYP3A4"). The most potent direct inhibitors of CYP1A2 (i.e., K_i or IC$_{50}$ < 0.1 μM) are small (i.e., <300 Da), planar, polycyclic compounds such as flavonoids (e.g., galangin, α-naphthoflavone, kaempferol). Potent direct CYP2A6 inhibitors (i.e., K_i or IC$_{50}$ < 1 μM) also include small molecules such as tranylcypromine, 2-(p-tolyl)-ethylamine and 4-methylbenzaldehyde as well as certain azoles (e.g., clotrimazole, letrozole, and miconazole). CYP2B6 is most potently inhibited (i.e., K_i or IC$_{50}$ < 2 μM) by azoles (e.g., sulconazole, tioconazole) and polycyclic, nitrogen-containing compounds such as sertraline, memantine, raloxifene, paroxetine, amlodipine, and N,N',N''-triethylenethiophosphamide (thio-TEPA). CYP2C8 is most potently inhibited in a direct manner (i.e., K_i or IC$_{50}$ <1 μM) by large (i.e., >400 Da) acidic drugs such as montelukast, zafirlukast, and candesartan, as well as the corticosteroid, mometasone, and the platinum-containing drug, satraplatin, and in a mechanism-based manner by the acyl glucuronide of gemfibrozil (Ogilvie et al., 2006). CYP2C9 is most potently inhibited (i.e., K_i or IC$_{50}$ <0.1 μM) by azoles (fluconazole, sulconazole, sulfaphenazole), acidic drugs, and also by sulfonarmides such as sulfaphenazole and sulfadiazine. Azoles are also some of the most potent direct inhibitors of CYP2C19 (i.e., K_i or IC$_{50}$ < 0.5 μM), as are compounds such as fluvoxamine, ($-$)-N-3-benzyl-phenobarbital, ($+$)-N-3-benzyl-nirvanol, and nootkatone. CYP2D6 is generally inhibited with high potency (i.e., K_i or IC$_{50}$ value < 0.1 μM) by compounds that contain a basic nitrogen (e.g., quinidine, ezlopitant, ajmalicine, terbinafine, propafenone, etc.). Direct inhibitors (i.e., K_i or IC$_{50}$ 1–6 μM) of CYP2E1 are generally small compounds (i.e., 79–150 Da) such as 4-methylpyrazole, pyridine, tranylcypromine, and diethyldithiocarbamate. However, a few larger compounds such as lasofoxifene and tioconazole can inhibit CYP2E1 with K_i or IC$_{50}$ values <0.5 μM. As noted above for several other CYPs, some of the most potent inhibitors of CYP enzymes are azole antifungals. This is especially true for CYP3A4, for which the most potent inhibitors (i.e., K_i or IC$_{50}$ values <0.1 μM) are azole antifungal drugs, with clotrimazole, ketoconazole, and itraconazole demonstrating K_i or IC$_{50}$ values from 0.00025 to 0.016 μM (K_i and IC$_{50}$ values obtained from http://www.druginteractioninfo.org).

As the name implies, metabolism-dependent inhibition is when cytochrome P450 converts a xenobiotic to a metabolite that is a more potent inhibitor than the parent compound. In some cases, the metabolite, once formed, functions as a potent, reversible inhibitor, as occurs when fluoxetine is N-demethylated to norfluoxetine. In other cases, however, the metabolite functions as an irreversible inhibitor (which occurs when the metabolite alkylates the heme or apoprotein moiety of cytochrome P450) or a quasi-irreversible inhibitor (which occurs when the metabolite coordinates tightly but not covalently with the ferrous heme to form what is known as a metabolite-inhibitory complex or MIC). Metabolism-dependent inhibitors that cause irreversible inactivation of cytochrome P450 include furafylline (CYP1A2), 8-methoxypsoralen (CYP2A6), clopidogrel (CYP2B6), tienilic acid (CYP2C9), and ticlopidine (CYP2C19), all of which contain a furan or thiophene that is activated by cytochrome P450 to a reactive metabolite that in-

activates the enzyme (suicide inactivation). Metabolism-dependent inhibitors that form metabolite inhibitory complexes and cause quasi-irreversible inhibition include the CYP3A4 inhibitor troleandomycin, which contains a tertiary amine (R–N(CH$_3$)$_2$) that is converted by several successive oxidative N-demethylation reactions to a nitroso metabolite (R–N=O) that coordinately binds to the ferrous heme iron. This interaction resembles the binding of carbon monoxide to the ferrous heme iron, and indeed compounds that form inhibitory metabolite complexes with cytochrome P450 can be detected spectrophotometrically based on an absorbance peak at around 455 nm (which is similar to the peak at ~450 nm when carbon monoxide binds to cytochrome P450). The chemical structures commonly associated with metabolism-dependent inhibition of cytochrome P450 are shown in Table 6-13.

In some cases, the metabolism-dependent inhibition involves metabolism by enzymes other than the affected CYP enzyme. For example, the inhibition of CYP2C8 by gemfibrozil requires the formation of gemfibrozil glucuronide by UGT, after which gemfibrozil glucuronide functions as a metabolism-dependent inhibitor of CYP2C8 (Ogilvie et al., 2006).

There are cases where inhibition of cytochrome P450 has proved advantageous, as in the case of certain combinations of anti-HIV drugs. For example, by inhibiting CYP3A4, the HIV protease inhibitor ritonavir improves the pharmacokinetic profile of saquinavir and lopinavir, protease inhibitors that are otherwise cleared so rapidly by CYP3A4 that blood levels easily fall below therapeutically effective concentrations.

Induction of Cytochrome P450—Xenosensors The induction (upregulation) of xenobiotic-biotransforming enzymes and transporters is a receptor-mediated, adaptive process that augments xenobiotic elimination during periods of high xenobiotic exposure. It is not a toxicological or pathological response, but enzyme induction is often associated with liver enlargement (due to both hepatocellular hypertrophy and hyperplasia), and it may be associated with toxicological and pharmacological consequences, especially for the safety evaluation of drug candidates in laboratory animals and for clinical practice in humans. In animals, enzyme induction may be associated with pharmacokinetic tolerance, whereby the xenobiotic induces its own elimination. During safety testing in animals, auto-induction may require increasing dosages of drug candidate to achieve the same degree of systemic exposure. In rodents, lifetime exposure to enzyme inducers may be associated with liver or thyroid tumor formation, as discussed later in this section. In humans, enzyme induction may also be associated with pharmacokinetic tolerance (autoinduction). Long-term treatment of humans with enzyme inducers can cause osteomalacia due to increased inactivation of 1α,25-dihydroxyvitamin D$_3$, the active metabolite of vitamin D (discussed later in this section), but it is not associated with liver or thyroid tumor formation. However, in humans, enzyme induction by one drug (the perpetrator) can augment the clearance of a concomitantly administered drug (the victim), which is a cause of drug–drug interactions.

As an underlying cause of serious adverse events, enzyme induction is generally less important than enzyme inhibition because the latter can cause a rapid and profound increase in blood levels of a victim drug, which can cause an exaggerated pharmacological or toxicological effect. In contrast, enzyme induction lowers blood levels, which does not cause an exaggerated pharmacological or toxicological response to the drug. However, enzyme induction may be associated with a loss of therapeutic effectiveness, which

Table 6-13

Structures Associated with Metabolism-Dependent Inhibition of Cytochrome P450 (CYP) Enzymes

CHEMICAL GROUPS (EXAMPLES)	STRUCTURES
Terminal (ω) and ω-1 acetylenes (Gestodene)	R—≡— R—≡
Furans and thiophenes (Furafylline and tienilic acid)	(furan O ring) (thiophene S ring)
Epoxides (R-Bergamottin-6′,7′-epoxide)	R—(epoxide O)—R_1
Dichloro- and trichloro-ethylenes (1,2,-Dichloroethylene and trichloroethylene)	Cl/Cl C=C H/Cl H/Cl C=C H/Cl Cl/Cl C=C H/H
Secondary amines (Nortriptyline)	H, R on N—R_1
Benzodioxoles (Paroxetine)	(benzodioxole ring, O–CH$_2$–O)
Isothiocyanates (Phenethyl isothiocyanate)	R–N=C=S
Thioamides (Methimazole)	H$_3$C–C(=S)–S–N(H)–R
Dithiocarbamates (Disulfiram)	R–N(H)–C(=S)–SH
Conjugated structures (Rhapontigenin)	R–CH=CH–CH=CH–R
Terminal alkenes (Tiamulin)	R–CH=CH$_2$

Data adapted from Fontana E, Dansette PM, Poli SM: Cytochrome p450 enzymes mechanism based inhibitors: Common sub-structures and reactivity. *Curr Drug Metab* 6:413–454, 2005.

is a particular concern when it compromises the therapeutic effectiveness of drugs that have a narrow therapeutic index and are being used to treat a life-threatening illness, such as anti-HIV drugs, antirejection drugs (like cyclosporine and tacrolimus), and oral anticoagulants (like warfarin), or when it is used with drugs that exhibit a quantal (all-or-nothing) dose–response relationship, such as oral contraceptive steroids (which either block or don't block ovulation and thereby provide or don't provide protection against unwanted pregnancy).

CYP induction does not necessarily enhance the biotransformation of the inducer, in which case the induction is said to be gratuitous. Consequently, lack of autoinduction cannot be taken as evidence that a xenobiotic does not cause enzyme induction. For example, in humans, omeprazole induces CYP1A2, even though the disposition of this acid-suppressing drug is largely determined by CYP2C19 and, to a lesser extent, CYP3A4. Some of the most effective inducers of cytochrome P450 are polyhalogenated aromatic hydrocarbons (PHAHs), such as polychlorinated derivatives of dibenzo-p-dioxin (PCDDs), dibenzofurans (PCDFs), azobenzenes and azoxybenzenes, biphenyl (PCBs), and naphthalene. In general, highly chlorinated compounds are resistant to biotransformation and cause a prolonged induction of CYP and other enzymes. Some in-

ducers are potent direct-acting or metabolism-dependent inhibitors such that they mask the activity of one or more of the enzymes they induce. Such dual-acting xenobiotics include macrolide antibiotics (e.g., erythromycin and troleandomycin), methylenedioxy-containing compounds (e.g., tadalafil [Cialis®], safrole, isosafrole), and imidazole antimycotics (e.g., clotrimazole, ketoconazole, and miconazole). In the case of dual-acting drugs (such as the induction/inhibition of CYP3A4 by ritonavir and several other HIV protease inhibitors, and the induction/inhibition of CYP2E1 by isoniazid), the initial effect—and often the effect observed during the period of drug treatment—is CYP inhibition, with induction becoming evident after prolonged drug treatment or following drug cessation. However, when ritonavir induces CYP3A4, for example, it also induces several other CYP enzymes, as well as conjugating enzymes and transporters that are regulated by CAR/PXR. Ritonavir does not inhibit all of the enzymes it induces. For example, in the presence of 2–20 μM ritonavir for 72 hours, CYP2B6 activity is increased by 4- to 6-fold in primary cultures of human hepatocytes, conditions that cause CYP3A4 inhibition (Faucette *et al.*, 2004). Some dual-acting xenobiotics, like allylisopropylacetamide, cause certain types of porphyria (a disorder of heme synthesis) because they induce CYP enzymes and destroy the CYP heme moiety, which greatly increases the demand for heme synthesis (discussed later in this section).

In general, CYP induction is mediated by four ligand-activated receptors, namely, AhR, CAR, PXR, and PPARα, as summarized in Table 6-14 (adapted from Tirona and Kim, 2005). These so-called xenosensors resemble other nuclear receptors, such as steroid and thyroid hormone receptors, which has consequences for receptor interactions (cross-talk among xenosensors and cross-talk between xenosensors and other nuclear receptors), the role that some xenosensors play in responding to endobiotics and regulating their metabolism (e.g., bilirubin, bile acids, and 1α,25-dihydroxyvitamin D_3), and the role that some nuclear receptors (such as FXR, VDR, SHP, NF-κB) play in inducing or suppressing the expression of xenobiotic-biotransforming enzymes and transporters, as discussed later in this section. Xenosensors have a ligand-binding domain (LBD) and a DNA-binding domain (DBD). In general, CYP induction involves the following steps (with steps 2 and 3 reversed in the case of AhR): (1) Binding of ligand (xenobiotic) to the receptor, which triggers conformational changes that promote its dissociation from accessory proteins (such as co-repressors, chaperones, and cytoplasm-retention proteins) and/or promote its association with co-activators; (2) dimerization of the ligand-bound receptor with a partner protein to form a DNA-binding heterodimer (which is analogous to the two halves of a clothes peg coming together to form a functional unit); (3) translocation of the functional receptor heterodimer from the cytoplasm to the nucleus; (4) binding of the functional receptor heterodimer to discrete regions of DNA (response elements) that are typically located in the 5′-promoter region of the gene (which is analogous to a clothes peg being fastened to a clothes line); (5) recruitment of other transcription factors and RNA-polymerase to form a transcription complex; and (6) gene transcription, which leads to increased levels of CYP mRNA and CYP enzyme (as well as other xenobiotic-biotransforming enzymes and transporters).

As shown in Table 6-14, the major ligand-activated receptors mediating CYP induction are (1) AhR (the aryl hydrocarbon receptor), which partners with ARNT to induce CYP1A1, 1A2, 1B1, and 2S1; (2) CAR (the constitutive androstane receptor; a.k.a. the constitutively active receptor), which partners with RXRα (the retinoid X receptor, which binds 9-cis-retinoic acid) to induce several members of the CYP2A, 2B, 2C, and 3A subfamilies; (3) PXR (the pregnane X receptor, a.k.a. SXR, the steroid X receptor) which, like CAR, partners with RXRα and induces several members of the CYP2A, 2B, 2C, and 3A subfamilies; and (4) PPARα (the peroxisome proliferator activated receptor-alpha), which partners with RXRα and induces CYP4A enzymes. The response elements (a.k.a. consensus sequences) to which xenosensors bind are generally a pair of hexanucleotide sequences in a direct repeat (DR), inverted repeated (IR), or everted repeat (ER) orientation, separated by a 0–8 nucleotide spacer. As shown in Table 6-14, activation of a xenosensor leads to the induction of multiple enzymes, which is called a pleiotypic response. However, in terms of fold induction, CYP enzymes tend to be the most inducible and, consequently, the most studied enzymes. Like induction of CYP enzymes, induction of conjugating and other non-CYP enzymes is an important mechanism of drug–drug and drug–endobiotic interactions. For example, induction of various conjugating enzymes (both SULT and UGT enzymes) plays a key role in the induction of oral contraceptive steroid metabolism in humans, which is associated with a loss of therapeutic effect, and the induction of thyroid hormone metabolism in rodents, which is associated with thyroid follicular cell hyperplasia and tumor forma-

tion. As shown in Table 6-14, AhR, CAR, PXR, and PPARα are not the only receptors that regulate CYP expression in response to xenobiotics (or certain endobiotics). Nrf2 plays a key role in regulating the induction of several enzymes in response to electrophilic metabolites, oxidative stress, or glutathione depletion, as discussed previously (see Point 8 and sections "Epoxide Hydrolases" and "Quinone Reduction—NQO1 and NQO2"). The enzymes regulated by Nrf2 include several conjugating but few CYP enzymes (notable exceptions are CYP2C55 and 2U1 in mice), whereas those regulated by AhR, CAR, PXR, and PPARα include both conjugating and CYP enzymes, for which reason xenobiotics that activate the former are known as *monofunctional inducers* whereas xenobiotics that activate the latter are known as *bifunctional inducers*, as described previously (see "Quinone Reduction—NQO1 and NQO2"). Some of the other receptors listed in Table 6-14 are discussed later in this section. CYP induction can also involve mechanisms other than receptor-mediated transcriptional activation. Increased translation of preexisting mRNA is the mechanism by which several xenobiotics increase the levels of CYP2E1, and increased translational efficiency and protein stabilization play important roles in the induction of several CYP enzymes including CYP1A2, 2E1, and 3A enzymes.

It might be assumed that xenobiotics can be divided into four categories of inducers represented by the four xenosensors (AhR, CAR, PXR, and PPARα). This is largely true of rats where 3-methylcholanthrene, phenobarbital, pregnenolone-16α-carbonitrile (PCN), and clofibric acid are prototypical inducers of CYP1A, 2B, 3A, and 4A by virtue of their ability to activate AhR, CAR, PXR, and PPARα, respectively. In fact, rats have five classes of inducible CYP enzymes with the fifth class represented by CYP2E1, which is inducible by the prototypical inducer isoniazid. However, the situation in other species (including rats on a xenobiotic-by-xenobiotic basis) is not so straightforward because (1) CAR and PXR have similar but not identical LBDs such that ligands that activate one receptor activate the other and vice versa, and (2) CAR and PXR have similar but not identical DBDs such that, once activated, CAR and PXR bind to some of the same response elements and induce the same enzymes. It was once thought that CYP2B induction was mediated only by CAR, and that CYP3A induction was only mediated by PXR. However, the PXR agonist dexamethasone can maximally induce both CYP2B10 and CYP3A11 in wild-type and CAR knock-out mice, indicating that PXR can maximally induce both CYP2B and 3A enzyme in mice. Similarly, the CAR activator phenobarbital can maximally induce CYP2B10 and induce CYP3A11 (albeit submaximally) in wild-type and PXR knockout mice, indicating that CAR can also induce both CYP2B and 3A enzymes (Kodama and Negishi, 2006). The same is true of humans: PXR can maximally induce both CYP2B6 and CYP3A4, whereas CAR can maximally induce CYP2B6 and induce CYP3A4 (albeit submaximally) (Faucette *et al.*, 2006). Furthermore, there are species and strain differences in the LBDs, the DBDs, and the DNA-response elements that give rise to species and strain differences in enzyme induction, and even interindividual differences in humans. Some species differences in enzyme induction reflect differences in the catalytic activity of CYP enzymes. For example, although 7-methoxy- and 7-ethoxyresorufin are useful substrates to study CYP1A enzyme induction in all mammalian species (with some subtle differences, as noted in the section "CYP1A1/2"), 7-pentoxyresorufin is useful for studying CYP2B only in mouse and rat (not hamster, dog, monkey, or humans). However, many species, strain, and individual differences in enzyme induction reflect differences in xenosensor

Table 6-14

Receptors Mediating the Induction (or Suppression) of Cytochrome P450 Enzymes and Other Xenobiotic Biotransforming Enzymes

NUCLEAR RECEPTOR	RESPONSE ELEMENT(S)	RECEPTOR ACTIVATORS	REGULATED GENES[a]
AhR	XRE	PAHs, TCDD (other PHAHs), β-naphthoflavone, indigoids, tryptophan metabolites, omeprazole, lansoprazole	CYP1A1, 1A2, 1B1, 2S1, UGT1A1, UGT1A6
CAR	DR-3 DR-4 ER-6	Phenobarbital, phenytoin, carbamazepine, CITCO (human), TCPOBOP (mouse), clotrimazole, Yin Zhi Wuang (many PXR agonists are also CAR agonists, and vice versa)	CYP2A6, 2B6, 2C8, 2C9, 2C19, 3A4, UGT1A1, SULT1A1, ALAS, MRP2, MRP3
PXR	DR-3 DR-4 ER6 ER-8	Amprenavir, avasimibe, bosentan, bile acids, carbamazepine, clindamycin, clotrimazole, cortisol, cyproterone acetate, dicloxacillin, efavirenz, etoposide, dexamethasone, griseofulvin, guggulsterone, hyperforin (SJW), indinavir, lovastatin, mifepristone, nafcillin, nelfinavir, nifedipine, omeprazole, paclitaxel, PCBs, phenobarbital, phthalate monoesters, 5β-pregnane-3,20-dione, rifabutin, rifampin, ritonavir, saquinavir, simvastatin, spironolactone, sulfinpyrazole, TAO, tetracycline, topotecan, transnanoclor, troglitazone, verapamil, vitamin E, vitamin K_2	CYP2B6, 2C8, 2C9, 2C19, 3A4, 3A7, 7A1↓, SULT2A1, UGT1A1, 1A3, 1A4, PAPSS2, ALAS, MDR1, AhR
PPARα	DR-1	Fibrates, WY-14,643, perfluorodecanoic acid	CYP4A, UGT1A9, 2B4
Nrf2	ARE	β-Naphthoflavone, oltipraz, phenolic antioxidants (e.g., BHA and BHT) and various glutathione depletors	NQO1, mEH, AKR7A, UGTs, GSTA1, γ-GCL, MRP1
GR	GRE	Glucocorticoids	CYP2C9, 2B6, 3A4, 3A5, CAR, PXR
FXR	IR-1	Bile acids, GW4064, AGN29, AGN31	BSEP, I-BABP, MDR3, UGT2B4, SULT2A1, OATP8, PPARα, SHP
LXRα	DR-4	GW3965, T0901317, paxiline, F$_3$methylAA,[b] acetyl-podocarpic dimer (APD)	LRH1, SHP, CYP7A, LXRα, CYP3A4↓↓, 2B6↓
VDR	DR-3 ER-6 IR-0	1α,25-Dihydroxyvitamin D$_3$, lithocholate	CYP2B6, 2C9, 3A4, SULT2A1
HNF1α	c		OATP-C, OATP8, CYP7A1, UGT1A6, 1A8, 1A9, 1A10, HNF4α, PXR
HNF4α	DR		CYP2A6, 2B6, 2C9, 2D6, 3A4, DD4, MDR1, PXR, CAR, FXR, PPARα, HNF1α
LRH-1	DR-4		CYP7A, ASBT
SHP	None		Targets of PPARα ↓, AhR↓, PXR↓, CAR↓, LRH-1↓, HNF4α↓, LXRα↓, GR↓

[a] A downward arrow indicates downregulation (suppression). All others are upregulated (induced).

[b] [3-Chloro-4-(3-(7-propyl-3-trifluoromethyl-6-(4,5)-isoxazolyl)propylthio)-phenylacetic acid].

[c] The HNF1α consensus sequence is GTTTAATNATTAAC.

Data adapted from Tirona RG , Kim RB: Nuclear receptors and drug disposition gene regulation. *J Pharm Sci* 94:1169–1186, 2005.

function, as discussed below (this section). The following descriptions of the individual xenosensors focus largely on the mouse and human receptors; studies of the latter have been driven by the desire to investigate drug–drug interactions whereas studies of the former have been facilitated by the ability to create transgenic mice in which a particular xenosensor has been deleted (so-called knockout or null mice) or replaced with the human receptor (so-called humanized mice).

The Aryl Hydrocarbon Receptor (AhR)   AhR and ARNT are cytosolic and nuclear transcription factors, respectively, that are expressed in most tissues and many cell lines. The binding of an agonist like 2,3,7,8-tetrachlorodibenzo-p-dioxin (TCDD, the structure of which is shown in Table 6-15), to AhR initiates a number of changes (such as dissociation from heat-shock protein [hsp90] and other chaperones, dissociation from proteins that retain the unbound receptor in the cytoplasm, phosphorylation by tyrosine kinase) that culminate in (1) the translocation of AhR to the nucleus, (2) the dimerization of AhR with ARNT (which is somewhat misnamed as the *aryl hydrocarbon receptor nuclear translocator* because it is a nuclear not a cytoplasmic protein that complexes with AhR after it translocates to the nucleus), (3) the binding of AhR–ARNT to DNA-response elements known as XRE, and (4) the increased transcription of CYP1A1 and numerous other genes listed in Table 6-14. Whereas members of the nuclear receptor superfamily (such as CAR, PXR, and PPARα) are "zinc-finger" proteins, AhR and ARNT are "bHLH-PAS" proteins, so-named because they belong to the per-arnt-sim (PAS) class of receptors and they have a basic helix-loop-helix (bHLH) domain near their N-terminus, which is involved in protein–protein interactions.

TCDD is a high affinity ligand for AhR (K_D values tend to be in the nanomolar-to-submicromolar range), and AhR mediates the toxicity of TCDD and related PHAHs (such as various chlorinated or brominated dibenzodioxins, dibenzofurans, and biphenyls), which is characterized by a wasting syndrome (progressive weight loss or cachexia resulting in death), immunosuppression (thymic atrophy), tumor promotion, fetal abnormalities (cleft palate and other teratogenic disorders) and, in some species, liver enlargement and a skin condition called chloracne. TCDD binds to AhR and induces CYP1A1 in all mammalian species, but it causes lethal cachexia in some species (such as guinea pig, where the LD_{50} is ~1 µg/kg) but not others (such as hamsters, where the LD_{50} exceeds 1000 µg/kg). This species difference in toxicity but not in CYP1A1 induction raised the possibility that AhR does not mediate the toxicity of TCDD, but several lines of evidence established that AhR does in fact mediate many, perhaps all, of the toxic effects of TCDD and related compounds. First, naturally occurring strain differences in the responsiveness of mice (such as so-called responsive C57 and nonresponsive DBA mice) and rats (such as responsive Long–Evans and nonresponsive Han/Wistar rats) to TCDD toxicity are associated with polymorphisms in AhR (Pohjanvirta *et al.*, 1999). Second, AhR knockout mice are resistant to TCDD-induced toxicity, whereas transgenic mice that express a constitutively active form of AhR (CA-AhR mice) spontaneously display numerous signs of TCDD toxicity (even though the CYP1A1 levels in the liver of CA-AhR mice are elevated to a lesser extent than those in TCDD-treated wild-type mice) (Brunnberg *et al.*, 2006). Third, the AhR antagonist CH-223191 (see Table 6-15) blocks the enzyme-inducing effects and various toxic effects of TCDD (Kim *et al.*, 2006). Nevertheless, it remains to be determined why prolonged activation of AhR by TCDD and related compounds causes an irreversible cachexia that leads to death after a certain time (after a latency period that varies from one species to the next but that cannot be shortened by administering "super-lethal" doses of TCDD).

AhR agonists include PHAHs (like TCDD), PAHs (like 3-methylcholanthrene and benzo[*a*]pyrene), flavonoids (like β-naphthoflavone), and various acid-catalyzed condensation products or UV-induced derivatives of naturally occurring indoles (such as indole-3-carbinol and tryptophan). In general, AhR agonists induce CYP1A1 and other enzymes across all mammalian and many nonmammalian species. A notable exception is a class of benzimidazole-containing compounds that includes the proton-pump inhibitors omeprazole and lansoprazole. These drugs are not typical AhR agonists for two reasons. First, they do not bind to the ligand-binding domain of AhR but activate AhR either directly (by binding to a second site on AhR) or indirectly (by activating a tyrosine kinase that phosphorylates AhR). Second, they activate AhR and induce CYP1A enzymes in humans but not in rats or mice,

which is one of the few species differences in AhR activation by xenobiotics (Diaz *et al.*, 1990). An endogenous AhR ligand is suspected to exist because AhR function is so well conserved from fish to humans and because of developmental abnormalities observed in AhR knockout mice. However, an endogenous AhR ligand has yet to be identified.

Several compounds can disrupt AhR signaling at a variety of levels. CH-223191 (Table 6-15) and α-naphthoflavone are receptor antagonists that bind to the ligand-binding domain of AhR without activating the receptor. Omeprazole sulfide (which forms by reduction of the sulfoxide group in omeprazole [see Table 6-15]) antagonizes CYP1A1 induction by omeprazole by stabilizing AhR in an inactive conformation (Gerbal-Chaloin *et al.*, 2005). After AhR is activated, its translocation to the nucleus is blocked by 3'-methoxy-4-nitroflavone, its binding to XRE is blocked by salicylamide, and its ability to recruit transcription factors and initiate gene transcription is blocked by resveratrol (an antioxidant in red wine) (Gerbal-Chaloin *et al.*, 2005). The presence of exogenous (and perhaps endogenous) AhR antagonists is one of the many factors that are known or suspected of causing clinically observed interindividual differences in CYP1A induction. These factors have been reviewed by Ma and Lu (2003), who have documented that differences in the magnitude of CYP1A induction in humans can be attributed to (1) genetic polymorphisms in AhR, ARNT, or XRE; (2) altered levels or function of accessory proteins (some of which are associated with inflammation and other disease states that activate NF-κB, as discussed later in this section); (3) gender differences in basal CYP1A2 activity (which tends to be lower in females compared with males); and (4) variation in the intracellular concentration of the inducing drug, as exemplified by variation in the metabolism of omeprazole. The clearance of omeprazole is largely determined by its rate of metabolism by the polymorphically expressed enzyme CYP2C19. Based on measurements of caffeine metabolism, a daily dose of 40 mg omeprazole causes CYP1A2 induction in CYP2C19 PMs but not in CYP2C19 EMs, which require higher doses (120 mg) to achieve CYP1A2 induction. In a clinical setting, the formation of omeprazole sulfide (an AhR antagonist) does not prevent CYP1A induction by omeprazole (an agonist). However, it is possible that the formation of rabeprazole sulfide, which occurs rapidly and extensively (by nonenzymatic means), explains why rabeprazole is one of the proton-pump inhibitors that does not induce CYP1A.

Although strain differences in CYP1A inducibility have been linked to genetic polymorphisms in the mouse and rat AhR gene, species differences have been attributed either to the unusual interaction of AhR with benzimidazole-containing compounds like omeprazole and lansoprazole or to species differences in the location of XRE. For example, rat UGT1A6 and 1A7 are highly inducible (> 20-fold) enzymes because these conjugating genes are under the control of XRE in rats but in few other species.

Constitutive Androstane Receptor (CAR) and Pregnane X Receptor (PXR) CAR and PXR are members of the nuclear receptor family 1 (NR1I2 and NR1I3, respectively). In contrast to AhR, which is expressed in most tissues and several cell lines, CAR and PXR are expressed in relatively few organs—liver, small intestine, and colon—and in few cell lines. CAR and PXR are both activated by some of the same compounds, and both dimerize with RXRα to form DNA-binding proteins that recognize some of the same response elements, as shown in Table 6-14. Consequently, there is considerable cross-talk between these two xenosensors, and it can sometimes be difficult to ascertain whether induction is mediated

Table 6-15

Examples of Agonists and Antagonists for the Receptors that Mediate Enzyme Induction (AhR, CAR, and PXR)

	AGONISTS			ANTAGONISTS		

AhR — TCDD (agonist); CH-223191 (antagonist)

Omerprazole (agonist); Omerprazole sulfide (antagonist)

CAR		Human	Mouse		Human	Mouse
	Agonists			Inverse agonists		
	Chlorpromazine	No	Yes	Chlorpromazine	Yes	No
	Clotrimazole	No	Yes	Meclizine	Yes	No
	Meclizine	No	Yes			
	Indirect activators	Yes	Yes			
	Phenobarbital	Yes	Yes			
	Phenytoin					
PXR	Agonists	Human	Mouse	Antagonists	Human	Mouse
	Artemisinin	Yes	No	Ketoconazole	Yes	Unknown
	Clotrimazole	Yes	No	Trabectedin (ET-743)	Yes	Unknown
	Hyperforin	Yes	Yes			
	Nicardipine	Yes	No			
	Nifedipine	Yes	No			
	Phenobarbital	Yes	Yes			
	PCN	Weak	Yes			
	Rifampin	Yes	No			

PCN, Pregnenolone-16α-carbonitrile; TCDD, 2,3,7,8-tetrachlorodibenzo-*p*-dioxin.

by CAR, PXR, or both receptors. As shown in Table 6-14, three factors combine to make CAR and PXR the most important human xenosensors in terms of drug–drug interactions. First, CAR and PXR regulate several CYP enzymes (e.g., CYP2B6, 2C8, 2C9, 2C19, and 3A4), conjugating enzymes (several UGTs and SULTs), and transporters (such as *P*-glycoprotein [MDR1 or ABCB1]). Second, a large number of xenobiotics (drugs and the herbal preparations, St. John's wort and Yin Zhi Wuang) and certain endobiotics (such as bilirubin, bile acids, and 1α,25-dihydroxyvitamin D$_3$) activate CAR and/or PXR. Third, some of the genes regulated by CAR and PXR encode proteins with broad substrate specificities, such as CYP3A4 and *P*-glycoprotein, such that the induction mediated by CAR and PXR impacts the disposition of a large number of xenobiotics and certain endobiotics (see Table 6-11). In terms of drug–drug interactions, human xenosensors can be rank-ordered (from most important to least) as follows: CAR/PXR > AhR > "CYP2E1" > PPARα. PPARα is ranked last because its activation in humans, in contrast to its activation in rodents, does not lead to CYP4 induction (a family of enzymes that plays a limited role in drug metabolism compared with CYP1, 2, and 3 enzymes). CYP2E1 is an inducible enzyme in humans (by mechanisms that do not appear to involve any of the xenosensors listed in Table 6-15), but relatively few drugs are in-

ducers of—or substrates for—CYP2E1. AhR is less important than CAR/PXR because there are relatively few drugs that activate AhR and because the major hepatic enzyme regulated by AhR, namely, CYP1A2, plays a more limited role in drug metabolism than the hepatic and intestinal CYP enzymes regulated by CAR/PXR, namely, CYP2B6, 2C8, 2C9, 2C19, and 3A4.

The activation of PXR follows the canonical steps outlined above (this section), beginning with ligand binding, dissociation from cytoplasmic retention protein and co-repressors (like SMRT), and association with co-activators (like RAC3), dimerization with RXRα, translocation to the nucleus and binding to various DNA-response elements (multiple PXREs known as DR-3, DR-4, ER-6, and ER-8), which culminates in transcriptional activation of multiple genes, as shown in Table 6-14 (Chang and Waxman, 2006; Stanley *et al.*, 2006). Species differences in the LBD of PXR account for certain species differences in CYP3A induction. For example, PCN is a prototypical inducer of CYP3A in rats and mice, but not humans, whereas the opposite is true of rifampin. Transgenic mice with human PXR in place of mouse PXR (PXR-humanized mice) lose the ability to respond to PCN and gain the ability to respond to rifampin. Rifampin can also bind and activate rat PXR once the opening to the LBD is slightly widened (by changing a phenylalanine to a leucine residue). As shown in Table 6-14, rifampin, artemisinin, clotrimazole, nicardipine, and nifedipine are agonists for human PXR but not mouse PXR, which exemplifies why enzyme induction studies in rodents often fail to predict enzyme induction in humans. Some agonists bind to human PXR with relatively high affinity (with K_D values in the [sub]micromolar range), including rifampin and hyperforin, the inducing agent in St. John's wort. In general, activation of CAR/PXR shows little or no stereospecificity, although the C-cyclopropylalkylamide known as S20 is a rare exception: $(-)$-C20 preferentially activates mouse PXR whereas $(+)$-C20 preferentially activates human PXR. This difference further underscores the lack of predictability of rodent data to the human situation.

Tang *et al.* (2005) have reviewed the factors that give rise to differences in the magnitude of enzyme induction by PXR/CAR agonists in humans; such differences can be attributed to (1) genetic polymorphisms or splicing variation in PXR or CAR and/or polymorphism in their DNA-response elements; (2) altered levels or function of accessory proteins (some of which are associated with inflammation and other disease states that activate NF-κB, as discussed later in this section); (3) gender differences in basal CYP3A4 activity (which tends to be lower in males compared with females); and (4) variation in the intracellular concentration of the inducing drug, as exemplified by variation in the metabolism of propafenone and celecoxib. Propafenone is metabolized by CYP2D6, 3A4, and 1A2. In CYP2D6 EMs, the clearance of propafenone is determined by CYP2D6, and treatment with rifampin causes no induction of propafenone metabolism. However, in CYP2D6 PMs, CYP3A4 plays a significant role in the clearance of propafenone, and treatment of CYP2D6 PMs with rifampin causes a doubling of propafenone clearance. The COX-2 inhibitor celecoxib is a PXR agonist whose in vivo clearance is largely determined by CYP2C9. There is evidence to suggest that, at recommended clinical doses, celecoxib induces CYP3A4 in CYP2C9 PMs but not in CYP2C9 EMs due to the higher levels of celecoxib in the poor metabolizers (Rodrigues *et al.*, 2006).

The activation of CAR is considerably more complex than that of PXR (Chang and Waxman, 2006; Kodama and Negishi, 2006; Stanley *et al.*, 2006). CAR is constitutively active, meaning that, in the absence of an exogenous ligand, it can complex with RXRα, translocate to the nucleus, bind to DNA-response elements (known as PBREM [for phenobarbital response elements] or Barbie boxes), and activate gene transcription, which is what generally happens when CAR is expressed in cell lines in vitro. In the in vivo situation (such as occurs in hepatocytes), CAR is prevented from being transcriptionally active by its retention in the cytoplasm by cytoplasmic CAR-retention protein (CCRP) and chaperones such as hsp90, and possibly by its binding to an endogenous reverse agonist such as androstanol (5α-androstan-3α-ol) and androstenol (5α-androst-16-en-3α-ol), the androstanes for which CAR is named (reverse agonists are discussed later in this section). The release of CAR from CCRP can be triggered either by *direct activators*, which bind directly to CAR, or by *indirect activators*, which trigger the phosphorylation of CAR by AMP-activated protein kinase (AMPK) (Rencurel *et al.*, 2006). The classical inducer phenobarbital is an indirect activator of CAR, which leads to induction of CYP2B and, to a lesser extent, CYP3A enzymes. The ability of phenobarbital to induce CYP2B10 and CYP3A11 is abolished in transgenic mice lacking either CAR or the α-subunit of AMPK, which is compelling evidence that activation of AMPK is the mechanism by which phenobarbital activates CAR (Rencurel *et al.*, 2006). AMPK is sensitive to energy charge; consequently it is activated by an increase in the ratio of AMP to ATP.

Consequently, AMPK is activated by fasting, which has been shown to induce CYP2B10 in mice. Metformin, a drug used to lower fasting blood glucose levels in patients with noninsulin-dependent (Type 2) diabetes, also activates AMPK, and metformin has been shown to induce CYP2B6 and 3A4 in human hepatocytes. It is interesting that, like metformin, phenobarbital also lowers glucose levels in patients with Type 2 diabetes (Rencurel *et al.*, 2006). This glucose-lowering effect appears to involve, at least in part, the following steps: (1) activation of AMPK by phenobarbital or metformin; (2) activation of CAR by AMPK-dependent phosphorylation; (3) binding of activated CAR to FoxO1, a transcription factor that binds to insulin-response sequences (IRS), which are DNA-response elements in the promoter region of gluconeogenic genes such as phosphoenolpyruvate carboxykinase-1 (PEPCK1) and glucose-6-phosphatase and (4) decreased gluconeogenesis (i.e., decreased glucose synthesis) as a result of FoxO1 repression by CAR (Kodama and Negishi, 2006; Rencurel *et al.*, 2006). Consistent with this mechanism of action, phenobarbital decreases glucose levels in wild-type mice but not in CAR knockout mice.

The interaction between CAR and FoxO1 has opposing effects on transcriptional activity: CAR is a *co-repressor* of FoxO1 whereas FoxO1 is a *co-activator* of CAR. Activation of FoxO1 by diabetes increases CYP2B and 3A expression in rats and mice, and this effect is reversed by insulin treatment (which stimulates the phosphorylation of FoxO1 and thereby decreases its activity). By inactivating FoxO1 (which removes a co-activator for CAR), insulin blunts the induction of CYP2B enzymes by phenobarbital (Kodama and Negishi, 2006).

Phosphorylation is required for both the retention of CAR in the cytoplasm and the release of CAR from CCRP, which seems paradoxical. However, the paradox is resolved by the fact that phosphorylation for CAR retention and phosphorylation for CAR activation occur at different sites. Phosphorylation of serine-202 in mouse CAR and of serine-192 in human CAR is required for the retention of CAR in the cytoplasm, and dephosphorylation by protein phosphatase 2A is an important step in CAR activation (as evidenced by the observation that the protein phosphatase 2A inhibitor okadaic acid blocks CAR translocation in mouse hepatocytes). In addition to dephosphorylation, activation of CAR also requires phosphorylation by AMPK, which occurs at sites other than serine-202 in mouse CAR and serine-192 in human CAR (Rencurel *et al.*, 2006).

Because CAR is constitutively active but retained in the cytoplasm, ligands can function as agonists, reverse agonists, or antagonists. Agonists activate CAR by displacing endogenous reverse agonists (e.g., androstanes) or by promoting the dissociation of co-repressors (such as NcoR) and the recruitment of co-activators (such as SRC-1, Sp1, ASC-2, and PBP). Reverse agonists have the opposite effect: they promote the dissociation of co-activators and the recruitment of co-repressors, and they may also decrease the transcriptional activity of CAR. Antagonists bind to the same LBD as agonists and reverse agonists; they neither activate nor deactivate CAR, but they block the binding of other ligands.

As shown in Table 6-15, xenobiotics can function as CAR agonists or antagonists in a species-specific manner. For example, chlorpromazine and meclizine are agonists for mouse CAR, but they are inverse agonists for human CAR. TCPOBOP and CITCO are potent direct activators of CAR, but they function as CAR agonists in a species-specific manner: TCPOBOP is a potent agonist for mouse CAR whereas CITCO is a potent agonist for human CAR. The use of these selective CAR agonists must be used in a species-specific manner, as underscored by the fact that the mouse CAR agonist

TCPOBOP is *not* an agonist for human CAR but it *is* an agonist for human PXR. Phenobarbital is an indirect activator of mouse and human CAR, but it is also an activator of human PXR (but not mouse or rat PXR). In contrast, another enzyme-inducing antiepileptic drug (EIAED) phenytoin does not activate human PXR and, like CITCO, is a selective activator of human CAR. These species differences in CAR, like those described earlier in this section for PXR, illustrate why, during the safety evaluation of drug candidates, enzyme induction studies in rodents are often of limited value in predicting enzyme induction in humans.

CAR and PXR are activated by certain endobiotics, and the enzymes regulated by these xenosensors play important roles in terminating the hormonal activity of $1\alpha,25$-dihydroxyvitamin D_3 ($1,25$-$(OH)_2$-D_3 and attenuating the toxicity of high levels of bilirubin and bile acids. The active form of vitamin D, namely, $1,25$-$(OH)_2$-D_3, binds to the vitamin D receptor (VDR) to induce the synthesis of calbindin-D9K, a calcium-binding protein that facilitates the uptake of calcium from the intestinal lumen to blood. VDR also induces CYP enzymes that further hydroxylate and thereby inactivate $1,25$-$(OH)_2$-D_3, which establishes a negative feedback loop. Two VDR-inducible CYP enzymes have been shown to inactivate $1,25$-$(OH)_2$-D_3 by hydroxylating the active hormone in the 24- and, to a lesser extent, the 23-position. The first is CYP24A1, which is expressed mainly in the kidney, and which catalyzes the $24R$-hydroxylation of $1,25$-$(OH)_2$-D_3. The second is CYP3A4, which is expressed mainly in intestine and liver, and which catalyzes the $24S$-hydroxylation of $1,25$-$(OH)_2$-D_3. The stereochemical differences in the 24-hydroxylation reaction helped to establish that CYP3A4 is the principal inactivator of $1,25$-$(OH)_2$-D_3 in the intestine, with little or no contribution from CYP24A1. These findings are important for two reasons. First, the ability of VDR to mimic PXR/CAR and induce CYP3A4 is an example of the cross-talk that can occur between a xenosensor and other nuclear receptors. Second, the key role played by CYP3A4 in the inactivation of $1,25$-$(OH)_2$-D_3 in the intestine provides an explanation for the clinical observation that long-term treatment of patients with rifampin, phenobarbital, phenytoin, or carbamazepine can lead to osteomalacia, a bone disorder that is symptomatic of vitamin D deficiency. These PXR/CAR agonists are thought to cause osteomalacia by inducing CYP3A4 in the intestine, which accelerates the inactivation of $1,25$-$(OH)_2$-D_3 and thereby impairs calcium absorption (Xu *et al.*, 2006; Zhou *et al.*, 2006a).

CAR plays an important role in detoxifying high levels of bilirubin, as might occur in patients with hemolytic anemia. Like phenobarbital, bilirubin is an indirect activator of CAR. When activated, CAR induces UGT1A1, the major hepatic enzyme responsible for glucuronidating bilirubin, as well as transporters of bilirubin/bilirubin glucuronide. When hemolytic anemia is induced by treating mice with phenylhydrazine, bilirubin levels rise to a greater extent in CAR knockout mice compared with wild-type mice, which demonstrates the important role CAR plays in responding to high levels of bilirubin. Phenobarbital was once used to treat neonatal jaundice, and the Chinese herbal Yin Zhi Wuang is still used for this purpose. Phenobarbital and scoparone (6,7-dimethylesculetin), the active ingredient in Yin Zhi Wuang, are CAR activators that, like bilirubin itself, induces the major bilirubin-conjugating enzyme UGT1A1 and related transporters (Chang and Waxman, 2006; Kodama and Negishi, 2006). In contrast, CAR appears to play a role in acetaminophen hepatotoxicity by allowing acetaminophen to induce its own activation to a toxic quinoneimine. CAR knockout mice are relatively resistant to acetaminophen hepatotoxicity compared with both wild-type and CAR-humanized mice, which suggests early treatment with a CAR agonist might be a useful adjunct treatment for acetaminophen overdose.

CAR and PXR appear to act as backup receptors to prevent bile acid accumulation and toxicity when the principal bile acid sensor, FXR (the farnesoid X receptor), is overloaded. High concentrations of bile acids activate FXR, which suppresses the expression of CYP7A1, the cholesterol 7α-hydroxylase that catalyzes the rate-limiting step in bile acid synthesis, and which induces the expression of bile acid conjugating enzymes (UGT2B4 and SULT2A1) and bile acid transporters (such as BSEP, the bile salt export pump). When hepatocytes contain low concentrations of bile acids, FXR is inactive and the expression of CYP7A1 is stimulated by LRH-1 (liver receptor homolog-1), a constitutively active nuclear receptor. When hepatocytes contain high concentrations of bile acids, FXR is activated, and it inactivates LRH-1 by inducing the synthesis of small heterodimer partner-1 (SHP), so named because it lacks a DNA-binding domain (hence its small size) and because it forms heterodimers with LRH-1 and numerous other nuclear receptors including AhR, CAR, PXR, LXRα, HNF4α, and the glucocorticoid receptor (GR). Because it lacks a DBD, SHP inactivates all of these receptors; in the case of LRH-1, this results in a loss of CYP7A1 expression and a decrease in bile acid synthesis, which represents a negative feedback loop. FXR knockout mice are more sensitive than wild-type mice to bile acid toxicity, and treatment with the FXR ligand GW4064 further protects wild-type mice against experimentally induced extra- and intrahepatic cholestasis. Cholic acid is both an FXR and PXR agonist; it suppresses CYP7A1 expression first by activating FXR and then PXR. In contrast to the situation in wild-type or single receptor knockout mice, 1% dietary cholic acid is lethal to FXR/PXR double knockout mice. PXR and CAR play a similar role in attenuating the toxicity of lithocholic acid, which is both a PXR agonist and a substrate for many of the enzymes regulated by PXR, including CYP3A, SULT, and transporters involved in the hepatic uptake and efflux of lithocholic acid. In PXR/CAR double knockout mice, lithocholic acid causes lethal hepatotoxicity at doses that are well tolerated by wild-type mice. The mouse PXR agonist PCN can markedly suppress CYP7A1 expression and bile acid synthesis in mice, and the human PXR agonist rifampin can markedly suppress CYP7A1 expression in human hepatocytes. The ability of PXR/CAR to function as a backup system for FXR may be compromised by the expression of SHP, which represses the activity of these xenosensors. This complex interplay is one of the likely reasons why there are some conflicting results from studies of the role of PXR/CAR in bile acid detoxication.

As the preceding examples in this section illustrate, there is a complex interplay between many of the nuclear receptors listed in Table 6-14. Some nuclear receptors, such as the hepatic nuclear factors HNF1α and HNF4α, play a critical permissive role in gene regulation by CAR, PXR, and other receptors, whereas others, such as SHP, play a widespread role in suppressing nuclear receptor activity. HNF1α is instrumental for the expression of high levels of CYP2E1 mRNA in liver, although it is not the only factor because disruption of the β-catenin gene in mice greatly reduces CYP2E1 mRNA levels in the liver in the absence of changes in HNF1α expression (Gonzalez, 2007). The glucocorticoid receptor (GR) plays an important role in inducing the synthesis of CAR and PXR (and individual xenobiotic-biotransforming enzymes like CYP2C9). The role of GR in regulating the synthesis of xenosensors and the interplay among nuclear receptors are instrumental to the mechanism by which infections and inflammatory diseases suppress the expression and blunt the induction of xenobiotic-biotransforming enzymes and, conversely, the mechanism by which PXR agonists cause immuno-suppression.

The expression and induction of xenobiotic-biotransforming enzymes by AhR, CAR, PXR, and PPARα are all suppressed by infection (viral, bacterial, and parasitic), vaccination, inflammation, and treatment with endotoxin (lipopolysaccharide or LPS) or inflammatory cytokines such as interleukin-1β (IL-1β) and IL-6. The suppression involves (1) a decrease in the *levels* of PXR and CAR due to a decrease in GR activity, and (2) a decrease in the *activity* of GR, PXR, CAR, AhR, PPARα, and several other nuclear receptors including the androgen, estrogen, and mineralocorticoid receptors (De Bosscher *et al.*, 2006; Pascual and Glass, 2006; Zhou *et al.*, 2006b). The decrease in receptor activity is caused by NF-κB (nuclear factor kappa-B), which is activated during infection and inflammatory disease, and which induces the synthesis of COX-2, TNFα, ICAM-1, and several interleukins. NF-κB binds to the DBD of RXRα and thereby decreases the transcriptional activity of all nuclear receptors that form heterodimers with RXRα (such as PXR, CAR, PPARα, GR, etc.). It also decreases the transcriptional activity of AhR even though AhR forms heterodimers with ARNT, not RXRα. By lowering the levels and/or inhibiting the activity of the major xenosensors and numerous other nuclear factors, NF-κB mediates the widespread suppression of xenobiotic-biotransforming enzymes associated with infection and inflammatory disease. However, the converse is also true inasmuch as certain nuclear receptors, when activated, can complex NF-κB and thereby repress the expression of NF-κB-regulated genes (COX-2, TNFα, ICAM-1, interleukins). This is the basis, at least in part, for the immunosuppressive effect of corticosteroids, which activate GR, and the immunosuppressive effect of PXR ligands such as rifampin and mifepristone (RU-486). PXR appears to play an important role in suppressing NF-κB activity in the small intestine. PXR knockout mice show signs of inflammation of the small intestine, and certain genetic polymorphisms and splicing variants of PXR are associated with inflammatory bowel disease. The role of PXR in regulating NF-κB activity, responding to high levels of bile acids, terminating the actions of 1,25-(OH)$_2$-D$_3$, and the role of CAR in responding to high level of bilirubin and the activation of CAR by FoxO1 and food deprivation all illustrate that these so-called xenosensors do not simply respond to xenobiotics but play key roles in endobiotic homeostasis.

Peroxisome Proliferator Activated Receptor-Alpha (PPARα) The distinction between xenobiotic- and endobiotic-sensing functions is particularly blurred in the case of PPARα, which is activated by endogenous fatty acids (e.g., arachidonic acid), eicosanoids and conjugated steroids such as dehydroepiandrosterone sulfate, as well as numerous acidic xenobiotics such as hypolipidemic fibrate drugs (e.g., clofibrate, fenofibrate, ciprofibrate), various NSAIDs, aspirin, leukotriene receptor antagonists (MK-0571 and RG 7512), organic solvents (trichloroacetic acid), phthalate ester plasticizers, herbicides (haloxyfab, lactyofen, 2,4-dichlorophenoxyacetic acid or 2,4-D), perfluorodecanoic acid, nicotinic acid, and the potent and widely used experimental PPARα agonist Wy-14643. Some of these ligands bind to PPARα stereoselectively; therefore, the enantiomers of certain drugs differ in their ability to activate PPARα. When activated with ligand and complexed with RXRα, PPARα activates the transcription of several genes that encode peroxisomal enzymes involved in the β-oxidation of fatty acids, including fatty acyl-CoA oxidase, bifunctional enzyme (enoyl-CoA hydratase/3-hydroxyacyl-CoA dehydrogenase), and fatty acid binding protein.

In rodents, this is associated with a proliferation of peroxisomes and hepatomegaly, which is why xenobiotics that activate PPARα are often called peroxisome proliferators. Increased peroxisomal fatty acid degradation is the mechanism by which the hypolipidemic fibrate drugs decrease the pool of fatty acyl-CoA required for triglyceride synthesis, but it is not clear where in the body this increased peroxisomal fatty acid degradation occurs. It appears to occur in the kidney, skeletal muscle, and heart, and it may also occur in the liver, although in humans fatty acids are thought to be degraded mainly by mitochondrial, not peroxisomal, β-oxidation. The limited role of liver peroxisomal fatty acid oxidation in mediating the hypolipidemic effects of fibrate drugs is further suggested by the observation that the levels of PPARα in human liver are relatively low (about one-tenth those in rodent liver), and in contrast to the situation in rodents, activation of human PPARα does not result in the induction of microsomal CYP4A enzymes or liver enlargement due to a proliferation of peroxisomes. In contrast to agonists for other xenosensors, PPARα agonists are not a concern as perpetrators of drug–drug interactions, but they are a concern from a tumor promotion perspective, as outlined in the next section.

Enzyme Induction and Chemical Carcinogenesis   In humans, induction of CYP2E1 and the associated increased activation of acetaminophen to *N*-acetylbenzoquinoneimine (NAPQI) is one of the mechanisms by which alcohol consumption and fasting potentiate acetaminophen hepatotoxicity (other contributing mechanisms include the impaired conjugation of acetaminophen due to lowered levels of UDPGA and PAPS and the impaired detoxication of NAPQI due to lowered levels of glutathione). By analogy, induction of CYP enzymes would be expected to increase the activation of procarcinogens to DNA-reactive metabolites, leading to increased tumor formation. However, contrary to expectation, treatment of rodents with a CYP inducer prior to treatment with a known proximate carcinogen (tumor initiators like aflatoxin, various nitrosamines, or polycyclic aromatic hydrocarbons) is generally associated with a decrease, not an increase, in tumor incidence (Parkinson and Hurwitz, 1991). The route of exposure to the carcinogen can affect the impact of enzyme induction; it protects against orally administered drugs but may increase the tumorigenicity of carcinogens applied directly to their site of action (Nebert *et al.*, 2004). Although treatment of rats and mice with a CYP inducer *before* treatment with an initiator (a genotoxic carcinogen) generally decreases tumor incidence, treatment with a CYP inducer *after* the initiator (such as diethylnitrosamine) generally increases tumor incidence because CYP inducers generally function as tumor promoters in rodents.

Phenobarbital is representative of a large number of compounds that appear to promote liver tumor formation in rats or mice by an epigenetic mechanism, including phenytoin, carbamazepine, chlordecone, butylated hydroxytoluene, DDT, dieldrin, hexachlorocyclohexane, certain polychlorinated and polybrominated biphenyls, loratadine, doxylamine, lansoprazole, musk xylene, and fenbuconazole (Williams and Iatropoulos, 2002; Juberg *et al.*, 2006). Although the exact mechanism of tumor formation remains unknown, it is critically dependent on CAR activation, as evidenced by the finding that phenobarbital and related compounds do not function as tumor promoters in CAR knockout mice (Gonzalez and Yu, 2006). Furthermore, phenobarbital and related compounds only cause liver tumors at doses that cause liver enlargement due to an increase in cell number (hepatocellular hyperplasia) and cell size (hepatocellular hypertrophy). The liver changes induced by phenobarbital, including an increase in DNA synthesis within 24 hours, a wave of mitotic activity after 1–3 days, enzyme induction (e.g., CYP2B enzymes) and a progressive increase in liver weight, all exhibit nonlinear dose–response relationships, suggesting that there is a threshold dose below which no activation of CAR and no liver tumor promotion occur.

Although induction of CYP2B enzymes (and other xenobiotic-biotransforming enzymes and transporters) is a common feature of phenobarbital and related tumor-promoting chemicals, the two events do not appear to be mechanistically linked (Williams and Iatropoulos, 2002). After CAR activation, the key downstream events leading to liver tumor formation are not known in great detail, but the downregulation (suppression) of gap junctions, which impedes intercellular communication, is one such critical downstream event, as evidenced by the lack of tumor-promoting activity by phenobarbital in transgenic mice lacking connexin 32, a component of gap junctions, even though CYP2B10 and other enzymes can be induced in these knockout mice.

The mechanism of thyroid tumor formation is better understood. In rodents, CAR (and PPARα) agonists induce UGT and SULT enzymes and transporters that accelerate the conjugation and elimination of thyroid hormones, which triggers a compensatory increase in thyroid-stimulating hormone (TSH). Sustained stimulation of the thyroid gland by TSH leads to the development of thyroid follicular tumors, the development of which can be blocked by administering thyroxine, which blocks the release of TSH and thereby abrogates the hormonal stimulation of the thyroid gland. It is not clear why sustained stimulation of the thyroid gland by TSH results in tumor formation in rodents, but such tumors develop in other rodent organs following prolonged hormonal stimulation: LH causes Leydig cell tumors, gastrin causes stomach tumors, and corticosteroids cause pancreatic tumors. In addition, just as proliferation of the hepatic endoplasmic reticulum and peroxisomes by phenobarbital and Wy-14643 is associated with liver tumor formation, so the proliferation of hepatic lysosomes by Ponceau-S and the proliferation of mitochondria by methapyrilene are also associated with liver tumor formation (Grasso et al., 1991).

Epidemiological studies of epileptic patients treated for more than 35 years with phenobarbital or phenytoin have established that chronic liver microsomal enzyme induction in humans does not increase the incidence of liver or thyroid tumor formation (Singh et al., 2005). Prolonged elevation of TSH in humans does not lead to tumor formation but causes goiter, a reversible enlargement of the thyroid gland associated with iodide deficiency and treatment with drugs that block thyroid hormone synthesis. In humans and monkeys, circulating thyroxine (T4) is largely bound to thyroxine-binding globulin (TBG). This high-affinity binding protein is not present in rodents, for which reason T4 is rapidly conjugated and excreted in bile. Accordingly, the plasma half-life of thyroxine in rats (12–24 h) is considerably shorter than in humans (5–9 d). Similar differences are observed for triiodothyronine (T3). To compensate for the increased turnover of thyroid hormones, the rat pituitary secretes more TSH. Whereas baseline serum TSH levels in humans are ~2.2 μU/mL, TSH levels in rats range from 55.5 to 65 μU/mL in males and 36.5 to 41 in females (Hill et al., 1989). It is estimated that rats require a tenfold higher rate of thyroxine production (on a per kilogram body weight basis) than do humans to maintain physiological T4 levels. These differences in plasma half-life, protein binding, thyroid hormone metabolism, and TSH secretion between rats and humans are thought to be one reason for the greater sensitivity of rats to developing hyperplastic and/or neoplastic nodules in response to chronic TSH stimulation (Capen, 1997).

PPARα plays a critical role in tumor formation by peroxisome proliferators as evidenced by the finding that Wy-14643 does not function as a tumor promoter in PPARα knockout mice (Gonzalez and Yu, 2006). Furthermore, there is excellent agreement between the potency with which agonists activate PPARα and the potency with which they promote liver tumor formation in rodents (which in turn is correlated with their ability to induce the proliferation of peroxisomes, induce peroxisomal enzymes involved in the β-oxidation of fatty acids, and induce microsomal CYP4A enzymes). Like CAR agonists, PPARα agonists are considered epigenetic (nongenotoxic) tumorigens because they are not mutagenic and they are not known to be converted to mutagenic metabolites. However, induction of acyl-CoA oxidase by Wy-14643 and other peroxisome proliferators leads to increased production of hydrogen peroxide, which can cause oxidative stress and DNA damage that possibly play a role in some of the downstream events leading to tumor promotion.

Activation of PPARα is required but apparently not sufficient to lead to liver tumor formation. Other key events include increased oxidant production (such as increased peroxisomal H_2O_2 production), increased cell proliferation (which fixes mutations), and suppression of apoptosis (which prevents the removal of genetically damaged cells and permits clonal expansion) (Klaunig et al., 2003; Lai, 2004; Bosgra et al., 2005). Kupffer cells appear to play an important role in liver tumor formation by releasing mitogenic cytokines and possibly by contributing to oxidative stress by releasing superoxide anion, although it is not clear how PPARα agonists trigger these events. Inhibition of gap junctional intercellular communication appears to play an important role in liver tumor formation by PPARα agonists, just as it does in the promotion of liver tumors by phenobarbital-type inducers.

Epidemiological studies designed to assess the human cancer risk posed by PPARα agonists have produced inconclusive results. Clofibrate has been reported to cause a statistically significant increase in cancer mortality rate during a 5- to 8-year treatment period. However, there were no significant increase in cancer rate in a follow-up study, which included a posttreatment period (Lai, 2004). Two compelling lines of evidence suggest that PPARα agonists will not cause liver tumors in humans. First, PPARα agonists do not cause peroxisome proliferation and microsomal CYP4A induction in human hepatocytes in vitro or in primates in vivo. Second, treatment of PPARα-humanized mice (transgenic mice with human PPARα in place of mouse PPARα) with Wy-14643 or fenofibrate does not result in the hepatocellular proliferation characteristic of wild-type mice (Gonzalez and Yu, 2006).

Enzyme Induction and Porphyria Due to the increased demand for heme, persistent induction of cytochrome P450 can lead to porphyria, a disorder characterized by excessive accumulation of intermediates in the heme biosynthetic pathway. In 1956, widespread consumption of wheat contaminated with the fungicide hexachlorobenzene caused an epidemic of porphyria cutanea tarda in Turkey. Another outbreak occurred in 1964 among workers at a factory in the United States manufacturing 2,4,5-trichlorophenoxyacetic acid (the active ingredient in several herbicides and in the defoliant, Agent Orange). The outbreak of porphyria cutanea tarda was caused not by the herbicide itself but by a contaminant, namely, TCDD. Drugs that cause P450 induction have not been shown to cause porphyria cutanea tarda under normal circumstances, but phenobarbital, phenytoin, and alcohol are recognized as *precipitating factors* because they cause episodes of porphyria in individuals with an inherited deficiency in the heme-biosynthetic enzyme, uroporphyrinogen decarboxylase.

CONJUGATION

Conjugation reactions include glucuronidation, sulfonation (often called sulfation), acetylation, methylation, conjugation with glutathione (mercapturic acid synthesis), and conjugation with amino acids (such as glycine, taurine, and glutamic acid). The cofactors for these reactions, which are shown in Fig. 6-49, react with functional groups that are either present on the xenobiotic or introduced/exposed during oxidation, reduction, or hydrolysis. With the exception of methylation and acetylation, conjugation reactions result in a large increase in xenobiotic hydrophilicity, so they greatly promote the excretion of foreign chemicals. Glucuronidation, sulfonation, acetylation, and methylation involve reactions with activated or "high-energy" cofactors, whereas conjugation with amino acids or glutathione involves reactions with activated xenobiotics. Most conjugation enzymes are located in the cytosol; a notable exception is the UDP–glucuronosyltransferases, which are microsomal enzymes (Table 6-1).

Glucuronidation

Glucuronidation is a major pathway of xenobiotic biotransformation in mammalian species except for members of the cat family (lions, lynxes, civets, and domestic cats) (Tukey and Strassburg, 2000). Glucuronidation requires primarily the cofactor UDPGA, but can also use UDP–glucose, UDP–xylose, and UDP–galactose. The reaction is catalyzed by UDP–glucuronosyltransferases (UGTs), which are located predominantly in the endoplasmic reticulum of liver and other tissues, such as the kidney, gastrointestinal tract, lungs, prostate, mammary glands, skin, brain, spleen, and nasal mucosa (Fig. 6-50). Examples of xenobiotics that are glucuronidated are shown in Fig. 6-51. The site of glucuronidation is generally an electron-rich nucleophilic O, N, or S heteroatom. Therefore, substrates for glucuronidation contain functional groups such as aliphatic alcohols and phenols (which form O-glucuronide ethers), carboxylic acids (which form O-glucuronide esters), primary and secondary aromatic and aliphatic amines (which form N-glucuronides), and free sulfhydryl groups (which form S-glucuronides). In humans and monkeys, more than 30 tertiary amines (including tripelennamine, cyclobenzaprine, and imipramine) are substrates for N-glucuronidation, which leads to the formation of positively charged quaternary glucuronides, some of which may be carcinogenic (see below) (Hawes, 1998). Certain xenobiotics, such as phenylbutazone, sulfinpyrazone, suxibuzone, ethchlorvynol, Δ^6- tetrahydrocannabinol, and feprazone, contain carbon atoms that are sufficiently nucleophilic to form C-glucuronides. The C-glucuronidation of the enolic form of phenylbutazone is catalyzed specifically by UGT1A9 (Nishiyama et al., 2006). Coumarin and certain other carbonyl-containing compounds are glucuronidated to form arylenol-glucuronides. In spite of the broad and overlapping substrate specificities of the UGT1As, some generalities can be made regarding certain types of substrates and the UGT1A enzymes that can glucuronidate them. For instance, UGT1A3 and 1A4 are largely responsible for glucuronidating tertiary amines (Vashishtha et al., 2001). For UGT1A1 and 1A4, the site of glucuronidation is always adjacent to a hydrophobic region of the substrate, with another hydrophobic region 6–8 Å from the position that is glucuronidated (Smith et al., 2004). UGT1A9 is similar,

except that the distal hydrophobic region also contains a hydrogen-bond acceptor (Smith et al., 2004). In a series of twenty four 4-substituted phenols, a methyl or ether in any position increases the rate of glucuronidation compared with phenol itself. UGT1A9 catalyzed the glucuronidation of all 24 substrates, whereas UGT1A6 tended only to glucuronidate less bulky phenolic substrates (Smith et al., 2004).

In addition to the typical conjugation reactions above, UGTs can form unusual conjugates: (1) bisglucuronides (e.g., bilirubin and morphine), where two different functional groups on the same molecule are glucuronidated; (2) diglucuronides (e.g., 5α-dihydrotestosterone), where two glucuronides are attached in tandem to a single site; (3) N-carbamoyl glucuronides (e.g., sertraline and varenicline), where carbonate is incorporated in the glucuronide; and (4) glycosidation with UDP–sugars other than UDP–glucuronic acid (e.g., glucosidation of barbiturates). Two examples are shown in Fig. 6-52. These reactions will be covered in greater detail later in this chapter. In addition to numerous xenobiotics, substrates for glucuronidation include several endogenous compounds, such as bilirubin, steroid hormones, and thyroid hormones. Table 6-16 provides examples of marker substrates for the major human UGTs. A listing of over 350 UGT substrates is available at http://arjournals.annualreviews.org/doi/suppl/10.1146/annurev.pharmtox.40.1.581 (Tukey and Strassburg, 2000). A review by Kiang and colleagues (2005) also provides an extensive table of UGT substrates along with corresponding K_m and V_{max} values.

Glucuronide conjugates of xenobiotics and endogenous compounds are polar, water-soluble metabolites that are eliminated from the body in urine or bile. Whether glucuronides are excreted from the body in bile or urine depends, in part, on the size of the aglycone (parent compound or unconjugated metabolite). In rat, glucuronides are preferentially excreted in urine if the molecular weight of the aglycone is less than 250, whereas glucuronides of larger molecules (aglycones with molecular weight >350) are preferentially excreted in bile. Molecular weight cutoffs for the preferred route of excretion vary among mammalian species. The carboxylic acid moiety of glucuronic acid, which is ionized at physiological pH, promotes excretion because (1) it increases the aqueous solubility of the xenobiotic and (2) it is recognized by the biliary and renal organic anion transport systems, which enable glucuronides to be secreted into urine and bile.

The cofactor for glucuronidation, UDPGA, is synthesized from glucose-1-phosphate, and the linkage between glucuronic acid and UDP has an α-configuration, as shown in Fig. 6-50. This configuration protects the cofactor from hydrolysis by β-glucuronidase. However, glucuronides of xenobiotics have a β-configuration. This inversion of configuration occurs because glucuronides are formed by nucleophilic attack by an electron-rich atom (usually O, N, or S) on UDPGA, and this attack occurs on the opposite side of the linkage between glucuronic acid and UDP, as shown in Fig. 6-50. In contrast to the UDPGA cofactor, xenobiotics conjugated with glucuronic acid are substrates for β-glucuronidase. Although present in the lysosomes of some mammalian tissues, considerable β-glucuronidase activity is present in the intestinal microflora. The intestinal enzyme can release the aglycone, which can be reabsorbed and thereby enters a cycle called *enterohepatic circulation*, which delays the elimination of xenobiotics. N-Glucuronides are more slowly hydrolyzed by β-glucuronidase than O- or S-glucuronides, whereas O-glucuronides tend to be more stable to acid-catalyzed hydrolysis than N- or S-glucuronides. The potential for glucuronides to be hydrolyzed in the presence of an acid or a base complicates the

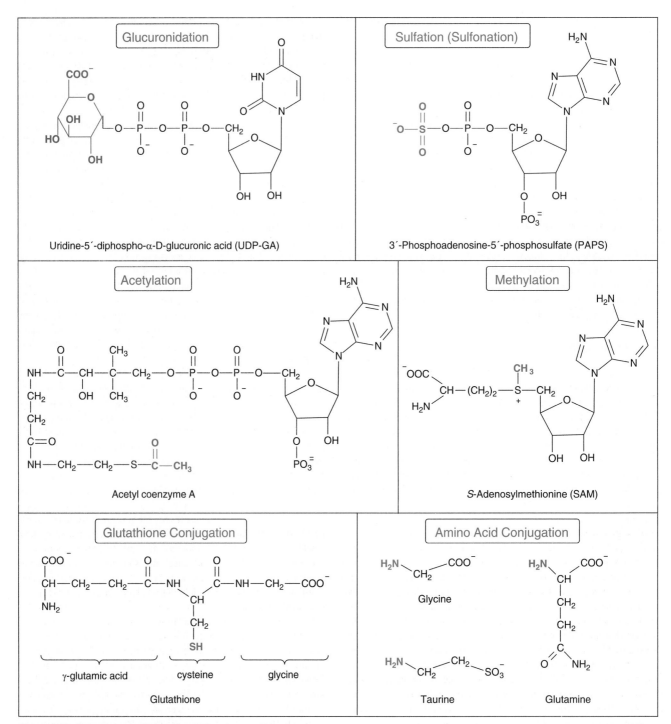

Figure 6-49. *Structures of cofactors for conjugation reactions.*

The functional group that reacts with or is transferred to the xenobiotic is shown in blue.

analysis of conjugates in urine or feces, and has implications for the tumorigenicity of N-glucuronides of compounds such as benzidine (discussed later in this section).

The C-terminus of all UGTs contains a membrane-spanning domain that anchors the enzyme in the endoplasmic reticulum. The enzyme faces the lumen of the endoplasmic reticulum, where it is ideally placed to conjugate lipophilic xenobiotics and their metabolites generated by oxidation, reduction, or hydrolysis. The lumenal orientation of UGT poses a problem because UDPGA is

a water-soluble cofactor synthesized in the cytoplasm. Several nucleotide sugar transporters (NSTs) have been postulated to shuttle UDPGA from the cytoplasm to the lumen of the endoplasmic reticulum, and they may also shuttle UDP (the byproduct of glucuronidation) back into the cytoplasm for synthesis of UDPGA, as shown in Fig. 6-50. Kobayashi and colleagues (2006) showed that, when expressed in V79 cells, three human NSTs, namely hUGTrel1 (SLC35B1), huYEA4 (SLC35B4), and huYEA4S (a transcript variant of SLC35B4), all transported UDPGA into the lumen

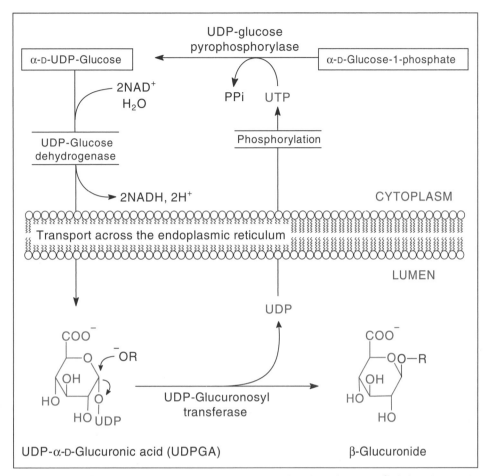

Figure 6-50. *Synthesis of UDP–glucuronic acid and inversion of configuration ($\alpha \rightarrow \beta$) during glucuronidation of a phenolic xenobiotic (designated RO^-).*

of microsomes prepared from these Chinese hamster fibroblasts, and they further showed that this microsomal transport was entirely dependent on the presence of UDP-N-acetylgalactosamine (a feature of many NSTs). They also demonstrated that the uptake of UDPGA into rat liver microsomes is partially dependent ($\sim$50%) on the presence of UDP-N-acetylgalactosamine, which suggests that NSTs may only be partially responsible for the transport of UDPGA from the cytoplasm to the lumen of the endoplasmic reticulum of rat liver (although they could be entirely responsible for such transport if 50% of the microsomal vesicles were inside out, which is possible).

In addition to UDPGA, the glucuronide metabolites are transported either across the bile canalicular membrane for excretion in bile or back across the endoplasmic reticulum and across the sinusoidal membrane into the blood for excretion in urine. Transport of glucuronides across the sinusoidal membrane into the blood is mediated by MRP1 (ABCC1), MRP3 (ABCC3), and MRP4 (ABCC4). The transport of glucuronides across the canalicular membrane into bile is mediated by MRP2 (ABCC2) and BCRP (ABCG2). Glucuronides can also be taken up by hepatocytes through the action of OATP1B1 (OATP2) and OATP1B3 (OATP8) on the sinusoidal membrane (Giacomini and Sugiyama, 2006). In rats, the hepatic uptake of estradiol-17β-glucuronide is mediated by OATP1A1, 1A4, and 1B2, whereas the biliary excretion of estradiol 3-sulfate-17β-glucuronide (see below, this section) is mediated by MRP2 and possibly BCRP (Sun *et al.*, 2006). Saturable ATP-independent, bidirectional carrier-mediated transport of estradiol-17β-glucuronide

across rat liver microsomal vesicles has also been demonstrated (Battaglia and Gollan, 2001). Other studies have shown that sulfoconjugates, phenolphthalein glucuronide, and estradiol 3-glucuronide are transported across the rat liver endoplasmic reticulum by facilitated diffusion, whereas 4-nitrophenyl glucuronide and 4-acetamidophenyl glucuronide are not, which suggests the presence of at least three microsomal glucuronide transporters with partially overlapping substrate specificity (Csala *et al.*, 2004).

In vitro, the glucuronidation of xenobiotics by liver microsomes can be stimulated by detergents (e.g., CHAPS and Brij-58), which disrupt the lipid bilayer of the endoplasmic reticulum and allow UGTs free access to UDPGA. High concentrations of detergent can inhibit UGTs, presumably by disrupting their interaction with phospholipids, which are important for catalytic activity. Detergents can inhibit certain UGTs, hence, they can affect UGT activity directly in addition to their indirect effects through interaction with phospholipids. Consequently, detergents, especially nonionic detergents such as Brij-58, can alter the kinetics of UGT reactions (Fisher *et al.*, 2000). Treatment of microsomes with detergents also virtually eliminates CYP activity; hence, detergents cannot be used to study the possible coupling of oxidation reactions catalyzed by cytochrome P450 with conjugation reactions catalyzed by UGT. This is not a limitation of alamethicin, a pore-forming peptide that activates UGT activity, like detergent, but which does not inhibit cytochrome P450. Furthermore, in contrast to certain detergents, alamethicin appears to increase V_{max} without affecting K_m.

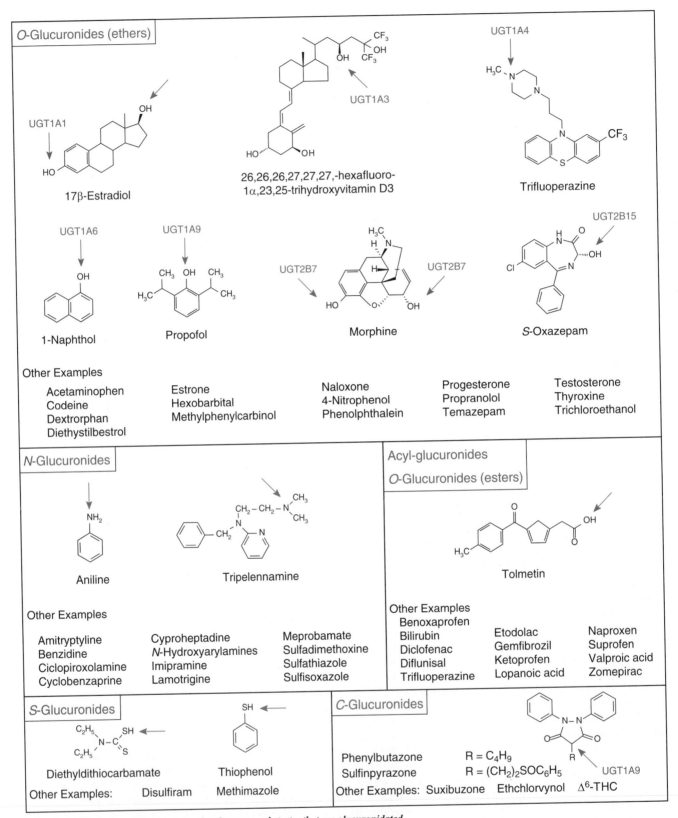

Figure 6-51. *Examples of xenobiotics and endogenous substrates that are glucuronidated.*

The arrow indicates the site of glucuronidation, with the UGT enzyme if selective.

Table 6-16

Major Human UDP-Glucuronosyltransferase Enzymes

UGT	PRESENT IN LIVER?	TISSUE	EXAMPLE SUBSTRATES
1A1	Yes	Liver, small intestine, colon	**Bilirubin, 17β-estradiol (3-glucuronidation)**, raloxifene, ethinyl estradiol, carvedilol, levothyroxine, acetaminophen
1A3	Yes	Liver, small intestine, colon	**Hexafluoro-1α,23(s),25-trihydroxyvitamin D3**, tertiary amines, antihistamines, 17β-estradiol, ketotifen, naproxen, ketoprofen, ibuprofen, fenoprofen, valproic acid, ezetimibe, norbuprenorphine
1A4	Yes	Liver, small intestine, colon	**Trifluoperazine**, tertiary amines, antihistamines, lamotrigine, amitriptyline, cyclobenzaprine, olanzapine
1A5	Yes	Liver	Unknown
1A6	Yes	Liver, small intestine, colon, stomach	**1-Naphthol, serotonin**, 4-nitrophenol, 4-methylumbelliferone, ibuprofen, acetaminophen, SN-38, diclofenac
1A7	No	Esophagus, stomach, lung	Octylgallate, arylamines, 4-hydroxybiphenyl, 4-hydroxyestrone, mycophenolic acid, SN-38
1A8	No	Colon, small intestine, kidney	Entacapone, troglitazone, anthraquinone, 8-hydroxyquinoline, furosemide, raloxifene, niflumic acid, ciprofibric acid, clofibric acid, valproic acid, mycophenolic acid, diflunisal, furosemide
1A9	Yes	Liver, colon, kidney	**Propofol**, thyroid hormones, entacapone, salicylic acid, scopoletin, fenofibrate, acetaminophen, ketoprofen, ibuprofen, fenoprofen, naproxen, furosemide, diflunisal, diclofenac, bumetanide
1A10	No	Stomach, small intestine, colon	1-Naphthol, mycophenolic acid, estrogen, raloxifene, troglitazone, furosemide
2A1	No	Olfactory	Valproic acid, ibuprofen
2A2	Unknown	Unknown	Unknown
2A3	Unknown	Unknown	Unknown
2B4	Yes	Liver, small intestine	Hyodeoxycholate, estriol, codeine, androsterone, carvedilol
2B7	Yes	Kidney, small intestine, colon	**Zidovudine (AZT), morphine (6-glucuronidation[a])**, ibuprofen, ketoprofen, diclofenac, opioids, oxazepam, carvedilol, clofibric acid, naloxone, valproic acid, tiaprofenic, zomepirac, benoxaprofen
2B10	Yes	Liver, ileum, prostate	Unknown
2B11	Yes	Mammary, prostate, others	4-Nitrophenol, naphthol, estriol, 2-aminophenol, 4-hydroxybiphenyl
2B15	Yes	Liver, small intestine, prostate	**S-Oxazepam**, androgens, flavonoids, 4-hydroxytamoxifen, estriol, entacapone, SN-38, tolcapone, diclofenac
2B17	Yes	Liver, prostate	Androgens, eugenol, scopoletin, galangin, ibuprofen
2B28	Yes	Liver, mammary	17β-Estradiol, testosterone

Bold text represents selective substrates (or reactions).

[a]UGT2B7 also catalyzes the 3-glucuronidation of morphine, but this reaction is also catalyzed by other UGTs.

Data adapted from Miners JO, Knights KM, Houston JB, Mackenzie PI: In vitro–in vivo correlation for drugs and other compounds eliminated by glucuronidation in humans: Pitfalls and promises. *Biochem Pharmacol* 71:1531–1539, 2006; Kiang TKL, Ensom MHH, Chang TKH: UDP-glucuronosyltransferases and clinical drug–drug interactions. *Pharmacol Ther* 106:97–132, 2005; Williams JA, Hyland R, Jones BC, et al.: Drug–drug interactions for UDP-glucuronosyltransferase substrates: a pharmacokinetic explanation for typically observed low exposure (AUCi/AUC) ratios. *Drug Metab Dispos* 32:1201–1208, 2004; Fisher M, Campanale K, Ackermann B, VandenBranden M, Wrighton S: In vitro glucuronidation using human liver microsomes and the pore-forming peptide alamethicin. *Drug Metab Dispos* 28:560–566, 2000.

From a review of the literature, Miners and colleagues report that alamethicin and nonionic detergents like Brij-58 generally result in the highest UGT activity and that alamethicin is the preferred activator because the effects of detergents are not reproducible between substrates (Miners *et al.*, 2006). However, in incubations designed strictly to measure UGT activity (and not both UGT and cytochrome P450 activity), the zwitterionic detergent, CHAPS, can activate certain UGT activities to a comparable or even greater extent than alamethicin.

The in vitro activity of UGT enzymes is highly dependent not only on the substance used to activate the microsomal membranes, but also on incubation conditions. The kinetic properties of UGTs have been demonstrated to vary with the concentration of cofactor, membrane composition, type of buffer, ionic strength, and pH (Miners *et al.*, 2006). In vitro intrinsic clearance (CL_{int}) values (measured

as V_{max}/K_m) for zidovudine (AZT) glucuronidation in human liver microsomes were shown to vary sixfold depending on incubation conditions, but even under conditions that produced the greatest CL_{int}, the in vivo clearance rate was under-predicted by three- to fourfold (Miners *et al.*, 2006). This in vitro under-prediction of the in vivo rate of clearance of drugs that are glucuronidated is typical when human liver microsomal kinetic data are used to assess CL_{int}, and is likely due to a number of factors including the presence or absence of albumin, correction for nonspecific binding, atypical in vitro kinetics, active uptake into hepatocytes, and significant extrahepatic expression of various UGTs (Miners *et al.*, 2006). The prediction of the in vivo clearance of drugs that are glucuronidated by hepatocytes appears to be more accurate than for predictions made with microsomes, but under-prediction is still the likely outcome. The case of zidovudine appears to be an exception to this rule, as in

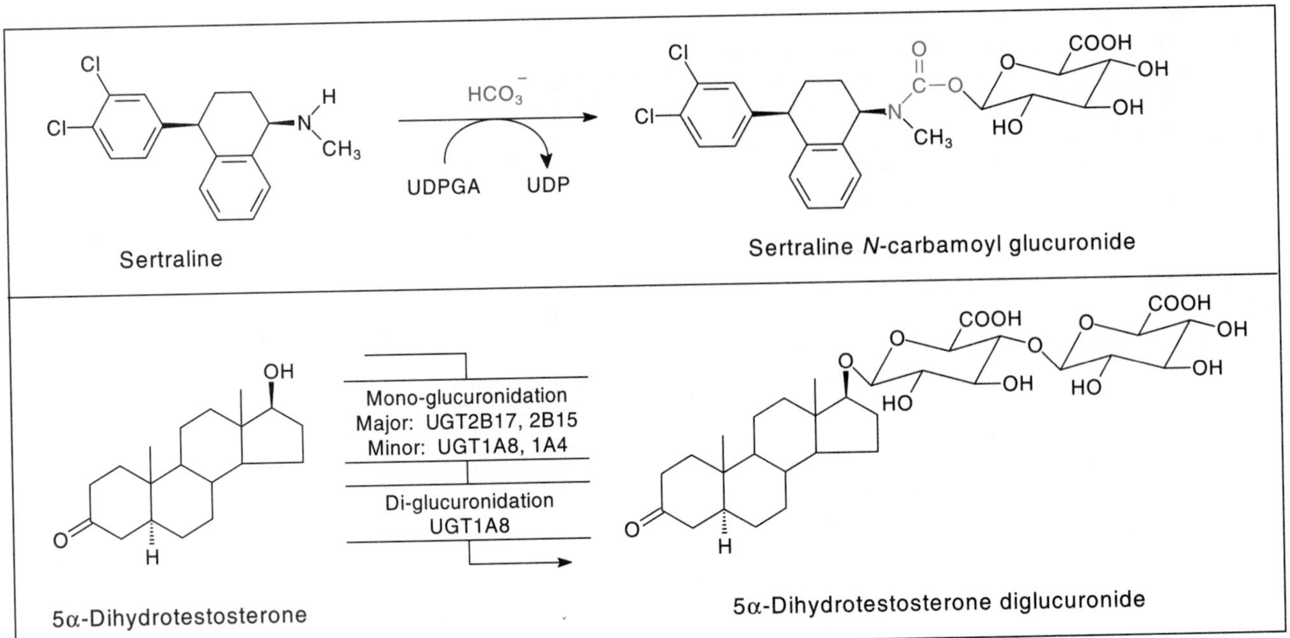

Figure 6-52. Examples of unusual glucuronide conjugates.

vivo clearance values were well-predicted with hepatocytes (Miners *et al.*, 2006). The use of either microsomes or recombinant UGT2B7 also appears to under-predict the in vivo magnitude of the *inhibitory* interaction between fluconazole and zidovudine by five- to tenfold (Miners *et al.*, 2006). However, when 2% bovine serum albumin (BSA) is added to either systems, there is a decrease in the K_i value of 85% which results in a much improved prediction of the in vivo interaction (Miners *et al.*, 2006). The effect of BSA is not due to nonspecific binding; it may involve the removal of inhibitory fatty acids or some as yet unidentified mechanism.

The kinetic properties of UGTs are possibly influenced by the formation of homo- and heterodimers among UGT enzymes and by the formation of heterodimers with other microsomal enzymes such as various CYP enzymes or epoxide hydrolase (Miners *et al.*, 2006). For instance, it has been demonstrated that the ratio of morphine 3-glucuronide to morphine 6-glucuronide formed by UGT2B7 is altered by the presence of CYP3A4 (Miners *et al.*, 2006). It is not known whether dimerization between UGT2B7 and CYP3A4, if it occurs, also alters the substrate specificity of other individual UGTs, which would have implications for studies designed to determine the substrate specificity of recombinant enzymes, which are invariably expressed individually. Additionally, there is currently no universally accepted method to quantify UGTs in a recombinant preparation, which precludes the accurate determination of relative activity factors, as for recombinant CYP enzymes. Finally, posttranslational modifications to UGTs that occur in vivo in humans (e.g., phsophorylation and N-glycosylation) may not occur in the cell expression system chosen to produce the recombinant UGTs (i.e., bacterial systems), which can impact activity in a substrate-dependent manner (Miners *et al.*, 2006). All of these findings suggest that the use of recombinant human UGT enzymes may not provide accurate indications of the extent to which a given UGT can glucuronidate a given substrate.

Cofactor availability can limit the rate of glucuronidation of drugs that are administered in high doses and are conjugated exten-

sively, such as aspirin and acetaminophen. In experimental animals, the glucuronidation of xenobiotics can be impaired in vivo by factors that reduce or deplete UDPGA levels, such as diethyl ether, borneol, and galactosamine. The lowering of UDPGA levels by fasting, such as might occur during a severe toothache or oral cancer, is thought to predispose individuals to the hepatotoxic effects of acetaminophen, although even then hepatotoxicity only occurs with higher-than-recommended doses of this analgesic (Whitcomb and Block, 1994; Rumack, 2004).

The existence of multiple forms of UGT was first suggested by the observation that in rats developmental changes in glucuronidation rates were substrate-dependent, and the glucuronidation of xenobiotics could be differentially affected by the treatment of rats with chemicals known to induce CYP. Based on their ontogeny and inducibility, the UGT activities in rat liver microsomes were categorized into four groups. The activity of enzyme(s) in the first group peaks 1 to 5 days *before* birth, and it is inducible by 3-methylcholanthrene and other CYP1A enzyme inducers. Substrates for the group 1 enzyme(s) tend to be planar chemicals, such as 1-naphthol, 4-nitrophenol, and 4-methylumbelliferone. The activity of enzyme(s) in the second group peaks ~5 days *after* birth and is inducible by phenobarbital and other CYP2B enzyme inducers. Substrates for the group 2 enzyme(s) tend to be bulky chemicals, such as chloramphenicol, morphine, 4-hydroxybiphenyl, and monoterpenoid alcohols. The activity of enzyme(s) in the third group peaks around the time of puberty (~1 month) and is inducible by PCN and other CYP3A enzyme inducers. Substrates for the group 3 enzyme(s) include digitoxigenin monodigitoxoside (dt_1), a metabolite of digitoxin formed by CYP3A (see Fig. 6-47), and possibly bilirubin. The activity of enzyme(s) in the fourth group also peak around the time of puberty (~1 month) and is inducible by clofibrate and other CYP4A enzyme inducers. Substrates for the group 4 enzyme(s) include bilirubin but not dt_1, which distinguishes group 3 from group 4 UGTs.

Although this classification system still has some practical value, it has become evident that the four groups of UGTs do not simply represent four independently regulated enzymes with different substrate specificities. This realization stems from various studies, including those conducted with Gunn rats that are hyperbilirubinemic due to a genetic defect in bilirubin conjugation. The glucuronidation defect in Gunn rats is substrate-dependent in a manner that does not match the categorization of UGTs into the four aforementioned groups. For example, in Gunn rats the glucuronidation of the group 2 substrates, morphine and chloramphenicol, is not impaired, whereas the glucuronidation of 1-naphthol, dt_1 and bilirubin (group 1, 3, and 4 substrates), is low or undetectable. The induction of UGT activity by 3-methylcholanthrene, PCN, and clofibric acid is impaired in Gunn rats, whereas the induction by phenobarbital is normal. (Although phenobarbital does not induce the conjugation of bilirubin in Gunn rats, it does so in normal Wistar rats.)

Only when the UGTs were cloned did it become apparent why the genetic defect in Gunn rats affects three of the four groups of UGTs that are otherwise independently regulated as a function of age and xenobiotic treatment (Owens and Ritter, 1992). It is now apparent that the UGTs expressed in rat liver microsomes belong to two large gene families, UGT1 and UGT2. The former gene family contains at least eight enzymes, all of which belong to the same subfamily designated UGT1A. The individual members of the rat UGT1A subfamily are UGT1A1, 1A2, 1A3, 1A5, 1A6, 1A7, 1A8, and 1A10. Rat UGT1A4 and 1A9 are pseudogenes and are not a member of the rat UGT1A subfamily, although additional members may yet be identified. Additional members of the rat UGT1A subfamily are thought to exist, including the one that glucuronidates digitoxigenin monodigitoxoside (dt_1), a metabolite of digitoxin. The second UGT gene family in rats is divided into two subfamilies, UGT2A and UGT2B; the former contains at least three members (UGT2A1, 2A2, and 2A3) whereas the second contains at least seven members (UGT2B1, 2B2, 2B3, 2B6, 2B8, 2B12, and 2B34). Unlike the UGT1 enzymes (see below), members of the gene family 2 are composed of six exons that are not shared between members, with the exception of UGT2A1, and 2A2. UGT2A1, and 2A2 are encoded by six exons, and the two enzymes arise by differential splicing of the variable first exon to the same set of five exons that lie downstream, similar to UGT1A enzymes (Mackenzie *et al.*, 2005). In contrast, members of family 1 are formed from a single gene with multiple copies of the first exon, each of which can be connected in cassette fashion with a common set of exons (exons 2–5). This arrangement is illustrated in Fig. 6-53 for the human UGT1 gene locus, and will be discussed later in this section. A simplified view of the UGT1A gene locus is that the multiple UGT1A enzymes are constructed by linking different substrate binding sites (encoded by multiple copies of exon 1) to a constant portion of the enzyme (encoded by exons 2–5). This constant region is involved in cofactor binding and membrane insertion. This method of generating multiple forms of an enzyme from a single gene locus is economical, but it is also the genetic equivalent of putting all of one's eggs in the same basket. Whereas a mutation in any one of the UGT2 enzymes affects a single enzyme, a mutation in the constant region of the UGT1 gene affects all enzymes encoded by this locus. In the Gunn rat, a mutation at codon 415 introduces a premature stop signal, so that all forms of UGT encoded by the UGT1 locus are truncated and functionally inactive. The UGTs known to be encoded by the rat UGT1 locus include the 3-methylcholanthrene-inducible enzyme that conjugates planar molecules such as 1-naphthol (UGT1A6 and UGT1A7), the phenobarbital- and clofibric acid-inducible enzyme that conjugates bilirubin (UGT1A1), and the PCN-inducible en-

zyme that conjugates dt_1. All these UGT1 enzymes are defective in Gunn rats.

As mentioned previously, the second family of rat UGTs, which share less than 50% of amino acid sequence identity with the first family, are divided into two subfamilies (UGT2A and UGT2B). UGT2A1 is expressed specifically in olfactory epithelium where it conjugates a wide variety of substrates. Members of the rat UGT2B subfamily are expressed in liver and various extrahepatic tissues. Members of the UGT2B subfamily are named in the order they are cloned, regardless of the species of origin (much like the nomenclature system for most of the CYP enzymes). UGT2B enzymes have been cloned from rat (forms 1, 2, 3, 6, 8, 12, and 34), humans (forms 4, 7, 10, 11, 15, 17, and 28), mouse (forms 1, 5, 34, 35, 36, 37, and 38), and rabbits (forms 13, 14, and 16). A rabbit UGT has been classified as UGT2C1; however, UGT2C genes in other mammalian species have not been identified.

In rats, at least one UGT2B enzyme (UGT2B1) is inducible by phenobarbital. The gene encoding this enzyme is not defective in Gunn rats; therefore, treatment of Gunn rats with phenobarbital induces the glucuronidation of substrates for UGT2B1. However, UGT2B1 does not conjugate bilirubin (a reaction mainly catalyzed by UGT1A1 and/or UGT1A4), which is why phenobarbital cannot induce the conjugation of bilirubin in Gunn rats. UGT2B1 is the main enzyme responsible for catalyzing the 3-O-glucuronidation of morphine, which is markedly increased by treating of rats with phenobarbital. Whereas Gunn rats are genetically defective in all UGT1A enzymes, LA rats are selectively defective in UGT2B2, which allowed this enzyme to be identified as the principal enzyme responsible for glucuronidating androsterone and triiodothyronine (T_3) in rats (Burchell, 1999).

The mammalian UGT gene superfamily contains four families, UGT1, UGT2, UGT3, and UGT8. To date, at least 22 human UGT enzymes have been identified. The current UGT nomenclature may be found at: http://som.flinders.edu.au/FUSA/ClinPharm/ UGT/index.html. Families 1 and 2 preferentially utilize UDPGA as the cofactor, but may use other UDP sugars such as UDP-glucose and UDP-xylose (Mackenzie *et al.*, 2005). UGT3A1 and 3A2 were identified in the human genome, and are ~30% similar to UGT1 and 2 sequences (Mackenzie *et al.*, 2005). The sugar specificity, localization, and activity of UGT3A1 and 3A2 are currently unknown and these enzymes will not be covered in this chapter. Likewise, UGT2A2 and 2A3 have not yet been characterized beyond their gene structure. UGT8A1 utilizes UDP-galactose and is involved in the synthesis of membrane components, which is therefore beyond the scope of this chapter.

The multiple forms of the major drug-metabolizing human UGT are products of either a single UGT1A gene locus (see Fig. 6-52) or multiple UGT2 genes (with the exception of UGT2A1 and 2A2, see below). The human UGT1A locus contains two unique first exons, 1A1 and 1A6, with two clusters of additional exons, 1A2–5 and 1A7–1A13. The polypeptides encoded by the first exons, 1A1 and 1A6, are ~50% identical to one another and to the other polypeptides encoded by the remaining exons, whereas the polypeptides within a cluster are 75–92% identical and this arrangement has been conserved in the rat (Mackenzie *et al.*, 2005). This arrangement allows for 13 potential transcripts (i.e., UGT1A1, 1A2, 1A3, 1A4, 1A5, 1A6, 1A7, 1A8, 1A9, 1A10, 1A11, 1A12, and 1A13), but only nine are translated in vivo into functional enzymes. The genes that are not translated into functional enzymes lack an open reading frame, and are therefore pseudogenes (i.e., UGT1A2, 1A11, 1A12, and 1A13).

The UGT2 genes expressed in humans are UGT2A1, 2A2, 2A3, 2B4, 2B7, 2B10, 2B11, 2B15, 2B17, and 2B28. UGT2B24–27 and 2B29 are pseudogenes. The UGT2 genes are made up of six exons each, which are not shared between subfamily members, with the exception of UGT2A1 and 2A2, and these two genes are >70% similar (Mackenzie *et al.*, 2005). UGT2A1 and 2A2 share five exons with a variable first exon, similar to the UGT1A enzymes, whereas UGT2A3 is made up of six unique exons.

A summary of the current understanding of the tissue distribution and substrate specificity of the human UGT1 and UGT2 enzymes can be found in Table 6-16. Suffice it to say that these enzymes are expressed in a wide variety of tissues, and some enzymes—including UGT1A7, 1A8, 1A10, and 2A1—are expressed only in extrahepatic tissues, which has implications for the common practice of using human liver microsomes to investigate the role of glucuronidation in drug metabolism. Of the hepatically expressed UGT enzymes, UGT1A1, 1A3, 1A4, 1A6, 1A9, 2B7, and 2B15 are considered to be the UGT enzymes most important for hepatic drug metabolism because UGT1A5, 2B4, 2B10, 2B11, 2B17, and 2B28 are reported to have low or negligible activity toward xenobiotics (Miners *et al.*, 2006). UGT1A7, 1A8, and 1A10 expressed in the gastrointestinal tract may also be important for prehepatic elimination of various orally administered drugs. Numerous UGT1 and UGT2 enzymes are expressed throughout the gastrointestinal tract, where they contribute significantly to the first pass elimination of numerous xenobiotics. Several UGT2B enzymes are expressed in steroid-sensitive tissues, such as prostate and mammary gland, where they presumably terminate the effects of steroid hormones.

Probe drugs have been identified for some but not all of the human UGTs, including UGT1A1 (17β-estradiol 3-glucuronidation and bilirubin), UGT1A3 (hexafluoro-1α,25-trihydroxyvitamin D3), UGT1A4 (trifluoperazine), UGT1A6 (serotonin and 1-naphthol), UGT1A9 (propofol), UGT2B7 (morphine 6-glucuronidation and zidovudine [AZT]), and UGT2B15 (*S*-oxazepam) (Miners *et al.*, 2006). The glucuronidation of morphine by UGT2B7 involves conjugation of the phenolic 3-hydroxyl and the alcoholic 6-hydroxyl group in a 7:1 ratio. The 6-*O*-glucuronide is 600 times more potent an analgesic than the parent drug, whereas the 3-*O*-glucuronide is devoid of analgesic activity. UGT2B7 is present in the brain, where it might facilitate the analgesic effect of morphine through formation of the 6-*O*-glucuronide, which presumably does not readily cross the blood–brain barrier and may be retained in the brain longer than morphine (Tukey and Strassburg, 2000). Only UGT2B7 catalyzes the 6-glucuronidation of morphine, whereas several UGTs including UGT1A1, 1A3, 1A6, 1A8, 1A9, 1A10 as well as 2B7 can catalyze the 3-glucuronidation (Stone *et al.*, 2003). Selective probe inhibitors have only been characterized for UGT1A4 (hecogenin) and 2B7 (fluconazole) (Miners *et al.*, 2006).

Drug–drug interactions that are at least partly due to inhibition of UGTs have been reported. For instance, plasma levels of indomethacin are increased about twofold upon coadministration of diflunisal, and in vitro studies indicate that this interaction is due in part to inhibition of indomethacin glucuronidation in the intestine (Gidal *et al.*, 2003; Mano *et al.*, 2006). Valproic acid coadministration increases the AUC of lorazepam and lamotrigine by 20% and 160%, respectively (Williams *et al.*, 2004). In contrast to the situation with CYP enzymes, there are fewer inhibitory drug–drug interactions caused by the inhibition of UGT enzymes, and AUC increases are rarely greater than twofold (Williams *et al.*, 2004), whereas dramatic AUC increases have been reported for CYP enzymes, such as the 190-fold increase in AUC reported for the

CYP1A2 substrate ramelteon (Rozerem™) upon coadministration of fluvoxamine (Rozerem™ prescribing information, 2005). The low magnitude of UGT-based inhibitory interactions is partly due to the fact that most drugs that are primarily cleared by glucuronidation are metabolized by several UGTs. Drug–drug interactions due to induction of UGT enzymes have also been observed. Rifampin coadministration increases mycophenolic acid clearance by 30%, and increases the AUC of its acyl glucuronide (formed by UGT2B7) and its 7-*O*-glucuronide (formed by various UGT1 enzymes) by more than 100% and 20%, respectively (Naesens *et al.*, 2006).

As mentioned above and as shown in Fig. 6-52, UGTs can form unusual conjugates including bisglucuronides, diglucuronides, *N*-carbamoyl glucuronides, *N*-glucosides, and other glycoside conjugates. Bisglucuronides (i.e., a glucuronide in which two separate functional groups on the aglycone are glucuronidated) are more common than diglucuronides, and include the bisglucuronides of bilirubin, morphine, octylgallate, diosmetin, phenolphthalein, and hydroxylated polycyclic aromatic hydrocarbons (such as hydroxylated chrysene and benzo[*a*]pyrene) (Murai *et al.*, 2006). A diglucuronide is a glucuronide in which a single functional group on the aglycone is conjugated twice resulting in two glucuronosyl groups in tandem (Murai *et al.*, 2006). Diglucuronides of the xenobiotics nalmefene and 4-hydroxybiphenyl, and of the endogenous steroids androsterone, 5α-dihydrotestosterone, 17β-estradiol, estriol, estrone, and testosterone have previously been detected in dogs. Rat liver microsomes do not form diglucuronides of these steroids, whereas monkey liver microsomes form detectable levels of the 5α-dihydrotestosterone, testosterone, and 17β-estradiol diglucuronides, with human liver microsomes forming only the diglucuronide of 5α-dihydrotestosterone (see Fig. 6-52) (Murai *et al.*, 2005). In all cases, it is the 2′-hydroxyl group of the first glucuronide moiety that is subject to additional glucuronidation. In the case of 5α-dihydrotestosterone, only human UGT1A8 (an intestinal UGT) has been found to produce the diglucuronide from 5α-dihydrotestosterone itself, although UGT1A4, 2B15, and 2B17 can produce the monoglucuronide, and UGT1A1 and 1A9 can produce the diglucuronide when the monoglucuronide is the substrate (Murai *et al.*, 2006). Human intestinal microsomes form the diglucuronide more efficiently than human liver microsomes, reflecting the fact that UGT1A8, an extrahepatic UGT, is the predominant enzyme involved in the diglucuronidation of 5α-dihydrotestosterone.

N-Carbamoyl glucuronidation has been reported for relatively few primary amines, or the demethylated metabolites of secondary and tertiary amines, and includes drugs such as sertraline (Fig. 6-52), carvedilol, varenicline, mofegiline, garenoxacin, tocainide, and sibutramine (Gipple *et al.*, 1982; Tremaine *et al.*, 1989; Beconi *et al.*, 2003; Hayakawa *et al.*, 2003; Link *et al.*, 2006; Obach *et al.*, 2006). Marked species difference have been found in the formation of *N*-carbamoyl glucuronides, and humans have only been found to produce these conjugates from even fewer drugs, including sertraline, varenicline, and mofegiline. To form this type of conjugate in vitro, the incubation must be performed under a CO_2 atmosphere, in a carbonate buffer. Although not directly demonstrated, it has been hypothesized that a transient carbamic acid intermediate is formed by the interaction of the amine with the dissolved CO_2, followed by glucuronidation (Obach *et al.*, 2005). Because the intermediate is not stable, the hypothesis that UGT also catalyzes the formation of the carbamic acid cannot be disproved. However, in the case of sertraline, and varenicline it is predominantly UGT2B7 that forms the *N*-carbamoyl glucuronide, which also conjugates various carboxylic acids (Obach *et al.*, 2005, 2006). Given that the in vitro

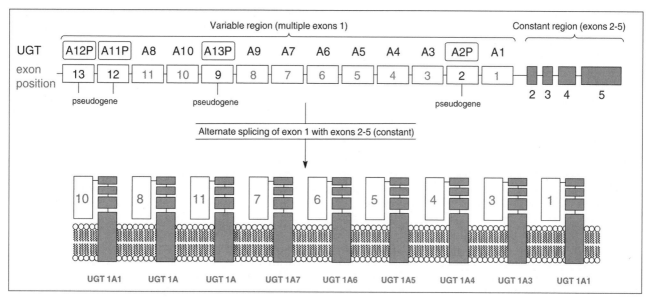

Figure 6-53. Structure of the human UGT1 locus which encodes multiple forms of UDP–glucuronosyltransferase.

Note that these microsomal enzymes face the lumen of the endoplasmic reticulum.

formation of N-carbamoyl glucuronides occurs only under special incubation conditions that are not typically employed, it is possible that many other primary and secondary amines or their oxidative metabolites can be converted to such conjugates but have not been detected because of the unusual incubation conditions required to support the formation of N-carbamoyl glucuronides.

Finally, although human UGTs typically are highly selective in the use of UDPGA as a sugar donor, they can accommodate the use of other sugar donors such as UDP-glucose, UDP-galactose, and UDP-xylose in an aglycone-dependent manner, as mentioned previously (Tang and Ma, 2005). For instance, recombinant human UGT1A1 can utilize UDPGA, UDP-xylose, or UDP-glucose to form glycosides, but only with bilirubin (Tang and Ma, 2005). It has also been demonstrated that recombinant human UGT2B7 can glycosidate an endothelin ET_A receptor antagonist with UDPGA, UDP-glucose, and UDP-galactose, but can glycosidate diclofenac with only UDPGA (Tang and Ma, 2005). In the case of an aldose-reductase inhibitor (AS-3201), Toide and colleagues (2004) found that UGT2B4, 2B7, and especially 2B15 all *preferentially* utilize UDP-glucose over UDPGA. Several other compounds have been found to be glucosidated in mammals, including 5-aminosalicylic acid, bromfenac, pranoprofen, pantothenic acid, hyodeoxycholic acid, mycophenolic acid, sulphadimidine, sulphamerazine, sulphamethoxazole, and various barbiturates (e.g., phenobarbital and amobarbital) (Tang and Carro-Ciampi, 1980; Nakano *et al.*, 1986; Arima, 1990; Kirkman *et al.*, 1998; Toide *et al.*, 2004; Picard *et al.*, 2005). In the case of the carboxyl-containing amine, bromfenac, the aglycone was observed in rat bile after base hydrolysis, and it was concluded that it was formed by hydrolysis of an acyl glucuronide (Kirkman *et al.*, 1998). In later studies to characterize the stability of the putative acyl glucuronide, an N-glucoside was detected (Kirkman *et al.*, 1998). 5-Aminosalicylic acid is structurally similar to bromfenac in that both NSAIDs contain a primary amine near the carboxyl group, and both are converted to N-glucosides (Kirkman *et al.*, 1998). In the human metabolism of barbiturates, N-glucosides are the major metabolites found in urine, and glucuronides have not been detected. Accordingly, it was theorized that enzymes other

than UGTs may be involved in the conjugation of barbiturates in humans (Toide *et al.*, 2004). This latter theory is interesting because liver homogenates from cats, which lack UGT activity, can N-glucosidate amobarbital (however, it should be noted that glucose conjugates can sometimes form nonenzymatically) (Carro-Ciampi *et al.*, 1985). However, Toide and colleagues (2004) have demonstrated that the N-glucosidation of amobarbital in human liver microsomes correlates highly with the N-glucosidation of AS-3201, but not its N-glucuronidation, indicating that UGT2B15 is probably the predominant human UGT responsible for the glucosidation of amobarbital.

In humans, Crigler–Najjar syndrome (type I and II) and Gilbert disease are congenital defects in bilirubin conjugation. The diseases have historically been differentiated largely on the basis of the severity of symptoms and total plasma concentrations of bilirubin (e.g., Crigler–Najjar Type I: 310–855 μM, Crigler–Najjar Type II: 100–430 μM, and Gilbert disease: 20–100 μM). The major bilirubin-conjugating enzyme in humans is UGT1A1. Genetic polymorphisms in exons 2-5 (which affect all enzymes encoded by the UGT1A locus), in exon 1 (which affect only UGT1A1), in the promoter regions, and in introns 1 and 3 have been identified in patients with Crigler–Najjar syndrome or Gilbert disease. More than 60 genetic polymorphisms are associated with these diseases. A current list of all UGT polymorphisms and phenotypes (when known) can be found at http://galien.pha.ulaval.ca/alleles/alleles.html. Some polymorphisms cause the introduction of a premature stop codon in one of the exons 2-5 (which causes a loss of all UGT1A enzymes, analogous to the Gunn rat) and are associated with type I Crigler–Najjar syndrome, a severe form of the disease characterized by a complete loss of bilirubin-conjugating activity and marked hyperbilirubinemia. Type I Crigler–Najjar syndrome is also associated with various frameshifts and deletions in exons 1-5, and in at least three cases, with changes in introns 1 and 3 that affect splice donor or acceptor sites. Other polymorphisms are associated with the less severe type II Crigler–Najjar syndrome (i.e., UGT1A1*7–9, 12, 26, 30, 33–38, 42, 48, 51, 52, 59, and 64). Individuals with Gilbert disease have an occasionally transient, and generally mild hyperbilirubinemia which is often caused by the addition of one "TA" segment in the TATA promoter region (i.e., UGT1A1*28: A(TA)$_6$TAA → A(TA)$_7$TAA). There is some overlap between Crigler–Najjar Type II and Gilbert disease, not only in terms of the plasma concentrations of bilirubin, but also in the type of polymorphism that underlies the disease. In addition to the *28 allele, the *6, *27, *29, *60, and *62 alleles are associated with Gilbert disease, and some of these polymorphisms affect coding regions of the UGT1A1 gene. In addition, the UGT1A1*37 allele produces a A(TA)$_8$TAA promoter defect which results in Crigler–Najjar Type II. A Korean individual heterozygous for three UGT1A1 alleles associated with Gilbert disease (i.e., likely *6, *28, and *60), was found to have total bilirubin concentrations as high as 193 μM (Seok Seo et al., 2007), which is a concentration typically associated with Crigler–Najjar Type II. Crigler–Najjar Type II and Gilbert disease (in contrast to Crigler–Najjar Type I) typically respond to some extent to phenobarbital treatment, which stimulates bilirubin conjugation presumably by inducing UGT1A1. Type I Crigler–Najjar syndrome is also associated with impaired glucuronidation of propofol, ethinylestradiol, and various phenolic substrates for UGT1A enzymes. Polymorphisms that might affect the other UGT1A enzymes have not been thoroughly characterized in vivo, but there are data to suggest that polymorphisms in these enzymes may modify the risk of developing certain types of cancer (Nagar and Remmel, 2006).

The UGT1A1*28 allele has received widespread attention in recent years due to the impact this variant has on the toxicity of the topoisomerase I inhibitor, irinotecan, that is used primarily to treat colorectal cancer. The disposition of irinotecan is complex, with conversion to the active metabolite, SN-38, occurring mainly in the liver by hydrolysis by carboxylesterase. The active metabolite SN-38 is subsequently glucuronidated primarily by UGT1A1, with potential contribution from UGT1A6, 1A7, 1A9, and 1A10 (Nagar and Blanchard, 2006). The UGT1A1*28 variant has now been referenced in the Camptosar® prescribing information, which notes that patients with reduced UGT1A1 activity have a higher exposure to SN-38 (which is 50–100 times more toxic than the glucuronide), and that the dose of irinotecan should be adjusted downward accordingly (Nagar and Blanchard, 2006). The toxicity of SN-38 primarily manifests as severe diarrhea and myelosuppression (in the form of leucopenia, severe thrombocytopenia, severe anemia, or grade 3–4 neutropenia) (Nagar and Blanchard, 2006). Several studies have demonstrated grade 3–4 neutropenia and/or grade 3–4 diarrhea upon irinotecan administration in patients with at least one UGT1A1*28 or *27 allele, and one study implicated high activity variants of UGT1A7 and 1A9 with diarrhea (Nagar and Blanchard, 2006). In at least one study, the UGT1A1*28 allele has also been reported to increase the risk of invasive breast cancer in premenopausal women by 1.8-fold, which was attributed to decreased glucuronidation of estradiol, but other studies appear to contradict this finding (Nagar and Remmel, 2006).

Polymorphisms have been identified in UGT2B4, 2B7, 2B15, and 2B28. For example, oxazepam is glucuronidated by UGT2B15, which preferentially glucuronidates S-oxazepam over its R-enantiomer. Ten percent (10%) of the population appear to be poor glucuronidators of S-oxazepam, and one study has implicated the low activity UGT2B15*2 allele as a possible determinant of such variation (Nagar and Remmel, 2006). Such polymorphisms also appear to be the underlying cause of alterations in hyodeoxycholate glucuronidation in gastric mucosa (Tukey and Strassburg, 2000).

Human UGT1A6 glucuronidates acetaminophen and the glucuronidation of acetaminophen in humans is enhanced by cigarette smoking and dietary cabbage and Brussels sprouts, which suggests that human UGT1A6 is inducible by polycyclic aromatic hydrocarbons and derivatives of indole 3-carbinol (Bock et al., 1994). Ligands for the Ah receptor, such as those present in cigarette smoke, induce CYP1A2, which would be expected to enhance the hepatotoxicity of acetaminophen. Increased acetaminophen glucuronidation may explain why cigarette smoking does not enhance the hepatotoxicity of acetaminophen. Conversely, decreased glucuronidation may explain why some individuals with Gilbert's syndrome are predisposed to the hepatotoxic effects of acetaminophen (de Morais et al., 1992). Low rates of glucuronidation predispose newborns to jaundice and to the toxic effects of chloramphenicol; the latter was once used prophylactically to prevent opportunistic infections in newborns until it was found to cause severe cyanosis and even death (gray baby syndrome).

Glucuronidation generally detoxifies xenobiotics and potentially toxic endobiotics, such as bilirubin, for which reason glucuronidation is generally considered a beneficial process. However, steroid hormones glucuronidated on the D-ring (but not the A-ring) cause cholestasis, and induction of UGT activity has been implicated as an epigenetic mechanism of thyroid tumor formation in rodents (McClain, 1989; Curran and DeGroot, 1991). Inducers of UGTs cause a decrease in serum thyroid hormone levels, which triggers a compensatory increase in thyroid stimulating hormone (TSH). During sustained exposure to the enzyme-inducing agent, prolonged stimulation of the thyroid gland by TSH (>6 months) results in the development of thyroid follicular cell neoplasia. Glucuronidation followed by biliary excretion is a major pathway of thyroxine biotransformation in rodents whereas deiodination is the major pathway (up to 85%) of thyroxine metabolism in humans. In contrast to the situation in rodents, prolonged stimulation of the thyroid gland by TSH in humans will result in malignant tumors only in exceptional circumstances and possibly only in conjunction with some thyroid abnormality. Therefore, chemicals that cause thyroid tumors in rats or mice by inducing UGT activity are unlikely to cause such tumors in humans. In support of this conclusion, extensive epidemiological data in epileptic patients suggest that phenobarbital and other anticonvulsants do not function as thyroid (or liver) tumor promoters in humans (Parkinson et al., 2006).

In some cases, glucuronidation represents an important event in the toxicity of xenobiotics. For example, the aromatic amines that cause bladder cancer (such as benzidine, 2-aminonaphthalene, and 4-aminobiphenyl) undergo N-hydroxylation in the liver followed by N-glucuronidation of the resultant N-hydroxyaromatic amine, although direct N-glucuronidation also occurs, and is a competing pathway of hepatic metabolism. In the case of 4-aminobiphenyl, the competing pathways of ring hydroxylation and O-esterification (i.e., O-glucuronidation, O-sulfonation, or O-acetylation) are detoxication pathways, whereas N-esterification catalyzed by UGTs, SULTs, or NATs represent activating pathways (see section entitled Acetylation) (Cohen et al., 2006). Benzidine and 2-aminonaphthalene are particularly tumorigenic; with accumulating data which demonstrates that the risk of bladder cancer may increase by up to 100-fold in workers exposed to these substances in the course of their occupation in various manufacturing processes (Al-Zoughool et al., 2006). The N-glucuronides of such carcinogens, which accumulate in the urine of the bladder, are unstable in acidic pH and thus are hydrolyzed to the corresponding unstable, tumorigenic N-hydroxyaromatic amine, as shown in Fig. 6-54. N-Hydroxyaromatic amines can give rise to highly electrophilic aromatic nitrenium ions that can bind to DNA and other macromolecules, or they can be

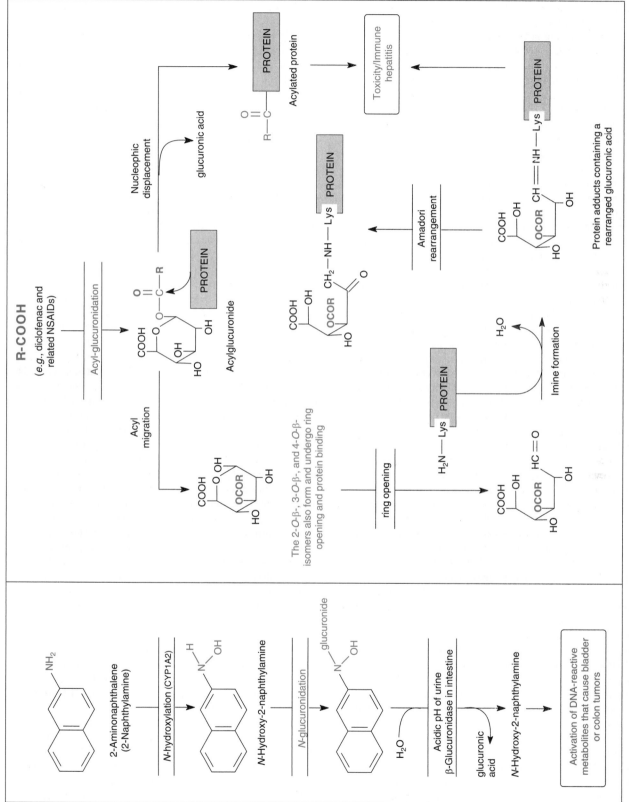

Figure 6-54. Role of glucuronidation in the activation of xenobiotics to toxic metabolites.

converted to reactive acetoxy metabolites directly in the bladder epithelium via NAT-mediated O-acetylation, which also leads to the formation of aromatic nitrenium ions (Al-Zoughool *et al.*, 2006). Because N-glucuronidation of aromatic amines can also occur directly without a prior oxidation, this reaction competes with oxidation, and therefore a decrease in UGT activity in the liver would favor N-hydroxylation, with subsequent O-acetylation by NAT and spontaneous formation of aromatic nitrenium ions in the liver, rather than the bladder. In contrast, decreased acetylation with normal UGT activity would lead to a greater accumulation of *N*-hydroxyaromatic amines in the bladder with increased bladder tumor formation. Concordant with this scenario, benzidine has been shown to induce predominantly liver tumors in rats (fast acetylators) but bladder cancer in dogs (poor acetylators) (Al-Zoughool *et al.*, 2006). In humans, there are sex differences in aromatic amine carcinogenicity. Irrespective of ethnicity or race, men are 2.5–5 times more likely to develop bladder cancer than women in general, and in particular male smokers, hairdressers, dye and textile workers who are exposed to aromatic amines have several times increased risk relative to their female counterparts. Male mice, which *N*-glucuronidate 4-aminobiphenyl faster than females, were found during the treatment with this carcinogen to have a 2.2-fold higher rate of DNA-adduct formation, and increased rates of bladder tumor formation relative to females, and female mice were found to have tumors only in the liver (Al-Zoughool *et al.*, 2006). In mice, coadministration of 4-aminobiphenyl with hecogenin, which in humans has been found to inhibit hepatic UGT1A4 (Uchaipichat *et al.*, 2006), was found to increase DNA-adduct formation in a statistically significant manner in the livers of male mice, and to slightly decrease adduct formation in the bladders of both male and female mice (Al-Zoughool *et al.*, 2006). The available literature regarding sex differences in human UGT activity is conflicting. On the one hand, glucuronidation of temazepam, oxazepam, propranolol, and salicylic acid were 20–60% higher in men than in women (Al-Zoughool *et al.*, 2006), whereas 4-methyumbelliferone glucuronidation in cryopreserved human hepatocytes was found to be an average of 40% higher in female samples ($n = 33$), than in male samples ($n = 31$). The carcinogenicity of aromatic amines is multifactorial, and involves not only hepatic N-glucuronidation but also hepatic oxidation, hepatic and bladder acetylation, and possibly peroxidation of *N*-hydroxy-*N*-acetyl aromatic amines in the bladder (Al-Zoughool *et al.*, 2006). Therefore, sex differences in UGT activity alone may not fully explain the sex differences observed in the carcinogenicity of aromatic amines. A similar mechanism may be involved in colon tumor formation by aromatic amines, although in this case hydrolysis of the *N*-glucuronide is probably catalyzed by β-glucuronidase in intestinal microflora.

Some acylglucuronides are reactive intermediates that bind covalently to protein by mechanisms that may or may not result in cleavage of the glucuronic acid moiety, as shown in Fig. 6-54. Several drugs, including the NSAIDs benoxaprofen, bromfenac, diclofenac, diflunisal, etodolac, fenoprofen, flurbiprofen, indoprofen, ketoprofen, ketorolac, loxoprofen, sulindac, suprofen (very similar to the diuretic, tienilic acid), tiaprofenic acid, tolmetin, and zomepirac, contain a carboxylic acid moiety that can be glucuronidated to form a reactive acylglucuronide that can form covalent adducts with proteins. Acyl glucuronides vary widely in their reactivity, from the highly reactive zomepirac and tolmetin acyl glucuronides to the less reactive acyl glucuronides of ibuprofen and salicylic acid (Shipkova *et al.*, 2003). A relationship between the reactivity of acyl glucuronides and the substitution near the carboxylic acid has been found. In general, α-unsubstituted acetic acid

derivatives such as zomepirac, tolmetin, and diclofenac exhibit the highest degree of covalent binding, while mono-α-substituted acetic acids such as fenoprofen show intermediate levels, and fully substituted α-acetic acids such as furosemide, ketoprofen, ibuprofen, and suprofen exhibit lower levels of covalent binding (Bolze *et al.*, 2002). However, a direct correlation between the ability of acyl glucuronides to give rise to covalent adducts with proteins such as albumin and their ability to cause drug-related toxicity has not been firmly established, and other mechanisms may come into play. For instance, diclofenac is still a widely used drug in spite of the fact that its acyl glucuronide is very reactive, whereas zomepirac, which is less reactive than these other drugs, was withdrawn from the market in 1983 (Chen *et al.*, 2006).

Neoantigens formed by binding of acylglucuronides to protein might be the cause of rare cases of NSAID-induced immune hepatitis. Covalent adducts with proteins in the liver, kidneys, colon, small intestine, skeletal muscle, and bladder were detected in rats administered diflunisal, and in the liver, lungs, and spleen of rats administered diclofenac of UGT activity (Shipkova *et al.*, 2003). Covalent binding of acyl glucuronides appears to be selective, with diclofenac acyl glucuronide forming adducts with dipeptidyl peptidase in rat liver, and with aminopeptidase *N* and sucrase-isomaltase in rat intestine (Shipkova *et al.*, 2003). Human and rat liver UGTs are themselves targets of adducts formed by ketoprofen acyl glucuronide, which may cause nonspecific irreversible inhibition (Shipkova *et al.*, 2003). Binding of acyl glucuronides to protein can involve isomerization reactions that lead to the retention of a rearranged glucuronide moiety (Fig. 6-54). Formation of a common neoantigen (i.e., one that contains a rearranged glucuronic acid moiety) might explain the allergic cross reactivities (cross sensitization) observed among different NSAIDs (Spahn-Langguth and Benet, 1992; Kretz-Rommel and Boelsterli, 1994). There are reports of the detection of antibodies to acyl glucuronide–protein adducts in rats administered diflunisal, and in humans treated with valproic acid (Shipkova *et al.*, 2003). The inherent reactivity of acyl glucuronides (covered above) can be investigated by determining the rate of disappearance of the acyl glucuronide in aqueous buffers at various pH levels (determination of hydrolysis and intramolecular rearrangement), by including human serum albumin to assess the formation of covalently bound adducts, or by the use of a lysine–phenylalanine dipeptide (Lys-Phe) to assess adduct formation. The use of the lysine–phenylalanine dipeptide allows for the rapid quantitative LC/MS/MS analysis of adducts produced by Schiff's base formation (Wang *et al.*, 2004). The rank order of the reactivity of the acyl glucuronides of some carboxylic acid-containing drugs determined by this approach is as follows: tolmetin > zomepirac > diclofenac > ketoprofen > fenoprofen > ibuprofen > furosemide (Wang *et al.*, 2004).

Some glucuronide conjugates have been found to act as substrates for further biotransformation by oxidation or even by further conjugation. For instance, in male Wag/Rij rats, estradiol 17β-glucuronide can be sulfonated by one or more SULTs to estradiol 3-sulfate-17β-glucuronide (Sun *et al.*, 2006). In addition, the acyl glucuronide of 4'-hydroxydiclofenac can be formed either by glucuronidation of the oxidative metabolite of diclofenac, 4'-hydroxydiclofenac (an example of conjugation following oxidation, as historically conceptualized), or the acyl glucuronide of the parent can be 4'-hydroxylated by CYP2C8 (Kumar *et al.*, 2002), (an example of oxidative metabolism occurring after conjugation). Glucuronidation has been shown to convert several other CYP2C9 substrates into CYP2C8 substrates or inhibitors. For instance, CYP2C8 has been shown to catalyze the oxidation of several glucuronides, the aglycones of which are CYP2C9 substrates, including

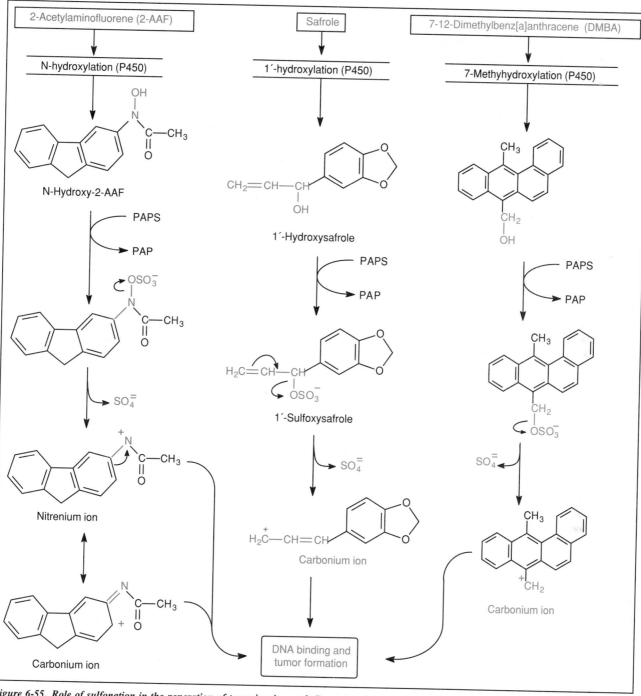

Figure 6-55. Role of sulfonation in the generation of tumorigenic metabolites (nitrenium or carbonium ions) of 2-acetylaminofluorene, safrole, and 7,12-dimethylbenz[a]anthracene (DMBA).

estradiol 17β-glucuronide and the acyl glucuronides of naproxen, the PPAR-α/agonist MRL-C, and gemfibrozil (Delaforge *et al.*, 2005; Kochansky *et al.*, 2005; Ogilvie *et al.*, 2006). In the case of gemfibrozil, the CYP2C8-mediated hydroxylation of its 1-O-β-glucuronide can apparently lead to the formation of a reactive product that causes irreversible inhibition of this enzyme (Ogilvie *et al.*, 2006). The formation of a hydroxylated gemfibrozil acyl glucuronide by CYP2C8 leads to the irreversible inactivation of this enzyme, which leads to significant drug–drug interactions with drugs such as repaglinide and cerivastatin (Ogilvie *et al.*, 2006). Kumar and colleagues demonstrated that formation of the acyl glucuronide of 4'-hydroxydiclofenac leads to an underestimation of

hepatic clearance of diclofenac when it is not accounted for. It may also be that oxidation of glucuronide metabolites can lead to toxicity. A case report described the formation of an IgM antibody that bound erythrocytes, but only in the presence of the 4'-hydroxydiclofenac acyl glucuronide in a patient that developed hemolysis during diclofenac treatment (Shipkova *et al.*, 2003). A determination of the absolute amount of diclofenac acyl glucuronide formed in vivo relative to the amount of 4'-hydroxydiclofenac formed in vivo would be confounded by the rapid hydrolysis of the glucuronide to the aglycone, and it would therefore be likely that detection of 4'-hydroxydiclofenac acyl glucuronide would be attributed to oxidative metabolism occurring prior to conjugation. Two recent reports suggest that direct glucuronidation with subsequent oxidation (by a combination of UGT2B7 and CYP2C8 in humans) may be the major determinants of diclofenac clearance in humans (possibly as high as 75%) and monkeys (>90%) (Kumar et al., 2002; Prueksaritanont et al., 2006), as opposed to earlier in vivo data that suggested oxidative metabolism by CYP2C9 alone is the major determinant of clearance (Stierlin and Faigle, 1979; Stierlin et al., 1979). Prueksaritanont and colleagues (2006) further note that there are no clinical reports that implicate pharmacokinetic interactions between diclofenac and potent CYP2C9 inhibitors or inducers. Taken together, these observations suggest that the CYP-mediated oxidation of glucuronide metabolites has implications not only for the prediction of in vivo drug–drug interactions from in vitro data (i.e., gemfibrozil), but also for the prediction of in vivo clearance (i.e., diclofenac), and possibly also toxicity, as in the case of immune-mediated toxicity of diclofenac.

Sulfonation

Many of the xenobiotics and endogenous substrates that undergo O-glucuronidation also undergo sulfonation, as illustrated in Fig. 6-34 for acetaminophen (Mulder, 1981; Paulson et al., 1986). Sulfonation generally produces a highly water-soluble sulfuric acid ester. The reaction is catalyzed by sulfotransferases (SULT), a large multigene family of enzymes found primarily in the liver, kidney, intestinal tract, lung, platelets, and brain. In mammals, there are two major classes of SULTs: (1) membrane-bound SULTs in the Golgi apparatus, and (2) soluble SULTs in the cytoplasm (Gamage et al., 2006). The membrane-bound SULTs are responsible for the sulfonation of glycosaminoglycans, proteins, and peptides such as cholecystokinin, factors V and VIII, α-2-glycoprotein, gastrin, and p-selective glycoprotein ligand-1, thereby modulating their structure and function. At least five different Golgi-resident N-acetylglucosamine 6-O-sulfotransferases have been identified in humans. They are important for many biological processes including cell–cell adhesion, axon function, T-cell response, cell proliferation, and modulation of viral and bacterial infection (reviewed by Grunwell and Bertozzi, 2002), but they have no activity toward xenobiotics (Wang and James, 2006). Brachymorphic mice are undersized because the defect in PAPS synthesis prevents the normal sulfonation of glycosaminoglycans and proteoglycans, such as heparin and chondroitin, which are important components of cartilage. These particular sulfonation reactions are catalyzed by membrane-bound sulfotransferase, which are thought not to play a role in xenobiotic sulfonation. This section will focus on the cytosolic SULTs, which are known for the sulfonation of various drugs, mutagens, flavonoids, and other xenobiotics, as well as endogenous substrates such as bile acids, thyroid hormones, catecholamine neurotransmitters, and steroids.

The cofactor for the sulfonation reaction is 3'-phosphoadenosine-5'-phosphosulfate (PAPS), the structure of which is shown in Fig. 6-49. The sulfonation of aliphatic alcohols and phenols, R-OH, proceeds as follows:

Sulfonation involves the transfer of sulfonate not sulfate (i.e., SO_3^- not SO_4^-) from PAPS to the xenobiotic. SULTs are single α/β globular proteins that contain a PAPS-binding site which is present on a characteristic five-stranded β-sheet along with the core of the catalytic site. The central β-sheet is surrounded by α-helices (Wang and James, 2006). The sulfonate donor PAPS is synthesized from inorganic sulfate (SO_4^{2-}) and ATP in a two-step reaction. The first reaction is catalyzed by ATP sulfurylase, which converts ATP and SO_4^{2-} to adenosine-5'-phosphosulfate (APS) and pyrophosphate. The second reaction is catalyzed by APS kinase, which transfers a phosphate group from ATP to the 3'-position of APS. The major source of sulfate required for the synthesis of PAPS appears to be derived from cysteine through a complex oxidation sequence. Because the concentration of free cysteine is limited, the cellular concentrations of PAPS (4–80 μM) are considerably lower than those of UDP-glucuronic acid (200–350 μM) and glutathione (5–10 mM). This topic has been thoroughly reviewed, and is outside the scope of this chapter (Klaassen and Boles, 1997). The relatively low concentration of PAPS limits the capacity for xenobiotic sulfonation. In general, sulfonation is a high-affinity but low-capacity pathway of xenobiotic conjugation, whereas glucuronidation is a low-affinity but high-capacity pathway. Acetaminophen is one of the several xenobiotics that are substrates for both sulfotransferases and UDP-glucuronosyltransferases (see Fig. 6-34). The relative amount of sulfonate and glucuronide conjugates of acetaminophen is dependent on dose. At low doses, acetaminophen sulfonate is the main conjugate formed due to the high affinity of sulfotransferases. As the dose increases, the proportion of acetaminophen conjugated with sulfonate decreases, whereas the proportion conjugated with glucuronic acid increases. In some cases, even the absolute amount of xenobiotic conjugated with sulfonate can decrease at high doses apparently because of substrate inhibition of sulfotransferase.

Sulfonation is not limited to phenols and aliphatic alcohols (which are often the products of oxidative or hydrolytic biotransformation), although these represent the largest groups of substrates for sulfotransferases. Certain aromatic amines, such as aniline and 2-aminonaphthalene, can undergo sulfonation to the corresponding sulfamates. The primary amines in cisapride and DPC423 can also be directly N-sulfonated. The N-oxide group in minoxidil and the N-hydroxy group in N-hydroxy-2-aminonaphthalene and N-hydroxy-2-acetylaminofluorene can also be sulfonated. In all cases, the conjugation reaction involves nucleophilic attack of oxygen or nitrogen on the electrophilic sulfur atom in PAPS with cleavage of the phosphosulfate bond. Table 6-17 lists some examples of xenobiotics and endogenous compounds that are sulfonated without prior biotransformation by oxidative enzymes. An even greater number of xenobiotics are sulfonated after a hydroxyl group is exposed or introduced during oxidative or hydrolytic biotransformation.

Carboxylic acids can be conjugated with glucuronic acid but not with sulfonate. However, a number of carboxylic acids, such as benzoic acid, naphthoic acid, naphthylacetic acid, salicylic acid, and naproxen, are competitive inhibitors of sulfotransferases (Rao and Duffel, 1991). Pentachlorophenol and 2,6-dichloro-4-nitrophenol are potent sulfotransferase inhibitors because they bind to the enzyme but cannot initiate a nucleophilic attack on PAPS due to the presence of electron-withdrawing substituents in the ortho- and para-positions on the aromatic ring.

Sulfonate conjugates of xenobiotics are excreted mainly in urine. Those excreted in bile may be hydrolyzed by aryl sulfatases present in gut microflora, which contributes to the enterohepatic circulation of certain xenobiotics. Sulfatases are also present in the endoplasmic reticulum and lysosomes, where they primarily hydrolyze sulfonates of endogenous compounds presumably in a

Table 6-17

Properties of the Human Cytosolic Sulfotransferases (SULTs)

HUMAN SULT	MAJOR TISSUE DISTRIBUTION	MAJOR SUBSTRATES[a]
SULT1A1	Liver (very high), platelets. placenta, adrenals, endometrium, colon, jejunum, brain leukocytes	**4-Nitrophenol**, 4-ethylphenol, 4-cresol, 2-naphthol, other phenols, acetaminophen, minoxidil, N-hydroxy-PhIP, T2, T3, 17β-estradiol (and other phenolic steroids), dopamine, benzylic alcohols, 2-nitropropane, aromatic amines, hydroxylamines, hydroxamic acids, apomorphine, troglitazone,
SULT1A2	Liver, bladder tumors	4-Nitrophenol, N-hydroxy-2-acetylaminofluorene, 2-naphthol, aromatic hydroxylamines, hydroxamic acids
SULT1A3	Jejunum and colon mucosa (very high), platelets, placenta, brain, leukocytes	**Dopamine**, 4-nitrophenol, 1-hydroxymethylpyrene, norepinephrine, salbutamol, dobutamine
SULT1A4	Liver, pancreas, colon, brain[b]	Not characterized. Likely similar to SULT1A3
SULT1B1	Colon (highest), liver, leukocytes	4-Nitrophenol, T2, T3, r-T3, T4, dopamine, benzylic alcohols
SULT1C2	Fetal lung and kidney, kidney, stomach, thyroid gland	4-Nitrophenol, N-hydroxy-2-AAF, aryl hydroxylamines, thyroid hormones
SULT1C4	Kidney, ovary, spinal cord, fetal kidney, fetal lung	4-Nitrophenol, N-hydroxy-2-AAF, 17β-estrone, bisphenol-A, 4-octylphenol, nonylphenol, diethylstilbestrol, 1-hydroxymethylpyrene
SULT1E1	Liver (highest), endometrium, jejunum, adrenals, mammary epithelial cells, fetal liver	**17β-Estradiol**, estrone, ethinyl estradiol, 17β-estrone, equilenin, 2-hydroxy-estrone, 2-hydroxy-estradiol, 4-hydroxy-estrone, 4-hydroxy-estradiol, diethylstilbestrol, tamoxifen, thyroid hormones, 4-hydroxylonazolac, pregnenolone, dehydroepiandrosterone, 1-naphthol, naringenin
SULT2A1	Liver (highest), adrenals, jejunum, brain	**Dehydroepiandrosterone (DHEA)**, 1-hydroxymethylpyrene, 6-hydroxymethylbenzo[a]pyrene, hycanthone, bile acids, pregnenolone, testosterone, androgens, estrone, 17β-estradiol, other hydroxysteroids, budenoside
SULT2B1_v1	Placenta (highest), prostate, trachea, skin	Dehydroepiandrosterone, pregnenolone, oxysterols, other hydroxysteroids
SULT2B1_v2		**Cholesterol**, dehydroepiandrosterone, other hydroxysteroids
SULT4A1_v1	Brain: cortex, globus pallidus, islands of Calleja, septum, thalamus, red nucleus, substantia nigra and pituitary	Endogenous: 4 unidentified compounds from mouse brain homogenate.[c] Other: T3, T4, estrone, 4-nitrophenol, 2-naphthylamine, 2-naphthol[d]
SULT4A1_v2		

Substrates in bold are reported to be selective probe substrates for the SULT listed (Coughtrie and Fisher, 2005).

[a]T4 is thyroxine. T2 and T3 are di- and tri-iodothyronine.

[b]Data from Bradley, Benner (2005).

[c]Sakakibara *et al.*: Reported that recombinant human SULT4A1 expressed in *E. coli* (and subsequently purified) sulfonated four distinct endogenous substances from mouse brain homogenate (2002).

[d]Sakakibara *et al.*: Reported that recombinant human SULT4A1 expressed in *E. coli* (and subsequently purified) sulfonated these prototypical SULT substrates (2002).

Adapted from Gamage N, Barnett A, Hempel N, *et al.*: Human sulfotransferases and their role in chemical metabolism. *Toxicol Sci* 90:5–22, 2006; Wang LQ, James MO: Inhibition of sulfotransferases by xenobiotics. *Curr Drug Metab* 7:83–104, 2006; Blanchard RL, Freimuth RR, Buck J, Weinshilboum RM, Coughtrie MW: A proposed nomenclature system for the cytosolic sulfotransferase (SULT) superfamily. *Pharmacogenetics* 14:199–211, 2004.

manner analogous to that described for microsomal β-glucuronidase (Dwivedi *et al.*, 1987) (see comments on egasyn in section "Carboxylesterases"). Sulfonation facilitates the deiodination of thyroxine and triiodothyronine and can determine the rate of elimination of thyroid hormones in some species. Inhibition of SULTs can occur with exposure to drugs such as mefenamic acid, salicylic acid, clomiphene, danazol, environmental chemicals, such as hydroxylated PCBs, hydroxylated PAHs, pentachlorophenol, triclosan, and bisphenol A, and dietary constituents, such as catechins, colorants, phytoestrogens, and flavonoids. Adverse effects on human health can potentially result from SULT inhibition, such as the thyroid hormone disruption that occurs with exposure to hydroxylated PCBs (Wang and James, 2006). In contrast, given that some sulfonate conjugates are chemically reactive, inhibition of their formation may be protective. There are a few reports of drug–drug interactions due to SULT inhibition. It has been reported that the sulfonation rates of both acetaminophen and salicylamide are decreased when these drugs are coadministered, and dapsone and lamivudine have been found to decrease acetaminophen sulfonation (Wang and James, 2006). Coadministration of acetaminophen with ethinyl estradiol increases its AUC by up to 54% and decreases the AUC of ethinyl estradiol sulfate by ~40%, indicating that acetaminophen may directly inhibit one or more SULTs (Rogers *et al.*, 1987). Drug–drug interactions involving induction of SULT are detailed later in this section.

Sulfonation may represent a benign metabolic pathway compared with competing pathways that can lead to the activation of promutagens and procarcinogens. For instance, sulfonation of hydroquinones, phenols, and aminophenols can prevent or reduce the formation of reactive quinones, semiquinones, and quinnone amines. Sulfonation of aromatic amines such as 2-amino-3,8-dimethylimidazo-[4,5-f]quinoxaline (MelQx), which leads to sulfamate formation can compete with activation by N-O-acetylation or sulfonation (Wang and James, 2006).

Like glucuronide conjugates, some sulfonate conjugates are substrates for further biotransformation. For instance, the 7- and 4-sulfates of daidzein and genistein can be sulfonated by SULT1E1 to disulfates (Nakano *et al.*, 2004). Other examples include the oxidation of sulfonate conjugates of testosterone and estrogens. Dehydroepiandrosterone-3-sulfate is 16α-hydroxylated by CYP3A7, the major CYP enzyme expressed in human fetal liver (Ingelman-Sundberg *et al.*, 1975; Kitada *et al.*, 1987; Ohmori *et al.*, 1998). CYP2C12, which is expressed in female but not male rats, catalyzes the oxidation of a steroid *di*-sulfate (namely, 5α-androstane-3α,17β-diol-3,17-disulfate) (Ryan *et al.*, 1984).

Multiple sulfotransferases have been identified in all mammalian species examined. An international workshop approved the abbreviation "SULT" for sulfotransferase (although ST remains a common abbreviation) and developed a nomenclature system based on amino acid sequences (and, to some extent, function). SULT nomenclature is available on line at: http://www.fccc.edu/research/labs/blanchard/sult/accessions.html. The SULTs are arranged into gene families that share at least 45% amino acid sequence identity. The nine gene families identified to date (vertebrate: SULT1–SULT6; insect: SULT101; and plant: SULT201–SULT202) are subdivided into subfamilies that are at least 60% identical (Blanchard *et al.*, 2004; Gamage *et al.*, 2006). For example, SULT1 is divided into five subfamilies designated SULT1A–SULT1E. Two SULTs that share more than 60% similarity are considered individual members of the same subfamily. For example, SULT1A1, SULT1A2, SULT1A3, and SULT1A4 are four individual members of the human SULT1A subfamily. In general, the first published sequence in a subfamily is designated as enzyme 1 and subsequent enzymes within that subfamily are assigned on the basis of percentage amino acid identity relative to the "1" enzyme (Blanchard *et al.*, 2004). Exceptions to this rule have been made to maintain historical use of a name (e.g., SULT2A1). Variant forms with different amino acid sequences encoded by the same gene are designated by "vn" at the end. For instance, the SULTs initially referenced as SULT2B1a and SULT2B1b are now called SULT2B1_v1 and SULT2B1_v2. Although nine SULT gene families have been identified, these have not been identified in all mammalian species. Currently, SULT1 and SULT2 are the only gene families subdivided into multiple subfamilies (five in the case of SULT1 [SULT1A–1E]; two in the case of SULT2 [SULT2A and SULT2B]).

Most of the SULTs cloned belong to one of the two families, SULT1 and SULT2. These two families are functionally different; the SULT1 enzymes catalyze the sulfonation of phenols, isoflavones, the procarcinogen *N*-OH-2-acetylaminofluorene, endogenous compounds such as 17β-estradiol (including its glucuronide conjugate; see section "Glucuronidation"), and other steroids, iodothyronines, endogenous catecholamines, and eicosanoids. The SULT2 enzymes catalyze the sulfonation of the 3β-hydroxy groups of steroids with unsaturated A rings, bile acids, benzylic alcohols of polycyclic aromatic hydrocarbons, and other primary and secondary alcohols. A sulfotransferase that catalyzes the sulfonation of heterocyclic amines such as 2-naphthylamine, desipramine, and aniline (to form sulfamates) has been cloned from rabbit and mouse (SULT3A1).

SULT4A1 has been identified in rat, mouse, and human. These enzymes are expressed in the cerebral cortex, cerebellum, pituitary, and brainstem and do not sulfonate typical SULT substrates (Blanchard *et al.*, 2004; Gamage *et al.*, 2006). These SULTs share $\sim$97% amino acid sequence identity across species, which suggests that SULT4A1 likely serves a critical endogenous function. The SULT4A1 sequence has also been identified as SULT5A1,

but the 4A1 nomenclature has been retained. A separate gene, SULT5A1, has been cloned from mouse, but no information on its function is available. SULT6A1 has been cloned from chicken liver, and the recombinant enzyme was found to sulfonate 17β-estradiol and corticosterone (Blanchard *et al.*, 2004). SULT201 and 202 represent two families of plant SULTs. SULTT101A1 is an insect SULT cloned from *Spodoptera frugiperda* and converts retinol to anhydroretinol via a retinyl sulfate intermediate (Blanchard *et al.*, 2004). SULT101A also exhibits sulfotransferase activity toward ethanol, dopamine, vanillin, 4-nitrophenol, serotonin, and hydroxybenzylhydrazine (Blanchard *et al.*, 2004). Thirteen cytosolic SULTs have been cloned from rat, and they belong either to the SULT1, SULT2, or SULT4 gene families. The individual rat enzymes are SULT1A1, 1B1, 1C1, 1C2, 1C3, 1D1, 1E1, 1E2, 2A1, 2A2, 2A3, 2A4, and 4A1.

Eleven genes encoding 13 cytosolic SULTs have been identified in humans, and they belong either to the SULT1, SULT2, or SULT4 gene families. The individual human enzymes are listed in Table 6-17. Various single-nucleotide polymorphisms have been reported in most of the SULT genes with rare single-base deletions in SULT1A2 and 4A1 (Glatt and Meinl, 2004). With a few exceptions, the functional consequences of most of these polymorphisms remain unknown. Several of the human SULT genes have multiple initiation sites for transcription, which produces different mRNA transcripts. Consequently, in some cases, different versions of the same human SULT gene have been cloned several times. For example, there are three alternative first exons (exons 1a, 1b, and 1c) in the human SULT1A3 gene (none of which contains a coding region), and five SULT1A3 cDNAs have been cloned from various human tissues, each with a unique 5′-region (Nagata and Yamazoe, 2000).

Historically, human liver cytosol was found to contain two phenol sulfotransferase activities (PST) that could be distinguished by their thermal stability; hence, they were known as TS-PST (*thermally stable*) and TL-PST (*thermally labile*) (Weinshilboum, 1992a; Weinshilboum *et al.*, 1997). It is now known that TS-PST actually reflects the activity of two SULTs, namely, SULT1A1 and SULT1A2 which share 93% identity, whereas TL-PST reflects the activity of SULT1A3 (and likely SULT1A4), which is 60% similar to both SULT1A1 and 2 (Gamage *et al.*, 2006). Hence, the four members of the SULT1A gene subfamily in human were represented functionally by TS-PST and TL-PST activity. SULT1A1 and SULT1A2 function as homo- and heterodimers, and are coregulated. Although these two individual SULTs are not catalytically identical, they are sufficiently similar to consider them as the single activity traditionally known as TS-PST. Because of differences in their substrate specificity, SULT1A1/2 and 1A3 were also known as phenol-PST and monoamine-PST, respectively. SULT1A3 preferentially catalyzes the sulfonation of dopamine, epinephrine, and levodopa, whereas SULT1A1 and 1A2 preferentially catalyze the sulfonation of simple phenols, such as phenol, 4-nitrophenol, minoxidil, and acetaminophen. SULT1A1 and 1A2 also catalyze the *N*-sulfonation of 2-aminonaphthalene. SULT1A1/2 and SULT1A3 can also be distinguished by differences in their sensitivity to the inhibitory effects of 2,6-dichloro-4-nitrophenol.

The expression of SULT1A1 and 1A2 in human liver is largely determined by genetic factors, which also determines the corresponding sulfotransferase activity in blood platelets. Inherited variation in platelet SULT1A1 and 1A2 largely reflects genetic polymorphisms in these enzymes. One allelic variant of SULT1A1 known as SULT1A1*2 ($Arg_{213} \rightarrow His_{213}$) is associated with decreased activity in platelets but not liver, and decreased thermal stability (Glatt and Meinl, 2004). This particular genetic polymorphism is common in both Caucasians and Nigerians (with an allele frequency of 0.31 and 0.37, respectively), and is correlated with interindividual variation in the sulfonation of acetaminophen. Low SULT1A1 and 1A2 activity predisposes individuals to diet-induced migraine headaches, possibly due to impaired sulfonation of unidentified phenolic compounds in the diet that cause such headaches. A fourth member of the human SULT1A subfamily, SULT1A4, has been recently described, which appears to be a duplication of SULT1A3, and these two enzymes share >99% sequence identity (Bradley and Benner, 2005; Gamage *et al.*, 2006). The genes for both of these SULTs lie on chromosome 16p, which contains a segmental duplication that results in two nearly identical, transcriptionally active copies of SULT1A3 and SULT1A4. Each copy shares exons with an adjacent copy of SULT1A1. Four nonsynonymous SNPs were reported for these genes, which show different enzyme activities (Gamage *et al.*, 2006).

Human SULT1B1, like the corresponding enzyme in other species, catalyzes the sulfonation of thyroid hormones, 2-naphthol, and dopamine. SULT1B1 levels in human liver cytosol vary widely, possibly due to polymorphisms (e.g., $Glu_{186} \rightarrow Gly_{186}$ and $Glu_{204} \rightarrow Asp_{204}$) (Glatt and Meinl, 2004). SULT1B1 is also expressed in human colon, small intestine, and blood leukocytes. Humans have two SULT1C enzymes (SULT1C2 and SULT1C4). Their function has not been determined, although the corresponding rat enzyme (SULT1C1) catalyzes the sulfonation of *N*-hydroxy-2-acetylaminofluorene (see Fig. 6-55). SULT1C2 is expressed at high levels in the thyroid, stomach, and kidneys (Blanchard *et al.*, 2004). High levels of SULT1C4 are expressed in fetal liver and kidney, with hepatic levels declining in adulthood, but it is also present in adult ovary and brain.

Human SULT1E1 has been identified as a high affinity estrogen sulfotransferase. SULT1A1 also catalyzes the sulfonation of estrogens, such as 17β-estradiol, but it does so with a much lower affinity than does SULT1E1. The sulfonation of ethinyl estradiol in human hepatocytes is inducible by rifampin (Li *et al.*, 1999), which raises the possibility that SULT1E1 is an inducible enzyme. In addition to human liver, SULT1E1 is expressed in placenta, breast, brain, testes, adrenal glands, and uterine tissue. SULT1E1 has been studied in SULT1E1-deficient mice, and it was shown that these mice had spontaneous fetal loss caused by placental thrombosis, which was reversible by administration of antiestrogens (Gamage *et al.*, 2006).

SULT2A1 is the human alcohol sulfotransferase, long known as DHEA-ST (for its ability to sulfonate dehydroepiandrosterone). In addition to DHEA, substrates for SULT2A1 include steroid hormones, bile acids, and cholesterol. Furthermore, SULT2A1 converts several procarcinogens to electrophilic metabolites, including hydroxymethyl polycyclic aromatic hydrocarbons, *N*-hydroxy-2-acetylaminofluorene, and 1′-hydroxysafrole, as shown in Fig. 6-55. The thermal stability of SULT2A1 is intermediate between that of the four phenol SULTs (SULT1A1/2 and 1A3/4), and the enzyme is resistant to the inhibitory effects of 2,6-dichloro-4-nitrophenol. SULT2A1 is not expressed in blood platelets, but the activity of this enzyme has been measured in human liver cytosol. SULT2A1 is also expressed in adrenal cortex, brain, and intestine (Blanchard *et al.*, 2004). SULT2A1 is bimodally distributed, possibly due to a genetic polymorphism that apparently lies outside of the coding region, and perhaps outside of the *SULT2A1* gene itself, with a high activity group composed of ~25% of the population (Glatt and Meinl,

2004). Several SULT2A1 SNPs have been identified, but the underlying basis for the high activity group remains to be determined as these polymorphisms appear to be too rare to explain the bimodal distribution.

Human SULT2B1 is also a DHEA-sulfotransferase. It is expressed in placenta, prostate, and trachea. The SULT2B1 gene can be transcribed from one of the two exons, both of which contain coding sequences, hence, two forms of SULT2B1 (known as 2B1_v1 and 2B1_v2) with different N-terminal amino acid sequences can be transcribed by alternate splicing of precursor mRNA. This situation is analogous to the alternative splicing of multiple exons 1 in the UGT1 gene family (see Fig. 6-53). SULT2B1_v1 appears to catalyze the sulfonation of pregnenolone, and SULT2B1_v2 can catalyze the sulfonation of both pregnenolone and cholesterol (Blanchard *et al.*, 2004).

The SULT enzymes were previously categorized into five classes based on their catalytic activity. These five functional classes were: *Arylsulfotransferase*, which sulfonates numerous phenolic xenobiotics; *alcohol sulfotransferase*, which sulfonates primary and secondary alcohols including nonaromatic hydroxysteroids (for which reason these enzymes are also known as hydroxysteroid SULTs); *estrogen sulfotransferase*, which sulfonates estrone and other aromatic hydroxysteroids; *tyrosine ester sulfotransferase*, which sulfonates tyrosine methyl ester and 2-cyanoethyl-*N*-hydroxythioacetamide, and *bile salt sulfotransferase*, which sulfonates conjugated and unconjugated bile acids. The *arylsulfotransferase* and *estrogen sulfotransferase* are composed largely of SULT1 enzymes, which catalyze the sulfonation of phenolic xenobiotics, catechols, and aromatic (phenolic) steroids. The *alcohol sulfotransferase* and *bile salt sulfotransferase* are composed largely of SULT2 enzymes, which catalyze the sulfonation of a variety of primary and secondary alcohols, bile acids, and hydroxysteroids (such as dehydroepiandrosterone or DHEA).

In rats, sulfotransferase activity varies considerably with the sex and age. In mature rats, phenol sulfotransferase activity (SULT1A activity) is higher in males, whereas alcohol sulfotransferase and bile acid sulfotransferase activities (SULT2 activities) are higher in females. Sex differences in the developmental expression of individual sulfotransferases are the result of a complex interplay between gonadal, thyroidal, and pituitary hormones, which similarly determine sex differences in CYP enzyme expression. However, compared with CYP enzymes, the SULTs are refractory or only marginally responsive to the enzyme-inducing effects of 3-methylcholanthrene and phenobarbital, although one or more individual SULT2 enzymes are inducible by PCN. Likewise, SULT1A1, 2A1, or 2E1 expressed in Caco-2 cells are refractory to various polycyclic aromatic hydrocarbons, and 3-methylcholanthrene has no effect on SULT1A1 and 1A3 mRNA levels in primary human hepatocytes (Gamage *et al.*, 2006). From rodent studies, it is generally held that AhR agonists have suppressive effects on SULT regulation. 2-AAF, TCDD, 3-methylcholanthrene, and β-naphthoflavone markedly suppress SULT1A1 and 2A activities and mRNA levels in rat livers (Gamage *et al.*, 2006). In contrast, there is evidence that the rat liver hydroxysteroid SULTs (SULT2s) may be inducible by tamoxifen and estrogens (Gamage *et al.*, 2006). For mouse SULT2A2, a functional nuclear response element responsive for CAR has been reported (Gamage *et al.*, 2006). Human SULT2A1 has been reported to be regulated by FXR, PXR, VDR, and PPARα, whereas SULT1A1, 2A1, and 2A9 genes in mice are regulated by CAR (Tirona and Kim, 2005; Gamage *et al.*, 2006). There are conflicting data regarding the influence of CAR ligands on

SULT1A1 and 1A3. One study reports an 11-fold increase in SULT1A1 mRNA in primary human hepatocytes by the CAR ligand, CITCO, whereas another study could not reproduce these results for either SULT1A1 or 1A3 (Gamage et al., 2006). The glucocorticoid, dexamethasone, has been reported to induce both murine and human SULT2A1 through PXR and GR activation (Gamage et al., 2006). Human SULT2A1 mRNA and protein have also been reported to be induced by rifampin, vitamin D_3, phenobarbital, TCPOBOP, and the PPARα-agonist, ciprofibrate (Runge-Morris and Kocarek, 2005).

Induction of SULTs by rifampin, on the other hand, may be clinically relevant. Rifampin (600 mg q.d.) has been reported to cause up to a 190% increase in the clearance of ethinyl estradiol (35 μg q.d.) (Barditch-Crovo et al., 1999). The interaction between ethinyl estradiol-containing oral contraceptives and antibiotics such as rifampin is often attributed to the induction of CYP3A4, which is the major CYP involved in the *oxidative* metabolism of ethinyl estradiol (e.g., Ortho-Evra® prescribing information, 2005). Several lines of evidence suggest that induction of CYP3A4 is not the predominant mechanism by which rifampin increases the clearance of ethinyl estradiol. First, Li and colleagues (1999) reported that treatment of primary cultures of human hepatocytes with rifampin (33.3 μM) caused up to a 3.3-fold increase in ethinyl estradiol 3-*O*-sulfate formation. Second, SULTs 1A1, 1A2, 1A3, 1E1, and 2A1 catalyze the 3-*O*-sulfonation of ethinyl estradiol with K_m values ranging from 6.7 to 4500 nM, nearer the pharmacologically relevant concentrations (Schrag et al., 2004). Finally, it is known that ethinyl estradiol is predominantly excreted in bile and urine as the 3-sulfate and, to a lesser extent, the 3-glucuronide (Li et al., 1999), which suggests that 3-sulfonation is the major pathway of ethinyl estradiol metabolism. Taken together, these data suggest that induction of SULTs can be clinically relevant at least for low-dose drugs that can be sulfonated with high affinity.

Extrapolation of animal data with regard to biotransformation by SULTs is confounded by the number of SULTs, the expression pattern of SULTs and pronounced sexual dimorphisms in many rodents (Gamage et al., 2006). For instance, expression of SULTs in humans appears to have a largely extrahepatic pattern, whereas rodent SULT expression is predominantly hepatic. For instance, based on RT-PCR measurements of mRNA levels in human tissues, SULT1A3 is expressed at the greatest level in the small intestine, 1B1 in the colon, 2B1 in the placenta, and 4A1 in the brain (Nishimura and Naito, 2006). Of the SULTs that have been characterized by RT-PCR in various human tissues, only SULT1A1, 1E1, and 2A1 are predominantly expressed in the liver (Nishimura and Naito, 2006).

Additionally, humans have four members of the SULT1A subfamily whereas rodents have only one. In contrast, rats have four members of the SULT2A subfamily, whereas humans have only a single SULT2A gene. Human equivalents of mouse SULT3A1 and 5A1 have not yet been identified in humans (Gamage et al., 2006). There are also significant differences between other mammalian species. For instance, sulfotransferase activity is low in pigs but high in cats. The high sulfotransferase activity in cats offsets their low capacity to conjugate xenobiotics with glucuronic acid.

In general, sulfonation is an effective means of decreasing the pharmacological and toxicological activity of xenobiotics. There are cases, however, in which sulfonation increases the toxicity of foreign chemicals because certain sulfonate conjugates are chemically unstable and degrade to form potent electrophilic species. As shown in Fig. 6-55, sulfonation plays an important role in the activation of aromatic amines, methyl-substituted polycyclic aromatic hydrocarbons, and safrole to tumorigenic metabolites. To exert its tumorigenic effect in rodents, safrole must be hydroxylated by CYP to 1'-hydroxysafrole, which is then sulfonated to the electrophilic and tumor-initiating metabolite, 1'-sulfooxysafrole (Boberg et al., 1983). 1'-Hydroxysafrole is a more potent hepatotumorigen than safrole. Two lines of evidence support a major role for sulfonation in the hepatotumorigenic effect of 1'-hydroxysafrole. First, the hepatotumorigenic effect of 1'-hydroxysafrole can be inhibited by treating mice with the sulfotransferase inhibitor, pentachlorophenol. Second, the hepatotumorigenic effect of 1'-hydroxysafrole is markedly reduced in brachymorphic mice, which have a diminished capacity to sulfonate xenobiotics because of a genetic defect in PAPS synthesis. The sulfo-conjugates of benzylic and allylic alcohols, aromatic hydroxylamines, and hydroxamic acids (including those in cooked meat) are short-lived electrophiles capable of reacting with nucleophilic substances including proteins and DNA (Wang and James, 2006). Sulfonation can also convert procarcinogens and promutagens to electrophilic nitrenium or carbocation intermediates such as N-hydroxy-2-acetylaminofluorene (N-OH-AAF), 1-hydroxymethylpyrene (1-HMP), 1'-hydroxysafrole, and the cooked food mutagen N-hydroxy-2-amino-1-methyl-6-phenylimidazo(4,5-b)pyridine (N-OH-PhIP) (Wang and James, 2006).

Some drugs must be converted to a sulfonate conjugate to exert their desired effect, including triamterene, cicletanine, and minoxidil (Wang and James, 2006). Sulfonation (as well as glucuronidation) converts morphine to more potent analgesics than the parent, with morphine 6-sulfate being 30 times more potent and with morphine-6-glucuronide being 45–800 times more potent than morphine itself in rats (Wang and James, 2006). Similarly, several sulfonated steroids such as pregnenolone sulfate and DHEA sulfate interact directly with neurotransmitter receptors. It has been found that pregnenolone sulfate and DHEA sulfate enhance memory in mice. Prevention of hydrolysis of these sulfates by the steroid sulfatase inhibitor, (*para-O*-sulfamoyl)-*N*-tetradecanoyl tyramine, increases the memory enhancement caused by DHEA sulfate in rats, which suggests there is an important role of these sulfates in the central nervous system (Wang and James, 2006).

Polymorphisms with consequences for the bioactivation of xenobiotics have been reported. For instance, the human SULT1A*Arg (*1) allelozyme expressed in *Salmonella typhinurium* is 12- to 350-fold more active in the sulfonation of 2-acetylamino-4-hydroxyaminotoluene, 2-nitropropoane, 2,4-dinitrobenzylalcohol, (−)-1-(α-hydroxyethyl) pyrene, and 1-hydroxymethylpyrene to mutagens than are cells expressing SULT1A1*His (Gamage et al., 2006). Enantioselective sulfonation of promutagens has been reported, as in the case of 1-(α-hydroxyethyl) pyrene, for which SULT2A1 exhibits a 15-fold preference for the (+)-enantiomer, and SULT1E1 exhibits a 160-fold preference for the (−)-enantiomer (Gamage et al., 2006).

Methylation

Methylation is a common but generally minor pathway of xenobiotic biotransformation. Methylation differs from most other conjugation reactions because it generally decreases the water solubility of xenobiotics and masks functional groups that might otherwise be metabolized by other conjugating enzymes. One exception to this rule is the N-methylation of pyridine-containing xenobiotics, such as nicotine, which produces quaternary ammonium ions that are water soluble and readily excreted. Another exception is the S-methylation of thioethers to form positively charged sulfonium ions, a reaction catalyzed by thioether methyltransferase (TEMT), which has only been identified in mice (Weinshilboum *et al.*, 1999). The cofactor for methylation is *S*-adenosylmethionine (SAM), the structure of which is shown in Fig. 6-49. The methyl group bound to the sulfonium ion in SAM has the characteristics of a carbonium ion and is transferred to xenobiotics and endogenous substrates by nucleophilic attack from an electron-rich heteroatom (*O*, *N*, or *S*). Consequently, the functional groups involved in methylation reactions are phenols, catechols, aliphatic and aromatic amines, *N*-heterocyclics, and sulfhydryl-containing compounds. The conversion of benzo[*a*]pyrene to 6-methylbenzo[*a*]pyrene is a rare example of C-methylation. Another reaction that appears to involve C-methylation, the conversion of cocaine to ethylcocaine, is actually a transesterification reaction, as shown in Fig. 6-4. Metals can also be methylated. Inorganic mercury and arsenic can both be dimethylated, and inorganic selenium can be trimethylated. The selenium atom in ebselen is methylated following the ring opening of this antiinflammatory drug. Some examples of xenobiotics and endogenous substrates that undergo O-, N-, or S-methylation are shown in Fig. 6-56. During these methylation reactions, SAM is converted to *S*-adenosyl-L-homocysteine (SAH). This section will cover the following methyltransferases: AS3MT, COMT, GNMT, HNMT, INMT, NNMT, PNMT, POMT (TMT), TEMT, and TPMT. Other methyltransferases that have been implicated as drug metabolizing enzymes include GAMT and PEMT (Nishimura and Naito, 2006).

The O-methylation of phenols and catechols is catalyzed by two different enzymes known as catechol-*O*-methyltransferase (COMT) and the enzyme historically termed phenol *O*-methyltransferase (POMT) (Weinshilboum, 1989, 1992b). POMT is a microsomal enzyme that methylates phenols but not catechols, and COMT is both a cytosolic and microsomal enzyme with the converse substrate specificity, i.e., an absolute requirement for catechol substrates (Weinshilboum, 2006). COMT plays a greater role in the biotransformation of catechols than POMT plays in the biotransformation of phenols. It should be noted that there is strong evidence to suggest that the membrane-bound POMT is the same enzyme as TMT (Weinshilboum, 2006). COMT was originally described as a cytosolic, Mg^{2+}-requiring, monomeric enzyme (Mr 25,000). However, in rats and humans, the enzyme is encoded by the COMT gene (on chromosome 22 in humans) with two different promoters and transcription initiation sites. Transcription at one site produces a cytosolic form of COMT, whereas transcription from the other site produces a membrane-bound form by adding 50 hydrophobic amino acids to the N-terminal of the microsomal COMT, which targets this form to the endoplasmic reticulum (Weinshilboum *et al.*, 1999; Weinshilboum, 2006). The microsomal COMT is expressed at high levels in the brain and lymphocytes (Weinshilboum, 2006). The cytosolic form of COMT is present in virtually all tissues, including erythrocytes, but the highest concentrations are found in liver and kidney. The membrane-bound form is more highly expressed in brain.

Substrates for COMT include several catecholamine neurotransmitters, such as epinephrine, norepinephrine, and dopamine; and catechol drugs, such as the anti-Parkinson's disease agent L-dopa (3,4-dihydroxyphenylalanine) and the antihypertensive drug methyldopa (α-methyl-3,4-dihydroxyphenylalanine). Catechol estrogens, which are formed by 2- or 4-hydroxylation of the steroid A-ring, are substrates for COMT, as are drugs that are converted

to catechols either by two consecutive hydroxylation reactions (as in the case of phenobarbital and diclofenac), by ring opening of a methylenedioxy group (as in the case of stiripentol and 3,4-methylenedioxymethamphetamine), or by hydrolysis of vicinal esters (as in the case of ibopamine). Formation of catechol estrogens, particularly 4-hydroxyestradiol, has been suggested to play an important role in estrogen-induced tumor formation in hamster kidney, rat pituitary, and mouse uterus (Zhu and Liehr, 1993) (see section "CYP1B1"). These tissues contain high levels of epinephrine or dopamine, which inhibit the O-methylation of 4-hydroxyestradiol by COMT. Nontarget tissues do not contain high levels of catecholamines, which suggests that 4-hydroxyestradiol induces tumor formation in those tissues that fail to methylate and detoxify this catechol estrogen. These observations in animals are especially intriguing in view of subsequent epidemiological evidence demonstrating that low COMT activity appears to increase the risk of breast cancer, with odds ratios ranging from 1.7 to 3.0 (Weinshilboum, 2006).

In the 1970s, when COMT levels in erythrocytes (predominantly the cytosolic form) were measured in human subjects, it was apparent that there was a subpopulation that displayed low levels of this enzyme. Segregation analysis indicated that erythrocyte COMT activity was an autosomal codominant trait, and that erythrocyte levels correlated with relative COMT levels in liver and lymphocyte cytosol (Weinshilboum, 2006). It was subsequently found that COMT is encoded by a single gene with alleles for a low activity form (COMT^L) and high activity form (COMT^H) (Weinshilboum, 1989, 1992b, 2006; Weinshilboum *et al.*, 1999). This polymorphism results from a single G → A transition in exon 4 that results in the substitution Val^{108}Met in cytosolic COMT and Val^{158}Met in microsomal COMT (Weinshilboum *et al.*, 1999; Weinshilboum, 2006). The presence of methionine at position 108 in the cytosolic enzyme not only decreases the catalytic activity of COMT, but it decreases the thermal stability of the enzyme, which has long been used to differentiate COMT^L (thermolabile) from COMT^H (thermostable). In Caucasians, these allelic variants are expressed with equal frequency, so that 25% of the population is homozygous for either the low or high activity enzyme, and 50% is heterozygous and have intermediate COMT activity. COMT activity is generally higher in Asians and African Americans due to a higher frequency of the COMT^H allele (~0.75 for Asians and African Americans vs. ~0.5 for Caucasians [McLeod *et al.*, 1994]). Subsequent resequencing of the COMT gene has revealed numerous single-nucleotide polymorphisms, with at least eight that occur with a frequency >10% in Caucasians, and 11 such SNPs in African Americans. Several of these SNPs are found in the intronic regions. A list of current COMT (and many other) alleles can be found at http://alfred.med.yale.edu/alfred/index.asp.

The genetically determined levels of COMT in erythrocytes correlate with individual differences in the proportion of L-dopa converted to 3-*O*-methyldopa and the proportion of methyldopa converted to its 3-*O*-methyl metabolite. O-Methylation is normally a minor pathway of L-dopa biotransformation, but 3-*O*-methyldopa is the major metabolite when L-dopa is administered with a dopa decarboxylase inhibitor, such as carbidopa or benserazide, which is common clinical practice. High COMT activity, resulting in extensive O-methylation of L-dopa to 3-*O*-methyldopa, has been associated with poor therapeutic management of Parkinson's disease and an increased incidence of drug-induced toxicity (dyskinesia). A large number of epidemiological studies have been performed to examine the effects of the COMT Val$^{108/158}$Met polymorphism, and there is no evidence that the genetic polymorphism in COMT represents a risk modifier for the development of Parkinson's disease

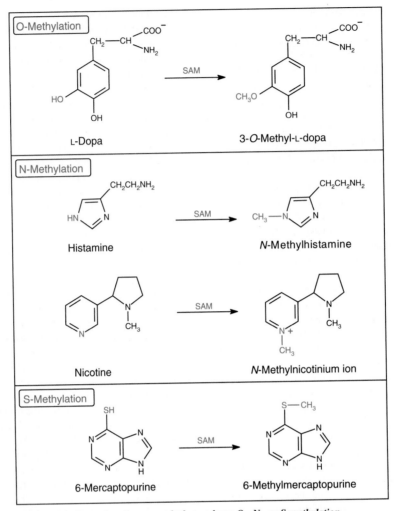

Figure 6-56. *Examples of compounds that undergo O-, N-, or S-methylation.*

(Weinshilboum *et al.*, 1999). However, Egan and colleagues have demonstrated that COMT genotype was related in an allele-dosage manner to cognitive performance, with individuals homozygous for Met[108] (COMT[L] phenotype) demonstrating increased executive cognition, as measured by the Wisconsin Card Sorting Test (Egan *et al.*, 2001). The impact of the Met[108] allele was attributed to decreased dopamine catabolism in the prefrontal cortex, which results in enhanced neuronal function. Conversely, those individuals who are homozygous for Val[108] (COMT[H] phenotype) appear to have decreased executive cognition, and may be at a slightly increased risk of developing schizophrenia (Egan *et al.*, 2001).

Several *N*-methyltransferases have been described in humans and other mammals, including phenylethanolamine *N*-methyltransferase (PNMT), which catalyzes the N-methylation of the neurotransmitter norepinephrine to form epinephrine; histamine *N*-methyltransferase (HNMT), which specifically methylates the imidazole ring of histamine and closely related compounds (Fig. 6-56); and nicotinamide *N*-methyltransferase (NNMT), which methylates compounds containing a pyridine ring, such as nicotinamide, or an indole ring, such as tryptophan and serotonin (Weinshilboum, 1989, 1992b; Weinshilboum *et al.*, 1999). PNMT is a cytosolic enzyme expressed at high levels in adrenal medullary chromafin cells, and in neurons of the medulla oblongata, hypothalamus, as well as in sensory nuclei of the vagus nerve and the retina,

and is not thought to play a significant role in the biotransformation of xenobiotics (Ji *et al.*, 2005).

Histamine *N*-methyltransferase is a cytosolic enzyme (Mr 33,000) which is highly expressed in kidney, liver, colon, prostate, ovary, and spinal cord cells (Horton *et al.*, 2005). Its activity (which can be measured in erythrocytes) varies sixfold among individuals due to a genetic polymorphism (C → T) that results in a point mutation, namely Thr[115]Ile. The latter allele (Ile[115]) is quite common in Caucasians and Han Chinese (10% frequency) and encodes a variant of HNMT with decreased catalytic activity and thermal stability. HNMT may influence efficacy of some drugs by a mechanism that is not yet fully understood. For instance, individuals who are heterozygous for the Ile[115] allele have been found to exhibit significantly decreased methylprednisolone-induced cortisol suppression relative to (Thr[115])-homozygous individuals (Hon *et al.*, 2006). Several other polymorphisms in the noncoding region of the HNMT gene have also been identified. HNMT can be inhibited by several antihistamines, quinacrine, amodiaquine, metoprine, and tacrine (Horton *et al.*, 2005).

NNMT is a monomeric, cytosolic enzyme (Mr ~30,000) that appears to be a member of a family of methyltransferases that includes PNMT and TEMT (the thioether *S*-methyltransferase present in mouse lung). NNMT catalyzes the N-methylation of nicotinamide and structurally related pyridine compounds (including pyridine itself) to form positively charged pyridinium ions. Nicotinic acid (niacin), a commonly used lipid-lowering agent, is converted to nicotinamide in vivo, which is then methylated by NNMT (or it is incorporated into nicotinamide adenine dinucleotide, NAD). In contrast to many other methyltransferases, NNMT is not expressed in erythrocytes.

Nicotinamide N-methyltransferase activity in human liver, like HNMT activity in erythrocytes, varies considerably from one individual to the next, and has a trimodal distribution dependent on variations in mRNA and protein levels, and up to 25% of the general population have high NNMT levels (Souto *et al.*, 2005; Williams *et al.*, 2005). It is not known to what extent genetic polymorphisms account for this variation. However, 10 SNPs in the untranslated regions of the gene have been detected in a Spanish population (Souto *et al.*, 2005). A genome-wide scan for genes associated with plasma homocysteine levels determined that there was a statistically significant association with the NNMT gene, and, moreover that one SNP (dbSNP ID#: rs694539), has a greater statistically significant association with homocysteine levels ($p = 0.017$) (Souto *et al.*, 2005). Homocysteine plasma levels are an independent intermediate risk marker for osteoporotic fractures, congestive heart failure, venous thrombosis, myocardial infarction, stroke, and Alzheimer's disease (Souto *et al.*, 2005). In humans, the only source of homocysteine is from the demethylation of methionine in a multistep pathway that involves SAM-dependent methyltransferases to form S-adenosylhomocysteine, the immediate precursor to homocysteine. Taken together, these data suggest that high methyltransferase activity could contribute to hyperhomocysteinemia. Of the many SAM-dependent methyltransferase genes examined for an association with homocysteine levels, only NNMT (which is highly expressed in the liver) was found to show a significant association (Souto *et al.*, 2005). NNMT is reported to be expressed in the brain and has been implicated as a component of the etiology of idiopathic Parkinson disease because it can convert 4-phenylpyridine to MPP$^+$, which is known to cause Parkinson's disease symptoms due to its toxic effect on neuronal mitochondria (see section "Monoamine Oxidase, Diamine Oxidase, and Polyamine Oxidase" and Fig. 6-28) (Williams *et al.*, 2005).

There are numerous other human N-methyltransferases (as well as O-, S-, and C-methyltransferases) that appear to play relatively specific roles in the methylation of endogenous compounds, and most have not been well-characterized with regard to their capability to methylate xenobiotics (there are at least 39 SAM-dependent methyltransferases in humans [Souto *et al.*, 2005]). For instance, indolethylamine N-methyltransferase (INMT) catalyzes the N-methylation of tryptamine and structurally related compounds (Thompson *et al.*, 1999). Other such enzymes that were initially thought to play a role only in the N-methylation of endogenous compounds were later found to play a role, albeit a minor one, in the N-methylation of one or more xenobiotics. Amine N-methyltransferase (AMNT, also called arylamine N-methyltransferase or nicotine N-methyltransferase), which is highly expressed in human thyroid and is also found in adrenal gland and lung, exhibits some activity toward tryptamine and has been also found to preferentially methylate the pyridine nitrogen of R-nicotine, which gives rise to nicotine isomethonium ions (Hukkanen *et al.*, 2005). Glycine N-methyltransferase (GNMT) is thought to play an important role in the regulation of methyl group metabolism in the liver and pancreas through regulation of the ratio between S-adenosyl-L-methionine and S-adenosyl-L-homocysteine. Rat data show that the tetrameric form of the GNMT has catalytic activity,

and the dimeric form binds polycyclic aromatic hydrocarbons. There is also evidence that the dimeric form of human GNMT sequesters benzo[*a*]pyrene, and thereby decreases its cytotoxic effects (Chen *et al.*, 2004b; Lee *et al.*, 2006).

The system that is used to classify human N-methyltransferases may not be appropriate for other species. In guinea pigs, for example, nicotine and histamine are both methylated by a common N-methyltransferase. Guinea pigs have an unusually high capacity to methylate histamine and xenobiotics. The major route of nicotine biotransformation in the guinea pig is methylation, although R-nicotine is preferentially methylated over its S-enantiomer (Cundy *et al.*, 1985). Guinea pigs also methylate the imidazole ring of cimetidine.

S-Methylation is an important pathway in the biotransformation of sulfhydryl-containing xenobiotics, such as the antihypertensive drug captopril, the antirheumatic agent D-penicillamine, the antineoplastic and immunosuppressive drugs 6-mercaptopurine, 6-thioguanine, and azathioprine, metabolites of the alcohol deterrent disulfiram, and the deacetylated metabolite of the antidiuretic, spironolactone. In humans, S-methylation is catalyzed by at least two enzymes, thiopurine methyltransferase (TPMT) and thiol methyltransferase (TMT, which may be the same enzyme as POMT).

TPMT is a cytoplasmic enzyme that preferentially methylates aromatic and heterocyclic compounds such as the thiopurine drugs 6-mercaptopurine, 6-thioguanine, and azathioprine. TMT is a microsomal enzyme that preferentially methylates aliphatic sulfhydryl compounds such as captopril, D-penicillamine, and disulfiram derivatives. TMT has also been found to methylate the heterocyclic thiol-containing leaving groups of some cephalosporins (Wood *et al.*, 2002), the thiazolidinedione drug, MK-0767, a dual α/γ peroxisome proliferator-activated receptor (PPAR) agonist (Karanam *et al.*, 2004; Kochansky *et al.*, 2006), dithiothreitol (Weinshilboum, 2006), and some thiofuran flavoring agents (Lake *et al.*, 2003). Although a gene that encodes TMT has not yet been definitively identified, there is strong evidence to suggest that the membrane-bound POMT is the same enzyme as TMT, which means that TMT could also catalyze the O-methylation of phenols (Weinshilboum, 2006).

Both TMT and TPMT are present in erythrocytes at levels that reflect the expression of TPMT and TMT in liver and other tissues. Although TPMT and TMT are independently regulated, their expression in erythrocytes is largely determined by genetic factors. TPMT is encoded by a single gene with alleles for a low activity form (TPMT^L) and for a high activity form (TPMT^H). The allele frequency of TPMT^L and TPMT^H are 0.06 and 0.94, respectively, which produces a tri-modal distribution of TPMT activity with low, intermediate, and high activity expressed in 0.3, 11.1, and 88.6% of Caucasians, respectively. At least 21 separate genetic polymorphisms are associated with low TPMT activity, with the *2, *3A, and *3C alleles accounting for greater than 95% of the TPMT^L phenotype (Weinshilboum, 2006). In Caucasians, the allele that is most commonly associated with the TPMT^L phenotype is TPMT*3A (5%), which contains two nonsynonymous single-nucleotide polymorphisms: Ala$_{154}$Thr and Tyr$_{240}$Cys (Weinshilboum, 2006). These amino acid changes (and those in the TPMT*3B and *3C variants) lead to aggregation and rapid degradation of expressed TPMT by a ubiquitin/proteasome-dependent mechanism (Wang *et al.*, 2005a).

Cancer patients with low TPMT activity are at increased risk for thiopurine-induced myelotoxicity, in contrast to the potential need for higher-than-normal doses to achieve therapeutic levels of thiopurines in patients with high TPMT activity (Weinshilboum, 1989, 1992b). The thiopurine drugs metabolized by TPMT have a relatively narrow therapeutic index, and are used to treat life-threatening illnesses such as acute lymphoblastic leukemia or organ-transplant patients. The thiopurines are also oxidized by xanthine oxidase, but since there is extensive variation in TPMT activity and xanthine oxidase is not present in hematopoietic tissues, TPMT activity in these tissues is more important in the avoidance of life-threatening myelosuppression at standard doses (Weinshilboum, 2006). Phenotyping for the TPMT genetic polymorphism represents one of the first examples in which testing for a genetic variant has entered standard clinical practice (Weinshilboum *et al.*, 1999). The clinical relevance of TPMT polymorphisms is reflected by the inclusion of TPMT as a "valid biomarker" for pharmacogenomics, along with CYP2D6 polymorphisms, in the FDA's 2005 "Guidance for Pharmacogenomic Data Submission." TPMT can be inhibited by benzoic acid derivatives, which also complicates therapy with drugs that are metabolized by TPMT. Patients with inflammatory bowel disorders such as Crohn disease are often treated with thiopurine drugs, which are metabolized by TPMT, and with sulfasalazine or olsalazine, which are potent TPMT inhibitors. The combination of these drugs can lead to thiopurine-induced myelosuppression.

A genetic polymorphism for TMT also has been described, but its pharmacological and toxicological significance remain to be determined. The molecular basis for the polymorphism has not been determined, but studies have shown that 98% of the five-fold individual variation in erythrocyte TMT activity is due to inheritance, with an allele for high TMT activity having a frequency of 0.12. TMT is relatively specific for aliphatic sulfhydryl compounds such as 2-mercatoethanol, captopril, D-penicillamine, and *N*-acetylcysteine. TMT also rapidly methylates a dihydro-metabolite of ziprasidone that is formed by aldehyde oxidase as shown in Fig. 6-3 (Obach and Walsky, 2005). TMT is present at high levels in the colonic mucosa and is also expressed in liver microsomes and erythrocyte membranes. TMT is not inhibited by benzoic acid derivatives, but it is inhibited by the cytochrome P450 inhibitor proadifen (a.k.a. SKE-525A) (Weinshilboum *et al.*, 1999).

Some of the hydrogen sulfide produced by anaerobic bacteria in the intestinal tract is converted by *S*-methyltransferases to methane thiol and then to dimethylsulfide. Another source of substrates for *S*-methyltransferases is the thioethers of glutathione conjugates. Glutathione conjugates are hydrolyzed to cysteine conjugates, which can either be acetylated to form mercapturic acids or cleaved by cysteine-conjugate β-lyase (CCBL1). This β-lyase pathway converts the cysteine conjugate to pyruvate, ammonia, and a sulfhydryl-containing xenobiotic, which is a potential substrate for S-methylation.

Methylation can also lead to increased toxicity. A recently characterized methyltransferase, AS3MT (previously called Cyt19), methylates inorganic arsenic to form methylarsonic and dimethylarsonic acids, which are more cytotoxic and genotoxic than arsenate and arsenite (Wood *et al.*, 2006). As many as 27 polymorphisms have been identified in this gene, with two rare alleles that cause markedly decreased activity and immunoreactive protein levels, and one frequent allele (i.e., ~10% in both African Americans and Caucasians) that causes increased activity and immunoreactive protein levels (Wood *et al.*, 2006). Up to 1% of African Americans and Caucasians would be expected to be homozygous for the allele that encodes the high activity AS3MT, and this may potentially lead to increased arsenic toxicity in such individuals.

Acetylation

N-Acetylation is a major route of biotransformation for xenobiotics containing an aromatic amine ($R-NH_2$) or a hydrazine group ($R-NH-NH_2$), which are converted to aromatic amides ($R-NH-COCH_3$) and hydrazides ($R-NH-NH-COCH_3$), respectively (Evans, 1992). Xenobiotics containing primary aliphatic amines are rarely substrates for N-acetylation, a notable exception being cysteine conjugates, which are formed from glutathione conjugates and converted to mercapturic acids by N-acetylation in the kidney (see section "Glutathione Conjugation"). Like methylation, N-acetylation masks an amine with a nonionizable group, so that many *N*-acetylated metabolites are less water soluble than the parent compound. Nevertheless, N-acetylation of certain xenobiotics, such as isoniazid, facilitates their urinary excretion.

The N-acetylation of xenobiotics is catalyzed by *N*-acetyltransferases (NATs) and requires the cofactor acetyl-coenzyme A (acetyl-CoA), the structure of which is shown in Fig. 6-49. The reaction occurs in two sequential steps according to a *ping-pong Bi–Bi* mechanism (Hein, 1988). In the first step, the acetyl group from acetyl-CoA is transferred to a cysteine residue in the NAT active site with release of coenzyme A (E-SH + CoA-S-COCH$_3$ → E-S-COCH$_3$ + CoA-SH). In the second step, the acetyl group is transferred from the acylated enzyme to the amino group of the substrate with regeneration of the enzyme. For strongly basic amines, the rate of N-acetylation is determined by the first step (acetylation of the enzyme), whereas the rate of N-acetylation of weakly basic amines is determined by the second step (transfer of the acetyl group from the acylated enzyme to the acceptor amine). In certain cases (discussed below), *N*-acetyltransferases can catalyze the O-acetylation of xenobiotics.

N-Acetyltransferases are cytosolic enzymes found in liver and many other tissues of most mammalian species, with the notable exception of the dog and fox, which are unable to acetylate xenobiotics. In contrast to other xenobiotic-biotransforming enzymes, the number of *N*-acetyltransferases known to play a role in xenobiotic metabolism is limited (Vatsis *et al.*, 1995; Boukouvala and Fakis, 2005). NAT activities are distinguishable from other *N*-acetyltransferases such as those involved in melatonin synthesis and serotonin metabolism (arylalkylamine *N*-acetyltransferases) but are indistinguishable from the group of bacterial enzymes termed *N*-hydroxyarylamine *O*-acetyltransferases (Boukouvala and Fakis, 2005). Rabbits and hamsters express only two *N*-acetyltransferases, known as NAT1 and NAT2, whereas mice and rats express three enzymes, namely, NAT1, NAT2, and NAT3. The Human Genome Organisation (HUGO) Gene Nomenclature Committee (http://www.gene.ucl.ac.uk/nomenclature) has designated NAT as the official symbol for arylamine *N*-acetyltransferases. The two well-known and characterized xenobiotic-acetylating human enzymes are NAT1 and NAT2, which are encoded by two highly polymorphic genes located on chromosome 8. Other HUGO-approved human NAT gene symbols include NAT5–6 and NAT8–14, located on other chromosomes. The activities and expression pattern of these enzymes have not yet been definitively characterized, although some of these genes have been associated with atopic dermatitis or psoriasis (NAT9) and nasopharyngeal cancer (NAT6) (Helms *et al.*, 2003; Bowcock and Cookson, 2004; Duh *et al.*, 2004; Yamada and Ymamoto, 2005; Morar *et al.*, 2006). Individual NATs and their allelic variants were named in the order of their description in the literature, which makes for a somewhat confusing nomenclature system (Vatsis *et al.*, 1995). For example, in humans, the "wild-type" NAT1 and NAT2 alleles are designated NAT1*4 and NAT2*4, respectively, because they are the most common alleles in some but not all ethnic groups (Hein, 2006).For NAT enzymes, the term "wild-type" may be somewhat arbitrary because it depends on the particular ethnic group that is studied. The official website for maintaining and updating NAT allele nomenclature is http://www.louisville.edu/medschool/pharmacology/NAT.html. The frequency of some SNPs and alleles in various ethnic groups is available online from the National Cancer Institute's SNP500Cancer database (http://snp500cancer.nci.nih.gov).

In each species examined, NAT1 and NAT2 are closely related proteins (79–95% identical in amino acid sequence) with an active site cysteine residue (Cys_{68}) in the N-terminal region (Grant et al., 1992; Vatsis et al., 1995). Human NAT1 and NAT2 genes are composed of intronless open reading frames of 870 bp on the same chromosome with a NAT pseudogene (NATP1) between them, and encode proteins of 290 amino acids that share 87% homology in the coding region (Boukouvala and Fakis, 2005; Hein, 2006). In spite of this apparently simple structure, NAT genes are fairly complex. For instance, comparisons of genomic and cDNA clones of the human NAT2 gene performed in the early 1990s revealed that the 5′ untranslated region is contained in a "noncoding exon," 8 kb upstream of the coding region (Boukouvala and Fakis, 2005). A similar type of unusual structure was later revealed for NAT2 genes in rabbit, hamster, mouse, and rat. More recent sequence alignments of expressed sequence tags with genomic sequences reveal that the presence of one or more upstream "noncoding exons" is typical for all vertebrate NAT genes, with the contiguous coding region contained in a single exon in the 3′ untranslated region (Boukouvala and Fakis, 2005). Furthermore, the splice site nearest the coding region appears to be universally conserved at position-6, relative to the first codon. The primary transcript of both NAT1 and 2 genes are also subject to alternative intron splicing in human, rat, and possibly chicken, whereas alternative splicing for NAT2 has been observed in rabbit and hamster. Alternative splicing in the case of NATs generates mRNAs with variable 5′ untranslated regions. The presence of "noncoding exons" lying upstream of higher eukaryotic genes (especially intronless genes) is common, and their transcription is likely required for transport of the entire transcript to the cytoplasm (Boukouvala and Fakis, 2005). The differential transcription of upstream noncoding exons has been frequently associated with cell-specific regulation of transcription and translation, and recent studies show that certain noncoding NAT exons are present to different extents in different tissues (Boukouvala and Fakis, 2005). There is also evidence of differential utilization of multiple tandem poly-adenosine repeats in the 3′ untranslated regions in different species, but the precise effect of polyadenylation of NATs remains unknown (Boukouvala and Fakis, 2005).

Despite their coexistence on the same chromosome, NAT1 and NAT2 are independently regulated proteins. For instance, human NAT1 protein and/or mRNA has been detected in every tissue examined (e.g., liver, gastrointestinal tract, leukocytes, erythrocytes, bladder, uroepithelial cells, mammary, lung, placenta, kidney, pineal gland, skeletal muscle, heart, brain, and pancreas) and are present from the blastocyst stage, whereas NAT2 is thought to be mainly expressed in liver and intestine. However, most (but not all) of the tissues that express NAT1 also appear to express low levels of NAT2, at least at the level of mRNA (Debiec-Rychter et al., 1999). Hein has also challenged the hypothesis that NAT2 is expressed mainly in the liver and intestine, and noted that the O-acetylation of N-hydroxy-4-aminobiphenyl in human urinary bladder cytosol did not correlate with NAT1 activity (4-aminobenzoic acid N-acetylation) consistent with acetylation by both enzymes (Hein, 2006). Regulation of human NAT1 is complex, and involves a promoter region composed of an AP1-box flanked by two TCATT boxes (Boukouvala and Fakis, 2005). The 3′ TCATT box is required for expression whereas the 5′-box attenuates promoter activity. Transcription factors such as c-Fos/Fra, c-Jun, and YY1 bind to the NAT1 promoter (Boukouvala and Fakis, 2005). In addition, because transcription of human NAT1 can begin with different upstream "noncoding exons," it is likely that there are additional promoters that regulate expression.

NAT1 and NAT2 also have different but overlapping substrate specificities, although no substrate is exclusively N-acetylated by one enzyme or the other. Substrates preferentially N-acetylated by human NAT1 include 4-aminobenzoic acid (PABA), 4-aminosalicylic acid, sulfamethoxazole, and sulfanilamide, whereas substrates preferentially N-acetylated by human NAT2 include isoniazid, hydralazine, procainamide, dapsone, aminoglutethimide, and sulfamethazine. Some investigators have used 4-aminobenzoic acid as a selective probe substrate for wild-type NAT1, and either sulfamethazine or sulfadiazine as selective probe substrates for wild-type NAT2 (Winter and Unadkat, 2005). Some xenobiotics, such as the carcinogenic aromatic amine, 2-aminofluorene, are N-acetylated equally well by NAT1 and NAT2. Other drugs that are substrates for either NAT1 or NAT2 include acebutolol, amantadine, amonafide, amrinone, benzocaine, declopramide, metamizole, and phenelzine (Gonzalez and Tukey, 2006; Sirot et al., 2006).

Several drugs are N-acetylated following their biotransformation by hydrolysis, reduction, or oxidation. For example, caffeine is N3-demethylated by CYP1A2 to paraxanthine (Fig. 6-44), which is then N-demethylated to 1-methylxanthine and N-acetylated to 5-acetylamino-6-formylamino-3-methyluracil (AFMU) by NAT2. Other drugs converted to metabolites that are N-acetylated by NAT2 include sulfasalazine, nitrazepam, and clonazepam. Examples of drugs that are N-acetylated by NAT1 and NAT2 are shown in Fig. 6-57. It should be noted, however, that there are species differences in the substrate specificity of N-acetyltransferases. For example, 4-aminobenzoic acid is preferentially N-acetylated by NAT1 in humans and rabbits but by NAT2 in mice and hamsters.

Genetic polymorphisms for N-acetylation have been documented in humans, hamsters, rabbits, and mice (Evans, 1992; Grant et al., 1992; Vatsis et al., 1995; Hirvonen, 1999; Hein et al., 2000). A series of clinical observations in the 1950s established the existence of slow and fast acetylators of the antitubercular drug isoniazid. In general, ~50% of patients treated with isoniazid have adverse events such as peripheral neuropathy and hepatotoxicity. Slow acetylators also exhibit a higher incidence of adverse events with clonazepam, hydralazine, procainamide, and sulfonamides (Sirot et al., 2006). The incidence of the slow acetylator phenotype is high in Middle Eastern populations (e.g., ~92% in Egyptians), intermediate in Caucasian and African populations (e.g., ~50–59% in Caucasian Americans, Australians, and Europeans; ~41% in African Americans; ~50–60% in black Africans), and low in Asian populations (e.g., <20% in Chinese; ~8–10% in Japanese) (Sirot et al., 2006). Many studies have demonstrated the typical bimodal distribution of fast and slow acetylators with drugs such as isoniazid, but the use of other drugs such as caffeine or sulfamethazine exhibit slow, intermediate, and fast acetylators (Hein, 2006). Parkin and colleagues (1997) also demonstrated that isoniazid elimination is trimodal, and that phenotype and genotype were concordant.

The slow acetylator phenotype is caused by various mutations in the NAT2 gene that either decrease NAT2 activity or enzyme

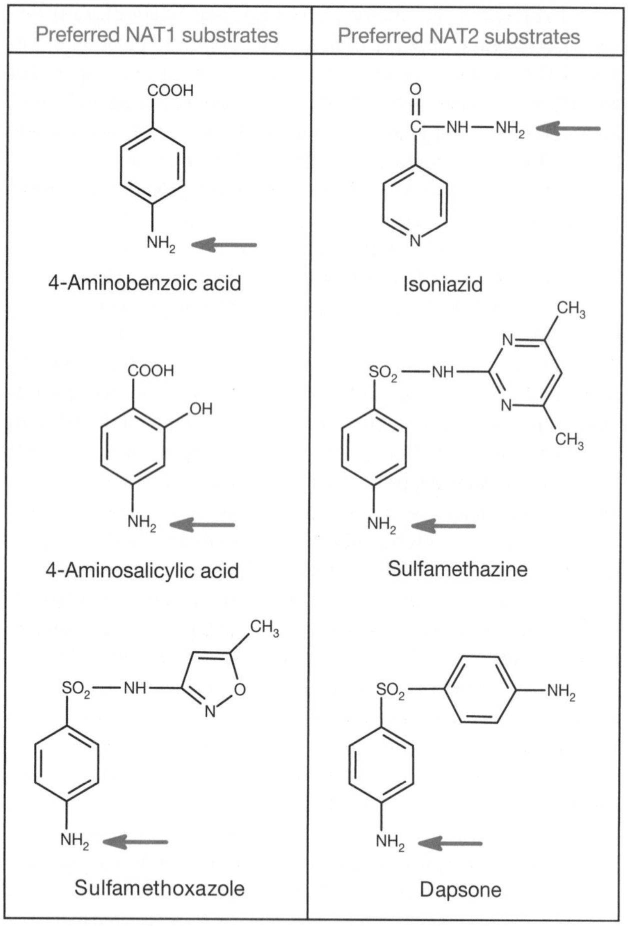

Figure 6-57. *Examples of substrates for the human N-acetyltransferases, NAT1, and the highly polymorphic NAT2.*

stability (at least 36 allelic variants of human NAT2 have been documented). For example, a point mutation $T^{341}C$ (which causes the amino acid substitution $Ile^{114}Thr$) decreases V_{max} for N-acetylation without altering the K_m for substrate binding or the stability of the enzyme. This mutation (which is the basis for the NAT2*5 allele) is the most common cause of the slow acetylator phenotype in Caucasians (e.g., frequency >50% in the U.K.) but is rarely observed in Koreans (i.e., <5%) (Hein, 2006). (Note: There are 10 known NAT2*5 alleles, designated NAT2*5A through NAT*5J.) The alleles containing only the $Ile^{114}Thr$ substitution are NAT2*5A (which also contains a silent $C^{481}T$ nucleotide change) and NAT2*5D. The others contain this and at least one other nucleotide and/or amino acid substitution, and NAT2*5B confers the "slowest acetylator" phenotype (Patin *et al.*, 2006). The NAT2*7 allele is more prevalent in Asians than Caucasians or Africans (Hein, 2006), and involves either a point mutation $G^{857}A$ (i.e., NAT2*7A) or both this change and $C^{282}T$ (i.e., NAT2*7B). Both of these changes cause the amino acid substitution $Gly^{286}Glu$, which decreases the stability, rather than the activity, of NAT2. NAT2*6 (more common in southern India) and NAT2*14 (present mainly in Africa and Spain) also result in one or more amino acid changes that lead to decreased NAT2 activity, whereas the amino acid change in NAT2*12 (present mainly in Africa and Spain) does not decrease activity (Hein, 2006). Within the slow NAT2 acetylator phenotype there is considerable variation in rates of xenobiotic N-acetylation. This is partly because different

mutations in the NAT2 gene have different effects on NAT2 activity and/or enzyme stability, heterozygotes retain moderate NAT2 activity, and because the N-acetylation of "NAT2-substrates" by NAT1 becomes significant in slow acetylators.

The slowest acetylator haplotype (NAT2*5B, which has the strongest association with bladder cancer) appears to have been positively selected for in only the last 6500 years in western and central Eurasians, which suggests that slow acetylation conferred an evolutionary advantage within this population, contrary to much of the recent epidemiological data (Patin *et al.*, 2006). Moreover, because most of the NAT2 polymorphisms that lead to slow acetylation are present at high frequencies in various populations, it would seem that varied rates of acetylation may be an important human adaptation to environmental variables. Because acetylation can be so important in the determination of the interaction between human populations and many xenobiotics in their particular environment (e.g., through different diets and lifestyles), it is not surprising that they are recent targets for natural selection.

NAT1 and NAT2 used to be referred to as *monomorphic* and *polymorphic* N-acetyltransferases because only the latter enzyme was thought to be genetically polymorphic. However, at least 26 allelic variants have now been documented for the human NAT1 gene, although these variants are less prevalent than the NAT2 allelic variants, hence, there is less genetically determined variation in the metabolism of "NAT1 substrates." Nevertheless, there is evidence that phenotypic differences in the N-acetylation of 4-aminosalicylic acid are distributed bimodally, consistent with the existence of low and high activity forms of NAT1. Furthermore, an extremely slow acetylator of 4-aminosalicylic acid has been identified with mutations in both NAT1 alleles; one that decreases NAT1 activity and stability and one that encodes a truncated and catalytically inactive form of the enzyme. It has also been demonstrated that NAT1*16 but not NAT1*10 or NAT1*11 cause a 50% decrease in NAT1 activity and NAT1 protein levels in COS-1 cell cytosol (Soucek *et al.*, 2004). The incidence and pharmacological/toxicological significance of genetic polymorphisms in NAT1 that produce phenotypically discernible alterations in NAT1 activity remain to be determined. Cascorbi and colleagues (2001) found that individuals who express NAT1*10 and NAT2*4 (i.e., low NAT1 activity and normal NAT2 activity) were at a significantly lower risk of bladder cancer, especially when exposed to environmental carcinogens. It is therefore likely that the interplay between NAT1 and NAT2 phenotypes is relevant to the susceptibility to certain carcinogens.

Genetic polymorphisms in NAT2 have a number of pharmacological and toxicological consequences for drugs that are N-acetylated by this enzyme. The pharmacological effects of the antihypertensive drug hydralazine are more pronounced in slow NAT2 acetylators. Slow NAT2 acetylators are predisposed to several drug toxicities, including nerve damage (peripheral neuropathy) from isoniazid and dapsone, systemic lupus erythematosus from hydralazine and procainamide, and the toxic effects of coadministration of the anticonvulsant phenytoin with isoniazid. Slow NAT2 acetylators that are deficient in glucose-6-phosphate dehydrogenase are particularly prone to hemolysis from certain sulfonamides. HIV-infected individuals of the slow acetylator phenotype suffer more often from adverse drug events and, among patients with Stevens–Johnson syndrome, the overwhelming majority are slow acetylators. Fast NAT2 acetylators are predisposed to the myelotoxic effects of amonafide because N-acetylation retards the clearance of this antineoplastic drug.

Some epidemiological studies suggest that rapid NAT2 acetylators are at increased risk for the development of isoniazid-induced liver toxicity, although several other studies contradict these findings and provide convincing evidence that slow NAT2 acetylation is a risk modifier for isoniazid-induced hepatotoxicity. Following its acetylation by NAT2, isoniazid can be hydrolyzed to isonicotinic acid and acetylhydrazine ($CH_3CO–NHNH_2$). This latter metabolite can be N-hydroxylated by FMO or CYP to a reactive intermediate, as shown in Fig. 6-37a. The generation of a reactive metabolite from acetylhydrazine would seem to provide a mechanistic basis for enhanced isoniazid hepatotoxicity in fast acetylators. However, acetylhydrazine can be further acetylated to diacetlyhydrazine ($CH_3CO–NHNH–COCH_3$), and this detoxication reaction is also catalyzed by NAT2. Therefore, acetylhydrazine is both produced and detoxified by NAT2, hence slow acetylation, not fast acetylation, becomes the risk modifier for isoniazid-induced hepatotoxicity, just as it is for isoniazid-induced peripheral neuropathy. Rifampin and alcohol have been reported to enhance the hepatotoxicity of isoniazid. These drug interactions are probably the result of increased N-hydroxylation of acetylhydrazine due to CYP induction rather than to an alteration in NAT2 activity. Isoniazid is an antitubercular drug, and its inactivation by NAT2 is interesting from the perspective that several organisms, including *M. tuberculosis*, express a NAT2-like enzyme, which has implications for isoniazid-resistance in tuberculosis.

Aromatic amines can be both activated and deactivated by N-acetyltransferases (Kato and Yamazoe, 1994; Hirvonen, 1999; Hein *et al.*, 2000). The N-acetyltransferases detoxify aromatic amines by converting them to the corresponding amides because aromatic amides are less likely than aromatic amines to be activated to DNA-reactive metabolites by CYP, PHS, and UGTs. However, NATs can activate aromatic amines if they are first N-hydroxylated by CYP because N-acetyltransferases can also function as O-acetyltransferases and convert N-hydroxyaromatic amines (hydroxylamines) to acetoxy esters. As shown in Fig. 6-11, the acetoxy esters of N-hydroxyaromatic amines, like the corresponding sulfonate esters (Fig. 6-55), can break down to form highly reactive nitrenium and carbonium ions that bind to DNA. N-Acetyltransferases catalyze the O-acetylation of N-hydroxyaromatic amines by two distinct mechanisms. The first reaction, which is exemplified by the conversion of N-hydroxyaminofluorene to N-acetoxyaminofluorene, requires acetyl-CoA and proceeds by the same mechanism previously described for N-acetylation. The second reaction is exemplified by the conversion of 2-acetylaminofluorene to N-acetoxyaminofluorene, which does not require acetyl-CoA but involves an intramolecular transfer of the N-acetyl group from nitrogen to oxygen. These reactions are shown in Fig. 6-58.

Genetic polymorphisms in NAT2 have been reported to influence susceptibility to aromatic amine-induced bladder and colon cancer (see section "Glucuronidation") (Evans, 1992; Kadlubar, 1994; Hirvonen, 1999; Hein *et al.*, 2000). Bladder cancer is thought to be caused by bicyclic aromatic amines (benzidine, 2-aminonaphthalene, and 4-aminobiphenyl), whereas colon cancer is thought to be caused by heterocyclic aromatic amines, such as the products of amino acid pyrolysis (e.g., 2-amino-6-methylimidazo[4,5-*b*]pyridine or PhIP, and others listed in Table 6-12). Epidemiological studies suggest that slow NAT2 acetylators are more likely than fast NAT2 acetylators to develop bladder cancer from cigarette smoking and from occupational exposure to bicyclic aromatic amines. The possibility that slow NAT2 acetylators are at increased risk for aromatic amine-induced cancer is supported by the finding that dogs, which are poor acetylators, are highly prone to aromatic amine-induced bladder cancer. By comparison, fast NAT2 acetylators appear to be at increased risk for colon cancer from heterocyclic aromatic amines.

looseness1The influence of acetylator phenotype on susceptibility to aromatic amine-induced cancer can be rationalized on the ability of N-acetyltransferases to activate and detoxify aromatic amines and by differences in the substrate specificity and tissues distribution of NAT1 and NAT2 (recall that NAT1 is expressed in virtually all tissues, whereas NAT2 is expressed mainly in the liver and intestinal tract). Both NAT1 and NAT2 catalyze the O-acetylation (activation) of N-hydroxy bicyclic aromatic amines, whereas the O-acetylation of N-hydroxy heterocyclic aromatic amines is preferentially catalyzed by NAT2. Bicyclic aromatic amines can also be N-acetylated (detoxified) by NAT1 and NAT2, but heterocyclic aromatic amines are poor substrates for both enzymes. Therefore, the fast acetylator phenotype protects against aromatic amine-induced bladder cancer because NAT2 (as well as NAT1) catalyzes the N-acetylation (detoxication) of bicyclic aromatic amines in the liver. In slow acetylators, a greater proportion of the bicyclic aromatic amines are activated through N-hydroxylation by CYP1A2. These N-hydroxylated aromatic amines can be activated by O-acetylation, which can be catalyzed in the bladder itself by NAT1. Recent evidence suggests that a high level of NAT1 in the bladder is a risk modifier for aromatic amine-induced bladder cancer. In addition, the fast acetylator phenotype potentiates the colon cancer-inducing effects of heterocyclic aromatic amines. These aromatic amines are poor substrates for NAT1 and NAT2, so that high levels of NAT2 in the liver do little to prevent their N-hydroxylation by CYP1A2. The N-hydroxylated metabolites of heterocyclic aromatic amines can be activated by O-acetylation, which can be catalyzed in the colon itself by NAT2. The presence of NAT2 (and NAT1) in the colons of fast acetylators probably explains why this phenotype is a risk modifier for the development of colon cancer.

Whether fast acetylators are protected from or predisposed to the cancer-causing effects of aromatic amines depends on the nature of the aromatic amine (bicyclic vs. heterocyclic) and on other important risk modifiers. For example, CYP1A2 plays an important role in the N-hydroxylation of both bicyclic and heterocyclic amines, and high CYP1A2 activity has been shown to be a risk modifier for aromatic amine-induced bladder and colon cancer. A single nucleotide polymorphism in intron 1 of CYP1A2 is associated with high inducibility, and this allelic variant is a risk modifier for bladder cancer in smokers or in people who are slow NAT2 acetylators (Brockmöller *et al.*, 1998). The activation of aromatic amines by N-glucuronidation and the activation of N-hydroxy aromatic amines by sulfonation are both suspected of playing an important role in the incidence of bladder and colon cancer. These and other risk modifiers may explain why some epidemiological studies, contrary to expectation, have shown that slow NAT2 acetylators are at increased risk for aromatic amine-induced bladder cancer, as was demonstrated for benzidine manufacturers in China (Hayes *et al.*, 1993).

The N-acetylation of aromatic amines (a detoxication reaction) and the O-acetylation of N-hydroxy aromatic amines (an activation reaction) can be reversed by a microsomal enzyme called arylacetamide deacetylase (gene symbol AADAC) (Probst *et al.*,

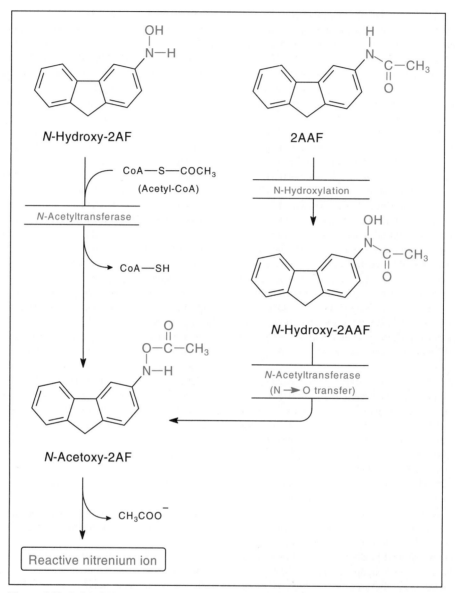

Figure 6-58. *Role of N-acetyltransferase in the O-acetylation of N-hydroxy-2-aminofluorene (N-hydroxy-2AF) and the intramolecular rearrangement of N-hydroxy-2-acetylaminofluorene (N-hydroxy-2-AAF).*

1994). This enzyme is similar to but distinct from the microsomal carboxylesterases that hydrolyze esters and amides. Arylacetamide deacetylase can potentially alter the overall balance between detoxication and activation of aromatic amines.

Overall, it would appear that low NAT2 activity increases the risk of bladder, breast, liver and lung cancers, and decreases the risk of colon cancer, whereas low NAT1 activity increases the risk of bladder and colon cancers and decreases the risk of lung cancer (Hirvonen, 1999). The individual risks associated with particular NAT1 and/or NAT2 acetylator genotypes are small, but they increase when considered in conjunction with other susceptibility genes and/or exposure to carcinogenic aromatic and heterocyclic amines. Because of the relatively high frequency of allelic variants of NAT1 and NAT2, the attributable risk of cancer in the population may be high (Hein *et al.*, 2000).

Amino Acid Conjugation

There are two principal pathways by which xenobiotics are conjugated with amino acids, as illustrated in Fig. 6-59. The first involves conjugation of xenobiotics containing a carboxylic acid group with the *amino group* of amino acids such as glycine, glutamine, and taurine (see Fig. 6-49). This pathway involves activation of the xenobiotic by conjugation with CoA, which produces an acyl-CoA thioether that reacts with the *amino group* of an amino acid to form an amide linkage. The second pathway involves conjugation of xenobiotics containing an aromatic hydroxylamine (*N*-hydroxy aromatic amine) with the *carboxylic acid group* of such amino acids as serine and proline. This pathway involves activation of an amino acid by aminoacyl-tRNA-synthetase, which reacts with an aromatic hydroxylamine to form a reactive *N*-ester (Kato and Yamazoe, 1994).

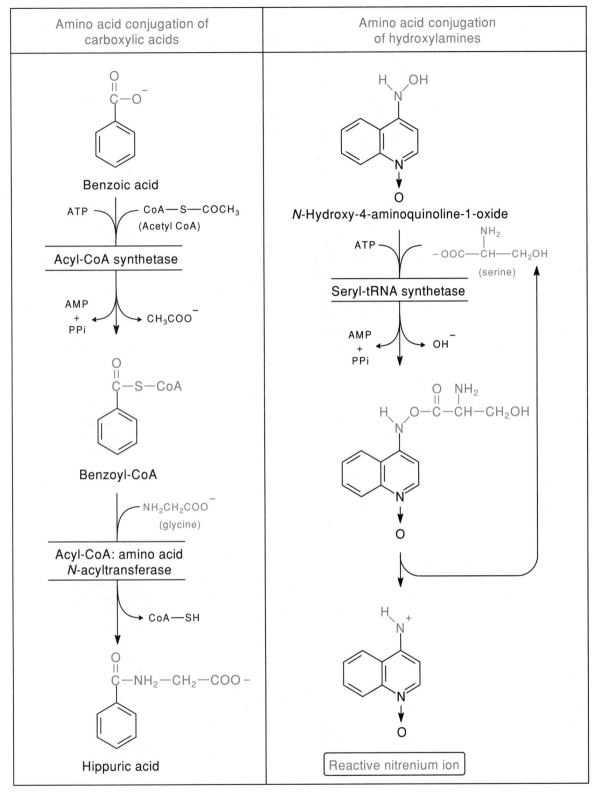

Figure 6-59. Conjugation of xenobiotics with amino acids.

The conjugation of benzoic acid with glycine to form hippuric acid (see Fig. 6-1) was discovered in 1842, making it the first biotransformation reaction discovered (Paulson *et al.*, 1986). The first step in this conjugation reaction involves activation of benzoic acid to an acyl-CoA thioester. This reaction requires ATP and is catalyzed by acyl-CoA synthetase (ATP-dependent acid:CoA ligase). The second step is catalyzed by acyl-CoA:amino acid *N*-acyltransferase, which transfers the acyl moiety of the xenobiotic to the amino group of the acceptor amino acid. The reaction proceeds by a *ping-pong Bi–Bi* mechanism, and involves transfer of the xenobiotic to a cysteine residue in the enzyme with release of coenzyme A, followed by transfer of the xenobiotic to the acceptor amino acid with regeneration of the enzyme. The second step in amino acid conjugation is analogous to amide formation during the acetylation of aromatic amines by *N*-acetyltransferase. Substrates for amino acid conjugation are restricted to certain aliphatic, aromatic, heteroaromatic, cinnamic, and arylacetic acids.

The ability of xenobiotics to undergo amino acid conjugation depends on steric hindrance around the carboxylic acid group, and by substituents on the aromatic ring or aliphatic side chain. In rats, ferrets, and monkeys, the major pathway of phenylacetic acid biotransformation is amino acid conjugation. However, due to steric hindrance, diphenylacetic acid cannot be conjugated with an amino acid, so the major pathway of diphenylacetic acid biotransformation in these three species is acylglucuronidation. Bile acids are endogenous substrates for glycine and taurine conjugation. However, the activation of bile acids to an acyl-CoA thioester is catalyzed by a microsomal enzyme, cholyl-CoA synthetase, and conjugation with glycine or taurine is catalyzed by bile acid-CoA:amino acid *N*-acyltransferase (BACAT, gene symbol BAAT) (Falany *et al.*, 1994). BACAT is expressed at high levels in the liver, kidney, gallbladder, and intestine, with lower levels in the adrenal gland, muscle, lung, and brain, which suggests that it may have substrates other than bile acids (O'Byrne *et al.*, 2003). In vitro studies show that BACAT can form glycine conjugates of long-chain fatty acids, and also possesses thioesterase activity toward the same substrates (O'Byrne *et al.*, 2003). In contrast to bile acids, the activation of xenobiotics occurs mainly in mitochondria, which appear to contain multiple acyl-CoA synthetases. The second step in the conjugation of xenobiotics with amino acids is catalyzed by cytosolic and/or mitochondrial forms of *N*-acyltransferase. Amino acid conjugation is apparently catalyzed by separate *N*-acyltransferases specific for each amino acid (Gopaul *et al.*, 2003). Glycine-*N*-acyltransferase and glutamine-*N*-phenylacetyltransferase have been isolated from human hepatic mitochondria (Gopaul *et al.*, 2003). Another important difference between the amino acid conjugates of xenobiotics and bile acids is their route of elimination: Bile acids are secreted into bile whereas amino acid conjugates of xenobiotics are eliminated primarily in urine. The addition of an endogenous amino acid to xenobiotics may facilitate this elimination by increasing their ability to interact with the tubular organic anion transport system in the kidney.

In addition to glycine, glutamine, and taurine, acceptor amino acids for xenobiotic conjugation include ornithine, arginine, histidine, serine, aspartic acid, and several dipeptides, such as glycylglycine, glycyltaurine, and glycylvaline. The acceptor amino acid used for conjugation is both species- and xenobiotic-dependent. For benzoic, heterocyclic, and cinnamic acids, the acceptor amino acid is glycine, except in birds and reptiles, which use ornithine. Arylacetic acids are also conjugated with glycine except in primates, which use glutamine. In mammals, taurine is generally an alternative acceptor to glycine. Taurine conjugation is well developed in nonmammalian species and carnivores. Whereas most species conjugate bile acids with both glycine and taurine, cats and dogs conjugated bile acids only with taurine.

Conjugation of carboxylic acid-containing xenobiotics is an alternative to glucuronidation. Conjugation with amino acids is a detoxication reaction, whereas the glucuronidation of carboxylic acid-containing xenobiotic produces potentially toxic acylglucuronides (see Fig. 6-54). Amino acid conjugation of ibuprofen and related *profens* (2-substituted propionic acid NSAIDs) is significant for two reasons: It limits the formation of potentially toxic acylglucuronides, and it leads to chiral inversion (the interconversion of *R*- and *S*-enantiomers) (Shirley *et al.*, 1994). This latter reaction requires conversion of the profen to its acyl-CoA thioester, which undergoes chiral inversion by 2-arylpropionyl-CoA epimerase (this involves the intermediacy of a symmetrical, conjugated enolate anion). Chiral inversion explains why the *R*- and *S*-enantiomers of several profen NSAIDs have comparable anti-inflammatory effects in vivo, even though the *S*-enantiomers are considerably more potent than their antipodes as inhibitors of cyclooxygenase (the target of NSAID therapy). In general, amino acid conjugation is a high affinity–low capacity reaction, whereas glucuronidation is a high capacity–low affinity reaction. At low substrate concentrations, amino acid conjugation would presumably be the more important reaction.

In contrast to amino acid conjugation of carboxylic acid-containing xenobiotics, which is a detoxication reaction, amino acid conjugation of *N*-hydroxy aromatic amines (hydroxylamines) is an activation reaction because it produces *N*-esters that can degrade to form electrophilic nitrenium and carbonium ions (Anders, 1985; Kato and Yamazoe, 1994). Conjugation of hydroxylamines with amino acids is catalyzed by cytosolic aminoacyl-tRNA synthetases and requires ATP (Fig. 6-59). Hydroxylamines activated by aminoacyl-tRNA synthetases include *N*-hydroxy-4-aminoquinoline 1-oxide, which is conjugated with serine, and *N*-hydroxy-Trp-P-2, which is conjugated with proline. (*N*-hydroxy-Trp-P-2 is the *N*-hydroxylated metabolite of Trp-P-2, a pyrolysis product of tryptophan [see Table 6-12]). It is now apparent that the hydroxylamines formed by the cytochrome P450-dependent N-hydroxylation of aromatic amines can potentially be activated by numerous reactions, including N-glucuronidation by UGTs (Fig. 6-54), O-acetylation by *N*-acetyltransferase (Fig. 6-11), O-sulfonation by sulfotransferase (Fig. 6-55), and conjugation with amino acids by seryl- or prolyl-tRNA synthetase (Fig. 6-59).

Various amino acid conjugates of valproic acid, including glutamine-, glutamate-, and glycine-conjugates, have been detected in the urine, serum, and cerebrospinal fluid of patients administered this antiepleptic (Gopaul *et al.*, 2003). CSF concentrations of the glutamine and glutamate conjugates of valproic acid were five and nine times higher than in serum, which suggests that these conjugation reactions in the brain decrease levels of the excitatory neurotransmitter glutamic acid and decrease the incidence of seizure (Gopaul *et al.*, 2003). Taken together, these data suggest that amino acid conjugation in the brain may play a role in the mechanism of action of valproic acid.

Glutathione Conjugation

The preceding section described the conjugation of xenobiotics with certain amino acids, including some simple dipeptides, such as glycyltaurine. This section describes the conjugation of xenobiotics with the tripeptide glutathione (GSH), which is composed of glycine, cysteine, and glutamic acid (the latter being linked to cysteine via the γ-carboxyl group, not the usual α-carboxyl group, as shown in Fig. 6-49). Glutathione transferase activity was first discovered as the enzyme-catalyzed conjugation of glutathione with halogenated compounds such as chloronitrobenzenes and bromosulfophthalein (Mannervik et al., 2005). The activity was initially designated GSH S-aryltransferase, and glutathione transferase activities toward other substrates such as alkyl halides and epoxides were called S-alkyl and S-epoxide transferases. The original names were later replaced with letter designations once the overlapping substrate specificity was described, especially toward 1-chloro-2,4-dinitrobenzene (Mannervik et al., 2005). Although the abbreviation "GST" has survived, the term "glutathione transferase" is technically incorrect because the glutathionyl group is transferred rather than a single sulfur atom (Mannervik et al., 2005) (the correct term is glutathione transferase). GSTs function endogenously as part of a defense mechanism against reactive oxygen species which reduces the formation of hydroperoxides of fatty acids, phospholipids, cholesterol, and against the redox-cycling of some quinone-containing compounds, by conjugation with glutathione (Hayes et al., 2005). GSTs also play a role in other endogenous functions such as the degradation of aromatic amino acids, steroid hormone synthesis, eicosanoid synthesis and inactivation, and modulation of signaling pathways (Hayes et al., 2005). Conjugation of xenobiotics with glutathione is fundamentally different from their conjugation with other amino acids and dipeptides (Mantle et al., 1987; Sies and Ketterer, 1988). Substrates for glutathione conjugation include an enormous array of electrophilic xenobiotics, or xenobiotics that can be biotransformed to electrophiles. In contrast to the amides formed by conjugation of xenobiotics to other amino acids, glutathione conjugates are thioethers, which form by nucleophilic attack of glutathione thiolate anion (GS$^-$) with an electrophilic carbon atom in the xenobiotic. Glutathione can also conjugate xenobiotics containing electrophilic heteroatoms (O, N, and S).

The synthesis of glutathione involves formation of the peptide bond between cysteine and glutamic acid, followed by peptide bond formation with glycine. The first reaction is catalyzed by γ-glutamylcysteine synthetase (γ-GCL); the second by glutathione synthetase. At each step, ATP is hydrolyzed to ADP and inorganic phosphate. The first reaction is inhibited by buthionine-S-sulfoximine, which can be used in vivo to decrease glutathione levels in experimental animals.

The conjugation of xenobiotics with glutathione is catalyzed by glutathione transferases (GSTs), found in cytosolic, microsomal (i.e., the MAPEG family), and mitochondrial cell fractions (Hayes et al., 2005). Most GSTs were originally found in the soluble cell fraction, and those GSTs that are found in the cytoplasm are referred to as cytosolic or soluble GSTs, even though they may also be found in the nucleus or peroxisomes (Mannervik et al., 2005). The only mitochondrial GST found to date has traditionally been referred to as Kappa GST, and although it dimerizes (as do the cytosolic GSTs), Kappa GST has a structure that is distinct from the cytosolic GSTs and is also present in peroxisomes, which suggests that it is involved in fatty acid β-oxidation (Hayes et al., 2005; Mannervik et al., 2005). The microsomal GSTs are an independent group of proteins termed "membrane-associated proteins in eicosanoid and glutathione metabolism" (MAPEG), and are integral microsomal and mitochondrial membrane components. It should also be noted that some GSTs have nonenzymatic functions such as binding of zeaxanthin in the retina and c-Jun N-terminal kinase1 by GST P1-1, and

were initially designated by other names (Mannervik et al., 2005). There are also other proteins that are homologous to some GSTs but are not yet known to serve as detoxication enzymes, such as the chloride intracellular channels (CLIC) (Mannervik et al., 2005). Hence, proteins that are already characterized and named may eventually be designated as GSTs, as was the case with glutathione-dependent prostaglandin D_2 synthase, now determined to be GST S1-1 due to similarities with the Sigma class GSTs expressed in nonmammalian organisms. The GSTs are present in most tissues, with high concentrations in the liver, intestine, kidney, testis, adrenal, and lung.

Substrates for glutathione transferase share three common features: they are hydrophobic, they contain an electrophilic atom, and they react nonenzymatically with glutathione at some measurable rate. The mechanism by which glutathione transferase increases the rate of glutathione conjugation involves deprotonation of GSH to GS$^-$ by an active site tyrosine or serine, which functions as a general base catalyst (Atkins et al., 1993; Dirr, 1994). In the case of the Omega class GSTs, the active site contains a cysteine residue (Mukherjee et al., 2006). The concentration of glutathione in liver is extremely high ($\sim$5–10 mM); hence, the nonenzymatic conjugation of certain xenobiotics with glutathione can be significant. However, some xenobiotics are conjugated with glutathione stereoselectively, indicating that the reaction is largely catalyzed by glutathione transferase. Like glutathione, the glutathione transferases are themselves abundant cellular components, accounting for up to 10% of the total cellular protein. These enzymes bind, store, and/or transport a number of compounds that are not substrates for glutathione conjugation. The cytoplasmic protein formerly known as ligandin, which binds heme, bilirubin, steroids, azo-dyes and polycyclic aromatic hydrocarbons, and thyroid hormones is an Alpha class GST.

As shown in Fig. 6-60, substrates for glutathione conjugation can be divided into two groups: those that are sufficiently electrophilic to be conjugated directly, and those that must first be biotransformed to an electrophilic metabolite prior to conjugation. The second group of substrates for glutathione conjugation includes reactive intermediates produced during conjugation and other biotransformations such as oxiranes (arene oxides and alkene epoxides), nitrenium ions, carbonium ions, and free radicals. The conjugation reactions themselves can be divided into two types: displacement reactions, in which glutathione displaces an electron-withdrawing group, and addition reactions, in which glutathione is added to an activated double bond or strained ring system. Table 6-18 provides examples of typical substrates for each of the characterized GSTs.

The displacement of an electron-withdrawing group by glutathione typically occurs when the substrate contains halide, sulfate, sulfonate, phosphate, or a nitro group (i.e., good leaving groups) attached to an allylic or benzylic carbon atom. Displacement of an electron-withdrawing group from aromatic xenobiotics is decreased by the presence of other substituents that donate electrons to the aromatic ring (–NH$_2$, –OH, –OR, and –R). Conversely, such displacement reactions are increased by the presence of other electron-withdrawing groups (–F, –Cl, –Br, –I, –NO$_2$, –CN, –CHO, and –COOR). This explains why 1,2-dichloro-4-nitrobenzene and 1-chloro-2,4-dinitrobenzene, each of which contains three electron-withdrawing groups, are commonly used as substrates for measuring glutathione transferase activity in vitro, and one or more members of all three GST families can catalyze this conjugation (Hayes et al., 2005). Glutathione transferase can catalyze the O-demethylation of dimethylvinphos and other methylated organophosphorus compounds. The reaction is analogous to the

Table 6-18
Human Glutathione Transferase Enzymes

GST FAMILY	CLASS	GENE	EXAMPLE ENZYMES	EXAMPLE SUBSTRATES
Cytosolic	Alpha	GSTA1	GST A1-1	Δ^5-ADD, BCDE, BPDE, busulfan, chlorambucil, DBADE, DBPDE, BPhDE, N-a-PhIP
		GSTA2	GST A2-2	CuOOH, DBPDE, 7-chloro-4-nitrobenz-2-oxa-1,3-diazole
		GSTA3	GST A3-3	Δ^5-ADD, Δ^5-pregnene-3,20-dione, DBPDE
		GSTA4	GST A4-4	COMC-6, EA, 4-hydroxynonenal, 4-hydroxydecenal
		GSTA5	GST A5-5	Unknown
	Mu	GSTM1	GST M1-1	$trans$-4-Phenyl-3-buten-2-one, BPDE, CDE, DBADE, $trans$-stilbene oxide, styrene-7,8-oxide
		GSTM2	GST M2-2	COMC-6, 1,2-dichloro-4-nitrobenzene, aminochrome, dopa O-quinone, PGH$_2$ $\rightarrow$ PGE$_2$
		GSTM3	GST M3-3	BCNU, PGH$_2$ $\rightarrow$ PGE$_2$
		GSTM4	GST M4-4	CDNB
		GSTM5	GST M5-5	CDNB
	Pi	GSTP1	GST P1-1	Acrolein, base propenals, BPDE, CDE, Chlorambucil, COMC-6, EA, Thio-TEPA
	Sigma	PGDS	GST S1-1[a]	PGH$_2$ $\rightarrow$ PGD$_2$
	Theta	GSTT1	GST T1-1	BCNU, butadiene epoxide, CH$_2$Cl$_2$, EPNP, ethylene oxide
		GSTT2	GST T2-2	CuOOH, menaphthyl sulfonate
	Zeta	GSTZ1	GST Z1-1	Dichloroacetate, fluoroacetate, 2-chloropropionate, maleylacetoacetate
	Omega	GSTO1	GST O1-1	Monomethylarsonic acid, dehydroascorbic acid
		GSTO2	GST O2-2	Monomethylarsonic acid, dehydroascorbic acid
Mitochondrial	Kappa	GSTK1	GST K1-1	CDNB, CuOOH, (S)-15-hydroperoxy-5,8,11,13-eicosatetraenoic acid
Microsomal (MAPEGs)	gp I	MGST2	MGST2	CDNB, LTA$_4$ $\rightarrow$ LTC$_4$, (S)-5-hydroperoxy-8,11,14-cis-6-$trans$-eicosatetraenoic acid
		ALOX5AP	FLAP	Arachidonic acid binding (nonenzymatic)
		LTC4S	LTC$_4$S	LTA$_4$ $\rightarrow$ LTC$_4$
	gp II	MGST3	MGST3	CDNB, LTA$_4$ $\rightarrow$ LTC$_4$, (S)-5-hydroperoxy-8,11,14-cis-6-$trans$-eicosatetraenoic acid
	gp IV	MGST1	MGST1	CDNB*, CuOOH, hexachlorobuta-1,3-diene
		PTGEs	PGES1	PGH$_2$ $\rightarrow$ PGE$_2$

[a] GST S1-1 is also the glutathione-dependent prostaglandin D$_2$ synthase.

Δ^5-ADD, Δ^5-androstene-3,17-dione; BCDE, benzo[g]chrysene diol epoxide; BCNU, 1,3-bis(2-chloroethyl)-1-nitrosourea; BPDE, benzo[a]pyrene diol epoxide; BPhDE, benzo[c]phenanthrene diol epoxide; CDE, chrysene-1,2-diol 3,4-epoxide; CDNB, 1-chloro-2,4-dinitrobenzene; COMC-6, crotonyloxymethyl-2-cyclohexenone; CuOOH, cumene hydroperoxide; DBADE, dibenz[a,h]anthracene diol epoxide; DBPDE, dibenzo[a,l]pyrene diol epoxide; EA, ethacrynic acid; EPNP, 1,2-epoxy-3-(p-nitrophenoxy)propane; N-a-PhIP, N-acetoxy-2-amino-1-methyl-6-phenylimidazo[4,5-b]pyridine.

Data adapted from Hayes JD, Flanagan JU, Jowsey IR: Glutathione transferases. *Annu Rev Pharmacol Toxicol* 45:51–88, 2005; Mannervik B, Board PG, Hayes JD, Listowsky I, Pearson WR: Nomenclature for mammalian soluble glutathione transferases. *Methods Enzymol* 401:1–8, 2005.

interaction between methyliodide and glutathione, which produces methylglutathione and iodide ion (GS$^-$ + CH$_3$I $\rightarrow$ GS-CH$_3$ + I$^-$). In this case, iodide is the leaving group. In the case of dimethylvinphos, the entire organophosphate molecule (minus the methyl group) functions as the leaving group.

The addition of glutathione to a carbon–carbon double bond is also facilitated by the presence of a nearby electron-withdrawing group; hence, substrates for this reaction typically contain a double bond attached to –CN, –CHO, –COOR, or –COR. The double bond in diethyl maleate is attached to two electron-withdrawing groups and readily undergoes a Michael addition reaction with glutathione, as shown in Fig. 6-60. Diethyl maleate reacts so well with glutathione that it is often used in vivo to decrease glutathione levels in experimental animals. The loop diuretic, ethacrynic acid, contains an α/β-unsaturated ketone that readily reacts with glutathione and other sulfhydryls by Michael addition. The conver-

sion of acetaminophen to a glutathione conjugate involves addition of glutathione to an activated double bond, which is formed during the CYP-dependent dehydrogenation of acetaminophen to N-acetylbenzoquinoneimine, as shown in Fig. 6-34.

Arene oxides and alkene epoxides, which are often formed by CYP-dependent oxidation of aromatic hydrocarbons and alkenes, are examples of strained ring systems that open during the addition of glutathione (Fig. 6-60). In many cases, conjugation of arene oxides with glutathione proceeds stereoselectively, as shown in Fig. 6-61 for the 1,2-oxides of naphthalene. The glutathione conjugates of arene oxides may undergo rearrangement reactions, which restore aromaticity and possibly lead to migration of the conjugate to the adjacent carbon atom (through formation of an episulfonium ion), as shown in Fig. 6-61. Conjugation of quinones and quinoneimines with glutathione also restores aromaticity, as shown in Fig. 6-34 for N-acetylbenzoquinoneimine, the reactive

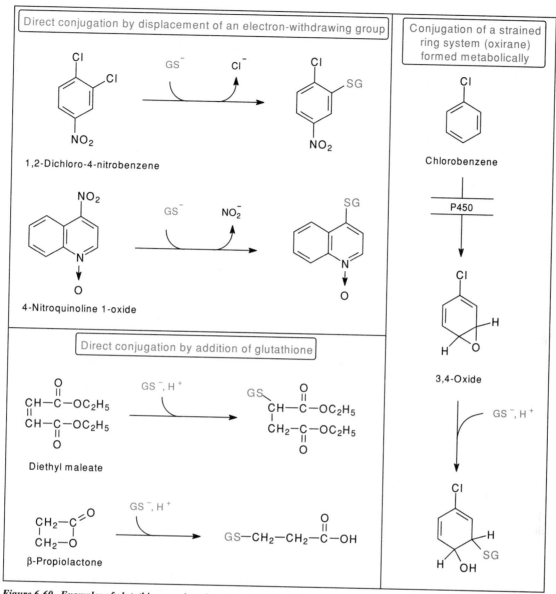

Figure 6-60. *Examples of glutathione conjugation of xenobiotics with an electrophilic carbon.*

GS⁻ represents the anionic form of glutathione.

metabolite of acetaminophen. Compared with glucuronidation and sulfonation, conjugation with glutathione is a minor pathway of acetaminophen biotransformation, even though the liver contains high levels of both glutathione and glutathione transferases. The relatively low rate of glutathione conjugation reflects the slow rate of formation of *N*-acetylbenzoquinoneimine, which is catalyzed by CYP (Fig. 6-34).

Glutathione can also conjugate xenobiotics with an electrophilic heteroatom (*O*, *N*, and *S*), as shown in Fig. 6-62. In each of the examples shown in Fig. 6-62, the initial conjugate formed between glutathione and the heteroatom is cleaved by a second molecule of glutathione to form oxidized glutathione (GSSG). The initial reactions shown in Fig. 6-62 are catalyzed by glutathione transferase, whereas the second reaction (which leads to GSSG formation) generally occurs nonenzymatically. Analogous reactions leading to the reduction and cleavage of disulfides have been described previously (see Fig. 6-13). Some of the reactions shown in

Fig. 6-62, such as the reduction of hydroperoxides to alcohols, can also be catalyzed by glutathione peroxidase, which is a selenium-dependent enzyme. For their role in the reduction of hydroperoxides, the glutathione transferases are sometimes called nonselenium-requiring glutathione peroxidases. For instance, one or more members of the mammalian cytosolic, microsomal, and mitochondrial GSTs exhibit glutathione peroxidase activity toward cumene hydroperoxide (Hayes *et al.*, 2005). The Omega class GSTs also play a role in the reduction of monomethyl arsenate from an oxidation state of +V to +III, which represents the rate-limiting step in arsenic biotransformation in humans as it occurs after methylation of inorganic arsenic (Mukherjee *et al.*, 2006). Cleavage of the nitrate esters of nitroglycerin releases nitrite, which can be converted to the potent vasodilator, nitric oxide. The ability of sulfhydryl-generating chemicals to partially prevent or reverse tolerance to nitroglycerin suggests that glutathione-dependent denitration may play a role in nitroglycerin-induced vasodilation.

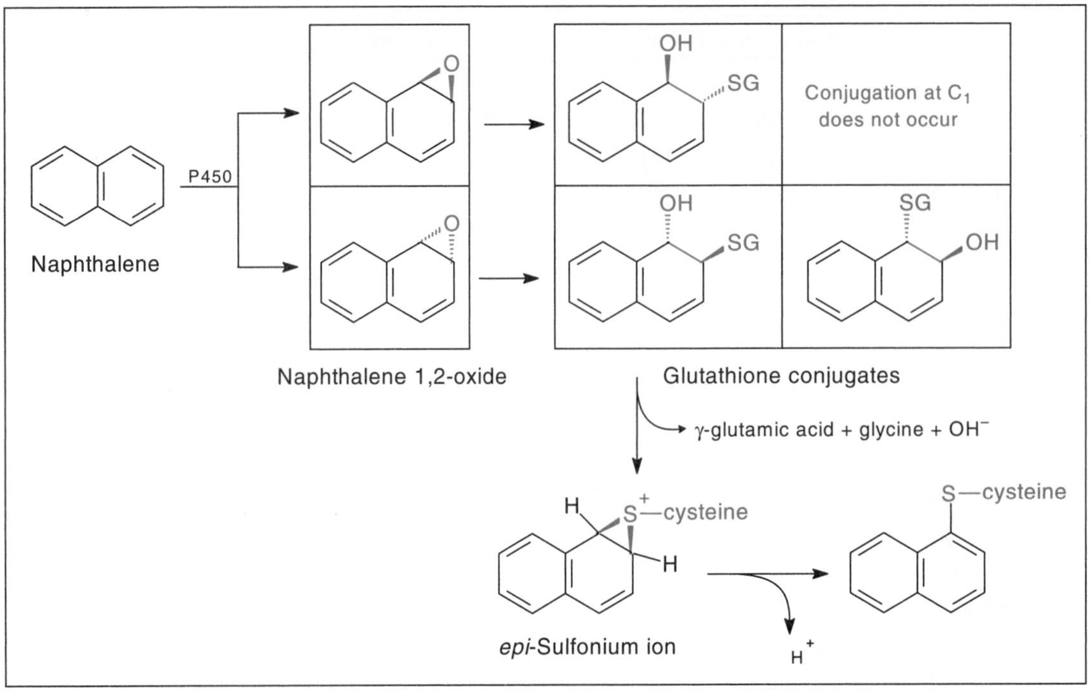

Figure 6-61. *Stereoselective conjugation of naphthalene 1,2-oxide and rearrangement of 2-naphthyl to 1-naphthyl conjugates.*

Cytosolic or mitochondrial glutathione transferases catalyze two important isomerization reactions, namely, the conversion of the endoperoxide, PGH_2, to the prostaglandins PGD_2 and PGE_2, and the conversion of Δ^5 steroids to Δ^4 steroids, such as the formation of androstenedione from androst-5-ene-3,17-dione. Another physiological function of glutathione transferase is the synthesis of leukotriene C_4, which is catalyzed by the microsomal GSTs, namely, MGST2, MGST3, and LTC_4S (see Table 6-18).

Glutathione conjugates formed in the liver can be effluxed into bile by MRP2, into the blood by MRP3 and 4, and they can be converted to mercapturic acids in the kidney and excreted in urine (Giacomini and Sugiyama, 2006). As shown in Fig. 6-63, the conversion of glutathione conjugates to mercapturic acids involves the sequential cleavage of glutamic acid and glycine from the glutathione moiety, followed by N-acetylation of the resulting cysteine conjugate. The first two steps in mercapturic acid synthesis are catalyzed by γ-glutamyltransferase (GGT1) and membrane alanyl aminopeptidase (ANPEP). The glutathione conjugate, leukotriene C_4, is similarly hydrolyzed by γ-glutamyltransferase to form leukotriene D_4, which is hydrolyzed by membrane alanyl aminopeptidase to form leukotriene E_4.

Cytosolic glutathione transferases are dimers, typically composed of identical subunits (Mr 23–29 kDa), although some forms are heterodimers. Each subunit contains 199–244 amino acids and one catalytic site. Mitochondrial GSTs are also dimeric with 226 amino acids per subunit. The microsomal GSTs vary in their ability to form complex aggregates across the three groups of human MAPEGs. Numerous subunits have been cloned and sequenced, which forms the basis of a nomenclature system for naming the glutathione transferases (Mannervik *et al.*, 1992, 2005; Hayes and Pulford, 1995; Whalen and Boyer, 1998; Hayes *et al.*, 2005), as shown in Table 6-18. Each cytosolic and mitochondrial enzyme is assigned a two-digit number to designate its subunit composition. For example, the homodimers of subunits 1 and 2 are designated

1-1 and 2-2, respectively, whereas the heterodimer is designated 1-2. The soluble glutathione transferases were initially arranged into four classes designated A, M, P, and T (which refer to Alpha, Mu, Pi, and Theta). More recently, four additional classes have been identified, namely, K (Kappa; the mitochondrial form), S (Sigma), Z (Zeta), and O (Omega) (Hayes and Pulford, 1995; Whalen and Boyer, 1998; Strange *et al.*, 2000; Hayes *et al.*, 2005). None of these eight gene classes corresponds to the microsomal glutathione transferases, which appear to have evolved independently. By definition, the subunits in the different classes share less than 50% amino acid sequence identity. Generally, the subunits within a class are ~70% identical, but can share up to 90% sequence identity, and can form heterodimers, whereas the subunits in different classes are generally only ~30% identical. Members of the Alpha and Mu classes can also form heterodimers with each other (Hayes *et al.*, 2005). Affinity labeling studies with rat Alpha GSTs demonstrated the presence of a high-affinity, nonsubstrate binding sites within the cleft between the two subunits of the dimer. Presumably, the cleft in heterodimers would be different from that in homodimers, which suggests the possibility that there is an evolutionary reason that the formation of heterodimers between Alpha and Mu subunits has been conserved (Hayes *et al.*, 2005).

The rat genome database (http://rgd.mcw.edu) indicates that rats express at least three GSTA genes, GSTA3, GSTA4, and Yc_2 (provisional). Humans express five subunits belonging to the Alpha class of glutathione transferases, designated GSTA1–GSTA5. Human GSTA1 and 2 are polymorphic, with at least two and five alleles identified, respectively, which affect the amount or the activity of expressed protein (Hayes *et al.*, 2005). Members of the alpha class of glutathione transferases have basic isoelectric points. They are the major glutathione transferases in liver and kidney.

A single Kappa subunit (the mitochondrial GST) is expressed in mouse, rat, and humans. The three-dimensional structure of

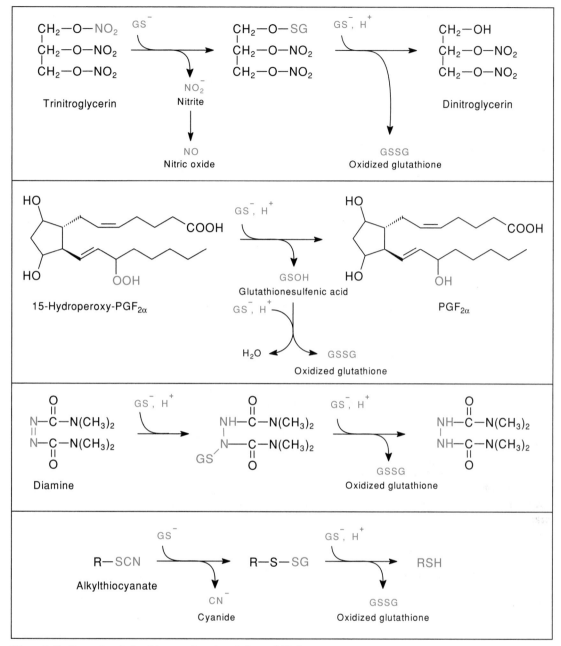

Figure 6-62. Examples of glutathione conjugation of electrophilic heteroatoms.

the Kappa subunit is more similar to bacterial GSH-dependent and disulfide-bond-forming oxidoreductase, than to the cytosolic GSTs (Hayes *et al.*, 2005). GSTK1 appears to be widely and uniformly expressed in humans, whereas in mice and rats it is present at high levels in the liver, kidney, stomach, and heart.

Rats express at least six functional Mu subunits, designated GSTM1–6. Humans express five subunits belonging to the Mu class of glutathione transferases, designated GSTM1. Human GSTM1, 3, and 4 are known to be polymorphic. In the case of GSTM1, the *A and *B allelic variants differ by a single amino acid; *A is a "basic variant" with lysine at residue 173, whereas *B is an "acidic variant" with asparagine at the corresponding site. There is also a GSTM1 deletion (*0) and a duplication (*1×2) (Hayes *et al.*, 2005).

The incidence of the GSTM1 deletion is high in Pacific Islander and Malaysian populations (i.e., 62–100%), intermediate in several other populations (i.e., 35–62% in those of European descent; 32–53% for those of Asian descent; 40–53% for those of Hispanic descent), and low in those of African descent (i.e., 23–41%) (Geisler and Olshan, 2001). GSTM1*0 appears to have only a modest effect on the incidence of lung, head, and neck cancers consistent with its high prevalence in various populations. The GSTM1*0 polymorphism has been linked to an increased susceptibility to certain inflammatory diseases (e.g., asthma) (Hayes *et al.*, 2005). At least two allelic variants of GSTM3 and 4 have also been identified. Members of the Mu class of glutathione transferases have neutral isoelectric points. Human GSTM2 and M3 are expressed in muscle and brain, respectively.

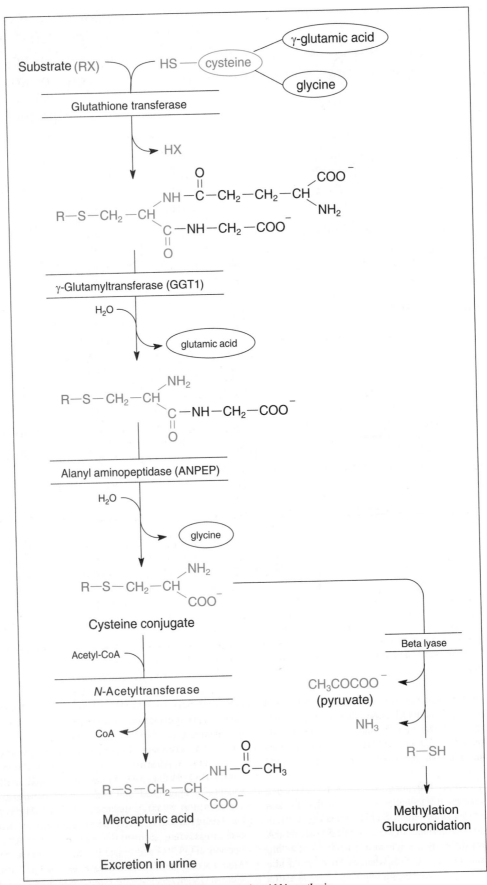

Figure 6-63. Glutathione conjugation and mercapturic acid biosynthesis.

Humans express one subunit belonging to the Pi class of glutathione transferases, GSTP1, and whereas rats are also known to express only one subunit (GSTP1), five other GSTP-like sequences have been mapped. The human Pi enzyme is polymorphic, with at least four allelic variants reported (Hayes *et al.*, 2005). The subunit encoded by GSTP1*B is seven times more active than that encoded by GSTP1*A in conjugating diol epoxides of polycyclic aromatic hydrocarbons (Strange *et al.*, 2000). GSTP polymorphisms are known to influence susceptibility to carcinogens (including some pesticides), affect the response to chemotherapy used in the treatment of metastatic colon cancer and multiple myeloma, and to modify the risk of acute myeloid leukemia which results from the successful treatment of Hodgkin's disease, non-Hodgkin's lymphoma, breast, and ovarian cancer (Hayes *et al.*, 2005; Liu *et al.*, 2006b). GSTP polymorphisms that result in decreased activity have also been implicated in an increased susceptibility to certain inflammatory diseases (e.g., asthma) (Hayes *et al.*, 2005). Members of the Pi class of glutathione transferases have acidic isoelectric points. They are expressed in the placenta, lung, gut, and other extrahepatic tissues. In rats, GSTP1 is one of several proteins (so-called preneoplastic antigens) that are overexpressed in chemical-induced tumors.

Rats also express a single GSTS-like protein (GSTS1) from the gene PTGDS2 (glutathione-dependent prostaglandin D_2 synthase) (Mannervik *et al.*, 2005). Humans appear to express one subunit that belongs to the Sigma class of glutathione transferases (GSTS1, also known as the glutathione-dependent prostaglandin D_2 synthase). At least two allelic variants of GSTS have been identified, but their functional significance remains to be elucidated (Hayes *et al.*, 2005).

Humans appear to express two subunits belonging to the Theta class of glutathione transferases (GSTT1 and GSTT2), and rats also appear to express two subunits, with a third GSTT-like sequence mapped. A GSTT1 deletion has been identified (GSTT1*0), which appears to have a modest effect on the incidence of lung, head, and neck cancers, and has also been implicated in an increased susceptibility to certain inflammatory diseases (e.g., asthma) (Hayes *et al.*, 2005).

A single Zeta subunit is expressed in mice and humans (GSTZ1), with a GSTZ-like sequence identified in rats. GSTZ1-1 has maleylacetoacetate isomerase activity and, as such, it catalyzes the penultimate step in tyrosine and phenylalanine catabolism (Hayes *et al.*, 2005). At least four GSTZ alleles have been identified, although their significance in humans is unknown. However, GSTZ1 knockout mice have increased levels of GSTA1, A2, M1, P1, P2, and NQO1 in the liver, and undergo rapid weight loss which results in death when provided 2% phenylalanine in drinking water (Hayes *et al.*, 2005).

Two Omega subunits have been identified in mice, rats, and humans (GSTO1 and 2). The GSTOs differ from the other cytosolic GSTs in that they do not display the typical activity toward substrates such as 1-chloro-2,4-dinitrobenzene, dichloromethane, or ethacrynic acid, but have some characteristics of glutaredoxins (GLRXs) (Mukherjee *et al.*, 2006). Additionally, whereas most GSTs have a tyrosine or serine at the active site, GSTOs have a cysteine and an additional 19 amino acids at the N-terminus (Mukherjee *et al.*, 2006). Many polymorphisms have been detected in both GSTO1 and 2, with five and four polymorphisms that result in amino acid changes, respectively (Mukherjee *et al.*, 2006). A wide variation in expression of these alleles was found, with potential implications for the toxicity of arsenic because of the role played by Omega GSTs, role in the metabolism of arsenic.

The microsomal glutathione transferases are distinct from the soluble enzymes. Six human microsomal glutathione transferases divided into three groups have been identified (see Table 6-18), which differ in their ability to form aggregates. For instance, MGST1 exists as a trimer, as does the other group IV MAPEG, namely, PTGEs, whereas the group I MAPEGs can function as monomers, dimers, trimers, or more complex aggregates (Hayes *et al.*, 2005). MGST1 conjugates xenobiotics with glutathione and probably functions solely as a detoxication enzyme, whereas MGST2 and 3 contribute to detoxication and synthesis of leukotriene C_4 (Hayes *et al.*, 2005). 5-Lipoxygenase-activating protein (FLAP) does not have catalytic activity, but binds arachidonic acid and is essential for leukotriene synthesis. LTC_4S and PGES1 do not appear to be involved in xenobiotic metabolism (Hayes *et al.*, 2005). Many SNPs have been identified in MGST1 and FLAP as well as diallelic variants in MGST3 in certain populations, but the biological significance has not yet been determined (Hayes *et al.*, 2005).

The conjugation of certain xenobiotics with glutathione is catalyzed by most classes of glutathione transferase. For example, members of the Alpha, Kappa, Mu, and Pi classes of human cytosolic GSTs, as well as several of the MAPEG GSTs all catalyze the conjugation of 1-chloro-2,4-dinitrobenzene. Other reactions are fairly specific for one class of enzymes (Hayes and Pulford, 1995). For example, the Alpha glutathione transferases preferentially isomerize Δ^5 steroids to Δ^4 steroids and reduce linoleate and cumene hydroperoxide to their corresponding alcohols. The Mu glutathione transferases preferentially conjugate certain arene oxides and alkene epoxides, such as styrene-7,8-epoxide. The Pi glutathione transferases preferentially conjugate ethacrynic acid. (For additional examples, see Table 6-18.) However, individual members within a class of glutathione transferases can differ markedly in their substrate specificity. In mice, for example, the Alpha glutathione transferases composed of Yc subunits can rapidly conjugate aflatoxin B_1 8,9-epoxide, whereas those composed of Ya subunits are virtually incapable of catalyzing this reaction (Eaton and Gallagher, 1994).

In rodents, individual members of the Alpha and Mu class of glutathione transferases are inducible (generally two- to threefold) by 3-methylcholanthrene, phenobarbital, corticosteroids, oltipraz, and various antioxidants (such as ethoxyquin and butylated hydroxyanisole). Several glutathione transferase substrates (i.e., Michael acceptors) are glutathione transferase inducers, as are certain nonsubstrates, such as hydrogen peroxide and other reactive oxygen species (Rushmore *et al.*, 1991; Daniel, 1993; Nguyen *et al.*, 1994; Hayes and Pulford, 1995; Hayes *et al.*, 2005). Induction is usually associated with increased levels of mRNA due to transcriptional activation of the gene encoding a subunit of glutathione transferase. Not all subunits are induced to the same extent.

The enhancer regions of the genes encoding some of the rodent glutathione transferases (such as rat GSTA2-2) have been shown to contain a xenobiotic (dioxin)-responsive element (XRE), a putative phenobarbital-responsive element, a glucocorticoid-responsive element (GRE), and an antioxidant responsive element (ARE, which is also known as the electrophile-responsive element [see Point 8]). Accordingly, in rodents, certain glutathione transferase subunits are regulated by both *monofunctional* and *bifunctional* agents, as described previously for DT-diaphorase (see sections "Quinone Reduction—NQO1 and NQO2" and "Induction of Cytochrome P450"). Induction of glutathione transferases by the monofunctional agent sulforaphane, which induces one or more GSTs in mice, is thought to be responsible, at least in part, for the anticancer effects of broccoli (Zhang *et al.*, 1992). GSTA4 is induced in mice administered α-angeliclactone, butylated hydroxyanisole, ethoxyquin, indole-3-carbinol, limettin, and oltipraz (Hayes *et al.*, 2005). In addition to inducing one or more GSTs, activation of Nrf-2 by oxidative stress or exposure to electrophiles induces. -GCL, which increases GSH levels in response to an initial decrease in GSH levels (see "Point 8").

Factors that regulate the expression of glutathione transferases in rodents may have similar effects in humans, but some differences have been noted. For example, the 5′ promoter region of Alpha glutathione transferase in humans (GSTA1) lacks the ARE and XRE consensus sequences through which the corresponding rat enzyme is induced. However, such sequences appear to be present in the promoter region of human GSTM4 and GSTP1 genes (Hayes and Pulford, 1995; Whalen and Boyer, 1998). (A functional ARE is also present in the promoter region of human DT-diaphorase [NQO1].) Therefore, certain subunits of glutathione transferases are inducible by a variety of mechanisms in rats, and other subunits appear to be inducible by similar mechanisms in humans. Species differences in glutathione transferase regulation may also stem from differences in xenobiotic biotransformation, especially differences in the formation of electrophiles, Michael acceptors, and/or the production of oxidative stress. For example, coumarin is thought be an inducer of GSTP1 in rats because it is converted in rat liver to reactive metabolites, namely, coumarin 3,4-epoxide and *ortho*-hydroxyphenylacetaldehyde (see Fig. 6-42). In contrast, the major route of coumarin biotransformation in humans is by 7-hydroxylation, which would not be expected to be associated with glutathione transferase induction.

Conjugation with glutathione represents an important detoxication reaction because electrophiles are potentially toxic species that can bind to critical nucleophiles, such as proteins and nucleic acids, and cause cellular damage and genetic mutations. All the enzymes involved in xenobiotic biotransformation have the potential to generate reactive intermediates, most of which are detoxified to some extent by conjugation with glutathione. Glutathione is also a cofactor for glutathione peroxidases (GPXs), which play an important role in protecting cells against lipid and hemoglobin peroxidation. Resistance to toxic compounds is often associated with an over-expression of glutathione transferase. Examples include the resistance of insects to DDT (see Fig. 6-20), of corn to atrazine, and of cancer cells to chemotherapeutic agents.

Glutathione transferase is the major determinant of certain species differences in chemical-induced toxicity. For example, low doses of aflatoxin B_1 cause liver toxicity and tumor formation in rats but not mice, even though rats and mice convert aflatoxin B_1 to the highly reactive 8,9-epoxide at similar rates (this reaction is shown in Fig. 6-33). This species difference arises because mice express high levels of an Alpha class glutathione transferase (Yc) enabling them to conjugate aflatoxin B_1 8,9-epoxide with glutathione up to 50 times faster than rats (or humans, which are also considered a susceptible species) (Eaton and Gallagher, 1994). Mice become sensitive to the adverse effects of aflatoxin B_1 following treatment with chemicals that decrease glutathione levels, such as diethyl maleate (which depletes glutathione) or buthionine-*S*-sulfoximine (which inhibits glutathione synthesis). Conversely, treatment of rats with inducers of certain GSTs, such as ethoxyquin, BHA, oltipraz, and phenobarbital, protects them from the hepatotoxic/tumorigenic action of aflatoxin B_1 (Hayes *et al.*, 1994).

The conjugation of aflatoxin B_1 8,9-epoxide with glutathione provides an interesting example of the stereospecificity with which certain glutathione conjugation reactions can occur. CYP converts aflatoxin B_1 to a mixture of *exo-* and *endo-*8,9-epoxides (only a generic 8,9-epoxide is shown in Fig. 6-33; meaning the figure does not indicate whether the oxygen atom is above or below the plane of the ring system). Both enantiomeric epoxides are formed by liver microsomes from mice, rats, and humans, but only the *exo*-epoxide binds extensively to DNA (where it binds to the N^7 position of guanine). One or more mouse Alpha GSTs rapidly conjugate the *exo*-epoxide, which accounts for the resistance of this species to aflatoxin-induced hepatotoxicity and tumorigenicity (as described above). Rat and human GSTAs do not rapidly conjugate either the *exo-* or the *endo*-epoxide (with the exception of the inducible rat glutathione transferase, which is not constitutively expressed in rats to any great extent). However, human GSTM1-1 can conjugate aflatoxin B_1 8,9-epoxide, but it preferentially conjugates the relatively innocuous *endo*-isomer (Wang *et al.*, 2000).

Species differences in the detoxication of aflatoxin B_1 8,9-epoxide suggest that individual differences in glutathione transferase may determine susceptibility to the toxic effects of certain chemicals. In support of this interpretation, a genetic polymorphism for GSTM1 has been identified, and individuals who are homozygous for the null allele (i.e., those with low glutathione transferase activity due to complete deletion of the GSTM1 gene) appear to be at a moderately increased risk for cigarette smoking-induced lung cancer, head and neck, and possibly bladder cancer (Hayes and Pulford, 1995; Whalen and Boyer, 1998; Strange *et al.*, 2000; Hayes *et al.*, 2005). Depending on the ethnic group, 22 to 100% of the population is homozygous for the GSTM1 null genotype, which results in a complete lack of GSTM1 activity in all tissues. On the other hand, there is evidence that GSTM1 confers significant protection from breast cancer in individuals homozygous for a functional GSTM1 allele (Hayes *et al.*, 2005). GSTT1 activity is absent from 11 to 58% of the population (depending on ethnicity) due to deletion of the GSTT1 gene, which appears to increase susceptibility to development of astrocytoma, meningioma, and myelodysplasia. When examined for their individual effect, these null genotypes generally have a small effect on susceptibility, with an odds ratio of 2 or less. However, the odds ratio can increase dramatically when these null glutathione transferase genotypes are examined in conjunction with other genotypes or with environmental factors (such as exposure to carcinogens). For example, when the GSTM1 null genotype is combined with cigarette smoking and a particular CYP1A1 allele, the odds ratio can increase to 8.9 (in one study) or 21.9 (in another study). Polymorphisms that result in amino substitutions have been reported for most human glutathione transferase genes; some of which alter glutathione transferase function. Some of these polymorphisms may also be risk modifiers for certain diseases in an analogous manner to the GSTM1 and GSTT1 null genotypes.

In some cases, conjugation with glutathione enhances the toxicity of a xenobiotic (Monks *et al.*, 1990; Dekant and Vamvakas, 1993). Five mechanisms of glutathione-dependent activation of xenobiotics have been identified, with the first four shown in Fig. 6-64. These mechanisms are (1) formation of glutathione conjugates of haloalkanes, organic thiocyanates, and nitrosoguanides that release a toxic metabolite; (2) formation of glutathione conjugates of vicinal dihaloalkanes that are inherently toxic because they can form electrophilic sulfur mustards; (3) formation of glutathione conjugates of halogenated alkenes that are degraded to toxic metabolites by β-lyase in the kidney, (4) formation of glutathione conjugates of quinones, quinoneimines, and isothiocyanates that are degraded to toxic metabolites by γ-glutamyltransferase and alanyl aminopeptidase (ANPEP) in the kidney, and (5) cyclical glutathione conjugation which leads to glutathione depletion.

The first mechanism is illustrated by dichloromethane, which is conjugated with glutathione to form the highly unstable S-chloromethyl-glutathione, which then breaks down to formaldehyde. Both formaldehyde and the glutathione conjugate are reactive metabolites, and either or both may be responsible for dichloromethane-induced tumorigenesis in sensitive species. The rate of conjugation of dichloromethane with glutathione is considerably faster in mice, which are susceptible to dichloromethane-induced tumorigenesis, than in rats or hamsters, which are resistant species.

The second mechanism accounts for the toxicity of dichloroethane and dibromoethane. These vicinal dihaloalkanes are converted to glutathione conjugates that can rearrange to form mutagenic and nephrotoxic episulfonium ions (sulfur half-mustards) (Fig. 6-64). Dichloroethane and dibromoethane can also be oxidized by CYP to chloroacetaldehyde and bromoacetaldehyde (by reactions analogous to those shown in Fig. 6-48). Either pathway can potentially account for the toxic and tumorigenic effects of these dihaloalkanes. However, the toxicity and DNA-binding of dihaloalkanes are increased by factors that decrease their oxidation by CYP and increase their conjugation with glutathione.

The third mechanism accounts for the nephrotoxicity of several halogenated alkenes. Several halogenated alkenes, such as hexachlorobutadiene, cause damage to the kidney tubules in rats, which leads to carcinoma of the proximal tubules. These nephrotoxic halogenated alkenes are conjugated with glutathione and transported to the kidney for processing to mercapturic acids. The cysteine conjugates, which form by removal of glutamic acid and glycine, are substrates for N-acetyltransferase, which completes the synthesis of mercapturic acids, and cysteine-conjugate β-lyase, which removes pyruvate and ammonia from the cysteine conjugate to produce thionylacyl halides, thiiranes, thiolactones, and thioketenes. The early damage to renal mitochondria caused by halogenated alkenes is probably because cysteine-conjugate β-lyase is a mitochondrial enzyme.

The fourth mechanism accounts for the nephrotoxicity of bromobenzene, which causes damage to the proximal tubules in rats. Bromobenzene is oxidized by CYP in the liver to bromohydroquinone, which is conjugated with glutathione and transported to the kidney (Fig. 6-64). The glutathione conjugate is converted to the cysteine derivative by γ-glutamyltransferase and membrane alanyl aminopeptidase. Substitution of bromohydroquinones with cysteine lowers their redox potential and thereby facilitates their oxidation to toxic quinones. The cysteine conjugates of bromohydroquinone are thought to undergo redox cycling and cause kidney damage through the generation of reactive oxygen species. 4-Aminophenol is thought to cause kidney damage by a similar mechanism, except a benzoquinoneimine is involved in conjugation with glutathione and subsequent damage to proximal tubules of the kidney. Treatment of rats with the glutathione depletor, buthionine-S-sulfoximine, protects them against the nephrotoxic effects of 4-aminophenol, which implicates glutathione conjugation in the activation of this compound.

The fifth mechanism occurs with moderately toxic allyl-, benzyl-, and phenethyl-isothiocyantes as well as sulforaphane formed from plant glucosinolates. These compounds are reversibly conjugated with glutathione to form thiocarbamates which spontaneously degrade to their isothiocyanates upon export from the cell, which releases glutathione. The isothiocyanate is then taken up by the cells again and the cycle can repeat until intracellular glutathione is depleted. Once glutathione levels are low, the compounds will tend to thiocarbamylate proteins, which can lead to cell death (Hayes *et al.*, 2005).

The ability of GSTs to form reactive metabolites has been exploited with the development of cancer therapies that specifically target cells that overexpress GSTP1-1, which is often associated with a poor prognosis and chemotherapeutic resistance in ovarian, nonsmall cell lung, breast, and colorectal cancers. For instance, Telcyta™ (TLK286: Confosfamide (not yet approved) is a modified glutathione analog that can be metabolized by GSTP1-1, which results in the release of two electrophilic fragments, glutathione vinyl sulfone, and a tetrakis (chloroethyl) phosphorodiamidate which leads to apoptosis (Townsend and Tew, 2003; Rosen *et al.*, 2004; Gonzalez and Tukey, 2006). Other drugs have also been recently developed to take advantage of activation by GSTP1-1, which is present in some tumor cells at 2–4 times the level found in normal cells.

Thiosulfate Sulfurtransferase (Rhodanese)

Cyanide forms naturally in leucocytes and neural cells, and also as a result of vitamin B12 metabolism, and is also encountered as a xenobiotic in plants containing cyanogenic glycosides, such as cassava, and tobacco smoke (Billaut-Laden *et al.*, 2006). Thiosulfate sulfurtransferase is a mitochondrial enzyme encoded by the TST gene that converts cyanide to the far less toxic metabolite, thiocyanate. The reaction involves transfer of sulfur from thiosulfate (or another sulfur donor) as follows:

$$\underset{\text{cyanide}}{CN^-} \; + \; \underset{\text{thiosulfate}}{S_2O_3{}^{2-}} \; \rightarrow \; \underset{\text{thiocyanate}}{SCN^-} \; + \; \underset{\text{sulfite}}{SO_3{}^{2-}}$$

The sulfite produced by this reaction can be converted to sulfate by the molybdozyme, sulfite oxidase. Cyanide can also be "detoxified" by binding to methemoglobin (the oxidized or ferric form of hemoglobin). 4-Dimethylaminophenol is used to induce methemoglobinemia as an antidote to cyanide poisoning because methemoglobin competes with cytochrome oxidase for the cyanide ion. However, 4-dimethylaminophenol is nephrotoxic to rats, presumably by a mechanism similar to that described above for the structural analog, 4-aminophenol (see preceding section and "Peroxidase-Dependent Cooxidation").

In humans, TST is expressed at high levels in the colon, where it plays a major role in the detoxification of hydrogen sulfide (which can reach concentrations of 3.4 mM) produced by anaerobic bacteria (Billaut-Laden *et al.*, 2006). TST is also widely distributed in the central nervous system. Six allelic variants of TST have been identified, namely, TST*1B–*1F and TST*2, with the latter showing significantly reduced intrinsic clearance for thiocyanate formation (Billaut-Laden *et al.*, 2006). TST polymorphisms that decrease cyanide and hydrogen sulfide detoxification may ultimately become important in understanding certain diseases, such as ulcerative colitis and amyotrophic lateral sclerosis (ALS). For instance, hydrogen sulfide release has been found to be 3–4 times higher in patients with ulcerative colitis when compared with normal subjects, and is positively correlated with disease severity (Billaut-Laden *et al.*, 2006). Finally, it has been postulated that individuals with ALS display a disorder in cyanide metabolism because of the higher blood and urine levels of cyanide

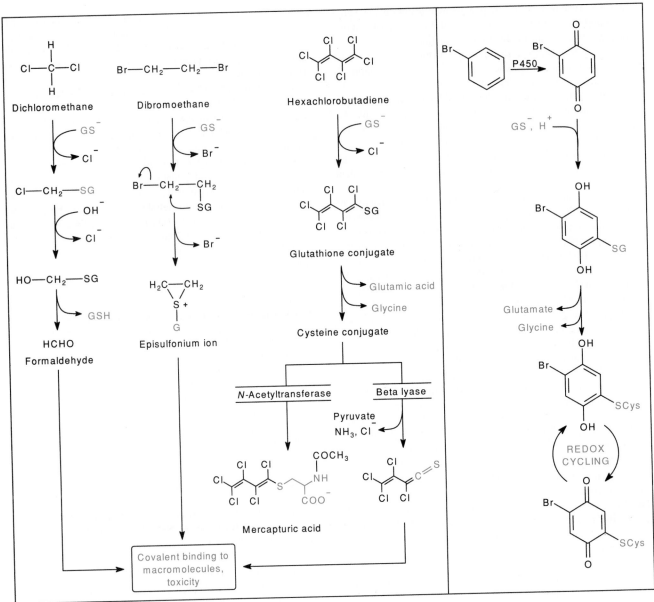

Figure 6-64. Role of glutathione conjugation in the activation of xenobiotics to toxic metabolites.

(Billaut-Laden *et al.*, 2006). Mimori and colleagues (1984) also reported significantly decreased TST activity in cervical and thoracic spinal cords of patients with ALS, compared with normal subjects.

Phosphorylation—The Dog That Did Not Bark

Some drugs are intentionally designed to be phosphorylated by intracellular enzymes. For example, the anti-HIV drug zidovudine (AZT) is converted to a triphosphate nucleoside by enzymes in the salvage pathway (nucleoside kinase, nucleoside monophosphate kinase or NMK, and nucleoside diphosphate kinase or NDK). However, phosphorylation of xenobiotics is the exception rather than the rule. All conjugation reactions ultimately require ATP, either to activate the xenobiotic for conjugation with glutathione or amino acids, or to synthesize high-energy cofactors such as UDPGA and

PAPS. The process is inefficient in that several ATP molecules (or their equivalent) are used to synthesize each cofactor molecule. The question arises: Why is ATP not used directly by conjugating enzymes? In other words, why are xenobiotics never phosphorylated directly (with the exception of drugs such as zidovudine), which would require less ATP and would achieve the goal of converting xenobiotics to water-soluble conjugates? It is difficult to be certain why this does not occur, but four reasons suggest themselves. First, if xenobiotics could be phosphorylated, high intracellular levels of a xenobiotic might consume so much ATP as to jeopardize cell viability, whereas UDPGA and PAPS can be depleted without killing cells. Second, phosphorylation of endogenous substrates, such as glucose, is a mechanism for trapping endogenous substrates inside a cell. This works because the plasma membrane of all cells is a barrier to the passage of polar compounds by virtue of its hydrophobic properties (lipid bilayer) and its general lack of transporters that pump phosphorylated compounds out of the cell. The same is true for the phosphorylated metabolites of zidovudine and related antiviral drugs; they are retained inside the cell that forms them. A lipid bilayer is also a physical barrier to other water-soluble conjugates, such as glucuronides and sulfonates, but these are transported out of the cell by various transporters. Third, phosphorylation of both small molecules (such as inositol) and proteins (such as membrane-bound receptors and various transcription factors) plays an important role in intracellular and intranuclear signaling. It is possible that some xenobiotics, if they

were phosphorylated, might interfere with these regulatory systems and thereby disrupt cellular homeostasis. Fourth, even if xenobiotics were phosphorylated in the liver and excreted in bile, they would be rapidly hydrolyzed by high levels of alkaline phosphatase lining the surface of enterocytes in the small intestine, which would promote reabsorption of the xenobiotic (by the very process exploited in the design of phosphorylated prodrugs like fosamprenavir). Whatever the reason, there appears to be strong evolutionary pressure against the conjugation of xenobiotics with phosphoric acid.

REFERENCES

Adamson RH, Bridges JW, Evans ME, Williams RT: Species differences in the aromatization of quinic acid in vivo and the role of gut bacteria. *Biochem J* 116:437–443, 1970.

Agarwal DP: Pharmacogenetics of alcohol dehydrogenase, in Kalow W (ed.): *Pharmacogenetics of Drug Metabolism*. New York: Pergamon, 1992, pp. 263–280.

Agostinelli E, Arancia G, Vedova LD, et al.: The biological functions of polyamine oxidation products by amine oxidases: Perspectives of clinical applications. *Amino Acids* 27:347–358, 2004.

Agundez JA, Gallardo L, Ledesma MC, et al.: Functionally active duplications of the CYP2D6 gene are more prevalent among larynx and lung cancer patients. *Oncology* 61:59–63, 2001.

Al-Zoughool M, Succop P, Desai: Effect of *N*-glucuronidation on urinary bladder genotoxicity of 4-aminobiphenyl in male and female mice. *Environ Toxicol Pharmacol* 22:153–159, 2006.

Aldridge WN: Serum esterases. I. Two types of esterase (A and B) hydrolysing *p*-nitrophenyl acetate, propionate and butyrate, and a method for their determination. *Biochem J* 53:110–117, 1953.

Amano T, Ochi N, Sato H, Sakaki S: Oxidation reaction by xanthine oxidase: theoretical study of reaction mechanism. *J Am Chem Soc* 129:8131–8138, 2007.

Anders MW (ed.): *Bioactivation of Foreign Compounds*. New York: Academic, 1985a.

Anders MW, Ratnayake JH, Hanna PE, Fuchs JA: Thioredoxin-dependent sulfoxide reduction by rat renal cytosol. *Drug Metab Dispos* 9:307–310, 1981.

Arima N: Acyl glucuronidation and glucosidation of pranoprofen, a 2-arylpropionic acid derivative, in mouse liver and kidney homogenates. *J Pharmacobiodyn* 13:724–732, 1990.

Arimitsu E, Aoki S, Ishikura S, et al.: Cloning and sequencing of the cDNA species for mammalian dimeric dihydrodiol dehydrogenases. *Biochem J* 342(3):721–728, 1999.

Armstrong RN: Kinetic and chemical mechanism of epoxide hydrolase. *Drug Metab Rev* 31:71–86, 1999.

Atkins WM, Wang RW, Bird AW, Newton DJ, Lu AY: The catalytic mechanism of glutathione *S*-transferase (GST): Spectroscopic determination of the p*K*a of Tyr-9 in rat alpha 1-1 GST. *J Biol Chem* 268:19188–19191, 1993.

Augustinsson KB: The nature of an "anionic" site in butyrylcholinesterase compared with that of a similar site in acetylcholinesterase. *Biochim Biophys Acta* 128:351–362, 1966.

Ayesh R, Smith RL: Genetic polymorphism of trimethylamine *N*-oxidation, in Kalow W (ed.): *Pharmacogenetics of Drug Metabolism*. New York: Pergamon, 1992, pp. 315–332.

Banhegyi G, Garzo T, Fulceri R, Benedetti A, Mandl J: Latency is the major determinant of UDP-glucuronosyltransferase activity in isolated hepatocytes. *FEBS Lett* 328:149–152, 1993.

Barditch-Crovo P, Trapnell CB, Ette E, et al.: The effects of rifampin and rifabutin on the pharmacokinetics and pharmacodynamics of a combination oral contraceptive. *Clin Pharmacol Ther* 65:428–438, 1999.

Battaglia E, Gollan J: A unique multifunctional transporter translocates estradiol-17 beta-glucuronide in rat liver microsomal vesicles. *J Biol Chem* 276:23492–23498, 2001.

Beconi MG, Mao A, Liu DQ, et al.: Metabolism and pharmacokinetics of a dipeptidyl peptidase IV inhibitor in rats, dogs, and monkeys with selective carbamoyl glucuronidation of the primary amine in dogs. *Drug Metab Dispos* 31:1269–1277, 2003.

Beedham C: Molybdenum hydroxylases, in Ioannides C (ed.): *Enzyme Systems that Metabolise Drugs and Other Xenobiotics*. New York: John Wiley & Sons, 2002, pp. 147–187.

Beedham CPM, Miceli JJP, Obach RSP: Ziprasidone metabolism, aldehyde oxidase, and clinical implications. *J Clin Psychopharmacol* 23:229–232, 2003.

Beetham J, Grant D, Arand M, et al.: Gene evolution of epoxide hydrolases and recommended nomenclature. *DNA Cell Biol* 14:61–71, 1995.

Bendotti C, Prosperini E, Kurosaki M, Garattini E, Terao M: Selective localization of mouse aldehyde oxidase mRNA in the choroid plexus and motor neurons. *Neuroreport* 8:2343–2349, 1997.

Benedetti M, Dostert P: Contribution of amine oxidases to the metabolism of xenobiotics. *Drug Metab Rev* 26:507–535, 1994.

Benedetti MS: Biotransformation of xenobiotics by amine oxidases. *Fundam Clin Pharmacol* 15:75–84, 2001.

Billaut-Laden I, Allorge D, Crunelle-Thibaut A, et al.: Evidence for a functional genetic polymorphism of the human thiosulfate sulfurtransferase (Rhodanese), a cyanide and H_2S detoxification enzyme. *Toxicology* 225:1–11, 2006.

Bjornsson TD, Callaghan JT, Einolf HJ, et al.: The conduct of in vitro and in vivo drug–drug interaction studies: A Pharmaceutical Research and Manufacturers of America (PhRMA) perspective. *Drug Metab Dispos* 31:815–832, 2003.

Blanchard RL, Freimuth RR, Buck J, Weinshilboum RM, Coughtrie MW: A proposed nomenclature system for the cytosolic sulfotransferase (SULT) superfamily. *Pharmacogenetics* 14:199–211, 2004.

Boberg E, Miller E, Miller J, Poland A, Liem A: Strong evidence from studies with brachymorphic mice and pentachlorophenol that 1′-sulfooxysafrole is the major ultimate electrophilic and carcinogenic metabolite of 1′-hydroxysafrole in mouse liver. *Cancer Res* 43:5163–5173, 1983.

Bock K, Schrenk D, Forster A, et al.: The influence of environmental and genetic factors on CYP2D6, CYP1A2 and UDP-glucuronosyltransferases in man using sparteine, caffeine, and paracetamol as probes. *Pharmacogenetics* 4:209–218, 1994.

Bolton J, Trush M, Penning TM, Dryhurst G, Monks T: Role of quinones in toxicology. *Chem Res Toxicol* 13:135–160, 2000.

Bolze S, Bromet N, Gay-Feutry C, Massiere F, Boulieu R, Hulot T: Development of an in vitro screening model for the biosynthesis of acyl glucuronide metabolites and the assessment of their reactivity toward human serum albumin. *Drug Metab Dispos* 30:404–413, 2002.

Bosgra S, Mennes W, Seinen W: Proceedings in uncovering the mechanism behind peroxisome proliferator-induced hepatocarcinogenesis. *Toxicology* 206:309–323, 2005.

Boukouvala S, Fakis G: Arylamine *N*-acetyltransferases: What we learn from genes and genomes. *Drug Metab Rev* 37:511–564, 2005.

Boulton DW, Fawcett JP: Pharmacokinetics and pharmacodynamics of single oral doses of albuterol and its enantiomers in humans. *Clin Pharmacol Ther* 62:138–144, 1997.

Bowcock AM, Cookson WO: The genetics of psoriasis, psoriatic arthritis and atopic dermatitis. *Hum Mol Genet* 13 Spec No 1:R43–55, 2004.

Boyd MA, Srasuebkul P, Ruxrungtham K, *et al.*: Relationship between hyperbilirubinaemia and UDP-glucuronosyltransferase 1A1 (UGT1A1) polymorphism in adult HIV-infected Thai patients treated with indinavir. *Pharmacogenet Genom* 16:321–329, 2006.

Bradley ME, Benner SA: Phylogenomic approaches to common problems encountered in the analysis of low copy repeats: The sulfotransferase 1A gene family example. *BMC Evol Biol* 5:22, 2005.

Bray RC, Bennett B, Burke JF, *et al.*: Recent studies on xanthine oxidase and related enzymes. *Biochem Soc Trans* 24:99–105, 1996.

Brennan P, Lewis S, Hashibe M, *et al.*: Pooled analysis of alcohol dehydrogenase genotypes and head and neck cancer: A HuGE review. *Am J Epidemiol* 159:1–16, 2004.

Brockmöller J, Cascorbi I, Kerb R, Sachse C, Roots I: Polymorphisms in xenobiotic conjugation and disease predisposition. *Toxicol Lett* 102–103:173–183, 1998.

Brunnberg S, Andersson P, Lindstam M, Paulson I, Poellinger L, Hanberg A: The constitutively active Ah receptor (CA-AhR) mouse as a potential model for dioxin exposure—Effects in vital organs. *Toxicology* 224:191–201, 2006.

Burchell B: Transformation reactions: Glucuronidation, in Woolf T (ed.): *Handbook of Drug Metabolism*. New York: Marcel Dekker, 1999, pp. 153–173.

Burczynski ME, Penning TM: Genotoxic polycyclic aromatic hydrocarbon ortho-quinones generated by Aldo-Keto reductases induce CYP1A1 via nuclear translocation of the aryl hydrocarbon receptor. *Cancer Res* 60:908–915, 2000.

Capen CC: Mechanistic data and risk assessment of selected toxic end points of the thyroid gland. *Toxicol Pathol* 25:39–48, 1997.

Carro-Ciampi G, Jurima M, Kadar D, Tang BK, Kalow W: *N*-Glucosidation of amobarbital in the cat. *Can J Physiol Pharmacol* 63:1263–1266, 1985.

Cascorbi I, Roots I, Brockmöller J: Association of NAT1 and NAT2 polymorphisms to urinary bladder cancer: Significantly reduced risk in subjects with NAT1*10. *Cancer Res* 61:5051–5056, 2001.

Cashman JR: Structural and catalytic properties of the mammalian flavin-containing monooxygenase. *Chem Res Toxicol* 8:166–181, 1995.

Cashman JR: In vitro metabolism: FMO and related oxygenations, in Woolf T (ed.): *Handbook of Drug Metabolism*. New York: Marcel Dekker, 1999, pp. 477–505.

Cashman JR, Akerman BR, Forrest SM, Treacy EP: Population-specific polymorphisms of the human FMO3 gene: Significance for detoxication. *Drug Metab Dispos* 28:169–173, 2000.

Cashman JR, Xiong Y, Lin J, *et al.*: In vitro and in vivo inhibition of human flavin-containing monooxygenase form 3 (FMO3) in the presence of dietary indoles. *Biochem Pharmacol* 58:1047–1055, 1999.

Cashman JR, Zhang J: Human flavin-containing monooxygenases. *Annu Rev Pharmacol Toxicol* 46:65–100, 2006.

Casida JE, Quistad GB: Serine hydrolase targets of organophosphorus toxicants. *Chem Biol Interact* 157–158:277–283, 2005.

Chang T, Waxman D: Synthetic drugs and natural products as modulators of constitutive androstane receptor (CAR) and pregnane X receptor (PXR). *Drug Metab Rev* 38:51–73, 2006.

Chandrasekharan NV, Dai H, Roos KL, *et al.*: COX-3, a cyclooxygenase-1 variant inhibited by acetaminophen and other analgesic/antipyretic drugs: Cloning, structure, and expression. *Proc Natl Acad Sci USA* 99:13926–13931, 2002.

Chen Q, Doss GA, Tung EC, *et al.*: Evidence for the bioactivation of zomepirac and tolmetin by an oxidative pathway: Identification of glutathione adducts in vitro in human liver microsomes and in vivo in rats. *Drug Metab Dispos* 34:145–151, 2006.

Chen Q, Tan E, Strauss JR, *et al.*: Effect of quinidine on the 10-hydroxylation of R-warfarin: Species differences and clearance projection. *J Pharmacol Exp Ther* 311:307–314, 2004a.

Chen S-Y, Lin J-RV, Darbha R, Lin P, Liu T-Y, Chen Y-MA: Glycine *N*-methyltransferase tumor susceptibility gene in the benzo(*a*)pyrene-detoxification pathway. *Cancer Res* 64:3617–3623, 2004b.

Chen S, Wu K, Knox R: Structure-function studies of DT-diaphorase (NQO1) and NRH:quinone oxidoreductase (NQO2). *Free Radic Biol Med* 29:276–284, 2000.

Cohen S, Boobis A, (Bette) Meek M, Preston R, McGregor D: 4-Aminobiphenyl and DNA reactivity: Case study within the context of the 2006 IPCS Human Relevance Framework for Analysis of a Cancer Mode of Action for Humans. *Crit Rev Toxicol* 36:803–819, 2006.

Conney AH: Induction of microsomal enzymes by foreign chemicals and carcinogenesis by polycyclic aromatic hydrocarbons. *Cancer Res* 42:4875–4917, 1982.

Coughtrie MW, Fisher MB: The role of sulfotransferases (SULTs) and UDP-glucuronosyltransferases (UGTs) in human drug clearance and bioactivation, in Lee JS, Obach RS, Fisher MB (eds.): *Drug Metabolizing Enzymes*. New York: Marcel Dekker, 2003, pp. 541–575.

Csala M, Staines AG, Banhegyi G, Mandl J, Coughtrie MWH, Burchell B: Evidence for multiple glucuronide transporters in rat liver microsomes. *Biochem Pharmacol* 68:1353–1362, 2004.

Cundy K, Sato M, Crooks P: Stereospecific in vivo *N*-methylation of nicotine in the guinea pig. *Drug Metab Dispos* 13:175–185, 1985.

Curran P, DeGroot L: The effect of hepatic enzyme-inducing drugs on thyroid hormones and the thyroid gland. *Endocr Rev* 12:135–150, 1991.

Daly AK: Pharmacogenetics, in Woolf T (ed.): *Handbook of Drug Metabolism*. New York: Marcel Dekker, 1999, pp. 175–202.

Daniel V: Glutathione *S*-transferases: Gene structure and regulation of expression. *Crit Rev Biochem Mol Biol* 28:173–207, 1993.

Dawson JH: Probing structure-function relations in heme-containing oxygenases and peroxidases. *Science* 240:433–439, 1988.

de Morais SM, Uetrecht JP, Wells PG: Decreased glucuronidation and increased bioactivation of acetaminophen in Gilbert's syndrome. *Gastroenterology* 102:577–586, 1992.

Debiec-Rychter M, Land SJ, King CM: Histological localization of acetyltransferases in human tissue. *Cancer Lett* 143:99–102, 1999.

De Bosscher K, Vanden Berghe W, Haegeman G: Cross-talk between nuclear receptors and nuclear factor kappaB. *Oncogene* 25:6868–6886, 2006.

Dekant W, Vamvakas S: Glutathione-dependent bioactivation of xenobiotics. *Xenobiotica* 23:873–887, 1993.

Delaforge M, Pruvost A, Perrin L, Andre F: Cytochrome P450-mediated oxidation of glucuronide derivatives: Example of estradiol-17β-glucuronide oxidation to 2-hydroxy-estradiol-17β-glucuronide by CYP 2C8. *Drug Metab Dispos* 33:466–473, 2005.

Diaz D, Fabre I, Daujat M, *et al.*: Omeprazole is an aryl hydrocarbon-like inducer of human hepatic cytochrome P450. *Gastroenterology* 99:737–747, 1990.

Dirr H, Reinemer, P, Huber, R: X-ray crystal structures of cytosolic glutathione *S*-transferases. *Eur J Biochem* 220:645–661, 1994.

Dolphin C, Janmohamed A, Smith R, Shephard E, Phillips I: Missense mutation in flavin-containing mono-oxygenase 3 gene, FMO3, underlies fish-odour syndrome. *Nat Genet* 17:491–494, 1997.

Dolphin CT, Beckett DJ, Janmohamed A, *et al.*: The flavin-containing monooxygenase 2 Gene (FMO2) of humans, but not of other primates, encodes a truncated, nonfunctional protein. *J Biol Chem* 273:30599–30607, 1998.

Dow J, Piriou F, Wolf E, Dulery BD, Haegele KD: Novel carbamate metabolites of mofegiline, a primary amine monoamine oxidase B inhibitor, in dogs and humans. *Drug Metab Dispos* 22:738–749, 1994.

Draganov DI, La Du BN: Pharmacogenetics of paraoxonases: A brief review. *Naunyn Schmiedebergs Arch Pharmacol* 369:78–88, 2004.

Duh FM, Fivash M, Moody M, *et al.*: Characterization of a new SNP c767A/T (Arg222Trp) in the candidate TSG FUS2 on human chromosome 3p21.3: Prevalence in Asian populations and analysis of association with nasopharyngeal cancer. *Mol Cell Probes* 18:39–44, 2004.

Dwivedi C, Downie AA, Webb TE: Net glucuronidation in different rat strains: Importance of microsomal β-glucuronidase. *FASEB J* 1:303–307, 1987.

Eaton DL, Gallagher EP: Mechanisms of aflatoxin carcinogenesis. *Annu Rev Pharmacol Toxicol* 34:135–172, 1994.

Edenberg HJ: Regulation of the mammalian alcohol dehydrogenase genes. *Prog Nucleic Acid Res Mol Biol* 64:295–341, 2000.

Edmondson DE, Mattevi A, Binda C, Li M, Hubalek F: Structure and mechanism of monoamine oxidase. *Curr Med Chem* 11:1983–1993, 2004.

Egan MF, Goldberg TE, Kolachana BS, *et al.*: Effect of COMT Val108/158 Met genotype on frontal lobe function and risk for schizophrenia. *Proc Natl Acad Sci USA* 98:6917–6922, 2001.

Ekins S, Stresser DM, Andrew Williams J: In vitro and pharmacophore insights into CYP3A enzymes. *Trends Pharmacol Sci* 24:161–166, 2003.

Ekroos M, Sjögren T: Structural basis for ligand promiscuity in cytochrome P450 3A4. *Proc Natl Acad Sci USA* 103:13682–13687, 2006.

Eriksson T, Björkman S, Roth B, Fyge Å, Höglun P: Enantiomers of thalidomide: Blood distribution and the influence of serum albumin on chiral inversion and hydrolysis. *Chirality* 10:223–228, 1998.

Evans D: *N*-Acetyltransferase, in Kalow W (ed.): *Pharmacogenetics of Drug Metabolism.* New York: Pergamon, 1992, pp. 95–178.

Falany CN, Johnson MR, Barnes S, Diasio RB: Glycine and taurine conjugation of bile acids by a single enzyme. Molecular cloning and expression of human liver bile acid CoA:amino acid *N*-acyltransferase. *J Biol Chem* 269:19375–19379, 1994.

Faucette SR, Sueyoshi T, Smith CM, Negishi M, LeCluyse EL, Wang H: Differential regulation of hepatic CYP2B6 and CYP3A4 genes by constitutive androstane receptor but not pregnane X receptor. *J Pharmacol Exp Ther* 317:1200–1209, 2006.

Faucette SR, Wang H, Hamilton GA, *et al.*: Regulation of CYP2B6 in primary human hepatocytes by prototypical inducers. *Drug Metab Dispos* 32:348–358, 2004.

Fisher M, Campanale K, Ackermann B, Vandenbrande M, Wrighton S: In vitro glucuronidation using human liver microsomes and the pore-forming peptide alamethicin. *Drug Metab Dispos* 28:560–566, 2000.

Fontana E, Dansette PM, Poli SM: Cytochrome p450 enzymes mechanism based inhibitors: Common sub-structures and reactivity. *Curr Drug Metab* 6:413–454, 2005.

Franks ME, Macpherson GR, Figg WD: Thalidomide. *Lancet* 363:1802–1811, 2004.

Fretland AJ, Omiecinski CJ: Epoxide hydrolases: Biochemistry and molecular biology. *Chem Biol Interact* 129:41–59, 2000.

Frezza M, di Padova C, Pazzato G, Terpin M, Baraona E, Lieber CS: High blood alcohol levels in women. The role of decreased gastric alcohol dehydrogenase activity and first-pass metabolism. *N Engl J Med* 322:95–99, 1990.

Fujikawa Y, Satoh T, Suganuma A, *et al.*: Extremely sensitive biomarker of acute organophosphorus insecticide exposure. *Hum Exp Toxicol* 24:333–336, 2005.

Fung M, Thornton A, Mybeck A, Wu JH-H, Hornbuckle K, Muniz E: Evaluation of the characteristics of safety withdrawal of prescription drugs from worldwide pharmaceutical markets—1960 to 1999. *Drug Inf J* 35:293–317, 2001.

Furukawa M, Nishimura M, Ogino D, *et al.*: Cytochrome P450 gene expression levels in peripheral blood mononuclear cells in comparison with the liver. *Cancer Sci* 95:520–529, 2004.

Furuta T, Shirai N, Sugimoto M, Nakamura A, Hishida A, Ishizaki T: Influence of CYP2C19 pharmacogenetic polymorphism on proton pump inhibitor-based therapies. *Drug Metab Pharmacokinet* 20:153–167, 2005.

Gamage N, Barnett A, Hempel N, *et al.*: Human sulfotransferases and their role in chemical metabolism. *Toxicol Sci* 90:5–22, 2006.

Garattini E, Mendel R, Ramao MJ, Wright R, Terao M: Mammalian molybdo-flavoenzymes, an expanding family of proteins: structure, genetics, regulation, function and pathophysiology. *Biochem J* 372:15–32, 2003.

Gasche Y, Daali Y, Fathi M, *et al.*: Codeine intoxication associated with ultrarapid CYP2D6 metabolism. *N Engl J Med* 351:2827–2831, 2004.

Geisler SA, Olshan AF: GSTM1, GSTT1, and the risk of squamous cell carcinoma of the head and neck: A mini-HuGE review. *Am J Epidemiol* 154:95–105, 2001.

Gerbal-Chaloin S, Pichard-Garcia L, Fabre JM, *et al.*: Role of CYP3A4 in the regulation of the aryl hydrocarbon receptor by omeprazole sulphide. *Cell Signal* 18:740–750, 2006.

Gerlach M, Riederer P, Przuntek H, Youdim MB: MPTP mechanisms of neurotoxicity and their implications for Parkinson's disease. *Eur J Pharmacol* 208:273–286, 1991.

Geshi E, Kimura T, Yoshimura M, *et al.*: A single nucleotide polymorphism in the carboxylesterase gene is associated with the responsiveness to imidapril medication and the promoter activity. *Hypertens Res* 28:719–725, 2005.

Giacomini KM, Sugiyama Y: Membrane transporters and drug response, in Goodman LS, Gilman A, Brunton LL, Lazo JS, Parker KL (eds.): *Goodman & Gilman's The Pharmacological Basis of Therapeutics.* New York: McGraw-Hill, 2006, pp. 41–70.

Gidal BE, Sheth R, Parnell J, Maloney K, Sale M: Evaluation of VPA dose and concentration effects on lamotrigine pharmacokinetics: Implications for conversion to lamotrigine monotherapy. *Epilepsy Res* 57:85–93, 2003.

Gipple KJ, Chan KT, Elvin AT, Lalka D, Axelson JE: Species differences in the urinary excretion of the novel primary amine conjugate: Tocainide carbamoyl O-β-D-glucuronide. *J Pharm Sci* 71:1011–1014, 1982.

Glatt H, Meinl W: Pharmacogenetics of soluble sulfotransferases (SULTs). *Naunyn Schmiedebergs Arch Pharmacol* 369:55–68, 2004.

Goedde HW, Agarwal D: Pharmacogenetics of aldehyde dehydrogenase, in Kalow W (ed.): *Pharmacogenetics of Drug Metabolism.* New York: Pergamon, 1992, pp. 281–311.

Goetz MP, Rae JM, Suman VJ, *et al.*: Pharmacogenetics of tamoxifen biotransformation is associated with clinical outcomes of efficacy and hot flashes. *J Clin Oncol* 23:9312–9318, 2005.

Goh BC, Lee SC, Wang LZ, *et al.*: Explaining interindividual variability of docetaxel pharmacokinetics and pharmacodynamics in Asians through phenotyping and genotyping strategies. *J Clin Oncol* 20:3683–3690, 2002.

Gonzalez FJ: Role of gene knockout and transgenic mice in the study of xenobiotic metabolism. *Drug Metab Rev* 35:319–335, 2003.

Gonzalez FJ: The 2006 Bernard B. Brodie award lecture: CYP2E1. *Drug Metab Dispos* 35:1–8, 2007.

Gonzalez FJ, Tukey RH: Drug metabolism, in Goodman LS, Gilman A, Brunton LL, Lazo JS, Parker KL (eds.): *Goodman & Gilman's the Pharmacological Basis of Therapeutics.* New York: McGraw-Hill, 2006, pp. 71–91.

Gonzalez FJ, Yu A-M: Cytochrome P450 and xenobiotic receptor humanized mice. *Annu Rev Pharmacol Toxicol* 46:41–64, 2006.

Gopaul VS, Tang W, Farrell K, Abbott FS: Amino acid conjugates: Metabolites of 2-propylpentanoic acid (valproic acid) in epileptic patients. *Drug Metab Dispos* 31:114–121, 2003.

Gorell JM, Rybicki BA, Johnson CC, Peterson EL: Smoking and Parkinson's disease: A dose-response relationship. *Neurology* 52:115–119, 1999.

Grant DM, Blum M, Meyer UA: Polymorphisms of *N*-acetyltransferase genes. *Xenobiotica* 22:1073–1081, 1992.

Grasso P, Sharratt M, Cohen AJ: Role of persistent, non-genotoxic tissue damage in rodent cancer and relevance to humans. *Annu Rev Pharmacol Toxicol* 31:253–287, 1991.

Grunwell JR, Bertozzi CR: Carbohydrate sulfotransferases of the GalNAc/Gal/GlcNAc6ST family. *Biochemistry* 41:13117–13126, 2002.

Guengerich FP: Reactions and significance of cytochrome P-450 enzymes. *J Biol Chem* 266:10019–10022, 1991.

Guengerich FP: Common and uncommon cytochrome P450 reactions related to metabolism and chemical toxicity. *Chem Res Toxicol* 14:611–650, 2001a.

Guengerich FP: Uncommon P450-catalyzed reactions. *Curr Drug Metab* 2:93–115, 2001b.

Guengerich FP, Kim DH, Iwasaki M: Role of human cytochrome P-450 IIE1 in the oxidation of many low molecular weight cancer suspects. *Chem Res Toxicol* 4:168–179, 1991.

Guengerich FP, Shimada T: Oxidation of toxic and carcinogenic chemicals by human cytochrome P-450 enzymes. *Chem Res Toxicol* 4:391–407, 1991.

Gupta E, Lestingi TM, Mick R, Ramirez J, Vokes EE, Ratain MJ: Metabolic fate of irinotecan in humans: Correlation of glucuronidation with diarrhea. *Cancer Res* 54:3723–3725, 1994.

Gutierrez PL: The role of NAD(P)H oxidoreductase (DT-diaphorase) in the bioactivation of quinone-containing antitumor agents: A review. *Free Radic Biol Med* 29:263–275, 2000.

Hamman M, Haehner-Daniels B, Wrighton S, Rettie A, Hall S: Stereoselective sulfoxidation of sulindac sulfide by flavin-containing monooxygenases. *Biochem Pharmacol* 60:7–17, 2000.

Hawes EM: *N*+-Glucuronidation, a common pathway in human metabolism of drugs with a tertiary amine group. *Drug Metab Dispos* 26:830–837, 1998.

Hayakawa H, Fukushima Y, Kato H, *et al.*: Metabolism and disposition of novel des-fluoro quinolone garenoxacin in experimental animals and an interspecies scaling of pharmacokinetic parameters. *Drug Metab Dispos* 31:1409–1418, 2003.

Hayes JD, Flanagan JU, Jowsey IR: Glutathione transferases. *Annu Rev Pharmacol Toxicol* 45:51–88, 2005.

Hayes JD, Nguyen T, Judah DJ, Petersson DG, Neal GE: Cloning of cDNAs from fetal rat liver encoding glutathione *S*-transferase Yc polypeptides. The Yc2 subunit is expressed in adult rat liver resistant to the hepatocarcinogen aflatoxin B1. *J Biol Chem* 269:20707–20717, 1994.

Hayes JD, Pulford DJ: The glutathione *S*-transferase supergene family: Regulation of GST and the contribution of the isoenzymes to cancer chemoprotection and drug resistance. *Crit Rev Biochem Mol Biol* 30:445–600, 1995.

Hayes RB, Bi W, Rothman N, *et al.*: *N*-Acetylation phenotype and genotype and risk of bladder cancer in benzidine-exposed workers. *Carcinogenesis* 14:675–678, 1993.

Hill RN, Erdreich LS, Paynter OE, Roberts PA, Rosenthal SL, Wilkinson CF: Thyroid follicular cell carcinogenesis. *Fundam Appl Toxicol* 12:629–697, 1989.

Hein DW: Acetylator genotype and arylamine-induced carcinogenesis. *Biochim Biophys Acta* 948:37–66, 1988.

Hein DW: *N*-Acetyltransferase 2 genetic polymorphism: Effects of carcinogen and haplotype on urinary bladder cancer risk. *Oncogene* 25:1649–1658, 2006.

Hein DW, Doll MA, Fretland AJ, *et al.*: Molecular genetics and epidemiology of the NAT1 and NAT2 acetylation polymorphisms. *Cancer Epidemiol Biomarkers Prev* 9:29–42, 2000.

Helms C, Cao L, Krueger JG, *et al.*: A putative RUNX1 binding site variant between SLC9A3R1 and NAT9 is associated with susceptibility to psoriasis. *Nat Genet* 35:349–356, 2003.

Hines RN, Hopp KA, Franco J, Saeian K, Begun FP: Alternative processing of the human FMO6 gene renders transcripts incapable of encoding a functional flavin-containing monooxygenase. *Mol Pharmacol* 62:320–325, 2002.

Hirvonen A: Polymorphic NATs and cancer predisposition, in Ryder W (ed.): *Metabolic Polymorphisms and Susceptibility to Cancer (IARC)*. Lyon: IARC Scientific Publications, 1999, pp. 251–270.

Hon YY, Jusko WJ, Spratlin VE, Jann MW: Altered methylprednisolone pharmacodynamics in healthy subjects with histamine *N*-methyltransferase C314T genetic polymorphism. *J Clin Pharmacol* 46:408–417, 2006.

Horton JR, Sawada K, Nishibori M, Cheng X: Structural basis for inhibition of histamine *N*-methyltransferase by diverse drugs. *J Mol Biol* 353:334–344, 2005.

Howgate EM, Rowland YK, Proctor NJ, Tucker GT, Rostami-Hodjegan A: Prediction of in vivo drug clearance from in vitro data. I: impact of inter-individual variability. *Xenobiotica* 36:473–497, 2006.

Hu R, Xu C, Shen G, *et al.*: Identification of Nrf2-regulated genes induced by chemopreventive isothiocyanate PEITC by oligonucleotide microarray. *Life Sci* 79:1944–1955, 2006.

Huang W, Lin YS, McConn DJ, II, *et al.*: Evidence of significant contribution from CYP3A5 to hepatic drug metabolism. *Drug Metab Dispos* 32:1434–1445, 2004.

Hukkanen J, Jacob P, III, Benowitz NL: Metabolism and disposition kinetics of nicotine. *Pharmacol Rev* 57:79–115, 2005.

Humphrey MJ, Ringrose PS: Peptides and related drugs: A review of their absorption, metabolism, and excretion. *Drug Metab Rev* 17:283–310, 1986.

Idle JR: Is environmental carcinogenesis modulated by host polymorphism? *Mutat Res* 247:259–266, 1991.

Ingelman-Sundberg M, Rane A, Gustafsson JA: Properties of hydroxylase systems in the human fetal liver active on free and sulfoconjugated steroids. *Biochemistry* 14:429–437, 1975.

Isin EM, Guengerich FP: Complex reactions catalyzed by cytochrome P450 enzymes. *Biochim Biophys Acta* 1770:314–329, 2007.

Iskander K, Jaiswal AK: Quinone oxidoreductases in protection against myelogenous hyperplasia and benzene toxicity. *Chem Biol Interact* 153–154:147–157, 2005.

Jez JM, Penning TM: The aldo-keto reductase (AKR) superfamily: An update. *Chem Biol Interact* 130–132:499–525, 2001.

Ji Y, Salavaggione OE, Wang L, *et al.*: Human phenylethanolamine *N*-methyltransferase pharmacogenomics: Gene re-sequencing and functional genomics. *J Neurochem* 95:1766–1776, 2005.

Josephy DP, Guengerich FP, Miners J: Phase I and phase II drug metabolism: Terminology that we should phase out? *Drug Metab Rev* 37:575–580, 2005.

Juberg DR, Mudra DR, Hazelton GA, Parkinson A: The effect of fenbuconazole on cell proliferation and enzyme induction in the liver of female CD1 mice. *Toxicol Appl Pharmacol* 214:178–187, 2006.

Kadlubar FF: Biochemical individuality and its implications for drug and carcinogen metabolism: Recent insights from acetyltransferase and cytochrome P4501A2 phenotyping and genotyping in humans. *Drug Metab Rev* 26:37–46, 1994.

Kalsotra A, Strobel HW: Cytochrome P450 4F subfamily: At the crossroads of eicosanoid and drug metabolism. *Pharmacol Ther* 112:589–611, 2006.

Kamataki T, Fujieda M, Kiyotani K, Iwano S, Kunitoh H: Genetic polymorphism of CYP2A6 as one of the potential determinants of tobacco-related cancer risk. *Biochem Biophys Res Commun* 338:306–310, 2005.

Kanamitsu SI, Ito K, Okuda H, *et al.*: Prediction of in vivo drug–drug interactions based on mechanism-based inhibition from in vitro data: Inhibition of 5-fluorouracil metabolism by (E)-5-(2-bromovinyl) uracil. *Drug Metab Dispos* 28:467–474, 2000.

Kaplowitz N: Idiosyncratic drug hepatotoxicity. *Nat Rev Drug Discov* 4:489–499, 2005.

Karanam BV, Hop CE, Liu DQ, *et al.*: In vitro metabolism of MK-0767 [(+/−)-5-[(2,4-dioxothiazolidin-5-yl)methyl]-2-methoxy-*N*-[[(4-trifluoromethyl) phenyl]methyl]benzamide], a peroxisome proliferator-activated receptor alpha/gamma agonist. I. Role of cytochrome P450, methyltransferases, flavin monooxygenases, and esterases. *Drug Metab Dispos* 32:1015–1022, 2004.

Karlgren M, Gomez A, Stark K, *et al.*: Tumor-specific expression of the novel cytochrome P450 enzyme, CYP2W1. *Biochem Biophys Res Commun* 341:451–458, 2006.

Kato R, Yamazoe Y: Metabolic activation of *N*-hydroxylated metabolites of carcinogenic and mutagenic arylamines and arylamides by esterification. *Drug Metab Rev* 26:413–429, 1994.

Kiang TKL, Ensom MHH, Chang TKH: UDP-glucuronosyltransferases and clinical drug–drug interactions. *Pharmacol Ther* 106:97–132, 2005.

Kim K-A, Kim M-J, Park J-Y, *et al.*: Stereoselective metabolism of lansoprazole by human liver cytochrome P450 enzymes. *Drug Metab Dispos* 31:1227–1234, 2003.

Kim S-H, Henry EC, Kim D-K, et al.: Novel compound 2-methyl-2H-pyrazole-3-carboxylic acid (2-methyl-4-O-tolylazo-phenyl)-amide (CH-223191) prevents 2,3,7,8-TCDD-induced toxicity by antagonizing the aryl hydrocarbon receptor. Mol Pharmacol 69:1871–1878, 2006.

Kinobe RT, Parkinson OT, Mitchell DJ, Gillam EMJ: P450 2C18 catalyzes the metabolic bioactivation of phenytoin. Chem Res Toxicol 18:1868–1875, 2005.

Kirkman SK, Zhang M-Y, Horwatt PM, Scatina J: Isolation and identification of bromfenac glucoside from rat bile. Drug Metab Dispos 26:720–723, 1998.

Kitada M, Kamataki T, Itahashi K, Rikihisa T, Kanakubo Y: P-450 HFLa, a form of cytochrome P-450 purified from human fetal livers, is the 16 alpha-hydroxylase of dehydroepiandrosterone 3-sulfate. J Biol Chem 262:13534–13537, 1987.

Klaassen CD, Boles JW: Sulfation and sulfotransferases 5: The importance of 3′-phosphoadenosine 5′-phosphosulfate (PAPS) in the regulation of sulfation. Faseb J 11:404–418, 1997.

Klaunig JE, Babich MA, Baetcke KP, et al.: PPARalpha agonist-induced rodent tumors: Modes of action and human relevance. Crit Rev Toxicol 33:655–780, 2003.

Kobayashi T, Sleeman JE, Coughtrie MW, Burchell B: Molecular and functional characterization of microsomal UDP-glucuronic acid uptake by members of the nucleotide sugar transporter (NST) family. Biochem J 400:281–289, 2006.

Kochansky CJ, Rippley RK, Yan KX, et al.: Absorption, metabolism, and excretion of [14C]MK-0767 (2-methoxy-5-(2,4-dioxo-5-thiazolidinyl)-N-[[4-(trifluoromethyl)phenyl] methyl]benzamide) in humans. Drug Metab Dispos 34:1457–1461, 2006.

Kochansky CJ, Xia Y-Q, Wang S, et al.: Species differences in the elimination of a peroxisome proliferator-activated receptor agonist highlighted by oxidative metabolism of its acyl glucuronide. Drug Metab Dispos 33:1894–1904, 2005.

Kodama S, Negishi M: Phenobarbital confers its diverse effects by activating the orphan nuclear receptor CAR. Drug Metab Rev 38:75–87, 2006.

Koivusalo M, Baumann M, Uotila L: Evidence for the identity of glutathione-dependent formaldehyde dehydrogenase and class III alcohol dehydrogenase. FEBS Lett 257:105–109, 1989.

Koren G, Cairns J, Chitayat D, Gaedigk A, Leeder SJ: Pharmacogenetics of morphine poisoning in a breastfed neonate of a codeine-prescribed mother. Lancet 368:704, 2006.

Kretz-Rommel A, Boelsterli UA: Mechanism of covalent adduct formation of diclofenac to rat hepatic microsomal proteins. Retention of the glucuronic acid moiety in the adduct. Drug Metab Dispos 22:956–961, 1994.

Kroetz DL, Loiseau P, Guyot M, Levy RH: In vivo and in vitro correlation of microsomal epoxide hydrolase inhibition by progabide. Clin Pharmacol Ther 54:485–497, 1993.

Krueger S, VanDyke J, Williams D, Hines R: The role of flavin-containing monooxygenase (FMO) in the metabolism of tamoxifen and other tertiary amines. Drug Metab Rev 38:139–147, 2006.

Kubo T, Kim SR, Sai K, et al.: Functional characterization of three naturally occurring single nucleotide polymorphisms in the CES2 gene encoding carboxylesterase 2 (HCE-2). Drug Metab Dispos 33:1482–1487, 2005.

Kumar S, Samuel K, Subramanian R, et al.: Extrapolation of diclofenac clearance from in vitro microsomal metabolism data: Role of acyl glucuronidation and sequential oxidative metabolism of the acyl glucuronide. J Pharmacol Exp Ther 303:969–978, 2002.

Kurian JR, Chin NA, Longlais BJ, Hayes KL, Trepanier LA: Reductive detoxification of arylhydroxylamine carcinogens by human NADH cytochrome b_5 reductase and cytochrome b_5. Chem Res Toxicol 19:1366–1373, 2006.

La Du B: Human serum paraoxonase/arylesterase, in Kalow W (ed.): Pharmacogenetics of Drug Metabolism. New York: Pergamon, 1992, pp. 51–91.

Lai DY: Rodent carcinogenicity of peroxisome proliferators and issues on human relevance. J Environ Sci Health C Environ Carcinog Ecotoxicol Rev 22:37–55, 2004.

Lake BG, Price RJ, Walters DG, Phillips JC, Young PJ, Adams TB: Studies on the metabolism of the thiofurans furfuryl mercaptan and 2-methyl-3-furanthiol in rat liver. Food Chem Toxicol 41:1761–1770, 2003.

Lasser KE, Allen PD, Woolhandler SJ, Himmelstein DU, Wolfe SM, Bor DH: Timing of new black box warnings and withdrawals for prescription medications. JAMA 287:2215–2220, 2002.

Lawton MP, Cashman JR, Cresteil T, et al.: A nomenclature for the mammalian flavin-containing monooxygenase gene family based on amino acid sequence identities. Arch Biochem Biophys 308:254–257, 1994.

Lazarou J, Pomeranz BH, Corey PN: Incidence of adverse drug reactions in hospitalized patients: A meta-analysis of prospective studies. JAMA 279:1200–1205, 1998.

Lecoeur S, Bonierbale E, Challine D, et al.: Specificity of in vitro covalent binding of tienilic acid metabolites to human liver microsomes in relationship to the type of hepatotoxicity: Comparison with two directly hepatotoxic drugs. Chem Res Toxicol 7:434–442, 1994.

Lee CM, Chen SY, Lee YC, Huang CY, Chen YM: Benzo[a]pyrene and glycine N-methyltransferase interactions: Gene expression profiles of the liver detoxification pathway. Toxicol Appl Pharmacol 214:126–135, 2006.

Lee JM, Johnson JA: An important role of Nrf2-ARE pathway in the cellular defense mechanism. J Biochem Mol Biol 37:139–143, 2004.

Lehman-McKeeman LD, Caudill D, Vassallo JD, Pearce RE, Madan A, Parkinson A: Effects of musk xylene and musk ketone on rat hepatic cytochrome P450 enzymes. Toxicol Lett 111:105–115, 1999.

Levitt MD: Review article: Lack of clinical significance of the interaction between H2-receptor antagonists and ethanol. Aliment Pharmacol Ther 7:131–138, 1993.

Li AP, Hartman NR, Lu C, Collins JM, Strong JM: Effects of cytochrome P450 inducers on 17α-ethinyloestradiol (EE2) conjugation by primary human hepatocytes. Br J Clin Pharmacol 48:733–742, 1999.

Li TK: Pharmacogenetics of responses to alcohol and genes that influence alcohol drinking. J Stud Alcohol 61:5–12, 2000.

Li Y, Yokoi T, Katsuki M, Wang JS, Groopman JD, Kamataki T: In vivo activation of aflatoxin B1 in C57BL/6N mice carrying a human fetus-specific CYP3A7 gene. Cancer Res 57:641–645, 1997.

Lieber CS: Microsomal ethanol-oxidizing system (MEOS): The first 30 years (1968–1998)—A review. Alcohol Clin Exp Res 23:991–1007, 1999.

Lieber CS: The discovery of the microsomal ethanol oxidizing system. Drug Metab Review 36:511–529, 2004.

Liederer BM, Borchardt RT: Enzymes involved in the bioconversion of ester-based prodrugs. J Pharm Sci 95:1177–1195, 2006.

Lillibridge J, Kalhorn T, Slattery J: Metabolism of lisofylline and pentoxifylline in human liver microsome and cytosol. Drug Metab Dispos 24:1174–1179, 1996.

Lin YS, Dowling ALS, Quigley SD, et al.: Co-regulation of CYP3A4 and CYP3A5 and contribution to hepatic and intestinal midazolam metabolism. Mol Pharmacol 62:162–172, 2002.

Lindberg RLP, Negishi M: Alteration of mouse cytochrome P450coh substrate specificity by mutation of a single amino-acid residue. Nature 339:632–634, 1989.

Link M, Hakala KS, Wsol V, Kostiainen R, Ketola RA: Metabolite profile of sibutramine in human urine: A liquid chromatography-electrospray ionization mass spectrometric study. J Mass Spectrom 41:1171–1178, 2006.

Liu K-H, Kim M-G, Lee D-J, et al.: Characterization of ebastine, hydroxyebastine, and carebastine metabolism by human liver microsomes and expressed cytochrome P450 enzymes: Major roles for CYP2J2 and CYP3A. Drug Metab Dispos 34:1793–1797, 2006a.

Liu Y-J, Huang P-L, Chang Y-F, et al.: GSTP1 genetic polymorphism is associated with a higher risk of DNA damage in pesticide-exposed fruit growers. Cancer Epidemiol Biomarkers Prev 15:659–666, 2006b.

Liu ZC, Uetrecht JP: Metabolism of ticlopidine by activated neutrophils: Implications for ticlopidine-induced agranulocytosis. Drug Metab Dispos 28:726–730, 2000.

Lockridge O: Genetic variants of human serum butyrylcholinesterase influence the metabolism of the muscle relaxant succinylcholine, in Kalow W (ed.): *Pharmacogenetics of Drug Metabolism*. New York: Pergamon, 1992, pp. 15–50.

Long RM, Rickert DE: Metabolism and excretion of 2,6-dinitro [^{14}C]-toluene in vivo and in isolated perfused rat livers. *Drug Metab Dispos* 10:455–458, 1982.

Lunam CA, Hall PM, Cousins MJ: The pathology of halothane hepatotoxicity in a guinea-pig model: A comparison with human halothane hepatitis. *Br J Exp Pathol* 70:533–541, 1989.

Ma Q, Lu AYH: Origins of individual variability in p4501a induction. *Chem Res Toxicol* 16:249–260, 2003.

Mackenzie PI, Walter BK, Burchell B, *et al.*: Nomenclature update for the mammalian UDP glycosyltransferase (UGT) gene superfamily. *Pharmacogenet Genomics* 15:677–685, 2005.

Macphee IAM, Fredericks S, Tai T, *et al.*: Tacrolimus pharmacogenetics: Polymorphisms associated with expression of cytochrome P4503A5 and p-glycoprotein correlate with dose requirement. *Transplantation* 74:1486–1489, 2002.

Madan A, Williams T, Faiman M: Glutatione- and glutathione *S*-transferase-dependent oxidative desulfuration of the thione xenobiotic, diethyldithiocarbamate methyl ester (DDTC-Me). *Mol Pharmacol* 46:1217–1225, 1994.

Maecker B, Sherr DH, Vonderheide RH, *et al.*: The shared tumor-associated antigen cytochrome P450 1B1 is recognized by specific cytotoxic T cells. *Blood* 102:3287–3294, 2003.

Mallal S, Nolan D, Witt C, *et al.*: Association between presence of HLA-B*5701, HLA-DR7, and HLA-DQ3 and hypersensitivity to HIV-1 reverse-transcriptase inhibitor abacavir. *Lancet* 359:727–732, 2002.

Mannervik B, Awasthi YC, Board PG, *et al.*: Nomenclature for human glutathione transferases. *Biochem J* 282:305–306, 1992.

Mannervik B, Board PG, Hayes JD, Listowsky I, Pearson WR: Nomenclature for mammalian soluble glutathione transferases. *Methods Enzymol* 401:1–8, 2005.

Mano Y, Usui T, Kamimura H: In vitro drug interaction between diflunisal and indomethacin via glucuronidation in humans. *Biopharmaceutics & Drug Disposition* 27:267–273, 2006.

Mantle TJ, Pickett CB, Hayes JD: Glutathione *S*-transferases and carcinogenesis, in *Glutathione S-Transferases and Carcinogenesis*. London: Taylor and Francis, 1987, pp. 1–267.

Matsunaga T, Shintani S, Hara A: Multiplicity of mammalian reductases for xenobiotic carbonyl compounds. *Drug Metab Pharmacokinet* 21:1–18, 2006.

McClain R: The significance of hepatic microsomal enzyme induction and altered thyroid function in rats: Implications for thyroid gland neoplasia. *Toxicol Pathol* 17:294–306, 1989.

McLeod HL, Fang L, Luo X, Scott EP, Evans WE: Ethnic differences in erythrocyte catechol-*O*-methyltransferase activity in black and white Americans. *J Pharmacol Exp Ther* 270:26–29, 1994.

Meyer UA: The molecular basis of genetic polymorphisms of drug metabolism. *J Pharm Pharmacol* 46:409–415, 1994.

Mimori Y, Nakamura S, Kameyama M: Regional and subcellular distribution of cyanide metabolizing enzymes in the central nervous system. *J Neurochem* 43:540–545, 1984.

Miners JO, Knights KM, Houston JB, Mackenzie PI: In vitro–in vivo correlation for drugs and other compounds eliminated by glucuronidation in humans: Pitfalls and promises. *Biochem Pharmacol* 71:1531–1539, 2006.

Mirsalis JC, Butterworth BE: Induction of unscheduled DNA synthesis in rat hepatocytes following in vivo treatment with dinitrotoluene. *Carcinogenesis* 3:241–245, 1982.

Miura M, Satoh S, Tada H, Habuchi T, Suzuki T: Stereoselective metabolism of rabeprazole-thioether to rabeprazole by human liver microsomes. *Eur J Clin Pharmacol* 62:113–117, 2006.

Molina MA, Sitja-Arnau M, Lemoine MG, Frazier ML, Sinicrope FA: Increased cyclooxygenase-2 expression in human pancreatic carcinomas and cell lines: Growth inhibition by nonsteroidal anti-inflammatory drugs. *Cancer Research* 59:4356–4362, 1999.

Monks TJ, Anders MW, Dekant W, Stevens JL, Lau SS, van Bladeren PJ: Glutathione conjugate mediated toxicities. *Toxicol Appl Pharmacol* 106:1–19, 1990.

Morar N, Bowcock AM, Harper JI, Cookson WO, Moffatt MF: Investigation of the chromosome 17q25 PSORS2 locus in atopic dermatitis. *J Invest Dermatol* 126:603–606, 2006.

Mordente A, Meucci E, Martorana GE, Giardina B, Minotti G: Human heart cytosolic reductases and anthracycline cardiotoxicity. *IUBMB Life* 52:83–88, 2001.

Morisseau C, Hammock BD: Epoxide hydrolases: Mechanisms, inhibitor designs, and biological roles. *Annu Rev Pharmacol Toxicol* 45:311–333, 2005.

Mukherjee B, Salavaggione OE, Pelleymounter LL, *et al.*: Glutathione *S*-transferase ω-1 and ω-2 pharmacogenomics. *Drug Metab Dispos* 34:1237–1246, 2006.

Mulder GJ (ed.): *Sulfation of Drugs and Related Compounds*. Boca Raton, FL: CRC, 1981.

Murai T, Iwabuchi H, Ikeda T: Repeated glucuronidation at one hydroxyl group leads to structurally novel diglucuronides of steroid sex hormones. *Drug Metab Pharmacokinet* 20:282–293, 2005.

Murai T, Samata N, Iwabuchi H, Ikeda T: Human UDP-glucuronosyltransferase, UGT1A8, glucuronidates dihydrotestosterone to a monoglucuronide and further to a structurally novel diglucuronide. *Drug Metab Dispos* 34:1102–1108, 2006.

Naesens M, Kuypers DR, Streit F, *et al.*: Rifampin induces alterations in mycophenolic acid glucuronidation and elimination: Implications for drug exposure in renal allograft recipients. *Clin Pharmacol Ther* 80:509–521, 2006.

Nagar S, Blanchard R: Pharmacogenetics of uridine diphosphoglucuronosyltransferase (UGT) 1A family members and its role in patient response to irinotecan. *Drug Metab Rev* 38:393–409, 2006.

Nagar S, Remmel RP: Uridine diphosphoglucuronosyltransferase pharmacogenetics and cancer. *Oncogene* 25:1659–1672, 2006.

Nagata K, Yamazoe Y: Pharmacogenetics of sulfotransferase. *Annu Rev Pharmacol Toxicol* 40:159–176, 2000.

Nakajima M, Itoh M, Sakai H, *et al.*: CYP2A13 expressed in human bladder metabolically activates 4-aminobiphenyl. *Int J Cancer* 119:2520–2526, 2006.

Nakano H, Ogura K, Takahashi E, *et al.*: Regioselective monosulfation and disulfation of the phytoestrogens daidzein and genistein by human liver sulfotransferases. *Drug Metab Pharmacokinet* 19:216–226, 2004.

Nakano K, Ohashi M, Harigaya S: The β-glucosidation and β-glucuronidation of pantothenic acid compared with p-nitrophenol in dog liver microsome. *Chem Pharm Bull (Tokyo)* 34:3949–3952, 1986.

Nebert DW, Dalton TP: The role of cytochrome P450 enzymes in endogenous signaling pathways and environmental carcinogenesis. *Nat Rev Cancer* 6:947–960, 2006.

Nebert DW, Dalton TP, Okey AB, Gonzalez FJ: Role of aryl hydrocarbon receptor-mediated induction of the CYP1 enzymes in environmental toxicity and cancer. *J Biol Chem* 279:23847–23850, 2004.

Nguyen T, Rushmore TH, Pickett CB: Transcriptional regulation of a rat liver glutathione *S*-transferase Ya subunit gene: Analysis of the antioxidant response element and its activation by the phorbol ester 12-*O*-tetra-decanoylphorbol-13-acetate. *J Biol Chem* 269:13656–13662, 1994.

Nichols WK, Mehta R, Skordos K, *et al.*: 3-Methylindole-induced toxicity to human bronchial epithelial cell lines. *Toxicol Sci* 71:229–236, 2003.

Nigg HN, Knaak JB: Blood cholinesterases as human biomarkers of organophosphorus pesticide exposure. *Rev Environ Contam Toxicol* 163:29–111, 2000.

Nishimura M, Naito S: Tissue-specific mRNA expression profiles of human ATP-binding cassette and solute carrier transporter superfamilies. *Drug Metab Pharmacokinet* 20:452–477, 2005.

Nishimura M, Naito S: Tissue-specific mRNA expression profiles of human phase I metabolizing enzymes except for cytochrome P450 and phase II metabolizing enzymes. *Drug Metab Pharmacokinet* 21:357–374, 2006.

Nishimura M, Naito S, Yokoi T: Tissue-specific mRNA expression profiles of human nuclear receptor subfamilies. *Drug Metab Pharmacokinet* 19:135–149, 2004.

Nishimura M, Yaguti H, Yoshitsugu H, Naito S, Satoh T: Tissue distribution of mRNA expression of human cytochrome p450 isoforms assessed by high-sensitivity real-time reverse transcription PCR. *Yakugaku Zasshi* 123:369–375, 2003.

Nishiyama T, Kobori T, Arai K, *et al.*: Identification of human UDP-glucuronosyltransferase isoform(s) responsible for the C-glucuronidation of phenylbutazone. *Arch Biochem Biophys* 454:72–79, 2006.

O'Brien PJ: Peroxidases. *Chem Biol Interact* 129:113–139, 2000.

O'Byrne J, Hunt MC, Rai DK, Saeki M, Alexson SE: The human bile acid-CoA:amino acid *N*-acyltransferase functions in the conjugation of fatty acids to glycine. *J Biol Chem* 278:34237–34244, 2003.

Obach RS: Potent inhibition of human liver aldehyde oxidase by raloxifene. *Drug Metab Dispos* 32:89–97, 2004.

Obach RS, Cox LM, Tremaine LM: Sertraline is metabolized by multiple cytochrome P450 enzymes, monoamine oxidases, and glucuronyl transferases in human: An in vitro study. *Drug Metab Dispos* 33:262–270, 2005.

Obach RS, Reed-Hagen AE, Krueger SS, *et al.*: Metabolism and disposition of varenicline, a selective $\alpha 4\beta 2$ acetylcholine receptor partial agonist, in vivo and in vitro. *Drug Metab Dispos* 34:121–130, 2006.

Obach RS, Walsky RL: Drugs that inhibit oxidation reactions catalyzed by aldehyde oxidase do not inhibit the reductive metabolism of ziprasidone to its major metabolite, *S*-methyldihydroziprasidone: An in vitro study. *J Clin Psychopharmacol* 25:605–608, 2005.

Obata T: Diabetes and semicarbazide-sensitive amine oxidase (SSAO) activity: A review. *Life Sci* 79:417–422, 2006.

Ogilvie BW, Usuki E, Yerino P, Parkinson A: In vitro approaches for studying the inhibition of drug-metabolizing enzymes and identifying the drug-metabolizing enzymes responsible for the metabolism of drugs (Reaction Phenotyping) with Emphasis on Cytochrome P450, in: Drug-Drug Interactions (Rodrigues AD, ed.), Informa Healthcare, New York, 2007.

Ogilvie BW, Zhang D, Li W, *et al.*: Glucuronidation converts gemfibrozil to a potent, metabolism-dependent inhibitor of CYP2C8: Implications for drug–drug interactions. *Drug Metab Dispos* 34:191–197, 2006.

Ogura K, Nishiyama T, Takubo H, *et al.*: Suicidal inactivation of human dihydropyrimidine dehydrogenase by (E)-5-(2-bromovinyl)uracil derived from the antiviral, sorivudine. *Cancer Lett* 122:107–113, 1998.

Ohmori S, Fujiki N, Nakasa H, *et al.*: Steroid hydroxylation by human fetal CYP3A7 and human NADPH-cytochrome P450 reductase coexpressed in insect cells using baculovirus. *Res Commun Mol Pathol Pharmacol* 100:15–28, 1998.

Okamoto K, Matsumoto K, Hille R, Eger BT, Pai EF, Nishino T: The crystal structure of xanthine oxidoreductase during catalysis: implications for reaction mechanism and enzyme inhibition. *Proc Natl Acad Sci USA* 101:7931–7936, 2004.

Oppermann UCT, Filling C, Jornvall H: Forms and functions of human SDR enzymes. *Chem Biol Interact* 130–132:699–705, 2001.

Oshima M, Dinchuk JE, Kargman SL, *et al.*: Suppression of intestinal polyposis in Apc[Δ]716 knockout mice by inhibition of cyclooxygenase 2 (COX-2). *Cell* 87:803–809, 1996.

Owens IS, Ritter JK: The novel bilirubin/phenol UDP-glucuronosyltransferase UGT1 gene locus: Implications for multiple nonhemolytic familial hyperbilirubinemia phenotypes. *Pharmacogenetics* 2:93–108, 1992.

Pacher P, Nivorozhkin A, Szabo C: Therapeutic effects of xanthine oxidase inhibitors: Renaissance half a century after the discovery of allopurinol. *Pharmacol Rev* 58:87–114, 2006.

Paine MF, Widmer WW, Hart HL, *et al.*: A furanocoumarin-free grapefruit juice establishes furanocoumarins as the mediators of the grapefruit juice-felodipine interaction. *Am J Clin Nutr* 83:1097–1105, 2006.

Pal D, Mitra AK: MDR- and CYP3A4-mediated drug–herbal interactions. *Life Sci* 78:2131–2145, 2006.

Parkin DP, Vandenplas S, Botha FJ, *et al.*: Trimodality of isoniazid elimination: Phenotype and genotype in patients with tuberculosis. *Am J Respir Crit Care Med* 155:1717–1722, 1997.

Parkinson A, Hurwitz A: Omeprazole and the induction of human cytochrome P-450: A response to concerns about potential adverse effects. *Gastroenterology* 100:1157–1164, 1991.

Parkinson A, Leonard N, Draper A, Ogilvie B: On the mechanism of hepatocarcinogenesis of benzodiazepines: Evidence that diazepam and oxazepam are CYP2B inducers in rats, and both CYP2B and CYP4A inducers in mice. *Drug Metab Rev* 38:235–259, 2006.

Parkinson A, Mudra DR, Johnson C, Dwyer A, Carroll KM: The effects of gender, age, ethnicity, and liver cirrhosis on cytochrome P450 enzyme activity in human liver microsomes and inducibility in cultured human hepatocytes. *Toxicol Appl Pharmacol* 199:193–209, 2004.

Pascual G, Glass CK: Nuclear receptors versus inflammation: Mechanisms of transrepression. *Trends Endocrinol Metab* 17:321–327, 2006.

Patin E, Barreiro LB, Sabeti PC, *et al.*: Deciphering the ancient and complex evolutionary history of human arylamine *N*-acetyltransferase genes. *Am J Hum Genet* 78:423–436, 2006.

Patki KC, von Moltke LL, Greenblatt DJ: In vitro metabolism of midazolam, triazolam, nifedipine, and testosterone by human liver microsomes and recombinant cytochromes P450: Role of CYP3A4 and CYP3A5. *Drug Metab Dispos* 31:938–944, 2003.

Paulson GD, Caldwell J, Hutson DH, Menn JJ (eds.): *Xenobiotic Conjugation Chemistry*. Washington DC: American Chemical Society, 1986.

Penning T: Molecular endocrinology of hydroxysteroid dehydrogenases. *Endocr Rev* 18:281–305, 1997.

Picard N, Ratanasavanh D, Premaud A, Le Meur Y, Marquet P: Identification of the UDP-glucuronosyl transferase isoforms involved in mycophenolic acid phase II metabolism. *Drug Metab Dispos* 33:139–146, 2005.

Plaa GL: Chlorinated methanes and liver injury: Highlights of the past 50 years. *Annu Rev Pharmacol Toxicol* 40:43–65, 2000.

Pohjanvirta R, Viluksela M, Tuomisto JT, *et al.*: Physicochemical differences in the AH receptors of the most TCDD-susceptible and the most TCDD-resistant rat strains. *Toxicol Appl Pharmacol* 155:82–95, 1999.

Pohl LR, Kenna JG, Satoh H, Christ D, Martin JL: Neoantigens associated with halothane hepatitis. *Drug Metab Rev* 20:203–217, 1989.

Port JL, Yamaguchi K, Du B, *et al.*: Tobacco smoke induces CYP1B1 in the aerodigestive tract. *Carcinogenesis* 25:2275–2281, 2004.

Probst MR, Beer M, Beer D, Jeno P, Meyer UA, Gasser R: Human liver arylacetamide deacetylase. Molecular cloning of a novel esterase involved in the metabolic activation of arylamine carcinogens with high sequence similarity to hormone-sensitive lipase. *J Biol Chem* 269:21650–21656, 1994.

Prochaska HJ, Talalay P: Regulatory mechanisms of monofunctional and bifunctional anticarcinogenic enzyme inducers in murine liver. *Cancer Res* 48:4776–4782, 1988.

Prueksaritanont T, Li C, Tang C, Kuo Y, Strong-Basalyga K, Carr B: Rifampin induces the in vitro oxidative metabolism, but not the in vivo clearance of diclofenac in rhesus monkeys. *Drug Metab Dispos* 34:1806–1810, 2006.

Quinn LP, Perren MJ, Brackenborough KT, *et al.*: A beam-walking apparatus to assess behavioural impairments in MPTP-treated mice: Pharmacological validation with R-(-)-deprenyl. *J Neurosci Methods* 164:43–49, 2007.

Rajagopalan KV: Xanthine oxidase and aldehyde oxidase, in Jakoby WB (ed.): *Enzymatic Basis of Detoxication*. New York: Academic, 1980, pp. 295–306.

Rao SI, Duffel MW: Inhibition of aryl sulfotransferase by carboxylic acids. *Drug Metab Dispos* 19:543–545, 1991.

Rasmussen BB, Brix TH, Kyvik KO, Brosen K: The interindividual differences in the 3-demthylation of caffeine alias CYP1A2 is determined by both genetic and environmental factors. *Pharmacogenetics* 12:473–478, 2002.

Ratnayake JH, Hanna PE, Anders MW, Duggan DE: Sulfoxide reduction. In vitro reduction of sulindac by rat hepatic cytosolic enzymes. *Drug Metab Dispos* 9:85–87, 1981.

Reiss J, Johnson JL: Mutations in the molybdenum cofactor biosynthetic genes *MOCS1*, *MOCS2*, and *GEPH*. *Human Mutat* 21:569–576, 2003.

Relling MV, Giacomini KM: Pharmacogenetics, in Goodman LS, Gilman A, Brunton LL, Lazo JS, Parker KL (eds.): *Goodman & Gilman's the Pharmacological Basis of Therapeutics.* New York: McGraw-Hill, 2006, pp. 93–115.

Rencurel F, Foretz M, Kaufmann MR, et al.: Stimulation of AMP-activated protein kinase is essential for the induction of drug metabolizing enzymes by phenobarbital in human and mouse liver. *Mol Pharmacol* 70:1925–1934, 2006.

Rettie AE, Fisher MB: Transformation enzymes: Oxidative; non-P450, in Woolf T (ed.): *Handbook of Drug Metabolism.* New York: Marcel Dekker, 1999, pp. 131–151.

Rettie AE, Jones JP: Clinical and toxicological relevance of CYP2C9: Drug–drug interactions and pharmacogenetics. *Annu Rev Pharmacol Toxicol* 45:477–494, 2005.

Rizzo WB: Sjögren-Larsson syndrome: Molecular genetics and biochemical pathogenesis of fatty aldehyde dehydrogenase deficiency. *Mol Genet Metab* 90:1–9, 2007.

Robert J, Morvan VL, Smith D, Pourquier P, Bonnet J: Predicting drug response and toxicity based on gene polymorphisms. *Crit Rev Oncol/Hematol* 54:171–196, 2005.

Rodrigues A: Integrated cytochrome P450 reaction phenotyping. *Biochem Pharmacol* 57:465–480, 1999.

Rodrigues AD: Comparison of levels of aldehyde oxidase with cytochrome P450 activities in human liver in vitro. *Biochem Pharmacol* 48:197–200, 1994.

Rodrigues AD, Yang Z, Chen C, Pray D, Kim S, Sinz M: Is celecoxib an inducer of cytochrome P450 3A4 in subjects carrying the CYP2C9*3 allele? *Clin Pharmacol Ther* 80:298–301, 2006.

Roessner V, Weber A, Becker A, et al.: Decreased serum semicarbazide sensitive aminooxidase (SSAO) activity in patients with major depression. *Prog Neuropsychopharmacol Biol Psychiatry* 30:906–909, 2006.

Rogers SM, Back DJ, Stevenson PJ, Grimmer SF, Orme ML: Paracetamol interaction with oral contraceptive steroids: Increased plasma concentrations of ethinyloestradiol. *Br J Clin Pharmacol* 23:721–725, 1987.

Rosemond MJ, Walsh J: Human carbonyl reduction pathways and a strategy for their study in vitro. *Drug Metab Rev* 36:335–361, 2004.

Rosen LS, Laxa B, Boulos L, et al.: Phase 1 study of TLK286 (Telcyta) administered weekly in advanced malignancies. *Clin Cancer Res* 10:3689–3698, 2004.

Ross D: Functions and distribution of NQO1 in human bone marrow: Potential clues to benzene toxicity. *Chem Biol Interact* 153–154:137–146, 2005.

Rowland-Yeo K, Rostami-Hodjean A, Tucker GT: Abundance of cytochromes P450 in human liver: A meta-analysis. *Br J Clin Pharmacol* 57:687, 2004.

Rumack BH: Acetaminophen misconceptions. *Hepatology* 40:10–15, 2004.

Runge-Morris M, Kocarek TA: Regulation of sulfotransferases by xenobiotic receptors. *Curr Drug Metab* 6:299–307, 2005.

Rushmore TH, Morton MR, Pickett CB: The antioxidant responsive element. Activation by oxidative stress and identification of the DNA consensus sequence required for functional activity. *J Biol Chem* 266:11632–11639, 1991.

Ryan DE, Dixon R, Evans RH, et al.: Rat hepatic cytochrome P-450 isozyme specificity for the metabolism of the steroid sulfate, 5α-androstane-3α,17β-diol-3,17-disulfate. *Arch Biochem Biophys* 233:636–642, 1984.

Sakakibara Y, Suiko M, Pai TG, et al.: Highly conserved mouse and human brain sulfotransferases: Molecular cloning, expression, and functional characterization. *Gene* 285:39–47, 2002.

Sano M, Ernesto C, Thomas RG, et al.: A controlled trial of selegiline, alpha-tocopherol, or both as treatment for Alzheimer's disease. *N Engl J Med* 336:1216–1222, 1997.

Satoh T, Hosokawa M: The mammalian carboxylesterases: From molecules to functions. *Annu Rev Pharmacol Toxicol* 38:257–288, 1998.

Satoh T, Hosokawa M: Structure, function and regulation of carboxylesterases. *Chem Biol Interact* 162:195–211, 2006.

Satoh T, Taylor P, Bosron WF, Sanghani SP, Hosokawa M, La Du BN: Current progress on esterases: From molecular structure to function. *Drug Metab Dispos* 30:488–493, 2002.

Saulter JY, Kurian JR, Trepanier LA, et al.: Unusual dehydroxylation of antimicrobial amidoxime prodrugs by cytochrome b5 and NADH cytochrome b5 reductase. *Drug Metab Dispos* 33:1886–1893, 2005.

Saunders MP, Patterson AV, Harris AL, Stratford IJ: NADPH:cytochrome c (P450) reductase activates tirapazamine (SR4233) to restore hypoxic and oxic cytotoxicity in an aerobic resistant derivative of the A549 lung cancer cell line. *Br J Cancer* 82:651–656, 2000.

Schrag ML, Cui D, Rushmore TH, Shou M, Ma B, Rodrigues AD: Sulfotransferase 1E1 is a low km isoform mediating the 3-*O*-sulfation of ethinyl estradiol. *Drug Metab Dispos* 32:1299–1303, 2004.

Seitz J, Oneta C: Gastrointestinal alcohol dehydrogenase. *Nutr Rev* 56:52–60, 1998.

Senter PD, Marquardt H, Thomas BA, Hammock BD, Frank IS, Svensson HP: The role of rat serum carboxylesterase in the activation of paclitaxel and camptothecin prodrugs. *Cancer Res* 56:1471–1474, 1996.

Seok Seo Y, Keum B, Park S, et al.: Gilbert's syndrome phenotypically expressed as Crigler-Najjar syndrome type II. *Scand J Gastroenterol* 42:540–541, 2007.

Seto Y, Guengerich FP: Partitioning between *N*-dealkylation and *N*-oxygenation in the oxidation of *N*,*N*-dialkylarylamines catalyzed by cytochrome P450 2B1. *J Biol Chem* 268:9986–9997, 1993.

Shi D, Yang J, Yang D, LeCluyse EL, et al.: Anti-influenza prodrug oseltamivir is activated by carboxylesterase human carboxylesterase 1, and the activation is inhibited by antiplatelet agent clopidogrel. *J Pharmacol Exp Ther* 319:1477–1484, 2006.

Shih J, Chen K, Tidd M: Monamine oxidase: From genes to behavior. *Annu Rev Neurosci* 22:197–217, 1999.

Shih P-S, Huang J-D: Pharmacokinetics of midazolam and 1′-hydroxymidazolam in Chinese with different CYP3A5 genotypes. *Drug Metab Dispos* 30:1491–1496, 2002.

Shipkova M, Armstrong VW, Oellerich M, Wieland E: Acyl glucuronide drug metabolites: Toxicological and analytical implications. *Ther Drug Monit* 25:1–16, 2003.

Shiraga T, Niwa T, Ohno Y, Kagayama A: Interindividual variability in 2-hydroxylation, 3-sulfation, and 3-glucuronidation of ethinylestradiol in human liver. *Biol Pharm Bull* 27:1900–1906, 2004.

Shirley MA, Guan X, Kaiser DG, Halstead GW, Baillie TA: Taurine conjugation of ibuprofen in humans and in rat liver in vitro. Relationship to metabolic chiral inversion. *J Pharmacol Exp Ther* 269:1166–1175, 1994.

Sies H, Ketterer B (eds.): *Glutathione Conjugation Mechanisms and Biological Significance.* London: Academic, 1988.

Singh G, Driever PH, Sander JW: Cancer risk in people with epilepsy: The role of antiepileptic drugs. *Brain* 128:7–17, 2005.

Sirot EJ, van der Velden JW, Rentsch K, Eap CB, Baumann P: Therapeutic drug monitoring and pharmacogenetic tests as tools in pharmacovigilance. *Drug Saf* 29:735–768, 2006.

Sládek NE: Human aldehyde dehydrogenases: Potential pathological, pharmacological, and toxicological impact. *J Biochem Mol Toxicol* 17:7–23, 2003.

Smith PA, Sorich MJ, Low LSC, McKinnon RA, Miners JO: Towards integrated ADME prediction: Past, present and future directions for modeling metabolism by UDP-glucuronosyltransferases. *J Mol Graph Model* 22:507–517, 2004.

Sorenson RC, Primo-Parmo SL, Kuo C, Adkins S, Lockridge O, Du BNL: Reconsideration of the catalytic center and mechanism of mammalian paraoxonase/arylesterase. *Proc Natl Acad Sci USA* 92:7187–7191, 1995.

Soucek P, Skjelbred CF, Svendsen M, Kristensen T, Kure EH, Kristensen VN: Single-track sequencing for genotyping of multiple SNPs in the *N*-acetyltransferase 1 (NAT1) gene. *BMC Biotechnol* 4:28, 2004.

Souto JC, Blanco-Vaca F, Soria JM, et al.: A genomewide exploration suggests a new candidate gene at chromosome 11q23 as the major determinant of plasma homocysteine levels: Results from the GAIT project. *Am J Hum Genet* 76:925–933, 2005.

Spahn-Langguth H, Benet L: Acyl glucuronides revisited: Is the glucuronidation process a toxification as well as a detoxification mechanism? *Drug Metab Rev* 24:5–47, 1992.

Spiecker M, Liao J: Cytochrome P450 epoxygenase CYP2J2 and the risk of coronary artery disease. *Trends Cardiovasc Med* 16:204–208, 2006.

Stanley L, Horsburgh B, Ross J, Scheer N, Roland Wolf C: PXR and CAR: Nuclear receptors which play a pivotal role in drug disposition and chemical toxicity. *Drug Metab Rev* 38:515–597, 2006.

Stierlin H, Faigle JW: Biotransformation of diclofenac sodium (Voltaren) in animals and in man. II. Quantitative determination of the unchanged drug and principal phenolic metabolites, in urine and bile. *Xenobiotica* 9:611–621, 1979.

Stierlin H, Faigle JW, Sallmann A, *et al.*: Biotransformation of diclofenac sodium (Voltaren) in animals and in man. I. Isolation and identification of principal metabolites. *Xenobiotica* 9:601–610, 1979.

Stone AN, Mackenzie PI, Galetin A, Houston JB, Miners JO: Isoform selectivity and kinetics of morphine 3- and 6-glucuronidation by human UDP-glucuronosyltransferases: Evidence for atypical glucuronidation kinetics by UGT2B7. *Drug Metab Dispos* 31:1086–1089, 2003.

Strange RC, Jones PW, Fryer AA: Glutathione S-transferase: Genetics and role in toxicology. *Toxicol Lett* 112–113:357–363, 2000.

Strelevitz TJ, Foti RS, Fisher MB: In vivo use of the P450 inactivator 1-aminobenzotriazole in the rat: Varied dosing route to elucidate gut and liver contributions to first-pass and systemic clearance. *J Pharm Sci* 95:1334–1341, 2006.

Subramanyam B, Woolf T, Castagnoli NJ: Studies on the in vitro conversion of haloperidol to a potentially neurotoxic pyridinium metabolite. *Chem Res Toxicol* 4:123–128, 1991.

Sugihara K, Kitamura S, Tatsumi K: Involvement of mammalian liver cytosols and aldehyde oxidase in reductive metabolism of zonisamide. *Drug Metab Dispos* 24:199–202, 1996.

Sugiura M, Iwasaki K, Kato R: Reduction of tertiary amine N-oxides by liver microsomal cytochrome P-450. *Mol Pharmacol* 12:322–334, 1976.

Sugiura M, Kato R: Reduction of tertiary amine N-oxides by rat liver mitochondria. *J Pharmacol Exp Ther* 200:25–32, 1977.

Sun H, Liu L, Pang KS: Increased estrogen sulfation of estradiol 17beta-D-glucuronide in metastatic tumor rat livers. *J Pharmacol Exp Ther* 319:818–831, 2006.

Tafazoli S, O'Brien PJ: Peroxidases: A role in the metabolism and side effects of drugs. *Drug Discov Today* 10:617–625, 2005.

Tang BK, Carro-Ciampi G: A method for the study of N-glucosidation in vitro—Amobarbital-N-glucoside formation in incubations with human liver. *Biochem Pharmacol* 29:2085–2088, 1980.

Tang C, Lin JH, Lu AYH: Metabolism-based drug-drug interactions: What determines individual variability in cytochrome P450 induction? *Drug Metab Dispos* 33:603–613, 2005.

Tang C, Ma B: Glycosidation of an endothelin ETA receptor antagonist and diclofenac in human liver microsomes: Aglycone-dependent UDP-sugar selectivity. *Drug Metab Dispos* 33:1796–1802, 2005.

Tang M, Mukundan M, Yang J, *et al.*: Antiplatelet agents aspirin and clopidogrel are hydrolyzed by distinct carboxylesterases, and clopidogrel is transesterificated in the presence of ethyl alcohol. *J Pharmacol Exp Ther* 319:1467–1476, 2006.

Terao M, Kurosaki M, Demontis S, Zanotta S, Garattini E: Isolation and characterization of the human aldehyde oxidase gene: Conservation of intron/exon boundaries with the xanthine oxidoreductase gene indicates a common origin. *Biochem J* 332:383–393, 1998.

Thomas JA: "Black Box" warning labels and drug withdrawals. *Toxicol Appl Pharmacol* 183:81–82, 2002.

Thompson MA, Moon E, Kim UJ, Xu J, Siciliano MJ, Weinshilboum RM: Human indolethylamine N-methyltransferase: cDNA cloning and expression, gene cloning, and chromosomal localization. *Genomics* 61:285–297, 1999.

Tijet N, Boutros PC, Moffat ID, Okey AB, Tuomisto J, Pohjanvirta R: Aryl hydrocarbon receptor regulates distinct dioxin-dependent and dioxin-independent gene batteries. *Mol Pharmacol* 69:140–153, 2006.

Tinguely JN, Wermuth B: Identification of the reactive cysteine residue (Cys227) in human carbonyl reductase. *Eur J Biochem* 260:9–14, 1999.

Tirona RG, Kim RB: Nuclear receptors and drug disposition gene regulation. *J Pharm Sci* 94:1169–1186, 2005.

Tiwawech D, Srivatanakul P, Karalak A, Ishida T: Cytochrome P450 2A6 polymorphism in nasopharyngeal carcinoma. *Cancer Lett* 241:135–141, 2006.

Tobin P, Clarke S, Seale JP, *et al.*: The in vitro metabolism of irinotecan (CPT-11) by carboxylesterase and β-glucuronidase in human colorectal tumours. *Brit J Clin Pharmacol* 62:122–129, 2006.

Toide K, Terauchi Y, Fujii T, Yamazaki H, Kamataki T: Uridine diphosphate sugar-selective conjugation of an aldose reductase inhibitor (AS-3201) by UDP-glucuronosyltransferase 2B subfamily in human liver microsomes. *Biochem Pharmacol* 67:1269–1278, 2004.

Townsend DM, Tew KD: The role of glutathione-S-transferase in anti-cancer drug resistance. *Oncogene* 22:7369–7375, 2003.

Tremaine LM, Stroh JG, Ronfeld RA: Characterization of a carbamic acid ester glucuronide of the secondary amine sertraline. *Drug Metab Dispos* 17:58–63, 1989.

Tsuchiya Y, Nakajima M, Takagi S, Taniya T, Yokoi T: MicroRNA regulates the expression of human cytochrome P450 1B1. *Cancer Res* 66:9090–9098, 2006.

Tucker GT: Clinical implications of genetic polymorphism in drug metabolism. *J Pharm Pharmacol* 46(Suppl 1):417–424, 1994.

Tucker GT, Houston JB, Huang SM: Optimizing drug development: strategies to assess drug metabolism/transporter interaction potential—Toward a consensus. *Pharm Res* 18:1071–1080, 2001.

Tukey RH, Strassburg C: Human UDP-glucuronosyltransferases: metabolism, expression, and disease. *Annu Rev Pharmacol Toxicol* 40:581–616, 2000.

U.S. Food and Drug Administration CfDEaR Guidance for Industry: *Drug Interaction Studies—Study Design, Data Analysis, and Implications for Dosing and Labeling.* Food and Drug Administration, Rockville, MD, 2006, pp 1–55.

Uchaipichat V, Mackenzie PI, Elliot DJ, Miners JO: Selectivity of substrate (trifluoperazine) and inhibitor (amitriptyline, androsterone, canrenoic acid, hecogenin, phenylbutazone, quinidine, quinine, and sulfinpyrazone) "probes" for human UDP-glucuronosyl transferases. *Drug Metab Dispos* 34:449–456, 2006.

Uetrecht J: Prediction of a new drug's potential to cause idiosyncratic reactions. *Curr Opin Drug Discov Devel* 4:55–59, 2001.

Umulis DM, Gurmen NM, Singh P, Fogler HS: A physiologically based model for ethanol and acetaldehyde metabolism in human beings. *Alcohol* 35:3–12, 2005.

van Kuilenburg A, Meinsma R, van Gennip A: Pyrimidine degradation defects and severe 5-fluorouracil toxicity. *Nucleoside Nucleotide Nucleic Acids* 23:1371–1375, 2004.

Vashishtha SC, Hawes EM, McKay G, McCann DJ: Quaternary ammonium-linked glucuronidation of 1-substituted imidazoles: Studies of human UDP-glucuronosyltransferases involved and substrate specificities. *Drug Metab Dispos* 29:1290–1295, 2001.

Vasiliou V, Pappa A, Estey T: Role of human aldehyde dehydrogenases in endobiotic and xenobiotic metabolism. *Drug Metab Rev* 36:279–299, 2004.

Vatsis KP, Weber WW, Bell DA, *et al.*: Nomenclature for N-acetyltransferases. *Pharmacogenetics* 5:1–17, 1995.

Walgren JL, Mitchell MD, Thompson DC: Role of metabolism in drug-induced idiosyncratic hepatotoxicity. *Crit Rev Toxicol* 35:325–361, 2005.

Walton MI, Wolf CR, Workman P: The role of cytochrome P450 and cytochrome P450 reductase in the reductive bioactivation of the novel benzotriazine di-N-oxide hypoxic cytotoxin 3-amino-1,2,4-benzotriazine-1,4-dioxide (SR 4233, WIN 59075) by mouse liver. *Biochem Pharmacol* 44:251–259, 1992.

Wang C, Bammler TK, Guo Y, Kelly EJ, Eaton DL: Mu-class GSTs are responsible for aflatoxin b1-8,9-epoxide-conjugating activity in the nonhuman primate Macaca fascicularis liver. *Toxicol Sci* 56:26–36, 2000.

Wang EY, Gao H, Salter-Cid L, *et al.*: Design, synthesis, and biological evaluation of semicarbazide-sensitive amine oxidase (SSAO) inhibitors with anti-inflammatory activity. *J Med Chem* 49:2166–2173, 2006a.

Wang J, Davis M, Li F, Azam F, Scatina J, Talaat RE: A novel approach for predicting acyl glucuronide reactivity via Schiff base formation: Development of rapidly formed peptide adducts for LC/MS/MS measurements. *Chem Res Toxicol* 17:1206–1216, 2004.

Wang L, Nguyen TV, McLaughlin RW, Sikkink LA, Ramirez-Alvarado M, Weinshilboum RM: Human thiopurine *S*-methyltransferase pharmacogenetics: Variant allozyme misfolding and aggresome formation. *Proc Natl Acad Sci USA* 102:9394–9399, 2005a.

Wang LQ, James MO: Inhibition of sulfotransferases by xenobiotics. *Curr Drug Metab* 7:83–104, 2006.

Wang MZ, Saulter JY, Usuki E, *et al.*: CYP4F enzymes are the major enzymes in human liver microsomes that catalyze the *O*-demethylation of the antiparasitic prodrug db289 [2,5-bis(4-amidinophenyl)furan-bis-*O*-methylamidoxime]. *Drug Metab Dispos* 34:1985–1994, 2006b.

Wang S-L, He X-Y, Hong J-Y: Human cytochrome P450 2S1: Lack of activity in the metabolic activation of several cigarette smoke carcinogens and an the metabolism of nicotine. *Drug Metab Dispos* 33:336–340, 2005b.

Wardman P, Dennis MF, Everett SA, Patel KB, Stratford MR, Tracy M: Radicals from one-electron reduction of nitro compounds, aromatic *N*-oxides and quinones: The kinetic basis for hypoxia-selective, bioreductive drugs. *Biochem Soc Symp* 61:171–194, 1995.

Watkins PB: Noninvasive tests of CYP3A enzymes. *Pharmacogenetics* 4:171, 1994.

Weinshilboum R: Methyltransferase pharmacogenetics. *Pharmacol Ther* 43:77–90, 1989.

Weinshilboum R: Sulfotransferase pharmacogenetics, in Kalow W (ed.): *Pharmacogenetics of Drug Metabolism*. New York: Pergamon, 1992a, pp. 227–242.

Weinshilboum R, Otterness D, Szumlanski C: Methylation pharmacogenetics: Catechol *O*-methyltransferase, thiopurine methyltransferase, and histamine *N*-methyltransferase. *Annu Rev Pharmacol Toxicol* 39:19–52, 1999.

Weinshilboum RM: Methylation pharmacogenetics: Thiopurine methyltransferase as a model system. *Xenobiotica* 22:1055–1071, 1992b.

Weinshilboum RM: Pharmacogenomics: Catechol *O*-methyltransferase to thiopurine *S*-methyltransferase. 2006.

Weinshilboum RM, Otterness DM, Aksoy IA, Wood TC, Her C, Raftogianis RB: Sulfation and sulfotransferases 1: Sulfotransferase molecular biology: cDNAs and genes. *FASEB J* 11:3–14, 1997.

Westlind-Johnsson A, Malmebo S, Johansson A, Otter C, Andersson TB, Johansson I, Edwards RJ, Boobis AR, Ingelman-Sundberg M: Comparative analysis of CYP3A expression in human liver suggests only a minor role for CYP3A5 in drug metabolism. *Drug Metab Dispos* 31:755–761, 2003.

Whalen R, Boyer TD: Human glutathione *S*-transferases. *Semin Liver Dis* 18:345–358, 1998.

Whitcomb D, Block G: Association of acetaminophen hepatoxicity with fasting and ethanol use. *JAMA* 272:1845–1850, 1994.

Whitfield JB, Pang D, Bucholz KK, Madden PA, Heath AC, Statham DJ, Martin NG: Monoamine oxidase: Associations with alcohol dependence, smoking and other measures of psychopathology. *Psychol Med* 30:443–454, 2000.

Wilkinson GR, Guengerich FP, Branch RA: Genetic polymorphism of S-mephenytoin hydroxylation. *Pharmacol Ther* 43:53–76, 1989.

Williams AC, Cartwright LS, Ramsden DB: Parkinson's disease: The first common neurological disease due to auto-intoxication? *QJM* 98:215–226, 2005.

Williams GM, Iatropoulos MJ: Alteration of liver cell function and proliferation: Differentiation between adaptation and toxicity. *Toxicologic Pathology* 30:41–53, 2002.

Williams JA, Cook J, Hurst SI: A significant drug-metabolizing role for CYP3A5? *Drug Metab Dispos* 31:1526–1530, 2003a.

Williams JA, Hurst SI, Bauman J, *et al.*: Reaction phenotyping in drug discovery: moving forward with confidence? *Curr Drug Metab* 4:527–534, 2003b.

Williams JA, Hyland R, Jones BC, *et al.*: Drug-drug interactions for UDP-glucuronosyltransferase substrates: a pharmacokinetic explanation for typically observed low exposure (AUCi/AUC) ratios. *Drug Metab Dispos* 32:1201–1208, 2004.

Williams RT: *Detoxication Mechanisms; the Metabolism and Detoxication of Drugs, Toxic Substances, and Other Organic Compounds*, 2nd edn. New York: Wiley, 1959.

Winter HR, Unadkat JD: Identification of cytochrome P450 and arylamine *N*-acetyltransferase isoforms involved in sulfadiazine metabolism. *Drug Metab Dispos* 33:969–976, 2005.

Wood TC, Johnson KL, Naylor S, Weinshilboum RM: Cefazolin administration and 2-methyl-1,3,4-thiadiazole-5-thiol in human tissue: Possible relationship to hypoprothrombinemia. *Drug Metab Dispos* 30:1123–1128, 2002.

Wood TC, Salavagionne OE, Mukherjee B, *et al.*: Human arsenic methyltransferase (AS3MT) pharmacogenetics: Gene resequencing and functional genomics studies. *J Biol Chem* 281:7364–7373, 2006.

Wu Z-L, Sohl CD, Shimada T, Guengerich FP: Recombinant enzymes overexpressed in bacteria show broad catalytic specificity of human cytochrome P450 2W1 and limited activity of human cytochrome P450 2S1. *Mol Pharmacol* 69:2007–2014, 2006.

Xu Y, Hashizume T, Shuhart MC, *et al.*: Intestinal and hepatic CYP3A4 catalyze hydroxylation of 1α,25-dihydroxyvitamin D3: Implications for drug-induced osteomalacia. *Mol Pharmacol* 69:56–65, 2006.

Yamada R, Ymamoto K: Recent findings on genes associated with inflammatory disease. *Mutat Res* 573:136–151, 2005.

Yan B, Yang D, Brady M, Parkinson A: Rat kidney carboxylesterase. Cloning, sequencing, cellular localization, and relationship to rat liver hydrolase. *J Biol Chem* 269:29688–29696, 1994.

Yao K-S, Hageboutros A, Ford P, O'Dwyer PJ: Involvement of activator protein-1 and nuclear factor-kappa B transcription factors in the control of the DT-diaphorase expression induced by mitomycin C treatment. *Mol Pharmacol* 51:422–430, 1997.

Yates CR, Zhang W, Song P, *et al.*: Effect of CYP3A5 genotype on cyclosporine disposition: A pilot study. *Clin Pharmacol Ther* 71(2):2, 2002.

Yoshida A, Rzhetsky A, Hsu L, Chang C: Human aldehyde dehydrogenase gene family. *Eur J Biochem* 251:549–557, 1998.

Yoshioka H, Kasai N, Ikushiro S, *et al.*: Enzymatic properties of human CYP2W1 expressed in Escherichia coli. *Biochem Biophys Res Commun* 345:169–174, 2006.

Zhang J, Cashman JR: Quantitative analysis of FMO gene mRNA levels in human tissues. *Drug Metab Dispos* 34:19–26, 2006.

Zhang Y, Talalay P, Cho C, Posner GH: A major inducer of anticarcinogenic protective enzymes from broccoli: Isolation and elucidation of structure. *Proc Natl Acad Sci USA* 89:2399–2403, 1992.

Zheng H, Webber S, Zeevi A, *et al.*: Tacrolimus dosing in pediatric heart transplant patients is related to CYP3A5 and *MDR1* gene polymorphisms. *Am J Transplant* 3:477–483, 2003.

Zhou C, Assem M, Tay JC, *et al.*: Steroid and xenobiotic receptor and vitamin D receptor crosstalk mediates CYP24 expression and drug-induced osteomalacia. *J Clin Invest* 116:1703–1712, 2006a.

Zhou C, Tabb MM, Nelson EL, *et al.*: Mutual repression between steroid and xenobiotic receptor and NF-kappaB signaling pathways links xenobiotic metabolism and inflammation. *J Clin Invest* 116:2280–2289, 2006b.

Zhu BT, Liehr JG: Inhibition of the catechol-*O*-methyltransferase-catalyzed *O*-methylation of 2- and 4-hydroxyestradiol by catecholamines: Implications for the mechanism of estrogen-induced carcinogenesis. *Arch Biochem Biophys* 304:248–256, 1993.

Ziegler DM: Recent studies on the structure and function of multisubstrate flavin-containing monooxygenases. *Annu Rev Pharmacol Toxicol* 33:179–199, 1993.

Ziegler DM: An overview of the mechanism, substrate specificities, and structure of FMOs. *Drug Metab Rev* 34:503–511, 2002.

Zineh I, Beitelshees AL, Gaedigk A, *et al.*: Pharmacokinetics and CYP2D6 genotypes do not predict metoprolol adverse events or efficacy in hypertension. *Clin Pharmacol Ther* 76:536–544, 2004.

CHAPTER 7

TOXICOKINETICS

Danny D. Shen

INTRODUCTION

Toxicokinetics is the quantitative study of the movement of an exogenous chemical from its entry into the body, through its distribution to organs and tissues via the blood circulation, and to its final disposition by way of biotransformation and excretion. The basic kinetic concepts for the absorption, distribution, metabolism, and excretion of chemicals in the body system initially came from the study of drug actions or pharmacology; hence, this area of study is traditionally referred to as pharmacokinetics. Toxicokinetics represents extension of kinetic principles to the study of toxicology and encompasses applications ranging from the study of adverse drug effects to investigations on how disposition kinetics of exogenous chemicals derived from either natural or environmental sources (generally refer to as xenobiotics) govern their deleterious effects on organisms including humans.

The study of toxicokinetics relies on mathematical description or modeling of the time course of toxicant disposition in the whole organism. The classic approach to describing the kinetics of drugs is to represent the body as a system of one or two compartments even though the compartments do not have exact correspondence to anatomical structures or physiologic processes. These empirical compartmental models are almost always developed to describe the kinetics of toxicants in readily accessible body fluids (mainly blood) or excreta (e.g., urine, stool, and breath). This approach is particularly suited for human studies, which typically do not afford organ or tissue data. In such applications, extravascular distribution, which does not require detail elucidation, can be represented simply by lumped compartments. An alternate and newer approach, physiologically based toxicokinetic modeling attempts to portray the body as an elaborate system of discrete tissue or organ compartments that are interconnected via the circulatory system. Physiologically based models are capable of describing a chemical's movements in body tissues or regions of toxicological interest. It also allows a pri-

ori predictions of how changes in specific physiological processes affect the disposition kinetics of the toxicant (e.g., changes in respiratory status on pulmonary absorption and exhalation of a volatile compound) and the extrapolation of the kinetic model across animal species to humans.

It should be emphasized that there is no inherent contradiction between the classic and physiologic approaches. The choice of modeling approach depends on the application context, the available data, and the intended utility of the resultant model. Classic compartmental model, as will be shown, requires assumptions that limit its application. In comparison, physiologic models can predict tissue concentrations; however, it requires much more data input and often the values of the required parameters cannot be estimated accurately or precisely, which introduces uncertainty in its prediction.

We begin with a description of the classic approach to toxicokinetic modeling, which offers an introduction to the basic kinetic concepts for toxicant absorption, distribution, and elimination. This will be followed by a brief review of the physiologic approach to toxicokinetic modeling that is intended to illustrate the construction and application of these elaborate models.

CLASSIC TOXICOKINETICS

Ideally, quantification of xenobiotic concentration at the site of toxic insult or injury would afford the most direct information on exposure–response relationship and dynamics of response over time. Serial sampling of relevant biological tissues following dosing can be cost-prohibitive during in vivo studies in animals and is nearly impossible to perform in human exposure studies. The most accessible and simplest means of gathering information on absorption, distribution, metabolism, and elimination of a compound is to examine the time course of blood or plasma toxicant concentration over time. If one assumes that the concentration

One Compartment Model

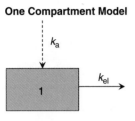

Two Compartment Model

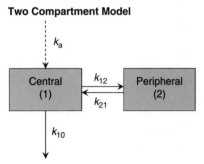

Figure 7-1. Compartmental toxicokinetic models.

Symbols for one-compartment model: k_a is the first-order absorption rate constant, and k_{el} is the first-order elimination rate constant. Symbols for two-compartment model: k_a is the first-order absorption rate constant into the central compartment (1), k_{10} is the first-order elimination rate constant from the central compartment (1), k_{12} and k_{21} are the first-order rate constants for distribution between central (1) and peripheral (2) compartment.

of a chemical in blood or plasma is in some describable dynamic equilibrium with its concentrations in tissues, then changes in plasma toxicant concentration should reflect changes in tissue toxicant concentrations and relatively simple kinetic models can adequately describe the behavior of that toxicant in the body system.

Classic toxicokinetic models typically consist of a central compartment representing blood and tissues that the toxicant has ready access and equilibration is achieved almost immediately following its introduction, along with one or more peripheral compartments that represent tissues in slow equilibration with the toxicant in blood (Fig. 7-1). Once introduced into the central compartment, the toxicant distributes between central and peripheral compartments. Elimination of the toxicant, through biotransformation and/or excretion, is usually assumed to occur from the central compartment, which should comprise the rapidly perfused visceral organs capable of eliminating the toxicant (e.g., kidneys, lungs, and liver). The obvious advantage of compartmental toxicokinetic models is that they do not require information on tissue physiology or anatomic structure. These models are useful in predicting the toxicant concentrations in blood at different doses, in establishing the time course of accumulation of the toxicant, either in its parent form or as biotransformed products during continuous or episodic exposures, in defining concentration–response (vs. dose–response) relationships, and in guiding the choice of effective dose and design of dosing regimen in animal toxicity studies (Rowland and Tozer, 1995).

One-Compartment Model

The most straightforward toxicokinetic assessment entails quantification of the blood or more commonly plasma concentrations of a toxicant at several time points after a bolus intravenous (iv) injection.

Often, the data obtained fall on a straight line when they are plotted as the logarithms of plasma concentrations versus time; the kinetics of the toxicant is said to conform to a one-compartment model (Fig. 7-2). Mathematically, this means that the decline in plasma concentration over time profile follows a simple exponential pattern as represented by the following mathematical expressions:

$$C = C_0 \times e^{-k_{el} \times t} \tag{7-1}$$

or its logarithmic transform

$$\text{Log } C = \text{Log } C_0 - \frac{k_{el} \times t}{2.303} \tag{7-2}$$

where C is the plasma toxicant concentration at time t after injection, C_0 is the plasma concentration achieved immediately after injection, and k_{el} is the exponential constant or elimination rate constant with dimensions of reciprocal time (e.g., min^{-1} or hr^{-1}). The constant 2.303 in Equation (7-2) is needed to convert natural logarithm to base-10 logarithm. It can be seen from Equation (7-2) that the elimination rate constant can be determined from the slope of the log C versus time plot (i.e., $k_{el} = -2.303 \times$ slope).

The elimination rate constant k_{el} represents the overall elimination of the toxicant, which includes biotransformation, exhalation, and/or excretion pathways. When elimination of a toxicant from the body occurs in an exponential fashion, it signifies a first-order process; that is, the rate of elimination at any time is proportional to the amount of toxicant remaining in the body (i.e., body load) at that time. This means that following an iv bolus injection, the absolute rate of elimination (e.g., mg of toxicant eliminated per minute) continually changes over time. Shortly after introduction of the dose, the rate of toxicant elimination will be at the highest. As elimination proceeds and body load of the toxicant is reduced, the elimination rate will decline in step. As a corollary, it also means that at multiple levels of the toxicant dose, the absolute rate of elimination at corresponding times will be proportionately more rapid at the higher doses. This mode of elimination offers an obvious advantage for the organism to deal with increasing exposure to a toxicant. First-order kinetics occur at toxicant concentrations that are not sufficiently high to saturate either metabolic or transport processes.

In view of the nature of first-order kinetics, k_{el} is said to represent a constant fractional rate of elimination. Thus, if the elimination rate constant is, for example, 0.3 h^{-1}, the percentage of plasma concentration remaining in the body ($C/C_0 \times 100$) and the percentage of the dose eliminated from the body after 1 hour, i.e., $1 - (C/C_0 \times 100)$, are 74% and 26%, respectively, regardless of the dose administered (Table 7-1). The percentage of the total dose eliminated at 1 hour is said to be independent of dose. It also means that the fractional rate of elimination of the toxicant remains constant over time after iv injection or any acute exposure. Because a constant percentage of toxicant present in the body is eliminated over a given time period regardless of dose or the starting concentration, it is more intuitive and convenient to refer to an elimination half-life ($T_{1/2}$); that is, the time it takes for the original blood or plasma concentration to fall by 50% or to eliminate 50% of the original body load. By substituting $C/C_0 = 0.5$ into Equation (7-1), we obtain the following relationship between $T_{1/2}$ and k_{el}:

$$T_{1/2} = \frac{0.693}{k_{el}} \tag{7-3}$$

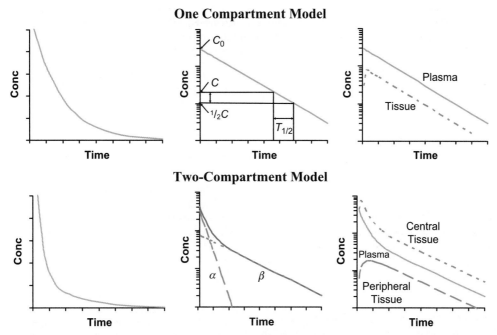

Figure 7-2. Plasma concentration versus time curves of toxicants exhibiting kinetic behavior conforming to a one-compartment model (top row) and a two-compartment model (bottom row) following intravenous bolus injection. Left and middle panels show the plots on a rectilinear and semilogarithmic scale, respectively. Right panels illustrate the relationship between tissue (dash lines) and plasma (solid line) concentration over time.

The right panel for the one-compartment model shows a typical tissue with a higher concentration than plasma. Note that tissue concentration can be higher, nearly the same, or lower than plasma concentration. Tissue concentration peaks almost immediately, and thereafter declines in parallel with plasma concentration. The right panel for the two-compartment model shows typical tissues associated with the central (1) and peripheral (2) compartments as represented by short and long dash lines, respectively. For tissues associated with the central compartment, their concentrations decline in parallel with plasma. For tissues associated with peripheral compartment, toxicant concentration rises, while plasma concentration declines rapidly during the initial phase; it then reaches a peak and eventually declines in parallel with plasma in the terminal phase. Elimination rate constant k_{el} for one-compartment model and the terminal exponential rate constant β are determined from the slope of the log-linear concentration versus time curve. Half-life ($T_{1/2}$) is the time required for plasma toxicant concentration to decrease by one-half. C_0 is the concentration of a toxicant for a one compartment model at $t = 0$ determined by extrapolating the log-linear concentration time curve to the Y-axis.

where 0.693 is the natural logarithm of 2. Simple calculations reveals that it would take about four half-lives for >90% (exactly 93.8%) of the dose to be eliminated, and about seven half-lives for >99% (exactly 99.2%) elimination. Thus, given the elimination $T_{1/2}$ of a toxicant, the length of time it takes for near complete washout of a toxicant after discontinuation of its exposure can easily be estimated. As will be seen in next section, the concept of $T_{1/2}$ is applicable to toxicants that exhibit multi-exponential kinetics.

We can infer from the mono-exponential decline of blood or plasma concentration that the toxicant equilibrates very rapidly between blood and the various tissues relative to the rate of elimination, such that extravascular equilibration is achieved nearly instantaneously and maintained thereafter. Depiction of the body system by a one-compartment model does not mean that the concentration of the toxicant is the same throughout the body, but it does assume that the changes that occur in the plasma concentration reflect proportional changes in tissue toxicant concentrations (Fig. 7-2 upper, right panel). In other words, toxicant concentrations in tissues are expected to decline with the same elimination rate constant or $T_{1/2}$ as in plasma.

Two-Compartment Model

After rapid iv administration of some toxicants, the semi-logarithmic plot of plasma concentration versus time does not yield a straight line but a curve that implies more than one dispositional phase (Fig. 7-2). In these instances, it takes some time for the toxicant to be taken up into certain tissue groupings, and to then reach an equilibration with the concentration in plasma; hence, a multi-compartmental model is needed for the description of its kinetics in the body (Fig. 7-1). The concept of tissue groupings with distinct uptake and equilibration rates of toxicant becomes apparent when we consider the factors that govern the uptake of a lipid-soluble, organic toxicant. Table 7-2 presents data on the volume and blood perfusion rate of various organs and tissues in a standard size human. From these data and assuming reasonable partitioning ratios of a typical lipid-soluble, organic compound in the various tissue types, we can estimate the uptake equilibration half-times of the toxicant in each organ or tissue region during constant, continuous exposure. The results suggest that the tissues can be grouped into rapid-equilibrating visceral organs, moderately slow-equilibrating lean body tissues (mainly skeletal muscle), and very slow-equilibrating body fat; these

Table 7-1

Elimination of a Toxicant that Follows First-Order Kinetics ($k_{el} = 0.3$ h^{-1}) by 1 Hour After IV Administration at Four Different Dose Levels

DOSE (mg)	TOXICANT REMAINING (mg)	TOXICANT ELIMINATED (mg)	TOXICANT ELIMINATED (% of dose)
10	7.4	2.6	26
30	22	8	26
90	67	23	26
250	185	65	26

groupings give rise to three distinct uptake phases; that is, half-times of <2 minutes for the rapid-equilibrating tissues, several tens of minutes for the moderately slow-equilibrating lean body tissues, and hours for the very slow-equilibrating body fat. By inference, three distinct phases of washout should also be evident following a brief exposure to the toxicant, such as after a bolus iv injection. The relative prominence of these distributional phases will vary depending on the average lipid solubility of the toxicant in each tissue grouping and any other sequestration and removal mechanisms of a toxicant in particular tissues (e.g., tight binding to tissue proteins, active influx into, or efflux transport out of the tissue cell types), as well as the competing influence of elimination from the visceral organs. For example, very rapid metabolism or excretion at the visceral organs would limit distribution into the slow or very slow tissue groupings. Also, there are times when equilibration rates of a toxicant into visceral organs overlaps with lean body tissues, such that the distribution kinetics of a toxicant into these two tissue groupings become indistinct with respect to the exponential decline of plasma concentration, in which case two instead of three tissue groupings may be observed. The concept of tissue groupings with respect to uptake or washout kinetics serves to justify the seemingly simplistic, yet pragmatic, mathematical description of extravascular distribution by the classic two- or three-compartment models.

Plasma concentration-time profile of a toxicant that exhibits multi-compartmental kinetics can be characterized by multi-exponential equations. For example, a two-compartment model can be represented by the following bi-exponential equation.

$$C = A \times e^{-\alpha \times t} + B \times e^{-\beta \times t} \tag{7-4}$$

where A and B are coefficients in units of toxicant concentration, and α and β are the respective exponential constants for the initial and terminal phases in units of reciprocal time. The initial (α) phase is often referred to as the distribution phase, and terminal (β) phase as the post-distributional or elimination phase. The lower, middle panel of Fig. 7-2 shows a graphical resolution of the two exponential phases from the plasma concentration-time curve. It should be noted that the α constant is the slope of the residual log linear plot and not the initial slope of the decline in the observed plasma toxicant concentration; that is, the initial rate of decline in plasma concentration approximates, but is not exactly equal, the α rate constant in Equation (7-4).

It should be noted that distribution into and out of the tissues and elimination of the toxicant are ongoing at all times; that is, elimination does occur during the "distribution" phase, and distribution between compartments is still ongoing during the "elimination" phase. As illustrated in Fig. 7-3, the dynamics of a

Table 7-2

Prediction of Equilibration Half-Times for Tissues in the Groupings of Highly Perfused Visceral Tissues, Poorly Perfused Lean Tissues, and Adipose Tissues for a Lipid-Soluble, Organic Toxicant with Assumed Typical Tissue-to-Blood Partitioning Ratios (P)[a]

GROUPING	TISSUE	PERFUSION (L/min)[b]	VOLUME (L)[b]	EQUILIBRATION $T_{1/2}$ (min)[c]
Highly perfused viceral tissues, $P = 1$	Heart	0.20	0.28	0.97
	Lungs	5.0	1.1	0.15
	Liver, Gut	1.4	2.8	1.4
	Kidneys	1.1	0.35	0.22
	Brain	0.70	1.4	1.4
Poorly perfused tissues, $P = 0.5$	Muscle (resting)	0.75	30	14
	Skin (cool weather)	0.30	7.7	9.0
Adipose tissue, $P = 5$	—	0.20	14	243

[a]Adapted from Rowland and Tozer (1995).

[b]Data taken from the compilation of Rowland and Tozer (1995), Table 10-1 on p. 138.

[c]Equilibration half-time is the predicted time it takes to achieve 50% of the eventual equilibrated concentration in a tissue when arterial toxicant concentration is held constant and assuming that distribution is perfusion rate-limited. It is calculated by $0.693 \times (V/Q)$, where Q = blood perfusion rate of the tissue, and V = tissue volume.

Note that the equilibration half-times for the highly perfused visceral tissues are predicted to be very short, <2 min. The equilibration half-times for poorly perfused lean tissues are estimated to be around 10–20 min. The equilibration half-time predicted for fat is the order of at least several hours. This tissue grouping in equilibration kinetics gives rise to multiphasic toxicokinetics that are describable by two or three compartment models.

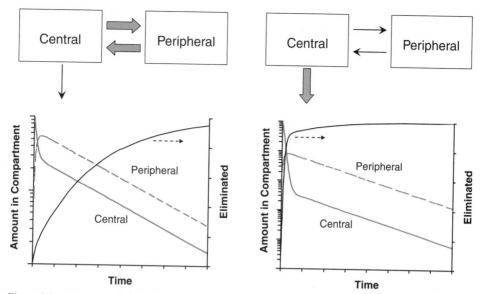

Figure 7-3. *Effects of interplay between kinetics of distribution and elimination processes on time course of exchange between body compartments and elimination from the body for toxicants whose disposition conforms to a two-compartment model.*

Left panel depicts the more common scenario of rapid distribution between compartments relative to elimination, in which case elimination from the body occurs largely during the terminal phase when a dynamic equilibrium between the central and peripheral compartment has been reached. Accordingly, half-life of the terminal phase is an appropriate measure of elimination. Right panel depicts the scenario of very slow distribution relative to elimination, in which case a substantial (>90% of dose) loss of toxicant occurs during the initial phase. The terminal phase reflects the slow redistribution of the toxicant sequestered in the peripheral site to the central site where it can be eliminated (i.e., washout is rate-limited by redistribution). Under this scenario, the initial phase reflects elimination kinetics, whereas the terminal phase reflects tissue distribution kinetics. (Adapted from Tozer and Rowland, 2006.)

multi-compartmental system is such that the governing factor, that is, be it inter-compartmental distribution or elimination, for each of the phases depends on the relative magnitude of the rate constants for inter-compartmental exchange and the elimination process. In the usual case, that of rapid distribution and relatively slow elimination (left panel of Fig. 7-3), the initial rapid phase indeed reflects extravascular distribution, and the later, slow phase reflects elimination after a dynamic equilibration between tissue and blood is attained. There are cases where distribution into some tissue group is much slower than elimination. Then, the initial phase is governed largely by elimination, and the later phase reflects the slow redistribution of the toxicant from the tissues associated with the peripheral compartment to the central compartment, where it is eliminated (i.e., washout in the terminal phase is rate-limited by redistribution from the peripheral compartment). The aminoglycoside antibiotic gentamicin is a case in point (Schentag and Jusko, 1977). Following an iv injection of gentamicin in patients with normal renal function, serum gentamicin concentration exhibits biphasic kinetics. Serum concentration of gentamicin initially falls very quickly with a half-life of around 2 hours; a slow terminal phase does not emerge until serum concentration has fallen to less than 10% of initial concentration. The terminal half-life of serum gentamicin is in the range of 4 to 7 days. This protracted terminal half-life reflects the slow turnover of gentamicin sequestered in the kidneys. In fact, repeated administration of gentamicin leads to accumulation of gentamicin in the kidneys, which is a risk factor for its nephrotoxicity. Because of the complication arising from the interplay of distribution and elimination kinetics, it has been recommended that multiphasic dis-

position should be simply described as consisting of early and late or rapid and slow phases; mechanistic labels of distribution and elimination should be applied with some caution. Lastly, the initial phase may last for only a few minutes or for hours. Whether multiphasic kinetics becomes apparent depends to some extent on how often and when the early blood samples are obtained, and on the relative difference in the exponential rate constants between the early and later phases. If the early phase of decline in toxicant concentration is considerably more rapid than the later phase or phases, the timing of blood sampling becomes critical in the ability to resolving two or more phases of washout.

Sometimes three or even four exponential terms are needed to fit a curve to the plot of log C versus time. Such compounds are viewed as displaying characteristics of three- or four-compartment open models. The principles underlying such models are the same as those applied to the two-compartment open model, but the mathematics is more complex and beyond the scope of this chapter.

Apparent Volume of Distribution

For a one-compartment model, a toxicant is assumed to equilibrate between plasma and tissues immediately following its entry into the systemic circulation. Thus, a consistent relationship should exist between plasma concentration and the amount of toxicant in each tissue and, by extension, to the entire amount in the body or body burden. The apparent volume of distribution (V_d) is defined as the proportionality constant that relates the total amount of the toxicant in the body to its concentration in plasma, and typically has units of liters or liters per kilogram of body weight (Rowland and Tozer, 1995). V_d is the apparent fluid space into which an amount of toxicant is distributed in the body to result in a given plasma concentration. As an illustration, envision the body as a tank containing an unknown volume (L) of well mixed water. If a known amount (mg) of dye is placed into the water, the volume of that water can be calculated indirectly by determining the dye concentration (mg/L) that resulted after the dye has equilibrated in the tank; that is, by dividing the amount of dye added to the tank by the resultant concentration of the dye in water. Analogously, the apparent volume of distribution of a toxicant in the body is determined after iv bolus administration, and is mathematically defined as the quotient of the amount of chemical in the body and its plasma concentration. V_d is calculated as

$$V_d = \frac{Dose_{iv}}{\beta \times AUC_0^\infty} \qquad (7\text{-}5)$$

where $Dose_{iv}$ is the intravenous dose or known amount of chemical in body at time zero; β is the elimination rate constant; and AUC_0^∞ is the area under the toxicant concentration versus time curve from time zero to infinity. AUC_0^∞ is estimated by numerical methods, the most common one being the trapezoidal rule (Gibaldi and Perrier, 1982). The product, $\beta \times AUC_0^\infty$, in unit of concentration, is the theoretical concentration of toxicant in plasma if dynamic equilibration were achievable immediately after introduction of the toxicant into the systemic circulation. For a one-compartment model, immediate equilibration of the toxicant between plasma and tissues after an acute exposure does hold true, in which case V_d can be calculated by a simpler and more intuitive equation

$$V_d = \frac{Dose_{iv}}{C_0} \qquad (7\text{-}6)$$

where C_0 is the concentration of toxicant in plasma at time zero. C_0 is determined by extrapolating the plasma disappearance curve after iv injection to the zero time point (Fig. 7-2).

For the more complex multi-compartmental models, V_d is calculated according to Equation (7-5) that involves the computation of area under the toxicant concentration-time curve. Moreover, the concept of an overall apparent volume of distribution is strictly applicable to the terminal exponential phase when equilibration of the toxicant between plasma and all tissue sites are attained. This has led some investigators to refer to the apparent volumes of distribution calculated by Equation (7-5) as V_β (for a two-compartment model) or V_z (for a general multi-compartmental model); the subscript designation refers to the terminal exponential phase (Gibaldi and Perrier, 1982). It should also be noted that when Equation (7-6) is applied to the situation of a multi-compartmental model, the resultant volume is the apparent volume of the central compartment, often times referred to as V_c. By definition, V_c is the proportionality constant that relates the total amount of the toxicant in the central compartment to its concentration in plasma. It has limited utility; for example, it can be used to calculate an iv dose of the toxicant to target an initial plasma concentration.

V_d is appropriately called the *apparent* volume of distribution because it does not correspond to any real anatomical volumes. The magnitude of the V_d term is toxicant-specific and represents the extent of distribution of toxicant out of plasma and into extravascular sites (Table 7-3). Equation (7-7) provides a more intuitive interpretation of an apparent volume of distribution:

$$V_d = V_p + \sum P_{t,i} \times V_{t,i} \qquad (7\text{-}7)$$

where V_p is the plasma volume and the $\sum$-term represents the summation of the apparent volume of each tissue region as represented by the product of $P_{t,i}$ (i.e., partition ratio or tissue-to-plasma concentration ratio at dynamic equilibrium) and $V_{t,i}$ (i.e., anatomical volume of tissue). At one extreme, a toxicant that predominantly remains in the vasculature will have a low V_d that approximates the volume of blood or plasma; that is, the minimum V_d for any toxicant is the plasma volume. For toxicants that distribute extensively into extravascular tissues, V_d exceeds physiological fluid spaces, such as plasma or blood volume, interstitial fluid or extracellular fluid. A toxicant that is highly sequestered in tissues (i.e., high $P_{t,i}$) can have a volume of distribution larger than average body size (>1 L/kg). The mechanisms of tissue sequestration include partitioning of a toxicant into tissue fat, high affinity binding to tissue proteins, trapping in specialized organelles (e.g., pH trapping of amine compounds in acidic lysozomes), and concentrative uptake by active transporters. In fact, the equation below is an alternate form of Equation (7-7), which features the interplay of binding to plasma and tissue proteins in determining the partitioning of a toxicant in that only free or unbound drug can freely diffuse across membrane and cellular barriers.

$$V_d = V_p + \sum \left(\frac{f_{up}}{f_{ut,i}} \right) \times V_{t,i} \qquad (7\text{-}8)$$

where f_{up} is the unbound fraction of toxicant in plasma (Table 7-3) and $f_{ut,i}$ is the effective unbound fraction in a tissue region. Here, $P_{t,i}$ is governed by the ratio $f_{up}/f_{ut,i}$. Thus, a toxicant that has high affinity for plasma proteins (e.g., albumin and/or α_1-acid glycoprotein) relative to tissue proteins has a restricted distribution volume; for example, the anticoagulant warfarin with a plasma-bound fraction of 0.995 or an f_{up} of 0.005 (Table 7-3). On the other hand, a toxicant that has a high affinity for tissue proteins and lesser affinity for plasma proteins can have a very high V_d. For example, the tricyclic antidepressant nortriptyline has a good affinity for plasma proteins with a bound fraction of 0.92 or an f_{up} of 0.08; however, binding of nortriptyline to tissues constituents is so much higher such that it has a V_d of 18 times the body weight in adult humans.

Table 7-3

Volume of Distribution (V_d) and Unbound or Free Fraction in Plasma (f_{up}) for Several Drugs that are of Clinical Toxicological Interest.[a] Volumes of Body Fluid Compartments in Healthy Human Adults are Included for Comparison.

CHEMICAL	V_d (L/kg)	f_{up}
Chloroquine	~200	~0.45
Nortriptyline	18	0.080
Oxycodone	2.0	0.55
	Body size = 1.0	
Acetaminophen	0.95	<0.20
	Total body water = 0.60	
Phenytoin	0.64	0.11
	Extracellular fluid = 0.27	
Warfarin	0.14	0.005
Epoetin alfa	0.05	–
	Plasma volume = 0.045	

[a]V_d and f_{up} values taken from Thummel *et al.* (2006).

In addition to its value as a parameter to indicate the extent of extravascular distribution of a toxicant, V_d also has practical utility. Once the V_d for a toxicant is known, it can be used to estimate the amount of toxicant remaining in the body at any time when the plasma concentration at that time is known; that is,

$$X_B = V_d \times C \qquad (7\text{-}9)$$

where X_B is the amount of toxicant in the body or body burden, and C is the plasma concentration at a given time.

Clearance

Toxicants are cleared from the body via various routes; for example, excretion by the kidneys into urine or via bile into the intestine, biotransformation by the liver, or exhalation by the lungs. Clearance is an important toxicokinetic parameter that relates the rate of toxicant elimination from the whole body in relation to plasma concentration (Wilkinson, 1987). Whereas terminal $T_{1/2}$ is reflective of the rate of removal of a toxicant from plasma or blood, as was explained earlier, it is also subject to the influence of distributional processes, especially for toxicants exhibiting multi-compartmental kinetics. Clearance, on the other hand, is a parameter that solely represents the rate of toxicant elimination.

A formal definition of total body clearance is the ratio of overall elimination rate of a toxicant divided by plasma concentration at any time after an acute exposure or during repetitive or continuous exposure (i.e., elimination rate/C); in effect, clearance expresses the overall efficiency of the elimination mechanisms. Because this measure of elimination efficiency is in reference to blood or plasma toxicant concentration, it is also named blood or plasma clearance. High values of clearance indicate efficient and generally rapid removal, whereas low clearance values indicate slow and less efficient removal of a toxicant from the body. By definition, clearance has the units of flow (e.g., mL/min or L/hr). In the classic compartmental context, clearance is portrayed as the apparent volume containing the toxicant that is cleared per unit of time. After intravenous bolus administration, total body clearance (Cl) is calculated by

$$Cl = \frac{Dose_{iv}}{AUC_0^\infty} \qquad (7\text{-}10)$$

Clearance can also be calculated if the volume of distribution and elimination rate constants are known; that is, $Cl = V_d \times k_{el}$ for a one-compartment model and $Cl = V_d \times \beta$ for a two-compartment model. It should be noted that the relationship is a mathematical derivation and does not imply that clearance is dependent upon the distribution volume (see later section for further commenting). A clearance of 100 mL/min can be visualized as having a 100 mL of blood or plasma completely cleared of toxicant in each minute during circulation.

The biological significance of total body clearance is better appreciated when it is recognized that it is the sum of clearances by individual eliminating organs (i.e., organ clearances):

$$Cl = Cl_r + Cl_h + Cl_p + \cdots \qquad (7\text{-}11)$$

where Cl_r depicts renal, Cl_h hepatic, and Cl_p pulmonary clearance. Each organ clearance is in turn determined by blood perfusion flow through the organ and the fraction of toxicant in the arterial inflow that is irreversibly removed, i.e., the extraction fraction (E_i). Various

organ clearance models have been developed to provide quantitative description of clearance that is related to blood perfusion flow (Q_i), free fraction in blood (f_{ub}), and intrinsic clearance ($Cl_{int,i}$) (Wilkinson, 1987). For example, for hepatic clearance (Cl_h), if the delivery of the toxicant to its intracellular site of removal is rate-limited by liver blood flow (Q_h) and the toxicant is assumed to have equal, ready access to all the hepatocytes within the liver (i.e., the so-called well-stirred model):

$$Cl_h = Q_h \times E_h = \frac{Q_h \times f_{ub} \times Cl_{int,h}}{f_{ub} \times Cl_{int,h} + Q_h} \qquad (7\text{-}12)$$

where $Cl_{int,h}$ is the hepatic intrinsic clearance that embodies a combination of factors that determines the access of the toxicant to the enzymatic sites (e.g., plasma protein binding and sinusoidal membrane transport) and the biochemical efficiency of the metabolizing enzymes (e.g., $\frac{V_{max}}{K_M}$ for an enzyme obeying Michaelis kinetics). Equation (7-12) dictates that hepatic clearance of a toxicant from the blood is bounded by either liver blood flow or intrinsic clearance (i.e., $f_{ub} \times Cl_{int,h}$). Note that when $f_{ub} \times Cl_{int,h}$ is very much higher than Q_h, E_h approaches unity (i.e., near complete extraction during each passage of toxicant through the hepatic sinusoid or high extraction) and Cl_h approaches Q_h. Put in another way, hepatic clearance cannot exceed the hepatic blood flow rate even if the maximum rate of metabolism in the liver is more rapid than the rate of hepatic blood flow, because the rate of overall hepatic clearance is limited by the delivery of the toxicant to the metabolic enzymes in the liver via the blood. At the other extreme, when $f_{ub} \times Cl_{int,h}$ is very much lower than Q_h, E_h becomes quite small (i.e., low extraction) and Cl_h nearly equals $f_{ub} \times Cl_{int,h}$ In this instance, the intrinsic clearance is relatively inefficient; hence, alteration in liver blood flow would have little, if any, influence on liver clearance of the toxicant. Thus, the concept of clearance is grounded in the physiological and biochemical mechanisms of an eliminating organ.

Relationship of Elimination Half-Life to Clearance and Volume

Elimination half-life ($T_{1/2}$) is probably the most easily understood pharmacokinetic concept and is an important parameter as it determines the persistence of a toxicant following discontinuation of exposure. As will be seen in a later section, elimination half-life also governs the rate of accumulation of a toxicant in the body during continuous or repetitive exposure. Elimination half-life is dependent upon both volume of distribution and clearance. $T_{1/2}$ can be calculated from V_d and Cl:

$$T_{1/2} = \frac{0.693 \times V_d}{Cl} \qquad (7\text{-}13)$$

The above relationship among $T_{1/2}$, V_d, and Cl is another illustration that care should be exercised in interpretation of data when relying upon $T_{1/2}$ as the sole representation of elimination of a chemical in toxicokinetic studies, since $T_{1/2}$ is influenced by both the volume of distribution for the chemical and the rate by which the chemical is cleared from the blood. For a fixed V_d, $T_{1/2}$ decreases as Cl increases, because the chemical is being removed from this fixed volume faster as clearance increases (Fig. 7-4). Conversely, as the V_d increases, $T_{1/2}$ increases for a fixed Cl since the volume of

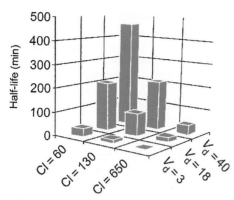

Figure 7-4. The dependence of $T_{1/2}$ on V_d and Cl.

Renal *Cl* values of 60, 130, and 650 mL/min represent partial reabsorption, glomerular filtration, and tubular secretion, respectively. Values for V_d of 3, 18, and 40 L represent approximate volumes of plasma water, extracellular fluid and total body water, respectively, for an average-sized person.

fluid that must be cleared of chemical increases but the efficiency of clearance does not.

Absorption and Bioavailability

For most chemicals in toxicology, exposure occurs by extravascular routes (e.g., inhalation, dermal, or oral), and absorption into the systemic circulation is often incomplete. The extent of absorption of a toxicant can be experimentally determined by comparing the plasma AUC_0^∞ after intravenous and extravascular dosing. Because intravenous dosing assures full (100%) delivery of the dose into the systemic circulation, the AUC ratio should equal the fraction of extravascular dose absorbed and reaches the systemic circulation in its intact form, and is called *bioavailability* (*F*). In acute toxicokinetic studies, bioavailability can be determined by using different iv and non-iv doses according to the following equation, provided that the toxicant does not display dose-dependent or saturable kinetics.

$$F = \left(\frac{AUC_{\text{non-iv}}}{Dose_{\text{non-iv}}} \right) \Big/ \left(\frac{AUC_{\text{iv}}}{Dose_{\text{iv}}} \right) \tag{7-14}$$

where $AUC_{\text{non-iv}}$, AUC_{iv}, $Dose_{\text{non-iv}}$, and $Dose_{\text{iv}}$ are the respective area under the plasma concentration versus time curves and doses for non-iv and iv administration. Bioavailabilities for various chemicals range in value between 0 and 1. Complete availability of chemical to the systematic circulation is demonstrated by $F = 1$. When $F < 1$, less than 100% of the dose is able to reach the systemic circulation. Because the concept of bioavailability is judged by how much of the dose reaches the systemic circulation, it is often referred to as systemic availability. Systemic availability is determined by how well a toxicant is absorbed from its site of application and any intervening processes that could remove or inactivate the toxicant between its point of entry and the systemic circulation. Specifically, systemic availability of an orally administered toxicant is governed by its absorption at the gastrointestinal barrier, metabolism within the intestinal mucosa, and metabolism and biliary excretion during its first transit through the liver. Metabolic inactivation and excretion of the toxicant at the intestinal mucosa and the liver prior to its entry into the systemic circulation is called pre-systemic extraction or first-pass effect. The following equation accounts for the action

of absorption and sequential first-pass extraction at the intestinal mucosa and the liver as determinants of the bioavailability of a toxicant taken orally:

$$F = f_{\text{g}} \times (1 - E_{\text{m}}) \times (1 - E_{\text{h}}) \tag{7-15}$$

where f_{g} is the fraction of the applied dose that is released and absorbed across the mucosal barrier along the entire length of the gut, E_{m} is the extent of loss due to metabolism within the gastrointestinal mucosa, and E_{h} is the loss due to metabolism or biliary excretion during first-pass through the liver. Note that E_{h} in this equation is same as the hepatic extraction E_{h} defined in Equation (7-12), which refers to hepatic extraction of a toxicant during recirculation. This means that poor oral bioavailability of a chemical can be attributed to multiple factors. The chemical may be absorbed to a limited extent because of low aqueous solubility preventing its effective dissolution in the gastrointestinal fluid or poor permeability across the brush-border membrane of the intestinal mucosa. Extensive degradation by metabolic enzymes residing at the intestinal mucosa and the liver may also hinder entry of the chemical in its intact form into the systemic circulation.

The rate of absorption of a toxicant via an extravascular route of entry is another critical determinant of outcome, particularly in acute exposure situations. As shown in Fig. 7-5, slowing the absorption rate of a toxicant, while maintaining the same extent of absorption or bioavailability, leads to a delay in time to peak plasma concentration (T_{p}) and a decrease in the maximum concentration (C_{max}) (compare case 2 to case 1). The converse is true; accelerating absorption shortens T_{p} and increases C_{max}. The dependence of T_{p} and C_{max} on absorption rate has obvious implication in the speed of onset and maximum toxic effects following exposure to a chemical. Case 3 in Fig. 7-5 illustrates the peculiar situation when the absorption rate is so much slower than the elimination rate (e.g., $k_{\text{a}} \ll k_{\text{el}}$ for a one-compartment model). The terminal rate of decline in plasma concentration reflects the absorption rate constant, instead of the elimination rate constant; that is, the washout of toxicant is rate-limited by slow absorption until the applied dose is completely absorbed or removed, beyond which time the toxicant remaining in the body will be cleared according the elimination rate-constant. This means that continual absorption of a chemical can affect the persistence of toxic effect following an acute exposure, and that it is important to institute decontamination procedure quickly after overdose or accidental exposure to a toxicant. This is especially a consideration in occupational exposure via dermal absorption following skin contact with permeable industrial chemicals.

Metabolite Kinetics

The toxicity of a chemical is in some cases attributed to its biotransformation product(s). Hence, the formation and subsequent disposition kinetics of a toxic metabolite is of considerable interest. As expected, the plasma concentration of a metabolite rises as the parent drug is transformed into the metabolite. Once formed, the metabolite is subject to further metabolism to a nontoxic by-product or undergoes excretion via the kidneys or bile; hence at some point in time, the plasma metabolite concentration peaks and falls thereafter. Figure 7-6 illustrates the plasma concentration time course of a primary metabolite in relation to its parent compound under contrasting scenarios. The left panel shows the case when the elimination rate constant of the metabolite is much greater than

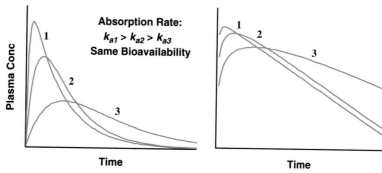

Figure 7-5. Influence of absorption rate on the time to peak (T_p) and maximum plasma concentration (C_{max}) of a toxicant that exhibit one-compartment kinetics.

The left panel illustrates the change in plasma concentration-time curves as the first-order absorption rate constant (k_a) decreases, while keep the extent of absorption or bioavailability (F), hence the AUC, constant. The right panel displays the same curves in a semi-logarithmic plot. Time to peak plasma concentration shows a progressive delay as k_a decreases, along with a decrease in C_{max}. In case 1 and 2, the terminal decline in plasma concentration is governed by elimination half-life; hence, the parallel decline in the semi-logarithmic plot. In case 3 where $k_a \ll k_{el}$, the absorption becomes so slow that decline in plasma concentration in the terminal phase reflects the absorption half-life; that is, washout of toxicant is rate-limited by absorption. Accordingly, the terminal decline is slower than in case 1 and 2.

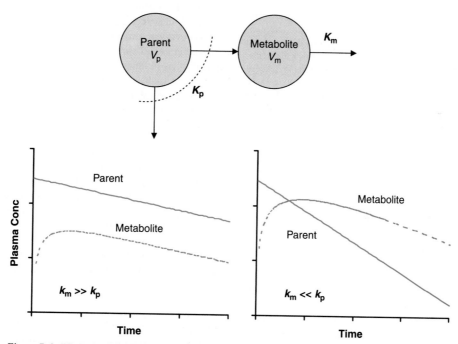

Figure 7-6. Plasma concentration time course of a primary metabolite and its parent compound under contrasting scenarios: when elimination of the metabolite is much more rapid than its formation ($k_m \gg k_p$, lower left panel) and when elimination of the metabolite is much slower than its formation ($k_m \ll k_p$, lower right panel). Semi-logarithmic plots are shown to compare the slope of the terminal decline of parent compound and its metabolite.

The top panel shows the model for conversion of the parent compound to a single metabolite. Note that the elimination rate constant for the parent compound (k_p) includes both the rate constant for metabolism and extra-metabolic routes of elimination. k_m is the elimination rate constant for the derived metabolite. When $k_m \gg k_p$, the terminal decline of the metabolite parallels that of the parent compound; i.e., metabolite washout is rate-limited by its formation. When $k_m \ll k_p$, the terminal decline of metabolite concentration is much slower than that of parent compound; i.e., metabolite washout is rate-limited by its elimination.

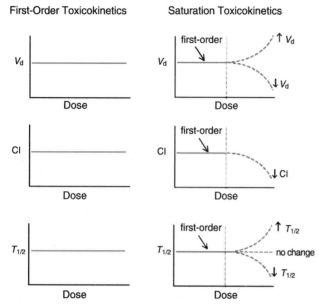

First-Order Toxicokinetics   **Saturation Toxicokinetics**

Figure 7-7. Changes in V_d, Cl ***and*** $T_{1/2}$ ***following first-order toxicokinetics (left panels) and following saturable toxicokinetics (right panels).***

Vertical dashed lines represent point of departure from first-order to saturation toxicokinetics. Pharmacokinetic parameters for toxicants that follow first-order toxicokinetics are independent of dose. When plasma protein binding or elimination mechanisms are saturated with increasing dose, pharmacokinetic parameter estimates become dose-dependent. V_d may increase, for example, when protein binding is saturated, allowing more free toxicant to distribute into extravascular sites. Conversely, V_d may decrease with increasing dose if tissue protein binding saturates. Then, chemical may redistribute more freely back into plasma. When chemical concentrations exceed the capacity for biotransformation by metabolic enzymes, overall clearance of the chemical decreases. These changes may or may not have effects on $T_{1/2}$ depending upon the magnitude and direction of changes in both V_d and Cl.

the overall elimination rate constant of the parent compound (i.e., $k_m \gg k_p$). The terminal decline of the metabolite parallels that of the parent compound; the metabolite is cleared as quickly as it is formed or its washout is rate-limited by conversion from the parent compound. The right panel shows the opposite case when the elimination rate constant of the metabolite is much lower than the overall elimination rate constant of the parent compound (i.e., $k_m \ll k_p$). The slower terminal decline of the metabolite compared to the parent compound simply reflects a longer elimination half-life of the metabolite. It should also be noted that the AUC_0^∞ of the metabolite relative to the parent compound is dependent on the partial clearance of the parent drug to the metabolite and clearance of the derived metabolite. A biologically active metabolite assumes toxicological significance when it is the major metabolic product and is cleared much less efficiently than the parent compound.

Saturation Toxicokinetics

As already mentioned, the distribution and elimination of most chemicals occurs by first-order processes. Under first-order elimination kinetics, the elimination rate constant, apparent volume of distribution, clearance and half-life are expected not to change with increasing or decreasing dose (i.e., dose independent). As a result, a semi-logarithmic display of plasma concentration versus time over a range of doses shows a set of parallel plots. Furthermore, plasma

concentration at a given time or the AUC_0^∞ is strictly proportional to dose; for example, a twofold change in dose results in an exact twofold change in plasma concentration or AUC_0^∞. However, for some toxicants, as the dose of a toxicant increases, its volume of distribution and/or clearance may change, as shown in Fig. 7-7. This is generally referred to as non-linear or dose-dependent kinetics. Biotransformation, active transport processes, and protein binding have finite capacities and can be saturated. For instance, most metabolic enzymes operate in accordance to Michaelis–Menten kinetics (Gibaldi and Perrier, 1982). As the dose is escalated and concentration of a toxicant at the site of metabolism approaches or exceeds the K_M (substrate concentration at one-half V_{max}, the maximum metabolic capacity), the increase in rate of metabolism becomes less than proportional to the dose and eventually approaches a maximum at exceedingly high doses. The transition from first-order to saturation kinetics is important in toxicology because it can lead to prolonged persistence of a compound in the body after an acute exposure and excessive accumulation during repeated exposures. Some of the salient characteristics of nonlinear kinetics include the following: (1) the decline in the levels of the chemical in the body is not exponential; (2) AUC_0^∞ is not proportional to the dose; (3) V_d, Cl, k_{el} (or β), or $T_{1/2}$ change with increasing dose; (4) the composition of excretory products changes quantitatively or qualitatively with the dose, and (5) dose–response curves show an abruptly steeper change in response with an increasing dose, starting at the dose at which saturation effects become evident.

Inhaled methanol provides an example of a chemical whose metabolic clearance changes from first-order kinetics at low level exposures to zero-order kinetics at near toxic levels (Burbacher et al., 2004). Figure 7-8 shows predicted blood methanol concentration-time profiles in female monkeys followed a 2-hour controlled exposure in an inhalation chamber at two levels of methanol vapor, 1200 ppm and 4800 ppm. Blood methanol kinetics at 1200 ppm exposure follows typical first-order kinetics. At 4800 ppm, methanol metabolism is fully saturated, such that the initial decline in blood methanol following the 2-hour exposure occurs at a constant rate (i.e., a fixed decrease in concentration per unit time independent of blood concentration), rather than a constant fractional rate. As a result, a rectilinear plot of blood methanol concentration versus time yields an initial linear decline, whereas a convex curve is observed in the semi-logarithmic plot (compare left and right panels of Fig. 7-8). In time, methanol metabolism converts to first-order kinetics when blood methanol concentration falls below K_M (i.e., the Michaelis constant for the dehydrogenase enzyme); at which time, blood methanol shows an exponential decline in the rectilinear plot and a linear decline in the semi-logarithmic plot. Moreover, Fig. 7-8 shows the greater than proportionate increase (i.e., > fourfold) in C_{max} and AUC_0^∞ as the methanol vapor concentration is raised from 1200 ppm to 4800 ppm. It should be noted that a constant $T_{1/2}$ or k_{el} does not exist during the saturation regime; it varies depending upon the saturating methanol dose.

In addition to the complication of dose-dependent kinetics, there are chemicals whose clearance kinetics changes over time (i.e., time-dependent kinetics). A common cause of time-dependent kinetics is auto-induction of xenobiotic metabolizing enzymes; that is, the substrate is capable of inducing its own metabolism through activation of gene transcription. The classic example of auto-induction is with the antiepileptic drug, carbamazepine. Daily administration of carbamazepine leads to a continual increase in clearance and shortening in elimination half-life over the first few weeks of therapy (Bertilsson et al., 1986).

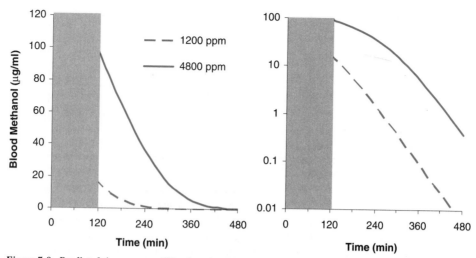

Figure 7-8. *Predicted time course of blood methanol concentration following a 120-minute exposure to 1200 and 4800 ppm of methanol vapor in the female monkey based on the toxicokinetic model reported by Burbacher et al. (2004) that features a saturable (Michaelis–Menten type) metabolic clearance.*

The left panel is a rectilinear plot of the simulated blood methanol concentration–time curves at the two exposure levels. The right panel shows the same simulation in a semi-logarithmic plot. The washout of blood methanol following the 120-min inhalation exposure at 1200 ppm follows a typical concave or exponential pattern in the rectilinear plot (left panel) and is linear in a semi-logarithmic plot (right panel). The post exposure profile at 4800 ppm shows a linear segment during the first 120 min of washout and becomes exponential thereafter in the rectilinear plot (left panel). The linear segment reflects saturation of alcohol dehydrogenase, which is the principal enzyme responsible for the metabolism of methanol. The in vivo K_M for this simulation was set at 32.7 μg/mL. At concentrations above K_M, the kinetics approach zero-order kinetics. At concentrations below K_M, washout kinetics become first-order with a half-life of about 60 min. The right panel shows a characteristic convex semi-logarithmic plot for the initial phase of zero-order kinetics and becomes linear as expected for first-order kinetics when the concentration falls below K_M. It should also be noted that the maximum blood methanol following 4800 ppm exposure is predicted to be 5.9-times higher than that following 1200 ppm. Also, the area under the blood concentration-time curve (AUC) from time zero to 480 min at 4800 ppm exposure is eightfold higher than at 1200 ppm. Under linear kinetics, the increase in maximum blood methanol and AUC ought to be proportionate to the dose increase, i.e., a fourfold increment. Here, we observe a more than proportionate increase in blood methanol concentration in relation to the dose, which is another hallmark of saturation kinetics.

Accumulation During Continuous or Intermittent Exposure

It stands to reason that continual or chronic exposure to a chemical leads to its cumulative intake and accumulation in the body. For a chemical that follows first-order elimination kinetics, the elimination rate increases as the body burden increases. Therefore, at a fixed level of continuous exposure, accumulation of a toxicant in the body eventually reaches a point when the intake rate of the toxicant equals its elimination rate, from thereon the body burden stays constant. This is referred to as the steady state. Figure 7-9 illustrates the rise of toxicant concentration in plasma over time during continuous exposure and the eventual attainment of a plateau or the steady-state. Steady-state concentration of a toxicant in plasma (C_{ss}) is related to the intake rate (R_{in}) and clearance of the toxicant.

$$C_{ss} = \frac{R_{in}}{Cl} \qquad (7\text{-}16)$$

For a one-compartment model, an exponential rise in plasma concentration is expected during continuous exposure and the time it takes for a toxicant to reach steady state is governed by its elimination half-life. It takes one half-life to reach 50%, four half-lives to reach 93.8%, and seven half-lives to reach 99.2% of steady state.

Time to attainment of steady state is not dependent on the intake rate of the toxicant. The left panel of Fig. 7-9 shows the same time to 50% steady state at three different rates of intake; on the other hand, the steady-state concentration is strictly proportional to the intake rate. Change in clearance of a toxicant often leads to a corresponding change in elimination half-life (see right panel of Fig. 7-9), in which case both the time to reach and magnitude of steady-state concentration are altered. The same steady-state principle applies to toxicants that exhibit multi-compartmental kinetics; except that, accumulation occurs in a multi-phasic fashion reflective of the multiple exponential half-lives for inter-compartmental distribution and elimination. Typically, the rise in plasma concentration is relatively rapid at the beginning, being governed by the early (distribution) half-life, and becomes slower at later times when the terminal (elimination) half-life takes hold.

The concept of accumulation applies to intermittent exposure as well. Figure 7-10 shows a typical occupational exposure scenario to volatile chemicals at the workplace over the course of a week. Whether accumulation occurs from day to day and further from week to week depends on the intervals between exposure and the elimination half-life of the chemicals involved. For a chemical with relatively short half-life compared to the interval between work shifts and the "exposure holiday" over the weekend, little accumulation is expected. In contrast, for a chemical with elimination

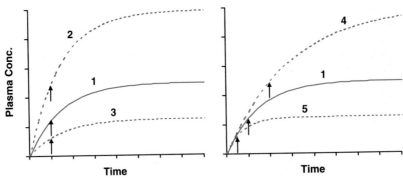

Figure 7-9. Accumulation of plasma toxicant concentration over time during constant, continuous exposure as a function of exposure level (left panel) and elimination half-life (right panel).

These simulations are based on a one-compartment model at a constant apparent volume of distribution. Case 1 serves as the reference with an elimination half-life set equal to one arbitrary time unit. In the left panel, which illustrates accumulation of toxicant as a function of exposure level, exposure level is raised by twofold in Case 2 and lowered by 50% in Case 3. The changes in eventual steady state concentration are proportional to the changes in exposure level, i.e., increased by twofold in Case 2 and decreased by 50% in Case 3. During continuous exposure, 50% of steady state is achieved in one half-life. Near plateau or steady-state (>90%) is reached after four half-lives. Since the elimination half-life is constant across Cases 1–3 in the left panel, the time it takes to attain 50% of steady-state concentration (see arrows) is the same, i.e., one time unit. Right panel illustrates the influence of elimination half-life and clearance on accumulation at a fixed constant rate of exposure. Case 4 represents a 50% decrease in clearance and a corresponding twofold increase in elimination half-life compared to Case 1. Case 5 represents a twofold increase in clearance and a corresponding 50% decrease in elimination half-life. Changes in both the time to attain steady-state and the steady-state concentration are evident. In Case 4, the steady-state concentration increased by twofold as a result of a 50% reduction in clearance, and the time to achieved 50% of steady state increased by twofold as a result of the prolonged elimination half-life. In Case 5, the steady-state concentration is reduced by 50%, while the time to reach 50% steady state is shortened by 50%.

half-life approaching or exceeding the between-shift intervals (>12 to 24 hours), progressive accumulation is expected over the successive workdays. Washout of the chemical may not be complete over the weekend and result in a significant carry forward of body burden into the next week. It should also be noted that the overall exposure as measured by the AUC over the cycle of a week is dependent on the toxicant clearance.

Conclusion

For many chemicals, blood or plasma chemical concentration versus time data can be adequately described by a one- or two-compartment, classic pharmacokinetic model when basic assumptions are made (e.g., instantaneous mixing within compartments and first-order kinetics). In some instances, more sophisticated models with increased numbers of compartments will be needed to describe blood or plasma toxicokinetic data; for example, if the chemical is preferentially sequestered and turns over slowly in select tissues. The parameters of the classic compartmental models are usually estimated by statistical fitting of data to the model equations using nonlinear regression methods. A number of software packages are available for both data fitting and simulations with classic compartmental models; examples include WinNonlin (Pharsight Corp., Palo Alto, CA), SAAM II (SAAM Institute, University of Washington, Seattle, WA), ADAPT II (University of Southern California, Los Angeles, CA), and PK Solutions (Summit Research Services, Montrose, CO).

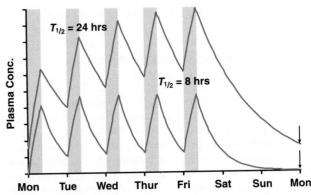

Figure 7-10. Simulated accumulation of plasma concentration from occupational exposure over the cycle of a work week compared between two industrial chemicals with short and long elimination half-lives.

Shading represents the exposure period during the 8-hour workday, Monday through Friday. Intake of the chemical into the systemic circulation is assumed to occur at a constant rate during exposure. Exposure is negligible over the weekend. For the chemical with the short elimination half-life of 8 hours, minimal accumulation occurs from day to day over the work days. Near complete washout of the chemical is observed when work resumes on Monday (see arrow). For the chemical with the long elimination half-life of 24 hours, progressive accumulation is observed over the five work days. Washout of the longer half-life chemical over the weekend is incomplete; a significant residual is carried into the next work week. Because of its lower clearance, the overall AUC of the long half-life chemical over the cycle of a week is higher by threefold.

Knowledge of toxicokinetic data and compartmental modeling are useful in deciding what dose or dosing regimen of chemical to use in the planning of toxicology studies (e.g., targeting a toxic level of exposure), in choosing appropriate sampling times for biological monitoring, and in seeking an understanding of the dynamics of a toxic event (e.g., what blood or plasma concentrations are achieved to produce a specific response, how accumulation of a chemical controls the onset and degree of toxicity, and the persistence of toxic effects following termination of exposure).

PHYSIOLOGIC TOXICOKINETICS

The primary difference between physiologic compartmental models and classic compartmental models lies in the basis for assigning the rate constants that describe the transport of chemicals into and out of the compartments (Andersen, 1991). In classic kinetics, the rate constants are defined by the data; thus, these models are often referred to as data-based models. In physiologic models, the rate constants represent known or hypothesized biological processes, and these models are commonly referred to as physiologically based models. The concept of incorporating biological realism into the analysis of drug or xenobiotic distribution and elimination is not new. For example, one of the first physiologic models was proposed by Teorell (1937). This model contained all the important determinants in chemical disposition that are considered valid today. Unfortunately, the computational tools required to solve the underlying equations were not available at that time. With advances in computer science, the software and hardware needed to implement physiological models are now well within the reach of toxicologists.

The advantages of physiologically based models compared with classic models are that (1) these models can describe the time course of distribution of toxicants to any organ or tissue, (2) they allow estimation of the effects of changing physiologic parameters on tissue concentrations, (3) the same model can predict the toxicokinetics of chemicals across species by allometric scaling, and (4) complex dosing regimes and saturable processes such as metabolism and binding are easily accommodated (Gargas and Andersen, 1988). The disadvantages are that (1) much more information is needed to implement these models compared with classic models, (2) the mathematics can be difficult for many toxicologists to handle, and (3) values for parameters are often ill defined in various species, strains, and disease states. Nevertheless, physiologically based toxicokinetic models are conceptually sound and are potentially useful tools for gaining rich insight into the kinetics of toxicants beyond what classic toxicokinetic models can provide.

Basic Model Structure

Physiologic models are fundamentally complex compartmental models; it generally consists of a system of tissue or organ compartments that are interconnected by the circulatory network. If necessary, each tissue or organ compartments can further be divided into extracellular and intracellular compartments to describe movement of toxicant at the cellular level. The exact model structure, or how the compartments are organized and linked together, depends on both the chemical and the organism being studied. For example, a physiologic model describing the disposition of a chemical in fish would require a description of the gills (Nichols *et al.*, 1994), whereas a model for the same chemical in mammals would require a lung compartment (Ramsey and Andersen, 1984). Model structures can also vary with the chemicals being studied. For

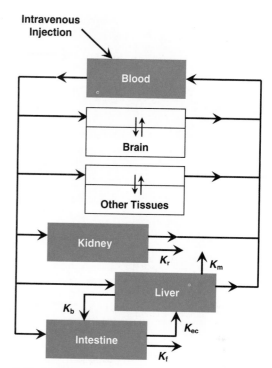

Figure 7-11. Physiologic model for a hypothetical toxicant that is soluble in water, has a low vapor pressure (not volatile), and has a relatively large molecular weight (MW > 100).

This hypothetical chemical is eliminated through metabolism in the liver (K_m), biliary excretion (K_b), renal excretion (K_r) into the urine, and fecal excretion (K_f). The chemical can also undergo enterohepatic circulation (K_{ec}). Perfusion-limited compartments are noted in blue and diffusion-limited compartments are noted in white.

example, a model for a non-volatile, water-soluble chemical, which might be administered by intravenous injection (Fig. 7-11), has a structure different from that of a model for a volatile organic chemical for which inhalation is the likely route of exposure (Fig. 7-12). The route of administration is not the only difference between these two models. For example, the first model has a compartment for the intestines, because biliary excretion, fecal elimination, and enterohepatic circulation are presumed important in the disposition of this chemical. The second model has a compartment for fat because fat is an important storage organ for organics. However, the models are not completely different. Both contain a liver compartment because the hepatic metabolism of each chemical is an important element of its disposition. It is important to realize that there is no generic physiologic model. Models are simplifications of reality and should contain elements believed to represent the essential disposition features of a chemical.

In view of the fact that physiologic modeling requires more effort than does classic compartmental modeling, what then accounts for the popularity of this approach among toxicologists? The answer lies in the potential predictive power of physiologic models. Toxicologists are constantly faced with the issue of extrapolation in risk assessments—from laboratory animals to humans, from high to low doses, from occasional to continuous exposure, and from single chemicals to mixtures. Because the kinetic constants in physiologic models represent measurable biological or chemical processes, the resultant physiologic models have the potential for extrapolation from observed data to predicted scenarios.

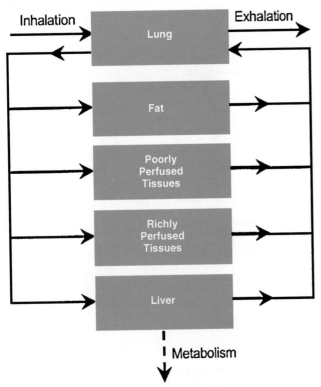

Figure 7-12. Physiological model for a typical volatile organic chemical.
Chemicals for which this model would be appropriate have low molecular weights (*MW* < 100), are soluble in organic solvents, and have significant vapor pressures (volatile). Transport of chemical throughout the body by blood is depicted by the black arrows. Elimination of chemical as depicted by the model includes metabolism (*dashed arrow*) and exhalation (*black arrow*). All compartments are perfusion-limited.

One of the best illustrations of the predictive power of physiologic models is their ability to extrapolate kinetic behavior from laboratory animals to humans. For example, physiologic models developed for styrene and benzene correctly simulate the concentration of each chemical in the blood of both rodents and humans (Ramsey and Andersen, 1984; Travis *et al.*, 1990). Simulations are the outcomes or results (such as a chemical's concentration in blood or tissue) of numerically solving the model equations over a time period of concern, using a set of initial conditions (such as intravenous dose) and parameter values appropriate for the species (such as organ weights and blood flow). Both styrene and benzene are volatile organic chemicals; thus, the model structures for the kinetics of both chemicals in rodents and humans are identical to that shown in Fig. 7-12. However, the parameter values for rodents and humans are different. Humans have larger body weights than rodents, and thus weights of organs such as the liver are larger. Because humans are larger, they also breathe more air per unit of time than do rodents, and a human heart pumps a larger volume of blood per unit of time than does that of a rodent, although the rodent's heart beats more times in the same period. The parameters that describe the chemical behavior of styrene and benzene, such as solubility in tissues, are similar in the rodents and human models. This is often the case because the composition of tissues in different species is similar.

For both styrene and benzene, there are experimental data for humans and rodents and the model simulations can be compared with the actual data to see how well the model has performed

(Ramsey and Andersen, 1984; Andersen *et al.*, 1984; Travis *et al.*, 1990). The conclusion is that the same model structure is capable of describing the chemicals' kinetics in two different species. Because the parameters underlying the model structure represent measurable biological and chemical determinants, the appropriate values for those parameters can be chosen for each species, forming the basis for successful interspecies extrapolation. Even though the same model structure is used for both rodents and humans, the simulated and the observed kinetics of both chemicals differ between rats and humans. The terminal half-life of both organics is longer in the human compared with the rat. This longer half-life for humans is due to the fact that clearance rates for smaller species are faster than those for larger ones. Even though the larger species breathes more air or pumps more blood per unit of time than does the smaller species, blood flows and ventilation rates per unit of body mass are greater for the smaller species. The smaller species has more breaths per minute or heartbeats per minute than does the larger species, even though each breath or stroke volume is smaller. The faster flows per unit mass result in a more efficient delivery of a chemical to organs responsible for elimination. Thus, a smaller species can eliminate the chemical faster than a larger one can. Because the parameters in physiologic models represent real, measurable values, such as blood flows and ventilation rates; the same model structure can resolve such disparate kinetic behaviors among species.

Compartments

The basic unit of the physiologic model is the lumped compartment, which is often depicted as a box in a graphical scheme (Fig. 7-13). A compartment represents a definable anatomical site or tissue type in the body that acts as a unit in effecting a measurable kinetic process (Rowland, 1984, 1985). A compartment may represent a particular structure or functional portion of an organ, a segment of blood vessel with surrounding tissue, an entire discrete organ such as the liver or kidney, or a widely distributed tissue type such as fat or skin. Compartments usually consist of three individual well-mixed regions, or sub-compartments, that correspond to specific physiologic spaces or regions of the organ or tissue. These sub-compartments are: (1) the vascular space through which the compartment is perfused with blood, (2) the interstitial space that forms the matrix for the cells, and (3) the intracellular space consisting of the cells in the tissue (Gerlowski and Jain, 1983).

As shown in Fig. 7-13, the toxicant enters the vascular sub-compartment at a certain rate in mass per unit of time (e.g., mg/h). The rate of entry is a product of the blood flow rate to the tissue (Q_t in L/h) and the concentration of the toxicant in the blood entering the tissue (C_{in} in mg/L). Within the compartment, the toxicant moves from the vascular space to the interstitial space at a certain net rate (*Flux$_1$*) and moves from the interstitial space to the intracellular space at different net rate (*Flux$_2$*). Some toxicants can bind to cell components; thus, within a compartment there may be both free and bound toxicants. The toxicant leaves the vascular space at a certain venous concentration (C_{out}). C_{out} is equal to the concentration of the toxicant in the vascular space assuming a well-mixed compartment.

Parameters

The most common types of parameters, or information required, in physiologic models are anatomic, physiologic, thermodynamic, and transport.

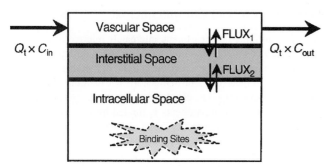

Figure 7-13. Schematic representation of a lumped tissue compartment in a physiologic model.

The blood capillary and cell membranes separating the vascular, interstitial, and intracellular sub-compartments are depicted in heavy black lines. The vascular and interstitial sub-compartments are often combined into a single extracellular sub-compartment. Q_t is blood flow, C_{in} is chemical concentration into the compartment, and C_{out} is chemical concentration out of the compartment.

Anatomic   Anatomic parameters are used to describe the physical size of various compartments. The size is generally specified as a volume (milliliters or liters), because a unit density is assumed even though weights of organs and tissues are most frequently obtained experimentally. If a compartment contains sub-compartments such as those in Fig. 7-13, those volumes also must be known. Volumes of compartments often can be obtained from the literature or from specific toxicokinetic experiments. For example, kidney, liver, brain, and lung can be weighed. Obtaining precise data for volumes of compartments representing widely distributed tissues such as fat or muscle is more difficult. If necessary, these tissues can be removed by dissection and weighed. Among the numerous sources of general information on organ and tissue volumes across species, Brown *et al.* (1997) is a good starting point.

Physiologic   Physiologic parameters encompass a wide variety of processes in biological systems. The most commonly used physiologic parameters are blood flows and lung ventilation. The blood flow rate (Q_t in volume per unit time, such as mL/min or L/h) to individual compartments must be known. Additionally, information on the total blood flow rate or *cardiac output* (Q_c) is necessary. If inhalation is the route for exposure to the chemical or is a route of elimination, the alveolar ventilation rate (Q_p) also must be known. Blood flow rates and ventilation rates can be taken from the literature or can be obtained experimentally.

Parameters for renal excretion and hepatic metabolism are another subset of physiologic parameters, and are required, if these processes are important in describing the elimination of a chemical. For example, glomerular filtration rate and renal tubular transport parameters are required to describe renal clearance. If a chemical is known to be metabolized via a saturable process, both V_{max} (the maximum rate of metabolism) and K_M (the concentration of chemical at one-half V_{max}) for each of the enzymes involved must be obtained so that elimination of the chemical by metabolism can be described in the model. In principle, these parameters can be determined from in vitro metabolism studies with cultured cells, tissue homogenates, or cellular fractions containing the metabolic enzymes (e.g., microsomes for cytochrome P450 enzymes and UDP-GTs), along with appropriate in vitro-in vivo scaling techniques (Iwatsubo *et al.*, 1997; MacGregor *et al.*, 2001; Miners *et al.*, 2006). Although there have

been examples of remarkable success with quantitative prediction of in vivo metabolic clearance based on in vitro biochemical data, there are also notable failures. Unfortunately, estimation of metabolic parameters from in vivo studies is also fraught with difficulties, especially when multiple metabolic pathways and enzymes are present. Estimation of metabolic parameters remains a challenging aspect of physiologically based toxicokinetic modeling.

Thermodynamic   Thermodynamic parameters relate the *total* concentration of a chemical in a tissue (C_t) to the concentration of *free* chemical in that tissue (C_f). Two important assumptions are that (1) total and free concentrations are in equilibrium with each other, and (2) only free chemical can be exchanged between the tissue sub-compartments (Lutz *et al.*, 1980). Most often, total concentration is measured experimentally; however, it is the free concentration that is available for passage across membrane barriers, binding to proteins, metabolism, or carrier-mediated transport. Various mathematical expressions describe the relationship between these two entities. In the simplest situation, the toxicant is a freely diffusible water-soluble chemical that does not bind to any molecules. In this case, free concentration of the chemical is equal to the total concentration of the chemical in the tissue: total = free, or $C_t = C_f$. The affinity of many chemicals for tissues of different composition varies. The extent to which a chemical partitions into a tissue is directly dependent on the composition of the tissue and independent of the concentration of the chemical. Thus, the relationship between free and total concentration becomes one of proportionality: total = free × partition coefficient, or $C_t = C_f \times P_t$. In this case, P_t is called a tissue partition coefficient, which is most often determined from tissue distribution studies in animals, ideally at steady-state during continuous intravenous infusion of the chemical. Estimation of P_t based on in vitro binding studies with human or animal tissues or tissue fractions has proven successful in some cases (Lin *et al.*, 1982; MacGregor *et al.*, 2001). Knowledge of the value of P_t permits an indirect calculation of the free concentration of toxicant in the tissue or $C_f = C_t/P_t$.

Table 7-4 compares the partition coefficients for a number of toxic volatile organic chemicals. The larger values for the fat/blood partition coefficients compared with those for other tissues suggests that these chemicals distribute into fat to a greater extent than they distribute into other tissues. This has been observed experimentally. Fat and fatty tissues, such as bone marrow, contain higher concentrations of benzene than do tissues such as liver and blood. Similarly, styrene concentrations in fatty tissue are higher than styrene concentrations in other tissues. It should be noted that lipophilic organic compounds often can bind to plasma proteins and/or blood cell constituents, in which case the observed tissue/blood partition coefficients will be a function of both the tissue and blood partition coefficient (i.e., P_t/P_b). Hence, partitioning or binding to blood

Table 7-4

Partition Coefficients for Four Volatile Organic Chemicals in Several Tissues

CHEMICAL	BLOOD/AIR	MUSCLE/BLOOD	FAT/BLOOD
Isoprene	3	0.67	24
Benzene	18	0.61	28
Styrene	40	1	50
Methanol	1350	3	11

constituents (P_b) must be known in order to estimate the true thermodynamic partitioning coefficient for a tissue or the free toxicant concentration at equilibrium. P_b can be determined from in vitro studies of blood cells to plasma distribution and plasma protein binding of the chemical.

A more complex relationship between the free concentration and the total concentration of a chemical in tissues is also possible. For example, the chemical may bind to saturable binding sites on tissue components. In these cases, nonlinear functions relating the free concentration in the tissue to the total concentration are necessary. Examples in which more complex binding has been used are physiologic models for dioxin and *tertiary*-amyl methyl ether (Andersen *et al.*, 1993; Collins *et al.*, 1999).

Transport Passage of a chemical across a biological membrane may occur by passive diffusion, carrier-mediated transport involving either facilitated or active transporters, or a combination thereof (Himmelstein and Lutz, 1979). The simplest of these processes—passive diffusion is a first-order process described by Fick's law of diffusion. Diffusion of a chemical occurs during its passage across the blood capillary membrane (*Flux₁* in Fig. 7-13) and across cell membrane (*Flux₂* in Fig. 7-13). *Flux* refers to the rate of transfer of a chemical across a boundary. For simple diffusion, the net flux (mg/h) from one side of a membrane to the other is governed by the barrier permeability and the chemical concentration gradient.

$$Flux = PA \times (C_1 - C_2) = PA \times C_1 - PA \times C_2 \qquad (7\text{-}17)$$

The term *PA* is often called the *permeability-area product* for the membrane or cellular barrier in flow units (e.g., L/h), and is a product of the barrier permeability coefficient (*P* in velocity units, e.g., μm/h) for the chemical and the total barrier surface area (*A*, in μm²). The permeability coefficient takes into account the diffusivity of the specific chemical and the thickness of the cell membrane. C_1 and C_2 are the respective *free* concentrations of the chemical in the originating and receiving compartments. Diffusional flux is enhanced when the barrier thickness is small, the barrier surface area is large, and a large concentration gradient exists. Membrane transporters offer an additional route of entry into cells, and allow more effective tissue penetration for chemicals that have limited passive permeability. Alternately, the presence of efflux transporters at epithelial or endothelial barriers can limit toxicant penetration into critical organs, even for highly permeable toxicant (e.g., P-glycoprotein mediated efflux functions as part of the blood–brain barrier). For both transporter-mediated influx and efflux processes, the kinetics is saturable and can be characterized by T_{max} (the maximum transport rate) and K_T (the concentration of toxicant at one-half T_{max}) for each of the transporters involved. In principle, kinetic parameters for passive permeability or carrier-mediated transport can be estimated from in vitro studies with cultured cell systems. However, the predictability and applicability of such in vitro approaches for physiologic modeling has not been systematically evaluated (MacGregor *et al.*, 2001). At this time, the transport parameters have to be estimated from in vivo data, which are at times difficult and carry some degree of uncertainty.

There are two limiting conditions for the uptake of a toxicant into tissues: perfusion-limited and diffusion-limited. An understanding of the assumptions underlying the limiting conditions is critical because the assumptions change the way in which the model equations are written to describe the movement of a toxicant into and out of the compartment.

Perfusion-Limited Compartments

A perfusion-limited compartment, alternately referred to as blood flow-limited or simply flow-limited compartment, describes the situation when permeability across the cellular or membrane barriers (*PA*) for a particular toxicant is much greater than the blood flow rate to the tissue (Q_t), i.e., $PA \gg Q_t$. In this case, uptake of toxicant by tissue sub-compartments is limited by the rate at which the toxicant is presented to the tissue via the arterial inflow, and not by the rate at which the toxicant penetrates through the vascular endothelium, which is fairly porous in most tissues, or gains passage across the cell membranes. As a result, equilibration of a toxicant between the blood in the tissue vasculature and the interstitial sub-compartment is maintained at all times, and the two sub-compartments are usually lumped together as a single extracellular compartment. An important exception to this vascular-interstitial equilibrium relationship is in the brain, where the capillary endothelium with its tight junctions poses a diffusional barrier between the vascular space and the brain interstitium. Furthermore, as indicated in Fig. 7-13, the cell membrane separates the extracellular compartment from the intracellular compartment. The cell membrane is the most crucial diffusional barrier in a tissue. Nonetheless, for molecules that are very small (molecular weight < 100) or lipophilic (log P > 2), cellular permeability generally does not limit the rate at which a molecule moves across cell membranes. For these molecules, flux across the cell membrane is fast compared with the tissue perfusion rate ($PA \gg Q_t$), and the molecules rapidly distribute throughout the sub-compartments. In this case, free toxicant in the intracellular compartment is always in equilibrium with the extracellular compartment, and these tissue sub-compartments can be lumped as a single compartment. Such a flow-limited tissue compartment is shown in Fig. 7-14. Movement into and out of the entire tissue compartment can be described by a single equation.

$$V_t \times \frac{dC_t}{dt} = Q_t \times (C_{in} - C_{out}) \qquad (7\text{-}18)$$

where V_t is the volume of the tissue compartment, C_t is the toxicant concentration in the compartment ($V_t \times C$ equals the amount of toxicant in the compartment), $V_t \times dC_t/dt$ is the change in the amount of toxicant in the compartment with time, expressed as mass per unit of time, Q_t is blood flow to the tissue, C_{in} is the toxicant concentration entering the compartment, and C_{out} is the toxicant

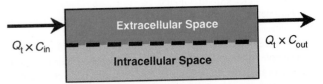

Figure 7-14. Schematic representation of a tissue compartment that features blood flow–limited uptake kinetics.

Rapid exchange of toxicant between the extracellular space (*blue*) and intracellular space (*light blue*), unhindered by a significant diffusional barrier as symbolized by the dashed line, allows equilibrium to be maintained between the two sub-compartments at all times. In effect, a single compartment represents the tissue distribution of the toxicant. Q_t is blood flow, C_{in} is the chemical concentration entering the compartment via the arterial inflow, and C_{out} is the chemical concentration leaving the compartment in the venous outflow.

concentration leaving the compartment. Equations of this type are called mass-balance differential equations. Differential refers to the term dC_t/dt. Mass balance refers to the requirement that the rate of change in the amount of toxicant in a compartment (left-hand side of Equation (7-18)) equals the difference in the rate of entry via arterial inflow and the rate of departure via venous outflow (right-hand side of Equation (7-18)).

In the perfusion-limited case, the concentration of chemical in the venous drainage from the tissue is equal to the free concentration of chemical in the tissue (i.e., $C_{out} = C_f$) when the chemical is not bound to blood constituents. As was noted previously, C_f (or C_{out}) can be related to the total concentration of chemical in the tissue through a simple linear partition coefficient, $C_{out} = C_f = C_t/P_t$. In this case, the differential equation describing the rate of change in the amount of a chemical in a tissue becomes

$$V_t \times dC_t/dt = Q_t \times [C_{in} - C_t/P_t] \qquad (7\text{-}19)$$

In the event the chemical does bind to blood constituents, blood partitioning coefficient needs to be recognized in the mass balance equation.

$$V_t \times dC_t/dt = Q_t \times [C_{in} - C_t/(P_t/P_b)] \qquad (7\text{-}20)$$

The physiologic model shown in Fig. 7-12, which was developed for volatile organic chemicals such as styrene and benzene, is a good example of a model in which all the compartments are described as flow-limited. Distribution of a toxicant in all the compartments is described by using equations of the type noted above. In a flow-limited compartment, the assumption is that the concentrations of a toxicant in all parts of the tissue are in equilibrium. For this reason, the compartments are generally drawn as simple boxes (Fig. 7-12) or boxes with dashed lines that symbolize the equilibrium between the intracellular and extracellular sub-compartments (Fig. 7-14). Additionally, with a flow-limited model, estimates of fluxes between sub-compartments are not required to develop the mass balance differential equation for the compartment. Given the challenges in measuring flux across the vascular endothelium and cell membrane, this is a simplifying assumption that significantly reduces the number of parameters required in the physiologic model.

Diffusion-Limited Compartments

When uptake of a toxicant into a compartment is governed by its diffusion or transport across cell membrane barriers, the model is said to be diffusion-limited or barrier-limited. Diffusion-limited uptake or release occurs when the flux, or the transport of a toxicant across cell membranes, is slow compared with blood flow to the tissue. In this case, the permeability-area product is small compared with blood flow, i.e., $PA \ll Q_t$. The distribution of large polar molecules into tissue cells is likely to be limited by the rate at which the molecules pass through cell membranes. In contrast, entry into the interstitial space of the tissue through the leaky capillaries of the vascular space is usually rapid even for large molecules. Figure 7-15 shows the structure of such a compartment. The toxicant concentrations in the vascular and interstitial spaces are in equilibrium and make up the extracellular sub-compartment, where uptake from the incoming blood is flow-limited. The rate of toxicant uptake across the cell membrane from the extracellular space into the intracellular space is limited by membrane permeability, and is thus diffusion-limited. Two mass balance differential equations are necessary to

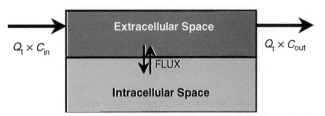

Figure 7-15. Schematic representation of a tissue compartment that features membrane-limited uptake kinetics.

Perfusion of blood into and out of the extracellular compartment is depicted by thick arrows. Transmembrane transport (flux) from the extracellular to the intracellular sub-compartment is depicted by thin double arrows. Q_t is blood flow, C_{in} is chemical concentration entering the compartment, and C_{out} is chemical concentration leaving the compartment.

describe the events in these two sub-compartments:

$$\textit{Extracellular: } V_{t1} \times dC_{t1}/dt = Q_t \times (C_{in} - C_{out})$$
$$- PA_t \times (C_{t1}/P_{t1}) + PA_t \times (C_{t2}/P_{t2}) \quad (7\text{-}21)$$

$$\textit{Intracellular: } V_{t2} \times dC_{t2}/dt = PA_t \times (C_{t1}/P_{t1})$$
$$- PA_t \times (C_{t2}/P_{t2}) \qquad (7\text{-}22)$$

Q_t is blood flow, and C is the chemical concentration in entering blood (in), exiting blood (out), tissue extracellular space (t1), or tissue intracellular space (t2). The subscript (t) for the PA term acknowledges the fact that PA, reflecting either via passive diffusion or carrier-mediated processes, can differ between tissues. Both equations feature fluxes or transfers across the cell membrane that are driven by free concentration. Hence, partition coefficients are needed to convert extracellular and intracellular tissue concentration to their corresponding free concentration. The physiologic model in Fig. 7-11 is composed of two diffusion-limited compartments each of which contain two sub-compartments—extracellular and intracellular space, and several perfusion-limited compartments.

Specialized Compartments

Lung   The inclusion of a lung compartment in a physiologic model is an important consideration because inhalation is a common route of exposure to many volatile toxic chemicals. Additionally, the lung compartment serves as an instructive example of the assumptions and simplifications that can be incorporated into physiologic models while maintaining the overall objective of describing processes and compartments in biologically relevant terms. For example, although lung physiology and anatomy are complex, Haggard (1924) developed a simple approximation that sufficiently describes the uptake of many volatile chemicals by the lungs. A diagram of this simplified lung compartment is shown in Fig. 7-16. The assumptions inherent in this compartment description are as follows: (1) ventilation is continuous, not cyclic; (2) conducting airways (nasal passages, larynx, trachea, bronchi, and bronchioles) function as inert tubes, carrying the vapor to the pulmonary or gas exchange region; (3) diffusion of vapor across the lung cell and capillary walls is rapid compared with blood flow through the lung; (4) all chemicals disappearing from the inspired air appears in the arterial blood (i.e., there is no hold-up of chemical in the lung tissue and insignificant lung mass); and (5) vapor in the alveolar air and arterial blood within the lung compartment are in rapid equilibrium and are related by $P_{b/a}$, the

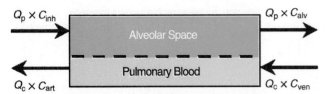

Figure 7-16. Simple model for exchange of volatile chemicals in the alveolar region of the respiratory tract.

Rapid exchange in the lumped lung compartment between the alveolar gas (*blue*) and the pulmonary blood (*light blue*) maintains the equilibrium between them as symbolized by the dashed line. Q_p is alveolar ventilation (L/h); Q_c is cardiac output (L/h); C_{inh} is inhaled vapor concentration (mg/L); C_{art} is concentration of vapor in the arterial blood; C_{ven} is concentration of vapor in the mixed venous blood. The equilibrium relationship between the chemical in the alveolar air (C_{alv}) and the chemical in the arterial blood (C_{art}) is determined by the blood/air partition coefficient $P_{b/a}$, i.e., $C_{alv} = C_{art}/P_{b/a}$.

blood/air partition coefficient (e.g., $C_{alv} = C_{art}/P_{b/a}$). $P_{b/a}$ is a thermodynamic parameter that quantifies the equilibrium partitioning of a volatile chemical between blood and air.

In the lung compartment depicted in Fig. 7-16, the rate of inhalation of a volatile chemical is controlled by the ventilation rate (Q_p) and the inhaled concentration (C_{inh}). The rate of exhalation of the chemical is a product of the ventilation rate and the chemical's concentration in the alveoli (C_{alv}). Chemical also can enter the lung compartment via venous blood returning from the heart, at a rate represented by the product of cardiac output (Q_c) and the concentration of chemical in venous blood (C_{ven}). Chemical leaving the lungs via the blood at a rate determined by both cardiac output and the concentration of chemical in arterial blood (C_{art}). Putting these four processes together, a mass balance differential equation can be written for the rate of change in the amount of chemical in the lung compartment (L):

$$\frac{dL}{dt} = Q_p \times (C_{inh} - C_{alv}) + Q_c \times (C_{ven} - C_{art}) \qquad (7\text{-}23)$$

Because of these assumptions, at steady-state the rate of change in the amount of chemical in the lung compartment becomes zero ($dL/dt = 0$). C_{alv} can be replaced by $C_{art}/P_{b/a}$, and the differential equation can be solved for the arterial blood concentration:

$$C_{art} = (Q_p \times C_{inh} + Q_c \times C_{ven})/(Q_c + Q_p/P_{b/a}) \qquad (7\text{-}24)$$

This algebraic equation is incorporated into physiologic models for many volatile organics. Because the lung is viewed here as a portal of entry and not as a target organ, the concentration of a chemical delivered to other organs by the arterial blood is of primary interest. The assumptions of continuous ventilation, dead space, rapid equilibration with arterial blood, and no hold-up of vapor in the lung tissues have worked extremely well with many volatile organics, especially relatively lipophilic volatile solvents. Indeed, the use of these assumptions simplifies and speeds model calculations and may be entirely adequate for describing the chemical behavior of relatively inert vapors with low water solubility.

Inspection of the equation for calculating the arterial concentration of the inhaled organic vapor indicates that the term $P_{b/a}$, the blood/air partition coefficient of the chemical, becomes an important term for simulating the uptake of various volatile organics. As the value for $P_{b/a}$ increases, the maximum concentration of the

chemical in the blood increases. Additionally, the time to reach the steady-state concentration and the time to clear the chemical also increase with increasing $P_{b/a}$. Fortunately, $P_{b/a}$ is readily measured by using in vitro techniques in which a volatile chemical in air is equilibrated with blood in a closed system, such as a sealed vial (Gargas and Andersen, 1988).

Liver The liver is almost always featured as a distinct compartment in physiologic models because biotransformation is an important route of elimination for many toxicants and the liver is considered the major organ for biotransformation of xenobiotics. A simple compartmental structure for the liver is depicted in Fig. 7-17, where uptake into the liver compartment is assumed to be flow-limited. This liver compartment is similar to the general tissue compartment in Fig. 7-14, except that the liver compartment contains an additional process for metabolic elimination. Under first-order elimination, the rate of hepatic metabolism (R) by the liver can be presented as:

$$R = Cl_l \times C_f \qquad (7\text{-}25)$$

where C_f is the free concentration of toxicant in the liver (mg/L), and Cl_l is the clearance of free toxicant within the liver (L/h). The latter parameter is conceptually the same as the intrinsic hepatic clearance term ($Cl_{int,h}$) in Equation (7-12). In the case of a single enzyme mediating the biotransformation and Michaelis–Menten kinetics are obeyed, Cl_l is related to the maximum rate of metabolism, V_{max} (in mg/h) and the Michaelis constant, K_M (in mg/L) (Andersen, 1981). As a result, the rate of hepatic metabolism can be expressed in terms of the Michaelis parameters.

$$R = [V_{max}/(K_M + C_f)] \times C_f \qquad (7\text{-}26)$$

Under non-saturating or first-order condition (i.e., $C_f \ll K_M$), Cl_l becomes equal to the ratio of V_{max}/K_M. Because many chemicals at toxic levels display saturable metabolism, the above equation is a key factor in the success of physiologic models for simulation of chemical disposition across a wide range of doses.

Other, more complex expressions for metabolism also can be incorporated into physiologic models. Bi-substrate second-order

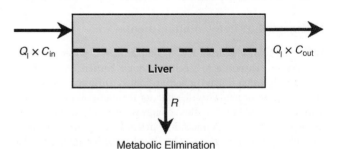

Metabolic Elimination

Figure 7-17. Schematic representation of a flow-limited liver compartment in which metabolic elimination occurs.

R, in milligrams per hour, is the rate of metabolism. Q_l is hepatic blood flow, C_{in} is chemical concentration entering the liver compartment, and C_{out} is chemical concentration out of the liver compartment. It should be noted that the liver receives blood from two sources, arterial inflow via hepatic artery and outflow from the upper mesentery via portal vein. This dual inflow is featured in the physiologic model featuring enterohepatic circulation in Fig. 7-11. Inflow via hepatic artery is often ignored, as in this case and in the physiologic model shown in Fig. 7-12, because of its relatively small flow rate compared to portal flow.

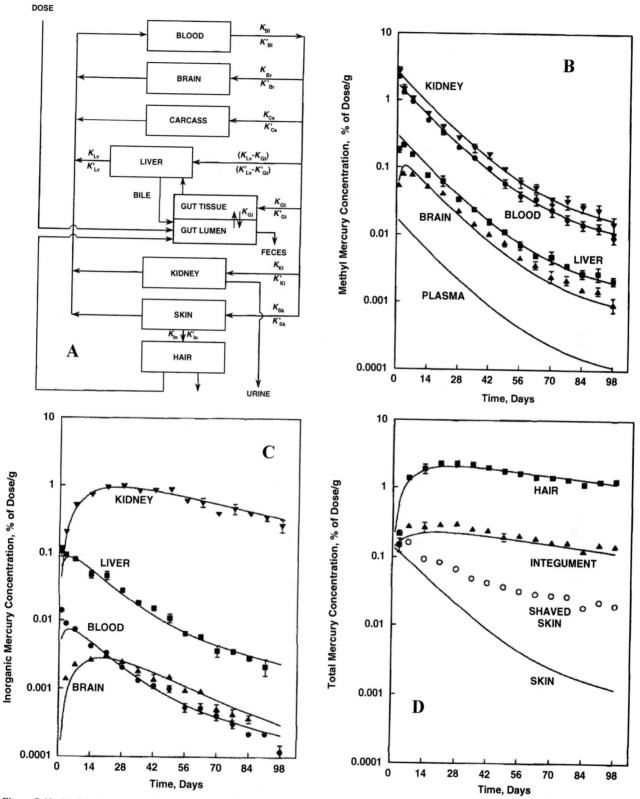

Figure 7-18. *Model simulations compared with experimental data obtained in growing adult rats dosed orally with ^{203}Hg-labelled methylmercury chloride.*

Panel A shows the physiologic model for methylmercury and its demethylated product, inorganic mercury. Primed symbols denote the parameters for inorganic mercury. Panels B and C show the respective time course of methylmercury and inorganic mercury concentration in blood, liver, kidneys and the brain. Panel C shows the slow accumulation of total mercury in hair and skin, or the integument (skin plus hair). Reprinted from Farris FF, Dedrick RL, Allen P, *et al.*: Physiological model for the pharmacokientics of methyl mercury in the growing rat. *Toxciol Appl Pharmacol* 119:74–90, 1993. With permission from Elsevier.

reactions, reactions involving the destruction of enzymes, inhibition of enzymes, or the depletion of cofactors, have been simulated using physiologic models. Metabolism can be also included in other compartments in much the same way as described for the liver.

Blood In a physiologic model, the tissue compartments are linked together by the circulatory network. Figures 7-11 and 7-12 represent different approaches toward describing the circulating blood in physiologic models. In general, the arterial system delivers a chemical into various tissues. Exceptions are the liver, which receives arterial and portal blood, and the lungs, which receive mixed venous blood from the right cardiac ventricle. In the body, the venous blood supplies draining from tissue compartments eventually merge in the vena cava and heart chambers to form mixed venous blood. In Fig. 7-11, a blood compartment is created in which the input is the sum of the toxicant outflow from each compartment ($Q_t \times C_{vt}$). Outflow from the blood compartment is a product of the blood concentration in the compartment and the total cardiac output ($Q_c \times C_{bl}$). The mass-balance differential equation for the blood compartment in Fig. 7-11 is as follows:

$$V_{bl} \times dC_{bl}/dt = (Q_{br} \times C_{vbr} + Q_{ot} \times C_{vot} + Q_k \times C_{vk} + Q_l C_{vl})$$
$$- Q_c \times C_{bl}, \qquad (7\text{-}27)$$

where V_{bl} is the volume of the blood compartment; C is concentration; Q is blood flow; bl, br, ot, k, and l represent the blood, brain, other tissues, kidney, and liver compartments, respectively; and vbr, vot, vk, and vl represent the venous blood leaving the organs. Q_c is the total blood flow equal to the sum of the venous blood flows from each organ.

In contrast, the physiologic model in Fig. 7-12 does not feature an explicit blood compartment. For simplicity, the blood volumes of the heart and the major blood vessels that are not within organs are assumed to be negligible. The venous concentration of a chemical returning to the lungs is simply the weighted average of the concentrations in the venous blood emerging from the tissues.

$$C_v = (Q_l \times C_{vl} \times Q_{rp} \times C_{vrp} + Q_{pp} \times C_{vpp} + Q_f \times C_{vf})/Q_c$$
$$(7\text{-}28)$$

where C is concentration; Q is blood flow; v, l, rp, pp, and f represent the venous blood entering the lungs, liver, richly perfused, poorly perfused, and fat tissue compartments, respectively; and vl, vrp, vpp, and vf represent the venous blood leaving the corresponding organs. Q_c is the total blood flow equal to the sum of the blood flows exiting each organ.

In the physiologic model in Fig. 7-12, the blood concentration entering each tissue compartment is the arterial concentration (C_{art}) that was calculated above for the lung compartment (Equation (7-24)). The decision to use one formulation as opposed to another to describe blood in a physiologic model depends on the role the blood plays in disposition and the type of application. If the toxicokinetics after intravenous injection is to be simulated or if binding to or metabolism by blood components is suspected, a separate compartment for the blood that incorporates these additional processes is required. A blood compartment is obviously needed if the model were developed to explain a set of blood concentration–time data for a toxicant. On the other hand, if blood is simply a conduit to the other compartments, as in the case for inhaled volatile organics shown in Fig. 7-12, the algebraic solution is acceptable.

Figure 7-18 shows the application of physiologic modeling in elucidating the disposition fate of methylmercury and its demethylated product, inorganic mercury following a single peroral administration in the growing adult rat (Farris *et al.*, 1993). The model scheme presented in Panel A for both the organic and inorganic forms of mercury has the following unique features: (1) increase in compartment size due to growth over the long duration of the tissue washout experiment; (2) mercury enters the gut lumen via biliary excretion and secretory transport from gut tissue to lumen, some of which is reabsorbed; (3) uptake of methylmercury from blood into tissues, except for the brain, is assumed to be rate-limited by plasma flow because of sequestration of mercury in rat erythrocytes and its slow release; (4) uptake of methylmercury across the blood brain barrier is rate-limited by transport; (5) uptake of inorganic mercury into all tissues, except the liver, is limited by permeability/transport; (6) mercury is transferred from skin into hair, where it is irreversibly bound; and (7) mercury in hair is either shed or ingested by the animal during grooming. The model simulations displayed in Panels B, C, and D show two prominent features of methylmercurcy disposition: (1) methylmercury is rapidly demethylated to inorganic mercury, which is slowly eliminated from the brain and the kidneys, two major sites of methylmercury toxicities; and (2) a significant portion of mercury is sequestered in hair and the ingestion of hair by the animal contributes to the remarkable persistence of mercury in the rat. This example illustrates the capability of physiologic models to deal with the varied and complex disposition kinetics of toxicants from a wide range of sources under a multitude of experimental and environmental exposure scenarios.

Conclusions

The second section provides an introduction to the simpler elements of physiologic models and the important assumptions that underlie model structures. For more detailed aspects of physiologic modeling, the readers can consult several in-depth and well-annotated reviews on physiologically based toxicokinetic models (Clewell and Anderson, 1994, 1996; O'Flaherty, 1998; Krishnan and Anderson, 2001; Krishnan *et al.*, 2002; Anderson, 2003). Computer softwares are available for numerically integrating the system of differential equations that form the models. Investigators have successfully used Advanced Continuous Simulation Language (Pharsight Corp., Palo Alto, CA), Simulation Control Program (Simulation Resources, Inc., Berrien Springs, MI), MATLAB (The MathWorks, Inc., Natick, MA), and SAS software applications to name a few. Choice of software depends on prior experience, familiarity with the computer language used, and cost of the software package.

The field of physiologic modeling is evolving as toxicologists and pharmacologists develop increasingly more sophisticated applications. Three-dimensional visualizations of xenobiotic transport in fish and vapor transport in the rodent nose, physiologic models of a parent chemical linked in series with one or more active metabolites, models describing biochemical interactions among xenobiotics, and more biologically realistic descriptions of tissues previously viewed as simple lumped compartments are just a few of the more sophisticated applications. Finally, physiologically based toxicokinetic models are beginning to be linked to biologically based toxicodynamic models to simulate the entire exposure → dose → response paradigm that is basic to the science of toxicology.

REFERENCES

Andersen ME: A physiologically based toxicokinetic description of the metabolism of inhaled gases and vapors: Analysis at steady state. *Toxicol Appl Pharmacol* 60:509–526, 1981.

Andersen ME: Physiological modeling of organic compounds. *Ann Occup Hyg* 35:309–321, 1991.

Andersen ME: Toxicokinetic modeling and its applications in chemical risk assessment. *Toxicol Lett* 138:9–27, 2003.

Andersen ME, Gargas ML, Ramsey JC: Inhalation pharmacokinetics: Evaluating systemic extraction, total *in vivo* metabolism, and the time course of enzyme induction for inhaled styrene in rats based on arterial blood:inhaled air concentration ratios. *Toxicol Appl Pharmacol* 73:176–187, 1984.

Andersen ME, Mills JJ, Gargas ML, *et al*.: Modeling receptor-mediated processes with dioxin: Implications for pharmacokinetics and risk assessment. *Risk Anal* 13:25–36, 1993.

Bertilsson L, Tomson T, Tybring G: Pharmacokinetics: time-dependent changes—autoinduction of carbamazepine epoxidation. *J Clin Pharmacol* 26:459–462, 1986.

Brown RP, Delp MD, Lindstedt SL, *et al*.: Physiological parameter values for physiologically based pharmacokinetic models. *Toxicol Ind Health* 13:407–484, 1997.

Burbacher TM, Shen DD, Lalovic B, *et al*.: Chronic maternal methanol inhalation in nonhuman primates (Macaca fascicularis): Exposure and toxicokinetics prior to and during pregnancy. *Neurotoxicol Teratol* 26:201–221, 2004.

Clewell HJ IIIrd, Andersen ME. Physiologically-based pharmacokinetic modeling and bioactivation of xenobiotics. *Toxicol Ind Health* 10:1–24, 1994.

Clewell HJ IIIrd, Andersen ME. Use of physiologically based pharmacokinetic modeling to investigate individual versus population risk. *Toxicology* 111:315–329, 1996.

Collins AS, Sumner SCJ, Borghoff SJ, *et al*.: A physiological model for tert-amyl methyl ether and *tert*-amyl alcohol: Hypothesis testing of model structures. *Toxicol Sci* 49:15–28, 1999.

Farris FF, Dedrick RL, Allen P, *et al*.: Physiological model for the pharmacokientics of methyl mercury in the growing rat. *Toxciol Appl Pharmacol* 119:74–90, 1993.

Gargas ML, Andersen ME: Physiologically based approaches for examining the pharmacokinetics of inhaled vapors, in Gardner DE, Crapo JD, Massaro EJ (eds): *Toxicology of the Lung.* New York: Raven Press, 1988, pp. 449–476.

Gerloski LE, Jain RK: Physiologically based pharmacokinetic modeling: Principles and applications. *J Pharm Sci* 72:1103–1127, 1983.

Gibaldi M, Perrier D: *Pharmacokinetics*, 2nd ed. New York: Marcel Dekker, 1982.

Haggard HW: The absorption, distribution, and elimination of ethyl ether: II. Analysis of the mechanism of the absorption and elimination of such a gas or vapor as ethyl ether. *J Biol Chem* 49:753–770, 1924.

Himmelstein KJ, Lutz RJ: A review of the applications of physiologically based pharmacokinetic modeling. *J Pharmacokinet Biopharm* 7:127–145, 1979.

Iwatsubo T, Hirota N, Ooie T, *et al*.: Prediction of in vivo drug metabolism in the human liver from in vitro metabolism data. *Pharmacol Ther* 73:147–171, 1997.

Krishnan K, Anderson ME: Physiologically based pharmacokinetic modeling in toxicology, in Hayes AW (ed): *Principles and Methods of Toxicology.* Philadelphia: Taylor & Francis, 2001, pp. 193–241.

Krishnan K, Haddad S, Beliveau M, *et al*.: Physiological modeling and extrapolation of pharmacokinetic interactions from binary to more complex chemical mixtures. *Environ Health Perspect* 110 (Suppl 6):989–994, 2002.

Lin JH, Sugiyama Y, Awazu S, *et al*.: In vitro and in vivo evaluation of the tissue-to-blood partition coefficient for physiological pharmacokinetic models. *J Pharmacokinet Biopharm* 10:637–647, 1982.

Lutz RJ, Dedrick RL, Zaharko DS: Physiological pharmacokinetics: An in vivo approach to membrane transport. *Pharmacol Ther* 11:559–592, 1980.

MacGregor JT, Collins JM, Sugiyama Y, *et al*.: In vitro human tissue models in risk assessment: report of a consensus-building workshop. *Toxicol Sci* 59:17–36, 2001.

Miners JO, Knights KM, Houston JB, *et al*.: In vitro-in vivo correlation for drugs and other compounds eliminated by glucuronidation in humans: pitfalls and promises. *Biochem Pharmacol* 71:1531–1539, 2006.

Nichols J, Rheingans P, Lothenbach D, *et al*.: Three-dimensional visualization of physiologically based kinetic model outputs. *Environ Health Perspect* 102:952–956, 1994.

O'Flaherty EJ. Physiologically based models of metal kinetics. *Crit Rev Toxicol* 28:271–317, 1998.

Ramsey JC, Andersen ME: A physiologically based description of the inhalation pharmacokinetics of styrene in rats and humans. *Toxicol Appl Pharmacol* 73:159–175, 1984.

Rowland M: Physiologic pharmacokinetic models and interanimal species scaling. *Pharmacol Ther* 29:49–68, 1985.

Rowland M: Physiologic pharmacokinetic models: Relevance, experience, and future trends. *Drug Metab Rev* 15:55–74, 1984.

Rowland M, Tozer TN: Clinical Pharmacokinetics. Baltimore: Williams & Wilkins, 1995.

Schentag JJ, Jusko WJ: Renal clearance and tissue accumulation of gentamicin. *Clin Pharmacol Ther* 22:364-70, 1977.

Teorell T: Kinetics of distribution of substances administered to the body: I. The extravascular modes of administration. *Arch Int Pharmacodyn Ther* 57:205–225, 1937.

Thummel KE, Shen DD, Isoherranen N, Smith HE: Appendix II. Design and optimization of dosage regimens: Pharmacokinetic data. In: Brunton LL, Parker KL, Buxton IOL, Blumenthal DK (eds.): *Goodman & Gilman's: The Pharmacological Basis of Therapeutics, 11th ed.* The McGraw-Hill Companies, 2006.

Tozer NT, Rowland M: *Introduction to Pharmacokinetics and Pharmacodynamics: The Quantitative Basis of Drug Therapy.* Lippincott Williams & Wilkins, 2006, p. 75.

Travis CC, Quillen JL, Arms AD: Pharmacokinetics of benzene. *Toxicol Appl Pharmacol* 102:400–420, 1990.

Wilkinson GR. Clearance approaches in Pharmacology. *Pharmacol Rev* 39:1–47, 1987.

UNIT 3

NON-ORGAN-DIRECTED TOXICITY

CHAPTER 8

CHEMICAL CARCINOGENESIS

James E. Klaunig and Lisa M. Kamendulis

OVERVIEW

Cancer is a disease of cellular mutation, proliferation, and aberrant cell growth. It ranks as one of the leading causes of death in the world. In the United States, cancer ranks as the second leading cause of death, with over one million new cases of cancer diagnosed and more than one half million Americans die from cancer annually. Multiple causes of cancer have been either firmly established or suggested, including infectious agents, radiation, and chemicals. Estimates suggest that 70–90% of all human cancers have a linkage to environmental, dietary, and behavioral factors (Fig. 8-1). While our understanding of the biology of the progression from a normal cell to a malignant one has advanced considerably in the past several decades, many aspects of the causes, prevention, and treatment of human cancers remain unresolved.

HISTORICAL BACKGROUND

A strong historical foundation for the linkage of the induction of cancer by chemicals has been documented (Table 8-1). In 1775, Percival Pott described a linkage between the increased occurrence of scrotal and nasal cancer among chimney sweepers and their profession. Pott (1775) concluded that chimney soot was the causative agent for cancer induction in these individuals. Other investigators also recognized an association between exposure to chemicals and the

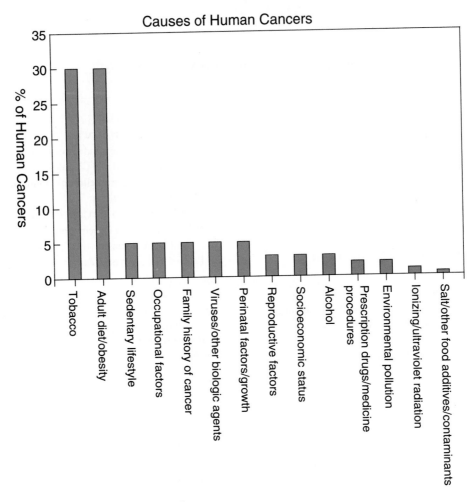

Figure 8-1. *Major causes of Human Cancers.*

Adapted from *Harvard Reports on Cancer Prevention volume* 1 (1996).

induction of human cancer. Thiersch (1875) described a relationship between sunlight exposure and skin cancer in humans. A linkage between an increased incidence of lung cancer and uranium mining was noted by Harting and Hesse (1879). Butlin, in a follow-up of Potts' observations, noted that scrotal cancer in chimney sweepers in the European continent was relatively rare compared to that seen in England (Butlin, 1892). He attributed this difference to better hygiene practices by the European sweepers as well as to the use of younger boys as sweeps in England, suggesting that the age of exposure and the duration of exposure influence the formation of the cancer. Rehn (1895) reported a linkage between the manufacturer of aniline dyes and the induction of bladder cancer in dye workers. Due to the increase in demand for synthetic dyes in the 19th century, production of the aniline-based dyes increased, as did the development of skin and bladder cancer in exposed workers. The specific chemicals in the dyes related to the cause of skin and bladder cancer were later determined to be the aromatic compounds 2-naphthylamine and benzidine (Hueper *et al.*, 1938). Exposure of workers to metals such as chromium (Alwens and Jonas, 1932), nickel (Stephens, 1932), as well as asbestos (Wood and Gloyne, 1934) was shown to be associated with an increased incidence of lung cancers in workers.

Based on these human observations, further investigations in the first half of the 20th century were performed to examine the role of these chemical mixtures and individual chemical compounds in the mixtures using animal models. Initial studies by Yamagiwa and Ichikawa (1915) examined the linkage between exposure to coal tar and its derivatives on cancer induction in humans by painting coal tar on rabbit ears. This resulted in skin cancer in the rabbits. Subsequently, Kennaway and Hieger (1930) purified the compound dibenz(*a,h*)anthracene from the coal tar extract, and determined that dibenz(*a,h*)anthracene was at least one compound in the coal tar mixture that was responsible for inducing skin cancer in mice. Cook *et al.* (1933) similarly isolated another polyaromatic hydrocarbon, benzo(*a*)pyrene, from the coal tar and showed this to also function as a carcinogen in rodents. In similar approaches with aromatic amines, Hueper *et al.* (1937) reported that 2-naphthylamine induced bladder tumors in dogs, and Yoshida and Kinosita (1936) found that feeding aminoazotoluene or aminoazobenzene to rodents induced liver cancer. Studies with the aromatic amine compounds in animal models correlated with the human epidemiological studies that had revealed an association between bladder cancer in humans and exposure to aniline dyes, and helped to define the specific chemicals in the dyes responsible for the cancer induction. These

Table 8-1

Historical Events in Chemically Induced Cancer

DATE	INVESTIGATOR(S)	CAUSATIVE AGENT(S)
1775	Pott	Soot and chimney sweeps
1822	Ayrton	Arsenic-containing metal
1875	Thiersch	Sunlight
1876	Manourriez	Coal tar
1879	Harting and Hesse	Lung cancer and uranium
1892	Butlin	Soot and chimney sweeps
1895	Rehn	Manufacture of aniline dyes
1902	Frieben	X-rays
1915	Davis	Pipe smokers and betel nut chewers
1915	Yamagiwa, Ichikawa, and Tsusui	Induction of skin cancer in rabbits and mice by coal tar
1920	Leitch and Seguina	Radium radiation
1928	Delore and Bergamo	Benzene
1930	Kennaway and Hieger	Tumor induction by dibenz[a,h] anthracene
1932	Stephens	Nickel
1932	Alwens	Chromium compounds
1933	Cook, Hewett, and Hieger	Isolation of the carcinogen benzo[a]pyrene from coal tar
1936	Yoshida and Kinosita	Induction of liver cancer in rats by o-aminoazotoluene
1934	Wood and Gloyne	Arsenicals, beryllium, and asbestos
1934	Neitzel	Mineral oil mists and radiation
1936	Kawahata	Coal tar fumes
1938	Hueper, Wiley, and Wolfe	Induction of urinary cancer in dogs by 2-naphthylamine
1941	Berenblum, Rous, MacKenzie, and Kidd	Initiation and promotion stages in skin carcinogenesis with benzo[a]pyrene
1951	Miller and Miller	Carcinogen binding to cellular macromolecule

epidemiological and experimental studies have shown a clear relationship between the induction of cancer in humans and rodents by a specific chemical or chemical mixture. In addition, this experimental work, demonstrated that animal models could be used as surrogates for humans in the study of chemical carcinogenesis.

Definitions

An understanding of the cellular and molecular aspects of the cancer process requires an understanding of the pathology and scientific terms involved in defining neoplasia (Table 8-2). Neoplasia is often defined as new growth or autonomous growth of tissue. The resulting neoplastic lesion is referred to as a neoplasm. Both benign and malignant neoplasms can be induced by chemical carcinogens. Benign neoplasms are lesions characterized by expansive growth, frequently exhibiting slow rates of proliferation that do not invade surrounding tissue or other organs. In contrast, a malignant neoplasm demonstrates invasive growth characteristics, capable of spreading throughout the organ of origin, and through metastasis to other tissues and organs. Metastases are

Table 8-2

Terminology

Neoplasia	New growth or autonomous growth of tissue
Neoplasm	The lesion resulting from the neoplasia
Benign	Lesions characterized by expansive growth, frequently exhibiting slow rates of proliferation that do not invade surrounding tissues
Malignant	Lesions demonstrating invasive growth, capable of metastases to other tissues and organs
Metastases	Secondary growths derived from a primary malignant neoplasm
Tumor	Lesion characterized by swelling or increase in size, may or may not be neoplastic
Cancer	Malignant neoplasm
Carcinogen	A physical or chemical agent that causes or induces neoplasia
Genotoxic	Carcinogens that interact with DNA resulting in mutation
Nongenotoxic	Carcinogens that modify gene expression but do not damage DNA

Table 8-3
Neoplasm Nomenclature

TISSUE OF ORIGIN	BENIGN NEOPLASM	MALIGNANT NEOPLASM
Connective tissue		
Bone	Osteoma	Osteosarcoma
Fibrous	Fibroma	Fibrosarcoma
Fat Lipid	Lipoma	Liposarcoma
Blood cells and related cells		
Hematopoietic cells		Leukemias
Lymphoid tissue		Lymphomas
Muscle		
Smooth	Leiomyoma	Leiomyosarcoma
Striated	Rhabdomyoma	Rhabdomyosarcoma
Endothelium	Hemangioma	Angiosarcoma
Mesothelium		Mesothelioma
Epithelial		
Squamous	Squamous cell papilloma	Squamous cell or carcinoma
Respiratory	Bronchial adenoma	Bronchogenic carcinoma
Renal epithelium	Renal tubular adenoma	Renal cell carcinoma
Liver cells	Liver cell adenoma	Hepatocellular carcinoma
Urinary epithelium	Transitional cell papilloma	Transitional cell carcinoma
Testicular epithelium		Seminoma
Melanocytes		Malignant melanoma

secondary growths derived from the cells of the primary malignant neoplasm.

The term "tumor" describes a lesion that may or may not be neoplastic, and is characterized by swelling or an increase in size. In classifying neoplasms, the nomenclature reflects both the tissue or cell of origin, and the characteristics of the type of tissue involved (Table 8-3). For benign neoplasms, the tissue of origin is frequently followed by the suffix "oma"; for example, a benign fibrous neoplasm would be termed *fibroma*, and a benign glandular epithelium termed an *adenoma*. Malignant neoplasms from epithelial origin are called *carcinomas* while those derived from mesenchymal origin are referred to as *sarcoma*. Thus, a malignant neoplasm of fibrous tissue would be a *fibrosarcoma*, whereas that derived from bone would be an *ostoesarcoma*. Similarly, a malignant neoplasm from the liver would be a *hepatocellular carcinoma*, whereas that derived from skin would be referred to as a *squamous cell carcinoma*. Preneoplastic lesions have also been observed in a number of target organs in both animal models and humans, and reflect an early reversible lesion in neoplasm progression. The characterization and study of preneoplastic cells has led to a further understanding of the process of cancer formation.

The term "cancer" describes the subset of neoplasia that represents malignant neoplasms. A *carcinogen* is an agent, chemical or physical, that causes or induces neoplasia. This definition has been more thoroughly defined as an agent whose administration to previously untreated animals leads to a statistically significant increased incidence of neoplasia of one or more histogenetic types, as compared with the incidence of the appropriate untreated control animals (Pitot, 1986). Thus, the induction of both benign and malignant neoplasms is included in this definition.

Carcinogens can be chemicals, viruses, hormones, radiation, or solid materials. Carcinogens either produce new neoplastic growth in a tissue or organ or increase the incidence and/or multiplicity of background spontaneous neoplastic formation in the target tissue.

Table 8-4
Features of Genotoxic and Nongenotoxic Carcinogens

Genotoxic carcinogens
  Mutagenic
  Can be complete carcinogens
  Tumorigenicity is dose responsive
  No theoretical threshold
Nongenotoxic carcinogens
  Nonmutagenic
  Threshold, reversible
  Tumorigenicity is dose responsive
  May function at tumor promotion stage
  No direct DNA damage
  Species, strain, tissue specificity

Carcinogens may be *genotoxic*, meaning that they interact physically with DNA to damage or change its structure. Other carcinogens may change how DNA expresses information without modifying or directly damaging its structure, or may create a situation in a cell or tissue that makes it more susceptible to DNA damage from other sources. Chemicals belonging to this latter category are referred to as *nongenotoxic* carcinogens. Common features of genotoxic and nongenotoxic carcinogens are shown in Table 8-4.

This knowledge has led to continued efforts, using both epidemiological information and experimental animal models, to assess chemical carcinogenicity of occupational, industrial, and environmental agents, to gain an understanding of the mechanisms of action for these agents, and to determine the relevance of human exposure to cancer risk.

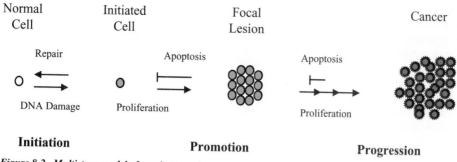

Figure 8-2. Multistage model of carcinogenesis.

MULTISTAGE CARCINOGENESIS

Through extensive experimental studies with animal models and evaluation of human cancers, it has been shown that the carcinogenesis process involves a series of definable and reproducible stages. Operationally, these stages have been defined as initiation, promotion, and progression (Fig. 8-2). These steps follow a temporal sequence of events that have been observed in a wide variety of target tissues. The defining characteristics of each of these stages are outlined in Table 8-5.

Initiation

The first stage of the cancer process involves initiation, a process that is defined as a stable, heritable change. This stage is a rapid, irreversible process that results in a carcinogen-induced mutational event. Chemical and physical agents that function at this stage are referred to as initiators or initiating agents. Initiating agents lead to genetic changes including mutations and deletions. Chemical carcinogens that covalently bind to DNA and form adducts that result in mutations are initiating agents. Included among chemicals classified as initiating carcinogens are compounds such as polycyclic hydrocarbons and nitrosamines, biological agents such as viruses, and physical agents such as X-rays and UV light. Most chemical carcinogens that function at the initiation stage of the cancer process are indirect-acting genotoxic compounds that require metabolic activation in the target cell to produce the DNA-damaging event. For indirect-acting genotoric compounds, the chemical must be taken into the target site and metabolized. The ultimate form of the carcinogen is then able to bind to nuclear DNA, resulting in adduct formation. The initiating event becomes "fixed" when the DNA adducts or other damage to DNA are not correctly repaired or are incompletely repaired prior to DNA synthesis. This event can lead to inappropriate base pairing and/or formation of a mutation.

Initiation by itself does not appear to be sufficient for neoplastic formation. Once initiated cells are formed, their fate has multiple potential outcomes: (1) the initiated cell can remain in a static nondividing state through influences by growth control via either normal surrounding cells or through endocrine influence; (2) the initiated cell may possess mutations incompatible with viability or normal function and be deleted through apoptotic mechanisms; or (3) the cell, through stimuli such as intrinsic factors or from chemical exposure, may undergo cell division resulting in the growth in the proliferation of the initiated cell. In some instances, typically following relatively high doses and/or repeated exposure to the genotoxic carcinogen, a chemical carcinogen may function as a complete carcinogen, i.e., it is capable of progressing through all stages of the cancer process.

Table 8-5
Characteristics of the Stages of the Carcinogenesis Process

Initiation
  DNA modification
  Mutation
  Genotoxic
  One cell division necessary to lock in mutation
  Modification is not enough to produce cancer
  Nonreversible
  Single treatment can induce mutation
Promotion
  No direct DNA modification
  Nongenotoxic
  No direct mutation
  Multiple cell divisions necessary
  Clonal expansion of the initiated cell population
  Increase in cell proliferation or decrease in cell death (apoptosis)
  Reversible
  Multiple treatments (prolonged treatment) necessary
  Threshold
Progression
  DNA modification
  Genotoxic event??
  Mutation, chromosome disarrangement
  Changes from preneoplasia to neoplasia benign/malignant
  Irreversible
  Number of treatments needed with compound unknown (may require only single treatment)

Promotion

Derived from either endogenous or exogenous stimuli of cell growth, the second stage of the carcinogenesis process involves the selective clonal expansion of initiated cells to produce a preneoplastic lesion. This is referred to as the promotion stage of the carcinogenesis process. Both exogenous and endogenous agents that function at this stage are referred to as tumor promoters. Tumor promoters are not mutagenic and generally are not able to induce tumors by themselves; rather they act through several mechanisms involving gene expression changes that result in sustained cell proliferation, either through increases in cell proliferation and/or the inhibition of apoptosis. Nongenotoxic carcinogens frequently function at the tumor promotion stage. The growth of preneoplastic lesions requires repeated applications of or continuous exposure to tumor-promoting compounds. While initial exposure to tumor promoters may result in an increase in cell proliferation and/or DNA synthesis in all tissues of the organ, this is usually a transient effect and with repeated applications of the tumor promoter only the initiated cells continue to clonally expand and divide (Fig. 8-2). Promotion is a reversible phenomenon whereby upon removal of the promoting agent, the focal cells may return to single initiated cell thresholds. In addition, these agents demonstrate a well-documented threshold for their effects, below a certain dose or frequency of application, tumor promoters are unable to induce cell proliferation. Multiple chemical compounds as well as physical agents have been linked to the tumor promotion stage of the cancer process. Tumor promoters in general show organ-specific effects, e.g., a tumor promoter of the liver, such as phenobarbital will not function as a tumor promoter in the skin or other tissues.

Progression

The final stage of the carcinogenesis process, progression, involves the conversion of benign preneoplastic lesions into neoplastic cancer. In this stage, due to increase in DNA synthesis cell proliferation in the preneoplastic lesions, additional genotoxic events may occur resulting in additional DNA damage including chromosomal aberrations and translocations. These events result in the transfer from preneoplastic, clonally derived cell populations into neoplastic cell populations. Chemicals that impact on the progression stage are usually genotoxic agents. By definition, the progression stage is an irreversible stage in that neoplasm formation, whether benign or malignant, occurs. With the formation of neoplasia, an autonomous growth and/or lack of growth control is achieved. Spontaneous progression can occur from spontaneous karyotypic changes that occur in mitotically active initiated cells during promotion. An accumulation of nonrandom chromosomal aberrations and karyotypic instability are hallmarks of progression. As such, chemicals that function as progressor agents are usually clastogenic and are capable of causing chromosomal abnormalities. Complete carcinogens have the ability to function at the initiation, promotion, and progression stages and hence by definition have genotoxic properties. In addition, a number of model systems are available to test for carcinogenicity and/or to study the multistep mechanisms involved in chemical carcinogenesis. The models are described in a later section of this chapter.

MECHANISMS OF ACTION OF CHEMICAL CARCINOGENS

The development of neoplasia requires two major events: the formation of an initiated, mutated cell and the selective proliferation of the mutated cell to form a neoplasm. Both these events can be induced or acted upon by chemical carcinogens. Chemicals that induce cancer have been broadly classified into one of two categories—genotoxic or DNA reactive, and nongenotoxic or epigenetic carcinogens—based on their relative abilities to interact with genomic DNA.

Genotoxic Carcinogens

Genotoxic carcinogens initiate tumors by producing DNA damage. Experimental and epidemiological observations made in the middle of the 20th century identified a number of chemicals that could cause cancer in humans or experimental animals. Coal tar carcinogens including benzo(*a*)pyrene, pesticides such as 2-acetylaminofluorine,

Table 8-6
Examples of Genotoxic Carcinogens

Direct-acting carcinogens
  Nitrogen or sulfur mustards
  Propane sulfone
  Methyl methane sulfonate
  Ethyleneimine
  B-Propiolactone
  1,2,3,4-Diepoxybutane
  Dimethyl sulfate
  Bis-(Chloromethyl) ether
  Dimethylcarbamyl chloride
Chemicals requiring activation (indirect-acting carcinogens)
  Polycyclic aromatic hydrocarbons and heterocyclic aromatics
  Aromatic amines
  N-Nitrosoamines
  Azo dyes
  Hydrazines
  Cycasin
  Safrole
  Chlorinated hydrocarbons
  Aflatoxin
  Mycotoxin
  Pyrrolizidine alkaloids
  Bracken fern
  Carbamates

and azo dyes such as diaminobenzamide were among the first chemical carcinogens to be studied. DNA reactive carcinogens can be further subdivided according to whether they are active in their parent form (i.e., direct-acting carcinogens—agents that can directly bind to DNA without being metabolized) and those that require metabolic activation (i.e., indirect-acting carcinogens—compounds that require metabolism in order to react with DNA). Examples of direct-acting and indirect-acting carcinogens are listed in Table 8-6.

Direct-Acting (Activation-Independent) Carcinogens A variety of carcinogens do not require metabolic activation or chemical modification to induce cancer, and are termed direct acting or activation-independent carcinogens. These chemicals are also defined as ultimate carcinogens. Examination of the chemical structure of these agents reveals that they are highly reactive electrophilic molecules that can interact with and bind to nucleophiles, such as cellular macromolecules including DNA. Common electrophilic species are shown in Fig. 8-3. Generally, chemicals containing these moieties are highly reactive and frequently result in tumor formation at the site of chemical exposure.

Direct-acting carcinogens include epoxides, imines, alkyl and sulfate esters, and mustard gases (Fox and Scott, 1980; Sontag, 1981). Direct-acting electrophilic carcinogenic chemicals typically test positive in the Ames test without additional bioactivation with a liver metabolic fraction. The relative carcinogenic strength of direct-acting carcinogens depends in part on the relative rates of interaction between the chemical and genomic DNA, as well as competing reactions with the chemical and other cellular nucleophiles. The relative carcinogenic activity of direct-acting carcinogens is dependent upon such competing reactions and also on detoxification reactions. Chemical stability, transport, and membrane permeability determine the carcinogenic activity of the chemical. Direct-acting

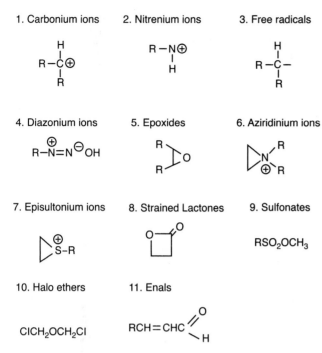

1. Carbonium ions   2. Nitrenium ions   3. Free radicals

4. Diazonium ions   5. Epoxides   6. Aziridinium ions

7. Episultonium ions   8. Strained Lactones   9. Sulfonates

RSO_2OCH_3

10. Halo ethers   11. Enals

$ClCH_2OCH_2Cl$

Figure 8-3. Structures of reactive carcinogenic electrophiles.

carcinogens are typically carcinogenic at multiple sites and in all species examined. A number of direct-acting alkylating agents, including a number of chemotherapeutic chemicals, are carcinogenic in humans (Vainio *et al.*, 1991).

Indirect-Acting Genotoxic Carcinogens   An important discovery in the understanding of chemical carcinogenesis came from the investigations of the Millers who established that many carcinogens are not intrinsically carcinogenic, but require metabolic activation to be carcinogenic. They demonstrated that azo dyes covalently bind to proteins in liver, leading to the conclusion that carcinogens may bind to proteins that are critical for cell growth control (Miller and Miller, 1947). Subsequent work with benzo(*a*)pyrene showed covalent binding of benzo(*a*)pyrene or the metabolites of benzo(*a*)pyrene in rodents (Miller, 1951). Additional investigations with other indirect-acting genotoxic carcinogens confirmed that metabolism of the parent compound was necessary to produce a metabolite (activation) that was able to interact with DNA (Miller, 1970).

It has since been shown that the majority of DNA reactive carcinogens are found as parent compounds, or procarcinogens. Procarcinogens are stable chemicals that require subsequent metabolism to be carcinogenic (Miller and Miller, 1981; Weisburger and Wiliams, in Becker, 1981; Conney, 1982; Miller *et al.*, 1983). The terms procarcinogen, proximate carcinogen, and ultimate carcinogen have been coined to define the parent compound (procarcinogen) and its metabolite form, either intermediate (proximate carcinogen) or final (ultimate carcinogen) that reacts with DNA (Fig. 8-4). The ultimate form of the carcinogen is most likely the chemical species that results in mutation and neoplastic transformation. The ultimate form of certain carcinogenic chemicals is not known, whereas for other chemicals there may be more than one ultimate carcinogenic metabolite depending on the metabolic pathway followed. It is important to note that besides activation of the procarcinogen to a DNA

reactive form, detoxification pathways may also occur resulting in inactivation of the carcinogen.

Indirect-acting genotoxic carcinogens usually produce their neoplastic effects, not at the site of exposure (as seen with direct-acting genotoxic carcinogens) but at the target tissue where the metabolic activation of the chemical occurs. Indirect-acting genotoxic carcinogens include the polycyclic aromatic hydrocarbons (PAHs), nitrosamines, aromatic amines, and aflatoxin B1. Figure 8-4 shows the parent (procarcinogen) and metabolites for several representative indirect-acting genotoxic carcinogens.

Mutagenesis

The reaction of a carcinogen with genomic DNA, either directly or indirectly, may result in DNA adduct formation or DNA damage, and frequently produces a mutation. Several mechanisms of mutagenesis are known to occur. Modification of DNA by electrophilic carcinogens can lead to a number of products. Modified DNA are dependent upon when in the cell cycle the adducts are formed; where the adducts are formed; and, the type of repair process used in response to the damage.

Transitions are a substitution of one pyrimidine by the other, or one purine by the other (changes within a chemical class), whereas a transversion occurs when a purine is replaced by a pyrimidine, or a pyrimidine is replaced by a purine (changes across a chemical class). Carcinogens can induce transitions and transversions several ways. In one scenario, when adducts (or apurinic or apyrmidinic sites) are encountered by the DNA replication processes, they may be misread. The polymerase may preferentially insert an adenine (A) in response to a noninformative site. Thus, the daughter strand of an A, C, G, or T adduct will have an adenine (A) and this change is fixed (mutation) and resistant to subsequent DNA repair. A second outcome, a shift in the reading frame (resulting in a frame-shift mutation) may also result from carcinogen–DNA adducts formation. Most frame-shift mutations are deletions and occur more frequently when the carcinogen–DNA adduct is formed on a nucleotide. In a third scenario, DNA strand breaks can also result from carcinogen DNA adducts. These may arise either as a result of excision–repair mechanisms that are incomplete during DNA replication or via direct alkylation of the phosphodiester backbone leading to backbone cleavage. Strand scission can lead to double-strand breaks, recombination, or loss of heterozygosity.

Damage by Alkylating Electrophiles

As noted above, most chemical carcinogens require metabolic activation to exert a carcinogenic effect. The ultimate carcinogenic forms of these chemicals are frequently strong electrophiles (Fig. 8-3) that can readily form covalent adducts with nucleophilic targets. Because of their unpaired electrons, S:, O:, and N: atoms are nucleophilic targets of many electrophiles. The extent of adducts formed is limited by the structure of DNA, where bulky electrophilic chemicals can bind, and size of the ultimate carcinogenic form. In general, the stronger electrophiles display a greater range of nucleophilic targets (i.e., they can attack weak and strong nucleophiles), whereas weak electrophiles are only capable of alkylating strong nucleophiles (e.g., S: atoms in amino acids). In addition, the metabolic capability of a target cell will dictate the extent and types of electrophiles generated from the procarcinogenic parent.

An important and abundant source of nucleophiles is contained not only in the DNA bases, but also in the phosphodiester

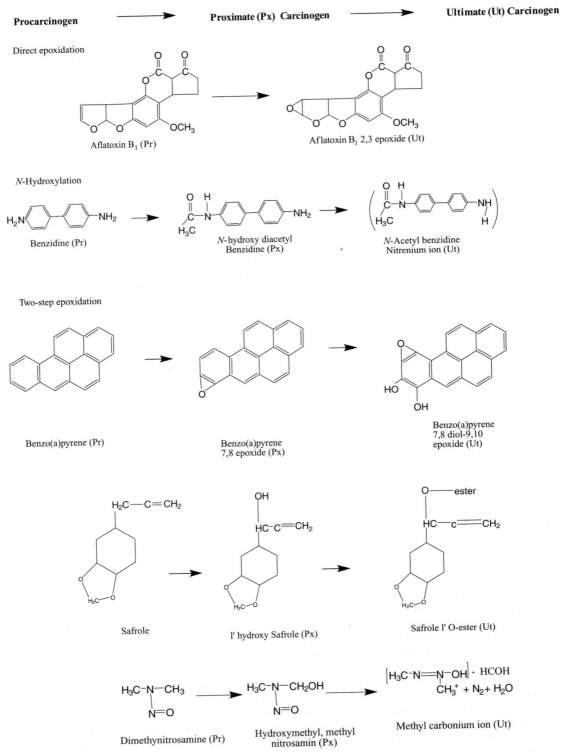

Procarcinogen ⟶ **Proximate (Px) Carcinogen** ⟶ **Ultimate (Ut) Carcinogen**

Direct epoxidation

Aflatoxin B₁ (Pr)

Aflatoxin B₁ 2,3 epoxide (Ut)

N-Hydroxylation

Benzidine (Pr)

N-hydroxy diacetyl Benzidine (Px)

N-Acetyl benzidine Nitrenium ion (Ut)

Two-step epoxidation

Benzo(a)pyrene (Pr)

Benzo(a)pyrene 7,8 epoxide (Px)

Benzo(a)pyrene 7,8 diol-9,10 epoxide (Ut)

Safrole

1′ hydroxy Safrole (Px)

Safrole 1′ O-ester (Ut)

Dimethynitrosamine (Pr)

Hydroxymethyl, methyl nitrosamin (Px)

Methyl carbonium ion (Ut)

Figure 8-4. Structures of representative indirect-acting carcinogens and their metabolic derivatives.

The proximate (Px) and ultimate (Ut) carcinogenic forms result from the metabolism of the procarcinogenic form (Pr).

backbone (Fig. 8-5). Whereas carcinogen DNA adducts may be formed at all sites in DNA, the most common sites of alkylation include the N^7 of guanine, the N^3 of adenine, the N^1 of adenine, the N^3 of guanine, and the O^6 of guanine. Alkylations of phosphate may also occur at a high frequency. Selective examples of carcinogen interactions with proteins and nucleic acids are shown in Fig. 8-6. Different electrophilic carcinogens will often display different preferences for nucleophilic sites in DNA and different spectra of damage. Dimethylnitrosamine and diethylnitrosamine, for example, are metabolized by P450 oxidation to yield a methyl carbonium ion

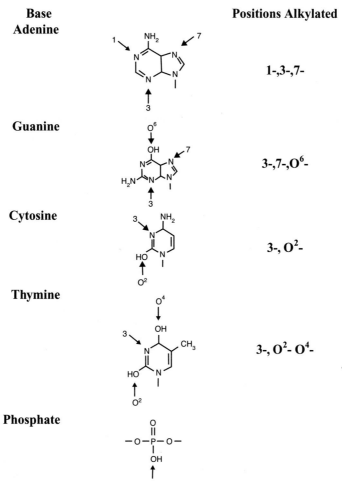

Figure 8-5. Examples of cellular nucleophiles and sites of possible adduct formation.

(CH_3^+) and an ethyl carbonium ion ($CH_3CH_2^+$), respectively. Despite the structural similarities of the ultimate electrophiles, they display significant differences in alkylation profiles (Pegg, 1984). The relative proportions of methylated bases present in DNA following reaction with carcinogen-methylating agents are shown in Table 8-7 (Pegg, 1984). The predominant adduct formed following exposure to methylating chemicals such as methylmethane sulfonate is 7-methylguanine. In contrast, ethylating agents produce adducts predominately in the phosphate backbone of DNA. The carcinogenic potential of the type of adducts formed is often debated; some believe that O^6-alkylguanine is the most carcinogenic adduct, while others report that O^4-alkylthymine is more important in the carcinogenic process, due to its persistence relative to other adducts (Pegg, 1984; Swenberg et al., 1984).

Another common modification to DNA is the hydroxylation of DNA bases. Oxidative DNA adducts have been identified in all four DNA bases (Fig. 8-7); however, 8-hydroxyguanine is among the most prevalent oxidative DNA adduct (Floyd, 1990). The source of oxidative DNA damage is typically formed from free radical reactions that occur endogenously in the cell or from exogenous sources (Floyd, 1990; Ames and Shigenaga, 1993; Klaunig and Kamendulis, 2004). Although a relatively large amount of oxidative DNA adducts have been proposed to be formed per day, repair mechanisms exist that maintain the cellular level at a low rate and keep endogenous mutations to a relatively low level. The role of oxidative

damage and oxidative stress is discussed in greater detail later in this chapter.

Methylation of deoxycytidine residues is a well-studied DNA adduct. This reaction occurs by the transfer of a methyl group from S-adenosylmethionine by DNA methyltransferases (Holliday, 1990). Methylation of DNA results in heritable expression or repression of genes, with hypomethylation associated with active transcription of genes, while hypermethylated genes tend to be rarely transcribed. Chemical carcinogens may inhibit DNA methylation by several mechanisms including forming covalent adducts, single strand breaks in the DNA, alteration of methionine pools, and inactivation of the DNA methyltransferase responsible for methylation (Riggs and Jones, 1983). The importance of DNA methylation in chemical carcinogenesis is discussed later in this chapter.

Although a large number of adducts can be formed following exposure to chemicals, whether a particular DNA adduct will result in mutation and participate in the carcinogenesis process is dependent in part on the persistence of the adduct through the process of DNA replication, which is also in part dependent upon DNA repair.

DNA Repair

Following the formation of a carcinogen DNA adduct, the persistence of the adduct is a major determinant of the outcome. This

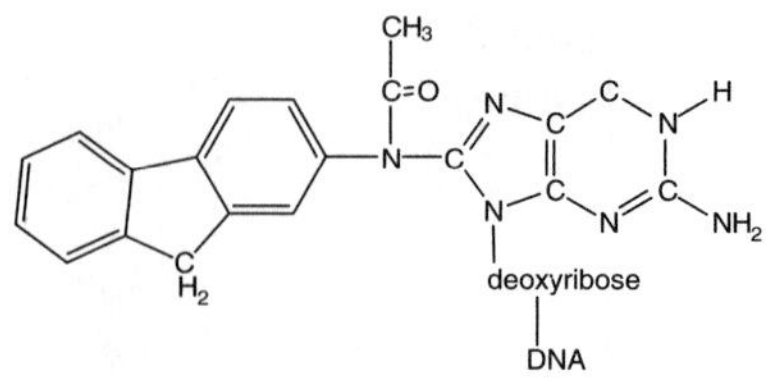

N-(deoxyguanosine-8-yl)-acetylaminofluorene in
DNA

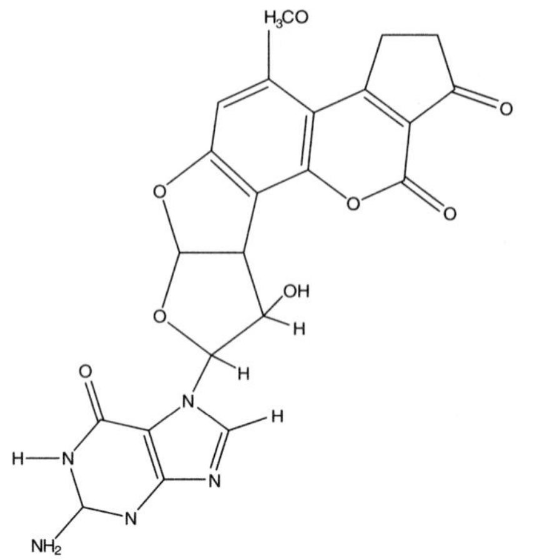

Aflatoxin B₁ N-⁷ guanine-adduct

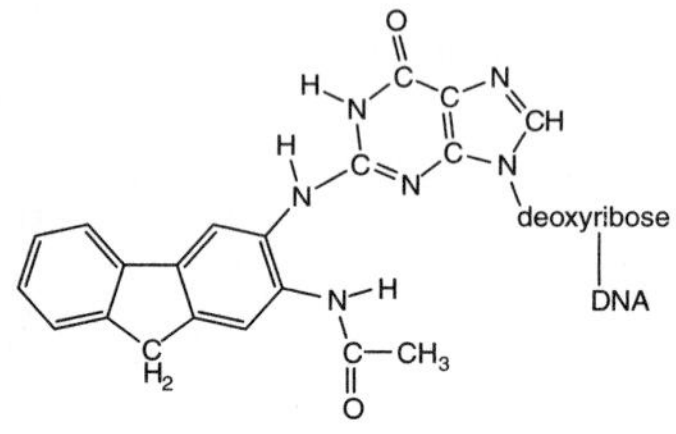

3-(deoxyguanosine N₂-yl)-acetylaminofluorene
in DNA

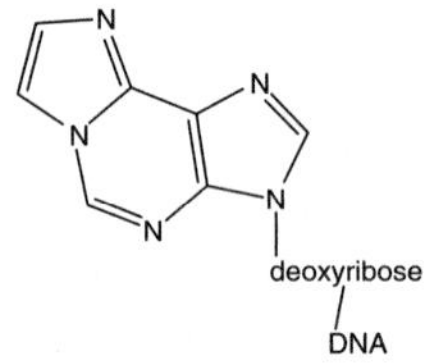

1, N⁶-ethenoadenine in
DNA

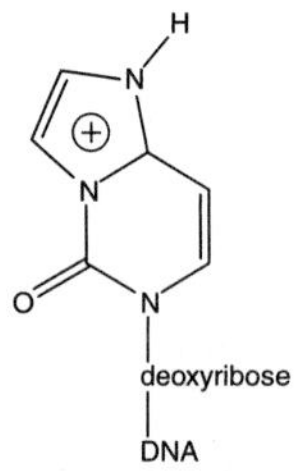

3,N⁴-ethenocytosine in DNA

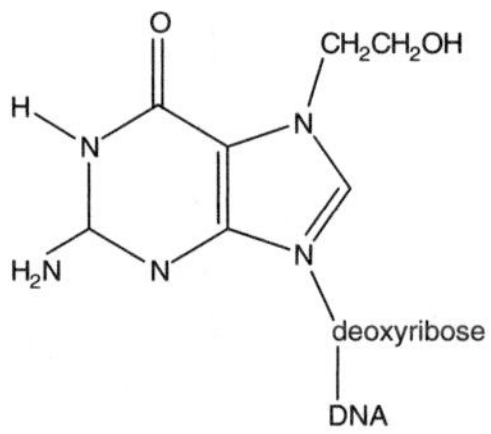

N-7-(2-hydroxyethyl) guanosine
in DNA

Figure 8-6. Select structures of protein and nucleic adducts of certain chemical carcinogens.

persistence depends on the ability of the cell to repair the altered DNA. The detection of unique DNA adducts has proven to be important in understanding the mechanism of action of specific carcinogens and has been correlated with carcinogenesis (Goth and Rajewsky, 1974; Kadlubar *et al.*, 1981; Becker and Shank, 1985; Swenberg *et al.*, 1985). However, the presence of a DNA adduct is not sufficient for the carcinogenesis process to proceed. The relative rates or persistence of particular DNA adducts may be an important determinant of carcinogenicity, for example, O^4-ethylthymine is relatively stable in DNA while O^6-ethylguanine does not persist in DNA after continuous exposure to diethylnitrosamine (Swenberg *et al.*, 1984). The persistence of DNA adducts of trans-4-aminostilbene does not correlate with organ carcinogenicity and/or tissue susceptibility. While the liver and kidney exhibited the greatest burden and persistence of the adduct and the Zymbals gland showed the least amount of DNA adducts, the latter tissue was more susceptible to carcinogenesis by this chemical (Neumann, 1983). As such, differences in susceptibility to carcinogenesis are likely the result of a number of factors, including DNA replication within a tissue and repair of a DNA adduct.

The quantification of covalent DNA adducts in tissues has been used to demonstrate exposure of humans to carcinogenic chemicals and to assess the relative risk from exposure to carcinogenic chemicals. For example, DNA adducts of carcinogenic polyaromatic hydrocarbons have been demonstrated at relatively high levels in tissues and blood of smokers and foundry workers compared with nonexposed individuals (Perera *et al.*, 1991). In addition, DNA adducts of aflatoxin B1 were seen in samples of human placenta and cord blood in individuals in Taiwan, an area that has a high incidence of liver cancer (Hsieh and Hsieh, 1993). The presence of macromolecular carcinogen adducts may be important to their mechanism of carcinogenicity, the presence and persistence of the adducts is only one factor in the process of cancer development.

Experimental and epidemiological evidence indicates that the development of cancer following exposure to chemical carcinogens is a relatively rare event. This can be explained by the ability of a cell to recognize and repair damaged DNA. During the DNA repair, the DNA region containing the adduct is removed and a new patch of DNA is synthesized, using the opposite intact strand as a template. The new DNA segment is then spliced into the DNA molecule in

Table 8-7

Relative Proportions of Methylated Bases Present in DNA after Reaction with Carcinogenic Alkylating Agents

	PERCENT OF TOTAL ALKYLATION BY	
	DIMETHYL-NITROSAMINE, N-METHYL-N-NITROSOUREA, OR 1,2-DIMETHYL-HYDRAZINE	DIETHYL-NITROSAMINE OR N-ETHYL-N-NITROSOUREA
1-Alkyladenine	0.7	0.3
3-Alkyladenine	8	4
7-Alkyladenine	1.5	0.4
3-Alkylguanine	0.8	0.6
7-Alkylguanine	68	12
O^6-Alkylguanine	7.5	8
3-Alkylcytosine	0.5	0.2
O^2-Alkylcytosine	0.1	3
3-Alkylthymine	0.3	0.8
O^2-Alkylthymine	0.1	7
O^4-Alkylthymine	0.1–0.7	1–4
Alkylphosphates	12	53

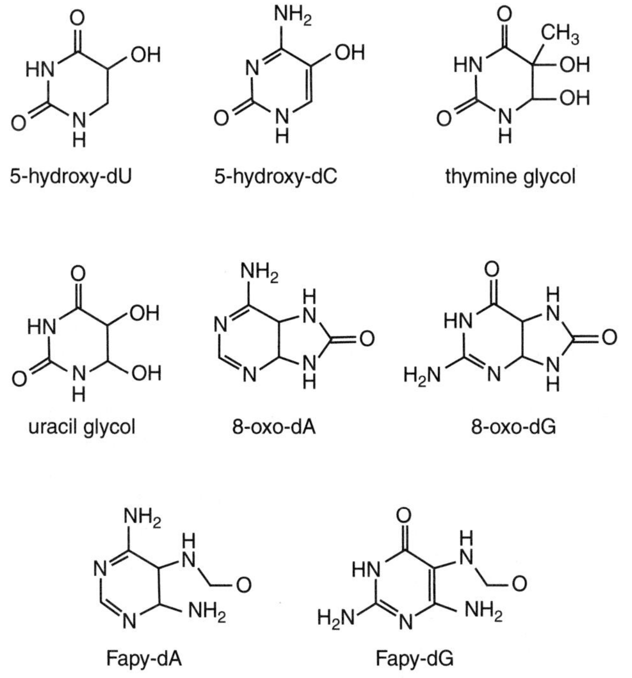

5-hydroxy-dU 5-hydroxy-dC thymine glycol

uracil glycol 8-oxo-dA 8-oxo-dG

Fapy-dA Fapy-dG

Figure 8-7. Structures of selected oxidative DNA bases.

DNA damage can lead to the insertion of an incorrect base during DNA replication, followed by transcription and translation of the mutated templates, ultimately leading to the synthesis of altered protein. Mutations in an oncogene, tumor-suppressor gene, or gene that controls the cell cycle can result in a clonal cell population with a survival advantage. The development of a cancer requires many such events, occurring over a long period of time, and for this reason human cancer induction often takes place within the context of chronic exposure to chemical carcinogens.

A number of structural alterations may occur in DNA as a result of interaction with reactive chemicals or radiation, and the more frequent types of damage are depicted in Fig. 8-8. The reaction of chemical species with DNA can produce adducts within the bases, sugar, and phosphate backbone of DNA. In addition, bifunctional alkylating agents (such as mustards) may cause DNA crosslinking between two opposing bases. Other structural changes such as pyrimidine dimer formation are specific for exposure to UV light, while double-stranded breaks in DNA are more commonly associated with ionizing radiation. A variety of mechanisms have evolved to effectively remediate and repair DNA damage. The more common types of DNA repair mechanisms seen in mammalians are listed in Table 8-8.

In addition to the proofreading activity of DNA polymerases that can correct miscopied bases during replication, cells have several mechanisms for repairing DNA damage. Repair of DNA

place of the defective one. To be effective in restoring a cell to normal, repair of DNA must occur prior to cell division; if repair is not complete prior to replication, the presence of the adducts can give rise to mispairing of bases and other genetic effects such as rearrangements and translocations of DNA segments. Thus, a chemical that alters the repair process or the rate of cell division can itself affect the frequency of neoplastic transformation.

DNA Repair Mechanisms

Although cells possess mechanisms to repair many types of DNA damage, these are not always completely effective, and residual

Table 8-8

DNA Repair Pathways

1. Direct reversal of DNA damage
2. Excision repair systems
   Base excision repair
   Nucleotide excision repair
   Mismatch repair
3. Postreplicational repair (recombination repair)
4. Nonhomologous-end-jointing (NHEJ): double-strand break repair

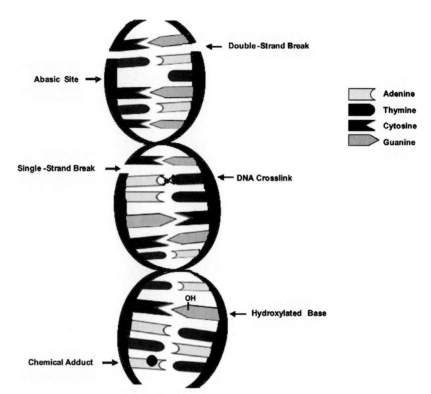

Figure 8-8. Common Forms of DNA Damage.

damage does not always occur prior to cell replication, and in addition, repair of DNA damage by some chemicals is relatively inefficient, as such, exposure to chemicals that cause DNA damage can increase the probability of acquiring mutations that ultimately lead to cancer development.

Mismatch Repair of Single-Base Mispairs   Spontaneous mutations may occur through normal cellular DNA replication errors. Many spontaneous mutations are point mutations, a change in a single base pair in the DNA sequence. The issue for mismatch repair is determining which is the normal DNA and which is the damaged DNA strand, and therefore repairing the mutated strand such that the correct base pairs are restored. Depurination is a fairly common occurrence and a spontaneous event in mammals, and results in the formation of apurinic sites. If these lesions are left unrepaired, mutations are generated during DNA replication since the DNA synthetic machinery is unable to determine the appropriate base with which to pair. All mammalian cells possess apurinic endonucleases that function to cut DNA near apurinic sites. The cut is then extended by exonucleases, and the resulting gap repaired by DNA polymerases and ligases.

Excision Repair   DNA regions containing chemically modified bases, or DNA chemical adducts, are typically repaired by excision repair processes. DNA adducts cause a distortion in the normal shape of DNA. Proteins that slide along the surface of a double-stranded DNA molecule recognize the irregularities in the shape of the double helix, and affect the repair of the lesion. DNA lesions that are repaired by excision repair processes include thymine–thymine dimers, produced following exposure to UV light; dimers that interfere with both replication and transcription of DNA. The repair

of DNA regions containing bases altered by the attachment of large chemical adducts such as benzo(*a*)pyrene are also effectively repaired by excision repair processes (Fig. 8-9).

End-Joining Repair of Nonhomologous DNA   A cell that has double-strand breaks can be repaired by joining the free DNA ends. The joining of broken ends from different chromosomes, however, will lead to the translocation of DNA pieces from one chromosome to another, translocations that have the potential to enable abnormal cell growth by placing a proto-oncogene next to, and therefore under the control of, another gene promoter. Double-strand breaks can be caused by ionizing radiation, and drugs such as anticancer drugs. Double-strand breaks are correctly repaired only when the free ends of DNA rejoin exactly. The repair of double-stranded DNA is therefore confounded by the absence of single-stranded regions that can signal the correct base pairing during the rejoining process. Homologous recombination is one of two mechanisms responsible for the repair of double-strand breaks. In this process, the double-strand break on one chromosome is repaired using the information on the homologous, intact chromosome.

The predominant mechanism for double-stranded DNA repair in multicellular organisms is nonhomologous repair, and involves the rejoining of the ends of the two DNA molecules. Although this process yields a continuous double-stranded molecule, several base pairs are lost at the joining point. This type of deletion may produce a possibly mutagenic coding change.

Classes of Genotoxic Carcinogens

Polyaromatic Hydrocarbons   Polyaromatic hydrocarbons are found at high levels in charcoal broiled foods, cigarette smoke,

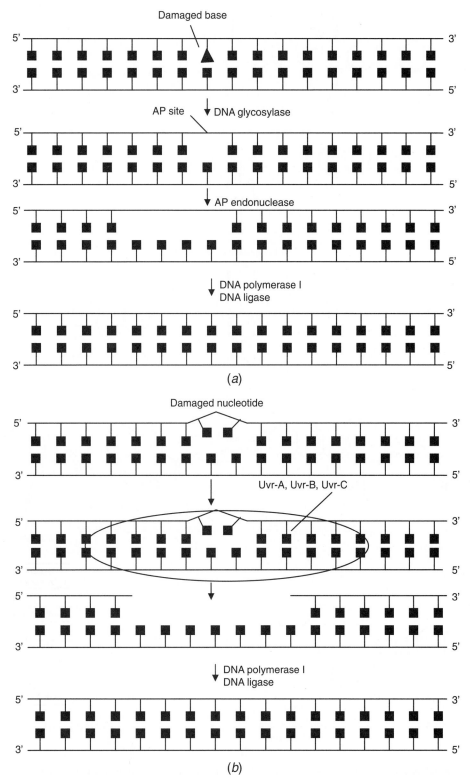

Figure 8-9. *(A) DNA repair by base excision. (B) DNA repair by nucleotide excision.*

and in diesel exhaust. Representative chemicals belonging to this class are shown in Fig. 8-10a. Benzo(*a*)pyrene is a representative polycyclic hydrocarbon that has been studied extensively. The metabolism and pathways that lead to tumor formation have been characterized through the work of a number of laboratories (Conney, 1982). The ultimate carcinogen is a diol epoxide of benzo(*a*)pyrene,

formed following three separate enzymatic reactions (Sims *et al.*, 1974). Benzo[*a*]pyrene is first oxidized by cytochrome P4501A1 to form benzo[*a*]pyrene 7,8-oxide, further metabolized by epoxide hydrolase, yielding the 7,8-dihydrodiol. And then further metabolism by cytochrome P4501A1 to yield the ultimate carcinogen, the 7,8-dihydrodiol-9,10-epoxide (Yang *et al.*, 1976; Lowe and

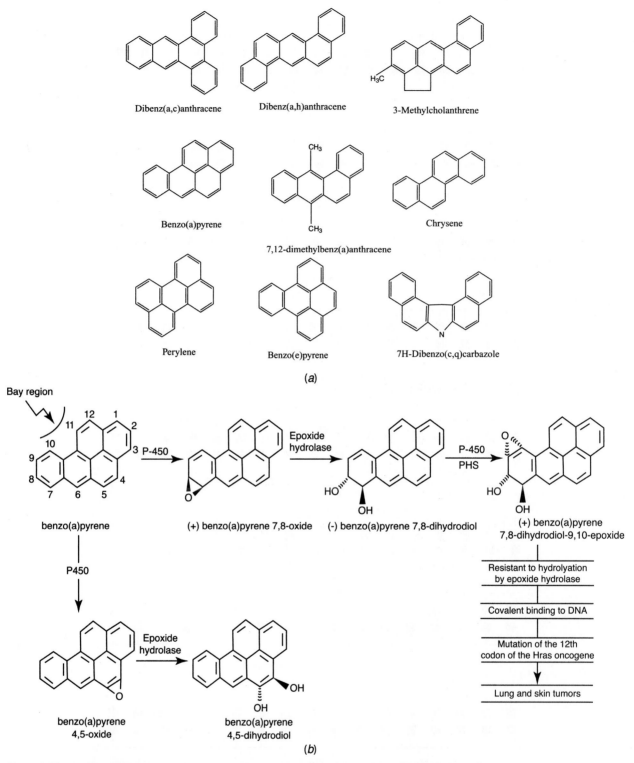

Figure 8-10. *(A) Chemical structures of selected carcinogenic polycyclic hydrocarbons. (B) Role of epoxide hydrolase in the activation of benzo[a]pyrene 4,5-oxide and in the conversion of benzo[a]pyrene to its tumorigenic bay-region diole poxide.*

Silverman, 1994). The Bay region or K region of the benzo(*a*)pyrene molecule is the site of metabolic targeting and DNA interaction (Fig. 8-10b). The importance of the bay region (K region) of the benzo(*a*) pyrene molecule was demonstrated from the understanding of the metabolism of the benzo(*a*)pyrene to its ultimate DNA reactive form. Similar regions (to the Bay region) have been iden-

tified in other carcinogenic polycyclic hydrocarbons and used to access and predict carcinogenic potential of other PAHs.

Alkylating Agents Alkylating chemicals represent an important class of chemical carcinogens. Whereas some alkylating chemicals are direct-acting genotoxic agents, many require

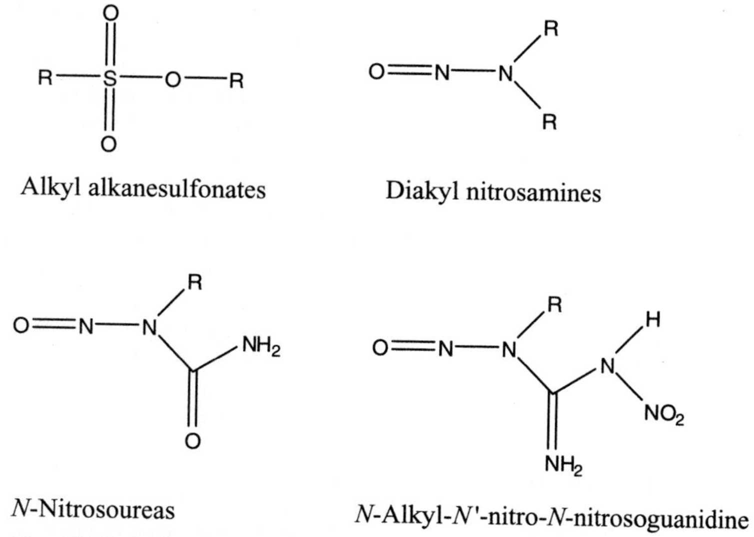

Alkyl alkanesulfonates   Diakyl nitrosamines

N-Nitrosoureas   *N*-Alkyl-*N'*-nitro-*N*-nitrosoguanidine

Figure 8-11. *Structures of representative methylating and ethylating agents.*

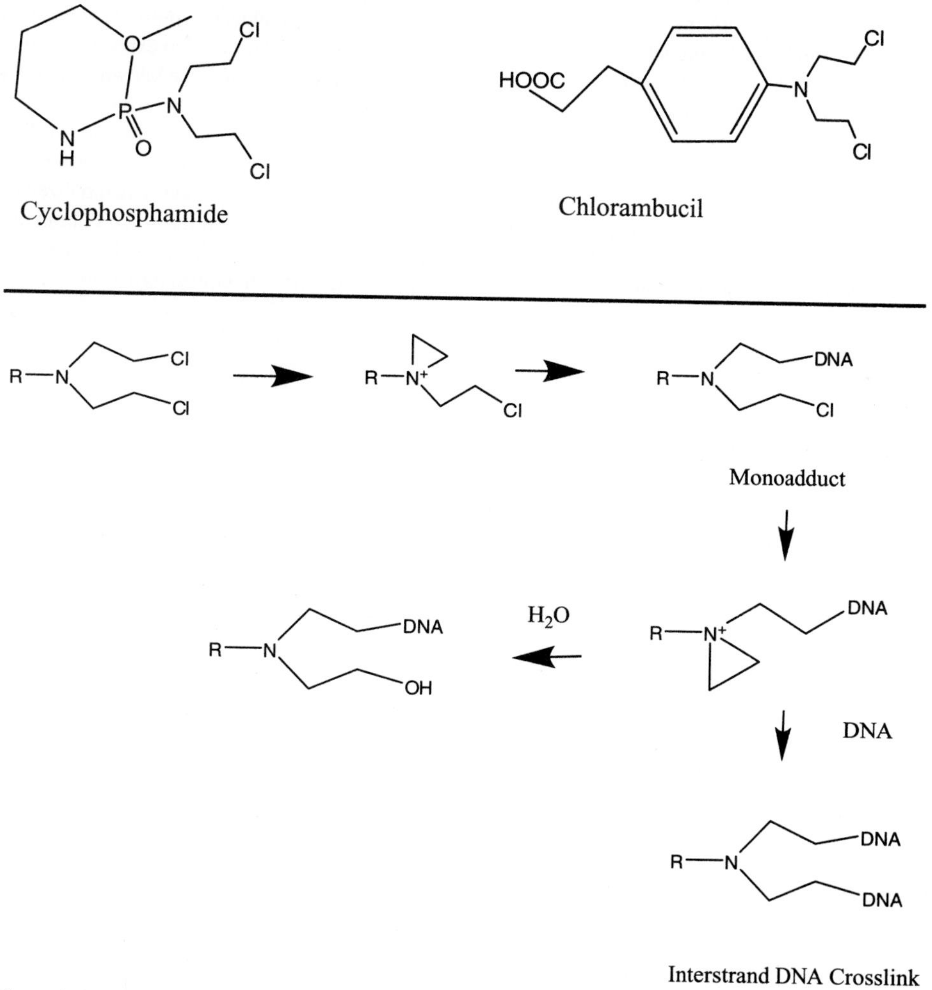

Cyclophosphamide   Chlorambucil

Monoadduct

Interstrand DNA Crosslink

Figure 8-12. *Nitrogen mustards and proposed mechanism for the reaction of nitrogen mustards with DNA.*

metabolic activation to produce electrophilic metabolites that can react with DNA. Alkylating agents can be classified into several groups including the direct-acting alkylalkanesulfonates (methyl- and ethyl methanesulfonate) and nitrosamides (*N*-methyl-*N*-nitrosourea,

N-ethyl-*N*-nitrosourea,   *N*-methyl-*N*-nitro-*N*-nitrosoguanidine, and the indirect-acting nitrosamides (dimethyl- and diethylnitrosamines) (Fig. 8-11). The alkylating compounds (or in the case of diethylnitrosamine and dimethylnitrosamine; their metabolites)

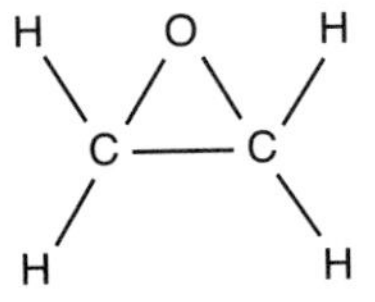

Ethylene oxide

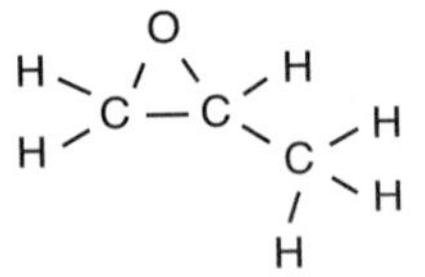

Propylene oxide

Figure 8-13. Chemical structures for ethylene and propylene oxide.

readily react with DNA at more than 12 sites. The N^7 position of guanine and the N^3 position of adenine are the most reactive sites in DNA for alkylating chemicals. DNA methylation reactions occur more readily and thus exhibit >20 more adducts than with ethylation reactions. However, ethylation reactions have a greater affinity for oxygen centers, an event that appears to correlate with the mutagenicity and carcinogenicity of these compounds. Nitrosamines were initially used as solvents in chemistry. Their toxic effects were identified when workers using the nitrosamines solvents developed jaundice and liver damage. Subsequent studies in animal models revealed that dimethylnitrosamine and diethylnitrosamine were highly hepatotoxic and hepatocarcinogenic.

Other alkylating chemicals including the nitrogen mustards (e.g., chlorambucil, cyclophosphamide) have been used in cancer chemotherapy. They produce DNA adducts as well as induce the formation of DNA strand breaks. The alkylation of DNA by nitrogen mustards requires the formation of highly reactive *N*-alkylazirdinium ions (Fig. 8-12). Nitrogen mustards can produce a wide spectrum of mutations including base pair substitutions (AT and GC) and deletions. In addition, nitrogen mustards are potent clastogens causing chromosomal aberrations and sister chromatid exchanges (SCEs), predominantly in GC-rich regions.

Ethylene oxide and propylene oxide are other examples of mutagenic and carcinogenic alkylating agents (Fig. 8-13). Ethylene oxide is a direct-acting alkylating carcinogen in rodents, and perhaps of human concern (Hogstedt *et al.*, 1986). Ethylene oxide is mutagenic in short term in vitro assays, and produces chromosomal aberrations and SCEs in eukaryotic cells (Ehrenberg and Hussain, 1981). Propylene oxide is also a mutagenic rodent carcinogen inducing nasal tumors in rodents following inhalation exposure (NTP, 1985). Alkylation of DNA by ethylene and propylene oxide occurs predominantly at the N^7 position of guanine, yielding 7-(2-hydroxyethyl)guanine and 7-(2-hydroxypropyl)guanine adducts, respectively. These adducts represent the major adducts formed following either in vitro or in vivo exposure (Walker *et al.*, 1992).

Vinyl chloride is another known rodent and human carcinogen, producing angiosarcomas in the liver and tumors in the lung and hematopoetic system in humans (Doll, 1985). Limited evidence also suggests that vinyl chloride exposure results in brain tumors. Vinyl chloride is mutagenic and is metabolized by cytochrome P450 to form chloroethylene oxide, which rearranges nonenzymatically to produce chloroacetaldehyde, both of which can alkylate DNA. Vinyl chloride and metabolites form several DNA adducts including

4-Aminobiphenyl (ABP)

Aniline

4-Aminoazobenzene

2-Aminophenanthrene

Benzidine

Diphenylamine

4,4'-Methylene-*bis*-2-chloroaniline

2-Naphthylamine

2-Acetylaminofluorene (2-AAF)

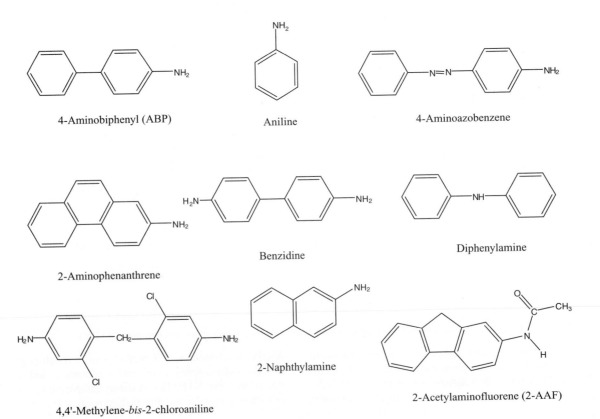

Figure 8-14. Chemical structures of selected carcinogenic aromatic amines.

Table 8-9
Carcinogenicity of Metals

| METAL | ANIMAL | | | HUMAN | |
	SPECIES	TUMOR SITE	TUMOR TYPE	EXPOSURE	TUMOR TYPE
Arsenic	Mice, dogs, rats	None observed	None observed	Cu refinery	Pulmonary carcinoma
				As pesticides	Lymphoma, leukemia
				Chemical plants	Dermal carcinoma
				Drinking water (oral)	Hepatic angiosarcoma
Beryllium	Mice, rats, monkeys	Bone Lung	Osteosarcoma Carcinoma	None observed	None observed
Cadmium	Mice, rats, chickens	Injection site Testes	Sarcoma Teratoma	CD refinery	Pulmonary carcinoma
Chromium	Mice, rats, rabbits	Injection site Lung	Sarcoma Carcinoma	CR refinery Chrome plating Chromate pigments	Pulmonary carcinoma Gastrointestinal carcinoma
Cobalt	Rats, rabbits	Injection site	Sarcoma	None observed	None observed
Iron	Hamsters, mice, rats, rabbits	Injection site	Sarcoma	None observed	None observed
Lead	Mice, rats	Kidney	Carcinoma	None observed	None observed
Nickel	Mice, rats, cats, hamsters, rabbits Guinea pigs, rats	Injection site Lung Kidney	Carcinoma Carcinoma Carcinoma	Ni refinery	Pulmonary carcinoma Nasolaryngeal carcinoma Gastric and renal carcinoma Sarcoma (?)
Titanium	Rats	Injection site	Sarcoma	None observed	None observed
Zinc	Chickens, rats, hamsters	Testes Testes	Carcinoma Teratoma	None observed	None observed

7-(2′-oxoethyl)guanine, N^2, 3-ethenoguaine, 3,N^4-ethenocytosine, and 1,N^6-ethenoadenine (Guengerich, 1994).

Aromatic Amines and Amides   Aromatic amines and amides encompass a class of chemicals with varied structures (aromatic amines, e.g. aniline dyes, 2-naphthylamine, benzidine, 2-acetylaminofluorene) (Fig. 8-14). Because of their use in the dye industry and other industrial processes their carcinogen potential in humans was realized as early as the late 19th century. While proper industrial hygiene processes have considerably reduced the human exposure to aromatic amines and amides in the workplace, exposure to these chemicals still occurs through cigarette smoke and environmental sources. The aromatic amines undergo both phase-I and phase-II metabolism. Phase-I reactions occur mainly by cytochrome P450-mediated reactions, yielding hydroxylated metabolites that are often associated with adduct formation in proteins and DNA, and produce liver and bladder carcinogenicity (Miller *et al.*, 1964). For example, metabolism of 2-acetylaminofluorene (AAF) results in the formation of N-hydroxy-AAF, which is a metabolite responsible for the liver tumorigenicity. Similarly, 1-napthylamine exhibits carcinogenic activity only in test systems capable of producing the N-hydroxy metabolite of naphthylamine. Aromatic amines are capable of forming adducts with several DNA bases.

Inorganic Carcinogens

Several metals exhibit carcinogenicity in experimental animals and/or exposed humans. Table 8-9 provides a listing of some common metals and their corresponding carcinogenicity in animals and humans. Additional details are provided below.

Arsenic   Arsenic compounds are poorly mutagenic in both bacterial and mammalian cell assays (Lofroth and Ames, 1978). Metallic arsenic, arsenic trioxide, sodium arsenite, sodium arsenate, potassium arsenite, lead arsenate, calcium arsenate, and pesticide mixtures containing arsenic have been tested for carcinogenicity in experimental animals (IARC, 1980, 1987). In the majority of studies in experimental animals—including oral exposure studies in mice, rats, and dogs; dermal exposure studies in mice; inhalation exposure studies in mice; injection studies in mice and rats; and intramedullary injection studies in rats and rabbits—no tumors were observed or the results were inconclusive, and thus it has previously been concluded that limited evidence exists for the carcinogenicity of inorganic arsenic compounds in experimental animals (IARC, 1987).

In contrast, inorganic arsenic compounds are known human carcinogens, based on sufficient evidence of carcinogenicity in humans. Epidemiological studies of humans exposed to arsenic compounds demonstrated that exposure to inorganic arsenic compounds increases the risk of cancer in the skin, lung, digestive tract, liver, bladder, kidney, and lymphatic and hematopoietic systems (IARC, 1973, 1980). Several of the epidemiological studies have reported dose–response relationships between arsenic in drinking water and several types of cancer, including bladder, kidney, lung, and skin cancer (Cantor, 1997; Ferreccio *et al.*, 2000). The mechanisms for cancer formation are unclear but possibly involve the induction of oxidative stress, altered cell signaling, modulation of apoptosis, and/or altered cell cycle (Harris and Shi, 2003; Quian and Shi, 2003; Hughes and Kitchin, 2006). The latency period in humans of arsenic-related carcinogenesis is considered to be 30–50 years. The first signs of chronic exposure, frequently seen in water supplies contaminated with arsenic, are skin pigmentation, depigmentation, hyperkeratosis of palms and soles, and skin lesions. A unique peripheral vascular disease associated with chronic arsenic exposure is black foot disease, starting with numbness and ulceration of extremities and ending in gangrene and spontaneous amputations (Chen *et al.*, 1988).

Beryllium   Beryllium and its salts are not mutagenic and do not appear to induce cellular transformation (IARC, 1993). Mechanistically, beryllium salts bind to nucleoproteins and inhibit enyzmes involved in DNA synthesis, resulting in infidelity of DNA synthesis and also induce gene mutations in cultured cells (Leonard and Lauwerys, 1987). Studies in animal models have consistently reported increases in lung tumors in rodents and nonhuman primates exposed to beryllium or beryllium compounds (IARC, 1993; Finch *et al.*, 1996; NTP, 1998). Beryllium metal and several beryllium compounds (e.g., beryllium–aluminum alloy, beryllium ore, beryllium chloride, beryllium hydroxide, beryllium sulfate tetrahydrate, and beryllium oxide) induced lung tumors in rats. Beryllium oxide and beryllium sulfate produced lung cancer (anaplastic carcinoma) in monkeys after intrabronchial implantation or inhalation. In rabbits, osteosarcomas were reported after exposure to beryllium metal, beryllium carbonate, beryllium oxide, beryllium phosphate, beryllium silicate, or zinc beryllium silicate (IARC, 1993).

Beryllium and beryllium compounds have been classified as human carcinogens based on animal studies and evidence of carcinogenicity in humans. Epidemiological studies indicate an increased risk of lung cancer in occupational groups exposed to beryllium or beryllium compounds (Steenland and Ward, 1991; Ward *et al.*, 1992). Further, an association with lung cancer has consistently been observed in occupational populations exposed to beryllium or beryllium compounds. Acute beryllium pneumonitis, a marker for exposure to beryllium has been shown to be associated with higher lung cancer rates (Steenland and Ward, 1991).

Cadmium   Animal studies have shown that cadmium and cadmium compounds induce tumor formation at various sites in multiple species of experimental animals, following multiple exposure routes, including the induction of prostate tumors in rats, testicular tumors in rats and mice, lymphoma in mice, adrenal-gland tumors in hamsters and mice, and lung and liver tumors in mice (IARC, 1993; Waalkes *et al.*, 1994, 1999). It has been suggested that ionic cadmium, or compounds that release ionic cadmium, is the cause of genetic damage and thus the carcinogenic species. Increased frequencies of chromosomal aberrations (changes in chromosome structure or number) have been observed in lymphocytes of workers occupationally exposed to cadmium. Many studies of cultured mammalian cells have shown that cadmium compounds cause genetic damage, including gene mutations, DNA strand breaks, chromosomal damage, cell transformation, and disrupted DNA repair (IARC, 1993).

Cadmium and cadmium compounds have been classified as known human carcinogens based on evidence of carcinogenicity in humans, including epidemiological and mechanistic information that indicate a causal relationship between exposure to cadmium and cadmium compounds and human cancer (IARC, 1993). Epidemiological studies of cadmium workers found that exposure to various cadmium compounds increased the risk of death from lung cancer (IARC, 1993). Follow-up analysis of some of these cohorts has confirmed that cadmium exposure is associated with elevated lung cancer risk under some industrial circumstances (Sorahan *et al.*, 1995; Sorahan and Lancashire, 1997). Some epidemiological evidence has also suggested an association between cadmium exposure and prostate cancer (Shigematsu *et al.*, 1982; van der Gulden *et al.*,

1995), kidney (Mandel *et al.*, 1995), and bladder (Siemiatycki *et al.*, 1994).

Chromium   Chromium has multiple oxidation states: from -2 to $+6$; however, the most common forms are the trivalent (III) and hexavalent (VI) forms. With regard to carcinogenicity, chromium III does not exhibit carcinogenicity in laboratory animals whereas chromium VI has been tested to be positive for genotoxicity and carcinogenicity in a variety of bioassays (Langard, 1988; IARC, 1990). Chromium VI compounds cause genetic damage including gene mutations and DNA damage in bacteria. Several chromium VI compounds also caused mutations in yeast and insects. Many chromium VI compounds caused genetic damage in cultured human and other animal cells and in experimental animals exposed in vivo, including SCE, chromosomal aberrations, and cell transformation. Chromosomal aberrations, SCE, and aneuploidy were observed in workers exposed to chromium VI compounds (IARC, 1990). Chromium VI (calcium chromate, chromium trioxide, sodium dichromate, lead chromates, strontium chromate, or zinc chromates) exposure in rats following inhalation, intrabronchial, intrapleural, intratracheal, intramuscular, or subcutaneous administration resulted in benign and malignant lung tumors in rats in a number of studies. In mice, calcium chromate caused benign lung tumors and chromium trioxide caused malignant lung tumors. Exposure of hamsters, guinea pigs, and rabbits to chromium VI compounds by intratracheal instillation did not cause lung tumors (IARC, 1980, 1990). While the mechanisms for chromium VI carcinogenicity remain unresolved, it has been speculated that the reduction of chromium VI by glutathione is involved (Connett and Whtterhahn, 1985; Kortenkamp and O'Brien, 1994).

Hexavalent chromium (chromium VI) compounds have been classified as known human carcinogens based on data from animal studies and human epidemiological studies. Human epidemiological studies have consistently reported increased risks of lung cancer among chromate workers. Chromate workers are exposed to a variety of chromium compounds, including chromium VI and trivalent (III) compounds. In addition, an increased risk of a rare cancer of the sinonasal cavity was observed in these workers (IARC, 1990). Some studies suggested that exposure to chromium among workers, such as chromium-exposed arc welders, chromate pigment workers, chrome platers, and chromium tanning workers, may be associated with leukemia and bone cancer (Costa, 1997).

Nickel   Many studies in cultured rodent and human cells have shown that a variety of nickel compounds, including both soluble and insoluble forms of nickel, exhibit genotoxicity, producing DNA strand breaks, mutations, chromosomal damage, cell transformation, and modulation of DNA repair. Soluble nickel salts can be complete carcinogens and/or initiators of carcinogenesis (Kasprzak *et al.*, 1990; Diwan *et al.*, 1992). In rats and mice, inhalation or intratracheal instillation of nickel subsulfide or nickel oxide produced dose-related increases of benign and malignant lung tumors (IARC, 1990; NTP, 1996). Inhalation of nickel compounds also caused malignant and benign pheochromocytoma in rats (NTP, 1996). Short-term intraperitoneal exposure during gestation to soluble nickel salt induced malignant pituitary tumors in the offspring. Additionally, exposure to nickel acetate through the placenta followed by exposure of the offspring to barbital (a known tumor promoter) produces kidney tumors (renal cortical and pelvic tumors) (Diwan *et al.*, 1992). In adult rats, injection of soluble nickel salts followed by exposure to a promoting carcinogen resulted in kidney cancer (renal cortical adenocarcinomas) that frequently metastasized to the lung, liver, and spleen (Kasprzak *et al.*, 1990). The carcinogenic properties of metallic nickel are believed to be due to ionic nickel, which can slowly dissolve in the body from nickel compounds.

Nickel compounds are classified as known human carcinogens (IARC, 1990) based on animal data and sufficient evidence of carcinogenicity from human studies. The IARC (1990) evaluation of nickel and nickel compounds concluded that nickel compounds are carcinogenic to humans based on sufficient evidence in the nickel refining industry and very strong evidence of carcinogenicity of a variety of nickel compounds in experimental studies in rodents. Several cohort studies of workers exposed to various nickel compounds showed an elevated risk of death from lung and nasal cancers (IARC, 1990). An excess risk of lung and nasal cancer was seen in nickel refinery workers exposed primarily to soluble nickel compounds (Anderson *et al.*, 1996).

Lead Lead compounds do not appear to cause genetic damage directly, but may do so through several indirect mechanisms, including inhibition of DNA synthesis and repair, oxidative damage, and interaction with DNA-binding proteins and tumor-suppressor proteins (NTP, 2003). Lead has exhibited conflicting results concerning its genotoxicity; it does not cause mutations in bacteria, but does cause chromosomal aberrations in vitro and in vivo, and causes DNA damage in vivo and in cell-free systems, whereas in mammalian systems, conflicting results were observed. Lead also inhibits the activity of DNA and RNA polymerase in cell-free systems and in mammalian cell cultures. Conflicting results were observed for SCE and micronucleus formation in mammalian test systems.

In studies with laboratory animals, carcinogenicity has been observed for soluble (lead acetate and lead subacetate) and insoluble (lead phosphate, lead chromate) inorganic lead compounds as well as for tetraethyl lead (an organic lead compound), following exposure via oral, injection, and in offspring exposed via the placenta or lactation. Although kidney tumors (including adenomas, carcinomas, and adenocarcinomas) were most frequently associated with lead exposure, tumors of the brain, hematopoietic system, and lung were reported in some studies (IARC, 1980, 1987; Waalkes *et al.*, 1995). Lead also appears to function as a tumor promoter, leading to increased incidence in kidney tumors initiated by *N*-ethyl-*N*-hydroxyethylnitrosamine and *N*-(4'-fluoro-4-biphenyl)acetamide (IARC, 1980, 1987). The mechanisms by which lead causes cancer are not understood.

Lead and lead compounds are classified as reasonably anticipated to be human carcinogens based on limited evidence from studies in humans and sufficient evidence from studies in experimental animals. Lead exposure has been associated with increased risk of lung, stomach, and bladder cancer in diverse human populations (Fu and Boffetta, 1995; Steenland and Boffetta, 2000; NTP, 2003). Epidemiological studies link lead exposure to increased risk for lung and stomach cancer. However, most studies of lead exposure and cancer reviewed had limitations, including poor exposure assessment and failure to control for confounding factors.

Nongenotoxic (Epigenetic) Carcinogens

A number of chemicals that produce tumors in experimental animals following chronic treatment appear to act via mechanisms not involving direct binding, damage, or interaction of the chemical or its metabolites with DNA (Williams and Whysner, 1996). Based on the lack of genotoxicity, yet their ability to induce tumors in rodent models, these agents have been labeled nongenotoxic carcinogens. The

organ and tissue targets induced by nongenotoxic carcinogens are many times in tissues where a significant incidence of background, spontaneous tumors is seen in the animal model. Prolonged exposure to relatively high levels of chemicals is usually necessary for the production of tumors. In addition, with nongenotoxic carcinogens, tumors are not theoretically expected to occur at exposures below a threshold at which relevant cellular effects are not observed. In contrast to DNA-reactive genotoxic effects, non-DNA reactive mechanisms may be unique to the rodent species used for testing. Certain chemical carcinogens have been well studied and provide examples for the use of mechanistic information in risk assessment. Further, the biochemical modes of action for non-DNA reactive carcinogens are diverse. Examples include agents that function via sustained cytotoxicity, receptor-mediated (e.g., CAR, PPARα, AhR) effects, hormonal perturbation, as well as the induction of oxidative stress and modulation of methylation status (Table 8-10). Each of these potential mechanisms is discussed in greater detail in the following sections.

Cytotoxicity Cytotoxicity and consequent regenerative hyperplasia is a well-documented mode of action for a variety of non-DNA reactive chemical carcinogens (Dietrich and Swenberg, 1991). Chloroform-induced liver and kidney tumors and melamine-induced bladder tumors are classic examples of chemical carcinogens that are classified as functioning via a cytolethal mode of action (Bull *et al.*, 1986; Butterworth, 1990; Larson *et al.*, 1994; Pereira, 1994; Andersen *et al.*, 1998). Chemicals that function through this mechanism produce sustained cell death, often related to metabolism of

Table 8-10

Proposed Modes of Action for Selected Nongenotoxic Chemical Carcinogens

MODE OF ACTION	EXAMPLE
Cytotoxicity	Chloroform
	Melamine
α_{2u}-*Globulin-binding*	D-limonene,
	1,4-dichlorobenzene
Receptor mediated CAR	Phenobarbital
PPARα	Trichloroethylene
	Perchloroethylene
	Diethylhexylphthalate
	Fibrates (e.g., clofibrate)
AhR	TCDD
	Polychlorinated biphenyls (PCBs)
	Polybrominated biphenyls (PBBs)
Hormonal	Biogenic amines
	Steroid and peptide hormones
	DES
	Phytoestrogens (bisphenol-A)
	Tamoxifen
	Phenobarbital
Altered methylation	Phenobarbital
	Choline deficiency
	Diethanolamine
Oxidative stress inducers	Ethanol
	TCDD
	Lindane
	Dieldrin
	Acrylonitrile

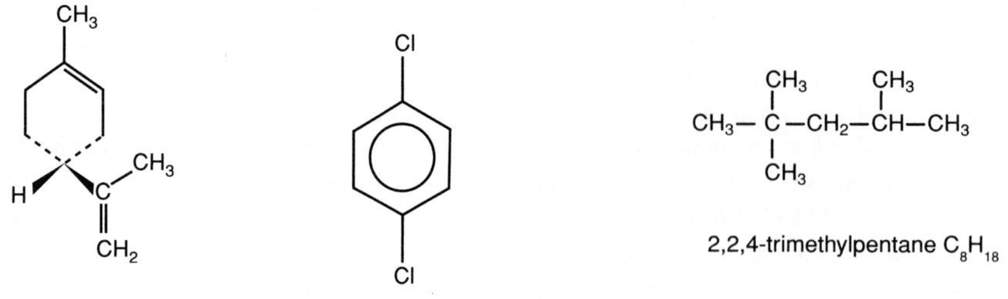

D-limonene   1,4-dichlorobenzene

Figure 8-15. Examples of selective α2u-globulin-binding chemicals.

the chemical, that is accompanied by persistent regenerative growth, resulting in the potential for the acquisition of "spontaneous" DNA mutations and allowing mutated cells to accumulate and proliferate. This process then gives rise to preoplastic focal lesions that upon further expansion can lead to tumor formation. Chloroform has been shown to induce mouse liver tumors only at doses that produce liver necrosis, thus demonstrating an association between necrosis with compensatory hyperplasia and the resulting tumorigenicity, and also supports that a threshold for the induction of tumors is likely at doses that do not produce toxicity. It is important to note that the induction of cytotoxicity may be observed with many carcinogens both genotoxic and nongenotoxic when high toxic exposures occur. Thus, the induction of cytotoxicity with compensatory hyperplasia may contribute to the observed tumorigenicity of many carcinogenic chemicals at high doses.

α_{2u}-**Globulin-Binding Chemicals**   The carcinogens D-limonene, 1,4-dichlorobenzene, and trimethylpentane (Fig. 8-15) induce renal tumors selectively in the male rat, and provide excellent examples of species, sex, and tissue specificity of non-DNA reactive carcinogens. The mechanism for the species and sex specificity is related to the ability of these compounds to bind to α_{2u}-globulin, a protein synthesized by the male rat liver at the onset of puberty, as the mechanism of tumorigenesis. α_{2u}-Globulin is filtered through the glomerulus, and only partially excreted (~50%) in the urine. The reabsorbed fraction accumulates in the lysosomes of the P2 segment of the proximal tubules, where it is hydrolyzed to amino acids (Melnick *et al.*, 1996). Chemicals with the ability to bind to α_{2u}-globulin prevent the digestion of α_{2u}-globulin and result in the accumulation in lysosomes, dysfunction of this organelle, and subsequent release of digestive enzymes and cell necrosis. The greater loss of tubule cells leads to increased cell proliferation in the P2 segment, which may be responsible for the tumor development and malignant transformation (Dietrich and Swenberg, 1991).

Receptor Mediated

P450 Inducers: Phenobarbital-like Carcinogens   Phenobarbital is a commonly studied non-DNA reactive compound that is known to cause tumors by a nongenotoxic mechanism involving liver hyperplasia (Williams and Whysner, 1996). One feature seen following phenobarbital exposure is the induction of P450 enzymes, particularly CYP2B (Nims and Lubet, 1996). Because a number of diverse chemicals are known to induce various members of the P450 system (e.g., dieldrin, ethanol, TCDD), the specificity of this effect to carcinogenesis has been questioned. Recent evidence has shown that

the induction of CYP2B is mediated by activation of the constitutive androstane receptor (CAR), a member of the nuclear receptor family (Honkakoski *et al.*, 1998; Ueda *et al.*, 2002; Kodama *et al.*, 2004). CAR-null mice show no induction of CYP2B following phenobarbital exposure (Wei *et al.*, 2000). Other phenobarbital responses that are critical for tumor formation include increased cell proliferation, inhibition of apoptosis, inhibition of gap junctional communication, hypertrophy, and development of preoplastic focal lesions in the liver (Whysner *et al.*, 1996), effects that have all been shown to be CAR-dependent (Wei *et al.*, 2000; Kodama *et al.*, 2004) (Fig. 8-16).

Peroxisome Proliferator Activated Receptor α (PPARα)   A wide array of chemicals are capable of increasing the number and volume of peroxisomes in the cytoplasm of cells. These chemicals, termed peroxisome proliferators, include chemicals such as herbicides, chlorinated solvents (e.g., trichloroethylene and perchloroethylene), plasticizers (e.g., diethylhexylphthalate and other phthalates), lipid lowering fibrate drugs (e.g., ciprofibrate, clofibrate), and natural products. In addition, many of these chemicals produce liver enlargement and hepatocellular carcinoma in rats and mice through non-DNA reactive mechanisms (Lake, 1995; Reddy and Rao, 1997). Two additional tumor types are also associated with exposure to peroxisome proliferating compounds: Leydig cell tumors and pancreatic acinar-cell tumors in the rat. Studies conducted either in vivo or in vitro in primary hepatocyte cultures have shown important interspecies differences in the hepatic peroxisome proliferation responses to chemicals within the class of compounds. The rat and mouse were clearly responsive species, whereas primates and the guinea pig proved to be nonresponders. The Syrian hamster exhibits an intermediate response (Bentley *et al.*, 1993; Lake, 1995). Due to the wide structural diversity of this chemical class, the mechanism(s) involved in peroxisome proliferation and tumorigenesis went unrecognized for years. The currently accepted mode of action for this class of chemicals involves agonist binding to the nuclear hormone receptor, peroxisome proliferator-activated receptor alpha (PPARα). Largely through the use of PPARα knockout mice, the activation of PPARα by agonists is needed for these chemicals to induce peroxisome proliferation and tumorigenesis in rodents (Issemann and Green, 1990; Lee *et al.*, 1995; Peters *et al.*, 1998, reviewed in Klaunig *et al.*, 2003). PPARα is highly expressed in cells that have active fatty acid oxidation capacity (e.g., hepatocytes, cardiomyocytes, enterocytes).

It is well documented that PPARα plays a central role in lipid metabolism and acts as a transcription factor to modulate gene expression following ligand activation. This latter effect arises through the heterodimerization of PPAR and RXRα, which results in binding

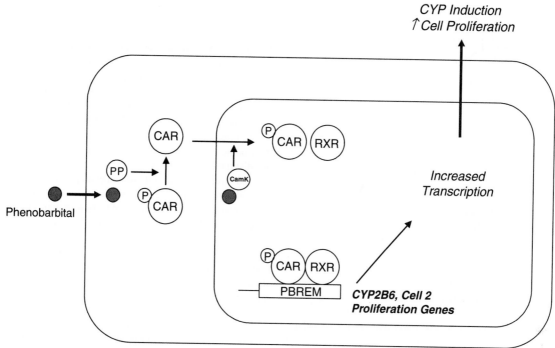

Figure 8-16. Proposed mechanism for the involvement of the constitutive androstane receptor (CAR) in phenobarbital-induced gene expression changes.

PP, protein phosphatase; CamK, CaM Kinase; RXR, retinoic acid receptor; PBREM, phenobarbital response element. Following dephosphorylation of CAR by protein phosphatase, CAR crosses the cell membrane and becomes phosphorylated by CaM kinase. CAR then forms a dimer with RXR and binds to PBREMs, resulting in increased gene expression.

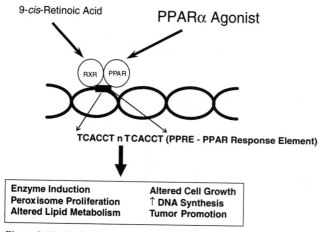

Figure 8-17. Mechanism for altered gene expression by peroxisome proliferator activated receptor α (PPARα) agonist binding.

Following agonist binding to PPARα, the receptor dimerizes with the retinoic acid receptor (RXR). This complex then binds to PPREs, resulting in enhanced gene transcription.

to response elements (PPREs) and subsequent modulation of target gene transcription (Fig. 8-17). Following this event is the induction of cell proliferation and suppression of apoptosis (Marsman *et al.*, 1988; James and Roberts, 1996; Burkhardt *et al.*, 2001). Both these events would then be expected to affect tumor development as these effects would enhance the rate of fixation of DNA damage in the genome, leading to changes in gene expression such as the silencing of tumor suppressor genes or increased expression of oncogenes,

or suppress apoptosis that may normally remove DNA-damaged, potentially tumorigenic, cells.

Because humans are exposed to a number of chemicals that are PPARα ligands, the relevance of this mode of action to humans has been evaluated (Klaunig *et al.*, 2003). Although the same events would be expected to occur in exposed humans, several species differences have been noted, including a lack of induction of cell proliferation in nonhuman primates (Pugh *et al.*, 2000), and the finding that the amount of PPARα in human liver is at least ten-fold lower compared with the rat or mouse (Palmer *et al.*, 1998; Tugwood *et al.*, 1998). Based on these kinetic and dynamic differences between species, it has been concluded that tumors are not likely to occur in humans (Klaunig *et al.*, 2003).

Aryl Hydrocarbon Receptor (AhR) Agonists of the AhR including TCDD and selective members of the polychlorinated- and brominated-biphenyl (PCBs and PBBs) class of compounds (Fig. 8-18) have been linked to tumor development, and appear to function as hepatic tumor promoters (Pitot *et al.*, 1982; IARC, 1997). The tumor response has been determined to be AhR dependent (Knutson and Poland, 1982) (Fig. 8-19). Upon ligand binding to the AhR, the ligand-bound AhR translocates to the nucleus, dimerizes with the Ah receptor nuclear translocator (ARNT), and binds to aryl hydrocarbon response elements [AREs also known as dioxin response elements (DRE) and xenobiotic response elements (XRE)] (for review see Nebert *et al.*, 2000). AhR-ARNT-dependent genes include cytochrome P450 family members, NAD(P)H:quinine oxidoreductase, a cytosolic aldehyde dehydrogenase 3, a UDP-glucuronosyltransferase, and a glutathione transferase (Nebert *et al.*, 2000), genes that are involved in metabolic

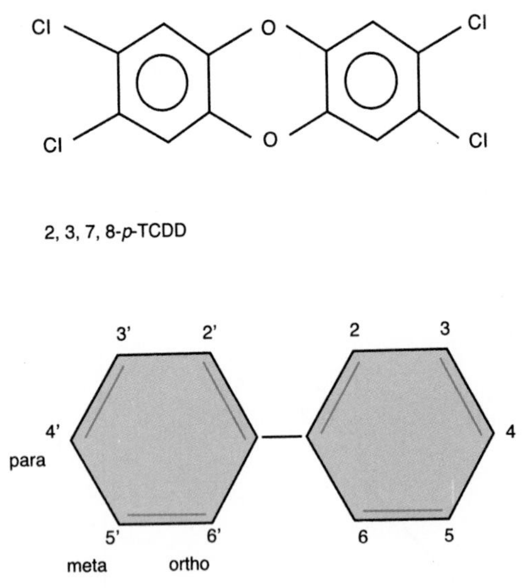

2, 3, 7, 8-*p*-TCDD

PCB*

*Prototypical structure for PCBs or PBBs. PCBs and PBB exhibit varying degrees of Chlorination or Bromination at all position of the biphenyl molecular

Figure 8-18. Selective examples of aryl hydrocarbon receptor-binding chemicals.

Prototypical structure for PCBs or PBBs. PCBs and PBBs exhibit varying degrees of chlorination or bromination at positions 2-6 and 2′-6′ of the biphenyl molecule.

activation as well as detoxification of chemicals. It has been hypothesized that there are additional AhR-ARNT-dependent genes (Nebert *et al.*, 2000). AhR knockout mice showed a diminished response to tumor induction by AhR ligands (Nakatsuru *et al.*, 2004), conversely, constitutively overexpressed AhR resulted in an increased incidence of liver tumors (Moennikes *et al.*, 2004). As seen with

other promoting chemicals, TCDD does inhibit apoptosis in hepatic foci (Stinchcombe *et al.*, 1995).

Hormonal Mode of Action Hormonally active chemicals include biogenic amines, steroids, and peptide hormones that cause tissue-specific changes through interaction with a receptor. In addition, a number of non-DNA reactive chemicals can induce neoplasms in rodents through receptor-mediated mechanisms, and/or perturbation of hormonal balance. Trophic hormones are known to induce cell proliferation at their target organs. This action may lead to the development of tumors when the mechanisms of hormonal control are disrupted and some or other hormone shows persistently increased levels. Several well-studied examples include the induction of ovarian neoplasms via decreased estradiol and increased LH levels (Capen *et al.*, 1995) and the induction of thyroid tumors in rats by phenobarbital-type P450 inducers (McClain, 1995; Williams, 1995).

Estrogenic agents can induce tumors in estrogen-dependent tissue. Selective estrogenic chemicals (agonists and antagonists) are shown in Fig. 8-20. Oral administration of 17β-estradiol to female mice increases the incidence of mammary tumors (Highman *et al.*, 1977; Welsch *et al.*, 1977), whereas subcutaneous administration of estradiol to young female mice produced tumors of the cervix and vagina (Pan and Gardner, 1948). Evidence that estrogenic chemicals are carcinogenic to humans comes from epidemiological data on breast and ovarian cancer, which indicates that individuals with higher circulating estrogen levels and those with exposure to the potent estrogenic agent diethylstilbesterol (DES) are at increased risk of cancer development. DES was first shown to induce mammary tumors in male mice following subcutaneous administration of the hormone. DES has been causally associated to the higher incidence of adenocarcinomas of the vagina and cervix in daughters of women treated with the hormone during pregnancy (Herbst and Scully, 1970; Herbst *et al.*, 1972; Noller *et al.*, 1972). The mechanism of action for DES is believed to function through its ability to induce

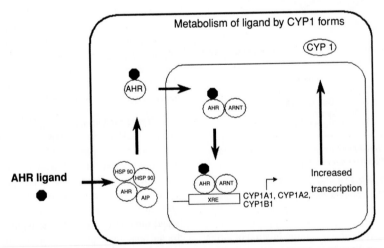

Figure 8-19. Proposed mechanism of aryl hydrocarbon receptor (AhR) mediated gene expression.

ARNT, AhR nuclear transporter; XRE, xenobiotic response element. Non-ligand bound AhR is maintained in the cytoplasm via association with chaperone proteins (e.g., AIP, Hsp90). Following ligand binding, chaperone proteins dissociate and AhR translocates to the nucleus where it binds with ARNT. The heterodimer binds to XREs resulting in an increase in gene transcription.

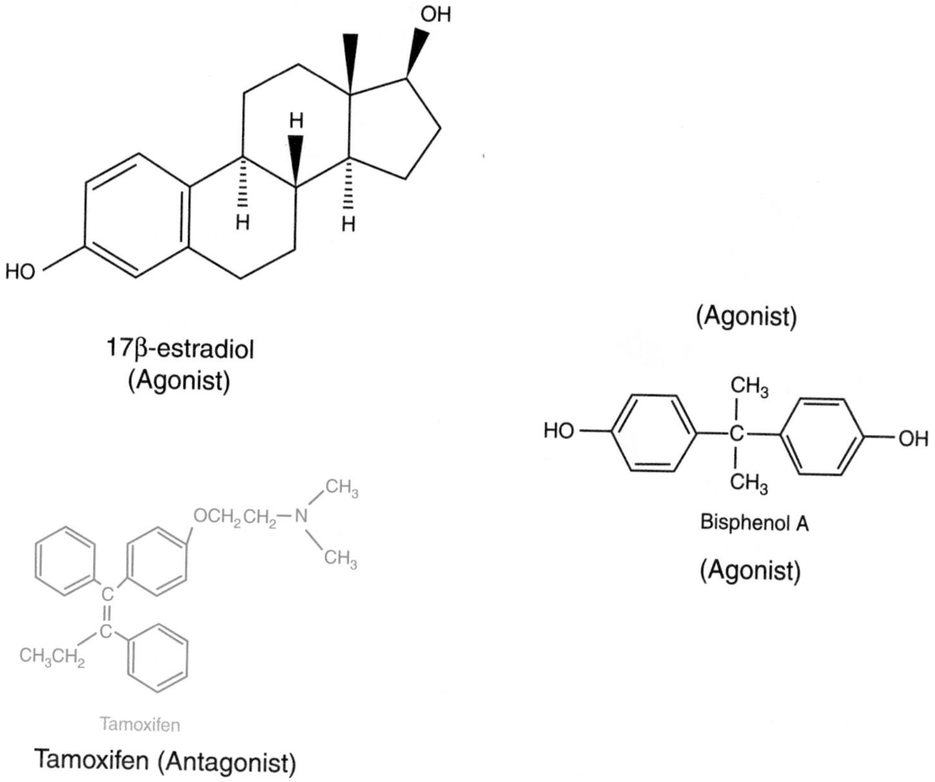

17β-estradiol
(Agonist)

Tamoxifen (Antagonist)

Bisphenol A
(Agonist)

Figure 8-20. Chemical examples of estrogenic agonists and antagonists.

aneuploidy (Li *et al.*, 1997; Tsutsui *et al.*, 1997). The effects of steroidal chemicals on the cell cycle (Sutherland *et al.*, 1995) and on microtubule assembly (Metzler *et al.*, 1996) may be important in the aneuploidy inducing effects of some hormonal agents (Li *et al.*, 1996).

Chronic exogenous administration of hormonally active chemicals, including synthetic estrogens and anabolic steroids, can increase hepatic adenoma incidence in rats (Li *et al.*, 1992) and in humans (IARC, 1997). Women of child-bearing age are sensitive to hepatic adenoma formation, which can be exacerbated by oral contraceptive use. These adenomas will regress upon hormone cessation (Edmondson *et al.*, 1977) and can progress with continued administration (Christopherson *et al.*, 1978). Chronic administration (>8 years) is required to detect this increased liver tumor risk from oral contraceptives (Tavani *et al.*, 1993).

Many substances in plants (phytoestrogens) have been described. These include compounds such as genestein, daidzein, glycetein, equol, and their metabolites found in soy products and various lignan derivatives (Adlercreutz and Mazur, 1997). In addition, a number of environmental nonsteroidal synthetic compounds have been identified that demonstrate apparent estrogenic activity (e.g., nonyl-phenol, bisphenol-A, chlorinated hydrocarbons) (Soto *et al.*, 1997). The potential for these chemicals to induce cancer in humans is an area of current investigation.

Species and tissue specificity in response to receptor and hormone-mediated carcinogenesis is often observed. As an example, tamoxifen is antiestrogenic in the chick oviduct, estrogenic in the mouse uterus with acute administration, but antiestrogenic with chronic administration in the same tissue, while it is estrogenic in the rat uterus. Whereas this may be in part due to tissue and species differences in coactivator and corepressor levels and availability,

many other pharmacokinetic and pharmacodynamic properties are likely to participate (Carthew *et al.*, 1995). To further exemplify the complexity of the role of estrogen in cancer development, estrogens have also been shown to be protective in prostate cancer.

Induction of ovarian tumors by dietary administration of nitrofurantoin in mice is an example of a tumorigenic effect secondary to drug-induced hormonal disturbance. Nitrofurantoin treatment resulted in ovarian atrophy with absence of graafian follicles and sterility. The reduction of follicles induced a reduction of sex steroids by the ovary, resulting in increased production of gonadotrophins, notably LH, presumably due to the decreased negative feedback on the hypothalamus–pituitary axis by estrogens. Persistent stimulation by LH of the ovary cells resulted in development of tumors (Capen *et al.*, 1995). A similar effect is known to occur with dopamine agonists. The induction of hypoprolactinemia changes the number of LH receptors and leads to enhanced sensitivity to LH and a higher stimulation by LH, similar to nitrofurantoin.

A number of chemicals that reduce thyroid hormone concentrations (T4 and/or T3) and increase thyroid-stimulating hormone (TSH) have been shown to induce neoplasia in the rodent thyroid. TSH demonstrates proliferative activity in the thyroid, with chronic drug-induced TSH increases leading to progression of follicular cell hypertrophy, hyperplasia, and eventually neoplasia. Inducers of metabolic enzymes in the liver, a classic and well-studied example being phenobarbital (Hood *et al.*, 1999), result in increased thyroid hormone metabolism and as such lead to increases in TSH levels (Fig. 8-21). It is this latter event that is associated with the development of thyroid tumors in rodents. Recent evidence suggests that the enhancement of metabolism and excretion of thyroid hormones by xenobiotics (via induction of Phase II enzymes) is a consequence of CAR (and presumably PXR) activation. Qualitatively, thyroid gland

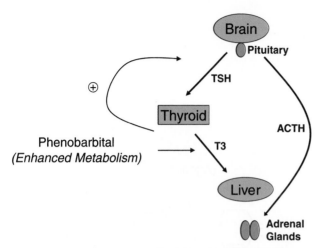

Figure 8-21. *Mechanism for phenobarbital-induced thyroid tumors.*

Through alteration of gene expression, phenobarbital enhances metabolism of thyroid hormone (T3) resulting in enhanced TSH production. Increased TSH then leads to increased cell proliferation in the thyroid.

DNA Methylation and Carcinogenesis Post-DNA synthetic methylation of the 5-position on cytosine (5-methylcytosine, 5mC) is a naturally occurring modification to DNA in higher eukaryotes that influences gene expression (Holliday, 1990) (Fig. 8-22). Under normal conditions, DNA is methylated symmetrically on both strands. Immediately following DNA replication, the newly synthesized double-stranded DNA contains hemimethylated sites that signal for DNA maintenance methylases to transfer methyl groups from *S*-adenosylmethionine to cytosine residues on the new DNA strand (Hergersberg, 1991). The degree of methylation within a gene inversely correlates with the expression of that gene; hypermethylation of genes is associated with gene silencing, whereas hypermethylation results in an enhanced expression of genes. Several chemical carcinogens are known to modify DNA methylation, methyltransferase activity, and chromosomal structure. During carcinogenesis, both hypomethylation and hypermethylation of the genome have been observed (Counts and Goodman, 1995; Baylin, 1997). Increased methylation of CpG islands have been observed in bladder cancer and tumor suppressor genes such as the retinoblastoma gene, $p16^{ink4a}$, and $p14^{ARF}$ have been reported to be hypermethylated in tumors (Stirzaker *et al.*, 1997; Belinsky *et al.*, 1998; Myöhänen *et al.*, 1998; Salem *et al.*, 2000; Esteller *et al.*, 2001). Hypomethylation has been associated with increased mutation rates. Most metastatic neoplasms in humans have significantly lower 5MeC than normal tissue (Gama-Sosa *et al.*, 1983); furthermore, many oncogenes are hypomethylated and their expression amplified.

Choline and methionine, which can be derived from dietary sources, provide a source of methyl groups used in methylation reactions. Rats exposed to choline and/or methionine-deficient

function in rodents is much more susceptible to disturbances of the thyroid hormone levels than it is in humans. In contrast to humans, rodents lack the thyroid-binding globulin, which is the predominant plasma protein responsible for thyroxin binding and transport in humans (McClain, 1995). A relatively higher level of functional activity is present in rat thyroid compared to humans.

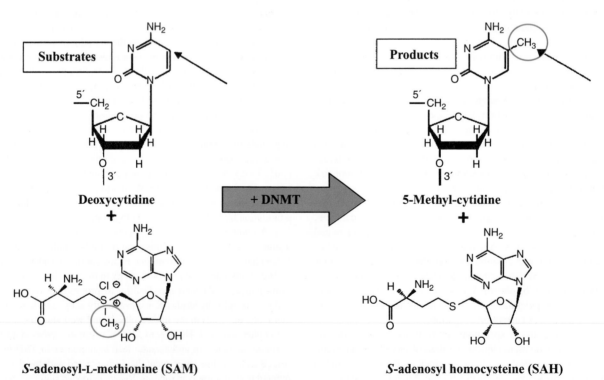

Figure 8-22. *Substrates and products involved in DNA methylation.*

Methylation of DNA occurs through an enzymatic reaction catalyzed by DNA methyltransferases (DNMTs). DNA is methylated at the 5-position of cytosine and requires the cofactor *S*-adenosyl methionine.

Table 8-11
Evidence for Choline Depletion in Hepatocarcinogenesis

CHOLINE	METHIONINE	FOLATE	HEPATOCELLULAR CARCINOMA	DURATION (MONTHS)	REFERENCE
−	+	+	100%	12	Nakae *et al.*, 1992
−	+	+	73%	12	Lombardi *et al.*, 1988
−	Low	−	100%	15	Henning *et al.*, 1996
−	−	+	51%	13	Ghoshal *et al.*, 1984

diets resulted in hepatocellular proliferation and neoplasia (Abanobi *et al.*, 1982; Wainfan and Poirier, 1992) (Table 8-11). In rodents fed choline or methyl donor groups deficient diets, the hepatic neoplasia is thought to arise from hypomethylation of *c-myc*, *c-fos*, and *c-H-ras* proto-oncogenes, due to the decreased availability of *S*-adenosyl-methionine (Newberne *et al.*, 1982; Wainfan and Poirier, 1992). Chemicals such as diethanolamine result in hepatic neoplasia, in part via mechanisms involving choline depletion, altered methylation, and modulation of gene expression (Kamendulis and Klaunig, 2005; Carnell *et al.*, 2006). Reactive oxygen species have also been shown to modify DNA methylation, resulting in changes in DNA methylation profiles through interfering with the ability of methyltransferases to interact with DNA leading to hypomethylation of CpG sites (Weitzman *et al.*, 1994; Turk *et al.*, 1995). Also, the presence of 8-OHdG in DNA can lead to hypomethylation of DNA, because this adduct if present in CpCpGpGp sequences will inhibit the methylation of adjacent C residues. Thus, oxidative DNA damage may be an important contributor to the carcinogenesis process brought about by the loss of DNA methylation, allowing the expression of normally quiescent genes. Also, the abnormal methylation pattern observed in cells transformed by chemical oxidants may contribute to an overall aberrant gene expression and promote the tumor process.

Oxidative Stress and Chemical Carcinogenesis Experimental evidence has shown that increases in reactive oxygen in the cell, through either physiological modification or through chemical carcinogen exposure, contribute to the carcinogenesis processes (Vuillaume, 1987; Trush and Kensler, 1991; Witz, 1991; Guyton and Kensler, 1993). Reactive oxygen species encompass a series of reactive compounds including the superoxide anion ($^{\bullet}O_2$-), hydroperoxyl radical ($HO_2^{\bullet}$.), hydrogen peroxide (H_2O_2), and the hydroxyl radical ($^{\bullet}OH$), all derived through the reduction of molecular oxygen (Table 8-12). Oxygen radicals can be produced by both endogenous and exogenous sources and are typically counterbalanced by antioxidants (Table 8-13). Antioxidant defenses are both enzymatic (e.g., superoxide dismutase, glutathione peroxidase, and catalase) and nonenzymatic (e.g., vitamin E, vitamin C, β-carotene, glutathione (Betteridge, 2000; Abuja and Albertini, 2001). Importantly, many of these antioxidants are provided through dietary intake (Clarkson and Thompson, 2000).

Endogenous sources of reactive oxygen species include oxidative phosphorylation, P450 metabolism, peroxisomes, and inflammatory cell activation (Table 8-13). Within the mitochondria, a small percentage of oxygen is converted into the superoxide anion via one-electron reduction of molecular oxygen. Superoxide can be dismutated by superoxide dismutase to yield hydrogen peroxide (Barber

Table 8-12
Pathways for Intercellular Oxidant Generation

Generation of reactive oxygen species via reduction of molecular oxygen
$$O_2 + e^- \rightarrow O_2^{-\bullet} \text{ (superoxide anion)}$$
$$O_2^{-\bullet} + H_2O \rightarrow HO_2^{\bullet} \text{ (hydroperoxyl radical)}$$
$$HO_2^{\bullet} + e^- + H \rightarrow H_2O_2 \text{ (hydrogen peroxide)}$$
$$H_2O_2 + e^- \rightarrow OH^- + {}^{\bullet}OH \text{ (hydroxyl radical)}$$

A series of oxygen radicals are produced by the reduction of molecular oxygen. Of the radicals produced, the hydroxyl radical, hydroperoxyl radical, and the superoxide anion are sufficiently reactive and may interact with biomolecules.

and Harris, 1994). In the presence of partially reduced metal ions, hydrogen peroxide is converted to the highly reactive hydroxyl radical through Fenton and Haber-Weiss reactions (Betteridge, 2000). Neutrophils, eosinophils, and macrophages represent another intracellular source of reactive oxygen species. Activated macrophages, through "respiratory burst" elicit a rapid increase in oxygen uptake that gives rise to a variety of reactive oxygen species including superoxide anion, hydrogen peroxide, and nitric oxide. The release of cytokines and reactive oxygen intermediates from activated Kupffer cells (the resident macrophage of the liver) has been implicated in hepatotoxicological and hepatocarcinogenic events (Rose *et al.*, 1999; Rusyn *et al.*, 1999); in particular, recent studies show that Kupffer cells may function at the promotion stage of carcinogenesis. Reactive oxygen species can also be produced by cytochrome P450-mediated mechanisms including: (1) redox cycling in the presence of molecular oxygen, (2) peroxidase-catalyzed single-electron drug oxidations, and (3) "futile cycling" of cytochromes P450 (Parke, 1994; Parke and Sapota, 1996). Ethanol, phenobarbital, and a number of chlorinated and nonchlorinated compounds such as dieldrin, TCDD, and lindane are among the xenobiotics shown to increase in reactive oxygen species through P450-mediated mechanisms (Eksrom and Ingleman-Sundberg, 1989; Rice *et al.*, 1994; Klaunig *et al.*, 1997). Chemicals classified as peroxisome proliferators activated receptor α (PPARα) agonists (e.g., clofibrate, phthalate esters) represent chemicals that induce cytochrome P4504A, and increase the formation of peroxisomes. As such, an increase in H_2O_2 production often accompanies exposure to chemicals that stimulate the number and activity of peroxisomes (Rao and Reddy, 1991; Wade *et al.*, 1992). Through these or other currently unknown mechanisms, a number of chemicals that induce cancer (e.g., chlorinated compounds, radiation, metal ions, barbiturates, and some PPARα agonists) induce reactive oxygen species formation and/or oxidative stress (Rice-Evans and Burdon, 1993; Klaunig *et al.*, 1997; Kamendulis and Klaunig, 2005).

Table 8-13

Reactive Oxygen Species Generation and Removal in the Cell

Cellular oxidants	
Endogenous	Exogenous
Mitochondria	Redox cycling compounds
$O_2^{-\bullet}$, H_2O_2, $^\bullet OH$	$O_2^{-\bullet}$
Cytochrome P450	Metals (Fenton reaction)
$O_2^{-\bullet}$, H_2O_2	$H_2O_2 + Fe^{2+} \rightarrow OH^- + {}^\bullet OH + Fe^{3+}$
Macrophage/inflammatory cells	Radiation
$O_2^{-\bullet}$, $^\bullet NO$, H_2O_2, OCl^-	$^\bullet OH$
Peroxisomes	
H_2O_2	
Cellular antioxidants	
Enzymatic	Non-enzymatic
Superoxide dismutase	Vitamin E
Catalase	Glutathione
Glutathione peroxidase	Vitamin C
Glutaredoxin	Catechins
Thioredoxin	
Oxidants > Antioxidants	Oxidative Damage (DNA, RNA, Lipid, Protein)

Oxidants can be produced via both endogenous and exogenous sources. Antioxidants function to maintain the cellular redox balancing. However, excess production of oxidants and or inadequate supplies of antioxidants result in damage to cellular biomolecules and may impact on neoplastic development.

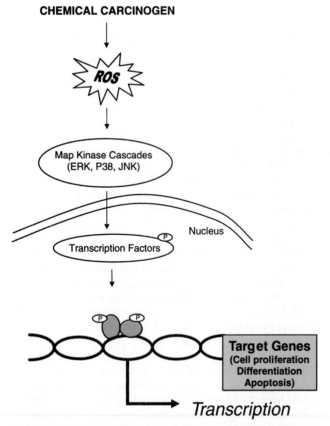

Figure 8-23. Role of reactive oxygen species (ROS) on altered gene expression.

Many chemical carcinogens increase ROS and activate signaling cascades, such as the mitogen activated (MAP) kinase family. These serene/threonine kinases activate transcription factors, leading to DNA binding and gene expression changes.

Oxidative Damage and Carcinogenesis   Reactive oxygen species left unbalanced by antioxidants can result in damage to cellular macromolecules. In DNA, reactive oxygen species can produce single- or double-stranded DNA breaks, purine, pyrimidine, or deoxyribose modifications, and DNA crosslinks (von Sonntag, 1987; Dizdaroglu, 1992; Demple and Harrison, 1994). Persistent DNA damage can result in either arrest or induction of transcription, induction of signal transduction pathways, replication errors, and genomic instability, events that are potentially involved in carcinogenesis. Oxidation of guanine at the C8 position results in the formation of 8-hydroxydeoxyguanosine (8-OHdG; see Fig. 8-7). This oxidative DNA adduct is mutagenic in bacterial and mammalian cells, produces dose-related increases in cellular transformation, and causes G $\rightarrow$ T transversions which are commonly observed in mutated oncogenes and tumor suppressor genes (Shibutani *et al.*, 1991; Moriya, 1993; Hussain and Haris, 1998; Zhang *et al.*, 2000). During DNA replication, 8-OHdG in the nucleotide pool can incorporate into the DNA template strand opposite dC or dA resulting in A:T to C:G transversions (Cheng *et al.*, 1992; Demple and Harrison, 1994). Oxidative damage to mitochondrial DNA and mutations in mitochondrial DNA have been identified in a number of cancers (Schumacher *et al.*, 1973; Horton *et al.*, 1996; Cavalli and Liang, 1998; Tamura *et al.*, 1999). Compared to nuclear DNA, mitochondrial genome is relatively susceptible to oxidative base damage due to (1) close proximity to the electron transport system, a major source of reactive oxygen species (Barber and Harris, 1994); (2) mitochondrial DNA is not protected by histones; and (3) DNA repair capacity is limited in the mitochondria (Bohr and Dianov, 1999; Sawyer and Van Houten, 1999). Although many pathways exist that enable the formation of oxidative DNA damage, mammalian cells also possess specific repair pathways for the remediation of oxidative DNA damage (Tchou and Grollman, 1993; Fortini *et al.*, 1999).

Apart from oxidized nucleic acids, oxygen radicals can damage cellular biomembranes resulting in lipid peroxidation. Peroxidation of biomembranes generates a variety of products, including reactive electrophiles, such as epoxides and aldehydes, including

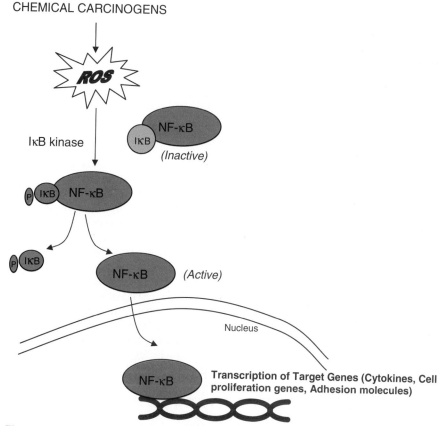

Figure 8-24. *Interaction between reactive oxygen species (ROS) and NFkB-induced gene expression.*

A number of chemicals that increase ROS have been shown to activate NFkB. It is proposed that ROS enhance the dissociation of IkB from the NFkB/IkB complex leading to active NFkB. NFkB can then translocate into the nucleus where it binds DNA and increases gene transcription.

malondialdehyde (MDA) (Janero, 1990). MDA is a highly reactive aldehyde and exhibits reactivity toward nucleophiles and can form MDA–MDA dimers. Both MDA and the MDA–MDA dimers are mutagenic in bacterial assays and the mouse lymphoma assay (Riggins and Marnett, 2001).

Oxidative Stress and Cell Growth Regulation   Reactive oxygen species production and oxidative stress can affect both cell proliferation and apoptosis (Cerutti, 1985; Burdon, 1995; Slater *et al.*, 1995). H_2O_2 and superoxide anion can induce cell proliferation in several mammalian cell types (D'Souza *et al.*, 1993). Conversely, high concentrations of reactive oxygen species can initiate apoptosis (Dypbukt *et al.*, 1994). It has clearly been demonstrated that low levels of reactive oxygen species influence signal transduction pathways and alter gene expression (Fiorani *et al.*, 1995). Many xenobiotics, by increasing cellular levels of oxidants, alter gene expression through activation of signaling pathways including cAMP-mediated cascades, calcium-calmodulin pathways, and transcription factors such as AP-1 and NF-κB as well as signaling through mitogen-activated protein (MAP) kinases, extracellular signal-regulated kinases (ERK), c-Jun N-terminal kinases (JNK), and the p38 kinases (Kerr, 1992; Muller *et al.*, 1997; Timblin *et al.*, 1997). Activation of these signaling cascades by reactive oxygen species induced by chemical carcinogens ultimately leads to altered gene expression for a number of genes including those affecting proliferation, dif-

ferentiation, and apoptosis (Hollander and Fornace, 1989; Amstad *et al.*, 1992; Pinkus, 1993; Zawaski, 1993; Brown *et al.*, 1998; Chang and Karin, 2001; Martindale and Holbrook, 2002) (Fig. 8-23). Activation of NFκB, a ubiquitously expressed transcription factor, is regulated, in part, by reactive oxygen species and the cellular redox status, and has been observed to occur following a wide variety of extracellular stimuli, including exposure to chemical carcinogens such as PPARα agonists (Rusyn *et al.*, 2003) and PCBs (Beauerle *et al.*, 1988; Li and Karin, 1998; Schulze-Oshoff *et al.*, 1998; Pahl, 1999; Nebreda and Porrai, 2000; Molina *et al.*, 2001; Glauert *et al.*, 2002) (Fig. 8-24).

Gap Junctional Intercellular Communication and Carcinogenesis

Cells within an organism communicate in a variety of ways including through gap junctions, which are aggregates of connexin proteins that form a conduit between two adjacent cells (Lowenstein *et al.*, 1981) (Fig. 8-25). Gap junctional intercellular communication appears to play an important role in the regulation of cell growth and cell death, in part through the ability to exchange small molecules (<1 kDa) between cells through gap junctions. Loss of gap junctions or decreased cell-to-cell communication is seen during liver regeneration following partial hepatectomy, a situation in which gap junction expression remains decreased until liver mass and

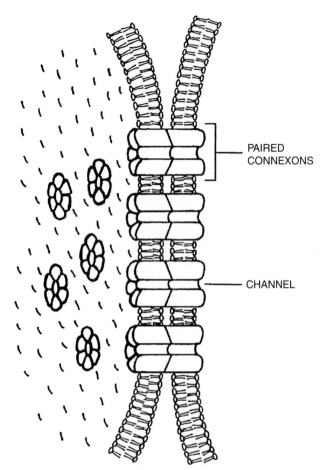

Figure 8-25.   Schematic diagram of a gap junction.

Gap junctions consist of connexin hexamers that form a pore between neighboring cells through which molecules <1 kDa can pass.

lobular conformation are restored. Aberrant growth control is an essential feature of cancer cells, and since the absence or reduction in cell-to-cell communication has been observed between cancer cells, between cancer and normal cells, and in transformed cells, it has been speculated that altered gap junctional cell communication is involved in carcinogenesis (Trosko and Chang, 1984). If cell communication is blocked between tumor and normal cells, the exchange of growth inhibitory signals from normal cells would be prevented from acting on initiated cells, thus allowing the potential for unregulated growth and clonal expansion of initiated cell populations. This would therefore allow for the acquisition of additional genetic changes that may lead to neoplastic transformation (Klaunig and Ruch, 1989).

Intercellular communication is also decreased by growth factor administration and following exposure to a variety of tumor-promoting compounds (e.g., phenobarbital, phthalates, dieldrin, phorbol esters). Tumor-promoting chemicals inhibit gap junctional intercellular communication in a number of cell types following exposure both in vivo and in vitro (Klaunig and Ruch, 1989). The ability of a tumor-promoting compound to block cell-to-cell communication in cultured cells correlates with its ability to induce rodent tumors (Klaunig and Ruch, 1987). In addition, the inhibition of gap junctional intercellular communication by tumor promotors appears to be tissue and species specific; they produce inhibition in target

organs and sensitive species, while they do not inhibit cell-to-cell communication in nontarget tissues for carcinogenicity (Klaunig and Ruch, 1987). The mechanisms by which tumor promoters inhibit intercellular communication are not clear but may be due to decreased synthesis and/or enhanced degradation of gap junction proteins in the cell, reducing the number of channels in cell membranes, or other changes that modulate gap junction function and/or protein expression (Sugie *et al.*, 1987; Klaunig and Ruch, 1989).

Modifiers of Chemical Carcinogenic Effects

Genetic and environmental factors have a significant impact on the way in which individuals and/or organisms respond to carcinogen exposure. As with most genes, enzymes that metabolize carcinogens are expressed in a tissue-specific manner. Within tissues, the enzymatic profile can vary with cell type or display differential localization within cells. Further, carcinogen-metabolizing enzymes are differentially expressed among species. These differences may represent an underlying factor explaining the differential responses to chemical carcinogens across species.

The expression of many carcinogen-metabolizing enzymes is highly inducible by foreign chemicals. For example, compounds such as benzo(*a*)pyrene highly induce P450 isozymes CYP1A1 and 1A2, enzymes which display catalytic activity toward a number of polycyclic aromatics. A number of other enzymes, e.g., GST isozymes, UDPGTs are also induced by PAHs, thus the net result is enhanced metabolism of PAHs. Numerous other chemical carcinogens are potent inducers of drug-metabolizing enzymes; examples include chemicals such as phenobarbital, DDT, ethanol, 17β-estradiol, PPARα agonists, each of which results in the up-regulation of a distinct set of phase I and phase II enzymes. Many chemicals produce inhibitory effects on drug metabolism enzymes, and could either increase the half-life of a chemical carcinogen or prevent or delay the formation of active metabolites of carcinogens.

Polymorphisms in Carcinogen Metabolism and DNA Repair

Genetic polymorphisms arise from human genetic variability. A genetic polymorphism is when a gene has more than one allele. In assessing variability in the human genome project, it was found that base variations occurred at approximately once in every 1000 base pairs. Therefore, more than 1 million genetic variations may be seen between any two individuals. A single nucleotide polymorphism (SNP) is a variant in DNA sequence found in greater than 1% of the population (Fig. 8-26). Thus, the definition of shift changes in DNA sequence goes from mutation to polymorphism when a unique genotype is seen in over 1% of the population. Over 3 million candidate SNPs have been identified to date with up to 10 million being estimated to be present within the human genome. In carcinogenesis, genetic polymorphisms may account for the susceptibility of some individuals to certain cancers. In particular, SNPs of genes involved in carcinogen metabolism (activation and detoxification) and DNA repair have, to date, received considerable attention. A number of polymorphisms have been described in carcinogen-metabolizing enzymes, with certain alleles linked to altered risk of selective cancers (Boddy and Ratain, 1997). Glutathione-*S*-transferases (GSTs), which are involved in detoxification of many chemical carcinogens and also in the remediation of oxidative stress, are highly polymorphic in humans. Polymorphisms of the GSTM1 phenotype have been related to bladder, gastric, and lung cancer in humans (Welfare

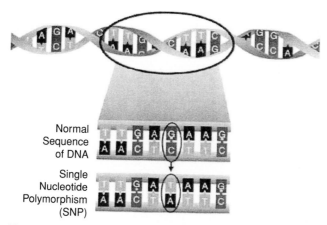

Normal
Sequence
of DNA

Single
Nucleotide
Polymorphism
(SNP)

Figure 8-26. Example of a single nucleotide polymorphism in DNA.

Single nucleotide polymorphisms are instances in which a single nucleotide is changed within a DNA sequence.

Table 8-14

Carcinogen Exposure and Cancer Risk in Humans

EXPOSURE	SUSCEPTIBILITY (GENOTYPE)	RESULT (DISEASE)
↓	↓	Low risk
↑	↓	Low risk
↓	↑	Mod risk
↑	↑	High risk

et al., 1999; Tsuchida and Sato, 1992). Individuals expressing the GSTM1 null genotype have a 1.5-fold higher risk for bladder cancer and 1.7-fold increased risk for gastric cancer, compared to individuals expressing the common genotype (Risch *et al.*, 2001; Ates *et al.*, 2005). The GSTM1 isoform is of particular importance in carcinogenesis, because this isoform exhibits the highest reactivity toward epoxides. GSTT1 null isoform individuals show a 3-fold increased risk in breast cancer, a 1.6-fold increased risk in gastric cancer, and a 4-fold increased risk in liver cancer compared to individuals having the common genotype (Bosch *et al.*, 2006).

Similarly in women (nonsmokers) with lung cancer, a higher level of PAH DNA adducts have been detected. Higher DNA adduct levels are also found to be associated with the expression of the cytochrome *P*4501*A*1 (CYP1A1) gene (Han *et al.*, 2003). This enzyme causes bioactivation of the carcinogen benzopyrene, and increased DNA adduct levels correlate with increased expression of CYP1A1. SNPs of DNA repair genes, in particular oxidative DNA repair, OGG1, involved in the repair of 8-OHdG-induced damage, have been linked to increase in lung cancer in individuals with lower OGG1 expression (Goode *et al.*, 2002).

In the case of prostate cancer, studies have suggested roles for a number of candidate SNPs. Recent evidence suggests that the presence of a genetic variant which is more prevalent in African-American men is less effective of clearing reactive oxygen species. Examples of candidate genes which likely contribute to prostate cancer carcinogenesis include the androgen receptor gene, steroid synthesis, and metabolism genes (*CYP17, CYP1B1, CYP3A4, CYP3A5, CYP3A43, SD5A2, HSD3B1, HSD3B2, CYP19*), transmembrane drug efflux genes (*ABCG2*), and reactive oxygen species metabolizing genes (*MnSOD, APE1, XRCC1, GSTP1*) (Dong, 2005). Individually, polymorphisms in each of these genes have been associated with an increased risk of prostate cancer.

The importance of SNPs, cancer susceptibility, and cancer risk are illustrated in Table 8-14. If exposure to a chemical carcinogen is low and the genetic susceptibility for genes related to the carcinogenic activity is low, then the risk for cancer will also be low. If exposure to a chemical carcinogen is high but the genetic susceptibility is low, then the risk for cancer development is likely to be low. However, if the genetic susceptibility is high, then exposure to a chemical carcinogen will result in a higher risk for cancer development.

Proto-Oncogenes and Tumor-Suppressor Genes

Proto-oncogenes and tumor-suppressor genes play a key role in cancer induction. These genes encode a wide array of proteins that function to control cell growth and proliferation. Common characteristics of oncogenes and tumor suppressor genes are shown in Table 8-15. Mutations in both oncogenes and tumor suppressor genes contribute to the progressive development of human cancers. Accumulated damage to multiple oncogenes and/or tumor suppressor genes can result in altered cell proliferation, differentiation, and/or survival of cancer cells.

Retroviruses   Evidence that specific genes (oncogenes) could cause cancer, first came from studies showing sarcomas could be produced in healthy chickens by injecting them with cell-free

Table 8-15

Characteristics of Proto-Oncogenes, Cellular Oncogenes, and Tumor Suppressor Genes

PROTO-ONCOGENES	ONCOGENES	TUMOR SUPPRESSOR GENES
Dominant	Dominant	Recessive
Broad tissue specificity for cancer development	Broad tissue specificity for cancer development	Considerable tissue specificity for cancer development
Germ line inheritance rarely involved in cancer development	Germ line inheritance rarely involved in cancer development	Germ line inheritance frequently involved in cancer development
Analogous to certain viral oncogenes	No known analogues in oncogenic viruses	No known analogues in oncogenic viruses
Somatic mutations activated during all stages of carcinogenesis	Somatic mutations activated during all stages of carcinogenesis	Germ line mutations may initiate, but mutation to neoplasia occurs only during progression stage

Table 8-16
Examples of Oncogenes and Cancer Association

	ONCOGENE	NEOPLASM
Tyrosine kinases	EGFR	Squamous cell carcinoma
	PDGF	Lung carcinoma
		Astrocytoma
	v-fms	Sarcoma
	v-kit	Sarcoma
	v-ros	Sarcoma
	v-fgr	Sarcoma
	v-fps	Sarcoma
	Src	Colon carcinoma
	Neu	Breast carcinoma
		Neuroblastoma
	Ret	Thyroid carcinoma
	Trk	Colon carcinoma
Serine/threonine kinases	v-raf	Sarcoma
	v-mos	Sarcoma
G Proteins	H-Ras	Colon and lung carcinoma
	K-Ras	Melanoma, AML, and thyroid carcinoma
	N-Ras	Carcinoma and melanoma
	NF-1	Neurofibromas
Nuclear proteins	c-Myc	CML, Burkitt's lymphoma
	N-Myc	AML, breast and lung carcinoma
	L-Myc	Neuroblastoma and lung carcinoma
	v-myb	Lung carcinoma
	v-jun	Sarcoma
	v-fos	Osteosarcoma
	v-rel	Leukemia
	v-ets	Myeloblastosis
	v-erbA	Erythroblastosis

extracts derived from chicken tumors (Rous, 1911). The transforming agent in the filtrate eventually was shown to be an RNA-type tumor virus, the *Rous sarcoma virus* (RSV) that is capable of transforming a normal cell and producing sarcomas within weeks of injection (Temin and Rubin, 1958). The genome of RSV and other retroviruses consists of two identical copies of mRNA, which is then reverse transcribed into DNA and incorporated into the host-cell genome. Oncogenic transforming viruses like RSV contain the v-*src* gene, a gene required for cancer induction. It was later demonstrated that normal cells from chickens and other species contain a gene closely related to v-*src* in RSV; the normal "proto-oncogene" commonly is distinguished from the viral gene by the prefix "c" (c-*src*; Oppermann *et al.*, 1979). This discovery showed that cancer may be induced by the action of normal, or nearly normal, genes.

DNA Viruses Six major classes of DNA tumor viruses have been identified: simian virus 40 (SV40), polyoma virus, hepatitis B virus, papilloma viruses, adenoviruses, herpes viruses, and poxviruses. Unlike retroviral oncogenes, which are derived from normal cellular genes and have no function for the virus, the known oncogenes of DNA viruses are integral parts of the viral genome required for viral replication. SV40 or polyoma viruses are not capable of inducing tumors in their natural host species (monkey and mice, respectively). Infection by small DNA viruses is lethal to most nonhost

animal cells; however, a small proportion integrates the viral DNA into the host-cell genome. The cells that survive infection become permanently transformed due to the presence of one or more oncogenes in the viral DNA. For example, SV40 codes for the large T antigen, which alone is capable of inducing transformation (Fried and Prives, 1986). Both SV40 and polyoma viruses use the host cells DNA synthetic apparatus for their own replication. Papilloma viruses can infect and cause tumors in rabbits, cows, and humans (Lancaster and Olson, 1982). Of the human papilloma viruses, types 6, 10, and 11 are associated with genital warts whereas types 16, 18, 31, and 33 are associated with human cervical cancers (Vousden, 1989). Herpes viruses are complex, and are capable of producing tumors in frogs, chickens, monkeys, and humans (Rapp, 1974). Included among this class is the Epstein–Barr virus, a causative agent in the development of Burkett's B-cell lymphomas and in nasopharyngeal carcincoma (de-Thé *et al.*, 1978), and is mediated by genes encoding *EBNA-1*, *EBNA-2*, and *latent membrane protein* (Fahreus *et al.*, 1990). Adenoviruses affect host and nonhost cells differently; in host cells, infection causes lysis, whereas in nonhost cells, infection results in transformation via *E1A* and *E1B* genes (Pettersson and Roberts, 1986). Hepatitis B viruses specifically infect the liver of ducks, woodchucks, and squirrels and is strongly associated with liver cancer development in humans; infected individuals exhibit a >100-fold risk for cancer development (Snyder *et al.*, 1982). Hepatitis B gene X is thus far the main gene implicated in the transformation process (Kim *et al.*, 1991). Poxviruses (e.g., Yaba monkey virus, Shope fibroma virus) replicate in the cytoplasm of infected cells and produce benign tumors (Niven *et al.*, 1961).

Proto-Oncogenes An oncogene is a gene encoding a protein that is capable of transforming cells in culture or inducing cancer in animals. Of the known oncogenes, the majority appear to have been derived from normal genes (i.e., proto-oncogenes), and are involved in cell signaling cascades (Table 8-16). Because most proto-oncogenes are essential for maintaining viability, they are highly conserved evolutionarily. It has been clearly demonstrated that altered expression of these genes results in unregulated control of cell growth. Activation of proto-oncogenes arises through mutational events occurring within proto-oncogenes (Alitalo and Schwab, 1986; Bos, 1989). It has been recognized that a number of chemical carcinogens are capable of inducing mutations in proto-oncogenes (Balmain and Pragnell, 1983).

Several oncogene products are associated with growth factors. The *sis* oncogene encodes for platelet-derived growth factor (PDGF), which consists of types A and B chains. Active PDGF can consist of homo- or heterodimers of the A and B chains. Only cells that express the PDGF receptor are susceptible to transformation by the *sis* oncogene (Doolittle *et al.*, 1983). Fibroblast growth factor (FGF), epidermal growth factor (EGF), and the *wnt* family also have oncogenes that encode for their production (Burgess and Maciag, 1989; Nusse and Varmus, 1992). Enhanced expression of these growth factor genes leads to transformation of cultured cells. In addition, lung carcinomas and astrocytomas in humans express both PDGF and its receptor.

In order for the growth factors listed above to induce cell growth, the cell must also express the appropriate growth factor receptors. Ligand binding to receptors in many cases results in the activation of signaling cascades, of which a number have protein kinase activity. Protein kinases can phosphorylate at tyrosine, serine, or threonine residues. Several oncogene products have been identified that have tyrosine kinase activity (e.g., *src*, *fps*, *fgr*, *fms*, *kit*, and *ros*) (Collett and Erickson, 1978). Growth factor receptors including EGF, PDGF, insulin, insulin-like growth factor, and FGF have tyrosine activity (Wells, 1999). An extensive number of protein kinases are serine or threonine kinases, some of which can be activated in tumor cells and lead to transformation. The protein kinase C family consists of serine/threonine kinases (Nishizuka, 1988). This family of proteins participates in the inositol-phospholipid second messenger pathway and can be activated by calcium and diacylglycerol, as well as phorbol ester tumor promoters. The *raf* and *mos* oncogenes are other examples of serine threonine kinases, that interact with mitogen-activated kinase pathways, leading to enhanced expression of "immediate-early" genes such as Myc and Fos/Jun heterodimers, which ultimately leads to enhanced cell growth (Su and Karin, 1996).

Guanine nucleotide-binding proteins are a subset of the GTP superfamily. The primary oncogenic members of this family are the *ras* genes (e.g., *Ha-*, *Ki-*, and *n-ras*), which were initially found in murine retroviruses, and are frequently activated in human tumors and in chemically induced tumors in rodent models (McCormick, 1994). The three ras forms differ by only 20 amino acids, and have a conserved cytosine-186, which is a site for posttranslational modification by a farnesyl, isoprenyl group, a modification that is needed for membrane localization (Hancock *et al.*, 1989). Mutations in *ras*

affect the association of the Ras with GTP, and because Ras is active when GTP is bound, constitutive Ras activation is often seen with mutated forms of *ras*. Many mutation sites are associated with activation of *ras* and include codons 12, 13, 61, 116, 117, 119, and 146 (de Vos *et al.*, 1988). Although a dominant gain-of-function mutation in the *ras* gene converts it into an oncogene, a recessive loss-of-function mutation in the *NF1* gene also leads to constitutive Ras activation. *NF1* encodes a GTPase-activating enzyme (GAP) that accelerates hydrolysis of GTP and the conversion of active GTP-bound Ras to inactive GDP-bound Ras. The loss of GAP leads to sustained Ras activation of downstream signal transduction proteins. Individuals with neurofibromatosis have inherited a single mutant *NF1* allele; subsequent somatic mutation in the other allele leads to formation of neurofibromas.

In addition to acting at the receptor level, some oncogene products are nuclear transcription factors and thus alter gene expression. One of the first to be identified was the erbA oncogene product, which is an altered form of the thyroid hormone receptor (Damm *et al.*, 1989). This altered form is unable to bind thyroid hormone and allows the oncogene protein to act in a dominant-negative manner, functioning as a constitutive repressor of normal expression of genes regulated by thyroid hormone. Another family of oncogenes encode for the AP-1 transcription factor, a complex consisting of *jun* and *fos*, as well as Jun family members with homology to c-jun (Jun B and Jun D) (Chiu *et al.*, 1988; Vogt, 2001). Phorbol esters and several other tumor-promoting compounds are able to rapidly induce gene expression of both *fos* and *jun*. Activation of both *fos* and *jun* results in the constitutive expression of the transcription factors and sustained stimulation of cell growth signals. The *myc* family (c-*myc*, N-*myc*, and L-*myc*) encodes for transcription factors that are found activated in a number of tumor types (Marcu *et al.*, 1992).

Tumor Suppressor Genes

Retinoblastoma (Rb) Gene In contrast to oncogenes, the proteins encoded by most tumor suppressor genes act as inhibitors of cell proliferation or cell survival (Table 8-17). The prototype tumor suppressor gene, *Rb*, was identified by studies of inheritance of retinoblastoma. Loss or mutational inactivation of *Rb* contributes to the development of a wide variety of human cancers. In its unphosphorylated form, Rb binds to the *E2F* transcription factors preventing E2F-mediated transcriptional activation of a number of genes whose products are required for DNA synthesis. In addition, the Rb–E2F complex acts as a transcriptional repressor for many of these same genes (Chellappan *et al.*, 1991). During the early G1 phase of the cell

Table 8-17

Examples of Tumor Suppressor Genes and Cancer Association

TUMOR SUPPRESSOR	DISORDER	NEOPLASM
Rb1	Retinoblastoma	Small-cell lung carcinoma
p53	Li-Fraumeni syndrome	Breast, Colon, Lung Cancers
BRCA1	Unknown	Breast carcinoma
WT-1	Wilm's tumor	Lung cancer
p16	Unknown	Melanoma

cycle, Rb is in an unphosphorylated state, but becomes phosphorylated during the late G1, causing dissociation from E2F—a process that allows E2F to induce synthesis of DNA replication enzymes, resulting in a commitment to the cell cycle. Rb phosphorylation is initiated by an active Cdk4–cyclin D complex, and is completed by other cyclin-dependent kinases (Sherr, 1993; Weinberg, 1995). Most tumors contain an oncogenic mutation of one of the genes in this pathway, such that cells enter the S phase of the cell cycle in the absence of the proper extracellular growth signals that regulate Cdk activity. In addition, Rb is bound and inactivated by the E1A protein of the adenoviruses (Whyte et al., 1988) and also by the large T antigen of SV40 and the E7 protein of the papilloma virus, suggesting that the elimination of Rb function may be an important mechanism in tumor development by viruses and/or mutations induced by chemical carcinogens.

p53 Gene   The p53 protein is a tumor suppressor gene that is essential for checkpoint control and arrests the cell cycle in G_1 in cells with damaged DNA. Cells with functional p53 arrest in G_1 when exposed to DNA damaging agents such as irradiation, whereas cells lacking functional p53 are unable to block the cell cycle. p53 is activated by a wide array of stressors including ultraviolet light, γ irradiation, heat, and several carcinogens. DNA damage by γ irradiation or by other stresses leads to the activation of certain kinases, including ATM, which is encoded by the gene mutated in ataxia telangiectasia, and a DNA-dependent protein kinase. Phosphorylation of p53 by these and other kinases results in stabilization of p53 and an increase in cell content of this protein (Finlay et al., 1989). The active form of p53 is a tetramer of four identical subunits. A missense point mutation in one *p53* of the two alleles in a cell can abrogate almost all p53 activity, because virtually all the oligomers will contain at least one defective subunit, and such oligomers cannot function as a transcription factor. Oncogenic *p53* mutations thus act as "dominant negatives," in contrast to tumor-suppressor genes such as *Rb* (Levine et al., 1991).

Virtually all p53 mutations abolish its ability to bind to specific DNA sequences and activate gene expression (El-Deiry et al., 1992). The transcription of cyclin-kinase inhibitor p21, which binds to and inhibits mammalian G_1 Cdk–cyclin complexes, is induced by p53. As a result, cells with damaged DNA are arrested in G_1 until the damage is repaired and the levels of p53 and p21 fall; the cells then can progress into the S phase. In most cells, accumulation of p53 also leads to induction of proteins that promote apoptosis, and therefore would prevent proliferation of cells that are likely to accumulate multiple mutations. When the p53 checkpoint control does not operate properly, damaged DNA can replicate, producing mutations and DNA rearrangements that contribute to the development of transformed cells. Proteins that interact with and regulate p53 are also altered in many human tumors. The gene encoding one such protein, MDM2, is amplified in many sarcomas and other human tumors that maintain functional p53 (Leach et al., 1993). Under normal conditions, MDM2 binds the N-terminus of p53, repressing the ability of p53 to activate transcription of *p21* and genes mediating p53 degradation. Thus, MDM2 normally inhibits the ability of p53 to block at G1 or induce apoptosis. Enhanced MDM2 levels in tumor cells therefore results in decreased functional p53 and prevents p53 from growth arrest in response to irradiation or chemical carcinogens. For example, benzo(*a*)pyrene produces inactivating mutations at codons 175, 248, and 273 of the *p53* gene in cultured cells; these same positions are mutational hot spots in human lung cancer (Nakayama et al., 1984). Aflatoxin exposure induces a G to T transversion at codon 249 of

p53, and methyl-N'-nitro-N-nitrosoguanidine (MNNG) can alter methylation of DNA leading to inactivation of p53 (Burns et al., 1987).

BRCA1 Gene   Genetic analysis of breast tumors has revealed an hereditary predisposition for breast cancer is linked to *BRCA1*, a tumor-suppressor gene. Mutation of a single *BRCA1* allele has a 60% probability of developing breast cancer by age 50. In families transmitting the mutant BRCA1 allele, the normal allele is often absent in tumors. A number of investigators have shown that germ line mutations lead to loss of function of the BRCA1 gene, perhaps by acting as a transcription factor through binding at a zinc finger domain. However, no mutations have been observed in sporadic breast cancers (Futreal et al., 1994), suggesting that BRCA1 gene silencing may occur through nonmutational mechanisms.

Wilm's Tumor Gene (WT1)   Wilm's tumor occurs in the developing kidney at a rate of approximately 1 per 10,000 children. The WT1 gene is believed to be responsible for tumor development and is thought to function as a transcription factor (Hastie, 1994). The DNA-binding region of the WT1 gene contains four zinc finger domains, and binds a consensus sequence shared with EGR1; however, WT1 acts as a transcriptional repressor at this site (Rauscher et al., 1990). Similar to p53, WT1 mutant alleles act in a dominant negative manner.

p16 Gene   The group of proteins that function as cyclin-kinase inhibitors play an important role in cell cycle regulation. Mutations, especially deletions of the *p16* gene, that inactivate the ability of p16 to inhibit cyclin D-dependent kinase activity are common in several human cancers including a high percentage of melanomas (Kamb et al., 1994). Loss of p16 would mimic cyclin D1 overexpression, leading to Rb hyperphosphorylation and release of active E2F transcription factor. Thus p16 normally acts as a tumor suppressor. As with the BRCA1 gene, relatively few mutations have been found in this gene, and some researchers have speculated that epigenetic mechanisms such as gene silencing by DNA methylation may occur during tumorigenesis (Merlo et al., 1995).

Hormesis and Carcinogenesis

Hormesis is defined as a dose–response curve in which a U, J, or inverted U-shaped dose–response is observed; with low-dose exposures often resulting in beneficial rather than harmful effects (Calabrese, 2002) (Fig. 8-27). One of the first reports establishing an hormetic response was observed with ionizing radiation, in which it was hypothesized to be due to adaptation to background radiation exposure, as well as enhanced metabolism and

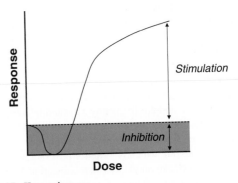

Figure 8-27. Hormesis curve.

Table 8-18
Classes of Chemopreventive Agents

INHIBITORS OF CARCINOGEN FORMATION	EXAMPLES
Reductive acids	Ascorbic acid
Phenols	Cafeic acid, ferulic acid, gallic acid
Sulfhydryl compounds	N-Acetylcysteine
Amino acids	Praline, thioproline
Blocking agents	
Inhibition of cytochrome P450	Dithiocarbamates, ellagic acid, diallyl sulfide, isothiocyanates
Induction of cytochrome P450	Indole-3-carbinol, B-naphthoflavone
Induction of phase II enzymes	
Glutathione S-transferase	Allyl sulfides, dithiolethiones, isothiocyanates
UDP-glucuronyltransferase	Polyphenols
Glutathione peroxidase	Selenium
Scavenge electrophiles	Ellagic acid, N-acetylcysteine
Scavenge free radicals	Sodium thiosulfate, polyphenols, vitamin E
Increase overall levels of DNA repair	Vanillin
Increase poly(ADP-ribosyl) transferase	N-acetylcysteine
Suppress error-prone DNA repair	Protease inhibitors
Suppressing agents	
Inhibit polyamine metabolism	DRv10, polyphenols, substituted putrescines
Induce terminal cell differentiation	Calcium, retinoids, vitamin D_3
Modulate signal transduction	Glycyrrhetinic acid, NSAIDSs, polyphenols, retinoids
Modulate hormonal/growth factor activity	NSAIDs, retinoids, tamoxifen
Inhibit oncogene activity	Genistein, NSAIDs, monoterpenes
Promote intracellular communication	Carotenois, polyphenols, retinoids
Restore immune response	NSAIDs, selenium, vitamin E
Induce apoptosis	Butyric acid, genistein, selenium, sulindac sulfone, retinoids
Correct DNA methylation imbalances	Folic acid, choline, methionine
Inhibit basement membrance degradation	Protease inhibitors
Inhibit arachidonic acid metabolism	Glycyrrhetinic acid, N-acetylcysteine, NSAIDs, polyphenols

detoxification (Calabrese, 2002; Parsons, 2003). Numerous examples exist that provide evidence for U- and J-shape dose relationships to different biomarkers of carcinogenesis, both for initiating and promoting carcinogens. For example, low-dose styrene treatment resulted in a decrease of chromosomal aberrations (Camurri *et al.*, 1983). A reduction in DNA strand breaks in human keratinocytes was seen following low-dose exposure to N-methyl-N'-nitro-N-nitrosoguanidine, while high doses markedly increased DNA strand breaks (Kleczkowska and Althaus, 1996). Several chronic bioassays for carcinogenicity in rats and mice have demonstrated a negative correlation between proliferative hepatocellular lesions and lymphomas at low and medium dose levels (Young and Gries, 1984). TCDD at hepatocarcinogenic doses caused dose-dependent reduction in mammary and uterine tumors (Kociba *et al.*, 1978). TCDD has also been shown to reduce tumor incidence after exposure to low doses of radiation and selenium (Nordberg and Andersen, 1981; Pollycove and Feinendegen, 2001). Evidence for a U-shaped dose–response curve has also been demonstrated for phenobarbital (Kitano *et al.*, 1998; Ito *et al.*, 2003; Kinoshita *et al.*, 2003). These investigators have shown that phenobarbital promoted the growth of diethylnitrosamine-induced hepatic lesions at doses between 60 and 500 ppm, while doses between 1 and 7.5 ppm decreased lesion growth, hepatocellular carcinoma, and tumor multiplicity.

Adaptive responses have been proposed to explain the hormetic effects observed by chemical carcinogens. When experimental an-

imals are exposed to chemicals, the initial response is an adaptive response to maintain homeostasis (Calabrese, 2002). Adaptive responses usually involve actions of the chemical on cellular signaling pathways that lead to changes in gene expression, resulting in enhanced detoxification and excretion of the chemical, as well as preserving the cell cycle and programmed cell death. It has been proposed that following very low doses of chemicals, the upregulation of these mechanisms overcompensates for cell injury such that a reduction in tumor promotion and/or tumor development is seen, and would explain the U- or J-shaped response curves obtained following carcinogen exposure.

A common feature of chemical carcinogens for which hormetic effects have been proposed is the formation of reactive oxygen species and the induction of cytochrome P450 isoenzymes. Inhibition of carcinogenesis by low levels of phenobarbital has been postulated to involve the suppression of 8-OHdG generation and cellular proliferation within areas of GST-P positive foci, possibly related to enhanced expression of the gene encoding the enzyme oxoguanine glycosylase 1 (Ogg1), which is involved in the repair of 8-OHdG lesions (Kinoshita *et al.*, 2003). Another explanation for the suppressive effect of low level phenobarbital on the development of preneoplastic lesions involves the stimulation of hepatic drug-metabolizing enzymes, which detoxify carcinogens (Pitot *et al.*, 1987). In a low-dose phenobarbital study, cDNA microarray analysis showed a suppression in mRNA expression MAP

Table 8-19
General Methods for Identification of Potential Carcinogens

METHOD	TIME FRAME
Short term	
Mutagenesis assays	Several wks
Transformation in cell culture	1–3 months
Medium term	
Qualitative and quantitative analysis of preneoplasia	2–8 months
Long term	
Chronic bioassay in animals	18–24 months

kinase p38, JNK1,2, and other intracellular kinases (Kinoshita *et al.*, 2003). Thus, suppression of gene expression of signal transduction modulators appears to be involved in the inhibitory effect of phenobarbital on cell proliferation.

Chemoprevention

The study of chemicals that prevent, inhibit, or slow down the process of cancer is referred to as chemoprevention. A number of chemicals, including drugs, antioxidants, foodstuffs, and vitamins have been found to inhibit or retard the components of the cancer process (Table 8-18) in both in vitro and in vivo models. Cancer chemopreventive agents may function at one or more of the steps in the carcinogenesis process. Cancer chemoprevention involves the administration or inclusion in the diet of natural or synthetic chemicals in an attempt to prevent, halt, or reverse the process of carcinogenesis. A basic assumption in chemoprevention is that treating early stages of malignant process will halt or delay the progression to neoplasia. Chemopreventive agents may function via one or several mechanisms; inhibitors of carcinogen formation, blocking agents, and/or as suppressing agents (Table 8-18). Blocking agents serve to prevent the metabolic activation of genotoxic or nongenotoxic carcinogens by either inhibiting its metabolism or by enhancing the detoxification mechanisms. In the case of reactive oxygen species generation by a carcinogen, antioxidants, such as, *N*-acetylcysteine, or vitamins E, A, and C serve as blocking agents by trapping the oxidative species before it can induce cellular damage. The drug oltipraz induces the phase II enzymes, in particular glutathione-*S*-transferase, has been shown to reduce the carcinogenicity of aflatoxin B1 by enhancing its detoxification (Jacobson *et al.*, 1997). Chemopreventive agents that increase tissue resistance function on the target tissue, usually an early preneoplastic lesion, by increasing tissue maturation and/or decreasing cell proliferation. Suppressing agents induce tissue differentiation, may counteract oncogenes, enhance tumor suppressor gene activities, inhibit proliferation of premalignant cells, or modify the effect of the carcinogen on the target tissue. Retinoic acid is a classic chemical that functions by inducing target tissue differentiation. Similarly, viral vectors containing wild-type p53 have been shown to negate the effects of tumor growth driven via p53 mutation. Extensive experimental evidence exists showing the inhibition or retardation of the cancer process by chemopreventive agents. These studies have been performed in animal models and cell systems. Whereas the human results of chemoprevention interventions are less convincing than the experimental models, considerable epidemiological evidence demonstrates an inverse relationship of some nutrient factors with cancer risks.

TEST SYSTEMS FOR CARCINOGENICITY ASSESSMENT

Numerous in vivo and in vitro experimental systems are available to assess the potential carcinogenicity of chemicals. The types of tests available to identify chemicals with carcinogenic potential can be classified into general categories, based on the duration required to conduct the test (Table 8-19). Short-term tests are typically of the duration of days to a few weeks, intermediate-term tests last from weeks up to a year, while chronic long-term tests usually encompass 6 months to 2 years exposure to a chemical. These bioassays use bacterial and mammalian targets.

Short-term Tests for Mutagenicity

Short-term tests for mutagenicity were developed to identify potentially carcinogenic chemicals based on their ability to induce mutations in DNA either in vivo or in vitro. A variety of in vivo and in vitro short-term tests are available to test the potential carcinogenicity of a chemical (Table 8-20). The majority of these tests measure the mutagenicity of chemicals as a surrogate for carcinogenicity. Therefore, while they are usually very predictive of indirect acting and direct acting (if a metabolic source is provided), these tests routinely fail to detect nongenotoxic carcinogens.

In Vitro Gene Mutation Assays   The most widely used short-term test is the Ames assay (Ames *et al.*, 1975). The relative simplicity and low cost of the test make it a valuable screening tool for mutagenic carcinogens. *Salmonella typhimurium* strains, deficient in DNA repair and unable to synthesize histidine, are used. In the presence of a mutagenic chemical, the defective histidine gene can be mutated back to a functional state (*back mutation*), resulting in a restoration of bacterial growth in a medium lacking histidine. The mutant colonies, which can make histidine, are referred to as "revertants." The Ames test in basic form can detect direct-acting genotoxic carcinogens. With the inclusion of a metabolic source, specifically the 9000g supernatant (S9) of a rat liver homogenate to promote metabolic conversion of the chemical, the Ames test can also detect indirect-acting genotoxic carcinogens. Figure 8-28 describes the standard method used for performing the Ames assay.

Genetically unique strains of the *S. typhimurium* bacterium have been developed for determining specific mutational targets. Strains TA100 and TA1535 are able to detect point mutations, whereas strains TA98, TA1537, and TA1538 are able to detect frameshift mutations. Chemicals are typically tested at several dose levels (usually five or more) and the mutation frequency (number of revertants) is calculated. Activation-independent (e.g., sodium azide and methyl methanesulfonate) and activation-dependent (e.g., 2-aminoanthracene) positive controls are included in each assay.

The mouse lymphoma assay is a mutagenicity assay used to determine whether a chemical is capable of inducing mutation in eukaryotic cells. Typically, mouse lymphoma L5178Y cells are used, and the ability of the cell cultures to acquire resistance to trifluorothymidine (the result of forward mutation at the thymidine kinase locus) is quantified. Another mammalian cell mutation assay, the Chinese hamster ovary (CHO) test, is also commonly used to assess the potential mutagenicity of chemicals. This assay uses the

Table 8-20

Short-Term Tests for Mutagenicity

TEST	ENDPOINT	REFERENCE
Gene mutation assays in vitro		
Prokaryote mutagenesis in vitro (Ames test, etc.)	Back or forth mutations in specific bacterial strains	Maron and Ames, 1983
Mouse lymphoma thymidine kinase (TK)	Mutations in TK	Majeska and Matheson, 1990
Chinese hamster ovary (CHO) and V79 hypoxanthine guanine phosphoribosyltranferase (HGPRT)	Mutations in HGPRT	Li et al., 1987
Gene mutation assays in vivo		
Dominant lethal assay	Death of fertilized egg in mammalian implanted species	Bateman, 1973 Lockhart et al., 1992
Sperm abnormality induction	Microscopically abnormal sperm	Wyrobek and Bruce, 1975
Mutation induction in transgenes in vivo		
LacZ mouse	Mutations in LacZ gene	Myhr, 1991
LacI mouse	Mutations in LacI gene	cf. Mirsalis et al., 1994
LacI rat	Mutations in LacI gene	de Boer et al., 1996
rpsL mouse	Mutations in rpsL gene	Gondo et al., 1996
Chromosomal alterations in vivo		
Heritable translocation test (mice)	Translocations induced in germ cells	Generoso et al., 1980
Rat bone marrow clastogenesis in vivo	Chromosomal aberrations in bone marrow cells in vivo	Ito et al., 1994
Micronucleus test	Appearance of micronuclei in bone marrow cells in vivo	Tinwell and Ashby, 1994 Heddle et al., 1983
Chromosomal alterations in vitro		
Mitotic recombination, mitotic crossing over, or mitotic gene conversion in yeast	Conversion of heterozygous alleles to homozygous state	Wintersberger and Klein, 1988
Induced chromosomal aberrations in cell lines	Visible alterations in karyotype	Galloway et al., 1985
Sister chromatid exchange	Visible exchange of differentially labeled sister chromatids	Latt, 1981 Murphy et al., 1992
Primary DNA damage		
DNA repair in vivo or in vitro	Unscheduled DNA synthesis and/or DNA strand breaks	Furihata and Matsushima, 1987
Rodent liver: unscheduled DNA synthesis induction	Unscheduled DNA synthesis in rodent cells in vivo and/or in vitro	Kennelly, 1995 Steinmetz et al., 1988

hypoxanthine-guanine phosphoribosyltransferase (HGPRT) gene as the end point. The basis for these assays is shown in Fig. 8-29. Cells are treated with the test chemical and then placed into suspension with selective medium for replication and fixation of induced mutations. Cells are then plated for colony growth, and after several days, colony numbers and colony size are recorded. The number of mutant colonies is a measure of the ability of the test chemical to induce a genetic change at the thymidine kinase or HGPRT loci in these transformed cells.

As with the Ames assay, these assays are frequently performed in the presence of an exogenous metabolic source (e.g., irradiated epithelial cell feeder layer). Because not all carcinogens are mutagens and/or directly damage the DNA, the concordance with the chronic in vivo bioassay for these mutagenicity assays is relatively low.

In Vivo Gene Mutation Assays For the assessment of the carcinogenic potential of chemicals, in vivo genotoxicity tests are important complement to in vitro mutagenicity tests. The in vivo tests have advantages over the in vitro test systems in that they take into account the whole animal processes such as absorption, tissue distribution, metabolism, and excretion of chemicals and their metabolites. The commonly used in vivo models include transgenic rodent mutation assay systems based on the genes of the lac operon, Muta™Mouse (Gossen et al., 1989), and Big Blue® (Kohler et al., 1991a,b).

The Muta™Mouse is a transgenic mouse in which a vector prepared from bacteriophage λDNA (λgt10) has been stably inserted into the genome and exists within every cell. Within the λDNA sequence, the bacterial gene lacZ, which encodes for β-galactosidase, was inserted at the single EcoRI restriction site. The entire vector contains ~47,000 bp, of which the lacZ gene comprises 3126 bp. The construction and analysis of Muta™Mouse have been previously described (Gossen et al., 1989). The Big Blue® transgenic mouse was developed using a 47.6 kb λshuttle vector containing the bacterial lacI gene (1080 bp), which encodes the repressor protein of the lacZ gene. As with the Muta™Mouse, this vector is stably inserted into the genome and exists in every cell. Details on the Big Blue® system are described elsewhere (Kohler et al., 1991a,b).

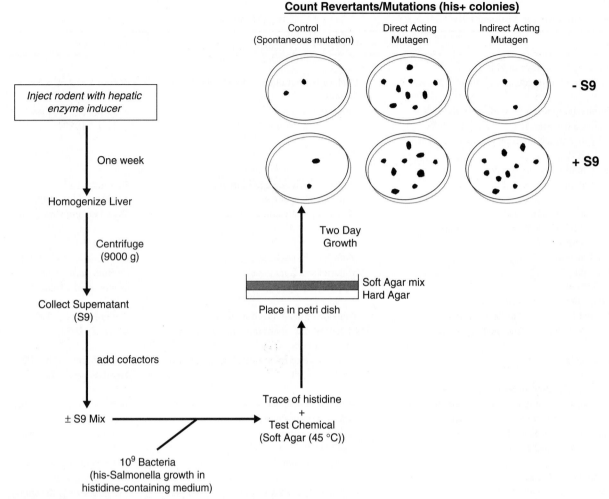

Figure 8-28. Ames tests for mutagenesis of chemicals in Salmonella typhimurium bacteria.

To detect mutations, following exposure of mice to test chemicals, mutations are analyzed in high molecular DNA isolated from the tissue under investigation. The next step is to isolate a viable λphage for the analysis of mutations in the *lacZ* or *lacI* genes from the mouse. The infectious λparticles are detected as plaques that form on a bacterial (*Escherichia coli* strain) lawn grown on an agar surface. In the case of Muta™Mouse, a positive selection system is used that involves the scoring of clear plaques on titration plates to determine the total number of plaque forming units and on selection plates to determine the number of mutants (Gossen and Vijg, 1993). For Big Blue®, a nonselectable color screening assay is used, scoring blue mutant plaques among the nonmutant clear plaques (Kohler *et al.*, 1991a). In each case the ratio of mutants to the total population will provide a mutation frequency for each chemical and each organ tested. As with the other short-term tests that have been discussed, it is unlikely that in vivo genotoxicity test systems will identify nongenotoxic/non-DNA reactive compounds.

Chromosomal Alterations Chromosomal alterations are quite common in malignant neoplasms, as such the detection of chromosomal abnormalities by test chemicals is considered an excellent test for the assessment of carcinogenic potential. Both in vivo and in vitro assays are available to assess chromosomal alterations. In mammalian cell lines, most of the test systems used the same lines as used in the mutation assay (Galloway *et al.*, 1985). To assess induction of chromosomal alterations, cells are harvested in their first mitotic division after the initiation of chemical exposure. Cells are stained with Giemsa and scored for completeness of karyotype (21 +/− 2 chromosomes). The classes of aberrations recorded include breaks and terminal deletions, rearrangements and translocations, as well as despiralized chromosomes, and cells containing 10 or more aberrations.

SCEs are a measure of DNA damage and increased levels of DNA damage, events that are associated with mutation induction and cancer. During metaphase, sister chromatids, each encompassing a complete copy of one chromosome, are bound together through specific protein interactions. SCEs are a reflection of an interchange of DNA between different chromatids at homologous loci within a replicating chromosome (Latt, 1981). Differential staining of chromatids is therefore used to assess SCEs. Typically, 5-bromodeoxyuridine (BrdU) is added along with the test chemical for one cell replication followed by replacement of the medium with a medium containing BrdU and colcemid, without test chemical.

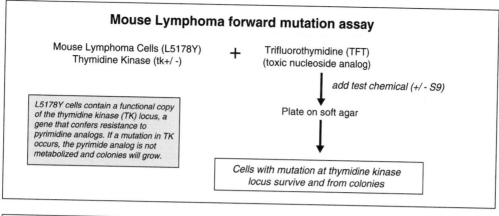

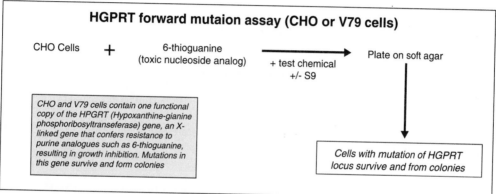

Figure 8-29. In vitro approaches for assessing forward mutations using the TK and HGPRT Assays.

Cells are then harvested, stained, and second-division metaphase cells scored to determine the frequency of SCE/cell for each dose level.

In vivo analysis of chromosomal alterations have been described since the 1980s (Generosso *et al.*, 1980). Disruption of the DNA replication process or damage to chromosomes by chemicals can alter the genetic material distributed to either of the two daughter nuclei. When this occurs, the genetic material that is not incorporated into a new nucleus may form its own "micronucleus," which is clearly visible with a microscope. For this assay, animals are exposed to chemicals and the frequency of micronucleated cells is determined at some specified time after treatment. Micronucleus tests must be performed on cells that are dividing, most typically in cells from bone marrow samples (Heddle *et al.*, 1983). As with other short-term tests, the micronucleus test provides complementary information to gene mutation data but the tests neither enhance the ability to detect genotoxic carcinogens nor are capable of detecting non-DNA reactive carcinogens. However, this assay does provide information on the ability of a chemical to disrupt mammalian chromosome structure and function.

DNA Damage   Primary DNA damage represents possible premutational events that can be detected, either directly or indirectly, by a number of techniques using mammalian cells in culture or using rodent tissue. Unscheduled DNA synthesis (UDS) is a commonly used assay that measures the ability of a chemical to induce DNA lesions by measuring the increase in DNA repair. Among the available techniques is the measurement of DNA strand breaks both in

vivo and in vitro (Miyamae *et al.*, 1997). Whereas a wide array of assays are available to assess DNA damage, the Comet Assay, or single-cell gel electrophoresis has become one of the standard methods for assessing DNA damage and repair at the individual cell level. Since its introduction in 1988, the alkaline comet assay has been modified to increase the utility of this technique for detecting various forms of DNA damage (e.g., single- and double-strand breaks, oxidative DNA base damage, and DNA-DNA/DNA-protein/DNA-drug crosslinking) and DNA repair in virtually any eukaryotic cell. Through the use of lesion-specific endonucleases, the levels of ultraviolet (UV)-induced pyrimidine dimers, oxidized bases, and alkylation damage can be assessed in biological samples (Collins, 2004).

Transformation Assays   A variety of in vitro test systems have been developed to assess the carcinogenic potential of chemicals. The C3H/10T$^{1/2}$ cell line has been widely used in the transformation assays. It was originally derived from fibroblasts taken from the prostate of a C3H mouse embryo. The cells are approximately tetraploid but the chromosome number in the cells varies widely. As such, these cells are chromosomally abnormal and have already passed through some of the stages that might be involved in the production of a cancerous cell. Upon plating these cells, they will stop growing when their density is sufficiently high (contact growth inhibition). However, the contact inhibition can fail, resulting in cell piling forming a transformed colony. Therefore, following exposure to xenobiotics, this assay

Table 8-21
Animal Models of Neoplastic Development

	ENDPOINT	REFERENCES
Chronic 2-year bioassay	Tumors in all organs	Sontag, 1977
Tissue-specific bioassays		
Liver, mouse	Hepatomas	Camichael et al., 1997
Lung, mouse	Pulmonary adenomas	Shimkin and Stoner, 1975
Brain, rat	Gliomas	Kroh, 1995
Mammary gland, rat/mouse	Adenomas and carcinomas	Dunnick et al., 1995
Medium-term bioassays		
Ito model	Hepatic adenomas and carcinomas	Ito et al., 1989
Newborn mouse	Neoplasms in liver, lung, lymphoid organs	Fujii, 1991
Multistage models of neoplastic development		
Bladder, rat	Papillomas/carcinomas	Hicks, 1980
Colon, rat	Aberrant crypt polyp	Sutherland and Bird, 1994
Epidermis, mouse	Papillomas	DiGiovanni, 1992
Liver, rat	Altered hepatic foci	Pitot et al., 1996
Transgenic mice		
Knockout of p53 tumor suppressor gene (p53[def])	Tumors in heterozygous animals having normal phenotype	Donehower, 1996
v-Ha-ras with zetaglobin promoter; tandem insertion on chromosome 11 (TG AC)	Induced transgene expression in skin leads to papilloma development	Spalding et al., 1993

assesses carcinogenic potential based on the percentage of colonies that are transformed (Reznikoff et al., 1973).

The most frequently used endpoint for cell transformation is morphological transformation of mammalian cell fibroblasts in culture. Transformation assays using BALB3T3 and Syrian Hamster Embryo (SHE) cells are available for the assessment of the carcinogenic potential of chemicals. BALB/3T3 transformation assay, however, has not gained full acceptance as a carcinogenic screening assay, mainly due to issues regarding its relatively low sensitivity, low reproducibility, and relatively long test period (Schectman et al., 1985; Sakai et al., 1989). The Syrian hamster embryo (SHE) cell assay, a diploid cell transformation assay, measures carcinogenic potential of xenobiotics by assessing transformed colonies based on morphological criteria. The SHE cell assay has several features that make it an appealing method to evaluate the carcinogenic potential of xenobiotics: (1) The assay has a >85% concordance with the 2-year rodent bioassay; (2) the stages involved in the clonal transformation of SHE cells (e.g., morphological transformation, immortalization, and tumorigenicity) closely resemble those associated with the classic defined stages of carcinogenesis (e.g., initiation, promotion, and progression); and (3) nongenotoxic/non-DNA reactive carcinogens elicit a positive response on morphological transformation in the SHE cell assay (Barrett and Lamb, 1985; LeBeouf et al., 1990; Isfort et al., 1994, 1996). The SHE assay offers an alternative, regulatory approved, means to check the validity of the positive result before embarking on potentially unnecessary and expensive chronic or subchronic testing protocols.

Chronic Testing for Carcinogenicity

The majority of in vivo carcinogenicity testing is performed in rodent models. The administration of chemicals in the diet, often for extended periods, for assessment of their safety and/or toxicity began in the 1930s (Sasaki and Yoshida, 1935). Animal testing today remains a standard approach for determining the potential carcinogenic activity of xenobiotics. In addition to the lifetime exposure rodent models, organ-specific model systems, multistage models, and transgenic models are being developed and used in carcinogen testing (Table 8-21).

Chronic (2-Year) Bioassay Two-year studies in laboratory rodents remain the primary method by which chemicals or physical agents are identified as having the potential to be hazardous to humans. The most common rodents used are the rat and mouse. Typically the bioassays are conducted over the lifespan of the rodents (2 years). Historically, selective rodent strains have been used in the chronic bioassay; however, each strain has both advantages and disadvantages. For example, the National Toxicology Program (NTP) typically uses Fisher 344 (F344) rats and B6C3F1 mice. The F344 rat has a high incidence of testicular tumors and leukemias, whereas the B6C3F1 mouse is associated with a high background of liver tumors (Table 8-22).

In the chronic bioassay, two or three dose levels of a test chemical and a vehicle control are administered to 50 males and 50 females (mice and rats), beginning at 8 weeks of age, continuing throughout their lifespan. The route of administration can be via oral (gavage), dietary (mixed in feed), or inhalation (via inhalation chambers) exposure. Typically a number of short-term in vivo tests are conducted prior to the chronic bioassay to determine acute toxicity profiles, appropriate route of administration, and the maximum tolerated dose (MTD). Generally, the MTD is used to set the high dose in the chronic study. The use of the MTD as the upper dose level has been questioned by many investigators, as it is recognized that the doses selected often represent doses that are considered unrealistically high for human exposure. Pharmacokinetics and metabolism at high dose are frequently unrepresentative of those at lower doses; in

Table 8-22

Spontaneous Tumor Incidence (Combined Benign and Malignant) in Selected Sites of the Two Species, B6C3F1 Mice and F344 Rats, Used in the NCI/NTP Bioassay

SITE	B6C3F1 MICE		F344 RATS	
	MALE	FEMALE	MALE	FEMALE
Liver				
Adenoma	10.3	4.0	3.4	3.0
Carcinoma	21.3	4.1	0.8	0.2
Pituitary	0.7	8.3	24.7	47.5
Adrenal	3.8	1.0	19.4	8.0
Thyroid	1.3	2.1	10.7	9.3
Hematopoietic	12.7	27.2	30.1	18.9
Mammary gland	0	1.9	2.5	26.1
Lung	17.1	7.5	2.4	1.2

addition, a general relationship between toxicity and carcinogenicity cannot be drawn for all classes of chemicals. During the study, food consumption and bodyweight gain should be monitored, and the animals observed clinically on a regular basis, and at necropsy the tumor number, location, and pathological diagnosis for each animal is thoroughly assessed.

Organ-Specific Bioassays and MultiStage Animal Models

Many tissue-specific bioassays have been developed with the underlying goal being to produce a sensitive and reliable assay that could be conduced in a time frame shorter in duration than the 2-year chronic bioassay. These assays are commonly used to detect carcinogenic activity of chemicals in various target organs (Weisburger and Williams, 1984). Of the many models available, three models, the liver, skin, and lung models are more widely used.

Carcinogenicity Testing in the Liver   The liver represents a major target organ for chemical carcinogens. It has been estimated that nearly half of the chemicals tested in the 2-year chronic bioassay by the National Toxicology Program showed an increased incidence of liver cancer. The rodent liver has been used as an animal model for carcinogenesis since the 1930s. Early pioneering work by Peraino and Pitot as well as Farber showed the multistaged process that occurs in the liver. The multistage nature of carcinogenesis is paralleled in the animal models; the system is characterized by well-defined changes including the formation of initiated cells by genotoxic agents that then progress to preneoplastic focal lesions, some of which subsequently convert into neoplasms. The use of preneoplastic lesions as endpoints in carcinogenicity testing may shorten the experiment from 2 years to a few months. Several rodent liver focus assays have been developed to assess the ability of a chemical to induce liver cancer, and study the mechanisms involved in tumor development (Williams, 1982; Bannasch, 1986a; Ito et al., 1989). Liver carcinogenesis assays have been developed to study and distinguish chemicals that affect the initiation or promotion stage of hepatocarcinogenesis. During the assay for initiating activity of a chemical, the test substance is given prior to exposure to a promoting chemical. Although a single initiating dose can result in the induction of focal lesions, exposure over several weeks is often used to increase

the sensitivity of the model (Williams, 1982; Parnell et al., 1988). Phenobarbital is a commonly used tumor promoter; however, a wide range of chemicals have also been used as promoting agents (Solt and Farber, 1976; Oesterle and Deml, 1988). To assess the promoting activity of a chemical, the liver is initiated with a genotoxic chemical, often diethylnitrosamine. The test chemical is then administered for a duration of weeks to several months, and chemical substances with promoting activity may stimulate the proliferation of initiated cells or may inhibit the proliferation of the surrounding putatively normal cells. The dose of the initiating carcinogen should represent a dose that will not itself induce liver tumors during the course of the experiment.

Another method commonly used was developed in Japan by Ito and coworkers (Ogiso et al., 1990; Ito et al., 1994; Shirai et al., 1999). The entire assay takes only 8 weeks to perform. Rats are initiated with a single dose of diethylnitrosamine, followed by a 2-week recovery period, after which point the animals are exposed to the test compound for 8 weeks. After 1 week of exposure to the test substance, the animals are given a 2/3 partial hepatectomy. The control group receives the same initiation and partial hepatectomy, but is not exposed to the test chemical. Hepatic focal lesions, while individually are clonal in nature express a number of phenotypic alterations in various enzyme markers. A common endpoint assessed is the formation of liver lesions that stain for glutathione-S-transferase pi (GST-P), a marker that stains many focal lesions in the rat. Using this assay, these investigators have demonstrated a significant correlation between the results obtained using this assay and the medium- and long-term study results (Ogiso et al., 1990). This group has also modified the original procedure to enable the detection of promoting agents. In this protocol, carcinogens are given over a 4-week period to initiate the formation of focal lesions, after which, test chemicals are administered for an additional 24- to 36-week period (Ito et al., 1996). In this manner, the ability of the test chemical to promote the growth of preneoplastic lesions can be assessed. The newborn mouse model originally described by Shubik and coworkers (Pietra et al., 1959) has also been used as a model for hepatocarcinogenesis (Vesselinovitch et al., 1978; Fujii, 1991). In this model, a single dose of diethylnitrosamine is administered to infant mice to initiate focal lesions. This step is then followed by exposure to test chemicals for several weeks to assess their potential to promote focal lesion development in the liver.

Identification of hepatic foci in H&E-stained sections is regarded as the most reliable approach for the diagnosis and quantification of preneoplastic liver lesions in rodents. Preneoplastic lesions are obligatory precursor lesions that can lead to liver tumors and will progress to benign and malignant liver cell tumors without further chemical exposure, and are used as endpoints in carcinogenicity testing (Pitot et al., 1987; Pereira and Herren-Freund, 1988; Ito et al., 1989; Maronpot et al., 1989; Williams, 1989). In addition to the sensitive detection of these preneoplastic lesions in conventional H&E staining, a number of histochemically detectable phenotypic alterations have been used for their quantification; however, these markers are only useful in the rat model, as focal lesions in mice to not exhibit these same phenotypic markers.

Carcinogenicity Testing in the Skin   The Mouse Skin model is one of the most extensively studied and used models for understanding multistage carcinogenesis. This model of carcinogenesis is an assay that has been used to dissect mechanisms of carcinogenesis and also is purported to be a useful intermediate-term cancer bioassay. The skin was the target organ of the first experimental induction

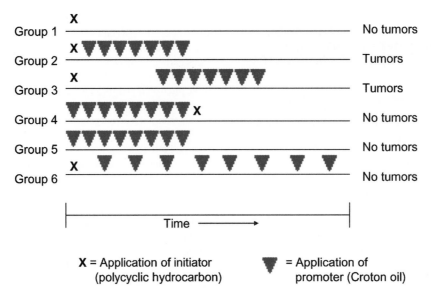

Figure 8-30. Experiments demonstrating the initiation and promotion phases of carcinogens in mice.

Group 2: Application of promoter repeated at twice-weekly intervals for several months. Group 3: Application of promoter delayed for several months and then applied twice weekly. Group 6: Promoter applied at monthly intervals.

of chemical carcinogenesis (Yamagiwa and Ichikawa, 1915). The early studies by Friedwald and Rous (1944) and Berenblum and Shubik (1947) introduced the two-stage concept of carcinogenesis in the skin (Fig. 8-30). This model exploits many of the unique properties of the mouse skin; one major being that the development of neoplasia can be followed visually. In addition, the number and relative size of papillomas and carcinomas can be quantified as the tumors progress.

Both initiating and promoting activities of chemical carcinogens can be assessed using this model. In the promotion assay, a number of chemical carcinogens have been used to initiate cells in the mouse skin including urethane, UV light, benzo(a)pyrene, and dimethylbenzanthracene, with the latter of more common usage. The requirement for all initiating agents is to induce a genotoxic event that upon failure to repair DNA damage results in the formation of a mutated cell. Grossly, initiated cells of the skin appear identical to normal skin. Initiation in skin is frequently linked with the mutation of the CHr gene. Since the terminally differentiated cells in the skin are no longer capable of undergoing cell division, only initiated cells retain their proliferative capacity and thus represent the cell populations that give rise to tumors. To assess promotion by a chemical, an initiating chemical is applied first and is followed by the administration of a test substance for several weeks on the shaved skin of mice (Slaga, 1984). The promotion of initiated karatinocytes is commonly assessed using the phorbol ester TPA, which is routinely included as a positive control in this assay. The current hypothesis is that during the initiation stage the expansion of initiated cells occurs as a result of inflammation and hyperplasia from either TPA or through mechanical wound healing mechanisms. Upon repeated application of tumor promoters, selective clonal expansion of initiated keratinocytes occurs, resulting in skin papillomas, which over time can progress to carcinomas. In the standard two-stage protocol for mouse skin, malignant progression is relatively rare with approximately 5% of the papillomas progressing to the carcinoma stage. For the detection of initiating activity,

the test substance is applied to skin prior to promotion with phorbol esters. Several mouse models are available, including hairless mice, SENCAR mice, both of which have enhanced sensitivity to induction of skin cancer (Brown and Balmain, 1995; Sundberg *et al.*, 1997).

Carcinogenicity Testing in the Lung   Strain A mice are genetically susceptible to the development of lung tumors, with lung tumors being observed in control animals as early as 3–4 weeks of age, with a steady increase to nearly 100% by 24 months of age (Shimkin and Stoner, 1975). Chemically induced tumors appear to be derived from hyperplastic lesions that progress to adenoma, carcinoma within adenoma, and ultimately, to carcinomas (Stoner *et al.*, 1993). In this model, carcinogenicity is typically assessed as an acceleration of tumor development, rather than an increase in the tumor incidence. The protocol currently used is that the chemical is administered for a period of 8 weeks, after which the animals remain on test for 4 additional months without chemical exposure. The strain A mouse lung tumor assay is sensitive to particular classes of chemicals, such as polycyclic aromatic hydrocarbons, nitrosamines, nitrosoureas, carbamates, aflatoxin, certain metals, and hydrazines (Stoner and Shimkin, 1985; Maronpot *et al.*, 1986; Stoner, 1991).

Carcinogenicity Testing in Other Organs   Test systems to examine the ability of a chemical to promote neoplastic development at organ sites other than liver, skin, and lung have also been developed. The available systems include animal models directed at examining carcinogenicity in the kidney, bladder, pancreas, stomach, colon, small intestine, and oral cavity. These models vary in the initiating carcinogen used, and frequency, duration, and site of application, as well as the duration of promoting chemical exposure. Table 8-23 provides an overview of the animal models available for these target organs.

Table 8-23

ORGAN	SPECIES	INITIATING CARCINOGEN	INITIATOR DURATION	CARCINOGEN (PROMOTER) DURATION	REFERENCES
Kidney	Rat[1]	N-ethyl-N-hydroxyethylnitrosamine	Single exposure	20 wks	Hiasa et al., 1991
Bladder	Rat	N-nitrosobutyl(4-hydroxybutyl)amine	4 wks	32 wks	Fukushima et al., 1983
Pancreas	Rat, Syrian Hamsters	N-nitrosobis(2-oxopropyl)amine, N-nitroso(2-hydroxypropyl)(2-oxopropyl)amine	Single exposure		Longnecker et al., 1984, 1985
Stomach (forestomach)	Rat	Benzo(a)pyrene	1–2x/week, 4 wks	40 wks	Silva et al., 1995
Stomach (glandular)	Rat	N-methyl-N'-nitro-N-nitronitrosoguanidine	Single exposure	40 wks	Takahashi et al., 1986
Colon	Rat	Azoxymethane	2 exposures	12 wks	Yamashita et al., 1994
Small intestine	Rat Mice	1,2-Dimethylhydrazine N-ethyl-N'-nitro-N-nitrosoguanidine	2–9 wks 4 wks	16–20 wks	Lindenschmidt et al., 1987; Jagadeesan et al., 1994
Oral cavity (lip, oral, nasal)	Rat	4-Nitroquinoline N-oxide	4 wks[2]		Johansson et al., 1989
Oral cavity (tongue)	Rat	4-Nitroquinoline N-oxide	8 wks[3]		Tanaka et al., 1995
Buccal cells (squamous cell carcinoma)	Syrian Hamster	—	—	Repeated application[4] 10–16 wks	Solt et al., 1987
Buccal cells (squamous cell carcinoma)	Syrian Hamster	dimethylbenz[a]anthracene	Single exposure	45 wks	Gimenez-Conti and Slaga, 1993

Transgenic Animals in Carcinogenicity Assessment

Due to the development of animal models with genetic alterations that invoke a susceptibility to carcinogenesis by chemical agents, the use of transgenic and knockout animals in carcinogenicity assessment is gaining more popularity. The common models that have been used include the Tg.AC and rasH2 transgenic mice, and p53[+/−] and XPA[−/−] knockout mice (Gulezian et al., 2000). Recently, the feasibility of the use of these animal models as alternative assays for the 2-year chronic bioassay was assessed by the Health and Environmental Sciences Institute (HESI) branch of the International Life Sciences Institute (ILSI). In this assessment, 21 chemicals were evaluated, encompassing genotoxic, nongenotoxic, and noncarcinogenic chemicals. The conclusions drawn from the scientific review suggested that these models appear to have usefulness as screening models for assessment of chemical carcinogenicity; however, they do not provide definitive proof of potential human carcinogenicity. Further the scientific panel suggested that these models could be used in place of the mouse 2-year bioassay (Tennant et al., 1998; Cohen et al., 2001). Coupled with information on genotoxicity, particularly DNA reactivity, structure–activity relationships, results from other bioassays, and the results of other mechanistic investigations including toxicokinetics, metabolism, and mechanistic information, these alternate mouse models for carcinogenicity appear to be useful models for assessing the carcinogenicity of chemical agents.

CHEMICAL CARCINOGENESIS IN HUMANS

A number of factors have been implicated in the induction of cancer in humans. Infectious agents, lifestyle, medical treatments, environmental and occupational exposure account either directly or indirectly for the majority of cancers seen in humans. Of these, the component that contributes the most to human cancer induction and progression is lifestyle: tobacco use, alcohol use, and poor diet (Fig. 8-1 and Table 8-24). Tobacco usage either through smoking tobacco, chewing tobacco, or tobacco snuff-type products is estimated to be responsible for 25–40% of all human cancers. In particular a strong correlation between tobacco usage and mouth, larynx, lung, esophageal, and bladder cancer exists. It has been estimated (Doll and Peto, 1981) that 85–90% of all lung cancer cases in the United States are a direct result of tobacco use. The induction of pancreatic cancer also appears to have a linkage to tobacco use. Alcohol

Table 8-24

Carcinogenic Factors Associated with Lifestyle

CHEMICAL(S)	NEOPLASM(S)
Alcohol beverage	Esophagus, liver, oropharynx, and larynx
Aflatoxins	Liver
Betel chewing	Mouth
Dietary intake (fat, protein, calories)	Breast, colon, endometrium, gallbladder
Tobacco smoking	Mouth, pharynx, larynx, lung, esophagus, bladder

Table 8-25

Occupational Human Carcinogens

AGENT	INDUSTRIAL PROCESS	NEOPLASMS
Asbestos	Construction, asbestos mining	Peritoneum, bronchus
Arsenic	Mining and smelting	Sking, bronchus, liver
Alkylating agents (mechloro-ethamine hydrochloride and bis[chloromethyl]ether)	Chemical manufacturing	Bronchus
Benzene	Chemical manufacturing	Bone marrow
Benzidine, beta-naphthylamine	Dye and textile	Urinary bladder
Chromium and chromates	Tanning, pigment making	Nasal sinus, bronchus
Nickel	Nickel refining	Nasal sinus, bronchus
Polynuclear aromatic hydrocarbons	Steel making, roofing, chimney cleaning	Skin, scrotum, bronchus
Vinyl chloride monomer	Chemical manufacturing	Liver
Wood dust	Cabinet making	Nasal sinus
Beryllium	Aircraft manufacturing, electronics	Bronchus
Cadmium	Smelting	Bronchus
Ethylene oxide	Production of hospital supplies	Bone marrow
Formaldehyde	Plastic, textile, and chemical	Nasal sinus, bronchus
Polychlorinated biphenyls	Electrical-equipment production and maintenance	Liver

Table 8-26

Human Carcinogenic Chemicals Associated with Medical Therapy and Diagnosis

CHEMICAL OR DRUG	ASSOCIATED NEOPLASMS
Alkylating agents (cyclophospamide, melphalan)	Bladder, leukemia
Azathioprine	Lymphoma, reticulum cell sarcoma, skin, Kaposi's sarcoma (?)
Chloramphenicol	Leukemia
Diethylstilbestrol	Vagina (clear cell carcinoma)
Estrogens	Liver cell adenoma, endometrium, skin
Phenacetin	Renal pelvis (carcinoma)
Phenytoin	Lymphoma, neuroblastoma
Thorotrast	Liver (angiosarcoma)

consumption contributes anywhere from 2 to 4% of cancers of the esophagus, liver, and larynx.

Poor diets whether high fat, low protein, high calories, or diets lacking in needed antioxidants and minerals account for anywhere from 10 to 70% of human cancers. Diet contaminated by molds such as Aspergillus flavis (which produces aflatoxin B1) have been linked epidemiologically to a higher incidence of liver cancer. It also appears that aflatoxin B1 exposure coupled with hepatitis B virus infection produces an increased incidence of liver cancer compared to aflatoxin B1 or hepatitis B exposure individually. Mold contaminated food stuffs have also been shown to produce nitroso compounds.

There is substantial evidence that over nutrition either through excess calories and/or high fat diets contribute to a number of human cancers (Doll and Peto, 1981). In particular high fat and high calorie diets have been linked to breast, colon, and gall bladder cancer in humans. Diets poor in antioxidants and/or vitamins such as vitamin A and vitamin E probably also contribute to the onset of cancer. The method of cooking may also influence the production of carcinogens produced in the cooking process. Carcinogenic heterocyclic amines and polycyclic aromatic hydrocarbons are formed during broiling and grilling of meat. Acrylamide, a suspected human carcinogen has been found in fried foods at low concentrations.

A number of occupations have been associated with the development of specific cancers (Table 8-25). As noted earlier, the linkage between chimney sweepers who as young boys in England were exposed to polyaromatic hydrocarbons through constant exposure to soot, developed scrotal cancer. The linkage between occupational

Table 8-27
IARC Classification of the Evaluation of Carcinogenicity for Human Beings

GROUP	EVIDENCE
1. Agent is carcinogenic to humans	Human data strong
	Animal data strong
2A. Agent is probably carcinogenic to humans	Human epidemiology data suggestive
	Animal data positive
2B. Agent is possibly carcinogenic to humans	Human epidemiology data weak
	Animal data positive
3. Agent is not classifiable as to carcinogenicity to humans	Human and animal data inadequate
4. Agent is probably not carcinogenic to humans	Human and animal data negative

exposure to asbestos and the development of bronchiogenic carcinoma and as well as malignant mesothelioma has been clearly established. The appearance of bronchiogenic carcinoma was much higher in shipyard workers who were exposed to both asbestos as well as cigarette smoking. Muscat and Wynder (1991) noted no association between cigarette smoking and mesothelioma formation. Similarly, asbestos exposure by itself (without smoking) does not seem to increase the risk of bronchiogenic carcinoma. Aromatic amines used in the chemical and dye industries have been shown to produce or induce bladder cancer in humans. Prolonged high exposure to benzene in an occupational setting has been linked to the formation of acute myelogenous leukemia in humans.

A number of medical therapy and medical diagnostic tools have also been linked to the induction of human cancer (Table 8-26). Cancer chemotherapeutic drugs, such as the alkylating agent cyclophos-

phamide, have been associated with bladder tumors and leukemia in patients receiving these treatments. The administration of the synthetic estrogenic compound diethylstilbestrol to pregnant women, in order to improve embryo implantation and prevent spontaneous abortion, has been shown to result in the formation of clear cell carcinomas of the vagina in the female offspring of mothers treated with diethylstilbestrol during pregnancy. The use of oral contraceptives containing synthetic estrogens as their major or only component has been implicated in the induction of liver cell adenomas. In addition, an association exists between prolonged use of estrogenic oral contraceptives and an increased incidence of premenopausal breast cancer. Androgenic steroids and synthetic testosterone compounds have been implicated in hepatocellular carcinoma induction. Therapeutic immunosuppression given to transplant patients or arising secondary to selective diseases such as acquired immune deficiency syndrome (AIDS) result in an increase in a variety of different neoplasms. These results further support the role of the immune system in identifying and removing early preneoplastic cells from the body. In addition, the previously used diagnostic tracer Thorotrast has been sufficiently linked to the formation of hemangiosarcomas in the liver.

Table 8-28
USEPA Cancer Guidelines Descriptors

Carcinogenic to humans
– strong evidence of human carcinogenicity, including convincing epidemiologic evidence of a causal association between human exposure and cancer.
– the mode(s) of carcinogenic action and associated key precursor events have been identified in animals, and there is strong evidence that the key precursor events in animals are anticipated to occur in humans.

Likely to be carcinogenic to humans
– weight of the evidence is adequate to demonstrate carcinogenic potential to an agent in animal experiments in more than one species, sex, strain, site, or exposure route, with or without evidence of carcinogenicity in humans

Suggestive evidence of carcinogenic potential
– the weight of evidence is suggestive of carcinogenicity; a concern for potential carcinogenic effects in humans is raised, but the data are judged not sufficient for a stronger conclusion.

Inadequate information to assess carcinogenic potential
– available data are judged inadequate for applying one of the other descriptors.

Not likely to be carcinogenic to humans
– This descriptor is appropriate when the available data are considered robust; there is no basis for human hazard concern, evidence in both humans and animals that the agent is not carcinogenic.

Classification Evaluation of Carcinogenicity in Humans

The assessment and designation of a chemical or a mixture of chemicals as carcinogenic in humans is evaluated by various agencies worldwide. The evaluation usually encompasses both epidemiological and experimental animal and in vitro data utilizing assays as described earlier in this chapter. One of the first devised schemes for the classification of an agent's carcinogenicity was devised by the International Agency for Research on Cancer (IARC) (Table 8-27). The IARC approach assigns the chemical or mixture to one of five groupings based upon strength of evidence for the

Table 8-29
USEPA Mode of Action Definitions

Mode of action: Key events and processes, starting with the interaction of an agent with a cell, through functional and anatomical changes, resulting in cancer or other health endpoints.

Key event: Empirically observable precursor step that is itself a necessary element of the mode of action or is a biologically based marker for such an element.

Table 8-30
US EPA Mode of Action Framework

Mode of action criteria
Summary description of the hypothesized mode of action
Identification of key events
Strength, consistency, specificity of association
Dose–response concordance
Temporal relationship
Biological plausibility and coherence
Consideration of the possibility of other MOAs
Is the mode of action sufficiently supported in the test animals?
Is the mode of action relevant to humans?
Which populations or life stages can be particularly susceptible to the mode or action?

agent's possible, probable, or definite carcinogenicity to humans. In Group 1 classification, the agent or mixture is classified as definitely carcinogenic to humans. The second grouping is Group 2A in which the agent is probably carcinogenic to humans. In Group 2B, the agent is classified as possibly carcinogenic to humans. In Group 3, the agent is not classifiable. In the last group, Group 4, the agent is not carcinogenic to humans. The IARC produces a series of monographs that describe the methodology for the evaluation of specific chemicals and the rationale for their final classification. Currently, more than 100 chemical agents or mixtures or exposure circumstances have been classified by IARC as falling in Group 1, which shows sufficient evidence for carcinogenicity to humans.

Similar classifications exist for the U.S. EPA, the Food & Drug Administration, and the European Community (EC). The classification of agents with regard to human carcinogenicity can many times be very difficult, in particular, when animal data and/or epidemiological data in humans are inconclusive or confounded.

New U.S. EPA Guidelines for Cancer Risk Assessment (2005) uses descriptors for defining the relative carcinogenic risk to humans (Table 8-28). These descriptors include: carcinogenic to humans; likely to be carcinogenic to humans; suggestive evidence of carcinogenic potential; inadequate information to access carcinogenic potential; and, not likely to be carcinogenic in humans. The EPA Guidelines take into account the understanding of the mode of carcinogenic action and associated key precursor events needed for the cancer to form (Table 8-29). Central to the U.S. EPA Guidelines for Cancer Risk Assessment is the utilization of the mode of action framework to define the key events in rodents, and assessment of whether those same key events and mode of action can occur in humans (Table 8-30). This approach is similar to that developed by the International Program on Chemical Safety and by panels in the International Life Sciences Institute.

SUMMARY

The induction of cancer by chemicals is well established in animal models as well as in humans. Linkages between chemicals found in human lifestyle, occupational exposure, and environmental exposure provides strong evidence for the induction or contribution of environmental occupational lifestyle carcinogens to human cancer. Cancer is a multistage process that involves a mutational event followed by the selected clonal proliferation of the mutated cell. The multistage nature of the process has been extensively examined with regard to molecular, cellular, tissue, and organ events.

REFERENCES

Abanobi SE, Lombardi B, Shinozuka H: Stimulation of DNA synthesis and cell proliferation in the liver of rats fed a choline-devoid diet and their suppression by phenobarbital. *Cancer Res* 41:412–415, 1982.

Abuja PM, Albertini R: Methods for monitoring oxidative stress, lipid peroxidation, and oxidation resistance of lipoproteins. *Clin Chim Acta* 306:1–17, 2001.

Adlercreutz H, Mazur W: Phyto-estrogens and western diseases. *Ann Med* 29:95–120, 1997.

Alitalo K, Schwab M: Oncogene amplication in tumor cells. *Adv Cancer Res* 47:235–281, 1986.

Alwens W, Jonas W: Chrome lung cancer. *Acta Unio Internationalis contra Cancrum* 3:1–114, 1938.

Ames BN, McCann J, Yamasaki E: Methods for detecting carcinogens and mutagens with the salmonella/mammalian-microsome mutagenicity test. *Mutat Res* 31:347–364, 1975.

Ames BN, Shigenaga MK: Oxidants are a major contributor to cancer and aging, in Halliwell B, Aruoma O (eds.): *DNA and Free Radicals*. London, England: Ellis Horwood Ltd., 1993, pp. 1–15.

Amstad PA, Krupitza G, Cerutti PA: Mechanisms of c-fos induction by active oxygen. *Cancer Res* 52:3952–3960, 1992.

Andersen A, Berge SR, Engeland A, Norseth T: Exposure to nickel compounds and smoking in relation to incidence of lung and nasal cancer among nickel refinery workers. *Occup Environ Med* 53(10):708–713, 1996.

Andersen M, Brusick D, Cohen S, *et al*.: U.S. Environmental Protection Agency's revised cancer guidelines for carcinogen risk assessment. *Toxicol Appl Pharmacol* 153:133–136, 1998.

Ates NA, Tamer L, Ates C, *et al*.: Glutathione S-transferase M1, T1, P1 genotypes and risk for development of colorectal cancer. *Biochem Genet* 43(3–4):149–163, 2005.

Bachman AN, Kamendulis LM, Goodman JI: Diethanolamine and phenobarbital produce an altered pattern of methylation in GC-rich regions of DNA in B6C3F1 mouse hepatocytes similar to that resulting from choline deficiency. *Toxicol Sci* 90:317–325, 2006.

Balmain A, Pragnell IB: Mouse skin carcinomas induced in vivo by chemical carcinogens have a transforming Harvey-ras oncogene. *Nature* 303:72–74, 1983.

Bannasch P: Preneoplastic lesions as end points in carcinogenicity testing I. Hepatic preneoplasia. *Carcinogenesis* 7(5):689–695, 1986a.

Bannasch P: Preneoplastic lesions as end points in carcinogenicity testing. II. Preneoplasia in various non-hepatic tissues. *Carcinogenesis* 7(6):849–852, 1986b.

Barber DA, Harris SR: Oxygen free radicals and antioxidants: A review. *Am Pharm* NS34:26–35, 1994.

Barrett JC, Lamb PW: Tests with the Syrian hamster embryo cell transformation assay, in Ashbey J, DeSerres FJ, Draper M, Ishidate M, Margolin BH, Matter BE, Shelby MD (eds.): *Progress in Mutation Research-Evaluation of Short Term Tests for Carcinogens*. New York: Elsevier, 1985, vol. 5, pp. 623–628.

Baylin SB: Tying it all together: epigenetics, genetics, cell cycle, and cancer. *Science* 277:1948–1949, 1997.

Beauerle PA, Lenardo M, Pierce JW, Baltimore D: Phorbol-ester-induced activation of the NF-$_K$B transcription factor involved dissociation of an apparently cytoplasmic Nf-$_K$B/inhibitor complex. *Cold Springs Harb Symp Quant Biol* 53:789–798, 1988.

Becker RA, Shank RC: Kinetics of formation and persistence of ethylguanines in dna of rats and hamsters treated with diethylnitrosamine. *Cancer Res* 45:2076–2084, 1985.

Bentley P, Calder I, Elcombe C, Grasso P, Stringer D, Wiegand HJ: Hepatic peroxisome proliferation in rodents and its significance for humans. *Food Chem Toxicol* 31:857–907, 1993.

Berenblub J, Shubik P: A new quantitative approach to the study of the stages of chemical carcinogenesis in the mouse's skin. *Br J Cancer* 1:389–391, 1947.

Betteridge DJ: What is oxidative stress? *Metabolism* 49:3–8, 2000.

Blaauboer BJ, Balls M, Barratt M, *et al.*: 13th meeting of the Scientific Group on Methodologies for the Safety Evaluation of Chemicals (SGOMSEC): alternative testing methodologies and conceptual issues. *Environ Health Perspect* 106(Suppl 2):413–418, 1998.

Boddy AV, Ratain MJ: Pharmacogenetics in cancer etiology and chemotherapy. *Clin Cancer Res* 3:1025–1030, 1997.

Bohr VA, Dianov GL: Oxidative DNA damage processing in nuclear and mitochondrial DNA. *Biochimie* 81:155–160, 1999.

Bos JL: Ras oncogene in human cancer: A review. *Cancer Res* 49:4682–4689, 1989.

Bosch TM, Meijerman I, Beijnen, JH, Schellens, JHM: Genetic polymorphisms of drug metabolising enzymes and drug transporters in relation to cancer risk. *Current Ther Rev* 2(2):137–155, 2006.

Bressac B, Kew M, Wands J, Ozturk M: Selective G to T mutations of p53 gene in hepatocellular carcinoma from southern Africa. *Nature* 350:429–431, 1991.

Brown JR, Nigh E, Lee RJ, *et al.*: Fos family members induce cell cycle entry by activating Cyclin D1. *Mol Cell Biol* 18:55609–55619, 1998.

Brown K, Balmain A: Transgenic mice and squamous multistage skin carcinogenesis. *Cancer Metastasis Rev* 14:113–124, 1995.

Bull RJ, Brown JM, Meierhenry EA, Jorgenson TA, Robinson M, Stober JA: Enhancement of the hepatotoxicity of chloroform in B6C3F1 mice by corn oil: Implications for chloroform carcinogenesis. *Environ Health Perspect* 69:49–58, 1986.

Burdon RH: Superoxide and hydrogen peroxide in relation to mammalian cell proliferation. *Free Radic Biol Med* 18:775–794, 1995.

Burgess WH, Maciag T: The heparin-binding (fibroblast) growth factor family of proteins. *Annu Rev Biochem* 575–606, 1989.

Burkhardt S, Mellert W, Reinacher M, Bahnenmann R: Zonal evaluation of proliferation and apoptosis in mice reveals newmechanistic data for PB, WY 14,643 and CH. *Toxicologist* 60:286, 2001.

Butlin HJ: Three lectures on cancer of the scrotum in chimney sweeps and others. I. Secondary cancer without primary cancer. II. Why foreign sweeps do not suffer from scrotal cancer. III. Tar and paraffin cancer. *Br Med J* 1:1341–1346, 2:1–6; 66–71, 1892.

Butterworth BE: Consideration of both genotoxic and nongenotoxic mechanisms in predicting carcinogenic potential. *Mutat Res* 239,117–132, 1990.

Calabrese EJ: Hormesis: Changing view of the dose–response, a personal account of the history and current status. *Mutat Res* 511:181–189, 2002.

Camurri L, Codeluppi S, Pedroni C, Scarduelli L: Chromosomal aberrations and sister-chromatid exchanges in workers exposed to styrene. *Mutat Res* 119:361–369, 1983.

Cantor KP: Drinking water and cancer. *Cancer Causes Control* 8(3):292–308, 1997.

Capen CC, Dayan AD, Green S: Receptor-mediated mechanisms in carcinogenesis: An overview. *Mutat Res* 333(1–2):215–224, 1995.

Carthew P, Martin EA, White IN, *et al.*: Tamoxifen induces short-term cumulative DNA damage and liver tumors in rats: Promotion by phenobarbital. *Cancer Res* 55(3):544–547, 1995.

Cavalli LR, Liang BD: Mutagenesis, tumorigenicity, and apoptosis: Are the mitochondria involved? *Mutat Res* 398:19–26, 1998.

Cerutti PA: Prooxidant states and tumor promotion. *Science* 227:375–381, 1985.

Chang L, Karin M: Mammalian MAP kinase signalling cascades. *Nature* 410:37–40, 2001.

Chellappan SP, Hiebert S, Mudryj M, Horowitz JM, Nevins JR: The E2F transcription factor is a cellular target for the RB protein. *Cell* 65:1053–1061, 1991.

Chen CJ, Wu MM, Lee SS, Wang JD, Cheng SH, Wu HY: Atherogenicity and carcinogenicity of high-arsenic artesian well water. Multiple risk factors and related malignant neoplasms of blackfoot disease. *Arteriosclerosis* 8:452–460, 1988.

Cheng KC, Cahill DS, Kasai H, Nishimura S, Loeb LA: 8-Hydroxyguanosine, an abundant form of oxidative DNA damage, causes G $\rightarrow$ T and A $\rightarrow$ C substitutions. *J Biol Chem* 267:166–172, 1992.

Chiu R, Boyle J, Meek J, *et al.*: The c-Fos protein interacts with c-Jun/AP-1 to stimulate transcription of AP-1 responsive genes. *Cell* 54:541–552, 1988.

Christopherson W, Mays E, Barrows G: Hepatocellular carcinoma in young women on oral contraceptives. *Lancet* 2:38, 1978.

Clarkson PM, Thompson HS: Antioxidants: what role do they play in physical activity and health? *Am J Clin Nutr* 72:637–646, 2000.

Cohen SM, Robinson D, MacDonald J: Alternative models for carcinogenicity testing. *Toxicol Sci* 64:14–19, 2001.

Collett MS, Erickson RL: Protein kinase activity associated with the avian sarcoma virus src gene product. *Proc Natl Acad Sci USA* 75:2021–2024, 1978.

Collins AR: The comet assay for DNA damage and repair: Principals, applications, and limitations. *Mol Biotech* 26:249–261, 2004.

Connett PH, Whtterhahn KE: In vitro reduction of the carcinogen chromate with cellular thiols and carboxylic acids. *J Am Chem Soc* 107:4282–4288, 1985.

Conney AH: Induction of microsomal enzymes by foreign chemicals and carcinogenesis by polycyclic aromatic hydrocarbons. *Cancer Res* 42:4875–4917, 1982.

Cook JW, Hewett CL, Hieger I: The isolation of a cancer-producing hydrocarbon from coal tar. *J Chem Soc* 395–405, 1933.

Costa M: Toxicity and carcinogenicity of Cr(VI) in animal models and humans. *Crit Rev Toxicol* 27(5):431–442, 1997.

Counts JL, Goodman JI: Alterations in DNA methylation may play a variety of roles in carcinogenesis. *Cell* 83:13–15, 1995.

D'Souza RJ, Philips EM, Jones PW, Strange RC, Aber GM: Interactions of hydrogen peroxide with interleukin-6 and platelet-derived growth factor in determining mesangial cell growth: Effect of repeated oxidant stress. *Clin Sci* 86:747–451, 1993.

Damm K, Thompson CC, Evans RM: Proteinencoded by v-erbA functions as a thyroid-hormone receptor antagonist. *Nature* 339:593–597, 1989.

de Vos AM, Tong L, Milburn MV, *et al.*: Three dimensional structure of an oncogene protein: Catalytic domain of human C-H-ras p21. *Science*: 239, 888–893, 1988.

Demple B, Harrison L: Repair of oxidative damage to DNA. *Annu Rev Biochem* 63:915–948, 1994.

de-Thé G, Geser A, Day NE, *et al.*: Epidemiological evidence for causal relationship between Epstein-Barr virus and Burkitt's lymphoma from Ugandan prospective study. *Nature* 274:756–761, 1978.

Dietrich DR, Swenberg JA: Preneoplastic lesions in rodent kidney induced spontaneously or by non-genotoxic agents: Predictive nature and comparison to lesions induced by genotoxic carcinogens. *Mutat Res* 248:239–260, 1991.

Diwan BA, Kasprzak KS, Rice JM: Transplacental carcinogenic effects of nickel(II) acetate in the renal cortex, renal pelvis and adenohypophysis in F344/NCr rats. *Carcinogenesis* 13(8):1351–1357, 1992.

Dizdaroglu M: Oxidative damage to DNA in mammalian chromatin. *Mutat Res* 275:331–342, 1992.

Doll R: Effects of exposure to vinyl chloride. An assessment of evidence. *Scan J Work Environ Health* 14:61–78, 1988.

Doll R, Peto R: The causes of cancer: quantitative estimates of avoidable risks of cancer in the United States today. *J Natl Cancer Inst* 66(6):1191–1308, 1981.

Dong J-T: Prevalent mutations in prostate cancer. *J Cell Biochem* 97(3):433–447, 2005.

Doolittle RF, Hunkapiller MW, Hood LE, *et al*.: Simian sarcoma virus oncogene, v-sis, is derived from the gene (or genes) encoding a platelet-derived growth factor. *Science* 221:275–277, 1983.

Dypbukt JM, Ankarcrona M, Burkitt M, *et al*.: Different prooxidant levels stimulate growth, trigger apoptosis, or produce necrosis of insulin-secreting RINm5F cells. The role of intracellular polyamines. *J Biol Chem* 269:30533–30560, 1994.

Edmondson H, Reynolds T, Henderson B, Benton B: Regression of liver cell adenomas associated with oral contraceptives. *Ann Intern Med* 86:180–182, 1977.

Ehrenberg L, Hussain S: Genetic toxicity of some important epoxides. *Mutat Res* 86:1–113, 1981.

Eksrom G, Ingleman-Sundberg M: Rat liver microsomal NADPH-supported oxidase activity and lipid peroxidation dependent on ethanol inducible cytochromes P-450. *Biochem Pharmacol* 38:1313–1319, 1989.

El-Deiry WS, Kern SE, Pietenpol JA, Kinzler KW, Vogelstein B: Definition of a consensus binding site for p53. *Nat Genet* 1:45–49, 1992.

Fahreus R, Rymo L, Rhim JS, *et al*.: Morphological transformation of human keratinocytes expressing the LMP gene of Epstein-Barr virus. *Nature* 345:447–449, 1990.

Ferreccio CC, Gonzalez V, Milosavjlevic G, Marshall AM, Sancha, Smith AH: Lung cancer and arsenic concentrations in drinking water in Chile. *Epidemiology* 11(6):673–679, 2000.

Finch GL, Hoover MD, Hahn FF, *et al*.: Animal models of beryllium-induced lung disease. *Environ Health Perspect* 104(Suppl 5):973–979, 1996.

Finlay CA, Hinds PW, Levine AJ: The p53 proto-oncogene can act as a suppressor of transformation. *Cell* 57:1083–1093, 1989.

Fiorani M, Cantoni O, Tasinto A, Boscoboinik D, Azzi A: Hydrogen peroxide- and fetal bovine serum-induced DNA synthesis in vascular smooth muscle cells; positive and negative regulation by protein kinase C isoforms. *Biochem Biophys Acta* 1269:98–104, 1995.

Floyd RA: 8-Hydoxy-2′-deoxyguanosine in carcinogenesis. *Carcinogenesis* 11:1447–1450, 1990.

Fortini P, Parlanti E, Sidorkina OM, Laval J, Dogliotti E: The type of DNA glycosylase determines the base excision repair pathway in mammalian cells. *J Biol Chem* 274:230–236, 1999.

Fox M, Scott D: The genetic toxicology of nitrogen and sulphur mustard. *Mutat Res* 75(2):131–168, 1980.

Fried M, Prives C: In Botchan M, Grodzicker T, Sharp PA (eds.): *Cancer Cells 4: DNA Tumor Viruses*. New York: Cold Spring Harbor, 1986, pp. 1–16.

Friedwald WF, Rous P: Initiating and promoting elements in tumor production; analysis of effects of tar, benzpyrene and methylcholanthrene on rabbit skin. *J Exp Med* 80:101–126, 1944.

Fu H, Boffetta, P: Cancer and occupational exposure to inorganic lead compounds: A meta-analysis of published data. *Occup Environ Med* 52(2):73–81, 1995.

Fujii K: Evaluation of the newborn mouse model for chemical tumorigenesis. *Carcinogenesis* 12(8):1409–1415, 1991.

Futreal PA, Liu Q, Shattuck-Eidens D, *et al*.: BRCA1 mutations in primary breast and ovarian carcinomas. *Science* 266(5182):120–122, 1994.

Gama-Sosa MA, Slagel VA, Trewyn RW, Oxenhandler R, Kuo KC, *et al*.: The 5-methylcytosine content of DNA from human tumors. *Nucleic Acids Res* 11:6883–6894, 1983.

Goode EL, Ulrich CM, Potter JD: Polymorphisms in DNA repair genes and associations with cancer risk. *Cancer Epidemiol Biomarkers Prev* 11:1513–1530, 2002.

Gossen JA, de Leeuw WJF, Tan CHT, *et al*.: Efficient rescue of integrated shuttle vectors from transgenic mice: A model for studying mutations in vivo. *Proc Natl Acad Sci USA* 86:7971–7975, 1989.

Gossen JA, Vijg J: A selective system for lacZ⁻ phage using a galactose-sensitive *E. coli* host. *Biotechniques* 14:326–330, 1993.

Goth R, Rajewsky MF: Persistence of O6-ethylguanine in rat-brain DNA: Correlation with nervous system-specific carcinogenesis by ethylnitrosourea. *Proc Natl Acad Sci USA* 71(3):639–643, 1974.

Guengerich FP: Mechanisms of formation of DNA adducts from ethylene dihalides, vinyl halides, and arylamines. *Drug Metab Rev* 26:47–66, 1994.

Gulezian D, Jacobson-Kram D, McCullough CB, *et al*.: Use of transgenic animals for carcinogenicity testing: Considerations for risk assessment. *Toxicol Pathol* 28(3):482–499, 2000.

Guyton KZ, Kensler TW: Oxidative mechanisms in carcinogenesis. *Br Med Bul* 49:523–544, 1993.

Han W, Pentecost BT, Spivack SD: Functional evaluation of novel single nucleotide polymorphisms and haplotypes in the promoter regions of *CYP1B1* and *CYP1A1* genes. *Mol Carcinogenesis* 37(3):158–169, 2003.

Hancock JF, Magee AI, Childs JE, *et al*.: All ras proteins are polyisoprenylated but only some are palmitoylated. *Cell* 57:1167–1177, 1989.

Harris GK, Shi X: Signaling by carcinogenic metals and metal-induced reactive oxygen species. *Mutat Res* 533:183–200, 2003.

Harting FH, Hesse W: Der lungenkrebs, die Bergkrankheit in den Schneeberger gruben. *Vjschr Gerichtl Med Offentl Gesundheitswesen* 31:102–132, 313–337, 1879.

Hastie ND: The genetics of Wilms' tumor—A case of disrupted development. *Annu Rev Genet* 28:523–558, 1994.

Heddle JA, Hite M, Kirkhart B, *et al*.: The induction of micronuclei as a measure of genotoxicity. A report of the US Environmental Protection Agency GENE-TOX program. *Mutat Res* 123:61–118, 1983.

Herbst AL, Scully RE: Adenocarcinoma of the vagina in adolescence: A report of 7 cases including 6 clear-cell carcinomas (so-called mesonephromas). *Cancer* 25:745–757, 1970.

Herbst AL, Kurman RJ, Scully RE, Poskanzer DC: Clear-cell adenocarcinoma of the genital tract in young females: Registry report. *N Engl J Med* 287:1259–1264, 1972.

Hergersberg M: Biological aspects of cytosine methylation in eukaryotic cells. *Experientia* 47:1171–1185, 1991.

Highman B, Norvell MJ, Shellenberger TE: Pathological changes in female C3H mice continuously fed diets contain-1:1–30, 1977.

Hogstedt C, Aringer L, Gustavsson A: Epidemiological support for ethylene oxide as a cancer-causing agent. *JAMA* 255:1575–1578, 1986.

Hollander MC, Fornace AJJ: Induction of fos RNA by DNA-damaging agents. *Cancer Res* 49:1687–1692, 1989.

Holliday R: Mechanisms for the control of gene activity during development. *Biol Rev* 65:431–471, 1990.

Hollstein M, Sidransky D, Vogelstein B, Harris CC: p53 mutations in human cancers. *Science* 253(5015):49–53, 1991.

Honkakoski P, Zelko I, Sueyoshi T, Negishi M: The nuclear orphan receptor CAR-retinoid X receptor heterodimer activates the phenobarbital-responsive enhancer module of the CYP2B gene. *Mol Cell Biol* 18:5652–5658, 1998.

Hood A, Liu J, Klaassen CD: Effects of phenobarbital, pregnenolone-16α-carbonitrile, and propylthiouracil on thyroid follicular cell proliferation. *Toxicol Sci* 50:45–53, 1999.

Horton TM, Petros JA, Heddi A, Shoffner J, Kaufman AE, *et al*.: Novel mitochondrial DNA deletion found in renal cell carcinoma. *Genes Chromosomes Cancer* 15:95–101, 1996.

Hsieh L-L, Hsieh T-T: Detection of aflatoxin B1-DNA adducts in human placenta and cord blood. *Cancer Res*, 53:1278–1280, 1993.

Hueper WC, Wiley FH, Wolfe HD: Experimental production of bladder tumors in dogs by administration of beta-naphthylamine. *J Ind Hyg Toxicol* 20:46–84, 1938.

Hughes MF, Kitchin KT: In: SKK (ed.): *Arsenic, Oxidative Stress and Carcinogenesis Oxidative Stress, Disease and Cancer*. London: Imperial College Press, 2006.

Hussain SP, Haris CC: Molecular epidemiology of human cancer: contribution of mutation spectra studies of tumor suppressor genes. *Cancer Res* 58:4023–4037, 1998.

IARC: Some inorganic and organometallic compounds. *IARC Monographs on the Evaluation of Carcinogenic Risk of Chemicals to Humans.* Lyon, France: International Agency for Research on Cancer, 1973, vol. 2, p 181.

IARC: Some metals and metallic compounds. *IARC Monographs on the Evaluation of Carcinogenic Risk of Chemicals to Humans.* Lyon, France: International Agency for Research on Cancer, 1980, vol. 23, p 438.

IARC: Overall evaluations of carcinogenicity. *IARC Monographs on the Evaluation of Carcinogenic Risk of Chemicals to Humans.* Lyon, France: International Agency for Research on Cancer, 1987, Supplement 7, p 440.

IARC: Chromium, nickel and welding. *IARC Monographs on the Evaluation of Carcinogenic Risk of Chemicals to Humans.* Lyon, France: International Agency for Research on Cancer, 1990, vol. 49, p 677.

IARC: Beryllium, cadmium, mercury and exposures in the glass manufacturing industry. *IARC Monographs on the Evaluation of Carcinogenic Risk of Chemicals to Humans..* Lyon, France: International Agency for Research on Cancer, 1993, vol. 58, p 444.

IARC: Polychlorinated dibenzo-para-dioxins and polychlorinated dibenzofurans. *IARC Monographs on the Evaluation of the Carcinogenic Risks to Humans*, no. 69. Lyon: IARC, 1997.

IARC: Polychlorinated dibenzofurans. *Monographs on the Evaluaiton of Carcinogenic Risks to humans.* Lyon: IARC, 1997, vol. 69.

Isfort RJ, Cody DB, Doersen CJ, Kerckaert GA, LeBoeuf RA: Alterations in cellular differentiation, mitogenesis, cytoskeleton and growth characteristics during Syrian hamster embryo cell multistep in vitro transformation. *Int J Cancer* 59:114–125, 1994.

Isfort RJ, Kerckaert GA, LeBoeuf RA: Comparison of the standard and reduced pH Syrian hamster embryo (SHE) cell in vivo transformation assays in predicting the carcinogenic potential of chemicals. *Mut Res* 356:11–63, 1996.

Issemann I, Green S: Activation of a member of the steroid hormone receptor superfamily by peroxisome proliferators. *Nature* 347:645–650, 1990.

Ito N, Hasegawa R, Imaida K, Takahashi S, Shirai T: Medium-term rat liver bioassay for rapid detection of carcinogens and modifiers of hepatocarcinogenesis. *Drug Metabol Rev* 26:431–442, 1994.

Ito N, Imaida K, Hasegawa R, Tsuda H: Rapid bioassay methods for carcinogens and modifiers of hepatocarcinogenesis. *Crit Rev Toxicol* 19:386–415, 1989.

Ito N, Tamano S, Shirai T: A medium-term rat liver bioassay for rapid in vivo detection of carcinogenic potential of chemicals. *Cancer Sci* 94:3–8, 2003.

Jacobson LP, Zhang BC, Zhu YR, et al.: Oltipraz chemoprevention trial in Qidong, People's Republic of China: Study design and clinical outcomes. *Cancer Epidemiol Biomarkers Prevention* 6(4):257–265, 1997.

James NH, Roberts RA: Species differences in response to peroxisome proliferators correlate in vitro with induction of DNA synthesis rather than suppression of apoptosis. *Carcinogenesis* 17:1623–1632, 1996.

Janero DR: Malondialdehyde and thiobarbituric acid reactivity as diagnostic indices of lipid peroxidation and peroxidative tissue injury. *Free Radic Biol Med* 9:515–540, 1990.

Kadlubar FF, Unruh LE, Flammang TJ, Sparks D, Mitchum RK, Mulder GJ: Alteration of urinary levels of the carcinogen, N-hydroxy-2-naphthylamine, and its N-glucuronide in the rat by control of urinary pH, inhibition of metabolic sulfation, and changes in biliary excretion. *Chem Biol Interact* 33:129–147, 1981.

Kamendulis LM, Klaunig JE: Species differences in the induction of hepatocellular DNA synthesis by diethanolamine. *Toxicol Sci* 87(2):328–336, 2005.

Kasprzak KS, Diwan BA, Konishi N, Misra M, Rice JM: Initiation by nickel acetate and promotion by sodium barbital of renal cortical epithelial tumors in male F344 rats. *Carcinogenesis* 11(4):647–652, 1990.

Kennaway E, Hieger I: Carcinogenic substances and their fluorescence spectra. *Br Med J* 1:1044–1046, 1930.

Kerr LD: Signal transduction: The nuclear target. *Curr Opin Cell Biol* 4:496–501, 1992.

Kim CM, Koike K, Saito I, et al.: HBx gene of hepatitis B virus induces liver cancer in transgenic mice. *Nature* 351:317–320, 1991.

Kinoshita A, Wanibuchi H, Morimura K, et al.: Phenobarbital at low dose exerts hormesis in rat hepatocarcinogenesis by reducing oxidative DNA damage, altering cell proliferation, apoptosis and gene expression. *Carcinogenesis* 24:1389–1399, 2003.

Kinosita R: Researches on the carcinogenesis of the various chemical substances. *Gann* 30:423–426, 1936 (in Japanese).

Kitano M, Ichihara T, Matsuda T, et al.: Presence of a threshold for promoting effects of phenobarbital on diethylnitrosamine-induced hepatic foci in the rat. *Carcinogenesis* 19:1475–1480, 1998.

Klaunig JE, Babich MA, Baetcke KP, et al.: PPARα agonist-induced rodent tumors: modes of action and human relevance. *Crit Rev Toxicol* 33:655–780, 2003.

Klaunig JE, Kamendulis LM: The role of oxidative stress in carcinogenesis. *Annu Rev Pharmacol Toxicol* 44:239–267, 2004.

Klaunig JE, Ruch RJ: Strain and species effects on the inhibition of hepatocyte intercellular communication by liver tumor promoters. *Cancer Lett*: 36:161–68, 1987.

Klaunig JE, Ruch RJ: Role of inhibition of intercellular communication in carcinogenesis. *Lab Invest* 62(2):135–146 1990.

Klaunig JE, Xu Y, Bachowski S, Jiang J: Free-radical oxygen-induced changes in chemical carcinogenesis, in Wallace KB (ed.): *Free Radical Toxicology*, London: Taylor & Francis, 1997, pp. 375–400.

Kleczkowska HE, Althaus FR: Response of human keratinocytes to extremely low concentrations of N-methyl-N′-nitro-N-nitrosoguanidine. *Mutat Res* 367, 151–159, 1996.

Knutson JC, Poland A: Response of murine epidermis to 2,3,7,8-tetrachlorodibenzo-p-dioxin: Interaction of the Ah and hr loci. *Cell* 30:225–234, 1982.

Kociba RJ, Keyes DG, Beyer JE, et al.: Results of a two-year chronic toxicity and oncogenicity study of 2,3,7,8-tetrachlorodibenzo-p-dioxin in rats. *Toxicol Appl Pharmacol* 46:279–303, 1978.

Kodama S, Koike C, Negishi M, Yamamoto Y: Nuclear receptors CAR and PXR cross talk with FOXO1 to regulate genes that encode drug-metabolizing and gluconeogenic enzymes. *Mol Cell Biol* 24:7931–7940, 2004.

Kohler SW, Provost GS, Fieck A, et al.: Spectra of spontaneous and mutagen-induced mutations in the lacI gene in transgenic mice. *Proc Natl Acad Sci USA* 88:7958–7962, 1991a.

Kohler SW, Provost GS, Fieck A, et al.: Spectra of spontaneous and induced mutations using a lambda ZAP/lacI shuttle vector. *Environ Mol Mutagen* 18:316–321, 1991b.

Kortenkamp A, O'Brien P: The generation of DNA single-strand breaks during the reduction of chromate by ascorbic acid and/or glutathione in vitro. *Environ Health Perspect* 102(3):237–241, 1994.

Lake BG: Mechanisms of hepatocarcinogenicity of peroxisome-proliferating drugs and chemicals. *Annu Rev Pharmacol Toxicol* 35:483–507, 1995.

Lancaster WD, Olson C: Animal papilloma-viruses. *Microbiol Rev* 46:191–207, 1982.

Langard S: Chromium carcinogenicity: a review of experimental animal data. *Sci Total Environ* 71:341–350, 1988.

Larson JL, Wolf DC, Butterworth BE: Induced cytolethality and regenerative cell proliferation in the livers and kidneys of male B6C3F1 mice given chloroform by gavage. *Fundam Appl Toxicol:* 23, 537–543, 1994.

Latt SA, Allen J, Bloom SE, et al.: Sister-chromatid exchanges: a report of the GENE-TOX program. *Mutat Res* 87(1):17–62, 1981.

Leach FS, Tokino T, Meltzer P, et al.: p53 Mutation and MDM2 amplification in human soft tissue sarcomas. *Cancer Res* 53(Suppl):2231–2234, 1993.

LeBoeuf RA, Kerckaert GA, Aardema MJ, Gibson DP: Multistage neoplastic transformation of Syrian hamster embryo cells cultured at pH 6.70. *Cancer Res* 50:3722–3729, 1990.

Lee SS, Pineau T, DragoJ, *et al.*: Targeted disruption of the alpha isoform of the peroxisome proliferators-activated receptor gene in mice results in abolishment of the pleiotropic effects of peroxisome proliferators. *Mol Cell Biol* 15:3012–3022, 1995.

Leonard A, Lauwerys R: Mutagenicity, carcinogenicity and teratogenicity of beryllium. *Mutat Res* 186:35–42, 1987.

Li J, Kirkman H, Li S: Synthetic estrogens and liver cancer: Risk analysis of animal and human data, in Li J, Nandi S, Li S (eds.): *Hormonal Carcinogenesis*, New York: Springer-Verlag, 1992, pp. 217–224.

Li N, Karin M: Ionizing radiation and short wavelength UV activate NF-$_K$B through two distinct mechanisms. *Proc Natl Acad Sci USA* 95:13012–13017, 1998.

Li R, Yerganian G, Duesberg P, Kraemer A, Willer D, Rausche C, Hehlmann R: Aneuploidy correlated 100% with chemical transformation of Chinese hamster cells. *Proc Natl Acad Sci* 94:14506–14511, 1997.

Li S, Hou X, Li J: Estrogen carcinogenesis: a sequential, epi-genetoxic, multistage process, in Li J, Nandi S, Li S (eds.): *Hormonal Carcinogenesis*. New York: Springer-Verlag, 1996, pp. 200–208.

Loewenstein WR: The cell-to-cell channel of gap junctions. *Cell* 48:725–726, 1987.

Lofroth G, Ames BN: Mutagenicity of inorganic compounds in *Salmonella typhimurium*: Arsenic, chromium and selenium. *Mutat Res* 53:65–66, 1978.

Lowe JP, Silverman BD: Predicting the carcinogenicity of polycyclic aromatic hydrocarbons. *J Am Chem Soc* 106:5955–5958, 1994.

Mandel, JS, McLaughlin JK, Schlehofer B, *et al.*: International renal-cell cancer study. IV. Occupation. *Int J Cancer* 61(5):601–605, 1995.

Marcu KB, Bossone SA, Patel AJ: Myc function and regulation. *Annu Rev Biochem* 61:809–860, 1992.

Maronpot RR, Pitot HC, Peraino C: Use of rat liver altered focus models for testing chemicals that have completed two-year carcinogenicity studies. *Toxicol Pathol* 17:651–662, 1989.

Maronpot RR, Shimkin MB, Witschi HP, Smith I, Cline JM: Strain A mouse pulmonary tumor test results for chemicals previously tested in National Cancer Institute carcinogenicity tests. *J Natl Cancer Inst* 76:1101–1112, 1986.

Marselos M, Vainio H: Carcinogenic properties of pharmaceutical agents evaluated in the IARC Monographs programme. *Carcinogenesis* 12:1751–1766, 1991.

Marsman DS, Goldsworthy TL, Popp JA: Contrasting hepatocytic peroxisome proliferation, lipofuscin accumulation and cell turnover for the hepatocarcinogens WY 14,643-14,643 and clofibric acid. *Carcinogenesis* 13:1011–1017, 1992.

Martindale JL, Holbrook NJ: Cellular response to oxidative stress: Signaling for suicide and survival. *J Cell Physiol* 192:1–15, 2002.

McClain RM: Mechanistic considerations for the relevance of animal data on thyroid neoplasia to human risk assessment. *Mutat Res* 333:131–142, 1995.

McCormick F: Activators and effecrtors of ras p21 proteins. *Curr Opin Genet Dev* 4:71–76, 1994.

Melnick RL, Kohn MC, Portier CJ: Implications for risk assessment of suggested nongenotoxic mechanisms of chemical carcinogenesis. *Environ Health Perspect* 104(S1):123–133, 1996.

Merlo A, Herman JG, Mao L, *et al.*: *Nat Med* 1:686–692, 1995.

Metzler M, Pfeiffer E, Schuler M, Rosenberg B: Effects of estrogens on microtubule assembly: significance for aneuploidy, in Li J, Li S, Gustafsson J-A, Nandi S, Seakely L (eds.): *Hormonal Carcinogenesis II*. New York: Springer-Verlag, 1996, pp. 193–199.

Miller EC: Studies on the formation of protein-bound derivatives of 3,4-benzpyrene in the epidermal fraction of mouse skin. *Cancer Res* 11:100–108, 1951.

Miller EC, Miller JA: The presence and significance of bound amino azodyes in the livers of rats fed p-dimethylaminoazobenzene. *Cancer Res* 7:468–480, 1947.

Miller EC, Miller JA: Searches for ultimate chemical carcinogens and their reactions with cellular macromolecules. *Cancer* 47(10):2327–2345, 1981.

Miller EC, Miller JA, Enomoto M: The comparative carcinogenicities of 2-acetylaminofluorene and its N-hydroxy metabolite in mice, hamsters, and guinea pigs. *Cancer Res* 24:2018–2031, 1964.

Miller EC, Swanson AB, Phillips DH, Fletcher TL, Liem A, Miller JA: Structure-activity studies of the carcinogenicities in the mouse and rat of some naturally occurring and synthetic alkenylbenzene derivatives related to safrole and estragole. *Cancer Res* 43:1124–1134, 1983.

Miller JA: Carcinogenesis by chemicals: An overview—G. H. A. Clowes memorial lecture. *Cancer Res* 3:559–576, 1970.

Miyamae Y, Iwasaki K, Kinae N, *et al.*: Detection of DNA lesions induced by chemical mutagens by the single cell gel electrophoresis (Comet) assay: Relationship between DNA migration and alkaline conditions. *Mutat Res* 393:107–113, 1997.

Moennikes O, Loeppen S, Buchmann A, *et al.*: Constitutively active dioxin/aryl hydrocarbon receptor promotes hepatocarcinogenesis in mice. *Cancer Res* 64(14):4707–4710, 2004.

Molina EP, Klatt P, Vasquez J, *et al.*: Glutathionylation of the p50 subunit of NF-$_K$B: A mechanism for redox-induced inhibition of DNA binding. *Biochemistry* 40:14134–14142, 2001.

Moriya M: Single-stranded shuttle phagemid for mutagenesis studies in mammalian cells: 8-Oxoguanine in DNA induces targeted G:C → T:A transversions in simian kidney cells. *Proc Natl Acad Sci USA* 90:1122–1126, 1993.

Mortelmans, Kristien, Zeiger E: The Ames Salmonella Microsome Mutagenicity Assay. *Mutat Res: Fund Mol Mech Mutagenesis* 455:29–60, 2000.

Muscat JE, Wynder EL: Diesel engine exhaust and lung cancer: An unproven association. *Environ Health Perspect* 103(9):812–818, 1995.

Myöhänen SK, Baylin SB, Herman JG: Hypermethylation can selectively silence individual p16^{ink4a} alleles in neoplasia. *Cancer Res* 58:591–593, 1998.

Nakatsuru Y, Wakabayashi K, Fuji-Kuriyama T, Kusuma K, Ide F: Dibenzo[A,L]pyrene-induced genotoxic and carcinogenic responses are dramatically suppressed in aryl hydrocarbon receptor-deficient mice. *Int J Cancer* 112(2):179–183, 2004.

Naoe T, Takeyama K, Yokozawa T, *et al.*: Analysis of genetic polymorphism in *NQO1*, *GST-M1*, *GST-T1*, and *CYP3A4* in 469 Japanese patients with therapy-related leukemia/myelodysplastic syndrome and de novo acute myeloid leukemia. *Clin Cancer Res* 6:4091–4095, 2000.

Nebert DW, Roe AL, Dieter MZ, Solis WA, Yang Y, Dalton TP: Role of the aromatic hydrocarbon receptor and [Ah] gene battery in the oxidative stress response, cell cycle control, and apoptosis. *Biochem Pharmacol* 59:65–85, 2000.

Nebreda AR, Porrai A: P38 MAP kinases: Beyond the stress response. *Trends Biochem Sci* 25:257–260, 2000.

Neumann HG: Role of extent and persistence of DNA modifications in chemical carcinogenesis by aromatic amines. *Recent Results Cancer Res* 84:77–89, 1983.

Newberne PM, deCanargo JLV, Clark AJ: Choline deficiency, partial hepatectomy, and liver tumors in rats and mice. *Toxicol Pathol* 10:95–106, 1982.

Nims RW, Lubet RA: The CYP2B subfamily, in Ioannides C (ed.): *Cytochromes P450: Metabolic and Toxicological Aspects*. Boca Raton, FL: CRC Press, 1996, pp. 135–160.

Nishizuka Y: The molecular heterogeneity of protein kinase C and its implications for cellular regulation. *Nature* 334:661–665, 1988.

Niven JSF, Armstrong JA, Andrews CH, *et al.*: Subcutaneous "growths" in monkeys produced by a poxvirus. *J Pathol Bacteriol* 81:1–14, 1961.

Noller KL, Decker DG, Lanier AP, Kurkland LT: Clear-cell adenocarcinoma of the cervix after maternal treatment with synthetic estrogens. *Mayo Clin Proc* 47:629–630, 1972.

Nordberg GF, Andersen O: Metal interactions in carcinogenesis: Enhancement, inhibition. *Environ Health Perspect* 40:65–81, 1981.

NTP: *Toxicology and Carcinogenesis Studies of Propylene Oxide (CAS No. 75-569) in F344/N Rats and B6C3F$_1$ Mice (Inhalation Studies)*, TR-267. Research Triangle Park, NC: National Toxicology Program, 1985.

NTP: *Toxicology and Carcinogenesis Studies of Nickel Subsulfide (CAS No. 12035-72-2) in F344 Rats and B6C3F1 Mice (Inhalation Studies)*, Technical Report Series No 453. Research Triangle Park, NC: National Toxicology Program, 1996, p 365.

NTP: *Report on Carcinogens Background Document for Lead and Lead Compounds*. National Toxicology Program, 2003. http://ntp-server.niehs.nih.gov/newhomeroc/roc11/Lead-Public.pdf

Nusse R, Varmus HE: Wnt genes. *Cell* 69:1073–1087, 1992.

Oesterle D, Deml E: Lack of initiating and promoting activity of thiourea in rat liver foci bioassay. *Cancer Lett* 41:245–249, 1988.

Ogiso T, Tatematsu M, Tamano S, Hasegawa R, Ito N: Correlation between medium-term liver bioassay system data and results of long-term testing in rats. *Carcinogenesis* 11:561–566, 1990.

Oppermann H, Levinson AD, Varmus HE, Levintow L, Bishop JM: Uninfected vertebrate cells contain a protein that is closely related to the product of the avian sarcoma virus transforming gene (src). *Proc Natl Acad Sci USA* 76:1804–1808, 1979.

Pahl HL: Activators and target genes of Rel/NF-κB transcription factors. *Oncogene* 18:6853–6866, 1999.

Palmer CN, Hsu MH, Griffin KJ, Raucy JL, Johnson EF: Peroxisome proliferator activated receptor-alpha expression in human liver. *Mol Pharmacol* 53:14–22, 1998.

Pan SC, Gardner WU: Carcinomas of the uterine cervix and vagina in estrogen- and androgen-treated hybrid mice. *Cancer Res* 8:337–341, 1948.

Parke DV: The cytochromes P450 and mechanisms of chemical carcinogenesis. *Environ Health Perspect* 102:852–853, 1994.

Parke DV, Sapota A: Chemical toxicity and reactive oxygen species. *Int J Occ Med Environ Health* 9:331–340, 1996.

Parnell MJ, Exon JH, Koller LD: Assessment of hepatic initiation-promotion properties of trichloroacetic acid. *Arch Environm Contam Toxicol* 17:429–436, 1988.

Parsons PA: Energy, stress and the invalid linear no-threshold premise: A generalization illustrated by ionizing radiation. *Biogerontology* 4:227–231, 2003.

Pegg AE: Methylation of the O6 position of guanine in DNA is the most likely initiating event in carcinogenesis by methylating agents. *Cancer Invest* 2(3):223–231, 1984.

Pereira MA: Route of administration determines whether chloroform enhances or inhibits cell proliferation in the liver of B6C3F1 mice. *Fundam Appl Toxicol* 23:87–92, 1994.

Pereira MA, Herren-Freund SL: Liver initiation assay, the rat liver foci bioassay of carcinogens and noncarcinogens, in Ashby J, de Serres FJ, Shelby MD, Margolin BH, Ishidate M, Becking GC (eds.): *Evaluation of Short-term Assays for Carcinogens*. Cambridge University Press, 1988, pp. 1.325–1.328.

Perera F, Mayer J, Santella RM, *et al.*: Biological markers in risk assessment for environmental carcinogens. *Environ Health Persp* 90:247–254, 1991.

Peters JM, Aoyama T, Cattley RC, Nobumitsu U, Hashimoto T, Gonzalez FJ: Role of peroxisome proliferator-activated receptor alpha in altered cell cycle regulation in mouse liver. *Carcinogenesis* 19:1989–1994, 1998.

Pettersson U, Roberts RJ: In Botchan M, Grodzicker T, Sharp PA (eds.): *Cancer Cells 4: DNA Tumor Viruses*. New York: Cold Spring Harbor, 1986, pp. 37–57.

Pietra G, Spencer K, Shubik P: Response of newly bornmice to a chemical carcinogen. *Nature* 183:1689, 1959.

Pinkus R: Phenobarbital induction of AP-1 binding activity mediate activation of glutathione S-transferase and quinine reductase gene expression. *Biochem J* 290:637–640, 1993.

Pitot HC: *Fundamentals of oncology*. New York: Marcel Dekker, Inc, 1986.

Pitot HC, Goldsworthy T, Moran S, Sirica J: Properties of incomplete carcinogens and promoters in hepatocarcinogenesis. *Carcinogen Compr Surv* 7:85–98, 1982.

Pitot HC, Goldsworthy TL, Moran S, *et al.*: A method to quantitate the relative initiating and promoting potencies of hepatocarcinogenic agents in their dose–response relationships to altered hepatic foci. *Carcinogenesis* 8:1491–1499, 1987.

Pollycove M, Feinendegen LE: Biologic responses to low doses of ionizing radiation: Detriment versus hormesis. Part 2. Dose responses of organisms. *J Nucl Med* 42:26N–32N, 37N, 2001.

Pott P: The chirurgical works. *Chirurgical Observations Relative to the Cataract, The Polypus of the Nose, The Cancer of the Scrotum, The Different Kinds of Ruptures, and The Mortification of the Toes and Feet*. London: Hawes, W. Clarke, and R. Collins, 1775, Ch. III, pp. 60–68.

Pugh G Jr, Isenberg JS, Kamendulis LM, *et al.*: Effects of diisononyl phthalate, di-2-ethylhexyl phthalate, and clofibrate in cynomolgus monkeys. *Toxicol Sci* 56:181–188, 2000.

Qian VC, Shi X: New perspectives in arsenic-induced cell signal transduction. *J Inorg Biochem* 96:271–278, 2003.

Rao MS, Reddy JK: An overview of peroxisome proliferator-induced hepatocarcinogenesis. *Environ Health Perspect* 93:205–209, 1991.

Rapp F: Herpesviruses and cancer. *Adv Cancer Res* 19:265–302, 1974.

Rauscher FJ, III, Morris JF, Tournay OE, Cook DM, Curran T: Binding of the Wilms tumor locus zinc finger protein to the EGR-1 consensus sequence. *Science* 250:1259–1262, 1990.

Reddy JK, Rao MS: Malignant tumors in rats fed nafenopin, a hepatic peroxisome proliferator. *JNCI* 59:1645–1650, 1997.

Rehn L: Blasengeschwülste bei Fuchsin-arbeitern. *Arch Klin Chir* 50:588–600, 1895.

Reznikoff CA, Brankow DW, Heidelberger C: Establishment and characterization of a cloned line of C3H mouse embryo cells sensitive to post-confluence inhibition of division. *Cancer Res* 33:3231–3238, 1973.

Rice JM, Diwan BA, Hu H, Ward JM, Nims RW, Lubet RA: Enhancement of hepatocarcinogenesis and induction of specific cytochromes P450-dependent monooxygenase activities by the barbiturates allobarbital, aprobarbital, pentobarbital, secobarbital, and 5-phenyl- and 5-ethylbarbituric acids. *Carcinogenesis* 15:395–402, 1994.

Rice-Evans C, Burdon R: Free radical-lipid interactions and their pathological consequences. *Prog Lipid Res* 32:71–110, 1993.

Riggins JN, Marnett LJ: Mutagenicity of the Malondialdehyde oligerimerization products 2-(3′oxo-1′-propeneyl)-malondialdehyde and 2,4-dyhydroxymethylene-3-(2,2-dimethoxyethyl)-gluteraldehyde in Salmonella. *Mutat Res* 497:153–157, 2001.

Riggs AD, Jones PA: 5-Methylcytosine, gene regulation and cancer. *Adv Cancer Res* 40:1–30, 1983.

Risch A, Wikman H, Thiel S, *et al.*: Glutathione-S-transferase M1, M3, T1 and P1 polymorphisms and susceptibility to non-small-cell lung cancer subtypes and hamartomas. *Pharmacogenetics* 1(9):757–764, 2001.

Rose ML, Rivera CA, Bradford BU, Graves LM, Cattley RC, Thurman, RG: Kupffer cell oxidant production is central to the mechanism of peroxisome proliferators. *Carcinogenesis* 20:27–33, 1999.

Rous P: A sarcoma of the foul transmissible by an agent separable from the tumor cells. *J Exper Med* 13(4):397–411, 1911.

Rusyn I, Bradham CA, Cohn L, Schoonhoven R, Swenberg JA, Thurman, RG: Corn oil rapidly activates nuclear factor-κB in hepatic Kupffer cells by oxidant-dependant mechanisms. *Carcinogenesis* 20:2095–2100, 1999.

Sakai A, Sato M: Improvement of carcinogen identification in BALB/3T3 cell transformation by the application of a 2-stage method. *Mutat Res* 214:289–296, 1989.

Salem C, Liang G, Tsai YC, *et al.*: Progressive increases in de novo methylation of CpG islands in bladder cancer. *Cancer Res* 60:2473–2476, 2000.

Sasaki MS: Chromosome aberration formation and sister chromatid exchange in relation to DNA repair in human cells, in Generoso WM, Shelby MD, De Serres FJ (eds.): *DNA Repair and Mutagenesis in Eukaryotes*. New York: Plenum Press, 1980, pp. 285–313.

Sasaki T, Yoshida T: Experimentelle Erzeugung des Lebercarcinoms durch Fütterung mit o-Amidoazotoluol. *Virchows Archiv, Pathologische Anatomie* 295:175–200, 1935.

Sawyer DE, Van Houten B: Repair of DNA damage in mitochondria. *Mutat Res* 434:161–176, 1999.

Schechtman LM: BALB/3T3 cell transformation: Protocols, problems and improvements. *IARC Sci Publ* 67:165–184, 1985.

Schulze-Oshoff K, Ferrari D, Los M, Wesselborg S, Peter ME: Apoptosis signaling by death receptors. *Eur J Biochem* 254:439–459, 1998.

Schumacher HR, Szelkely LE, Patel SB, Fisher DR: Mitochondria: A clue to oncogenesis? *Lancet* 2:327, 1973.

Sherr CJ: Mammalian G$_1$ cyclins. *Cell* 73:1059–1065, 1993.

Shibutani S, Takeshita M, Grollman AP: Insertion of specific bases during DNA synthesis past the oxidative-damage base 8-oxo-dG. *Nature* 349:431–434, 1991.

Shigematsu I, Kitamaru S, Takeuchi J, et al.: A retrospective mortality study on cadmium exposed populations in Japan, in Wilson D, Volpe RA (eds.): *Third International Cadmium Conference*. Cadmium Association/Cadmium Council.

Shimkin MB, Stoner GD: Lung tumors in mice: Application to carcinogenesis bioassay. *Adv Cancer Res* 21:1–58, 1975.

Shirai T, Hirose M, Ito N: Medium-term bioassays in rats for rapid detection of the carcinogenic potential of chemicals. *IARC Scientific Publ* 146:251–272, 1999.

Siemiatycki J, Dewar R, Nadon L, Gerin M: Occupational risk factors for bladder cancer: Results from a case-control study in Montreal, Quebec, Canada. *Am J Epidemiol* 140(12):1061–180, 1994.

Sims P, Grover PL, Swaisland A, Pal K, Hewer A: Metabolic activation of benzo[a]pyrene proceeds by a diol-epoxide. *Nature* 252:326–328, 1974.

Slaga TJ: Multistage skin carcinogenesis, a useful model for the study of the chemoprevention of cancer. *Acta Pharmacologica et Toxicologica* 55:107–124, 1984.

Slater AF, Stefan C, Nobel I, van den Dobbelsteen DJ, Orrenius S: Signalling mechanisms and oxidative stress in apoptosis. *Toxicol Lett* 82–83:149–53, 1995.

Solt D, Farber E: New principle for the analysis of chemical carcinogenesis. *Nature* 263:701–703, 1976.

Sontag J: Carcinogenicity of substituted-benzenediamines (phenylenediamines) in rats and mice. *J Natl Cancer Inst* 66:591–602, 1981.

Sorahan T, Lancashire RJ: Lung cancer mortality in a cohort of workers employed at a cadmium recovery plant in the United States: An analysis with detailed job histories. *Occup Environ Med* 54(3):194–201, 1997.

Sorahan T, Lister A, Gilthorpe MS, Harrington JM: Mortality of copper cadmium alloy workers with special reference to lung cancer and non-malignant diseases of the respiratory system, 1946–92. *Occup Environ Med* 52(12):804–812, 1995.

Soto AM, Fernandez MF, Luizzi MF, et al.: Developing a marker of exposure to xenoestrogen mixtures in hmn serum. *Environ Health Perspec* 105:647–654, 1997.

Steenland K, Boffetta P: Lead and cancer in humans: Where are we now? *Am J Ind Med* 38(3):295–299, 2000.

Steenland K, Ward E: Lung cancer incidence among patients with beryllium disease: A cohort mortality study. *J Natl Cancer Inst* 83(19):1380–1385, 1991.

Stinchcombe S, Buchmann A, Bock KW, Schwarz M: Inhibition of apoptosis during 2,3,7,8-tetrachlorodibenzo-p-dioxin-mediated tumour promotion in rat liver. *Carcinogenesis* 16(6):1271–1275, 1995.

Stirzaker C, Millar DS, Paul CL, et al.: Extensive DNA methylation spanning the RB promoter in retinoblastoma tumors. *Cancer Res* 57:2229–2237, 1997.

Stoner GD: Lung tumors in strain A mice as a bioassay for carcinogenicity of environmental chemicals. *Exper Lung Res* 17:405–423, 1991.

Stoner GD, Adam-Rodwell G, Morse MA: Lung tumors in strain A mice: Application for studies in cancer chemoprevention. *J Cell Biochem* 17F:95–103, 1993.

Stoner GD, Shimkin MB: Lung tumors in strain A mice for carcinogenesis bioassays, in Milman H, Weisburger EK (eds.): *Handbook of Carcinogen Testing*. Park Rigde, NJ: Noyes Publications, 1985, pp. 179–214.

Su B, Karin M: Mitogen-activated protein kinase cascades and regulation of gene expression. *Curr Opin Immunol* 8:402–411, 1996.

Sugie S, Mori H, Takahashi M: Effect of in vivo exposure to the liver tumor promoters phenobarbital or DDT on the gap junctions of rat hepatocytes: A quantitative freeze-fracture analysis. *Carcinogenesis* 8:45–51, 1987.

Sundberg JP, Sundberg BA, Beamer WG: Comparison of chemical carcinogen skin tumor induction efficacy in inbred, mutant, and hybrid strains of mice: Morphologic variations of induced tumors and absence of a papilloma virus. *Mol Carcinogenesis* 20:19–32, 1997.

Sutherland RL, Hamilton J, Sweeney K, Watts C, Musgrove E: Steroidal regulation of cell cycle progression. *Ciba Found Symp* 191:218–228, 1995.

Swenberg JA, Dyroff MC, Bedell MA, et al.: O^4-ethyldeoxythymidine, but not O^6-ethyldeoxyguanosine, Accumulates in Hepatocyte DNA of Rats Exposed Continuously to Diethylnitrosamine. *Proc Natl Acad Sci* 81(6):1692–1695, 1984.

Swenberg JA, Richardson FC, Boucheron JA, Dyroff MC: Relationships between DNA adduct formation and carcinogenesis. *Environ Health Persp* 62:177–183, 1985.

Synder RL, Tyler G, Summers J: Chronic hepatitis and hepatocellular carcinoma associated with woodchuck hepatitis virus. *Am J Pathol* 107:422–425, 1982.

Tamura G, Nishizuka S, Maesawa C, et al: Mutations in mitochondrial control region DNA in gastric tumors of Japanese patients. *Eur J Cancer* 35:316–319, 1999.

Tavani A, Negri E, Parazzini F, Franceschi S, La Vecchia C: Female hormone utilisation and risk of hepatocellular carcinoma. *Br J Cancer* 67(3):635–637, 1993.

Tchou J, Grollman AP: Repair of DNA containing the oxidatively damaged base, 8-oxoguanine. *Mutat Res* 299:277–287, 1993.

Temin HM, Rubin H: Characteristics of an assay for Rous sarcoma virus and Rous sarcoma cells in tissue culture. *Virology* 6:669–688, 1958.

Thiersch K: Der Epithelialkrebs, Namentliehlder Ausseren Haut. Leipzig, Germany.

Timblin CR, Janssen YMW, Mossman BT: Free-radical-mediated alterations of gene expression by xenobiotics, in Wallace KB (ed.): *Free Radical Toxicology*. London: Taylor & Francis, 1997, pp. 325–349.

Trosko JE, Ruch R: Cell-cell communication and carcinogenesis. *Front Biosci* 3:208–236, 1998.

Trush MA, Kensler TW: An overview of the relationship between oxidative stress and chemical carcinogenesis. *Free Radic Biol Med* 10:201–209, 1991.

Tsuchida S, Sato K: Glutathione transferases and cancer. *Crit Rev Biochem Mol Biol* 27:337–384, 1992.

Tsutsui T, Taguchi S, Tanaka Y, Barrett JC: 17beta-estradiol, diethylstilbesterol, tamoxifen, toremifene, and ICI 164384 induce morphological transformation and aneuploidy in cultured Syrian hamster cells. *Intl J Cancer* 70:188–193, 1997.

Tugwood JD, Holden PR, James NH, Prince RA, Roberts RA: A PPAR alpha cDNA cloned from guinea pig liver encodes a protein with similar properties to the mouse PPAR alpha: Implications for species differences in response to peroxisome proliferators. *Arch Toxicol* 72:169–177, 1998.

Turk PW, Laayoun A, Smith SS, Weitzman SA: DNA adduct 8-hydroxy-2′-deoxyguanosine (8-hydroxy-guanosine) affects function of human DNA methyltransferase. *Carcinogenesis* 16:1253–1256, 1995.

Ueda A, Hamadeh HK, Webb HK, et al.: Diverse roles of the nuclear orphan receptor CAR in regulating hepatic genes in response to phenobarbital. *Mol Pharmacol* 61:1–6, 2002.

van der Gulden JW, Kolk JJ, Verbeek AL: Work environment and prostate cancer risk. *Prostate* 27(5):250–257, 1995.

Vesselinovitch SD, Hacker HJ, Bannasch P: Histochemical characterization of focal hepatic lesions induced by single diethylnitrosamine treatment in infant mice. *Cancer Res* 45:2774–2780, 1985.

Vogt PK: Jun, the oncoprotein. *Oncogene* 20:2365–2377, 2001.

von Sonntag C: New aspects in the free-radical chemistry of pyrimidine nucleobases. *Free Radic Res Comm* 2:217–224, 1987.

Vousden KH: Human papillomavirus and cervical carcinoma. *Cancer Cells* 1:43–50, 1989.

Vuillaume M: Reduced oxygen species, mutation, induction and cancer initiation. *Mutat Res* 186:43–72, 1987.

Waalkes MP, Anver MR, Diwan BA: Chronic toxic and carcinogenic effects of oral cadmium in the Noble (NBL/Cr) rat: Induction of neoplastic and proliferative lesions of the adrenal, kidney, prostate, and testes. *J Toxicol Environ Health A* 58(4):199–214, 1999.

Waalkes MP, Diwan BA, Ward JM, Devor DE, Goyer RA: Renal tubular tumors and atypical hyperplasias in B6C3F1 mice exposed to lead acetate during gestation and lactation occur with minimal chronic nephropathy. *Cancer Res* 55(22):5265–5271, 1995.

Waalkes MP, Rehm S, Sass B, Kovatch R, Ward JM: Chronic carcinogenic and toxic effects of a single subcutaneous dose of cadmium in male NFS and C57 mice and male Syrian hamsters. *Toxic Subst J* 13:15–28, 1994.

Wade N, Marsman DS, Popp JA: Dose related effects of hepatocarcinogen Wy 14,263 on peroxisomes and cell replication. *Fundam Appl Toxicol* 18:149–54, 1992.

Wainfan E, Poirier LA: Methyl groups in carcinogenesis: Effects on DNA methylation and gene expression. *Cancer Res* 52(Suppl.):S2071–S2077, 1992.

Walker VE, Fennell TR, Upton PB, *et al.*: Molecular dosimetry of ethylene oxide: Formation and persistence of 7-(2-hydroxyethyl) guanine in DNA following repeated exposures of rats and rice. *Cancer Res* 52:5328–5334, 1992.

Ward E, Okun A, Ruder A, Fingerhut M, Steenland K: A mortality study of workers at seven beryllium processing plants. *Am J Ind Med* 22(6):885–904, 1992.

Wei P, Zhang J, Egan-Hafley M, Liang S, Moore DD: The nuclear receptor CAR mediates specific xenobiotic induction of drug metabolism. *Nature* 407:920–923, 2000.

Weinberg RA: The retinoblastoma protein and cell cycle control. *Cell* 81:323–330, 1995.

Weisburger JH, Williams GM: Metabolism of chemical carcinogens, in Becker FF (ed.): *Cancer: A Comprehensive Treatise*, 2nd edn. New York: Plenum, 1981, pp. 241–333.

Weisburger JH, Williams GM: Bioassay of carcinogens: In vitro and in vivo tests, in Searle CE (ed.): *Chemical Carcinogens*. Washington, DC: American Chemical Society, 1984, vol. 2, pp. 1323–1373.

Weitzman SA, Turk PW, Milkowski DH, Kozlowski K: Free radical adducts induce alterations in DNA cytosine methylation. *Proc Natl Acad Sci USA* 91:1261–1264, 1994.

Welfare M, Monesola AA, Bassendine MF, Daly AK: Polymorphisms in *GSTP1*, *GSTM1*, and *GSTT1* and susceptibility to colorectal cancer. *Cancer Epidemiol Biomarker Prevent* 8:289–292, 1999.

Wells: EGF receptor. *Int J Biochem Cell Biol* 31:637–643, 1999.

Welsch CW, Adams C, Lambrecht LK, Hassett CC, Brooks CL: 17b-Oestradiol and enovid mammary tumorigenesis in C3H/HeJ female mice: Counteraction by concurrent 2-bromo-a-ergocryptine. *Br J Cancer Res* 52:1–17, 1977.

Whysner J, Ross PM, Williams GM: Phenobarbital mechanistic data and risk assessment: Enzyme induction, enhanced cell proliferation, and tumor promotion. *Pharmacol Ther* 71:153–191, 1996.

Whyte P, Buchkovich FJ, Horowitz JM, *et al.*: Association between an oncogene and an anti-oncogene: The adenovirus E1A proteins bind to the retinoblastoma gene product. *Nature* 334:124–129, 1988.

Williams GM: In vivo and in vitro markers of liver cell transformation, in Smith GJ, Stewart BW (eds.): *In Vitro Epithelial Cell Differentiation and Neoplasia*. Cancer Forum, 1982, vol. 6, pp. 166–172.

Williams GM, Whysner J: Epigenetic carcinogens: Evaluation and risk assessment. *Exp Toxicol Pathol* 48:189–195, 1996.

Witz G: Active oxygen species as factors in multistage carcinogenesis. *Proc Soc Exp Biol Med* 198:675–682, 1991.

Wood WB, Gloyne SR: Pulmonary asbestosis. A review of one hundred cases. *Lancet* 2:1383–1385, 1934.

Yamagiwa K, Ichikawa K: Experimentelle Studie über die Pathogenese der Epithelialgeschwülste. *Mitt Med Fak Kaiserl Univ Tokio* 15:295–344, 1915.

Yang SK, McCourt DW, Roller PP, Gelboin HV: Enzymatic conversion of Benzo[a]pyrene leading predominantly to the diol-epoxide r-7, t-8-dihydroxy-t-9,10-oxy-7,8,9,10-tetrahydrobenzo[a]pyrene through a single enantiomer of r-7,t-8-dihydroxy-7,8-dihydrobenzo[a]pyrene. *Proc Nat Acad Sci USA* 73(8):2594–2598, 1976.

Yoshida T: Über die serienweise Verfolgung der Veränderungen der Leber der experimentellen Hepatomerzeugung durch o -Aminoazotoluol. *Trans Jpn Path Soc* 23:636–638, 1933.

Young SS, Gries CL: Exploration of the negative correlation between proliferative hepatocellular lesions and lymphoma in rats and mice—Establishment and implications. *Fundam Appl Toxicol* 4:632–640, 1984.

Zawaski K: Evidence for enhanced expression of c-fos, c-jun, and the CA2+-activated neutral protease in rat liver following carbon tetrachloride administration. *Biochem Biophys Res Commun* 197:585–590, 1993.

Zhang H, Kamendulis LM, Xu Y, Klaunig JE: The role of 8-hydroxy-2'-deoxyguanosine in morphological transformation of Syrian hamster embryo (SHE) Cells. *Toxicol Sci* 56:303–312, 2000.

GENETIC TOXICOLOGY

R. Julian Preston and George R. Hoffmann

WHAT IS GENETIC TOXICOLOGY?

Genetic toxicology is a branch of the field of toxicology that assesses the effects of chemical and physical agents on the hereditary material (DNA) and on the genetic processes of living cells. Such effects can be assessed directly by measuring the interaction of agents with DNA or more indirectly through the assessment of DNA repair or the production of gene mutations or chromosome alterations. Given the risk assessment framework of this chapter, it is important at the outset to distinguish between genotoxicity and mutagenicity. Genotoxicity covers a broader spectrum of endpoints than mutagenicity. For example, unscheduled DNA synthesis, sister chromatid exchanges, and DNA strand breaks are measures of genotoxicity, not mutagenicity, because they are not themselves transmissible from cell to cell or generation to generation. Mutagenicity on the other hand refers to the production of transmissible genetic alterations.

This chapter discusses the history of the development of the field of genetic toxicology, the use of genetic toxicology data in cancer and genetic risk assessments, the mechanisms underlying genetic toxicology assays, the assays that can be used for detecting genotoxic endpoints, the use of the same assays for better understanding mechanisms of mutagenesis, and new methods for the assessment of genetic alterations. The field is evolving rapidly, and the present snapshot will set the stage for considering this evolution.

HISTORY OF GENETIC TOXICOLOGY

The field of genetic toxicology can be considered to have its roots in the pioneering work of H.J. Muller (1927), who showed that X-rays could induce mutations in the fruit fly, *Drosophila*. In his studies he showed not only that radiation exposure could increase the overall frequencies of mutations but also that the types of mutations induced were exactly the same in effect, or phenotype, as those observed in the absence of radiation exposure. Thus, the induced mutagenic responses must be assessed in relation to background mutations. As a conclusion to this study of radiation-induced mutations, Muller predicted the utility of mutagenesis studies not only for the study of mutations themselves but also for gene mapping approaches.

Karl Sax (1938) built upon Muller's original studies of radiation-induced mutations by showing that X-rays could also induce structural alterations to chromosomes in *Tradescantia* pollen grains. Sax and his colleagues, notably in the absence of a knowledge of DNA structure and chromosomal organization, showed that at least two critical lesions in a nuclear target are required for the production of an exchange within (intrachromosome) or between (interchromosome) chromosomes. We know now that the lesions identified by Sax are DNA double-strand breaks, base damages, or multiply damaged sites (reviewed by Ward, 1988). In addition, Sax and colleagues (Sax, 1939; Sax and Luippold, 1952) showed that the yield of chromosome aberrations was reduced if the total dose of X-rays was delivered over extended periods of time or split into two fractions separated by several hours. These observations led to the concept of restitution of radiation-induced damage, which was later recognized as involving specific DNA repair processes (see below).

Consideration of the genetic effects of exogenous agents on cells was expanded to include chemicals in 1946, when Charlotte Auerbach and colleagues reported that mustard gas could induce mutations in *Drosophila* and that these mutations were phenotypically similar to those induced by X-rays (Auerbach and Robson, 1946). Thus, the field of chemical mutagenesis was initiated to run in parallel with studies of radiation mutagenesis. These original studies of Auerbach (actually conducted in 1941) are placed in a historical and biological perspective by the delightful review of Geoffrey Beale (1993).

Although the scientific value of the analysis of mutations in *Drosophila* was clear, there was an impression that the extrapolation to predict similar effects in human populations was too wide a step. Thus, a research effort of great magnitude was initiated to attempt to assess radiation-induced mutations in mice. This effort resulted in the publication by William Russell (1951) of data on X-ray-induced mutations using a mouse specific-locus mutation assay. These data clearly showed that the type of results obtained with *Drosophila* could be replicated in a mammalian system. The mouse tester strain developed for the specific-locus assay has recessive mutations at seven loci coding for visible mutations, such as coat color, eye color, and ear shape. This homozygous recessive tester strain can be used for identifying recessive mutations induced in wild-type genes at the same loci in mice treated with radiation or chemical mutagens. It was noteworthy that the mutation rate for X-ray-induced mutations in germ cells was similar in mouse and *Drosophila*. Subsequent studies by Liane Russell and colleagues showed that chemicals could induce mutations at the same seven loci (Russell *et al.*, 1981).

Over the next 20 years, genetic toxicologists investigated the induction of mutations and chromosomal alterations in somatic and germ cells largely following exposures to radiation. The ability to grow cells in vitro, either as primary cultures or as transformed cell lines, enhanced these quantitative studies. The in vitro culture of human lymphocytes, stimulated to reenter the cell cycle by phytohemagglutinin, greatly expanded the information on the assessment of chromosomal alterations in human cells [an excellent review by Hsu (1979) is recommended]. It also became feasible to use cytogenetic alterations in human lymphocytes as a biodosimeter for assessing human exposures to ionizing radiations (Bender and Gooch, 1962).

Two events during the 1970s served to expand the utility of mutagenicity data into the realm of risk assessment. The Millers and their colleagues (Miller and Miller, 1977) showed that chemical carcinogens could react to form stable, covalent derivatives with DNA, RNA, and proteins both in vitro and in vivo. In addition, they reported that these derivatives could require the metabolism of the parent chemical to form reactive metabolites. This metabolism is required for some chemicals to become mutagens and carcinogens. Metabolic capability is endogenous in vivo, but most cell lines in vitro have lost this capacity. To overcome this for in vitro mutagenicity studies, Heinrich Malling and colleagues developed an exogenous metabolizing system based upon a rodent liver homogenate (S9) (Malling and Frantz, 1973). Although this exogenous metabolism system has had utility, it does have drawbacks related to species and tissue specificity and loss of cellular compartmentalization. The development of transgenic cell lines containing inducible P450 genes has overcome this drawback to some extent (Crespi and Miller, 1999).

The second development in the 1970s that changed the field of genetic toxicology was the development by Bruce Ames *et al.* (1975) of a simple, inexpensive mutation assay with the bacterium *Salmonella typhimurium*. This assay can be used to detect chemically induced reverse mutations at the histidine locus and can include the exogenous metabolizing S9 system described above. The Ames assay, as it is generally called, has been expanded and modified to enhance its specificity as discussed below (under section "Gene Mutations in Prokaryotes"). The assay has been used extensively, especially for hazard identification, as part of the cancer risk assessment process. This use was based on the assumption that carcinogens were mutagens, given that cancer required mutation induction. This latter dogma proved to be somewhat inhibitory, in some ways, to the field of genetic toxicology because it provided a framework that was too rigid. Nonetheless, over the decade of the mid-1970s to mid-1980s somewhere on the order of 200 short-term genotoxicity and mutagenicity assays were developed for screening potentially carcinogenic chemicals. The screens included mutation induction, DNA damage, DNA repair, and cell killing or other genotoxic activities. Several international collaborative studies were organized to establish the sensitivity and specificity of a select group of assays as well as to assess interlaboratory variation (IPCS, 1988). In summary, most assays were able to detect carcinogens or noncarcinogens with an efficiency of about 70% as compared with the outcome of 2-year cancer bioassays. There are a number of possible reasons for the imperfect correspondence, the most likely being that there is a group of chemical carcinogens that do not induce cancer by a direct mutagenic action. The latter point was addressed to some extent by Tennant *et al.* (1987), who compared the effectiveness of a small standard battery of well-characterized short-term assays to identify carcinogens. Again, this battery predicted about 70% of known carcinogens. Subsequently, the lack of a tight correlation between carcinogenicity and mutagenicity (and the converse, noncarcinogenicity and nonmutagenicity) was found to be due to the fact that some chemicals were not directly mutagenic but instead induced the damage necessary for tumor development indirectly by, for example, clonally expanding preexisting mutant cells (i.e., tumor promotion) or through the production of reactive oxygen species. This class of chemicals has been given the rather unfortunate name of *nongenotoxic* to contrast them with genotoxic ones; the classification as *not directly mutagenic* is more appropriate. In the context of the mechanism of their mutagenicity, it is even more preferable to distinguish between DNA-reactivity and its correlate non-DNA-reactivity. In the past 10 years or so, emphasis has been placed on identifying mechanisms whereby nondirectly mutagenic chemicals can be involved in tumor production. Those identified include cytotoxicity with regenerative cell proliferation, mitogenicity, receptor-mediated processes, changes in methylation status, and alterations in cell–cell communication.

In the past 10 years or so, the field of genetic toxicology has moved away from the short-term assay approach for assessing carcinogenicity to a much more mechanistic approach, fueled to quite an extent by the advances in molecular biology. The ability to manipulate and characterize DNA, RNA, and proteins and to understand basic cellular processes and how they can be perturbed has advanced enormously over this period. Knowing how to take advantage of these technical developments is paramount. This chapter addresses current genetic toxicology: the assays for qualitative and quantitative assessment of cellular changes induced by chemical and physical agents, the underlying molecular mechanisms for these changes, and how such information can be incorporated into cancer and genetic risk assessments. In addition, the way forward for the field is addressed in the form of an epilogue. Thus, the preceding historical overview sets the stage for the rest of the chapter.

HEALTH IMPACT OF GENETIC ALTERATIONS

The importance of mutations and chromosomal alterations for human health is evident from their roles in genetic disorders, including birth defects and cancer. Therefore, mutations in both germ cells and somatic cells need to be considered when an overall risk resulting from mutations is concerned.

Somatic Cells

An association between mutation and cancer has long been evident, such as through the correlation between the mutagenicity and carcinogenicity of chemicals, especially in biological systems that have the requisite metabolic activation capabilities. Moreover, human chromosome instability syndromes and DNA repair deficiencies are associated with increased cancer risk (Friedberg, 1985). Cancer cytogenetics has greatly strengthened the association in that specific chromosomal alterations, including deletions, translocations, inversions, and amplifications, have been implicated in many human leukemias and lymphomas as well as in some solid tumors (Rabbitts, 1994).

Critical evidence that mutation plays a central role in cancer has come from molecular studies of oncogenes and tumor suppressor genes. Oncogenes are genes that stimulate the transformation of normal cells into cancer cells (Bishop, 1991). They originate when genes called proto-oncogenes, involved in normal cellular growth and development, are genetically altered. Normal regulation of cellular proliferation requires a balance between factors that promote growth and those that restrict it. Mutational alteration of proto-oncogenes can lead to overexpression of their growth-stimulating activity, whereas mutations that inactivate tumor suppressor genes, which normally restrain cellular proliferation, free cells from their inhibitory influence (Hanahan and Weinberg, 2000).

The action of oncogenes is genetically dominant in that a single active oncogene is expressed even though its normal allele is present in the same cell. Proto-oncogenes can be converted into active oncogenes by point mutations or chromosomal alterations. Base-pair substitutions in *ras* proto-oncogenes are found in many human tumors (Bishop, 1991; Barrett, 1993). Among chromosomal alterations that activate proto-oncogenes, translocations are especially prevalent (Rabbitts, 1994). For example, Burkitt's lymphoma involves a translocation between the long arm of chromosome 8, which is the site of the *c-MYC* oncogene, and chromosome 14 (about 90% of cases), 22, or 2. A translocation can activate a proto-oncogene by moving it to a new chromosomal location, typically the site of a T-cell receptor or immunoglobulin gene, where its expression is enhanced. A similar translocation-based mechanism also applies to various other hematopoietic cancers. Alternatively, the translocation may join two genes, resulting in a protein fusion that contributes to cancer development. Fusions have been implicated in other hematopoietic cancers and some solid tumors (Rabbitts, 1994). Like translocations, other chromosomal alterations can activate proto-oncogenes, and genetic amplification of oncogenes can magnify their expression (Bishop, 1991).

Mutational inactivation or deletion of tumor suppressor genes has been implicated in many cancers. Unlike oncogenes, the cancer-causing alleles that arise from tumor suppressor genes are typically recessive in that they are not expressed when they are heterozygous (Evans and Prosser, 1992). However, several genetic mechanisms, including mutation, deletion, chromosome loss, and mitotic recombination, can inactivate or eliminate the normal dominant allele, leading to the expression of the recessive cancer gene in a formerly heterozygous cell (Cavenee et al., 1983). The inactivation of tumor suppressor genes has been associated with various cancers, including those of the eye, kidney, colon, brain, breast, lung, and bladder (Fearon and Vogelstein, 1990; Marshall, 1991). Gene mutations in a tumor suppressor gene called *P53*, located on chromosome 17, occur in many different human cancers, and molecular characterization of *P53* mutations has linked specific human cancers to mutagen exposures (Harris, 1993; Aguilar et al., 1994; Royds and Iacopetta, 2006).

In the simplest model for the action of tumor suppressor genes, two events are considered to be required for the development of retinoblastoma, a tumor of the eye, because both normal alleles must be inactivated or lost (Knudson, 1997). In sporadic forms of the cancer (i.e., no family history), the two genetic events occur independently, but in familial forms (e.g., familial retinoblastoma), the first mutation is inherited, leaving the need for only a single additional event for expression. The strong predisposition to cancer in the inherited disease stems from the high likelihood that a loss of heterozygosity will occur by mutation, recombination, or aneuploidy in at least one or a few cells in the development of the affected organ. The simple model involving two events and a single pair of alleles cannot explain all observations concerning tumor suppressor genes because many cancers involve more than one tumor suppressor gene. For example, the childhood kidney tumor called Wilms' tumor can be caused by damage in at least three different genes (Marshall, 1991), and colorectal carcinomas are often found to have lost not only the wild-type *P53* tumor suppressor gene but also other tumor suppressor genes (Fearon and Vogelstein, 1990; Stoler et al., 1999). Moreover, a single mutation in a tumor suppressor gene, even though not fully expressed, may contribute to carcinogenesis. For example, a single *P53* mutation in a developing colorectal tumor may confer a growth advantage that contributes to the development of the disease (Venkatachalam et al., 1998). Subsequent loss of heterozygosity will increase the growth advantage as the tumor progresses from benign to malignant (Fearon and

Vogelstein, 1990). In this regard (mutation and selection), carcinogenesis has been likened to an evolutionary process, with genomic instability providing the substrate and with growth advantage as the selection pressure.

Many cancers involve both activation of oncogenes and inactivation of tumor suppressor genes (Fearon and Vogelstein, 1990; Bishop, 1991). The observation of multiple genetic changes supports the view that cancer results from an accumulation of genetic alterations and that carcinogenesis is a multistep process (Kinzler *et al.*, 1996; Hahn *et al.*, 1999; Stoler *et al.*, 1999). At least three stages have been defined in carcinogenesis: initiation, promotion, and progression (Barrett, 1993). *Initiation* involves the induction of a genetic alteration, such as the mutational activation of a *ras* proto-oncogene by a mutagen. It is an irreversible step that starts the process toward cancer. *Promotion* involves cellular proliferation in an initiated cell population. Promotion can lead to the development of benign tumors such as papillomas. Agents called promoters stimulate this process. Promoters may be mutagenic but are not necessarily so. *Progression* involves the continuation of cell proliferation and the accumulation of additional irreversible genetic changes; it is marked by increasing genetic instability and malignancy. More recent studies are beginning to change this view, leading to the concept of acquired capabilities (Hanahan and Weinberg, 2000). In their *Hallmarks of Cancer*, Hanahan and Weinberg describe a set of six acquired characteristics that are essential for the formation of all tumors irrespective of tumor type and species. These characteristics are broadly described as follows: self-sufficiency in growth signals, insensitivity to antigrowth signals, evading apoptosis, limitless replicative potential, sustained angiogenesis, and tissue invasion and metastasis. It seems probable that there is no specific order for obtaining these characteristics.

Gene mutations, chromosome aberrations, and aneuploidy are all implicated in the development of cancer. Mutagens and clastogens (chromosome breaking agents) contribute to carcinogenesis as initiators. Their role does not have to be restricted to initiation, however, in that mutagens, clastogens, and aneugens (agents that induce aneuploidy) may contribute to the multiple genetic alterations that characterize progression or the development of acquired capabilities. Other agents that contribute to carcinogenesis, such as promoters, need not be mutagens. However, the role of mutations is critical, and analyzing mutations and mutagenic effects is essential for understanding and predicting chemical carcinogenesis.

Germ Cells

The relevance of gene mutations to health is evident from the many disorders that are inherited as simple Mendelian characteristics (Mohrenweiser, 1991). About 1.3% of newborns suffer from autosomal dominant (1%), autosomal recessive (0.25%), or sex-linked (0.05%) genetic diseases (NRC, 1990; Sankaranarayanan, 1998). Molecular analysis of the mutations responsible for Mendelian diseases has revealed that almost half these mutations are base-pair substitutions; of the remainder, most are small deletions (Sankaranarayanan, 1998).

Many genetic disorders (e.g., cystic fibrosis, phenylketonuria, Tay-Sachs disease) are caused by the expression of recessive mutations. These mutations are mainly inherited from previous generations and are expressed when an individual inherits the mutant gene from both parents. New mutations make a larger contribution to the incidence of dominant diseases than to that of recessive diseases because only a single dominant mutation is required for expression.

Thus, new dominant mutations are expressed in the first generation. If a dominant disorder is severe, its transmission between generations is unlikely because of reduced fitness. For dominants with a mild effect, reduced penetrance, or a late age of onset, the contribution from previous generations is apt to be greater than that from new mutations. Estimating the proportion of all Mendelian genetic diseases that can be ascribed to new mutations is not straightforward; a rough estimate is 20% (Wyrobek, 1993; Shelby, 1994).

Besides causing diseases that exhibit Mendelian inheritance, gene mutations undoubtedly contribute to human disease through the genetic component of disorders with a complex etiology (Sankaranarayanan *et al.*, 1999). Some 3% (UNSCEAR, 2001) or 5–6% (Sankaranarayanan, 1998) of infants are affected by congenital abnormalities; if one includes multifactorial disorders that often have a late onset, such as heart disease, hypertension, and diabetes, the proportion of the population affected increases to more than 60% (Sankaranarayanan, 1998; UNSCEAR, 2001). Such frequencies are necessarily approximate because of differences among surveys in the reporting and classification of disorders. A higher prevalence would be found if less severe disorders were included in the tabulation. Nevertheless, such estimates provide a sense of the large impact of genetic disease.

Sensitive cytogenetic methods have led to the discovery of minor variations in chromosome structure that have no apparent effect. On the other hand, other relatively minor structural chromosome aberrations cause fetal death or serious abnormalities. Aneuploidy (gain or loss of one or more chromosomes) also contributes to fetal deaths and causes disorders such as Down syndrome. About 4 infants per 1000 live births have syndromes associated with chromosomal abnormalities, including translocations and aneuploidy. The majority of these syndromes (about 85%) result from trisomies (NRC, 1990). The majority of the adverse effects of chromosomal abnormalities occur prenatally. It has been estimated that 5% of all recognized pregnancies involve chromosomal abnormalities, as do about 6% of infant deaths and 30% of all spontaneous embryonic and fetal deaths (Mohrenweiser, 1991). Among the abnormalities that have been observed, aneuploidy is the most common, followed by polyploidy. Structural aberrations constitute about 5% of the total. Unlike gene mutations, many of which are inherited from the previous generation, about 85% of the chromosomal anomalies observed in newborns arose de novo in the germ cells of the parents (Mohrenweiser, 1991). The frequency of aneuploidy assessed directly in human sperm, initially by standard karyotyping and more recently by fluorescence in situ hybridization (FISH), is 3–4%; about 0.4% are sex chromosome aneuploidies (Martin *et al.*, 1991, 1996). The frequency of aneuploidy in human oocytes is about 18% (Martin *et al.*, 1991).

CANCER AND GENETIC RISK ASSESSMENTS

Cancer Risk Assessment

The formalized process for conducting a cancer risk assessment has many variations based upon national requirements and regulations. A summary of some of the different approaches can be found in Moolenaar (1994). There are ongoing attempts, for example, by the International Program on Chemical Safety (IPCS), to develop a harmonized approach to cancer (and genetic) risk assessments. However, no unified approach is currently available. Thus, for the purpose of this chapter, the formalized approach developed by the U.S. Environmental Protection Agency (EPA) based upon the paradigm presented by the National Research Council (NRC, 1983) is described here for depicting the use of genetic toxicology in the risk assessment process.

Genetic toxicology data have been used until recently solely for hazard identification. Namely, if a chemical is DNA-reactive, then tumors are considered to be produced by this chemical via direct mutagenicity. This has led, in turn, to the use of the default linear extrapolation from the rodent bioassay tumor data to exposure levels consistent with human environmental or occupational exposures (EPA, 1986). The assessment of risk requires the application of a series of default options, e.g., from laboratory animals to humans, from high to low exposures, from intermittent to chronic lifetime exposures, and from route to route of exposure. Default options are "generic approaches, based on general scientific knowledge and policy judgement that are applied to various elements of the risk assessment process when specific scientific information is not available" (NRC, 1994). The default options have been, in some ways, the Achilles' heel of the cancer risk-assessment process because they have a very significant impact on low exposure risk but are based on an uncertain database. This concern led the EPA (1996) to develop a very different approach, initially described in the *Proposed Guidelines for Carcinogen Risk Assessment*, now released as the *Guidelines for Carcinogen Risk Assessment* (EPA, 2005). In these guidelines, the emphasis is on using mechanistic data, when available, to inform the risk assessment process, particularly for dose–response assessment. The goal is to develop biologically based dose–response models for estimating cancer risk at low environmental exposures. This does, in general, bring the EPA approach into some harmony with those in other countries (Moolenaar, 1994), where a more narrative approach to risk assessment is preferred to a strictly quantitative one. The outcome of a more mechanistically based cancer risk assessment process is that there is a greater impetus to developing a database for mechanisms in addition to the yes/no output from genotoxicity assays. The same group of genotoxicity assays can be used for the collection of both types of information. The advent of molecular biology techniques has certainly aided in the pursuit of mechanisms of mutagenicity and carcinogenicity. It is anticipated that the cancer risk assessment process will evolve as new types of data are obtained.

In this regard, some of the issues that remain to be more firmly elucidated are (1) the relative sensitivities of different species (particularly rodent and human) to the induction of organ-specific mutations and tumors by chemicals and radiation; (2) the shape of the dose response for genetic alterations and tumors at low (environmental) exposure levels, especially for genotoxic chemicals; and (3) the relative sensitivity of susceptible subpopulations of all types. A better understanding of these major issues will greatly reduce the uncertainty in cancer risk assessments by, in part, replacing default options with biological data.

The recently released EPA (2005) Guidelines provide a framework for cancer risk assessment that utilizes a mode-of-action (MoA) as the means of describing the "necessary but not sufficient" steps required for a chemical to produce a tumor. A particular MoA can further be defined by a set of key events that are required for tumor development (Preston and Williams, 2005). In addition, the key events can be used to establish whether or not a particular MoA described for a rodent model is plausible in humans (the so-called Human Relevance Framework, Meek *et al.*, 2003). This more defined approach based on the use of the best available science can possibly be extended to include noncancer health effects (Seed *et al.*, 2005).

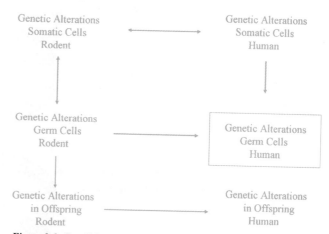

Figure 9-1. Parallelogram approach for genetic risk assessment.
Data obtained for genetic alterations in rodent somatic and germ cells and human somatic cells are used to estimate the frequency of the same genetic alterations in human germ cells. The final step is to estimate the frequency of these genetic alterations that are transmitted to offspring.

Genetic Risk Assessment

The approach for conducting a genetic risk assessment is less well defined than that for cancer risk. In fact, only a handful of genetic risk assessments have been conducted. An in-depth discussion of the topic can be found in the book *Methods for Genetic Risk Assessment* (Brusick, 1994). The reader is also referred to the genetic risk for ethylene oxide developed by the EPA (Rhomberg *et al.*, 1990) and the discussion of this and a recalculation presented by Preston *et al.* (1995). These two articles serve to highlight the difficulties with and uncertainties in genetic risk assessments.

The general approach is to use rodent germ cell and somatic cell data for induced genetic alterations and human data for induced genetic alterations in somatic cells (when available) to estimate the frequency of genetic alterations in human germ cells. This is the "parallelogram approach" (Fig. 9-1) first used by Brewen and Preston (1974) for X-irradiation and subsequently more fully developed for chemical exposures by Sobels (1982). The aim of this approach is to develop two sensitivity factors: (1) somatic to germ cell in the rodent and (2) rodent to human using somatic cells. These factors can then be used to estimate genetic alterations in human germ cells. Of course, for a complete estimate of genetic risk, it is necessary to obtain an estimate of the frequency of genetic alterations transmitted to the offspring (UNSCEAR, 2001). In addition, separate genetic risk assessments need to be conducted for males and females, given the considerable difference in germ cell development and observed and predicted sensitivity differences.

MECHANISMS OF INDUCTION OF GENETIC ALTERATIONS

DNA Damage

The types of DNA damage produced by ionizing radiations, non-ionizing radiations, and chemicals are many and varied, including single- and double-strand breaks in the DNA backbone, crosslinks between DNA bases or between DNA bases and proteins, and chemical addition to the DNA bases (adducts) (Fig. 9-2). The aim of this section is to introduce the topic of DNA damage because such

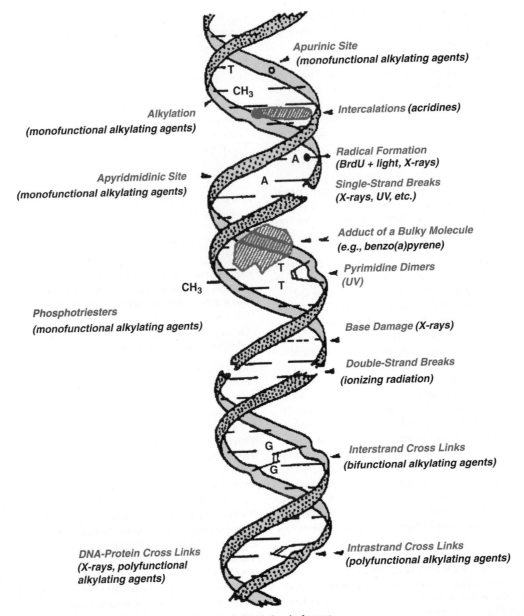

Figure 9-2. Spectrum of DNA damage induced by physical and chemical agents.

damage is the substrate for the formation of genetic alterations and genotoxicity in general. However, much greater detail can be found in recent reviews that are referenced at the appropriate places within each section. It should be noted that endogenous processes and exogenous agents can produce DNA damage, but mutations themselves are produced by errors in DNA repair or replication that are a consequence of the induced DNA damage.

Ionizing Radiations Ionizing radiations such as X-rays, gamma rays, and alpha particles produce DNA single- and double-strand breaks and a broad range of base damages (Goodhead, 1994; Wallace, 1994; Ward, 1994). In addition, it has been reported more recently that multiply damaged sites or clustered lesions can be formed that appear to be more difficult to repair. Such lesions consist of multi single lesions, including oxidized purine or pyrimidine bases, sites of base loss, and single-strand breaks. These multiple lesions can be formed in DNA from the same radiation energy depo-

sition event (Blaisdell *et al.*, 2001). The relative proportions of these different classes of DNA damage vary with type of radiation. For example, single-strand breaks and base damages predominate with X-rays, for which ionization density is sparse, whereas the frequencies of single- and double-strand breaks are more similar with alpha particles, for which ionization density is dense. The frequencies of individual base damages have been assessed using monoclonal antibodies, for example (Le *et al.*, 1998), but only a very few of the total spectrum have so far been studied. More recently, it has been demonstrated that the modified histone gamma-H2AX can be used as a sensitive marker of DNA double-strand breaks (Nakamura *et al.*, 2006).

Ultraviolet Light Ultraviolet light (a nonionizing radiation) induces two predominant lesions, cyclobutane pyrimidine dimers and 6,4-photoproducts. These lesions have been studied extensively because they can both be quantitated by chemical and immunological methods (Friedberg *et al.*, 1995). In part because of this feature, the repair of cyclobutane dimers and 6,4-photoproducts has been extremely well characterized, as discussed below.

Chemicals   Chemicals can produce DNA alterations either directly (DNA-reactive) as adducts or indirectly by intercalation of a chemical between the base pairs (e.g., 9-aminoacridine) (see Heflich, 1991, for a review). Many electrophilic chemicals react with DNA, forming covalent addition products (adducts). The DNA base involved and the positions on DNA bases can be specific for a given chemical. Such specificity of DNA damage can result in a spectrum of mutations that is chemical specific, i.e., a fingerprint of sorts (Dogliotti *et al.*, 1998). Some alkylated bases can mispair, causing mutations when DNA is replicated. Alkylated bases can also lead to secondary alterations in DNA. For example, the alkyl group of an N7-alkylguanine adduct, which is a major adduct formed by many alkylating agents, labilizes the bond that connects the base to deoxyribose, thereby stimulating base loss. Base loss from DNA leaves an apurinic or apyrimidinic site, commonly called an AP site. The insertion of incorrect bases into AP sites causes mutations (Laval *et al.*, 1990).

Bulky DNA adducts formed, for example, by metabolites of benzo(*a*)pyrene or *N*-2-acetylaminofluorene are recognized by the cell in a similar way to UV damages and are repaired similarly (see below). Such adducts can also hinder polymerases and cause mutation as a consequence of errors that they trigger in replication.

Endogenous Agents   Endogenous agents are responsible for several hundred DNA damages per cell per day (Lindahl, 2000). The majority of these damages are altered DNA bases (e.g., 8-oxoguanine and thymine glycol) and AP sites. The cellular processes that can lead to DNA damage are oxygen consumption that results in the formation of reactive oxygen species (e.g., superoxide $^{\bullet}O_2$, hydroxyl free radicals $^{\bullet}OH$, and hydrogen peroxide) and deamination of cytosines and 5-methylcytosines leading to uracils and thymines, respectively. The process of DNA replication itself is somewhat error-prone, and an incorrect base can be added by replication polymerases. The frequencies of these endogenously produced DNA damages can be increased by exogenous (genotoxic) agents.

DNA Repair

The cell is faced with the problem of how to cope with the quite extensive DNA damage that it sustains. In a general sense, two processes are present to achieve this. If the damage is extensive, the cell can undergo apoptosis (programmed cell death), effectively releasing it from becoming a mutant cell (Evan and Littlewood, 1998). If the damage is less severe, it can be repaired by a range of processes that are part of a generalized cellular DNA damage response network that returns the DNA to its undamaged state (error-free repair) or to an improved but still altered state (error-prone repair). As a feature of this error-prone repair, it has recently been demonstrated that a family of polymerases, the eukaryotic translesion synthesis polymerases (e.g., human Y-family polymerases eta, iota, kappa, and Rev1) can bypass lesions that otherwise would block replication by the normal processive polymerases (Rattray and Strathern, 2003; Prakash *et al.*, 2005). These polymerases have the ability to bypass specific DNA lesions or groups of lesions. The result of the bypass can be an incorrect DNA sequence or a correct one depending on the induced lesion and the particular bypass polymerase. The basic

principles underlying most repair processes (other than translesion synthesis) are damage recognition, removal of damage (except for strand breaks or cleavage of pyrimidine dimers), repair DNA synthesis, and ligation. In order to achieve this for different types of DNA lesions, cells have modified the protein complexes used for other housekeeping processes (e.g., transcription, replication, and recombination). This chapter presents a brief outline of the major classes of DNA repair; much greater detail can be found in the reviews provided for each section and general reviews by Van Houten and Albertini (1995), Friedberg (2000), and Wood *et al.* (2005).

Base Excision Repair   The major pathways by which DNA base damages are repaired involve a glycosylase that removes the damaged base, causing the production of an apurinic or apyrimidinic site that can be filled by the appropriate base or processed further (Demple and Harrison, 1994; Seeberg *et al.*, 1995; Wood, 1996; McCullough *et al.*, 1999; Sung and Demple, 2006). The resulting gap from this further processing can be filled by a DNA polymerase, followed by ligation to the parental DNA. The size of the gap is dependent upon the particular polymerase involved in the repair (i.e., polymerase β for short patches; polymerase δ or $\in$ for longer patches). Oxidative damage, either background or induced, are important substrates for base excision repair (Lindahl, 2000). The role of translesion bypass polymerases in the repair of DNA base alterations is discussed above.

Nucleotide Excision Repair   The nucleotide excision repair (NER) system provides the cell's ability to remove bulky lesions from DNA. In the past decade the NER process has been studied extensively, and a complete characterization of the genes and proteins involved has been obtained (Reardon and Sancar, 2006). NER uses about 30 proteins to remove a damage-containing oligonucleotide from DNA. The basic steps are damage recognition, incision, excision, repair synthesis, and ligation. The characterization of these steps has been enhanced by the use of rodent mutant cell lines and cells from individuals with the UV-sensitivity, skin cancer-prone syndrome xeroderma pigmentosum (XP, for which there are at least seven distinct genetic complementation groups). Of particular interest is the link between NER and transcription, for which the DNA damage in actively transcribing genes, and specifically the transcribed strand, is preferentially and thus more rapidly repaired than the DNA damage in the rest of the genome (Lommel *et al.*, 1995; Jiang and Sancar, 2006). Thus, the cell protects the integrity of the transcription process. This link between transcription and repair appears to be provided by two factors: (1) when a bulky lesion is located on the transcribed strand of an active gene, RNA polymerase II is blocked, thus providing a signal for recruiting the NER complex, and (2) a major component of the NER complex is the TFII H basal transcription factor. The involvement of TFII H in repair also provides some specificity to the incisions in the DNA required to remove the damaged nucleotide. An incision on the 3' side of the damage is made first by the XPG protein followed by one on the 5' side by the XPF-ERRC1 complex. The lesion is removed in the 27–30 nucleotide segment formed by the two incisions. The gap is filled by polymerase δ or $\in$ in the presence of replication factor C and proliferating cell nuclear antigen (PCNA). Ligation by DNA ligase I completes the process. This NER process has been reconstituted in vitro, allowing for complete characterization, kinetic studies, and estimates of fidelity (Aboussekhra *et al.*, 1995).

Double-Strand Break Repair   Cell survival is seriously compromised by the presence in the cell of broken chromosomes. Unrepaired double-strand breaks trigger one or more DNA damage response systems to either check cell-cycle progression or induce apoptosis. In order to reduce the probability of persistent DNA double-strand breaks, cells have developed an array of specific repair pathways. These pathways are largely similar across a broad range of species from yeast to humans, although the most frequently used one is different among species. There are two general pathways for repair of DNA double-strand breaks: homologous recombination and nonhomologous end-joining. These two can be considered as being in competition for the double-strand break substrate (Haber, 2000; Sonoda *et al.*, 2006).

Homologous Recombination   Eukaryotes undergo homologous recombination as part of their normal activities both in germ cells (meiotic recombination) and somatic cells (mitotic recombination). The repair of double-strand breaks (and single-strand gaps) basically uses the same process and complex of proteins, although some different protein–protein interactions are involved (Shinohara and Ogawa, 1995). In eukaryotes, the process has been characterized most extensively for yeast, but evidence is accumulating that a very similar process occurs in mammalian cells, including human (Johnson *et al.*, 1999; Cahill *et al.*, 2006). The basic steps in double-strand break repair are as follows. The initial step is the production of a 3'-ended single-stranded tail by exonucleases or helicase activity. Through a process of strand invasion, whereby the single-stranded tail invades an undamaged homologous DNA molecule, together with DNA synthesis, a so-called Holliday junction DNA complex is formed. By cleavage of this junction, two DNA molecules are produced (with or without a structural crossover), neither of which now contain a strand break. Additional models have been proposed but probably play a minor role in mammalian cells (Haber, 2000). A detailed description of the specific enzymes known to be involved can be found in Shinohara and Ogawa (1995) and Cahill *et al.* (2006).

Nonhomologous End-Joining (NHEJ)   The characterization of NHEJ in mammalian cells was greatly enhanced by the observation that mammalian cell lines that are hypersensitive to ionizing radiation are also defective in the V(D)J recombination process, which is the means by which the huge range of an antibody's antigen-binding sites and T-cell receptor proteins are generated during mammalian lymphoid cell development. V(D)J recombination requires the production of double-strand breaks, recombination of DNA pieces, and subsequent religation. A major component of the NHEJ repair complex is a DNA-dependent protein kinase (DNA-PK). This protein, a serine/threonine kinase, consists of a catalytic subunit (DNA-PK$_{cs}$) and a DNA-end-binding protein consisting of KU70 and KU80 subunits. The specific role of DNA-PK in the repair of double-strand breaks is unclear in mammalian cells; a detailed discussion of what is known and some possible models of NHEJ are presented in the reviews by Critchlow and Jackson (1998) and Burma *et al.* (2006). Perhaps the most viable role of DNA-PK is to align the broken DNA ends to facilitate their ligation. In addition, DNA-PK might serve as a signal molecule for recruiting other repair proteins known to be involved in yeast and to some extent in mammalian cells. The final ligation step is performed by DNA ligase IV in human cells.

Mismatch Repair   The study of DNA mismatch repair systems has received considerable attention over the past few years, in part because an association has been demonstrated between genetic defects in mismatch repair genes and the genomic instability associated with cancer susceptibility syndromes and sporadic cancers. In general, DNA mismatch repair systems operate to repair mismatched bases formed during DNA replication, genetic recombination, and as a result of DNA damage induced by chemical and physical agents. Detailed reviews can be found in Kolodner (1995), Jiricny (1998), Modrich and Lahue (1996), and Jun *et al.* (2006).

The principal steps in all cells from prokaryotes to human are damage recognition by a specific protein that binds to the mismatch, stabilizing of the binding by the addition of one or more proteins, cutting the DNA at a distance from the mismatch, excision past the mismatch, resynthesis, and ligation. In some prokaryotes, the cutting of the DNA (for DNA replication mismatches) is directed to the strand that contains the incorrect base by using the fact that recently replicated DNA is unmethylated at N^6-methyladenine at a GATC sequence. The question of whether or not strand-specific mismatch repair occurs in mammalian cells has not been resolved, although some evidence does point to its occurrence (Modrich, 1997). Strand specificity for DNA mismatches resulting from induced DNA damage has not been identified.

O^6-Methylguanine-DNA Methyltransferase Repair   The main role for O^6-methylguanine-DNA methyltransferase (MGMT) is to protect cells against the toxic effects of simple alkylating agents. The methyl group is transferred from O^6-methylguanine in DNA to a cysteine residue in MGMT. The adducted base is reverted to a normal one by the enzyme, which is itself inactivated by the reaction. Details of the MGMT enzyme properties and the gene isolation and characterization can be found in Tano *et al.* (1990), Grombacher *et al.* (1996), and Margison *et al.* (2003).

The probability that induced DNA damage can be converted into a genetic alteration is influenced by the particular repair pathway(s) recruited, the rate of repair of the damage, and the fidelity and completeness of the repair. The mechanisms of induction of gene mutations and chromosome alterations discussed in the following sections build upon the assessment of the probability of repair versus misrepair versus nonrepair that can be derived from a knowledge of the mechanism of action of the different DNA repair mechanisms. The preceding sections, together with the references provided, should assist in this assessment.

Formation of Gene Mutations

Somatic Cells   Gene mutations are considered to be small DNA sequence changes confined to a single gene; larger genomic changes are considered below, under section "Formation of Chromosomal Alterations." The general classes of gene mutations are base substitutions and small additions or deletions. More detailed classifications can be found in the review by Ripley (1991). Base substitutions are the replacement of the correct nucleotide by an incorrect one; they can be further subdivided as transitions where the change is purine for purine or pyrimidine for pyrimidine; and transversions where the change is purine for pyrimidine and vice versa. Frameshift mutations are strictly the addition or deletion of one or a few base pairs (not in multiples of three) in protein-coding regions. The definition is more generally expanded to include such additions and deletions in any DNA region. For the discussion of the mechanism of induction of gene mutations and chromosomal alterations, it is necessary to distinguish chemicals by their general mode of action. Chemicals that can produce genetic alterations with similar effectiveness in all stages of the cell cycle are called radiomimetic because they act like radiation in this regard. Chemicals that produce genetic alterations far more effectively in the S phase of the cell cycle are described as nonradiomimetic. The great majority of chemicals are nonradiomimetic; the radiomimetic group includes bleomycin, streptonigrin, neocarzinostatin, and 8-ethoxycaffeine.

Gene mutations can arise in the absence of specific exogenous exposures to radiations and chemicals. The great majority of so-called spontaneous (background) mutations arise from *replication* of an altered template. The DNA alterations that arise are either the result of oxidative damage or are produced from the deamination of 5-methylcytosine to thymine at CpG sites resulting in G:C → A:T transitions. Mutations induced by ionizing radiations tend to be deletions ranging in size from a few bases to multilocus events (Thacker, 1992). The rapid rate of repair of the majority of radiation-induced DNA damages greatly reduces the probability of DNA lesions being present at the time of DNA replication. Thus, mutations induced by ionizing radiations are generally the result of errors of *DNA repair* (Preston, 1992). The low frequencies of gene mutations are produced from any unrepaired DNA base damage present during DNA replication.

Gene mutations produced by a majority of chemicals and non-ionizing radiations are base substitutions, frameshifts, and small deletions. Of these mutations, a very high proportion is produced by errors of DNA *replication* on a damaged template. Thus, the probability of a DNA adduct, for example, being converted into a mutation is determined, to a significant extent by the number of induced DNA adducts that remain in the DNA at the time that it is replicated. Thus, relative mutation frequency will be the outcome of the race between repair and replication, i.e., the more repair that takes place prior to replication, the lower the mutation frequency for a given amount of induced DNA damage. Significant regulators

of the race are cell cycle checkpoint genes (e.g., *P53*) because if the cell is checked from entering the S phase at a G_1/S checkpoint, more repair can take place prior to the cell starting to replicate its DNA (Mercer, 1998).

The proportion of chemically induced gene mutations that result from DNA repair errors is low, given that the DNA repair processes involved are error-free, and that, as a generalization, repair of chemically induced DNA damage is slower than for ionizing radiation damage, leading to the balance tipping toward replication prior to repair, especially for cells in the S phase at the time of exposure. However, in the case of translesion bypass, discussed above, gene mutations can be produced at relatively high frequencies.

Germ Cells   The mechanism of production of gene mutations in germ cells is basically the same as in somatic cells. Ionizing radiations produce mainly deletions via errors of DNA repair; the majority of chemicals induce base substitutions, frameshifts, and small deletions by errors of DNA replication (Favor, 1999).

An important consideration for assessing gene mutations induced by chemicals in germ cells is the relationship between exposure and the timing of DNA replication. Figure 9-3 depicts the stages in oogenesis and spermatogenesis when DNA replicates. A few features are worthy of note. The spermatogonial stem cell in humans and rodents has a long cell cycle time, 8 days or longer, with only a small fraction being occupied by the S phase. Thus, the probability of DNA repair taking place prior to DNA replication is high, for both acute and chronic treatments. However, for considerations of genetic risk, it is the spermatogonial stem cell that is the major contributor because it is present, in general, throughout the reproductive lifetime of an individual. Each time a spermatogonial stem cell divides it produces a differentiating spermatogonium and a stem cell. Thus, the stem cell can accumulate genetic damage from chronic exposures. Differentiating spermatogonia, as far as the

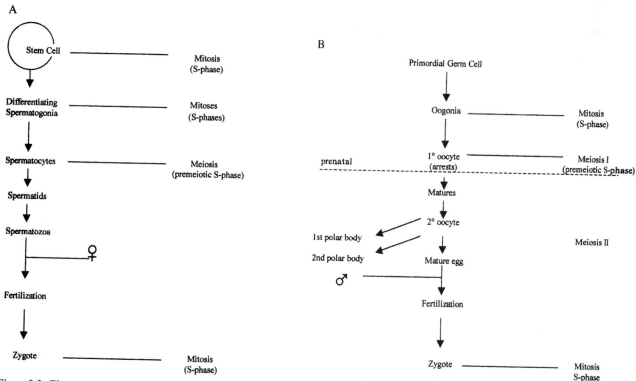

Figure 9-3. The stages of spermatogenesis (A) and oogenesis (B) indicating the periods of cell division and DNA replication (S phase).

induction of gene mutation is concerned, are the same as mitotically dividing somatic cells.

The first S phase after gametogenesis occurs in the zygote, formed following fertilization. This fact needs to be balanced by the lack of DNA repair in late spermatids and sperm. Thus, DNA damage induced in these stages will remain until the zygote. Postmeiotic germ cells are particularly sensitive to mutation induction by nonradiomimetic chemicals, especially following acute exposures (Russell, 2004). The fairly short duration of this stage (approximately 21 days in the mouse) means that their contribution to genetic risk following chronic exposures is quite small.

For oogenesis (Fig. 9-3) similar observations on gene mutation induction and timing of S phase can be made. In this case the primary oocyte arrests prior to birth, and there is no further S phase until the zygote. For this reason, the oocyte is resistant to the induction of gene mutations by nonradiomimetic chemicals but not to radiation, for which DNA repair is the mode of formation of mutations, and DNA repair occurs in oocytes (Brewen and Preston, 1982).

These mechanistic aspects of the production of gene mutations (and chromosome alterations described in the following two sections) by chemicals and radiations in somatic and germ cells are most important for considerations of the design of genetic toxicology assays, the interpretation of the data generated, and the incorporation of the data into cancer and genetic risk assessments.

Formation of Chromosomal Alterations

Somatic Cells

Structural Chromosome Aberrations   There are components of the formation of chromosome aberrations, sister chromatid exchanges (the apparently reciprocal exchange between the sister chromatids of a single chromosome), and gene mutations that are similar. In particular, damaged DNA serves as the substrate leading to all these events. However, chromosome aberrations induced by ionizing radiations are generally formed by errors of DNA repair, whereas those produced by nonradiomimetic chemicals are generally formed by errors of DNA replication on a damaged DNA template.

The DNA repair errors that lead to the formation of chromosome aberrations following ionizing radiation (and radiomimetic chemical) exposure arise from misligation of double-strand breaks or interaction of coincidentally repairing regions during nucleotide excision repair of damaged bases. The details of the DNA damage types and their repair are described above. Thus, the overall kinetics and fidelity of DNA repair influence the sensitivity of cells to the induction of chromosomal aberrations produced by misrepair. The broad outcomes of misrepair are that incorrect rejoining of chromosomal pieces during repair leads to chromosomal exchanges within (e.g., inversions and interstitial deletions) and between (e.g., dicentrics and reciprocal translocations) chromosomes. In fact, using fluorescence in situ hybridization, it can be shown that very complex rearrangements take place (Anderson et al., 2000). Failure to rejoin double-strand breaks or to complete repair of other types of DNA damage leads to terminal deletions.

Acentric fragments arise from interstitial deletions, terminal deletions, and the formation of dicentric chromosomes and rings. The failure to incorporate an acentric fragment into a daughter nucleus at anaphase/telophase, or the failure of a whole chromosome to segregate at anaphase to the cellular poles, can result in the formation of a membrane-bounded micronucleus that resides in the cytoplasm.

Errors of DNA replication on a damaged template can lead to a variety of chromosomal alterations. The majority of these involve deletion or exchange of individual chromatids (chromatid-type aberrations). Thus, nonradiomimetic chemicals induce only chromatid-type aberrations, whereas radiations and radiomimetic chemicals induce chromatid-type aberrations in the S and G_2 phases of the cell cycle, but chromosome-type aberrations affecting both chromatids in G_1. The reason for this latter observation is that the G_1 (or G_0) chromosome behaves as a single DNA molecule and aberrations formed in it will be replicated in the S phase and will involve both chromatids. This distinction is important for considerations of outcome of the aberrations and the probability of an effect on cells because for chromatid-type aberrations, one chromatid remains intact and genetically unaltered, in contrast to chromosome-type aberrations in which both chromatids are damaged (Preston et al., 1995).

Numerical Chromosome Changes   Numerical changes (e.g., monosomies, trisomies, and ploidy changes) can arise from errors in chromosomal segregation. The complexity of the control and the mechanics of the mitotic process means that alteration of various cellular components can result in failure to segregate the sister chromatids to separate daughter cells or in failure to segregate a chromosome to either pole (Bickel and Orr-Weaver, 1996; Preston, 1996; Hunt, 2006). The mechanisms underlying chromosomal loss are pertinent to those involved in the formation of micronuclei.

A limited set of chemicals has been demonstrated to cause aneuploidy through interaction with components of the structures that facilitate chromosome movement (Preston, 1996; Aardema et al., 1998). These include benomyl, griseofulvin, nocodazole, colchicine, colecemid, vinblastine, and paclitaxel. These chemicals affect tubulin polymerization or spindle microtubule stability. To date, other mechanisms of aneuploidy induction by chemicals have not been firmly identified.

Sister Chromatid Exchanges   Sister chromatid exchanges (SCEs) are produced during the S phase and are presumed to be a consequence of errors in the replication process, perhaps at the sites of stalled replication complexes (Painter, 1980; Heartlein et al., 1983; Preston, 1991). Because SCEs are apparently reciprocal exchanges, it is quite possible that they result from a recombination process occurring at the site of the stalled replication fork. It is, in fact, this mode of action that makes assays for SCE less than ideal for detecting effects due directly to a chemical exposure. The creation of intracellular conditions that slow the progress of DNA replication, for example, could lead to the formation of SCE.

Germ Cells   The formation of chromosomal alterations in germ cells is basically the same as that for somatic cells, namely, via misrepair for ionizing radiations and radiomimetic chemicals for treatments in G_1 and G_2, and by errors of replication for all radiations and chemicals for DNA damage present during the S phase. Also, the restrictions on the timing of formation of chromosomal alterations induced by nonradiomimetic chemicals in germ cells is as described above for gene mutations, namely at the specific stages where DNA synthesis occurs, as depicted in Fig. 9-3.

The types of aberrations formed in germ cells are the same as those formed in somatic cells (e.g., deletions, inversions, translocations), although their appearance in diplotene/diakinesis of meiosis I, where analysis is frequently conducted, is rather different because of the homologous chromosome pairing that takes place in meiotic cells (see the review by Leonard, 1973). The specific segregation of chromosomes during meiosis influences the probability of recovery of an aberration, particularly a reciprocal translocation, in the offspring of a treated parent. This is discussed in detail in Preston *et al.* (1995).

ASSAYS FOR DETECTING GENETIC ALTERATIONS

Introduction to Assay Design

Genetic toxicology assays are used to identify germ-cell mutagens, somatic-cell mutagens, and potential carcinogens. They detect diverse kinds of genetic alterations that are relevant for human health, including gene mutations, chromosome aberrations, and aneuploidy. Over the last three decades, hundreds of chemicals and complex mixtures have been evaluated for genotoxic effects. Genetic toxicology assays serve two interrelated but distinct purposes in the toxicologic evaluation of chemicals: (1) identifying mutagens for purposes of hazard identification and (2) characterizing dose–response relationships and mutagenic mechanisms, both of which contribute to an understanding of genetic and carcinogenic risks.

A common experience in surveying the mutagenicity literature is encountering a bewildering array of assays in viruses, bacteria, fungi, cultured mammalian cells, plants, insects, and mammals. More than 200 assays for mutagens have been proposed, and useful information has been obtained from many of them. Although most genetic toxicology testing and evaluation relies on relatively few assays, data from relatively obscure assays can sometimes contribute to a judgment about the genetic activity of a compound.

Table 9-1 lists key assays that have a prominent place in genetic toxicology. Table 9-2 is a more comprehensive list that provides literature citations to many of the assays that one might encounter in the genetic toxicology literature. Even this extensive table is not exhaustive, in that it emphasizes methods in applied genetic toxicology and not those assays whose use has been largely restricted to studies of mutational mechanisms. The commonly used assays rely on phenotypic effects as indicators of gene mutations or small deletions and on cytological methods for observing gross chromosomal damage. Detailed information on assay design, testing data, controls, sample sizes, and other factors in effective testing is found in the references cited.

Some assays for gene mutations detect forward mutations whereas others detect reversion. Forward mutations are genetic alterations in a wild-type gene and are detected by a change in phenotype caused by the alteration or loss of gene function. In contrast, a back mutation or reversion is a mutation that restores gene function in a mutant, bringing about a return to the wild-type phenotype. In principle, forward-mutation assays should respond to a broad spectrum of mutagens because any mutation that interferes with gene expression should confer the detectable phenotype. In contrast, a reversion assay might be expected to have a more restricted mutational response because only mutations that correct or compensate for the specific mutation in a particular mutant will be detected. In fact, some reversion assays respond to a broader spectrum of mutational changes than one might expect because mutations at a site other than that of the original mutation, either within the test gene or in a different gene (i.e., a suppressor mutation), can sometimes confer the selected phenotype. Both forward mutation assays and reversion assays are used extensively in genetic toxicology.

The simplest gene mutation assays rely on selection techniques to detect mutations. A selection technique is a means of imposing

Table 9-1

Principal Assays in Genetic Toxicology

I. Pivotal assays
  A. A well-characterized assay for gene mutations
    The *Salmonella*/mammalian microsome assay (Ames test)
  B. A mammalian assay for chromosome damage in vivo
    Metaphase analysis or micronucleus assay in rodent bone marrow

II. Other assays offering an extensive database or unique genetic endpoint
  A. Assays for gene mutations
    E. coli WP2 tryptophan reversion assay
    TK or *HPRT* forward mutation assays in cultured mammalian cells
    Drosophila sex-linked recessive lethal assay
  B. Cytogenetic analysis in cultured Chinese hamster or human cells
    Assays for chromosome aberrations and micronuclei
    Assays for aneuploidy
  C. Other indicators of genetic damage
    Mammalian DNA damage and repair assays
    Mitotic recombination assays in yeast and *Drosophila*
  D. Mammalian germ-cell assays
    Mouse specific-locus tests
    Assays for skeletal or cataract mutations in mice
    Cytogenetic analysis and heritable translocation assays
    DNA damage and repair in rodent germ cells
    Mutation analysis in tandem-repeat loci in mice

experimental conditions under which only cells or organisms that have undergone mutation can grow. Selection techniques greatly facilitate the identification of rare cells that have experienced mutation among the many cells that have not. Forward mutations and reversions can both be detected by selection techniques in microorganisms and cultured mammalian cells. Because of their speed, low cost, and ease of detecting events that occur at low frequency (i.e., mutation), assays in microorganisms and cell cultures have figured prominently in genetic toxicology.

Studying mutagenesis in intact animals requires assays of more complex design than the simple selection methods used in microorganisms and cultured cells. Genetic toxicology assays therefore range from inexpensive short-term tests that can be performed in a few days to complicated assays for mutations in mammalian germ cells. Even in multicellular organisms, there has been an emphasis on designing assays that detect mutations with great efficiency. Nevertheless, there remains a gradation in which an increase in relevance for human risk entails more elaborate and costly tests. The most expensive mammalian tests are typically reserved for agents of special importance in basic research or risk assessment, whereas the simpler assays can be applied more broadly.

Cytogenetic assays differ in design from typical gene mutation assays because of their reliance on cytological rather than genetic methods. The goal in cytogenetic methods is the unequivocal visual recognition of cells that have experienced genetic damage. The alterations measured include chromosome aberrations, micronuclei, SCEs, and changes in chromosome numbers (aneuploidy).

In all mutagenicity testing, one must be aware of possible sources of error. Factors to consider in the application of mutagenicity assays are the choice of suitable organisms and growth

Table 9-2
Overview of Genetic Toxicology Assays

ASSAYS	SELECTED LITERATURE CITATIONS
I. DNA Damage and Repair Assays	
A. Direct detection of DNA damage:	
Alkaline elution assays for DNA strand breakage	Elia *et al.*, 1994
Comet assay for DNA strand breakage	Fairbairn *et al.*, 1995; Singh, 2000; Tice *et al.*, 2000
Assays for chemical adducts in DNA	Chang *et al.*, 1994; Kriek *et al.*, 1998; Phillips *et al.*, 2000
B. Bacterial assays for DNA damage:	
Differential killing of repair-deficient and wild-type strains	Hamasaki *et al.*, 1992
Induction of the SOS system by DNA damage	Quillardet and Hofnung, 1993; Yasunaga *et al.*, 2004
C. Assays for repairable DNA damage in mammalian cells:	
Unscheduled DNA synthesis (UDS) in rat hepatocytes	Madle *et al.*, 1994
UDS in rodent hepatocytes in vivo	Madle *et al.*, 1994
II. Prokaryote Gene Mutation Assays	
A. Bacterial reverse mutation assays:	
Salmonella/mammalian microsome assay (Ames test)	Ames *et al.*, 1975; Kier *et al.*, 1986; Kirkland *et al.*, 1990; Maron and Ames, 1983; Mortelmans and Zeiger, 2000
E. coli WP2 tryptophan reversion assay	Kirkland *et al.*, 1990; Mortelmans and Riccio, 2000
Salmonella specific base-pair substitution assay	Gee *et al.*, 1994, 1998
(Ames-II assay)	
E. coli lacZ specific reversion assay	Cupples and Miller, 1989; Cupples *et al.*, 1990; Josephy, 2000
B. Bacterial forward mutation assays:	
E. coli lacI assay	Calos and Miller, 1981; Halliday and Glickman, 1991
Resistance to toxic metabolites or analogs in *Salmonella*	Jurado *et al.*, 1994; Vlasakova *et al.*, 2005
III. Assays in Nonmammalian Eukaryotes:	
A. Fungal assays:	
Forward mutations, reversion, and small deletions	Zimmermann *et al.*, 1984; Crouse, 2000
Mitotic crossing over and gene conversion in yeast	Zimmermann *et al.*, 1984; Zimmermann, 1992
Mitotic aneuploidy: chromosome loss or gain in yeast	Zimmermann *et al.*, 1984; Parry, 1993; Aardema *et al.*, 1998
Meiotic nondisjunction in yeast or Neurospora	Zimmermann *et al.*, 1984
B. Plant assays:	
Gene mutations affecting chlorophyll in seedlings or	Grant, 1994
waxy in pollen	
Tradescantia stamen hair color mutations	Grant, 1994
Chromosome aberrations or micronuclei in mitotic or	Grant, 1994
meiotic cells	
Aneuploidy detected by pigmentation or cytogenetics	Parry, 1993; Grant, 1994; Aardema *et al.*, 1998
C. Drosophila assays:	
Sex-linked recessive lethal test in germ cells	Lee *et al.*, 1983; Mason *et al.*, 1987
Heritable translocation assays	Mason *et al.*, 1987
Sex chromosome loss tests for aneuploidy	Aardema *et al.* 1998; Osgood and Cyr, 1998
Induction of mitotic recombination in eyes or wings	Vogel *et al.*, 1999
IV. Mammalian Gene Mutation Assays	
A. In vitro assays for forward mutations:	
tk mutations in mouse lymphoma or human cells	Kirkland *et al.*, 1990; Clements, 2000; Moore *et al.*, 2003
hprt or x*prt* mutations in Chinese hamster or human cells	DeMarini *et al.*, 1989
B. In vivo assays for gene mutations in somatic cells:	
Mouse spot test (somatic cell specific locus test)	Styles and Penman, 1985; Lambert *et al.*, 2005
hprt mutations (6-thioguanine-resistance) in rodent	Cariello and Skopek, 1993; Lambert *et al.*, 2005
lymphocytes	
C. Transgenic assays:	
Mutations in the bacterial *lacI* gene in "Big Blue®" mice	Mirsalis *et al.*, 1994; Lambert *et al.*, 2005
and rats	
Mutations in the bacterial *lacZ* gene in the "Muta™ Mouse"	Mirsalis *et al.*, 1994; Lambert *et al.*, 2005
Mutations in the phage *cII* gene in *lacI* or *lacZ* transgenic	Swiger, 2001; Lambert *et al.*, 2005
mice	
Point mutations and deletions in the *lacZ* plasmid mouse	Lambert *et al.*, 2005
Point mutations and deletions in *delta gpt* mice and rats	Okada *et al.*, 1999; Lambert *et al.*, 2005

Table 9-2
Overview of Genetic Toxicology Assays

ASSAYS	SELECTED LITERATURE CITATIONS
V. Mammalian Cytogenetic Assays	
A. Chromosome aberrations:	
Metaphase analysis in cultured Chinese hamster or human cells	Ishidate *et al.*, 1988; Kirkland *et al.*, 1990; Galloway *et al.*, 1994
Metaphase analysis of rodent bone marrow or lymphocytes in vivo	Preston *et al.*, 1981; Kirkland *et al.*, 1990; Tice *et al.*, 1994
B. Micronuclei:	
Cytokinesis-block micronucleus assay in human lymphocytes	Fenech, 2000; Fenech *et al.*, 2003
Micronucleus assay in mammalian cell lines	Kirsch-Volders *et al.*, 2000, 2003
In vivo micronucleus assay in rodent bone marrow or blood	Heddle *et al.*, 1991; Hayashi *et al.*, 2000; Krishna and Hayashi, 2000; Hamada *et al.*, 2001
C. Sister chromatid exchange:	
SCE in human cells or Chinese hamster cells	Tucker *et al.*, 1993a
SCE in rodent tissues, especially bone marrow	Tucker *et al.*, 1993a
D. Aneuploidy in mitotic cells:	
Mitotic disturbance seen by staining spindles and chromosomes	Parry, 1998
Hyperploidy detected by chromosome counting	Galloway and Ivett, 1986; Aardema *et al.*, 1998
Chromosome gain or loss in cells with intact cytoplasm	Natarajan, 1993
Micronucleus assay with centromere labeling	Lynch and Parry, 1993; Natarajan, 1993; Aardema *et al.*, 1998; Fenech, 2000
Hyperploid cells in vivo in mouse bone marrow	Aardema *et al.*, 1998
Mouse bone marrow micronucleus assay with centromere labeling	Heddle *et al.*, 1991; Adler *et al.*, 1994; Aardema *et al.*, 1998
VI. Germ Cell Mutagenesis	
A. Measurement of DNA damage	
Molecular dosimetry based on mutagen adducts	Russell and Shelby, 1985
UDS in rodent germ cells	Bentley *et al.*, 1994; Sotomayor and Sega, 2000
Alkaline elution assays for DNA strand breaks in rodent testes	Bentley *et al.*, 1994
B. Gene mutations	
Mouse specific locus test for gene mutations and deletions	Russell *et al.*, 1981; Kirkland *et al.*, 1990; Ehling, 1991; Russell and Russell, 1992
Mouse electrophoretic specific-locus test	Lewis, 1991
Dominant mutations causing mouse skeletal defects or cataracts	Ehling, 1991
Mouse tandem-repeat loci analysis	Yauk, 2004
C. Chromosomal aberrations	
Cytogenetic analysis in oocytes, spermatogonia, or spermatocytes	Kirkland *et al.*, 1990; Tease, 1992; Russo, 2000
Micronuclei in mouse spermatids	Hayashi *et al.*, 2000; Russo, 2000
Mouse heritable translocation test	Russell and Shelby, 1985
D. Dominant lethal mutations	
Mouse or rat dominant lethal assay	Adler *et al.*, 1994
E. Aneuploidy	
Cytogenetic analysis for aneuploidy arising by nondisjunction	Allen *et al.*, 1986; Adler, 1993; Aardema *et al.*, 1998
Sex chromosome loss test for nondisjunction or breakage	Russell and Shelby, 1985; Adler, 1993
Micronucleus assay in spermatids with centromere labeling	Aardema *et al.*, 1998
FISH with probes for specific chromosomes in sperm	Russo, 2000; Wyrobek *et al.*, 2005

conditions, appropriate monitoring of genotypes and phenotypes, effective experimental design and treatment conditions, inclusion of proper positive and negative controls, and sound methods of data analysis (Kirkland et al., 1990).

Many compounds that are not themselves mutagenic or carcinogenic can be activated into mutagens and carcinogens by metabolism. Such compounds are called promutagens and procarcinogens. Because microorganisms and mammalian cell cultures lack many of the metabolic capabilities of intact mammals, provision must be made for metabolic activation in order to detect promutagens in many genetic assays. Incorporating an in vitro metabolic activation system derived from a mammalian tissue homogenate is the most common means of adding metabolic activation to microbial or cell culture assays. For example, the promutagens dimethylnitrosamine and benzo[a]pyrene are not themselves mutagenic in bacteria, but they are mutagenic in bacterial assays if the bacteria are treated with the promutagen in the presence of a homogenate from mammalian liver.

The most widely used metabolic activation system in microbial and cell culture assays is a postmitochondrial supernatant from a rat liver homogenate, along with appropriate buffers and cofactors (Maron and Ames, 1983; Kirkland et al., 1990). The standard liver metabolic activation system is called an S9 mixture, designating a supernatant from centrifugation at 9000g (Malling and Frantz, 1973). Most of the short-term assays in Table 9-2 require exogenous metabolic activation to detect promutagens. Exceptions are assays in intact mammals and a few simpler assays that have a high level of endogenous cytochrome P450 metabolism, such as the detection of unscheduled DNA synthesis (UDS) in cultured hepatocytes (Madle et al., 1994).

Rat liver S9 provides a broad assemblage of metabolic reactions, but they are not necessarily the same as those of hepatic metabolism in an intact rat. Metabolic activation systems based on homogenates from other species or organs have found some use, but they may similarly differ from the species or organs of their origin. Therefore, alternative metabolic activation systems tend to be more useful if chosen for mechanistic reasons rather than simply testing another species or organ. For example, metabolism by intact hepatocytes (Langenbach and Oglesby, 1983) can preserve elements of the cellular compartmentalization of reactions that would be altered when tissues are made into homogenates. Likewise, a system that includes a reductive reaction not encompassed by standard S9 is required for detecting the mutagenicity of some azo dyes and nitro compounds (Dellarco and Prival, 1989). Despite their usefulness, in vitro metabolic activation systems, however well refined, cannot mimic mammalian metabolism perfectly. There are differences among tissues in reactions that activate or inactivate foreign compounds, and organisms of the normal flora of the gut can contribute to metabolism in intact mammals. Agents that induce enzyme systems or otherwise alter the physiological state can also modify the metabolism of toxicants, and the balance between activation and detoxication reactions in vitro may differ from that in vivo.

An interesting development with respect to metabolic activation is the incorporation of genes encoding human enzymes into microorganisms or cell cultures. For example, the expression of human cytochrome P4501A2 in Salmonella tester strains from the Ames assay permits the activation of such promutagens as 2-aminoanthracene and 2-aminofluorene without an S9 mixture (Josephy et al., 1995). Mammalian cell lines have also been genetically engineered to express human Phase-I and Phase-II en-zymes, including those catalyzing reactions of metabolic activation (Sawada and Kamataki, 1998). Many cell lines stably expressing a single form of P450 have been established. Mutagenesis can be measured through such endpoints as HPRT mutations and cytogenetic alterations, and the cells are well suited to analyzing the contribution of different enzymes to the activation of promutagens.

Metabolic activation is so central to genetic toxicology that all mutagenicity testing programs must provide for it in the choice of assays and procedures. In special circumstances, other forms of activation may be relevant, and assays are adapted accordingly. Some chemicals are subject to photochemical activation, such that genotoxic effects depend both on the chemical and on its being irradiated with ultraviolet or visible light. Many of the assays listed in Table 9-2, including gene-mutation assays in bacteria and cultured mammalian cells, cytogenetic assays, and the comet assay, have been adapted so that they can measure photogenotoxic effects (Brendler-Schwaab et al., 2004).

DNA Damage and Repair Assays

Some assays measure DNA damage itself, rather than mutational consequences of DNA damage. They may do so directly, through such indicators as chemical adducts or strand breaks in DNA, or indirectly, through the measurement of biological repair processes. Adducts in DNA are detected by ^{32}P-postlabeling, immunological methods using antibodies against specific adducts, or fluorometric methods in the case of such fluorescent compounds as polynuclear aromatic hydrocarbons and aflatoxins (Chang et al., 1994; Kriek et al., 1998; Phillips et al., 2000). The ^{32}P-postlabeling method is highly sensitive and applicable to diverse mutagens. The measurement of adducts after human chemical exposures has proven useful in human monitoring and molecular dosimetry (Chang et al., 1994; Kriek et al., 1998; Phillips et al., 2000). DNA strand breakage can be measured by alkaline elution and electrophoretic methods (Elia et al., 1994). The applicability of DNA damage assays to rodent testes (Bentley et al., 1994) makes these methods helpful in interpreting risks to germ cells.

Single-cell gel electrophoresis, also called the comet assay, is a widely used, rapid method of measuring DNA damage (Fairbairn et al., 1995; Singh, 2000; Tice et al., 2000). In this assay cells are incorporated into agarose on slides, lysed so as to liberate their DNA, and subjected to electrophoresis. The DNA is stained with a fluorescent dye for observation and image analysis. Because broken DNA fragments migrate more quickly than larger pieces of DNA, a blur of fragments (a "comet") is observed when the DNA is extensively damaged. The extent of DNA damage can be estimated from the length and other attributes of the comet tail. Variations in the procedure permit the general detection of DNA strand breakage under alkaline conditions (Fairbairn et al., 1995; Singh, 2000; Tice et al., 2000) or the preferential detection of double-strand breaks under neutral conditions (Fairbairn et al., 1995). Although the comet assay is relatively new and needs further evaluation, it appears to be a sensitive indicator of DNA damage with broad applicability. It has been used most commonly with human lymphocytes (Fairbairn et al., 1995; Singh, 2000) and other mammalian cells (Tice et al., 2000), but it can be adapted to diverse species, including plants, worms, mollusks, fish, and amphibians (Cotelle and Férard, 1999). This adaptability suggests that it will find diverse uses in environmental genetic toxicology.

The occurrence of DNA repair can serve as an easily measured indicator of DNA damage. Repair assays have been developed in microorganisms, cultured mammalian cells, and intact mammals (Table 9-2). Greater toxicity of a chemical in DNA-repair-deficient strains than in their repair-proficient counterparts has served as an indicator of DNA damage in bacteria (e.g., $polA^-$ and $polA^+$ in E. coli or rec^- and rec^+ in Bacillus subtilis) (Hamasaki et al., 1992). The induction of bacterial SOS functions, indicated by phage induction or by colorimetry in the SOS chromotest, can similarly serve as a general indicator of genetic damage (Quillardet and Hofnung, 1993). The most common repair assay in mammalian cells is the measurement of unscheduled DNA synthesis (UDS). UDS is a measure of excision repair, and its occurrence indicates that DNA had been damaged (Madle et al., 1994). The absence of UDS, however, does not provide clear evidence that DNA has not been damaged, because some classes of damage are not readily excised, and some excisable damage may not be detected as a consequence of assay insensitivity. Though bacterial repair assays have declined in usage over the years, UDS assays continue to be used because of their applicability to cultured hepatocytes with endogenous cytochrome P450 enzyme activities and to tissues of intact animals, including hepatocytes (Madle et al., 1994) and germinal tissue (Bentley et al., 1994; Sotomayor and Sega, 2000).

Gene Mutations in Prokaryotes

The most common means of detecting mutations in microorganisms is selecting for reversion in strains that have a specific nutritional requirement differing from wild-type members of the species; such strains are called auxotrophs. For example, the widely used assay developed by Bruce Ames and his colleagues is based on measuring reversion in several histidine auxotrophs in Salmonella enterica Serovar typhimurium, commonly called Salmonella typhimurium.

In the Ames assay one measures the frequency of histidine-independent bacteria that arise in a histidine-requiring strain in the presence or absence of the chemical being tested. Auxotrophic bacteria are treated with the chemical of interest by one of several procedures (e.g., the standard plate-incorporation assay) and plated on medium that is deficient in histidine (Ames et al., 1975; Maron and Ames, 1983; Kirkland et al., 1990; Mortelmans and Zeiger, 2000). The assay is conducted using genetically different strains so that reversion by base-pair substitutions and frameshift mutations in several DNA sequence contexts can be detected and distinguished. Because Salmonella does not metabolize promutagens in the same way as mammalian tissues, the assay is generally performed in the presence and absence of a rat liver S9 metabolic activation system. Hence, the Ames assay is also called the Salmonella/microsome assay.

The principal strains of the Ames test and their characteristics are summarized in Table 9-3. In addition to the histidine alleles that provide the target for measuring mutagenesis, the Ames tester strains contain other genes and plasmids that enhance the assay. Part I of the table gives genotypes, and Part II explains the rationale for including specific genetic characteristics in the strains. Part III summarizes the principal DNA target in each strain and their mechanisms of reversion. Taken together, the Ames strains detect a broad array of mutations, and they complement one another. For example, strains TA102 and TA104, which are sensitive to agents that cause oxidative damage in DNA, detect the A:T → G:C base-pair substitutions that are not detected by hisG46 strains (Mortelmans and Zeiger, 2000). TA102 also detects agents that cause DNA crosslinks because it has

an intact excision repair system whereas the other common tester strains do not.

The most common version of the Ames assay is the plate-incorporation test (Ames et al., 1975; Maron and Ames, 1983; Mortelmans and Zeiger, 2000). In this procedure, the bacterial tester strain, the test compound (or solvent control), and the S9 metabolic activation system (or buffer for samples without S9) are added to 2 mL of molten agar containing biotin and a trace of histidine to allow a few cell divisions, mixed, and immediately poured onto the surface of a petri dish selective for histidine-independent revertants. For general testing it is recommended to use at least 3 plates per dose, 5 doses, samples with and without S9, and appropriate concurrent positive and negative controls (Mortelmans and Zeiger, 2000). Variations on the standard plate-incorporation assay confer advantages for some applications. These include a preincubation assay that facilitates the detection of unstable compounds and short-lived metabolites; a desiccator assay for testing volatile chemicals and gases; a microsuspension assay for working with small quantities of test agent; assays incorporating reductive metabolism rather than the conventional S9 system; and assays under hypoxic conditions (Mortelmans and Zeiger, 2000).

Whereas simplicity is a great merit of microbial assays, it can also be deceptive. Even assays that are simple in design and application can be performed incorrectly. For example, in the Ames assay one may see very small colonies in the petri dishes at highly toxic doses (Maron and Ames, 1983; Kirkland et al., 1990; Mortelmans and Zeiger, 2000). Counting such colonies as revertants would be an error because they may actually be nonrevertant survivors that grew on the low concentration of histidine in the plates. Were there millions of survivors, the amount of histidine would have been insufficient to allow any of them (except real revertants) to form colonies. This artifact is easily avoided by checking that there is a faint lawn of bacterial growth in the plates; one can also confirm that colonies are revertants by streaking them on medium without histidine to be sure that they grow in its absence. Such pitfalls exist in all mutagenicity tests. Therefore, anyone performing mutagenicity tests must have detailed familiarity with the laboratory application and literature of the assay and be observant about the responsiveness of the assay.

Although information from the Ames assay has become a standard in genetic toxicology testing, equivalent information can be obtained from other bacterial assays. Like the Ames assay, the WP2 tryptophan reversion assay in Escherichia coli (Kirkland et al., 1990; Mortelmans and Riccio, 2000) incorporates genetic features that enhance assay sensitivity, can accommodate S9 metabolic activation, and performs well in many laboratories. Mutations are detected by selecting for reversion of a trpE allele from Trp⁻ to Trp⁺. Its responsiveness to mutagens most closely resembles TA102 among the Ames strains (Mortelmans and Riccio, 2000).

Bacterial reversion assays are commonly used for testing purposes, but they also provide information on molecular mechanisms of mutagenesis. The broader understanding of mutational mechanisms that comes from refined genetic assays and molecular analysis of mutations can contribute to the interpretation of mutational hazards. The primary reversion mechanisms of the Ames strains, summarized in Table 9-3, were initially determined by genetic and biochemical means (Maron and Ames, 1983). An ingenious method called allele-specific colony hybridization greatly facilitated the molecular analysis of revertants in the Ames assay (Koch et al., 1994), and many spontaneous and induced revertants have been cloned or amplified by the polymerase chain reaction (PCR) and sequenced (Levine et al., 1994; DeMarini, 2000).

Table 9-3

The Ames Assay: Tester Strains and Their Characteristics

I. STANDARD TESTER STRAINS OF *SALMONELLA TYPHIMURIUM*			
STRAIN	TARGET ALLELE	CHROMOSOMAL GENOTYPE	PLASMIDS
TA1535	*hisG46*	*hisG46 rfa ΔuvrB*	None
TA100	*hisG46*	*hisG46 rfa ΔuvrB*	pKM101 (*mucAB* Ap^r)
TA1538	*hisD3052*	*hisD3052 rfa ΔuvrB*	None
TA98	*hisD3052*	*hisD3052 rfa ΔuvrB*	pKM101 (*mucAB* Ap^r)
TA1537	*hisC3076*	*hisC3076 rfa ΔuvrB*	None
TA97	*hisD6610*	*hisD6610 hisO1242 rfa ΔuvrB*	pKM101 (*mucAB* Ap^r)
TA102	*hisG428*	*hisΔ(G)8476 rfa*	pKM101 (*mucAB* Ap^r) and pAQ1 (*hisG428* Tc^r)
TA104	*hisG428*	*hisG428 rfa ΔuvrB*	pKM101 (*mucAB* Ap^r)

II. GENETIC CHARACTERISTICS OF THE AMES TESTER STRAINS	
CHARACTERISTIC	RATIONALE FOR INCLUSION IN THE TESTER STRAIN
rfa	Alters the lipopolysaccharide wall, conferring greater permeability to mutagens.
ΔuvrB	Deletes the excision repair system, increasing sensitivity to many mutagens; retention of excision in TA102 permits the detection of DNA-crosslinking agents.
mucAB	Enhances sensitivity to some mutagens whose activity depends on the SOS system.
Ap^r	Permits selection for the presence of pKM101 by ampicillin resistance.
hisO1242	Affects regulation of histidine genes, enhancing revertibility of *hisD6610* in TA97.
hisΔ(G)8476	Eliminates the chromosomal *hisG* gene, allowing detection of the reversion of *hisG428* on pAQ1 in TA102.
Tc^r	Permits selection for the presence of pAQ1 in TA102 by tetracycline resistance.

III. MECHANISMS OF REVERSION DETECTED BY THE AMES TESTER STRAINS		
STRAIN	PRIMARY TARGET*	MUTATIONS DETECTED
TA1535, TA100	GGG/CCC	Base-pair substitutions, principally those beginning at G:C base pairs (G:C → A:T; G:C → T:A; G:C → C:G), but also A:T → C:G. These strains do not detect A:T → G:C.
TA1538, TA98	CGCGCGCG/GCGCGCGC	Frameshift mutations, especially −2 frameshifts (ΔGC or ΔCG), +1 frameshifts, other small deletions, and some complex mutations.
TA1537	GGGGG/CCCCC	Frameshift mutations, mainly −1 (ΔG or ΔC; less frequently ΔT), but also some +CG frameshifts.
TA97	GGGGGG/CCCCCC	Frameshift mutations, combining the specificity of TA1537 at the primary target and with some characteristics of TA98.
TA102, TA104	TAA/ATT	Base-pair substitutions, principally those beginning at A:T base pairs (A:T → G:C; A:T → T:A; A:T → C:G), but also G:C → T:A and G:C → A:T.

*The sequences before and after the backslash represent the two complementary strands of DNA.

Part III of Table 9-3 is by necessity a simplification with respect both to targets and mechanisms of reversion of the Ames strains. Some mutations that bring about reversion to histidine independence fall outside the primary target, and the full target has been found to be as much as 76 base pairs in *hisD3052* (DeMarini *et al.*, 1998). Other revertants can arise by suppressor mutations in other genes. It has been shown that *hisG46*, *hisG428*, *hisC3076*, *hisD6610*, and *hisD3052* all revert by multiple mechanisms and that the spectrum of classes of revertants may vary depending on the mutagen, experimental conditions, and other elements of the genotype (Cebula and Koch, 1990; Prival and Cebula, 1992; DeMarini *et al.*, 1998; Mortelmans and Zeiger, 2000).

The development of Salmonella strains that are highly specific with respect to mechanisms of reversion has made the identification of particular base-pair substitutions more straightforward. These strains (TA7001–TA7006) each revert from *his⁻* to *his⁺* by a single kind of mutation (e.g., G:C to T:A), and collectively they permit the specific detection of all six possible base-pair substitutions (Gee *et al.*, 1994, 1998; Mortelmans and Zeiger, 2000).

Specific reversion assays are also available in *E. coli*. A versatile system based on reversion of *lacZ* mutations in *E. coli* permits the specific detection of all six possible base-pair substitutions (Cupples and Miller, 1989; Josephy, 2000) and frameshift mutations for which one or two bases have been added or deleted in various sequence contexts (Cupples *et al.*, 1990; Josephy, 2000). The versatility of the *lacZ* assay has been expanded through the introduction of useful characteristics into the strains parallel to those incorporated into the Ames strains. Among the features added to the *lacZ* assay are DNA repair deficiencies, permeability alterations, plasmid-enhanced mutagenesis, and enzymes of mutagen metabolism (Josephy, 2000).

Bacterial forward mutation assays, such as selections for resistance to arabinose or to purine or pyrimidine analogs in Salmonella (Jurado *et al.*, 1994; Vlasakova *et al.*, 2005), are also used in research and testing, though less extensively than reversion assays. A versatile forward mutation assay that has contributed greatly to an understanding of mechanisms of mutagenesis is the *lacI* system in *E. coli* (Calos and Miller, 1981; Halliday and Glickman, 1991).

Mutations in the *lacI* gene, which encodes the repressor of the lactose operon, are easily identified by phenotype, cloned or amplified by PCR, and sequenced. The *lacI* gene is widely used as a target for mutagenesis both in *E. coli* and in transgenic mice, and more than 30,000 *lacI* mutants had been sequenced by the mid-1990s (Mirsalis *et al.*, 1994).

Genetic Alterations in Nonmammalian Eukaryotes

Gene Mutations and Chromosome Aberrations   Many early studies of mutagenesis used yeasts, mycelial fungi, plants, and insects as experimental organisms. Even though well-characterized genetic systems permit the analysis of a diverse array of genetic alterations in these organisms (Table 9-2), they have been largely supplanted in genetic toxicology by bacterial and mammalian systems. Exceptions are to be found where the assays in nonmammalian eukaryotes permit the study of genetic endpoints that are not readily analyzed in mammals or where the organism has special attributes that fit a particular application.

The fruit fly, Drosophila, has long occupied a prominent place in genetic research. In fact, the first unequivocal evidence of chemical mutagenesis was obtained in Scotland in 1941 when Charlotte Auerbach and J.M. Robson demonstrated that mustard gas is mutagenic in Drosophila. Drosophila continues to be used in modern mutation research (Potter and Turenchalk, 2000) but its role in genetic toxicology is now more limited. The Drosophila assay of greatest historical importance is the sex-linked recessive lethal (SLRL) test. A strength of the SLRL test is that it permits the detection of recessive lethal mutations at 600–800 different loci on the X chromosome by screening for the presence or absence of wild-type males in the offspring of specifically designed crosses (Mason *et al.*, 1987). The genetic alterations include gene mutations and small deletions. The spontaneous frequency of SLRL is about 0.2%, and a significant increase over this frequency in the lineages derived from treated males indicates mutagenesis. Although it requires screening large numbers of fruit fly vials, the SLRL test yields information about mutagenesis in germ cells, which is lacking in all microbial and cell culture systems. However, means of exposure, measurement of doses, metabolism, and gametogenesis in insects differ from those in mammalian toxicology, thereby introducing doubt about the relevance of Drosophila assays to human genetic risk. Drosophila assays are also available for studying the induction of chromosome abnormalities in germ cells, specifically heritable translocations (Mason *et al.*, 1987) and sex-chromosome loss (Osgood and Cyr, 1998).

Genetic and cytogenetic assays in plants (Grant, 1994) also occupy a more restricted niche in modern genetic toxicology than they did years ago. However, plant assays continue to find use in special applications, such as in situ monitoring for mutagens and exploration of the metabolism of promutagens by agricultural plants. In situ monitoring entails looking for evidence of mutagenesis in organisms that are grown in the environment of interest. Natural populations of organisms can also be examined for evidence of genetic damage (Klekowski *et al.*, 1994; Jha, 2004). For example, frequencies of chlorophyll mutations in red mangroves have been correlated with concentrations of polycyclic hydrocarbons in the sediments in which they were growing (Klekowski *et al.*, 1994). Although studies of natural populations are of obvious interest, they require utmost precaution when characterizing the environments and defining appropriate control populations.

Mitotic Recombination   Assays in nonmammalian eukaryotes continue to be important in the study of induced recombination. Recombinogenic effects in yeast have long been used as a general indicator of genetic damage (Zimmermann *et al.*, 1984), and interest in the induction of recombination has increased as recombinational events have been implicated in the etiology of cancer (Sengstag, 1994; Bishop and Schiestl, 2003). The widely used assays for recombinogens are those that detect mitotic crossing over and mitotic gene conversion in the yeast *Saccharomyces cerevisiae* (Zimmermann, 1992). Hundreds of chemicals have been tested for recombinogenic effects in straightforward yeast assays. In yeast strain D7, for example, mitotic crossing over involving the *ade2* locus is detected on the basis of pink and red colony color, and mitotic gene conversion at the *trp5* locus is detected by selection for growth without tryptophan. Strategies have also been devised to detect recombinogenic effects in human lymphocytes (Turner *et al.*, 2003), other mammalian cells, mice, plants, and mycelial fungi (Hoffmann, 1994). At least 350 chemicals have been evaluated in Drosophila somatic cell assays in which recombinogenic effects are detected by examining wings or eyes for regions in which recessive alleles are expressed in heterozygotes (Vogel *et al.*, 1999).

Gene Mutations in Mammals

Gene Mutations In Vitro   Mutagenicity assays in cultured mammalian cells have some of the same advantages as microbial assays with respect to speed and cost, and they use similar approaches. The most widely used assays for gene mutations in mammalian cells detect forward mutations that confer resistance to a toxic chemical. For example, mutations in the gene encoding hypoxanthine-guanine phosphoribosyltransferase (HPRT enzyme; *HPRT* gene) confer resistance to the purine analogue 6-thioguanine (Walker *et al.*, 1999), and thymidine kinase mutations (TK enzyme; *TK* gene) confer resistance to the pyrimidine analogue trifluorothymidine (Clements, 2000). HPRT and TK mutations may therefore be detected by attempting to grow cells in the presence of purine analogues and pyrimidine analogues, respectively. For historical reasons, HPRT assays have most commonly been conducted in Chinese hamster cells or human cells, while TK assays have used mouse lymphoma cells or human cells. Forward-mutation assays typically respond to diverse mechanisms of mutagenesis, but there are exceptions. For example, a specific alteration in the target gene confers resistance to ouabain, but alterations that eliminate the gene function are lethal (DeMarini *et al.*, 1989). Because the ability to detect various kinds of mutations is desirable, assays that do not do so, such as ouabain resistance, are not useful for general mutagenicity testing.

Gene Mutations In Vivo   In vivo assays involve treating intact animals and analyzing appropriate tissues for genetic effects. The choice of suitable doses, treatment procedures, controls, and sample sizes is critical in the conduct of in vivo tests. Mutations may be detected either in somatic cells or in germ cells. The latter are of special interest with respect to risk for future generations.

The mouse spot test is a traditional genetic assay for gene mutations in somatic cells (Styles and Penman, 1985; Lambert *et al.*, 2005). Visible spots of altered phenotype in mice heterozygous for coat color genes indicate mutations in the progenitor cells of the altered regions. Although straightforward in design, the spot test is less used today than other somatic cell assays or than its germ-cell counterpart, the mouse specific-locus test.

Cells that are amenable to positive selection for mutants when collected from intact animals form the basis for efficient in vivo mutation-detection assays analogous to those in mammalian cell cultures. Lymphocytes with mutations in the HPRT gene are readily detected by selection for resistance to 6-thioguanine. The *hprt* assay in mice and rats, and *HPRT* in monkeys (Casciano *et al.*, 1999; Walker *et al.*, 1999) is of special interest because it permits comparisons to the measurement of *HPRT* mutations in humans, an important assay in human mutational monitoring (Cole and Skopek, 1994; Albertini and Hayes, 1997).

Besides determining whether agents are mutagenic, mutation assays provide information on mechanisms of mutagenesis that contributes to an understanding of mutational hazards. Base-pair substitutions and large deletions, which may be indistinguishable on the basis of phenotype, can be differentiated through the use of probes for the target gene and Southern blotting, in that base substitutions are too subtle to be detectable on the blots, whereas gross structural alterations are visible (Cole and Skopek, 1994; Albertini and Hayes, 1997). Molecular analysis has been used to determine proportions of mutations ascribable to deletions and other structural alterations in several assays, including the specific-locus test for germ-cell mutations in mice (Favor, 1999) and the human *HPRT* assay (Cole and Skopek, 1994). Gene mutations have been characterized at the molecular level by DNA sequence analysis both in transgenic rodents (Mirsalis *et al.*, 1994; Lambert *et al.*, 2005) and in endogenous mammalian genes (Cariello and Skopek, 1993). Many *HPRT* mutations from human cells in vitro and in vivo have been analyzed at the molecular level and classified with respect to base-pair substitutions, frameshifts, small deletions, large deletions, and other alterations (Cole and Skopek, 1994).

Transgenic Assays   Transgenic animals are products of DNA technology in which the animal contains foreign DNA sequences that have been added to the genome. The foreign DNA is represented in all the somatic cells of the animal and is transmitted in the germ line to progeny. Mutagenicity assays in transgenic animals combine in vivo metabolic activation and pharmacodynamics with simple microbial detection systems, and they permit the analysis of mutations induced in diverse mammalian tissues (Mirsalis *et al.*, 1994; Lambert *et al.*, 2005).

The transgenic animals that have figured most heavily in genetic toxicology are rodents that carry *lac* genes from *E. coli*. The bacterial genes were introduced into mice or rats by injecting a vector carrying the genes into fertilized oocytes (Mirsalis *et al.*, 1994; Lambert *et al.*, 2005). The strains are commonly referred to by their commercial names—the "Big Blue® mouse" and "Big Blue® rat," which use *lacI* as a target for mutagenesis, and the "Muta™ Mouse," which uses *lacZ* (Lambert *et al.*, 2005). After mutagenic treatment of the transgenic animals, the *lac* genes are recovered from the animal, packaged in phage λ, and transferred to *E. coli* for mutational analysis. Mutant plaques are identified on the basis of phenotype, and mutant frequencies can be calculated for different tissues of the treated animals (Mirsalis *et al.*, 1994). The *cII* locus may be used as a second target gene in both the *lacZ* and *lacI* transgenic assays (Swiger, 2001; Lambert *et al.*, 2005). Its use offers technical advantages as a small, easily sequenced target in which mutations are detected by positive selection, and it permits interesting comparisons both within and between assays.

A *lacZ* transgenic mouse, which uses a plasmid-based system rather than a phage vector is available and has the advantage

that deletion mutants are more readily recovered than in the phage-based *lac* systems (Lambert *et al.*, 2005). Deletions may also be detected in the *gpt delta* mouse and rat using a phage vector system. These transgenic animals detect two kinds of genetic events in two targets—point mutations in *gpt* detected by resistance to 6-thioguanine and *spi* deletions that permit growth on P2 lysogens (Okada *et al.*, 1999; Lambert *et al.*, 2005). Other transgenic assays are under development and offer the prospect of expanding the versatility of such assays (Lambert *et al.*, 2005).

Various mutagens, including alkylating agents, nitrosamines, procarbazine, cyclophosphamide, and polycyclic aromatic hydrocarbons have been studied in transgenic mouse assays, and mutant frequencies have been analyzed in such diverse tissues as liver, skin, spleen, kidney, bladder, small intestine, bone marrow, and testis (Lambert *et al.*, 2005). Tissue-specific mutant frequencies can be compared to the distribution of adducts among tissues and to the site specificity of carcinogenesis (Mirsalis *et al.*, 1994). An important issue that remains to be resolved is the extent to which transgenes resemble endogenous genes. Although their mutational responses tend to be comparable (Lambert *et al.*, 2005), some differences have been noted (Burkhart and Malling, 1993; Lambert *et al.*, 2005), and questions have been raised about the relevance of mutations that might be recovered from dying or dead animal tissues (Burkhart and Malling, 1994). Therefore, transgenic animals offer promising models for the study of chemical mutagenesis, but they must be further characterized before their ultimate place in hazard assessment is clear.

Mammalian Cytogenetic Assays

Chromosome Aberrations   Cytogenetic assays rely on the use of microscopy for the direct observation of the effects of interest. This approach differs sharply from the indirectness of traditional genetic assays in which one observes a phenotype and reaches conclusions about genes. It is only through the addition of DNA sequencing that genetic assays can approach the directness of cytogenetic assays.

In conventional cytogenetics, metaphase analysis is used to detect chromosomal anomalies, especially unstable chromosome and chromatid aberrations. A key factor in the design of cytogenetic assays is obtaining appropriate cell populations for treatment and analysis (Preston *et al.*, 1981; Ishidate *et al.*, 1988; Kirkland *et al.*, 1990; Galloway *et al.*, 1994). Cells with a stable, well-defined karyotype, short generation time, low chromosome number, and large chromosomes are ideal for cytogenetic analysis. For this reason, Chinese hamster cells have been used widely in cytogenetic testing. Other cells are also suitable, and human cells, especially peripheral lymphocytes, have been used extensively. Cells should be treated during a sensitive period of the cell cycle (typically S), and aberrations should be analyzed at the first mitotic division after treatment so that the sensitivity of the assay is not reduced by unstable aberrations being lost during cell division. Examples of chromosome aberrations are shown in Fig. 9-4.

Cytogenetic assays require careful attention to growth conditions, controls, doses, treatment conditions, and time intervals between treatment and the sampling of cells for analysis (Kirkland *et al.*, 1990). Data collection is a critical part of cytogenetic analysis. It is essential that sufficient cells be analyzed because a negative result in a small sample is inconclusive. Results should be recorded for specific classes of aberrations, not just an overall index of aberrations per cell. The need for detailed data is all the more important because of nonuniformity in the classification of aberrations and

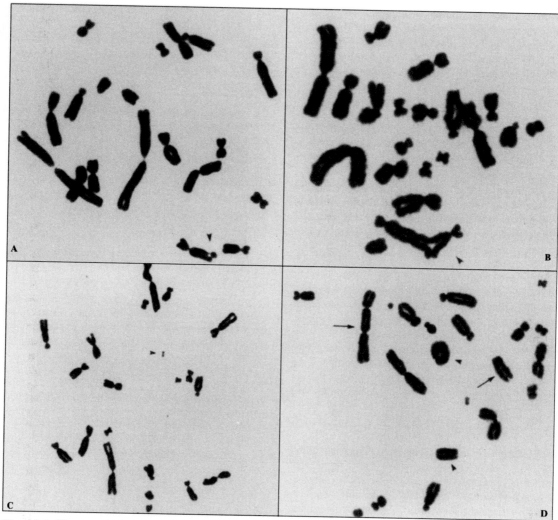

Figure 9-4. *Chromosome aberrations induced by X-rays in Chinese hamster ovary (CHO) cells.*

A. A chromatid deletion (▶). *B.* A chromatid exchange called a triradial (▶). *C.* A small interstitial deletion (▶) that resulted from chromosome breakage. *D.* A metaphase with more than one aberration: a centric ring plus an acentric fragment (▶) and a dicentric chromosome plus an acentric fragment (→).

disagreement on whether small achromatic (i.e., unstained) gaps in chromosomes are true chromosomal aberrations. Gaps should be quantified but not pooled with other aberrations.

In interpreting results on the induction of chromosome aberrations in cell cultures, one must be alert to the possibility of artifacts associated with extreme assay conditions because aberrations induced under such circumstances may not be a reflection of a chemical-specific genotoxicity (Scott *et al.*, 1991; Galloway, 2000). Questionable positive results have been found at highly cytotoxic doses (Galloway, 2000), high osmolality, and pH extremes (Scott *et al.*, 1991). The possibility that metabolic activation systems may be genotoxic also warrants scrutiny (Scott *et al.*, 1991). Although excessively high doses may lead to artifactual positive responses, the failure to test to a sufficiently high dose also undermines the utility of a test. Therefore, testing should be extended to a dose at which there is some cytotoxicity, such as a reduction in the mitotic index (the proportion of cells in division), or to an arbitrary limit of about 10 mM if the chemical is nontoxic (Kirkland *et al.*, 1990).

In vivo assays for chromosome aberrations involve treating intact animals and later collecting cells for cytogenetic analysis (Preston *et al.*, 1981; Kirkland *et al.*, 1990; Tice *et al.*, 1994). The main advantage of in vivo assays is that they include mammalian metabolism, DNA repair, and pharmacodynamics. The target is typically a tissue from which large numbers of dividing cells are easily prepared for analysis. Bone marrow from rats, mice, or Chinese hamsters is most commonly used. Peripheral lymphocytes are another suitable target when stimulated to divide with a mitogen such as phytohemagglutinin. Effective testing requires dosages and routes of administration that ensure adequate exposure of the target cells, proper intervals between treatment and collecting cells, and sufficient numbers of animals and cells analyzed (Kirkland *et al.*, 1990).

An important development in cytogenetic analysis is fluorescence in situ hybridization (FISH), in which a nucleic acid probe is hybridized to complementary sequences in chromosomal DNA. The probe is labeled with a fluorescent dye so that the chromosomal location to which it binds is visible by fluorescence microscopy. Composite probes have been developed from sequences unique to specific human chromosomes, giving a uniform fluorescent label over the entire chromosome. Slides prepared for standard metaphase analysis are suitable for FISH after they have undergone a simple denaturation procedure. The use of whole-chromosome probes is commonly called "chromosome painting" (Speicher and Carter, 2005).

Chromosome painting facilitates cytogenetic analysis, because aberrations are easily detected by the number of fluorescent regions in a painted metaphase. For example, if chromosome 4 were painted with a probe while the other chromosomes were counterstained in a different color, one would see only the two homologues of chromosome 4 in the color of the probe in a normal cell. However, if there were a translocation or a dicentric chromosome and fragment involving chromosome 4, one would see three areas of fluorescence—one normal chromosome 4 and the two pieces involved in the chromosome rearrangement. Aberrations are detected only in the painted portion of the genome, but this disadvantage can be offset by painting a few chromosomes simultaneously with probes of different colors (Tucker *et al.*, 1993b). FISH reduces the time and technical skill required to detect chromosome aberrations, and it permits the scoring of stable aberrations, such as translocations and insertions, that are not readily detected in traditional metaphase analysis without special labeling techniques. Using FISH, some chromosomal analysis can even be conducted in interphase cells. Although FISH is not routinely used in genotoxicity testing, it is a valuable research tool for studying clastogens and is having a substantial impact in monitoring human populations for chromosomal damage.

Micronuclei Metaphase analysis is time consuming and requires considerable skill, so simpler cytogenetic assays have been developed, of which micronucleus assays have become especially important. Micronuclei are membrane-bounded structures that contain chromosomal fragments, or sometimes whole chromosomes, that were not incorporated into a daughter nucleus at mitosis. Because micronuclei usually represent acentric chromosomal fragments, they are most commonly used as simple indicators of chromosomal damage. However, the ability to detect micronuclei containing whole chromosomes has led to their use for detecting aneuploidy as well. Micronucleus assays may be conducted in primary cultures of human lymphocytes (Fenech, 2000; Fenech *et al.*, 2003), mammalian cell lines (Kirsch-Volders *et al.*, 2000, 2003), or mammals in vivo (Heddle *et al.*, 1991; Hayashi *et al.*, 2000; Krishna and Hayashi, 2000; Hamada *et al.*, 2001).

Micronucleus assays in lymphocytes have been greatly improved by the cytokinesis-block technique in which cell division is inhibited with cytochalasin B, resulting in binucleate and multinucleate cells (Fenech, 2000; Kirsch-Volders *et al.*, 2000; Fenech *et al.*, 2003). In the cytokinesis-block assay in human lymphocytes, nondividing (G$_0$) cells are treated with ionizing radiation or a radiomimetic chemical and then stimulated to divide with the mitogen phytohemagglutinin. Alternatively, the lymphocytes may be exposed to the mitogen first, so that the subsequent mutagenic treatment with radiation or chemicals includes the S period of the cell cycle. In either case, cytochalasin B is added for the last part of the culture period, and micronuclei are counted only in binucleate cells so as to ensure that the cells have undergone a single nuclear division that is essential for micronucleus development. The assay thereby avoids confusion owing to differences in cellular proliferation kinetics. Although micronuclei resulting

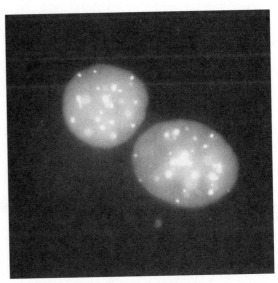

Figure 9-5. Micronucleus in a human lymphocyte.

The cytochalasin B method was used to inhibit cytokinesis that resulted in a binucleate nucleus. The micronucleus resulted from failure of an acentric chromosome fragment or a whole chromosome being included in a daughter nucleus following cell division. (Figure courtesy of James Allen, Jill Barnes, and Barbara Collins.)

from chromosome breakage comprise the principal endpoint in the cytokinesis-block micronucleus assay, the method can also provide evidence of aneuploidy, chromosome rearrangements that form nucleoplasmic bridges, inhibition of cell division, necrosis, apoptosis, and excision-repairable lesions (Fenech, 2000; Fenech *et al.*, 2003). Micronuclei in a binucleate human lymphocyte are shown in Fig. 9-5.

The in vivo micronucleus assay is most often performed by counting micronuclei in immature (polychromatic) erythrocytes in the bone marrow of treated mice, but it may also be based on peripheral blood (Heddle *et al.*, 1991; Hayashi *et al.*, 2000; Krishna and Hayashi, 2000; Hamada *et al.*, 2001). Micronuclei remain in the cell when the nucleus is extruded in the maturation of erythroblasts. In vivo micronucleus assays are increasingly used in genotoxicity testing as a substitute for bone marrow metaphase chromosome analysis. Micronucleus assays in mammalian tissues other than bone marrow and blood are useful for mechanistic studies and research but are less often applied to genotoxicity testing (Hayashi *et al.*, 2000).

Sister Chromatid Exchanges Sister chromatid exchanges (SCE), in which there has been an apparently reciprocal exchange of segments between the two chromatids of a chromosome, are visible cytologically through differential staining of chromatids. Figure 9-6 shows SCE in human cells. Many mutagens induce SCE in cultured cells and in mammals in vivo (Tucker *et al.*, 1993a). Despite the convenience and responsiveness of SCE assays, data on SCE are less informative than data on chromosome aberrations. There is uncertainty about the underlying mechanisms by which SCEs are formed and how DNA damage or perturbations of DNA synthesis stimulate their formation (Preston, 1991). SCE assays are therefore best regarded as general indicators of mutagen exposure, analogous to DNA damage and repair assays, rather than measures of a mutagenic effect.

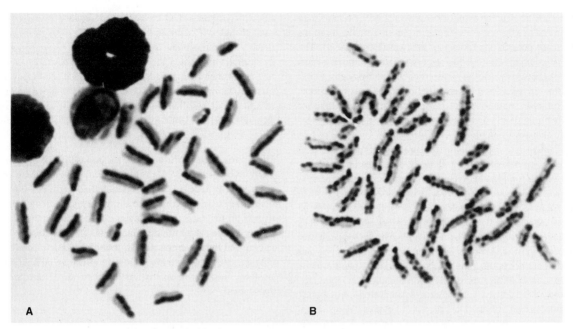

Figure 9-6. Sister chromatid exchanges (SCEs) in human lymphocytes.

A. SCE in untreated cell. *B*. SCE in cell exposed to ethyl carbamate. The treatment results in a very large increase in the number of SCE. (Figure courtesy of James Allen and Barbara Collins.)

Aneuploidy Although assays based on the underlying mechanisms of the induction of aneuploidy are not yet as refined as those for gene mutations and chromosome aberrations, they are being developed (Aardema *et al.*, 1998). Some of the methods are restricted to specific targets, such as the mitotic spindle in an assay for effects on the polymerization of tubulin in vitro (Parry, 1993). Most, however, measure aneuploidy itself and should therefore encompass all relevant cellular targets. Assays include chromosome counting (Aardema *et al.*, 1998), the detection of micronuclei that contain kinetochores (Natarajan, 1993; Aardema *et al.*, 1998; Fenech, 2000), and the observation of abnormal spindles or spindle–chromosome associations in cells in which spindles and chromosomes have been differentially stained (Parry, 1998). FISH-based assays have also been developed for the assessment of aneuploidy in interphase somatic cells (Rupa *et al.*, 1997) and in sperm (Russo, 2000; Wyrobek *et al.*, 2005).

A complication in chromosome counting is that a metaphase may lack chromosomes because they were lost during cell preparation for analysis, rather than having been absent from the living cell. To avoid this artifact, cytogeneticists generally use extra chromosomes (i.e., hyperploidy) rather than missing chromosomes (i.e., hypoploidy) as an indicator of aneuploidy in chromosome preparations from mammalian cell cultures (Galloway and Ivett, 1986; Aardema *et al.*, 1998) or mouse bone marrow (Adler, 1993). A possible means of circumventing this difficulty is growing and treating cells on a glass surface and then making chromosome preparations in situ, rather than dropping cells onto slides from a cell suspension. By counting chromosomes in intact cells, one can collect data for both hyperploidy and hypoploidy (Natarajan, 1993). It has been suggested that counting polyploid cells, which is technically straightforward, may be an efficient way to detect aneugens (Aardema *et al.*, 1998), but there remains some disagreement on the point (Parry, 1998).

Micronucleus assays can detect aneugens as well as clastogens. Micronuclei that contain whole chromosomes tend to be somewhat larger than those containing chromosome fragments, but the two categories are not readily distinguished in typically stained preparations (Natarajan, 1993). However, the presence of the spindle attachment region of a chromosome (kinetochore) or of centromeric DNA in a micronucleus can serve as an indicator that it contains a whole chromosome. Aneuploidy may therefore be detected by means of antikinetochore antibodies with a fluorescent label or FISH with a probe for centromere-specific DNA (Lynch and Parry, 1993; Natarajan, 1993; Fenech, 2000). Micronuclei containing kinetochores or centromeric DNA may be detected in cultured cells (Lynch and Parry, 1993; Aardema *et al.*, 1998; Fenech, 2000) and in mouse bone marrow in vivo (Heddle *et al.*, 1991; Adler, 1993). Frequencies of micronuclei ascribable to aneuploidy and to clastogenic effects may therefore be determined concurrently by tabulating micronuclei with and without kinetochores.

Germ Cell Mutagenesis

Gene Mutations Germ-cell mutagenesis assays are of special interest as indicators of genetic damage that can enter the gene pool and be transmitted through generations. Mammalian germ-cell assays provide the best basis for assessing risks to human germ cells and therefore hold a central place in genetic toxicology despite their relative complexity and expense. The design of the test must compensate for the fact that mutations occur at low frequency, and even the simplest animal systems face a problem of there being a sufficiently large sample size. One can easily screen millions of bacteria or cultured cells by selection techniques, but screening large numbers of mice poses practical limitations. Therefore, germ-cell assays must offer a straightforward, unequivocal identification of mutants with minimal labor.

The mouse specific-locus test detects recessive mutations that produce easily analyzed, visible phenotypes (coat pigmentation and ear size) conferred by seven genes (Russell and Shelby, 1985;

Ehling, 1991; Russell and Russell, 1992; Favor, 1999). Mutants may be classified as having point mutations or chromosomal alterations on the basis of genetic and molecular analysis (Favor, 1999). The assay has been important in assessing genetic risks of ionizing radiation and has been used to study various chemical mutagens. Other mouse germ-cell assays use different indicators of gene mutations, such as dominant mutations that cause skeletal abnormalities or cataracts (Ehling, 1991) and recessive mutations that cause electrophoretic changes in proteins (Lewis, 1991).

Mammalian assays permit the measurement of mutagenesis at different germ-cell stages (Favor, 1999). Late stages of spermatogenesis are often found to be sensitive to mutagenesis, but spermatocytes, spermatids, and spermatozoa are transitory. Mutagenesis in stem-cell spermatogonia and resting oocytes is of special interest in genetic risk assessment because of the persistence of these stages throughout reproductive life. Chemical mutagens show specificity with respect to germ-cell stages. For example, ethylnitrosourea and chlorambucil are both potent mutagens in the mouse specific-locus test, but the former induces primarily point mutations in spermatogonia, whereas the latter mostly induces deletions in spermatids (Russell and Russell, 1992). The ratio of deletions to point mutations is not only a function of the nature of the mutagen but depends on germ-cell stage, as some mutagens induce higher proportions of gross alterations in late stages of spermatogenesis than in spermatogonia (Lewis, 1991; Favor, 1999; Russell, 2004).

There is currently no unequivocal evidence of induced gene mutations in human germ cells, but studies in mice leave little doubt about the susceptibility of mammalian germ cells to mutagenesis by radiation and chemicals. New molecular methods, particularly those involving the assessment of changes in tandem repeat loci (reviewed in Yauk, 2004), hold great promise for the development of systems that will permit the efficient detection of germ-cell mutations in humans. The development of such methods in other species is also important, in that it permits in situ monitoring for environmental mutagens (Yauk, 2004) and the quantification of mutagenesis after controlled exposures of laboratory animals using systems parallel to those being developed for human monitoring (Wu et al., 2006).

Chromosomal Alterations Cytogenetic assays in germ cells are not routinely included in mutagenicity testing, but they are an important source of information for assessing risks to future generations posed by the induction of chromosome aberrations. Metaphase analysis of germ cells is feasible in rodent spermatogonia, spermatocytes, or oocytes (Kirkland et al., 1990; Tease, 1992; Russo, 2000). A germ-cell micronucleus assay, in which chromosomal damage induced in meiosis is measured by observation of rodent spermatids, has also been developed (Hayashi et al., 2000; Russo, 2000).

Aneuploidy originating in mammalian germ cells may be detected cytologically through chromosome counting for hyperploidy (Allen et al., 1986; Adler, 1993; Aardema et al., 1998) or genetically in the mouse sex-chromosome loss test (Russell and Shelby, 1985; Allen et al., 1986), but these methods are not widely used in toxicological testing. A promising development is the detection of aneuploidy in the sperm of mice or rats by FISH with chromosome-specific probes (Russo, 2000; Wyrobek et al., 2005). The presence of two fluorescent spots indicates the presence of an extra copy of the chromosome identified by the probe; probes for several chromosomes are used simultaneously so that aneuploid sperm are distinguishable from diploid sperm.

Besides cytological observation, indirect evidence for chromosome aberrations is obtained in the mouse heritable transloca-

tion assay, which measures reduced fertility in the offspring of treated males (Russell and Shelby, 1985). This presumptive evidence of chromosomal rearrangements can be confirmed through cytogenetic analysis. Data from the mouse heritable translocation test in postmeiotic male germ cells have been used in an attempt to quantify human germ-cell risk for ethylene oxide, a mutagen used as a fumigant, sterilizing agent, and reactant in chemical syntheses (Rhomberg et al., 1990; Preston et al., 1995).

Dominant Lethal Mutations The mouse or rat dominant lethal assay (Adler et al., 1994) offers an extensive database on the induction of genetic damage in mammalian germ cells. In the most commonly used version of the assay, males are treated on an acute or subchronic basis with the agent of interest and then mated with virgin females at appropriate intervals. The females are killed and necropsied during pregnancy so that embryonic mortality may be characterized and quantified. Most dominant lethal mutations, manifested as intrauterine deaths, are thought to arise from chromosomal anomalies.

Development of Testing Strategies

Concern about adverse effects of mutation on human health, principally carcinogenesis and the induction of transmissible damage in germ cells, has provided the impetus to identify environmental mutagens. Priorities must be set for testing, because it is not feasible to conduct multiple tests of all chemicals to which people are exposed. Such factors as production volumes, intended uses, the extent of human exposure, environmental distribution, and effects that may be anticipated on the basis of chemical structure or previous testing must be considered in order to ensure that compounds with the greatest potential for adverse effects receive the most comprehensive study. The most obvious use of genetic toxicology assays is screening chemicals to detect mutagens, but they are also used to obtain information on mutagenic mechanisms and dose–responses that contribute to an evaluation of hazards. Besides testing pure chemicals, environmental samples are tested because many mutagens exist in complex mixtures (DeMarini 1998; Ohe et al., 2003; White, 2004). The analysis of complex mixtures often requires a combination of mutagenicity assays and refined analytical methods (White, 2004; Hewitt and Marvin, 2005).

The first indication that a chemical is a mutagen often lies in chemical structure. Potential electrophilic sites in a molecule serve as an alert to possible mutagenicity and carcinogenicity, because such sites confer reactivity with nucleophilic sites in DNA (Tennant and Ashby, 1991). Attempts to formalize the structural prediction through automated computer programs have not yet led to an ability to predict mutagenicity and carcinogenicity of new chemicals with great accuracy (Richard, 1998; Snyder et al., 2004), but developmental work on such systems continues (Votano et al., 2004). Moreover, structural alerts in combination with critical interpretation are a valuable adjunct to mutagenicity testing (Tennant and Ashby, 1991; Ashby and Paton, 1993). Although informative, structural alerts cannot eliminate the need for biological data, and they must be used with cognizance of other factors that can influence the effects of a chemical. Factors that may reduce the likelihood of mutagenicity or carcinogenicity of a structurally alerting compound are steric hindrance of reactive or potentially reactive substituents, metabolism, toxicity, and substituents that enhance the chemical's excretion (Ashby, 1994). Moreover, some agents that lack structural alerts may stimulate mutagenesis indirectly by such mechanisms as the generation of radicals that cause oxidative DNA damage (Clayson *et al.*, 1994).

Assessment of a chemical's genotoxicity requires data from well-characterized assays. Assays are said to be validated when they have been shown to perform reproducibly and reliably with many compounds from diverse chemical classes in several laboratories. An evaluation of test performance, however, sometimes extends beyond determining whether the assay effectively detects the specific endpoint that it actually measures to whether it is predictive of other endpoints of interest. For example, there is great interest in the ability of mutagenicity tests, which do not measure carcinogenicity per se, to predict whether chemicals are carcinogens.

Mutagenicity testing, combined with an evaluation of chemical structure, has been found to identify a large proportion of trans-species, multiple-site carcinogens (Tennant and Ashby, 1991; Gold *et al.*, 1993). In contrast, some carcinogens are not detected as mutagens. Putatively nongenotoxic carcinogens often give responses that are more specific with respect to species, sites, and conditions (Ashby and Paton, 1993; Gold *et al.*, 1993). In predicting carcinogenicity, one should consider both the sensitivity and the specificity of an assay. Sensitivity refers to the proportion of carcinogens that are positive in the assay, whereas specificity is the proportion of noncarcinogens that are negative (Tennant *et al.*, 1987; McGregor *et al.*, 1999). Sensitivity and specificity both contribute to the predictive reliability of an assay. The commonly held view that deficiencies in the sensitivity or specificity of individual assays may be circumvented by using assays in complementary combinations called tiers or batteries has fallen into disfavor because, rather than offsetting each other's strengths and weaknesses, genetic toxicology assays are often consistent with one another (Tennant *et al.*, 1987; Ashby and Tennant, 1991; Kim and Margolin, 1999).

Strategies for testing have evolved over the last few decades, such that data from a few well-chosen assays are now considered sufficient (MacGregor *et al.*, 2000). Rather than trying to assemble extensive batteries of complementary assays, it is prudent to emphasize mechanistic considerations in choosing assays. Such an approach makes a sensitive assay for gene mutations (e.g., the Ames assay) and an assay for clastogenic effects in mammals pivotal in the evaluation of genotoxicity, and this is the basis for our highlighting these assays in Table 9-1. The Ames assay has performed reliably with hundreds of compounds in laboratories throughout the world. Other bacterial assays and mammalian cell assays also provide useful information on gene mutations. Beyond gene mutations, one should evaluate damage at the chromosomal level with a mammalian in vitro or in vivo cytogenetic assay. Cytogenetic assays in rodents are especially useful for this purpose because they combine a well-validated genetic assay with mammalian pharmacodynamics and metabolism. The other assays in Table 9-1 offer an extensive database on chemical mutagenesis (i.e., Drosophila SLRL), a unique genetic endpoint (i.e., aneuploidy; mitotic recombination), applicability to diverse organisms and tissues (i.e., DNA damage assays, such as the comet assay), or special importance in the assessment of genetic risk (i.e., germ cell assays). The more extensive listing of assays in Table 9-2 provides references that can be helpful in interpreting genetic toxicology data that can be found in the scientific literature.

HUMAN POPULATION MONITORING

For cancer risk assessment considerations, the human data utilized most frequently, in the absence of epidemiologic data, are those collected from genotoxicity/mutagenicity assessments in human populations. The studies conducted most frequently are for chromosome aberrations, micronuclei, and SCEs in peripheral lymphocytes. Cytogenetic alterations have also been assessed in a small number of bone marrow samples. Mutations at the *HPRT* locus have been assessed in peripheral lymphocytes, and glycophorin A variants have been studied in red blood cells.

An important component of any population monitoring study is the selection of the study groups, namely those individuals who are potentially exposed and the matched unexposed controls. The size of each study group should be sufficiently large to avoid any confounder having undue influence. Certain characteristics should be matched among exposed and unexposed groups. These include age, sex, smoking status, and general dietary features. Certain characteristics are exclusionary, namely current or recent medication, radiation exposure, and certain illnesses. It is possible to develop a lengthy list of additional possible confounders of response that would make the selection of suitable study groups very difficult indeed. Study groups of 20 or more individuals can be used as a reasonable substitute for exact matching because confounders will be less influential on chromosome alteration or mutation frequency in larger groups, as mentioned above (discussed in Au *et al.*, 1998). In some instances, it might be informative to compare exposed groups with a historical control, as well as to a concurrent control.

The magnitude of different known confounders varies considerably among studies, based in part on the size of the study populations. Some general indication of the magnitude of the effects of age and smoking status on the frequencies of chromosome aberrations and SCE is presented to illustrate the importance of accounting for confounders in the design of a population monitoring study. The comparisons presented are for large studies only. For chromosome aberrations, the frequency of aberrations has been reported in one large study to be about 50% higher in smokers (1.5 aberrations per 100 cells in smokers vs. 1.0 per 100 cells in the nonsmokers) (Galloway *et al.*, 1986) and in another no difference between smokers and nonsmokers (Bender *et al.*, 1988). The complete data set has been reviewed by Au *et al.* (1998). In general, the frequency of SCE is increased by about one SCE per cell in smokers compared with nonsmokers (Bender *et al.*, 1988; Barale *et al.*, 1998). The study by Barale *et al.* (1998) also reported a dose–response association between SCE frequency and smoking level.

The frequency of chromosome aberrations, particularly chromosome-type (reciprocal) exchanges, has been shown to increase with age of subject (Tucker and Moore, 1996). Galloway *et al.* (1986) reported an increase from 0.8 per 100 cells at about 25 years of age to about 1.5 at 60. Bender *et al.* (1988) reported an increase with age only for chromosome-type dicentric aberrations, but the increase over a broad age range was small and just statistically significant. Ramsey *et al.* (1995), using chromosome painting techniques, reported that individuals 50 years and older had frequencies of stable aberrations, dicentrics, and acentric fragments that were 10.6-fold, 3.3-fold, and 2.9-fold, respectively, greater than the frequency in cord bloods. Bender *et al.* (1998) did not find an increase in SCE frequency with the increasing age of the subject. The differences among the results from these large control studies emphasize the difficulty of adequately accounting for confounders (age and smoking presented here) when only a small control group is used, as is frequently the case.

Similar sources of variation have been identified for the monitoring of individuals for *HPRT* mutations. The data are reviewed in detail by Albertini and Hayes (1997). There is less information on sources of variation of glycophorin A (GPA) variants, although quite considerable interindividual variation exists (reviewed in Cole and Skopek, 1994; Kyoizumi *et al.*, 2005).

For cytogenetic assays (chromosome aberrations, SCEs, and micronuclei) the alterations are produced as a consequence of errors of DNA replication, as discussed in previous sections. From the nature of the alterations, assessed in traditional cytogenetic assays, in which nontransmissible alterations are analyzed, it can be established that these alterations were produced at the first in vitro S phase. Irrespective of the duration of exposure, the frequency of cytogenetic alterations will be proportional to that fraction of the DNA damage that remains at the time of in vitro DNA replication. All the DNA damage induced by potent clastogens that results in chromosome alterations is repaired within a relatively short time after exposure for G_0 human lymphocytes. Thus, for chronic exposures the lymphocyte cytogenetic assay as typically conducted is insensitive.

It is now possible to analyze reciprocal translocations using FISH methods (reviewed in Tucker *et al.*, 1997; Kleinerman *et al.*, 2006), and because this aberration type is transmissible from cell generation to generation, its frequency can be representative of an accumulation over time of exposure. The importance of this is that stable chromosome aberrations observed in peripheral lymphocytes exposed in vivo, but assessed following in vitro culture, are produced in vivo in hematopoietic stem cells or other precursor cells of the peripheral lymphocytes pool. To date, population cytogenetic monitoring studies involving the analysis of reciprocal translocations in chemically exposed individuals or radiation-exposed individuals have been conducted quite rarely (Lucas *et al.*, 1992; Smith *et al.*, 1998; Kleinerman *et al.*, 2006). The overall sensitivity of the FISH analysis of reciprocal translocations for assessing effects of chronic, low level of exposure to chemical clastogens has not been established. However, a cautionary note is provided by the study of Director *et al.* (1998), who showed that there was no increase in reciprocal translocations assessed by FISH following exposure to cyclophosphamide (0, 32, 64, or 96 ppm) or urethane (0, 5000, 10,000, or 15,000 ppm) for up to 12 weeks. In contrast, recent data on ethylene oxide (Preston *et al.*, unpublished) have shown that exposure of male mice to ethylene oxide at concentrations of 0, 25, 50, 100, 200 ppm for 6, 12, 24, or 48 weeks resulted in a time and concentration-dependent increase in reciprocal translocations assessed by FISH.

Another factor that certainly affects the utility of population monitoring data with reciprocal translocations using FISH is that the frequency of reciprocal translocations increases significantly with increasing age (Ramsey *et al.*, 1995), but to a lesser extent for nontransmissible aberrations (Bender *et al.*, 1988). Ramsey *et al.* (1995) provided data on the influence of other confounders on the frequency of reciprocal translocations in human groups. These confounders include smoking, consumption of diet drinks and/or diet sweeteners, exposure to asbestos or coal products, and having a previous major illness. This reemphasizes the point that the selection of study groups and accounting for confounders is essential for human population cytogenetic monitoring studies to be of utility.

Thus, very few of the published studies of cytogenetic population monitoring for individuals have analyzed the appropriate endpoint for detecting the genetic effects of long-term exposure to chemicals. It is quite surprising that positive responses have been reported for increases in unstable, chromatid aberrations because these are nontransmissible, and as noted above are induced at the first in vitro S phase. This anomaly is especially concerning when very low levels of exposure are reported (reviewed for ethylene oxide in Preston, 1999).

The *HPRT* mutation assay can assess the frequency of induced mutations in stem cells or other precursor cells, because a proportion of the mutations are induced as nonlethal events. The transmissible proportion will be greater for agents that do not induce large deletions; this will include the majority of nonradiomimetic chemicals. Induction of mutations in lymphocyte precursor cells will lead to clonal expansion of mutations in the peripheral pool. However, assessment of the T-cell antigen receptor status of the mutant clones permits a correction for clonal expansion. The population of cells derived from any particular stem cell has a unique antigen receptor status (Albertini and Hayes, 1997). The GPA assay can similarly be used for the assessment of chronic exposures or for estimating exposures at some long time after exposure (Albertini and Hayes, 1997). The predictive value of the assay for adverse health outcome appears to be limited, but it can provide an estimate of exposure.

The potential for cytogenetic endpoints being predictive of relative cancer risk has been addressed in recent reports from the European Study Group on Cytogenetic Biomarkers and Health (Hagmar *et al.*, 1998a,b; Bonassi *et al.*, 2004; Norppa *et al.*, 2006). The groups selected for cytogenetic studies consisted of individuals with reported occupational exposure and unexposed controls. The association between cancer and the frequency of unstable chromosome aberrations in the study groups was not based on exposure status, but rather on the relative frequency of chromosome aberrations, namely, low (1–33 percentiles), medium (34–66 percentiles), and high (67–100 percentiles). In general, the higher the relative frequency of unstable aberrations, the greater the risk of cancer death for all tumors combined. The authors make it clear that there is insufficient information on exposure for it to be used as a predictor of cancer development. In fact, the data indicate that individuals with higher frequencies of chromosome aberrations for whatever reason (genetic or environmental) are *as a group* at greater risk of dying from cancer. This is very different from concluding that exposures to mutagens that result in a higher frequency of chromosome aberrations in peripheral lymphocytes leads to an increased risk of cancer, especially for specific tumor types. The relevance of exposure to mutagenic chemicals in these studies by Hagmar *et al.* (1998a,b) is uncertain because there was no association between increased SCE frequencies and increased cancer mortality.

This latter concern was addressed by the same group (Bonassi *et al.*, 2000) in a more recent study. The study again showed that there was a significantly increased risk for subjects with a high level of chromosome aberrations compared to those with a low level in both Nordic and Italian cohorts. Of particular relevance to risk assessment was the observation that the relationships were not affected by the inclusion of occupational exposure level or smoking. The risk for high versus low levels of chromosome aberrations was similar in individuals heavily exposed to carcinogens and in those who had never, to their knowledge, been exposed to any specific environmental carcinogen. These data highlight the need to use caution when considering the relevance of chromosome aberration data in cancer risk assessment.

NEW APPROACHES FOR GENETIC TOXICOLOGY

In the past 15 or so years, the field of genetic toxicology has moved into the molecular era. The potential for advances in our understanding of basic cellular processes and how they can be perturbed is enormous. The ability to manipulate and characterize DNA, RNA, and proteins has been at the root of this advance in knowledge. However, the development of sophisticated molecular biology does not in itself imply a corresponding advance in the utility of genetic toxicology and its application to risk assessment. Knowing the types of studies to conduct and knowing how to interpret the data remain as fundamental as always. Measuring finer and finer detail can perhaps complicate the utility of the various mutagenicity assays. There is a need for genetic toxicology to avoid the temptation to use more and more sophisticated techniques to address the same questions and in the end make the same mistakes as have been made previously. How successful we are in designing informative studies based on the most recent molecular techniques perhaps cannot be judged at this time. However, the following examples of recent approaches to obtaining data for enhancing our ability to use noncancer (genotoxicity) data in a mechanistically based cancer (and genetic) risk assessment process provide some encouragement. Several recent developments (e.g., the use of transgenic animals, the comet assay for assessing DNA damages) have already been described in the appropriate assay sections above because they are currently in general use.

Advances in Cytogenetics

Until quite recently, the analysis of chromosome alterations relied on conventional chromosome staining with DNA stains such as Giemsa or on the process of chromosome banding. Both approaches require considerable expenditure of time and a rather high level of expertise. However, chromosome banding does allow for the assessment of transmissible aberrations such as reciprocal translocations and inversions with a fairly high degree of accuracy. Knowing the induction frequency of such aberrations is very important, given that they are generally not lethal to the cell and constitute by far the major class observed in inherited genetic defects and a significant fraction of the alterations observed in tumors. In addition, because stable aberrations are transmissible from parent to daughter cell, they represent accumulated effects of chronic exposures. The more readily analyzed but cell lethal, nontransmissible aberrations such as dicentrics and deletions reflect only recent exposures and then only when analyzed at the first division after exposure. A more detailed discussion of these factors can be found in Preston (1998).

The relative ease with which specific chromosomes, specific genes, and chromosome alterations can be detected has been radically enhanced by the development of FISH (Trask et al., 1993; Speicher and Carter, 2005). In principle, the technique relies on amplification of DNA from particular genomic regions such as whole chromosomes or gene regions and the hybridization of these amplified DNAs to metaphase chromosome preparations or interphase nuclei. Regions of hybridization can be determined by the use of fluorescent antibodies that detect modified DNA bases incorporated during amplification or by incorporating fluorescent bases themselves during amplification. The fluorescently labeled, hybridized regions are detected by fluorescence microscopy, and the signal can be increased in strength by computer-enhanced processes. The level of sophistication has increased so much that all 24 different human chromosomes (22 autosomes, X and Y) can be individually detected (Macville et al., 1997), as can all mouse chromosomes (Liyanage et al., 1996). Alterations in tumors can also be detected on a whole-genome basis (Coleman et al., 1997; Veldman et al., 1997). A recent example highlights the ability to construct breakpoint profiles of specific tumor types (Trost et al., 2006). In this example, a detailed analysis by spectral karyotyping of specific breakpoints in a set of primary myelodysplastic syndrome and acute myeloid leukemia samples revealed recurrent involvement of specific chromosome bands that contained oncogenes or tumor suppressor genes.

The aim will be to attempt to reveal the possible prognostic significance of the subgroups linked to these specific markers.

There is an extensive literature on the use of FISH for karyotyping tumors and in gene mapping but less on its utility for genetic toxicology studies, especially the assessment of stable chromosome aberrations at long periods after exposure or after long-term exposures. Three particular studies do, however, serve to exemplify the use of FISH in genetic toxicology.

Lucas et al. (1992) demonstrated that stable chromosomal aberrations could be detected in individuals decades after exposure to atomic bombs in Japan. How these frequencies relate to frequencies at the time of exposure is not known with any certainty, given the fact that induced frequencies were not measured because appropriate techniques were not available at that time.

Studies by Tucker et al. (1997, 2005) provided some assessment of the utility of FISH for the analysis of radiation-induced, stable chromosome alterations at various times after exposure. The frequency of reciprocal translocations induced by gamma rays in rat peripheral lymphocytes decreased with time after exposure, reaching a plateau at four days that was 55–65% of the induced frequency and with a dose dependency (Tucker et al., 1997). Similar results were obtained for human samples (Tucker et al., 2005). These results suggest that reciprocal translocations fall into two classes, stable and unstable (cell-lethal). It is quite possible that these "unstable" translocations are lost because of the presence of other cell-lethal damage in the same cell. Additional work is required to clarify this conclusion and to extend the studies to the effects of chemicals.

FISH methods have also allowed for an accurate and sensitive assessment of chromosomal alterations present in tumors. The particular advance that makes this assessment feasible is known as comparative genomic hybridization (CGH) (Kallioniemi et al., 1992). CGH results in the ability to identify the role of chromosomal structural and numerical alterations in tumor development. The genomic instability present in all tumor types appears to have a specific genetic basis, as shown elegantly for colon cancer by Vogelstein and colleagues (Cahill et al., 1998). For CGH, tumor and control DNAs are differentially labeled with fluorescence probes and cohybridized to normal metaphase chromosome preparations. The ratio of the fluorescence intensities of hybridized tumor and control DNA indicates regions of normal genomic content as well as those regions that are over- or underrepresented in tumors. The CGH method is being adapted for automated screening approaches using biochips (Solinas-Tolado et al., 1997; Hosoya et al., 2006). Assessing genetic alterations such as specific gene deletions in single metastatic tumor cells is feasible using a slightly different but complementary approach (Pack et al., 1997, 2005).

The types of FISH approaches described here undoubtedly indicate the direction in which cytogenetic analysis will proceed. The types of data collected will affect our understanding of how tumors develop. Data on the dose–response characteristics for a specific chromosomal alteration as a proximate marker of cancer can enhance the cancer risk assessment process by describing effects of low exposures that are below those for which tumor incidence can be reliably assessed. Cytogenetic data of the types described above can also improve extrapolation from data generated with laboratory animals to humans.

Molecular Analysis of Mutations and Gene Expression

With the advent of molecular biology techniques, the exact basis of a mutation at the level of the DNA sequence can be established.

In many cases, the genetic basis of human disease can be determined even though human genes have long DNA sequences and a complex genomic arrangement. Molecular biology techniques have also enabled a distinction to be made between background mutations and those induced by specific agents. The latter observations are addressed by analyzing the mutational spectra in target genes in laboratory animals and in humans (DeMarini, 2000; Hemminki and Thilly, 2004). For reasons of inherent sensitivity of available methods, the genes analyzed for mutations are ones for which mutated forms can be selected. The confounding factor of many normal cells, which far outnumber a few mutant cells in an exposed cellular population, can be removed by mutant selection approaches. Methods to overcome the drawback of only being able to study selectable genes are currently being developed, and particular ones such as ligation-mediated polymerase chain reaction (PCR) are close to the required sensitivity level (Albertini and Hayes, 1998; Makrigiorgos, 2004; Yeh et al., 2006).

A giant step forward in the ability to detect and characterize mutations at both the DNA and RNA level has been provided by the development of chip technology (Southern, 1996) and array-based assay systems (Woldicka et al., 1997). With hybridization of test DNAs to oligonucleotide arrays, specific genetic alterations or their cellular consequences can be determined rapidly and automatically (Houlston and Peto, 2004; Vissers et al., 2005). Cost remains a limiting factor, but the potential for assessing specific cellular changes following chemical exposure is enormous.

Until quite recently, alterations in gene expression following specific exposures or for specific genotypes were analyzed gene by gene. Such an approach makes it difficult to assess changes in gene expression that occur in a concerted fashion. Recent advances using cDNA microarray technologies have allowed the measurement of changes in expression of hundreds or even thousands of genes at one time (Harrington et al., 2000; Elvidge, 2006). The level of expression at the mRNA level is measured by the amount of hybridization of isolated cDNAs to oligonucleotide fragments from known genes or expressed sequence tags (ESTs) on a specifically laid out grid. Although this technique holds great promise for establishing a cell's response to exposure to chemical or physical agents in the context of normal cellular patterns of gene expression, it remains to be established how to analyze the vast amounts of data that can and are being obtained and what magnitude of change in gene expression constitutes an adverse effect as far as cellular phenotype is concerned. Extrapolating the responses to organs and whole animals represents a challenge still to be addressed.

There are parallel efforts in the area of proteomics and metabolomics whereby changes in a broad range of cellular proteins can be assessed in response to endogenous or exogenous factors, potentially leading to the development of biomarkers of effect (Aebersold et al., 2005; Robertson, 2005; Griffin, 2006; McGregor and Souza, 2006). The biggest hurdle currently is the relative paucity of sequence data available for the world of proteins and their multiple posttranslational modifications. Certainly progress is rapid, and so methodologies akin to gene expression microarrays are likely to be close at hand.

The move in the field of genetic toxicology is away from the "yes/no" approach to hazard identification and much more toward a mechanistic understanding of how a chemical or physical agent can produce adverse cellular and tissue responses. The move is clearly toward analysis at the whole genome level and away from single gene responses. The challenges are apparent and the solutions are being identified.

CONCLUSIONS

The field of genetic toxicology has had an overall life of about 70 years and has undergone several rebirths during this period. Genetic toxicology began as a basic research field with demonstrations that ionizing radiations and chemicals could induce mutations and chromosome alterations in plant, insect, and mammalian cells. The development of a broad range of short-term assays for genotoxicity served to identify many mutagens and address the relationship between mutagens and cancer-causing agents, or carcinogens. The inevitable failure of the assays to be completely predictive resulted in the identification of nongenotoxic carcinogens. In the 1980s, genetic toxicology began to move more toward gaining a better understanding of the mutagenic mechanisms underlying carcinogenicity and heritable effects. With this improved understanding, genetic toxicology studies began to turn away from hazard identification alone and move toward quantitative risk assessment. Major advances in our knowledge of mechanisms of cancer formation have been fueled by truly amazing progress in molecular biology. Genetic toxicology has begun to take advantage of the knowledge that cancer is a genetic disease with multiple steps, many of which require a mutation. The identification of chromosome alterations involved in tumor formation has been facilitated greatly by the use of FISH. The ability to distinguish between background and induced mutations can in some cases be achieved by mutation analysis at the level of DNA sequence. Key cellular processes related to mutagenesis have been identified, including multiple pathways of DNA repair, cell cycle controls, and the role of checkpoints in ensuring that the cell cycle does not proceed until the DNA and specific cellular structures are checked for fidelity. These observations have enhanced our knowledge of the importance of genotype in susceptibility to cancer. Recent developments in genetic toxicology have greatly improved our understanding of basic cellular processes and alterations that can affect the integrity of the genetic material and its functions. The ability to detect and analyze mutations in mammalian germ cells continues to improve and can contribute to a better appreciation for the long-term consequences of mutagenesis in human populations. Improvements in the qualitative assessment of mutation in somatic cells and germ cells have been paralleled by advances in the ability to assess genetic alterations quantitatively, especially in ways that enhance the cancer and genetic risk assessment process (Preston, 2005).

ACKNOWLEDGMENTS

We would like to recognize the outstanding secretarial support provided by Carolyn Fowler in the preparation of this chapter. The authors also thank Drs. David DeMarini, James Allen, and Les Recio for their valuable comments as part of the review of this chapter.

This document has been reviewed in accordance with the U.S. Environmental Protection Agency policy and approved for publication but does not necessarily reflect EPA policy. Mention of trade names or commercial products does not constitute endorsement or recommendation for use.

REFERENCES

Aardema MJ, Albertini S, Arni P, et al.: Aneuploidy: A report of an ECETOC task force. Mutat Res 410:3–79, 1998.

Adler I-D: Synopsis of the in vivo results obtained with the 10 known or suspected aneugens tested in the CEC collaborative study. Mutat Res 287:131–137, 1993.

Adler I-D, Shelby MD, Bootman J, et al.: Summary report of the working group on mammalian germ cell tests. Mutat Res 312:313–318, 1994.

Aebersold R, Anderson L, Caprioli R, et al.: Perspective: A program to improve protein biomarker discovery for cancer. Proteome Res 4:1104–1109, 2005.

Aguilar F, Harris CC, Sun T, et al.: Geographic variation of p53 mutational profile in nonmalignant human liver. Science 264:1317–1319, 1994.

Albertini RJ, Hayes RB: Somatic cell mutations in cancer epidemiology. IARC Sci Pub 142:159–184, 1997.

Allen JW, Liang JC, Carrano AV, Preston RJ: Review of literature on chemical-induced aneuploidy in mammalian germ cells. Mutat Res 167:123–137, 1986.

Ames BN, McCann J, Yamasaki E: Methods for detecting carcinogens and mutagens with the Salmonella/mammalian-microsome mutagenicity test. Mutat Res 31:347–364, 1975.

Anderson RM, Marsden SJ, Wright EG, et al.: Complex chromosome aberrations in peripheral blood lymphocytes as a potential biomarker of exposure to high-Let alpha-particles. Int J Radiat Biol 76:31–42, 2000.

Ashby J: Two million rodent carcinogens? The role of SAR and QSAR in their detection. Mutat Res 305:3–12, 1994.

Ashby J, Paton D: The influence of chemical structure on the extent and sites of carcinogenesis for 522 rodent carcinogens and 55 different human carcinogen exposures. Mutat Res 286:3–74, 1993.

Ashby J, Tennant RW: Definitive relationships among chemical structure, carcinogenicity and mutagenicity for 301 chemicals tested by the U.S. NTP. Mutat Res 257:229–306, 1991.

Au WW, Gajas-Salazar N, Salama S: Factors contributing to discrepancies in population monitoring studies. Mutat Res 400:467–478, 1998.

Auerbach C, Robson JM: Chemical production of mutations. Nature 157:302, 1946.

Barale R, Chelotti L, Davini T, et al.: Sister chromatid exchange and micronucleus frequency in human lymphocytes of 1,650 subjects in an Italian population: II. Contribution of sex, age, and lifestyle. Environ Mol Mutagen 31:228–242, 1998.

Barrett JC: Mechanisms of multistep carcinogenesis and carcinogen risk assessment. Environ Health Prospect 100:9–20, 1993.

Baumgarthner A, Van Hummelen P, Lowe XR, et al.: Numerical and structural chromosomal abnormalities detected in human sperm with a combination of multicolor FISH assays. Environ Mol Mutagen 33:49–58, 1999.

Beale G: The discovery of mustard gas mutagenesis by Auerbach and Robson in 1941. Genetics 134:393–399, 1993.

Bender MA, Gooch PC: Persistent chromosome aberrations in irradiated human subjects. Radiat Res 16:44–53, 1962.

Bender MA, Preston RJ, Leonard RC, et al.: Chromosomal aberration and sister-chromatid exchange frequencies in peripheral blood lymphocytes of a large human population sample. Mutat Res 204:421–433, 1988.

Bender MA, Preston RJ, Leonard RC, et al.: Chromosomal aberration and sister-chromatid exchange frequencies in peripheral blood lymphocytes of a large human population sample. II. Extension of age range. Mutat Res 212:149–154, 1988.

Bentley KS, Sarrif AM, Cimino MC, Auletta AE: Assessing the risk of heritable gene mutation in mammals: Drosophila sex-linked recessive lethal test and tests measuring DNA damage and repair in mammalian germ cells. Environ Mol Mutagen 23:3–11, 1994.

Bickel SE, Orr-Weaver TL: Holding chromatids together to ensure they go their separate ways. Bioessays 18:293–300, 1996.

Bishop AJR, Schiestl RH: Role of homologous recombination in carcinogenesis. Exp Mol Pathol 74:94–105, 2003.

Bishop JM: Molecular themes in oncogenesis. Cell 64:235–248, 1991.

Blaisdell JO, Harrison L, Wallace SS: Base excision repair processing of radiation-induced clustered DNA lesions. Radiat Prot Dosimetry 97:25–31, 2001.

Bonassi S, Hagmar L, Strömberg U, et al.: Chromosomal aberrations in lymphocytes predict human cancer independently of exposure to carcinogens. Cancer Res 60:1619–1625, 2000.

Bonassi S, Znaor A, Norppa H, Hagmar L: Chromosomal aberrations and risk of cancer in humans: An epidemiologic perspective. Cytogenet Genome Res 104:376–382, 2004.

Brendler-Schwaab S, Czich A, Epe B, et al.: Photochemical genotoxicity: Principles and test methods. Report of a GUM task force. Mutat Res 566:65–91, 2004.

Brewen JG, Preston RJ: Cytogenetic effects of environmental mutagens in mammalian cells and the extrapolation to man. Mutat Res 26:297–305, 1974.

Brewen JG, Preston RJ: Cytogenetic analysis of mammalian oocytes in mutagenicity studies, in Hsu TC (ed.): Cytogenetic Assays of Environmental Mutagens. Totowa, NJ: Allanheld, Osmun, 1982, pp. 277–287.

Brusick JD (ed.): Methods for Genetic Risk Assessment. Boca Raton, FL: CRC Press, 1994.

Burkhart JG, Malling HV: Mutagenesis and transgenic systems: Perspective from the mutagen, N-ethyl-N-nitrosourea. Environ Mol Mutagen 22:1–6, 1993.

Burkhart JG, Malling HV: Mutations among the living and the undead. Mutat Res 304:315–320, 1994.

Burma S, Chen BP, Chen DJ: Role of non-homologous end joining (NHEJ) in maintaining genomic integrity. DNA Repair Jul 3:[Epub ahead of print], 2006.

Cahill D, Connor B, Carney JP: Mechanisms of eukaryotic DNA double strand break repair. Front Biosci 11:1958–1976, 2006.

Cahill DP, Lengauer C, Yu J, et al.: Mutations of mitotic checkpoint genes in human cancers. Nature 392:300–303, 1998.

Calos MP, Miller JH: Genetic and sequence analysis of frameshift mutations induced by ICR-191. J Mol Biol 153:39–66, 1981.

Cariello NF, Skopek TR: Analysis of mutations occurring at the human hprt locus. J Mol Biol 231:41–57, 1993.

Casciano DA, Aidoo A, Chen T, et al.: Hprt mutant frequency and molecular analysis of Hprt mutations in rats treated with mutagenic carcinogens. Mutat Res 431:389–395, 1999.

Cavenee WK, Dryja TP, Phillips RA, et al.: Expression of recessive alleles by chromosomal mechanisms in retinoblastoma. Nature 305:779–784, 1983.

Cebula TA, Koch WH: Sequence analysis of Salmonella typhimurium revertants, in Mendelsohn ML, Albertini RJ (eds.): Mutation and the Environment, Part D. New York: Wiley-Liss, 1990, pp. 367–377.

Chang LW, Hsia SMT, Chan P-C, Hsieh L-L: Macromolecular adducts: Biomarkers for toxicity and carcinogenesis. Annu Rev Pharmacol Toxicol 34:41–67, 1994.

Clayson DB, Mehta R, Iverson F: Oxidative DNA damage—The effects of certain genotoxic and operationally non-genotoxic carcinogens. Mutat Res 317:25–42, 1994.

Clements J: The mouse lymphoma assay. Mutat Res 455:97–110, 2000.

Cole J, Skopek TR: Somatic mutant frequency, mutation rates and mutational spectra in the human population in vivo. Mutat Res 304:33–105, 1994.

Coleman AE, Schrock E, Weaver Z, et al.: Previously hidden chromosome aberrations in t(12;15)-positive BALB/c plasmacytomas uncovered by multicolor spectral karyotyping. Cancer Res 57:4585–4592, 1997.

Cotelle S, Férard JF: Comet assay in genetic ecotoxicology. *Environ Mol Mutagen* 34:246–255, 1999.

Crespi CL, Miller VP: The use of heterologously expressed drug metabolizing enzymes—State of the art and prospects for the future. *Pharmacol Ther* 84:121–131, 1999.

Critchlow SE, Jackson SP: DNA end-joining from yeast to man. *Trends Biochem Sci* 23:394–398, 1998.

Crouse GF: Mutagenesis assays in yeast. *Methods* 22:116–119, 2000.

Cupples CG, Cabrera M, Cruz C, Miller JH: A set of *lacZ* mutations in *Escherichia coli* that allow rapid detection of specific frameshift mutations. *Genetics* 125:275–280, 1990.

Cupples CG, Miller JH: A set of *lacZ* mutations in *Escherichia coli* that allow rapid detection of each of the six base substitutions. *Proc Natl Acad Sci U S A* 86:5345–5349, 1989.

Dellarco VL, Prival MJ: Mutagenicity of nitro compounds in *Salmonella typhimurium* in the presence of flavin mononucleotide in a preincubation assay. *Environ Mol Mutagen* 13:116–127, 1989.

DeMarini DM: Environmental mutagens/complex mixtures, in Li AP, Heflich RH (eds.): *Genetic Toxicology: A Treatise*. Boca Raton, FL: CRC Press, 1991, pp. 285–302.

DeMarini DM: Mutation spectra of complex mixtures. *Mutat Res* 411:11–18, 1998.

DeMarini DM: Influence of DNA repair on mutation spectra in S*almonella*. *Mutat Res* 450:5–17, 2000.

DeMarini DM, Brockman HE, de Serres FJ, *et al.*: Specific-locus mutations induced in eukaryotes (especially mammalian cells) by radiation and chemicals: A perspective. *Mutat Res* 220:11–29, 1989.

DeMarini DM, Shelton ML, Abu-Shakra A, *et al.*: Spectra of spontaneous frameshift mutations at the *his*D3052 allele of *Salmonella typhimurium* in four DNA repair backgrounds. *Genetics* 149:17–36, 1998.

Demple B, Harrison L: Repair of oxidative damage to DNA: Enzymology and biology. *Annu Rev Biochem* 63:915–948, 1994.

Director AE, Tucker JD, Ramsey MJ, Nath J: Chronic ingestion of clastogens by mice and the frequency of chromosome aberrations. *Environ Mol Mutagen* 32:139–147, 1998.

Dogliotti E, Hainant P, Hernandez T, *et al.*: Mutation spectra resulting from carcinogenic exposures: From model systems to cancer-related genes. *Recent Results Cancer Res* 154:97–124, 1998.

Ehling UH: Genetic risk assessment. *Annu Rev Genet* 25:255–280, 1991.

Elia MC, Storer R, McKelvey TW, *et al.*: Rapid DNA degradation in primary rat hepatocytes treated with diverse cytotoxic chemicals: Analysis by pulsed field gel electrophoresis and implications for alkaline elution assays. *Environ Mol Mutagen* 24:181–191, 1994.

Elvidge G: Microarray expression technology: From start to finish. *Pharmacogenomics* 7:123–134, 2006.

EPA (U.S. Environmental Protection Agency): Guidelines for carcinogen risk assessment. *Fed Reg* 51:33992–34003, 1986.

EPA (U.S. Environmental Protection Agency): *Proposed Guidelines for Carcinogen Risk Assessment*. EPA/600P/P-92/003c. Office of Research and Development. Washington DC: U.S. Environmental Protection Agency, 1996.

EPA (U.S. Environmental Protection Agency): *Guidelines for Carcinogen Risk Assessment*. Risk Assessment Forum. Washington, DC: U.S. Environmental Protection Agency, 2005. www.epa.gov/cancerguidelines.

Evan G, Littlewood T: A matter of life and cell death. *Science* 281:1317–1322, 1998.

Evans HJ, Prosser J: Tumor-suppressor genes: Cardinal factors in inherited predisposition to human cancers. *Environ Health Perspect* 98:25–37, 1992.

Fairbairn DW, Olive PL, O'Neill KL: The comet assay: A comprehensive review. *Mutat Res* 339:37–59, 1995.

Favor J: Mechanisms of mutation induction in germ cells of the mouse as assessed by the specific-locus test. *Mutat Res* 428:227–236, 1999.

Fearon ER, Vogelstein B: A genetic model for colorectal tumorigenesis. *Cell* 61:759–767, 1990.

Fenech M: The cytokinesis-block micronucleus technique: A detailed description of the method and its application to genotoxicity studies in human populations. *Mutat Res* 285:35–44, 1993.

Fenech M: The advantages and disadvantages of the cytokinesis-block micronucleus method. *Mutat Res* 392:11–18, 1997.

Fenech M: The in vitro micronucleus technique. *Mutat Res* 455:81–95, 2000.

Fenech M, Chang WP, Kirsch-Volders M, *et al.*: HUMN project: Detailed description of the scoring criteria for the cytokinesis-block micronucleus assay using isolated human lymphocyte cultures. *Mutat Res* 534:65–75, 2003.

Fischer AH, Young KA, DeLellis RA: Incorporating pathologists' criteria of malignancy into the evolutionary model for cancer development. *J Cell Biochem* 93:28–36, 2004.

Friedberg EC: *DNA Repair*. New York: Freeman, 1985.

Friedberg EC: Biological responses to DNA damage: A perspective in the new millennium. *Cold Spring Harb Symp Quant Biol* 65:593–602, 2000.

Friedberg EC, Walker GC, Siede W: *DNA Repair and Mutagenesis*. Washington, DC: ASM Press, 1995.

Galloway SM: Cytotoxicity and chromosome aberrations in vitro: Experience in industry and the case for an upper limit on toxicity in the aberration assay. *Environ Mol Mutagen* 35:191–201, 2000.

Galloway SM, Aardema MJ, Ishidate M Jr, *et al.*: Report from working group on in vitro tests for chromosomal aberrations. *Mutat Res* 312:241–261, 1994.

Galloway SM, Berry PK, Nichols WW, *et al.*: Chromosome aberrations in individuals occupationally exposed to ethylene oxide, and in a large control population. *Mutat Res* 170:55–74, 1986.

Galloway SM, Ivett JL: Chemically induced aneuploidy in mammalian cells in culture. *Mutat Res* 167:89–105, 1986.

Gatehouse D, Haworth S, Cebula T, *et al.*: Recommendations for the performance of bacterial mutation assays. *Mutat Res* 312:217–233, 1994.

Gatenby RA, Vincent TL: An evolutionary model of carcinogenesis. *Cancer Res* 63:6212–6220, 2003.

Gee P, Maron DM, Ames BN: Detection and classification of mutagens: A set of base-specific *Salmonella* tester strains. *Proc Natl Acad Sci U S A* 91:11606–11610, 1994.

Gee P, Sommers CH, Melick AS, *et al.*: Comparison of responses of base-specific *Salmonella* tester strains with the traditional strains for identifying mutagens: The results of a validation study. *Mutat Res* 412:115–130, 1998.

Gold LS, Slone TH, Stern BR, Bernstein L: Comparison of target organs of carcinogenicity for mutagenic and non-mutagenic chemicals. *Mutat Res* 286:75–100, 1993.

Goodhead DT: Initial events in the cellular effects of ionizing radiations: Clustered damage in DNA. *Int J Radiat Biol* 65:7–17, 1994.

Grant WF: The present status of higher plant bioassays for the detection of environmental mutagens. *Mutat Res* 310:175–185, 1994.

Griffin JL: Understanding mouse models of disease through metabolomics. *Curr Opin Chem Biol* 10:309–315, 2006.

Grombacher T, Mitra S, Kaina B: Induction of the alkyltransferase (MGMT) gene by DNA damaging agents and the glucocorticoid dexamethasone and comparison with the response of base excision repair. *Carcinogenesis* 17:2329–2336, 1996.

Haber JE: Partners and pathways: Repairing a double-strand break. *Trends Genet* 16:259–264, 2000.

Hagmar L, Bonassi S, Strömberg U, *et al.*: Cancer predictive value of cytogenetic markers used in occupational health surveillance programs: A report from an ongoing study by the European Study Group on Cytogenetic Biomarkers and Health. *Mutat Res* 405:171–178, 1998a.

Hagmar L, Bonassi S, Strömberg U, *et al.*: Chromosomal aberrations in lymphocytes predict human cancer: A report from the European Study Group on Cytogenetic Biomarkers and Health (ESCH). *Cancer Res* 58:4117–4121, 1998b.

Hahn WC, Counter CM, Lundberg AS, *et al.*: Creation of human tumor cells with defined genetic elements. *Nature* 400:464–468, 1999.

Halliday JA, Glickman BW: Mechanisms of spontaneous mutation in DNA repair-proficient *Escherichia coli. Mutat Res* 250:55–71, 1991.

Hamada S, Sutou S, Morita T, *et al.*: Evaluation of the rodent micronucleus assay by a 28-day treatment protocol: Summary of the 13th collaborative study by the collaborative study group for the micronucleus test (CSGMT)/environmental mutagen society of Japan (JEMS)-mammalian mutagenicity study group (MMS). *Environ Mol Mutagen* 37:93–110, 2001.

Hamasaki T, Sato T, Nagase H, Kito H: The genotoxicity of organotin compounds in SOS chromotest and rec-assay. *Mutat Res* 280:195–203, 1992.

Hanahan D, Weinberg RA: The hallmarks of cancer. *Cell* 100:57–70, 2000.

Harrington CA, Rosenow C, Retief J: Monitoring gene expression using DNA microarrays. *Curr Opin Microbiol* 3:285–291, 2000.

Harris CC: P53: At the crossroads of molecular carcinogenesis and risk assessment. *Science* 262:1980–1981, 1993.

Hayashi M, MacGregor JT, Gatehouse DG, *et al.*: In vivo rodent erythrocyte micronucleus assay: II. Some aspects of protocol design including repeated treatments, integration with toxicity testing, and automated scoring. *Environ Mol Mutagen* 35:234–252, 2000.

Hayashi M, Tice RR, MacGregor JT, *et al.*: In vivo rodent erythrocyte micronucleus assay. *Mutat Res* 312:293–304, 1994.

Heartlein MW, O'Neill JP, Preston RJ: SCE induction is proportional to substitution in DNA for thymidine by CldU. *Mutat Res* 107:103–109, 1983.

Heddle JA, Cimino MC, Hayashi M, *et al.*: Micronuclei as an index of cytogenetic damage: Past, present, and future. *Environ Mol Mutagen* 18:277–291, 1991.

Heddle JA, Dean S, Nohmi T, *et al.*: In vivo transgenic mutation assays. *Environ Mol Mutagen* 35:253–259, 2000.

Heflich RH: Chemical mutagens, in Li AP, Heflich RH (eds.): *Genetic Toxicology: A Treatise.* Boca Raton, FL: CRC Press, 1991, pp. 143–202.

Hemminki K, Thilly WG: Implications of results of molecular epidemiology on DNA adducts, their repair and mutations for mechanisms of human cancer. *IARC Sci Publ* 157:217–235, 2004.

Hewitt LM, Marvin CH: Analytical methods in environmental effects-directed investigations of effluents. *Mutat Res* 589:208–232, 2005.

Hoffmann GR: Induction of genetic recombination: Consequences and model systems. *Environ Mol Mutagen* 23(Suppl 24):59–66, 1994.

Hosoya N, Sanada M, Nannya Y, *et al.*: Genomewide screening of DNA copy number changes in chronic myelogenous leukemia with the use of high-resolution array-based comparative genomic hybridization. *Genes Chromosomes Cancer* 45:482–494, 2006.

Houlston RS, Peto J: The search for low-penetrance cancer susceptibility alleles. *Oncogene* 23:6471–6476, 2004.

Howlett NG, Schiestl RH: Simultaneous measurement of the frequencies of intrachromosomal recombination and chromosome gain using the yeast DEL assay. *Mutat Res* 454:53–62, 2000.

Hsu TC: *Human and Mammalian Cytogenetics: An Historical Perspective.* New York: Springer-Verlag, 1979.

Hunt PA: Meiosis in mammals: Recombination, non-disjunction and the environment. *Biochem Soc Trans* 34:574–577, 2006.

International Program on Chemical Safety (IPCS): in Ashby J, de Serres FJ, Shelby MD, *et al.* (eds.): *Evaluation of Short-Term Tests for Carcinogens*, vols. I and II. Cambridge, England: Cambridge University Press, 1988.

Ishidate M Jr, Harnois MC, Sofuni T: A comparative analysis of data on the clastogenicity of 951 chemical substances tested in mammalian cell cultures. *Mutat Res* 195:151–213, 1988.

Jha AN: Genotoxicological studies in aquatic organisms: An overview. *Mutat Res* 552:1–17, 2004.

Jiang G, Sancar A: Recruitment of DNA damage checkpoint proteins to damage in transcribed and nontranscribed sequences. *Mol Cell Biol* 26:39–49, 2006.

Jiricny J: Eukaryotic mismatch repair: An update. *Mutat Res* 409:107–121, 1998.

Johnson RD, Liu N, Jasin M: Mammalian XRCC2 promotes the repair of DNA double-strand breaks by homologous recombination. *Nature* 401:397–399, 1999.

Josephy PD: The *Escherichia coli lacZ* reversion mutagenicity assay. *Mutat Res* 455:71–80, 2000.

Josephy PD, DeBruin LS, Lord HL, *et al.*: Bioactivation of aromatic amines by recombinant human cytochrome P4501A2 expressed in Ames tester strain bacteria: A substitute for activation by mammalian tissue preparations. *Cancer Res* 55:799–802, 1995.

Jun SH, Kim TG, Ban C: DNA mismatch repair system. Classical and fresh roles. *FEBS J* 273:1609–1619, 2006.

Jurado J, Alejandre-Durán E, Pueyo C: Mutagenicity testing in *Salmonella typhimurium* strains possessing both the His reversion and Ara forward mutation systems and different levels of classical nitroreductase or o-acetyltransferase activities. *Environ Mol Mutagen* 23:286–293, 1994.

Kallioniemi A, Kallioniemi O-P, Sudar D, *et al.*: Comparative genomic hybridization for molecular cytogenetic analysis of solid tumors. *Science* 258:818–821, 1992.

Kier LE, Brusick DJ, Auletta AE, *et al.*: The *Salmonella typhimurium/* mammalian microsomal assay: A report of the U.S. Environmental Protection Agency Gene-Tox Program. *Mutat Res* 168:69–240, 1986.

Kim BS, Margolin BH: Prediction of rodent carcinogenicity utilizing a battery of in vitro and in vivo genotoxicity tests. *Environ Mol Mutagen* 34:297–304, 1999.

Kinzler KW, Vogelstein B: Lessons from hereditary colorectal cancer. *Cell* 87:159–170, 1996.

Kirkland DJ, Gatehouse DG, Scott D, *et al.* (eds.): *Basic Mutagenicity Tests: UKEMS Recommended Procedures.* New York: Cambridge University Press, 1990.

Kirsch-Volders M, Sofuni T, Aardema M, *et al.*: Report from the in vitro micronucleus assay working group. *Environ Mol Mutagen* 35:167–172, 2000.

Kirsch-Volders M, Sofuni T, Aardema M, *et al.*: Report from the in vitro micronucleus assay working group. *Mutat Res* 540:153–163, 2003.

Kleinerman RA, Romanyukha AA, Schauer DA, Tucker JD: Retrospective assessment of radiation exposure using biological dosimetry: Chromosome painting, electron paramagnetic resonance and the glycophorin a mutation assay. *Radiat Res* 166:287–302, 2006.

Klekowski EJ Jr, Corredor JE, Morell JM, Del Castillo CA: Petroleum pollution and mutation in mangroves. *Marine Pollution Bull* 28:166–169, 1994.

Knudson AG: Hereditary predisposition to cancer. *Ann NY Acad Sci* 833:58–67, 1997.

Koch WH, Henrikson EN, Kupchella E, Cebula TA: *Salmonella typhimurium* strain TA100 differentiates several classes of carcinogens and mutagens by base substitution specificity. *Carcinogenesis* 15:79–88, 1994.

Kolodner RD: Mismatch repair: Mechanisms and relationship to cancer susceptibility. *Trends Biochem Sci* 20:397–401, 1995.

Kriek E, Rojas M, Alexandrov K, Bartsch H: Polycyclic aromatic hydrocarbon-DNA adducts in humans: Relevance as biomarkers for exposure and cancer risk. *Mutat Res* 400:215–231, 1998.

Krishna G, Hayashi M: In vivo rodent micronucleus assay: Protocol, conduct and data interpretation. *Mutat Res* 455:155–166, 2000.

Kyoizumi S, Kusunoki Y, Hayashi T, *et al.*: Individual variation of somatic gene mutability in relation to cancer susceptibility: Prospective study on erythrocyte glycophorin a gene mutations of atomic bomb survivors. *Cancer Res* 65:5462–5469, 2005.

Lähdetie J, Keiski A, Suutari A, Toppari J: Etoposide (VP-16) is a potent inducer of micronuclei in male rat meiosis: Spermatid micronucleus test and DNA flow cytometry after etoposide treatment. *Environ Mol Mutagen* 24:192–202, 1994.

Lambert IB, Singer TM, Boucher SE, Douglas GR: Detailed review of transgenic rodent mutation assays. *Mutat Res* 590:1–280, 2005.

Langenbach R, Oglesby L: The use of intact cellular activation systems in genetic toxicology assays, in de Serres FJ (ed.): *Chemical Mutagens: Principles and Methods for Their Detection*, vol. 8. New York: Plenum Press, 1983, pp. 55–93.

Laval J, Boiteux S, O'Connor TR: Physiological properties and repair of apurinic/apyrimidinic sites and imidazole ring-opened guanines in DNA. *Mutat Res* 233:73–79, 1990.

Le XC, Xing JZ, Lee J, et al.: Inducible repair of thymine glycol detected by an ultrasensitive assay for DNA damage. *Science* 280:1066–1069, 1998.

Lee WR, Abrahamson S, Valencia R, et al.: The sex-linked recessive lethal test for mutagenesis in *Drosophila melangoaster*: A report of the U.S. Environmental Protection Agency Gene-Tox Program. *Mutat Res* 123:183–279, 1983.

Léonard A: Observations on meiotic chromosomes of the male mouse as a test of the potential mutagenicity of chemicals in mammals, in Hollaender A (ed.): *Chemical Mutagens: Principles and Methods for Their Detection*, vol. 3. New York: Plenum Press, 1973, p. 21.

Levine JG, Schaaper RM, DeMarini DM: Complex frameshift mutations mediated by plasmid pKM101: Mutational mechanisms deduced from 4-aminobiphenyl-induced mutation spectra in *Salmonella*. *Genetics* 136:731–746, 1994.

Lewis SE: The biochemical specific-locus test and a new multiple-endpoint mutation detection system: Considerations for genetic risk assessment. *Environ Mol Mutagen* 18:303–306, 1991.

Lewtas J: Environmental monitoring using genetic bioassays, in Li AP, Heflich RH (eds.): *Genetic Toxicology: A Treatise*. Boca Raton, FL: CRC Press, 1991, pp. 359–374.

Lindahl T: Suppression of spontaneous mutagenesis in human cells by DNA base excision-repair. *Mutat Res* 462:129–135, 2000.

Liyanage M, Coleman A, duManoir S, et al.: Multicolour spectral karyotyping of mouse chromosomes. *Nat Genet* 14:312–315, 1996.

Lommel L, Carswell-Crumpton C, Hanawalt PC: Preferential repair of the transcribed DNA strand in the dihydrofolate reductase gene throughout the cell cycle in UV-irradiated human cells. *Mutat Res* 366:181–192, 1995.

Lucas JN, Awa A, Straume T, et al.: Rapid translocation analysis in humans decades after exposure to ionizing radiation. *Int J Radiat Biol* 62:53–63, 1992.

Lynch AM, Parry JM: The cytochalasin-B micronucleus/kinetochore assay in vitro: Studies with 10 suspected aneugens. *Mutat Res* 287:71–86, 1993.

MacGregor JT, Casciano D, Muller L: Strategies and testing methods for identifying mutagenic risks. *Mutat Res* 455:3–20, 2000.

Macville M, Veldman T, Padilla-Nash H, et al.: Spectral karyotyping, a 24-colour FISH technique for the identification of chromosomal rearrangements. *Histochem Cell Biol* 108:299–305, 1997.

Madle S, Dean SW, Andrae U, et al.: Recommendations for the performance of UDS tests in vitro and in vivo. *Mutat Res* 312:263–285, 1994.

Malling HV, Frantz CN: In vitro versus in vivo metabolic activation of mutagens. *Environ Health Prospect* 6:71–82, 1973.

Margison GP, Povey AC, Kaina B, Santibanez Koref MF: Variability and regulation of O6-alkylguanine-DNA alkyltransferase. *Carcinogenesis* 24:625–635, 2003.

Maron DM, Ames BN: Revised methods for the *Salmonella* mutagenicity test. *Mutat Res* 113:173–215, 1983.

Marshall CJ: Tumor suppressor genes. *Cell* 64:313–326, 1991.

Martin RH, Ko E, Rademaker A: Distribution of aneuploidy in human gametes: Comparison between human sperm and oocytes. *Am J Med Genet* 39:321–331, 1991.

Martin RH, Spriggs E, Rademaker AW: Multicolor fluorescence *in situ* hybridization analysis of aneuploidy and diploidy frequencies in 225,846 sperm from 10 normal men. *Biol Reprod* 54:394–398, 1996.

Mason JM, Aaron CS, Lee WR, et al.: A guide for performing germ cell mutagenesis assays using *Drosophila melanogaster*. *Mutat Res* 189:93–102, 1987.

McCullough AK, Dodson ML, Lloyd RS: Initiation of base excision repair: Glycosylase mechanisms and structures. *Annu Rev Biochem* 68:255–285, 1999.

McGregor DB, Rice JM, Venitt S (eds.): *The Use of Short- and Medium-term Tests for Carcinogens and Data on Genetic Effects in Carcinogenic Hazard Evaluation*. IARC Sci Pub No. 146. Lyon, France: IARC, 1999.

McGregor E, De Souza A: Proteomics and laser microdissection. *Methods Mol Biol* 333:291–304, 2006.

Meek ME, Bucher JR, Cohen SM, et al.: A framework for human relevance analysis of information on carcinogenic modes of action. *Crit Rev Toxicol* 33:591–653, 2003.

Mercer WE: Checking on the cell cycle. *J Cell Biochem Suppl* 30–31:50–54, 1998.

Makrigiorgos GM: PCR-based detection of minority point mutations. *Hum Mutat* 23:406–412, 2004.

Miller B, Pötter-Locher F, Seelbach A, et al.: Evaluation of the in vitro micronucleus test as an alternative to the in vitro chromosomal aberration assay: Position of the GUM working group on the in vitro micronucleus test. *Mutat Res* 410:81–116, 1998.

Miller JA, Miller EC: Ultimate chemical carcinogens as reactive mutagenic electrophiles, in Hiatt HH, Watson JD, Winsten JA (eds.): *Origins of Human Cancer*. Cold Spring Harbor, NY: Cold Spring Harbor Laboratory Press, 1977, pp. 605–628.

Mirsalis JC, Monforte JA, Winegar RA: Transgenic animal models for measuring mutations *in vivo*. *Crit Rev Toxicol* 24:255–280, 1994.

Modrich P: Strand-specific mismatch repair in mammalian cells. *J Biol Chem* 272:24727–24730, 1997.

Modrich P, Lahue R: Mismatch repair in replication fidelity, genetic recombination, and cancer biology. *Annu Rev Biochem* 65:101–133, 1996.

Mohrenweiser HW: Germinal mutation and human genetic disease, in Li AP, Heflich RH (eds.): *Genetic Toxicology: A Treatise*. Boca Raton, FL: CRC Press, 1991, pp. 67–92.

Moolenaar RJ: Carcinogen risk assessment: International comparison. *Reg Tox Pharmacol* 20:302–336, 1994.

Moore MM, Honma M, Clements J, et al.: Mouse lymphoma thymidine kinase locus gene mutation assay: International workshop on genotoxicity test procedures workgroup report. *Environ Mol Mutagen* 35:185–190, 2000.

Moore MM, Honma M, Clements J, et al.: Mouse lymphoma thymidine kinase gene mutation assay: International workshop on genotoxicity tests workgroup report—Plymouth, UK 2002. *Mutat Res* 540:127–140, 2003.

Morrison V, Ashby J: A preliminary evaluation of the performance of the Muta^{TM}Mouse (*lacZ*) and Big Blue^{TM}(*lacI*) transgenic mouse mutation assays. *Mutagenesis* 9:367–375, 1994.

Mortelmans K, Riccio ES: The bacterial tryptophan reverse mutation assay with *Escherichia coli* WP2. *Mutat Res* 455:61–69, 2000.

Mortelmans K, Zeiger E: The Ames *Salmonella*/microsome mutagenicity assay. *Mutat Res* 455:29–60, 2000.

Muller HJ: Artificial transmutation of the gene. *Science* 66:84–87, 1927.

Nakamura A, Sedelnikova OA, Redon C, et al.: Techniques for gamma-H2AX detection. *Methods Enzymol* 409:236–250, 2006.

Natarajan AT: An overview of the results of testing of known or suspected aneugens using mammalian cells in vitro. *Mutat Res* 287:113–118, 1993.

Norppa H, Bonassi S, Hansteen IL, et al.: Chromosomal aberrations and SCEs as biomarkers of cancer risk. *Mutat Res* June 29:[Epub ahead of print], 2006.

NRC (National Research Council): *Risk Assessment in the Federal Government: Managing the Process*. Washington, DC: National Academy Press, 1983.

NRC (National Research Council): Committee on the Biological Effects of Ionizing Radiations. *Health Effects of Exposure to Low Levels of Ionizing Radiation: BEIR V*. Washington, DC: National Academy Press, 1990.

NRC (National Research Council): *Science and Judgment in Risk Assessment*. Washington, DC: National Academy Press, 1994.

Ohe T, White PA, DeMarini DM: Mutagenic characteristics of river waters flowing through large metropolitan areas in North America. *Mutat Res* 534:101–112, 2003.

Okada N, Masumura K, Nohmi T, Yajima N: Efficient detection of deletions induced by a single treatment of mitomycin C in transgenic mouse *gpt* delta using the Spi(-) selection. *Environ Mol Mutagen* 34:106–111, 1999.

Osgood CJ, Cyr K: Induction by nitriles of sex chromosome aneuploidy: Tests of mechanism. *Mutat Res* 403:149–157, 1998.

Pack S, Vortmeyer AO, Pak E, *et al.*: Detection of gene deletion in single metastatic tumor cells in lymph node tissue by fluorescent in-situ hybridization. *Lancet* 350:264–265, 1997.

Pack SD, Weil RJ, Vortmeyer AO, *et al.*: Individual adult human neurons display aneuploidy: Detection by fluorescence in situ hybridization and single neuron PCR. *Cell Cycle* 4:1758–1760, 2005.

Painter RB: A replication model for sister-chromatid exchange. *Mutat Res* 70:337–341, 1980.

Parry JM: An evaluation of the use of in vitro tubulin polymerisation, fungal and wheat assays to detect the activity of potential chemical aneugens. *Mutat Res* 287:23–28, 1993.

Parry JM: Detecting and predicting the activity of rodent carcinogens. *Mutagenesis* 9:3–5, 1994.

Parry JM: Detecting chemical aneugens: A commentary to 'Aneuploidy: A report of an ECETOC task force.' *Mutat Res* 410:117–120, 1998.

Phillips DH, Farmer PB, Beland FA, *et al.*: Methods of DNA adduct determination and their application to testing compounds for genotoxicity. *Environ Mol Mutagen* 35:222–233, 2000.

Potter CJ, Turenchalk GS, Xu T: *Drosophila* in cancer research. *Trends Genet* 16:33–39, 2000.

Prakash S, Johnson RE, Prakash L: Eukaryotic translesion synthesis DNA polymerases: Specificity of structure and function. *Annu Rev Biochem* 74:317–353, 2005.

Preston RJ: Mechanisms of induction of chromosomal alterations and sister chromatid exchanges, in Li AP, Heflich RF (eds.): *Genetic Toxicology: A Treatise*. Boca Raton, FL: CRC Press, 1991, pp. 41–66.

Preston RJ: A consideration of the mechanisms of induction of mutations in mammalian cells by low doses and dose rates of ionizing radiation. *Adv Radiat Biol* 16:125–135, 1992.

Preston RJ: Aneuploidy in germ cells: Disruption of chromosome mover components. *Environ Mol Mutagen* 28:176–181, 1996.

Preston RJ: Chromosomal changes, in McGregor DB, Rice JM, Venitt S (eds.): *The Use of Short- and Medium-Term Tests for Carcinogens and Data on Genetic Effects in Carcinogenic Hazard Evaluation*. IARC Sci Pub 146. Lyon, France: IARC, 1999, pp. 395–408.

Preston RJ: Cytogenetic effects of ethylene oxide, with an emphasis on population monitoring. *Crit Rev Toxicol* 29:263–282, 1999.

Preston RJ: Mechanistic data and cancer risk assessment: The need for quantitative molecular endpoints. *Environ Mol Mutagen* 45:214–221, 2005.

Preston RJ, Au W, Bender MA, *et al.*: Mammalian in vivo and in vitro cytogenetic assays: A report of the U.S. EPA's Gene-Tox Program. *Mutat Res* 87:143–188, 1981.

Preston RJ, Fennell TR, Leber AP, *et al.*: Reconsideration of the genetic risk assessment for ethylene oxide exposures. *Environ Mol Mutagen* 26:189–202, 1995.

Preston RJ, Williams GM: DNA-reactive carcinogens: Mode of action and human cancer hazard. *Crit Rev Toxicol* 35:673–683, 2005.

Prival MJ, Cebula TA: Sequence analysis of mutations arising during prolonged starvation of *Salmonella typhimurium*. *Genetics* 132:303–310, 1992.

Quillardet P, Hofnung M: The SOS chromotest: A review. *Mutat Res* 297:235–279, 1993.

Rabbitts TH: Chromosomal translocations in human cancer. *Nature* 372:143–149, 1994.

Ramsey MJ, Moore DH, Briner JF, *et al.*: The effects of age and lifestyle factors on the accumulation of cytogenetic damage as measured by chromosome painting. *Mutat Res* 338:95–106, 1995.

Rattray AJ, Strathern JN: Error-prone DNA polymerases: When making a mistake is the only way to get ahead. *Annu Rev Genet* 37:31–66, 2003.

Reardon JT, Sancar A: Nucleotide excision repair. *Prog Nuclei Acid Res Mol Biol* 79:183–235, 2005.

Rhomberg L, Dellarco VL, Siegel-Scott C, *et al.*: Quantitative estimation of the genetic risk associated with the induction of heritable translocations at low-dose exposure: Ethylene oxide as an example. *Environ Mol Mutagen* 16:104–125, 1990.

Richard AM: Structure-based methods for predicting mutagenicity and carcinogenicity: Are we there yet? *Mutat Res* 400:493–507, 1998.

Ripley LS: Mechanisms of gene mutations, in Li AP, Heflich RH (eds.): *Genetic Toxicology: A Treatise*. Boca Raton, FL: CRC Press, 1991, pp. 13–40.

Robertson DG: Metabonomics in toxicology: A review. *Toxicol Sci* 85:809–822, 2005.

Royds JA, Iacopetta B: p53 and disease: When the guardian angel fails. *Cell Death Differ* 13:1017–1026, 2006.

Rupa DS, Schuler M, Eastmond DA: Detection of hyperdiploidy and breakage affecting the 1cen-1q12 region of cultured interphase human lymphocytes treated with various genotoxic agents. *Environ Mol Mutagen* 29:161–167, 1997.

Russell LB: Effects of male germ-cell stage on the frequency, nature, and spectrum of induced specific-locus mutations in the mouse. *Genetica* 122: 25–36, 2004.

Russell LB, Russell WL: Frequency and nature of specific-locus mutations induced in female mice by radiations and chemicals: A review. *Mutat Res* 296:107–127, 1992.

Russell LB, Selby PB, Von Halle E, *et al.*: The mouse specific-locus test with agents other than radiations: Interpretation of data and recommendations for future work. *Mutat Res* 86:329–354, 1981.

Russell LB, Shelby MD: Tests for heritable genetic damage and for evidence of gonadal exposure in mammals. *Mutat Res* 154:69–84, 1985.

Russell WL: X-ray-induced mutations in mice. *Cold Spring Harb Symp Quant Biol* 16:327–336, 1951.

Russo A: In vivo cytogenetics: Mammalian germ cells. *Mutat Res* 455:167-189, 2000.

Sankaranarayanan K, Chakraborty R, Boerwinkle EA: Ionizing radiation and genetic risks. VI. Chronic multifactorial diseases: A review of epidemiological and genetical aspects of coronary heart disease, essential hypertension and diabetes mellitus. *Mutat Res* 436:21–57, 1999.

Sankaranarayanan K: Ionizing radiation and genetic risks: IX. Estimates of the frequencies of mendelian diseases and spontaneous mutation rates in human populations: A 1998 perspective. *Mutat Res* 411:129–178, 1998.

Sawada M, Kamataki T: Genetically engineered cells stably expressing cytochrome P450 and their application to mutagen assays. *Mutat Res* 411:19–43, 1998.

Sax K: Induction by X-rays of chromosome aberrations in *Tradescantia* microspores. *Genetics* 23:494–516, 1938.

Sax K: The time factor in X-ray production of chromosome aberrations. *Proc Natl Acad Sci U S A* 25:225–233, 1939.

Sax K, Luippold H: The effects of fractional x-ray dosage on the frequency of chromosome aberrations. *Heredity* 6:127–131, 1952.

Scott D, Galloway SM, Marshall RR, *et al.*: Genotoxicity under extreme culture conditions. *Mutat Res* 257:147–204, 1991.

Seeberg E, Eide L, Bjoras M: The base excision repair pathway. *Trends Biochem Sci* 20:391–397, 1995.

Seed J, Carney EW, Corley RA, *et al.*: Overview: Using mode of action and life stage information to evaluate the human relevance of animal toxicity data. *Crit Rev Toxicol* 35:674–672, 2005.

Sengstag C: The role of mitotic recombination in carcinogenesis. *Crit Rev Toxicol* 24:323–353, 1994.

Shelby MD: Human germ cell mutagens. *Environ Mol Mutagen* 23(Suppl 24):30–34, 1994.

Shinohara A, Ogawa T: Homologous recombination and the roles of double-strand breaks. *Trends Biochem Sci* 20:387–391, 1995.

Singh NP: Microgels for estimation of DNA strand breaks, DNA protein crosslinks and apoptosis. *Mutat Res* 455:111–127, 2000.

Smith MT, Zhang L, Wang Y, *et al.*: Increased translocations and aneusomy in chromosomes 8 and 21 among workers exposed to benzene. *Cancer Res* 58:2176–2181, 1998.

Snyder RD, Pearl GS, Mandakas G, *et al.*: Assessment of the sensitivity of the computational programs DEREK, TOPKAT, and MCASE in the prediction of the genotoxicity of pharmaceutical molecules. *Environ Mol Mutagen* 43:143–158, 2004.

Sobels FH: The parallelogram: An indirect approach for the assessment of genetic risks from chemical mutagens, in Bora KC, Douglas GR, Nestman ER (eds.): *Progress in Mutation Research*, vol. 3. 1982, pp. 323–327.

Solinas-Toldo S, Lampel S, Stilgenbauer S, *et al.*: Matrix-based comparative genomic hybridization: Biochips to screen for genomic imbalances. *Genes Chromosomes Cancer* 20:399–407, 1997.

Sonoda E, Hochegger H, Saberi A, *et al.*: Differential usage of non-homologous end-joining and homologous recombination in double strand break repair. *DNA Repair (Amst)* Jun 23:[Epub ahead of print], 2006.

Sotomayor RE, Sega GA: Unscheduled DNA synthesis assay in mammalian spermatogenic cells: An update. *Environ Mol Mutagen* 36:255–265, 2000.

Southern EM: DNA chips: Analyzing sequence by hybridization to oligonucleotides on a large scale. *Trends Genet* 12:110–115, 1996.

Speicher MR, Carter NP: The new cytogenetics: Blurring the boundaries with molecular biology. *Nat Rev Genet* 6:782–792, 2005.

Stoler DL, Chen N, Basik M, *et al.*: The onset and extent of genomic instability in sporadic colorectal tumor progression. *Proc Natl Acad Sci U S A* 96:15121–15126, 1999.

Styles JA, Penman MG: The mouse spot test: Evaluation of its performance in identifying chemical mutagens and carcinogens. *Mutat Res* 154:183–204, 1985.

Sung JS, Demple B: Roles of base excision repair subpathways in correcting oxidized abasic sites in DNA. *FEBS J* 273:1620–1629, 2006.

Swiger RR: Just how does the *cII* selection system work in Muta^{TM}Mouse? *Environ Mol Mutagen* 37:290–296, 2001.

Swiger RR, Cosentino L, Shima N, *et al.*: The *cII* locus in the Muta Mouse system. *Environ Mol Mutagen* 34:201–207, 1999.

Tano K, Shiota S, Collier J, *et al.*: Isolation and structural characterization of a cDNA clone encoding the human DNA repair protein for 0^6-alkylguanine. *Proc Natl Acad Sci U S A* 87:686–690, 1990.

Tease C: Radiation- and chemically-induced chromosome aberrations in mouse oocytes: A comparison with effects in males. *Mutat Res* 296:135–142, 1992.

Tennant RW, Ashby J: Classification according to chemical structure, mutagenicity to Salmonella and level of carcinogenicity of a further 39 chemicals tested for carcinogenicity by the U.S. National Toxicology Program. *Mutat Res* 257:209–227, 1991.

Tennant RW, Margolin BH, Shelby MD, *et al.*: Prediction of chemical carcinogenicity in rodents from in vitro genetic toxicity assays. *Science* 236:933–941, 1987.

Thacker J: Radiation-induced mutation in mammalian cells at low doses and dose rates. *Adv Radiat Biol* 16:77–124, 1992.

Tice RR, Agurell E, Anderson D, *et al.*: Single cell gel/comet assay: Guidelines for in vitro and in vivo genetic toxicology testing. *Environ Mol Mutagen* 35:206–221, 2000.

Tice RR, Hayashi M, MacGregor JT, *et al.*: Report from the working group on the in vivo mammalian bone marrow chromosomal aberration test. *Mutat Res* 312:305–312, 1994.

Trask BJ, Allen S, Massa H, *et al.*: Studies of metaphase and interphase chromosomes using fluorescence in situ hybridizaiton. *Cold Spring Harb Symp Quant Biol* 58:767–775, 1993.

Trost D, Hildebrandt B, Beier M, *et al.*: Molecular cytogenetic profiling of complex karyotypes in primary myelodysplastic syndromes and acute myeloid leukemia. *Cancer Genet Cytogenet* 165:51–63, 2006.

Tucker JD, Auletta A, Cimino M, *et al.*: Sister-chromatid exchange: Second report of the Gene-Tox program. *Mutat Res* 297:101–180, 1993.

Tucker JD, Breneman JW, Briner JF, *et al.*: Persistence of radiation-induced translocations in rat peripheral blood determined by chromosome painting. *Environ Mol Mutagen* 30:264–272, 1997.

Tucker JD, Cofield J, Matsumoto K, *et al.*: Persistence of chromosome aberrations following acute radiation: I, PAINT translocations, dicentrics, rings, fragments, and insertions. *Environ Mol Mutagen* 45:229–248, 2005.

Tucker JD, Moore DH 2nd: The importance of age and smoking in evaluating adverse cytogenetic effects of exposure to environmental agents. *Environ Health Perspect* 104:489–492, 1996.

Tucker JD, Ramsey MJ, Lee DA, Minkler JL: Validation of chromosome painting as a biodosimeter in human peripheral lymphocytes following acute exposure to ionizing radiation in vitro. *Int J Radiat Biol* 64:27–37, 1993.

Turner DR, Dreimanis M, Holt D, Firgaira FA, Morley AA: Mitotic recombination is an important mutational event following oxidative damage. *Mutat Res* 522:21–26, 2003.

UNSCEAR (United Nations Scientific Committee on the Effects of Atomic Radiation): *Hereditary Effects of Radiation*. UNSCEAR 2001 Report to the General Assembly, with Scientific Annex. New York: United Nations.

Van Houten B, Albertini R: DNA damage and repair, in Craighead JE (ed.): *Pathology of Environmental and Occupational Disease*. St. Louis: Mosby-Year Book, 1995, pp. 311–327.

Veldman T, Vignon C, Schrock E, *et al.*: Hidden chromosome abnormalities in haematological malignancies detected by multicolour spectral karyotyping. *Nat Genet* 15:406–410, 1997.

Venkatachalam S, Shi YP, Jones SN, *et al.*: Retention of wild-type p53 in tumors from p53 heterozygous mice: Reduction of p53 dosage can promote cancer formation. *EMBO J* 17:4657–4667, 1998.

Vijg J, van Steeg H: Transgenic assays for mutations and cancer: Current status and future perspectives. *Mutat Res* 400:337–354, 1998.

Vissers LE, Veltman JA, van Kessel AG, Brunner HG: Identification of disease genes by whole genome CGH arrays. *Hum Mol Genet* 14:R215–R223, 2005.

Vlasakova K, Skopek TR, Glaab WE: Induced mutation spectra at the *upp* locus in *Salmonella typhimurium*: Response of the target gene in the FU assay to mechanistically different mutagens. *Mutat Res* 578:225–237, 2005.

Vogel EW, Graf U, Frei HJ, Nivara MM: The results of assays in *Drosophila* as indicators of exposure to carcinogens. *IARC Sci Publ* 146:427–470, 1999.

Votano JR, Parham M, Hall LH, *et al.*: Three new consensus OSAR models for the prediction of Ames genotoxicity. *Mutagenesis* 19:365–377, 2004.

Walker VE, Jones IM, Crippen TL, *et al.*: Relationships between exposure, cell loss and proliferation, and manifestation of *Hprt* mutant T cells following treatment of preweanling, weanling, and adult male mice with N-ethyl-N-nitrosourea. *Mutat Res* 431:371–388, 1999.

Wallace SS: DNA damages processed by base excision repair: Biological consequences. *Int J Radiat Biol* 66:579–589, 1994.

Ward JF: The complexity of DNA damage: Relevance to biological consequences. *Int J Radiat Biol* 66:427–432, 1994.

Ward JF: DNA damage produced by ionizing radiation in mammalian cells: Identities, mechanisms of formation, and reparability. *Prog Nucl Acid Res Mol Biol* 35:95–125, 1988.

White PA (ed.): The sources and potential hazards of mutagens in complex environmental matrices. *Mutat Res* 567(2–3):105–479, 2004.

Wodicka L, Dong H, Mittmann M, *et al.*: Genome-wide expression monitoring in *Saccharomyces cerevisiae*. *Nature Biotech* 15:1359–1367, 1997.

Wood RD: DNA repair in eukaryotes. *Annu Rev Biochem* 65:135–167, 1996.

Wood RD, Mitchell M, Lindahl T: Human DNA repair genes, 2005. *Mutat Res* 577:275–283, 2005.

Wu J, Morimyo M, Hongo E, *et al.*: Radiation-induced germline mutations detected by a direct comparison of parents and first-generation offspring DNA sequences containing SNPs. *Mutat Res* 596:1–11, 2006.

Wyrobek AJ: Methods and concepts in detecting abnormal reproductive outcomes of paternal origin. *Reprod Toxicol* 7:3–16, 1993.

Wyrobek AJ, Schmid TE, Marchetti F: Cross-species sperm-FISH assays for chemical testing and assessing paternal risk for chromosomally abnormal pregnancies. *Environ Mol Mutagen* 45:271–283, 2005.

Yasunaga K, Kiyonari A, Oikawa T, *et al.*: Evaluation of the Salmonella *umu* test with 83 NTP chemicals. *Environ Mol Mutagen* 44:329–345, 2004.

Yauk CL: Advances in the application of germline tandem repeat instability for in situ monitoring. *Mutat Res* 566:169, 2004.

Yeh HC, Ho YP, Shih IeM, Wang TH: Homogeneous point mutation detection by quantum dot-mediated two-color fluorescence coincidence analysis. *Nuclei Acids Res* 34:e35, 2006.

Zimmermann FK: Tests for recombinogens in fungi. *Mutat Res* 284:147–158, 1992.

Zimmermann FK, von Borstel RC, von Halle ES, *et al.*: Testing of chemicals for genetic activity with *Saccharomyces cerevisiae:* A report of the U.S. Environmental Protection Agency Gene-Tox Program. *Mutat Res* 133:199–244, 1984.

CHAPTER 10

DEVELOPMENTAL TOXICOLOGY

John M. Rogers and Robert J. Kavlock

HISTORY

Developmental toxicology encompasses the study of pharmacokinetics, mechanisms, pathogenesis, and outcome following exposure to agents or conditions potentially leading to abnormal development. Manifestations of developmental toxicity include structural malformations, growth retardation, functional impairment, and/or death of the organism. Developmental toxicology so defined is a relatively new science, but teratology, or the study of structural birth defects, as a descriptive science precedes written language. A marble sculpture from southern Turkey, dating to 6500 B.C., depicts conjoined twins (Warkany, 1983), and Egyptian wall paintings of human conditions such as cleft palate and achondroplasia date to as early as 5000 years ago. It is believed that mythological figures such as the Cyclops and Sirens took their origin in the birth of malformed infants (Thompson, 1930; Warkany, 1977). The Babylonians, Greeks, and Romans believed that abnormal infants were reflections of celestial events and as such were considered to be portents of the future. Indeed, the Latin word *monstrum*, from *monstrare* (to show) or *monere* (to warn), is derived from this perceived ability of malformed infants to foretell the future. In turn, derivation of the word *teratology* is from the Greek word for monster, *teras*.

Hippocrates and Aristotle thought that abnormal development could originate in physical causes such as uterine trauma or pressure, but Aristotle also shared a widespread belief that maternal impressions and emotions could influence the development of the child. He advised pregnant women to gaze at beautiful statuary to increase their child's beauty. Though this theory may sound fanciful, it is present in diverse cultures throughout recorded history. Indeed, we now know that maternal stress can be deleterious to the developing conceptus (Chernoff *et al.*, 1989).

Another belief, the hybrid theory, held that interbreeding between humans and animals was a cause of congenital malformations (Ballantyne, 1904). Again, such hybrid creatures abound in mythology, including centaurs, minotaurs, and satyrs. Into the seventeenth century, cohabitation of humans with demons and witches was blamed for the production of birth defects. Birth defects were also viewed by some to represent God's retribution on the parents of the malformed infant and on society.

In 1649, the French surgeon Ambrois Paré expounded the theory of Aristotle and Hippocrates by writing that birth defects could result from narrowness of the uterus, faulty posture of the pregnant woman, or physical trauma, such as a fall. Amputations were thought to result from amniotic bands, adhesions, or twisting of the umbilical cord. This conjecture has proven to be accurate. With the blossoming of the biological sciences in the sixteenth and seventeenth centuries, theories of the causation of birth defects with bases in scientific fact began to emerge. In 1651, William Harvey put forth the theory of developmental arrest, which stated that malformations resulted from incomplete development of an organ or structure. An example given by Harvey was harelip in humans, a congenital malformation that represents a normal early developmental stage. Much later, the theory of developmental arrest was solidified by the experiments of Stockard (1921) using eggs of the minnow, *Fundulus heteroclitus*. By manipulating the chemical constituents and temperature of growth media, he produced malformations in the embryos, the nature of which depended on the stage of the insult. He concluded that developmental arrest explained all malformations except those of hereditary origin (Barrow, 1971).

With the advent of the germplasm theory elucidated by Weissmann in the 1880s and the rediscovery of Mendel's laws in 1900, genetics as the basis for some birth defects was accepted. In 1894, Bateson published his treatise on the study of variations in animals as a tool for understanding evolution, inferring that inheritance of such variations could be a basis for speciation (Bateson, 1894). His study contains detailed descriptions and illustrations of such human birth defects as polydactyly and syndactyly, supernumerary cervical and thoracic ribs, duplicated appendages, and horseshoe (fused) kidneys. Bateson coined the term *homeosis* to denote morphologic alterations in which one structure has taken on the likeness of another. Studies of such alterations in mutants of the fruit fly *Drosophila melanogaster* and, more recently, the mouse have served as the basis for much of the recent knowledge of the genetic control of development. *Homeobox genes* are found throughout the animal and plant kingdoms and direct embryonic pattern formation (Graham *et al.*, 1989; Deschamps and van Nes, 2005). Acceptance of a genetic basis of birth defects was furthered with studies of human inborn errors of metabolism in the first decade of the twentieth century.

Modern experimental teratology began in the early nineteenth century with the work of Etienne Geoffrey Saint-Hilaire. Saint-Hilaire produced malformed chick embryos by subjecting eggs to various environmental conditions including physical trauma (jarring, inversion, pricking) and toxic exposures. In the latter part of the nineteenth century, Camille Dareste experimented extensively with chick embryos, producing a wide variety of malformations by administering noxious stimuli, physical trauma, or heat shock at various times after fertilization. He found that timing was more important than the nature of the insult in determining the type of malformation produced. Among the malformations described and beautifully illustrated by Dareste (1877, 1891) were the neural tube defects anencephaly and spina bifida, cyclopia, heart defects, situs inversus, and conjoined twins. Many of the great embryologists of the nineteenth and twentieth centuries, including Loeb, Morgan, Driesch, Wilson, Spemann, and Hertwig performed teratological manipulations using various physical and chemical probes to deduce principles of normal development.

In the early twentieth century, a variety of environmental conditions (temperature, microbial toxins, drugs) were found to perturb development in avian, reptilian, fish, and amphibian species. In contrast, mammalian embryos were thought to be resistant to induction of malformations, protected from adverse environmental conditions by the maternal system. The first reports of induced birth defects in mammalian species were published in the 1930s and were the result of experimental maternal nutrient deficiencies. Hale (1935)

produced malformations including anophthalmia and cleft palate in offspring of sows fed a diet deficient in vitamin A. Beginning in 1940, Josef Warkany and co-workers began a series of experiments in which they demonstrated that maternal dietary deficiencies and other environmental factors could affect intrauterine development in rats (Warkany and Nelson, 1940; Warkany, 1945; Warkany and Schraffenberger, 1944; Wilson *et al.*, 1953). These experiments were followed by many other studies in which chemical and physical agents, e.g., nitrogen mustard, trypan blue, hormones, antimetabolites, alkylating agents, hypoxia, and x-rays, to name a few, were clearly shown to cause malformations in mammals (Warkany, 1965).

The first recognized human epidemic of malformations induced by an environmental agent was reported by Gregg (1941), who linked an epidemic of rubella virus infection in Australia to an elevation in the incidence of eye, heart, and ear defects as well as to mental retardation. Heart and eye defects predominated with maternal infection in the first or second months of pregnancy, whereas hearing and speech defects and mental retardation were most commonly associated with infection in the third month. Later, the risk of congenital anomalies associated with rubella infection in the first 4 weeks of pregnancy was estimated to be 61%; in weeks 5–8, 26%; and in weeks 9–12, 8% (Sever, 1967). It has been estimated that in the United States alone approximately 20,000 children were impaired as a consequence of prenatal rubella infections (Cooper and Krugman, 1966). While maternal rubella is now rare in developing countries due to vaccination programs, there are still rubella epidemics in developing countries (De Santis *et al.*, 2006).

Although embryos of mammals, including humans, were found to be susceptible to common external influences such as nutritional deficiencies and intrauterine infections, the impact of these findings was not great at the time (Wilson, 1973). That changed, however, in 1961, when the association between thalidomide ingestion by pregnant women and the birth of severely malformed infants was established (see section "Scope of the Problem," below).

SCOPE OF PROBLEM: THE HUMAN EXPERIENCE

Successful pregnancy outcome in the general population occurs at a surprisingly low frequency. Estimates of adverse outcomes include postimplantation pregnancy loss, 31%; major birth defects, 2–3% at birth and increasing to 6–7% at 1 year as more manifestations are diagnosed; minor birth defects, 14%; low birth weight, 7%; infant mortality (prior to 1 year of age), 1.4%; and abnormal neurological function, 16–17% (Schardein, 2000). Thus, less than half of all human conceptions result in the birth of a completely normal, healthy infant. Reasons for the adverse outcomes are largely unknown. Brent and Beckman (1990) attributed 15–25% of human birth defects to genetic causes, 4% to maternal conditions, 3% to maternal infections, 1–2% to *deformations* (e.g., mechanical problems such as umbilical cord limb amputations), <1% to chemicals and other environmental influences, and 65% to unknown etiologies. These estimates are not much different from those suggested by Wilson (1977). Regardless of the etiology, the sum total represents a significant health burden in light of the two million annual births in the United States.

It has been estimated that more that 4100 chemicals have been tested for teratogenicity, with approximately 66% shown to be nonteratogenic, 7% teratogenic in more than one species, 18% teratogenic in most species tested, and 9% producing equivocal experimental results (Schardein, 2000). In contrast, only about 50–60

Table 10-1

Human Developmental Toxicants

Radiation	Drugs and chemicals
Atomic fallout	Aminoglycosides
Radioiodine	Androgenic hormones
Therapeutic	Angiotensin converting enzyme
	inhibitors: captopril, enalapril
Infections	Angiotensin receptor antagonists:
Cytomegalovirus	sartans
Herpes simplex	Anticonvulsants:
virus I and II	Diphenylhydantoin,
Parvovirus B-19	trimethadione, valproic acid,
(erythema	carbamazepine
infectiosum)	Busulfan
Rubella virus	Carbon monoxide
Syphilis	Chlorambucil
Toxoplasmosis	Cocaine
Varicella virus	Coumarins
Venezuelan	Cyclophosphamide
equine	Cytarabine
encephalitis	Diethylstilbestrol
virus	Danazol
	Ergotamine
Maternal trauma	Ethanol
and metabolic	Ethylene oxide
imbalances	Fluconazole
Alcoholism	Folate antagonists: aminopterin,
Amniocentesis,	methotrexate
early	Iodides
Chorionic villus	Lead
sampling	Lithium
(before day 60)	Mercury, organic
Cretinism	Methimazole
Diabetes	Methylene blue
Folic acid	Misoprostal
deficiency	Penicillamine
Hyperthermia	Polychlorobiphenyls
Phenylketonuria	Quinine (high dose)
Rheumatic	Retinoids: Accutane, isotretinoin,
disease and	etretinate, acitretin
congenital	Tetracyclines
heart block	Thalidomide
Sjogren's	Tobacco smoke
syndrome	Toluene
Virilizing tumors	Vitamin A (high dose)

Adapted from Shepard (1998) and Schardein and Macina (2007).

chemicals, chemical classes, or conditions (Table 10-1) have been documented to alter prenatal development in humans (Schardein and Macina, 2007; Shepard, 1998). Review of selected human developmental toxicants provides both a historical view of the field of developmental toxicology and an illustration of some of the key principles presented below.

Thalidomide

In 1960, a striking increase in newborns with rare limb malformations was recorded in West Germany. The affected individuals had amelia (absence of the limbs) or various degrees of phocomelia

(reduction of the long bones of the limbs), usually affecting the arms more than the legs and usually involving both left and right sides, although to differing degrees. Congenital heart disease; ocular, intestinal, and renal anomalies; and malformations of the external and inner ears were also involved. However, the limb defects were characteristic. Limb reduction anomalies of this nature are exceedingly rare. At the university clinic in Hamburg, for example, no cases of phocomelia were reported between 1940 and 1959. In 1959 there was a single case; in 1960, there were 30 cases; and in 1961, a total of 154 cases (Taussig, 1962). The unusual nature of the malformations was key in unraveling the epidemic. In 1961, Lenz and McBride, working independently in Germany and Australia, identified the sedative thalidomide as the causative agent (McBride, 1961; Lenz, 1961, 1963). Thalidomide had been introduced in 1956 by Chemie Grunenthal as a sedative/hypnotic and was used throughout much of the world as a sleep aid and to ameliorate nausea and vomiting in pregnancy. It had no apparent toxicity or addictive properties in humans or adult animals at therapeutic exposure levels. The drug was widely prescribed at an oral dose of 50–200 mg/day. There were a few reports of peripheral neuritis attributed to thalidomide, but only in patients with long-term use for up to 18 months (Fullerton and Kermer, 1961). Following the association with birth defects, thalidomide was withdrawn from the market by Grunenthal in November 1961, and case reports ended in mid-1962 as exposed pregnancies were completed. All told, an estimated 5850 thalidomide exposed malformed infants were born worldwide during this period (Lenz, 1988). Quantitative estimates of malformation risks from exposure have been difficult to compile but are believed to be in the range of one in two to one in ten (Newman, 1985). Due to concerns regarding the severity of the peripheral neuritis and subsequent questions with regard to safety in pregnancy, thalidomide did not receive marketing approval by the U.S. Food and Drug Administration (FDA) prior to its removal from the world market following the epidemic.

As a result of the thalidomide catastrophe, regulatory agencies in many countries began developing animal testing requirements specifically for evaluating the effects of drugs during pregnancy (Stirling et al., 1997). In the United States, the discussions ultimately led to the development of the Segment I, II, and III testing protocols (Kelsey, 1988).

It is both ironic and telling that the chemical largely responsible for the advent of modern regulation of potential developmental toxicants presents a very complex pattern of effects in various animal species. It has been tested for prenatal toxicity in at least 19 laboratory species. Malformations and increased resorptions have been observed in some studies in rats, while generally no effects were reported in studies with hamsters or most mouse strains. Effects similar to those observed in humans have been reported for several rabbit strains and in eight of nine primate species. The teratogenic potency of thalidomide ranges from approximately 1–100 mg/kg among sensitive species. In this ranking the human sensitivity was estimated to be 1 mg/kg (Schardein, 1993).

Studies of the relationship between periods of drug use and type of malformation induced established that thalidomide was teratogenic between 20 and 36 days after *fertilization* (Lenz and Knapp, 1962). Because of its short half-life, teratogenic potency, and good records/recall of drug use, fairly concise timetables of susceptibility can be constructed (Lenz and Knapp, 1962; Neubert and Neubert, 1997; Miller and Stromland, 1999). During the susceptible period of 20–36 days postfertilization, anotia (missing ear) was the defect induced earliest, followed by thumb, upper extremity, lower extremity, and triphalangeal thumb (Miller and Stromland, 1999).

Despite extensive effort, research to understand the species and strain differences in response to thalidomide has met with limited success until recently. Extensive structure-activity studies involving analogs of thalidomide found strict structural requirements (e.g., an intact phthalimide or phthalimidine group) but shed little light on potential mechanisms (Jonsson, 1972; Schumacher, 1975; Helm, 1981). Stephens (1988) reviewed 24 proposed mechanisms, including biochemical alterations involving vitamin B, glutamic acid, acylation, nucleic acids, and oxidative phosphorylation; cellular mechanisms including cell death and cell-cell interactions; and tissue level mechanisms including inhibition of nerve and blood vessel outgrowth. None was considered sufficient by that reviewer. More recent hypotheses concerning the mechanism of thalidomide teratogenesis include effects on angiogenesis (D'Amato et al., 1994; Joussen et al., 1999; Sauer et al., 2000), integrin regulation (Neubert et al., 1996), oxidative DNA damage (Parman et al., 1999), TNF-α inhibition (Argiles et al., 1998), growth factor antagonism (Stephens et al., 1998; Stephens and Fillmore, 2000), and effects on glutathione and redox status (Hansen et al., 1999).

The idea that thalidomide exerts its teratogenicity in sensitive species by altering cellular redox status has been further explored by Wells and colleagues (Parman et al., 1999). These investigators compared the effects of thalidomide in the pregnant mouse (an insensitive species) and the pregnant rabbit (a sensitive species). First, they demonstrated increased DNA oxidation in rabbits, in both maternal and embryonal tissues, including a 380% increase in embryos. Pretreatment of pregnant rabbits with the spin-trapping (free-radical scavenging) agent alpha-phenyl-N-t-butylnitrone (PBN) reduced thalidomide-induced embryonal DNA oxidation by 73%. Thalidomide was teratogenic and embryotoxic in the rabbit, inducing characteristic limb defects as well as other malformations, embryo/fetal mortality, and reduced fetal weight. Almost all these effects on the rabbit embryos were abolished by maternal pretreatment with PBN. Taken together, these results indicate that, in the rabbit, thalidomide is activated to a free-radical intermediate that initiates the formation of reactive oxygen species that appear to be a key element of the mechanism of teratogenicity, because both oxidation and teratogenicity are largely reduced by PBN. Although oxidation of DNA may be part of the teratogenic mechanism of thalidomide, Hansen et al. (2004) have provided strong evidence to support their hypothesis that the limb defects induced by thalidomide are due to misregulation of the expression of genes critical for the outgrowth of the limb in the embryo. They too have shown that thalidomide causes oxidative stress in sensitive (rabbit) but not in resistant (rat) pregnant animals and their embryos, by comparing glutathione depletion following administration of thalidomide (Hansen et al., 2002). They further demonstrated that this shift in redox potential reduces binding of a key transcription factor, NF-κB, to its binding sites in DNA. Binding of NF-κB is required to turn on the expression of the genes twist and FGF-10 in the mesenchyme of the developing limb. In turn, absence of expression of these two genes results in loss of FGF-8 expression in the apical ectodermal ridge of the developing limb bud. Given our understanding of the importance of these genes for normal limb development, ablation of their expression by thalidomide would be predicted to cause the limb defects seen in sensitive species. That these genes are under the control of the redox-sensitive NF-κB explains the basis for the differences in teratogenicity of thalidomide in the sensitive rabbit (and, presumably, human) and the resistant mouse and rat.

Research on alterations in immune function and angiogenesis has opened the possibility of expanded use of thalidomide in diseases including HIV infection, arthritis, multiple myeloma, diabetic retinopathy, and macular degeneration (Adler, 1994; Calabrese and Fleischer, 2000; Schwab and Jagannath, 2006). Thalidomide has recently been approved by the FDA for oral ulcers associated with AIDS and for erythema nodosum leprosum, an inflammatory complication of Hansen's disease (leprosy). An unprecedented level of safeguards, embodied in the STEPS program (System of Thalidomide Education and Prescribing Safety), surrounds thalidomide use to prevent accidental exposure during pregnancy, including required registration of all prescribers, pharmacies, and patients, required use of contraception, and periodic pregnancy testing for patients of childbearing ability (Lary et al., 1999).

Diethylstilbestrol

Diethylstilbestrol (DES) is a synthetic nonsteroidal estrogen widely used from the 1940s to the 1970s in the United States to prevent threatened miscarriage by stimulating synthesis of estrogen and progesterone in the placenta. Between 1966 and 1969, seven young women between the ages of 15 and 22 were seen at Massachusetts General Hospital with clear cell adenocarcinoma of the vagina. This tumor had never before been seen in patients younger than 30. An epidemiologic case-control study subsequently found an association with first-trimester DES exposure (reviewed in Poskranzer and Herbst, 1977). The Registry of Clear Cell Adenocarcinoma of the Genital Tract of Young Females was established in 1971 to track affected offspring. Maternal use of DES prior to the 18th week of gestation appeared to be necessary for induction of the genital tract anomalies in offspring. The incidence of genital tract tumors peaked at age 19 and declined through age 22, with absolute risk of clear cell adenocarcinoma of the vagina and cervix estimated to be 0.14–1.4 per 1000 exposed pregnancies (Herbst et al., 1977). However, the overall incidence of noncancerous alterations in the vagina and cervix was estimated to be as high as 75% (Poskranzer and Herbst, 1977). Effects of developmental exposure on the female reproductive tract may be due to alterations in genetic pathways governing uterine differentiation (Huang et al., 2005). In male offspring of exposed pregnancies, a high incidence of epididymal cysts, hypotrophic testes, and capsular induration along with low ejaculated semen volume and poor semen quality were observed (Bibbo et al., 1977). The realization of the latent and devastating manifestations of prenatal DES exposure has broadened our concept of the magnitude and scope of potential adverse outcomes of intrauterine exposures. Yet, the impact of DES suggests even broader developmental targets; a recent study in mice by Newbold et al. (2006) suggests that the increased susceptibility to tumors and reproductive tract abnormalities conferred by DES exposure may be passed on to future generations (both males and females) of exposed mothers.

Ethanol

The developmental toxicity of ethanol has been a recurrent concern throughout history and can be traced to biblical times (e.g., Judges 13: 3–4). Yet, only since the description of the Fetal Alcohol Syndrome (FAS) by Jones and Smith in the early 1970s (Jones and Smith, 1973; Jones et al., 1973) has there been a clear recognition and acceptance of alcohol's developmental toxicity. Since that time, there have been hundreds of clinical, epidemiologic, and experimental studies of the effects of ethanol exposure during gestation (for review, see Rogers and Daston, 1997).

The FAS comprises craniofacial dysmorphism, intrauterine and postnatal growth retardation, retarded psychomotor and intellectual development, and other nonspecific major and minor abnormalities (Abel, 1982, 2006). The average IQ of FAS children has been reported to be 68 (Streissguth *et al.*, 1991a) and changes little over time (Streissguth *et al.*, 1991b). The craniofacial malformations as well as other morphological and anatomical effects of prenatal ethanol exposure may be due, at least in part, to interference with retinol metabolism in the early embryo, at a time when the anterior part of the embryo, including the brain, is just beginning to form (Yelin *et al.*, 2005). Oxidation of retinol to the signaling molecule, retinoic acid, is crucial for normal development of the embryo. Full-blown FAS has been observed only in children born to alcoholic mothers, and among alcoholics the incidence of FAS has been estimated at 25 per 1000 (Abel, 1984). Numerous methodological difficulties are involved in attempting to estimate the level of maternal ethanol consumption associated with FAS, but estimates of a minimum of 3–4 oz of alcohol per day have been made (Clarren *et al.*, 1987; Ernhart *et al.*, 1987).

In utero exposure to lower levels of ethanol has been associated with a wide range of effects, including isolated components of FAS and milder forms of neurological and behavioral disorders. The developmental effects of ethanol, including both FAS and lesser expressions of the toxicity of prenatal ethanol exposure have been termed Fetal Alcohol Spectrum Disorder (FASD) (Koren *et al.*, 2003; Sokol, 2003). Alcohol consumption can affect birth weight in a dose-related fashion even if the mother is not alcoholic. Little (1977) studied 800 women prospectively to evaluate the effects of drinking on birth weight. After adjusting for smoking, gestational age, maternal height, age, parity, and sex of the child, it was found that for each ounce of absolute ethanol consumed per day during late pregnancy there was a 160-gram decrease in birth weight. Effects of maternal alcohol consumption during pregnancy on attention, short-term memory, and performance on standardized tests have been noted in a longitudinal prospective study of 462 children (Streissguth *et al.*, 1994a,b). Alcohol intake was related to these effects, the number of drinks per drinking occasion being the strongest predictor. Recently, Streissguth and co-workers (Baer *et al.*, 2003) reported that prenatal alcohol exposure was significantly associated with alcohol drinking problems at age twenty-one, independent of family history or other environmental factors.

One animal model of FAS in which pathogenesis of the craniofacial effects has been extensively studied involves intraperitoneal injection of ethanol to pregnant C57Bl/6J mice in early pregnancy when embryos are undergoing *gastrulation* (Sulik *et al.*, 1981; Sulik and Johnston, 1983). Following such exposures, term fetuses exhibit many of the features of FAS, including microcephaly, microphthalmia, short palpebral fissures, deficiencies of the philtral region, and a long upper lip. The specific set of craniofacial malformations produced in offspring depends on the time of exposure. The mechanisms by which ethanol exerts its teratogenic effects are not understood but probably involve a complex combination of maternal factors and biochemical/cellular effects in the embryo (Rogers and Daston, 1997). Excess cell death in sensitive cell populations appears to be a common finding (Kotch and Sulik, 1992; Sulik, 2005).

Tobacco Smoke

Prenatal and early postnatal exposure to tobacco smoke or its constituents may well represent the leading cause of environmentally induced developmental disease and morbidity today. Approximately 25% of women in the United States continue to smoke during pregnancy, despite public health programs aimed at curbing this behavior. Because of the high number of pregnant smokers and the relative accuracy of assessing smoking during pregnancy, results of epidemiologic studies provide a well-characterized picture of the consequences of developmental tobacco smoke exposure. These include spontaneous abortions, perinatal deaths, increased risk of sudden infant death syndrome (SIDS), increased risk of learning, behavioral, and attention disorders, and lower birth weight (Slotkin, 1998; Fried *et al.*, 1998; Tuthill *et al.*, 1999; Haug *et al.*, 2000; Markussen Linnet *et al.*, 2006). In a recent review of smoking and sudden infant death syndrome (Mitchell and Milerad, 2006), the relative risk associated with maternal smoking was 2.86 (95% confidence interval 2.77–2.95) before prone-sleep-position intervention (putting infants on their backs for sleep reduces the overall risk of SIDS) and 3.93 (3.78–4.08) after intervention programs were started. The authors of the review estimated that about one-third of SIDS deaths might have been prevented if all fetuses had not been exposed in utero to maternal smoking.

Maternal smoking has not been associated with a high risk of structural malformations. However, maternal smoking is a known risk factor for orofacial clefts, and increased risk is associated with particular xenobiotic metabolizing gene polymorphisms (Lammer *et al.*, 2005; Honein *et al.*, 2007; Ramirez *et al.*, 2007). Pregnant smokers with variant alleles for N053, ICAM1, and/or NPPA may be at elevated risk for offspring with gastroschisis.

One component of tobacco smoke, nicotine, is a known neuroteratogen in experimental animals and can by itself produce many of the adverse neurodevelopmental outcomes associated with tobacco smoke (Slotkin, 1998). Perinatal exposure to tobacco smoke can also affect branching morphogenesis and maturation of the lung, leading to altered physiologic function (Pinkerton and Joad, 2000; Gilliland *et al.*, 2000). Dempsey and co-workers (2000) found that hypertonia among cocaine-exposed infants was associated not with maternal cocaine usage (as determined by fetal meconium analyses for the cocaine metabolite benzoylecgonine) but rather with maternal urine cotinine levels (a nicotine metabolite).

It is important to keep in mind that environmental (passive) tobacco smoke also represents a significant risk to the pregnant nonsmoker and her baby, and has been associated with many of the effects caused by active maternal smoking (e.g., Windham *et al.*, 2000; George *et al.*, 2006; Mitchell and Milerad, 2006). Inhaled doses in some situations are similar to those for light active smokers.

Cocaine

Cocaine, a plant alkaloid derived from coca, is a local anesthetic with vasoconstrictor properties. During the 1980s, as more potent forms became available, cocaine abuse became an epidemic health problem. It has been estimated that up to 45% of pregnancies at an urban teaching hospital and 6% in a suburban hospital had recent cocaine exposure. Effects on the fetus are complicated and controversial and demonstrate the difficulty of monitoring the human population for adverse reproductive outcomes (reviewed in Scanlon, 1991; Volfe, 1992). Accurate exposure ascertainment is difficult, as many confounding factors, including socioeconomic status and concurrent use of cigarettes, alcohol, and other drugs of abuse, may be involved. In addition, reported effects on the fetus and infant (neurological and behavioral changes) are difficult to identify and quantify. Nevertheless, adverse effects on pregnancy appear to be reliably associated with cocaine exposure in humans, including abruptio placentae; premature labor and delivery; microcephaly; altered prosencephalic development; decreased birth weight; a neonatal neurologic syndrome of abnormal sleep, tremor, poor feeding, irritability, and occasional seizures; and SIDS. Congenital malformations of the genitourinary tract have also been reported (Lutiger *et al.*, 1991), and kidney and bladder function is diminished in fetuses of pregnant women using cocaine (Mitra, 1999). Moreover, fetal cocaine exposure has been associated with impaired neonatal auditory processing (Potter *et al.*, 2000). Fetal cocaine exposure was estimated by chemical analysis of fetal meconium, which can provide a measure of developmental exposure to xenobiotic agents ranging from food additives to over-the-counter medications to drugs of abuse (Ostrea *et al.*, 1998).

Retinoids

The ability of excess vitamin A (retinol) to induce malformations has been known for over fifty years (Cohlan, 1954). Effects on the developing embryo include malformations of the face, limbs, heart, central nervous system, and skeleton. Similar malformations were later shown to be induced by retinoic acid administration in the mouse (Kochhar, 1967) and hamster (Shenefelt, 1972). Since those observations, knowledge relating to the effects of retinol, retinoic acid, and structurally related chemicals that bind to and activate specific nuclear receptors that regulate a variety of transcriptional events has been expanding rapidly (Chambon, 1994; Lohnes *et al.*, 1994; Mendelsohn *et al.*, 1994; Collins and Mao, 1999; Arafa *et al.*, 2000). The RXR-alpha receptor appears to play an important role in cleft palate induced by retinoic acid (Nugent *et al.*, 1999). The teratogenic effects of vitamin A and retinoids have been reviewed (Nau *et al.*, 1994; Collins and Mao, 1999). A link between retinoids and schizophrenia has been proposed, supported by three lines of evidence (Goodman, 1998). First, congenital anomalies similar to those caused by retinoid dysfunction are found in schizophrenics and their relatives; second, genetic loci that are putatively involved in schizophrenia are also the loci of genes in the retinoid cascade; and third, transcriptional activation of candidate schizophrenia genes as well as that of the dopamine D2 receptor is regulated by retinoic acid.

Beginning in 1982, one retinoid, 13-*cis*-retinoic acid (isotretinoin or Accutane), was marketed as an effective treatment of recalcitrant cystic acne. Despite clear warnings against use in pregnancy on the label of this prescription drug (FDA pregnancy category X), an extensive physician and patient education program, and restrictive requirements for prescription to women of childbearing potential, infants with pathognomonic malformations involving the ears, heart, brain, and thymus began to be reported as early as 1983 (Rosa, 1983; Lammer *et al.*, 1985). Among 115 exposed pregnancies not electively terminated, 18% ended in spontaneous abortion and 28% of the live-born infants had at least one major malformation (Dai *et al.*, 1992). In another prospective study, there was nearly a doubling of the risk for premature delivery after first-trimester exposure, and about 50% of the exposed children had full-scale IQ scores below 85 at age 5 (Lammer, 1992). In a recent study (Robertson *et al.*, 2005), almost 25% of women with an isotretinoin-exposed pregnancy did not recall having contraception counseling before starting their medication. Rates of recommended birth control and monthly pregnancy testing were low. Thus, voluntary pregnancy prevention programs for women receiving prescriptions for isotretinoin were not highly effective, resulting in fetal exposures.

Valproic Acid

Valproic acid, or 2-propylpentanoic acid, is an anticonvulsant first marketed in Europe in 1967 and in the United States in 1978. In 1982, Elizabeth Robert reported that of 146 cases of spina bifida aperta recorded in a birth defects surveillance system in Lyon, France, nine of the mothers had taken valproate during the first trimester. The odds ratio for this finding in a case-control study was 20.6, and the estimated risk of a valproate-exposed woman having a child with spina bifida was 1.2%, a risk similar to that for women with a previous child with a neural tube defect (Centers for Disease Control, 1982). The report was quickly confirmed in other areas of the world through the efforts of the International Clearinghouse of Birth Defect Registries (Centers for Disease Control, 1983). Because of the relatively low risk, the fact that epileptic women are already at elevated risk for birth defects, and that the majority of pregnant epileptics are on drug therapy (including several known teratogens), it was fortunate that several events came together to allow the determination of valproate as a human teratogen. These included the active birth defects registry, an interest by Robert in the genetics of spina bifida, a question on epilepsy and anticonvulsant use in Robert's survey, and the prevalence of valproate monotherapy for epilepsy in that region (Lammer *et al.*, 1987). Although these findings spurred a great deal of research on the effects of valproate in multiple species, including interesting results on the effects of enantiomers of valproate analogs, the mechanism of action, as for most developmental toxicants, remains elusive (Nau *et al.*, 1991; Ehlers *et al.*, 1992; Hauck and Nau, 1992). Use of inbred mouse strains differing in their sensitivity to valproate-induced teratogenesis has revealed several candidate genes conferring sensitivity in that species (Finnell *et al.*, 1997, 2000; Craig *et al.*, 2000; Bennett *et al.*, 2000).

Clinical management of women of childbearing age who have epilepsy is difficult. Although control of seizures during pregnancy is crucial, all of the current antiepileptic drugs (AEDs) carry risk of developmental toxicity including birth defects, cognitive impairment, and fetal death. As a class they are considered human teratogens. The interested reader is directed to several recent reviews (Tatum, 2006; Tomson and Battino, 2005; Ornoy, 2006).

Angiotensin Converting Enzyme Inhibitors and Angiotensin Receptor Antagonists

The renin-angiotensin system is a key controller of blood pressure. The final active signaling messenger of this system is angiotensin II, which binds to AT1 receptors to cause vasoconstriction and fluid retention, resulting in elevation of blood pressure. Antihypertensive agents acting on this system include the angiotensin converting enzyme (ACE) inhibitors and the angiotensin II (AT1) receptor blockers (collectively known as "sartans"). ACE inhibitors are widely prescribed and, when used in the second half of pregnancy, are known to cause oligohydramnios, fetal growth retardation, pulmonary hypoplasia, joint contractures, hypocalvaria, neonatal renal failure, hypotension, and death. Angiotensin II receptor antagonists taken during the same period (second or third trimester) in pregnancy cause a very similar spectrum of developmental toxicity (Friedman, 2006; Quan, 2006). These findings in the fetus can be related to reduced amniotic fluid volume, a consequence of impaired fetal renal function (Tabacova, 2005). While the developmental toxicity of first trimester use of ACE inhibitors and AT1 receptor antagonists has been somewhat controversial (Schaefer, 2003), a recent study found an increased risk of major congenital malformations following first trimester exposure to ACE inhibitors (Cooper *et al.*, 2006). These authors studied a cohort of 29,507 infants born between 1985 and 2000. Of these, 209 infants had exposure to ACE inhibitors in the first trimester alone. These infants exposed in the first trimester had an increased risk of major congenital malformations (relative risk = 2.71, 95% confidence interval 1.72–4.27). The risk ratio for malformations of the cardiovascular system and the central nervous system were 3.72 and 4.39, respectively. These authors conclude that exposure to ACE inhibitors during the first trimester cannot be considered safe and should be avoided. Because the fetal kidney is not functional at this time, it is likely that different mechanisms underlie the developmental toxicity of these drugs in the first trimester compared to their effects later in development.

PRINCIPLES OF DEVELOPMENTAL TOXICOLOGY

Principles of teratology were put forth by Jim Wilson in his watershed monograph *Environment and Birth Defects* (Wilson, 1973) (Table 10-2). Much progress has been made in the ensuing decades, yet these principles have withstood the test of time and remain basic to developmental toxicology.

Critical Periods of Susceptibility and Endpoints of Toxicity

Familiarity with principles of normal development is prerequisite to understanding abnormal development. Development is characterized by change: change in size, changes in biochemistry and physiology, changes in form and functionality. These changes are orchestrated by a cascade of factors regulating gene transcription, the first of which are maternally inherited and present in the egg prior to fertilization. In turn, these factors activate regulatory genes in the embryonic genome, and sequential gene activation continues throughout development. Intercellular and intracellular signaling pathways essential for normal development have been elucidated and rely on transcriptional, translational, and posttranslational controls.

Table 10-2

Wilson's General Principles of Teratology

I.	Susceptibility to teratogenesis depends on the genotype of the conceptus and the manner in which this interacts with adverse environmental factors.
II.	Susceptibility to teratogenesis varies with the developmental stage at the time of exposure to an adverse influence.
III.	Teratogenic agents act in specific ways (mechanisms) on developing cells and tissues to initiate sequences of abnormal developmental events (pathogenesis).
IV.	The access of adverse influences to developing tissues depends on the nature of the influence (agent).
V.	The four manifestations of deviant development are death, malformation, growth retardation, and functional deficit.
VI.	Manifestations of deviant development increase in frequency and degree as dosage increases, from the no effect to the totally lethal level.

SOURCE: Wilson JG: *Environment and Birth Defects*. New York: Academic Press, 1973, pp. 12–30, with permission from Elsevier.

Table 10-3

Timing of Key Developmental Events in Some Mammalian Species

	RAT	RABBIT	MONKEY	HUMAN
Blastocyst formation	3–5	2.6–6	4–9	4–6
Implantation	5–6	6	9	6–7
Organogenesis	6–17	6–18	20–45	21–56
Primitive streak	9	6.5	18–20	16–18
Neural plate	9.5	—	19–21	18–20
First somite	10	—	—	20–21
First branchial arch	10	—	—	20
First heartbeat	10.2	—	—	22
10 Somites	10–11	9	23–24	25–26
Upper limb buds	10.5	10.5	25–26	29–30
Lower limb buds	11.2	11	26–27	31–32
Testes differentiation	14.5	20	—	43
Heart septation	15.5	—	—	46–47
Palate closure	16–17	19–20	45–47	56–58
Urethral groove closed in male	—	—	—	90
Length of gestation	21–22	31–34	166	267

*Developmental ages are days of gestation.

SOURCE: Adapted from Shepard (1998), with permission.

Because of the rapid changes occurring during development, the nature of the embryo/fetus as a target for toxicity is also changing. While the basic tenets of toxicology discussed elsewhere in this text also apply during development, the principle of critical periods of sensitivity based on developmental stage of the conceptus is a primary and somewhat unique consideration. In this section we discuss normal developmental stages in the context of their known and potential susceptibility to toxicants. It should be made clear, however, that development is a continuum. Therefore, these stages are used for descriptive purposes and do not necessarily represent discrete developmental events. Timing of some key developmental events in humans and experimental animal species is presented in Table 10-3.

As a logical starting point, *gametogenesis* is the process of forming the haploid germ cells, the egg and sperm. These gametes fuse in the process of fertilization to form the diploid *zygote*, or one-celled embryo. Gametogenesis and fertilization are vulnerable to toxicants, but this is the topic of another chapter in this text. It is now known that the maternal and paternal genomes are not equivalent in their contributions to the zygotic genome. The process of *imprinting* occurs during gametogenesis, conferring to certain allelic genes a differential expressivity depending on whether they are of maternal or paternal origin (Latham, 1999). Because imprinting involves cytosine methylation and changes in chromatin conformation, this process may be susceptible to toxicants that affect these targets (Murphy and Jirtle, 2000). Jirtle and colleagues have demonstrated that both early nutrition (Waterland and Jirtle, 2003, 2004) and the estrogenic compound genistein (Dolinoy *et al.*, 2006) can modify the methylation patterns of specific genes and cause altered phenotypes in mice. Anway *et al.* (2006) demonstrated a transgenerational effect of the fungicide vinclozolin in rats, in which male offspring of treated F0 females had reduced spermatogenic capacity which was transmitted to subsequent generations (F2–F4). Toxic effects on imprinting and epigenetic gene regulation could conceivably play a role in paternally mediated developmental toxicity, a topic that is not discussed here but which has received increased attention (Olshan and Mattison, 1995).

Exposure to toxicants during a brief period (~6 hours) immediately following fertilization has been demonstrated to result in malformed fetuses for a few chemicals including ethylene oxide (Generoso et al., 1987), ethylmethane sulfonate, ethylnitrosourea, and triethylene melamine (Generoso et al., 1988). The mechanisms underlying these unexpected findings have not been elucidated but probably do not involve point mutations.

Following fertilization, the embryo moves down the fallopian tube (oviduct) and implants on the wall of the uterus. The *preimplantation* period comprises mainly an increase in cell number through a rapid series of cell divisions with little growth in size (*cleavage of the zygote*) and cavitation of the embryo to form a fluid-filled blastocoele. This stage, termed the *blastocyst,* consisting of about a thousand cells, may contain as few as three cells destined to give rise to the embryo proper (Markert and Petters, 1978), and these cells are within a region called the *inner cell mass.* The remainder of the blastocyst cells give rise to extraembryonic membranes and support structures (e.g., trophoblast and placenta). However, the fate of the cells in the early embryo are not completely determined at this stage. The relatively undifferentiated preimplantation embryo has great restorative (regulative) growth potential (Snow and Tam, 1979). Experiments of Moore et al. (1968) demonstrated that single cells from eight-celled rabbit embryos are capable of producing normal offspring.

Toxicity during preimplantation is generally thought to result in either no or slight effect on growth (because of regulative growth) or in death (through overwhelming damage or failure to implant). Preimplantation exposure to DDT, nicotine, or methylmethane sulfonate results in body and/or brain weight deficits and embryo lethality, but not malformations (Fabro, 1973; Fabro et al., 1984). However, there are also examples of toxic exposures during the preimplantation period leading to fetal malformations. Treatment of pregnant mice with methylnitrosourea on days 2.5, 3.5, and 4.5 of gestation resulted in neural tube defects and cleft palate (Takeuchi, 1984). Cyproterone acetate and medroxyprogesterone acetate are capable of producing malformations when administered on day 2 of gestation (Eibs et al., 1982). Rutledge and co-workers (Rutledge et al., 1994) produced hind-limb and lower body duplications by treating pregnant mice with all-*trans* retinoic acid on gestation day 4.5–5.5, at which time the embryos are at the late blastocyst and proamniotic stages. This finding suggests that patterning of the limbs and lower body may begin prior to gastrulation. Because of the rapid mitoses occurring during the preimplantation period, chemicals affecting DNA synthesis or integrity or those affecting microtubule assembly would be expected to be particularly toxic if given access to the embryo.

Following implantation the embryo undergoes gastrulation. Gastrulation is the process of formation of the three primary germ layers—the *ectoderm, mesoderm,* and *endoderm.* During gastrulation, cells migrate through a structure called the *primitive streak,* and their movements set up basic morphogenetic fields in the embryo (Smith et al., 1994). A prelude to *organogenesis,* the period of gastrulation is quite susceptible to teratogenesis. A number of toxicants administered during gastrulation produce malformations of the eye, brain, and face. These malformations are indicative of damage to the anterior *neural plate,* one of the regions defined by the cellular movements of gastrulation.

The formation of the neural plate in the ectoderm marks the onset of organogenesis, during which the rudiments of most bodily structures are established. This is a period of heightened susceptibility to malformations and extends from approximately the third to the eighth weeks of gestation in humans. Within this short period, the embryo undergoes rapid and dramatic changes. At 3 weeks of gestation, the human conceptus is in most ways indistinguishable from other mammalian and indeed other vertebrate embryos, consisting of only a few cell types in a trilaminar arrangement. By 8 weeks, the conceptus, which can now be termed a fetus, has a clearly recognizable human form. The rapid changes of organogenesis require cell proliferation, cell migration, cell-cell interactions, and morphogenetic tissue remodeling. These processes are exemplified by the *neural crest* cells. These cells originate at the border of the neural plate and migrate to form a wide variety of structures throughout the embryo. Neural crest cells derived from segments of the hindbrain (*rhombomeres*) migrate to form bone and connective tissues in the head (Krumlauf, 1993; Vaglia and Hall, 1999; Trainor and Krumlauf, 2001).

Within organogenesis, there are periods of peak susceptibility for each forming structure. This is nicely illustrated by the work of Shenefelt (1972), who studied the developmental toxicity of carefully timed exposures to retinoic acid in the hamster. The incidence of some of the defects seen after retinoic acid administration at different times in development are shown in Fig. 10-1. The peak incidence of each malformation coincides with the timing of key developmental events in the affected structure. Thus, the specification of developmental fields for the eyes is established quite early, and microphthalmia has an early critical period. Establishment of rudiments of the long bones of the limbs occurs later, as does susceptibility to shortened limbs. The palate has two separate peaks of susceptibility, the first corresponding to the early establishment of the palatal folds and the second to the later events leading to palatal closure. Notice also that the total incidence of malformations is lower prior to organogenesis but increases to 100% by gestation day $7^3/_4$. The processes underlying the development of normal structures are poorly understood but involve a number of key events. A given toxicant may affect one or several developmental events, so the pattern of sensitivity of a structure can change depending on the nature of the toxic insult. Cleft palate is induced in mouse fetuses following maternal exposure to methanol as early as day 5 of gestation, with a peak sensitivity at day 7 and little or no sensitivity after day 9 (Rogers and Mole, 1997). In contrast, the typical peak critical period for induction of cleft palate for most agents is between gestation days 11 and 13. In a large series of experiments in NMRI mice, Neubert's group found that the day of peak sensitivity to the induction of cleft palate was day 11 for TCDD, day 12 for 2,4,5-trichlorophenoxyacetic acid, and day 13 for dexamethasone (Neubert et al., 1973). Detection of unexpected critical periods like that for induction of cleft palate by methanol may provide clues to normal developmental processes not presently understood.

The end of organogenesis marks the beginning of the *fetal period* (starting at days 56–58 to birth in humans), characterized primarily by tissue differentiation, growth, and physiologic maturation. This is not to say that formation of the organs is complete but rather that almost all organs are present and grossly recognizable. Further development of organs proceeds during the fetal period to attain requisite functionality prior to birth, including fine structural morphogenesis (e.g., neurite outgrowth and synaptogenesis, branching morphogenesis of the bronchial tree and renal cortical tubules) as well as biochemical maturation (e.g., induction of tissue specific enzymes and structural proteins). One of the latest organogenetic events is closure of the urethral groove in the male, which occurs at

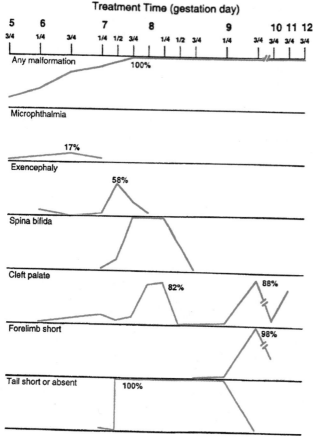

Figure 10-1. *Critical periods of sensitivity for induction of various defects by retinoic acid in the hamster.*

Incidence of defects are estimates for the embryo/fetal LD$_{50}$ maternal dosage. Note in the top panel that fewer malformations are induced on days 5–6, prior to organogenesis, indicating that during this period embryos for the most part either die or recover. Likelihood of malformation increases rapidly during gastrulation and reaches 100% during organogenesis. Peak incidence for each defect is enumerated and reflect timing of critical events in the development of each structure. [Modified from Shenefelt (1972), with permission.]

about gestation day 90. Failure of this event produces hypospadias, a ventral clefting of the penis.

Exposure during the fetal period is most likely to result in effects on growth and functional maturation. Functional anomalies of the central nervous system and reproductive organs—including behavioral, mental, and motor deficits as well as decreases in fertility—are among the possible adverse outcomes. These manifestations are not apparent prenatally and may require careful postnatal observation and testing. Such postnatal functional manifestations can be sensitive indicators of in utero toxicity, and reviews of postnatal functional deficits of the central nervous system (Rodier *et al.*, 1994), immune system (Holladay and Luster, 1994), and heart, lung, and kidneys (Lau and Kavlock, 1994) are available.

Major structural alterations can occur during the fetal period, but these generally result from deformations (disruption of previously normal structures) rather than malformations. The extremities may be affected by amniotic bands, wrapping of the umbilical cord, or vascular disruptions, leading to loss of distal structures.

Recently, the concept of "fetal programming" has emerged, in which the developmental environment is thought to determine,

in part, the metabolic parameters of the individual that will persist throughout life and may affect life-long risk of adult diseases (for review, see McMillen and Robinson, 2005). Much of the work on fetal programming has focused on the role of maternal nutrition. There is a paucity of data concerning the long-term effects of toxic exposures during the fetal period. Some effects could require years to become apparent (such as those noted for DES above), and others may even result in the premature onset of senescence and/or organ failure late in life. In rats, prenatal exposure to high dosages of ethanol during the second half of pregnancy shortens life span of the offspring, by about 20 weeks in females and 2.5–7 weeks in males (Abel *et al.*, 1987).

Dose–Response Patterns and the Threshold Concept

The major effects of prenatal exposure, observed at the time of birth in developmental toxicity studies, are lethality, malformations, and growth retardation. The relationships among these effects are complex and vary with the type of agent, the time of exposure, and the dose. For some agents these endpoints may represent a continuum of increasing toxicity, with low dosages producing growth retardation and increasing dosages producing malformations and then lethality. Malformations and/or death can occur in the absence of any effect on intrauterine growth, but this is unusual. Likewise, growth retardation and embryo lethality can occur without malformations. Chemicals producing the latter pattern of response would be considered embryotoxic or embryolethal but not teratogenic (unless it was established that death was due to a structural malformation).

Another key element of the dose–response relationship is the shape of the dose–response curve at low exposure levels. Because of the high restorative growth potential of the mammalian embryo, cellular homeostatic mechanisms, and maternal metabolic defenses, mammalian developmental toxicity has generally been considered a threshold phenomenon. Assumption of a threshold means that there is a maternal dosage below which an adverse response is not elicited. Daston (1993) summarized two approaches for establishing the existence of a threshold. The first, exemplified by a large teratology study on 2,4,5-T (Nelson and Holson, 1978), suggests that no study is capable of evaluating the dose–response at low response rates (e.g., 805 litters per dose would be necessary to detect a 5% increase in resorptions). The second approach is to determine whether a threshold exists for the mechanism responsible for the observed effect. Although relatively few mechanisms of abnormal development have been thoroughly studied, it is clear that cellular and embryonic repair mechanisms and dose-dependent kinetics both support the plausibility of a mechanistic threshold. Lack of a threshold implies that exposure to any amount of a toxic chemical, even one molecule, has the potential to cause developmental toxicity. One mechanism of abnormal development for which this might be the case is gene mutation. A point mutation in a critical gene could theoretically be induced by a single hit or single molecule, leading to a deleterious change in a gene product and consequent abnormal development. This, of course, carries the large assumption that the molecule could traverse the maternal system and the placenta and enter a critical progenitor cell in the embryo. An effect on a single cell might result in abnormal development at the zygote (one-cell) stage, the blastocyst stage (when only a few cells in the inner cell mass are embryo progenitors), or during organogenesis, when organ rudiments may consist of only a few cells.

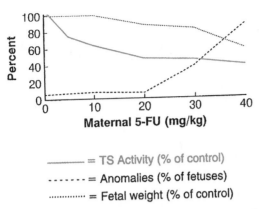

Figure 10-2. Relationship between inhibition of embryonal thymidy-late synthetase (TS) and adverse fetal outcome following maternal 5-fluorouracil (5-FU) administration on gestation day 14 in the rat.

5-FU inhibits embryonal TS activity at low dosages, with most of the inhibition occurring below 20 mg/kg. Fetal weight is affected at 20 mg/kg and above, while incidence of anomalies increases only at 30 mg/kg and above. Anomalies include edema, skull dysmorphology, orbital hemorrhage, wavy ribs, cleft palate, brachygnathia and hindlimb defects. [Based on Shuey *et al.* (1994), Lau *et al.* (1992) and unpublished observations.]

An apparent threshold for developmental toxicity based at least in part on cellular homeostatic mechanisms is demonstrated in studies of mechanisms underlying the developmental dose–response for 5-fluorouracil (Shuey *et al.*, 1994; see also "Safety Assessment" later in this chapter). This chemical inhibits the enzyme thymidylate synthetase (TS), thus interfering with DNA synthesis and cell proliferation. Significant embryonal TS inhibition can be measured at maternal dosages of an order of magnitude below those required to produce malformations and about fivefold below those affecting fetal growth (Fig. 10-2). The lack of developmental toxicity below 10 mg/kg despite significant TS inhibition probably reflects an ability of the embryo to compensate for imbalances in cellular nucleotide pool sizes.

In the context of human health risk assessment, it is also important to consider the distinction between individual thresholds and population thresholds. There is wide variability in the human population, and a threshold for a population is defined by the threshold of the most sensitive individual in the population (Gaylor *et al.*, 1988). Indeed, even though the biological target of a developmental toxicant may be thresholded, background factors such as health status or concomitant exposures may render an individual at or even beyond the threshold for failure of that biological process. Any further toxic impact on that process, even one molecule, would theoretically increase risk.

MECHANISMS AND PATHOGENESIS OF DEVELOPMENTAL TOXICITY

The term *mechanisms* is used here to refer to cellular-level events that initiate the process leading to abnormal development. *Pathogenesis* comprises the cell-, tissue-, and organ-level sequelae that are ultimately manifest in abnormality. Mechanisms of teratogenesis listed by Wilson (1977) include mutations, chromosomal breaks, altered mitosis, altered nucleic acid integrity or function, diminished supplies of precursors or substrates, decreased energy supplies, altered membrane characteristics, osmolar imbalance, and enzyme

inhibition. Although these cellular insults are not unique to development, they may relatively quickly trigger unique pathogenetic responses in the embryo, such as reduced cell proliferation, cell death, altered cell-cell interactions, reduced biosynthesis, inhibition of morphogenetic movements, or mechanical disruption of developing structures.

Experimental studies of cyclophosphamide (CP), a teratogenic chemotherapeutic drug, provide an example of current approaches to understanding teratogenic mechanisms and pathogenesis. Much of this and other mechanistic work was made possible by the advent of rodent whole embryo culture techniques, which involve removing rodent embryos from the uterus at the beginning of organogenesis and growing them in serum-containing culture media (New, 1978; Sadler and Warner, 1984). Embryos will grow normally for about 48 hours, completing most of organogenesis. The ability to grow embryos in isolation allows direct exposure, manipulation, and observation of the organogenesis-stage embryo.

Using the embryo culture system, Fantel *et al.* (1979) and Sanyal *et al.* (1979) showed that hepatic S9 fractions and cofactors were needed to elicit abnormal development by CP, demonstrating that it must be metabolically activated to be teratogenic. Activation of CP was inhibited by metyrapone or carbon monoxide, indicating involvement of P450 monooxygenases. Of the CP metabolites (Fig. 10-3), 4-hydroxycyclophosphamide (4OHCP) and aldophosphamide (AP) are unstable. A stable derivative of 4OHCP, 4-hydroperoxy-cyclophosphamide (4OOHCP) was tested in vivo (Hales, 1982) and in whole embryo culture (Mirkes, 1987). In the latter study, the morphology of the treated embryos was indistinguishable from that of embryos cultured with CP and an activating system. Spontaneous conversion of 4OOHCP to 4OHCP and then to phosphoramide mustard and acrolein occurs rapidly, and these further metabolites, as well as 4-ketocyclophosphamide (4-ketoCP) and carboxyphosphamide (CaP), have also been studied for their teratogenicity. It appears that 4OHCP is not teratogenic (Hales, 1983) and toxicity elicited by 4-ketoCP is dissimilar to that of activated CP (Mirkes *et al.*, 1981). Subsequent work centered on the two remaining metabolites, PM and AC. Mirkes *et al.* (1981) demonstrated that the effects of PM on cultured rat embryos were indistinguishable from those of activated CP. Hales (1982) administered CP, PM, or AC to gestation day 13 rat embryos by intraamniotic injection. CP and AC caused hydrocephaly, open eyes, cleft palate, micrognathia, omphalocele, and tail and limb defects, whereas PM produced only hydrocephaly and tail and limb defects. Thus, both PM and AC appear to be teratogenic metabolites of CP.

What are the cell and molecular targets of activated CP, and what is the nature of the interaction? Experiments with (^{3}H)CP show that approximately 87% of bound radioactivity is associated with protein, 5% with DNA, and 8% with RNA (Mirkes, 1985a). Using alkaline elution, it was demonstrated that CP and PM produce single-strand DNA breaks and DNA-DNA and DNA-protein cross-linking. To determine whether DNA cross-linking is essential for teratogenicity, a monofunctional derivative of PM, capable of producing single-strand breaks but not cross-links in DNA, was tested. Although higher concentrations were needed, this derivative produced the same spectrum of effects as PM (Mirkes *et al.*, 1985). Later, Little and Mirkes (1990) showed that 4-hydroperoxydechlorocyclophosphamide, a CP analog that yields AC and a nonalkylating derivative of PM, did not produce DNA damage when embryos were exposed in serum-containing medium. Using radiolabeled CP, they further found that AC preferentially binds to protein and shows high incorporation into the yolk sac,

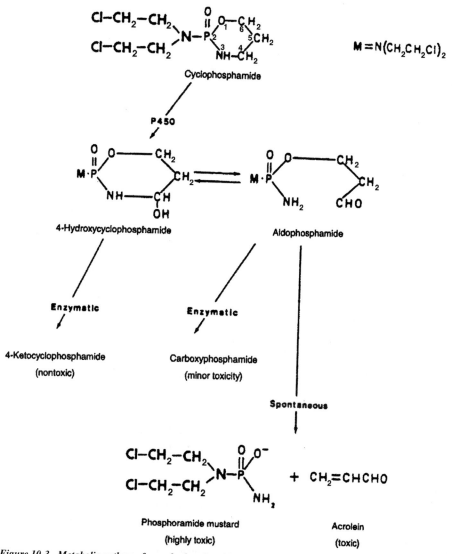

Figure 10-3. Metabolic pathway for cyclophosphamide. [From Mirkes (1985b), with permission.]

whereas PM binds preferentially to DNA. Hales (1989) showed that PM and AC have strikingly different effects on limb buds in culture. These results indicate that PM and AC have different targets in the embryo and that PM is responsible for CP-induced DNA damage.

How do chemical insults at the cell and molecular level translate to a birth defect? To illustrate pathogenesis, we will consider inhibition of cell cycle perturbations and cell death, and continue with our example of cyclophosphamide. Cell death plays a critical role in normal morphogenesis. The term *programmed cell death* (pcd) refers to a specific type of cell death, *apoptosis*, under genetic control in the embryo (Lavin and Watters, 1993). Apoptosis is necessary for sculpting the digits from the hand plate, for instance, and for assuring appropriate functional connectivity between the central nervous system and distal structures. Cell proliferation is obviously essential for development. Cells within the primitive streak of the gastrula-stage rat embryo have the shortest known cell cycle time of any mammalian cell, 3–3.5 hours (MacAuley *et al.*, 1993). Cell proliferation rates change both spatially and temporally during ontogenesis, as can be demonstrated by examining the proportion of cells in S phase over time in different tissues during mid- to late

gestation (Fig. 10-4). There is a delicate balance between cell proliferation, cell differentiation, and apoptosis in the embryo, and one molecular mechanism discussed above (DNA damage) might lead to the cell cycle perturbations and cell death induced by CP in specific cell populations.

Maternal cyclophosphamide treatment on gestation day 10 in the rat causes an S-phase cell cycle block as well as widespread cell death in the embryo (Fig. 10-5). In agreement with the S-phase cell cycle block, cell death is observed in areas of rapid cell proliferation (Chernoff *et al.*, 1989; Francis *et al.*, 1990). Similar blockage of the embryonal cell cycle and cell death were observed using activated CP in whole embryo culture (Little and Mirkes, 1992). The embryonal neuroepithelium is quite sensitive to CP-induced cell death, whereas the heart is resistant. Differences in cell cycle length may, in part, underlie this differential sensitivity. The neuroepithelium of the day 10 rat embryo has a cell cycle time of approximately 9.5 hours, whereas the cell cycle length in the heart was estimated to be 13.4 hours. This difference is due to a longer G_0/G_1 phase in the heart cells compared to the neuroepithelium (Mirkes *et al.*, 1989). Damage to DNA by PM occurs predominantly in S phase (Little and

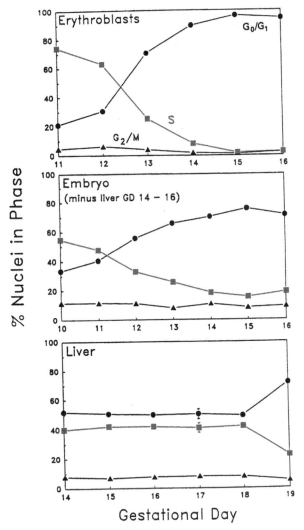

Figure 10-4. Normal developmental changes in cell cycle distributions in erythroblasts, embryo (minus the liver after GD 13), and fetal liver. Percentages of cells in: ● G_0/G_1; ■ S; and ▲ G_2/M are shown for rat embryos between gestation days 10 and 19 (note changing x-axis range).

The proportion of cells in S phase generally reflects proliferation rate, which decreases with developmental stage in the embryo and erythroblasts. The percentage of S-phase cells in the fetal liver remains fairly high and constant until near term, when a spurt of hypertrophy occurs. [From Elstein *et al.* (1993), with permission.]

Mirkes, 1992), which constitutes a relatively greater proportion of the cell cycle in the heart than in the neuroepithelium.

Damage to DNA can inhibit cell cycle progression at the G_1-S transition, through the S phase, and at the G_2-M transition. If DNA damage is repaired, the cell cycle can return to normal, but if damage is too extensive or cell cycle arrest too long, apoptosis may be triggered. The relationship between DNA damage and repair, cell cycle progression, and apoptosis is depicted in Fig. 10-6 in a greatly simplified form. A large number of genes play a role in apoptosis (White, 1993). The p53 gene, which may function as a tumor suppressor, can promote apoptosis or growth arrest. Apoptosis occurring during normal development does not require this gene, as p53-deficient embryos develop normally. However, p53 may be critical for induction of growth arrest or apoptosis in re-

sponse to DNA damage. The incidence of benzo[a]pyrene-induced fetal resorptions and postpartum death were increased threefold and over tenfold, respectively, in offspring of heterozygous p53-deficient (p/+) pregnant mice compared to normal homozygous (+/+) controls (Harrison *et al.*, 1994). Growth factors and some cytokines (IL-3, IL-6) can prevent p53-dependent apoptosis. Expression of c-myc produces continued DNA synthesis, which may precipitate apoptosis in the face of DNA damage. Bcl-2 functions as a repressor of apoptosis and functions in conjunction with Bax, a homolog that dimerizes with itself or with Bcl-2. Bax homodimers favor cell death whereas Bcl-2/Bax heterodimers inhibit cell death (Oltvai and Korsmeyer, 1994).

From the multiple checkpoints and factors present to regulate the cell cycle and apoptosis, it is clear that different cell populations may respond differently to a similar stimulus, in part because cellular predisposition to apoptosis can vary. In regard to the induction of cell death in the neuroepithelium but not the heart by CP, it may be relevant that a portion of the cells from the neuroepithelium undergoes apoptosis normally during this stage of development, indicating competence to respond to an appropriate signal. Conversely, although diverse environmental agents including ethanol, 13-*cis* retinoic acid, ionizing radiation, and hyperthermia are able to induce characteristic patterns of cell death in the embryo (Sulik *et al.*, 1988), none of them effect cell death in the heart. Mirkes and Little (1998) have shown that treatment of postimplantation mouse embryos with hyperthermia, cyclophosphamide, or sodium arsenate induced DNA fragmentation, activation of caspase-3, and cleavage of poly (ADP-ribose) polymerase (PARP) along with apoptosis in some embryonal tissues, but none of these events occurred in the heart. Subsequently, these investigators demonstrated that these chemicals can induce changes in embryonal mitochondria resulting in release of cytochrome *c* and activation of caspase-9, the upstream activator of caspase-3 (Mirkes and Little, 2000). Additional downstream caspases including caspase 6 and caspase 7, are also induced by the active metabolite of CP (Little *et al.*, 2003). In agreement with the observed lack of apoptosis in the heart, this tissue was also refractory to teratogen-induced cytochrome *c* release from mitochondria and caspase activation.

In addition to affecting proliferation and cell viability, molecular and cellular insults can affect essential processes such as cell migration, cell-cell interactions, differentiation, morphogenesis, and energy metabolism. Although the embryo has compensatory mechanisms to offset such effects, production of a normal or malformed offspring will depend on the balance between damage and repair at each step in the pathogenetic pathway.

Advances in the Molecular Basis of Dysmorphogenesis

Our still limited understanding of normal development, combined with the small size and inaccessibility of the mammalian embryo, have made the elucidation of mechanisms of abnormal development a daunting task. However, advances in molecular biology, genomics, and proteomics are bringing new understanding of mechanisms of normal and abnormal development. A key approach, targeted gene disruption by homologous recombination (gene "knockout"), has been used to study the function of the retinoic acid receptor (RAR) family of nuclear ligand-inducible transcription factors that bind retinoic acid and 9-*cis* retinoic acid. Chambon and colleagues have produced mice lacking several of these receptors either singly or as multiple knockouts. Single-receptor isoform mutants were often

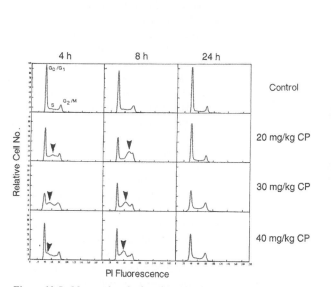

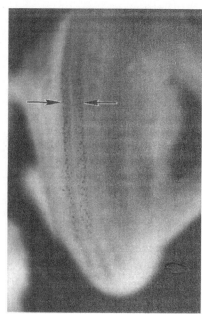

Figure 10-5. Maternal cyclophosphamide (CP) administration on gestation day 10 in CD-1 mice produces perturbations of the embryonal cell cycle and cell death in areas of rapid proliferation.

Left: Cells are inhibited from progressing through the S (DNA synthetic) phase of the cell cycle, indicated by the abnormal population of cells (*arrowheads*) accumulating at progressively earlier stages of S phase 4 hours and 8 hours after increasing maternal CP dosages. The upper panels show the normal GD 10-11 distributions, with the G_0/G_1, S, and G_2/M peaks identified in the upper left panel. By 24 hour postdosing, cell cycle distributions have returned to normal at 20 mg/kg, but remain abnormal at higher dosages. *Right*: Nile blue sulfate staining of a mouse embryo 24 hours after maternal CP dosing shows cell death (*stippling along either side of the midline, arrows*) in the neural tube, one of the most sensitive target sites for CP. [Adapted from Chernoff *et al.* (1989), and Francis *et al.* (1990).]

unaffected, suggesting functional redundancy, whereas double mutants were invariably nonviable and presented widespread malformations of the skeleton and viscera (Lohnes *et al.*, 1994; Mendelsohn *et al.*, 1994). The compound RARγ-RARβ null mouse exhibits syndactyly, indicating that retinoic acid plays a role in interdigital cell death (Dupe *et al.*, 1999). The rexinoid receptors (RXRα, β, and γ) bind 9-*cis* retinoic acid exclusively, and it is now understood that RAR/RXR heterodimers are involved in retinoic acid signaling via transcriptional control in the embryo (Mark *et al.*, 2006).

The use of synthetic antisense oligonucleotides allows temporal and spatial restriction of gene ablation. In this technique, 15-25-mer oligonucleotides are synthesized that are complimentary to the mRNA to be disrupted (Helene *et al.*, 1990). These probes can enter embryonal cells, and hybridization with cellular mRNA causes disruption of native message. In this way, gene function can be turned off at specific times. Added advantages of the antisense approach are the ability to ablate multiple gene family members (by making the antisense probes to regions of sequence homology) and the much shorter time frame for the experiments (Sadler and Hunter, 1994). The proto-oncogenes Wnt-1 and Wnt-3a have been implicated in the development of the midbrain and hindbrain. Augustine *et al.* (1993) attenuated Wnt-1 expression using antisense oligonucleotide inhibition in mouse embryos developing in culture. Exposure during neurulation produced mid- and hindbrain malformations similar to those seen in Wnt-1 null mutant mice, as well as cardiac anomalies not observed in Wnt-1 knockouts created by homologous recombination. Antisense attenuation of Wnt-3a caused anomalies of the forebrain, midbrain, and spinal cord. Simultaneously attenuating both Wnt-1 and Wnt-3a targeted all brain regions and worsened the

effect on the spinal cord, suggesting that these genes may serve a complementary function in the development of the central nervous system.

Gain of gene function can also be studied by engineering genetic constructs with an inducible promoter attached to the gene of interest. Ectopic gene expression can be made ubiquitous or site-specific depending on the choice of promoter to drive expression. Ectopic expression of the Hoxa-7 gene induced in mouse embryos by attaching it to the chicken β-actin promoter resulted in a phenotype exhibiting multiple craniofacial and cervical vertebral malformations (Balling *et al.*, 1989; Kessel *et al.*, 1990). Transient overexpression of specific genes can be accomplished by adding extra copies using adenoviral transduction. In proof-of-concept, Hartig and Hunter (1998) injected the adenoviral vector containing either the bacterial beta-galactosidase or green fluorescent protein reporter gene under the control of the human cytomegalovirus early gene promoter into the intraamniotic space of neurulation-stage mouse embryos and achieved intense gene expression in the neuroepithelium.

Advances in gene targeting and transgenic strategies now allow modification of gene expression at specific points in development and in specific cell types. Conditional knockouts or knock-ins, inducible gene expression and other techniques are being used to study the effects of specific gene products on development in great detail (Mikkola and Orkin, 2005).

Reporter transgenes contain a gene with a readily detectable product fused downstream of a selected regulatory region. The *Escherichia coli lacZ* (β-galactosidase) gene is commonly used for this purpose. Cell lineage studies can be carried out by fusing *lacZ*

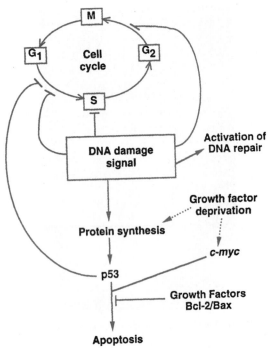

Figure 10-6. Relationships between DNA damage and the induction of cell cycle arrest or apoptosis.

DNA damage can signal inhibition of the cell cycle between G_1 and S, in S phase or between G_2 and mitosis. The signal(s) can also activate DNA repair mechanisms and synthesis of proteins, including p53, that can initiate apoptosis. Growth factors and products of the proto-oncogene *c-myc* and the Bcl-2/Bax gene family, as well as differentiation state and cell cycle phase, are important determinants of the ultimate outcome of embryonal DNA damage.

to a constitutive regulatory sequence and introducing the construct into a somatic cell early in ontogenesis. The reporter gene will then be expressed in and mark all progeny of the transfected cell. This method has been used to study postimplantation development in the mouse embryo (Sanes *et al.*, 1986), although intracellular injection of fluorescent dyes has also proven highly reliable for cell lineage studies (e.g., Smith *et al.*, 1994). The pattern of expression of a particular gene of interest can be discriminated by fusing upstream regulatory elements of the gene to *lacZ*, which will then be transcribed under control of those upstream elements (Zakany *et al.*, 1990).

Retinoic acid (RA) can activate hox genes in vitro, and the 3′ hox genes have multiple RA response elements (RAREs). Evidence that RA-induced malformations in mouse embryos are related to changes in hox expression was first provided by staining of hox-*lacZ* transgenic embryos (Marshall, 1992). Within a few hours of RA treatment, hoxb-1 expression extends anteriorly, suggesting that hox genes could be direct targets of RA induction. Regions of altered hox expression could be manifest as abnormal cell fate and morphogenesis (Marshall, 1996; Collins and Mao, 1999).

PHARMACOKINETICS AND METABOLISM IN PREGNANCY

The manner in which chemicals are absorbed during pregnancy and the extent to and form in which they reach the conceptus are important determinants of whether the chemical can impact development.

The maternal, placental, and embryonic compartments are distinct yet interacting systems that undergo profound changes during the course of pregnancy. Changes in maternal physiology during pregnancy involve hepatic metabolism, the gastrointestinal tract, cardiovascular system, excretory system, and the respiratory system (Hytten, 1984; Krauer, 1987; Mattison *et al.*, 1991). While these physiologic changes are necessary to support the growing needs of the conceptus in terms of energy supply and waste elimination, the alterations can have significant impact on the uptake, distribution, metabolism, and elimination of xenobiotics. For example, decreases in intestinal motility and increases in gastric emptying time result in longer retention time of ingested chemicals in the upper gastrointestinal tract. Cardiac output increases by 50% during the first trimester in humans and remains elevated throughout pregnancy, while blood volume increases and plasma proteins and peripheral vascular resistance decrease. The relative increase in blood volume over red cell volume leads to borderline anemia and a generalized edema with a 70% elevation of extracellular space. Thus, the volume of distribution of a chemical and the amount bound by plasma proteins may change considerably during pregnancy. Renal blood flow and glomerular filtration are also increased in many species during pregnancy. Increase in tidal volume, minute ventilation, and minute O_2 uptake can result in increased pulmonary distribution of gases and decrease in time to reach alveolar steady state.

In addition to changes in maternal physiology, limited available evidence suggests that relative rates of drug metabolizing enzymes also change during pregnancy (Juchau, 1981; Juchau and Faustman-Watts, 1983). Decreased hepatic monooxygenase activity has been observed during pregnancy in rats and has been attributed to decreased enzyme levels and to competitive inhibition by circulating steroids (Neims, 1976). Another factor that contributes to lower monooxygenase activity is that pregnant rats appear to be less responsive to induction of hepatic monooxygenases by phenobarbital (but not 3-methylcholanthrene) than are nonpregnant females (Guenther and Mannering, 1977). Despite the absence of a comprehensive literature on this subject, there appears to be an overall decrease in hepatic xenobiotic biotransformation during pregnancy. Clearly, maternal handling of a chemical bears considerable weight in determining the extent of embryotoxicity. In one of the few studies of its type, a linear combination of the 45-minute and the 24-hour maternal blood concentrations was able to predict the litter response rate for pregnant rats dosed with 500 mg/kg sodium salicylate on gestation day 11 (Kimmel and Young, 1983). These two kinetic parameters probably reflect the influence of the peak drug concentration as well as the cumulative area under the concentration-time curve in inducing developmental disturbances.

The placenta plays a central role in influencing embryonic exposure by helping to regulate blood flow, by offering a transport barrier, and by metabolizing chemicals (Slikker and Miller, 1994). Functionally, the placenta acts as a lipid membrane that permits bidirectional transfer of substances between maternal and fetal compartments. The extent of transfer depends on three major elements: the type of placentation, the physicochemical properties of the chemical, and rates of placental metabolism. Although there are marked species differences in types of placentas, orientation of blood vessels, and numbers of exchanging layers, these do not seem to play a dominant role in placental transfer of most chemicals. It is important to note that virtually any substance present in the maternal plasma will cross the placenta to some extent. The passage of most drugs across the placenta seems to occur by simple passive diffusion, the rate of which is proportional to the diffusion constant of the drug, the concentration gradient between the maternal and embryonic plasma, the area of exchange, and the inverse of the membrane thickness (Nau, 1992). Important modifying factors to the rate and extent of transfer include lipid solubility, molecular weight, protein binding, the type of transfer (passive diffusion, facilitated or active transport), the degree of ionization, and placental metabolism. Weak acids appear to be rapidly transferred across the placenta, due in part to the pH gradient between the maternal and embryonic plasma which can trap ionized forms of the drug in the slightly more acidic embryonic compartment (Nau and Scott, 1986). Placental blood flow probably constitutes the major rate-limiting step for more lipid-soluble compounds.

Quantifying the form, amount, and timing of chemical delivery to the embryonic compartment relative to concurrent developmental processes is an important component of understanding mechanisms of embryotoxicity and species differences in embryonic sensitivity (Nau, 1986). The small size of the conceptus during organogenesis and the fact that the embryo is changing at a rapid rate during this period makes assessment of toxicokinetics difficult. Nevertheless, there has been considerable progress in this area (Nau and Scott, 1987; Clark, 1993; Corley et al., 2003). Increasingly sensitive analytical methods are now providing evidence to challenge the historical view, particularly for cytochrome P450-dependent monooxygenases, that the early embryo has low metabolic capabilities (Juchau et al., 1992). Using an embryo culture system, Juchau and co-workers demonstrated that the rat conceptus was able to generate sufficient amounts of metabolites of the proteratogen 2-acetylaminofluorene (2-AAF) to induce dysmorphogenesis, and that the proximate toxicant, the 7-hydroxy metabolite, was different from the metabolite responsible for 2-AAF mutagenesis and carcinogenesis. Prior exposure of the dams to 3-methylcholanthrene increased the sensitivity of the cultured embryos to 2-AAF, thus demonstrating the inducibility of at least some cytochromes in the conceptus. These investigators later showed that embryos could further metabolize the 7-hydroxy metabolite to an even more toxic catechol. No previous induction was necessary for this activation step, demonstrating the presence of constitutive metabolizing enzymes in the embryo. Although the rates of metabolism for these activation steps may be low relative to the maternal liver, they occur close to the target site of the embryo or even within it, and thus are significant in terms of inducing embryotoxicity.

Physiologically based pharmacokinetic models provide the framework to integrate what is known about physiologic changes during pregnancy, both within and between species, with aspects of drug metabolism and embryonic development into a quantitative description of the events. Gabrielson and co-workers (Gabrielson and Paalkow, 1983; Gabrielson and Larsson, 1990) were among the first investigators to develop physiologically based models of pregnancy, and others (Fisher et al., 1989; O'Flaherty et al., 1992; Clark et al., 1993; Luecke et al., 1994, 1997; Young, 1998) have added to their comprehensiveness. The pregnancy model of O'Flaherty and coworkers describes the entire period of gestation, and consists of the uterus, mammary tissue, maternal fat, kidney, liver, other well-perfused maternal tissues, embryo/fetal tissues and yolk sac, and chorioallantoic placentas. It takes into account the growth of various compartments during pregnancy (including the embryo itself), as well as changes in blood flow and the stage-dependent pH gradients between maternal and embryonic plasma. Transfer across the placenta in the model is diffusion limited. The utility of the model was evaluated using 5,5'-dimethyloxazolidine-2,4-dione (DMO), a weak acid that is not appreciably bound to plasma proteins and is eliminated by excretion in the urine. The model demonstrated that the whole body disposition of DMO, including distribution to the embryo, can be accounted for solely on the basis of its pKa and of the pH and volumes of body fluid spaces. Differences between the disposition of DMO by the pregnant mouse and rat are consistent simply with differences in fluid pH.

The solvent 2-methoxyethanol is embryotoxic and teratogenic in all species tested to date. The proximate teratogen appears to be the metabolite 2-methoxyacetic acid (2-MAA). A physiologically based pharmacokinetic model has been developed for the pregnant mouse (Terry et al., 1995). Pharmacokinetics and tissue partition coefficients for 2-MAA were determined at different stages of embryonal development, and various models were tested based on the alternative hypotheses involving (1) blood-flow limited delivery of 2-MAA to model compartments, (2) pH trapping of ionized 2-MAA within compartments, (3) active transport of 2-MAA into compartments, and (4) reversible binding of 2-MAA within compartments. Although the blood-flow limited model best predicted gestation day 8 dosimetry, the active transport models better described dosimetry on gestation days 11 and 13. Using published data on biotransformation of 2-methoxyethanol to ethylene glycol and 2-MAA in rats, Hays et al. (2000) have adapted the pregnant mouse PBPK model to the pregnant rat and successfully predicted tissue levels of 2-MAA following oral or intravenous administration of 2-methoxyethanol. The next step was to extrapolate this model to the inhalation route of exposure, and to model both rats and humans (Gargas et al., 2000). The extrapolation of the model enabled predictions of the exposures needed for pregnant women to reach blood concentrations (C_{max} or AUC) equivalent to those in pregnant rats exposed to the no observed adverse effect level (NOAEL) or LOAEL for developmental toxicity. The body of work on PBPK modeling of 2-methoxyethanol is exemplary of the power of these techniques for extrapolating across dose, developmental stage, route, and species.

Maternal metabolism of xenobiotics is an important and variable determinant of developmental toxicity. As for other health endpoints, the developing field of pharmacogenomics offers hope for increasing our ability to predict susceptible subpopulations based on empirical relationships between maternal genotype and fetal phenotype. These relationships will hopefully guide further work to elucidate mechanisms of toxicant-induced abnormal development.

RELATIONSHIPS BETWEEN MATERNAL AND DEVELOPMENTAL TOXICITY

Although all developmental toxicity must ultimately result from an insult to the conceptus at the cellular level, the insult may occur through a direct effect on the embryo/fetus, indirectly through toxicity of the agent to the mother and/or the placenta, or a combination of direct and indirect effects. Maternal physiological conditions capable of adversely affecting the developing organism include decreased uterine blood flow, maternal anemia, altered nutritional status, toxemia, altered organ function, autoimmune states, diabetes, electrolyte or acid-base disturbances, decreased milk quantity or quality, and abnormal behavior (Chernoff et al., 1989; Daston, 1994). Induction or exacerbation of such maternal conditions by toxic agents and the degree to which they manifest in abnormal development are dependent on maternal genetic background, age, parity, size, nutrition, disease, stress, and other health parameters and exposures (DeSesso, 1987; Chernoff et al., 1989; Rogers et al., 2005). These relationships are depicted in Fig. 10-7. In this section

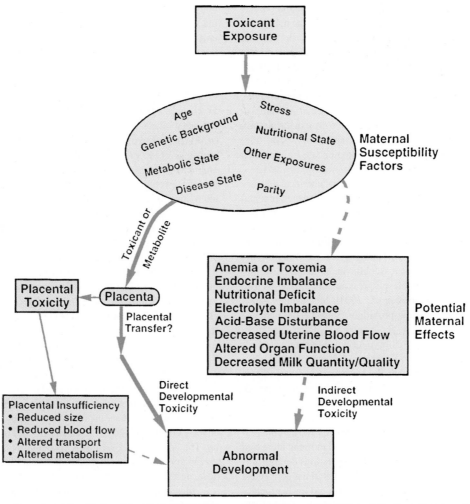

Figure 10-7. Interrelationships between maternal susceptibility factors, metabolism, induction of maternal physiologic or functional alterations, placental transfer and toxicity, and developmental toxicity.

A developmental toxicant can cause abnormal development through any one or a combination of these pathways. Maternal susceptibility factors determine the predisposition of the mother to respond to a toxic insult, and the maternal effects listed can adversely affect the developing conceptus. Most chemicals traverse the placenta in some form, and the placenta can also be a target for toxicity. In most cases, developmental toxicity is probably mediated through a combination of these pathways.

we will discuss maternal conditions known to adversely affect the conceptus, as well as examples of xenobiotics whose developmental toxicity results completely or in large part from maternal or placental toxicity.

The distinction between direct and indirect developmental toxicity is important for interpreting safety assessment results in pregnant animals, as the highest dosage levels in these experiments are chosen based on their ability to produce some maternal toxicity (e.g., decreased food or water intake, weight loss, clinical signs). However, maternal toxicity defined only by such crude manifestations gives little insight to the toxic actions of a xenobiotic. When developmental toxicity is observed only in the presence of maternal toxicity, the developmental effects may be indirect; however, understanding of the physiologic changes underlying the observed maternal toxicity and elucidation of the association with developmental effects is needed before one can begin to address the relevance of the observations to human safety assessment. Many known human developmental toxicants, including ethanol and cocaine, adversely affect

the embryo/fetus predominately at maternally toxic levels, and part of their developmental toxicity may be ascribed to secondary effects of maternal physiological disturbances. For example, the nutritional status of alcoholics is generally poor, and effects on the conceptus may be exacerbated by effects of alcohol on placental transfer of nutrients. Effects of chronic alcohol abuse on maternal folate and zinc metabolism may be particularly important in the induction of fetal alcohol syndrome (Dreosti, 1993).

MATERNAL FACTORS AFFECTING DEVELOPMENT

Genetics

The genetic makeup of the pregnant female has been well documented as a determinant of developmental outcome in both humans and animals. The incidence of cleft lip and/or palate [CL(P)], which occurs more frequently in whites than in blacks, has been investigated in offspring of interracial couples in the United States (Khoury *et al.*, 1983). Offspring of white mothers had a higher incidence of CL(P) than offspring of black mothers after correcting for paternal race, while offspring of white fathers did not have a higher incidence of CL(P) than offspring of black fathers after correcting for maternal race.

Among experimental animals, the "A" family of inbred mice has a high spontaneous occurrence of cleft lip and palate (Kalter, 1979). Two related mouse strains, A/J and CL/Fr, produce spontaneous CL(P) at 8–10% and 18–26% frequencies, respectively. The incidence of CL(P) in offspring depends on the genotype of the mother rather than that of the embryo (Juriloff and Fraser, 1980). The response to vitamin A of murine embryos heterozygous for the curly-tail mutation depends on the genotype of the mother (Seller *et al.*, 1983). The teratogenicity of phenytoin has been compared in several inbred strains of mice. The susceptibility of offspring of crosses between susceptible A/J mice and resistant C57BL/6J mice was determined by the maternal, but not the embryonic genotype (Hansen and Hodes, 1983). New genomic approaches have begun to identify genes associated with differential susceptibility of mouse strains to valproic acid (Finnell *et al.*, 1997; Craig *et al.*, 2000; Bennett *et al.*, 2000; Faiella *et al.*, 2000; Okada *et al.*, 2004, 2005).

Disease

Chronic hypertension is a risk factor for the development of preeclampsia, eclampsia, and toxemia of pregnancy, and hypertension is a leading cause of pregnancy-associated maternal deaths. Uncontrolled maternal diabetes mellitus is a significant cause of prenatal morbidity. Certain maternal infections can adversely affect the conceptus (e.g., rubella virus, discussed earlier), either through indirect disease-related maternal alterations or direct transplacental infection. Cytomegalovirus infection is associated with fetal death, microcephaly, mental retardation, blindness, and deafness (MacDonald and Tobin, 1978) and maternal infection with *Toxoplasma gondii* is known to induce hydrocephaly and chorioretinitis in infants (Alford *et al.*, 1974).

One factor common to many disease states is hyperthermia. Hyperthermia is a potent experimental animal teratogen (Edwards, 1986), and there is a body of evidence associating maternal febrile illness during the first trimester of pregnancy with birth defects in humans, most notably malformations of the central nervous system (Warkany, 1986; Milunsky, *et al.*, 1992).

Nutrition

A wide spectrum of dietary insufficiencies ranging from protein-calorie malnutrition to deficiencies of vitamins, trace elements, and/or enzyme cofactors is known to adversely affect pregnancy (Keen *et al.*, 1993). Among the most significant findings related to human nutrition and pregnancy outcome in recent years are results of studies in which pregnant women at risk for having infants with neural tube defects (NTDs) were supplemented with folate (Wald, 1993). The largest and most convincing study is the Medical Research Council (MRC) Vitamin Study, in which supplementation with 4 mg of folic acid reduced NTD recurrence by over 70% (MRC, 1991). Results of these studies have prompted the U.S. Centers for Disease Control and Prevention to recommend folate supplementation for women of childbearing age and folate supplementation of some foodstuffs. In 1996, The United States Food and Drug Administration mandated enrichment of cereal grain products with folate

by 1998. One study has demonstrated more than a doubling of mean serum folate concentrations across all sex and age groups since then (Dietrich *et al.*, 2005). Yet, in the same population, less than 10% of women of childbearing age reached the recommended erythrocyte folate concentration of greater than 906 nmol/L that has been shown to be associated with a reduction in the risk of neural tube defects (NTDs). The Centers for Disease Control and Prevention (2004) estimated that the number of NTD-affected pregnancies in the United States declined from 4000 in 1995–1996 to 3000 in 1999–2000. While this survey indicates partial success of the folate fortification program, women capable of becoming pregnant were urged to continue to follow the U.S. Public Health Service recommendation to consume 400 μg folate daily. Mills and Signore (2004) compared the rates of antenatal detection of NTDs in the United States (incomplete ascertainment and underprediction of NTDs) and Canada (more complete antenatal ascertainment) and determined that the studies that best identify cases of NTDs show that folic acid fortification is preventing upto 54% of NTDs. These authors estimate that the percentage of folate-preventable NTDs in the United States is about 50–60%, suggesting that we may be close to achieving optimum protection.

Stress

Diverse forms of maternal toxicity may have in common the induction of a physiologic stress response. Understanding potential effects of maternal stress on development may help interpret developmental toxicity observed in experimental animals at maternally toxic dosages. Various forms of physical stress have been applied to pregnant animals in attempts to isolate the developmental effects of stress. Subjecting pregnant rats or mice to noise stress throughout gestation can produce developmental toxicity (Kimmel *et al.*, 1976; Nawrot *et al.*, 1980, 1981). Restraint stress produces increased fetal death in rats (Euker and Riegle, 1973) and cleft palate (Barlow *et al.*, 1975), fused and supernumerary ribs, and encephaloceles in mice (Beyer and Chernoff, 1986).

Objective data on effects of stress in humans are difficult to obtain. Nevertheless, studies investigating the relationship of maternal stress and pregnancy outcome have indicated a positive correlation between stress and adverse developmental effects, including low birth weight and congenital malformations (Stott, 1973; Gorsuch and Key, 1974).

Placental Toxicity

The placenta is the interface between the mother and the conceptus, providing attachment, nutrition, gas exchange, and waste removal. The placenta also produces hormones critical to the maintenance of pregnancy, and it can metabolize and/or store xenobiotics. Placental toxicity may compromise these functions and produce or contribute to untoward effects on the conceptus. Slikker and Miller (1994) list 46 toxicants known to be toxic to the yolk sac or chorioallantoic placenta, including metals such as cadmium (Cd), arsenic, or mercury, cigarette smoke, ethanol, cocaine, endotoxin, and sodium salicylate (Daston, 1994; Slikker and Miller, 1994). Cd is among the best studied of these, and it appears that the developmental toxicity of Cd during mid- to late gestation involves both placental toxicity (necrosis, reduced blood flow) and inhibition of nutrient transport across the placenta. Maternal injection of Cd during late gestation results in fetal death in rats, despite little cadmium entering the fetus (Parizek, 1964; Levin and Miller, 1980). Fetal death occurs concomitant with reduced uteroplacental blood flow within 10 hours (Levin and Miller, 1980). The authors' conclusion that fetal death was caused by placental toxicity was supported by experiments in which fetuses were directly injected with Cd. Despite fetal Cd burdens almost tenfold higher than those following maternal administration, only a slight increase in fetal death was observed.

Cd is a transition metal similar in its physicochemical properties to the essential metal zinc (Zn). Cadmium interferes with Zn transfer across the placenta (Ahokas *et al.*, 1980; Sorell and Graziano, 1990), possibly via metallothionein (MT), a metal-binding protein induced in the placenta by Cd. Because of its high affinity for Zn, MT may sequester Zn in the placenta, impeding transfer to the conceptus (induction of maternal hepatic MT by Cd or other agents can also induce fetal Zn deficiency, as discussed below). Cadmium inhibits Zn uptake by human placental microvesicles (Page *et al.*, 1992) suggesting that Cd may also compete directly with Zn for membrane transport. Cadmium may also competitively inhibit other Zn-dependent processes in the placenta. Coadministration of Zn ameliorates the developmental toxicity of administered Cd, further indicating that interference of Cd with Zn metabolism is a key to its developmental toxicity (Ferm and Carpenter, 1967; Daston, 1982).

Maternal Toxicity

A retrospective analysis of relationships between maternal toxicity and specific prenatal effects found species-specific associations between maternal toxicity and adverse developmental effects. Yet, among rat, rabbit, and hamster studies, 22% failed to show any developmental toxicity in the presence of significant maternal toxicity (Khera, 1984, 1985). The approach of tabulating literature data suffers from possible bias in the types of studies published (e.g., negative results may not be published), incomplete reporting of maternal and developmental effects, and lack of standard criteria for the evaluation of maternal and developmental toxicity. In a study designed to test the potential of maternal toxicity to affect development, Kavlock *et al.* (1985) acutely administered 10 structurally unrelated compounds to pregnant mice at maternotoxic dosages. Developmental effects were agent-specific, ranging from complete resorption to lack of effect. An exception was an increased incidence of supernumerary ribs (ribs on the first lumbar vertebra), which occurred with 7 of the 10 compounds. Chernoff *et al.* (1990) dosed pregnant rats for 10 days with a series of compounds chosen because they exhibited little or no developmental toxicity in previous studies. When these compounds were administered at high dosages producing maternal toxicity (weight loss or lethality), a variety of adverse developmental outcomes was noted, including increased intrauterine death (two compounds), decreased fetal weight (two compounds), supernumerary ribs (two compounds), and enlarged renal pelves (two compounds). In addition, two of the compounds produced no developmental toxicity despite substantial maternal toxicity. These diverse developmental responses led the authors to conclude that maternal toxicity defined by weight loss or mortality is not associated with any consistent syndrome of developmental effects in the rat.

There have been a number of studies directly relating specific forms of maternal toxicity to developmental toxicity, including those in which the test chemical causes maternal effects that exacerbate the agent's developmental toxicity, as well as instances in which developmental toxicity is thought to be the direct result of adverse maternal effects. However, clear delineation of the relative role(s) of indirect maternal and direct embryo/fetal toxicity is difficult.

Acetazolamide inhibits carbonic anhydrase and is teratogenic in mice (Hirsch and Scott, 1983). Although maternal weight loss is not correlated with malformation frequency, maternal hypercapnia potentiates the teratogenicity of acetazolamide. In C57Bl/6J mice, maternal hypercapnia alone results in right forelimb ectrodactyly, the characteristic malformation induced by acetazolamide. Correction of maternal acidosis failed to reduce developmental toxicity, suggesting that the primary teratogenic factor was elevated maternal plasma CO_2 tension (Weaver and Scott, 1984a,b).

Diflunisal, an analgesic and anti-inflammatory drug, causes axial skeletal defects in rabbits. Developmentally toxic dosages resulted in severe maternal anemia (hematocrit = 20–24% vs. 37% in controls) and depletion of erythrocyte ATP levels (Clark *et al.*, 1984). Teratogenicity, anemia, and ATP depletion were unique to the rabbit among the species studied. A single dose of diflunisal on day 5 of gestation was teratogenic and produced a maternal anemia that lasted through day 15. Concentration of the drug in the embryo was less than 5% of the peak maternal blood level, and diflunisal was cleared from maternal blood before day 9, the critical day for induction of similar axial skeletal defects by hypoxia. Thus, the teratogenicity of diflunisal in the rabbit was probably due to hypoxia resulting from maternal anemia.

Phenytoin, an anticonvulsant, can affect maternal folate metabolism in experimental animals, and these alterations may play a role in the teratogenicity of this drug (Hansen and Billings, 1985). Further, maternal heart rates were monitored on gestation day 10 after administration to susceptible A/J mice and resistant C57Bl/6J mice (Watkinson and Millikovsky, 1983). Heart rates were depressed by phenytoin in a dose-related manner in the A/J mice but not in C57Bl/6J mice. A mechanism of teratogenesis was proposed relating depressed maternal heart rate and embryonic hypoxia. Supporting studies have demonstrated that hyperoxia reduces the teratogenicity of phenytoin in mice (Millicovsky and Johnston, 1981). Reduced uterine blood flow has been proposed as a mechanism of teratogenicity caused by hydroxyurea, which produces elevated systolic blood pressure, altered heart rate, decreased cardiac output, severely decreased uterine blood flow, and increased vascular resistance in pregnant rabbits (Millicovsky *et al.*, 1981). Embryos exhibited craniofacial and pericardial hemorrhages immediately after treatment (Millicovsky and DeSesso, 1980a), and identical embryopathies were achieved by clamping the uterine vessels of pregnant rabbits for 10 minutes (Millicovsky and DeSesso, 1980b).

Metallothionein synthesis is inducible by a wide variety of chemical and physical agents including metals, alcohols, urethane, endotoxin, alkylating agents, hyper- or hypothermia, and ionizing radiation (Daston, 1994). MT synthesis is also induced by endogenous mediators such as glucocorticoids and certain of the cytokines (Klaassen and Lehman-McKeeman, 1989). A mechanism common to the developmental toxicity of these diverse agents may be Zn deficiency of the conceptus secondary to induction of maternal MT. Induction of MT synthesis can produce hepatic MT concentrations over an order of magnitude higher than normal, leading to substantial sequestration of circulating Zn in maternal liver, lowered plasma Zn concentrations, and reduced Zn availability to the conceptus. Embryofetal zinc deficiency secondary to maternal hepatic MT induction has been demonstrated for diverse chemicals including valproic acid (Keen *et al.*, 1989), 6-mercaptopurine (Amemiya *et al.*, 1985, 1989), urethane (Daston *et al.*, 1991), ethanol, and α-hederin (Taubeneck *et al.*, 1994). In a study combining data for

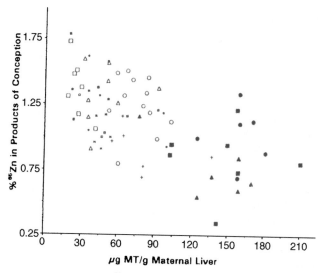

***Figure 10-8. Transfer of ^{65}Zn to the products of conception as a function
of maternal hepatic metallothionein (MT) concentration.***

Pregnant rats were dosed on gestation day 11 with: ● α-hederin; ◻ dimethyl-
sulfoxide; ◻ ethanol; ▲ urethane; + melphalan; ♦ acidified alcohol; or ◻
styrene, or were ○ food-deprived or △ food-restricted. ◻: Saline control.
Eight hours after dosing, dams were orally gavaged with a diet slurry containing ^{65}Zn. The amount of ^{65}Zn transferred to the conceptuses was inversely correlated with the degree of treatment-related maternal hepatic MT
induction. [Adapted from Taubeneck *et al.* (1994) with permission.]

many of these compounds, Taubeneck and coworkers (1994) found
a strong positive relationship between maternal hepatic MT induction and maternal hepatic ^{65}Zn retention, and a negative relationship
between maternal MT induction and ^{65}Zn distribution to the litter
(Fig. 10-8).

DEVELOPMENTAL TOXICITY OF ENDOCRINE-DISRUPTING CHEMICALS

One of the most pressing environmental issues facing developmental
and reproductive toxicology in recent years has been the concern that
exposure to chemicals that can interact with the endocrine system
may pose a serious health hazard (Toppari *et al.*, 1996; Kavlock
et al. 1996). An "endocrine disruptor" has been broadly defined
as "an exogenous agent that interferes with the production, release,
transport, metabolism, binding, action, or elimination of natural hormones responsible for the maintenance of homeostasis and the regulation of developmental processes" (Kavlock *et al.*, 1996). Due to
the critical role of hormones in directing differentiation in many
tissues, the developing organism is particularly vulnerable to fluctuations in the timing or intensity of exposure to chemicals with
hormonal (or antihormonal) activity. Chemicals from a wide variety of chemical classes (e.g., pesticides, herbicides, fungicides,
plasticizers, surfactants, organometals, halogenated polyaromatic
hydrocarbons, phytoestrogens) have been shown to induce developmental toxicity via at least three modes of action involving the
endocrine system: (1) by serving as steroid receptor ligands; (2) by
altering steroid hormone metabolizing enzymes; and (3) by perturbing hypothalamic-pituitary release of trophic hormones. Interactions
with the functions of estrogens, androgens, and thyroid hormones
have been the most studied.

Laboratory Animal Evidence

Chemicals with estrogenic activity are a well-described class of developmental toxicants based on standard criteria of causing specific
malformations during critical developmental periods of relatively
short duration (Schardein, 2000). Estrogens induce pleiotropic effects, acting on many types of cells with estrogen receptors, and
can display cell and organ-specific agonist and antagonist actions.
The pattern of outcomes is generally similar across different estrogens. Diethylstilbestrol (DES) provides one of the most well-
characterized examples of the effects of an estrogen on development.
Manifestations include malformations and functional alterations
of the male and female reproductive tract and brain. In the CD-
1 mouse, effective exposures are in the range of 0.1–100 μg/kg
on GD 9-16 (Newbold, 1995). At the higher end of the exposure range (10–100 μg/kg), total sterility of female offspring is
noted, due in part to structural abnormalities of the oviduct, uterus,
cervix, and vagina and to depletion and abnormalities of ovarian
follicles. In adulthood, male offspring show hypospadias, while females exhibit excessive vaginal keratinization and epidermoid tumors of the vagina. Vaginal adenocarcinoma is seen at dosages as
low as 2.5 μg/kg and benign uterine tumors (leiomyomas) are seen
at as low as 0.1 μg/kg. In male offspring, sterility is observed
at high doses, the result of retained rete testes and Mullerian
duct remnants, abnormal sperm morphology and motility, cryptorchidism, abnormal reproductive tract secretions, and inflammation (Newbold, 1995). Other estrogenic (or anti-estrogenic) developmental toxicants include estradiol (Biegel *et al.*, 1998; Cook *et al.*,
1998), ethynyl estradiol, antiestrogenic drugs such as tamoxifen and
clomiphene citrate (Branham *et al.*, 1988), and pesticides and industrial chemicals such as methoxychlor (Gray *et al.*, 1989), *o,p'*-DDT
(Heinrichs *et al.*, 1971), kepone (Gellert, 1978; Guzelian, 1982),
dioxins (Mably *et al.*, 1992; Gray *et al.*, 1997a, b), bisphenol A
(Nagel *et al.*, 1997), and phytoestrogens such as genistein and
coumestrol (Medlock *et al.*, 1995). Female offspring are generally
more sensitive than males and altered pubertal development, reduced
fertility, and reproductive tract anomalies are common findings.

   Although most of the studies on estrogens have indicated traditional dose–response patterns of effect, with severity and incidence increasing with dose, vom Saal and coworkers (vom Saal
et al., 1997; Nagel *et al.*, 1997) have reported that unusual dose–
response patterns may occur for endocrine effects on some endpoints. In their studies, a 50% elevation in fetal serum estradiol
concentration resulting from implantation of estradiol-containing
Silastic capsules on days 13–19 of gestation in mice caused a 30%
increase in adult prostate weight in male offspring, whereas higher
maternal serum concentrations were associated with decreased adult
prostate weight. A similar U-shaped dose–response pattern was observed for DES given on days 11–17 of gestation, as increased
adult prostate weights were seen between 0.02 and 20 ng/kg/day,
whereas 200 ng/kg/day resulted in smaller prostates. Bisphenol A
(2 or 20 μg/kg/day on gestation days 11–17) also increased adult
prostate weight in these mice. However, the issue is controversial,
as other researchers using similar testing paradigms have not seen
this pattern (e.g., Cagen *et al.*, 1999). Vom Saal and colleagues (vom
Saal and Hughes, 2005; Welshons *et al.*, 2006) argue that bisphenol
A exerts estrogenic effects at low doses and exhibits an inverted U-
shaped dose–response. Naciff *et al.* (2005) observed changes in gene
expression in response to in utero exposure to three estrogen receptor
agonists, 17α-ethynyl estradiol, genistein, or bisphenol A. Expression of 50 genes was changed by all three chemicals, suggesting

that these chemicals have a consistent mode of action. Further, the dose–response for these gene expression changes was monotonic, arguing against the existence of a U-shaped dose–response for these chemicals.

Antiandrogens represent another major class of endocrine disrupting chemicals. Principal manifestations of developmental exposure to an antiandrogen are generally restricted to males, and include hypospadias, retained nipples, reduced testes and accessory sex gland weights, and decreased sperm production. Examples of chemicals known to affect development via an antiandrogenic mechanism include pharmaceuticals such as the androgen receptor antagonist flutamide (Imperato-McGinley et al., 1992) and the 5α-reductase inhibitor finasteride (Clark et al., 1990), and environmentally relevant compounds such as the fungicide vinclozolin (Gray et al., 1994) and the DDT metabolite p,p′-DDE (Kelce et al., 1995; You et al., 1998) which are both androgen receptor antagonists. A phthalate ester (dibutylphthalate) has been shown to induce an antiandrogen phenotype in developing rats, but the effect does not appear to be mediated by direct interaction with the androgen receptor (Mylchreest et al., 1998, 1999). The critical developmental window for these effects of dibutylphthalate appears to be gestation days 16–18 in the rat (Carruthers and Foster, 2005). A similar phenotype has been observed in offspring of dibutylphthalate treated rabbits (Higuchi et al., 2003).

Hypothyroidism causes growth retardation, cognitive deficits, delayed eye opening, hyperactivity, and auditory defects in rodents. Polychlorinated biphenyls (PCBs) may act at several sites to lower thyroid hormone levels during development and cause body weight and auditory deficits (Goldey et al., 1995; Goldey and Crofton, 1998). PCBs also cause learning deficits and alter locomotor activity patterns in rodents (Eriksson et al., 1991; Schantz et al., 1995) and monkeys (Bowman, 1982; Schantz et al., 1991).

Human Evidence

Despite the biological plausibility of effects demonstrated in numerous laboratory studies, it is not clear that human health is being adversely impacted from exposures to environmental endocrine disruptors. It is extraordinarily difficult to demonstrate cause-and-effect relationships in epidemiologic studies where the signals may be weak, the effects evident only long after an exposure, and the endpoints sensitive to a number of other factors. Reports in humans which are or may be relevant are of two types: (1) Observations of adverse effects on reproductive system development and function following exposure to chemicals with known endocrine activities that are present in medicines, contaminated food, or the workplace. These have tended to involve relatively high exposures to chemicals with known endocrine effects. (2) Epidemiologic evidence of increasing trends in adverse reproductive and developmental outcomes having an endocrine basis. With the exception of the classic case of DES (Herbst and Bern, 1981), evidence is either lacking to support a definitive link to an exposure, or appears to be variable across study populations as to whether the responses are observed at all. For example, secular trends have been reported for cryptorchidism (Toppari et al., 1996); hypospadias (Toppari et al., 1996; Pauluzzi et al., 1997; Pauluzzi, 1999); semen quality (Carlsen et al., 1992; Skakkebaek and Keiding, 1994; Olsen et al., 1995; Swann et al., 1997; Auger et al., 1995; de Mouzon et al., 1996; Irvine et al., 1996; Vierula et al., 1996; Bujan et al., 1996; Fisch and Goluboff, 1996), and testicular cancer (Toppari et al., 1996), but due to the

lack of exposure assessment, such studies provide limited evidence of a cause and effect relationship.

The most convincing evidence for effects of endocrine disrupting chemicals in humans comes from reports of neurobehavioral changes and learning deficits in children exposed to PCBs in utero or lactationally, either through their mothers' consumption of PCB-contaminated fish (Jacobson et al., 1990; Jacobson and Jacobson, 1996) or through exposure to background levels of PCBs in the United States (Rogan and Gladen, 1991) or the Netherlands (Koopman-Esseboom et al., 1996). In addition, there have been two occurrences of high level exposure to contaminated rice oil (in Japan in 1968 and in Taiwan in 1979) in which alterations in development of ectodermal tissues and delays in neurological development were seen (Hsu et al., 1985; Yu et al., 1991; Guo et al., 1994; Schecter et al., 1994). In these cases, there was coexposure to polychlorinated dibenzofurans as well as PCBs. The precise mode of action of the developmental neurotoxicity of PCBs is, however, not yet understood.

Impact on Screening and Testing Programs

The findings of altered reproductive development following early life stage exposures to endocrine disrupting chemicals helped prompt revision of traditional safety evaluation tests such as those issued by the EPA (US EPA, 1997). These now include assessments of female estrous cyclicity, sperm parameters (total number, percent progressively motile and sperm morphology in both the parental and F1 generations), the age at puberty in the F1 (vaginal opening in the female, preputial separation in the males); an expanded list of organs for either pathology, gravimetric analysis, and/or histopathology to identify and characterize effects at the target organ; as well as some triggered endpoints including ano-genital distance in the F2 and primordial follicular counts in the parental and F1 generations. For the prenatal developmental toxicity test guidelines, one important modification aimed at improved detection of endocrine disruptors was the expansion of the period of dosing from the end of organogenesis (i.e., palatal closure) to the end of pregnancy in order to include the developmental period of urogenital differentiation.

MODERN SAFETY ASSESSMENT

Experience with chemicals that have the potential to induce developmental toxicity indicates that both laboratory animal testing and surveillance of the human population (i.e., epidemiologic studies) are necessary to provide adequate public health protection. Laboratory animal investigations are guided both by regulatory requirements for drug or chemical marketing as well as by the basic desire to understand mechanisms of toxicity.

Regulatory Guidelines for In Vivo Testing

Prior to the thalidomide tragedy, safety evaluations for reproductive effects were limited in both the types of chemicals evaluated and the sophistication of the endpoints. Subsequently, the FDA issued more extensive testing protocols (termed Segments I, II, and III) for application to a broader range of chemicals (US FDA, 1966). These testing protocols, with minor variations, were adopted by a variety of regulatory agencies around the world and remained similar for nearly thirty years. Several factors including the historical experience of testing thousands of chemicals, increased knowledge of basic reproductive processes, the ever-increasing cost of testing,

Table 10-4

Summary of In Vivo Regulatory Protocol Guidelines for Evaluation of Developmental Toxicity

STUDY	EXPOSURE	ENDPOINTS COVERED	COMMENTS
Segment I: Fertility and general reproduction study	Males: 10 weeks prior to mating Females: 2 weeks prior to mating	Gamete development, fertility, pre- and post implantation viability, parturition, lactation	Assesses reproductive capabilities of male and female following exposure over one complete spermatogenic cycle or several estrous cycles.
Segment II: Teratogenicity test	Implantation (or mating) through end of organogenesis (or term)	Viability, weight, and morphology (external, visceral, and skeletal) of conceptuses just prior to birth	Shorter exposure to prevent maternal metabolic adaptation and to provide high exposure to the embryo during gastrulation and organogenesis. Earlier dosing option for bioaccumulative agents or those impacting maternal nutrition. Later dosing option covers male reproductive tract development and fetal growth and maturation.
Segment III: Perinatal study	Last trimester of pregnancy through lactation	Postnatal survival, growth and external morphology	Intended to observe effects on development of major organ functional competence during the perinatal period, and thus may be relatively more sensitive to adverse effects at this time.
ICH 4.1.1: Fertility protocol	Males: 4 weeks prior to mating Females: 2 weeks prior to mating	Males: Reproductive organ weights and histology, sperm counts and motility Females: Viability of conceptuses at mid-pregnancy or later	Improved assessment of male reproductive endpoints; shorter treatment duration than Segment I.
ICH 4.1.2: Effects on prenatal and postnatal development, including maternal function	Implantation through end of lactation	Relative toxicity to pregnant versus non-pregnant female; postnatal viability, growth, development and functional deficits (including behavior, maturation, and reproduction)	
ICH 4.1.3: Effects on embryo/fetal development	Implantation through end of organogenesis	Viability and morphology (external, visceral, and skeletal) of fetuses just prior to birth.	Similar to Segment II study. Usually conducted in two species (rodent and nonrodent).
OECD 414 Prenatal developmental	Implantation (or mating) through day prior to cesarean section	Viability and morphology (external, visceral, and skeletal) of fetuses just prior to birth.	Similar to Segment II study. Usually conducted in two species (rodent and nonrodent).

the acknowledged redundancy and overlap of required protocols, a growing divergence in study design requirements of various countries, and the expanding international presence of the pharmaceutical industry have succeeded in producing streamlined testing protocols that have been accepted internationally (US FDA, 1994). These guidelines, the result of the International Conference of Harmonization of Technical Requirements for Registration of Pharmaceuticals for Human Use (ICH), specifically include considerable flexibility in implementation depending on the particular circumstances of the agent under evaluation. Rather than specify study and technical details, they rely on the investigator to meet the primary goal of detecting and bringing to light any indication of toxicity to reproduction. Key elements of the FDA Segment I, II, and III studies, the ICH protocols, and the OECD equivalent of the FDA Segment II test

are provided in Table 10-4. In each protocol, guidance is provided on species/strain selection, route of administration, number and spacing of dosage levels, exposure duration, experimental sample size, observational techniques, statistical analysis, and reporting requirements. Details are available in the original publications as well as in several reviews (e.g., Manson, 1994; Claudio et al., 1999; Reuter et al., 2003). Variations of these protocols also exist that include extensions of exposure to early or later time points in development and extensions of observations to postnatal ages with more sophisticated endpoints. For example, the EPA has developed a Developmental Neurotoxicity Protocol for the rat that includes exposure from gestation day 6 though lactation day 10, and observation of postnatal growth, developmental landmarks of puberty (balanopreputial separation, vaginal opening), motor activity, auditory startle, learning and memory, and neuropathology at various ages through postnatal day 60 (US EPA, 1998).

The general goal of these regulatory studies is to identify the No Observed Adverse Effect Level (NOAEL), which is the highest dosage level that does not produce a significant increase in adverse effects in the offspring. These NOAELs are then used in the risk assessment process (see below) to assess the likelihood of effects in humans given certain exposure conditions.

Multigeneration Tests

Information pertaining to developmental toxicity can also be obtained from studies in which animals are exposed to the test substance continuously over one or more generations. For additional information on this approach, see Chap. 20.

Children's Health and the Food Quality Protection Act

In 1993, the National Academy of Sciences published a report entitled "Pesticides in the Diets of Infants and Children," which brought to light the fact that infants and children differ both qualitatively and quantitatively from adults in their exposure to pesticide residues in food because of different dietary composition and intake patterns and different activities (NRC, 1993). This report, along with the report from the International Life Sciences Institute entitled "Similarities and Differences between Children and Adults" (Guzelian et al., 1992) provided background and impetus for passage of the Food Quality Protection Act (FQPA) of 1996. The FQPA incorporates an additional tenfold safety factor for children, cumulative effects of toxicants acting through a common mode of action, aggregate exposure (i.e., same toxicant from different sources), and endocrine disruption (see above). The inclusion (at the discretion of the EPA) of the tenfold factor for calculating allowable intakes for children affects most strongly the pesticide industry, whose products appear as residues in food. The application of this safety factor is controversial, in part because its opponents claim that developmental susceptibility is already considered in other tests, such as the Segment II test for prenatal toxicity, the two-generation test, and the developmental neurotoxicity test. On the other hand, proponents applaud the measure and point to the numerous factors that may increase the exposure of infants and children to environmental toxicants and their susceptibility to harm from these exposures. Children have different diets than adults and also have activity patterns that change their exposure profile compared to adults, such as crawling on the floor or ground, putting their hands and foreign objects in their mouths, and raising dust and dirt during play. Even the level of their activity (i.e., closer to the ground) can affect their exposure to some toxicants. In addition to exposure differences, children are growing and developing, which makes them more susceptible to some types of insults. Effects of early childhood exposure, including neurobehavioral effects and cancer, may not be apparent until later in life. Debate continues over the approach to be used in risk assessment in consideration of infants and children.

In the last few years, a proposal has been developed for a large prospective study on children's health in the United States, the National Children's Study (NCS) (Branum et al., 2003; Needham et al., 2005; Kimmel et al., 2005). For this longitudinal birth cohort, families would be identified and children followed from before birth through 21 years of age. Among many parameters and endpoints to be assessed, exposure to environmental contaminants would be assessed, including those present in breast milk. In this unique study, because the children will be followed to adulthood, the opportunity exists to assess the full range of potentially adverse developmental consequences of environmental exposures.

Alternative Testing Strategies

A variety of alternative test systems have been proposed to refine, reduce, or replace reliance on the standard regulatory mammalian tests for assessing prenatal toxicity (Table 10-5). These can be grouped into assays based on cell cultures, cultures of embryos in vitro (including submammalian species), and short-term in vivo tests. Some effort has been made to qualitatively and quantitatively compile results across both the standard and the alternative tests (Faustman, 1988; Kavlock, et al., 1991). Daston (1996) has discussed the theoretical and empirical underpinnings supporting the use of a number of these systems. Yet, validation of these alternative tests continues to be a major issue (Neubert, 1989; Welsch, 1990). Assessing the significance of the sensitivity and specificity of results from the tests has been problematic. While it was initially hoped that the alternative approaches would become generally applicable to all chemicals, and help prioritize full-scale testing, this has not yet been accomplished. Indeed, given the complexity of embryogenesis and the multiple mechanisms and target sites of potential teratogens, it was perhaps unrealistic to have expected a single test, or even a small battery, to accurately prescreen the activity of chemicals in general. To date, their primary success has come from evaluating the relative potency of series of congeners when the prototype chemical has demonstrated appropriate concordance with in vivo results (Kavlock, 1993). Over the past several years, a validation study of three in vitro embryotoxicity assays, the rat embryo limb bud micromass assay, the mouse embryonic stem cell test, and the rat embryo culture test, has been carried out (Genschow et al., 2000, 2002, 2004; Brown, 2002; Piersma et al., 2004; Seiler et al., 2004; Spielmann et al., 2004). This study involves interlaboratory blind trials to validate these assays, and the approach involves the development of "prediction models" which mathematically combine assay endpoints to determine which combinations and formulations are most predictive of mammalian in vivo results.

Submammalian species have been used for many years in the study of normal developmental biology, and among these animal models, the African clawed frog, *Xenopus laevis* or *X. tropicalis* (Bantle, 1995; Fort et al., 2000, 2004; Fort and Paul, 2002), and the zebrafish, *Danio rerio* (Fraysse et al., 2006; Love et al., 2004; Ton et al., 2006), have been used for developmental toxicology to a number of advantages. Chief among the features of these species is the rapid external development of the embryos, the large historical and recent literature on their normal development, and the availability of genetic mutants and molecular biological tools for studying these embryos. In addition, they can be bred to produce large numbers of embryos in a relatively short period and are easy and inexpensive to maintain.

Important to the consideration of all these alternative test models is the application of new genomic and proteomic screening approaches, especially those amenable to high throughput screening. These techniques offer for the future the potential to develop highly automated, rapid, and specific tests for developmental toxicity.

An exception to the limited acceptance to date of alternate tests for prescreening for developmental toxicity is the in vivo test developed by Chernoff and Kavlock (1982). In this test, pregnant

Table 10-5

Brief Survey of Alternative Test Methodologies for Developmental Toxicity

ASSAY	BRIEF DESCRIPTION AND ENDPOINTS EVALUATED	CONCORDANCE*	REFERENCE(S)
Micromass culture	Midbrain or limb bud cells dissociated from rat embryos and grown in micromass culture for 5 days. Cell proliferation and biochemical markers of differentiation assessed.	Sensitivity: 25/27; 20/33; 11/15 Specificity: 17/19; 18/18; 8/10 Accuracy: 79%	Flint and Orton, 1984 Renault *et al.*, 1989 Uphill *et al.*, 1990 Genschow *et al.*, 2000 Spielmann *et al.*, 2004
Mouse embryonic stem cell (EST) test	Mouse ESTs and 3T3 cells in 96-well plates assessed for viability after 3 and 5 days. ESTs grown for 3 days in hanging drops form embryoid bodies which are plated and examined after 10 days for differentiation into cardiocytes.	Sensitivity: 84% Specificity: 68% Accuracy: 79%	Scholz *et al.*, 1999 Genschow *et al.*, 2000, 2004
Chick embryo neural retina cell culture	Neural retinas of day 6.5 chick embryos dissociated and grown in rotating suspension culture for 7 days. Endpoints include cellular aggregation, growth, differentiation, and biochemical markers.	Sensitivity: 36/41 Specificity: 14/17	Daston *et al.*, 1991 Daston *et al.*, 1995a (concordances combined)
Drosophila	Fly larvae grown from egg disposition through hatching of adults. Adult flies examined for specific structural defects (bent bristles and notched wing).	Sensitivity: 10/13 Specificity: 4/5	Lynch *et al.*, 1991 Palermo *et al.*, 2004
FETAX	Mid-blastula stage *Xenopus* embryos exposed for 96 h and evaluated for viability, growth, morphology.	Sensitivity: 6/7 Specificity: 2/2	Bantle, 1995 Fort *et al.*, 2000 Fort and Paul, 2002
Rodent whole embryo culture	Postimplantation rodent embryos grown in vitro for up to two days and evaluated for growth and development.	Accuracy: 88%	Webster *et al.*, 1997 Genschow *et al.*, 2000 Piersma *et al.*, 2004
Zebrafish	Zebrafish eggs or blastulae exposed to chemical in water (can be in multi-well plates) for up to four days and evaluated for growth, development and (in some cases) gene expression.	Sensitivity: ND Specificity: ND	Fraysse *et al.*, 2006 Love *et al.*, 2004
Chernoff/Kavlock assay	Pregnant mice or rats exposed during organogenesis and allowed to deliver. Postnatal growth, viability and gross morphology of litters assessed.	Sensitivity: 49/58 Specificity: 28/34	Hardin *et al.*, 1987

*Authors interpretation. Sensitivity: correct identification of "positive" chemicals. Specificity: correct identification of "negative" compounds. Accuracy: correct classification of test agents as non-, weakly, or strongly teratogenic. Accuracy values are from Genschow *et al.* (2004), Piersma *et al.* (2004) and Spielmann *et al.*(2004). ND: Not Determined (too few chemicals tested to determine these values).

females are exposed during the period of major organogenesis to a limited number of dosage levels near those inducing maternal toxicity, and offspring are evaluated over a brief neonatal period for external malformations, growth, and viability. It has proven reliable over a large number of chemical agents and classes (Hardin *et al.*, 1987), and a regulatory testing guideline (US EPA, 1985).

Epidemiology

Reproductive epidemiology is the study of associations between specific exposures of the father or pregnant woman and her conceptus and the outcome of pregnancy. In rare situations, such as rubella, thalidomide, and isotretinoin, where a relatively high risk exists and the outcome is a rare event, formal studies may not be needed to identify causes of abnormal birth outcomes. The likelihood of linking a particular exposure with a series of case reports increases with the rarity of the defect, the rarity of the exposure

in the population, a small source population, a short time span for study, and biological plausibility for the association (Khoury *et al.*, 1991). In other situations, such as those with ethanol and valproic acid, associations are sought through either a case-control or a cohort approach. Both approaches require accurate ascertainment of abnormal outcomes and exposures, and a large enough effect and study population to detect an elevated risk. Therein lies one of the difficulties for epidemiologists studying abnormal reproductive outcomes. For example, it has been estimated that the monitoring of more than 1 million births would have been necessary to detect a statistically significant increase in the frequency of spina bifida following the introduction of valproic acid in the United States, where the frequency of exposure was less than 1 in 1000 pregnancies and the risk was only a doubling over the background incidence (Khoury *et al.*, 1987). Another challenge to epidemiologists is the high percentage of human pregnancy wastage, perhaps as much as 31% in the peri-implantation period (Wilcox *et al.*, 1988) and an additional 15% that are clinically recognized. Therefore, pregnancy failures related to a particular exposure may go undetected in the general population. Furthermore, with the availability of prenatal diagnostic procedures, additional pregnancies of malformed embryos (particularly neural tube defects) are electively aborted. Thus, the incidence of abnormal outcomes at birth may not reflect the true rate of abnormalities, and the term prevalence, rather than incidence, is preferred when the denominator is the number of live births rather than total pregnancies.

Epidemiologic studies of abnormal reproductive outcomes are usually undertaken with three objectives in mind: the first is scientific research into the causes of abnormal birth outcomes and usually involves analysis of case reports or clusters; a second aim is prevention and is targeted at broader surveillance of trends by birth defect registries around the world; and the last objective is informing the public and providing assurance. In this regard, it is informative to consider the review by Schardein (1993) of the method and year by which humans teratogens were detected. For 23 of 28 chemicals (including nine cancer therapeutics, androgenic hormones, antithyroid drugs, aminoglycoside antibiotics, coumarin anticoagulants, diethylstilbestrol, methylmercury, hydantoins, primidone, penicillamine, lithium, vitamin A, and retinoic acid), case reports presented the first evidence in humans. For two of these (diethylstilbestrol and lithium), the case reports were soon followed by registries that provided confirmation, while for two others (methyl mercury and hydantoins) follow-up epidemiology studies added support. For only four chemicals, alcohol, PCBs, carbamazepine, and cocaine, did an analytical epidemiological study provide the first human evidence. Evidence for one chemical, valproic acid, was first obtained by analysis of a birth defect registry. For the 28 chemicals in that review, human evidence of developmental toxicity preceded published animal evidence in eleven instances. Cohort studies, with their prospective exposure assessment and ability to monitor both adverse and beneficial outcomes, may be the most methodologically robust approach to identifying human developmental toxicants. The lack of cohort studies demonstrating risk for pregnancy may be in part due to the difficulty in making such associations, but may also reflect the fact that use in pregnancy is not associated with increased risk for the majority of drugs (Irl and Hasford, 2000).

Concordance of Data

There have been several extensive reviews of the similarity of responses of laboratory animals and humans to developmental toxicants. In general, these studies support the assumption that results from laboratory tests are predictive of potential human effects. Concordance is strongest when there are positive data from more than one test species. In a quantitative sense, the few comparisons that have been made suggest that humans tend to be more sensitive to developmental toxicants than is the most sensitive test species. While concordance among species for agents reported as positive is high, often special steps must be taken retrospectively to produce an animal model that reflects the nature of outcome in humans (e.g., valproic acid, Ehlers et al., 1992).

Frankos (1985) reviewed data for 38 compounds having demonstrated or suspect activity in humans; all except tobramycin, which caused otologic defects, were positive in at least one test species and 76% were positive in more than one test species. Predictiveness was highest in the mouse (85%) and rat (80%), with lower rates for rabbits (60%), and hamsters (40%). Frankos identified 165 chemicals with no evidence of human effects; only 29%

were negative in all species tested while 51% were negative in more than one species. Schardein and Keller (1989) examined concordance by species and developmental manifestation for 51 potential human developmental toxicants that had adequate animal data (three human developmental toxicants did not). Thalidomide received the widest testing, with data from 19 species; 53% had data from 3 species, whereas 18% had data from four or five species. Across all chemicals, the most common findings in humans, rabbits, and monkeys were spontaneous abortion and fetal/neonatal death, followed by malformations and then growth retardation. In the rat, prenatal death, growth retardation, and then malformations was the typical pattern. The concordance of results is presented in Table 10-6. All species showed at least one positive response for 64% of the human developmental toxicants and, with only one exception, all of the potential human developmental toxicants showed a positive response in at least one species. Overall, the match to the human, regardless of the nature of the developmental response, was rat, 98%; mouse, 91%; hamster, 85%; monkey, 82%; and rabbit, 77%. Jelovsek et al. (1989) reviewed the predictiveness of animal data for 84 negative human developmental toxicants, 33 with unknown activity, 26 considered suspicious, and 32 considered positive. Variables considered included the response of each species, the number of positive and negative species, percent positive and negative species, and mutagenicity and carcinogenicity. The compounds were correctly classified 63–91% of the time based on animal data, depending upon how the suspect and unknown human toxicants were considered. The various models had a sensitivity of 62–75%, a positive predictive value of 75–100%, and a negative predictive value of 64–91%.

Schardein and Macina (2007) reviewed 50 human developmental toxicants. They reported that 49/50 showed developmental toxicity in at least one common test species. However, the specific endpoint of toxicity was often different in humans than those of the test species. When adverse outcomes were placed in the categories, such as growth retardation, death, malformation and functional deficit, the concordance of outcome category for humans and animal test species was observed for 48% of toxicants in rat, 26% in mouse, 16% in rabbit and 8% in primates. Overall, 27/50 (54%) of the agents evaluated had at least one species exhibiting the same endpoint as did humans.

In addition to qualitative comparisons among species, several attempts at quantitative comparisons of potencies have been developed, although these have been based upon administered dosage and have not attempted to factor in pharmacokinetic differences. Schardein and Keller (1989) estimated the human and animal "threshold" dosages for 21 chemicals. In only two cases, aminopterin and carbon disulfide, were developmental effects seen at lower dosages in animal studies than were believed to cause effects in humans. For the other chemicals, ratios of the "threshold" dosages in the most sensitive animals to those in humans ranged from 1.2–200. Newman et al. (1993) looked at the data for four well-characterized human developmental toxicants: valproic acid, isotretinoin, thalidomide, and methotrexate. The monkey was the most sensitive test species for the first three chemicals, whereas the rabbit was the most sensitive to methotrexate. Base upon the NOAEL of the most sensitive test species, human embryos were 0.9 to approximately 10 times more sensitive.

Elements of Risk Assessment

The extrapolation of animal test data for developmental toxicity follows two basic directions, one for drugs where exposure is voluntary

Table 10-6

Predictiveness of Animal Data for 51 Potential Human Developmental Toxicants

		MOUSE	RAT	MONKEY	RABBIT	HAMSTER
Potential human developmental toxicants tested (%)		86	96	33	61	26
Concordance by class	G[1]	61	57	65	39	39
	D	75	71	53	52	54
	M	71	67	65	65	62
	All	91	98	82	77	85
False positives	G	25	33	6	19	8
	D	11	16	18	10	0
	M	14	12	6	7	15
False negatives	G	10	14	29	39	54
	D	14	12	29	39	46
	M	11	25	29	29	23

KEY: G, growth retardation; D, death of conceptus; M, malformation; All, either growth, death, or malformations.
SOURCE: Adapted from Schardein and Keller (1989), with permission.

and usually to high (biologically effective) dosages, the other for environmental agents where exposure is generally involuntary and to low levels. For drugs, a use-in-pregnancy rating is utilized (US FDA, 1979). In this system the letters A, B, C, D, and X are used to classify the evidence that a chemical poses a risk to the human conceptus. For example, drugs are placed in category A if adequate, well-controlled studies in pregnant humans have failed to demonstrate a risk, and in category X (contraindicated for pregnancy) if studies in animals or humans, or investigational or postmarketing reports have shown fetal risk which clearly outweighs any possible benefit to the patient. The default category is C (risks cannot be ruled out), assigned when there is a lack of human studies and animal studies are either lacking or are positive for fetal risk, but the benefits may justify the potential risk. Categories B and D represent areas of relatively lesser, or greater concern for risk, respectively. Manson (1994) reviewed the 1992 Physicians' Desk Reference and found 7% of the 1033 drugs belonged to category X, 66% to category C, and only 0.7% to category A. The FDA categorization procedure has been criticized (Teratology Society, 1994) as being too reliant on risk/benefit comparisons, especially given that the magnitude of risk is often unknown, or the benefits are not an issue (e.g., after the drug in question has been taken during early pregnancy, the question is then directed to the management of the exposed pregnancy). The FDA system has also been criticized for demanding an unrealistically high quality of data for assignment to category A (negative controlled studies in pregnant women) and overuse of category C, interpreted as "risks cannot be ruled out" (Sannerstedt *et al.*, 1996). This is an important issue, because presently the perception of teratogenic risk is strong among both patients and prescribers even for safe drugs (Pole *et al.*, 2000). The often necessary reliance on studies conducted in animals has also been criticized, and acceptance by clinicians of these studies as reflective of human risks/benefits may be limited (Doering *et al.*, 2002).

For environmental agents, the purpose of the risk assessment process for noncancer endpoints such as developmental toxicity is generally to define the dose, route, timing, and duration of exposure that induces effects at the lowest level in the most relevant laboratory animal model (US EPA, 1991a,b). The exposure associated with this "critical effect" is then subjected to a variety of safety or uncertainty factors in order to derive an exposure level for humans

that is presumed to be relatively safe (see Chap. 4). The principal uncertainty factors include one for interspecies extrapolation and one for variability in the human population. The default value for each of these factors is 10. In the absence of firm evidence upon which to base decisions on whether or not to extrapolate animal test data, certain default assumptions are generally made. They include: (1) an agent that produces an adverse developmental effect in experimental animals will potentially pose a hazard to humans following sufficient exposure during development; (2) all four manifestations of developmental toxicity (death, structural abnormalities, growth alterations, and functional deficits) are of concern; (3) the specific types of developmental effects seen in animal studies are not necessarily the same as those that may be produced in humans; (4) the most appropriate species is used to estimate human risk when data are available (in the absence of such data, the most sensitive species is appropriate); and (5) in general, a threshold is assumed for the dose–response curve for agents that produce developmental toxicity.

One of the more troubling and subjective aspects of risk assessment for developmental toxicants is distinguishing between adverse effects (defined as an unwanted effect determined to be detrimental to health) and lesser effects, which while different than those observed in control groups, may not be considered significant to human health. Considerations relevant to this issue can be categorized into two areas: (1) the observance of the finding and related events in the same or associated experiments; and (2) the understanding of the biology of the effect. The interpretation of reduced fetal growth in developmental toxicity studies illustrates most of the issues. While we have accepted definitions of low birth weight in humans and understand how intrauterine growth retardation translates to an elevated risk of infant mortality and mental retardation, we do not have similar knowledge for fetal weight in rodents, and we seldom even know if reduced fetal weight recorded in prenatal toxicity studies persists beyond birth. Further complicating matters, recent epidemiological evidence suggests that birth weight in humans is inversely related to risk of adult-onset diseases including hypertension, cardiovascular disease, and diabetes (Rich-Edwards, *et al.*, 1999; Osmond and Barker, 2000; McMillen and Robinson, 2005). Exposure to poor nutrition perinatally is also predictive of insulin resistance in adulthood (Stocker *et al.*, 2005), obesity at

50 years of age in women (Ravelli *et al.*, 1999), and obstructive airway disease in adulthood (Lopuhaa *et al.*, 2000). Animal models of the long-term latent effects of prenatal toxic exposures are just now being developed (Lau and Rogers, 2004).

Contemporary Approaches

The Benchmark-Dose Approach   The use of safety or uncertainty factors applied to an experimentally derived NOAEL to arrive at a presumed safe level of human exposure is predicated on the risk assessment assumption that a threshold for developmental toxicity exists (see section "Principles of Developmental Toxicology," above). A threshold should not be confused with the NOAEL, as the NOAEL is dependent entirely on the power of the study and, as will be seen later, is associated with risks perhaps on the order of 5% over the control incidence in typical studies. Also, the value obtained by the application of uncertainty factors to the NOAEL should not be confused with a threshold, as this exposure is only assumed to be without appreciable added risk.

The use of the NOAEL in the risk assessment process has been criticized for several reasons. For example, because it is dependent on statistical power to detect pair-wise differences between a treated and a control group, the use of larger sample sizes and more dose groups (which might better characterize the dose–response relationship) can only yield lower NOAELs, and thus better experimental designs are actually penalized by this approach. In addition, the NOAEL is limited to an experimental dose level, and an experiment might need to be repeated to develop a NOAEL for risk assessment. A final point relates to the fact that, given varying experimental designs and variability of control values, NOAELs actually represent different levels of risk across studies.

Crump (1984) proposed using a mathematical model to estimate the lower confidence bounds on a predetermined level of risk [the "benchmark dose" (BMD)] as a means of avoiding many of the disadvantages of the NOAEL. The application of this approach to a large compilation of Segment II type data sets (Faustman *et al.*, 1994; Allen *et al.*, 1994a,b; Kavlock, 1995) demonstrated that a variety of mathematical models, including those that incorporate developmental-specific features such as litter size and intra-litter correlations, can be readily applied to standard test results. On average, benchmark doses based on a 5% added risk of effect calculated on quantal endpoints (e.g., whether an implant was affected or not) were approximately equivalent to traditionally determined NOAELs. When the litter was used as the unit of response (did it contain at least one affected implant?), benchmarks calculated for a 10% added risk were most similar to the correspondingly determined NOAEL. Discrepancies between the benchmark dose and the NOAEL were most pronounced when one or more of the following conditions were present: a shallow dose–response, small sample sizes, wide spacing of experimental dosage levels, or more than the typical number of dose levels. These features tend to make determination of the NOAEL more problematic (usually higher) and the confidence limits around the maximum likelihood estimate broader (resulting in lower BMDs).

Biologically Based Dose–Response Modeling   The introduction of statistical dose–response models for noncancer endpoints is the first step in developing quantitative, mechanistic models that will help reduce the major uncertainties of high-to-low dose and species-to-species extrapolation of experimental data. These biologically based dose–response models integrate pharmacokinetic information on target tissue dosimetry with molecular/biochemical responses, cellular/tissue responses, and developmental toxicity (O'Flaherty, 1997; Lau and Setzer, 2000; Lau *et al.*, 2001; Setzer *et al.*, 2001). Gaylor and Razzaghi (1992) proposed a model that related induction of cleft palate to fetal growth inhibition, and Gaylor and Chen (1993) proposed a model relating fetal weight and the probability of fetal abnormality. Shuey *et al.* (1994) presented a model using the cancer chemotherapeutic 5-fluorouracil (Fig. 10-9). They postulated that the developmental toxicity observed in the term fetus was due to an active metabolite (FdUMP) inhibiting the enzyme thymidylate synthetase, with subsequent depletion of thymidine, decreased DNA synthetic rates, reduced cell proliferation, and ultimately, reduced tissue growth and differentiation. Each step in the process was determined experimentally and the relationships were described by Hill equations. The individual equations were then linked in an integrated model to describe the entire relationship between administered dose and the incidence of hind limb defects. While this is still an empirically based model, the process clearly demonstrated the utility of the approach in understanding the relative importance of various pathways of abnormal development in the ultimate manifestation and in providing a basis for models which could incorporate species-specific response parameters. Leroux and coworkers (1996) took a more theoretical approach, using a cell kinetic model in which a progenitor cell would either divide, differentiate, or die, each event proceeding at a certain rate. These authors constructed a stochastic model based on the premise that a malformation occurs when the number of differentiated cells is less than a critical number for a given stage of development. Ultimately, BBDR models will need to be generalizable across dose, route of exposure, species, and perhaps even chemicals of similar mechanistic classes.

Understanding the mode of action for any toxicant, including developmental toxicants, can greatly inform the human risk assessment process. Although the construction of BBDR models exemplifies the extent of sophistication and quantification to which such exercises can be pursued, even more qualitative information on modes of action can have a great impact on the interpretation of developmental toxicity test results. For excellent examples of the utility of mode of action information, the reader is referred to an issue of Critical Reviews in Toxicology (Volume 35, September–October, 2005) devoted to this topic. Developmental toxicants for which mode of action is discussed include ethylene glycol (Corley *et al.*, 2005), nicotine (Slikker *et al.*, 2005), phthalate esters (Foster, 2005), vinclozolin (Kavlock and Cummings, 2005), valproic acid (Wiltse, 2005), hemoglobin-based oxygen carriers (Holson *et al.*, 2005), ACE inhibitors (Tabacova, 2005), and propylthiouracil (Zoeller and Crofton, 2005).

PATHWAYS TO THE FUTURE

In 2000, a committee assembled by the National Research Council released its report, "Scientific Frontiers in Developmental Toxicology and Risk Assessment" (NRC, 2000). The report presents a number of exciting findings and ideas, and serves as a framework to help advance the field of developmental toxicology in the next decade.

The NRC committee reports that major discoveries have been made about mechanisms of normal development, that these mechanisms are conserved in diverse animals, many of which have been used extensively in developmental biology and genetics, including the fruit fly, roundworm, zebrafish, frog, chick, and mouse.

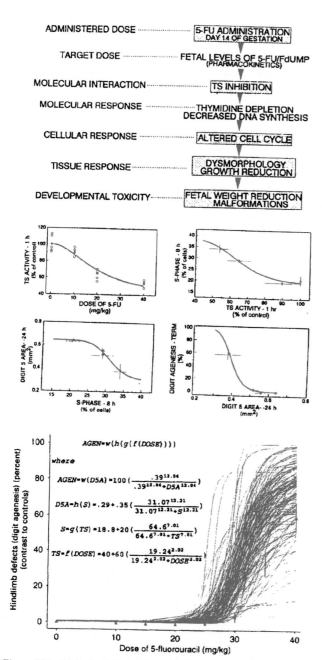

Figure 10-9. Biologically based dose–response modeling of the developmental toxicity of 5-fluorouracil (5-FU) following maternal administration on gestation day 14.

Top: Proposed model for the developmental toxicity of 5-FU based on thymidylate synthetase (TS) inhibition, decreased DNA synthesis, cell cycle alterations, and growth deficits and hind-limb dysmorphogenesis. Shaded events were measured experimentally. *Middle:* Relationships between successive endpoints are shown in these four panels (hind-limb bud TS activity versus 5-FU dose, S-phase accumulation versus TS activity, limb digit 5 area at 24 hour postdose versus proportion of cells in S phase, and digit agenesis at term versus limb digit 5 area at 24 hours). Data were fitted with Hill equations. *Bottom:* Model for induction of hind-limb defects induced by 5-FU, generated by integration of the individual Hill equations describing the relationships between successive model endpoints as presented in the middle panels. These individual equations are listed here, and the curves were generated by Monte Carlo simulation to estimate variability around the predicted relationship. The simulation results indicate that variability in the intermediate endpoints can account for differences between the predicted and actual dose–response. AGEN: digit agenesis at term; D5A: digit 5 area; S: % of cells in S phase. [Adapted from Shuey *et al.* (1994).]

Table 10-7

The 17 Intercellular Signaling Pathways Used in Development by Most Metazoans

PERIOD DURING DEVELOPMENT	SIGNALING PATHWAY
Before organogenesis; later for growth and tissue renewal	1. Wingless-Int pathway
	2. Transforming growth factor β pathway
	3. Hedgehog pathway
	4. Receptor tyrosine kinase pathway
	5. Notch-Delta pathway
	6. Cytokine pathway (STAT pathway)
Organogenesis and cytodifferentiation; later for growth and tissue renewal	7. Interleukin-1-toll nuclear factor-kappa B pathway
	8. Nuclear hormone receptor pathway
	9. Apoptosis pathway
	10. Receptor phosphotyrosine phosphatase pathway
Larval and adult physiology	11. Receptor guanylate cyclase pathway
	12. Nitric oxide receptor pathway
	13. G-protein coupled receptor (large G proteins) pathway
	14. Integrin pathway
	15. Cadherin pathway
	16. Gap junction pathway
	17. Ligand-gated cation channel pathway

SOURCE: Modified from NRC (2000).

Seventeen conserved intercellular signaling pathways are described which are used repeatedly at different times and locations during development of these and other animal species, as well as in humans (Table 10-7). The conserved nature of these key pathways provides a strong scientific rationale for using these animal models to advantage for developmental toxicology. Not only are these organisms advantageous for developmental toxicity studies due to their well-known genetics and embryology and their rapid generation time, but they are also amenable to genetic manipulation to enhance the sensitivity of specific developmental pathways or to incorporate human genes, such as those of drug metabolizing enzymes, to answer questions of interspecies extrapolation.

The Hedgehog signaling pathway serves as an example of the exciting linkages being made between embryology, genetics, and toxicology. This pathway, first discovered in *Drosophila*, is also present in vertebrates and is important in the development of a number of organs including the central nervous system, the limbs, and the face. Ligands for the hedgehog family receptors require proteolytic cleavage and addition of cholesterol for activation, and this pathway is exemplified by the Sonic Hedgehog (SHH) pathway in Fig. 10-10. The receptor for the SHH ligand, called *patched (ptc)*, is associated with and normally represses function of the membrane protein *smoothened (smo)*. Binding of SHH to *ptc* derepresses

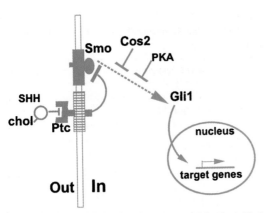

Figure 10-10. Diagram showing the transduction of the Sonic Hedgehog (SHH) signal through the patched (ptc) and smoothened (smo) receptor complex.

The SHH protein requires proteolytic cleavage and covalent binding to cholesterol (*chol*) prior to binding to *ptc*. Binding to *ptc* derepresses *smo*, which activates a signal cascade of transcription factor (*gli*) activation and target-gene transcription.

function of *smo*, leading to activation of specific transcription factors and transcription of target genes. Mutations of the SHH gene lead to holoprosencephaly (a malformation involving the forebrain and associated structures) in mice and humans. Toxicologically, cyclopamine and jervine, plant alkaloids that bind to *ptc*, can induce holoprosencephaly in animals. Further, covalent binding of cholesterol is required for SHH activity, and cholesterol synthesis inhibitors have also been shown to cause holoprosencephaly. Understanding of the biochemistry and function of this signaling pathway in normal development elucidates the mechanisms of toxicity leading to holoprosencephaly. Conversely, use of such specific toxicants as pharmacological probes allows confirmation of the role of this pathway in brain development.

As our knowledge of the genetic control of normal development has advanced immensely in the past few years, so has the technology to examine gene expression and its control, networks of interrelated gene products, and changes in gene expression induced by alterations in the developmental environment. Advances in genomics, proteomics, metabolomics, and bioinformatics are being used to advance our understanding of health and disease, including normal and abnormal development. One of the current pioneering efforts in this arena is the Birth Defects Systems Manager website (http://systems analysis.louisville.edu) being developed at the University of Louisville. Among a number of approaches in this system is the construction of a microarray database with various teratogens, doses, time intervals, and stages for congenital malformations. It is hoped that such a database will enable generation of hypotheses about the mechanisms underlying toxicant-inducted birth defects. Hypotheses can then be tested with laboratory experiments using genetic expression profiling or other powerful approaches. The investigators putting together this new approach for investigating the physiological state of the embryo have called the in silico aspects of this approach "cyber-teratology."

REFERENCES

Abel EL: Consumption of alcohol during pregnancy: A review of effects on growth and development of offspring. *Hum Biol* 54:421–453, 1982.

Abel EL: Factors affecting the outcome of maternal alcohol exposure: I. Parity. *Neurobehav Toxicol Teratol* 3:49–51, 1984.

Abel EL: Fetal alcohol syndrome: A cautionary note. *Curr Pharm Des* 12:1521–1529, 2006.

Abel EL, Church MW, Dintcheff BA: Prenatal alcohol exposure shortens life span in rats. *Teratology* 36:217–220, 1987.

Adler T: The return of thalidomide. *Sci News* 146:424–425, 1994.

Ahokas RA, Dilts PV Jr, LaHaye EB: Cadmium-induced fetal growth retardation: Protective effect of excess dietary zinc. *Am J Obstet Gynecol* 136:216–221, 1980.

Alford CA, Stagno S, Reynolds DW: Perinatal infections caused by viruses, *Toxoplasma*, and *Treponema pallidum*, in Aldjem S, Brown AK (eds.): *Clinical Perinatology.* St. Louis: Mosby, 1974, p. 31.

Allen BC, Kavlock RJ, Kimmel CA, Faustman EM: Dose response assessment for developmental toxicity: II. Comparison of generic benchmark dose models with no observed adverse effect levels. *Fundam Appl Toxicol* 23:487–495, 1994a.

Allen BC, Kavlock RJ, Kimmel CA, Faustman EM: Dose response assessment for developmental toxicity: III. Statistical models. *Fundam Appl Toxicol* 23:496–509, 1994b.

Amemiya K, Hurley LS, Keen CL: Effect of the anticarcinogenic drug 6-mercaptopurine on mineral metabolism in the mouse. *Toxicol Lett* 25:55–62, 1985.

Amemiya K, Hurley LS, Keen CL: Effect of 6-mercaptopurine on 65Zn distribution in the pregnant rat. *Teratology* 39:387–393, 1989.

Anway MD, Memon MA, Uzumcu M, Skinner MK: Transgenerational effect of the endocrine disruptor vinclozolin on male spermatogenesis. *J Androl* 27:868–879, 2006.

Arafa HM, Elmazar MM, Hamada FM, et al.: Selective agonists of retinoic acid receptors: Comparative toxicokinetics and embryonic exposure. *Arch Toxicol* 73:547–556, 2000.

Argiles JM, Carbo N, Lopez-Soriano FJ: Was tumour necrosis factor-alpha responsible for the fetal malformations associated with thalidomide in the early 1960's? *Med Hypotheses* 50:313–318, 1998.

Auger J, Kunstmann JM, Czyglik F, Jouannet P: Decline in semen quality among fertile men in Paris during the past 20 years. *N Engl J Med* 332:281–285, 1995.

Augustine K, Liu ET, Sadler TW: Antisense attenuation of Wnt-1 and Wnt-3a expression in whole embryo culture reveals roles for these genes in craniofacial, spinal cord, and cardiac morphogenesis. *Dev Genet* 14:500–520, 1993.

Baer JS, Sampson PD, Barr HM, Connor PD, Streissguth AP: A 21-year longitudinal analysis of the effects of prenatal alcohol exposure on young adult drinking. *Arch Gen Psychiatry* 60:377–385, 2003.

Ballantyne JW: *Manual of Antenatal Pathology and Hygiene: The Embryo.* Edinburgh: Green and Sons, 1904.

Balling R, Mutter G, Gruss P, Kessel M: Craniofacial abnormalities induced by ectopic expression of the homeobox gene Hox-1.1 in transgenic mice. *Cell* 58:337–347, 1989.

Bantle JA: FETAX: A developmental toxicity assay using frog embryos, in Rand G (ed.): *Fundamentals of Aquatic Toxicology: Effects, Environmental Fate, Risk Assessment,* 2nd ed. Washington, DC: Taylor and Francis, 1995, pp. 207–230.

Barlow SM, McElhatton PR, Sullivan FM: The relation between maternal restraint and food deprivation, plasma corticosterone, and cleft palate in the offspring of mice. *Teratology* 12:97–103, 1975.

Barrow MV: A brief history of teratology to the early 20th century. *Teratology* 4:119–130, 1971.

Bateson W: *Materials for the Study of Variation Treated with Especial Regard to Discontinuity in the Origin of Species.* London: Macmillan, 1894.

Bennett GD, Wlodarczyk B, Calvin JA, *et al.*: Valproic acid-induced alterations in growth and neurotrophic factor. *Reprod Toxicol* 14:1–11, 2000.

Beyer PE, Chernoff N: The induction of supernumerary ribs in rodents: Role of maternal stress. *Teratog Carcinog Mutagen* 6:419–429, 1986.

Bibbo M, Gill W, Azizi F, *et al.*: Follow-up study of male and female offspring of DES-exposed mothers. *Obstet Gynecol* 49:1–8, 1977.

Biegel LB, Hirshfield AN, Flaws JA, *et al.*: 90-day feeding and one-generation reproduction study in Crl:CR BR rat with 17β-estradiol. *Toxicol Sci* 44:116–142, 1998.

Bowman RE: Behavioral sequelae of toxicant exposure during neurobehavioral development, in Hunt VR, Smith MK, Worth D (eds.): *Banbury Report 11: Environmental Factors in Human Growth and Development.* Cold Spring Harbor, NY: Cold Spring Harbor Laboratory Press, 1982, pp. 283–294.

Branham WS, Zehr DR, Chen JJ, Sheehan DM: Uterine abnormalities in rats exposed neonatally to diethylstilbestrol, ethynylestradiol, or clomiphene citrate. *Toxicology* 51:201–212, 1988.

Branum AM, Collman GW, Correa A, *et al.*: The National Children's Study of environmental effects on child health and development. *Environ Health Perspect* 111:642–646, 2003.

Brent RL, Beckman DA: Environmental teratogens. *Bull NY Acad Med* 66:123–163, 1990.

Brown NA: Selection of test chemicals for the ECVAM international validation study on in vitro embryotoxicity tests. European Centre for the Validation of Alternative Methods. *Altern Lab Anim* 30:177–198, 2002.

Bujan L, Mansat A, Pontonnier F, Mieusset R: Time series analysis of sperm concentration in fertile men in Toulouse, France between 1977 and 1992. *Br Med J* 312:471–472, 1996.

Cagen SZ, Waechter JM, Dimond SS, *et al.*: Normal reproductive organ development in CF-1 mice following prenatal exposure to Bisphenol A. *Toxicol Sci* 50:36–44, 1999.

Calabrese L, Fleischer AB: Thalidomide: Current and potential clinical applications. *Am J Med* 108:487–495, 2000.

Carlsen E, Giwercman A, Keiding N, Skakkebaek NE: Evidence for decreasing quality of semen during past 50 years. *Br Med J* 305:609–613, 1992.

Carruthers CM, Foster PM: Critical window of male reproductive tract development in rats following gestational exposure to di-n-butyl phthalate. *Birth Defects Res B Dev Reprod Toxicol* 74:277–285, 2005.

Centers for Disease Control: *MMWR Morb Mortal Wkly Rep* 31(42):565–566, 1982.

Centers for Disease Control: *MMWR Morb Mortal Wkly Rep* 32(33):438–439, 1983.

Centers for Disease Control and Prevention (CDC): Use of vitamins containing folic acid among women of childbearing age—United States, 2004. *MMWR Morb Mortal Wkly Rep* 36:847–850, 2004.

Chambon P: The retinoid signaling pathway: Molecular and genetic analyses. *Semin Cell Biol* 5:115–125, 1994.

Chernoff N, Kavlock RJ: An in vivo teratology screen utilizing pregnant mice. *J Environ Toxicol Health* 10:541–550, 1982.

Chernoff N, Rogers JM, Alles AJ, *et al.*: Cell cycle alterations and cell death in cyclophosphamide teratogenesis. *Teratog Carcinog Mutagen* 9:199–209, 1989.

Chernoff N, Setzer RW, Miller DM, *et al.*: Effects of chemically-induced maternal toxicity on prenatal development in the rat. *Teratology* 42:651–658, 1990.

Clark DO: Pharmacokinetic studies in developmental toxicology: Practical considerations and approaches. *Toxicol Meth* 3:223–251, 1993.

Clark DO, Elswick BA, Welsch F, Conolly R: Pharmacokinetics of 2-methoxyethanol and 2-methoxyacetic acid in the pregnant mouse: A physiologically based mathematical model. *Toxicol Appl Pharmacol* 121:239–252, 1993.

Clark RL, Antonello JM, Grosman SJ, *et al.*: External genitalia abnormalities in male rats exposed in utero to finasteride, a 5α-reductase inhibitor. *Teratology* 42:91–100, 1990.

Clark RL, Robertson RT, Minsker DH, *et al.*: Diflunisal-induced maternal anemia as a cause of teratogenicity in rabbits. *Teratology* 30:319–332, 1984.

Clarren SK, Sampson PD, Larsen J, *et al.*: Facial effects of fetal alcohol exposure: Assessment by photographs and morphometric analysis. *Am J Med Genet* 26:651–666, 1987.

Claudio L, Bearer CF, Wallinga D: Assessment of the US Environmental Protection Agency methods for identification of hazards to developing organisms: Part II. The developmental toxicity testing guideline. *Am J Ind Med* 35:554–563, 1999.

Cohlan SQ: Congenital anomalies in the rat produced by excessive intake of vitamin A during pregnancy. *Pediatrics* 13:556–567, 1954.

Collins MD, Mao GE: Teratology of retinoids. *Annu Rev Pharmacol Toxicol* 39:399–430, 1999.

Cook JC, Johnson L, O'Connor JC, *et al.*: Effects of dietary 17β-estradiol exposure on serum hormone concentrations and testicular parameters in male Crl:CD BR rats. *Toxicol Sci* 44:155–168, 1998.

Cooper LZ, Krugman S: Diagnosis and management: Congeneital rubella. *Pediatrics* 37:335–342, 1966.

Cooper WO, Hernandez-Diaz S, Arbogast PG, *et al.*: Major congenital malformations after first-trimester exposure to ACE inhibitors. *N Engl J Med* 354:2443–2451, 2006.

Corley RA, Mast TJ, Carney EW, Rogers JM, Daston GP: Evaluation of physiologically based models of pregnancy and lactation for their application in children's health risk assessments. *Crit Rev Toxicol* 33:137–211, 2003.

Corley RA, Meek ME, Carney EW: Mode of action: Oxalate crystal-induced renal tubule degeneration and glycolic acid-induced dysmorphogenesis–renal and developmental effects of ethylene glycol. *Crit Rev Toxicol* 35:691–702, 2005.

Craig JC, Bennett GD, Miranda RC, *et al.*: Ribonucleotide reductase subunit R1: A gene conferring sensitivity to valproic acid-induced neural tube defects in mice. *Teratology* 61:305–313, 2000.

Crump K: A new method for determining allowable daily intakes. *Fundam Appl Toxicol* 4:854–871, 1984.

D'Amato RJ, Loughman MS, Flynn E, Folkman J: Thalidomide is an inhibitor of angiogenesis. *Proc Natl Acad Sci U S A* 91:4082–4085, 1994.

Dai WS, LaBraico JM, Stern RS: Epidemiology of isotretinoin exposure during pregnancy. *J Am Acad Dermatol* 26:599–606, 1992.

Dareste C: *Récherches sur la production artificielle des monstruosités, ou essais de tératogénie expérimentale.* Paris: Reinwald, 1877.

Dareste C: *Récherches sur la production artificielle des monstruosités, ou essais de tératogénie expérimentale,* 2nd ed. Paris: Reinwald, 1891.

Daston GP: Fetal zinc deficiency as a mechanism for cadmium-induced toxicity to the developing rat lung and pulmonary surfactant. *Toxicology* 24:55–63, 1982.

Daston GP: Do thresholds exist for developmental toxicants? A review of the theoretical and experimental evidence, in Kalter H (ed.): *Issues and Review in Teratology.* New York: Plenum Press, 1993, pp. 169–197.

Daston GP: Relationships between maternal and developmental toxicity, in Kimmel CA, Buelke-Sam J (eds.): *Developmental Toxicology,* 2nd ed. New York: Raven Press, 1994, pp. 189–212.

Daston GP: The theoretical and empirical case for in vitro developmental toxicity screens, and potential applications. *Teratology* 53:339–344, 1996.

Daston GP, Baines D, Elmore E, *et al.*: Evaluation of chick embryo neural retina cell culture as a screen for developmental toxicants. *Fundam Appl Toxicol* 26:203–210, 1995.

Daston GP, Baines D, Yonker JE: Chick embryo neural retinal cell culture as a screen for developmental toxicity. *Toxicol Appl Pharmacol* 109:352–366, 1991.

de Mouzon J, Thonneau P, Spira A, Multigner L: Semen quality has declined among men born in France since 1950. *Br Med J* 313:43, 1996.

Dempsey DA, Hajnal BL, Partridge JC, *et al.*: Tone abnormalities are associated with maternal cigarette smoking during pregnancy in in utero cocaine-exposed infants. *Pediatrics* 106:79–85, 2000.

De Santis M, Cavaliere AF, Straface G, Caruso A: Rubella infection in pregnancy. *Reprod Toxicol* 21:390–398, 2006.

Deschamps J, van Nes J: Developmental regulation of the Hox genes during axial morphogenesis in the mouse. *Development* 132:2931–2942, 2005.

DeSesso JM: Maternal factors in developmental toxicity. *Teratog Carcinog Mutagen* 7:225–240, 1987.

Dietrich M, Brown CJ, Block G: The effect of folate fortification of cereal-grain products on blood folate status, dietary folate intake, and dietary folate sources among adult non-supplement users in the United States. *J Am Coll Nutr* 24:266–274, 2005.

Doering PL, Boothby LA, Cheok M: Review of pregnancy labeling of prescription drugs: Is the current system adequate to inform of risks? *Am J Obstet Gynecol* 187:333–339, 2002.

Dolinoy DC, Weidman JR, Waterland RA, Jirtle RL: Maternal genistein alters coat color and protects Avy mouse offspring from obesity by modifying the fetal epigenome. *Environ Health Perspect* 114:567–572, 2006.

Dreosti IE: Nutritional factors underlying the expression of the fetal alcohol syndrome. *Ann NY Acad Sci* 678:193–204, 1993.

Dupe V, Ghyselinck NB, Thomazy V, *et al.*: Essential roles of retinoic acid signaling in interdigital apoptosis and control of BMP-7 expression in mouse autopods. *Dev Biol* 208:30–43, 1999.

Edwards MJ: Hyperthermia as a teratogen: A review of experimental studies and their clinical significance. *Teratog Carcinog Mutag* 6:563–582, 1986.

Ehlers K, Sturje H, Merker H-J, Nau H: Spina bifida aperta induced by valproic acid and by all-*trans*-retinoic acid in the mouse: Distinct differences in morphology and periods of sensitivity. *Teratology* 46:117–130, 1992.

Eibs HG, Speilman H, Hagele M: Teratogenic effects of cyproterone acetate and medroxyprogesterone treatment during the pre- and postimplantation period of mouse embryos. *Teratology* 25:27–36, 1982.

Elstein KH, Zucker RM, Andrews JE, *et al.*: Effects of developmental stage and tissue type on embryo/fetal DNA distributions and 5-fluorouracil-induced cell-cycle perturbations. *Teratology* 48:355–363, 1993.

Eriksson P, Lundkvist U, Fredriksson A: Neonatal exposure to 3,4,3′,4′-tetrachlorobiphenyl: Changes in spontaneous behavior and cholinergic muscarinic receptors in the adult mouse. *Toxicology* 69:27–34, 1991.

Ernhart CB, Sokol RJ, Martier S, *et al.*: Alcohol teratogenicity in the human: A detailed assessment of specificity, critical period and threshold. *Am J Obstet Gynecol* 156:33–39, 1987.

Euker JS, Riegle GD: Effect of stress on pregnancy in the rat. *J Reprod Fertil* 34:343–346, 1973.

Fabro S: Passage of drugs and other chemicals into the uterine fluids and preimplantation blastocyst, in Boreus L (ed.): *Fetal Pharmacology.* New York: Raven Press, 1973, pp. 443–461.

Fabro S, McLachlan JA, Dames NM: Chemical exposure of embryos during the preimplantation stages of pregnancy: Mortality rate and intrauterine development. *Am J Obstet Gynecol* 148:929–938, 1984.

Faiella A, Wernig M, Consalez GG, *et al.*: A mouse model for valproate teratogenicity: Parental effects, homeotic transformations, and altered HOX expression. *Hum Mol Genet* 9:227–236, 2000.

Fantel AG, Greenaway JC, Juchau MR, Shepard TH: Teratogenic bioactivation of cyclophosphamide in vitro. *Life Sci* 25:67–72, 1979.

Faustman EM: Short-term tests for teratogens. *Mutat Res* 205:355–384, 1988.

Faustman EM, Allen BC, Kavlock RJ, Kimmel CA: Dose response assessment for developmental toxicity: I. Characterization of database and determination of no observed adverse effect levels. *Fundam Appl Toxicol* 23:478–486, 1994.

Ferm VH, Carpenter SJ: Teratogenic effect of cadmium and its inhibition by zinc. *Nature* 216:1123, 1967.

Finnell RH, Wlodarczyk BC, Craig JC, *et al.*: Strain-dependent alterations in the expression of folate pathway genes following teratogenic exposure to valproic acid in a mouse model. *Am J Med Genet* 70:303–311, 1997.

Fisch H, Goluboff ET: Geographic variation in sperm counts: A potential cause of bias in studies of semen quality. *Fertil Steril* 65:1044–1046, 1996.

Fisher JW, Whitaker TA, Taylor DH, *et al.*: Physiologically based pharmacokinetic modeling of the pregnant rat: A multiroute exposure model for trichloroethylene and its metabolite, trichloroacetic acid. *Toxicol Appl Pharmacol* 99:395–414, 1989.

Flint OP, Orton TC: An in vitro assay for teratogens with culture of rat embryo midbrain and limb bud cells. *Toxicol Appl Pharmacol* 76:383–395, 1984.

Fort DJ, Paul RR: Enhancing the predictive validity of frog embryo teratogenesis assay—Xenopus (FETAX*). J Appl Toxicol* 22:185–191, 2002.

Fort DJ, Rogers RL, Thomas JH, Buzzard BO, Noll AM, Spaulding CD: Comparative sensitivity of Xenopus tropicalis and Xenopus laevis as test species for the FETAX model. *J Appl Toxicol* 24:443–457, 2004.

Fort DJ, Stover EL, Farmer DR, Lemen JK: Assessing the predictive validity of frog embryo teratogenesis assay—*Xenopus* (FETAX). *Teratog Carcinog Mutagen* 20:87–98, 2000.

Foster PM: Mode of action: Impaired fetal leydig cell function–effects on male reproductive development produced by certain phthalate esters. *Crit Rev Toxicol* 35:713–719, 2005.

Francis BM, Rogers JM, Sulik KK, *et al.*: Cyclophosphamide teratogenesis: Evidence for compensatory responses to induced cellular toxicity. *Teratology* 42:473–482, 1990.

Frankos VH: FDA perspectives on the use of teratology data for human risk assessment. *Fundam Appl Toxicol* 5:615–622, 1985.

Fraysse B, Mons R, Garric J: Development of a zebrafish 4-day embryo-larval bioassay to assess toxicity of chemicals. *Ecotoxicol Environ Saf* 63:253–267, 2006.

Fried PA, Watkinson B, Gray R: Differential effects on cognitive functioning in 9- to 12-year olds prenatally exposed to cigarettes and marihuana. *Neurotoxicol Teratol* 20:293–306, 1998.

Friedman JM: ACE inhibitors and congenital anomalies. *N Engl J Med* 354:2498–2500, 2006.

Fullerton PM, Kermer M: Neuropathy after intake of thalidomide. *Br Med J* 2:855–858, 1961.

Gabrielson JL, Larson KS: Proposals for improving risk assessment in reproductive toxicology. *Pharmacol Toxicol* 66:10–17, 1990.

Gabrielson JL, Paalkow LK: A physiological pharmacokinetic model for morphine disposition in the pregnant rat. *J Pharmacokinet Biopharm* 11:147–163, 1983.

Gargas ML, Tyler TR, Sweeney LM, *et al.*: A toxicokinetic study of inhaled ethylene glycol monomethyl ether (2-ME) and validation of a physiologically based pharmacokinetic model for the pregnant rat and human. *Toxicol Appl Pharmacol* 165:53–62, 2000.

Gaylor DW, Chen JJ: Dose response models for developmental malformations. *Teratology* 47:291–297, 1993.

Gaylor DW, Razzaghi M: Process of building biologically based dose response models for developmental defects. *Teratology* 46:573–581, 1992.

Gaylor DW, Sheehan DM, Young JF, Mattison DR: The threshold dose question in teratogenesis. *Teratology* 38:389–391, 1988.

Gellert RJ: Kepone, mirex, dieldrin and aldrin: Estrogenic activity and the induction of persistent vaginal estrus and anovulation in rats following prenatal treatment. *Environ Res* 16:131–138, 1978.

Generoso WM, Rutledge JC, Cain KT, *et al.*: Exposure of female mice to ethylene oxide within hours after mating leads to fetal malformations and death. *Mutat Res* 176:269–274, 1987.

Generoso WM, Rutledge JC, Cain KT, *et al.*: Mutagen-induced fetal anomalies and death following treatment of females within hours after mating. *Mutat Res* 199:175–181, 1988.

Genschow E, Scholz G, Brown N, *et al.*: Development of prediction models for three in vitro embryotoxicity tests in an ECVAM validation study. *In Vitr Mol Toxicol* 13:51–65, 2000.

Genschow E, Spielmann H, Scholz G, *et al.*: The ECVAM international validation study on in vitro embryotoxicity tests: Results of the definitive phase and evaluation of prediction models. European Centre for the Validation of Alternative Methods. *Altern Lab Anim* 30:151–176, 2002.

Genschow E, Spielmann H, Scholz G, *et al.*: Validation of the embryonic stem cell test in the international ECVAM validation study on three in vitro embryotoxicity tests. *Altern Lab Anim* 32:209–244, 2004.

George L, Granath F, Johansson AL, Anneren G, Cnattingius S: Environmental tobacco smoke and risk of spontaneous abortion. *Epidemiology* 17:500–505, 2006.

Gilliland FD, Berhane K, McConnell R, *et al.*: Maternal smoking during pregnancy, environmental tobacco smoke exposure and childhood lung function. *Thorax* 55:271–276, 2000.

Goldey ES, Crofton KM: Thyroxine replacement attenuates hypothyroxinemia, hearing loss and motor deficits following developmental exposure to Arochlor 1254 in rats. *Toxicol Sci* 45:94–105, 1998.

Goldey ES, Kehn LS, Lau C, *et al.*: Developmental exposure to polychlorinated biphenyls (Arochlor 1254) reduces circulating thyroid hormone concentrations and causes hearing deficits in rats. *Toxicol Appl Pharmacol* 135:77–88, 1995.

Goodman AB: Three independent lines of evidence suggest retinoids as causal to schizophrenia. *Proc Natl Acad Sci U S A* 95:7240–7244, 1998.

Gorsuch RL, Key MK: Abnormalities of pregnancy as a function of anxiety and life stress. *Psychosom Med* 36:352–362, 1974.

Graham A, Papoalopulu N, Krumlauf R: The murine and *Drosophila* homeobox gene complexes have common features of organization and expression. *Cell* 57:367–378, 1989.

Gray LE, Ostby J, Ferrell J, *et al.*: A dose–response analysis of methoxychlor-induced alterations of reproductive development and function in the rat. *Fundam Appl Toxicol* 12:92–108, 1989.

Gray LE, Ostby JS, Kelce WR: Developmental effects of an environmental anti-androgen: The fungicide vinclozolin alters sex differentiation of the male rat. *Toxicol Appl Pharmacol* 129:46–52, 1994.

Gray LE, Ostby J, Kelce WR: A dose–response analysis of the reproductive effects of a single gestational dose of 2,3,7,8-tetrachloro-*p*-dioxin (TCDD) in male Long Evans Hooded rat offspring. *Toxicol Appl Pharmacol* 146:11–20, 1997a.

Gray LE, Wold C, Mann P, Ostby JS: In utero exposure to low doses of 2,3,7,8-tetrachloro-p-dioxin (TCDD) alters reproductive development of female Long Evans Hooded rat offspring. *Toxicol Appl Pharmacol* 146:237–244, 1997b.

Gregg NM: Congenital cataract following German measles in the mother. *Trans Ophthalmol Soc Aust* 3:35–40, 1941.

Guenther TM, Mannering GT: Induction of hepatic monooxygenase systems of pregnant rats with phenobarbital and 3-methylcholanthrene. *Biochem Pharmacol* 26:577–584, 1977.

Guo YL, Lin CJ, Yao WJ, Ryan JJ, Hsu CC: Musculoskeletal changes in children prenatally exposed to polychlorinated biphenyls and related compounds (Yu-Cheng children). *J Toxicol Environ Health* 41:83–93, 1994.

Guzelian PS: Comparative toxicology of chlordecone (kepone) in humans and experimental animals. *Annu Rev Pharmacol Toxicol* 22:89–113, 1982.

Guzelian PS, Henry CJ, Olin SS (eds.): *Similarities and Differences Between Children & Adults: Implications for Risk Assessment.* Washington, DC: ILSI Press, 1992.

Hale F: Pigs born without eyeballs. *J Hered* 27:105–106, 1935.

Hales B: Comparison of the mutagenicity of cyclophosphamide and its active metabolites, 4-hydroxycyclophosphamide, phosphoramide mustard and acrolein. *Cancer Res* 42:3018–3021, 1982.

Hales B: Relative mutagenicity and teratogenicity of cyclophosphamide and two of its structural analogs. *Biochem Pharmacol* 32:3791–3795, 1983.

Hales BF: Effects of phosphoramide mustard and acrolein, cytotoxic metabolites of cyclophosphamide, on mouse limb development in vitro. *Teratology* 40:11–20, 1989.

Hansen DK, Billings RE: Phenytoin teratogenicity and effects on embryonic and maternal folate metabolism. *Teratology* 31:363–371, 1985.

Hansen JM, Carney EW, Harris C: Differential alteration by thalidomide of the glutathione content of rat vs rabbit conceptuses in vitro. *Reprod Toxicol* 13:547–554, 1999.

Hansen JM, Harris C: A novel hypothesis for thalidomide-induced limb teratogenesis: Redox misregulation of the NF-kappaB pathway. *Antioxid Redox Signal* 6:1–14, 2004.

Hansen JM, Harris KK, Philbert MA, Harris C: Thalidomide modulates nuclear redox status and preferentially depletes glutathione in rabbit limb versus rat limb. *J Pharmacol Exp Ther* 300:768–776, 2002.

Hansen DK, Hodes ME: Comparative teratogenicity of phenytoin among several inbred strains of mice. *Teratology* 28:175–179, 1983.

Hardin BD, Becker RJ, Kavlock RJ, *et al.*: Overview and summary: Workshop on the Chernoff/Kavlock preliminary developmental toxicity test. *Teratogenesis Carcinog Mutagen* 7:119–127, 1987.

Harrison ML, Nicol CJ, Wells PJ: Tumor supressor genes and chemical teratogenesis: Benzo[a]pyrene embryopathy and cytochromes p-450 activities in p53-deficient transgenic mice. *Toxicologist* 14:246, 1994.

Hartig PC, Hunter ES III: Gene delivery to the neurulating embryo during culture. *Teratology* 58:103–112, 1998.

Hauck R-S, Nau H: The enantiomers of the valproic acid analogue 2-*n*-propylpentyoic acid (4-yn-VPA): Asymmetric synthesis and highly stereoselective teratogenicity in mice. *Pharm Res* 9:850–854, 1992.

Haug K, Irgens LM, Skjaerven R, *et al.*: Maternal smoking and birthweight: Effect modification of period, maternal age and paternal smoking. *Acta Obstet Gynecol Scand* 79:485–489, 2000.

Hays SM, Elswick BA, Blumenthal GM, *et al.*: Development of a physiologically based pharmacokinetic model of 2-methoxyethanol and 2-methoxyacetic acid disposition in pregnant rats. *Toxicol Appl Pharmacol* 163:67–74, 2000.

Heinrichs WL, Gellert RJ, Bakke JL, Lawrence NL: DDT administered to neonatal rats induces persistent estrus syndrome. *Science* 173:642–643, 1971.

Helene C, Toulme JJ: Specific regulation of gene expression by antisense, sense and antigene nucleic acids. *Biochim Biophys Acta* 1049:99–125, 1990.

Helm FC, Frankus E, Friderichs E, *et al.*: Comparative teratological investigation of compounds structurally related to thalidomide. *Arnz Forsch Drug Res* 31:941–949, 1981.

Herbst AL, Bern HA: *Developmental Effects of Diethylstibestrol in Pregnancy.* New York: Thieme-Stratton, 1981.

Herbst AL, Cole P, Colton T, *et al.*: Age-incidence and risk of diethylstilbestrol-related clear cell adenocarcinoma of the vagina and cervix. *Am J Obstet Gynecol* 128:43–50, 1977.

Higuchi TT, Palmer JS, Gray LE Jr, Veeramachaneni DN: Effects of dibutyl phthalate in male rabbits following in utero, adolescent, or postpubertal exposure. *Toxicol Sci* 72:301–13, 2003.

Hirsch KS, Scott WJ Jr: Searching for the mechanism of acetazolamide teratogenesis, in Kalter H (ed.): Vol 1. *Issues and Reviews in Teratology.* New York: Plenum Press, 1983, pp. 309–347.

Holladay SD, Luster MI: Developmental immunotoxicology, in Kimmel CA, Buelke-Sam J (eds.): *Developmental Toxicology*, 2nd ed. New York: Raven Press, 1994, pp. 93–117.

Holson JF, Stump DG, Pearce LB, Watson RE, DeSesso JM: Mode of action: Yolk sac poisoning and impeded histiotrophic nutrition–HBOC-related congenital malformations. *Crit Rev Toxicol* 35:739–745, 2005.

Honein MA, Rasmussen SA, Reefhuis J, Romitti PA, Lammer EJ, Sun L, Correa A: Maternal smoking and environmental tobacco smoke exposure and the risk of orofacial clefts. *Epidemiology* 18:226–233, 2007.

Hsu S-T, Ma C-I, Hsu SK, *et al.*: Discovery and epidemiology of PCB poisoning in Taiwan: A four-year followup. *Environ Health Perspect* 59:5–10, 1985.

Huang WW, Yin Y, Bi Q, *et al.*: Developmental diethylstilbestrol exposure alters genetic pathways of uterine cytodifferentiation. *Mol Endocrinol* 19:669–682, 2005.

Hytten FE: Physiologic changes in the mother related to drug handling, in Krauer B, Hytten F, del Pozo E (eds.): *Drugs and Pregnancy.* New York: Academic Press, 1984, pp. 7–17.

Imperato-McGinley J, Sanchez R, Spencer JR, Yee B, Vaughan ED: Comparison of the effects of the 5α-reductase inhibitor finasteride and the antiandrogen flutamide on prostate and genital differentiation: Dose–response studies. *Endocrinology* 131:1149–1156, 1992.

Irl C, Hasford J: Assessing the safety of drugs in pregnancy: The role of prospective cohort studies. *Drug Saf* 22:169–177, 2000.

Irvine S, Cawood E, Richardson D, *et al.*: Evidence of deteriorating semen quality in the United Kingdom: Birth cohort study in 577 men in Scotland over 11 years. *Br Med J* 312:467–471, 1996.

Jacobson J, Jacobson S: Intellectual impairment in children exposed to polychlorinated biphenyls in utero. *N Engl J Med* 335:783–789, 1996.

Jacobson J, Jacobson S, Humphrey H: Effects of exposure to PCBs and related compounds on growth and activity in children. *Neurotoxicol Teratol* 12:319–326, 1990.

Jelovsek FR, Mattison DR, Chen JJ: Prediction of risk for human developmental toxicity: How important are animal studies for hazard identification? *Obstet Gynecol* 74:624–636, 1989.

Jones KL, Smith DW: Recognition of the fetal alcohol syndrome in early infancy. *Lancet* 2:999–1001, 1973.

Jones KL, Smith DW, Ulleland CN, Streissguth AP: Pattern of malformation in offspring of chronic alcoholic mothers. *Lancet* 1:1267–1271, 1973.

Jonsson NA: Chemical structure and teratogenic properties. *Acta Pharm Sueccia* 9:521–542, 1972.

Joussen AM, Germann T, Kirchhof B: Effect of thalidomide and structurally related compounds on cornela angiogenesis is comparable to their teratological potency. *Graefes Arch Clin Exp Ophthalmol* 237:952–961, 1999.

Juchau MR: Enzymatic bioactivation and inactivation of chemical teratogens and transplacental carcinogens/mutagens, in Juchau MR (ed.): *The Biochemical Basis of Chemical Teratogenesis*. New York: Elsevier/ North Holland, 1981, pp. 63–94.

Juchau MR, Faustman-Watts EM: Pharmacokinetic considerations in the maternal-placental unit. *Clin Obstet Gynecol* 26:379–390, 1983.

Juchau MR, Lee QP, Fantel AG: Xenobiotic biotransformation/bioactivation in organogenesis-stage conceptual tissues: Implications for embryotoxicity and teratogenesis. *Drug Metab Rev* 24:195–238, 1992.

Juriloff DM, Fraser FC: Genetic maternal effects on cleft lip frequency in A/J and CL/Fr mice. *Teratology* 21:167–175, 1980.

Kalter H: The history of the A family of inbred mice and the biology of its congenital malformations. *Teratology* 20:213–232, 1979.

Kavlock RJ: Structure-activity approaches in the screening of environmental agents for developmental toxicity. *Reprod Toxicol* 7:113–116, 1993.

Kavlock RJ, Allen BC, Faustman EM, Kimmel CA: Dose response assessment for developmental toxicity: IV. Benchmark doses for fetal weight changes. *Fundam Appl Toxicol* 26:211–222, 1995.

Kavlock RJ, Chernoff N, Rogers EH: The effect of acute maternal toxicity on fetal development in the mouse. *Teratog Carcinog Mutagen* 5:3–13, 1985.

Kavlock R, Cummings A: Mode of action: Inhibition of androgen receptor function–vinclozolin-induced malformations in reproductive development. *Crit Rev Toxicol* 35:721–726, 2005.

Kavlock RJ, Daston GP, DeRosa D, *et al.*: Research needs for the risk assessment of health and environmental effects of endocrine disruptors: A report of the US EPA-sponsored workshop. *Environ Health Perspect* 104(Suppl 4):715–740, 1996.

Kavlock RJ, Greene JA, Kimmel GL, *et al.*: Activity profiles of developmental toxicity: Design considerations and pilot implementation. *Teratology* 43:159–185, 1991.

Keen CL, Bendich A, Willhite CC (eds.): Maternal nutrition and pregnancy outcome. *Ann NY Acad Sci* 678:1–372, 1993.

Keen CL, Peters JM, Hurley LS: The effect of valproic acid on ^{65}Zn distribution in the pregnant rat. *J Nutr* 119:607–611, 1989.

Kelce WR, Stone CR, Laws SC, *et al.*: Persistent DDT metabolite p,p'-DDE is a potent androgen receptor antagonist. *Nature* 375:581–585, 1995.

Kelsey FO: Thalidomide update: Regulatory aspects. *Teratology* 38:221–226, 1988.

Kessel M, Balling R, Gruss P: Variations of cervical vertebrae after expression of a Hox-1.1 transgene in mice. *Cell* 61:301–308, 1990.

Khera KS: Maternal toxicity—A possible factor in fetal malformations in mice. *Teratology* 29:411–416, 1984.

Khera KS: Maternal toxicity: A possible etiological factor in embryo/fetal deaths and fetal malformations of rodent-rabbit species. *Teratology* 31:129–153, 1985.

Khoury MJ, Erickson JD, James LM: Maternal factors in cleft lip with or without palate: Evidence from interracial crosses in the United States. *Teratology* 27:351–357, 1983.

Khoury MJ, Holtzman NA: On the ability of birth defects monitoring systems to detect new teratogens. *Am J Epidemiol* 126:136–143, 1987.

Khoury MJ, James LM, Lynberg MC: Quantitative analysis of associations between birth defects and suspected human teratogens. *Am J Med Genet* 40:500–505, 1991.

Kimmel CA, Collman GW, Fields N, Eskenazi B: Lessons learned for the National Children's Study from the National Institute of Environmental Health Sciences/U.S. Environmental Protection Agency Centers for Children's Environmental Health and Disease Prevention Research. *Environ Health Perspect* 113:1414–1418, 2005.

Kimmel CA, Cook RO, Staples RE: Teratogenic potential of noise in rats and mice. *Toxicol Appl Pharmacol* 36:239–245, 1976.

Kimmel CA, Young JF: Correlating pharmacokinetics and teratogenic endpoints. *Fundam Appl Toxicol* 3:250–255, 1983.

Klaassen CD, Lehman-McKeeman LD: Induction of metallothionein. *J Am Coll Toxicol* 8:1315–1321, 1989.

Kochhar DM: Teratogenic activity of retinoic acid. *Acta Pathol Microbiol Scand* 70:398–404, 1967.

Koopman-Esseboom C, Weisglas-Kuperus N, de Ridder MAJ, *et al.*: Effects of polychlorinated biphenyl/dioxin exposure and feeding type on infant's mental and psychomotor development. *Pediatrics* 97:700–706, 1996.

Koren G, Nulman I, Chudley AE, Loocke C: Fetal alcohol spectrum disorder. *CMAJ* 169:1181–1185, 2003.

Kotch LE, Sulik KK: Experimental fetal alcohol syndrome: Proposed pathogenic basis for a variety of associated facial and brain anomalies. *Am J Med Genet* 44:168–176, 1992.

Krauer B: Physiological changes and drug disposition during pregnancy, in Nau H, Scott WJ (eds.): *Pharmacokinetics in Teratogenesis* Vol 1. Boca Raton, FL: CRC Press, 1987, pp. 3–12.

Krumlauf R: *Hox* genes and pattern formation in the branchial region of the vertebrate head. *Trends Genet* 9:106–112, 1993.

Lammer EJ: Retinoids: Interspecies comparisons and clinical results, in Sundwall A, Danielsson BR, Hagberg O, *et al.* (eds.): *Developmental Toxicology—Preclinical and Clinical Data in Retrospect*. Stockholm: Tryckgruppen, 1992, pp. 105–109.

Lammer EJ, Chen DT, Hoar RM, *et al.*: Retinoic acid induced embryopathy. *N Engl J Med* 313:837–841, 1985.

Lammer EJ, Sever LE, Oakley GP Jr: Teratogen update: Valproic acid. *Teratology* 35:465–473, 1987.

Lammer EJ, Shaw GM, Iovannisci DM, Finnell RH: Maternal smoking, genetic variation of glutathione s-transferases, and risk for orofacial clefts. *Epidemiology* 16:698–701, 2005.

Lary JM, Daniel KL, Erickson JD, *et al.*: The return of thalidomide: Can birth defects be prevented? *Drug Saf* 21:161–169, 1999.

Latham KE: Epigenetic modification and imprinting of the mammalian genome during development. *Curr Top Dev Biol* 43:1–49, 1999.

Lau C, Kavlock RJ: Functional toxicity in the developing heart, lung and kidney, in Kimmel CA, Buelke-Sam J (eds.): *Developmental Toxicology*, 2nd ed. New York: Raven Press, 1994, pp. 119–188.

Lau C, Mole ML, Copeland MF, *et al.*: Toward a biologically based dose-response model for developmental toxicity of 5-fluorouracil in the rat: Acquisition of experimental data. *Toxicol Sci* 59:37–48, 2001.

Lau C, Rogers JM: Embryonic and fetal programming of physiological disorders in adulthood. *Birth Defects Res C Embryo Today* 72:300–312, 2004.

Lau C, Setzer RW: Biologically based risk assessment models for developmental toxicity, in Tuan RS, Lo CW (eds.): *Developmental Biology Protocols*. Vol II. Totowa, NJ: Humana Press, 2000, pp. 271–281.

Lavin M, Watters D (eds.): *Programmed Cell Death: The Cellular and Molecular Biology of Apoptosis.* Chur, Switzerland: Harwood Academic Publishers, 1993.

Lenz W: Kindliche Missbildungen nach Medikament-Einnahme während der Gravidität? *Dtsch Med Wochenschr* 86:2555–2556, 1961.

Lenz W: Das thalidomid-syndrom. *Fortschr Med* 81:148–153, 1963.

Lenz W: A short history of thalidomide embryopathy. *Teratology* 38:203–215, 1988.

Lenz W, Knapp K: Die thalidomide-embryopathie. *Dtsch Med Wochenschr* 87:1232–1242, 1962.

Leroux BG, Leisenring WM, Moolgavkar SH, Faustman EM: A biologically-based dose–response model for developmental toxicology. *Risk Anal* 16:449–458, 1996.:

Levin AA, Miller RK: Fetal toxicity of cadmium in the rat: Maternal vs. fetal injections. *Teratology* 22:1–5, 1980.

Little RE: Moderate alcohol use during pregnancy and decreased infant birth weight. *Am J Public Health* 67:1154–1156, 1977.

Little SA, Kim WK, Mirkes PE: Teratogen-induced activation of caspase-6 and caspase-7 in early postimplantation mouse embryos. *Cell Biol Toxicol* 19:215–226, 2003.

Little SA, Mirkes PE: Relationship of DNA damage and embryotoxicity induced by 4-hydroperoxydichlorocyclophosphamide in postimplantation rat embryos. *Teratology* 41:223–231, 1990.

Little SA, Mirkes PE: Effects of 4-hydroperoxycyclophosphamide (4-OOH-CP) and 4-hydroperoxydichlorocyclophosphamide (4-OOH-deClCP) on the cell cycle of postimplantation rat embryos. *Teratology* 45:163–173, 1992.

Lohnes D, Mark M, Mendelsohn C, *et al.*: Function of the retinoic acid receptors (RARs) during development: I. Craniofacial and skeletal abnormalities in RAR double mutants. *Development* 120:2723–2748, 1994.

Lopuhaa CE, Roseboom TJ, Osmond C, *et al.*: Atopy, lung function, and obstructive airways disease after prenatal exposure to famine. *Thorax* 55:555–561, 2000.

Love DR, Pichler FB, Dodd A, Copp BR, Greenwood DR: Technology for high-throughput screens: The present and future using zebrafish. *Curr Opin Biotechnol* 15:564–571, 2004.

Luecke RH, Wosilait WD, Pearce BA, Young JF: A physiologically based pharmacokinetic computer model for human pregnancy. *Teratology* 49:90–103, 1994.

Luecke RH, Wosilait WD, Young JF: Mathematical analysis for teratogenic sensitivity. *Teratology* 55:373–380, 1997.

Lutiger B, Graham K, Einarson TR, Koren G: Relationship between gestational cocaine use and pregnancy outcome: A meta-analysis. *Teratology* 44:405–414, 1991.

Lynch DW, Schuler RL, Hood RD, Davis DG: Evaluation of *Drosophila* for screening developmental toxicants: Test results with eighteen chemicals and presentation of new *Drosophila* bioassay. *Teratogenesis Carcinog Mutagen* 11:147–173, 1991.

Mably TA, Bjerke DL, Moore RW, *et al.*: In utero and lactational exposure of male rats to 2,3,7,8-tetrachlorodibenzo-p-dioxin. 3. Effects on spermatogenesis and reproductive capability. *Toxicol Appl Pharmacol* 114:118–126, 1992.

MacAuley AM, Werb Z, Mirkes PE: Characterization of the unusually rapid cell cycles during rat gastrulation. *Development* 117:873–883, 1993.

MacDonald H, Tobin JOH: Congenital cytomegalovirus infection: A collaborative study on epidemiological, clinical and laboratory findings. *Dev Med Child Neurol* 20:271–282, 1978.

Manson JM: Testing of pharmaceutical agents for reproductive toxicity, in Kimmel CA, Buelke-Sam J (eds.): *Developmental Toxicology,* 2nd ed. New York: Raven Press, 1994, pp. 379–402.

Mark M, Ghyselinck NB, Chambon P: Function of retinoid nuclear receptors: Lessons from genetic and pharmacological dissections of the retinoic acid signaling pathway during mouse embryogenesis. *Annu Rev Pharmacol Toxicol* 46:451–480, 2006.

Markert CL, Petters RM: Manufactured hexaparental mice show that adults are derived from three embryonic cells. *Science* 202:56–58, 1978.

Markussen Linnet K, Obel C, Bonde E, *et al.*: Cigarette smoking during pregnancy and hyperactive-distractible preschoolers: A follow-up study. *Acta Paediatr* 95:694–700, 2006.

Marshall H, Morrison A, Studer M, *et al.*: Retinoids and hox genes. *FASEB J* 10:969–978, 1996.

Marshall H, Nonchev S, Sham MH, *et al.*: Retinoic acid alters hindbrain Hox code and induces transformation of rhombomeres 2/3 into a 4/5 identity. *Nature* 360:737–741, 1992.

Mattison DR, Blann E, Malek A: Physiological alterations during pregnancy: Impact on toxicokinetics. *Fundam Appl Toxicol* 16:215–218, 1991.

McBride WG: Thalidomide and congenital anomalies. *Lancet* 2:1358, 1961.

McMillen IC, Robinson JS: Developmental origins of the metabolic syndrome: Prediction, plasticity, and programming. *Physiol Rev* 85:571–633, 2005.

Medlock KL, Branham WS, Sheehan DM: Effects of coumestrol and equol on the developing reproductive tract of the rat. *Proc Soc Exp Biol Med* 208:67–71, 1995.

Mendelsohn C, Lohnes D, Décimo D, *et al.*: Function of the retinoic acid receptors (RARs) during development: II. Multiple abnormalities at various stages of organogenesis in RAR double mutants. *Development* 120:2749–2771, 1994.

Mikkola HK, Orkin SH: Gene targeting and transgenic strategies for the analysis of hematopoietic development in the mouse. *Methods Mol Med* 105:3–22, 2005.

Miller MT, Stromland K: Teratogen update: Thalidomide: A review with a focus on ocular findings and new potential uses. *Teratology* 60:306–321, 1999.

Millicovsky G, DeSesso JM: Cardiovascular alterations in rabbit embryos in situ after a teratogenic dose of hydroxyurea: An in vivo microscopic study. *Teratology* 22:115–124, 1980.

Millicovsky G, DeSesso JM: Differential embryonic cardiovascular responses to acute maternal uterine ischemia: An in vivo microscopic study of rabbit embryos with either intact or clamped umbilical cords. *Teratology* 22:335–343, 1980.

Millicovsky G, DeSesso JM, Kleinman LI, Clark KE: Effects of hydroxyurea on hemodynamics of pregnant rabbits: A maternally mediated mechanism of embryotoxicity. *Am J Obstet Gynecol* 140:747–752, 1981.

Millicovsky G, Johnston MC: Maternal hyperoxia greatly reduces the incidence of phenytoin-induced cleft lip and palate in A/J mice. *Science* 212:671–672, 1981.

Mills JL, Signore C: Neural tube defect rates before and after food fortification with folic acid. *Birth Defects Res A Clin Mol Teratol* 70:844–845, 2004.

Milunsky A, Ulcickas M, Rothman KJ, *et al.*: Maternal heat exposure and neural tube defects. *JAMA* 268:882–885, 1992.

Mirkes PE: Cyclophosphamide teratogenesis: A review. *Teratog Carcinog Mutagen* 5:75–88, 1985b.

Mirkes PE: Simultaneous banding of rat embryo DNA, RNA and protein in cesium trifluoroacetate gradients. *Anal Biochem* 148:376–383, 1985a.

Mirkes PE: Molecular and metabolic aspects of cyclophosphamide teratogenesis, in Welsch F (ed.): *Approaches to Elucidate Mechanisms in Teratogenesis.* Washington, DC: Hemisphere, 1987, pp. 123–147.

Mirkes PE, Fantel AG, Greenaway JC, Shepard TH: Teratogenicity of cyclophosphamide metabolites: Phosphoramide mustard, acrolein, and 4-ketocyclophosphamide on rat embryos cultured in vitro. *Toxicol Appl Pharmacol* 58:322–330, 1981.

Mirkes PE, Greenaway JC, Hilton J, Brundrett R: Morphological and biochemical aspects of monofunctional phosphoramide mustard teratogenicity in rat embryos cultured in vitro. *Teratology* 32:241–249, 1985a.

Mirkes PE, Little SA: Teratogen-induced cell death in postimplantation mouse embryos: Differential tissue sensitivity and hallmarks of apoptosis. *Cell Death Differ* 5:592–600, 1998.

Mirkes PE, Little SA: Cytochrome c release from mitochondria of early postimplantation murine embryos exposed to 4-hydroperoxycyclophosphamide, heat shock, and staurosporine. *Toxicol Appl Pharmacol* 62:197–206, 2000.

Mirkes PE, Ricks JL, Pascoe-Mason JM: Cell cycle analysis in the cardiac and neuroepithelial tissues of day 10 rat embryos and the effects of phosphoramide mustard, the major teratogenic metabolite of cyclophosphamide. *Teratology* 39:115–120, 1989.

Mitchell EA, Milerad J: Smoking and the sudden infant death syndrome. *Rev Environ Health* 21:81–103, 2006.

Mitra SC: Effects of cocaine on fetal kidney and bladder function. *J Matern Fetal Med* 8:262–269, 1999.

Moore NW, Adams CE, Rowson LEA: Developmental potential of single blastomeres of the rabbit egg. *J Reprod Fertil* 17:527–531, 1968.

MRC Vitamin Study Research Group [prepared by Wald N with assistance from Sneddon J, Frost C, Stone R]: Prevention of neural tube defects: Results of the MRC vitamin study. *Lancet* 338:132–137, 1991.

Murphy SK, Jirtle RL: Imprinted genes as potential genetic and epigenetic toxicologic targets. *Environ Health Perspect* 108(Suppl 1):5–11, 2000.

Mylchreest E, Cattley RC, Foster PM: Male reproductive tract malformations in rats following gestational and lactational exposure to di(n-butyl)phthalate: An anti-androgenic mechanism? *Toxicol Sci* 43:67–60, 1998.

Mylchreest E, Sar M, Cattley RC, Foster PM: Disruption of androgen-regulated male reproductive development by di(*n*-butyl)phthalate during late gestation in rats is different from flutamide. *Toxicol Appl Pharmacol* 156:81–95, 1999.

Naciff JM, Hess KA, Overmann GJ, *et al.*: Gene expression changes induced in the testis by transplacental exposure to high and low doses of 17{alpha}-ethynyl estradio, genistein, or bisphenol A. *Toxicol Sci* 86:396–416, 2005.

Nagel SC, vom Saal FS, Thayer KA, *et al.*: Relative binding affinity–serum modified access (RBA–SMA) assay predicts the relative in vivo bioactivity of the xenoestrogens bisphenol A and octylphenol. *Environ Health Perspect* 105:70–76, 1997.

National Research Council: *Pesticides in the Diets of Infants and Children.* Washington, DC: National Academy Press, 1993.

National Research Council: *Hormonally Active Agents in the Environment.* Washington, DC: National Academy Press, 1999.

National Research Council: *Scientific Fromtiers in Developmental Toxicology and Risk Assessment.* Washington, DC: National Academy Press, 2000.

Nau H: Species differences in pharmacokinetics and drug teratogenesis. *Environ Health Perspect* 70:113–129, 1986.

Nau H: Physicochemical and structural properties regulating placenta drug transfer, in Polin RA, Fox WW (eds.): *Fetal and Neonatal Physiology.* Vol 1. Philadelphia: WB Saunders, 1992, pp. 130–149.

Nau H, Chahoud I, Dencker L, *et al.*: Teratogenicity of vitamin A and retinoids, in Blomhoff R (ed.): *Vitamin A in Health and Disease.* New York: Marcel Dekker, 1994, pp. 615–664.

Nau H, Hauck R-S, Ehlers K: Valproic acid induced neural tube defects in mouse and human: Aspects of chirality, alternative drug development, pharmacokinetics and possible mechanisms. *Pharmacol Toxicol* 69:310–321, 1991.

Nau H, Scott WJ: Weak acids may act as teratogens by accumulating in the basic milieu of the early mammalian embryo. *Nature* 323:276–278, 1986.

Nau H, Scott WJ: *Pharmacokinetics in Teratogenesis.* Vols I and II. Boca Raton, FL: CRC Press, 1987.

Nawrot PS, Cook RO, Hamm CW: Embryotoxicity of broadband high-frequency noise in the CD-1 mouse. *J Toxicol Environ Health* 8:151–157, 1981.

Nawrot PS, Cook RO, Staples RE: Embryotoxicity of various noise stimuli in the mouse. *Teratology* 22:279–289, 1980.

Needham LL, Ozkaynak H, Whyatt RM, *et al.*: Exposure assessment in the National Children's Study: Introduction. *Environ Health Perspect* 113:1076–1082, 2005.

Neims AH, Warner M, Loughnan PM, Aranda JV: Developmental aspects of the hepatic cytochrome P_{450} monooxygenase system. *Annu Rev Pharmacol Toxicol* 16:427–444, 1976.

Nelson CJ, Holson JF: Statistical analysis of teratologic data: Problems and recent advances. *J Environ Pathol Toxicol* 2:187–199, 1978.

Neubert D: In-vitro techniques for assessing teratogenic potential, in Dayan AD, Paine AJ (eds.): *Advances in Applied Toxicology.* London: Taylor and Francis, 1989, pp. 191–211.

Neubert R, Neubert D: Peculiarities and possible mode of actions of thalidomide, in Kavlock RJ, Daston GP (eds.): *Drug Toxicity in Embryonic Development, II.* Berlin/Heidelberg: Springer-Verlag, 1997, pp. 41–119.

Neubert R, Hinz N, Thiel R, Neubert D: Down-regulation of adhesion receptors on cells of primate embryos as a probable mechanism of the teratogenic action of thalidomide. *Life Sci* 58:295–316, 1996.

Neubert D, Zens P, Rothenwallner A, Merker H-J: A survey of the embryotoxic effects of TCDD in mammalian species. *Environ Health Perspect* 5:63–79, 1973.

New DAT: Whole embryo culture and the study of mammalian embryos during organogenesis. *Biol Rev* 5:81–94, 1978.

Newbold RR: Cellular and molecular effects of developmental exposure to diethylstilbestrol: Implications for other environmental estrogens. *Environ Health Perspect* 103(Suppl 7):83–87, 1995.

Newbold RR, Padilla-Banks E, Jefferson WN: Adverse effects of the model environmental estrogen diethylstilbestrol are transmitted to subsequent generations. *Endocrinology* 147:S11–S17, 2006.

Newman CGH: Teratogen update: Clinical aspects of thalidomide embryopathy—A continuing preoccupation. *Teratology* 32:133–144, 1985.

Newman LM, Johnson EM, Staples RE: Assessment of the effectiveness of animal developmental toxicity testing for human safety. *Reprod Toxicol* 7:359–390, 1993.

Nugent P, Sucov HM, Pisano MM, Greene RM: The role of RXR-alpha in retinoic acid–induced cleft palate as assessed with the RXR-alpha knockout mouse. *Int J Dev Biol* 43:567–570, 1999.

O'Flaherty EJ: Pharmacokinetics, pharmacodynamics, and prediction of developmental abnormalities. *Reprod Toxicol* 11:413–416, 1997.

O'Flaherty EJ, Scott WJ, Shreiner C, Beliles RP: A physiologically based kinetic model of rat and mouse gestation: Disposition of a weak acid. *Toxicol Appl Pharmacol* 112:245–256, 1992.

Okada A, Aoki Y, Kushima K, Kurihara H, Bialer M, Fujiwara M: Polycomb homologs are involved in teratogenicity of valproic acid in mice. *Birth Defects Res A Clin Mol Teratol* 70:870–879, 2004.

Okada A, Kushima K, Aoki Y, Bialer M, Fujiwara M: Identification of early-responsive genes correlated to valproic acid-induced neural tube defects in mice. *Birth Defects Res A Clin Mol Teratol* 73:229–238, 2005.

Olsen GW, Bodner KM, Ramlow JM, Ross CE, Lipshultz LI: Have sperm counts been reduced 50 percent in 50 years? A statistical model revisited. *Fertil Steril* 63:887–893, 1995.

Olshan A, Mattison D (eds.): *Male-Mediated Developmental Toxicity.* New York: Plenum Press, 1995.

Oltvai ZN, Korsmeyer SJ: Checkpoints of dueling dimers foil death wishes. *Cell* 79:189–192, 1994.

Ornoy A: Neuroteratogens in man: An overview with special emphasis on the teratogenicity of antiepileptic drugs in pregnancy. *Reprod Toxicol* 22:214–26 [Epub], 2006.

Osmond C, Barker DJ: Fetal, infant, and childhood growth are predictors of coronary heart disease, diabetes, and hypertension in adult men and women. *Environ Health Perspect* 108(Suppl 3):545–553, 2000.

Ostrea EM Jr, Matias O, Keane C, *et al.*: Spectrum of gestational exposure to illicit drugs and other xenobiotic agents in newborn infants meconium analysis. *J Pediatr* 133:513–515, 1998.

Page K, Abramovich D, Aggett P *et al.*: Uptake of zinc by the human placenta microvillus border membranes and characterization of the effects of cadmium on the process. *Placenta* 13:151–162, 1992.

Palermo AM, Reynoso AS, Lopez Nigro M, Carballo MA, Mudry MD: Teratogenic evaluation of metronidazole and ornidazole using Drosophila melanogaster as an experimental model. *Birth Defects Res A Clin Mol Teratol* 70:157–162, 2004.

Parizek J: Vascular changes at sites of estrogen biosynthesis produced by parenteral injection of cadmium salts: The destruction of the placenta by cadmium salts. *J Reprod Fertil* 7:263–265, 1964.

Parman T, Wiley MJ, Wells PG: Free radical-mediated oxidative DNA damage in the mechanism of thalidomide teratogenicity. *Nat Med* 5:582–585, 1999.

Paulozzi LJ: International trends in rates of hypospadias and cryptorchidism. *Environ Health Perspect* 107:297–302, 1999.

Paulozzi LJ, Erickson JD, Jackson RJ: Hypospadias trends in two American surveillance systems. *Pediatrics* 100:831–834, 1997.

Piersma AH, Genschow E, Verhoef A, et al.: Validation of the postimplantation rat whole-embryo culture test in the international ECVAM validation study on three in vitro embryotoxicity tests. *Altern Lab Anim* 32:275–307, 2004.

Pinkerton KE, Joad JP: The mammalian respiratory system and critical windows of exposure for children's health. *Environ Health Perspect* 108(Suppl 3):457–462, 2000.

Pole M, Einarson A, Pairaudeau N, et al.: Drug labeling and risk perceptions of teratogenicity: A survey of pregnant Canadian women and their health professionals. *J Clin Pharmacol* 40:573–577, 2000.

Poskanzer D, Herbst AL: Epidemiology of vaginal adenosis and adenocarcinoma associated with exposure to stilbestrol in utero. *Cancer* 39:1892–1895, 1977.

Potter SM, Zelazo PR, Stack DM, Papageorgiou AN: Adverse effects of fetal cocaine exposure on neonatal auditory information processing. *Pediatrics* 105:E40, 2000.

Quan A: Fetopathy associated with exposure to angiotensin converting enzyme inhibitors and angiotensin receptor antagonists. *Early Hum Dev* 82:23–8, 2006.

Ravelli AC, van Der Meulen JH, Osmond C, et al.: Obesity at the age of 50 y in men and women exposed to famine prenatally. *Am J Clin Nutr* 70:811–816, 1999.

Renault J-Y, Melcion C, Cordier A: Limb bud cell culture for in vitro teratogen screening: Validation of an improved assessment method using 51 compounds. *Teratog Carcinog Mutagen* 9:83–96, 1989.

Reuter U, Heinrich-Hirsch B, Hellwig J, Holzum B, Welsch F: Evaluation of OECD screening tests 421 (reproduction/developmental toxicity screening test) and 422 (combined repeated dose toxicity study with the reproduction/developmental toxicity screening test). *Regul Toxicol Pharmacol* 38:17–26, 2003.

Rich-Edwards JW, Colditz GA, Stampfer MJ, et al.: Birthweight and the risk of type 2 diabetes in adult women. *Ann Intern Med* 130:278–284, 1999.

Robertson J, Polifka JE, Avner M, et al.: A survey of pregnant women using isotretinoin. *Birth Defects Res A Clin Mol Teratol* 73:881–887, 2005.

Rodier PM, Cohen IR, Buelke-Sam J: Developmental neurotoxicology: Neuroendocrine manifestations of CNS insult, in Kimmel CA, Buelke-Sam J (eds.): *Developmental Toxicology,* 2nd ed. New York: Raven Press, 1994, pp. 65–92.

Rogan WJ, Gladen BC: PCBs, DDE and child development at 18 and 24 months. *Am J Epidemiol* 1:407–413, 1991.

Rogers JM, Chernoff N, Keen CL, Daston GP: Evaluation and interpretation of maternal toxicity in Segment II studies: Issues, some answers, and data needs. *Toxicol Appl Pharmacol* 207:367–374, 2005.

Rogers JM, Daston GP: Alcohols: Ethanol and methanol, in Kavlock RJ, Daston GP (eds.): *Drug Toxicity in Embryonic Development II.* Berlin/Heidelberg: Springer-Verlag, 1997, pp. 333–405.

Rogers JM, Mole ML: Critical periods of sensitivity to the developmental toxicity of inhaled methanol in the CD-1 mouse. *Teratology* 55:364–372, 1997.

Rosa FW: Teratogenicity of isotretinoin. *Lancet* 2:513, 1983.

Rutledge JC, Shourbaji AG, Hughes LA, et al.: Limb and lower-body duplications induced by retinoic acid in mice. *Proc Natl Acad Sci U S A* 91:5436–5440, 1994.

Sadler TW, Hunter ES: Principles of abnormal development: Past, present and future, in Kimmel CA, Buelke-Sam J (eds.): *Developmental Toxicology,* 2nd ed. New York: Raven Press, 1994, pp. 53–63.

Sadler TW, Warner CW: Use of whole embryo culture for evaluating toxicity and teratogenicity. *Pharmacol Rev* 36:145S–150S, 1984.

Sanes JR, Rubenstein LR, Nicolas JF: Use of a recombinant retrovirus to study postimplantation cell lineage in mouse embryos. *EMBO J* 5:3133–3142, 1986.

Sannerstedt R, Lundborg P, Danielsson BR, et al.: Drugs during pregnancy: An issue of risk classification and information to prescribers. *Drug Saf* 14:69–77, 1996.

Sanyal MK, Kitchin KT, Dixon RL: Anomalous development of rat embryos cultured in vitro with cyclophosphamide and microsomes. *Pharmacologist* 21:A231, 1979.

Sauer H, Gunther J, Hescheler J, Wartenberg M: Thalidomide inhibits angiogenesis in embryoid bodies by the generation of hydroxyl radicals. *Am J Pathol* 56:151–158, 2000.

Scanlon JW: The neuroteratology of cocaine: Background, theory, and clinical implications. *Reprod Toxicol* 5:89–98, 1991.

Schaefer C: Angiotensin II-receptor-antagonists: Further evidence of fetotoxicity but not teratogenicity. *Birth Defects Res A Clin Mol Teratol* 67:591–594, 2003.

Schantz SL, Levin ED, Bowman RE: Long-term neurobehavioral effects of perinatal PCB exposure in monkeys. *J Environ Toxicol Chem* 10:747–756, 1991.

Schantz SL, Moshtaghian J, Ness DK: Spatial learning deficits in adult rats exposed to ortho-substituted PCB congeners during gestation and lactation. *Fundam Appl Toxicol* 26:117–126, 1995.

Schardein JL: *Chemically Induced Birth Defects,* 2d ed. New York: Marcel Dekker, 1993.

Schardein JL: *Chemically Induced Birth Defects,* 3d ed. New York: Marcel Dekker, 2000.

Schardein JL, Keller KA: Potential human developmental toxicants and the role of animal testing in their identification and characterization. *CRC Crit Rev Toxicol* 19:251–339, 1989.

Schardein JL, Macina OT: *Human Developmental Toxicants: Aspects of Toxicology and Chemistry.* Boca Raton, FL: CRC Press, Taylor and Francis Group, 2007, p. 427.

Schecter A, Ryan JJ, Masuda Y, et al.: Chlorinated and brominated dioxins and dibenzofurans in human tissue following exposure. *Environ Health Perspect* 102(Suppl 1):135–147, 1994.

Scholz G, Pohl I, Genschow E, et al.: Embryotoxicity screening using embryonic stem cells in vitro: Correlation to in vivo teratogenicity. *Cells Tissues Organs* 165:203–211, 1999.

Schumacher HJ: Chemical structure and teratogenic properties, in Shepard T, Miller R, Marois M (eds.): *Methods for Detection of Environmental Agents That Produce Congenital Defects.* New York: American Elsevier, 1975, pp. 65–77.

Schwab C, Jagannath S: The role of thalidomide in multiple myeloma. *Clin Lymphoma Myeloma* 7:26–9, 2006.

Seiler A, Visan A, Buesen R, Genschow E, Spielmann H: Improvement of an in vitro stem cell assay for developmental toxicity: The use of molecular endpoints in the embryonic stem cell test. *Reprod Toxicol* 18:231–240, 2004.

Seller MJ, Perkins KJ, Adinolfi M: Differential response of heterozygous curly-tail mouse embryos to vitamin A teratogenesis depending on maternal genotype. *Teratology* 28:123, 1983.

Setzer RW, Lau C, Mole ML, Copeland MF, Rogers JM, Kavlock RJ: Toward a biologically based dose-response model for developmental toxicity of 5-fluorouracil in the rat: A mathematical construct. *Toxicol Sci* 59:49–58, 2001.

Sever JL: Rubella as a teratogen. *Adv Teratol* 2:127–138, 1967.

Shenefelt RE: Morphogenesis of malformations in hamsters caused by retinoic acid: Relation to dose and stage of treatment. *Teratology* 5:103–118, 1972.

Shepard TH: *Catalog of Teratogenic Agents,* 9th ed. Baltimore: The Johns Hopkins University Press, 1998.

Shepard TH: *Catalog of Teratogenic Agents,* 7th ed. Baltimore: The Johns Hopkins University Press, 1992.

Shuey DL, Lau C, Logsdon TR, *et al.*: Biologically based dose–response modeling in developmental toxicology: Biochemical and cellular sequelae of 5-fluorouracil exposure in the developing rat. *Toxicol Appl Pharmacol* 126:129–144, 1994.

Skakkebaek NE, Keiding N: Changes in semen and the testis. *Br Med J* 309:1316–1317, 1994.

Slikker W, Miller RK: Placental metabolism and transfer: Role in developmental toxicology, in Kimmel CA, Buelke-Sam J (eds.): *Developmental Toxicology*, 2nd ed. New York: Raven Press, 1994, pp. 245–283.

Slikker W Jr, Xu ZA, Levin ED, Slotkin TA: Mode of action: disruption of brain cell replication, second messenger, and neurotransmitter systems during development leading to cognitive dysfunction–developmental neurotoxicity of nicotine. *Crit Rev Toxicol* 35:703–711, 2005.

Slotkin TA: Fetal nicotine or cocaine exposure: Which one is worse? *J Pharmacol Exp Ther* 285:931–945, 1998.

Smith JL, Gesteland KM, Schoenwolf GC: Prospective fate map of the mouse primitive streak at 7.5 days of gestation. *Dev Dynam* 201:279–289, 1994.

Snow MHL, Tam PPL: Is compensatory growth a complicating factor in mouse teratology? *Nature* 279:555–557, 1979.

Sokol RJ, Delaney-Black V, Nordstrom B: Fetal alcohol spectrum disorder. *JAMA* 290:2996–2999, 2003.

Sorrell TL, Graziano JH: Effect of oral cadmium exposure during pregnancy on maternal and fetal zinc metabolism in the rat. *Toxicol Appl Pharmacol* 102:537–545, 1990.

Spielmann H, Genschow E, Brown NA, *et al.*: Validation of the rat limb bud micromass test in the international ECVAM validation study on three in vitro embryotoxicity tests. *Altern Lab Anim* 32:245–74, 2004.

Stephens TD: Proposed mechanisms of action in thalidomide embryopathy. *Teratology* 38:229–239, 1988.

Stephens TD, Bunde CJW, Torres RD, *et al.*: Thalidomide inhibits limb development through its antagonism of IFG-I+FGF-2+heparin (abstr). *Teratology* 57:112, 1998.

Stephens TD, Fillmore BJ: Hypothesis: thalidomide embryopathy: Proposed mechanism of action. *Teratology* 61:189–195, 2000.

Stirling DI, Sherman M, Strauss S: Thalidomide: A surprising recovery. *J Am Pharmacol Assoc* NS37:307–313, 1997.

Stockard CR: Developmental rate and structural expression: An experimental study of twins, "double monsters," and single deformities, and the interaction among embryonic organs during their origin and development. *Am J Anat* 28:115–277, 1921.

Stocker CJ, Arch JR, Cawthorne MA: Fetal origins of insulin resistance and obesity. *Proc Nutr Soc* 64:143–151, 2005.

Stott DH: Follow-up study from birth of the effects of prenatal stress. *Dev Med Child Neurol* 15:770–787, 1973.

Streissguth AP, Aase JM, Clarren SK, *et al.*: Fetal alcohol syndrome in adolescents and adults. *JAMA* 265:1961–1967, 1991a.

Streissguth AP, Barr HM, Olson HC, *et al.*: Drinking during pregnancy decreases word attack and arithmetic scores on standardized tests: Adolescent data from a population-based prospective study. *Alcohol Clin Exp Res* 18:248–254, 1994a.

Streissguth AP, Randels SP, Smith DF: A test-retest study of intelligence in patients with fetal alcohol syndrome: Implications for care. *J Am Acad Child Adolesc Psychiatry* 30:584–587, 1991b.

Streissguth AP, Sampson PD, Olson HC, *et al.*: Maternal drinking during pregnancy: Attention and short-term memory in 14-year-old offspring: A longitudinal prospective study. *Alcohol Clin Exp Res* 18:202–218, 1994b.

Sulik KK: Genesis of alcohol-induced craniofacial dysmorphism. *Exp Biol Med* 230:366–375, 2005.

Sulik KK, Cook CS, Webster WS: Teratogens and craniofacial malformations: Relationships to cell death. *Development* 103(Suppl):213–231, 1988.

Sulik KK, Johnston MC: Sequence of developmental alterations following acute ethanol exposure in mice: Craniofacial features of the fetal alcohol syndrome. *Am J Anat* 166:257–269, 1983.

Sulik KK, Johnston MC, Webb MA: Fetal alcohol syndrome: Embryogenesis in a mouse model. *Science* 214:936–938, 1981.

Swann SH, Elkin EP, Fenster L: Have sperm counts declined? A reanalysis of global trend data. *Environ Health Perspect* 105:1228–1232, 1997.

Tabacova S: Mode of action: Angiotensin-converting enzyme inhibition–developmental effects associated with exposure to ACE inhibitors. *Crit Rev Toxicol* 35:747–755, 2005.

Takeuchi IK: Teratogenic effects of methylnitrosourea on pregnant mice before implantation. *Experientia* 40:879–881, 1984.

Tatum WO: Use of antiepileptic drugs in pregnancy. *Expert Rev Neurother* 6:1077–1086, 2006.

Taubeneck MW, Daston GP, Rogers JM, Keen CL: Altered maternal zinc metabolism following exposure to diverse developmental toxicants. *Reprod Toxicol* 8:25–40, 1994.

Taussig HB: A study of the German outbreak of phocomelia: The thalidomide syndrome. *JAMA* 180:1106, 1962.

Teratology Society: FDA classification system of drugs for teratogenic risk. *Teratology* 49:446–447, 1994.

Terry KK, Elswick BA, Welsch F, Connolly RB: Development of a physiologically based pharmacokinetic model describing 2-methoxyacetic acid disposition in the pregnant mouse. *Toxicol Appl Pharmacol* 132:103–114, 1995.

Thompson CJS: *Mystery and Lore of Monsters*. London: Williams and Norgate, 1930.

Tomson T, Battino D: Teratogenicity of antiepileptic drugs: State of the art. *Curr Opin Neurol* 18:135–40, 2005.

Ton C, Lin Y, Willett C: Zebrafish as a model for developmental neurotoxicity testing. *Birth Defects Res A Clin Mol Teratol* 76:553–567, 2006.

Toppari J, Larsen JC, Christiansen P, *et al.*: Male reproductive health and environmental xenoestrogens. *Environ Health Perspect* 104(Suppl 4):741–776, 1996.

Trainor PA, Krumlauf R: Hox genes, neural crest cells and branchial arch patterning. *Curr Opin Cell Biol* 13:698–705, 2001.

Tuthill DP, Stewart JH, Coles EC, *et al.*: Maternal cigarette smoking and pregnancy outcome. *Paediatr Perinatol Epidemiol* 13:245–253, 1999.

U.S. FDA: *Guidelines for Reproduction Studies for Safety Evaluation of Drugs for Human Use*. Rockville, MD: US FDA, 1966.

U.S. FDA: Labeling and prescription drug advertising: Content and format for labeling for human prescription drugs. *Fed Reg* 44:37434–37467, 1979.

U.S. EPA: Toxic Substance Control Act Testing Guidelines. Final rules: Preliminary developmental toxicity screen. *Fed Reg* 50:39428–39429, 1985.

U.S. EPA: Guidelines for developmental toxicity risk assessment; notice. *Fed Reg* 56:63798–63826, 1991.

U.S. EPA: *Pesticide Assessment Guidelines, subdivision F, Hazard Evaluation: human and domestic animals, addendum 10: neurotoxicity*. Series 81, 82, and 83. EPA 540/09-91-123 PB 91-154617, 1991.

U.S. FDA: International conference on harmonization; Guideline on detection of toxicity to reproduction for medicinal products; availability; notice. *Fed Reg* 59:48746–48752, 1994.

U.S. EPA: *Special Report on Environmental Endocrine Disruption: An Effects Assessment and Analysis*. US Environmental Protection Agency, EPA/630/R-012., Washington, DC: US EPA, February, 1997.

U.S. Environmental Protection Agency: Health Effects Test Guidelines. OPPTS 870.3700. Prenatal Developmental Toxicity Study. EPA 712-C-98-207, 1998.

U.S. EPA: Endocrine screening program: statement of policy. *Fed Reg* 63(248):71542–71568, 1998.

Uphill PF, Wilkins SR, Allen JA: In vitro micromass teratogen test: Results from a blind trial of 25 compounds. *Toxicol in Vitro* 4:623–626, 1990.

Vaglia JL, Hall BK: Regulation of neural crest cell populations: Occurrence, distribution and underlying mechanisms. *Int J Dev Biol* 43:95–110, 1999.

Vierula M, Niemi M, Keiski A, *et al.*: High and unchanged sperm counts of Finnish men. *Int J Androl* 19:11–17, 1996.

Volfe JJ: Effects of cocaine on the fetus. *N Engl J Med* 327:399–407, 1992.

vom Saal FS, Hughes C: An extensive new literature concerning low-dose effects of bisphenol A shows the need for a new risk assessment. *Environ Health Perspect* 113:926–33, 2005.

vom Saal FS, Timms BG, Montano MM, *et al.*: Prostate enlargement in mice due to fetal exposure to low doses of estradiol or diethylstilbestrol and opposite effects at high doses. *Proc Natl Acad Sci U S A* 94:2056–2061, 1997.

Wald N: Folic acid and the prevention of neural tube defects, in Keen CL, Bendich A, Willhite CC (eds.): Maternal Nutrition and Pregnancy Outcome. *Ann NY Acad Sci* 678:112–129, 1993.

Warkany J: Manifestations of prenatal nutritional deficiency. *Vit Horm* 3:73–103, 1945.

Warkany J: Development of experimental mammalian teratology, in Wilson JG, Warkany J (eds.): *Teratology: Principles and Techniques.* Chicago: University of Chicago Press, 1965, pp. 1–11.

Warkany J: History of teratology, in *Handbook of Teratology.* Vol 1. New York: Plenum Press, 1977, pp. 3–45.

Warkany J: Teratology: Spectrum of a science, in Kalter H (ed.): *Issues and Reviews in Teratology.* Vol 1. New York: Plenum Press, 1983, pp. 19–31.

Warkany J: Teratogen update: Hyperthermia. *Teratology* 33:365–371, 1986.

Warkany J, Nelson RC: Appearance of skeletal abnormalities in the offspring of rats reared on a deficient diet. *Science* 92:383–384, 1940.

Warkany J, Schraffenberger E: Congenital malformations induced in rats by roentgen rays. *Am J Roentgenol Radium Ther* 57:455–463, 1944.

Waterland RA, Jirtle RL: Transposable elements: targets for early nutritional effects on epigenetic gene regulation. *Mol Cell Biol* 23:5293-300, 2003.

Waterland RA, Jirtle RL: Early nutrition, epigenetic changes at transposons and imprinted genes, and enhanced susceptibility to adult chronic diseases. *Nutrition* 20:63–68, 2004.

Watkinson WP, Millicovsky G: Effects of phenytoin on maternal heart rate in A/J mice: Possible role in teratogenesis. *Teratology* 28:1–8, 1983.

Weaver TE, Scott WJ Jr: Acetazolamide teratogenesis: Association of maternal respiratory acidosis and ectrodactyl in C57BL/6J mice. *Teratology* 30:187–193, 1984a.

Weaver TE, Scott WJ Jr: Acetazolamide teratogenesis: Interactions of maternal metabolic and respiratory acidosis in the induction of ectrodactyly in C57BL/6J mice. *Teratology* 30:195–202, 1984b.

Webster WS, Brown-Woodman PD, Ritchie HE: A review of the contribution of whole embryo culture to the determination of hazard and risk in teratogenicity testing. *Int J Dev Biol* 41:329–335, 1997.

Welsch F: Short term methods of assessing developmental toxicity hazard, in Kalter H (ed): *Issues and Review in Teratology.* Vol 5. New York: Plenum Press, 1990, pp. 115–153.

Welshons WV, Nagel SC, vom Saal FS: Large effects from small exposures. III. Endocrine mechanisms mediating effects of bisphenol A at levels of human exposure. *Endocrinology* 147:S56–69, 2006.

White E: Death defying acts: A meeting review on apoptosis. *Genes Dev* 7:2277–2284, 1993.

Wilcox AJ, Weinberg CR, O'Connor JF, *et al.*: Incidence of early loss of pregnancy. *N Engl J Med* 319:189–194, 1988.

Wilson JG, Roth CB, Warkany J: An analysis of the syndrome of malformations induced by maternal vitamin A deficiency: Effects of restoration of vitamin A at various times during gestation. *Am J Anat* 92:189–217, 1953.

Wilson JG: *Environment and Birth Defects.* New York: Academic Press, 1973.

Wilson JG: Embryotoxicity of drugs in man, in Wilson JG, Fraser FC (eds): *Handbook of Teratology.* New York: Plenum Press, 1977, pp. 309–355.

Wiltse J: Mode of action: Inhibition of histone deacetylase, altering WNT-dependent gene expression, and regulation of beta-catenin–developmental effects of valproic acid. *Crit Rev Toxicol* 35:727–738, 2005.

Windham GC, Hopkins B, Fenster L, Swan SH: Prenatal active or passive tobacco smoke exposure and the risk of preterm delivery or low birth weight. *Epidemiology* 11:427–433, 2000.

Yelin R, Schyr RB, Kot H, Zins S, Frumkin A, Pillemer G, Fainsod A: Ethanol exposure affects gene expression in the embryonic organizer and reduces retinoic acid levels. *Dev Biol* 279:193–204, 2005.

You L, Casanova M, Archibeque-Engel S, *et al.*: Impaired male sexual development in perinatal Sprague-Dawley and Long-Evans Hooded rats exposed in utero and lactationally to pp'-DDE. *Toxicol Sci* 45:162–173, 1998.

Young JF: Physiologically-based pharmacokinetic model for pregnancy as a tool for investigation of developmental mechanisms. *Comput Biol Med* 28:359–364, 1998.

Yu M-L, Hsu C-C, Gladen B, Rogan WJ: In utero PCB/PCDF exposure: Relation of developmental delay to dysmorphology and dose. *Neurotoxicol Teratol* 13:195–202, 1991.

Zakany J, Tuggle CK, Nguyen-Huu CM: The use of *lacZ* gene fusions in the studies of mammalian development: Developmental regulation of mammalian homeobox genes in the CNS. *J Physiol Paris* 84:21–26, 1990.

Zoeller RT, Crofton KM: Mode of action: Developmental thyroid hormone insufficiency–neurological abnormalities resulting from exposure to propylthiouracil. *Crit Rev Toxicol* 35:771–781, 2005.

UNIT 4

TARGET ORGAN TOXICITY

CHAPTER 11

TOXIC RESPONSES OF THE BLOOD

John C. Bloom and John T. Brandt

BLOOD AS A TARGET ORGAN

Hematotoxicology is the study of adverse effects of drugs, nontherapeutic chemicals and other agents in our environment on blood and blood-forming tissues (Bloom, 1997). This subspecialty draws on the discipline of hematology and the principles of toxicology. Scientific understanding of the former began with the contributions of Leeuwenhoek and others in the seventeenth century with the microscopic examination of blood (Wintrobe, 1985). Hematology was later recognized as an applied laboratory science but limited to quatification of formed elements of the blood and the study of their morphology, along with that of bone marrow, spleen, and lymphoid tissues. It is now a diverse medical specialty, which, perhaps more than any other discipline, has made tremendous contributions to molecular medicine (Kaushansky, 2000).

The vital functions that blood cells perform, together with the susceptibility of this highly proliferative tissue to intoxication, makes the hematopoietic system unique as a target organ. Accordingly, it ranks with liver and kidney as one of the most important considerations in the risk assessment of individual patient populations exposed to potential toxicants in the environment, workplace, and medicine cabinet.

The delivery of oxygen to tissues throughout the body, maintenance of vascular integrity, and provision of the many affector and effector immune functions necessary for host defense, requires a prodigious proliferative and regenerative capacity. The various blood cells (erythrocytes, granulocytes, and platelets) are each produced at a rate of approximately 1–3 million per second in a healthy adult and up to several times that rate in conditions where demand for these cells is high, as in hemolytic anemia or suppurative inflammation (Kaushansky, 2006). As with intestinal mucosa and gonads, this characteristic makes hematopoietic tissue a particularly sensitive target for cytoreductive or antimitotic agents, such as those used to treat cancer, infection, and immune-mediated disorders. This tissue is also susceptible to secondary effects of toxic agents that affect the supply of nutrients, such as iron; the clearance of toxins and metabolites, such as urea; or the production of vital growth factors, such as erythropoietin and granulocyte colony stimulating factor (G-CSF).

The consequences of direct or indirect damage to blood cells and their precursors are predictable and potentially life-threatening. They include hypoxia, hemorrhage, and infection. These effects may be subclinical and slowly progressive or acute and fulminant, with dramatic clinical presentations. Hematotoxicity is usually assessed in the context of risk versus benefit. It may be used to define dosage in treatment modalities in which these effects are limiting, such as those employing certain anticancer, antiviral, and antithrombotic agents.

Hematotoxicity is generally regarded as unacceptable, however, in treatments for less serious illnesses, such as mild hypertension or arthritis or following exposure to contaminated foods or environmental contaminants. Risk-versus-benefit decisions involving hematotoxicity may be controversial, especially when the incidence of these effects is very low. Whether the effect is linked to the pharmacologic action of the agent, as with cytoreductive or thrombolytic chemicals, or unrelated to its intended action, the right balance between risk and benefit is not always clear.

Hematotoxicity may be regarded as *primary*, where one or more blood components are directly affected, or *secondary*, where the toxic effect is a consequence of other tissue injury or systemic disturbances. Primary toxicity is regarded as among the more common serious effects of xenobiotics, particularly drugs (Vandendries and Drews, 2006). Secondary toxicity is exceedingly common, due to the propensity of blood cells to reflect a wide range of local and systemic effects of toxicants on other tissues. These secondary effects on hematopoietic tissue are often more reactive or compensatory than toxic, and provide the toxicologist with an important and accessible tool for monitoring and characterizing toxic responses.

HEMATOPOIESIS

The production of blood cells, or hematopoiesis, is a highly regulated sequence of events by which blood cell precursors proliferate and differentiate to meet the relentless needs of oxygen transport, host defense and repair, hemostasis, and other vital functions described previously. The bone marrow is the principal site of hematopoiesis in humans and most laboratory and domestic animals. The spleen has little function in blood cell production in the healthy human, but plays a critical role in the clearance of defective or senescent cells, as well in host defense. In the human fetus, hematopoiesis can be found in the liver, spleen, bone marrow, thymus, and lymph nodes. The bone marrow is the dominant hematopoietic organ in the latter half of gestation and the only blood cell producing organ at birth (Moore, 1975). All marrow is active, or "red marrow," at birth (Hudson, 2006). During early childhood, hematopoiesis recedes in long bones and, in adults, is confined to the axial skeleton and proximal humerus and femur (Custer and Ahlfeldt, 1932). The marrow in the distal long bones becomes "yellow" or fatty. When demand for blood cell production is great, as with certain disease states, fatty marrow can be reactivated as sites of hematopoiesis (Fig. 11-1). This can be useful in toxicology studies as a marker of sustained hematopoietic stress, as exemplified in studies on the hematopathology of cephalosporin toxicity in the dog (Bloom *et al.*, 1987). Under extreme conditions, embryonic patterns of hematopoiesis may reappear as *extramedullary hematopoiesis* (Young and Weiss, 1997).

Whereas the central function of bone marrow is hematopoiesis and lymphopoiesis, bone marrow is also one of the sites of the mononuclear phagocyte system (MPS), contributing monocytes that differentiate into a variety of MPS cells located in liver (Kupffer cells), spleen (littoral cells), lymph nodes, and other tissues. Conventional histologic and cytologic sampling of bone marrow reveals a very limited picture of an exceedingly complex tissue containing erythroid, granulocytic, megakaryocytic, MPS, and lymphoid precursors in varied stages of maturation; stromal cells; and vasculature all encased by bone (Fig. 11-1). Routine examinations of such specimens in our pathology and toxicology laboratories cannot possibly reveal the sophisticated interactions that mediate lineage commitment, proliferation, differentiation, acquisition of functional characteristics, and trafficking that result in the delivery of mature

cells to the circulation, as required in sickness and in health. Exactly how the process of hematopoietic progenitor cell differentiation and maturation, and subsequent release into the peripheral circulation is so tightly regulated is not fully known. Early and elegant morphologic studies revealed a complex interplay of developing cells with stromal cells, extracellular matrix components, and cytokines that make up the *hematopoietic inductive microenvironment*, or HIM (Young and Weiss, 1997). More recent studies have shown that each lineage, and even stage of maturation, is supported within a specific niche that is maintained by the surrounding stromal cells (Heissig *et al.*, 2005). An array of cytokines and chemokines direct a particular progenitor cell to the appropriate niche (Lataillade *et al.*, 2004). Today's powerful research tools, that include the use of knock-out mice, have begun to define how hematopoietic growth factors, cytokines and chemokines interact with the HIM and other tissues to control the production and trafficking of blood cells (Kaushansky, 2006; Laurence, 2006). These understandings are providing opportunities to develop promising therapies that are now presenting new pharmacologic and toxicologic challenges.

TOXICOLOGY OF THE ERYTHRON

The Erythrocyte

Erythrocytes (red blood cells, or RBCs) make up 40–45% of the circulating blood volume and serve as the principal vehicle of transportation of oxygen from the lungs to the peripheral tissues. In addition, erythrocytes are involved in the transport of carbon dioxide from tissues to the lung, maintenance of a constant pH in blood and regulation of blood flow to tissues (Hsia, 1998; Kim-Shapiro *et al.*, 2005). Erythrocytes help modulate the inflammatory response through clearance of immune complexes containing complement components and through interaction with nitric oxide, a potent vasodilator (Kim-Shapiro *et al.*, 2005; Lindorfer *et al.*, 2001). An area of developing interest is the role of erythrocytes as a carrier and/or reservoir for drugs and toxins (Schrijvers *et al.*, 1999). The effect of xenobiotics on erythrocytes has been extensively evaluated, both because of the ready access to the tissue and the frequency with which xenobiotics cause changes in this critical tissue.

Xenobiotics may affect the production, function and/or survival of erythrocytes. These effects are most frequently manifest as a change in the circulating red cell mass, usually resulting in a decrease (anemia). Occasionally, agents that increase oxygen affinity lead to an increase in red cell mass (erythrocytosis), but this is distinctly less common. Shifts in plasma volume can alter the relative concentration of erythrocytes/hemoglobin and can be easily confused with true anemia or erythrocytosis.

There are two general mechanisms that lead to true anemia—either decreased production or increased erythrocyte destruction. Both mechanisms may be operative in some disorders, or a combination may arise due to the imposition of a second disorder on a compensated underlying problem. For example, patients with compensated congenital hemolytic anemias are very susceptible to additional insults that may precipitate an acute drop in a previously stable red cell mass, such as parvovirus-infection-associated suppression of erythropoiesis.

Evaluation of a peripheral blood sample can provide evidence for the underlying mechanism of anemia (Prchal, 2006). The usual parameters of a complete blood count (CBC)—including the red blood cell (RBC) count, hemoglobin concentration (Hbg) and hematocrit (also referred to as packed cell volume, or PCV)—can

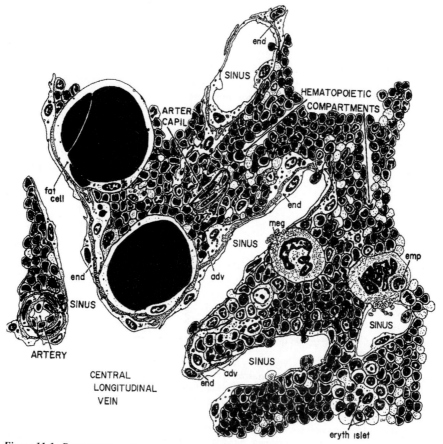

Figure 11-1. Bone marrow schema.

Several venous sinuses (SINUS), cut longitudinally, drain into the central longitudinal vein, cut in cross section. A branch of the nutrient artery (ARTERY) and an arterial capillary (ARTER CAPIL) are present. The circulation in the bone marrow, as in the other tissues of the body save the spleen, is "closed," that is, there is endothelial continuity from artery into vein. Veins in bone marrow have in common with veins elsewhere the primary function of returning blood to the heart. Marrow veins, in addition, possess the distinctive function of receiving blood cells produced and stored in the marrow and carrying them to thymus or spleen, or into the general circulation, for further maturation, widespread distribution and function. The hematopoietic compartments of the bone marrow consist of hematopoietic cells in varying stages of differentiation supported by a fibroblastic stroma. They lie between the most proximal veins, termed venous sinuses or vascular sinuses. When hematopoiesis is rather quiet and few nascent blood cells cross the wall of vascular sinuses, moving from hematopoietic compartments into the sinus lumen, the wall of the sinus tends to be trilaminar, consisting of endothelium (end), wispy basement membrane (in stipple), and adventitial reticular cells (adv) that form an incomplete outermost layer and branch out into the hematopoietic compartment, forming a scaffolding enclosing and supporting the hematopoietic cells. Thus, adventitial reticular cells are both vascular, as the outermost wall of the vascular sinus, and stromal, branching into the perivascular hematopoietic space, holding the vascular sinus in place and supporting hematopoietic cells. Where hematopoietic cell traffic across the wall of the venous sinus is heightened, the adventitial cell cover is retracted and a larger expanse of endothelium, covered only by wisps of basement membrane, is exposed to the hematopoietic cells, facilitating their transmural cell passage. Where transmural cell passage is greatly reduced, adventitial cells accumulate fat and become rounded and bulky, now termed adipocytes, impeding hematopoietic cell passage, and occupying space in the hematopoietic compartment which, when they transform again to adventitial cells flattened upon veins, they yield to hematopoiesis. These fibroblastic stromal cells in the marrow of central bones can modulate readily to and from adventitial cell and adipocyte and retain their granulocyte inductive capacities in either form. In the distal limb and tail bones, where there is little hematopoiesis, they assume the adipocyte form in such large numbers that the marrow is grossly yellow. These adipocytes lose fat only in marked hematopoietic stress, as in spherocytic and other severe anemias where this marrow becomes hematopoietic and grossly red. In such stress, moreover, barrier cells may augment or replace adventitial reticular cells and even endothelial cells. Thus, adventitial cells/adipocytes, by their disposition and bulk, mechanically regulate hematopoiesis and blood cell delivery. In addition, they do so in a subtle manner, through paracrine secretion of several small-protein regulatory factors termed cytokines, which include interleukins. [Reprinted from Young and Weiss (1997) with permission from the authors and Elsevier Science.]

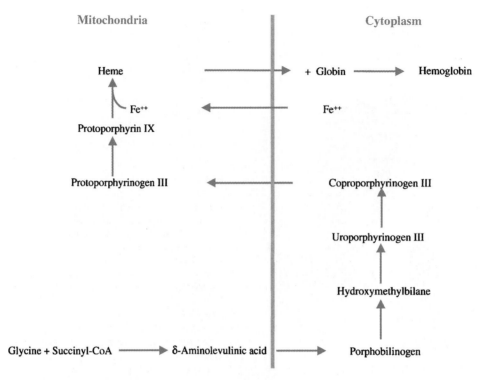

Figure 11-2. The synthesis of heme involves a series of reactions that occur in the cytoplasm and mitochondria of erythroblasts. The initial step in the pathway is the mitochondria synthesis of δ-aminolevulinic acid, a step that is commonly affected by xenobiotics, including lead. Ferrochelatase catalyzes the incorporation of ferrous iron into the tetrapyrrole protoporphyrin IX. Inhibition of the synthetic pathway leading to protoporphyrin IX, as occurs in the sideroblastic anemias, can cause an imbalance between iron concentration and ferrochelatase activity, resulting in iron deposition within mitochondria. Mitochondrial accumulation of iron is the hallmark lesion of the sideroblastic anemias.

establish the presence of anemia. Two additional parameters helpful in classifying an anemia are the mean corpuscular volume (MCV) and the reticulocyte count. Increased destruction is usually accompanied by an increase in reticulocytes (young erythrocytes containing residual RNA), which are easily enumerated using appropriate stains. The introduction of automated methods has improved the precision of reticulocyte counting and introduced new parameters which aid in characterization of red cell production (Brugnara, 2000). With these new methods, reticulocyte counting may also be useful in conditions associated with decreased production, particularly when assessing response to therapy. Other readily performed parameters helpful in the evaluation of the human erythron include: erythrocyte morphology (e.g., megaloblastic changes, erythrocyte fragmentation, sickled RBCs); serum concentration of haptoglobin, lactic dehydrogenase (LD), free hemoglobin, vitamin B12, folate, iron, and ferritin; direct and indirect red cell antiglobulin tests; and bone marrow morphology (Prchal, 2006; Ryan, 2006).

Alterations in Red Cell Production

Erythrocyte production is a continuous process that is dependent on frequent cell division and a high rate of hemoglobin synthesis. Adult hemoglobin (hemoglobin A), the major constituent of the erythrocyte cytoplasm, is a tetramer composed of two α- and two β-globin chains, each with a heme residue located in a stereospecific pocket of the globin chain. Synthesis of hemoglobin is dependent on coordinated production of globin chains and heme moieties. Abnormalities that lead to decreased hemoglobin synthesis are relatively common

(e.g., iron deficiency) and are often associated with a decrease in the MCV and hypochromasia (increased central pallor of RBCs on stained blood films due to the low hemoglobin concentration).

An imbalance between α- and β-chain production is the basis of congenital thalassemia syndromes and results in decreased hemoglobin production and microcytosis (Weatherall, 2006). Xenobiotics can affect globin-chain synthesis and alter the composition of hemoglobin within erythrocytes. This is perhaps best demonstrated by hydroxyurea, which has been found to increase the synthesis of γ-globin chains. The γ-globin chains are a normal constituent of hemoglobin during fetal development, replacing the β chains in the hemoglobin tetramer (hemoglobin F, $\alpha_2\gamma_2$). Hemoglobin F has a higher affinity for oxygen than hemoglobin A and can protect against crystallization (sickling) of deoxyhemoglobin S in sickle cell disease (Steinberg, 2006).

Synthesis of heme requires incorporation of iron into a porphyrin ring (Fig. 11-2) (Napier *et al.*, 2005; Ponka, 1997). Iron deficiency is usually the result of dietary deficiency or increased blood loss. Any drug that contributes to blood loss, such as nonsteroidal anti-inflammatory drugs, with their increased risk of gastrointestinal ulceration and bleeding, may potentiate the risk of developing *iron deficiency anemia*. Defects in the synthesis of the porphyrin ring of heme can lead to *sideroblastic anemia*, with its characteristic accumulation of iron in bone marrow erythroblasts. The accumulated iron precipitates within mitochondria in a complex with mitochondria ferritin, causing the characteristic staining pattern of ringed sideroblasts evident on iron stains such as Prussian blue (Cazzola *et al.*, 2003). A number of xenobiotics (Table 11-1) can interfere

Table 11-1

Xenobiotics Associated with Sideroblastic Anemia

Ethanol	Chloramphenicol
Isoniazid	Cooper chelation/deficiency
Pyrazinamide	Zinc intoxication
Cycloserine	Lead intoxication

Table 11-2

Laboratory Features of Megaloblastic Anemia

MORPHOLOGY	BIOCHEMISTRY
Peripheral blood	Peripheral blood
Pancytopenia	Decreased B_{12} and/or folate
Macrocytosis ($\uparrow$MCV)	Increased LD
Oval macrocytes	Antiparietal cell antibodies
Hypersegmented neutrophils	Antibody to intrinsic factor
Variation in RBC shape	Increased serum iron
Bone marrow	Hypokalemia
Erythroid hyperplasia	
Megaloblastic anemia	
Giant band neutrophils	
Giant metamyelocytes	

Table 11-3

Xenobiotics Associated with Megaloblastic Anemia

B_{12} DEFICIENCY	FOLATE DEFICIENCY
Paraminosalicylic acid	Phenytoin
Colchicine	Primidone
Neomycin	Carbamazepine
Ethanol	Phenobarbital
Omeprazole	Sulfasalazine
Hemodialysis	Cholestyramine
Zidovudine	Triamterine
Fish tapeworm	Malabsorption syndromes
	Antimetabolites

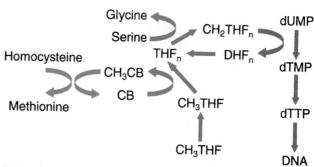

Figure 11-3. *Both tetrahydrofolate (THF) and cobalamin (CB, or vitamin B_{12}) are necessary for the synthesis of thymidine (dTMP) for incorporation into DNA. Folate enters the cell as a monoglutamate (CH₃THF) but is transformed to a polyglutamate within the cell, a step that helps prevent leakage of folate back across the cell membrane. However, CH₃THF cannot be conjugated with glutamate. CB is necessary for demethylation of the folate, allowing formation of conjugated (polyglutamate) folate (THFₙ). In the absence of CB, folate levels within the cell drop, causing a functional deficiency of folate and impairing synthesis of thymidine.*

other therapeutic proteins, there is a risk of antibody formation in response to administration of these proteins; if the antibody reacts with the endogenous growth factor it may cause profound cytopenia (Bennett *et al.*, 2004; Li *et al.*, 2001).

Erythropoietin is commonly used to support red cell production in patients undergoing chemotherapy and with renal failure. Following a change in formulation, a series of cases of red cell aplasia associated with erythropoietin use was reported (Bennett *et al.*, 2004). The etiology was antibodies to the synthetic protein that cross-reacted with endogenous erythropoietin. A change in formulation in combination with the nature of the storage container and route of administration is thought to have promoted the formation of protein aggregates, a phenomenon known to be associated with an increased risk of antibody formation (Koren *et al.*, 2002). The incidence of red cell aplasia appears to have diminished following a change in packaging and administration of erythropoietin by intravenous injection (Bennett *et al.*, 2004).

Drug-induced *aplastic anemia* may represent either a predictable or idiosyncratic reaction to a xenobiotic. This life-threatening disorder is characterized by peripheral blood pancytopenia, reticulocytopenia, and bone marrow hypoplasia (Vandendries and Drews, 2006; Young, 1999, 2000). Chemicals such as benzene and radiation have a *predictable* effect on hematopoietic progenitors, and the resulting aplastic anemia corresponds to the magnitude of the exposure to these chemicals. In contrast, idiosyncratic aplastic anemia does not appear to be related to the dose of the chemical initiating the process. A long list of chemicals has been associated with the development of aplastic anemia (Table 11-4), many of which have been reported in only a few patients. The mechanism(s) of aplasia in affected patients is (are) still unknown. Immune mechanisms have long been thought to contribute to the development of the idiosyncratic form of drug-induced aplastic anemia. However, it has been difficult to obtain definitive evidence for humoral and/or cellular mechanisms of marrow suppression (Vandendries and Drews, 2006; Young, 2000).

Pure red cell aplasia is a syndrome in which the decrease in marrow production is limited to the erythroid lineage (Djaldetti *et al.*, 2003; Fisch *et al.*, 2000). Pure red cell aplasia is an uncommon disorder that may be due to genetic defects, infection (parvovirus B19), immune-mediated injury, myelodysplasia, drugs

with one or more of the steps in erythroblast heme synthesis and result in sideroblastic anemia (Alcindor and Bridges, 2002; Beutler, 2006a,b; Fiske *et al.*, 1994).

Hematopoiesis requires active DNA synthesis and frequent mitoses. Folate and vitamin B_{12} are necessary to maintain synthesis of thymidine for incorporation into DNA (Fig. 11-3). Deficiency of folate and/or vitamin B_{12} results in *megaloblastic anemia*, with its characteristic morphologic and biochemical changes (Table 11-2), which commonly affect erythroid, myeloid, and megakaryocytic lineages. A number of xenobiotics may contribute to a deficiency of vitamin B_{12} and/or folate (Table 11-3), leading to megaloblastic anemia (Babior, 2006).

Many of the antiproliferative drugs used in the treatment of malignancy predictably inhibit hematopoiesis, including erythropoiesis. The resulting bone marrow toxicity may be dose-limiting, as previously discussed. New chemicals, such as amifostine, are being developed that may help protect against the marrow toxicity of these agents (Phillips, 2002). The development of recombinant forms of some of the growth factors that regulate hematopoiesis has helped shorten the duration of bone marrow suppression. As with

Table 11-4

Drugs and Chemicals Associated with the Development of Aplastic Anemia

Chloramphenicol	Organic arsenicals	Quinacrine
Methylphenylethylhydantoin	Trimethadione	Phenylbutazone
Gold	Streptomycin	Benzene
Penicillin	Allopurinol	Tetracycline
Methicillin	Sulfonamides	Chlortetracycline
Sulfisoxazole	Sulfamethoxypyridazine	Amphotericin B
Mefloquine	Ethosuximide	Felbamate
Carbimazole	Methylmercaptoimidazole	Potassium perchlorate
Propylthiouracil	Tolbutamide	Pyrimethamine
Chlorpropamide	Carbutamide	Tripelennamine
Indomethacin	Carbamazepine	Diclofenac
Meprobamate	Chlorpromazine	Chlordiazepoxide
Mepazine	Chlorphenothane	Parathion
Thiocyanate	Methazolamide	Dinitrophenol
Bismuth	Mercury	Chlordane
Carbon tetrachloride	Cimetidine	Metolazone
Azidothymidine	Ticlopidine	Isoniazid
Trifluoperazine	D-penicillamine	

or other toxicants. As pure red cell aplasia occurs sporadically and infrequently, the linkage between drug exposure and pathogenesis of the aplasia remains speculative for some chemicals. The drugs most clearly implicated and for which there are multiple case reports, include isoniazid, phenytoin, and azathioprine. The mechanism of drug-induced pure red cell aplasia is unknown, but some evidence suggests that it may be immune-mediated. Patients with drug-induced red cell aplasia should not be re-exposed to the purported offending chemical. As noted above, pure red aplasia may also occur as a consequence of an immune response to therapeutic erythropoietin.

Alterations in the Respiratory Function of Hemoglobin

Hemoglobin is necessary for effective transport of oxygen and carbon dioxide between the lungs and tissues. The respiratory function of hemoglobin has been studied in detail, revealing an intricately balanced system for the transport of oxygen from lungs to the tissues (Hsia, 1998). Electrostatic charges hold the globin chains of deoxyhemoglobin in a "tense" (T) conformation, characterized by a relatively low affinity for oxygen. Binding of oxygen alters this conformation to a "relaxed" (R) conformation that is associated with a 500-fold increase in oxygen affinity. Thus the individual globin units show cooperativity in the binding of oxygen, resulting in the familiar sigmoid shape of the oxygen dissociation curve (Fig. 11-4). The ability of hemoglobin to safely and efficiently transport oxygen is dependent on both intrinsic (homotropic) and extrinsic (heterotropic) factors that affect the performance of this system.

Homotropic Effects One of the most important homotropic properties of oxyhemoglobin is the slow but consistent oxidation of heme iron to the ferric state to form methemoglobin (Percy *et al.*, 2005). Methemoglobin is not capable of binding and transporting oxygen. In addition, the presence of methemoglobin in a hemoglobin tetramer has allosteric effects that increase the affinity of oxyhemoglobin for oxygen, resulting in a leftward shift of the oxygen dissociation curve (Fig. 11-4). The combination of decreased oxy-

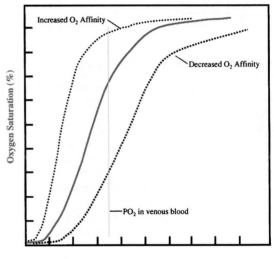

Figure 11-4. *The normal oxygen dissociation curve (solid line) has a sigmoid shape due to the cooperative interaction between the four globin chains in the hemoglobin molecule. Fully deoxygenated hemoglobin has a relatively low affinity for oxygen. Interaction of oxygen with one heme-iron moiety induces a conformational change in that globin chain. Through surface interactions, that conformational change affects the other globin chains, causing a conformational change in all of the globin chains that increases their affinity for oxygen. Homotropic and heterotropic parameters also affect the affinity of hemoglobin for oxygen. An increase in oxygen affinity results in a shift to the left in the oxygen-dissociation curve. Such a shift may decrease oxygen delivery to the tissues. A decrease in oxygen affinity results in a shift to the right in the oxygen dissociation curve, facilitating oxygen delivery to the tissues.*

gen content and increased affinity impairs delivery of oxygen to tissues when the concentration of methemoglobin rises beyond critical levels (Hsia, 1998; Percy *et al.*, 2005).

Not surprisingly, the normal erythrocyte has metabolic mechanisms for reducing heme iron back to the ferrous state; these

Table 11-5

Xenobiotics Associated with Methemoglobinemia

THERAPEUTIC AGENTS	ENVIRONMENTAL AGENTS
Benzocaine	Nitrites
Lidocaine	Nitrates
Prilocaine	Nitrobenzenes
Dapsone	Aniline dyes and aniline derivatives
Amyl nitrate	Butyl nitrite
Isobutyl nitrite	Potassium chlorate
Nitroglycerine	Gasoline additives
Primaquine	Aminobenzenes
Sulfonamide	Nitrotoluenes
Phenacetin	Trinitrotoluene
Nitric oxide	Nitroethane
Phenazopyridine	Ortho-toluidine
Metoclopramide	Paratoluidine
Flutamide	Betanaphthol disulfonate
Silver nitrate	
Quinones	
Methylene blue	

mechanisms are normally capable of maintaining the concentration of methemoglobin at less than 1% of the total hemoglobin (Percy *et al.*, 2005). The predominant pathway is cytochrome b_5 methemoglobin reductase, which is dependent on reduced nicotine adenine dinucleotide (NADH) and is also known as NADH-diaphorase. An alternate pathway involves a reduced nicotine adenine dinucleotide phosphate (NADPH) diaphorase that reduces a flavin that in turn reduces methemoglobin. This pathway usually accounts for less than 5% of the reduction of methemoglobin, but its activity can be greatly enhanced by methylene blue, which is reduced to leukomethylene blue by NADPH-diaphorase. Leukomethylene blue then reduces methemoglobin to deoxyhemoglobin.

A failure of these control mechanisms leads to increased levels of methemoglobin, or *methemoglobinemia*. The most common cause of methemoglobinemia is exposure to an oxidizing xenobiotic that overwhelms the NADH-diaphorase system. A large number of chemicals and therapeutic chemicals may cause methemoglobinemia (Table 11-5) (Bradberry *et al.*, 2001; Bradberry, 2003; Coleman and Coleman, 1996). These chemicals may be divided into direct oxidizers, which are capable of inducing methemoglobin formation when added to erythrocytes in vitro or in vivo, and indirect oxidizers, which do not induce methemoglobin formation when exposed to erythrocytes in vitro, but do so after metabolic modification in vivo. Nitrites appear to be able to interact directly with heme to facilitate oxidation of heme iron, but the precise mechanism that leads to methemoglobin formation is unknown for many of the other substances listed in Table 11-5.

The development of methemoglobinemia may be slow and insidious or abrupt in onset, as with the use of some topical anesthetics (Bradberry *et al.*, 2001; Bradberry, 2003; Khan and Kruse, 1999; Nguyen *et al.*, 2000). Most patients tolerate low levels (<10%) of methemoglobin without clinical symptoms. Cyanosis is often evident when the methemoglobin concentration exceeds 5–10%. Levels above 20% are generally clinically significant and some patients may begin to manifest symptoms related to tissue hypoxemia at methemoglobin levels between 10 and 20%. The severity of clinical manifestations increases as the concentration rises above

20–30%, with methemoglobin levels above 70% being life-threatening. Intravenous administration of 1–2 mg/kg methylene blue is effective in rapidly reversing methemoglobinemia through activation of the NADPH diaphorase pathway (Clifton and Leikin, 2003). The effect of methylene blue is dependent on an adequate supply of NADPH. Consequently, methylene blue is not effective in patients with glucose-6-phosphate dehydrogenase (G-6-PD) deficiency, because of the decreased capacity to form NADPH (Bradberry, 2003; Coleman and Coleman, 1996).

Heterotropic Effects   There are three major heterotropic effectors of hemoglobin function: pH, erythrocyte 2,3-bisphosphoglycerate (2,3-BPG, formerly designated 2,3-diphosphoglycerate) concentration, and temperature (Hsia, 1998). A decrease in pH (e.g., lactic acid, carbon dioxide) lowers the affinity of hemoglobin for oxygen; that is, it causes a right-shift in the oxygen dissociation curve, facilitating the delivery of oxygen to tissues (Fig. 11-4). As bicarbonate and carbon dioxide equilibrate in the lung, the hydrogen ion concentration decreases, increasing the affinity of hemoglobin for oxygen and facilitating oxygen uptake. Thus the buffering capacity of hemoglobin also serves to improve oxygen uptake and delivery.

The binding site for 2,3-BPG is located in a pocket formed by the two β chains of a hemoglobin tetramer. Binding of 2,3-BPG to deoxyhemoglobin results in stabilization of the "T" conformation, with reduced oxygen affinity (a shift to the right of the oxygen dissociation curve). The conformational change induced by binding of oxygen alters the binding site for 2,3-BPG and results in release of 2,3-BPG from hemoglobin. This facilitates uptake of more oxygen for delivery to tissues. The concentration of 2,3-BPG increases whenever there is tissue hypoxemia but may decrease in the presence of acidosis or hypophosphatemia. Thus hypophosphatemia may result in a left shift of the oxygen dissociation curve.

Clofibric acid and bezafibrate are capable of lowering the oxygen affinity of hemoglobin, analogous to 2,3-BPG (Poyart *et al.*, 1994). However, the association constant of bezafibrate for hemoglobin is too low for there to be a meaningful effect in vivo. Work continues on bezafibrate derivatives that may lower oxygen affinity and enhance tissue oxygenation. In contrast, some aromatic benzaldehydes have been shown to increase oxygen affinity and shift the dissociation curve to the left. It was thought that these compounds may be useful in preventing the sickling of deoxyhemoglobin S in patients with sickle cell disease. However, these and other chemicals evaluated for their effect on hemoglobin oxygen affinity have not progressed into clinical usage (Papassotiriou *et al.*, 1998; Poyart *et al.*, 1994).

The oxygen affinity of hemoglobin decreases as the body temperature increases (Hsia, 1998). This facilitates delivery of oxygen to tissues during periods of extreme exercise, and febrile illnesses associated with increased temperature. Correspondingly, oxygen affinity increases during hypothermia, which may lead to decreased oxygen delivery under these conditions. This must be taken into consideration during surgical procedures during which there is induction of deep hypothermia.

The respiratory function of hemoglobin may also be impaired by blockade of the ligand binding site following interaction with other substances, most notably carbon monoxide (Hsia, 1998). Carbon monoxide has a relatively low rate of association with deoxyhemoglobin but has high affinity once bound. The affinity is about 200 times that of oxygen, and thus persistent exposure to a low level of carbon monoxide (for example, 0.1%) may lead to 50% saturation of hemoglobin. Binding of carbon monoxide also results in stabilization of the hemoglobin molecule in the high-affinity "R" conformation. Consequently, the oxygen dissociation curve is shifted to the left, further compromising oxygen delivery to the tissues. Carbon monoxide is produced at low levels by the body through the metabolism of heme and equilibrates across the pulmonary capillary/alveolar bed. Low concentrations of carboxyhemoglobin can be cytoprotective during inflammatory stress or ischemia/reperfusion injury, and the therapeutic use of low concentrations of carbon monoxide is being explored (Kao and Nanagas, 2005; Ryter and Otterbein, 2004).

The major sources of significant exogenous exposure to carbon monoxide are smoking and burning of fossil fuels (including automobiles), particularly in enclosed spaces. Heavy smoking during pregnancy may result in significant levels of carboxyhemoglobin in fetal blood and diminished oxygenation of fetal tissues. Symptoms of carbon monoxide toxicity, such as dizziness, shortness of breath and headache begin to appear when carboxyhemoglobin levels reach 20%. Levels of 50–80% carboxyhemoglobin may be lethal. In addition to effects due to interaction with hemoglobin, CO may cause toxicity through effects on myoglobin, cytochromes, guanylate cyclase or nitric oxide. The key to therapy is removal from the source of carbon monoxide and provision of an adequate supply of oxygen; hyperbaric hyperoxia may be used in serious cases (Kao and Nanagas, 2005; Ryter and Otterbein, 2004).

Methemoglobin can combine reversibly with a variety of chemical substances, including cyanide, sulfides, peroxides, fluorides, and azides. The affinity of methemoglobin for cyanide is utilized in two settings. First, nitrites are administered in cyanide poisoning to form methemoglobin, which then binds free cyanide, sparing other critical cellular respiratory enzymes (Cummings, 2004). Second, formation of cyanmethemoglobin by reaction of hemoglobin with potassium ferricyanide is a standard method for measurement of hemoglobin concentration.

Nitric oxide, an important vasodilator that modulates vascular tone, binds avidly to heme iron. An additional function of erythrocytes is related to this interaction, which can influence the availability of nitric oxide in parts of the circulation (Hsia, 1998; Lundberg and Weitzberg, 2005). Solutions of hemoglobin have been evaluated as a potential replacement for red blood cell transfusions. However, these trials have been halted due to the toxicity associated with administration of hemoglobin solutions. Vascular instability is one of the complications associated with infusion of hemoglobin solutions and is thought to be related to the scavenging of essential nitric oxide by the administered hemoglobin (Moore et al., 2005; Rother et al., 2005).

Alterations in Erythrocyte Survival

The normal survival of erythrocytes in the circulation is about 120 days (Dessypris, 1999). During this period, the erythrocytes are exposed to a variety of oxidative injuries and must negotiate the tortuous passages of the microcirculation and the spleen. This requires a deformable cell membrane and energy to maintain the sodium-potassium gradients and repair mechanisms (Van Wijk and van Solinge, 2005). Very little protein synthesis occurs during this time, as erythrocytes are anucleate when they enter the circulation and residual mRNA is rapidly lost over the first 1–2 days in the circulation. Consequently, senescence occurs over time until the aged erythrocytes are removed by the spleen, where the iron is recov-

ered for reutilization in heme synthesis. Any insult that increases oxidative injury, decreases metabolism, or alters the membrane may cause a decrease in erythrocyte concentration and a corresponding anemia.

Nonimmune Hemolytic Anemia

Microangiopathic Anemias Intravascular fragmentation of erythrocytes gives rise to the *microangiopathic hemolytic anemias* (Baker, 2006). The hallmark of this process is the presence of schistocytes (fragmented RBCs) in the peripheral blood. These abnormal cellular fragments are usually promptly cleared from the circulation by the spleen. Thus their presence in peripheral blood samples indicates either an increased rate of formation or abnormal clearance function of the spleen. The formation of fibrin strands in the microcirculation is a common mechanism for RBC fragmentation. This may occur in the setting of disseminated intravascular coagulation, sepsis, the hemolytic-uremic syndrome, and thrombotic thrombocytopenic purpura. The erythrocytes are essentially sliced into fragments by the fibrin strands that extend across the vascular lumen and impede the flow of erythrocytes through the vasculature. Excessive fragmentation can also be seen in the presence of abnormal vasculature, as occurs with damaged cardiac valves, arteriovenous malformations, vasculitis, and widely metastatic carcinoma (Baker, 2006). The high shear associated with malignant hypertension may also lead to RBC fragmentation.

Other Mechanical Injuries March hemoglobinuria is an episodic disorder characterized by destruction of RBCs during vigorous exercise or marching (Abarbanel et al., 1990; Sagov, 1970). The erythrocytes appear to be destroyed by mechanical trauma in the feet. Sufficient hemoglobin may be released to cause hemoglobinuria. The disorder should be distinguished from other causes of intermittent hemoglobinuria such as paroxysmal nocturnal hemoglobinuria. The introduction of improved footgear for athletes and soldiers has significantly decreased the incidence of this problem.

Major thermal burns are also associated with a hemolytic process. The erythrocyte membrane becomes unstable as the temperature increases. With major burns there can be significant heat-dependent lysis of erythrocytes. Small RBC fragments break off, with resealing of the cell membrane. These cell fragments usually assume a spherical shape and are not as deformable as normal erythrocytes. Consequently, these abnormal cell fragments are removed in the spleen, leading to anemia. The burden of RBC fragments may impair the phagocytic function of the spleen, contributing to the increased susceptibility to endotoxic shock following major burns (Hatherill et al., 1986; Schneidkraut and Loegering, 1984).

Infectious Diseases A variety of infectious diseases may be associated with significant hemolysis, either by direct effect on the erythrocyte or development of an immune-mediated hemolytic process (Berkowitz, 1991; Beutler, 2006a,b). The most common agents that directly cause hemolysis include malaria, babesiosis, clostridial infections, and bartonellosis. Erythrocytes are parasitized in malaria and babesiosis, leading to their destruction. Clostridial infections are associated with release of hemolytic toxins that enter the circulation and lyse erythrocytes. The hemolysis can be severe with significant hemoglobinuria, even with apparently localized infections. *Bartonella bacilliformis* is thought to adhere to the erythrocyte, leading to rapid removal from the circulation. The hemolysis can be severe and the mortality rate in this disorder (Oroya fever) is high.

Oxidative Hemolysis Molecular oxygen is a reactive and potentially toxic chemical species; consequently, the normal respiratory function of erythrocytes generates oxidative stress on a continuous basis. The major mechanisms that protect against oxidative injury in erythrocytes include NADH-diaphorase, superoxide dismutase, catalase, and the glutathione pathway (Coleman and Coleman, 1996; Njalsson and Norgren, 2005). As indicated previously, a small amount of methemoglobin is continuously formed during the process of loading and unloading of oxygen from hemoglobin. Formation of methemoglobin is associated with formation of superoxide free radicals, which must be detoxified to prevent oxidative injury to hemoglobin and other critical erythrocyte components. Under physiologic conditions, superoxide dismutase converts superoxide into hydrogen peroxide, which is then metabolized by catalase and glutathione peroxidase (Fig. 11-5).

A number of xenobiotics, particularly compounds containing aromatic amines, are capable of inducing oxidative injury in erythrocytes (Table 11-6) (Bradberry, 2003; Percy *et al.*, 2005). These agents appear to potentiate the normal redox reactions and are capable of overwhelming the usual protective mechanisms. The interaction between these xenobiotics and hemoglobin leads to the formation of free radicals that denature critical proteins, including hemoglobin, thiol-dependent enzymes, and components of the erythrocyte membrane. In the presence of hydrogen peroxide and xenobiotics such as hydroxylamine, hydroxamic acid, and phenolic compounds, a reactive ferryl (Fe^{+4}) hemoglobin intermediate may be formed according to the following reaction:

$$H_2O_2 + Hgb - Fe^{3+} \rightarrow H_2O + Hgb(\bullet+) - Fe^{4+} - O^-$$

In this intermediate, referred to as compound 1, tyrosine may donate the extra electron, turning it into a reactive free radical. Compound 1 may undergo further reaction with organic compounds (AH_2 in equations below) to yield additional free radicals according to the following reactions:

$$Hgb(\bullet+) - Fe^{4+} - O + AH_2 \rightarrow Hgb - Fe^{4+} - O^- + AH\bullet + H^+$$
$$Hgb - Fe^{4+} - O^- + AH_2 + H^+ \rightarrow Hgb - Fe^{3+} + AH\bullet + H_2O$$

Hemoglobin contains exposed free cysteines ($\beta93$) that are critical for the structural integrity of the molecule. Oxidation of these groups can denature hemoglobin and decrease its solubility. The oxidized, denatured hemoglobin species comprise what has been designated sulfhemoglobin. The denatured hemoglobin can form aggregates that bind to the cell membrane to form inclusions called *Heinz bodies*, a hallmark of oxidative injury to erythrocytes (Jandl, 1987). Heinz bodies can be visualized by use of phase-contrast microscopy or supravital stains such as crystal violet. These membrane-associated inclusions impair the deformability of the erythrocyte membrane and thus impede movement of erythrocytes through the microcirculation and spleen. Heinz bodies are effectively removed from the erythrocyte by the spleen, so they are not often observed in peripheral blood samples from patients despite ongoing oxidative injury. However, the culling of Heinz bodies can alter the morphology of the affected cells, giving rise to what are called "bite" cells and "blister" cells, which may provide an important clue as to the ongoing process (Yoo and Lessin, 1992). These

Table 11-6
Xenobiotics Associated with Oxidative Injury

Acetanilide	Phenylhydrazine
Naphthalene	Nitrobenzene
Nitrofurantoin	Phenacetin
Sulfamethoxypyridazine	Phenol
Aminosalicylic acid	Hydroxylamine
Sodium sulfoxone	Methylene blue
Dapsone	Toluidine blue
Phenazopyridine	Furazolidone
Primaquine	Nalidixic acid
Chlorates	Sulfanilamide
Sulfasalazine	

$$HgbFe^{++}O_2 \rightleftharpoons HgbFe^{++} + O_2 \quad (1)$$

$$HgbFe^{++}O_2 \rightleftharpoons HgbFe^{+++} + O_2^- \quad (2)$$

$$2O_2^- + 2H^+ \xrightarrow[\text{Dismutase}]{\text{Superoxide}} O_2 + H_2O_2 \quad (3)$$

$$2 H_2O_2 \xrightarrow{\text{Catalase}} H_2O + O_2 \quad (4)$$

$$H_2O_2 + GSH \xrightarrow[\text{Peroxidase}]{\text{Glutathione}} GSSH + H_2O \quad (5)$$

$$O_2^- + GSH \xrightarrow[\text{Peroxidase}]{\text{Glutathione}} GSSH + H_2O \quad (6)$$

Figure 11-5. Oxygen normally exchanges with the ferrous iron of deoxyhemoglobin [Eq. (1)]. Oxygen can "capture" one of the iron electrons, resulting in the generation of methemoglobin ($HgbFe^{3+}$) and superoxide (O_2-) [Eq. (2)]. Superoxide must be detoxified or it can lead to oxidative injury within the cell. The pathways involved include superoxide dismutase [Eq. (3)], catalase [Eq. (4)], and glutathione peroxidase [Eqs. (5 and 6)]. A supply of reduced glutathione (GSH) is necessary to prevent excessive oxidative injury.

cells look as though a portion of the cytoplasm had been cut away. Heinz body formation can be induced by in vitro exposure to oxidizing agents and patients with oxidative hemolysis often show increased in vitro formation of Heinz bodies.

Oxidative denaturation of the globin chain decreases its affinity for the heme group, which may dissociate from the globin chain during oxidative injury (Kumar and Bandyopadhyay, 2005). Free heme itself is toxic to cells and can induce tissue injury through formation of reactive oxygen species. The ferric iron in the heme ring may react with chloride to form a complex called hemin. Hemin is hydrophobic and intercalates into the erythrocyte membrane from which it is removed by interaction with albumin. However, if the rate of hemin formation exceeds the rate of removal by albumin, hemin accumulates in the membrane, where it can cause rapid lysis of the erythrocyte.

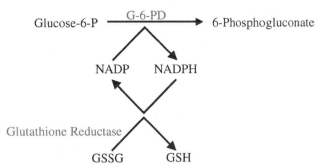

Figure 11-6. *The hexose monophosphate shunt in the erythrocyte is critical for generation of NADPH, which helps maintain an intracellular supply of reduced glutathione (GSH). With a deficiency of glucose-6-phosphate dehydrogenase (G-6-PD), the rate-limiting step in this pathway, the cellular levels of GSH are reduced. Such cells show increased susceptibility to oxidative injury. Acute exposure of such cells to an oxidizing agent can result in rapid hemolysis.*

The generation of free radicals may also lead to peroxidation of membrane lipids (Jandl, 1987; Kumar and Bandyopadhyay, 2005). This may affect the deformability of the erythrocyte and the permeability of the membrane to potassium. The alteration of the Na^+/K^+ gradient is independent of injury to the Na^+/K^+ pump and is potentially lethal to the affected erythrocyte. Oxidative injury also impairs the metabolic machinery of the erythrocyte, resulting in a decrease in the concentration of ATP (Tavazzi *et al.*, 2000). Damage to the membrane can also permit leakage of denatured hemoglobin from the cell. Such free denatured hemoglobin can be toxic on its own. Free hemoglobin may irreversibly bind nitric oxide, resulting in vasoconstriction. Released hemoglobin may form nephrotoxic hemoglobin dimers, leading to kidney damage.

Oxidative injury thus results in a number of changes that decrease the viability of erythrocytes. Protection against many of the free radical-induced modifications is mediated by reduced glutathione (Njalsson and Norgren, 2005). Formation of reduced glutathione is dependent on NADPH and the hexose monophosphate shunt (Fig. 11-6). Significant oxidative injury usually occurs when the concentration of the xenobiotic is high enough (either due to high exposure or decreased metabolism of the xenobiotic) to overcome the normal protective mechanisms, or, more commonly, when there is an underlying defect in the protective mechanisms.

The most common enzyme defect associated with oxidative hemolysis is glucose-6-phosphate dehydrogenase (G-6-PD) deficiency, a relatively common sex-linked disorder characterized by alterations in the primary structure of G-6-PD that diminish its functional activity(Beutler, 1996). It is often clinically asymptomatic until the erythrocytes are exposed to oxidative stress. The stress may come from the host response to infection or exposure to xenobiotics. The level of G-6-PD normally decreases as the erythrocytes age. In the African type of G-6-PD deficiency, the enzyme is less stable than normal; thus the loss of activity is accelerated compared to the normal level. In the Mediterranean type of G-6-PD deficiency, the rate of loss of enzyme activity is even higher. Consequently, the older erythrocytes with the lowest levels of G-6-PD are most susceptible to hemolysis, with the degree of hemolysis affected by the residual amount of enzyme activity as well as the magnitude of the oxidative injury.

Erythrocyte reduced glutathione is rapidly depleted upon exposure to an oxidizing chemical in patients with G-6-PD deficiency. This leads to the series of oxidative injuries described above with

the development of intra- and extravascular hemolysis. Oxidative hemolysis is usually reversible if the process is promptly recognized and the offending chemical is removed. Occasionally the hemolysis may be sufficiently severe to result in death or serious morbidity (e.g., renal failure). Hemolytic anemia may occur in patients with deficiency of glutathione synthetase due to the reduced intracellular concentration of glutathione (Njalsson and Norgren, 2005).

Nonoxidative Chemical-Induced Hemolysis   Exposure to some xenobiotics is associated with hemolysis without significant oxidative injury (Beutler, 2006a,b). Arsenic hydride is a gas that is formed during several industrial processes. Inhalation of the gas can result in severe hemolysis, with anemia, jaundice, and hemoglobinuria. The mechanism of hemolysis in arsine toxicity is not understood. Lead poisoning is associated with defects in heme synthesis and a shortening of erythrocyte survival. The cause of the hemolysis is uncertain, but lead can cause membrane damage and interfere with the Na^+/K^+ pump. These effects may cause premature removal of erythrocytes from the circulation. Excess copper has been associated with hemolytic anemia. The pathogenesis may relate to inhibitory effects on the hexose monophosphate shunt and the Embden-Meyerhof pathway. Ingestion of excess chromium may result in a hemolytic anemia and thrombocytopenia, although the mechanism is not known (Cerulli *et al.*, 1998). Significant hemolysis may also occur with biologic toxins found in insect and snake venoms (Beutler, 2006a,b).

Immune Hemolytic Anemia   Immunologic destruction of erythrocytes is mediated by the interaction of IgG or IgM antibodies with antigens expressed on the surface of the erythrocyte. In the case of autoimmune hemolytic anemia the antigens are intrinsic components of the patient's own erythrocytes. A large number of drugs have been associated with enhanced binding of immunoglobulin to the erythrocyte surface and shortened RBC survival (Arndt and Garratty, 2005).

A number of mechanisms have been implicated in xenobiotic-mediated antibody binding to erythrocytes (Arndt and Garratty, 2005). Some drugs, of which penicillin is a prototype, appear to bind to the surface of the cell, with the "foreign" drug acting as a *hapten* and eliciting an immune response. The antibodies that arise in this type of response only bind to drug-coated erythrocytes. Other drugs, of which quinidine is a prototype, bind to components of the erythrocyte surface and induce a conformational change in one or more components of the membrane. This type of interaction can give rise to a confusing array of antibody specificities. Some of the antibodies recognize only the *drug-membrane component* complex; others are specific for the membrane component, but only when drug is present; whereas still others may recognize the membrane component in the presence or absence of the drug. A third mechanism, for which α-methyldopa is a prototype, results in production of a *drug-induced autoantibody* that cannot be distinguished from the antibodies arising in idiopathic autoimmune hemolytic anemia. The mechanism for induction of this group of antibodies is not understood, but may be related to development of an autoimmune response. A variant of this type of response is the augmentation of autoimmune hemolytic anemia that may occur during therapy of some lymphoproliferative disorders. Autoimmune phenomena, including autoimmune hemolytic anemia, are known to occur in lymphoproliferative disorders such as chronic lymphocytic leukemia. Treatment of these disorders with some chemicals has been associated with worsening of the hemolytic anemia (Gonzalez *et al.*, 1998). It has been hypothesized that therapy further disrupts regulation of the autoimmune phenomenon, allowing increased antibody production.

Some xenobiotics are associated with *nonspecific deposition of proteins* on erythrocytes. This was first associated with cephalosporins but has also been seen with other drugs, including cisplatin and the beta-lactamase inhibitors sulbactam and clavulanate (Arndt and Garratty, 2005). Immunoglobulin and complement proteins may be among the proteins deposited on the erythrocyte surface. These proteins may cause a positive direct antiglobulin test, suggesting a drug-induced antibody response. However, there is no evidence of a drug-dependent antibody in the patient's serum, and drug-treated erythrocytes may bind antibody from normal nondrug exposed serum. This form of antibody deposition is generally not associated with hemolysis, although the possibility of hemolysis related to this type of reaction has been raised.

Drug-induced intravascular hemolysis is often a dramatic clinical event and may be associated with fever, chills, back pain, hypotension, a rapid fall in hemoglobin concentration, a decrease in serum haptoglobin, a marked increase in serum LD, and hemoglobinuria (Arndt and Garratty, 2005). The clinical picture of extravascular hemolysis depends on the rate of hemolysis but is usually less dramatic. Often there is evidence of reticulocytosis, polychromasia, spherocytosis, a moderate increase in serum LD, and an increase in serum bilirubin. Serologic studies usually show evidence of IgG and/or complement on the surface of erythrocytes, although it may be difficult to document that antibody binding is drug-dependent. The mainstay of therapy in patients with drug-induced hemolytic anemia is removal of the offending drug and avoidance of re-exposure.

TOXICOLOGY OF THE LEUKON

Components of Blood Leukocytes

The leukon consists of leukocytes, or white blood cells. They include granulocytes (which may be subdivided into neutrophils, eosinophils, and basophils), monocytes, and lymphocytes. Granulocytes and monocytes are nucleated ameboid cells that are phagocytic. They play a central role in the inflammatory response and host defense. Unlike the RBC, which resides exclusively within blood, granulocytes and monocytes generally pass through the blood on their way to the extravascular tissues, where they reside in large numbers; although it is now understood that senescent neutrophils that remain in the circulation return to the bone marrow through the SDF-1α/CXCR4 chemokine axis (Martin *et al.*, 2003).

Granulocytes are defined by the characteristics of their cytoplasmic granules as they appear on a blood smear stained with a polychromatic (Romanovsky) stain. Neutrophils, the largest component of blood leukocytes, are highly specialized in the mediation of inflammation and the ingestion and destruction of pathogenic microorganisms. The turnover of the neutrophil is enormous and increases dramatically in times of inflammation and infection, elevating the number of these cells released from the bone marrow. Eosinophils and basophils modulate inflammation through the release of various mediators and play an important role in other homeostatic functions. All these are influenced by humoral immunity, as discussed in greater detail in Chap. 12.

In the world of clinical and experimental toxicology, the neutrophil is the focus of concern when evaluating granulocytes

as possible targets for drug and nontherapeutic chemical effects. Eosinophils and basophils are far more difficult to study, with changes in these populations most frequently associated with reactions to other target organ or systemic toxicity. Examples include the eosinophilia observed with the toxic oil syndrome in northwestern Spain that resulted from exposure to rapeseed oil denatured with aniline (Kilbourne *et al.*, 1991); and the eosinophilia-myalgia syndrome associated with λ-tryptophan preparations contaminated with 1, 1-ethylidene-bis [tryptophan] (Varga *et al.*, 1992). Peripheral eosinophilia is often but not reliably observed with hypersensitivity reactions to drugs (Roujeau, 2005), while tissue eosinophilia can be diagnostic, in the context of a suggestive clinical course, in conditions such as drug-induced cutaneous vasculitis (Bahrami *et al.*, 2006) and eosinophilic pneumonia (Flieder and Travis, 2004). This variability in systemic response can be genetically predisposed, as demonstrated in studies using transgenic mice on genetic restrictions in people afflicted by the aforementioned toxic oil syndrome (Gallardo *et al.*, 2005). The time course of the reaction can also influence whether eosinophilia can be demonstrated in hypersensitivity disease (Roujeau, 2005).

Evaluation of Granulocytes

The most informative test to assess the neutrophil compartment is the blood neutrophil count. Accurate interpretation requires an understanding of neutrophil kinetics and the response of this tissue to physiologic and pathologic changes. In the blood, neutrophils are distributed between *circulating* and *marginated* pools, which are of equal size in humans and in constant equilibrium (Athens *et al.*, 1961). A blood neutrophil count assesses only the circulating pool, which remains between 1800 and 7500 μL^{-1} in a healthy adult human (Dale, 2006).

This constancy is remarkable, considering that as many as 10^{11} neutrophils are released from the marrow daily, and this circulating pool represents only 1% of the total body neutrophils (Semerad *et al.*, 2002), and that the circulating half life of these cells is only approximately 6 hours (Cartwright *et al.*, 1964). How this extraordinary regulation is achieved is only partially understood. Recent studies using knock-out mice suggest that G-CSF is an essential regulator of both granulopoiesis and neutrophil release from the bone marrow (Semerad *et al.*, 2002). It is induced by the T-cell derived cytokine IL-17 which, in turn, is controlled by IL-23 that is provided by dendritic cells and macrophages (Stark *et al.*, 2005). The latter is down regulated by the phagocytosis of apoptotic neutrophils in the tissues, which provides an important negative feedback loop. The up and down regulation of chemokine receptors further controls the release of neutrophils from the bone marrow (as discussed below) and their return following senescence (Martin *et al.*, 2003). Pharmaceutical companies are currently developing recombinant proteins that function as agonists and inhibitors of these mediators, which have great potential as exciting new therapies. Many will also be shown to cause unacceptable immunotoxicity and hematotoxicity, which portends exciting times for the academic and industrial hematopathologist and toxicologist.

Neutrophil kinetics and response to disease will vary substantially among animal species (Feldman, 2000). Thus, a thorough understanding of these features in any animal model used in investigative toxicology is required before informed interpretations can be made. In humans, clinically significant neutropenia occurs when the blood neutrophil count is less than 1000 μL^{-1}, but serious recurrent infections do not usually occur until counts fall below 500 μL^{-1}

(Dale, 2006). Morphologic assessment of peripheral blood granulocytes can be helpful in characterizing neutropenia. In humans and most healthy animal species, mature (segmented) and a few immature (band) neutrophils can be identified on blood films stained with Wright or Giemsa stain. During inflammation, a "shift to the left" may occur, which refers to an increased number of immature (nonsegmented) granulocytes in the peripheral blood, which may include bands, metamyelocytes, and occasionally myelocytes. During such times, neutrophils may also show "toxic" granulation, Döhle bodies, and cytoplasmic vacuoles. These morphologic changes may be prominent in sepsis or as a result of drug or chemical intoxication. In order to fully characterize such changes or understand the pathogenesis of the abnormality, bone marrow must be examined using marrow aspirates and biopsies. These provide information on rates of production, bone marrow reserves, abnormalities in cell distribution and occasionally specific clues as to etiology. In vitro stem cell assays may be used to assess the granulocyte progenitor cell compartment, which may include granulocyte-monocyte colony-forming cells (CFU-GM) performed in a semisolid medium, such as agar or methylcellulose, that contains appropriate growth factors, as discussed later in this chapter. Normal human marrow specimens contain approximately 50–1000 CFU-GM per 10^6 nucleated cells cultured (Liesveld and Lichtman, 1997). Marrow stem cell reserves can be assessed in vitro after administration of G-CSF (Demirer and Bensinger, 1995), which stimulates increased production and release of neutrophil precursors. Glucocorticoids (Peters *et al.*, 1972) and epinephrine (Babior and Golde, 1995) may also be used for this purpose but are rarely used in a clinical setting.

The recent understanding that the CXC-chemokine ligand CXCL12/CXCL4 mediates the retention of granulopoietic stem cells within their bone marrow niche (Laurence, 2006), as well as mature neutrophils within the bone marrow pool (Semerad *et al.*, 2002), has led to the development of an inhibitor of this ligand which, when administered with G-CSF, can cause a transient release of neutrophils and CD34+ (stem) cells into the circulation (Liles *et al.*, 2005). The latter can be collected and re-engrafted to form new functioning bone marrow (Broxmeyer *et al.*, 2005). The ability to manipulate this system in this way will likely provide important research, diagnostic and therapeutic tools for the hematologist, oncologist, and toxicologist.

The degree of proliferation in the granulocyte compartment can also be assessed using older techniques that employ ^{3}H-thymidine suicide assays or DNA binding dyes with fluorescence-activated cell sorting analyses (Keng, 1986).

Toxic Effects on Granulocytes

The toxicologist is concerned with the effect of xenobiotics on granulocytes as relates to proliferation (granulopoiesis) and kinetics, the extent to which a drug or chemical contaminant can impair the vital functions these cells perform, and how neutrophils mediate or exacerbate inflammatory disease or other target organ toxicity. The latter two areas are discussed in Chap. 12, as they relate to their role as important effector cells of the immune system. However, it is difficult to separate effects on granulopoiesis and neutrophil kinetics from that of function. Both are complex and highly regulated through an array of growth factors, chemokines, cytokines and interactions with monocytes, dendritic cells and lymphocytes in a bidirectional, multicompartmental manner (Nathan, 2006). Such complexity is not surprising, given the daunting task these cells perform, which is elegantly described in a recent review (Nathan, 2006): *"The [neu-*

trophil] must remain nonsticky as it hurtles through the arterial and arteriolar circulation; then it must squeeze through capillaries smaller in diameter than itself, without allowing collision, friction or distortion to activate it. A fraction of the population must adhere tightly enough to the normal endothelium of post-capillary venules to resist being washed away in the circulation, but loosely enough to roll while scouting for evidence of tissue damage and microbial infection. If such evidence is received, the cell must crawl to a boundary between endothelial cells, penetrate the junctions and the underlying basement membrane without damaging these structures, move up the chemotactic gradient and decide whether its original information remains valid. If the answer is negative, the cell must execute itself by apoptosis. If the answer is positive, the cell must attempt to engulf and destroy microbes. If it cannot locate microbes quickly, it must attempt to destroy them at a distance by releasing every weapon at its disposal." Many of the mediators and interactions that enable this feat have now become targets for the therapeutic dysregulation of these processes, which has led to the development of candidate drugs that may prove to be uniquely efficacious and/or toxic, as discussed below.

Effects on Proliferation   As with other hematopoietic tissue, the high rate of proliferation of neutrophils makes their progenitor and precursor granulocyte pool particularly susceptible to inhibitors of mitosis. Such effects by cytotoxic drugs are generally nonspecific, as they similarly affect cells of the dermis, gastrointestinal tract, and other rapidly dividing tissues. Chemicals that affect both neutrophils and monocytes pose a greater risk for toxic sequelae, such as infection (Dale, 2006). Such effects tend to be dose-related, with mononuclear phagocyte recovery preceding neutrophil recovery (Arneborn and Palmblad, 1982).

Myelotoxicity in clinical medicine and preclinical safety studies today is most commonly seen with cytoreductive cancer chemotherapy agents. The toxicity is often dose-limiting with the most serious manifestation being febrile neutropenia associated with life-threatening infections (Kuderer *et al.*, 2002). These chemicals vary in terms of their mechanism, the kinetics of the cytopenias they induce and how individual patients or animals respond. Most act to inhibit DNA synthesis or directly attack its integrity through the formation of DNA adducts or enzyme-mediated breaks (Chabner *et al.*, 2006). Whereas cytoreductive drugs like alkylating agents, cisplatin and nitrosureas can be toxic to both resting and actively dividing cells, nonproliferating cells such as metamyelocytes, bands and mature neutrophils are relatively resistant (Friberg and Karlsson, 2003). Generally, stem cells cycle slowly and are therefore minimally affected by a single administration of a cytotoxic drug like 5-fluorouracil; however, such exposure can stimulate cycling activity, making these cells more vulnerable to doses administered 3–5 days later (Harrison and Lerner, 1991). Cytokines have long been thought to enhance these effects by driving cells into the S phase (Smith *et al.*, 1994). Sustained exposure to drugs affecting slowly cycling stem cells are believed to cause more prolonged myelosuppression, similar to that observed with idiosyncratic toxic neutropenia (Tannock, 1986).

Finally, there is considerable variation among individuals as regards susceptibility to bone marrow toxicity; this can relate to how the drug is metabolized as with 5-fluorouracil (Sundman-Engberg *et al.*, 1998) and 6-mercaptopurine (Chabner *et al.*, 2006). Based on these and other data, including plasma drug concentrations, "semi-mechanistic" prarmacokinetic/pharmacodynamic models of myelosuppression have been developed to tailor doses and treatment regimens to individual patients (Friberg and Karlsson, 2003). Pharmacokinetic monitoring is now routinely performed with some anticancer treatment regimens, particularly high-dose methotrexate (Chabner *et al.*, 2006).

Two innovations have had a dramatic impact on cancer chemotherapy and the dose-limiting myelotoxicity associated with these drugs: 1) the development of drugs with cancer-cell-specific molecular targets that are relatively bone marrow sparing, such as those relating to aberrant growth factor receptor signaling, apoptosis or angiogenesis; and 2) the use of hematopoietic growth factors, the co-treatment with which mitigates or successfully rescues patients from the affects of myelosuppression. Most notable of the latter has been the development and application of the granulocyte colony stimulating factors (G-CSFs), filgrastim and the longer acting peg filgrastim, the action of which was discussed previously. Treatment with these recombinant proteins can substantially reduce the incidence, severity, and duration of neutropenia and its complications (Rader, 2006). Antagonists to the aforementioned chemokine ligand CXCR4 are also under development for treatment alone or in combination with G-CSF, which have been shown to be effective in mobilizing both stem cells and mature neutrophils (De Clercq, 2005; Larochelle *et al.*, 2006). Cytokine-induced differentiation therapy of leukemias is also emerging as an exciting treatment modality (Leung *et al.*, 2005). The prospect of exaggerated pharmacology and off-target effects of these sophisticated interventions should provide the preclinical toxicologist and oncologist with interesting hematotoxicologic challenges.

The effects of epinephrine and glucocorticoids on granulocyte kinetics were also referred to previously. Dexamethasone has long been known to cause neutrophilia through enhanced release of mature neutrophils from the bone marrow and demargination, with the latter being the largest contributor to the expanded circulating pool (Nakagawa *et al.*, 1998). It is now clear that the reduced margination of neutrophils is mediated by multiple effects, including altered chemotaxis, expression of adhesion molecules, and the release of mediators from other cells (Barnes, 2006; Caramori and Adcock, 2005). It is widely assumed that inhibition of margination and homing are among the important mechanisms of the anti-inflammatory and immunosuppressive effects of these widely-used drugs. The development of drugs with more selective effects on neutrophils is among the most active areas of investigative pharmacology and toxicology today.

Lindane, an insecticide used to treat seeds and soil, has been associated with leukopenia (Parent-Massin *et al.*, 1994). It is cytotoxic for human CFU-GMs at concentrations observed in blood and adipose tissue from exposed human subjects. An example of chemicals affecting mature cells is methylmethacrylate monomer, which has been used in orthopedic surgical procedures and is cytotoxic to both neutrophils and monocytes at clinically relevant concentrations (Dahl *et al.*, 1994).

Effects on Function While there are a variety of disorders associated with defects in the parameters of neutrophil function discussed above, demonstrable in vivo effects associated with drugs and nontherapeutic chemicals are surprisingly few (Borregaard and Boxer, 2006). Examples include ethanol and glucocorticoids, which impair phagocytosis and microbe ingestion in vitro and in vivo (Brayton *et al.*, 1970). Iohexol and ioxaglate, components of radiographic contrast media, have also been reported to inhibit phagocytosis

(Lillevang *et al.*, 1994). Superoxide production, required for microbial killing and chemotaxis, has been reported to be reduced in patients using parenteral heroin as well as in former opiate abusers on long-term methadone maintenance (Mazzone *et al.*, 1994).

In addition to glucocorticoids, several drugs and nontherapeutic chemicals have been shown to inhibit neutrophil chemotaxis. Examples include macrolide antibiotics, which suppress the expression of the adhesion molecule ICAM (Tamaoki, 2004); zinc salts, which are found in antiacne preparations (Dreno *et al.*, 1992); the inorganic pollutant chlordane (Miyagi *et al.*, 1998), and mercuric chloride/methylmecuric chloride (Contrino *et al.*, 1988). More common is the activation of neutrophils with the potential for proinflammatory consequences, specifically through increased phagocytosis, O_2^- production or both. Examples include the environmental contaminants sodium sulfite, mercuric chloride, chlordane and toxaphene (Girard, 2003). This toxicologic potential of xenobiotics will be discussed in more detail in Chap. 12.

Idiosyncratic Toxic Neutropenia Of greater concern are chemicals that unexpectedly damage neutrophils and granulocyte precursors—particularly to the extent of inducing *agranulocytosis*, which is characterized by a profound depletion in blood neutrophils to less than 500 μL^{-1} (Pisciotta, 1973). Such injury occurs in specifically conditioned individuals, and is therefore termed "idiosyncratic." Mechanisms of idiosyncratic damage often do not relate to pharmacologic properties of the parent drug, which makes managing this risk a particular challenge to hematologists and toxicologists, as discussed later in this chapter. Preclinical toxicology is rarely predictive of these effects, which are generally detected and characterized following exposure of a large population to the chemical (Dieckhaus *et al.*, 2002; Szarfman *et al.*, 2002). Idiosyncratic drug-induced neutropenia may be dose-related and involve a nonselective disruption of protein synthesis or cell replication resulting in agranulocytosis, as discussed below. Alternatively, it may not be dose dependent, in which case it is usually thought to be allergic or immunologic in origin. The latter has been observed with many drugs, and is more frequently observed in women, older patients, and patients with a history of allergies (Dale, 2006).

Idiosyncratic xenobiotic-induced agranulocytosis may involve a sudden depletion of circulating neutrophils concomitant with exposure, which may persist as long as the chemical or its metabolites persist in the circulation. Hematopoietic function is usually restored when the chemical is detoxified or excreted. Suppression of granulopoiesis, however, is more prevalent than peripheral lysis of neutrophils and is asymptomatic unless sepsis supervenes (Pisciotta, 1973). The onset of leukopenia in the former is more gradual, but may be precipitous if lysis of circulating neutrophils also occurs. The pattern of the disease varies with the stage of granulopoiesis affected, which has been well defined for several agents that cause bone marrow toxicity (Table 11-7). Toxicants affecting uncommitted stem cells induce total marrow failure, as seen in aplastic anemia, which generally carries a worse prognosis than chemicals affecting more differentiated precursors, such as CFU-G. It is thought that, in the latter case, surviving uncommitted stem cells eventually produce recovery, provided that the risk of infection is successfully managed during the leukopenic episodes (Pisciotta, 1973).

The incidence of drug-induced idiosyncratic agranulocytosis ranges from 2–15 cases per million patients exposed to drugs per year (Andres *et al.*, 2002). The severity of the neutropenia often causes severe sepsis or localized infections, such as sore throat,

Table 11-7

Stages of Granulocytopoiesis: Site of Xenobiotic-Induced Cellular Damage

STAGE OF DEVELOPMENT	DISEASE	OFFENDING DRUGS
Uncommitted (totipotential) stem cell	Aplastic anemia	Chloramphenicol
CFU-S		Gold salts
		Phenylbutazone
		Phenytoin
		Mephenytoin
		Carbamazepine
Committed stem cell	Aplastic anemia	Carbamazepine
	Agranulocytosis	Chlorpromazine
CFU-G		Carbamazepine
		Clozapine
CFU-E	Pure red cell aplasia	
BFU-E		Phenytoin
Morphologically recognizable precursors	Hypoplastic marrow	Most cancer chemo—therapy agents
Dividing pool	Hypoplastic marrow	Chloramphenicol
Promyelocyte		Alcohol
Myelocyte		
Nondividing pool	Agranulocytosis	Clozapine
Metamyelocytes, bands		Phenothiazines, etc.
PMNs		
Peripheral blood lysis	Agranulocytosis	Clozapine, etc.
PMNs		Aminopyrine
Tissue pool		

Modified from Pisciotta AV: Response of granulocytes to toxic injury, in Sipes IG, McQueen CA, Gandolfi AJ (eds.): *Comprehensive Toxicology*. Vol 4. Oxford, England: Pergamon Press, 1997, pp. 146, with permission from Elsevier Science.

pneumonia or various cutaneous infections. While all drugs may be causative, the most commonly incriminated drugs include antithyroid drugs and antibiotics, particularly sulfonamides (Andres *et al.*, 2002; Berliner *et al.*, 2004). Some drugs commonly implicated in the past, such as phenylbutazone, chloramphenicol and ticlopidine, are used less commonly today due to this and other toxicities. Prior to the use of hematopoietic growth factors, the mortality was 10–20% (Julia *et al.*, 1991); with appropriate management it is now approximately 5% (Andres *et al.*, 2002).

Clozapine-induced agranulocytosis is unique, as a genetic predisposition has been established (Turbay *et al.*, 1997; Yunis *et al.*, 1995). Prior to an aggressive risk management program that included careful screening of prospective patients and early detection through hematologic monitoring, the incidence of agranulocytosis with this highly efficacious atypical antipsychotic was as high as 1–2%. This measure reduced the incidence to 0.38% and the mortality by 90% (Honigfeld *et al.*, 1998).

Mechanisms of Toxic Neutropenia   Because cases of drug-induced neutropenia are relatively rare, sporadic or transient, studies on the pathogenesis of this hematotoxicity have been limited. Toxic neutropenia may be classified according to mechanism as *immune-mediated* or *nonimmune-mediated*. The incidence of xenobiotic-induced immune neutropenia, is considerably less than that of immune hemolytic anemias (Vandendries and Drews, 2006). In immune-mediated neutropenia, antigen-antibody reactions lead to destruction of peripheral neutrophils, granulocyte precursors, or

both. As with RBCs, an immunogenic xenobiotic can act as a hapten, where the chemical must be physically present to cause cell damage, or may induce immunogenic cells to produce antineutrophil antibodies that do not require the drug to be present (Salama *et al.*, 1989). Also like immune hemolytic anemia, drug-induced *autoimmune* neutropenia has been observed (Capsoni *et al.*, 2005). Examples of chemicals that have been implicated include fludarabine (Stern *et al.*, 1999), propylthiouracil (Sato *et al.*, 1985), and rituximab (Voog *et al.*, 2003). Xenobiotic-induced immune-mediated damage may also be cell-mediated (Pisciotta, 1973).

Detection of xenobiotic induced neutrophil antibodies is also considerably more difficult than those of RBCs or platelets. This is because the neutrophil is relatively fragile, short-lived and becomes easily activated (Palmblad *et al.*, 2001). There is no good test for direct antigranulocyte antibodies comparable to the Coombs' (antiglobulin) test. Several assays have been used, which can be grouped into four categories: those measuring endpoints of leukoagglutination, cytotoxic inhibition of neutrophil function, immunoglobulin binding and those using cell-mediated mechanisms. Among the specific challenges these assays pose are the tendency of neutrophils to stick to each other in vitro, attract immunoglobulin nonspecifically to their surface, and reflect membrane damage through indirect and semi quantitative changes (Pisciotta, 1973). The reader is referred elsewhere for a more detailed discussion of assays for immune-mediated neutrophil damage (Hagen *et al.*, 1993; Nifli *et al.*, 2006; Palmblad *et al.*, 2001).

Some nonimmune-mediated toxic neutropenias have long been known to have a genetic predisposition (Pisciotta, 1973). Direct

Table 11-8

Examples of Toxicants That Cause Immune and Non-immune Idiopathic Neutropenia

DRUGS ASSOCIATED WITH WBC ANTIBODIES	DRUGS NOT ASSOCIATED WITH WBC ANTIBODIES
Aminopyrine	INH
Propylthiouracil	Rifampicin
Ampicillin	Ethambutol
Metiamide	Allopurinol
Dicloxacillin	Phenothiazines/CPZ
Phenytoin	Flurazepam
Aprindine	HCTZ
Azulfidine	
Chlorpropamide	
CPZ/Phenothiazines	
Procainamide	
Nafcillin	
Tolbutamide	
Lidocaine	
Methimazole	
Levamisole	
Gold	
Quinidine	
Clozapine	

Modified from Pisciotta AV: Response of granulocytes to toxic injury, in Sipes IG, McQueen CA, Gandolfi AJ (eds.): *Comprehensive Toxicology*. Vol 4. Oxford, England: Pergamon Press, 1997, pp. 150, with permission from Elsevier Science.

damage may cause inhibition of granulopoiesis or neutrophil function. It may entail failure to detoxify or excrete a xenobiotic or its metabolites, which subsequently build up to toxic proportions (Gerson and Meltzer, 1992; Gerson et al., 1983; Uetrecht, 1990). Some studies suggest that a buildup of toxic oxidants generated by leukocytes can result in neutrophil damage, as with the reactive intermediates derived from the interaction between clozapine and neutrophils. The resulting superoxide and hypochlorous acid production by the myeloperoxidase system are thought to contribute to clozapine-induced neutropenia (Uetrecht, 1990). Accumulation of nitrenium ion, a metabolite of clozapine which causes a depletion of ATP and a reduction of glutathione, rendering the neutrophil highly susceptible to oxidant-induced apoptosis, is now thought to be the principal mechanism of this disorder (Williams et al., 2000).

Examples of chemicals associated with immune and nonimmune neutropenia/ agranulocytosis are listed in Table 11-8.

LEUKEMOGENESIS AS A TOXIC RESPONSE

Human Leukemias

Leukemias are proliferative disorders of hematopoietic tissue that are monoclonal in origin and thus originate from individual bone marrow cells. Historically they have been classified as myeloid or lymphoid, referring to the major lineages for erythrocytes/granulocytes/thrombocytes or lymphocytes, respectively. Because the degree of leukemic cell differentiation has also loosely correlated with the rate of disease progression, poorly differentiated phenotypes have been designated as "acute," whereas well-differentiated ones are referred to as "chronic" leukemias. The classification of human leukemias proposed by the French-American-

British (FAB) Cooperative Group has become convention, based on the above and other morphologic features (Bennett and Sanger, 1982; Bennett et al., 1985; Levine and Bloomfield, 1992). It provides the diagnostic framework for classifying chronic lymphocytic leukemia (CLL), chronic myelogenous leukemia (CML), acute lymphoblastic leukemia (ALL), acute myelogenous leukemia (AML), and the myelodysplastic syndromes (MDS), along with various subtypes of these disorders. The WHO has incorporated into these parameters more recent discoveries regarding the genetics and phenotypic features of disorders like AML in order to define subtypes that are biologically homogenous and that have prognostic and therapeutic relevance (Altucci et al., 2005). These early correlations imply that the biology and clinical features of these proliferative disorders relate to the stage of differentiation of the target cell, which is now being linked to individual gene alterations, as well as epigenetic factors such as cytokine stimulation (Altucci et al., 2005; Look, 2005).

There is considerable evidence supporting the notion that leukemogenesis is a multievent progression (Look, 2005; Pedersen-Bjergaard et al., 1995; Varmus and Weinberg, 1993; Vogelstein et al., 1988; Williams and Whitaker, 1990). These studies suggest that factors involved in the regulation of hematopoiesis also influence neoplastic transformation. Such factors include cellular growth factors (cytokines), protooncogenes and other growth-promoting genes, as well as additional genetic and epigenetic factors that govern survival, proliferation, and differentiation.

Mechanisms of Toxic Leukemogenesis

The understanding that certain chemicals and radiation can dysregulate hematopoiesis, resulting in leukemogenesis, is a relatively recent one. While suggested by Hunter as early as 1939, following his observations on benzene exposure and AML (Hunter, 1939), it was not until the introduction of radiation and chemotherapy as treatments for neoplasia that these agents became associated with blood dyscrasias that included (or led to) AML (Andersen et al., 1981; Casciato and Scott, 1979; Foucar et al., 1979). The notion emerged that myelotoxic chemicals, under certain circumstances, can be leukemogenic.

Curiously, AML is the dominant leukemia associated with drug or chemical exposure, followed by MDS (Andersen et al., 1981; Casciato and Scott, 1979; Irons, 1997). The evidence that this represents a continuum of one toxic response is compelling (Irons, 1997; Look, 2005). This has also been linked to cytogenetic abnormalities, particularly nonrandom deletions that include $7q^-$, $5q^-$, $20q^-$, $6q^-$, $11q^-$, and 13^-, which activate tumor suppressor genes required for normal myeloid cell development (Bench et al., 1998). The frequency of at least one of these deletions in patients who develop MDS and/or AML after treatment with alkylating or other antineoplastic chemicals has historically run from 67–95% , depending on the study (Bitter et al., 1987; Johansson et al., 1991; Le Beau et al., 1986; Pedersen-Bjergaard et al., 1984; Rowley et al., 1981). The cytogenetic classification known as *complex karyotypes*, or complex chromosomal aberrations (CCAs, defined as more than 3 aberrations), has been shown to occur in up to 50% of therapy-related AML and MDS cases (Mauritzson et al., 2000; Rossi et al., 2000). CAAs are also associated with the most unfavorable prognosis among the subtypes of MDS and AML (Look, 2005).

Larson and LeBeau reported the results of cytogenetic analyses on 306 consecutive patients with treatment-related AML, which were largely consistent with the above understandings (Larson and

Hypothetical Changes Occurring During the Evolution of Secondary AML

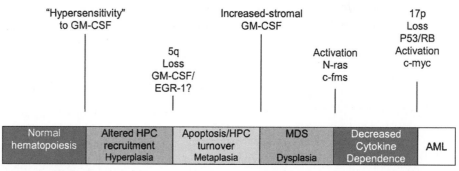

Figure 11-7. Hypothetical model for the evolution of s-AML involving 5q-. Schematic representation of one model for tumor progression consistent with frequently observed events in the development of AML secondary to drug or chemical exposure. Altered myeloid progenitor cell proliferation leads to increased division in the target cell population, which results in clonal loss of heterozygosity due to nondysjunction (e.g., 5q-). The resulting haploinsufficiency of a gene, such as GM-CSF, results in increased cell turnover, abnormal maturation, and ineffective hematopoiesis (i.e., MDS) in the abnormal clone. This is subsequently followed by activation of additional proto-oncogenes that result in progressive growth and survival independence in successive subclones and the development of overt AML. [Adapted from Irons (1997), with permission from Elsevier Science.]

Le Beau, 2005; Look, 2005). They went on, however, to perform gene expression profiling of CD34+ hematopoietic progenitor cells from these patients, through which they were able to identify distinct subtypes of AML with characteristic gene expressions. Not surprisingly, these early progenitor cells showed expression patterns typical of arrested differentiation. Through this work they positioned treatment-related AML as an important model that provides a unique opportunity to examine the effects of mutagens on carcinogenesis in humans, as well as the role of genetic susceptibility.

Some of the same chromosomal deletion changes described with treatment-related AML have been observed in AML patients occupationally exposed to benzene (Bitter et al, 1987; Cuneo *et al.*, 1992; Fagioli *et al.*, 1992; Golomb *et al.*, 1982; Mitelman *et al.*, 1978, 1981), who also show aneuploidy with a high frequency of involvement of chromosome 7 (Irons, 1997). Molecular mechanisms for benzene-induced hematotoxicity, which include both leukemogenesis and aplastic anemia (Hoffmann *et al.*, 2001), are thought to include the bioactivation of reactive metabolites (Powley and Carlson, 2001), the formation of reactive oxygen species (Kolachana *et al.*, 1993), and activation of the aryl hydrocarbon receptor (AhR) and the oncogene C-Myb (Wan *et al.*, 2005). Recent studies have also suggested that polymorphisms in genes involved in DNA double strand break repair might influence susceptibility to these effects (Shen *et al.*, 2006). The relatively low frequency of deletions in chromosomes 5 and 7 in de novo, as compared with secondary AML, have made these cytogenetic markers useful in discriminating between toxic exposures and other etiologies of this leukemia. These observations, together with the understandings on the pathogenesis of leukemia previously discussed, have further corroborated the model proposed by Irons ten years ago for the evolution of toxic leukemogenesis, which is illustrated in Fig. 11-7 (Irons, 1997).

Other forms of leukemia—including CML, CLL, ALL, and multiple myeloma—have shown weak correlations with occupational exposure or treatment with alkylating agents (Irons, 1997). The latter has been repeatedly associated with exposure to benzene,

although a causal relationship has yet to be demonstrated (Bergsagel *et al.*, 1999).

Leukemogenic Agents

The overwhelming majority of toxic or secondary leukemias seen today are therapy-related (Godley and Larson, 2001). Putative chemicals can be classified by mechanism, as discussed previously, and include alkylating agents, topoisomerase II inhibitors, antimetabolite and antitubulin drugs. The clinical syndrome is a late complication of these cytotoxic therapies, with a latency period between primary diagnosis and treatment-related disease ranging from months to years. While the morphologic abnormalities may vary (Godley and Larson, 2001; Jaffe, 2001; Thirman and Larson, 1996), there is a continuum in the percentage of marrow blasts from a myelodysplastic syndrome to overt AML (Larson and Le Beau, 2005).

Most *alkylating agents* used in cancer chemotherapy can cause MDS and/or AML, including cyclophosphamide, melphalan, busulfan, chlorambucil, and nitrosurea compounds such as carmustine, or BCNU (Casciato and Scott, 1979; Greene *et al.*, 1986). Other oncolytic agents implicated include azathioprine, procarbazine, doxorubicin, and bleomycin (Carver *et al.*, 1979; Valagussa *et al.*, 1979; Vismans *et al.*, 1980). The risk these drugs pose varies considerably with the therapeutic regimen. The incidence of MDS/AML in patients treated with alkylating agents has been reported to be 0.6–17%, with an average of 100-fold relative risk. Moreover, treatment-related MDS is associated with a substantially higher rate of transformation to AML than is primary or spontaneous MDS (Bitter *et al.*, 1987; Kantarjian *et al.*, 1986).

Treatment with *topoisomerase II inhibitors*, particularly the epipodophyllotoxins etoposide and teniposide, can induce AML, the clinical course of which has the following distinguishing characteristics: (1) the absence of a preleukemic phase, (2) a short latency period, (3) frequent involvement of an M4/5 subtype, and (4) balanced chromosome aberrations involving chromosomes 11q23 and 21q22, among others (Larson and Le Beau, 2005;

Murphy, 1993). Similar cytogenetic features have been observed following treatment with doxorubicin or dactinomycin (intercalating topoisomerase II inhibitors) in conjunction with alkylating agents and irradiation (Sandoval *et al.*, 1993).

Of the *aromatic hydrocarbons*, only benzene has been proven to be leukemogenic. While substituted aromatic hydrocarbons have long been suspected to be causative, due to the fact that preparations of xylene and toluene in the past contained as much as 20% benzene (Browning, 1965), clinical or experimental evidence for that is lacking (Irons, 1997).

Exposure to *high-dose γ- or x-ray radiation* has long been associated with ALL, AML, and CML, as demonstrated in survivors of the atom bombings of Nagasaki and Hiroshima (Cartwright *et al.*, 1964; Shimizu *et al.*, 1989). Less clear is the association of these diseases with low-dose radiation secondary to fallout or diagnostic radiographs (Cartwright *et al.*, 1964).

Other *controversial agents* include 1,3-butadiene, nonionizing radiation (electromagnetic, microwave, infrared, visible, and the high end of the ultraviolet spectrum), and cigarette smoking, for which published studies on the relationship to leukemia incidence is confusing, contradictory, or difficult to interpret based on dose response (Irons, 1997). Data suggesting that formaldehyde may be leukemogenic in humans has also been recently reviewed (Golden *et al.*, 2006). The results were similarly inconclusive.

TOXICOLOGY OF PLATELETS AND HEMOSTASIS

Hemostasis is a multicomponent system responsible for preventing the loss of blood from sites of vascular injury and maintaining circulating blood in a fluid state. Loss of blood is prevented by formation of stable hemostatic plugs mediated by the procoagulant arm of hemostasis. This procoagulant response is normally limited to sites of vascular injury by the multicomponent regulatory arm of hemostasis. The dynamically modulated balance between procoagulant and regulatory pathways permits a rapid, localized response to injury. The major constituents of the hemostatic system include circulating platelets, a variety of plasma proteins, and vascular endothelial cells. More recently the role of other cells in hemostasis, especially leukocytes, has become apparent (Lane *et al.*, 2005; Monroe and Hoffman, 2005). Alterations in these components or systemic activation of this system can lead to the clinical manifestations of deranged hemostasis, including excessive bleeding and thrombosis. The hemostatic system is a frequent target of therapeutic intervention as well as inadvertent expression of the toxic effect of a variety of xenobiotics. This section briefly reviews the inadvertent effects of xenobiotics on hemostasis and the toxic effects of agents used to manipulate the hemostatic system.

Toxic Effects on Platelets

The Thrombocyte Platelets are essential for formation of a stable hemostatic plug in response to vascular injury. Platelets initially adhere to the damaged wall through binding of von Willebrand factor (vWF) with the platelet glycoprotein Ib/IX/V (GP Ib/IX/V) receptor complex (Jurk and Kehrel, 2005). Ligand binding to GP Ib/IX/V or interaction of other platelet agonists (e.g., thrombin, collagen, ADP, thromboxane A_2) with their specific receptors initiates biochemical response pathways that lead to shape change, platelet contraction, platelet secretion of granule contents, activation of the GP IIb/IIIa receptor, and externalization of phosphatidylserine (Jurk and Kehrel,

2005). Activation of the GP IIb/IIIa receptor permits fibrinogen and other multivalent adhesive molecules to form cross-links between nearby platelets, resulting in platelet aggregation (Jurk and Kehrel, 2005). Xenobiotics may interfere with the platelet response by causing thrombocytopenia or interfering with platelet function; some chemicals are capable of affecting both platelet number and function.

Thrombocytopenia Like anemia, thrombocytopenia may be due to decreased production or increased destruction. Thrombocytopenia is a common side effect of intensive chemotherapy, due to the predictable effect of antiproliferative drugs on hematopoietic precursors, including those of the megakaryocytic lineage. Thrombocytopenia is a clinically significant component of idiosyncratic xenobiotic-induced aplastic anemia. Indeed, the initial manifestation of aplastic anemia may be mucocutaneous bleeding secondary to thrombocytopenia.

Exposure to xenobiotics may cause increased immune-mediated platelet destruction through any one of several mechanisms (Table 11-9) (Aster, 2005; van den Bemt *et al.*, 2004). Some drugs function as haptens, binding to platelet membrane components and eliciting an immune response that is specific for the hapten. The responding antibody then binds to the hapten on the platelet surface, leading to removal of the antibody-coated platelet from the circulation. This type of antibody interaction can often be blocked in vitro by excess soluble drug that binds to the antibody and prevents its interaction with the platelet surface (van den Bemt *et al.*, 2004).

A second mechanism of immune thrombocytopenia is initiated by xenobiotic-induced exposure of a neoepitope on a platelet membrane glycoprotein. This elicits an antibody response, with the responding antibody binding to this altered platelet antigen in the presence of drug, resulting in removal of the platelet from the circulation by the mononuclear phagocytic system. The epitope specificity can be quite selective, as there is often little or no cross-reactivity between drugs having a very similar structure (e.g., quinine and quinidine). This type of interaction is not inhibited in vitro by excess soluble drug, as the antibody target is a platelet-dependent epitope. Quinidine is a prototype of this type of mechanism and can induce antibodies directed at GP Ib/IX/V, GP IIb/IIIa and/or platelet endothelial cell adhesion molecule-1 (PECAM-1) (van den Bemt *et al.*, 2004).

The diagnosis of drug-dependent antiplatelet antibodies can be quite difficult. A number of assays have been described for measurement of platelet-associated immunoglobulin, but the sensitivity and specificity of these assays have not been established. Therefore, these assays are not used in routine clinical practice. Consequently, the diagnosis is usually established by observing the resolution of thrombocytopenia following discontinuation of the offending drug. In most cases, the platelet count returns to normal within 5–10 days of drug discontinuation. Although a large number of chemicals have been implicated in the development of immune thrombocytopenia, the supporting evidence in many cases is weak (van den Bemt *et al.*, 2004).

Thrombocytopenia is an uncommon but serious complication of inhibitors of GP IIb/IIIa such as abciximab (Huxtable *et al.*, 2006). The mechanism appears to be related to exposure of epitopes on GP IIb/IIIa that react with naturally occurring antibodies. Because the reaction is dependent on antibodies formed prior to exposure to drug, it may occur shortly after the first exposure to the drug. Ligand binding is known to alter the conformation of GP IIb/IIIa.

Table 11-9
Mechanism of Immune-Mediated Thrombocytopenia

MECHANISM	PROTOTYPIC AGENT	ANTIGEN/EPITOPE	PLATELET EFFECT	CLINICAL EFFECT
Hapten-directed antibody	Penicillin	Drug	Opsonization ↑ Clearance	Bleeding
Acquired antibody to drug-induced epitope	Quinidine	Drug-GP Ib/IX/V Drug-GP IIb/IIIa	Opsonization ↑ Clearance	Bleeding
Natural antibody to drug-induced epitope	Abciximab	GP IIb/IIIa	Opsonization ↑ Clearance	Bleeding
Induction of autoimmune antibodies	Gold	Platelet membrane	Opsonization ↑ Clearance	Bleeding
Immune complex	Heparin	PF 4–heparin complex	Platelet activation and aggregation ↑ Clearance	Thrombosis
Thrombotic thrombocytopenic purpura (TTP)	Ticlopidine	VWF-cleaving protease	Platelet activation Platelet aggregation ↑ Clearance	Microvascular thrombosis Microangiopathic hemolytic anemia
Hemolytic-uremic syndrome	Mitomycin	Unknown	Platelet activation and aggregation ↑ Clearance	Microvascular thrombosis Microangiopathic hemolytic anemia Renal failure

The GP IIb/IIIa inhibitors bind at the ligand binding site and also cause a conformational change in GP IIb/IIIa, permitting naturally occurring antibodies to bind to and initiate clearance of platelets by the mononuclear phagocytic system.

Heparin-induced thrombocytopenia (HIT) represents another mechanism of immune-mediated platelet destruction. This disorder is due to the development of antibodies that react with a multimolecular complex formed by the interaction between heparin and a protein, usually platelet factor 4 (PF 4) (Davoren and Aster, 2006; Warkentin and Greinacher, 2004). When the relative concentration of heparin to PF 4 is appropriate, formation of this complex is associated with exposure of a neoepitope on PF 4 (or another target protein) and development of an IgG response to the neoepitope. The IgG then binds to the PF 4-heparin complex to form an immune complex that binds to the platelet Fc receptor, FcγRIIa. Clustering of platelet FcγRIIa by the immune complex activates biochemical signaling pathways mediated by the cytoplasmic domain of FcγRIIa. This results in platelet activation and aggregation. During the process of platelet activation, platelet microparticles that promote thrombin generation are released. Consequently, HIT is associated with both thrombocytopenia and an increased risk of arterial and venous thrombosis. Other drug-antibody complexes (e.g., streptokinase-IgG) may trigger platelet activation and thrombocytopenia through a similar mechanism (Deckmyn et al., 1998; McRedmond et al., 2000).

Thrombotic thrombocytopenic purpura (TTP) is a syndrome characterized by the sudden onset of thrombocytopenia, a microangiopathic hemolytic anemia, and multisystem organ failure, which often includes neurologic dysfunction. The syndrome tends to occur following an infectious disease but may also occur following administration of some drugs. The pathogenesis of TTP appears to be related to the ability of unusually large vWF multimers to activate platelets, even in the absence of significant vascular damage (Lian, 2005). Although these large multimers are normally secreted into blood by endothelial cells, they are rapidly processed into smaller multimers by a protease (ADAMTS13) present in plasma. Acquired TTP is associated with the development of an antibody that inhibits this protease, permitting the very large vWF multimers to persist in the circulation (Lian, 2005; Veyradier and Meyer, 2005). Consequently, these multimers bind to platelet GP Ib/IX/V and induce platelet activation and aggregation. The organ failure and hemolysis in TTP is due to the formation of platelet-rich microthrombi throughout the circulation. The development of TTP or TTP-like syndromes has been associated with drugs such as ticlopidine, clopidogrel, cocaine, mitomycin, and cyclosporine (Veyradier and Meyer, 2005; Zakarija and Bennett, 2005). In some cases, drug-induced TTP is related to development of antibodies to ADAMTS13; whereas in other cases it may be due to direct endothelial cell toxicity from the drug.

The hemolytic uremic syndrome (HUS) is a disorder characterized by clinical features similar to those of TTP, with microangiopathic hemolytic anemia, thrombocytopenia, and renal failure (Zakarija and Bennett, 2005). Neurologic complications tend to be less severe, while renal failure often dominates the clinical picture. Sporadic cases of HUS have been linked to infection with verocytotoxin-producing Escherichia coli, but they may also occur during therapy with some drugs, including mitomycin. In contrast to TTP, the vWF-cleaving protease is normal in patients with HUS (Furlan et al., 1998). The pathogenesis of the thrombocytopenia and microangiopathic changes in HUS is still uncertain, but there is experimental evidence suggesting that it is related to endothelial cell injury, with subsequent platelet activation and thrombus formation.

Desmopressin, a vasopressin analog, is an example of nonimmune-mediated increased platelet destruction. Desmopressin induces a two- to five-fold increase in the plasma concentration of vWF and factor VIII. It is commonly used in the treatment of patients with von Willebrand's disease and other mild bleeding syndromes. Desmopressin has been associated with the development or accentuation of thrombocytopenia in some patients with type 2B von Willebrand disease. The thrombocytopenia in such cases is related to the release of an abnormal vWF from endothelial cells. The abnormal vWF has enhanced affinity for GP Ib/IX/V and the interaction of the vWF with its receptor leads to platelet clearance from the circulation (Mannucci, 1998).

Toxic Effects on Platelet Function Platelet function is dependent on the coordinated interaction of a number of biochemical response pathways. A variety of drugs and foods have been found to inhibit platelet function, either in vivo or in vitro (Abrams, 2006). Major drug groups that affect platelet function include nonsteroidal anti-inflammatory agents, β-lactam-containing antibiotics, cardiovascular drugs, particularly beta blockers, psychotropic drugs, anesthetics, antihistamines, and some chemotherapeutic agents. The effect of these drugs can vary between individuals, perhaps due to subclinical variations in underlying platelet function.

Xenobiotics may interfere with platelet function through a variety of mechanisms. Some drugs inhibit the phospholipase A_2/cyclooxygenase pathway and synthesis of thromboxane A_2 (e.g., nonsteroidal anti-inflammatory agents). Other chemicals appear to interfere with the interaction between platelet agonists and their receptors (e.g., antibiotics, ticlopidine, clopidogrel). As the platelet response is dependent on a rapid increase in cytoplasmic calcium, any agent that interferes with translocation of calcium may inhibit platelet function (e.g., calcium channel blockers). Occasionally, drug-induced antibodies will bind to a critical platelet receptor and inhibit its function. The functional defect induced by such antibodies may potentiate the bleeding risk associated with the xenobiotic-induced thrombocytopenia. In some cases, the mechanism of inhibition is not known.

The effect of xenobiotics on platelet function can often be studied following in vitro exposure of platelets to the agent of interest. However, evaluation following in vivo exposure is preferred, as metabolites of the parent compound may contain the platelet inhibitory activity. The most common method of assessing platelet function is turbidometric platelet aggregation using platelet-rich plasma, but alternate techniques are available, including the PFA 100 analyzer, flow cytometry, and whole-blood impedance aggregometry (Cesar et al., 2005; Matzdorff, 2005).

Toxic Effects on Fibrin Clot Formation

Coagulation Fibrin clot formation is the result of sequential activation of a series of serine proteases that culminates in the formation of thrombin (Lane et al., 2005; Monroe and Hoffman, 2005). Thrombin is a multifunctional enzyme that converts fibrinogen to fibrin; activates factors V, VIII, XI, XIII, protein C, and platelets; and interacts with a variety of cells (e.g., leukocytes and endothelial cells), activating cellular signaling pathways (Lane et al., 2005).

The most common toxic effects of xenobiotics on fibrin clot formation are related to a decreased level of one or more of the critical proteins necessary for this process. The decrease in clotting factor activity may be due to decreased synthesis of the protein(s) or increased clearance from the circulation. Decreased synthesis is most often a reflection of hepatocellular damage or interference with vitamin K metabolism, as discussed below, whereas increased clearance is usually associated with the development of an antibody to a specific coagulation factor.

Decreased Synthesis of Coagulation Proteins The majority of proteins involved in the coagulation cascade are synthesized in the

Table 11-10

Conditions Associated with Abnormal Synthesis of Vitamin K—Dependent Coagulation Factors

Warfarin and analogues	Intravenous α-tocopherol
Rodenticides (e.g., brodifacoum)	Dietary deficiency
	Cholestyramine resin
Broad-spectrum antibiotics	Malabsorption syndromes
N-methyl-thiotetrazole cephalosporins	

liver. Therefore, any chemical that impairs liver function may cause a decrease in production of coagulation factors. The common tests of the coagulation cascade, the prothrombin time (PT) and activated partial thromboplastin time (aPTT), may be used to screen for liver dysfunction and a decrease in clotting factors. These assays are often performed as part of the safety evaluation of a new chemical entity. The half-life of clotting factors in the circulation varies significantly, with factor VII having the shortest half-life (3–4 hours). Therefore, with acute toxicity (e.g., acetaminophen overdose), the effect on blood coagulation may be first seen as a decrease in the level of factor VII. Such a decrease would lead to prolongation of the PT with a normal aPTT. With a more chronic process, the PT, the aPTT or both may be affected.

Factors II, VII, IX, and X are dependent on vitamin K for their complete synthesis (Stafford, 2005). Anything that interferes with vitamin K metabolism may lead to a deficiency of these factors and a bleeding tendency. This may occur with chemicals that interfere with absorption of vitamin K from the intestine or with chemicals that interfere with the reduction of vitamin K epoxide (Table 11-10). The combination of antibiotic therapy and limited oral intake is a common cause of acquired deficiency of vitamin K-dependent proteins among hospitalized patients (Chakraverty et al., 1996). The "super rodenticides" are another cause of acquired vitamin K deficiency (Berry et al., 2000; Chua and Friedenberg, 1998). These chemicals have a very prolonged half-life in vivo; thus the coagulation defect may persist for weeks or months following exposure. Rodenticide exposure may occur accidentally, as part of a Munchausen syndrome, in association with a suicide attempt, or as part of a homicide attempt. At times it may be important to distinguish between a true vitamin K deficiency and interference with the reduction of vitamin K epoxide. This is most readily accomplished by quantifying the level of vitamin K and vitamin K epoxide in serum or plasma. In the case of vitamin K deficiency, vitamin K and vitamin K epoxide are both decreased; whereas in the case of inhibition of vitamin K reduction, vitamin K epoxide is significantly increased. Specific rodenticides may be measured using HPLC techniques, but it is important to specify which active agent (e.g., brodifacoum) should be measured, as the assays may not show cross-reactivity between chemicals.

Increased Clearance of Coagulation Factors Idiosyncratic reactions to xenobiotics include the formation of antibodies that react with coagulation proteins. These antibodies bind to the coagulation factor, forming an immune complex that is rapidly cleared from the circulation and results in deficiency of the factor. The antibody is often reversible over time if the initiating chemical is withdrawn. However, during the acute phase, these patients may have life-threatening bleeding. The factors that are most often affected include factor VIII, factor V, factor XIII, vWF, prothrombin, and thrombin (Table 11-11)

Table 11-11

Relationship Between Xenobiotics and the Development of Specific Coagulation Factor Inhibitors

COAGULATION FACTOR	XENOBIOTIC
Thrombin	Topical bovine thrombin
	Fibrin glue
Factor V	Streptomycin
	Penicillin
	Gentamicin
	Cephalosporins
	Topical bovine thrombin
Factor VIII	Penicillin
	Ampicillin
	Chloramphenicol
	Phenytoin
	Methyldopa
	Nitrofurazone
	Phenylbutazone
Factor XIII	Isoniazid
	Procainamide
	Penicillin
	Phenytoin
	Practolol
Von Willebrand Factor	Ciprofloxacin
	Hydroxyethyl starch
	Valproic acid
	Griseofulvin
	Tetracycline
	Pesticides

(Lollar, 2004, 2005). Many of these antibodies inhibit the functional activity of the coagulation factor in addition to increasing the rate of clearance. Other antibodies have been demonstrated to have catalytic activity, resulting in proteolysis of the target coagulation factor (Ananyeva *et al.*, 2004).

Lupus anticoagulants are antibodies that interfere with in vitro phospholipid-dependent coagulation reactions (Bertolaccini *et al.*, 2004). Although it was once hypothesized that these antibodies were directed against phospholipid, it is now evident that lupus anticoagulants are directed against phospholipid binding proteins, including prothrombin and β_2-glycoprotein 1. These antibodies usually do not cause a deficiency of any specific coagulation factor. However, in vivo, these antibodies can potentiate procoagulant mechanisms and interfere with the protein C system. Consequently, these antibodies have been associated with an increased risk of thrombosis (Bertolaccini *et al.*, 2004). The development of lupus anticoagulants has been seen in association with a variety of medications, including procainamide, chlorpromazine, and hydralazine.

Toxicology of Agents Used to Modulate Hemostasis

Patients with bleeding or thrombotic problems are commonly encountered in clinical practice. A variety of drugs are available to treat such patients, ranging from recombinant hemostatic proteins to chemical entities that modulate the activity of the coagulation system. The major toxicologic reactions to plasma-derived products are infectious diseases (e.g., hepatitis C) and allergic reactions, which can be severe. The use of some products, such as activated concentrates of vitamin K-dependent proteins (e.g., Autoplex and FEIBA), has been associated with the development of disseminated intravascular coagulation and/or thrombosis in some patients (Mannucci, 1998).

Oral Anticoagulants   Oral anticoagulants (warfarin) interfere with vitamin K metabolism by preventing the reduction of vitamin K epoxide, resulting in a functional deficiency of reduced vitamin K (Ansell *et al.*, 2004). These drugs are widely used for prophylaxis and therapy of venous and arterial thrombosis. The therapeutic window for oral anticoagulants is relatively narrow, and there is considerable interindividual variation in the response to a given dose. A number of factors, including concurrent medications and genetics, affect the individual response to oral anticoagulants (Ansell *et al.*, 2004; D'Andrea *et al.*, 2005; Rojas *et al.*, 2005). For these reasons, therapy with these drugs must be routinely monitored to maximize both safety and efficacy. This is routinely performed with the PT, with results expressed in terms of the international normalized ratio (INR).

A number of xenobiotics, including foods, have been found to affect the response to oral anticoagulants (Ansell *et al.*, 2004). Perhaps the most common mechanism for interference with oral anticoagulants is mediated by inhibition of CYP2C9 (Rojas *et al.*, 2005). Other mechanisms of interference include induction of CYP2C9, which tends to diminish the effect of warfarin by shortening its half-life; interference with absorption of warfarin from the gastrointestinal tract; displacement of warfarin from albumin in plasma, which temporarily increases the bioavailability of warfarin until equilibrium is reestablished; diminished vitamin K availability, either due to dietary deficiency or interference with the absorption of this lipid-soluble vitamin; and inhibition of the reduction of vitamin K epoxide, which potentiates the effect of oral anticoagulants.

Just as other drugs interfere with the action of oral anticoagulants, administration of oral anticoagulants may affect the activity of other medications, particularly those that are metabolized by CYP2C9. Dicumarol administration prolongs the half-life of chlorpropamide and phenytoin, resulting in hypoglycemia in the case of chlorpropamide and an increased plasma drug concentration in the case of phenytoin. Bis-hydroxycoumarin, but not warfarin, potentiates the activity of tolbutamide, resulting in enhanced hypoglycemia (Harder and Thurmann, 1996).

Oral anticoagulants have been associated with the development of warfarin-induced skin necrosis (Ansell *et al.*, 2004). This disorder is due to the development of extensive microvascular thrombosis in the affected skin. This uncommon toxic effect is thought to be related to a rapid drop in protein C following administration of the drug, resulting in impaired protein C function. The risk of developing warfarin-induced skin necrosis increases with the dose of warfarin used to initiate therapy, particularly when the initial dose exceeds 10 mg per day. This is one of the reasons that loading doses of warfarin are no longer recommended.

Vitamin K is necessary for the synthesis of proteins other than the coagulation-related factors, including osteocalcin, a major component of bone. Perhaps because of this, long-term administration of warfarin has been associated with bone demineralization (Ansell *et al.*, 2004; Stafford, 2005). This effect can be important in patients with borderline bone density. Administration of warfarin during pregnancy, particularly the first 12 weeks of pregnancy, is associated with congenital anomalies in 25–30% of exposed infants (Bates *et al.*, 2004). Many of the anomalies are related to abnormal bone formation. It is thought that warfarin may interfere with synthesis of proteins critical for normal structural development.

Heparin Heparin is a widely used anticoagulant for both prophylaxis and therapy of acute venous thromboembolism (Hirsh and Raschke, 2004). In many hospitals, the majority of patients are exposed to this potent anticoagulant at some point during their hospitalization. The major complication associated with heparin therapy is bleeding, a direct manifestation of its anticoagulant activity. The risk of bleeding is related to the intensity of therapy, the patient's body mass and underlying condition, and the presence of other hemostatic defects (e.g., thrombocytopenia).

As discussed in the section on platelets, heparin administration is also associated with the development of HIT. For unknown reasons, this complication occurs more frequently with heparin derived from bovine sources than with that derived from porcine sources. The incidence of HIT is also significantly higher in patients receiving unfractionated heparin than it is in patients receiving low-molecular-weight heparin (Davoren and Aster, 2006; Warkentin and Greinacher, 2004).

Long term administration of heparin is associated with an increased risk of clinically significant osteoporosis (Dinwoodey and Ansell, 2006; Hirsh and Raschke, 2004). The mechanism underlying the development of osteoporosis in these patients is not known. Patients may suffer from spontaneous vertebral fractures and demineralization of long bones of the arms and legs. The risk of osteoporosis may be less with low-molecular-weight heparin as compared to unfractionated heparin.

Heparin administration may also cause a transient rise in serum transaminases, suggesting significant liver dysfunction (Guevara et al., 1993). However, the rise is rapidly reversible upon discontinuation of heparin and may reverse even before heparin is discontinued. The elevation of serum transaminases has not been associated with chronic liver dysfunction. The mechanism of heparin-induced increase in transaminases is not known.

Fibrinolytic Agents Fibrinolytic drugs are used in the treatment of acute thromboembolic disease with the goal of dissolving the pathogenic thrombus (Collen and Lijnen, 2005). Each of these drugs works by converting plasminogen, an inactive zymogen, to plasmin, an active proteolytic enzyme. Plasmin is normally tightly regulated and is not freely present in the circulation. However, administration of fibrinolytic drugs regularly results in the generation of free plasmin leading to systemic fibrin(ogen)olysis. The toxicology of the fibrinolytic drugs can be divided into toxic effects of systemic plasmin activation and toxic effects of the activators themselves.

Systemic fibrinolysis is associated with the development of a complex coagulopathy characterized by a decrease in fibrinogen, factor V, factor VIII, α_2-antiplasmin; an increase in circulating fibrin split products; degradation of platelet GP Ib/IX/V and IIb/IIIa; degradation of endothelial cell glycoproteins; degradation of fibronectin and thrombospondin; and prolongation of the PT, APTT, and thrombin time (Hajjar, 2006). All of these effects potentiate the risk of bleeding. Anatomic locations that are frequently involved in bleeding complications include the cerebral circulation and sites of recent vascular access. As systemic plasmin can lyse physiologic as well as pathologic thrombi, reactivation of bleeding from sites of vascular access is not uncommon. Platelet inhibitors and heparin are commonly used in conjunction with fibrinolytic therapy to prevent recurrent thrombosis. As one might expect, the concurrent use of

anticoagulants with systemic fibrinolysis may contribute to the risk of bleeding (Menon et al., 2004).

Another complication associated with fibrinolysis is recurrent thrombosis at the site of pathologic thrombosis. Whereas rethrombosis may be related to underlying damage to the vascular wall, there is some evidence that fibrinolytic therapy may contribute to this process. For example, plasmin, in appropriate concentrations can actually induce platelet activation (McRedmond et al., 2000). This process may be mediated by plasmin or streptokinase/plasminogen cleavage of the platelet thrombin receptor (protease activated receptor-1). Cleavage of the receptor is associated with activation of the platelet biochemical signaling pathways. There is sufficient "cross talk" between the fibrinolytic system and the contact system of coagulation that one could also anticipate increased thrombin generation occurring as a result of fibrinolytic therapy (Schmaier et al., 1999).

Streptokinase is a protein derived from group C β-hemolytic streptococci and is antigenic in humans. Antibody formation to streptokinase occurs commonly in association with streptococcal infections as well as due to exposure to streptokinase. Acute allergic reactions may occur in 1–5% of patients exposed to streptokinase, and these allergic reactions may consist of minor symptoms such as hives and fever as well as major, life-threatening anaphylactic reactions. In addition, delayed hypersensitivity reactions associated with severe morbidity may occur (Curzen et al., 1998; Siebert et al., 1992). Allergic reactions also occur with other fibrinolytic agents containing streptokinase (e.g., anisoylated plasminogen-streptokinase complex) or streptokinase-derived peptides. The immune complex formed by IgG and streptokinase is capable of binding to and clustering platelet FcγRIIa, initiating platelet activation and aggregation (McRedmond et al., 2000).

Urokinase and recombinant tissue plasminogen activator (t-PA) are generally not associated with allergic reactions. However, work is progressing on a number of genetically engineered forms of t-PA. Whether or not such mutant forms of t-PA are immunogenetic has not been firmly established (Collen and Lijnen, 2005).

Inhibitors of Fibrinolysis Inhibitors of fibrinolysis are commonly used to control bleeding in patients with congenital abnormalities of hemostasis, such as von Willebrand disease. Tranexamic acid and ε-aminocaproic acid are small molecules that block the binding of plasminogen and plasmin to fibrin and other substrate proteins through interaction with lysine binding sites on plasmin(ogen). Although relatively well tolerated, there is some evidence that administration of these chemicals may increase the risk of thrombosis, due to the inhibition of the fibrinolytic system (Mannucci, 1998). In a single case, intravenous infusion of ε-aminocaproic in a patient with chronic renal failure was associated with acute hyperkalemia (Perazella and Biswas, 1999).

Aprotinin is a naturally occurring polypeptide inhibitor of serine proteases. It is usually derived from bovine material and consequently is immunogenic when administered to humans. Aprotinin is given by intravenous infusion, as it is inactive when given orally. Allergic reactions in response to aprotinin have been reported, ranging from minor cutaneous manifestations to anaphylactic reactions (Peters and Noble, 1999). A recent observational study compared clinical outcomes after cardiac surgery performed with aprotinin, tranexamix acid or aminocaproic acid to outcomes after cardiac surgery without an inhibitor of fibrinolysis (Mangano et al., 2006). In this study, use of antifibrinolytics was associated with decreased blood loss. However, use of aprotinin was associated with a significant increase in end-organ damage, including renal, cardiac, and cerebral events. The design and results of this study have been questioned, with calls for prospective randomized comparative studies (Sedrakyan *et al.*, 2006). The results also point out the intricate balance within the hemostatic system and the potential for problems when modulating the activity of one portion of this system.

RISK ASSESSMENT

Assessing the risk that exposure to new drugs, chemical products, and other agents pose to humans, in terms of significant toxic effects on hematopoiesis and the functional integrity of blood cells and hemostatic mechanisms, can be logistically and intellectually challenging. This is due in part to the complexity of hematopoiesis and the range of important tasks that these components perform, as previously discussed. A central issue in drug and nontherapeutic chemical development is the *predictive value* of preclinical toxicology data and the expansive but inevitably limited preregistration clinical database for the occurrence of significant hematotoxicity upon broad exposure to human populations. Appropriately, this area of well-resourced applied toxicology is highly regulated yet provides unique and exciting opportunities for sophisticated, well-controlled research (Bloom, 1993).

Preclinical Risk Assessment

Most preclinical studies that assess the potential for candidate drugs or nontherapeutic chemicals to induce hematotoxicity in humans are performed in industry as part of the routine safety evaluation of these molecules. These studies are largely prescribed by government regulatory bodies of the various countries and regions, including the United States, the European Union, and Japan (Federal Register, 2000; Hall, 1992, 1997). The issues relating to the assessment of blood as a target organ that confront the industrial toxicologist are largely similar to those of other target organs and include the selection of the appropriate animal model, how to best monitor for hematotoxicity, and the appreciation of species differences in responding to hematotoxic insults.

Animal Models and Hematologic Monitoring Selection of a species that is practical to study and predictive for hematotoxicity in humans is always a challenge. While this is driven in part by the aforementioned regulatory requirements, the selection is influenced by other considerations, including having a pharmacokinetic profile comparable to that of humans; prior information on sensitivity of a particular species to a class of compounds; the ability to fully characterize effects on peripheral blood and bone marrow; and practical considerations, such as logistics and economics (Bloom, 1993). These become of particular importance in choosing a model to fully characterize the toxicity of a chemical known to have a hematotoxic potential.

Of the commonly used animal species, rats and mice offer the advantage of their small size, which favorably impacts test compound requirements and number of subjects that can be economically housed and tested. Both have been well characterized hematologically (Moore, 2000a,b; Valli and McGrath, 1997). Blood volume limitations, however, often prohibit the frequent, or serial, evaluation of blood and bone marrow required to characterize the progression of a hematotoxic effect. Whereas this can be addressed in part through serial sacrifices, the inability to fully characterize individ-

Table 11-12

Examples of Problem-Driven Tests Used to Characterize Hematologic Observations in Preclinical Toxicology

Reticulocyte count
Heinz body preparation
Cell-associated antibody assays (erythrocyte, platelet, neutrophil)
Erythrocyte osmotic fragility test
Erythrokinetic/ferrokinetic analyses
Cytochemical/histochemical staining
Electron microscopy
In vitro hematopoietic clonogenic assays
Platelet aggregation
Plasma fibrinogen concentration
Clotting factor assays
Thrombin time
Bleeding time

ual animals poses a significant disadvantage. Test results will also vary in accordance with the phlebotomy site and method, particularly in rodents (Suber and Kodell, 1985), and with the physical and chemical restraint employed (Loomis *et al.*, 1980).

Serial blood and bone marrow sampling is practical in larger species, such as the dog and monkey. These models offer the additional advantage of being hematologically more similar to humans, as regards hematopoiesis and blood cell kinetics, which in the monkey extends to immunohematologic features (Ladiges *et al.*, 1990; Shifrine and Wilson, 1980). The latter species, however, presents more interanimal hematologic variability, particularly in wild-caught primates, due to temperment, vascular access, and other influences, that include nutritional status and infection.

Tests used to assess blood and bone marrow in preclinical toxicology studies will vary with the phase or objective of the evaluation (acute, subacute, chronic), the intended use of the chemical, and what is understood or suspected regarding the toxicologic profile of the xenobiotic. Ideally, the studies in aggregate should provide information on the effects of single- and multiple-dose exposure on erythrocyte parameters (RBC, Hbg, PCV, MCV, MCHC), leukocyte parameters (WBC and absolute differential counts), thrombocyte counts, screening coagulation tests (PT, aPTT), peripheral blood cell morphology, and bone marrow cytologic and histologic features (Bloom, 1993; Lund, 2000; Weingand *et al.*, 1996). Additional tests should be employed in a problem-driven fashion, as required to better characterize findings from the aforementioned screening efforts or to more fully explore a class-specific effect or other hematotoxicologic potential of concern (Bloom, 1993). Examples of these tests are listed in Table 11-12. While much progress has been made in validating many of the more specialized assays in our principal animal models, additional validation that addresses laboratory- and species-specific preanalytic and analytic variables is often required.

Because hematologic features and response to disease can vary substantially among animal species, it is essential that the toxicologist fully understands the hematology of the animal model used for preclinical risk assessment. Whereas complete and accurate reference data are helpful, they do not provide information on pathophysiology that may be species-specific and required to accurately interpret the preclinical data. Examples of these features include the relative influence of preanalytic variables (blood collection technique, nutritional status, sample stability), response to blood loss or hemolysis, stress effects on the leukogram, susceptibility to secondary effects associated with other target organ toxicity, etc. It is beyond the scope of this chapter to fully discuss the comparative hematology of laboratory animals, which is provided in several excellent reviews (Feldman, 2000; Valli and McGrath, 1997).

Applications of In Vitro Bone Marrow Assays As with other target-organ risk assessment, in vitro methods for assessing potential hematotoxicity are attractive in that they are faster and less expensive than in vivo studies, while providing data that often suggest or clarify the mechanism of a toxic effect. Drug- or chemical-induced bone marrow suppression can result from effects on specific hematopoietic stem cells or on the hematopoietic microenvironment. These effects can be distinguished and confirmed using short-term clonogenic assays and long-term functional assays, respectively (Deldar, 1994; Naughton et al., 1992; Williams et al., 1988). The former include burst-forming-unit erythroid (BFU-E), colony-forming-unit erythroid (CFU-E), colony-forming-unit granulocyte/monocyte (CFU-GM), colony-forming-unit megakaryocyte (CFU-MK), and colony-forming-unit granulocyte, erythroid, megakaryocyte, monocyte (CFU-GEMM), which have been developed for several laboratory animal species (Deldar and Parchment, 1997; Pessina et al., 2005). It is therefore possible to examine effects on the myeloid, erythroid, and megakaryocytic lineages in a fashion where concentrations of the chemical are tightly controlled, as is duration of exposure to it.

In vitro clonogenic assays are best used in a preclinical setting in combination with in vivo testing. Used in this way, the predictive value of these assays is enhanced. This has been particularly true for anticancer and antiviral drugs, where the in vitro component of risk assessment has been used for therapeutic index-based screening to identify less myelosuppressive analogs, structure-toxicity relationships, and new-drug lead candidates (Deldar and Stevens, 1993; Parchment et al., 1993; Pessina et al., 2003). Other advantages of the in vitro hematopoietic stem cell assays include the opportunities they provide to test combinations of chemicals as well as their metabolites and effects of serum and other cell components, such as lymphocytes (Deldar and Parchment, 1997). Most important is the ability to test human hematopoietic cells directly in a preclinical setting, thus obviating extrapolation considerations. Concern for possible metabolic activation can be addressed by culturing the target cells in question with metabolizing systems in a cell-free extract (s9), with isolated hepatocytes, or with other CYP450-expressing cell types (Frazier, 1992; Negro et al., 2001).

Perhaps the most interesting use of these in vitro clonogenic assays in risk assessment has been their role in making practical interspecies comparisons regarding sensitivity to a particular chemical or group of drugs or chemicals. Comparisons to the sensitivity of human cells can be made that have implications for the relative predictive value of various animal models for hematotoxicity in humans. Examples include the resistance of murine CFU-GM to the anticancer drug topotecan relative to that of the canine and human cells (Deldar and Stevens, 1993). This is consistent with the early observations of Marsh, that the dog is a particularly predictive model for the myelosuppression associated with anticancer drugs in humans (Marsh, 1985). Thus, whereas some agents show comparable suppressive activity across species lines (doxorubicin, pyrazoloacridine, hepsulfan, cyclopentenyl cytosine), others, such as camptothecins, carboxyamidotriazole and

fostriecin, show differences of as much as three log concentrations (Du et al., 1991; Horikoshi and Murphy Jr., 1982; Reagan et al., 1993).

Because myelotoxicity, and particularly suppression of granulopoiesis, is a major limitation in administering anticancer drugs, and is often used to determine the optimal dose, the clonogenic assay for CFU-GM has received the most attention as a preclinical tool for predicting this response. It is the only assay that has been validated by an international study supported by the European Centre for Validation of Alternative Methods (Pessina et al., 2003). Analytical validation was completed for human and mouse assays, and a predictive model was developed to calculate the maximum tolerated dose (MTD) in humans using data from the mouse assay that is adjusted for the established interspecies variation (Pessina et al., 2001). The model was applied in an international blind trial to 20 drugs that included 14 antineoplastic drugs, the antiviral drugs zidovudine and acyclovir, and the pesticide lindane (Pessina et al., 2003). It predicted the MTD for all 20 agents, although extrapolation on the regression curve out of the range of the actual drug doses tested was required to derive the IC90 for 10 of these drugs.

Whereas this discussion has focused on in vitro hematopoietic clonogenic assays in the context of risk assessment, these assays have also proven to be extraordinarily useful tools for investigating mechanisms of toxic cytopenia in humans (Deldar, 1994). Parchment and Murphy reviewed the application of these to four categories of hematologic toxicity observed clinically: (1) the reversible cytopenia following acute exposure to a cytotoxic or cytostatic agent; (2) the permanent loss in the production of a mature blood cell type(s); (3) cytosis, or the dramatic increase in blood cell counts following single or repeated toxicant exposure; and (4) the progressive loss of one or more blood cell lineages during chronic exposure to a toxicant (Parchment and Murphy, 1997). In all these circumstances, in vitro and ex vivo hematopoietic clonogenic assays have proven useful in understanding the mechanism(s) of these toxic effects and formulating strategies for risk management and treatment.

Emerging Technologies As discussed previously, the well controlled and resource intensive preclinical toxicology and safety studies prescribed for candidate drugs and non-therapeutic chemicals provide unique opportunities for studies on mechanisms of xenobiotic-induced hematoxicity (Bloom, 1993; Deldar and Parchment, 1997). Together with the traditional biomarkers for toxicity, mechanism-based technologies such as toxicogenomics, proteomics, and metabonomics are now available to the toxicologist and are increasingly helpful in both predicting toxicity and determining whether a particular finding is relevant to man (Todd and Ulrich, 1999). Challenges that the application of these tools present relate to informatics, standardization and validation (Reynolds, 2005).

Clinical Trials and Risk Assessment

As with preclinical risk assessment, most of the clinical research on hematotoxicity is driven by regulatory requirements and supported by the drug, cosmetic, and chemical industries. The challenges and opportunities this presents are similar to those in preclinical development with the following differences. First, most clinical studies involve actual patients with the targeted disease, in contrast to the inbred, healthy, well-defined animals employed in preclinical

Table 11-13
WHO Grading Criteria for Subacute and Acute Hematotoxicity

HEMATOLOGICAL PARAMETERS (ADULTS)	GRADE 0	GRADE 1	GRADE 2	GRADE 3	GRADE 4
Hemoglobin (g dL^{-1}) (nmol/L)	11.0 (6.8)	9.5–10.5 (6.5–6.7)	8.0–9.4 (4.95–5.8)	6.5–7.9 (4.0–4.9)	6.5 (4.0)
Leukocytes (1000 µL^{-1})	4.0	3.0–3.9	2.0–2.9	2.0–1.9	1.0
Granulocytes (1000 µL^{-1})	2.0	1.5–1.9	1.0–1.4	0.5–0.9	0.5
Platelets (1000 µL^{-1})	100	75–99	50–74	25–49	<25
Hemorrhage, blood loss	None	Petechiae	Mild	Gross	Debilitating

Data from WHO, 1979.

studies. This presents additional variables and challenges to manage. Second, the scale of clinical trials, the volume of data produced, and the resources required exceed by orders of magnitude those of preclinical studies. Third, many clinical trials involve research cooperative groups that represent a network of clinical scientists from academic medical centers, such as the Eastern Cooperative Oncology Group (ECOG), the AIDS Clinical Trial Group (ACTG), Thrombolysis in Myocardial Infarction (TIMI), and others. Most of the information on drug- or chemical-induced hematotoxicity in humans is collected through this industry-sponsored and highly-regulated clinical research.

It is well understood that the ways in which drugs and nontherapeutic chemicals affect the hematopoietic system are influenced by both the nature of the chemical and the response of the subject or target population. As discussed previously, many chemicals are known to induce dose-dependent hematotoxicity in a fashion that is highly predictable. Others cause toxicity in a small number of susceptible individuals, and these often include chemicals not otherwise hematotoxic in most individuals (Dieckhaus *et al.*, 2002; Patton and Duffull, 1994). These *idiosyncratic reactions* present the biggest challenge as regards detection and characterization before human patients or populations are broadly exposed. They include aplastic anemia, thrombocytopenia, hemolysis, and leukopenia, which may or may not be immune-mediated (Salama *et al*, 1989).

Prevailing theories today, as regards mechanisms for these idiosyncratic reactions, include drug or reactive metabolite alkylation of endogenous proteins forming a hapten-protein complex that ultimately initiates an immune response. The latter may entail presentation of cryptic antigens by the major histocompatibility complex (MHC) and the subsequent induction of a response to self protein and an irreversible autoimmune reaction (Uetrecht, 1999). Another theory suggests that hapten-protein formation is not requited for a reaction to occur. This "direct metabolism-independent T-cell stimulation" theory involves direct binding of a drug to peptide-loaded MHC on antigen presenting cells for T-cell receptor cell recognition (Zanni *et al.*, 1998). While there is evidence supporting both theories, the first is most widely accepted.

The chemical structure can be a risk factor if it is similar to that of other known toxicants. Patient or population-related risk factors include pharmacogenetic variations in drug metabolism and detoxification that lead to reduced clearance of the chemical or production of novel intermediate metabolites (Cunningham *et al.*, 1974; Gerson *et al.*, 1983; Mason and Fischer, 1992), histocompatibility antigens (Frickhofen *et al.*, 1990), interaction with drugs or other chemicals (West *et al.*, 1988), increased sensitivity of hematopoietic precursors to damage (Vincent, 1986), preexisting disease of the bone marrow,

and metabolic defects that predispose to oxidative or other stresses associated with the chemical (Stern, 1989).

In drug development, the clinical evaluation of candidate molecules is usually performed in three phases: *Phase I* examines the effect of single and multiple increasing doses in small numbers of normal and/or patient volunteers. Pharmacokinetic properties are usually addressed, as well as the routes of excretion and metabolism; and the assessment of active and inactive metabolites. The emphasis is usually on safety assessment. *Phase II* includes controlled studies in the target patient population that examine both safety and efficacy. They explore dose response and usually provide the first indication of benefit versus risk. *Phase III* entails larger studies designed to confirm efficacy in an expanded patient population and evaluate less frequent adverse effects, such as the aforementioned idiosyncratic blood dyscrasias.

Development of a demonstrably hematotoxic drug is usually stopped in phase I or II, unless the indication includes life-threatening conditions where toxicity is acceptable (e.g., anticancer drugs). Thus, drugs tested in phase III generally show an acceptable safety profile in most subjects at the doses used. Even phase III studies, however, are not usually powered to detect the low incidence of idiosyncratic hematotoxicity previously discussed (Levine and Szarfman, 1996). In order to detect one adverse event affecting 1% of an exposed patient population at a 95% confidence level, a trial must include approximately 300 subjects (O'Neill, 1988). Clinical databases supporting new drug applications generally cannot be used to detect adverse events that occur below 1 per 1000 exposures (Federal Register, 2001), and most will not rule out events with a frequency of less than 1 per 500 (Szarfman *et al.*, 1997). Thus, rare, delayed or cumulative toxicity is often missed in preregistration clinical trials.

Detection of low-incidence hematotoxicity is usually achieved through postmarketing surveillance, such as the Med Watch program introduced by the FDA in 1993 (Szarfman *et al.*, 1997). Other countries that practice comprehensive postmarketing surveillance include Canada, the United Kingdom, Sweden, Germany, France, Australia, and New Zealand. Adverse event data, including serious hematotoxicity, are provided to the WHO, this information is compiled by a computer-based recording system employing WHO terminology, and system and organ classifications for adverse reactions (Edwards *et al.*, 1990). Examples of iatrogenic blood dyscrasias detected through postmarketing surveillance include the hemolysis and thrombocytopenia associated with the antibiotic temafloxacin; the aplastic anemia linked to the antiepileptic felbamate; the hemolysis caused by the antidepressant nomifensine; and the agranulocytosis associated with the antiarrhythmic aprindine.

The WHO has also established criteria for grading hemato-toxicity (WHO, 1979), which is summarized in Table 11-13. These have been particularly useful in establishing and communicating treatment strategies and guidelines for chemicals known to suppress hematopoiesis (cytoreductive oncolytic, immunosuppressive, and antiviral agents, etc.) and for which this limiting toxicity is used to establish maximum tolerated doses for individual patients.

Greater risk is acceptable with these drugs due to the life-threatening conditions they are used to treat. Similar risk–benefit decisions are also made regarding the use of drugs that cause blood dyscrasias in an idiosyncratic fashion, as previously discussed. Some are used to treat nonmalignant or life-threatening conditions, the risk of which is managed through rigorous laboratory monitoring. Examples include felbamate, ticlopidine, and clozapine, as discussed previously. Postmarketing surveillance plays a critical role in measuring the effectiveness of such monitoring.

Critical to the effectiveness of such surveillance by manufacturers and government regulatory agencies is the ability to detect a "signal," such as that related to life-threatening idiosyncratic hematotoxicity. Over the past 5 years, regulatory agencies and drug monitoring centers have been developing computerized data mining methods to better identify reporting relationships in spontaneous reporting databases that have enabled and optimized such signal detection (Almenoff et al., 2005). This includes the use of screening algorithms and computer systems that efficiently signal higher-than-expected combinations of drugs and events in the FDA's spontaneous reports database, such as aplastic anemia, agranulocytosis and idiopathic thrombocytopenic purpura. Examples include the Multi-Item Gamma Poison Shrinker (MGPS) program, which computes signal scores for pairs, and for higher-order (e.g. triplet, quadruplet) combinations of xenobiotics and events that are significantly more frequent than their pair-wise associations would predict (Szarfman et al., 2002). Such tools provide an objective and unprecedented systematic and simultaneous view of these large databases and alert government and manufacturers to critically important new safety signals that inform the toxicologist.

REFERENCES

Abarbanel J, Benet AE, Lask D, et al.: Sports hematuria. J Urol 143:887–890, 1990.

Abrams CS: Acquired qualitive platelet disorders, in Lichtman MA, Beutler E, Kipps TJ, Seligsohn U, Kaushansky K, Prchal JT (eds): Williams Hematology, 7th edn. New York: McGraw Hill, 2006, pp. 1833–1855.

Alcindor T, Bridges KR: Sideroblastic anaemias. Br J Haematol 116:733–743, 2002.

Almenoff J, Tonning JM, Gould AL, et al.: Perspectives on the use of data mining in pharmaco-vigilance. Drug Saf 28:981–1007, 2005.

Altucci L, Clarke N, Nebbioso A, et al.: Acute myeloid leukemia: Therapeutic impact of epigenetic drugs. Int J Biochem Cell Biol 37:1752–1762, 2005.

Ananyeva NM, Lacroix-Desmazes S, Hauser CA, et al.: Inhibitors in hemophilia A: Mechanisms of inhibition, management and perspectives. Blood Coagul Fibrinolysis 15:109–124, 2004.

Andersen RL, Bagby Jr. GC, Richert-Boe K: Therapy-related preleukemic syndrome. Cancer 47:1867–1871, 1981.

Andres E, Kurtz JE, Martin-Hunyadi C, et al.: Nonchemotherapy drug-induced agranulocytosis in elderly patients: The effects of granulocyte colony-stimulating factor. Am J Med 112:460–464, 2002.

Ansell J, Hirsh J, Poller L, et al.: The pharmacology and management of the vitamin K antagonists: The Seventh ACCP Conference on Antithrombotic and Thrombolytic Therapy. Chest 126:204S–233S, 2004.

Arndt PA, Garratty G: The changing spectrum of drug-induced immune hemolytic anemia. Semin Hematol 42:137–144, 2005.

Arneborn P, Palmblad J: Drug-induced neutropenia—a survey for Stockholm 1973–1978. Acta Med Scand 212:289–292, 1982.

Aster RH: Drug-induced immune cytopenias. Toxicology 209:149–153, 2005.

Athens JW, Haab OP, Raab SO, et al.: Leukokinetic studies. IV. The total blood, circulating and marginal granulocyte pools and the granulocyte turnover rate in normal subjects. J Clin Invest 40:989–995, 1961.

Babior BM: Folate, cobalamin, and myeloblastic anemias, in Lichtman MA, Beutler E, Kipps TJ, Seligsohn U, Kaushansky K, Prchal JT (eds.): Williams Hematology, 7th edn. New York: McGraw-Hill, 2006, pp. 477–509.

Babior BM, Golde DW: Production, distribution and fate of neutrophils, in Beutler E, Lichtman MA, Coller BS, Kipps TJ (eds.): Williams Hematology, 5th edn. New York: McGraw Hill, 1995, pp. 773–779.

Bahrami S, Malone JC, Webb KG, et al.: Tissue eosinophilia as an indicator of drug-induced cutaneous small-vessel vasculitis. Arch Dermatol 142:155–161, 2006.

Baker KR: Hemolytic anemia resulting from physical injury to red cells, in Lichtman MA, Beutler E, Kipps TJ, Seligsohn U, Kaushansky K, Prchal JT (eds.): Williams Hematology. New York: McGraw-Hill, 2006, pp. 709–716.

Barnes PJ: Corticosteroids: The drugs to beat. Eur J Pharmacol 533:2–14, 2006.

Bates SM, Greer IA, Hirsh J, et al.: Use of antithrombotic agents during pregnancy: The Seventh ACCP Conference on Antithrombotic and Thrombolytic Therapy. Chest 126:627S–644S, 2004.

Bench AJ, Nacheva EP, Champion KM, et al.: Molecular genetics and cytogenetics of myeloproliferative disorders. Baillieres Clin Haematol 11:819–848, 1998.

Bennett A, Sanger GJ: Pinane thromboxane A2 analogues are non-selective prostanoid antagonists in rat and human stomach muscle. Br J Pharmacol 77:591–596, 1982.

Bennett CL, Luminari S, Nissenson AR, et al.: Pure red-cell aplasia and epoetin therapy. N Engl J Med 351:1403–1408, 2004.

Bennett JM, Catovsky D, Daniel MT, et al.: Proposed revised criteria for the classification of acute myeloid leukemia. A report of the French-American-British Cooperative Group. Ann Intern Med 103:620–625, 1985.

Bergsagel DE, Wong O, Bergsagel PL, et al.: Benzene and multiple myeloma: Appraisal of the scientific evidence. Blood 94:1174–1182, 1999.

Berkowitz FE: Hemolysis and infection: Categories and mechanisms of their interrelationship. Rev Infect Dis 13:1151–1162, 1991.

Berliner N, Horwitz M, Loughran Jr. TP: Congenital and acquired neutropenia, in Broudy VC, Berliner N, Larson RA, Leung LL (eds.): American Society of Hematology Education Program Book. Washington, D.C.: American Society of Hematology, 2004, pp. 63–79.

Berry RG, Morrison JA, Watts JW, et al.: Surreptitious superwarfarin ingestion with brodifacoum. South Med J 93:74–75, 2000.

Bertolaccini ML, Hughes GR, Khamashta MA: Revisiting antiphospholipid antibodies: From targeting phospholipids to phospholipid binding proteins. Clin Lab 50:653–665, 2004.

Beutler E: Hemolytic anemias resulting from infections with microorganisms, in Lichtman MA, Beutler E, Kipps TJ, Seligsohn U, Kaushansky K, Prchal JT (eds.): Williams Hematology, 7th ed. New York: McGraw-Hill, 2006, pp. 723–727.

Beutler E: G6PD: Population genetics and clinical manifestations. Blood Rev 10:45–52, 1996.

Beutler E: Hemolytic anemias resulting from chemical and physical agents, in Lichtman MA, Beutler E, Kipps TJ, Seligsohn U, Kaushansky K, Prchal JT (eds.): *Williams Hematology, 7th ed.* New York: McGraw-Hill, 2006a, pp. 717–721.

Beutler E: Hereditary and acquired sideroblastic anemias, in Lichtman MA, Beutler E, Kipps TJ, Seligsohn U, Kaushansky K, Prchal JT (eds.): *Williams Hematology, 7th ed.* New York: McGraw-Hill, 2006b, pp. 823–828.

Bitter MA, Le Beau MM, Rowley JD, *et al.*: Associations between morphology, karyotype, and clinical features in myeloid leukemias. *Hum Pathol* 18:211–225, 1987.

Bloom JC: Principles of hematotoxicology: Laboratory assessment and interpretation of data. *Toxicol Pathol* 21:130–134, 1993.

Bloom JC: Introduction to hematoxicology, in Sipes IG, McQueen CA, Gandolfi AJ (eds.): *Comprehensive Toxicology.* Oxford, UK: Pergamon Press, 1997, pp. 1–10.

Bloom JC, Lewis HB, Sellers TS, *et al.*: The hematopathology of cefonicid- and cefazedone-induced blood dyscrasias in the dog. *Toxicol Appl Pharmacol* 90:143–155, 1987.

Borregaard N, Boxer LA: Disorders of neutrophil function, in Lichtman MA, Beutler E, Kipps TJ, Seligsohn U, Kaushansky K, Prchal JT (eds.): *Williams Hematology, 7th ed.* New York: McGraw-Hill, 2006, pp. 921–957.

Bradberry SM: Occupational methaemoglobinaemia. Mechanisms of production, features, diagnosis and management including the use of methylene blue. *Toxicol Rev* 22:13–27, 2003.

Bradberry SM, Aw TC, Williams NR, *et al.*: Occupational methaemoglobinaemia. *Occup Environ Med* 58:611–615, 2001.

Brayton RG, Stokes PE, Schwartz MS, *et al.*: Effect of alcohol and various diseases on leukocyte mobilization, phagocytosis and intracellular bacterial killing. *N Engl J Med* 282:123–128, 1970.

Browning E: *Toxicity and Metabolism of Industrial Solvents.* London: Elsevier, 1965.

Broxmeyer HE, Orschell CM, Clapp DW, *et al.*: Rapid mobilization of murine and human hematopoietic stem and progenitor cells with AMD3100, a CXCR4 antagonist. *J Exp Med* 201:1307–1318, 2005.

Brugnara C: Reticulocyte cellular indices: A new approach in the diagnosis of anemias and monitoring of erythropoietic function. *Crit Rev Clin Lab Sci* 37:93–130, 2000.

Capsoni F, Sarzi-Puttini P, Zanella A: Primary and secondary autoimmune neutropenia. *Arthritis Res Ther* 7:208–214, 2005.

Caramori G, Adcock I: Anti-inflammatory mechanisms of glucocorticoids targeting granulocytes. *Curr Drug Targets Inflamm Allergy* 4:455–463, 2005.

Cartwright GE, Athens JW, Wintrobe MM: The kinetics of granulopoiesis in normal man. *Blood* 24:780–803, 1964.

Carver JH, Hatch FT, Branscomb EW: Estimating maximum limits to mutagenic potency from cytotoxic potency. *Nature* 279:154–156, 1979.

Casciato DA, Scott JL: Acute leukemia following prolonged cytotoxic agent therapy. *Medicine* 58:32–47, 1979.

Cazzola M, Invernizzi R, Bergamaschi G, *et al.*: Mitochondrial ferritin expression in erythroid cells from patients with sideroblastic anemia. *Blood* 101:1996–2000, 2003.

Cerulli J, Grabe DW, Gauthier I, *et al.*: Chromium picolinate toxicity. *Ann Pharmacother* 32:428–431, 1998.

Cesar JM, de Miguel D, Garcia AA, *et al.*: Platelet dysfunction in primary thrombocythemia using the platelet function analyzer, PFA-100. *Am J Clin Pathol* 123:772–777, 2005.

Chabner BA, Wilson W, Supko J: Pharmacology and toxicity of antineoplastic drugs, in Lichtman MA, Beutler E, Kipps TJ, Seligsohn U, Kaushansky K, Prchal JT (eds.): *Williams Hematology, 7th ed.* New York: McGraw-Hill, 2006, pp. 247–274.

Chakraverty R, Davidson S, Peggs K, *et al.*: The incidence and cause of coagulopathies in an intensive care population. *Br J Haematol* 93:460–463, 1996.

Chua JD, Friedenberg WR: Superwarfarin poisoning. *Arch Intern Med* 158:1929–1932, 1998.

Clifton J, Leikin JB: Methylene blue. *Am J Ther* 10:289–291, 2003.

Coleman MD, Coleman NA: Drug-induced methaemoglobinaemia. Treatment issues. *Drug Safety* 14:394–405, 1996.

Collen D, Lijnen HR: Thrombolytic agents. *Thromb Haemost* 93:627–630, 2005.

Contrino J, Marucha P, Ribaudo R, *et al.*: Effects of mercury on human polymorphonuclear leukocyte function in vitro. *Am J Pathol* 132:110–118, 1988.

Cummings TF: The treatment of cyanide poisoning. *Occup Med* 54:82–85, 2004.

Cuneo A, Fagioli F, Pazzi I, *et al.*: Morphologic, immunologic and cytogenetic studies in acute myeloid leukemia following occupational exposure to pesticides and organic solvents. *Leuk Res* 16:789–796, 1992.

Cunningham JL, Leyland MJ, Delamore IW, *et al.*: Acetanilide oxidation in phenylbutazone-associated hypoplastic anaemia. *Br Med J* 3:313–317, 1974.

Curzen N, Haque R, Timmis A: Applications of thrombolytic therapy. *Intensive Care Med* 24:756–768, 1998.

Custer RP, Ahlfeldt FE: Studies on the structure and function of bone marrow. *J Lab Clin Med* 17:960–962, 1932.

D'Andrea G, D'Ambrosio RL, Di Perna P, *et al.*: A polymorphism in the VKORC1 gene is associated with an interindividual variability in the dose-anticoagulant effect of warfarin. *Blood* 105:645–649, 2005.

Dahl OE, Garvik LJ, Lyberg T: Toxic effects of methylmethacrylate monomer on leukocytes and endothelial cells in vitro. *Acta Orthop Scand* 65:147–153, 1994.

Dale DC: Neutropenia and neutrophilia, in Lichtman MA, Beutler E, Kipps TJ, Seligsohn U, Kaushansky K, Prchal JT (eds.): *Williams Hematology, 7th ed.* New York: McGraw-Hill, 2006, pp. 907–955.

Davoren A, Aster RH: Heparin-induced thrombocytopenia and thrombosis. *Am J Hematol* 81:36–44, 2006.

De Clercq E: Potential clinical applications of the CXCR4 antagonist bicyclam AMD3100. *Mini Rev Med Chem* 5:805–824, 2005.

Deckmyn H, Vanhoorelbeke K, Peerlinck K: Inhibitory and activating human antiplatelet antibodies. *Baillieres Clin Haematol* 11:343–359, 1998.

Deldar A: Drug-induced blood disorders: Review of pathogenetic mechanisms and utilization of bone marrow cell culture technology as an investigative approach. *Curr Topics Vet Res* 1:83–101, 1994.

Deldar A, Parchment RE: Preclinical risk assessment for hematotoxicity: Animal models and in vitro systems, in Sipes IG MAGA (ed.): *Comprehensive Toxicology.* Oxford: Pergamon Press, 1997, pp. 321–333.

Deldar A, Stevens CE: Development and application of in vitro models of hematopoiesis to drug development. *Toxicol Pathol* 21:231–240, 1993.

Demirer T, Bensinger WI: Optimization of peripheral blood stem cell collection. *Curr Opin Hematol* 2:219–226, 1995.

Dessypris EN: Erythropoiesis, in Lee CR, Foerster J, Lukens J, Paraskevas P, Greer JP, Rodgers GM (eds.): *Wintrobe's Clinical Hematology, 10th ed.* Philadelphia: Lippincott Williams & Wilkins, 1999, pp. 169–192.

Dieckhaus CM, Thompson CD, Roller SG, *et al.*: Mechanisms of idiosyncratic drug reactions: The case of felbamate. *Chem Biol Interact* 142:99–117, 2002.

Dinwoodey DL, Ansell JE: Heparins, low-molecular-weight heparins, and pentasaccharides. *Clin Geriatr Med* 22:1–15, vii, 2006.

Djaldetti M, Blay A, Bergman M, *et al.*: Pure red cell aplasia—a rare disease with multiple causes. *Biomed Pharmacother* 57:326–332, 2003.

Dreno B, Trossaert M, Boiteau HL, *et al.*: Zinc salts effects on granulocyte zinc concentration and chemotaxis in acne patients. *Acta Derm Venereol* 72:250–252, 1992.

Du DL, Volpe DA, Grieshaber CK, *et al.*: Comparative toxicity of fostriecin, hepsulfam and pyrazine diazohydroxide to human and murine hematopoietic progenitor cells in vitro. *Invest New Drugs* 9:149–157, 1991.

Edwards IR, Lindquist M, Wiholm BE, *et al.*: Quality criteria for early signals of possible adverse drug reactions. *Lancet* 336:156–158, 1990.

Fagioli F, Cuneo A, Piva N, *et al.*: Distinct cytogenetic and clinicopathologic features in acute myeloid leukemia after occupational exposure to pesticides and organic solvents. *Cancer* 70:77–85, 1992.

Federal Register: Note for Guidance on Non-Clinical Safety Studies for the Conduct of Human Clinical Trials for Pharmaceuticals. 2000.

Federal Register: Safety Pharmacology Studies for Human Pharmaceuticals. 2001.

Feldman BF: *Schalm's Veterinary Hematology.* Ames, Iowa: Blackwell Publishing, 2000.

Fisch P, Handgretinger R, Schaefer HE: Pure red cell aplasia. *Br J Haematol* 111:1010–1022, 2000.

Fiske DN, McCoy HE, III, Kitchens CS: Zinc-induced sideroblastic anemia: Report of a case, review of the literature, and description of the hematologic syndrome. *Am J Hematol* 46:147–150, 1994.

Flieder DB, Travis WD: Pathologic characteristics of drug-induced lung disease. *Clin Chest Med* 25:37–45, 2004.

Foucar K, McKenna RW, Bloomfield CD, *et al.*: Therapy-related leukemia: A panmyelosis. *Cancer* 43:1285–1296, 1979.

Frazier JM: In vitro toxicity testing: Applications to safety evaluation, in Frazier JM (ed.): *In Vitro Toxicity Testing Applications to Safety Evaluation.* New York: Marcel Dekker, 1992, pp. 5–7.

Friberg LE, Karlsson MO: Mechanistic models for myelosuppression. *Invest New Drugs* 21:183–194, 2003.

Frickhofen N, Liu JM, Young NS: Etiologic mechanisms of hematopoietic failure. *Am J Pediatr Hematol Oncol* 12:385–395, 1990.

Furlan M, Robles R, Galbusera M, *et al.*: von Willebrand factor-cleaving protease in thrombotic thrombocytopenic purpura and the hemolytic-uremic syndrome. *N Engl J Med* 339:1578–1584, 1998.

Gallardo S, Cardaba B, Posada M, *et al.*: Toxic oil syndrome: Genetic restriction and immunomodulatory effects due to adulterated oils in a model of HLA transgenic mice. *Toxicol Lett* 159:173–181, 2005.

Gerson SL, Meltzer H: Mechanisms of clozapine-induced agranulocytosis. *Drug Safety* 7 Suppl 1:17–25, 1992.

Gerson WT, Fine DG, Spielberg SP, *et al.*: Anticonvulsant-induced aplastic anemia: Increased susceptibility to toxic drug metabolites in vitro. *Blood* 61:889–893, 1983.

Girard D: Activation of human polymorphonuclear neutrophils by environmental contaminants. *Rev Environ Health* 18:75–89, 2003.

Godley LA, Larson RA: The syndrome of therapy-related myelodysplasia and myeloid leukemia, in Bennett JM (ed.): *The Myelodysplastic Syndromes: Pathobiology and Clinical Management.* New York: Dekker, 2001, pp. 139–176.

Golden R, Pyatt D, Shields PG: Formaldehyde as a potential human leukemogen: An assessment of biological plausibility. *Crit Rev Toxicol* 36:135–153, 2006.

Golomb HM, Alimena G, Rowley JD, *et al.*: Correlation of occupation and karyotype in adults with acute nonlymphocytic leukemia. *Blood* 60:404–411, 1982.

Gonzalez H, Leblond V, Azar N, *et al.*: Severe autoimmune hemolytic anemia in eight patients treated with fludarabine. *Hematol Cell Ther* 40:113–118, 1998.

Greene MH, Harris EL, Gershenson DM, *et al.*: Melphalan may be a more potent leukemogen than cyclophosphamide. *Ann Intern Med* 105:360–367, 1986.

Guevara A, Labarca J, Gonzalez-Martin G: Heparin-induced transaminase elevations: A prospective study. *Int J Clin Pharmacol Ther Toxicol* 31:137–141, 1993.

Hagen EC, Ballieux BE, van Es LA, *et al.*: Antineutrophil cytoplasmic autoantibodies: A review of the antigens involved, the assays, and the clinical and possible pathogenetic consequences. *Blood* 81:1996–2002, 1993.

Hajjar A: Fibrinolysis and thrombolysis, in Lichtman MA, Beutler E, Kipps TJ, Seligsohn U, Kaushansky K, Prchal JT (eds.): *Williams Hematology, 7th ed.* New York: McGraw-Hill, 2006, pp. 1833–1855.

Hall RL: Clinical pathology for preclinical safety assessment: Current global guidelines. *Toxicol Pathol* 20:472–476, 1992.

Hall RL: Evaluation and interpretation of hematologic data in preclinical toxicology, in Sipes IG, McQueen AC, Gandolfi AJ (eds.): *Comprehensive Toxicology.* Oxford: Pergamon Press, 1997, pp. 321–333.

Harder S, Thurmann P: Clinically important drug interactions with anticoagulants. An update. *Clin Pharmacokinet* 30:416–444, 1996.

Harrison DE, Lerner CP: Most primitive hematopoietic stem cells are stimulated to cycle rapidly after treatment with 5-fluorouracil. *Blood* 78:1237–1240, 1991.

Hatherill JR, Till GO, Bruner LH, *et al.*: Thermal injury, intravascular hemolysis, and toxic oxygen products. *J Clin Invest* 78:629–636, 1986.

Heissig B, Ohki Y, Sato Y, *et al.*: A role for niches in hematopoietic cell development. *Hematology* 10:247–253, 2005.

Hirsh J, Raschke R: Heparin and low-molecular-weight heparin: The Seventh ACCP Conference on Antithrombotic and Thrombolytic Therapy. *Chest* 126:188S–203S, 2004.

Hoffmann MJ, Sinko PJ, Lee YH, *et al.*: Pharmacokinetic studies in Tg.AC and FVB mice administered [14C] benzene either by oral gavage or intradermal injection. *Toxicol Appl Pharmacol* 174:139–145, 2001.

Honigfeld G, Arellano F, Sethi J, *et al.*: Reducing clozapine-related morbidity and mortality: 5 years of experience with the Clozaril National Registry. *J Clin Psychiatry* 59 Suppl 3:3–7, 1998.

Horikoshi A, Murphy Jr. MJ: Comparative effects of chemotherapeutic drugs on human and murine hematopoietic progenitors in vitro. *Chemotherapy* 28:480–501, 1982.

Hsia CC: Respiratory function of hemoglobin. *N Engl J Med* 338:239–247, 1998.

Hudson G: Bone-marrow volume in the human foetus and newborn. *Br J Haematol* 446–452, 2006.

Hunter FT: Chronic exposure of benzene. II. The clinical effects. *J Ind Hyg Toxicol* 21:331–354, 1939.

Huxtable LM, Tafreshi MJ, Rakkar AN: Frequency and management of thrombocytopenia with the glycoprotein IIb/IIIa receptor antagonists. *Am J Cardiol* 97:426–429, 2006.

Irons RD: Leukemogenesis as a toxic response, in Sipes IG, McQueen AC, Gandolfi AJ (eds.): *Comprehensive Toxicology,* Oxford: Pergamon Press, 1997, pp. 175–199.

Jaffe ES: *World Health Organization Classification of Tumours: Tumours of Haematopoietic and Lymphoid Tissues Pathology and Genetics.* Lyon: IARC Press, 2001.

Jandl JH: *Blood.* Boston: Little Brown & Co., 1987.

Johansson B, Mertens F, Heim S, *et al.*: Cytogenetics of secondary myelodysplasia (sMDS) and acute nonlymphocytic leukemia (sANLL). *Eur J Haematol* 47:17–27, 1991.

Julia A, Olona M, Bueno J, *et al.*: Drug-induced agranulocytosis: Prognostic factors in a series of 168 episodes. *Br J Haematol* 79:366–371, 1991.

Jurk K, Kehrel BE: Platelets: Physiology and biochemistry. *Semin Thromb Hemost* 31:381–392, 2005.

Kantarjian HM, Keating MJ, Walters RS, *et al.*: Therapy-related leukemia and myelodysplastic syndrome: Clinical, cytogenetic, and prognostic features. *J Clin Oncol* 4:1748–1757, 1986.

Kao LW, Nanagas KA: Carbon monoxide poisoning. *Med Clin North Am* 89:1161–1194, 2005.

Kaushansky K: Blood: New designs for a new millennium. *Blood* 95:1–6, 2000.

Kaushansky K: Lineage-specific hematopoietic growth factors. *N Engl J Med* 354:2034–2045, 2006.

Keng PC: Use of flow cytometry in the measurement of cell mitotic cycle. *Int J Cell Cloning* 4:295–311, 1986.

Khan NA, Kruse JA: Methemoglobinemia induced by topical anesthesia: A case report and review. *Am J Med Sci* 318:415–418, 1999.

Kilbourne EM, Posada de la PM, Abaitua B, I, *et al.*: Toxic oil syndrome: A current clinical and epidemiologic summary, including comparisons with the eosinophilia-myalgia syndrome. *J Am Coll Cardiol* 18:711–717, 1991.

Kim-Shapiro DB, Gladwin MT, Patel RP, *et al.*: The reaction between nitrite and hemoglobin: The role of nitrite in hemoglobin-mediated hypoxic vasodilation. *J Inorg Biochem* 99:237–246, 2005.

Kolachana P, Subrahmanyam VV, Meyer KB, *et al.*: Benzene and its phenolic metabolites produce oxidative DNA damage in HL60 cells in vitro and in the bone marrow in vivo. *Cancer Res* 53:1023–1026, 1993.

Koren E, Zuckerman LA, Mire-Sluis AR: Immune responses to therapeutic proteins in humans—clinical significance, assessment and prediction. *Curr Pharm Biotechnol* 3:349–360, 2002.

Kuderer NM, Cosler L, Crawford J: Cost and mortality associated with febrile neutropenia in adult cancer patients. *Proc Am Soc Clin Oncol* 21:250a, 2002.

Kumar S, Bandyopadhyay U: Free heme toxicity and its detoxification systems in human. *Toxicol Lett* 157:175–188, 2005.

Ladiges WC, Storb R, Thomas ED: Canine models of bone marrow transplantation. *Lab Anim Sci* 40:11–15, 1990.

Lane DA, Philippou H, Huntington JA: Directing thrombin. *Blood* 106:2605–2612, 2005.

Larochelle A, Krouse A, Metzger M, *et al.*: AMD3100 mobilizes hematopoietic stem cells with long-term repopulating capacity in nonhuman primates. *Blood* 107:3772–3778, 2006.

Larson RA, Le Beau MM: Therapy-related myeloid leukaemia: A model for leukemogenesis in humans. *Chem Biol Interact* 153–154:187–195, 2005.

Lataillade JJ, Domenech J, Le Bousse-Kerdiles MC: Stromal cell-derived factor-1 (SDF-1)\CXCR4 couple plays multiple roles on haematopoietic progenitors at the border between the old cytokine and new chemokine worlds: Survival, cell cycling and trafficking. *Eur Cytokine Netw* 15:177–188, 2004.

Laurence AD: Location, movement and survival: The role of chemokines in haematopoiesis and malignancy. *Br J Haematol* 132:255–267, 2006.

Le Beau MM, Albain KS, Larson RA, *et al.*: Clinical and cytogenetic correlations in 63 patients with therapy-related myelodysplastic syndromes and acute nonlymphocytic leukemia: Further evidence for characteristic abnormalities of chromosomes no. 5 and 7. *J Clin Oncol* 4:325–345, 1986.

Leung KN, Mak NK, Fung MC: Cytokines in the differentiation therapy of leukemia: From laboratory investigations to clinical applications. *Crit Rev Clin Lab Sci* 42:473–514, 2005.

Levine EG, Bloomfield CD: Leukemias and myelodysplastic syndromes secondary to drug, radiation, and environmental exposure. *Semin Oncol* 19:47–84, 1992.

Levine JG, Szarfman A: Standardized data structures and visualization tools: A way to accelerate the regulatory review of the integrated summary of safety of new drug applications. *Biopharm Rep* 4:1996.

Li J, Yang C, Xia Y, *et al.*: Thrombocytopenia caused by the development of antibodies to thrombopoietin. *Blood* 98:3241–3248, 2001.

Lian EC: Pathogenesis of thrombotic thrombocytopenic purpura: ADAMTS13 deficiency and beyond. *Semin Thromb Hemost* 31:625–632, 2005.

Liesveld JL, Lichtman MA: Evaluation of granulocytes and mononuclear phagocytes, in Sipes IG, McQueen CA, Gandolfi AJ (eds.): *Comprehensive Toxicology*. Oxford: Pergamon Press, 1997, pp. 123–144.

Liles WC, Rodger E, Broxmeyer HE, *et al.*: Augmented mobilization and collection of CD34+ hematopoietic cells from normal human volunteers stimulated with granulocyte-colony-stimulating factor by single-dose administration of AMD3100, a CXCR4 antagonist. *Transfusion* 45:295–300, 2005.

Lillevang ST, Albertsen M, Rasmussen F, *et al.*: Effect of radiographic contrast media on granulocyte phagocytosis of Escherichia coli in a whole blood flow cytometric assay. *Invest Radiol* 29:68–71, 1994.

Lindorfer MA, Hahn CS, Foley PL, *et al.*: Heteropolymer-mediated clearance of immune complexes via erythrocyte CR1: Mechanisms and applications. *Immunol Rev* 183:10–24, 2001.

Lollar P: Pathogenic antibodies to coagulation factors. Part one: Factor VIII and factor IX. *J Thromb Haemost* 2:1082–1095, 2004.

Lollar P: Pathogenic antibodies to coagulation factors. Part II. Fibrinogen, prothrombin, thrombin, factor V, factor XI, factor XII, factor XIII, the protein C system and von Willebrand factor. *J Thromb Haemost* 3:1385–1391, 2005.

Look AT: Molecular Pathogenesis of MDS, in Berliner N, Lee SJ, Linenberger M, Vogelsang GB (eds.): *American Society of Hematology Education Program Book*. Washington, D.C.: American Society of Hematology, 2005, pp. 156–160.

Loomis MR, Henrickson RV, Anderson JH: Effects of ketamine hydrochloride on the hemogram of rhesus monkeys (Macaca mulatta). *Lab Anim Sci* 30:851–853, 1980.

Lund JE: Toxicologic effects on blood and bone marrow, in Feldman BF, Zinkl JG, Jain NC (eds.): *Schalm's Veterinary Hematology*, 5th ed. Ames, Iowa: Blackwell Publishing, 2000, pp. 44–50.

Lundberg JO, Weitzberg E: NO generation from nitrite and its role in vascular control. *Arterioscler Thromb Vasc Biol* 25:915–922, 2005.

Mangano DT, Tudor IC, Dietzel C: The risk associated with aprotinin in cardiac surgery. *N Engl J Med* 354:353–365, 2006.

Mannucci PM: Hemostatic drugs. *N Engl J Med* 339:245–253, 1998.

Marsh JC: Correlation of hematologic toxicity of antineoplastic agents with their effects on bone marrow stem cells: Interspecies studies using an in vivo assay. *Exp Hematol* 16(suppl 13):16–22, 1985.

Martin C, Burdon PC, Bridger G, *et al.*: Chemokines acting via CXCR2 and CXCR4 control the release of neutrophils from the bone marrow and their return following senescence. *Immunity* 19:583–593, 2003.

Mason RP, Fischer V: Possible role of free radical formation in drug-induced agranulocytosis. *Drug Safety* 1(suppl 7):45–50, 1992.

Matzdorff A: Platelet function tests and flow cytometry to monitor antiplatelet therapy. *Semin Thromb Hemost* 31:393–399, 2005.

Mauritzson N, Johansson B, Albin M, *et al.*: Survival time in a population-based consecutive series of adult acute myeloid leukemia—the prognostic impact of karyotype during the time period 1976–1993. *Leukemia* 14:1039–1043, 2000.

Mazzone A, Mazzucchelli I, Fossati G, *et al.*: Granulocyte defects and opioid receptors in chronic exposure to heroin or methadone in humans. *Int J Immunopharmacol* 16:959–967, 1994.

McRedmond JP, Harriott P, Walker B, *et al.*: Streptokinase-induced platelet activation involves antistreptokinase antibodies and cleavage of protease-activated receptor-1. *Blood* 95:1301–1308, 2000.

Menon V, Harrington RA, Hochman JS, *et al.*: Thrombolysis and adjunctive therapy in acute myocardial infarction: The Seventh ACCP Conference on Antithrombotic and Thrombolytic Therapy. *Chest* 126:549S–575S, 2004.

Mitelman F, Brandt L, Nilsson PG: Relation among occupational exposure to potential mutagenic/carcinogenic agents, clinical findings, and bone marrow chromosomes in acute nonlymphocytic leukemia. *Blood* 52:1229–1237, 1978.

Mitelman F, Nilsson PG, Brandt L, *et al.*: Chromosome pattern, occupation, and clinical features in patients with acute nonlymphocytic leukemia. *Cancer Genet Cytogenet* 4:197–214, 1981.

Miyagi T, Lam KM, Chuang LF, *et al.*: Suppression of chemokine-induced chemotaxis of monkey neutrophils and monocytes by chlorinated hydrocarbon insecticides. *In Vivo* 12:441–446, 1998.

Monroe DM, Hoffman M: What does it take to make the perfect clot? *Arterioscler Thromb Vasc Biol* 25:2463–2469, 2005.

Moore DM: Hematology of the mouse, in Feldman BF, Zinkl JG, Jain NC (eds.): *Schalm's Veterinary Hematology*, 5th ed. Ames, Iowa: Blackwell Publishing, 2000a, pp. 1219–1224.

Moore DM: Hematology of the rat, in Feldman BF, Zinkl JG, Jain NC (eds.): *Schalm's Veterinary Hematology*, 5th ed. Ames, Iowa: Blackwell Publishing, 2000b, pp. 1210–1218.

Moore EE, Johnson JL, Cheng AM, *et al.*: Insights from studies of blood substitutes in trauma. *Shock* 24:197–205, 2005.

Moore MAS: Embryologic and phylogenetic development of the haematopoietic system. *Adv Biosci* 16:87–103, 1975.

Murphy SB: Secondary acute myeloid leukemia following treatment with epipodophyllotoxins. *J Clin Oncol* 11:199–201, 1993.

Nakagawa M, Terashima T, D'yachkova Y, *et al.*: Glucocorticoid-induced granulocytosis: Contribution of marrow release and demargination of intravascular granulocytes. *Circulation* 98:2307–2313, 1998.

Napier I, Ponka P, Richardson DR: Iron trafficking in the mitochondrion: Novel pathways revealed by disease. *Blood* 105:1867–1874, 2005.

Nathan C: Neutrophils and immunity: Challenges and opportunities. *Nat Rev Immunol* 6:173–182, 2006.

Naughton BA, Sibanda B, Azar L, et al.: Differential effects of drugs upon hematopoiesis can be assessed in long-term bone marrow cultures established on nylon screens. *Proc Soc Exp Biol Med* 199:481–490, 1992.

Negro GD, Bonato M, Gribaldo L: In vitro bone marrow granulocyte-macrophage progenitor cultures in the assessment of hematotoxic potential of the new drugs. *Cell Biol Toxicol* 17:95–105, 2001.

Nguyen ST, Cabrales RE, Bashour CA, et al.: Benzocaine-induced methemoglobinemia. *Anesth Analg* 90:369–371, 2000.

Nifli AP, Notas G, Mamoulaki M, et al.: Comparison of a multiplex, bead-based fluorescent assay and immunofluorescence methods for the detection of ANA and ANCA autoantibodies in human serum. *J Immunol Methods* 311:189–197, 2006.

Njalsson R, Norgren S: Physiological and pathological aspects of GSH metabolism. *Acta Paediatr* 94:132–137, 2005.

O'Neill R: Assessment of safety, in Peace KE (ed.): *Biopharmaceutical Statistics for Drug Development*. New York: Marcel Dekker, 1988, pp. 543–604.

Palmblad J, Papadaki HA, Eliopoulos G: Acute and chronic neutropenias. What is new? *J Intern Med* 250:476–491, 2001.

Papassotiriou I, Kister J, Griffon N, et al.: Modulating the oxygen affinity of human fetal haemoglobin with synthetic allosteric modulators. *Br J Haematol* 102:1165–1171, 1998.

Parchment RE, Huang M, Erickson-Miller CL: Roles for in vitro myelotoxicity tests in preclinical drug development and clinical trial planning. *Toxicol Pathol* 21:241–250, 1993.

Parchment RE, Murphy MJ: Human hematopoietic stem cells: Laboratory assessment and response to toxic injury, in Sipes IG MAGA (ed.): *Comprehensive Toxicology*. Oxford: Pergamon Press, 1997, pp. 303–320.

Parent-Massin D, Thouvenot D, Rio B, et al.: Lindane haematotoxicity confirmed by in vitro tests on human and rat progenitors. *Hum Exp Toxicol* 13:103–106, 1994.

Patton WN, Duffull SB: Idiosyncratic drug-induced haematological abnormalities. Incidence, pathogenesis, management and avoidance. *Drug Safety* 11:445–462, 1994.

Pedersen-Bjergaard J, Pedersen M, Roulston D, et al.: Different genetic pathways in leukemogenesis for patients presenting with therapy-related myelodysplasia and therapy-related acute myeloid leukemia. *Blood* 86:3542–3552, 1995.

Pedersen-Bjergaard J, Philip P, Pedersen NT, et al.: Acute nonlymphocytic leukemia, preleukemia, and acute myeloproliferative syndrome secondary to treatment of other malignant diseases. II. Bone marrow cytology, cytogenetics, results of HLA typing, response to antileukemic chemotherapy, and survival in a total series of 55 patients. *Cancer* 54:452–462, 1984.

Perazella MA, Biswas P: Acute hyperkalemia associated with intravenous epsilon-aminocaproic acid therapy. *Am J Kidney Dis* 33:782–785, 1999.

Percy MJ, McFerran NV, Lappin TR: Disorders of oxidised haemoglobin. *Blood Rev* 19:61–68, 2005.

Pessina A, Albella B, Bayo M, et al.: Application of the CFU-GM assay to predict acute drug-induced neutropenia: An international blind trial to validate a prediction model for the maximum tolerated dose (MTD) of myelosuppressive xenobiotics. *Toxicol Sci* 75:355–367, 2003.

Pessina A, Albella B, Bueren J, et al.: Prevalidation of a model for predicting acute neutropenia by colony forming unit granulocyte/macrophage (CFU-GM) assay. *Toxicol In Vitro* 15:729–740, 2001.

Pessina A, Malerba I, Gribaldo L: Hematotoxicity testing by cell clonogenic assay in drug development and preclinical trials. *Curr Pharm Des* 11:1055–1065, 2005.

Peters DC, Noble S: Aprotinin: An update of its pharmacology and therapeutic use in open heart surgery and coronary artery bypass surgery. *Drugs* 57:233–260, 1999.

Peters WP, Holland JF, Senn H, et al.: Corticosteroid administration and localized leukocyte mobilization in man. *N Engl J Med* 286:342–345, 1972.

Phillips GL: The potential of amifostine in high-dose chemotherapy and autologous hematopoietic stem cell transplantation. *Semin Oncol* 29:53–56, 2002.

Pisciotta AV: Immune and toxic mechanisms in drug-induced agranulocytosis. *Semin Hematol* 10:279–310, 1973.

Ponka P: Tissue-specific regulation of iron metabolism and heme synthesis: Distinct control mechanisms in erythroid cells. *Blood* 89:1–25, 1997.

Powley MW, Carlson GP: Hepatic and pulmonary microsomal benzene metabolism in CYP2E1 knockout mice. *Toxicology* 169:187–194, 2001.

Poyart C, Marden MC, Kister J: Bezafibrate derivatives as potent effectors of hemoglobin. *Methods Enzymol* 232:496–513, 1994.

Prchal JT: Clinical manifestations and classification of erythrocyte disorders, in Lichtman MA, Beutler E, Kipps TJ, Seligsohn U, Kaushansky K, Prchal JT (eds.): *Williams Hematology, 7th ed.* New York: McGraw Hill, 2006, pp. 411–418.

Rader M: Granulocyte colony-stimulating factor use in patients with chemotherapy-induced neutropenia: Clinical and economic benefits. *Oncology* 20:16–21, 2006.

Reagan WJ, Handy V, McKamey A, et al.: Effects of doxorubicin on the canine erythroid and myeloid progenitor cells and bone marrow microenvironment. *Comp Haematol* 3:96–101, 1993.

Reynolds VL: Applications of emerging technologies in toxicology and safety assessment. *Int J Toxicol* 24:135–137, 2005.

Rojas JC, Aguilar B, Rodriguez-Maldonado E, et al.: Pharmacogenetics of oral anticoagulants. *Blood Coagul Fibrinolysis* 16:389–398, 2005.

Rossi G, Pelizzari AM, Bellotti D, et al.: Cytogenetic analogy between myelodysplastic syndrome and acute myeloid leukemia of elderly patients. *Leukemia* 14:636–641, 2000.

Rother RP, Bell L, Hillmen P, et al.: The clinical sequelae of intravascular hemolysis and extracellular plasma hemoglobin: A novel mechanism of human disease. *JAMA* 293:1653–1662, 2005.

Roujeau JC: Clinical heterogeneity of drug hypersensitivity. *Toxicology* 209:123–129, 2005.

Rowley JD, Golomb HM, Vardiman JW: Nonrandom chromosome abnormalities in acute leukemia and dysmyelopoietic syndromes in patients with previously treated malignant disease. *Blood* 58:759–767, 1981.

Ryan DH: Examination of the blood, in Lichtman MA, Beutler E, Kipps TJ, Seligsohn U, Kaushansky K, Prchal JT (eds.): *Williams Hematology, 7th ed.* New York: McGraw-Hill, 2006, pp. 11–19.

Ryter SW, Otterbein LE: Carbon monoxide in biology and medicine. *Bioessays* 26:270–280, 2004.

Sagov SE: March hemoglobinuria treated with rubber insoles: Two case reports. *J Am Coll Health Assoc* 19:146–1970.

Salama A, Schutz B, Kiefel V, et al.: Immune-mediated agranulocytosis related to drugs and their metabolites: Mode of sensitization and heterogeneity of antibodies. *Br J Haematol* 72:127–132, 1989.

Sandoval C, Pui CH, Bowman LC, et al.: Secondary acute myeloid leukemia in children previously treated with alkylating agents, intercalating topoisomerase II inhibitors, and irradiation. *J Clin Oncol* 11:1039–1045, 1993.

Sato K, Miyakawa M, Han DC, et al.: Graves' disease with neutropenia and marked splenomegaly: Autoimmune neutropenia due to propylthiouracil. *J Endocrinol Invest* 8:551–555, 1985.

Schmaier AH, Rojkjaer R, Shariat-Madar Z: Activation of the plasma kallikrein/kinin system on cells: A revised hypothesis. *Thromb Haemost* 82:226–233, 1999.

Schneidkraut MJ, Loegering DJ: Effect of extravascular hemolysis on the RES depression following thermal injury. *Exp Mol Pathol* 40:271–279, 1984.

Schrijvers D, Highley M, De BE, et al.: Role of red blood cells in pharmacokinetics of chemotherapeutic agents. *Anticancer Drugs* 10:147–153, 1999.

Sedrakyan A, Atkins D, Treasure T: The risk of aprotinin: A conflict of evidence. *Lancet* 367:1376–1377, 2006.

Semerad CL, Liu F, Gregory AD, et al.: G-CSF is an essential regulator of neutrophil trafficking from the bone marrow to the blood. *Immunity* 17:413–423, 2002.

Shen M, Lan Q, Zhang L, *et al.*: Polymorphisms in genes involved in DNA double strand break repair pathway and susceptibility to benzene-induced hematotoxicity. *Carcinogenesis* 2006.

Shifrine M, Wilson FD: *The Canine As a Biomedical Research Model: Immunological, Hematological and Oncological Aspects*. Springfield: US Department of Commerce Technical Information Center, 1980.

Shimizu Y, Kato H, Schull WJ, *et al.*: Studies of the mortality of A-bomb survivors. 9. Mortality, 1950–1985: Part 1. Comparison of risk coefficients for site-specific cancer mortality based on the DS86 and T65DR shielded kerma and organ doses. *Radiat Res* 118:502–524, 1989.

Siebert WJ, Ayres RW, Bulling MT, *et al.*: Streptokinase morbidity—more common than previously recognised. *Aust N Z J Med* 22:129–133, 1992.

Smith MA, Smith JG, Provan AB, *et al.*: The effect of rh-cytokines on the sensitivity of normal human CFU-GM progenitors to Ara-C and on the S-phase activity of light density human bone marrow cells. *Leuk Res* 18:105–110, 1994.

Stafford DW: The vitamin K cycle. *J Thromb Haemost* 3:1873–1878, 2005.

Stark MA, Huo Y, Burcin TL, *et al.*: Phagocytosis of apoptotic neutrophils regulates granulopoiesis via IL-23 and IL-17. *Immunity* 22:285–294, 2005.

Steinberg MH: Pathophysiologically based drug treatment of sickle cell disease. *Trends Pharmacol Sci* 27:204–210, 2006.

Stern A: Drug-induced oxidative denaturation in red blood cells. *Semin Hematol* 26:301–306, 1989.

Stern SC, Shah S, Costello C: Probable autoimmune neutropenia induced by fludarabine treatment for chronic lymphocytic leukaemia. *Br J Haematol* 106:836–837, 1999.

Suber RL, Kodell RL: The effect of three phlebotomy techniques on hematological and clinical chemical evaluation in sprague-dawley rats. *Vet Clin Pathol* 14:23–30, 1985.

Sundman-Engberg B, Tidefelt U, Paul C: Toxicity of cytostatic drugs to normal bone marrow cells in vitro. *Cancer Chemother Pharmacol* 42:17–23, 1998.

Szarfman A, Machado SG, O'Neill RT: Use of screening algorithms and computer systems to efficiently signal higher-than-expected combinations of drugs and events in the US FDA's spontaneous reports database. *Drug Safety* 25:381–392, 2002.

Szarfman A, Talarick L, Levine JG: Analysis and risk assessment of hematological data from clinical trials, in Sipes IG, MAGA (ed.): *Comprehensive Toxicology*. Oxford: Pergamon Press, 1997, pp. 363–379.

Tamaoki J: The effects of macrolides on inflammatory cells. *Chest* 125:41S–50S, 2004.

Tannock IF: Experimental chemotherapy and concepts related to the cell cycle. *Int J Radiat Biol Relat Stud Phys Chem Med* 49:335–355, 1986.

Tavazzi B, Di PD, Amorini AM, *et al.*: Energy metabolism and lipid peroxidation of human erythrocytes as a function of increased oxidative stress. *Eur J Biochem* 267:684–689, 2000.

Thirman MJ, Larson RA: Therapy-related myeloid leukemia. *Hematol Oncol Clin North Am* 10:293–320, 1996.

Todd MD, Ulrich RG: Emerging technologies for accelerated toxicity evaluation of potential drug candidates. *Curr Opin Drug Disc Res* 2:58–68, 1999.

Turbay D, Lieberman J, Alper CA, *et al.*: Tumor necrosis factor constellation polymorphism and clozapine-induced agranulocytosis in two different ethnic groups. *Blood* 89:4167–4174, 1997.

Uetrecht J: Drug metabolism by leukocytes and its role in drug-induced lupus and other idiosyncratic drug reactions. *Crit Rev Toxicol* 20:213–235, 1990.

Uetrecht JP: New concepts in immunology relevant to idiosyncratic drug reactions: The "danger hypothesis" and innate immune system. *Chem Res Toxicol* 12:387–395, 1999.

Valagussa P, Kenda R, Fossati F, *et al.*: Incidence of 2d malignancies in Hodgkin's-Disease (HD) after various forms of treatment (abstr). *Proc Am Soc Clin Oncol* 20:360, 1979.

Valli VE, McGrath JP: Comparative leukocyte biology and toxicology, in Sipes IG, MAGA (ed.): *Comprehensive Toxicology*. Oxford: Pergamon Press, 1997, pp. 201–215.

van den Bemt PM, Meyboom RH, Egberts AC: Drug-induced immune thrombocytopenia. *Drug Safety* 27:1243–1252, 2004.

Van Wijk R, van Solinge WW: The energy-less blood cell is lost: Erythrocyte enzyme abnormalities of glycolysis. *Blood* 106:4034–4042, 2005.

Vandendries ER, Drews RE: Drug-associated disease: Hematologic dysfunction. *Crit Care Clin* 22:347–355, 2006.

Varga J, Uitto J, Jimenez SA: The cause and pathogenesis of the eosinophilia-myalgia syndrome. *Ann Intern Med* 116:140–147, 1992.

Varmus H, Weinberg RA: *Genes and the Biology of Cancer*. New York: Scientific American Library, 1993.

Veyradier A, Meyer D: Thrombotic thrombocytopenic purpura and its diagnosis. *J Thromb Haemost* 3:2420–2427, 2005.

Vincent PC: Drug-induced aplastic anaemia and agranulocytosis. Incidence and mechanisms. *Drugs* 31:52–63, 1986.

Vismans JJ, Briet E, Meijer K, *et al.*: Azathioprine and subacute myelomonocytic leukemia. *Acta Med Scand* 207:315–319, 1980.

Vogelstein B, Fearon ER, Hamilton SR, *et al.*: Genetic alterations during colorectal-tumor development. *N Engl J Med* 319:525–532, 1988.

Voog E, Morschhauser F, Solal-Celigny P: Neutropenia in patients treated with rituximab. *N Engl J Med* 348:2691–2694, 2003.

Wan J, Badham HJ, Winn L: The role of c-MYB in benzene-initiated toxicity. *Chem Biol Interact* 153–154, 171–178, 2005.

Warkentin TE, Greinacher A: Heparin-induced thrombocytopenia: Recognition, treatment, and prevention: The Seventh ACCP Conference on Antithrombotic and Thrombolytic Therapy. *Chest* 126:311S-337S, 2004.

Weatherall D: Disorders of globin synthesis in the thalassemias, in Lichtman MA, Beutler E, Kipps TJ, Seligsohn U, Kaushansky K, Prchal JT (eds.): *Williams Hematology, 7th ed*. New York: McGraw-Hill, 2006, pp. 663–666.

Weingand K, Brown G, Hall R, *et al.*: Harmonization of animal clinical pathology testing in toxicity and safety studies. *Fundam Appl Toxicol* 29:198–201, 1996.

West BC, DeVault Jr. GA, Clement JC, *et al.*: Aplastic anemia associated with parenteral chloramphenicol: Review of 10 cases, including the second case of possible increased risk with cimetidine. *Rev Infect Dis* 10:1048–1051, 1988.

WHO: *World Health Organization Handbook for Reporting Results of Cancer Treatments*. Offset Publication No. 48. Geneva: WHO, 1979.

Williams CL, Whitaker MH: The molecular biology of acute myeloid leukemia. Proto-oncogene expression and function in normal and neoplastic myeloid cells. *Clin Lab Med* 10:769–796, 1990.

Williams DP, Pirmohamed M, Naisbitt DJ, *et al.*: Induction of metabolism-dependent and -independent neutrophil apoptosis by clozapine. *Mol Pharmacol* 58:207–216, 2000.

Williams LH, Udupa KB, Lipschitz DA: Long-term bone marrow culture as a model for host toxicity: The effect of methotrexate on hematopoiesis and adherent layer function. *Exp Hematol* 16:80–87, 1988.

Wintrobe MM: *Hematology, The Blossoming of Science: A Story of Inspiration and Effort*. New York: Lea & Febiger, 1985.

Yoo D, Lessin LS: Drug-associated "bite cell" hemolytic anemia. *Am J Med* 92:243–248, 1992.

Young NS: Acqired aplastic anemia. *JAMA* 282:271–278, 1999.

Young NS: Hematopoietic cell destruction by immune mechanisms in acquired aplastic anemia. *Semin Hematol* 37:14, 2000.

Young KM, Weiss L: Hematopoiesis: Structure-function relationships in bone marrow and spleen, in Sipes IG, McQueen AC, Gandolfi AJ (eds.): *Comprehensive Toxicology*. Oxford: Pergamon Press, 1997, pp. 11–34.

Yunis JJ, Corzo D, Salazar M, *et al.*: HLA associations in clozapine-induced agranulocytosis. *Blood* 86:1177–1183, 1995.

Zakarija A, Bennett C: Drug-induced thrombotic microangiopathy. *Semin Thromb Hemost* 31:681–690, 2005.

Zanni MP, Schnyder B, von GS, *et al.*: Involvement of T cells in drug-induced allergies. *Trends Pharmacol Sci* 19:308–310, 1998.

CHAPTER 12

TOXIC RESPONSES OF THE IMMUNE SYSTEM

Norbert E. Kaminski, Barbara L. Faubert Kaplan, and Michael P. Holsapple

Immunotoxicology can be most simply defined as the study of adverse effects on the immune system resulting from occupational, inadvertent, or therapeutic exposure to drugs, environmental chemicals, and, in some instances, biological materials. Studies in animals and humans have indicated that the immune system comprises potential target organs, and that damage to this system can be associated with morbidity and even mortality. Indeed, in some instances, the immune system has been shown to be compromised (decreased lymphoid cellularity, alterations in lymphocyte subpopulations, decreased host resistance, and altered specific immune function responses) in the absence of observed toxicity in other organ systems. These studies coupled with tremendous advances made in immunology and molecular biology have led to a steady and exponential growth in our understanding of immunotoxicology during the past 25 years. Recognition by regulatory agencies that the immune system is an important, as well as sensitive, target organ for chemical- and drug-induced toxicity (as described in greater detail later in this chapter) is another indication of the growth of this subdiscipline of toxicology. With the availability of sensitive, reproducible, and predictive tests, it is now apparent that the inclusion of immunotoxicity testing represents a significant adjunct to routine safety evaluations for therapeutic agents, biological agents, and chemicals now in development.

Understanding the impact of toxic responses on the immune system requires an appreciation of its role, which may be stated succinctly as the preservation of integrity. It is a series of delicately balanced, complex, multicellular, and physiological mechanisms that allow an individual to distinguish foreign material (i.e., "nonself") from "self," and to neutralize, eliminate, and/or coexist with the foreign matter. Examples of self are all the tissues, organs, and cells of the body. Examples of nonself are a variety of opportunistic pathogens, including bacteria and viruses, and transformed cells or tissues (i.e., tumors). The immune system is characterized by a virtually infinite repertoire of specificities, highly specialized effectors, complex regulatory mechanisms, and an ability to travel throughout the body. The great complexity of the mammalian immune system is an indication of the importance, as well as the difficulty, of its role. If the immune system fails to recognize as nonself an infectious entity or neoantigens expressed by a newly arisen tumor, then the host is in danger of rapidly succumbing to the unopposed invasion. This aspect of immunocompetence is the reason why the immune system is often made synonymous with "host defense." Alternatively, if some integral bodily tissue is not identified as self, then the immune system is capable of turning its considerable defensive capabilities against that tissue, and an autoimmune disease may be the end result. This aspect of immunocompetence emphasizes the tremendous destructive potential that is associated with the host defense mechanisms of the immune system. The cost to the host of these mistakes, made in either direction, may be quite high. The fact that mistakes can occur in either direction is an indication that immunotoxicology should be considered as a continuum (Fig. 12-1). At the center of the concept of the continuum is the recognition that immune responses in the normal human population can vary by more than two standard deviations (Luebke *et al.*, 2004), as described in greater detail in the section "Approaches to the Assessment of Human Immunotoxicity." Treatment-related effects that are not clearly manifested as adverse are depicted in Fig. 12-1 as the lightly shaded areas both above and below the normal range. Because the cost of mistakes in immunocompetence can be so high, and because of the tremendous diversity involved in the identification of self versus nonself, a complex array of organs, cells, soluble factors, and their interactions has evolved to regulate this system and minimize the frequency of errors in either direction. Due to the potentially profound effects resulting from disruption of the delicately balanced immune system, there is a need to understand the cellular, biochemical, and molecular mechanisms of xenobiotic-induced immune modulation.

This chapter provides (1) an overview of basic concepts in immunology (structure, components, and functions), which are important to the understanding of the impact xenobiotics may have on the exposed individual; (2) a summary of selected current methods utilized to assess immune function; and (3) a brief review of current information on the immune modulation (immune suppression, immune enhancement, hypersensitivity, and autoimmunity) induced by a variety of xenobiotics. This chapter is not meant to be an immunology textbook, nor an exhaustive review of the mechanisms

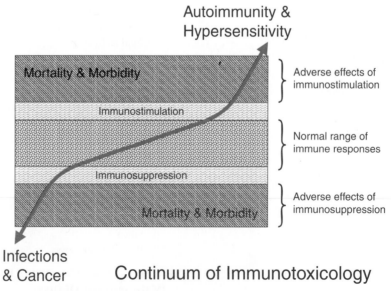

Figure 12-1. The continuum of immunotoxicology.

Table 12-1

Organization of the Immune System: Lymphoid Tissue

CLASSIFICATION	LYMPHOID ORGANS
Primary	Bone marrow
	Thymus
Secondary	Spleen
	Lymph nodes
	Peyer's patches
Tertiary	Skin-associated lymphoid tissue (SALT)
	Mucosal lamina propria (MALT)
	Gut-associated lymphoid tissue (GALT)
	Bronchial-associated lymphoid tissue (BALT)
	Nasal-associated lymphoid tissue (NALT)
	Cells lining the genitourinary tract

of immunotoxicity of a myriad of xenobiotics. For detailed information on immunology, the reader is referred to three texts: the first edited by Paul (5th edition, 2003), *Fundamental Immunology*, the second edited by Roitt, Brostoff, and Male (10th edition, 2003), *Immunology*, and the third edited by Janeway, Travers, Walport, and Capra, (6th edition, 2004), *Immunobiology, The Immune System in Health and Disease*. For a more comprehensive review of immunotoxicology, the reader is referred to two texts: the first edited by Vohr *et al.* (2005), *Encyclopedic Reference of Immunotoxicology*; and the second edited by Luebke, House, and Kimber (2nd edition, 2006), *Immunotoxicology and Immunopharmacology, Target Organ Toxicity Series*.

THE IMMUNE SYSTEM

Unlike most organ systems, the immune system has the unique quality of not being confined to a single site within the body. It comprises

numerous lymphoid organs (Table 12-1) and numerous different cellular populations with a variety of functions. The bone marrow and thymus are referred to as primary lymphoid organs because they contain the microenvironments capable of supporting the production of mature B- and T cells, respectively. In addition, the bone marrow is the site of origin of the pluripotent stem cell, a self-renewing cell from which all other hematopoietic cells are derived (Figs. 12-2 and 12-6). During gestation, this cell is found in the embryonic yolk sac and fetal liver; eventually, it migrates to the bone marrow. Within the bone marrow, the cells of the immune system developmentally "commit" to either the lymphoid or myeloid lineages. Cells of the lymphoid lineage make a further commitment to become either T- or B cells. Because of their critical role in initiation and regulation of immune responses, T-cell precursors are programmed to leave the bone marrow and migrate to the thymus, where they undergo "thymic education" for recognition of self and nonself.

Mature, naive, or virgin lymphocytes (those T- and B cells that have never undergone antigenic stimulation) are first brought into contact with exogenously derived antigens within the highly organized microenvironment of the spleen and lymph nodes, otherwise known as the secondary lymphoid organs. These organs can be thought of as biological sieves. The spleen serves as a filter for the blood, removing both foreign antigens and any circulating dead cells and cellular debris. The lymph nodes are part of a network of lymphatic veins that filter antigens from the fluid surrounding the tissues of the body.

Lymphoid tissues associated with the skin, mucosal lamina propria, gut, bronchioles, or nasal cavity are classified as tertiary lymphoid tissues and are referred to as associated lymphoid tissues (abbreviated SALT, MALT, GALT, BALT, and NALT, respectively). Peyer's patches, which are specialized structures in the small intestine that collect antigens from the gastrointestinal tract, are also tertiary lymphoid tissues. Tertiary lymphoid tissues are primarily effector sites where memory and effector cells exert immunologic

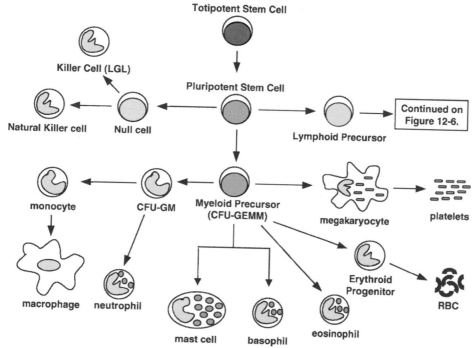

Figure 12-2. Development of the cellular components of the immune system.

Table 12-2

Innate versus Acquired Immunity

CHARACTERISTIC	INNATE IMMUNITY	ACQUIRED IMMUNITY
Cells involved	Polymorphonuclear cells (PMN)	T cells
	Monocytes/macrophages	B cells
	NK/NKT cells	Macrophages
Primary soluble mediators	Complement	Antibody
	Perforin/granzyme	Cytokines
	Acute phase proteins	Perforin/granzyme
	Interferon-α/β	
	Other cytokines	
Specificity of response	Limited to antigen-receptor binding (TLR, Fc, complement receptors)	Yes (very high specificity)
Response enhanced by repeated antigen challenge	No	Yes

Table 12-3

Properties of Immunoglobulin Classes and Subclasses

CLASS	MEAN SERUM CONCENTRATION (mg/mL)	HUMAN HALF-LIFE (DAYS)	BIOLOGICAL PROPERTIES
IgG			Complement fixation (selected subclasses)
			Crosses placenta
			Heterocytotropic antibody
Subclasses			
IgG$_1$	9	21	
IgG$_2$	3	20	
IgG$_3$	1	7	
IgG$_4$	1	21	
IgA	3	6	Secretory antibody
IgM	1.5	10	Complement fixation
			Efficient agglutination
IgD	0.03	3	Possible role in antigen-triggered lymphocyte differentiation
IgE	0.0001	2	Allergic responses (mast-cell degranulation)

and immunoregulatory functions. Although in a broad interpretation this would include essentially all tissues of the body, tertiary lymphoid tissues are defined as those tissues that have direct access to the external environment.

Antigen Recognition

Immunity   Mammalian immunity can be classified into two functional divisions: innate immunity and acquired (adaptive) immunity (Table 12-2). Innate immunity has historically been characterized as a nonspecific first-line defense response with no associated immunologic memory. Therefore, in a normal healthy adult, the magnitude of the innate immune response to a foreign organism is the same for a secondary or tertiary challenge as it is for the primary exposure. Acquired (adaptive) immunity, however, is characterized by both specificity and memory. Thus, in a normal healthy adult, the speed and magnitude of the acquired immune response to a foreign organism is greater for a secondary challenge than it is for the primary challenge.

Antigen   The primary determinant in either type of immune response is the ability of the immune system components to recognize self versus nonself. In one recent review, the definition of nonself, essentially, is anything other than that encoded in one's own germ line genome (Nathan, 2006). Given this broad interpretation of nonself, this includes foreign DNA, RNA, protein, and carbohydrates, and may even include aberrantly expressed or mutated self-proteins, since those are likely not contained in one's own germ line genome. A nonself substance that can be recognized by the immune system is called an antigen (also referred to as an immunogen or allergen). Although antigens were originally defined as substances that elicit antibody production, some antigens do not. Antigens are usually (but not absolutely) biological molecules that can be cleaved and rearranged for presentation to other immune cells. Generally, antigens are about 10 kDa or larger in size. Smaller antigens are termed "haptens" and must be conjugated with carrier molecules (larger antigens) in order to elicit a specific response. However, once an initial response is made, the hapten can induce subsequent responses in the absence of the carrier.

Antibodies   Antibodies are produced by B cells and are defined functionally by the antigen with which they react, and by their subtype (IgM, IgG and subsets, IgE, IgD, and IgA; Table 12-3). Thus, an IgM antibody directed against sheep red blood cells (sRBCs) is

Antigen-Binding Regions

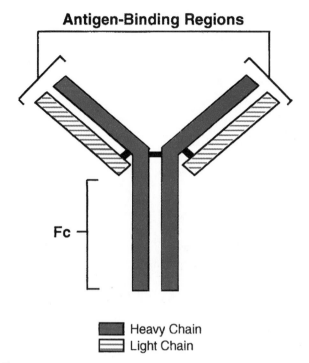

Fc —

▰ Heavy Chain
▤ Light Chain

Figure 12-3. Immunoglobulin structure.

called anti-sRBC IgM. Because the immune system generates antibody to thousands of antigens with which the host may or may not ever come into contact, general antibody of unknown specificity is referred to as immunoglobulin (e.g., serum immunoglobulin or serum IgM) until it can be defined by its specific antigen (e.g., anti-sRBC IgM). A simple way to view this point is that an antibody is an immunoglobulin, but an immunoglobulin is not necessarily an antibody.

The ability of the immune system to generate antibody to thousands of antigens is the result of somatic recombination, in which the germ line DNA that encodes for antibodies is rearranged in B cells. All immunoglobulins are made up of heavy and light chains and of constant and variable regions. For the light chain genes, two separate gene segments (V and J) are combined to form the variable region, which is then joined to one constant region. For the heavy chain genes, three separate gene segments (V, D, and J) are combined to form the variable region, which is then joined to one constant region. There are several light chain V and J genes, and several heavy chain V, D, and J genes, which when rearranged in various combinations, contribute to the immense genetic diversity of the immunoglobulin genes. Finally, the five types of immunoglobulin are dependent on which heavy chain constant region is transcribed and translated (heavy chain genes μ, γ, ε, δ, or α encode for the IgM, IgG, IgE, IgD, or IgA proteins, respectively).

The variable regions determine antibody specificity and interact with antigen (Fig. 12-3). The Fc region mediates various effector functions, such as complement activation (IgM and some IgG subclasses) and phagocyte binding (via Fc receptors). Antibodies possess several functions: (1) opsonization, which is coating of a pathogen with antibody to enhance Fc receptor-mediated endocytosis by phagocytic cells; (2) initiation of the classic pathway of complement-mediated lysis; (3) neutralization of viral infection by binding to viral particles and preventing further infection; and (4) enhancement of the specificity of effectors of

cell-mediated immunity (CMI) by binding to specific antigens on target cells, which are then recognized and eliminated by effector cells such as natural killer cells (NK cells), or cytotoxic T lymphocytes (CTL).

Complement   One of the consequences of antigen–antibody binding is initiation of the classical pathway of complement-mediated lysis. The complement system is a series of about 30 serum proteins whose primary functions are the destruction of membranes of infectious agents and the promotion of an inflammatory response (see section "Inflammation"). Complement activation occurs with each component sequentially acting on others, in a manner similar to the blood-clotting cascade (Fig. 12-4). Proximal components of the cascade are often modified serine proteases, which activate the system but have limited substrate specificity. Several components are capable of binding to microbial membranes and serve as ligands for complement receptors associated with the membrane. The final components, which are related structurally, are also membrane-binding proteins that can enter into the membrane and disrupt membrane integrity, termed the membrane attack complex (MAC).

Specifically, three pathways have been identified in activation of the complement cascade. The classical complement pathway is initiated when antibody binds antigen on the microorganism. The classical pathway then proceeds by activating a C1 subunit serine protease, subsequently recruiting C4, C2, and C3. Various cleavages ultimately result in C3b surface binding to the microorganism and release of C3a, a pro-inflammatory mediator (see section "Inflammation"). Microorganism-bound C3b can then be recognized by complement receptors on phagocytic cells, which engulf and destroy the microorganism. It is also at this point that the alternative pathway can be activated and amplifies the complement-mediated killing of the microorganism. Finally, C3b mediates recruitment of C5, which is cleaved, generating C5b on the surface and releasing C5a, another pro-inflammatory mediator (see section "Inflammation"). Microorganism-bound C5b recruits C6 and C7, the three of which form a complex and recruit C8. C9 is ultimately recruited, polymerizes, and forms a pore in the membrane of the microorganism, causing its death. In addition to the classical and alternative pathways, complement-mediated lysis is also activated through the lectin pathway, in which binding of mannin-binding lectin to the surface of the microorganism activates the pathway and converges with the classical pathway at C4.

Antigen Processing   In order to elicit an acquired immune response to a particular antigen, that antigen must be taken up and processed by accessory cells for presentation to lymphocytes. Accessory cells that perform this function are termed antigen-presenting cells (APC) and include the macrophage, follicular dendritic cell (FDC), Langerhans-dendritic cell, and B cells. Unique among the APCs is the FDC. Unlike hematopoietic cells, the FDC is not derived from the bone marrow stem cell. It is found in secondary lymphoid organs and binds antigen–antibody complexes, but it does not internalize and process the antigen. Instead, the primary function of the FDC is the presentation of antigen to B cells, which is dependent on the persistence of antigen within the secondary lymphoid tissue. This is believed to be critical for the maintenance of memory for B cells and the induction of high-affinity B-cell clones. Although thought of more for its ability to produce immunoglobulin, the B cell can also serve as an APC, and in low antigen concentrations this cell

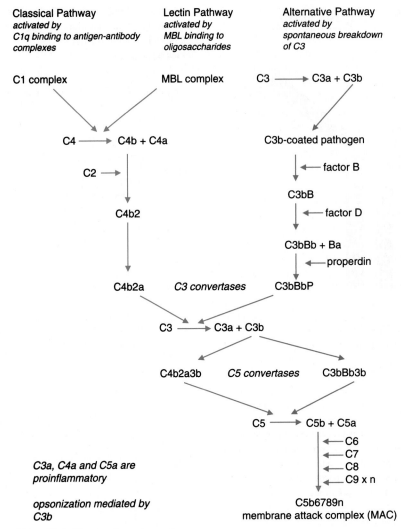

Classical Pathway
activated by
C1q binding to antigen-antibody complexes

Lectin Pathway
activated by
MBL binding to oligosaccharides

Alternative Pathway
activated by
spontaneous breakdown of C3

C1 complex   MBL complex   C3 → C3a + C3b

C4 → C4b + C4a   C3b-coated pathogen

C2 →   ← factor B

C4b2   C3bB

          ← factor D

          C3bBb + Ba

          ← properdin

C4b2a   *C3 convertases*   C3bBbP

C3 → C3a + C3b

C4b2a3b   *C5 convertases*   C3bBb3b

C5 → C5b + C5a

          ← C6
          ← C7
          ← C8
          ← C9 x n

C3a, C4a and C5a are proinflammatory

opsonization mediated by C3b

C5b6789n
membrane attack complex (MAC)

Figure 12-4. The complement cascade.

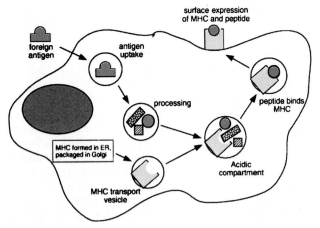

Figure 12-5. General schematic of antigen processing and presentation by the MHC class II pathway.

is equally as competent as the macrophage in serving this function. The Langerhans-dendritic cell is also a bone marrow-derived cell, but its lineage is distinct from that of the macrophage. It is found primarily in the epidermis, mucosal epithelium, and lymphoid tissues. The Langerhans-dendritic cell can migrate into the lymphatic system, where it serves as an APC in the lymph nodes. This cell plays a primary role in contact sensitization.

The interaction of APCs and lymphocytes is critical for the development of an acquired immune response. With the exception of the FDC, APCs internalize the antigen either by phagocytosis, pinocytosis, or receptor-mediated endocytosis (via antigen, Fc, or complement receptors). Following internalization, antigen is processed (intracellular denaturation and catabolism) through several cytoplasmic compartments, and a piece of the antigen (peptide fragments about 20 amino acids in length) becomes physically associated with major histocompatibility complex (MHC) class II (Fig. 12-5). This MHC class II–peptide complex is then transported to the surface of the cell and can interact in a specific manner with T lymphocytes. For most APCs, an immunogenic determinant is expressed on the surface of the APC within an hour after internalization, although this is slightly longer for B cells (3–4 hours). In addition to processing and presentation, pieces of processed antigen may be expelled into the extracellular space. These pieces of processed antigen can then bind in the peptide groove of empty MHC class II on the surface of other APCs for the presentation of that peptide fragment to lymphocytes.

In addition to antigen processing and presentation via MHC class II, some antigens may be processed and presented via MHC class I. Although the pathways share some similarities in that short peptide fragments of antigens are generated, loaded onto MHC class I, and presented on the surface of cells to T lymphocytes, major differences between the MHC class I and II pathways are (1) antigens processed and presented via MHC class I are not limited to professional APC; (2) all nucleated cells express MHC class I; (3) the mechanisms by which the antigen is processed and loaded on to MHC class I is slightly different than MHC class II ; (4) the MHC class I antigenic peptides are usually smaller, often 8–10 amino acids in length; (5) the MHC class I antigens to be processed are usually aberrantly expressed proteins, such as viral-associated proteins or mutated proteins. MHC class I antigen processing and presentation is the major pathway by which virally infected cells are detected and killed by the acquired immune system.

Regardless of the MHC utilized to present antigens to lymphocytes, T cells are able to recognize antigen in the context of MHC with their T-cell receptor (TCR). Similar to immunoglobulin, the ability of T cells to specifically recognize thousands of antigens is again due to somatic recombination. All TCRs are comprised of two different subunits, each encoded from a distinct gene (the most abundant T-cell populations express α/β, but γ/δ also exist). All TCR subunits are made up of constant and variable regions. For α subunits, two separate gene segments (V and J) are combined to form the variable region, which is then joined to one constant region. For β subunits, three separate gene segments (V, D, and J) are combined to form the variable region, which is then joined to one of two constant regions. Similar to the immunoglobulin genes, there are several light chain V and J genes, and several heavy chain V, D, and J genes.

With regard to T- and B cells, key events that occur following antigen encounter are: (1) specific antigen recognition either in the context of MHC class I or II for T cells or through the immunoglobulin receptor for B cells; (2) cellular activation and initiation of intracellular signaling cascades that contribute to production and release of cytokines and other cellular mediators; (3) clonal expansion (proliferation) of antigen-specific cells; and (4) differentiation of antigen-stimulated lymphocytes into effector and memory cells.

Antigen-specific Receptors Although historically antigens were thought to only bind either antibody or TCR in the context of MHC, it is now clear that antigen-specific receptors exist. One such family of receptors is the toll-like receptors (TLRs). For instance, lipopolysaccharide, a component in the cell wall of gram-negative bacteria, has been determined to be a ligand for at least two different TLRs. Since these TLRs are expressed by a variety of cell types, and their ligands include components of bacteria, fungi, and viruses (reviewed in Xu *et al.*, 2004), it is likely that they play critical roles in the initiation of the innate immune response. TLRs also contribute to sustaining and regulating the adaptive immune response to various antigens.

Innate Immunity

As stated above, innate immunity acts as a first line of defense against anything nonself. With respect to infectious agents, the innate immune system eliminates most potential pathogens before significant infection occurs. The innate immune system includes physical and biochemical barriers both inside and outside the body, as well as immune cells designed for host defense responses.

Externally, the skin provides an effective barrier, as most organisms cannot penetrate intact skin. Most infectious agents enter the body through the respiratory system, gut, or genitourinary tract. Innate defenses present to combat infection from pathogens entering through the respiratory system include mucus secreted along the nasopharynx, the presence of lysozyme in most secretions, and cilia lining the trachea and main bronchi. In addition, reflexes such as coughing, sneezing, and elevation in body temperature are also a part of innate immunity. Pathogens that enter the body via the digestive tract are met with severe changes in pH (acid) within the stomach and a host of microorganisms living in the intestines.

Cellular Components: NK, NKT, PMN, Macrophage Two general types of cells are involved in innate host resistance: NK cells and professional phagocytes (Table 12-4). Like other immune cells, NK cells are derived from the bone marrow stem cell. It is not yet clear exactly how the NK lineage progresses; however, NK precursor cells have been identified recently (reviewed in Colucci *et al.*, 2003). There are two major NK functions: cytokine production and cytolysis. NK cells are located primarily in blood, all lymphoid organs, and liver and lungs. The vast majority of cytolytic NK cells express CD16 (Fc receptor for IgG) and the killer cell immunoglobulin receptor. NK cells mediate antibody-dependent cellular cytotoxicity via CD16. The primary mediators of cell death are perforin and granzyme. These mediators are expelled onto the surface of the target cell, which subsequently undergoes apoptosis (or programmed cell death, as characterized by DNA fragmentation, membrane blebbing, and cellular disintegration).

NKT cells have been described relatively recently (reviewed in Kronenberg, 2005). Although their lineage is ill-defined at this point, they express cell surface markers characteristic of both NK cells and T cells, as their name implies. NKT cells are considered important for innate immunity because they are activated fairly early in an immune response and they do not possess immunologic memory. Much information exists regarding NKT cell surface markers, but most prominent are expression of a TCR and a C-lectin-type NK receptor, to which glycolipids may bind. Functionally, NKT cells are similar to NK cells in that they produce cytokines and mediate cytolysis of target cells.

Phagocytic cells include polymorphonuclear cells (PMN; neutrophil) and the monocyte/macrophage. The precursors of the macrophage and PMN develop from pluripotent stem cells that have become committed to the myeloid lineage (Fig. 12-2). Evidence exists that there are bipotentiating reactive precursors for PMN and macrophage and that differentiation into one or the other is dependent on the interaction with specific colony-stimulating factors (CSFs) such as macrophage-CSF (M-CSF), granulocyte-CSF (G-CSF), granulocyte-macrophage-CSF (GM-CSF), interleukin (IL)-3, and others (Unanue, 1993). Within the bone marrow, both cell types undergo several rounds of replication before entering the bloodstream where they circulate for about 10 hours and then enter the tissues where they perform effector functions for about 1–2 days. PMNs are capable of passing through the cell membrane of the blood vessels and thereby represent a primary line of defense against infectious agents. They are excellent phagocytic cells and can eliminate most microorganisms through the release of various reactive oxygen species, such as superoxide, singlet oxygen, ozone, hydrogen peroxide, and hydroxyl radicals. Their phagocytic activity is greatly enhanced by the presence of complement and antibody deposited on the surface of the foreign target. They are also important in the induction of an inflammatory response (see section "Inflammation").

Macrophages are terminally differentiated monocytes. Upon exiting the bone marrow, monocytes circulate within the bloodstream for about 1 day. At that time, they begin to distribute to the

Table 12-4
Characteristics of Selected Immune Cells

PROPERTIES	MONOCYTE/MACROPHAGE	T CELLS	B CELLS	NK CELLS
Phagocytosis	Yes	No	No	No
Adherence	Yes	No	No	No
Surface receptors:				
Antigen receptors	No	Yes	Yes	No
Complement	Yes	No	Yes	Yes
Fc region of Ig	Yes	Some	Yes	Yes
Surface markers	CD64	CD4	Ig	CD16
	CD11b	CD8		Asialo-GM1
		CD3		(mouse)
		Thy-1(mouse)		CD11b
Proliferation in response to:				
Allogeneic cells (MLR)	No	Yes	No	No
Lipopolysaccharide (LPS)	No	No	Yes	No
Phytohemagglutinin (PHA)	No	Yes	No	No
Concanavalin A (Con A)	No	Yes	No	No
Anti-Ig + IL-4	No	No	Yes	No
Anti-CD3 + IL-2	No	Yes	No	No
Effector functions:				
Antibody production	No	No	Yes	No
Cytokine production	Yes	Yes	Yes	Yes
Bactericidal activity	Yes	No	No	No
Tumor cell cytotoxicity	Yes	Yes	No	Yes
Immunologic memory	No	Yes	Yes	No
Suppressor activity	No	Yes	No	No

SOURCE: Modified from Dean JH, Murray MJ: Toxic responses of the immune system, in Amdur MO, Doull J, Klaassen CD (eds): *Casarett and Doull's Toxicology: The Basic Science of Poisons,* 4th ed. New York: Pergammon Press, 1991, p. 286.

various tissues, where they can then differentiate into macrophages. Macrophages can be found in all tissues, most notably in the liver, lung, spleen, kidney, peritoneum, and brain. Within different tissues, macrophages have distinct properties and vary in extent of surface receptors, oxidative metabolism, and expression of MHC class II. This is likely due to the factors present within the microenvironment in which the monocyte differentiates. The liver macrophages, or Kupffer cells, are primarily responsible for particulate and microbial clearance from the blood. They express high levels of MHC class II, are actively phagocytic, and release several soluble mediators. Thus, they are the primary cells responsible for the acute phase response. Alveolar (lung) macrophages remove foreign particulate matter from the alveolar space. They are self-renewing and have a particularly long life span. These cells can be harvested by bronchoalveolar lavage and actively secrete proteases and bactericidal enzymes, such as lysozyme. Splenic macrophages also phagocytose particulate material and polysaccharides from the blood and tissue. However, unlike other tissue macrophages, they are more diverse within the tissue and their level of expression of MHC class II and their stage of differentiation appears to be dependent on where within the splenic architecture the macrophages are located. Mononuclear phagocytes within the central nervous system (CNS) are known as microglia and are responsible for antigen presentation in immunologic diseases of the CNS. Microglia have a very slow turnover time, and thus recruitment of monocytes to areas of inflammation within the CNS is also slow.

In addition to the cellular components of innate immunity, there are several soluble components (Table 12-2). These include the complement cascade, acute phase proteins, granzyme and perforin, and various cytokines, chemokines, and interferons. Although the complement cascade is described elsewhere in this chapter (see sections "Antigen Recognition" and "Inflammation"), it is also important in innate immunity because of its activation through the lectin pathway. Furthermore, C3a and C5a, which are chemokines generated during the cascade, recruit phagocytic cells to the site of complement activation. Acute phase proteins, such as serum amyloid A, serum amyloid P, and C-reactive protein, participate in an acute phase response to infection by binding bacteria and facilitating complement activation. Granzyme and perforin work in conjunction, with perforin disrupting the target cell membrane, allowing granzyme to enter and mediate cell lysis by several mechanisms.

Cytokines, chemokines, and interferons are also critical soluble components of the innate immune system. Although a partial list of cytokines and a brief description of the cell types that release and are acted upon by these various mediators is provided in Table 12-5, there are also several shared characteristics of cytokines, chemokines, and inteferons that merit discussion for the purposes of understanding immunotoxicological mechanisms. First, the primary function of cytokines, chemokines, and interferons is cell–cell interactions. The consequences of various interactions as dictated by cytokines, chemokines, or interferons include cellular activation, initiation or termination of intracellular signaling events, proliferation, differentiation, migration, trafficking, or effector functions. Second, although some of these molecules might be constitutively expressed, most are inducible in response to

Table 12-5

Cytokines: Sources and Functions in Immune Regulation

CYTOKINE	SOURCE	PHYSIOLOGIC ACTIONS
IL-1	Macrophages	Activation and proliferation of T cells (Th2 > Th1)
	B cells	Proinflammatory
	Several nonimmune cells	Induces fever and acute-phase proteins
		Induces synthesis of IL-8 and TNF-α
IL-2	T cells	Primary T-cell growth factor
		Growth factor for B cells and NK cells
		Enhances lymphokine production
IL-3	T cells	Stimulates the proliferation and differentiation of stromal cells,
		progenitors of the macrophage, granulocyte, and erythroid lineages
	Mast cells	
IL-4	T cells	Proliferation of activated T (Th2 > Th1) and B cells
	Mast cells	B-cell differentiation and isotype switching may inhibit some
	Stromal cells	macrophage functions
	Basophils	Antagonizes IFN-γ
	CD4$^+$/NK1.1$^+$ cells	Inhibits IL-8 production
IL-5	T cells	Proliferation and differentiation of eosinophils
	Mast cells	Promotes B cell isotype switching
		Synergizes with IL-4 to induce secretion of IgE
IL-6	Macrophages	Enhances B-cell differentiation and immunoglobulin secretion
	Activated T cells	Induction of acute phase proteins by liver
	B cells	
	Fibroblasts	Proinflammatory
	Keratinocytes	Proliferation of T cells and increased IL-2 receptor expression
	Endothelial cells	Synergizes with IL-4 to induce secretion of IgE
	Hepatocytes	
IL-7	Stromal cells	Proliferation of thymocytes (CD4$^-$/CD8$^-$)
	Epithelial cells	Proliferation of pro- and pre-B cells (mice)
		T-cell growth
IL-8	Macrophages	Activation and chemotaxis of monocytes, neutrophils, basophils and
	Platelets	T cells
	Fibroblasts	Proinflammatory
	NK cells	
	Keratinocytes	
	Hepatocytes	
	Endothelial cells	
IL-9	Th cells	T-cell growth factor (primarily CD4$^+$ cells)
		Enhances mast-cell activity
		Stimulates growth of early erythroid progenitors
IL-10	T cells	Inhibits macrophage cytolytic activity and macrophage activation
	Macrophages	of T cells
	B cells	General inhibitor of cytokine synthesis by Th1 cells
		(in presence of APCs)
		Enhances CD8$^+$ T cell cytolytic activity
		Enhances proliferation of activated B cells
		Mast-cell growth
		Anti-inflammatory
		Inhibits endotoxin shock
Interferon-α/β	Leukocytes	Induction of class I expression
(IFN-α/β)	Epithelial cells	Antiviral activity
(Type 1 IFN)	Fibroblasts	Stimulation of NK cells
Interferon-γ	T cells	Induction of class I and II
(IFN-γ)	NK cells	Activates macrophages (as APC and cytolytic cells)
	Epithelial cells	Improves CTL recognition of virally infected cells
	Fibroblasts	
Tumor necrosis factor (TNF-α)	Macrophages	Induces inflammatory cytokines
and lymphotoxin (TNF-β)		

Table 12-5
Continued.

CYTOKINE	SOURCE	PHYSIOLOGIC ACTIONS
	Lymphocytes	Increases vascular permeability
	Mast cells	Activates macrophages and neutrophils
		Tumor necrosis (direct action)
		Primary mediator of septic shock
		Interferes with lipid metabolism (result is cachexia)
		Induction of acute phase proteins
Transforming	Macrophages	Enhances monocyte/macrophage chemotaxis
growth factor-β	Megakaryocytes	Enhances wound healing: angiogenesis, fibroblast proliferation,
(TGF-β)		deposition of extracellular matrix
	Chondrocytes	Inhibits T- and B-cell proliferation
		Inhibits macrophage cytokine synthesis
		Inhibits antibody secretion
		Primary inducer of isotype switch to IgA
GM-CSF	T cells	Stimulates growth and differentiation of monocytes and granulocytes
	Macrophages	
	Endothelial cells	
	Fibroblasts	
Migration inhibitory	T cells	Inhibits macrophage migration
factor (MIF)	Anterior pituitary cells	Proinflammatory (induces TNF-α production by macrophages)
	Monocytes	Appears to play a role in delayed hypersensitivity responses
		May be a counterregulator of glucocorticoid activity

SOURCE: Information on selected cytokines taken from Ruddle (1992), Quesniaux (1992), Paul and Seder (1994), Zurawski and de Vries (1994), Lawrence (1997), and Paul (1999).

antigens, cellular stressors, or other cytokines. Thus many cytokines, chemokines, and interferons are not stored in the cell, but rather are tightly regulated, often at the transcriptional level, so that they are quickly generated on demand. An example of a cytokine important in innate immunity is IL-1, which is rapidly transcribed in response to various stimulants using the critical transcription factor nuclear factor κB (NF-κB). Third, many cytokines share common receptor subunits such that should one particular subunit of a receptor be adversely affected by an immunotoxic agent, the functional outcome might be amplified. An example would be the common γ chain, which is shared by the IL-2, IL-4, IL-7, IL-9, IL-13, IL-15, and IL-21 receptors. Although a compound might "only" affect transcription of the common γ chain, the immunologic consequences of affecting this target could be quite destructive. Specifically for innate immunity, there are several cytokines, chemokine, and interferons that play critical roles, such as the proinflammatory cytokines IL-1, IL-6, and TNF-α (see section "Inflammation") and the type I interferons, α and β, which are themselves anti-viral.

Acquired (Adaptive) Immunity

If the primary defenses against infection (innate immunity) are breached, the acquired arm of the immune system is activated and produces a specific immune response to each infectious agent, which usually eliminates the infection. This branch of immunity is also capable of remembering the pathogen, and can protect the host from future infection by the same agent. Therefore, the two key features that define acquired immunity are specificity and memory. Acquired immunity may be further subdivided into humoral immunity and CMI. Humoral immunity is directly dependent on the production of antigen-specific antibody by B cells and involves the coordinated interaction of APCs, T cells, and B cells. CMI is that part of the acquired immune system in which effector cells, be they phagocytic cells, helper cells, regulatory cells, APC, cytotoxic cells, or memory cells, play the critical role(s) without antibody involvement.

Cellular Components: APCs, T Cells, and B Cells   APCs, which were discussed previously in the "Antigen Processing" section, include professional APCs such as B cells, macrophages, and dendritic cells. Although all cells may act as APCs with internal antigen processing through the MHC class I pathway, what distinguishes a professional APC is the ability to internalize external antigens and process them through the MHC class II pathway for presentation to T cells.

B lymphocytes are not only capable of serving as professional APCs, but they are also the effector cells of humoral immunity, producing a number of isotypes of immunoglobulin with varying specificities and affinities. Like other immune cells, the B cell develops in the bone marrow from the pluripotent stem cell and becomes committed to the B-cell lineage when the cell begins to rearrange its immunoglobulin genes, as described in "Antigen Recognition" (Fig. 12-6). Following successful immunoglobulin rearrangement, these cells express heavy chains in their cytoplasm and are termed pre-B cells. Expression of surface IgM and IgD indicates a mature B cell. Mature B cells are found in the lymph nodes, spleen, and peripheral blood. Upon antigen binding to surface immunoglobulin (part of the B-cell receptor), the mature B cell becomes activated and, after proliferation, undergoes differentiation into either a memory B cell or an antibody-forming plasma cell [plaque-forming cell (PFC)], actively secreting antigen-specific antibody. A

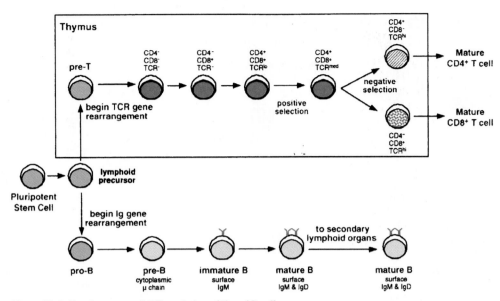

Figure 12-6. Development and differentiation of T- and B cells.

broad description of several B-cell characteristics can be found in Table 12-4.

At a specified time following their commitment to the T-cell lineage, pre-T cells migrate from the bone marrow to the thymus where, in a manner analogous to their B-cell cousins, they begin to rearrange their TCRs, as described in section "Antigen Recognition" (Fig. 12-6). This receptor consists of two chains (α/β or γ/δ) and is critical for the recognition of MHC plus peptide on APCs. At this time, the T cells begin to express the surface marker cluster of differentiation antigen (CD) 8. CD8 (and CD4) are coreceptors expressed by T cells and are involved in the interaction of the T cell with the APC. T cells bearing the γ/δ TCR subsequently lose expression of CD8 and proceed to the periphery. T cells with the α/β TCR gain surface expression of both the TCR and the CD4 and are termed immature double-positive cells (CD4$^+$/CD8$^+$). These immature cells then undergo positive selection to eliminate cells that do not recognize MHC. Following this interaction, TCR expression increases. Any of these T cells that interact with MHC plus self-peptide are then eliminated (termed negative selection). The double-positive cells then undergo another selection process whereby they lose expression of either CD4 or CD8 and then proceed to the periphery as mature single-positive cells (CD4$^+$ or CD8$^+$) with a high level of TCR expression. This rigorous selection process produces T cells that can recognize MHC plus foreign peptides and eliminates autoreactive T cells. Generally, T cells that express CD8 mediate cell killing (CTL); whereas T cells that express CD4 mediate helper functions through coordinated interactions with other cells. A relatively recently described population of T cells, the T-regulatory cells, are a subset of CD4$^+$ T cells that express CD25 and the transcription factor Foxp3. These cells act to suppress T-cell function and prevent uncontrolled immune responses (reviewed in Hoglund, 2006). Mature T cells are found in the lymph nodes, spleen, and peripheral blood. Upon MHC plus antigen binding to the TCR, the mature T cell becomes activated and, after proliferation, undergoes differentiation into either an effector cell or a memory T cell. Effector T-helper cells can subsequently differentiate into either a Th1 or a Th2 phenotype. Th1 cells predominantly express IL-2 and IFN-γ and promote CMI and delayed-type hypersensitivity (DTH). Th2

cells predominantly express IL-4, IL-5, IL-6, IL-10, and IL-13 and promote humoral immune responses. Although the two populations are not mutually exclusive, they do negatively regulate each other, such that a strong Th1 response suppresses a Th2 response and vice versa. A broad description of several T-cell characteristics can be found in Table 12-4.

The ability of APCs, B cells, and T cells to communicate with each other is dependent on a variety of receptor–ligand interactions between cell types. These interactions dictate the type of immune response (i.e., humoral immunity vs. CMI) and the magnitude of the immune response. For example, antigen presented in the context of MHC binding to a TCR is the major interaction that must occur between APCs and T cells to initiate an acquired immune response. Subsequent to this initial interaction, costimulatory molecules must be engaged on both the T cells and APCs to sustain and direct the immune response. One of the best-characterized interactions occur between CD28 on the T cells and CD80 (or CD86) on the APCs, which provide a more robust immune response as measured by clonal expansion and cytokine production, such as IL-2. Later in the response (2–3 days), T cells express Cytotoxic T lymphocyte antigen 4 (CTLA-4), which exhibits higher affinity for CD80 and CD86 than does CD28, and the CTLA-4–CD80 (or CD86) interaction serves to suppress the immune response. Other important interactions between cells include CD40–CD40 ligand (on APC–T cell, respectively), which sustains clonal expansion and differentiation of the T cells, and provides activation signals to the APC; ICOS-ligand for ICOS (on T cell–APC, respectively), which also sustains clonal expansion and differentiation of the T cells, and induces IL-10 production; and 4-1BB–4-1BB ligand (on T cell–APC, respectively), which, similar to CD40–CD40 ligand, helps to sustain an immune response and activate the APCs.

Humoral and Cell-Mediated Immunity As described earlier, humoral immunity is that part of the acquired immune system in which antibody is involved. In general, B cells produce antibodies specific to an antigen, which may act to opsonize or neutralize the invader, or the antibodies act to recruit other factors, such as the complement

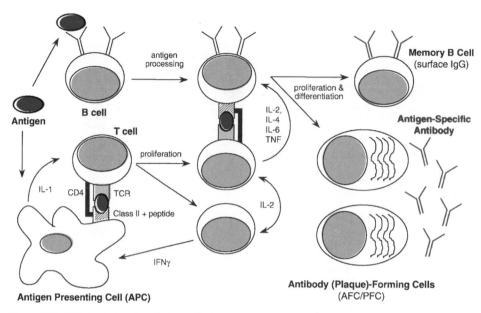

Figure 12-7. Cellular interactions in the antibody response.

cascade. CMI is that part of the immune system in which various effector cells perform a wide variety of functions to eliminate invaders. Often, these two branches are coordinated, such as activation of CMI in the form of a T-helper cell produces specific cytokines that enhance B-cell proliferation and differentiation to produce more antibody. A general diagram of the cellular interactions involved in a humoral immune response is given in Fig. 12-7. The production of antigen-specific IgM requires 3–5 days after the primary (initial) exposure to antigen (Fig. 12-8). Upon secondary antigenic challenge, the B cells undergo isotype switching, producing primarily IgG antibody, which is of higher affinity. In addition, there is a higher serum antibody titer associated with a secondary antibody response. Other CMI functions include DTH and cell-mediated cytotoxicity. DTH is discussed in the section "Immune-Mediate Disease, Hypersensitivity." Cell-mediated cytotoxicity responses may occur in numerous ways: (1) MHC-dependent recognition of specific antigens (such as viral particles or tumor proteins) by CTL; (2) indirect antigen-specific recognition by the binding of antibody-coated target cells to NK cells via Fc receptors on the latter; and (3) receptor-mediated recognition of complement-coated foreign targets by macrophages.

In cell-mediated cytotoxicity, the CD8$^+$ T cells (CTL) or NK effector cell binds in a specific manner to the target cell (Fig. 12-9). The majority of CTLs express CD8 and recognize either foreign MHC class I on the surface of allogeneic cells, or antigen in association with self-MHC class I (e.g., viral particles). NK cell recognition of target cells may be considered antigen specific because the mechanism of recognition involves the binding of the Fc portion of antigen-specific antibody coating a target cell to the NK cell via its Fc receptors. Once the CTL or NK cells interact with the target cell, the effector cell undergoes cytoplasmic reorientation so that cytolytic granules are oriented along the side of the effector, which is bound to the target. The effector cell then releases the contents of these granules onto the target cell. The target cell may be damaged by the perforins or enzymatic contents of the cytolytic granules. In addition, the target is induced to undergo apoptosis. Once it has degranulated, the effector cell can release the dying target and move on to kill other target cells. Macrophage-dependent

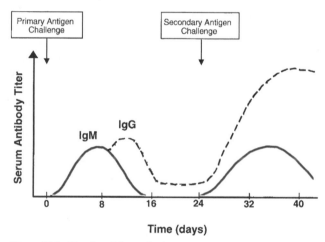

Figure 12-8. Kinetics of the antibody response.

cytotoxicity occurs via complement receptors present on the surface of the macrophage, which recognize complement-coated invaders. In response, the macrophages release various mediators, including reactive oxygen species and proteases, which act to kill the infected cell. Finally, it is clear that many of the soluble factors critical to the innate immune system are also primary effectors in the acquired immune system, including reactive oxygen species, granzyme, perforin, cytokines, and interferons, again demonstrating the interplay among the various arms of the immune system.

Inflammation

Inflammation, simply defined, refers to a complex reaction to injury, irritation, or foreign invaders – collectively referred to as an 'insult' – that is characterized by pain, swelling, redness, and heat. Briefly, inflammation involves various stages, including release of chemotactic factors following the insult, increased blood flow, increased capillary permeability allowing for cellular infiltration, followed by either an acute resolution of tissue damage or persistence of the

1. Identification and engagement of target by effector.

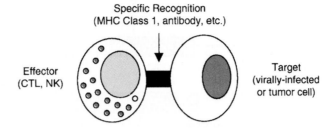

2. Strengthening of interaction and cytoplasmic reorientation of effector.

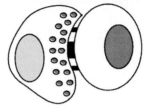

3. Degranulation of effector onto target.

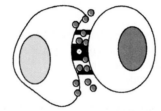

4. Disengagement of effector and death of target.

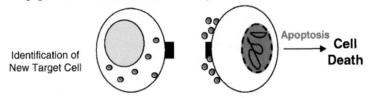

Figure 12-9. Cell-mediated cytotoxicity.

response that might contribute to fibrosis or subsequent organ failure (Serhan and Savill, 2005). Again, it is important to emphasize that whereas inflammation is a natural reaction to repair tissue damage or attack foreign invaders, the process often results in destruction of adjacent cells and/or tissues. Thus, there is overwhelming evidence that inflammation plays a critical role in many diseases, including asthma, multiple sclerosis, cardiovascular disease, Alzheimer's disease, bowel disorders, and cancer. In addition, recent studies have suggested that inflammation exacerbates idiosyncratic reactions to drugs and other chemicals (reviewed in Ganey *et al.*, 2004).

Cellular Components: Macrophages, PMN, and T cells Many of the cellular components described in the sections above are critical to initiation and maintenance of an inflammatory response. Major cellular contributors to an inflammatory response are macrophages, neutrophils, and T cells. Neutrophils are often the first, and most numerous, responders to sites of insult. In response to either host- or pathogen-derived signals, neutrophils secrete chemotactic factors to recruit professional APCs, such as macrophages, to the area. In addition, neutrophils induce apoptosis of cells at the site of in-

sult through the release of reactive oxygen species, and they can activate the Th1 lineage of T cells through IFN-γ release and B cells through B-lymphocyte stimulator (BlyS) production (reviewed in Nathan, 2006). Macrophages can be activated by a variety of mechanisms at the site of insult, such as activation via TLR, pro-inflammatory cytokines, or recognition of opsonized particles by Fc receptors or complement receptors. Macrophages also induce apoptosis of cells in the insult area through the release of nitric oxide and other reactive oxygen species, resulting in disruption of extracellular structures that compromise tissue structure and function (reviewed in Duffield, 2003). Both neutrophils and macrophages are phagocytic cells and can contribute to clearing of apoptotic cells. Later in the inflammatory response, T cells are critical for generating an adaptive immune response, primarily through recruitment and activation of CD4$^+$ or CD8$^+$ T cells. There is much evidence that particularly in asthma, cytokines produced by Th2 lymphocytes contribute to inflammation, mucus production, and airway hyperresponsiveness, although the Th1 cytokine IFN-γ undoubtedly also plays a critical role (reviewed in Georas *et al.*, 2005). T cells are attracted to the insult area by adhesion molecules and integrins, and are activated in response to antigen presented in the context

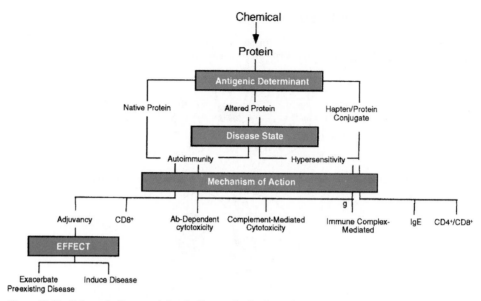

Figure 12-10. *Schematic diagram of chemical interaction leading to hypersensitivity reactions or autoimmunity.*

of MHC, often by a professional APC, such as a macrophage. Depending on the differentiation signals that the T cell receives, it may secrete cytokines that either mediate direct cell killing (Th1) or recruit other cells (Th2), such as B cells, to aid in resolution of the insult.

Although many soluble factors that contribute to inflammation were mentioned above, there are several others that warrant discussion as well. As previously mentioned, reactive oxygen species are released from both macrophages and neutrophils to compromise membrane integrity and interact with several macromolecules in the insulted cells. A plethora of cytokines and chemokines also contribute to the inflammatory process, not only by acting as chemotactic factors, but also by dictating differentiation processes of T cells. Furthermore, there are "pro-inflammatory" cytokines such as IL-1, IL-6, and TNF-α, which act to induce fever (IL-1), activate T cells (IL-1), stimulate T-cell proliferation (IL-6), stimulate proliferation of B cells (IL-6), activate macrophages (IL-1), increase vascular permeability (TNF-α), or induce apoptosis (TNF-α). Furthermore, many of these mediators induce expression of others (i.e., TNF-α induces expression of IL-1 and IL-6) such that an inflammation cascade is established. Many of these pro-inflammatory cytokines also induce acute phase proteins, such as C-reactive protein. C-reactive protein binds to several ligands, including phosphatidylcholine on the membranes of cells, Fc receptors, and C1q (part of the complement C1 complex), which activates the classical complement cascade (reviewed in Marnell *et al.*, 2005). Complement participates in inflammation through inappropriate and sustained activation of the cascade, ultimately leading to destruction of cells through the MAC (Fig. 12-4). Furthermore, complement fragments, such as C3a and C5a, act as chemotactic factors to recruit other phagocytic cells to sites of insult (reviewed in Roozendaal and Carroll, 2006). Finally, prostaglandins and other eicosinoids possess various pro-inflammatory actions, including T-cell proliferation (thromboxane A2), Th1/Th2 polarization (prostaglandin E2), and increase vascular permeability (prostacyclin I2) (reviewed in Hata and Breyer, 2004). In addition, prostaglandins contribute to hyperalgesia and it is for this reason that cyclooxygenase-2, which converts arachidonic acid to other bioactive prostaglandins, is an attractive therapeutic target

to reduce inflammation and pain (see section "Immunomodulation by Xenobiotics, Anti-Inflammatory Agents").

Immune-Mediated Disease

As stated earlier, the purpose of the immune system is to preserve the integrity of the individual from disease states, whether infectious, parasitic, or cancerous, through both cellular and humoral mechanisms. In so doing, the ability to distinguish self from nonself plays a predominant role. However, situations arise in which the individual's immune system responds in a manner producing tissue damage, resulting in a self-induced disease. These disease states fall into two categories (1) hypersensitivity, or allergy, and (2) autoimmunity. Figure 12-10 is a schematic delineating the possible cascade of effects that can occur when a chemical produces an immune-mediated disease. Hypersensitivity reactions result from the immune system responding in an exaggerated or inappropriate manner. These reactions have been subdivided by Coombs and Gell (1975) into four types, which represent four different mechanisms leading to tissue damage. In the case of autoimmunity, mechanisms of self-recognition break down and immunoglobulins and TCR react with self-antigens, resulting in tissue damage and disease.

Hypersensitivity

Classification of Hypersensitivity Reactions   One characteristic common to all four types of hypersensitivity reactions is the necessity of prior exposure leading to sensitization in order to elicit a reaction upon subsequent challenge. In the case of types I, II, and III, prior exposure to antigen leads to the production of specific antibody (IgE, IgM, or IgG) and, in the case of type IV, to the generation of memory T cells. Figure 12-11 illustrates the mechanisms of hypersensitivity reactions as classified by Coombs and Gell. Although not completely understood, regulation of immunoglobulin production is dependent in part on the characteristics of the antigen, the genetics of the individual, and environmental factors. The mechanisms of antibody production in hypersensitivity reactions are identical to those described earlier in the chapter (Fig. 12-7). A brief

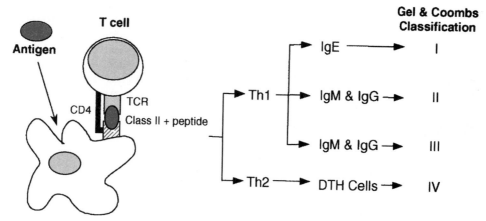

Figure 12-11. *Schematic of classification for hypersensitivity reactions.*

description of the four types of hypersensitivity reactions is presented below.

Type I (Immediate Hypersensitivity)

Using penicillin as an example, Fig. 12-12 depicts the major events involved in a type I hypersensitivity reaction. Sensitization occurs as the result of exposure to appropriate antigens through the respiratory tract, dermally, or by exposure through the gastrointestinal tract. IgE production is highest in lymphatic tissues that drain sites of exposure (i.e., tonsils, bronchial lymph nodes, and intestinal lymphatic tissues, including Peyer's patches). It is low in the spleen. Serum concentration of IgE is low compared to other immunoglobulins, and serum half-life is short (Table 12-3). Once produced, IgE binds to local tissue mast cells before entering the circulation, where it binds to circulating mast cells, basophils, and tissue mast cells at distant sites. Once an individual is sensitized, reexposure to the antigen results in degranulation of the mast cells with the release of preformed mediators and cytokines typical of Th2 cells. Synthesis of leukotrienes and thromboxanes is also induced. These mediators promote vasodilation, bronchial constriction, and inflammation. Clinical manifestations can vary from urticarial skin reactions (wheals and flares) to signs of hay fever, including rhinitis and conjuctivitis, to more serious diseases, such as asthma and potentially life-threatening anaphylaxis. These responses may begin within minutes of reexposure to the offending antigen; therefore, type I hypersensitivity is often referred to as immediate hypersensitivity.

Type II (Antibody-Dependent Cytotoxic Hypersensitivity)

Type II hypersensitivity is IgG mediated. Figure 12-13 shows the mechanisms of action of a complement-independent cytotoxic reaction and complement-dependent lysis. Tissue damage may result from the direct action of cytotoxic cells, such as macrophages, neutrophils, or eosinophils, linked to immunoglobulin-coated target cells through the Fc receptor on the antibody or by antibody activation of the classic complement pathway. Complement activation may result in C3b binding to the target cell surface. This acts as a recognition site for effector cells. Alternatively, the C5b-9 MAC may be bound to the target cell surface, resulting in cell lysis (Fig. 12-4).

Type III (Immune Complex-Mediated Hypersensitivity)

Type III hypersensitivity reactions also involve IgG immunoglobulins. The distinguishing feature of type III is that, unlike type II, in which immunoglobulin production is against specific tissue-associated

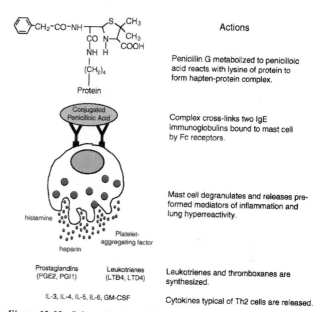

	Actions
	Penicillin G metabolized to penicilloic acid reacts with lysine of protein to form hapten-protein complex.
	Complex cross-links two IgE immunoglobulins bound to mast cell by Fc receptors.
	Mast cell degranulates and releases preformed mediators of inflammation and lung hyperreactivity.
	Leukotrienes and thromboxanes are synthesized.
	Cytokines typical of Th2 cells are released.

Figure 12-12. *Schematic of type I hypersensitivity reaction.*

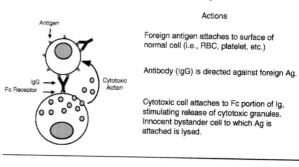

Complement-Independent Cytotoxic Lysis

Actions

Foreign antigen attaches to surface of normal cell (i.e., RBC, platelet, etc.)

Antibody (IgG) is directed against foreign Ag.

Cytotoxic cell attaches to Fc portion of Ig, stimulating release of cytotoxic granules. Innocent bystander cell to which Ag is attached is lysed.

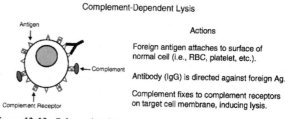

Complement-Dependent Lysis

Actions

Foreign antigen attaches to surface of normal cell (i.e., RBC, platelet, etc.).

Antibody (IgG) is directed against foreign Ag.

Complement fixes to complement receptors on target cell membrane, inducing lysis.

Figure 12-13. *Schematic of type II hypersensitivity reactions.*

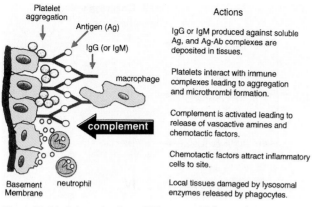

Figure 12-14. *Schematic of type III hypersensitivity reaction.*

antigen, immunoglobulin production is against soluble antigen in the serum (Fig. 12-14). This allows for the formation of circulating immune complexes composed of a lattice of antigen and immunoglobulin, which may result in widely distributed tissue damage in areas where immune complexes are deposited. The most common location is the vascular endothelium in the lung, joints, and kidneys. The skin and circulatory systems may also be involved. Pathology results from the inflammatory response initiated by the activation of complement. Macrophages, neutrophils, and platelets attracted to the deposition site contribute to the tissue damage.

Type IV (Cell-Mediated Hypersensitivity) Type IV, or DTH responses, can be divided into two classes: contact hypersensitivity and tuberculin-type hypersensitivity. A classical example of contact hypersensitivity is that seen following poison ivy exposure. Contact hypersensitivity is initiated by topical exposure, and the associated pathology is primarily epidermal. It is characterized clinically by an eczematous reaction at the site of allergen contact and, like type I through III responses, consists of two phases: sensitization and elicitation. However, in this case sensitization is the result of the de-

velopment of activated and memory T cells as opposed to antibody production (Figs. 12-15 and 12-16). Sensitization occurs when a hapten penetrates the epidermis and forms a complex with a protein carrier. The hapten–carrier complex is processed by Langerhans-dendritic cells that migrate out of the epidermis to the local lymph nodes. There, the APC presents the processed antigen to CD4$^+$ T cells, leading to clonal expansion and the generation of memory T cells.

Upon second contact, Langerhans-dendritic cells present the processed hapten–carrier complex to memory T cells in either the skin or the lymph nodes. These activated T cells then secrete cytokines that bring about further proliferation of T cells and induce the expression of adhesion molecules on the surface of keratinocytes and endothelial cells in the dermis. Both the expression of adhesion molecules and the secretion of pro-inflammatory cytokines by T cells and keratinocytes facilitate the movement of inflammatory cells into the skin, resulting in erythema and the formation of papules and vesicles. CD8$^+$ cells may play a role in tissue damage. In cases where chemicals are lipid soluble and can therefore readily cross the cell membrane, they can modify intracellular proteins. These cells then present modified peptides on their cell surface in conjunction with MHC class I molecules. CD8$^+$ cells recognize these foreign peptides and cause tissue damage by either direct cytotoxic action or secretion of cytokines that further promote the inflammatory response.

Autoimmunity Autoimmune disease occurs when the reactions of the immune system are directed against the body's own tissues, and, for hypersensitivity, is characterized by a genetic susceptibility. Autoimmune diseases may be tissue specific, where the damage is associated with a specific type of tissue or a specific organ, or tissue nonspecific, where the signs and symptoms are associated with several organs and tissues. The targets from the perspective of the primary sites of tissue damage in autoimmune disease are many and varied. The following organs, cells, and organelles have all been determined to be the site of autoimmune reactions:

Induction of Sensitization

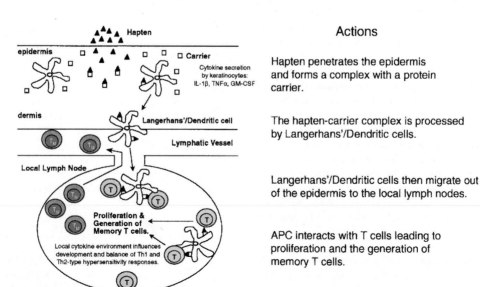

Figure 12-15. *Schematic of sensitization phase for type IV hypersensitivity reaction.*

Elicitation

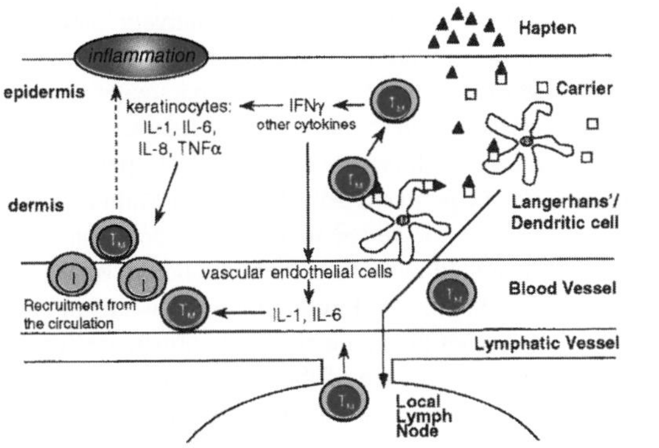

Actions

Upon subsequent contact, some Langerhans'/Dendritic cells (LDC) migrate to local lymph node as before. Other LDC can present processed hapten-carrier to memory T cells in skin.

Activated memory T cells then secrete cytokines which induce release of inflammatory cytokines from other cell types.

Memory T cells and inflammatory cells are recruited from the circulation via local chemoattractant cytokines and expression of adhesion molecules.

These cells migrate to the epidermis and elicit the characteristic local inflammatory response.

Figure 12-16. Schematic of elicitation phase for type IV hypersensitivity reaction.

nuclei (specifically histones and/or single-stranded DNA—one of the hallmark indicators of certain types of autoimmune disease is the expression of antinuclear antibodies), red blood cells, lymphocytes, neutrophils, platelets, immunoglobulins (primarily IgG), striated muscle (cholinergic receptors), smooth muscle, mitochondria, skin (basement membranes), thyroid (thyoglobulin), kidney (glomerular and tubular basement membrane), CNS (myelin), connective tissue (synovial lining of joints), lung, and liver. Both humoral immunity and CMI can be involved as effector mechanisms in causing the damage in autoimmune conditions. Examples of autoimmune diseases include: (1) myasthenia gravis, in which cholinergic receptors, especially those associated with neuromuscular junctions, are targeted; (2) multiple sclerosis, in which myelin is targeted; and (3) rheumatoid arthritis, in which connective tissue, especially the synovial lining of joints, is targeted. The terms "hypersensitivity" and "autoimmunity" are often confused and are certainly interrelated. Based on their definitions, a hypersensitivity response can be a mechanism by which an autoimmune disease is produced.

In the section on hypersensitivity presented above, two mechanisms, types II and III, were discussed by which host tissues are damaged by the host's own immune system, creating autoimmune-like disease. In these situations, unaltered self-antigens are not the target of the immune mechanisms but damage occurs to cells bearing hapten on membranes or to innocent bystander cells in close proximity to antigen–antibody complexes. For example, damage produced in autoimmune Goodpasture's disease is similar to that seen in type III hypersensitivity reactions in the lung due to trimellitic anhydride. Although the resulting pathology may be the same for autoimmune reactions and hypersensitivity, mechanisms of true autoimmune disease are distinguished from hypersensitivity. In cases of autoimmunity, self-antigens are the target, and in the case of chemical-induced autoimmunity, the disease state is induced by a modification of host tissues or immune cells by the chemical and not the chemical acting as an antigen/hapten.

Mechanisms of Autoimmunity Various aspects of the immunopathogenesis of autoimmune disease have been reviewed (Ayensu *et al.*, 2004; Lee and Sinha, 2005; Veldman *et al.*, 2006) and are described briefly below as background information for understanding how chemicals may induce autoimmunity. Two major

types of B- and T cells are produced that play a role in autoimmunity. B cells expressing CD5 predominate in embryonic life and are later found mostly in the intestinal mucosa. These cells produce high levels of IgM, and much of which are autoantibodies. Although most B cells do not express CD5 prior to class switching, they do express high levels of IgM. Influenced by cytokines produced by interacting T cells following antigen stimulation, these cells produce primarily IgG, IgA, or IgE. Similarly, T cells develop from one of two lineages: those with α/βTCRs and those with γ/δTCRs. Although most mature T cells express α/βTCRs, γ/δTCRs are predominant on mucosal surfaces. As described earlier in the chapter, α/βTCRs continue differentiation into CD4[+] or CD8[+] T cells. CD4[+] cells have primarily helper and inducer functions and recognize antigens in the context of MHC class II molecules. CD8[+] T lymphocytes are mainly cytotoxic cells and recognize antigenic determinants in conjunction with MHC class I molecules. As discussed earlier, the rearrangement and combination of the genes that comprise immunoglobulin and TCR results in tremendous diversity of potential antigen recognition by B- and T cells, respectively. Ideally, those lymphocytes that recognize self-antigens are deleted through negative and positive selection for T cells.

The process of negative selection against autoreactive T cells in the thymus is important in the prevention of autoimmune disease. T cells expressing α/βTCRs that fit self-MHC molecules with high affinity undergo apoptosis at an accelerated rate, whereas those with a low affinity for self-antigen and a high affinity for foreign antigen undergo positive selection and proliferate in the thymus, eventually migrating to the peripheral lymphatics. Although negative selection greatly reduces the numbers of self-reactive T cells, some of these cells do leave the thymus and remain in circulation in a state of anergy, or unresponsiveness. These cells are able to bind their designated antigen but do not undergo proliferation owing to a lack of necessary second signal. This second signal is generally provided by CD80 (or CD86) on the APC interacting with CD28 on the T cell. The inability of self-reactive T cells that escape negative selection to proliferate in response to self-antigen is termed "self-tolerance."

Several mechanisms are involved with the break down of self-tolerance, leading to autoimmunity. The first is exposure to antigens not available in the thymus during embryonic development. Therefore, the antigen-specific T-cell-reactive lymphocytes not subjected to negative selection could induce an autoimmune reaction. Examples include myelin- and organ-specific antigens such as thyroglobulin. Break down of self-tolerance to these antigens may be induced by exposure to adjuvants or to another antigenically related protein. The second is the overcoming of T-cell anergy by chronic lymphocyte stimulation. Finally, there is interference with normal immunoregulation by T-regulatory cells, which may create an environment conducive to the development of autoimmune disease.

Effector mechanisms involved in autoimmune disease can be the same as those described earlier for types II and III hypersensitivity or, in the case of pathology associated with solid tissues, including organs, they may involve CD8+ CTL. Tissue damage associated with CTL may be the result of direct cell membrane damage and lysis, or the result of cytokines produced and released by the T cell. TNF-β has the ability to kill susceptible cells and IFN-γ may increase the expression of MHC class I on cell surfaces, making them more susceptible to CD8+ cells. Cytokines may also be chemotactic for macrophages, which can cause tissue damage directly or indirectly through the release of pro-inflammatory cytokines. As is the case with hypersensitivity reactions, autoimmune disease is often the result of more than one mechanism working simultaneously. Therefore, pathology may be the result of antibody-dependent cytotoxicity, complement-dependent antibody-mediated lysis, or direct or indirect effects of CTL.

Developmental Immunology

A sequential series of carefully timed and coordinated developmental events, beginning early in embryonic/fetal life and continuing through the early postnatal period is required to establish a functional immune system in all mammals, including humans. The immune system develops initially from a population of pluripotent hematopoietic stem cells that are generated early in gestation from uncommitted mesenchymal stem cells in the intraembryonic splanchnoplure surrounding the heart. This early population of hematopoietic stem cells gives rise to all circulating blood cell lineages, including cells of the immune system, via migration through an orderly series of tissues, and a dynamic process that involves continual differentiation of lineage-restricted stem cells. Lymphoid–hematopoietic progenitor cells are established via the migration of these cells from intraembryonic mesenchyme to fetal liver and fetal spleen, and ultimately, the relocation of these cells in late gestation to bone marrow and thymus. The latter two organs are the primary sites of lymphopoiesis and appear to be unique in providing the microenvironment factors necessary for the development of functionally competent immune cells. These lineage-restricted stem cells expand to form a pool of highly proliferative progenitor cells that are capable of a continual renewal of short-lived functional immunocompetent cells, and that ultimately provide the necessary cellular capacity for effective immune responsiveness, and the necessary breadth of the immune repertoire (Good, 1995).

It is important to recognize that immune system development does not cease at birth, and that immunocompetent cells continue to be produced from proliferating progenitor cells in the bone marrow and thymus. Mature immunocompetent cells leave these primary immune organs and migrate via the blood to the secondary immune organs: spleen, lymph nodes, and mucosal lymphoid tissues. Because birth occurs at various stages of fetal maturity, the significance of parturition as a landmark in the development of the immune system can vary from species to species (Holsapple et al., 2003). As such, direct comparison of immune functional development between humans and animals is complicated by differences in the maturity of the immune system before and after partution. This difference has been linked to the length of gestation (Holladay and Smialowicz, 2000) in that animals with short gestation periods (e.g., mice, rats, rabbits, and hamsters) have relatively immature immune systems at birth compared to humans. The onset of functional immune competence depends on the specific parameter being measured, and varies across species with striking differences noted between rodents and humans (Holsapple et al., 2003). Exposure to specific antigens during the perinatal period results in a rapidly expanding accumulation of lymphocyte specificities in the pool of memory cells in secondary lymphoid tissues. As thymic function wanes and thymocytes are no longer produced in that tissue, it is this pool of memory B- and T cells that maintains immunocompetence for the life of the individual. Senescence of the immune responses is not well understood, but it is clear that both innate and acquired immune responses to antigens are different in the last quartile of life. This failure of the immune response is due, in part, to a continual reduction in the production of newly formed cells, and to the decreased survival of long-lived memory cells in lymphoid tissues.

One feature of the developing immune system that clearly distinguishes it from the mature immune system, especially during gestation, is the role played by organogenesis. Defects in the development of the immune system due to heritable changes in the lymphoid elements have provided clinical and experimental examples of the devastating consequences of impaired immune development (Rosen et al., 1995). Therefore, the effects of chemicals on the genesis of critical immune organs in the developing fetus may be more important than effects on these tissues after they have been populated by hematopoietic and lymphoid cells. However, a chemical that induces the formation of this kind of developmental abnormality in the fetus would legitimately be classified as a teratogen, prompting the question as to how many known teratogens would have an impact on organs essential to the normal functioning of the immune system. Interestingly, immune organs, like the thymus, spleen, and/or bone marrow, are not typically assessed in routine developmental and reproductive toxicology studies, and it has been noted that this failure to assess developmental damage to the immune system in standard developmental and reproductive toxicology protocols should be reevaluated (Holsapple et al., 2003).

Neuroendocrine Immunology

There is overwhelming evidence that cytokines, neuropeptides, neurotransmitters, and hormones, as well as their receptors, are an integral and interregulated part of the CNS, the endocrine system, and the immune system (reviewed in Sanders and Kohm, 2002). Because receptors for neuropeptides, neurotransmitters, and hormones are present on lymphoid cells, it is reasonable to suspect that some chemicals may exert their immunomodulatory effects indirectly on the immune system by acting to modulate the activity of the nervous or endocrine systems. In addition, immune cells are capable of secreting, and do secrete, peptide hormones and neurotransmitters, which can have autocrine (immune system) and paracrine (endocrine and nervous systems) effects. Similar to the complexity of the cytokine network, the effects of various hormones and neurotransmitters are too vast to discuss here. However, it is evident, even from this brief overview of the immune system and its potential interaction with other biological systems, that immune responses are complex processes involving multiple cell types and mediators. It is not difficult to imagine then, that perturbation of the cell types or

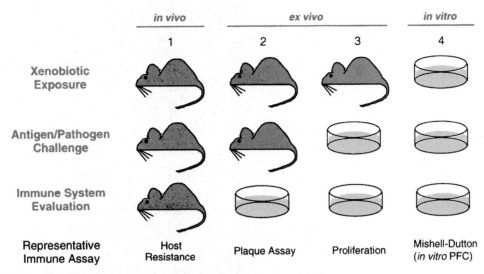

Figure 12-17. Approaches for assessing the immunotoxicity of xenobiotics.

mediators by drugs or chemicals could contribute to the mechanisms by which a compound is immunotoxic.

ASSESSMENT OF IMMUNOLOGIC INTEGRITY

For many years, it has been widely established that xenobiotics can have significant effects on the immune system. More recently, and during the establishment of the subdiscipline of immunotoxicology, a significant emphasis was placed on the development of a standardized battery of tests to evaluate immune competence. Among the unique features of the immune system is the ability of immune cells to be removed from the body and to function in vitro. This unique quality makes it possible to comprehensively evaluate the actions of xenobiotics on the immune system employing in vivo, ex vivo, and in vitro approaches to dissect the cellular, biochemical, and molecular mechanisms of action of xenobiotics. While standard toxicological end points such as organ weights, cellularity, and enumeration of cell subpopulations are important components in assessing when an agent is capable of altering the immune system, by far the most sensitive indicators of immunotoxicity are the tests that challenge the various immune cells to respond functionally to exogenous stimuli (reviewed in White, 1992). Employing such a battery of functional assays whereby different cell types can be evaluated not only for their effector functions, but also in certain cases for their ability to participate as accessory cells in an immune response, can provide important mechanistic information concerning which cell type(s) within the immune system are, in fact, targeted by a xenobiotic. This section focuses on selected in vivo, ex vivo, and in vitro tests currently used for evaluating immunotoxicity, as well as models and approaches that can be utilized for elucidation of the mechanism of action.

Methods to Assess Immunocompetence

General Assessment Central to any series of studies evaluating immunocompetence is the inclusion of standard toxicological studies, because any immunologic finding should be interpreted in conjunction with effects observed on other target organs. Standard toxicological studies that are usually evaluated include body and selected

organ weights, general observations of overall animal health, selected serum chemistries, hematologic parameters, and status of the bone marrow (ability to generate specific colony-forming units). In addition, histopathology of lymphoid organs, such as the spleen, thymus, and lymph nodes, may provide insight into potential immunotoxicants. Because of the unique nature of the immune system, there are several experimental approaches that may be taken to assess immunotoxicity and to evaluate the mechanisms of action of xenobiotics. These are depicted in Fig. 12-17 and vary with respect to in vivo or in vitro exposure, immunologic challenge, or immunologic evaluation (immune assay). As an example, the PFC assay [Fig. 12-17 (2)] is an ex vivo assay where xenobiotic exposure and antigen challenge occur in vivo and the immune response is evaluated in vitro. In contrast [as depicted in Fig. 12-17 (3)], splenocytes can be isolated after in vivo treatment with a xenobiotic, sensitized with an antigen in vitro and evaluated in vitro; or [as depicted in Fig. 12-17 (4)], splenocytes can be removed from a naive animal, exposed to xenobiotic and antigen in vitro, and evaluated in vitro. An example of this would be the in vitro-generated PFC response (Mishell–Dutton assay; Mishell and Dutton, 1967).

Functional Assessment

Innate Immunity As described earlier, innate immunity encompasses all those immunologic responses that do not require prior exposure to an antigen and that are nonspecific in nature. These responses include recognition of tumor cells by NK cells, phagocytosis of pathogens by macrophages, and the lytic activity of the components of the complement cascade.

To evaluate phagocytic activity, macrophages are harvested from the peritoneal cavity (peritoneal exudate cells) and are allowed to adhere in tissue culture plates. The cells are then incubated with chromated chicken red blood cells (^{51}Cr-cRBCs). Following incubation, the supernatant, containing ^{51}Cr-cRBCs that have not been bound by macrophages, is removed. The cRBCs which are bound to the macrophages, but which have not been phagocytized, are removed by a brief incubation with ammonium chloride. Finally, macrophages are lysed with NaOH and radioactivity in the lysate is counted to determine the amount of phagocytosis that occurred. A set of control wells is needed to determine DNA content for each set of wells. Data are presented as a specific activity for adherence and phagocytosis (adhered or phagocytized counts per minute (cpm)/DNA content) because xenobiotics altering adherence will have a significant effect on the results.

Another method to evaluate phagocytosis, but which does not require radioactivity, begins similarly to the ^{51}Cr-cRBC assay. Peritoneal macrophages are allowed to adhere to each chamber of a tissue culture slide. After adherence, macrophages are washed and incubated with latex covaspheres. At the end of incubation, cells are fixed in methanol and stained in methylene chloride. Macrophages containing five covaspheres or more are counted as positive and data are expressed as a percentage of phagocytosis (the ratio of macrophages with ≥5 covaspheres to total macrophages counted).

The previous macrophage assays are conducted in vitro after chemical exposure either in vivo or in vitro. If an in vivo assay to assess the ability of tissue macrophages to phagocytose a foreign antigen is required, the functional activity of the reticuloendothelial system can be evaluated. Intravenously injected radiolabeled sRBCs (^{51}Cr-sRBCs) are removed by the tissue macrophage from the circulation and sequestered for degradation in organs such as the liver, spleen, lymph nodes, lung, and thymus. Clearance of the ^{51}Cr-sRBCs is monitored by sampling of the peripheral blood. When steady state has been attained, animals are killed and organs are removed and counted in a gamma counter to assess uptake of the ^{51}Cr-sRBCs.

Evaluation of the ability of NK cells to lyse tumor cells is achieved using the YAC-1 cell line as a tumor target for an in vitro cytotoxicity assay. YAC-1 cells are radiolabeled with ^{51}Cr and incubated (in microtiter plates) in specific effector-to-target ratios with splenocytes from xenobiotic-exposed and xenobiotic-nonexposed animals. During an incubation step, splenic NK cells (effectors) lyse the ^{51}Cr-YAC-1 cells, releasing ^{51}Cr into the supernatant. At the end of the incubation, plates are centrifuged and the supernatant is removed and counted on a gamma counter. After correcting for spontaneous release (which should be <10%), specific release of ^{51}Cr is calculated for each effector-to-target ratio and compared to the specific release from control animals.

Acquired Immunity—Humoral The plaque (antibody)-forming cell (PFC or AFC) assay is a sensitive indicator of immunologic integrity for several reasons. It is a test of the ability of the host to mount an antibody response to a specific antigen. When the particulate T-dependent antigen (an antigen that requires T cells to help B cells make antibody) sRBCs is used, this response requires the coordinated interaction of several different immune cells: macrophages, T cells, and B cells. Therefore, an effect on any of these cells (e.g., antigen processing and presentation, cytokine production, proliferation, or differentiation) can have a profound impact on the ability of B cells to produce antigen-specific antibody. Other antigens, termed T-cell-independent antigens, such as dinitrophenyl-ficoll or trinitrophenyl-lipopolysaccharide, can be used that bypass the requirement for T cells in eliciting antibody production by B cells.

A standard PFC assay involves immunizing control and xenobiotic-exposed mice either intravenously or intraperitoneally with sRBCs. The antigen is taken up in the spleen and an antibody response occurs. At 4 days after immunization, spleens are removed and splenocytes are mixed with sRBC, complement, and agar. This mixture is plated onto Petri dishes and covered with a cover slip. After the agar hardens the plates are incubated for 3 hours at 37°C. During this time, the B cells that have been appropriately activated by the antigen and have differentiated into plasma cells secrete anti-

1. Bind antigen to plate. Wash.

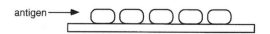

2. Add test sera and incubate. Wash.

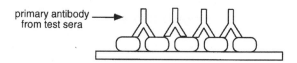

3. Add enzyme-coupled secondary antibody. Wash.

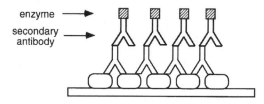

4. Add chromogen and develop color.

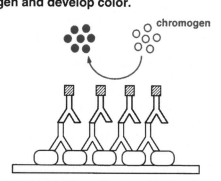

Figure 12-18. Schematic diagram of a standard enzyme-linked immunosorbent assay (ELISA).

sRBC IgM antibody. When the complement and the secreted IgM coat the surrounding sRBCs, areas of hemolysis (plaques) appear that can be enumerated. At the center of each plaque is a single B cell (antibody- or plaque-forming cell; AFC or PFC). Data are usually presented as IgM PFC per million splenocytes. IgG PFC can also be enumerated by slight modifications of this same assay. This isotype switching (from IgM to IgG) is important in secondary responses in which memory B cells respond more quickly to an antigen.

More recently, it has become evident that the PFC assay can be evaluated ex vivo using serum from peripheral blood of immunized mice and an enzyme-linked immunosorbent assay (ELISA; Fig. 12-18). Although the optimal response is delayed by 1–2 days (compared to the PFC assay), this assay takes into account antigen-specific antibody secreted by B cells in the spleen, as well as B cells residing in the bone marrow. Like the PFC assay, mice (or other experimental animals) are immunized with sRBCs and 6 days later peripheral blood is collected. Serum from each sample is serially diluted and incubated in microtiter plates that have been coated with sRBC membranes. The membranes serve as the antigen to which sRBC-specific IgM or IgG will bind. After incubation of the test sera and a wash step, an enzyme-conjugated monoclonal antibody (the secondary antibody) against IgM (or IgG) is added. This antibody recognizes the IgM (or IgG) and binds specifically to that antibody. After incubation and a wash step, the enzyme substrate (chromogen) is added. When the substrate comes into contact with the enzyme on the secondary antibody, a color change occurs which can be detected by measuring absorbance with a plate reader. Because this is a kinetic assay (color develops over time and is dependent on concentration of anti-sRBC antibody in the test sera), it is important to establish control concentration–response curves so that data can be evaluated in the linear range of the curve. Data are usually expressed in arbitrary optical density units. An advantage of the ELISA over the PFC assay is the ability to attain a greater degree of flexibility, because serum samples can be stored frozen for analysis at a later date.

One final assay measures the ability of B cells to undergo blastogenesis and proliferation, which are critical steps in the generation of an antibody response. This is achieved in microtiter plates by stimulating splenocytes with a monoclonal antibody to surface immunoglobulin in the presence of IL-4, or with the B-cell mitogen lipopolysaccharide. Proliferation is evaluated 2–3 days after stimulation by measuring uptake of ^{3}H-thymidine into DNA of the cultured cells. Data are usually expressed as mean cpm for each treatment group. These studies are usually done in conjunction with T-cell proliferative responses described below.

Acquired Immunity—Cell Mediated   While there are numerous assays used to assess CMI, three primary tests are used routinely in the National Toxicology Program (NTP) test battery (see "The National Toxicology Program Tier Approach" later in this chapter). The test battery includes the CTL assay, DTH response, and the T-cell proliferative responses to antigens (anti-CD3 + IL-2), mitogens (phytohemagluttinin and concanavalin A), and allogeneic cell antigens [mixed lymphocyte responses (MLRs)].

The CTL assay measures the in vitro ability of splenic T cells to recognize allogeneic target cells by evaluating the ability of the CTLs to proliferate and then lyse the target cells. Splenocytes are incubated with P815 mastocytoma cells, which serve as target cells. These target cells are pretreated with mitomycin C so that they cannot proliferate themselves. During this sensitization phase, the CTLs recognize the targets and undergo proliferation. At 5 days after sensitization, the CTLs are harvested and incubated in microtiter plates with radiolabeled (^{51}Cr) P815 mastocytoma cells. During this elicitation phase, the CTLs that have acquired memory recognize the foreign MHC class I on the P815 cells and lyse the targets. At the end of the incubation, plates are centrifuged, the supernatant is removed, and radioactivity released into the supernatant is counted on a gamma counter. After correcting for spontaneous release, the percent cytotoxicity is calculated for each effector-to-target ratio and compared to that from control animals.

The DTH response evaluates the ability of memory T cells to recognize foreign antigen, proliferate and migrate to the site of the antigen, and secrete cytokines and chemokines, which result in the influx of other inflammatory cells. The assay itself quantifies the influx of radiolabeled monocytes into the sensitization site. During xenobiotic exposure, mice are sensitized twice with keyhole limpet hemocyanin subcutaneously between the shoulders. On the last day of exposure, mononuclear cells are labeled in vivo with an IV injection of ^{125}I-5-iododeoxyuridine. One day later, mice are challenged intradermally in one ear with keyhole limpet hemocyanin. Twenty-four hours after challenge, animals are killed, the ears are biopsied, and radiolabeled cells are counted in a gamma counter. Data are expressed as a stimulation index, which represents the cpm

of ^{125}I activity in the challenged ear divided by the cpm in the unchallenged ear.

T cells play a central role in CMI and the ability of T cells to undergo blastogenesis and proliferation is critical to this role. Several mechanisms exist to evaluate proliferative capacity. The MLR measures the ability of T cells to recognize foreign MHC class I on splenocytes from an MHC-incompatible mouse (allogeneic cells) and undergo proliferation. For example, splenocytes from B6C3F1 mice (responders) are incubated with splenocytes from mitomycin C-treated DBA/2 mice (stimulators). Proliferation is evaluated 4–5 days after stimulation by measuring uptake of ^{3}H-thymidine into the DNA of the cultured responder cells. Cells are collected from each well using a cell harvester and counted in a scintillation counter. Data may be expressed as either the mean cpm for each treatment group or as a stimulation index where the index is calculated by dividing the cpm of wells containing responders and stimulators by the cpm of wells containing responders alone.

General T-cell proliferation can be evaluated in a manner similar to that described above for B cells (Table 12-4). Splenocytes are stimulated in microtiter plates with a monoclonal antibody to the CD3 complex of the TCR (anti-CD3) in the presence of IL-2, or with the T-cell mitogens concanavalin A or phytohemagluttinin. Proliferation is evaluated 2–3 days after stimulation by measuring uptake of ^{3}H-thymidine into the DNA of the cultured T cells. Data are usually expressed as mean cpm for each treatment group. These studies are usually done in conjunction with B-cell proliferative responses described above.

Flow Cytometric Analysis   One of the most rapidly advancing areas and powerful tools in immunotoxicology has been the application of fluorescence-activated cell sorting, or more commonly referred to as flow cytometry. In the most general sense, flow cytometry is a method that employs light scatter, fluorescence, and absorbance measurements to analyze large numbers of cells (typically 5000–20,000/sample) on an individual basis. Most commonly, fluorochrome-conjugated monoclonal antibodies raised against a specific protein of interest are employed for detection. The strength of the approach is that a wide variety of measurements can be made on large numbers of cells, rapidly, and with a high level of precision. In addition, methods are now available that allow for the analysis of specific proteins in cell-free preparations such as cell lysates and culture supernatants. A broad selection of monoclonal antibodies is now available to cell surface markers, intracellular proteins, and secreted proteins (Table 12-4).

The most common application of flow cytometry in immunotoxicology is to enumerate specific leukocyte populations and subpopulations. For example, antibodies are available to the T-cell surface markers CD4, CD8, and CD3 (among others). Because flow cytometers can detect light emission of multiple wavelengths simultaneously, multiple-colored fluorochromes can be used concurrently facilitating an analysis of more than one protein simultaneously in a given sample. In this manner, the number of CD4$^+$ and CD8$^+$ cells can be determined simultaneously on a single sample of cells. In the thymus, dual staining can be used to assess T-cell maturation by determining the number of CD4$^+$/CD8$^+$ (double positive), CD4$^-$/CD8$^-$ (double negative), CD4$^+$/CD8$^-$ (single positive), and CD4$^-$/CD8$^+$ (single positive) cells residing in this organ (Fig. 12-19). This approach can be used to provide insight into which specific T-cell subsets are targeted after exposure to a xenobiotic, and to identify putative effects on T-cell maturation. Similarly, antibodies are readily available to identify other leukocyte

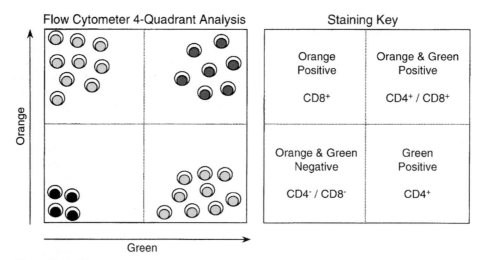

Figure 12-19. Flow cytometry.

In this example, cells from the thymus are stained simultaneously with a fluorescent PE-conjugated (orange) antibody to CD8 and a fluorescent FITC-conjugated (green) antibody. When analyzed on a flow cytometer, the instrument is requested to display a four-quadrant analysis (*left*). Increasing fluorescent intensity (brightness) is indicated by the arrows on each axis. The key to this analysis is displayed on the right. Cells that possess only CD8 fluoresce orange (CD8$^+$) and are displayed in the upper left quadrant (*light blue*). Cells that possess only CD4 fluoresce green (CD4$^+$) and are displayed in the lower right quadrant (*medium blue*). Cells that possess both CD8 and CD4 fluoresce both orange and green (CD4$^+$/CD8$^+$; double positives) and are displayed in the upper right *quadrant* (*dark blue*). Cells that do not possess either CD8 or CD4 do not fluoresce (CD4$^-$/CD8$^-$; double negatives) and are displayed in the lower left quadrant (*black*). The instrument can then be requested to determine the percentage of cells in each quadrant. In a typical mouse thymus, there are approximately 8–13% CD4$^+$, 2–5% CD8$^+$, 80–85% CD4$^+$/CD8$^+$, and 2–5% CD4$^-$/CD8$^-$ cells.

subpopulations including to surface immunoglobulin and to B220 (the CD45 phosphatase on B cells) for enumerating B cells, Mac1, and F4/80 for macrophages, CD16/CD56 for NK cells in humans and CD161 (NK-1.1) in mice. Surface marker analysis of heterogenous cell preparations can reveal significant alterations in lymphoid subpopulations, and in many instances this is indicative of alterations in immunologic integrity. Indeed, an indicator of AIDS is the changes observed in CD4$^+$ T-cell numbers. Luster *et al.*, (1992) reported that, in conjunction with two or three functional tests, the enumeration of lymphocyte subsets can greatly enhance the detection of immunotoxic chemicals. However, it is important to emphasize that although surface marker analysis can identify changes in leukocyte populations, functional analysis of the immune system is more definitive for the detection of immunotoxicity because the ability of immunocompetent cells to mount an effector response is assessed directly.

With technical advancements of flow cytometers (i.e., an increased number of wavelengths that can be simultaneously detected, enhanced sensitivity of detection and more rapid analysis) coupled with a steady growth of applications, reagents, and methods, flow cytometry has become an integral tool in elucidating the cellular and molecular mechanisms of action produced by immunotoxicants. Current applications go well beyond strictly evaluating cell surface markers and include measurements of cell cycle, intracellular free calcium, cellular viability, induction of apoptosis, DNA strand breaks (TUNEL assay), intracellular proteins, membrane potential, intracellular pH, oxidative stress, and membrane lipophilicity (reviewed in Burchiel *et al.*, 1997, 1999). A major recent advancement in flow cytometry-based analyses has been the development of fluorescent microspheres that are individually identified by the instrument. By coating the surface of microspheres with various

concentrations of two fluorescent dyes, sets of microspheres can be generated with each set possessing a unique spectral signature. Subsequently, various materials (i.e., proteins, antibodies, or nucleic acids) can be covalently conjugated to the surface of these microspheres in order to create unique detection systems. This technology is being widely applied for analyzing a broad variety of soluble cellular components including proteins in cell-free preparations by flow cytometry. For example, up to 15 different cytokines can be measured simultaneously in cell supernatants or biological fluids (e.g., bronchoalveolar lavage). A major advantage of this method over more traditional approaches, such as ELISA-based assays, is that only small amounts of biological samples and reagents are required as multiple proteins are assayed simultaneously. The same technology is also being applied for analyzing cell lysates for changes in protein phosphorylation in investigations of cell signaling. In addition, flow cytometry is routinely used to purify and isolate leukocyte subpopulation from heterogeneous cellular preparations. Thus, flow cytometry has become a powerful tool for characterizing the cellular and molecular mechanisms associated with immunotoxicants.

Measurements of Cytokines and Cytokine Profiling   As discussed in the earlier part of this chapter, development, maturation, differentiation, and effector responses of the immune system are highly dependent on a multitude of small secreted proteins termed cytokines. In most cases, these immunologic processes are controlled by the production of multiple cytokines, some of which are released simultaneously, whereas others are released in a very defined temporal sequence. Many of these cytokines are produced by T cells and are the mechanism by which a wide variety of functions by T cells are mediated. Due to the importance of cytokines in regulating the immune system, xenobiotics that alter the production and

Table 12-6
Models of Host Resistance

PRIMARY FACTORS INVOLVED IN CHALLENGE MODEL	PATHOGEN	HOST RESISTANCE
Bacterial	*Listeria monocytogenes*	Macrophage, T cell, NK cell
	Streptococcus pneumoniae	Complement, PMN, macrophage, B cell
Parasite	*Plasmodium yoelii*	T cell
Viral	Influenza A2	Cytotoxic T cell, antibody, complement
Tumor	B16F10 melanoma	NK cell, macrophage

SOURCE: From Bradley and Morahan (1982), with permission. See also for an extensive review of host-resistance models.

release of these mediators can significantly affect immune competence. Therefore measurement of multiple cytokines, often referred to as cytokine profiling, has become routine in immunotoxicology and can provide significant insights into the mechanisms by which a xenobiotic produces its immunotoxicity. For example, cytokine profiling has been explored more recently as an approach for identifying chemical allergens, either contact sensitizers, which typically induce a Th1 profile of cytokines (IL-2, IFN-γ, and TNF-β), or respiratory sensitizers, which typically produce a strong Th2 cytokine profile (IL-4, IL-5, IL-6, and IL-10) (Mosmann and Coffman, 1989; Mosmann *et al.*, 1991). Cytokines are most commonly measured in cell culture supernatants or biological fluids (i.e., serum or bronchoalveolar lavage) by ELISA (see Fig. 12-18). Quantification of test samples is accomplished by comparison to a standard curve employing recombinant cytokine standards. There is also a relatively new ELISA-type assay, the ELISPOT, which measures the number of cells producing the cytokine of interest. Cytokines in media or biological fluids can also be accurately assayed and quantified by flow cytometery with the main advantage being that many cytokines can be assayed simultaneously from one sample (see section "Flow Cytometric Analysis"). Because cytokines are regulated transcriptionally and then actively synthesized by cells at the time they are secreted, rather than existing as stored proteins, measurements of cytokine mRNA levels has become another common approach of assessing which cytokines are being expressed at a given time and the putative effects xenobiotics exert on their regulation and expression. Real-time polymerase chain reaction is most commonly used for quantifying mRNA levels of specific cytokines, as well as for other genes of interest in cells or tissues but other approaches including RNase protection and microarrays are also being more widely employed. Major advantages to quantifying cytokine expression at the mRNA rather than protein level include significantly greater sensitivity, the ability to quantify expression in solid tissues, and the capability to rapidly design appropriate reagents (PCR primers) specific for any cytokine. The major disadvantage is that changes at the mRNA level for a given cytokine may not necessarily correlate with changes in protein. One additional limitation to cytokine measurements by ELISA or via quantification of cytokine mRNA levels is that neither of these approaches provide information concerning the biological activity of the proteins being measured.

Host Resistance Assays   Host resistance assays represent a way of assessing how xenobiotic exposure affects the ability of the host to combat infection by a variety of pathogens. Although host resistance studies provide significant insight into the mechanisms by

which an immunotoxicant is acting, these assays are not used as a first or only choice for evaluating immunocompetence. The results from host resistance assays are typically more variable than other immune function assays already discussed, and therefore require markedly greater numbers of animals in order to obtain statistical power. The increased number of animals required also raises ethical considerations as well as cost. In addition, as with other immune function tests, no single host resistance model can predict overall immunocompetence of the host, primarily because each model uses different mechanisms for elimination of various pathogens. A representative list of host resistance models is shown in Table 12-6, as well as some of the cells involved in the immune response to these pathogens. Typically, three challenge levels of pathogen (approximating the LD_{20}, LD_{50}, and LD_{80}) for each concentration of xenobiotic are used in order to be able to detect both increases and decreases in resistance. End point analyses are lethality (for bacterial and viral pathogens), changes in tumor burden, and increased or decreased parasitemia. In host resistance studies, it is also important to consider the following: (1) strain, route of administration, and challenge size of the pathogen; (2) strain, age, and sex of the host; (3) physiological state of the host and the pathogen; and (4) time of challenge with the pathogen (prior to, during, or after xenobiotic exposure). All of these can have significant effects on the results from any individual study.

Assessment of Developmental Immunotoxicology   Interest in developmental immunotoxicology is predicated on the recognition that the developing immune system represents a novel target for xenobiotic-induced toxicity that presents some special considerations when it comes to assessment. The concept that any of a number of dynamic changes associated with the developing immune system may provide periods of unique susceptibility to chemical perturbation has been previously reviewed (Dietert *et al.*, 2000; Holladay and Smialowicz, 2000). This unique susceptibility may be manifested as a qualitative difference, in the sense that a chemical could affect the developing immune system without affecting the adult immune system, or as a quantitative difference, in the sense that a chemical could affect the developing immune system at lower doses than the adult immune system, or as a temporal difference, in the sense that a chemical could produce either a more persistent effect in younger animals than adults, or trigger a delayed effect (i.e., the consequences of early exposure are not manifested until early adulthood). As a result, while effective assessment of developmental immunotoxicology should certainly draw upon the prior experience with adult-exposure immunotoxicity assessment, it is important to examine the database of known immune changes that reflect the potential for unique susceptibility, and are specific for the developing immune (Dietert and Piepenbrink, 2006).

One of the most comprehensive reports to date attempted to compare the immunotoxicity following developmental or adult exposure to the following compounds: diethylstilbestrol, diazepam, lead, 2,3,7,8-tetrachlorodibenzo-p-dioxin (TCDD) and tributyltin oxide (Luebke *et al.*, 2006a). The selection of these five compounds was reported to be based on the availability of some human data. The authors concluded that for all five chemicals, the developing immune system was found to be at greater risk than the adult, either because lower doses produced immunotoxicity, adverse effects were persistent, or both.

A better understanding of the developing immune system, and in particular, an understanding of critical developmental landmarks has prompted some to speculate about the existence of five critical "windows" of vulnerability (Dietert *et al.*, 2000). The first window encompasses a period of hematopoietic stem cell formation from undifferentiated mesenchymal cells. Exposure of the embryo to toxic chemicals during this period could result in failures of stem cell formation, abnormalities in production of all hematopoietic lineages, and immune failure. The second window is characterized by migration of hematopoietic cells to the fetal liver and thymus, differentiation of lineage-restricted stem cells, and expansion of progenitor cells for each leukocyte lineage. This developmental window is likely to be particularly sensitive to agents that interrupt cell migration, adhesion, and proliferation. The critical developmental events during the third window are the establishment of bone marrow as the primary hematopoietic site and the establishment of the bone marrow and the thymus as the primary lymphopoietic sites for B- and T cells, respectively. The fourth window addresses the critical periods of immune system functional development, including the initial period of perinatal immunodeficiency, and the maturation of the immune system to adult levels of competence. The final window, addresses the subsequent period during which mature immune responses are manifest, and functional pools of protective memory cells are established.

Most recently, considerable attention has been focused on the perinatal period (i.e., prior to and just after birth) because this window of development is known to be replete with dynamic immune changes, many of which do not occur in adults (Dietert and Piepenbrink, 2006). Indeed, one reality associated with developmental immunotoxicology windows is that the developing immune system exists in an unbalanced state through the latter portion of gestation with certain functional CMI capacities deliberately impaired. In fact, Taylor *et al.* (2006) demonstrated that placentally induced immune skewing via the release of Fas-ligand-containing exosomes is one hallmark of a successful pregnancy brought to full term. Upon birth, restoring effective immune balance through the enhancement of Th1 capacity in the newborn is critical for protecting childhood health (Holt *et al.*, 2005; Yun and Lee, 2005). Prenatal maturation and functional skewing of the fetal immune system followed by the rapid reversal of the imbalance at birth has features that are not effectively modeled using adult exposure–assessment (Dietert and Piepenbrink, 2006), and developmental immunotoxicity is best viewed as a continuum of alterations. Suppression of the developing immune system, manifested as increased susceptibility to infections and cancer, is not the only concern, and immunotoxic changes that increase the risk for allergic or autoimmune responses in later life should also be considered (Edwards and Cooper, 2006; Selgrade *et al.*, 2006; Yeatts *et al.*, 2006). Adding to the complexity is the demonstration that some developmental immunotoxicants seem capable of inducing targeted immune suppression while at the same time elevating the risk of allergy and/or autoimmunity (Haggqvist *et al.*, 2005). Because either significant immune suppression or disrupted immune regulation is a concern and needs to be detected, the most effective methodology for assessing developmental immunotoxicity must also be capable of assessing significant changes in immune balance.

In spite of the increased interest in assessing the potential for developmental immunotoxicity, it must be emphasized that neither validated nor widely accepted methods currently exist for evaluating the effects of a chemical on the developing immune system. Several recent workshops and groups have summarized consensus thinking concerning developmental immunotoxicity evaluation (Luster *et al.*, 2003; Van Loveren and Piersma, 2004). Additionally, other reviews have dealt with issues concerning immunotoxicity evaluation across various life stages (Germolec *et al.*, 2004; Holsapple *et al.*, 2005; Ladics *et al.*, 2005; Ravel and Descotes, 2005). In light of the fact that neither validated nor established protocols presently exist to comprehensively assess whether a xenobiotic is a developmental immunotoxicant, below is a brief discussion of critical issues requiring consideration in establishing a testing framework.

In constructing a developmental immunotoxicity testing framework, one of the first points to consider is the selection of an animal model. Consistently, the rat has been identified as the preferred species for evaluations of developmental immunotoxicity, largely due to the fact that the rat has been utilized extensively in guideline developmental and reproductive toxicology testing. A recent review compared the anatomical and functional differences in the immune systems of the mouse, rat, dog, primate, and human, and their use as models for developmental immunotoxicity testing (Holsapple *et al.*, 2003). The review concluded that the developing immune systems of mice and humans have been best characterized to date. In addition, the review also concluded that immune ontogeny in the mouse and rat is likely similar. Another important consideration when selecting a species is that the development of the immune system in the rodent is delayed relative to the human, and how this differential maturation will impact data extrapolation for predicting human risk. For example, some developmental landmarks observed in utero in humans, occur after parturition in the rat.

A second consideration when constructing a framework for assessing developmental immunotoxicity concerns gender-specific effects. Results from perinatal exposure to xenobiotics suggest that significant sex-based differences in immunotoxic sensitivity are common and are at least as prevalent, if not more frequent, compared with the incidence observed following adult exposure–assessment (Dietert and Piepenbrink, 2006; Luebke *et al.*, 2006a). As such, for the evaluation of developmental immunotoxicity, testing of both sexes is critical.

A third major consideration in a developmental immunotoxicology testing framework is a consideration of exposure. There is general agreement that the best exposure protocol is one where exposure occurs across all non-adult developmental windows followed either by immediate assessment or assessment after a few weeks (Luster *et al.*, 2003; Holsapple *et al.*, 2005; Ladics *et al.*, 2005). Exposure to pregnant dams has been a hallmark feature of most developmental immunotoxicology protocols, and the maternal influences on exposure to the fetus/newborn pups would be dependent on transfer of the xenobiotic either across the placenta or via lactation. The gestational (e.g., transplacental) and lactational periods in the rat would result in exposure from conception to early postweaning in the pup, approximately 3 weeks of age. Direct exposure of pups via the diet would generally commence at about 3 weeks after birth. An unresolved issue is whether direct exposure of the pups, which is generally accepted as a routine procedure at around postnatal Day 7, should occur during the lactational period as well (Ladics *et al.*, 2005); however, any decisions concerning this issue will require consideration of how humans would be exposed and the specific properties of the chemical being studied. For example, if exposure is only oral and there is no reason to believe that the lactational transfer differs significantly for a class of compounds between rat and human, then direct dosing of pups could be initiated postweaning. In addition, information on pharmacokinetic and dosimetry could be useful in determining whether any direct dosing of pups during lactation is necessary. However, it is important to emphasize that this type of information is not routinely available for most xenobiotics.

A fourth consideration in creating a developmental immunotoxicology testing framework concerns which specific end points to measure. As discussed above, immune organs, like the thymus, spleen, and/or bone marrow, are not typically assessed in routine developmental and reproductive toxicology studies, and it has been the consensus of recent workshops that histopathological evaluation of these immune organs could be easily integrated into these protocols (Luster *et al.*, 2003; Holsapple *et al.*, 2005). However, presently, there is uncertainty whether routine histopathology is sufficiently sensitive to detect all potential immunotoxic effects, especially when the unique characteristics of the developing immune system, as discussed above, are considered. Indeed, there are examples where morphometric histopathologic findings do not predict functional impairments due to toxicity produced on the developing immune system (Hussain *et al.*, 2005). Ultimately, while the use of specific rather than general histopathology has been recommended, it has been also suggested that functional tests be employed in the assessment of developmental immunotoxicity. Unfortunately, few if any functional assays have been validated for detection of developmental immunotoxicity, even for routine assays like the T-cell-dependent antibody response, which has largely been confined to adult exposure protocols. Results published on several chemicals and drugs in recent years suggest that functional tests are a front-line priority for perinatal immunotoxicity detection and that a combination of at least two functional tests, such as a multi-isotype T-cell-dependent antibody response, and a cell-mediated immune response assay, such as the DTH assay and/or CTL or NK cytotoxicity assays, should be paired with histopathological analysis and phenotypic analysis of lymphocyte subsets using flow cytometry (Dietert and Piepenbrink, 2006).

One final point regarding the evaluation of developmental immunotoxicity needs to be considered. As developmental immunotoxicity protocols are inserted into exising toxicology testing regimes, such as developmental and reproductive toxicology protocols, it is likely to be necessary to incorporate immunization protocols. This approach has raised concerns among those evaluating other physiological systems (e.g., reproductive and neurological) in terms of potential immunization-induced changes. However, investigations addressing this potential by determining the impact of the incorporation of immunotoxicological functional assays on standard toxicological studies in rats have been largely negative. Ladics *et al.* (1995) showed that immunization did not significantly alter the weights or morphology of routine protocol tissues with the exception of the spleen (i.e., which manifested the anticipated increases in the numbers and size of germinal centers) In a subsequent study by this same group, immunization did not alter any hematological or clinical chemistry parameters, nor lymphocyte subset numbers (i.e., measured on peripheral blood with a flow cytometer), and did not mask the anticipated hepatotoxic effects of subchronic exposure to carbon tetrachloride (Ladics *et al.*, 1998a). An additional component of this discussion is the reality that the species being modeled, the human, has immunizations as a routine lifelong component of preventative medicine. As such, to avoid all immunizations in animal evaluation protocols does not closely simulate the childhood experience. Additionally, until the immune system is asked to respond specifically to a foreign antigen, the capacity to detect immunotoxicity may be severely limited. Therefore, immunization and a range of functional T-cell-dependent immune response evaluations seem necessary as components of an effective developmental immunotoxicity assessment.

Assessment of Hypersensitivity Responses As noted above, a primary role of the immune system is the discrimination of self versus nonself, and immunotoxicology can be thought of as a continuum with immunotoxic effects occurring in either direction (Fig. 12-1). The adverse consequences of exaggerated immune function would reflect an inability to recognize self, and are generally depicted as hypersensitivity and autoimmunity.

Drugs and chemicals that are capable of eliciting an immune response are generally low molecular weight substances possessing some inherent reactivity. There is a genetic susceptibility to hypersensitivity responses in that not all individuals react to the same drugs and chemicals. For the most part, the xenobiotic cannot be considered an antigen, simply because in itself it is not capable of stimulating an immune response. Instead, the xenobiotic often forms a hapten, which triggers the immune response in some tissue in the host. This property is called the sensitizing potential of the hapten and is associated with its inherent reactivity. Hapten-specific immune responses are therefore triggered only in the presence of the hapten–carrier complex and can be mediated either by humoral immunity or CMI. The damage associated with either type of hypersensitivity response can be directed against the tissue that is bound by the hapten. One of the most important and challenging problems in the field of immunotoxicology is determining the potential for chemicals to induce immune modulation and, in the current context, to demonstrate the sensitizing potential of xenobiotics. Thus, it becomes essential to have validated predictive animal models and to understand the underlying mechanisms of action. The following is a discussion of the currently used methods of predicting the most frequently occurring hypersensitivity reactions to chemicals, type I and type IV, which are most often manifested as respiratory hypersensitivity and contact sensitization, respectively.

Assessment of Respiratory Hypersensitivity in Experimental Animals Methods for assessing the potential to induce respiratory hypersensitivity were recently reviewed (Holsapple *et al.*, 2006). The objectives of this review were to describe the appropriate methods for identifying and characterizing respiratory hazards and risks and to identify the key data gaps and related research needs. The review addressed these objectives from the perspectives of proteins, chemicals, and drugs; and emphasized the important roles played by IgE and Th2 cell-mediated responses, while recognizing that damage to the respiratory tract can be triggered either by nonspecific irritation or by other specific (i.e., non-IgE/Th2) immune-mediated mechanisms.

The current state-of-the-science of animal models for respiratory hypersensitivity was also recently reviewed (Pauluhn, 2005). Current assays utilize two phases: induction/sensitization and

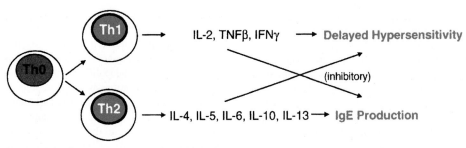

Figure 12-20. Schematic of cytokines involved in hypersensitivity reactions.

challenge/elicitation. The induction phase usually includes multiple exposures to the test compound (sensitization) via the respiratory tract (i.e., intranasal or intratracheal instillations or by inhalation) or by dermal contact. There are advantages and disadvantages to each. Inhalation more closely represents environmental exposure by allowing for chemical contact with the upper as well as the lower respiratory tract. However, the equipment required is expensive and difficult to maintain. Exposure via the intranasal route is easily accomplished and allows for distribution of antigen to the upper and lower respiratory tract; however, studies have shown that a large proportion of the material can be recovered from the stomach (Robinson *et al.*, 1996). In contrast, intratracheal instillation results in exposure to the lower respiratory tract only. The observation that a predominant respiratory sensitizer would still trigger an IgE response when applied topically has suggested an important interplay between type I hypersensitivity reactions, manifested primarily as respiratory sensitization, and type IV hypersensitivity reactions, manifested primarily as contact sensitization. The basis for this observation can be accounted for by a cytokine network model, which involves important cross-talk between humoral immunity and CMI (Fig. 12-20). Basically, a chemical with the capability of being a respiratory sensitizer will trigger an IgE response regardless of its route of exposure because it "selects" or supports the development of a Th2-dependent response, with the associated cytokine profile: IL-4, IL-5, IL-10, and IL-13. In contrast, a chemical which lacks the capability of being a respiratory sensitizer; but which can still trigger contact dermatitis, will select or support a Th1-dependent response, with the associated cytokine profile: IL-2 and IFN-γ.

The challenge (elicitation) phase involves exposure to the chemical (hapten), the homologous protein conjugate of the hapten, or the antigen. End points to characterize a positive response range from the induction of immunoglobulins (i.e., total IgE for chemicals or specific IgE for protein antigens), cytokines or lymphokines in serum, to pathophysiological responses, including the influx of inflammatory cells and the onset of bronchoconstriction along with the associated changes in respiratory functional parameters. The latter may be accomplished by visual inspection of the animals' respiratory pattern or more quantitatively by plethysmography. With plethysmography, changes in the respiratory rate, tidal volume, and plethysmographic pressure can be measured. However, plethysmography in guinea pigs, rats, and mice can be technically challenging and labor intensive. In addition, there is some controversy over the interpretation of measurements made from whole body plethysmography, and whether these measurements truly reflect changes in airway mechanics (Lundblad *et al.*, 2002; Mitzner and Tankersley, 2003).

None of the currently applied animal models duplicate all features of human asthma, and most of the current animal models were developed for studying specific hypersensitivity responses to high-molecular weight protein allergens (Pauluhn, 2005). Fewer animal models have been developed for use in the area of chemically induced respiratory allergy, which was one of the key data gaps identified in the review by Holsapple *et al.* (2006). One of the challenges associated with low-molecular weight models is that often these compounds must conjugate with body proteins to become antigenic (i.e., form hapten–carrier complexes). Often, a challenge with the conjugated chemical is necessary to induce a pulmonary response. Adding this variable can make the analysis of test results more difficult. False-negative results may occur due to variability in test article conjugation. Chemical conjugates are also necessary to measure specific immunologic responses.

The majority of the current animal models are based on antibody-mediated events occurring as a reflection of the induction phase (Pauluhn, 2005). In certain cases, immunologic sensitization may be confirmed by the detection of antigen-specific antibody; however, subsequent challenge does not produce clinical signs of respiratory distress. It is also possible to detect pulmonary sensitization in animal models, where there is no detectable antigen-specific antibody production. In these cases, CMI or other mechanisms may be involved, or there may be difficulty in antibody detection.

Guinea pig models have been most frequently used for detection of pulmonary reactions to chemicals because this species is known to respond vigorously to appropriate stimuli by developing an asthmatic-like bronchial spasm. In guinea pigs, as in humans, the lung is the major shock organ for anaphylactic response. Like humans, the guinea pig also demonstrates immediate- and late-onset allergic reactions as well as bronchial hyperreactivity and eosinophil influx and inflammation. The major difference in the mechanism of pulmonary responses between humans and guinea pigs is that the antibody involved in type I reactions in humans is IgE and in guinea pigs is predominantly IgG1. The key features of this animal model involve protocols using single or repeated inhalation or cutaneous (i.e., primarily topical or intradermal) exposures followed by a rest period until Day 21 (Pauluhn, 2005). After the rest period, inhalation challenge with the hapten or antigen is performed, thereby focusing on a measurement of the elicitation phase of the response (Karol *et al.*, 1994). Respiratory patterns are often measured in whole-body plethysmographs, as discussed above. A common pathologic accompaniment of increased airway hyperactivity is prolonged eosinophil-rich inflammatory leukocyte infiltration into the lungs of guinea pigs after inhalation challenge of the protein or hapten conjugate. One of the disadvantages of using guinea pigs is the lack of reagents needed to identify cells and mediators in respiratory allergy, which has hampered mechanistic studies.

Murine models, in which the reagent availability is not an issue, are becoming more frequently utilized in the evaluation of respiratory hypersensitivity, and two approaches have been described. The first approach capitalizes on the fact that, like humans, IgE is the major anaphylactogenic antibody in mice, and focuses on the induction of total serum IgE (Dearman *et al.*, 1998). The second approach capitalizes on the aforementioned cytokine network and has been referred to as "cytokine fingerprinting" (Dearman *et al.*, 2002, 2003; Plitnick *et al.*, 2002, 2003). Both approaches have relied on dermal application of potential allergens/sensitizers, and on the theoretical foundation that chemical allergens induce divergent immune responses characteristic of the selective activation of discrete T-cell subpopulations (Pauluhn, 2005). Contact allergens, such as 2,4-dinitrochlorobenzene, are considered not to cause sensitization of the respiratory tract, and trigger an immune response in mice that is consistent with the preferential activation of Th1 cells (i.e., little to no increase in total serum IgE and the production of IL-2 and IFN-γ in the draining lymph nodes). In contrast, topical sensitization to chemical respiratory allergens, such as trimellitic anhydride, triggers an immune response in mice that is consistent with the preferential activation of Th2 cells (i.e., moderate-to-marked increase in total serum IgE and the production of IL-4, IL-5, IL-10, and IL-13 in the draining lymph nodes). It is important to emphasize that while both the mouse total serum IgE test and cytokine profiling hold much promise, neither approach can be considered validated at this time.

Assessment of IgE-Mediated Hypersensitivity Responses in Humans Described below are methods of human type I hypersensitivity testing. These test results, in conjunction with a relevant history and physical exam, can be diagnostic of IgE-mediated pulmonary disease. Two skin tests are available for immediate hypersensitivity testing. In both, the measured end point is a "wheal and flare" reaction (i.e., the result of edema and erythema subsequent to the release of preformed inflammatory mediators). The prick–puncture test introduces very small amounts of antigen under the skin and, owing to the reduced chance of systemic reaction, is recommended as a screening test. For test compounds not eliciting a reaction in the less sensitive test, the intradermal test using dilute concentrations of antigen may be used, but there is a higher risk of systemic reactions. The reader is referred to an additional text for a more detailed description of testing methods (Demoly *et al.*, 1998).

In vitro serologic tests, ELISAs, and radioallergosorbent tests may also be used to detect the presence of antigen-specific antibody in the patient's serum. These tests do not pose a risk of adverse reactions and may be used in situations where standardized reagents for skin testing are not available. Serologic testing is often used in population-based epidemiologic studies.

Bronchial provocation tests may be performed by having the patient inhale an antigen into the bronchial tree and evaluating his or her pulmonary response. In some cases this may be the only way to demonstrate that a test article is capable of producing an asthmatic response. Care must be taken in these test situations in that it is possible to produce severe asthmatic reactions or anaphylaxis in sensitized individuals.

Assessment of Contact Hypersensitivity in Experimental Animals Classically, the potential for a chemical to produce contact hypersensitivity has been assessed by the use of guinea pig models. These tests vary in their method of application of the test article, in the dosing schedule, and in the utilization of adjuvants. For a description of methods employed in representative tests, see Klecak (1987). The two most commonly utilized guinea pig models, the Büehler test (Buehler, 1965) and the guinea pig maximiza-

tion test (Magnusson and Kligman, 1969), are described briefly below.

In the Büehler test, the test article is applied to the shaven flank and covered with an occlusive bandage for 6 hours. This procedure is repeated on Days 7 and 14. On Day 28, a challenge dose of the test article is applied to a shaven area on the opposite flank and covered with an occlusive dressing for 24 hours. At 24 and 48 hours after the patch is removed, test animals are compared with vehicle-treated controls for signs of edema and erythema. The guinea pig maximization test differs in that the test article is administered by intradermal injection, an adjuvant is employed, and irritating concentrations are used. Animals are given pairs of intradermal injections at a shaven area on the shoulders. One pair of injections contains adjuvant alone, one pair contains test article alone, and one pair contains the test article mixed with adjuvant. After 7 days following injection, after the area is reshaven, the test article is applied topically and an occluded patch is applied for 48 hours. In cases where the test article at the given concentration is nonirritating, the area is pretreated with 10% sodium lauryl sulfate 24 hours before the patch is applied to produce a mild inflammatory response. At 2 weeks following topical application, the animals are challenged on the shaven flank with a nonirritating concentration of the test article, which remains under an occluded patch for 24 hours. Then, after 24 and 48 hours, the test site is examined for signs of erythema and edema, two well-recognized indicators of cutaneous inflammation and contact dermatitis. However, the end points for evaluation in the guinea pig assays are subjective, and it is difficult to assess irritating or colored compounds using these models.

Over the past 20 years, efforts have been made to develop and establish more quantitative and immunologically based assay methods in other species, focusing mainly on the mouse, again primarily because of the availability of reagents and techniques to conduct mechanistic studies. Gad *et al.* (1986) developed the mouse ear-swelling test, which uses a quantitative measurement of ear thickness as an end point. Animals are sensitized by topical application of the test article for 4 consecutive days to abdominal skin that has been prepared by intradermal injection of adjuvant and tape stripping. On Day 10, the animals are challenged by topical application of the test article to one ear and vehicle to the contralateral ear. Measurements are made of ear thickness 24 and 48 hours later. A positive response is considered anything above a 20% percent increase in thickness of the treated ear over the control ear. Thorne *et al.* (1991) showed that dietary supplementation with vitamin A enhanced the mouse ear-swelling assay in the absence of adjuvants, injections, or occlusive patches.

The assays described above evaluate the elicitation phase of the response in previously sensitized animals. In contrast, the mouse local lymph node assay (LLNA) identifies contact allergens as a function of the events occurring during the induction (sensitization) phase of a hypersensitivity response. The origins, development, evaluation, and eventual validation of the LLNA have recently been described in a comprehensive review (Kimber *et al.*, 2002). In this assay, the induction phase of contact sensitization is measured by the incorporation of ^{3}H-thymidine into proliferating lymphocytes in lymph nodes draining the site where the test article has been applied. Animals are dosed by topical application of the test article to the ears for 3 consecutive days. The animals are rested for 2 days and then injected intravenously with 20 μCi of ^{3}H-thymidine. After 5 hours, animals are sacrificed, the draining lymph nodes are dissected out, and single-cell suspensions are prepared and radioassayed.

With consideration of dose–response and statistical significance, a three-fold increase in ^{3}H-thymidine cpm in chemically exposed animals over vehicle control animals (i.e., the stimulation index) is considered to be a positive response.

The LLNA offers several advantages over the guinea pig assays in that (1) it has the potential to reduce the number of animals required and reduces animal distress; (2) it provides quantitative data that allow for statistical analysis; and (3) it provides dose–response data. The latter qualities of the LLNA have facilitated its integration into comparisons of potency across individual chemicals and/or within a chemical class. These additional advantages of the LLNA have facilitated its integration into risk assessments for contact dermatitis (Felter *et al.*, 2003). Additionally, because the LLNA evaluates the induction phase of the immune response, it is more applicable to mechanistic studies. As an example, some compounds capable of producing contact sensitization also induce IgE production and subsequent respiratory hypersensitivity. Using three known allergenic diisocyanates—diphenylmethane-4,4′,-diisocyanate; dicyclohexylmethane-4,4′-diisocyanate; and isophorone diisocyanate—Dearman *et al* (1992), showed that all three known contact sensitizers induced lymphocyte proliferation in the draining lymph node but that only diphenylmethane-4,4′,-diisocyanate, a known respiratory sensitizer, induced elevated levels of serum IgE and IgG2b. These types of results have prompted a number of investigators to propose that the LLNA could be considered as the first step in a safety evaluation process for allergenic potential (i.e., as a method to identify sensitization potential of a chemical) with other methods being deployed to distinguish between skin and respiratory sensitizing activity (Holsapple *et al.*, 2006).

Assessment of Contact Hypersensitivity in Humans Human testing for contact hypersensitivity reactions is by skin patch testing. Patch testing allows for the diagnostic production of acute lesions of contact hypersensitivity by the application of a suspected allergen to the skin. Patches containing specified concentrations of the allergen in the appropriate vehicle are applied under an occlusive patch for 48 hours in most test protocols. Once the patch is removed and enough time elapses for the signs of mechanical irritation to resolve (approximately 30 minutes), the area is read for signs of erythema, papules, vesicles, and edema. Generally, the test is read again at 72 hours and in some cases signs may not appear for up to 1 week or more. Detailed information on patch testing has been reviewed in Mydlarski *et al.* (1998).

Human repeat insult patch tests are available as predictive tests in humans. Like predictive testing in animal models, there are many variations in attempts to increase the sensitivity of these procedures. These include preparation of the induction site by either tape stripping, the application of an irritating concentration of sodium lauryl sulfate, or use of high concentrations of the test article for induction of sensitization. In general, the application of multiple occlusive patches, up to 10 for 48 hours each at the same site, is followed by a rest period and then challenge takes place under an occlusive patch at a different site. Positive reactions are scored in the same manner as for diagnostic patch tests.

Assessment of Autoimmune Responses As described in the preceding section, exaggerated immune responses can be mediated by two entirely different types of interactions between the immune system and xenobiotics. One type of interaction was described in the preceding section in which the xenobiotic is a hapten and the immune system plays an active role in eliciting a hypersensitivity response. The immune system can also be a passive target for the enhancing effects of drugs and chemicals, such as occurs when a xenobiotic mimics or causes the aberrant production of immunomodulatory cytokines, or when a xenobiotic disrupts the regulatory mechanisms that serve to protect self (i.e., disrupt a suppressor mechanism). Additional mechanisms were presented above in the section "Autoimmunity."

Another way that xenobiotics can enhance immune function is by acting as an adjuvant, which is defined as any substance that nonspecifically enhances the immune response to an antigen. The classic adjuvant is complete Freund's adjuvant, which is a water-in-oil emulsion containing killed mycobacteria. The effectiveness of adjuvants in enhancing immune responses can be demonstrated by the fact that animals are often injected with complete Freund's adjuvant to increase the production of antigen-specific antibodies, and by the desire to develop an adjuvant that is safe in humans (i.e., complete Freund's adjuvant produces severe side effects) that could be used in conjunction with vaccines or immunotherapy. The specific mechanisms for the actions of adjuvants, including complete Freund's adjuvant, are not known. Moreover, the existence of environmental adjuvants is controversial and/or poorly studied.

In the context of testing strategies, the situation with autoimmunity is much more complex than with hypersensitivity responses. Animal models exist for a number of autoimmune diseases, and autoimmunity has been clearly demonstrated in humans, although it is a relatively infrequent occurrence. Therefore, the existence of autoimmune disease, and the expected consequences cannot be denied. However, the ability of drugs and chemicals to exacerbate or trigger autoimmune disease in either animal models or humans is poorly understood. In fact, of all the possible consequences of immunotoxicity, autoimmunity is unquestionably the least understood. Primarily because of the strong genetic component in the susceptibility to autoimmunity, deciphering the exact role of xenobiotics in the induction of these conditions has proven to be very difficult. The following is a review of the currently used methods of predicting the potential of a xenobiotic to trigger or exacerbate autoimmunity leading to an inappropriate immune response to self-tissue antigens that can be associated with the generation of autoantibodies and/or autoreactive T cells.

As emphasized throughout this chapter, immunotoxicology has evolved to the point where an ever-increasing number of studies are being conducted to characterize the immunotoxicity of a variety of xenobiotics using standard immunotoxicological parameters. Depending on the specific drug/chemical, the exposure conditions, the species being tested and the immune parameter being measured, the outcomes can be manifested as decreases, increases, or no effect. Whereas there is no question that the most frequent observation has been immune suppression, there is also no doubt that some examples of immune stimulation have been reported, a profile consistent with the concept of immunotoxicology existing as a continuum (Fig. 12-1). However, this observation can trigger some important questions. Should a treatment-related increase in an immune parameter such as the T-cell-dependent antibody response be considered an adverse response? Should an increase in the antibody response to a neo-antigen be considered a harbinger of autoimmune potential? There simply is no consensus regarding the correct way to interpret an increase in immune parameters such as the T-cell-dependent antibody response, which were primarily developed to characterize the immunosuppressive potential of xenobiotics.

An assay that was specifically developed to characterize the immunostimulatory capacity of low-molecular weight compounds (i.e., in particular, pharmaceuticals) is the popliteal lymph node assay (PLNA) (Kammuller et al., 1989). The concept for this assay was originally proposed by Gleichmann et al., (1984) who speculated that graft-versus-host reactions might be the basis for the pathogenetic mechanisms behind the development of drug-induced allergy and autoimmunity. The primary approach to the PLNA is to inject compounds subcutaneously into the hind footpad of either mice or rats. After 6–8 days, the draining PLNs are excised and compared with PLNs from vehicle-treated animals. Differences (e.g., increase) in the weight or cellularity of the treated nodes are an indication of the immunostimulatory potential of the test compound. Over the last 20–25 years, more than 130 chemicals have been tested in the PLNA (Pieters and Albers, 1999), yet the assay can still not be considered as validated. One of the first intralaboratory studies with the PLNA was recently reported (Weaver et al., 2005). These investigators concluded that this method might be able to detect drugs capable of causing human drug hypersensitivity with high prevalence; but that additional development is needed to increase the reproducibility of the PLNA and to increase detection of drugs that require metabolic activation to become allergenic, or drugs for which there is dose-limiting toxicity. The interpretability of the PLNA was increased by the integration of reporter antigens, trinitrophenyl-ficoll and trinitrophenyl-ovalbumin (Albers et al., 1997; Gutting et al., 1999). The reporter antigen-PLNA differs from the standard PLNA in two ways. First, the reporter antigens are injected with the test substance under investigation. Second, anti-trinitrophenyl-specific antibodies are measured via ELISPOT, in addition to the comparisons of the PLNs. The profile of antibody production against the T-cell-independent antigen, trinitrophenyl-ficoll, and against trinitrophenyl-ovalbumin, an antigen recognized by T- and B cells, enables the discrimination between immunosensitizing, and mere adjuvant or irritant potential of compounds.

The state-of-the-science of animal models of autoimmune disease was recently summarized (Germolec, 2005). This review emphasized that, while a wide variety of animal species have been studied, rodents have been most common, and concluded that rodent models fall into three categories: genetically predisposed animal models; animal models in which the autoimmune disease is produced by immunization with specific antigens; and animal models in which the disease is chemically induced.

Examples of genetically predisposed animal models include the non-obese diabetic (NOD) mouse, the F1 cross between the New Zealand black (NZB) and New Zealand white (NZW) mouse, and the MRL/lpr mouse. The NOD model has been used to study type 1 diabetes, specifically the T-cell autoimmune response, the role of B-cell antigen presentation and the role of cytokines in the disease progression. The NZB × NZW F1 and the MRL/lpr mouse models have been used to study human systemic lupus erythematosus. The NZB × NZW F1 model has been used to map the specific susceptibility loci and to assess the importance of B-cell hyperactivity and T-cell involvement in autoantibody production in the development of systemic lupus erythematosus (reviewed in Germolec, 2005), whereas the important role of apoptosis in negative selection has been studied in the MRL/lpr mouse model, in which a genetic defect results in a mutation in the Fas gene. While both models exhibit characteristics of human systemic lupus erythematosus including high levels of serum immunoglobulins (i.e., antinuclear and anti-DNA antibodies), as well as the immune-mediated nephritis, the MRL/lpr mouse model also exhibits rheumatoid factor autoantibodies and inflammatory joint disease characteristic of an arthritic response.

Arthritis can also be induced in susceptible rat strains by immunization with complete Freund's adjuvant containing killed Mycobacterium tuberculosis in oil. Immunization of susceptible mouse strains (i.e., those containing H-2^q or H-2^r alleles of the MHC) with type II collagen or cartilage glycoproteins, in the presence of adjuvant, can induce pathology similar to human rheumatoid arthritis. In collagen-induced models of arthritis, the immune response is directed against specific connective tissue antigens, whereas the complete Freund's adjuvant-induced response is directed against a mycobacterium heat shock protein, with the observed pathology resulting from cross-reactive destruction of a proteoglycan found in joints (Germolec, 2005). Experimental autoimmune encephalomyelitis can be induced in a number of species by immunization with myelin basic protein and complete Freund's adjuvant. This model has been used in rodents to characterize the role of T-helper cell-mediated autoimmune disease characterized by perivascular lymphocyte infiltration of the CNS and the destruction of the myelin nerve sheath resulting in paralysis, similar to human multiple sclerosis.

One of the most commonly used models of chemically induced autoimmunity is the Brown Norway rat model, where animals are injected with mercuric chloride. Whereas the selection of doses is such that exposure produces no overt signs of toxicity, Brown Norway rats develop an immunologically mediated disease characterized by T-cell polyclonal B-cell activation, autoantibodies to laminin, collagen IV, and other components of the glomerular basement membrane similar to human autoimmune glomerulonephritis. Numerous mouse strains have also been used to evaluate the development of autoantibodies following exposure to mercury, gold, and cadmium (Selgrade et al., 1999). Other examples of xenobiotics that have been demonstrated to be associated with autoimmune disease will be provided below.

Molecular Biology Approaches to Immunotoxicology As in all the biological sciences, the continuing evolution of molecular biology-based methods and technologies have vastly expanded the tools available to immunotoxicologists. In general, molecular biology approaches have been thus far employed primarily in the investigation and elucidation of mechanisms of immunotoxicity rather than for identifying immunotoxicants. As these approaches become more refined and sophisticated with time, their application will surely expand. The primary application of molecular biology presently in immunotoxicology has been to identify genes whose expression has been altered by a xenobiotic, often termed gene expression profiling, and/or to quantify the magnitude to which gene expression has been changed due to some treatment. As already discussed, methods for assessing changes in gene expression have been particularly useful for studies of the immune system, due to the fact that many of the immunologic mediators produced by leukocytes (e.g., cytokines, chemokines, and immunoglobulins) are regulated transcriptionally (i.e., synthesized and secreted on demand) rather than being maintained in cells as stored products. Toward this end, quantitative reverse transcriptase-polymerase chain reaction (RT-PCR) has been the principal method currently used to assess changes in mRNA levels for specific genes in tissues and cells. With the development of real-time PCR, accurate quantification of gene specific mRNA levels is readily achieved through the analysis of PCR kinetics by detecting products as they accumulate in "real-time" through the application of fluorogenic probes or double-stranded DNA-binding dyes. Significant advantages of RT-PCR over traditional methods for analysis of mRNA levels, principally Northern blotting, includes accuracy; sensitivity; markedly less RNA required to conduct the analysis; and less time required to complete the analysis. Recent advances in thermocycler technology and the availability of commercial reagents currently permit the quantification of up to 384 genes from one RNA sample by employing what are termed "low-density" arrays. The technology takes advantage of plates comprised of 384 wells that have been pre-coated with primers for up to 384 specific genes of interest.

Another approach for conducting gene expression profiling by assessing changes in mRNA levels for multiple genes simultaneously has been through the use of cDNA microarrays. The approach facilitates the analysis of hundreds up to tens of thousands of genes from a single RNA sample. The principal advantage of microarrays is the ability to assay mRNA levels for a large number of genes simultaneously. The primary disadvantages are the cost associated with microarray analysis, the complexity associated with data analysis and bioinformatics, and the sensitivity of the methodology to assess moderate changes in mRNA levels. In spite of these challenges, the application of microarray analysis in immunotoxicology has been increasing (Luebke *et al.*, 2006b).

A routinely employed methodology for characterizing effects on gene transcription has been the use of reporter assays. Reporter assays are being widely used to discern whether xenobiotic-induced changes in mRNA levels for specific genes are due to alterations at the level of transcription versus mRNA stability. Likewise, reporters can be used to characterize the effects of xenobiotics on specific transcription factors acting through defined regulatory elements. The approach involves construction of a DNA plasmid possessing the 5′ untranslated regulatory region of the gene of interest that has been ligated to the translated region of a reporter gene. Commonly used reporter genes are typically enzymes, because their expression can be easily assayed. Moreover, studies in mammalian systems commonly employ reporter genes of insect or bacterial origin, thus eliminating the need to differentiate between endogenous and ectopic expression. The most widely used reporter genes are firefly luciferase and bacterial β-galactosidase. Most often, reporter assays are performed by transient transfection into cell lines. This approach has been extensively used to study the effects of leukocyte activation stimuli and xenobiotics on the regulation of promoter and enhancer regions of cytokine and immunoglobulin genes. In spite of the important mechanistic information that can be gained from these types of studies, significant challenges often arise in utilizing reporter assays to study leukocytes. Transfection of primary leukocytes, especially lymphocytes, yielding both high transfection efficiency and good cell viability is extremely difficult. An additional complicating factor concerns the fact that primary lymphocytes can only be maintained viable in culture for short periods (approximately 24 hours) in the absence of activation, which limits the duration the cells can be given to recover after transfection. Likewise, it is not uncommon for T- and B-cell-derived lines to be resistant to transfection in spite of the many commercial transfection reagents presently available and new refinements made to electroporators. In most cases, transfection conditions must be optimized for transfection efficiency and cell viability for each cell line or preparation using a control plasmid (i.e., a plasmid possessing strong constitutive expression).

RNA interference employing small interfering double-stranded RNAs (siRNA) to achieve posttranscriptional gene-specific silencing is a relatively new technology that is beginning to be applied to

investigations aimed at elucidation of mechanism of immunotoxicity. A total of 21 nucleotide RNA duplexes possessing two to three nucleotide 3′ overhanging ends once transfected into the cell incorporate into a nuclease complex known as the RNA-induced silencing complex (RISC). Through an ATP-dependent mechanism, the duplexes are unwound and separated into their sense and antisense strands. RISC is directed by the unwound antisense siRNA strand homologous to the target mRNA, which then undergoes cleavage by an endonuclease termed Slicer. The ensuing destruction of the target gene mRNA results in the posttranscriptional silencing of gene expression. This approach provides a rapid mechanism by which the involvement of a specific gene product can be linked to biochemical and functional events induced by a xenobiotic in a given cell type, including leukocytes (Sandy *et al.*, 2005). Major challenges in the application of this methodology can exist. First, identification of an effective siRNA is critical, as not all sites of a given mRNA being targeted will result in gene silencing. Numerous strategies and criteria have been developed to assist in the rationale design of siRNA (Khvorova *et al.*, 2003; Schwarz *et al.*, 2003; Jia *et al.*, 2006). Second, as with the transient transfection of reporters discussed above, leukocytes, and especially lymphocytes, are often resistant to transfection resulting either in poor delivery of the siRNA into the desired cell preparation or low viability. Because siRNA are most often used in cell lines, the doubling rate of the cells can significantly affect the level of knock down achieved, based on the fact that each time a cell undergoes replication, the cellular siRNA is diluted by half. The half-life of the protein can also significantly impact on the level of knock down achieved even if large amounts of siRNA are delivered into the cells. Also, genes that are highly expressed can be difficult to effectively knock down due to the large amount of mRNA that must be destroyed. Likewise, genes with very low expression can be difficult to silence as the odds of the RISC complex finding rare mRNAs in the cell may be low. Lastly, antibodies must be available to the gene product being targeted for knock down so that the magnitude of knock down can be confirmed at the protein level. In spite of these many potential challenges, the ability to effectively achieve gene-specific silencing, in some cases of a magnitude greater than 90%, is a remarkably powerful tool when elucidating biological mechanisms for which knockout mice are not available.

A relatively new area of research that has not yet had broad application to the field of immunotoxicology is proteomics. Proteomics can be defined as research that aims to identify, quantify, and classify the function of proteins produced by given genomes. In addition to the systematic identification and characterization of proteins, a potentially important application of proteomics is in the characterization of protein–protein interactions, especially as they relate to the elucidation of signal transduction mechanisms. Recently, strategies have been proposed for the functional analysis of signal transduction, termed phosphoproteomics (Morandell *et al.*, 2006). Unfortunately, a major drawback in the application of proteomics includes the lack of an experimental platform currently available to systematically measure the diverse properties of proteins in a high throughput approach. Presently, most proteomic methods are based on mass spectrometry and require expensive instrumentation, information-technology infrastructure and highly specialized personnel. In addition, the complexity of the proteosome is enormous as recently illustrated by Aebersold when he compared the human genome, which is comprised of approximately 30,000 genes, to human serum, which alone has been estimated to contain approximately 500,000 different protein species

(Aebersold, 2003). Nevertheless, the application of proteomics to study specific defined proteins is occurring routinely in cell-based systems.

As stated above, the use of molecular biology-based methods in immunotoxicology to date has been primarily for understanding of the mechanisms of action of known immunotoxicants. Much research is currently focused on quantifying changes in mRNA levels (e.g., cytokines) and elucidating mechanism responsible for those xenobiotic-induced changes. Similarly, changes in mRNA expression profiles may be useful as possible biomarkers of exposure. Proteomics and genomics, combined with bioinformatics, are making it possible to evaluate chemically induced alterations in entire pathways and signaling networks. The utility of molecular biology tools such as proteomics and genomics in elucidating mechanisms of action is obvious. More challenging will be the application of these tools for identifying new or suspected immunotoxicants (Luebke *et al.*, 2006b).

Mechanistic Approaches to Immunotoxicology   Once an agent has been identified as being an immunotoxicant, it may be necessary to further characterize the mechanism by which it exerts its effects on the immune system. Toward this end, a unique aspect of the immune system that greatly facilitates investigations aimed at delineating the underlying mechanisms of action is the ability to study the immune system in the intact animal, as well as remove immune cells from the intact animal and have them function in vitro. Using a combination of these two approaches, a general strategy that has been successfully employed by a wide number of laboratories for characterizing mechanisms of immunotoxic action by xenobiotics and involves the following steps: (1) identifying the cell type(s) targeted by the agent; (2) determining whether the effects are mediated by the parent compound or by a metabolite of the parent; (3) determining whether the effects are mediated directly or indirectly by the xenobiotic; and (4) elucidating the molecular events responsible for altered leukocyte function. The significance of each and the experimental strategies typically employed are discussed below.

Identification of the Cell Type or Type(s) Targeted   With few exceptions, the first objective toward elucidation of the mechanism(s) responsible for immunotoxicity is the identification of the cell type(s) affected by the xenobiotic. The rationale is that the immune system is comprised of a wide variety of cell types with broad, and often, overlapping effector functions. Therefore, identification of specific cell type(s) affected allows for the selection of appropriate approaches and techniques to employ to further elucidate the mechanism of action.

The approaches available for the identification of which cell types are targeted by a specific agent are numerous but typically originate with the employment of one or more of the functional assays within the immunotoxicology tier testing battery (see section "The National Toxicology Program Tier Approach" later in this chapter). Each of the functional assays in the immunotoxicology tier testing battery provides information on accessory and/or effector cell function. For example, the PFC response to the T-cell-dependent antigen, sRBC, requires macrophages and CD4$^+$ T cells (helper T cells) to function as accessory cells, and B cells to serve as the effector cells. Therefore, if any one of these three cell types is adversely affected by an immunotoxicant, changes in the magnitude of the PFC response would be observed as compared to control (i.e., enhancement or sup-

pression). Similarly, the CTL response requires macrophages and CD4$^+$ T cells as accessory cells and CD8$^+$ CTL as the effector cells. Functional assays can be further refined to provide additional information concerning the targeted cell types by employment of various defined antigens requiring different cellular cooperativity to elicit an effector response. The PFC response has been especially useful in this respect. In addition to using a T-cell-dependent sensitizing antigen such as sRBC, T-cell-independent antigens can be employed including dinitrophenyl-ficoll or trinitrophenyl-lipopolysaccharide, which require macrophages, but do not require T cells to elicit an antibody response. Likewise, B cells can be driven to differentiate into PFC in the absence of accessory cells using polyclonal B-cell activators such as lipopolysaccharide. By employing the three different types of antigens in order to characterize a xenobiotic, a profile of activity emerges that can distinguish between affects on the B cell, T cell, and macrophage.

As described in the examples above, when accessory cells are required in the elicitation of an immune response, it is often difficult to discern whether alteration of an immune response is due to the xenobiotic targeting the effector cell population or one or more of the accessory cell populations. Under such circumstances, another strategy utilized for identifying the cellular targets is a cell fractionation–reconstitution approach. Specifically, leukocytes can be isolated from treated and vehicle control animals, typically mice, and fractionated into their respective subpopulations. The fractioned cell populations from vehicle and treated animals can then be reconstituted in various combinations to be used in functional assays to determine the population of cells that has been altered. A comprehensive discussion of the various methods that can be used to fractionate leukocyte populations and subpopulations is beyond the scope of this chapter; however, two of the most common approaches to fractionate leukocyte populations are briefly described here. The first is by cell sorting using flow cytometry. The primary advantage of this approach is that it yields an exceptionally high purity of cell populations and subpopulations. The primary disadvantages include: (1) access to a high-end flow cytometer; (2) cost of reagents and trained personnel capable of operating a flow cytometer; (3) practical limitations concerning the total number of cells that can be collected within a reasonable period of time due to the rate at which the instrument analyzes and collects the cells; and (4) positive selection is used for identifying the desired cell population being collected. The second and more commonly used approach utilizes antibodies directed at surface antigens unique to specific leukocyte populations and subpopulations that have been covalently conjugated to magnetic beads. Using the conjugated magnetic beads and a magnet, large numbers of highly pure cell populations can be isolated rapidly, by positive or negative selection, without requirements for expensive instrumentation. As with the cell sorting approach, purified population of cells isolated from vehicle and treated animals can be isolated and reconstituted in various combinations for evaluation in functional assays.

Determination of Whether Immunotoxicity is Mediated by the Parent or by a Metabolite of the Parent Compound   A critical aspect in the elucidation of the mechanism of toxicity for any compound, regardless of the target tissue is whether the adverse effects are mediated by the parent form of the compound or by a metabolite of the parent. An understanding of the role of metabolism is especially critical when studying immunotoxicants, as it will dictate the experimental approaches that can be utilized. In general, leukocytes possess very modest levels of drug metabolizing

Table 12-7
Possible Mechanisms of Chemically Induced Immune Modulation

TYPES OF EFFECT	MECHANISM	EXAMPLES
Direct	Functional changes	Altered antibody-mediated responses
		Altered cell-mediated responses
		Altered release of preformed mediators
		Altered host resistance
		Inability of one or more cell types to perform a required activity, e.g.:
		Production of antibody
		Release of cytokines
		Processing and presentation of antigen
		Proliferation and differentiation
		Receptor-mediated signal transduction
	Structural changes	Alterations in surface receptors or ligands
		Alteration in expression of receptors or ligands
		Histopathologic changes in lymphoid organs
	Compositional changes	Alterations in $CD3^+$, $CD4^+$, $CD8^+$, $B220^+$, and/or Ig^+ in spleen
		Alterations in $CD4^+$, $CD8^+$, $CD4^+/CD8^+$, and/or $CD4^-/CD8^-$ in thymus
		Changes in hematologic cellular parameters
		Alterations in circulating Ig
		Alterations in CFU profile in bone marrow
	Metabolic activation	Conversion to a toxic metabolite
Indirect	Effects secondary to other target organ toxicity	Induction of acute phase proteins as a result of liver injury
		Increased corticosteroid release from the adrenal gland
	Hormonal changes	Alteration in neuroendocrine regulation
		Alteration in autonomic output from the CNS
		Altered release of steroids from sex organs

enzymes, especially those within the cytochrome P-450 family. Therefore, those agents that are metabolically bioactivated to an immunosuppressive form will in most cases not exhibit their immunotoxic profile of activity when added directly to cultured leukocytes. In fact, an important indication that metabolic activation may be a requisite mechanistic event is the observation that an agent is immunotoxic following in vivo administration while exhibiting no immunotoxic activity when added directly to cultured leukocytes. An example of such an agent is the therapeutic, cyclophosphamide. When administered in vivo, cyclophosphamide is a potent immunosuppressant that preferentially suppresses humoral immune responses while having no effect when directly added to cultured leukocytes.

In order to assess whether metabolic bioactivation is required for immunotoxicity, several different approaches can be employed. One approach is to determine whether pre- or co-treatment with either an inducer or inhibitor of the enzymes known to be involved in the metabolism of the agent, modify the immunotoxicity produced in vivo. Similarly, in vitro approaches have also been used to assess the role of metabolism for an immunotoxicant. Specifically, these approaches utilize various in vitro metabolic activation systems such as S9 liver homogenates or isolated liver microsomes, which can activate the xenobiotic when incorporated with leukocyte cultures. Alternatively, freshly isolated primary hepatocytes can be co-cultured with leukocytes in the presence of the xenobiotic. Although primary hepatocytes most closely simulate the metabolic activity observed in vivo, this approach is also the most technically challenging metabolic activation system because the approach is critically dependent on the isolation of viable and metabolically

active hepatocytes. Cyclophosphamide is typically employed as a positive control in all three of the aforementioned in vitro activation systems to confirm metabolic activity. The metabolic activation systems discussed above can also be employed for conducting mechanistic studies in vitro that cannot be performed in the intact animal to further characterize immunotoxicants requiring metabolic bioactivation.

Determination of Whether the Effects are Mediated Directly or Indirectly by the Xenobiotic or a Metabolite of the Xenobiotic In most instances, immunotoxicants mediate their effects by interacting directly with the immune system. These direct actions may include structural alterations in lymphoid organs or on the cellular composition of lymphoid organs, on the expression of regulatory molecules on the immune cell surface, and/or by altering intracellular biochemical or molecular events (Table 12-7). However, some xenobiotics mediate changes in immune competence through an indirect action on the immune system. Under these circumstances, changes in immune competence are mediated through the release of an immunomodulatory factor resulting from the actions of the immunotoxicant on cells or tissues other than the immune system. One tissue most often implicated in indirectly modulating the immune system is the liver, as it is the source of a broad and extremely diverse group of proteins including acute phase proteins. Acute phase proteins are a family of serum proteins produced by the liver in response to inflammation or infection (see section "Inflammation"). Acute phase proteins are believed to have evolved as part of an immediate survival response to systemic infection. In general, acute phase proteins are associated with downregulation of the immune system and are therefore believed to play a role in maintaining immune homeostasis. The acute phase proteins most extensively characterized with respect to immune modulating properties include alpha-fetoprotein, serum amyloid A, and C-reactive protein. Another important group of regulatory proteins involved in indirectly modulating the immune system are those that contribute to the repair and regeneration of the liver after acute injury; specifically, transforming growth factor-β1 (TGF-β_1) and hepatocyte growth factor. Another example of indirect actions on the immune system is stress, as well as chemicals that alter the regulation of the hypothalamic–pituitary–adrenal axis, thus leading to changes in hormonal homeostasis. Deregulation of hormonal homeostasis, especially increased circulating levels of glucocorticoids, can markedly decrease immune competence and are yet another example of indirect modulation of the immune system.

The elucidation of indirect mechanisms of action by an immunotoxicant can be challenging by virtue that the effect is indirect and mediated by one or more circulating immunomodulatory serum factors. The involvement of an immunomodulatory serum factor can be partially deduced by two distinguishing features. First, the profile of immunotoxicity observed after in vivo administration of the causative chemical is different from that produced by its direct addition to leukocytes in culture. Second, the profile of immunotoxicity observed after in vivo administration of the chemical can be mimicked by direct addition of serum from the treated animal to naive leukocytes in culture. Third, the involvement of a metabolite of the parent form of the chemical has been ruled out. Confirmation of the involvement of a specific serum factor is most often accomplished in vitro by abrogating the immunotoxic activity produced by serum from treated animals using neutralizing antibodies directed against the suspected serum factor.

Elucidation of the Molecular Mechanism   Numerous methodologies are available to evaluate cellular and molecular mechanisms of action and those continue to increase with the availability of new "omics" technologies, new animal models including transgenic and knockouts, and an ever-expanding list of reagents and molecular probes. Due to the broad nature of this topic area, this section is devoted to a general discussion of considerations and strategies aimed at the elucidation of molecular mechanisms. The discussion will be directed at B- and T cells for illustrative purposes but is certainly applicable to other cell types comprising the immune system.

When considering the molecular mechanism by which a xenobiotic alters the function of a mature lymphocyte, a practical strategy is to first identify at which stage of leukocyte function the chemical is acting, antigen recognition/signaling through the antigen receptor, activation, proliferation, or differentiation. As discussed in the earlier sections of this chapter, lymphocytes have evolved a number of specialized mechanisms by which B- and T cells recognize antigen. Common to both cell types is that immediately after recognition of an antigen there are a number of biochemical events triggered including changes in protein phosphorylation and activation of a variety of kinases, fluxes in ions, and changes in the level of cyclic nucleotides. Since lymphocytes undergo a rapid and robust rise in intracellular calcium almost immediately after triggering through the antigen receptor, changes in calcium flux prior to and immediately following stimulation by an antigen provide important insights on whether a chemical alters the most proximal stage of leukocyte function. Similarly changes in the phosphorylation status of the intracellular domain of membrane-associated proteins (CD3 complex, CD4 and CD8 on T cells, and CD79, CD45, and CD22 on B cells)

and the kinases that mediate the phosphorylation (e.g., lyk and fyn) can be investigated to study the most proximal events associated with triggering of antigen receptors. In order to activate large numbers of lymphocytes simultaneously facilitating the evaluation of changes in these early biochemical events, often polyclonal activators are employed. For B cells antibodies directed against the B-cell receptor in combination with CD40 ligand can be used. Conversely, for T cells antibodies directed against the TCR/CD3 complex and the coreceptor, CD28 can be used.

The stage termed lymphocyte activation is functionally defined and refers to that period that begins when the T cell has initiated a response to an activation stimulus and ends when there is robust transcription of the T-cell autocrine/paracrine growth factor, IL-2. In B cells it is the period that begins with the cell responding to an activation signal and ends with the upregulation of immunoglobulin gene transcription. In the case of B- and T cells, the events leading up to and resulting in the initiation of robust transcription of the immunoglobulin genes and IL-2, respectively, are complex and involve the activation of multiple signal transduction events initiated at the cell membrane culminating in the binding of transcription factors to regulatory regions of genes coding for the immunoglobulin heavy and light chains in B cells, and IL-2 in T cells. Investigations directed at elucidating the molecular events deregulated by xenobiotics during lymphocyte activation represent one of the most intensively studied areas presently in immunotoxicology as many different immunotoxicants affect this stage of lymphocyte function.

Clonal expansion is a critical phase of the immune response as it insures that a sufficient number of antigen-specific B- and T-effector cells are generated to respond effectively to combat a pathogen. In light of the importance of clonal expansion in mounting an effective immune response, the effect xenobiotics exert on lymphocyte proliferation has been widely used to determine whether a xenobiotic has immunotoxic properties. As with measurements directed at other stages of the immune response, it is often convenient to employ polyclonal B- and T-cell activators for investigating effects on proliferative responses. Due to a significant increase in the understanding of the cell cycle, coupled with the availability of reagents for measuring specific proteins involved in the regulation of cell cycle, it is now possible to functionally characterize and dissect the mechanism and specific intracellular targets affected by xenobiotics that disrupt lymphocyte proliferation. Measurements of changes on cell cycle-associated regulatory proteins are most commonly achieved by employing flow cytometric approaches.

The final stage of the immune response involves differentiation into a mature effector or memory cell. For B- and T cells, terminal differentiation into effector cells can be best assessed by measurements of effector function in conjunction with the upregulation and downregulation of proteins on the cell surface. In the case of B cells, measurements of antibody production and the case of T cells, either cytokine production (helper T cells and CTL) or lysis of target cells expressing viral or tumor proteins (CTL) are most often employed. A number of commonly used immune function methods for assessing B- and T-cell effector functions were described earlier in this section.

Once the specific stage of lymphocyte function being altered by a specific xenobiotic has been established, experiments can be designed to identify the specific intracellular proteins affected by the xenobiotic and the molecular mechanism by which it is modulated. Cell line models can be invaluable tools for studies involving cell signaling and gene regulation.

Table 12-8
Celluar Models for Immunotoxciology

CELL LINE	CELL TYPE	SPECIES	EFFECTOR RESPONSE	STIMULUS
EL4	T cell	Mouse	IL-2	Phorbol ester
Jurkat E6	T cell	Human	IL-2	Phorbol ester + Ca ionophore or αCD3 + αCD28
CHI2.LX	B cell	Mouse	IgM	Lipopolysaccharide
BCL-1	B cell	Mouse	IgM	Lipopolysaccharide
SKW	B cell	Human	IgM	Lipopolysaccharide Or αIgM + CD40L
Daudi	B cell	Human	None (signal transduction)	αIgM
RAW 264.7	Macrophage	Mouse	Nitric oxide, IL-1	Lipopolysaccharide
J774.1	Macrophage	Mouse	Nitric oxide, IFN-γ	Lipopolysaccharide
U937	Macrophage	Human	TNF-α, IL-1α, IL-6, IL-8	Lipopolysaccharide

Cell Line Models in Immunotoxicology   Cell line-based models are being widely used for identifying agents possessing the potential of producing immunotoxicity, as well as for conducting indepth investigations aimed at elucidating molecular mechanisms for immunotoxicity. Significant advantages and disadvantages exist when applying cell line-based models, some of which are unique to investigations of the immune system. A brief discussion of the strengths and limitations of cell line-based models in the context of studies of immunotoxicants is provided below.

Although there are many advantages to cell line-based models, the most important characteristic is that all the cells are derived from the same clone, thus providing a homogenous cellular preparation. The homogeneity of the model is especially useful for studies directed at characterizing signal transduction pathways as well as gene expression profiling due to the greater likelihood of obtaining reproducible results. There are a number of advantages of cell line-based models that are especially useful in immunotoxicology. Primary leukocytes, whether isolated from blood or lymphoid organs, are highly heterogeneous in their cellular composition. Purification of these primary cell preparations into specific cell types is expensive, can be labor intensive, and with most isolation methods typically yielding 50–75% efficiency (i.e., 25–50% of the desired cells are lost during the purification process). Purification efficiency can become a critical issue when utilizing small rodents such as mice where the number of animals per assay can be significantly increased due to the loss of cells being recovered in the cell isolation procedure. When employing cell line models, typically there is no limitation on the number of cells available for a given study. Another important consideration in the case of primary lymphocytes is that they can only be maintained viable in culture for relatively brief periods of time (approximately 24 hours) in the absence of receiving an activation signal. Therefore, extended pre-incubation periods in culture with an immunotoxicant or other response modifiers that do not activate primary lymphocytes cannot be performed. Primary leukocytes, especially lymphocytes, are also difficult to transfect, often yielding poor transfection efficiency and/or viability. The combination of poor transfection efficiency and limited duration, where they can be maintained in culture in the absence of activation make reporter assays, transient ectopic gene expression, and utilization of siRNA to silence gene expression extremely challenging in primary lymphocytes. Conversely, cell line-based models, especially of the lymphoid lineage, in most cases can be readily transfected with suitable efficiency and viability to conduct reporter assays, ectopic gene expression, and gene silencing with siRNA. It is noteworthy that primary cells of the myeloid lineage are more suited for long-

term culture and transfection-based experimental approaches as they have less stringent requirements for activation to be maintained in culture for extended periods. In such instances, it may be more advantageous to employ primary cells. Lastly, cell line-based models are also now being widely adapted for high throughput screening due to the reproducibility of results obtained with these models and the ease in which cell lines can be maintained and manipulated.

In spite of the advantages discussed above, there are numerous disadvantages and limitations inherent in utilizing cell line models for characterizing immunotoxicants. The most important consideration when utilizing cell lines is that by definition, a cell line is an abnormal population of cells that has undergone a change rendering it capable of dividing indefinitely in culture. Because cell lines are continuously dividing, in most cases they are not good models for studying immunotoxicants that act by altering cell proliferation and/or regulators of the cell cycle. The aberrant nature of cell lines may also extend to a loss of function through one or more of its cognate receptors. Lastly, it is critical that cell lines are carefully monitored and characterized for changes in function and morphology after repeated passage in culture.

Additional important considerations when selecting a cell line for mechanistic studies are the capacity of the cell line to perform a given effector function and the stimuli to which the model will respond. Toward this end a number of cell lines have been extensively characterized and widely utilized that are capable of induced effector functions including cytokine production, antibody secretion, and release of a wide variety of mediators. Table 12-8 provides examples of some commonly used cell lines in immunotoxicology. As discussed above, with some cell lines, induction of an effector function may only be achievable by using pharmacological activators (e.g., phorbol ester plus calcium ionophore) that bypass extracellular receptors or by agents that are polyclonal activators (e.g., lipopolysaccharide) that do not activate directly through antigen receptors. Again these are characteristics of the models that need to be considered in the context of how the models will be used and for what specific purpose. In most cases, the utilization of cell line-based models can be extremely useful but results should always be confirmed, when possible, in primary leukocytes because cell lines are aberrant models.

Animal Models: Transgenics, Knockouts, and Humanized/Severe Combined Immunodeficient   The developments in molecular biology have not only permitted the evaluation of specific genes or arrays of genes, but have also allowed for the manipulation of the embryonic genome, creating transgenic and knockout mice (reviewed in IPCS, 1996). As a consequence of transgenic technology, complex immune responses can be dissected into their components. In this way, the mechanisms by which immunotoxicants act can be better understood. Mice engineered to express nonself genes (e.g., human MHC class I) or overexpress self-genes (e.g., constitutively active transcription factors) are termed "transgenic," and can be used to address the role of a certain protein in immunotoxicology. In contrast, mice lacking certain proteins (e.g., receptors, transcription factors, or cytokines), are termed "knockouts," and can be used for similar mechanistic studies. Numerous transgenic and knockout mice have been created and are available to investigators worldwide. Of particular interest and potential utility in the area of immunotoxicology is what has been termed "humanized" mice. Humanized mice refer to immune-deficient mice that have been reconstituted either with human hematopoietic cells to support a fully human immune system, or with mature cells to evaluate immune regulation, hematopoiesis, hypersensitivity, and autoimmunity. Severe combined immunodeficient (SCID) mice, which are mouse T- and B-cell deficient due to a VDJ recombination defect, are a major strain into which human immune cells/system are established. In addition, SCID mice are backcrossed with other strains in order to eliminate various arms of the immune system (i.e., β2M^{null}/SCID eliminate MHC class I interactions) prior to reconstitution with human cells (reviewed in Thomsen *et al.*, 2005). Although their use in mechanistic studies is obvious, SCID/hu mice have also been utilized for evaluation of efficacy of antiviral drugs for HIV/AIDS (reviewed in Taggart *et al.*, 2004). There are still considerations, however, for broader application of these humanized mouse models for immunotoxicological assessment of compounds. For instance, one must consider how these animals compare with standard animal models with respect to time course of action, dose–response, pharmacokinetics, and other factors of chemical toxicity. With the hope that these humanized mouse models can be used to identify new or suspected immunotoxicants, and mechanisms of action, one must also consider whether they are as sensitive, predictive, and/or cost-effective as traditional animal models.

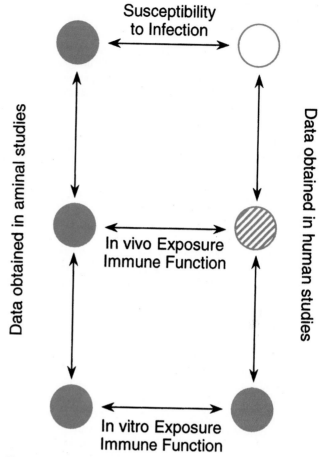

Figure 12-21. *Parallelogram approach in immunotoxicology for relating animal data to human data.* SOURCE: *Modified from Selgrade (1999), with permission.*

Approaches to the Assessment of Human Immunotoxicity As emphasized throughout this chapter, animal models have been extensively utilized to characterize immunotoxicity, and it is widely recognized that chemicals that produce immunotoxicity in animals have the potential to produce immune effects in the human population. The increasing emphasis on human risk assessment requires that those potential health hazards be identified whenever possible. The significant homology of the rodent and human immune systems has facilitated our ability to make decisions on the immunotoxic potential of test materials based on the results of these experimental models (House, 1997). One of the obvious and most important goals of an experimental immunotoxicity testing strategy is to enable the best extrapolations between the results generated in the animal models and the potential risk of immunotoxicity in humans. A parallelogram approach has been used to assess relationships between animal data and human data (Fig. 12-21) (van Loveren *et al.*, 1995; Selgrade, 1999). In this approach, filled circles represent data that can be readily obtained in vivo or in vitro. Unfilled circles represent data that cannot be obtained experimentally. Data that may occasionally be obtained, but must sometimes be extrapolated, are represented by circles filled with blue lines. This approach has been used to extrapolate animal-to-human data in an initial quantitative assessment of the risk for deleterious effects of UV radiation (van

Loveren *et al.*, 1995), and of the immunotoxicity associated with exposure to bis(tri-*n*-butyltin)oxide (Van Loveren *et al.*, 1998). A dual parallelogram approach has also been used to propose that data for ozone suggest that effects of in vivo human exposure to phosgene on alveolar macrophages phagocytosis may be predicted based on effects of in vitro exposure and in vivo animal data (reviewed in Selgrade *et al.*, 1995).

In spite of these successful applications of the parallelogram approach, it is recognized that extrapolations of alterations in immune function observed in animals to human health is associated with various uncertainties (House, 1997). For example, experimental animals are often inbred, which certainly lessens inter-animal variability, thereby simplifying the statistical evaluation of observations. Additionally, laboratory studies in rodents are highly controlled for environment, diet, and health status. In contrast, humans are a highly outbred species with a high degree of interindividual variability in immune response, and any human study must take into account extreme variability in all the controlled parameters. In fact, it has been estimated that the overall immunocompetence of the individual is affected by age, gender, genetic factors, use of certain medications, drug/alcohol use, smoking history, stress, and nutritional status, and that these factors can account for variability more than 2 standard deviations in the "normal" human population (Luebke *et al.*, 2004).

Nonetheless, there is a clear association between suppression of immune function and an increased incidence of infectious and neoplastic disease in humans (reviewed in Biagini, 1998). In the context of xenobiotics, the majority of such data comes from immunotherapeutic drugs, which were intentionally designed to influence the immune system. The aforementioned association has been established primarily with a standard battery of parameters used extensively in clinical immunology studies, including the following: routine complete blood counts and differentials, phenotypic characterization of surface markers and more detailed analysis of cellular subsets using a flow cytometer, lymphoproliferative assays (i.e., using a number of stimuli including mitogens like concanavalin A and phytohemagluttinin, recall antigens like tetanus toxoid, anti-CD3 monoclonal antibody, and allogeneic lymphocytes in an MLR), and DTH responses using a test panel of recall antigens. In contrast with the clear association demonstrated for drugs used to deliberately suppress immune function or treat cancer, the assessment of immunotoxicity in humans exposed to potentially immunotoxic chemicals is much more complicated than in experimental animals (reviewed in IPCS, 1996). This observation has been attributed in part to the inherent variability of the human population, and in part to the moderate immune suppression associated with these chemicals. One of the fallouts of this observation has been the recognition that the historic approaches that have been used in clinical immunology may not have much use in human immunotoxicology. While these end points are sufficient to detect immunodeficiencies associated with either congenital disorders or immunosuppressive drug therapy, they do not possess the necessary sensitivity to detect the more subtle consequences of xenobiotic-induced immunotoxicity. Interestingly, Luebke *et al.* (2004) noted that in contrast to individuals with severe forms of primary or secondary immunodeficiency, where infections to opportunistic pathogens (i.e., members of the herpes viruses family, certain protozoans, *Candida albicans*, a yeast, and *Pneumocystis carinii*, a fungus) are seen, humans with low-to-moderate suppression of immune function are more susceptible to infection with pathogens associated with infections common in the general population (i.e., encapsulated bacteria like *Streptococcus*, and the viruses which cause influenza). As a result, several recent proposals have been put forth to reevaluate the way that we measure immune function in humans. Most of these testing strategies have incorporated plans to measure the primary response to a new antigen, and several of these testing strategies have recommended using newly developed vaccines as the new antigen (Van Loveren *et al.*, 2001). Vaccine response rates have been successfully used to characterize the impact of chronic stress on human immunocompetence (Kiecolt-Glaser *et al.*, 1996; Glaser *et al.*, 2000).

It is anticipated that the development, validation, and utilization of human immunotoxicology methods will be increasingly important in the future. Of particular importance is the fact that few biomarkers for the immune system currently exist, which can provide specific information on the impact of changes in immunocompetence on the susceptibility for disease associated with drug or chemical exposure. The development of biomarkers would not only have applicability in studies to characterize the impact of environmental chemicals, but could also facilitate the progression from preclinical studies to clinical studies in drug development.

Regulatory Approaches to the Assessment of Immunotoxicity

The maturity and acceptance of any subdiscipline of toxicology can frequently be directly correlated to the level of interest being demon-

Table 12-9

Tier Approach for Immunotoxicology Testing

TESTING LEVEL	PROCEDURES
Tier I	Hematology
	Body weight
	Organ weights (spleen, thymus, kidney, liver)
	Spleen cellularity
	Bone marrow cellularity and CFU
	Immunopathology
	PFC assay
	Proliferative responses
	NK assay
Tier II	Surface marker analysis
	Secondary (IgG) PFC assay
	CTL assay
	DTH response
	Host-resistance studies

strated by the regulatory community. This section will provide a brief review of the history of regulatory approaches to immunotoxicity. As regulatory approaches to immunotoxicity have evolved with the science, specific guidelines have been promulgated only relatively recently. Because of the importance of the evolution of the science, this section will begin with an overview of one of the most comprehensive databases for immunotoxicology.

The National Toxicology Program (NTP) Tier Approach   Although the concept of required immunotoxicity testing is a relatively recent development, the recognition that the immune system is a potential target organ has prompted a consideration of the need to assess the potential of immunotoxicity for some time. All testing strategies to date have recognized the complexity of the immune system as a target organ, and that no single immune parameter can be used with sufficient confidence to test for the hazard of immunotoxicity. Therefore, historically, immunotoxicity has been assessed by a battery of assays usually structured in a multitiered approach. However, recent studies, most notably studies conducted by the NTP, have indicated that immunotoxicity can be assessed with a finite number of assays. Luster *et al.* (1988) have described the selection of a battery of tests used by the NTP to screen for potential immunotoxic chemicals. The result was a tier approach to assessing immunotoxicity, which is summarized in Table 12-9.

Tier I provides assessment of general toxicity (immunopathology, hematology, and body and organ weights), as well as end line functional assays (proliferative responses, the T-cell-dependent antibody response assay, measured as PFC assay, and the NK assay). Tier I was designed to detect potential immunotoxic compounds at concentrations that do not produce overt toxicity. Tier II was designed to further define an immunotoxic effect, and included tests for CMI (CTL and DTH), secondary antibody responses, enumeration of lymphocyte populations, and host resistance models.

In the NTP effort, over 50 chemicals were studied, and included a variety of chemical classes, such as catalysts, solvents, dyes, lubricants, pesticides, disinfectants, drugs, food additives, and natural products (Luster *et al.*, 1988). It is important to emphasize that the chemicals selected for study by the NTP were nominated for testing because of a suspicion that they would target the immune system. These studies were conducted in young adult rodents, principally the

Table 12-10

Suggested Testing Configurations: Three Tests with 100 percent Concordance

PFC	DHR	Surface markers
PFC	NK	DHR
PFC	NK	Thymus: body weight
PFC	DHR	Thymus: body weight
Surface markers	NK	DHR
Surface markers	DHR	T-cell mitogens
Surface markers	DHR	Thymus: body weight
Surface markers	DHR	LPS response

SOURCE: Luster *et al.* (1988), modified, with permission.

mouse, and involved comparative studies across multiple labs. The experimental design emphasized that regardless of the specific immune parameters included in a testing strategy, the interpretation for immunotoxicity can only be made in the context of a well-designed study from the perspective of the dose–response relationship. The approach by Luster and coworkers also emphasized the importance of avoiding high doses (i.e., triggered less than a 10% reduction in body weight), as these types of exposures will increase the likelihood that indirect mechanisms of immunotoxicity may be involved.

Several testing configurations were ultimately defined that would minimize the number of immune tests needed, yet still provide a high degree of sensitivity for detecting potential immunotoxicants. These configurations are depicted in Table 12-10. Specifically, the results indicated that whereas none of the assays measured were 100% predictive alone, the T-cell-dependent antibody response, an assessment of lymphocyte subpopulations by cytofluorometric analysis, and an assessment of NK cell activity were the most valuable in terms of predicting immunotoxicity (Luster *et al.*, 1992). Subsequent analysis indicated that an application of the full extent of the tiered approach was not necessary. The NTP studies indicated that several combinations of only two tests could give >90% concordance, and that a number of combinations of just three tests gave 100% concordance. Subsequent results also indicated a good correlation between the results from functional tests and host resistance models (Luster *et al.*, 1993), which indicated that the latter were not necessary to adequately identify immunosuppressive potential. The impacts of the NTP database are clear, and one only needs to consider the recently established immunotoxicity guidelines. Specifically, after several years of international debate, the importance of including functional immunotoxicity assessments in regulatory studies has been emphasized, as opposed to relying solely on histopathology as an indicator of further testing needs.

Regulatory Guidance in Immunotoxicology   The history of regulatory guidance in immunotoxicology was recently reviewed by House (2005). The Office of Prevention, Pesticides and Toxic Substances (OPPTS) of the U.S. Environmental Protection Agency (EPA) published guidelines entitled, *"Biochemicals Test Guidelines: OPPTS 880.3550 Immunotoxicity"* in 1996. These guidelines described the preferred study design for an exceptionally thorough evaluation of the potential immunotoxicity in biochemical pest control agents. This guideline described a panel of tests that included standard toxicology tests, as well as immune functional tests assessing both humoral immunity and CMI. OPPTS 880.3550 clearly presented a very comprehensive approach to immunotoxicity; but a second document, *"Biochemicals Test Guide-*

lines: OPPTS 880.3800 Immune Response," was needed to provide the rationale for when these studies should be conducted. The 880 series of immunotoxicity guidelines would arguably detect any type of immunotoxic potential by pesticides. However, the comprehensive nature of these guidelines rendered them prohibitively expensive and time consuming. The EPA released the *"Health Effects Test Guidelines: OPPTS 870.7800 Immunotoxicity"* in 1998. These guidelines described the approach to immunotoxicology testing for nonbiochemical chemicals regulated by the EPA. The testing approach in OPPTS 870.7800 reflected the continued evolution of the science of immunotoxicology and reflected a more limited, case-by-case approach than previously described by the earlier more comprehensive guidelines. The cornerstone of OPPTS 870.7800 was a functional test, a primary T-dependent antibody response. If the chemical produced significant suppression of the humoral response, surface marker assessment by flow cytometry may be performed. If the chemical produces no suppression of the humoral response, an assessment of innate immunity (NK cell activity assay) may be performed. Specific criteria for the conduct of these "optional" tests have never been identified. The tests do not represent a comprehensive assessment of immune function but are intended to complement assessment made in routine toxicity testing (hematological assessments, lymphoid organ weights, and histopathology).

Internationally, the Organization for Economic Cooperation and Development (OECD) has not as yet adopted specific guidelines for immunotoxicity assessment. As reviewed by (House, 2005), the OECD Guideline 407, entitled, *"Repeated Dose 28-day Oral Toxicity Study in Rodents,"* while not specific for immunotoxicology, includes a variety of toxicological end points that can provide early evidence of immune system alterations. House (2005) also noted that over 10 years ago, an international immunology working group recommended that functional assessments be included in standard toxicology studies when desired or when suggested by expanded histopathological results on other standard toxicology studies. However, to date, the OECD Guideline 407 has not been modified in accord with these recommendations.

The earliest immunotoxicity guidelines from the Food and Drug Administration (FDA) were centered on food additives as the *"Draft Redbook II"* in 1993. This document, although never finalized, contained an extensive description of immunotoxicology testing. In general, the Redbook guidelines reflected the tiered approach to immunotoxicology (Fig. 12-9), as described in greater detail above. Specifically, the Redbook emphasized a stepwise approach that began with expanded studies utilizing data obtained in standard toxicology testing as initial indicators of immunotoxicity. Progressively more complicated immunologic tests were prescribed using an approach that was very much case by case, with each new level of testing predicated on positive results in the preceding level. The FDA Center for Drug Evaluation and Research (CDER) released its document entitled, *"Guidance for Industry: Immunotoxicology Evaluation of Investigational New Drugs,"* in 2002. This document is arguably the most comprehensive description of approaches to immunotoxicology. Not only does the FDA CDER *"Guidance for Industry"* describe all of the spectrum of adverse events associated with the immunotoxicology continuum, including immune suppression, immunogenicity, hypersensitivity, autoimmunity, and adverse immune stimulation, this document provides approaches at the level of specific methodology for evaluating each event. As with the earlier document from the FDA, the new *"Guidance for Industry"* advocating the use of information derived from standard repeat-dose toxicity studies to provide the earliest indicators of immunotoxicity.

The review by House (2005) also addresses the current status of regulatory guidance for biologicals, vaccines, devices, and radiological agents within the FDA.

Internationally, perhaps one of the most significant advances in our approach to the assessment of immunotoxicity with human pharmaceuticals has been a guidance entitled, "*S8 Immunotoxicity Studies for Human Pharmaceuticals*," which was prepared under the auspices of the International Conference on Harmonization (ICH) of Technical Requirements for Registration of Pharmaceutical for Human Use and made available in 2006. The objectives of this guideline are two-fold: to provide recommendations on nonclinical testing approaches to identify compounds which have the potential for immunotoxicity; and to provide guidance on a weight-of-evidence decision-making approach for immunotoxicity testing. The guidance applies to unintended immune suppression and immune enhancement, excluding allergenicity or drug-specific autoimmunity. The ICH S8 guideline is based on a cause for concern approach using a review of factors such as the following: results from Standard Toxicity Studies, pharmacological properties of the drug, the intended patient population, structural similarities to known immune modulators, the disposition of the drug, and clinical information.

As emphasized in the Introduction, immunotoxicity exists in a continuum (Fig. 12-1). By and large, more effort has been invested in the validation of studies to address the immunosuppressive part of the continuum, and there is no doubt that much attention is paid to immune suppression in the majority of guidance documents (House, 2005). Nonetheless, it is important to measure xenobiotic-induced changes in immune function in both directions. As noted by House (2005), it is hypersensitivity that is the most common type of immune modulation resulting from exposure to xenobiotics. One of the most significant advances in our approach to assessing the potential of xenobiotics has been the LLNA. As discussed above, the LLNA was the first assay to be judged by the Interagency Coordinating Committee for the Validation of Alternative Methods (ICCVAM). The impact of this decision by ICCVAM is that the LLNA is now covered in considerable detail in both the OECD 429 Guideline, "*Skin Sensitization: Local Lymph Node Assay*," and the EPA document, "*OPPTS 870.2600 Skin Sensitization*."

Biomarkers True biomarkers indicate exposure to a specific chemical as well as susceptibility to adverse effect, and/or are predictive of disease associated with chemical exposure. Although the tier approach for assessing whether a compound is immunotoxic has been used for several years, there is no accepted panel of biomarkers that one can use to determine whether, and to what extent, exposure to an immunotoxic agent has occurred. A biomarker, or, more likely, biomarkers, must be sensitive, specific, relevant, and measurable in the population. Various studies have been conducted to ascertain the feasibility, predictablity, and accuracy of various biomarkers of immune modulation (Karmaus *et al.*, 2005; Luster *et al.*, 2005; Schwab *et al.*, 2005). Potential biomarkers include cytokine gene expression patterns, cell population quantification using flow cytometry, and serum antibody titers. In addition, the relatively recent discovery and assessment for the presence of single nucleotide polymorphisms in various genes make it possible to determine whether small populations of individuals might be more susceptible to immunotoxicants. It is clear from the small number of studies currently available that biomarkers can be predictive and accurate, but limitations of their use exist. For example, suppression of CD4$^+$ T cells certainly indicates immune suppression, but it would be challenging

to determine which agent(s) correlate with the magnitude of suppression, and how the exposure to multiple chemicals affects that magnitude. Certainly these issues are not unique to immunotoxicology, and it should also be noted that immunologic biomarkers might be affected by other physiological processes, such as stress (Schwab *et al.*, 2005).

IMMUNE MODULATION BY XENOBIOTICS

The very nature of the immune system with the different cell types, the presence of various cell types in every tissue of the body, the dependence on proliferation and differentiation for effector functions, and the necessity to maintain immune function homeostasis, renders it susceptible to modulation by a wide variety of xenobiotics. Although many of the xenobiotics immediately following exhibit immunosuppressive actions, it is important to realize that many of these chemicals are actually immunomodulatory; that is, they might produce both immune suppression and immune enhancement (in the absence of true hypersensitivity or autoimmunity). Of course, one cannot ignore the chemicals that do produce true hypersensitivity and/or autoimmunity and some examples of these are discussed later in the section "Xenobiotic-Induced Hypersensitivity and Autoimmunity." Regardless of the end effect (suppression, enhancement, hypersensitivity, or autoimmunity) of a particular xenobiotic on the immune system, several common themes exist regarding the mechanism by which these chemicals act. First, the mechanisms by which a xenobiotic affects immune function are likely to be multifaceted, involving several proteins, signaling cascades, or receptors. In fact, for several of the xenobiotics discussed below, there is evidence to suggest that immune system effects are both xenobiotic-specific receptor dependent and receptor independent. Second, whether a xenobiotic produces a particular immune effect might depend on the concentration or dose of the xenobiotic, the mode and/or magnitude of cellular stimulation, and the kinetic relationship between exposure to the xenobiotic and exposure to the stimulant (i.e., antigen, mitogen, and pharmacological agent). Third, xenobiotic exposures rarely occur one chemical at a time; thus, the effects and/or mechanisms observed might be attributable to several chemicals or classes of chemicals. Finally, determination of immune system effects and/or mechanisms by xenobiotics in humans might be further confounded by the physiological or immunologic state of the individual. Despite these variables, the application of general, functional, and mechanistic tools discussed above have driven the determination of some of the effects and mechanisms for several xenobiotics.

Halogenated Aromatic Hydrocarbons

Few classes of xenobiotics have been as extensively studied for immunotoxicity as the halogenated aromatic hydrocarbons (HAHs; reviewed by Kerkvliet and Burleson, 1994; Holsapple, 1996; Kerkvliet, 2002). The prototypical and most biologically potent member of this family of chemicals, which includes the polychlorinated biphenyls (PCBs), the polybrominated biphenyls (PBBs), the polychlorinated dibenzofurans (PCDFs), and the polychlorinated dibenzodioxins (PCDDs), is 2,3,7,8-tetrachlorodibenzo-*p*-dioxin (TCDD). Substantial evidence has accumulated that demonstrates the immune system to be a sensitive target for toxicity for these chemicals. Derived from a variety of animal models, primarily rodents, this evidence includes thymic atrophy, pancytopenia, cachexia, immune suppression, and tumor promotion. There is also epidemiological evidence suggesting that immunotoxicity by the HAHs can also occur in humans (Weisglas-Kuperus *et al.*, 1995, 2000, 2004); however, significant immune suppression has not been associated conclusively with specific alterations of human immune function.

The majority of the biochemical and toxic effects produced by the HAHs are mediated via HAH binding to the cytosolic aryl hydrocarbon receptor (AHR). The AHR is a 95–110-kDa basic helix–loop–helix type of ligand-activated transcription factor (Burbach *et al.*, 1992; Ema *et al.*, 1992), which is associated with at least two heat shock proteins (hsp90) in the absence of ligand (Denis *et al.*, 1988; Perdew, 1988; Pongratz *et al.*, 1992). Ligand binding induces conformational changes in the AHR, enabling the receptor–ligand complex to translocate to the nucleus where it sheds its hsp90 and is transformed into a DNA-binding protein (Okey *et al.*, 1980; Cuthill *et al.*, 1987; Denis *et al.*, 1988; Perdew, 1988; Pongratz *et al.*, 1992; Probst *et al.*, 1993; Pollenz *et al.*, 1994). This transformation involves dimerization of the receptor–ligand complex with a structurally related 87-kDa basic helix–loop–helix protein termed the aryl hydrocarbon receptor nuclear translocator (ARNT) (Hoffman *et al.*, 1991; Reyes *et al.*, 1992; Probst *et al.*, 1993). The ligand-AHR/ARNT complex acts as a transcription factor by binding to DNA at the dioxin-responsive element (DRE) in the promoter and enhancer region of sensitive genes such as cytochrome *P*-4501A1, ALDH-3, glutathione *S*-transferase, and menadione oxidoreductase (Poland and Knutson, 1982; Fujisawa-Sehara *et al.*, 1987; Dunn *et al.*, 1988; Elferink *et al.*, 1990; Whitlock, 1990; Hoffman *et al.*, 1991; Reyes *et al.*, 1992; Sutter and Greenlee, 1992; Watson and Hankinson, 1992). Numerous lines of evidence have supported the involvement of the AHR in mediation of toxicity including immunotoxicity by HAHs. Structure–activity relationship studies have demonstrated that with few exceptions, high-affinity AHR ligands are more immunosuppressive than low-affinity ligands (Davis and Safe, 1988). In mice, allelic variation at the *Ah* locus has been described. These alleles code for AHR with differential binding affinities for TCDD. For example, the C57BL/6 mouse represents a strain of mice (*Ah*^bb), which is exquisitely sensitive to TCDD (TCDD responsive), while the DBA/2 mouse strain (*Ah*^dd) is much less sensitive to the toxic effects of TCDD (TCDD nonresponsive or TCDD low responsive). More recently, AHR null mice and cell lines that do not express the AHR have collectively provided compelling evidence supporting the role of AHR in the immunotoxicity mediated by HAHs (Sulentic *et al.*, 2000; Vorderstrasse *et al.*, 2001).

Polychlorinated Dibenzodioxins By far the majority of the investigations into the immunotoxic potential and mechanisms of action of the HAHs have focused on TCDD, primarily because this chemical is the most potent of the HAHs, binding the AHR with the highest affinity. The effects of TCDD on immune function have been demonstrated to be among the earliest and most sensitive indicators of TCDD-induced toxicity (reviewed Holsapple *et al.*, 1991a,b; Kerkvliet and Burleson, 1994; Holsapple, 1996; Kerkvliet, 2002). TCDD is not produced commercially, except in small amounts for research purposes. Rather, it is an environmental contaminant formed primarily as a by-product of the manufacturing process that uses chlorinated phenols or during the combustion of chlorinated materials. It is usually associated with the production of herbicides such as 2,4,5-trichlorophenoxyacetic acid (2,4,5-T), and Agent Orange [a 1:1 combination of 2,4-dichlorophenoxyacetic acid (2,4-D) and 2,4,5-T]. Other sources include pulp and paper manufacturing (chlo-

rine bleaching), automobile exhaust (leaded gasoline), combustion of municipal and industrial waste, and the production of PCBs.

Like other HAHs, exposure to TCDD results in severe lymphoid atrophy. Because thymus-derived cells play an integral role in tumor surveillance and host resistance, the earliest studies on TCDD-induced immunotoxicity focused on changes in CMI. Studies on CMI have shown that this branch of acquired immunity is sensitive to the toxic effects of TCDD after in vivo administration. CTL development and activity has been shown by numerous investigators to be significantly decreased after exposure to TCDD, an effect that appeared to be age dependent (e.g., the younger the mice when exposed, the greater the sensitivity to TCDD). More recently, in an in vivo acute graft-versus-host model of T-cell immunity, the direct AHR-dependent effects of TCDD on T cells were demonstrated. In this model, T cells from C57BL/6 mice were injected into C57BL/6 × DBA/2 F1 host mice resulting in the generation of an anti-host CTL response (Kerkvliet *et al.*, 2002). By comparing the ability of TCDD to suppress the CTL response of T cells obtained from AHR^+/+ and AHR^−/− C57BL/6 mice, the role for AHR expression in T cells was assessed. These studies showed that the CTL response was suppressed by TCDD through direct effects on CD4^+ and CD8^+ T cells via an AHR-dependent mechanism (Kerkvliet *et al.*, 2002). The findings are consistent with the identification of AHR expression in T cells (Lawrence *et al.*, 1996) and structure–activity relationship studies showing a positive correlation between AHR-binding affinity of dioxin-like PCBs and suppression of in vivo CTL responses (Kerkvliet *et al.*, 1990). More recently using the same graft-versus-host model, TCDD treatment resulted in a significant increase in the percentage of donor CD4^+ cells that expressed high levels of CD25, low levels of CD62L as well as glucocorticoid-induced TNFR and cytotoxic T lymphocyte antigen 4(CTLA-4), a phenotype associated with some types of T-regulatory cells suggesting that an important component of the immune suppression of the CTL response induced by TCDD may be the generation of regulatory T cells (Funatake *et al.*, 2005). In addition to suppression of CTL function, TCDD exposure also results in decreases in phytohemagluttinin- and concanavalin A-induced proliferative responses, and DTH responses. Enhanced proliferative responses in juvenile mice have also been observed (Lundberg *et al.*, 1990).

Consistent with the observation that mice exposed perinatally or postnatally (developmentally younger animals) are more sensitive to the effects of TCDD, it has been determined that thymic involution is a result of TCDD-induced terminal differentiation of the thymic epithelium and, thus, T cells do not have a proper nutrient-filled microenvironment in which to develop (Greenlee *et al.*, 1984, 1985). This conclusion is consistent with observations that TCDD significantly decreased the number of immature T cells (CD4^+/CD8^+) in the thymus (Kerkvliet and Brauner, 1990). More recently, it was reported that TCDD administration in mice induced apoptosis in thymocytes (Kamath *et al.*, 1999) and that the mechanism involved a TCDD-induced increase in Fas ligand in thymic stromal but not thymic T cells (Camacho *et al.*, 2005). In these experiments it was demonstrated that when TCDD-exposed stromal cells were mixed with untreated thymic T cells, increased apoptosis was detected in T cells that involved Fas–Fas ligand interactions. In addition the TCDD-mediated apoptosis of thymic T cells was demonstrated to occur via an AHR-dependent mechanism, which also involved NF-κB-mediated upregulation of Fas ligand promoter activity in the thymic stromal cells (Camacho *et al.*, 2005).

Numerous investigations have demonstrated humoral immunity, as assessed by the PFC response to be exquisitely sensitive to the toxic effects of TCDD. This effect segregates with the *Ah* locus (Vecchi *et al.*, 1983; Sulentic *et al.*, 2000) and appears to be dependent on duration and conditions of exposure. Although TCDD induces profound changes in the PFC assay, no changes have been observed in splenic cellularity (numbers of Ig$^+$, CD4$^+$, or Thy-1$^+$ cells) either before or after antigen challenge. Cell fraction/reconstitution of splenocytes from in vivo TCDD and/or vehicle-treated mice identify the B cell as the primary cell type impaired in the PFC response, with only modest changes observed in T-cell accessory function (Dooley and Holsapple, 1988). Interestingly, unlike CMI-mediated responses, which were only affected when TCDD treatment was performed in vivo, direct addition of TCDD to leukocyte cultures was found to strongly suppress humoral immune responses to a variety of B-cell antigens and activators (i.e., lipopolysaccharide, dinitrophenyl-ficoll, and sRBC) demonstrating the ability of TCDD to directly target B cells (Holsapple *et al.*, 1986). Investigations using AHR null mice and cell lines that differentially express AHR have demonstrated definitively that suppression of primary humoral immune responses by TCDD is dependent on AHR activation (Sulentic *et al.*, 2000; Vorderstrasse *et al.*, 2001). More recently, motif searches of regulatory regions of genes involved in immunoglobulin regulation lead to the identification of several DRE in the 3'α enhancer of the immunoglobulin heavy chain. The 3'α enhancer plays a crucial role in mediating high-level immunoglobulin heavy chain expression and immunoglobulin class switching. Electrophoretic mobility shift assays identified TCDD-induced AHR DNA binding and transient transfection experiments demonstrated strong suppression of 3'α enhancer reporter activity by TCDD in a cell line model of B-cell differentiation (Sulentic *et al.*, 2000, 2004a,b). In addition, TCDD was also found to block Pax5 downregulation, a transcriptional repressor of the immunoglobulin heavy chain, immunoglobulin light chain and immunoglobulin J chain by targeting the 3'α immunoglobulin heavy chain enhancer and like enhancers controlling the immunoglobulin light chain and immunoglobulin J chain (Yoo *et al.*, 2004). Collectively, the aforementioned findings suggest that humoral immune responses are suppressed through the direct actions of TCDD on B cells via a AHR-dependent mechanism that leads to impairment of B-cell terminal differentiation and transcription repression of the Ig chains.

The effects of TCDD on innate immunity are less well studied. TCDD has been shown to inhibit some functions of PMNs, including cytolytic and cytostatic activities. This inhibition has been postulated to be related to PMN development in the bone marrow. Results by several investigators have shown TCDD-induced alterations in serum C3, indicating soluble mediators of innate immunity may also be targeted (White and Anderson, 1985; White *et al.*, 1986). There have been no observed effects on macrophage-mediated cytotoxicity, NK function, or interferon production. In host resistance models, TCDD exposure has been shown to increase susceptibility to several bacterial, viral, and tumor models. The most extensively employed model of host resistance for assessing the effects of TCDD on immune competence has been influenza virus. Uniformly, all of these studies have shown impaired resistance to influenza after TCDD treatment as evidenced typically by increased mortality (Burleson *et al.*, 1996; Warren *et al.*, 2000; Nohara *et al.*, 2002). However, it is noteworthy that significant differences have been reported between laboratories concerning the magnitude of impairment produced by TCDD, which may be due in part to differences in the strain of influenza virus used. In this model of host resistance, lymphocyte migration to the lung and the production of virus-specific IgG2a, IgG1, and IgG2b antibodies were markedly diminished

while IgA and neutrophilia were increased in TCDD-treated mice (Vorderstrasse *et al.*, 2003). Conversely, in this same study, no significant TCDD-associated effects were found on T-cell expansion in the lymph nodes and on the production of IFN-γ and IL-12. Collectively, the results suggested that the increase in mortality to influenza in TCDD-treated mice was due to decreased antibody production and increased pulmonary inflammation (Vorderstrasse *et al.*, 2003).

TCDD has also been identified as a potent immunohematopoietic toxicant with the ability to alter the number of Lin-Sca-1$^+$cKit$^+$ (LSK) bone marrow cells, a population enriched for murine hematopoietic stem cells. Assessment of bone marrow cells from TCDD-treated C57BL/6J mice for hematopoietic alterations revealed increases in the number of bone marrow LSK cells, relative to control, over 24 hours through 31 days following TCDD treatment. These findings suggest that proliferation and/or differentiation processes of hematopoietic stem cells are affected by TCDD and that these effects contribute to a reduced capacity of bone marrow to generate pro-T lymphocytes (Murante and Gasiewicz, 2000). Activation of the AHR by TCDD was also found to elicit disruptions in the circadian rhythms of hematopoietic precursors as evidenced by an abnormal in vivo rhythm of the percentage of total number of LSK cells in G$_0$ phase of the cell cycle, suggesting disruption of stem cell quiescence (Garrett and Gasiewicz, 2006). In addition, expression of AHR and ARNT mRNA within enriched hematopoietic precursors oscillated with a circadian period. Taken together, these findings demonstrate that activation of the AHR by TCDD alters the profile of hematopoietic precursors as well as the circadian rhythms associated with these precursors.

There is little doubt that TCDD and related PCDDs are immunotoxic, particularly in mice. However, extrapolation to human exposure has proven to be difficult. There are a few instances in which accidental human exposure to TCDD and related congeners has afforded the opportunity to study exposure-related human immunologic responses. In children exposed to PCDDs in Seveso, Italy (1976), nearly half of the exposed study group exhibited chloracne (a hallmark of high-level human exposure to PCDDs) 3 years after the accident. Immune parameters measured at that time were unaffected. In a second study conducted 6 years later on different subjects, there was an increase in complement, which correlated with the incidence of chloracne, an increase in circulating T- and B cells, and an increase in peripheral blood lymphocyte (PBL) mitogenic responses. In 2002, follow-up studies, in which the population in the most highly exposed zone was randomly sampled, revealed modestly decreased median serum IgG but not in IgM, IgA, C3, and C4 concentrations as compared to human subjects in the surrounding noncontaminated area (Baccarelli *et al.*, 2002). A second incident occurred in 1971 in Times Beach, Missouri, when wastes containing TCDD were sprayed on roads to prevent dust formation. Both low- and high-risk individuals from this area were examined for DTH responses. Slight, but statistically nonsignificant alterations were observed in high-risk compared to low-risk individuals. In addition, there was a low-level increase in mitogenic responsiveness in high-risk persons. In a second study conducted 12 years later, no alterations were observed in DTH or mitogenic responses between exposed or control individuals. In studies undertaken to evaluate the in vitro effects of TCDD on human cells, TCDD suppressed IgM secretion by human B cells in response to the superantigen toxic shock syndrome toxin-1 and the proliferation and IgG secretion of human tonsillar B cells in response to lipopolysaccharide and cytokines (Wood and Holsapple, 1993; Wood *et al.*, 1993).

Polychlorinated Dibenzofurans Like the PCDDs, PCDFs are not produced commercially but are true environmental contaminants associated with the production of chlorophenoxy acids, pentachlorophenol, and other PCB mixtures. Although higher concentrations are required to achieve observable effects, the immunotoxic profile of the PCDFs is similar in nature to that described for TCDD. In fact, most of what is known regarding the immunotoxicity of the PCDFs in animal models has been learned during structure–activity relationship studies comparing TCDD to congeners of the dibenzofurans. TCDF (tetrachlorodibenzofuran) exposure in most species is associated with thymic atrophy and in guinea pigs it has been shown to suppress the DTH and lymphoproliferative responses to phytohemagluttinin and lipopolysaccharide. Suppression of the PFC response to sRBC after exposure to several PCDF congeners has also been reported.

Two important case studies of human immunotoxicology involved populations accidentally exposed to HAHs. There is evidence that the PCDFs were the primary contributors to the observed toxic effects. More than 1850 individuals in Japan (in 1968) and in excess of 2000 people in Taiwan (in 1979) were affected when commercial rice oil was found to be contaminated with HAHs. PCDFs were observed in the tissues of the exposed populations and subsequent studies on immune status revealed a decrease in total circulating T cells, decreased DTH response, and enhanced lymphoproliferative responses to phytohemagluttinin and pokeweed mitogen. In addition, many of the exposed individuals suffered from recurring respiratory infections, suggesting that host resistance mechanisms had been compromised.

Polychlorinated Biphenyls PCBs have seen extensive commercial use for over half a century. Their unique physical and chemical properties make PCB mixtures ideal for use as plasticizers, adhesives, and as dielectric fluids in capacitors and transformers. Mixtures of PCBs (e.g., Aroclors) have been commonly used to evaluate the immunotoxicity of PCBs and have been reported to suppress immune responses and decrease host resistance (reviewed in Holsapple, 1996). The first indication that PCBs produced immunotoxic effects was the observation of severe atrophy of the primary and secondary lymphoid organs in general toxicity tests and the subsequent demonstration of the reduction in numbers of circulating lymphocytes. Studies to characterize the immunotoxic action of the PCBs have primarily focused on the antibody response. This parameter is by far the one most consistently affected by PCB exposure and effects on antibody response have been demonstrated in guinea pigs, rabbits, mice, and rhesus monkeys. PCB-exposed monkeys exhibit chloracne, alopecia, and facial edema, all classical symptoms of HAH toxicity. In an extensive characterization of the effects of PCBs on non-human primates, Tryphonas *et al.* (1991a,b) exposed rhesus monkeys to Aroclor 1254 for 23–55 months. The only immune parameter consistently suppressed was the PFC response to sRBC (both IgM and IgG). In addition, after 55 months of exposure, lymphoproliferative responses were dose-dependently suppressed and serum complement levels were significantly elevated. The observed elevation in serum complement has also been reported in PCDD-exposed children from Seveso, Italy (Tognoni and Boniccorsi, 1982) and in B6C3F1-exposed mice (White *et al.*, 1986).

The effects of PCBs on CMI are far less clear and both suppression and enhancement have been reported. Exposure to Aroclor 1260 has been demonstrated to suppress DTH responses in guinea

pigs, whereas exposure to Aroclor 1254 was reported to enhance lymphoproliferative responses in rats. In a similar study in Fischer 344 rats (Aroclor 1254), thymic weight was decreased, NK cell activity was suppressed, phytohemagluttinin-induced proliferative responses were enhanced, and there was no effect on the MLR proliferative response or CTL activity. Other investigators (Silkworth and Loose, 1978, 1979) have reported enhancement of graft-versus-host reactivity and the MLR proliferative response. The augmentation of selected CMI assays may reflect a PCB-induced change in T-cell subsets (as described above), which contributes to immune regulation.

Studies on host resistance following exposure to PCBs indicate that the host defenses against hepatitis virus (ducks) and to herpes simplex virus, *Plasmodium berghei*, *Listeria monocytogenes*, and *Salmonella typhimurium* (mice) are suppressed (reviewed by Dean *et al.* (1985). PCB-induced changes in tumor defenses have not been well defined and both augmentation and suppression have been reported. This probably reflects the variability in observed responses in CMI.

The immunotoxicological effects of PCBs in humans are unclear. There are four separate reports of a longitudinal study in a cohort of Dutch children suggesting that the developing human immune system may be susceptible to immunotoxic alterations from exposure to Western European environmental levels of dioxin-like compounds, primarily PCBs (Weisglas-Kuperus *et al.*, 1995, 2000, 2004; ten Tusscher *et al.*, 2003). Three industrial areas were compared to a rural area with about 20% less PCBs in maternal plasma. The Dutch study measured the major PCB congeners in plasma in the mother and the newborn, and all dioxin-like compounds in maternal breast milk at 2 weeks after birth. The results showed an association between dioxin-like compound exposure and immunologic changes which included an increased number of lymphocytes, γ/δ T cells, CD3$^+$HLA-DR$^+$ (activated) T cells, CD8$^+$ cells, CD4$^+$CD45RO$^+$ (memory T cells), and lower antibody levels to mumps and measles vaccination at preschool age. In addition, an association was found between dioxin/PCB prenatal exposure and decreased shortness of breath with wheeze, and current PCB burden was associated with a higher prevalence of recurrent middle-ear infections and chicken pox and a lower prevalence of allergic reactions. It is notable that although an association between dioxin/PCB exposure and changes in immune status was observed, all infants were found to be in the normal range. In a second study, modest but persistent changes in immune status were reported in children with perinatal exposure to dioxin-like compounds, as evidenced by a decrease in allergy and increased CD4$^+$ T cells and increased CD45RA$^+$ cell counts in a longitudinal subcohort of 27 healthy 8-year-old children with documented perinatal dioxin exposure (ten Tusscher *et al.*, 2003). The original cohort at 42 months demonstrated an association between reduced vaccine titers, increased incidence of chicken pox, and increased incidence of otitis media with higher exposure to toxicity equivalents of dioxin. However, by 8 years of age the more frequent recurrent ear infections were still apparent (overall), although the chicken pox frequency showed an inverse correlation with PCB/dioxin levels.

Polybrominated Biphenyls The PBBs have been used primarily as flame retardants (Firemaster BP-6 and FF-1). While it is assumed that their profile of activity is similar to that of the PCBs, few studies have actually evaluated the action of the PBBs on immunocompetence. In Michigan (in 1973) Firemaster BP-6 was inadvertently substituted for a nutrient additive in cattle feed, resulting in widespread exposure of animals and humans to PBBs. Studies conducted on livestock following the incident indicated little if any PBB-induced alterations in immunocompetence (Kately and Bazzell, 1978; Vos and Luster, 1989). Like CMI observations involving PCBs, CMI responses in PBB-exposed individuals are not conclusive, showing both a reduction in circulating numbers of T- and B cells and a suppression of selected CMI parameters or no effect on CMI at all.

Polycyclic Aromatic Hydrocarbons

The polycyclic aromatic hydrocarbons (PAHs) are a ubiquitous class of environmental contaminants. They enter the environment through many routes including the burning of fossil fuels and forest fires. In addition to being carcinogenic and mutagenic, the PAHs have been found to be potent immunosuppressants. Effects have been documented on immune system development, humoral immunity, CMI, and on host resistance. The most extensively studied PAHs are 7,12-dimethylbenz anthracene (DMBA) and benzo pyrene (BaP).

Early immunotoxicology studies of PAHs such as BaP, DMBA, and 3-methylcholanthrene demonstrated suppression of the antibody response to a variety of T-cell-dependent and T-cell-independent antigens. In addition, mice treated with BaP exhibit suppressed lymphoproliferative responses to mitogens but not alloantigens (Dean et al., 1983). In Dean's studies, host resistance to the PYB6 tumor and to L. monocytogenes were unaffected by BaP exposure, as was the DTH response and allograft rejection, suggesting that the T cell (and CMI) was only minimally affected by BaP. In contrast to BaP, DMBA (a more potent PAH) significantly suppresses not only PFC responses, but also NK cell activity, CTL responses, DTH responses, and alloantigen-induced lymphoproliferative responses. Therefore, DMBA exposure seems to result in long-lasting immune suppression of humoral immunity, CMI, and tumor resistance mechanisms in mice. In addition, both BaP and DMBA also produced significant effects on the bone marrow as evidenced by suppression of pre-B-cell formation.

Significant progress has been made toward elucidation of the mechanism(s) by which PAHs exert their toxicological effects including those on the immune system. Biologic and toxicological activity of PAHs is generally dependent on two factors, AHR activation and the metabolism of PAHs to active metabolites by cytochrome P-450 isozymes, CYP1A1, CYP1A2, and CYP1B1, which are transcriptionally induced by AHR DNA binding to DRE in the promoter region of the genes that code for the aforementioned isozymes. Although leukocytes in general possess modest cytochrome P-450 drug metabolizing activity, in in vitro studies splenocytes from naive untreated mice were found to metabolize exogenously added DMBA via P-450 enzymes (Ladics et al., 1991). In addition, Ladics et al. (1992a,b) demonstrated that macrophages were the primary cell type in a splenic leukocyte preparation capable of metabolizing BaP to 7,8-dihydroxy-9,10-epoxy-7,8,9,10-benzo[a]pyrene (BPDE), the reactive metabolite proposed to be the ultimate carcinogenic and immunotoxic form of BaP. These data are consistent with other studies demonstrating the presence and inducibility of CYP1A1, CYP1A2, and most importantly in leukocytes, CYP1B1 (Gao et al., 2005a).

PAHs, including BaP, have also been shown to induce AHR-independent biochemical changes in lymphocytes leading to oxidative stress, activation of tyrosine kinases, and increased intracellular calcium (Mounho and Burchiel, 1998; Pessah et al., 2001). The elevation in intracellular calcium in B- and T lymphocytes was recently shown to be mediated by BaP-7,8-dione and blocked by high concentrations of ryanodine suggesting the involvement of ryanodine receptors (Gao et al., 2005b).

Significant progress has also been made on the elucidation of the mechanism by which BaP and DMBA mediate bone marrow toxicity, specifically suppression of pre-B-cell formation. In vitro models demonstrated that BaP and DMBA rapidly induced apoptosis in primary pre-B cells and in the pro/pre-B-cell line, BU-11 (Yamaguchi et al., 1997). The mechanism for pre-B cells apoptosis by PAHs was shown to be dependent on bone marrow-derived stromal cells (Yamaguchi et al., 1997), CYP1B1 metabolism (Heidel et al., 1998), to be AHR dependent (Yamaguchi et al., 1997), and coincide with induction of p53 (Yamaguchi et al., 1997). More recently, it was demonstrated that DMBA-mediated bone marrow cytotoxicity was absent in p53 null mice and apoptosis of primary bone marrow progenitor B cells cocultured with bone marrow stromal cells and DMBA was p53 dependent (Page et al., 2003). Collectively, these and other studies suggest that PAHs are metabolized by bone marrow stromal cells, which in turn release active PAH metabolites as part of a metabolite protein complex that induce pre-B cells to apoptosis (Allan et al., 2003).

Pesticides

Pesticides include all xenobiotics whose specific purpose is to kill another form of life, including insects (insecticides), small rodents (rodenticides), or even vegetation (herbicides). As such, these chemicals have clear biological activity and many pesticides have been studied for their effects on the immune system. The effects of the following four classes of pesticides will be summarized: organophosphates, organochlorines, organotins, and carbamates. The herbicide, atrazine, is also discussed. While there is evidence that certain pesticides can produce alterations in immune function in animal models, studies in humans, both mechanistic and epidemiological, have been conducted in order to determine whether the effects seen in animal models also occur in humans (reviewed in Colosio et al., 2005). Exposure to pesticides occurs most often in occupational settings, in which manufacturers, those applying the pesticides, or those harvesting treated agricultural products, are exposed.

Organophosphates   Organophosphates include malathion, parathion, methyl parathion, and diazinon. Although the neurotoxic effects of organophosphates are well understood to occur via the inhibition of acetylcholinesterase, the mechanism by which these compounds suppress the immune system is not as well-defined. Furthermore, it is still unclear how the "lymphocytic cholinergic system" (Tarkowski et al., 2004) contributes to immunotoxicity. Despite these uncertainties, there are several established immune system effects of the various organophosphates (reviewed in Galloway and Handy, 2003).

Malathion exhibits both immune suppressive and immune enhancing effects. Malathion has been shown to suppress humoral immunity as measured by the PFC response to sRBC following a subacute exposure in mice (Casale et al., 1983). In contrast, acute oral exposure has been shown to enhance humoral immunity and mitogenic proliferative responses with no other immune-related effects. In vitro exposure of either human mononuclear cells or murine splenocytes to malathion results in decreased lymphoproliferative responses, suppressed CTL generation, and a decrease in the stimulus-induced respiratory burst in peritoneal cells (Rodgers and Ellefson, 1990). There is also evidence that the mechanism by which malathion is immunotoxic involves induction of apoptosis in thymocytes (Olgun *et al.*, 2004).

Parathion has attracted more attention than malathion, probably because it is more acutely toxic. This pesticide suppresses both humoral immunity and CMI. Following exposure to methyl parathion, decreased germinal centers after antigen challenge, thymic atrophy, and suppressed DTH responses have been reported. Other experiments have shown suppression of lymphoproliferative responses as well as increased susceptibility to pathogens. In vitro exposure to parathion or paraoxon, a primary metabolite of parathion, suppresses CMI in murine splenocytes, IL-2 production in rat splenocytes, and proliferative responses in human lymphocytes. However, there was no alteration of the parathion-induced suppression of the PFC response following exposure to phenobarbitol, which induces metabolism of parathion (Kim *et al.*, 2005), indicating that the phenobarbitol-sensitive metabolizing enzymes are not involved in parathion-induced suppression of humoral immunity.

Fewer studies exist that describe the immunotoxicity of diazinon. Recently, it has been shown that diazinon produced gross changes in the spleen and thymus in response to acute doses in mice (Handy *et al.*, 2002; Neishabouri *et al.*, 2004). Diazinon also suppressed humoral immunity as measured by the PFC response to sRBC and CMI as measured by the DTH response following subchronic exposure to mice (Neishabouri *et al.*, 2004).

Organochlorines The organochlorines include chemicals such as chlordane, dichlorodiphenyltrichloroethane (DDT), mirex, pentachlorophenol, aldrin, dieldrin, and hexachlorobenzene. Although technically this class of compounds also includes the herbicides 2,4-D and 2,4,5-T, these compounds are considered separately under section "Halogenated Aromatic Hydrocarbons." The organochlorines are among the longer-lived pesticides and they have an increased propensity for contamination of soil and groundwater, thus providing an additional route of exposure to the general population. Many organochlorine compounds also act as xenoestrogens although it is unclear as to whether the estrogenic effects of these compounds contribute to immunotoxicity.

Although DDT has been banned in several countries, it is still used to control malaria, typhoid, and dengue infections in some places of the world. DDT suppresses both humoral immunity and CMI. Early studies demonstrated suppression of humoral immunity following oral gavage in mice (Wiltrout *et al.*, 1978). Studies by Street indicated that chickens exposed to DDT or mirex had suppressed levels of circulating IgM and IgG, although specific antibody titers were normal. In addition, DDT exposure resulted in decreased antigen-induced germinal centers, thymic atrophy, and suppressed CMI (Street, 1981). More recently, DDT has been shown to suppress IL-2 production from a human T-cell line and that the mechanism involved suppression of the critical transcription factor NF-κB (Ndebele *et al.*, 2004). In another study in which occupationally exposed individuals were evaluated for cytokine levels, DDE, a primary metabolite of DDT, was associated with suppression of IL-2 and IFN-γ, and enhancement of IL-4, suggesting an imbalance of Th1/Th2 populations (Daniel *et al.*, 2002). Finally, there is a correlation between DDE levels in breast milk and incidence of infant ear infections, suggesting increased susceptibility to infection following DDT exposure (Dewailly *et al.*, 2000). An increased susceptibility to infection might also involve suppression of macrophage function by DDT (Nunez *et al.*, 2002).

The humoral immune response to both T-cell-dependent and T-cell-independent antigens is suppressed following exposure to dieldrin (Bernier *et al.*, 1987), and macrophage functions from dieldrin-exposed animals are depressed. The apparent effect of dieldrin on macrophages correlates with the increased susceptibility of dieldrin-exposed animals to murine hepatitis virus, which targets macrophages (Krzystyniak *et al.*, 1985). CMI was also suppressed in mice following dieldrin exposed as measured by a suppression of the mixed lymphocyte reaction and graft-versus-host disease (Hugo *et al.*, 1988a,b). As discussed above for other immunotoxic chemicals, dieldrin is also immunostimulatory under certain conditions as dieldrin enhanced the pro-inflammatory cytokine IL-8 in vitro and induced neutrophilic inflammation in vivo (Pelletier *et al.*, 2001).

Chlordane refers to a group of structurally related chemicals used to control termites. The principal constituents of chlordane are heptachlor, α-chlordane, γ-chlordane, α-nonachlor, β-nonachlor, α-chlordene, β-chlordene and γ-chlordene. Definitive immune suppression produced by chlordane was first reported in 1982 by Spyker-Cranmer *et al.* (1982). In utero exposure resulted in decreased DTH responses in mice with no deficit in antibody production to sRBC. This effect correlated with an increase in resistance to influenza infection because the DTH contributes to the pathology of the infection (Menna *et al.*, 1985). In contrast to observations from mice exposed in utero, exposure of adult mice to chlordane did not result in any changes to several immune parameters, including PFC response to sRBC, MLR, DTH response, or mitogenic lymphoproliferation. In vitro, however, chlordane suppressed several immunologic end points. The discrepancy between chlordane's effects in vitro versus in vivo was attributed to nonspecific binding of chlordane to serum proteins in vivo (Johnson *et al.*, 1987a). In rats, immunomodulatory effects of three constituents of chlordane were noted following 28-day oral dosing (technical chlordane, *cis*-nonachlor, and *trans*-nonachlor), the most profound being increased lymphocyte numbers with a decrease NK cell activity and proliferation in response to *S. typhimurium* (Tryphonas *et al.*, 2003).

Many organochlorine pesticides have also been associated with increased cancer incidence (reviewed in Dich *et al.*, 1997). The mechanism by which this occurs is unclear but is likely multifaceted, including, in part, organochlorine-induced modulation of the immune system. For instance, chlordane suppressed expression of the tumor suppressor, retinoblastoma in a human B-cell/T-cell hybrid cell line (Rought *et al.*, 1999). Furthermore, several organochlorine pesticides were demonstrated in vitro to suppress NK cell activity, which play a role in defense against tumor formation (Reed *et al.*, 2004).

Organotins Trisubstituted organotins such as tributyltin oxide are widely used as biocides and have recently been recognized as producing some immunotoxic effects. The most outstanding action of tributyltin oxide is the induction of profound but reversible thymic atrophy. One study suggested that anti-proliferative effects of tributyltin oxide on lymphocytes, as opposed to apoptosis, might account for the thymic atrophy (Vandebriel *et al.*, 1999). In addition, the developing immune system appears to be more sensitive to the effects of tributyltin oxide than does the immune system of the adult animal (reviewed in Luebke *et al.*, 2006a). Studies by Vos and colleagues demonstrated a decrease in cellularity in the spleen, bone marrow, and thymus. The decrease in splenic cellularity was associated with a concomitant loss of T lymphocytes. More specifically, oral tributyltin oxide exposure resulted in decreased serum

IgG, increased serum IgM, and suppression of DTH responses to tuberculin and ovalbumin. In those studies, host resistance to *L. monocytogenes* was diminished. Cytotoxicity by adherent peritoneal cells was suppressed but there was no observed effect on NK cytotoxicity (Vos *et al.*, 1984). In contrast, Van Loveren *et al.* (1990) observed suppressed lung NK cytotoxicity in rats exposed orally to tributyltin oxide. In addition, the lymphoproliferative response of thymocytes to phytohemagglutinin (PHA), concanavalin A, and pokeweed mitogen (PWM) was significantly suppressed. Recent studies also demonstrated that tributyltin oxide modestly suppressed proliferation from lymph nodes in mice sensitized with dinitrochlorobenzene and that the suppression was associated with a modest shift toward a Th2 population (van den Berg *et al.*, 2005).

Carbamates   Carbamate insecticides, which include carbaryl (Sevin), aldicarb, mancozeb, and sodium methyldithiocarbamate, are used primarily as insecticides. Similar to the organophosphates, the mechanism of action of the neurotoxic effects involves inhibition of acetylcholinesterase. In an evaluation of humoral immunity following a 2-week exposure to carbaryl in rats, suppression of the IgM PFC response to sRBC was observed following inhalation exposure, but not oral or dermal exposure (Ladics *et al.*, 1994). Conflicting results have been observed in animals exposed to aldicarb or methyl isocyanate, an intermediate in carbamate pesticide production. Deo *et al.* (1987) reported alterations in T cells and lymphoproliferative responses in humans accidentally exposed to methyl isocyanate. In contrast, mice exposed to the same compound showed no significant alterations in immune status (Luster *et al.*, 1986).

Pruett *et al.* (1992a) evaluated the immunotoxicity of sodium methyldithiocarbamate, and observed decreased thymus weight, depletion of the CD4$^+$/CD8$^+$ population of thymocytes, and profound suppression of NK cell activity following both oral and dermal exposure. They also determined that the mechanism by which sodium methyldithiocarbamate altered cytokine production from peritoneal macrophages involves inhibition of MAP kinase activity via TLR4 (Pruett *et al.*, 2005). Pruett *et al.* (2006) further determined that the mechanism of cytokine alteration involved depletion of glutathione, alteration of copper-dependent proteins, and induction of stress.

Atrazine   Atrazine is an herbicide applied to various agricultural crops to control broad leaf weeds. It is widely used in the United States and it has been detected in soils and groundwater because of its resistance to degradation. Similar to other chemicals discussed, atrazine exhibits immunomodulatory effects. Using offspring of female mice treated with atrazine and challenged with antigen, atrazine induced elevations in T-cell proliferation, cytolytic activity, and antigen-specific B cells (Rowe *et al.*, 2006). In contrast, using young mice directly administered atrazine orally for 14 days, it was determined that atrazine suppressed thymic weight, spleen and thymic cellularity, and B-cell fractions, although CD4+ T-cell numbers increased (Filipov *et al.*, 2005). Similarly, in adult mice, it was confirmed that atrazine suppressed thymic weight, and also suppressed splenic weight and decreased the host resistance of the mice to B16F10 melanoma tumors (Karrow *et al.*, 2005). Although the mechanism by which atrazine-induced immune suppression occurred is unclear, atrazine treatment of mice does induce corticosterone levels, indicating that activation of the hypothalamic–pituitary–adrenal axis might be involved (Pruett *et al.*, 2003).

Metals

Generally speaking, metals target multiple organ systems and exert their toxic effects via an interaction of the free metal with the target: enzyme systems, membranes, or cellular organelles. Although specific immunotoxic consequences of metal exposure are well documented in the literature (reviewed in Zelikoff and Thomas, 1998), this section focuses on the four best-studied immunotoxic metals: lead, arsenic, mercury, and cadmium. In considering the immunotoxicity of most metals, it is important to remember that at high concentrations, metals usually exert immunosuppressive effects; however, at lower concentrations, immune enhancement is often observed (Koller, 1980; Vos, 1977). Furthermore, as with most immunotoxic chemicals, it is important to note that exposures to metals are likely not single exposures, although one metal might dominate depending on the exposure conditions (e.g., high levels of mercury in fish or high levels of lead from paint).

Lead   By far the most consistent finding in studies evaluating the effects of metals on immune responses is increased susceptibility to pathogens. For lead, decreased resistance to the bacterial pathogens *S. typhimurium*, *Escherichia coli*, and *L. monocytogenes* has been observed. One study suggested that the decreased resistance to *L. monocytogenes* involves a lack of functional IL-12 in lead-exposed mice, which, subsequently, could be related to increased stress in response to infection (Kishikawa *et al.*, 1997).

Studies on the specific effects of lead on functional immunity have demonstrated that lead is immunomodulatory. In rodents exposed to lead, lower antibody titers have been observed (Luster *et al.*, 1978). In addition, children environmentally exposed to lead and infected naturally with *Shigella dysenteriae* had prolonged diarrhea, and occupationally exposed persons reported more colds and influenza, and exhibited suppressed secretory IgA levels, demonstrating lead-induced suppression of humoral immunity. Following in vivo exposure to lead, splenocytes displayed consistently suppressed IgM PFC responses to sRBC. Separation and reconstitution experiments indicated that this suppression is likely due to an effect on macrophage function.

In mechanistic studies (reviewed in McCabe, 1994), an alteration in the ability of the macrophage to process and present antigen to antigen-primed T cells confirmed the previous observation and suggested that lead alters immune recognition. In contrast to other reports concerning the immunosuppressive action of lead on PFC responses, enhancement of the in vitro-generated PFC response appears to be the result of enhancement of B-cell differentiation. This effect may occur at the level of B-cell activation or cytokine responsiveness. And finally, in vitro addition studies indicate that lead shifts the T-cell balance from Th1 to Th2, which can result in either immune enhancement or immune suppression (reviewed in Lawrence and McCabe, 2002). Interestingly, it has been hypothesized that lead exposure might contribute to the development of asthma (Dietert *et al.*, 2004), a predominantly Th2-mediated disease. This theory is consistent with the observation that lead activates the transcription factor NF-κB (Pyatt *et al.*, 1996), which is an important regulator of several pro-inflammatory cytokines.

Arsenic   The literature concerning arsenic-induced immune modulation is fraught with inconsistencies due to differences in speciation of arsenic (which plays a significant role in arsenic toxicity), the route of administration, the concentrations used, and the various species and strains of animals utilized. As with many other metals, exposure to low concentrations of arsenic often leads to enhanced immune responses, whereas exposure to higher concentrations results in immune suppression (reviewed in Burns *et al.*, 1994d). Exposure of mice to sodium arsenite in the drinking water or subcutaneously was shown to decrease resistance to viral pathogens. Interestingly, host resistance studies, conducted after exposure to the semiconductor material gallium arsenide, revealed that gallium arsenide afforded modest protection against infection with both *Streptococcus pneumoniae* and *L. monocytogenes,* although resistance to the B16F10 melanoma was reduced. It was subsequently determined that the arsenic concentrations in the blood of these animals was high enough to offer a chemotherapeutic effect against the bacterial pathogens (arsenicals are again gaining favor as chemotherapeutic agents). These studies are important because they are among the first to demonstrate the intricate interplay between the host, the pathogen, and the xenobiotic (Burns *et al.*, 1993).

In addition to these holistic immune alterations, exposure has been shown to inhibit both the PFC response in animal models and PBL proliferation in humans. Also, substantial mechanistic information exists regarding the immunotoxicity of intratracheally instilled gallium arsenide. Exposure results in suppression of the PFC, CTL, DTH, and MLR responses. Mechanistic studies revealed that all cell types involved in the generation of an antibody response (macrophage, T-, and B cells) are affected by gallium arsenide exposure (Sikorski *et al.*, 1991). Sodium arsenate administered in the drinking water to mice also attenuated the DTH response to dinitrochlorobenzene (Patterson *et al.*, 2004). Part of the mechanism by which arsenic compounds are immunosuppressive might be induction of apoptosis, as demonstrated in human monocytes (Lemarie *et al.*, 2006).

Mercury Exposure to mercury includes organic (often methyl mercury) or inorganic compounds. Both organic and inorganic mercury have been shown to decrease immunologic responses (reviewed in Sweet and Zelikoff, 2001). Early studies demonstrated increased susceptibility to encephalomyocarditis virus (Gainer, 1977). Similar to arsenic, the mechanism by which mercury compounds are immunomodulatory might be induction of apoptosis, but mercury also depletes glutathione (Mondal *et al.*, 2005). In contrast to immune suppression, several studies have demonstrated that mercury compounds induce autoimmunity and might play a role in the pathogenesis of autism (see mercury discussion under section "Autoimmunity"). Interestingly, in one genetically susceptible mouse model of autoimmunity, subcutaneous administration of methyl mercury reduced T- and B-cell numbers prior to autoimmunity induction, demonstrating the immunomodulatory actions of mercury in vivo (Haggqvist *et al.*, 2005).

Cadmium Like other metals, cadmium exhibits immunomodulatory effects. Early studies demonstrated that oral administration of cadmium to mice increased susceptibility to herpes simplex type 2 virus, suppressed T- and B-cell proliferation, but enhanced macrophage phagocytosis (Thomas *et al.*, 1985). An evaluation of school-aged children exposed to cadmium revealed decreased levels of hypersensitivity and IgG antibody titers (Ritz *et al.*, 1998). As with many other immunotoxic agents, it has been suggested that the stress response, a shift to a Th2 cell population, and induction of apoptosis all contribute to the mechanism by which cadmium suppresses humoral immunity and CMI (Lall and Dan, 1999; Hemdan

et al., 2006; Pathak and Khandelwal, 2006). Interestingly, the ability of cadmium to modulate cytokine production was associated with the mode of cellular activation (Hemdan *et al.*, 2006).

It has long been known that cadmium (and mercury) bind to a protein called metallothionein, which is a small, cysteine-rich protein that complexes normally with divalent cations, such as copper and zinc. The role of metallothionein in metal-induced immunotoxicity has been recently reviewed (Lynes *et al.*, 2006) and there are several mechanisms by which the cadmium (or mercury)–metallothionein complex might contribute to immune modulation. The binding of cadmium (or mercury) to metallothionein could displace copper or zinc, altering the availability of the latter cations for biochemical processes. Alternatively, metallothionein is induced in response to several stimuli, including cadmium and mercury, and it has been demonstrated that metallothionein influences lymphocyte proliferation, differentiation, and various effector functions. Finally, because metallothionein is a cysteine-rich protein, it also plays a role in the oxidative homeostasis of the cell, which could be compromised under conditions of oxidative stress.

Solvents and Related Chemicals

There is limited but substantive evidence that exposure to organic solvents and their related compounds can produce immune suppression. Chemicals to be discussed are aromatic hydrocarbons, such as benzene, haloalkanes, and haloalkenes, glycols and glycol ethers, and nitrosamines.

Aromatic Hydrocarbons By far the best-characterized immunotoxic effects by an organic solvent are those produced by benzene. In animal models, benzene induces anemia, lymphocytopenia, and hypoplastic bone marrow. In addition, it has recently been suggested that this myelotoxicity may be a result of altered differentiative capacity in bone marrow-derived lymphoid cells. Benzene (oral and inhaled) exposure has been reported to alter both humoral and cell-mediated immune parameters including suppression of the anti-sRBC antibody response, decreased T- and B-cell lymphoproliferative responses (mitogens and alloantigens), and inhibition of CTL activity. Benzene exposure also appears to increase the production of both IL-1 and TNF-α and to inhibit the production of IL-2. With these dramatic effects on immune responses, it is not surprising that animals exposed to benzene exhibit reduced resistance to a variety of pathogens. In terms of a possible mechanism of action, Pyatt *et al.* (1998) demonstrated that hydroquinone, a reactive metabolite of benzene, inhibited the activity of NF-κB, a transcription factor known to regulate the expression of a number of genes critical for normal T cells. The authors concluded that NF-κB might be an important molecular mediator of the immunotoxicity of hydroquinone (and benzene).

A number of compounds structurally related to benzene have also been studied for their potential effects on the immune system. For example, nitrobenzene (an oxidizing agent used in the synthesis of aniline and benzene compounds) has been previously reported to also produce immunotoxic effects (Burns *et al.*, 1994b), with the primary targets being the peripheral blood erythrocyte and the bone marrow. Immunomodulating activity has also been observed for toluene, although most effects occur at markedly high concentrations. When compared with benzene, toluene has little to no effect on immunocompetence. However, it is noteworthy that toluene exposure effectively attenuates the immunotoxic effects of benzene (probably because of competition for metabolic enzymes).

In contrast to the parent toluene, the monosubstituted nitrotoluenes (*para-* and *meta-*nitrotoluene) do significantly alter the immune system (Burns *et al.*, 1994a,c). Exposure to *p*-nitrotoluene has been demonstrated to suppress the antibody response to sRBC, to decrease the number of CD4$^+$ splenic T cells, and to inhibit the DTH response to keyhole limpet hemocyanin. In addition, host resistance to *L. monocytogenes* was impaired, suggesting the T cell as a primary target. Similarly, *m*-nitrotoluene suppresses the antibody response to sRBC, the DTH response to keyhole limpet hemocyanin, T-cell mitogenesis, and host resistance to *L. monocytogenes*, again suggesting the T cell as the cellular target. The di-substituted nitrotoluene (2,4-dinitrotoluene) is also immunosuppressive (Burns *et al.*, 1994c), with exposure resulting in suppressed humoral immunity, NK cell activity, and phagocytosis by splenic macrophages. Host resistance to bacterial challenge was also impaired. It would appear that 2,4-dinitrotoluene might perturb the differentiation and maturation of leukocytes.

Haloalkanes and Haloalkenes Carbon tetrachloride is widely recognized as hepatotoxic. Studies in mice revealed that carbon tetrachloride is also immunosuppressive. Mice exposed for 7–30 days to carbon tetrachloride (orally or intraperitoneally) exhibited a decreased T-cell-dependent antibody response (sRBC), suppressed MLR response, and lower lymphoproliferative capacity (T- and B cells) (Kaminski *et al.*, 1989a). Ex vivo activation of splenic T cells isolated from carbon tetrachloride-treated mice revealed a marked enhancement in IL-2 production. Moreover, the effect on IL-2 by carbon tetrachloride was associated with the serum of treated animals as direct addition of serum from carbon tetrachloride-treated mice also produced strong enhancement of IL-2 in naive-activated splenic T cells. Carbon tetrachloride-dependent induction and release of TGF-β_1 from the liver was readily induced concomitantly with the onset of immune suppression. Addition of anti-TGF-β_1-neutralizing antibodies abrogated IL-2 enhancement by serum isolated from carbon tetrachloride-treated mice; suggesting that the enhancing effects on IL-2 were mediated indirectly through TGF-β_1 released from the liver (Delaney *et al.*, 1994; Jeon *et al.*, 1997). Induction or inhibition of liver cytochrome *P*-450 activity augmented and blocked, respectively, the immunotoxic actions of carbon tetrachloride, suggesting a requirement for metabolism in order for carbon tetrachloride to be immunosuppressive (Kaminski *et al.*, 1990). More recently, it was demonstrated that TGF-β_1 produces profound effects on IL-2 regulation. Specifically, results in mouse spleen cells showed that TGF-β_1 exerts bifunctional effects on IL-2 as evidenced by the fact that TGF-β_1 stimulates IL-2 production at low concentrations (0.1–1 pg/mL) and conversely inhibits IL-2 production at high concentrations (1–10 ng/mL), when activated using monoclonal antibodies directed against the CD3 complex and CD28 (McKarns and Kaminski, 2000). Additionally, concentrations of TGF-β_1 that stimulated IL-2 production concomitantly inhibited splenocyte proliferation under similar conditions. Recent studies have revealed that IL-2 regulation by TGF-β_1 is mediated, at least in part, via a mechanism dependent on SMAD3, a transcription factor involved in signaling through the TGF-β receptor (McKarns *et al.*, 2004). In studies comparing acute versus subchronic carbon tetrachloride administration, acute carbon tetrachloride treatment enhanced phagocytosis and NK cell activity, whereas subchronic treatment significantly impaired phagocytosis and NK cell activity (Jirova *et al.*, 1996). In contrast, Fischer 344 rats exposed orally for 10 days exhibited no immunotoxic effects, despite signs of liver

toxicity (Smialowicz *et al.*, 1991c). The difference in sensitivity between studies in the mouse and rat may represent differences in the metabolic capabilities between these two species, as well as the degree of liver injury induced, and hence the magnitude of TGF-β_1 production.

There is relatively little new information on solvents and other chemicals structurally related to carbon tetrachloride. Some early studies were conduced to assess the potential immunotoxicity of a number of drinking water contaminants. Exposure to dichloroethylene (in drinking water for 90 days) has been reported to suppress the anti-sRBC antibody response in male CD-1 mice and to inhibit macrophage function in their female counterparts (Shopp *et al.*, 1985). Similarly, exposure to trichloroethylene (in the drinking water for 4–6 months) was reported to inhibit both humoral immunity and CMI and bone marrow colony-forming activity (Sanders *et al.*, 1982). In those experiments, females were more sensitive than males. Exposure to 1,1,2-trichloroethane resulted in suppression of humoral immunity in both sexes. In addition, macrophage function was inhibited (males only) (Sanders *et al.*, 1985). Inhalation studies with dichloroethane, dichloromethane, tetrachloroethane, and trichloroethene indicated that the pulmonary host resistance to *Klebsiella pneumoniae* was suppressed (Aranyi *et al.*, 1986; Sherwood *et al.*, 1987), suggesting that alveolar macrophages may be affected. The most recent work with this series of solvents indicated that exposure to trichloroethylene may be an effective developmental immunotoxicant in B6C3F1 mice, suggesting that additional studies are required to determine the health risks associated with developmental exposure to this chemical (Peden-Adams *et al.*, 2006).

Glycols and Glycol Ethers Exposure to glycol ethers has been associated with adverse effects in laboratory animals, including thymic atrophy and mild leukopenia. Oral administration of ethylene glycol monomethyl ether for 1–2 weeks (House *et al.*, 1985; Kayama *et al.*, 1991) or its metabolite methoxyacetic acid for 2 weeks (House *et al.*, 1985) produced decreased thymic weight, thymic atrophy, and a selective depletion of immature thymocytes in mice. No alterations in humoral immunity, CMI, macrophage function, or host resistance to *L. monocytogenes* were observed (House *et al.*, 1985). It has also been suggested that perinatal exposure to ethylene glycol monomethyl ether may produce thymic hypocellularity and inhibition of thymocyte maturation, and that it may affect pro-lymphocytes in fetal liver (Holladay *et al.*, 1994).

Oral studies (5–10 days) on the glycol ether 2-methoxyethanol have consistently shown a decrease in thymus weight in the rat (Smialowicz *et al.*, 1991a; Williams *et al.*, 1995). This decrease is often accompanied by alterations in lymphoproliferative responses, although suppression is seen in some cases and stimulation in others, with no clear reason for the differences in response. Alterations in spleen weight and splenic cell populations have also been observed, as well as suppression of trinitrophenyl-lipopolysaccharide and anti-sRBC PFC responses. Similar results have been obtained following dermal exposure to 2-methoxyethanol (Williams *et al.*, 1995). A decrease in IL-2 production has also been reported (Smialowicz *et al.*, 1991a). Studies using the metabolites of 2-methoxyethanol (methoxyacetaldehyde and methoxyacetic acid) or specific metabolic pathway inhibitors have shown that methoxyacetaldehyde and methoxyacetic acid are more immunotoxic than 2-methoxyethanol alone (methoxyacetaldehyde > methoxyacetic acid > 2-methoxyethanol) (Smialowicz *et al.*, 1991a,b; Kim and

Smialowicz, 1997), suggesting a role for metabolism in the observed alterations in immunocompetence. Although there was no effect following 10-day oral exposures to 2-methoxyethanol (50–200 mg/kg/d) (Smialowicz *et al.*, 1991a), subchronic exposure for 21 days to 2000–6000 ppm (males) or 1600–4800 ppm (females) did produce an enhanced NK cell response (Exon *et al.*, 1991) in addition to suppression of the PFC response and a decrease in IFN-γ production. In that study, it was also determined that 2-methoxyethanol produced greater immunotoxic effects than 2-butoxyethanol. 2-Butoxyethanol was observed to enhance NK cell activity, but only at the low doses.

Nitrosamines   The nitrosamine family comprises the nitrosamines, nitrosamides, and C-nitroso compounds. Exposure to nitrosamines, especially N-nitrosodimethylamine (dimethylnitrosamine, the most prevalent nitrosamine) comes primarily through industrial and dietary means, and minimally through environmental exposure. N-nitrosodimethylamine is used commonly as an industrial solvent in the production of dimethylhydrazine. It is currently used as an antioxidant, as an additive for lubricants and gasolines, and as a softener of copolymers. The toxicity and immunotoxicity of N-nitrosodimethylamine have been extensively reviewed (Myers and Schook, 1996). Single or repeated exposure to N-nitrosodimethylamine inhibits T-dependent humoral immune responses (IgM and IgG), but not T-independent responses. Other symmetrical nitrosamines, such as diethylnitrosamine, dipropylnitrosamine, and dibutylnitrosamine, demonstrated similar effects on humoral immunity but were not as potent as N-nitrosodimethylamine (Kaminski *et al.*, 1989b). In fact, as the length of the aliphatic chain increased, the dose required to suppress the anti-sRBC PFC response by 50% (ED_{50}) also increased. In contrast, nonsymmetrical nitrosamines suppressed humoral immunity at comparable concentrations. Overall, the rank order of ED_{50} values paralleled their LD_{50} values. T-cell-mediated lymphoproliferative responses (mitogens or MLR) and DTH response are also suppressed following N-nitrosodimethylamine exposure. In vivo exposure to N-nitrosodimethylamine followed by challenge with several pathogens did not produce a pattern of effects that was consistent (decreased resistance to *Streptococcus zooepidemicus* and influenza, no effects on resistance to herpes simplex types 1 or 2 or *Trichinella spiralis,* and increased resistance to *L. monocytogenes*). In contrast, antitumor activity in N-nitrosodimethylamine-exposed animals was consistently enhanced. N-Nitrosodimethylamine-exposed animals also have altered development of hematopoietic cells (increased macrophage precursors). Together these data suggest the macrophage (or its developmental precursors) as a primary target. Mechanistic studies have demonstrated that N-nitrosodimethylamine alterations in CMI are associated with enhanced macrophage activity, increased myelopoietic activity, and alterations in TNF-α transcriptional activity. It has been postulated that N-nitrosodimethylamine may cause the enhanced production of GM-CSF, which can have autocrine (enhanced tumoricidal and bactericidal activity) and paracrine (induced secretion of T-cell-suppressing cytokines by macrophages) activities.

Mechanistic studies have also indicated a critical role for metabolism in the immune suppression by N-nitrosodimethylamine (Johnson *et al.*, 1987b; Kim *et al.*, 1988; Haggerty and Holsapple, 1990). It is known that N-nitrosodimethylamine is metabolized by the liver cytochrome P-450 system to a strong alkylating agent, and studies have shown that there is a relationship between N-nitrosodimethylamine-induced immune suppression, and the anticipated hepatotoxicity. Interestingly, a molecular dissection of N-nitrosodimethylamine-induced hepatotoxicity by mRNA differential display demonstrated an increase in transcripts for the complement protein C3 and serum amyloid A (Bhattacharjee *et al.*, 1998). Previous work by Kaminski and Holsapple (1987) demonstrated the potential immune suppression associated with an increase in serum amyloid A.

Mycotoxins   The immunotoxicity of mycotoxins, structurally diverse secondary metabolites of fungi that grow on feed, has been reviewed (IPCS, 1996; Bondy and Pestka, 2000). This class of chemicals comprises such toxins as aflatoxin, ochratoxin, and the tricothecenes, notably T-2 toxin and deoxynivalenol (vomitoxin). As a class, these toxins can produce cellular depletion in lymphoid organs, alterations in T- and B-lymphocyte function, suppression of antibody responses, suppression of NK cell activity, decreased DTH responses, and an apparent increase in susceptibility to infectious disease. T-2 toxin has also been implicated as a developmental immunotoxicant, targeting fetal lymphocyte progenitors leading to the thymic atrophy often observed with these mycotoxins (Holladay *et al.*, 1993). For ochratoxin, at least, the dose, the route of administration, and the species appear to be critical factors in results obtained in immunotoxicity studies. Past studies with aflatoxin B1 suggest that CMI and phagocytic cell functions are affected as evidenced by decreased proliferative responses to PHA and suppression of DTH responses (Raisuddin *et al.*, 1993). In addition, in vitro experiments demonstrated that aflatoxin B1 required metabolic bioactivation in order to produce suppression of antibody responses and mitogen-induced lymphoproliferation (Yang *et al.*, 1986). Studies in laboratory animals have also shown increased risk to secondary infection after aflatoxin B1 treatment. The effects of aflatoxins on the human immune system have not been characterized but are of concern in light of the fact that in many parts of the world, such as in West Africa, exposure to aflatoxins is widespread as recent studies in Benin and Togo found that 99% of children possessed measurable aflatoxin–albumin adducts in blood (Gong *et al.*, 2003).

For the extensively studied tricothecenes, the mechanism of immune impairment is related in part to inhibition of protein synthesis. Interestingly, trichothecenes at high doses induce leukocyte apoptosis concomitantly with immune suppression (Pestka *et al.*, 1994). Conversely, at low doses trichothecenes promote expression of a diverse array of cytokines including IL-1, IL-2, IL-5, and IL-6. In addition, tricothecenes activate mitogen-activated protein kinases in vivo and in vitro via a mechanism known as the ribotoxic stress response (Moon and Pestka, 2002; Chung *et al.*, 2003; Zhou *et al.*, 2003). Prolonged consumption of deoxynivalenol by mice was shown to induce elevation of IgA and IgA immune complex formation, and kidney mesangial IgA deposition (Pestka, 2003). It has been postulated that the enhancement in IgA production induced by deoxynivalenol may be associated with the increase in cytokine production described above. The tricothecenes are currently considered among the most potent small-molecule inhibitors of protein synthesis in eukaryotic cells.

Adverse health effects have been associated with damp indoor environments following building envelope breech resulting from heavy rains and/or flooding, as occurred during Hurricanes Katrina and Rita in the Gulf Coast of the United States. The adverse health effects have been attributed, at least in part, to the presence of molds, most notably *Stachybotrys chartarum*, also known as black mold.

S. chartarum produces the macrocyclic trichothecene toxin, satratoxin G, which like many of the trichothecenes is a potent inhibitor of protein synthesis. In a recent study, satratoxin G exposure of mice, 100 μg/kg for 5 consecutive days by intranasal instillation, induced apoptosis of olfactory sensory neurons, and neutrophilic rhinitis (Islam *et al.*, 2006). Elevated mRNA levels for pro-inflammatory cytokines TNF-α, IL-6, and IL-1, and the chemokine, MIP-2, were detected in nasal airways and the adjacent olfactory bulb of the brain. By Day 7, marked atrophy of the olfactory nerve and glomerular layer of the olfactory bulb was detected. These finding suggest that neurotoxicity and inflammation within the nose may be potential adverse health effects associated with *Stachybotrys* exposure in indoor air.

Natural and Synthetic Hormones

It is well established that a sexual dimorphism exists in the immune system. Females have higher levels of circulating immunoglobulins, a greater antibody response, and a higher incidence of autoimmune disease than do males. Males appear to be more susceptible to the development of sepsis and the mortality associated with soft tissue trauma and hemorrhagic shock. Specific natural sex hormones in this dichotomy have been implicated. Immune effects of androgens and estrogens appear to be very tightly controlled within the physiological range of concentrations, and profound changes in immune activity can result for very slight changes in concentrations of hormones.

Estrogens Diethylstilbestrol is a synthetic nonsteroidal compound possessing estrogenic activity. Diethylstilbestrol was used in men to treat prostatic cancer and in women to prevent threatened abortions, as an estrogen replacement, and as a contraceptive drug. Extensive functional and host resistance studies on diethylstilbestrol (mg/kg/d range) have indicated that exposure to this chemical results in alterations in CMI and/or macrophage function and are believed to be mediated by the presence of the estrogen receptor on immune cells (Kalland, 1980; Luster *et al.*, 1980, 1984; Holsapple *et al.*, 1983). Targeted sites of action include the thymus (thymic depletion and alteration in T-cell maturation process), T cells (decreased MLR, DTH, and lymphoproliferative responses), and macrophage (enhanced phagocytic, antitumor, and suppressor function). Pre- and neonatal exposures (mg/kg/d dose range) have also demonstrated immunotoxic effects related to T-cell dysfunction. DTH and inflammatory responses associated with diethylstilbestrol exposure in adult mice have been shown to be reversible upon cessation of exposure (Luster *et al.*, 1980; Holsapple *et al.*, 1983). However, effects from in utero and neonatal exposures appear to have more lasting, possibly permanent effects on immune responses (Kalland *et al.*, 1979; Luster *et al.*, 1979; Ways *et al.*, 1980).

Exposure to 17β-estradiol in male rats (63 days of age) intraperitoneally for 15 days (1–50 μg/kg/d) did not alter spleen weight, spleen cellularity, or the humoral immune response to sRBC (Ladics *et al.*, 1998b). As observed with other estrogenic chemicals, thymic weight was decreased following exposure. Serum androgens and luteinizing hormone and male accessory organ weights were depressed, while serum estradiol and prolactin were increased. Dietary exposure (2.5–50 ppm) of male and female rats for 90 days resulted in decreased spleen weights and alterations in hematologic elements suggestive of bone marrow effects. Body weights were also affected. No histological alterations were noted. Decreases in splenic T- and B-cell populations were observed at the higher concentrations. These data suggest the possibility that exposure to

17β-estradiol may have resulted in altered normal immune cell trafficking and distribution, the mechanism of which is not clear. This hypothesis is supported by recent data indicating that the observed anti-inflammatory effects of estrogens may be related to a combination of alterations in homing and the activation of inflammatory cells and their production of TNF-α and IFN-γ (Salem *et al.*, 2000). Recent findings suggest that 17β-estradiol can drive the expansion of the CD4$^+$CD25$^+$ regulatory T-cell compartment as evidenced by an increase in Foxp3 expression levels in these cells (Polanczyk *et al.*, 2004). Foxp3 is a transcriptional repressor required for the development and function of T-regulatory cells and in combination with surface expression of CD4 and CD25, is currently the most definitive marker of T-regulatory cells.

Bisphenol A, a monomer in polycarbonate plastics and a constituent of epoxy and polystyrene resins possessing weak binding affinity for the estrogen receptor, has been recently evaluated by a number of laboratories for its potential to affect various aspects of immune function. The majority of studies to date demonstrate that leukocytes cultured in the presence of very high concentrations (>1 μM) of bisphenol A exhibit a number of alterations, primarily in innate immune function responses, including suppression of lipopolysaccharide-induced nitric oxide production and TNF-α secretion by macrophages (Kim and Jeong, 2003). The effects on nitric oxide production where shown to be correlated with a decrease in NF-κB DNA-binding activity, a transcription factor critically involved in the regulation of inducible nitric oxide synthase and TNF-α. In this study, suppression by bisphenol A of lipopolysaccharide-induced nitric oxide production was blocked by the estrogen receptor antagonist, ICI 182,780. Bisphenol A (10–50 μM) has also been reported to enhance IL-4 production in a model of a secondary immune response (Lee *et al.*, 2003). In vivo treatment of mice with bisphenol A (2.5 mg/kg) for 7 days produced a decrease in ex vivo concanavalin A-induced proliferation and IFN-γ secretion, but had no effect on the number of CD4$^+$, CD8$^+$, and CD19$^+$ cells in the spleen (Sawai *et al.*, 2003). Presently, the putative effects of bisphenol A on immune function are poorly defined and based on the current literature it is unclear whether the majority of the immunomodulatory effects reported are mediated through an estrogen receptor-dependent mechanism.

While it appears that estrogens can affect the maturation and function of the thymus and its components, it has recently been observed that estrogen receptor knockout mice have significantly smaller thymi than do their wild-type littermates, apparently due to the lack of the estrogen receptor-alpha (ERα) (Staples *et al.*, 1999). In addition, it has been suggested that the effects of estrogens on the thymus appear to be mediated not only through ERαs but also through an ERα-independent pathway yet to be elucidated.

Androgens Oxymetholone is a synthetic androgen structurally related to testosterone and used in the past in the treatment of pituitary dwarfism and as an adjunctive therapy in osteoporosis. Its current use is limited to treatment of certain anemias. Oxymetholone was administered orally to male mice daily for 14 consecutive days (50–300 mg/kg/d) (Karrow *et al.*, 2000). In male mice, oxymetholone exposure resulted in a minimal decrease in CMI (MLR and CTL response); but did not alter the ability of the animals to resist infection in host resistance assays. In contrast, anabolic androgenic steroids have been shown to significantly inhibit the sRBC PFC response and to increase the production of pro-inflammatory cytokines from human PBLs.

No comprehensive studies evaluating the effects of testosterone on immune parameters have been conducted. However, it is clear that testosterone is capable of contributing to the suppression of immune function; in particular, CMI responses and macrophage activity. There are numerous reports in the clinical literature that males are more susceptible than females to infection following soft tissue trauma and hemorrhagic shock (reviewed in Catania and Chaudry, 1999). Treatment of males with chemicals that block testosterone (e.g., flutamide) can prevent the trauma- and hemorrhage-induced depression of immunity. Similarly, treatment of females with dihydrotestosterone prior to trauma–hemorrhage results in depression of CMI, similar to that of males. Furthermore, gonadectomized mice of either sex have elevated immune responses to endotoxin, which can be attenuated in either sex by the administration of testosterone. The mechanisms in these cases, including influences of the neuroendocrine system, are not clear. Other investigators have reported that, like estrogenic agents, testosterone and other androgens are capable of influencing host defense by altering lymphocyte trafficking in the body and altering the ability of the macrophage to participate in immune responses.

Glucocorticoids The immunosuppressive actions of corticosteroids have been known for years. Following binding to a cytosolic receptor, these chemicals produce profound lymphoid cell depletion in rodent models. In non-human primates and humans, lymphopenia associated with decreased monocytes and eosinophils and increased PMNs are seen. Corticosteroids induce apoptosis in rodents, and T cells are particularly sensitive. In addition, these chemicals inhibit macrophage accessory cell function, the production of IL-1 from macrophages, and the subsequent synthesis of IL-2 by T cells. In general, corticosteroids suppress the generation of CTL responses, MLR, NK cell activity, and lymphoproliferation. Whereas it is clear that these drugs inhibit T-cell function, their effects on B cells are not completely clear. Corticosteroids inhibit humoral responses, but this appears to be due to effects on T cells, as antigen-specific antibody production by B cells to T-independent antigens does not appear to be affected by corticosteroid treatment.

In spite of the wide therapeutic use of glucocorticoids, the mechanism of action by which glucocorticoids mediate their anti-inflammatory/immunosuppressive activity is not well understood. Several mechanisms have been proposed all of which involve activation of the glucocorticoid receptor. Binding of glucocorticoids to the cytosolic glucocorticoid receptor induces the receptor to function as a ligand-activated transcription factor that undergoes homodimerization and DNA binding to glucocorticoid response elements (GRE) in the regulatory regions of glucocorticoid-responsive genes. Depending on the gene, GRE can either positively or negatively regulate transcription. For example, glucocorticoids induce annexin 1 (lipocortin 1), a calcium and phospholipid-binding protein, which acts to inhibit PLA2 (Goulding and Guyre, 1992; Taylor et al., 1997). Inhibition of PLA2 results in a decrease in arachidonate formation, the precursor in the biosynthesis of inflammatory prostaglandin and leukotriene. Similarly, glucocorticoids induce transcription of IκB, which is the endogenous inhibitor of the transcription factor, NF-κB (Auphan et al., 1995; Scheinman et al., 1995). As transcription of many key inflammatory cytokines is regulated positively by NF-κB, induction of IκB results in retention of NF-κB in the cytosol and thus suppression of inflammatory cytokine production. Ligand-activated glucocorticoid receptors have also been found to physically interact with other transcription factors including AP-1 (Schule et al.,

1990) and NF-κBg (Ray and Prefontaine, 1994), to inhibit DNA binding and/or their transcriptional activity. Presently, it is believed that all the above mechanisms contribute to the anti-inflammatory and immunosuppressive properties of glucocorticoids.

Therapeutics

Historically speaking, very few drugs used today as immunosuppressive drugs were actually developed for that purpose. In fact, if one looks closely enough, most therapeutic agents possess some degree of immunomodulatory activity at some dose (Descotes, 1986). The recent explosion of knowledge regarding the function and regulation of the immune system (at the cellular, biochemical, and molecular levels) has provided investigators with a relatively new avenue for specific drug development. The following discussion focuses on those drugs used primarily for modulating the immune system: the immunosuppressants (corticosteroids are described in the section "Natural and Synthetic Hormones"), AIDS therapeutics, "biologics" (i.e., monoclonal antibodies, recombinant cytokines, and interferons), and anti-inflammatory drugs.

Immunosuppressive Drugs Several immunosuppressive drugs are efficacious simply due to their ability to inhibit cellular proliferation, since proliferation is required for lymphocyte clonal expansion and, subsequently, differentiation. Other drugs inhibit specific intracellular proteins that are critical in the activation of the immune response.

Originally developed as an antineoplastic agent, cyclophosphamide (Cytoxan, CYP) is the prototypical member of a class of drugs known as alkylating agents. Upon entering the cell, the inactive drug is metabolically cleaved into phosphoramide mustard, a powerful DNA alkylating agent that leads to blockade of cell replication, and acrolein, a compound known to primarily bind to sulfhydral groups. Clinically, CYP has found use in reducing symptoms of autoimmune disease and in the pretreatment of bone marrow transplant recipients. Experimentally, this drug is often used as a positive immunosuppressive control in immunotoxicology studies because it can suppress both humoral immunity and CMI responses. There appears to be preferential inhibition of B-cell responses, possibly due to decreased production and surface expression of immunoglobulins. CMI activities that are suppressed include the DTH response, CTL, graft-versus-host disease, and the MLR. Adminsitration of low doses of CYP prior to antigenic stimulation can produce immune enhancement of cell-mediated and humoral immune responses, which has been attributed, in part, to an inhibition of suppressor T-cell activity (Limpens et al., 1990; Limpens and Scheper, 1991). The immune enhancing properties of CYP where demonstrated to be mediated by acrolein but not by phosphoramide mustard (Kawabata and White, 1988).

Azathioprine, one of the antimetabolite drugs, is a purine analog that is more potent than the prototype, 6-mercaptopurine, as an inhibitor of cell replication. Immune suppression likely occurs because of the ability of the drug to inhibit purine biosynthesis. It has found widespread use in the inhibition of allograft rejection, although it is relatively ineffective in attenuating acute rejection reactions. It can also act as an anti-inflammatory drug and can reduce the number of PMNs and monocytes. Clinical use of the drug is limited by bone marrow suppression and leukopenia. Azathioprine inhibits humoral immunity, but secondary responses (IgG) appear more sensitive than primary responses (IgM). Several CMI activities are also reduced by azathioprine treatment, including DTH response,

MLR, and graft-versus-host disease. Although T-cell functions are the primary targets for this drug, inhibition of NK function and macrophage activities has also been reported.

Leflunomide, an isoxazole derivative, is another drug that suppresses cellular proliferation, which has been used in the treatment of rheumatic disease and transplantation (Xiao et al., 1994). Leflunomide inhibits de novo pathways of pyrimidine synthesis, thereby blocking progression from G_1 to S of the cell cycle. Thus, direct inhibition of B-cell proliferation may account for the drug's ability to inhibit both T-cell-dependent and T-cell-independent specific antibody production. Leflunomide can also directly inhibit T-cell proliferation induced by mitogens, antibody directed against CD3, or IL-2.

Cyclosporin A (Sandimmune, CsA) is a cyclic undecapeptide isolated from fungal organisms found in the soil. Important to its use as an immunosuppressant is the relative lack of secondary toxicity (e.g., myelotoxicity) at therapeutic concentrations (Calne et al., 1981). However, hepatotoxicity and nephrotoxicity are limiting side effects. CsA acts preferentially on T cells by inhibiting the biochemical signaling pathway emanating from the TCR (reviewed in Ho et al., 1996). The result is inhibition of IL-2 gene transcription and subsequent inhibition of T-cell proliferation and clonal expansion of effector T cells. More specifically, CsA interacts with the intracellular molecule cyclophilin, an intracellular protein with peptidyl proline isomerase activity (although this enzymatic activity has nothing to do with the immunosuppressive effect of CsA). The CsA–cyclophilin complex inhibits the serine/threonine phosphatase activity of a third molecule, calcineurin. The function of calcineurin is to dephosphorylate the cytoplasmic form of the transcription factor, nuclear factor of activated T cells (NFAT), therefore facilitating the transport of NFAT into the nucleus, where it can couple with nuclear components and induce the transcription of the IL-2 gene. Inhibition of calcineurin phosphatase activity by the CsA–cyclophillin complex prevents nuclear translocation of NFAT and the resulting IL-2 gene transcription.

FK506 is a cyclic macrolide which is structurally distinct from CsA, but which possesses a nearly identical mechanism of action (reviewed in Ho et al., 1996). Like CsA, FK506 binds intracellularly to proteins with peptidyl proline isomerase activity, the most abundant of which is FK506-binding protein-12 (FKBP12). The FK506–FKBP12 complex also binds to and inhibits calcineurin activity, thereby inhibiting IL-2 gene transcription. Clinically, FK506 inhibits T-cell proliferation, lacks myelotoxicity (although, like CsA, it does cause nephrotoxicity), and induces transplantation tolerance. In addition, the minimum effective dose appears to be approximately one-tenth than that of CsA.

Rapamycin (RAP) is also a cyclic macrolide, which is structurally related to FK506. However, the mechanism by which it produces inhibition of proliferation is strikingly distinct. Unlike CsA and FK506, RAP does not inhibit TCR-dependent signaling events and IL-2 gene transcription. Rather, this compound inhibits IL-2-stimulated T-cell proliferation by blocking cell-cycle progression from late G_1 into S phase (Morice et al., 1993; Terada et al., 1993). Like FK506, RAP binds to the intracellular protein FKBP12. But this RAP–FKBP12 complex does not bind calcineurin. Rather, the RAP–FKBP12 complex binds to the target of rapamycin (TOR) (Sabers et al., 1995), inhibiting its function. Inhibition of TOR results in reduced cell growth, suppression of cell cycle progression and proliferation (reviewed in Fingar and Blenis, 2004). Unlike both CsA and FK506, RAP does not appear to be nephrotoxic. Due to its mechanisms of action, a significant advantage of RAP over CsA and

FK506 is that it is an effective immune suppressant even after T cells have been activated, due to the fact that it blocks signaling through the IL-2 receptor. Conversely, for CsA and FK506 to be effective, T cells must encounter the drug prior to activation, as once IL-2 transcription begins, neither therapeutic provides effective suppression of the already activated T cells and IL-2 production.

AIDS Therapeutics Traditionally, antiviral therapies have not been extremely successful in their attempt to rid the host of viral infection. This may be due to the fact that these organisms target the DNA of the host. Thus, eradication of the infection means killing infected cells, which for HIV are primarily CD4$^+$ T cells. Numerous strategies have been developed to combat HIV, including targeting viral reverse transcriptase, viral protease, stimulating immune responses, and targeting the virus-T-cell interaction proteins. The multidrug therapy used currently is referred to as highly active antiretroviral therapy (HAART). However, eradication of this virus, and subsequently AIDS, remains a challenge because the very nature of the infection has significant immunosuppressive consequences. In addition, some of the current therapies also exhibit immunosuppressive actions. One such antiviral drug is zidovudine.

Zidovudine (3′-azido-3′-deoxythymidine) is a pyrimidine analog that inhibits viral reverse transcriptase. It was the first drug shown to have any clinical efficacy in the treatment of HIV-1 infection. Unfortunately, its use is limited by myelotoxicity (macrocytic anemia and granulocytopenia) (Luster et al., 1989). Early studies confirmed that the primary action of zidovudine is on innate immunity, although changes in both humoral immunity and CMI have also been observed (reviewed in Feola et al., 2006). In addition, it was shown that oral administration of high doses of zidovudine caused thymic involution and decreased responsiveness of T cells to the HIV protein, gp120 (McKallip et al., 1995). Clinically, zidovudine increases the number of circulating CD4$^+$ cells and can transiently stimulate cell-mediated immune responses (lymphoproliferation, NK cell activity, and IFN-γ production). A final consideration for the immunotoxicity associated with AIDS therapeutics like zidovudine is that they are rarely administered alone and thus, drug interactions likely contribute to various immune effects.

Biologics Biologics refers to those therapies that are derived in some manner from living organisms and include monoclonal antibodies, recombinant proteins, and adoptive cell therapies. By its very nature, the immune system is often both the intended therapeutic target and unintended toxicological target of various biologics. Overall, manifestations of toxicity may include exaggerated pharmacology, effects due to biochemical cross-talk, and disruptions in immune regulation by cytokine networks. Monoclonal antibodies can bind normal as well as targeted tissues, and any foreign protein may elicit the production of neutralizing antibodies against the therapeutic protein (i.e., the therapeutic protein may be immunogenic). While certainly many biologics are being utilized safely, the immunotoxicological aspects of an example of a monoclonal antibody (anti-CD3) and a recombinant protein (IFN-α) will be discussed.

Monoclonal antibodies have been designed in general to suppress immune function, and include antibodies directed against certain molecules that are critical for inducing or sustaining an immune response (CD3, IL-2 receptor, CD52, or TNF-α), or directed to stimulate certain molecules critical for downregulating activated T cells and in turn the immune response (CTLA-4). Monoclonal antibodies directed against CD3 (OKT3), part of the TCR complex, have been used for acute transplant rejection. As all T cells express CD3 as part of the TCR complex, anti-CD3 blockage potently suppresses immune function. Acutely, an adverse effect of OKT3 is "cytokine release syndrome," in which soon after initial administration, flu-like symptoms, pulmonary edema and hematological disorders have been reported (reviewed in Sgro, 1995). Although rare, anaphylactic reactions to the antibody can occur, as it is a murine monoclonal antibody.

The majority of recombinant proteins have been used as immunostimulants, including IFN-α, IFN-γ, GM-CSF, erythropoietin, IL-2, and IL-12. IFN-α, which is used as an antiviral drug, is used to treat Hepatitis C and other chronic viral illnesses. The mechanism of the antiviral action of IFN-α involves, in part, direct suppression of viral replication, enhancement of expression of MHC class I on virally infected cells, thus increasing the likelihood of recognition by virus-specific T cells, and activation of NK cells. Administration of IFN-α has been associated with autoimmune diseases, including autoimmune hypothyroidism and lupus (Vial and Descotes, 1995) and hematologic disorders stemming from bone marrow suppression.

Anti-inflammatory Agents Anti-inflammatory agents include nonsteroidal anti-inflammatory drugs (NSAIDs), which suppress the production of pro-inflammtory soluble factors, such as prostaglandins and thromboxanes. This mechanism of action has also been demonstrated for other anti-inflammatory drugs, such as aspirin, acetaminophen, and cyclooxygenase (COX) inhibitors, such as rofecoxib or celecoxib. This section also includes a brief discussion of anti-inflammatory biologics, such as anti-TNF-α monoclonal antibodies (adalimumab or infliximab), or recombinant TNF-α receptors (entanercept).

Aspirin irreversibly modifies COX enzymes 1 and 2, preventing the formation of prostaglandins and thromboxanes. Aspirin is especially effective as an antiplatelet because platelets possess little biosynthesizing capacity and therefore, aspirin will inhibit COX for the life of the platelet (8–11 days). Acetaminophen and other COX inhibitors are reversible inhibitors of COX enzymes. The COX-2 enzyme, in particular, is induced in response to inflammatory cytokines and mediators and therefore, represents an attractive target to combat inflammatory diseases. Although COX-2 inhibitors are currently available (rofecoxib or celecoxib), their use has been limited due to increased risk of cardiovascular effects in some patients (reviewed in Grosser et al., 2006).

Etanercept, adalimumab, and infliximab are a fairly recently developed class of anti-inflammatory drugs that are also biologics. All three drugs target TNF-α, a critical pro-inflammatory cytokine (see "Inflammation"). Etanercept is a recombinant TNF-α receptor, which binds circulating TNF-α levels and prevents TNF-α binding to the endogenous TNF-α receptor. Adalimumab and infliximab, however, are monoclonal antibodies directed against TNF-α, which neutralizes circulating TNF-α and prevents interaction of TNF-α with its receptor. All three drugs suppress TNF-α signaling to prevent (1) induction of other pro-inflammatory cytokines such as IL-1 and IL-6; (2) leukocyte migration to inflammation sites; (3) neutrophil activation; (4) fibroblast activation; and (5) induction of other acute phase proteins.

Drugs of Abuse

Drug abuse is a social issue with far-reaching effects on the abuser as well as on friends and family. Whereas drug paraphernalia has been directly associated with the spread of HIV, in recent years the actual abuse of some drugs has been linked to the progression, and possibly the onset, of AIDS, suggesting that drugs of abuse may exhibit immunosuppressive actions. Indeed, many studies do suggest that drugs of abuse alter immune competence. Several classes of drugs will be discussed, including cannabinoids, opioids, cocaine, methamphetamine, and ethanol. Reports regarding the immune system effects of many of these drugs, particularly opioids, are often contradictory, so it should be noted that the mechanisms by which drugs of abuse suppresses immune function might depend on the development of tolerance or addiction to the drugs, or the immune, withdrawal, and pain status of the individual as endogenous molecules (i.e., endorphins or endocannabinoids) play critical roles in all of these physiological processes.

Cannabinoids Much attention has been focused on the immunomodulatory effects of the cannabinoids, which can be defined as plant derived (i.e., from the marijuana plant), synthetic, or endogenous. Therapeutically, the primary psychoactive congener of marijuana, Δ^9-tetrahydrocannabinol is approved for use as an antiemetic in patients undergoing cancer chemotherapy and as an appetite stimulant for cachexia associated with advanced AIDS disease. The mechanism by which Δ^9-tetrahydrocannabinol produces the high in the CNS is mediated through a G protein-coupled cannabinoid receptor, CB1 (Varvel et al., 2005). Peripheral tissues also express CB1, in addition to a second cannabinoid receptor, CB2. Although both receptors are expressed on immune system cells and are coupled to suppression of adenylate cyclase activity (Schatz et al., 1997), it is not entirely clear the extent to which the receptors and/or suppression of adenylate cyclase activity contributes to immune system effects by cannabinoids.

Early studies showed that exposure to Δ^9-tetrahydrocannabinol decreases host resistance to bacterial and viral pathogens (reviewed in Kaminski, 1994). For example, mice treated with Δ^9-tetrahydrocannabinol exhibited higher mortalities to the opportunistic brain infection Acanthamoeba (Cabral and Marciano-Cabral, 2004). In addition, Δ^9-tetrahydrocannabinol treatment of mice prior to primary infection with Legionella pneumophila pneumophilia increased mortality following secondary infection (Newton et al., 1994). Recent evidence demonstrates that the mechanism of decreased host resistance to L. pneumophila might involve suppression of dendritic cell function (Lu et al., 2006).

Cannabinoids alter both humoral and cell-mediated immune responses as evidenced by suppression of the T-cell-dependent PFC response both in vivo and in vitro (Schatz et al., 1993) and direct suppression of T-cell function (Condie et al., 1996). With respect to the mechanism of T-cell suppression, many plant-derived compounds suppress IL-2 at the transcriptional level which is due, in part, to suppression of transcription factor activation (AP-1, NFAT, and NF-κB) and ERK MAPK activity (Condie et al., 1996; Herring et al., 1998; Faubert and Kaminski, 2000). Although both cannabinoid receptors are expressed on T cells (Galiegue et al., 1995), many of the direct T-cell effects of cannabinoids have been demonstrated to occur independently of either cannabinoid receptor (Kaplan et al., 2003). Interestingly, although endogenous cannabinoids, such as anandamide and 2-arachidonoyl-glycerol, also suppress IL-2, their mechanism has been determined to involve a COX-2 metabolite that activates the peroxisome proliferator-activated receptor-γ (Rockwell and Kaminski, 2004; Rockwell et al., 2006).

Cannabinoid compounds have also been demonstrated to suppress innate immunity, particularly suppression of macrophage function. Δ^9-Tetrahydrocannabinol exposure impaired lysosomal or cytochrome c processing in macrophages (McCoy et al., 1995; Matveyeva et al., 2000). Interestingly, suppression of macrophage function by Δ^9-tetrahydrocannabinol seems to be mediated via the CB2 receptor (Buckley et al., 2000; Chuchawankul et al., 2004). Together these studies demonstrate that cannabinoid compounds alter immune function, and the mechanisms involve both cannabinoid receptor-dependent and receptor-independent actions.

Opioids Similar to cannabinoids, opioids refer to plant-derived, synthetic, or endogenous (endorphins) compounds that bind opioid receptors. Although technically "opioid" refers to drugs derived from the poppy plant, and "opiate" refers to agonists and antagonists with morphine-like activity (including plant-derived and synthetic compounds), they are often used interchangeably. It is well established that opioids suppress immune responses (reviewed in Dinda et al., 2005). It is not established, however, whether this action is a direct effect of the drug on immune cells or an indirect effect, and whether the effects are mediated through an opioid receptor (Wei et al., 2003; Sharp, 2006). There are at least three opioid receptors, μ, κ (and subtypes), and δ, which are all G protein coupled. Although many reports have identified opioid receptors on immune cells, controversy still exists as to which receptors and/or subtypes are present on the various immune cell populations and to what extent these receptors mediate immune responses to opioids. Nevertheless, a few reports will be discussed that describe some of the effects and mechanisms of opioid-induced immune modulation, and the reader is referred to several recent reviews for further information (Dinda et al., 2005; Page, 2005; Sharp, 2006).

Early studies evaluating the immune competence of heroin addicts revealed a decrease in total T cells and E-rosette capability, which was reversed with the general opioid receptor antagonist, naloxone, suggesting a role for an opioid receptor in mediating immune suppression (McDonough et al., 1980). Later studies demonstrated that although morphine suppressed several immune parameters, there was no dose–response, suggesting the effects were not receptor mediated, but were the result of increased circulating corticosteroids (which were significantly elevated in those animals; LeVier et al., 1994). This conclusion is supported by the findings of other investigators as well (Pruett et al., 1992b).

Several investigators have reported decreased host resistance to viral and bacterial infections in opioid-treated animals or heroin addicts. In one recent study, morphine treatment of mice infected with S. pneumoniae demonstrated increased bacterial burden in the lungs and increased mortality. The mechanism by which the immune response was compromised involved, in part, suppression of NF-κB gene transcription, which likely contributes to decreased expression of inflammatory mediators, such as chemokines, reducing recruitment of neutrophils to the infection site (Wang et al., 2005). There is also evidence that opioid use increases susceptibility to HIV infection. Although morphine and/or heroin use is associated with risk of HIV infection through shared needles, opioid use may contribute to progression of AIDS through immune suppression. Specifically, there is evidence that morphine treatment increases CCR5 expression, which is a primary receptor for HIV entry into macrophages (Guo et al., 2002). In addition, chronic morphine treatment shifts the T-cell balance toward Th2 (Roy et al., 2004). Further evidence for

compromised immunity toward HIV is the observation that morphine inhibited the anti-HIV activity in CD8$^+$ cells in an opioid receptor-dependent manner (Wang et al., 2005).

Opioids also modulate innate immunity. Earlier studies demonstrated that chronic treatment of mice with morphine suppressed bone marrow cell stimulation in response to macrophage colony-stimulating factor (Roy et al., 1991). Consistent with the observations that morphine and/or heroin use contributes to the progression of AIDS, Kupffer cells infected with HIV maintained in vitro in the presence of morphine resulted in a higher number of viral particles relative to untreated HIV-infected cells (Schweitzer et al., 1991). More recent studies demonstrate either suppression (Sacerdote, 2003) or enhancement (Peng et al., 2000) of cytokine production from macrophages. The differences might be due to agonist used, in vitro versus in vivo administration, and dosing regimen (i.e., whether tolerance was induced or not). Overall, it is clear that opioids suppress immune function and that the mechanism by which this occurs is complex and likely involves the CNS, the autonomic nervous system, the hypothalamic–pituitary–adrenal axis, and one or more opioid receptors (Alonzo and Bayer, 2002).

Cocaine Cocaine is a potent local anesthetic and CNS stimulant. This drug and its derivatives have been shown to alter several measures of immunocompetence, including humoral and cell-mediated immune responses and host resistance (Watson et al., 1983; Ou et al., 1989; Starec et al., 1991). Jeong et al. (1996) evaluated the effect of acute in vivo cocaine exposure on the generation of the anti-sRBC PFC, and determined that immune suppression was due to a cytochrome P-450 metabolite of cocaine. Further studies demonstrated that sex, strain and age differences can be detected in cocaine-induced immunodulation as assessed by the anti-SRBC PFC response (Matulka et al., 1996). Similar to other immunotoxic agents, the mechanism by which cocaine alters immune function involves a disruption of the Th1/Th2 balance and the stress response (Stanulis et al., 1997a,b). Cocaine also induces the secretion of TGF-β, which has been linked to the observation that cocaine exposure enhances replication of the HIV-1 virus in human peripheral blood mononuclear cells (Chao et al., 1991; Peterson et al., 1991). More recently, and in agreement with the above studies, cocaine was demonstrated to cause an increased HIV viral burden in a human PBL–SCID animal model, which was mediated through σ1 receptors, which are informally referred to as psychoactive drug receptors (Roth et al., 2005). Although the function and role of σ1 receptors still remain to be elucidated, additional studies also suggest that cocaine effects are mediated through these receptors (Maurice and Romieu, 2004).

Methamphetamine Methamphetamine use has been growing over the past several years. Methamphetamine is a stimulant that is similar to amphetamine, although highly addictive. Only recently has the immunotoxicity of methamphetamine been explored (In et al., 2005). Following oral administration to mice, methamphetamine suppressed the anti-sRBC PFC response, IgG production and mitogenic stimulation of T-cell proliferation. Even more striking was the suppression of GM-CSF-stimulated bone marrow colony growth by methamphetamine. These results indicate suppression of both CMI and humoral immunity in vivo following methamphetamine administration.

Ethanol Ethanol exposure has been studied both in alcoholic patients and in animal models of binge drinking. In humans, alcoholism is associated with an increased incidence of, and mortality from, pulmonary infection and mortality from it (reviewed in Happel and Nelson, 2005). There is also an increased incidence of bacterial infection and spontaneous bacteremia in alcoholics with cirrhosis of the liver (reviewed in Leevy and Elbeshbeshy, 2005). A consistent finding in abusers of ethanol is the significant change in the mononuclear cells of the peripheral blood. In animal models, this is observed as depletion of T- and B cells in the spleen and the T cells in the thymus, particularly $CD4^+/CD8^+$ cells. The latter effect may be related in part to increased levels of corticosteroids (Han *et al.*, 1993).

More recently, in a binge-drinking model, ethanol suppresses innate immunity through an inhibition of TLR3 signaling in peritoneal macrophages. The authors also demonstrated suppression of pro-inflammatory cytokines (Pruett *et al.*, 2004a). In addition to suppression of TLR3, ethanol suppresses signaling through other TLRs, contributing to pielotropic effects of ethanol on innate immunity (Pruett *et al.*, 2004b).

Medical Devices and Silicon-Based Materials

As reviewed in Rodgers *et al.* (1997), many of these devices may have intimate and prolonged contact with the body and possible immunologic consequences of this contact could be envisioned to include immune suppression, immune stimulation, inflammation, and sensitization. Concern over the influence of medical devices on the immune system reached a peak during the scientific, medical, social, and legal debate in the late 1990s about the potential impact of silicon breast implants on human health. As such, this section will emphasize studies that have focused on silicon-based materials.

Silicon-based materials have known uses in consumer products such as cosmetics, toiletries, food stuffs, household products, and paints as well as in the medical field (e.g., as lubricants in tubing and syringes and as components in numerous implantable devices). Significant interest was focused on the biocompatibility of certain silicon-based materials (silicones) and the potential for these products to produce immunotoxic effects, because of persistent, unsubstantiated speculation that breast implants made with silicone materials were able to provoke connective tissue disease. A committee formed by the Institute of Medicine concluded in 2000 that "a review of the toxicology studies of silicones and other substances known to be in breast implant does not provide a basis for health concerns" (IOM, 2000).

Two studies were conducted which extensively evaluated immune status following exposure to dimethylpolysiloxanes used in medical practice (Bradley *et al.*, 1994a,b). In the first study, mice were implanted for 10 days with dimethylpolysiloxane fluid, gel, and elastomer as well as polyurethane as a control. There were no observable alterations in innate or acquired immune function. In fact, the materials tested afforded modest protection to an approximate LD_{50} challenge with *L. monocytogenes*. Implantation of the same materials for 180 days resulted in a modest suppression of NK cell activity that did not correlate with altered susceptibility to challenge with B16F10 melanoma. No other alterations in host resistance have been observed.

Studies have also been conducted on two low-molecular weight cyclic siloxanes: octamethylcyclotetrasiloxane and decamethylcyclotetrasiloxane. One-month inhalation exposures of rats to high concentrations of octamethylcyclotetrasiloxane (up to 540 ppm) and decamethylcyclotetrasiloxane (up to a maximum 160 ppm) did not result in alterations in humoral immunity (Burns-Naas *et al.*, 1998; Klykken *et al.*, 1999). Inhalation exposure of human volunteers to octamethylcyclotetrasiloxane at 10 ppm for 1 hour revealed no effects on several immune parameters (Looney *et al.*, 1998).

Finally, under highly specific experimental conditions that do not mimic human exposure, a few silicon-based materials have been observed to act as immunologic adjuvants (reviewed in Potter and Rose, 1996). Under typical exposure conditions, neither octamethylcyclotetrasiloxane, a combination of octamethylcyclotetrasiloxane and decamethylcyclotetrasiloxane, nor dimethylpolysiloxane acts as an immunologic adjuvant (Bradley *et al.*, 1994a,b; Klykken and White, 1996; Klykken *et al.*, 1999). Overall, the studies to date have been largely negative and no link between exposure to silicones and human disease has been established.

Inhaled Substances

Pulmonary defenses against inhaled gases and particulates are dependent on both physical and immunologic mechanisms. Immune mechanisms primarily involve the complex interactions between PMNs and alveolar macrophages and their abilities to phagocytize foreign material and produce cytokines, which not only act as local inflammatory mediators, but also serve to attract other cells into the airways.

Oxidant Gases It is becoming increasingly clear that exposure to oxidant gases—such as ozone (O_3), sulfur dioxide (SO_2), nitrogen dioxide (NO_2), and phosgene—alters pulmonary immunologic responses and may increase the susceptibility of the host to bacterial infections (reviewed by Selgrade and Gilmour, 1994). Infiltration of both PMNs and macrophages has been observed, resulting in the release of cellular enzyme components and free radicals, which contribute to pulmonary inflammation, edema, and vascular changes. Exposure to O_3 has been demonstrated to impair the phagocytic function of alveolar macrophages and to inhibit the clearance of bacteria from the lung. This correlated with decreased resistance to *S. zooepidemicus* and suggests that other extracellular bacteriostatic factors may be impaired following exposure to these oxidant gases. Short-term NO_2 exposure decreases killing of several bacterial pathogens and, like O_3, this decreased resistance is probably related to changes in pulmonary macrophage function. A role for the products of arachidonic acid metabolism (specifically, the prostaglandins) has recently been implied and is supported by the facts that decreased macrophage functions are associated with increased PGE_2 production and that pretreatment with indomethacin inhibits O_3-induced pulmonary hyperresponsiveness and related inflammatory responses.

It is clear that exposure to oxidant gases can also augment pulmonary allergic reactions. This may be a result of increased lung permeability (leading to greater dispersion of the antigen) and to the enhanced influx of antigen-specific IgE-producing cells in the lungs. In studies involving O_3 exposure and challenge with *L. monocytogenes*, decreased resistance to the pathogen correlated not only with changes in macrophage activity, but also with alterations in T-cell-derived cytokine production (which enhances phagocytosis). In support of an effect on T cells, other cell-mediated changes were observed including changes in the T- to B-cell ratio in the lung, decreased DTH response, enhanced allergic responses, and changes in T-cell proliferative responses.

Particles: Asbestos and Silica It is believed that alterations in both humoral immunity and CMI occur in individuals exposed to asbestos and exhibiting asbestosis. Decreased DTH response and fewer T cells circulating in the periphery as well as decreased T-cell proliferative responses have been reported to be associated with asbestosis (reviewed in Miller and Brown, 1985; Warheit and Hesterberg, 1994). Autoantibodies and increased serum immunoglobulin levels have also been observed. Within the lung, alveolar macrophage activity has been implicated as playing a significant role in asbestos-induced changes in immune competence. Fibers of asbestos that are deposited in the lung are phagocytized by macrophages, resulting in macrophage lysis and release of lysosomal enzymes and subsequent activation of other macrophages. Recently, it has been hypothesized that the development of asbestosis in animal models occurs by the following mechanism: Fibers of asbestos deposited in the alveolar space recruit macrophages to the site of deposition. Some fibers may migrate to the interstitial space where the complement cascade becomes activated, releasing C5a, a potent macrophage activator and chemoattractant for other inflammatory cells. Recruited interstitial and resident alveolar macrophages phagocytize the fibers and release cytokines, which cause the proliferation of cells within the lung and the release of collagen. A sustained inflammatory response could then contribute to the progressive pattern of fibrosis, which is associated with asbestos exposure.

The primary adverse consequence of silica exposure, like that to asbestos, is the induction of lung fibrosis (silicosis). However, several immune alterations have been associated with silica exposure in experimental animals, including decreased antibody- and cell-mediated immune parameters (reviewed in IPCS, 1996). Alterations in both T- and B-cell parameters have been reported, although T-cell-dependent responses appear to be more affected than B-cell-dependent responses. Dose and route of antigen exposure appear to be important factors in determining silica-induced immunomodulation. Silica is toxic to macrophages and PMNs, and exposure is correlated with increased susceptibility to infectious pathogens. The significance of these immunologic alterations for the pathogenesis of silicosis remains to be determined. The association of this disease with the induction of autoantibodies is covered elsewhere in this chapter.

Pulmonary Irritants Chemicals such as formaldehyde, silica, and ethylenediamine have been classified as pulmonary irritants and may produce hypersensitivity-like reactions. Macrophages from mice exposed to formaldehyde vapor exhibit increased synthesis of hydroperoxide (Dean et al., 1984). This may contribute to enhanced bactericidal activity and potential damage to local tissues. Although silica is usually thought of for its potential to induce silicosis in the lung (a condition similar to asbestosis), its immunomodulatory effects have also been documented (Levy and Wheelock, 1975). Silica decreased reticuloendothelial system clearance and suppressed both humoral immunity (PFC response) and the cell-mediated response (CTL) against allogeneic fibroblasts. Both local and serum factors were found to play a role in silica-induced alterations in T-cell proliferation. Silica exposure may also inhibit phagocytosis of bacterial antigens (related to reticuloendothelial system clearance) and inhibit tumoricidal activity (Thurmond and Dean, 1988).

Ultraviolet Radiation

Ultraviolet radiation (UVR) is an important environmental factor affecting human health with both beneficial effects, such as vitamin D production, tanning, and adaptation to UV, and adverse effects, such as sunburn, skin cancer, and ocular damage. UVR has also been demonstrated to modulate immune responses in animals and humans, and the effects of UV exposure on the immune system have been reviewed (Garssen and van Loveren, 2001). UV-induced immunomodulation has been shown to have some beneficial effects on some skin diseases, such as psoriasis, and has been demonstrated to impair some allergic and autoimmune diseases in both animals and humans. However, UV-induced immunomodulation can also lead to several adverse health consequences, including a pivotal role during the process of skin carcinogenesis. UV-induced immunomodulation has been demonstrated in experimental animal studies and human studies utilizing vaccine response rates to impair the resistance to a number of infectious agents, including bacteria, parasites, viruses, and fungi (reviewed in Sleijffers et al., 2004). As noted in the section "Approaches to the Assessment of Human Immunotoxicity," the parallelogram approach has been used to extrapolate animal to human data in an initial quantitative assessment of the risk for deleterious effects of UV radiation (van Loveren et al., 1995). Importantly, the effects of UVR on host resistance are not limited to skin-associated infections, but are also apparent in systemic infections.

There have been a number of recent studies to characterize the mechanism of action for UV-induced immunomodulation. The first step is the absorption of UV photons by chromophores, the so-called "photoreceptors", such as DNA and urocanic acid (Garssen et al., 1997). As a consequence of UV absorption by chromophores, epidermal and dermal cells, including keratinocytes, melanocytes, Langerhans cells, mast cells, dermal fibroblasts, endothelial cells, as well as skin-infiltrating cells (i.e., granulocytes and macrophages) produce and/or release many immunoregulatory mediators, including cytokine, chemokines, and neurohormones (Sleijffers et al., 2004). The mediators include both pro- and anti-inflammatory cytokines, such as TNF-α, IL-1, IL-6, and IL-10, which can modify directly or indirectly the function of APCs. Langerhans cells, the major APC in the skin, change phenotypically and functionally, which ultimately impacts the activity of T cells at the time of antigen presentation, both locally and systemically. One early explanation for UV-induced immunomodulation is that UVR induced a switch from a predominantly Th1 response (favoring DTH responses) to a Th2 response (favoring antibody responses). This hypothesis was supported by findings of altered cytokine secretion patterns indicative of a Th1 to Th2 switch (Araneo et al., 1989; Simon et al., 1990). Indeed, the majority of studies dealing with the effects of UVR indicated that Th1-mediated immune responses are especially sensitive to UV exposure. However, as noted above, UVR has been demonstrated to be associated with a suppression of certain allergic and autoimmune reactions. Indeed, more recent studies have demonstrated that Ig isotypes that are linked to either Th1 or Th2 cells can be suppressed by UVR and that UV exposure not only impairs Th1 responses; but also some Th2 responses (Sleijffers et al., 2004).

XENOBIOTIC-INDUCED HYPERSENSITIVITY AND AUTOIMMUNITY

Hypersensitivity

Polyisocyanates Polyisocyanates have a widespread use in industry and are responsible for more cases of occupationally related lung disease than any other class of low-molecular weight compounds. These chemicals are used in the production of adhesives, paint hardeners, elastomers, and coatings. Occupational exposure is by inhalation and skin contact. Members of the group are known to induce the full spectrum of hypersensitivity responses, types I–IV, as well as nonimmune inflammatory and neuroreflex reactions in the lung (Grammer, 1985; Bernstein and Bernstein, 1994). Sensitized individuals have shown cross-reactivity between compounds in this group.

Toluene diisocyanate is among the most widely used and most studied members of this group. Pulmonary sensitization to this compound can occur through either topical or inhalation exposure. It is a highly reactive compound that readily conjugates with endogenous protein. Laminin, a 70,000-kDa protein, has been identified as one protein that toluene diisocyanate conjugates in the airways, presumably forming one of the neoantigens responsible for hypersensitivity. Studies with guinea pigs have confirmed the need for a threshold level of exposure to be reached in order to obtain pulmonary sensitization. This finding supports the human data in which pulmonary sensitization is frequently the result of exposure to a spill, whereas workers exposed to low levels of vapors for long periods of time fail to develop pulmonary sensitization. Unlike the case in many hypersensitivity reactions, where removal of the antigen alleviates the symptoms of disease, symptoms may persist for years after cessation of exposure in many toluene diisocyanate-induced asthma patients.

The molecular mechanism, in part, involves the recognition of neoantigens formed via covalent binding of toluene diisocyanate to airway-associated proteins and their recognition as nonself. The neoantigens drive the clonal expansion of Th2 cells, which upon secondary antigenic stimulation induce a strong Th2 cytokine response involving the production of IL-4, IL-5, and IL-13. Production of IL-4 is especially critical to the hypersensitivity response as it is involved in immunoglobulin class switching by B cells to form IgE, one of the principal mediators responsible for mast cell degranulation and the ensuing airway hyperreactivity typically associated with type I hypersensitivity. In murine models employing intranasal or intratracheal sensitization and challenge with toluene diisocyanate, significant induction of Th2 cytokines, IgE, and eosinophilia has been demonstrated (Matheson et al., 2005; Plitnick et al., 2005; Ban et al., 2006).

Acid Anhydrides The acid anhydrides make up another group of compounds for which nonimmune and IgE, cytotoxic, immune complex, and cell-mediated reactions have been reported (Grammer, 1985; Bernstein and Bernstein, 1994). These reactive organic compounds are used in the manufacturing of paints, varnishes, coating materials, adhesives, and casting and sealing materials. Trimellitic acid anhydride is one of the most widely used compounds in this group. Inhaled trimellitic acid anhydride fumes may conjugate with serum albumin or erythrocytes leading, to type I (trimellitic acid anhydride-asthma), type II (pulmonary disease–anemia), or type III (hypersensitivity pneumonitis) hypersensitivity reactions upon subsequent exposure. Topical exposure to trimellitic acid anhydride may lead to type IV hypersensitivity reactions, resulting in contact dermatitis. Also, re-exposure by inhalation may lead to a cell-mediated immune response in the lung, which plays a role in the pathology seen in conjunction with type II and III pulmonary disease. Human and animal testing has supported the clinical findings in trimellitic acid anhydride-exposed workers. Levels of serum IgE can be measured in exposed workers and are predictive of the occurrence of type I pulmonary reactions. Serum titers of IgA, IgG, and IgM have been detected in patients with high levels of exposure

to trimellitic acid anhydride. Similar findings have been reported in studies with rhesus monkeys, in which exposed animals showed IgA, IgG, and IgM titers to trimellitic acid anhydride-haptenized erythrocytes. Inhalation studies with rats have produced a model corresponding to human trimellitic acid anhydride-induced pulmonary pneumonitis. Other anhydrides known to induce immune-mediated pulmonary disease include phthalic anhydride, himic anhydride, and hexahydrophthalic anhydride. The mechanism responsible for respiratory hypersensitivity by trimellitic acid anhydride is believed to be similar to that described above for toluene diisocyanate and involves induction of Th2 cytokines, IL-4, IL-5, and IL-3, formation of allergen-specific IgE, and eosinophilia. In a murine model, intranasal sensitization and challenge with trimellitic acid anhydride-induced Th2 cytokine expression in nasal airways and allergic rhinitis as well as mucous cell metaplasia in nasal and pulmonary airways that was not detected in mice only sensitized or challenged with trimellitic acid anhydride. Similarly, intranasal sensitization and challenge with contact sensitizers, dinitrochlorobenzene, or oxazolone, did not induce Th2 cytokines, IgE or mucus cell metaplasia in airways (Farraj et al., 2004). More recent studies compared topical versus intranasal sensitization in mice with trimellitic acid anhydride, in light of the fact that dermal exposure is likely to occur in the occupational setting (Farraj et al., 2006). Intranasal challenge with trimellitic acid anhydride in mice that were either topically or via intranasal sensitized with trimellitic acid anhydride produced a marked allergic rhinitis, of similar severity, characterized by an influx of eosinophils and lymphocytes. Both the topical and the intranasal routes of sensitization also produced significant increases in total serum IgE after intranasal challenge with trimellitic acid anhydride. In addition, both the topical and the intranasal routes of sensitization induced significant increases in the mRNA expression of the Th2 cytokines, IL-4, IL-5, and IL-13 (Farraj et al., 2006). These findings are significant as they suggest that dermal exposure represent a potential route of sensitization of the respiratory tract to chemical allergens. Based on the strong Th2 cytokine responses induced by several model respiratory sensitizers, such as toluene diisocyanate and trimellitic acid anhydride in rodent models, cytokine profiling has been proposed as an approach for identifying potential respiratory sensitizers (Dearman et al., 1996).

Metals Metals and metallic substances, including metallic salts, are responsible for producing contact and pulmonary hypersensitivity reactions. Metallic salts have been implicated in numerous immunologic and nonimmunologic pulmonary diseases. Exposure to these compounds may occur via inhalation or due to their solubility in aqueous media (they can be dissociated and transported into the lungs, where damage due to sensitization or nonimmunologic events takes place). Platinum, cobalt, chromium, nickel, and beryllium (and their salts) are the most commonly implicated allergenic metals.

Platinum Exposure to plantinum salts, such as hexachloroplatic acid, occurs occupationally in the mining, and metallurgic industries, in chemical industries where platinum is used as a catalyst, and in the production of catalytic converters. Platinum salts are highly allergenic and induce hypersensitivity reactions such as contact dermatitis and respiratory symptoms. Platinum-reactive T cells and increased IgE have been detected in the peripheral blood of platinum-sensitized patients (Raulf-Heimsoth et al., 2000).

Cobalt Cobalt exposure comes from metal-on-metal replacement prostheses, or occupationally in superalloy production and pigment manufacturing. Cobalt induces allergic contact dermatitis. Cobalt-reactive lymphocytes can be detected in patients with metal prostheses and the reactivity of the lymphocytes positively correlated with serum levels of cobalt (Hallab *et al.*, 2004).

Chromium Chromium is another metal in which exposure occurs either from metal-on-metal prostheses, or occupationally in the electroplating, leather tanning, and paint, cement, and paper pulp production industries. Chromium eczema is a type IV hypersensitivity reaction and is the most common form of allergic contact dermatitis to chromium. Chromium exists in several oxidation states and chromium eczema is associated most often with exposure to either chromium (III) or chromium (VI). Evidence of IgE-mediated reactions to chromium has been supported by immediate bronchial hyperreactivity after challenge and the identification of antigen-specific IgE antibodies.

Nickel Exposure to nickel occurs via body piercings or clothing fasteners, or occupationally in the mining, milling, smelting, and refinishing industries. Nickel is a common contact sensitizer, but pulmonary hypersensitivity reactions are rare. Nickel-reactive T cells can be identified in subjects with contact dermatitis (Sinigaglia *et al.*, 1985) and there is recent evidence that regulatory T cells act to suppress nickel-specific effector T cells in healthy individuals but not in nickel-allergic patients (Moed *et al.*, 2005).

Beryllium Beryllium exposure occurs most frequently in high-technology ceramics and dental alloy manufacturing, and in the electronics, nuclear, and aerospace industries. Although its use in the manufacturing of fluorescent bulbs has been discontinued, chronic beryllium disease was originally identified in 1946 in a group of fluorescent lamp-manufacturing workers. Beryllium is capable of producing both contact and tuberculin type IV hypersensitivity reactions. Skin contact has been found to produce lesions of contact hypersensitivity, whereas lesions produced by penetration of splinters of beryllium under the skin are granulomatous in nature. Inhalation of beryllium can result in disease ranging from acute pneumonitis, tracheobronchitis, and chronic beryllium disease to an increase in the risk of lung cancer.

Chronic beryllium disease still exists today with 2–16% of exposed workers developing the disease (reviewed in Fontenot and Maier, 2005). Unlike most hypersensitivity reactions in which removal of the sensitizing agent abates the disease, chronic beryllium disease mortality changes little following lower beryllium exposure. The mechanism of beryllium-induced hypersensitivity involves a pulmonary influx of CD4$^+$ T cells. Th2 and CD8$^+$ cells have minimal roles in chronic beryllium disease. Bronchoalveloar lavage fluid from chronic beryllium disease patients contains CD4$^+$ T cells, which in mouse models, precedes the development of granulomas. The frequency of beryllium-specific T cells in the blood of sensitized individuals is lower than that of chronic beryllium disease patients. Although still unclear at this time, these CD4$^+$ T cells are often from an oliogclonal T-cell population in which the predominant TCRβ chain is encoded by the Vβ3 gene. In addition, there is some evidence that people with a certain MHC class II allele (DPB1*0201) are more susceptible to the development of chronic beryllium disease.

Therapeutic Agents Hypersensitivity responses to therapeutic drugs are among the major types of unpredictable drug reactions, accounting for up to 10% of all adverse effects. Drugs that commonly induce hypersensitivity include sulfa drugs, barbiturates, anticonvulsants, insulin, iodine (used in many X-ray contrast dyes), and platinum-containing chemotherapeutics. Penicillin is the most common agent involved in drug allergy and is discussed here as an example. Exposure to penicillin is responsible for 75% of the deaths due to anaphylaxis in the United States. The route of administration, dosage, and length of treatment all appear to play a role in the type and severity of hypersensitivity reaction elicited. Severe reactions are less likely following oral administration as compared to parenteral, and prolonged treatment with high doses increases the risk of acute interstitial nephritis and immune hemolytic anemia. The high incidence of allergic reaction to penicillin is in part due to widespread exposure to the compound. Not only has there been indiscriminant use of the drug, but exposure also occurs through food products including milk from treated animals and the use of penicillin as an antimicrobial in the production of vaccines. Efforts are still being made to reduce unnecessary exposure.

The mechanism by which hypersensitivity to penicillin, and likely other drugs, occurs is through the formation of a neo-antigen, which is then recognized by the immune system as nonself. The formation of the primary penicillin neo-antigen occurs during the break down of penicillin, in which the β-lactam ring opens, forming a reactive intermediate that reacts with other proteins. The resultant penicilloylated protein now acts as a hapten to which the immune system mounts a response. As is the case with other haptens, subsequent exposures to penicillin may not absolutely require the formation of penicilloylated proteins to elicit secondary responses.

Reactions to penicillin are varied and may include any of the four types of hypersensitivity reactions. The most commonly seen clinical manifestation of type I reactions is urticaria; however, anaphylactic reactions occur in about 10–40 of every 100,000 patients receiving injections. Clinical signs of rhinitis and asthma are much less frequently observed. Blood dyscrasias can occur due to the production of IgG against penicillin metabolites bound to the surface of red blood cells (type II reaction). Penicillin has also been implicated in type III reactions leading to serum-sickness-like symptoms. Owing to the high frequency of type IV reactions when penicillin is applied topically, especially to inflamed or abraded skin, products are no longer available for topical application. Type IV reactions generally result in an eczematous skin reaction, but a rare, life-threatening form of dermal necrosis may result. In these cases there is severe erythema and a separation of the epidermis at the basal layer. This reaction, which gives the clinical appearance of severe scalding, is thought to be a severe delayed reaction.

Latex Natural rubber latex is derived from the rubber tree *Hevea brasiliensis* and is used in the manufacture of over 40,000 products including examination and surgical gloves, among other medical products. Allergic reactions to natural rubber latex products have become an important occupational health concern over the past decade with increased use of universal precautions, particularly latex gloves, to combat the spread of bloodborne pathogens. Hypersensitivity to latex usually occurs via a type I or type IV reaction. Dermatologic reactions to latex include irritant dermatitis due to chemical additives or mechanical abrasion and the occlusive conditions caused by wearing gloves; contact dermatitis (which represents approximately 80% of the allergic responses) due to the chemical additives used in the glove manufacturing (e.g., thiurams, carbamates, mercapto compounds, and phenylenediamines), and potentially more serious IgE-mediated responses due to residual latex proteins that remained in the finished products. The IgE responses may manifest as urticaria, asthma, or life-threatening anaphylaxis. Several latex proteins have been identified and antibodies to most can be detected in latex-allergic individuals (Ahmed *et al.*, 2004).

Food and Genetically Modified Organisms   Awareness of hypersensitivity reactions to foods and genetically modified organisms (or crops; GMOs) has increased in the last several years. The most common food allergens are milk, egg, peanuts and other tree nuts, fish, shellfish, soy, and wheat. Peanut allergies are relatively common, can be severe, and there is much interest sociologically to reduce even airborne exposures to peanuts; thus, current information regarding the mechanism of peanut hypersensitivity is provided as an example. Although many food allergies that develop in infancy or childhood might be outgrown, peanut allergy is often life long. Hypersensitivity to peanuts occurs primarily via a type I reaction and the IgE responses may include shortness of breath, asthma, and anaphylaxis. Several peanut proteins have been identified and antibodies to most can be detected in peanut-allergic patients (reviewed in Palmer and Burks, 2006). The stability of peanut proteins and their ability to interact with IgE contribute to the antigenicity of a particular protein over another. In addition, peanut-reactive T cells have been isolated from the blood of peanut-allergic individuals, suggesting the hypersensitivity to peanuts also involves a type IV reaction (de Jong *et al.*, 1996).

Exposure to GMOs are becoming more widespread as biotechnological advances in food production are used, for example, to confer insect resistance or provide desired nutrients. Allergenic determinants in GMOs result from the expression of novel proteins that might be recognized as nonself by the immune system. There are several considerations in determining potential hypersensitivity to a GMO. It is critical to establish whether the introduced protein is allergenic and/or whether its amino acid sequence is similar enough to known allergens to be considered potentially allergenic. In addition, the appropriate test must be selected (e.g., radioallergosorbent tests and immunoglobulin levels) in order to avoid false positives or false negatives. Finally, ideally, hypersensitivity to GMOs will be tested on subjects prior to release, but it is also important to survey reactions in the general public following widespread availability (reviewed in Germolec *et al.*, 2003).

Enzymes   Detergent enzymes have been implicated in occupationally induced hypersensitivity. Subtilin, a proteolytic enzyme derived from *Bacillus subtilis,* is used in laundry detergents to enhance their cleaning ability. Both individuals working in the environment where the product is made and those using the product may become sensitized. Subsequent exposure may produce signs of rhinitis, conjunctivitis, and asthma. An alveolar hypersensitivity reaction associated with precipitation antibodies and a type III Arthus reaction from skin testing has also been seen. Papain is another enzyme known to induce IgE-mediated disease. It is a high-molecular weight sulfhydryl protease obtained from the fruit of the papaya tree and most commonly used as a meat tenderizer and a clearing agent in the production of beer. However, it is also used in the production of tooth powders, laxatives, and contact lens cleaning solutions.

As emphasized in the section "Assessment of Hypersensitivity Responses," there is a strong genetic component, and the specific nature of the genetic susceptibility and of the T-cell responses to detergent enzymes is largely unknown. In a recent study, transgenic mice with the following human haplotypes, HLA-DQ6, HLA-DQ8, HLA-DR2, HLA-DR3, and HLA-DR4, were generated and used to study the immune and inflammatory components involved in the response to subtilisin. Their results demonstrated that only DQ8 mice showed consistent T-cell responses to subtilisin, developed allergic eosinophilic inflammatory reactions in the airways following intranasal instillations of the enzyme, and responded with a significant IgG1 and IgE production. As noted by the authors, these results offer promise for the use of HLA Class II transgenic mice as models to study the allergenic responses to enzymes in humans, and for the potential to develop modified enzymes to maintain efficient detergent qualities without the allergenic properties (Xue *et al.*, 2005).

Sarlo and Kirchner (2002), reviewed the latest developments in the control of enzyme-induced occupational asthma and allergy in the detergent industry. Guidelines have been developed for the safe handling of enzymes, and those manufacturing facilities that follow all of the guidelines enjoy very low or no cases of asthma and allergy among workers exposed to enzymes. The key to the success of these guidelines is the prospective surveillance for the development of enzyme-specific IgE antibody before the onset of allergic symptoms. The results to date have shown that workers with IgE to enzymes can still continue to work in the industry symptom free for their entire career. Mechanistically, these observations suggest that exposures needed to induce sensitization are different, and probably lower, than exposures needed to elicit enzyme allergic symptoms (Sarlo and Kirchner, 2002). More recently, Sarlo (2003) provided an overview of how a comprehensive preclinical, clinical, and industrial hygiene program has been used successfully to control allergy and asthma to enzymes in the detergent industry. These guidelines and industrial hygiene programs designed to minimize sensitization to enzymes and the development of disease can be applied to other industries where occupational allergy and asthma to proteins are common.

Formaldehyde   Formaldehyde exposure occurs in the cosmetic industry, the dental industry, and the textile industry, where it is used to improve wrinkle resistance, and in the furniture, auto upholstery, and resins industries. The general public may be exposed to low levels of formaldehyde in products as ubiquitous as newspaper dyes and photographic films and paper. This low-molecular weight compound is extremely soluble in water and forms haptens with human proteins easily (Maibach, 1983). Human predictive testing with 1–10% formalin (formalin is 37% formaldehyde) for induction and 1% formalin for challenge showed sensitization rates of 4.5–7.8% (Marzulli and Maibach, 1987). Occupational exposure to formaldehyde has been associated with the occurrence of asthma, although it has proven difficult to demonstrate antibodies to formaldehyde in the affected individuals.

Animal studies have confirmed the sensitization potential of formaldehyde. Frankild *et al.* (2000), demonstrated that formaldehyde was a strong sensitizer in both the Buehler test and the guinea pig maximization test. More recently, Basketter *et al.* (2001) compared 10 aldehydes of varying degrees of allergenicity in man using the LLNA. The results confirmed that the interpolation of the LLNA dose–response data to define the effective concentration of the test chemical required to induce a three-fold stimulation of proliferation (EC3) offers the prospect of a quantitative index of the relative potency of a contact allergen. The comparative study showed that

Table 12-11

Chemical Agents Known to be Associated with Autoimmunity

PROPOSED ANTIGENIC CHEMICAL	CLINICAL MANIFESTATIONS	DEPARTMENT	REFERENCES
Drugs			
Methyl dopa	Hemolytic anemia	Rhesus antigens	Murphy and Kelton (1991)
Hydralazine	SLE-like syndrome	Myeloperoxidase	Cambridge et al. (1994)
Isoniazid	SLE-like syndrome	Myeloperoxidase	Jiang et al. (1994)
Procainamide	SLE-like syndrome	DNA	Totoritis et al. (1988)
Halothane	Autoimmune hepatitis	Liver microsomal proteins	Kenna et al. (1987)
Nondrug chemicals			
Vinyl chloride	Scleroderma-like syndrome	Abnormal protein synthesized in liver	Ward et al. (1976)
Mercury	Glomerular neuropathy	Glomerular basement membrane protein	Pelletier et al. (1994)
Silica	Scleroderma	Most likely acts as an adjuvant	Pernis and Paronetto (1962)

formaldehyde had the lowest EC3 value, an observation consistent with the fact that it is regarded as the strongest allergen in man.

Taken together, the evidence is clear that formaldehyde is a contact sensitizer. It has also been demonstrated to irritate the skin, eyes, and respiratory system, and it is considered a typical air pollutant. One of ongoing debates surrounding formaldehyde is whether it should also be considered to be a respiratory sensitizer. A study by Arts et al. (1997) used the LLNA and serum IgE test in Brown Norway rats to compare the profiles of activity of trimellitic anhydride, a dermal and respiratory sensitizer, dinitrochlorobenzene, a dermal sensitizer with no or limited potential to cause respiratory allergy, formaldehyde, described by the authors as a skin irritant and dermal sensitizer with equivocal evidence for respiratory sensitizing potential, and methyl salicylate, a skin irritant devoid of sensitizing properties. Their results indicated that only exposure to trimellitic anhydride resulted in a significant increase in serum IgE concentration, and that formaldehyde, but not methyl salicylate, caused a dose-dependent activation of the draining lymph nodes. These results would suggest that formaldehyde is not a respiratory sensitizer. Other studies have demonstrated that formaldehyde can augment or enhance the respiratory allergic response to other stimuli. For example, Sadakane et al. (2002) showed that formaldehyde exposure (0.5% mist once a week for 4 weeks) in ICR mice enhanced the eosinophilic airway inflammation following the intratracheal instillation with Der f, the dust mite allergen. Fujimaki and colleagues exposed C3H/He mice to formaldehyde at 0-, 80-, 400-, or 2000-ppb formaldehyde for 12 weeks. When mice were immunized

with ovalbumin and then exposed to formaldehyde, the total number of bronchoalveolar lavage cells, macrophages, and eosinophils were significantly increased at the highest concentration (Fujimaki et al., 2004). Exposure to 400-ppb formaldehyde induced significant decreases in anti-ovalbumin IgG1 and IgG3 antibodies; but there was no effect on anti-ovalbumin IgE antibody. In addition, the ovalbumin-induced increase in plasma nerve growth factor was decreased by 80- and 400-ppb formaldehyde. The authors concluded that this was the first experimental evidence that low levels of long-term formaldehyde inhalation can induce differential immunogenic and neurogenic responses in allergic mice.

Autoimmunity

There are numerous reports of xenobiotics that have been associated with autoimmunity. However, firm evidence for their involvement is difficult to obtain, and there are very few human autoimmune diseases for which an environmental trigger has been definitely identified (Rose, 2005). These relationships may be causative through direct mechanisms, or they may be indirect, acting as an adjuvant. In the area of xenobiotic-induced autoimmunity, exact mechanisms of action are not always known. Chemical exposure may also serve to exacerbate a pre-existing autoimmune state (Coleman and Sim, 1994; Kilburn and Warshaw, 1994). Table 12-11 lists chemicals known to be associated with autoimmunity, showing the proposed self-antigenic determinant or stating adjuvancy as the mechanism of action. Table 12-12 shows chemicals that have been implicated

Table 12-12

Chemicals Implicated in Autoimmunity

MANIFESTATION	IMPLICATED CHEMICAL	REFERENCES
Scleroderma	Solvents (toluene, xylene)	Walder (1983)
	Tryptophan	Silver et al. (1990)
	Silicones	Fock et al. (1984)
Systemic lupus erythrematosus	Phenothiazines	Canoso et al. (1990)
	Penicillamine	Harpey et al. (1971)
	Propylthiouracil	DeSwarte (1985)
	Quinidine	Jiang et al. (1994)
	L-Dopa	DeSwarte (1985)
	Lithium carbonate	Ananth et al. (1989)
	Trichloroethylene	Kilburn and Washaw (1992)
	Silicones	Fock et al. (1984)

in autoimmune reactions, but in these cases the mechanism of autoimmunity has not been as clearly defined or confirmed. The list includes both drug and nondrug chemicals. The heterogeneity of these structures and biological activities illustrate the breadth of potential for the induction of chemically mediated autoimmune disease. A number of recent papers have reviewed some specific examples of xenobiotics associated with autoimmune disease, including drugs/immunotherapeutics (D'Cruz, 2000; Vial *et al.*, 2002; Pichler, 2003), vaccines (Descotes *et al.*, 2002; Vial and Descotes, 2004), environmental chemicals (D'Cruz, 2000; Hess, 2002), and pesticides (Holsapple, 2002). A brief discussion of selected drug and nondrug chemicals is provided.

Therapeutic Agents

Methyldopa Methyldopa is a centrally acting sympatholytic drug that has been widely used for the treatment of essential hypertension; but with the advent of newer antihypertensive drugs, the use of methyldopa has declined. Platelets and erythrocytes are targeted by the immune system in individuals treated with this drug. In the case of thrombocytopenia, antibodies are detected against platelets, which are indicative of immune recognition of a self- or altered self-antigen. Hemolytic anemia occurs in at least 1% of individuals treated with methyldopa, and up to 30% of these individuals develop antibodies to erythrocytes as manifest in a positive Coombs test. Interestingly, the antibodies are not directed against the chemical or a chemical membrane conjugate.

Hydralazine, Isoniazid, and Procainamide Hydralazine is a direct-acting vasodilator drug used in the treatment of hypertension. Isoniazid is an antimicrobial drug used in the treatment of tuberculosis. Procainamide is a drug that selectively blocks sodium channels in myocardial membranes, making it useful in the treatment of cardiac arrhythmias. All three drugs produce autoimmunity, which is manifested as a sytemic lupus erythematosus-like syndrome. Indeed, procainamide represents one of the best examples for a clear association between exposure to a xenobiotic and the onset or progression of an autoimmune disease. The association between procainamide and the sytemic lupus erythematosus-like condition is based on the finding that the disease remits when the drug is discontinued and recurs when the drug is re-administered. Antibodies to DNA have been detected in individuals showing this syndrome. Studies with hydralazine and isoniazid indicate that the antigenic determinant is myeloperoxidase. Immunoglobulins are produced against myeloperoxidase in individuals treated with these drugs. DNA is the apparent antigenic determinant for procainamide. For these three drugs, there is no evidence indicating that the immune system is recognizing the chemical or a chemical conjugate. In addition, these drugs have also been shown to produce hypersensitivity responses not associated with the sytemic lupus erythematosus syndrome.

Halothane Halothane, one of the most widely studied of the drugs inducing autoimmunity, is an inhalation anesthetic that can induce autoimmune hepatitis. The incidence of this iatrogenic disease in humans is about one in 20,000. The pathogenesis of the hepatitis results from the chemical altering a specific liver protein to such a degree that the immune system recognizes the altered protein and antibodies are produced. Studies using rat microsomes show that halothane has to be oxidized by cytochrome P-450 enzymes to trifluoroacetylhalide before it binds to the protein. Investigations indicate that in affected individuals antibodies to specific microsomal proteins are produced.

Vinyl Chloride Vinyl chloride, which is used in the plastics industry as a refrigerant and in the synthesis of organic chemicals, is a known carcinogen and is also associated with a scleroderma-like syndrome. The disease affects multisystemic collagenous tissues, manifesting itself as pulmonary fibrosis, skin sclerosis, and/or fibrosis of the liver and spleen. Ward *et al.* (1976) reported on 320 exposed workers, showing that 58 (18%) had a scleroderma-like syndrome. The individuals who showed the disease were in a group genetically similar (i.e., HLA-DR5) to patients with classic idiopathic scleroderma patients. Although the exact mechanism whereby this chemical produces autoimmunity is unclear, it is presumed that vinyl chloride acts as an amino acid and is incorporated into protein. Because this would produce a structurally abnormal protein, which would be antigenic, an immune response would be directed against tissues with the modified protein present.

Other occupational exposures suspected to induce scleroderma-like reactions include solvents, particularly organic solvents; but the evidence is still limited. Although several epidemiological studies found an increased relative risk when compared to the general population, the association was weak and not reproduced in other studies, and these studies frequently assessed exposure to solvents in general without providing details on specific solvents (Garabrant and Dumas, 2000; Garabrant *et al.*, 2003).

Mercury This widely used metal is now known to have several target systems, including the CNS and renal system. Mercury also has two different actions with respect to the immune system. The first action is direct injury, described previously in the section "Immunomodulation by Xenobiotics, Metals." The second action was highlighted in the section "Assessment of Autoimmune Responses" as an example of a model in which the autoimmune disease is chemically induced. Indeed, mercury produces an autoimmune disease that is manifested as glomerular nephropathy. Antibodies produced to laminin are believed to be responsible for damage to the basement membrane of the kidney. Mice and rats exposed to mercury also show antinuclear antibodies. The role of these antibodies in the autoimmune disease is not clear; however, they represent a known biomarker of autoimmunity. Studies in the Brown Norway rat point to a mercury-induced autoreactive CD4[+] cell as being responsible for the polyclonal antibody response. Mercury chloride induces an increase in the expression of MHC class II molecules on B lymphocytes, as well as shifting the T-helper cell population along the Th2 line. It is the Th2 cell that promotes antibody production. The imbalance between Th1 and Th2 cells is believed to be caused by the depletion of cysteine and the reduced form of gluthathione in Th1 cells. These chemical groups are known to be important in the synthesis of and responsiveness to IL-2 in T cells. Thus, Th1 cells that synthesize and respond to IL-2 would be at a greater risk than Th2 cells.

Mercury-induced autoimmunity has a strong genetic component. This has been extensively studied in the rat. Some strains of rats, such as the Lewis rat, are completely resistant, while others, such as the Brown Norway, are exquisitely sensitive. Susceptibility appears to be linked to three or four genes, one of which is the MHC. A number of reviews addressing the role of mercury in autoimmunity have been prepared (Pelletier *et al.*, 1994; Bigazzi, 1999).

Silica   Crystalline silica (silicon dioxide) is a primary source of elemental silicon and is used commercially in large quantities as a constituent of building materials, ceramics, concretes, and glasses. Experimental animals as well as humans exposed to silica may have perturbations in the immune system. Depending on the length of exposure, dose, and route of administration of silica, it may kill macrophages or may act as an immunostimulant. Silica has been shown to be associated with an increase in scleroderma in silica-exposed workers (Kilburn and Warshaw, 1994). This effect is believed to be mediated via an adjuvant mechanism. Adjuvancy as a mechanism of causing autoimmunity has been implicated with a number of other chemicals, including paraffin and silicones. Inherent in adjuvancy as a mechanism of producing autoimmunity is that the population affected by these chemicals must already be at risk for the autoimmune disease. This is supported by the data indicating a genetic component to many autoimmune diseases.

More recently, Brown and colleagues have developed a model in which apoptosis plays a critical role in silica-induced autoimmune diseases. As described by the authors, inhalation of crystalline silica results in concurrent activation and apoptosis of the alveolar macrophage resulting in an environment of inflammation and apoptosis (Brown *et al.*, 2004). This environment may provide excess antigen that is further ingested by activated macrophages or dendritic cells that are able to migrate to local lymph nodes. Within these local lymph nodes, these APCs, laden with apoptotic material, activate T- and B cells thereby inducing an autoimmune response.

Hexachlorobenzene   As noted above, a critical review of the state-of-the-science of autoimmunity by pesticides was prepared (Holsapple, 2002). There is little doubt that the pesticide that has been most extensively studied in the context of autoimmunity is hexachlorobenzene. Hexachlorobenzene is a low-molecular weight compound that was used in the past as a fungicide for seed grains. Even though its use as a pesticide was prohibited in most countries in the 1970s, it is still generated as a by product of several industrial processes and trace amounts of hexachlorobenzene are present as contaminants in some chlorine-containing pesticides. Finally, although emissions of hexachlorobenzene have decreased dramatically compared to the 1970s, residues can still be found throughout the environment due to its stability and persistence.

One of the drivers for including hexachlorobenzene in this brief presentation of examples of xenobiotics associated with autoimmune disease is based on an accidental poisoning incident that occurred in Turkey in 1955–1959. Approximately 3000–5000 people ingested seed grain contaminated with the fungicide, hexachlorobenzene. Patients developed a disease characterized by hepatic porphyria, called *porphyria turcica*, which was manifested as bullous skin lesions, mainly in sun-exposed skin that ultimately healed with severe scars. The skin lesions have been attributed to the phototoxicity associated with the elevated levels of porphyrins. In addition to the dermatological changes, other clinical manifestations included neurologic symptoms, hepatomegaly, enlarged thyroid, splenomegaly, hyperpigmentation, hirsutism, enlarged lymph nodes and painful arthritis of the hands. For many of the clinical symptoms exhibited by the victims of the hexachlorobenzene poisoning incident in Turkey, an immune etiology was considered.

Indeed, the autoimmunogenic potential of hexachlorobenzene has been characterized in a number of laboratory studies, which have been reviewed (Michielsen *et al.*, 1999; Ezendam *et al.*, 2004). The former review emphasized a striking difference in the profile

of activity in rats, where the predominant effect was immune enhancement, and in mice, where the predominant effect was immune suppression (Michielsen *et al.*, 1999). Only the former results will be discussed further in this chapter. Exposure to a variety of strains of rats produced increases in the following types of parameters: peripheral blood counts, serum IgM and IgG levels, autoantibodies, spleen and lymph node weights, marginal zones and follicles of spleens, and primary and secondary antibody responses to tetanus toxoid. Interestingly, exposure to hexachlorobenzene caused opposite effects on two induced autoimmune models in Lewis rats, causing an increase in the severity of experimental allergic encephalomyelitis, and a decrease in the severity of adjuvant arthritis (Michielsen *et al.*, 1999). This finding suggests that comparative studies using different genetically autoimmune-prone models may be needed to investigate the role of xenobiotics in the onset and progression of autoimmunity.

In terms of a possible mechanism of action, Ezendam *et al.* (2004) proposed that after exposure to hexachlorobenzene, its deposition can directly induce cell damage or elicit damage by interfering with the integrity of cell membranes due to its lipophilic nature. Ultimately, hexachlorobenzene exposure triggers pro-inflammatory mediators, such as TNF-α, IL-1, IL-6, reactive oxygen species, and chemokines. These pro-inflammatory mediators serve as adjuvant signals that induce a systemic inflammatory response with influxes of neutrophils and macrophages into various nonimmune and immune organs. Subsequently, this leads to polyclonal activation of T- and B cells, eosinophilia, and eventually to visible clinical effects.

NEW FRONTIERS AND CHALLENGES IN IMMUNOTOXICOLOGY

As noted throughout this chapter, the immune system has unquestionably been identified as a potential target organ for drugs and chemicals. With the demonstration that (1) chemicals can perturb the immune system of animals; (2) perturbation of immune function is correlated with an increased risk of infectious disease; and (3) perturbations in immune function can occur in the absence of any clinically observable effect, attention has focused, and will continue to focus, on the risk to the human population following exposure to chemicals that can alter immune function in animals. In fact, the characterization of the risk associated with xenobiotic-induced immunotoxicity arguably represents one of the key challenges for this discipline in the immediate future.

Risk can be defined as the probability that an adverse event/effect will manifest itself. Risk must also incorporate the hazard, including dose–response relationships, and exposure. Exposure is a function of the amount of chemical involved and the time of its interaction with people and/or the environment. As such, assessment of risk is often an assessment of the probability for exposure. However, most papers in the immunotoxicology literature that are identified as "risk assessment" papers have focused on just one of the above components, most often, hazard identification. Thus, risk assessment in immunotoxicology must still be considered a "New Frontier."

The science of immunotoxicology continues to evolve, and any overview, including this chapter, must consider the discipline as a "snapshot" in time. Just during the period of time since this chapter was last published, immunotoxicology has experienced significant advancement. This, in part, has been driven by the tremendous growth in knowledge within immunology and cell biology coupled with an explosion in methodological and technological capabilities.

New tests reflecting a variety of potential impacts of immunotoxicity have emerged, and traditional tests have been improved. In spite of these advances, significant challenges remaining to be addressed within the discipline of immunotoxicology and include: (1) how to interpret the significance of minor or moderate immunotoxic effects in animal models in relation to human risk assessment; (2) how to better integrate a consideration of exposure, especially to multiple agents simultaneously, into immunotoxicological risk assessment; (3) how to design better human studies to assess the impact on the immune system in the species of greatest interest in the context of risk assessment; (4) how to identify and establish sensitive human biomarkers of immunotoxicity; and (5) how to gain a better understanding of the role of genetics in identifying sensitive subpopulations to immune-altering agents. Many of the challenges identified above are not unique to immunotoxicology, but nevertheless are critical, and will need to be addressed through concerted and systematic efforts to improve human immune testing strategies.

REFERENCES

99-4494 NPN (1999) in National Institute of Environmental Health Sciences NIoH (ed.): *The Murine Local Lymph Node Assay: A Test Method for Assessing the Allergic Contact Dermatitis Potential of Chemicals/Compounds.* U.S. Public Health Service, Department of Health and Human Services.

Aebersold R: Constellations in a cellular universe. *Nature* 422:115–116, 2003.

Ahmed SM, Aw TC, Adisesh A Toxicological and immunological aspects of occupational latex allergy. *Toxicol Rev* 23:123–134, 2004.

Albers R, Broeders A, van der Pijl A, Seinen W, Pieters R: The use of reporter antigens in the popliteal lymph node assay to assess immunomodulation by chemicals. *Toxicol Appl Pharmacol* 143:102–109, 1997.

Allan LL, Mann KK, Matulka RA, Ryu HY, Schlezinger JJ, Sherr DH: Bone marrow stromal-B cell interactions in polycyclic aromatic hydrocarbon-induced pro/pre-B cell apoptosis. *Toxicol Sci* 76:357–365, 2003.

Alonzo NC, Bayer BM: Opioids, immunology, and host defenses of intravenous drug abusers. *Infect Dis Clin North Am* 16:553–569, 2002.

Araneo BA, Dowell T, Moon HB, Daynes RA: Regulation of murine lymphokine production in vivo. Ultraviolet radiation exposure depresses IL-2 and enhances IL-4 production by T cells through an IL-1-dependent mechanism. *J Immunol* 143:1737–1744, 1989.

Aranyi C, O'Shea WJ, Graham JA, Miller FJ: The effects of inhalation of organic chemical air contaminants on murine lung host defenses. *Fundam Appl Toxicol* 6:713–720, 1986.

Arts JH, Droge SC, Spanhaak S, Bloksma N, Penninks AH, Kuper CF: Local lymph node activation and IgE responses in brown Norway and Wistar rats after dermal application of sensitizing and non-sensitizing chemicals. *Toxicology* 117:229–234, 1997.

Auphan N, DiDonato JA, Rosette C, Helmberg A, Karin M: Immunosuppression by glucocorticoids: Inhibition of NF-kappa B activity through induction of I kappa B synthesis. *Science* 270:286–290, 1995.

Ayensu WK, Tchounwou PB, McMurray RW: Molecular and cellular mechanisms associated with autoimmune diseases. *Int J Environ Res Public Health* 1:39–73, 2004.

Baccarelli A, Mocarelli P, Patterson DG, Jr., *et al.*: Immunologic effects of dioxin: New results from Seveso and comparison with other studies. *Environ Health Perspect* 110:1169–1173, 2002.

Ban M, Morel G, Langonne I, Huguet N, Pepin E, Binet S: TDI can induce respiratory allergy with Th2-dominated response in mice. *Toxicology* 218:39–47, 2006.

Basketter DA, Wright ZM, Warbrick EV, *et al.*: Human potency predictions for aldehydes using the local lymph node assay. *Contact Dermatitis* 45:89–94, 2001.

Bernier J, Hugo P, Krzystyniak K, Fournier M: Suppression of humoral immunity in inbred mice by dieldrin. *Toxicol Lett* 35:231–240, 1987.

Bernstein JA, Bernstein IL: Clinical aspects of respiratory hypersensitivity to chemicals, in Dean JH, Luster MI, Munson AE, Kimber I (eds.):

Immunotoxicology and Immunopharmacology. New York: Raven Press, 1994, pp. 617–642.

Bhattacharjee A, Lappi VR, Rutherford MS, Schook LB: Molecular dissection of dimethylnitrosamine (DMN)-induced hepatotoxicity by mRNA differential display. *Toxicol Appl Pharmacol* 150:186–195, 1998.

Biagini RE: Epidemiology studies in immunotoxicity evaluations. *Toxicology* 129:37–54, 1998.

Bigazzi PE: Metals and kidney autoimmunity. *Environ Health Perspect* 107(suppl 5):753–765, 1999.

Bondy GS, Pestka JJ: Immunomodulation by fungal toxins. *J Toxicol Environ Health B Crit Rev* 3:109–143, 2000.

Bradley SG, Munson AE, McCay JA, *et al.*: Subchronic 10 day immunotoxicity of polydimethylsiloxane (silicone) fluid, gel and elastomer and polyurethane disks in female B6C3F1 mice. *Drug Chem Toxicol* 17:175–220, 1994a.

Bradley SG, White KL, Jr., McCay JA, *et al.*: Immunotoxicity of 180 day exposure to polydimethylsiloxane (silicone) fluid, gel and elastomer and polyurethane disks in female B6C3F1 mice. *Drug Chem Toxicol* 17:221–269, 1994b.

Brown JM, Pfau JC, Pershouse MA, Holian A: Silica, apoptosis, and autoimmunity. *J Immunotoxicol* 1:177–188, 2004.

Buckley NE, McCoy KL, Mezey E, *et al.*: Immunomodulation by cannabinoids is absent in mice deficient for the cannabinoid CB(2) receptor. *Eur J Pharmacol* 396:141–149, 2000.

Buehler EV: Delayed contact hypersensitivity in the guinea pig. *Arch Dermatol* 91:171–177, 1965.

Burbach CM, Poland A, Bradfield CA: Cloning of the Ah-receptor cDNA reveals a distinctive ligand-activated transcription factor. *Proc Natl Acad Sci USA* 89:8185–8189, 1992.

Burchiel SW, Kerkvliet NL, Gerberick GF, Lawrence DA, Ladics GS: Assessment of immunotoxicity by multiparameter flow cytometry. *Fundam Appl Toxicol* 38:38–54, 1997.

Burchiel SW, Lauer FT, Gurule D, Mounho BJ, Salas VM: Uses and future applications of flow cytometry in immunotoxicity testing. *Methods* 19:28–35, 1999.

Burleson GR, Lebrec H, Yang YG, Ibanes JD, Pennington KN, Birnbaum LS: Effect of 2,3,7,8-tetrachlorodibenzo-p-dioxin (TCDD) on influenza virus host resistance in mice. *Fundam Appl Toxicol* 29:40–47, 1996.

Burns LA, Bradley SG, White KL, Jr., *et al.*: Immunotoxicity of mononitrotoluenes in female B6C3F1 mice: I. Para-nitrotoluene. *Drug Chem Toxicol* 17:317–358, 1994a.

Burns LA, Bradley SG, White KL, Jr., *et al.*: Immunotoxicity of nitrobenzene in female B6C3F1 mice. *Drug Chem Toxicol* 17:271–315, 1994b.

Burns LA, Bradley SG, White KL, *et al.*: Immunotoxicity of 2,4-diaminotoluene in female B6C3F1 mice. *Drug Chem Toxicol* 17:401–436, 1994c.

Burns LA, LeVier DG, Munson AE: Immunotoxicology of arsenic, in Dean JH, Luster MI, Munson AE, Kimber I (eds.): *Immunotoxicology and Immunopharmacology*. New York: Raven Press, 1994d, pp. 213–225.

Burns LA, McCay JA, Brown R, Munson AE: Arsenic in the sera of gallium arsenide-exposed mice inhibits bacterial growth and increases host resistance. *J Pharmacol Exp Ther* 265:795–800, 1993.

Burns-Naas LA, Mast RW, Meeks RG, Mann PC, Thevenaz P: Inhalation toxicology of decamethylcyclopentasiloxane (D5) following a 3-month nose-only exposure in Fischer 344 rats. *Toxicol Sci* 43:230–240, 1998.

Cabral GA and Marciano-Cabral F: Cannabinoid-mediated exacerbation of brain infection by opportunistic amebae. *J Neuroimmunol* 147:127–130, 2004.

Calne RY, Rolles K, White DJ, *et al.*: Cyclosporin-A in clinical organ grafting. *Transplant Proc* 13:349–358, 1981.

Camacho IA, Singh N, Hegde VL, Nagarkatti M, Nagarkatti PS: Treatment of mice with 2,3,7,8-tetrachlorodibenzo-p-dioxin leads to aryl hydrocarbon receptor-dependent nuclear translocation of NF-kappaB and expression of Fas ligand in thymic stromal cells and consequent apoptosis in T cells. *J Immunol* 175:90–103, 2005.

Casale GP, Cohen SD, DiCapua RA: The effects of organophosphate-induced cholinergic stimulation on the antibody response to sheep erythrocytes in inbred mice. *Toxicol Appl Pharmacol* 68:198–205, 1983.

Catania RA and Chaudry IH: Immunological consequences of trauma and shock. *Ann Acad Med Singapore* 28:120–132, 1999.

Chao CC, Molitor TW, Gekker G, Murtaugh MP, Peterson PK: Cocaine-mediated suppression of superoxide production by human peripheral blood mononuclear cells. *J Pharmacol Exp Ther* 256:255–258, 1991.

Chuchawankul S, Shima M, Buckley NE, Hartmann CB, McCoy KL: Role of cannabinoid receptors in inhibiting macrophage costimulatory activity. *Int Immunopharmacol* 4:265–278, 2004.

Chung YJ, Zhou HR, Pestka JJ: Transcriptional and posttranscriptional roles for p38 mitogen-activated protein kinase in upregulation of TNF-alpha expression by deoxynivalenol (vomitoxin). *Toxicol Appl Pharmacol* 193:188–201, 2003.

Coleman JW, Sim E: Autoallergic responses to drugs: Mechanistic aspects, in JH D, MI L, AE M, I K (eds.): *Immunotoxicology and Immunopharmacology*. New York: Raven Press, 1994, pp. 553–572.

Colosio C, Birindelli S, Corsini E, Galli CL, Maroni M: Low level exposure to chemicals and immune system. *Toxicol Appl Pharmacol* 207:320–328, 2005.

Colucci F, Caligiuri MA, Di Santo JP: What does it take to make a natural killer? *Nat Rev Immunol* 3:413–425.

Condie R, Herring A, Koh WS, Lee M, Kaminski NE: Cannabinoid inhibition of adenylate cyclase-mediated signal transduction and interleukin 2 (IL-2) expression in the murine T-cell line, EL4.IL-2. *J Biol Chem* 271:13175–13183, 1996.

Coombs RRA, Gell PGH: Classification of allergic reactions responsible for clinical hypersensitivity and disease, in Gell PGH, Coombs RRA, Lachmann PJ (eds.): *Clinical Aspects of Immunology*. Oxford, England: Oxford University Press, 1975, p. 761.

Cuthill S, Poellinger L, Gustafsson JA: The receptor for 2,3,7,8-tetrachlorodibenzo-p-dioxin in the mouse hepatoma cell line Hepa 1c1c7. *J Biol Chem* 262:3477–3481, 1987.

D'Cruz D: Autoimmune diseases associated with drugs, chemicals and environmental factors. *Toxicol Lett* 112–113:421–432, 2000.

Daniel V, Huber W, Bauer K, Suesal C, Conradt C, Opelz G: Associations of dichlorodiphenyltrichloroethane (DDT) 4.4 and dichlorodiphenyldichloroethylene (DDE) 4.4 blood levels with plasma IL-4. *Arch Environ Health* 57:541–547, 2002.

Davis D, Safe S: Immunosuppressive activities of polychlorinated dibenzofuran congeners: Quantitative structure activity relationships and interactive effects. *Toxicol Appl Pharmacol* 94:141–149, 1988.

de Jong EC, Spanhaak S, Martens BP, Kapsenberg ML, Penninks AH, Wierenga EA: Food allergen (peanut)-specific TH2 clones generated from the peripheral blood of a patient with peanut allergy. *J Allergy Clin Immunol* 98:73–81.

Dean JH, Lauer LD, House RV, *et al.*: Studies of immune function and host resistance in B6C3F1 mice exposed to formaldehyde. *Toxicol Appl Pharmacol* 72:519–529, 1984.

Dean JH, Luster MI, Boorman GA, Lauer LD, Leubke RW, Lawson L: Selective immunosuppression resulting from exposure to the carcinogenic congener of benzopyrene in B6C3F1 mice. *Clin Exp Immunol* 52:199–206, 1983.

Dean JH, Luster MI, Munson AE, Amos H: *Immunotoxicology and Immunopharmacology*. New York: Raven Press, 1985.

Dearman RJ, Basketter DA, Blaikie L, *et al.*: The mouse IgE test: Interlaboratory evaluation and comparison of BALB/c and C57BL/6 strain mice. *Toxicol Meth* 8:69–85, 1998.

Dearman RJ, Betts CJ, Humphreys N, *et al.*: Chemical allergy: Considerations for the practical application of cytokine profiling. *Toxicol Sci* 71:137–145, 2003.

Dearman RJ, Moussavi A, Kemeny DM, Kimber I: Contribution of CD4+ and CD8+ T lymphocyte subsets to the cytokine secretion patterns induced in mice during sensitization to contact and respiratory chemical allergens. *Immunology* 89:502–510, 1996.

Dearman RJ, Spence LM, Kimber I: Characterization of murine immune responses to allergenic diisocyanates. *Toxicol Appl Pharmacol* 112:190–197, 1992.

Dearman RJ, Warbrick EV, Skinner R, Kimber I: Cytokine fingerprinting of chemical allergens: Species comparisons and statistical analyses. *Food Chem Toxicol* 40:1881–1892, 2002.

Delaney B, Strom SC, Collins S, Kaminski NE: Carbon tetrachloride suppresses T-cell-dependent immune responses by induction of transforming growth factor-beta 1. *Toxicol Appl Pharmacol* 126:98–107, 1994.

Demoly P, Michel F, Bousquet J: In vivo methods for study of allergy skin tests, techniques and interpretation, in Middleton EJ, Reed C, Ellis E (eds.): *Allergy Principles and Practice*. St. Louis: Mosby, 1998, pp. 430–439.

Denis M, Cuthill S, Wikstroem AC, Poellinger L, Gustafsson JA: Association of the dioxin receptor with the Mr 90,000 heat shock protein. *Biochem Biophys Res Commun* 155:801–807, 1988.

Deo MG, Gangal S, Bhisey AN, *et al.*: Immunological, mutagenic & genotoxic investigations in gas exposed population of Bhopal. *Indian J Med Res* 86(suppl):63–76, 1987.

Descotes J (ed.): *Immunotoxicology and Drugs and Chemicals*. Amsterdam: Elsevier, 1986.

Descotes J, Ravel G, Ruat C: Vaccines: Predicting the risk of allergy and autoimmunity. *Toxicology* 174:45–51, 2002.

Dewailly E, Ayotte P, Bruneau S, Gingras S, Belles-Isles M, Roy R: Susceptibility to infections and immune status in Inuit infants exposed to organochlorines. *Environ Health Perspect* 108:205–211, 2000.

Dich J, Zahm SH, Hanberg A, Adami HO: Pesticides and cancer. *Cancer Causes Control* 8:420–443, 1997.

Dietert RR, Etzel RA, Chen D, *et al.*: Workshop to identify critical windows of exposure for children's health: Immune and respiratory systems work group summary. *Environ Health Perspect* 108(suppl 3):483–490, 2000.

Dietert RR, Lee JE, Hussain I, Piepenbrink M: Developmental immunotoxicology of lead. *Toxicol Appl Pharmacol* 198:86–94, 2004.

Dietert RR, Piepenbrink MS: Perinatal immunotoxicity: Why adult exposure assessment fails to predict risk. *Environ Health Perspect* 114:477–483, 2006.

Dinda A, Gitman M, Singhal PC: Immunomodulatory effect of morphine: Therapeutic implications. *Expert Opin Drug Saf* 4:669–675, 2005.

Dooley RK, Holsapple MP: Elucidation of cellular targets responsible for tetrachlorodibenzo-*p*-dioxin (TCDD)-induced suppression of antibody responses: I. The role of the B lymphocyte. *Immunopharmacology* 16:167–180, 1988.

Duffield JS: The inflammatory macrophage: A story of Jekyll and Hyde. *Clin Sci (London)* 104:27–38, 2003.

Dunn TJ, Lindahl R, Pitot HC: Differential gene expression in response to 2,3,7,8-tetrachlorodibenzo-*p*-dioxin (TCDD). *J Biol Chem* 263:10878–10886, 1988.

Edwards CJ, Cooper C: Early environmental factors and rheumatoid arthritis. *Clin Exp Immunol* 143:1–5, 2006.

Elferink CJ, Gasiewicz TA, Whitlock JP: Protein–DNA interactions at a dioxin-responsive enhancer. *J Biol Chem* 265:20708–20712, 1990.

Ema M, Sogawa K, Watanabe N, *et al.*: cDNA cloning and structure of mouse putative Ah receptor. *Biochem Biophys Res Commun* 184:246–253, 1992.

Exon JH, Mather GG, Bussiere JL, Olson DP, Talcott PA: Effects of subchronic exposure of rats to 2-methoxyethanol or 2-butoxyethanol: Thymic atrophy and immunotoxicity. *Fundam Appl Toxicol* 16:830–840, 1991.

Ezendam J, Vos JG, Pieters R: Mechanisms of hexachlorobenzene-induced adverse immune effects in Brown Norway rats. *J Immunotoxicol* 1:167–176, 2004.

Farraj AK, Harkema JR, Kaminski NE: Allergic rhinitis induced by intranasal sensitization and challenge with trimellitic anhydride but not with dinitrochlorobenzene or oxazolone in A/J mice. *Toxicol Sci* 79:315–325, 2004.

Farraj AK, Harkema JR, Kaminski NE: Topical application versus intranasal instillation: A qualitative comparison of the effect of the route of sensitization on trimellitic anhydride-induced allergic rhinitis in A/J mice. *Toxicol Sci* 92:321–328, 2006.

Faubert BL, Kaminski NE: AP-1 activity is negatively regulated by cannabinol through inhibition of its protein components, c-fos and c-jun. *J Leukoc Biol* 67:259–266, 2000.

Felter SP, Ryan CA, Basketter DA, Gilmour NJ, Gerberick GF: Application of the risk assessment paradigm to the induction of allergic contact dermatitis. *Regul Toxicol Pharmacol* 37:1–10, 2003.

Feola DJ, Thornton AC, Garvy BA: Effects of antiretroviral therapy on immunity in patients infected with HIV. *Curr Pharm Des* 12:1015–1022, 2006.

Filipov NM, Pinchuk LM, Boyd BL, Crittenden PL: Immunotoxic effects of short-term atrazine exposure in young male C57BL/6 mice. *Toxicol Sci* 86:324–332, 2005.

Fingar DC, Blenis J: Target of rapamycin (TOR): An integrator of nutrient and growth factor signals and coordinator of cell growth and cell cycle progression. *Oncogene* 23:3151–3171, 2004.

Fontenot AP, Maier LA: Genetic susceptibility and immune-mediated destruction in beryllium-induced disease. *Trends Immunol* 26:543–549, 2005.

Frankild S, Volund A, Wahlberg JE, Andersen KE: Comparison of the sensitivities of the Buehler test and the guinea pig maximization test for predictive testing of contact allergy. *Acta Derm Venereol* 80:256–262, 2000.

Fujimaki H, Kurokawa Y, Kunugita N, Kikuchi M, Sato F, Arashidani K: Differential immunogenic and neurogenic inflammatory responses in an allergic mouse model exposed to low levels of formaldehyde. *Toxicology* 197:1–13, 2004.

Fujisawa-Sehara A, Sogawa K, Yamane M, Fujii-Kuriyama Y: Characterization of xenobiotic responsive elements upstream from the drug metabolizing cytochrome P450c gene: A similarity to glucocorticoid response elements. *Nucl Acids Res* 15:4179–4191, 1987.

Funatake CJ, Marshall NB, Steppan LB, Mourich DV, Kerkvliet NI: Cutting edge: Activation of the aryl hydrocarbon receptor by 2,3,7,8-tetrachlorodibenzo-*p*-dioxin generates a population of CD4+ CD25+ cells with characteristics of regulatory T cells. *J Immunol* 175:4184–4188, 2005.

Gad SC, Dunn BJ, Dobbs DW, Reilly C, Walsh RD: Development and validation of an alternative dermal sensitization test: The mouse ear swelling test (MEST). *Toxicol Appl Pharmacol* 84:93–114, 1986.

Gainer JH: Effects of heavy metals and of deficiency of zinc on mortality rates in mice infected with encephalomyocarditis virus. *Am J Vet Res* 38:869–872, 1977.

Galiegue S, Mary S, Marchand J, *et al.*: Expression of central and peripheral cannabinoid receptors in human immune tissues and leukocyte subpopulations. *Eur J Biochem* 232:54–61, 1995.

Galloway T, Handy R: Immunotoxicity of organophosphorous pesticides. *Ecotoxicology* 12:345–363, 2003.

Ganey PE, Luyendyk JP, Maddox JF, Roth RA: Adverse hepatic drug reactions: Inflammatory episodes as consequence and contributor. *Chem Biol Interact* 150:35–51, 2004.

Gao J, Lauer FT, Dunaway S, Burchiel SW: Cytochrome P450 1B1 is required for 7,12-dimethylbenz(a)-anthracene (DMBA) induced spleen cell immunotoxicity. *Toxicol Sci* 86:68–74, 2005a.

Gao J, Voss AA, Pessah IN, Lauer FT, Penning TM, Burchiel SW: Ryanodine receptor-mediated rapid increase in intracellular calcium induced by 7,8-benzo(a)pyrene quinone in human and murine leukocytes. *Toxicol Sci* 87:419–426, 2005b.

Garabrant DH, Dumas C: Epidemiology of organic solvents and connective tissue disease. *Arthritis Res* 2:5–15, 2000.

Garabrant DH, Lacey JV, Jr., Laing TJ, *et al.*: Scleroderma and solvent exposure among women. *Am J Epidemiol* 157:493–500, 2003.

Garrett RW, Gasiewicz TA: The aryl hydrocarbon receptor agonist 2,3,7,8-tetrachlorodibenzo-*p*-dioxin alters the circadian rhythms, quiescence, and expression of clock genes in murine hematopoietic stem and progenitor cells. *Mol Pharmacol* 69:2076–2083, 2006.

Garssen J, van Loveren H: Effects of ultraviolet exposure on the immune system. *Crit Rev Immunol* 21:359–397, 2001.

Garssen J, Vandebriel RJ, van Loveren H: Molecular aspects of UVB-induced immunosuppression. *Arch Toxicol Suppl* 19:97–109, 1997.

Georas SN, Guo J, De Fanis U, Casolaro V: T-helper cell type-2 regulation in allergic disease. *Eur Respir J* 26:1119–1137, 2005.

Germolec D: Autoimmune disease, animal models, in vohr H-W (ed.): *Encyclopedic Reference of Immunotoxicology*. Springer, 2005, pp. 75–79.

Germolec DR, Kashon M, Nyska A, *et al.*: The accuracy of extended histopathology to detect immunotoxic chemicals. *Toxicol Sci* 82:504–514, 2004.

Germolec DR, Kimber I, Goldman L, Selgrade M: Key issues for the assessment of the allergenic potential of genetically modified foods: Breakout group reports. *Environ Health Perspect* 111:1131–1139, 2003.

Glaser R, Sheridan J, Malarkey WB, MacCallum RC, Kiecolt-Glaser JK: Chronic stress modulates the immune response to a pneumococcal pneumonia vaccine. *Psychosom Med* 62:804–807, 2000.

Gleichmann E, Pal ST, Rolink AG, Radasziewicz T, Gleichmann H: Graft versus host reactions: Clues to the etiopathology of a spectrum of immunological diseases. *Immunol Today* 5: 1984.

Gong YY, Egal S, Hounsa A, *et al.*: Determinants of aflatoxin exposure in young children from Benin and Togo, West Africa: the critical role of weaning. *Int J Epidemiol* 32:556–562, 2003.

Good RA: Organization and development of the immune system. Relation to its reconstruction. *Ann NY Acad Sci* 770:8–33, 1995.

Goulding NJ, Guyre PM: Regulation of inflammation by lipocortin 1. *Immunol Today* 13:295–297, 1992.

Grammer LC: Occupational immunologic lung disease, in Patterson R (ed.): *Allergic Diseases, Diagnosis and Management*. Philadelphia: Lippincott, 1985, pp. 691–708,.

Greenlee WF, Dold KM, Irons RD, Osborne R: Evidence for direct action of 2,3,7,8-tetrachlorodibenzo-*p*-dioxin (TCDD) on thymic epithelium. *Toxicol Appl Pharmacol* 79:112–120, 1985.

Greenlee WF, Dold KM, Osborne R: *A Proposed Model for the Actions of TCDD on Epidermal and Thymic Epithelial Target Cells in Poland A*. Cold Spring Harbor: Cold Harbor Spring, 1984.

Grosser T, Fries S, FitzGerald GA: Biological basis for the cardiovascular consequences of COX-2 inhibition: Therapeutic challenges and opportunities. *J Clin Invest* 116:4–15, 2006.

Guo CJ, Li Y, Tian S, Wang X, Douglas SD, Ho WZ: Morphine enhances HIV infection of human blood mononuclear phagocytes through modulation of beta-chemokines and CCR5 receptor. *J Investig Med* 50:435–442, 2002.

Gutting BW, Schomaker SJ, Kaplan AH, Amacher DE: A comparison of the direct and reporter antigen popliteal lymph node assay for the detection of immunomodulation by low molecular weight compounds. *Toxicol Sci* 51:71–79, 1999.

Haggerty HG, Holsapple MP: Role of metabolism in dimethylnitrosamine-induced immunosuppression: a review. *Toxicology* 63:1–23, 1990.

Haggqvist B, Havarinasab S, Bjorn E, Hultman P: The immunosuppressive effect of methylmercury does not preclude development of autoimmunity in genetically susceptible mice. *Toxicology* 208:149–164, 2005.

Hallab NJ, Anderson S, Caicedo M, Skipor A, Campbell P, Jacobs JJ: Immune responses correlate with serum-metal in metal-on-metal hip arthroplasty. *J Arthroplasty* 19:88–93, 2004.

Han YC, Lin TL, Pruett SB: Thymic atrophy caused by ethanol in a mouse model for binge drinking: Involvement of endogenous glucocorticoids. *Toxicol Appl Pharmacol* 123:16–25, 1993.

Handy RD, Abd-El Samei HA, Bayomy MF, *et al.*: Chronic diazinon exposure: Pathologies of spleen, thymus, blood cells, and lymph nodes are modulated by dietary protein or lipid in the mouse. *Toxicology* 172:13–34, 2002.

Happel KI, Nelson S: Alcohol, immunosuppression, and the lung. *Proc Am Thorac Soc* 2:428–432, 2005.

Hata AN, Breyer RM: Pharmacology and signaling of prostaglandin receptors: Multiple roles in inflammation and immune modulation. *Pharmacol Ther* 103:147–166, 2004.

Heidel SM, Czuprynski CJ, Jefcoate CR: Bone marrow stromal cells constitutively express high levels of cytochrome P4501B1 that metabolize 7,12-dimethylbenz[a]anthracene. *Mol Pharmacol* 54:1000–1006, 1998.

Hemdan NY, Emmrich F, Sack U, *et al.*: The in vitro immune modulation by cadmium depends on the way of cell activation. *Toxicology* 222:37–45, 2006.

Herring AC, Koh WS, Kaminski NE: Inhibition of the cyclic AMP signaling cascade and nuclear factor binding to CRE and kappaB elements by cannabinol, a minimally CNS-active cannabinoid. *Biochem Pharmacol* 55:1013–1023, 1998.

Hess EV: Environmental chemicals and autoimmune disease: Cause and effect. *Toxicology* 181–182:65–70, 2002.

Ho S, Clipstone N, Timmermann L, *et al.*: The mechanism of action of cyclosporin A and FK506. *Clin Immunol Immunopathol* 80:S40–S45, 1996.

Hoffman EC, Reyes H, Chu FF, *et al.*: Cloning of a factor required for activity of the Ah (dioxin) receptor. *Science* 252:954–958, 1991.

Hoglund P: Induced peripheral regulatory T cells: The family grows larger. *Eur J Immunol* 36:264–266, 2006.

Holladay S, Smialowicz R: Development of the murine and human immune system: Differential effects of immunotoxicants depent on time of exposure. *Environ Health* 108(Suppl):463–473, 2000.

Holladay SD, Blaylock BL, Comment CE, Heindel JJ, Luster MI: Fetal thymic atrophy after exposure to T-2 toxin: selectivity for lymphoid progenitor cells. *Toxicol Appl Pharmacol* 121:8–14, 1993.

Holladay SD, Comment CE, Kwon J, Luster MI: Fetal hematopoietic alterations after maternal exposure to ethylene glycol monomethyl ether: prolymphoid cell targeting. *Toxicol Appl Pharmacol* 129:53–60, 1994.

Holsapple MP: Immunotoxicity of halogenated aromatic hydrocarbons, in Smialowicz RJ, Holsapple MP (eds.): *Experimental Immunotoxicology*. Boca Raton: CRC Press, 1996, pp. 257–297.

Holsapple MP: Autoimmunity by pesticides: A critical review of the state of the science. *Toxicol Lett* 127:101–109, 2002.

Holsapple MP, Burns-Naas LA, Hastings KL, *et al.*: A proposed testing framework for developmental immunotoxicology (DIT). *Toxicol Sci* 83:18–24, 2005.

Holsapple MP, Dooley RK, McNerney PJ, McCay JA: Direct suppression of antibody responses by chlorinated dibenzodioxins in cultured spleen cells from (C57BL/6 × C3H)F1 and DBA/2 mice. *Immunopharmacology* 12:175–186, 1986.

Holsapple MP, Jones D, Kawabata TT, *et al.*: Assessing the potential to induce respiratory hypersensitivity. *Toxicol Sci* 91:4–13, 2006.

Holsapple MP, Morris DL, Wood SC, Snyder NK: 2,3,7,8-tetrachlorodibenzo-*p*-dioxin-induced changes in immunocompetence: Possible mechanisms. *Annu Rev Pharmacol Toxicol* 31:73–100, 1991a.

Holsapple MP, Munson AE, Munson JA, Bick PH: Suppression of cell-mediated immunocompetence after subchronic exposure to diethylstilbestrol in female B6C3F1 mice. *J Pharmacol Exp Ther* 227:130–138, 1983.

Holsapple MP, Snyder NK, Wood SC, Morris DL: A review of 2,3,7,8-tetrachlorodibenzo-*p*-dioxin-induced changes in immunocompetence: 1991 update. *Toxicology* 69:219–255, 1991b.

Holsapple MP, West LJ, Landreth KS: Species comparison of anatomical and functional immune system development. *Birth Defects Research (Part B)* 68:321–334, 2003.

Holt PG, Upham JW, Sly PD: Contemporaneous maturation of immunologic and respiratory functions during early childhood: Implications for development of asthma prevention strategies. *J Allergy Clin Immunol* 116:16–24, 2005; quiz 25.

House R: Immunotoxicology methods, in Massaro E (ed.): *Handbook of Human Toxicology*. Boca Raton: CRC Press, 1997, pp. 677–708.

House R: Regulatory guidance in immunotoxicology, in Vohr H-W (ed.): *Encyclopedic Reference of Immunotoxicology*. New York: Springer, 2005, pp. 551–555.

House RV, Laurer LD, Murray MJ: Immunological studies in B6C3F1 mice following exposure to ethylene glycol monomethyl ether and its principal metabolite methoxyacetic acid. *Toxicol Appl Pharmacol* 77:358–362, 1985.

Hugo P, Bernier J, Krzystyniak K, Fournier M: Transient inhibition of mixed lymphocyte reactivity by dieldrin in mice. *Toxicol Lett* 41:1–9, 1988a.

Hugo P, Bernier J, Krzystyniak K, Potworowski EF, Fournier M: Abrogation of graft-versus-host reaction by dieldrin in mice. *Toxicol Lett* 41:11–22, 1988b.

Hussain I, Piepenbrink MS, Fitch KJ, Marsh JA, Dietert RR: Developmental immunotoxicity of cyclosporin-A in rats: Age-associated differential effects. *Toxicology* 206:273–284, 2005.

In SW, Son EW, Rhee DK, Pyo S: Methamphetamine administration produces immunomodulation in mice. *J Toxicol Environ Health A* 68:2133–2145, 2005.

IOM: Safety of silicone breast implants, in Bondurant S, Ernster V, Herdman R (eds.). Washington, DC: National Academy Press, 2000.

(IPCS) IPoCS: *Environmental Health Criteria 180: Principles and Methods for Assessing Direct Immunotoxicity Associated with Exposure to Chemicals*, in, World Health Organization, Geneva, Switzerland, 1996.

Islam Z, Harkema JR, Pestka JJ: Satratoxin G from the black mold *Stachbotrys chartarum* evokes olfactory sensory neuron loss and inflammation in the murine nose and brain. *Environ Health Perspect* 114:1099–1107, 2006.

Jeon YJ, Han SH, Yang KH, Kaminski NE: Induction of liver-associated transforming growth factor beta 1 (TGF-beta 1) mRNA expression by carbon tetrachloride leads to the inhibition of T helper 2 cell-associated lymphokines. *Toxicol Appl Pharmacol* 144:27–35, 1997.

Jeong TC, Jordan SD, Matulka RA, Stanulis ED, Park SS, Holsapple MP: Immunosuppression induced by acute exposure to cocaine is dependent on metabolism by cytochrome P-450. *J Pharmacol Exp Ther* 276:1257–1265, 1996.

Jia P, Shi T, Cai Y, Li Y: Demonstration of two novel methods for predicting functional siRNA efficiency. *BMC Bioinformatics* 7:271, 2006.

Jirova D, Sperlingova I, Halaskova M, Bendova H, Dabrowska L: Immunotoxic effects of carbon tetrachloride—the effect on morphology and function of the immune system in mice. *Cent Eur J Public Health* 4:16–20, 1996.

Johnson KW, Kaminski NE, Munson AE: Direct suppression of cultured spleen cell responses by chlordane and the basis for differential effects on in vivo and in vitro immunocompetence. *J Toxicol Environ Health* 22:497–515, 1987a.

Johnson KW, Munson AE, Kim DH, Holsapple MP: Role of reactive metabolites in suppression of humoral immunity by *N*-nitrosodimethylamine. *J Pharmacol Exp Ther* 240:847–855, 1987b.

Kalland T: Alterations of antibody response in female mice after neonatal exposure to diethylstilbestrol. *J Immunol* 124:194–198, 1980.

Kalland T, Strand O, Forsberg JG: Long-term effects of neonatal estrogen treatment on mitogen responsiveness of mouse spleen lymphocytes. *J Natl Cancer Inst* 63:413–421, 1979.

Kamath AB, Camacho I, Nagarkatti PS, Nagarkatti M: Role of Fas-Fas ligand interactions in 2,3,7,8-tetrachlorodibenzo-*p*-dioxin (TCDD)-induced immunotoxicity: Increased resistance of thymocytes from Fas-deficient (lpr) and Fas ligand-defective (gld) mice to TCDD-induced toxicity. *Toxicol Appl Pharmacol* 160:141–155, 1999.

Kaminski NE: Mechanisms of immune modulation by cannabinoids, in Dean JH, Luster MI, Munson AE, Kimber I (eds.): *Immunotoxicology and Immunopharmacology*. New York: Raven Press, 1994, pp. 349–362.

Kaminski NE, Barnes DW, Jordan SD, Holsapple MP: The role of metabolism in carbon tetrachloride-mediated immunosuppression: In vivo studies. *Toxicol Appl Pharmacol* 102:9–20, 1990.

Kaminski NE, Holsapple MP: Cell type responsible for SAA-induced immunosuppression in casein-treated preamyloid mice. *J Immunol* 139:1804–1811, 1987.

Kaminski NE, Jordan SD, Holsapple MP: Suppression of humoral and cell-mediated immune responses by carbon tetrachloride. *Fundam Appl Toxicol* 12:117–128, 1989a.

Kaminski NE, Jordan SD, Page D, Kim BS, Holsapple MP: Suppression of humoral immune responses by dialkylnitrosamines: Structure–activity relationships. *Fundam Appl Toxicol* 12:321–332, 1989b.

Kammuller ME, Thomas C, De Bakker JM, Bloksma N, Seinen W: The popliteal lymph node assay in mice to screen for the immune disregulating potential of chemicals—a preliminary study. *Int J Immunopharmacol* 11:293–300, 1989.

Kaplan BL, Rockwell CE, Kaminski NE: Evidence for cannabinoid receptor-dependent and -independent mechanisms of action in leukocytes. *J Pharmacol Exp Ther* 306:1077–1085, 2003.

Karmaus W, Brooks KR, Nebe T, Witten J, Obi-Osius N, Kruse H: Immune function biomarkers in children exposed to lead and organochlorine compounds: A cross-sectional study. *Environ Health* 4:5, 2005.

Karol MH, Cormier Y, Donham KJ, et al.: Animal models. *Am J Ind Med* 25:135–138, 1994.

Karrow NA, McCay JA, Brown R, Musgrove D, Munson AE, White KL, Jr.: Oxymetholone modulates cell-mediated immunity in male B6C3F1 mice. *Drug Chem Toxicol* 23:621–644, 2000.

Karrow NA, McCay JA, Brown RD, et al.: Oral exposure to atrazine modulates cell-mediated immune function and decreases host resistance to the B16F10 tumor model in female B6C3F1 mice. *Toxicology* 209:15–28, 2005.

Kately JR, Bazzell SJ: Immunological studies in cattle exposed to polybrominated biphenyl. *Environ Health Perspect* 23:750, 1978.

Kawabata TT, White KL, Jr.: Enhancement of in vivo and in vitro murine immune responses by the cyclophosphamide metabolite acrolein. *Cancer Res* 48:41–45, 1988.

Kayama F, Yamashita U, Kawamoto T, Kodama Y: Selective depletion of immature thymocytes by oral administration of ethylene glycol monomethyl ether. *Int J Immunopharmacol* 13:531–540, 1991.

Kerkvliet NI: Recent advances in understanding the mechanisms of TCDD immunotoxicity. *Int Immunopharmacol* 2:277–291, 2002.

Kerkvliet NI, Baecher-Steppan L, Smith BB, Youngberg JA, Henderson MC, Buhler DR: Role of the Ah locus in suppression of cytotoxic T lymphocyte activity by halogenated aromatic hydrocarbons (PCBs and TCDD): Structure–activity relationships and effects in C57Bl/6 mice congenic at the Ah locus. *Fundam Appl Toxicol* 14:532–541, 1990.

Kerkvliet NI, Brauner JA: Flow cytometric analysis of lymphocyte subpopulations in the spleen and thymus of mice exposed to an acute immunosuppressive dose of 2,3,7,8-tetrachlorodibenzo-p-dioxin (TCDD). *Environ Res* 52:146–154, 1990.

Kerkvliet NI, Burleson GR: Immunotoxicity of TCDD and related halogenated aromatic hydrocarbons, in Dean JH, Luster MI, Munson AE, Kimber I (eds.): *Immunotoxicology and Immunopharmacology*. New York: Raven Press, 1994, pp. 97–121.

Kerkvliet NI, Shepherd DM, Baecher-Steppan L: T lymphocytes are direct, aryl hydrocarbon receptor (AhR)-dependent targets of 2,3,7,8-tetrachlorodibenzo-*p*-dioxin (TCDD): AhR expression in both CD4[+] and CD8[+] T cells is necessary for full suppression of a cytotoxic T lymphocyte response by TCDD. *Toxicol Appl Pharmacol* 185:146–152, 2002.

Khvorova A, Reynolds A, Jayasena SD: Functional siRNAs and miRNAs exhibit strand bias. *Cell* 115:209–216, 2003.

Kiecolt-Glaser JK, Glaser R, Gravenstein S, Malarkey WB, Sheridan J: Chronic stress alters the immune response to influenza virus vaccine in older adults. *Proc Natl Acad Sci U S A* 93:3043–3047, 1996.

Kilburn KH, Warshaw RH: Chemical-induced autoimmunity, in (Dean JH, Luster MI, Munson AE, Kimber I (eds.): *Immunotoxicology and Immunopharmacology*. New York: Raven Press, 1994, pp. 523–538.

Kim BS, Smialowicz RJ: The role of metabolism in 2-methoxyethanol-induced suppression of in vitro polyclonal antibody responses by rat and mouse lymphocytes. *Toxicology* 123:227–239, 1997.

Kim DH, Yang KH, Johnson KW, Holsapple MP: Role of the transfer of metabolites from hepatocytes to splenocytes in the suppression of in vitro antibody response by dimethylnitrosamine. *Biochem Pharmacol* 37:2765–2771, 1988.

Kim DO, Lee SK, Jeon TW, et al.: Role of metabolism in parathion-induced hepatotoxicity and immunotoxicity. *J Toxicol Environ Health A* 68:2187–2205, 2005.

Kim J, Jeong H: Suppression of inducible nitric oxide synthase and tumor necrosis a expression by bisphenol A via nuclear factor-κB inactivation in macrophages. *Toxicol Sci* 71:153–154, 2003.

Kimber I, Dearman RJ, Basketter DA, Ryan CA, Gerberick GF: The local lymph node assay: Past, present and future. *Contact Dermatitis* 47:315–328, 2002.

Kishikawa H, Song R, Lawrence DA: Interleukin-12 promotes enhanced resistance to *Listeria monocytogenes* infection of lead-exposed mice. *Toxicol Appl Pharmacol* 147:180–189, 1997.

Klecak G: Identification of contact allergens: Predicitive tests in animals, in Marzulli FN, Maibach HI (eds.): *Dermatotoxicology*. Washington, DC: Hemisphere, 1987, pp. 227–290.

Klykken PC, Galbraith TW, Kolesar GB, et al.: Toxicology and humoral immunity assessment of octamethylcyclotetrasiloxane (D4) following a 28-day whole body vapor inhalation exposure in Fischer 344 rats. *Drug Chem Toxicol* 22:655–677, 1999.

Klykken PC, White KL, Jr.: The adjuvancy of silicones: Dependency on compartmentalization. *Curr Top Microbiol Immunol* 210:113–121, 1996.

Kronenberg M: Toward an understanding of NKT cell biology: Progress and paradoxes. *Annu Rev Immunol* 23:877–900, 2005.

Krzystyniak K, Hugo P, Flipo D, Fournier M: Increased susceptibility to mouse hepatitis virus 3 of peritoneal macrophages exposed to dieldrin. *Toxicol Appl Pharmacol* 80:397–408, 1985.

Ladics GS, Chapin RE, Hastings KL, et al.: Developmental toxicology evaluations—issues with including neurotoxicology and immunotoxicology assessments in reproductive toxicology studies. *Toxicol Sci* 88:24–29, 2005.

Ladics GS, Kawabata TT, Munson AE, White KL, Jr.: Generation of 7,8-dihydroxy-9,10-epoxy-7,8,9,10-tetrahydrobenzo[a]pyrene by murine splenic macrophages. *Toxicol Appl Pharmacol* 115:72–79, 1992a.

Ladics GS, Kawabata TT, Munson AE, White KL, Jr.: Metabolism of benzo[a]pyrene by murine splenic cell types. *Toxicol Appl Pharmacol* 116:248–257, 1992b.

Ladics GS, Kawabata TT, White KL, Jr.: Suppression of the in vitro humoral immune response of mouse splenocytes by 7,12-dimethylbenz[a]anthracene metabolites and inhibition of immunosuppression by alpha-naphthoflavone. *Toxicol Appl Pharmacol* 110:31–44, 1991.

Ladics GS, Smith C, Elliott GS, Slone TW, Loveless SE: Further evaluation of the incorporation of an immunotoxicological functional assay for assessing humoral immunity for hazard identification purposes in rats in a standard toxicology study. *Toxicology* 126:137–152, 1998a.

Ladics GS, Smith C, Heaps K, Elliott GS, Slone TW, Loveless SE: Possible incorporation of an immunotoxicological functional assay for assessing humoral immunity for hazard identification purposes in rats on standard toxicology study. *Toxicology* 96:225–238, 1995.

Ladics GS, Smith C, Heaps K, Loveless SE: Evaluation of the humoral immune response of CD rats following a 2-week exposure to the pesticide carbaryl by the oral, dermal, or inhalation routes. *J Toxicol Environ Health* 42:143–156, 1994.

Ladics GS, Smith C, Nicastro SC, Loveless SE, Cook JC, O'Connor JC: Evaluation of the primary humoral immune response following exposure of male rats to 17beta-estradiol or flutamide for 15 days. *Toxicol Sci* 46:75–82, 1998b.

Lall SB, Dan G: Role of corticosteroids in cadmium induced immunotoxicity. *Drug Chem Toxicol* 22:401–409, 1999.

Lawrence BP, Leid M, Kerkvliet NI: Distribution and behavior of the Ah receptor in murine T lymphocytes. *Toxicol Appl Pharmacol* 138:275–284, 1996.

Lawrence DA, McCabe MJ, Jr.: Immunomodulation by metals. *Int Immunopharmacol* 2:293–302, 2002.

Lee E, Sinha AA: T cell targeted immunotherapy for autoimmune disease. *Autoimmunity* 38:577–596, 2005.

Lee MH, Chung SW, Kang BY, *et al.*: Enhanced interleukin-4 production in CD4$^+$ T cells and elevated immunoglobulin E levels in antigen-primed mice by bisphenol A and nonylphenol, endocrine disruptors: involvement of nuclear factor-AT and Ca2$^+$. *Immunology* 109:76–86, 2003.

Leevy CB, Elbeshbeshy HA: Immunology of alcoholic liver disease. *Clin Liver Dis* 9:55–66, 2005.

Lemarie A, Morzadec C, Merino D, Micheau O, Fardel O, Vernhet L: Arsenic trioxide induces apoptosis of human monocytes during macrophagic differentiation through nuclear factor-kappaB-related survival pathway down-regulation. *J Pharmacol Exp Ther* 316:304–314, 2006.

LeVier DG, McCay JA, Stern ML, *et al.*: Immunotoxicological profile of morphine sulfate in B6C3F1 female mice. *Fundam Appl Toxicol* 22:525–542, 1994.

Levy MH, Wheelock EF: Effects of intravenous silica on immune and non-immune functions of the murine host. *J Immunol* 115:41–48, 1975.

Limpens J, Garssen J, Scheper RJ: Local administration of cytostatic drugs enhances delayed-type hypersensitivity to Sendai virus in mice. *Clin Immunol Immunopathol* 54:161–165, 1990.

Limpens J, Scheper RJ: Inhibition of T suppressor cell function by local administration of an active cyclophosphamide derivative at the sensitization site. *Clin Exp Immunol* 84:383–388, 1991.

Looney RJ, Frampton MW, Byam J, *et al.*: Acute respiratory exposure of human volunteers to octamethylcyclotetrasiloxane (D4): Absence of immunological effects. *Toxicol Sci* 44:214–220, 1998.

Lu T, Newton C, Perkins I, Friedman H, Klein TW: Cannabinoid treatment suppresses the T helper cell polarizing function of mouse dendritic cells stimulated with Legionella pneumophila infection. *J Pharmacol Exp Ther* 2006.

Luebke RW, Chen DH, Dietert R, Yang Y, King M, Luster MI: The comparative immunotoxicity of five selected compounds following developmental or adult exposure. *J Toxicol Environ Health B Crit Rev* 9:1–26, 2006a.

Luebke RW, Holsapple MP, Ladics GS, *et al.*: Immunotoxicogenomics: The potential of genomics technology in the immunotoxicity risk assessment process. *Toxicol Sci* 2006b.

Luebke RW, Parks C, Luster MI: Suppression of immune function and susceptibility to infections in humans: Association of immune function with clinical disease. *J Immunotoxicol* 1:15–24, 2004.

Lundberg K, Grovnick K, Goldschmidt TJ: 2,3,7,8-tetrachlorodibenzo-*p*-dioxin (TCDD) alters intrathymic T cell development in mice. *Chem Biol Interact* 74:179, 1990.

Lundblad LK, Irvin CG, Adler A, Bates JH: A reevaluation of the validity of unrestrained plethysmography in mice. *J Appl Physiol* 93:1198–1207, 2002.

Luster MI, Boorman GA, Dean JH: Effect of in utero exposure of diethylstilbestrol on the immune response in mice. *Toxicol Appl Pharmacol* 47:287–293, 1979.

Luster MI, Boorman GA, Dean JH, Luebke RW, Lawson LD: The effect of adult exposure to diethylstilbestrol in the mouse: Alterations in immunological functions. *J Reticuloendothel Soc* 28:561–569, 1980.

Luster MI, Dean JH, Germolec DR: Consensus workshop on methods to evaluate developmental immunotoxicity. *Environ Health Perspect* 111:579–583, 2003.

Luster MI, Faith RE, Kimmel CA: Depression of humoral immunity in rats following chronic developmental lead exposure. *J Environ Pathol Toxicol* 1:397–402, 1978.

Luster MI, Germolec DR, White KL, Jr., *et al.*: A comparison of three nucleoside analogs with anti-retroviral activity on immune and hematopoietic functions in mice: In vitro toxicity to precursor cells and microstromal environment. *Toxicol Appl Pharmacol* 101:328–339, 1989.

Luster MI, Hayes HT, Korach K, *et al.*: Estrogen immunosuppression is regulated through estrogenic responses in the thymus. *J Immunol* 133:110–116, 1984.

Luster MI, Johnson VJ, Yucesoy B, Simeonova PP: Biomarkers to assess potential developmental immunotoxicity in children. *Toxicol Appl Pharmacol* 206:229–236, 2005.

Luster MI, Munson AE, Thomas PT, *et al.*: Development of a testing battery to assess chemical-induced immunotoxicity: National Toxicology Program's guidelines for immunotoxicity evaluation in mice. *Fundam Appl Toxicol* 10:2–19, 1988.

Luster MI, Portier C, Pait DG, *et al.*: Risk assessment in immunotoxicology. II. Relationships between immune and host resistance tests. *Fundam Appl Toxicol* 21:71–82, 1993.

Luster MI, Portier C, Pait DG, *et al.*: Risk assessment in immunotoxicology. I. Sensitivity and predictability of immune tests. *Fundam Appl Toxicol* 18:200–210, 1992.

Luster MI, Tucker JA, Germolec DR: Immunotoxicity studies in mice exposed to methyl isocyanate. *Toxicol Appl Pharmacol* 86:140–144, 1986.

Lynes MA, Fontenot AP, Lawrence DA, Rosenspire AJ, Pollard KM: Gene expression influences on metal immunomodulation. *Toxicol Appl Pharmacol* 210:9–16, 2006.

Magnusson B, Kligman AM: The identification of contact allergens by animal assay. The guinea pig maximization test. *J Invest Dermatol* 52:268–276, 1969.

Maibach H: Formaldehyde: Effects on animal and human skin, in Gibson J (ed.): *Formaldehyde Toxicity*. Washington, DC: Hemisphere, 1983, pp. 166–174.

Marnell L, Mold C, Du Clos TW: C-reactive protein: Ligands, receptors and role in inflammation. *Clin Immunol* 117:104–111, 2005.

Marzulli FN, Maibach HI: Contact allergy: Predictive testing in humans, in Marzulli FN, Maibach HI (eds.): *Dermatotoxicology*. Washington, DC: Hemishpere, 1987, pp. 319–340.

Matheson JM, Johnson VJ, Vallyathan V, Luster MI: Exposure and immunological determinants in a murine model for toluene diisocyanate (TDI) asthma. *Toxicol Sci* 84:88–98, 2005.

Matulka RA, Jordan SD, Stanulis ED, Holsapple MP: Evaluation of sex- and strain-dependency of cocaine-induced immunosuppression in B6C3F1 and DBA/2 mice. *J Pharmacol Exp Ther* 279:12–17, 1996.

Matveyeva M, Hartmann CB, Harrison MT, Cabral GA, McCoy KL: Delta(9)-tetrahydrocannabinol selectively increases aspartyl cathepsin D proteolytic activity and impairs lysozyme processing by macrophages. *Int J Immunopharmacol* 22:373–381, 2000.

Maurice T and Romieu P: Involvement of the sigma1 receptor in the appetitive effects of cocaine. *Pharmacopsychiatry* 37(Suppl 3):S198–S207, 2004.

McCabe MJJ: Mechanisms and consequences of immunomodulation by lead, in Dean JH, Luster MI, Munson AE, Kimber I (eds.): *Immunotoxicology and Immunopharmacology*. New York: Raven Press, 1994, pp. 143–162.

McCoy KL, Gainey D, Cabral GA: delta 9-Tetrahydrocannabinol modulates antigen processing by macrophages. *J Pharmacol Exp Ther* 273:1216–1223, 1995.

McDonough RJ, Madden JJ, Falek A, *et al.*: Alteration of T and null lymphocyte frequencies in the peripheral blood of human opiate addicts: In vivo evidence for opiate receptor sites on T lymphocytes. *J Immunol* 125:2539–2543, 1980.

McKallip RJ, Nagarkatti M, Nagarkatti PS: Immunotoxicity of AZT: inhibitory effect on thymocyte differentiation and peripheral T cell responsiveness to gp120 of human immunodeficiency virus. *Toxicol Appl Pharmacol* 131:53–62, 1995.

McKarns SC, Kaminski NE: TGF-beta 1 differentially regulates IL-2 expression and [^{3}H]-thymidine incorporation in CD3 epsilon mAb- and CD28 mAb-activated splenocytes and thymocytes. *Immunopharmacology* 48:101–115, 2000.

McKarns SC, Schwartz RH, Kaminski NE: Smad3 is essential for TGF-beta 1 to suppress IL-2 production and TCR-induced proliferation, but not IL-2-induced proliferation. *J Immunol* 172:4275–4284, 2004.

Menna JH, Barnett JB, Soderberg LS: Influenza type A virus infection of mice exposed in utero to chlordane; survival and antibody studies. *Toxicol Lett* 24:45–52, 1985.

Michielsen CC, van Loveren H, Vos JG: The role of the immune system in hexachlorobenzene-induced toxicity. *Environ Health Perspect* 107(suppl 5):783–792, 1999.

Miller K, Brown RC: The immune system and asbestos-associated disease, in Dean JH, Luster MI, Munson AE, Amos H (eds.): *Immunotoxicology and Immunopharmacology*. New York: Raven Press, 1985, pp. 429–440.

Mishell RI, Dutton RW: Immunization of dissociated mouse spleen cell culture from normal mice. *J Exp Med* 126:423–442, 1967.

Mitzner W, Tankersley C: Interpreting Penh in mice. *J Appl Physiol* 94:828–831, 2003; author reply 831–822.

Moed H, von Blomberg BM, Bruynzeel DP, Scheper RJ, Gibbs S, Rustemeyer T: Regulation of nickel-induced T-cell responsiveness by CD4$^+$CD25$^+$ cells in contact allergic patients and healthy individuals. *Contact Dermatitis* 53:71–74, 2005.

Mondal TK, Li D, Swami K, Dean JK, Hauer C, Lawrence DA: Mercury impairment of mouse thymocyte survival in vitro: Involvement of cellular thiols. *J Toxicol Environ Health A* 68:535–556, 2005.

Moon Y, Pestka JJ: Vomitoxin-induced cyclooxygenase-2 gene expression in macrophages mediated by activation of ERK and p38 but not JNK mitogen-activated protein kinases. *Toxicol Sci* 69:373–382, 2002.

Morandell S, Stasyk T, Grosstessner-Hain K, *et al.*: Phosphoproteomics strategies for the functional analysis of signal transduction. *Proteomics* 2006.

Morice WG, Brunn GJ, Wiederrecht G, Siekierka JJ, Abraham RT: Rapamycin-induced inhibition of p34cdc2 kinase activation is associated with G1/S-phase growth arrest in T lymphocytes. *J Biol Chem* 268:3734–3738, 1993.

Mosmann TR, Coffman RL: Heterogeneity of cytokine secretion patterns and functions of helper T cells. *Adv Immunol* 46:111–147, 1989.

Mosmann TR, Schumacher JH, Street NF, *et al.*: Diversity of cytokine synthesis and function of mouse CD4$^+$ T cells. *Immunol Rev* 123:209–229, 1991.

Mounho BJ, Burchiel SW: Alterations in human B cell calcium homeostasis by polycyclic aromatic hydrocarbons: Possible associations with cytochrome P450 metabolism and increased protein tyrosine phosphorylation. *Toxicol Appl Pharmacol* 149:80–89, 1998.

Murante FG, Gasiewicz TA: Hemopoietic progenitor cells are sensitive targets of 2,3,7,8-tetrachlorodibenzo-*p*-dioxin in C57BL/6J mice. *Toxicol Sci* 54:374–383, 2000.

Mydlarski P, Katz A, Sauder D: Contact dermatitis, in Middleton EJ, Reed C, Ellis E (eds.): *Allergy Principles and Practice*. St. Louis: Mosby, 1998, pp. 1141–1143.

Myers MJ, Schook LB: Immunotoxicity of nitrosamines, in Smialowicz RJ, Holsapple MP (eds.): *Experimental Immunotoxicology*. Boca Raton: CRC Press, 1996, pp. 351–366.

Nathan C: Neutrophils and immunity: Challenges and opportunities. *Nat Rev Immunol* 6:173–182, 2006.

Ndebele K, Tchounwou PB, McMurray RW: Coumestrol, bisphenol-A, DDT, and TCDD modulation of interleukin-2 expression in activated CD^{+4} Jurkat T cells. *Int J Environ Res Public Health* 1:3–11, 2004.

Neishabouri EZ, Hassan ZM, Azizi E, Ostad SN: Evaluation of immunotoxicity induced by diazinon in C57bl/6 mice. *Toxicology* 196:173–179, 2004.

Newton CA, Klein TW, Friedman H: Secondary immunity to *Legionella pneumophila* and Th1 activity are suppressed by delta-9-tetrahydrocannabinol injection. *Infect Immun* 62:4015–4020, 1994.

Nohara K, Izumi H, Tamura S, Nagata R, Tohyama C: Effect of low-dose 2,3,7,8-tetrachlorodibenzo-*p*-dioxin (TCDD) on influenza A virus-induced mortality in mice. *Toxicology* 170:131–138, 2002.

Nunez GM, Estrada I, Calderon-Aranda ES: DDT inhibits the functional activation of murine macrophages and decreases resistance to infection by *Mycobacterium microti*. *Toxicology* 174:201–210, 2002.

Okey AB, Bondy GP, Mason M, *et al.*: Temperature-dependent cytosol-to-nuclear translocation of the Ah receptor for 2,3,7,8-tetrachlorodibenzo-*p*-dioxin in continuous cell culture lines. *J Biol Chem* 255:11415–11422, 1980.

Olgun S, Gogal RM, Jr., Adeshina F, Choudhury H, Misra HP: Pesticide mixtures potentiate the toxicity in murine thymocytes. *Toxicology* 196:181–195, 2004.

Ou DW, Shen ML, Luo YD: Effects of cocaine on the immune system of Balb/C mice. *Clin Immunol Immunopathol* 52:305–312, 1989.

Page GG: Immunologic effects of opioids in the presence or absence of pain. *J Pain Symptom Manage* 29:S25–S31, 2005.

Page TJ, O'Brien S, Holston K, MacWilliams PS, Jefcoate CR, Czuprynski CJ: 7,12-Dimethylbenz[a]anthracene-induced bone marrow toxicity is p53-dependent. *Toxicol Sci* 74:85–92, 2003.

Palmer K, Burks W: Current developments in peanut allergy. *Curr Opin Allergy Clin Immunol* 6:202–206, 2006.

Pathak N, Khandelwal S: Oxidative stress and apoptotic changes in murine splenocytes exposed to cadmium. *Toxicology* 220:26–36, 2006.

Patterson R, Vega L, Trouba K, Bortner C, Germolec D: Arsenic-induced alterations in the contact hypersensitivity response in Balb/c mice. *Toxicol Appl Pharmacol* 198:434–443, 2004.

Pauluhn J: Animal models for respiratory hypersensitivity, in Vohr H-W (ed.): *Encyclopedic Reference of Immunotoxicology*. New York: Springer, 2005, pp. 15–21.

Peden-Adams MM, Eudaly JG, Heesemann LM, *et al.*: Developmental immunotoxicity of trichloroethylene (TCE): studies in B6C3F1 mice. *J Environ Sci Health A Tox Hazard Subst Environ Eng* 41:249–271, 2006.

Pelletier L, Castedo M, Bellon B, Druet P: Mercury and autoimmunity, in Dean JH, Luster MI, Munson AE, Kimber I (eds.): *Immunotoxicology and Immunopharmacology*. New York: Raven Press, 1994, pp. 539–552.

Pelletier M, Roberge CJ, Gauthier M, Vandal K, Tessier PA, Girard D: Activation of human neutrophils in vitro and dieldrin-induced neutrophilic inflammation in vivo. *J Leukoc Biol* 70:367–373, 2001.

Peng X, Mosser DM, Adler MW, Rogers TJ, Meissler JJ, Jr., Eisenstein TK: Morphine enhances interleukin-12 and the production of other pro-inflammatory cytokines in mouse peritoneal macrophages. *J Leukoc Biol* 68:723–728, 2000.

Perdew GH: Association of the Ah receptor with the 90-kDa heat shock protein. *J Biol Chem* 263:13802–13805, 1988.

Pessah IN, Beltzner C, Burchiel SW, Sridhar G, Penning T, Feng W: A bioactive metabolite of benzo[a]pyrene, benzo[a]pyrene-7,8-dione, selectively alters microsomal Ca^{2+} transport and ryanodine receptor function. *Mol Pharmacol* 59:506–513, 2001.

Pestka JJ: Deoxynivalenol-induced IgA production and IgA nephropathy-aberrant mucosal immune response with systemic repercussions. *Toxicol Lett* 140–141:287–295, 2003.

Pestka JJ, Yan D, King LE: Flow cytometric analysis of the effects of in vitro exposure to vomitoxin (deoxynivalenol) on apoptosis in murine T, B and IgA$^+$ cells. *Food Chem Toxicol* 32:1125–1136, 1994.

Peterson PK, Gekker G, Chao CC, Schut R, Molitor TW, Balfour HH, Jr.: Co-caine potentiates HIV-1 replication in human peripheral blood mononuclear cell cocultures. Involvement of transforming growth factor-beta. *J Immunol* 146:81–84, 1991.

Pichler WJ: Drug-induced autoimmunity. *Curr Opin Allergy Clin Immunol* 3:249–253, 2003.

Pieters R, Albers R: Screening tests for autoimmune-related immunotoxicity. *Environ Health Perspect* 107(Suppl 5):673–677, 1999.

Plitnick LM, Loveless SE, Ladics GS, Holsapple MP, Selgrade MJ, Sailstad DM and Smialowicz RJ (2002) Cytokine profiling for chemical sensitizers: application of the ribonuclease protection assay and effect of dose. *Toxicol Appl Pharmacol* 179:145–154.

Plitnick LM, Loveless SE, Ladics GS, *et al.*: Identifying airway sensitizers: Cytokine mRNA profiles induced by various anhydrides. *Toxicology* 193:191–201, 2003.

Plitnick LM, Loveless SE, Ladics GS, *et al.*: Cytokine mRNA profiles for isocyanates with known and unknown potential to induce respiratory sensitization. *Toxicology* 207:487–499, 2005.

Polanczyk MJ, Carson BD, Subramanian S, *et al.*: Cutting edge: Estrogen drives expansion of the CD4$^+$CD25$^+$ regulatory T cell compartment. *J Immunol* 173:2227–2230, 2004.

Poland A, Knutson JC: 2,3,7,8-tetrachlorodibenzo-*p*-dioxin and related aromatic hydrocarbons: Examination of the mechanism of toxicity. *Annu Rev Pharmacol Toxicol* 22:517–554, 1982.

Pollenz RS, Sattler CA, Poland A: The aryl hydrocarbon receptor and aryl hydrocarbon receptor nuclear translocator protein show distinct subcellular localizations in Hepa 1c1c7 cells by immunfluorescence microscopy. *Mol Pharmacol* 45:428–438, 1994.

Pongratz IG, Masson GF, Poellinger L: Dual roles of the 90-kDa heat shock protein hsp90 in modulating functional activities of the dioxin receptor. *J Biol Chem* 267:13728–13734, 1992.

Potter M, Rose N: *Immunology of Silicones*. New York: Springer-Verlag, 1996.

Probst MP, Reisz-Porszasz S, Agbunag RV, Ong MS, Hankinson O: Role of the aryl hydrocarbon receptor nuclear translocator protein in aryl hydrocarbon (dioxin) receptor action. *Mol Pharmacol* 44:511–518, 1993.

Pruett SB, Barnes DB, Han YC, Munson AE: Immunotoxicological characteristics of sodium methyldithiocarbamate. *Fundam Appl Toxicol* 18:40–47, 1992a.

Pruett SB, Fan R, Zheng Q: Involvement of three mechanisms in the alteration of cytokine responses by sodium methyldithiocarbamate. *Toxicol Appl Pharmacol* 213:172–178, 2006.

Pruett SB, Fan R, Zheng Q, Myers LP, Hebert P: Modeling and predicting immunological effects of chemical stressors: Characterization of a quantitative biomarker for immunological changes caused by atrazine and ethanol. *Toxicol Sci* 75:343–354, 2003.

Pruett SB, Han YC, Fuchs BA: Morphine suppresses primary humoral immune responses by a predominantly indirect mechanism. *J Pharmacol Exp Ther* 262:923–928, 1992b.

Pruett SB, Schwab C, Zheng Q, Fan R: Suppression of innate immunity by acute ethanol administration: A global perspective and a new mechanism beginning with inhibition of signaling through TLR3. *J Immunol* 173:2715–2724, 2004a.

Pruett SB, Zheng Q, Fan R, Matthews K, Schwab C: Acute exposure to ethanol affects Toll-like receptor signaling and subsequent responses: An overview of recent studies. *Alcohol* 33:235–239, 2004b.

Pruett SB, Zheng Q, Schwab C, Fan R: Sodium methyldithiocarbamate inhibits MAP kinase activation through toll-like receptor 4, alters cytokine production by mouse peritoneal macrophages, and suppresses innate immunity. *Toxicol Sci* 87:75–85, 2005.

Pyatt DW, Stillman WS, Irons RD: Hydroquinone, a reactive metabolite of benzene, inhibits NF-kappa B in primary human CD4$^+$ T lymphocytes. *Toxicol Appl Pharmacol* 149:178–184, 1998.

Pyatt DW, Zheng JH, Stillman WS, Irons RD: Inorganic lead activates NF-kappa B in primary human CD4$^+$ T lymphocytes. *Biochem Biophys Res Commun* 227:380–385, 1996.

Raisuddin S, Singh KP, Zaidi SI, Paul BN, Ray PK: Immunosuppressive effects of aflatoxin in growing rats. *Mycopathologia* 124:189–194, 1993.

Raulf-Heimsoth M, Merget R, Rihs HP, *et al.*: T-cell receptor repertoire expression in workers with occupational asthma due to platinum salt. *Eur Respir J* 16:871–878, 2000.

Ravel G, Descotes J: Popliteal lymph node assay: Facts and perspectives. *J Appl Toxicol* 25:451–458, 2005.

Ray A, Prefontaine KE: Physical association and functional antagonism between the p65 subunit of transcription factor NF-kappa B and the glucocorticoid receptor. *Proc Natl Acad Sci U S A* 91:752–756, 1994.

Reed A, Dzon L, Loganathan BG, Whalen MM: Immunomodulation of human natural killer cell cytotoxic function by organochlorine pesticides. *Hum Exp Toxicol* 23:463–471, 2004.

Reyes H, Reisz-Porszasz S, Hankinson O: Identification of the Ah receptor nuclear translocator protein (ARNT) as a component of the DNA binding form of the Ah receptor. *Science* 256:1193–1195, 1992.

Ritz B, Heinrich J, Wjst M, Wichmann E, Krause C: Effect of cadmium body burden on immune response of school children. *Arch Environ Health* 53:272–280, 1998.

Robinson MK, Babcock LS, Horn PA, Kawabata TT: Specific antibody responses to subtilisin Carlsberg (Alcalase) in mice: Development of an intranasal exposure model. *Fundam Appl Toxicol* 34:15–24, 1996.

Rockwell CE, Kaminski NE: A cyclooxygenase metabolite of anandamide causes inhibition of interleukin-2 secretion in murine splenocytes. *J Pharmacol Exp Ther* 311:683–690, 2004.

Rockwell CE, Snider NT, Thompson JT, Vanden Heuvel JP, Kaminski NE: Interleukin-2 suppression by 2-arachidonyl glycerol is mediated through peroxisome proliferator-activated receptor {gamma} independently of cannabinoid receptors 1 and 2. *Mol Pharmacol* 70:101–111, 2006.

Rodgers K, Klykken P, Jacobs J, Frondoza C, Tomazic V, Zelikoff J: Immunotoxicity of medical devices. Symposium overview. *Fundam Appl Toxicol* 36:1–14, 1997.

Rodgers KE, Ellefson DD: Modulation of respiratory burst activity and mitogenic response of human peripheral blood mononuclear cells and murine splenocytes and peritoneal cells by malathion. *Fundam Appl Toxicol* 14:309–317, 1990.

Roozendaal R, Carroll MC: Emerging patterns in complement-mediated pathogen recognition. *Cell* 125:29–32, 2006.

Rose NR: 2005Autoimmunity, autoimmune diseases, in Vohr H-W (ed.): *Encyclopedic Reference of Immunotoxicology*. New York: Springer, 2005, pp. 79–82.

Rosen F, Cooper M, Wedgewood R: The primary immunodeficiencies. *N Engl J Med* 333:431–440, 1995.

Roth MD, Whittaker KM, Choi R, Tashkin DP, Baldwin GC: Cocaine and sigma-1 receptors modulate HIV infection, chemokine receptors, and the HPA axis in the huPBL–SCID model. *J Leukoc Biol* 78:1198–1203, 2005.

Rought SE, Yau PM, Chuang LF, Doi RH, Chuang RY: Effect of the chlorinated hydrocarbons heptachlor, chlordane, and toxaphene on retinoblastoma tumor suppressor in human lymphocytes. *Toxicol Lett* 104:127–135, 1999.

Rowe AM, Brundage KM, Schafer R, Barnett JB: Immunomodulatory effects of maternal atrazine exposure on male Balb/c mice. *Toxicol Appl Pharmacol* 214:69–77, 2006.

Roy S, Ramakrishnan S, Loh HH, Lee NM: Chronic morphine treatment selectively suppresses macrophage colony formation in bone marrow. *Eur J Pharmacol* 195:359–363, 1991.

Roy S, Wang J, Gupta S, Charboneau R, Loh HH, Barke RA: Chronic morphine treatment differentiates T helper cells to Th2 effector cells by modulating transcription factors GATA 3 and T-bet. *J Neuroimmunol* 147:78–81, 2004.

Sabers CJ, Martin MM, Brunn GJ, *et al.*: Isolation of a protein target of the FKBP12–rapamycin complex in mammalian cells. *J Biol Chem* 270:815–822, 1995.

Sacerdote P: Effects of in vitro and in vivo opioids on the production of IL-12 and IL-10 by murine macrophages. *Ann NY Acad Sci* 992:129–140, 2003.

Sadakane K, Takano H, Ichinose T, Yanagisawa R, Shibamoto T: Formaldehyde enhances mite allergen-induced eosinophilic inflammation in the murine airway. *J Environ Pathol Toxicol Oncol* 21:267–276, 2002.

Salem ML, Hossain MS, Nomoto K: Mediation of the immunomodulatory effect of beta-estradiol on inflammatory responses by inhibition of recruitment and activation of inflammatory cells and their gene expression of TNF-alpha and IFN-gamma. *Int Arch Allergy Immunol* 121:235–245, 2000.

Sanders VM, Kohm AP: Sympathetic nervous system interaction with the immune system. *Int Rev Neurobiol* 52:17–41, 2002.

Sanders VM, Tucker AN, White KL, Jr., *et al.*: Humoral and cell-mediated immune status in mice exposed to trichloroethylene in the drinking water. *Toxicol Appl Pharmacol* 62:358–368, 1982.

Sanders VM, White KL, Jr., Shopp GM, Jr., Munson AE: Humoral and cell-mediated immune status of mice exposed to 1,1,2-trichloroethane. *Drug Chem Toxicol* 8:357–372, 1985.

Sandy P, Ventura A, Jacks T: Mammalian RNAi: Aa practical guide. *Biotechniques* 39:215–224, 2005.

Sarlo K: Control of occupational asthma and allergy in the detergent industry. *Ann Allergy Asthma Immunol* 90:32–34, 2003.

Sarlo K, Kirchner DB: Occupational asthma and allergy in the detergent industry: New developments. *Curr Opin Allergy Clin Immunol* 2:97–101, 2002.

Sawai C, Anderson K, Walser-Kuntz D: Effect of bisphenol A on murine immune function: Modulation of interferon-gamma, IgG2a, and disease symptoms in NZB × NZW F1 mice. *Environ Health Perspect* 111:1883–1887, 2003.

Schatz AR, Koh WS, Kaminski NE: Delta 9-tetrahydrocannabinol selectively inhibits T-cell dependent humoral immune responses through direct inhibition of accessory T-cell function. *Immunopharmacology* 26:129–137, 1993.

Schatz AR, Lee M, Condie RB, Pulaski JT, Kaminski NE: Cannabinoid receptors CB1 and CB2: A characterization of expression and adenylate cyclase modulation within the immune system. *Toxicol Appl Pharmacol* 142:278–287, 1997.

Scheinman RI, Cogswell PC, Lofquist AK, Baldwin AS, Jr.: Role of transcriptional activation of I kappa B alpha in mediation of immunosuppression by glucocorticoids. *Science* 270:283–286, 1995.

Schule R, Umesono K, Mangelsdorf DJ, Bolado J, Pike JW, Evans RM: Jun-Fos and receptors for vitamins A and D recognize a common response element in the human osteocalcin gene. *Cell* 61:497–504, 1990.

Schwab CL, Fan R, Zheng Q, Myers LP, Hebert P, Pruett SB: Modeling and predicting stress-induced immunosuppression in mice using blood parameters. *Toxicol Sci* 83:101–113, 2005.

Schwarz DS, Hutvagner G, Du T, Xu Z, Aronin N, Zamore PD: Asymmetry in the assembly of the RNAi enzyme complex. *Cell* 115:199–208, 2003.

Schweitzer C, Keller F, Schmitt MP, *et al.*: Morphine stimulates HIV replication in primary cultures of human Kupffer cells. *Res Virol* 142:189–195, 1991.

Selgrade MK: Use of immunotoxicity data in health risk assessments: uncertainties and research to improve the process. *Toxicology* 133:59–72, 1999.

Selgrade MK, Cooper GS, Germolec DR, Heindel JJ: Linking environmental agents and autoimmune disease: An agenda for future research. *Environ Health Perspect* 107 Suppl 5:811–813, 1999.

Selgrade MK, Cooper KD, Devlin RB, van Loveren H, Biagini RE, Luster MI: Immunotoxicity—bridging the gap between animal research and human health effects. *Fundam Appl Toxicol* 24:13–21, 1995.

Selgrade MK, Gilmour MI: Effects of gaseous air pollutants on immune responses and susceptibility to infectious and allergic diseases, in Dean JH, Luster MI, Munson AE, Kimber I (eds.): *Immunotoxicology and Immunopharmacology*. New York: Raven Press, 1994, pp. 395–411.

Selgrade MK, Lemanske RF, Jr., Gilmour MI, *et al.*: Induction of asthma and the environment: What we know and need to know. *Environ Health Perspect* 114:615–619, 2006.

Serhan CN, Savill J: Resolution of inflammation: The beginning programs the end. *Nat Immunol* 6:1191–1197, 2005.

Sgro C: Side-effects of a monoclonal antibody, muromonab CD3/orthoclone OKT3: Bibliographic review. *Toxicology* 105:23–29, 1995.

Sharp BM: Multiple opioid receptors on immune cells modulate intracellular signaling. *Brain Behav Immun* 20:9–14, 2006.

Sherwood RL, O'Shea W, Thomas PT, Ratajczak HV, Aranyi C, Graham JA: Effects of inhalation of ethylene dichloride on pulmonary defenses of mice and rats. *Toxicol Appl Pharmacol* 91:491–496, 1987.

Shopp GM, Jr., Sanders VM, White KL, Jr., Munson AE: Humoral and cell-mediated immune status of mice exposed to trans-1,2-dichloroethylene. *Drug Chem Toxicol* 8:393–407, 1985.

Sikorski EE, Burns LA, Stern ML, Luster MI, Munson AE: Splenic cell targets in gallium arsenide-induced suppression of the primary antibody response. *Toxicol Appl Pharmacol* 110:129–142, 1991.

Silkworth JB, Loose LD: Cell-mediated immunity in mice fed either Aroclor 1016 or hexachlorobenzene. *Toxicol Appl Pharmacol* 45:326–327, 1978.

Silkworth JB, Loose LD: PCB and HCB induced alteration of lymphocyte blastogenesis. *Toxicol Appl Pharmacol* 49:86, 1979.

Simon JC, Cruz PD, Jr., Bergstresser PR, Tigelaar RE: Low dose ultraviolet B-irradiated Langerhans cells preferentially activate CD4+ cells of the T helper 2 subset. *J Immunol* 145:2087–2091, 1990.

Sinigaglia F, Scheidegger D, Garotta G, Scheper R, Pletscher M, Lanzavecchia A: Isolation and characterization of Ni-specific T cell clones from patients with Ni-contact dermatitis. *J Immunol* 135:3929–3932, 1985.

Sleijffers A, Garssen J, Vos JG, Van Loveren H: Ultraviolet light and resistance to infectious diseases. *J Immunol* 1:3–14, 2004.

Smialowicz RJ, Riddle MM, Luebke RW, *et al.*: Immunotoxicity of 2-methoxyethanol following oral administration in Fischer 344 rats. *Toxicol Appl Pharmacol* 109:494–506, 1991a.

Smialowicz RJ, Riddle MM, Rogers RR, Copeland CB, Luebke RW, Andrews DL: Evaluation of the immunotoxicity of orally administered 2-methoxyacetic acid in Fischer 344 rats. *Fundam Appl Toxicol* 17:771–781, 1991b.

Smialowicz RJ, Simmons JE, Luebke RW, Allis JW: Immunotoxicologic assessment of subacute exposure of rats to carbon tetrachloride with comparison to hepatotoxicity and nephrotoxicity. *Fundam Appl Toxicol* 17:186–196, 1991c.

Spyker-Cranmer JM, Barnett JB, Avery DL, Cranmer MF: Immunoteratology of chlordane: Cell-mediated and humoral immune responses in adult mice exposed in utero. *Toxicol Appl Pharmacol* 62:402–408, 1982.

Stanulis ED, Jordan SD, Rosecrans JA, Holsapple MP: Disruption of Th1/Th2 cytokine balance by cocaine is mediated by corticosterone. *Immunopharmacology* 37:25–33, 1997a.

Stanulis ED, Matulka RA, Jordan SD, Rosecrans JA, Holsapple MP: Role of corticosterone in the enhancement of the antibody response after acute cocaine administration. *J Pharmacol Exp Ther* 280:284–291, 1997b.

Staples JE, Gasiewicz TA, Fiore NC, Lubahn DB, Korach KS, Silverstone AE: Estrogen receptor alpha is necessary in thymic development and estradiol-induced thymic alterations. *J Immunol* 163:4168–4174, 1999.

Starec M, Rouveix B, Sinet M, *et al.*: : Immune status and survival of opiate- and cocaine-treated mice infected with Friend virus. *J Pharmacol Exp Ther* 259:745–750, 1991.

Street JC: Pesticides and the immune system, in Sharma RP (ed.): *Immunologic Considerations in Toxicology*. Boca Raton: CRC Press, 1981, pp. 46–66.

Sulentic CE, Holsapple MP, Kaminski NE: Putative link between transcriptional regulation of IgM expression by 2,3,7,8-tetrachlorodibenzo-*p*-dioxin and the aryl hydrocarbon receptor/dioxin-responsive enhancer signaling pathway. *J Pharmacol Exp Ther* 295:705–716, 2000.

Sulentic CE, Kang JS, Na YJ, Kaminski NE: Interactions at a dioxin responsive element (DRE) and an overlapping kappaB site within the hs4 domain of the 3′alpha immunoglobulin heavy chain enhancer. *Toxicology* 200:235–246, 2004a.

Sulentic CE, Zhang W, Na YJ, Kaminski NE: 2,3,7,8-tetrachlorodibenzo-*p*-dioxin, an exogenous modulator of the 3′alpha immunoglobulin heavy chain enhancer in the CH12.LX mouse cell line. *J Pharmacol Exp Ther* 309:71–78, 2004b.

Sutter TR, Greenlee WF: Classification of members of the Ah gene battery. *Chemosphere* 25:223, 1992.

Sweet LI, Zelikoff JT: Toxicology and immunotoxicology of mercury: A comparative review in fish and humans. *J Toxicol Environ Health B Crit Rev* 4:161–205, 2001.

Taggart BR, Harrington P, Hollingshead M: HIV hollow fiber SCID model for antiviral therapy comparison with SCID/hu model. *Antiviral Res* 63:1–6, 2004.

Tarkowski M, Lutz W, Birindelli S: The lymphocytic cholinergic system and its modulation by organophosphorus pesticides. *Int J Occup Med Environ Health* 17:325–337, 2004.

Taylor AD, Christian HC, Morris JF, Flower RJ, Buckingham JC: An anti-sense oligodeoxynucleotide to lipocortin 1 reverses the inhibitory actions of dexamethasone on the release of adrenocorticotropin from rat pituitary tissue in vitro. *Endocrinology* 138:2909–2918, 1997.

Taylor DD, Akyol S, Gercel-Taylor C: Pregnancy-associated exosomes and their modulation of T cell signaling. *J Immunol* 176:1534–1542, 2006.

ten Tusscher GW, Steerenberg PA, van Loveren H, et al.: Persistent hematologic and immunologic disturbances in 8-year-old Dutch children associated with perinatal dioxin exposure. *Environ Health Perspect* 111:1519–1523, 2003.

Terada N, Lucas JJ, Szepesi A, Franklin RA, Domenico J, Gelfand EW: Rapamycin blocks cell cycle progression of activated T cells prior to events characteristic of the middle to late G1 phase of the cycle. *J Cell Physiol* 154:7–15, 1993.

Thomas PT, Ratajczak HV, Aranyi C, Gibbons R, Fenters JD: Evaluation of host resistance and immune function in cadmium-exposed mice. *Toxicol Appl Pharmacol* 80:446–456, 1985.

Thomsen M, Yacoub-Youssef H, Marcheix B: Reconstitution of a human immune system in immunodeficient mice: models of human alloreaction in vivo. *Tissue Antigens* 66:73–82, 2005.

Thorne PS, Hawk C, Kaliszewski SD, Guiney PD: The noninvasive mouse ear swelling assay. I. Refinements for detecting weak contact sensitizers. *Fundam Appl Toxicol* 17:790–806, 1991.

Thurmond LM, Dean JH: Immunological responses following inhalation exposure to chemical hazards, in E GE, Crapo JD, Massaro EJ (eds.): *Toxicology of the Lung*. New York: Raven Press, 1988, pp. 375–406.

Tognoni G, Boniccorsi A: Epidemiological problems with TCDD. A critical review. *Drug Metab Rev* 13:447–469, 1982.

Tryphonas H, Bondy G, Hodgen M, et al.: Effects of cis-nonachlor, trans-nonachlor and chlordane on the immune system of Sprague–Dawley rats following a 28-day oral (gavage) treatment. *Food Chem Toxicol* 41:107–118, 2003.

Tryphonas H, Luster MI, Schiffman G, et al.: Effect of chronic exposure of PCB (Aroclor 1254on specific and nonspecific immune parameters in the rhesus (Macaca mulatta) monkey. *Fundam Appl Toxicol* 16:773–786, 1991a.

Tryphonas H, Luster MI, White KL, Jr., et al.: Effects of PCB (Aroclor 1254on non-specific immune parameters in rhesus (*Macaca mulatta*) monkeys. *Int J Immunopharmacol* 13:639–648, 1991b.

van den Berg FA, Baken KA, Vermeulen JP, Gremmer ER, van Steeg H, van Loveren H: Use of the local lymph node assay in assessment of immune function. *Toxicology* 211:107–114, 2005.

Van Loveren H, De Jong WH, Vandebriel RJ, Vos JG, Garssen J: Risk assessment and immunotoxicology. *Toxicol Lett* 102–103:261–265, 1998.

van Loveren H, Goettsch W, Slob W, Garssen J: Risk assessment of the harmful effects of UVB radiation on the immunological resistance to infectious diseases. *Arch Toxicol Suppl* 18:21–28, 1995.

Van Loveren H, Krajnc EI, Rombout PJ, Blommaert FA, Vos JG: Effects of ozone, hexachlorobenzene, and bis(tri-n-butyltin)oxide on natural killer activity in the rat lung. *Toxicol Appl Pharmacol* 102:21–33, 1990.

Van Loveren H, Piersma A: Immunotoxicological consequences of perinatal chemical exposures. *Toxicol Lett* 149:141–145, 2004.

Van Loveren H, Van Amsterdam JG, Vandebriel RJ, et al.: Vaccine-induced antibody responses as parameters of the influence of endogenous and environmental factors. *Environ Health Perspect* 109:757–764, 2001.

Vandebriel RJ, Spiekstra SW, Hudspith BN, Meredith C, Van Loveren H: In vitro exposure effects of cyclosporin A and bis(tri-n-butyltin)oxide

on lymphocyte proliferation, cytokine (receptor) mRNA expression, and cell surface marker expression in rat thymocytes and splenocytes. *Toxicology* 135:49–66, 1999.

Varvel SA, Bridgen DT, Tao Q, Thomas BF, Martin BR, Lichtman AH: Delta9-tetrahydrocannbinol accounts for the antinociceptive, hypothermic, and cataleptic effects of marijuana in mice. *J Pharmacol Exp Ther* 314:329–337, 2005.

Vecchi A, Sironi M, Canegrati MA, Recchia M, Garattini S: Immunosuppressive effects of 2,3,7,8-tetrachlorodibenzo-p-dioxin in strains of mice with different susceptibility to induction of aryl hydrocarbon hydroxylase. *Toxicol Appl Pharmacol* 68:434–441, 1983.

Veldman C, Nagel A, Hertl M: Type I regulatory T cells in autoimmunity and inflammatory diseases. *Int Arch Allergy Immunol* 140:174–183, 2006.

Vial T, Choquet-Kastylevsky G, Descotes J: Adverse effects of immunotherapeutics involving the immune system. *Toxicology* 174:3–11, 2002.

Vial T, Descotes J: Immune-mediated side-effects of cytokines in humans. *Toxicology* 105:31–57, 1995.

Vial T, Descotes J: Autoimmune diseases and vaccinations. *Eur J Dermatol* 14:86–90, 2004.

Vorderstrasse BA, Bohn AA, Lawrence BP: Examining the relationship between impaired host resistance and altered immune function in mice treated with TCDD. *Toxicology* 188:15–28, 2003.

Vorderstrasse BA, Steppan LB, Silverstone AE, Kerkvliet NI: Aryl hydrocarbon receptor-deficient mice generate normal immune responses to model antigens and are resistant to TCDD-induced immune suppression. *Toxicol Appl Pharmacol* 171:157–164, 2001.

Vos JG, de Klerk A, Krajnc EI, Kruizinga W, van Ommen B, Rozing J: Toxicity of bis(tri-n-butyltin)oxide in the rat. II. Suppression of thymus-dependent immune responses and of parameters of nonspecific resistance after short-term exposure. *Toxicol Appl Pharmacol* 75:387–408, 1984.

Vos JG, Luster MI: Immune alterations, in Kimbrough RD, Jensen AA (eds.): *Halogenated Biphenyls, Terphenyls, Napthalenes, Dibenzodioxins, and Related Products*: Amsterdam: Elsevier, 1989, pp. 295–322.

Wang J, Barke RA, Charboneau R, Roy S: Morphine impairs host innate immune response and increases susceptibility to *Streptococcus pneumoniae* lung infection. *J Immunol* 174:426–434, 2005.

Ward AM, Udnoon S, Watkins J, Walker AE, Darke CS: Immunological mechanisms in the pathogenesis of vinyl chloride disease. *Br Med J* 1:936–938, 1976.

Warheit DB, Hesterberg TW: Asbestos and other fibers in the lung, in (Dean JH, Luster MI, Munson AE, Kimber I (eds.): *Immunotoxicology and Immunopharmacology*. New York: Raven Press, 1994, pp. 363–376.

Warren TK, Mitchell KA, Lawrence BP: Exposure to 2,3,7,8-tetrachlorodibenzo-p-dioxin (TCDD) suppresses the humoral and cell-mediated immune responses to influenza A virus without affecting cytolytic activity in the lung. *Toxicol Sci* 56:114–123, 2000.

Watson AJ, Hankinson O: Dioxin and Ah receptor-dependent protein binding to xenobiotic responsive elements and G-rich DNA studied by in vivo footprinting. *J Biol Chem* 266:6874–6878, 1992.

Watson ES, Murphy JC, ElSohly HN, ElSohly MA, Turner CE: Effects of the administration of coca alkaloids on the primary immune responses of mice: Interaction with delta 9-tetrahydrocannabinol and ethanol. *Toxicol Appl Pharmacol* 71:1–13, 1983.

Ways SC, Blair PB, Bern HA, Staskawicz MO: Immune responsiveness of adult mice exposed neonatally to diethylstilbestrol, steroid hormones, or vitamin A. *J Environ Pathol Toxicol* 3:207–220, 1980.

Weaver JL, Chapdelaine JM, Descotes J, et al.: Evaluation of a lymph node proliferation assay for its ability to detect pharmaceuticals with potential to cause immune-mediated drug reactions. *J Immunotoxicol* 2:11–20, 2005.

Wei G, Moss J, Yuan CS: Opioid-induced immunosuppression: Is it centrally mediated or peripherally mediated? *Biochem Pharmacol* 65:1761–1766, 2003.

Weisglas-Kuperus N, Patandin S, Berbers GA, et al.: Immunologic effects of background exposure to polychlorinated biphenyls and dioxins in Dutch preschool children. *Environ Health Perspect* 108:1203–1207, 2000.

Weisglas-Kuperus N, Sas TC, Koopman-Esseboom C, *et al.*: Immunologic effects of background prenatal and postnatal exposure to dioxins and polychlorinated biphenyls in Dutch infants. *Pediatr Res* 38:404–410, 1995.

Weisglas-Kuperus N, Vreugdenhil HJ, Mulder PG: Immunological effects of environmental exposure to polychlorinated biphenyls and dioxins in Dutch school children. *Toxicol Lett* 149:281–285, 2004.

White KL, Jr.: Specific immune function assays, in Miller K, Turk JL, Nicklin S (eds.): *Principles and Practice of Immunotoxicology*. Boston: Blackwell, 1992, pp. 304–323.

White KL, Jr., Anderson AC: Suppression of mouse complement activity by contaminants of technical grade pentachlorophenol. *Agents Actions* 16:385, 1985.

White KL, Jr., Lysy HH, McCay JA, Anderson AC: Modulation of serum complement levels following exposure to polychlorinated dibenzo-*p*-dioxins. *Toxicol Appl Pharmacol* 84:209–219, 1986.

Whitlock JP, Jr.: Genetic and molecular aspects of 2,3,7,8-tetrachlorodibenzo-*p*-dioxin action. *Annu Rev Pharmacol Toxicol* 30:251–277, 1990.

Williams WC, Riddle MM, Copeland CB, Andrews DL, Smialowicz RJ: Immunological effects of 2-methoxyethanol administered dermally or orally to Fischer 344 rats. *Toxicology* 98:215–223, 1995.

Wiltrout RW, Ercegovich CD, Ceglowski WS: Humoral immunity in mice following oral administration of selected pesticides. *Bull Environ Contam Toxicol* 20:423–431, 1978.

Wood SC, Holsapple MP: Direct suppression of superantigen-induced IgM secretion in human lymphocytes by 2,3,7,8-TCDD. *Toxicol Appl Pharmacol* 122:308–313, 1993.

Wood SC, Jeong HG, Morris DL, Holsapple MP: Direct effects of 2,3,7,8-tetrachlorodibenzo-*p*-dioxin (TCDD) on human tonsillar lymphocytes. *Toxicology* 81:131–143, 1993.

Xiao F, Chong AS-F, Bartlett RR, Williams JW: A promising immunosuppressant in transplantation, in Thomas AW, Starzyl TE (eds.): *Immuno-suppressive Drugs: Developments in Anti-Rejection Therapy*. Boston: Edward Arnold, 1994, pp. 203–212.

Xu D, Liu H, Komai-Koma M: Direct and indirect role of Toll-like receptors in T cell mediated immunity. *Cell Mol Immunol* 1:239–246, 2004.

Xue A, Chapoval SP, Finn ES, *et al.*: HLA-DQ8 is a predisposing molecule for detergent enzyme subtilisin BPN'-induced hypersensitivity. *Clin Immunol* 117:302–315, 2005.

Yamaguchi K, Matulka RA, Shneider AM, *et al.*: Induction of PreB cell apoptosis by 7,12-dimethylbenz[a]anthracene in long-term primary murine bone marrow cultures. *Toxicol Appl Pharmacol* 147:190–203, 1997.

Yang KH, Kim BS, Munson AE, Holsapple MP: Immunosuppression induced by chemicals requiring metabolic activation in mixed cultures of rat hepatocytes and murine splenocytes. *Toxicol Appl Pharmacol* 83:420–429, 1986.

Yeatts K, Sly P, Shore S, *et al.*: A brief targeted review of susceptibility factors, environmental exposures, asthma incidence, and recommendations for future asthma incidence research. *Environ Health Perspect* 114:634–640, 2006.

Yoo BS, Boverhof DR, Shnaider D, Crawford RB, Zacharewski TR, Kaminski NE: 2,3,7,8-Tetrachlorodibenzo-*p*-dioxin (TCDD) alters the regulation of Pax5 in lipopolysaccharide-activated B cells. *Toxicol Sci* 77:272–279, 2004.

Yun AJ, Lee PY: The link between T helper balance and lymphoproliferative disease. *Med Hypotheses* 65:587–590, 2005.

Zelikoff JT, Thomas P: *Immunotoxicology of Environmental and Occupational Metals*. Bristol, PA: Taylor & Francis, 1998.

Zhou HR, Islam Z, Pestka JJ: Rapid, sequential activation of mitogen-activated protein kinases and transcription factors precedes proinflammatory cytokine mRNA expression in spleens of mice exposed to the trichothecene vomitoxin. *Toxicol Sci* 72:130–142, 2003.

CHAPTER 13

TOXIC RESPONSES OF THE LIVER

Hartmut Jaeschke

INTRODUCTION

The liver is the main organ where exogenous chemicals are metabolized and eventually excreted. As a consequence, liver cells are exposed to significant concentrations of these chemicals, which can result in liver dysfunction, cell injury, and even organ failure. If an industrial chemical, e.g., carbon tetrachloride, bromobenzene, or vinyl chloride, is identified as a hepatotoxant, the use of the chemical may be restricted, the exposure may be minimized by mandating protective clothing and respirators, and attempts are made to replace it with a safer alternative. In the pharmaceutical industry, adverse effects on the liver are one of the most frequently cited reasons for discontinuing the development of drug candidates. In addition, hepatotoxicity recognized during the postmarketing phase is one of the main causes for withdrawing drugs from the market (Temple and Himmel, 2002). Troglitazone (Rezulin®), a new antidiabetic drug, was removed from the market after close to 100 of the 1.9 million patients treated with the drug suffered from liver failure (Chojkier, 2005). Thus, predictable and idiosyncratic hepatotoxicities severely restrict drug discovery efforts and drug development (Lee and Senior, 2005). Furthermore, the increasing popularity of herbal medicines, which are generally plant extracts, enhances the incidence of drug-induced liver injury and liver failure (Stickel *et al.*, 2005). Since these medicines are mixtures of sometimes hundreds of compounds, it remains a difficult task to identify the causative agent and the mechanism of injury (Lee and Senior, 2005). Basic science and clinical aspects of drug- and chemical-induced liver injury was discussed in detail in several monographs and reviews (McCuskey and Earnest, 1997; Zimmerman, 1999; Jaeschke *et al.*, 2002; Kaplowitz and DeLeve, 2002; Boyer *et al.*, 2006b).

Given the unprecedented speed of drug discovery and the increasing demand and use of "natural products" as food supplements and medicine, the early identification of hepatotoxins remains a formidable challenge for the future. The liver, with its multiple cell types and numerous functions, can respond in many different ways to acute and chronic insults. To recognize potential liver cell dysfunction and injury, it is necessary to have a general knowledge of basic liver functions, the structural organization of the liver, the processes involved in the excretory functions of the liver, and mechanisms of cell and organ injury. Each of these aspects can contribute to mechanisms of drug- and chemical-induced hepatotoxicities.

LIVER PHYSIOLOGY

Hepatic Functions

The liver's strategic location between intestinal tract and the rest of the body facilitates the performance of its enormous task of maintaining metabolic homeostasis of the body (Table 13-1). Venous blood from the stomach and intestine flows into the portal vein and then through the liver before entering the systemic circulation. Thus the liver is the first organ to encounter ingested nutrients, vitamins, metals, drugs, and environmental toxicants as well as waste products of bacteria that enter portal blood. Efficient scavenging or uptake processes extract these absorbed materials from the blood for catabolism, storage, and/or excretion into bile.

All the major functions of the liver can be detrimentally altered by acute or chronic exposure to toxicants (Table 13-1). When toxicants inhibit or otherwise impede hepatic transport and synthetic processes, dysfunction can occur without appreciable cell damage. Loss of function also occurs when toxicants kill an appreciable number of cells and when chronic insult leads to replacement of cell mass by nonfunctional scar tissue. Alcohol abuse is the major cause of liver disease in most western countries (Crawford, 1999); thus ethanol provides a highly relevant example of a toxicant with multiple functional consequences (Lieber, 1994). Early stages of ethanol abuse are characterized by lipid accumulation (fatty liver) due to diminished use of lipids as fuels and impaired ability to synthesize the lipoproteins that transport lipids out of the liver. As alcohol-induced liver disease progresses, appreciable cell death occurs, the functioning mass of the liver is replaced by scar tissue, and hepatic capacity for biotransformation of certain drugs progressively declines. People with hepatic cirrhosis due to chronic alcohol abuse frequently become deficient at detoxifying both the ammonia formed by catabolism of amino acids and the bilirubin derived from breakdown of hemoglobin. Uncontrollable hemorrhage due to

Table 13-1
Major Functions of Liver and Consequences of Impaired Hepatic Functions

TYPE OF FUNCTION	EXAMPLES	CONSEQUENCES OF IMPAIRED FUNCTIONS
Nutrient homeostasis	Glucose storage and synthesis	Hypoglycemia, confusion
	Cholesterol uptake	Hypercholesterolemia
Filtration of particulates	Products of intestinal bacteria (e.g., endotoxin)	Endotoxemia
Protein synthesis	Clotting factors	Excess bleeding
	Albumin	Hypoalbuminemia, ascites
	Transport proteins (e.g., very low density lipoproteins)	Fatty liver
Bioactivation and detoxification	Bilirubin and ammonia	Jaundice, hyperammonemia-related coma
	Steroid hormones	Loss of secondary male sex characteristics
	Xenobiotics	Diminished drug metabolism
		Inadequate detoxification
Formation of bile and biliary secretion	Bile acid–dependent uptake of dietary lipids and vitamins	Fatty diarrhea, malnutrition, Vitamin E deficiency
	Bilirubin and cholesterol	Jaundice, gallstones, hypercholesterolemia
	Metals (e.g., Cu and Mn)	Mn-induced neurotoxicity
	Xenobiotics	Delayed drug clearance

inadequate synthesis of clotting factors is a common fatal complication of alcoholic cirrhosis. A consequence of liver injury that merits emphasis is that loss of liver functions can lead to aberrations in other organ systems and to death.

Structural Organization

Two concepts exist for organization of the liver into operational units, namely, the lobule and the acinus (McCuskey, 2006b). Classically, the liver was divided into hexagonal lobules oriented around terminal hepatic venules (also known as central veins). At the corners of the lobule are the portal triads (or portal tracts), containing a branch of the portal vein, a hepatic arteriole, and a bile duct (Fig. 13-1). Blood entering the portal tract via the portal vein and hepatic artery is mixed in the penetrating vessels, enters the sinusoids, and percolates along the cords of parenchymal cells (hepatocytes), eventually flows into terminal hepatic venules, and exits the liver via the hepatic vein. The lobule is divided into three regions known as centrolobular, midzonal, and periportal. The acinus is the preferred concept for a functional hepatic unit. The terminal branches of the portal vein and hepatic artery, which extend out from the portal tracts, form the base of the acinus. The acinus has three zones: zone 1 is closest to the entry of blood, zone 3 abuts the terminal hepatic vein, and zone 2 is intermediate. Despite the utility of the acinar concept, lobular terminology is still used to describe regions of pathologic lesions of hepatic parenchyma. Fortunately, the three zones of the acinus roughly coincide with the three regions of the lobule (Fig. 13-1).

Acinar zonation is of considerable functional consequence regarding gradients of components both in blood and in hepatocytes (Jungermann and Kietzmann, 2000). Blood entering the acinus consists of oxygen-depleted blood from the portal vein (60–70% of hepatic blood flow) plus oxygenated blood from the hepatic artery (30–40%). Enroute to the terminal hepatic venule, oxygen rapidly leaves the blood to meet the high metabolic demands of the parenchymal cells. Approximate oxygen concentrations in zone 1 are 9–13%, compared with only 4–5% in zone 3. Therefore, hepatocytes in zone 3 are exposed to substantially lower concentrations of oxygen than

hepatocytes in zone 1. In comparison to other tissues, zone 3 is hypoxic. Another well-documented acinar gradient is that of bile salts (Groothuis et al., 1982). Physiologic concentrations of bile salts are efficiently extracted by zone 1 hepatocytes with little bile acids left in the blood that flows past zone 3 hepatocytes.

Heterogeneities in protein levels of hepatocytes along the acinus generate gradients of metabolic functions. Hepatocytes in the mitochondria-rich zone 1 are predominant in fatty acid oxidation, gluconeogenesis, and ammonia detoxification to urea. Gradients of enzymes involved in the bioactivation and detoxification of xenobiotics have been observed along the acinus by immunohistochemistry (Jungermann and Katz, 1989). Notable gradients for hepatotoxins are the higher levels of glutathione in zone 1 and the greater amounts of cytochrome P450 proteins in zone 3, particularly the CYP2E1 isozyme inducible by ethanol (Tsutsumi et al., 1989).

Hepatic sinusoids are the channels between cords of hepatocytes where blood percolates on its way to the terminal hepatic vein. Sinusoids are larger and more irregular than normal capillaries. The three major types of cells in the sinusoids are endothelial cells, Kupffer cells, and stellate cells (Fig. 13-2) (McCuskey, 2006b). In addition, there are rare pit cells, which are liver-associated lymphocytes with natural killer (NK) activity (Bouwens and Wisse, 1992). Sinusoids are lined by thin, discontinuous endothelial cells with numerous fenestrae (or pores) that allow molecules smaller than 250 kDa to cross the interstitial space (known as the space of Disse) between the endothelium and hepatocytes. Sinusoidal endothelial cells are separated from the hepatocytes by a basement membrane-like matrix, which is not as electron-dense as a regular basement membrane (Friedman, 2000). However, this subendothelial extracellular matrix is important for the normal function of all resident liver cells (Friedman, 2000). The numerous fenestrae and the lack of basement membrane facilitate exchanges of fluids and molecules, such as albumin, between the sinusoid and hepatocytes, but hinder movement of particles larger than chylomicron remnants. Endothelial cells are important in the scavenging of lipoproteins via the apo E receptor and of denatured proteins and advanced glycation endproducts by the scavenger receptor (Smedsrod et al., 1994). Hepatic endothelial cells also secrete cytokines, prostanoids, nitric

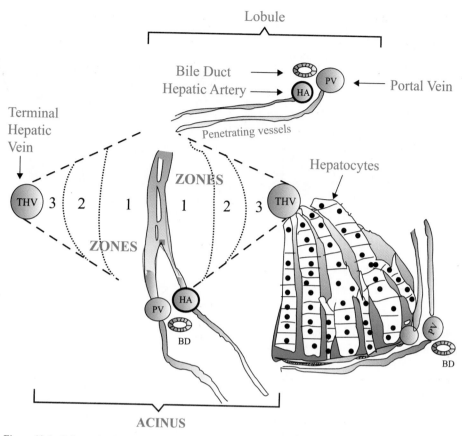

Figure 13-1. Schematic of liver operational units, the classic lobule and the acinus.

The lobule is centered around the terminal hepatic vein (central vein), where the blood drains out of the lobule. The acinus has as its base the penetrating vessels, where blood supplied by the portal vein and hepatic artery flows down the acinus past the cords of hepatocytes. Zones 1, 2, and 3 of the acinus represent metabolic regions that are increasingly distant from the blood supply.

oxide, and endothelins (Smedsrod *et al.*, 1994) and express inter-cellular adhesion molecule-1 (ICAM-1) and vascular cell adhesion molecule-1 (VCAM-1) on the cell surface (Jaeschke, 1997).

Kupffer cells are the resident macrophages of the liver and constitute approximately 80% of the fixed macrophages in the body (McCuskey, 2006b). Kupffer cells are situated within the lumen of the sinusoid. The primary function of Kupffer cells is to ingest and degrade particulate matter. Also, Kupffer cells are a major source of cytokines and eicosanoids and can act as antigen-presenting cells (Laskin, 1990). Hepatic stellate cells (also known as Ito cells or by the more descriptive terms of *fat-storing cells*) are located between endothelial cells and hepatocytes (Wake, 1980). Stellate cells are the major sites for vitamin A storage in the body (Wake, 1980). Upon activation, these cells can synthesize and excrete collagen and other extracellular matrix proteins and express smooth muscle actin (Friedman, 2000).

Bile Formation

Bile is a yellow fluid containing bile acids, glutathione, phospholipids, cholesterol, bilirubin and other organic anions, proteins, metals, ions, and xenobiotics (Klaassen and Watkins, 1984). Formation of this fluid is a specialized function of the liver. Adequate bile formation is essential for uptake of lipid nutrients from the small

intestine (Table 13-1), for protection of the small intestine from oxidative insults (Aw, 1994), and for excretion of endogenous and xenobiotic compounds. Hepatocytes begin the process of bile formation by transporting bile acids, glutathione, and other osmolytically active compounds including xenobiotics and their metabolites into the canalicular lumen. These molecules are the major driving force for the passive movement of water and electrolytes across the tight junctions and the hepatocyte epithelium. The canalicular lumen is a space formed by specialized regions of the plasma membrane between adjacent hepatocytes (Fig. 13-2). The canaliculi are separated from the intercellular space between hepatocytes by tight junctions, which form a barrier permeable only to water, electrolytes, and to some degree to small organic cations. Under physiological conditions, tight junctions are impermeable to organic anions allowing the high concentrations of bile acids, glutathione, bilirubin-diglucuronide, and other organic anions in bile. The structure of the biliary tract is analogous to the roots and trunk of a tree, where the tips of the roots equate to the canalicular lumens. Canaliculi form channels between hepatocytes that connect to a series of larger and larger channels or ducts within the liver. The large extrahepatic bile ducts merge into the common bile duct. Bile can be stored and concentrated in the gallbladder before its release into the duodenum. However, the gallbladder is not essential to life and is absent in several species, including the horse, whale, and rat.

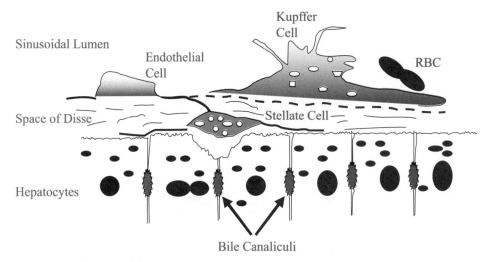

Figure 13-2. Schematic of liver sinusoidal cells.

Note that the Kupffer cell resides within the sinusoidal lumen. The stellate cell is located in the space of Disse between the thin, fenestrated endothelial cells and the cord of hepatocytes.

With the identification of specific transporters, substantial progress has been made in the understanding of the molecular mechanisms of bile formation (reviewed in Jansen and Groen, 2006; Pauli-Magnus and Meier, 2006). On the basolateral (sinusoidal) side of the hepatocytes, there are sodium-dependent and sodium-independent uptake systems. Most conjugated bile acids (taurine- and glycine-conjugates) and some of the unconjugated bile acids are transported into hepatocytes by NTCP (sodium-dependent taurocholate cotransporting polypeptide) (Fig. 13-3) (Trauner and Boyer, 2003; Hagenbuch and Dawson, 2004; Stieger *et al.*, 2007). Sodium-independent uptake of conjugated and unconjugated bile acids is performed by members of the organic anion-transporting polypeptides (OATPs) (Hagenbuch and Meier, 2004). OATP1B1 and OATP1B3, which are predominantly expressed in the liver and OATP1A2 are all capable of transporting conjugated and unconjugated bile acids and steroids, bromosulfophthalein and many other organic anions (Hagenbuch and Meier, 2004). Furthermore, the OATPs are transporting numerous drugs and also some hepatotoxins, e.g., phalloidin, microcystin, and amanitin (Pauli-Magnus and Meier, 2006). In addition to the uptake systems, there are ATP-dependent efflux pumps located on the basolateral membrane of hepatocytes. These carriers are members of the multidrug resistance-associated proteins (MRPs; ABCC), which are multispecific transporters for many different anions (Homolya *et al.*, 2003) (Fig. 13-3).

All unconjugated bile acids in hepatocytes are conjugated before being transported by the bile salt export pump (BSEP) across the canalicular membrane. Bile acid excretion is a major driving force of bile formation (bile salt-dependent bile flow). Other constituents of bile are transported by members of the multidrug resistance (MDR) *P*-glycoprotein family such as MDR3 (ABCC2), which transports phospholipids, and the heterodimeric transporters ABCG5/ABCG8, which transport cholesterol and plant sterols into bile (Pauli-Magnus and Meier, 2006). In addition, MRP2 (a member of the multidrug resistance-associated proteins) transports glutathione (GSH), which is the main compound responsible for the bile salt-independent bile flow, as well as sulfated and glucuronidated bile acids, glutathione disulfide and glutathione conjugates, bilirubin diglucuronide, and many other conjugated drugs and chemicals (Gerk and Vore, 2002; Borst *et al.*, 2000). Other transport systems of the canalicular membrane include the breast cancer resistance protein (BCRP; ABCG2), which can contribute to the biliary excretion of bile acids and xenobiotics.

Metals are excreted into bile by a series of processes that include (1) uptake across the sinusoidal membrane by facilitated diffusion or receptor-mediated endocytosis; (2) storage in binding proteins or lysosomes; and (3) canalicular secretion via lysosomes, a glutathione-coupled event, or use of specific canalicular membrane transporter, e.g. MRP2 (Ballatori, 2002). Biliary excretion is important in the homeostasis of multiple metals, notably copper, manganese, cadmium, selenium, gold, silver, and arsenic (Klaassen, 1976; Gregus and Klaassen, 1986). Species differences are known for biliary excretion of several toxic metals; for example, dogs excrete arsenic into bile much more slowly than rats. Inability to export Cu into bile is a central problem in Wilson's disease, a rare autosomal recessive inherited disorder characterized by a defect or the absence of a copper transporting P-type ATPase (ATP7B). This carrier is located in the trans-Golgi network and transports copper into the secretory pathway for binding to ceruloplasmin and then exretion into bile (Loudianos and Gitlin, 2000). Because biliary excretion is the only way to eliminate Cu, a defect in ATP7B results in excessive Cu accumulation in hepatocytes, which causes chronic hepatitis and cirrhosis (Loudianos and Gitlin, 2000).

Canalicular lumen bile is propelled forward into larger channels by dynamic, ATP-dependent contractions of the pericanalicular cytoskeleton (Watanabe *et al.*, 1991). Bile ducts, once regarded as passive conduits, modify bile by absorption and secretion of solutes (Lira *et al.*, 1992). Bile acids are taken up into biliary epithelial cells (cholangiocytes) by OATP1A2 (sodium-independent uptake) and by the sodium-dependent bile acid transporter (Hagenbuch and Dawson, 2004; Hagenbuch and Meier, 2004). These bile acids are then excreted on the basolateral side mainly by MRP3 and heterodimeric organic solute transporter (OSTα/OSTβ) (Ballatori *et al.*, 2005). The bile acids excreted from cholangiocytes return to the portal circulation via the peribiliary plexus (cholehepatic shunt pathway). Biliary epithelial cells also express a variety of phase I and phase II enzymes, which may contribute to the biotransformation of chemical toxicants present in bile (Lakehal *et al.*, 1999).

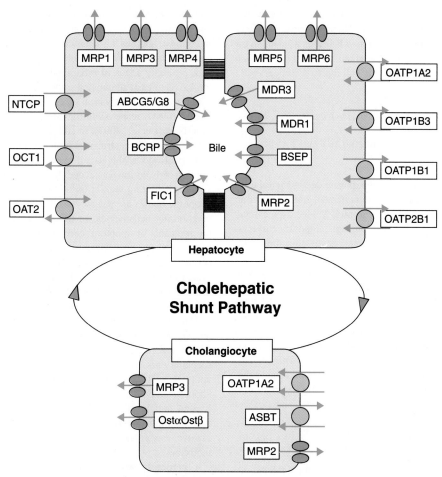

Figure 13-3. Transport proteins in human hepatocytes and cholangiocytes.

Efflux transporters (blue symbols): BSEP, bile salt export pump; MDR, multidrug resistance protein; MRP, multidrug resistance-associated protein; ABCG5/8; BCRP, breast cancer resistance protein; Ostα/Ostβ. Uptake transporters (red symbols): ASBT, apical sodium dependent bile salt transporter; NTCP, sodium taurocholate cotransporting polypeptide; OATP, organic anion-transporting polypeptide; OCT, organic cation transporter; OAT, organic anion transporter. Transporters localized to the sinusoidal membrane extract solutes from the blood. Exporters localized to canalicular membrane move solutes into the lumen of the canaliculus. Exporters of particular relevance to canalicular secretion of toxic chemicals and their metabolites are the canalicular multiple organic anion transporter (MOAT) system and the family of multiple-drug resistant (MDR) P-glycoproteins. (From Pauli-Magnus C, Meier PJ: Hepatobiliary transporters and drug-induced cholestasis. *Hepatology* 44:778–787, 2006. Reprinted with permission of John Wiley & Sons, Inc.)

Secretion into biliary ducts is usually but not always a prelude to toxicant clearance by excretion in feces or urine. Exceptions occur when compounds such as arsenic are repeatedly delivered into the intestinal lumen via bile, efficiently absorbed from the intestinal lumen, and then redirected to the liver via portal blood, a process known as *enterohepatic cycling.* A few compounds, such as methyl mercury, are absorbed from the biliary tract; the extensive reabsorption of methyl mercury from the gallbladder is thought to contribute to the long biological half-life and toxicity of this toxicant (Dutczak *et al.*, 1991). Alternatively, secretion into bile of toxicant metabolites can be a critical prelude to the development of injury in extrahepatic tissues. A clinically relevant example of bile as an important delivery route for a proximate toxicant is that of diclofenac, a widely prescribed nonsteroidal anti-inflammatory drug (NSAID) that causes small intestinal ulceration. Experiments with mutant rats lacking a functional MRP2 exporter (Fig. 13-3) have shown that these mutants secrete little of the presumptive proximate toxicant metabolite into bile and are resistant to the intestinal toxicity of diclofenac (Seitz and Boelsterli, 1998).

Toxicant-related impairments of bile formation are more likely to have detrimental consequences in populations with other conditions where biliary secretion is marginal. For example, neonates exhibit delayed development of multiple aspects of bile formation, including synthesis of bile acids and the expression of sinusoidal and canalicular transporters (Arrese *et al.*, 1998). Neonates are more prone to develop jaundice when treated with drugs that compete with bilirubin for biliary clearance. Individuals with genetic deficiency of certain transporters are not only at risk for chronic liver injury and fibrosis but may also be more susceptible to drugs and hepatotoxins (Jansen and Sturm, 2003; Jansen and Groen, 2006). Patients with sepsis frequently develop cholestasis, which is mainly caused by downregulation of multiple canalicular transport systems (Geier *et al.*, 2006). In addition, direct inhibition of BSEP, as was shown for the endothelin receptor antagonist bosentan, can lead to retention of bile acids in the liver and potentially cell injury (Fattinger *et al.*, 2001).

LIVER PATHOPHYSIOLOGY

Mechanisms and Types of Toxin-induced Liver Injury

The response of the liver to chemical exposure depends on the intensity of the insults, the cell population affected, and the duration of the chemical exposure (acute vs. chronic). Milder stresses may just cause reversible cellular dysfunction, e.g., temporary cholestasis after exposure to estrogens. However, acute poisoning with acetaminophen or carbon tetrachloride triggers parenchymal cell necrosis. Exposure to ethanol induces steatosis, which may enhance the susceptiblity to subsequent inflammatory insults (Table 13-2). Note that the representative hepatotoxins listed in Table 13-2 include pharmaceuticals (valproic acid, cyclosporin A, diclofenac, acetaminophen, tamoxifen), recreational drugs (ethanol, ecstasy), a vitamin (vitamin A), metals (Fe, Cu, Mn), hormones (estrogens, androgens), industrial chemicals (dimethylformamide, methylene diailine), compounds found in teas (germander) or foods (phalloidin, pyrrolidine alkaloids), and toxins produced by fungi (sporidesmin) and algae (microcystin).

Cell Death Based on morphology, liver cells can die by two different modes, oncotic necrosis ("necrosis") or apoptosis. Necrosis is characterized by cell swelling, leakage of cellular contents, nuclear disintegration (karyolysis), and an influx of inflammatory cells. Because necrosis is generally the result of an exposure to a toxic chemical or other traumatic conditions, e.g., ischemia, large numbers of contiguous hepatocytes and nonparenchymal cells may be affected. Cell contents released during oncotic necrosis includes proteins such a high mobility group box-1 (HMGB1) and other alarmins, which are a subset of the larger class of damage-associated molecular patterns (DAMPs) (Bianchi, 2007). These molecules are recognized by cells of the innate immune system including Kupffer cells through their toll-like receptors and trigger cytokine formation, which orchestrate the inflammatory response after tissue injury (Scaffidi *et al.*, 2002). Thus, an ongoing oncotic necrotic process can be identified by the release of liver-specific enzymes such as alanine (ALT) or aspartate (AST) aminotransferase into the plasma and by histology, where areas of necrosis with loss of nuclei and inflammatory infiltrates are easily detectable in H&E sections. In contrast, apoptosis is characterized by cell shrinkage, chromatin condensation, nuclear fragmentation, formation of apoptotic bodies, and, generally a lack of inflammation. The characteristic morphological features of apoptosis are caused by the activation of caspases, which trigger the activation of enzymes such as caspase-activated DNase (CAD) responsible for internucleosomal DNA fragmentation (Nagata *et al.*, 2003). In addition, caspases can directly cleave cellular and nuclear structural proteins (Fischer *et al.*, 2003). Apoptosis is always a single cell event with the main purpose of removing cells no longer needed during development or eliminating aging cells during regular tissue turnover. Under these conditions, apoptotic bodies are phagocytosed by Kupffer cells or taken up by neighboring hepatocytes. In the absence of cell contents release, the remnants of apoptotic cells disappear without causing an inflammatory response. Because of effective regeneration, apoptotic cell death during normal tissue turnover or even a moderately elevated rate of apoptosis is of limited pathophysiological relevance in the liver. However, if the rate of apoptosis is substantially increased, the apoptotic process cannot be completed. In this case, cells undergo secondary necrosis with breakdown of membrane potential, cell swelling, and cell contents release (Ogasawara *et al.*, 1993). The fundamental difference between oncotic necrosis and secondary necrosis is the fact that during secondary necrosis many apoptotic cells can still be identified based on morphology, many apoptotic characteristics such as activation of various caspases are present, and the process can be completely inhibited by potent pan-caspase inhibitors (Jaeschke *et al.*, 2004). Oncotic necrosis does not involve relevant caspase activation and is not inhibitable by caspase inhibitors.

In recent years, signaling mechanisms of apoptosis were elucidated in great detail (Fig. 13-4) (reviewed in Jaeschke, 2006a; Malhi *et al.*, 2006; Schulze-Bergkamen *et al.*, 2006). In the extrinsic pathway of apoptosis, ligands (e.g., Fas ligand, TNF-α) bind to their respective death receptor (Fas receptor, TNF receptor type I), which triggers the trimerization of the receptor followed by recruitment of various adapter molecules and procaspases to the cytoplasmic tail of the receptor. The assembly of this death-inducing signaling complex (DISC) leads to the activation of initiator caspases (caspase-8 or -10). In hepatocytes, the active initiator caspase cleaves Bid, a member of the Bcl-2 family of proteins, and the truncated Bid (tBid) translocates together with other Bcl-2 family members such as Bax to the mitochondria. These proteins form pores in the outer membrane of the mitochondria and cause the release of intermembrane proteins such as cytochrome *c* and the second mitochondria-derived

Table 13-2
Types of Hepatobiliary Injury

TYPE OF INJURY OR DAMAGE	REPRESENTATIVE TOXINS
Fatty liver	Amiodarone, CCl$_4$, ethanol, fialuridine, tamoxifen, valproic acid
Hepatocyte death	Acetaminophen, allyl alcohol, Cu, dimethylformamide, ethanol
Immune-mediated response	Diclofenac, ethanol, halothane, tienilic acid
Canalicular cholestasis	Chlorpromazine, cyclosporin A, 1,1-dichloroethylene, estrogens, Mn, phalloidin
Bile duct damage	Alpha-naphthylisothiocyanate, amoxicillin, methylene dianiline, sporidesmin
Sinusoidal disorders	Anabolic steroids, cyclophosphamide, microcystin, pyrrolizidine alkaloids
Fibrosis and cirrhosis	CCl$_4$, ethanol, thioacetamide, vitamin A, vinyl chloride
Tumors	Aflatoxin, androgens, arsenic, thorium dioxide, vinyl chloride

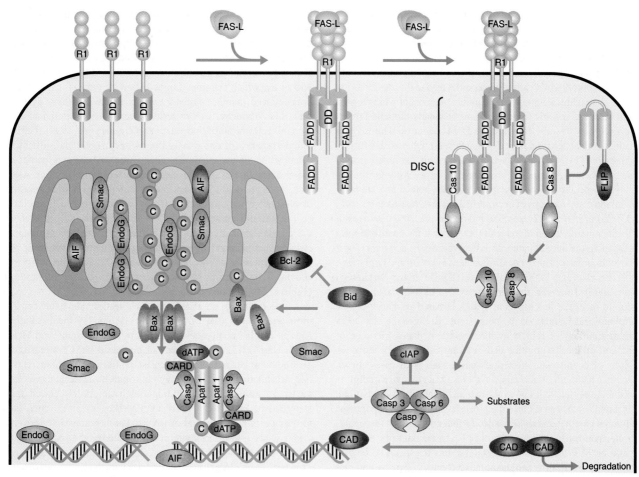

Figure 13-4. Fas receptor-mediated apoptotic signaling pathways in hepatocytes.

AIF, apoptosis-inducing factor; Apaf1, apoptosis protease-activating factor-1; CARD, caspase-activating and -recruiting domain; Casp, caspase; c, cytochrome *c*; cIAP, cellular inhibitor of apoptosis proteins; DD, death domain; Smac, second mitochondria-derived activator of caspases; DISC, death-inducing signaling complex; EndoG, endonuclease G; FADD, Fas-associated death domain; FAS-L, Fas-ligand; FLIP, FLICE-inhibitory protein. (Adapted from Jaeschke H: Mechanisms of liver cell destruction, in Boyer TD, Wright TL, Manns M (eds): *Zakim and Boyer's Hepatology*. 5th edn. Philadelphia: Saunders-Elsevier, 2006a, p 37.)

activator of caspases (Smac). Cytochrome *c*, together with apoptosis protease activating factor-1 (APAF-1), ATP, and procaspase-9, forms the apoptosome causing the activation of caspase-9, which then processes (and activates) downstream effector caspases, e.g. caspase-3. The effector caspases can propagate the apoptosis signal by activating CAD to initiate nuclear DNA fragmentation and by cleaving numerous cellular proteins critical to cellular function and the structural integrity of the cell and the nucleus (Fischer *et al.*, 2003; Nagata *et al.*, 2003). In addition to downstream substrates, caspase-3 can also process more procaspase-8 and further amplify the apoptotic signal. Although hepatocytes constitutively express Fas and TNF receptors, the death signal generated with ligation of the receptor is clearly insufficient to trigger apoptosis. Inhibitor studies and experiments with gene-deficient mice support the hypothesis that only the amplification of the receptor-derived signal through multiple mitochondrial cycles can successfully induce apoptosis in hepatocytes (Yin *et al.*, 1999; Bajt *et al.*, 2000, 2001). In addition to the direct propagation of the apoptosis signal by mitochondrial cytochrome *c* release, the simultaneous release of Smac ensures that the cytosolic inhibitors of apoptosis proteins (IAPs) are inactivated and do not interfere with the promotion of apoptosis (Li *et al.*,

2002). Thus, mitochondria are an indispensable part of the extrinsic (receptor-mediated) apoptotic signal transduction pathway in liver cells.

In contrast to the extrinsic pathway, the intrinsic or mitochondrial pathway of apoptosis is initiated independent of the TNF receptor family, caspase-8 activation, and formation of the DISC. Despite the upstream differences, the postmitochondrial effects are largely similar to the extrinsic pathway. The intrinsic pathway is generally triggered by a cytotoxic stress or DNA damage, which activates the tumor suppressor p53 (Sheikh and Fornace, 2000). This protein acts as transcription factor to promote the formation of pro-apoptotic Bcl-2 family members, e.g., Bax. The increased Bax translocation to the mitochondria induces the release of mitochondrial intermembrane proteins including cytochrome *c*, Smac, endonuclease G, and apoptosis-inducing factor (AIF) (Saelens *et al.*, 2004). An intrinsic mechanism of apoptosis has been discussed for cell death in aging livers (Zhang *et al.*, 2002), prolonged treatment with alcohol (Ishii *et al.*, 2003), or toxicity of benzo(*a*)pyrene and acetaminophen in hepatoma cells (Boulares *et al.*, 2002; Ko *et al.*, 2004). For other hepatotoxic chemicals, such as carbon tetrachloride (Cai *et al.*, 2005), galactosamine (Gomez-Lechon *et al.*, 2002), and microcystin (Ding *et al.*, 2000), evidence for mitochondria-dependent apoptosis has been reported in cultured hepatocytes and relevant apoptotic cell death was observed after in vivo exposure to these chemicals (Shi *et al.*, 1998; Hooser, 2000; Gujral *et al.*, 2003b).

The dramatically increased knowledge of the signaling mechanisms of apoptotic cell death in hepatocytes lead to the identification of many biochemical "apoptosis" parameters, most of which turned out to be not as specific for apoptosis as originally thought. Prominent examples of these tests are the DNA ladder on agarose gels and the terminal deoxynucleotidyl transferase-mediated dUTP nick-end labeling (TUNEL) assay, which demonstrate internucleosomal DNA fragmentation and DNA strandbreaks, respectively. Originally thought to specifically identify apoptotic cells, both assays are positive for most mechanisms of necrotic cell death (Grasl-Kraupp *et al.*, 1995; Gujral *et al.*, 2002; Jaeschke and Lemasters, 2003). As a result of the misinterpretation of many of these assays, the contribution of apoptosis to the overall pathophysiology processes and toxicological liver injuries is controversially debated (Jaeschke and Lemasters, 2003; Jaeschke *et al.*, 2004; Malhi *et al.*, 2006; Schulze-Bergkamen *et al.*, 2006). However, the controversy can be avoided if the decision to label the process as apoptosis is based primarily on the morphological features of the dying cells. Because the characteristic morphology is caused by the caspase-mediated cleavage of structural proteins within the cell, relevant caspase activation, especially of downstream effector caspases such as caspase-3 or -6, is another hallmark of apoptosis. As a result, pancaspase inhibitors can effectively prevent apoptosis-induced liver injury in vivo and in isolated hepatocytes. Once the process is identified as apoptosis, additional parameters can be used to further characterize the signaling mechanism. In addition, the use of positive controls, e.g., Fas ligand- or TNF-mediated hepatocellular apoptosis, can be helpful in assessing qualitative and quantitative changes of many parameters relative to a proven apoptotic process (Jaeschke *et al.*, 2004). Another critical issue to consider is the model system that is being used. For example, both the antidiabetic drug troglitazone and the analgesic acetaminophen clearly induce apoptosis in hepatoma cell lines (Yamamoto *et al.*, 2001; Boulares *et al.*, 2002). However, there is no evidence for a relevant role of apoptotic cell death in animals or patients for both drugs (Gujral *et al.*, 2002; Jaeschke *et al.*, 2004; Chojkier, 2005). Thus, characterization of cell death after chemical exposure has to be primarily based on morphology and a number of additional biochemical parameters, which need to quantitatively correlate with the number of apoptotic cells. In addition, the relevance of the model system for the human pathophysiology needs to be considered.

The mechanisms of oncotic necrosis are more diverse and depend on the chemical insult to the cell (a detailed example of the mechanism of acetaminophen-induced hepatocellular necrosis is discussed later). However, a general trend is emerging. Independent of the initial insult and signaling pathways, mitochondria are almost always involved in the pathophysiology. The opening of the mitochondrial membrane permeability transition pore with collapse of the membrane potential and depletion of cellular ATP is a common final step of the mechanism of necrotic cell death (Kim *et al.*, 2003). The loss of ATP inhibits ion pumps of the plasma membrane resulting in the loss of cellular ion homeostasis, which causes the characteristic swelling of oncotic necrosis.

Canalicular Cholestasis This form of liver dysfunction is defined physiologically as a decrease in the volume of bile formed or an impaired secretion of specific solutes into bile. Cholestasis is characterized biochemically by elevated serum levels of compounds normally concentrated in bile, particularly bile salts and bilirubin. When biliary excretion of the yellowish bilirubin pigment is impaired, this pigment accumulates in skin and eyes, producing jaundice, and spills into urine, which becomes bright yellow or dark brown. Because drug-induced jaundice reflects a more generalized liver dysfunction, it is considered a more serious warning sign in clinical trials than mild elevations of liver enzymes (Zimmerman, 1999). The histologic features of cholestasis can be very subtle and difficult to detect without ultrastructural studies. Structural changes include dilation of the bile canaliculus and the presence of bile plugs in bile ducts and canaliculi. Toxicant-induced cholestasis can be transient or chronic; when substantial, it is associated with cell swelling, cell death, and inflammation. Cell injury is generally caused by the accumulation of chemicals in the liver, i.e., the cholestasis-causing chemical and, as a consequence, potentially cytotoxic bile acids, bilirubin, and other bile constituents. Many different types of chemicals, including metals, hormones, and drugs, cause cholestasis (Table 13-2) (Zimmerman, 1999).

The molecular mechanisms of cholestasis are related to expression and function of transporter systems in the basolateral and canalicular membranes (reviewed by Pauli-Magnus and Meier, 2006) (Fig. 13-3). In principle, an increased hepatic uptake, decreased biliary excretion, and increased biliary reabsorption (cholehepatic shunting) of a drug may contribute to its accumulation in the liver. Although no case of drug toxicity has been reported in response to modifications of basolateral uptake, OATPs can contribute to the liver injury potential of toxins. The hepatotoxicity of phalloidin, microcystin, and amanitin is facilitated by the uptake through OATPs (Pauli-Magnus and Meier, 2006). Furthermore, there is a growing list of drugs including rifampicin, bosentan, and troglitazone, which are known to directly inhibit BSEP (Stieger *et al.*, 2000; Fattinger *et al.*, 2001). However, estrogen and progesterone metabolites inhibit BSEP from the canalicular side after excretion by MRP2 (Stieger *et al.*, 2000). A substantial inhibition of bile salt excretion can lead to accumulation of these compounds in hepatocytes and may directly cause cell injury (Palmeira and Rolo, 2004). In addition, the initial tissue injury can be aggravated by the subsequent inflammatory response (Gujral *et al.*, 2003a). However, the increased bile acid levels can trigger compensatory mechanisms, which limit the injury potential of cholestasis (Zollner *et al.*, 2006). Bile acids are substrates for the nuclear receptor farnesoid X receptor (FXR). FXR activation stimulates the small heterodimeric partner 1 (SHP1), which downregulates NTCP and limits bile acid uptake (Denson *et al.*, 2001). In addition, FXR activation causes the increased expression of BSEP and MDR3, which enhances the transport capacity for bile acids and phospholipids, respectively, at the canalicular membrane (Ananthanarayanan *et al.*, 2001; Huang *et al.*, 2003). Furthermore, the FXR-independent upregulation of the basolateral transporters MRP3 and MRP4 reduces intracellular bile acid and drug concentrations (Schuetz *et al.*, 2001; Wagner *et al.*, 2003; Fickert *et al.*, 2006). Recent findings indicate that agonists of the nuclear xenobiotic receptors constitutive androstane receptor (CAR) and pregnane X receptor (PXR) can not only induce MRP3 and -4 expression but also induce bile acid hydroxylation by Cyp3a11 and Cyp2b10 resulting in improved export and detoxification of bile acids during cholestasis (Wagner *et al.*, 2005). In cholangiocytes, OSTα/OSTβ is upregulated at the basolateral membrane during cholestasis (Boyer *et al.*, 2006a). This response, which is dependent on FXR, mediates the enhanced return of bile acids from bile to the plasma (Boyer *et al.*, 2006a). Thus, the pharmacological modulation of transporter expression may counteract some of the detrimental effects of cholestasis with various etiologies (Zollner *et al.*, 2006).

Bile Duct Damage   Another name for damage to the intrahepatic bile ducts is *cholangiodestructive cholestasis* (Cullen and Ruebner, 1991; Zimmerman, 1999). A useful biochemical index of bile duct damage is a sharp elevation in serum activities of enzymes localized to bile ducts, particularly alkaline phosphatase. In addition, serum levels of bile acids and bilirubin are elevated, as observed with canalicular cholestasis. Initial lesions following a single dose of cholangiodestructive chemicals include swollen biliary epithelium, debris of damaged cells within ductal lumens, and inflammatory cell infiltration of portal tracts. Chronic administration of toxins that cause bile duct destruction can lead to biliary proliferation and fibrosis resembling primary biliary cirrhosis (PBC). A number of drugs have been implicated to cause prolonged cholestasis with features of PBC (Zimmerman, 1999). However, only in rare cases will there be permanent damage or even loss of bile ducts, a condition known as *vanishing bile duct syndrome*. Cases of this persisting problem have been reported in patients receiving antibiotics (Davies *et al.*, 1994), anabolic steroids, contraceptive steroids, or the anticonvulsant carbamazepine (Zimmerman, 1999).

Sinusoidal Damage   The sinusoid is, in effect, a specialized capillary with numerous fenestrae for high permeability (Braet and Wisse, 2002). The functional integrity of the sinusoid can be compromised by dilation or blockade of its lumen or by progressive destruction of its endothelial cell wall. Dilation of the sinusoid will occur whenever efflux of hepatic blood is impeded. The rare condition of primary dilation, known as *peliosis hepatis*, has been associated with exposure to anabolic steroids and the drug danazol. Blockade will occur when the fenestrae enlarge to such an extent that red blood cells become caught in them or pass through with entrapment in the interstitial space of Disse. Endothelial cell gaps and injury have been shown after exposure to acetaminophen (Ito *et al.*, 2005), galactosamine/endotoxin (Ito *et al.*, 2006), or an anti-Fas antibody (Ogasawara *et al.*, 1993). These gaps can be caused by direct injury to endothelial cells by acetaminophen (DeLeve *et al.*, 1997) and the Fas antibody (Bajt *et al.*, 2000) or could be just the result of detachment from the extracellular matrix (Ito *et al.*, 2006). In general, matrix metalloproteinase inhibitors prevent the gap formation (McCuskey, 2006a). A consequence of endothelial cell injury is the loss of barrier function with extensive blood accumulation in the liver resulting in hypovolemic shock. Microcystin produces this effect within hours in rodents (Hooser *et al.*, 1989). Microcystin dramatically deforms hepatocytes by altering cytoskeleton actin filaments, but it does not affect sinusoidal cells (Hooser *et al.*, 1991). Thus, the deformities that microcystin produces on the cytoskeleton of hepatocytes likely produce a secondary change in the structural integrity of the sinusoid owing to the close proximity of hepatocytes and sinusoidal endothelial cells (Fig. 13-2).

Progressive destruction of the endothelial wall of the sinusoid will lead to gaps and then ruptures of its barrier integrity, with entrapment of red blood cells. These disruptions of the sinusoid are considered the early structural features of the vascular disorder known as veno-occlusive disease (DeLeve *et al.*, 1999). Well established as a cause of veno-occlusive disease are the pyrrolizidine alkaloids (e.g., monocrotaline, retrorsine, and seneciphylline) found

in some plants used for herbal teas and in some seeds that contaminate food grains. Numerous episodes of human and animal poisoning by pyrrolizidine alkaloids have been reported around the world, including massive problems affecting thousands of people in Afghanistan in 1976 and 1993 (Huxtable, 1997). Veno-occlusive disease is also a serious complication in about 15% of the patients given high doses of chemotherapy (e.g., cyclophosphamide) as part of bone-marrow transplantation regimens (DeLeve *et al.*, 1999). Selective depletion of glutathione within sinusoidal endothelial cells and activation of matrix metalloproteinases are critical events in the mechanism of endothelial cell injury in the pathophysiology of veno-occlusive disease (Wang *et al.*, 2000; DeLeve *et al.*, 2003b). Endothelial cell gap formation and injury and the resulting microcirculatory disturbances have been well established as the cause of veno-occlusive disease (DeLeve *et al.*, 2003a).

Disruption of the Cytoskeleton   Phalloidin and microcystin disrupt the integrity of hepatocyte cytoskeleton by affecting proteins that are vital to its dynamic nature. The detrimental effects of these two potent hepatotoxicants are independent of their biotransformation and are exclusive for hepatocytes, because there is no appreciable uptake of either toxin into other types of cells. Tight binding of phalloidin to actin filaments prevents the disassembly phase of the normally dynamic rearrangement of the actin filament constituent of the cytoskeleton. Phalloidin uptake into hepatocytes leads to striking alterations in the actin-rich web of cytoskeleton adjacent to the canalicular membrane; the actin web becomes accentuated and the canalicular lumen dilates (Phillips *et al.*, 1986). Experiments using time-lapse video microscopy have documented dose-dependent declines in the contraction of canalicular lumens between isolated hepatocyte couplets after incubation with a range of phalloidin concentrations (Watanabe and Phillips, 1986).

Microcystin uptake into hepatocytes leads to hyperphosphorylation of cytoskeletal proteins secondary to this toxicant's covalent binding to the catalytic subunit of serine/threonine protein phosphatases (Runnegar *et al.*, 1995b). Reversible phosphorylations of cytoskeletal structural and motor proteins are critical to the dynamic integrity of the cytoskeleton. Extensive hyperphosphorylation produced by large amounts of microcystin leads to marked deformation of hepatocytes due to a unique collapse of the microtubular actin scaffold into a spiny central aggregate (Hooser *et al.*, 1991). Lower doses of microcystin, insufficient to produce the gross structural deformations, diminish uptake and secretory functions of hepatocytes in association with preferential hyperphosphorylation of the cytoplasmic motor protein dynein (Runnegar *et al.*, 1999). Dynein is a mechanicochemical protein that drives vesicles along microtubules using energy from ATP hydrolysis; central to the hydrolysis of the dynein-bound ATP is a cycle of kinase phosphorylation and phosphatase dephosphorylation. Thus, hyperphosphorylation of dynein freezes this motor pump. Chronic exposure to low levels of microcystin has raised new concerns about the health effects of this water contaminant. Specifically, low levels of microcystin promote liver tumors and kill hepatocytes in the zone 3 region, where microcystin accumulates (Solter *et al.*, 1998).

Information about the binding of phalloidin and microcystin to specific target molecules is valuable for two reasons. First, the linkages of specific binding to loss of target protein functions provide compelling evidence that such binding constitutes a defined molecular mechanism of injury. Second, the demonstrations of high-affinity binding to a target molecule without confounding effects on other processes or tissues have *translated* into applications of these toxins as tools for cell biology research. For example, phalloidin complexed with a fluorochrome (e.g., rhodamine phalloidin or Texas Red phalloidin) is used to visualize the actin polymer component of the cytoskeleton in all types of permeabilized cells. The collapse of actin filaments into spiny aggregates after microcystin treatment was visualized by fluorescence microscopy of cells stained with rhodamine phalloidin (Hooser et al., 1991). Low levels of microcystin are being used to discriminate the roles of dynein from other cytoskeletal motor proteins (Runnegar et al., 1999).

Fatty Liver Fatty liver (steatosis) is defined biochemically as an appreciable increase in the hepatic lipid (mainly triglyceride) content, which is <5% by weight in normal human liver. Histologically, in standard paraffin-embedded and solvent-extracted sections, hepatocytes containing excess fat appear to have multiple round, empty vacuoles that displace the nucleus to the periphery of the cell. Use of frozen sections and special stains is needed to document the contents of the vesicles as fat. Based on the size of the fat droplets, one can distinguish between macrovesicular and microvesicular steatosis.

Currently, the most common cause of hepatic steatosis is insulin resistance due to central obesity and sedentary lifestyle. However, acute exposure to many hepatotoxins, e.g., carbon tetrachloride, and drugs can induce steatosis (Zimmerman, 1999). Compounds that produce prominent steatosis associated with lethality include the antiepileptic drug valproic acid (Scheffner et al., 1988) and the antiviral drug fialuridine (Honkoop et al., 1997). Ethanol is by far the most relevant drug or chemical leading to steatosis in humans and in experimental animals. Often, drug-induced steatosis is reversible and does not lead to death of hepatocytes. The metabolic inhibitors ethionine, puromycin, and cycloheximide cause fat accumulation without causing cell death. Although steatosis alone may be benign, it can develop into steatohepatitis (alcoholic or nonalcoholic), which is associated with significant liver injury (Farrell, 2002; Pessayre et al., 2002; Stravitz and Sanyal, 2003; Neuschwander-Tetri, 2006; Saito et al., 2007). Steatohepatitis can progress to fibrosis and even hepatocellular carcinoma. Livers with steatosis are more susceptible to additional insults such as hepatotoxins (Donthamsetty et al., 2007) or hepatic ischemia (Selzner and Clavien, 2001).

Free fatty acids (FFAs) can be newly synthesized in hepatocytes (mainly from carbohydrate-derived acetyl-coenzyme A). FFAs released from adipose tissue can be taken up into hepatocytes or they are generated in the liver from hydrolysis of absorbed fat (chylomicrons). Once in the cytosol, FFAs can be imported into mitochondria for degradation (β-oxidation), or esterified into triglycerides for incorporation into very low density lipoproteins (VLDL), which transports the FFAs to the peripheral adipose tissue. FFA uptake into mitochondria depends on the activity of the mitochondrial enzyme carnitine palmitoyl transferase 1, which can be downregulated by malonyl-coenzyme A, the first intermediate of FFA synthesis. Thus, FFA synthesis, consumption, and storage are in a state of equilibrium with no relevant accumulation of triglycerides in the liver (Pessayre et al., 2002). However, if there is chronic excess food consumption with obesity and insulin resistance, excess uptake of FFAs derived from adipose tissue and food into hepatocytes leads to an overload of FFAs, which cannot be degraded and are therefore esterified to triglycerides. One part of the excess triglycerides is incorporated into VLDL and the other part is stored in the liver gradually leading to steatosis (Pessayre et al., 2002). Drug-induced steatosis is mainly caused by compounds such

as 4,4'-diethylaminoethoxyhexestrol, amiodarone, tamoxifen, perhexiline, amineptine, doxycycline, tetracycline, tianeptine, and pirprofen, which accumulate in mitochondria and inhibit β-oxidation and mitochondrial respiration (Berson et al., 1998; Larosche et al., 2007). This effect does not only lead to steatosis but also to increased reactive oxygen formation and lipid peroxidation. In addition, amineptine, amiodarone, tetracycline, pirprofen, and tianeptine can inhibit directly microsomal triglyceride transfer protein, which lipidates apolipoprotein B to form triglyceride-rich VLDL particles (Letteron et al., 2003). Drugs with this dual effect on β-oxidation and VLDL secretion are generally most steatogenic.

Fibrosis and Cirrhosis Hepatic fibrosis (scaring) occurs in response to chronic liver injury and is characterized by the accumulation of excessive amounts of fibrous tissue, specifically fibril-forming collagens type I and III, and a decrease in normal plasma membrane collagen type IV (reviewed in Bataller and Brenner, 2005; Rockey and Friedman, 2006; Gutierrez-Ruiz and Gomez-Quiroz, 2007). Fibrosis can develop around central veins and portal tracts or within the space of Disse. The excessive extracellular matrix protein deposition and the loss of sinusoidal endothelial cell fenestrae and of hepatocyte microvilli limit exhange of nutrients and waste material between hepatocytes and sinusoidal blood. With continuing collagen deposition, the architecture of the liver is disrupted by interconnecting fibrous scars. When the fibrous scars subdivide the remaining liver mass into nodules of regenerating hepatocytes, fibrosis has progressed to cirrhosis and the liver has limited residual capacity to perform its essential functions. The primary cause of hepatic fibrosis/cirrhosis in humans worldwide is viral hepatitis. However, biliary obstruction and in particular alcoholic and nonalcoholic steatohepatitis are of growing importance for the development of hepatic fibrosis (Bataller and Brenner, 2005). In addition, fibrosis can be induced by chronic exposure to drugs and chemicals including ethanol and by heavy metal overload (Gutierrez-Ruiz and Gomez-Quiroz, 2007). Repeated treatment with carbon tetrachloride, thioacetamide, dimethylnitrosamine, aflatoxin, or other chemicals has been associated with hepatic fibrosis in experimental animals and humans (Zimmerman, 1999).

Central to the development of fibrosis is the activation of hepatic stellate cells (HSC) (Fig. 13-2), which are the main cell type producing extracellular matrix proteins (Bataller and Brenner, 2005; Gressner and Weiskirchen, 2006; Rockey and Friedman, 2006). Products formed during liver cell injury initiate HSC activation. Activating signals can be reactive oxygen species and lipid peroxidation products generated in injured hepatocytes. In addition, Kupffer cells can release reactive oxygen and proinflammatory cytokines during the phagocytosis of cell debris or apoptotic bodies thereby recruiting more inflammatory cells and enhancing the injury and oxidant stress (Tsukamoto, 2002). Damaged sinusoidal endothelial cells contribute to the activation of HSC by generating a splice variant of cellular fibronectin and by release of urokinase-type plasminogen activator, which processes latent transforming growth factor-β1 (TGF-β1) (Friedman, 2000). Furthermore, accumulating platelets at the site of injury can produce TGF-β1 and growth factors such as platelet-derived growth factor (PDGF) (Rockey and Friedman, 2006). Together these stimuli cause the activation of HSC, which undergo phenotypic changes including proliferation, fibrogenesis and matrix remodeling, chemotaxis and proinflammatory mediator formation, and contractility (Rockey and Friedman, 2006). The proliferation of HSC is induced by the formation of mitogens such as PDGF. In addition, it also involves the upregulation of the PDGF receptor, which further enhances the responsiveness of HSC to this mitogen (Pinzani, 2002). Another hallmark of HSC activation is enhanced contractility due to the increased expression of α-smooth muscle actin. Increased expression of endothelin-1 receptors on HSC together with the general imbalance between vasodilator (nitric oxide, carbon monoxide) and vasoconstrictor (ET-1) formation contribute to the development of portal hypertension during fibrosis (Rockey, 2003). The increased accumulation of HSC at sites of injury is caused by migration and proliferation of HSC. PDGF, monocyte chemotactic protein 1 (MCP-1), and other chemokines have been shown to be HSC chemoattractants (Marra, 2002). One of the central events in HSC activation is the excessive formation of extracellular matrix proteins induced mainly by TGF-β1. The effects of TGF-β1, which is generated to a large degree by HSCs, are amplified by the increased expression of TGF-β receptors on HSC (Gressner and Weiskirchen, 2006). However, during fibrogenesis there is not only an overall increase in extracellular matrix deposition but also a change from the basement membrane-like matrix dominated by non-fibril-forming collagens (type IV, VI, and XIV) to a basement membrane-type matrix involving fibril-forming collagens type I and III. The effect is caused by the differential expression and release of matrix metalloproteinases (MMPs) and their inhibitors (TIMPs) from HSC and Kupffer cells. TIMP1 and TIMP2 are upregulated and MMP1 (collagenase I) is downregulated during fibrogenesis leading to the reduced degradation of fibril-forming collagens, e.g., type I. At the same time, MMP2 and -9 (collagenase IV) are activated causing the accelerated degradation of non-fibril-forming collagens (Arthur, 2000). Previously, it was assumed that fibrotic changes, especially the state of cirrhosis, were irreversible. However, more recent insight into the pathophysiology indicated the possibility for reversal of fibrosis. Stimulation of apoptosis in activated HSC and the expression of different MMPs and TIMPs can reduce matrix deposition and enhance degradation resulting in a gradual reversal of fibrosis (Arthur, 2000; Bataller and Brenner, 2005; Rockey and Friedman, 2006). This area is of considerable interest for pharmaceutical intervention.

Tumors Chemically induced neoplasia can involve tumors that are derived from hepatocytes, bile duct cells, or the rare, highly malignant angiosarcomas derived from sinusoidal lining cells. Hepatocellular cancer has been linked to chronic abuse of androgens, alcohol, and a high prevalence of aflatoxin-contaminated diets. In addition, viral hepatitis, metabolic diseases such as hemochromatosis and α_1-antitrypsin deficiency, and nonalcoholic steatohepatitis are major risk factors for hepatocellular carcinoma (Zimmerman, 1999; McKillop et al., 2006; Wands and Moradpour, 2006). The synergistic effect of co-exposure to aflatoxin and hepatitis virus B is well recognized (Henry et al., 2002). The prevalence of hepatitis B and C viruses and environmental factors make hepatocellular carcinoma one of the most common malignant tumors worldwide (Bosch et al., 2005). Angiosarcomas have been associated with occupational exposure to vinyl chloride and arsenic (Zimmerman, 1999). Exposure to Thorotrast (radioactive thorium dioxide used as contrast medium for radiology) has been linked to tumors derived from hepatocytes, sinusoidal cells, and bile duct cells (cholangiocarcinoma) (Zimmerman, 1999). The compound accumulates in Kupffer cells and emits radioactivity throughout its extended half-life. One study of Danish patients exposed to Thorotrast found that the risk for bile duct and gallbladder cancers was increased 14-fold and

that for liver cancers more than 100-fold (Andersson and Storm, 1992).

The molecular pathogenesis of hepatocellular carcinoma is complex and poorly understood. The malignant transformation of hepatocytes occurs as a result of increased cell turnover due to chronic liver injury, persistent inflammation, regeneration, and cirrhosis (Wands and Moradpour, 2006). Direct DNA binding of carcinogens or their reactive metabolites (e.g., aflatoxin metabolites) or indirect DNA modifications by reactive oxygen species generated during inflammation and cell injury can lead to genetic alterations in hepatocytes resulting in impaired DNA repair, the activation of cellular oncogenes, and inactivation of tumor suppressor genes. An overall imbalance between stimulation of proliferation and inhibition of apoptosis in the liver leads to the survival and expansion of these preneoplastic cells (Fabregat et al., 2007). This concept is supported by the observation that 30% of hepatocellular carcinomas show mutations in the tumor suppressor gene p53; the mutation rate is up to 70% in areas with high aflatoxin exposure (Wands and Moradpour, 2006). The functional inactivation of p53 by mutations prevents the induction of apoptosis. Because most chemotherapeutic agents require p53 to induce apoptosis in these cancer cells, hepatocellular carcinomas are mostly resistant to conventional chemotherapy (Bruix et al., 2006). However, p53 mutations alone are not sufficient to initiate carcinogenesis. It was shown that telomere dysfunction and chromosomal instability in combination with p53 mutations are critical for the progression from neoplasms to malignant carcinomas (Farazi et al., 2006). Because telomere dysfunction (shortening) limits the capacity of cancer cells to proliferate, the activity of the telomere-synthesizing enzyme telomerase is activated in advanced hepatocellular carcinomas (Satyanarayana et al., 2004). Stabilization and repair of telomeres promotes the expansion of the tumor. Additional tumor cell survival mechanisms include the disruption of TGF-β apoptosis signaling and activation of phosphatidylinositol-3-kinase/AKT survival pathways (Thorgeirsson et al., 1998). Furthermore, NF-κB activation during inflammation is responsible for induction of prosurvival genes such as Bcl-X_L and XIAP, the downregulation of the Fas receptor on hepatocytes and the reduced expression of the proapoptotic Bax gene (Fabregat et al., 2007). These effects are combined with the overexpression and dysregulated signaling of pro-mitogenic and anti-apoptotic growth factors such as insulin-like growth factor (IGF), hepatocyte growth factor (HGF), wingless (Wnt), and transforming growth factor-α (TGF-α)/epidermal growth factor (EGF) (Breuhahn et al., 2006). Many of these pathways may offer novel therapeutic targets to prevent or eliminate hepatocellular carcinoma.

Critical Factors in Toxicant-Induced Liver Injury

Why is the liver the target site for many chemicals of diverse structure? Why do many hepatotoxicants preferentially damage one type of liver cell? Our understanding of these fundamental questions is incomplete. Influences of several factors are of obvious importance (Table 13-3). Location and specialized processes for uptake and biliary secretion produce higher exposure levels in the liver than in other tissues of the body, and strikingly high levels within certain types of liver cells. Then the abundant capacity for bioactivation reactions influences the rate of exposure to proximate toxicants. Subsequent events in the pathogenesis appear to be critically influenced by responses of sinusoidal cells and the immune system. Discussion of the evidence for the contributions of these factors to the

Table 13-3
Factors in the Site-Specific Injury of Representative Hepatotoxicants

SITE	REPRESENTATIVE TOXICANTS	POTENTIAL EXPLANATION FOR SITE-SPECIFICITY
Zone 1 hepatocytes (versus zone 3)	Fe (overload)	Preferential uptake and high oxygen levels
	Allyl alcohol	Higher oxygen levels for oxygen-dependent bioactivation
Zone 3 hepatocytes (versus zone 1)	CCl_4	More P450 isozyme for bioactivation
	Acetaminophen	More P450 isozyme for bioactivation and less GSH for detoxification
	Ethanol	More hypoxic and greater imbalance in bioactivation/detoxification reactions
Bile duct cells	Methylene dianiline, Sporidesmin	Exposure to the high concentration of reactive metabolites in bile
Sinusoidal endothelium (versus hepatocytes)	Cyclophosphamide, monocrotaline	Greater vulnerability to toxic metabolites and less ability to maintain glutathione levels
Kupffer cells	Endotoxin, $GdCl_3$	Preferential uptake and then activation
Stellate cells	Vitamin A	Preferential site for storage and then engorgement
	Ethanol (chronic)	Activation and transformation to collagen-synthesizing cell

hepatotoxicity of representative compounds requires commentary about mechanistic events.

In vitro systems using tissue slices, the isolated perfused liver, primary isolated cultured liver cells, and cell fractions allow observations at various levels of complexity without the confounding influences of other systems. Models using cocultures or chemicals that inactivate a given cell type can document the contributions and interactions between cell types. A limitation of these in vitro systems is the fact that the artificial cell culture conditions will modify the basal gene expression profile (Boess *et al.*, 2003) and may influence or even dominate the response of cells to a chemical. Whole-animal models are essential for assessment of the progression of injury and responses to chronic insult and the confirmation of in vitro results. Use of chemicals that induce, inhibit, deplete, or inactivate gene products can define roles of specific processes, although potential influences of nonspecific actions can confound interpretations. Application of molecular biology techniques for gene transfection or repression attenuates some of these interpretive problems. Gene knockout animals are extremely useful models to study complex aspects of hepatotoxicity. However, it is critical that the relevance of in vivo systems for the human pathophysiology is being established.

Uptake and Concentration Hepatic "first pass" uptake of ingested chemicals is facilitated by the location of the liver downstream of the portal blood flow from the gastrointestinal tract. Lipophilic compounds, particularly drugs and environmental pollutants, readily diffuse into hepatocytes because the fenestrated epithelium of the sinusoid enables close contact between circulating molecules and hepatocytes. Thus, the membrane-rich liver concentrates lipophilic compounds. Other toxins are rapidly extracted from blood because they are substrates for transporters located on the sinusoidal membrane of hepatocytes.

Phalloidin and microcystin are illustrative examples of hepatotoxins that target the liver as a consequence of extensive uptake into hepatocytes by sinusoidal transporters (Frimmer, 1987; Runnegar *et al.*, 1995a). Ingestion of the mushroom *Amanita phalloides* is a common cause of severe, acute hepatotoxicity in continental Europe

and North America. Microcystin has produced numerous outbreaks of hepatotoxicity in sheep and cattle that drank pond water containing the blue-green alga *Microcystis aeruginosa*. An episode of microcystin contamination of the water source used by a hemodialysis center in Brazil led to acute liver injury in 81% of the 124 exposed patients and the subsequent death of 50 of these (Jochimsen *et al.*, 1998). Microcystin contamination was verified by analysis of samples from the water-holding tank at the dialysis center and from the livers of patients who died. This episode indicates the vulnerability of the liver to toxicants regardless of the route of administration. Because of its dual blood supply from both the portal vein and the hepatic artery, the liver is presented with appreciable amounts of all toxicants in the systemic circulation.

An early clue to preferential uptake as a factor in phalloidin's target-organ specificity was the observation that bile duct ligation, which elevates systemic bile acid levels, protects rats against phalloidin-induced hepatotoxicity in association with an 85% decrease in hepatic uptake of phalloidin (Walli *et al.*, 1981). Subsequent studies found that co-treatment with substrates (e.g., cyclosporin A, rifampicin) known to prevent the in vivo hepatotoxicity of phalloidin or microcystin would also inhibit their uptake into hepatocytes by sinusoidal transporters for bile acids and other organic anions (Ziegler and Frimmer, 1984; Runnegar *et al.*, 1995a).

Accumulation within liver cells by processes that facilitate uptake and storage is a determining factor in the hepatotoxicity of vitamin A and several metals. Vitamin A hepatotoxicity initially affects stellate cells, which actively extract and store this vitamin. Early responses to high-dose vitamin A therapy are stellate cell engorgement, activation, increase in number, and protrusion into the sinusoid (Geubel *et al.*, 1991). Cadmium hepatotoxicity becomes manifest when the cells exceed their capacity to sequester cadmium as a complex with the metal-binding protein metallothionein. This protective role for metallothionein (MT) was definitively documented by observations with MT transgenic and knock-out mice. Overexpression of MT in the transgenic mice rendered them more resistant than wild-type animals to the hepatotoxicity and lethality of cadmium poisoning (Liu *et al.*, 1995). In contrast, MT gene knock-out mice were dramatically more susceptible to cadmium heptatotoxicity (Liu *et al.*, 1996).

Iron poisoning produces severe liver damage. Hepatocytes contribute to the homeostasis of iron by extracting this essential metal from the sinusoid by a receptor-mediated process and maintaining a reserve of iron within the storage protein ferritin. Acute Fe toxicity is most commonly observed in young children who accidentally ingest iron tablets. The cytotoxicity of free iron is attributed to its function as an electron donor for the Fenton reaction, where hydrogen peroxide is reductively cleaved to the highly reactive hydroxyl radical, an initiator of lipid peroxidation. Accumulation of excess iron beyond the capacity for its safe storage in ferritin is initially evident in the zone 1 hepatocytes, which are closest to the blood entering the sinusoid. Thus, the zone 1 pattern of hepatocyte damage after iron poisoning is attributable to location for (1) the preferential uptake of iron and (2) the higher oxygen concentrations that facilitate the injurious process of lipid peroxidation (Table 13-3). Chronic hepatic accumulation of excess iron in cases of hemochromatosis is associated with a spectrum of hepatic disease including a greater than 200-fold increased risk for liver cancer.

Bioactivation and Detoxification   One of the vital functions of the liver is to eliminate exogenous chemicals and endogenous intermediates. Therefore, hepatocytes contain high levels of phase-I enzymes, which have the capacity to generate reactive electrophilic metabolites. Hepatocytes also have a wide variety of phase-II enzymes, which enhance the hydrophilicity by adding polar groups to lipophilic compounds and target these conjugates to certain carriers in the canalicular or plasma membrane for excretion. Generally, phase-II reactions yield stable, nonreactive metabolites. Although electrophiles may be effectively conjugated and excreted, if the intermediate is highly reactive, some of these compounds can react with proteins and other target molecules before an interaction with a phase-II enzyme is possible. In contrast, if the amount of the reactive metabolite exceeds the capacity of the hepatocyte to detoxify it, covalent binding to cellular macromolecules will occur and potentially result in cell injury. Thus, the balance between phase-I reactions, which generate the electrophile, and conjugating phase-II reactions determines whether a reactive intermediate is safely detoxified or may cause cell dysfunction or injury. Because the expression of phase-I and -II enzymes and of the hepatic transporters can be influenced by genetics (e.g., polymorphism of drug-metabolizing enzymes) and lifestyle (e.g., diet, consumption of other drugs and alcohol), the susceptibility to potential hepatotoxins can vary markedly between individuals. Several prominent and important examples are discussed.

Acetaminophen   One of the most widely used analgesics, acetaminophen (APAP) is a safe drug when used at therapeutically recommended doses. However, an overdose can cause severe liver injury and even liver failure in experimental animals and in humans (Lee, 2004). About half of all overdose cases are caused by suicide attempts but an increasing number of cases are reported with unintentional overdosing (Larson *et al.*, 2005). Although the toxicity is a rare event compared to the millions of patients taking the drug daily, APAP-mediated liver injury represents a significant clinical problem. During the last ten years, APAP-induced hepatotoxicity became the most frequent cause of drug-induced liver failure in the US and the UK (Lee, 2004; Larson *et al.*, 2005).

Because >90% of a therapeutic dose of APAP is conjugated with sulfate or glucuronide, the limited formation of a reactive metabolite, i.e., *N*-acetyl-*p*-benzoquinone imine (NAPQI), poses no risk for liver injury. In fact, long-term studies with acetaminophen in osteoarthritis patients did not reveal any evidence of liver dysfunction or cell injury even in patients consuming the maximal recommended daily dose of APAP for 12 months (Kuffner *et al.*, 2006; Temple *et al.*, 2006). In contrast, after an overdose, the formation of large amounts of NAPQI leads first to depletion of cellular glutathione (GSH) stores and subsequently causes covalent binding of NAPQI to intracellular proteins (Jollow *et al.*, 1973; Mitchell *et al.*, 1973) (Fig. 13-5). The generally higher levels of P450 enzymes combined with the lower GSH content in centrilobular hepatocytes are the main reasons for the predominant centrilobular necrosis observed after APAP poisoning. Consistent with the critical role of protein binding for cell injury are the findings that APAP protein adducts are located only in centrilobular hepatocytes undergoing necrosis (Roberts *et al.*, 1991) and that no APAP hepatotoxicity is observed without protein binding (Nelson, 1990). Because protein binding can be prevented by conjugation of NAPQI with GSH, any manipulation that reduces hepatic GSH levels, e.g., fasting or protein malnutrition, potentially enhances the toxicity of APAP. In contrast, interventions such as the supply of cysteine, the rate-limiting amino acid for GSH synthesis, promote the detoxification of NAPQI and limits cell injury (Mitchell *et al.*, 1973). Based on this fundamental insight into the mechanism of APAP hepatotoxicity, *N*-acetylcysteine was introduced in the clinic as intervention therapy (Smilkstein *et al.*, 1988). This highly successful approach, which saved the lives of many patients who took an APAP overdose, is still the most effective treatment available (Lee, 2004).

A significant factor in APAP hepatotoxicity can be the consumption of alcoholic beverages. In addition to potential malnutrition in alcoholics, ethanol is a potent inducer of CYP2E1, which is the main enzyme responsible for the metabolic activation of APAP in humans (Gonzalez, 2007). Whereas the simultaneous exposure of ethanol and APAP competitively inhibits NAPQI formation and therefore prevents APAP-induced toxicity (Sato and Lieber, 1981), the increased expression of CYP2E1 can enhance APAP toxicity after ethanol metabolism (Gonzalez, 2007). In addition, the presence of higher-chain alcohols, e.g., isopentanol, in alcoholic beverages can induce additional P450 isoenzymes such as CYP3A, which can significantly enhance APAP hepatotoxicity (Sinclair *et al.*, 2000; Guo *et al.*, 2004). Despite the clear experimental evidence that alcohol consumption can increase the susceptibility to APAP (Sato *et al.*, 1981) and the clinical observation of severe APAP hepatotoxicity in alcoholics, it remains controversial whether alcohol can actually induce hepatotoxicity at therapeutic doses of APAP as suggested by some case reports (Zimmerman and Maddrey, 1995). However, extensive review of the literature involving APAP consumption in alcoholics suggests no relevant risk for APAP hepatotoxicity at therapeutic levels in this patient population (Dart *et al.*, 2000). In addition, a randomized, double-blind, placebo-controlled trial with multiple therapeutic doses of APAP showed no evidence of liver dysfunction or cell injury in alcoholics (Kuffner *et al.*, 2001). Thus, alcohol consumption does not increase the risk for liver injury after therapeutic doses of APAP. This finding may apply to the potential interaction with other drugs and dietary chemicals. Nevertheless, consistent with experimental data and clinical experience, inducers of CYPs aggravate liver injury after a hepatotoxic dose of APAP.

Although the focus of early mechanistic investigations was on the role of covalent binding in APAP-induced hepatotoxicity, it became apparent during the last decade that protein adduct formation

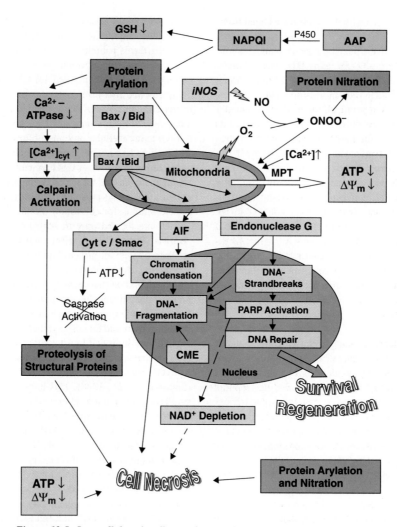

Figure 13-5. *Intracellular signaling pathways of acetaminophen-induced liver cell necrosis.*

Proposed sequence of events leading to acetaminophen (APAP)-induced hepatotoxicity (see text for details). Abbreviations: AIF, apoptosis-inducing factor; CME, nuclear Ca^{2+}/Mg^{2+}-dependent endonuclease (DNAS1L3); cyt, cytosolic; cyt c, cytochrome c; $\Delta\Psi_m$, mitochondrial membrane potential; GSH, reduced glutathione; iNOS, inducible NO synthase; MPT, mitochondrial membrane permeability transition; NAPQI, N-acetyl-p-benzoquinone imine; NO, nitric oxide; O_2^-, superoxide; ONOO$^-$, peroxynitrite; PARP, poly(ADP-ribose) polymerase; Smac, second mitochondria-derived activator of caspases; tBid, truncated form of Bid. (Adapted from Jaeschke H, Bajt ML: Intracellular signaling mechanisms of acetaminophen-induced liver cell death. *Toxicol Sci* 89:31–41, 2006, with permission from Oxford University Press.)

is an important biomarker for APAP overdose (Davern *et al.*, 2006), but protein binding alone was not sufficient to explain cell injury (Fig. 13-5). Because no APAP-induced cell injury is observed without covalent binding of NAPQI to cellular proteins, in particular mitochondrial proteins (Tirmenstein and Nelson, 1989), it is considered a critical initiating event of the toxicity that requires amplification (Jaeschke *et al.*, 2003). Mitochondrial protein binding causes inhibition of mitochondrial respiration, a selective mitochondrial oxidant stress, mitochondrial peroxynitrite formation, and declining ATP levels in the liver (Jaeschke and Bajt, 2006). The early mitochondrial translocation of Bax and Bid, members of the Bcl-2 family of proteins, trigger the release of mitochondrial intermembrane proteins including endonuclease G and apoptosis-inducing factor (AIF) (Jaeschke and Bajt, 2006). These endonucle-

ases, which translocate to the nucleus after APAP exposure, cause the initial nuclear DNA fragmentation (Bajt *et al.*, 2006). Recent findings suggest that activation of c-Jun N-terminal kinase could induce the mitochondrial Bax translocation (Gunawan *et al.*, 2006). However, the continued exposure of GSH-depleted mitochondria to peroxynitrite results in nitration of mitochondrial proteins and mitochondrial DNA modifications (Cover *et al.*, 2005). The continued oxidant stress will eventually trigger the mitochondrial membrane permeability transition (MPT) pore opening with breakdown of the membrane potential, mitochondrial swelling, and rupture of the outer membrane (Kon *et al.*, 2004). These events lead to the loss of mitochondrial ATP synthesis capacity, more extensive nuclear DNA fragmention, and eventually oncotic necrosis (Gujral *et al.*, 2002). In addition to these intracellular signaling mechanisms leading to cell death, additional events may expand the area of necrosis. The release of calpains, which are Ca^{2+}-activated proteases, during necrosis can promote further cell injury in neighboring cells (Limaye et al., 2003). Likewise, the release of DNase-1 enhances nuclear DNA fragmentation in adjacent cells and aggravates the injury after APAP overdose (Napirei et al., 2006). Also, the release of intracellular proteins such as the nuclear protein HMGB-1 from necrotic cells can stimulate macrophages to produce proinflammatory cytokines (Scaffidi et al., 2002). This way, the necrotic cell death during APAP hepatotoxicity can promote an innate immune response with recruitment of neutrophils and other inflammatory leukocytes, which may clear cell debris and prepare for regeneration of the lost tissue (Jaeschke, 2005; Cover et al., 2006) but, under certain conditions, may cause additional injury (see section "Inflammation").

Although many details of the mechanism still remain to be elucidated, the newly gained insight into signaling events in response to APAP overdose suggests two fundamentally new developments: First, necrotic cell death is in most cases not caused by a single catastrophic event but can be the result of a cellular stress, which is initiated by metabolic activation and triggers sophisticated signaling mechanisms culminating in cell death (Fig. 13-5). Second, the multitude of events following the initial stress offers many opportunities for therapeutic interventions at later time points. Because these events are not occurring in all cells to the same degree and at the same time, delayed interventions may not completely prevent cell damage but limit the area of necrosis enough to prevent liver failure. Delayed treatment with GSH to accelerate the recovery of mitochondrial GSH levels effectively scavenged peroxynitrite, reduced the area of necrosis, and promoted regeneration resulting in improved survival after APAP overdose (Bajt et al., 2003). Overexpression of calpastatin, an inhibitor of calpains, attenuated APAP-induced liver injury and enhanced survival (Limaye et al., 2006). A similar effect on the progression of APAP-induced liver injury was also observed in animals deficient in DNase-1 (Napirei et al., 2006). Furthermore, inhibiting the innate immune response exerted beneficial effects against APAP hepatotoxicity (Liu et al., 2004). Together these findings underscore the concept that the later stages of APAP-induced liver injury can be affected at the level of intracellular signaling in hepatocytes, during the propagation of the injury to neighboring cells and the inflammatory response.

Ethanol   Morbidity and mortality associated with the consumption of alcohol is mainly caused by the toxic effects of ethanol on the liver (Stewart and Day, 2006). This targeted toxicity is due to the fact that >90% of a dose of ethanol is metabolized in the liver. Three principal pathways of ethanol metabolism are known (Fig. 13-6). Alcohol dehydrogenase (ADH) oxidizes ethanol to acetaldehyde with a Km of 1 mM; the electrons are transferred to NAD^+, which leads to the production of NADH. Acetaldehyde is further oxidized to acetate in a NAD-dependent reaction by acetaldehyde dehydrogenase (ALDH). This pathway is mainly regulated by the mitochondrial capacity to utilize NADH and regenerate NAD^+ (Stewart and Day, 2006). The formation of excess reducing equivalents and acetate stimulates fatty acid synthesis and is a major factor in the development of alcohol-induced steatosis. Both ADH and ALDH exhibit genetic polymorphisms and ethnic variations, which play a role in the development of alcoholism and liver damage (Agarwal, 2001; Day, 2006). A toxicologically relevant polymorphism involves the mitochondrial ALDH2, where the ALDH2*2 form shows little or no catalytic activity. The increased levels of acetaldehyde present in individuals that carry this polymorphism is thought to cause the

"flushing" syndrome after ethanol exposure. The inactive form of ALDH is found in 50% of Asians but is absent in Caucasians. This may be the reason for the overall reduced incidence of alcoholism in Asia compared to Europe and North America (Chen et al., 1999). However, heterozygotes of ALDH2*2 were found to develop more severe liver injury in response to lower alcohol consumption, suggesting a higher susceptibility to alcoholic liver disease (Enomoto et al., 1991). These findings underscore the importance of acetaldehyde in the pathophysiology.

The second major pathway involves the alcohol-inducible enzyme CYP2E1, which oxidizes ethanol to acetaldehyde (Fig. 13-6). The enzyme is located predominantly in hepatocytes of the centrilobular region and requires oxygen and NADPH. Because the Km of CYP2E1 for ethanol is >10 mM, this reaction is most relevant for high doses of ethanol and, due to the enzyme's inducibility, for chronic alcoholism (Stewart and Day, 2006). The third pathway involves catalase in peroxisomes. In this reaction, ethanol functions as electron donor for the reduction of hydrogen peroxide to water. Thus, the capacity of this pathway is limited due to the low levels of hydrogen peroxide. It is estimated that <2% of an ethanol dose is metabolized through this pathway (Stewart and Day, 2006).

The mechanisms of alcohol-induced liver disease are complex and still incompletely understood. Steatosis is a common feature of chronic alcohol consumption. It is caused by the excessive supply of acetate and NADH, which promotes fatty acid synthesis. In addition, ethanol and acetaldehyde inhibit the DNA binding of peroxisome proliferator-activated receptor-α (PPAR-α), which regulates constitutive and inducible expression of mitochondrial and peroxisomal fatty acid metabolizing enzymes (Aoyama et al., 1998). In addition to the enhanced synthesis and reduced consumption of fatty acids, ethanol exposure inhibits the transfer of triglycerides from liver to adipose tissue. Acetaldehyde inhibits the microsomal triglyceride transfer protein, which incorporates triglycerides into VLDL (Lin et al., 1997), and disrupts the export mechanism of VLDL by interfering with microtubular function (Kannarkat et al., 2006). These effects of ethanol and its metabolites can be compounded in the presence of a high-fat diet. Although steatosis alone does generally not develop into more severe liver disease, it has been clearly established that it plays a critical role in the advancement of the disease process (Day and James, 1998). Steatosis is considered the "first hit," which requires a "second hit" to progress to severe alcoholic liver disease (Day and James, 1998). Based on extensive experimental studies, oxidant stress and lipid peroxidation are currently considered important factors in the pathophysiology of alcohol-induced liver disease. CYP2E1 is a relevant source of reactive oxygen formation during ethanol metabolism (Dey and Cederbaum, 2006). This intracellular oxidant stress in hepatocytes can ultimately induce mitochondrial dysfunction and cell death of hepatocytes, but also activate stellate cells and promote fibrosis (Dey and Cederbaum, 2006). In addition to the intracellular events, alcohol exposure causes an inflammatory response, which contributes to the oxidant stress (Arteel, 2003; Hines and Wheeler, 2004). Gut-derived endotoxin can activate Kupffer cells to produce reactive oxygen species and cytokines such as TNF-α. The formation of these mediators can be further amplified by feedback loops, which enhance cytokine and chemokine formation through priming of the redox-sensitive transcription factor NF-κB in Kupffer cells (Arteel, 2003). In addition, TNF-α can induce the inducible nitric oxide synthase (iNOS, NOS2) leading to the formation of peroxynitrite, a potent oxidant and nitrating species (Arteel, 2003). TNF-α can also directly promote cell death by acting on hepatocytes, which are primed by ethanol-induced depletion of mitochondrial glutathione (Colell et al., 1998). Inhibition of the

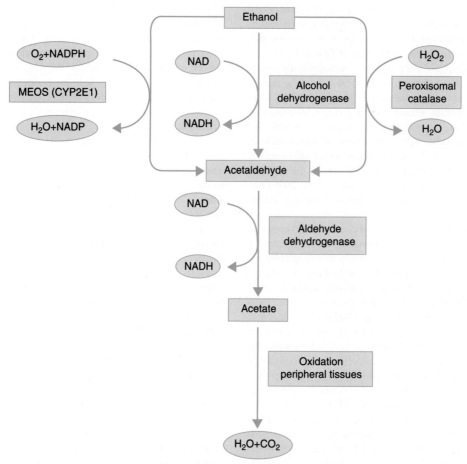

Figure 13-6. Three pathways of alcohol oxidation: ADH, MEOS, and Catalase.

ADH, alcohol dehydrogenase; MEOS, microsomal ethanol-oxidizing system; NADPH, nicotinamide-adenine dinucleotide phosphate (From Stewart SF, Day CP: Alcoholic liver disease, in Boyer TD, Wright TL, Manns M (eds): *Zakim and Boyer's Hepatology.* 5th edn. Philadelphia: Saunders-Elsevier, 2006, p. 579.)

proteasome pathway, a well-recognized feature of chronic alcohol exposure, can enhance chemokine formation in hepatocytes and promote inflammatory liver injury (McClain *et al.*, 2005). Additional proinflammatory mediators and immune responses can be triggered by protein adducts of acetaldehyde and malondialdehyde (Tuma, 2002; Freeman *et al.*, 2005).

Allyl Alcohol An industrial chemical used in the production of resins, plastics, and fire retardants, allyl alcohol is primarily used as a model hepatotoxin due to its preferential periportal (zone 1) hepatotoxicity. The alcohol is metabolized by ADH to acrolein, a highly reactive aldehyde, which is then further oxidized by ALDH to acrylic acid. The fact that the toxicity depends on depletion of hepatic GSH levels is prevented by inhibitors of ADH but enhanced by inhibitors of ALDH suggests that acrolein formation is the critical event in liver injury (Jaeschke *et al.*, 1987; Rikans, 1987). Age and gender differences in allyl alcohol hepatotoxicity can be explained by variations in the balance between ADH and ALDH expression (Rikans and Moore, 1987). The preferential occurrence of allyl alcohol injury in zone 1 hepatocytes (Table 13-3) is caused by the predominant uptake of allyl alcohol in the periportal region and the oxygen dependence of the toxicity (Badr *et al.*, 1986). Although protein binding of the reactive metabolite acrolein and subsequent adduct formation appears to be the main cause of liver cell death

(Kaminskas *et al.*, 2004), lipid peroxidation can become a relevant mechanism of cell injury under conditions of a compromised antioxidant status (Jaeschke *et al.*, 1987). Lipid peroxidation is caused by a reductive stress where the excessive NADH formation leads to mobilization of redox-active iron from storage proteins (Jaeschke *et al.*, 1992).

Carbon Tetrachloride Cytochrome P450-dependent conversion of CCl_4 to $\bullet CCl_3$ and then to $CCl_3OO\bullet$ is the classic example of xenobiotic bioactivation to a free radical that initiates lipid peroxidation by abstracting a hydrogen atom from the polyunsaturated fatty acid of a phospholipid (Recknagel *et al.*, 1989; Weber *et al.*, 2003). The metabolic activation of CCl_4 involves primarily CYP2E1 in vivo as indicated by the absence of toxicity in CYP2E1 knockout mice (Wong *et al.*, 1998). CCl_4-induced lipid peroxidation increases the permeability of the plasma membrane to Ca^{2+}, leading to severe disturbances of the calcium homeostasis and necrotic cell death (Weber *et al.*, 2003). In addition, the $\bullet CCl_3$ radical can directly bind to tissue macromolecules and some of the lipid peroxidation products are reactive aldehydes, e.g., 4-hydroxynonenal, which can form adducts with proteins (Weber *et al.*, 2003). In addition to the intracellular events, Kupffer cell activation can contribute to liver injury (elSisi *et al.*, 1993). Kupffer cells may enhance the injury by oxidant stress (elSisi *et al.*, 1993) or TNF-α generation, which may lead to apoptosis (Shi *et al.*, 1998). In support of these different components of the mechanism of CCl$_4$-mediated cell and organ damage, beneficial effects were shown with inhibition of CYPs, preservation of Ca^{2+} homeostasis, antioxidants, and anoxia (Weber *et al.*, 2003). In contrast, treatments with chemicals that induce CYP2E1, e.g., ethanol or acetone, enhance the injury. This was confirmed in humans. A case report showed the higher vulnerability of workers with a history of alcohol abuse to CCl$_4$ vapors compared to similarly exposed moderately drinking coworkers (Manno *et al.*, 1996). Although the use of CCl$_4$ is restricted and human exposure is limited, it is still a popular model hepatotoxin to study mechanism of cell injury and fibrosis.

Regeneration   The liver has a high capacity to restore lost tissue and function by regeneration. Loss of hepatocytes due to hepatectomy or cell injury triggers proliferation of all mature liver cells. This process is capable of restoring the original liver mass (Fausto, 2000). However, if hepatocyte replication is blocked, hepatic stem cells or oval cells may proliferate to replace the lost parenchyma (Dabeva and Shafritz, 1993; Fausto, 2000). This effect is caused by the reduced sensitivity of oval cells to the proliferation-inhibiting cytokine transforming growth factor-β (TGF-β) (Nguyen *et al.*, 2007). Hepatocytes are normally quiescent, i.e., are in G0 phase of the cell cycle. In order to proliferate, they need to enter the cell cycle. The process is initiated by cytokines (TNF-α, IL-6), which prime hepatocytes to respond to essential growth factors such as hepatocyte growth factor (HGF) and transforming growth factor-α (TGF-α) (Fausto, 2000). Both cytokines and growth factors are involved in the activation of transcription factors and ultimately expression of cell cycle-regulating proteins, i.e., cyclins, the activators of cyclin-dependent kinases (CDK), and p18, p21, and p27, inhibitors of CDKs (Taub, 2004; Trautwein, 2006). The coordinated expression of individual cyclins and inhibitors of CDKs guide the cell through the different phases of the cell cycle including DNA synthesis (S-phase) and mitosis (M-phase). For details on the intracellular signal mechanisms of hepatocyte regeneration, the reader is referred to excellent reviews on this subject (Taub, 2004; Trautwein, 2006).

In recent years, work from Mehendale and coworkers demonstrated extensively that regeneration is not just a response to cell death but is a process that actively determines the final injury after exposure to hepatotoxic chemicals such as thioacetamide, APAP, chloroform, CCl$_4$, galactosamine, and allyl alcohol (Mehendale, 2005). Inhibition of mitosis with colchicine prevented tissue repair and aggravated liver injury after thioacetamide (Mangipudy *et al.*, 1996) and other chemicals (Mehendale, 2005). In contrast, stimulation of repair by exposure to a moderate dose of a hepatotoxicant strongly attenuates tissue damage of a subsequent high dose of the same chemical (autoprotection) or a different hepatotoxin (heteroprotection) (Mehendale, 2005). Tissue repair follows a dose–response up to a threshold where the injury is getting too severe and cell proliferation is inhibited (Mangipudy *et al.*, 1995). In addition to the dose of the hepatotoxin, other factors such as age, nutritional status, and disease state may influence tissue repair (Mehendale, 2005). Of particular interest is the potential increased susceptibility of diabetic animals to hepatotoxins. Streptozotocin-induced diabetes reduced liver injury after APAP overdose in rats (Price and Jollow, 1982) and in mice (Shankar *et al.*, 2003). The mechanism of protection included the faster clearance of APAP due to enhanced sulfation and glucuronidation and stimulated tissue re-

pair (Price and Jollow, 1982; Shankar *et al.*, 2003). However, it remains to be evaluated if the reduced susceptibility is caused by the chemical streptozotocin rather than diabetes. In a genetic model of diabetes and obesity, acetaminophen hepatotoxicity is actually enhanced (Kon *et al.*, 2005). This may have been caused by the increased oxidant stress and the impaired regenerative capacity in these steatotic livers (Aoyama *et al.*, 2006).

Inflammation   The activation of resident macrophages (Kupffer cells), NK and NKT cells and the migration of activated neutrophils, lymphocytes, and monocytes into regions of damaged liver is a well-recognized feature of the hepatotoxicity produced by many chemicals. The main reason for an inflammatory response is to remove dead and damaged cells. However, under certain circumstances these inflammatory cells can aggravate the existing injury by release of directly cytotoxic mediators or by formation of pro- and anti-inflammatory mediators (Fig. 13-7).

Kupffer cells and neutrophils are potent phagocytes, which have a vital function in host defense and removal of cell debris. Formation of reactive oxygen species by NADPH oxidase is a critical tool for these cells. Upon activation, Kupffer cells generate mainly hydrogen peroxide, which can diffuse into neighboring liver cells and create an intracellular oxidant stress leading to cellular stress and injury (Bilzer *et al.*, 1999). Kupffer cells can be activated by bacterial products, opsonized particles and activated complement factors to cause oxidant stress and cell injury (Bilzer *et al.*, 2006). A detrimental role of Kupffer cells in the pathogenesis of toxicant-induced liver injury has been suggested for a number of chemicals including ethanol (Knecht *et al.*, 1995), acetaminophen (Laskin *et al.*, 1995), CCl$_4$ (elSisi *et al.*, 1993) and 1,2-dichlorobenzene (Hoglen *et al.*, 1998). Despite the capacity to directly cause cell damage, a prominent function of Kupffer cells is to generate inflammatory mediators (Decker, 1990). Recent evidence suggests that not only bacterial products but also intracellular proteins, e.g., HMGB-1, which are released during necrotic cell death, can bind to toll-like receptors on Kupffer cells and trigger cytokine and chemokine formation (Schwabe *et al.*, 2006). These mediators may aggravate injury by recruiting cytotoxic neutrophils into the liver (Bajt *et al.*, 2001), directly cause apoptotic cell death in susceptible hepatocytes (Nagai *et al.*, 2002), or promote cytotoxic mechanisms such as induction of iNOS during acetaminophen hepatotoxicity (Bourdi *et al.*, 2002). However, Kupffer cells can also generate anti-inflammatory mediators such as prostaglandin E$_2$ and interleukin-10 (Decker *et al.*, 1990), which downregulate formation of proinflammatory cytokines and attenuate toxin-induced liver injury (Bourdi *et al.*, 2002; Ju *et al.*, 2002). Thus, Kupffer cells can promote or inhibit an injury process and assist in removal of cell debris and apoptotic bodies. In addition, newly recruited mononuclear cells (macrophages) can function in a similar way as Kupffer cells in liver. Although there is a capacity for additional damage by these cells, in general, the recruitment of macrophages into the damaged liver and even the formation of proinflammatory mediators are important signals for inducing regeneration and repair of the damaged tissue (Chiu *et al.*, 2003).

Neutrophils are activated and accumulate in the liver vasculature in response to extensive cell injury or bacterial infection (Fig. 13-7). The main purpose of hepatic neutrophil recruitment is to remove bacteria and cell debris, at least in part through interactions with the resident macrophages (Gregory and Wing, 2002). Neutrophils generate the aggressive oxidant and chlorinating species

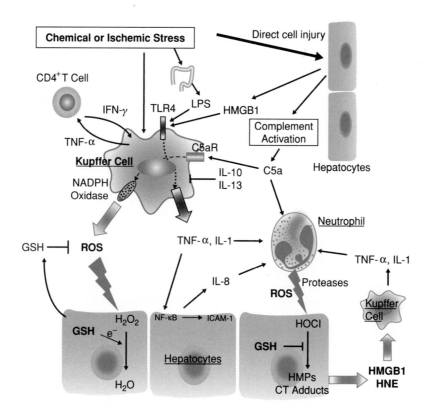

Figure 13-7. Self-perpetuating inflammatory response after chemical or ischemic stress.

C5aR, C5a complement receptor; CT, chlorotyrosine protein adducts; GSH, reduced glutathione; HMGB1, high mobility group box-1; HMPs, hypochlorous acid modified proteins; HNE, hydroxynonenal; HOCl, hypochlorous acid; ICAM-1, intercellular adhesion molecule-1; IFN-γ, Interferon-γ; IL-1, interleukin-1; LPS, lipopolysaccharide; NF-κB, nuclear factor-κB; ROS, reactive oxygen species; TLR4, toll-like receptor-4; TNF, tumor necrosis factor.

hypochlorous acid through NADPH oxidase and myeloperoxidase (El-Benna *et al.*, 2005). In addition, neutrophils can release a large number of proteolytic enzymes and bacteriocidal proteins (Wiedow *et al.*, 2005). The capability of neutrophils to migrate out of the vasculature, adhere to and generate potent cytotoxins in close proximity to its target makes this leukocyte an effective killer of invading microorganisms and remover of dead or dying cells. However, if the cytotoxicity is directed against still viable liver cells, this can cause additional tissue injury or even liver failure (Jaeschke and Smith, 1997). Recent insight into the pathomechanisms revealed that neutrophil-induced liver cell injury is a multistep process (Jaeschke and Hasegawa, 2006) (Fig. 13-7). It requires exposure to inflammatory mediators, which upregulate adhesion molecules such as Mac-1 (CD11b/CD18) on the surface, prime the neutrophils for reactive oxygen formation and cause their accumulation in vascular beds of the liver. If a chemotactic signal is received from the parenchyma, neutrophils will extravasate and adhere to the target. In contrast to other vascular beds, in the liver this process can take place in both sinusoids (capillaries) and in venules (portal and/or postsinusoidal venules). However, extravasation from sinusoids is most critical for parenchymal cell injury (Chosay *et al.*, 1997). At this time, the neutrophil becomes fully activated, i.e., initiates a prolonged adherence-dependent oxidant stress and releases proteolytic enzymes (Jaeschke and Hasegawa, 2006). Cell killing is predominantly caused by hypochlorous acid diffusing into the target cell

and causing an intracellular oxidant stress (Jaeschke, 2006b). Although proteases can also be directly involved in the injury process, the main function of neutrophil-derived proteases appears to be the promotion of the inflammatory process by generation of inflammatory mediators and facilitation of neutrophil migration (Jaeschke and Hasegawa, 2006). It has previously been assumed that the killing of "innocent bystanders" mainly caused the aggravation of liver injury by neutrophils during the attack on dying hepatocytes (Jaeschke and Smith, 1997). More recent findings suggest that neutrophils only attack distressed or damaged but not healthy cells (Gujral *et al.*, 2004). Thus, the aggravation of liver injury by neutrophils is mainly caused by the killing of distressed cells, which would actually survive the original insult (Jaeschke, 2006b). Neutrophils have been shown to be involved in the injury process during hepatic ischemia-reperfusion (Jaeschke *et al.*, 1990), alcoholic hepatitis (Bautista, 1997), alpha-naphthylisothiocyanate hepatotoxicity (Dahm *et al.*, 1991; Kodali *et al.*, 2006), obstructive cholestasis (bile acid toxicity) (Gujral *et al.*, 2003a) and halothane-induced liver injury (You *et al.*, 2006). The recently reported involvement of neutrophils in acetaminophen hepatotoxicity is controversial (Cover *et al.*, 2006; Liu *et al.*, 2006; Jaeschke, 2006c). Although many chemicals cause liver injury without neutrophil participation or do not cause injury at moderate doses, the initiation of an inflammatory response with endotoxin triggers a neutrophil-induced injury or aggravates the existing injury after ethanol, allyl alcohol, aflatoxin B₁, monocrotaline, ranitidine, and

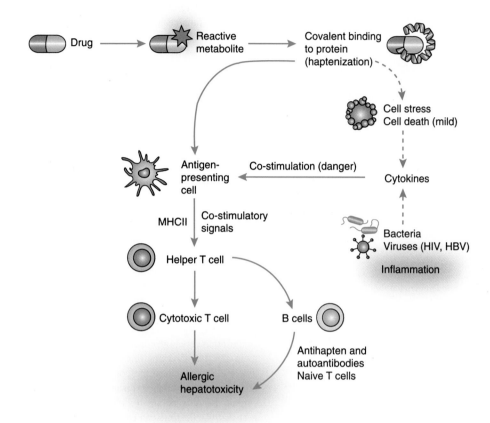

Figure 13-8. The danger hypothesis for immune-mediated idiosyncratic hepatotoxicity.

Hapten formation leading to major histocompatibility complex class II (MHCII) presentation of haptenized peptide by antigen-presenting cells (APCs) along with co-stimulation of APC signalling molecules by mild injury, inflammation or infection promotes helper T-cell activation leading to T-cell responses to the antigen. The cytotoxic T cells are then targeted against hepatocytes that express haptenized protein or MHCI presentation of haptenized peptides on the cell surface. Antibody to haptenized protein or concomitant autoantibodies could theoretically mediate and promote antibody-dependent cell-mediated hepatotoxicity (From Kaplowitz N: Idiosyncratic drug hepatotoxicity. *Nat Rev Drug Discov* 4:489–499, 2005.)

diclofenac (Ganey and Roth, 2001; Apte *et al.*, 2005; Luyendyk *et al.*, 2005; Deng *et al.*, 2006). Thus, a detrimental effect of neutrophils only occurs when activated neutrophils are recruited to the site of injury and if a relevant number of distressed cells, which are killed by neutrophils, would survive without the neutrophil attack (Jaeschke, 2006b).

Immune Responses In addition to the activation of an inflammatory response, immune-mediated reactions may also lead to severe liver injury (Ju, 2005). Drugs and chemicals that have been suggested to cause immune-mediated injury mechanisms in the liver include halothane, tienilic acid, and dihydralazine (Ju, 2005; Uetrecht, 2007). A delay in onset of the injury or the requirement for repeated exposure to the drug and the formation of antibodies against drug-modified hepatic proteins are characteristic features of immune reactions (Ju, 2005). However, the mechanisms of these

immune-mediated liver injuries are not well understood. The *hapten hypothesis* assumes that a reactive metabolite covently binds to cellular proteins and the drug-modified protein is taken up by antigen presenting cells (APCs), cleaved to peptide fragments, which are then presented within the major histocompatibility complex (MHC) to T cells (Ju, 2005; Uetrecht, 2007). In support of the hapten hypothesis, antibodies against drug-modified proteins were detected in the serum of patients with halothane hepatitis (Vergani *et al.*, 1980; Satoh *et al.*, 1989) or with liver injury caused by ethanol, tienilic acid, and dihydralazine (Bourdi *et al.*, 1994; Lecoeur *et al.*, 1996; Tuma, 2002). However, the hapten hypothesis does not explain why other drugs (e.g., acetaminophen), which also form reactive metabolites and drug-modified proteins, do not trigger an immune response. This suggests that additional activating factors may be necessary to induce immune-mediated liver injury. The *danger hypothesis* (Fig. 13-8) postulates that damaged cells release danger

Table 13-4
Examples of Drugs with Known Idiosyncratic Hepatotoxicity

A. *Immune-mediated (allergic) idiosyncratic hepatotoxicity*
  Diclofenac (analgesic)
  Halothane (anesthetic)
  Nitrofurantoin (antibiotic)
  Phenytoin (anticonvulsant)
  Tienilic acid (diuretic)
B. *Nonimmune-mediated (non-allergic) idiosyncratic*
  hepatotoxicity
  Amiodarone (antiarrhythmic)
  Bromfenac (alagesic)—withdrawn from market
  Diclofenac (analgesic)
  Disulfiram (alcoholism)
  Isoniazid (antituberculosis)
  Ketoconazole (antifungal)
  Rifampicin (antimicrobial)
  Troglitazone (antidiabetes)—withdrawn from market
  Valproate (anticonvulsant)

SOURCE: Kaplowitz N: Idiosyncratic drug hepatotoxicity. *Nat Rev Drug Discov* 4:489–499, 2005, and Zimmerman HJ: *Hepatotoxicity.* 2nd edn, Philadelphia: Lippincott Williams & Wilkins, 1999.

signals, which induce the upregulation of B7 on APCs and, the interaction of B7 with CD28 on T cells generates a co-stimulatory signal (Uetrecht, 2007). A cytotoxic immune response occurs only when the T-cell receptor stimulation with the antigen is accompanied by an independent co-stimulation of the T cell. In the absence of this co-stimulatory signal, the antigens derived from drug-modified proteins induce immune tolerance (Ju, 2005; Uetrecht, 2007). Both liver sinusoidal endothelial cells and Kupffer cells can function as APCs in the liver and can be inducers of tolerance to hapten-induced immunological responses (Knolle *et al.*, 1999; Ju *et al.*, 2003). More recently another mechanism of tolerance has been proposed. Hepatotoxic doses of acetaminophen caused a loss of lymphocytes from spleen, thymus, and draining hepatic lymph node and immunesuppression (Masson *et al.*, 2007). These mechanisms could be the reason that tolerance appears to be the default reaction to drug-induced protein modifications in most people. However, impairment of these mechanisms in a limited number of patients can make them susceptible to the immune-mediated liver disease (Ju, 2005; Uetrecht, 2007).

Idiosyncratic Liver Injury Idiosyncratic drug hepatoxicity is a rare but potentially serious adverse event, which is not clearly dose-dependent, is at this point unpredictable and affects only very few of the patients exposed to a drug or other chemicals. However, idiosyncratic toxicity is a leading cause for failure of drugs in clinical testing and it is the most frequent reason for posting warnings, restricting use, or even withdrawal of the drug from the market (Li, 2002; Kaplowitz, 2005) (Table 13-4). In addition, idiosyncratic hepatotoxicity is observed after consumption of herbal remedies and food supplements (Stickel *et al.*, 2005). There are no known mechanisms of cell injury specific for idiosyncratic hepatotoxins. A number of drugs including halothane (anesthetic), nitrofurantoin (antibiotic), and phenytoin (anticonvulsant) are thought to cause injury mainly by immune (allergic) mechanisms as described in the previous paragraph (Kaplowitz, 2005; Uetrecht, 2007). Other drugs, e.g., isoni-

azid (antituberculosis), disulfiram (alcoholism), valproic acid (anticonvulsant), or troglitazone (antidiabetic), are considered nonimmune (nonallergic) idiosyncratic hepatotoxins (Kaplowitz, 2005). Diclofenac (analgesic) can elicit allergic and nonallergic mechanisms of toxicity (Boelsterli, 2003). Because only very few patients (1 in 10,000 or less) treated with these drugs actually experience significant hepatotoxicity, the prevailing opinion at the present time is that an enhanced individual susceptibility with the failure to adapt to a mild adverse drug reaction is a key factor in the pathogenesis (Watkins, 2005). Thus, only small subsets of patients who show elevated plasma ALT levels during drug treatment actually develop severe tissue damage or liver failure (Watkins, 2005). In support of this concept, it was reported that 10–20% of patients treated with isoniazid show increased levels of plasma ALT levels as an indicator of hepatocellular injury (Mitchell *et al.*, 1975). However, only a small subgroup of these patients develops severe hepatotoxicity (Mitchell *et al.*, 1975). This raises the possibility that one or several gene defects, which prevent effective adaption to drug-induced cellular stress, may be involved in idiosyncratic reactions (Watkins, 2005). Recent findings appear to support this hypothesis. The antidiabetic drug troglitazone (Rezulin®) was withdrawn from the market due to idiosyncratic hepatotoxicity. In preclinical studies troglitazone did not cause any relevant liver toxicity and despite extensive investigations since withdrawal of the drug, the mechanism of toxicity remains unclear (Chojkier, 2005). Several studies suggest that very high concentrations of troglitazone can induce mitochondrial dysfunction in vitro (Haskins *et al.*, 2001; Tirmenstein *et al.*, 2002). Because the conditions applied in these studies are not relevant for human exposure, the proposed mechanism cannot explain the idiosyncratic toxicity in humans. However, the data suggest that troglitazone can cause a subclinical mitochondrial stress, which could sensitize hepatocytes to troglitazone. In fact, mice partially deficient in mitochondrial manganese superoxide dismutase (Mn-SOD; SOD2) showed mitochondrial dysfunction and mild liver injury after treatment with 30 mg/kg troglitazone for 28 days (Ong *et al.*, 2007). Although the animals did not develop severe hepatic injury as observed in humans, the injury in mice occurred also after a lag time, which is consistent with the hypothesis that a certain threshold of mitochondrial stress has to be reached to cause cell injury (Ong *et al.*, 2007). Overall, these findings support the concept that a clinically silent genetic deficiency in individuals can trigger the hepatotoxicity of a drug, which by itself may only cause a mild and clinically silent cellular stress. This recent insight indicates the need for a paradigm shift for preclinical toxicity studies (Jaeschke, 2007). The assumption in traditional toxicity studies is that an adverse effect of a drug can be detected by progressively increasing the dose. The experience with troglitazone suggests that this is not always the case. It may be necessary to include experiments with genetically deficient animals in these studies if there is any evidence for clinically silent adverse effects of these drugs. In addition to the genetic makeup, which may render individuals more susceptible to stress induced by the metabolism of drugs or chemicals, a second "hit" such as a systemic inflammatory response can also contribute to the unmasking of the toxicity at least in experimental models (Ganey and Roth, 2001). Because idiosyncratic hepatotoxicity is a rare event for most drugs, it is likely that a combination of gene defects and adverse events need to be present simultaneously in an individual to trigger the severe liver injury. A detailed genomic analysis of patients with idiosyncratic responses to drug exposure may give additional insight what gene expression profile renders a patient susceptible (Watkins, 2005).

FUTURE DIRECTIONS

Continued progress in the understanding of drug- and chemical hepatotoxicity will depend on the use of relevant in vivo and in vitro models including human hepatocytes and analysis of human liver tissue. Traditional mechanistic investigations in combination with genomic and proteomic approaches have the greatest potential to yield important new insight into pathomechanisms. Progress in the understanding of the liver's response to known hepatotoxins and other adverse conditions will not only aid in the development of therapies to limit and reverse acute and chronic liver injury but also improve the predictability of the potential hepatotoxicity of new drugs and other chemicals (Guengerich and MacDonald, 2007).

REFERENCES

Agarwal DP: Genetic polymorphisms of alcohol metabolizing enzymes. *Pathol Biol (Paris)* 49:703–709, 2001.

Ananthanarayanan M, Balasubramanian N, Makishima M, *et al.*: Human bile salt export pump promoter is transactivated by the farnesoid X receptor/bile acid receptor. *J Biol Chem* 276:28857–28865, 2001.

Andersson M, Storm HH: Cancer incidence among Danish thorotrast-exposed patients. *J Natl Cancer Inst* 84:1318–1325, 1992.

Aoyama T, Ikejima K, Okumura K, *et al.*: Liver regeneration after partial hepatectomy is impaired in obese and diabetic KK-AY mice (abstract). *Hepatology* 44(Suppl 1):667A, 2006.

Aoyama T, Peters JM, Iritani N, *et al.*: Altered constitutive expression of fatty acid-metabolizing enzymes in mice lacking the peroxisome proliferator-activated receptor alpha (PPARalpha). *J Biol Chem* 273:5678–5684, 1998.

Apte UM, Banerjee A, McRee R, *et al.*: Role of osteopontin in hepatic neutrophil infiltration during alcoholic steatohepatitis. *Toxicol Appl Pharmacol* 207:25–38, 2005.

Arrese M, Ananthananarayanan M, Suchy FJ: Hepatobiliary transport: Molecular mechanisms of development and cholestasis. *Pediatr Res* 44:141–147, 1998.

Arteel GE: Oxidants and antioxidants in alcohol-induced liver disease. *Gastroenterology* 124:778–790, 2003.

Arthur MJ: Fibrogenesis II. Metalloproteinases and their inhibitors in liver fibrosis. *Am J Physiol Gastrointest Liver Physiol* 279:G245–G249, 2000.

Aw TY: Biliary glutathione promotes the mucosal metabolism of lumenal peroxidized lipids by rat small intestine in vivo. *J Clin Invest* 94:1218–1225, 1994.

Badr MZ, Belinsky SA, Kauffman FC, *et al.*: Mechanism of hepatotoxicity to periportal regions of the liver lobule due to allyl alcohol: Role of oxygen and lipid peroxidation. *J Pharmacol Exp Ther* 238:1138–1142, 1986.

Bajt ML, Cover C, Lemasters JJ, *et al.*: Nuclear translocation of endonuclease G and apoptosis-inducing factor during acetaminophen-induced liver injury. *Toxicol Sci* 94:217–225, 2006.

Bajt ML, Farhood A, Jaeschke H. Effects of CXC chemokines on neutrophil activation and sequestration in hepatic vasculature. *Am J Physiol Gastrointest Liver Physiol* 281:G1188–G1195, 2001.

Bajt ML, Knight TR, Farhood A, *et al.*: Scavenging peroxynitrite with glutathione promotes regeneration and enhances survival during acetaminophen-induced liver injury in mice. *J Pharmacol Exp Therap* 307:67–73, 2003.

Bajt ML, Lawson JA, Vonderfecht SL, *et al.*: Protection against Fas receptor-mediated apoptosis in hepatocytes and nonparenchymal cells by a caspase-8 inhibitor in vivo: Evidence for a postmitochondrial processing of caspase-8. *Toxicol Sci* 58:109–117, 2000.

Bajt ML, Vonderfecht SL, Jaeschke H: Differential protection with inhibitors of caspase-8 and caspase-3 in murine models of tumor necrosis factor and Fas receptor-mediated hepatocellular apoptosis. *Toxicol Appl Pharmacol* 175:243–252, 2001.

Ballatori N: Transport of toxic metals by molecular mimicry. *Environ Health Perspect* 110(Suppl 5):689–694, 2002.

Ballatori N, Christian WV, Lee JY, *et al.*: OSTalpha-OSTbeta: A major basolateral bile acid and steroid transporter in human intestinal, renal, and biliary epithelia. *Hepatology* 42:1270–1279, 2005.

Bataller R, Brenner DA: Liver fibrosis. *J Clin Invest* 115:209–218, 2005.

Bautista AP: Chronic alcohol intoxication induces hepatic injury through enhanced macrophage inflammatory protein-2 production and intercellular adhesion molecule-1 expression in the liver. *Hepatology* 25:335–342, 1997.

Berson A, De Beco V, Letteron P, *et al.*: Steatohepatitis-inducing drugs cause mitochondrial dysfunction and lipid peroxidation in rat hepatocytes. *Gastroenterology* 114:764–774, 1998.

Bianchi ME: DAMPs, PAMPs and alarmins: all we need to know about danger. *J Leukoc Biol* 81:1–5, 2007.

Bilzer M, Jaeschke H, Vollmar AM, *et al.*: Prevention of Kupffer cell-induced oxidant injury in rat liver by atrial natriuretic peptide. *Am J Physiol* 276:G1137–G1144, 1999.

Bilzer M, Roggel F, Gerbes AL: Role of Kupffer cells in host defense and liver disease. *Liver Int* 26:1175–1186, 2006.

Boelsterli UA: Diclofenac-induced liver injury: a paradigm of idiosyncratic drug toxicity. *Toxicol Appl Pharmacol* 192:307–322, 2003.

Boess F, Kamber M, Romer S, *et al.*: Gene expression in two hepatic cell lines, cultured primary hepatocytes, and liver slices compared to the in vivo liver gene expression in rats: Possible implications for toxicogenomics use of in vitro systems. *Toxicol Sci* 73:386–402, 2003.

Borst P, Evers R, Kool M, *et al.*: A family of drug transporters: The multidrug resistance-associated proteins. *J Natl Cancer Inst* 92:1295–1302, 2000.

Bosch FX, Ribes J, Cleries R, Diaz M: Epidemiology of hepatocellular carcinoma. *Clin Liver Dis* 9:191–211, 2005.

Boulares AH, Zoltoski AJ, Stoica BA, *et al.*: Acetaminophen induces a caspase-dependent and Bcl-XL sensitive apoptosis in human hepatoma cells and lymphocytes. *Pharmacol Toxicol* 90:38–50, 2002.

Bourdi M, Masubuchi Y, Reilly TP, *et al.*: Protection against acetaminophen-induced liver injury and lethality by interleukin 10: role of inducible nitric oxide synthase. *Hepatology* 35:289–298, 2002.

Bourdi M, Tinel M, Beaune PH, *et al.*: Interactions of dihydralazine with cytochromes P4501A: a possible explanation for the appearance of anti-cytochrome P4501A2 autoantibodies. *Mol Pharmacol* 45:1287–1295, 1994.

Bouwens L, Wisse E: Pit cells in the liver. *Liver* 12:3–9, 1992.

Boyer JL, Trauner M, Mennone A, *et al.*: Upregulation of a basolateral FXR-dependent bile acid efflux transporter OSTalpha-OSTbeta in cholestasis in humans and rodents. *Am J Physiol Gastrointest Liver Physiol* 290:G1124–G1130, 2006a.

Boyer TD, Wright TL, Manns M: *Zakim and Boyer's Hepatology*, 5th edn. Philadelphia: Saunders-Elsevier, 2006b.

Braet F, Wisse E: Structural and functional aspects of liver sinusoidal endothelial cell fenestrae: a review. *Comp Hepatol* 1:1, 2002.

Breuhahn K, Longerich T, Schirmacher P: Dysregulation of growth factor signaling in human hepatocellular carcinoma. *Oncogene* 25:3787–3800, 2006.

Bruix J, Hessheimer AJ, Forner A, *et al.*: New aspects of diagnosis and therapy of hepatocellular carcinoma. *Oncogene* 25:3848–3856, 2006.

Cai Y, Gong LK, Qi XM, et al.: Apoptosis initiated by carbon tetrachloride in mitochondria of rat primary cultured hepatocytes. Acta Pharmacol Sin 26:969–975, 2005.

Chen CC, Lu RB, Chen YC, et al.: Interaction between the functional polymorphisms of the alcohol-metabolism genes in protection against alcoholism. Am J Hum Genet 65:795–807, 1999.

Chiu H, Gardner CR, Dambach DM, et al.: Role of tumor necrosis factor receptor 1 (p55) in hepatocyte proliferation during acetaminophen-induced toxicity in mice. Toxicol Appl Pharmacol 193:218–227, 2003.

Chojkier M: Troglitazone and liver injury: in search of answers. Hepatology 41:237–246, 2005.

Chosay JG, Essani NA, Dunn CJ, et al.: Neutrophil margination and extravasation in sinusoids and venules of liver during endotoxin-induced injury. Am J Physiol 272:G1195–G1200, 1997.

Colell A, Garcia-Ruiz C, Miranda M, et al.: Selective glutathione depletion of mitochondria by ethanol sensitizes hepatocytes to tumor necrosis factor. Gastroenterology 115:1541–1551, 1998.

Cover C, Liu J, Farhood A, et al.: Pathophysiological role of the acute inflammatory response during acetaminophen hepatotoxicity. Toxicol Appl Pharmacol 216:98–107, 2006.

Cover C, Mansouri A, Knight TR, et al.: Peroxynitrite-induced mitochondrial and endonuclease-mediated nuclear DNA damage in acetaminophen hepatotoxicity. J Pharmacol Exp Therap 315:879–887, 2005.

Crawford JM: The liver and the biliary tract, in Cotran RS, Kumar V, Collins T (eds.): Robbins: Pathologic Basis of Disease, 6th edn. Philadelphia: WB Saunders, 1999, pp. 845–901.

Cullen JM, Ruebner BH: A histopathologic classification of chemical-induced injury of the liver, in Meeks RG, Harrison SD, Bull RJ (eds.): Hepatotoxicology. Boca Raton, FL: CRC Press, 1991, pp. 67–92.

Dabeva MD, Shafritz DA: Activation, proliferation, and differentiation of progenitor cells into hepatocytes in the D-galactosamine model of liver regeneration. Am J Pathol 143:1606–1620, 1993.

Dahm LJ, Schultze AE, Roth RA: An antibody to neutrophils attenuates alpha-naphthylisothiocyanate-induced liver injury. J Pharmacol Exp Ther 256:412–420, 1991.

Dart RC, Kuffner EK, Rumack BH: Treatment of pain or fever with paracetamol (acetaminophen) in the alcoholic patient: A systematic review. Am J Ther 7:123–134, 2000.

Davern TJ 2nd, James LP, Hinson JA, et al.: Acute Liver Failure Study Group. Measurement of serum acetaminophen-protein adducts in patients with acute liver failure. Gastroenterology 130:687–694, 2006.

Davies MH, Harrison RF, Elias E, et al.: Antibiotic-associated acute vanishing bile duct syndrome: A pattern associated with severe, prolonged intrahepatic cholestasis. J Hepatol 20:112–116, 1994.

Day CP: Genes or environment to determine alcoholic liver disease and non-alcoholic fatty liver disease. Liver Int 26:1021–1028, 2006.

Day CP, James OF: Hepatic steatosis: innocent bystander or guilty party? Hepatology 27:1463–1466, 1998.

Decker K: Biologically active products of stimulated liver macrophages (Kupffer cells). Eur J Biochem 192:245–261, 1990.

DeLeve LD, Ito Y, Bethea NW, et al.: Embolization by sinusoidal lining cells obstructs the microcirculation in rat sinusoidal obstruction syndrome. Am J Physiol Gastrointest Liver Physiol 284:G1045–G1052, 2003a.

DeLeve LD, McCuskey RS, Wang X, et al.: Characterization of a reproducible rat model of hepatic veno-occlusive disease. Hepatology 29:1779–1791, 1999.

DeLeve LD, Wang X, Kaplowitz N, et al.: Sinusoidal endothelial cells as a target for acetaminophen toxicity. Direct action versus requirement for hepatocyte activation in different mouse strains. Biochem Pharmacol 53:1339–1345, 1997.

Deleve LD, Wang X, Tsai J, et al.: Sinusoidal obstruction syndrome (veno-occlusive disease) in the rat is prevented by matrix metalloproteinase inhibition. Gastroenterology 125:882–890, 2003b.

Deng X, Stachlewitz RF, Liguori MJ, et al.: Modest inflammation enhances diclofenac hepatotoxicity in rats: Role of neutrophils and bacterial translocation. J Pharmacol Exp Ther 319:1191–1199, 2006.

Denson LA, Sturm E, Echevarria W, et al.: The orphan nuclear receptor, shp, mediates bile acid-induced inhibition of the rat bile acid transporter, ntcp. Gastroenterology 121:140–147, 2001.

Dey A, Cederbaum AI: Alcohol and oxidative liver injury. Hepatology 43(2 Suppl 1):S63–S74, 2006.

Donthamsetty S, Bhave VS, Mitra MS, et al.: Nonalcoholic fatty liver sensitizes rats to carbon tetrachloride hepatotoxicity. Hepatology 45:391–403, 2007.

Ding WX, Shen HM, Ong CN: Critical role of reactive oxygen species and mitochondrial permeability transition in microcystin-induced rapid apoptosis in rat hepatocytes. Hepatology 32:547–555, 2000.

Dutczak WJ, Clarkson TW, Ballatori N: Biliary-hepatic recycling of a xenobiotic: Gallbladder absorption of methyl mercury. Am J Physiol 260:G873–G880, 1991.

El-Benna J, Dang PM, Gougerot-Pocidalo MA, et al.: Phagocyte NADPH oxidase: A multicomponent enzyme essential for host defenses. Arch Immunol Ther Exp (Warsz) 53:199–206, 2005.

elSisi AE, Earnest DL, Sipes IG: Vitamin A potentiation of carbon tetrachloride hepatotoxicity: Role of liver macrophages and active oxygen species. Toxicol Appl Pharmacol 119:295–301, 1993.

Enomoto N, Takase S, Takada N, et al.: Alcoholic liver disease in heterozygotes of mutant and normal aldehyde dehydrogenase-2 genes. Hepatology 13:1071–1075, 1991.

Fabregat I, Roncero C, Fernandez M: Survival and apoptosis: a dysregulated balance in liver cancer. Liver Int 27:155–162, 2007.

Farazi PA, Glickman J, Horner J, et al.: Cooperative interactions of p53 mutation, telomere dysfunction, and chronic liver damage in hepatocellular carcinoma progression. Cancer Res 66:4766–4773, 2006.

Farrell GC. Drugs and steatohepatitis: Semin Liver Dis 22:185–194, 2002.

Fattinger K, Funk C, Pantze M, et al.: The endothelin antagonist bosentan inhibits the canalicular bile salt export pump: A potential mechanism for hepatic adverse reactions. Clin Pharmacol Ther 69:223–231, 2001.

Fausto N: Liver regeneration. J Hepatol 32(1 Suppl):19–31, 2000.

Fickert P, Fuchsbichler A, Marschall HU, et al.: Lithocholic acid feeding induces segmental bile duct obstruction and destructive cholangitis in mice. Am J Pathol 168:410–422, 2006.

Fischer U, Janicke RU, Schulze-Osthoff K: Many cuts to ruin: a comprehensive update of caspase substrates. Cell Death Differ 10:76–100, 2003.

Freeman TL, Tuma DJ, Thiele GM, et al.: Recent advances in alcohol-induced adduct formation. Alcohol Clin Exp Res 29:1310–1316, 2005.

Friedman SL: Molecular regulation of hepatic fibrosis, an integrated cellular response to tissue injury. J Biol Chem 275:2247–2250, 2000.

Frimmer M: What we have learned from phalloidin. Toxicol Lett 35:169–182, 1987.

Ganey PE, Roth RA: Concurrent inflammation as a determinant of susceptibility to toxicity from xenobiotic agents. Toxicology 169:195–208, 2001.

Geier A, Fickert P, Trauner M: Mechanisms of disease: Mechanisms and clinical implications of cholestasis in sepsis. Nat Clin Pract Gastroenterol Hepatol 3:574–585, 2006.

Gerk PM, Vore M: Regulation of expression of the multidrug resistance-associated protein 2 (MRP2) and its role in drug disposition. J Pharmacol Exp Ther 302:407–415, 2002.

Geubel AP, De Galocsy C, Alves N, et al.: Liver damage caused by therapeutic vitamin A administration: Estimate of dose-related toxicity in 41 cases. Gastroenterology 100:1701–1709, 1991.

Gomez-Lechon MJ, O'Connor E, Castell JV, et al.: Sensitive markers used to identify compounds that trigger apoptosis in cultured hepatocytes. Toxicol Sci 65:299–308, 2002.

Gonzalez FJ: The 2006 Bernard B. Brodie Award Lecture. Cyp2e1. Drug Metab Dispos 35:1–8, 2007.

Grasl-Kraupp B, Ruttkay-Nedecky B, Koudelka H, et al.: In situ detection of fragmented DNA (TUNEL assay) fails to discriminate among apoptosis, necrosis, and autolytic cell death: A cautionary note. Hepatology 21:1465–1468, 1995.

Gregory SH, Wing EJ: Neutrophil-Kupffer cell interaction: A critical component of host defenses to systemic bacterial infections. *J Leukoc Biol* 72:239–248, 2002.

Gregus Z, Klaassen CD: Disposition of metals in rats: A comparative study of fecal, urinary, and biliary excretion and tissue distribution of eigh-teen metals. *Toxicol Appl Pharmacol* 85:24–38, 1986.

Gressner AM, Weiskirchen R: Modern pathogenetic concepts of liver fibrosis suggest stellate cells and TGF-beta as major players and therapeutic targets. *J Cell Mol Med* 10:76–99, 2006.

Groothuis GMM, Hardonk MJ, Keulemans KPT, *et al.*: Autoradiographic and kinetic demonstration of acinar heterogeneity of taurocholate transport. *Am J Physiol* 243:G455–G462, 1982.

Guengerich FP, MacDonald JS: Applying mechanisms of chemical toxicity to predict drug safety. *Chem Res Toxicol* 20:344–369, 2007.

Gujral JS, Farhood A, Bajt ML, *et al.*: Neutrophils aggravate acute liver injury during obstructive cholestasis in bile duct-ligated mice. *Hepatology* 38:355–363, 2003a.

Gujral JS, Farhood A, Jaeschke H: Oncotic necrosis and caspase-dependent apoptosis during galactosamine-induced liver injury in rats. *Toxicol Appl Pharmacol* 190:37–46, 2003b.

Gujral JS, Hinson JA, Farhood A, *et al.*: NADPH oxidase-derived oxidant stress is critical for neutrophil cytotoxicity during endotoxemia. *Am J Physiol Gastrointest Liver Physiol* 287:G243–G252, 2004.

Gujral JS, Knight TR, Farhood A, *et al.*: Mode of cell death after acetaminophen overdose in mice: apoptosis or oncotic necrosis? *Toxicol Sci* 67:322–328, 2002.

Gunawan BK, Liu ZX, Han D, *et al.*: c-Jun N-terminal kinase plays a major role in murine acetaminophen hepatotoxicity. *Gastroenterology* 131:165–178, 2006.

Guo GL, Moffit JS, Nicol CJ, *et al.*: Enhanced acetaminophen toxicity by activation of the pregnane X receptor. *Toxicol Sci* 82:374–380, 2004.

Gutierrez-Ruiz MC, Gomez-Quiroz LE: Liver fibrosis: searching for cell model answers. *Liver Int* 27:434–439, 2007.

Hagenbuch B, Dawson P: The sodium bile salt cotransport family SLC10. *Pflugers Arch* 447:566–570, 2004.

Hagenbuch B, Meier PJ: Organic anion transporting polypeptides of the OATP/ SLC21 family: phylogenetic classification as OATP/ SLCO superfamily, new nomenclature and molecular/functional properties. *Pflugers Arch* 447:653–665, 2004.

Haskins JR, Rowse P, Rahbari R, *et al.*: Thiazolidinedione toxicity to isolated hepatocytes revealed by coherent multiprobe fluorescence microscopy and correlated with multiparameter flow cytometry of peripheral leukocytes. *Arch Toxicol* 75:425–438, 2001.

Henry SH, Bosch FX, Bowers JC: Aflatoxin, hepatitis and worldwide liver cancer risks. *Adv Exp Med Biol* 504:229–233, 2002.

Hines IN, Wheeler MD: Recent advances in alcoholic liver disease III. Role of the innate immune response in alcoholic hepatitis. *Am J Physiol Gastrointest Liver Physiol* 287:G310–G314, 2004.

Hoglen NC, Younis HS, Hartley DP, *et al.*: 1,2-Dichlorobenzene-induced lipid peroxidation in male Fischer 344 rats is Kupffer cell dependent. *Toxicol Sci* 46:376–385, 1998.

Homolya L, Varadi A, Sarkadi B: Multidrug resistance-associated proteins: Export pumps for conjugates with glutathione, glucuronate or sulfate. *Biofactors* 17:103–114, 2003.

Honkoop P, Scholte HR, de Man RA, Schalm SW: Mitochondrial injury: Lessons from the fialuridine trial. *Drug Saf* 17:1–7, 1997.

Hooser SB: Fulminant hepatocyte apoptosis in vivo following microcystin-LR administration to rats. *Toxicol Pathol* 28:726–733, 2000.

Hooser SB, Beasley VR, Lovell RA, *et al.*: Toxicity of microcystin LR, a cyclic heptapeptide hepatotoxin from *Microcystis aeruginosa*, to rats and mice. *Vet Pathol* 26:246–252, 1989.

Hooser SB, Beasley VR, Waite LL, *et al.*: Actin filament alterations in rat hepatocytes induced in vivo and in vitro by microcystin-LR, a hepatotoxin from the blue green alga *Microcystis aeruginosa*. *Vet Pathol* 28:259–266, 1991.

Huang L, Zhao A, Lew JL, *et al.*: Farnesoid X receptor activates transcription of the phospholipid pump MDR3. *J Biol Chem* 278:51085–51090, 2003.

Huxtable RJ: Pyrrolizidine alkaloids, in Sipes IG, McQueen CA, Gandolfi AJ (eds.): *Comprehensive Toxicology*, vol. 9. New York: Pergamon Press, 1997, pp. 423–431.

Ishii H, Adachi M, Fernandez-Checa JC, *et al.*: Role of apoptosis in alcoholic liver injury. *Alcohol Clin Exp Res* 27:1207–1212, 2003.

Ito Y, Abril ER, Bethea NW, *et al.*: Inhibition of matrix metalloproteinases minimizes hepatic microvascular injury in response to acetaminophen in mice. *Toxicol Sci* 83:190–196, 2005.

Ito Y, Abril ER, Bethea NW, *et al.*: Mechanisms and pathophysiological implications of sinusoidal endothelial cell gap formation following treatment with galactosamine/endotoxin in mice. *Am J Physiol Gastrointest Liver Physiol* 291:G211–G218, 2006.

Jaeschke H: Cellular adhesion molecules: Regulation and role in the pathogenesis of liver disease. *Am J Physiol Gastrointest Liver Physiol* 273:G602–G611, 1997.

Jaeschke H: Role of inflammation in the mechanism of acetaminophen-induced hepatotoxicity. *Expert Opin Drug Metab Toxicol* 1:389–397, 2005.

Jaeschke H: Mechanisms of liver cell destruction, in Boyer TD, Wright TL, Manns M (eds.): *Zakim and Boyer's Hepatology*, 5th edn. Philadelphia: Saunders-Elsevier, 2006a, p. 37.

Jaeschke H: Mechanisms of Liver Injury. II. Mechanisms of neutrophil-induced liver cell injury during hepatic ischemia-reperfusion and other acute inflammatory conditions. *Am J Physiol Gastrointest Liver Physiol* 290:G1083–G1088, 2006b.

Jaeschke H: How relevant are neutrophils for acetaminophen hepatotoxicity? *Hepatology* 43:1191–1194, 2006c.

Jaeschke H: Troglitazone Hepatotoxicity: Are we getting closer to understanding idiosyncratic liver injury? *Toxicol Sci* 97:1–3, 2007.

Jaeschke H, Bajt ML: Intracellular signaling mechanisms of acetaminophen-induced liver cell death. *Toxicol Sci* 89:31–41, 2006.

Jaeschke H, Farhood A, Smith CW: Neutrophils contribute to ischemia/reperfusion injury in rat liver in vivo. *FASEB J* 4:3355–3359, 1990.

Jaeschke H, Gores GJ, Cederbaum AI, *et al.*: Mechanisms of hepatotoxicity. *Toxicol Sci* 65:166–176, 2002.

Jaeschke H, Gujral JS, Bajt ML: Apoptosis and necrosis in liver disease. *Liver Int* 24:85–89, 2004.

Jaeschke H, Hasegawa T: Role of neutrophils in acute inflammatory liver injury. *Liver Int* 26:912–919, 2006.

Jaeschke H, Kleinwaechter C, Wendel A: The role of acrolein in allyl alcohol-induced lipid peroxidation and liver cell damage in mice. *Biochem Pharmacol* 36:51–57, 1987.

Jaeschke H, Kleinwaechter C, Wendel A: NADH-dependent reductive stress and ferritin-bound iron in allyl alcohol-induced lipid peroxidation in vivo: The protective effect of vitamin E. *Chem Biol Interact* 81:57–68, 1992.

Jaeschke H, Knight TR, Bajt ML: The role of oxidant stress and reactive nitrogen species in acetaminophen hepatotoxicity. *Toxicol Lett* 144:279–288, 2003.

Jaeschke H, Lemasters JJ: Apoptosis versus oncotic necrosis in hepatic ischemia/reperfusion injury. *Gastroenterology* 125:1246–1257, 2003.

Jaeschke H, Smith CW: Mechanisms of neutrophil-induced parenchymal cell injury. *J Leukoc Biol* 61:647–653, 1997.

Jansen PL, Groen AK: Mechanisms of bile secretion, in Boyer TD, Wright TL, Manns M (eds.): *Zakim and Boyer's Hepatology*, 5th edn. Philadelphia: Saunders-Elsevier, 2006, p. 67.

Jansen PL, Sturm E: Genetic cholestasis, causes and consequences for hepatobiliary transport. *Liver Int* 23:315–322, 2003.

Jochimsen EM, Carmichael WW, An J, *et al.*: Liver failure and death after exposure to microcystins at a hemodialysis center in Brazil. *N Engl J Med* 338:873–878, 1998.

Jollow DJ, Mitchell JR, Potter WZ, *et al.*: Acetaminophen-induced hepatic necrosis. II. Role of covalent binding in vivo. *J Pharmacol Exp Ther* 187:195–202, 1973.

Ju C: Immunological mechanisms of drug-induced liver injury. *Curr Opin Drug Discov Dev* 8:38–43, 2005.

Ju C, McCoy JP, Chung CJ, *et al.*: Tolerogenic role of Kupffer cells in allergic reactions. *Chem Res Toxicol* 16:1514–1519, 2003.

Ju C, Reilly TP, Bourdi M, *et al.*: Protective role of Kupffer cells in acetaminophen-induced hepatic injury in mice. *Chem Res Toxicol* 15:1504–1513, 2002.

Jungermann K, Katz N: Functional specialization of different hepatocyte populations. *Physiol Rev* 69:708–764, 1989.

Jungermann K, Kietzmann T: Oxygen: Modulator of metabolic zonation and disease of the liver. *Hepatology* 31:255–260, 2000.

Kaminskas LM, Pyke SM, Burcham PC: Strong protein adduct trapping accompanies abolition of acrolein-mediated hepatotoxicity by hydralazine in mice. *J Pharmacol Exp Ther* 310:1003–1010, 2004.

Kannarkat GT, Tuma DJ, Tuma PL: Microtubules are more stable and more highly acetylated in ethanol-treated hepatic cells. *J Hepatol* 44:963–970, 2006.

Kaplowitz N: Idiosyncratic drug hepatotoxicity. *Nat Rev Drug Discov* 4:489–499, 2005.

Kaplowitz N, DeLeve LD: *Drug-induced Liver Disease*. New York: Marcel Dekker, Inc., 2002.

Kim JS, He L, Lemasters JJ: Mitochondrial permeability transition: A common pathway to necrosis and apoptosis. *Biochem Biophys Res Commun* 304:463–470, 2003.

Klaassen CD: Biliary excretion of metals. *Drug Metab Rev* 5:165–193, 1976.

Klaassen CD, Watkins JB: Mechanisms of bile formation, hepatic uptake, and biliary excretion. *Pharmacol Rev* 36:1–67, 1984.

Knecht KT, Adachi Y, Bradford BU, *et al.*: Free radical adducts in the bile of rats treated chronically with intragastric alcohol: inhibition by destruction of Kupffer cells. *Mol Pharmacol* 47:1028–1034, 1995.

Knolle PA, Schmitt E, Jin S, *et al.*: Induction of cytokine production in naive CD4(+) T cells by antigen-presenting murine liver sinusoidal endothelial cells but failure to induce differentiation toward Th1 cells. *Gastroenterology* 116:1428–1440, 1999.

Ko CB, Kim SJ, Park C, *et al.*: Benzo(a)pyrene-induced apoptotic death of mouse hepatoma Hepa1c1c7 cells via activation of intrinsic caspase cascade and mitochondrial dysfunction. *Toxicology* 199:35–46, 2004.

Kodali P, Wu P, Lahiji PA, *et al.*: ANIT toxicity toward mouse hepatocytes in vivo is mediated primarily by neutrophils via CD18. *Am J Physiol Gastrointest Liver Physiol* 291:G355–G363, 2006.

Kon K, Ikejima K, Okumura K, *et al.*: Acetaminophen induces severe liver injury in obese and diabetic KK-AY mice (abstract). *Hepatology* 42(Suppl 1):512A, 2005.

Kon K, Kim JS, Jaeschke H, *et al.*: Mitochondrial permeability transition in acetaminophen-induced necrotic and apoptotic cell death to cultured mouse hepatocytes. *Hepatology* 40:1170–1179, 2004.

Kuffner EK, Dart RC, Bogdan GM, *et al.*: Effect of maximal daily doses of acetaminophen on the liver of alcoholic patients: A randomized, double-blind, placebo-controlled trial. *Arch Intern Med* 161:2247–2252, 2001.

Kuffner EK, Temple AR, Cooper KM, *et al.*: Retrospective analysis of transient elevations in alanine aminotransferase during long-term treatment with acetaminophen in osteoarthritis clinical trials. *Curr Med Res Opin* 22:2137–2148, 2006.

Lakehal F, Wendum D, Barbu V, *et al.*: Phase I and phase II drug-metabolizing enzymes are expressed and heterogeneously distributed in the biliary epithelium. *Hepatology* 30:1498–1506, 1999.

Larosche I, Letteron P, Fromenty B, *et al.*: Tamoxifen inhibits topoisomerases, depletes mitochondrial DNA, and triggers steatosis in mouse liver. *J Pharmacol Exp Ther* 2007 Feb 2; [Epub ahead of print].

Larson AM, Polson J, Fontana RJ, *et al.*: Acute Liver Failure Study Group. Acetaminophen-induced acute liver failure: Results of a United States multicenter, prospective study. *Hepatology* 42:1364–1372, 2005.

Laskin DL: Nonparenchymal cells and hepatotoxicity. *Semin Liver Dis* 10:293–304, 1990.

Laskin DL, Gardner CR, Price VF, *et al.*: Modulation of macrophage functioning abrogates the acute hepatotoxicity of acetaminophen. *Hepatology* 21:1045–1050, 1995.

Lecoeur S, Andre C, Beaune PH: Tienilic acid-induced autoimmune hepatitis: Anti-liver and -kidney microsomal type 2 autoantibodies recognize a three-site conformational epitope on cytochrome P4502C9. *Mol Pharmacol* 50:326–333, 1996.

Lee WM: Acetaminophen and the U.S. Acute Liver Failure Study Group: Lowering the risks of hepatic failure. *Hepatology* 40:6–9, 2004.

Lee WM, Senior JR: Recognizing drug-induced liver injury: Current problems, possible solutions. *Toxicol Pathol* 33:155–164, 2005.

Letteron P, Sutton A, Mansouri A, *et al.*: Inhibition of microsomal triglyceride transfer protein: Another mechanism for drug-induced steatosis in mice. *Hepatology* 38:133–140, 2003.

Li AP: A review of the common properties of drugs with idiosyncratic hepatotoxicity and the "multiple determinant hypothesis" for the manifestation of idiosyncratic drug toxicity. *Chem Biol Interact* 142:7–23, 2002.

Li S, Zhao Y, He X, *et al.*: Relief of extrinsic pathway inhibition by the Bid-dependent mitochondrial release of Smac in Fas-mediated hepatocyte apoptosis. *J Biol Chem* 277:26912–26920, 2002.

Lieber CS: Alcohol and the liver: 1994 update. *Gastroenterology* 106:1085–1105, 1994.

Limaye PB, Apte UM, Shankar K, *et al.*: Calpain released from dying hepatocytes mediates progression of acute liver injury induced by model hepatotoxicants. *Toxicol Appl Pharmacol* 191:211–226, 2003.

Limaye PB, Bhave VS, Palkar PS, *et al.*: Upregulation of calpastatin in regenerating and developing rat liver: Role in resistance against hepatotoxicity. *Hepatology* 44:379–388, 2006.

Lin MC, Li JJ, Wang EJ, *et al.*: Ethanol down-regulates the transcription of microsomal triglyceride transfer protein gene. *FASEB J* 11:1145–1152, 1997.

Lira M, Schteingart CD, Steinbach JH, *et al.*: Sugar absorption by the biliary ductular epithelium of the rat: Evidence for two transport systems. *Gastroenterology* 102:563–571, 1992.

Liu ZX, Govindarajan S, Kaplowitz N: Innate immune system plays a critical role in determining the progression and severity of acetaminophen hepatotoxicity. *Gastroenterology* 127:1760–1774, 2004.

Liu ZX, Han D, Gunawan B, *et al.*: Neutrophil depletion protects against murine acetaminophen hepatotoxicity. *Hepatology* 43:1220–1230, 2006.

Liu Y, Liu J, Iszard MB, *et al.*: Transgenic mice that overexpress metallothionein-1 are protected from cadmium lethality and hepatotoxicity. *Toxicol Appl Pharmacol* 135:222–228, 1995.

Liu J, Liu Y, Michalska AE, *et al.*: Metallothionein plays less of a protective role in cadmium-metallothionein-induced nephrotoxicity than in cadmium chloride-induced hepatotoxicity. *J Pharmacol Exp Ther* 276:1216–1223, 1996.

Loudianos G, Gitlin JD: Wilson's disease. *Semin Liver Dis* 20:353–364, 2000.

Luyendyk JP, Shaw PJ, Green CD, *et al.*: Coagulation-mediated hypoxia and neutrophil-dependent hepatic injury in rats given lipopolysaccharide and ranitidine. *J Pharmacol Exp Ther* 314:1023–1031, 2005.

Malhi H, Gores GJ, Lemasters JJ: Apoptosis and necrosis in the liver: A tale of two deaths? *Hepatology* 43(2 Suppl 1):S31–44, 2006.

Mangipudy RS, Chanda S, Mehendale HM: Tissue repair response as a function of dose in thioacetamide hepatotoxicity. *Environ Health Perspect* 103:260–267, 1995.

Mangipudy RS, Rao PS, Mehendale HM: Effect of an antimitotic agent colchicine on thioacetamide hepatotoxicity. *Environ Health Perspect* 104:744–749, 1996.

Manno M, Rezzadore M, Grossi M, *et al.*: Potentiation of occupational carbon tetrachloride toxicity by ethanol abuse. *Hum Exp Toxicol* 15:294–300, 1996.

Marra F: Chemokines in liver inflammation and fibrosis. *Front Biosci* 7:d1899–914, 2002.

Masson MJ, Peterson RA, Chung CJ, *et al.*: Lymphocyte loss and immunosuppression following acetaminophen-induced hepatotoxicity in mice as a potential mechanism of tolerance. *Chem Res Toxicol* 20:20–26, 2007.

McClain C, Barve S, Joshi-Barve S, *et al.*: Dysregulated cytokine metabolism, altered hepatic methionine metabolism and proteasome dysfunction in alcoholic liver disease. *Alcohol Clin Exp Res* 29(11 Suppl):180S–188S, 2005.

McCuskey RS: Sinusoidal endothelial cells as an early target for hepatic toxicants. *Clin Hemorheol Microcirc* 34:5–10, 2006a.

McCuskey RS: Anatomy of the liver, in Boyer TD, Wright TL, Manns M (eds.): *Zakim and Boyer's Hepatology*, 5th edn. Philadelphia: Saunders-Elsevier, 2006b, p. 37.

McCuskey RS, Earnest DL: Hepatic and gastrointestinal toxicology, in Sipes IG, McQueen CA, Gandolfi AJ (eds.): *Comprehensive Toxicology*, Vol 9. New York: Pergamon Press, 1997.

McKillop IH, Moran DM, Jin X, *et al.*: Molecular pathogenesis of hepatocellular carcinoma. *J Surg Res* 136:125–135, 2006.

Mehendale HM: Tissue repair: An important determinant of final outcome of toxicant-induced injury. *Toxicol Pathol* 33:41–51, 2005.

Mitchell JR, Jollow DJ, Potter WZ, *et al.*: Acetaminophen-induced hepatic necrosis. IV. Protective role of glutathione. *J Pharmacol Exp Ther* 187:211–217, 1973.

Mitchell JR, Thorgeirsson UP, Black M, *et al.*: Increased incidence of isoniazid hepatitis in rapid acetylators: Possible relation to hydranize metabolites. *Clin Pharmacol Ther* 18:70–79, 1975.

Nagai H, Matsumaru K, Feng G, *et al.*: Reduced glutathione depletion causes necrosis and sensitization to tumor necrosis factor-alpha-induced apoptosis in cultured mouse hepatocytes. *Hepatology* 36:55–64, 2002.

Nagata S, Nagase H, Kawane K, *et al.*: Degradation of chromosomal DNA during apoptosis. *Cell Death Differ* 10:108–116, 2003.

Napirei M, Basnakian AG, Apostolov EO, *et al.*: Deoxyribonuclease 1 aggravates acetaminophen-induced liver necrosis in male CD-1 mice. *Hepatology* 43:297–305, 2006.

Nelson SD: Molecular mechanisms of the hepatotoxicity caused by acetaminophen. *Semin Liver Dis* 10:267–278, 1990.

Neuschwander-Tetri BA: NASH, in Boyer TD, Wright TL, Manns M (eds.): *Zakim and Boyer's Hepatology*, 5th edn. Philadelphia: Saunders-Elsevier, 2006, p. 1031.

Nguyen LN, Furuya MH, Wolfraim LA, *et al.*: Transforming growth factor-beta differentially regulates oval cell and hepatocyte proliferation. *Hepatology* 45:31–41, 2007.

Ogasawara J, Watanabe-Fukunaga R, Adachi M, *et al.*: Lethal effect of the anti-Fas antibody in mice. *Nature* 364:806–809, 1993.

Ong MM, Latchoumycandane C, Boelsterli UA: Troglitazone-induced hepatic necrosis in an animal model of silent genetic mitochondrial abnormalities. *Toxicol Sci* 97:205–213, 2007.

Palmeira CM, Rolo AP: Mitochondrially-mediated toxicity of bile acids. *Toxicology* 203:1–15, 2004.

Pauli-Magnus C, Meier PJ: Hepatobiliary transporters and drug-induced cholestasis. *Hepatology* 44:778–787, 2006.

Pessayre D, Mansouri A, Fromenty B: Nonalcoholic steatosis and steatohepatitis. V. Mitochondrial dysfunction in steatohepatitis. *Am J Physiol Gastrointest Liver Physiol* 282:G193–G199, 2002.

Phillips MJ, Poucell S, Oda M: Mechanisms of cholestasis. *Lab Invest* 54:593–608, 1986.

Pinzani M: PDGF and signal transduction in hepatic stellate cells. *Front Biosci* 7:d1720–d1726, 2002.

Price VF, Jollow DJ: Increased resistance of diabetic rats to acetaminophen-induced hepatotoxicity. *J Pharmacol Exp Ther* 220:504–513, 1982.

Recknagel RO, Glende EA Jr, Dolak JA, *et al.*: Mechanisms of carbon tetrachloride toxicity. *Pharmacol Ther* 43:139–154, 1989.

Rikans LE: The oxidation of acrolein by rat liver aldehyde dehydrogenases. Relation to allyl alcohol hepatotoxicity. *Drug Metab Dispos* 15:356–362, 1987.

Rikans LE, Moore DR: Effect of age and sex on allyl alcohol hepatotoxicity in rats: Role of lirer alcohol and aldehyde dehydrogenase activities. *J Pharmacol Exp Ther* 243:20–26, 1987.

Roberts DW, Bucci TJ, Benson RW, *et al.*: Immunohistochemical localization and quantification of the 3-(cystein-S-yl)-acetaminophen protein adduct in acetaminophen hepatotoxicity. *Am J Pathol* 138:359–371, 1991.

Rockey DC: Vascular mediators in the injured liver. *Hepatology* 37:4–12, 2003.

Rockey DC, Friedman SL: Hepatic fibrosis and cirrhosis, in Boyer TD, Wright TL, Manns M (eds.): *Zakim and Boyer's Hepatology*, 5th edn. Philadelphia: Saunders-Elsevier, 2006, p. 87.

Runnegar MT, Berndt N, Kaplowitz N: Microcystin uptake and inhibition of protein phosphatases: Effects of chemoprotectants and self-inhibition in relation to known hepatic transporters. *Tox Appl Pharmacol* 134:264–272, 1995a.

Runnegar MT, Berndt N, Kong S-M, *et al.*: In vivo and in vitro binding of microcystin to protein phosphatases 1 and 2A. *Biochem Biophys Res Commun* 216:162–169, 1995b.

Runnegar MT, Wei X, Hamm-Alvarez SF: Increased protein phosphorylation of cytoplasmic dynein results in impaired motor function. *Biochem J* 342:1–6, 1999.

Saelens X, Festjens N, Vande Walle L, *et al.*: Toxic proteins released from mitochondria in cell death. *Oncogene* 23:2861–2874, 2004.

Saito T, Misawa K, Kawata S: 1. Fatty liver and non-alcoholic steatohepatitis. *Intern Med* 46:101–103, 2007.

Sato C, Matsuda Y, Lieber CS: Increased hepatotoxicity of acetaminophen after chronic ethanol consumption in the rat. *Gastroenterology* 80:140–148, 1981.

Sato C, Lieber CS: Mechanism of the preventive effect of ethanol on acetaminophen-induced hepatotoxicity. *J Pharmacol Exp Ther* 218:811–815, 1981.

Satoh H, Martin BM, Schulick AH, *et al.*: Human anti-endoplasmic reticulum antibodies in sera of patients with halothane-induced hepatitis are directed against a trifluoroacetylated carboxylesterase. *Proc Natl Acad Sci U S A* 86:322–326, 1989.

Satyanarayana A, Manns MP, Rudolph KL: Telomeres and telomerase: A dual role in hepatocarcinogenesis. *Hepatology* 40:276–283, 2004.

Scaffidi P, Misteli T, Bianchi ME: Release of chromatin protein HMGB1 by necrotic cells triggers inflammation. *Nature* 418:191–195, 2002.

Scheffner D, Konig S, Rauterberg-Ruland I, *et al.*: Fatal liver failure in 16 children with valproate therapy. *Epilepsia* 29:530–542, 1988.

Schuetz EG, Strom S, Yasuda K, *et al.*: Disrupted bile acid homeostasis reveals an unexpected interaction among nuclear hormone receptors, transporters, and cytochrome P450. *J Biol Chem* 276:39411–39418, 2001.

Schulze-Bergkamen H, Schuchmann M, Fleischer B, *et al.*: The role of apoptosis versus oncotic necrosis in liver injury: Facts or faith? *J Hepatol* 44:984–993, 2006.

Schwabe RF, Seki E, Brenner DA: Toll-like receptor signaling in the liver. *Gastroenterology* 130:1886–1900, 2006.

Seitz S, Boelsterli UA: Diclofenac acyl glucuronide, a major biliary metabolite, is directly involved in small intestinal injury in rats. *Gastroenterology* 115:1476–1482, 1998.

Selzner M, Clavien PA: Fatty liver in liver transplantation and surgery. *Semin Liver Dis* 21:105–113, 2001.

Shankar K, Vaidya VS, Apte UM, *et al.*: Type 1 diabetic mice are protected from acetaminophen hepatotoxicity. *Toxicol Sci* 73:220–234, 2003.

Sheikh MS, Fornace AJ Jr: Role of p53 family members in apoptosis. *J Cell Physiol* 182:171–181, 2000.

Shi J, Aisaki K, Ikawa Y, *et al.*: Evidence of hepatocyte apoptosis in rat liver after the administration of carbon tetrachloride. *Am J Pathol* 153:515–525, 1998.

Sinclair JF, Szakacs JG, Wood SG, *et al.*: Acetaminophen hepatotoxicity precipitated by short-term treatment of rats with ethanol and isopentanol: Protection by triacetyloleandomycin. *Biochem Pharmacol* 59:445–454, 2000.

Smedsrod B, DeBleser PJ, Braet F, *et al.*: Cell biology of liver endothelial and Kupffer cells. *Gut* 35:1509–1516, 1994.

Smilkstein MJ, Knapp GL, Kulig KW, *et al.*: Efficacy of oral N-acetylcysteine in the treatment of acetaminophen overdose. Analysis of the national multicenter study (1976 to 1985). *N Engl J Med* 319:1557–1562, 1988.

582

Solter PF, Wollenberg, GK, Huang X, *et al.*: Prolonged sublethal exposure to the protein phosphatase inhibitor microcystin-LR results in multiple dose-dependent hepatotoxic effects. *Toxicol Sci* 44: 87–96, 1998.

Stewart SF, Day CP: Alcoholic liver disease, in Boyer TD, Wright TL, Manns M (eds.): *Zakim and Boyer's Hepatology*, 5th edn. Philadelphia: Saunders-Elsevier, 2006, p. 579.

Stickel F, Patsenker E, Schuppan D: Herbal hepatotoxicity. *J Hepatol* 43:901–910, 2005.

Stieger B, Fattinger K, Madon J, *et al.*: Drug- and estrogen-induced cholestasis through inhibition of the hepatocellular bile salt export pump (Bsep) of rat liver. *Gastroenterology* 118:422–430, 2000.

Stieger B, Meier Y, Meier PJ: The bile salt export pump. *Pflugers Arch* 453:611–620, 2007.

Stravitz RT, Sanyal AJ: Drug-induced steatohepatitis. *Clin Liver Dis* 7:435–451, 2003.

Taub R: Liver regeneration: From myth to mechanism. *Nat Rev Mol Cell Biol* 5:836–847, 2004.

Temple AR, Benson GD, Zinsenheim JR, *et al.*: Multicenter, randomized, double-blind, active-controlled, parallel-group trial of the long-term (6-12 months) safety of acetaminophen in adult patients with osteoarthritis. *Clin Ther* 28:222–235, 2006.

Temple RJ, Himmel MH: Safety of newly approved drugs: Implications for prescribing. *JAMA* 287:2273–2275, 2002.

Thorgeirsson SS, Teramoto T, Factor VM: Dysregulation of apoptosis in hepatocellular carcinoma. *Semin Liver Dis* 18:115–122, 1998.

Tirmenstein MA, Hu CX, Gales TL, *et al.*: Effects of troglitazone on HepG2 viability and mitochondrial function. *Toxicol Sci* 69:131–138, 2002.

Tirmenstein MA, Nelson SD: Subcellular binding and effects on calcium homeostasis produced by acetaminophen and a nonhepatotoxic regioisomer, 3′-hydroxyacetanilide, in mouse liver. *J Biol Chem* 264:9814–9819, 1989.

Trauner M, Boyer JL: Bile salt transporters: Molecular characterization, function, and regulation. *Physiol Rev* 83:633–671, 2003.

Trautwein C. Liver regeneration, in Boyer TD, Wright TL, Manns M (eds.): *Zakim and Boyer's Hepatology*, 5th edn. Philadelphia: Saunders-Elsevier, 2006, p. 23.

Tsukamoto H: Redox regulation of cytokine expression in Kupffer cells. *Antioxid Redox Signal* 4:741–748, 2002.

Tsutsumi M, Lasker JM, Shimizu M, *et al.*: The intralobular distribution of ethanol-inducible P450IIE1 in rat and human liver. *Hepatology* 10:437–446, 1989.

Tuma DJ: Role of malondialdehyde-acetaldehyde adducts in liver injury. *Free Radic Biol Med* 32:303–308, 2002.

Uetrecht J: Idiosyncratic drug reactions: Current understanding. *Annu Rev Pharmacol Toxicol* 47:513–539, 2007.

Vergani D, Mieli-Vergani G, Alberti A, *et al.*: Antibodies to the surface of halothane-altered rabbit hepatocytes in patients with severe halothane-associated hepatitis. *N Engl J Med* 303:66–71, 1980.

Wagner M, Fickert P, Zollner G, *et al.*: Role of farnesoid X receptor in determining hepatic ABC transporter expression and liver injury in bile duct-ligated mice. *Gastroenterology* 125:825–838, 2003.

Wagner M, Halilbasic E, Marschall HU, *et al.*: CAR and PXR agonists stimulate hepatic bile acid and bilirubin detoxification and elimination pathways in mice. *Hepatology* 42:420–430, 2005.

Wake K: Perisinusoidal stellate cells (fat-storing cells, interstitial cells, lipocytes), their related structure in and around liver sinusoids, and vitamin A-storing cells in extrahepatic organs. *Int Rev Cytol* 66:303–353, 1980.

Walli AK, Wieland E, Wieland TH: Phalloidin uptake by the liver of cholestatic rats in vivo, in isolated perfused liver and isolated hepatocytes. *Naunyn-Schmiedeberg's Arch Pharmacol* 316:257–261, 1981.

Wands JR, Moradpour D: Molecular pathogenesis of hepatocellular carcinoma, in Boyer TD, Wright TL, Manns M (eds.): *Zakim and Boyer's Hepatology*, 5th edn. Philadelphia: Saunders-Elsevier, 2006, p. 165.

Wang X, Kanel GC, DeLeve LD: Support of sinusoidal endothelial cell glutathione prevents hepatic veno-occlusive disease in the rat. *Hepatology* 31:428–434, 2000.

Watanabe S, Phillips MJ: Acute phalloidin toxicity in living hepatocytes: Evidence for a possible disturbance in membrane flow and for multiple functions for actin in the liver cell. *Am J Pathol* 122:101–111, 1986.

Watanabe N, Tsukada N, Smith CR, *et al.*: Permeabilized hepatocyte couplets: Adenosine triphosphate-dependent bile canalicular contractions and a circumferential pericanalicular microfilament belt demonstrated. *Lab Invest* 65:203–213, 1991.

Watkins PB: Idiosyncratic liver injury: Challenges and approaches. *Toxicol Pathol* 33:1–5, 2005.

Weber LW, Boll M, Stampfl A: Hepatotoxicity and mechanism of action of haloalkanes: Carbon tetrachloride as a toxicological model. *Crit Rev Toxicol* 33:105–136, 2003.

Wiedow O, Meyer-Hoffert U: Neutrophil serine proteases: Potential key regulators of cell signalling during inflammation. *J Intern Med* 257(4):319–328, 2005.

Wong FW, Chan WY, Lee SS: Resistance to carbon tetrachloride-induced hepatotoxicity in mice which lack CYP2E1 expression. *Toxicol Appl Pharmacol* 153:109–118, 1998.

Yamamoto Y, Nakajima M, Yamazaki H, *et al.*: Cytotoxicity and apoptosis produced by troglitazone in human hepatoma cells. *Life Sci* 70:471–482, 2001.

Yin XM, Wang K, Gross A, *et al.*: Bid-deficient mice are resistant to Fas-induced hepatocellular apoptosis. *Nature* 400:886–891, 1999.

You Q, Cheng L, Reilly TP, *et al.*: Role of neutrophils in a mouse model of halothane-induced liver injury. *Hepatology* 44:1421–1431, 2006.

Zhang Y, Chong E, Herman B: Age-associated increases in the activity of multiple caspases in Fisher 344 rat organs. *Exp Gerontol* 37:777–789, 2002.

Ziegler K, Frimmer M: Cyclosporin A protects liver cells against phalloidin: Potent inhibition of the inward transport by cholate and phallotoxins. *Biochim Biophys Acta* 805:174–180, 1984.

Zimmerman HJ: *Hepatotoxicity*, 2nd edn. Philadelphia: Lippincott, Williams & Wilkins, 1999.

Zimmerman HJ, Maddrey WC: Acetaminophen (paracetamol) hepatotoxicity with regular intake of alcohol: Analysis of instances of therapeutic misadventure. *Hepatology* 22:767–773, 1995.

Zollner G, Marschall HU, Wagner M, *et al.*: Role of nuclear receptors in the adaptive response to bile acids and cholestasis: Pathogenetic and therapeutic considerations. *Mol Pharm* 3:231–251, 2006.

CHAPTER 14

TOXIC RESPONSES OF THE KIDNEY

Rick G. Schnellmann

The functional integrity of the mammalian kidney is vital to total body homeostasis because the kidney plays a principal role in the excretion of metabolic wastes and in the regulation of extracellular fluid volume, electrolyte composition, and acid–base balance. In addition, the kidney synthesizes and releases hormones, such as renin and erythropoietin, and metabolizes vitamin D_3 to the active 1,25-dihydroxy vitamin D_3 form. A toxic insult to the kidney therefore could disrupt any or all of these functions and could have profound effects on total body metabolism. Fortunately, the kidneys are equipped with a variety of detoxification mechanisms and have considerable functional reserve and regenerative capacities. Nonetheless, the nature and severity of the toxic insult may be such that these detoxification and compensatory mechanisms are overwhelmed, and kidney injury ensues. The outcome of renal failure can be profound; permanent renal damage may result, requiring chronic dialysis treatment or kidney transplantation.

FUNCTIONAL ANATOMY

Gross examination of a sagittal section of the kidney reveals three clearly demarcated anatomic areas: the cortex, medulla, and papilla (Figs. 14-1 and 14-2). The cortex constitutes the major portion of the kidney and receives a disproportionately higher percentage (90%) of blood flow compared to the medulla ($\sim$6–10%) or papilla (1–2%). Thus, when a blood-borne toxicant is delivered to the kidney, a high percentage of the material will be delivered to the cortex and will have a greater opportunity to influence cortical rather than medullary or papillary functions. However, medullary and papillary tissues are exposed to higher luminal concentrations of toxicants for prolonged periods of time, a consequence of the more concentrated tubular fluid and the more sluggish flow of blood and filtrate in these regions.

The functional unit of the kidney, the nephron, may be considered in three portions: the vascular element, the glomerulus, and the tubular element.

Renal Vasculature and Glomerulus

The renal artery branches successively into interlobar, arcuate, and interlobular arteries (Fig. 14-1). The last of these give rise to the afferent arterioles, which supply the glomerulus; blood then leaves the glomerular capillaries via the efferent arteriole. Both the afferent and efferent arterioles, arranged in a series before and after the glomerular capillary tuft, respectively, are ideally situated to control

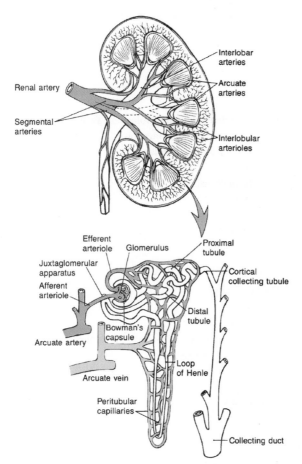

Figure 14-1. Schematic of the human kidney showing the major blood vessels and the microcirculation and tubular components of each nephron. [From Guyton AC, Hall JE (eds.): Textbook of Medical Physiology. Philadelphia: WB Saunders, 1996, p. 318, with permission from Elsevier.]

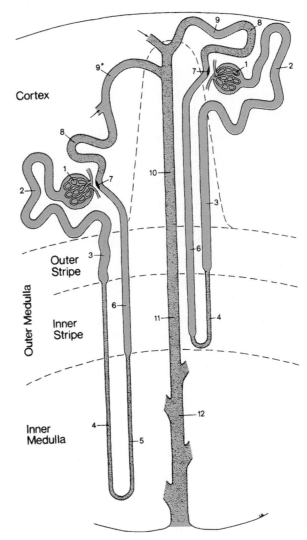

Figure 14-2. Schematic of short- and long-looped nephrons and the collecting system.

A medullary ray is delineated by a dashed line within the cortex. (1) Renal corpuscle including Bowman's capsule and the glomerulus; (2) proximal convoluted tubule; (3) proximal straight tubule; (4) descending thin limb; (5) thin ascending limb; (6) thick ascending limb; (7) macula densa, located within the final portion of the thick ascending limb; (8) distal convoluted tubule; (9) connecting tubule; (9*) connecting tubule of the juxtamedullary nephron, which forms an arcade; (10) cortical collecting duct; (11) outer medullary collecting duct; (12) inner medullary collecting duct. [From Kriz W: Standard nomenclature for structures of the kidney. *Am J Physiol* 254:F1–F8, 1988, with permission.]

glomerular capillary pressure and glomerular plasma flow rate. Indeed, these arterioles are innervated by the sympathetic nervous system and contract in response to nerve stimulation, angiotensin II, vasopressin, endothelin, adenosine, and norepinehrine, affecting glomerular pressures and blood flow. The efferent arterioles draining the cortical glomeruli branch into a peritubular capillary network, whereas those draining the juxtamedullary glomeruli form a capillary loop, the vasa recta, supplying the medullary structures. These postglomerular capillary loops provide an efficient arrangement for delivery of nutrients to the postglomerular tubular structures, delivery of wastes to the tubule for excretion, and return of reabsorbed electrolytes, nutrients, and water to the systemic circulation.

The glomerulus is a complex, specialized capillary bed composed primarily of endothelial cells that are characterized by an attenuated and fenestrated cytoplasm, visceral epithelial cells characterized by a cell body (podocyte) from which many trabeculae and pedicles (foot processes) extend, and a glomerular basement membrane (GBM), which is a trilamellar structure sandwiched between the endothelial and epithelial cells (Fig. 14-3). A portion of the blood entering the glomerular capillary network is fractionated into a virtually protein-free and cell-free ultrafiltrate, which passes through Bowman's space and into the tubular portion of the nephron. The formation of such an ultrafiltrate is the net re-

sult of the Starling forces that determine fluid movement across capillary beds, that is, the balance between transcapillary hydrostatic pressure and colloid oncotic pressure (Maddox and Brenner, 1991). Filtration is therefore favored when transcapillary hydrostatic pressure exceeds plasma oncotic pressure. An additional determinant of ultrafiltration is the effective hydraulic permeability of the glomerular capillary wall, in other words, the ultrafiltration coefficient (K_f), which is determined by the total surface area available for filtration and the hydraulic permeability of the capillary wall. Consequently, chemically induced decreases in glomerular filtration rate (GFR) may be related to decreases in transcapillary

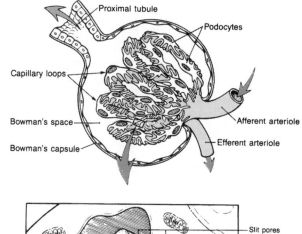

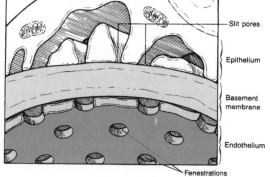

Figure 14-3. A. Schematic of the ultrastructure of the glomerular capillaries. B. Cross-section of the glomerular capillary membrane with the capillary endothelium, basement membrane, and epithelium podocytes. [From Guyton AC, Hall JE (eds.): Textbook of Medical Physiology. Philadelphia: WB Saunders, 1996, p. 32, with permission from Elsevier.]

hydrostatic pressure and glomerular plasma flow due to increased afferent arteriolar resistance or to decreases in the surface area available for filtration, resulting from decreases in the size and/or number of endothelial fenestrae or detachment or effacement of foot processes.

Although the glomerular capillary wall permits a high rate of fluid filtration (approximately 20% of blood entering the glomerulus is filtered), it provides a significant barrier to the transglomerular passage of macromolecules. Experiments using a variety of charged and neutral tracers have established that this barrier function is based on the ability of the glomerulus to act as a size-selective and charge-selective filter (Brenner *et al.*, 1977). In general, the filtration of macromolecules is inversely proportional to the molecular weight of a substance; thus, small molecules, such as inulin (MW 5,500), are freely filtered, whereas large molecules, such as albumin (MW 56,000–70,000), are restricted. Filtration of anionic molecules tends to be restricted compared to that of neutral or cationic molecules of the same size. These permselective properties of the glomerulus appear to be directly related to the physicochemical properties of the different cell types within the glomerulus (Kanwar *et al.*, 1991). In particular, charge-selective properties of the glomerulus appear to be related to the anionic groups of the GBM coupled with the anionic coating of the epithelial and endothelial cells (Fig. 14-3). These highly anionic components produce electrostatic repulsion and hinder the circulation of polyanionic macromolecules, thereby markedly retarding passage of these molecules across the filtration barrier. Toxicants that neutralize or reduce the number of fixed an-

ionic charges on glomerular structural elements therefore will impair the charge- and/or size-selective properties of the glomerulus, resulting in urinary excretion of polyanionic and/or high-molecular-weight proteins.

Proximal Tubule

The proximal tubule consists of three discrete segments: the S_1 (pars convoluta), S_2 (transition between pars convoluta and pars recta), and S_3 (the pars recta) segments (Fig. 14-2). The S_1 segment is the initial portion of the proximal convoluted tubule and is characterized by a tall brush border and a well-developed vacuolar lysosomal system. The basolateral membrane is extensively interdigitated and many long mitochondria fill the basal portion of the cell, characteristic of Na^+-transporting epithelia. The S_2 segment comprises the end of the convoluted segment and the initial portion of the straight segment. These cells possess a shorter brush border, fewer apical vacuoles and mitochondria, and less basolateral interdigitation compared to the S_1 cells. The S_3 segment comprises the distal portion of proximal segments and extends to the junction of the outer and inner stripe of the outer medulla. The S_3 cells have a well-developed brush border but fewer and smaller lysosomes and mitochondria than S_1 and S_2 cells.

The formation of urine is a highly complex and integrated process in which the volume and composition of the glomerular filtrate is progressively altered as fluid passes through each of the different tubular segments. The proximal tubule is the workhorse of the nephron, as it reabsorbs approximately 60–80% of solute and water filtered at the glomerulus. Toxicant-induced injury to the proximal tubule therefore will have major consequences to water and solute balance. Water reabsorption is through a passive iso-osmotic process, driven primarily by Na^+ reabsorption, mediated by the Na^+, K^+-ATPase localized in the basolateral plasma membrane. In addition to active Na^+ reabsorption, the proximal tubule reabsorbs other electrolytes, such as K^+, HCO_3^-, Cl^-, PO_4^{3-}, Ca^{2+}, and Mg^{2+}. The proximal tubule contains numerous transport systems capable of driving concentrative transport of many metabolic substrates, including amino acids, glucose, and citric acid cycle intermediates. The proximal tubule also reabsorbs virtually all the filtered low-molecular-weight proteins by specific endocytotic protein reabsorption processes. In addition, small linear peptides may be hydrolyzed by peptidases associated with the proximal tubular brush border. An important excretory function of the proximal tubule is secretion of weak organic anions and cations by specialized transporters that drive concentrative movement of these ions from postglomerular blood into proximal tubular cells, followed by secretion into tubular fluid. Toxicant-induced interruptions in the production of energy for any of these active transport mechanisms or the function of critical membrane-bound enzymes or transporters can profoundly affect proximal tubular and whole-kidney function.

The different segments of the proximal tubule exhibit marked biochemical and physiologic heterogeneity (Goldstein, 1993). For example, filtered HCO_3^-, low-molecular-weight proteins, amino acids, and glucose are primarily reabsorbed by the S_1 segment. Transport capacities for these substances in the S_2 and S_3 segments are appreciably less; for example, glucose reabsorption in the S_2 and S_3 segments is about 50% and 10% of that in the S_1 segment, respectively. In contrast, the principal site of organic anion and cation secretion is in the S_2 and S_1/S_2 segments, respectively. Oxygen consumption, Na^+, K^+-ATPase activity, and gluconeogenic capacity are greater in the S_1 and S_2 segments than in the S_3 segment.

Table 14-1
Filtration, Reabsorption, and Excretion Rates of Different Substances by the Kidneys*

	FILTERED (meq/24 h)	REABSORBED (meq/24 h)	EXCRETED (meq/24 h)	REABSORBED (%)
Glucose (g/day)	180	180	0	100
Bicarbonate (meq/day)	4320	4318	2	>99.9
Sodium (meq/day)	25,560	25,410	150	99.4
Chloride (meq/day)	19,440	19,260	180	99.1
Water (L/day)	169	167.5	1.5	99.1
Urea (g/day)	48	24	24	50
Creatinine (g/day)	1.8	0	1.8	0

*Glomerular filtration rate: 125 mL/min = 180 L/24 h.

Catabolism and apical transport of glutathione (GSH) occurs to a much greater extent in the S_3 segment, where the brush-border enzyme γ-glutamyl transpeptidase is present in greater amounts. Chemically induced injury to distinct proximal tubular segments therefore may be related in part to their segmental differences in biochemical properties (see section "Site-Selective Injury").

Loop of Henle

The thin descending and ascending limbs and the thick ascending limb of the loop of Henle are critical to the processes involved in urinary concentration (Fig. 14-2). Approximately 25% of the filtered Na^+ and K^+ and 20% of the filtered water are reabsorbed by the segments of the loop of Henle. The tubular fluid entering the thin descending limb is iso-osmotic to the renal interstitium; water is freely permeable and solutes, such as electrolytes and urea, may enter from the interstitium. In contrast, the thin ascending limb is relatively impermeable to water and urea, and Na^+ and Cl^- are reabsorbed by passive diffusion. The thick ascending limb is impermeable to water, and active transport of Na^+ and Cl^- is mediated by the Na^+/K^+-$2Cl^-$ cotransport mechanism, with the energy provided by the Na^+, K^+-ATPase. The relatively high rates of Na^+, K^+-ATPase activity and oxygen demand, coupled with the meager oxygen supply in the medullary thick ascending limb, are believed to contribute to the vulnerability of this segment of the nephron to hypoxic injury. The close interdependence between metabolic workload and tubular vulnerability has been demonstrated, revealing that selective damage to the thick ascending limb in the isolated perfused kidney can be blunted by reducing tubular work and oxygen consumption (via inhibition of the Na^+, K^+-ATPase with ouabain) or by increasing oxygen supply (via provision of an oxygen carrier, hemoglobin) (Brezis and Epstein, 1993). Conversely, increasing the tubular workload (via the ionophore amphotericin B) exacerbates hypoxic injury to this segment (Brezis et al., 1984).

Distal Tubule and Collecting Duct

The macula densa comprises specialized cells located between the end of the thick ascending limb and the early distal tubule, in close proximity to the afferent arteriole (Fig. 14-2). This anatomic arrangement is ideally suited for a feedback system whereby a stimulus received at the macula densa is transmitted to the arterioles of the same nephron. Under normal physiologic conditions, increased solute delivery or concentration at the macula densa triggers a signal resulting in afferent arteriolar constriction leading to decreases in GFR (and hence decreased solute delivery). Thus, increases in fluid/solute out of the proximal tubule, due to impaired tubular re-

absorption, will activate this feedback system, referred to as tubuloglomerular feedback (TGF) and resulting in decreases in the filtration rate of the same nephron. This regulatory mechanism is viewed as a powerful volume-conserving mechanism, designed to decrease GFR in order to prevent massive losses of fluid/electrolytes due to impaired tubular reabsorption. Humoral mediation of TGF by the renin-angiotensin system has been proposed, and evidence suggests that other substances may be involved. The distal tubular cells contain numerous mitochondria but lack a well-developed brush border and an endocytotic apparatus characteristic of the pars convoluta of the proximal tubule. The early distal tubule reabsorbs most of the remaining intraluminal Na^+, K^+, and Cl^- but is relatively impermeable to water.

The late distal tubule, cortical collecting tubule, and medullary collecting duct perform the final regulation and fine-tuning of urinary volume and composition. The remaining Na^+ is reabsorbed in conjunction with K^+ and H^+ secretion in the late distal tubule and cortical collecting tubule. The combination of medullary and papillary hypertonicity generated by countercurrent multiplication and the action of antidiuretic hormone (vasopressin, ADH) serve to enhance water permeability of the medullary collecting duct. Agents that interfere with ADH synthesis, secretion, or action therefore may impair concentrating ability. Additionally, because urinary concentrating ability is dependent upon medullary and papillary hypertonicity, agents that increase medullary blood flow may impair concentrating ability by dissipating the medullary osmotic gradient.

Table 14-1 illustrates the efficiency of the nephrons in the conservation of electrolytes, substrates, and water and excretion of nitrogenous wastes (urea). The reader may refer Brenner and Rector's *The Kidney* (2004) and *Diseases of the Kidney and Urinary Tract* (2006) for further review of renal physiology.

PATHOPHYSIOLOGIC RESPONSES OF THE KIDNEY

Acute Kidney Injury

One of the most common manifestations of nephrotoxic damage is acute renal failure—an abrupt decline in kidney function secondary to an injury that leads to a functional or structural change in the kidney (American Society of Nephrology, 2005). While *acute renal failure* is the commonly used terminology, it has numerous definitions; the American Society of Nephrology Research Report (2005) recently suggested that the term *acute kidney injury* (AKI) be used to describe the entire spectrum of the disease. AKI is defined as a complex disorder that comprises multiple causative factors and occurs

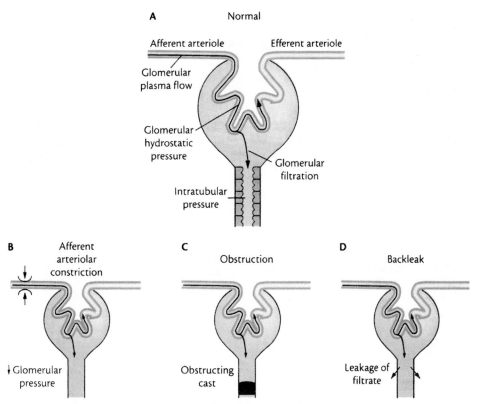

Figure 14-4. Mechanisms of reduction of the GFR.

A. GFR depends on four factors: (1) adequate blood flow to the glomerulus; (2) adequate glomerular capillary pressure; (3) glomerular permeability; and (4) low intratubular pressure. *B.* Afferent arteriolar constriction decreases GFR by reducing blood flow, resulting in diminished capillary pressure. *C.* Obstruction of the tubular lumen by cast formation increases tubular pressure; when tubular pressure exceeds glomerular capillary pressure, filtration decreases or ceases. *D.* Back-leak occurs when the paracellular space between cells increases and the glomerular filtrate leaks into the extracellular space and bloodstream. [From Molitoris BA, Bacallao R: Pathophysiology of ischemic acute renal failure: Cytoskeletal aspects, in Berl T, Bonventre JV (eds.): *Atlas of Diseases of the Kidney.* Philadelphia: Current Medicine, 1999, p. 13.5, with permission.]

in a variety of settings with varied clinical manifestations ranging from a minimal elevation in serum creatinine to anuric renal failure.

Any decline in GFR is complex and may result from prerenal factors (renal vasoconstriction, intravascular volume depletion, and insufficient cardiac output), postrenal factors (ureteral or bladder obstruction), and intrarenal factors (glomerulonephritis, tubular cell injury, death, and loss resulting in back leak; renal vasculature damage, interstitial nephritis) (Fig. 14-4). Figure 14-5 illustrates the pathways that lead to diminished GFR following chemical exposure. As discussed above, pre- and postrenal factors can lead to decreased GFR. If a chemical causes tubular damage directly, then tubular casts can cause tubular obstruction, increased tubular pressure, and decreased GFR. The tubular damage may result in epithelial cell death/loss, leading to back leak of glomerular filtrate and a decrease in GFR. If a chemical causes intrarenal vascular damage with hemodynamic alterations that lead to vasoconstriction, the resulting medullary hypoxia may cause tubular damage and/or decreases in perfusion pressure, glomerular hydrostatic pressure, and GFR. If a chemical causes intrarenal inflammation, then tubular and vascular damage may follow with decreases in GFR. Finally, a chemical may disrupt glomerular function, resulting in decreased glomerular ultrafiltration and GFR. It has been estimated that prerenal factors are responsible for AKI in 55–60% of patients, intrare-

nal factors are responsible for AKI in 35–40% of patients, and postrenal factors are responsible for AKI in <5% of patients (Brady *et al.*, 2004). Further, it is thought that more than 90% of AKI mediated by intrarenal factors is the result of ischemia/reperfusion injury or nephrotoxicity. Table 14-2 provides a partial list of chemicals that produce AKI through these different mechanisms.

The maintenance of tubular integrity is dependent on cell-to-cell and cell-to-matrix adhesion; these interactions are mediated in part by integrins and cell adhesion molecules (Fig. 14-6). It has been hypothesized that after a chemical or hypoxic insult, adhesion of nonlethally damaged, apoptotic, and oncotic cells to the basement membrane is compromised, leading to their detachment from the basement membrane and appearance in the tubular lumen (Goligorksy *et al.*, 1993). Morphologically, such an event would lead to gaps in the epithelial cell lining, potentially resulting in back leak of filtrate and diminished GFR. These detached cells may aggregate in the tubular lumen (cell-to-cell adhesion) and/or adhere or reattach to adherent epithelial cells downstream, resulting in tubular obstruction. Further, the loss of expression of integrins on the basolateral membrane may be responsible for the exfoliation of tubular cells, and the redistribution of integrins from the basolateral to the apical membrane facilitates adhesion of detached cells to the in situ epithelium.

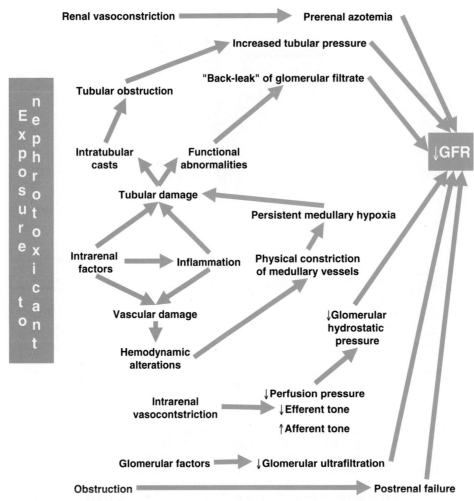

Figure 14-5. Mechanisms that contribute to decreased GFR in acute renal failure.

After exposure to a nephrotoxicant, one or more mechanisms may contribute to a reduction in the GFR. These include renal vasoconstriction resulting in prerenal azotemia and obstruction due to precipitation of a drug or endogenous compound within the kidney. Intrarenal factors include direct tubular obstruction and dysfunction, with or without inflammation, resulting in tubular back-leak and increased tubular pressure. Vascular damage, with or without inflammation, leading to hemodynamic changes. Alterations in the levels of a variety of vasoactive mediators may result in decreased renal perfusion pressure or efferent arteriolar tone and increased afferent arteriolar tone, leading to decreased glomerular hydrostatic pressure. [Modified from Schnellmann RG, Kelly KJ: Pathophysiology of nephrotoxic acute renal failure, in Berl T, Bonventre JV (eds.): *Atlas of Diseases of the Kidney*. Philadelphia: Current Medicine, 1999, p. 15.4, with permission.]

Increasing evidence supports the idea that inflammatory cells (T cells, B cells, neutrophils, and macrophages) play a role in ischemia-induced AKI. Injury to the renal vasculature endothelium results in chemokine and proinflammatory cytokine production and neutrophil adhesion (Fig. 14-7). Neutrophil adhesion leads to capillary damage/leakage and vascular congestion. Bonventre and colleagues have demonstrated that treatment of rats with either monoclonal antibodies against the integrins, CD11a and CD11b, or a monoclonal antibody against ICAM-1 (a ligand for CD11a) conferred significant protection against renal ischemic injury (Kelly *et al.*, 1994; Rabb *et al.*, 1994; Bonventre and Zuk, 2004; Friedewald and Rabb, 2004), suggesting a critical role for leukocyte-endothelial adhesion in the pathophysiology of ischemic AKI. More recently, Rabb and colleagues provided evidence that T cells and B cells play a role in AKI (Rabb *et al.*, 2000; Burne *et al.*, 2001; Burne-Taney *et al.*, 2003; Ikeda *et al.*, 2006). Double CD4-CD8 knockout, CD4 knock-

out and T-cell deficient mice subjected to ischemia/reperfusion injury exhibited less AKI compared to wild-type mice. Further, B-cell deficient mice exhibited less AKI compared to wild-type mice. Thus, while inflammatory cells play a role in AKI, the specific role of each inflammatory cell remains to be elucidated and studies are needed to determine the role of inflammatory cells in chemical-induced AKI.

While chemically induced ARF can be initiated by proximal tubular cell injury, nephrotoxicants may also delay the recovery of renal function by inhibiting cellular repair and regeneration. For example, Leonard *et al.* (1994) demonstrated that cisplatin impaired tubular regeneration resulting in prolonged renal dysfunction, effects that were in contrast to the regenerative response and renal functional recovery following tobramycin-induced nephrotoxicity. Using an in vitro model, Counts *et al.* (1995) reported that following mechanically induced injury to a proximal tubular monolayer, proliferation and migration were inhibited by the heavy metal

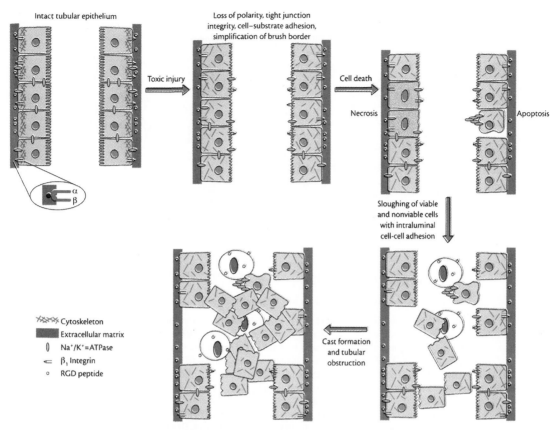

Figure 14-6. *After injury, alterations can occur in the cytoskeleton and in the normal distribution of membrane proteins such as* Na^+, K^+*-ATPase, and* β_1 *integrins in sublethally injured renal tubular cells.*

These changes result in loss of cell polarity, tight junction integrity, and cell-substrate adhesion. Lethally injured cells undergo oncosis or apoptosis, and both dead and viable cells may be released into the tubular lumen. Adhesion of released cells to other released cells and to cells remaining adherent to the basement membrane may result in cast formation, tubular obstruction, and further compromise the GFR. [From Schnellmann RG, Kelly KJ: Pathophysiology of nephrotoxic acute renal failure, in Berl T, Bonventre JV (eds.): *Atlas of Diseases of the Kidney.* Philadelphia: Current Medicine, 1999, p. 15.5, with permission.]

$HgCl_2$, the mycotoxin fumonisin B_1, and dichlorovinyl-L-cysteine (DCVC), suggesting that nephrotoxicants may inhibit/delay the regenerative process.

Adaptation Following Toxic Insult

Fortunately, the kidney has a remarkable ability to compensate for a loss in renal functional mass. Micropuncture studies have revealed that following unilateral nephrectomy, GFR of the remnant kidney increases by approximately 40–60%, an effect associated with early compensatory increases in glomerular plasma flow rate and glomerular hydraulic pressure. Compensatory increases in single-nephron GFR are accompanied by proportionate increases in proximal tubular water and solute reabsorption; glomerulotubular balance is therefore maintained and overall renal function appears normal by standard clinical tests. Consequently, chemically induced changes in renal function may not be detected until these compensatory mechanisms are overwhelmed by significant nephron loss and/or damage.

There are a number of cellular and molecular responses to a nephrotoxic insult. After a population of tubular epithelial cells are exposed to a toxicant, a fraction of the cells will be severely injured and will undergo cell death by apoptosis or oncosis (see below) (Fig. 14-8). Those cells that are nonlethally injured may undergo cell repair and/or adaptation, and contribute to the recovery of the

nephron (Fig. 14-9). In addition, there is a population of cells that are uninjured and may undergo compensatory hypertrophy, adaptation, and proliferation. Current evidence supports the hypothesis that tubular epithelial cells are primarily responsible for the structural and functional recovery of the nephron following injury and that bone marrow-derived stem cells do not play a significant role (Lin *et al.*, 2005; Duffield *et al.*, 2005). Surviving tubular epithelial cells replace dead and detached cells through dedifferentiation, proliferation, migration, and redifferentiation. Growth factors delivered to tubular epithelial cells from local and systemic sources may help orchestrate the proliferative response of the nephron. Several growth factors such as epidermal growth factor (EGF), heparin-binding epidermal growth factor (HB-EGF), insulin-like growth factor-1 (IGF-1), hepatocyte growth factor (HGF), fibroblast growth factors, and transforming growth factors α and β have been implicated in proximal tubular regeneration (Hammerman and Miller, 1994). Interestingly, exogenous administration of EGF, HGF, or IGF-1 accelerates renal repair following ischemic-, gentamicin-, bromohydroquinone-, and/or $HgCl_2$-induced ARF. However, it is not clear which endogenous growth factors are required for tubular regeneration.

Two of the most notable cellular adaptation responses are metallothionein induction (see section "Cadmium") and stress protein induction. Heat-shock proteins (Hsps) and glucose-regulated proteins (Grps) are two examples of stress protein families that are

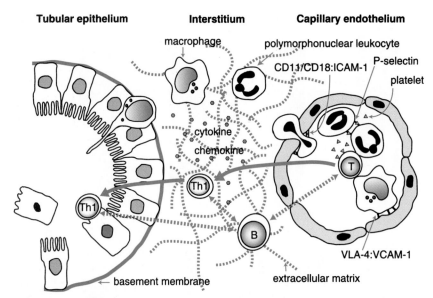

Tubular epithelium   Interstitium   Capillary endothelium

Figure 14-7. Ischemia acute tubular injury and inflammatory cells.

Initially ischemia causes injury of endothelial cells, followed by leukocyte activation and formation of platelet-leukocyte plugs. Chemokines and cytokines produced by both leukocytes and tubular cells lead to the recruitment of inflammatory cells from the microvasculature to the interstitium, allowing inflammatory cells to be able to interact with tubular epithelial cells. Renal inflammation is associated with the shortened microvilli of tubular epithelial cells and to the denuded epithelium. The sloughed cells adhere to each other and in turn form intratubule casts. Abbreviations: B, B cells; ICAM-1, intercellular adhesion molecule-1; T, CD4+ T cells; Th1, T helper 1 cells; VCAM-1, vascular cell adhesion molecule-1; VLA-4, very late antigen-4. [From Ikeda M *et al.*: Ischemic acute tubular necrosis models and drug discovery: A focus on cellular inflammation, *Drug Discov Today* 11:364–370, 2006, with permission from Elsevier.]

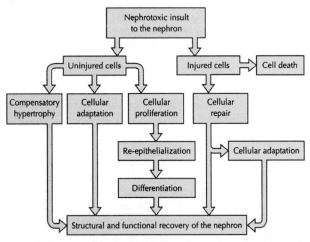

Figure 14-8. The response of the nephron to a nephrotoxic insult.

After a population of cells is exposed to a nephrotoxicant, the cells respond; ultimately the nephron recovers function or, if cell death and loss are extensive, nephron function ceases. Terminally injured cells undergo cell death through oncosis or apoptosis. Cells injured sublethally undergo repair and adaptation in response to the nephrotoxicant. Cells not injured and adjacent to the injured area may undergo dedifferentiation, proliferation, migration or spreading, and differentiation. Cells not injured may also undergo compensatory hypertrophy in response to the cell loss and injury. Finally the uninjured cells also may undergo adaptation in response to a nephrotoxicant exposure. [From Schnellmann RG, Kelly KJ: Pathophysiology of nephrotoxic acute renal failure, in Berl T, Bonventre JV (eds.): *Atlas of Diseases of the Kidney*. Philadelphia: Current Medicine, 1999, p. 15.4, with permission.]

induced in response to a number of pathophysiologic states such as heat shock, anoxia, oxidative stress, toxicants, heavy metal exposure, and tissue trauma (Kelly, 2005; van de Water *et al.*, 2006). The distribution of individual stress proteins varies between different cell types in the kidney and within subcellular compartments (Goering *et al.*, 2000). These proteins play important roles in protein folding, translocation of proteins across organelle membranes, prevention of aggregation of damaged proteins, repair and degradation of damaged proteins, and thereby provide a defense mechanism against toxicity and/or for the facilitation of recovery and repair. Hsp induction in renal tissue has been demonstrated following treatment with nephrotoxicants such as gentamicin (Komatsuda *et al.*, 1993), haloalkane cysteine conjugates (Chen *et al.*, 1992), and $HgCl_2$ (Goering *et al.*, 1992). Interestingly, proximal tubular HSP60 and mitochondrial HSP70 and HSP27 have been identified as molecular targets of the reactive metabolites of the haloalkane cysteine conjugate tetrafluoroethyl-L-cysteine (TFEC) and DCVC, respectively, an effect that could alter the normal housekeeping functions of the proximal tubule and thereby potentially contribute to and exacerbate nephrotoxicity (Bruschi *et al.*, 1993; van de Water *et al.*, 2006). HSP70 induction in the kidney is cytoprotective and renoprotective following injury and HSP70 blocks apoptosis upstream of mitochondrial events.

Chronic Renal Failure

Progressive deterioration of renal function may occur with long-term exposure to a variety of chemicals (e.g., analgesics, lithium, and cyclosporine). It is generally believed that progression to end-stage

Site-Selective Injury

Many nephrotoxicants have their primary effects on discrete segments or regions of the nephron. For example, the proximal tubule is the primary target for most nephrotoxic antibiotics, antineoplastics, halogenated hydrocarbons, mycotoxins, and heavy metals, whereas the glomerulus is the primary site for immune complexes, the loop of Henle/collecting ducts for fluoride ions, and the medulla/papilla for chronically consumed analgesic mixtures. The reasons underlying this site-selective injury are complex but can be attributed in part to site-specific differences in blood flow, transport and accumulation of chemicals, physicochemical properties of the epithelium, reactivity of cellular/molecular targets, balance of bioactivation/detoxification reactions, cellular energetics, and/or regenerative/repair mechanisms.

Glomerular Injury

The glomerulus is the initial site of chemical exposure within the nephron, and a number of nephrotoxicants produce structural injury to this segment. In certain instances, chemicals alter glomerular permeability to proteins by altering the size- and charge-selective functions. Both puromycin aminonucleoside and doxorubicin target glomerular epithelial cells, resulting in changes in size and charge selectivity and proteinuria. The decrease in charge selectivity is thought to result from a decrease in negatively charged sites, while the loss of size selectivity is thought to result from focal detachment of podocytes from the GBM.

Cyclosporine, amphotericin B, and gentamicin are examples of chemicals that impair glomerular ultrafiltration without significant loss of structural integrity and decrease GFR. Amphotericin B decreases GFR by causing renal vasoconstriction and decreasing the glomerular capillary ultrafiltration coefficient (K_f), an effect probably mediated through the endothelial cells. Because of its polycationic nature, the aminoglycoside gentamicin interacts with the anionic sites on the endothelial cells, decreasing K_f and GFR. Finally, cyclosporine not only causes renal vasoconstriction and vascular damage but is injurious to the glomerular endothelial cell.

Chemically induced glomerular injury may also be mediated by extrarenal factors. Circulating immune complexes may be trapped within the glomeruli; binding of complement, attraction of neutrophils, and phagocytosis may result. Neutrophils and macrophages are commonly observed within glomeruli in membranous glomerulonephritis, and the local release of cytokines and reactive oxygen species (ROS) may contribute to glomerular injury. Heavy metals (e.g., $HgCl_2$, gold, cadmium), hydrocarbons, penicillamine, and captopril can produce this type of glomerular injury. A chemical may function as a hapten attached to some native protein (e.g., tubular antigens released secondary to toxicity) or as a complete antigen—particularly if it is sequestered within the glomerulus via electrostatic interactions—and elicit an antibody response. Antibody reactions with cell-surface antigens (e.g., GBM) lead to immune deposit formation within the glomeruli, mediator activation, and subsequent injury to glomerular tissue. Volatile hydrocarbons, solvents, and $HgCl_2$ have been implicated in this type of glomerulonephritis.

Proximal Tubular Injury

The proximal tubule is the most common site of toxicant-induced renal injury. The reasons for this relate in part to the selective accumulation of xenobiotics into this segment of the nephron. For example, in contrast to the distal tubule, which is characterized by a relatively tight epithelium with high electrical resistance, the proximal tubule has a leaky epithelium, favoring the flux of compounds into proximal tubular cells. More importantly, tubular transport of organic anions and cations, low-molecular-weight proteins and peptides, GSH conjugates, and heavy metals is localized primarily if not exclusively to the proximal tubule. Thus, transport of these molecules will be greater in the proximal tubule than in other segments, resulting in proximal tubular accumulation and toxicity. Indeed, segmental differences in transport and accumulation appear to play a significant role in the onset and development of proximal tubular toxicity associated with certain drugs such as aminoglycosides, β-lactam antibiotics, and cisplatin; environmental chemicals such as ochratoxin, haloalkene S-conjugates, d-limonene, and 2,4,4-trimethylpentane; and metals such as cadmium and mercury. Although correlations between proximal tubular transport, accumulation, and toxicity suggest that the site of transport is a crucial determinant of the site of toxicity, transport is unlikely to be the sole criterion. For example, the S_2 segment is the primary site of transport and toxicity of cephaloridine, and several lines of evidence suggest a strong correlation between the transport, accumulation, and nephrotoxicity of this antibiotic. However, when a variety of cephalosporins are considered, the rank order of accumulation does not follow the rank order of nephrotoxicity; for example, renal cortical concentrations of the potent nephrotoxicant cephaloglycin are comparable to those of the relatively nontoxic cephalexin. Thus, site-specific transport and accumulation are necessary but not sufficient to cause proximal tubular toxicity of cephalosporins. Once taken up and sequestered by the proximal tubular cell, the nephrotoxic potential of these drugs ultimately may be dependent upon the intrinsic reactivity of the drug with subcellular or molecular targets.

In addition to segmental differences in transport, segmental differences in cytochrome P450 and cysteine conjugate β-lyase activity also are contributing factors to the enhanced susceptibility of the proximal tubule. Both enzyme systems are localized almost exclusively in the proximal tubule, with negligible activity in the glomerulus, distal tubules, or collecting ducts. Thus, nephrotoxicity requiring P450 and β-lyase-mediated bioactivation will most certainly be localized in the proximal tubule. Indeed, the site of proximal tubular bioactivation contributes at least in part to the proximal tubular lesions produced by chloroform (via cytochrome P450) and by haloalkene S-conjugates (via cysteine β-lyase).

Finally, proximal tubular cells appear to be more susceptible to ischemic injury than are distal tubular cells. Therefore, the proximal tubule likely will be the primary site of toxicity for chemicals that interfere with RBF, cellular energetics, and/or mitochondrial function.

Loop of Henle/Distal Tubule/Collecting Duct Injury

Chemically induced injury to the more distal tubular structures, compared to the proximal tubule, is an infrequent occurrence. Functional abnormalities at these sites manifest primarily as impaired concentrating ability and/or acidification defects. Drugs that have been associated with acute injury to the more distal tubular structures include amphotericin B, cisplatin, and methoxyflurane. Each of these drugs induces an ADH-resistant polyuria, suggesting that the concentrating defect occurs at the level of the medullary thick ascending limb and/or the collecting duct. However, the mechanisms mediating these drug-induced concentrating defects appear to be different.

Amphotericin B is highly lipophilic and interacts with lipid sterols such as cholesterol, resulting in the formation of transmembrane channels or pores and disrupting membrane permeability (Bernardo and Branch, 1997). Thus, amphotericin effectively transforms the tight distal tubular epithelium into one that is leaky to water and ions and impairs reabsorption at these sites. The mechanisms mediating cisplatin-induced polyuria are not completely understood, but the first phase is responsive to vasopressin and inhibitors of prostaglandin synthesis (Safirstein and Deray, 1998). The second phase is not responsive to vasopressin or prostaglandin synthesis inhibitors but is associated with decreased papillary solute content. Methoxyflurane nephrotoxicity is associated with the inhibitory effects of the metabolite fluoride on solute and water reabsorption (Jarnberg, 1998). Fluoride inhibits sodium chloride reabsorption in the thick ascending limb and inhibits ADH-mediated reabsorption of water, possibly due to disruption in adenylate cyclase.

Papillary Injury

The renal papilla is susceptible to the chronic injurious effects of abusive consumption of analgesics. The initial target is the medullary interstitial cells, followed by degenerative changes in the medullary capillaries, loops of Henle, and collecting ducts (Bach, 1997). Although the exact mechanisms underlying selective damage to the papilla by analgesics are not known, the intrarenal gradient for prostaglandin H synthase activity has been implicated as a contributing factor. This activity is greatest in the medulla and least in the cortex, and the prostaglandin hydroperoxidase component metabolizes phenacetin to reactive intermediates capable of covalent binding to cellular macromolecules. Other factors may contribute to this site-selective injury, including high papillary concentrations of potential toxicants and inhibition of vasodilatory prostaglandins, compromising RBF to the renal medulla/papilla and resulting in tissue ischemia. The lack of animal models that mimic the papillary injury observed in humans has limited mechanistic research in this area (Schnellmann, 1998).

ASSESSMENT OF RENAL FUNCTION

Evaluation of the effects of a chemical on the kidney can be accomplished using a variety of both in vivo and in vitro methods. Initially, nephrotoxicity can be assessed by evaluating serum and urine chemistries following treatment with the chemical in question. The standard battery of noninvasive tests includes measurement of urine volume and osmolality, pH, and urinary composition (e.g., electrolytes, glucose, and protein). Although specificity is often lacking in such an assessment, urinalysis provides a relatively easy and noninvasive assessment of overall renal functional integrity and can provide some insight into the nature of the nephrotoxic insult. For example, chemically induced increases in urine volume accompanied by decreases in osmolality may suggest an impaired concentrating ability, possibly via a defect in ADH synthesis, release, and/or action. To determine whether the impaired concentrating ability is due to an altered tubular response to ADH, concentrating ability can be determined before and after an exogenous ADH challenge. Glucosuria may reflect chemically induced defects in proximal tubular reabsorption of sugars; however, because glucosuria also may be secondary to hyperglycemia, measurement of serum glucose concentrations also must be evaluated. Urinary excretion of high-molecular-weight proteins, such as albumin, is suggestive of glomerular damage, whereas excretion of low-molecular-weight proteins, such as β_2-microglobulin, suggests proximal tubular injury. Urinary excretion of enzymes localized in the brush border (e.g., alkaline phosphatase, γ-glutamyl transpeptidase) may reflect brush-border damage, whereas urinary excretion of other enzymes (e.g., lactate dehydrogenase) may reflect more generalized cell damage. Enzymuria is often a transient phenomenon, as chemically induced damage may result in an early loss of most of the enzyme available. Thus, the absence of enzymuria does not necessarily reflect an absence of damage.

The simultaneous analysis of cellular metabolites in sera and urine using nuclear magnetic analysis (metabonomics) has matured over the past few years and may provide an additional technology to identify and monitor nephrotoxicity (Lindon et al., 2006). For example, rats treated with the nephrotoxicant $HgCl_2$ exhibited increased levels of threonine, isobutyric acid, glutamate, and lysine in renal cortical tissue (Wang et al., 2006) and increased levels of isoleucine and lysine and decreased levels of fumarate in the urine, and that these changes are associated with renal dysfunction (Holmes et al., 2006). However, this technology will require further development and validation using different species and renal insults in the presence and absence of underlying diseases prior to greater use.

GFR can be measured directly by determining creatinine or inulin clearance. Creatinine is an endogenous compound released from skeletal muscle at a constant rate under most circumstances. Further, it is completely filtered with limited secretion. Inulin is an exogenous compound that is completely filtered with no reabsorption or secretion. Following the injection of inulin, inulin serum and urinary concentrations and urine volume are determined over time. If creatinine is being used, then serum and urinary creatinine concentrations and urine volume are determined over time. Creatinine or inulin clearance is determined by the following formula:

$$\text{Inulin clearance(mL/min)} =$$
$$\frac{\text{inulin concentration in urine (mg/L)} \times \text{urine volume (mL/min)}}{\text{inulin concentration in serum (mg/L)}}$$

Indirect markers of GFR are serial blood urea nitrogen (BUN) and serum creatinine concentrations. However, both serum creatinine and BUN are rather insensitive indices of GFR; a 50–70% decrease in GFR must occur before increases in serum creatinine and BUN develop (Fig. 14-10). Chemically induced increases in BUN and/or serum creatinine may not necessarily reflect renal damage but rather may be secondary to dehydration, hypovolemia, and/or protein catabolism. These extrarenal events should be taken into consideration in evaluating BUN/serum creatinine as potential endpoints of renal toxicity and/or when correlating these endpoints with renal histopathology.

Cystatin C, a 13-kDa endogenous protein that inhibits cysteine proteases, is a viable candidate to replace creatinine in the measurement of GFR (Filler et al., 2005; Stevens and Levey, 2005; Hart and Kinter, 2005). It is produced at a constant rate by all tissues, freely filtered by the glomerulus and catabolized by the tubular epithelial cells; thus, its use is limited to serum levels and not urinary levels. Serum cystain C levels appear to be independent of height, gender, age, muscle mass, and coexisting diseases, and are more sensitive than creatinine in mildly impaired GFR.

Histopathologic evaluation of the kidney following treatment is crucial in identifying the site, nature, and severity of the nephrotoxic lesion. Assessment of chemically induced nephrotoxicity therefore should include urinalysis, serum clinical chemistry, and

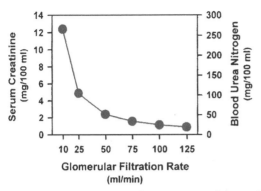

Figure 14-10. Relationships among GFR, serum creatinine, and BUN concentrations in the determination of renal function.

In general, approximately 50% of renal function must be lost before serum creatinine or BUN increases. [From Tarloff JB, Kinter LB: In vivo methodologies used to assess renal function, in Sipes IG, McQueen CA, Gandolfi AJ (eds.): *Comprehensive Toxicology,* Oxford, England: Elsevier, 1997, Vol 7, pp. 99–120, with permission.]

Table 14-3
Models to Study Renal Function

In Vivo
Continuous microperfusion
Stopped-flow microperfusion
Free-flow micropuncture
Confocal microscopy

Ex Vivo
Isolated perfused kidney
Isolated perfused tubules

In Vitro
Renal slices
Freshly isolated and purified glomeruli
Freshly isolated and purified tubular segments
Freshly isolated and purified proximal tubular epithelial cells
Primary cultures of renal cells
   Tubular epithelial cells
   Glomerular cells
   Fibroblasts
Immortalized renal epithelial cell lines
   LLC-PK1
   MDCK
   NRK-52E
   OK
   HK-2

histopathology to provide a reasonable profile of the functional and morphologic effects of a chemical on the kidney. Further, information on the biotransformation and toxicokinetics of the chemical should be used to direct further in vivo and in vitro studies; in particular, what metabolites are found in the kidney and what are the concentrations of parent compound and metabolites in the kidney over time.

Once a chemical has been identified as a nephrotoxicant in vivo, a variety of in vitro techniques may be used to elucidate underlying mechanisms (Table 14-3). Tissue obtained from naive animals may be used in the preparation of isolated perfused kidneys, kidney slices, isolated suspensions of renal tubules, cells, or subcellular organelles, primary cultures of renal cells, and established renal cell lines. For example, freshly prepared isolated perfused kidneys, kidney slices, and renal tubular suspensions and cells exhibit the greatest degree of differentiated functions and similarity to the in vivo situation. However, these models have limited life spans of 2–24 hours. In contrast, primary cultures of renal cells and established renal cell lines exhibit longer life spans (>2 weeks), but—by comparison to the in vivo condition—exhibit differentiated functions and similarity to a lesser degree; this is particularly true of immortalized renal cell lines. The reader is referred to several excellent reviews for further details on the utility and limitations of these preparations (Tarloff and Kinter, 1997; Ford, 1997; Hart and Kinter, 2005; Kirkpatrick and Gandolfi, 2005; Ford, 2005). Such approaches may be used to distinguish between an effect on the kidney due to a direct chemical insult and one caused by extrarenal effects such as extrarenally generated metabolites, hemodynamic effects, immunologic effects, and so forth. Care must be taken to ensure that the cell type affected in the in vitro model is the same as that affected in vivo. In addition, concentrations of the nephrotoxicant to be used in the in vitro preparations must be comparable to those observed in vivo, as different mechanisms of toxicity may be operative at concentrations that saturate metabolic pathways or overwhelm detoxification mechanisms. Once a mechanism has been identified in vitro, the postulated mechanism must be tested in vivo. Thus, appropriately designed in vivo and in vitro studies should provide a complete characterization of the biochemical, functional, and morphologic effects of a chemical on the kidney and an understanding of the underlying mechanisms in the target cell population(s).

BIOCHEMICAL MECHANISMS/MEDIATORS OF RENAL CELL INJURY

Cell Death

In many cases, renal cell injury may culminate in cell death. In general, cell death is thought to occur through either oncosis or apoptosis (Levin *et al.*, 1999). The morphologic and biochemical characteristics of oncosis ("necrotic cell death") and apoptosis are very different. For example, apoptosis is a tightly controlled, organized process that usually affects scattered individual cells. The organelles retain integrity while cell volume decreases. Ultimately, the cell breaks into small fragments that are phagocytosed by adjacent cells or macrophages without producing an inflammatory response. In contrast, oncosis often affects many contiguous cells; the organelles swell, cell volume increases, and the cell ruptures with the release of cellular contents, followed by inflammation. The reader is encouraged to see Brady *et al.* (2004) and Cummings and Schnellmann (2006) for additional details of apoptosis and oncosis. With many toxicants, lower but injurious concentrations produce cell death through apoptosis (Fig. 14-11). As the concentration of the toxicant increases, oncosis plays a predominant role. However, because apoptosis is an ATP-dependent process, for those toxicants that target the mitochondrion, oncosis may be the predominant pathway with only limited apoptosis occurring. In general, nephrotoxicants produce cell death through apoptosis and oncosis, and it is likely that both forms of cell death contribute to AKI.

Mediators of Toxicity

A chemical can initiate cell injury by a variety of mechanisms (Fig. 14-12). In some cases the chemical may initiate toxicity due to its intrinsic reactivity with cellular macromolecules. For example,

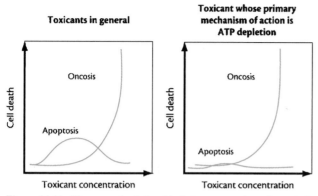

Figure 14-11. *The general relationship between oncosis and apoptosis after nephrotoxicant exposure.*

For many toxicants, low concentrations primarily cause apoptosis and oncosis occurs principally at higher concentrations. When the primary mechanism of action of the nephrotoxicant is ATP depletion, oncosis may be the predominant cause of cell death, with limited apoptosis occurring. [From Schnellmann RG, Kelly KJ: Pathophysiology of nephrotoxic acute renal failure, in Berl T, Bonventre JV (eds.): *Atlas of Diseases of the Kidney.* Philadelphia: Current Medicine, 1999, p. 15.6, with permission.]

amphotericin B reacts with plasma membrane sterols, increasing membrane permeability; fumonisin B_1 inhibits sphinganine (sphingosine) *N*-acyltransferase; and Hg^{2+} binds to sulfhydryl groups on cellular proteins. In contrast, some chemicals are not toxic until they are biotransformed to a reactive intermediate. Biologically reactive intermediates, also known as alkylating agents, are electron-deficient compounds (electrophiles) that bind to cellular nucleophiles (electron-rich compounds) such as proteins and lipids. For example, acetaminophen and chloroform are metabolized in the mouse kidney by cytochrome P450 to the reactive intermediates, *N*-acetyl-*p*-benzoquinoneimine and phosgene, respectively (see sections "Chloroform" and "Acetaminophen"). The covalent binding of the reactive intermediate to critical cellular macromolecules is thought to interfere with the normal biological activity of the macromolecule and thereby initiate cellular injury. In other instances, extrarenal biotransformation may be required prior to the delivery of the penultimate nephrotoxic species to the proximal tubule, where it is metabolized further to a reactive intermediate.

Finally, chemicals may initiate injury indirectly by inducing oxidative stress via increased production of ROS, such as superoxide anion, hydrogen peroxide, and hydroxyl radicals. ROS can react with a variety of cellular constituents to induce toxicity. For example, ROS are capable of inducing lipid peroxidation, which may result in altered membrane fluidity, enzyme activity, and membrane permeability and transport characteristics; inactivating cellular enzymes by directly oxidizing critical protein sulfhydryl or amino groups; depolymerizing polysaccharides; and inducing DNA strand breaks and chromosome breakage. Each of these events could lead to cell injury and/or death. Oxidative stress has been proposed to contribute, at least in part, to the nephrotoxicity associated with ischemia/reperfusion injury, gentamicin, cyclosporine, cisplatin, and haloalkene cysteine conjugates (Chen *et al.*, 1990; Groves *et al.*, 1991; Ueda *et al.*, 2001).

While nitric oxide is an important second messenger in a number of physiologic pathways, recent studies suggest that in the presence of oxidative stress, nitric oxide can be converted into reactive nitrogen species that contribute to cellular injury and death. For

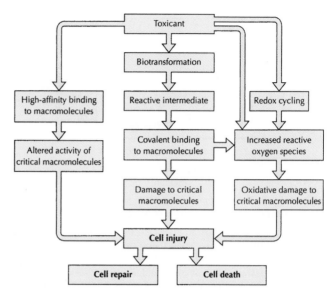

Figure 14-12. *Covalent and noncovalent binding versus oxidative stress mechanisms of cell injury.*

Nephrotoxicants are generally thought to produce cell injury and death through one of two mechanisms, either alone or in combination. In some cases the toxicant may have a high affinity for a specific macromolecule or class of macromolecules that results in altered activity (increase or decrease) of these molecules and cell injury. Alternatively, the parent nephrotoxicant may not be toxic until it is biotransformed into a reactive intermediate that binds covalently to macromolecules and, in turn, alters their activity, resulting in cell injury. Finally, the toxicant may increase ROS in the cells directly, after being biotransformed into a reactive intermediate or through redox cycling. The resulting increase in ROS results in oxidative damage and cell injury. [From Schnellmann RG, Kelly KJ: Pathophysiology of nephrotoxic acute renal failure, in Berl T, Bonventre JV (eds.): *Atlas of Diseases of the Kidney.* Philadelphia: Current Medicine, 1999, p. 15.7, with permission.]

example, in the presence of superoxide anion, nitric oxide can be transformed into peroxynitrite ($ONOO^-$), a strong oxidant and nitrating species (Pryor and Squadrito, 1995). Proteins, lipids, and DNA are all targets of peroxynitrite. The primary evidence for a role of peroxynitrite in renal ischemia/reperfusion injury is the formation of nitrotyrosine-protein adducts and the attenuation of renal dysfunction through the inhibition of the inducible form of nitric oxide synthase (Ueda *et al.*, 2001).

Cellular/Subcellular and Molecular Targets

A number of cellular targets have been identified to play a role in cell death. It is generally thought that an intracellular interaction (e.g., an alkylating agent or ROS with a macromolecule) initiates a sequence of events that leads to cell death. In the case of oncosis, a "point of no return" is reached in which the cell will die regardless of any intervention. The idea of a single sequence of events is probably simplistic for most toxicants, given the extensive number of targets available for alkylating species and ROS. Rather, multiple pathways, with both distinct and common sequences of events, may lead to cell death.

Cell Volume and Ion Homeostasis

Cell volume and ion homeostasis are tightly regulated and are critical for the reabsorptive properties of the tubular epithelial cells.

Toxicants generally disrupt cell volume and ion homeostasis by interacting with the plasma membrane and increasing ion permeability or by inhibiting energy production. The loss of ATP, for example, results in the inhibition of membrane transporters that maintain the internal ion balance and drive transmembrane ion movement. Following ATP depletion, Na$^+$, K$^+$-ATPase activity decreases, resulting in K$^+$ efflux, Na$^+$ and Cl$^-$ influx, cell swelling, and ultimately cell membrane rupture. Miller and Schnellmann (1993, 1995) have proposed that ATP depletion in rabbit renal proximal tubule segments initially results in K$^+$ efflux and Na$^+$ influx followed by a lag period before Cl$^-$ influx occurs. Cl$^-$ influx occurs during the late stages of cell injury produced by a diverse group of toxicants and appears to be due to the volume-sensitive, outwardly rectifying (VSOR) Cl$^-$ channel (Okada et al., 2004). Cl$^-$ influx may be a trigger for cell swelling, because decreasing Cl$^-$ influx decreased cell swelling and cell death, and inhibition of cell swelling decreased cell lysis but not Cl$^-$ influx. Meng and Reeves (2000) have reported similar findings using hydrogen peroxide as the toxicant and LLC-PK$_1$ cells. In contrast, the cell shrinkage that occurs during apoptosis is mediated by K$^+$ and Cl$^-$ efflux through respective channels and inhibition of these channels is cytoprotective (Okada et al., 2004).

Cytoskeleton and Cell Polarity

Toxicants may cause early changes in membrane integrity such as loss of the brush border, blebbing of the plasma membrane, or alterations in membrane polarity. These changes can result from toxicant-induced alterations in cytoskeleton components and cytoskeletal-membrane interactions, or they may be associated with perturbations in energy metabolism or calcium and phospholipid homeostasis. Marked changes in the polarity of tubular epithelium occur following an ischemic insult. Under controlled conditions, the tubular epithelial cell is polarized with respect to certain transporters and enzymes. During in vivo ischemia and in vitro ATP depletion there is a dissociation of Na$^+$, K$^+$-ATPase from the actin cytoskeleton and redistribution from the basolateral membrane to the apical domain in renal proximal tubule cells (Molitoris, 1997). The redistribution of this enzyme has been postulated to explain decreased Na$^+$ and water reabsorption during ischemic injury.

Mitochondria

Many cellular processes depend on mitochondrial ATP and thus become compromised simultaneously with inhibition of respiration. Conversely, mitochondrial dysfunction may be a consequence of some other cellular process altered by the toxicant. Numerous nephrotoxicants cause mitochondrial dysfunction (Schnellmann and Griner, 1994). For example, following an in vivo exposure, HgCl$_2$ altered isolated renal cortical mitochondrial function and mitochondrial morphology prior to the appearance of tubular necrosis (Weinberg et al., 1982a). Furthermore, HgCl$_2$ produced similar changes in various respiratory parameters when added to isolated rat renal cortical mitochondria (Weinberg et al., 1982b). Different toxicants also produce different types of mitochondrial dysfunction. For example, pentachlorobutadienyl-L-cysteine initially uncouples oxidative phosphorylation in renal proximal tubular cells by dissipating the proton gradient, whereas TFEC does not uncouple oxidative phosphorylation but rather inhibits state 3 respiration by inhibiting sites I and II of the electron transport chain (Schnellmann et al., 1987, 1989; Wallin et al., 1987; Hayden and Stevens, 1990).

Whether toxicants target mitochondria directly or indirectly, it is clear that mitochondria play a critical role in determining whether cells die by apoptosis or oncosis. The mitochondrial permeability transition (MPT) is characterized by the opening of a high-conductance pore that allows solutes of <1500 molecular weight to pass (Lemasters et al., 1999). It is thought that the MPT occurs during cell injury and ultimately progresses to apoptosis if sufficient ATP is available or oncosis if ATP is depleted. Further, the release of apoptotic proteins such as apoptosis inducing factor (AIF), cytochrome c, Smac/Diablo, Omi and Endonuclease G following MPT play a key role in activating downstream caspases and executing apoptosis.

Ca^{2+} Homeostasis

Ca^{2+} is a second messenger and plays a critical role in a variety of cellular functions. The distribution of Ca^{2+} within renal cells is complex and involves binding to anionic sites on macromolecules and compartmentation within subcellular organelles. The cytosolic free Ca^{2+} concentration of this pool is approximately 100 nM and is maintained at this level against a large extracellular/intracellular gradient (10,000:1) by a series of pumps and channels located on the plasma membrane and endoplasmic reticulum (ER). Because the proximal tubular cells reabsorb approximately 50–60% of the filtered load of Ca^{2+}, they must maintain low cytosolic Ca^{2+} concentrations during a large Ca^{2+} flux.

Sustained elevations or abnormally large increases in cytosolic free Ca^{2+} can exert a number of detrimental effects on the cell. For example, an increase in cytosolic free Ca^{2+} can activate a number of degradative Ca^{2+}-dependent enzymes, such as phospholipases and proteinases (e.g., calpains), and can produce aberrations in the structure and function of cytoskeletal elements. While the precise role of Ca^{2+} in toxicant-induced injury remains unclear, release of ER Ca^{2+} stores may be a key step in initiating the injury process and increasing cytosolic free Ca^{2+} concentrations (Harriman et al., 2002). For example, prior depletion of ER Ca^{2+} stores protects renal proximal tubules from extracellular Ca^{2+} influx and cell death produced by mitochondrial inhibition and hypoxia (Waters et al., 1997b). Further, the release of ER Ca^{2+} activates calpains which leads to further disruption of ion homeostasis, cleavage of cytoskeleton proteins, cell swelling, and, ultimately oncosis (Waters et al., 1997a; Liu and Schnellmann 2003). Mitochondria are known to accumulate Ca^{2+} in lethally injured cells through a low-affinity, high-capacity Ca^{2+} transport system. While this system plays a minor role in normal cellular Ca^{2+} regulation, under injurious conditions the uptake of Ca^{2+} may facilitate ROS formation and damage.

Phospholipases

Phospholipase A$_2$ (PLA$_2$) consists of a family of enzymes that hydrolyze the acyl bond at the sn-2 position of phospholipids, resulting in the release of arachidonic acid and lysophospholipid. The enzymes within this family have different biochemical characteristics, substrate preferences, and Ca^{2+} dependencies. PLA$_2$ activation has been suggested to play a role in various forms of cell injury through a variety of mechanisms (Cummings et al., 2000). A supraphysiologic increase in PLA$_2$ activity could result in the loss of membrane phospholipids and consequently impair membrane function. The increase in PLA$_2$ activity may be secondary to an increase in cytosolic Ca^{2+}, because some PLA$_2$ enzymes translocate to membranes following increases in cytosolic free Ca^{2+}. Cell membranes are rich with polyunsaturated fatty acids and as such are susceptible to lipid peroxidation. Peroxidized lipids are predisposed to degradation by PLA_2, resulting in increased PLA_2 activity and the formation of peroxidized arachidonic acid metabolites and lysophospholipids. Lysophospholipids can be toxic to cells and alter membrane permeability characteristics and uncouple mitochondrial respiration. Furthermore, the eicosanoid products of arachidonic metabolism are chemotactic for neutrophils, which may also contribute to tissue injury.

The actual role of PLA_2 in renal cell injury has been controversial and it now appears that different PLA_2 isoforms have different roles following different toxicants. Sapirstein et al. (1996) showed that cytosolic Ca^{2+}-dependent PLA_2 ($cPLA_2$) contributed to oxidant-induced oncosis by overexpressing $cPLA_2$ or secretory PLA_2 in LLC-PK_1 cells and demonstrated that cells overexpressing $cPLA_2$ were more susceptible to H_2O_2 toxicity, whereas overexpression of $sPLA_2$ did not increase H_2O_2 toxicity. In contrast, inhibition of a Ca^{2+}-independent $PLA_2\gamma$ ($iPLA_2\gamma$) resident in the endoplasmic reticulum and mitochondria potentiates oxidant-induced oncosis and decreases cisplatin-induced apoptosis in rabbit renal proximal tubular cells (Cummings et al., 2002, 2004a; Kinsey et al., 2006). Thus, the role of PLA_2s in oncosis depends upon the PLA_2 isoform and stimulus of injury.

Endonucleases

Endonucleases have been suggested to play a role in renal cell oncosis and apoptosis. Endonuclease activation with associated DNA cleavage produces a "ladder" pattern following gel electrophoresis and is a well-characterized late event in apoptosis, though not considered a specific marker. In contrast, DNA cleavage during oncosis typically results in a "smear" pattern following gel electrophoresis. With respect to oncosis, Ueda et al. (1995) and Basnakian et al. (2005) reported DNA damage and the activation of an endonuclease G by ceramide in rat renal proximal tubules or NRK-52E cells subjected to hypoxia/reoxygenation.

Proteinases

Calpains are likely candidates for a role in cell death because they are cysteine proteinases; they are activated by calcium; and they have cytoskeletal proteins, membrane proteins, and enzymes as substrates. For example, calpain activity increased in rat proximal tubules subjected to hypoxia, and calpain inhibitors were cytoprotective (Edelstein et al., 1996). Calpain inhibitors with different mechanisms of action decreased cell death produced by a variety of toxicants, suggesting that calpains may play an important role in the cell death produced by a diverse range of toxicants (Waters et al., 1997a; Schnellmann and Williams, 1998; Liu et al., 2004). Finally, Takaoka et al. (1999) reported that treatment with calpeptin increased renal function in rats subjected to ischemia-reperfusion.

Recent data reveal that mitochondria have a resident calpain, calpain 10, and that mitochondrial Ca^{2+} accumulation results in mitochondrial calpain 10 activation which causes mitochondrial dysfunction (Arrington et al., 2006). Further, Ca^{2+}-induced inhibition of complex 1 of the electron transport chain was blocked by calpain inhibitors and the complex 1 proteins NDUFV2 and ND6 were identified as substrates of mitochondrial calpain 10. Additional cellular and in vivo studies are needed to completely elucidate the role of calpain 10 in AKI.

Caspases are another class of cysteine proteinases that play a role in the initiation and execution of renal cell apoptosis. A number of caspases have been identified in the rat kidney (e.g., caspases 1, 2, 3, 6, 9), and rat kidneys subjected to ischemia/reperfusion injury exhibit differential expression of caspases with marked increases in caspases 1 and 3 (Kaushal et al., 1998). The administration of a pan-caspase inhibitor blocked the increase in caspase activities and renal injury following ischemia/reperfusion injury (Daemen et al., 1999). Using renal cell models, many studies have demonstrated that nephrotoxicants induce apoptosis that is sensitive to caspase inhibitors. However, it should be noted that caspase activity is not required for apoptosis to occur (Cummings et al., 2004b).

Signaling Kinases

Signaling kinases such as protein kinase C, mitogen activated protein kinases (e.g., ERK1/2, p38, JNK/SAPK), protein kinase B (Akt), src, and phosphoinositide-3-kinase phosphorylate other proteins and, thereby, alter their activity, expression, or localization. Numerous recent studies reveal critical roles for signaling kinases in renal cell death and in the recovery of renal cells after toxicant injury (Table 14-4) (Schnellmann and Cummings, 2006). For example, PKC mediates fumonision-B1- and TNF-induced toxicity in human renal cells and in LLC-PK1 cells (Nowak, 2002; Gopee et al., 2003; Woo et al., 1996). However, the exact role of PKC in renal cell death depends on the toxicant and the specific isoform(s) involved (Nowak, 2002, 2003; Nowak et al., 2004). Activation of $PKC\alpha$ contributes to mitochondrial dysfunction and cell death in rabbit RPTC exposed to cisplatin while PKC-ζ mediates RPTC repair after exposure to tert-butylhdyroperoxide. Interestingly, cisplatin-induced PKC activation was followed by ERK1/2 activation, which decreased mitochondrial membrane potential and caused caspase 3 activation, and apoptosis. In vitro studies using LLC-PK1 cells exposed to 2,3,5-tris-(glutathion-S-yl)hydroquinone (TGHQ) and in vivo studies in mice exposed to cisplatin support a role for ERK in renal cell death (Ramachandiran et al., 2002; Arany et al., 2004; Dong et al., 2004; Sheikh-Hamad et al., 2004; van de Water et al., 2000). However, the role of MAPK in toxicant-induced renal cell death is toxicant-specific because ERK activation prevented cell death following oxidant exposure (Arany et al., 2004).

SPECIFIC NEPHROTOXICANTS

Heavy Metals

Many metals, including cadmium, chromium, lead, mercury, platinum, and uranium, are nephrotoxic. It is important to recognize that the nature and severity of metal nephrotoxicity varies with respect to its form. For example, salts of inorganic mercury produce a greater degree of renal injury and a lesser degree of neurotoxicity than do organic mercury compounds, an effect that has been associated with the greater degree of lipophilicity of organic mercury compounds (Conner and Fowler, 1993; Zalups and Lash, 1994). In addition, different metals have different primary targets within the kidney. For example, potassium dichromate and cadmium primarily affect the S_1 and S_2 segments of the proximal tubule, whereas mercuric chloride affects the S_2 and S_3 segments (Zalups and Lash, 1994; Zalups and Diamond, 2005).

Metals may cause toxicity through their ability to bind to sulfhydryl groups. For example, the affinity of mercury for sulfhydryl groups is very high and is about ten orders of magnitude

Table 14-4

Selected Signaling Kinases Involved in Renal Cell Injury, Survival or Repair*

KINASE	LOCATION	NEPHROTOXICANT	REFERENCE
Protein kinase C (PKC)			
Conventional PKC			
PKCα	Proximal tubules	Cisplatin DCVC[†]	Nowak, 2002; Liu *et al.*, 2004
Atypical PKC			
PKCζ	Proximal tubules	*t*-butylhydroperoxide	Nowak *et al.*, 2004
Mitogen activated protien kianse (MAPK)			
ERK1/2	Proximal tubules	Cisplatin H$_2$O$_2$ TGHQ[‡]	Nowak, 2002; Arany *et al.*, 2004; Ramachandiran *et al.*, 2002; Dong *et al.*, 2004; Zhuang and Schnellmann, 2004
JNK/SAPK[†]	Proximal tubules	Cisplatin	Arany *et al.*, 2004
P38	Proximal tubules	Cisplatin H$_2$O$_2$ TGHQ[‡]	Arany *et al.*, 2004; Ramachandiran *et al.*, 2002; Dong *et al.*, 2004; Zhuang and Schnellmann, 2004
Other kinases			
Protein kinase B[§]	LLC-PK1 Proximal tubules	Cisplatin mechanical injury H$_2$O$_2$	Zhuang *et al.*, 2003; Zhuang and Schnellmann, 2004
Phosphoinositide-3-kinase	LLC-PK1 Proximal tubules	Cisplatin mechanical injury	Zhuang *et al.*, 2003

*Taken from Schnellmann and Cummings, 2006.

[†] *S*-(1,2)-dichlorovinyl-L-cysteine.

[‡] 2,3,5-*tris*-(glutathion-*S*-yl)hydroquinone.

Also known as AKT.

higher than the affinity of mercury for carbonyl or amino groups (Ballatori, 1991). Thus, metals may cause renal cellular injury through their ability to bind to sulfhydryl groups of critical proteins within the cells and thereby inhibit their normal function.

Mercury Humans and animals are exposed to elemental mercury vapor, inorganic mercurous and mercuric salts, and organic mercuric compounds through the environment. Administered elemental mercury is rapidly oxidized in erythrocytes or tissues to inorganic mercury, and thus the tissue distribution of elemental and inorganic mercury is similar. Due to its high affinity for sulfhydryl groups, virtually all of the Hg^{2+} found in blood is bound to cells— albumin, other sulfhydryl-containing proteins, glutathione, and cysteine.

The kidneys are the primary target organs for accumulation of Hg^{2+}, and the S$_3$ segment of the proximal tubule is the initial site of toxicity. As the dose or duration of treatment increases, the S$_1$ and S$_2$ segments may be affected. Renal uptake of Hg^{2+} is very rapid with as much as 50% of a nontoxic dose of Hg^{2+} found in the kidneys within a few hours of exposure. Considering the fact that virtually all of the Hg^{2+} found in blood is bound to an endogenous ligand, it is likely that the luminal and/or basolateral transport of Hg^{2+} into the proximal tubular epithelial cell is through cotransport of Hg^{2+} with an endogenous ligand such as glutathione, cysteine, or albumin, or through some plasma membrane Hg^{2+}-ligand complex (Zalups and Diamond, 2005). Current evidence indicates that at least two mechanisms are involved in the proximal tubular uptake of Hg^{2+} (Fig. 14-13) (Zalups and Diamond, 2005). One mechanism appears to involve the apical activity of γ-glutamyl transpeptidase, cysteinylglycinase, and the transport of Cys-S-Hg-S-Cys through one of more amino acid transporters. Basolateral membrane transport is likely to be mediated by the organic anion transport system.

The acute nephrotoxicity induced by HgCl$_2$ is characterized by proximal tubular necrosis and ARF within 24–48 hours after administration (Zalups, 1997). Early markers of HgCl$_2$-induced renal dysfunction include an increase in the urinary excretion of brush-border enzymes such as alkaline phosphatase and γ-GT, suggesting that the brush border may be an initial target of HgCl$_2$. As injury progresses, tubular reabsorption of solutes and water decreases and there is an increase in the urinary excretion of glucose, amino acids, albumin, and other proteins. Associated with the increase in injured proximal tubules is a decrease and progressive decline in the GFR. For example, GFR was reduced 35% in rats within 6 hours of HgCl$_2$ administration and continued to decline to 32% and 16% of controls at 12 and 24 hours, respectively (Eknoyan *et al.*, 1982). The reduction in GFR results from the glomerular injury, tubular injury, and/or vasoconstriction. Interestingly, there is an early decrease in RBF secondary to the vasoconstriction. RBF may return to normal within 24–48 hours, while GFR continues to decline. If the decline in renal function is not too severe, the remaining proximal tubular cells undergo a proliferative response and renal function returns over time. Chelation therapy with 2,3-dimercaptopropane-1-sulfonate or 2,3-mesodimercaptosuccinic acid is used for the treatment for mercury-induced nephrotoxicity (Zalups and Diamond, 2005).

As stated above, inorganic mercury has a very high affinity for protein sulfhydryl groups, and this interaction is thought to play an important role in the toxicity of mercury at the cellular level. Changes in mitochondrial morphology and function are very early events following HgCl$_2$ administration, supporting the hypothesis that mitochondrial dysfunction is an early and important contributor to inorganic mercury-induced cell death along the proximal tubule. Other studies have suggested that oxidative stress and disregulation of Ca^{2+} homeostasis plays an important role in HgCl$_2$-induced renal injury (Fukino *et al.*, 1984; Smith *et al.*, 1987; Lund *et al.*, 1993).

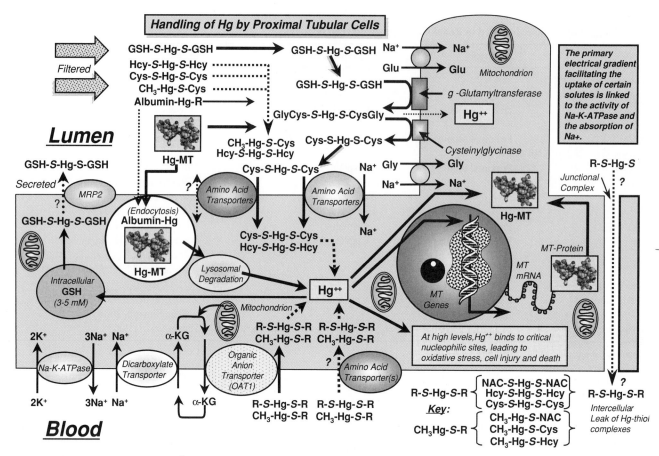

Figure 14-13. *Cellular transport of Hg*$^{2+}$.

Proximal tubular uptake of inorganic mercury is thought to be the result of the transport of Hg^{2+} conjugates [e.g., diglutathione-Hg^{2+} conjugate (GSH-Hg-GSH), dicysteine-Hg^{2+} conjugate (CYS-HG-CYS)]. At the luminal membrane, GSH-Hg-GSH is metabolized by γ-GT and a dipeptidase to form CYS-HG-CYS. CYS-HG-CYS may be taken up by amino acid transporters. It is not clear whether albumin-Hg-R conjugates are transported across the liminal membrane in vivo. At the basolateral membrane, Hg^{2+}-conjugates appear to be transported by organic anion transporters OAT1 and OAT3. (Courtesy of Dr. R.K. Zalups.) [From Zalups RK, Diamond GL: Nephrotoxicology of Metals, in Tarloff JB, Lash LH (eds.): *Toxicology of the Kidney (3rd)*. Boca Raton: CRC Press, 2005, p. 954, with permission.]

Several animal studies have shown that chronic exposure to inorganic mercury results in an immunologically mediated membranous glomerular nephritis secondary to the production of antibodies against the GBM and the deposition of immune complexes (Zalups and Diamond, 2005).

Cadmium   Chronic exposure of nonsmoking humans and animals to cadmium is primarily through food and results in nephrotoxicity (Kido and Nordberg, 1998; Zalups and Diamond, 2005). In the workplace, inhalation of cadmium-containing dust and fumes is the major route of exposure. Cadmium has a half-life of greater than 10 years in humans and thus accumulates in the body over time. Approximately 50% of the body burden of cadmium can be found in the kidney and nephrotoxicity can be observed when Cd concentrations exceed 50 μg/gm kidney wet weight (Zalups and Diamond, 2005). Lauwerys and coworkers (1994) suggested that cadmium concentrations in the urine greater than 5 and 2 nmol/mmol creatinine for adult male workers and the general population, respectively, are associated with tubular dysfunction. Cadmium produces proximal tubule dysfunction (S$_1$ and S$_2$ segments) and injury characterized by increases in urinary excretion of glucose, amino acids, calcium, and cellular enzymes. This injury may progress to a chronic interstitial nephritis.

A very interesting aspect of cadmium nephrotoxicity is the role of metallothioneins (Klaassen *et al.*, 1999). Metallothioneins are a family of low-molecular-weight, cysteine-rich metal-binding proteins that have a high affinity for cadmium and other heavy metals. In general, the mechanism by which metallothionein is thought to play a role in cadmium and heavy metal toxicity is through its ability to bind to a heavy metal and thereby render it biologically inactive. This assumes that the unbound or "free" concentration of the metal is the toxic species. Metallothionein production can be induced by low, nontoxic concentrations of metals. Subsequently, animals challenged with a higher dose of the metal will not exhibit toxicity compared to naive animals.

Following an oral exposure to CdCl$_2$, Cd^{2+} is thought to reach the kidneys both as Cd^{2+} and as a Cd^{2+}-metallothionein complex formed and released either from intestinal cells or hepatocytes. The Cd^{2+}-metallothionein complex is freely filtered by the glomerulus and reabsorption by the proximal tubule is probably by endocytosis and is limited (Zalups and Diamond, 2005). Inside the tubular cells it is thought that lysosomal degradation of the Cd^{2+}-metallothionein results in the release of "free" Cd^{2+}, which, in turn, induces renal metallothionein production. Once the renal metallothionein pool is saturated, "free" Cd^{2+} initiates injury. It is also likely that Cd is reabsorbed luminally and basolaterally as a cysteine conjugate (Zalups and Diamond, 2005). The mechanism by which Cd^{2+} produces injury at the cellular level is not clear; however, low concentrations of Cd^{2+} have been shown to interfere with the normal function of several cellular signal transduction pathways.

Chemically Induced α2u-Globulin Nephropathy

A diverse group of chemicals, including unleaded gasoline, d-limonene, 1,4-dichlorobenzene, tetrachloroethylene, decalin, and lindane, cause α_{2u}-globulin nephropathy or hyaline droplet nephropathy (Lehman-McKeeman, 1997). This nephropathy occurring in male rats, is characterized by the accumulation of protein droplets in the S_2 segment of the proximal tubule, and results in single-cell necrosis, the formation of granular casts at the junction of the proximal tubule and the thin loop of Henle, and cellular regeneration. Chronic exposure to these compounds results in progression of these lesions and ultimately in chronic nephropathy. With compounds such as unleaded gasoline, chronic exposure results in an increased incidence of renal adenomas/carcinomas by nongenotoxic mechanisms.

As the name implies, the expression of this nephropathy requires the presence of the α_{2u}-globulin protein. α_{2u}-Globulin is synthesized in the liver of male rats and is under androgen control. Due to its low molecular weight (18.7 kDa), α_{2u}-globulin is freely filtered by the glomerulus with approximately half being reabsorbed via endocytosis in the S_2 segment of the proximal tubule. Many of the compounds that cause α_{2u}-globulin nephropathy bind to α_{2u}-globulin in a reversible manner and decrease the ability of lysosomal proteases in the proximal tubule to breakdown α_{2u}-globulin. This results in the accumulation of α_{2u}-globulin in the proximal tubule with an increase in the size and number of lysosomes and the characteristic protein-droplet morphology. A proposed mechanism of α_{2u}-globulin nephropathy is that cellular necrosis secondary to lysosomal overload leads to a sustained increase in cell proliferation, which, in turn, results in the promotion of spontaneously or chemically initiated cells to form preneoplastic and neoplastic foci (Lehman-McKeeman, 1997; Melnick, 1992).

α_{2u}-Globulin nephropathy appears to be sex- and species-specific. That is, it occurs in male rats but not female rats and in male or female mice, rabbits, or guinea pigs because they do not produce α_{2u}-globulin (Lehman-McKeeman, 1997). Furthermore, it does not occur in male Black Reiter rats that lack α_{2u}-globulin. Considering the diversity of compounds that cause α_{2u}-globulin nephropathy and renal tumors and the fact that humans are exposed to these compounds regularly, the question arises whether humans are at risk for α_{2u}-globulin nephropathy and renal tumors when exposed to these compounds. Current data suggest that humans are not at risk because (1) humans do not synthesize α_{2u}-globulin, (2) humans secrete less proteins in general and in particular less low-molecular-weight proteins in urine than the rat, (3) the low-molecular-weight proteins in human urine are either not related structurally to α_{2u}-globulin, do not bind to compounds that bind to α_{2u}-globulin, or are similar to proteins in female rats, male Black Reiter rats, rabbits, or guinea pigs that do not exhibit α_{2u}-globulin nephropathy, and (4) mice excrete a low-molecular-weight urinary protein that is 90% homologous to α_{2u}-globulin, but they do not exhibit α_{2u}-globulin-nephropathy and renal tumors following exposure to α_{2u}-globulin-nephropathy-inducing agents.

Halogenated Hydrocarbons

Halogenated hydrocarbons are a diverse class of compounds and are used extensively as chemical intermediates, solvents, and pesticides. Consequently, humans are exposed to these compounds not only in the workplace but also through the environment. Numerous toxic effects have been associated with acute and chronic exposure to halogenated hydrocarbons, including nephrotoxicity (Elfarra, 1997). The two examples provided below illustrate the importance of biotransformation in the nephrotoxicity of halogenated hydrocarbons (Dekant, 2005; Rankin and Valentovic, 2005).

Chloroform Chloroform produces nephrotoxicity in a variety of species, with some species being more sensitive than others. The primary cellular target is the proximal tubule, with no primary damage to the glomerulus or the distal tubule. Proteinuria, glucosuria, and increased BUN levels are all characteristic of chloroform-induced nephrotoxicity. The nephrotoxicity produced by chloroform is linked to its metabolism by renal cytochrome P450 and the formation of a reactive intermediate that binds covalently to nucleophilic groups on cellular macromolecules. Cytochrome P450 biotransforms chloroform to trichloromethanol, which is unstable and releases HCl to form phosgene. Phosgene can react with (1) water to produce $2HCl + CO_2$, (2) two molecules of glutathione to produce diglutathionyl dithiocarbonate, (3) cysteine to produce 2-oxothizolidine-4-carboxylic acid, or (4) cellular macromolecules to initiate toxicity. The sex differences observed in chloroform nephrotoxicity appear to be related to differences in renal cytochrome P450 isozyme contents. For example, castration of male mice decreased renal cytochrome P450 and chloroform-induced nephrotoxicity (Smith *et al.*, 1984). Likewise, testosterone pretreatment of female mice increased cytochrome P450 content and rendered female mice susceptible to the nephrotoxic effects of chloroform. Cytochrome P450 isozyme 2E1 is present in male mice and expressed in female mice treated with testosterone (Lock and Reed, 1997). Thus, these isozymes may play a role in chloroform-induced nephrotoxicity.

Tetrafluoroethylene Tetrafluoroethylene is metabolized in the liver by GSH-S-transferases to S-(1,1,2,2-tetrafluoroethyl)-glutathione. The GSH conjugate is secreted into the bile and small intestine where it is degraded to the cysteine S-conjugate (TFEC), reabsorbed, and transported to the kidney. The mercapturic acid may also be formed in the small intestine and reabsorbed. Alternatively, the glutathione conjugate can be transported to the kidney and biotransformed to the cysteine conjugate by γ-GT and a dipeptidase located on the brush border (Fig. 14-14). The mercapturic acid is transported into the proximal tubule cell by the organic anion transporter, whereas cysteine conjugates are transported by the organic anion transporter and the sodium-independent L and T transport systems. The cysteine S-conjugate of these compounds is thought to be the penultimate nephrotoxic species. Following transport into the proximal tubule, which is the primary cellular target for haloalkenes and haloalkanes, the cysteine S-conjugate is a substrate for the cytosolic and mitochondrial forms of the enzyme cysteine conjugate β-lyase. In the case of the N-acetyl-cysteine S-conjugate, the N-acetyl group must be removed by a deacetylase for it to be a substrate for cysteine conjugate β-lyase. The products of the reaction are ammonia, pyruvate, and a reactive thiol that is capable of binding covalently to cellular macromolecules. There is a correlation

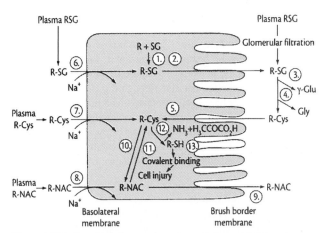

Figure 14-14. Renal tubular uptake and metabolism of GSH conjugates.

(1) Intracellular formation of GSH conjugates (R-SG) catalyzed by renal GSH S-transferase(s); (2) Secretion of the R-SG into the lumen; (3) γ-GT-mediated catabolism of R-SG and formation of the corresponding S-cysteinylglycine conjugate; (4) formation of the corresponding cysteine conjugate (R-Cys); (5) Na$^+$-coupled transport of R-Cys into the renal proximal tubular cell; (6) Na$^+$-coupled transport of RSG across the basolateral membrane; (7) Na$^+$-coupled transport of R-Cys across the basolateral membrane; (8) Na$^+$-coupled and probenecid-sensitive transport of the mercapturate (R-NAC) across the basolateral membrane; (9) secretion of R-NAC into the lumen; (10) deacetylation of R-NAC to R-Cys and (11) acetylation of R-Cys to R-NAC; (12) reactive thiol formation via β-lyase; (13) binding of the reactive thiol to cellular macromolecules and initiation of cell injury. [From TJ Monks and SS Lau: Renal transport processes and glutathione conjugate-mediated nephrotoxicity, *Drug Metab Dispos* 1987 15:437–441, with permission.]

between the covalent binding of the reactive thiol of the cysteine conjugate with renal protein and nephrotoxicity. Hayden and colleagues (1991) and Bruschi and coworkers (1993) have shown that biotransformation of TFEC results in difluorothioamidyl-L-lysine-protein adducts in mitochondria and that two of the targeted proteins may belong to the heat shock family of proteins. Hayden and colleagues (1992) have also shown that halogenated thioamide adducts of phosphatidylethanolamine are formed in mitochondria following cysteine conjugate β-lyase biotransformation of TFEC.

The nephrotoxicity produced by haloalkenes is characterized morphologically by proximal tubular necrosis, primarily affecting the S$_3$ segment, and functionally by increases in urinary glucose, protein, cellular enzymes, and BUN. Following in vivo and in vitro exposures to TFEC, the mitochondrion appears to be a primary target. In rabbit renal proximal tubules and isolated mitochondria, there is a marked decrease in state 3 respiration (respiration associated with maximal ATP formation) following TFEC exposure (Groves *et al.*, 1993). Furthermore, the decrease in mitochondrial function occurs prior to the onset of cell death. Oxidative stress may also play a contributing role in TFEC-induced cell death because lipid peroxidation products were formed prior to the onset of cell death, and antioxidants and iron chelators decreased cytotoxicity (Chen *et al.*, 1990; Groves *et al.*, 1991).

Mycotoxins

Mycotoxins are products of molds and fungi and a number of mycotoxins produce nephrotoxicity such as aflatoxin B$_1$, citrinin, ochratoxins, fumonisins, and patulin (O'Brien and Dietrich, 2005). Two

examples of nephrotoxic mycotoxins will be discussed. Citrinin nephrotoxicity is characterized by decreased urine osmolality, GFR and RBF, and increased urinary enzyme excretion. Interestingly, the location of citrinin-induced tubular damage (proximal, distal) varies among species. Whereas the mechanism of citrinin toxicity to the tubules remains unresolved, citrinin enters the cells through the organic anion transporter and causes mitochondrial dysfunction. While acute exposures of ochratoxin A produce similar effects on the kidney as citrinin, chronic exposures result in progressive tubular atrophy and fibrosis. One or both of these mycotoxins have been implicated in Balkan nephropathy in humans, although the data to support this are less than clear.

Fumonisins B$_1$ and B$_2$ are commonly found on corn and corn products and produce nephrotoxicity in rats and rabbits (Bucci *et al.*, 1998). Histologic examination of the kidney revealed disruption of the basolateral membrane, mitochondrial swelling, increased numbers of clear and electron-dense vacuoles, and apoptosis in proximal tubular cells at the junction of the cortex and medulla. Changes in renal function included increased urine volume, decreased osmolality, and increased excretion of low- and high-molecular-weight proteins. The fumonisins are structurally similar to sphingoid bases and are thought to produce their toxicity through the inhibition of sphinganine (sphingosine) N-acyltransferase. Inhibition of this enzyme results in an increase in the ratio of free sphinganine to free sphingosine and a decrease in complex sphingolipids. However, the mechanism by which these sphingolipid alterations results in cell death is unknown.

Therapeutic Agents

Acetaminophen Large doses of the antipyretic and analgesic acetaminophen (APAP) are commonly associated with hepatoxicity (Tarloff, 2005). However, large doses of APAP can also cause nephrotoxicity in humans and animals. APAP nephrotoxicity is characterized by proximal tubular necrosis with increases in BUN and plasma creatinine; decreases in GFR and clearance of *para*-aminohippurate; increases in the fractional excretion of water, sodium, and potassium; and increases in urinary glucose, protein, and brush-border enzymes. There appears to be a marked species difference in the nature and mechanism of APAP nephrotoxicity (Emeigh Hart *et al.*, 1994; Tarloff, 1997). Morphologically, the primary targets in the mouse kidney are the S$_1$ and S$_2$ segments of the proximal tubule, whereas in the rat kidney the S$_3$ segment is the target. In the mouse, renal cytochrome P450 2E1 has been associated with APAP biotransformation to a reactive intermediate, N-acetyl-*p*-amino-benzoquinoneimine, that arylates proteins in the proximal tubule and initiates cell death. Two of the proteins that are targets of N-acetyl-*p*-amino-benzoquinoneimine are a selenium-binding protein and a glutamine synthetase (Emeigh Hart *et al.*, 1994; Tarloff, 1997). However, the mechanism by which protein adducts initiate proximal tubular cell death and ultimately nephrotoxicity remains to be determined. While renal cytochrome P450 plays a role in APAP activation and nephrotoxicity, glutathione conjugates of APAP may also contribute to APAP nephrotoxicity. Evidence for this pathway was provided by experiments in which γ-GT or organic anion transport was inhibited and APAP-induced nephrotoxicity decreased (Emeigh Hart *et al.*, 1990). In contrast to its effects in the mouse, a critical and early step in APAP nephrotoxicity in the rat is the conversion of APAP to *para*-aminophenol (PAP) (Tarloff, 1997). The steps following PAP formation and the expression of nephrotoxicity are less clear.

Nonsteroidal Anti-Inflammatory Drugs (NSAIDs) NSAIDs such as aspirin, ibuprofen, naproxen, indomethacin, and cyclooxygenase-2 inhibitors (e.g., celecoxib) are extensively used as analgesics and anti-inflammatory agents and produce their therapeutic effects through the inhibition of prostaglandin synthesis. At least three different types of nephrotoxicity have been associated with NSAID administration (Tarloff, 2005; Palmer and Heinrich, 2004). ARF may occur within hours of a large dose of a NSAID, is usually reversible upon withdrawal of the drug, and is characterized by decreased RBF and GFR and by oliguria. When the normal production of vasodilatory prostaglandins is inhibited by NSAIDs, vasoconstriction induced by circulating catecholamines and angiotensin II is unopposed, resulting in decreased RBF and ischemia. A number of risk factors (e.g., congestive heart failure, hepatic cirrhosis, hemorrhage, hypertension, sepsis, diabetes) are known to facilitate the development of ARF following NSAIDs consumption.

In contrast, chronic consumption of combinations of NSAIDs and/or APAP (>3 years) results in an often irreversible form of nephrotoxicity known as analgesic nephropathy (Palmer and Heinrich, 2004; Tarloff, 2005; De Broe, 2005). The incidence of analgesic nephropathy varies widely in the western world, ranging from less than 2–5% of all end-stage renal disease patients in countries where analgesic consumption is low (e.g., U.S. Canada), and up to 20% of all end-stage renal disease patients in countries with the highest analgesic consumption (e.g., Australia, Sweden). Impaired urinary concentration and acidification are the earliest clinical manifestations. The primary lesion in this nephropathy is papillary necrosis with chronic interstitial nephritis. Initial changes are to the medullary interstitial cells and are followed by degenerative changes to the medullary loops of Henle and medullary capillaries. Well-defined clinical signs have been associated with analgesic nephropathy and are helpful in the diagnosis thereof. De Broe (2005) and colleagues have developed an effective computed tomography (CT) protocol that does not use contrast media to diagnose analgesic nephropathy. While analgesic nephropathy is associated with a number of well-defined effects, the mechanism by which NSAIDs produce analgesic nephropathy is not known, but may result from chronic medullary/papillary ischemia secondary to renal vasoconstriction. Other studies have suggested that a reactive intermediate is formed in the cells that, in turn, initiates an oxidative stress, or binds covalently to critical cellular macromolecules.

The third albeit rare type of nephrotoxicity associated with NSAIDs is an interstitial nephritis with a mean time of NSAID exposure to development of approximately 5 months (Tarloff, 2005; Palmer and Heinrich, 2004). This nephrotoxicity is characterized by a diffuse interstitial edema with mild to moderate infiltration of inflammatory cells. Patients normally present with elevated serum creatinine, proteinuria, and nephritic syndrome. If NSAIDs are discontinued, renal function improves in 1–3 months.

Aminoglycosides

The aminoglycoside antibiotics are so named because they consist of two or more amino sugars joined in a glycosidic linkage to a central hexose nucleus. Whereas they are drugs of choice for many gram-negative infections, their use is primarily limited by their nephrotoxicity. The incidence of renal dysfunction following aminoglycoside administration ranges from 5 to 25%, but seldom leads to a fatal outcome (Servais et al., 2005; Palmer and Heinrich, 2004).

Renal dysfunction by aminoglycosides is characterized by a nonoliguric renal failure with reduced GFR and an increase in serum creatinine and BUN. Polyuria is an early event following aminoglycoside administration and may be due to inhibition of chloride transport in the thick ascending limb (Kidwell et al., 1994). Within 24 hours, increases in urinary brush-border enzymes, glucosuria, aminoaciduria, and proteinuria are observed. Histologically, lysosomal alterations are noted initially, followed by damage to the brush border, endoplasmic reticulum, mitochondria, and cytoplasm, ultimately leading to tubular cell necrosis. Interestingly, proliferation of renal proximal tubule cells can be observed early after the onset of nephrotoxicity.

Aminoglycosides are highly polar cations; they are almost exclusively filtered by the glomerulus and excreted unchanged. Filtered aminoglycosides undergo proximal tubular reabsorption by binding to anionic phospholipids in the brush border, followed by endocytosis and sequestration in lysosomes of the S_1 and S_2 segments of proximal tubules (Fig. 14-15). Basolateral membrane binding and uptake also may occur, but this is a minor contribution to the total proximal tubular uptake of aminoglycosides. The earliest lesion observed following clinically relevant doses of aminoglycosides is an increase in the size and number of lysosomes. These lysosomes contain *myeloid bodies,* which are electron-dense lamellar structures containing undergraded phospholipids. The renal phospholipidosis produced by the aminoglycosides is thought to occur through their inhibition of lysosomal hydrolases, such as sphingomyelinase and phospholipases. Whereas phospholipidosis plays an important role in aminoglycoside nephrotoxicity, the steps between the phospholipid accumulation in the lysosomes and tubular cell death are less clear. One hypothesis suggests that the lysosomes become progressively distended until they rupture, releasing lysosomal enzymes and high concentrations of aminoglycosides into the cytoplasm (Fig. 14-15). The released lysosomal contents can interact with various membranes and organelles and trigger cell death. Another mechanism of aminoglycoside nephrotoxicity includes a decrease in K_f and GFR (see above).

Amphotericin B Amphotericin B is a very effective antifungal agent whose clinical utility is limited by its nephrotoxicity (Bernardo and Branch, 1997; Palmer and Heinrich, 2004). Renal dysfunction associated with amphotericin B treatment is dependent on cumulative dose and is due to both hemodynamic and tubular effects. With respect to hemodynamics, Amphotericin B administration is associated with decreases in RBF and GFR secondary to renal arteriolar vasoconstriction or activation of TGF. Amphotericin B nephrotoxicity is characterized by ADH-resistant polyuria, renal tubular acidosis, hypokalemia, and either acute or chronic renal failure. Amphotericin B nephrotoxicity is unusual in that it impairs the functional integrity of the glomerulus and of the proximal and distal portions of the nephron.

Some of the renal tubular cell effects of amphotericin B are due to the ability of this polyene to bind to cholesterol in the plasma membrane and form aqueous pores. In the presence of amphotericin B, cells of the turtle and rat distal tubule do not produce a normal net outward flux of protons due to an increase in proton permeability (Steinmetz and Husted, 1982; Gil and Malnic, 1989). This results in impaired proton excretion and renal tubular acidosis. The hypokalemia observed with amphotericin B may be due to an increase in luminal potassium ion permeability in the late distal tubule and the cortical collecting duct and the loss of potassium ions in the urine.

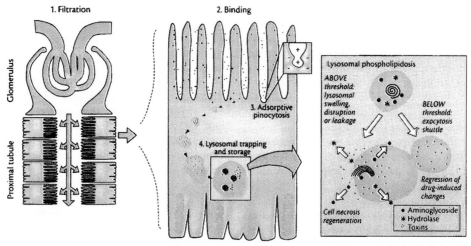

Figure 14-15. *Renal handling of aminoglycosides: (1) glomerular filtration, (2) binding to the brush-border membranes of the proximal tubule, (3) pinocytosis, and (4) storage in the lysosomes. [From De Broe ME: Renal injury due to environmental toxins, drugs, and contrast agents, in Berl T, Bonventre JV (eds.): Atlas of Diseases of the Kidney. Philadelphia: Current Medicine, 1999, p. 11.4, with permission.]*

Cyclosporine   Cyclosporine is an important immunosuppressive agent and is widely used to prevent graft rejection in organ transplantation (Charney *et al.*, 2005; Palmer and Heinrich, 2004). Cyclosporine is a fungal cyclic polypeptide and acts by selectively inhibiting T-cell activation. Nephrotoxicity is a critical side effect of cyclosporine, with nearly all patients who receive the drug exhibiting some form of nephrotoxicity. Clinically, cyclosporine-induced nephrotoxicity may manifest as (1) acute reversible renal dysfunction, (2) acute vasculopathy, and (3) chronic nephropathy with interstitial fibrosis (Mason and Moore, 1997; Dieperink *et al.*, 1998).

Acute renal dysfunction is characterized by dose-related decreases in RBF and GFR and increases in BUN and serum creatinine. These effects are lessened by reducing the dosage or by cessation of therapy. The decrease in RBF and GFR is related to marked vasoconstriction induced by cyclosporine; and it is probably produced by a number of factors, including an imbalance in vasoconstrictor and vasodilatory prostaglandin production. In particular, increased production of the vasoconstrictor thromboxane A_2 appears to play a role in cyclosporine-induced ARF. Endothelin may contribute to constriction of the afferent arteriole because endothelin receptor antagonists inhibit cyclosporine-induced vasoconstriction (Lanese and Conger, 1993). Whereas cyclosporine can produce proximal tubular epithelial changes (many small equally sized vacuoles in the cytosol), it is still not clear whether a direct effect of cyclosporine on tubular cells plays a significant role in the nephrotoxicity.

Acute vasculopathy or thrombotic microangiopathy is a rather unusual nephrotoxic lesion that affects arterioles and glomerular capillaries, without an inflammatory component, following cyclosporine treatment. The lesion consists of fibrin-platelet thrombi and fragmented red blood cells occluding the vessels (Charney *et al.*, 2005). The pathogenesis of this lesion is poorly understood. Whereas the characteristics of this lesion differ from the vascular changes of acute rejection, a variety of factors may contribute to this lesion in the clinical transplant setting.

Long-term treatment with cyclosporine can result in chronic nephropathy with interstitial fibrosis and tubular atrophy. Modest elevations in serum creatinine and decreases in GFR occur along with hypertension, proteinuria, and tubular dysfunction. Histologic changes are profound; they are characterized by arteriolopathy,

global and segmental glomerular sclerosis, striped interstitial fibrosis, and tubular atrophy. These lesions may not be reversible if cyclosporine therapy is discontinued and may result in end-stage renal disease. Whereas the mechanism of chronic cyclosporine nephropathy is not known, vasoconstriction probably plays a contributing role. Studies by Wang and Salahudeen (1994, 1995) indicated that rats treated with cyclosporine and an antioxidant lazaroid for 30 days exhibited increased GFR and RBF and less tubulointerstitial fibrosis and lipid peroxidation than rats treated with cyclosporine alone, suggesting that oxidative stress plays a role in cyclosporine nephrotoxity in rats. The marked interstitial cell proliferation and increased procollagen secretion that occurs following cyclosporine administration may contribute to the interstitial fibrosis (Racusen and Solez, 1993).

Tacrolimus (FK-506) is a newer immunosuppressive agent that also exhibits nephrotoxicity. At this time, the degree and incidence of nephrotoxicity and morphologic changes associated with tacrolimus exposure are similar to that exhibited with cyclosporine, suggesting similar modes of toxic action.

Cisplatin   Cisplatin is a valuable drug in the treatment of solid tumors, with nephrotoxicity limiting its clinical use. The kidney is not only responsible for the majority of cisplatin excreted but is also the primary site of accumulation. The effects of cisplatin on the kidney are several, including acute and chronic renal failure, renal magnesium wasting, and polyuria and patients treated with cisplatin regimens permanently lose 10–30% of their renal function (Bonegio and Lieberthal, 2005).

Early effects of cisplatin are decreases in RBF and GFR produced by vasoconstriction and is followed by tubular injury with enzymuria. The early polyuria, has been suggested, to result from the inhibition of vasopressin release (Clifton *et al.*, 1982). Although the primary cellular target associated with ARF is the proximal tubule S_3 segment in the rat, in humans the S_1 and S_2 segments, distal tubule, and collecting ducts can also be affected. The chronic renal failure observed with cisplatin is due to prolonged exposure and is characterized by focal necrosis in numerous segments of the nephron without a significant effect on the glomerulus. Considerable effort has been expended in the development of measures to prevent cisplatin nephrotoxicity. These efforts include the use of extensive hydration and mannitol diuresis and the development of less nephrotoxic platinum compounds such as carboplatin.

The mechanism by which cisplatin produces cellular injury is not known but may involve metabolites of cisplatin. For example, in a mouse model of cisplatin-induced nephrotoxicity the inhibition of γ-glutamyl transpeptidase or cysteine S-conjugate β-lyase blocked toxicity, suggesting that cisplatin-glutathione conjugates may be important in targeting cisplatin to the kidney and its resulting nephrotoxicity (Townsend and Hanigan, 2002). Interestingly, the *trans* isomer of cisplatin is not nephrotoxic even though similar concentrations of platinum are observed in the kidney after dosing. Thus, it is not the platinum atom per se that is responsible for the toxicity but rather the geometry of the complex or a metabolite. The antineoplastic and perhaps the nephrotoxic effects of cisplatin may be due to its intracellular hydrolysis to the reactive mono-chloro-mono-aquo-diammine-platinum or diaquo-diammine-platinum species and the ability of these metabolites to alkylate purine and pyrimidine bases.

In vitro studies using primary cultures of mouse proximal tubular cells revealed that the type of cell death produced by cisplatin is dependent on the concentration (Lieberthal *et al.*, 1996). At cisplatin concentrations less than 100 μM, the primary form of cell death is apoptosis. As the concentration increases above 100 μM, a greater percentage of the cells die by oncosis. Using rabbit renal proximal tubule cells, Courjault *et al.* (1993) showed that while DNA synthesis, protein synthesis, glucose transport, Na^+, K^+-ATPase activity,

and cell viability were all inhibited by cisplatin, DNA synthesis was the most sensitive. These results suggest that cisplatin may produce nephrotoxicity through its ability to inhibit DNA synthesis as well as transport functions. Finally, primarily through the use of antioxidants, in vivo and in vitro studies support a role for oxidative stress in cisplatin-induced nephrotoxicity (Bonegio and Lieberthal, 2005). The lack of complete return of renal function following cisplatin treatment in vivo may result from the interference of cisplatin with the normal proliferative response that occurs after injury.

Radiocontrast Agents Iodinated contrast media are used for the imaging of tissues, with two major classes of compounds currently in use. The ionic compounds, diatrizoate derivatives, are (1) ionized at physiologic pH, (2) not significantly bound to protein, (3) restricted to the extracellular space, (4) almost entirely eliminated by the kidney, and (5) freely filtered by the glomerulus and neither secreted nor reabsorbed. These agents have a very high osmolality (>1200 mOsm/L) and are potentially nephrotoxic, particularly in patients with existing renal impairment, diabetes, or heart failure or who are receiving other nephrotoxic drugs. The newer contrast agents (e.g., iotrol, iopamidol) are nonionic owing to the addition of an organic side chain, their low osmolality, and their lower nephrotoxicity. The nephrotoxicity of these agents is due to both hemodynamic alterations (vasoconstriction) and proximal tubular injury (Kaperonis *et al.*, 2005). The vasoconstriction is prolonged and is probably produced by more than one mediator while ROS are thought to play a role in the proximal tubular injury.

REFERENCES

American Society of Nephrology: Renal research report. *J Am Soc Nephrol* 16:1886–1903, 2005.

Arany I, Megyesi JK, Kaneto H, *et al.*: Cisplatin-induced cell death is EGFR/src/ERK signaling dependent in mouse proximal tubule cells. *Am J Physiol Renal Physiol* 87:F543, 2004.

Arrington D, Van Vleet T, Schnellmann RG: Calpain 10: A mitochondrial calpain and its role in calcium-induced mitochondrial dysfunction. *Am J Physiol* 291:C1159–C1171, 2006.

Bach PH: The renal medulla and distal nephron toxicity, in Sipes IG, McQueen CA, Gandolfi AJ (eds.): *Comprehensive Toxicology,* Vol 7. Oxford, England: Elsevier, 1997, pp. 279–298.

Ballatori N: Mechanisms of metal transport across liver cell plasma membrane. *Drug Metab Rev* 23:83–132, 1991.

Basnakian AG, Ueda N, Hong X, Galitovsky VE, Yin X, Shah SV: Ceramide synthase is essential for endonuclease-mediated death of renal tubular epithelial cells induced by hypoxia-reoxygenation. *Am J Physiol* 288:F308, 2005.

Bernardo JF, Branch RA: Amphotericin B, in Sipes IG, McQueen CA, Gandolfi AJ (eds.): *Comprehensive Toxicology,* Vol 7. Oxford, England: Elsevier, 1997, pp. 475–494.

Bonegio R, Lieberthal W: Cisplatin-induced nephrotoxicity, in Tarloff JB, Lash LH (eds.): *Toxicology of the Kidney,* 3rd ed. Boca Raton, FL: CRC Press, 2005, pp. 779–815.

Bonventre JV, Zuk A: Ischemic acute renal failure: An inflammatory disease? *Kidney Int* 66:480–485, 2004.

Brady HR, Clarkson W, Lieberthal W: Acute renal failure, in Brenner BM (ed.): *Brenner and Rector's The Kidney,* 7th ed., Philadelphia: WB Saunders, 2004, pp. 1215–1292.

Brenner BM (ed.): *Brenner and Rector's The Kidney,* 7th ed., Philadelphia: WB Saunders, 2004.

Brenner BM, Bohrer MP, Baylis C, Deen WM: Determinants of glomerular permselectivity: Insights derived from observations in vivo. *Kidney Int* 12:229–237, 1977.

Brenner BM, Meyer TH, Hotstetter TH: Dietary protein intake and the progressive nature of kidney disease: The role of hemodynamically mediated glomerular injury in the pathogenesis of glomerular sclerosis in agina, renal ablation and intrinsic renal disease. *N Engl J Med* 307:652–659, 1982.

Brezis M, Epstein FH: Pathophysiology of acute renal failure, in Hook JB, Goldstein RS (eds.): *Toxicology of the Kidney,* 2nd ed. New York: Raven Press, 1993, pp. 129–152.

Brezis M, Rosen S, Silva P: Transport activity modifies thick ascending limb damage in isolated perfused kidney. *Kidney Int* 25:65–72, 1984.

Bruschi SA, West K, Crabb JW, *et al.*: Mitochondrial HSP60 (P1 protein) and a HSP-70 like protein (mortalin) are major targets for modification during S-(1,1,2,2-tetrafluorethyl)-L-cysteine induced nephrotoxicity. *J Biol Chem* 268:23157–23161, 1993.

Bucci TJ, Howard PC, Tolleson WH, *et al.*: Renal effects of fumonisin mycotoxins in animals. *Toxicol Pathol* 26:160–164, 1998.

Burne MJ, Daniels F, El Ghandour A, *et al.*: Identification of the CD4(+) T cell as a major pathogenic factor in ischemic acute renal failure. *J Clin Invest* 108:1065–1073, 2001.

Burne-Taney MJ, Ascon DB, Daniels F, Racusen L, Baldwin W, Rabb H: B cell deficiency confers protection from renal ischemia reperfusion injury. *J Immunol* 171:3210–3215, 2003.

Charney D, Solez K, Racusen LC: Nephrotoxicity of cyclosporine and other immunosuppressive and immunotherapeutic agents, in Tarloff JB, Lash LH (eds.): *Toxicology of the Kidney,* 3rd ed., Boca Raton, FL: CRC Press, 2005, pp. 687–777.

Chen Q, Jones TW, Brown PC, Stevens JL: The mechanism of cysteine conjugate cytotoxicity in renal epithelial cells. *J Biol Chem* 265:21603–21611, 1990.

Chen Q, Yu K, Stevens JL: Regulation of the cellular stress response by reactive electrophiles: The role of covalent binding and cellular thiols in transcriptional activation of the 70-kDa heat shock protein gene by nephrotoxic cysteine conjugates. *J Biol Chem* 267:24322–24327, 1992.

Clifton GG, Pearce C, O'Neill WM Jr, Wallin JD: Early polyuria in the rat following single-dose cis-dichlorodiammineplatinum (II): Effects on plasma vasopressin concentration and posterior pituitatary function. *J Lab Clin Med* 100:659–670, 1982.

Conner EA, Fowler BA: Mechanisms of metal-induced nephrotoxicity, in Hook JB, Goldstein RS (eds.): *Toxicology of the Kidney,* 2nd ed. New York: Raven Press, pp. 437–457, 1993.

Counts RS, Nowak G, Wyatt RD, Schnellmann RG: Nephrotoxicants inhibition of renal proximal tubule cell regeneration. *Am J Physiol* 269:F274–F281, 1995.

Courjault F, Leroy D, Coquery I, Toutain H: Platinum complex-induced dysfunction of cultured renal proximal tubule cells. *Arch Toxicol* 67:338–346, 1993.

Cummings BS, Kinsey GR, Bolchoz LJ, Schnellmann RG: Identification of caspase-independent apoptosis in epithelial and cancer cells. *J Pharmacol Exp Ther* 310:126, 2004a.

Cummings BS, McHowat J, Schnellmann RG: Phospholipase A_2s in cell injury and death. *J Pharmacol Exp Ther* 294(3):793–799, 2000.

Cummings BS, McHowat J, Schnellmann RG: Role of an endoplasmic reticulum Ca^{2+}-independent phospholipase A_2 in oxidant-induced renal cell death. *Am J Physiol* 283:F492, 2002.

Cummings BS, McHowat J, Schnellmann RG: Role of an endoplasmic reticulum Ca^{2+}-independent phospholipase A_2 in cisplatin-induced renal cell apoptosis. *J Pharmacol Exp Ther* 308:921, 2004b.

Cummings BS, Schnellmann RG: Pathophysiology of nephrotoxic cell injury, in Schrier RW (ed.): *Diseases of the Kidney and Urinary Tract,* 8th ed. Philadelphia: Lippincott, 2006, pp. 962–985.

Daemen MARC, van 'tVeer C, Denecker G, *et al.*: Inhibition of apoptosis induced by ischemia-reperfusion prevents inflammation. *J Clin Invest* 104:541–549, 1999.

De Broe ME: Renal injury due to environmental toxins, drugs, and contrast agents, in Berl T, Bonventre JV (eds.): *Atlas of Diseases of the Kidney.* Philadelphia: Current Medicine, 1999, pp. 11.2–11.14.

De Broe ME: Anagesic nephropathy, in Tarloff JB, Lash LH (eds.): *Toxicology of the Kidney,* 3rd ed., CRC Press: Boca Raton, FL, 2005, pp. 619–634.

Dekant W: Chemical-induced nephrotoxicity mediated by glutathione S-conjugate formation, in Tarloff JB, Lash LH (eds.): *Toxicology of the Kidney,* 3rd ed., Boca Raton, FL: CRC Press, 2005, pp. 995–1020.

Dieperink H, Perico N, Nielsen FT, Remuzzi G: Cyclosporine/tacrolimus (FK-506), in DeBroe ME, Porter GA, Bennett AM, Verpooten GA (eds.): *Clinical Nephrotoxicants, Renal Injury from Drugs and Chemicals.* The Netherlands: Kluwer, 1998, pp. 275–300. Schrier RW (ed.): *Diseases of the Kidney and Urinary Tract,* 8th ed., Philadelphia: Lippincott, 2006.

Dong J, Ramachandiran S, Tikoo K, Jia Z, Lauu SS, Monks TJ: EGFR-independent activation of p38 MAPK and EGFR-dependent activation of ERK1/2 are required for ROS-induced renal cell death. *Am J Physiol Renal Physiol* 287:F1049–1058, 2004.

Duffield JS, Park KW, Hsiao LL, *et al.*: Restoration of tubular epithelial cells during repair of the postischemic kidney occurs unependently of bone marrow-derived stem cells. *J Clin Invest* 115:1743–1755, 2005.

Dunn RB, Anderson S, Brenner B: The hemodynamic basis of progressive renal disease. *Semin Nephrol* 6:122–138, 1986.

Edelstein CL, Yaqoob MM, Schrier RW: The role of calcium-dependent enzymes nitric oxide synthase and calpain in hypoxia-induced proximal tubule injury. *Ren Fail*, 501–511, 1996.

Eknoyan G, Bulger RE, Dobyan DC: Mercuric chloride-induced acute renal failure in the rat: I. Correlation of functional and morphologic changes and their modification by clonidine. *Lab Invest* 46:613–620, 1982.

Elfarra AA: Halogenated hydrocarbons, in Sipes IG, McQueen CA, Gandolfi AJ (eds.): *Comprehensive Toxicology,* Vol 7. Oxford, England: Elsevier, 1997, pp. 601–616.

Emeigh Hart SG, Wyand DS, Khairallah EA, Cohen SD: A role for the glutathione conjugate and renal cytochrome P450 in acetaminophen (APAP) induced nephrotoxicity in the CD-1 mouse. *Toxicologist* 11:57, 1990.

Emeigh Hart SGE, Beierschmitt WP, Wyand DS, *et al.*: Acetaminophen nephrotoxicity in CD-1 Mice. I. Evidence of a role for in situ activation in selective covalent binding and toxicity. *Toxicol Appl Pharmacol* 126:267–275, 1994.

Filler G, Bokenkamp A, Hofmann W, Le Bricon T, Martinez-Bru C, Grubb A: Cystatin C as a maker of GFR-history, indications and future research. *Clin Biochem* 38:1–8, 2005.

Ford SM: *In vitro* toxicity systems, in Sipes IG, McQueen CA, Gandolfi AJ (eds.): *Comprehensive Toxicology.* Vol 7. Oxford, England: Elsevier, 1997, pp. 121–142.

Ford SM: In vitro techniques in screening and mechanistic studies: Cell culture, cell-free systems, and molecular and cell biology, in Tarloff JB,Lash LH (eds.): *Toxicology of the Kidney,* 3rd ed., Boca Raton, FL: CRC Press, 2005, pp. 191–213.

Friedewald JJ, Rabb H: Inflammatory cells in ischemic acute renal failure. *Kidney Int* 66:486–491, 2004.

Fukino H, Hirai M, Hsueh YM, Yamane Y: Effect of zinc pretreatment on mercuric chloride–induced lipid peroxidation in the rat kidney. *Toxicol Appl Pharmacol* 73:395–401, 1984.

Gil FZ, Malnic G: Effect of amphotericin B on renal tubular acidification in the rat. *Pflugers Arch* 413:184–286, 1989.

Goering PL, Fisher BR, Chaudhary PP, Dick CA: Relationship between stress protein induction in rat kidney by mercuric chloride and nephrotoxicity. *Toxicol Appl Pharmacol* 113:184–191, 1992.

Goering PL, Fisher BR, Noren BT, et al: Mercury induces regional and cell-specific stress protein expression in rat kidney. *Toxicol Sci* 53:447–457, 2000.

Goldstein RS: Biochemical heterogeneity and site-specific tubular injury, in Hook JB, Goldstein RS (eds.): *Toxicology of the Kidney,* 2nd ed. New York: Raven Press, 1993, pp. 201–248.

Goligorsky MS, Lieberthal W, Racusen L, Simon EE: Integrin receptors in renal tubular epithelium: New insights into pathophysiology of acute renal failure. *Am J Physiol* 264:F1–F8, 1993.

Gopee NV, He Q, Sharma RP: Fumonisin B1-induced apoptosis is associated with delayed inhibition of protein kinase C, nuclear factor-kappaB and tumor necrosis factor alpha in LLC-PK1 cells. *Chem Biol Interact* 146:131–145, 2003.

Groves CE, Hayden PJ, Lock EA, Schnellmann RG: Differential cellular effects in the toxicity of haloalkene and haloalkane cysteine conjugates to rabbit renal proximal tubules. *J Biochem Toxicol* 8:49–56, 1993.

Groves CE, Lock EA, Schnellmann RG: The role of lipid peroxidation in renal proximal tubule cell death induced by haloalkene cysteine conjugates. *J Toxicol Appl Pharmacol* 107:54–62, 1991.

Hammerman MR, Miller SB: Therapeutic use of growth factors in renal failure. *J Am Soc Nephrol* 5:1–11, 1994.

Harriman JF, Liu XL, Aleo MD, Machaca K, Schnellmann RG: Endoplasmic reticulum Ca2+ signaling and calpains mediate renal cell death. *Cell Death Differ* 9:734–741, 2002.

Hart SE, Kinter LB: Assessing renal effects of toxicants in vivo, in Tarloff JB, Lash LH (eds.): *Toxicology of the Kidney,* 3rd ed., Boca Raton, FL: CRC Press, 2005, pp. 81–147.

Hayden PJ, Stevens JL: Cysteine conjugate toxicity, metabolism and binding to macro-molecules in isolated rat kidney mitochondria. *Mol Pharmacol* 37:468–476, 1990.

Hayden PJ, Welsh CJ, Yang Y, *et al.*: Formation of mitochondrial phospholipid adducts by nephrotoxic cysteine conjugate metabolites. *Chem Res Toxicol* 5:231–237, 1992.

Hayden PJ, Yang Y, Ward AJ, *et al.*: Formation of diflourothionoacetyl-protein adducts by S-(1,1,2,2-tetrafluoroethyl)-L-cysteine metabolites: Nucleophilic catalysis of stable lysyl adduct formation by histidine and tyrosine. *Biochemistry* 30:5935–5943, 1991.

Holmes E, Cloarec O, Nicholson JK: Probing latent biomarker signatures and in vivo pathway activity in experimental disease states via statistical total correlation spectroscopy (STOCSY) of biofluids: Application to HgCl2 toxicity. *J Proteome Res* 5:1313–1320, 2006.

Ikeda M, Prachasilchai W, Burner-Taney MJ, Rabb H, Yokota-Ikeda N: Ischemic acute tubular necrosis models and drug discovery: A focus on cellular inflammation. *Drug Discov Today* 11:364–370, 2006.

Jarnberg P: Renal toxicity of anesthetic agents, in DeBroe ME, Porter GA, Bennett AM, Verpooten GA (eds.): *Clinical Nephrotoxicants, Renal Injury from Drugs and Chemicals.* The Netherlands: Kluwer, 1998, pp. 413–418.

Kanwar YS, Liu ZZ, Kashihara N, Wallner EI: Current status of the structural and functional basis of glomerular filtration and proteinuria. *Semin Nephrol* 11:390–413, 1991.

Kaperonis N, Krause M, Bakris GL: The pathogenesis and prevention of radiocontrast medium induced renal dysfunction, in Tarloff JB, Lash LH (eds.): *Toxicology of the Kidney*, 3rd ed. Boca Raton, FL: CRC Press, 2005, pp. 817–860.

Kaushal GP, Singh AB, Shah SV: Identification of gene family cf caspases in rat kidney and altered expression in ischemia-reperfusion injury. *Am J Physiol* 274:F587–F595, 1998.

Kelly KJ: Heat shock (stress response) proteins and renal ischemia/reperfusion injury. *Contrib Nephrol* 148:86–106, 2005.

Kelly KJ, Williams WW, Colvin RB, Bonventre JV: Antibody to intercellular adhesion molecule 1 protects the kidney against ischemic injury. *Proc Natl Acad Sci U S A* 91:812–816, 1994.

Kido T, Nordberg G: Cadmium-induced renal effects in the general environment, in DeBroe ME, Porter GA, Bennett AM, Verpooten GA (eds.): *Clinical Nephrotoxicants, Renal Injury from Drugs and Chemicals.* The Netherlands: Kluwer, 1998, pp. 345–362.

Kidwell DT, KcKeown JW, Grider JS, *et al.*: Acute effects of gentamicin on thick ascending limb function in the rat. *Eur J Pharmaco Environ Toxicol Pharmacol Section* 270:97–103, 1994.

Kinsey GR, McHowat J, Beckett C, Schnellmann RG: Identification of calcium-independent phospholipase A2γ in mitochondria and its role in mitochondrial oxidative stress. *Am J Physiol* 292:F853–F860, 2007.

Kirkpatrick DS, Gandolfi AJ: In vitro techniques in screening and mechanistic studies: Organ perfusion, slices, and nephron components, in Tarloff JB, Lash LH (eds.): *Toxicology of the Kidney*, 3rd ed., Boca Raton, FL: CRC Press, 2005, pp. 149–189.

Klaassen CD, Liu J, Choudhuri S: Metallothionein: An intracellular protein to protect cadmium toxicity. *Ann Rev Pharmacol Toxicol* 39:267–294, 1999.

Komatsuda A, Wakui H, Satoh K, *et al.*: Altered localization of 73-kilodalton heat shock protein in rat kidneys with gentamicin–induced acute tubular injury. *Lab Invest* 68:687–695, 1993.

Lanese DM, Conger JD: Effects of endothelin receptor antagonist on cyclosporine-induced vasoconstriction in isolated rat renal arterioles. *J Clin Invest* 91:2144–2149, 1993.

Lauwerys RR, Bernard AM, Roels HA, Buchet JP: Cadmium: Exposure markers as predictors of nephrotoxic effects. *Clin Chem* 40:1391–1394, 1994.

Lehman-McKeeman LD: α_{2u}-globulin nephropathy, in Sipes IG, McQueen CA, Gandolfi AJ (eds.): *Comprehensive Toxicology,* Vol 7. Oxford, England: Elsevier, 1997, pp. 677–692.

Leiberthal W, Triaca V, Levine J: Mechanisms of death induced by cisplatin in proximal tubular epithelial cells: Apoptosis vs. necrosis. *Am J Physiol* 270:F700–F708, 1996.

Lemasters JJ, Qian T, Bradham CA, *et al.*: Mitochondrial dysfunction in the pathogenesis of necrotic and apoptotic cell death. *J Bioenerg Biomembr* 31:305–319, 1999.

Leonard I, Zanen J, Nonclercq D, *et al.*: Modification of immunoreactive EGF and EGF receptor after acute tubular necrosis induced by tobramycin or cisplatin. *Ren Fail* 16(5):583–608, 1994.

Levin S, Bucci TJ, Cohen SM, *et al.*: The nomenclature of cell death: Recommendations of an *ad hoc* committee of the society of toxicologic pathologists. *Tox Pathol* 27:484–490, 1999.

Lin F, Moran A, Igarashi P: Intrarenal cells, not bone marrow-derived cells, are the major source for regeneration in postischemic kidney. *J Clin Invest* 115:1756–1764, 2005.

Lindon JC, Holmes E, Nicholson JK: Metabonomics techniques and applications to pharmaceutical research and development. *Pharm Res* 23:1075–1088, 2006.

Liu X, Van Vleet T, Schnellmann RG: The role of calpain in oncotic cell death. *Ann Rev Pharmacol Toxicol* 44:349–370, 2004.

Liu X, Schnellmann RG: Calpain mediates progressive plasma membrane permeability and proteolysis of cytoskeleton-associated paxillin, talin, and vinculin during renal cell death. *J Pharmacol Exp Ther* 304:63–70, 2003.

Lock EA, Reed CJ: Renal xenobiotic metabolism, in Sipes IG, McQueen CA, Gandolfi AJ (eds.): *Comprehensive Toxicology,* Vol 7. Oxford, England: Elsevier, 1997, pp. 77–98.

Lund BO, Miller DM, Woods JS: Studies in Hg(II)-induced H_2O_2 formation and oxidative stress in vivo and in vitro in rat kidney mitochondria. *Biochem Pharmacol* 45:2017–2024, 1993.

Maddox DA, Brenner BM: Glomerular ultrafiltration, in Brenner BM, Rector FC (eds.): *The Kidney,* 4th ed. Philadelphia: WB Saunders, 1991, pp. 205–244.

Mason J, Moore LC: Cyclosporine, in Sipes IG, McQueen CA, Gandolfi AJ (eds.): *Comprehensive Toxicology.* Vol 7 Oxford, England: Elsevier, 1997, pp. 567–582.

Melnick R: An alternative hypothesis on the role of chemically induced protein droplet (α_{2u}-globulin) nephropathy in renal carcinogenesis. *Reg Toxicol Pharmacol* 16:111–125, 1992.

Meng X, Reeves WB: Effects of chloride channel inhibitors on H_2O_2-induced renal epithelial cell injury. *Am J Physiol Renal Physiol* 278:F83–F90, 2000.

Miller GW, Schnellmann RG: Cytoprotection by inhibition of chloride channels: The mechanism of action of glycine and strychnine. *Life Sci* 53:1211–1215, 1993.

Miller GW, Schnellmann RG: Inhibitors of renal chloride transport do not block toxicant-induced chloride influx in the proximal tubule. *Toxicol Lett* 76:179–184, 1995.

Molitoris BA: Alterations in surface membrane composition and fluidity: Role in cell injury, in Sipes IG, McQueen CA, Gandolfi AJ (eds.): *Comprehensive Toxicology.* Vol 7. Oxford, England: Elsevier, 1997, pp. 317–328.

Nowak G: Protein kinase C-alpha and ERK1/2 mediate mitochondrial dysfunction, decreases in active Na+ transport, and cisplatin-induced apoptosis in renal cells. *J Biol Chem* 277:43377–43388, 2002.

Nowak G: Protein kinase C mediates repair of mitochondrial and transport functions after toxicant-induced injury in renal cells. *J Pharmacol Exp Ther* 306:157–165, 2003.

Nowak G, Bakajsova D, Clifton GL: Protein kinase C-{epsilon} modulates mitochondrial function and active Na+ transport after oxidant injury in renal cells. *Am J Physiol Renal Physiol* 286:F307, 2004.

O'Brien E, Dietrich DR: Mycotoxins affecting the kidney, in Tarloff JB, Lash LH (eds.): *Toxicology of the Kidney*, 3rd ed., Boca Raton, FL: CRC Press, 2005, pp. 895–936.

Okada Y, Maeno E, Shimizu T, Manabe K, Mori S, Nabekura T: Dual roles of plasmalemmal chloride channels in induction of cell death. *Pflugers Arch* 448:287–295, 2004.

Palmer BF, Heinrich WL: Toxic nephropathy, in Brenner BM (ed.): *Brenner and Rector's The Kidney*, 7th ed., Philadelphia: WB Saunders, 2004, pp. 1625–1658.

Pryor WA, Squadrito GL: The chemistry of peroxynitrite: A product from the reaction of nitric oxide with superoxide *Am J Physiol* 268:L699–L722, 1995.

Rabb H, Daniels F, O'Donnell M, *et al.*: Pathophysiological role of T lymphocytes in renal ischemia-reperfusion injury in mice. *Am J Physiol* 279:F525–F531, 2000.

Rabb H, Mendiola CC, Dietz J, *et al.*: Role of CD11a and CD11b in ischemic acute renal failure in rats. *Am J Physiol* 267:F1052–F1058, 1994.

Racusen LC, Solez K: Nephrotoxicity of cyclosporine and other immunotherapeutic agents, in Hook JB, Goldstein RS (eds.): *Toxicology of the Kidney,* 2nd ed. New York: Raven Press, 1993, pp. 319–360.

Ramachandiran S, *et al.*: Mitogen-activated protein kinases contribute to reactive oxygen species-induced cell death in renal proximal tubule epithelial cells. *Chem Res Toxicol* 15:1635, 2002.

Rankin GO, Valentovic MA: Role of xenobiotic metabolism, in Tarloff JB, Lash LH (eds.): *Toxicology of the Kidney,* 3rd ed. Boca Raton, FL: CRC Press, 2005, pp. 217–243.

Safirstein R, Deray G: Anticancer, cisplatin/carboplatin, in DeBroe ME, Porter GA, Bennett AM, Verpooten GA (eds.): *Clinical Nephrotoxicants, Renal Injury from Drugs and Chemicals.* The Netherlands: Kluwer, 1998, pp. 261–272.

Sapirstein A, Spech RA, Witzgall R, *et al.*: Cytosolic phospholipase A_2 (PLA_2) but not secretory PLA_2, potentiates hydrogen peroxide cytotoxicity in kidney epithelial cells. *J Biol Chem* 271(35):21505–21513, 1996.

Servais H, Mingeot-Leclercq M-P, Tulkens PM: Antibiotic-induced nephrotoxicity, in Tarloff JB, Lash LH (eds.): *Toxicology of the Kidney,* 3rd ed. Boca Raton, FL: CRC Press: 2005 pp. 635–685.

Schnellmann RG: Analgesic nephropathy in rodents. *J Toxicol Environ Health, Part B* 1:81–90, 1998.

Schnellmann RG, Cross TJ, Lock EA: Pentachlorabutadienyl-L-cysteine uncouples oxidative phosphorylation by dissipating the proton gradient. *Toxicol Appl Pharmacol* 100:498–505, 1989.

Schnellmann RG, Cummings BS: Pathophysiology of nephrotoxic cell injury, in Schrier RW (ed.): *Diseases of the Kidney and Urinary Tract,* 8th ed. Philadelphia: Lippincott, 2006, pp. XXX-YYY.

Schnellmann RG, Griner RD: Mitochondrial mechanisms of tubular injury, in Goldstein RS (ed.): *Mechanisms of Injury in Renal Disease and Toxicity.* Boca Raton, FL: CRC, 1994, pp. 247–265.

Schnellmann RG, Lock EA, Mandel LJ: A mechanism of *S*-(1,2,3,4,4-pentachloro-1,3-butadienyl)-L-cysteine toxicity to rabbit renal proximal tubules. *Toxicol Appl Pharmacol* 90:513–521, 1987.

Schnellmann RG, Williams SW: Proteases in renal cell death: Calpains mediate cell death produced by diverse toxicants. *Ren Fail* 20(5):679–686, 1998.

Sheikh-Hamad D, Cacini W, Buckley AR, *et al.*: Cellular and molecular studies on cisplatin-induced apoptotic cell death in rat kidney. *Arch Toxicol* 78:147–155, 2004.

Smith JH, Maita K, Sleight SD, Hook JB: Effect of sex hormone status on chloroform nephrotoxicity and renal mixed function oxidases in mice. *Toxicology* 30:305–316, 1984.

Smith MW, Ambudkar IS, Phelps PC, *et al.*: $HgCl_2$-induced changes in cytosolic Ca^{2+} of cultured rabbit renal tubular cells. *Biochem Biophys Acta* 931:130–142, 1987.

Steinmetz PR, Husted RF: Amphotericin B toxicity for epithelial cells, in Porter GA (ed.): *Nephrotoxic Mechanisms of Drugs and Environmental Toxins.* New York, London: Plenum, 1982, pp. 95–98.

Stevens LA, Levey AS: Measurement of Kidney Function. *Med Clinics of North America* 89:457–473, 2005.

Takaoka M, Itoh M, Hayashi S, Kuro T, Matsumura Y: Proteasome participates in the pathogenesis of ischemic acute renal failure in rats. *Eur J Pharmacol* 384:43–46, 1999.

Tarloff JB: Analgesics and nonsteroidal anti-inflammatory drugs, in Sipes IG, McQueen CA, Gandolfi AJ (eds.): *Comprehensive Toxicology.* Vol 7. Oxford, England: Elsevier, 1997, pp. 583–600.

Tarloff JB: Analgesics and nonsteroidal anti-inflammatory drugs, in Tarloff JB, Lash LH (eds.): *Toxicology of the Kidney,* 3rd ed., Boca Raton, FL: CRC Press, 2005, pp. 861–894.

Tarloff JB, Kinter LB: *In vivo* methodologies used to assess renal function, in Sipes IG, McQueen CA, Gandolfi AJ (eds.): *Comprehensive Toxicology.* Vol 7. Oxford, England: Elsevier, 1997, pp. 99–120.

Townsend DM, Hanigan MH: Inhibition of γtglutamyl transpeptidase or cysteine S-conjugate β-lyase activity blocks the nephrotoxicity of cisplain in mice. *J Pharmacol Exptl Ther* 300:142–148, 2002.

Ueda N, Mayeux PR, Baglia R, Shah SV: Oxidant mechanisms in acute renal failure, in Molitoris BA, Finn W (eds.): *Acute Renal Failure: A Companion to Brenner's and Rector's The Kidney.* St. Louis: WB Saunders, 2001, pp. F853–F860.

Ueda N, Walker PD, Hsu SM, Shah SV: Activation of a 15-kDa endonuclease in hypoxia/reoxygenation injury without morphologic features of apoptosis. *Proc Natl Acad Sci USA* 92:7202–7206, 1995.

van de Water B, de Graauw M, Le Devedec S, Alderliesten M: Cellular stress responses and molecular mechanisms of nephrotoxicity. *Toxicol Lett* 162:83–93, 2006.

van de Water B, Tijdens IB, Verbrugge A, *et al.*: Cleavage of the actin-capping protein alpha -adducin at Asp-Asp-Ser-Asp633-Ala by caspase-3 is preceded by its phosphorylation on serine 726 in cisplatin-induced apoptosis of renal epithelial cells. *J Biol Chem* 275:25805–25813, 2005.

Wallin A, Jones TW, Vercesi AE, *et al.*: Toxicity of *S*-pentacorobutadienyl-L-cysteine studied with isolated rat renal cortical mitochondria. *Arch Biochem Biophys* 258:365–372, 1987.

Wang C, Salahudeen AK: Cyclosporine nephrotoxicity: Attenuation by an antioxidant-inhibitor of lipid peroxidation in vitro and in vivo. *Transplantation* 58:940–946, 1994.

Wang C, Salahudeen AK: Lipid peroxidation accompanies cyclosporine nephrotoxicity: Effects of vitamin E. *Kidney Int* 47:927–934, 1995.

Wang Y, Bollard ME, Nicholson JK, Holmes E: Exploration of the direct metabolic effects of mercury II chloride on the kidney on Sprague-Dawley rats using high-resolution magic angle spinning 1H NMR spectroscopy of intact tissue and patter recognition. *J Pharm Biomed Anal* 40:375–381, 2006.

Waters SL, Sarang SS, Wang KKW, Schnellmann RG: Calpains mediate calcium and chloride influx during the late phase of cell injury. *J Pharmacol Exp Ther* 283:1177–1184, 1997a.

Waters SL, Wong JK, Schnellmann RG: Depletion of endoplasmic reticulum calcium stores protects against hypoxia- and mitochondrial inhibitor–induced cellular injury and death. *Biochem Biophys Res Commun* 240:57–60, 1997b.

Weinberg JM, Harding PG, Humes HD: Mitochondrial bioenergetics during the initiation of mercuric chloride-induced renal injury: I. Direct effects of in vitro mercuric chloride on renal cortical mitochondrial function. *J Biol Chem* 257:60–67, 1982b.

Weinberg JM, Harding PG, Humes HD: Mitochondrial bioenergetics during the initiation of mercuric chloride-induced renal injury: II. Functional alterations of renal cortical mitochondria isolated after mercuric chloride treatment. *J Biol Chem* 257:68–74, 1982a.

Woo KR, Shu WP, Kong L, Liu BC: Tumor necrosis factor mediates apoptosis via Ca++/Mg++ dependent endonuclease with protein kinase C as a possible mechanism for cytokine resistance in human renal carcinoma cells. *J Urol* 155:1779–1783, 1996.

Zalups RK: Renal toxicity of mercury, in Sipes IG, McQueen CA, Gandolfi AJ (eds.): *Comprehensive Toxicology.* Vol 7. Oxford, England: Elsevier, 1997, pp. 633–652.

Zalups RK, Diamond GL: Nephrotoxicology of metal, in Tarloff JB, Lash LH (eds.): *Toxicology of the Kidney,* 3rd ed. Boca Raton, FL: CRC Press, 2005, pp. 937–994.

Zalups RK, Lash LH: Advances in understanding the renal transport and toxicity of mercury. *J Toxicol Environ Health* 42:1–44, 1994.

CHAPTER 15

TOXIC RESPONSES OF THE RESPIRATORY SYSTEM

Hanspeter R. Witschi, Kent E. Pinkerton, Laura S. Van Winkle, and Jerold A. Last

Lung injury caused by chemicals was first recognized as an occupational disease. In 1713, the Italian physician Bernardino Ramazzini provided detailed and harrowing accounts of the sufferings of miners. Two of his quotations remain noteworthy. With regard to miners of metals, he stated, "the lungs and brains of that class of workers are badly affected, the lungs especially, since they take in with the air mineral spirits and are the first to be keenly aware of injury." Ramazzini was also aware of the important concept of exposure: "They (workers who shovel, melt, cast and refine mined material) are liable of the same diseases, though in less acute form, because they perform their tasks in open air (Ramazzini, 1964)." Thus, exposure to chemicals by inhalation can have two effects: on the lung tissues and on distant organs that are reached after chemicals enter the body by means of inhalation. Indeed, "inhalation toxicology" refers to the route of exposure, whereas "respiratory tract toxicology" refers to target organ toxicity, in this case abnormal changes in the respiratory tract produced by airborne (and occasionally blood-borne) agents.

We now know of numerous lung diseases prompted by occupational exposures, many crippling and some fatal. Examples include black lung in coal miners, silicosis and silicotuberculosis in sandblasters and tunnel miners, and asbestosis in shipyard workers and asbestos miners. Occupational exposures to asbestos or metals such as nickel, beryllium, and cadmium can also cause lung cancer. In the twentieth century, it has become obvious that disease caused by airborne agents may not be limited to certain trades. The ubiquitous presence of airborne chemicals is a matter of concern, since "air pollution" adversely affects human health and may be an important contributor to morbidity and mortality.

To better understand environmental lung disease, we need more precise knowledge about the doses of toxic inhalants delivered to specific sites in the respiratory tract and an understanding of the extent to which repeated and often intermittent low-level exposures eventually may initiate and propagate chronic lung disease. Inhalation and respiratory tract toxicology cover a field in which

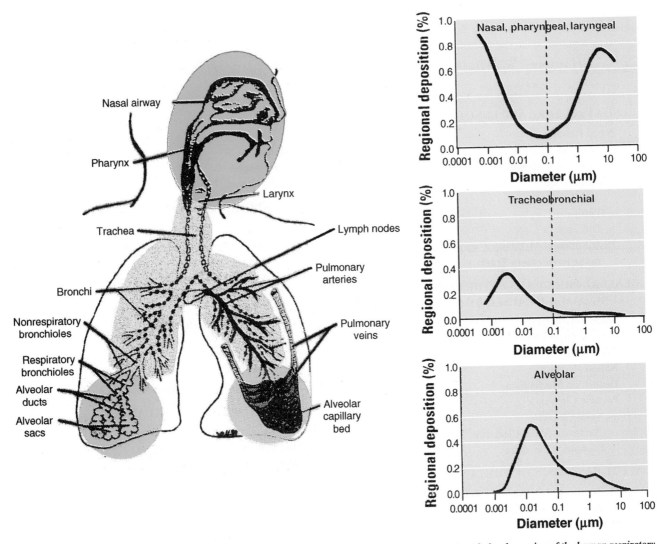

Figure 15-1. *Predicted fractional deposition of inhaled particles in the nasopharyngeal, tracheobronchial, and alveolar region of the human respiratory tract during nose breathing. Based on data from the International Commission on Radiological Protection (1994). (Drawing courtesy of J. Harkema.) [From Fig. 8 in Oberdorster et al., 2005a. Nanotoxicology: An emerging discipline evolving from studies of ultrafine particles. Environ Health Perspect Vol. 113, No 7. 823–839, 2005.]*

epidemiologists, physiologists, toxicologists, and cell and molecular biologists must closely work together. Epidemiologists now use a variety of pulmonary function tests to assess decrements in lung function in people. Many of these tests have been adapted for animal studies. Bronchoalveolar lavage is widely utilized in experimental animals and human subjects to examine airways contents after exposure. When similar data can be obtained in both experimental animals and humans, these direct comparisons assist in extrapolation and modeling. Progress has been made in understanding some mechanisms that underlie the response of the lung to toxic agents. In response to toxic insult, pulmonary cells are known to release a variety of potent chemical mediators that may critically affect lung function. Biochemical data from the study of cells taken from exposed animals and in vitro exposure of cells are also useful in assessing the toxic potential of many agents. This chapter will discuss how pulmonary toxicologists profit from these methods to study the biochemical, structural, and functional changes produced by the inhalation of gases and particles in both humans and experimental animals.

LUNG STRUCTURE AND FUNCTION

Nasal Passages

Figure 15-1 shows a schematic overview of the different regions of the respiratory tract. Air enters the respiratory tract through the nasal and oral regions. Many species, particularly small laboratory rodents, are obligate nose breathers in which air passes almost exclusively through the nasal passages. Other species, including humans, monkeys, and dogs can inhale air through both the nose and the mouth (oronasal breathers). Air is warmed and humidified while passing through the nose. The nasal passages function as a filter for particles, which may be collected by diffusion or impaction on the nasal mucosa. Highly water soluble gases are absorbed efficiently in the nasal passages, which reach from the nostril to the pharynx. The nasal turbinates thus form a first defensive barrier against many toxic inhalants.

The nasal passages are lined by distinctive epithelia: stratified-squamous epithelium in the vestibule, nonciliated cuboidal/

columnar epithelium in the anterior chamber, and ciliated pseudos-stratified respiratory epithelium. Located in the superior part is the olfactory epithelium, which contains sensory cells. Nerve endings in the nasal passages are associated mostly with the fifth cranial (trigeminal) nerve. Nasal epithelia are competent to metabolize foreign compounds and P-450 isozymes have been localized in the nose of several species by immunohistochemical procedures. The nasal cavity is thus a ready target site for metabolite-induced lesions.

Conducting Airways

The proximal airways (trachea and bronchi) of humans have a pseudostratified epithelium containing ciliated cells and two types of nonciliated cells: mucous and serous cells. Mucous cells (and glandular structures) produce respiratory tract mucus, a family of high-molecular-weight glycoproteins with a sugar content of 80% or more. They coat the epithelium with a viscoelastic sticky protective layer that traps pollutants and cell debris. Serous cells produce a fluid in which mucus may be dissolved, or upon which a mucus layer may be floated. The action of the respiratory tract cilia continuously drives the mucus layer toward the pharynx, where it is removed from the respiratory system by swallowing or expectoration. The mucus layer is also thought to have antioxidant, acid-neutralizing, and free radical scavenging functions that protect the epithelial cells (Cross *et al.*, 1998).

Conducting airways have a characteristic branched bifurcating structure, with successive airway generations containing approximately twice the number of bronchi progressively decreasing in internal diameter. Thus, the conducting airways contain a continuously increasing total surface area from the trachea to the distal airways. Bifurcations are flow dividers and airway branch points serve as sites of impaction for particles. Successively narrower diameters also favor the collection of gases and particles on airway walls. Eventually a transition zone is reached where cartilaginous airways (bronchi) give way to noncartilaginous airways (bronchioles), which in turn give way to gas exchange regions, respiratory bronchioles, and alveoli. In the bronchiolar epithelium, mucus-producing cells and glands give way to Clara cells.

Gas Exchange Region

Human lungs are divided into five lobes: the superior and inferior left lobes and the superior, middle, and inferior right lobes. In small laboratory animals such as rats, mice, and hamsters, the left lung consists of a single lobe, whereas the right lung is divided into four lobes: cranial, middle, caudal, and ancillary. In the guinea pig and rabbit, the left lung is divided into two lobes. Dogs have two left and four right lobes. The lung can be further subdivided at the periphery of the bronchial tree into distinct anatomic bronchopulmonary segments, then into lobules, and finally into acini. An acinus includes a terminal bronchiole and all its respiratory bronchioles, alveolar ducts, and alveolar sacs. An acinus may be made up of 2–8 ventilatory units. A ventilatory unit is defined as an anatomical region that includes all alveolar ducts and alveoli distal to each bronchiolar-alveolar duct junction (Mercer and Crapo, 1991). The ventilatory unit is important because it represents the smallest common denominator when the distribution of inhaled gases to the gas-exchanging surface of the lung is modeled (Fig. 15-2).

Gas exchange occurs in the alveoli, which comprise approximately 80–90% of the total parenchymal lung volume; adult human lungs contain an estimated 300 million alveoli. The ratio of total

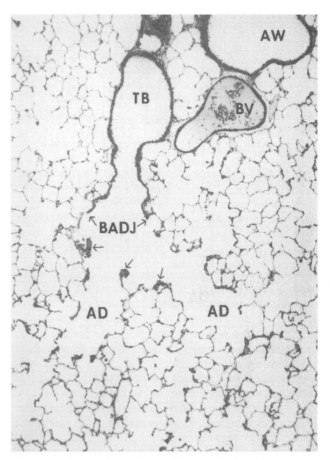

Figure 15-2. Centriacinar region (ventilatory unit) of the lung.

An airway (AW) and an arteriole [blood vessel (BV)] are in close proximity to the terminal bronchiole (TB) opening into alveolar ducts (AD) at the bronchiole–alveolar duct junction (BADJ). A number of the alveolar septal tips (*arrows*) close to the BADJ are thickened after a brief (4 hour) exposure to asbestos fibers, indicating localization of fiber deposition. Other inhalants, such as ozone, produce lesions in the same locations. (Photograph courtesy of Dr. Kent E. Pinkerton, University of California, Davis.)

capillary surface to total alveolar surface is slightly less than 1. Capillaries, blood plasma, and formed blood elements are separated from the air space by a thin layer of tissue formed by epithelial, interstitial, and endothelial components (Fig. 15-3).

Type I and type II alveolar cells represent approximately 25% of all the cells in the alveolar septum (Fig. 15-3). Type I cells cover a large surface area (approximately 90% of the alveolar surface). They have an attenuated cytoplasm and appear to be poor in organelles but probably are as metabolically competent as are the more compact type II cells. Preferential damage to type I cells by various agents may be explained by the fact that they constitute a large percentage of the total target (surface of the epithelium). Type II cells are cuboidal and show abundant perinuclear cytoplasm. They produce surfactant and, in the case of damage to the type I epithelium, may undergo mitotic division and replace damaged cells (Witschi, 1997). The shape of type I and type II cells is independent of alveolar size and is remarkably similar in different species. A typical rat alveolus (14,000 μm^2 surface area) contains an average of two type I cells and three type II cells, whereas a human alveolus with a surface area of 200,000–300,000 μm^2 contains an average of 32 type I cells and 51 type II cells (Pinkerton *et al.*, 1991).The mesenchymal

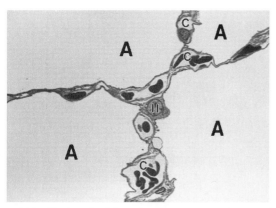

Figure 15-3. Micrograph of four alveoli (A) separated by the alveolar septum.

The thin air-to-blood tissue barrier of the alveolar septal wall is composed of squamous alveolar type I cells and occasional alveolar type II cells (II), a small interstitial space, and the attenuated cytoplasm of the endothelial cells that form the wall of the capillaries (C). (Photograph courtesy of Dr. Kent E. Pinkerton, University of California, Davis.)

interstitial cell population consists of fibroblasts and myofibroblasts that produce collagen and elastin as well as other cell matrix components and various effector molecules. Pericytes, monocytes, and lymphocytes also reside in the interstitium and so do macrophages before they enter the alveoli. Endothelial cells have a thin cytoplasm and cover about one-fourth of the area covered by type I cells.

Gas Exchange

The principal function of the lung is gas exchange, which consists of ventilation, perfusion, and diffusion. The lung is superbly equipped to handle its main task: bringing essential oxygen to the organs and tissues of the body and eliminating its most abundant waste product, CO_2 (Weibel, 1983).

Ventilation   During inhalation, fresh air is moved into the lung through the upper respiratory tract and conducting airways and into the terminal respiratory units when the thoracic cage enlarges and the diaphragm moves downward; the lung passively follows this expansion. After diffusion of oxygen into the blood and that of CO_2 from the blood into the alveolar spaces, the air (now enriched in CO_2) is expelled by exhalation. Relaxation of the chest wall and diaphragm diminishes the internal volume of the thoracic cage, the elastic fibers of the lung parenchyma contract, and air is expelled from the alveolar zone through the airways. Any interference with the elastic properties of the lung, for example, the decrease in elastic fibers that occurs in emphysema, adversely affects ventilation, as do the decrease in the diameters of, or blockage of, the conducting airways, as in asthma.

The total volume of air in an inflated human lung, approximately 5700 cm^3, represents the total lung capacity (TLC). After a maximum expiration, the lung retains approximately 1200 cm^3 of air, the residual volume (RV). The air volume moved into and out of the lung with a maximum inspiratory and expiratory movement, which is called the vital capacity (VC), is thus approximately 4500 cm^3. Under resting conditions, only a fraction of the VC, the tidal volume (TV), is moved into and out of the lung. In resting humans, the TV measures approximately 500 cm^3 with each breath (Fig. 15-4). The respiratory frequency, or the number of breaths per minute, is approximately 12–20. If an augmented metabolic demand of the body requires the delivery of increased amounts of oxygen, for example, during heavy and prolonged exercise, both the TV and the respiratory rate can be greatly increased. The amount of air moved into and out of the human lung may increase to up to 60 L/min. Increased ventilation in a polluted atmosphere increases the deposition of inhaled toxic material. For this reason, it is often stated that people, particularly children, should not exercise during episodes of heavy air pollution.

The TLC, as well as the ratio of RV to VC, changes when the lung is diseased. In emphysema, the alveoli overextend and more air is trapped. While the TLC may stay the same or even increase, the volume of air that is actually moved during breathing is diminished.

RESPONSES OF THE RESPIRATORY SYSTEM TO TOXIC AGENTS

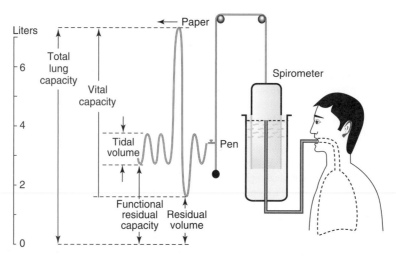

Figure 15-4. Lung volumes.

Note that the functional residual capacity and RV cannot be measured with spirometer but require special procedures (e.g., nitrogen or helium outwash).

This results in decreased VC with a concomitant increase in RV. If part of the lung collapses or becomes filled with edema fluid, TLC and VC are reduced. Pulmonary function tests give quantitative information on such changes.

Perfusion The lung receives the entire output from the right ventricle, approximately 70–80 cm^3 of blood per heartbeat, and thus may be exposed to substantial amounts of toxic agents carried in the blood. A chemical placed onto or deposited under the skin (subcutaneous injection) or introduced directly into a peripheral vein (intravenous injection) travels through the venous system to the right ventricle and then comes into contact with the pulmonary capillary bed before distribution to other organs or tissues in the body.

Diffusion Gas exchange takes place across the entire alveolar surface. Contact to an airborne toxic chemical thus occurs over a surface of approximately 140 m^2. This surface area is second only to the small intestine (approximately 250 m^2) and considerably larger than the skin (approximately 1.75 m^2), two other organs that are in direct contact with the outside world. A variety of abnormal processes may severely compromise the unhindered diffusion of oxygen to the erythrocytes. Acute events may include collection of liquid or of inflammatory cells in the alveolar space. Chronic toxicity can impair diffusion due to abnormal increase in formation and deposition of extracellular substances such as collagen in the interstitium or through interstitial accumulation of edema fluid.

Distribution of Metabolic Competence in the Respiratory Tract

Often overlooked as an organ involved in metabolism of chemicals, in favor of the liver, the lung has substantial capabilities for both metabolic activation as well as detoxification. Total lung P-450 activity is roughly one-tenth to one-third of that in the liver. However, when specific activity in a few cell types is considered, the difference is only twofold for many enzymes and in the case of nasal mucosa higher enzyme activity is reported per cell. Metabolic competence in the lung and nasal tissues is concentrated in a few cell types and these have a defined, and sometimes limited, distribution in the respiratory tract that can vary substantially by species (Table 15-1). The balance of activation and detoxification is a critically important determinant of lung protection as well as of lung injury (Buckpitt and Cruikshank, 1997). Protection from oxidation is another important ongoing function of detoxifying enzymes in light of the high tissue oxygen concentration that occurs in the respiratory tract. Other factors that can influence the role of Phase-I and Phase-II systems in lung toxicity include: age, sex, diet, local inflammation, and the history of prior exposure (Plopper et al., 2001a). Interestingly, many xenobiotic metabolizing enzymes have different patterns of induction (less) in the respiratory tract than in the liver, leading to the concept that regulation of these systems may be different depending on where they are located (Buckpitt and Cruikshank, 1997).

The major Phase-I enzyme system, the cytochrome P-450 monooxygenases, are concentrated into a few lung cells: nonciliated bronchiolar (Clara) cells, Type 2 cells, macrophages and endothelial cells, predominantly. Of these cell types, the Clara cell has the most P-450 followed by the Type 2 cell. The amount of total lung P-450 contributed by Clara cells is species dependent, with humans having less P-450 in their lungs from Clara cells than rats or mice. Further, the isoforms of P-450 present and their loca-

tion also vary by species. Nasal epithelia also metabolize foreign compounds via the cytochrome P-450 monooxygenase system. Cytochrome P-450s are expressed at some of the highest levels for an extrahepatic tissue in the nasal mucosa and this pattern of expression varies by nasal region and cell type (Ding and Kaminsky, 2003). The olfactory mucosa is considered to be a "metabolic hot spot." Most species have P-450 in nasal tissue and some of these P-450s are predominantly, possibly even solely, expressed in the olfactory mucosa (e.g., CYP2G1, CYP2A3, and CYP2A13) (Ling et al., 2004). Metabolism by the olfactory epithelium may play a role in providing, or preventing, access of inhalants directly to the brain; for example, inhaled xylene may be converted to metabolites that move to the brain by axonal transport. The presence of the following cytochrome P-450 isozymes in the respiratory tract of at least one species has been reported: CYP1A1, CYP1B1, CYP2A3, CYP2A10/2A11, CYP2B1/4, CYP2B6, CYP2B7, CYP2E1, CYP2F1/2/4, CYP2S1, CYP2J2, CYP2G1, CYP3A, and CYP4B1 (for a review of CYP expression in human lung see Hukkanen et al., 2002).

Other enzymes found in lung tissue include epoxide hydrolases, flavin monooxygenases, prostaglandin synthases, glucuronsyl transferases, sulfotransferases, and glutathione S-transferases (alpha, mu, and pi). The only constant feature of the expression of these enzymes is lack of uniformity in their expression by cell type and airway level throughout the lung and their tendency to concentrate in epithelia. Both microsomal and cytosolic epoxide hydrolases are found in the lung and nasal tissues and the activity of microsomal epoxide hydrolase can be greater in the distal airways of the lung than even in the liver (Bond et al., 1988). Flavin monooxygenase activity (FMO1 and FMO2) is found in rodent and human lung and nasal tissue. The isoforms present in the lung (FMO2) are different from that found in the liver (FMO1). FM01 is the predominant isoform in the nasal mucosa (Shehin-Johnson et al., 1995). There are polymorphisms in the expression of FMO2 in humans. The gene for FMO2 in human lung contains a premature stop codon encoding production of an inactive protein, but some ethnic groups have at least one copy of an allele that expresses the full length protein (Whetstine et al., 2000). Prostaglandin synthases (aka cyclooxygenases) oxidize substrates at a much lower rate than the cytochrome P-450 monooxygenases but may have a role in human pulmonary metabolism due to the relatively lower P-450 activity in human lung tissue compared to rodents (Smith et al., 1991). Despite the fact that activity of glucuronosyl transferase has been reported in both rodent and human pulmonary tissues, these proteins have received little attention. An olfactory-specific glucoronosyl transferase has been reported and is suggested to have a role in termination of odorant signals (Lazard et al., 1991). There is little information on sulfotransferases in respiratory tract tissues although some studies have demonstrated immunochemical localization of these enzymes to the conducting airway epithelium (He et al., 2005) and activity has been demonstrated in human bronchoscopy samples (Gibby and Cohen, 1984). Sulphotransferases have been localized to the sustentacular cells of the olfactory epithelium and some isoforms may be specific to the olfactory epithelium (Miyawaki et al., 1996; Tamura et al., 1998). Glutathione S-transferases (and glutathione) play a major role in the modulation of both acute and chronic chemical toxicity in the lung (West et al., 2003). A major determinant of the potential for detoxification may also be the cellular localization of, and ability to synthesize, glutathione in the lung (Plopper et al., 2001b, West et al., 2000). Pulmonary glutathione S-transferase activity is 5–15% that of the liver in rodents and about 30% of that in human liver (Buckpitt and Cruikshank, 1997). The distribution of

Table 15-1
Distribution of Xenobiotic Metabolizing Enzymes in the Respiratory Tract

ENZYME	NASAL TISSUE	PROXIMAL AIRWAYS TRACHEA, BRONCHIAL (EPITHELIUM)	DISTAL AIRWAYS (BRONCHIOLAR EPITHELIUM)	ALVEOLI	OTHER
Cytochrome P450s	+++ Olfactory mucosa: sustentacular cells and Bowmans glands +/− Trasitional epithelium Respiratory epithelium + Other glands/ducts	++ Secretory cell types (2J2 only is ++ in ciliated cells)	+++ Clara cells and secretory cell types	++ Type II cells	++ Macrophages Endothelium (3A5, 1A1)
Miceosomal Epoxide Hydrolases	+++	++ Clara cells, ciliated cells	+++ Clara cells, ciliated cells	++	+ Macrophages ++ Blood vessels
Flavin Monooxygenases	+	++ Clara cells + Ciliated cells	+++ Clara cells + Ciliated cells	++ Type II cells + Type I cells	+ Capillary endothelial cells
Prostaglandin synthase (Cyclooxygenase-1,-2)	++ Basal and ciliated cells (cox-1 and cox-2)	++ Basal cells, columnar epithelial cells (Cox-1 > Cox2)	++ Clara cells	+/− Type II cells, alveolar septa	+++ Macrophages (Cox-1 < Cox2), mast cells (Cox2) eosinophils and neutrophils (Cox2), vascular smooth muscle (Cox1), endothelium (Cox1)
Glutathione S-Transferases	+ Olfactory epithelium	++ Cell types vary with isoform & include ciliated and Clara cells	+++ Cell types vary with isoform & include ciliated and Clara cells	+ Type II cells	?
Glucuronsyl Transferases	+ Olfactory epithelium	?	++ Clara cells, Ciliated cells	+ Type II cells	?
Sulfotransferases	++ Olfactory epithelium, sustentacular cells	+	+	+/−	?

Code for labels: +++, most isoforms expressed highly; +/−, some expression in some studies but not in others, generally low; ++, some isoforms expressed highly; ?, unknown/not found; +, low level of expression.

the isoforms of glutathione S-transferase varies by lung region with the alpha, mu, and pi isoforms (the most abundant) and the alpha and pi classes predominate in the airway epithelia of human lung. In nasal tissue, glutathione S-transferases are found in the olfactory mucosa. The mu isoform demonstrates a zonal pattern of expression increased in the lateral olfactory turbinates of the mouse (Whitby-Logan *et al.*, 2004). The glutathione transferases have recently been the focus of acute interest because of widespread polymorphisms in their expression in humans and the potential for correlation of this with lung cancer, particularly in smokers. A key point to keep in mind is that these enzyme systems work in concert with one another (i.e., a decrease in one enzyme may result in a concomitant increase in another) and it is the balance of all of them, and their location, that determines toxicity.

GENERAL PRINCIPLES IN THE PATHOGENESIS OF LUNG DAMAGE CAUSED BY CHEMICALS

Toxic Inhalants, Gases, and Dosimetry

The sites of deposition of gases in the respiratory tract define the pattern of toxicity of those gases. Water solubility is the critical factor in determining how deeply a given gas penetrates into the lung. Highly soluble gases such as SO_2 do not penetrate farther than the nose unless doses are very high, and are therefore relatively nontoxic to animals, especially obligatory nose breathers, such as the rat. Relatively insoluble gases such as ozone and NO_2 penetrate deeply into the lung and reach the smallest airways and the alveoli (centriacinar region), where they can elicit toxic responses. Mathematical models of gas entry and deposition in the lung that are based solely on the aqueous solubility of a gas predict sites of lung lesions fairly accurately. These models may be useful for extrapolating findings made in laboratory animals to humans (Kimball and Miller, 1999; Medinsky *et al.*, 1999). Very insoluble gases such as CO and H_2S efficiently pass through the respiratory tract and are taken up by the pulmonary blood supply to be distributed throughout the body.

Particle Deposition

Particle size is usually the critical factor that determines the region of the respiratory tract in which a particle or an aerosol will be deposited. Deposition of particles on the surface of the lung and airways is brought about by a combination of lung anatomy and the patterns of airflow in the respiratory system (Raabe, 1999; Miller, 1999).

Particle Size

The median diameter that is determined may reflect the number of particles, as in the count median diameter (CMD), or reflect mass, as in the mass median aerodynamic diameter (MMAD). If more particles actually reach the deep lung, the higher is the probability of a toxic effect. Particle surface area is of special importance when toxic materials are adsorbed on particles and thus are carried into the lung.

Large particles (larger than 5 μm MMAD) are usually trapped in the upper respiratory tract (nasopharyngeal region and large conducting airways), whereas smaller particles (0.2–5 μm MMAD) can be transported to the smaller airways and the alveoli (Fig. 15-5). Patterns of breathing can change the site of deposition of a particle of

a given size. Inhaled ambient particles and aerosols are most frequently polydisperse in size. The size distribution of many aerosols approximates a log-normal distribution that may be described by the median or geometric mean and the geometric standard deviation. A plot of the frequency of occurrence of a given size against the log of the size produces a bell-shaped probability curve. Particle data frequently are analyzed by plotting the cumulative percentage of particles smaller than a stated size on log-probability paper. This results in a straight line that may be fitted by eye or mathematically. In actual practice, it is not unusual to have some deviation from a straight line at the largest or smallest particle sizes measured. The geometric mean is the 50% size as the mean bisects the curve. The geometric standard deviation (σ_g) is calculated as

$$\sigma_g = 84.1\% \text{ size}/50\% \text{ size}$$

The σ_g of the particle size distribution is a measure of the polydispersity of the aerosol. In the laboratory, values for σ_g of 1.8–3.0 are encountered frequently. In the field, value for σ_g may range up to 4.5. An aerosol with a σ_g below 1.2 may be considered monodispersed.

Particles that are nonspherical in shape are frequently characterized in terms of equivalent spheres on the basis of equal mass, volume, or aerodynamic drag. The MMAD takes into account both the density of the particle and aerodynamic drag. It represents the diameter of a unit density sphere with the same terminal settling velocity as the particle, regardless of its size, shape, and density. Aerodynamic diameter is the proper measurement for particles that are deposited by impaction and sedimentation. For very small particles, which are deposited primarily by diffusion, the critical factor is particle size, not density. It must be kept in mind that the size of a particle may change before its deposition in the respiratory tract. Materials that are hygroscopic, such as sodium chloride, sulfuric acid, and glycerol, take on water and grow in size in the warm, saturated atmosphere of the upper and lower respiratory tract.

Nanotoxicology

There is intense current interest in the lung toxicity of nanoparticles, particles with diameters of <100 nm (Oberdorster *et al.*, 2005a,b). Ultrafine particles of this size range are increasingly being used in manufactured products, and synthesis and release of particles of this size to the environment, and exposure of individuals in the workplace, is increasing exponentially. In addition, emissions control devices on internal combustion engines, diesel engines, and industrial furnaces and burners can efficiently trap larger particles; however, technology that decreases emissions of larger particles (which contain most of the mass of the particulate fraction) generally produces greater amounts of ultrafine particles (on a particle number basis). The toxicological concerns reflect three major issues: (1) the enormous surface area of these nanoparticles relative to their mass, especially with regard to the adsorption of co-pollutants and the presence of reactive metals on their surfaces, (2) commercially important forms of nanoparticles include nanotubes, which are high axial ratio rods that provoke concerns that they might be far more toxic than spheres of the same MMAD, and (3) the question of whether normal host defenses are effective against particles this small, which can be readily transported through and out of the lung to other tissues via pathways that are not normally accessible to larger particles.

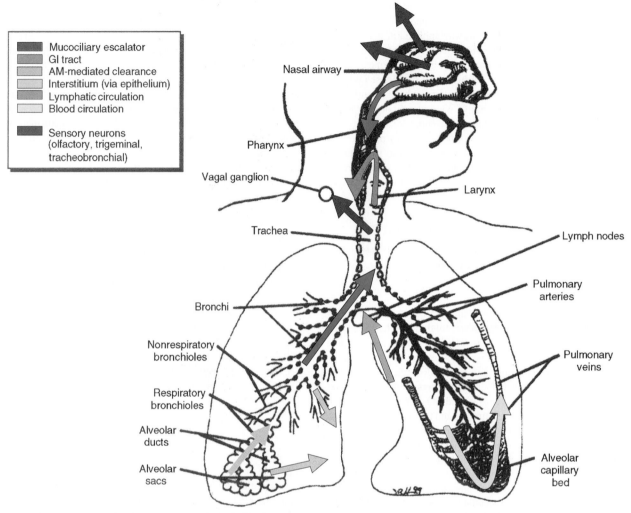

Figure 15-5. Pathways of particle clearance (disposition) in and out of the respiratory tract. There are significant differences between nanosized particles (NSPs) and larger particles for some of these pathways. (Drawing courtesy of J. Harkema.) [From Fig. 9 in Oberdorster et al., 2005. Nanotoxicology: An emerging discipline evolving from studies of ultrafine particles. Environ Health Perspect. Vol 113, No 7. 823–839, 2005a.]

A major technical issue in interpretation of the emerging literature that tries to address this topic is whether intratracheally (IT) administered nanoparticles behave similarly to inhaled nanoparticles (Warheit *et al.*, 2004), as most of the studies thus far of "nanotoxicology" have used IT instillation as the mode of delivery. Conflicting results have been observed with nanoparticles administered IT: transient inflammatory responses that suggest no greater toxicity than observed with larger particles (Huczko *et al.*, 2001; Warheit *et al.*, 2004, 2006) or much greater toxicity than observed with larger particles (Lam *et al.*, 2004). Several major working groups have been convened to formulate appropriate strategies for risk assessment of nanoparticles, and their recommendations provide guidance for future studies in this area (Oberdorster *et al.*, 2005a, b).

Additional concern about potential toxicity of nanoparticles is triggered by the large body of epidemiological evidence linking exposure to ultrafine particles as air pollutants and increased mortality in sensitive populations (Dockery *et al.*, 1993; Pope *et al.*, 2004). There is, as yet, no defined mechanistic basis for the observed epidemiological associations, and this is a very active field of current research in inhalation toxicology.

Deposition Mechanisms

Deposition of particles occurs primarily by interception, impaction, sedimentation, and diffusion (Brownian movement). Interception occurs when the trajectory of a particle brings it near enough to a surface so that an edge of the particle contacts the airway surface. Interception is important for the deposition of fibers. Whereas fiber diameter determines the probability of deposition by impaction and sedimentation, interception is dependent on fiber length. Thus, a fiber with a diameter of 1 μm and a length of 200 μm will be deposited in the bronchial tree primarily by interception rather than impaction.

As a result of inertia, particles suspended in air tend to continue to travel along their original path. In an airstream that is not straight, such as at an airway bifurcation, a particle may be impacted on the surface. At relatively symmetrical bifurcations, which typically occur in the human lung, the deposition rate is likely to be high for particles that move in the center of the airway. In the average adult, most particles larger than 10 μm in aerodynamic diameter are deposited in the nose or oral pharynx and cannot penetrate to tissues distal to the larynx. Very fine particles (0.01 μm and smaller) are also trapped relatively efficiently in the upper airways by diffusion. Particles that penetrate beyond the upper airways are available to be deposited in the bronchial region and the deep-lying airways. Therefore, the alveolar region has significant deposition efficiencies for particles smaller than 5 μm and larger than 0.01 μm (Fig. 15-5).

Sedimentation brings about deposition in the smaller bronchi, the bronchioles, and the alveolar spaces, where the airways are small and the velocity of airflow is low. As a particle moves through air, buoyancy and the resistance of air act on the particle in an upward direction while gravitational force acts on the particle in a downward direction. Eventually, the gravitational force equilibrates with the sum of the buoyancy and the air resistance, and the particle continues to settle with a constant velocity known as the terminal settling velocity. Sedimentation is not a significant route of particle deposition when the aerodynamic diameter is below 0.5 μm.

Diffusion is an important factor in the deposition of submicrometer particles. A random motion is imparted to these particles by the impact of gas molecules. This Brownian motion increases with decreasing particle size, so diffusion is an important deposition mechanism in the nose and in other airways and alveoli for particles smaller than about 0.5 μm.

An important factor in particle deposition is the pattern of breathing. During quiet breathing, in which the TV is only two to three times the volume of the anatomic dead space (i.e, the volume of the conducting airways where gas exchange does not occur), a large proportion of the inhaled particles may be exhaled. During exercise, when larger volumes are inhaled at higher velocities, impaction in the large airways and sedimentation and diffusion in the smaller airways and alveoli increase. Breath holding also increases deposition from sedimentation and diffusion. Factors that modify the diameter of the conducting airways can alter particle deposition. In patients with chronic bronchitis, the mucous layer is greatly thickened and extended peripherally and may partially block the airways in some areas. Jets formed by air flowing through such partially occluded airways have the potential to increase the deposition of particles by impaction and diffusion in the small airways. Irritant materials that produce bronchoconstriction tend to increase the tracheobronchial deposition of particles. Cigarette smoking has been shown experimentally to produce such an effect.

Particle Clearance

The clearance of deposited particles is an important aspect of lung defense (see Fig. 15-5). Rapid removal lessens the time available to cause damage to the pulmonary tissues or permit local absorption. It is important to emphasize that clearance of particles from the respiratory tract is not synonymous with clearance from the body. The only mechanisms by which deposited particles can truly be removed from the respiratory system are coughing and blowing of the nose.

Nasal Clearance Particles deposited in the nose are cleared depending on their site of deposition and solubility in mucus. Particles deposited in the anterior portion of the nose are removed by extrinsic actions such as wiping and blowing. The other regions of the nose are largely covered by a mucociliary epithelium that propels mucus toward the glottis, where it is swallowed. Insoluble particles generally are cleared from this region in healthy adults and swallowed within an hour of deposition. Particles that are soluble in mucus may dissolve and enter the epithelium and/or blood before they can be mechanically removed.

Tracheobronchial Clearance The mucus layer covering the tracheobronchial tree is moved upward by the beating of the underlying cilia. This mucociliary escalator transports deposited particles and particle-laden macrophages upward to the oropharynx, where they are swallowed and pass through the GI tract. Mucociliary clearance is relatively rapid in healthy individuals and is completed within 24–48 hours for particles deposited in the lower airways. Infection and other injuries can greatly impair clearance.

Pulmonary Clearance There are several ways by which particulate material is removed from the lower respiratory tract once it has been deposited:

1. Particles may be directly trapped on the lining layer of the conducting airways by impaction and cleared upward in the tracheobronchial tree via the mucociliary escalator.
2. Particles may be phagocytized by macrophages and cleared via the mucociliary escalator.
3. Particles may be phagocytized by alveolar macrophages and removed via the lymphatic drainage.
4. Materials may dissolve from the surfaces of particles and be removed via the bloodstream or lymphatics.
5. Small particles may directly penetrate epithelial membranes.
6. Minutes after particles are inhaled, they may be found in alveolar macrophages. Insoluble particles, especially long narrow fibers, may be sequestered in the lung for very long periods, often in macrophages located in the interstitium.

ACUTE RESPONSES OF THE LUNG TO INJURY

Mechanisms of Respiratory Tract Injury

Airborne agents can come in contact with cells lining the respiratory tract from the nostrils to the gas-exchanging region. The sites of interaction of toxicants in the respiratory tract have important implications for evaluation of the risk to humans posed by inhalants. For example, rats have much more nasal surface on a per body weight basis than do humans. Measurement of DNA-protein cross-links formed in nasal tissue by the highly reactive gas formaldehyde has demonstrated that rats, which readily develop nasal tumors, have many more DNA cross-links per unit of exposure (concentration of formaldehyde × duration of exposure) than do monkeys. Because the breathing pattern of humans resembles that of monkeys more than that of rats, it was concluded that extrapolation of tumor data from rats to humans on the basis of formaldehyde concentration may overestimate doses of formaldehyde to humans. Patterns of animal activity can affect dose to the lung; nocturnally active animals such as rats receive a greater dose per unit of exposure at night than during the day, whereas humans show the opposite diurnal relationships of exposure concentration to dose.

Certain gases and vapors stimulate nerve endings in the nose, particularly those of the trigeminal nerve (Alarie *et al.*, 1998). The result is holding of the breath or changes in breathing patterns, to avoid or reduce further exposure. If continued exposure cannot be avoided, many acidic or alkaline irritants produce cell necrosis and increased permeability of the alveolar walls. Other inhaled chemicals can be more insidious; inhalation of high concentrations of HCl, NO_2, NH_3, or phosgene may at first produce very little apparent damage in the respiratory tract. The epithelial barrier in the alveolar zone, after a latency period of several hours, begins to leak, flooding the alveoli and producing a delayed pulmonary edema that is often fatal.

A different pathogenetic mechanism is typical of highly reactive molecules such as ozone. It is unlikely that ozone as such can penetrate beyond the layer of fluid covering the cells of the lung. Instead, ozone lesions are propagated by a cascade of secondary reaction products, such as aldehydes and hydroxyperoxides produced by ozonolysis of fatty acids and other substrates in the lung lining fluid, and by reactive oxygen species arising from free radical reactions.

Metabolism of foreign compounds can be involved in the pathogenesis of lung injury. The balance of activation and detoxification plays a key role in determining whether a given chemical ultimately will cause damage. The lung contains most of the enzymes involved in xenobiotic metabolism that have been identified in other tissues, such as the liver (Cascorbi, 2006). These enzymes are highly concentrated in specific cell populations of the respiratory tract and the content of particular cytochrome P-450 isozymes may be much higher in lung. Thus, the turnover of a particular substrate by a lung P-450 may be far more rapid than occurs in liver. Many isozymes of the cytochrome P-450 complex have been identified in and isolated from the lungs of rabbits, rats, hamsters, and humans. Cytochrome P-450 1A1 is present in low amounts in normal rat and rabbit lungs but is highly inducible by polycyclic aromatic hydrocarbons, flavones, and mixtures of polyhalogenated biphenyls. By inference, this P-450 isozyme may play a role in the pathogenesis of lung cancer. Cytochrome P-450 2B1, which is readily inducible in rat liver by phenobarbital, is not inducible in lung tissue. Other isozymes identified in human lung are cytochrome P-450 2F1, 4B1, and 3A4, as well as NADPH cytochrome P-450 reductase, epoxide hydrolase, and flavin-containing monoxygenases. Two important cytosolic enzymes involved in lung xenobiotic metabolism are glutathione-S-transferases and glutathione peroxidase.

Oxidative Burden

An undue oxidative burden that often is mediated by free radicals, such as those generated by ozone, NO_2, tobacco smoke, and lung defense cells (Rahman, 2003), can directly and indirectly cause lung damage. Numerous studies have reported increases in the activity of free radical scavenging enzymes in the lungs of animals exposed to O_3, NO_2, and other toxicants, indirectly supporting this hypothesis.

Theories of lung oxidant toxicity suggest the formation of reactive and unstable free radicals and active oxygen species. Subsequent chain reactions can lead to uncontrolled destructive oxidation. Recent work has emphasized the pivotal roles of superoxide, nitric oxide, peroxynitrite, hydroxyl radicals, hydrogen peroxide, and even possibly singlet oxygen in mediating tissue damage. Reduction of O_2 to active O_2 metabolites normally occurs as a by-product of cellular metabolism during both microsomal and mitochondrial electron transfer reactions; considerable amounts of superoxide anion are generated by NADPH cytochrome P-450 reductase reactions. Because these oxidant species are potentially cytotoxic, they may mediate or promote the actions of various pneumotoxicants. Such mechanisms have been proposed for paraquat- and nitrofurantoin-induced lung injury.

Among mammalian cells, neutrophils, monocytes, and macrophages are particularly adept at converting molecular O_2 to reactive O_2 metabolites; this is likely related to their phagocytotic and antimicrobial activities. As a by-product of this capability, toxic O_2 species are released into surrounding tissues. As most forms of toxic pulmonary edema are accompanied by phagocyte accumulation in the lung microcirculation (pulmonary leukostasis) and parenchyma, oxidative damage may represent a significant component of pneumotoxic lung injury.

Chemotactic and phagocytic activation processes result in a substantial increase in the release of potent oxidants by stimulated phagocytes; these radicals cause oxidative damage to the surrounding tissues. A key role of hydrogen peroxide as the mediator of the extracellular cytotoxic mechanism of activated phagocytes has been well documented. In addition, hydrogen peroxide is a potent intracellular signaling molecule that readily crosses cell membranes, and can thereby amplify cell damage. Phagocytic production of active oxygen species causes inactivation of proteinase inhibitors and degranulation of mast cells. Platelets (and platelet microthrombi) also have the ability to generate activated O_2 species.

The lung can respond with specific defense mechanisms that may be stimulated by constant exposure to airborne microorganisms, as well as by a variety of low- and high-molecular- weight antigenic materials. The immune system can mount either cellular or humorally mediated responses to these inhaled antigens. Direct immunologic effects occur when inhaled foreign material sensitizes the respiratory system to further exposure to the same material. Lymphocytes reside in the hilar or mediastinal lymph nodes, lymphoid aggregates, and lymphoepithelial nodules, as well as in aggregates or as single cells throughout the airways. Bronchoconstriction and chronic pulmonary disease can result from the inhalation of materials that appear to act wholly or partly through an allergic response. Frequently, chemical components of the sensitizing dusts or gases are responsible for the allergic response. Low-molecular-weight compounds can act as haptens that combine with native proteins to form a complex that is recognized as an antigen by the immune system. Further exposure to the sensitizing compound can result in an allergic reaction that is characterized by the release of various inflammatory mediators that produce an early and/or a late bronchoconstrictor response. Such a response is observed in sensitized workers exposed to toluene diisocyanate (TDI), a chemical widely used in the manufacture of polyurethane plastics (Matheson *et al.*, 2001).

Increased susceptibility of asthmatic individuals to air pollutants such as ozone and sulfur dioxide may be mediated by indirect immune effects.

Mediators of Lung Toxicity

Interleukin 1 (IL-1β), transforming growth factor (TGF-beta), and tumor necrosis factor (TNF-alpha) have all been implicated in the cascade of reactions that are thought to be responsible for the pathogenesis of pulmonary fibrosis (Zhang and Phan, 1999). Several members of the interleukin family, especially IL-1, IL-2, IL-5, IL-8, and IL-13, are thought to be essential components of the lung's response to epithelial cell injury. Various specific prostaglandins, especially PGE$_2$, and leukotrienes have been implicated in intracellular signaling pathways in the lung. The roles of cell surface adhesion molecules and their interaction with cell matrix components and with control of inflammatory cell migration (particularly neutrophil influx to the lung) have been studied intensively.

Analysis of normal lung homogenates suggests that the lung contains large amounts of endogenous cytokines and inflammatory mediators, far more than enough for these potent compounds to elicit effects. Thus, these agents must be compartmentalized in a healthy lung to control their potent bioactivity. How these processes are regulated normally, what exactly goes wrong with homeostasis in a damaged lung, the temporal and geographic relationship of different cytokines in the amplification of an initial injurious event, and detailed mechanisms of resolution of lung injury are not well understood and represent the current focus of much research on mechanisms of lung injury by toxic agents.

Airway Reactivity

Large airways are surrounded by bronchial smooth muscle, which helps maintain airway tone and diameter during expansion and contraction of the lung. Bronchial smooth muscle tone is normally regulated by the autonomic nervous system. Bronchoconstriction can be provoked by irritants such as cigarette smoke and air pollutants, and by cholinergic drugs such as acetylcholine. This phenomenon serves as the basis for a sensitive measure of whether a toxicant can cause bronchoconstriction in animals or humans primed by a prior dose of an acetylcholine-like agent (bronchoprovocation testing). These chemicals bind to cell surface receptors (cholinergic receptors) and trigger an increase in the intracellular concentration of cyclic guanosine monophosphate (cGMP), which in turn facilitates smooth muscle contraction. The actions of cGMP can be antagonized by cyclic adenosine monophospate (cAMP), which has bronchodilatory activity, and can be increased by agents that bind to beta-adrenergic receptors on the cell surface. Other important mediators of airway smooth muscle tone include histamine, various prostaglandins and leukotrienes, substance P, and nitric oxide. The bronchial smooth muscles of individuals with asthma contract with much less provocation than do those of normal subjects.

Bronchoconstriction causes a decrease in airway diameter and a corresponding increase in resistance to airflow. Characteristic associated symptoms include wheezing, coughing, a sensation of chest tightness, and dyspnea. Exercise potentiates these problems. Because the major component of airway resistance usually is contributed by large bronchi, inhaled chemicals that cause reflex bronchoconstriction are generally irritant gases with moderate solubility. Asthmatic individuals may represent a population that is particularly susceptible to the adverse health effects of ambient air pollution, especially ozone, other respiratory irritant gases, and respirable particles.

Pulmonary Edema

Toxic pulmonary edema represents an acute, exudative phase of lung injury that generally produces a thickening of the alveolar-capillary barrier. Edema fluid alters ventilation-perfusion relationships and limits diffusive transfer of O_2 and CO_2 even in otherwise structurally normal alveoli.

Toxic pulmonary edema may not only induce acute compromise of lung structure and function but may also cause abnormalities that remain after resolution of the edematous process. After exposure to some toxic chemicals in which the alveolar-capillary surface is denuded (such as alloxan), recovery is unlikely, whereas in situations of more modest injury (such as histamine administration), full recovery is readily achievable. Between these two extremes there are forms of severe lung injury accompanied by amplified inflammatory damage and/or exaggerated restorative-reparative processes (e.g., after paraquat ingestion). In these severe forms, the extensive interstitial and intraalveolar inflammatory exudate resolves via fibrogenesis, an outcome that may be beneficial or damaging to the lung. Accumulation and turnover of inflammatory cells and related

immune responses in an edematous lung probably play a role in eliciting both mitogenic activity and fibrogenic responses.

Pulmonary edema is customarily quantified in experimental animals by measurement of lung water content. Very commonly, the wet (undesiccated) weight of the whole lung or that of a single lung lobe is determined. This value is often normalized to the weight of the animal from which the lung was taken. Alternatively, some investigators determine lung water content by weighing whole lungs or lung slices before and after complete drying in an oven or desiccator. Commonly used methods for expressing such data include (1) percentage water content [100 × (wet weight − dry weight)/(wet weight)], (2) percentage dry weight [100 × (dry weight)/(wet weight)], and (3) water content [(mL of water)/(dry weight)].

CHRONIC RESPONSES OF THE LUNG TO INJURY

Emphysema

Emphysema is commonly defined as "an abnormal enlargement of the airspaces distal to the terminal bronchiole accompanied by destruction of the walls without obvious fibrosis" (Snider *et al.*, 1985). Destruction of the gas-exchanging surface area results in a distended, hyperinflated lung that no longer effectively exchanges oxygen and carbon dioxide as a result of both loss of tissue and air trapping (Fig. 15-6). The major cause of human emphysema is, by far, cigarette smoke inhalation, although other toxicants also can elicit this response. A feature of toxicant-induced emphysema is severe or recurrent inflammation.

A unifying hypothesis that explains the pathogenesis of emphysema has emerged from studies by several investigators. Early clinical research on screening blood protein phenotypes identified a rare mutation giving rise to a hereditary deficiency of the serum globulin alpha$_1$-antitrypsin. Homozygotes for this mutation had no circulating levels of this protein, which can prevent the proteolytic activity of serine proteases such as trypsin, and tended to get emphysema at a very young age. Alpha$_1$-antitrypsin (now called alpha$_1$-antiprotease) is one of the body's main defenses against uncontrolled proteolytic digestion by this class of enzymes, which includes elastase. Studies in smokers led to the hypothesis that neutrophil (and perhaps alveolar macrophage) elastases can break down lung elastin and thus cause emphysema; these elastases usually are kept in check by alpha$_1$-antiprotease that diffuses into the lung from the blood. As an individual ages, an accumulation of random elastolytic events can cause the emphysematous changes in the lungs that are normally associated with aging. Toxicants that cause inflammatory cell influx and thus increase the burden of neutrophil elastase can accelerate this process. In accord with this hypothesis are a large number of experimental studies in animals instilled intratracheally with pancreatic or neutrophil elastase or with other proteolytic enzymes that can digest elastin. A pathological condition then develops that has some of the characteristics of emphysema, including destruction of alveolar walls and airspace enlargement in the lung parenchyma.

Mice with defects in genes that code for elastin and collagen modifying enzymes develop emphysema (O'Byrne and Postma, 1999). These observations suggest that problems with elastin synthesis may play an important role in the pathogenesis of emphysema, and that in its simplest form the elastase-antiprotease model alone cannot fully explain the detailed biochemical mechanisms that underlie the etiology of emphysema.

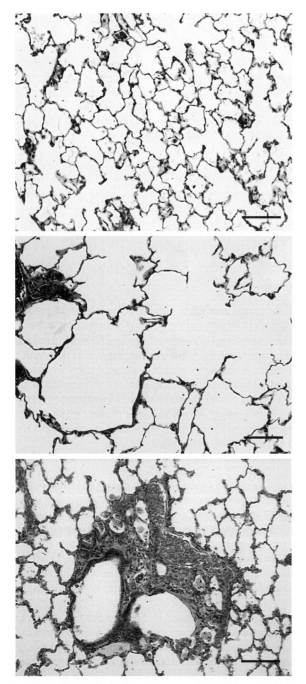

Figure 15-6. Top panel: Light micrograph of a normal rat lung. Middle panel: Lung of a spontaneously hypertensive (SH) rat 12 weeks after inhalation of tobacco smoke at a concentration of 90 mg/m^3 of total suspended particulate material. Note extensive distension of alveoli (emphysema). Bottom panel: Lung of a rat one year after exposure (8 h/d, 5 days a week for 12 months) to chrysotile asbestos. Note accumulation of connective tissue around blood vessel and airways (fibrosis). Bar length: 100 μm. (Photograph courtesy of Dr. Kent E. Pinkerton, University of California, Davis.)

Fibrosis

The pathological hallmark of pulmonary fibrosis is increased focal staining of collagen fibers in the alveolar interstitium. Fibrotic lungs from humans with acute or chronic pulmonary fibrosis contain increased amounts of collagen as evaluated biochemically.

In lungs damaged by toxicants, the response resembles adult or infant respiratory distress syndrome more closely than it resembles chronic interstitial fibrosis. Excess lung collagen is usually observed not only in the alveolar interstitium but also throughout the centriacinar region, including the alveolar ducts and respiratory bronchioles (Fig. 15-6). The relationship between increased collagen deposition around small airways and lung mechanics is not understood either theoretically or empirically.

Types I and III collagen are major lung interstitial components, representing about 90% or more of the total lung collagen, that are found in the normal lungs of all mammals in an approximate ratio of 2:1. There is an increase in type I collagen relative to type III collagen in patients with idiopathic pulmonary fibrosis and in patients dying of acute respiratory distress syndrome. It is not known whether shifts in collagen types, compared with absolute increases in collagen content, account for the increased stiffness of fibrotic lungs. Type III collagen is more compliant than is type I; thus, increasing type I relative to type III collagen may result in a stiffer lung. Changes in collagen cross-linking in fibrotic lungs also may contribute to the increased stiffness. Increased collagen type I:type III ratios and altered collagen cross-linking have been observed in collagen in several animal models of acute pulmonary fibrosis.

Asthma

Asthma is becoming increasingly prevalent in the United States and Europe especially in crowded urban areas. The clinical literature describes "an epidemic" of childhood asthma, with prevalence rates reportedly as high as 40% in children living in the inner city. This alarming increase in reported asthma in children has stimulated public health concerns, many of which have focused on air pollution (especially ultrafine particulate air pollution) as a possible cause of the observed increase in asthma. Asthma is characterized clinically by attacks of shortness of breath, which may be mild or severe. The clinical hallmark of asthma is increased airway reactivity: the smooth muscle around the large airways contracts in response to exposure to irritants. There are well-established links between occupational and environmental exposure to antigens or to chemicals that can act as haptens and the pathogenesis of asthma. There may be common mechanisms, which are shared between asthma and pulmonary fibrosis, especially with regard to the role of recurrent or chronic inflammation in disease pathogenesis (Quan *et al*., 2006).

Lung Cancer

At the begining of the twentieth century, lung cancer was an extremely rare disease. It is now the leading cause of death from cancer among both men and women. Retrospective and, more conclusively, prospective epidemiological studies unequivocally show an association between tobacco smoking and lung cancer. It has been estimated that approximately 80–90% of lung cancers (and several other cancers, such as cancer of the bladder, esophagus, oral cavity, and pancreas) are caused by cigarette smoking. Average smokers have a 10-fold, and heavy smokers a 20-fold, increased risk of developing lung cancer compared with nonsmokers. Quitting the habit will reduce the risk (IARC 2004).

Exposure to many chemicals encountered in industrial settings also pose a lung cancer risk. Inhalation of asbestos fibers and metallic dusts or fumes, such as arsenic, beryllium, cadmium, chromium, and nickel, encountered in smelting and manufacturing operations has been associated with cancer of the respiratory tract (IARC 1993).

Workers who manufacture chloromethyl ether or mustard gas have an increased risk of developing lung cancers, as do workers exposed to effluent gases from coke ovens. Radon gas is a known human lung carcinogen. Formaldehyde is a probable human respiratory carcinogen. Silica, human-made fibers, and welding fumes are suspected carcinogens. Smokers who inhale radon or asbestos fibers increase their risk of developing lung cancer severalfold, suggesting a synergistic interaction between the carcinogens. To what extent common air pollutants such as ozone, nitrogen dioxide, sulfur dioxide, and fumes emanating from power plants, oil refineries, and from diesel fuel powered trucks and cars contribute to the development of lung cancer in the general population remains an open question. Some evidence suggests that respirable particulates suspended in polluted air are a risk factor (Beeson *et al.*, 1998). Indoor air pollution, including environmental tobacco smoke, increases the risk of developing lung cancer in nonsmokers (IARC 2004).

Human lung cancers may have a latency period of 20–40 years, making the relationship to specific exposures difficult to establish. Many lung cancers in humans originate from the cells lining the airways (lung cancer originating from such sites is often referred to as bronchogenic carcinoma), but during the last two decades a significant increase in peripheral adenocarcinomas has occurred. Compared with cancer in the lung, cancer in the upper respiratory tract is less common. Malignant lesions of the nasal passages, which are seen frequently in experimental animals, are comparatively rare in humans. They are associated with certain occupations, including chromate workers, nickel refiners, mustard gas makers, isopropyl alcohol workers, makers of wooden furniture, and boot and shoe workers. Possible carcinogens include hexavalent chromium compounds, metallic nickel and nickel subsulfide, nickel oxide, formaldehyde, and certain wood and leather dusts.

The potential mechanisms of lung carcinogenesis have been studied extensively by means of analysis of tumor material and in studies of human bronchial cells maintained in culture. Damage to DNA is thought to be a key mechanism. An activated carcinogen or its metabolic product, such as alkyldiazonium ions derived from N-nitrosamines, may interact with DNA. Persistence of O^6-alkyldeoxyguanosine in DNA appears to correlate with carcinogenicity (Hecht, 1999). However, tumors do not always develop when adducts are present, and adduct formation may be a necessary but not sufficient condition for carcinogenesis. DNA damage caused by active oxygen species is another potentially important mechanism. Ionizing radiation leads to the formation of superoxide, which is converted through the action of superoxide dismutase to hydrogen peroxide. In the presence of Fe and other transition metals, hydroxyl radicals may be formed which then cause DNA strand breaks. Cigarette smoke contains high quantities of active oxygen species and other free radicals. Additional oxidative stress may be placed on the lung tissue of smokers by the release of superoxide anions and hydrogen peroxide by activated macrophages, metabolism of carcinogens, and lipid peroxidation caused by reactive aldehydes.

Epithelial lung cancers develop in a sequence of distinct morphological changes. Initially, cell numbers in the epithelium lining the airways increase (hyperplasia) and eventually display abnormal nuclei and changes in shape (dysplasia), often assuming squamous cell characteristics (squamous metaplasia). The lesions then progress to first carcinoma in situ, an accumulation of cancerous cells in small foci and then into large tumor masses. Eventually tumor cells invade adjacent local tissues, blood vessels, and lymphatics, leading to the formation of distant metastases. The histolog-

ically visible sequential development is accompanied by multiple molecular lesions that have been characterized in detail (Wistuba and Gazdar, 2003). Genomic instability is a hallmark of lung cancer. Chromosomal deletions expressed as loss of heterozygygosity, microsatellite alterations, and aberrant methylation seem to progress from the earliest lesions to full tumor development. Overexpression of MYC, TP53, and K-ras mutations are later events and many mutations in both dominant and recessive oncogenes have to develop until the cancers become fully invasive.

In laboratory animals, spontaneously occurring malignant lung tumors are uncommon unless the animals reach a very advanced age (Haschek *et al.*, 2002). Exposure to carcinogens by the inhalation route, by intratracheal instillation or by systemic administration readily produces lung tumors in many laboratory species, such as mice, rats, hamsters, and dogs. There are several differences between lung tumors in animals and bronchogenic cancer in humans. In animals, particularly rodents, most tumors are in the periphery rather than arising from the bronchi. The incidence of benign lung tumors such as adenomas is often very high, and carcinomas seem to require more time to develop. Lung tumors in animals do not metastasize as aggressively, if they do so at all, as do human lung cancers. This has been illustrated in animal inhalation studies with tobacco smoke. Tobacco smoke produces highly malignant lung tumors in man that metastasize aggressively to distant organs. In rats and mice exposed for lifetime to tobacco smoke concentrations approximating exposure of active human smokers, the majority of lung tumors failed to develop frank malignant features and distant metastasis were practically not observed (Mauderly *et al.*, 2004; Hutt *et al.*, 2005). Thus, tobacco smoke induced lung tumors in small laboratory rodents do not faithfully mimic the lesions seen in man.

In addition to peripherally located adenomas and adenocarcinomas, rats on occasion develop lung tumors that are characterized by an epithelium surrounding a space filled with keratin. The mass may compress the adjacent lung parenchyma and occasionally invades it. These lesions are classified by some pathologists as bona fide tumors, whereas other pathologists characterize this type of lesion as a cyst filled with keratin. Classification of such a lesion is important because these lesions often are found in long-term tests in animals that have been exposed to agents that are not considered carcinogens, such as carbon black, titanium dioxide, and certain human-made fibers (ILSI 2000). A unifying hypothesis postulates that clearance mechanisms in the deep lung depend predominantly if not completely on phagocytosis and migration of pulmonary alveolar macrophages and can be overwhelmed by quantities of respirable dusts far in excess of physiological loads (Morrow, 1992). As a consequence, lung burdens of these dusts persist for months or years, and completely unphysiological mechanisms of disease pathogenesis may come into play. In rats, lung tumors have been produced by particles such as diesel exhaust that carry mutagens and carcinogens on their surface, and also by inert carbon black particles. The issue of whether particle overloading defines a threshold in such experiments remains unresolved.

The Developing Lung

The increase in the prevalence of childhood asthma, observed in many countries during the last two decades, is one of the most dramatic developments indicating that infants and small children may be a particularly sensitive subpopulation to suffer from untoward health effects caused by air pollutants. It is now being recognized that the developing lung is uniquely sensitive to many airborne and blood-borne toxicants. One of the most striking examples is the perinatal effect of the complex mixture tobacco smoke. Children living in the homes of active smokers have been found to suffer from smoke-related health effects such as increased occurrence of middle ear infections and infections of the lower respiratory tract (bronchitis and pneumonia). They are also more prone to develop asthma or to suffer from exacerbation of this disease (NCI 1999). Sudden infant death syndrome (SIDS) has also been related to exposure to tobacco smoke. Of particular importance is the observation that both exposure of the fetus, while in utero, and then postnatal exposure is needed to trigger the event. For example, smoking by fathers seemed to increase the risk of SIDS only when the mothers had smoked during pregnancy. Although the mechanisms causing SIDS are not known with certainty, airway narrowing may be one critical event. Infants born to mothers who smoked had thickened and narrower airways compared to infants of nonsmoking mothers. In experimental animals it was found that only animals exposed to tobacco smoke while in utero and postnatally showed markedly increased airway hyperreactivtiy to methacholine, whereas no such changes occurred in animals that had been exposed while in utero or during the immediate postnatal period only. An increase in neuroendocrine cells in the airway was also only seen in animals exposed both while in utero and postnatally. Remarkably, the changes persisted well into young adulthood even after exposure to tobacco smoke was discontinued (Joad, 2004). Additional studies in experimental animals have also shown the developing lung to be susceptible to alterations in normal growth through altered signaling pathways such as NF-kB. Increased cell death is seen within the lung parenchyma, while sparing the developing airways (Zhong et al., 2006). These early-life alterations may play an important role in lung structure and function in later life. Further studies using environmental scenarios also continue to suggest that the developing lung deserves special attention for several reasons that impact early life changes (Fanucchi, 2004; Fanucchi and Plopper, 2004; Smiley-Jewell and Van Winkle, 2004). Differentiation and development of lung cells as well as maturation of metabolic competence occurs during both the prenatal and postnatal periods, usually occurring in a proximal to distal manner. Differentiation and development of the phase-I and phase-II metabolizing enzyme systems show a distinct spatial and temporal pattern. The stage of development (prenatal and/or postnatal) may greatly influence the severity of the lesion upon exposure to a toxicant or the capability for repair or, on occasion, prevent the development of damage. These different "windows of vulnerability" thus determine the eventual outcome. On occasion, toxic insults to a developing lung may become manifest only late in life. Prenatal (in utero) exposure to carcinogens such as benzo[a]pyrene or ethylnitrosourea have been found to produce cancers later in the life of experimental animals. Similarly, the development of asthma may be favored later in life by sensitization to allergens or exposure to air pollutants early in lung development. The study of perinatal lung toxicology is a developing field that promises to have considerable impact on future hazard evaluations and risk assessment of environmental pollutants for infants and young children.

AGENTS KNOWN TO PRODUCE LUNG INJURY IN HUMANS

The prevention and treatment of acute and chronic lung disease will eventually be based on knowledge of the cellular and molecular events that determine lung injury and repair. During the past 20 years, a large body of evidence has accumulated. Table 15-2 lists common toxicants that are known to produce acute and chronic lung injury in humans. In the following sections, a few examples of our current understanding of lung injury at the mechanistic level are discussed, with emphasis on agents directly responsible for human lung disease.

Airborne Agents That Produce Lung Injury in Humans

Asbestos   The term asbestos describes silicate minerals in fiber form. The most commonly mined and commercially used asbestos fibers include the serpentine chrysotile asbestos and the amphiboles crocidolite, anthophyllite, amosite, actinolite, and tremolite. Exposure to asbestos fibers occurs in mining operations and in the construction and shipbuilding industries, where asbestos was at one time widely used for its highly desirable insulating and fireproofing properties. During the last few decades, concern about asbestos in older buildings has led to the removal of asbestos-based insulating material; abatement workers may now represent an additional population at risk.

The hazards associated with asbestos exposure depend on fiber length. Fibers 2 μm in length may produce asbestosis; mesothelioma is associated with fibers 5 μm long, and lung cancer with fibers larger than 10 μm. Fiber diameter is another critical feature. Fibers with diameters larger than approximately 3 μm do not readily penetrate into the peripheral lung. For the development of mesothelioma, fiber diameter must be less than 0.5 μm, because thinner fibers may be translocated from their site of deposition via the lymphatics to other organs, including the pleural surface.

Once asbestos fibers have been deposited in the lung, they may become phagocytized by alveolar macrophages. Short fibers are completely ingested and subsequently removed via the mucociliary escalator. Longer fibers are incompletely ingested, and the macrophages become unable to leave the alveoli. Activated by the fibers, macrophages release mediators such as lymphokines and growth factors, which in turn attract immunocompetent cells or stimulate collagen production. Asbestos-related lung disease thus may be mediated through the triggering of an inflammatory sequence of events or the production of changes that eventually lead to the initiation (DNA damage caused by reactive molecular species) or promotion (increased rate of cell turnover in the lung) of the carcinogenic process.

The surface properties of asbestos fibers appear to be an important mechanistic element in toxicity. The protection afforded by superoxide dismutase or free radical scavengers in asbestos-related cell injury in vitro suggests that the generation of active oxygen species and concomitant lipid peroxidation are important mechanisms in asbestos toxicity. The interaction of iron on the surface of asbestos fibers with oxygen may lead to the production of hydrogen peroxide and the highly reactive hydroxyl radical—events that have been associated with asbestos toxicity (Upadhya and Kamp, 2003).

In humans, asbestos causes three forms of lung disease: asbestosis, lung cancer, and malignant mesothelioma. Asbestosis is characterized by a diffuse increase of collagen in the alveolar walls (fibrosis) and the presence of asbestos fibers, either free or coated with a proteinaceous material (asbestos bodies). Lung cancer develops in workers in the asbestos mining industry and smoking of cigarettes greatly enhances risk. Malignant mesothelioma (a rare tumor of the cells covering the surface of the visceral and parietal pleura) is unequivocally associated with asbestos exposure; in

Table 15-2

Industrial Toxicants That Produce Lung Disease

TOXICANT	COMMON NAME OF DISEASE	OCCUPATIONAL SOURCE	ACUTE EFFECT	CHRONIC EFFECT
Asbestos	Asbestosis	Mining, construction, shipbuilding, manufacture of asbestos-containing material		Fibrosis, pleural calcification, lung cancer, pleural mesothelioma
Aluminum dust	Aluminosis	Manufacture of aluminum products, fireworks, ceramics, paints, electrical goods, abrasives	Cough, shortness of breath	Interstitial fibrosis
Aluminum abrasives	Shaver's disease, corundum smelter's lung, bauxite lung	Manufacture of abrasives, smelting	Alveolar edema	Interstitial fibrosis, emphysema
Ammonia		Ammonia production, manufacture of fertilizers, chemical production, explosives	Upper and lower respiratory tract irritation, edema	Chronic bronchitis
Arsenic		Manufacture of pesticides, pigments, glass, alloys	Bronchitis	Lung cancer, bronchitis, laryngitis
Beryllium	Berylliosis	Ore extraction, manufacture of alloys, ceramics	Severe pulmonary edema, pneumonia	Fibrosis, progressive dyspnea, interstitial granulomatosis, lung cancer, cor pulmonale
Cadmium oxide		Welding, manufacture of electrical equipment, alloys, pigments, smelting	Cough, pneumonia	Emphysema, cor pulmonale
Carbides of tungsten, titanium, tantalum	Hard metal disease	Manufacture of cutting edges on tools	Hyperplasia and metaplasia of bronchial epithelium	Peribronchial and perivascular fibrosis
Chlorine		Manufacture of pulp and paper, plastics, chlorinated chemicals	Cough, hemoptysis, dyspnea, tracheobronchitis, bronchopneumonia	
Chromium (VI)		Production of Cr compounds, paint pigments, reduction of chromite ore	Nasal irritation, bronchitis	Lung cancer, fibrosis
Coal dust	Pneumoconiosis	Coal mining		Fibrosis
Cotton dust	Byssinosis	Manufacture of textiles	Chest tightness, wheezing, dyspnea	Reduced pulmonary function, chronic bronchitis
Hydrogen fluoride		Manufacture of chemicals, photographic film, solvents, plastics	Respiratory irritation, hemorrhagic pulmonary edema	
Iron oxides	Siderotic lung disease; silver finisher's lung, hematite miner's lung, arc welder's lung	Welding, foundry work, steel manufacture, hematite mining, jewelry making	Cough	Silver finisher's lung: subpleural and perivascular aggregations of macrophages; hematite miner's lung: diffuse fibrosislike pneumoconiosis; arc welder's lung: bronchitis
Isocyanates		Manufacture of plastics, chemical industry	Airway irritation, cough, dyspnea	Asthma, reduced pulmonary function
Kaolin	Kaolinosis	Pottery making		Fibrosis
Manganese	Manganese pneumonia	Chemical and metal industries	Acute pneumonia, often fatal	Recurrent pneumonia

(Continued)

Table 15-2
(Continued)

TOXICANT	COMMON NAME OF DISEASE	OCCUPATIONAL SOURCE	ACUTE EFFECT	CHRONIC EFFECT
Nickel		Nickel ore extraction, smelting, electronic electroplating, fossil fuels	Pulmonary edema, delayed by 2 d (NiCO)	Squamous cell carcinoma of nasal cavity and lung
Oxides of nitrogen		Welding, silo filling, explosive manufacture	Pulmonary congestion and edema	Bronchiolitis obliterans
Ozone		Welding, bleaching flour, deodorizing	Pulmonary edema	Fibrosis
Phosgene		Production of plastics, pesticides, chemicals	Edema	Bronchitis, fibrosis
Perchloro-ethylene		Dry cleaning, metal degreasing, grain fumigating	Edema	Cancer, liver and lung
Silica	Silicosis, pneumoconiosis	Mining, stone cutting, construction, farming, quarrying, sand blasting	Acute silicosis	Fibrosis, silicotuberculosis
Sulfur dioxide		Manufacture of chemicals, refrigeration, bleaching, fumigation	Bronchoconstriction, cough, chest tightness	Chronic bronchitis
Talc	Talcosis	Rubber industry, cosmetics		Fibrosis
Tin	Stanosis	Mining, processing of tin		Widespread mottling of X-ray without clinical signs
Vanadium		Steel manufacture	Airway irritation and mucus production	Chronic bronchitis

the general population. It is only very rarely found. There is some discrepancy between observations in case of humans and the findings in animals that inhale asbestos fibers. In animal experiments, chrysotile produces mesothelioma much more readily than do the amphibole fibers. In humans, amphibole fibers are implicated more often even when the predominant exposure is to chrysotile asbestos. Chrysotile breaks down much more readily than do the amphiboles. It is possible that in small laboratory animals chrysotile fibers, even if broken down, are retained longer relative to the life span of the animal than they are in humans, thus explaining the higher rate of mesothelioma developed.

Silica Inhaled particles of silicon dioxide (silica) cause a characteristic human lung disease. The disease may be acute or chronic; this distinction is important conceptually because the pathological consequences are manifested quite differently. Acute silicosis occurs only in subjects exposed to a very high level of aerosol containing silicon dioxide particles (most often in form of quartz or sand) small enough to be respirable (usually less than 5 μm) over a relatively short period, generally a few months to a few years. These patients have worsening dyspnea, fever, cough, and weight loss. There is rapid progression of respiratory failure, usually ending in death within a year or two. No known treatment modality influences the relentless course of acute silicosis.

Chronic silicosis has a long latency period, usually more than 10 years. Uncomplicated silicosis is almost entirely asymptomatic; little alteration is shown on routine pulmonary function tests even after the disease is radiographically demonstrable. The X-ray picture

presents fibrotic nodules, generally in the apical portion of lung. The hilar lymph nodes have peripheral calcifications known as eggshell calcifications. Simple silicosis may progress into complicated silicosis, which is defined as the presence of conglomerate nodules larger than 1 cm in diameter. These nodules usually occur in the upper and midlung zones. At an advanced stage they may be surrounded by emphysematous bullae. Chronic silicosis is associated with an increased incidence of tuberculosis.

Crystalline silica is a major component of the earth's crust; after oxygen, silicon is the most common element. As a pure mineral, silicon exists primarily in the form of its dioxide, silica (SiO_2), which has a crystalline form in which a central silicon atom forms a tetrahedron with four shared oxygen atoms. The three principal crystalline isomeric forms are quartz, tridymite, and cristobalite. The tetrahedral structure is linked to fibrogenic potential. Stishovite, a rare crystalline variant without the tetrahedral conformation, is biologically inert. Amorphous forms of silica such as kieselguhr and vitreous silica have very low fibrogenic potential. The ubiquitous presence of silica has made it an occupational hazard ever since humans began shaping tools from stone, and silicosis remains a significant industrial hazard throughout the world in occupations such as mining and quarrying, sandblasting, and foundry work. The main factors that affect the pathogenicity of silica both in vivo and in vitro, in addition to its structure, are particle size and concentration. Many studies have examined the relationship of silica particle size to fibrogenicity. In studies with humans, the most fibrogenic particle size appears to be about 1 μm (range 0.5–3 μm). In animal experiments (rats, hamsters), the comparable values appear to be 1–2 μm (range 0.5–5 μm). In animal models, there appears to be a direct relationship between the concentration of silica dust to which an animal is exposed and the intensity and rapidity of the histological reaction in the lung.

The pathophysiological basis of pulmonary fibrosis in chronic silicosis is probably better understood than is the etiology of any other form of lung fibrosis. The role of pulmonary alveolar macrophages in the ingestion of silica as an initiating event has been established. Apparently, as part of the cytotoxic response of a macrophage to silica ingestion, the macrophage may release cytokines and other substances that cause fibroblasts to replicate and/or increase their rate of collagen biosynthesis. The role of inflammatory cells other than alveolar macrophages in this process is unknown. Also not understood is the role of the host's immune response and the roles of lymphocyte factors in stimulating fibroblast proliferation and/or collagen synthesis by fibroblasts in lung fibrogenesis (Barbarin *et al.*, 2004).

Naphthalene Naphthalene occurs in tars and petroleum and is a widely used precursor chemical for synthetic tanning agents, phthalic acid anhydride, carbaryl, and 2-naphthol. It is present in ambient air. Smokers inhale substantial amounts of naphthalene in cigarette smoke. In experimental animals, inhaled or parenterally administered naphthalene has shown remarkable species and tissue specificity: it produces extensive and selective necrosis in the bronchiolar epithelium of the mouse but much less necrosis in the airways of rats and hamsters.

Animals treated with small doses of naphthalene along with inhibitors of cytochrome P-450s show little or no tissue damage, implicating metabolism in the toxicity of this chemical. Metabolism to the naphthalene oxide is mediated primarily through CYP-2F2 in mice (Shultz *et al.*, 1999). In rats and other species, including monkeys, conversion of naphthalene is less stereospecific and the rates of formation of the epoxide are much slower than in mice. This may explain the species differences that were noted previously. Naphthalene epoxides may subsequently be conjugated with glutathione and form adducts that are eliminated as mercapturic acids. The epoxide can undergo rearrangement to 1-naphthol with subsequent metabolism to quinones, which are potentially toxic compounds. Naphthalene metabolites bind covalently to cellular proteins that are important in normal cellular homeostasis and protein folding and this may be related to the mechanism of toxicity by this chemical. Interestingly, in both mice and rhesus monkeys the total amount of adducted protein is similar (Lin *et al.*, 2005, 2006).

Blood-borne Agents That Cause Pulmonary Toxicity in Humans

Bleomycin Bleomycin, a mixture of several structurally similar compounds, is a widely used cancer chemotherapeutic agent. Pulmonary fibrosis, often fatal, represents the most serious form of toxicity. The sequence of damage includes necrosis of capillary endothelial and type I alveolar cells, edema formation and hemorrhage, delayed (after 1–2 weeks) proliferation of type II epithelial cells, and eventually thickening of the alveolar walls by fibrotic changes.

In many tissues, the cytosolic enzyme bleomycin hydrolase inactivates bleomycin. In lung and skin, two target organs for bleomycin toxicity, the activity of this enzyme is low compared with that in other organs. Bleomycin stimulates the production of collagen in the lung. Before increased collagen biosynthesis, steady-state levels of mRNA coding for fibronectin and procollagens are

increased, presumably subsequent to a bleomycin-mediated release of cytokines such as TGF beta and TNF alpha. Bleomycin also combines with Fe (II) and molecular oxygen; when it combines with DNA, single- and double-strand breaks are produced by a free radical reaction. Animal models of belomycin-induced pulmonary fibrosis have been used to study the efficacy of promising antifibrotic drugs (Giri, 2003).

Cyclophosphamide and 1,3 Bis (2-Chloroethyl)-1-Nitrosourea (BCNU) Cyclophosphamide is widely used as an anticancer and immunosuppressive drug. The undesirable side effects include hemorrhagic cystitis and pulmonary fibrosis. Cyclophosphamide is metabolized by the cytochrome P-450 system to two highly reactive metabolites: acrolein and phosphoramide mustard. In the lung, cooxidation with the prostaglandin H synthase system, which has high activity in the lung, is a possibility. Although the exact mechanism of action for causing lung damage has not been established, studies with isolated lung microsomes have shown that cyclophosphamide and its metabolite acrolein initiate lipid peroxidation. Carmustine (BCNU) is an effective chemotherapeutic agent that exerts its antitumor properties by reacting with cellular macromolecules and forms inter- and intrastrand cross-links with DNA. In humans, a dose-related pulmonary toxicity is often noticed first by a decrease in diffusion capacity. Pulmonary fibrosis caused by this drug can be fatal. The mechanism of action is not entirely clear. It is possible that BCNU inhibits pulmonary glutathione disulfide reductase, an event that may lead to a disturbed GSH/GSSG state in pulmonary cells. Eventually, this state leaves the cell unable to cope with oxidant stress. High concentrations of oxygen in the inspired air may enhance the pulmonary toxicity of BCNU and also that of the other anticancer drugs known to affect lung tissue: cyclophosphamide and bleomycin. Several other chemotherapeutic drugs can produce lung damage and pulmonary toxicity in patients treated with these drugs can be a significant problem (Ramu and Kehrer, 1997).

EVALUATION OF TOXIC LUNG DAMAGE

Studies Being Done in Humans

While the lung is susceptible to multiple toxic injuries, it is also amenable to a number of tests that allow evaluation of proper functioning (Rennard and Spurzen, 2006; Frampton *et al.*, 2006). Commonly used tests include measurement of VC, TLC, functional RV, tidal volume, airway resistance, and maximum flow. Additional tests evaluate the distribution of ventilation, lung and chest wall compliance, diffusion capacity, and the oxygen and carbon dioxide content of the arterial and venous blood.

Many pulmonary function tests require active collaboration by the subject examined, for example, the so-called FEV_1 (forced expiratory volume) during the first second of an active exhalation. This is an easy test to administer to humans, does not require sophisticated equipment or a hospital setting, and is completely noninvasive. The subject is asked first to inhale deeply and then to exhale the air as quickly as possible. The test is often used in epidemiological studies or controlled clinical studies designed to assess the potential adverse effects of air pollutants. A reduction in FEV_1 is usually indicative of impaired ventilation such as that found in restrictive (increased lung stiffness) or obstructive (obstructed airflow) lung disease.

To accomplish proper oxygenation of venous blood and elimination of CO_2, the gases have to diffuse across the air-blood barrier. Gas exchange may be hindered by the accumulation of fluids or cellular elements in the alveoli (edema, pneumonic infiltrates), thickening of the alveolar wall (fibrosis), insufficient ventilation of the alveolar region (emphysema), or insufficient presence of oxygen transport elements (reduced alveolar blood volume or reduced amount of hemoglobin in the blood). Gas exchange can be evaluated by measuring the arterial partial pressure of both oxygen and CO_2.

In general, blood gas analysis is a comparatively insensitive assay for disturbed ventilation because of the organisms' buffering and reserve capacities, but may be a useful tool in clinical medicine. Measurement of diffusion capacity with CO, a gas that binds with 250 times higher affinity to hemoglobin than does oxygen, is more sensitive. The test is easy to perform in humans and laboratory animals and is widely used in clinical studies.

Proper lung function in humans can be evaluated with several additional techniques. Computed tomography provides detailed roentgenographic information of airways and lung parenchyma. Increased concentrations of nitric oxide are often found in exhaled air when inflammatory processes have led to induction of iNOS. Fiberoptic bronchoscopy has become one of the most valuable tools for the detection of toxic lung injury. The procedure allows direct visual inspection of the major lobar and segmental airways; the depth of penetration is limited by the external diameter of the bronchoscope, usually 5 mm. Bronchoscopy also allows the introduction and retrieval of saline solutions into the lung and subsequent analysis for cellular and molecular constituents (broncholveolar lavage). Excision of small tissue samples (biopsies) during bronchoscopy is an additional diagnostic tool, most helpful in the evaluation and staging of precancerous and cancerous lesions.

Studies Being Done in Animals

The toxicology of inhaled materials has been and continues to be extensively studied in experimental animals. In such studies, selection of animals with a respiratory system similar to that of humans is particularly desirable. The respiratory system of monkeys most closely resembles that of humans. However, the availability and cost of these animals and the necessity for special facilities for housing monkeys and performing long-term exposures, along with ethical considerations, including the confinement of primates in small exposure chambers for prolonged periods, severely limit the use of primates. Rats and mice are widely used, although fundamental differences in respiratory anatomy (for example, lack of respiratory bronchioles) and function (rats and mice are obligate nose breathers) can complicate the extrapolation of effects to humans. Experimental studies with guinea pigs and rabbits provided the first conclusive evidence that sulfuric acid and SO_2 may damage human lungs (Amdur, 1989). The following techniques are used to study the effects of inhaled toxicants in animals.

Inhalation Exposure Systems

In inhalation studies, animals are kept within a chamber that is ventilated with a defined test atmosphere. Generation of such an atmosphere is comparatively easy for gases that are available in high purity in a compressed tank, for example, SO_2, O_2, or NO_2. Metering and dilution produce appropriate concentrations for exposure. Final concentrations within the chamber need to be monitored with suitable detectors (e.g., UV for ozone or infrared for CO_2) that need frequent calibration (and usually a computer to process the tremendous amount of data generated). Alternatively, labor-intensive wet chemical analysis procedures are applied after sampled gases from the chambers are bubbled through traps. More challenging is the generation of complex mixtures, such as tobacco smoke, diesel, and gasoline exhaust or residual oil fly ash, particularly because of the possibility of interactions between individual mixture constituents and the possibility of formation of artifacts (Pauluhn, 2005).

Exposure chambers must allow for the rapid attainment of the desired concentrations of toxicants, maintenance of desired toxicant levels homogeneously throughout the chamber, adequate capacity for experimental animals, and minimal accumulation of undesired products associated with animal occupancy (usually ammonia, dander, heat, and carbon dioxide). As a general rule, the total body volume of the animals should not exceed 5% of the chamber volume. Nose-only exposure chambers avoid some of these problems. However, nose-only exposure systems create different problems, including a great deal of stress on the animals due to confinement during exposure, and the very labor intensive handling that is required for exposures by this route. The proper selection of exposure techniques for a given chemical is ultimately a decision that must be made on a case-by-case basis. Finally, concern for the environment and the safety of facility personnel suggest prudence in how chambers are exhausted.

Pulmonary Function Tests in Experimental Animals

Conducting pulmonary function tests in experimental animals poses distinct challenges. Experimental animals cannot be made to maximally inhale or exhale at the investigators will. For example, FEV_1 can be obtained in experimental animals only under anesthesia. Expiration is forced by applying external pressure to the thorax or negative pressure to the airways. On the other hand, analysis of pressure-volume curves is a comparatively easy test to perform in animals, requiring little as far as specialized apparatus is concerned. The test provides some indication of lung compliance. Compliance (volume/pressure) is calculated as the slope of the volume-pressure curve; it gives some indication of the intrinsic elastic properties of the lung parenchyma and, when measured in vivo, the thoracic cage. Cannulation of excised lungs and attachment to a syringe and manometer to quantify volume and pressure are all that is needed. Volume-pressure curves can be obtained from lungs filled with air or physiological saline. The latter test is much more sensitive to structural changes in lung parenchyma, as the effects of surfactant are eliminated in a saline-filled lung. Another test widely used is analysis of breathing patterns (respiratory frequency). This technique allows one to differentiate between sensory upper airway irritants and "pulmonary" irritants. Highly water soluble irritants such as ammonia, chlorine, and formaldehyde produce upper respiratory tract irritation, whereas less soluble gases such as nitrogen dioxide and ozone generate pulmonary irritation. The sensory irritant pattern has been described as slowing down respiratory frequency while increasing TV. Pulmonary irritants usually increase respiratory frequency and decrease minute volume. The result is rapid, shallow breathing.

Morphologic Techniques

The pathology of acute and chronic injury may be described after examination of the respiratory tract by gross inspection and under the microscope. Morphologic evaluation should not be limited to the peripheral lung; nasal passages, the larynx, and major airways must be examined as carefully as is the lung parenchyma.

Careful consideration must be given to tissue fixation and preparation. Nasal passages must be flushed with fixative. After decalcification, cross sections should be cut at multiple levels; the regional distribution of lesions may vary from agent to agent. Proper fixation of the lung is done by vascular perfusion with fixative through the pulmonary artery or by instillation of fixative through the trachea. Perfusion fixation does not dislodge material (lining fluid, deposited particles) or cells in the lumen of the airways or the alveoli from their original position. Fixation by instillation does this, but it also keeps the alveoli open. It is done under controlled pressure, usually 30 cm H_2O, and is required if semiquantitative or quantitative measurements are to be made. The choice of fixative depends on how the lung will be further analyzed. Formalin-based fixatives are satisfactory for routine histopathology, whereas the use of more sophisticated techniques such as electron microscopy, immunohistochemistry, and in situ hybridization require careful selection of the fixative.

Ordinary paraffin sections of respiratory tract tissue are suitable for routine histopathologic analysis; gross pathologic changes such as inflammation and the presence of cancerous tissue can be detected easily. Plastic or Epon sections about 1 μm thick are required for proper identification of different cell types lining the airways or alveoli and for recognition of cytoplasmic changes in damaged Clara cells. Other structural alterations, such as degenerative changes or necrosis of type I epithelial cells or capillary endothelial cells, usually are detected by transmission electron microscopy (TEM). TEM is essential for an unequivocal identification of cells in the alveolar interstitium and is used mainly in morphometric analysis of the lung. Scanning electron microscopy allows visualization of the surface of interior lung structures, reveals alterations in the tissue surface, and detects rearrangement of the overall cell population. Confocal microscopy, consisting of a laser microscope coupled to a computer, allows examination of thick sections and discovery of specific cell types deep within the tissue labeled with fluorescent markers; it is an ideal tool for three-dimensional reconstruction of normal and damaged lung.

Morphometry, the quantitative description of structure, refers to a quantitative analysis of tissue (Gehr *et al.*, 1993). Measurements made in two dimensions on photographs taken under the microscope allow one to measure areas, the thickness of a structure, and numerical density. With the help of appropriate formulas, values such as the volume occupied by a specific cell population in the entire lung parenchyma can be calculated.

Additional tools for the study of toxic lung injury include immunohistochemistry, in situ hybridization, analysis of cell kinetics and gene expression profiling. Antibodies to a variety of enzymes, mediators, and other proteins are available. It is possible to identify cell types that carry certain enzymes and their anatomic locations. In situ hybridization allows one to visualize anatomic sites where a specific gene product is expressed, for example, collagen production in a fibrotic lung. Ascribing a given metabolic capability to a specific cell type requires evaluation of gene expression and/or protein production in specific cells in situ. The normal adult lung is an organ for which under normal circumstances very few cells appear to die and to be replaced. When damaged by a toxic insult, the lung parenchyma is capable of repairing itself in an efficient manner (Witschi, 1997). Type I cell damage is followed by proliferation of type II epithelial cells which eventually transform into new type I

cells; in the airways, the Clara cells proliferate and divide following injury to ciliated cells. Quantitative data can be obtained by either injection of the DNA precursors tritated thymide, bromodeoxyuridine or visualization of proliferating cell nuclear antigen (PCNA). Flow cytometry is valuable in the study of cell populations prepared from the lung.

Pulmonary Lavage

Pulmonary edema and/or pulmonary inflammation appear to be obligate early events in acute and chronic lung injury. The fluid lining the pulmonary epithelium can be recovered by bronchoalveolar lavage. Analysis of the lavage fluid is a useful tool to detect respiratory tract toxicity (Henderson, 2005). Generally, the lungs of exposed and control animals are washed with multiple small volumes of isotonic saline. This technique has the further advantage of allowing direct comparisons with data accessible from normal human volunteers or patients undergoing bronchopulmonary lavage for therapeutic purposes. Influx of neutrophils or other leukocytes such as lymphocytes or eosinophils into the lavage fluid is the most sensitive sign of inflammation. Additional measurements include secretory products of macrophages and epithelial cells such as tumor necrosis factor alpha, fibronectin, interleukin-1, various chemotactic factors such as IL-8 and MIP-2. Reduced glutathione levels may be an indicator of oxidative stress. Lactate dehydrogenase activity (and its substituent isoenzymes), N-acetylglucosaminidase, acid or alkaline phosphatase, other lysosomal hydrolases, lavageable total protein and/or albumin, and sialic acid add additional information.

In Vitro Approaches

In vitro systems with materials originally obtained either from human tissues or from experimental animals are particularly suited for the study of mechanisms that cause lung injury. The following systems are widely used (Aufderheide, 2005; Allen, 2006).

Isolated Perfused Lung

The isolated perfused lung method is applicable to lungs from many laboratory animal species (rabbit, rat, mouse, guinea pig). The lung, in situ or excised, is perfused with blood or a blood substitute through the pulmonary arterial bed. At the same time, the lung is actively (through rhythmic inflation-deflation cycles with positive pressure) or passively (by creating negative pressure with an artificial thorax in which the lung is suspended) ventilated. Toxic agents can be introduced into the perfusate or the inspired air. Repeated sampling of the perfusate allows one to determine the rate of metabolism of drugs and the metabolic activity of the lung.

Microdissection

Many inhalants act in circumscribed regions of the respiratory tract, such as the terminal bronchioles, a region especially rich in the highly metabolically competent Clara cells. Microdissection of the airways consists of the stripping of the surrounding parenchyma away from the small bronchi and terminal bronchioli (Plopper *et al.*, 1991; Fanucchi *et al.*, 1999). This facilitates study of the metabolically active Clara cells found in the airways. Microdissected airways can be maintained in culture for up to 1 week (Van Winkle *et al.*, 1996), can be used to study site specific gene expression, morphologic changes in response to toxicants or during repair or can be used for biochemical reactions including enzyme activity measures and determination of native antioxidant concentrations (such as glutathione).

Organotypic Cell Culture Systems

Tissue culture systems have been developed in which epithelial cells maintain their polarity, differentiation, and normal function similar to what is observed in vivo. Epithelial cell surfaces are exposed to air (or a gas phase containing an airborne toxic agent), while the basal portion is bathed by a tissue culture medium. Maintenance of the epithelial cells at the air–liquid interface is important to maintain polarity and differentiation. Epithelial cells may be seeded on top of a suitable supporting material (e.g., collagen or nitrocellulose membranes) with mesenchymal cells seeded on the other side to observe epithelial cell–fibroblast interactions.

Isolated Lung Cell Populations

Many specific lung cell types have been isolated and maintained as primary cultures in vitro. Alveolar macrophages are easily obtained from human and animal lungs by lavage. Their function can be examined in vitro with or without exposure to appropriate toxic stimuli. Type II alveolar epithelial cells are isolated after digestion of the lung. Direct isolation of type I epithelial cells has also been successful. Systems for the isolation and culture of Clara cells and neuroepithelial cells are available. Lung fibroblasts are easily grown and have been studied in coculture with epithelial cells. Multiple primary cell cultures and cell lines have been established from lung tumors found in experimental animals and humans. Isolated cell techniques suffer from possible enzymatic digestion of critical cellular components and the loss of the normal integration of the many cell types within the tissue layers which may be important for maintenance of normal function. Caution should be exercised in the final interpretation of experiments utilizing this approach.

REFERENCES

Alarie Y, Nielsen GD, Abraham MD: A theoretical approach to the Ferguson principle and its use with nonreactive and reactive airborne chemicals. *Pharmacol Toxicol* 83:270–279, 1998.

Allen CB: In vitro models for lung toxicology, in Gardner DE (ed.): *Toxicology of the Lung*, 4th ed. Boca Raton: CRC Press, Taylor & Francis, 2006, pp. 107–150.

Amdur MO: Sulfuric acid: The animals tried to tell us. 1989 Herbert Stokinger Lecture. *Appl Ind Hyg* 4:189–197, 1989.

Aufderheide M: Direct exposure methods for testing native atmospheres. *Exp Toxicol Pathol* 57 (Suppl 1):213–226, 2005.

Barbarin V, Arras M, Misson P, *et al.*: Characterization of the effect of interleukin-10 on silica-induced lung fibrosis in mice. *Am J Respir Cell Mol Biol* 31:78–85, 2004.

Beeson WL, Abbey DE, Knutsen SF: Long-term concentrations of ambient air pollutants and incident lung cancer in California adults: Results from the ASHMOG study. *Environ Health Persp* 106:813–823, 1998.

Bond J A, Harkema J R, Russell V I: Regional distribution of xenobiotic metabolizing enzymes in respiratory airways of dogs. *Drug Metab Dispos* 16:116–124, 1988.

Buckpitt AR, Cruikshank MK: Biochemical function of the respiratory tract: Metabolism of xenobiotics, in Sipes IG, McQueen CA, Gandolfi JA (eds.): *Comprehensive Toxicology, Vol 8, Toxicology of the Respiratory System*. Oxford: Elsevier Science, 1997, pp. 159–186.

Cascorbi I: Genetic basis of toxic reactions to drugs and chemicals. *Toxicol Lett* 162:16–28, 2006.

Cross CE, van der Vliet A, Louie S, Thiele JJ, Halliwell B: Oxidative stress and antioxidants at biosurfaces: Plants, skin, and respiratory tract surfaces. *Environ Health Persp* 106 (Suppl 5):1241–1251, 1998.

Ding X, Kaminsky LS: Human extrahepatic cytochromes P450: Function in xenobiotic metabolism and tissue-selective chemical toxicity in the respiratory and gastrointestinal tracts. *Annu Rev Pharmacol Toxicol* 43:149–173, 2003.

Dockery DW, Pope III CA, Xu X, *et al.*: An association between air pollution and mortality in six U.S. cities. *N Engl J Med* 329:1753–1759, 1993.

Fanucchi M: Development of antioxidant and xenobiotic metabolizing enzyme systems, in Harding R, Pinkerton KE, Plopper CG (eds.): *The Lung. Development, Aging and the Environment*. Holland: Elsevier, 2004, pp. 177–185.

Fanucchi MV, Plopper CG: Environmental toxicants and lung development in experimental models, in Harding R, Pinkerton KE, Plopper CG (eds.): *The Lung. Development, Aging and the Environment*. Holland: Elsevier, 2004, pp. 345–351.

Fanucchi MV, Plopper CG, Harkema JR, Hotchkiss JA: In vitro culture of microdissected rat nasal airway tissues. *Am J Respir Cell Mol Biol* 20:1274–1285, 1999.

Frampton MW, Pietropaoli AP, Morrow PE, Utell MJ: Human clinical studies of airborne pollutants, in Gardner DE (ed.): *Toxicology of the Lung*, 4th ed. Boca Raton: CRC Press, Taylor & Francis, 2006, pp. 1–28.

Gehr P, Geiser M, Stone KC, Crapo JD: Morphometric analysis of the gas exchange region of the lung, in Gardner DE, Crapo JD, McClellan RO (eds.): *Toxicology of the Lung*, 2nd ed. New York: Raven Press, 1993, pp. 111–154.

Gibby EM, Cohen GM: Conjugation of 1-naphthol by human bronchus and bronchoscopy samples. *Biochem Pharmacol* 33:739–743, 1984.

Giri SN: Novel pharmacological approaches to manage interstitial lung fibrosis in the twenty-first century. *Annu Rev Pharmacol Toxicol* 43:73–95, 2003.

Haschek WM, Witschi HP, Nikula K: Respiratory System, in Haschek WM, Rousseaux CG, Wallig MA (eds.): *Handbook of Toxicologic Pathology*, 2nd ed., Vol 2. Academic Press, 2002, pp. 3–83.

He D, Frost AR, Falany CN: Identification and immunohistochemical localization of Sulfotransferase 2B1b (SULT2B1b) in human lung. *Biochim Biophys Acta* 1724:119–126, 2005.

Hecht SS: Tobacco smoke carcinogens and lung cancer. *J Natl Cancer Inst* 91:1194–1210, 1999.

Henderson RF: Use of bronchoalveolar lavage to detect respiratory tract toxicity of inhaled material. *Exp Toxicol Pathol* 57 (Suppl 1):155–159, 2005.

Huczko A, Lange H, Clko E, Grubeck-Jaworska H, Droszcz P: Physiological testing of carbon nanotubules: Are they asbestos like? *Fullerene Sci Technol* 9:251–254, 2001.

Hukkanen J, Pelkonen O, Hakkola J, Raunio H: Expression and regulation of xenobiotic-metabolizing cytochrome P450 (CYP) enzymes in human lung. *CRC Crit Rev Toxicol* 32:391–411, 2002.

Hutt JA, Vuillemenot BR, Barr EB, *et al.*: Life-span inhalation exposure to mainstream cigarette smoke induces lung cancer in B6C3F1 mice through genetic and epigenetic pathways. *Carcinogenesis* 26:1999–2009, 2005.

IARC (International Agency for Research on Cancer): IARC monographs on the evaluation of carcinogenic risks to humans, in *Beryllium, Cadmium, Mercury and Exposures in the Glass Manufacturing Industry*, Vol 58. Lyon, France: IARC, 1993.

IARC (International Agency for Research on Cancer): IARC monographs on the evaluation of the carcinogenic risk of chemicals to humans, in *Tobacco Smoke and Involuntary Smoking*, Vol 83. Lyon, France: IARC, 2004.

ILSI Risk Science Institute Workshop: The relevance of the rat lung response to particle overload for human risk assessment. *Inhal Toxicol* 12:1–148, 2000.

Joad J: Effects of environmental tobacco smoke on lung development, in Harding R, Pinkerton KE, Plopper CG (eds.): *The Lung. Development, Aging and the Environment*. Holland: Elsevier, 2004, pp. 291–299.

Kimball JS, Miller F: Regional respiratory-tract absorption of inhaled reactive gases: A modeling approach, in Gardner DE, Crapo JD, McClellan RO (eds.): *Toxicology of the Lung,* 3rd ed. Philadelphia: Taylor & Francis, 1999, pp. 557–597.

Lam CW, James JT, McCluskey R, Hunter RL: Pulmonary toxicity of single-wall carbon nanotubes in mice 7 and 90 days after intratracheal instillation. *Toxicol Sci* 77:126–134, 2004.

Lazard D, Zupko K, Poria Y, et al.: Odorant signal termination by olfactory UDP glucuronosyl transferase. *Nature* 349:790–793, 1991.

Lin CY, Boland BC, Lee YJ, et al.: Identification of proteins adducted by reactive metabolites of naphthalene and 1-nitronaphthalene in dissected airways of rhesus macaques. *Proteomics* 6:972–982, 2006.

Lin CY, Isbell MA, Morin D, et al.: Characterization of a structurally intact in situ lung model and comparison of naphthalene protein adducts generated in this model vs lung microsomes. *Chem Res Toxicol* 18:802–813, 2005.

Ling G, Gu J, Genter MB, Zhuo X, Ding X: Regulation of cytochrome P450 gene expression in the olfactory mucosa. *Chem Biol Interact* 147:247–258, 2004.

Matheson JM, Lange RW, Lemus R, Karol MH, Luster MI: Importance of inflammatory and immune components in a mouse model of airway reactivity to toluene diisocyanate (TDI). *Clin Exp Allergy* 31:1067–1076, 2001.

Mauderly JL, Gigliotti AP, Barr EB, et al.: Chronic inhalation exposure to mainstream cigarette smoke increases lung and nasal tumor incidence in rats. *Toxicol Sci* 81:280–292, 2004.

Medinsky MA, Bond JA, Schlosser PM, Morris JB: Mechanisms and models for respiratory-tract uptake of volatile organic chemicals, in Gardner DE, Crapo JD, McClellan RO (eds.): *Toxicology of the Lung*, 3rd ed. Philadelphia: Taylor & Francis, 1999, pp. 483–512.

Mercer RR, Crapo JD: Architecture of the acinus, in Parent RA (ed.): *Treatise on Pulmonary Toxicology: Comparative Biology of the Normal Lung*. Boca Raton, FL: CRC Press, 1991, pp. 109–120.

Miller F: Dosimetry of particles in laboratory animals and humans, in Gardner DE, Crapo JD, McClellan RO (eds.): *Toxicology of the Lung*, 3rd ed. Philadelphia: Taylor & Francis, 1999, pp. 513–555.

Miyawaki A, Homma H, Tamura H, Matsui M, Mikoshiba K: Zonal distribution of sulfotransferase for phenol in olfactory sustentacular cells. *Embo J* 15:2050–2055, 1996.

Morrow PE: Dust overloading in the lungs: Update and appraisal. *Toxicol Appl Phamacol* 113:1–12, 1992.

NCI (National Cancer Institute): *Health Effects of Exposure to Environmental Tobacco Smoke: The Report of the California Environmental Protection Agency*. Smoking and Tobacco Control Monograph No. 10. Bethesda, MD: U.S. Department of Health and Human Services, National Institutes of Health, National Cancer Institute, NIH Pub. No. 99-4645, 1999.

O'Byrne PM, Postma DS: The many faces of airway inflammation. *Am J Respir Crit Care Med* 159:541–566, 1999.

Oberdorster G, Oberdorster E, Oberdorster J: Nanotoxicology: An emerging discipline evolving from studies of ultrafine particles. *Environ Health Perspect* 113:823–839, 2005a.

Oberdorster G, Maynard A, Donaldson K, et al.: ILSI Research Foundation/Risk Science Institute Nanomaterial Toxicity Screening Working Group. Principles for characterizing the potential human health effects from exposure to nanomaterials: Elements of a screening strategy. *Part Fibre Toxicol* 2:8, 2005b.

Pauluhn J: Overview of inhalation exposure techniques: Strengths and weaknesses. *Exp ToxicolPathol* 57 (Suppl 1):111–128, 2005.

Pinkerton KE, Gehr P, Crapo JD: Architecture and cellular composition of the air-blood barrier, in Parent RA (ed.): *Treatise on Pulmonary Toxicology: Comparative Biology of the Normal Lung*. Boca Raton, FL: CRC Press, 1991, pp. 121–128.

Plopper C, Winkle LV, Fanucchi M, et al.: Early events in naphthalene-induced acute Clara cell toxicity: II. Comparison of glutathione depletion and histopathology by airway location. *Am J Resp Cell Mol Biol* 24:272–281, 2001a.

Plopper CG, Chang AM, Pang A, Buckpitt AR: Use of microdissected airways to define metabolism and cytotoxicity in murine bronchiolar epithelium. *ExpLung Res* 17:197–212, 1991.

Plopper CG, Buckpitt A, Evans M, et al.: Factors modulating the epithelial response to toxicants in tracheobronchial airways. *Toxicology* 160:173–80, 2001b.

Pope III CA, Burnett RT, Thurston GD, et al.: Cardiovascular mortality and longterm exposure to particulate air pollution: Epidemiological evidence of general pathophysiological pathways of disease. *Circulation* 109:71–77, 2004.

Quan TE, Cowper SE, Bucala R: The role of circulating fibrocytes in fibrosis. *Curr Rheumatol Rep* 8:145–150, 2006.

Raabe OG: Respiratory exposure to air pollutants, in Swift DL, Foster WM (eds.): *Air Pollutants and the Respiratory Tract*. New York: Marcel Dekker, 1999, pp. 39–73.

Rahman I: Oxidative stress, chromatin remodeling and gene transcription inflammation and chronic lung diseases. *J Biochem Mol Biol* 36:95–109, 2003.

Ramazzini B: *Disease of Workers*. Transl. from the Latin text *De Morbis Artificum* by Wright WC. New York, London: Hafner, 1964.

Ramu K, Kehrer JP.: The pulmonary toxicity of chemotherapeutic agents, in Sipes IG, McQueen CA, Gandolfi JA (eds.): *Comprehensive Toxicology,* Vol 8, *Toxicology of the Respiratory System*. Oxford: Elsevier Science, 1997, pp. 521–541.

Rennard SI, Spurzen JR: Methods for evaluating the lung in human subjects, in Gardner DE (ed.): *Toxicology of the Lung*, 4th ed. Boca Raton: CRC Press, Taylor & Francis, 2006, pp. 1–28.

Shehin-Johnson SE, Williams DE, Larsen-Su S, Stresser DM, Hines RN: Tissue specific expression of flavin-containing monooxygenase (FMO) forms 1 and 2 in the rabbit. *J Pharmacol Exp Ther* 272:1293–1299, 1995.

Shultz MA, Choudary PV, Buckpitt AR: Role of murine cytochrome P-450 2F2 in metabolic activation of naphthalene and metabolism of other xenobiotics. *J Exp Ther* 290:281–288, 1999.

Smiley-Jewell S, Van Winkle LS: Repair of environmental lung injury during development, in Harding R, Pinkerton KE, Plopper CG (eds.): *The Lung. Development, Aging and the Environment*. Holland: Elsevier, 2004, pp. 353–362.

Smith BJ, Curtis JF, Eling TE: Bioactivation of xenobiotics by prostaglandin H synthase. *Chem Biol Interact* 79:245–264, 1991.

Snider GL, Kleinerman J, Thurlbeck WM, Bengali ZH: The definition emphysema: Report of a National Heart, Lung, and Blood Institute workshop. *Am Rev Respir Dis* 132:182–185, 1985.

Tamura HO, Harada Y, Miyawaki A, Mikoshiba K, Matsui M: Molecular cloning and expression of a cDNA encoding an olfactory-specific mouse phenol sulphotransferase. *Biochem J* 331 (Pt 3): 953–958, 1998.

Upadhyay D, Kamp DW: Asbestos-induced pulmonary toxicity: Role of DNA damage and apoptosis. *Exp Biol Med* (Maywood) 228:650–659, 2003.

Van Winkle LS, Buckpitt AR, Plopper CG: Maintenance of differentiated murine Clara cells in microdissected airway cultures. *Am J Respir Cell Mol Biol* 14:586–598, 1996.

Warheit DB, Laurence BR, Reed KL, Roach DH, Reynolds GA, Webb TR: Comparative pulmonary toxicity assessment of single-wall carbon nanotubes in rats. *Toxicol Sci* 77:117–125, 2004.

Warheit DB, Webb TR, Sayes CM, Colvin VL, Reed KL: Pulmonary instillation studies with nanoscale TiO2 rods and dots in rats: Toxicity is not dependent upon particle size and surface area. *Toxicol Sci* 91:227–236, 2006.

Weibel ER: Is the lung built reasonably? The 1983 J. Burns Anderson lecture. *Am Rev Respir Dis* 128:752–760, 1983.

West JA, Chichester CH, Buckpitt AR, *et al.*: Heterogeneity of clara cell glutathione. A possible basis for differences in cellular responses to pulmonary cytotoxicants. *Am J Respir Cell Mol Biol* 23:27–36, 2000.

West JA, Van Winkle LS, Morin D, *et al.*: Repeated inhalation exposures of the bioactivated cytotoxicant naphthalene (NA) produce airway specific clara cell tolerance in mice. *Toxicol Sci* 190:286–293, 2003.

Whetstine JR, Yueh MF, McCarver DG, *et al.*: Ethnic differences in human flavin-containing monooxygenase 2 (FMO2) polymorphisms: Detection of expressed protein in African-Americans. *Toxicol Appl Pharmacol* 168:216–224, 2000.

Whitby-Logan GK, Weech M, Walters E: Zonal expression and activity of glutathione S-transferase enzymes in the mouse olfactory mucosa. *Brain Res* 995:151–157, 2004.

Wistuba II, Gazdar AF: Charactetristic genetic alterations in lung cancer, in Driscoll B (ed.): *Lung Cancer Volume 1: Molecular Pathology Methods and Reviews*. Totowa NJ: Humana Press, 2003, pp. 3–28.

Witschi HP: Cell damage and cell renewal in the lung, in Sipes IG, McQueen CA, Gandolfi JA (eds.): *Comprehensive Toxicology* Vol 8, ed. RA Roth, *Toxicology of the Respiratory System*. Oxford Elsevier Science, 1997, pp. 231–248.

Zhang HY, Phan S: Inhibition of myofibroblast apoptosis by transforming growth factor β_1, *Am J Respir Cell Mol Biol* 21:658–665, 1999.

Zhong CY, Zhou YM, Joad FP, Pinkerton KE: Environmental tobacco smoke suppresses NF-KB signaling to increase apoptosis in infant moneky lungs. *Am J Resp Crit Care Med* 174:428–436, 2006.

TOXIC RESPONSES OF THE NERVOUS SYSTEM

Virginia C. Moser, Michael Aschner, Rudy J. Richardson, and Martin A. Philbert

OVERVIEW OF THE NERVOUS SYSTEM

Neurotoxicants and toxins have been extensively studied, both because of their toxic effects on humans and because of their utility in the study of the nervous system (NS). Many insights into the organization and function of the NS are based on observations derived from the action of neurotoxicants. The binding of exogenous compounds to membranes has been the basis for the definition of specific receptors within the brain; an understanding of the roles of different cell types in the function of the NS has stemmed from the selectivity of certain toxicants in injuring specific cell types while sparing others; and important differences in basic metabolic requirements of different subpopulations of neurons have been inferred from the effects of toxicants.

It is estimated that millions of people worldwide are exposed to known neurotoxicants each year, a fact underscored by repeated outbreaks of neurologic disease (Federal Register, 1994). An even larger potential problem stems from the incomplete information on many compounds that may have neurotoxic effects. Unknown is the extent to which neurologic disability may be related to chronic low-level exposures, nor do we understand the overall impact of environmental contaminants on brain function.

In order to study neurotoxicologic consequences of chemical exposures, one must understand the structure, function, and development of the NS. These features can be quite complex, with dif-

ferential anatomy, physiology, and cell types specific for location and function. Several general aspects modulate the NS response to chemicals, including (1) the privileged status of the NS with the maintenance of a biochemical barrier between the brain and the blood, (2) the importance of the high energy requirements of the brain, (3) the spatial extensions of the NS as long cellular processes and the requirements of cells with such a complex geometry, (4) the maintenance of an environment rich in lipids, (5) the transmission of information across extracellular space at the synapse, (6) the distances over which electrical impulses must be transmitted, coordinated and integrated, and (7) development and regenerative patterns of the nervous system. Each of these features of the NS carries with it specialized metabolic/physiological requirements and unique vulnerabilities to toxic compounds.

Blood–Brain Barrier

The NS is protected from the adverse effects of many potential toxicants by an anatomic barrier. In 1885, Ehrlich noticed that dyes did not distribute into the brain and spinal cord, while other tissues became stained. Conversely, when injected into the brain, the dye did not appear in the periphery. This observation pointed to the existence of an interface between the blood and the brain, or a "blood–brain barrier." Most of the brain, spinal cord, retina, and peripheral NS

(PNS) maintain this barrier with the blood, with selectivity similar to the interface between cells and the extracellular space. The principal basis of the blood–brain barrier is thought to be specialized endothelial cells in the brain's microvasculature, aided, at least in part, by interactions with glia (Kniesel and Wolburg, 2000). In addition to this interface with blood, the brain, spinal cord, and peripheral nerves are also completely covered with a continuous lining of specialized cells that limits the entry of molecules from adjacent tissue. In the brain and spinal cord, this is the meningeal surface; in peripheral nerves, each fascicle of nerve is surrounded by perineurial cells.

Among the unique properties of endothelial cells in the NS is the presence of tight junctions between cells (Kniesel and Wolburg, 2000; Rubin and Staddon, 1999). Thus, molecules must pass through membranes of endothelial cells, rather than between them, as they do in other tissues. The blood–brain barrier also contains transporters, such as the multidrug-resistant protein, which transport some xenobiotics that have diffused through endothelial cells back into the blood. If not actively transported into the brain, the penetration of toxicants is largely related to their lipid solubility and to their ability to pass through the plasma membranes of the cells forming the barrier (Pardridge, 1999; Stewart, 2000). There are, however, important exceptions to this general rule. In the mature NS, the spinal and autonomic ganglia as well as a small number of other sites within the brain, called *circumventricular organs,* do not contain specialized endothelial tight junctions and are not protected by blood-tissue barriers. Rather, a somewhat less tight barrier is provided by several layers of overlapping astrocytic foot processes. Indeed, it is this cellular anatomical arrangement that allows the endocrine-regulating components of the circumventricular organs to sense changes in blood hormone levels and respond accordingly. This discontinuity of the barrier allows entry of some chemicals, for example, the anticancer drug doxorubicin, into the sensory ganglia. This is the basis for the selective neurotoxicity of this compound to ganglionic neurons (Spencer, 2000). The blood–brain barrier is incompletely developed at birth and even less so in premature infants. This predisposes the premature infant to brain injury by toxins, such as unconjugated bilirubin or hexachlorophene, that later in life are excluded from the NS (Lucey *et al.*, 1964; Mullick, 1973).

Energy Requirements

Neurons and cardiac myocytes share the property of conduction of electrical impulses, and their critical dependence on aerobic respiration is due to the high metabolic demand associated with the maintenance and repetitive reinstitution of ion gradients. Membrane depolarizations and repolarizations occur with such frequency that these cells must be able to produce large quantities of high-energy phosphates even in a resting state. That the energy requirements of the brain are related to membrane depolarizations is supported by the fact that hyperactivity, as in epileptic foci, increases the energy requirements by as much as fivefold (Plum and Posner, 1985). The dependence on a continual source of energy, in the absence of energy reserves, places the neuron in a vulnerable position. To meet these high energy requirements, the brain utilizes aerobic glycolysis and, therefore, is extremely sensitive to even brief interruptions in the supply of oxygen or glucose.

Exposure to toxicants that inhibit aerobic respiration (e.g., cyanide) or to conditions that produce hypoxia (e.g., carbon monoxide, or CO poisoning) leads to the early signs of dysfunction in the myocardium and neurons. Damage to the NS under these conditions is a combination of direct toxic effects on neurons and secondary damage from systemic hypoxia or ischemia. For example, acute CO poisoning damages those structures in the central nervous system (CNS) that are most vulnerable to hypoxia: the neurons in specific regions of the basal ganglia and hippocampus, certain layers of the cerebral cortex, and the cerebellar Purkinje cells. Experiments utilizing several different laboratory animal species have shown that systemic hypotension is the best predictor of these lesions following CO poisoning; however, CO poisoning may also produce white matter damage, and this leukoencephalopathy may result from a primary effect of CO in the CNS (Penny, 1990). As with CO, survivors of cyanide poisoning may develop lesions in the CNS that are characteristic of systemic hypoxic or ischemic injury, and experiments in rats and monkeys have led to the conclusion that global hypoperfusion, rather than direct histotoxicity, is the major cause of CNS damage (Auer and Benveniste, 1997). 3-Nitropropionic acid (3-NP), a naturally occurring mycotoxin, is an irreversible inhibitor of succinate dehydrogenase that produces adenosine triphosphate (ATP) depletion in cerebral cortical explants and is associated with motor disorders in livestock and humans that have ingested contaminated food (Ludolph *et al.*, 1991, 1992). Some investigators removed the complication of systemic toxicity by directly injecting 3-NP into specific regions of the brain. They have observed neuron degeneration mediated in part by excitotoxic mechanisms (Brouillet *et al.*, 1993a). These examples demonstrate the exquisite sensitivity of neurons to energy depletion and also underscore the complex relationships between direct neurotoxicity and the effects of systemic toxicity on the NS.

Axonal Transport

In the NS, impulses are conducted over great distances at rapid speed, and provide information about the environment to the organism in a coordinated manner that allows an organized response to be carried out at a specific site. However, the intricate organization of such a complex network places an unparalleled demand on the cells of the NS. Single cells, rather than being spherical and a few micrometers in diameter, are elongated and may extend over a meter in length.

The anatomy of such a complex cellular network creates features of metabolism and cellular geometry that are peculiar to the NS. The two immediate demands placed on the neuron are the maintenance of a larger cellular volume and the transport of intracellular materials over great distances. The length of neurons may exceed 200,000 times the dimensions of most other cells. For example, the cell body of a lower motor neuron is located in the spinal cord and the axon extends to the site of innervation of a muscle at a distant location. In spite of the smaller diameter of the axon, the length of the axon translates to an axonal volume that is hundreds of times greater than that of the cell body itself (Schwartz, 1991). The cellular machinery which provides protein synthesis to maintain this volume is readily visible in large neurons through the light microscope, as the Nissl substance, which is formed by clusters of ribosomal complexes for the synthesis of proteins (Parent, 1996). In fact, neurons are the only cell type with such a Nissl substance, reflecting the unusual demand for protein synthesis.

In addition to the increased burden of protein synthesis, the neuron is dependent on the ability to distribute materials over the distances encompassed by its processes. Protein synthesis occurs in the cell body, and the products are then transported to the appropriate site through the process of axonal transport. The assembly of the

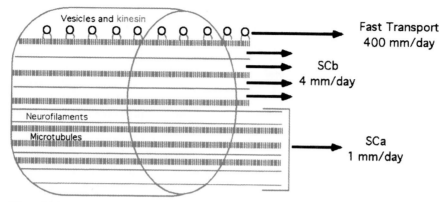

Figure 16-1. Axonal transport.

Fast axonal transport is depicted as spherical vesicles moving along microtubules with intervening microtubule-associated motors. The slow component A (SCa) represents the movement of the cytoskeleton, composed of neurofilaments and microtubules. Slow component b (SCb) moves at a faster rate than SCa and includes soluble proteins, which are apparently moving between the more slowly moving cytoskeleton.

cytoskeleton at tremendous distances from their site of synthesis in the cell body represents a formidable challenge (Nixon, 1998). Through studies of the movement of radiolabeled amino acid precursors, several major components of axonal transport are known (Grafstein, 1995). The fastest component, known as *fast axonal transport,* carries a large number of proteins, many of which are associated with vesicles (Grafstein, 1995). This ATP-dependent process reaches a rate of 400 mm/d (Fig. 16-1) and is dependent on microtubule-associated ATPase activity and motor proteins. These proteins, kinesin and dynein being the prototypes of a class of microtubule-associated motors, provide both the mechanochemical force in the form of a microtubule-associated ATPase and the interface between microtubules as the track and vesicles as the cargo. Vesicles are transported rapidly in an anterograde direction by kinesin and in a retrograde direction by dynein (Schnapp and Reese, 1989). In the axon, multiple waves of transport can be detected in the fast component of axonal transport (Mulugeta *et al.,* 2000).

The transport of some organelles, including mitochondria, constitutes an intermediate component of axonal transport, moving at 50 mm/d (Grafstein, 1995). As with the fast component, the function is apparently the continuous replacement of organelles within the axon. The slowest component of axonal transport represents the movement of the cytoskeleton itself (Fig. 16-1). The cytoskeleton is composed of structural elements, including microtubules formed by the association of tubulin subunits and neurofilaments formed by the association of three neurofilament protein subunits. Dynamic exchange of subunits of the filamentous structure has now been observed with high-resolution microscopy of living cells, indicating that stationary filamentous structures exchange subunits that move rapidly once dissociated (Wang *et al.,* 2000).

Neurofilaments and microtubules move at a rate of approximately 1 mm/d and make up the majority of SCa, which is the slowest-moving component of axonal transport (Hoffman and Lasek, 1975). Subunit structures appear to migrate and reassemble in a process that is dependent on nucleoside triphosphates, kinases, and phosphatases (Koehnle and Brown, 1999; Nixon, 1998). Moving at only a slightly more rapid rate of 2–4 mm/d in an anterograde direction, is SCb (Grafsteinx, 1995). Included in SCb are several structural proteins, such as the components of microfilaments (actin) and

several microfilament-associated proteins (M2 protein and fodrin), as well as clathrin and many soluble proteins.

This continual transport of proteins from the cell body through the various components of axonal transport is the mechanism through which the neuron provides the distal axon with its complement of functional and structural proteins. Some vesicles are also moving in a retrograde direction and provide the cell body with information concerning the status of the distal axon. The evidence for such a dynamic interchange of materials and information stems not only from the biochemical detection of these components of axonal transport, but also from the observations of the effects of terminating this interchange by severing the axon from its cell body. The result of transection of an axon is that the distal axon is destined to degenerate, a process known as axonal degeneration which is unique to the NS. The cell body of the neuron responds to the transection of the axon as well and undergoes a process of chromatolysis.

Axonal Degeneration

Current concepts of axonal degeneration were initially derived from nerve transections reported by Augustus Waller over a hundred years ago. Accordingly, the sequence of events that occur in the distal stump of an axon following transection is referred to as *Wallerian degeneration.* Because the axonal degeneration associated with chemical agents and some disease states is thought to occur through a similar sequence of events, it is often referred to as *Wallerian-like* axonal degeneration.

Following axotomy, there is degeneration of the distal nerve stump, followed by generation of a microenvironment supportive of regeneration and involving the distal axon, ensheathing glial cells and the blood nerve barrier. Initially there is a period during which the distal stump survives and maintains relatively normal structural, transport, and conduction properties. The duration of survival is proportional to the length of the axonal stump (Chaudry and Cornblath, 1992), and this relationship appears to be maintained across species. An exception has been noted in the C57/BL6/01a mouse, in which transected nerve fibers function electrically for 14–28 days (Lunn *et al.,* 1989). Although the underlying reason for slow degeneration in this mutant is unknown, the trait is transmitted by a dominant gene on chromosome 4 (Lyon *et al.,* 1993) and is an intrinsic

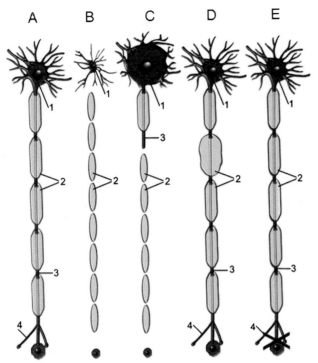

Figure 16-2. Patterns of neurotoxic injury.

(A) Normal neuron showing (1) cell body and dendrites, (2) myelinating cells, encircling the (3) axon, and (4) synapse. (B) A neuronopathy resulting from the death of the entire neuron. Astrocytes often proliferate in response to the neuronal loss, creating both neuronal loss and gliosis. (C) An axonopathy occurs when the axon is the primary site of injury, the axon degenerates, and the surviving neuron shows only chromatolysis with margination of its Nissl substance and nucleus to the cell periphery. (D) Myelinopathy resulting from disruption of myelin or from selective injury to the myelinating cells. To prevent cross-talk between adjacent axons, myelinating cells divide and cover the denuded axon rapidly; however, the process of remyelination is much less effective in the CNS than in the PNS. (E) Some forms of toxicity are due to interruption of the process of neurotransmission, either through blocking excitation or by excessive stimulation, rather than actual cell death.

property of the neuron that does not involve macrophages or Schwann cells (Glass *et al.*, 1993).

These dynamic relationships between the neuronal cell body and its axon are important in understanding the basic pathological responses to some axonal and neuronal injuries caused by neurotoxicants (Fig. 16-2). When the neuronal cell body has been lethally injured, it degenerates, in a process called *neuronopathy*. This is characterized by the loss of the cell body and all of its processes, with no potential for regeneration. However, when the injury is at the level of the axon, the axon may degenerate while the neuronal cell body continues to survive, a condition known as an *axonopathy*. In this setting, there is a potential for regeneration and recovery from the toxic injury as the axonal stump sprouts and regenerates.

Terminating the period of survival is an active proteolysis that digests the axolemma and axoplasm, leaving only a myelin sheath surrounding a swollen degenerate axon. Digestion of the axon appears to be an all-or-none event effected through endogenous proteases (Schlafer and Zimmerman, 1984) that are activated through increased levels of intracellular free Ca^{2+} (George *et al.*, 1995). Although it is established that degeneration of the most terminal portion of the axon occurs first, whether degeneration of the remainder

of the stump occurs from proximal to distal, distal to proximal, or simultaneously along its entire length remains a matter of debate. The active proteolysis phase occurs so rapidly in mammals that it has been difficult to define a spatial distribution.

In the PNS, Schwann cells respond to loss of axons by decreasing synthesis of myelin lipids, down-regulating genes encoding myelin proteins, and dedifferentiating to a premyelinating mitotic Schwann cell phenotype (Stoll and Muller, 1999). The proliferating Schwann cells align along the original basal lamina, which creates a tubular structure referred to as a band of Bungner. In addition to providing physical guidance for regenerating axons, these tubes provide trophic support from nerve growth factor, brain-derived nerve growth factor, insulin-like growth factor, and corresponding receptors produced by the associated Schwann cells. Resident macrophages distributed along the endothelium within the endoneurium and the denervated Schwann cells assist in clearing myelin debris, but the recruitment of hematogenous macrophages accounts for the removal of the majority of myelin. Infiltrating macrophages express complement receptor 3, and the presence of complement 3 on the surface of degenerating myelin sheaths facilitates opsonization. Another essential role of recruited circulating macrophages is the secretion of interleukin-1, which is responsible for stimulating production of nerve growth factor by Schwann cells. In contrast to the proteolysis of the axon, processing of myelin breakdown products proceeds in an established proximal-to-distal progression.

Investigations have shown that degeneration of the distal axonal stump after transection is an active, synchronized process that can be delayed experimentally through decreasing temperature, preventing the entry of extracellular Ca^{2+}, or inhibiting proteolysis by calpain II (George *et al.*, 1995). Accompanying events in glial cells and macrophages direct and facilitate the sprouting neurite originating from the surviving proximal axon that also undergoes changes in protein expression resembling a less differentiated state. The facilitation of regeneration in the peripheral nervous system by Schwann cells distinguishes it from the CNS, in which oligodendrocytes secrete inhibitory factors that impede neurite outgrowth. Eventually, though, even in the PNS, if axonal contact is not restored, Schwann cell numbers will decrease, bands of Bungner will disappear, and increased fibroblast collagen production will render regeneration increasingly unlikely.

Thus, a critical difference exists in the significance of axonal degeneration in the CNS compared with that in the PNS: peripheral axons can regenerate whereas central axons cannot. In the PNS, glial cells and macrophages create an environment supportive of axonal regeneration, and Schwann cells transplanted to the CNS maintain this ability. In the CNS, release of inhibitory factors from damaged myelin and astrocyte scarring actually interfere with regeneration (Qiu, 2000). Interestingly, when this glial interference is removed through transplantation of CNS neurons to the PNS, the neurons are capable of extending neurites. But there appears to be more than just glial interference to account for the lack of CNS regeneration. The observation that embryonic neurons can overcome glial interference when placed into the adult NS is consistent with the development of an intrinsic sensitivity to inhibitory factors during maturation. Therefore, the inability of the CNS to regenerate appears to be due to both unfavorable environmental glial factors and properties of the mature neuron. The clinical relevance of the disparity between the CNS and PNS is that partial recovery, or, in mild cases, complete recovery, can occur after axonal degeneration in the PNS, whereas the same event is irreversible in the CNS.

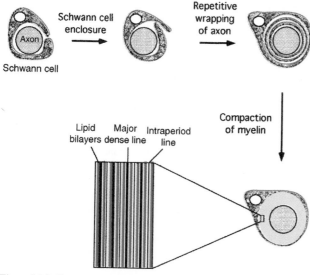

Figure 16-3. Process of myelination.

Myelination begins when a myelinating cell encircles an axon, either Schwann cells in the peripheral nervous system or oligodendrocytes in the central nervous system. Simple enclosure of the axon persists in unmyelinated axons. Myelin formation proceeds by a progressive wrapping of multiple layers of the myelinating cell around the axon, with extrusion of the cytoplasm and extracellular space to bring the lipid bilayers into close proximity. The intracellular space is compressed to form the major dense line of myelin, and the extracellular space is compressed to form the intraperiod line.

Myelin Formation and Maintenance

Myelin is formed in the CNS by oligodendrocytes and in the PNS by Schwann cells. Both these cell types form concentric layers of lipid-rich myelin by the progressive wrapping of their cytoplasmic processes around the axon in successive loops (Fig. 16-3). Ultimately, these cells exclude cytoplasm from the inner surface of their membranes to form the major dense line of myelin (Quarles *et al.*, 1997; Monuki and Lemke, 1995; Parent, 1996). In a similar process, the extracellular space is reduced on the extracellular surface of the bilayers, and the lipid membranes stack together, separated only by a proteinaceous intraperiod line existing between successive layers.

The formation and maintenance of myelin requires metabolic and structural proteins that are unique to the NS. Myelin basic protein, an integral protein of CNS myelin, is closely associated with the intracellular space (at the major dense line of myelin) (Quarles *et al.*, 1997; Monuki and Lemke, 1995), and an analogous protein, P1 protein, is located in the PNS. On the extracellular surface of the lipid bilayers is the CNS protein, proteolipid protein, at the intraperiod line of myelin. Mutation of this protein in several species, including humans, or overexpression of the wild-type gene in transgenic mice, results in disorders in which myelin of the CNS does not form normally (Pham-Dinh *et al.*, 1991; Readhead *et al.*, 1994).

There are a variety of hereditary disorders where myelin is either poorly formed from the outset or maintained after its formation. In addition to mutation of proteolipid protein, there are a variety of inherited abnormalities of myelin proteins and myelin-specific lipid catabolism. These genetic defects have provided some insight into the special processes required to maintain the lipid-rich environment of myelin. It is now known that the maintenance of myelin is dependent on a number of membrane-associated proteins and on

metabolism of specific lipids present in myelin bilayers. Some toxic compounds interfere with this complex process of the maintenance of myelin and result in the toxic "myelinopathies" (Fig. 16-2). In general, the loss of myelin with the preservation of axons is referred to as *demyelination*.

Neurotransmission

Intercellular communication is achieved in the NS through the synapse. Neurotransmitters released from one axon to another act as the first messenger. Binding of the transmitter to the postsynaptic receptor is followed by modulation of an ion channel or activation of a second messenger system, leading to changes in the responding cell. In the case of neuromuscular transmission, acetylcholine crosses the synaptic cleft to bind the cholinergic receptor of the myocyte and leads to muscle contraction. Chemically induced dysfunction of neurotransmission may occur in the absence of altered cellular structures; rather, the neurotoxicity expresses itself in terms of altered behavior or impaired performance on neurologic tests.

Chemicals acting on neurotransmission may interrupt the transmission of impulses, block or accentuate transsynaptic communication, block reuptake of neurotransmitters or precursors, or interfere with second-messenger systems. The structural similarity of many compounds with similar actions has led to the recognition of specific categories of drugs and toxins. For example, some drugs mimic the process of neurotransmission of the sympathetic nervous system and are termed sympathomimetic compounds. As the targets of these drugs are located throughout the body, the responses are not localized; however, the responses are stereotyped in that each member of a class tends to have similar biological effects. At times, altered neurotransmission is beneficial to an individual, for example, by stabilizing a disease-induced imbalance, and it is this aspect of biological response that is studied in the field of neuropharmacology. However, excessive or inappropriate exposure to compounds that alter neurotransmission may result in responses considered as neurotoxic. The therapeutic index is a measure of the margin between the desirable (therapeutic) and toxic effects of a chemical.

In terms of toxicity, most of the side effects of neurological drugs may be viewed as short-term interactions that are reversible with time or that may be counteracted by the use of appropriate antagonists. However, some of the toxicity associated with long-term use is irreversible. For example, phenothiazines, which have been used to treat chronic schizophrenia for long periods of time, may lead to the condition of tardive dyskinesia, in which the patient is left with a permanent disability of prominent facial grimaces (DeVeaugh-Geiss, 1982).

Development of the Nervous System

The nervous system begins development during gestation (first month in humans, day 7 in mice, day 9.5 in rats) and continues through adolescence (Bayer *et al.*, 1993; Rice and Barone, 2000). Proliferation, migration, differentiation, synaptogenesis, apoptosis, and myelination are the basic processes that underlie development of the NS, and these occur in a tightly choreographed sequence that depends on the region, cell type, and neurotrophic signals. Both neuronal and glial precursors replicate in a discrete zone near the inner surface of the neural tube. The proliferation and migration of these cells occur in waves that are specific for brain regions, but in general, the brain develops in a caudal to rostral direction (with cerebellar development being a notable exception). During differentiation (phenotype expression) and synaptogenesis (formation of functional synaptic connections), the circuitry of the NS is established. Chemicals such as nerve growth factors, adhesive molecules, and neurotransmitters serve as morphogenic signals; neurotransmitter developmental signals are separate from their synaptic transmission function (Lauder, 1993). Selected cells are also removed during ontogeny via apoptosis (programmed cell death) which results in the appropriate cell types in the correct regions. The glial supportive cells develop last, and myelination is protracted. The (mostly postnatal) period of rapid proliferation of glial cells is known as the brain growth spurt, during which time it is particularly vulnerable to insult (Dobbing and Sands, 1979; Dobbing and Smart, 1974).

The immature NS is especially vulnerable to certain agents (Rodier, 1995), and there are several factors that make the developing NS uniquely susceptible. Cell sensitivity differs with the developmental stage, leading to critical windows of vulnerability (Adams et al., 2000; Bayer et al., 1993). Chemicals which alter the timing and formation of neural connections could result in permanent malformations, the consequences of which may be quite unlike the chemical's effects in the adult NS. Furthermore, while synaptogenesis can continue throughout life, proliferation cannot; therefore, the CNS is unique in that damaged neural cells are not readily replaced. Finally, there are kinetic differences in the developing organism that may profoundly influence its sensitivity, including the slow formation of the blood–brain barrier and lack of key metabolic enzymes to protect the brain and eliminate toxicants (Makri et al., 2004).

While the developing NS is often more sensitive to insult (depending on the stage of development), the high rate of proliferation and regeneration in the developing NS may also lead to greater recovery or plasticity (an ability of one portion of the NS to assume the function of an injured area), which could attenuate some injuries (Goldberger and Murray, 1985). An example is the faster recovery from organophosphorus pesticide-induced acetylcholinesterase inhibition observed in younger laboratory rats, which is probably due to the rapid formation of the esterase enzyme and replacement of the phosphorylated form (Moser and Padilla, 1998). Some developmental changes may appear transient due to this plasticity and compensation, but underlying changes in the NS development could become manifest with aging or some form of challenge (e.g., Barone et al., 1995; Rice, 1996).

In evaluating developmental neurotoxicity, chemical exposure or treatment may occur during critical windows of susceptibility, or may cover the entire developmental process (i.e., during gestation, lactation, and adolescence). In general, injurious exposures early in gestation impact development of major brain regions whereas later exposures alter biochemical, morphological, or functional features of the neural systems. Functional, neurochemical, morphometric, or neuroanatomical endpoints are often used to assess the impact of developmental exposures; multiple measures are often needed to assess the wide array of potential outcomes. The ontogeny of specific behaviors, reflexes, and motor functions has been established for laboratory rats and mice, and compared to human developmental patterns (e.g., Altman and Sudershan, 1975; Fox, 1965; Wood et al., 2003). Markers of synaptic proteins, assays of synaptic enzymes, or challenges with pharmacologically specific chemicals are but a few methods by which to test synaptic function. While frank neuropathology is not as common with developmental neurotoxicants, measurements of layer widths in synaptic zones may reflect physical malformations.

Environmental Factors Relevant to Neurodegenerative Diseases

Individuals exposed to insufficient 1,2,3,6-tetrahydro-1-methyl-4-phenylpyridine (MPTP) to result in immediate Parkinsonism have developed early signs of the disease years later (Calne et al., 1985). This observation presents the possibility that the onset of a neurotoxic problem may follow toxic exposure for many years (Landrigan et al., 2005). It does not seem likely that an early sublethal injury to DAergic neurons later becomes lethal. Rather, smaller exposures to MPTP may cause a decrement in the population of dopaminergic (DAergic) neurons within the substantia nigra. Such a loss would most likely be silent, because the symptoms of PD do not develop until approximately 80–90% of the substantia nigra neurons are lost. These individuals with a diminished number of neurons may be more vulnerable to further loss of DAergic neurons. The neurologic picture of PD develops at an earlier age than in unexposed individuals, as a further loss of catecholaminergic neurons occurs during the process of aging.

The relationship between MPTP intoxication and Parkinsonism has stimulated investigations into the role that environmental and occupational exposures may play in the pathogenesis of Parkinson's disease. While several families with early-onset Parkinson's disease demonstrate autosomal dominant inheritance, with identification of candidate genes (Polymeropoulos et al., 1997; Agundez et al., 1995; Kurth and Kurth, 1993), twin studies indicate that environmental exposures play a more significant role than genetics in the vast majority of Parkinson's disease patients, particularly those with late-onset disease (Tanner et al., 1999; Kuopio et al., 1999). Epidemiologic studies implicate exposure to herbicides, pesticides, and metals as risk factors for Parkinson's disease (Gorell et al., 1998, 1999; Liou et al., 1997). Several studies suggest that dithiocarbamates also play an important role (Miller, 1982; Ferraz et al., 1988; Bachurin et al., 1996). Some studies suggest that cigarette smoking may have a protective effect against both Alzheimer's disease and Parkinson's disease, but alternative explanations have been offered (Riggs, 1992).

An epidemic of dialysis-related dementia with some pathologic resemblance to Alzheimer's disease appears to have been related to aluminum in the dialysate, and its removal has prevented further instances of dialysis dementia. However, there is no substantial evidence to date that aluminum is in any way related to sporadic Alzheimer's disease in the general population (Letzel et al., 2000).

The expanding field of the excitotoxic amino acids embodies many of the same attributes that characterize the entire discipline of neurotoxicology. Neurotoxicology is generally viewed as the study of compounds that are deleterious to the NS, and the effects of glutamate and kainate may be viewed as examples of this type of deleterious toxicity. Exposure to these excitotoxic amino acids leads to neuronal injury and—when of sufficient degree—may kill neurons. Many of these neurotoxic compounds have become tools for neurobiologists who seek to explore the anatomy and function of the NS. Kainate, through its selective action on neuronal cell bodies, has provided a greater understanding of the functions of cells within a specific region of the brain, while previous lesioning techniques addressed only regional functions. Finally, the questions surrounding domoic acid poisoning and the Guamanian neurodegenerative complex serve to remind the student of neurotoxicology and that the causes of many neurologic diseases remain unknown. This void in understanding and the epidemiologic evidence that some neurodegenerative diseases may have environmental contributors provide a heightened desire to appreciate more fully the effects of elements of our environment on the NS.

FUNCTIONAL MANIFESTATIONS OF NEUROTOXICITY

While knowledge of a toxicant's complete biochemical or molecular mechanism(s) is the ultimate goal of neurotoxicology, a full understanding of the toxicity also requires knowledge of the functional outcomes of those changes. Being the final output or manifestation of the NS, function includes motor, sensory, autonomic, and cognitive capabilities. The strength of functional assessments has been exploited by many investigators and regulatory agencies, and they are now routinely used in the assessment of the neurological effects of chemicals. Tilson (1993) has proposed two distinct tiers of functional testing of neurotoxicants: a first tier in which observational batteries or motor activity tests may be used to identify the presence of a neurotoxic substance, and a second tier that involves more complete description of the effects.

An overall assessment of behavior may be described using a series, or battery, of tests. These tests typically evaluate a variety of neurological functions, and are often used to screen for potential neurotoxicity in regulatory and safety pharmacology testing (Tilson and Moser, 1992; Moser, 2000). Specific methods include functional observational batteries (FOBs), Irwin screens, tests of motor activity, and expanded clinical observations. These tests have the advantage over biochemical and pathologic measures in that they permit evaluation of a single animal over longitudinal studies to determine the onset, progression, duration, and reversibility of a neurotoxic injury. Comparisons of defined protocols of FOBs with limited numbers of compounds (Moser *et al.*, 1997a,b) suggest that these methods can identify neurotoxic compounds reliably.

Some functional tests are more specific than observations and motor activity, and may be used to more fully characterize neurotoxic effects. Many of these functions have a clinical or behavioral correlate in humans, thus improving extrapolation of the outcomes. Measures of sensory function tap specific neuronal pathways that govern stimuli-dependent reflexes. For example, the acoustic startle response is a sensory-evoked motor reflex with a defined neuronal pathway (Davis *et al.*, 1982). Treatment effects could indicate sensory, motor, or muscle fiber alterations with little or no central involvement. Autonomic function includes evaluations of cardiovascular status and cholinergic/adrenergic balance. Acetylcholinesterase-inhibiting pesticides produce marked effects on multiple aspects of cholinergic homeostasis.

Deficits in cognitive function, especially in the context of developmental toxicity, represent an endpoint of great public concern and rhetoric. Behavioral toxicologists have incorporated methodologies from behavioral pharmacology and psychology to develop a range of tests of learning and memory for laboratory animals. These procedures include spatial navigation of mazes, associations with shock, conditioned responses, and appetite-motivated operant responses. In most cases, deficits in human cognitive function may be detected in laboratory animals as well, although the affected cognitive domain may vary. For example, in humans, exposure to lead in early childhood is known to lower IQ and alter behavioral control. Studies in rats have reported deficits in spatial learning, sustained attention, activity levels, and other behaviors (e.g., Morgan *et al.*, 2001; Nihei *et al.*, 2000). Detailed assessments such as these provide valuable insights into the damage caused by neurotoxicants. Ultimately, neurotoxicants identified by behavioral methods are evaluated at a cellular and molecular level to provide an understanding of the events in the NS that cause the neurological dysfunction.

MECHANISMS OF NEUROTOXICITY

Efforts to understand the mechanism of action of individual neurotoxic compounds have begun with the identification of the cellular target. In the nervous system, this has most often been one of four targets: the neuron, the axon, the myelinating cell, or the neurotransmitter system. As a result, neurotoxic compounds may be identified which cause neuronopathies, axonopathies, myelinopathies, or neurotransmitter-associated toxicity (Fig. 16-2). This is the classification system that is utilized here to organize the discussion of neurotoxic compounds and their mechanisms of action.

Neuronopathies

Certain toxicants are specific for neurons, or sometimes a particular group of neurons, resulting in their injury or, when intoxication is severe enough, their death. The loss of a neuron is irreversible and includes degeneration of all of its cytoplasmic extensions, dendrites and axons, and of the myelin ensheathing the axon (Fig. 16-2). Although the neuron is similar to other cell types in many respects, some features of the neuron are unique, placing it at risk for the action of cellular toxicants. Some of the unique features of the neuron include a high metabolic rate, a long cellular process that is supported by the cell body, and an excitable membrane that is rapidly depolarized and repolarized. Because many neurotoxic compounds act at the site of the cell body, when massive loss of axons and myelin are discovered in the PNS or CNS, the first question is whether the neuronal cell bodies themselves have been destroyed.

Although a large number of compounds are known to result in toxic neuronopathies (Table 16-1), all these toxicants share certain features. Each toxic condition is the result of a cellular toxicant that has a predilection for neurons, most likely due to one of the neuron's peculiar vulnerabilities. The initial injury to neurons is followed by apoptosis or necrosis, leading to permanent loss of the neuron. These chemicals tend to be diffuse in their action, although they may show some selectivity in the degree of injury of different neuronal subpopulations or at times an exquisite selectivity for such a subpopulation. The expression of these cellular events is often a diffuse encephalopathy, with global dysfunctions; however, the symptomatology reflects the injury to the brain, so neurotoxicants that are selective in their action and affect only a subpopulation of neurons may lead to interruption of only a particular functionality.

Doxorubicin Doxorubicin (Adriamycin), a quinone-containing anthracycline antibiotic, is one of the most effective antimitotics in cancer chemotherapy. Unfortunately, clinical application of doxorubicin is greatly limited by its acute and chronic cardiotoxicity. In addition to its cardiac toxicity that limits the quantity of doxorubicin that can be given to cancer patients, doxorubicin also injures neurons in the PNS, specifically those of the dorsal root ganglia and autonomic ganglia (Spencer, 2000). This selective vulnerability of peripheral ganglion cells is particularly dramatic in experimental animals. Doxorubicin's antineoplastic properties derive from its ability to intercalate into grooves of DNA, interfering with transcription. Other important mechanisms of action of doxorubicin include its interaction with topoisomerase II, which forms a DNA-cleavable complex (Chuang and Chuang, 1979; Cheng *et al.*, 1992) and generation of reactive oxygen species (ROS) by enzymatic

Table 16-1

Compounds Associated with Neuronal Injury (Neuronopathies)

NEUROTOXICANT	NEUROLOGIC FINDINGS	CELLULAR BASIS OF NEUROTOXICITY	REFERENCE
Aluminum	Dementia, encephalopathy (humans), learning deficits	Spongiosis cortex, neurofibrillary aggregates, degenerative changes in cortex	Chang and Dyer, 1995; Graham and Lantos, 1997; Spencer and Schaumburg, 2000
6-Amino-nicotinamide	Not reported in humans; hind limb paralysis (experimental animals)	Spongy (vacuolar) degeneration in spinal cord, brainstem, cerebellum; axonal degeneration of the peripheral nervous system (PNS)	Graham and Lantos, 1997; Spencer and Schaumburg, 2000
Arsenic	Encephalopathy (acute), peripheral neuropathy (chronic)	Brain swelling and hemorrhage (acute), axonal degeneration in PNS (chronic)	Graham and Lantos, 1997; Spencer and Schaumburg, 2000
Azide	Insufficient data (humans); convulsions, ataxia (primates)	Neuronal loss in cerebellum and cortex	Graham and Lantos, 1997; Spencer and Schaumburg, 2000
Bismuth	Emotional disturbances, encephalopathy, myoclonus	Neuronal loss, basal ganglia and Purkinje cells of cerebellum	Spencer and Schaumburg, 2000
Carbon monoxide	Encephalopathy, delayed parkinsonism/dystonia	Neuronal loss in cortex, necrosis of globus pallidus, focal demyelination; blocks oxygen binding site of hemoglobin and iron-binding sites of brain	Spencer and Schaumburg, 2000
Carbon tetrachloride	Encephalopathy (secondary to liver failure)	Enlarged astrocytes in striatum, globus pallidus	Spencer and Schaumburg, 2000
Chloramphenicol	Optic neuritis, peripheral neuropathy	Neuronal loss (retina), axonal degeneration (PNS)	Graham and Lantos, 1997; Spencer and Schaumburg, 2000
Cyanide	Coma, convulsions, rapid death; delayed parkinsonism/dystonia	Neuronal degeneration, cerebellum and globus pallidus; focal demyelination; blocks cytochrome oxidase/ATP production	Graham and Lantos, 1997; Spencer and Schaumburg, 2000
Doxorubicin	Insufficient data (humans); progressive ataxia (experimental animals)	Degeneration of dorsal root ganglion cells, axonal degeneration (PNS)	Graham and Lantos, 1997; Spencer and Schaumburg, 2000
Ethanol	Mental retardation, hearing deficits (prenatal exposure)	Microcephaly, cerebral malformations	Graham and Lantos, 1997
Lead	Encephalopathy (acute), learning deficits (children), neuropathy with demyelination (rats)	Brain swelling, hemorrhages (acute), axonal loss in PNS (humans)	Chang and Dyer, 1995; Graham and Lantos, 1997; Spencer and Schaumburg, 2000
Manganese	Emotional disturbances, parkinsonism/dystonia	Degeneration of striatum, globus pallidus	Chang and Dyer, 1995; Graham and Lantos, 1997
Mercury, inorganic	Emotional disturbances, tremor, fatigue	Insufficient data in humans (may affect spinal tracts; cerebellum)	Chang and Dyer, 1995; Graham and Lantos, 1997; Spencer and Schaumburg, 2000
Methanol	Headache, visual loss or blindness, coma (severe)	Necrosis of putamen, degeneration of retinal ganglion cells	Graham and Lantos, 1997; Spencer and Schaumburg, 2000
Methylazoxymethanol acetate (MAM)	Microcephaly, retarded development (rats)	Developmental abnormalities of fetal brain (rats)	Abou-Donia, 1993

(Continued)

Table 16-1
(Continued)

NEUROTOXICANT	NEUROLOGIC FINDINGS	CELLULAR BASIS OF NEUROTOXICITY	REFERENCE
Methyl bromide	Visual and speech impairment; peripheral neuropathy	Insufficient data	Spencer and Schaumburg, 2000
Methyl mercury (organic mercury)	Ataxia, constriction of visual fields, paresthesias (adult)	Neuronal degeneration, visual cortex, cerebellum, ganglia	Chang and Dyer, 1995; Graham and Lantos, 1997; Spencer and Schaumburg, 2000
	Psychomotor retardation (fetal exposure)	Spongy disruption, cortex and cerebellum	Graham and Lantos, 1997; Spencer and Schaumburg, 2000
1-Methyl-4-phenyl-1,2,3,6-tetrahydropyridine (MPTP)	Parkinsonism, dystonia (acute exposure)	Neuronal degeneration in substantia nigra	Graham and Lantos, 1997; Spencer and Schaumburg, 2000
	Early onset parkinsonism (late effect of acute exposure)	Neuronal degeneration in substantia nigra	Graham and Lantos, 1997; Spencer and Schaumburg, 2000
3-Nitropropionic acid	Seizures, delayed dystonia/grimacing	Necrosis in basal ganglia	Graham and Lantos, 1997; Spencer and Schaumburg, 2000
Phenytoin (diphenyl-hydantoin)	Nystagmus, ataxia, dizziness	Degeneration of Purkinje cells (cerebellum)	Graham and Lantos, 1997; Spencer and Schaumburg, 2000
Quinine	Constriction of visual fields	Vacuolization of retinal ganglion cells	Spencer and Schaumburg, 2000
Streptomycin (aminoglycosides)	Hearing loss	Degeneration of inner ear (organ of Corti)	Spencer and Schaumburg, 2000
Thallium	Emotional disturbances, ataxia, peripheral neuropathy	Brain swelling (acute), axonal degeneration in PNS	Graham and Lantos, 1997; Spencer and Schaumburg, 2000
Trimethyltin	Tremors, hyperexcitability (experimental animals	Loss of hippocampal neurons, amygdala pyriform cortex	Graham and Lantos, 1997

electron reduction of doxorubicin by variety of oxidases, reductases, and dehydrogenases (Gutierrez, 2000; Kappus, 1987). The neurotoxicity of doxorubicin is quite limited in its extent, despite the fact that all neurons are dependent on the ability to transcribe DNA. The particular vulnerability of sensory and autonomic neurons appears to reflect the lack of protection of these neurons by a blood-tissue barrier within ganglia. If the blood–brain barrier is temporarily opened by the use of mannitol, the toxicity of doxorubicin is expressed in a much more diffuse manner, with injury of neurons in the cortex and subcortical nuclei of the brain (Spencer, 2000).

Methyl Mercury The neuronal toxicity of organomercurial compounds, such as methyl mercury (MeHg), was tragically revealed in large numbers of poisonings in Japan and Iraq. The residents of Minamata Bay in Japan, whose diet was largely composed of fish from the bay, were exposed to massive amounts of methyl mercury when mercury-laden industrial effluent was rerouted into the bay (Kurland et al., 1960; Takeuchi et al., 1962). Methyl mercury injured even more people in Iraq, with more than 400 deaths and 6000 people hospitalized. In this epidemic, as well as in several smaller ones, the effects occurred after the consumption of grain that had been dusted with methyl mercury as an inexpensive pesticide (Bakir et al., 1973). Typically, environmental exposure to mercury occurs via the food chain due to accumulation of MeHg in fish. Latest statistics in the United States indicate that 46 states have fish consumption advisories covering 40% of the nation's rivers, lakes, and streams. In addition, mercury is a common pollutant in hazardous waste sites in the nation (US EPA, 2001). It is estimated that 3–4 million children live within one mile of at least one of the 1300+ active hazardous waste sites in the United States (US EPA, 2001).

The clinical picture of MeHg poisoning varies both with the severity of exposure and the age of the individual at the time of exposure. In adults, the most dramatic sites of injury are the neurons of the visual cortex and the small internal granular cell neurons of the cerebellar cortex, whose massive degeneration results in blindness and marked ataxia. In children, developmental disabilities, retardation, and cognitive deficits occur. Such age-related differences are seen also in other mammals, although the specific areas damaged may differ. It has been suggested that these differences are caused by an immature blood–brain barrier causing a more generalized distribution of mercury in the developing brain. Recent studies in rats show that the neurons that are most sensitive to the toxic effects of methyl mercury are those that reside in the dorsal root ganglia, perhaps again reflecting the vulnerability of neurons not shielded by blood-tissue barriers (Schionning *et al.*, 1998).

The mechanism of MeHg toxicity has been the subject of intense investigation. However, it remains unknown whether the ultimate toxicant is methyl mercury or the liberated mercuric ion. Whereas Hg^{2+} is known to bind strongly to sulfhydryl groups, it is not clear that MeHg results in cell death through sulfhydryl binding. A variety of aberrations in cellular function have been noted, including impaired glycolysis, nucleic acid biosynthesis, aerobic respiration, protein synthesis (Cheung and Verity, 1985), and neurotransmitter release (Atchison and Hare, 1994). In addition, there is evidence for enhanced oxidative injury (LeBel *et al.*, 1992; Shanker *et al.*, 2002) and altered calcium homeostasis (Marty and Atchison, 1997). Exposure to MeHg leads to widespread neuronal injury and subsequently to a diffuse encephalopathy. However, there is relative selectivity of the toxicant for some groups of neurons over others. The distribution of neuronal injury does not appear to be related to the tissue distribution of either MeHg or ionic mercury but rather to particular vulnerabilities of these neurons. Susceptibility of different brain regions or cell types to MeHg (Clarkson, 1997) may also be dependent on factors such as the intracellular reduced glutathione (GSH) concentration and the ability to increase glycolytic flux in the face of mitochondrial damage. These observations are consistent with morphological observations in which astrocytes that accumulate MeHg appear normal, while neurons that are found in their proximity and are void of MeHg undergo cell death (Garman *et al.*, 1975). It seems likely that MeHg toxicity is mediated by numerous reactions and that no single critical target will be identified. As these toxic events occur, the injured neurons eventually die.

Trimethyltin   Organotins are used industrially as plasticizers, antifungal agents, or pesticides. Intoxication with trimethyltin has been associated with a potentially irreversible limbic-cerebellar syndrome in humans and similar behavioral changes in primates (Besser *et al.*, 1987; Reuhl *et al.*, 1985). Trimethyltin gains access to the nervous system where, by an undefined mechanism, it leads to diffuse neuronal injury. Trimethyltin triggers selective apoptosis in specific subregions of the mammalian CNS and specific subsets of immune system cells (Balaban *et al.*, 1988; Patanow *et al.*, 1997). The hippocampus is particularly vulnerable to this process. Following acute intoxication, the cells of the fascia dentata degenerate; with chronic intoxication, the cells of the corpus ammonis are lost. Ganglion cells and hair cells of the cochlea are similarly sensitive (Liu and Fechter, 1996). Several hypotheses are suggested for the mechanism of trimethyltin neurotoxicity, including energy deprivation and excitotoxic damage. Evidence to date suggests that organotins, such as trimethyltin, interact with the CXC region of stannin, and that trimethyltin treatment significantly alters its expression (Toggas *et al.*, 1993). Stannin is located on human chromosome 16p13, and has a syntenic relationship to the murine chromosomal homolog (Dejneka *et al.*, 1998).

Axonopathies

The neurotoxic disorders termed *axonopathies* are those in which the primary site of toxicity is the axon itself. The axon degenerates, and with it the myelin surrounding that axon; however, the neuron cell body remains intact (Fig. 16-2). John Cavanagh coined the term *dying-back neuropathy* as a synonym for *axonopathy* (Cavanagh,

1964). The concept of "dying back" postulated that the focus of toxicity was the neuronal cell body itself and that the distal axon degenerated progressively from the synapse, back toward the cell body with increasing injury. It now appears that, in the best-studied axonopathies, a different pathogenetic sequence occurs; the toxicant results in a "chemical transection" of the axon at some point along its length, and the axon distal to the transection, biologically separated from its cell body, degenerates.

Because longer axons have more targets for toxic damage than shorter axons, one would predict that longer axons would be more affected in toxic axonopathies. Indeed, such is the case. The involvement of long axons of the CNS, such as ascending sensory axons in the posterior columns or descending motor axons, along with long sensory and motor axons of the PNS, prompted Spencer and Schaumburg (1976) to suggest that the toxic axonopathies in which the distal axon was most vulnerable be called *central peripheral distal axonopathies*, which, though cumbersome, accurately depicts the pathologic loci.

Axonopathies can be considered to result from a chemical transection of the axon. The number of axonal toxicants is large and increasing in number (Table 16-2); however, they may be viewed as a group, all of which result in the pathologic loss of distal axons with the survival of the cell body. Because the axonopathies pathologically resemble the actual physical transection of the axon, axonal transport appears to be a likely target in many of the toxic axonopathies. Furthermore, as these axons degenerate, the result is most often the clinical condition of peripheral neuropathy, in which sensations and motor strength are first impaired in the most distal extent of the axonal processes, the feet and hands. With time and continued injury, the deficit progresses to involve more proximal areas of the body and the long axons of the spinal cord. The potential for regeneration is great when the insult is limited to peripheral nerves and may be complete in axonopathies in which the initiating event can be determined and removed.

Gamma-Diketones   It was first noted in the late 1960s that humans with chronic high exposures to *n*-hexane, a simple alkane, in a work setting develop a progressive sensorimotor distal axonopathy (Yamamura, 1969). Intentional inhalation of materials containing *n*-hexane is also common, and produces the same neurotoxic effects. An identical axonopathy was also produced by methyl *n*-butyl ketone (2-hexanone), leading to the discovery of the mechanism by which these two compounds are similarly metabolized. The carbon chain undergoes ω-1 oxidation, resulting in 2,5-hexanedione, a γ-diketone. This metabolite is ultimately the toxic species produced from *n*-hexane and 2-hexanone. Other γ-diketones or precursors also produced the same axonopathy, whereas α- or β-diketones are not toxic to the nervous system (Krasavage *et al.*, 1980).

γ-Diketones, including 2,5-hexanedione, react with amino groups on all proteins, forming pyrrole adducts. This is an important step in development of axonopathy, as evidenced by the inability of 3,3-dimethyl-2,5-hexanedione, a γ-diketone which is unable to form pyrrole adducts, to cause neurotoxicity (Sayre *et al.*, 1986). After forming, these pyrroles are oxidized and cross-linking occurs between neurofilament subunits. The inability of 3-acetyl-2,5-hexanedione to cross-link prevents toxicity, suggesting that pyrrole oxidation and cross-linking is a necessary step in the development of axonopathy (St. Clair *et al.*, 1988). Neurofilaments accumulate in the distal axon, usually just proximal to a node of Ranvier, and form massive axonal swellings leading to retraction of

Table 16-2
Compounds Associated with Axonal Injury (Axonopathies)

NEUROTOXICANT	NEUROLOGIC FINDINGS	BASIS OF NEUROTOXICITY	REFERENCE
Acrylamide	Peripheral neuropathy (often sensory)	Axonal degeneration, axon terminal affected in earliest stages	Graham and Lantos, 1997; Spencer and Schaumburg, 2000
p-Bromophenylacetyl urea	Peripheral neuropathy	Axonal degeneration in the peripheral nervous system (PNS) and central nervous system (CNS)	Spencer and Schaumburg, 2000
Carbon disulfide	Psychosis (acute), peripheral neuropathy (chronic)	Axonal degeneration, early stages include neurofilamentous swelling	Graham and Lantos, 1997; Spencer and Schaumburg, 2000
Chlordecone (Kepone)	Tremors, in coordination (experimental animals)	Insufficient data (humans); axonal swelling and degeneration	Spencer and Schaumburg, 2000
Chloroquine	Peripheral neuropathy, weakness	Axonal degeneration, inclusions in dorsal root ganglion cells; also vacuolar myopathy	Graham and Lantos, 1997; Spencer and Schaumburg, 2000
Clioquinol	Encephalopathy (acute), subacute myelooptic neuropathy (subacute)	Axonal degeneration, spinal cord, PNS, optic tracts	Graham and Lantos, 1997; Spencer and Schaumburg, 2000
Colchicine	Peripheral neuropathy	Axonal degeneration, neuronal perikaryal filamentous aggregates; vacuolar myopathy	Graham and Lantos, 1997; Spencer and Schaumburg, 2000
Dapsone	Peripheral neuropathy, predominantly motor	Axonal degeneration (both myelinated and unmyelinated axons)	Graham and Lantos, 1997
Dichlorophenoxyacetate	Peripheral neuropathy (delayed)	Insufficient data	Spencer and Schaumburg, 2000
Dimethylaminopropionitrile	Peripheral neuropathy, urinary retention	Axonal degeneration (both myelinated and unmyelinated axons)	Spencer and Schaumburg, 2000
Ethylene oxide	Peripheral neuropathy	Axonal degeneration	Graham and Lantos, 1997
Glutethimide	Peripheral neuropathy (predominantly sensory)	Insufficient data	Spencer and Schaumburg, 2000
Gold	Peripheral neuopathy (may have psychiatric problems)	Axonal degeneration, some segmental demyelination	Graham and Lantos, 1997; Spencer and Schaumburg, 2000
n-Hexane	Peripheral neuropathy, severe cases have spasticity	Axonal degeneration, early neurofilamentous swelling, PNS and spinal cord	Graham and Lantos, 1997; Spencer and Schaumburg, 2000
Hydralazine	Peripheral neuropathy	Insufficient data	Spencer and Schaumburg, 2000
β,β′-Iminodipropionitrile	No data in humans; excitatory movement disorder (rats)	Proximal axonal swellings, degeneration of olfactory epithelial cells, vestibular hair cells	Graham and Lantos, 1997
Isoniazid	Peripheral neuropathy (sensory), ataxia (high doses)	Axonal degeneration	Graham and Lantos, 1997; Spencer and Schaumburg, 2000
Lithium	Lethargy, tremor, ataxia (reversible)	Insufficient data	Spencer and Schaumburg, 2000
Methyl n-butyl ketone	Peripheral neuropathy	Axonal degeneration, early neurofilamentous swelling, PNS and spinal cord	Graham and Lantos, 1997; Spencer and Schaumburg, 2000
Metronidazole	Sensory peripheral neuropathy, ataxia, seizures	Axonal degeneration, mostly affecting myelinated fibers; lesions of cerebellar nuclei	Graham and Lantos, 1997; Spencer and Schaumburg, 2000
Misonidazole	Peripheral neuropathy	Axonal degeneration	Graham and Lantos, 1997; Spencer and Schaumburg, 2000

(Continued)

Table 16-2

(Continued)

NEUROTOXICANT	NEUROLOGIC FINDINGS	BASIS OF NEUROTOXICITY	REFERENCE
Nitrofurantoin	Peripheral neuropathy	Axonal degeneration	Spencer and Schaumburg, 2000
Organophosphorus compounds (NTE inhibitors)	abdominal pain (acute); Peripheral neuropathy	Axonal degeneration	Chang and Dyer, 1995; Graham and Lantos, 1997; Spencer and Schaumburg, 2000
Paclitaxel (taxoids)	Delayed peripheral neuropathy (motor), spasticity	Axonal degeneration (delayed after single exposure), PNS and spinal cord	Chang and Dyer, 1995; Graham and Lantos, 1997; Spencer and Schaumburg, 2000; Abou-Donia, 1993
Platinum (cisplatin)	Peripheral neuropathy	Axonal degeneration; microtubule accumulation in early stages	Graham and Lantos, 1997; Spencer and Schaumburg, 2000
Pyridinethione (pyrithione)	Movement disorders (tremor, choreoathetosis)	Axonal degeneration (variable)	Chang and Dyer, 1995; Spencer and Schaumburg, 2000
Vincristine (vinca alkaloids)	Cranial (most often trigeminal) neuropathy	Insufficient data	Spencer and Schaumburg, 2000
	Peripheral neuropathy, variable autonomic symptoms	Axonal degeneration (PNS), neurofibrillary changes (spinal cord, intrathecal route)	Graham and Lantos, 1997; Spencer and Schaumburg, 2000

myelin from the nodes (Graham *et al.*, 1982). In addition to swelling, axonal atrophy is also a pathological feature of γ-diketone neurotoxicity.

This axonal atrophy was previously thought to occur secondary to swelling; however, more recent studies have suggested that it may be the more relevant pathophysiologic feature. In one study, rats dosed at a lower rate (100–250 mg/kg/d) developed axonal swelling and atrophy, and rats given a higher dose rate (400 mg/kg/d) failed to consistently develop swellings, while atrophy and behavioral alterations were nearly universal. These data suggest that axonal atrophy is the pathologic change that leads to nerve dysfunction and behavioral changes (Lehning *et al.*, 2000). The mechanism responsible for axonal atrophy is still unknown; however, a depletion of tubulin subunits has been reported, and is a likely contributor to the overall neuropathologic picture (LoPachin *et al.*, 2005).

The dimethyl analog of HD, 3,4-dimethyl-2,5-hexanedione (DMHD), produces a similar neuropathy. However, due to the methyl groups, DMHD forms the cyclic adduct much more rapidly than HD, forming pyrrole adducts that oxidize and lead to cross-linking faster than HD. DMHD is more potent than HD, and produces proximal axonal swellings similar to those seen in β,β′-iminodipropionitrile, and is thought to be the product of faster rates of adduct formation (Anthony *et al.*, 1983).

Carbon Disulfide   The most significant exposures of humans to CS_2 have occurred in the vulcan rubber and viscose rayon industries. Manic psychoses were observed in the former setting and were correlated with very high levels of exposure (Seppaleinen and Haltia, 1980). In recent decades, interest in the human health effects has been focused on the NS and the cardiovascular system, where injury has been documented in workers exposed to much higher levels than those that are allowed today.

What is clearly established is the capacity of CS_2 to cause a distal axonopathy that is identical pathologically to that caused by *n*-hexane. There is growing evidence that covalent cross-linking of neurofilaments also underlies CS_2 neuropathy through a series of reactions that parallel the sequence of events in *n*-hexane neuropathy. While *n*-hexane requires metabolism to 2,5-hexanedione, CS_2 is itself the ultimate toxicant, reacting with protein amino groups to form dithiocarbamate adducts (Lam and DiStefano, 1986). The dithiocarbamate adducts of lysyl amino groups undergo decomposition to isothiocyanate adducts, electrophiles that then react with protein nucleophiles to yield covalent cross-linking (Fig. 16-4). The reaction of the isothiocyanate adducts with cysteinyl sulfhydryls to form *N,S*-dialkyldithiocarbamate ester cross-links is reversible, while the reaction with protein amino functions forms thiourea cross-links irreversibly. Over time, the thiourea cross-links predominate and are most likely the most biologically significant (Amarnath *et al.*, 1991; Valentine *et al.*, 1992, 1995; Graham *et al.*, 1995).

As with *n*-hexane neuropathy, it has been postulated that the stability and long transport distance of neurofilaments determine that the neurofilament subunit proteins are the toxicologically relevant targets in chronic CS_2 intoxication. Nonetheless, proteins throughout the organism are derivatized and cross-linked as well. Cross-linking has been identified in erythrocyte-associated proteins including spectrin and globin as well as in the putative neurotoxic target neurofilament subunit proteins (Valentine *et al.*, 1993, 1997). Analysis of cross-linking in erythrocyte proteins has verified that cross-linking occurs through thiourea bridges that accumulate with continuing exposure (Erve *et al.*, 1998a,b). Neurofilament cross-linking involves all three subunits and also demonstrates a cumulative dose response and temporal relationship consistent with a contributing event in the development of the axonal neurofilamentous swellings. The correlation of protein cross-linking in erythrocyte

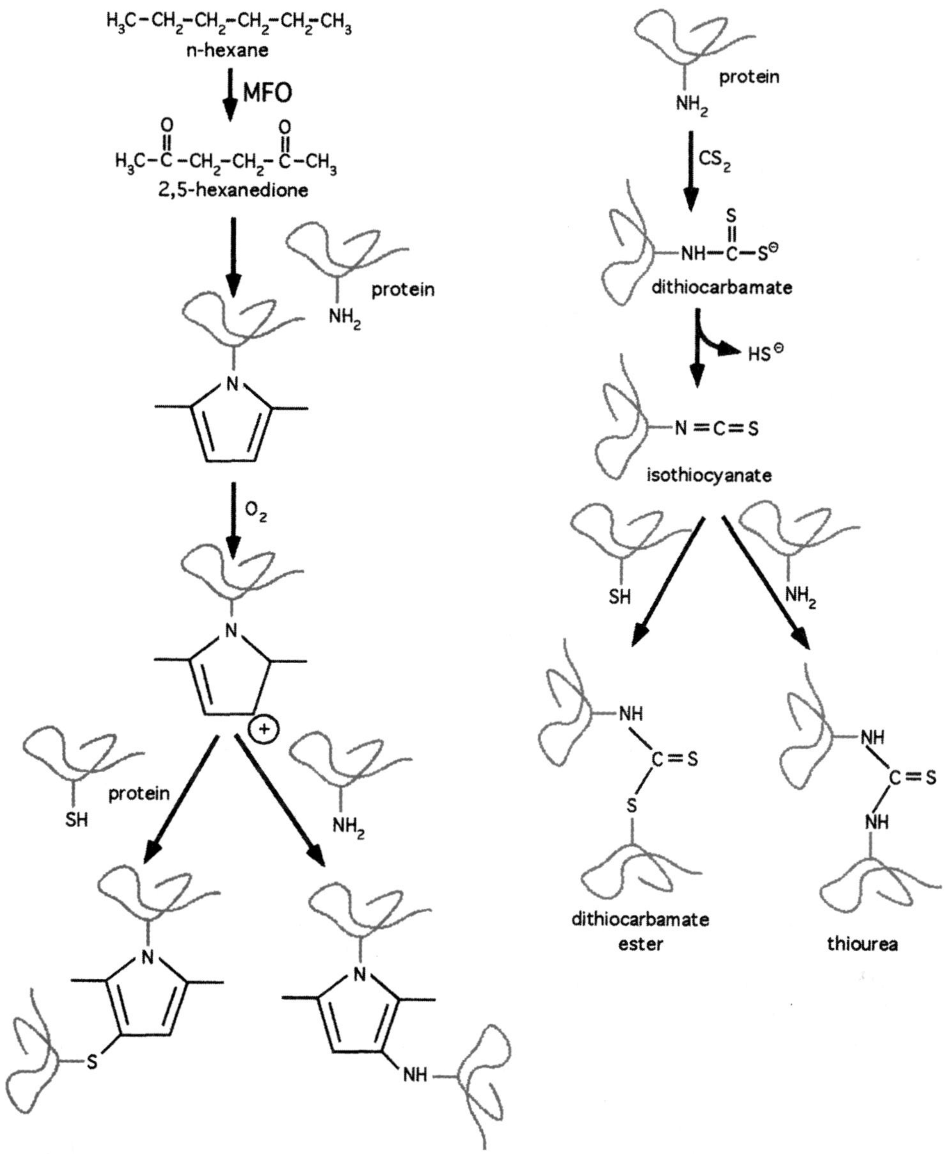

Figure 16-4. Molecular mechanisms of protein cross-linking in the neurofilamentous neuropathies.

Both 2,5-hexanedione, produced from hexane via ω-1 oxidation function of mixed function oxidase (MFO), and CS2 are capable of cross-linking proteins. Pyrrole formation from 2,5-hexanedione is followed by oxidation and reaction with adjacent protein nucleophiles. Dithiocarbamate formation from CS2 is followed by formation of the protein-bound isothiocyanate and subsequent reaction with adjacent protein nucleophiles.

proteins and axonal proteins together with the ability to detect covalent modifications on peripheral proteins at subneurotoxic levels and at preneurotoxic time points suggests that modifications on peripheral proteins can be used as biomarkers of effect for CS_2 exposure. These biomarkers together with morphologic changes have been used to establish CS_2 as the ultimate neurotoxic species in the peripheral neuropathy produced by oral administration of N,N-diethyldithiocarbamate (Johnson *et al.*, 1998).

The clinical effects of exposure to CS_2 in the chronic setting are very similar to those of hexane exposure, with the development of sensory and motor symptoms occurring initially in a stocking-and-glove distribution. In addition to this chronic axonopathy, CS_2 can also lead to aberrations in mood and signs of diffuse encephalopathic disease. Some of these are transient at first and subsequently

become more long lasting, a feature that is common in vascular insufficiency in the nervous system. This fact, in combination with the knowledge that CS_2 may accelerate the process of atherosclerosis, suggests that some of the effects of CS_2 on the CNS are vascular in origin.

β,β′-Iminodipropionitrile (IDPN) β,β′-iminodipropionitrile (IDPN) is a synthetic, bifunctional nitrile that causes a "waltzing syndrome" in rats and other mammals, although human exposure has never been documented. Features of this "waltzing syndrome" include excitement, circling, head twitching, and over-alertness, and are observed after a single large intraperitoneal injection to rats (1.5–2.0 g/kg) (Chou and Hartmann, 1964). While the cause of this behavior has not been conclusively determined, it has been suggested that degeneration of vestibular sensory hair cells is responsible (Llorens et al., 1993).

Pathologic changes also follow administration of IDPN, most notably in large caliber axons, the primary target of neurotoxicity. The accumulation of neurofilaments in the proximal axon occurs, leading to swelling without degeneration in most animals (Gold, 2000). Quails deficient in neurofilaments demonstrate no swellings when administered IDPN, suggesting that the toxicity is due to a selective effect on neurofilaments (Mitsuishi et al., 1993). These neurofilament swellings are similar to those observed in carbon disulfide or γ-diketones toxicity. Repeated exposure to IDPN leads to demyelination and onion bulb formation, and eventually can produce distal axonal atrophy due to a reduction in anterograde neurofilament transport to the distal axon (Clark et al., 1980).

This impairment of axonal transport results from the disruption of the association between microtubules and neurofilaments by IDPN, causing neurofilament accumulation (Griffin et al., 1983). This leads to complete disturbance of the cytoskeleton of the axon. Although unclear, the mechanism responsible for this interference is hypothesized to result from the direct alteration of neurofilament proteins by IDPN, possibly by changing their chemical properties and causing aggregation (Anderson et al., 1991).

Acrylamide Acrylamide is a vinyl monomer used widely in water purification, paper manufacturing, mining, and waterproofing. It is also used extensively in biochemical laboratories, and is present in many foods prepared at high temperatures. Although it can be dangerous if not handled carefully, most toxic events in humans have been observed as peripheral neuropathies in factory workers exposed to high doses (Garland and Peterson, 1967; Kesson et al., 1977; Collins et al., 1989; Myers and Macun, 1991).

Early studies of acrylamide neuropathy revealed a distal axonopathy characterized by multiple axonal swellings (Spencer and Schaumburg, 1976). Although a single large dose is enough to produce toxicity, the process appears the same in multiple smaller doses, suggesting that acrylamide neurotoxicity is not due to an accumulation of the toxicant in the brain (Crofton et al., 1996). Repeated dosing results in a more proximal axonopathy, in a "dying back" process. The first changes are seen in Pacinian corpuscles, followed by muscle spindles and the nerve terminal. These changes are caused by accumulations of neurofilaments at the nerve terminal. Paranodal swellings develop, leading to the retraction of myelin (Schaumburg et al., 1974; Spencer and Schaumburg, 1974). A decrease in the number of synaptic vesicles and mitochondria at the nerve terminal is also characteristic, probably due to inhibition of retrograde and anterograde axonal transport (DeGrandchamp et al., 1990; Padilla et al., 1993; Harris et al., 1994). Recently it has been observed that nerve terminal degeneration occurs prior to development of axonopathy, suggesting that this degeneration is the primary lesion (LoPachin et al., 2002).

Many early studies investigating acrylamide neurotoxicity noted nerve terminal degeneration, but for three decades the distal axonopathy was believed to be the lesion responsible for neurologic symptoms (ataxia, numbness in extremities, etc.). However, in more recent studies, neurologic symptoms and nerve terminal degeneration were similarly observed in both short-term high dose and long-term low dose animals in the rat PNS, while axonal degeneration occurred only in low-dose studies subsequent to neurologic alteration (LoPachin et al., 2002).

Organophosphorus (OP) Compounds OP compounds are used not only as insecticides and chemical warfare agents, but also as chemical intermediates, flame retardants, fuel additives, hydraulic fluids, lubricants, pharmaceuticals, and plasticizers. The OP insecticides and nerve agents are designed to inhibit acetylcholinesterase (AChE), thereby causing accumulation of acetylcholine in cholinergic synapses resulting in cholinergic toxicity and death (Thompson and Richardson, 2004). However, apart from the insecticides, nerve agents, and some of the pharmaceuticals, OP compounds produced for other applications often have little or no anti-AChE activity (Richardson, 2005).

Some OP compounds, such as tri-o-cresyl phosphate (TOCP), are neuropathic and can cause a severe sensorimotor central peripheral distal axonopathy called OP compound-induced delayed neurotoxicity (OPIDN) without inducing cholinergic poisoning. This condition is also referred to as a delayed neuropathy or delayed polyneuropathy (OPIDP) (Lotti and Moretto, 2005). However, neuropathy usually connotes peripheral nerve disease, whereas OPIDN also involves degeneration of ascending and descending spinal cord tracts (Richardson, 2005).

An OPIDN epidemic of massive proportions occurred during Prohibition in the United States, when Jamaica Ginger extract (Ginger Jake), a popular source of alcohol, was adulterated with TOCP. Another outbreak occurred in Morocco where olive oil was contaminated with TOCP. Human cases have also occurred after exposure to certain formerly used OP insecticides, such as EPN (O-ethyl-O-4-nitrophenyl phenylphosphonothionate) and leptophos [O-(4-bromo-2,5-dichlorophenyl)-O-methyl phenylphosphonothionate] (Lotti and Moretto, 2005).

Many OP compounds are hydrophobic and readily enter the NS. If the parent compound and/or metabolites have suitable reactivity, they can phosphorylate neural target proteins, such as various serine hydrolases (Casida and Quistad, 2005). When the principal target is acetylcholinesterase (AChE), cholinergic toxicity can ensue, either because of suprathreshold levels of inhibition or inhibition plus aging (Fig. 16-5). A substantial level of AChE inhibition on its own is sufficient to produce cholinergic toxicity and death. When aging of inhibited AChE also occurs (net loss of a ligand from the phosphorus of the OP-enzyme conjugate, leaving a negatively charged phosphoryl moiety attached to the active site), the qualitative nature of the toxicity does not change. Instead, the inhibited AChE becomes intractable to reactivation, rendering therapy with oximes, such as 2-pralidoxime methiodide (2-PAM) ineffective (Fig. 16-5) (Thompson and Richardson, 2004).

When the principal target is neuropathy target esterase (neurotoxic esterase, NTE), OPIDN can result only if both suprathreshold (>70%) inhibition occurs and the inhibited enzyme undergoes aging. Thus, in the case of NTE and OPIDN, inhibition alone is insufficient to precipitate toxicity. It appears that the biochemical lesion is not simply a blockade of the active site. Instead, axonopathy is triggered by specific chemical modification of the NTE protein (Fig. 16-6). Neuropathic (aging) inhibitors of NTE include compounds from the phosphate, phosphonate, and phosphoramidate classes of OP compounds (Richardson, 1992; Kropp et al., 2004) (Fig. 16-7).

Certain NTE inhibitors, including members of the phosphinate, carbamate, and sulfonylfluoride classes, do not age and do not cause OPIDN (Fig. 16-7). However, pretreatment with a nonaging NTE inhibitor prevents OPIDN from occurring after a challenge dose of a neuropathic (aging) NTE inhibitor. It has been proposed that these nonaging compounds protect against OPIDN by blocking the

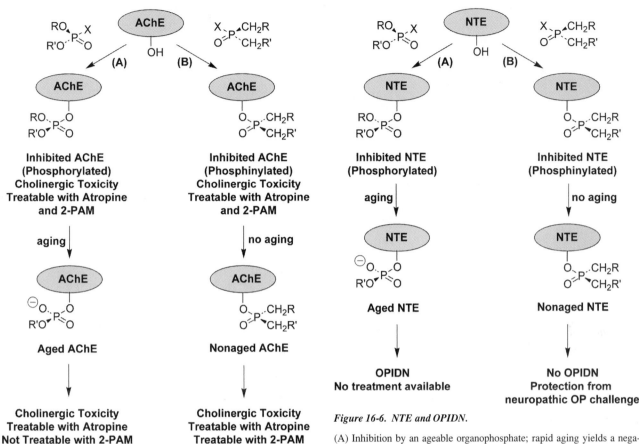

Figure 16-5. AChE and cholinergic toxicity.

(A) Inhibition by an ageable organophosphate produces cholinergic toxicity, treatable with atropine and 2-PAM. Aging does not alter the type of toxicity, but it obviates 2-PAM therapy. (B) Inhibition by a nonageable phosphinate produces cholinergic toxicity, treatable with atropine and 2-PAM. R, R': substituted or unsubstituted alkyl or aryl groups; X: primary leaving group displaced by the AChE active site serine.

Figure 16-6. NTE and OPIDN.

(A) Inhibition by an ageable organophosphate; rapid aging yields a negatively charged phosphoryl conjugate resulting in OPIDN. (B) Inhibition by a nonageable phosphinate does not produce OPIDN but provides protection against neuropathic (ageable) NTE inhibitors. R, R': substituted or unsubstituted alkyl or aryl groups. X: primary leaving group displaced by the NTE active site serine.

active site of NTE, and preventing inhibition and aging by a subsequent dose of a neuropathic (aging) inhibitor (Richardson, 2005) (Fig. 16-6).

In contrast, when protective NTE inhibitors are administered following exposure to a near-threshold subclinical dose of a neuropathic OP compound, OPIDN is fully expressed (Pope *et al.*, 1993). Because the initial treatment involves a compound that can produce OPIDN on its own and the disease is likely to be incipient rather than absent, this effect should be called *potentiation*; however, some authors refer to the phenomenon as *promotion* (Lotti, 2002). Although the potentiating agents inhibit NTE, this enzyme is not thought to be the target of potentiation. The level of NTE inhibition produced by the potentiator is not related to the level of potentiation observed, and these potentiators appear to exacerbate axonopathies from other causes as well, such as trauma and 2,5-hexanedione exposure. These results have been interpreted to indicate that potentiation enhances progression of the axonopathic process, inhibits repair, or both (Lotti, 2002; Randall *et al.*, 1997).

Axonal degeneration does not commence immediately after acute exposure to a neuropathic OP compound, but is delayed for at least 8 days between the acute high-dose exposure and clinical signs of axonopathy. Some effective regeneration of axons occurs in the PNS, for example, excitatory inputs to skeletal muscle from lower motor neurons in the spinal cord. In contrast, axonal degeneration is progressive and persistent in long tracts of the spinal cord, for example, inhibitory pathways from upper motor neurons in the motor cortex to lower motor neurons in the spinal cord anterior horn. Accordingly, the clinical picture of OPIDN changes from flaccid to spastic paralysis during a course of months to years (Lotti and Moretto, 2005; Richardson, 2005).

Fortunately, studies of the initiation steps of OPIDN and structure-activity relationships of neuropathic OP compounds have led to highly accurate prediction of the neuropathic potential of these chemicals. Consequently, human cases of OPIDN are now rare and usually arise from intentional ingestion of massive doses of OP insecticides in suicide attempts. Nevertheless, the fact remains that OPIDN is a debilitating and incurable condition. Moreover, the mechanism linking aged NTE to axonopathy is unknown. Accordingly, research continues in order to enhance mechanistic understanding that could be applied to improving biosensors and biomarkers of exposure, high-throughput testing of new compounds, and prophylaxis and treatment for OPIDN (Makhaeva *et al.*, 2003; Malygin *et al.*, 2003; Richardson, 2005).

The foregoing discussion has been limited to organic compounds of pentacovalent phosphorus, which are by far the most common and best studied of the OP compounds. However, organic

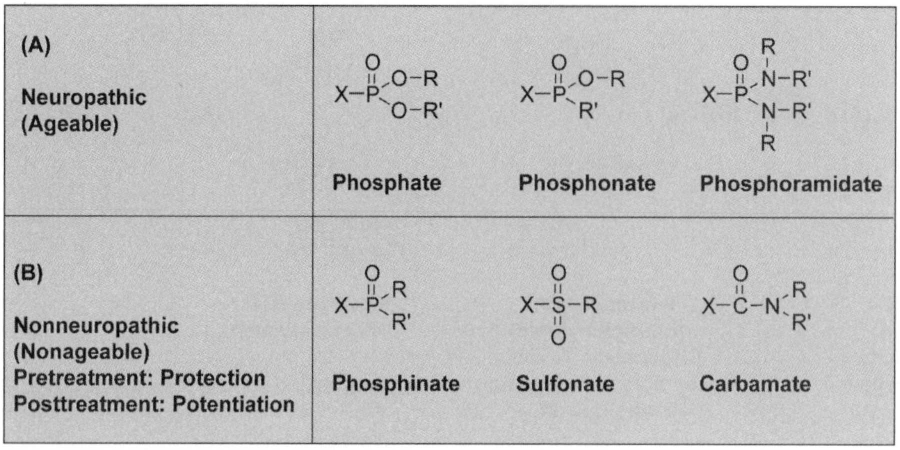

Figure 16-7. NTE inhibitors.

(A). Neuropathic (ageable). (B) Nonneuropathic (nonageable). R, R′: substituted or unsubstituted alkyl or aryl groups; X: primary leaving group displaced by the NTE active site serine.

compounds of trivalent phosphorus, such as triphenylphosphine (TPPn) and triphenylphosphite (TPPi), have relatively widespread use, particularly as antioxidants, chemical intermediates, and polymer enhancers. Both TPPn and TPPi produce axonal degeneration in the CNS and PNS, but the spatial-temporal distributions of lesions are different from that of classical OPIDN produced by organic pentacovalent phosphorus compounds and the pathogenic mechanisms are unknown (Abou-Donia, 1992). In particular, it appears that the mechanism of initiation of axonopathy by TTPn is independent of NTE inhibition and aging (Davis et al., 1999), and this relationship is unclear for TPPi (Padilla et al., 1987).

Pyridinethione This compound is a chelating agent that is usually encountered as the zinc complex. Two molecules of pyridinethione are complexed with zinc to form bis[1-hydroxy-2(1H)-pyridinethionato] zinc, commonly known as zinc pyridinethione or zinc pyrithione (ZPT) (Bond et al., 2002; Lewis et al., 2005).

ZPT is a biocide that has antibacterial and antifungal properties. It is the active ingredient in shampoos and other preparations for the treatment of seborrheic dermatitis and dandruff. ZPT is also used as an antifouling agent for ship paints, drywall, and tarps, and as an antibacterial agent for incorporation into cleaning sponges. Thus, the intended uses of ZPT can lead to human exposures through direct dermal contact and potential exposure to biota through leaching into marine and freshwater environments (Grunnet and Dahllof, 2005; Pierard-Franchimont et al., 2002).

Because the compound is directly applied to the human scalp in antidandruff shampoos, the finding that ZPT produced limb weakness and peripheral neuropathy in rodents after oral administration raised concern about potential neurotoxicity in humans (Sahenk and Mendell, 1979). Rats, rabbits, and guinea pigs all develop a distal axonopathy when exposed to ZPT in the diet. Fortunately, however, dermal absorption of ZPT is minimal, and there have been no reports of neurological findings in humans attributable to occupational or consumer ZPT exposures (Sahenk and Mendell, 2000).

Although the zinc ion appears to be an important component of the therapeutic action of ZPT, only the pyridinethione moiety is absorbed following ingestion, with the majority of zinc eliminated in the feces. In addition, oral sodium pyridinethione is also neurotoxic, indicating that the pyridinethione moiety is responsible for the neurotoxicity. Pyridinethione chelates zinc, copper, and other metal ions and, once oxidized to the disulfide, may lead to the formation of protein-pyridinethione mixed disulfides. However, which of these properties, if any, is responsible for the molecular mechanism of its neurotoxicity remains unknown (Sahenk and Mendell, 2000).

Although these molecular issues remain to be resolved, pyridinethione appears to interfere with the fast axonal transport systems. While the fast anterograde system is less affected, pyridinethione impairs the turnaround of rapidly transported vesicles and slows their retrograde transport (Sahenk and Mendell, 1980). This aberration of the fast axonal transport systems is the most likely physiologic basis of the accumulation of tubulovesicular structures in the distal axon. As these materials accumulate in one region of the axon, they distend the axonal diameter, resulting in axonal swellings filled with membranous profiles. As in many other distal axonopathies, the axon degenerates in its more distal regions beyond the accumulated structures. The earliest signs are diminished grip strength and electrophysiologic changes of the axon terminal, with normal conduction along the proximal axon in the early stages of exposure (Ross and Lawhorn, 1990).

Microtubule-Associated Neurotoxicity A number of plant alkaloids alter the assembly and depolymerization of microtubules in nerve axons, causing neurotoxicity. The oldest known of these are colchicine and the vinca alkaloids, which bind to tubulin and cause depolymerization of microtubules. Colchicine is an alkaloid pharmaceutical used in the treatment of gout, familial Mediterranean fever, and other disorders. A common side effect of treatment in patients with abnormal renal function is a peripheral axonal neuropathy. While this neuropathy is generally mild, it is often accompanied by a disabling myopathy that can lead to the inability to walk (Riggs et al., 1986).

A number of vinca alkaloids, including vincristine and vinblastine, both chemotherapeutic agents, produce a peripheral axonopathy very similar to that induced by colchicine. Vincristine is commonly used to treat leukemias and lymphomas, and also has greater potential for adverse toxic effects than vinblastine. The agent binds to tubulin subunits and prevents the polymerization into microtubules (Prakash and Timasheff, 1992). Nearly all evidence of vincristine-induced neuropathy has been observed in humans. Most treated patients develop neurotoxicity to some extent, beginning with parasthesias of the fingers. General weakness and clumsiness is common, but this improves quickly with removal of treatment. Parasthesias may persist, however, and some distal sensory loss may be permanent (Schaumburg, 2000).

More recently paclitaxel (Taxol), another plant alkaloid, has become a popular chemotherapeutic agent used to treat a variety of neoplasms. However, side effects include a predominantly sensory neuropathy, beginning in the hands and feet (Sahenk et al., 1994). Like colchicine and the vinca alkaloids, paclitaxel binds to tubulin; however, instead of leading to depolymerization, it promotes the formation of microtubules. Once formed, these microtubules remain stabilized by paclitaxel even in conditions that normally lead to dissociation of tubulin subunits, including cold temperatures or the presence of calcium (Schiff and Horowitz, 1981). When paclitaxel is injected directly into the sciatic nerve of rats, microtubules aggregate along the axon, causing axonal degeneration, demyelination, and impairment of regeneration (Lipton et al., 1989; Mielke et al., 2006).

The pathologies of the axon induced by these drugs are different. While colchicine leads to atrophy of the axon and a decrease in the number of microtubules, paclitaxel causes the aggregation to form a matrix that may inhibit fast axonal transport, which has been demonstrated with both colchicine and paclitaxel. A change in the number of microtubules has been observed in some reports and absent from others (Roytta et al., 1984; Nakata and Yorifuji, 1999). While the mechanisms may differ slightly, both exposures result in a peripheral neuropathy which must be taken into account in medical treatments.

Myelinopathies

Myelin provides electrical insulation of neuronal processes, and its absence leads to a slowing of and/or aberrant conduction of impulses between adjacent processes, so-called ephaptic transmission. Toxicants exist that result in the separation of the myelin lamellae, termed *intramyelinic edema,* and in the selective loss of myelin, termed *demyelination.* Intramyelinic edema may be caused by alterations in the transcript levels of myelin basic protein-mRNA (Veronesi et al., 1991) and early in its evolution is reversible. However, the initial stages may progress to demyelination, with loss of myelin from the axon. Demyelination may also result from direct toxicity to the myelinating cell. Remyelination in the CNS occurs to only a limited extent after demyelination. However, Schwann cells in the PNS are capable of remyelinating the axon after a demyelinating injury. Interestingly, remyelination after segmental demyelination in peripheral nerve involves multiple Schwann cells and results, therefore, in internodal lengths (the distances between adjacent nodes of Ranvier) that are much shorter than normal and a permanent record of the demyelinating event.

The compounds in Table 16-3 all lead to a myelinopathy. Some of these compounds have created problems in humans, and many have been used as tools to explore the process of myelination of the NS and the process of remyelination following toxic disruption of myelin. In general, the functional consequences of demyelination depend on the extent of the demyelination and whether it is localized within the CNS or the PNS or is more diffuse in its distribution. Those toxic myelinopathies in which the disruption of myelin is diffuse generate a global neurological deficit, whereas those that are limited to the PNS produce the symptoms of peripheral neuropathy.

Hexachlorophene Hexachlorophene, or methylene 2,2′-methyl-enebis(3,4,6-trichlorophenol), resulted in human neurotoxicity when newborn infants, particularly premature infants, were bathed with the compound to avoid staphylococcal skin infections (Mullick, 1973). Following skin absorption of this hydrophobic compound, hexachlorophene enters the NS and results in intramyelinic edema, splitting the intraperiod line of myelin in both the CNS and the PNS. The intramyelinic edema leads to the formation of vacuoles, creating a "spongiosis" of the brain (Purves et al., 1991). Experimental studies with erythrocyte membranes show that hexachlorophene binds tightly to cell membranes, resulting in the loss of ion gradients across the membrane (Flores and Buhler, 1974). This loss of the ability to exclude ions from between the layers of myelin leads to water and ion entry, which separates the myelin layers as "edema." Another, perhaps related, effect is the uncoupling of mitochondrial oxidative phosphorylation by hexachlorophene (Cammer and Moore, 1972), because this process is dependent on a proton gradient. Intramyelinic edema is reversible in the early stages, but with increasing exposure, hexachlorophene causes segmental demyelination. Swelling of the brain causes increased intracranial pressure, which may be fatal. With high-dose exposure, axonal degeneration is seen, along with degeneration of photoreceptors in the retina. It has been postulated that the pressure from severe intramyelinic edema may also injure the axon, leading to axonal degeneration; endoneurial pressure measurements support this idea (Myers et al., 1982). The toxicity of hexachlorophene expresses itself functionally in diffuse terms that reflect the diffuse process of myelin injury. Humans exposed acutely to hexachlorophene may have generalized weakness, confusion, and seizures. Progression may occur to include coma and death.

Tellurium Although human exposures have not been reported, neurotoxicity of tellurium has been demonstrated in animals. Young rats exposed to tellurium in their diet develop a severe peripheral neuropathy. Within the first 2 days of dietary exposure, the synthesis of myelin lipids in Schwann cells displays striking changes (Harry et al., 1989). These include decreased synthesis of cholesterol and cerebrosides (lipids richly represented in myelin), and down-regulated myelin protein mRNA (Morell et al., 1994). However, the synthesis of phosphatidylcholine, a more ubiquitous membrane lipid, is unaffected. The synthesis of free fatty acids and cholesterol esters increases to some degree, and there is a marked elevation of squalene, a precursor of cholesterol. These biochemical findings demonstrate a variety of lipid abnormalities, and the simultaneous increase in squalene and decrease in cholesterol suggest that tellurium or one of its derivatives may interfere with the normal conversion of squalene to cholesterol. Squalene epoxidase, a microsomal monooxygenase that utilizes NAPDH cytochrome P450 reductase, has been strongly implicated as the target of tellurium, because its inhibition by tellurium as well as certain other oranotellurium compounds shows a correlation between the potency of enzyme inhibition and demyelination in vivo (Goodrum, 1998).

In conjunction with these biochemical changes, lipids accumulate in Schwann cells within intracytoplasmic vacuoles; shortly afterwards, these Schwann cells lose their ability to maintain myelin. Axons and the myelin of the CNS are impervious to the effects of tellurium. However, individual Schwann cells in the PNS disassemble their concentric layers of myelin membranes, depriving the adjacent intact axon of its electrically insulated status. Not all Schwann cells are equally affected by the process; rather, those Schwann cells that encompass the greatest distances appear to be the most affected.

Table 16-3

Compounds Associated with Injury of Myelin (Myelinopathies)

NEUROTOXICANT	NEUROLOGIC FINDINGS	BASIS OF NEUROTOXICITY	REFERENCE
Acetylethyltetramethyl tetralin (AETT)	Not reported in humans; hyperexcitability, tremors (rats)	Intramyelinic edema; pigment accumulation in neurons	Graham and Lantos, 1997; Spencer and Schaumburg, 2000
Amiodarone	Peripheral neuropathy	Axonal degeneration and demyelination; lipid-laden lysosomes in Schwann cells	Graham and Lantos, 1997; Spencer and Schaumburg, 2000
Cuprizone	Not reported in humans; encephalopathy (experimental animals)	Status spongiosis of white matter, intramyelinic edema (early stages); gliosis (late)	Graham and Lantos, 1997; Spencer and Schaumburg, 2000
Disulfiram	Peripheral neuropathy, predominantly sensory	Axonal degeneration, swellings in distal axons	Graham and Lantos, 1997
Ethidium bromide	Insufficient data (humans)	Intramyelinic edema, status spongiosis of white matter	Spencer and Schaumburg, 2000
Hexachlorophene	Irritability, confusion, seizures	Brain swelling, intramyelinic edema in CNS and PNS, late axonal degeneration	Graham and Lantos, 1997; Spencer and Schaumburg, 2000
Lysolecithin	Effects only on direct injection into PNS or CNS (experimental animals)	Selective demyelination	Graham and Lantos, 1997
Perhexilene	Peripheral neuropathy	Demyelinating neuropathy, membrane-bound inclusions in Schwann cells	Graham and Lantos, 1997; Spencer and Schaumburg, 2000
Tellurium	Hydrocephalus, hind-limb paralysis (experimental animals)	Demyelinating neuropathy, lipofuscinosis (experimental animals)	Graham and Lantos, 1997
Triethyltin	Headache, photophobia, vomiting, paraplegia (irreversible)	Brain swelling (acute) with intramyelinic edema, spongiosis of white matter	Chang and Dyer, 1995; Graham and Lantos, 1997; Spencer and Schaumburg, 2000

These cells are associated with the largest-diameter axons, encompass the longest intervals of myelination, and provide the thickest layers of myelin. Thus, it appears that the most vulnerable cells are those with the largest volume of myelin to support (Bouldin et al., 1988).

As the process of remyelination begins, several cells cooperate to reproduce the myelin layers that were previously formed by a single Schwann cell. Perhaps this diminished demand placed upon an individual cell is the reason that remyelination occurs even in the presence of continued exposure to tellurium (Bouldin et al., 1988). The expression of the neurological impairment is also short in duration, reflecting the transient cellular and biochemical events. The animals initially develop severe weakness in the hind limbs but then recover their strength after 2 weeks on the tellurium-laden diet.

Lead   Lead exposure in animals results in a peripheral neuropathy with prominent segmental demyelination, a process that bears a strong resemblance to tellurium toxicity (Dyck et al., 1977). However, the neurotoxicity of lead is much more variable in humans than in rats, and there are also a variety of manifestations of lead toxicity in other organ systems.

The neurotoxicity of lead has been appreciated for centuries. In current times, adults are exposed to lead in occupational settings through lead smelting processes and soldering and in domestic settings through lead pipes or through the consumption of "moonshine" contaminated with lead. In addition, some areas contain higher levels of environmental lead, resulting in higher blood levels in the inhabitants. Children, especially those below 5 years of age, have higher blood levels of lead than adults in the same environment, due to the mouthing of objects and the consumption of substances other than food. In addition, children absorb lead more readily, and the very young do not have the protection of the blood–brain barrier. The most common acute exposure in children, however, has been through the consumption of paint chips containing lead pigments (Perlstein and Attala, 1966), a finding that has led to public efforts to prevent the use of lead paints in homes with children.

In young children, acute massive exposures to lead result in severe cerebral edema, perhaps from damage to endothelial cells. Children seem to be more susceptible to this lead encephalopathy than adults (Johnston and Goldstein, 1998); however, adults may also develop an acute encephalopathy in the setting of massive lead exposure.

Chronic lead intoxication in adults results in peripheral neuropathy, often accompanied by manifestations outside the NS, such as gastritis, colicky abdominal pain, anemia, and the prominent deposition of lead in particular anatomic sites, creating lead lines in the gums and in the epiphyses of long bones in children. The effects of lead on the peripheral nerve of humans (lead neuropathy) are not entirely understood. Electrophysiologic studies have demonstrated

Table 16-4

Compounds Associated with Neurotransmitter-Associated Toxicity

NEUROTOXICANT	NEUROLOGIC FINDINGS	BASIS OF NEUROTOXICITY	REFERENCE
Amphetamine and methamphetamine	Tremor, restlessness (acute); cerebral infarction and hemorrhage; neuropsychiatric disturbances	Bilateral infarcts of globus pallidus, abnormalities in dopaminergic, serotonergic, cholinergic systems Acts at adrenergic receptors	Spencer and Schaumburg, 2000; Hardman *et al.*, 1996
Atropine	Restlessness, irritability, hallucinations	Block cholinergic receptors (anticholinergic)	Spencer and Schaumburg, 2000; Hardman *et al.*, 1996
Cocaine	Increased risk of stroke and cerebral atrophy (chronic users); increased risk of sudden cardiac death; movement and psychiatric abnormalities, especially during withdrawal	Infarcts and hemorrhages; alteration in striatal dopamine neurotransmission	Spencer and Schaumburg, 2000; Hardman *et al.*, 1996
	Decreased head circumference (fetal exposure)	Structural malformations in newborns	
Domoic acid	Headache, memory loss, hemiparesis, disorientation, seizures	Neuronal loss, hippocampus and amygdala, layers 5 and 6 of neocortex Kainate-like pattern of excitotoxicity	Graham and Lantos, 1997; Spencer and Schaumburg, 2000
Kainate	Insufficient data in humans; seizures in animals (selective lesioning compound in neuroscience)	Degeneration of neurons in hippocampus, olfactory cortex, amygdala, thalamus Binds AMPA/kainate receptors	Graham and Lantos, 1997
β-*N*-Methylamino-ʟ-alanine (BMAA)	Weakness, movement disorder (monkeys)	Degenerative changes in motor neurons (monkeys) Excitotoxic probably via NMDA receptors	Graham and Lantos, 1997; Spencer and Schaumburg, 2000
Muscarine (mushrooms)	Nausea, vomiting, headache	Binds muscarinic receptors (cholinergic)	Hardman *et al.*, 1996
Nicotine	Nausea, vomiting, convulsions	Binds nicotinic receptors (cholinergic) low-dose stimulation; high-dose blocking	Spencer and Schaumburg, 2000; Hardman *et al.*, 1996
β-*N*-Oxalylamino-ʟ-alanine (BOAA)	Seizures	Excitotoxic probably via AMPA class of glutamate receptors	Graham and Lantos, 1997; Spencer and Schaumburg, 2000

a slowing of nerve conduction. Whereas this observation is consistent with the segmental demyelination that develops in experimental animals, pathologic studies in humans with lead neuropathy typically have demonstrated an axonopathy. Another finding in humans is the predominant involvement of motor axons, creating one of the few clinical situations in which patients present with predominantly motor symptoms. The basis for the effect on the brain (lead encephalopathy) is also unclear, although an effect on the membrane structure of myelin and myelin membrane fluidity has been shown (Dabrowska-Bouta *et al.*, 1999). The etiologies associated with the pathogenesis of peripheral neuropathy are, like that of central neuropathy, rather speculative. One hypothesis postulates that the effects of lead on the blood–nerve–barrier are similar to those on

the blood–brain barrier, providing a unitary mechanism for lead's effects on both the peripheral and central nervous systems. Another theory on the mechanisms associated with lead-induced effects on the peripheral nervous system suggests a toxic effect on Schwann cells, and the ensuing demyelination of nerves (Powell *et al.*, 1982). Although the manifestations of acute and chronic exposures to lead have been long established, the effects of low level exposures on infants and children have also become known. Initial reports noted a relationship between mild elevations of blood lead in children and school performance; more recently, correlations between elevated lead levels in decidual teeth and performance on tests of verbal abilities, attention, and behavior (nonadaptive) have been demonstrated (Needleman and Gatsonis, 1990; Needleman, 1994).

Although there is a clear association between lead level and intellectual performance, there has been some discussion as to whether lead is causal. Children with higher blood levels tend to share certain other environmental factors, such as socioeconomic status and parental educational level. However, in spite of these complex social factors, it appears that lead exposure has an adverse effect on the intellectual abilities of children (Needleman, 1994), although a threshold for these effects has not yet been determined.

Astrocytes

Rather than being the passive glue described by Virchow and other pathologists, astrocytes are now known to perform and regulate a wide range of physiological functions in the central nervous system. Perturbations in the function of these important cells are frequently reflected in abnormal neuronal physiology, even in the absence of altered nerve cell morphology. Indeed, the astrocyte appears to be a primary means of defense in the CNS following exposure to neurotoxicants, as a spatial buffering system for osmotically active ions, and as a depot for the sequestration and metabolic processing of endogenous molecules and xenobiotics. While in its relative infancy, investigations into the role of astrocytes in normal/abnormal function of the nervous system will be crucial to a better understanding of neurotoxicity and its pathological sequelae.

Ammonia   Hepatic encephalopathy (HE) or congenital and acquired hyperammonemia lead to excessive brain ammonia (ammonium, NH_4^+) accumulation. The condition results from liver failure. The effects of ammonia on the CNS vary with its concentration. At high CNS concentrations ammonia produces seizures, resulting from its depolarizing action on cell membranes, whereas, at lower concentrations, ammonia produces stupor and coma, consistent with its hyperpolarizing effects. Ammonia intoxication is associated with astrocytic swelling and morphological changes, yielding the so-called Alzheimer type II astrocytes, which precede any other morphological change (Mossakowski et al., 1970). The exclusive site for brain detoxification of glutamate to glutamine occurs within the astrocytes. This process requires ATP-dependent amidation of glutamate to glutamine, and it is mediated by the astrocyte-specific enzyme, glutamine synthetase (GS) and catalyzed by ammonia. Increased intracellular ammonia concentrations have also been implicated in the inhibition of neuronal glutamate precursor synthesis, resulting in diminished glutamatergic neurotransmission, changes in neurotransmitter uptake (glutamate), and changes in receptor-mediated metabolic responses of astrocytes to neuronal signals (Albrecht, 1996).

Nitrochemicals   The therapeutic potential of organic nitrates has been recognized for more than a century and began with the use of nitroglycerine for the management of acute anginal episodes. The resulting peripheral vasodilation and reduction in blood pressure, while useful in treating cardiovascular disease, has recently been shown to be only one of the pharmacologic properties of this class of chemicals. The mitochondrion features prominently as a target for nitrochemicals; however, the causal relationship between mitochondrial dysfunction and initiation of the neurotoxic state remains to be established for many of the chemicals.

The dinitrobenzenes are important synthetic intermediates in the industrial production of dyes, plastics, and explosives. The neurotoxic compound, 1,3-dinitrobenzene (DNB), produces gliovascular lesions that specifically target astrocytes in the periaqueductal gray matter of the brainstem and deep cerebellar roof nuclei (Philbert et al., 1987). Though the molecular basis for the remarkable sensitivity of this cell population is unclear, it has been proposed that bioactivation of DNB by NADPH-dependent cytochrome c reductase (Hu et al., 1997; Romero et al., 1991) and subsequent induction of oxidative stress underlies its toxicity (Romero et al., 1995; Ray et al., 1992, 1994; Hu et al., 1999). Brainstem nuclei with high glucose requirements, such as the vestibular and deep cerebellar roof nuclei are affected more severely than forebrain and mesencephalic structures that have similar or higher requirements for glucose and oxygen (Calingasan et al., 1994; Bagley et al., 1989; Mastrogiacomo et al., 1993). The molecular basis of the susceptibility of brainstem astrocytes is unknown but growing evidence suggests that differences in mitochondrial respiratory capacity, cellular antioxidant levels, and the expression of proteins that regulate the mitochondrial permeability transition pore all contribute to the observed regional and cellular differences in susceptibility. In vitro studies indicate that DNB is a potent inducer of the mitochondrial permeability transition pore (mtPTP) (for reviews of the mtPTP see Lemasters et al., 1998; Crompton, 1999) in cultured C6 glioma cells (Tjalkens et al., 2000). Mitochondrial inner membrane permeabilization in an in vitro model of DNB exposure is dependent on generation of reactive oxygen species, in agreement with the reported capacity of DNB to deplete reduced pyridine nucleotides and glutathione due to redox-cycling (Romero et al., 1995).

Metronidazole, a 5-nitroimidazole [1-(2-hydroxyethyl)-2-methyl-5-nitroimidazole], is an antimicrobial, antiprotozoal agent that is commonly used for the treatment of a wide variety of infections. Prolonged treatment with metronidazole is associated with a peripheral neuropathy characterized by paraesthesias and dysaesthesias. In addition, headaches, glossitis, urticaria, pruritis, and other somatosensory disorders are also seen. Long-term administration of mitronidazole produces an irreversible sensorimotor deficit in the lower extremities of humans (Kapoor et al., 1999). Metronidazole is readily reduced to the highly reactive and toxic hydroxylamine intermediate and binds to cellular macromolecules including proteins and DNA (Coxon and Pallis, 1976). Use of higher intravenous doses of metronidazole for extended periods results in the expression of epileptiform seizures, hallucination, and attendant encephalopathy. The distribution of lesions is similar to preceding descriptions for DNB with the exception that both neurons and glia appear to be equally susceptible to the effects of metronidazole (Schentag, 1982). The mechanism of toxicity is well linked to the fact that metronidazole and its reduced metabolites bear close structural resemblance to the antineuritic nutrient, thiamine. Thiamine triphosphate (Vitamin B1) is an essential coenzyme in the mitochondrial metabolism of α-ketoglutarate and pyruvate, and also modulates the activity of sodium channels. Given the similarity in the lesions produced by metronidazole and pyrithiamine, a common antimetabolite mode of action has been proposed as the primary mechanism of neurotoxicity (Evans et al., 1975; Watanabe and Kanabe, 1978; Kapoor et al., 1999).

Methionine Sulfoximine   Methionine sulfoximine (MSO) is an irreversible inhibitor of the astrocyte-specific enzyme, glutamine synthetase (GS) (Albrecht and Norenberg, 1990). Ingestion of large amounts of MSO leads to neuronal cell loss in the hippocampal fascia dentata and pyramidal cell layer, in the short association fibers and lower layers of the cerebral cortex, and in cerebellar

Purkinje cells. MSO also leads to large increases of glycogen levels (Folbergrova, 1973), primarily within astrocytic cell bodies (Phelps, 1975), as well as swollen and damaged astrocytic mitochondria (Hevor, 1994). Although it is generally accepted that MSO inhibits GS, it remains unclear whether this inhibition represents the primary mechanism of MSO neurotoxicity. The relationship between inhibition of GS by MSO and seizure generation is also not well understood but is believed to be associated with inhibition of glutamate and GABA in seizure generation, since glutamine provides the precursor for these neurotransmitters. Rothstein and Tabakoff (1986) have demonstrated that the calcium-dependent, potassium-stimulated release of glutamate and aspartate is inhibited in striatal tissue after intracerebroventricular injection of MSO, and that their release correlates over time with the inhibition of GS.

Fluroacetate and Fluorocitrate The Krebs cycle inhibitor fluorocitrate (FC) and its precursor fluoroacetate (FA) are preferentially taken up by glia. FA occurs naturally in a number of plants, and has been used as a rodenticide (Compound 1080). It is prevalent in the South African plant *Dichapetalum cymosum*, commonly referred to as the Gifblaar plant. Exposure to FA may also occur via exposure to the anticancer drug 5-fluorouracil (Okeda *et al.*, 1990). Ingestion of large amounts of FA results in ionic convulsions. Animals consuming FA commonly seize within minutes, and those surviving these episodes frequently die later on due to respiratory arrest or heart failure. The actions of FC and FA have been attributed to both the disruption of carbon flux through the Krebs cycle and to impairment of ATP production (Swanson and Graham, 1994). FA can be metabolized to fluoroacetyl CoA, followed by condensation with oxaloacetate to form FC by citrate synthase. A second hypothesis implies that FA toxicity is associated with the inhibition of a bi-directional citrate carrier in mitochondrial membranes, which leads to elevated intramitochondrial citrate and could affect citrate-dependent ATP synthesis (Kirsten *et al.*, 1978). Finally, it has been suggested that elevated citrate, secondary to inhibition of aconitase, is associated with the cytotoxicity of these compounds. FA selectively lowers the level of glutamine and inhibits glutamine formation in the brain, not by depleting glial cells of ATP, but by causing a rerouting of 2-oxoglutarate from glutamine synthesis into the TCA cycle during inhibition of aconitase (Hassel *et al.*, 1994). After the inhibition of aconitase, citrate accumulates, whereas the levels of isocitrate and α-ketoglutarate decrease. The reversible enzyme glutamate dehydrogenase begins to work in the opposite direction feeding more α-ketoglutarate into the TCA cycle (Martin and Waniewski, 1996).

Neurotransmission-Associated Neurotoxicity

A wide variety of naturally occurring toxins, as well as synthetic chemicals, alters specific mechanisms of intercellular communication. Some chemicals that have neurotransmitter-associated toxicity are listed in Table 16-4.

Whereas neurotransmitter-associated actions may be well understood for some chemicals, the specificity of the mechanisms should not be assumed. For example, organophosphorus (OP) and carbamate pesticides produce their insecticidal actions by inhibiting acetylcholinesterase, the catalytic enzyme that ends the postsynaptic action of acetylcholine. The resultant cholinergic overstimulation produces signs of acute toxicity ranging from flu-like symptoms to gastrointestinal distress, ataxia, twitching, convulsions, coma, and death. These effects are not as well correlated with acetyl-cholinesterase inhibition as might be expected for all such pesticides, leading to suggestions of additional mechanisms of actions that have since been verified in animal and in vitro studies. These include direct actions on pre- and postsynaptic cholinergic receptors and altered reuptake of choline; such actions serve to modulate the downstream impact of cholinergic overstimulation (reviewed in Pope, 1999). Thus, multiple neurotransmitter targets may be more common than was once expected.

Nicotine Widely available in tobacco products and in certain pesticides, nicotine has diverse pharmacologic actions and may be the source of considerable toxicity. These toxic effects range from acute poisoning to more chronic effects. Nicotine exerts its effects by binding to a subset of cholinergic receptors, the nicotinic receptors. These receptors are located in ganglia, at the neuromuscular junction, and also within the CNS, where the psychoactive and addictive properties most likely reside. Smoking and "pharmacologic" doses of nicotine accelerate heart rate, elevate blood pressure, and constrict blood vessels within the skin. Because the majority of these effects may be prevented by the administration of α- and β-adrenergic blockade, these consequences may be viewed as the result of stimulation of the ganglionic sympathetic nervous system (Benowitz, 1986). At the same time, nicotine leads to a sensation of "relaxation" and is associated with alterations of electroencephalographic (EEG) recordings in humans. These effects are probably related to the binding of nicotine with nicotinic receptors within the CNS, and the EEG changes may be blocked with mecamylamine, a nicotinic antagonist.

Acute overdose of nicotine has occurred in children who accidentally ingest tobacco products, in tobacco workers exposed to wet tobacco leaves (Gehlbach *et al.*, 1974), and in workers exposed to nicotine-containing pesticides. In each of these settings, the rapid rise in circulating levels of nicotine leads to excessive stimulation of nicotinic receptors, a process that is followed rapidly by ganglionic paralysis. Initial nausea, rapid heart rate, and perspiration are followed shortly by marked slowing of heart rate with a fall in blood pressure. Somnolence and confusion may occur, followed by coma; if death results, it is often the result of paralysis of the muscles of respiration.

Such acute poisoning with nicotine fortunately is uncommon. Exposure to lower levels for longer duration, in contrast, is very common, and the health effects of this exposure are of considerable epidemiologic concern. In humans, however, it has been difficult to separate the effects of nicotine from those of other components of cigarette smoke. The complications of smoking include cardiovascular disease, cancers (especially malignancies of the lung and upper airway), chronic pulmonary disease, and attention deficit disorders in children of women who smoke during pregnancy. Nicotine may be a factor in some of these problems. For example, an increased propensity for platelets to aggregate is seen in smokers, and this platelet abnormality correlates with the level of nicotine. Nicotine also places an increased burden on the heart through its acceleration of heart rate and blood pressure, suggesting that nicotine may play a role in the onset of myocardial ischemia (Benowitz, 1986). In addition, nicotine also inhibits apoptosis and may play a direct role in tumor promotion and tobacco-related cancers (Wright *et al.*, 1993).

Cocaine and Amphetamines While nicotine is a legal and readily available addictive compound, cocaine and amphetamines are illegal, although still widely used. The number of adults using these drugs in the United States was approximately 9 million in 1972. That number grew to near 33 million in 1982, and in the 2001 National Household Survey on Drug Abuse it was reported that just over 10% of those surveyed had ever used cocaine, while approximately 2.6% claimed to have used it in the past 12 months (Fishburne *et al.*, 1983; U.S. Department of Health and Human Services, 2001). Cocaine use is abundant in urban settings. It is estimated that from 10–45% of pregnant women take cocaine (Volpe, 1992), and metabolites can be detected in up to 6% of newborns in suburban hospitals (Schutzman *et al.*, 1991).

Cocaine blocks the reuptake of dopamine, norepinephrine, and serotonin at the nerve terminal in the CNS, and also causes release of dopamine from storage vesicles. The primary event responsible for the addictive properties and euphoric feeling when intoxicated is a block on the dopamine reuptake transporter (DAT) (Giros *et al.*, 1996). This leads to enhanced dopaminergic transmission, and can result in a variety of symptoms in the user. Many individuals report a euphoric feeling and increased self-confidence, in addition to racing thoughts and a feeling of pressure. In other users, a period of paranoid psychosis ensues. The mechanism of altered neurotransmission has been linked to the dopamine D1 receptor, as mice lacking this receptor fail to exhibit many of the same characteristic behaviors as wild-type mice (Xu *et al.*, 2000).

Cocaine abuse also puts individuals at risk for cerebrovascular defects. Habitual users exhibit a greater degree of cerebral atrophy, compared by CT scan, and are more at risk of stroke and intracranial hemorrhage (Berliner, 2000). Cerebrovascular resistance assessed by Doppler sonography has also been found to be higher in cocaine abusers than controls (Herning *et al.*, 1999). In chronic cocaine users, neurodegenerative disorders have been observed, similar to those observed with amphetamine use.

Amphetamines also affect catecholamine neurotransmission in the CNS, but also have the potential to damage monoaminergic cells directly. Amphetamines, including methylenedioxymethamphetamine (MDMA, or "ecstasy"), have become popular with young adults in recent decades due to the belief that it is a "safe" drug, and its ability to increase energy and sensation in adults. However, they also exert serious side effects. Similar to cocaine, the most pronounced effect of amphetamines is on the dopaminergic neurons, but they can also damage 5-HT axons and axon terminals (McCann and Ricaurte, 2004). The result is a distal axotomy of DA and 5-HT neurons.

The exact mechanism of amphetamine neurotoxicity is still unknown, but several clues have emerged recently. It seems that oxidative stress plays a key role in toxicity. Following amphetamine-triggered dopamine release from the neuron, the dopamine is oxidized to produce free radicals (Lotharius and O'Malley, 2001). Chronic use can affect superoxide dismutase and catalase balance in rodents (Frey *et al.*, 2006), and amphetamine neurotoxicity is attenuated by antioxidants (DeVito and Wagner, 1989). It also induces hyperthermia when given at ambient temperatures, and it has been shown that increasing environmental temperature increases the associated neurotoxicity (Miller and O'Callaghan, 2003).

Because drug use and HIV infection have been linked, the effect of cocaine and amphetamine use on toxicity induced by HIV-1 proteins Tat and gp120 has also been investigated recently. HIV associated dementia (HAD) is a neurological disorder afflicting many AIDS patients. Exposure to cocaine and amphetamines in AIDS patients results in a synergistic neurotoxicity, which is attenuated by

β-estradiol (Turchan *et al.*, 2001). Oxidative stress has been implicated in this mechanism as well. When a normally nontoxic dose of cocaine is administered, Tat-induced oxidative stress is enhanced (Aksenov *et al.*, 2006).

Excitatory Amino Acids   Glutamate and certain other acidic amino acids are excitatory neurotransmitters. The discovery that these excitatory amino acids can be neurotoxic at concentrations that can be achieved in the brain has generated a great amount of interest in these "excitotoxins." In vitro systems have established that the toxicity of glutamate can be blocked by certain glutamate antagonists (Rothman and Olney, 1986), and the concept has emerged that the toxicity of excitatory amino acids may be related to such divergent conditions as hypoxia, epilepsy, and neurodegenerative diseases (Meldrum, 1987; Choi, 1988; Lipton and Rosenberg, 1994; Beal, 1992, 1995, 1998).

Glutamate is the main excitatory neurotransmitter of the brain and its effects are mediated by several subtypes of receptors (Fig. 16-8) called *excitatory amino acid receptors* (EAARs) (Schoepfer *et al.*, 1994; Hollmann and Heinemann, 1994; Lipton and Rosenberg, 1994). The two major subtypes of glutamate receptors are those that are ligand-gated directly to ion channels (ionotropic) and those that are coupled with G proteins (metabotropic). Ionotropic receptors may be further subdivided by their specificity for binding kainate, quisqualate, α-amino-3-hydroxy-5-methylisoxazole-4-propionic acid (AMPA), and *N*-methyl-D-aspartate (NMDA). The entry of glutamate into the CNS is regulated at the blood–brain barrier and, following an injection of a large dose of glutamate in infant rodents, glutamate exerts its effects in the area of the brain in which the blood–brain barrier is least developed, the circumventricular organ. Within this site of limited access, glutamate injures neurons, apparently by

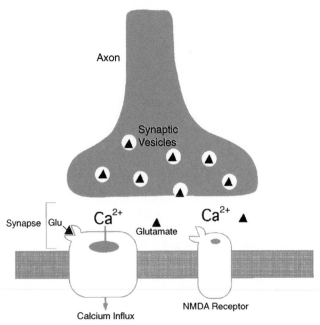

Figure 16-8. Excitatory synapse.

Synaptic vesicles are tranported to the axonal terminus, and released across the synaptic cleft to bind to the postsynaptic receptors. Glutamate, as an excitatory neurotransmitter, binds to its receptor and opens a calcium channel, leading to the excitation of the postsynaptic cell.

opening glutamate-dependent ion channels, ultimately leading to neuronal swelling and neuronal cell death (Olney, 1978; Coyle, 1987). The toxicity affects the dendrites and neuronal cell bodies but seems to spare axons. The only known related human condition is the "Chinese restaurant syndrome," in which consumption of large amounts of monosodium glutamate as a seasoning may lead to a burning sensation in the face, neck, and chest in sensitive individuals.

The cyclic glutamate analog kainate was initially isolated in Japan from seaweed as the active component of a herbal treatment of ascariasis. Kainate is extremely potent as an excitotoxin, being 100-fold more toxic than glutamate and is selective at a molecular level for the kainate receptor (Coyle, 1987). Like glutamate, kainate selectively injures dendrites and neurons and shows no substantial effect on glia or axons. As a result, this compound has found use in neurobiology as a tool. Injected into a region of the brain, kainate can destroy the neurons of that area without disrupting the fibers that pass through the same region. Neurobiologists, with the help of this neurotoxic tool, are able to study the role of neurons in a particular area independent of the axonal injuries that occur when similar lesioning experiments are performed by mechanical cutting.

Development of permanent neurological deficits in individuals accidentally exposed to high doses of an EAAR agonist has underscored the potential importance of excitatory amino acids in disease (Perl et al., 1990; Teitelbaum et al., 1990). A total of 107 individuals in the Maritime Provinces of Canada were exposed to domoic acid, an analog of glutamate, and suffered an acute illness that most commonly presented as gastrointestinal disturbance, severe headache, and short-term memory loss. A subset of the more severely afflicted patients was subsequently shown to have chronic memory deficits and motor neuropathy. Neuropathologic investigation of patients who died within 4 months of intoxication showed neurodegeneration that was most prominent in the hippocampus and amygdala but also affected regions of the thalamus and cerebral cortex.

Other foci of unusual neurodegenerative diseases also have been evaluated for being caused by dietary exposure to EAARs. Perhaps the best known of these is the complex neurodegenerative disease in the indigenous population of Guam and surrounding islands that shares features of amyotrophic lateral sclerosis, Parkinson's disease, and Alzheimer's disease. Early investigations of this Guamanian neurodegenerative complex suggested that the disorder may be related to an environmental factor, perhaps consumption of seeds of *Cycas circinalis* (Kurland, 1963). Subsequently, α-amino-methylaminopropionic acid (or B-*N*-methylamino-L-alanine, BMAA) was isolated from the cycad and was shown to be neurotoxic in model systems. The toxicity of BMAA is similar to that of glutamate in vitro and can be blocked by certain EAAR antagonists (Nunn et al., 1987). Studies in vivo, however, have not demonstrated a relationship between BMAA and the Guamanian neurodegenerative complex (Spencer et al., 1987; Hugon et al., 1988; Seawright et al., 1990; Duncan, 1992). Therefore, it remains unresolved what role cycad consumption and environmental factors play in this cluster of atypical neurodegenerative disease.

Models of Neurodegenerative Disease

MPTP Because of an error on the part of a so-called designer chemist, people who injected themselves with a meperidine derivative that was intended to serve as a substitute for heroin also received a contaminant, 1-methyl-4-phenyl-1,2,3,6-tetrahydropyridine (MPTP) (Fig. 16-9) (Langston et al., 1983). Over hours to days, dozens of these patients developed the signs and symptoms of irreversible Parkinson's disease (PD), some becoming immobile with rigidity (Langston and Irwin, 1986). Autopsy studies demonstrated marked degeneration of dopaminergic neurons in the substantia nigra, with degeneration continuing many years after exposure (Langston et al., 1999).

It was initially surprising to find not only that MPTP is neurotoxic, but also that it is a substrate for the B isozyme of monoamine oxidase (MAO-B) (Gerlach et al., 1991). MPTP, an uncharged species at physiologic pH, crosses the blood–brain barrier (BBB) and diffuses into cells, including astrocytes. The MAO-B of astrocytes catalyzes a two-electron oxidation to yield MPDP$^+$, the corresponding dihydropyridinium ion. A further two-electron oxidation yields the pyridinium ion, MPP$^+$ (Fig. 16-9). MPP$^+$ enters DAergic neurons of the substantia nigra via the dopamine (DA) uptake system, resulting in injury or death of the neuron. Noradrenergic neurons of the locus ceruleus are also vulnerable to repeated exposures of MPTP (Langston and Irwin, 1986), although they are less affected by single exposures than the DAergic neurons are. Once inside neurons, MPP$^+$ acts as a general mitochondrial toxin, blocking respiration at complex I (Di Monte and Langston, 2000). MPP$^+$ may also lead to the production of reactive oxygen species (ROS) and the release of DA from vesicles due to the higher pH environment of the cytosol, where the neurotransmitter undergoes autoxidation (Lotharius and O'Malley, 2000).

Consistent with the role of MAO-B in the bioactivation of MPTP to MPP$^+$, inhibitors of this enzyme, such as L-(-)-deprenyl (selegiline) protect against MPTP neurotoxicity. However, the protection afforded by deprenyl does not appear to arise from its inhibition of MAO-B alone, but also upon other properties, including its ability to act as an antioxidant and free-radical scavenger (Ebadi et al., 2002; Magyar and Szende, 2004; Mandel et al., 2003; Muralikrishnan et al., 2003). Thus, mice deficient in Cu,Zn-superoxide dismutase or glutathione peroxidase show increased vulnerability to MPTP neurotoxicity (Zhang et al., 2000), while overexpression of Mn-superoxide dismutase attenuates the toxicity (Klivenyi et al., 1998).

It should be noted that the general toxicity of the proximate neurotoxicant, MPP$^+$, is considerable when it is administered to animals, although systemic exposure to MPP$^+$ does not result in neurotoxicity, because it does not cross the BBB. Moreover, compared to primates, rats are relatively resistant to DAergic neurotoxicity from systemic administration of the parent compound, MPTP, even when the compound is injected directly in the cerebral circulation via the carotid artery. This resistance appears to be conferred, at least in part, by a high level of biotransformation of MPTP by rat endothelial cells to MPP$^+$ and other polar metabolites, such as MPTP-*N*-oxide, that are retained in endothelial cells and do not readily traverse the BBB (Mushiroda et al., 2001; Riachi et al., 1990; Scriba and Borchardt, 1989).

Although not identical, MPTP neurotoxicity and PD are strikingly similar. The symptomatology of each reflects a disruption of the nigrostriatal pathway. Thus, masked facies, difficulties in initiating and terminating movements, resting "pill-rolling" tremors, rigidity (including characteristic "cogwheel rigidity"), and bradykinesias are all features of both conditions. Pathologically, there is an unusually selective degeneration of neurons in the substantia nigra and depletion of striatal DA in both diseases (Di Monte and Langston, 2000). However, positron emission tomography (PET)

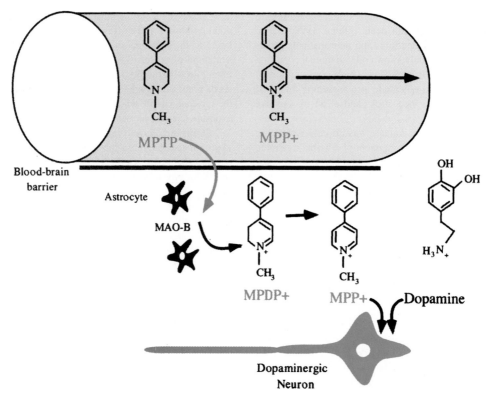

Figure 16-9. MPTP toxicity.

MPP$^+$, either formed elsewhere in the body following exposure to MPTP or injected directly into the blood, is unable to cross the blood–brain barrier. In contrast, MPTP gains access and is oxidized in situ to MPDP$^+$ and MPP$^+$. The same transport system that carries dopamine into the dopaminergic neurons also transports the cytotoxic MPP$^+$.

scanning studies employing the DAergic probe, [^{18}F]-fluorodopa, show that while patients with idiopathic PD demonstrate greater loss of DAergic function in the putamen than the caudate nucleus, the loss from these two nuclei was the same in patients who had taken MPTP (Snow *et al.*, 2000).

The discovery of the relationship between MPTP intoxication and Parkinsonism provided researchers with a new model for studying the pathogenic mechanism of PD and prompted investigations to reveal environmental and occupational exposures that might be associated with the disease (Dauer and Przedborski, 2003). Thus, epidemiological studies have implicated exposures to herbicides, other pesticides, or metals as risk factors for PD (Ferraz *et al.*, 1988; Gorell *et al.*, 1997, 1998, 1999; Liou *et al.*, 1997). Accordingly, the scope of neurotoxicants employed in experimental studies of PD has been enlarged beyond 6-hydroxydopamine (6-OHDA) and MPTP to include agricultural chemicals such as maneb, paraquat, and rotenone (Bove *et al.*, 2005; Uversky, 2004).

Epidemiological studies have also found apparent protective effects of cigarette smoking or coffee consumption on the development of PD (Lai *et al.*, 2002; Logroscino, 2005), and experimental studies indicate that nicotine and caffeine are protective in animal models of PD (Quik, 2004; Quik *et al.*, 2006; Ross and Petrovitch, 2001). It is interesting that PET studies of smokers show a marked reduction in brain MAO-B activity, similar to that produced by administration of the MAO-B inhibitor, L-deprenyl (Fowler *et al.*, 1996). Other MAO-B inhibitors are being developed as anti-PD drugs (Mandel *et al.*, 2005), and MAO-B inhibitors have been isolated from tobacco smoke (Khalil *et al.*, 2006). However, it appears that MAO-B inhibition is not essential for the neuropro-

tective activity of these agents; instead, their effectiveness stems from their overall ability to preserve mitochondrial integrity and function.

Although several families with early-onset PD demonstrate autosomal dominant inheritance and candidate genes have been identified (Agundez *et al.*, 1995; Kurth *et al.*, 1993; Polymeropoulos *et al.*, 1997), environmental exposures play a more significant role than genetics in the vast majority of PD patients, particularly those with late-onset disease (Kuopio *et al.*, 1999; Tanner *et al.*, 1999). Nevertheless, the delineation of specific genes involved in familial forms of PD (e.g., those encoding α-synuclein, parkin, ubiquitin C-terminal hydrolase L1, DJ-1, PTEN-induced putative kinase 1, and leucine-rich repeat kinase 2) has provided a rational basis for research concerning gene-environment interactions in the etiology of sporadic PD (Benmoyal-Segal and Soreq, 2006; Gosal *et al.*, 2006).

Several hypotheses on the loss of DAergic neurons in PD suggest that mitochondrial damage is a primary cause of DAergic neuronal death (Mandel *et al.*, 2005; Abou-Sleiman *et al.*, 2006). These include the following: (1) mitochondria of DAergic neurons are selectively vulnerable to environmental contaminants that cause mitochondrial dysfunction (Przedborski *et al.*, 2004; Amiry-Moghaddam *et al.*, 2005), (2) DAergic neurons produce an endogenous mitochondrial toxin (Naoi *et al.*, 2002), and (3) mitochondria harbor defects in enzymes, such as complex I, that lead to impaired energy metabolism (Greene *et al.*, 2005; Gu *et al.*, 1998). The centrality of mitochondria in these hypotheses arises primarily from findings that mitochondrial poisons, such as MPP$^+$ and rotenone can induce a Parkinson-like syndrome in humans, non-human primates, and rodents. These neurotoxicants are all capable of in-hibiting mitochondrial complex I and appear to model the pathology of PD. Moreover, neuropathological studies reveal a ~30% decrease in complex I function in deceased PD patients, as compared with age-matched controls (Adam-Vizi, 2005).

Mitochondrial complex I inhibitors, such as MPP^+ and rotenone, damage nigral neurons by mechanisms involving oxidation. Oxidative damage also plays a significant role in DAergic neuronal cell death induced by intracranial injection of 6-OHDA, another experimental model of PD (Cannon et al., 2006). Both enzymatic and auto-oxidation of 6-OHDA generate ROS, including H_2O_2, superoxide ions, and hydroxyl radicals (reactive oxygen species, or ROS). These ROS and the direct inhibition of complex I lead to lipid peroxidation, protein denaturation, and a decrease in reduced glutathione: all hallmark features of post mortem PD (Jenner, 2003).

It is remarkable that the poisoning of drug addicts by MPTP has led to major advances in our understanding of PD, which is the second most prevalent neurodegenerative disorder in the western world (Alzheimer's disease being first) (Landrigan et al., 2005). Although much remains to be done, knowing that most cases of PD arise from environmental exposures that promote mitochondrial dysfunction and oxidative damage provides us with promising avenues for prevention and treatment of this debilitating disease.

Manganese Manganese (Mn) is an essential metal in both humans and animals. Although Mn is present in almost all diets, animals maintain stable tissue Mn levels by tightly regulating absorption and excretory processes. As an essential trace metal that is found in all tissues, Mn is required for normal metabolism of amino acids, proteins, lipids, and carbohydrates. Mn acts as a cofactor for a variety of enzymes, such as manganese metalloenzymes and Mn-dependent enzyme families. Mn metalloenzymes include arginase, glutamine synthetase, phosphoenolpyruvate decarboxylase, and Mn superoxide dismutase (Mn-SOD). Mn-dependent enzymes include oxidoreductases, transferases, hydrolases, lyases, isomerases, and ligases. Therefore, Mn is necessary for the function of many organ systems. In rare Mn deficiencies, clinical manifestations can be seizures, impaired growth, skeletal abnormalities, and impaired reproductive function (Critchfield et al., 1993; Wedler, 1993).

At the other end of the spectrum, it is well established that excessive exposure to Mn causes neurotoxicity (McMillan, 1999; Aschner et al., 2005). The most common commercial sources of Mn include the fuel additive methylcyclopentadienyl manganese tricarbonyl (MMT), pesticides such as Maneb, steel factories, welding and mining plants. Occupational exposure to toxic levels of Mn in industrial workers results in psychological and neurological disturbances, including delusions, hallucinations, depression, disturbed equilibrium, compulsive or violent behavior, weakness and apathy, followed by extrapyramidal motor system defects such as tremors, muscle rigidity, ataxia, bradykinesia, and dystonia. Although Mn toxicity has been under investigation for many years, the underlying primary molecular mechanisms of its neurotoxicity remain to be elucidated. Very few potential biomarkers have been established with no early detection markers available.

The epidemiological associations and similarities in symptoms between Mn neurotoxicity and dopamine (DA) neuropathology suggest that exposure and accumulation of this metal may be an environmental factor that contributes to idiopathic Parkinson's disease (IPD). Mn toxicity causes a loss of DA neurons in the substantia nigra, and as in Parkinson's disease (PD), oxidative stress appears to play a significant role in the disorder (Oestreicher et al., 1994; Kienzl et al., 1995; Montgomery, 1995). The brain areas most susceptible to Mn injury are also highly sensitive to oxidative stress. Many metabolically active cell types, particularly tonically active motor neurons in the substantia nigra (SN), require high levels of ATP for optimal function and survival. Mn accumulates in the SN, globus pallidus (GP) and striatum and interferes with ATP synthesis, analogous to effects seen with mitochondrial inhibitors or ischemia. Appraisal of the literature strongly suggests that in addition to targeting similar brain areas, dopaminergic (DAergic) neurodegeneration associated with PD and Mn exposure share multiple common mechanisms, namely mitochondrial dysfunction, aberrant signal transduction, oxidative stress, protein aggregation, and the activation of cell death pathways. The accumulation of Mn in the striatum causes damage to the SN, reduction in tyrosine hydroxylase (TH) activity, and loss of DA neurons (Parenti et al., 1988; Tomas-Camardiel et al., 2002). Intracellular Mn is sequestered by mitochondria through the Ca^{2+} uniporter (Gavin et al., 1999). Intrastriatal injections of Mn result in excitotoxic brain injury similar to that caused by mitochondrial poisons, such as aminooxyacetic acid and 1-methyl-4-phenyl-pyridinium (Brouillet et al., 1993b). The specificity for Mn accumulation in GP and striatum likely correlates with Mn transporter distribution and the metabolic activity of these basal ganglia nuclei.

Guamanian Cycad-Induced Parkinsonism/ALS syndrome An unusual prevalence of "hereditary paralysis" among the native Guam Chamorros was first reported in the early 1900s. This led to the formation of the National Institute of Neurological and Communicative Disorders and Stroke Research Center on Guam in 1939 (Rodgers-Johnson et al. 1986). In the mid-1950s the incidence of amyotrophic lateral sclerosis (ALS) and parkinsonism–dementia complex (PDC) was up to 100 times higher in Guam than anywhere else in the world (Hirano et al. 1961a). While Guam ALS is clinically indistinguishable from ALS that occurs elsewhere in the world, Guam PDC is a distinct neurodegenerative disorder where parkinsonism and dementia may occur simultaneously in affected Chamorros.

Hirano and colleagues first described the clinical features and pathology in 1961 (Hirano et al., 1961a,b). The main clinical features included mental deterioration, parkinsonism, and evidence of motor neuron involvement. The duration of clinical symptoms was about 4 years with the average age of diagnosis being approximately 52 years and a higher incidence in men. The main macroscopic neuropathological features are the presence of cortical atrophy and depigmentation of the substantia nigra. Microscopic evaluations revealed widespread ganglion cell degeneration and neurofibrillary tangles throughout the central nervous system. The lack of uniformity in the clinical presentation of these diseases has made it difficult to determine a possible causative agent.

Through the years, the focus has shifted from a genetic to an environmental causative agent. Due to the formation of the case registrar, established in 1958, entire pedigrees have been developed using Chamorros from the same village as controls. Although several investigators have reported a high degree of familial occurrence, no definitive inheritance pattern has been established (Plato et al., 2002). Support for an environmental hypothesis includes a decrease in the incidence of the diseases and an increase in the age of onset with the westernization of Guam (Plato et al., 2003).

Cycads are primitive plants that contain several toxins, including cycasin and L-β-methylaminoalanine (BMAA) (Schneider et al., 2002). Cycasin, which is metabolized to methylazoxymethanol (MAM), is known to be carcinogenic and cause hepatotoxicity (Sieber et al., 1980). BMAA is a nonprotein amino acid that functions as a glutamate excitotoxin (Rakonczay et al., 1991). In 1987, Spencer and colleagues reported that BMAA, when fed to primates in high concentrations (>100 mg/kg), produced a syndrome that closely resembled the neurological disorder observed in Guam. Traditionally, native Chamorros prepare food from cycads by washing the seeds several times, then grinding them into flour (Kisby et al., 1992). However, it appears that the washing process is sufficient to remove the cycad toxins (Duncan et al., 1990).

In 2002, Cox and Sacks suggested "the Chamorro population of Guam ingested large quantities of cycad toxins indirectly by eating flying foxes." This study demonstrated that the sharp decrease in the flying fox population was followed by a sharp decrease in the incidence of ALS. The flying fox, Pteropus mariannus, is a fruit bat with a wing span of 3 feet and is known to eat three times its weight in fruit, cycad seeds, or beetles which are known to bioaccumulate cycad toxins for protective purposes (Schneider et al., 2002). The consumption of the flying foxes by the Chamorros is not only included in social, but ceremonial settings (Banack and Cox, 2003). Traditionally, the men consume the animal in its entirety, while the women only consume the breast meat.

Accumulation of the neurotoxin, BMAA, in the flying fox, Pteropus mariannus, may result in concentrations that are sufficient to cause behavioral and neuropathological changes in primates similar to those observed in the Guam ALS-PDC. Furthermore, BMAA-induced neurodegeneration may occur by an excitotoxic mechanism involving the mitochondria permeability transition pore (mtPTP). It has been shown that BMAA increases the intracellular calcium concentration through the formation of a β-carbamate intermediate (Brownson et al., 2002). This intermediate can act as a glutamate agonist and induce glutamate excitotoxicity. Studies have also demonstrated that an increase in intracellular calcium (Dubinsky and Levi, 1998) and glutamate excitotoxicity are able to induce mtPTP (Schinder et al., 1996).

Developmentally Neurotoxic Chemicals

Replication, migration, differentiation, myelination, and synapse formation are the basic processes that underlie development of the NS. There are a variety of insults known to disrupt NS development, the outcomes of which may be very different depending on the time of exposure, including exposures to certain metals, solvents, antimetabolites, persistent organic pollutants, pesticides, pharmaceuticals, and ionizing radiation. Multiple mechanisms of action may be present, producing a wide array of effects in the offspring. The impact on the developing NS may be very different, and often cannot be predicted, from effects observed in adults.

Ethanol exposure during pregnancy can result in abnormalities in the fetus, including abnormal neuronal migration and facial development, and diffuse abnormalities in the development of neuronal processes, especially the dendritic spines (Stoltenburg-Didinger and Spohre, 1983). While the exposure may be of little consequence to the mother, it can be devastating to the fetus. There is an effect on NMDA glutamate receptors and excessive activation of GABA receptors, with induction of apoptosis throughout the brain (Ikonomidou et al., 2000). The clinical result of fetal alcohol exposure is often mental retardation, with malformations of the brain and delayed myelination of white matter (Riikonen et al., 1999). Although there remains a great deal of uncertainty concerning the molecular basis of this developmental aberration, it occurs in a variety of experimental animals, and it appears that acetaldehyde, a product of ethanol catabolism, can produce migration defects in developing animals similar to those that occur in the fetal alcohol syndrome (O'Shea and Kaufman, 1979).

Some developmental neurotoxicants have been revealed by human studies or tragic poisoning occurrences. The methyl mercury contamination of fish in Minamata Bay, Japan, led to the birth of many children with developmental disabilities, including cerebral palsy, mental retardation, and seizures. Since then, it was shown that children exposed to methyl mercury in utero show widespread neuronal loss, disruption of cellular migration, profound mental retardation, and paralysis (Costa et al., 2004; Reuhl and Chang, 1979). Studies on primates exposed in utero also have demonstrated abnormal social development (Burbacher et al., 1990). The earlier the exposure, the more generalized the damage that is observed. As with methyl mercury, ethanol and lead are known to produce frank neuropathology in highly exposed populations. However, in recent years the concept has emerged that extremely low levels of exposure to these substances in "asymptomatic" children may have an effect on their behavioral and cognitive development. The association between lead exposure and brain dysfunction has received experimental support in animal models and has prompted screening for lead in children (Benjamin and Platt, 1999). There is no proven safe lower limit for lead, and recent studies have attributed lower IQ scores to blood lead levels less than 5–10 μg/dl (Canfield et al., 2003; Winneke et al., 1994). Similarly, the debate regarding "safe" level of drinking during pregnancy is ongoing, with recent reports of no threshold for subtle cognitive effects (Sampson et al., 2000).

There is considerable evidence that chronic exposure to nicotine has effects on the developing fetus (reviewed in Slikker et al., 2005). Along with decreased birth weights, attention deficit disorders are more common in children whose mothers smoke cigarettes during pregnancy, and nicotine has been shown to lead to analogous neurobehavioral abnormalities in animals exposed prenatally to nicotine (Lichensteiger et al., 1988). Nicotinic receptors are expressed early in the development of the NS, beginning in the developing brainstem and later expressed in the diencephalon. The role of these nicotinic receptors during development is unclear; however, it appears that prenatal exposure to nicotine alters the development of nicotinic receptors in the CNS (van de Kamp and Collins, 1994)—changes that may be related to subsequent attention and cognitive disorders in animals and children.

Cocaine use during pregnancy is a major concern, especially in urban areas, where use can lead to a variety of acute and chronic adverse events in offspring. Cocaine is able to cross the placental barrier and the fetal blood–brain barrier, and also causes reduced blood flow in the uterus. In severe events at large doses taken by the mother, the fetus may develop hypoxia, leading to a higher rate of birth defects (Woods et al., 1987). Maternal cocaine use is associated with low birth weight and behavioral defects, including a decreased awareness of the surroundings and altered response to stress and pain sensitivity (Chasnoff et al., 1985; Huber et al., 2001).

Several epidemiological studies have reported deficits in neurodevelopment and psychological performance in children exposed to polychlorinated hydrocarbons (PCBs) and/or dioxins

(Seegal, 1996). Research in animals has shown that these persistent pollutants produce endocrine disruptions, cognitive deficits, and changes in activity levels in exposed offspring; however, the specific outcomes depend on the congener or mixture tested as well as the timing of exposure. Changes in estrogen or thyroid hormone, neurotransmitter function, and second messenger systems have been proposed as cellular bases for PCB toxicity (Seegal, 1996; Tilson and Kodavanti, 1998). Recent studies with another persistent class of hydrocarbons, polybrominated diphenyl ethers (PBDEs), have shown similarities in altering thyroid hormone metabolism and cholinergic function, and it has thus been proposed that this chemical class would also be developmentally neurotoxic (Branchi et al., 2003). Thyroid hormone is critical to NS development, and animal studies have suggested that the developing brain may be vulnerable to environmental thyrotoxicants of all sorts (Porterfield, 1994). Finally, it has been shown that even reversible changes in neurotransmission, such as those produced by nicotine or cholinesterase inhibitors, may alter specific growth processes and produce long-lasting deficits (Slotkin, 2004).

CHEMICALS THAT INDUCE DEPRESSION OF NERVOUS SYSTEM FUNCTION

Generalized depression of central nervous system function is produced by a variety of volatile solvents. These solvents include several chemical classes—aliphatic and aromatic hydrocarbons, halogenated hydrocarbons, ketones, esters, alcohols, and ethers—that are small, lipophilic molecules. They are widely found in industry, medicine, and commercial products. Human exposures range from chronic low-level concentrations encountered in environmental or occupational setting to high-level concentrations intentionally generated through solvent abuse.

There are several theories as to the mechanism of this generalized depression, but none is fully explanatory. Solvent potency correlates well with the olive oil:water or octanol:water partition coefficients, leading to the once-popular Meyer-Overton hypothesis that CNS depressants exert their actions through nonspecific disruption of the lipid portions of cell membranes (e.g., Janoff et al., 1981). Anesthesia could occur as a consequence of membrane expansion or perturbations of mitochondrial calcium transport. More recent research has implicated interactions with ligand-gated ion channels as well as voltage-gated calcium channels. Specific receptors regulating these channels include gamma-aminobutyric acid type A (GABA$_A$), N-methyl-D-aspartate (NMDA), and glycine receptors. These actions relate the effects of solvents to those of pharmaceutical agents such as barbiturates and benzodiazepines. While these targets have been demonstrated mostly for ethanol (Davies, 2003), recent in vitro studies have extended this generality to other volatile solvents (e.g., Cruz et al., 2000).

The CNS maintains balance via interplay between inhibitory and excitatory influences. With general depressants, initial suppression of inhibitory systems at low doses produces excitation, such as intoxication observed with ethanol. Thus, acutely, solvents produce a continuum of effects from excitation to sedation, motor impairment, coma, and ultimately death by depression of respiratory centers. A syndrome known as solvent-induced chronic toxic encephalopathy has been described for some populations with long-term and/or high-level exposure. Somewhat vague presenting symptoms include irritability, fatigue, impaired memory or concentration, leading to the need for widely-accepted diagnostic criteria (van der Hoek et al., 2000). The absence of corroborating animal studies have prevented studies of molecular changes which may underlie these long-term effects, and indeed, have raised doubt as to the existence of such a syndrome (Ridgway et al., 2003). Specific solvents also produce other neurotoxicological actions, such as peripheral neuropathy, which are described elsewhere in this text.

REFERENCES

Abou-Donia MB: Triphenyl phosphite: A Type II organophosphorus compound-induced delayed neurotoxic agent, in Chambers JE, Levi PE (eds.): *Organophosphates: Chemistry, Fate, and Effects*. San Diego: Academic Press, 1992, pp. 327–351.

Abou-Donia MB, ed: *Neurotoxicology*. Boca Raton, FL: CRC Press, 1993.

Abou-Sleiman PM, Muqit MM, Wood NW: Expanding insights of mitochondrial dysfunction in Parkinson's disease. *Nat Rev Neurosci* 7:207–219, 2005.

Adams J, Barone Jr. S, LaMantia A, et al.: Workshop to identify critical windows of exposure for children's health: Neurobehavioral work group summary. *Environ Health Perspect* 108 (Suppl 3):535–544, 2000.

Adam-Vizi V: Production of reactive oxygen species in brain mitochondria: Contribution by electron-transport chain and non-electron transport chain sources. *Antioxid Redox Signal* 7:1140–1149, 2005.

Agundez JA, Jimenez JF, Luengo A, et al.: Association between the oxidative polymorphism and early onset of Parkinson's disease. *Clin Pharmacol Ther* 57:291–298, 1995.

Aksenov MY, Aksenov MV, Nath A, et al.: Cocaine-mediated enhancement of Tat toxicity in rat hippocampal cell cultures: The role of oxidative stress and D1 dopamine receptor. *Neurotoxicology* 27:217–228, 2006.

Albrecht J: Astrocytes and ammonia neurotoxicity, in Aschner M, Kimelberg HK (eds.): *The Role of Glia in Neurotoxicity*. Boca Raton: CRC Press, 1996, pp. 137–153.

Albrecht J, Norenberg MD: L-methionine-DL-sulfoximine induces massive efflux of glutamine from cortical astrocytes in primary culture. *Eur J Pharmacol* 182:587–599, 1990.

Altman J, Sudarshan K: Postnatal development of locomotion in the laboratory rat. *Anim Behav* 23:896–920, 1975.

Amarnath V, Anthony DC, Valentine WM, et al.: The molecular mechanism of the carbon disulfide mediated crosslinking of proteins. *Chem Res Toxicol* 4:148–150, 1991.

Amiry-Moghaddam M, Lindland H, Zelenin S, et al.: Brain mitochondria contain aquaporin water channels: Evidence for the expression of a short AQP9 isoform in the inner mitochondrial membrane. *FASEB J* 19:1459–1467, 2005.

Anderson JP, Carroll Z, Smulowitz M, et al.: A possible mechanism of action of the neurotoxic agent iminodipropionitrile (IDPN): A selective aggregation of the medium and heavy neurofilament polypeptides (NF-M and NF-H). *Brain Res* 547:353–357, 1991.

Anthony DC, Boekelheide K, Graham DG: The effect of 3,4-dimethyl substitution on the neurotoxicity of 2,5-hexanedione: I. Accelerated clinical neuropathy is accompanied by more proximal axonal swellings. *Toxicol Appl Pharmacol* 71:362–371, 1983.

Aschner M, Erikson KM, Dorman DC: Manganese dosimetry: Species differences and implications for neurotoxicity. *Crit Rev Toxicol* 35:1–32, 2005.

Atchison WD, Hare MF: Mechanisms of methylmercury-induced neurotoxicity. *FASEB J* 8:622–629, 1994.

Auer RN, Benveniste H: Hypoxia and related conditions, in Graham DI, Lantos PL (eds.): *Greenfield's Neuropathology,* 6th ed. New York: Arnold, 1997, pp. 263–314.

Bachurin SO, Shevtzove EP, Lermontova NN, *et al.*: The effect of dithiocarbamates on neurotoxic action of 1-methyl-4-phenyl-1,2,3,6-tetrahydropyridine (MPTP) and on mitochondrial respiration chain. *Neurotoxicology* 17:897–903, 1996.

Bagley PR, Tucker SP, Nolan C, *et al.*: Anatomical mapping of glucose transporter protein and pyruvate dehydrogenase in rat brain: An immunogold study. *Brain Res* 499:214–224, 1989.

Bakir F, Damluji SF, Amin-Zaki L, *et al.*: Methylmercury poisoning in Iraq. *Science* 181:230–241, 1973.

Balaban CD, O'Callaghan JP, Billingsley ML: Trimethyltin-induced neuronal damage in the rat brain: Comparative studies using silver degeneration stains, immunocytochemistry and immunoassay for neuronotypic and gliotypic proteins. *Neuroscience* 26:337–361, 1988.

Banack SA, Cox PA: Biomagnification of cycad neurotoxins in flying foxes: Implications for ALS-PDC in Guam. *Neurology* 61:387–389, 2003.

Barone Jr. S, Stanton ME, Mundy WR: Neurotoxic effects of triethyltin (TET) exposure are exacerbated with aging. *Neurobio Aging* 16:723–735, 1995.

Bayer SA, Altman J, Russo RJ, *et al.*: Timetables of neurogenesis in the human brain based on experimentally determined patterns in the rat. *Neurotoxicology* 14:83–144, 1993.

Beal MF: Does impairment of energy metabolism result in excitotoxic neuronal death in neurodegenerative illnesses? *Ann Neurol* 31:119–130, 1992.

Beal MF: Aging, energy, and oxidative stress in neurodegenerative diseases. *Ann Neurol* 38:357–366, 1995.

Beal MF: Excitotoxicity and nitric oxide in Parkinson's disease pathogenesis. *Ann Neurol* 44:S110–S114, 1998.

Benjamin JT, Platt C: Is universal screening for lead in children indicated? An analysis of lead results in Augusta, Georgia in 1997. *J Med Assoc Ga* 88:24–26, 1999.

Benmoyal-Segal L, Soreq H: Gene-environment interactions in sporadic Parkinson's disease. *J Neurochem* 97:1740–1755, 2006.

Benowitz NL: Clinical pharmacology of nicotine. *Annu Rev Med* 37:21–32, 1986.

Berliner R: Cocaine, in Spencer PS, Schaumburg HH (eds.): *Experimental and Clinical Neurotoxicology*. New York: Oxford University Press, 2000, pp. 408–413.

Besser R, Kramer G, Thumler R, *et al.*: Acute trimethyltin limbic-cerebellar syndrome. *Neurology* 37:945–950, 1987.

Bond AD, Benevellit F, Jones W: Modification of the solid-state structure of bis(1-hydroxy-2(1H)-pyridine-S²,O)zinc(II): Synthesis and characterization of a molecular solid solution incorporating 3-hydroxy-4-methyl-2-3H)-thiazolethione. *J Mater Chem* 12:324–332, 2002.

Bouldin TW, Samsa G, Earnhardt TS, *et al.*: Schwann cell vulnerability to demyelination is associated with internodal length in tellurium neuropathy. *J Neuropathol Exp Neurol* 47:41–47, 1988.

Bove J, Prou D, Perier C, *et al.*: Toxin-induced models of Parkinson's disease. *NeuroRx* 2:484–494, 2005.

Branchi I, Capone F, Alleva E, *et al.*: Polybrominated diphenyl ethers: Neurobehavioral effects following developmental exposure. *Neurotoxicology* 24:449–462, 2003.

Brouillet E, Jenkins BG, Hyman BT, *et al.*: Age-dependent vulnerability of the striatum to the mitochondrial toxin 3-nitropropionic acid. *J Neurochem* 60:356–359, 1993a.

Brouillet EP, Shinobu L, McGarvey U, *et al.*: Manganese injection into the rat striatum produces excitotoxic lesions by impairing energy metabolism. *Exp Neurol* 120:89–94, 1993b.

Brownson DM, Mabry TJ, Leslie SW: The cycad neurotoxic amino acid, beta-N-methylamino-L-alanine (BMAA), elevates intracellular calcium levels in dissociated rat brain cells. *J Ethnopharmacol* 82:159–167, 2002.

Burbacher TM, Sackett GP, Mottet NK: Methylmercury effects on the social behavior of Macaca fascicularis. *Neurotoxicol Teratol* 12:65–71, 1990.

Calingasan NY, Baker H, Sheu KF, *et al.*: Selective enrichment of cholinergic neurons with the alpha-ketoglutarate dehydrogenase complex in rat brain. *Neurosci Lett* 168:209–212, 1994.

Calne DB, Langston JW, Martin WR, *et al.*: Positron emission tomography after MPTP: Observations relating to the cause of Parkinson's disease. *Nature* 317:246–248, 1985.

Cammer W, Moore CL: The effect of hexachlorophene on the respiration of brain and liver mitochondria. *Biochem Biophys Res Commun* 46:1887–1894, 1972.

Canfield RL, Henderson Jr. CR, Cory-Slechta DA, *et al.*: Intellectual impairment in children with blood lead concentrations below 10 microg per deciliter. *N Engl J Med* 348:1517–1526, 2003.

Cannon JR, Keep RF, Schallert T, *et al.*: Protease-activated receptor-1 mediates protection elicited by thrombin preconditioning in a rat 6-hydroxydopamine model of Parkinson's disease. *Brain Res.* 1116:177–186, 2006.

Casida JE, Quistad GB: Serine hydrolase targets of organophosphorus toxicants. *Chem Biol Interact* 157–158:277–283, 2005.

Cavanagh JB: The significance of the "dying-back" process in experimental and human neurological disease. *Int Nat Rev Exp Pathol* 7:219–267, 1964.

Chang LW, Dyer RS, eds: *Handbook of Neurotoxicology*. New York: Marcel Dekker, 1995.

Chasnoff IJ, Burns WJ, Schnoll SH, *et al.*: Cocaine use in pregnancy. *N Engl J Med* 313:666–669, 1985.

Chaudry V, Cornblath DR: Wallerian degeneration in human nerves: Serial electrophysiological studies. *Muscle Nerve* 15:687–693, 1992.

Cheng KC, Cahill DS, Kasai H, *et al.*: 8-Hydroxyguanine, an abundant form of oxidative DNA damage, causes G–T and A–C substitutions. *J Biol Chem* 267:166–172, 1992.

Cheung MK, Verity MA: Experimental methyl mercury neurotoxicity: Locus of mercurial inhibition of brain protein synthesis in vivo and in vitro. *J Neurochem* 44:1799–1808, 1985.

Choi DW: Glutamate neurotoxicity and diseases of the nervous system. *Neuron* 1:623–634, 1988.

Chou SM, Hartmann HA: Axonal lesions and waltzing syndrome after IDPN administration in rats: with a concept "axostasis." *Acta Neuropathol* 3:428–450, 1964.

Chuang RY, Chuang LF: Inhibition of chicken myeloblastosis RNA polymerase II activity by adriamycin. *Biochemistry* 18:2069–2073, 1979.

Clark AW, Griffin JW, Price DL: The axonal pathology in chronic IDPN intoxication. *J Neuropathol Exp Neurol* 39:42–55, 1980.

Clarkson TW: The toxicology of mercury. *Crit Rev Clin Lab Sci* 34:369–403, 1997.

Collins JJ, Swaen GMH, Marsh GM, *et al.*: Mortality patterns among workers exposed to acrylamide. *J Occup Med* 31:614–617, 1989.

Costa LG, Aschner M, Vitalone A, *et al.*: Developmental neuropathology of environmental agents. *Ann Rev Pharmacol Toxicol* 44:87–110, 2004.

Cox PA, Sacks OW: Cycad neurotoxins, consumption of flying foxes, and ALS-PDC disease in Guam. *Neurology* 58:956–959, 2002.

Coxon A, Pallis CA: Metronidazole neuropathy. *J Neurol Neurosurg Psychiat* 36:403–405, 1976.

Coyle JT: Kainic acid: Insights into excitatory mechanisms causing selective neuronal degeneration, in Bock G, O'Connor M (eds.): *Selective Neuronal Death*. New York: Wiley, 1987, pp. 186–203.

Critchfield JW, Carl FG, Keen CL: Anticonvulsant-induced changes in tissue manganese, zinc, copper, and iron concentrations in Wistar rats. *Metabolism* 42:907–910, 1993.

Crofton KM, Padilla S, Tilson HA, *et al.*: The impact of dose rate on the neurotoxicity of acrylamide: The interaction of administered dose, target tissue concentrations, tissue damage, and functional effects. *Toxicol Appl Pharmacol* 139:163–176, 1996.

Crompton M: The mitochondrial permeability transition pore and its role in cell death. *Biochem J* 341:233–249, 1999.

Cruz SL, Balster RL, Woodward JJ: Effects of volatile solvents on recombinant N-methyl-D-aspartate receptors expressed in Xenopus oocytes. *Br J Pharmacol* 131:1303–1308, 2000.

Dabrowska-Bouta G, Sulkowski G, Bartosz G, *et al.*: Chronic lead intoxication affects the myelin membrane status in the central nervous system of adult rats. *J Mol Neurosci* 13:127–139, 1999.

Dauer W, Prezedborski S: Parkinson's disease: Mechanisms and models. *Neuron* 39:889–909, 2003.

Davies M: The role of GABAA receptors in mediating the effects of alcohol in the central nervous system. *J Psychiatry Neurosci* 28:263–274, 2003.

Davis M, Gendelman DS, Tischler MD, *et al.*: A primary acoustic startle circuit: Lesion and stimulation studies. *J Neurosci* 2:791–805, 1982.

Davis SL, Tanaka Jr D, Aulerich RJ, *et al.*: Organophosphorus-induced neurotoxicity in the absence of neuropathy target esterase inhibition: The effects of triphenyl phosphine in the European ferret. *Toxicol Sci* 49:78–85, 1999.

DeGrandchamp RL, Reuhl KR, Lowndes HE: Synaptic terminal degeneration and remodeling at the rat neuromuscular junction resulting from a single exposure to acrylamide. *Toxicol Appl Pharmacol* 105:422–433, 1990.

Dejneka NS, Polavarapu R, Deng X, *et al.*: Chromosomal localization and characterization of the stannin (Snn) gene. *Mamm Genome* 9:556–564, 1998.

DeVeaugh-Geiss J: Tardive dyskinesia: Phenomenology, pathophysiology, and pharmacology, in *Tardive Dyskinesia and Related Involuntary Movement Disorders.* Boston: John Wright PSG, 1982, pp. 1–18.

DeVito MJ, Wagner GC: Methamphetamine-induced neuronal damage: A possible role for free radicals. *Neuropharmacology* 28:1145–1150, 1989.

Di Monte DA, Langston JW: MPTP and analogs, in Spencer PS, Schaumburg HH (eds.): *Experimental and Clinical Neurotoxicology.* New York: Oxford University Press, 2000, pp. 812–818.

Dobbing J, Sands J: Comparative aspects of the brain growth spurt. *Early Hum Dev* 3:79–83, 1979.

Dobbing J, Smart JL: Vulnerability of developing brain and behaviour. *Br Med Bull* 30:164–168, 1974.

Dubinsky JM, Levi Y: Calcium-induced activation of the mitochondrial permeability transition in hippocampal neurons. *J Neurosci Res* 53:728–741, 1998.

Duncan MW: β-Methylamino-L-alanine (BMAA) and amyotrophic lateral sclerosis-parkinsonism dementia of the western Pacific. *Ann NY Acad Sci* 648:161–168, 1992.

Duncan MW, Steele JC, Kopin IJ, *et al.*: 2-Amino-3-(methylamino)-propanoic acid (BMAA) in cycad flour: An unlikely cause of amyotrophic lateral sclerosis and parkinsonism-dementia of Guam. *Neurology* 40:767–772, 1990.

Dyck PJ, O'Brien PC, Ohnishi A: Lead neuropathy: 2. Random distribution of segmental demyelination among "old internodes" of myelinated fibers. *J Neuropathol Exp Neurol* 36:570–575, 1977.

Ebadi M, Sharma S, Shavali S, *et al.*: Neuroprotective actions of selegiline. *J Neurosci Res* 67:285–289, 2002.

Erve JCL, Amarnath V, Graham D, *et al.*: Carbon disulfide and *N,N*-diethyldithiocarbamate generate thiourea cross-links on erythrocyte spectrin. *Chem Res Toxicol* 11:544–549, 1998a.

Erve JCL, Amarnath V, Sills RC, *et al.*: Characterization of a valine-lysine thiourea cross-link on rat globin produced by carbon disulfide or *N,N*-diethyldithiocarbamate in vivo. *Chem Res Toxicol* 11:1128–1136, 1998b.

Evans WC, Evans IA, Humphreys DJ, *et al.*: Induction of thiamine deficiency in sheep with lesions similar to those of cerebro-cortical necrosis. *J Comp Pathol* 85:253–267, 1975.

Federal Register: *Principles of Neurotoxicity Risk Assessment. Environmental Protection Agency Final Report*, Vol 59, no 158. Washington, DC: U.S. Government Printing Office, 1994, pp. 42360–42404.

Ferraz HB, Bertolucci PH, Pereira JS, *et al.*: Chronic exposure to the fungicide maneb may produce symptoms and signs of CNS manganese intoxication. *Neurology* 38:550–553, 1988.

Fishburne PM, Abelson HI, Cisin I: *National Household Survey on Drug Abuse: National Institute of Drug and Alcohol Abuse Capsules*, 1982. Washington, DC: Department of Health and Human Services, 1983.

Flores G, Buhler DR: Hemolytic properties of hexachlorophene and related chlorinated biphenols. *Biochem Pharmacol* 23:1835–1843, 1974.

Folbergrova J: Glycogen and glycogen phosphorylase in the cerebral cortex of mice under the influence of methionine sulfoximine. *J Neurochem* 20:547–557, 1973.

Fowler JS, Volkow ND, Wang GJ, *et al.*: Inhibition of monoamine oxidase B in the brains of smokers. *Nature* 379:733–736, 1996.

Fox WM: Reflex-ontogeny and behavioural development of the mouse. *Anim Behav* 13:234–241, 1965.

Frey BN, Valvassori SS, Reus GZ, *et al.*: Changes in antioxidant defense enzymes after D-amphetamine exposure: Implications as an animal model of mania. *Neurochem Res* 31:699–703, 2006.

Garland TO, Paterson MWH: Six cases of acrylamide poisoning. *Brit Med J* 4:134–138, 1967.

Garman RH, Weiss B, Evans HL: Alkylmercurial encephalopathy in the monkey: A histopathologic and autoradiographic study. *Acta Neuropathol (Berl)* 32:61–74, 1975.

Gavin CE, Gunter KK, Gunter TE: Manganese and calcium transport in mitochondria: Implications for manganese toxicity. *Neurotoxicology* 20:445–453, 1999.

Gehlbach SH, Williams WA, Perry LD, *et al.*: Green-tobacco sickness: An illness of tobacco harvesters. *JAMA* 229:1880–1883, 1974.

George EB, Glass JD, Griffin JW: Axotomy-induced axonal degeneration is mediated by calcium influx through ion-specific channels. *J Neurosci* 15:6445–6452, 1995.

Gerlach M, Riederer P, Przuntek H, *et al.*: MPTP mechanisms of neurotoxicity and their implications for Parkinson's disease. *Eur J Pharmacol* 12:273–286, 1991.

Giros B, Jaber SR, Wightman RM, *et al.*: Hyperlocomotion and indifference to cocaine and amphetamine in mice lacking the dopamine transporter. *Nature* 379:606–612, 1996.

Glass JD, Brushart TM, George EB, *et al.*: Prolonged survival of transected fibers in C57BL/Ola mice is intrinsic characteristic of the axon. *J Neurocytol* 22:311–321, 1993.

Gold BG.: β,β′-iminodipropionitrile, in Spencer PS, Schaumburg HH (eds.): *Experimental and Clinical Neurotoxicology.* New York: Oxford University Press, 2000, pp. 678–679.

Goldberger ME, Murray M: Recovery of function and anatomical plasticity after damage to the adult and neonatal spinal cord, in Cotman CW (ed.): *Synaptic Plasticity.* New York: Guilford Press, 1985, pp. 77–110.

Goodrum JF: Role of organotellurium species in tellurium neuropathy. *Neurochem Res* 23:1313–1319, 1998.

Gorell JM, Johnson CC, Rybicki BA, *et al.*: Occupational exposures to metals as risk factors for Parkinson's disease. *Neurology* 48:650–658, 1997.

Gorell JM, Johnson CC, Rybicki BA, *et al.*: The risk of Parkinson's disease with exposure to pesticides, farming, well water and rural living. *Neurology* 59:1346–1350, 1998.

Gorell JM, Johnson CC, Rybicki BA, *et al.*: Occupational exposure to manganese copper, lead, iron, mercury and zinc and the risk of Parkinson's disease. *Neurotoxicology* 20:239–247, 1999.

Gosal D, Ross OA, Toft M: Parkinson's disease: The genetics of a heterogeneous disorder. *Eur J Neurol* 13:616–627, 2006.

Grafstein B: Axonal transport: Function and mechanisms, in Waxman SG, Kocsis JD, Stys PK (eds.): *The Axon: Structure, Function, and Pathophysiology.* New York: Oxford University Press, 1995, pp. 185–199.

Graham DG, Amarnath V, Valentine WM, *et al.*: Pathogenetic studies of hexane and carbon disulfide neurotoxicity. *CRC Crit Rev Toxicol* 25:91–112, 1995.

Graham DG, Anthony DC, Boekelheide K, *et al.*: Studies of the molecular pathogenesis of hexane neuropathy. II. Evidence that pyrrole derivatization of lysyl residues leads to protein crosslinking. *Toxicol Appl Pharmacol* 64:415–422, 1982.

Graham DI, Lantos PL, eds: *Greenfield's Neuropathology,* 6th ed. New York: Arnold, 1997.

Greene JG, Dingledine R, Greenmyre JT: Gene expression profiling of rat midbrain dopamine neurons: Implications for selective vulnerability in parkinsonism. *Neurobiol Dis* 18:19–31, 2005.

Griffin JW, Fahnestock KE, Price DL, *et al.*: Microtubule-neurofilament segregation produced by β,β′-iminodipropionitrile: Evidence for the association of fast axonal transport with microtubules. *J Neurosci* 3:557–566, 1983.

Grunnet KS, Dahllof I: Environmental fate of the antifouling compound zinc pyrithione in seawater. *Environ Toxicol Chem* 24:3001–3006, 2005.

Gu M, Cooper JM, Taanman JW, *et al.*: Mitochondrial DNA transmission of the mitochondrial defect in Parkinson's disease. *Ann Neurol* 44:177–186, 1998.

Gutierrez PL: The role of NAD(P)H oxidoreductase (DT-Diaphorase) in the bioactivation of quinone-containing antitumor agents: A review. *Free Radic Biol Med* 29:263–275, 2000.

Hardman JG, Limbird LE, Molinoff PB, Ruddon RW, eds: *Goodman and Gilman's The Pharmacologic Basis of Therapeutics,* 9th ed. New York: McGraw-Hill, 1996.

Harris CH, Gulati AK, Friedman MA, *et al.*: Toxic neurofilamentous axonopathies and fast axonal transport: V. Reduced bidirectional vesicle transport in cultured neurons by acrylamide and glycidamide. *J Toxicol Environ Health* 42:343–456, 1994.

Harry GJ, Goodrum JF, Bouldin TW, *et al.*: Tellurium-induced neuropathy: Metabolic alterations associated with demyelination and remyelination in rat sciatic nerve. *J Neurochem* 52:938–945, 1989.

Hassel B, Sonnewald U, Unsgard G, *et al.*: NMR spectroscopy of cultured astrocytes: Effects of glutamine and the gliotoxin fluorocitrate. *J Neurochem* 62:2187–2194, 1994.

Herning R, King D, Better W, *et al.*: Neurovascular deficits in cocaine abusers. *Neuropsychopharmacology* 21:110–118, 1999.

Hevor TK: Some aspects of carbohydrate metabolism in the brain. *Biochimie* 76:111–120, 1994.

Hirano A, Kurland LT, Krooth RS, *et al.*: Parkinsonism-dementia complex, an endemic disease on the island of Guam. I. Clinical features. *Brain* 84:642–661, 1961a.

Hirano A, Malamud N, Kurland LT: Parkinsonism-dementia complex, an endemic disease on the island of Guam. II. Pathological features. *Brain* 84:662–679, 1961b.

Hoffman PN, Lasek RJ: The slow component of axonal transport: Identification of major structural polypeptides of the axon and their generality among mammalian neurons. *J Cell Biol* 66:351–366, 1975.

Hollmann M, Heinemann S: Cloned glutamate receptors. *Ann Rev Neurosci* 17:31–108, 1994.

Hu HL, Bennett N, Holton JL, *et al.*: Glutathione depletion increases brain susceptibility to m-dinitrobenzene neurotoxicity. *Neurotoxicology* 20:83–90, 1999.

Hu HL, Bennett N, Lamb JH, *et al.*: Capacity of rat brain to metabolize m-dinitrobenzene: An in vitro study. *Neurotoxicology* 18:363–370, 1997.

Huber JD, Darling SF, Park K, *et al.*: The role of NMDA receptors in neonatal cocaine-induced neurotoxicity. *Pharmacol Biochem Behav* 69:451–459, 2001.

Hugon J, Ludolph A, Roy DN, *et al.*: Studies on the etiology and pathogenesis of motor neuron diseases: II. Clinical and electrophysiologic features of pyramidal dysfunction in macaques fed *Lathyrus sativus* and IDPN. *Neurology* 38:435–442, 1988.

Ikonomidou C, Bittigau P, Ishimaru MJ, *et al.*: Ethanol-induced apoptotic neurodegeneration and fetal alcohol syndrome. *Science* 287:1056–1060, 2000.

Janavs JL, Aminoff MJ: Dystonia and chorea in acquired systemic disorders. *J Neurol Neurosurg Psychiatr* 65:436–445, 1998.

Janoff AS, Pringle MJ, Miller KW: Correlation of general anesthetic potency with solubility in membranes. *Biochim Biophys Acta* 649:125–128, 1981.

Jenner P: Oxidative stress in Parkinson's disease. *Ann Neurol* 53 (Suppl 3):S26–S36, 2003.

Johnson DJ, Graham DG, Amarnath V, *et al.*: Release of carbon disulfide is a contributing mechanism in the axonopathy produced by *N,N*-diethyldithiocarbamate. *Toxicol Appl Pharmacol* 148:288–296, 1998.

Johnston MV, Goldstein GW: Selective vulnerability of the developing brain to lead. *Curr Opin Neurol* 11:689–693, 1998.

Kapoor K, Chandra M, Nag D, *et al.*: Evaluation of metronidazole toxicity: A prospective study. *Int J Clin Pharmacol Res* 19:83–88, 1999.

Kappus H: Oxidative stress in chemical toxicity. *Arch Toxicol* 60:144–149, 1987.

Kesson CM, Baird AW, Lawson DH: Acrylamide poisoning. *Postgrad Med J* 53:16–17, 1977.

Khalil AA, Davies B, Castagnoli Jr. N: Isolation and characterization of a monoamine oxidase B selective inhibitor from tobacco smoke. *Bioorg Med Chem* 14:3392–3398, 2006.

Kienzl E, Puchinger L, Jellinger K, *et al.*: The role of transition metals in the pathogenesis of Parkinson's disease. *J Neurol Sci* 134:69–78, 1995.

Kirsten E, Sharma ML, Kun E: Molecular toxicology of (-)erythro-fluorocitrate: Selective inhibition of citrate transport I mitochondria and the binding of fluorocitrate to mitochondrial proteins. *Mol Pharmacol* 14:172–184, 1978.

Kisby GE, Ellison M, Spencer PS: Content of the neurotoxins cycasin (methylazoxymethanol beta-D-glucoside) and BMAA (beta-N-methylamino-L-alanine) in cycad flour prepared by Guam Chamorros. *Neurology* 42:1336–1340, 1992.

Klivenyi P, Clair D, Wermer M, *et al.*: Manganese superoxide dismutase overexpression attenuates MPTP toxicity. *Neurobiol Dis* 5:253–258, 1998.

Kniesel U, Wolburg H: Tight junctions of the blood-brain barrier. *Cell Mol Neurobiol* 20:57–76, 2000.

Koehnle TJ, Brown A: Slow axonal transport of neurofilament protein in cultured neurons. *J Cell Biol* 144:447–458, 1999.

Krasavage WJ, O'Donoghue JL, DiVincenzo GD, *et al.*: The relative neurotoxicity of MnBk, *n*-hexane, and their metabolites. *Toxicol Appl Pharmacol* 52:433–441, 1980.

Kropp TJ, Glynn P, Richardson RJ: The mipafox-inhibited catalytic domain of human neuropathy target esterase ages by reversible proton loss. *Biochemistry* 43:3716–3722, 2004.

Kuopio AM, Marttila RJ, Helenius H, *et al.*: Changing epidemiology of Parkinson's disease in southwestern Finland. *Neurology* 52:302–308, 1999.

Kurland LT, Faro SN, Siedler J: Minamata disease. *World Neurol* 1:370–395, 1960.

Kurland LT: Epidemiological investigations of neurological disorders in the Mariana islands, in Pemberton J (ed.): *Epidemiology Reports on Research and Teaching.* Oxford and New York: Oxford University Press, 1963, pp. 219–223.

Kurth MC, Kurth JH: Variant cytochrome P450 CYP2D6 allelic frequencies in Parkinson's disease. *Am J Med Genet* 48:166–168, 1993.

Lai BC, Marion SA, Teschke K, *et al.*: Occupational and environmental risk factors for Parkinson's disease. *Parkinsonism Relat Disord* 8:297–309, 2002.

Lam G-W, DiStefano V: Characterization of carbon disulfide binding in blood and to other biological substances. *Toxicol Appl Pharmacol* 86:235–242, 1986.

Landrigan PJ, Sonawane B, Butler RN, *et al.*: Early environmental origins of neurodegenerative disease in later life. *Environ Health Perspect* 113:1230–1233, 2005.

Langston JW, Ballard P, Tetrud JW, *et al.*: Chronic Parkinsonism in humans due to a product of meperidine-analog synthesis. *Science* 219:979–980, 1983.

Langston JW, Forno LS, Tetrud J, *et al.*: Evidence of active nerve cell degeneration in the substantia nigra of humans years after 1-methyl-4-phenyl-1,2,3,6-tetrahydropyridine exposure. *Ann Neurol* 46:598–605, 1999.

Langston JW, Irwin I: MPTP: Current concepts and controversies. *Clin Neuropharmacol* 9:485–507, 1986.

Lauder JM: Neurotransmitters as growth regulatory signals: Role of receptors and second messengers. *Trends Neurosci* 16:233–240, 1993.

LeBel CP, Ali SF, Bondy SC: Deferoxamine inhibits methyl mercury-induced increases in reactive oxygen species formation in rat brain. *Toxicol Appl Pharmacol* 112:161–165, 1992.

Lehning EJ, Jortner BS, Fox JH, et al.: γ-Diketone peripheral neuropathy. I. Quantitative morphometric analyses of axonal atrophy and swelling. *Toxicol Appl Pharmacol* 165:127–40, 2000.

Lemasters JJ, Nieminen AL, Qian T, et al.: The mitochondrial permeability transition in cell death: A common mechanism in necrosis, apoptosis and autophagy. *Biochim Biophys Acta* 366:177–196, 1998.

Letzel S, Lang CJ, Schaller KH, et al.: Longitudinal study of neurotoxicity with occupational exposure to aluminum dust. *Neurology* 54:997–1000, 2000.

Lewis JA, Tran BL, Puerta DT, et al.: Synthesis, structure and spectroscopy of new thiopyrone and hydroxypyridine transition-metal complexes. *Dalton Trans* 7:2588–2596, 2005.

Lichensteiger W, Ribary U, Schlumpf M, et al.: Prenatal adverse effects of nicotine on the developing brain, in Boer GJ, Feenstra MGP, Mirmiran M, et al. (eds.): *Progress in Brain Research.* Vol 73. Amsterdam: Elsevier, 1988, pp. 137–157.

Liou HH, Tsai MC, Chen CJ, et al.: Environmental risk factors and Parkinson's disease: A case-control study in Taiwan. *Neurology* 48:1583–1588, 1997.

Lipton RB, Apfel SC, Dutcher JP, et al.: Taxol produces a predominantly sensory neuropathy. *Neurology* 39:368–373, 1989.

Lipton SA, Rosenberg PA: Excitatory amino acids as a final common pathway for neurologic disorders. *N Engl J Med* 330:613–622, 1994.

Liu Y, Fechter LD: Comparison of the effects of trimethyltin on the intracellular calcium levels in spiral ganglion cells and outer hair cells. *Acta Otolaryngol* 116:417–421, 1996.

Llorens J, Dememes D, Sans A: The behavioral syndrome caused by 3,3'-iminodipropionitrile and related nitriles in the rat is associated with degeneration of the vestibular sensory hair cells. *Toxicol Appl Pharmacol* 123:199–210, 1993.

Logroscino G: The role of early life environmental risk factors in Parkinson disease: What is the evidence? *Environ Health Perspect* 113:1234–1238, 2005.

LoPachin RM, Jortner BS, Reid ML, et al.: γ-Diketone central neuropathy: Quantitative analyses of cytoskeletal components in myelinated axons of the rat rubrospinal tract. *Neurotoxicology* 26:1021–1030, 2005.

LoPachin RM, Ross JF, Reid ML, et al.: Neurological evaluation of toxic axonopathies in rats: Acrylamide and 2,5-hexanedione. *Neurotoxicology* 23:95–110, 2002.

Lotharius J, O'Malley KL: The parkinsonian-inducing drug 1-methyl-4-phenylpyridinium triggers intracellular dopamine oxidation. *J Biol Chem* 275:38581–38588, 2000.

Lotharius J, O'Malley KL: Role of mitochondrial dysfunction and dopamine-dependent oxidative stress in amphetamine-induced toxicity. *Ann Neurol* 49:79–89, 2001.

Lotti M: Promotion of organophosphate induced delayed polyneuropathy by certain esterase inhibitors. *Toxicology* 181–182:245–248, 2002.

Lotti M, Moretto A: Organophosphate-induced delayed polyneuropathy. *Toxicol Rev* 24:37–49, 2005.

Lucey JF, Hibbard E, Behrman RE, et al.: Kernicterus in asphyxiated newborn rhesus monkeys. *Exp Neurol* 9:43–58, 1964.

Ludolph AC, He F, Spencer PS, et al.: 3-Nitropropionic acid: Exogenous animal neurotoxin and possible human striatal toxin. *Can J Neurol Sci* 18:492–498, 1991.

Ludolph AC, Seelig M, Ludolf A, et al.: 3-Nitropropionic acid decreases cellular energy levels and causes neuronal degeneration in cortical explants. *Neurodegeneration* 1:155–161, 1992.

Lunn ER, Perry VH, Brown MC, et al.: Absence of Wallerian degeneration does not hinder regeneration in peripheral nerve. *Eur J Neurosci* 1:27–33, 1989.

Lyon MF, Ogunkolade BW, Brown MC, et al.: A gene affecting Wallerian nerve degeneration maps distally on mouse chromosome 4. *Proc Nat Acad Sci USA* 90:9717–9720, 1993.

Magyar K, Szende B: (-)-Deprenyl, a selective MAO-B inhibitor, with apoptotic and anti-apoptotic properties. *Neurotoxicology* 25:233–242, 2004.

Makhaeva GF, Sigolaeva LV, Zhuravleva LV, et al.: Biosensor detection of neuropathy target esterase in whole blood as a biomarker of exposure to neuropathic organophosphorus compounds. *J Toxicol Environ Health A* 66:599–610, 2003.

Makri A, Goveia M, Balbus J, et al.: Children's susceptibility to chemicals: A review by developmental stage. *J Toxicol Environ Health Part B* 7:417–435, 2004.

Malygin VV, Sokolov VB, Richardson RJ, et al.: Quantitative structure-activity relationships predict the delayed neurotoxicity potential of a series of O-alkyl-O-methylchloroformimino phenylphosphonates. *J Toxicol Environ Health A* 66:611–625, 2003.

Mandel S, Grunblatt E, Riederer P, et al.: Neuroprotective strategies in Parkinson's disease: An update on progress. *CNS Drugs* 17:729–762, 2003.

Mandel S, Weinreb O, Amit T, et al.: Mechanism of neuroprotective action of the anti-Parkinson drug rasagiline and its derivatives. *Brain Res Brain Res Rev* 48:379–387, 2005.

Martin DL, Waniewski RA: Precursor synthesis and neurotransmitter uptake by astrocytes as targets of neurotoxicants, in Aschner M, Kimelberg HK (eds.): *The Role of Glia in Neurotoxicity.* Boca Raton: CRC Press, 1996, pp. 335–357.

Marty MS, Atchison WD: Pathways mediating Ca^{2+} entry in rat cerebellar granule cells following in vitro exposure to methyl mercury. *Toxicol Appl Pharmacol* 147:319–330, 1997.

Mastrogiacomo F, Bergeron C, Kish SJ: Brain alpha-ketoglutarate dehydrogenase complex activity in Alzheimer's disease. *J Neurochem* 61:2007–2014, 1993.

McCann UD, Ricaurte GA: Amphetamine neurotoxicity: Accomplishments and remaining challenges. *Neurosci Behav Rev* 27:821–826, 2004.

McMillan DE: A brief history of the neurobehavioral toxicity of manganese: Some unanswered questions. *Neurotoxicology* 20:499–507, 1999.

Meldrum B: Excitatory amino acid antagonists as potential therapeutic agents, in Jenner P (ed.): *Neurotoxins and Their Pharmacological Implications.* New York: Raven Press, 1987, pp. 33–53.

Mielke S, Sparreboom A, Mross K: Peripheral neuropathy: A persisting challenge in paclitaxel-based regimes. *Eur J Cancer* 42:24–30, 2006.

Miller DB: Neurotoxicity of the pesticidal carbamates. *Neurobehav Toxicol Teratol* 4:779–787, 1982.

Miller DB, O'Callaghan JP: Elevated environmental temperature and methamphetamine neurotoxicity. *Environ Res* 92:48–53, 2003.

Mitsuishi K, Takahashi A, Mizutani M, et al.: Beta, beta'-iminodipropionitrile toxicity in normal and congenitally neurofilament-deficient Japanese quails. *Acta Neuropathol* 86:578–581, 1993.

Montgomery Jr. EB: Heavy metals and the etiology of Parkinson's disease and other movement disorders. *Toxicology* 97:3–9, 1995.

Monuki ES, Lemke G: Molecular biology of myelination, in Waxman SG, Kocsis JD, Stys PK (eds.): *The Axon: Structure, Function, and Pathophysiology.* New York: Oxford University Press, 1995, pp. 144–163.

Morell P, Toews AD, Wagner M, et al.: Gene expression during tellurium-induced primary demyelination. *Neurotoxicology* 15:171–180, 1994.

Morgan RE, Garavan H, Smith EG, et al.: Early lead exposure produces lasting changes in sustained attention, response initiation, and reactivity to errors. *Neurotoxicol Teratol* 23:519–531, 2001.

Moser VC: Observational batteries in neurotoxicity testing. *Int J Toxicol* 19:407–411, 2000.

Moser VC, Becking GC, Cuomo V, et al.: The IPCS collaborative study on neurobehavioral screening methods: V. Results of chemical testing. *Neurotoxicology* 18:969–1055, 1997a.

Moser VC, Becking GC, Cuomo V, et al.: The IPCS collaborative study on neurobehavioral screening methods. III. Results of proficiency studies. *Neurotoxicology* 18:939–946, 1997b.

Moser VC, Padilla S: Age- and gender-related differences in the time-course of behavioral and biochemical effects produced by oral chlorpyrifos in rats. *Toxicol Appl Pharmacol* 149:107–119, 1998.

Mossakowski MJ, Renkawek K, Krasnicka Z, et al.: Morphology and histochemistry of Wilsonian and hepatic gliopathy in tissue culture. *Acta Neuropathol (Berl)* 16:1–16, 1970.

Mullick FG: Hexachlorophene toxicity: Human experience at the AFIP. *Pediatrics* 51:395–399, 1973.

Mulugeta S, Ciavarra RP, Maney RK, *et al.*: Three subpopulations of fast axonally transported retinal ganglion cell proteins are differentially trafficked in the rat optic pathway. *J Neurosci Res* 59:247–258, 2000.

Muralikrishnan D, Samantaray S, Mohanakumar KP: D-deprenyl protects nigrostriatal neurons against 1-methyl-4-1,2,3,6-tetrahydropyridine-induced dopaminergic neurotoxicity. *Synapse* 50:7–13, 2003.

Mushiroda T, Ariyoshi N, Yokoi T, *et al.*: Accumulation of the 1-methyl-4-pyridinium ion in suncus (Suncus murinus) brain: Implication for flavin-containing monooxygenase activity in brain microvessels. *Chem Res Toxicol* 14:228–232, 2001.

Myers JE, Macun I: Acrylamide neuropathy in a South African factory: An epidemiologic investigation. *Am J Ind Med* 19:487–493, 1991.

Myers RR, Mizisin AP, Powell HC, *et al.*: Reduced nerve blood flow in hexachlorophene neuropathy: Relationship to elevated endoneurial pressure. *J Neuropathol Exp Neurol* 41:391–399, 1982.

Nakata T, Yorifuji H: Morphological evidence of the inhibitory effect of taxol on the fast axonal transport. *Neurosci Res* 35:113–122, 1999.

Naoi M, Maruyama W, Akao Y, *et al.*: Dopamine-derived endogenous *N*-methyl-(*R*)-solsolinol: Its role in Parkinson's disease. *Neurotoxicol Teratol* 24:579–591, 2002.

Needleman HL: Childhood lead poisoning. *Curr Opin Neurol* 7:187–190, 1994.

Needleman HL, Gatsonis CA: Low-level lead exposure and the IQ of children. A meta-analysis of modern studies. *JAMA* 263:673–678, 1990.

Nihei MK, Desmond NL, McGlothan JL, *et al.*: N-methyl-D-aspartate receptor subunit changes are associated with lead-induced deficits of long-term potentiation and spatial learning. *Neurosci* 99:233–242, 2000.

Nixon RA: Dynamic behavior and organization of cytoskeleton proteins in neurons: Reconciling old and new findings. *Bioessays* 20:798–807, 1998.

Nunn PB, Seelig M, Zagoren JC, *et al.*: Stereospecific acute neurotoxicity of "uncommon" plant amino acids linked to human motor system diseases. *Brain Res* 410:375–379, 1987.

Oestreicher E, Sengstock GJ, Riederer P, *et al.*: Degeneration of nigrostriatal dopaminergic neurons increases iron within the substantia nigra: Ahistochemical and neurochemical study. *Brain Res* 660:8–18, 1994.

Okeda R, Shibutani M, Matsuo T, *et al.*: Experimental neurotoxicity of 5-fluorouracil and its derivatives is due to poisoning by the monofluorinated organic metabolites, monofluoroacetic acid and alpha-fluorobeta-alanine. *Acta Neuropathol (Berl)* 81:66–73, 1990.

Olney JW: Neurotoxicity of excitatory amino acids, in McGeer EG, Olney JW, McGeer PL (eds.): *Kainic Acid as a Tool in Neurobiology.* New York: Raven Press, 1978, pp. 95–122.

O'Shea KS, Kaufman MH: The teratogenic effect of acetaldehyde: Implications for the study of fetal alcohol syndrome. *J Anat* 128:65–76, 1979.

Padilla S, Atkinson MB, Breuer AC: Direct measurement of fast axonal organelle transport in the sciatic nerve of rats treated with acrylamide. *J Toxicol Environ Health* 39:429–445, 1993.

Padilla S, Grizzle TB, Lyerly D: Triphenyl phosphite: In vivo and in vitro inhibition of rat neurotoxic esterase. *Toxicol Appl Pharmcol* 87:249–256, 1987.

Pardridge WM: Blood-brain barrier biology and methodology. *J Neurovirol* 5:556–569, 1999.

Parent A: *Carpenter's Human Neuroanatomy,* 9th ed. Baltimore: Williams & Wilkins, 1996, pp. 131–198.

Parenti M, Rusconi L, Cappabianca V, *et al.*: Role of dopamine in manganese neurotoxicity. *Brain Res* 473:236–240, 1988.

Patanow CM, Day JR, Billingsley ML: Alterations in hippocampal expression of SNAP-25, GAP-43, stannin and glial fibrillary acidic protein following mechanical and trimethyltin-induced injury in the rat. *Neuroscience* 76:187–202, 1997.

Penny DG: Acute carbon monoxide poisoning: Animal models: A review. *Toxicology* 62:123–160, 1990.

Perl TM, Bedard L, Kosatsky T, *et al.*: An outbreak of toxic encephalopathy caused by eating mussels contaminated with domoic acid. *N Engl J Med* 322:1775–1780, 1990.

Perlstein MA, Attala R: Neurologic sequelae of plumbism in children. *Clin Pediatr* 5:292–298, 1966.

Pham-Dinh D, Popot JL, Boespflug-Tanguy O, *et al.*: Pelizaeus-Merzbacher disease: A valine to phenylalanine point mutation in a putative extracellular loop of myelin proteolipid. *Proc Natl Acad Sci U S A* 88:7562–7566, 1991.

Phelps CH: An ultrastructural study of methionine sulphoximine-induced glycogen accumulation in astrocytes of the mouse cerebral cortex. *J Neurocytol* 4:479–490, 1975.

Philbert MA, Nolan CC, Cremer JE, *et al.*: 1,3-Dinitrobenzene-induced encephalopathy in rats. *Neuropathol Appl Neurobiol* 13:371–389, 1987.

Pierard-Franchimont C, Goffin V, Decroix J, *et al.*: A multicenter randomized trial of ketoconazole 2% and zinc pyrithione 1% shampoos in severe dandruff and seborrheic dermatitis. *Skin Pharmacol Appl Skin Physiol* 15:434–441, 2002.

Plato CC, Galasko D, Garruto R, *et al.*: ALS and PDC of Guam: Forty-year follow-up. *Neurology* 58:765–773, 2002.

Plato CC, Garruto RM, Galasko D, *et al.*: Amyotrophic lateral sclerosis and parkinsonism-dementia complex of Guam: Changing incidence rates during the past 60 years. *Am J Epidemiol* 157:149–157, 2003.

Plum F, Posner JB: Neurobiologic essentials, in Smith Jr. LH, Thier SO (eds.): *Pathophysiology: The Biological Principles of Disease.* Philadelphia: WB Saunders, 1985, pp. 1009–1036.

Polymeropoulos MH, Lavedan C, Leroy E, *et al.*: Mutation in the alphasynuclein gene identified in families with Parkinson's disease. *Science* 276:2045–2047, 1997.

Pope CN: Organophosphorus pesticides: Do they all have the same mechanism of toxicity? *J Toxicol Environ Health B* 2:161–181, 1999.

Pope CN, Tanaka Jr. D, Padilla S: The role of neurotoxic esterase (NTE) in the prevention and potentiation of organophosphorus-induced delayed neurotoxicity (OPIDN). *Chem Biol Interact* 87:395–406, 1993.

Porterfield SP: Vulnerability of the developing brain to thyroid abnormalities: Environmental insults to the thyroid system. *Environ Health Perspect* 102 (Suppl 2):125–130, 1994.

Powell HC, Myers RR, Lampert PW: Changes in Schwann cells and vessels in lead neuropathy. *Am J Pathol* 109:193–205, 1982.

Prakash V, Timasheff SN: Aging of tubulin at neutral pH: The destabilizing effect of Vinca alkaloids. *Arch Biochem Biophys* 295:137–145, 1992.

Przedborski S, Tieu K, Perier C, *et al.*: MPTP as a mitochondrial neurotoxic model of Parkinson's disease. *J Bioenerg Biomembr* 36:375–379, 2004.

Purves DC, Garrod IJ, Dayan AD: A comparison of spongiosis induced in the brain by hexachlorophene, cuprizone, and triethyl tin in the Sprague-Dawley rat. *Hum Exp Toxicol* 10:439–444, 1991.

Qiu J, Cai D, Filbin MT: Glial inhibition of nerve regeneration in mature mammalian CNS. *Glia* 29:166–174, 2000.

Quarles RH, Farrer RG, Yim SH: Structure and function of myelin, an extended and biochemically modified cell surface membrane, in Juurlink BHJ, Devon RM, Doucette JR, *et al.* (eds.): *Cell Biology and Pathology of Myelin: Evolving Biological Concepts and Therapeutic Approaches.* New York: Plenum Press, 1997, pp. 1–12.

Quik M: Smoking, nicotine and Parkinson's disease. *Trends Neurosci* 27:561–568, 2004.

Quik M, Parameswaran N, McCallum SE, *et al.*: Chronic oral nicotine treatment protects against striatal degeneration in MPTP-treated primates. *J Neurochem* 98:1866–1875, 2006.

Rakonczay Z, Matsuoka Y, Giacobini E: Effects of L-beta-N-methylamino-L-alanine (L-BMAA) on the cortical cholinergic and glutamatergic systems of the rat. *J Neurosci Res* 29:121–126, 1991.

Randall JC, Yano BL, Richardson RJ: Potentiation of organophosphorus compound-induced delayed neurotoxicity (OPIDN) in the central and peripheral nervous system of the adult hen: Distribution of axonal lesions. *J Toxicol Environ Health* 51:571–590, 1997.

Ray DE, Abbott NJ, Chan MW, *et al.*: Increased oxidative metabolism and oxidative stress in m-dinitrobenzene neurotoxicity. *Biochem Soc Trans* 22:407S, 1994.

Ray DE, Brown AW, Cavanagh JB, *et al.*: Functional/metabolic modulation of the brain stem lesions caused by 1,3-dinitrobenzene in the rat. *Neurotoxicology* 13:379–388, 1992.

Readhead C, Schneider A, Griffiths I, *et al.*: Premature arrest of myelin formation in transgenic mice with increased proteolipid protein gene dosage. *Neuron* 12:583–595, 1994.

Reuhl KR, Chang LW: Effects of methylmercury on the development of the nervous system: A review. *Neurotoxicology* 1:21–55, 1979.

Reuhl KR, Gilbert SG, Mackenzie BA, *et al.*: Acute trimethyltin intoxication in the monkey *(Macaca fascicularis)*. *Toxicol Appl Pharmacol* 79:436–452, 1985.

Riachi NJ, Dietrich WD, Harik SI: Effects of internal carotid administration of MPTP on rat brain and blood-brain barrier. *Brain Res* 533:6–14, 1990.

Rice D, Barone Jr. S: Critical periods of vulnerability for the developing nervous system: Evidence from humans and animal models. *Environ Health Perspect* 108 (Suppl 3):511–533, 2000.

Rice DC: Evidence for delayed neurotoxicity produced by methylmercury. *Neurotoxicology* 17:583–596, 1996.

Richardson RJ: Interactions of organophosphorus compounds with neurotoxic esterase, in Chambers JE, Levi PE (eds.): *Organophosphates: Chemistry, Fate, and Effects*. San Diego: Academic Press, 1992, pp. 299–323.

Richardson RJ: Organophosphate poisoning, delayed neurotoxicity, In Wexler P (ed.): *Encyclopedia of Toxicology, 2nd Edn*. Oxford: Elsevier Ltd., 2005, pp. 302–306.

Ridgway P, Nixon TE, Leach JP: Occupational exposure to organic solvents and long-term nervous system damage detectable by brain imaging, neurophysiology or histopathology. *Food Chem Toxicol* 41:153–187, 2003.

Riggs JE: Cigarette smoking and Parkinson's disease: The illusion of a neuroprotective effect. *Clin Neuropharmacol* 15:88–99, 1992.

Riggs JE, Schochet SS, Gutmann L, *et al.*: Chronic human colchicine neuropathy and myopathy. *Arch Neurol* 43:521–523, 1986.

Riikonen R, Salonen I, Partanen K, *et al.*: Brain perfusion SPECT and MRI in foetal alcohol syndrome. *Dev Med Child Neurol* 41:652–659, 1999.

Rodgers-Johnson P, Garruto RM, Yanagihara R, *et al.*: Amyotrophic lateral sclerosis and parkinsonism-dementia on Guam: A 30-year evaluation of clinical and neuropathologic trends. *Neurology* 36:7–13, 1986.

Rodier PM: Developing brain as a target of toxicity. *Environ Health Perspect* 103 (Suppl 6):73–76, 1995.

Romero I, Brown AW, Cavanagh JB, *et al.*: Vascular factors in the neurotoxic damage caused by 1,3-dinitrobenzene in the rat. *Neuropathol Appl Neurobiol* 17:495–508, 1991.

Romero IA, Lister T, Richards HK, *et al.*: Early metabolic changes during m-dinitrobenzene neurotoxicity and the possible role of oxidative stress. *Free Rad Biol Med* 18:311–319, 1995.

Ross JF, Lawhorn GT: ZPT-related distal axonopathy: Behavioral and electrophysiologic correlates in rats. *Neurotoxicol Teratol* 12:153–159, 1990.

Ross GW, Petrovitch H: Current evidence for neuroprotective effects of nicotine and caffeine against Parkinson's disease. *Drugs Aging* 18:797–806, 2001.

Rothman SM, Olney JM: Glutamate and the pathophysiology of hypoxic-ischemic brain damage. *Ann Neurol* 19:105–111, 1986.

Rothstein JD, Tabakoff B: Regulation of neurotransmitter aspartate metabolism by glial glutamine synthetase. *J Neurochem* 46:1923–1928, 1986.

Roytta M, Horwitz SB, Raine CS: Taxol-induced neuropathy: Short-term effects of local injection. *J Neurocytol* 13:685–701, 1984.

Rubin LL, Staddon JM: The cell biology of the blood-brain barrier. *Annu Rev Neurosci* 22:11–28, 1999.

Sahenk Z, Barohn R, New P, *et al.*: Taxol neuropathy: Electrodiagnostic and sural nerve biopsy findings. *Arch Neurol* 51:726–729, 1994.

Sahenk Z, Mendell JR: Ultrastructural study of zinc pyridinethione-induced peripheral neuropathy. *J Neuropathol Exp Neurol* 38:532–550, 1979.

Sahenk Z, Mendell JR: Axoplasmic transport in zinc pyridinethione neuropathy: Evidence for an abnormality in distal turn-around. *Brain Res* 186:343–353, 1980.

Sahenk Z, Mendell JR: Pyrithione, In Spencer PS, Schaumburg HH (eds.): *Experimental and Clinical Neurotoxicology*. New York: Oxford University Press, 2000, pp. 1050–1054.

Sampson PD, Streissguth AP, Bookstein FL, *et al.*: On categorizations in analyses of alcohol teratogenesis. *Environ Health Perspect* 108 (Suppl 3):421–428, 2000.

Sayre LM, Shearson CM, Wongmongkolrit T, *et al*: Structural basis of γ-diketone neurotoxicity: Non-neurotoxicity of 3,3-dimethyl-2,5-hexanedione a γ-diketone incapable of pyrrole formation. *Toxicol Appl Pharmacol* 84:36–44, 1986.

Schaumburg HH: Vinca Alkaloids, in Spencer PS, Schaumburg HH (eds.): *Experimental and Clinical Neurotoxicology*. New York: Oxford University Press, 2000, pp. 1232–1236.

Schaumburg HH, Wisniewski HM, Spencer PS: Ultrastructural studies of the dying-back process I. Peripheral nerve terminal and axon degeneration in systemic acrylamide intoxication. *J Neuropathol Exp Neurol* 33:260–284, 1974.

Schentag JJ: Mental confusion in a patient treated with metronidazole—a concentration-related effect? *Pharmacotherapy* 2:384–387, 1982.

Schiff PB, Horwitz SB: Taxol assembles tubulin in the absence of exogenous guanosine 59-triphosphate or microtubule-associated proteins. *Biochemistry* 20:3242–3252, 1981.

Schinder AF, Olson EC, Spitzer NC, *et al.*: Mitochondrial dysfunction is a primary event in glutamate neurotoxicity. *J Neurosci* 16:6125–6133, 1996.

Schionning JD, Larsen JO, Tandrup T, *et al.*: Selective degeneration of dorsal root ganglia and dorsal nerve roots in methyl mercury intoxicated rats: A stereological study. *Acta Neuropathol* 96:191–201, 1998.

Schlafer WW, Zimmerman U-JP: Calcium-activated protease and the regulation of the axonal cytoskeleton, in Elam JS, Cancalon P (eds.): *Advances in Neurochemistry*. New York: Plenum Press, 1984, pp. 261–273.

Schnapp BJ, Reese TS: Dynein is the motor for retrograde axonal transport of organelles. *Proc Natl Acad Sci U S A* 86:1548–1552, 1989.

Schneider D, Wink M, Sporer F, *et al.*: Cycads: Their evolution, toxins, herbivores and insect pollinators. *Naturwissenschaften* 89:281–294, 2002.

Schoepfer R, Monyer H, Sommer B, *et al.*: Molecular biology of glutamate receptors. *Prog Neurobiol* 42:353–357, 1994.

Schutzman DL, Frankenfield-Chernicoff M, Clatterbaugh HE, *et al.*: Incidence of intrauterine cocaine exposure in a suburban setting. *Pediatrics* 88:825–827, 1991.

Schwartz JH: The cytology of neurons, in Kandel ER, Schwartz JH, Jessell TM (eds.): *Principles of Neural Science*. 3rd ed. Norwalk, CT: Appleton & Lange, 1991, pp. 37–48.

Scriba GK, Borchardt RT: Metabolism of 1-methyl-4-phenyl-1,2,3,6-tetrahydropyridine (MPTP) by bovine brain microvessel endothelial cells. *Brain Res* 501:175–178, 1989.

Seawright AA, Brown AW, Nolan CC, *et al.*: Selective degeneration of cerebellar cortical neurons caused by cycad neurotoxin, L-beta-methylaminoalanine (L-BMAA), in rats. *Neuropathol Appl Neurobiol* 16:153–164, 1990.

Seegal RF: Epidemiological and laboratory evidence of PCB-induced neurotoxicity. *Crit Rev Toxicol* 26:709–737, 1996.

Seppaleinen AM, Haltia M: Carbon disulfide, in Spencer PS, Schaumburg HH (eds.): *Experimental and Clinical Neurotoxicology*. Baltimore: Williams & Wilkins, 1980, pp. 356–373.

Shanker G, Mutkus LA, Walker S, *et al.*: Methylmercury enhances arachidonic acid release and cytosolic phospholipase A_2 expression in primary cultures of neonatal astrocytes. *Mol Brain Res* 106:1–11, 2002.

Sieber SM, Correa P, Dalgard DW, *et al.*: Carcinogenicity and hepatotoxicity of cycasin and its aglycone methylazoxymethanol acetate in nonhuman primates. *J Natl Cancer Inst* 65:177–189, 1980.

Slikker Jr. W , Xu ZA, Levin ED, *et al.*: Mode of action: Disruption of brain cell replication, second messenger, and neurotransmitter systems during development leading to cognitive dysfunction—developmental neurotoxicity of nicotine. *Crit Rev Toxicol* 35:703–711, 2005.

Slotkin TA: Cholinergic systems in brain development and disruption by neurotoxicants: Nicotine, environmental tobacco smoke, organophosphates. *Toxicol Appl Pharmacol* 15:132–151, 2004.

Snow BJ, Vingerhoets FJ, Langston JW, *et al.*: Pattern of dopaminergic loss in the striatum of humans with MPTP induced parkinsonism. *J Neurol Neurosurg Psychiatr* 68:313–316, 2000.

Spencer PS: Doxorubicin and related anthracyclines, in Spencer PS, Schaumburg HH (eds.): *Experimental and Clinical Neurotoxicology.* New York: Oxford University Press, 2000, pp. 529–533.

Spencer PS, Nunn PB, Hugon J, *et al.*: Guam amyotrophic lateral sclerosis-parkinsonism-dementia linked to a plant excitant neurotoxin. *Science* 237:517–522, 1987.

Spencer PS, Schaumburg HH: Ultrastructural studies of the dying-back process III. The evolution of experimental peripheral giant axonal degeneration. *J Neuropathol Exp Neurol* 36:276, 1974.

Spencer PS, Schaumburg HH: Central-peripheral distal axonopathy: The pathology of dying-back polyneuropathies, in Zimmerman H (ed.): *Progress in Neuropathology.* Vol 3. New York: Grune & Stratton, 1976, pp. 253–295.

Spencer PS, Schaumburg HH, eds: *Experimental and Clinical Neurotoxicology,* 2nd ed. New York: Oxford University Press, 2000.

St. Clair MBG, Amarnath V, Moody MA, *et al.*: Pyrrole oxidation and protein crosslinking are necessary steps in the development of γ-diketone neuropathy. *Chem Res Toxicol* 1:179–185, 1988.

Stewart PA: Endothelial vesicles in the blood-brain barrier: Are they related to permeability? *Cell Mol Neurobiol* 20:149–163, 2000.

Stoll G, Muller HW: Nerve injury, axonal degeneration and neural regeneration: Basic insights. *Brain Pathol* 9:313–325, 1999.

Stoltenburg-Didinger G, Spohr HL: Fetal alcohol syndrome and mental retardation: Spine distribution of pyramidal cells in prenatal alcohol exposed rat cerebral cortex. *Brain Res* 11:119–123, 1983.

Swanson RA, Graham SH: Fluorocitrate and fluoroacetate effects on astrocyte metabolism in vitro. *Brain Res* 664:94–100, 1994.

Takeuchi T, Morikawa H, Matsumoto H, *et al.*: A pathological study of Minamata disease in Japan. *Acta Neuropathol* 2:40–57, 1962.

Tanner CM, Ottman R, Goldman SM, *et al.*: Parkinson disease in twins: An etiologic study. *JAMA* 281:341–346, 1999.

Teitelbaum JS, Zatorre RJ, Carpenter S, *et al.*: Neurologic sequelae of domoic acid intoxication due to the ingestion of contaminated mussels. *N Engl J Med* 322:1781–1787, 1990.

Thompson CM, Richardson RJ: Anticholinesterase insecticides, in Marrs TC, Ballantyne, B (eds.): *Pesticide Toxicology and International Regulation.* Chichester: John Wiley & Sons Ltd., 2004, pp. 89–127.

Tilson HA: Neurobehavioral methods used in neurotoxicological research. *Toxicol Lett* 68:231–240, 1993.

Tilson HA, Kodavanti PR: The neurotoxicity of polychlorinated biphenyls. *Neurotoxicology* 19:517–525, 1998.

Tilson HA, Moser VC: Comparison of screening approaches. *Neurotoxicology* 13:1–14, 1992.

Tjalkens RB, Ewing MM, Philbert MA: Differential cellular regulation of the mitochondrial permeability transition in an in vitro model of 1,3-dinitrobenzene-induced encephalopathy. *Brain Res* 874:165–177, 2000.

Toggas SM, Krady JK, Thompson TA, *et al.*: Molecular mechanisms of selective neurotoxicants: Studies on organotin compounds. *Ann NY Acad Sci* 679:157–177, 1993.

Tomas-Camardiel M, Herrera AJ, Venero JL, *et al.*: Differential regulation of glutamic acid decarboxylase mRNA and tyrosine hydroxylase mRNA expression in the aged manganese-treated rats. *Brain Res Mol Brain Res* 103:116–129, 2002.

Turchan J, Anderson C, Hauser KF, *et al.*: Estrogen protects against the synergistic toxicity by HIV proteins, methamphetamine and cocaine. *BMC Neurosci* 2:3–13, 2001.

U.S. Department of Health and Human Services, Substance Abuse and Mental Health Services Administration, Office of Applied Studies: *National Household Study on Drug Abuse, 2001*. Washington, DC.

U.S. Environmental Protection Agency Water Quality Criterion for the Protection of Human Health: Methylmercury, Office of Science and Technology, Office of Water, Environmental Protection Agency Washington, DC 20460, EPA-823-R-01-001, 2001.

Uversky VN: Neurotoxicant-induced animal models of Parkinson's disease: Understanding the role of rotenone, maneb and paraquat in neurodegeneration. *Cell Tissue Res* 318:225–241, 2004.

Valentine WM, Amarnath V, Amarnath K, *et al.*: Carbon disulfide-mediated protein cross-linking by N,N-diethyldithiocarbamate. *Chem Res Toxicol* 8:96–102, 1995.

Valentine WM, Graham DG, Anthony DC: Covalent cross-linking of erythrocyte spectrin in vivo. *Toxicol Appl Pharmacol* 121:71–77, 1993.

Valentine WM, Amarnath V, Graham DG, *et al.*: Covalent cross-linking of proteins by carbon disulfide. *Chem Res Toxicol* 5:254–262, 1992.

Valentine WM, Amarnath V, Graham DG, *et al.*: CS_2 mediated cross-linking of erythrocyte spectrin and neurofilament protein: Dose response and temporal relationship to the formation of axonal swellings. *Toxicol Appl Pharmacol* 142:95–105, 1997.

Van de Kamp JL, Collins AC: Prenatal nicotine alters nicotinic receptor development in the mouse brain. *Pharmacol Biochem Behav* 47:889–900, 1994.

Van der Hoek JA, Verberk MM, Hageman G: Criteria for solvent-induced chronic toxic encephalopathy: A systematic review. *Int Arch Occup Environ Health* 73:362–368, 2000.

Veronesi B, Jones K, Gupta S, *et al.*: Myelin basic protein-messenger RNA (MBP-mRNA) expression during triethyltin-induced myelin edema. *Neurotoxicology* 12:265–276, 1991.

Volpe JJ: Effect of cocaine use on the fetus. *N Engl J Med* 327:399–407, 1992.

Wang L, Ho CL, Sun D, *et al.*: Rapid movement of axonal neurofilaments interrupted by prolonged pauses. *Nat Cell Biol* 2:137–141, 2000.

Watanabe I, Kanabe S: Early edematous lesion of pyrithiamine-induced acute thiamine deficient encephalopathy in the mouse. *J Neuropathol Exp Neurol* 37:401–413, 1978.

Wedler FC: Biological significance of manganese in mammalian systems. *Prog Med Chem* 30:89–133, 1993.

Winneke G, Altmann L, Kramer U, *et al.*: Neurobehavioral and neurophysiological observations in six-year-old children with low lead levels in East and West Germany. *Neurotoxicology* 15:705–713, 1994.

Wood SL, Beyer BK, Cappon GD: Species comparison of postnatal CNS development: Functional measures. *Birth Defects Res (Part B)* 68:391–407, 2003.

Woods JR, Plessinger MA, Clark KE: Effect of cocaine on uterine blood flow and fetal oxygenation. *JAMA* 257:957–961, 1987.

Wright SC, Zhong J, Zheng H, *et al.*: Nicotine inhibition of apoptosis suggests a role in tumor production. *FASEB J* 7:1045–1051, 1993.

Xu M, Guo Y, Vorhees CV, *et al.*: Behavioral responses to cocaine and amphetamine administration in mice lacking the dopamine D1 receptor. *Brain Res* 852:198–207, 2000.

Yamamura Y: n-Hexane polyneuropathy. *Folia Psychiatr Neurol* 23:45–57, 1969.

Zhang J, Graham DG, Montine TS, *et al.*: Enhanced N-methyl-4-tetrahydropyridine toxicity in mice deficient in CuZn-superoxide dismutase or glutathione peroxidase. *J Neuropathol Exp Neurol* 59:53–61, 2000.

CHAPTER 17

TOXIC RESPONSES OF THE OCULAR AND VISUAL SYSTEM

Donald A. Fox and William K. Boyes

INTRODUCTION TO OCULAR AND VISUAL SYSTEM TOXICOLOGY

Environmental and occupational exposure to toxic chemicals, gases, and vapors as well as side effects resulting from systemic and ocular therapeutic drugs frequently result in structural and functional alterations in the eye and central visual system (Grant, 1986; Anger and Johnson, 1985; Grant and Schuman, 1993; Otto and Fox, 1993; Jaanus *et al.*, 1995; Fox, 1998; Santaella and Fraunfelder, 2007). Almost half of all neurotoxic chemicals affect some aspect of sensory function (Crofton and Sheets, 1989). The most frequently reported sensory system alterations occur in the visual system (Anger and Johnson, 1985; Crofton and Sheets, 1989; Fox, 1998; Grant and Schuman, 1993). Grant (1986) lists approximately 2800 substances that are reportedly toxic to the eye. In many cases, alterations in visual function are the initial symptoms following chemical exposure (Hanninen *et al.*, 1978; Damstra, 1978; Baker *et al.*, 1984; Mergler *et al.*, 1987; Iregren *et al.*, 2002a). Even more relevant is the fact that these alterations often occur in the absence of any clinical signs of toxicity (Baker *et al.*, 1984; Anger and Johnson, 1985). This suggests that sensory systems, and in particular the retina and central visual system, may be especially vulnerable to toxic insult. In fact, alterations in the structure and/or function of the eye or central visual system are among the criteria utilized for setting permissible occupational or environmental exposure levels for many different chemicals in the United States (http://www.cdc.gov/niosh/npg/, http://www.epa.gov/iris/index.html). In addition, numerous new drugs used for the treatment of ocular diseases or ocular complications of systemic diseases recently entered the marketplace (Novack, 2003). Moreover, subtle alterations in visual processing of information (e.g., visual perceptual, visual motor) can have profound immediate, long-term, and—in some cases—delayed effects on the mental, social, and physical health and performance of an individual. Finally, ocular and visual system impairments can lead to increased occupational injuries, loss of productive work time, costs for providing medical and social services, lost

Table 17-1
Ocular and Central Visual System Sites of Action of Selected Xenobiotics Following Systemic Exposure

XENOBIOTIC	CORNEA	LENS	OUTER RETINA: RPE	OUTER RETINA: RODS AND CONES	INNER RETINA: BCS, ACS, IPCS	RGCS, OPTIC NERVE OR TRACT	LGN, VISUAL CORTEX
Acrylamide				−	−	++	++
Amiodarone	+	+				+	
Carbon disulfide				+	−	++	+
Chloroquine	+		+	+		+	
Chlorpromazine	+	+	+	+			
Corticosteroids		++				+	
Digoxin and digitoxin	+	+	+	++		+	+
Ethambutol				+		++	
Hexachlorophene				+		+	+
Indomethacin	+		+	+			
Isotretinoin	+						
Lead	+		+	++	+	+	+
Methanol			+	++	−	++	+
Methyl mercury, mercury				+	−	−	++
n-Hexane			+	+		+	
Naphthalene		+		+			
Organic solvents				+			+
Organophosphates		+		+		+	+
Styrene				+			
Tamoxifen	+			+		+	

KEY: RPE = retinal pigment epithelium; BC = bipolar cell; AC = amacrine cell; IPC = interplexiform cell; RGC = retinal ganglion cell; LGN = lateral geniculate nucleus. "+" indicates that this site of action was cited in one or more case reports, review articles, clinical or animal studies. "−" indicates that this site of action showed no adverse effect as cited in one or more case reports, review articles, clinical or animal studies.

productivity, and a distinct decrease in the overall quality of life.

The overall goal of this chapter is to review the structural and functional alterations in the mammalian eye and central visual system commonly produced by environmental and workplace chemicals, gases, and vapors and by therapeutic drugs. Except where noted, all these compounds are referred to as chemicals and drugs. The adverse effects of these agents on the different compartments of the eye [i.e., cornea, lens, retina, and retinal pigment epithelium (RPE)], central visual pathway [i.e., optic nerve and optic tract], and the central processing areas [i.e., lateral geniculate nucleus (LGN), visual cortex] are addressed (Table 17-1). To further understand the disposition and effects of these chemicals and drugs on the eye and central visual system, the pharmacodynamics and pharmacokinetics of these compartments are briefly reviewed (Table 17-2). Furthermore, the ophthalmologic evaluation of the eye and the testing of visual function are discussed, as the results from these clinical, behavioral, and electrophysiologic studies form the basis of our diagnosis and understanding of adverse visual system effects in patients and animals. Many of the chemicals discussed below initially appear to have a single site and, by inference, mechanism of action, whereas others have several sites and corresponding mechanisms of action. However, a more in-depth examination reveals that, depending upon dose (concentration), many of these chemicals have multiple sites of action. A few examples illustrate the point. First, as described below in more detail, carbon disulfide produces optic nerve and optic tract degeneration and also adversely affects the neurons and vasculature of the retina, resulting in photoreceptor and retinal ganglion cell (RGC) structural and functional alterations (Hotta et al., 1971; Raitta et al., 1974; Palacz et al., 1980; Seppalainen et al., 1980; Raitta et al., 1981; De Rouck et al.,

1986; Eskin et al., 1988; Merigan et al., 1988; Fox, 1998). Second, gestational and postnatal exposure to inorganic lead clearly affects rod photoreceptors in developing and adult mammals, resulting in rod-mediated (or scotopic) vision deficits; however, structural and functional deficits at the level of the RGCs, visual cortex, and oculomotor system are also observed (Fox and Sillman, 1979; Costa and Fox, 1983; Fox, 1984; Glickman et al., 1984; Lilienthal et al., 1988, 1994; Reuhl et al., 1989; Ruan et al., 1994; Fox et al., 1997; Rice, 1998; Rice and Hayward, 1999; He et al., 2000; and see reviews by Otto and Fox, 1993; Fox, 1998; Rothenberg et al., 2002). Although both gestational and postnatal lead exposure produce scotopic electroretinographic (ERG) deficits, the amplitude changes are in opposite directions and their underlying mechanisms are distinctly different. Finally, some environmental and occupational neurotoxicants (e.g., acrylamide, lead) have been utilized for in vivo and in vitro animal models to examine the pathogenesis of selected retinal, neuronal, or axonal diseases; the basic functions of the retinocortical pathways; and/or the molecular mechanisms of apoptosis (Fox and Sillman, 1979; Vidyasagar, 1981; Lynch et al., 1992; He et al., 2000).

The conceptual approach, format, and overall organization of this chapter on ocular and visual system toxicology for the 7th edition of Casarett and Doull's *Toxicology: The Basic Science of Poisons* were designed in anticipation that the main audience would be graduate and medical school students, ophthalmologists and occupational physicians, basic and applied science researchers interested in ocular and visual system toxicology, and those interested in having a basic reference source. To write this chapter, information was synthesized and condensed from several excellent resources on different aspects of ocular, retinal, and visual system anatomy, biochemistry, cell and molecular biology, histology, pharmacology,

Table 17-2
Distribution of Ocular Xenobiotic-Biotransforming Enzymes

	ENZYMES	TEARS	CORNEA	IRIS/CILIARY BODY	LENS	RETINA	CHORIOD
Phase I reactions	Acetylcholinesterase (AChE)	+		+		+	+
	Alcohol dehydrogenase		+		–	+	+
	Aldehyde dehydrogenase		+		+	+	+
	Aldehyde reductase		+	+	+	+	+
	Aldose reductase		+		+	+	
	Carboxylesterase	+	+	+		+	+
	Catalase	–	+	+	+	+	+
	Cu/Zn superoxide dismutase	+	+		–/+	+	
	CYP1A1 or CYP1A2	+	+	+	–	+	+
	CYP1B1		+	+	+	+	
	CYP2B1 or CYP2B2				+	+	
	CYP2C11				+		
	CYP3A1				+	+	
	CYP4A1 or CYP4B2		+	+		+	
	CYP27A1					+	
	MAO-A or MAO-B	+		+		+	+
Phase II reactions	Glutathione peroxidase	–	+	+	+	+	+
	Glutathione reductase		+		+	+	
	Glutathione-S-transferase		+	+	+	+	
	Sulfotransferases				+	+	
	UDP-glucuronosyl transferases				+	+	
	N-Acetyltransferase		+	+	+	+	+

KEY: "+" and "–" indicate that the enzyme was present (localized by immunohistochemistry, immunogold electron microscopy, Western blot or gene expression) or absent, respectively, in human, monkey or rodent tissues.

physiology, and toxicology (Hogan *et al.*, 1971; Merigan and Weiss, 1980; Fox *et al.*, 1982; Sears, 1984; Dayhaw-Barker *et al.*, 1986; Grant, 1986; Dowling, 1987; Fraunfelder and Meyer, 1989; Ogden and Schachat, 1989; Berman, 1991; Boyes, 1992; Chiou, 1992; Hart, 1992; Hockwin *et al.*, 1992; Bartlett and Jaanus, 1995; Herr and Boyes, 1995; Potts, 1996; Fox, 1998; Rodieck, 1998; Ballantyne, 1999; Kaufman and Alm, 2002; Schuman and Grant, 2003). The interested reader should consult these sources for more detail than is provided below. We gratefully acknowledge the use of the information in these sources as well as those cited in the text below.

EXPOSURE TO THE EYE AND VISUAL SYSTEM

Ocular Pharmacodynamics and Pharmacokinetics

Toxic chemicals and systemic drugs can affect all parts of the eye (Fig. 17-1; Table 17-1). Several factors determine whether a chemical can reach a particular ocular site of action, including the physiochemical properties of the chemical, concentration and duration of exposure, route of exposure, and the movement of the chemical into and across the different ocular compartments and barriers. The cornea and external adnexa of the eye, including the conjunctiva (the delicate membranes covering the inner surface of the eyelids and the exposed surface of the sclera) and eyelids are often exposed directly to chemicals (i.e., acids, bases, solvents), gases and particles, and drugs. The first site of action is the tear film—a three-layered structure with both hydrophobic and hydrophilic properties.

The outermost tear film layer is a thin (0.1 μm) hydrophobic layer that is secreted by the meibomian (sebaceous) glands. This superficial lipid layer protects the underlying thicker (7 μm) aqueous layer that is produced by the lacrimal glands. The third layer, which has both hydrophobic and hydrophilic properties, is the very thin (0.02 to 0.05 μm) mucoid layer. It is secreted by the goblet cells of the conjunctiva and acts as an interface between the hydrophilic layer of the tears and the hydrophobic layer of the corneal epithelial cells. Thus, the aqueous layer is the largest portion of the tear film, and therefore water-soluble chemical compounds more readily mix with the tears and gain access to the cornea. However, a large proportion of the compounds that are splashed into the eyes is washed away by the tears and thus not absorbed.

The cornea, an avascular tissue, is considered the external barrier to the internal ocular structures. Once a chemical interacts with the tear film and subsequently contacts the cornea and conjunctiva, the majority of what is absorbed locally enters the anterior segment by passing across the cornea. In contrast, a greater systemic absorption and higher blood concentration occurs through contact with the vascularized conjunctiva (Sears, 1984; Pepose and Ubels, 1992; Fig. 17-2). The human cornea, which is approximately 500 μm thick, has several distinct layers, or barriers, through which a chemical must pass in order to reach the anterior chamber (see discussion on the cornea, below). The first is the corneal epithelium. It is a stratified squamous, nonkeratinized, and multicellular hydrophobic layer. These cells have a relatively low ionic conductance through apical cell membranes, and due to the tight junctions (desmosomes), they have a high resistance paracellular pathway. The primary barrier to chemical penetration of the cornea is the set of tight junctions

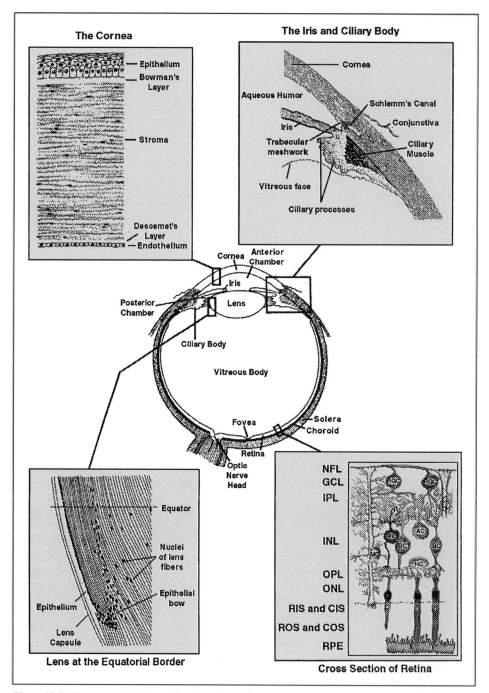

Figure 17-1. Diagrammatic horizontal cross section of the eye, with medium-power enlargement of details for the cornea, iris and ciliary body, lens, and retina.

The morphologic features, their role in ocular pharmacodynamics, pharmacokinetics, drug metabolism, and the adverse effects of drugs and chemical agents on these sites are discussed in the text.

at the superficial layer of the corneal epithelial cells. Thus, the permeability of the corneal epithelium as a whole is low and only lipid soluble chemicals readily pass through this layer. Bowmann's membrane separates the epithelium from the stroma. The corneal stroma makes up 90% of the corneal thickness and is composed of water, collagen, and glycosaminoglycans. It contains approximately 200 lamellae, each about 1.5 to 2.0 μm thick. Due to the composition and structure of the stroma, hydrophilic chemicals eas-

ily dissolve in this thick layer, which can also act as a reservoir for these chemicals. The inner edge of the corneal stroma is bounded by a thin, limiting basement membrane, called Descemet's membrane, which is secreted by the corneal endothelium. The innermost layer of the cornea, the corneal endothelium, is composed of a single layer of large diameter hexagonal cells connected by terminal bars and surrounded by lipid membranes. The endothelial cells have a relatively low ionic conductance through apical cell surface and

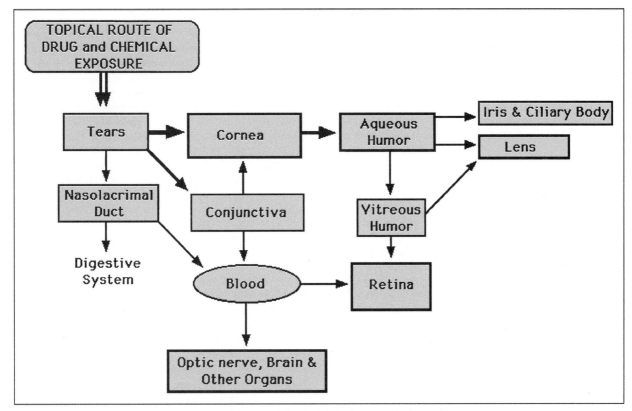

Figure 17-2. Ocular absorption and distribution of drugs and chemicals following the topical route of exposure.

The details for movement of drugs and chemicals between compartments of the eye and subsequently to the optic nerve, brain, and other organs are discussed in the text. The conceptual idea for this figure was obtained from Lapalus and Garaffo (1992).

a high-resistance paracellular pathway. Although, the permeability of the corneal endothelial cells to ionized chemicals is relatively low, it is still 100 to 200 times more permeable than the corneal epithelium. The Na^+,K^+-pump is located on the basolateral membrane while the energy-dependent Na^+,HCO_3^--transporter is located on the apical membrane (Sears, 1984; Pepose and Ubels, 1992).

There are two separate vascular systems in the eye: (1) the uveal blood vessels, which include the vascular beds of the iris, ciliary body, and choroid, and (2) the retinal vessels (Hogan, 1971; Alm, 1992). In humans, the ocular vessels are derived from the ophthalmic artery, which is a branch of the internal carotid artery. The ophthalmic artery branches into (1) the central retinal artery, which enters the eye and then further branches into four major vessels serving each of the retinal quadrants; (2) two posterior ciliary arteries; and (3) several anterior arteries. In the anterior segment of the eye, there is a blood–aqueous barrier that has relatively tight junctions between the endothelial cells of the iris capillaries and nonpigmented cells of the ciliary epithelium (Hogan, 1971; Alm, 1992). The major function of the ciliary epithelium is the production of aqueous humor from the plasma filtrate present in the stroma of the ciliary processes.

In humans and several widely used experimental animals (e.g., monkeys, pigs, dogs, rats, mice), the retina has a dual circulatory supply: choroidal and retinal. The retinal blood vessels are distributed within the inner or proximal portion of the retina, which consists of the outer plexiform layer (OPL), inner nuclear layer (INL), inner plexiform layer (IPL), and ganglion cell layer (GCL). The endothelial cells of capillaries of the retinal vessels have tight junctions similar to those that form the blood–brain barrier in the cerebral capillaries. These capillaries form the blood-retinal barrier

and under normal physiologic conditions, they are largely impermeable to chemicals such as glucose and amino acids (Alm, 1992). However, at the level of the optic disk, the blood-retinal barrier lacks these tight-junction types of capillaries and thus hydrophilic molecules can enter the optic nerve head by diffusion from the extravascular space (Alm, 1992) and cause selective damage at this site of action. The outer or distal retina, which consists of the retinal pigment epithelium (RPE), rod, and cone photoreceptor outer segments (ROS, COS) and inner segments (RIS, CIS), and the photoreceptor outer nuclear layer (ONL), are avascular. These areas of the retina are supplied by the choriocapillaris: a dense, one-layered network of fenestrated vessels formed by the short posterior ciliary arteries and located next to the RPE. Consistent with their known structure, these capillaries have loose endothelial junctions and abundant fenestrae; they are highly permeable to large proteins. Thus, the extravascular space contains a high concentration of albumin and γ-globulin (Sears, 1992).

Following systemic exposure to drugs and chemicals by the oral, inhalation, dermal, or parenteral route, these compounds are distributed to all parts of the eye by the blood in the uveal blood vessels and retinal vessels (Fig. 17-3). Most of these drugs and chemicals can rapidly equilibrate with the extravascular space of the choroid where they are separated from the retina and vitreous body by the RPE and endothelial cells of the retinal capillaries, respectively. Hydrophilic molecules with molecular weights less than 200 to 300 Da can cross the ciliary epithelium and iris capillaries and enter the aqueous humor (Sears, 1992). Thus, the corneal endothelium—the cells responsible for maintaining normal hydration and transparency of the corneal stroma—could be exposed to chemical compounds by the aqueous humor and limbal capillaries.

Similarly, the anterior surface of the lens can also be exposed as a result of its contact with the aqueous humor. The most likely retinal target sites following systemic drug and chemical exposure appear to be the RPE and photoreceptors in the distal retina because the endothelial cells of the choriocapillaris are permeable to proteins smaller than 50 to 70 kDa. However, the cells of the RPE are joined on their basolateral surface by tight junctions—zonula occludens—that limit the passive penetration of large molecules into the neural retina.

The presence of intraocular melanin plays a special role in ocular toxicology. First, it is found in several different locations in the eye: pigmented cells of the iris, ciliary body, RPE, and uveal tract. Second, it has a high binding affinity for polycyclic aromatic hydrocarbons, electrophiles, calcium, and toxic heavy metals such as aluminum, iron, lead, and mercury (Meier-Ruge, 1972; Potts and Au, 1976; Dräger, 1985; Ulshafer et al., 1990; Eichenbaum and Zheng, 2000). Although this initially may play a protective role, it also results in the excessive accumulation, long-term storage, and slow release of numerous drugs and chemicals from melanin. For example, atropine binds more avidly to pigmented irides and thus its duration of action is prolonged (Bartlett and Jaanus, 1995). In addition, the accumulation of chloroquine in the RPE produces an 80-fold higher concentration of chloroquine in the retina relative to liver (Meier-Rouge, 1972). Similarly, lead accumulates in the human retina such that its concentration is 5 to 750 times that in other ocular tissues (Eichenbaum and Zheng, 2000).

Ocular Drug Metabolism

Metabolism of xenobiotics occurs in all compartments of the eye by well-known Phase I and II xenobiotic-biotransforming enzymes. Drug metabolizing enzymes such as acetylcholinesterase, carboxylesterase (also known as pseudocholinesterase: see chap. 6 entitled "Biotransformation of Xenobiotics"), alcohol and aldehyde dehydrogenase, aldehyde and aldose reductase, catalase, monoamine oxidase A and/or B, and Cu^{2+}/Zn^{2+} superoxide dismutase as well as several types of proteases are present in the tears, iris-ciliary body, choroid, and retina of many different species (Shanthaverrappa and Bourne, 1964; Waltmann and Sears, 1964; Bausher, 1976; Anderson, 1980; Puro, 1985; Atalla et al., 1998; Berman, 1991; Crouch et al., 1991; Watkins et al., 1991; Gondhowiardjo and van Haeringen, 1993; Downes and Holmes, 1995; Gaudet et al., 1995; Behndig et al., 1998; King et al., 1999; Table 17-2). Although there are new data on the number and activity of cytochrome P450 (CYP) isoforms (Phase I metabolism) and Phase II conjugating enzymes in ocular tissues since our first edition of this chapter, there is still less known about xenobiotic metabolism in ocular tissues than in other tissues (Shichi et al., 1975; Shichi and Nebert, 1982; Sears, 1992; Zhao and Shichi, 1995; Shichi, 1996; Srivastava et al., 1996; Schwartzman, 1997; Singh and Shichi, 1998; Mastyugin et al., 1999; Nakamura et al., 2005; Doshi et al., 2006; Lee et al., 2006). CYP1A1 and CYP1A2—previously known as aryl hydrocarbon hydroxylase activity—are found in all bovine and mouse ocular tissues except the lens and can be induced by 3-methylcholanthrene and β-naphthoflavone (Shichi et al., 1975; Shichi et al., 1982; Zhao and Shichi, 1995). Moreover, a CYP4 family member—CYP4A1 in the mouse and CYP4B1 in the rabbit—is present in corneal epithelium and can be induced by phenobarbital and the peroxisome proliferator clofibrate (Zhao et al., 1996; Mastyugin et al., 1999). This corneal epithelial CYP monooxygenase metabolizes arachidonic acid to two of its major metabolites: 12(R)-HETE [12(R)-hydroxy-5,8,10,14-

eicosatrienoic acid] and 12(R)-HETrE [12(R)-hydroxy-5,8,14-eicosatrienoic acid] (Schwartzman, 1987; Asakura et al., 1994; Mastyugin et al., 1999). In the corneal epithelium, 12(R)-HETE is a potent inhibitor of Na^+,K^+-ATPase, whereas 12(R)-HETrE is a potent angiogenic and chemotactic factor (Schwartzman, 1997).

The Phase II conjugating enzymes found in bovine, rabbit, and rat ocular tissues include UDP glucuronosyltransferase, glutathione peroxidase, glutathione reductase, glutathione S-transferase, and N-acetyltransferase (Awasthi et al., 1980; Shichi and Nebert, 1982; Penn et al., 1987; Watkins et al., 1991: Srivastava et al., 1996; Singh and Shichi, 1998; Nakamura et al., 2005; see Table 17-2). Whereas the activity of these enzymes varies between species and ocular tissues, the whole lens appears to have low biotransformational activity. Metabolically, the lens is a heterogeneous tissue, with glutathione S-transferase activity found in the lens epithelium and not in the lens cortex or nucleus (Srivastava et al., 1996). Overall, these findings suggest that ocular tissues that contact the external environment have a blood supply possessing both CYPs and Phase II conjugating enzymes, especially those enzymes related to glutathione conjugation. The presence and need for a competent glutathione conjugation system is clearly understandable in ocular tissues that directly interact with UV radiation, light, and xenobiotics and that have high rates of metabolism and high lipid content. Further work is needed to determine the presence and activity of other CYP family members in ocular tissue, the various factors (i.e., age, gender, tissue-specific, xenobiotics, etc.) that regulate their expression, and their endogenous and exogenous substrates.

Central Visual System Pharmacokinetics

The penetration of potentially toxic compounds into visual areas of the central nervous system (CNS) is governed, like other parts of the CNS, by the blood–brain barrier (Fig. 17-3). The blood–brain barrier is formed through a combination of tight junctions in brain capillary endothelial cells and foot processes of astrocytic glial cells that surround the brain capillaries. Together these structures serve to limit the penetration of blood-borne compounds into the brain and in some cases actively exclude compounds from brain tissue. The concept of an absolute barrier is not correct, however, because the blood–brain barrier is differentially permeable to compounds depending on their size, charge, and lipophilicity. Compounds that are large, highly charged, or otherwise not very lipid soluble tend to be excluded from the brain, whereas smaller, uncharged, and lipid-soluble compounds more readily penetrate into the brain tissue. In addition to entering the CNS through this nonspecific semipermeable diffusion barrier, some specific nutrients including, ions, amino acids, and glucose enter the CNS through selective transport mechanisms. In some cases, toxic compounds may be actively transported into the brain by mimicking the natural substrates of active transport systems. A few areas of the brain lack a blood–brain barrier; consequently, blood-borne compounds readily penetrate into the brain tissue in these regions. Interestingly, one such area is the optic nerve near the lamina cribrosa (Alm, 1992), which could cause this part of the central visual system to be vulnerable to exposures that do not affect much of the remainder of the brain.

TESTING VISUAL FUNCTION

Testing for potential toxic effects of compounds on the eye and visual system can be divided into tests of ocular toxicity and tests of visual function. Alternatively, such tests could be grouped according

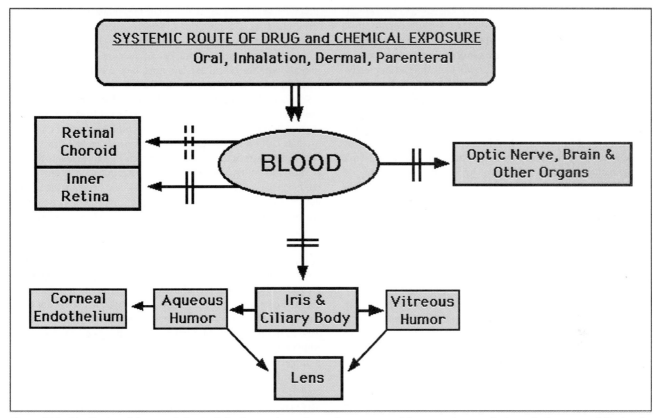

Figure 17-3. Distribution of drugs and chemicals in the anterior and posterior segments of the eye, optic nerve, brain, and other organs following the systemic route of exposure.

The details for movement of drugs and chemicals between compartments of the eye are discussed in the text. The conceptual idea for this part of the figure was obtained from Lapalus and Garaffo (1992). The solid and dotted double lines represent the different blood–tissue barriers present in the anterior segment of the eye, retina, optic nerve, and brain. The solid double lines represent tight endothelial junctions, whereas the dotted double lines represent loose endothelial junctions.

to the professional training of the individual conducting the evaluation. Such a categorization might include tests of contact irritancy or toxicity akin to dermatologic procedures, ophthalmologic evaluations, neurophysiologic studies of the function of the visual system, and behavioral or psychophysical evaluations of visual thresholds and aspects of perception.

Evaluation of Ocular Irritancy and Toxicity

Standard procedures for evaluating ocular irritation have been based on a method originally published by Draize *et al.* over a half a century ago (Draize *et al.*, 1944). Over this time, the Draize test with some additions and revisions formed the basis of safety evaluations in data submitted to several government regulatory bodies including the European Economic Community and several federal agencies within the United States. Traditionally, albino rabbits were the subjects evaluated in the Draize test, although the Environmental Protection Agency (EPA) protocol allows different test species to be used if sufficient justification is provided. The standard procedure involves instillation of 0.1 mL of a liquid or 100 mg of a solid into the conjunctival sac of one eye and then gently holding the eye closed for 1 second. The untreated eye serves as a control. Both eyes are evaluated at 1, 24, 48, and 72 hours, respectively, after treatment. If there is evidence of damage in the treated eye at 72 hours, the examination time may be extended. The cornea, iris, and conjunc-

tiva are evaluated and scored according to a weighted scale. The cornea is scored for both the degree of opacity and area of involvement, with each measure having a potential range from 0 (none) to 4 (most severe). The iris receives a single score (0 to 2) for irritation, including degree of swelling, congestion, and degree of reaction to light. The conjunctiva is scored for the redness (0 to 3), chemosis (swelling: 0 to 4), and discharge (0 to 3). The individual scores are then multiplied by a weighting factor: 5 for the cornea, 2 for the iris, and 5 for the conjunctiva. The results are summed for a maximum total score of 110. Photographic examples of lesions receiving each score are provided in Datson and Freeberg (1991). In this scale, the cornea accounts for 80 (73%) of the total possible points, in accordance with the severity associated with corneal injury. The Draize test, although a standard for decades, has been criticized on several grounds, including high interlaboratory variability, the subjective nature of the scoring, poor predictive value for human irritants, and most significantly, for causing undue pain and distress to the tested animals. These criticisms have spawned a concerted effort to develop alternative methods or strategies to evaluate compounds for their potential to cause ocular irritation. These alternatives include modifications of the traditional Draize test to reduce the number of test animals required, reduce the volume of the compound administered, and increase objectivity of scoring (e.g., Kennah *et al.*, 1989; Bruner *et al.*, 1992; Lambert *et al.*, 1993). In addition, several alternative test procedures have been proposed, including the use of skin irritancy tests as substitutes for ocular irritancy and the use of in vitro assays (Datson and Freeberg, 1991; Chamberlain *et al.*, 1997; Kruszewski *et al.*, 1997). Additional research efforts are developing quantitative structure activity relationships to better predict ocular irritancy (Barratt, 1995; Sugai *et al.*, 1990; Kulkarni and Hopfinger, 1999). To date, there is no general consensus as to which of the alternative test strategies, alone or in combination, provides a suitable alternative to the Draize procedure.

The Interagency Coordinating Committee on the Validation of Alternative Methods (ICCVAM), a committee representing 14 agencies of the U.S. Federal government, has established criteria for validating methods to substitute for whole animal testing of ocular corrosiveness or irritancy (NIEHS, 1997). ICCVAM was established in 1997 by the Director of the National Institute of Environmental Health Sciences (NIEHS) to implement NIEHS directives in Public Law 103-43 (http://iccvam.niehs.nih.gov/home.htm). In March of 2005, ICCVAM released a summary evaluation of the current status of validation of in vitro test methods for identifying ocular corrosives and irritants (http://iccvam. niehs.nih.gov/methods/ocudocs/EPreport/ocureport.htm). The report considered methods that utilize isolated rabbit, chicken, or bovine eyes and one that utilized the hen egg chorioallantoic membrane (ICCVAM, 2005). Among the most important concerns in developing alternative test approaches is the predictive ability of the assay as compared to the existing results of the Draize test. The Draize results are used as a standard because information available from human ocular exposures almost invariably comes from accidental exposure episodes in which the dose levels, durations and conditions of exposure are unknown. However, the Draize test cannot be considered a "gold standard" due to the variability of results within and between studies, subjectivity of scoring outcomes, and inter-species differences in the ability to predict human ocular toxic potency from testing rabbit eyes. On the positive side, however, a large number of substances have been assessed using the Draize test and consequently, there is an ample list of chemicals against which alternative test procedures can be assessed. A list of positive and negative control substances against which alternative tests can be assessed was reviewed by ICCVAM. Factors considered included the presence of important classes of substances, quality and reliability of the data, ready availability of the chemicals in a reasonably pure form, and the range and types of lesions produced. None of the alternative tests reviewed reproduced injurious responses that produced an inflammatory response, nor did they reflect the time course of lesion development and recovery, as does the Draize test. On the other hand, most of the alternative tests were reasonably consistent with the Draize test at identifying irritant or corrosive substances. The alternative tests were less consistent with regard to classification of surfactants, alcohols, organic solvents, or solids.

Ophthalmologic Evaluations

There are many ophthalmologic procedures for evaluating the health of the eye. These should be conducted by a trained ophthalmologist or optometrist experienced in evaluating the species of interest. Procedures available range from fairly routine clinical screening evaluations to sophisticated techniques for very targeted purposes, the latter of which are beyond the scope of this chapter. A clinical evaluation of the eye addresses the adnexa and both the anterior and posterior structures in the eye. Examination of the adnexa includes evaluating the eyelids, lacrimal apparatus, and palpebral (covering the eyelid) and bulbar (covering the eye) conjunctiva. The anterior

structures or anterior segment include the cornea, iris, lens, and anterior chamber. The posterior structures, referred to as the *ocular fundus,* include the retina, retinal vasculature, choroid, optic nerve, and sclera. The adnexa and surface of the cornea can be examined initially with the naked eye and a hand-held light. Closer examination requires a slit-lamp biomicroscope, using a mydriatic drug (causes pupil dilation) if the lens is to be observed. The width of the reflection of a thin beam of light projected from the slit lamp is an indication of the thickness of the cornea and may be used to evaluate corneal edema. Lesions of the cornea can be better visualized with the use of fluorescein dye, which is retained where there is an ulceration of the corneal epithelium. Examination of the fundus requires use of a mydriatic drug. Fundoscopic examination is conducted using a direct or an indirect ophthalmoscope, as described (Gelatt, 1981; Harroff, 1991; Hockwin *et al.*, 1992). Several recently developed techniques are described in Peiffer *et al.* (2000).

An ophthalmologic examination of the eye may also involve, prior to introducing mydriatics, an examination of the pupillary light reflex. The direct pupillary reflex involves shining a bright light into the eye and observing the reflexive pupil constriction in the same eye. The consensual pupillary reflex is observed in the eye not stimulated. Both the direct and consensual pupillary light reflexes are dependent on function of a reflex arc involving cells in the retina, which travel through the optic nerve, optic chiasm, and optic tract to project to neurons in the pretectal area. Pretectal neurons travel to both ipsilateral (for the direct reflex) and contralateral (for the consensual reflex) parasympathetic neurons of the midbrain accessory oculomotor (Edinger–Westphal) nucleus. Preganglion neurons from the Edinger–Westphal nucleus project through the oculomotor nerve to the ciliary ganglion. Postganglionic neurons from the ciliary ganglion then innervate the smooth muscle fibers of the iridal pupillary sphincter. The absence of a pupillary reflex is indicative of damage somewhere in the reflex pathway, and differential impairment of the direct or consensual reflexes can indicate the location of the lesion. The presence of a pupillary light reflex, however, is not synonymous with normal visual function. Pupillary reflexes can be maintained even with substantial retinal damage. In addition, lesions in visual areas outside of the reflex pathway, such as in the visual cortex, may also leave the reflex function intact.

Electrophysiologic Techniques

Many electrophysiologic or neurophysiologic procedures are available for testing visual function in a toxicologic context. In a simple sense, most of these procedures involve stimulating the eyes with visual stimuli and electrically recording potentials generated by visually responsive neurons. Different techniques and stimuli are used to selectively study the function of specific retinal or visual cortical neurons. In the study of the effects of potential toxic substances on visual function, the most commonly used electrophysiologic procedures are the flash-evoked ERG, visual-evoked potentials (VEPs), and, less often, the electrooculogram (EOG).

ERGs are typically elicited with a brief flash of light and recorded from an electrode placed in contact with the cornea. A typical ERG waveform (see Fox and Farber, 1988; Rosolen *et al.*, 2005) includes an initial negative-going waveform, called the a-wave, that reflects the activation of photoreceptors, and a following positive b-wave that reflects the activity of retinal bipolar cells and associated membrane potential changes in Müller cells—a type of retinal glial cell that buffers extracellular potassium ions and glutamate (Dowling, 1987; Rodieck, 1998). In addition, a series of oscillatory potentials can be observed overriding the b-wave, of which the neural generators are somewhat uncertain, but they presumably reflect various stages of intraretinal signal processing. A standard set of ERG procedures has been recommended and updated for screening assessments of human clinical patients (Marmor *et al.*, 1989; Marmor and Zrenner, 1995). These procedures include the recording of (1) a response reflective of only rod photoreceptor function in the dark-adapted eye, (2) the maximal response in the dark-adapted eye, (3) a response developed by cone photoreceptors, (4) oscillatory potentials, and (5) the response to rapidly flickered light. These recommendations were used to create a protocol for screening the retinal function of dogs in toxicologic studies (Jones *et al.*, 1994). For testing retinal function beyond a screening level evaluation, ERG amplitude and latency versus log stimulus intensity functions are very useful (e.g., Fox and Farber, 1988; Rosolen *et al.*, 2005). Although flash-evoked ERGs do not reflect the function of the RGC layer, ERGs elicited with pattern-reversal stimuli (PERGs) do reflect the activation of RGCs. To date, PERGs have not been used widely in toxicological evaluations.

VEPs are elicited with stimuli similar to those used to evoke ERGs; however, VEPs are recorded from electrodes overlying visual (striate) cortex. Consequently, VEPs reflect the activity of the retinogeniculostriate pathway and the activity of cells in the visual cortex. Flash-elicited VEPs have been used in a number of studies of potentially neurotoxic compounds in laboratory animals (Fox *et al.*, 1977, 1982; Dyer *et al.*, 1982; Rebert, 1983; Dyer, 1985; Boyes, 1992; Mattsson *et al.*, 1992; Herr and Boyes, 1995). Pattern-elicited VEPs (PEPs) are more widely used in human clinical evaluations because of their diagnostic value. However, they are infrequently used in laboratory animals because albino rats do not produce usable PEPs (Boyes and Dyer, 1983). Recording PEPs and conducting psychophysical studies with pigmented Long-Evans hooded rats, Fox (1984) found that the PEP spatial frequency functions yielded almost the same visual acuity values (1.4 cycles per degree) as the psychophysically determined spatial resolution limit values (1.8 cycles per degree). These values are in good agreement with those obtained by others using single-cell electrophysiological and behavioral techniques (Powers and Green, 1978; Birch and Jacobs, 1979; Dean, 1981). Moreover, PEPs and flash-elicited VEPs have exhibited differential sensitivity to some neurotoxic agents (Boyes and Dyer, 1984; Fox, 1984). The U.S. Environmental Protection Agency has published guidelines for conducting visual evoked potential testing in a toxicological context, along with analogous sensory evoked potential procedures for evaluating auditory and somatosensory function (EPA, 1998a).

The EOG is generated by a potential difference between the front and back of the eye, which originates primarily within the RPE (Berson, 1992). Metabolic activity in the RPE generates a light-insensitive potential (the standing potential) and a light-sensitive potential; the difference in amplitude between these two potentials is easily measured as the EOG. The magnitude of the EOG is a function of the level of illumination and health status of the RPE. Electrodes placed on the skin on a line lateral or vertical to the eye measure potential changes correlated with eye movements as the relative position of the ocular dipole changes. Thus, the EOG finds applications in assessing both RPE status and measuring eye movements. The EOG is also used in monitoring eye movements during the recording of other brain potentials, so that eye movement artifacts are not misinterpreted as brain generated electrical activity (Berson, 1992). In addition, EOG measurements have been used to detect eye movement deficits caused by exposures to toxic

substances, such as those altering the function of the cerebellum (reviewed by Geller *et al.*, 1995).

As noted in the introduction to this chapter, there is a clear need for testing visual function as a component of the toxicological evaluation of commercial chemicals. The magnitude of the potential threat posed by visual system toxicity is not known, because sensory function has not been evaluated in a systematic fashion. Currently, the EPA screening batteries for neurotoxicological evaluation of laboratory animals include only minimal evaluations of visual function. Standard screening procedures such as those included in EPA's neurotoxicity screening battery (EPA, 1998b) include a functional observational battery (FOB)—an automated measurement of motor activity and neuropathology. Of the screening procedures, only the FOB evaluates visual function and the extent of these measures is very limited. The entire assessment of visual function includes observing the animal's response to an approaching object such as a pencil and observing the pupil's response to a light. These procedures are limited in not exploring responsiveness over a range of stimulus features such as luminance, color, spatial frequency, and temporal frequency. In addition, they do not evaluate rod or cone sensory thresholds, nor do they isolate potential motor or integrative contributions to task performance. Despite these shortcomings, the FOB has been successful at detecting visual deficits produced by exposure to 3,3′-iminodipropionitrile (Moser and Boyes, 1993) or carbon disulfide (Moser *et al.*, 1998), which illustrates the importance of conducting at least this level of visual function screening in routine testing programs. Some studies include ophthalmologic and/or ocular pathologic evaluations. Comprehensive visual toxicity studies should include ophthalmologic and pathologic evaluation of ocular tissues and assessments of visual function.

Another potentially limiting problem in product safety testing is the routine use of albino animals, whose capacity for visual function is limited at best. The toxicity of many polycyclic aromatic compounds is mediated through interactions with melanin (Potts, 1964, 1996; Meier-Ruge, 1972; see discussion of the retina, below), which is absent in the eyes of albino strains. Furthermore, light-related ocular lesions, including cataracts and retinal degeneration, are often observed in control albino rats and mice used in 2-year product-safety evaluations. It is well known that normal photoreceptor physiology and susceptibility to chemical damage in rats and mice are mediated by light (LaVail, 1976; Williams *et al.*, 1985; Williams, 1986; Penn and Williams, 1986; LaVail *et al.*, 1987; Penn *et al.*, 1987, 1989; Rapp *et al.*, 1990; Backstrom *et al.*, 1993). For example, one study showed that the proportion of Fisher 344 rats in the control group with photoreceptor lesions ranged from less than 10% of rats housed on the bottom row of the cage racks to over 55% of rats housed on the top row, where the luminance was greater (Rao, 1991). Even under reduced light levels, the incidence of these effects was as high as 15%. If albino animals are used as the test subjects, it is important to control the overall level of illumination in the animal colony and also to periodically rotate the animals among the rows of the cage racks. Even under these conditions, it is extremely difficult to interpret pathologic changes in albino rats and mice exposed to test compounds against such high rates of background retinal lesions.

Sensory dysfunction can confound other measures of neurotoxicity. Many behavioral and observational evaluations of neurotoxicity involve presentation of sensory stimuli to human or animal subjects followed by the observation or measurement of a behavioral or motor response. In many cases, the inferences drawn from such measures are stated in terms of the cognitive abilities of the test subject, such as whether learning or memory have been compromised as a function of exposure to the test compound. If the subject was unable to clearly and precisely perceive the test stimuli, which are often complex patterns or contain color, task performance may be affected independently of any effect on cognition. Controlling for visual deficits may alter the interpretation of performance or cognitive tasks (Anger *et al.*, 1994; Hudnell *et al.*, 1996; Walkowiak *et al.*, 1998; Cestnick and Coltheart, 1999).

Behavioral and Psychophysical Techniques

Behavioral and psychophysical testing procedures typically vary the parameters of the visual stimulus and then determine whether the subject can discriminate or perceive the stimulus (Woodhouse and Barlow, 1982; Maurissen, 1995). Many facets of visual function in humans and laboratory animals have been studied using these procedures. Often, the goal of these procedures is to resolve the spatial or temporal limits of visual discrimination; however, most visual scenes and targets in our daily life involve discrimination of objects with low to middle spatial and temporal frequencies (Woodhouse and Barlow, 1982). Contrast sensitivity functions are used to assess these parameters. In addition, as discussed below, other visual parameters also have been investigated.

Contrast sensitivity refers to the ability to resolve small differences in luminance contrast, such as the difference between subtle shades of gray. Contrast sensitivity should be measured for a series of visual patterns that differ in pattern size. Typically, such patterns are a series of sine-wave gratings (striped patterns where the luminance changes across the pattern in a sinusoidal profile) where the spatial frequency of the sinusoidal pattern (i.e., the width of the bars in the pattern) varies in octave steps. The contrast of the patterns (i.e., the difference between the brightest and darkest parts of the pattern that is adjusted for mean luminance) also varies. The resulting data, when plotted on log/log coordinates, forms a contrast sensitivity function that is representative of the ability to detect visual patterns over the range of visible pattern sizes. Contrast sensitivity functions are dependent primarily on the neural as opposed to the optical properties of the visual system. The contrast sensitivity functions generally form an inverted U-shaped profile with highest sensitivity to contrast at intermediate spatial frequencies. Sensitivity to high spatial frequencies is equivalent to a measure of visual acuity, whereas sensitivity to mid-range spatial frequencies is important for facial recognition (Ginsburg, 2003). The peak of the function as well as the limits of resolution on both the spatial frequency and contrast axes vary across species. For example, at relatively mesopic (rod- and cone-mediated) luminance levels, the peak of the spatial contrast sensitivity function for the albino rat, hooded rat, cat, and human are 0.1, 0.3, 0.3, and 2 cycles per degree, respectively (Birch and Jacobs, 1979; Fox, 1984).

Some of the visual parameters that have been investigated include: (1) the absolute luminance threshold, which is the threshold value for detecting an illuminated target by a dark-adapted subject in a dark-adapted environment; (2) visual acuity, which is the spatial resolution of the visual system [approximately 50 cycles per degree in humans (Woodhouse and Barlow, 1982) and 1.1 to 1.8 cycles per degree in albino and hooded rats (Fox, 1984; Birch and Jacobs, 1979; Dean, 1981)]; (3) color and spectral discriminations (Porkony *et al.*, 1979); (4) critical flicker fusion frequency, which is the threshold value for detecting a flickering light at different luminance intensities; and (5) the peak of the spatial and temporal contrast sensitivity functions at different luminance levels (Wood-

house and Barlow, 1982). Most of these tests are dependent upon the quality of the ocular optics and the ability to obtain a sharply focused visual image on the retina. Thresholds for detecting luminance, contrast, flicker, and color are primarily dependent on retinal and central mechanisms of neural function, although optical impairments (e.g., cataracts) interfere with these functions. The assessment of visual acuity and contrast sensitivity has been recommended for field studies of humans potentially exposed to neurotoxic substances (ATSDR, 1992).

Color vision deficits are either inherited or acquired. Hereditary red-green color deficits occur in about 8% of males (X-linked), while only about 0.5% of females show similar congenital deficits (Porkony *et al.*, 1979). Inherited color deficiencies take two common forms: protan, a red-green confusion caused by abnormality or absence of the long-wavelength (red) sensitive cones; and deutan, concomitant confusion of red-green and blue-yellow caused by abnormality or absence of the middle-wavelength (green) sensitive cones. Congenital loss of short-wavelength cones, resulting in a blue-yellow confusion (tritanopia, or type III), is extremely rare. Most acquired color vision deficits, such as those caused by drug and chemical exposure, begin with a reduced ability to perform blue-yellow discriminations (Porkony *et al.*, 1979; Jaanus *et al.*, 1995). With increased or prolonged low-level exposure, the color confusion can progress to the red-green axis as well. Because of the rarity of inherited tritanopia, it is generally assumed that blue-yellow deficits, when observed, are acquired deficits. Köllner's rule of thumb states that disorders of the outer retina produce blue-yellow deficits, whereas disorders of the inner retina and optic nerve produce red-green perceptual deficits (Porkony *et al.*, 1979). Bilateral lesions in the area V4 of visual cortex can also lead to color blindness (prosopagnosia). Several reviews discuss and/or list the effects of drugs and chemicals on color vision (Lyle, 1974; Porkony, 1979; Grant, 1986; Mergler, 1990; Grant and Schuman, 1993; Jaanus *et al.*, 1995; Lessel, 1998).

Recently, the assessment of color vision by rapid screening procedures has been used to evaluate occupationally and environmentally exposed populations (Mergler, 1990; Geller and Hudnell, 1997; Iregren *et al.*, 2002a; Iregren *et al.*, 2002b: see discussion below of the retina and optic nerve/tract for specific references and details). Color vision may be evaluated using several different testing procedures. Commonly used procedures in human toxicologic evaluations include the Ishihara color plates and chip arrangement tests such as the Farnsworth–Munson 100 Hue (FM-100) test and the simplified 15-chip tests using either the saturated hues of the Farnsworth D-15 or the desaturated hues of the Lanthony Desaturated Panel D-15. The Ishihara plates involve a series of colored spots arranged in patterns that take advantage of perceived difference in shades resulting from congenital protan or deutan anomalies. Normal observers perceive different sets of embedded numbers than do those with color vision deficits. The Farnsworth–Munson procedure involves arrangement of 85 chips in order of progressively changing color. The relative chromatic value of successive chips induces those with color perception deficits to abnormally arrange the chips. The pattern is indicative of the nature of the color perception anomaly. The FM-100 is considered more diagnostically reliable but takes considerably longer to administer than the similar but more efficient Farnsworth and Lanthony tests. The desaturated hues of the Lanthony D-15 are designed to better identify subtle acquired color vision deficits. For this reason, and because it requires only a few minutes to administer, the Lanthony D-15 was recommended as the procedure for color vision screening of potentially occupationally and environmentally exposed populations (ATSDR, 1992). A critical review of this procedure, its test–retest reliability and its use in toxicologic applications should be consulted prior to its use (see Geller and Hudnell, 1997; Good *et al.*, 2005).

TARGET SITES AND MECHANISMS OF ACTION: CORNEA

The cornea provides the anterior covering of the eye and as such must provide three essential functions. First, it must provide a clear refractive surface. The air-to-fluid/tissue interface at the cornea is the principal refractive surface of the eye, providing approximately 48 diopters of refraction. The curvature of the cornea must be correct for the visual image to be focused at the retina. Second, the cornea provides tensile strength to maintain the appropriate shape of the globe. Third, the cornea protects the eye from external factors, including potentially toxic chemicals. The anatomy is reviewed in the discussion of ocular pharmacodynamics and pharmacokinetics above.

The cornea is transparent to wavelengths of light ranging between 310 nm (UV) to 2500 nm (IR) in wavelengths. Exposure to UV light below this range can damage the cornea. It is most sensitive to wavelengths of approximately 270 nm. Excessive UV exposure leads to photokeratitis and corneal pathology, the classic example being welder's arc burns.

The cornea can be damaged by topical or systemic exposure to drugs and chemicals. Reports of such adverse reactions have been catalogued and reviewed by Diamante and Fraunfelder (1998). One summary analysis, of approximately 600 agricultural and industrial chemicals (raw materials, intermediates, formulation components, and sales products), evaluated using the Draize procedure, reported that over half of the materials tested caused no (18–31%) or minimal (42–51%) irritation. Depending on the chemical category, 9–17% of compounds were graded as slightly irritant, whereas 1–6% were graded as strong or extreme irritants (Kobel and Gfeller, 1985).

Direct chemical exposure to the eye requires emergency medical attention. Acid and alkali chemicals that come into contact with the cornea can be extremely destructive. Products at pH extremes ≤2.5 or ≥11.5 are considered as extreme ocular irritants (Potts, 1996). They can cause severe ocular damage and permanent loss of vision. Damage that extends to the corneal endothelium is associated with poor repair and recovery. The most important therapy is immediate and adequate irrigation with large amounts of water or saline, whichever is most readily available. The extent of damage to the eye and the ability to achieve a full recovery are dependent upon the nature of the chemical, the concentration and duration of exposure, and the speed and magnitude of the initial irrigation.

Acids

Strong acids with a pH ≤2.5 can be highly injurious. Among the most significant acidic chemicals in terms of the tendency to cause clinical ocular damage are hydrofluoric acid, sulfurous acid, sulfuric acid, chromic acid, hydrochloric acid and nitric acid and acetic acid (McCulley, 1998). Injuries may be mild if contact is with weak acids or with dilute solutions of strong acids. Compounds with a pH between 2.5 and 7, produce pain or stinging; but with only brief contact, they will cause no lasting damage (Grant and Schuman, 1993). Following mild burns, the corneal epithelium may become turbid as the corneal stroma swells. Mild burns are typically followed by rapid regeneration of the corneal epithelium and full recovery.

In more severe burns, the epithelium of the cornea and conjunctiva become opaque and necrotic and may disintegrate over the course of a few days. In severe burns, there may be no sensation of pain because the corneal nerve endings are destroyed (Grant, 1986; Potts, 1996).

Acid chemical burns of the cornea occur through hydrogen ion–induced denaturing and coagulation of proteins. As epithelial cell proteins coagulate, glycosaminoglycans precipitate and stromal collagen fibers shrink. These events cause the cornea to become cloudy. The protein coagulation and shrinkage of the collagen is protective in that it forms a barrier and reduces further penetration of the acid. The collagen shrinkage, however, contracts the eye and can lead to a dangerous acute increase in intraocular pressure. The pH of the acid is not the only determinant of the severity of injury; however, as equimolar solutions of several chemicals adjusted to the same pH of 2 produce a wide range of outcomes. Both the hydrogen ion and anionic portions of the acid molecules contribute to protein coagulation and precipitation. The tissue proteins also tend to act as buffers (Grant, 1986; Potts, 1996).

Bases or Alkalies

Compounds with a basic pH are potentially even more damaging to the eye than are strong acids. Among the compounds of clinical significance in terms of frequency and severity of injuries are ammonia or ammonium hydroxide, sodium hydroxide (lye), potassium hydroxide (caustic potash), calcium hydroxide (lime), and magnesium hydroxide (McCulley, 1998). One of the reasons that caustic agents are so dangerous is their ability to rapidly penetrate the ocular tissues. This is particularly true for ammonia, which has been measured in the aqueous humor just seconds after application to the cornea. The toxicity of these substances is a function of their pH, being more toxic with increasing pH values. As with acid burns, the concentration of the solution and the duration of contact with the eye are important determinants of the eventual clinical outcome. Rapid and extensive irrigation after exposure and removal of particles, if present, is the immediate therapy of choice (Grant, 1986; Potts, 1996).

A feature of caustic burns that differentiates them from acid burns is that two phases of injury may be observed. There is an acute phase from exposure up to 1 week. Depending on the extent of injury, direct damage from exposure is observed in the cornea, adnexia, and possibly in the iris, ciliary body, and lens. The presence of strong hydroxide ions causes rapid necrosis of the corneal epithelium and, if sufficient amounts are present, penetration through and/or destruction of the successive corneal layers. Strong alkali substances attack membrane lipids, causing necrosis and enhancing penetration of the substance to deeper tissue layers. The cations also react with the carboxyl groups of glycosaminoglycans and collagen, the latter reaction leading to hydration of the collagen matrix and corneal swelling. The cornea may appear clouded or become opaque immediately after exposure as a result of stromal edema and changes to, or precipitation of, proteoglycans. The denaturing of the collagen and loss of protective covering of the glycosoaminoglycans is thought to make the collagen fibrils more susceptible to subsequent enzymatic degradation. Intraocular pressure may increase as a result of initial hydration of the collagen fibrils and later through the blockage of aqueous humor outflow. Conversely, if the alkali burn extends to involve the ciliary body, the intraocular pressure may decrease due to reduced formation of aqueous humor. The acute phase of damage is typically followed by initiation of corneal repair. The repair process may involve corneal neovascularization along with regeneration of the corneal epithelium. Approximately, 2 to 3 weeks after alkali burns, however, damaging ulceration of the corneal stroma often occurs. The formation of these lesions is related to the inflammatory infiltration of polymorphonuclear leukocytes and fibroblasts and the release of degratory proteolytic enzymes. Clinically, anti-inflammatory therapy limits ulcerative damage. Stromal ulceration usually stops when the corneal epithelium is restored (Grant, 1986; Potts, 1996).

Organic Solvents

When organic solvents are splashed into the eye, the result is typically a painful immediate reaction. As in the case of acids and bases, exposure of the eye to solvents should be treated rapidly with abundant water irrigation. Highly lipophilic solvents can damage the corneal epithelium and produce swelling of the corneal stroma. Most organic solvents do not have a strongly acid or basic pH and therefore cause little in the way of chemical burns to the cornea. In most cases, the corneal epithelium will be repaired over the course of a few days and there will be no residual damage. Exposure to solvent vapors may produce small transparent vacuoles in the corneal epithelium, which may be asymptomatic or associated with moderate irritation and tearing (Grant, 1986; Potts, 1996).

Surfactants

These compounds have water-soluble (hydrophilic) properties at one end of the molecule and lipophilic properties at the other end that help to dissolve fatty substances in water and also serve to reduce water surface tension. The widespread use of these chemicals in soaps, shampoos, detergents, cosmetics, and similar consumer products leads to abundant opportunities for exposure to ocular tissues. Many of these agents may be irritating or injurious to the eye. The hydrophilic portion of these compounds may be anionic, cationic, or neutral. In general, the cationic substances tend to be stronger irritants and more injurious than the other types, and anionic compounds more so than neutral ones (Grant, 1986; Potts, 1996). Because these compounds are by design soluble in both aqueous and lipid media, they readily penetrate the sandwiched aqueous and lipid barriers of the cornea (see discussion of ocular pharmacodynamics and pharmacokinetics, above). This property has implications in drug delivery; for example, low concentrations of the preservative benzalkonium chloride to ophthalmic solutions enhance ocular penetration of topically applied medications (Jaanus et al., 1995).

TARGET SITES AND MECHANISMS OF ACTION: LENS

The lens of the eye plays a critical role in focusing the visual image on the retina. While the cornea is the primary refractive surface for bending incoming light rays, the lens is capable of being reshaped to adjust the focal point to adapt for the distance of visual objects. The lens is a biconvex transparent body, encased in an elastic capsule, and located between the pupil and the vitreous humor (Fig. 17-1). The mature lens has a dense inner nuclear region surrounded by the lens cortex. The high transparency of the lens to visible wavelengths of light is a function of its chemical composition, approximately two-thirds water and one-third protein, and the special organizational structure of the lenticular proteins. The water-soluble crystallins are a set of proteins particular to the lens that, through their close inter-

molecular structure, give the lens both transparency and the proper refractive index. The lens fibers are laid down during development, as the epithelial cells grow and elongate along meridian pathways between the anterior and posterior poles of the lens. As the epithelial cells continue to grow, the nuclei recede and, in the central portions of the lens, disappear, such that the inner lens substance is composed of nonnucleated cells that form long proteinaceous fibers. The lens fibers are arranged within the lens in an onion-like fashion of concentric rings that have a prismatic arrangement in cross section. The regular geometric organization of the lens fibers is essential for the refractive index and transparency of the lens. At birth, the lens has no blood supply and no innervation. Nutrients are provided from the aqueous and vitreous fluids, and are transported into the lens substance through a system of intercellular gap-type junctions. The lens is a metabolically active tissue that maintains careful electrolyte and ionic balance. The lens continues to grow throughout life, with new cells added to the epithelial margin of the lens as the older cells condense into a central nuclear region. The dramatic growth of the lens is illustrated by increasing its weight, from approximately 150 mg at 20 years of age to approximately 250 mg at 80 years of age (Patterson and Delamere, 1992).

Cataracts are decreases in the optical transparency of the lens that ultimately can lead to functional visual disturbances. They are the leading cause of blindness worldwide, affecting an estimated 30 to 45 million people. In the United States, approximately 400,000 people develop cataracts each year. This accounts for about 35% of existing visual impairments (Patterson and Delamere, 1992). Cataracts can occur at any age; they can also be congenital (Rogers and Chernoff, 1988). However, they are much more frequent with advancing age. Senile cataracts develop most frequently in the cortical or nuclear regions of the lens and less frequently in the posterior subcapsular region. Senile cataracts in the cortical region of the lens are associated with disruptions of water and electrolyte homeostasis, whereas nuclear cataracts are characterized by an increase in the water-insoluble fraction of lens proteins (Patterson and Delamere, 1992).

Recent studies indicate that both genetic and environmental factors contribute to age-related and environmentally mediated cataracts and that these involve several different mechanisms of action (Hammond et al., 2000; Ottonello et al., 2000; Spector, 2000). Risk factors for the development of cataracts include aging, diabetes, low antioxidant levels, and exposure to a variety of environmental factors. Environmental factors include exposure to UV radiation and visible light, trauma, smoking, and exposure to a large variety of topical and systemic drugs and chemicals (e.g., Grant, 1986; Leske et al., 1991; Taylor and Nowell, 1997; Spector, 2000). Several different mechanisms of action have been hypothesized to account for the development of cataracts. These include the disruption of lens energy metabolism, hydration and/or electrolyte balance, the occurrence of oxidative stress due to the generation of free radicals and reactive oxygen species, and the occurrence of oxidative stress due a decrease in antioxidant defense mechanisms such as glutathione, superoxide dismutase, catalase, ascorbic acid, or vitamin E (Giblin, 2000; Ottonello et al., 2000; Spector, 2000). The generation of reactive oxygen species leads to oxidation of lens membrane proteins and lipids. A critical pathway in the development of high-molecular-weight aggregates involves the oxidation of protein thiol groups, particularly in methionine or cysteine amino acids, that leads to the formation of polypeptide links through disulfide bonds, and in turn, high-molecular-weight protein aggregates (Patterson and Delamere, 1992; Ottonello et al., 2000; Spector, 2000). These large aggregations of proteins can attain a size sufficient to scatter light, thus reducing lens transparency. Oxidation of membrane lipids and proteins may also impair membrane transport and permeability.

Light and Phototoxicity

The most important oxidizing agents are visible light and UV radiation, particularly UV-A (320 to 400 nm) and UV-B (290 to 320 nm), and other forms of electromagnetic radiation. Light- and UV-induced photooxidation leads to generation of reactive oxygen species, and oxidative damage that can accumulate over time. Higher-energy UV-C (100 to 290 nm) is even more damaging. At sea level, the atmosphere filters out virtually all UV-C and all but a small fraction of UV-B derived from solar radiance (AMA Report, 1989). The cornea absorbs about 45% of light with wavelengths below 280 nm, but only about 12% between 320 and 400 nm. The lens absorbs much of the light between 300 and 400 nm and transmits 400 nm and above to the retina (Patterson and Delamere, 1992). Absorption of light energy in the lens triggers a variety of photoreactions, including the generation of fluorophores and pigments that lead to the yellow-brown coloration of the lens. Sufficient exposure to infrared radiation, as occurs to glassblowers, or microwave radiation will also produce cataracts through direct heating of the ocular tissues.

Drugs and other chemicals can serve as mediators of photoinduced toxicity in the cornea, lens or retina (Dayhaw-Barker et al., 1986; Roberts, 2001; Glickman, 2002; Roberts, 2002). This occurs when the chemical structure allows absorption of light energy in the UV or visible spectrum and the subsequent generation of activated intermediates, free radicals and reactive oxygen species. Chemical structures likely to participate in such phototoxic mechanisms include those with tricyclic, heterocyclic or porphyrin ring structures because, with light, they produce stable triplet reactive molecules leading to free radicals and reactive oxygen species. The propensity of chemicals to cause phototoxic reactions can be predicted using photo-physical and in vitro procedures (Roberts, 2001; Glickman, 2002; Roberts, 2002).

Corticosteroids

Systemic treatment with corticosteroids causes cataracts (Urban and Cotlier, 1986). Observable opacities begin in the posterior subcapsular region of the lens and progress into the cortical region as the size of the lesion increases. Development of cataracts in individuals varies as a function of total dose of the drug, age, and the nature of the individual's underlying disease. It was estimated that 22% of patients receiving corticosteroid immunosuppressive therapy for renal transplants experienced cataracts as a side effect of therapy (Veenstra et al., 1999). The use of inhaled corticosteroids—commonly prescribed asthma therapy—was once thought to be without this risk, but subsequent epidemiologic evidence documented a significant association between inhaled steroidal therapy and development of nuclear and posterior subcapsular cataracts (Cumming et al., 1997; Cumming and Mitchell, 1999). There are two proposed mechanisms through which corticosteroids might cause cataracts. One proposal involves disruption of the lens epithelium electrolyte balance through inhibition of Na^+,K^+-ATPase. The regular hexagonal array structure of normal lens epithelial cells is disrupted and appears reticulated, while gaps appear between the lateral epithelial cell borders in lenses of humans with steroid-induced cataracts (Karim et al., 1989). Another theory is that cor-

ticosteroid molecules react with lens crystallin proteins through Schiff base reactions between the carbonyl group of the steroid and protein amino groups, with subsequent rearrangement into stable products (Urban and Cotlier, 1986). The resulting covalent corticosteroid–crystallin adducts would be high-molecular-weight light-scattering complexes. Whatever mechanism is responsible, these results illustrate the importance of routine ophthalmologic screening of patients receiving chronic corticosteroid therapy.

Naphthalene

Accidental exposure to naphthalene results in cortical cataracts and retinal degeneration (Grant, 1986; Potts, 1996). Naphthalene itself is not cataractogenic; instead, the metabolite 1,2-dihydro-1,2-dihydroxynaphthalene (naphthalene dihydrodiol) is the cataract-inducing agent (van Heyningen and Pirie, 1967). Subsequent studies using biochemical and pharmacologic techniques, in vitro assays, and transgenic mice showed that aldose reductase in the rat lens is a major protein associated with naphthalene dihydrodiol dehydrogenase activity and that lens aldose reductase is the enzyme responsible for the formation of naphthalene dihydrodiol (Sato, 1993; Lee and Chung, 1998; Sato et al., 1999). In addition, in vivo and in vitro studies have shown that aldose reductase inhibitors prevent naphthalene-induced cataracts (Lou et al., 1993; Sato et al., 1999). Finally, there is a difference in naphthalene-induced cataract formation between albino and pigmented rats, with the latter showing a faster onset and more uniform cataract (Murano et al., 1993).

Phenothiazines

It has been known since the 1950s that schizophrenics receiving phenothiazine drugs as anti-psychotic medication develop pigmented deposits in their eyes and skin (Grant, 1986; Potts, 1996). The pigmentation begins as tiny deposits on the anterior surface of the lens and progresses, with increasing dose, to involve the cornea as well. The phenothiazines combine with melanin to form a photosensitive product that reacts with sunlight, causing formation of the deposits. The amount of pigmentation is related to the dose of the drug, with the annual yearly dose being the most predictive dose metric (Thaler et al., 1985). More recent epidemiologic evidence demonstrates a dose-related increase in the risk of cataracts from use of phenothiazine-like drugs, including both antipsychotic drugs such as chlorpromazine and nonantipsychotic phenothiazines (Isaac et al., 1991).

TARGET SITES AND MECHANISMS OF ACTION: RETINA

The adult mammalian retina is a highly differentiated tissue containing nine distinct layers plus the RPE, ten major types of neurons, and three cells with glial functions (Fig. 17-1). The nine layers of the neural retina, which originate from the cells of the inner layer of the embryonic optic cup, are the nerve fiber layer (NFL), ganglion cell layer (GCL), inner plexiform layer (IPL), inner nuclear layer (INL), outer plexiform layer (OPL), outer nuclear layer (ONL), rod and cone photoreceptor inner segment layer (RIS; CIS), and the rod and cone photoreceptor outer segment layer (ROS; COS). The RPE, which originates from the cells of the outer layer of the embryonic optic cup, is a single layer of cuboidal epithelial cells that lies on Bruch's membrane adjacent to the vascular choroid. Between the RPE and photoreceptor outer segments lies the subretinal space, which is similar to the brain ventricles. The ten major types of neurons are the rod (R) and cone (C) photoreceptors, (depolarizing) ON-rod and ON-cone bipolar cells (BC), (hyperpolarizing) OFF-cone bipolar cells, horizontal cells (HC), numerous subtypes of amacrine cells (AC), an interplexiform cell (IPC), and ON-RGCs and OFF-RGCs. The three cells with glial functions are the Müller cells (MC), fibrous astrocytes, and microglia. The somas of the MCs are in the INL. The end feet of the MCs in the proximal or inner retina along with a basal lamina form the internal limiting membrane (ILM) of the retina, which is similar to the pial surface of the brain. In the distal retina, the MC end feet join with the photoreceptors and zonula adherens to form the external limiting membrane (ELM), which is located between the ONL and RIS/CIS. The interested reader is referred to the excellent references in the Introduction as well as to numerous outstanding websites devoted exclusively to the retina (e.g., http://webvision.umh.es/webvision/intro.html; http://cvs.anu.edu.au/; http://retina.anatomy.upenn.edu/~lance/retina/retina.html) for basic information on the anatomic, biochemical, cell and molecular biological, and physiologic aspects of retinal structure and function.

The mammalian retina is highly vulnerable to toxicant-induced structural and/or functional damage due to (1) the presence of a highly fenestrated choriocapillaris that supplies the distal or outer retina as well as a portion of the inner retina; (2) the very high rate of oxidative mitochondrial metabolism, especially that in the photoreceptors (Linsenmeier, 1986; Ahmed et al., 1993; Medrano and Fox, 1994, 1995; Braun et al., 1995; Winkler, 1995; Shulman and Fox, 1996); (3) high daily turnover of rod and cone outer segments (LaVail, 1976; Rodieck, 1998); (4) high susceptibility of the rod and cones to degeneration due to inherited retinal dystrophies as well as associated syndromes and metabolic disorders (Ogden and Schachat, 1989; Hart, 1992; von Soest et al., 1999); (5) presence of specialized ribbon synapses and synaptic contact sites (Dowling, 1987; Ogden and Schachat, 1989; Cohen, 1992; Rodieck, 1998); (6) presence of numerous neurotransmitter and neuromodulatory systems, including extensive glutamatergic, GABAergic and glycinergic systems (Rauen et al., 1996; Brandstätter et al., 1998; Rodieck, 1998; Kalloniatis and Tomisich, 1999; Winkler et al., 1999); (7) presence of numerous and highly specialized gap junctions used in the information signaling process (Cohen, 1992; Cook and Becker, 1995; Rodieck, 1998); (8) presence of melanin in the choroid and RPE and also in the iris (Meier-Rouge, 1972; Potts, 1996); (9) a very high choroidal blood flow rate, as high as ten times that of the gray matter of the brain (Alm, 1992; Cohen, 1992); and (10) the additive or synergistic toxic action of certain chemicals with light (Dayhaw-Barker et al., 1986; Backstrom et al., 1993; Roberts, 2001; Glickman, 2002; Roberts, 2002).

The retina is also an excellent model system for studying the effects of chemicals on the developing and mature CNS. Its structure–function relations are well established. The histogenic steps of development of the neurons and glial components are well characterized. The development of the CNS and most retinal cells occurs early during gestation in humans (Hendrickson, 1992; Hendrickson and Drucker, 1992) and continues for an additional 7 to 14 days postnatally in the rat (Dobbing and Sands, 1979; Raedler and Sievers, 1975). Therefore, toxicological effects in the rodent retina have relevance for chemical exposure during the early gestation period in humans as well as during early postnatal development. The retina contains a wide diversity of synaptic transmitters and second messengers whose developmental patterns are well described.

Moreover, the rodent retina is easily accessible, it has most of the same anatomical and functional features found in the developing and mature human retina, and the rat rod pathway is similar to that in other mammals (Dowling, 1987; Finlay and Sengelbaub, 1989; Berman, 1991; Chun et al., 1993). Finally, rat rods have similar dimensions, photochemistry, and photocurrents as human and monkey rods (Baylor et al., 1984; Schnapf et al., 1988). These general and specific features underscore the relevance and applicability of using the rodent retina to investigate the effects of chemicals on this target site as well as a model to investigate the neurotoxic effects of chemicals during development.

Each of the retinal layers can undergo specific as well as general toxic effects. These alterations and deficits include, but are not limited to visual field deficits, scotopic vision deficits such as night blindness and increases in the threshold for dark adaptation, cone-mediated (photopic) deficits such as decreased color perception, decreased visual acuity, macular and general retina edema, retinal hemorrhages and vasoconstriction, and pigmentary changes. The list of chemicals and drugs that cause retinal alterations is extensive, as evidenced by an examination of Grant's *Toxicology of the Eye* (Grant, 1986) and Dr. Potts' chapter entitled "Toxic Responses of the Eye" in an earlier edition of this volume (1996). In addition, a review by Jaanus et al. (1995) discusses the adverse retinal effects of therapeutic systemic drugs. Another review by Wolfensberger (1998) concentrates on toxic effects on the retinal pigment epithelium. The main aim of this section is to discuss in detail several chemicals and drugs (1) that are currently used as pharmacological agents or environmentally relevant neurotoxicants; (2) whose behavioral, physiologic, and/or pathologic effects on retina are known; and (3) whose retinal site(s) and/or mechanism of action are well characterized. In addition, the effects of organic solvents and organophosphates on retinal function and vision are discussed, as these are emerging areas of concern.

The chemical- and drug-induced alterations in retinal structure and function are grouped into two major categories. The first category focuses on retinotoxicity of systemically administered therapeutic drugs. Four major drugs are discussed in detail: chloroquine/hydroxychloroquine, digoxin/digitoxin, indomethacin, and tamoxifen. The second category focuses on well-known neurotoxicants that produce retinotoxicity: inorganic lead, methanol, selected organic solvents, and organophosphates. See chapters 16 and 23 entitled "Toxic Responses of the Nervous System" and "Toxic Effects of Metals" for information on the effects of lead on the brain and other target organs and chapter 24 entitled "Toxic Effects of Solvents and Vapors," for additional information on methanol and the organic solvents discussed below.

Retinotoxicity of Systemically Administered Therapeutic Drugs

Cancer Chemotherapeutics Ocular toxicity is a common side effect of cancer chemotherapy (Imperia et al., 1989; Schmid et al., 2006). Symptoms include blurred vision, diplopia, decreased color vision, decreased visual acuity, optic/retrobular neuritis, transient cortical blindness, and demyelination of the optic nerves (Imperia et al., 1989; Schmid et al., 2006). The retina due to its high metabolic activity and choroidal circulation (vide infra) appears to be particularly vulnerable to numerous cytotoxic agents such as the alkylating agents cisplatin, carboplatin, and carmustine; the antimetabolites cytosine arabinoside, 5-fluorouracil and methotrexate; and the mitotic inhibitors such as docetaxel. The ocular toxicity of different drugs is dependent upon the dose, duration of dosage, and route of administration. However, if not detected at an early stage of toxicity, the ocular complications are often irreversible even after chemotherapy is discontinued (Imperia *et al.*, 1989; Schmid *et al.*, 2006). One strategy to avoid such retinal complications is to conduct prospective ophthalmological exams as well as scotopic and photopic ERG testing prior to the onset and during chemotherapy. The ocular side effects of tamoxifen, an estrogen antagonist used in oncology, are discussed below.

Chloroquine and Hydroxychloroquine   Two of the most extensively studied retinotoxic drugs are chloroquine (Aralen) and hydroxychloroquine (Plaquenil). The first case of chloroquine-induced retinopathy was reported more than 40 years ago (Jaanus *et al.*, 1995; Potts, 1996). These 4-aminoquinoline derivatives are used as antimalarial and anti-inflammatory drugs. The low-dose therapy used for malaria is essentially free from toxic side effects; however, the chronic, high-dose therapy used for rheumatoid arthritis, and discoid and systemic lupus erythematosus (initially 400 to 600 mg/day for 4 to 12 weeks and then 200 to 400 mg/day; Ellsworth *et al.*, 1999) can cause irreversible loss of retinal function. Chloroquine, its major metabolite desethylchloroquine, and hydroxychloroquine have high affinity for melanin, which results in very high concentrations of these drugs accumulating in the choroid and RPE, ciliary body, and iris during and following drug administration (Rosenthal *et al.*, 1978; Potts, 1996). Prolonged exposure of the retina to these drugs, especially chloroquine, may lead to an irreversible retinopathy. In fact, small amounts of chloroquine and its metabolites were excreted in the urine years after cessation of drug treatment (Bernstein, 1967). Approximately, 20–30% of patients who received high doses of chloroquine exhibited some type of retinal abnormality, while 5–10% showed severe changes in retinal function (Burns, 1966; Potts, 1996; Shearer and Dubois, 1967; Sassaman *et al.*, 1970; Krill *et al.*, 1971). Hydroxychloroquine is now the drug of choice for treatment of rheumatic diseases because it has fewer side effects and less ocular toxicity. Doses less than 400 mg per day appear to produce little or no retinopathy even after prolonged therapy (Johnson and Vine, 1987).

The clinical findings accompanying chloroquine retinopathy can be divided into early and late stages. The early changes include (1) the pathognomonic "bull's-eye retina" visualized as a dark, central pigmented area involving the macula, surrounded by a pale ring of depigmentation, which, in turn, is surrounded by another ring of pigmentation; (2) a diminished EOG; (3) possible granular pigmentation in the peripheral retina; and (4) visual complaints such as blurred vision and problems discerning letters or words. Late-stage findings, which can occur during or even following cessation of drug exposure, include (1) a progressive scotoma, (2) constriction of the peripheral fields commencing in the upper temporal quadrant, (3) narrowing of the retinal artery, (4) color and night blindness, (5) absence of a typical retinal pigment pattern, and (6) very abnormal EOGs and ERGs. These late-stage symptoms are irreversible. Interestingly, dark adaptation is relatively normal even during the late stages of chloroquine retinopathy, which helps distinguish the peripheral retinal changes from those observed in patients with retinitis pigmentosa (Bernstein, 1967).

In humans and monkeys, long-term chloroquine administration results in sequential degeneration of the RGCs, photoreceptors, and RPE and the eventual migration of RPE pigment into the ONL and OPL. In addition, in the RPE there is a thickening of the RPE layer, an increase in the mucopolysaccharide and sulfhydryl group content, and a decrease in activity of several enzymes (Potts, 1996; Ramsey

and Fine, 1972; Rosenthal *et al.*, 1978). Although the molecular mechanism of action is unknown, it has been suggested that the primary biochemical mechanism is inhibition of protein synthesis (Bernstein, 1967).

Digoxin and Digitoxin   The cardiac glycosides digoxin (Lanoxin) and digitoxin (Crystodigin) are digitalis derivatives used in the treatment of congestive heart disease and in certain cardiac arrhythmias. As part of the extract of the plant foxglove, digitalis was recommended for heart failure (dropsy) over 200 years ago. Digitalis-induced visual system abnormalities such as decreased vision, flickering scotomas, and altered color vision were documented during that time (Withering, 1785). Approximately, 20–60% of patients with cardiac glycoside serum levels in the therapeutic range and 50–80% of the patients with cardiac glycoside serum levels in the toxic range complain of visual system disturbances within 2 weeks after the onset of therapy (Robertson *et al.*, 1966a; Aronson and Ford, 1980; Rietbrock and Alken, 1980; Haustein *et al.*, 1982; Piltz *et al.*, 1993; Duncker *et al.*, 1994). Digoxin produces more toxicity than digitoxin due to its greater volume of distribution and plasma protein binding (Haustein and Schmidt, 1988). The most frequent visual complaints are color vision impairments and hazy or snowy vision, although complaints of flickering light, colored spots surrounded by bright halos, blurred vision, and glare sensitivity also are reported. The color vision disturbances have been confirmed with the Farnsworth-Munsell 100 Hue Test (Aronson and Ford, 1980; Rietbrock and Alken, 1980; Haustein *et al.*, 1982; Haustein and Schmidt, 1988; Duncker and Krastel, 1990). Clinical examinations show that these patients have decreased visual acuity and central scotomas but no funduscopic changes. ERG analysis revealed reduced rod and cone amplitudes, increased rod and cone implicit times, and elevated rod and cone thresholds (Robertson *et al.*, 1966a; Robertson *et al.*, 1966b; Alken and Belz, 1984; Duncker and Krastel, 1990; Madreperla *et al.*, 1994). Taken together, these ophthalmologic, behavioral, and electrophysiologic findings demonstrate that the photoreceptors are a primary target site of the cardiac glycosides digoxin and digitoxin.

The above results suggest that cone photoreceptors are more susceptible to the effects of cardiac glycosides than rod photoreceptors. To directly test this hypothesis, Madreperla *et al.* (1994) conducted electrophysiologic (suction electrode) experiments with isolated tiger salamander (*Ambystoma tigrinum*) rods and cones exposed to different physiologically and toxicologically relevant concentrations of digoxin in the bathing solution. Following a single light flash of saturating intensity, rods and cones exhibited concentration-dependent decreases in the peak light (current) response. The cones, however, were about 50 times more sensitive to digoxin and were impaired to a greater degree at the same digoxin concentration than the rods. Neither the rods nor the cones recovered to their dark-adapted baseline following the short-duration saturating light flash. The rods, however, appeared to recover faster and more completely than the cones. Moreover, following a return to control Ringer's solution, the photoreceptors still did not recover to their dark-adapted baseline response level. This latter finding correlates with the slow recovery of the ERG seen in patients following termination of digoxin exposure (Robertson *et al.*, 1966b; Duncker and Krastel, 1990; Madreperla *et al.*, 1994) and is most likely due to the high affinity and slow off-rate of digoxin binding to the cardiac glycoside site located on the extracellular side of the catalytic α-subunit of the Na^+,K^+-ATPase enzyme (Sweadner, 1989).

Digitalis glycosides, like ouabain, are potent inhibitors of retinal Na^+,K^+-ATPase (Winkler and Riley, 1977; Fox et al., 1991b; Ottlecz et al., 1993; Shulman and Fox, 1996). Digoxin binding studies show that the retina has the highest number of Na^+,K^+-ATPase sites of any ocular tissue, even higher than those of brain (Lissner et al., 1971; Lufkin et al., 1967). There are three different isoforms of the α subunit of Na^+,K^+-ATPase (i.e., $\alpha1$, $\alpha2$, and $\alpha3$), and they differ significantly in their sensitivity to cardiac glycoside inhibition (Sweadner, 1989). In the rat retina, the $\alpha1$-low and $\alpha3$-high ouabain affinity isoforms of the enzyme account for $\geq 97\%$ of the Na^+,K^+-ATPase mRNA. The $\alpha3$ isoform is localized to rat photoreceptors, horizontal cells, and bipolar cells. Photoreceptors predominantly express the $\alpha3$ mRNA (approximately 85%), a small amount of $\alpha1$ mRNA (approximately 15%), and almost no detectable $\alpha2$ mRNA. Electron microscopic immunocytochemistry studies reveal that the $\alpha3$ isoform is localized exclusively to the plasma membrane of the rat photoreceptor inner segments (McGrail and Sweadner, 1989; Schneider and Kraig, 1990; Schneider et al., 1990). The $\alpha3$ isozyme accounts for most of the rod Na^+,K^+-ATPase activity (Shulman and Fox, 1996). The rat rod photoreceptor Na^+,K^+-ATPase–specific activity is approximately threefold higher than whole retinal (Fox et al., 1991b; Shulman and Fox, 1996) or whole brain values (Marks and Seeds, 1978). This is also reflected in the two- to threefold greater ouabain-sensitive oxygen consumption in the dark-adapted outer retina relative to the whole or inner retina, respectively (Medrano and Fox, 1995; Shulman and Fox, 1996).

Indomethacin Indomethacin is a nonsteroidal anti-inflammatory drug with analgesic and antipyretic properties that is frequently used for the management of arthritis, gout, and musculoskeletal discomfort. It inhibits prostaglandin synthesis by inhibiting cyclooxygenase. The first cases of indomethacin-induced retinopathy were reported approximately 30 years ago (Jaanus et al., 1995; Potts, 1996). Chronic administration of 50 to 200 mg per day of indomethacin for 1 to 2 years has been reported to produce corneal opacities, discrete pigment scattering of the RPE perifoveally, paramacular depigmentation, decreases in visual acuity, altered visual fields, increases in the threshold for dark adaptation, blue-yellow color deficits, and decreases in ERG and EOG amplitudes (Burns, 1966; Burns, 1968; Henkes et al., 1972; Koliopoulos and Palimeris, 1972; Palimeris et al., 1972). Decreases in the ERG a- and b-wave amplitudes, with larger changes observed under scotopic dark-adapted than light-adapted conditions, have been reported. Upon cessation of drug treatment, the ERG waveforms and color vision changes return to near normal, although the pigmentary changes are irreversible (Burns, 1968; Henkes et al., 1972; Palimeris et al., 1972). The mechanism of retinotoxicity is unknown; however, it appears likely that the RPE is a primary target site.

Sildenafil Citrate Sildenafil citrate (Viagra) is a cGMP-specific phosphodiesterase (PDE) type 5 inhibitor that is utilized in the treatment of erectile dysfunction (Corbin et al., 2002). Sildenafil is also a weak cGMP PDE type 6 inhibitor, which is present in rod and cone photorecepotrs (Corbin et al., 2002; Zhang et al., 2005). Transient visual symptoms such as a blue tinge to vision, increased brightness of lights and blurry vision as well as alterations in scotopic and photopic ERGs have been reported following sildenafil usage (Laties and Zrenner, 2002; Jagle et al., 2004). More recently, sildenafil has been associated with the occurrence of nonarteritic anterior

ischemic optic neuropathy (NAION) in at-risk patients (i.e., those with small cup-to-disc ratios and/or arteriosclerotic risk profiles) within minutes to hours after the ingestion of the drug (Fraunfelder et al., 2006). However, available data suggest that the risk of occurrence of NAION in patients taking sildenafil is not significantly different from the general population (Laties and Zrenner, 2002; Fraunfelder et al., 2006; Gorkin et al., 2006).

Tamoxifen Tamoxifen (Nolvadex, Tamoplex), a triphenylethylene derivative, is a nonsteroidal antiestrogenic drug that competes with estrogen for its receptor sites. It is a highly effective antitumor agent used for the treatment of metastatic breast carcinoma in postmenopausal women. Tamoxifen-induced retinopathy following chronic high-dose therapy (180 to 240 mg per day for approximately 2 years) was first reported 20 years ago (Kaiser-Kupfer et al., 1981). At this dose, there is widespread axonal degeneration in the macular and perimacular area, as evidenced by the presence of different sized yellow–white refractile opacities in the IPL and NFL observed during fundus examination. Macular edema may or may not be present. Clinical symptoms include a permanent decrease in visual acuity and abnormal visual fields, as the axonal degeneration is irreversible (reviewed by Jaanus et al., 1995; Potts, 1996; Ah-Song and Sasco, 1997). Several prospective studies, with sample sizes ranging from 63 to 303 women with breast cancer, have shown that chronic low-dose tamoxifen (20 mg per day) can result in a small but significant increase in the incidence ($\leq 10\%$) of keratopathy (Pavlividis et al., 1992; Gorin et al., 1998; Lazzaroni et al., 1998; Noureddin et al., 1999). In addition, these studies showed that retinopathy is much less frequently observed than with high-dose therapy and, except for a few reports of altered color vision and decreased visual acuity, there were no significant alterations in visual function. Following cessation of low-dose tamoxifen therapy, most of the keratopathy and retinal alterations except the corneal opacities and retinopathy were reversible (Pavlividis et al., 1992; Gorin et al., 1998; Noureddin et al., 1999).

Retinotoxicity of Known Neurotoxicants

Inorganic Lead Inorganic lead is probably the oldest known and most studied environmental toxicant. For almost 100 years, it has been known that overt lead poisoning [mean blood lead (BPb) ≥ 80 $\mu g/dL$] in humans produces visual system pathology and overt visual symptoms (Grant, 1986; Otto and Fox, 1993; Fox, 1998). Clinical manifestations include amblyopia, blindness, optic neuritis or atrophy, peripheral and central scotomas, paralysis of eye muscles, and decreased visual function. Moderate to high level lead exposure produces scotopic and temporal visual system deficits in occupationally exposed factory workers and developmentally lead-exposed monkeys and rats (Bushnell et al., 1977; Guguchkova, 1972; Cavelleri et al., 1982; Betta et al., 1983; Signorino et al., 1983; Campara et al., 1984; Jeyaratnam et al., 1986; Fox and Farber, 1988; Lilienthal et al., 1988; Fox et al., 1991a; Fox and Katz, 1992; Otto and Fox, 1993; Lilienthal et al., 1994; Fox, 1998; Rice, 1998). Early work in monkeys exposed to moderate to high levels of lead during and following gestation reveal that this lead exposure regimen produces irreversible retinal deficits (Lilienthal et al., 1988; Lilienthal et al., 1994; Kohler et al., 1997). A recent study in 7–10 year old children reveals that low-level gestational lead exposure produces long-lasting scotopic supernormal ERG deficits (Rothenberg et al., 2002). However, relatively little effort has been made to understand the impact of lead-induced alterations on retinal and central visual information processing on learning and memory in children. These types of visual deficits can adversely affect learning and memory as well as experimental procedures used to assess these cognitive parameters (Anger *et al.*, 1994; Hudnell *et al.*, 1996; Walkowiak *et al.*, 1998; Cestnick and Coltheart, 1999).

Studies in Occupationally Exposed Lead Workers Clinical and electrophysiological studies in lead-exposed factory workers have assessed both the site of action and extent of injury. Several cases of retrobulbar optic neuritis and optic nerve atrophy have been observed following chronic moderate-level or acute high-level lead exposure (Sherer, 1935; Baghdassarian, 1968; Baloh *et al.*, 1979; Karai *et al.*, 1979). Most of these cases presented with fundus lesions, peripheral or paracentral scotomas while the most severe cases also had a central scotoma. Generally, the scotomas were not observed until approximately 5 years of continuous lead exposure. Interestingly, the earliest observable scotomas were not detected under standard photopic viewing conditions but became evident only under scotopic or mesopic (rod- and cone-mediated) viewing conditions. These ophthalmologic findings correlate directly with the ERG data observed in similarly exposed lead workers. No alterations in the critical flicker fusion threshold (i.e., temporal resolution) were observed when the test was conducted under photopic conditions or when using red lights. However, consistent decreases in temporal resolution were observed when the test was conducted under scotopic conditions or when green lights were used (Cavelleri *et al.*, 1982; Betta *et al.*, 1983; Signorino *et al.*, 1983; Campara *et al.*, 1984; Jeyaratnam *et al.*, 1986). Moreover, in occupationally lead-exposed workers with or without visual acuity deficits or no observable alterations following ophthalmologic examination, the sensitivity and amplitude of the a-wave and/or b-wave of the dark-adapted ERG were decreased (Guguchkova, 1972; Scholl and Zrenner, 2000). In other lead-exposed workers, one funduscopic study noted the presence of a grayish lead pigmentary deposit in the area peripheral to the optic disk margins (Sonkin, 1963).

In addition to the retinal deficits, oculomotor deficits occur in chronically lead-exposed workers who have no observable ophthalmologic abnormalities. Results from three independent studies, including a follow-up, show that the mean accuracy of saccadic eye movements is lower in lead-exposed workers and the number of overshoots is increased (Baloh *et al.*, 1979; Spivey *et al.*, 1980; Specchio *et al.*, 1981; Glickman *et al.*, 1984). In addition, these studies also revealed that the saccade maximum velocity was decreased. Moreover, one study also observed abnormal smooth pursuit eye movements in lead-exposed workers (Specchio *et al.*, 1981). Although the site and mechanism of action underlying these alterations are unknown, they most likely result from CNS-mediated deficits.

In summary, these results suggest that occupational lead exposure produces concentration- and time-dependent alterations in the retina such that higher levels of lead directly and adversely affect both the retina and optic nerve, whereas lower levels of lead appear to primarily affect the rod photoreceptors and their pathway. Interestingly, these latter clinical findings showing preferential lead-induced rod-selective deficits in sensitivity and temporal resolution are observed in both in vivo and in vitro animal studies (see below). Furthermore, these retinal and oculomotor alterations were, in most cases, correlated with the blood lead levels and occurred in the absence of observable ophthalmologic changes, CNS symptoms, and abnormal performance test scores. Thus, these measures of temporal visual function may be among the most sensitive for the early detection of the neurotoxic effects of inorganic lead.

In Vivo and in Vitro Animal Studies Lead exposure to adult animals and postnatally developing animals produces retinal damage and functional deficits. The degree and extent of these alterations depends upon the dose, age, and duration of lead exposure. High-level lead exposure to adult rabbits for 60 to 300 days (Hass *et al.*, 1964; Brown, 1974; Hughes and Coogan, 1974) and to newborn rats for 60 days (Santos-Anderson *et al.*, 1984) resulted in focal necrosis of the rod inner and outer segments, necrosis in the inner nuclear layer and Müller cells, and lysosomal inclusions in the RPE. In addition, high-level lead exposure to mice and rats from birth to weaning resulted in hypomyelination of the optic nerve and a reduction in its diameter; but, interestingly, there were no changes in the sciatic nerve (Tennekoon *et al.*, 1979; Toews *et al.*, 1980). Newborn monkeys exposed to high levels of lead for 6 years had no changes in optic nerve diameter or myelination, although visual cortex neuronal volume and branching were decreased (Reuhl *et al.*, 1989). Rhesus monkeys exposed prenatally and postnatally to moderate or high levels of lead for 9 years, followed by almost 2 years of no lead exposure, had decreased tyrosine hydroxylase immunoreactivity in the large dopaminergic amacrine cells and a complete loss of tyrosine hydroxylase immunoreactivity in small subset of amacrine cells (Kohler *et al.*, 1997). These results suggest that long-term lead exposure produces a decrease in tyrosine hydroxylase synthesis, a finding consistent with other studies (Lasley and Lane, 1988; Jadhav and Ramesh, 1997), and/or a loss of a subset of tyrosine hydroxylase–positive amacrine cells, a finding consistent with recent in vitro work (Scortegagna and Hanbauer, 1997). In contrast to these studies, 6 weeks of moderate-level lead exposure to adult rats (Fox *et al.*, 1997) and 3 weeks of low- or moderate-level lead exposure to neonatal rats from birth to weaning produced rod- and bipolar cell–selective apoptotic cell death (Fox and Chu, 1988; Fox *et al.*, 1997). Moreover, recent results reveal that brief (15-min) exposure of isolated adult rat retinas to nanomolar to micromolar Pb^{2+}, concentrations regarded as pathophysiologically relevant (Cavalleri *et al.*, 1984; Al-Modhefer *et al.*, 1991), resulted in rod-selective apoptosis (He *et al.*, 2000). By extension, these results suggest that the triggering event (initiating phase) and the execution phase of rod and bipolar cell death share common underlying biochemical mechanisms.

Results from several studies suggest that an elevated level of rod photoreceptor Ca^{2+} and/or Pb^{2+} plays a key role in the process of apoptotic rod cell death in humans and animals during inherited retinal degenerations, retinal diseases and injuries, chemical exposure, and lead exposure. These include patients with retinitis pigmentosa and cancer-associated retinopathy (Thirkill *et al.*, 1987; van Soest *et al.*, 1999), mice with retinal degeneration (*rd*) (Chang *et al.*, 1993; Fox *et al.*, 1999), rats injected with antirecoverin monoclonal antibodies (Adamus *et al.*, 1998), rats with hypoxic-ischemic injury (Crosson *et al.*, 1990), rats with light-induced damage (Edward *et al.*, 1991), and lead-exposed rats (Fox and Chu, 1988; Fox *et al.*, 1997, 1999). In addition, moderate-level Pb^{2+} exposure produces apoptotic neuronal cell death in primary cultured cells (Oberto *et al.*, 1996; Scortegagna *et al.*, 1997). In vivo and in vitro data suggest that Pb^{2+} produces a dose (concentration)- dependent inhibition of rod cGMP phosphodiesterase (PDE), a resultant elevation of rod cGMP (Fox and Farber, 1988; Fox *et al.*, 1991a; Srivastava *et al.*, 1995a; Srivastava *et al.*, 1995b; Fox *et al.*, 1997), which gates the nonselective cation channel of the rod photoreceptor outer segments (Yau and

Baylor, 1989), and an elevation of the rod Ca^{2+} concentration (Fox and Katz, 1992; Medrano and Fox, 1994; He *et al.*, 2000). Detailed kinetic analysis revealed that picomolar Pb^{2+} competitively and directly inhibits rod cGMP PDE relative to millimolar concentrations of Mg^{2+} (Srivastava *et al.*, 1995a, 1995b). In addition, nanomolar Pb^{2+} can elevate the rod Ca^{2+} (and Pb^{2+}) concentration via its competitive inhibition of retinal Na^+,K^+-ATPase relative to MgATP (Fox *et al.*, 1991b). Once inside the rod, both Ca^{2+} and Pb^{2+} enter the mitochondria via the ruthenium red-sensitive Ca^{2+} uniporter and induce mitochondrial depolarization, swelling, and cytochrome *c* release (He *et al.*, 2000). The effects of Ca^{2+} and Pb^{2+} were additive and blocked completely by the mitochondrial permeability transition pore inhibitor cyclosporin A. Following cytochrome *c* release, caspase-9 and caspase-3 are sequentially activated. There was no evidence of caspase-8, oxidative stress or lipid peroxidation in this model. These results demonstrate that rod mitochondria are the target site for Ca^{2+} and Pb^{2+}. This is consistent with numerous studies from different tissues demonstrating that lead is preferentially associated with mitochondria and particularly with the inner membrane and matrix fractions (Barltrop *et al.*, 1971; Bull, 1980; Pounds, 1984). Taken together, the results suggest that Ca^{2+} and Pb^{2+} bind to the internal divalent metal binding site of the mitochondrial permeability transition pore (Szabo *et al.*, 1992) and subsequently open it, which initiates the cytochrome *c*–caspase cascade of apoptosis in rods (He *et al.*, 2000).

In vitro extracellular and intracellular electrophysiologic recordings in isolated whole retinas or photoreceptors reveal that nanomolar to micromolar Pb^{2+} selectively depress the amplitude and absolute sensitivity of the rod but not cone photoreceptor potential (Fox and Sillman, 1979; Sillman *et al.*, 1982; Tessier-Lavigne *et al.*, 1985; Frumkes and Eysteinsson, 1988). These electrophysiologic results are similar to the ERG alterations observed in occupationally lead-exposed workers (Cavelleri *et al.*, 1982; Betta *et al.*, 1983; Signorino *et al.*, 1983; Campara *et al.*, 1984; Jeyaratnam *et al.*, 1986) and in adult rats exposed to low and moderate levels of lead only during development (Fox and Farber, 1988; Fox and Rubinstein, 1989; Fox *et al.*, 1991a; Fox and Katz, 1992). In addition, these postnatally lead-exposed rats exhibit rod-mediated increases in dark and light adaptation time, decreases in critical flicker fusion frequency (i.e., temporal resolution), decreases in relative sensitivity, and increases in a- and b-wave latencies (Fox and Farber, 1988; Fox and Rubinstein, 1989; Fox *et al.*, 1991a; Fox and Katz, 1992) and decreases in the temporal response properties of both sustained (X-type) and transient (Y-type) RGCs, such as decreased optimal temporal frequency and temporal resolution (Ruan *et al.*, 1994). By extension, these results suggest that there is a common underlying biochemical mechanism responsible for these rod-mediated deficits. In vivo and in vitro data suggest that lead-induced inhibition of cGMP PDE and resultant elevation of rod Ca^{2+} underlies the ERG deficits (Fox and Katz, 1992; Medrano and Fox, 1994; Fox *et al.*, 1997; He *et al.*, 2000). Finally, rod-mediated alterations in dark adaptation and b-wave amplitude are also observed in adult rats and monkeys with prenatal and lifetime moderate- and high-level lead exposure (Hennekes *et al.*, 1987; Lilienthal *et al.*, 1988; Lilienthal *et al.*, 1994). In the gestationally and postnatally lead-exposed monkeys and children, the amplitude of the scotopic b-wave was increased (Lilienthal *et al.*, 1988; Lilienthal *et al.*, 1994; Rothenberg *et al.*, 2002): an effect hypothesized to result from the loss of dopaminergic amacrine cells or their processes (Kohler *et al.*, 1997). If rods and blue-sensitive cones in humans exhibit the same sensitivity to a lead-induced inhibition of cGMP-PDE as

they do to the drug-induced inhibition of cGMP-PDE (Zrenner and Gouras, 1979; Zrenner *et al.*, 1982), Fox and Farber (1998) predicted that blue-cone color vision deficits as well as scotopic deficits may be found in adults and children exposed to lead. S- (or blue-) cone deficits have been observed in an occupationally lead-exposed worker (Scholl and Zrenner, 2000).

Methanol   Methanol is a low-molecular-weight (32), colorless, and volatile liquid that is widely used as an industrial solvent; a chemical intermediate; a fuel source for picnic stoves, racing cars, and soldering torches; an antifreeze agent; and an octane booster for gasoline. The basic toxicology and references can be found in two thorough reviews (Tephly and McMartin, 1984; Eells, 1992). Briefly, methanol is readily and rapidly absorbed from all routes of exposure (dermal, inhalation, and oral), easily crosses all membranes, and thus is uniformly distributed to organs and tissues in direct relation to their water content. Following different routes of exposures, the highest concentrations of methanol are found in the blood, aqueous and vitreous humors, and bile as well as the brain, kidneys, lungs, and spleen. In the liver, methanol is oxidized sequentially to formaldehyde by alcohol dehydrogenase in human and nonhuman primates or by catalase in rodents and then to formic acid. It is excreted as formic acid in the urine or oxidized further to carbon dioxide and then excreted by the lungs. Formic acid is the toxic metabolite that mediates the metabolic acidosis as well as the retinal and optic nerve toxicity observed in humans, monkeys, and rats with a decreased capacity for folate metabolism (Tephly and McMartin, 1984; Murray *et al.*, 1991; Eells, 1992; Lee *et al.*, 1994a; Lee *et al.*, 1994b; Garner *et al.*, 1995a; Garner *et al.*, 1995b; Eells *et al.*, 1996; Seme *et al.*, 1999).

Human and nonhuman primates are highly sensitive to methanol-induced neurotoxicity due to their limited capacity to oxidize formic acid. The toxicity occurs in several stages. It first occurs as a mild CNS depression, followed by an asymptomatic 12- to 24-hour latent period, then by a syndrome consisting of formic acidemia, uncompensated metabolic acidosis, ocular and visual toxicity, coma, and possibly death (Tephly and McMartin, 1984; Eells, 1992). The treatment of methanol poisoning involves both combating acidosis and preventing methanol oxidation, but it is not discussed further here. Experimental rats were made as sensitive to acute methanol exposure as primates by using two different, but related, procedures that effectively reduce the levels of hepatic tetrahydrofolate. One study acutely inhibited methionine synthase and reduced the level of hepatic tetrahydrofolate (Murray *et al.*, 1991; Eells *et al.*, 1996; Seme *et al.*, 1999), while the other fed rats a folate-deficient diet for 18 weeks (Lee *et al.*, 1994a; Lee *et al.*, 1994b). Administration of methanol to rats with a decreased capacity for folate metabolism resulted in toxic blood formate concentrations of 8 to 16 mM (Murray *et al.*, 1991; Lee *et al.*, 1994a; Lee *et al.*, 1994b; Garner *et al.*, 1995a; Garner *et al.*, 1995b; Eells *et al.*, 1996; Seme *et al.*, 1999). Permanent visual damage occurred in humans and monkeys when the blood folate levels exceeded 7 mM (Tephly and McMartin, 1984; Eells, 1992).

Acute methanol poisoning in humans, monkeys, and experimental rats resulted in profound and permanent structural alterations in the retina and optic nerve and visual impairments ranging from blurred vision to decreased visual acuity and light sensitivity to blindness. Ophthalmologic studies of exposed humans and monkeys reveal varying degrees of edema of the papillomacular bundle and optic nerve head (Benton and Calhoun, 1952; Potts, 1955;

Baumbach *et al.*, 1977; Hayreh *et al.*, 1980). Histopathologic and ultrastructural investigations in methanol-exposed monkeys and folate-modified rats showed retinal edema, swollen and degenerated photoreceptors, degenerated RGCs, swollen retinal pigment epithelial cells, axonal (optic nerve) swelling, and mitochondrial swelling and disintegration in each of these cells but especially in the photoreceptors and optic nerve (Baumbach *et al.*, 1977; Hayreh *et al.*, 1980; Murray *et al.*, 1991; Seme *et al.*, 1999). Considering the differences in species, methanol exposures, time course of analysis, and procedures utilized, the overall data for the acute effects of methanol on the ERG are remarkably consistent. Following methanol exposure, the ERG b-wave amplitude in humans, monkeys, and folate-modified rats starts to decrease significantly when the blood formate concentration exceeded 7 mM (Potts, 1955; Ruedeman, 1961; Ingemansson, 1983; Murray *et al.*, 1991; Lee *et al.*, 1994b). These ERG b-wave alterations, as well as flicker-evoked ERG alterations (Seme *et al.*, 1999), occur at lower formate concentrations than those associated with structural changes in the retina and optic nerve, as discussed above. Decreases in the a-wave amplitude are delayed, relative to the b-wave and occur when blood formate concentrations further increase (Ruedeman, 1961; Ingemansson, 1983; Murray *et al.*, 1991; Eells *et al.*, 1996). In addition, it has been shown that intraretinal metabolism of methanol is necessary for the formate-mediated alterations in the ERG (Garner *et al.*, 1995a), although intravenous infusion of formate in monkeys does induce optic nerve edema (Martin-Amat *et al.*, 1978). Finally, in the folate-modified rats, it appears that photoreceptors that respond to a 15-Hz flicker/510-nm wavelength mesopic-photopic stimulus [i.e., rods and middle wavelength–sensitive (M) cones] are more sensitive to methanol than the ultraviolet-sensitive (UV) cones (Seme *et al.*, 1999).

The retinal sources of the ERG a-wave and b-wave were previously discussed. Thus, the data from the ERG b-wave methanol studies suggest that the initial effect of formate is directly on the ON-type rod bipolar cells, Müller glial cells, and/or synaptic transmission between the photoreceptors and bipolar cells. A well-designed series of pharmacologic, ERG, and potassium-induced Müller cell depolarization studies using several controls and folate-modified rats revealed a direct toxic effect of formate on Müller glial cell function (Garner *et al.*, 1995a; Garner *et al.*, 1995b). These studies also provided evidence that formate does not directly affect depolarizing rod bipolar cells or synaptic transmission between the photoreceptors and bipolar cells. Formate also appears to directly and adversely affect the rod and cone photoreceptors as evidenced by the markedly decreased ERG a-wave and flicker response data (Ruedeman, 1961; Ingemansson, 1983; Murray *et al.*, 1991; Eells *et al.*, 1996; Seme *et al.*, 1999).

Although there are no direct data on the underlying molecular mechanism responsible for the toxic effects of formate on Müller glial cells and photoreceptors, several findings suggest that the mechanism involves a disruption in oxidative energy metabolism. First, the whole retinal ATP concentration is decreased in folate-deficient rats 48 hour following methanol exposure, the time point when the b-wave was lost (Garner *et al.*, 1995b). Second, both formate (10 to 200 mM) and formaldehyde (0.5 to 5 mM) inhibited oxygen consumption in isolated ox retina, and formaldehdye was considerably more potent (Kini and Cooper, 1962). Third, similar concentrations of formaldehyde inhibited oxidative phosphorylation of isolated ox retinal mitochondria, with greater effects observed using FAD-linked than NADH-linked substrates (Kini and Cooper, 1962). Unfortunately, the effects of formate were not exam-

ined. Fourth, and consistent with the above results, formate inhibits succinate-cytochrome *c* reductase and cytochrome oxidase activity (Ki = 5 to 30 mM), but not NADH-cytochrome *c* reductase activity in isolated beef heart mitochondria and/or submitochondrial particles (Nicholls, 1976). Fifth, ultrastructural studies reveal swollen mitochondria in rat photoreceptor inner segment and optic nerve 48 to 72 hour after nitrous oxide/methanol exposure (Murray *et al.*, 1991; Seme *et al.*, 1999). To date, there are no such studies conducted on the Müller glial cells. Taken together, these results suggest formate is a mitochondrial poison that inhibits oxidative phosphorylation of photoreceptors, Müller glial cells, and optic nerve. The evidence for this hypothesis and establishment of subsequent steps resulting in retinal and optic nerve cell injury and death remain to be elucidated.

Organic Solvents: *n*-Hexane, Perchloroethylene, Styrene, Toluene, Trichloroethylene, Xylene and Mixtures The neurotoxicity of organic solvents is well established. However, there is a paucity of mechanistic studies on the adverse effects of organic solvents on the retina and visual system despite findings of structural alterations in rods and cones as well as functional alterations such as color vision deficits, decreased contrast sensitivity, and altered visual-motor performance (Raitta *et al.*, 1978; Odkvist *et al.*, 1983; Baker and Fine, 1986; Larsby *et al.*, 1986; Mergler, 1990; Arlien-Söborg, 1992; Backstrom and Collins, 1992; Backstrom *et al.*, 1993; Broadwell *et al.*, 1995; Fox, 1998; Iregren *et al.*, 2002a; Paramei *et al.*, 2004; Benignus *et al.*, 2005; chapter 24 entitled "Toxic Effects of Solvents and Vapors").

Dose-response color vision loss (acquired dyschromatopsia) and decreases in the contrast sensitivity function occur in workers exposed to organic solvents such as alcohols, *n*-hexane, toluene, trichlorethylene, xylene, and mixtures of these and others. Adverse effects usually occur only at concentrations above the occupational exposure limits (Raitta *et al.*, 1978; Baird *et al.*, 1994; Mergler *et al.*, 1987, 1988, 1991; Nakatsuka *et al.*, 1992). A large percentage of workers in microelectronic plants, print shops, and paint manufacturing facilities, who were exposed to concentrations of solvents that exceeded the threshold limit values, had acquired dyschromatopsia as assessed by the Lanthony D-15 desaturated color arrangement panel (Mergler *et al.*, 1987, 1988, 1991). These workers had no observable clinical abnormalities as assessed by biomicroscopy, funduscopy, and peripheral visual field tests. The color vision losses were mainly blue-yellow losses, although more severe red-green losses were reported. As a rule, acquired blue-yellow losses generally result from lens opacification or outer retinal alterations, whereas red-green losses are associated with inner retinal, retrobular, or central visual pathway alterations (Porkony *et al.*, 1979). Moreover, these occupationally exposed workers also exhibited lower contrast sensitivity at intermediate spatial frequencies, which likely reflects alterations in neural function (Mergler *et al.*, 1991). The data from the Mergler *et al.* (1987, 1988, 1991) studies appear to show gender differences in these adverse visual effects. A study of female workers, where the Lanthony D-15 desaturated test was used to assess color vision, showed a trend toward increased prevalence of color vision impairment following exposure to low to moderate concentrations of toluene (Zavalic *et al.*, 1996). Similar blue–yellow deficits as well as macular changes were observed in workers exposed to *n*-hexane for 5 to 21 years (Raitta *et al.*, 1978). These findings correlate with the rod and cone degeneration observed in rats exposed to 2,5-hexanedione (Backstrom and Collins, 1992; Backstrom *et al.*, 1993). Clearly more detailed, well-designed, and well-executed studies are needed to determine (1) which solvent(s) cause alterations in color vision, (2) are spatial and temporal contrast sensitivity affected, (3) the dose (concentration)-response relations between exposure and effects, (4) possible gender differences, and (5) whether these deficits are reversible.

Perchloroethylene Deficits in visual function, such as contrast sensitivity, have been observed in residents of neighborhoods containing dry cleaners using perchloroethylene (Altmann *et al.*, 1995), and in residents of apartment buildings with co-located dry cleaners (Schreiber *et al.*, 2002). For both of these residential studies, the atmospheric concentrations of perchloroethylene were well below those typical of occupational settings. Laboratory experiments with human subjects exposed to perchloroethylene for four hours for four days revealed increased peak latency delays in the N75, P100, and N150 of the VEP as well as decreases in contrast sensitivity at low and intermediate spatial frequencies (Altmann *et al.*, 1990). Interestingly, there were no changes in the brainstem auditory evoked potential during the exposure period. Moreover, gestational exposure to perchloroethylene produced clinical red-green color loss and decreased visual acuity in the children of occupationally exposed mothers (Till *et al.*, 2001). The above results reveal that perchloroethylene is toxic to both the developing and adult visual system.

Styrene Six independent studies report that workers exposed to mean atmospheric concentrations of styrene ranging from 20 to 70 ppm exhibit concentration-dependent alterations in color vision (Gobba *et al.*, 1991; Fallas *et al.*, 1992; Chia *et al.*, 1994; Eguchi *et al.*, 1995; Campagna *et al.*, 1995: Iregren *et al.*, 2005). A combined data analysis from two of the above studies (Gobba *et al.*, 1991; Campagna *et al.*, 1995) suggests that the threshold for color visual impairments is ≤4 ppm styrene (Campagna *et al.*, 1996). This is well below the threshold limit value–time weighted average (TLV-TWA) value for any country: range 20 to 50 ppm. The findings of similar blue-yellow color vision deficits by five different groups of investigators in different countries argue convincingly for the reproducibility and validity of these styrene-induced color vision deficits. The reversibility of these impairments has not been thoroughly studied, although in one study no recovery was found after a 1-month period of no exposure (Gobba *et al.*, 1991). The findings reveal the potential sensitivity of the visual system and especially the photoreceptors to toxicant exposure. The results overall demonstrate that the Lanthony D-15 desaturated test can be a sensitive and reliable test for detecting color vision abnormalities in solvent-exposed workers. In summary, the evidence indicates that organic solvents can produce color vision deficits in occupationally exposed workers.

In addition to these articles, two meta-analyses of the solvent literature have been presented. Paramei *et al.* (2004) focused on color confusion index (CCI) measures, and evaluated studies of CCI scores from workers exposed to toluene, styrene, or mixed solvents from a total of 15 studies. To combine the data for their meta-analysis a z-score transformation was conducted on the CCI values. While 13 of the original 15 studies reported CCI values indicative of poorer performance in the exposed group than in controls, the meta-analysis showed large variations among the effect sizes across studies. This obscured any statistically significant association between the level of exposure and CCI values for toluene

and mixtures, however, a borderline significant difference was found for styrene. Benignus *et al.* (2005) only focused on styrene exposure from six independent studies. They conducted a meta-analysis on behavioral reaction time data as well as CCI values. Z-score transformations were not conducted under the rationale that z-score transformations confound the magnitude of an outcome with its variability. Instead, Benignus *et al.* (2005) used proportional changes with respect to the control group as a measure of the effect magnitude and utilized the data variability to estimate confidence limits around the estimates of association between cumulative exposure and CCI. Using this approach, the meta-analysis revealed statistically significant relationships in the digitized individual subject data between cumulative styrene exposure and increased CCI scores, as well as between cumulative styrene exposure and prolonged choice reaction times.

In summary, the above studies indicate that occupational styrene exposure causes long-lasting color vision deficits in humans. The severity of such impairments needs to be considered, especially in relation to public health and regulatory issues. An example is to compare the loss of visual function from occupational styrene exposure to that associated with normal aging. Thus, it was estimated that loss of visual function from 8 years of occupational exposure to 20 ppm styrene would be equivalent to 1.7 additional years of aging (Benignus *et al.*, 2005). Analyses such as this may lead to better understanding of the severity of subtle changes in visual function. The mechanism of action underlying these color vision changes is unknown. One rodent study suggests that a styrene-induced loss of tyrosine hydroxylase immunoreactive amacrine cells and subsequent decrease in retinal dopamine may contribute to this deficit (Vettori *et al.*, 2000). At present, it is not clear how this mechanism would work.

Organophosphates The neurotoxicity of organophosphates is well established (see chapter 16 entitled "Toxic Responses of the Nervous System"); however, the link between organophosphate exposure and retinotoxicity is presently unresolved. Clinical studies conducted in Japan, report on ocular toxicity from laboratory animals exposed to organophosphates, and reports to the EPA by pesticide manufacturers suggest that various organophosphates produce retinotoxicity and chronic ocular damage (Ishikawa, 1973; Dementi, 1994). However, many of the early clinical reports were poorly designed and remain unconfirmed. The evidence for organophosphate-induced retinal toxicity is strongest for fenthion (dimethyl 3-methyl-4-methylthiophenyl phosphorothionate) (Imai *et al.*, 1983; Misra *et al.*, 1985; Boyes *et al.*, 1994; Tandon *et al.*, 1994). Two recent epidemiologic studies of licensed pesticide applicators and their spouses in two states, North Carolina and Iowa, did not find a statistically increased risk of retinal degeneration from use of organophosphate insecticides as a class, but risks were increased for some individual members of the chemical class (Kamel *et al.*, 2000; Kirrane *et al.*, 2005). Interestingly, both studies identified an increased risk of retinal degeneration in individuals exposed to fungicides. One report cites a high incidence of myopia in Japanese children exposed to organophosphates (Ko *et al.*, 1988) and one experimental study found that visual control of ocular growth was impaired in the eyes of chicks exposed to the organophosphate insecticide chlorpyrifos (Geller *et al.*, 1998). Until further detailed, well-designed, and replicated clinical and basic science studies are conducted; an adequate discussion of the sites and mechanisms of action of organophosphates must be delayed. In the interim, the references noted above will provide the interested reader with a synopsis of the current status in this area.

TARGET SITES AND MECHANISMS OF ACTION: OPTIC NERVE AND TRACT

The optic nerve consists primarily of RGC axons carrying visual information from the retina to several distinct anatomic destinations in the CNS. Both myelinated and nonmyelinated axons are present and grouped into bundles of axons that maintain a topographic distribution with respect to the site of origin in the retina. At the optic chiasm, the fibers split, so that, in humans and other primates, those fibers originating from the temporal retina continue in the optic tract toward the ipsilateral side of the brain, while those fibers originating in the nasal half of the retina, cross the midline and project to the contralateral side of the brain. In species with sideward-facing eyes such as the rat, a larger proportion of the optic nerve fibers (up to 90%) cross the midline. Fibers from the optic nerve terminate in the dorsal LGN, the superior colliculus, and pretectal areas. Information passing through the LGN to visual cortex gives rise to conscious visual perception. Information traveling to the superior colliculus is used to generate eye movements. Pathways leading to the pretectal areas subserve the pupil response. The LGN of primates contains six histologic layers that are alternately innervated by cells from the contralateral and ipsilateral eyes. The cells projecting to and from the ventral two layers of the LGN have large cell bodies, and consequently, this pathway is referred to as the magnocellular system. Retinal ganglion cells projecting to the magnocellular layers of the LGN are referred to as either M-type or P_α cells. Magnocellular neurons are sensitive to fast moving stimuli and to low levels of luminance contrast, but are insensitive to differences in color. The cells from the magnocellular pathway are involved in motion perception. On the dorsal side of the LGN, the cells are smaller and form the parvocellular pathway. Retinal ganglion cells projecting to the parvocellular layers of the LGN are referred to as P-type or P_β cells. Parvocellular neurons are sensitive to color and to fine detailed patterns, have slower conduction velocities, and are involved in perception of color and form (Horton, 1992; Rodieck, 1998).

Disorders of the optic nerve may be termed optic neuritis, optic neuropathy, or optic nerve atrophy, referring to inflammation, damage, or degeneration, respectively, of the optic nerve. Retrobulbar optic neuritis refers to inflammation of the portion of the optic nerve posterior to the globe. Among the symptoms of optic nerve disease are reduced visual acuity, contrast sensitivity, and color vision. Toxic effects observed in the optic nerve may originate from damage to the optic nerve fibers themselves or to the RGC somas that provide axons to the optic nerve. A number of nutritional disorders can adversely affect the optic nerve. Deficiency of thiamine, vitamin B_{12}, or zinc results in degenerative changes in optic nerve fibers. Nutritional and toxic factors can interact to produce optic nerve damage. A condition referred to as alcohol–tobacco amblyopia or simply as toxic amblyopia is observed in habitually heavy users of these substances and is associated nutritional deficiency. Dietary supplementation with vitamin B_{12} is therapeutically helpful, even when patients continue to consume large amounts of alcohol and tobacco (Grant, 1986; Anderson and Quigley, 1992; Potts, 1996).

Acrylamide

Acrylamide monomer is used in a variety of industrial and laboratory applications, where it serves as the basis for the production of polyacrylamide gels and other polyacrylamide products. Exposure to acrylamide produces a distal axonopathy in large-diameter axons of the peripheral nerves and spinal cord that is well documented in humans and laboratory animals (Spencer and Schaumburg, 1974a, 1974b). Visual effects of acrylamide exposure occur at dose levels sufficient to cause substantial peripheral neuropathy, but the selective nature of the visual deficits and associated neuropathology is very instructive. Whereas the large-diameter and long axons are most vulnerable to acrylamide in the peripheral nerve and spinal cord, this is not the case in the optic tract. The middle diameter axons of the P_β-type RGCs that project to the parvocellular layers of the LGN of New- and Old-World primates degenerate after prolonged treatment with acrylamide (Eskin and Merigan, 1986; Lynch et al., 1989). The larger-diameter P_α-type RGCs that project to the magnocellular layers of the LGN are apparently spared. Visual function testing in these primates, without a functional parvocellular system, revealed selective perceptual deficits in detecting visual stimuli with high spatial-frequency components (i.e., fine visual patterns) and low temporal-frequency components (i.e., slowly modulating sine waves) (Merigan and Eskin, 1986). However, the monkeys' perception of larger visual patterns, modulated at higher temporal rates, was not impaired. These toxicologic experiments helped elucidate the functional differentiation of primate parvocellular and magnocellular visual systems. Why the axons of the optic nerve and tract show a different size-based pattern of vulnerability than do axons of the peripheral nerve and spinal cord is not currently understood.

Carbon Disulfide

Carbon disulfide (CS_2) is used in industry to manufacture viscose rayon, carbon tetrachloride, and cellophane. The neurotoxicity of CS_2 is well known and involves damage to the peripheral and central nervous systems as well as profound effects on vision (Beauchamp et al., 1983). The peripheral neuropathy results from a distal axonal degeneration of the large-caliber and long axons of the peripheral nerves and spinal cord, probably through the reactions with the sulfhydryl groups of axonal neurofilament proteins, yielding covalent cross linkages that lead to filamentous tangles and axonal swellings (Graham and Valantine, 2000). The mechanism of action through which inhalation of high concentrations of CS_2 vapors leads to psychotic mania is not currently established but may result from alterations in catecholamine synthesis or neuronal degeneration in several brain areas (Beauchamp et al., 1983). Workers exposed to CS_2 experience loss of visual function accompanied by observable lesions in the retinal vasculature. Among the changes in visual function reported in viscose rayon workers are central scotoma, depressed visual sensitivity in the peripheral visual field, optic atrophy, pupillary disturbances, blurred vision, and disorders of color perception. A workplace study of 123 Belgian viscose rayon workers found a statistical association between a weighted cumulative CS_2 exposure score, deficits in color vision measured using the Farnsworth-Munsell 100-HUE test, and observations of excess microaneurysms observed ophthalmoscopically and in fundus photographs (Vanhoorne et al., 1996). This association was not observed in the 42 workers who were never exposed to levels above the TLV value of 31 mg/m^3. The coexistence of retinal microaneurysms with functional loss has led to the presumption that the visual deficits were a secondary consequence of vascular disease and perhaps of retinal hemorrhages. This association was addressed in carbon disulfide–exposed macaque monkeys used in visual psychophysical, fluorescein angiography, and fundus photography studies as well as postmortem neuropathologic evaluations (Merigan et al., 1988; Eskin et al., 1988). They observed markedly decreased contrast sensitivity functions, decreased visual acuity, and degeneration of the RGCs, all of which occurred in the absence of retinal microaneurysms or hemorrhages. There was little evidence of effects on the other retinal neurons. These findings indicate that the retinal and optic nerve pathology produced by CS_2 are likely a direct neuropathologic action and not the indirect result of vasculopathy. Interestingly, and importantly, after cessation of exposure, the visual acuity measures recovered temporarily in two of the CS_2-treated monkeys; however, the contrast sensitivity measures did not recover. This demonstrates the independence of these two measures and the utility and importance of independent evaluations of contrast sensitivity and visual acuity.

Cuban Epidemic of Optic Neuropathy

During 1992 and 1993, an epidemic occurred in Cuba in which over 50,000 people suffered from optic neuropathy, sensory and autonomic peripheral neuropathy, high-frequency neural hearing loss, and myelopathy. This is the largest epidemic of neurologic disease in the twentieth century (Roman, 1998). The affected individuals were characterized as having bilateral low visual acuity, impaired color perception, impaired visual contrast sensitivity, central scotoma, optic disk pallor, and, in particular, loss of nerve fibers from the papillomacular bundle (Sadun et al., 1994a; Hedges et al., 1997). Individuals with neurologic findings demonstrated stocking-glove sensory deficits, leg cramps, sensory ataxia, altered reflexes, and complaints of memory loss (Mojon et al., 1997). Various authors noticed similarities between the Cuban cases and nutritional or alcohol–tobacco amblyopia, Leber's hereditary optic neuropathy, and Strachan's disease (Hedges et al., 1994; Hirano et al; 1994; Espinosa et al., 1994; Sadun et al., 1994b; Mojon et al., 1997). The optic neuropathy resembled methanol poisoning (Roman, 1998; Sadun, 1998). The outbreak of the epidemic was linked to nutritional deficiencies (Hedges et al., 1997; Mojon et al., 1997; Roman, 1998). In most cases, aggressive supplementation of the diet with B vitamins and folic acid led to a significant clinical improvement (Mojon et al., 1997). Nutritional deficiencies were a primary contributor to the epidemic; however, it was not clear whether they were solely responsible or whether dietary insufficiency served to make individuals more susceptible to other factors. Genetic susceptibility factors and viral exposures have been considered (Johns et al., 1994; Johns and Sadun, 1994; Newman et al., 1994; Mas et al., 1997; Hedges et al., 1997). One likely contributing factor was co-exposure to low levels of neurotoxic compounds that would otherwise have been tolerated (Sadun, 1998). In addition to low food intake, risk factors for the development of optic neuropathy included use of tobacco, in particular the frequent smoking of cigars, and high cassava consumption (Roman, 1998). The mitochondrial toxicant cyanide may be a contaminant of both cassava and tobacco products. Moderate to severe folic acid deficiency was observed in more than half of the cases (Roman, 1998). Samples of local home-brewed rum showed approximately 1 percent contamination with methanol, a level that would not produce optic nerve toxicity in normal healthy individuals (Sadun et al., 1994). However, one-quarter of the Cuban patients showed elevated serum formate concentrations, probably a result of folic acid deficiency. The maximum serum formate concentrations observed (approximately 4 mM) were similar to levels that produce retinal and optic nerve toxicity in a rodent model of methanol toxicity (Eells et al., 1996). Sadun (1998) postulated that mitochondrial impairment, created by the combination of low nutritional status and toxic exposures, was responsible for the neurologic impairments. The nutritional deficiency would lead to ATP depletion. Exposure to either cyanide or formic acid, the toxic metabolite of methanol, causes inhibition of cytochrome oxidase, which further depletes ATP levels (Nicholls, 1976; also see retinal section for additional references and details). Because axoplasmic transport of new mitochondria from nerve cell bodies to distal axonal segments is energy-dependent (Vale et al., 1992), the lowered ATP levels would be expected to impair mitochondrial transport and start a cycle of further ATP depletion and reduced mitochondrial transport to the nerve terminal regions. Sadun proposed that the nerve fibers most sensitive to this type of damage would be the long peripheral nerve axons, which have high transport demands, and the small caliber fibers of the optic nerve, in particular at the papillomacular bundle, which have physical constrictions to transporting mitochondria. Exposure to toxicants could not be documented in most of the people identified late in the epidemic, suggesting nutritional deficit as the principal cause. However, co-exposure to low levels of mitochondrial toxicants or other factors may have pushed individuals over a threshold for causing nerve damage.

Ethambutol

The dextro isomer of ethambutol is widely used as an antimycobacterial drug for the treatment of tuberculosis. It is well known that ethambutol produces dose-related alterations in the visual system, such as blue-yellow and red-green dyschromatopsias, decreased contrast sensitivity, reduced visual acuity, and visual field loss. The earliest visual symptoms appear to be a decrease in contrast sensitivity and color vision, although impaired red-green color vision is the most frequently observed and reported complaint. However, the loss of contrast sensitivity may explain why some patients with normal visual acuity and color perception still complain of visual disturbance. These visual system alterations can occur with a few weeks of doses equal to or greater than 20 mg/kg body weight; however, they usually become manifest after several months of treatment (Koliopoulos and Palimeris, 1972; Polak et al., 1985; Salmon et al., 1987; Jaanus et al., 1995). The symptoms are primarily associated with one of two forms of retrobulbar optic neuritis (i.e., optic neuropathy). The most common form, seen in almost all cases, involves the central optic nerve fibers and typically results in a central or paracentral scotoma in the visual field and is associated with impaired red-green color vision and decreased visual acuity, whereas the second form involves the peripheral optic nerve fibers and typically results in a peripheral scotoma and visual field loss (Jaanus et al., 1995; Lessell, 1998).

In experimental animals, ethambutol causes RGC and optic nerve degeneration, discoloration of the tapetum lucidum (in dogs), retinal detachment (in cats), and possibly amacrine and bipolar cell alterations (van Dijk and Spekreijse, 1983; Grant and Schuman, 1993; Sjoerdsma et al., 1999). Although the mechanism responsible for producing the RGC and optic nerve degeneration is unknown, recent in vivo studies in rats and in vitro rat RGC cell culture experiments suggest that ethambutol causes RGC death secondary to glutamate-induced excitotoxicity (Heng et al., 1999). Pharmacologic studies, using the in vivo and in vitro models, show that although ethambutol is not a direct NMDA-receptor agonist, it makes RGCs more sensitive to endogenous levels of glutamate. Using the fluorescent Ca^{2+} dyes calcium green 1-AM and rhod-2, Heng *et al.* (1999) showed that following application of ethambutol in the presence, but not absence, of glutamate to isolated RGCs, there was a decrease in cytosolic Ca^{2+} and a subsequent increase in mitochondrial Ca^{2+}. Interestingly, the increase in mitochondrial Ca^{2+} resulted in an increase in the mitochondrial membrane potential as measured by the mitochondrial membrane potential sensitive dye JC-1. The authors (Heng *et al.*, 1999) postulate that this latter phenomenon occurs as a result of an ethambutol-mediated chelation of Zn^{2+} from the mitochondrial ATPase inhibitor protein IF1 (Rouslin *et al.*, 1993) that subsequently results in the inhibition of mitochondrial ATP synthesis and elevation of mitochondrial membrane potential. These intriguing ideas have merit; however, many additional experiments will be needed to prove this hypothesis. In addition, the authors suggest that some glutamate antagonists may be useful in decreasing the side effects of ethambutol—a practical suggestion that appears worthy of clinical investigation.

TARGET SITES AND MECHANISMS OF ACTION: THE CENTRAL VISUAL SYSTEM

Many areas of the cerebral cortex are involved in the perception of visual information. The primary visual cortex—called V1, Brodmann's area 17, or striate cortex—receives the primary projections of visual information from the LGN and also from the superior colliculus. Neurons from the LGN project to visual cortex maintaining a topographic representation of the receptive field origin in the retina. The receptive fields in the left and right sides of area 17 reflect the contralateral visual world and representations of the upper and lower regions of the visual field are separated below and above, respectively, the calcarine fissure. Cells in the posterior aspects of the calcarine fissure have receptive fields located in the central part of the retina. Cortical cells progressively deeper in the calcarine fissure have retinal receptive fields that are located more and more peripherally in the retina. The central part of the fovea has tightly packed photoreceptors for resolution of fine detailed images, and the cortical representation of the central fovea is proportionately larger than the peripheral retina in order to accommodate a proportionately larger need for neural image processing. The magnocellular and parvocellular pathways project differently to the histologically defined layers of primary striate visual cortex and then to extrastriate visual areas. The receptive fields of neurons in visual cortex are more complex than the circular center-surround arrangement found in the retina and LGN. Cortical cells respond better to lines of a particular orientation than to simple spots. The receptive fields of cortical cells are thought to represent computational summaries of a number of simpler input signals. As the visual information proceeds from area V1 to extrastriate visual cortical areas, the representation of the visual world reflected in the receptive fields of individual neurons becomes progressively more complex (Horton, 1992).

Lead

In addition to the well-documented retinal effects of lead (see above), lead exposure during adulthood or perinatal development produces structural, biochemical, and functional deficits in the visual cortex of humans, nonhuman primates, and rats (Fox *et al.*, 1977; Winneke, 1979; Costa and Fox, 1983; Sborgia *et al.*, 1983; Fox, 1984; Otto *et al.*, 1985; Lilienthal *et al.*, 1988; Reuhl *et al.*, 1989; Murata *et al.*, 1993; Otto and Fox, 1993; Altmann *et al.*, 1994,

1998; Winneke *et al.*, 1994). Quantitative morphometric studies in monkeys exposed to either high levels of lead from birth or infancy to 6 years of age revealed a decrease in visual cortex (areas V1 and V2), cell volume density, and a decrease in the number of initial arborizations among pyramidal neurons (Reuhl *et al.*, 1989). The former results may be due to an absolute decrease in total cell numbers, possibly resulting from lead-induced apoptosis as observed in the retina (Fox *et al.*, 1997; He *et al.*, 2000). This may also account for the decreased density of cholinergic muscarinic receptors found in the visual cortex of adult rats following moderate level developmental lead exposure (Costa and Fox, 1983). The morphometric results on neuronal branching are reminiscent of earlier findings in the neocortex of rats following high level developmental lead exposure (Petit and LeBoutillier, 1979), and recent findings in the somatosensory cortex of rats following low or moderate level developmental lead exposure (Wilson *et al.*, 2000). These alterations could partially contribute to the decreases in contrast sensitivity observed in lead-exposed rats and monkeys (Fox, 1984; Rice, 1998), the alterations in the amplitude and latency measures of the flash and pattern-reversal evoked potentials in lead-exposed children, workers, monkeys, and rats (Fox *et al.*, 1977; Winneke, 1979; Sborgia *et al.*, 1983; Otto *et al.*, 1985; Lilienthal *et al.*, 1988; Murata *et al.*, 1993; Altmann *et al.*, 1994, 1998; Winneke *et al.*, 1994), and the alterations in tasks assessing visual function in lead-exposed children (Winneke *et al.*, 1983; Hansen *et al.*, 1989; Muñoz *et al.*, 1993).

Methylmercury

Methyl mercury became notorious in two episodes of mass poisoning (see chapter. 16 entitled "Toxic Responses of the Nervous System"). In the 1950s, industrial discharges of mercury into Minamata Bay in Japan became biomethylated to form methyl mercury, which then accumulated in the food chain and reached toxic concentrations in the fish and shellfish consumed in the surrounding communities. Hundreds of people were poisoned, showing a combination of sensory, motor, and cognitive deficits. A more widespread episode of methyl mercury poisoning affected thousands of Iraqi citizens who mistakenly ground wheat grain into flour that had been treated with methyl mercury as a fungicide and that was intended for planting and not for direct human consumption.

Visual deficits are a prominent feature of methyl mercury intoxication in adult humans, along with several other neurologic manifestations such as difficulties with sensation, gait, memory, and cognition. Methyl mercury poisoned individuals experienced a striking and progressive constriction of the visual field (peripheral scotoma) as patients became progressively less able to see objects in the visual periphery (Iwata, 1977). The narrowing of the visual field gives impression of looking through a long tunnel, hence the term tunnel vision. Visual field constrictions also have been observed in methyl mercury–poisoned monkeys (Merigan, 1979). On autopsy of some of the Minamata patients, focal neurologic degeneration was observed in several brain regions including motor cortex, cerebellum, and calcarine fissure of visual cortex (Takeuchi and Eto, 1977). The histopathologic feature was a destruction of the cortical neural and glial cells, with sparing of the subcortical white matter, optic radiations, and LGN. Monkeys and dogs that were treated experimentally with methyl mercury showed greater damage in the calcarine fissure, associated with higher regional concentrations of protein-bound mercury, than in other brain regions (Yoshino *et al.*, 1966; Berlin *et al.*, 1975). In the Minamata patients, there was a regional distribution of damage observed within striate cortex, such that the most extensive damage occurred deep in the calcarine fissure and was progressively less in the more posterior portions. Thus, the damage was most severe in the regions of primary visual cortex that subserved the peripheral visual field, with relative sparing of the cortical areas representing the central vision. This regional distribution of damage corresponded with the progressive loss of peripheral vision while central vision was relatively preserved. Methyl mercury–poisoned individuals also experienced poor night vision (i.e., scotopic vision deficits), also attributable to peripheral visual field losses. Similar changes were observed in adult monkeys exposed to methyl mercury (Berlin *et al.*, 1975). Mercury also accumulates in the retina of animals exposed to methylmercury (DuVal *et al.*, 1987). Acute exposure of isolated retinas to mercury or methylmercury produces rod-selective electrophysiologic and morphologic alterations (Fox and Sillman, 1979; Braekevelt, 1982), whereas subacute dosing with methylmercury alters the photopic ERG prior to the scotopic ERG (Goto *et al.*, 2001). The neurologic damage in adult cases of Minamata disease was focally localized in the calcarine cortex and other areas but was more globally distributed throughout the brain in those developmentally exposed.

The levels of methyl mercury exposure experienced by people in Minamata Bay were undoubtedly high. Studies of visual function in nonhuman primates exposed to methyl mercury during perinatal development demonstrate a decrease in visual contrast sensitivity, visual acuity, and temporal flicker resolution at dose levels lower than those associated with constriction of the visual fields (Rice and Gilbert, 1982; Rice and Gilbert, 1990; Rice, 1996). Monkeys exposed to methyl mercury from birth onward or in utero plus postnatally exhibited spatial vision deficits under both high and low luminance conditions, although the deficits were greater under scotopic illumination (Rice and Gilbert, 1982; Rice, 1990). The effects on temporal vision were different. That is, monkeys exposed from birth displayed superior low-luminance temporal vision, whereas high-luminance temporal vision was not impaired. In contrast, monkeys exposed to methyl mercury in utero plus postnatally exhibited deficits in low-frequency high-luminance temporal vision, while low-luminance temporal vision was superior to that of control monkeys (Rice, 1990). These data indicate that the spatial and temporal vision deficits produced by developmental exposure to methyl mercury are different from those produced during adulthood. The underlying mechanisms have yet to be determined.

ACKNOWLEDGEMENTS

We thank Dr. Andrew M. Geller and Jean-Claude Mwanza for review and editorial comments. Partial support for writing this chapter came from a NIEHS RO1 Grant ES012482 to Donald A. Fox. This chapter has been reviewed by the National Health and Environmental Effects Research Laboratory, U.S. EPA, and approved for publication. Mention of trade names and commercial products does not constitute endorsement or recommendation for use.

REFERENCES

Adamus G, Machnicki M, Elerding H, *et al.*: Antibodies to recoverin induce apoptosis of photoreceptor and bipolar cells in vivo. *J Autoimmun* 11:523–533, 1998.

Agency for Toxic Substances and Disease Registry (ATSDR). *Neurobehavioral Test Batteries for Use in Environmental Health Field Studies.* Atlanta, GA: U.S. Department of Health, Public Health Service, 1992.

Ahmed J, Braun RD, Dunn R Jr, Linsenmeier RA: Oxygen distribution in the macaque retina. *Invest Ophthalmol Vis Sci* 34:516–521, 1993.

Ah-Song R, Sasco AJ: Tamoxifen and ocular toxicity. *Cancer Detect Prev* 21:522–531, 1997.

Al-Modhefer AJA, Bradbury MWB, Simons TJB: Observations on the chemical nature of lead in human blood serum. *Clin Sci* 81:823–829, 1991.

Alken RG, Belz GG: A comparative dose-effect study with cardiac glycosides assessing cardiac and extracardiac responses in normal subjects. *J Cardiovasc Pharmacol* 6:634–640, 1984.

Alm A: Ocular circulation, in Hart WM (ed): *Adler's Physiology of the Eye,* 9th ed. St. Louis: Mosby–Year Book, 1992, pp. 198–227.

Altmann L, Bottger A, Wiegand H: Neurophysiological and psychophysical measurements reveal acute low-level organic solvent exposure in humans. *Int Arch Occup Environ Health* 62:493–499, 1990.

Altmann L, Gutowski M, Wiegand H: Effects of maternal lead exposure on functional plasticity in the visual cortex and hippocampus of immature rats. *Brain Res Dev Brain Res* 81:50–56, 1994.

Altmann L, Florian Neuhann H, Kramer U, Witten J, Jermann E: Neurobehavioral and neurophysiological outcomes of chronic low-level tetrachloroethene exposure measured in neighborhoods of dry cleaning shops. *Environ Res* 69:83–89, 1995.

Altmann L, Sveinsson K, Kramer U, *et al.*: Visual functions in 6-year-old children in relation to lead and mercury levels. *Neurotoxicol Teratol* 20:9–17, 1998.

American Medical Association, Council on Scientific Affairs: Harmful effects of ultraviolet radiation. *JAMA* 262:380–384, 1989.

Anderson DR, Quigley HA: The optic nerve, in Hart WM (ed): *Adler's Physiology of the Eye,* 9th ed. St. Louis: Mosby–Year Book, 1992, pp. 616–640.

Anderson JA, Davis WL, Wei CP: Site of ocular hydrolysis of a prodrug, dipivefrin, and a comparison of its ocular metabolism with that of the parent compound, epinephrine. *Invest Ophthalmol Vis Sci* 19:817–823, 1980.

Anger WK, Johnson BL: Chemicals affecting behavior, in O'Donoghue JL (ed): *Neurotoxicity of Industrial and Commercial Chemicals.* Boca Raton, FL: CRC Press, 1985, pp. 51–148.

Anger WK, Letz R, Chrislip DW, *et al.*: Neurobehavioral test methods for environmental health studies of adults. *Neurotoxicol Teratol* 16:489–497, 1994.

Arlien-Söborg P: *Solvent Neurotoxicity.* Boca Raton, FL: CRC Press, 1992.

Aronson JK, Ford AR: The use of colour vision measurement in the diagnosis of digoxin toxicity. *Q J Med* 49:273–282, 1980.

Asakura T, Matsuda M, Matsuda S, Shichi H: Synthesis of 12(R)- and 12(S)-hydroxyeicosatetraenoic acid by porcine ocular tissues. *J Ocul Pharmacol* 10:525–535, 1994.

Atalla LR, Sevanian A, Rao NA: Immunohistochemical localization of glutathione peroxidase in ocular tissue. *Curr Eye Res* 7:1023–1027, 1988.

Awasthi YC, Saneto RP, Srivastava SK: Purification and properties of bovine lens glutathione S-transferase. *Exp Eye Res* 30:29–39, 1980.

Backstrom B, Collins VP: The effects of 2,5-hexanedione on rods and cones of the retina of albino rats. *Neurotoxicology* 13:199–202, 1992.

Backstrom B, Nylen P, Hagman M, *et al.*: Effect of exposure to 2,5-hexanediol in light or darkness on the retina of albino and pigmented rats. I. Morphology. *Arch Toxicol* 67:277–283, 1993.

Baghdassarian SA: Optic neuropathy due to lead poisoning. *Arch Ophthalmol* 80:721–723, 1968.

Baird B, Camp J, Daniell W, Antonelli J: Solvents and color discrimination ability. *J Occup Med* 36:747–751, 1994.

Baker EL, Feldman RG, White RA, *et al.*: Occupational lead neurotoxicity: A behavioral and electrophysiological evaluation. *Br J Ind Med* 41:352–361, 1984.

Baker EL, Fine LJ: Solvent neurotoxicity. The current evidence. *J Occup Med* 28:126–129, 1986.

Ballantyne B: Toxicology related to the eye, in Ballantyne B, Marrs TC, Syversen T (eds): *General and Applied Toxicology.* New York: McGraw-Hill, 1999, pp. 737–774.

Baloh RW, Langhofer L, Brown CP, Spivey GH: Quantitative tracking tests in lead workers. *Am J Med* 1:109–113, 1980.

Baloh RW, Spivey GH, Brown CP, *et al.*: Subclinical effects of chronic increased lead absorption—A prospective study. II. Results of baseline neurologic testing. *J Occup Med* 21:490–496, 1979.

Barltrop D, Barrett AJ, Dingle JT: Subcellular distribution of lead in the rat. *J Lab Clin Med* 77:705–712, 1971.

Barratt MD: A quantitative structure-activity relationship for the eye irritation potential of neutral organic chemicals. *Toxicol Lett* 80:69–74, 1995.

Bartlett JD, Jaanus SD: *Clinical Ocular Pharmacology,* 3rd ed. Boston: Butterworth-Heinemann, 1995.

Baumbach GL, Cancilla PA, Martin-Amat G, *et al.*: Methyl alcohol poisoning: IV. Alterations of the morphological findings of the retina and optic nerve. *Arch Ophthalmol* 95:1859–1865, 1977.

Bausher LP: Identification of A and B forms of monoamine oxidase in the iris-ciliary body, superior cervical ganglion, and pineal gland of albino rabbits. *Invest Ophthalmol* 15:529–537, 1976.

Baylor DA, Nunn BJ, Schnapf JL: The photocurrent, noise and spectral sensitivity of rods of the monkey *Macaca fascicularis. J Physiol* 357:575–607, 1984.

Beauchamp RO Jr, Bus JS, Popp JA, *et al.*: A critical review of the literature on carbon disulfide toxicity. *CRC Crit Rev Toxicol* 11:168–277, 1983.

Behndig A, Svensson B, Marklund SL, Karlsson K: Superoxide dismutase isoenzymes in the human eye. *Invest Ophthalmol Vis Sci* 39:471–475, 1998.

Benignus VA, Geller AM, Boyes WK, Bushnell PJ: Human neurobehavioral effects of long-term exposure to styrene: a meta-analysis. *Environ Health Perspect* 113:532–538, 2005.

Benton CD, Calhoun FP: The ocular effects of methyl alcohol poisoning: Report of a catastrophe involving three hundred and twenty persons. *Trans Am Acad Ophthalmol* 56:875–883, 1952.

Berlin M, Grant CA, Hellberg J, *et al.*: Neurotoxicity of methyl mercury in squirrel monkeys. Cerebral cortical pathology, interference with scotopic vision, and changes in operant behavior. *Arch Environ Health* 30:340–348, 1975.

Berman ER: *Biochemistry of the Eye.* New York: Plenum Press, 1991.

Bernstein HN: Chloroquine ocular toxicity. *Surv Ophthalmol* 12:415–477, 1967.

Berson EL: Electrical phenomena in the retina, in Hart WM (ed): *Adler's Physiology of the Eye,* 9th ed. St. Louis: Mosby–Year Book, 1992, pp. 641–707.

Betta A, De Santa A, Savonitto C, D'Andrea F: Flicker fusion test and occupational toxicology performance evaluation in workers exposed to lead and solvents. *Hum Toxicol* 2:83–90, 1983.

Birch D, Jacobs GH: Spatial contrast sensitivity in albino and pigmented rats. *Vision Res* 19:933–937, 1979.

Boyes WK: Testing visual system toxicity using visual evoked potential technology, in Isaacson RL, Jensen KF (eds): *The Vulnerable Brain and Environmental Risk: Malnutrition and Hazard Assessment.* Vol 1. New York: Plenum Press, 1992, pp. 193–222.

Boyes WK, Dyer RS: Chlordimeform produces profound but transient changes in visual evoked potentials of hooded rats. *Exp Neurol* 86:434–447, 1984.

Boyes WK, Dyer RS: Pattern reversal visual evoked potentials in awake rats. *Brain Res Bull* 10:817–823, 1983.

Boyes WK, Tandon P, Barone S Jr, Padilla S: Effects of organophosphates on the visual system of rats. *J Appl Toxicol* 14:135–143, 1994.

Braekevelt CR: Morphological changes in rat retinal photoreceptors with acute methyl mercury intoxication, in Hollyfield JG (ed): *The Structure of the Eye.* New York: Elsevier, 1982, pp. 123–131.

Brandstätter JH, Koulen P, Wässle H: Diversity of glutamate receptors in the mammalian retina. *Vision Res* 38:1385–1397, 1998.

Braun RD, Linsenmeier RA, Goldstick TK: Oxygen consumption in the inner and outer retina of the cat. *Invest Ophthalmol Vis Sci* 36:542–554, 1995.

Broadwell DK, Darcey DJ, Hudnell HK, *et al.*: Worksite clinical and neurobehavioral assessment of solvent-exposed workers. *Am J Indust Med* 27:677–698, 1995.

Brown DVL: Reaction of the rabbit retinal pigment epithelium to systemic lead poisoning. *Tr Am Ophthalmol Soc* 72:404–447, 1974.

Bruner LH, Parker RD, Bruce RD: Reducing the number of rabbits in the low-volume eye test. *Fundam Appl Toxicol* 19:330–335, 1992.

Bruner LH, Shadduck J, Essex-Sorlie D: Alternative methods for assessing the effects of chemicals in the eye, in Hobson DW (ed): *Dermal and Ocular Toxicity: Fundamentals and Methods.* Boca Raton, FL: CRC Press, 1991, pp. 585–606.

Bull RJ: Lead and energy metabolism, in Singhal RL, Thomas JA (eds): *Lead Toxicity.* Baltimore: Urban and Schwarzenberg, 1980, pp. 119–168.

Burns CA: Indomethacin, reduced retinal sensitivity and corneal deposits. *Am J Ophthalmol* 66:825–835, 1968.

Burns CA: Ocular effects of indomethacin. Slit lamp and electroretinographic: ERG study. *Invest Ophthalmol* 5:325–331, 1966.

Bushnell PJ, Bowman RE, Allen JR, Marlar RJ: Scotopic vision deficits in young monkeys exposed to lead. *Science* 196:333–335, 1977.

Campagna D, Gobba F, Mergler D, *et al.*: Color vision loss among styrene-exposed workers: Neurotoxicological threshold assessment. *Neurotoxicology* 17:367–373, 1996.

Campagna D, Mergler D, Huel G, *et al.*: Visual dysfunction among styrene-exposed workers. *Scand J Work Environ Health* 21:382–390, 1995.

Campara P, D'Andrea F, Micciolo R, *et al.*: Psychological performance of workers with blood-lead concentration below the current threshold limit value. *Int Arch Occup Environ Health* 53:233–246, 1984.

Cavalleri A, Minoia C, Ceroni A, Poloni M: Lead in cerebrospinal fluid and its relationship to plasma lead in humans. *J Appl Toxicol* 4:63–65, 1984.

Cavelleri A, Trimarchi F, Gelmi C, *et al.*: Effects of lead on the visual system of occupationally exposed subjects. *Scand J Work Environ Health* 8(suppl 1):148–151, 1982.

Cestnick L, Coltheart M: The relationship between language-processing and visual-processing deficits in developmental dyslexia. *Cognition* 71:231–255, 1999.

Chamberlain M, Gad SC, Gautheron P, Prinsen MK: IRAG working group 1. Organotypic models for the assessment/prediction of ocular irritation. Interagency Regulatory Alternatives Group. *Food Chem Toxicol* 35:23–37, 1997.

Chang GQ, Hao Y, Wong F: Apoptosis: Final common pathway of photoreceptor death in rd, rds, and rhodopsin mutant mice. *Neuron* 11:595–605, 1993.

Chia SE, Jeyaratnam J, Ong CN, *et al.*: Impairment of color vision among workers exposed to low concentrations of styrene. *Am J Ind Med* 26:481–488, 1994.

Chiou GCY: *Ophthalmic Toxicology.* New York: Raven Press, 1992.

Chun MH, Han SH, Chung JW, Wässle H: Electron microscopic analysis of the rod pathway of the rat retina. *J Comp Neurol* 332:421–432, 1993.

Cohen AI: The retina, in Hart WM (ed): *Adler's Physiology of the Eye,* 9th ed. St. Louis: Mosby–Year Book, 1992, pp. 579–615.

Cook JE, Becker DL: Gap junctions in the vertebrate retina. *Microsc Res Tech* 31:408–419, 1995.

Corbin JD, Francis SH, Webb DJ: Phosphodiesterase type 5 as a pharmacologic target in erectile dysfunction. *Urology* 60:4–11, 2002.

Costa LG, Fox DA: A selective decrease in cholinergic muscarinic receptors in the visual cortex of adult rats following developmental lead exposure. *Brain Res* 276:259–266, 1983.

Crofton KM, Sheets LP: Evaluation of sensory system function using reflex modification of the startle response. *J Am Coll Toxicol* 8:199–211, 1989.

Crosson CE, Willis JA, Potter DE: Effect of the calcium antagonist, nifedipine, on ischemic retinal dysfunction. *J Ocul Pharmacol* 6:293–299, 1990.

Crouch RK, Goletz P, Snyder A, Coles WH: Antioxidant enzymes in human tears. *J Ocul Pharmacol* 7:253–258, 1991.

Cumming RG, Mitchell P: Alcohol, smoking, and cataracts: The Blue Mountains Eye Study. *Arch Ophthalmol* 115:1296–1303, 1997.

Cumming RG, Mitchell P: Inhaled corticosteroids and cataract: Prevalence, prevention and management. *Drug Safety* 20:77–84, 1999.

Cumming RG, Mitchell P, Leeder SR: Use of inhaled corticosteroids and the risk of cataracts. *N Engl J Med* 337:8–14, 1997.

Damstra T: Environmental chemicals and nervous system dysfunction. *Yale J Biol Med* 51:457–468, 1978.

Datson GP, Freeberg FE: Ocular irritation testing, in Hobson DW (ed): *Dermal and Ocular Toxicity: Fundamentals and Methods.* Boca Raton, FL: CRC Press, 1991, pp. 509–539.

Dayhaw-Barker P, Forbes D, Fox DA, *et al.*: Drug photoxicity and visual health, in Waxler M, Hitchins VM (eds): *Optical Radiation and Visual Health.* Boca Raton, FL: CRC Press, 1986, pp. 147–175.

Dean P: Visual pathways and acuity hooded rats. *Behav Brain Res* 3:239–271, 1981.

Delcourt C, Carriere I, Ponton-Sanchez A, *et al.*: Light exposure and the risk of cortical, nuclear, and posterior subcapsular cataracts: The Pathologies Oculaires Liees a l'Age (POLA) study. *Arch Ophthalmol* 118:385–392, 2000.

Dementi B: Ocular effects of organophosphates: A historical perspective of Saku disease. *J Appl Toxicol* 14:119–129, 1994.

De Rouck A, De Laey JJ, Van Hoorne M, *et al.*: Chronic carbon disulfide poisoning: A 4-year follow-up study of the ophthalmological signs. *Int Ophthalmol* 9:17–27, 1986.

Diamante GG, Fraunfelder FT: Adverse effects of therapeutic agents on cornea and conjunctiva, in Leibowitz HM, Waring GO (eds): *Corneal Disorders, Clinical Diagnosis and Management,* 2nd ed. Philadelphia: Saunders, 1998, pp. 736–769.

Dobbing J, Sands J: Comparative aspects of the brain growth spurt. *Early Hum Dev* 3:79–91, 1979.

Doshi M, Marcus C, Bejjani BA, Edward DP: Immunolocalization of CYP1B1 in normal, human, fetal and adult eyes. *Exp Eye Res* 82:24–32, 2006.

Dowling JE: *The Retina: An Approachable Part of the Brain.* Cambridge, MA: Belknap Press, 1987.

Downes JE, Holmes RS: Purification and properties of murine corneal alcohol dehydrogenase. Evidence for class IV ADH properties. *Adv Exp Med Biol* 372:349–354, 1995.

Dräger UC: Calcium binding in pigmented and albino eyes. *Proc Natl Acad Sci USA* 82:6716–6720, 1985.

Draize JH, Woodard G, Calvery HO: Methods for the study of irritation and toxicity of substances applied topically to the skin and mucous membranes. *J Pharmacol Exp Ther* 82:377–389, 1944.

Duncker G, Krastel H: Ocular digitalis effects in normal subjects. *Lens Eye Tox Res* 7:281–303, 1990.

Duncker GI, Kisters G, Grille W: Prospective, randomized, placebo-controlled, double-blind testing of colour vision and electroretinogram at therapeutic and subtherapeutic digitoxin serum levels. *Ophthalmologica* 208:259–261, 1994.

DuVal G, Grubb BR, Bentley PJ: Mercury accumulation in the eye following administration of methyl mercury. *Exp Eye Res* 44:161–164, 1987.

Dyer RS: The use of sensory evoked potentials in toxicology. *Fundam Appl Toxicol* 5:24–40, 1985.

Dyer RS, Howell WE, Wonderlin WF: Visual system dysfunction following acute trimethyltin exposure in rats. *Neurobehav Toxicol Teratol* 4:191–195, 1982.

Edward DP, Lam TT, Shahinfar S, *et al.*: Amelioration of light-induced retinal degeneration by a calcium overload blocker: flunarizine. *Arch Ophthalmol* 109:554–562, 1991.

Eells, JT: Methanol, in Thurman RG, Kauffman FC (eds): *Browning's Toxicity and Metabolism of Industrial Solvents: Alcohols and Esters.* Vol 3. Amsterdam: Elsevier, 1992, pp. 3–20.

Eells JT, Salzman MM, Lewandowski MF, Murray TG: Formate-induced alterations in retinal function in methanol-intoxicated rats. *Toxicol Appl Pharmacol* 140:58–69, 1996.

Eguchi T, Kishi R, Harabuchi I, *et al.*: Impaired colour discrimination among workers exposed to styrene: Relevance of a urinary metabolite. *Occup Environ Med* 52:534–538, 1995.

Eichenbaum JW, Zheng W: Distribution of lead and transthyretin in human eyes. *Clin Toxicol* 38:371–381, 2000.

Ellsworth AJ, Witt DM, Dugdale DC, Oliver LM: *Mosby's 1999–2000 Medical Drug Reference.* St. Louis: Mosby, 1999, pp. 184–185.

Eskin TA, Merigan WH: Selective acrylamide-induced degeneration of color opponent ganglion cells in macaques. *Brain Res* 378:379–384, 1986.

Eskin TA, Merigan WH, Wood RW: Carbon disulfide effects on the visual system: II. Retinogeniculate degeneration. *Invest Ophthalmol Vis Sci* 29:519–527, 1988.

Espinosa A, Alvarez F, Vazquez L, Ordunez PO: Optic and peripheral neuropathy in Cuba. *JAMA* 271:664, 1994.

Fallas C, Fallas J, Maslard P, Dally S: Subclinical impairment of colour vision among workers exposed to styrene. *Br J Ind Med* 49:679–682, 1992.

Finlay BL, Sengelaub DR: *Development of the Vertebrate Retina.* New York: Plenum Press, 1989.

Fox DA: Psychophysically and electrophysiologically determined spatial vision deficits in lead-exposed rats have a cholinergic component, in Narahashi T (ed): *Cellular and Molecular Basis of Neurotoxicity.* New York: Raven Press, 1984, pp. 123–140.

Fox DA: Sensory system alterations following occupational exposure to chemicals, in Manzo L, Costa LG (eds): *Occupational Neurotoxicology.* Boca Raton, FL: CRC Press, 1998, pp. 169–184.

Fox DA, Campbell ML, Blocker YS: Functional alterations and apoptotic cell death in the retina following developmental or adult lead exposure. *Neurotoxicology* 18:645–665, 1997.

Fox DA, Chu LWF: Rods are selectively altered by lead: II. Ultrastructure and quantitative histology. *Exp Eye Res* 46:613–625, 1988.

Fox DA, Farber DB: Rods are selectively altered by lead: I. Electrophysiology and biochemistry. *Exp Eye Res* 46:579–611, 1988.

Fox DA, Katz LM: Developmental lead exposure selectively alters the scotopic ERG component of dark and light adaptation and increases rod calcium content. *Vision Res* 32:249–252, 1992.

Fox DA, Katz LM, Farber DB: Low-level developmental lead exposure decreases the sensitivity, amplitude and temporal resolution of rods. *Neurotoxicology* 12:641–654, 1991a.

Fox DA, Lewkowski JP, Cooper GP: Acute and chronic effects of neonatal lead exposure on the development of the visual evoked response in rats. *Toxicol Appl Pharmacol* 40:449–461, 1977.

Fox DA, Lowndes HE, Bierkamper GG: Electrophysiological techniques in neurotoxicology, in Mitchel CL (ed): *Nervous System Toxicology.* New York: Raven Press, 1982, pp. 299–335.

Fox DA, Poblenz AT, He L: Calcium overload triggers rod photoreceptor apoptotic cell death in chemical-induced and inherited retinal degenerations. *Ann NY Acad Sci* 893:282–286, 1999.

Fox DA, Rubinstein SD: Age-related changes in retinal sensitivity, rhodopsin content and rod outer-segment length in hooded rats following low level lead exposure during development. *Exp Eye Res* 48:237–249, 1989.

Fox DA, Rubinstein SD, Hsu P: Developmental lead exposure inhibits adult rat retinal, but not kidney, Na+,K+-ATPase. *Toxicol Appl Pharmacol* 109:482–493, 1991b.

Fox DA, Sillman AJ: Heavy metals affect rod, but not cone photoreceptors. *Science* 206:78–80, 1979.

Fraunfelder FT, Meyer SM: *Drug-Induced Ocular Side Effects and Drug Interactions,* 3rd ed. Philadelphia: Lea & Febiger, 1989.

Fraunfelder FW, Pomeranz HD, Egan RA: Nonarteritic anterior ischemic optic neuropathy and sildenafil. *Arch Ophthalmol* 124:733–734, 2006.

Frumkes TE, Eysteinsson T: The cellular basis for suppressive rod-cone interaction. *Vis Neurosci* 1:263–273, 1988.

Garner CD, Lee EW, Louis-Ferdinand RT: Muller cell involvement in methanol-induced retinal toxicity. *Toxicol Appl Pharmacol* 130:101–107, 1995b.

Garner CD, Lee EW, Terzo TS, Louis-Ferdinand RT: Role of retinal metabolism in methanol-induced retinal toxicity. *J Toxicol Environ Health* 44:43–56, 1995a.

Gaudet SJ, Razavi P, Caiafa GJ, Chader GJ: Identification of arylamine *N*-acetyltransferase activity in the bovine lens. *Curr Eye Res* 14:873–877, 1995.

Gelatt KN: *Veterinary Ophthalmology.* Philadelphia: Lea & Febiger, 1981.

Geller AM, Abdel-Rahman AA, Abou-Donia MB, *et al.*: The organophosphate pesticide chlorpyrifos affects form deprivation myopia. *Invest Ophthalmol Vis Sci* 39:1290–1294, 1998.

Geller AM, Hudnell HK: Critical issues in the use and analysis of the Lanthony desaturate color vision test. *Neurotoxicol Teratol* 19:455–465, 1997.

Geller AM, Osborne C, Peiffer RL: The ERG, EOG and VEP in rats, in Weisse I *et al.* (eds): *Ocular Toxicology.* New York, NY: Plenum Press, 1995, pp. 7–25.

Giblin FJ: Glutathione: A vital lens antioxidant. *J Ocul Pharmacol Ther* 16:121–135, 2000.

Ginsburg AP: Contrast sensitivity and functional vision. *Int Ophthalmol Clin* 43:5–15, 2003.

Glickman L, Valciukas JA, Lilis R, Weisman I: Occupational lead exposure. Effects on saccadic eye movements. *Int Arch Occup Environ Health* 54:115–125, 1984.

Glickman RD: Phototoxicity to the retina: mechanisms of damage. *Int J Toxicol* 21:473–490, 2002.

Gobba F, Galassi C, Imbriani M, *et al.*: Acquired dyschromatopsia among styrene-exposed workers. *J Occup Med* 33:761–765, 1991.

Gondhowiardjo TD, van Haeringen NJ: Corneal aldehyde dehydrogenase, glutathione reductase, and glutathione *S*-transferase in pathologic corneas. *Cornea* 12:310–314, 1993.

Good GW, Schepler A, Nichols JJ: The reliability of the Lanthony Desaturated D-15 test. *Optom Vis Sci* 82:1054–1059, 2005.

Gorin MB, Day R, Costantino JP, *et al.*: Long-term tamoxifen citrate use and potential ocular toxicity. *Am J Ophthalmol* 125:493–501, 1998.

Gorkin L, Hvidsten K, Sobel RE, Siegel R: Sildenafil citrate use and the incidence of nonarteritic anterior ischemic optic neuropathy. *Int J Clin Pract* 60:500–503, 2006.

Goto Y, Shigematsu J, Tobimatsu S, Sakamoto T, Kinukawa N, Kato M: Different vulnerability of rat retinal cells to methylmercury exposure. *Curr Eye Res* 23:171–178, 2001.

Graham DG, Valentine WM: Carbon disulfide, in Spencer PS, Schaumburg HH (eds): *Experimental and Clinical Neurotoxicology,* 2nd ed. New York: Oxford University Press, 2000, pp. 315–317.

Grant WM: *Toxicology of the Eye,* 3rd ed. Springfield, IL: Charles C Thomas, 1986.

Grant WM, Schuman JS: *Toxicology of the Eye,* 4th ed. Springfield, IL: Charles C Thomas, 1993.

Guguchkova PT: Electroretinographic and electrooculographic examinations of persons occupationally exposed to lead. *Vestnik Oftalmolog* 85:60–65, 1972.

Hammond CJ, Snieder H, Spector TD, Gilbert CE: Genetic and environmental factors in age-related nuclear cataracts in monozygotic twins. *N Engl J Med* 342:1786–1790, 2000.

Hanninen H, Nurminen M, Tolonen M, Martelin T: Psychological tests as indicators of excessive exposure to carbon disulfide. *Scand J Work Environ* 19:163–174, 1978.

Hansen ON, Trillingsgaard A, Beese I, *et al.*: A neuropsychological study of children with elevated dentine lead level: Assessment of the effect of lead in different socioeconomic groups. *Neurotoxicol Teratol* 11:205–213, 1989.

Harroff HH: Pathological processes of the eye related to chemical exposure, in Hobson DW (ed): *Dermal and Ocular Toxicity: Fundamentals and Methods.* Boca Raton, FL: CRC Press, 1991, pp. 493–508.

Hart WM: *Adler's Physiology of the Eye,* 9th ed. St. Louis: Mosby–Year Book, 1992.

Hass GM, Brown DVL, Eisenstein R, Hemmens A: Relation between lead poisoning in rabbit and man. *Am J Pathol* 45:691–727, 1964.

Haustein KO, Oltmanns G, Rietbrock N, Alken RG: Differences in color vision impairment caused by digoxin, digitoxin, or pengitoxin. *J Cardiovasc Pharmacol* 4:536–541, 1982.

Haustein KO, Schmidt C: Differences in color discrimination between three cardioactive glycosides. *Int J Clin Pharmacol Ther Toxicol* 26:517–520, 1988.

Hayreh MM, Hayreh SS, Baumbach GL, *et al.*: Ocular toxicity of methanol: An experimental study, in Merigan WH, Weiss B (eds): *Neurotoxicity of the Visual System.* New York: Raven Press, 1980, pp. 33–53.

He L, Poblenz AT, Medrano CJ, Fox DA: Lead and calcium produce photoreceptor cell apoptosis by opening the mitochondrial permeability transition pore. *J Biol Chem* 275:12175–12184, 2000.

Hedges TR III, Hirano M, Tucker K, Caballero B: Epidemic optic and peripheral neuropathy in Cuba: A unique geopolitical public health problem. *Surv Ophthalmol* 41:341–353, 1997.

Hedges TR III, Sokol S, Tucker K: Optic and peripheral neuropathy in Cuba. *JAMA* 271:662–663, 1994.

Hendrickson A: A morphological comparison of foveal development in man and monkey. *Eye* 6:136–144, 1992.

Hendrickson A, Drucker D: The development of parafoveal and mid-peripheral human retina. *Behav Brain Res* 49:21–31, 1992.

Heng JE, Vorwerk CK, Lessell E, *et al.*: Ethambutol is toxic to retinal ganglion cells via an excitotoxic pathway. *Invest Ophthalmol Vis Sci* 40:190–196, 1999.

Henkes HE, van Lith GHM, Canta LR: Indomethacin retinopathy. *Am J Ophthalmol* 73:846–856, 1972.

Hennekes R, Janssen K, Munoz C, Winneke G: Lead-induced ERG alterations in rats at high and low levels of exposure. *Concepts Toxicol* 4:193–199, 1987.

Herr DW, Boyes WK: Electrophysiological analysis of complex brain systems: Sensory evoked potentials and their generators, in Chang LW, Slikker W (eds): *Neurotoxicology: Approaches and Methods.* New York: Academic Press, 1995, pp. 205–221.

Herr DW, Boyes WK, Dyer RS: Alterations in rat flash and pattern evoked potentials after acute or repeated administration of carbon disulfide. *Fund Appl Toxicol* 18:328–342, 1992.

Hirano M, Odel JG, Lincoff NS: Optic and peripheral neuropathy in Cuba. *JAMA* 271:663, 1994.

Hockwin O, Green K, Rubin LF: *Manual of Oculotoxicity Testing of Drugs.* Stuttgart, Germany: Gustav Fischer Verlag, 1992.

Hogan MJ, Alvarado JA, Weddell JE: *Histology of the Human Eye.* Philadelphia: Saunders, 1971.

Horton JC: The central visual pathways, in Hart WM (ed): *Adler's Physiology of the Eye,* 9th ed. St. Louis: Mosby–Year Book, 1992, pp. 728–772.

Hotta R, Gotto S: A fluorescein angiographic study on micro-angiopathia sulfocarbonica. *Jpn J Ophthalmol* 15:132–139, 1971.

Hudnell HK, Otto DA, House DE: The influence of vision on computerized neurobehavioral test scores: A proposal for improving test protocols. *Neurotoxicol Teratol* 18:391–400, 1996.

Hughes WF, Coogan PS: Pathology of the pigment epithelium and retina in rabbits poisoned with lead. *Am J Pathol* 77:237–254, 1974.

Imai H, Miyata M, Uga S, Ishikawa S: Retinal degeneration in rats exposed to an organophosphate pesticide (fenthion). *Environ Res* 30:453–465, 1983.

Ingemansson SO: Studies on the effect of 4-methylpyrazole on retinal activity in the methanol poisoned monkey by recording the electroretinogram. *Acta Ophthalmol Suppl* 158:1–24, 1983.

Imperia PS, Lazarus HM, Lass JH: Ocular complications of systemic cancer chemotherapy. *Surv Ophthalmol* 34:209–230, 1989.

Interagency Coordinating Committee on the Validation of Alternative Methods (ICCVAM). Expert Panel Evaluation of the Current Validation Status of In Vitro Test Methods for Identifying Ocular Corrosives and Severe Irritants. National Toxicology Program (NTP) Interagency Center for the Evaluation of Alternative Toxicological Methods (NICEATM) National Institute of Environmental Health Sciences National Institutes of Health. U.S. Public Health Service. Department of Health and Human Services. Expert Panel Final Report, March 2005. This document is available electronically at: *http://iccvam.niehs.nih.gov/methods/ ocudocs/EPreport/ocureport.htm.*

Iregren A, Andersson M, Nylén P: Color vision and occupational chemical exposures: I. An overview of tests and effects. *Neurotoxicology* 23:719–733, 2002a.

Iregren A, Andersson M, Nylén P: Color vision and occupational chemical exposures. II. Visual functions in non-exposed subjects. *Neurotoxicology* 23:735–745, 2002b.

Iregren A, Johnson, A-C, Nylén, P: Low-level styrene exposure and color vision in Swedish styrene workers. *Environ Toxicol Pharmacol* 19:511–516, 2005.

Isaac NE, Walker AM, Jick H, Gorman M: Exposure to phenothiazine drugs and risk of cataract. *Arch Ophthalmol* 109:256–260, 1991.

Ishikawa S: Chronic optica-neuropathy due to environmental exposure of organophosphate pesticides (Saku disease): clinical and experimental study. *Nippon Ganka Gakkai Zasshi* 77:1835–1886, 1973.

Ito M, Nishibe Y, Inoue YK: Isolation of Inoue-Melnick virus from cerebrospinal fluid of patients with epidemic neuropathy in Cuba. *Arch Pathol Lab Med* 122:520–522, 1998.

Iwata K: Neuro-ophthalmological findings and a follow-up study in the Agano area, Niigata Pref, in Tsubaki T, Irukayama K (eds): *Minamata Disease: MethylMercury poisoning in Minamata and Niigata, Tokyo.* Tokyo: Kodansha, 1977, pp. 166–185.

Jaanus SD, Bartlett JD, Hiett JA: Ocular effects of systemic drugs, in Bartlett JD, Jaanus SD (eds): *Clinical Ocular Pharmacology,* 3rd ed. Boston: Butterworth-Heinemann, 1995, pp. 957–1006.

Jadhav AL, Ramesh GT: Pb-induced alterations in tyrosine hydroxylase activity in rat brain. *Mol Cell Biochem* 175:137–141, 1997.

Jagle H, Jagle C, Serey L, *et al.*: Visual short-term effects of Viagra: double-blind study in healthy young subjects. *Am J Ophthalmol* 137:842–849, 2004.

Jeyaratnam J, Boey KW, Ong CN, *et al.*: Neuropsychological studies on lead workers in Singapore. *Br J Ind Med* 43:626–629, 1986.

Johns DR, Neufeld MJ, Hedges TR III: Mitochondrial DNA mutations in Cuban optic and peripheral neuropathy. *J Neuroophthalmol* 14:135–140, 1994.

Johns DR, Sadun AA: Cuban epidemic optic neuropathy. Mitochondrial DNA analysis. *J Neuroophthalmol* 14:130–134, 1994.

Johnson MW, Vine AK: Hydroxychloroquine therapy in massive total doses without retinal toxicity. *Am J Ophthalmol* 104:139–144, 1987.

Jones RD, Brenneke CJ, Hoss HE, Loney ML: An electroretinogram protocol for toxicological screening in the canine model. *Toxicol Lett* 70:223–234, 1994.

Kaiser-Kupfer MI, Kupfer C, Rodriques MM: Tamoxifen retinopathy. A clinocopathologic report. *Ophthalmology* 88:89–93, 1981.

Kalloniatis M, Tomisich G: Amino acid neurochemistry of the vertebrate retina. *Prog Retinal Eye Res* 18:811–866, 1999.

Kamel F, Boyes WK, Gladen BC, *et al.*: Retinal degeneration in licensed pesticide applicators. *Am J Ind Med* 37:618–628, 2000.

Karai I, Horiguchi SH, Nishikawa N: Optic atrophy with visual field defect in workers occupationally exposed to lead for 30 years. *J Toxicol Clin Toxicol* 19:409–418, 1982.

Karim AKA, Jacob TJC, Thompson GM: The human lens epithelium, morphological and ultrastructural changes associated with steroid therapy. *Exp Eye Res* 48:215–224, 1989.

Kaufman PL, Alm A: *Adler's Physiology of the Eye,* 10th ed. New York: Mosby Press, 2002.

Kennah HE II, Hignet S, Laux PE, Dorko JD, Barrow CS: An objective procedure for quantitating eye irritation based upon changes of corneal thickness. *Fundam Appl Toxicol* 12:258–268, 1989.

King G, Hirst L, Holmes R: Human corneal and lens aldehyde dehydrogenases. Localization and function(s) of ocular ALDH1 and ALDH3 isozymes. *Adv Exp Med Biol* 463:189–198, 1999.

Kini MM, Cooper JR: Biochemistry of methanol poisoning. 4. The effect of methanol and its metabolites on retinal metabolism. *Biochem J* 82:164–172, 1962.

Kirrane EF, Hoppin JA, Kamel F, *et al.*: Retinal degeneration and other eye disorders in wives of farmer pesticide applicators enrolled in the Agricultural Health Study. *Am J Epidem* 161:1020–1029, 2005.

Klein BE, Klein RE, Lee KE: Incident cataract after a five-year interval and lifestyle factors: The Beaver Dam eye study. *Ophthalm Epidemiol* 6:247–255, 1999.

Ko LS, Shum JT, Chen YL, Wang YS: Pesticides and myopia, a working hypothesis. *Acta Ophthalmol Suppl* 185:145–146, 1988.

Kobel W, Gfeller W: Distribution of eye irritation scores of industrial chemicals. *Food Chem Toxicol* 23:311–312, 1985.

Kohler K, Lilienthal H, Guenther E, *et al.*: Persistent decrease of the dopamine-synthesizing enzyme tyrosine hydroxylase in the rhesus monkey retina after chronic lead exposure. *Neurotoxicology* 18:623–632, 1997.

Koliopoulos J, Palimeris G: On acquired colour vision disturbances during treatment with ethambutol and indomethacin. *Mod Probl Ophthalmol* 11:178–184, 1972.

Krill AE, Potts AM, Johanson CE: Chloroquine retinopathy. Investigation of discrepancy between dark adaptation and electroretinographic findings in advanced stages. *Am J Ophthalmol* 71:530–543, 1971.

Kruszewski FH, Walker TL, DiPasquale LC: Evaluation of a human corneal epithelial cell line as an in vitro model for assessing ocular irritation. *Fundam Appl Toxicol* 36:130–140, 1997.

Kulkarni AS, Hopfinger AJ: Membrane-interaction QSAR analysis: Application to the estimation of eye irritation by organic compounds. *Pharm Res* 16:1245–1253, 1999.

Lambert LA, Chambers WA, Green S, *et al.*: The use of low-volume dosing in the eye irritation test. *Food Chem Toxicol* 31:99–103, 1993.

Lapalus P, Garaffo RG: Ocular pharmacokinetics, in Hockwin O, Green K, Rubin LF (eds): *Manual of Oculotoxicity Testing of Drugs.* Stuttgart, Germany: Gustav Fischer Verlag, 1992, pp. 119–136.

Larsby B, Tham R, Eriksson B, *et al.*: Effects of trichloroethylene on the human vestibulo-oculomotor system. *Acta Otololaryngol (Stockholm)* 101:193–199, 1986.

Lasley SM, Lane JD: Diminished regulation of mesolimbic dopaminergic activity in rat after chronic inorganix lead exposure. *Toxicol Appl Pharmacol* 95:474–483, 1988.

Laties A, Zrenner E: Viagra (sildenafil citrate) and ophthalmology. *Prog Retin Eye Res* 21:485–506, 2002.

LaVail MM: Rod outer segment disk shedding in rat retina: Relationship to cyclic lighting. *Science* 194:1071–1074, 1976.

LaVail MM, Gorrin GM, Repaci MA, Yasumura D: Light-induced retinal degeneration in albino mice and rats: Strain and species differences. *Prog Clin Biol Res* 247:439–454, 1987.

Lazzaroni F, Scorolli L, Pizzoleo CF, *et al.*: Tamoxifen retinopathy: Does it really exist? *Graefes Arch Clin Exp Ophthalmol* 236:669–673, 1998.

Lee AY, Chung SS: Involvement of aldose reductase in naphthalene cataract. *Invest Ophthalmol Vis Sci* 39:193–197, 1998.

Lee EW, Garner CD, Terzo TS: A rat model manifesting methanol-induced visual dysfunction suitable for both acute and long-term exposure studies. *Toxicol Appl Pharmacol* 128:199–206, 1994b.

Lee EW, Garner CD, Terzo TS: Animal model for the study of methanol toxicity: Comparison of folate-reduced rat responses with published monkey data. *J Toxicol Environ Health* 41:71–82, 1994a.

Lee JW, Fuda H, Javitt NB, Strott CA, Rodriguez IR. Expression and localization of sterol 27-hydroxylase (CYP27A1) in monkey retina. *Exp Eye Res* 83:465–469, 2006.

Leske MC, Chylack LT Jr, Wu SY: The lens opacities case-control study. Risk factors for cataract. *Arch Ophthalmol* 109:244–251, 1991.

Lessell S: Toxic and deficiency optic neuropathies, in Miller NR, Newman NJ (eds): *Walsh and Hoyt's Clinical Neuro-Ophthalmology,* 5th ed. Baltimore: Williams & Wilkins, 1998.

Lilienthal H, Kohler K, Turfeld M, Winneke G: Persistent increases in scotopic b-wave amplitudes after lead exposure in monkeys. *Exp Eye Res* 59:203–209, 1994.

Lilienthal H, Lenaerts C, Winneke G, Hennekes R: Alteration of the visual evoked potential and the electroretinogram in lead-treated monkeys. *Neurotoxicol Teratol* 10:417–422, 1988.

Linsenmeier RA: Effects of light and darkness on oxygen distribution and consumption in the cat retina. *J Gen Physiol* 88:521–542, 1986.

Lissner W, Greenlee JE, Cameron JD, Goren SB: Localization of tritiated digoxin in the rat eye. *Am J Ophthalmol* 72:608–614, 1971.

Lou MF, Xu GT, Zigler S Jr, York B Jr: Inhibition of naphthalene cataract in rats by aldose reductase inhibitors. *Curr Eye Res* 15:423–432, 1996.

Lufkin MW, Harrison CE, Henderson JW, Ogle KN: Ocular distribution of digoxin-3H in the cat. *Am J Ophthalmol* 64:1134–1140, 1967.

Lyle WM: Drugs and conditions which may affect color vision: Part 1. Drugs and chemicals. *J Am Ophthalmol Soc* 45:47–60, 1974.

Lynch JJ III, Eskin TA, Merigan WH: Selective degeneration of the parvocellular-projecting retinal ganglion cells in a New World monkey, Saimiri sciureus. *Brain Res* 499:325–332, 1989.

Lynch JJ III, Silveira LC, Perry VH, Merigan WH: Visual effects of damage to P ganglion cells in macaques. *Vis Neurosci* 8:575–583, 1992.

Madreperla SA, Johnson MA, Nakatani K: Electrophysiological and electroretinographic evidence for phototreceptor dysfunction as a toxic effect of digoxin. *Arch Ophthalmol* 112:807–812, 1994.

Marks MJ, Seeds NW: A heterogeneous ouabain-ATPase interaction in mouse brain. *Life Sci* 23:2735–2744, 1978.

Marmor MF, Arden GB, Nilsson SEG, Zrenner E: International standardization committee. Standards for clinical electroretinography. *Arch Ophthalmol* 107:816–819, 1989.

Marmor MF, Zrenner E: Standard for clinical electroretinography (1994 update). *Doc Ophthalmol* 89:199–210, 1995.

Martin-Amat G, McMartin KE, Hayreh SS, et al.: Methanol poisoning: Ocular toxicity produced by formate. *Toxicol Appl Pharmacol* 45:201–208, 1978.

Mas P, Pelegrino JL, Guzman MG, et al.: Viral isolation from cases of epidemic neuropathy in Cuba. *Arch Pathol Lab Med* 121:825–833, 1997.

Mastyugin V, Aversa E, Bonazzi A, et al.: Hypoxia-induced production of 12-hydroxyeicosanoids in the corneal epithelium: Involvement of a cytochrome P-4504B1 isoform. *J Pharmacol Exp Ther* 289:1611–1619, 1999.

Mattsson JL, Boyes WK, Ross JF: Incorporating evoked potentials into neurotoxicity test schemes, in Tilson HA, Mitchell CL (eds): *Target Organ Toxicology Series: Neurotoxicity.* New York: Raven Press, 1992, pp. 125–145.

Maurer JK, Parker RD: Light microscopic comparison of surfactant-induced eye irritation in rabbits and rats at three hours and recovery at day 35. *Toxicol Pathol* 24:403–411, 1996.

Maurer JK, Parker RD, Carr GJ: Ocular irritation: Microscopic changes occurring over time in the rat with surfactants of known irritancy. *Toxicol Pathol* 26:217–225, 1998.

Maurissen JPJ: Neurobehavioral methods for the evaluation of sensory functions, in Chang LW, Slikker W (eds): *Neurotoxicology: Approaches and Methods.* New York: Academic Press, 1995, pp. 239–264.

McCulley JP: Chemical injuries of the eye, in Leibowitz HM, Waring GO (eds): *Corneal Disorders, Clinical Diagnosis and Management,* 2nd ed. Philadelphia: Saunders, 1998, pp. 770–790.

McGrail KM, Sweadner KJ: Complex expression patterns for Na+, K+-ATPase isoforms in retina and optic nerve. *Eur J Neurosci* 2:170–176, 1989.

Medrano CJ, Fox DA: Oxygen consumption in rat outer and inner retina: Light- and pharmacologically induced inhibition. *Exp Eye Res* 61:273–284, 1995.

Medrano CJ, Fox DA: Substrate-dependent effects of calcium on rat retinal mitochondria respiration: Physiological and toxicological studies. *Toxicol Appl Pharmacol* 125:309–321, 1994.

Meier-Ruge W: Drug induced retinopathy. *CRC Toxicol* 1:325–360, 1972.

Mergler D: Color vision loss: A sensitive indicator of the severity of optic neuropathy, in Anger WK (ed): *Advances in Neurobehavioral Toxicology: Applications in Environmental and Occupational Health.* Chelsea, MI: Lewis Publishers, 1990, pp. 175–183.

Mergler D, Belanger S, Grosbois S, Vachon N: Chromal focus of acquired chromatic discrimination loss and slovent exposure among printshop workers. *Toxicology* 49:341–348, 1988.

Mergler D, Blain L, Lagace JP: Solvent related colour vision loss: An indicator of damage? *Int Arch Occup Environ Health* 59:313–321, 1987.

Mergler D, Huel G, Bowler R, et al.: Visual dysfunction among former microelectronics assembly workers. *Arch Environ Health* 46:326–334, 1991.

Merigan WH: Effects of toxicants on visual systems. *Neurobehav Toxicol* 1(suppl 1):15–22, 1979.

Merigan WH, Weiss B: *Neurotoxicity of the Visual System.* New York: Raven Press, 1980.

Merigan WH, Eskin TA: Spatio-temporal vision of macaques with severe loss of P beta retinal ganglion cells. *Vision Res* 26:1751–1761, 1986.

Merigan WH, Wood RW, Zehl D, Eskin TA: Carbon disulfide effects on the visual system: I. Visual thresholds and ophthalmoscopy. *Invest Ophthalmol Vis Sci* 29:512–518, 1988.

Misra UK, Nag D, Misra NK, et al.: Some observations on the macula of pesticide workers. *Hum Toxicol* 4:135–145, 1985.

Mojon DS, Kaufmann P, Odel JG, et al.: Clinical course of a cohort in the Cuban epidemic optic and peripheral neuropathy. *Neurology* 48:19–22, 1997.

Möller C, Odkvist L, Larsby B, et al.: Otoneurological findings in workers exposed to styrene. *Scand J Work Environ Health* 16:189–194, 1990.

Moser VC, Boyes WK: Prolonged neurobehavioral and visual effects of short-term exposure to 3,3'-iminodipropionitrile (IDPN) in rats. *Fund Appl Toxicol* 21:277–290, 1993.

Moser VC, Phillips PM, Morgan DL, Sills RC: Carbon disulfide neurotoxicity in rats: VII. Behavioral evaluations using a functional observational battery. *Neurotoxicology* 19:147–158, 1998.

Muñoz H, Romiew I, Palazuelos E, et al.: Blood lead level and neurobehavioral development among children living in Mexico City. *Arch Environ Health* 48:132–139, 1993.

Murano H, Kojima M, Sasaki K: Differences in naphthalene cataract formation between albino and pigmented rat eyes. *Ophthalm Res* 25:16–22, 1993.

Murata K, Araki S, Yokoyama K, et al.: Assessment of central, peripheral, and autonomic nervous system functions in lead workers: Neuroelectrophysiological studies. *Environ Res* 61:323–336, 1993.

Murray TG, Burton TC, Rajani C, et al.: Methanol poisoning. A rodent model with structural and functional evidence for retinal involvement. *Arch Ophthalmol* 109:1012–1016, 1991.

Nakamura K, Fujiki T, Tamura HO: Age, gender and region-specific differences in drug metabolising enzymes in rat ocular tissues. *Exp Eye Res* 81:710–715, 2005.

Nakatsuka H, Watanabe T, Takeuchi Y, et al.: Absence of blue-yellow color vision loss among workers exposed to toluene or tetrachloroethylene, mostly at levels below occupational exposure limits. *Int Arch Occup Environ Health* 64:113–117, 1992.

National Institute of Environmental Health Sciences (NIEHS): Corrositex: *An In Vitro Test Method for Assessing Dermal Corrosivity Potential of Chemicals: The Results of an Independent Peer Review Evaluation.* NIH Publication No. 99-4495. Research Triangle Park, NC: NIEHS, 1999. Also at: *http://iccvam.niehs.nih.gov/corprrep.htm.*

National Institute of Environmental Health Sciences (NIEHS): *Validation and Regulatory Acceptance of Toxicological Test Methods: A Report of the ad hoc Interagency Coordinating Committee on the Validation of Alternative Methods.* NIH Publication No. 97-3981. Research Triangle Park, NC: NIEHS, 1997. Also at: *http://ntp-server.niehs. nih.gov/htdocs/ICCVAM/iccvam.html.*

Newman NJ, Torroni A, Brown MD, et al.: Epidemic neuropathy in Cuba not associated with mitochondrial DNA mutations found in Leber's hereditary optic neuropathy patients. Cuba Neuropathy Field Investation Team. *Am J Ophthalmol* 118:158–168, 1994.

Nicholls P: The effect of formate on cytochrome aa3 and on electron transport in the intact respiratory chain. *Biochim Biophys Acta* 430:13–29, 1976.

Niklasson M, Tham R, Larsby B, Eriksson B: Effects of toluene, styrene, trichloroethylene, and trichloroethane on the vestibulo- and opto-oculomotor system in rats. *Neurotoxicol Teratol* 15:327–334, 1993.

Noureddin BN, Seoud M, Bashshur Z, et al.: Ocular toxicity in low-dose tamoxifen: A prospective study. *Eye* 13:729–733, 1999.

Novack GD: Emerging drugs for ophthalmic diseases. *Expert Opin Emerg Drugs* 8:251–266, 2003.

Oberto A, Marks N, Evans HL, Guidotti A: Lead promotes apoptosis in newborn rat cerebellar neurons: Pathological implications. *J Pharmacol Exp Ther* 279:435–442, 1996.

Odkvist L, Larsby B, Tham R, Hyden D: Vestibulo-oculomotor disturbances caused by industrial solvents. *Otololaryngol Head Neck Surg* 91:537–539, 1983.

Ogden TE, Schachat AP: *Retina. Basic Science and Inherited Diseases.* Vol 1. St. Louis: Mosby, 1989.

Ottlecz A, Garcia CA, Eichberg J, Fox DA: Alterations in retinal Na+,K+-ATPase in diabetes: Streptozotocin-induced and Zucker diabetic fatty rats. *Curr Eye Res* 12:1111–1121, 1993.

Otto DA: The assessment of neurotoxicity in children. Electrophysiological methods. *Monogr Am Assoc Ment Defic* 8:139–158, 1987.

Otto DA, Fox DA: Auditory and visual dysfunction following lead exposure. *Neurotoxicology* 14:191–208, 1993.

Otto DA, Robinson G, Baumann S, et al.: 5-year follow-up study of children with low-to-moderate lead absorption: Electrophysiological evaluation. *Environ Res* 38:168–186, 1985.

Ottonello S, Foroni C, Carta A, et al.: Oxidative stress and age-related cataract. *Ophthalmologica* 214:78–85, 2000.

Palacz O, Szymanska K, Czepita D: Studies on the ERG in subjects with chronic exposure to carbon disulfide: I. Assessment of the condition of the visual system taking into account ERG findings depending on the duration of exposure to CS2. *Klin Oczna* 82:65–68, 1980.

Palimeris G, Koliopoulos J, Velissaropoulos P: Ocular side effects of indomethacin. *Ophthalmologica* 164:339–353, 1972.

Patterson CA, Delamere NA: The lens, in Hart WM (ed): *Adler's Physiology of the Eye,* 9th ed. St. Louis: Mosby–Year Book, 1992, pp. 348–390.

Paramei GV, Meyer-Baron M, Seeber A: Impairments of colour vision induced by organic solvents: A meta-analysis study. NeuroToxicology 25:803–816, 2004.

Pavlidis NA, Petris C, Briassoulis E, et al.: Clear evidence that long-term, low-dose tamoxifen treatment can induce ocular toxicity. A prospective study of 63 patients. *Cancer* 69:2961–2964, 1992.

Peiffer RL, McCary B, Bee W, et al.: Contemporary methods in ocular toxicology. *Toxicol Methods* 10:17–39, 2000.

Penn JS, Naash MI, Anderson RE: Effect of light history on retinal antioxidants and light damage susceptibility in the rat. *Exp Eye Res* 44:779–788, 1987.

Penn JS, Thum LA, Naash MI: Photoreceptor physiology in the rat is governed by the light environment. *Exp Eye Res* 49:205–215, 1989.

Penn JS, Williams TP: Photostasis: Regulation of daily photon-catch by rat retinas in response to various cyclic illuminances. *Exp Eye Res* 43:915–928, 1986.

Pepose JS, Ubels JL: The Cornea, in Hart WM (ed): *Adler's Physiology of the Eye,* 9th ed. St. Louis: Mosby–Year Book, 1992, pp. 29–70.

Petit TL, LeBoutillier JC: Effects of lead exposure during development on neocortical dendritic and synaptic structure. *Exp Neurol* 64:482–492, 1979.

Piltz JR, Wertenbaker C, Lance SE, et al.: Digoxin toxicity. Recognizing the varied visual presentations. *J Clin Neuroophthalmol* 13:275–280, 1993.

Polak BC, Leys M, van Lith GH: Blue-yellow colour vision changes as early symptoms of ethambutol oculotoxicity. *Ophthalmologica* 191:223–226, 1985.

Porkony J, Smith VS, Verriest G, Pinckers A: *Congenital and Acquired Color Vision Defects.* New York: Grune & Stratton, 1979.

Potts AM: The reaction of uveal pigment in vitro with polycyclic compounds. *Invest Ophthalmol* 3:405–416, 1964.

Potts AM: The visual toxicity of methanol: VI. The clinical aspects of experimental methanol poisoning treated with base. *Am J Ophthalmol* 39:76–82, 1955.

Potts AM: Toxic responses of the eye, in Klaassen CD (ed): *Casarett and Doull's Toxicology: The Basic Science of Poisons,* 5th ed. New York: McGraw-Hill, 1996, pp. 583–615.

Potts AM, Au PC: The affinity of melanin for inorganic ions. *Exp Eye Res* 22:487–491, 1976.

Pounds, JG: Effect of lead intoxication on calcium homeostasis and calcium-mediated cell function: A review. *Neurotoxicology* 5:295–332, 1984.

Powers MK, Green DG: Single retinal ganglion cell responses in the dark-reared rat: Grating acuity, contrast sensitivity, and defocusing. *Vision Res* 18:1533–1539, 1978.

Puro DG: Cholinergic systems, in Morgan WW (ed): *Retinal Transmitters and Modulators: Models for the Brain.* Vol 1. Boca Raton, FL: CRC Press, 1985.

Raedler A, Sievers J: The development of the visual system of the albino rat. *Adv Anat Embryol Cell Biol* 50:7–87, 1975.

Raitta C, Seppalainen AN, Huuskonen MS: *n*-hexane maculopathy in industrial workers. *Von Graefes Arch Klin Exp Ophthalmol* 209:99–110, 1978.

Raitta C, Teir H, Tolonen M, Nurminen M, Helpio E, Malmstrom S: Impaired color discrimination among viscose rayon workers exposed to carbon disulfide. *J Occup Med* 23:189–192, 1981.

Raitta C, Tolonen M, Nurminen M: Microcirculation of ocular fundus in viscose rayon workers exposed to carbon disulfide. *Arch Klin Exp Ophthalmol* 191:151–164, 1974.

Ramsey MS, Fine BS: Chloroquine toxicity in the human eye. Histopathologic observations by electron microscopy. *Am J Ophthalmol* 73:229–235, 1972.

Rao GN: Light intensity-associated eye lesions of Fisher 344 rats in long-term studies. *Toxicol Pathol* 19:148–155, 1991.

Rapp LM, Tolman BL, Koutz CA, Thum LA: Predisposing factors to light-induced photoreceptor cell damage: Retinal changes in maturing rats. *Exp Eye Res* 51:177–184, 1990.

Rauen T, Rothstein JD, Wässle H: Differential expression of three glutamate transporters subtypes in the rat retina. *Cell Tissue Res* 286:325–336, 1996.

Rebert CS: Multisensory evoked potentials in experimental and applied neurotoxicology. *Neurobehav Toxicol Teratol* 5:659–671, 1983.

Reuhl KR, Rice DC, Gilbert SG, Mallett J: Effects of chronic developmental lead exposure on monkey neuroanatomy: Visual system. *Toxicol Appl Pharmacol* 99:501–509, 1989.

Rice DC: Effects of lifetime lead exposure on spatial and temporal visual function in monkeys. *Neurotoxicology* 19:893–902, 1998.

Rice DC: Sensory and cognitive effects of developmental methylmercury exposure in monkeys, and a comparison to effects in rodents. *Neurotoxicology* 17:139–154, 1996.

Rice DC, Gilbert SG: Early chronic low-level methylmercury poisoning in monkeys impairs spatial vision. *Science* 216:759–761, 1982.

Rice DC, Gilbert SG: Effects of developmental exposure to methylmercury on spatial and temporal visual function in monkeys. *Toxicol Appl Pharmacol* 102:151–163, 1990.

Rice DC, Hayward S: Comparison of visual function at adulthood and during aging in monkeys exposed to lead or methylmercury. *Neurotoxicology* 20:767–784, 1999.

Rietbrock N, Alken RG: Color vision deficiencies: A common sign of intoxication in chronically digoxin-treated patients. *J Cardiovasc Pharmacol* 2:93–99, 1980.

Roberts JE: Ocular phototoxicity. *J Photochem Photobiol B* 64:136–43, 2001.

Roberts JE: Screening for ocular phototoxicity. *Int J Toxicol* 21:491–500, 2002.

Robertson DM, Hollenhorst RW, Callahan JA: Ocular manifestations of digitalis toxicity. *Arch Ophthalmol* 76:640–645, 1966a.

Robertson DM, Hollenhorst RW, Callahan JA: Receptor function in digitalis toxicity. *Arch Ophthalmol* 76:852–857, 1966b.

Rodieck RW: *The First Steps in Seeing.* Sunderland, MA: Sinuaer, 1998.

Rogers JM, Chernoff N: Chemically induced cataracts in the fetus and neonate, in Kacew S, Lock S (eds): *Toxicologic and Pharmacologic Principles in Pediatrics.* New York: Hemisphere, 1988, pp. 255–275.

Roman G: Tropical myeloneuropathies revisited. *Curr Opin Neurol* 11:539–544, 1998.

Rosenthal AR, Kolb H, Bergsma D, et al.: Chloroquine retinopathy in the Rhesus monkey. *Invest Ophthalmol Vis Sci* 17:1158–1175, 1978.

Rosolen SG, Rigaudiere F, Le Gargasson JF, Brigell MG: Recommendations for a toxicological screening ERG procedure in laboratory animals. *Doc Ophthalmol* 110:57–66, 2005.

Rothenberg SJ, Schnaas L, Salgado-Valladares M, et al.: Increased ERG a- and b-wave amplitudes in 7–10 year old children resulting from prenatal lead exposure. *Invest Ophthalmol Vis Sci* 43:2036–2044, 2002.

Rouslin W, Broge CW, Chernyak BV: Effects of Zn$_{2+}$ on the activity and binding of the mitochondrial ATPase inhibitor protein, IF1. *J Bioenerg Biomembr* 25:297–306, 1993.

Ruan DY, Tang LX, Zhao C, Guo YJ: Effects of low-level lead on retinal ganglion sustained and transient cells in developing rats. *Neurotoxicol Teratol* 16:47–53, 1994.

Ruedeman AD: The electroretinogram in chronic methyl alcohol poisoning in human beings. *Trans Am Ophthalmol Soc* 59:480–529, 1961.

Sadun AA, Martone JF, Muci-Mendoza R, et al.: Epidemic optic neuropathy in Cuba. Eye findings. *Arch Ophthalmol* 112:691–699, 1994a.

Sadun AA, Martone JF, Reyes L, et al.: Optic and peripheral neuropathy in Cuba. *JAMA* 271:663–664, 1994b.

Sadun AA: Acquired mitochondrial impairment as a cause of optic nerve disease. *Trans Am Ophthalmol Soc* 96:881–923, 1998.

Salmon JF, Carmichael TR, Welsh NH: Use of contrast sensitivity measurement in the detection of subclinical ethambutol toxic optic neuropathy. *Br J Ophthalmol* 71:192–196, 1987.

Santaella RM, Fraunfelder FW: Ocular adverse effects associated with systemic medications: Recognition and management. *Drugs* 67:75–93, 2007.

Santos-Anderson RM, Tso MOM, Valdes JJ, Annau Z: Chronic lead administration in neonatal rats. Electron microscopy of the retina. *J Neuropathol Exp Neurol* 43:175–187, 1984.

Sassaman FW, Cassidy JT, Alpern M, Maaseidvaag F: Electroretinography in patients with connective tissue diseases treated with hydroxychloroquine. *Am J Ophthalmol* 70:515–523, 1970.

Sato S: Aldose reductase the major protein associated with naphthalene dihydrodiol dehydrogenase activity in rat lens. *Invest Ophthalmol Vis Sci* 34:3172–3178, 1993.

Sato S, Sugiyama K, Lee YS, Kador PF: Prevention of naphthalene-1,2-dihydrodiol-induced lens protein modifications by structurally diverse aldose reductase inhibitors. *Exp Eye Res* 68:601–608, 1999.

Sborgia G, Assennato G, L'Abbate N, et al.: Comprehensive neurophysiological evaluation of lead-exposed workers, in Gilioli R, Cassito M, Foa V (eds): *Neurobehavioral Methods in Occupational Health.* New York: Pergamon Press, 1983, pp. 283–294.

Schmid KE, Kornek GV, Scheithauer W, Binder S: Update on ocular complications of systemic cancer chemotherapy. *Surv Ophthalmol* 51:19-40, 2006.

Schnapf JL, Kraft TW, Nunn BJ, Baylor DA: Spectral sensitivity of primate photoreceptors. *Vis Neurosci* 1:255–261, 1988.

Schneider BG, Kraig E: Na+,K+-ATPase of the photoreceptor: Selective expression of α3 and β2 isoforms. *Exp Eye Res* 51:553–564, 1990.

Schneider BG, Shygan AW, Levinson R: Co-localization and polarized distribution of Na, K-ATPase: α3 and β2 subunits in photoreceptor cells. *J Histochem Cytochem* 39:507–517, 1991.

Scholl HPN, Zrenner E: Electrophysiology in the investigation of acquired retinal disorders. *Surv Ophthalmol* 45:29–47, 2000.

Schreiber JS, Hudnell HK, Geller AM, et al.: Apartment residents' and day care workers' exposures to tetrachloroethylene and deficits in visual contrast sensitivity. *Environ Health Perspect* 110:655–664, 2002.

Schwartzmann ML: Cytochrome P450 and arachidonic acid metabolism in the corneal epithelium, in Green K, Edelhauser HF, Hackett RB, et al. (eds): *Advances in Ocular Toxicology.* New York: Plenum Press, 1997, pp. 3–20.

Schwartzman ML, Balazy M, Masferrer J, et al.: 12(R)-hydroxyicosatetraenoic acid: A cytochrome-P450–dependent arachidonate metabolite that inhibits Na+,K+-ATPase in the cornea. *Proc Natl Acad Sci USA* 84:8125–8129, 1987.

Scortegagna M, Hanbauer I: The effect of lead exposure and serum deprivation on mesencephalic primary cultures. *Neurotoxicology* 18:331–340, 1997.

Sears ML: *Pharmacology of the Eye.* Berlin: Springer-Verlag, 1984.

Seme MT, Summerfelt P, Henry MM, et al.: Formate-induced inhibition of photoreceptor function in methanol intoxication. *J Pharmacol Exp Ther* 289:361–370, 1999.

Seppalainen AM, Haltia M: Carbon disulfide, in Spencer PS, Schaumberg HH (eds): *Experimental and Clinical Neurotoxicology.* Baltimore: William & Wilkins, 1980, pp. 356–373.

Shanthaverrappa TR, Bourne GH: Monoamine oxidase distribution in the rabbit eye. *J Histochem Cytochem* 12:281–287, 1964.

Shearer RV, Dubois EL: Ocular changes induced by long-term hydroxychloroquine (Plaqenil) therapy. *Am J Ophthalmol* 64:245–252, 1967.

Sherer JW: Lead ablyopia with cataract from the same source. *J Missouri State Med Assoc* 32:275–277, 1935.

Shichi H, Atlas SA, Nebert DW: Genetically regulated aryl hydrocarbon hydroxylase induction in the eye: Possible significance of the drug-metabolizing enzyme system for the retinal pigmented epithelium-choroid. *Exp Eye Res* 21:557–567, 1975.

Shichi H, Nebert DW: Genetic differences in drug metabolism associated with ocular toxicity. *Environ Health Perspect* 44:107–117, 1982.

Shichi H: Immunocytochemical study of cytochrome P450 4A induction in mouse eye. *Exp Eye Res* 63:747–751, 1996.

Shulman LM, Fox DA: Dopamine inhibits mammalian photoreceptor Na+,K+-ATPase activity via a selective effect on the α3 isozyme. *Proc Natl Acad Sci USA* 93:8034–8039, 1996.

Signorino M, Scarpino O, Provincialli L, et al.: Modification of the electroretinogram and of different components of the visual evoked potentials in workers exposed to lead. *Ital Electroencephalogr J* 10:51P, 1983.

Sillman AJ, Bolnick DA, Bosetti JB, et al.: The effects of lead and cadmium on the mass photoreceptor potential the dose-response relationship. *Neurotoxicology* 3:179–194, 1982.

Singh AK, Shichi H: A novel glutathione peroxidase in bovine eye. Sequence analysis, mRNA level, and translation. *J Biol Chem* 273:26171–26178, 1998.

Sjoersdma T, Kamermans M, Spekreijse H: Effect of the tuberculostaticum ethambutol and stimulus intensity on chromatic discrimination in man. *Vision Res* 39:2955–2962, 1999.

Sonkin N: Stippling of the retina: A new physical sign in the early dignosis of lead poisoning. *N Engl J Med* 269:779–780, 1963.

Specchio LM, Bellomo R, Dicuonzo F, et al.: Smooth pursuit eye movements among storage battery workers. *Clin Toxicol* 18:1269–1276, 1981.

Spector A: Oxidative stress and disease. *J Ocul Pharmacol Ther* 16:193–201, 2000.

Spencer PS, Schaumburg HH: A review of acrylamide neurotoxicity: Part I. Properties, uses and human exposure. *Can J Neurol Sci* 1:145–150, 1974a.

Spencer PS, Schaumburg HH: A review of acrylamide neurotoxicity: Part II. Experimental animal neuorotoxicity and pathologic mechanisms. *Can J Neurol Sci* 1:152–169, 1974b.

Spivey GH, Baloh RW, Brown CP, et al.: Subclinical effects of chronic increased lead absorption—a prospective study: III. Neurologic findings at follow-up examination. *J Occup Med* 22:607–612, 1980.

Srivastava D, Fox DA, Hurwitz RL: Effects of magnesium on cyclic GMP hydrolysis by the bovine retinal rod cyclic GMP phosphodiesterase. *Biochem J* 308:653–658, 1995a.

Srivastava D, Hurwitz RL, Fox DA: Lead- and calcium-mediated inhibition of bovine rod cGMP phosphodiesterase: Interactions with magnesium. *Toxicol Appl Pharmacol* 134:43–52, 1995b.

Srivastava SK, Singhal SS, Awasthi S, et al.: A glutathione S-transferases isozyme (bGST 5.8) involved in the metabolism of 4-hydroxy-2-trans-nonenal is localized in bovine lens epithelium. Exp Eye Res 63:329–337, 1996.

Sugai S, Murata K, Kitagaki T, Tomita I: Studies on eye irritation caused by chemicals in rabbits—1. A quantitative structure-activity relationships approach to primary eye irritation of chemicals in rabbits. J Toxicol Sci 15:245–262, 1990.

Sweadner KJ: Isozymes of Na+/K+-ATPase. Biochem Biophys Acta 989:185–220, 1989.

Szabo I, Bernardi P, Zoratti M: Modulation of the mitochondrial megachannel by divalent cations and protons. J Biol Chem 267:2940–2946, 1992.

Takeuchi T, Eto K: Pathology and pathogenesis of Minamata disease, in Tsubaki T, Irukayama K (eds): Minamata Disease: Methylmercury poisoning in Minamata and Niigata, Japan. Tokyo: Kodansha; Amsterdam: Elsevier, 1977, pp. 103–141.

Tandon P, Padilla S, Barone S Jr, et al.: Fenthion produces a persistent decrease in muscarinic receptor function in the adult rat retina. Toxicol Appl Pharmacol 125:271–280, 1994.

Taylor A, Nowell T: Oxidative stress and antioxidant function in relation to risk for cataract. Adv Pharmacol 38:515–536, 1997.

Tennekoon G, Aitchison CS, Frangia J, et al.: Chronic lead intoxication: Effects on developing optic nerve. Ann Neurol 5:558–564, 1979.

Tephly TR, McMatin KE: Methanol metabolism, in Stegnik LD, Filer LJ Jr (eds): Aspartame: Physiology and Biochemistry. New York: Marcel Dekker, 1984, pp. 111–140.

Tessier-Lavigne M, Mobbs P, Attwell D: Lead and mercury toxicity and the rod light response. Invest Ophthalmol Vis Sci 26:1117–1123, 1985.

Thaler JS, Curinga R, Kiracofe G: Relation of graded ocular anterior chamber pigmentation to phenothiazine intake in schizophrenics—Quantification procedures. Am J Optom Physiol Ophthalmol 62:600–604, 1985.

Tham R, Bunnfors I, Eriksson B, et al.: Vestibulo-ocular disturbances in rats exposed to organic solvents. Acta Pharmacol Toxicol 54:58–63, 1984.

Thirkill CE, Roth AM, Keltner JL: Cancer-associated retinopathy. Arch Ophthalmol 105: 372–375, 1987.

Till C, Rovet JF, Koren G, Westall CA. Assessment of visual functions following prenatal exposure to organic solvents. Neurotoxicology 24:725–731, 2003.

Toews AD, Krigman MR, Thomas DJ, Morell P: Effect of inorganic lead exposure on myelination in the rat. Neurochem Res 5:605–616, 1980.

Ulshafer RJ, Allen CB, Rubin ML: Distributions of elements in the human retinal pigment epithelium. Arch Ophthalmol 108:113–117, 1990.

United States Environmental Protection Agency (EPA): Prevention, Pesticides and Toxic Substances (7101). EPA 712-C-98-242. Health Effects Test Guideline. OPPTS 870.6855. Neurophysiology: Sensory Evoked Potentials. August 1998a. Also at: http://www.epa.gov/docs/OPPTS_Harmonized/870_Health_Effects_Test_Guidelines/Series/.

United States Environmental Protection Agency (EPA): Prevention, Pesticides and Toxic Substances (7101). EPA 712–C–98–238. Health Effects Test Guideline. OPPTS 870.6200. Neurotoxicity Screening Battery. August 1998b. Also at: http://www.epa.gov/docs/OPPTS_Harmonized/870_Health_Effects_Test_Guidelines/Series/.

Urban RC, Cotlier E: Corticosteroid-induced cataracts. Surv Ophthalmol 31:102–110, 1986.

Vale RD, Banker G, Hall ZW: The neuronal cytoskeleton, in Hall ZW (ed): An Introduction to Molecular Neurobiology. Sunderland, MA: Sinauer, 1992, pp. 247–280.

van Dijk BW, Spekreijse H: Ethambutol changes the color coding of carp retinal ganglion cells reversibly. Invest Ophthalmol Vis Sci 24:128–133, 1983.

van Heyningen R, Pirie A: The metabolism of naphthalene and its toxic effect on the eye. Biochem J 102:842–852, 1967.

Vanhoorne M, De Rouck A, Bacquer D: Epidemiological study of the systemic ophthalmological effects of carbon disulfide. Arch Environ Health 51:181–188, 1996.

van Soest S, Westerveld A, de Jong PT, et al.: Retinitis pigmentosa: Defined from a molecular point of view. Surv Ophthalmol 43:321–334, 1999.

Veenstra DL, Best JH, Hornberger J, et al.: Incidence and long-term cost of steroid-related side effects after renal transplantation. Am J Kidney Dis 33:829–839, 1999.

Vettori MV, Corradi D, Coccini T, et al.: Styrene-induced changes in amacrine retinal cells: an experimental study in the rat. Neurotoxicology 21:607–614, 2000.

Vidyasagar TR: Optic nerve components may not be equally susceptible to damage by acrylamide. Brain Res 224:452–455, 1981.

Walkowiak J, Altmann L, Kramer U, et al.: Cognitive and sensorimotor functions in 6-year-old children in relation to lead and mercury levels: Adjustment for intelligence and contrast sensitivity in computerized testing. Neurotoxicol Teratol 20:511–521, 1998.

Waltman S, Sears ML: Catechol-O-methyltransferase and monoamine oxidase activity in the ocular tissues of albino rabbits. Invest Ophthalmol 3:601–605, 1964.

Watkins JB III, Wirthwein DP, Sanders RA: Comparative study of Phase II biotransformation in rabbit ocular tissues. Drug Metab Dispos 19:708–713, 1991.

Williams RA, Howard AG, Williams TP: Retinal damage in pigmented and albino rats exposed to low levels of cyclic light following a singlemydriatic treatment. Curr Eye Res 4:97–102, 1985.

Wilson MA, Johnston MV, Goldstein GW, Blue ME: Neonatal lead exposure impairs development of rodent barrel field cortex. Proc Natl Acad Sci USA 97:5540–5545, 2000.

Winkler BS, Kapousta-Bruneau N, Arnold MJ, Green DG: Effects of inhibiting glutamine synthetase and blocking glutamate uptake on b-wave generation in the isolated rat retina. Vis Neurosci 16:345–353, 1999.

Winkler BS, Riley MV: Na+,K+ and HCO3 ATPase activity in retina: Dependence on calcium and sodium. Invest Ophthalmol Vis Sci 16:1151–1154, 1977.

Winkler BS: A quantitative assessment of glucose metabolism in the rat retina, in Christen Y, Doly M, Droy-Lefaix MT (eds):Vision and Adaptation, Les Seminaires Ophtamologiques d'IPSEN. Vol 6. Paris: Elsevier, 1995, pp. 78–96.

Winneke G: Modification of visual evoked potentials in rats after long-term blood lead elevation. Act Nerv Sup (Praha) 4:282–284, 1979.

Winneke G, Beginn U, Ewert T, et al.: Study to determine the subclinical effects of lead on the nervous system in children with known prenatal exposure in Nordenham. Schr-Reine Verein Wabolu 59:215–230, 1984.

Winneke G, Kramer U, Brockhaus A, et al.: Neuropsychological studies in children with elevated tooth-lead concentrations: II. Extended study. Int Arch Occup Environ Health 51:231–252, 1983.

Winneke G, Altmann L, Krämer U, Turfeld M, Behler R, Gutsmuths FJ, Mangold M: Neurobehavioral and neurophysiological observations in six year old children with low lead levels in East and West Germany. Neurotoxicology 15:705–713, 1994.

Withering W: An Account of the Foxglove and Some of Its Medicinal Uses: With Practical Remarks on Dropsy and Other Diseases. London: Broomsleigh Press, 1785.

Wolfensberger TJ: Toxicology of the retinal pigment epithelium. In Marmor MF, Wolfensberger TJ (eds): The Retinal Pigment Epithelium Function and Disease. New York, NY. Oxford University Press, 1998, pp. 621–647.

Woodhouse JM, Barlow HB: Spatial and temporal resolution and analysis, in Barlow HB, Mollon JD (eds): The Senses. Cambridge: Cambridge University Press, 1982, pp. 133–164.

Yau KW, Baylor DA: Cyclic GMP-activated conductance of retinal photoreceptor cells. Annu Rev Neurosci 12:289–327, 1989.

Yoshino Y, Mozai T, Nako K: Distribution of mercury in the brain and its subcellular units in experimental organic mercury poisonings. J Neurochem 13:397–406, 1966.

Zavalic M, Turk R, Bogadi-Sare A, Skender L: Colour vision impairment in workers exposed to low concentrations of toluene. Arh Hig Rada Toksikol 47:167–175, 1996.

Zhao C, Schwartzman ML, Shichi H: Immunocytochemical study of cytochrome P450 4A induction in mouse eye. Exp Eye Res 63:747–751, 1996.

Zhao C, Shichi H: Immunocytochemical study of cytochrome P450 (1A1/1A2) induction in murine ocular tissues. *Exp Eye Res* 60:143–152, 1995.

Zhang X, Feng Q, Cote RH: Efficacy and selectivity of phosphodiesterase-targeted drugs in inhibiting photoreceptor phosphodiesterase (PDE6) in retinal photoreceptors. *Invest Ophthalmol Vis Sci* 46:3060–3066, 2005.

Zrenner E, Gouras P: Blue-sensitive cones of the cat produce a rod like electroretinogram. *Invest Ophthalmol Vis Sci* 18:1076–1081, 1979.

Zrenner E, Kramer W, Bittner C, *et al.*: Rapid effects on colour vision following intravenous injection of a new, non-glycoside positive ionotropic substance (AR-L 115BS). *Doc Ophthalmol Proc Ser* 33:493–507, 1982.

TOXIC RESPONSES OF THE HEART AND VASCULAR SYSTEM

Y. James Kang

INTRODUCTION

Cardiovascular toxicology is concerned with the adverse effects of extrinsic and intrinsic stresses on the heart and vascular system. Extrinsic stress involves exposure to therapeutic drugs, natural products, and environmental toxicants. Intrinsic stress refers to exposure to toxic metabolites derived from nontoxic compounds such as those found in food additives and supplements. The intrinsic exposures also include secondary neurohormonal disturbance such as overproduction of inflammatory cytokines derived from pressure overload of the heart and counter-regulatory responses to hypertension. These toxic exposures result in alterations in biochemical pathways, defects in cellular structure and function, and pathogenesis of the affected cardiovascular system. The manifestations of toxicologic response of the heart include cardiac arrhythmia, hypertrophy, and overt heart failure. The responses of the vascular system include changes in blood pressure and lesions in blood vessels in the form of atherosclerosis, hemorrhage, and edema.

This chapter is divided into two parts: the heart and the vascular system. For a better understanding of the toxic manifestations of the cardiovascular system, an overview of the physiology and biochemistry of the heart and the vascular system is presented in relation to toxicologic concerns. The toxicologic responses of the heart and the vascular system and the mechanisms of these responses are the major focus of this chapter. This chapter also presents a brief discussion of chemicals that affect the heart and the vascular system.

OVERVIEW OF THE HEART

Overview of Cardiac Structural and Physiological Features

Cardiac muscle, along with nerve, skeletal muscle, and smooth muscle, is one of the excitable tissues of the body. It shares many bioelectrical properties with other excitable tissues, but also has unique features associated with cardiac structural and physiological specificities. Figure 18-1 illustrates the basic anatomy of the heart. With regard to cardiac toxicology, this section will only review some features of cardiac physiology and structures. There are many textbooks of cardiac anatomy and physiology that provide extensive knowledge basis of cardiac physiology and structural properties, which will not be repeated in this section.

Review of Cardiac Structure   The primary contractile unit within the heart is the cardiac muscle cell, or cardiac myocyte. Cardiac myocytes are composed of several major structural features and organelles, as illustrated in Fig. 18-2. A primary component is the contractile elements known as the myofibril. Each myofibril consists of a number of smaller filaments (the thick and thin myofilaments). The thick filaments are special assemblies of the protein myosin, whereas the thin filaments are made up primarily of the protein actin. Cardiac myosin is a hexamer composed of one pair of myosin heavy chains (MHCs) and two pairs of myosin light chains (MLC). Two isoforms of MHC, α and β, are expressed in cardiac muscle; the expression of these is under developmental control and may be altered by a variety of physiologic, pathologic, and pharmacologic stimuli (Martin *et al.*, 1996; Metzger *et al.*, 1999). In addition, the predominant isoform expressed in normal adult cardiac tissue also depends on the species examined. Similarly, two isoforms of actin are expressed in the heart (cardiac and skeletal α-actin), and, as with MHC, actin isoform expression is influenced by developmental, physiologic, pathologic, and pharmacologic stimuli, and the primary isoform of actin found in normal adult cardiac muscle also depends on the species examined.

Under electron microscopy, these essential structural components of myocardial contractile proteins display alternating dark bands (A bands, predominantly composed of myosin) and light bands (I bands, predominantly composed of actin). Visible in the middle of the I band is a dense vertical Z line. The area between two Z lines is called a sarcomere, the fundamental unit of muscle contraction. Although cardiac and skeletal muscle share many similarities, a major difference lies in the organization of cardiac myocytes into a functional syncytium where cardiac myocytes are joined end-to-end by dense structures known as intercalated disks. Within these, there are tight gap junctions that facilitate action potential propagation and intercellular communication. About 50% of each cardiac myocyte is composed of myofibrils. The rest of the intracellular space contains the remaining major components of the cell: mitochondria (33%), one or more nuclei (5%), the sarcoplasmic reticulum (SR) (2%), lysosomes (very low), glycogen granules, a Golgi network, and cytosol (12%) (Opie, 1996).

Cardiac myocyte is the largest cell in the heart and contributes to the majority of cardiac mass. However, cardiac myocytes make

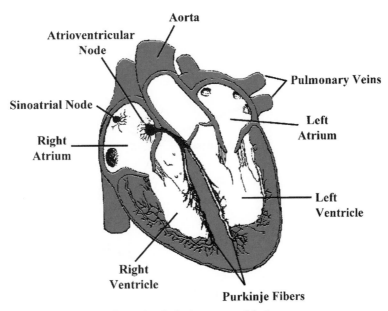

Figure 18-1. Diagram illustrating the basic anatomy of the heart.

up only about one-quarter of all the cells in the heart. Cardiac fibroblasts, vascular cells, Purkinje cells, and other connective tissue cells make up the majority of cell number in the heart. Cardiac fibroblasts make up approximately 90% of these "nonmuscle" cells. Cardiac myocytes are generally considered to be terminally differentiated, although this view has been challenged recently (Anversa *et al.*, 2006). These cells may be multinucleated, but they may not divide after birth unless under certain circumstances in some species such as mice (Anversa *et al.*, 2006). The heart undergoes a significant increase in size and mass throughout growth of the organism, but the increase in heart size and mass is produced by enlargement (or hypertrophy) of preexisting cardiac myocytes (Li *et al.*, 1996). With regard to this developmental period, cardiac hypertrophy is considered to be a normal physiological process. Under pathological conditions, hypertrophy of remaining cardiac myocytes is a hallmark of cardiac remodeling following myocardial injuries, such as myocardial infarction. Cardiac fibroblasts may continue to proliferate after birth, particularly in response to injury. Cardiac fibroblasts also contribute to cardiac remodeling following myocardial infarction and are believed to promote fibrosis and scarring of injured cardiac tissue. Thus, from a toxicologic perspective, the heart is vulnerable to injury because of limited proliferative capacity of cardiac myocytes, and promotion of cardiac fibroblast proliferation and remodeling following injury.

Electrophysiology The electrophysiology of the heart is concerned with bioelectricity and its related cardiac physiological function. Bioelectricity is the result of charge generated from the movement of positively and negatively charged ions in tissues. In cardiac myocytes, three major positively charged ions make a significant contribution to the bioelectricity of the heart; calcium (Ca^{2+}), sodium (Na^+), and potassium (K^+). Each of the ions has specific channels and transporters (pumps) on the membrane of cardiac myocytes. Through the movement of these ions across the cell membrane, an action potential is generated and propagated from one cell to another, so that electric conductance is produced in the heart.

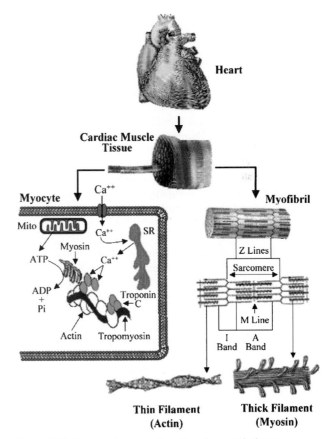

Figure 18-2. Structural organization of cardiac muscle tissue.

Action Potential Cardiac myocytes produce an action potential when activated. In the resting state, the resting potential of a myocyte is about −60 to −90 mV relative to the extracellular fluid potential. A sudden depolarization changes the membrane potential from negative inside to positive inside, followed by a repolarization

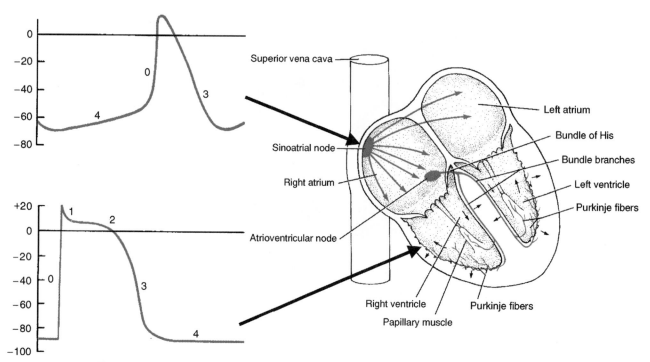

Figure 18-3. Characteristic cardiac action potential recorded from sinoatrial node and Purkinje fibers as indicated. (From Berne RM, Levy MN (eds.), Physiology pp. 454–457, 1983. With permission from Elsevier.)

to reset the resting potential. The process of an action potential from depolarization to the completion of repolarization is divided into five phases in cardiac Purkinje fibers as shown in Fig. 18-3. Phase 0 represents a rapid depolarization due to the inward current of Na^+. Phase 1 is associated with an immediate rapid repolarization, during which the Na^+ inward current is inactivated and a transient K^+ outward current is activated, followed by an action potential plateau or phase 2, which is dominated by slowly decreasing inward Ca^{2+} current and a slow activation of an outward K^+ current. Phase 3 reflects a fast K^+ outward current and inactivation of the plateau Ca^{2+} inward current, and phase 4 is the diastolic interval for the resetting of resting potential.

Automaticity   A group of specialized cells in the heart are capable of repetitively spontaneous self-excitation, which generate and distribute each impulse through the heart in a highly coordinated manner to control the normal heart beat. These cells include the sinus node P cells and Purkinje fibers in the ventricles. Other cells such as atrial-specialized fibers under normal conditions do not have automaticity, but can become automatic under abnormal conditions. The sinus node P cells or pacemaker cells have only three distinct phases of action potential (Fig. 18-3): phase 0, rapid depolarization; phase 3, plateau and repolarization; and phase 4, slow depolarization or often referred to as *pacemaker potential*. It is the pacemaker potential that brings the membrane potential to a level near the threshold for activation of the inward Ca^{2+} current, which triggers the phase 0 rapid depolarization and makes the pacemaker cells of automaticity. In pacemaker cells, phase 0 is mediated almost entirely by increased conductance of Ca^{2+} ions.

Contractility   Cardiac myocytes like other muscle cells have a unique functional feature, contractility. Myocyte contraction occurs when an action potential causes the release of Ca^{2+} from the SR

as well as the entry of extracellular Ca^{2+} into the cell. This action potential-triggered Ca^{2+} increase in the plasma and myocyte contraction is called *excitation–contraction coupling* (Fig. 18-4). The increase in Ca^{2+} concentrations in the cell allows Ca^{2+} to bind to troponin and tropomysin leading to some conformational change in the contractile unit of the cardiac myocyte, thin filament. This conformational change permits interaction between the actin and myosin filaments through the crossbridges (myosin heads). ATP is hydrolyzed by ATPase present in the crossbridges to release energy for the movement of the crossbridges in a ratchet-like fashion. This action increases the overlap of the actin and myosin filaments, resulting in shortening of the sarcomeres and contraction of the myocardium.

Electrotonic Cell-to-Cell Coupling   Myocardium as a whole has to synchronize the contraction and relaxation of individual myocytes in order to perform its pump function. This is achieved by a special structural feature of cell-to-cell interaction, electrotonic cell-to-cell coupling via the gap junction. Through the gap junction, major ionic fluxes between adjacent cardiomyocytes are spread, thus allowing electrical synchronization of contraction. Each single gap junction is composed of 12 connexin 43 (Cx43) units, assembled in two hexametric connexons (hemichannels) that are contributed, one each, by the two participating cells. The connexins interact with other proteins within the cell so that connexons are not only important for cell-to-cell coupling, but also involved in cell signaling and volume regulation. An important feature of the connexon-controlled electrotonic cell-to-cell coupling is the electrotonic current flow that attenuates the differences in action potential duration of individual cardiac myocytes.

Electrocardiograph   The electrophysiological features of cardiac myocytes and the electrotonic cell-to-cell coupling give rise to

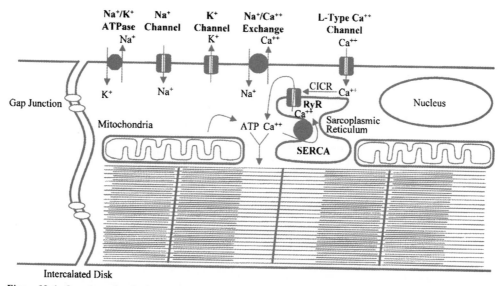

Figure 18-4. Overview of excitation–contraction coupling in cardiac myocytes.

Upon rapid depolarization (rapid influx of Na$^+$ through fast channels; phase 0 of the action potential), L-type Ca^{2+} channels are opened allowing a slower but sustained influx of Ca^{2+} down the electrochemical gradient (phase 2 of the action potential). During the process of Ca^{2+}-induced Ca^{2+} release (CICR), slight elevation in intracellular-free Ca^{2+} stimulates Ca^{2+} release from the sarcoplasmic reticulum (SR) through ryanodine receptors (RyR). The SR provides the majority of Ca^{2+} required for contraction. The mitochondria provide energy for contraction in the form of ATP. Repolarization of the cell occurs largely by activation of K$^+$ channels and efflux of K$^+$ (phase 3 of the action potential). For relaxation, the SR Ca^{2+} ATPase (SERCA) actively pumps Ca^{2+} back into the SR, although some Ca^{2+} may be removed by the Na$^+$/Ca^{2+} exchanger or by sarcolemmal Ca^{2+} pumps.

charge at any given locus in the heart with a magnitude and a direction. Therefore, at any given moment in the cardiac cycle, there is a complex pattern of electrical charges across the membranes of myriad cells in the heart. The sum of all the individual cells that exist at any given time within the heart is the *resultant cardiac vector*. The changes in the resultant cardiac vector throughout the cardiac cycle can be recorded as a *vector cardiograph*. Lead systems are used to record certain projections of the resultant cardiac vector. The potential difference between two recoding electrodes represents the projection of the vector on the line between the two leads. Components of vectors projected on such lines eliminate their directions and have a sum of magnitude, being scalar quantities. Thus, a recording of the changes with time in the potential differences between two points on the surface of the skin is the so-called *scalar electrocardiograph*.

In general, the pattern of the scalar electrocardiograph consists of P, QRS, and T waves, as shown in Fig. 18-5. The PR interval is a measure of the time from the onset of atrial activation to the onset of ventricular activation. The QRS complex represents the conduction pathways through the ventricles. The ST segment is the interval during which the entire ventricular myocardium is depolarized, and lies on the isoelectric line under normal conditions. The QT interval is sometimes referred to as the period of "electrical systole" of the ventricles, and reflects the action potential duration. The QT interval prolongation is recognized as a major life-threatening factor of drug cardiac toxicity, which is brought about by a reduction of outward currents and/or enhanced inward currents during phase 2 and 3 of the action potential.

Neurohormonal Regulation Although the heartbeat is governed by the automaticity of the sinus node P cells, neurohormonal regu-

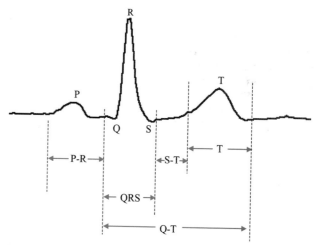

Figure 18-5. A typical electrocardiogram (ECG) with the illustration of important deflections and intervals.

lation of cardiac electrophysiology and contraction controls cardiac function under normal and abnormal conditions. Toxicants often exert their effects on the cardiac system through interference with the neurohormonal regulation, thus this regulatory system is of significant relevance to cardiac toxicology. There are many neurohormonal systems that have significant impact on the heart. A detailed description of the regulatory system will be provided in the following sections in association with specific discussion of cardiac functional regulation, compensatory and maladaptive responses to toxic exposures.

Overview of Cardiac Energy Metabolism and Biochemistry

ATP and the Heart   It is easy to understand that the need of energy for the heart is high. The chemical energy in the form of ATP is absolutely needed to support the systolic and diastolic work of the heart (Ventura-Clapier *et al.*, 2004). In the heart, the primary ATP-utilizing reactions are catalyzed by actomyosin ATPase in the myofibril, the Ca^{2+}-ATPase in the SR, and the Na^{+},K^{+}-ATPase in the sarcolemma (Ingwall and Weiss, 2004). ATP is also needed for molecular synthesis and degradation in the heart as in other organ systems. ATP synthesis by oxidative phosphorylation in the mitochondria is usually sufficient to support the normal needs of the heart, even when the work output of the heart increases three- to five-fold (Ingwall and Weiss, 2004). In addition, the glycolytic pathway and the tricarboxylic acid cycle also make small contributions to ATP synthesis. The concentration of ATP does not define the energetic state of the heart. The amount of ATP made and used at any given time is many times greater than the size of the measurable ATP pool (Ingwall and Weiss, 2004). Thus, cardiac myocytes contain high concentrations of mitochondria, which ensure that ATP remains constant through oxidation of a variety of carbon-based fuels for ATP synthesis under different conditions.

Phosphocreatine and the Heart   A unique feature in energy metabolism of the heart is the use of energy reserve systems, such as phosphocreatine (PCr), to maintain a high phosphorylation potential to drive ATPase reactions under highly demanding conditions (Ingwall *et al.*, 1985). PCr exists in the heart at twice the ATP concentration (Bittl and Ingwall, 1985). The enzyme creatine kinase (CK) transfers the phosphoryl group between ATP and PCr at a rate about 10 times faster than the rate of ATP synthesis by oxidative phosphorylation. The reaction catalyzed by CK is: PCr + ADP + H^{+} ↔ creatine + ATP. Under the conditions when ATP demand exceeds ATP supply, the use of PCr is a major pathway to maintain a constant supply of ATP. The CK reaction is also important to maintain low ADP and Pi concentrations, thereby retaining high phosphorylation potential (Saupe *et al.*, 2000). Creatine is not made in the heart but accumulates against a large concentration gradient facilitated by a creatine transporter. In the normal heart, about two-thirds of the total creatine pool is phosphorylated through the CK reaction to form PCr (Wallimann *et al.*, 1998; Neubauer *et al.*, 1999).

Metabolic Pathways   The continuous synthesis of ATP via mitochondrial oxidative phosphorylation is mandatory for the work of the heart (Huss and Kelly, 2005). Under normal conditions, the oxidation of fatty acid (FA) is the major pathway, providing about 65% of the total energy demand. In contrast, the oxidation of glucose provides about 30% of the total energy demand (Shipp *et al.*, 1961; Wisneski *et al.*, 1987). In hypertrophic and failing hearts, there is a metabolic shift from FA- to glucose-dependent energy supply. Thus, decreased FA oxidation and increased glucose utilization in association with depressed FA deposition and increased glucose uptake are observed in hypertrophic and failing hearts (van Bilsen *et al.*, 2004). This shift enhances the glycolytic pathway, and thus increases the anaerobic metabolism. However, it remains debated whether this metabolic shift to the so-called "fetal phenotype" is adaptive or maladaptive. It is important to note that the "shift" is only partial, and even when the proportion of ATP synthesized from glucose increases many fold, aerobic metabolism still remains dominant (van Bilsen *et al.*, 2004). With regard to the concern of cardiac toxicology, the metabolic shift is often observed with mitochondrial dysfunction. In response to toxic exposure, mitochondrial damage leads to impaired oxidative phsphorylation and a metabolic shift from aerobic to anaerobic and a reliance on glucose utilization.

Calcium and Calcineurin   The role of calcium in cardiac toxic responses has been extensively investigated. However, our understanding of the role of calcium in cardiac toxicity remains superficial. When carefully examining the current literature, one can find that there are very few mechanistic studies that specifically probe the role of calcium in cardiac toxicity, although numerous studies have implicated intracellular Ca^{2+} as a signal for cardiac responses to environmental toxic insults (Shier *et al.*, 1992; Toraason *et al.*, 1997; Buck *et al.*, 1999). In response to myocardial stress by environmental toxic exposures, calcium concentrations are increased in the myocardial cells (Sleight, 1996). This is consistent with the speculation that Ca^{2+} coordinates physiological responses to stresses. There are many other speculations that are derived from the studies examining the role of calcium in toxicologic responses in other systems. The unique action of calcium in cardiac toxicity, however, has to be studied specifically.

The role of calcium in mediating myocardial hypertrophic signals has been extensively studied (Stemmer and Klee, 1994). A sustained increase in intracellular Ca^{2+} concentrations activates calcineurin. Calcineurin is a ubiquitously expressed serine/threonine phosphatase that exists as a heterodimer, comprises a 59-kDa calmodulin (CaM)-binding catalytic A subunit and a 19-kDa Ca^{2+}-binding regulatory B subunit (Molkentin *et al.*, 1998). Activation of calcineurin is mediated by binding of Ca^{2+} to the regulatory subunit and CaM to the catalytic subunit (Fig. 18-6). Of toxicologic relevance is that calcineurin is activated by a sustained increase in Ca^{2+} concentration and is insensitive to transient Ca^{2+} fluxes, such as in response to cardiomyocyte contraction (Stemmer and Klee, 1994).

Numerous studies have demonstrated important roles for Ras, mitogen-activated protein kinase (MAPK), and protein kinase C (PKC) signaling pathways in myocardial responses to hypertrophic stimuli (Jalili *et al.*, 1999). All of these signal transduction pathways are associated with increase in intracellular Ca^{2+} concentrations (Ho *et al.*, 1998). The coordinating role of calcium in cardiac hypertrophic response has been demonstrated (Stemmer and Klee, 1994) as follows. Hypertrophic stimuli, such as angiotensin II and phenylephrine, cause an elevation of intracellular Ca^{2+} that results in activation of calcineurin. A series of reactions occur through activated calcineurin, including dephosphorylation of nuclear factor of activated T-cell (NFAT) and its translocation to nucleus, where it interacts with GATA4 (Fig. 18-6). Calcineurin also acts through an NFAT-independent mechanism to regulate hypertrophic gene expression.

AMP-Activated Protein Kinase   Activation of AMP-activated protein kinase (AMPK) often occurs when the myocardial metabolic phenotype shifts to the fetal form. Activation of AMPK occurs with changes in high-energy phosphate metabolism in hypertrophic and failing hearts. The increase in AMP/ATP ratio occurs when the PCr/ATP ratio decreases due to a decrease in PCr, with or without a concomitant decrease in ATP. The decrease in PCr/ATP ratio is an index of decreased energy reserve and correlates with the severity of heart failure and is of prognostic value (Neubauer *et al.*, 1997).

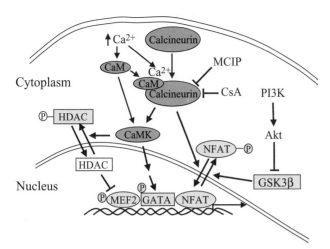

Figure 18-6. Calcineurin signal transduction pathways in regulation of transcription factors involved in hypertrophic growth of cardiac myocytes.

Sustained increases in intracellular Ca^{2+} concentrations, along with calmodulin (CaM), activate calcineurin, which in turn causes dephosphorylation of nuclear factor of activated T cells (NFAT), enabling NFAT to translocate to the nucleus where it interacts with GATA4 to regulate gene expression. Phosphorylation of NFAT is stimulated by glycogen synthase kinase 3β (GSK3β), whose activity is inhibited by activation of the phosphoinositide 3-kinase (PI3K)/Akt pathway. Calcineurin also regulates CaM activation of CaM-dependent kinase (CaMK), which activates GATA transcription factor. CaMK also phosphorylates histone deacetylases (HDAC), leading to HDAC translocation from nucleus to cytoplasm. Otherwise, HDAC in the nucleus inhibits myocyte-enhancer factor 2 (MEF2) transcription activity. Cyclosporine A (CsA) and modulatory calcineurin-interacting protein (MCIP) inhibit calcineurin activation.

Activation of AMPK leads to translocation of the insulin-dependent glucose transporter (GLUT4) from intracellular stores to the sarcolemma (Russell *et al.*, 1999). Mice overexpressing an active form of AMPK suffer from pathological cardiac glucogen accumulation (Arad *et al.*, 2003). Furthermore, the AMPK-dependent phosphorylation of the enzyme 6-phosphofructo-2-kinase stimulates glycolysis (Marsin *et al.*, 2000). These pathways indicate the importance of AMPK activation for the cardiac metabolic shift to the energy supply reliance on glucose metabolism.

Mitogen-Activated Protein Kinases MAPKs play a major role in cardiac response to toxic insults. A generalized diagram for MAPK signaling is presented in Fig. 18-7. The MAPKs consist of a series of successively acting kinases and three major branches are involved in the classic MAKP signaling pathway. These branches are divided based on their terminal effector kinases: the extracellular signal-regulated protein kniases (ERK), the c-jun NH2-terminal kinases (JNK), and p38 MAPKs (Sugden and Clerk, 1998). Each branch of the MAPKs has a hierarchy control system beginning at the MAPK kinase kinase (MAPKKK), as shown in Fig. 18-7. Among the MAPKs, p38 MAPKs have been extensively studied in myocardial apoptosis. This subfamily consists of p38α, p38β, p38γ, and p38δ (Sugden and Clerk, 1998). Several studies have identified p38 MAPKs as an important group of signaling molecules that mediate environmental stress responses in various cell types (Tibbles and Woodgett, 1999). In noncardiac cells, p38 MAPKs have been implicated in gene expression, morphological changes, and cell death in response to endotoxin, cytokines, physical stress, and chemical

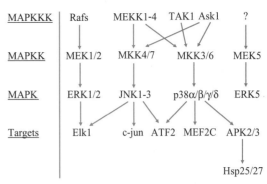

Figure 18-7. Schematic representation of the hierarchy constituents of the MAPK signaling pathways.

MAPK, mitogen-activated protein kinase; MAPKK, MAPK kinase; MAPKKK, MAPK kinase kinase.

insults (Tan *et al.*, 1996; Wang and Ron, 1996). In cardiac cells, p38 MAPKs are associated with the onset of apoptosis in ischemia–reperfusion (Yin *et al.*, 1997). In particular, transfection experiments using primary cultures of neonatal rat cardiomyocytes have shown that p38α is critically involved in myocyte apoptosis (Wang *et al.*, 1998).

Adriamycin is a cardiac toxicant and two observations indicate that the p38 MAPK is involved in Adriamycin-induced myocyte apoptosis (Kang *et al.*, 2000a). First, a time–course analysis revealed that p38 MAPK activation preceded the onset of apoptosis. As early as 30 minutes after Adriamycin administration, myocyte apoptosis occurs, detected by a sensitive method of fluorescein isothiocyanate (FITC) conjugation of Annexin V (Annexin V-FITC). However, p38 MAPK activation detected by the FITC-conjugated anti-phospho-p38 antibody and confocal microscopy is observed 20 minutes after Adriamycin treatment (Kang *et al.*, 2000a). Second, SB203580, a specific inhibitor of p38 MAPKs, inhibits Adriamycin-induced myocyte apoptosis (Kang *et al.*, 2000a). Because SB203580 acts as a specific inhibitor of p38α and p38β, but not p38γ and p38δ, the involvement of the former specific isoforms of the p38 MAPK in the Adriamycin-induced myocyte apoptosis are implicated. p38α is involved in apoptosis of neonatal rat cardiomyocytes in primary cultures and p38β mediates hypertrophy of these cells (Wang *et al.*, 1998).

Protein Kinase C PKC is among the most extensively studied signaling molecules in the heart. Many cardiac toxicologic studies have examined the role of PKC in mediating toxic signals. Several excellent reviews on PKC in myocardial signaling pathways leading to cardiac hypertrophy and heart failure are available (Puceat and Vassort, 1996). PKC is a ubiquitously expressed serine/threonine kinase, which is activated predominantly by G_q/G_{11}-coupled receptors. The PKC family consists of 11 isoforms, which are divided into three subgroups: conventional PKCs (cPKCs) including α, β (I and II), and γ, novel PKCs (nPKCs) including ε, δ, η, ζ, and θ, and atypical PKCs (aPKCs) including ι, λ, and μ (Newton, 1995). The cPKCs are activated by Ca^{2+} and diacylglycerol (DAG), as well as phorbol esters. The nPKCs do not bind Ca^{2+}, but respond to DAG and phorbol ester stimulation. The aPKCs do not respond to either Ca^{2+}, DAG, or phorbol esters. PKC has been demonstrated to participate in the regulation of transcription, the maintenance of cell growth and membrane structure, and modulation of immune responses. Disturbances in PKC signaling pathways lead to cardiac hypertrophy and heart failure, which is of toxicologic significance.

Transcription Factors   Transcription factors activate or deactivate myocardial gene expression, which affects the function and phenotype of the heart. Many transcription factors have been studied in myocardial tissue. Several of them are of toxicologic significance as described below:

Activator Protein-1   AP-1 is a transcription factor composed of *Jun* and *Fos* gene family members (McMahon and Monroe, 1992). The AP-1-binding site is the TRE (12-*O*-tetradecanoyl phorbol 13-acetate response element), and the binding of AP-1 to the TRE initiates transcription of the target genes (Diamond *et al.*, 1990). Elevated levels of c-Jun are seen in cardiomyocytes with ischemia–reperfusion (Brand *et al.*, 1992). In volume-overload hypertrophy, AP-1 plays an important role in the regulation of Fas and FasL activities (Wollert *et al.*, 2000). Over-stretching of myocardium induces Fas expression (Cheng *et al.*, 1995). Subsequently, Fas-dependent signaling pathways can lead to myocardial cell apoptosis. However, there are other studies that indicate activation of AP-1 is not associated with the induction of apoptosis (Lenczowski *et al.*, 1997). AP-1 has been implicated in transcriptional regulation of several genes associated with a hypertrophic response (Paradis *et al.*, 1996).

Myocyte-Enhancer Factor-2   MEF-2 is a transcription factor that binds to A-/T-rich DNA sequences within the promoter regions of a number of cardiac genes, including muscle CK gene, β-MHC, MLC1/3, MLC2v, skeletal α-actin, SR Ca^{2+}-ATPase, cardiac troponin T, C, and I, desmin, and dystrophin (Black and Olsen, 1998). MEF2 is critically involved in the regulation of inducible gene expression during myocardial hypertrophy. The activation of MEF2 involves phosphorylation of the transcription factor by p38 MAPK or ERK5-MAPK. The ERK5-MEF2 pathway has been observed in the generation of cardiac hypertrophy. An important function of MEF2 is the convergence in the binary downstream pathway of Ca^{2+} signaling. Increased intracellular Ca^{2+} binds to and activates Ca^{2+}-binding proteins including CaM, which regulates calcineurin and Ca^{2+}/CaM-dependent protein kinase (CaMKs). Activation of either calcineurin or CaMKs induces cardiac hypertrophy. CaMKs stimulate MEF2 through phosphorylation of the transcriptional suppressor, histone deacetylases (HDACs). CaMK is considered as HDAC kinase whose activity is enhanced by calcineurin. Thus, MEF2 converges the stimulating signaling of both CaMKs and calcineurin leading to activation of hypertrophic gene expression (Fig. 18-6).

Nuclear Factor of Activated T Cells 3   NFAT3 is a member of a multigene family that contains four members, NFATc, NFATp, NFAT3, and NFAT4 (Rao *et al.*, 1997). These transcription factors bind to the consensus DNA sequence GGAAAAT as monomers or dimers through a Rel homology domain (Rooney *et al.*, 1994). Unlike the other three members that are restricted in their expression to T cells and skeletal muscle, NFAT3 is expressed in a variety of tissues including the heart. NFAT3 plays a major role in cardiac hypertrophy (Pu *et al.*, 2003). Hypertrophic stimuli, such as angiotensin II and phenylephrine, cause an increase in intracellular Ca^{2+} levels in myocardial cells. This elevation in turn results in activation of calcineurin. NFAT3 is localized within the cytoplasm and is dephosphorylated by the activated calcineurin. This dephosphorylation enables NFAT3 to translocate to the nucleus where it interacts with GATA4 (Fig. 18-6). NFAT3 can also activate some hypertrophic responsive genes through mechanisms independent of GATA4.

GATA   GATA factors are a family of nuclear transcriptional regulatory proteins that are related structurally within a central DNA-binding domain, but are restricted in expression to distinct sets of cell types (Yamamoto *et al.*, 1990). Currently, six different family members have been characterized in vertebrate species. They are GATA1, 2, 3, 4, 5, and 6. Each protein contains two similar repeats of a highly conserved zinc finger of the form $CXNCX_6LWRRX_7CNAC$. The c-terminal repeat constitutes a minimal DNA-binding domain sufficient for sequence-specific recognition of a "GATA" *cis*-element, usually (A/T)GATA(A/G) or a related DNA sequence, present in promoters and/or enhancers of target genes (Evans *et al.*, 1988). It has been shown that GATA-1/2/3 regulate various aspects of hematopoiesis (Orkin, 1992), whereas GATA 4/5/6 regulates cardiogenesis (Yamamoto *et al.*, 1990). The significance of GATA-4 in regulation of hypertrophic response in myocardial cells has been demonstrated (Evens, 1997). Cardiac hypertrophy induced by angiotensin II is mediated by an angiotensin II type$_{1α}$ receptor ($AT_{1α}R$). A GATA motif exists in the $AT_{1α}R$ promoter. Mutations introduced to the consensus-binding site for GATA factor abolished the pressure overload response (Evens, 1997). Moreover, interactions between AP-1 and GATA-4, and between NFAT3 and GATA-4 are essential in myocardial hypertrophic responses.

CARDIAC TOXIC RESPONSES

Basic Concepts and Definitions

The ultimate functional effect of cardiac toxic manifestations is decreased cardiac output and peripheral tissue hypoperfusion, resulting from alterations in biochemical pathways, energy metabolism, cellular structural and function, electrophysiology, and contractility of the heart. These morphological and functional alterations induced by toxic exposure are referred to as toxicologic cardiomyopathy. The critical cellular event leading to toxicologic cardiomyopathy is myocardial cell death and extracellular matrix (ECM) remodeling. The recognition of the role of apoptosis in the development of heart failure during the last decade has significantly enhanced our knowledge of myocardial cell death (James, 1994; Haunstetter and Izumo, 1998; Sabbah and Sharov, 1998).

Manipulation of genes responsible for cardiac function began in the mid-1990s (Robbins, 2004). The most important conclusion of these studies is that a sustained expression of any single mutated functional gene, either in the form of gain-of-function or loss-of-function, can lead to a significant phenotype, often in the form of cardiac hypertrophy and heart failure (Robbins, 2004; Olson, 2004). However, it is difficult to apply this knowledge to patients: first, acquired cardiac disease such as heart failure is the result of interaction between environmental factors and genetic susceptibility, indicating the role of polymorphisms. Second, extrinsic and intrinsic stresses produce lesions that cannot be explained by a single gene or a single pathway, suggesting complexity between deleterious factors and the heart. Cardiac toxicity is the critical link between environmental factors and myocardial pathogenesis.

For a better understanding of cardiac toxicology, a triangle model of cardiac toxicity is presented in Fig. 18-8. In this model, complexity of the interaction between environmental stresses and the heart, and the balance between myocardial protection and

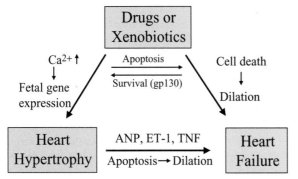

Figure 18-8. Triangle analytical model of cardiac responses to drugs and xenobiotics.

Drugs or xenobiotics can directly cause both heart failure and heart hypertrophy. Under severe acute toxic insults, myocardial cell death becomes the predominant response leading to cardiac dilation and heart failure. In most cases, myocardial survival mechanisms can be activated so that myocardial apoptosis is inhibited. The survived cardiomyocytes often become hypertrophy through activation of calcium-mediated fetal gene expression and other hypertrophic program. If toxic insult continues, the counter-regulatory mechanisms against heart hypertrophy such as activation of cytokine-mediacted pathways eventually lead to myocardial cell death through apoptosis or necrosis, dilated cardiomyopathy, and heart failure.

deleterious dose and time effects are considered. First, it is important to recognize that chemicals can lead to heart failure without heart hypertrophy. Second, a chemical can lead to activation of both protective and destructive responses in the myocardium. Third, long-term toxicologic responses often result in maladaptive hypertrophy, which primes the heart for malignant arrhythmia, leading to sudden death or transition to heart failure.

In the study of cardiac toxicology, the manifestations of cardiac toxicity in human patients and animal models are critical parameters serving as indices of cardiac toxicity. These manifestations are expressed in the forms of cardiac arrhythmia, hypertrophy, and heart failure. These abnormal changes reflect myocardial functional alterations resulting from both acute and chronic cardiac toxicity. Although some changes, such as cardiac hypertrophy, was viewed as a compensatory response to hemodynamic changes in the past, more recent studies suggest that cardiac hypertrophy is a maladaptive process of the heart in response to intrinsic and extrinsic stresses (van Empel *et al.*, 2004; Berenji *et al.*, 2005; Dorn and Force, 2005). Cardiac hypertrophy is a risk factor for sudden cardiac death and has a high potential to progress to overt heart failure. Therefore, a distinction between compensatory and maladaptive responses is critical for treatment of patients with toxicologic cardiomyopathy.

Cardiac Arrhythmia Cardiac rhythms under physiological conditions are set by pacemaker cells that are normally capable of developing spontaneous depolarization and responsible for generating the cardiac rhythm, the so-called automatic rhythm. A cardiac rhythm that deviates from the normal automatic rhythm is called cardiac arrhythmia, often manifested in the form of tachycardia (fast heart rate). There are several classes of tachycardia, including sinus tachycardia, atrial tachycardia, ventricular tachycardia, and torsade de pointes (TdP) (a life-threatening ventricular tachycardia). In addition, subclasses such as atrial fibrillation, atrial flutter, and accelerated idioventricular rhythm provide further description of the manifestations of arrhythmia. Mechanisms for different classes

of arrhythmia will be discussed in the section of QT-prolongation and sudden cardiac death. According to the cause of the tachycardia, it is divided into abnormal automatic arrhythmia and triggered arrhythmia, which will be discussed in other sections.

Cardiac Hypertrophy There are two basic forms of cardiac hypertrophy: concentric hypertrophy, which is often observed during pressure overload and is characterized by new contractile-protein units assembled in parallel resulting in a relative increase in the width of individual cardiac myocytes (De Simone, 2003). By contrast, eccentric hypertrophy is characterized by the assembly of new contractile-protein units in series resulting in a relatively greater increase in the length than in the width of individual myocytes, occurring in human patients and animal models with dilated cardiomyopathy (Kass *et al.*, 2004). Toxicologic cardiomyopathy is often manifested in the form of eccentric hypertrophy. The development of cardiac hypertrophy can be divided into three stages: Developing hypertrophy, during which period the cardiac workload exceeds cardiac output; compensatory hypertrophy, in which the workload/mass ratio is normalized and normal cardiac output is maintained; decompensatory hypertrophy, in which ventricular dilation develops and cardiac output progressively declines, and overt heart failure occurs (Richey and Brown, 1998).

Heart Failure A traditional definition of heart failure is the inability of the heart to maintain cardiac output sufficient to meet the metabolic and oxygen demands of peripheral tissues. This definition has been modified recently to include changes in systolic and diastolic function that reflect specific alterations in ventricular function and abnormalities in a variety of subcellular processes (Piano *et al.*, 1998). Therefore, a detailed analysis to distinguish right ventricular from left ventricular failure can provide a better understanding of the nature of the heart failure and predicting the prognosis.

Acute Cardiac Toxicity Acute cardiac toxicity is referred to as cardiac response to a single exposure to a high dose of cardiac toxic chemicals. It is often manifested by cardiac arrhythmia. However, myocardial apoptosis is also involved in acute cardiac toxicity. It is not difficult to define acute cardiac toxicity; however, it sometimes is technically difficult to measure acute cardiac toxicity. In particular, the impact of acute cardiac toxicity on the ultimate outcome of cardiac function is not often easily recognized. For instance, a single high dose of arsenic can lead to cardiac arrhythmia and sudden cardiac death, which is easy to measure (Goldsmith and From, 1980). However, that a single oral dose of monensin (20 mg/kg) leads to a diminished cardiac function progressing to heart failure in calves requires a long-term observation; often a few months for clinical signs of heart failure (van Vleet, *et al.*, 1983; Litwak *et al.*, 2005), which is difficult to measure. As shown in Fig. 18-8, toxic exposure can directly lead to heart failure, which is different from an often-observed hypertrophic response, which may or may not progress to heart failure.

Chronic Cardiac Toxicity Chronic cardiac toxicity is the cardiac response to long-term exposure to chemicals, which is often manifested by cardiac hypertrophy and the transition to heart failure. About 25% of human patients with cardiomyopathy are categorized as having idiopathic cardiomyopathy. At least a portion of these patients with idiopathic cardiomyopathy are due to chemical exposure. Environmental exposure to particulate matter (PMs) in the air can lead to cardiomyopathy, which has only been recognized recently (Dockery, 2001; Gordon and Reinman, 2002). Recognition of chronic cardiac toxicity in the pathogenesis of cardiomyopathy is of clinical relevance, and this knowledge can be used to prevent and treat patients with toxicologic cardiomyopathy.

Myocardial Degeneration and Regeneration

Myocardial degeneration is the ultimate response of the heart to toxic exposure, which can be measured by both morphological and functional degenerative phenotypes. However, myocardial degeneration should not be considered an irreversible toxic response. In the past, the heart has been considered incapable of regenerating, so that cardiac injury in the form of cell loss or scar tissue formation was considered permanent damage to the heart. However, evidence now indicates myocardial regeneration and recovery from cardiomyopathy. Cardiac toxic responses or damage are now divided into reversible and irreversible.

Myocardial Degenerative Responses Myocardial cell death, fibrosis (scar tissue formation), and contractile dysfunction are considered as degenerative responses, which can result in cardiac arrhythmia, hypertrophy, and heart failure. If acute cardiac toxicity does not affect the capacity of myocardial regeneration, the degenerative phenotype is reversible. Both acute and chronic toxic stresses can lead to irreversible degeneration, depending on whether or not the cardiac repair mechanisms are overwhelmed. Cell death is the most common phenotype of myocardial degeneration. Both apoptosis and necrosis occur in the process of myocardial cell death, which will be discussed in the next section. Myocardial cell death is accompanied by hypertrophy of the remaining cardiac myocytes so that in the hypertrophic heart, the total number of cardiac myocytes is reduced but the size or volume of individual cells is increased.

During myocardial remodeling after cell death, not only is there an increase in the size of cardiac myocytes, but also cardiac fibrosis occurs. Myocardial fibrosis results from excess accumulation of ECM, which is mainly composed of collagens. The net accumulation of ECM connective tissue results from enhanced synthesis or diminished break down of the matrix, or both. Collagen, predominately type I and III, are the major fibrous proteins in ECM and their synthesis may increase in response to toxic insults. The degradation of ECM is dependent on the activity of matrix metalloproteinases (MMPs). According to their substrate specificity, MMPs fall into five categories: collagenases (MMP-1, MMP-8, and MMP-13), gelatinases (MMP-2 and MMP-9), stromelysins (MMP-3, MMP-7, MMP-10, and MMP-11), membrane-type MMPs (MMP-14, MMP-15, MMP-16, MMP-17, MMP-24, and MMP-25), and metalloelastase (MMP-12). These MMPs are organ specific so that not all are present in the heart. The activities of these enzymes are altered during the processes of fibrogenesis and fibrinolysis. Under toxic stress condition, the imbalance between fibrogenesis and fibrinolysis leads to enhanced fibrogenesis and excess collagen accumulation—fibrosis.

Toxic Effect on Myocardial Regeneration The mainstay of cardiac medicine and therapy has centered on the concept that the heart is a terminally differentiated organ and that cardiac myocytes are incapable of proliferating. Thus, cell death would lead to a permanent loss of the total number of cardiac myocytes. However, this view has been challenged recently due to the identification of cardiac progenitor cells (Anversa *et al.*, 2006). These cells are characterized and proposed to be responsible for cardiac repair because these cells can make myocytes and vascular structures. These cells possess the fundamental properties of stem cells, therefore, they are also called cardiac stem cells. They are self-renewing, clonogenic, and multipotent, as demonstrated by reconstitution of infarcted heart by intramyocardial injection of cardiac progenitor cells or the local activation of these cells by growth factors. It is important to note that toxicologic studies of the cardiac progenitor cells have not been done and it is important to determine the potential of cardiac stem cells to help recover from toxic insults. The effect of chemicals on the cardiac progenitor cells is unknown. One speculation is that when severe damage to cardiac progenitor cells occurs, the potential for recovery from severe cardiac injury would be limited.

The removal of scar tissue or fibrosis in the myocardium in the past has been considered impossible. Although there are no studies that have shown scar tissue is removable, there are observations in animal models of hypertensive heart disease that myocardial fibrosis is recoverable (Weber, 2005).

Myocardial vascularization is required for myocardial regeneration. Many toxic insults affect the capacity of angiogenesis in the myocardium, so that cardiac ischemia occurs. The combination of cardiac ischemia and the direct toxic insults to cardiomyocytes constitute synergistic damage to the heart. During regeneration, coronary arterioles and capillary structures are formed to bridge the dead tissue (scar tissue) and supply nutrients for the survival of the regenerated cardiomyocytes. There is an orderly organization of myocytes within the myocardium and a well-defined relationship between the myocytes and the capillary network. This proportion is altered under cardiac toxic conditions; either toxicologic hypertrophy or diminished capillary formation can lead to hypoperfusion of myocytes in the myocardium. Unfortunately, our understanding of the toxic effects on myocardial angiogenesis is limited.

Reversible and irreversible toxic response. Cardiomyopathy was viewed not to be recoverable in the past, but there is cumulative evidence that demonstrates reversibility of cardiomyopathy. The issue related to whether or not toxicologic cardiac lesions are reversible has not been explored. However, it can be speculated that there would be reversible and irreversible manifestations of the cardiac response to toxic insults.

Myocardial Cell Death and Signaling Pathways

Apoptosis and Necrosis Toxic insults trigger a series of reactions in cardiac cells leading to measurable changes. Mild injuries can be repaired. However, severe injuries will lead to cell death in the modes of apoptosis and necrosis. If the cell survives the insults, structural and functional adaptations will take place.

Apoptosis was found to be involved in cardiomyopathy in 1994 (Gottlieb *et al.*, 1994). The loss of cardiac myocytes is a fundamental part of myocardial injury, which initiates or aggravates cardiomyopathy. An important mode of myocardial cell loss is apoptosis, which has been demonstrated in heart failure patients (Olivetti *et al.*, 1997). Myocardial apoptosis has been shown to play an important role in cardiac toxic effects induced by Adriamycin (Kang *et al.*, 2000a; Wang *et al.*, 2001a), an important anticancer drug whose clinical application is limited by its major toxic effect, cardiotoxicity. Exposure of primary cultures of cardiomyocytes to cadmium also induces apoptosis (El-Sherif *et al.*, 2000).

Many in vivo studies have shown that only a very small percentage of myocardial cell populations undergo apoptosis under pathological conditions. For example, less than 0.5% of cells appeared apoptotic in myocardial tissue under the stress of dietary copper deficiency in mice (Kang *et al.*, 2000b). At first glance, this number seems to be too insignificant to account for myocardial pathogenesis. In a carefully designed time–course study (Kajstura *et al.*, 1996), it was estimated that cardiomyocyte apoptosis is completed in less than 20 hours in rats. Myocytes that undergo apoptosis are lost and may not be replaced under toxicologic conditions. Although the possibility of myocardial regeneration has been identified (Anversa *et al.*, 2006), xenobiotics often cause degenerative effect through apoptosis as well as inhibitory effect on regeneration. Adriamycin-induced cardiomyopathy is a good example for the pathogenesis resulting from both degeneration and inhibition of regeneration. If apoptosis occurs at a constant rate of about 0.5% myocytes a day (Kang *et al.*, 2000b), the potential contribution of apoptosis to the overall loss of myocytes over a long period of time is significant under Adrimaycin toxic exposure.

Necrosis is a term that had been widely used to describe myocardial cell death in the past. Myocardial infarction, in particular, had been considered as a consequence of necrosis (Eliot *et al.*, 1977). It is now recognized that apoptosis contributes significantly to myocardial infarction (Yaoita *et al.*, 2000). However, the importance of necrosis in myocardial pathogenesis cannot be underestimated. The contribution of necrosis to cardiomyopathy induced by environmental toxicants and pollutants is particularly important. A critical issue is how to distinguish apoptosis from necrosis.

Apoptosis and necrosis were originally described as two distinct forms of cell death that can be clearly distinguished (Wyllie, 1994). However, these two modes of cell death can occur simultaneously in tissues and cultured cells. The intensity and duration of insults may determine the outcome. Triggering events can be common for both types of cell death. A downstream controller, however, may direct cells toward a programmed execution of apoptosis. If the apoptotic program is aborted before this control point and the initiating stimulus is severe, cell death may occur by necrosis (Leist *et al.*, 1997).

To distinguish apoptosis from necrosis, specific oligonucleotide probes have been developed to recognize different aspects of DNA damage (Didenko *et al.*, 1998), and have been successfully applied, in combination with confocal microscopy, to identify apoptotic and necrotic cell death in the heart with different pathogenic challenges.

Single-Strand DNA Breaks A monoclonal mouse anti-ssDNA antibody has been developed that is specifically reactive with ssDNA, but does not recognize dsDNA. An immunohistochemical assay for detection of ssDNA using this antibody in combination with a terminal deoxynucleotidyl-transferase-mediated dUTP nick end labeling(TUNEL) assay can distinguish repairable ssDNA breaks from apoptotic DNA damage in the heart.

Apoptotic DNA damage produces end products that are fragments of double-strand DNA cleavage with 3′ overhang (Didenko *et al.*, 1998), which can be specifically identified by *Tag* polymerase-generated probe (Didenko *et al.*, 1998). The specificity of this molecular probe to identify apoptosis has been confirmed by other methods such as dual labeling of TdT and caspase-3 (Frustaci *et al.*, 2000). In addition, this apoptotic specific probe in combination with fluorescence labeling of different cellular components allows quantitative detection of apoptotic cells, with the possibility of identifying the origin of the apoptotic cells, such as myocytes (stained with α-sarcomeric actin), endothelial cells (stained with factor VIII),

and fibroblasts (stained with vimentin) in the heart (Anversa, 2000).

Necrotic DNA damage is characterized by double-strand DNA cleavage with blunt ends. That is because during necrosis, the release of lysosomal proteases degrades histones, resulting in loss of DNA protection and exposure to endonucleases and exonucleases. Endonucleases produce double-strand DNA cleavage with 3′ overhangs, but exonucleases remove terminal nucleotides, leading to a bunt end of the damaged DNA. A probe generated by *pfu* polymerase can specifically recognize these blunt-end DNAs (Anversa, 2000). Its specific reaction with necrotic DNA has been confirmed by other methods such as the permeability of myosin antibody into necrotic cells (Guerra *et al.*, 1999), and the disruption of the sarcolemma by vinculin staining, which can clearly define the continuity of the sarcolemmal surface (Yamashita *et al.*, 2001).

Proportion of apoptotic and necrotic cell death in the heart can be estimated by the combination of the above procedures. First, a conventional TUNEL procedure can be used to identify the total TUNEL-positive cells. Second, the procedure to define double-strand DNA breaks with blunt ends can be used to quantify the proportion of necrotic cells in the total TUNEL-positive population. Finally, the combination of the procedure to identify double-strand DNA breaks with 3′ overhangs, and the specific antibody to identify total ssDNA breaks can distinguish the proportion of apoptotic cells from those with ssDNA breaks only.

Distinguishing apoptotic myocytes from non-myocytes in the myocardium is another problem to overcome. An in situ TUNEL assay in combination with a dual immunohistochemical detection of α-sarcomeric actin has been used to distinguish apoptotic myocytes from non-myocytes (Kang *et al.*, 2000a). Apoptotic myocytes are dually stained by TUNEL and α-sarcomeric actin, and apoptotic non-myocytes are stained only by TUNEL. Another procedure is immuno-gold TUNEL and electron microscopic examination of the apoptotic cells (Kang *et al.*, 2000a). The gold standard for identification of apoptotic cells is morphological examination by electron microscopy. The immuno-gold TUNEL and electron microscopic procedure defines cell type and morphological characteristics of apoptotic cells.

Mitochondrial Control of Cell Death The role of mitochondria in myocardial response to toxicants as well as therapeutic drugs has long been a focus of investigation. Mitochondrial control of cell death is an important topic of apoptotic research during the last decade. Factors affecting mitochondrial control of cell death is presented in Fig. 18-9. These factors have the same target effect: modification of mitochondrial permeability transition (MPT).

Mitochondrial permeability transition occurs under toxic insults (Kroemer *et al.*, 1997). This MPT behaves like a membrane pore that allows diffusion of solutes <1500 Da in size. Although MPT can occur as a temporary event, it can rapidly become irreversible, with the resulting loss of mitochondrial homeostasis and high-amplitude mitochondrial swelling. Because the inner membrane has a larger surface area than the outer membrane, mitochondrial swelling can cause the rupture of the outer membrane, releasing intermembrane proteins into the cytosol (Reed *et al.*, 1998). Among the intermembrane proteins is cytochrome *c*. Another possible mechanism that leads to mitochondrial cytochrome *c* release is the action of Bax, a proapoptotic protein of the Bcl-2 family (Adams and Cory, 1998). Overexpression of Bax under oxidative stress conditions has been observed in a number of studies using different

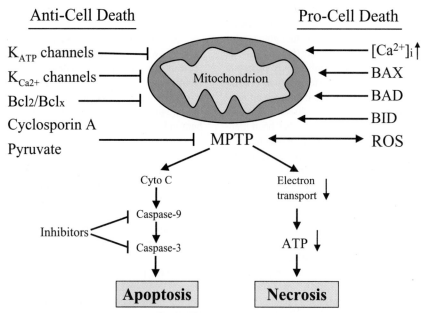

Figure 18-9. Major factors affecting mitochondrial MPTP and myocardial cell death.

Mitochondrial cytochrome *c* release is a critical factor controlling cardiomyocyte apoptosis. Mitochondrial permeability transition pore (MPTP) opening is a determinant factor for cytochrome *c* release, as well as for electron transport collapsing leading to decreases in ATP production. The factors affecting MPTP thus are classified as pro-cell death and anti-cell death. Many other factors also affect cell death programs such as apoptosis inducing factor (AIF) released from mitochondria, but the involvement of MPTP is not evidenced.

tissues including the heart (Cook *et al.*, 1999). It has been shown that Bax is translocated from cytosol to mitochondria and forms pores in mitochondrial outer membranes, leaving the inner membranes intact (Jurgensmeier *et al.*, 1998). This mechanism implies that Bax-mediated cytochrome *c* release is independent of MPT (Saikumar *et al.*, 1998). The release of cytochrome *c* from mitochondria into the cytosol is a critical initiation step in myocardial apoptosis. Cytochrome *c* aggregates with apoptotic protease activating factor-1 (apaf-1, another factor released from mitochondria under oxidative stress), procaspase-9, and dATP, and subsequently activates caspase-9, which activates caspase-3. The apoptotic pathway involving mitochondrial cytochrome *c* release and caspase-3 activation is presented in Fig. 18-10. To determine the significance of the caspase-3-activated apoptotic pathway in the pathogenesis of toxicologic cardiomyopathy, a caspase-3-specific inhibitor, Ac-DEVD-cmk, is often used. For instance, treatment of cultured cardiomyocytes isolated from neonatal mice with Ac-DEVD-cmk efficiently suppressed caspase-3 activity and reduced the number of apoptotic cells in cultures under treatment with Adriamycin (Wang *et al.*, 2001a).

Defective mitochondrial oxidative phosphorylation has been extensively investigated ever since the identification of mitochondrial oxidative phosphorylation. The link between defective oxidative phosphorylation and pathogenesis of cardiomyopathy has been revealed recently. The early phase of defects in oxidative phosphorylation increases mitochondrial outer membrane permeability, leading to cytochrome *c* release, thus resulting in cytochrome *c*-mediated caspase-9 activation and thereby caspase-3 activation, leading to apoptosis (Fosslien, 2001). The defective oxidative phosphorylation also leads to depletion of cellular ATP levels, resulting in necrosis

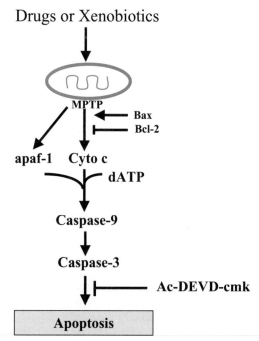

Figure 18-10. Mitochondrial control of myocardial apoptotic pathway.

Exposure to drugs or xenobiotics can cause mitochondrial MPTP opening and cytochrome *c* release, which in association with apaf-1 and in the presence of dATP, activates caspase-9. Caspase-9 consequently activates caspase-3 leading to apoptosis. Factors regulating the apoptotic pathway include those listed in Fig. 18-9, such as Bax and Bcl-2. Ac-DEVD-cml is a selective inhibitor of caspase-3.

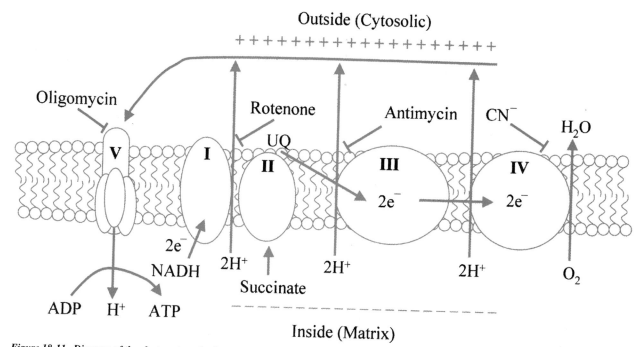

Figure 18-11. *Diagram of the electron-transferring complexes I, II, III, and IV and the ATPase (V) present in the inner mitochondrial membrane.*

The respective complexes are I, NADH: ubiquinone oxidoreductase; II, succinate: ubiquinone oxidoreductase; III, ubiquinol: ferrocytochrome c oxidoreductase; IV, ferrocytochrome c: oxygen oxidoreductase; V, ATP synthesase. UQ 5 ubiquinone or coenzyme Q. The mitochondrial electron transport chain is coupled at three points so that the electron transfer between carriers is sufficiently exergonic to drive the transport of protons and to establish an electrochemical proton gradient upon which ATP formation depends. Various inhibitors and their sites are also noted.

(Fosslien, 2001). Figure 18-11 presents a generalized mitochondrial oxidative phosphorylation process, including electron-transferring complexes and ATP production. Detection of mutated or otherwise defective components in oxidative phosphorylation is important for understanding the myocardial cell death by xenobiotics.

Abnormal mitochondrial biosynthesis is also linked to myocardial pathogenesis. Nuclear DNA encodes mitochondrial proteins, and thus nuclear DNA damage can lead to mutated products and abnormal mitochondrial biosynthesis. However, mitochondrial DNA encodes essential elements for mitochondrial function. Mitochondrial DNA is subjected to far more oxidative injury than nuclear DNA due to the lack of histones and high exposure to reactive oxygen species (ROS) generated by the electron transport chain. Mitochondrial DNA repair exists, although the repair is not as efficient as that of nuclear DNA repair. Due to these unique characteristics of mitochondrial DNA, cumulative mitochondrial DNA damage under oxidative stress conditions such as Adriamycin treatment, leads to irreversible mitochondrial dysfunction in the heart (Zhou *et al.*, 2001). This cumulative and relatively irreversible oxidative mitochondrial dysfunction concept has an important impact on our understanding of chronic as well as late-onset cardiomyopathy of anthracyclines. These drugs cause cardiomyopathy sometimes months to years after cessation of the drug therapy. During this time period, subtle pathological changes that may not be detectable but may continue to accumulate and lead to an overt toxic event. The cumulative and irreversible mitochondrial dysfunction might explain such a phenomenon, and may contribute to the delayed myocardial pathogenesis by Adriamycin.

Generation of reactive oxygen species has been ascribed as an "unwanted" function of mitochondria. Drugs and other chemicals have been studied individually to determine how they produce

ROS; however, debate continues regarding the importance of each identified pathway as well as the site of ROS generation in mitochondria. In general, it is accepted that changes in mitochondrial membrane potential are critically involved in ROS generation. There are two important potassium channels that play important roles in mitochondrial membrane permeability. The first is the mitochondrial ATP-sensitive potassium channel (Akao *et al.*, 2001), and the second is the Ca^{2+}-activated potassium channel in the cardiac inner mitochondrial membrane (Xu *et al.*, 2002). It has been shown that diazoxide opens mitochondrial ATP-sensitive potassium channels and preserves mitochondrial integrity, as well as suppresses hydrogen peroxide-induced apoptosis in cardiomyocytes (Akao *et al.*, 2001). The Ca^{2+}-activated potassium channels, in contrast, contribute to mitochondrial potassium uptake of myocytes, and opening of these channels protects the heart from infarction (Xu *et al.*, 2002).

Death Receptors and Signaling Pathways Death receptor-mediated apoptotic signaling pathway has been one of the focuses of cardiotoxicity research. In this regard, cytokines that trigger the death receptor signaling pathways have been studied. Among these cytokines is tumor necrosis factor-α (TNF-α) (Kubota *et al.*, 2001), the most studied cytokine in myocardial cell death signaling pathways. The pathway leading to TNF-α-induced myocardial apoptosis is mediated by TNF receptors, TNFR1, and TNFR2. TNF-α-binding of these receptors leads to activation of caspase 8, which in turn cleaves BID, a BH3 domain-containing proapoptotic Bcl2 family member. The truncated BID is translocated from cytosol to mitochondria, inducing first the clustering of mitochondria around the nuclei and release of cytochrome c, and then the loss of mitochondrial membrane potential, cell shrinkage, and nuclear condensation,

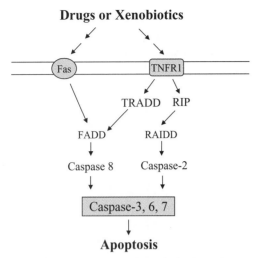

Figure 18-12. Simplified presentation of death receptors-mediated myocardial apoptosis.

The cardiotoxicity-related death receptors include Fas and tumor necrotic factor receptor 1 (TNFR1), as shown. Other death receptors such as DR3 and DR4/5 are not included in the figure. Both Fas- and TNFR1-activated apoptotic pathways can be altered by drugs and xenobiotics directly or indirectly through changes in the production of Fas ligand (FasL) or TNF-α. Fas activation activates caspase-8 through Fas-associated death domain (FADD). TNFR1 activates TNF-R1-associated death domain (TRADD), leading to activation of FADD. TNFR1 also activates a receptor-interacting protein (RIP), which activates caspase-2 through the adaptor protein, RIP-associated ICH-1/CED-3 homologous protein with a death domain (RAIDD). Both caspase-8 and caspase-3 activate the apoptosis executor proteins, caspase-3, -6 and -7.

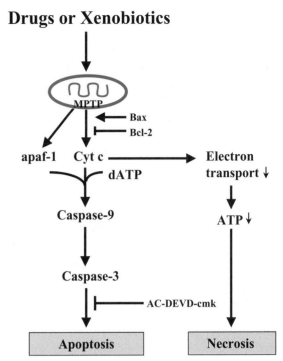

Figure 18-13. Interchange between apoptotic and necrotic cell death pathways regulated by mitochondrial MPTP.

Mitochondrial MPTP opening leads to cytochrome *c*-mediated activation of apoptotic pathway, which is ATP dependent. However, MPTP formation also leads to electron transport collapse and reduced ATP production, which eventually leads to necrosis. Inhibition of caspase-3 also potentially switches the cell death program from apoptotic to necrotic if the exposure to drugs or xenobiotics is persistent.

i.e., apoptosis. Caspase 8 also directly activates caspase-3, leading to apoptosis (Fig. 18-12). Besides TNF-α, Fas ligand is also able to induce apoptosis of cardiomyocytes through the death receptor-mediated signaling pathway (Hayakawa *et al.*, 2002).

The death receptor-mediated apoptosis thus can be divided into mitochondrion-dependent and mitochondrion-independent signaling pathways. There is a bewildering diversity of programmed cell death paradigms related to the mitochondrion-controlled process, eventually leading to caspase-3 activation and apoptosis. Under chronic toxic insults, the relative importance of mitochondrial MPT pore opening, cytochrome *c* release, and electron transport defects needs to be critically examined in order to understand the process or mode of cell death.

There are two important questions that need to be carefully addressed. First, how important is apoptosis in the overall pathogenesis of cardiomyopathy under different conditions? It essentially is a universal observation that apoptosis is involved in the cardiotoxicity of drugs and chemicals; however, there is very limited information regarding its significance in a quantitative manner in contribution to cardiomyopathy. This concern is followed by the second important question: can caspase inhibitors offer long-term protection against myocardial cell death leading to prevention of cardiomyopathy? It is important to note that apoptosis and necrosis are linked phenomena sharing common triggers, such as MPT pore opening, as depicted in Fig. 18-13. For instance, some studies have shown that caspase inhibitors effectively inhibit apoptosis, but cell death occured by necrosis instead of apoptosis (Suzuki *et al.*, 2001). It is thus important to define the most efficient approach to blocking myocardial cell

death rather than inhibiting a particular cell death program (Kang, 2001).

It is important to note that apoptosis is an energy-dependent process and that the switch in the decision between apoptosis and necrosis depends on ATP concentrations (Eguchi *et al.*, 1997), as depicted in Fig. 18-13. In particular, conditions causing ischemia by many drug and chemical exposures to myocardial cells result in significant reduction and eventual depletion of adenine nucleotides. Loss of more than 70% of the total ATP pool present in myocardial cells results in a switch from apoptosis to necrosis (Leist *et al.*, 1999). This extent of ATP depletion is observed in myocardial infarction.

Cardiac Hypertrophy and Heart Failure

Adaptive and Maladaptive Responses Myocardial adaptation refers to the general process by which the ventricular myocardium changes in structure and function. This process is often referred to as "remodeling." During maturation, myocardial remodeling is a normal feature for adaptation to increased demands. However, in response to pathological stimuli, such as exposure to environmental toxicants, myocardial remodeling is adaptive in the short term, but is maladaptive in the long term, and often results in further myocardial dysfunction. The central feature of myocardial remodeling is an increase in myocardial mass associated with a change in the shape of the ventricle (Frey and Olson, 2003).

At the cellular level, the increase in myocardial mass is reflected by cardiac myocyte hypertrophy, which is characterized by enhanced protein synthesis, heightened organization of the sarcomere, and the eventual increase in cell size. At the molecular level, the phenotype changes in cardiac myocytes are associated with reintroduction of the so-called fetal gene program, characterized by the patterns of gene expression mimicking those seen during embryonic development. These cellular and molecular changes are observed in both adaptive and maladaptive responses, thus distinguishing adaptive from maladaptive responses is difficult.

Adaptive Response   There is both physiological hypertrophy and pathological hypertrophy of the heart. Physiological hypertrophy is considered an adaptive response, which is an adjustment of cardiac function for an increased demand of cardiac output. Such an adaptive hypertrophy is the increase in cardiac mass after birth and in response to exercise. A biochemical distinction of the adaptive hypertrophy is that myocardial accumulation of collagen does not accompany the hypertrophy. Functionally, the increased mass is associated with enhanced contractility and cardiac output. In response to toxicologic stresses, the heart also often increases its mass, which has been viewed as an adaptive response as well. However, most recent evidence suggests that cardiac hypertrophy is a maladaptive process of the heart in response to intrinsic and extrinsic stresses.

Maladaptive Response   Although toxic stress-induced hypertrophy can normalize wall tension, it is a risk factor for sudden death and has a high potential to progress to overt heart failure. A distinction between adaptive and maladaptive hypertrophy is whether the hypertrophy is necessary for the compensatory function of the heart under physiological and pathological stress conditions. Many studies using genetically manipulated mouse models, either in the form of gain-of-function or loss-of-function, have supported the hypothesis that cardiac hypertrophy is neither required nor necessarily compensatory. For instance, forced expression of a dominant-negative calcineurin mutant confers protection against hypertrophy and fibrosis after abdominal aortic construction (Zou *et al.*, 2001). Also, the elimination of hypertrophy in animals by calcineurin suppression did not cause compromised hemodynamic changes over a period of several weeks (Hill *et al.*, 2000). Therefore, in these experimental approaches, hypertrophic growth could be abolished in the presence of continuous pressure overload, but the compensatory response could not be compromised. An interesting observation is that an almost complete lack of cardiac hypertrophy in response to aortic banding in a transgenic mouse model was accompanied with a significant slower pace of deterioration of systolic function (Esposito *et al.*, 2002). These observations indicate that cardiac hypertrophy in response to extrinsic and intrinsic stress is not a compensatory response. However, cardiac hypertrophy increases the risk for malignant arrhythmia and heart failure, and thus is now viewed as a maladaptive response.

Hypertrophic Signaling Pathways   Extrinsic and intrinsic stresses activate signaling transduction pathways leading to fetal gene program activation, enhanced protein synthesis of adult cardiomyocytes, and the eventual hypertrophic phenotype. The signaling pathways include several components: G-protein-coupled receptors, protein kinases including MAPK, PKC, and AMPK, calcium and calcineurin, and phosphoinositide 3-kinase (PI3K)/glycogen synthase kinase 3β (GSK3β), and transcription factors. Activation of each of the components is sufficient to induce myocardial hypertrophic growth. These components also affect each other through crosstalk. The diagram presented in Fig. 18-14 briefly summaries these pathways and their interactions. Among these pathways, protein kinases, calcium/calcineurin, and transcription factors have been discussed above. A brief summary for the G-protein-coupled receptors and the PI3K/GSK3 pathway is presented as follows:

G-Protein-Coupled Receptors   Myocardial adrenergic, angiotensin, and endothelin (ET-1) receptors belong to G-protein-coupled receptors, which are coupled to three major classes of heterotrimeric GTP-binding proteins, $G_{\alpha s}$, $G_{\alpha q}/G_{\alpha 11}$, and $G_{\alpha i}$. Activation of $G_{\alpha q}$-coupled receptors is sufficient to induce myocyte hypertrophy in vitro (Adams *et al.*, 1998). Cardiac-specific ablation of $G_{\alpha q}/G_{\alpha 11}$ in adult animals causes an almost complete lack of cardiac hypertrophy in response to aortic banding (Wettschureck *et al.*, 2001). Overexpression of a dominant-negative mutant of $G_{\alpha q}$ in transgenic mouse hearts suppresses pressure–overload hypertrophy (Akhter *et al.*, 1998). Cardiac overexpression of $G_{\alpha s}$, the downstream effector of β1-adenergic receptors in the heart, initially increases contractility, but eventually results in cardiac hypertrophy, fibrosis, and heart failure (Bisognano *et al.*, 2000).

Phosphoinositide 3-Kinase/Glycogen Synthase Kinase3β Pathway   Activation of PI3K is found in both physiological and pathological hypertrophy. Insulin-like growth factor (IGF) is involved in the growth of the heart after birth (Shioi *et al.*, 2002). Overexpression of IGF induces cardiac hypertrophy (Delaughter *et al.*, 1999). IGF signals through PI3K to the serine/threonine kinase Akt or protein kinase B. Both PI3K and the Akt induce hypertrophic growth of adult hearts. Overexpression of constitutively active PI3K mutant in the heart leads to increased heart size in mice, and expression of dominant-negative PI3K results in a small heart (Shioi *et al.*, 2000). Overexpression of Akt induces cardiac hypertrophy in transgenic mice without adverse effects on systolic function (Matsui *et al.*, 2002). Akt phsophorylates GSK3β, thus inhibits the activation of GSK3β. Otherwise, the activated GSK3β phosphorelates transcription factors of the NFAT family (Fig. 18-14). As discussed above, activation of calcineurin dephosphorylates NFAT3 in the cytoplasm, which enables NFAT3 to translocate to the nucleus where it can activate hypertrophic gene expression dependent on or independent of GATA4. Phosphorylation of NFAT3 in the nucleus by GSK3β promotes NFAT3 translocation to the cytoplasm, becoming inactive. Hypertrophic stimuli such as β-adrenergic agonist isoproterenol, ET-1, and phenylepherine all induce GSK3β phosphorylation in a PI3K-dependent fashion, indicating possible requirement of inactivation of GSK3β through phosphorylation in hypertrophic growth of the heart.

Transition from Cardiac Hypertrophy to Heart Failure   Pathological hypertrophy is a risk factor for malignant arrhythmia and heart failure. The link of heart hypertrophy to malignant arrhythmia will be discussed in the next section. The critical cellular event of this transition is myocardial apoptosis triggered by inflammatory cytokines, such as TNF-α, and neurohormonal factors, such as atrial natriuretic peptide (ANP), leads to dilated cardiomyopathy and deterioration of cardiac function. Toxicologic exposures may cause dilated cardiomyopathy or heart failure without an intermediate hypertrophic stage. Myocardial cell death also plays an essential role in direct cardiac dilation pathogenesis. Figure 18-15 illustrates the process of xenobiotic-induced transition from cardiac hypertrophy to heart failure.

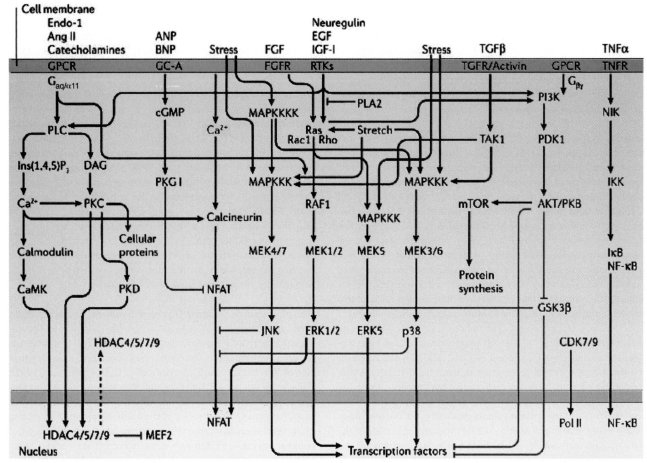

Figure 18-14. *Overview of signaling transduction pathways involved in cardiac hypertrophic growth and their cross-talk interactions.*

The signalling that occurs at the sarcolemmal membrane is shown at the top and the intermediate transduction of signals by various kinases and phosphatases is shown in the middle. The nucleus is shown at the bottom. ANP, atrial natriuretic peptide; Ang II, angiotensin II; BNP, B-type natriuretic peptide; CaMK, calmodulin-dependent kinase; CDK, cyclin-dependent kinase; DAG, diacylglycerol; EGF, epidermal growth factor; Endo-1, endothelin-1; ERK, extracellular signal-regulated kinase; FGF, fibroblast growth factor; FGFR, FGF receptor; GC-A, guanyl cyclase-A; GPCR, G-protein-coupled receptors; GSK3β, glycogen synthase kinase-3β; HDAC, histone deacetylases; IκB, inhibitor of NF-κB; IGF-I, insulin-like growth factor-I; IKK; inhibitor of NF-κB kinase; Ins(1,4,5)P3, inositol-1,4,5-trisphosphate; JNK, c-Jun N-terminal kinase; MAPKKK, mitogen-activated protein kinase kinase kinase; MAPKKKK, MAPKKK kinase; MEF, myocyte-enhancer factor; MEK, mitogen-activated protein kinase kinase; mTOR, mammalian target of rapamycin; NFAT, nuclear factor of activated T cells; NF-κB, nuclear factor-κB; NIK, NF-κB-inducing kinase; PDK, phosphoinositide-dependent kinase; PI3K, phosphatidylinositol 3-kinase; PKB, protein kinase B; PKC, protein kinase C; PKD, protein kinase D; PLA2, phospholipase A2; PLC, phospholipase C; Pol II, RNA polymerase II; RTK, receptor tyrosine kinase; TAK, TGFβ-activated kinase; TGF-β, transforming growth factor-beta; TGFR, TGF receptor; TNFα, tumour necrosis factor-α; TNFR, TNFα receptor. (Copied from *Nature Reviews of Molecular Cell Biology*, 7:589–600, 2006).

Alterations of biochemical reactions in the myocardium are often seen soon after exposure to environmental toxicants. These include alterations in ionic homeostasis, such as changes in intracellular calcium concentrations, which occur in most exposures to environmental toxicants (Symanski and Gettes, 1993). Aberrant energy metabolism is another early response to environmental toxicants in the heart, resulting in decreased production and/or enhanced consumption of ATP (Abas *et al.*, 2000). Alterations in enzymatic reactions are often described in cardiac toxic responses (Depre and Taegtmeyer, 2000). The early signaling pathways leading to myocardial toxic responses are the focus of current cardiac toxicology research (Piano, 1994). Detailed descriptions of these pathways and their role in cardiotoxicity are yet to be explored. It is likely that activation of signaling pathways is a critical response of myocardial cells to environmental toxic insults (Cheng *et al.*, 1999a). The crosstalk between signaling pathways determines the ultimate outcome of myocardial responses to chemicals.

Physiological alterations occur both as early responses to environmental toxicants and as subsequent events in the late development of cardiomyopathy. The most obvious myocardial dysfunction that occurs in the early responses to toxicants is cardiac arrhythmia (Peters *et al.*, 2000), which often results from the changes in intracellular calcium concentrations and other biochemical alterations, leading to miscommunication between cells and misconduction of electricity (Rosen, 1995). These changes, if not accompanied by cardiomyopathy, do not involve myocardial cell death and are reversible. In contrast, the late phase of cardiac dysfunction and arrhythmia, however, often result from cardiomyopathy.

Changes in myocardial morphology take place when extensive toxic insults are imposed on the heart and/or toxic exposures persist (He *et al.*, 1996). Cardiac hypertrophy is often observed as a

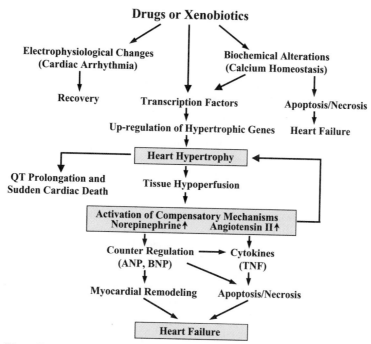

Figure 18-15. *Acute and chronic toxic exposure-induced heart failure and the transition from heart hypertrophy to heart failure.*

Acute exposure to drugs or xenobiotics can cause cardiac arrhythmia, which is often observed. But if the toxic insult is so severe, myocardial apoptosis and necrosis become predominant leading to dilated cardiomyopathy and heart failure. However, the heart often survives from toxic insults through adaptive mechanisms involving upregulation of hypertrophic genes and heart hypertrophy. Heart hypertrophy increases the risk for QT prolongation and sudden cardiac death, and also activates neurohormonal regulatory mechanisms including elevation of plasma concentration of sympathetic neural transmitters and angiotensins. These compensatory mechanisms in turn activate counter-regulatory mechanisms such as ANP, BNP, and TNF-α. A long-term action of the counter-regulatory mechanisms leads to myocardial remodeling and the transition from heart hypertrophy to heart failure.

consequence of long-term toxic insults. From cardiac hypertrophy to heart failure, activation of compensatory mechanisms, including the sympathetic nervous system and the renin–angiotensin system occurs (Holtz, 1993). The compensatory response in turn activates counter-regulatory mechanisms such as upregulation of ANP expression (Francis and Chu, 1995) and increase in cytokines, such as TNF-α production. Extensive biochemical, physiological, and molecular changes result in myocardial remodeling (Swynghedauw, 1999) and remarkable cell death, ultimately leading to heart failure.

QT prolongation and Sudden Cardiac Death

Recognition of QT prolongation and its associated adverse effects on the heart has been a major focus in drug discovery and development during the last decade. A number of drugs have been found to cause QT prolongation and Torsade de pointes (TdP), and thus were removed from the market or relabeled for restricted use. It has been known for a long time that quinidine causes sudden cardiac death; however, the severe and lethal side effect of QT prolongation did not draw sufficient attention until the last decade, due to the lack of knowledge and experimental approaches to obtain a comprehensive understanding of QT prolongation. Knowledge on QT prolongation has accumulated and regulatory guidelines for a battery of preclinical tests to assess QT liability of a potential drug are recommended.

Definition of QT Prolongation A simple definition for QT prolongation is that the length of QT interval observed from a typical electrocardiogram is prolonged. Clinically, long QT syndrome is defined when the QT interval is longer than 460 mseconds. However, TdP occurs with an average increase in QT interval by approximately 200 mseconds (a normal QT interval is about 300 mseconds). A human study has found that TdP does not occur with a QT interval shorter than 500 mseconds (Joshi *et al.*, 2004). In general, the long QT syndrome can be divided into two classes: congenital and acquired. Congenital long QT syndrome is rare and acquired is the major concern of drug cardiac toxicity in pharmaceutical discovery and development.

Molecular Basis of QT Prolongation Prolongation of the QT interval on the electrocardiogram is caused by prolongation of the action potential of ventricular myocytes. In cardiac action potential, phase 0 represents depolarization of myocytes and the depolarization of all ventricular myocytes is measurable as the QRS complex on the electrocardiogram. Phase 1 of the cardiac action potential is recognized as a partial repolarization of the membrane due to inactivation of cardiac sodium channels, and activation of transit outward potassium channels. Phase 2 of the action potential is generated primarily by slowly decreasing inward calcium currents through

L-type calcium channels, and gradually increasing outward currents through several types of potassium channels. This phase is sensitive to small changes in ion currents and is a critical determinant of the duration of the action potential. At this point, the cardiac cycle of the electrocardiogram has returned to baseline. Phase 3 of the cardiac action potential represents myocardial cell repolarization due to outward potassium currents. There are two critical potassium channels that terminate the plateau phase (phase 2) and initiate the final repolarization phase 3: I_{kr} and I_{ks}. I_{kr} is the rapidly activating delayed rectifier potassium current, and I_{ks} is the slowly activating delayed rectifier potassium current. The repolarization phase correlates with the T wave on the electrocardiogram. Therefore, the duration of the QT interval is related to the length of the ventricular action potentials.

A reduction in net outward current and/or an increase in inward current are potential contributors to the prolongation of cardiac action potential, thereby QT prolongation on the electrocardiogram. Although many channels are potentially involved in the prolongation of the cardiac action potential, current studies have identified three important channels that play a critical role in the plateau phase (phase 2) of the cardiac action potential, sodium inward channels, and potassium outward channels (I_{kr} and I_{ks}).

Sodium channel dysfunction in congenital long QT syndrome is related to mutations in *SCN5A* gene that encodes the α-subunits of sodium channels. Mutational analyses have found 14 distinct mutations of *SCN5A* associated with long QT syndrome (Splawski *et al.*, 2000). It has been hypothesized that gain-of-function mutations in *SCN5A* would cause long QT syndrome because reopening of the sodium channels during the plateau phase of action potential, even in a small inward current, would lengthen the duration of the cardiac action potential. Sodium channel inactivation immediately following depolarization (phase 1) is important for the transition to phase 2 of the action potential. A mutation of *SCN5A* has been found to destabilize the inactivation gate (Bennett *et al.*, 1995). Activation of these mutant sodium channels is normal and the rate of inactivation appears slightly faster than normal, but these mutant channels can reopen during the plateau phase of the action potential, leading to a prolonged plateau phase.

The I_{kr} potassium channels critically affect the length of the plateau phase of the cardiac action potential. The human *ether-à-go-go*-related gene (*HERG*) is expressed primarily in the heart and encodes the α-subunit of the cardiac I_{kr} potassium channel. There are 94 mutations of *HERG*, which have been identified to represent 45% of the total number of mutations related to long QT syndrome to date (Splawski *et al.*, 2000). The HERG α-subunits assemble with MiRP1 β-subunits to form cardiac I_{kr} channels. The I_{kr} potassium channel is one of the two channels that are primarily responsible for termination of the plateau phase of the action potential. During the repolarization of the action potential, the I_{kr} channels open, resulting in an increase in the magnitude of I_{kr} current during the first-half of phase 3 repolarization. Many *HERG* mutations occur around the membrane-spanning domains and the pore region of the channel. Most of these mutations have a loss-of-function effect and many long QT syndrome-associated mutations in *HERG* are missense mutations, which lead to a dominant-negative effect on I_{kr} channels because the functional I_{kr} potassium channels are composed of heteromultimers including several HERG subunits. Therefore, the loss-of-function mutations in *HERG* make a critical contribution to the long QT syndrome due to the prolonged plateau phase of cardiac potential.

The I_{ks} potassium channel is the other one of the two channels primarily responsible for the termination of the plateau phase of the action potential. The I_{ks} potassium channel is assembled from KVLQT1 α-subunits and the minK β-subunits. There are two molecular mechanisms that possibly account for reduced KVLQT1 function in the long QT syndrome (Wollnik *et al.*, 1997). First, intragenic deletions of one *KVLQT1* allele result in synthesis of abnormal α-subunits that do not assemble with normal subunits, leading to a 50% reduction in the number of the functional channels. Second, missense mutations result in synthesis of KVLQT1 subunits with structural abnormalities, which can assemble with normal subunits. Channels formed from the mutant KVLQT1 subunits have reduced or no function. Both of these mutations result in a dominant-negative effect. Interestingly, both *KVLQT1* and *minK* are expressed in the inner ear, in which the channels function to produce a potassium-rich fluid known as endolymph that bathes the organ of Corti, the cochlear organ responsible for hearing. Individuals with Jervell and Lange–Nielsen syndrome have homozygous mutations of *KVLQT1* or minK, thus having no functional I_{ks} channels. These individuals have severe arrhythmia susceptibility and congenital neural deafness.

Therefore, the molecular basis of the QT prolongation on the electrocardiogram is the prolongation of cardiac action potential. In this regard, the inward sodium channels and outward potassium channels play an important role in increasing the length of the plateau phase of action potentials. Congenital long QT syndrome is related to gain-of-function mutations in sodium channels and/or loss-of-function mutations in potassium channels. Acquired long QT syndrome is also related to altered function of these channels; however, many other factors that affect the phenotype of long QT syndrome and the clinical manifestations.

Torsade De Pointes and Sudden Cardiac Death   The abnormalities of different channels in different regions of the heart at varying levels result in channel dysfunction with regional variability. The regional abnormalities of cardiac repolarization or conductance provide a substrate for arrhythmia. Under these conditions, arrhythmia is induced if a trigger mechanism is implanted. The trigger for arrhythmia in the long QT syndrome is believed to be spontaneous secondary depolarization that arises during or just following the plateau of the action potential. This small action potential is the so-called early afterdepolarization, which occurs preferentially in M cells and Purkinje cells due to reactivation of the L-type calcium channels and/or activation of the sodium–calcium exchange current. When the spontaneous depolarization is accompanied by a marked increase in dispersion of repolarization, the likelihood to trigger an arrhythmia is increased. Once triggered, the arrhythmia is maintained by a regenerative circuit of electrical activity around relatively inexcitable tissue, a phenomenon known as reentry. The development of multiple reentrant circuits within the heart causes ventricular arrhythmia, or TdP, leading to sudden cardiac death. Drugs causing TdP are considered severe cardiac toxic agents. There are several drugs that were removed from the market due to their TdP effect. These drugs include those recently removed cyclo-oxygenase-2 (COX-2) inhibitors, Vioxx and Bextra, which will be discussed in the "Cardiac Toxic Chemicals" section. QT prolongation effect is now a required test by the U.S. Food and Drug Administration for drug development.

Parameters Affecting QT Prolongation and Torsadogenesis
Alterations in the function of cardiac channels, or "cardiac chan-nelopathies" occur at the cellular level. However, electrotonic cell-to-cell coupling influences the dispersion of repolarization. If my-ocardial cells with intrinsically different duration of action potential are well coupled, electrotonic current flow attenuates the differences in action potential duration in individual cardiomyocytes. Therefore, torsadogenesis results from not only cardiomyocytes, but also other types of cells and the interaction among these cells. There are many factors that affect the clinical manifestations of QT prolongation and torsadogenesis. Genetic polymorphisms and female gender are two distinct risk factors. The mechanism of the polymorphisms and the rationale for high susceptibility of females to QT prolongation and torsadogenesis are yet to be determined. The following factors are more descriptable.

Drugs and Environmental Toxicants   Drug-induced QT prolon-gation is a major acquired long QT syndrome. Selective blockers of potassium channels, including the drugs so-called class III anti-arrhythmics, have been developed for the treatment of various atrial arrhythmias. However, these drugs predictably produce long QT syndrome, which is sufficient to cause TdP in 5–7% of recipients. Environmental exposure to PM pollution in air is a risk factor for QT prolongation in elders, children, and individuals with compromised hearts.

Disturbances in Ion Homeostasis   Hypokalemia in combination with torsadogenic drugs is a most recognized risk factor for QT prolongation and TdP. It is also shown that sodium supplementa-tion can diminish the long QT syndrome due to the gain-of-function mutations in sodium channels. Stress-induced Ca^{2+} overload in my-ocardial cells increases the likelihood of arrhythmia. The electrode imbalance exerts more effect on compromised hearts.

Abnormal Gap Junction   Gap junction-mediated intercellular communication is essential in the propagation of electrical impulse in the heart. The gap junction is composed of connexons, as de-scribed in the cardiac physiology and structural features section. Under normal conditions, the gap junction electrotonic current flow attenuates the differences in action potential duration of myocardial cells. Toxicologic exposures cause damage to connexons leading to disruption of electrotonic cell-to-cell coupling, thus the differences in the action potential duration would be dominant, in particular under the influence of torsadogenic drugs or conditions.

Myocardial Ischemic Injury   Acute myocardial ischemia can cause immediate arrhythmia due to disturbance in ionic homeosta-sis, which is often transient. However, acute ischemia induces my-ocardial infarction can lead to block of cardiac conductance. Under the myocardial infarction, the areas separated by the scar tissue would be uncoupled, making the differences in the duration of ac-tion potential of myocardial cells in different regions apparent. The infarct heart thus is more susceptible to drug-induced QT prolonga-tion and TdP.

Cardiac Hypertrophy   Purkinje fibers are derived from myogenic precursors during embryonic development. The normal distribution of Purkinje fibers in the myocardium is proportional to the mass of the heart. Cardiac hypertrophy resulting from the hypertrophic growth of cardiac myocytes would lead to unbalanced distribution

of Purkinje fibers in the remodeling heart. The conduction of pace-maker potentials would thus be interrupted.

Myocardial Fibrosis   Dilated cardiomyopathy in alcoholics often involves myocardial fibrosis, which simulates the effect of myocar-dial infarction on the electrical conduction in the heart and the block of cardiac conductance.

Heart Failure   Most individuals with failing hearts die suddenly of cardiac arrhythmias. Heart failure presents a common, acquired form of the long QT syndrome. In human heart failure, selective downregulation of two potassium channels, I_{to1} and I_{k1}, has been shown to be involved in action potential prolongation. The I_{to1} cur-rent is involved in phase 1 of action potential and opposes the de-polarization. The increase in depolarization may be adaptive in the short term because it provides more time for excitation–contraction coupling, mitigating the decrease in cardiac output. However, down-regulation of potassium channels becomes maladaptive in the long term because it predisposes the individual to early afterdepolariza-tion, inhomogeneous repolarization, and polymorphic ventricular tachycardia.

Biomarkers for Cardiac Toxicity

Myocardial injury can be divided into two major classes: struc-tural and nonstructural injuries. The structural damage of the heart includes cell death and the associated histopathological changes such as myocardial infarction. Functional deficits often accompany the structural injury. Nonstructural damage represents functional deficits without apparent structural alterations. Myocardial adapta-tion to intrinsic and extrinsic stress leading to myocardial structural changes such as hypertrophy should be in the category of structural damage because the progression of hypertrophy leads to heart fail-ure in which cell death is a major determinant factor. Myocardial structural changes and functional alterations can be indirectly mea-sured by echocardiography and electrocardiogram in combination with stress testing. The data generated from these measurements can be considered in a broad sense as biomarkers. However, in clinical practice and experimental approach, biomarkers are referred to as indexes of myocardial injury measured from blood samples. The fundamental principle of the biomarkers is that molecules that are released from the myocardium under various injury conditions are readily detectable from blood samples.

Validation of Biomarkers   For a biomarker to be indicative of myocardial damage, an important question needs to be ad-dressed is what characteristics are required for a valid biomarker. In 2000, an Expert Working Group (EWG) on biomarkers of drug-induced cardiac toxicity was established under the Advisory Committee for Pharmaceutical Sciences of the Center for Drug Evaluation and Research of the U.S. Food and Drug Administra-tion. The report from this EWG has summarized the characteris-tics of ideal cardiac toxic injury biomarkers (Wallace *et al.*, 2004). These characteristics include cardiac specificity, sensitivity, predic-tive value, robust, bridge preclinical to clinical, and noninvasive procedure/accessibility. These characteristics are adapted as a stan-dard for development and validation of a biomarker of myocardial injury.

Availability of Biomarkers   Currently validated biomarkers that are included in clinical diagnostic testing guidelines are all related to myocardial structural injury. Developing biomarkers for non-structural injury is most challenging and demands implantation of more advanced technologies such as functional genomics and proteomics. In addition, currently available biomarkers have limitations, although they are useful.

Creatine Kinase   There are three major CK isoenzymes identified; CK-MM is the principal form in skeletal muscle, CK-MB presents in myocardium in which CK-MM is also found, and CK-BB is the predominant form in brain and kidney. Elevation of serum CK-MB is considered a reasonably specific marker of acute myocardial infarction.

Myoglobin   Myoglobin is found in all muscle types and its value as a biomarker of myocardial injury is based on the fact that serum concentrations of myoglobin increase rapidly following myocardial tissue injury, with peak values observed 1–4 hours after acute myocardial infarction. Elevation of serum myoglobin is likely reflective of the extent of myocardial damage.

B-Type Natriuretic Peptide   BNP is a cardiac neurohormone secreted by the ventricular myocardium in response to volume and pressure overload, and the release of BNP appears to be directly correlated with the degree of ventricular wall tension. BNP is now accepted as a biomarker for congestive heart failure and is included in the European guideline for the diagnosis of chronic heart failure.

C-Reactive Protein   The acute phase reactant CRP is a marker of systemic and vascular inflammation, which appears to predict future cardiac events in asymptomic individuals. In particular, inflammation has been shown to play a pivotal role in the inception, progression, and destabilization of atheromas. A predictive value of CRP for the prognosis of coronary heart disease is thus proposed. The measurement of CRP appears to provide additional prognostic information when cTnT is measured at the same time.

Cardiac Troponins   Cardiac troponin T (cTnT) and I (cTnI) are constituents of the myofilaments and expressed exclusively in cardiomyocytes. It is thus of absolute myocardial tissue specificity. In healthy persons, serum cTnT or cTnI are rarely detectable. Therefore, any measurable concentrations of serum cTnT or cTnI reflect irreversible myocardial injury such as myocardial infarction. The clinical experience has arrived at a recommendation that cTn measurement becomes the "gold standard" for diagnosis of acute myocardial infarction.

Biomarker Applications and Limitations   All the biomarkers described above have been used as indices of myocardial injury in clinical practice and experimental studies. The major concern of most of the biomarkers is their specificity. CK-MB is present in small quantities in skeletal muscle and other tissues, thus elevations of CK-MB occur in some diseases involving skeletal muscle injury. Myoglobin is found in all muscle types and its concentrations vary significantly between species and even within species. BNP has been proposed to use as a prognostic indicator of disease progression and outcome of congestive heart failure. However, the actual utility of this biomarker is untested. BNP is involved in the counter-regulation of heart hypertrophy, thus the changes in serum BNP concentrations

as a function of time in the transition from cardiac hypertrophy to heart failure needs to be understood comprehensively. Higher levels of BNP may not necessarily indicate more severity of the heart disease, indicating that more scrutiny to analysis is needed. CRP is a biomarker of inflammation and its use in myocardial injury is more supplementary to other tests than having independently predictive value.

Considering all of the limitations above, more reliable biomarkers are needed. A significant advance in the development and validation of biomarkers for myocardial injury is the promising clinical experience with cTn, which has absolute myocardial tissue specificity and high sensitivity. It is now accepted by the clinical community that cTn as the biomarker of choice for assessing myocardial damage in humans. Its preclinical value for monitoring drug cardiac toxicity and in drug development need to be evaluated.

CARDIAC TOXIC CHEMICALS

Many substances can cause cardiac toxic responses directly or indirectly. However, only chemicals that primarily act on the heart or whose cardiac toxicity is the primary concern should be categorized as cardiac toxic chemicals. Clinically, the most recognized toxicologic cardiomyopathy is found in alcoholic heart muscle disease, which is often referred to as alcoholic cardiomyopathy (ACM). In this section, ACM will be discussed as a prototype of toxicologic cardiomyopathy. However, cardiomyopathy induced by therapeutic drugs is also well recognized, but it is often referred to as cardiomyopathy induced by specific chemicals, such as anthracycline cardiomyopathy. In this context, the chemicals that cause cardiac toxicity can be classified in multiple ways, however, this chapter will category them into (1) pharmaceutical chemicals, (2) natural products, and (3) environmental and industrial chemicals. Because general mechanisms of cardiotoxicity have been discussed above, these cardiac toxic chemicals will be briefly discussed.

Alcohol and Alcoholic Cardiomyopathy

ACM has been recognized for a long time (Klatsky, 1998) and the prevalence of ACM in selected populations ranges from 23% to 40% (Fauchier *et al.*, 2000; Mckenna *et al.*, 1998). Alcohol is believed to be the causal chemical in up to 40% of all patients with nonischemic, dilated cardiomyopathy (Gavazzi *et al.*, 2000). ACM is characterized by an increase in myocardial mass, dilation of the ventricles, wall thinning, ventricular dysfunction, and heart failure (Piano, 2002).

The pathogenesis of ACM is not completely understood. However, it is clear that the duration of heavy alcohol use in patients is a critical factor. Clinical data have shown that ACM typically is seen after a long term of consistent consumption of at least 80 g of alcohol per day (Regan, 1990; Lazarevic *et al.*, 2000). In general, asymptomatic ACM patients with changes in cardiac structure and function had a history of consuming >90 g/d of alcohol for more than 5 years (Lazarevic *et al.*, 2000). For the symptomatic ACM, some limited data have shown that more than 10 years of excessive alcohol consumption in alcoholics produces congestive heart failure (Mathews *et al.*, 1981).

The pathogenesis of heart failure begins after an index event such as alcohol-induced cardiac muscle injury that produces an initial decline in pumping capacity of the heart. Following this initial decline, a variety of compensatory mechanisms are activated, including the adrenergic nervous system, the renin–angiotensin system, and the cytokine system. Some of these compensatory changes have been detected in alcoholic patients (Adams and Hirst, 1986). However, with time, the sustained activation of these systems can lead to secondary end-organ damage within the ventricle by activating and accelerating the left ventricle remodeling and subsequent cardiac decompensation, resulting in the transition from asymptomatic to symptomatic heart failure (Mathews et al., 1981).

It was proposed that the metabolite acetaldehyde is responsible for some of the cardiac injury associated with ethanol consumption. The metabolic enzyme responsible for the conversion of ethanol to acetaldehyde is alcohol dehydrogenase, which is absent in cardiac myocytes. Studies have indicated that the impaired liver function of alcoholics may be sufficient to generate quantities of acetaldehyde that can reach the heart. The direct effects of acetaldehyde on the myocardium include inhibition of protein synthesis, inhibition of Ca^{2+} sequestration by the SR, alterations in mitochondrial respiration, and disturbances in the association of actin and myosin. The exact mechanism of ACM is unresolved. It has been suggested that a combination of multiple factors is involved, including malnutrition, cigarette smoking, systemic hypertension, and beverage additives, in addition to a long-term consumption of alcohol in the ACM patients (Ahmed and Regan, 1992).

The generation of reactive oxidative metabolites from the biotransformation of ethanol has been suggested to be a major contributing factor for ACM, because these metabolites lead to lipid peroxidation of cardiac myocytes or oxidation of cytosolic and membraneous protein thiols (Ribiere et al., 1992; Kannan et al., 2004). Most experimental approaches involve alcohol-containing liquid diet feeding to rodent models of ACM for several weeks to several months. However, a key factor for the development of ACM in humans is the duration of excessive consumption of alcohol. The simulation of daily excessive amount of alcohol consumption in rodents without disturbances in the food intake to produce nutritional deficiency is a constant challenge. One of the difficulties in using rodent models is that the short life span of the animals does not allow a sufficient long period of alcohol exposure to produce some of the critical pathological changes such as myocardial fibrosis observed in humans.

A recent study using a mouse model in which alcohol-induced heart hypertrophy and fibrosis were all produced, may have been a breakthrough. In this mouse model, a zinc-regulatory protein, metallothionein (MT), is genetically deleted and when zinc was exogenously added to the alcohol-containing liquid diet, alcohol-induced cardiac fibrosis, but not heart hypertrophy, in the MT knockout (MT-KO) mice was prevented (Wang et al., 2005). Zinc deficiency is an important feature in alcoholic patients and animal models (McClain and Su, 1983; Bogden et al., 1984). Zinc homeostasis within the cell is dependant on MT, which under physiological conditions binds 7 atoms of zinc (Kagi, 1991). The role of MT in the regulation of zinc homeostasis has been revealed only recently (Maret, 2000; Kang, 2006). The most important feature of MT is that under oxidative stress conditions, it releases zinc (Maret, 2000; Kang, 2006). In the MT-KO mice, alcohol-induced myocardial pathological changes are either accelerated or severely altered relative to those in WT mice. These pathological changes, in particular the myocardial fibrosis, resemble the pathology observed in patients with ACM.

There are several interesting clues that have been provided from the MT-KO mouse studies. First, the link between the deficiency in endogenously stored zinc due to the lack of MT and the alcohol-induced myocardial fibrosis is suggested by the fact that supplementation with zinc inhibits alcoholic myocardial fibrosis.

Second, the dissociation between alcohol-induced heart hypertrophy and myocardial fibrosis is suggested by the fact that supplementation with zinc only inhibits fibrosis but heart hypertrophy. Third, possible involvement of oxidative stress in the fibrogenesis is suggested by the fact that MT functions as an antioxidant (Kang, 1999) and zinc release from MT is an essential response of MT to oxidative stress (Maret, 2000; Kang, 2006), suggesting that oxidative stress is involved in the fibrogenesis. Further studies following the same direction will provide more comprehensive insights into the pathogenesis of ACM.

Pharmaceutical Chemicals

Cardiac toxicity of pharmaceutical chemicals is a major problem in drug development and their clinical application. The pharmaceutical chemicals that cause cardiac toxic responses can be simply classified as drugs that are used to treat cardiac disease, and others that are used to treat noncardiac disease. In the category of drugs used to treat cardiac disease, cardiac toxicity is often produced by overexpression of the principal pharmaceutical effects. Although overdosing of these drugs can be a major factor for untoward effects, cardiac toxicity is often inevitable for this group of drugs. Drugs such as digitalis, quinidine, and procainamide often cause acute cardiac toxicity in the form of arrhythmia, which is reversible upon cessation of their use. Other cardiac drugs that may cause cardiac toxicity by mechanisms different from that of the therapeutic action. For instance, catecholamines may cause cardiac toxicity through oxidative stress, rather than by their pharmaceutical action on the sympathetic nervous system. The other category is noncardiac drugs that produce cardiac toxicity. For instance, anthracyclines, such as Adriamycin, are effective anticancer drugs, but their ability to produce severe cardiac toxicity limits their use in cancer patients. Vioxx is a selective COX-2 inhibitor used as an anti-inflammatory drug, but it causes QT prologation and increases the risk for sudden cardiac death.

Antiarrhythmic Agents Antiarrhythmic drugs have historically been classified based upon a primary mechanism of action: Na^+ channel blockers (class I), β-adrenergic blockers (class II), drugs that prolong action potential duration, especially K^+ channel blockers (class III), and Ca^{2+} channel blockers (class IV). However, this classification is artificial because most of the drugs have multiple mechanisms of action.

Class I antiarrhythmic agents are primarily Na^+ channel blockers, including disopyramide, encainide, flecainide, lidocaine, mexiletine, moricizine, phenytoin, procainamide, propafenone, quinidine, and tocainide. Blockade of cardiac Na^+ channels results in reduction of conduction velocity, prolonged QRS duration, decreased automaticity, and inhibition of triggered activity from delayed afterdepolarizations or early afterdepolarizations (Roden, 1996). The primary concern of Na^+ channel blocker toxicity is that proarrhythmic effects are seen at a much higher incidence in those patients with a previous history of myocardial infarction or with acute myocardial ischemia (Nattel, 1998). The proarrhythmic effects of these drugs would also be more prevalent in patients with other cardiac complications.

Class II antiarrhythmic drugs are β-adrenergic receptor-blocking drugs, including acebutolol, esmolol, propranolol, and sotalol. The catecholamines increase contractility, heart rate, and conduction through activation of β-adrenergic receptors in the heart. These effects can be explained by increased adenylyl cyclase activity, increased cyclic AMP, activation of protein kinase A, and phosphorylation and activation of L-type Ca^{2+} channels, thereby increasing intracellular Ca^{2+}, and particularly the amplitude of the Ca^{2+} transient. Therefore, antagonists of β-adrenergic receptors in the heart lead to effects that are opposite that of catecholamines, and are useful for the treatment of supraventricular tachycardia. The main adverse cardiovascular effect of β-adrenergic receptor antagonists is hypotension. These drugs may also exacerbate AV conduction deficits (e.g., heart block) and promote arrhythmias during bradycardia.

Class III antiarrhythmic drugs are primarily K^+ channel blockers. These drugs include amiodarone, bretylium, dofetilide, ibutilide, quinidine, and sotalol. Blockade of K^+ channels increases action potential duration and increases refractoriness. Prolonged action potential duration contributes to the development of early afterdepolarizations and promotion of tachycardia, especially polymorphic ventricular tachycardia (torsades de pointes). The most noticeable adverse effect of these drugs is QT prolongation and torsadogenesis. Most of the drugs in this class also affect other ion channels and/or receptors. Amiodarone and quinidine also block Na^+ channels, whereas sotalol inhibits β-adrenergic receptors in the heart. Amiodarone prolongs action potential duration and effective refractory period of Purkinje fibers and ventricular myocytes, and the most common adverse cardiovascular effect of amiodarone is bradycardia. Amiodarone may also have cardiotoxic effects by stimulating excessive Ca^{2+} uptake, especially in the presence of procaine (Gotzsche and Pedersen, 1994).

Class IV antiarrhythmic drugs are Ca^{2+} channel blockers and include diltiazem and verapamil. The dihydropyridine Ca^{2+} channel blockers are not used to treat arrhythmias because they have a greater selectivity for vascular cells; however, these drugs may also alter cardiac ion homeostasis when plasma concentrations of the drugs are elevated. The dihydropyridines interact with Ca^{2+} channels in the inactivated state of the channel, and because vascular smooth muscle resting potentials are lower than cardiac cells, the time spent in the inactivated state is relatively longer in vascular smooth muscle, thus providing some preference of dihydropyridines for the vasculature (Galan *et al.*, 1998). Bepridil, verapamil, and diltiazem exert negative inotropic and chronotropic effects. These drugs also exert a negative chronotropic effect, thus they may produce bradycardia. In contrast, the dihydropyridine Ca^{2+} channel blockers typically induce a reflex tachycardia subsequent to peripheral vascular dilation and baroreceptor reflex leading to increased sympathetic outflow from the medulla.

Inotropic Drugs Drugs involved in this category include the cardiac glycosides, Ca^{2+} sensitizing agents, catecholamines, and other sympathomimetic drugs. As with the antiarrhythmic drugs, inotropic drugs may exert cardiotoxic effects through extensions of their pharmacologic action.

Cardiac glycosides (digoxin and digitoxin) are inotropic drugs used for the treatment of congestive heart failure. Ouabain is a cardiac glycoside commonly used in the laboratory for electrophysiological experiments in cardiac myocytes. The mechanism of inotropic action of cardiac glycosides involves inhibition of Na^+, K^+-ATPase, elevation of intracellular Na^+, activation of Na^+/Ca^{2+} exchange, and increased availability of intracellular Ca^{2+} for contraction. Consequently, cardiotoxicity may result from Ca^{2+} overload, potentially including reduction in resting membrane potential (less negative), delayed afterdepolarizations, and premature ventricular contraction or ectopic beats. Cardiac glycosides also exhibit parasympatho-mimetic activity through vagal stimulation and facilitation of muscarinic transmission; however, at higher doses, sympathomimetic effects may occur as sympathetic outflow is enhanced. The principal adverse cardiac effects of cardiac glycosides include slowed AV conduction with potential block, ectopic beats, and bradycardia. During overdose, when the resting membrane potential is significantly altered and ectopic beats are prevalent, ventricular tachycardia may develop and can progress to ventricular fibrillation. A wide variety of drug interactions with digoxin have been reported, including both pharmacokinetic interactions (drugs that alter serum concentrations of digoxin) and pharmacodynamic interactions (drugs that alter the cardiac effects of digoxin).

Ca^{2+}-sensitizing drugs including adibendan, levosimendan, and pimobendan are useful as inotropic drugs for the treatment of heart failure. In contrast to the main mechanism by which many other inotropic drugs act through elevating intracellular-free Ca^{2+} ($[Ca^{2+}]_i$) during the Ca^{2+} transient (i.e., increase the amplitude of the Ca^{2+} transient), these Ca^{2+}-sensitizing drugs increase Ca^{2+} sensitivity of cardiac myocytes, thereby avoiding Ca^{2+} overload (Lee and Allen, 1997). Although cardiotoxicity resulting from Ca^{2+} overload would not be expected following administration of these new drugs, some experimental data suggest that they may still exert proarrhythmic effects (Lee and Allen, 1997). The possibility that such Ca^{2+}-sensitizing drugs interfere with diastolic function (relaxation) requires further investigation but may contribute to the ventricular arrhythmias associated with these drugs. Other Ca^{2+}-sensitizing drugs include the xanthine oxidase inhibitors allopurinol and oxypurinol, which have been shown to increase contractile force but decrease Ca^{2+} transient amplitude (Perez *et al.*, 1998).

Catecholamines and sympathomimetics Catecholamines represent a chemical class of neurotransmitters synthesized in the adrenal medulla (epinephrine and norepinephrine) and in the sympathetic nervous system (norepinephrine). These neurotransmitters exert a wide variety of cardiovascular effects. Because of their ability to activate α- and β-adrenergic receptors, especially in the cardiovascular system, a number of synthetic catecholamines have been developed for the treatment of cardiovascular disorders and other conditions such as asthma and nasal congestion. Inotropic and chronotropic catecholamines used to treat bradycardia, cardiac decompensation following surgery, or to increase blood pressure (e.g., hypotensive shock) include epinephrine, isoproterenol, and dobutamine, and these drugs typically display nonselective activation of adrenergic receptors. More selective β_2-adrenergic receptor agonists used for bronchodilatory effects in asthma include albuterol, bitolterol, fenoterol, formoterol, metaproterenol, pirbuterol, procaterol, salmeterol, and terbutaline. High oral doses of albuterol or terbutaline or inhalation doses (i.e., enhanced delivery to the stomach instead of the lungs with subsequent systemic absorption) of these drugs may lead to nonselective activation of β_1-adrenergic receptors in the heart with subsequent tachycardia.

Sympathomimetic drugs that are more selective for α-adrenergic receptors include the nasal decongestants ephedrine, phenylephrine, phenylpropanolamine, and pseudoephedrine. As with the asthma drugs, at high doses these nasal decongestants can produce tachycardia, and a number of deaths have been reported. Of particular interest is the high concentration of ephedra alkaloids that may be present in some herbal remedies or "neutraceuticals," especially in products containing ma huang (Gurley *et al.*, 1998). Tachycardia may occur from the consumption of large amounts of ephedra alkaloids, which may predispose the myocardium to ventricular arrhythmias.

High circulating concentrations of epinephrine (adrenaline) and norepinephrine (noradrenaline) and high doses of synthetic catecholamines, such as isoproterenol, may cause cardiac myocyte death. Many of the catecholamines and related drugs have been shown to induce cardiac myocyte hypertrophic growth in vitro. Catecholamine-induced cardiotoxicity involves pronounced pharmacologic effects, including increased heart rate, enhanced myocardial oxygen demand, and an overall increase in systolic arterial blood pressure.

Other possible mechanisms for the cardiotoxicity of high concentrations of catecholamines include coronary insufficiency resulting from coronary vasospasm, decreased levels of high-energy phosphate stores caused by mitochondrial dysfunction, increased sarcolemmal permeability leading to electrolyte alterations, altered lipid metabolism resulting in the accumulation of FAs, and intracellular Ca^{2+} overload (Dhalla *et al.*, 1992).

Central Nervous System Acting Drugs Some of central nervous system (CNS)-acting drugs have considerable effects on the cardiovascular system, including tricyclic antidepressants (TCAs), general anesthetics, some of the opioids, and antipsychotic drugs.

TCAs including amitriptyline, desipramine, doxepin, imipramine, and protriptyline have significant cardiotoxic effects, particularly in cases of overdose. The effects of TCAs on the heart include ST segment elevation, QT prolongation, supraventricular and ventricular arrhythmias (including torsades de pointes), and sudden cardiac death. In addition, as a result of peripheral α-adrenergic blockade, TCAs cause postural hypotension—the most prevalent cardiovascular effect. Although many of these adverse effects are related to the quinidine-like actions, anticholinergic effects, and adrenergic actions of these drugs, the tricyclics also have direct actions on cardiac myocytes and Purkinje fibers, including depression of inward Na^+ and Ca^{2+} and outward K^+ currents (Pacher *et al.*, 1998). Furthermore, the risk of TCA-induced cardiotoxicity is significantly enhanced in children and by concomitant administration of other drugs that alter ion movement or homeostasis in the heart (e.g., the Na^+ channel-blocking class I antiarrhythmic agents), or use in patients with cardiovascular disease.

Antipsychotic drugs include the phenothiazines (acetophenazine, chlorpromazine, fluphenazine, mesoridazine, perphenazine, thioridazine, and trifluoperazine), chlorprothixene, thiothixene, and other heterocyclic compounds (clozapine, haloperidol, loxapine, molindone, pimozide, and risperidone). As with TCAs, the most prominent adverse cardiovascular effect of antipsychotic drugs is orthostatic hypotension. However, the phenothiazines (e.g., chlorpromazine and thioridazine) may exert direct effects on the myocardium, including negative inotropic actions and quinidine-like effects (Baldessarini, 1996). Some ECG changes induced by these drugs include prolongation of the QT and PR intervals, blunting of T waves, and depression of the ST segment. Through anticholinergic actions, clozapine can produce substantial elevations in heart rate (tachycardia).

General anesthetics as exemplified by enflurane, desflurane, halothane, isoflurane, methoxyflurane, and sevoflurane have adverse cardiac effects, including reduced cardiac output by 20–50%, depression of contractility, and production of arrhythmias (generally benign in healthy myocardium but more serious in cardiac dis-

ease). These anesthetics may sensitize the heart to the arrhythmogenic effects of endogenous epinephrine or to β-receptor agonists. Halothane has been found to block the L-type Ca^{2+} channel by interacting with dihydropyridine-binding sites, to disrupt Ca^{2+} homeostasis associated with the SR, and to modify the responsiveness of the contractile proteins to activation by Ca^{2+} (Bosnjak, 1991). Propofol is an intravenously administered general anesthetic that also decreases cardiac output and blood pressure. In addition, propofol causes a negative inotropic effect by its direct action on cardiac myocytes. Propofol has been shown to antagonize β-adrenergic receptors, inhibit L-type Ca^{2+} current, and reduce Ca^{2+} transients (Zhou *et al.*, 1997, 1999; Guenoun *et al.*, 2000).

Local Anesthetics In general, local anesthetics have few undesirable cardiac effects. However, when high systemic concentrations of cocaine and procainamide are attained, these chemicals may have prominent adverse effects on the heart.

Cocaine acts as a local anesthetic agent by blocking conduction in nerve fibers through reversibly inhibiting Na^+ channels and stopping the transient rise in Na^+ conductance. In the heart, cocaine decreases the rate of depolarization and the amplitude of the action potential, slows conduction speed, and increases the effective refractory period. The other major pharmacologic action of cocaine is its ability to inhibit the reuptake of norepinephrine and dopamine into sympathetic nerve terminals (sympathomimetic effect). Cocaine also, indirectly through its actions on catecholamine reuptake, stimulates β- and α-adrenergic receptors, leading to increased cyclic AMP and inositol triphosphate levels. These second messengers will, in turn, provoke a rise in cytosolic Ca^{2+}, which causes sustained action potential generation and extrasystoles. The net effect of these pharmacologic actions is to elicit and maintain ventricular fibrillation. In addition, cocaine causes cardiac myocyte death and myocardial infarction, but the mechanism of action remains to be elucidated.

Other local anesthetic drugs include benzocaine, bupivacaine, etidocaine, lidocaine, mepivacaine, pramoxine, prilocaine, procaine, procainamide, proparacaine, ro-pivacaine, and tetracaine. Lidocaine and procainamide are also used as antiarrhythmic drugs. Extremely high doses of these drugs cause decreases in electrical excitability, conduction rate, and force of contraction likely through inhibition of cardiac Na^+ channels (Catterall and Mackie, 1996).

Anthracyclines and Other Antineoplastic Agents Cardiotoxicity is recognized as a serious side effect of chemotherapy for malignant cancers, especially with well-known antitumor agents such as doxorubicin, daunorubicin, 5-fluorouracil, and cyclophosphamide (Havlin, 1992).

Anthracyclines (doxorubicin or Adriamycin and daunorubicin) are widely used antineoplastic drugs for the treatment of breast cancer, leukemias, and a variety of other solid tumors. Unfortunately, the clinical usefulness of these drugs is limited because of acute and chronic cardiotoxic effects. The acute effects mimic anaphylactic-type responses, such as tachycardia and various arrhythmias. These effects are usually manageable and most likely are due to the potent release of histamine from mast cells sometimes observed in acute dosing. In addition, large acute doses can also cause left ventricular failure. The greatest limiting factor of the anthracyclines is associated with long-term exposure, which usually results in the development of cardiomyopathies and, in severe cases, congestive heart failure (Havlin, 1992).

Two new anthracyclines were introduced to the U.S. market in 1999, and a lipid formulation of doxorubicin (liposomal doxorubicin) is under development. *Valrubicin* is a semisynthetic derivative of doxorubicin approved for treatment of carcinoma in situ of the bladder. It is administered locally for bladder cancer and therefore induces only mild systemic toxicities; however, systemic absorption from the bladder may occur, but valrubicin seems to exhibit a lower propensity for cardiotoxicity than doxorubicin (Hussar, 2000). *Epirubicin* is a semisynthetic derivative of daunorubicin approved for treatment of breast cancer. Like doxorubicin, epirubicin is given systemically and may induce cardiotoxicity. However, epirubicin is more lipophilic than doxorubicin and is biotransformed by the conjugative pathways in the liver, resulting in a shorter half-life and a lower incidence of cardiotoxicity than with doxorubicin (Hussar, 2000).

Several major hypotheses have been suggested to account for the onset of anthracycline-induced cardiomyopathy: (1) oxidative stress from redox cycling or mitochondrial Ca^{2+} cycling, (2) defects in mitochondrial integrity and subsequent deterioration of myocardial energetics, (3) alterations in both SR Ca^{2+} currents and mitochondrial Ca^{2+} homeostasis, and (4) altered cardiac myocyte gene expression and induction of apoptosis. The cause-and-effect relationships of the proposed mechanisms of cardiotoxicity have not been determined, and no single theory adequately explains the exact mechanism for anthracycline-induced cardiomyopathy.

The free radical hypothesis has received the most attention in the understanding of anthrocycline-induced cardiotoxicity. The formation of ROS by doxorubicin (Fig. 18-16) has been attributed to redox cycling of the drug (Powis, 1989). Doxorubicin can undergo futile redox cycling that results in the production of oxygen free radicals; these ROS may then oxidize proteins, lipids, and nucleic acids and potentially cause DNA strand scission. The quinone-like structure of doxorubicin permits this molecule to accept an electron and form a semiquinone radical. Oxidation of the semiquinone back to the parent quinone by molecular oxygen results in the formation of superoxide radical ions that are believed to initiate oxidative stress. The enzymatic reduction that is believed to be responsible for the generation of superoxide by doxorubicin has been proposed to occur between complexes I and III of the mitochondrial respiratory chain. Doxorubicin has high affinity for cardiolipin, a phospholipid found on the inner mitochondrial membrane, where NADH dehydrogenase converts the drug to a semiquinone radical (Marcillat *et al.*, 1989). In the presence of oxygen, this radical is responsible for the generation of ROS, which then may peroxidize unsaturated membrane lipids and initiate myocardial cell injury.

Several alternate hypotheses to explain the cardiotoxicity of doxorubicin have been proposed and tested. For example, several studies have tested the hypothesis that doxorubicin induces a cycling of mitochondrial Ca^{2+} that is associated with the production of ROS and dissipation in the mitochondrial membrane potential, which in turn may result in depletion of cellular ATP (Chacon and Acosta, 1991; Solem *et al.*, 1994). It is important to note that the observed changes in ROS accumulation, disruption of Ca^{2+} homeostasis, and mitochondrial damage are not isolated, but rather these changes occur sequentially or simultaneously. It is extremely difficult to dissect the sequences of these changes, leading to several alternate hypotheses, which may in fact occur sequentially. One of the ultimate consequences of these changes is myocardial cell death. Many studies have demonstrated that anthracycline-induced cardiotoxicity includes induction of apoptosis (Kang *et al.*, 2000a; Wang *et al.*,

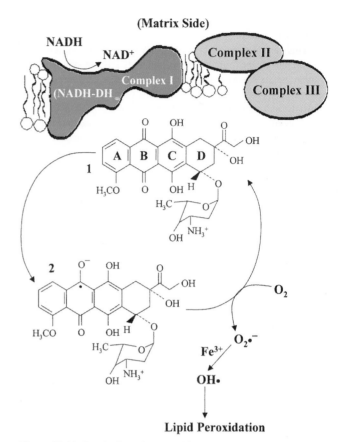

Figure 18-16. *Production of superoxide anions by oxidation-reduction cycling of doxorubicin at the level of the mitochondria.*

NADH dehydrogenase (NAD-DH), which is located within complex I, has been proposed as the enzyme that catalyzes the one-electron reduction of doxorubicin (1) to a semiquinone radical (2). The semiquinone then may be reoxidized back to the parent compound by means of the reduction of molecular oxygen (O_2) to the superoxide anion (O_2^-).

2001a; Sawyer *et al.*, 1999; Andrieu-Abadie *et al.*, 1999; Arola *et al.*, 2000).

5-Fluorouracil Clinical evidence of 5-fluorouracil cardiotoxicity ranges from mild precordial pain and ECG abnormalities (ST segment elevation, high peaked T waves, T-wave inversions, and sinus tachycardia) to severe hypotension, atrial fibrillation, and abnormalities of ventricular wall motion. The mechanism of cardiotoxicity of fluorouracil is unknown, but it may relate to impurities present in commercial products of the drug, one of which is metabolized to fluoroacetate, a compound that might participate in fluorouracil-induced cardiotoxicity.

Cyclophosphamide High doses of cyclophosphamide given to cancer or transplant patients may lead to severe hemorrhagic cardiac necrosis. The mechanism of the cardiotoxicity of this drug is not clear, but there is suggestive evidence that the toxic metabolite of cyclophosphamide, 4-hydroperoxycyclophosphamide, may alter the ion homeostasis in cardiac myocytes, resulting in increased Na^+ and Ca^{2+} content and reduced K^+ levels (Levine *et al.*, 1993).

Antimicrobial and Antiviral Agents Cardiotoxicity associated with the clinical use of antimicrobial and antiviral drugs is often observed in overdosage and in patients with preexisting cardiovascular dysfunction.

Aminoglycosides include amikacin, gentamicin, kanamycin, netilmicin, streptomycin, and tobramycin. Gentamicin is a representative aminoglycoside and has an inhibitory action on slow inward Ca^{2+} channels in heart muscle. Aminoglycosides inhibit the uptake or binding of Ca^{2+} at sarcolemmal sites, thus reducing the concentration of membrane-bound Ca^{2+} available for movement into the myoplasm during depolarization of the sarcolemma. The principle mechanism of cardiodepression by gentamicin is the dislocation of Ca^{2+} from slow-channel-binding sites on the external surface of the sarcolemma, which results in a blockade of the channels (Hino *et al.*, 1982).

Macrolides include azithromycin, clarithromycin, dirithromycin, and erythromycin. Erythromycin is associated with QT prolongation and cardiac dysrhythmias characterized by polymorphic ventricular tachycardia (torsades de pointes). These effects occur primarily in patients with underlying cardiac disease.

Fluoroquinolones are a group of rapid growing antibacterial chemicals in terms of numbers of new drugs released into the market in the United States. Fluoroquinolone antibacterial drugs include ciprofloxacin, enoxacin, gatifloxacin, gemifloxacin, grepafloxacin, levofloxacin (levo-rotatory isomer of ofloxacin), lomefloxacin, moxifloxacin, norfloxacin, ofloxacin, sparfloxacin, and trovafloxacin (Pickerill *et al.*, 2000). Grepafloxacin, moxifloxacin, and sparfloxacin are associated with QT prolongation in perhaps a higher incidence than macrolides. In fact, grepafloxacin was voluntarily removed from the U.S. market because of the relatively high incidence of QT prolongation and risk of torsades de pointes.

Tetracycline and chloramphenicol have been reported to depress myocardial contractility by direct cardiac myocyte interaction or an indirect effect that lowers Ca^{2+} concentrations in the plasma or extracellular spaces. Tetracyclines are Ca^{2+} chelating agents, which explain the action of tetracyclines on myocardial contractility.

Antifungal agents, such as amphotericin B, may depress myocardial contractility by blocking activation of slow Ca^{2+} channels and inhibiting the influx of Na^+. Ventricular tachycardia and cardiac arrest have been reported in patients treated with amphotericin B. Flucytosine is another antifungal drug that has been associated with cardiotoxicity. In fungal cells, flucytosine is converted to 5-fluorouracil, which then exerts antifungal effects. However, flucytosine may be converted to 5-fluorouracil by gastrointestinal microflora in humans, which then may be absorbed systemically and induce cardiotoxicity as discussed above. Cardiac arrest has been reported in individuals receiving flucytosine.

Antiviral drugs that are potentially cardiotoxic include the nucleoside analog reverse transcriptase inhibitors used for the treatment of human immunodeficiency virus (HIV) infections. Clinical studies of direct cardiotoxicity of these drugs in HIV patients are complicated by cardiomyopathy related to disease progression. The direct evidence for cardiotoxicity of zidovudine (AZT) has been obtained from a study using transgenic mice expressing replication-incompetent HIV (Lewis *et al.*, 2000). AZT-induced cardiotoxicity in this model is related to alteration in Ca^{2+} homeostasis and/or mitochondrial toxicity. The mitochondrial toxicity of AZT has also been shown in skeletal muscle biopsy samples from AIDS patients (Dalakas, *et al.*, 1990).

Although cardiotoxicity of individual antiviral drugs is rare in clinical setting, the combination of several antiviral drugs for highly active anti-retroviral therapy (HAART) has generated a major concern of cardiotoxicity (Bozkurt, 2004). HAART has dramatically improved the life expectancy of patients with HIV. The majority of the studies examining the incidence of cardiac effects demonstrated an increase in cardiac adverse event rate with HAART in the HIV-infected population. Overall, the cardiotoxicity risk appears to be greater in the HIV-infected population than in the general population, and the increased cardiac risk is associated with HAART, particularly with protease inhibitor use. However, there is general consensus that the benefits of HAART far outweigh toxicity-related risks of the treatment with HAART.

Anti-Inflammatory Agents Nonsteroidal anti-inflammatory drugs (NSAIDs) include aspirin, Motrin, and Naprosyn, which are classified as nonselective NSAIDs because they are inhibitors for both COX-1 and COX-2. Inhibition of COX-1 is associated with gastrointestinal toxicity because COX-1 exerts a protective effect on the lining of the stomach. A newer class of NSAIDs has been developed; including rofecoxib (Vioxx), celecoxib (Celebrex), and valdecoxib (Bextra), witch are selective inhibitors of COX-2. In September 2004, Vioxx was voluntarily withdrawn from the market based upon the data from a clinical trial that showed after 18 months of use Vioxx increased the relative risk for cardiovascular events, such as heart attack and stroke (Arellano, 2005). In April 2005, Bextra was removed from the market based on the potential increased risk for serious cardiovascular adverse events and increased risk of serious skin reactions (e.g., toxic epidermal necrolysis, Stevens–Johnson syndrome, erythema multiforme) (Talhari *et al.*, 2005). Emerging information indicates the risk of cardiovascular events may be increased in patients receiving Celebrex (Solomon *et al.*, 2005). The cardiovascular events induced by COX-2 inhibitors are presumably related to thrombotic events. Studies have also indicated the link of Vioxx to long QT syndrome and the increased risk for TdP and sudden cardiac death (Arellano 2005; Fitzgerald 2004).

Antihistamines The most severe adverse effect of the second-generation histamine H_1 receptor antagonists (antihistamines) is their association with life-threatening ventricular arrhythmias and sudden cardiac death (Simons, 1994). Terfenadine and astemizole cause altered repolarization, notched inverted T waves, prominent TU waves, prolonged QT interval, first- and second-degree AV block, ventricular tachycardia or fibrillation, and torsades de pointes. These antihistamines produce cardiac arrhythmias by blocking the delayed rectifier K^+ channel and prolonging action potential duration in cardiac myocytes. The prolonged action potential duration promotes early afterdepolarizations and predisposes the myocardium to ventricular arrhythmias. However, terfenadine also inhibits L-type Ca^{2+} channels in rat ventricular myocytes at concentrations near or below that required to inhibit delayed rectifier K^+ current (Liu *et al.*, 1997). Therefore, both inhibition of Ca^{2+} and inhibition of K^+ current likely contribute to the cardiotoxic actions of terfenadine. As a result of cardiotoxicity, both astemizole and terfenadine have been removed from the United States market. However, the understanding of astemizole- and terfenadine-induced cardiotoxicity continues to be an important consideration in drug development, and other drugs have demonstrated similar clinical limitations (e.g., cisapride and fluoroquinolone antibacterial agents).

Immunosuppressants Rapamycin and tacrolimus may produce adverse cardiovascular effects, including hypertension, hypokalemia, and hypomagnesemia. Rapamycin and tacrolimus (FK506) interact with a protein that associates with ryanodine receptors (RyRs), and the protein carries the tacrolimus- or FK506-binding protein (FKBP). When rapamycin or tacrolimus binds to

FKBP in cardiac myocytes, RyR becomes destabilized, resulting in Ca^{2+} leak from the SR (Marks, 1997). Tacrolimus has been shown to be associated with hypertrophic cardiomyopathy in pediatric patients, a condition that was reversed by discontinuation of tacrolimus and administration of cyclosporin A; some of these patients developed severe heart failure (Atkison *et al.*, 1995).

Miscellaneous Drugs   Several drugs that are not included in the categories discussed above have significant cardiotoxic concerns and are briefly discussed below, including cisapride, methylxanthines, and sildenafil.

Cisapride is a chemical that has been used as a prokinetic drug for gastrointestinal hypomotility. However, cisapride has been removed from the U.S. market because of risk of potentially life-threatening arrhythmias (torsades de pointes) associated with its use. Like astemizole and terfenadine, cisapride inhibits delayed rectifier K^+ current, prolongs action potential duration, prolongs the QT interval, and predisposes the heart to ventricular arrhythmias.

Methylxanthines (including caffeine, theobromine, and theophylline), can be found in significant quantities in coffee, tea, chocolate, soft-drinks, and other foods. Theophylline has been used for many decades for the treatment of asthma, although the mechanism of action has not been fully understood. Overdose of theophylline or rapid intravenous administration of therapeutic doses of aminophylline (theophylline complexed with ethylenediamine to increase water solubility) may produce life-threatening ventricular arrhythmias; these effects may in part be explained by direct actions of theophylline on cardiac myocyte SR or by inhibition of phosphodiesterase and elevation of cyclic AMP. The cardiac effects of methylxanthines observed in vivo (including increases in cardiac output and heart rate) may also be explained by elevated catecholamines, as theophylline has been shown to increase plasma epinephrine concentrations (Vestal *et al.*, 1983). High concentrations of caffeine stimulate massive release of Ca^{2+} from the SR, an effect that is often utilized experimentally to determine SR function. Although it rarely occurs, caffeine-associated ventricular arrhythmias have been reported.

Sildenafil is a relatively specific inhibitor of phosphodiesterase 5, which is responsible for the degradation of cyclic GMP (a vasodilatory second messenger). Interestingly, sildenafil was originally developed as a potential drug for treating angina; however, it was not very effective for this purpose and was subsequently developed for treatment of erectile dysfunction, where it produces vasodilation and filling of the corpus cavernosum. The primary concern regarding adverse effects of sildenafil is nonspecific inhibition of PDE3 in the heart and vasculature (Hussar, 1999). In vitro studies have revealed that sildenafil increases cyclic AMP in cardiac tissue without significant effects on cyclic GMP (Stief *et al.*, 2000); however, whether these effects are associated with cardiotoxicity is not known.

Natural Products

Natural products include naturally occurring catecholamines, hormones, and cytokines, as well as animal and plant toxins. Many of these products have been shown to cause cardiac toxic responses. However, it is difficult to define whether or not the cardiac toxicity results directly from the action of these products in vivo, although these products cause deleterious effects on cultured cardiomyocytes. The exposure levels of these chemicals tested in vitro in general are much higher than the concentration reached in cardiac tissue under in vivo exposure conditions. Therefore, extrapolation of in vitro data related to cardiac toxicity of natural products to in vivo conditions is challenging. However, there are some products that have clearly demonstrated cardiac toxic effects, and mechanisms of action of these products have been determined.

Catecholamines   The naturally occurring sympathomimetic amines, such as epinephrine and norepinepherine, are potent and can cause deleterious effects to the heart. The synthetic catecholamine, isoproterenol, is able to cause massive necrotic changes in the myocardium and is often used as a prototype compound for the study of catecholamine cardiotoxicity, which has been discussed in the therapeutic drugs that cause cardiotoxicity.

Steroids and Related Hormones   Estrogens, progestins, androgens, and adrenocortical steroids are major steroid hormones produced by mammals including humans. Myocardial tissue contains steroid receptors; therefore the heart serves as a target organ for steroid effects. It also has been shown that cardiac tissue can synthesize steroid hormones, although the capacity for synthesis may be much lower than more classic steroid synthesizing tissues. There are two major mechanisms of action of the hormones: the first is to alter gene expression and the second is to change signaling transduction pathways.

Estrogens are synthesized in ovaries, testes, and adrenal glands, and estrogen is an active metabolite of testosterone. Endogenous estrogens include 17β-estradiol (E_2), estrone, and estriol. Synthetic estrogens include diethylstilbestrol (nonsteroidal), equilin, esterified versions of E_2, ethinyl estradiol, mestranol, and quinestrol. In addition, many other synthetic chemicals have been shown to exert estrogenic activity, including the pesticides DDT and methoxychlor, the plasticizer bisphenol A, other industrial chemicals including polychlorinated biphenyls, and some compounds found in soybeans and tofu (e.g., phytoestrogens). Estrogens (frequently in combination with progestins) have been used for over 40 years as oral contraceptive drugs. The older versions of estrogenic oral contraceptives that contained high amounts of estrogens were associated with increased risk of coronary thrombosis and myocardial infarction; however, lower doses of estrogens have been found by numerous investigators to impart protective effects on the cardiovascular system, including antiapoptotic effects, and beneficial effects on lipid metabolism such as decreased low-density lipoproteins (LDL cholesterol) and increased high-density lipoproteins (HDL cholesterol). Estrogens alter cardiac fibroblast proliferation, but they can either increase or decrease proliferation of these cells.

Progestins are also synthesized in the ovaries, testes, and adrenal glands. Naturally occurring and synthetic progestins include desogestrel, hydroxyprogesterone, medroxyprogesterone, norethindrone, norethynodrel, norgestimate, norgestrel, and progesterone. As part of hormone replacement therapy, progestins serve an opposing role to estrogens. Unfortunately, estrogen treatment opposed with progestins may negate the cardiovascular benefits of estrogens on lipid metabolism (Kalin and Zumoff, 1990). Very little is known about the direct effects of progestins on the heart. Although progestins could exert deleterious effects on the heart, more studies are required to investigate mechanisms.

Androgens cause adverse cardiovascular effects (Rockhold, 1993; Melchert and Welder, 1995). The principal androgens are testosterone and its active metabolite dihydrotestosterone.

Testosterone is synthesized in the testes, ovaries, and adrenal glands and dihydrotestosterone mediates most androgen actions. Synthetic anabolic-androgenic steroids include the alkylated and orally available drugs danazol, fluoxymesterone, methandrostenolone, methenolone, methyltestosterone, oxandrolone, oxymetholone, and stanozolol. The nonalkylated drugs with poor oral bioavailability include androstenedione and dehydroepiandrosterone (both sold in various "nutraceutical" formulations), boldenone (veterinary product), nandrolone (19-nortestosterone), and testosterone. Nearly all of these chemicals have received significant illicit use, particularly in extremely high doses with attempts to improve physical appearance or performance. Anabolic-androgenic steroids have been associated with alterations in lipid metabolism, including increased LDL cholesterol and decreased HDL cholesterol; therefore these chemicals may predispose individuals to atherosclerosis (Melchert and Welder, 1995). Evidence indicating the direct cardiac toxic effect of anabolic-androgenic steroids includes alteration of Ca^{2+} fluxes in cardiac myocytes induced by testosterone (Koenig *et al.*, 1989), hypertrophic growth of neonatal rat cardiac myocytes stimulated by testosterone and dihydrotestosterone (Marsh *et al.*, 1998), and mitochondrial abnormalities and myofibrillar lesions induced by methandrostenolone given intramuscularly to rats (Behrendt and Boffin, 1977). In humans, high-dose anabolic-androgenic steroid use has been associated with cardiac hypertrophy and myocardial infarction. However, the mechanisms responsible for the cardiotoxic effects of anabolic-androgenic steroids remain poorly understood.

Glucocorticoids and mineralocorticoids are primarily synthesized in the adrenal glands. Naturally occurring glucocorticoids include corticosterone, cortisone, and hydrocortisone (cortisol), and the mineralocorticoid is aldosterone. A large number of synthetic glucocorticoids are used for treatment of various autoimmune and inflammatory diseases. These drugs include alclometasone, amcinonide, beclomethasone, betamethasone, clobetasol, desonide, desoximetasone, dexamethasone, diflorasone, fludrocortisone, flunisolide, fluocinolone, fluocinonide, fluorometholone, flurandrenolide, halcinonide, medrysone, methylprednisolone, mometasone, paramethasone, prednisolone, prednisone, and triamcinolone. Most of these agents are primarily used topically, intranasally, or inhalationally. The primary glucocorticoids used systemically include cortisone, hydrocortisone, dexamethasone, methylprednisolone, prednisolone, and prednisone. The mineralocorticoid aldosterone is not used clinically; however, the aldosterone receptor antagonist spironolactone has been used for years to treat hypertension and is now thought to decrease morbidity and mortality associated with congestive heart failure. Both aldosterone and glucocorticoids appear to stimulate cardiac fibrosis by regulating cardiac collagen expression independently of hemodynamic alterations (Young *et al.*, 1994; Robert *et al.*, 1995). Furthermore, aldosterone and glucocorticoids induce hypertrophic growth and alter expression of Na^+, K^+-ATPase, Na^+/H^+ antiporter, and chloride/bicarbonate exchanger of cardiac myocytes in vitro. Clinically relevant cardiac hypertrophy has been observed in premature infants undergoing dexamethasone treatment. The mechanisms responsible for the direct effects of these chemicals remain poorly understood.

Thyroid hormones include thyroxine (T_4) and triiodothyronine (T_3). These hormones exert profound effects on the cardiovascular system. Hypothyroid states are associated with decreased heart rate, contractility, and cardiac output; whereas hyperthyroid states are associated with increased heart rate, contractility, cardiac output,

ejection fraction, and heart mass. Patients with underlying cardiovascular disease may display arrhythmias under the treatment of thyroid hormones. Thyroid hormones also alter expression of cardiac SR Ca^{2+} handling proteins including increased expression of SR Ca^{2+} ATPase (SERCA) and decreased expression of phospholamban, an inhibitory protein of SERCA (Kaasik *et al.*, 1997).

Cytokines More than 100 different cytokines have been found, and the cardiovascular effects of these substances can be classified as proinflammatory, anti-inflammatory, or cardioprotective (Pulkki, 1997). Members of the proinflammatory class include TNF-α; interleukin-1β (IL-1β), interleukin-2 (IL-2), interleukin-6 (IL-6), interleukin-8 (IL-8), Fas ligand, and chemokines (e.g., C-C chemokines such as MCP-1, macrophage chemoattractant protein-1; MIP-1α, macrophage inflammatory protein-1α; and RANTES, regulated on activation normally T-cell-expressed and secreted). Members of the anti-inflammatory class typically down-regulate expression of proinflammatory cytokines and include interleukin-4 (IL-4), interleukin-10 (IL-10), interleukin-13 (IL-13), and transforming growth factor-beta (TGF-β). The cardioprotective cytokines include cardiotrophin-1 (CT-1) and leukemia inhibitor factor, which have been shown to inhibit cardiac myocyte apoptosis from a number of different stimuli. Many of these cytokines are elevated during cardiovascular diseases such as I/R injury, myocardial infarction, and congestive heart failure.

IL-1β is known to exert negative inotropic actions and induce apoptosis of cardiac myocytes. The effects of IL-1β on cardiac myocytes are likely mediated through induction of nitric oxide synthase (NOS) and/or increased production of nitric oxide (NO) (Arstall *et al.*, 1999). Superoxide anion and peroxynitrite formation was associated with reduced left ventricular ejection fraction in dogs treated with microspheres containing IL-1β, suggesting that involvement of peroxynitrite in IL-1β cardiotoxicity (Cheng *et al.*, 1999b).

TNF-α induces apoptotic cell death in myocardium (Krown *et al.*, 1996). The mechanisms responsible for TNF-α-induced apoptosis of cardiac myocytes are not entirely clear. TNF-α also exerts negative inotropic effects on cardiac myocytes at least potentially through increased production of sphingosine (Sugishita *et al.*, 1999). However, it has been shown TNF-α is essential for the cardiac protective response to stresses such as ischemic cardiac injury (Kurrelmeyer *et al.*, 2000).

IL-6 has been shown to induce negative inotropic effects on cardiac myocytes, possibly through induction of NOS expression and increased NO production (Sugishita *et al.*, 1999).

IL-2 may decrease the mechanical performance and metabolic efficiency of the heart, and these myocardial effects may be related to changes in NO synthesis and Na^+/H^+ exchange.

Interferon may result in cardiac arrhythmias, dilated cardiomyopathy, and signs of myocardial ischemia. Interferon-γ acts synergistically with IL-1β to increase NO formation in the heart, and induce Bax expression and apoptosis in cardiac myocyte cultures (Arstall *et al.*, 1999).

Animal and Plant Toxins Animal toxins in the venom of snakes, spiders, scorpions, and marine organisms have profound effects on the cardiovascular system. There are also a number of plants—such as foxglove, oleander, and monkshood—that contain toxic constituents and have adverse effects on the cardiovascular system.

Environmental Pollutants and Industrial Chemicals

There are many chemicals classified in this category that cause cardiac toxicity. Metals and metalloids can be found both in environmental pollutants and industrial chemicals. Some heavy metals, such as cadmium, block calcium channels that affect cardiac rhythm leading to arrhythmia, others such as arsenic have high affinity for sulfhydryl groups, and interfere with sulfhydryl-containing proteins, such as receptors, regulatory proteins, and transporters. During the last decade, epidemiological and experimental studies have identified an association of air pollution of PMs (particulate matters) and cardiac toxicity, however, mechanistic insights into cardiac toxicity induced by PM remain elusive. In this section, a brief discussion of selected industrial agents with their prominent cardiotoxic effects and proposed mechanisms of cardiotoxicity is presented. For a more comprehensive review of industrial chemicals and their cardiotoxic potential, the reader is referred to Zakhari (1992).

Particulate Matters   There are several obstacles in the systemic study of cardiac toxicity caused by particulate air pollution. One of the major challenges is the complexity of the particulate components of air pollution. Current consensus in the field is to divide the airborne particulates into classes according to aerodynamic diameters. There are three major classes: coarse (PM_{10}, 2.5–10 μm), fine ($PM_{2.5}$, <2.5 μm), and ultrafine ($PM_{0.1}$, <0.1 μm). However, ambient air PM consists of a mixture of combustive byproducts and resuspended crystal materials, of which the contents are highly related to geographic regions. Thus studying mechanisms by which particulate air pollution causes cardiovascular toxicity is extremely challenging, although attempts have been made to provide insights into the mechanistic link between particulate air pollution and cardiac toxicity. The documented cardiac toxic effects of particulate air pollution have been limited to electrocardiographic changes, including arrhythmia, decreased heart rate variability, and the exacerbation of ST-segment changes in experimental models of myocardial infarction.

Solvents   Industrial solvents can exert adverse effects on the heart directly or indirectly; both are related to their inherent lipohilicity. Solvents may affect cardiac physiological functions such as contraction and energy production by directly dispersing into plasma membranes. However, the effects of solvents on the heart would be more related to their actions on the neuro-hormonal regulation of cardiac function. Solvents may disrupt sympathetic and parasympathetic control of the heart as well as cause release of circulating hormones such as catecholamines, vasopressin, and serotonin, which in turn affects cardiac function.

Alcohols and Aldehydes   On a molar basis, there is a relationship between increased carbon chain length of the alcohol and cardiotoxicity. Metabolic oxidation of alcohols yields aldehydes. Aldehydes have sympathomimetic activity as a result of their effect on releasing catecholamines. Unlike alcohols, the sympathomimetic activity of aldehydes decreases with increased chain length. The acute cardiodepressant effects of alcohols and aldehydes may be related to inhibition of intracellular Ca^{2+} transport and/or generation of oxidative stress. Chronic alcoholic cardiotoxicity is more related to a long-term consumption of alcohol, referred to as ACM,

which was discussed above. The environmental exposure to alcohols is more lated to acute cardiaotoxicity, including a negative dromotropic effect (reduced conductivity) and a decreased threshold for ventricular fibrillation. The common inductrial alcohols include methanol (methyl alcohol or wood alcohol) and isopropyl alcohol (isopropanol). Methanol is metabolized by alcohol dehydrogenase and aldehyde dehydrogenase to formaldehyde and formic acid, and often causes reduction in heart rate. Isopropanol is metabolized to acetone, and both isopropanol and its metabolite are potent CNS depressants. Acetone is metabolized to formic acid and acetic acid, which have the potential to induce mild acidosis. Tachycardia is the most prominent clinical finding of isopropanol exposure.

Halogenated Alkanes   The highly lipophilic nature of halogenated alkanes allows them to cross the blood–brain barrier readily. This action, coupled with their CNS-depressant activity, makes these compounds ideally suited for anesthetics (halothane, methoxyfluorane, and enflurane). Halogenated hydrocarbons depress heart rate, contractility, and conduction. In addition, some of these agents sensitize the heart to the arrhythmogenic effects of β-adrenergic receptor agonists such as endogenous epinephrine. Fluorocarbons (freons) have been reported to have this sensitizing effect on the myocardium. Chronic exposure to halogenated hydrocarbons may cause myocardial degenerative response.

Metals and Metalloids   The most common heavy metals that have been associated with cardiotoxicity are cadmium, lead, and cobalt. These metals exhibit negative inotropic and dromotropic effects and can also produce structural changes in the heart. Chronic exposure to cadmium has been reported to cause cardiac hypertrophy. Lead has an arrhythmogenic sensitizing effect on the myocardium. In addition, lead has been reported to cause degenerative changes in the heart. Cobalt has been reported to cause cardiomyopathy. The cardiotoxic effects of heavy metals are attributed to their ability to form complexes with intracellular macromolecules and their ability to antagonize intracellular Ca^{2+}.

Other metals that have been reported to affect cardiac function are manganese, nickel, and lanthanum. Their mechanism of action appears to block Ca^{2+} channels. However, high concentrations are required to block Ca^{2+} channels (e.g., millimolar range). Barium is another metal that can affect cardiac function. Barium chloride given intravenously in high doses to laboratory animals has been reported to induce arrhythmias. This arrhythmogenic effect of barium chloride has been utilized to screen antirrhythmic agents.

Arsenic is a metalloid, which has been shown to cause cardiotoxicity directly. Arsenic has a high affinity for sulfhydryl proteins, which are involved in multiple cellular metabolism and function. Besides environmental exposure to arsenic such as through drinking water contamination, therapeutic use of arsenic in the form of arsenic trioxide for the treatment of acute promyelocytic leukemia (APL) is another important route of exposure. Clinical reports have shown serious ventricular tachycardia at the therapeutic doses of arsenic trioxide in APL patients. Experimetnal studies using a dose regiment that has been shown to produce plasma concentrations of arsenic within the range of those present in arsenic-treated APL patients have shown that arsenic causes myocardial cell death through apoptosis, and results in decreased systolic and diastolic function of the heart (Li *et al.*, 2002).

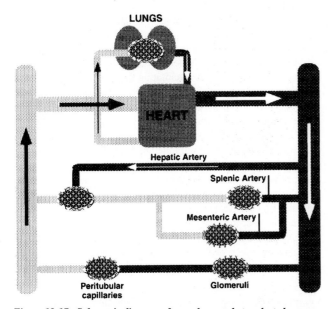

Figure 18-17. Schematic diagram of vascular supply to selected organs.

The capillary beds represented by a meshwork connnecting the arteries (right) with the veins (left); the distribution of the vasculature in several organs (liver, kidney, and lung) indicates the importance of the vascular system in toxicology.

OVERVIEW OF VASCULAR SYSTEM

Vascular Physiology and Structural Features

The vascular system consists of blood vessels of varying size and different cellular composition. Blood vessels can be divided into arterial, venous, and capillary systems. In addition, the lymphatic system belongs to the vascular system, but it only carries plasma. Although blood is the content of the vascular system and changes in the status of blood and circulation are associated with the functional alteration and toxicity of the vascular system, the blood is not included in this chapter because Chap. 11 specifically addresses the toxic responses of the blood. The main function of the vascular system is to provide oxygen and nutrients to and remove carbon dioxide and metabolic products from organ systems (Fig. 18-17). In

addition, the vascular system is a conduit that delivers hormones and cytokines to target organs. The vascular system also has regulatory functions to manipulate organ system responses under certain toxicologic conditions. For instance, endothelins produced by vascular endothelial cells alter cardiac rhythm and affect myocardial contractility. Many regulatory systems control the physiological function of the vascular system, so that the changes in the vascular system reflect either local action of chemicals or disruption of the regulatory systems, or both. The distinction between primary and secondary vascular toxic responses is challenging. To better understand the toxic responses of the vascular system, the following presents an overview of physiology and regulatory mechanism of the vascular system.

Arterial System and Physiological Function   The arterial system is composed of the aorta, major arteries, and small arterioles. The aorta and major arteries are thick-walled structures with vascular smooth muscle, elastic, and connective tissues (Fig. 18-18). Blood flow within the arterial system is initiated by contraction of the heart and begins at the ascending aorta. The ascending aorta receives all of the output of the heart with the exception of the coronary blood flow. Blood is distributed to the organ systems of the body through the major arteries that branch from the aorta. All these arteries further branch to give rise to smaller arteries and become arterioles that connect to capillaries for the delivery of oxygen and nutrients to target tissues.

The Aorta and Large Arteries   The aorta and the large arteries provide supporting structures and maintain the blood flow from the heart to the target organs. Therefore, these vessels function primarily as conduits. The driving force for the blood flow is derived from the contraction of the heart and the elasticity of the aorta and large arteries under the regulation of the neurohormonal system and the resistance of the target organs. Chemicals can affect directly the arterial systems leading to alterations in blood flow or indirectly act through the regulatory system to change the blood flow.

Arterioles and Vascular Resistance   The arterioles are composed of a tube of endothelial cells, surrounded by connective tissue basement membrane, a single or double layer of vascular smooth muscle cells, and a thin outer adventitial layer. The vascular smooth

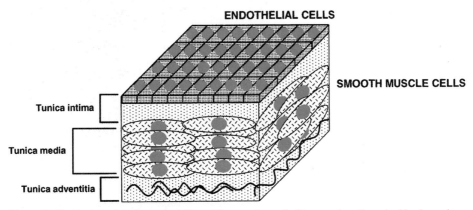

Figure 18-18. Cross-sectional representation of the vascular wall of large and medium-size blood vessels.

The tunica intima is composed of endothelial cells, facing the vessel lumen, which rest on a thin basal lamina. The tunica media consists mainly of vascular smooth muscle cells interwoven with collagen and elastin. The tunica adventia is a layer of fibroblasts, collagen, elastin, and glycosaminoglycans.

muscle cells are critical for the regulation of vascular resistance. The tension developed by the vascular smooth muscle cells alters the vessel diameter. Therefore, arterioles are primarily responsible for regulation of peripheral vascular resistance and blood flow. Toxic agents affecting the structure and function of the vascular smooth muscle cells can thus change the physiological regulation of the vascular resistance, leading to excess dilation or restriction.

Coronary Arteries and Circulation   Coronary arteries branch from the aorta immediately past the mitral valve. Supply of oxygen and nutrients to the heart is primarily supported by the coronary arteries. The coronary blood flow can increase about four-fold to supply additional oxygen needed by the heart muscle under demanding conditions, such as during exercise. However, even when the body is at rest, the oxygen supply through the coronary arteries to the heart is more than the supply to an equal mass of skeletal muscle during vigorous exercise. Heart tissue extracts most of the oxygen from blood during resting conditions the, and coronary blood flow increases with the workload demands on the heart. Increase in blood flow is the major mechanism of the heart to increase energy production. Coronary vasculature disruption both anatomically and physiologically leads to reduction in cardiac blood flow and cardiac work, which is an important effect of xenobiotics. In fact, pathology of the coronary vasculature is the cause of death in about one-third of the population in industrialized societies. Recent studies indicate that PMs in the air are associated with coronary heart disease (Dockery, 2001; Gordon and Reibman, 2000).

Capillaries and Microcirculation   Capillaries directly connect to the distal portion of the arterioles serving as the communication site between blood and tissues, and constitute the major part of the microcirculation where nutrients, water, gases, hormones, cytokines, and waste products are exchanged between blood and tissues. In other parts of the vascular system, blood is separated from tissues by the walls of arterial and venous vessels. In contrast, capillaries are only one cell layer thick. The passage of molecules through the capillary wall can occur both between and through the endothelial cells. Lipid-soluble molecules such as oxygen and carbon dioxide readily pass through the endothelial cell membranes. Water-soluble molecules diffuse between endothelial cells. The other pathway for water-soluble molecules is the cell membrane vesicle formation via pinocytosis (inward) and exocytosis (outward) on both the luminal and the tissue side of the capillary wall. This pathway can transfer even the largest molecules. The endothelial cells are targets of xenobiotics, whose effects can be measured by accumulation of toxic metabolites in the target organs and the pathophysiological changes in the microcirculation.

In general, there is some capillary reserve in tissues so that a particular area of a tissue can be perfused by more than one capillary, but not all of the capillaries open up at any given time. This capillary reserve serves two important functions: one is to meet the increase in metabolic demands. Under the condition that metabolic demands increase, more capillaries can open up. The other is to compensate for lesions or disruption of certain capillaries. For instance, if an occlusion occurs due to a thrombus, capillaries in close proximity can open to provide perfusion to the vulnerable area. However, in the brain, this capillary reserve appears absent so that any occlusion may result in damage.

Venous System and Physiological Function   The venous system is composed of venules, veins, and vena cava. The blood flow in the venous system starts from the thin-walled venules that collect the blood from the target tissues of the body. These vessels have a relatively large surface area facilitating the reabsorption of filtered plasma from the tissue. The venules merge to veins and eventually drain into the vena cava, returning blood to the heart. Therefore, the important physiological function of the venous system is collecting blood from organ systems of the body and returning the blood to the heart. The other important function of the venous system is the capacitance of the circulatory system. This is an important protective mechanism of the circulatory system. The large veins contain vascular smooth muscle cells that can increase the blood return to the heart by constriction and increase the capacitance by dilation. If hemorrhage occurs, the circulatory system can rapidly adjust the capacitance and maintain perfusion of the tissues. Xenobiotics can exert adverse effects on the vascular smooth muscle cells so that the capacitance function of the venous system can be compromised.

Lymphatic System and Physiological Function   Lymphatic vessels are endothelial tubes within tissues. The lymphatic system begins as blind-ended lymphatic end bulbs that drain into a meshwork of interconnected lymphatic vessels. This is a low-pressure system that collects excess tissue water and plasma proteins that have not been reabsorbed by the venous system. In general, in all organ systems with the exception of the CNS, more fluid is filtered than reabsorbed by the venous system. Therefore, removal of the excess fluid as well as plasma proteins that diffuse into the interstitial spaces by lymphatic system is essential. All the lymphatics ultimately drain into the vena cava. Therefore, the physiological function of the lymphatic system is to maintain a negative interstitial pressure by removing any excess fluid and plasma proteins. Toxic insults to the lymphatic system can lead to elevated interstitial pressures and subsequent tissue edema.

Regulatory Mechanisms of the Vascular System

The vascular system includes conduits and microcirculation. This system under physiological conditions is regulated by the demands of tissue metabolism. The mechanisms controlling vascular physiology can be divided into neural, hormonal, and local controls. However, this categorization is artificial because the performance of the vascular system at any given time is the result of the integration of all three controlling mechanisms, and each of the three mechanisms affects the other two. The controlling mechanisms can be divided into remote or systemic, and local regulation. The remote regulation includes both neural and hormonal mechanisms.

Neurohormonal Regulation   Most arteries, arterioles, venules, and veins, with the exception of those of the external genitalia, receive sympathetic innervation only. Norepinephrine is the usual transmitter that binds to α_1-adrenergic receptors. These receptors are distributed to vascular smooth muscle cells, and activation of the receptors leads to contraction of the vascular smooth muscle and thus the constriction of blood vessels. There are also β_2-adrenergic receptors in vascular smooth muscle cells, to which binds the circulating epinephrine released from the adrenal medulla. Activation of the β_2-adrenergic receptors leads to vascular smooth muscle relaxation and vasodilation. Coronary and skeletal muscle arteries are highly responsive to the epinephrine-induced vasodilation. In addition, the blood vessels of skeletal muscles receive sympathetic cholinergic innervation in addition to their sympathetic adrenergic innervation, whose activation leads to vascular smooth muscle relaxation and vasodilation. The CNS regulates the activity of the autonomic nerves at several levels. Interactions between the central and autonomic nerves take place in the spinal cord, medulla, and hypothalamus. These central nervous regulations are reviewed in many physiology textbooks and not covered in this chapter.

There are many hormones that control the vascular system. Catecholamines, renin–angiotensin–aldosterone, antidiuretic hormone (ADH), and atrial natriuretic peptide (ANP) are important hormones that affect the vascular system and will be briefly reviewed.

Catecholamines are primarily secreted from the adrenal medulla. During the activation of the sympathetic nervous system, the adrenal medulla releases epinephrine (>90%) and norepinephrine (<10%) into the blood. As discussed above, the increase in circulating epinephrine activates the β_2-adrenergic receptors localized in the coronary and skeletal muscle arteries leading to vascular smooth muscle relaxation and vasodilation. This occurs during defense and exercise.

The renin–angiotensin–aldosterone system is critically involved in the regulation of blood pressure and volume. Renin is released from the kidney in response to reduced arterial pressure and blood volume, which catalyzes the conversion of a plasma protein angiotensinogen to angiotensin I. Angiotensin I is further converted to angiotensin II by an angiotensin-converting enzyme. Angiotensin II is a powerful arteriolar vasoconstrictor and also causes the release of aldosterone from the adrenal cortex. One of the important actions of the aldosterone is to reduce renal sodium excretion, resulting in retention of water and increase in blood volume.

ADH is released from the posterior pituitary gland under the control of the hypothalamus. ADH is a vasoconstrictor but is not present in plasma in high concentrations under physiological conditions. However, ADH release is increased under the conditions of hemorrhage, decreased atrial stretch receptor firing, and increased plasma osmolarity. The effect of ADH on the vascular system is to increase the retention of water by the kidney, and thus increasing blood volume.

ANP is released from atrial muscle cells when they are stimulated by stretch. ANP increases the excretion of sodium so that it decreases the blood volume. Therefore, ANP regulation of blood volume is a counter-regulatory mechanism of the renin–angiotensin–aldosterone system and ADH.

Local Metabolic Regulation   The local regulation of the vascular system is primarily referred to as the control of microcirculation. The microcirculation is also controlled by the above neurohormonal system. This section will focus on the local metabolic regulation of microcirculation. In addition, chemicals released from endothelial cells are major local regulators of microcirculation and highly toxicologically relevant.

Oxygen is a major regulator of microcirculation. Oxygen is not stored in the end organs, and has to be replenished constantly from the blood flow. Therefore, change in metabolic rate in the end organ will require a parallel change in oxygen supply from the blood flow. The change in oxygen tension signals vascular muscles to relax or constrict. The vascular smooth muscle is not sensitive enough to respond to changes in oxygen tension except for extremely low or high oxygen tensions. However, decrease in oxygen tension along with increases in metabolic rate causes the release of adenine nucleotides, free adenosine, and Krebs cycle intermediates. In addition, lactic acid accumulates under hypoxia conditions. All these cause vasodilation at physiological concentrations.

An important mechanism of local regulation of microcirculation is the substance released by endothelial cells, endothelium-derived relaxing factor. This substance is NO generated from arginine by NOS. The mechanism of action of the endothelium-derived relaxing factor involves the increase in cyclic guanosine monophosphate (cGMP) and the subsequent activation of intracellular signaling pathways leading to relaxation of vascular smooth muscle cells. The endothelium-derived relaxing factor also suppresses platelet activation and reduces adhesion of leukocytes to endothelial cells.

VASCULAR SYSTEM TOXIC RESPONSES

Mechanisms of Vascular Toxicity

The effects of chemicals on the vascular system have been studied for some time, but the significance of the toxic responses of this system in affecting physiological function and pathogenesis of other organ systems is not fully understood. The potential effects of vascular toxicity on overall health and disease status are most likely underestimated. All chemicals, after absorption, contact the vascular system. Vascular endothelial cells are the immediate targets of the chemicals and are of the most frequent risk for toxic insults. These cells are the major component of the microcirculation system. Vascular smooth muscle cells are the next important targets of the chemicals.

Responses of Vascular Endothelial Cells to Toxic Insults   Vascular endothelial cells play a critical role in both vascular protection from toxic insults and triggering detrimental cascade in response to toxic insults. Damage to vascular endothelial cells is a critical starting point for vascular injury. In response to toxic insults, production of NO and ROS increases in endothelial cells. Substances mimicking agonists activate the receptors on the endothelial cells and trigger intracellular signaling transduction, leading to activation of nuclear factor kappa-B (NFκB) and MAPK activity. The downstream signaling transduction pathways triggered by NFκB, MAPK, NO, and ROS then activate gene expression and regulate posttranslational modification of proteins leading to cytoprotective action against toxic insults, or the production of cytokines, chemokines, and adhesion molecules to protect the circulatory system and the affected organ systems.

Angiogenesis is an adaptive response to damages that follow toxic insults. This process helps form new blood vessels and deliver nutrients and oxygen to damaged tissue to repair the lesion. Vascular endothelial cells are both central to initiating and promoting the formation of new blood vessels and essential for blood vessel formation by forming initial tube-like structures. Xenobiotics can both promote and suppress angiogenesis, and the primary target is the vascular endothelial cell. Apoptosis is a major mechanism for cell death of the vascular endothelial cells and mechanisms and molecular signaling pathways leading to apoptosis are basically the same as described for cardiomyocytes. Until recently, it was thought that preexisting endothelial cells are the sole cellular source for angiogenesis in adults. Recent results indicate the existence of endothelial progenitor cells. The injured endothelial monolayer can be regenerated by circulating bone marrow-derived endothelial progenitor cells, which accelerates re-endothelialization and limits atherosclerotic lesion formation. These endothelial progenitor cells may be important targets of xenobiotics, although no data are available.

Lesions to endothelial cells can result in atherosclerosis. Injury to endothelial cells results in increased production of endothelin-1 (ET-1) and increased release of prostacyclins. The endothelial cells are also involved in the recruitment of inflammatory cells to the lesion site. Activated lymphocytes secrete cytokines, such as TGF-β, which leads to a cascade of signaling transduction and a series of injurious responses including deposition of collagen.

ET-1 secreted by endothelial cells is a major mediator of vascular toxicity. ET is a peptide composed of 21 amino acids, derived from a large precursor, the big-ET, by the action of the endothelin-converting enzyme family. There are three isoforms of ET that have been identified, ET-1, ET-2, and ET-3. ET-1 is produced mainly by vascular endothelial cells and acts through two receptor subtypes, ET-A and ET-B. The ET receptors belong to the G-protein-coupled family. ET-1 is a potent vasoconstrictive chemical and plays an important role in the maintenance of vascular tone and blood pressure in healthy subjects. ET-1 contributes to the pathogenesis of myocardial disease. In failing hearts, activation of the ET system occurs; myocardial tissue levels of ET-1 are increased along with increased density of ET receptors, mainly in the form of ET-A due to upregulation in the myocardium (Ito *et al.*, 1993). In addition, circulating levels of both ET-1 and big-ET-1 are elevated in the patients with failing hearts. The elevation in serum levels of ET-1 thus has been used as an important marker of heart failure in humans (Monge, 1998). ET-1 mediated myocardial response is involved in air pollution PM-induced cardiac toxicity (Bouthillier *et al.*, 1998).

Responses of Smooth Muscle Cells to Toxic Insults   The consequence of damage to vascular smooth muscle cells involves changes in the vascular tone and atherosclerosis. Receptors localized on the plasma membrane of smooth muscle cells mediate the environmental changes and change the contractility of the blood vessels. The activation of these receptors leads to signaling transduction and changes in calcium conductance. Elevation of intracellular calcium activates the contractile apparatus, leading to alteration of vascular tone. Toxic substances influence calcium homeostasis in multiple ways. Calcium homeostasis is regulated by several regulatory mechanisms as well as affects many downstream actions. Toxic targets include the calcium-binding proteins, the calcium homeostasis regulatory proteins, the calcium-activated proteins such as calcineurin, and calcium storing and releasing process.

Proliferation and migration of medial smooth muscle cells are primarily responsible for the formation of sclerosis. Under certain circumstances, smooth muscle cells lose most of their contractility and become transformed smooth muscle cells. In most cases, this transformation is reversible. These new form of smooth muscle cells synthesize collagen and accumulate low-density lipoproteins along with a loss in the number of myofilaments. This phenotype transformation of the smooth muscle cells occurs in atherosclerosis. The mechanism and factors involved in the transformation are not fully understood, but the involvement of platelet activation has been indicated. Toxic substances affect the phenotype transformation of smooth muscle cells through multiple pathways. However, the growth-promoting effect is apparently a major action involved in the atherosclerotic lesion.

Oxidative Stress and Vascular Injury   Many xenobiotics generate ROS during their biotransformation. Both endothelial and smooth muscle cells are capable of producing ROS and the subsequent oxidative injury (Gurtner and Burke-Wolin, 1991). The mechanism of ROS generation from xenobiotics involves enzymatic and nonenzymatic reactions. Enzymes involved in the generation of ROS in vascular cells include amine oxidase, cytochrome $P450$ monooxygenases and prostaglandin synthetase. These enzymes use a diversity of substrates to produce ROS. The nonenzymatic reaction involves free iron and copper in the circulation system, which catalyze the Fenton' reaction to produce ROS.

Increase in ROS in endothelial cells is related to the stimulation by angiotensin II, as well as other neurohormonal factors and cyctokines. Angiotensin II binds to the AT1 receptor on the plasma membrane of endothelial cells. In response to receptor activation, cGMP production increases, leading to activation of endothelial CaM-dependent NOS and the production of NO. Stimulation of the AT1 receptor also leads to release of superoxide anion ($O_2^{\bullet-}$), through activation of a tyrosine phosphatase pathway. The release of both NO and $O_2^{\bullet-}$ is a major oxidative stress response of endothelial cells. The NO and $O_2^{\bullet-}$ production and release cause damage not only to endothelial cells, but also to other cells in the vascular system.

Vascular smooth muscle cells in response to angiotensin II markedly increase the production of $O_2^{\bullet-}$. The source of $O_2^{\bullet-}$ in these cells likely comes from NADPH oxidase, although NADH is also indicated in the production of $O_2^{\bullet-}$ in these cells. Xenobiotics, as discussed in the "Vascular System Toxic Chemicals" section, can activate the enzyme system and lead to more extensive production of $O_2^{\bullet-}$, or inhibit the antioxidant system including superoxide dismutase, catalase, glutathione peroxidase, and glutathione reductase resulting in accumulation of ROS in the cells.

Inflammatory Lesions   Inflammatory lesions of the vascular system are a common response of the vascular system. Inflammatory lesions are also called vasculitis. The pathogenesis of vasculitis has been studied both in vivo and in vitro, but the causes of many types of vasculitis are unknown. The initial injury to endothelial cells and the release of chemicals from the injured cells are responsible for the initiation of the inflammatory response, including recruitment of inflammatory cells to the injured site. Cytokines released from the activated inflammatory cells further propagate the inflammatory response leading to eventual lesion or vasculitis.

Toxic Responses of Blood Vessels

Hypertension and Hypotension   The vasculature pressure change is a major phenotype of vascular injury. Hypertension results from excessive constriction of the arterial vasculatures and/or increased resistance of the microcirculation system. However, the primary problem of sustained hypertension is an elevated vascular resistance in all organs. Once hypertension is established it becomes a disease of the microvasculature, particularly the arteriolar microvasculature. An increased incidence of temporary or, in some cases, permanent closure of small arterioles is associated with increased resistance of the end organs. The vascular smooth muscle cells become hypertrophied. However, the most predominant change is that all vascular smooth muscle cells are exceptionally responsive to norepinephrine. Sustained hypertension is a major complication of primary cardiovascular diseases. Complications include accelerated atherosclerosis and overload of the left ventricular muscle due to high arterial pressure. Toxic substances may directly or indirectly affect the sympathetic nervous system or alter the turnover of catecholamines in the circulation, resulting in hypertension. However, sustained hypertension by xenobiotics may involve more complicated metabolic changes in the end organs and thus changes in microcirculation also take place. For example, chemicals may enhance the renin–angiotensin system as well as renal toxicity, which may cause hypertension.

Hypotension is practically defined as the symptoms caused by low blood pressure. There are several regulatory mechanisms in the vascular system and the integration of these regulations that maintain blood flow and blood pressure within normal range. Baroreceptors, volume receptors, chemoreceptors, and pain receptors are all involved in the integrated regulatory action to maintain adequate blood pressure. During chemical exposure, these mechanisms may be affected individually or jointly resulting in a disturbance in the integration of the regulatory mechanisms. Both transient and sustained hypotension can be produced by xenobiotics. The most common adverse effect of antihypertension drugs is hypotension. Another major cause of hypotension is hemorrhage. Alcohol overdose also causes hypotension.

Atherosclerosis The most frequent vascular structural injury is atherosclerosis. The primary problem is the mechanical occlusion of the blood vessels so that blood flow is inadequate for the metabolic demands of the organs. As discussed above, activation of vascular smooth muscle cells is critically involved in atherosclerosis. Once stimulated, the vascular smooth muscle cells proliferate and migrate to the lesion site. These cells undergo phenotype transformation and increase the production of type I and II collagen, dermatan sulfate, proteoglycan, and stromelysins. In addition, the smooth muscle cells produce cytokines including macrophage colony-stimulating factor, TNF-α, and monocyte chemoatractant protein-1. The recruitment of inflammatory cells to the lesion site is the perpetuation process of atherosclerosis.

The classic definition of atherosclerotic plaque is a combination of changes in the intima of arteries consisting of local accumulation of lipids, complex carbohydrates, blood and blood products, fibrous tissue, and calcium deposits. However, this classic definition does not sufficiently describe the advanced atherosclerotic plaques that invade the media and produce bulging or enlarged arteries, cellular infiltration, and neovascularization. During the early development of atherosclerotic plaques, the lipid core has been described as the starting step of atherosclerosis. A lipid core develops and accumulates in the deep layer of the lesions before fibrous plaque formation begins. Inflammation and immune response are involved in both the early deposition of the lipid core and the late stage of fibrous accumulation. The inflammatory response includes cytokines, such as IL-6 and TNF-α. These cytokines are produced by vascular smooth muscle cells and infiltrated inflammatory cells. Many chemicals affect the oxidative metabolism of lipids in the circulatory system to trigger the formation and development of the lipid core of atherosclerosis. Toxic effects on smooth muscle cells can also initiate the formation of atherosclerotic plaques, which may be different from the lipid core mediated atherosclerosis. In addition, macrophages and monocytes are also targets for xenobiotics and have been shown to be importantly involved in the progression of atherosclerosis.

Hemorrhage A direct mechanical injury to blood vessels causes bleeding. Chemical-induced hemorrhages are seen when damage to

capillaries takes place. In addition, toxic effects on blood-clotting increases the probability of hemorrhage. A classic example of chemical-induced hemorrhage is observed in snake venom poisoning. Zinc-dependent metalloproteinases are major components of snake venom and responsible for the hemorrhage. Snake venom metalloproteinases degrade various components of the basement membrane and hydrolyze endothelial cell membrane proteins, such as integrins and cadherins, involved in cell–matrix and cell–cell adhesion. These actions weaken the capillary wall and perturb the interactions between endothelial cells and the basement membrane. Thus the transmural pressure acting on the weakened capillary wall causes distention. As a consequence, endothelial cells become very thin and eventually, the integrity of the capillary wall is lost. In addition, endothelial cells become more susceptible to blood flow-dependent shear stress, further contributing to the capillary wall disruption.

Edema The capillary exchange of fluid is bidirectional and capillaries and venules may alter the balance of hydrostatic and colloid osmotic pressure. Filtration occurs most likely at the arteriolar end of capillaries, where filtration forces exceed absorption forces. The absorption of water occurs in the venular end of the capillary and small venules. The capillary pressure is determined by both the resistance of, and the blood pressure in arterioles and venules. Xenobiotics can change the pressure gradient and cause more filtration than reabsorption of the extracellular liquid by the capillary system. In addition, more fluid is filtered than is reabsorbed by the venous system under physiological conditions. Therefore, the removal of excess fluid as well as plasma proteins that diffuse into the interstitial space is essential. This is accomplished by the lymphatic system. The lymphatics ultimately drain into the vena cava. Toxic insults to the lymphatic system can lead to elevated interstitial pressures and the subsequent tissue edema.

VASCULAR SYSTEM TOXIC CHEMICALS

Chemicals that cause vascular toxicity can also be classified into pharmaceutical chemicals, natural products, and environmental pollutants and industrial chemicals. Blood vessels are the target organ of these chemicals. However, some of these chemicals affect both the blood vessels and the heart. For instance, blood vessels in the heart belong to the vascular system, so that the toxicity of vascular toxic chemicals may express their toxicity in the form of cardiac toxic manifestations. Endothelial cells are major target cells of the chemicals affecting the vascular system, which are also found in the heart and make a contribution to cardiac toxicity. The same principle applies to other organ systems. Due to the distribution of vascular system in the end organs, vascular toxicity affects the organs in which the vessels are localized and is often accompanied with functional defects of the organ.

Pharmaceutical Chemicals

Vascular toxicity of pharmaceutical chemicals that are used to treat vascular disease or used to treat nonvascular disease is well-known clinically. The major manifestation and mechanisms of action of selected therapeutic agents are briefly discussed below.

Sympathomimetic Amines The sympathomimetic amines, including epinephrine, norepinephrine, dopamine, and isoproterenol, can damage the arterial vasculature by a variety of mechanisms.

Large doses of norepinephrine produce toxic effects on the endothelium of the thoracic aorta of rabbits, including degenerative changes in the aortic arch in the form of increased numbers of microvilli and many focal areas of unusual endothelial cytoarchitecture. Repeated exposure to catecholamines induces atherosclerotic lesions in several animal species. Experimetnal data suggest that catecholamines cause the proliferative disturbances in vascular cells via α-receptors because prazocin, an α-receptor antagonist, effectively prevents the toxic response (Nakaki et al., 1989). Smooth muscle cells subjected to increased stress by diabetes, hypertension, and balloon injury are more susceptible to the effects of catecholamines. Thus, the formation of arteriosclerotic lesions in certain forms of hypertension may be initiated and/or potentiated by high levels of circulating catecholamines.

Nicotine   Nicotine is an alkaloid found in various plants and mimics the actions of acetylcholine at nicotinic receptors throughout the body. At pharmacologic concentrations, nicotine increases heart rate and blood pressure as a result of stimulation of sympathetic ganglia and the adrenal medulla. Epidemiologic and experimental studies have suggested that nicotine is a causative or aggravating factor in myocardial and cerebral infarction, gangrene, and aneurysm. The effects of nicotine are related to competitive inhibition of cyclooxygenase.

Cocaine   The central actions of cocaine are to increase the circulating levels of catecholamines and cause a generalized state of vasoconstriction. Hypertension and cerebral strokes are common vascular complications. In pregnant women, cocaine-induced vascular changes have been associated with abortions and abruptio placentae. Studies have shown that cocaine enhances leukocyte migration across the cerebral vessel wall during inflammatory conditions. This effect is exerted through a cascade of augmented expression of inflammatory cytokines and endothelial adhesion molecules and may in fact underlie the cerebrovascular complications associated with cocaine abuse (Gan et al., 1999).

Psychotropic Agents   Trifluoperazine and chlorpromazine among the psychotropic drugs have been shown to cause intracellular cholesterol accumulation in cultured cells of the aortic intima (Iakushkin et al., 1992). Enalapril has been shown to cause angioedema in humans. Aside from the atherogenic effects, postural hypotension has been identified as the most common cardiovascular side effect of TCAs.

Antineoplastic Agents   The vasculotoxic responses elicited by antineoplastic drugs range from asymptomatic arterial lesions to thrombotic microangiopathy. Pulmonary veno-occlusive disease has been reported after the administration of various drugs, including 5-fluorouracil, doxorubicin, and mitomycin. Cyclophosphamide causes cerebrovascular and viscerovascular lesions, resulting in hemorrhages. Chronic infusions of 5-fluoro-2-deoxyuridine into the hepatic artery in dogs resulted in gastrointestinal hemorrhage and portal vein thrombosis.

Analgesics and Nonsteroidal Anti-Inflammatory Agents   Aspirin can produce endothelial damage as part of a pattern of gastric erosion. Studies in rats have shown early changes in the basement membrane of endothelial cells of the capillaries and postcapillary venules, leading to obliteration of small vessels and ischemic infarcts in the large intestine. Regular use of analgesics containing phenacetin has been associated with an increased risk of hypertension and cardiovascular morbidity. NSAIDs may induce glomerular and vascular renal lesions.

Oral Contraceptives   Oral contraceptive steroids can produce thromboembolic disorders. Epidemiologic studies have shown that oral contraceptive users have an increased risk of myocardial infarction relative to nonusers, a correlation that is markedly exacerbated by smoking, and oral contraceptive users experience an increased risk of cerebral thrombosis, hemorrhage, venous thrombosis, and pulmonary embolism (Stolley et al., 1989). However, the mechanism by which oral contraceptives increase the risk of vascular disease is unclear.

Natural Products

Natural products that cause vascular toxicity include those discussed for drugs causing cardiotoxicity. In addition, many other drugs also cause vascular leasions and toxicity such as bacterial endotoxins and homocysteines, which have unique vascular toxic effects.

Bacterial Endotoxins   Bacterial endotoxins are potent toxic agents to vascular system and cause a variety of toxic effects in many vascular beds. In the liver, they cause swelling of endothelial cells and adhesion of platelets to sinusoid walls. In the lung, endotoxins produce increased vascular permeability and pulmonary hypertension. Infusion of endotoxin into experimental animals produces thickening of endothelial cells and the formation of fibrin thrombi in small veins. The terminal phase of the effects of endotoxin on the systemic vasculature results in marked hypotension. The ability of vitamin E to prevent disseminated intravascular coagulation induced by bacterial endotoxins in the rat suggests that that action of these agents is somehow related to oxidative stress mechanisms.

Homocysteine   Moderately elevated levels of homocysteine have been associated with atherosclerosis and venous thrombosis. Conditions including increases in the circulating homocysteine involve cardiac complications such as hypertrophic cardiomyopathy and heart failure. Toxicity may involve oxidative injury to vascular endothelial and/or smooth muscle cells, leading to deregulation of vascular smooth muscle growth, synthesis and deposition of matrix proteins, and adverse effects on anticoagulant systems (Harpel, 1997).

Hydrazinobenzoic Acid   Hydrazinobenzoic acid is a nitrogen–nitrogen bonded chemical that is present in the cultivated mushroom *Agaricus bisporus*. This hydrazine derivative causes smooth muscle cell tumors in the aorta and large arteries of mice when administered over the life span of the animals (McManus et al., 1987). These tumors have the characteristic appearance and immunocytochemical features of vascular leiomyomas and leiomyosarcomas. Smooth muscle cell lysis with vascular perforation apparently precedes malignant transformation.

T-2 Toxin   Trichothecene mycotoxins, commonly classified as tetracyclic sesquiterpenes, are naturally occurring cytotoxic metabolites of *Fusarium* species. These mycotoxins, including T-2 toxin   [4β,15-diacetoxy-8α-(3-methylbutyryloxy)-3α-hydroxy-12,13-epoxytrichothec-9-ene], are major contaminants of foods and animal feeds and may cause illness in animals and humans. Intravenous infusion of T-2 toxin in rats causes an initial decrease in heart rate and blood pressure, followed by tachycardia and hypertension and finally by bradycardia and hypotension (Mcmanus *et al.*, 1987). Acute T-2 toxin exposure causes extensive destruction of myocardial capillaries, while repeated dosing promotes thickening of large coronary arteries.

Vitamin D The toxic effects of vitamin D may be related to its structural similarity to 25-hydroxycholesterol, a potent vascular toxin. The manifestions of vitamin D hypervitaminosis include medial degeneration, calcification of the coronary arteries, and smooth muscle cell proliferation in laboratory animals.

β-Amyloid Accumulation of β-amyloid is a major lesion in the brain of Alzheimer's patients. Studies have shown that administration of β-amyloid produces extensive vascular disruption, including endothelial and smooth muscle damage, adhesion and migration of leukocytes across arteries and venules (Thomas *et al.*, 1997). Most importantly, the vascular actions of β-amyloid appear to be distinct from the neurotoxic properties of the peptide. It appears that vascular toxicity of β-amyloid makes contributions to Alzheimer's dementia.

Environmental Pollutants and Industrial Chemicals

The environmental pollutants and industrial chemicals discussed in cardiac toxicity section all have toxic effects on the vascular system. As discussed above, the cardiac effect of some of these agents and pollutants may result primarily from the vascular effect. The by-products of vascular tissue damage or the secreted substances, such as cytokines derived from vascular injury, can affect the heart either directly because of the residual of the vascular system in the heart, or indirectly through blood circulation. In this context, some of the chemicals discussed in the cardiotoxicity will not be further described. Some unique vascular toxicity will be presented.

Carbon Monoxide Carbon monoxide induces focal intimal damage and edema in laboratory animals at a concentration (180 ppm) to which humans may be exposed from environmental sources such as automobile exhaust, tobacco smoke, and fossil fuels. However, it is difficult to distinguish the direct effects of carbon monoxide from those of chemicals such as sulfur oxides, nitrogen oxides, aldehydes, and hydrocarbons on humans because most sources of carbon monoxide are complex mixtures of chemicals. Degenerative changes of myocardial arterioles have been produced experimentally in dogs forced to smoke. Similar changes have also been detected in humans who were heavy smokers and died of noncardiac causes (Wald and Howard, 1975). Tobacco smoke not only exerts a direct atherogenic effect (endothelial injury, changes in lipid profiles, and proliferation of smooth muscle cells), but also facilitates thrombosis by modulation of platelet function and vascular spasm.

Short-term exposure to carbon monoxide is associated with direct damage to vascular endothelial and smooth muscle cells. Injury to endothelial cells increases intimal permeability and allows the interaction of blood constituents with underlying components of the vascular wall. This response may account in part for the ability of carbon monoxide to induce atherosclerotic lesions in several animal species. The toxic effects of carbon monoxide have been attributed to its reversible interaction with hemoglobin. As a result of this interaction, carboxyhemoglobin decreases the oxygen-carrying capacity of blood, eventually leading to functional anemia. In addition, carbon monoxide interacts with cellular proteins such as myoglobin and cytochrome *c* oxidase and elicits a direct vasodilatory response of the coronary circulation.

Carbon Disulfide Carbon disulfide (dithiocarbonic anhydride) occurs in coal tar and crude petroleum and is commonly used in the manufacture of rayon and soil disinfectants. This chemical has been identified as an atherogenic agent in laboratory animals. The mechanism for carbon disulfide-atheroma production may involve direct injury to the endothelium coupled with hypothyroidism, because thiocarbamate (thiourea), a potent antithyroid substance, is a principal urinary metabolite of carbon disulfide. Carbon disulfide also modifies low-density lipoprotein in vitro and enhances arterial fatty deposits induced by a high-fat diet in mice (Lewis *et al.*, 1999).

1,3-Butadiene Studies have shown that 1,3-butadiene, a chemical used in the production of styrene-butadiene, increases the incidence of cardiac hemangiosarcomas, which are tumors of endothelial origin (Miller and Boorman, 1990). Although hemangiosarcomas have also been observed in the liver, lung, and kidney, cardiac tumors are a major cause of death in animals exposed to this chemical. The toxic effects of 1,3-butadiene are dependent on its metabolic activation by cytochrome *P*450 to toxic epoxide metabolites. The ultimate outcomes of exposure probably are influenced by the rates of glutathione-mediated detoxification of oxidative metabolites.

Metals and Metalloids The vascular toxicity of food- and water-borne elements (selenium, chromium, copper, zinc, cadmium, lead, and mercury) as well as airborne elements (vanadium and lead) involves reactions of metals with sulfhydryl, carboxyl, or phosphate groups. Metals such as cobalt, magnesium, manganese, nickel, cadmium, and lead also interact with and block calcium channels. Intracellular calcium-binding proteins, such as CaM, are biologically relevant targets of heavy metals, including cadmium, mercury and lead, although the contribution of this mechanism to the toxic effects of metals has been fully understood.

Cadmium effects on the vascular system have been studied in the greatest detail. Although cadmium is not preferentially localized in blood vessels relative to other tissues, when present, cadmium is localized in the elastic lamina of large arteries, with particularly high concentrations at arterial branching points (Perry *et al.*, 1989). A large portion of the cadmium that accumulates in the body is tightly bound to hepatic and renal MT. The low MT levels in vascular tissue may actually predispose a person to the toxic effects of cadmium (Perry *et al.*, 1989). Long-term exposure of laboratory animals to low levels of cadmium has been associated with the development of atherosclerosis and hypertension in the absence of other toxic effects. Selenium and zinc inhibit, whereas lead potentiates the hypertensive effects of cadmium. Calcium has antagonistic effect on cadmium-induced high blood pressure. Cadmium increases sodium retention, induces vasoconstriction, increases cardiac output, and produces hyperreninemia. Any one of these mechanisms could account for the putative hypertensive effects of cadmium.

Lead has been shown from epidemiologic studies to be associated with essential hypertension in a large percentage of patients (Batuman *et al.*, 1983). Elevated blood pressure has also been observed during childhood lead poisoning. The direct vasoconstrictor effect of lead may be related to the putative hypertensive response. This effect can be complemented by the ability of lead to activate the renin–angiotensin–aldosterone system. Lead also directly affects vascular endothelial and smooth muscle cells. For instance, lead inhibits the repair process in damaged endothelial cells (Fujiwara *et al.*, 1997) and modulates spontaneous release of fibrinolytic proteins from subendothelial cells through intracellular calcium-independent pathways (Yamamoto *et al.*, 1997). Acute lead-induced neuropathy may be due to cerebral capillary dysfunction. Inorganic lead alters arterial elasticity and causes sclerosis of renal vessels.

Mercury produces vasoconstriction of preglomerular vessels and disrupts the integrity of the blood–brain barrier. The opening of the blood–brain barrier results in extravasation of plasma protein across vascular walls into adjoining brain tissues. Mercury added to platelet-rich plasma causes a marked increase in platelet thromboxane B_2 production and platelet responsiveness to arachidonic acid.

Arsenic poisoning causes vasodilation and capillary dilation. These actions have been associated with extravasation, transudation of plasma, and decreased intravascular volume. A severe form of arteriosclerosis, blackfoot disease, in Taiwan has beens shown to be associated with high levels of arsenic in the soil and water. Blackfoot disease is an endemic peripheral vascular occlusive disease that exhibits arteriosclerosis obliterans and thromboangiitis. The ability of arsenic to induce these changes has been attributed to its effects on vascular endothelial cells. Arsenic has been reported to cause noncirrhotic portal hypertension in humans.

Aromatic Hydrocarbons   Aromatic hydrocarbons, including polycyclic aromatic hydrocarbons and polychlorinated dibenzopdioxins, are persistent toxic environmental contaminants. Aromatic hydrocarbons have been identified as vascular toxins that can initiate and/or promote the atherogenic process in experimental animals (Ou and Ramos, 1992). The atherogenic effect is associated with cytochrome $P450$–mediated conversion of the parent compound to toxic metabolic intermediates, but aromatic hydrocarbons can also initiate the atherogenic process. However, studies have also shown that treatment with several polycyclic hydrocarbons increases the size but not the frequency of atherosclerotic lesions (Albert *et al.*, 1977; Penn and Synder, 1988), suggesting that polycyclic aromatic hydrocarbons act as promoters of the atherosclerotic process. Although additional studies are required to define the "initiating" versus "promotional" actions of polycyclic aromatic hydrocarbons, their ability to readily associate with plasma lipoproteins may play a critical role in vascular toxicity.

Particulate Air Pollution   Recent epidemiological studies have provided a strong body of evidence that elevated levels of ambient particulate air pollution (PM) are associated with increased cardiovascular and respiratory morbidity and mortality. Besides the PM effects on cardiomyocytes such as alterations in ion channel function leading to cardiac malfunction, available clinical and experimental evidence lends support to the vascular effects of inhaled ambient particles, including endothelial dysfunction and promotion of atherosclerotic lesions. Importantly, these lesions lead to release or secretion of cytokines and chemokines, worsening cardiac complications. For instance, PM exposure significantly increases serum total endothelin concentrations and worsens premature ventricular complexes of the electrocardiograms that occurr in the myocardial infaret rats (Kang *et al.*, 2002). The PM effects on vascular system and the consequences are important health-related topics and further studies are needed to substantiate our current understanding of mechanisms for PM adverse vascular effects.

REFERENCES

Abas L, Bogoyevitch MA, Guppy M: Mitochondrial ATP production is necessary for activation of the extracellular-signal-regulated kinases during ischaemia/reperfusion in rat myocyte-derived H9c2 cells. *Biochem J* 349(Pt 1):119–126, 2000.

Adams JM, Cory S: The Bcl-2 protein family: Arbiters of cell survival. *Science* 281(5381):1322–1326, 1998.

Adams JW, Sakata Y, Davis MG, *et al.*: Enhanced Galphaq signaling: A common pathway mediates cardiac hypertrophy and apoptotic heart failure. *Proc Natl Acad Sci U S A* 95(17):10140–10145, 1998.

Adams MA, Hirst M: Ethanol-induced cardiac hypertrophy: Correlation between development and the excretion of adrenal catecholamines. *Pharmacol Biochem Behav* 24(1):33–38, 1986.

Ahmed SS, Regan TJ: Cardiotoxicity of acute and chronic ingestion of various alcohols, in Acosta D (ed.): *Cardiovascular Toxicology*, 2nd ed. New York: Raven Press, 1992, pp. 345–407.

Akao M, Ohler A, O'Rourke B, *et al.*: Mitochondrial ATP-sensitive potassium channels inhibit apoptosis induced by oxidative stress in cardiac cells. *Circ Res* 88(12):1267–1275, 2001.

Akhter SA, Luttrell LM, Rockman HA, *et al.*: Targeting the receptor-Gq interface to inhibit in vivo pressure overload myocardial hypertrophy. *Science* 280(5363):574–577, 1998.

Albert RE, Vanderlaan M, Burns FJ, *et al.*: Effect of carcinogens on chicken atherosclerosis. *Cancer Res* 37(7 Pt 1):2232–2235, 1977.

Andrieu-Abadie N, Jaffrezou JP, Hatem S, *et al.*: L-Carnitine prevents doxorubicin-induced apoptosis of cardiac myocytes: Role of inhibition of ceramide generation. *FASEB J* 13(12):1501–1510, 1999.

Anversa P: Myocyte death in the pathological heart. *Circ Res* 86(2):121–124, 2000.

Anversa P, Leri A, Kajstura J: Cardiac regeneration. *J Am Coll Cardiol* 47(9):1769–1776, 2006.

Arad M, Moskowitz IP, Patel VV, *et al.*: Transgenic mice overexpressing mutant PRKAG2 define the cause of Wolff–Parkinson–White syndrome in glycogen storage cardiomyopathy. *Circulation* 107(22):2850–2856, 2003.

Arellano FM: The withdrawal of rofecoxib. *Pharmacoepidemiol Drug Saf* 14:213–217, 2005.

Arola OJ, Saraste A, Pulkki K, *et al.*: Acute doxorubicin cardiotoxicity involves cardiomyocyte apoptosis. *Cancer Res* 60(7):1789–1792, 2000.

Arstall MA, Sawyer DB, Fukazawa R, *et al.*: Cytokine-mediated apoptosis in cardiac myocytes: The role of inducible nitric oxide synthase induction and peroxynitrite generation. *Circ Res* 85(9):829–840, 1999.

Atkison P, Joubert G, Barron A, *et al.*: Hypertrophic cardiomyopathy associated with tacrolimus in paediatric transplant patients. *Lancet* 345(8954):894–896, 1995.

Baldessarini RJ: drugs and the treatment of psychiatric disorders, in Hardman JG, Limbird LE, Molinoff PB, et al. (eds.): *Goodman & Gilman's The Pharmacological Basis Of Therapeutics*, 9th ed. New York: Mcgraw-Hill, 1996, pp. 399–430.

Batuman V, Landy E, Maesaka JK, et al.: Contribution of lead to hypertension with renal impairment. *N Engl J Med* 309(1):17–21, 1983.

Behrendt H, Boffin H: Myocardial cell lesions caused by an anabolic hormone. *Cell Tissue Res* 181(3):423–426, 1977.

Bennett PB, Yazawa K, Makita N, et al.: Molecular mechanism for an inherited cardiac arrhythmia. *Nature* 376(6542):683–685, 1995.

Berenji K, Drazner MH, Rothermel BA, et al.: Does load-induced ventricular hypertrophy progress to systolic heart failure? *Am J Physiol Heart Circ Physiol* 289(1):H8–H16, 2005.

Bisognano JD, Weinberger HD, Bohlmeyer TJ, et al.: Myocardial-directed overexpression of the human beta(1)-adrenergic receptor in transgenic mice. *J Mol Cell Cardiol* 32(5):817–830, 2000.

Bittl JA, Ingwall JS: Reaction rates of creatine kinase and ATP synthesis in the isolated rat heart. A 31P NMR Magnetization Transfer Study. *J Biol Chem* 260(6):3512–3517, 1985.

Black BL, Olson EN: Transcriptional control of muscle development by myocyte enhancer factor-2 (MEF2) proteins. *Annu Rev Cell Dev Biol* 14:167–196, 1998.

Bogden JD, Al Rabiai S, Gilani SH: Effect of chronic ethanol ingestion on the metabolism of copper, iron, manganese, selenium, and zinc in an animal model of alcoholic cardiomyopathy. *J Toxicol Environ Health* 14(2–3):407–417, 1984.

Bosnjak ZJ: Cardiac effects of anesthetics, in Blank TJJ, Wheeler DM (eds.): *Mechanisms of Anesthetic Action in Skeletal, Cardiac and Smooth Muscle*. New York: Plenum Press, 1991, pp. 91–96.

Bouthillier L, Vincent R, Goegan P, et al.: Acute effects of inhaled urban particles and ozone: Lung morphology, macrophage activity, and plasma endothelin-1. *Am J Pathol* 153(6):1873–1884, 1998.

Bozkurt B: Cardiovascular toxicity with highly active antiretroviral therapy: Review of clinical studies. *Cardiovas Toxicol* 4:243–260, 2004.

Brand T, Sharma HS, Fleischmann KE, et al.: Proto-oncogene expression in porcine myocardium subjected to ischemia and reperfusion. *Circ Res* 71(6):1351–1360, 1992.

Buck ED, Lachnit WG, Pessah IN: Mechanisms of delta-hexachlorocyclohexane toxicity: I. Relationship between altered ventricular myocyte contractility and ryanodine receptor function. *J Pharmacol Exp Ther* 289(1):477–485, 1999.

Catterall W, Mackie K: Local anesthetics, in Hardman JG, Limbird LE, Molinoff PB, et al. (eds.): *Goodman & Gilman's The Pharmacological Basis Of Therapeutics*, 9th ed. New York: Mcgraw-Hill, 1996, pp. 331–347.

Chacon E, Acosta D: Mitochondrial regulation of superoxide by Ca^{2+}: An alternate mechanism for the cardiotoxicity of doxorubicin. *Toxicol Appl Pharmacol* 107(1):117–128, 1991.

Cheng TH, Shih NL, Chen SY, et al.: Reactive oxygen species modulate endothelin-i-induced c-fos gene expression in cardiomyocytes. *Cardiovasc Res* 41(3):654–662, 1999a.

Cheng W, Li B, Kajstura J, et al.: Stretch-induced programmed myocyte cell death. *J Clin Invest* 96(5):2247–2259, 1995.

Cheng XS, Shimokawa H, Momii H, et al.: Role of superoxide anion in the pathogenesis of cytokine-induced myocardial dysfunction in dogs in vivo. *Cardiovasc Res* 42(3):651–659, 1999b.

Cook SA, Sugden PH, Clerk A: Regulation of Bcl-2 family proteins during development and in response to oxidative stress in cardiac myocytes: Association with changes in mitochondrial membrane potential. *Circ Res* 85(10):940–949, 1999.

Dalakas MC, Illa I, Pezeshkpour GH, et al.: Mitochondrial myopathy caused by long-term zidovudine therapy. *N Engl J Med* 322(16):1098–1105, 1990.

De Simone G: Left ventricular geometry and hypotension in end-stage renal disease: a mechanical perspective. *J Am Soc Nephrol* 14(10):2421–2427, 2003.

Delaughter MC, Taffet GE, Fiorotto ML, et al.: Local insulin-like growth factor i expression induces physiologic, then pathologic, cardiac hypertrophy in transgenic mice. *FASEB J* 13(14):1923–1929, 1999.

Depre C, Taegtmeyer H: Metabolic aspects of programmed cell survival and cell death in the heart. *Cardiovasc Res* 45(3):538–548, 2000.

Dhalla NS, Yates JC, Maimark B, et al.: Cardiotoxicity of catecholamines and related agents, in Acosta D (ed.): *Cardiovascular Toxicology*, 2d ed. New York: Raven Press, 1992, pp. 239–282.

Diamond MI, Miner JN, Yoshinaga SK, et al.: Transcription factor interactions: selectors of positive or negative regulation from a single DNA element. *Science* 249(4974):1266–1272, 1990.

Didenko VV, Tunstead JR, Hornsby PJ: Biotin-labeled hairpin oligonucleotides: Probes to detect double-strand breaks in DNA in apoptotic cells. *Am J Pathol* 152(4):897–902, 1998.

Dockery DW: Epidemiologic evidence of cardiovascular effects of particulate air pollution. *Environ Health Perspect* 109(suppl 4):483–486, 2001.

Dorn GW, Force T: Protein kinase cascades in the regulation of cardiac hypertrophy. *J Clin Invest* 115(3):527–537, 2005.

Eguchi Y, Shimizu S, Tsujimoto Y: Intracellular ATP levels determine cell death fate by apoptosis or necrosis. *Cancer Res* 57(10):1835–1840, 1997.

EL-Sherif L, Wang GW, Kang YJ: Suppression of cadmium-induced apoptosis in metallothionein-overexpressing transgenic mouse cardiac myocytes. *FASEB J* 14:1193, 2000.

Eliot RS, Clayton FC, Pieper GM, et al.: Influence of environmental stress on pathogenesis of sudden cardiac death. *Fed Proc* 36(5):1719–1724, 1977.

Esposito G, Rapacciuolo A, Naga Prasad SV, et al.: Genetic alterations that inhibit in vivo pressure–overload hypertrophy prevent cardiac dysfunction despite increased wall stress. *Circulation* 105(1):85–92, 2002.

Evans T, Reitman M, Felsenfeld G: An erythrocyte-specific DNA-binding factor recognizes a regulatory sequence common to all chicken globin genes. *Proc Natl Acad Sci U S A* 85(16):5976–5980, 1988.

Evens T: Regulation of cardiac gene expression by GATA-4/5/6. *Trends Cardiovasc Med* 7:75–83, 1997.

Fauchier L, Babuty D, Poret P, et al.: Comparison of long-term outcome of alcoholic and idiopathic dilated cardiomyopathy. *Eur Heart J* 21(4):306–314, 2000.

Fitzgerald GA: Coxibs and cardiovascular disease. *N Engl J Med*, 351:1709–1711, 2004.

Fosslien E: Mitochondrial medicine—molecular pathology of defective oxidative phosphorylation. *Ann Clin Lab Sci* 31(1):25–67, 2001.

Francis GS, Chu C: Compensatory and maladaptive responses to cardiac dysfunction. *Curr Opin Cardiol* 10(3):260–267, 1995.

Frey N, Olson EN: Cardiac hypertrophy: The good, the bad, and the ugly. *Annu Rev Physiol* 65:45–79, 2003.

Frustaci A, Kajstura J, Chimenti C, et al.: Myocardial cell death in human diabetes. *Circ Res* 87(12):1123–1132, 2000.

Fujiwara Y, Kaji T, Sakurai S, et al.: Inhibitory effect of lead on the repair of wounded monolayers of cultured vascular endothelial cells. *Toxicology* 117(2–3):193–198, 1997.

Galan L, Talavera K, Vassort G, et al.: Characteristics of Ca^{2+} channel blockade by oxodipine and elgodipine in rat cardiomyocytes. *Eur J Pharmacol* 357(1):93–105, 1998.

Gan X, Zhang L, Berger O, et al.: Cocaine enhances brain endothelial adhesion molecules and leukocyte migration. *Clin Immunol* 91(1):68–76, 1999.

Gavazzi A, De Maria R, Parolini M, et al.: alcohol abuse and dilated cardiomyopathy in men. *Am J Cardiol* 85(9):1114–1118, 2000.

Goldsmith S, From AH: Arsenic-induced atypical ventricular tachycardia. *N Engl J Med* 303(19):1096–1098, 1980.

Gordon T, Reibman J: Cardiovascular toxicity of inhaled ambient particulate matter. *Toxicol Sci* 56(1):2–4, 2000.

Gottlieb RA, Burleson KO, Kloner RA, et al.: Reperfusion injury induces apoptosis in rabbit cardiomyocytes. *J Clin Invest* 94(4):1621–1628, 1994.

Gotzsche LS, Pedersen EM: Dose-dependent cardiotoxic effect of amiodarone in cardioplegic solutions correlates with loss of dihydropyridine binding sites: In vitro evidence for a potentially lethal interaction with procaine. *J Cardiovasc Pharmacol* 23(1):13–23, 1994.

Guenoun T, Montagne O, Laplace M, *et al*.: Propofol-Induced modifications of cardiomyocyte calcium transient and sarcoplasmic reticulum function in rats. *Anesthesiology* 92(2):542–549, 2000.

Guerra S, Leri A, Wang X, *et al*.: Myocyte death in the failing human heart is gender dependent. *Circ Res* 85(9):856–866, 1999.

Gurley BJ, Gardner SF, White LM, *et al*.: Ephedrine pharmacokinetics after the ingestion of nutritional supplements containing Ephedra Sinica (Ma Huang). *Ther Drug Monit* 20(4):439–445, 1998.

Gurtner GH, Burke-Wolin T: Interactions of oxidant stress and vascular reactivity. *Am J Physiol* 260(4 Pt 1):L207–L211, 1991.

Havlin KA: Cardiotoxicity of anthracyclines and other antineoplastic agents, in Acosta D (ed.): *Cardiovascular Toxicology*, 2nd ed. New York: Raven Press, 1992, pp. 143–164.

Harpel PC: Homocysteine, atherogenesis and thrombosis. *Fibrinolysis Proteolysis* 11(suppl 1):77–80, 1997.

Haunstetter A, Izumo S: Apoptosis: Basic mechanisms and implications for cardiovascular disease. *Circ Res* 82(11):1111–1129, 1998.

Hayakawa K, Takemura G, Koda M, *et al*.: Sensitivity to apoptosis signal, clearance rate, and ultrastructure of fas ligand-induced apoptosis in in vivo adult cardiac cells. *Circulation* 105(25):3039–3045, 2002.

He SY, Matoba R, Sodesaki K, *et al*.: Morphological and morphometric investigation of cardiac lesions after chronic administration of methamphetamine in rats. *Nippon Hoigaku Zasshi* 50(2):63–71, 1996.

Hill JA, Karimi M, Kutschke W, *et al*.: Cardiac hypertrophy is not a required compensatory response to short-term pressure overload. *Circulation* 101(24):2863–2869, 2000.

Hino N, Ochi R, Yanagisawa T: Inhibition of the slow inward current and the time-dependent outward current of mammalian ventricular muscle by gentamicin. *Pflugers Arch* 394(3):243–249, 1982.

Ho PD, Zechner DK, He H, *et al*.: The Raf-MEK-ERK Cascade represents a common pathway for alteration of intracellular calcium by Ras and protein kinase C in cardiac myocytes. *J Biol Chem* 273(34):21730–21735, 1998.

Holtz J: Pathophysiology of heart failure and the renin–angiotensin–system. *Basic Res Cardiol* 88(suppl 1):183–201, 1993.

Huss JM, Kelly DP: Mitochondrial energy metabolism in heart failure: A question of balance. *J Clin Invest* 115(3):547–555, 2005.

Hussar DA: New drugs of 1998. *J Am Pharm Assoc (Wash)* 39(2):151–206, 1999.

Hussar DA: New drugs of 1999. *J Am Pharm Assoc (Wash)* 40(2):181–221, 2000.

Iakushkin VV, Baldenkov GN, Tertov VV, *et al*.: Atherogenic properties of phenothiazine drugs manifesting in cultured cells of the human aortic intima. *Kardiologiia* 32(6):66–68, 1992.

Ingwall JS, Kramer MF, Fifer MA, *et al*.: The creatine kinase system In normal and diseased human myocardium. *N Engl J Med* 313(17):1050–1054, 1985.

Ingwall JS, Weiss RG: Is the failing heart energy starved? On using chemical energy to support cardiac function. *Circ Res* 95(2):135–145, 2004.

Ito H, Hirata Y, Adachi S, *et al*.: Endothelin-1 is an autocrine/paracrine factor in the mechanism of angiotensin II-induced hypertrophy in cultured rat cardiomyocytes. *J Clin Invest* 92(1):398–403, 1993.

Jalili T, Takeishi Y, Walsh RA: Signal transduction during cardiac hypertrophy: The role of G alpha Q, PLC Beta I, and PKC. *Cardiovasc Res* 44(1):5–9, 1999.

James TN: Normal and abnormal consequences of apoptosis in the human heart. from postnatal morphogenesis to paroxysmal arrhythmias. *Circulation* 90(1):556–573, 1994.

Joshi A, Dimino T, Vohra Y, *et al*.: Preclinical strategies to assess QT liability and torsadogenic potential of new drugs: The role of experimental models. *J Electrocardiol* 37(Suppl):7–14, 2004.

Jurgensmeier JM, Xie Z, Deveraux Q, *et al*.: Bax directly induces release of cytochrome *c* from isolated mitochondria. *Proc Natl Acad Sci U S A* 95(9):4997–5002, 1998.

Kaasik A, Minajeva A, Paju K, *et al*.: Thyroid hormones differentially affect sarcoplasmic reticulum function in rat atria and ventricles. *Mol Cell Biochem* 176(1–2):119–126, 1997.

Kagi JH: Overview of metallothionein. *Methods Enzymol* 205:401–414, 1991.

Kajstura J, Cheng W, Reiss K, *et al*.: Apoptotic and necrotic myocyte cell deaths are independent contributing variables of infarct size in rats. *Lab Invest* 74(1):86–107, 1996.

Kalin MF, Zumoff B: Sex hormones and coronary disease: A review of the clinical studies. *Steroids* 55(8):330–352, 1990.

Kang YJ: The antioxidant function of metallothionein in the heart. *Proc Soc Exp Biol Med* 222:263–273, 1999.

Kang YJ: Molecular and cellular mechanisms of cardiotoxicity. *Environ Health Perspect* 109(suppl 1):27–34, 2001.

Kang YJ: Metallothionein redox cycle and function. *Exp Biol Med (Maywood)* 231(9):1459–1467, 2006.

Kang YJ, Li Y, Zhou Z, *et al*.: Elevation of serum endothelins and cardiotoxicity induced by particulate matter (PM2.5) in rats with acute myocardial infarction. *Cardiovasc Toxicol* 2(4):253–261, 2002.

Kang YJ, Zhou ZX, Wang GW, *et al*.: Suppression by metallothionein of doxorubicin-induced cardiomyocyte apoptosis through inhibition of P38 mitogen-activated protein kinases. *J Biol Chem* 275(18):13690–13698, 2000a.

Kang YJ, Zhou ZX, Wu H, *et al*.: Metallothionein inhibits myocardial apoptosis in copper-deficient mice: Role of atrial natriuretic peptide. *Lab Invest* 80(5):745–757, 2000b.

Kannan M, Wang L, Kang YJ: Myocardial oxidative stress and toxicity induced by acute ethanol exposure in mice. *Exp Biol Med (Maywood)* 229(6):553–559, 2004.

Kass DA, Saavedra WF, Sabbah HN: Reverse Remodeling and enhanced inotropic reserve from the cardiac support device in experimental cardiac failure. *J Card Fail* 10(6 Suppl):S215–S219, 2004.

Klatsky AL: Alcohol and cardiovascular diseases: A historical overview. *Novartis Found Symp* 216:2–12, 1998.

Koenig H, Fan CC, Goldstone AD, *et al*.: Polyamines mediate androgenic stimulation of calcium fluxes and membrane transport in rat heart myocytes. *Circ Res* 64(3):415–426, 1989.

Kroemer G, Zamzami N, Susin SA: Mitochondrial control of apoptosis. *Immunol Today* 18(1):44–51, 1997.

Krown KA, Page MT, Nguyen C, *et al*.: Tumor necrosis factor alpha-induced apoptosis in cardiac myocytes. involvement of the sphingolipid signaling cascade in cardiac cell death. *J Clin Invest* 98(12):2854–2865, 1996.

Kubota T, Miyagishima M, Frye CS, *et al*.: Overexpression of tumor necrosis factor- alpha activates both anti- and pro-apoptotic pathways in the myocardium. *J Mol Cell Cardiol* 33(7):1331–1344, 2001.

Kurrelmeyer KM, Michael LH, Baumgarten G, *et al*.: Endogenous tumor necrosis factor protects the adult cardiac myocote against ischemic-induced apoptosis in a murine model of acute myocardial infarction. *Proc Natl Acad Sci U S A* 97:5456–5461, 2000.

Lazarevic AM, Nakatani S, Neskovic AN, *et al*.: Early changes in left ventricular function in chronic asymptomatic alcoholics: Relation to the duration of heavy drinking. *J Am Coll Cardiol* 35(6):1599–1606, 2000.

Lee JA, Allen DG: Calcium sensitisers: Mechanisms of action and potential usefulness as inotropes. *Cardiovasc Res* 36(1):10–20, 1997.

Leist M, Single B, Castoldi AF, *et al*.: Intracellular adenosine triphosphate (ATP) concentration: A switch in the decision between apoptosis and necrosis. *J Exp Med* 185(8):1481–1486, 1997.

Leist M, Single B, Naumann H, *et al*.: Inhibition of mitochondrial ATP generation by nitric oxide switches apoptosis to necrosis. *Exp Cell Res* 249(2):396–403, 1999.

Lenczowski JM, Dominguez L, Eder AM, *et al*.: Lack of a role for jun kinase and AP-1 in Fas-induced apoptosis. *Mol Cell Biol* 17(1):170–181, 1997.

Levine ES, Friedman HS, Griffith OW, *et al*.: Cardiac cell toxicity induced by 4-hydroperoxycyclophosphamide is modulated by glutathione. *Cardiovasc Res* 27(7):1248–1253, 1993.

Lewis JG, Graham DG, Valentine WM, *et al*.: Exposure of C57BL/6 mice to carbon disulfide induces early lesions of atherosclerosis and enhances arterial fatty deposits induced by a high fat diet. *Toxicol Sci* 49(1):124–132, 1999.

Lewis W, Grupp IL, Grupp G, *et al*.: cardiac dysfunction occurs in The HIV-1 transgenic mouse treated with zidovudine. *Lab Invest* 80(2):187–197, 2000.

Li F, Wang X, Capasso JM, *et al*.: Rapid transition of cardiac myocytes from hyperplasia to hypertrophy during postnatal development. *J Mol Cell Cardiol* 28(8):1737–1746, 1996.

Li Y, Sun X, Wang L, *et al*.: Myocardial toxicity of arsenic trioxide in a mouse model. *Cardiovasc Toxicol* 2(1):63–73, 2002.

Litwak KN, Mcmahan A, Lott KA, *et al*.: Monensin toxicosis in the domestic bovine calf: A large animal model of cardiac dysfunction. *Contemp Top Lab Anim Sci* 44(3):45–49, 2005.

Liu S, Melchert RB, Kennedy RH: Inhibition of L-type Ca^{2+} channel current in rat ventricular myocytes by terfenadine. *Circ Res* 81(2):202–210, 1997.

Marcillat O, Zhang Y, Davies KJ: Oxidative and non-oxidative mechanisms in the inactivation of cardiac mitochondrial electron transport chain components by doxorubicin. *Biochem J* 259(1):181–189, 1989.

Maret W: The function of zinc metallothionein: A link between cellular zinc and redox state. *J Nutr* 130(5S Suppl):1455S–1458S, 2000.

Marks AR: Intracellular calcium-release channels: Regulators of cell life and death. *Am J Physiol* 272(2 Pt 2):H597–H605, 1997.

Marsh JD, Lehmann MH, Ritchie RH, *et al*.: Androgen receptors mediate hypertrophy in cardiac myocytes. *Circulation* 98(3):256–261, 1998.

Marsin AS, Bertrand L, Rider MH, *et al*.: Phosphorylation and activation of heart PFK-2 by AMPK has a role in the stimulation of glycolysis during ischaemia. *Curr Biol* 10(20):1247–1255, 2000.

Martin XJ, Wynne DG, Glennon PE, *et al*.: Regulation of expression of contractile proteins with cardiac hypertrophy and failure. *Mol Cell Biochem* 157(1–2):181–189, 1996.

Mathews EC, Jr., Gardin JM, Henry WL, *et al*.: Echocardiographic abnormalities in chronic alcoholics with and without overt congestive heart failure. *Am J Cardiol* 47(3):570–578, 1981.

Matsui T, Li L, Wu JC, *et al*.: Phenotypic spectrum caused by transgenic overexpression of activated Akt in the heart. *J Biol Chem* 277(25):22896–22901, 2002.

Mcclain CJ, Su LC: Zinc deficiency in the alcoholic: A review. *Alcohol Clin Exp Res* 7(1):5–10, 1983.

Mckenna CJ, Codd MB, Mccann HA, *et al*.: Alcohol consumption and idiopathic dilated cardiomyopathy: a case control study. *Am Heart J* 135(5 Pt 1):833–837, 1998.

Mcmahon SB, Monroe JG: Role of primary response genes in generating cellular responses to growth factors. *FASEB J* 6(9):2707–2715, 1992.

Mcmanus BM, Toth B, Patil KD: Aortic rupture and aortic smooth muscle tumors in mice. Induction by P-hydrazinobenzoic acid hydrochloride of the cultivated mushroom *Agaricus Bisporus*. *Lab Invest* 57(1):78–85, 1987.

Melchert RB, Welder AA: Cardiovascular effects of androgenic-anabolic steroids. *Med Sci Sports Exerc* 27(9):1252–1262, 1995.

Metzger JM, Wahr PA, Michele DE, *et al*.: Effects of myosin heavy chain isoform switching on Ca^{2+}-activated tension development in single adult cardiac myocytes. *Circ Res* 84(11):1310–1317, 1999.

Miller RA, Boorman GA: Morphology of neoplastic lesions induced by 1,3-butadiene in B6C3F1 mice. *Environ Health Perspect* 86:37–48, 1990.

Molkentin JD, Lu JR, Antos CL, *et al*.: A calcineurin-dependent transcriptional pathway for cardiac hypertrophy. *Cell* 93(2):215–228, 1998.

Monge JC: Neurohormonal markers of clinical outcome in cardiovascular disease: Is endothelin the best one? *J Cardiovasc Pharmacol* 32(suppl 2):S36–S42, 1998.

Nakaki T, Nakayama M, Yamamoto S, *et al*.: Alpha 1-adrenergic stimulation and beta 2-adrenergic inhibition of DNA synthesis in vascular smooth muscle cells. *Mol Pharmacol* 37(1):30–36, 1990.

Nattel S: Experimental evidence for proarrhythmic mechanisms of antiarrhythmic drugs. *Cardiovasc Res* 37(3):567–577, 1998.

Neubauer S, Horn M, Cramer M, *et al*.: Myocardial phosphocreatine-to-ATP ratio is a predictor of mortality in patients with dilated cardiomyopathy. *Circulation* 96(7):2190–2196, 1997.

Neubauer S, Remkes H, Spindler M, *et al*.: Downregulation of the Na(+)-creatine cotransporter in failing human myocardium and in experimental heart failure. *Circulation* 100(18):1847–1850, 1999.

Newton AC: Protein kinase C: Structure, function, and regulation. *J Biol Chem* 270(48):28495–28498, 1995.

Olivetti G, Abbi R, Quaini F, *et al*.: Apoptosis in the failing human heart. *N Engl J Med* 336(16):1131–1141, 1997.

Olson EN: A decade of discoveries in cardiac biology. *Nat Med* 10(5):467–474, 2004.

Opie L: Heart cells and organells, in Opie L (ed.): *The Heart*. New York: Harcourt Brace Jovanovich, 1996, pp. 15–29.

Orkin SH: GATA-binding transcription factors in hematopoietic cells. *Blood* 80(3):575–581, 1992.

Ou X, Ramos KS: Modulation of aortic protein phosphorylation by benzo(A)pyrene: Implications in PAH-induced atherogenesis. *J Biochem Toxicol* 7(3):147–154, 1992.

Pacher P, Ungvari Z, Kecskemeti V, *et al*.: Review of cardiovascular effects of fluoxetine, a selective serotonin reuptake inhibitor, compared to tricyclic antidepressants. *Curr Med Chem* 5(5):381–390, 1998.

Paradis P, Maclellan WR, Belaguli NS, *et al*.: Serum response factor mediates AP-1-dependent induction of the skeletal alpha-actin promoter in ventricular myocytes. *J Biol Chem* 271(18):10827–10833, 1996.

Penn A, Snyder C: Arteriosclerotic plaque development is "promoted" by polynuclear aromatic hydrocarbons. *Carcinogenesis* 9(12):2185, 1988.

Perez NG, Gao WD, Marban E: Novel myofilament Ca^{2+}-sensitizing property of xanthine oxidase inhibitors. *Circ Res* 83(4):423–430, 1998.

Perry HM, Jr., Erlanger MW, Gustafsson TO, *et al*.: Reversal of cadmium-induced hypertension by D-myo-inositol-1,2,6-trisphosphate. *J Toxicol Environ Health* 28(2):151–159, 1989.

Peters A, Liu E, Verrier RL, *et al*.: Air pollution and incidence of cardiac arrhythmia. *Epidemiology* 11(1):11–17, 2000.

Piano MR: Cellular and signaling mechanisms of cardiac hypertrophy. *J Cardiovasc Nurs* 8(4):1–26, 1994.

Piano MR: Alcoholic cardiomyopathy: Incidence, clinical characteristics, and pathophysiology. *Chest* 121(5):1638–1650, 2002.

Piano MR, Bondmass M, Schwertz DW: The molecular and cellular pathophysiology of heart failure. *Heart Lung* 27(1):3–19, 1998.

Pickerill KE, Paladino JA, Schentag JJ: Comparison of the fluoroquinolones based on pharmacokinetic and pharmacodynamic parameters. *Pharmacotherapy* 20(4):417–428, 2000.

Powis G: Free radical formation by antitumor quinones. *Free Radic Biol Med* 6(1):63–101, 1989.

Pu WT, Ma Q, Izumo S: NFAT transcription factors are critical survival factors that inhibit cardiomyocyte apoptosis during phenylephrine stimulation in vitro. *Circ Res* 92(7):725–731, 2003.

Puceat M, Vassort G: Signalling by protein kinase C isoforms in the heart. *Mol Cell Biochem* 157(1–2):65–72, 1996.

Pulkki KJ: Cytokines and cardiomyocyte death. *Ann Med* 29(4):339–343, 1997.

Rao A, Luo C, Hogan PG: Transcription factors of the NFAT family: Regulation and function. *Annu Rev Immunol* 15:707–747, 1997.

Reed JC, Jurgensmeier JM, Matsuyama S: Bcl-2 family proteins and mitochondria. *Biochim Biophys Acta* 1366(1–2):127–137, 1998.

Regan TJ: Alcohol and the cardiovascular system. *JAMA* 264(3):377–381, 1990.

Ribiere C, Hininger I, Rouach H, *et al*.: Effects of chronic ethanol administration on free radical defence in rat myocardium. *Biochem Pharmacol* 44(8):1495–1500, 1992.

Richey PA, Brown SP: Pathological versus physiological left ventricular hypertrophy: A review. *J Sports Sci* 16(2):129–141, 1998.

Robbins J: Genetic modification of the heart: Exploring necessity and sufficiency in the past 10 years. *J Mol Cell Cardiol* 36(5):643–652, 2004.

Robert V, Silvestre JS, Charlemagne D, *et al*.: Biological determinants of aldosterone-induced cardiac fibrosis in rats. *Hypertension* 26(6 Pt 1):971–978, 1995.

Rockhold RW: Cardiovascular toxicity of anabolic steroids. *Annu Rev Pharmacol Toxicol* 33:497–520, 1993.

Roden DM: Antiarrhythmic drugs, in Hardman JG, Limbird LE, Molinoff PB, *et al.* (eds.): *Goodman & Gilman's The Pharmacological Basis Of Therapeutics*, 9th ed. New York: Mcgraw-Hill, 1996, pp. 839–874.

Rooney JW, Hodge MR, Mccaffrey PG, *et al.*: A common factor regulates both th1- and th2-specific cytokine gene expression. *EMBO J* 13(3):625–633, 1994.

Rosen MR: Cardiac arrhythmias and antiarrhythmic drugs: recent advances in our understanding of mechanism. *J Cardiovasc Electrophysiol* 6(10 Pt 2):868–879, 1995.

Russell RR, III, Bergeron R, Shulman GI, *et al.*: Translocation of myocardial GLUT-4 and increased glucose uptake through activation of AMPK by AICAR. *Am J Physiol* 277(2 Pt 2):H643–H649, 1999.

Sabbah HN, Sharov VG: Apoptosis in heart failure. *Prog Cardiovasc Dis* 40(6):549–562, 1998.

Saikumar P, Dong Z, Patel Y, *et al.*: Role of hypoxia-induced bax translocation and cytochrome *c* release in reoxygenation injury. *Oncogene* 17(26):3401–3415, 1998.

Saupe KW, Spindler M, Hopkins JC, *et al.*: Kinetic, thermodynamic, and developmental consequences of deleting creatine kinase isoenzymes from the heart. Reaction kinetics of the creatine kinase isoenzymes in the intact heart. *J Biol Chem* 275(26):19742–19746, 2000.

Sawyer DB, Fukazawa R, Arstall MA, *et al.*: Daunorubicin-induced apoptosis in rat cardiac myocytes is inhibited by dexrazoxane. *Circ Res* 84(3):257–265, 1999.

Shier WT, Dubourdieu DJ: Sodium- and calcium-dependent steps in the mechanism of neonatal rat cardiac myocyte killing by ionophores. I. The sodium-carrying ionophore, monensin. *Toxicol Appl Pharmacol* 116(1):38–46, 1992.

Shioi T, Kang PM, Douglas PS, *et al.*: The conserved phosphoinositide 3-kinase pathway determines heart size in mice. *EMBO J* 19(11):2537–2548, 2000.

Shioi T, Mcmullen JR, Kang PM, *et al.*: Akt/protein kinase B promotes organ growth in transgenic mice. *Mol Cell Biol* 22(8):2799–2809, 2002.

Shipp JC, Opie LH, Challoner D.: Fatty acid and glucose metabolism in the perfused heart. *Nature* 189(4769):1018–1019, 1961.

Simons FE: The therapeutic index of newer H1-receptor antagonists. *Clin Exp Allergy* 24(8):707–723, 1994.

Sleight P: Calcium antagonists during and after myocardial infarction. *Drugs* 51(2):216–225, 1996.

Solem LE, Henry TR, Wallace KB: Disruption of mitochondrial calcium homeostasis following chronic doxorubicin administration. *Toxicol Appl Pharmacol* 129(2):214–222, 1994.

Solomon SD, McMurray JJ, Pfeffer MA, *et al.*,: Cardiovascular risk associated with celecoxib in a clinical trual for colorectal adenoma prevntion. *N Engl J Med* 352:1071–1080, 2005.

Splawski I, Shen J, Timothy KW, *et al.*: Spectrum of mutations in long-QT syndrome genes. KVLQT1, HERG, SCN5A, KCNE1, and KCNE2. *Circulation* 102(10):1178–1185, 2000.

Stemmer PM, Klee CB: Dual calcium ion regulation of calcineurin by calmodulin and calcineurin B. *Biochemistry* 33(22):6859–6866, 1994.

Stief CG, Uckert S, Becker AJ, *et al.*: Effects of sildenafil on camp and cgmp levels in isolated human cavernous and cardiac tissue. *Urology* 55(1):146–150, 2000.

Stolley PD, Strom BL, Sartwell PE: Oral contraceptives and vascular disease. *Epidemiol Rev* 11:241–243, 1989.

Sugden PH, Clerk A: "Stress-responsive" mitogen-activated protein kinases (C-Jun N-terminal kinases and P38 mitogen-activated protein kinases) in the myocardium. *Circ Res* 83(4):345–352, 1998.

Sugishita K, Kinugawa K, Shimizu T, *et al.*: Cellular basis for the acute inhibitory effects of IL-6 and TNF-alpha on excitation–contraction coupling. *J Mol Cell Cardiol* 31(8):1457–1467, 1999.

Suzuki K, Kostin S, Person V, *et al.*: Time course of the apoptotic cascade and effects of caspase inhibitors in adult rat ventricular cardiomyocytes. *J Mol Cell Cardiol* 33(5):983–994, 2001.

Swynghedauw B: Molecular mechanisms of myocardial remodeling. *Physiol Rev* 79(1):215–262, 1999.

Symanski JD, Gettes LS: Drug effects on the electrocardiogram. A review of their clinical importance. *Drugs* 46(2):219–248, 1993.

Talhari C, lauceviciute I, Enderlein E, *et al.*: COX-2-selective inhibitor valdecoxib induces severe allergic skin reactions. *J Allergy Clin Immunol* 115:1089–1090. 2005.

Tan Y, Rouse J, Zhang A, *et al.*: FGF and stress regulate CREB and ATF-1 via A pathway involving P38 MAP kinase and MAPKAP kinase-2. *EMBO J* 15(17):4629–4642, 1996.

Thomas R, Sutton ET, Bryant MW, *et al.*: In vivo vascular damage, leukocyte activation and inflammatory response induced by beta-amyloid. *J Submicrosc Cytol Pathol* 29(3):293–304, 1997.

Tibbles LA, Woodgett JR: The stress-activated protein kinase pathways. *Cell Mol Life Sci* 55(10):1230–1254, 1999.

Toraason M, Wey HE, Richards DE, *et al.*: Altered Ca^{2+} Mobilization during excitation–contraction in cultured cardiac myocytes exposed to antimony. *Toxicol Appl Pharmacol* 146(1):104–115, 1997.

Van Bilsen M, Smeets PJ, Gilde AJ, *et al.*: Metabolic remodelling of the failing heart: The cardiac burn-out syndrome? *Cardiovasc Res* 61(2):218–226, 2004.

Van Empel VP, De Windt LJ: Myocyte hypertrophy and apoptosis: A balancing act. *Cardiovasc Res* 63(3):487–499, 2004.

Van Vleet JF, Amstutz HE, Weirich WE, *et al.*: Clinical, clinicopathologic, and pathologic alterations in acute monensin toxicosis in cattle. *Am J Vet Res* 44(11):2133–2144, 1983.

Ventura-Clapier R, Garnier A, Veksler V: Energy metabolism in heart failure. *J Physiol* 555(Pt 1):1–13, 2004.

Vestal RE, Eiriksson CE, Jr., Musser B, *et al.*: Effect of intravenous aminophylline on plasma levels of catecholamines and related cardiovascular and metabolic responses in man. *Circulation* 67(1):162–171, 1983.

Wald N, Howard S: Smoking, carbon monoxide and arterial disease. *Ann Occup Hyg* 18(1):1–14, 1975.

Wallace KB, Hausner E, Herman E, *et al.*: Serum troponins as biomarkers of drug-induced cardiac toxicity. *Toxicol Pathol* 32(1):106–121, 2004.

Wallimann T, Dolder M, Schlattner U, *et al.*: Some new aspects of creatine kinase (CK): Compartmentation, structure, function and regulation for cellular and mitochondrial bioenergetics and physiology. *Biofactors* 8(3–4):229–234, 1998.

Wang GW, Klein JB, Kang YJ: Metallothionein inhibits doxorubicin-induced mitochondrial cytochrome *c* release and caspase-3 activation in cardiomyocytes. *J Pharmacol Exp Ther* 298(2):461–468, 2001a.

Wang GW, Zhou Z, Klein JB, *et al.*: Inhibition of hypoxia/reoxygenation-induced apoptosis in metallothionein-overexpressing cardiomyocytes. *Am J Physiol Heart Circ Physiol* 280(5):H2292–H2299, 2001b.

Wang L, Zhou Z, Saari JT, *et al.*: Alcohol-induced myocardial fibrosis in metallothionein-null mice: Prevention by zinc supplementation. *Am J Pathol* 167(2):337–344, 2005.

Wang XZ, Ron D: Stress-induced phosphorylation and activation of the transcription factor CHOP (GADD153) By P38 MAP Kinase. *Science* 272(5266):1347–1349, 1996.

Wang Y, Huang S, Sah VP, *et al.*: Cardiac muscle cell hypertrophy and apoptosis induced by distinct members of the p38 mitogen-activated protein kinase family. *J Biol Chem* 273(4):2161–2168, 1998.

Weber KT: Are myocardial fibrosis and diastolic dysfunction reversible in hypertensive heart disease? *Congest Heart Fail* 11(6):322–324, 2005.

Wettschureck N, Rutten H, Zywietz A, *et al.*: Absence of pressure overload induced myocardial hypertrophy after conditional inactivation of Galphaq/Galpha11 in cardiomyocytes. *Nat Med* 7(11):1236–1240, 2001.

Wisneski JA, Gertz EW, Neese RA, *et al.*: Myocardial metabolism of free fatty acids. Studies with 14C-labeled substrates in humans. *J Clin Invest* 79(2):359–366, 1987.

Wollert KC, Heineke J, Westermann J, *et al.*: The cardiac Fas (APO-1/CD95) receptor/Fas ligand system: Relation to diastolic wall stress in volume-overload hypertrophy in vivo and activation of the transcription factor AP-1 in cardiac myocytes. *Circulation* 101(10):1172–1178, 2000.

Wollnik B, Schroeder BC, Kubisch C, *et al.*: Pathophysiological mechanisms of dominant and recessive KVLQT1 K$^+$ channel mutations found in inherited cardiac arrhythmias. *Hum Mol Genet* 6(11):1943–1949, 1997.

Wyllie AH: Death from inside out: An overview. *Philos Trans R Soc Lond B Biol Sci* 345(1313):237–241, 1994.

Wyllie AH: Death from inside out: An overview. *Philos Trans R Soc Lond B Biol Sci* 345(1313):237–241, 1994.

Xu W, Liu Y, Wang S, *et al.*: Cytoprotective role of Ca^{2+}-activated K$^+$ channels in the cardiac inner mitochondrial membrane. *Science* 298(5595):1029–1033, 2002.

Yamamoto C, Miyamoto A, Sakamoto M, *et al.*: Lead perturbs the regulation of spontaneous release of tissue plasminogen activator and plasminogen activator inhibitor-1 from vascular smooth muscle cells and fibroblasts in culture. *Toxicology* 117(2–3):153–161, 1997.

Yamamoto M, Ko LJ, Leonard MW, *et al.*: Activity and tissue-specific expression of the transcription factor NF-E1 multigene family. *Genes Dev* 4(10):1650–1662, 1990.

Yamashita K, Kajstura J, Discher DJ, *et al.*: Reperfusion-activated Akt kinase prevents apoptosis in transgenic mouse hearts overexpressing insulin-like growth factor-1. *Circ Res* 88(6):609–614, 2001.

Yaoita H, Ogawa K, Maehara K, *et al.*: Apoptosis in relevant clinical situations: Contribution of apoptosis in myocardial infarction. *Cardiovasc Res* 45(3):630–641, 2000.

Yin T, Sandhu G, Wolfgang CD, *et al.*: Tissue-specific pattern of stress kinase activation in ischemic/reperfused heart and kidney. *J Biol Chem* 272(32):19943–19950, 1997.

Young M, Fullerton M, Dilley R, *et al.*: Mineralocorticoids, hypertension, and cardiac fibrosis. *J Clin Invest* 93(6):2578–2583, 1994.

Zakhari S: Cardiovascular toxicology of halogenated hydrocarbons and other solvents, in Acosta D (ed.): *Cardiovascular Toxicology.* New York: Raven Press, 1992, pp. 409–454.

Zhou S, Starkov A, Froberg MK, *et al.*: Cumulative and irreversible cardiac mitochondrial dysfunction induced by doxorubicin. *Cancer Res* 61(2):771–777, 2001.

Zhou W, Fontenot HJ, Liu S, *et al.*: Modulation of cardiac calcium channels by propofol. *Anesthesiology* 86(3):670–675, 1997.

Zhou W, Fontenot HJ, Wang SN, *et al.*: Propofol-induced alterations in myocardial beta-adrenoceptor binding and responsiveness. *Anesth Analg* 89(3):604–608, 1999.

Zou Y, Hiroi Y, Uozumi H, *et al.*: Calcineurin plays a critical role in the development of pressure overload-induced cardiac hypertrophy. *Circulation* 104(1):97–101, 2001.

CHAPTER 19

TOXIC RESPONSES OF THE SKIN

Robert H. Rice and Theodora M. Mauro

As the body's first line of defense against external insult, the skin's enormous surface area (1.5–2 m^2) is exposed routinely to chemicals and may inadvertently serve as a portal of entry for topical contactants. Recognizing the potential hazards of skin exposure, the National Institute of Occupational Safety and Health (NIOSH) characterized skin disease as one of the most pervasive occupational health problems in the United States. In 1982, NIOSH placed skin disease in the top ten leading work-related diseases based on frequency, severity, and the potential for prevention. Data from the Bureau of Labor Statistics indicate that in 2004, skin disease attributed to workplace exposures accounted for nearly 16% of the reported nonfatal occupational disease in private industry; incidence data indicate a rate of 4.4 cases per 10,000 or nearly 39,000 new cases per year. Substantial reduction in the reported incidence has occurred in recent years thanks to workplace cleanup and better personal protective equipment. Nevertheless, improvements in prevention and management are needed for continued progress (Emmett, 2003). Skin conditions resulting from exposures to consumer products or occupational illnesses not resulting in work time loss are poorly recorded and tracked. Hence the incidence of such skin diseases appears greatly underestimated.

SKIN AS A BARRIER

A large and highly accessible human organ, the skin protects the body against external insults to maintain internal homeostasis. Its biological sophistication allows it to perform a myriad of functions above and beyond that of a suit of armor. Physiologically, the skin participates directly in thermal, electrolyte, hormonal, metabolic, and immune regulation, without which a human would perish. Rather than merely repelling noxious physical agents, the skin may react to them with a variety of defensive mechanisms that prevent internal or widespread cutaneous damage. If an insult is severe or sufficiently intense to overwhelm the protective function of the skin, acute or chronic injury becomes readily manifest in various ways. The specific presentation depends on a variety of intrinsic and extrinsic factors including body site, duration of exposure, and other environmental conditions (Table 19-1).

Skin Histology

The skin consists of two major components: the outer epidermis and the underlying dermis, which are separated by a basement membrane (Fig. 19-1). The junction ordinarily is not flat but has an undulating appearance (rete ridges). In addition, epidermal appendages (hair follicles, sebaceous glands, and eccrine glands) span the epidermis and are embedded in the dermis. In thickness, the dermis comprises approximately 90% of the skin and has mainly a supportive function. It has a high content of collagen and elastin secreted by scattered fibroblasts, thus providing the skin with elastic properties. Separating the dermis from the underlying tissues is a layer of adipocytes, whose accumulation of fat has a cushioning action. The blood supply to the epidermis originates in the capillaries located in the rete ridges at the dermal–epidermal junction. Capillaries also supply the bulbs of the hair follicles and the secretory cells of the eccrine (sweat) glands. The ducts from these glands carry a dilute salt solution to the surface of the skin, where its evaporation provides cooling.

    The interfollicular epidermis is a stratified squamous epithelium consisting primarily of keratinocytes. These cells are tightly attached to each other by desmosomes and to the basement membrane by hemidesmosomes. Melanocytes are interspersed among the basal cells and distributed in the papilla of hair follicles. In the epidermis, these cells are stimulated by ultraviolet light to produce melanin granules. The granules are extruded and taken up by the surrounding keratinocytes, which thereby become pigmented. Migrating through the epidermis are numerous Langerhans cells, which

Table 19-1
Factors Influencing Cutaneous Responses

VARIABLE	COMMENT
Body site	
Palms/soles	Thick stratum corneum—good physical barrier
	Common site of contact with chemicals
	Occlusion with protective clothing
Intertriginous areas (axillae, groin, neck, finger webs, umbilicus, genitalia)	Moist, occluded areas
	Chemical trapping
	Enhanced percutaneous absorption
Face	Exposed frequently
	Surface lipid interacts with hydrophobic substances
	Chemicals frequently transferred from hands
Eyelids	Poor barrier function—thin epidermis
	Sensitive to irritants
Postauricular region	Chemical trapping
	Occlusion
Scalp	Chemical trapping
	Hair follicles susceptible to metabolic damage
Predisposing cutaneous illnesses	
Atopic dermatitis	Increased sensitivity to irritants
	Impaired barrier function
Psoriasis	Impaired barrier function
Genetic factors	Predisposition to skin disorders
	Variation in sensitivity to irritants
	Susceptibility to contact sensitization
Temperature	Vasodilation—improved percutaneous absorption
	Increased sweating—trapping
Humidity	Increased sweating—trapping
Season	Variation in relative humidity
	Chapping and wind-related skin changes

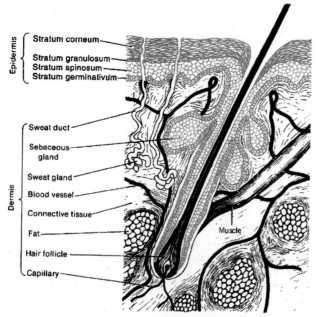

Figure 19-1. Diagram of a crosssection of human skin.

The epidermis and pilosebaceous unit are shown in blue.

are important participants in the immune response of skin to foreign agents.

Keratinocytes of the basal layer comprise the germinative compartment. When a basal cell divides, one of the progeny detaches from the basal lamina and migrates outward. As cells move toward the skin surface, they undergo a remarkable program of terminal differentiation. They gradually express new protein markers and accumulate keratin proteins, from which the name of this cell type is derived. The keratins form insoluble intermediate filaments accounting for nearly 40% of the total cell protein in the spinous layer. At the granular layer, the cells undergo a striking morphological transformation, becoming flattened and increasing in volume by nearly 40-fold. Lipid granules fuse with the plasma membrane at the granular layer/stratum corneum interface, filling the intercellular spaces of the stratum corneum with lipid, as opposed to the aqueous intercellular solution in the viable epidermis. Meanwhile, the plasma membranes of these cells become permeable, resulting in the loss of their reducing environment and consequently in extensive disulfide bonding among keratin proteins. Cell organelles are degraded, while a protein envelope is synthesized immediately beneath the plasma membrane. The membrane is altered characteristically by the loss of phospholipid and the addition of sphingolipid.

This program of terminal differentiation, beginning as keratinocytes leave the basal layer, produces the outermost layer of the skin, the stratum corneum. No longer viable, the mature cells (called *corneocytes*) are ~80% keratin in content. They are gradually shed from the surface and replaced from beneath. The process typically takes 2 weeks for basal cells to reach the stratum corneum and another 2 weeks to be shed from the surface. In the skin disease psoriasis, the migration of cells to the surface is nearly tenfold faster than normal, resulting in a stratum corneum populated by cells that are not completely mature. In instances in which the outer layer is deficient due to disease or physical or chemical trauma, the barrier to the environment that the skin provides is inferior to that provided by normal, healthy skin.

Percutaneous Absorption

Until a century ago, the skin was thought to provide an impervious barrier to exogenous substances. Gradually, the ability of substances to penetrate the skin, though this process generally is very slow, became appreciated. During the past 50 years, the stratum corneum has been recognized as the primary barrier (Scheuplein and Blank, 1971). Diseases (e.g., psoriasis) or other conditions (e.g., abrasion, wounding) in which this barrier is compromised can permit greatly increased uptake of poorly permeable substances, as does removal of the stratum corneum by tape stripping or organic solvents such as acetone. The viable layer of epidermis provides a much less effective barrier, because hydrophilic chemicals readily diffuse into the intercellular water, while hydrophobic chemicals can partition into cell membranes, and each can diffuse readily to the blood supply in the rete ridges of the dermis.

Probably the best-known biological membrane barrier for this purpose, the stratum corneum, prevents water loss from underlying tissues by evaporation. Its hydrophobic character reflects the lipid content of the intercellular space, ~15% of the total volume (Elias, 1992). The lipids, a major component being sphingolipids, have a high content of long-chain ceramides, removal of which seriously compromises barrier function as measured by transepidermal water loss. The stratum corneum ordinarily is hydrated (typically 20% water) with the moisture residing in corneocyte protein; however, it can take up a great deal more water upon prolonged immersion, thereby reducing the effectiveness of the barrier to chemicals with a hydrophilic character. Indeed, occlusion of the skin with plastic wrap, permitting the retention of perspiration underneath, is a commonly employed technique to enhance uptake of chemicals applied to the skin surface. Although penetration from the air is generally too low to be of concern, protection from skin uptake may be advisable for some compounds (e.g., nitrobenzene) at concentrations high enough to require respirator use.

Finding the rate at which the uptake of chemicals through the skin occurs is important for estimating the consequences of exposure we encounter in the environment. Indeed, a regulatory strategy permitting bathing in water considered barely unfit for drinking was revised when it was realized that exposure from dermal/inhalation uptake during bathing could be comparable to that from drinking 2 L of the water (Brown *et al.*, 1984). Uptake through the skin is now incorporated in pharmacokinetic modeling to estimate potential risks from exposures. The degree of uptake depends upon the details of exposure conditions, being proportional to solute concentration (assuming it is dilute), time, and the amount of skin surface exposed. In addition, two intrinsic factors contribute to the absorption rate of a given compound: its hydrophobicity, which affects its ability to partition into epidermal lipid, and its rate of diffusion through this barrier. A measure of the first property is the com-

monly used octanol/water partitioning ratio (K_{ow}). This is particularly relevant for exposure to contaminated water, as occurs during bathing or swimming. However, partitioning of a chemical into the skin is greatly affected by its solubility in or adhesion to the medium in which it is applied (including soil). Similarly, very hydrophobic compounds, once in the stratum corneum, may diffuse only very slowly into less hydrophobic regions below. The second property is an inverse function of molecular weight (MW) or molecular volume. Thus, hydrophobic agents of low MW permeate the skin better than those of high MW or those that are hydrophilic. For small molecules, hydrophobicity is a dominant factor in penetration.

Although only small amounts of chemicals may penetrate the stratum corneum, those of high potency may still be very dangerous. For example, hydrophobic organophosphorus and carbamate pesticides can be neurotoxic to humans and domestic animals by skin contact. Children and adolescents harvesting tobacco are especially susceptible to poisoning by contact with nicotine, a natural pesticide present in moisture on the leaves (McKnight and Spiller, 2005). Conditions of topical treatment of livestock for pest control must take into consideration not only the tolerance of the animals but also residues in meat and milk resulting from skin penetration. High-level skin exposure to chemicals considered safe at low levels can be dangerous, evident from the nervous system toxicity and deaths of babies exposed to hexachlorophene mistakenly added to talcum powder for their diapers (Martin-Bouyer *et al.*, 1982). Previous findings of *N*-nitrosamines that penetrate skin well (such as *N*-nitrosodiethanolamine) in cutting oils and cosmetics raised concern and led to their monitoring and to reduction of exposure.

Considerable empirical information has been collected on some chemicals of special interest (including pharmaceuticals, pesticides, and pollutants) for use in quantifying structure/penetration relationships. From such information, relations can be obtained for skin penetration (P_{cw}) using empirically derived constants (C_1, C_2, C_3) that have the form shown below (Potts and Guy, 1992). Such relations describe steady-state conditions, in which a chemical

$$\log P_{cw} = C_1 - C_2(\text{MW}) + C_3 \log K_{ow}$$

leaves the stratum corneum at the same rate it enters. Because rates of transfer of very hydrophobic agents into the aqueous phase of the spinous layer are slow, saturation of the stratum corneum provides a depot, leading to continued penetration into the body for relatively long time periods after external exposure to a chemical stops. More recent modeling efforts have taken into account vehicles and additives to improve predictability of complex chemical mixtures (Riviere and Brooks, 2005).

Diffusion through the epidermis is considerably faster at some anatomical sites than others. A list in order of decreasing permeability gives the following hierarchy: foot sole > palm > forehead > abdomen (Scheuplein and Blank, 1971). Scrotal skin reportedly has the highest permeability for some topical chemicals (Fisher, 1989). Under ordinary conditions, absorption through the epidermal appendages is generally neglected, despite the ability of chemicals to bypass the stratum corneum by this route, because the combined appendageal surface area is such a small fraction of the total available for uptake. However, because loading of the stratum corneum is slow, penetration through the appendages can constitute an appreciable fraction of the total for short exposures. In some cases, the effects of appendages can even be dominant. For instance, benzo(*a*)pyrene penetrates the skin of haired mice several-fold faster than that of hairless strains (Kao and Hall, 1987). As indicated below, in some cases these properties have been exploited for therapeutic uses.

Transdermal Drug Delivery The ability of the stratum corneum to serve as a reservoir for exogenously applied chemicals is well illustrated by the recent development of methods for the delivery of pharmaceuticals. Application of drugs to the skin can produce systemic effects, a phenomenon observed unintentionally before the ability of the skin to serve as a delivery system was appreciated. For example, topical exposure of young girls to estrogens has led to reports of pseudoprecocious puberty, whereas in young or adult males, such exposure has produced gynecomastia (Amin et al., 1998). Specially designed patches are currently in use to deliver estradiol, testosterone, nitroglycerin, scopolamine, clonidine, fentanyl, and nicotine for therapeutic purposes, and others are under development. The advantages of this approach over oral dosing include providing a steady infusion for extended periods (typically 1–7 days), thereby avoiding large variations in plasma concentration, preventing exposure to the acidic pH of the stomach, and avoiding biotransformation in the gastrointestinal tract or from first-pass removal by the liver. The contrast in plasma concentration kinetics between different methods of delivery is particularly evident for agents that are rapidly metabolized, such as nitroglycerin, which has a half-life of a few minutes. A variety of chemicals, chosen carefully to minimize irritation or allergenicity, have been incorporated into pharmaceutical preparations to enhance absorption and penetration. In addition, encapsulating a drug in small vesicles of phospholipid or nonionic surfactant can be effective at least in part by targeting hair follicles (Choi and Maibach, 2005).

Measurements of Penetration For many purposes, including risk assessment and pharmaceutical design, the most useful subject for experimentation is human skin. Volunteers are dosed, plasma and/or urine concentrations are quantified at suitable intervals, and amounts excreted from the body are estimated. Previous measurements of penetration often used ^{14}C-labeled agents. This approach is not preferred, but use of isotopic labels now is readily feasible when coupled to ultrasensitive detection by accelerator mass spectrometry (Buchholz et al., 1999). For in vitro work, excised split-thickness skin can be employed in special diffusion chambers, though care is needed to preserve the viability of the living layer of epidermis. The chemical is removed for quantification from the underside by a fluid into which it partitions, thereby permitting continued penetration. Commonly employed is a simpler set up, using cadaver skin with the lower dermis removed. This lacks biotransformation capability but retains the barrier function of the stratum corneum. The phamacokinetic approach with intact subjects is most commonly employed with experimental animals. Without verification using human skin, such measurements are subject to large uncertainties due to species differences in density of epidermal appendages, stratum corneum properties (e.g., thickness, lipid composition), and biotransformation rates. Because penetration through rodent skin is usually faster than through human skin, the former can provide an overestimate for the behavior of the latter. To simplify determination of penetration kinetics, skin flaps may be employed and the capillary blood flow monitored to measure penetration. For this purpose, pig skin has particular utility (Riviere and Brooks, 2005). A promising variation minimizing species differences is to use skin grafts on experimental animals for these measurements. Human skin persists well

on athymic mice and retains its normal barrier properties (Krueger and Pershing, 1993). More recently, penetration of chemicals can be tracked through the skin using confocal microscopy (Alvarez-Roman et al., 2004). In any case, accurate testing of percutaneous absorption of poorly soluble agents from environmental substrates requires attention to details of particle size, component complexes, application rate and skin contact.

Biotransformation

The ability of the skin to metabolize chemicals that diffuse through it contributes to its barrier function. This influences the potential biological activity of xenobiotics and topically applied drugs, leading to their degradation or their activation as skin sensitizers or carcinogens (Hotchkiss, 1998). To this end, the epidermis and pilosebaceous units are the most relevant and, indeed, are the major sources of such activity in the skin. On a body-weight basis, phase I metabolism in this organ usually is only a small fraction (~2%) of that in the liver, but its importance should not be underestimated. For example, when the epidermis of the neonatal rat is treated with benzo(a)pyrene or Aroclor 1254, the arylhydrocarbon hydroxylase (P450) activity in the skin can exceed 20% of that in the whole body (Mukhtar and Bickers, 1981). As illustrated in this example, cytochrome P4501A1 is inducible in the epidermis by chemicals that are inducers in other tissues—TCDD (tetrachlorodibenzo-p-dioxin), polycyclic aromatic hydrocarbons, PCBs (polychlorinated biphenyls), and crude coal tar, which is used in dermatological therapy. Thus, exposure to such inducers could influence skin biotransformation and even sensitize epidermal cells to other chemicals that are not good inducers themselves, a phenomenon observable in cell culture (Walsh et al., 1995).

Biotransformation of a variety of compounds in the skin has been detected, including arachidonic acid derivatives, steroids, retinoids, and 2-amino-anthracene, suggesting that multiple P450 activities are expressed. With the advent of DNA microarray and real-time polymerase chain reaction technologies, it is now evident that over a dozen distinct isozymes are expressed at widely varying levels. A recent survey of those in the CYP1-4 families indicated that half were expressed at substantially higher levels in differentiating keratinocytes (similar to spinous cells) than in basal-like cells (Du et al., 2006). In addition to influencing our response to the natural environment, these activities are also important in influencing our response to pharmaceuticals used in clinical dermatology inasmuch as a large fraction of the latter are P450 inducers, inhibitors, or substrates (Ahmad and Mukhtar, 2004). Species differences are apparent in the amounts of P450 activities detectable. For example, measured ethoxycoumarin-O-deethylase activity is 20-fold higher in mouse than human (or rat) skin. Differences of such magnitude help rationalize the observation that the rate of penetration of ethoxycoumarin is sufficient to saturate its metabolism in some species (e.g., the human) but not in others (e.g., the mouse or guinea pig) (Storm et al., 1990). To the extent that phase I (and II) metabolism influences sensitization to exogenous chemicals (Merk et al., 2004), they may also help rationalize species differences in allergic response.

Enzymes participating in phase II metabolism are expressed in skin. For example, multiple forms of epoxide hydrolase and UDP-glucuronosyl transferase have been detected in human and rodent skin. In general, this activity occurs at a much lower rate than observed in the liver, but exceptions are evident, as in the case of quinone reductase (Khan et al., 1987). Human and rodent skin exhibit qualitatively similar phase II reactions, but rodent skin often has a higher level of activity. An additional consideration is that different species express different relative amounts of the various isozymes, which could alter resulting target specificities or degree of responsiveness. Glutathione transferase, for instance, catalyzes the reaction of glutathione with exogenous nucleophiles or provides intracellular transport of bound compounds in the absence of a reaction. It also facilitates the reaction of glutathione with endogenous products of arachidonate lipoxygenation (leukotrienes) to yield mediators of anaphylaxis and chemotaxis, which are elements of the inflammatory response in the skin. Of the first three major transferase forms characterized in the liver, the major form in the skin of humans and rodents is the P isozyme. Human skin also expresses the A isozyme, whereas rat and mouse skin express the M isozyme and, in much smaller amounts, the A isozyme (Raza *et al.*, 1992).

A variety of other metabolic enzyme activities have also been detected in human epidermal cells, including sulfatases, β-glucuronidase, *N*-acetyl transferases, esterases, and reductases (Hotchkiss, 1998). The intercellular region of the stratum corneum has catabolic activities (e.g., proteases, lipases, glycosidases, phosphatases) supplied by the lamellar bodies along with their characteristic lipid (Elias, 1992). The report that cholesterol sulfotransferase is regulated by ligands of LXR and PPAR illustrates the potential for exogenous agents, including pharmaceuticals, to influence such activities and thereby the barrier function of the skin (Jiang *et al.*, 2005), where penetration can be influenced by cell differentiation and biotransformation. For example, methyl salicylate readily diffuses through the epidermis and is detected in the dermis, but only as de-esterified salicylate, illustrating first-pass metabolism (Cross *et al.*, 1997). The influence of hydroxysteroid dehydrogenases and microsomal reductase activities during percutaneous absorption is evident in studies on mouse skin in organ culture. In one study (Kao and Hall, 1987), 8 hours after topical application of testosterone, 59% of the permeated steroid was collected unchanged and the rest was transformed into metabolites. In parallel, estrone was converted substantially to estradiol (67%), while only 23% was collected as the parent compound. By contrast, estradiol was metabolized to a much lower extent (21%).

CONTACT DERMATITIS

In the occupational arena, where records are compiled on large workforces, contact dermatitis is by far the largest category ($\sim$90%) of compensated skin disease. Using eczema of the hand as a sentinel condition, since 80% of the total reported dermatitis occurs at that location (10% on the face), reveals a prevalence of 7–10% among workers. Attributed to better diagnosis, more accurate identification of offending chemicals, and more effective prevention and worker education, the fraction of afflicted workers recovering without impairment has improved nearly to 80% with proper management (Belsito, 2005). However, whereas certain conditions carry a favorable prognosis, others (e.g., chronic cumulative irritant contact dermatitis or contact allergy to nickel, chromate, formaldehyde, or rubber) frequently result in chronic disease in which changing jobs is of limited or no benefit (Emmett, 2003; Belsito, 2005). Overall, contact dermatitis falls into the two major categories of irritant and allergic forms. Both involve inflammatory processes and can have indistinguishable clinical characteristics of erythema (redness), induration (thickening and firmness), scaling (flaking), and vesiculation (blistering) in areas of direct contact with the chemical. Biopsies from affected sites reveal a mixed-cell inflammatory infiltrate of lymphocytes and eosinophils and spongiosis (intercellular edema), but are insufficient to distinguish the two conditions from each other or from certain other common syndromes.

Irritant Dermatitis

Accounting for $\sim$80% of contact dermatitis cases, this condition arises from the direct action of chemicals on the skin. A chemical in this category is anticipated to give an adverse reaction to anyone if the concentration is high enough and the exposure time long enough. Certain chemicals at sufficient concentration produce an acute irritation, sometimes called a second-degree chemical burn, which can even result in scarring in serious cases. These include strong acids and alkalies and powerful oxidizing and reducing agents that substantially disrupt the cornified layer, produce cytotoxicity directly, and stimulate release of proinflammatory cytokines. More common is chronic cumulative irritation from repeated exposures to mild irritants such as soaps, detergents, solvents, and cutting oils. An example of eczema from cutting oil is shown in Fig. 19-2A. The chronic friction and production of small-scale trauma can wear away the lipid barrier of the stratum corneum, leading gradually to further damage (loss of cohesion, desquamation) that facilitates penetration of exogenous chemicals, and may be detectable as increased transepidermal water loss. In some cases, epidermal thickening occurs without much inflammation. In any case, increased penetrance can facilitate exposure to chemicals that elicit a subsequent allergic reaction. For example, because wet cement is alkaline and often contains chromates (commonly allergenic), chronic exposure can produce a composite response.

The skin at some anatomic sites is more sensitive than at other sites. Eyelids have a thin epidermis and are quite sensitive, for example, and the back is more sensitive than the forearm or the scalp of individuals with male pattern baldness (Zhai *et al.*, 2004). Individuals vary greatly in sensitivity to irritant dermatitis. Figure 19-2B shows an irritant reaction on the inside of the elbow on an atopic person. Comprising up to 20% of school children (Laughter *et al.*, 2000), atopic individuals are the most sensitive to irritants and exhibit a propensity to produce specific IgE antibodies to allergens. They typically suffer from hay fever but do not seem more prone to allergic contact dermatitis (Belsito, 2005). These individuals usually have a poorer prognosis than nonatopics and have a higher frequency of persistent dermatitis. The best preventive measure for atopics and others is to avoid exposure to contact irritants, but in practice this strategy is difficult to implement. Lipid-rich moisturizers and barrier creams containing dimethicone or perfluoropolyethers may be useful in protecting skin from offending agents (Saary *et al.*, 2005).

Information on the irritancy of chemicals toward human skin may be obtained as part of differential diagnosis by patch testing for allergic response. The skin of laboratory animals (mice, rats, rabbits, guinea pigs) can be used for testing, but it is thinner and more sensitive than human skin to irritants. For development of new pharmaceuticals, cosmetics, and other consumer products, a great need exists for an in vitro system to determine the potential for irritant responses. Use of human epidermal cell cultures has been increasing as reconstructed epidermal and skin models come closer to the native differentiated state. For example, a recent study compared 50 chemicals for which data on 30 are available from patch testing (Tornier *et al.*, 2006). The tests provided useful comparative data and, judging by viability (mitochondrial function), histology, and release of inflammatory mediators (IL-1α) suggested a parallel with natural skin. Such models offer advantages in convenience

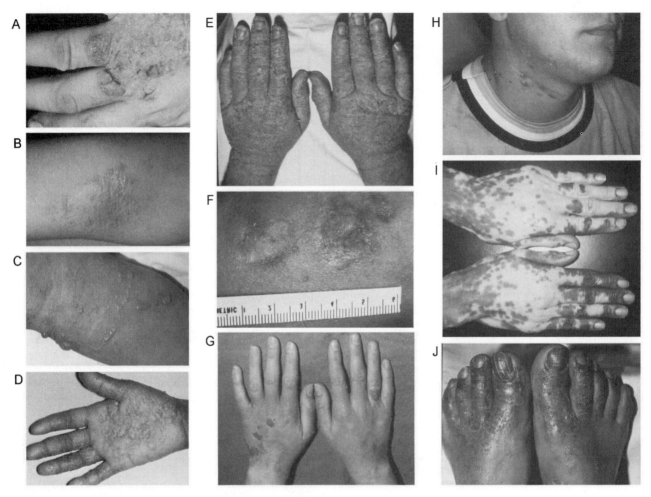

Figure 19-2. Examples of occupational skin toxicity. (See the colored insert.)

The panels, available at the NIOSH website (http://www.cdc.gov/niosh/ocderm1.html), are a small selection from the 140-slide NIOSH program "Occupational Dermatoses—A Program for Physicians" prepared by Drs. E. Shmunes, M.M. Key, J.B. Lucas, and J.S. Taylor. (A, eczema from cutting oil; B, atopic irritant dermatitis; C, burn from ethylene oxide; D, burn from alkali exposure; E, sensitization to dichromate; F, beryllium granulomas; G, phototoxicity from lime juice; H, acne from cutting oil; I, leukoderma from rubber antioxidants; J, hyperpigmentation from mercaptobenzothiazole.)

and cost, appear applicable to photoxicity as well, and are more uniform in response than skin in the human population. Though advanced, the state of maturation in such culture models is not complete, as seen by histology and barrier function, resulting in their greater sensitivity than the skin (Netzlaff *et al.*, 2005). In addition, extrapolation of the models to cumulative insult dermatitis presents a challenge.

Chemical Burns

A chemical that is extremely corrosive can produce immediate coagulative necrosis resulting in considerable tissue damage with ulceration and sloughing. Sometimes referred to as a third-degree chemical burn, the damage does not have a primary inflammatory component and thus may not be classified as an irritant reaction. Examples of burns from ethylene oxide and alkali are shown in Fig. 19-2C and 2D. If the chemical is not quickly and completely removed, damage to the skin may continue and, with increased access to the circulation, systemic injury can occur. Table 19-2 lists some important corrosive compounds giving chemical burns in the occupational arena. Certain chemical warfare agents first used in

combat nearly a century ago and intermittently since, such as bis-(2-chloroethyl)sulfide (sulfur mustard) or 2-chlorovinyl dichloroarsine (Lewisite), are potent vesicants upon skin contact and produce considerable damage when inhaled. Exposure today is rare, but the threat of use remains (McManus and Huebner, 2005).

Allergic Contact Dermatitis

Allergic contact dermatitis is a delayed (T-cell mediated) hypersensitive reaction. To induce sensitization through the skin, chemical haptens generally penetrate the lipid barrier and, to be detected by the immune system, become attached to carrier proteins. The complete antigens are then processed by Langerhans cells (resident macrophages) and displayed on their surfaces with major histocompatibility complex II molecules. The Langerhans cells present the processed peptides to T helper type 1 cells in regional lymph nodes, thereby stimulating interleukin release and proliferation of the sensitive T helper cells. Over a 1–3 week period, memory T cells are thus generated and enter the circulation. Upon subsequent exposure to a specific antigen previously encountered, allergen presentation by the Langerhans cells results in a much greater response due to

Table 19-2

Selected Chemicals Causing Skin Burns

CHEMICAL	COMMENT
Ammonia	Potent skin corrosive
	Contact with compressed gas can cause frostbite
Calcium oxide (CaO)	Severe chemical burns
	Extremely exothermic reaction—dissolving in water can cause heat burns
Chlorine	Liquid and concentrated vapors cause cell death and ulceration
Ethylene oxide	Solutions and vapors may burn
	Compressed gas can cause frostbite
Hydrogen chloride (HCl)	Severe burning with scar formation
Hydrogen fluoride (HF)	Severe, painful, slowly healing burns from high concentration
	Lower concentration causes delayed cutaneous injury
	Systemic absorption can lead to electrolyte abnormalities and death
	Calcium-containing topical medications and quaternary ammonium compounds are used to limit damage
Hydrogen peroxide	High concentration causes severe burns and blistering
Methyl bromide	Liquid exposure produces blistering, deep burns
Nitrogen oxides	Moist skin facilitates the formation of nitric acid causing severe yellow-colored burns
Phosphorus	White phosphorus continues to burn on skin in the presence of air
Phenol	Extremely corrosive even in low concentrations
	Systemic absorption through burn sites may result in cardiac arrhythmias, renal disease, and death
Sodium hydroxide	High concentration causes deep burns, readily denatures keratin
Toluene diisocyanate	Severe burns with contact
	Skin contact rarely may result in respiratory sensitization

homing by the memory cells to the skin, their clonal proliferation and their release of cytokines chemotactic for inflammatory cells and stimulatory for their further production. Because this process takes time, the characteristic dermal infiltration and spongiosis result after a delay (latent period) of 0.5–2 days (Mark and Slavin, 2006).

Thousands of chemicals have been reported to give rise to allergic contact dermatitis, many across a variety of occupations and consumer products. Table 19-3 lists some common contact allergens, several of which are shown in Fig 19-3. Because most compounds in the chemical universe are only weakly active or infrequently encountered, much effort has focused on finding the major allergens in the population by systematic patch testing of dermatology patients.

Although not measuring sensitivity in the population at large, the results are quite useful. The panel of compounds tested can vary with geographic location to accommodate local usage, or it can be directed to specific anatomic sites such as the foot (Holden and Gawkrodger, 2005). Panels also are adapted to emerging trends as new products appear and others decline in use. Table 19-4 lists the chemicals (22) giving positive reactions in at least 3% of the subjects in a recent test from the North American Contact Dermatitis Group (Pratt *et al.*, 2004). Other testing groups show similar results but often include some different chemicals or use them at different concentrations, which can affect the measured frequencies (Wetter *et al.*, 2005). A number of these chemicals (nickel, dichromate, *p*-phenylenediamine, formaldehyde) have shown high prevalences

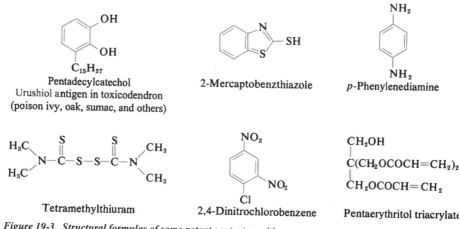

Figure 19-3. Structural formulas of some potent contact sensitizers.

Table 19-3
Common Contact Allergens

SOURCE	COMMON ALLERGENS	
	Antibiotics	**Therapeutics**
Topical medications/ hygiene products	Bacitracin	Benzocaine
	Neomycin	
	Polymyxin	Idoxuridine
	Aminoglycosides	α-Tocopherol (vitamin E)
	Sulfonamides	Corticosteroids
	Preservatives	**Others**
	Benzalkonium chloride	Cinnamic aldehyde
	Formaldehyde	Ethylenediamine
	Formaldehyde releasers	Lanolin
	Quaternium-15	p-Phenylenediamine
	Imidazolidinyl urea	Propylene glycol
	Diazolidinyl urea	Benzophenones
	DMDM Hydantoin	Fragrances
	Methylchloroisothiazolone	Thioglycolates
Plants and trees	Abietic acid	Pentadecylcatechols
	Balsam of Peru	Sesquiterpene lactone
	Rosin (colophony)	Tuliposide A
Antiseptics	Chloramine	Glutaraldehyde
	Chlorhexidine	Hexachlorophene
	Chloroxylenol	Thimerosal (Merthiolate)
	Dichlorophene	Mercurials
	Dodecylaminoethyl glycine HCl	Triphenylmethane dyes
Rubber products	Diphenylguanidine	Resorcinol monobenzoate
	Hydroquinone	Benzothiazolesulfenamides
	Mercaptobenzothiazole	Dithiocarbamates
	p-Phenylenediamine	Thiurams
Leather	Formaldehyde	Potassium dichromate
	Glutaraldehyde	
Paper products	Abietic acid	Rosin (Colophony)
	Formaldehyde	Triphenyl phosphate
	Nigrosine	Dyes
Glues and bonding agents	Bisphenol A	Epoxy resins
	Epichlorohydrin	p-(t-Butyl)formaldehyde resin
	Formaldehyde	Toluene sulfonamide resins
	Acrylic monomers	Urea formaldehyde resins
	Cyanoacrylates	
Metals	Chromium	Mercury
	Cobalt	Nickel

of reactivity for several decades, whereas others (e.g., gold salts), once thought innocuous, have recently become recognized as reactive (Cohen, 2004). An example of contact allergy to dichromate in cement is shown in Fig. 19-2E. Reduction in use of the most prevalent allergenic chemicals and their replacement by less allergenic substitutes is now advocated. Caution in using less characterized agents as replacements must be exercised, however, because their allergenicity may not become evident until they reach large populations of users, as has happened in several prominent cases (Uter *et al.*, 2005). For example, methylchloroisothiazolinone/methylisothiazolinone, used in cosmetics, was replaced with the biocide methyldibromo glutaronitrile, which did not cause allergic contact dermatitis in initial screens. Upon widespread use, however, the latter also was shown to be a potent contact allergen (Kynemund Pedersen *et al.*, 2004).

Unlike contact irritants, where the response is generally proportional to the applied dose and time, contact allergens can elicit reactions at very small doses. Nevertheless, careful analysis from human and animal testing (Boukhman and Maibach, 2001; Arts *et al.*, 2006) shows that a higher dose confers a greater likelihood of sensitization and that doses below a threshold for sensitization can have a cumulative effect. In addition, the dose required to elicit a reaction is lower after sensitization with a higher dose. Moreover, the dose dependence for sensitization displays nonlinearity, suggesting that the response of individual dendritic cells is sublinear, probably sigmoidal. Thus, more stimulation can produce a more than proportionally larger response, although at high doses saturation and sometimes even inhibition of the response become evident. This result emphasizes the importance of minimizing individual exposures. The findings also reveal a wide variation in human

Table 19-4
Prevalence of Positive Reactions in Patch Test Patients

ALLERGEN	PATIENTS WITH POSITIVE PATCH TESTS (%)
Nickel sulfate	16.7
Neomycin	11.6
Balsam of Peru	11.6
Fragrance mix	10.4
Thimerosal	10.2
Sodium gold thiosulfate	10.2
Quaternium-15	9.3
Formaldehyde	8.4
Bacitracin	7.9
Cobalt chloride	7.4
Methyldibromoglutaronitrile/ phenoxy ethanol	5.8
Carba mix	4.9
p-Phenylenediamine	4.8
Thiuram mix	4.5
Potassium dichromate	4.3
Benzalkonium chloride	4.3
Propylene glycol	4.2
2-Bromo-2-nitropropane	3.3
Diazolidinyl urea	3.2
Imidazolidinyl urea	3.0
Tixocortol-21-pivalate	3.0
Disperse blue 106	3.0

SOURCE: Data from Pratt *et al.* (2004).

Table 19-5
Common Cross-Reacting Chemicals

CHEMICAL	CROSS REACTOR
Abietic acid	Pine resin (colophony)
Balsam of Peru	Pine resin, cinnamates, benzoates
Bisphenol A	Diethylstilbestrol, hydroquinone monobenzyl ether
Canaga oil	Benzyl salicylate
Chlorocresol	Chloroxylenol
Diazolidinyl urea	Imidazolidinyl urea, formaldehyde
Ethylenediamine di-HCl	Aminophylline, piperazine
Formaldehyde	Arylsulfonamide resin, chloroallyl-hexaminium chloride
Hydroquinone	Resorcinol
Methyl hydroxybenzoate	Parabens, hydroquinone monobenzyl ether
p-Aminobenzoic acid	p-Aminosalicylic acid, sulfonamide
Phenylenediamine	Parabens, p-aminobenzoic acid
Propyl hydroxybenzoate	Hydroquinone monobenzyl ether
Phenol	Resorcinol, cresols, hydroquinone
Tetramethylthiuram disulfide	Tetraethylthiuram mono- and disulfide

response to sensitization, which appears to have at least in part a genetic basis.

Diagnosis and Testing When a patient exhibits allergic contact dermatitis, finding the responsible chemical is important to avoid continued exposure. For this purpose, patch testing is commonly employed by procedures refined over many years of practice since it was first employed a century ago (Mark and Slavin, 2006). On the washed backs of patients, who are not currently exhibiting contact dermatitis or using corticosteroids or other immunosuppressives, are placed patches each containing a small amount of a potential allergen. Conveniently, many of the materials are commercially available at standardized concentrations too low to produce irritant reactions. Certain chemicals normally are not tested because they induce too strong a response (urushiol from poison ivy) or might produce sensitization (beryllium). After 2–3 days, during which time a maximal reaction usually develops, the patches are removed and sites of exposure are scored for degree of response. Relevance to the pa-

tient's actual environment must be considered so that exposure in daily life can be minimized to appropriate chemicals. Interpretation of the results and environmental modification should take into account the phenomenon of cross-sensitivity, where reactivity to a compound may be evident if it shares functional groups that have provoked sensitization in another compound. Figure 19-4 illustrates the principle with three amine compounds, and Table 19-5 lists some common cross-reacting chemicals.

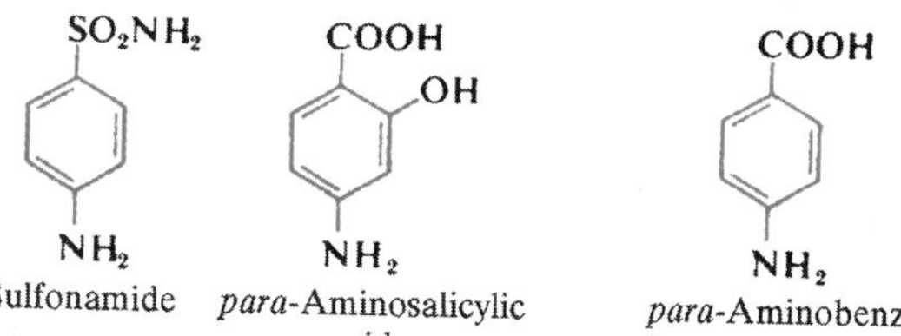

Animal testing to predict allergenicity has an extended history. A chemical is applied to intact or abraded skin or through intradermal injection with or without adjuvant to enhance sensitization. The reaction of the skin to subsequent challenge with the chemical is then observed and graded. This approach has successfully identified some strong sensitizers relevant to human exposures, but detection of weak sensitizers on a large scale is hampered by the usual difficulties in animal testing, including small animal numbers and limited experiment time to reduce expense. In addition, extrapolation of sensitivity measurements from laboratory animals to humans presents large uncertainties. Nevertheless, the local lymph node assay performed in mice has gained attention as a way to measure the pool of sensitized T cells by their proliferation in draining lymph nodes, illustrated by a comparison of potencies of Disperse Blue 106 and 2,4-dinitrochlorobenzene (Betts *et al.*, 2005). Because sensitizers differ in potency by at least four orders of magnitude, a quantitative assay has a distinct advantage. Other steps in the sensitization process (e.g., percutaneous absorption) would be expected to influence the potency, but incorporation of structure–activity data may improve the validity of predictions for certain chemicals (Uter *et al.*, 2005). To this end, a structure–activity study to streamline testing of new chemical products has identified

Figure 19-4. Structural formulas of selected para-amino compounds that show cross-reactions in allergic contact sensitization.

15 classes of reactive functional groups, as well as several subject to activation by metabolism, as especially suspect of bestowing allergenicity (Gerner *et al.*, 2004). That water solubility, octanol/water partitioning, and molecular weight (<1000) were not found to be diagnostic indicators for this endpoint suggests that the rate of stratum corneum penetration is not a decisive factor. If instead dendritic cell responses to chemicals are critical, the possibility of routine prediction of allergic potential from them is attractive (Ryan *et al.*, 2005). A number of parameters need further development such as determining appropriate endpoints, the dynamic range of the measurements and the possible need for interactions with or biotransformation by other cell types (e.g., keratinocytes). Using a minimally deviated continuous dendritic cell line could solve the problem of limited supply of human cells and the variability in responsiveness among donors, while finding the basis of the individual variability itself would be important.

GRANULOMATOUS DISEASE

Foreign body reactions, isolating invading substances that cannot be readily removed, occur infrequently toward a variety of agents introduced into the skin through injection or after laceration or abrasion. These can produce persistent lesions with abundant inflammatory cells resembling chronic infectious conditions (e.g., tuberculosis, leprosy, leishmaniasis, syphilis) and present diagnostic challenges (Del Rosario *et al.*, 2005). In the case of silica or talc (a magnesium silicate), a resulting hard nodule may appear after a latent period of months or years as the original large particles disaggregate to assume a colloidal state. Injection of paraffin or mineral oil in the skin or contamination of wounds with starch powder cross linked with epichlorohydrin for use in surgical gloves may also result in granulomatous reactions. Delayed allergic sensitization may occur with beryllium analogous to the reaction in the lung, and skin lesions have even been reported in individuals with life-threatening pulmonary exposure. An example of beryllium granuloma of the skin is shown in Fig. 19-2F. Metallic mercury, zirconium compounds formerly used in deodorants, and tattoo dye constituents (cobalt, chromium compounds) are also known to induce such reactions.

PHOTOTOXICOLOGY

The ultraviolet and visible spectra of solar radiation reaching the earth extend from 290 nm to 700 nm. Wavelengths beyond this range are either filtered by the earth's atmosphere or are insufficiently energetic to cause cutaneous pathology. Adequate doses of artificially produced UVC (<290 nm) or X-rays can produce profound physical and toxicologic skin changes. The protective skin pigment melanin, synthesized in melanocytes, absorbs a broad range of radiation from UVB (290–320 nm) through the visible spectrum. Other chromophores in the skin include amino acids, primarily tryptophan and to a lesser extent tyrosine, and their breakdown products (e.g., urocanic acid), which absorb light in the UVB range. Biologically, the most significant chromophore is DNA, because damage from radiation can have lasting effects on the genetic information in target cells.

Adverse Responses to Electromagnetic Radiation

The most evident acute feature of ultraviolet radiation exposure is erythema (redness or sunburn). The minimal erythema dose (MED),

the smallest dose of ultraviolet light needed to induce an erythematous response, varies greatly from person to person. Vasodilation responsible for the color change is accompanied by significant alterations in a variety of inflammatory mediators from injured keratinocytes and local inflammatory cells that may be responsible for some systemic symptoms associated with sunburn such as fever, chills, and malaise. UVB (290–320 nm) is the most effective solar band to cause erythema in human skin. A substantially greater dosage of UVA (320–400) reaches the earth compared to UVB (up to 100-fold); however, its efficiency in generating erythema in humans is about 1000-fold less than that of UVB. Both UVA and UVB have been implicated in the development of melanoma and nonmelanoma skin cancers. Because of its longer wavelength and greater depth of skin penetration, UVA is likely more responsible for long-term UV effects such as wrinkling, skin atrophy, and easy bruisibility. Overt pigment darkening is another typical response to ultraviolet exposure. This may be accomplished by enhanced melanin production by melanocytes or by photooxidation of melanin. Tanning or increased pigmentation usually occurs within 3 days of ultraviolet light exposure, because photooxidation is evident immediately. The tanning response is most readily produced by exposure to UVB and may be induced, along with erythema and DNA repair, by DNA damage. Tanning serves to augment the protective effects of melanin in the skin, but the protection afforded appears insufficient to balance the damage sustained in acquiring it, especially in fair-skinned individuals (Sheehan *et al.*, 2002).

Chronic exposure to radiation induces a variety of characteristic skin changes. For ultraviolet light, these changes accelerate or mimic aging, but the rate depends greatly on the baseline skin pigmentation of the individual. Lighter-skinned people suffer from chronic skin changes with greater frequency than darker individuals, and locations such as the head, neck, hands, and upper chest are more readily involved due to their routine exposures. Pigmentary changes such as freckling and hypomelanotic areas, wrinkling, telangiectasias (fine superficial blood vessels), actinic keratoses (precancerous lesions), and malignant skin lesions such as basal and squamous cell carcinomas and malignant melanomas are all consequences of chronic exposure to ultraviolet light exposure. One significant pathophysiologic response of chronic exposure to ultraviolet light is the pronounced decrease of epidermal Langerhans cells. Chronically sun exposed skin may have up to 50% fewer epidermal Langerhan cells compared to photoprotected areas. This decrease may result in lessened immune surveillance of neoantigens on malignant cells and thus allow such transformation to proceed unabated. For these reasons, gaining a tan, either naturally or through tanning salons, is not recommended (Spencer and Amonette, 1998). Exposures to ionizing radiation may produce a different spectrum of disease depending upon the dose delivered. Large acute exposures will result in local redness, blistering, swelling, ulceration, and pain. After a latent period or following subacute chronic exposures, characteristic changes such as epidermal thinning, freckling, telangiectasias, and nonhealing ulcerations may occur. Also, a variety of skin malignancies have been described years after skin exposure to radiation.

Apart from the toxic nature of electromagnetic radiation, natural and environmental exposures to certain bands of light are vital for survival. Ultraviolet radiation is critical for the conversion of 7-dehydrocholesterol to pre-vitamin D3, without which normal endogenous production of vitamin D would not take place. Blue light in the 420–490 nm range can be lifesaving due to its capacity to photo-isomerize bilirubin (a red blood cell breakdown product) in the skin. Infants with elevated serum bilirubin, potentially neurotoxic, have difficulty clearing this byproduct because of its low water solubility, but treatment with blue light renders bilirubin more water soluble and markedly augments excretion. In addition, the toxic effects of ultraviolet light have been exploited for decades through artificial light sources for treatment of hyperproliferative skin disorders such as psoriasis.

Photosensitivity

An abnormal sensitivity to ultraviolet and visible light, photosensitivity may result from endogenous or exogenous factors. Illustrating the former, a variety of genetic diseases, such as xeroderma pigmentosum, impair the cell's ability to repair ultraviolet light-induced damage. The autoimmune disease lupus erythematosus also features abnormal sensitivity to ultraviolet light. In hereditary or chemically induced porphyrias, enzyme abnormalities disrupt the biosynthetic pathways producing heme, the prosthetic building block for hemoglobin, myoglobin, catalases, peroxidases, and cytochromes, leading to accumulation of porphyrin precursors or derivatives throughout the body, including the skin. These compounds in general fluoresce when exposed to light of 400–410 nm (Soret band), and in this excited state interact with cellular macromolecules or with molecular oxygen to generate toxic free radicals. A "constitutional" sensitivity to light (porphyria cutanea tarda) can be precipitated by alcohol, estrogens, or certain antibiotics in individuals with hereditary abnormalities in porphyrin synthesis, and an "acquired" sensitivity in general by hexachlorobenzene and mixtures of polyhalogenated aromatic hydrocarbons (Kimbrough, 1987; van Birgelen *et al.*, 1996).

Phototoxicity Phototoxic reactions from exogenous chemicals may be produced by systemic or topical administration or exposure. In acute reactions, the skin can become red and blister within minutes to hours after ultraviolet light exposure. In an occupational setting, for example, exposing the skin to coal tar and sunlight can quickly produce a stinging sensation and elicit damage resembling a bad sunburn with hyperpigmentation. Phototoxic chemicals most commonly absorb ultraviolet light in the range of 320–400 nm (UVA), thereby assuming a higher energy excited triplet state and either transfer an electron to another molecule or become reduced to form highly reactive free radicals (DeLeo, 2004; Moan and Peng, 2004). An oxygen-dependent photodynamic reaction commonly occurs as these excited molecules, returning to the ground state, transfer their energy to oxygen to form highly reactive singlet oxygen. These reactive products are capable of damaging cellular macromolecules (notably unsaturated membrane lipids) and causing cell death. The resulting damage stimulates the release of a variety of immune mediators from keratinocytes and local white blood cells that recruit more inflammatory cells to the skin and thus yield the clinical signs of phototoxicity. Chemicals most often associated with phototoxic reactions are listed in Table 19-6.

Psoralens are good examples of agents that produce phototoxicity largely without requiring oxygen radicals. Upon entering cells, they intercalate with the DNA and then form covalent adducts and cross-links when activated by UVA. The result is to inhibit DNA synthesis and repair and cell growth or survival. Psoralens (and other phototoxins) can be encountered in a variety of food plants, including limes and celery, producing phytophotodermatitis in occupational settings where such food is routinely handled. An example

Table 19-6
Selected Phototoxic Chemicals

Furocoumarins
   8-Methoxypsoralen
   5-Methoxypsoralen
   Trimethoxypsoralen
Polycyclic aromatic hydrocarbons
   Anthracene
   Fluoranthene
   Acridine
   Phenanthrene
Drugs
   Tetracyclines
   Sulfonamides
   Sulfonylureas
   Nalidixic acid
   Thiazides
   Phenothiazines
   Nonsteroidal anti-inflammatories
Dyes
   Disperse blue 35
   Eosin
   Acridine orange
Porphyrin derivatives
   Hematoporphyrin

of phototoxicity from lime juice is given in Fig. 19-2G. Psoralens in combination with UVA (PUVA) are used therapeutically to inhibit the growth of keratinocytes and lymphocytes in hyperproliferative conditions such as psoriasis and T-cell lymphomas. In analogous fashion, though generating reactive oxygen, photodynamic therapy is a new approach that takes advantage of the selective uptake of a photosensitizing agent, usually a porphyrin derivative, into rapidly dividing cells such as in neoplasms. The photosensitizing agent is activated by laser or continuous wave light sources ranging from 400 to 600 nm or more, resulting in selective destruction of the neoplasm (Zeitouni *et al.*, 2003).

Nails often suffer toxic reactions to drugs, most commonly to systemically administered chemicals, such as antibiotics, and less commonly to topically applied chemicals. Whereas various types of nail pathology may result from therapy-induced changes in cell growth or division, changes in pigmentation, or detachment of the various layers of the nail plate from each other (onycholysis) often result from photosensitive reactions, commonly phototoxic and less commonly photoallergic. Chemicals, such as topical or systemic porphyrins, coal tar, and drugs, such as the tetracycline family of antibiotics, produce photodynamic toxicity, which requires generation of oxygen radicals. In contrast, topical or systemic psoralens produce onycholysis by a nonphotodynamic mechanism that does not require oxygen.

Photoallergy A photoallergen elicits an allergic response by forming a complete antigen upon absorbing ultraviolet or visible light. Light stimulates the chemical either to assume an excited state that can bind directly to a carrier protein or to yield a stable photoproduct that becomes conjugated to a carrier. As in the case of allergic contact dermatitis, the complete antigen formed then is processed by Langerhans cells and presented to T cells. Upon recurrent exposure to an exogenous chemical and light, a delayed hypersensitivity (Type IV) reaction ensues, leading typically to eczema (erythema, vesiculation, itching). Like phototoxins, most photoallergens respond to light in the range of 320–400 nm (UVA). Light sensitivity usually subsides within days but may persist for several weeks if the chemical is retained in the epidermis. Rarely, a person may display chronic actinic dermatitis with continued reaction to sunlight long after removal of the chemical (Goossens, 2004).

Use of halogenated salicylanilides and related antimicrobial chemicals in widely used consumer personal care products, such as soap, led to many thousands of cases of photoallergy in the 1960s and 1970s (Epstein, 1999). When the most active agents were removed from the market, fragrances in cosmetics and sunscreens then became conspicuous sources of photoallergy a decade later. Currently, active ingredients in sunscreens appear to be the most frequently recognized causes. Although of low risk, these chemicals have become widely used as the risks of extensive sun exposure have become appreciated. *p*-Aminobenzoate and derivatives in the original sunscreen formulations have been replaced with chemicals of lower risk, sensitivity to which are now being detected, although proper diagnosis must take into account contact dermatitis from fragrances and preservatives in these products (Cook and Freeman, 2001).

Photoallergy generally is distinguishable from phototoxicity, because the former results from delayed hypersensitivity, and amounts of chemical too low to give a toxic response still suffice to elicit allergy. Chemicals causing phototoxicity, because reactivity is generated upon light exposure, may also be photoallergenic, but the latter type of response is much less common. Among individuals with a history of photosensitivity, an estimated 10–20% exhibit photoallergy (DeLeo, 2004). Diagnosis is best performed by patch testing with and without light exposure of the treated surface to distinguish photocontact from contact allergy. Because the offending chemical may not be obvious from the patient history due to the delay between exposure to the chemical and sunlight and the symptoms, a panel of test chemicals may include some 30 common photoallergens as well as the patient's own sunscreen and personal care products. To assist in predicting risks of photoallergy, efforts have been made to derive important chemical features among existing photoallergens that account for their reactivity toward proteins. This information, coupled with assessment of physical properties such as aqueous/lipid partitioning, is anticipated to streamline testing of new products (Barratt, 2004).

ACNE

Acne is a common affliction of the pilosebaceous units in the face, upper chest, and upper back. Found in many forms, this condition typically arises from blockage of the sebaceous duct leading from the gland to the hair follicle, resulting in retention of sebum, and enlargement of the gland (Toyoda and Morohashi, 2001). In the most common form (acne vulgaris), androgen stimulation at puberty leads to excess sebum production and, likely as a result of the high local fatty acid concentration, excessive cornification of the ductal cells to plug the orifice. Proliferation of resident bacteria and inflammation typically result. Long chain fatty acids can give an acne-like response in animal models and appear to do so in sensitive individuals exposed to them in cosmetics. Likely acting in a similar fashion, petroleum products (oils, coal tar) in the workplace can give rise to acneiform eruptions. Insoluble cutting oils used in machining may have this effect, as illustrated in Fig. 19-2H. Such chemicals appear

to stimulate excessive stratification of the ductal cells, preventing their disaggregation and blocking the flow of sebum.

Chloracne

The most disfiguring form of acne in humans, chloracne, is caused by exposure to halogenated aromatic hydrocarbons. Chloracnegenic chemicals such as polychlorinated biphenyls and naphthalenes are often accompanied by the highly potent polychlorinated dibenzofurans and dioxins readily formed during synthesis of these chemicals or chlorinated phenolic pesticides, and can arise from combustion of the latter in fires and explosions. Chloracne is a rare disease; however, its recalcitrant nature and preventability make it an important occupational and environmental illness. Typically, comedones and straw-colored cysts are present behind the ears, around the eyes, shoulders, back, and genitalia. In addition to acne, hypertrichosis (increased hair in atypical locations), hyperpigmentation, brown discoloration of the nail, conjunctivitis, and eye discharge may be present. Because chloracne is a marker of systemic exposure, concurrent effects in the liver and nervous system may accompany the integumentary findings. Chloracne exhibits progressive degeneration of sebaceous units, transition of sebaceous gland cells to keratinizing cells, and prominent hyperkeratosis in the follicular canal.

Since the original recognition of the syndrome a century ago, effects of chloracnegens on humans have been clearly demonstrated over the past five decades through industrial disasters. In 1953 a chemical plant in Ludwigshafen exploded, discharging 2,4,5 trichlorophenol; in 1976 in Seveso, Italy, a reactor explosion liberated tetrachlorodibenzo-*p*-dioxin (TCDD); and in 1968 and 1979 in Japan and Taiwan, respectively, rice cooking oil was contaminated with polychlorinated biphenyls (PCBs), polychlorinated dibenzofurans, and related polychlorinated aromatic hydrocarbons. As in the Seveso accident (Baccarelli *et al.*, 2005), chloracne is noted within months after exposure and, depending on the severity, may either be cleared quickly or remain manifest even decades after exposure ceases, reflecting the high lipid solubility, recalcitrance to metabolic clearance, and thus long half-life in humans of the responsible chemicals. The highly potent TCDD has a half-life in humans of ~8 years (Geyer *et al.*, 2002), and highly chlorinated dibenzofurans and biphenyls are similarly persistent.

Chlorinated dioxins and dibenzofurans have significant and reproducible effects on cellular function. TCDD is one of the most potent known inducers of CYP1A1 by virtue of its high affinity for the Ah receptor stimulating its expression. The fate of individuals afflicted with chloracne has been of particular interest in view of the suggestion that they may be more prone to other adverse health effects of exposure. So far, however, chloracne has not proven to be such a "sentinel" biomarker (Baccarelli *et al.*, 2005). Because polymorphisms in Ah receptor sequence confer differences in sensitivity to health effects in animals, analogous polymorphisms have been sought in the human population; Ah receptor polymorphisms have been identified, but as yet they have not been shown to affect responses to the receptor ligands (Okey *et al.*, 2005). In mice, skin symptoms analogous to chloracne in humans are dependent on the hr locus, where the (–/–) genotype is susceptible (Poland and Knutson, 1982). An analogous locus has been identified in humans that governs hair loss, where mutations give a phenocopy of the generalized atrichia from loss of vitamin D receptor activity (Miller *et al.*, 2001), but a functional allele does not prevent susceptibility to chloracne.

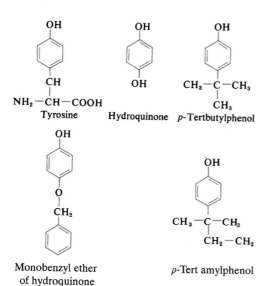

Figure 19-5. *Chemical structure of tyrosine and of selected hypopigmenting and depigmenting agents.*

PIGMENTARY DISTURBANCES

Melanocytes help protect the skin from harmful effects of ultraviolet light by producing the insoluble polymeric pigment melanin, starting with the action of tyrosine hydroxylase. As indicated in Table 19-7, a variety of chemicals can interfere with normal pigmentation to yield either excessive or reduced amounts of melanin. A rare acquired condition of generalized pigmentation loss (leukoderma or vitiligo) has a genetic basis but is triggered by environmental influences, largely obscure (Spritz, 2006). Thought likely to be of an autoimmune origin, this condition is characterized by the loss of melanocytes. In the occupational arena, depigmentation is well known to occur through exposure to phenols, catechols, quinones, and related compounds, several of which are shown in Fig 19-5, that appear toxic to melanocytes. An illustration of depigmentation caused by antioxidant exposure in rubber manufacture is given in Fig. 19-2I. In case reports, the cancer chemotherapeutic imatinib mesylate has been found to give pigment loss, probably through its inhibition of c-Kit tyrosine kinase signaling essential for melanocyte survival (Legros *et al.*, 2005). In sub-Saharan Africa and Asia, use of skin lightening creams containing hydroquinone, corticosteroids, or mercurials is common among women. The desired cosmetic effect, often nonuniform, is frequently accompanied by undesirable cutaneous consequences such as facial acne and hypertrichosis and carries the risk of systemic effects (del Giudice and Yves, 2002). By contrast, hyperpigmentation is well known to result from exposure to phototoxic agents including coal tar, coumarin derivatives found in perfumes and certain food such as limes (shown in Fig. 19-2G) and food plants (parsely, celery), dyes in cosmetics, and elements such as lead, bismuth, and arsenic (Table 19-7). An example of excessive pigmentation from mercaptobenzothiazole is shown in Fig. 19-2J.

URTICARIA

For those allergens to which IgE antibodies have been elicited by previous or ongoing exposure, subsequent contact can lead to development of hives, typically in minutes, through an immediate type I hypersensitivity reaction (Lipozencic and Wolfe, 2005). Hives are raised wheals that usually itch or sting and may appear reddish.

Table 19-7

Selected Causes of Cutaneous Pigmentary Disturbances

I. Hyperpigmentation
    Ultraviolet light exposure
    Postinflammatory changes (melanin and/or
        hemosiderin deposition)
    Hypoadrenalism
    Internal malignancy
    Chemical exposures
        Coal tar volatiles
        Anthracene
        Picric acid
        Mercury
        Lead
        Bismuth
        Furocoumarins (psoralens)
        Hydroquinone (paradoxical)
Drugs
        Chloroquine
        Amiodarone
        Bleomycin
        Zidovudine (AZT)
        Minocycline
II. Hypopigmentation/depigmentation/leukoderma
    Postinflammatory pigmentary loss
    Vitiligo
    Chemical leukoderma/hypopigmentation
        Hydroquinone
        Monobenzyl, monoethyl, and monomethyl ethers
            of hydroquinone
        p-(*t*-Butyl)phenol
        Mercaptoamines
        Phenolic germicides
        p-(*t*-Butyl)catechols
        Butylated hydroxytoluene

Generally disappearing within hours and rarely lasting longer than a day or two, the symptoms result from degranulation of cutaneous mast cells by liganded IgE, leading to release of histamine and other vasoactive substances. Food allergies and pharmaceuticals are major causes of acute urticaria, but many other causes are known (Table 19-8). Some chemicals (e.g., opiates) can bring about direct release of histamine from mast cells without antibody mediation, while others (nonsteroidal anti-inflammatories) may do so through effects on arachidonic acid metabolism or by uncertain mechanisms. Responses lasting longer than 6 weeks, if not attributable to allergen exposure, frequently have an autoimmune basis such as development of autoantibodies to IgE.

Contact urticaria in an occupational setting can arise from exposure to plant or animal proteins and appears more common in atopic individuals, who are especially sensitive to irritants. Among the numerous occupations where this response occurs include hairdressers and those involving routine handling of food, plant, or animal products (Doutre, 2005). A major problem in the health care industry involves allergy to latex protein, where the response can range from a mild skin reaction to anaphylaxis and death (Reines and Seifert, 2005). The widespread use of latex rubber in medical supplies and devices, notably in gloves, has resulted in widespread sensitization. In addition, powder used in the gloves can adsorb

Table 19-8
Selected Substances Reported to Elicit Contact Urticaria

CHEMICALS	FOODS
Anhydrides	Animal viscera
Methylhexahydrophthalic	Apple
Hexahydrophthalic	Artichoke
Maleic	Asparagus
Antibiotics	Beef
Bacitracin	Beer
Streptomycin	Carrot
Cephalosporins	Chicken
Penicillin	Deer
Rifamycin	Egg
Benzoic acid	Fish
Cobalt chloride	Lamb
Butylhydroxyanisol (BHA)	Mustard
Butylhydroxytoluene (BHT)	Paprika
Carboxymethylcellulose	Potato
Cyclopentolate hydrochloride	Pork
Diphenyl guanidine	Rice
Epoxy resin	Strawberry
Formaldehyde	Turkey
Fragrances	
Balsam of Peru	
Cinnamic aldehyde	
Isocyanates	
Diphenylmethane-4,4-diisocyanate	
Menthol	
Plants, woods, trees, and weeds	
Latex	
Phenylmercuric acetate	
Xylene	

the allergenic proteins and distribute them through the air, a phenomenon leading to use of powderless gloves and those made of nitrile.

A life-threatening response of anaphylactic shock, as from latex allergy, may occur from IgE-mediated massive release of histamine and other vasoactive agents from the mast cells upon systemic exposure to allergens. Certain food allergies (e.g., nuts, fish, and shellfish) are capable of producing this extreme response. Among pharmaceuticals, the best-known example is penicillin, where adverse reactions must be managed carefully to avoid serious consequences (Gruchalla and Pirmohamed, 2006). Other antibiotics that can produce anaphylaxis include cephalosporins, sulfonamides, macrolides, vancomycin, tetracyclines, and fluoroquinolines; all but the last two can also produce toxic epidermal necrolysis. Insect allergens such as those in bee and wasp stings are well known to be capable of giving an anaphylactic response.

TOXIC EPIDERMAL NECROLYSIS

Toxic epidermal necrolysis is a rare life-threatening skin disease with an incidence of ~1 case per million person-years. At the most severe end of a spectrum of adverse cutaneous hypersensitivity reactions to drugs, this syndrome involves detachment of ≥30% of the epidermal surface from the dermis, accompanied by severe erosions of the mucous membranes and often pulmonary, intestinal, and ocular damage. Sepsis and pulmonary manifestations are the most common causes of death, the fate of at least 30% of those afflicted. The Stevens–Johnson (sometimes called Lyell's) syndrome is a milder but still serious version of nearly the same phenomenon with up to 10% of the skin surface area affected and with a proportionally lower fatality rate. The two syndromes overlap when 10–30% of the skin surface is involved. Toxic epidermal necrolysis commonly resembles an upper respiratory tract infection in the first several days (fever, cough, malaise), but prompt diagnosis when the cutaneous lesions become evident several days later improves survival chances. Exposure to the offending drug is stopped and treatment is initiated similar to that for burns, where fluid and electrolyte replacement, protection from infection and nutritional assistance are critical. Responsible for at least 70% of the cases, nearly 100 drugs have been reported to cause this syndrome including sulfonamides and other antibiotics, anticonvulsants, nonsteroidal anti-inflammatories, allopurinol, and nevirapine (Roujeau, 2005; Wolf et al., 2005). Mechanisms leading to this idiosyncratic drug reaction are under scrutiny to prevent its occurrence or at least to optimize treatment. A characteristic feature of the syndrome is the large-scale apoptosis of epidermal keratinocytes. Candidates for mediating apoptosis through cell surface death receptors include tumor necrosis factor and FAS ligand, which appear elevated; alternatively, drug-sensitized cytotoxic T lymphocytes could be responsible for granzyme-induced cytolysis. The rare individuals susceptible to the syndrome may suffer from an autostimulation of death receptor pathways by the action of the cytotoxic T cells. Effective treatment may involve judicious immunosuppression, possibly with cyclosporine (Chave et al., 2005), or blockage of death receptors using intravenous immunoglobulin therapy (French et al., 2006).

SKIN CANCER

Radiation

Skin cancer is the most common neoplasm in humans, accounting for nearly one-third of all cancers diagnosed each year. At present, the major cause of skin cancer (half a million new cases per year in the United States) is sunlight, which damages epidermal cell DNA. UVB (290–320 nm) induces pyrimidine dimers and 8-oxoguanine modifications, thereby eliciting mutations in critical genes (Melnikova and Ananthaswamy, 2005; Nishigori, 2006). The p53 tumor suppressor gene is a major target in which damage occurs early and is detectable in most resulting squamous cell carcinomas. Because the p53 protein arrests cell cycling until DNA damage is repaired and may induce apoptosis, its loss destabilizes the genome of initiated cells and gives them a growth advantage. UV light also has immunosuppressive effects that may help skin tumors survive. Nonmelanoma skin cancer incidence is highest in the tropics and is highest in pale-complexioned whites, particularly at sites on the head and neck that receive the most intense exposure. Individuals with xeroderma pigmentosum, who are deficient in repair of pyrimidine dimers, must scrupulously avoid sun exposure to prevent the occurrence of premalignant lesions that progress with continued exposure. Even when it does not cause cancer in normal individuals, sun exposure leads to premature aging of the skin. For this reason, sunbathing is discouraged and the use of sunblock lotions is encouraged, especially those that remove wavelengths up to 400 nm. Protection from solar (and other) radiation as well as chemical carcinogens is important in the occupational arena (Gawkrodger, 2004).

In the past, ionizing radiation was an important source of skin cancer. With the discovery of radioactive elements at the turn of the twentieth century came the observation that X-rays can cause severe burns and squamous cell carcinomas of the skin. By the 1920s, basal cell carcinomas were also noted. For several decades thereafter, ionizing radiation was used to treat a variety of skin ailments (acne, atopic dermatitis, psoriasis, and ringworm) and for hair removal. The levels of exposure led to an increased risk of skin cancer and sometimes produced atrophy of the dermis (radiodermatitis) from the death or premature aging of fibroblasts which secrete elastic supporting fibrous proteins.

Polycyclic Aromatic Hydrocarbons

A landmark epidemiological investigation by Percival Pott in 1775 connected soot with the scrotal cancer prevalent among chimney sweepers in England. Since that time, substances rich in polycyclic aromatic hydrocarbons (coal tar, creosote, pitch, and soot) have become recognized as skin carcinogens in humans and animals. The polycyclic aromatic compounds alone are relatively inert chemically, but they would tend to accumulate in membranes and thus perturb cell function if they were not removed. They are hydroxylated by a number of cytochrome P450 isozymes, primarily 1A1 and 1B1 in epidermal cells, and conjugated for disposal from the body. Oxidative biotransformation, however, produces electrophilic epoxides that can form DNA adducts. Phenols, produced by rearrangement of the epoxides, can be oxidized further to electrophilic quinones that generate reactive oxygen species and lead to DNA adducts, oxidized bases, and abasic sites (Park et al., 2006). Occupations at risk of skin cancer from exposure to these compounds (e.g., roofing) often involve considerable sun exposure, an additional risk factor. Concern persists regarding the use of coal tar for pharmaceutical purposes (Thami and Sarkar, 2004). The combination of coal tar and UV light is useful in treating severe psoriasis, because the toxicity reduces the excessive turnover rate of keratinocytes that characterizes this disease. Repeated treatments are necessary, however, and carry with them an elevated risk of nonmelanoma skin cancer. Using longer wave UVA with phototoxic psoralen derivatives (PUVA) in place of coal tar in such protocols is much less messy and avoids UVB but produces DNA adducts and an elevation of nonmelanoma skin cancer risk as well. Although one large study suggested that PUVA also increased the risk of melanoma skin cancer (Stern et al., 1997), these findings have not been replicated in subsequent studies (Lindelof et al., 1999).

As a major regulator of induction of CYP1A1, and to a lesser extent CYP1B1, the aryl hydrocarbon receptor (AhR) plays a critical role in the response of epidermal cells to polycyclic aromatic hydrocarbons (Swanson, 2004). For example, mice in which the AhR gene has been functionally ablated are insensitive to skin cancer from topical application of benzo(a)pyrene (Shimizu et al., 2000). By contrast, a constitutively active AhR expressed in mouse epidermal keratinocytes was not seen to induce neoplasia, but it did result in inflammatory skin lesions reminiscent of contact dermatitis elicited by polycyclic aromatic hydrocarbons in humans (Tauchi et al., 2005). A common AhR polymorphism reduces the sensitivity in mice by an order of magnitude to toxic effects of ligands for this receptor, while in the rat an AhR variant with more subtle transactivation properties bestows dramatic resistance to lethal effects of TCDD without altering CYP1A1 inducibility (Okey et al., 2005). Screening efforts in humans have not yet revealed AhR polymorphisms that alter human responses to receptor ligands, but polymorphisms in cytochromes P450 do exist that are regulated by the AhR

and could plausibly affect skin sensitivity or function. An example is CYP2S1, which metabolizes retinoic acid (Saarikoski et al., 2005).

Mouse Skin Tumor Promotion

Through the work of numerous investigators over the past century, initially studying substances rich in polycyclic aromatic hydrocarbons, mouse skin has been developed as an important target for carcinogenicity testing (Rubin, 2001). The observed incidence of squamous cell carcinomas has been helpful in providing a biological basis for conclusions from epidemiological studies. For instance, mouse skin carcinogenicity of tobacco smoke condensate and constituents strongly supported the conclusion that tobacco smoke is carcinogenic in humans. Carcinogenicity in mouse skin is taken as evidence of a carcinogenic risk for humans, although not necessarily for our epidermis. Much has been learned about the pathogenesis of squamous cell carcinomas in mouse skin that does have general applicability to human squamous cell carcinomas of the skin or other anatomic sites, a learning process now augmented with mouse strains engineered for overexpression or ablation of genes of interest.

Initial fractionation of coal tar showed that the carcinogenic polycyclic aromatic hydrocarbons, thereby purified and identified, accounted for only a small fraction of the total carcinogenicity (Rubin, 2001). This puzzling observation led to the realization that other constituents, by themselves not carcinogenic, acted as cocarcinogens. Some chemicals, called tumor promoters, were found effective even when applied to the mouse skin long after a single treatment with a carcinogen applied at a dose too low to give cancer alone. The latter, inducing tumors by itself at sufficiently high doses, was a "complete" carcinogen with the salient property of being genotoxic. One explanation for the commonly observed nonlinear response is that a large dose of a complete carcinogen does more than initiate cancer by damaging the DNA in cells. It is also toxic, killing some cells and thereby stimulating a regenerative response in the surviving basal cells. Tumor promoters are chemicals that do not cause cancer themselves but induce tumor development in skin that has been initiated by a low dose of a carcinogen. Their promoting power generally is parallel to their ability to give sustained hyperplasia of the epidermis with continued treatment. Selective stimulation of tumor growth is envisioned to occur from differential stimulation of initiated cells or due to the insensitivity of initiated cells to toxicity or to terminal differentiation induced in uninitiated cells by the promoter. Continuing efforts to understand the promotion process are envisioned to assist development of short-term tests that predict promoting potential (Curtin et al., 2006).

An advantage of the experimental model of mouse skin carcinogenesis is the ability to separate the neoplastic process into stages of initiation, promotion, and progression, and the analysis can be extended to more complicated multihit, multistage models (Owens et al., 1999). In the simplest model, the skin is treated once with a low dose of an initiator, a polycyclic aromatic hydrocarbon, for example. The skin does not develop tumors unless it is subsequently treated with a promoter, which must be applied numerous times at frequent intervals (e.g., twice per week for 3 months). Application of the promoter need not start immediately after initiation, but if it is not continued long enough, or if it is applied before or without the initiator, tumors do not develop. A consequence of promotion then is a tendency to linearize the dose–response curve for the initiator. Although an important aspect of promotion is its epigenetic nature, papillomas arising from promotion characteristically are aneuploid.

Mutations in the *c-Ha-ras* gene are commonly found in papillomas, particularly those initiated by polycyclic aromatic hydrocarbons. Eventually some of the resulting papillomas become autonomous, continuing to grow without the further addition of the promoter. Genetic damage accumulates in the small fraction of tumors that progress to malignancy.

A number of natural products are tumor promoters, many of which alter phosphorylation pathways. The best-studied example, and one of the most potent, is the active ingredient of croton oil, 12-*O*-tetradecanoylphorbol-13-acetate. This is a member of a diverse group of compounds that give transitory stimulation followed by chronic depletion of protein kinase C in mouse epidermis (Fournier and Murray, 1987). Another group of chemicals, an example of which is okadaic acid, consists of phosphatase inhibitors. Compounds acting by other routes are known, including thapsigargin (calcium channel modulator) and benzoyl peroxide (free radical generator). Sensitivity to tumor promotion is an important factor in the relative sensitivity to skin carcinogenesis among different mouse strains and even among other laboratory animal species. An intriguing example, TCDD is 100-fold more potent than tetradecanoylphorbol acetate in certain hairless mouse strains but virtually inactive in some non-hairless strains (Poland *et al.*, 1982). Much effort is currently being focused on the signal transduction pathways that are perturbed by treatment with such chemicals.

The finding that chromate (a human lung carcinogen) in the drinking water enhances tumor yield from ultraviolet light in mouse skin suggests that generation of reactive oxygen can be effective and raises concern about the Cr(VI) drinking water standard (Davidson *et al.*, 2004).

The desire to reduce the cost and improve the effectiveness of cancer testing in animals has led to development of transgenic mice with useful properties. The Tg.AC strain, for example, exhibits a genetically initiated epidermis (Humble *et al.*, 2005). Integrated in this mouse genome is a v-Ha-ras oncogene driven by part of the ζ-globin promoter, which in this context fortuitously drives expression only in epidermis that is wounded or treated with tumor promoters. The mice display enhanced skin sensitivity to a number of nongenotoxic carcinogens and have low backgrounds of spontaneous tumors over a 26-week treatment period. They also respond to genotoxic carcinogens, which target genes that cooperate with the ras oncogene in neoplastic development (Owens *et al.*, 1995). Tg.AC mice can be employed for testing in combination with a different mouse strain that has one p53 allele inactivated, and thus displays enhanced sensitivity to genotoxic carcinogens in other tissues in addition to the skin. These genetically modified mice promise to speed up testing using fewer animals and to reduce false–positive results arising from either strain/species-specific idiosyncrasies or high doses that could elicit secondary responses not relevant to human exposures. Although replacement of the very expensive 2-year rodent carcinogenesis assay is not yet feasible, these genetically modified mice have reduced the number of such assays and assisted pharmaceutical evaluation (Jacobs, 2005).

Arsenic

An abundant element in the earth's crust, arsenic is encountered routinely in small doses in the air, water, and food. In earlier times, high exposures occurred from medications such as Fowler's solution (potassium arsenite) and from pesticides such as sodium arsenite and lead arsenate; the latter pesticides have been phased out in the United States but monomethylarsenate is still used in considerable (though decreasing) volumes in agriculture. Around the world, substantial exposures can occur as a result of mining operations to individuals from breathing dust from the ore or fumes from subsequent smelting or to communities encountering leachate from tailings into waterways. Glass manufacture and food dried using coal with high arsenic content can also contribute to high exposures, and the environmental burden is increased by disposal of large volumes of wood preserved with chromated copper arsenate and of litter from poultry fed organic arsenical antibiotics. Well water derived from geological formations with high arsenic content is now recognized as a major health concern, highlighted by populations in the tens of millions at risk in Bangladesh and India (Tapio and Grosche, 2006). Previous studies of populations in southwestern Taiwan revealed an association of high arsenic exposure with altered skin pigmentation and hyperkeratosis of the palms and soles, blackfoot disease from impaired circulation reflecting endothelial cell damage, and carcinomas of the skin and several other organs (bladder, lung, liver). More recent concentration dependence studies in West Bengal, India, show skin hyperpigmentation and keratoses occurring with drinking water concentrations close to 50 ppb (Mazumdur *et al.*, 1998), the former USA drinking water standard. In such regions, reduced lung function in men (von Ehrenstein *et al.*, 2005), stillbirths in women (von Ehrenstein *et al.*, 2006), and bronchiectasis in both sexes (Mazumdur *et al.*, 2005) are found at elevated rates among individuals with arsenic-induced skin lesions. Recognition that carcinomas of the skin and internal organs occur in humans imbibing drinking water with concentrations less than an order of magnitude higher than 50 ppb (Tapio and Grosche, 2006) contributed to reducing the U.S. standard to 10 ppb as of 2006.

Due to continuing debate over the dependence of health effects on arsenic at low concentration, which has regulatory implications (Schoen *et al.*, 2004), much effort is devoted to understanding arsenic action. Numerous mechanisms have been proposed by which arsenic serves as a carcinogen and gives other pathological effects, of which the majority could plausibly involve binding of trivalent forms to protein sulfhydryls (Kitchen and Wallace, 2005). Methylation has been considered a detoxification method, because the observed pentavalent mono- and dimethyl arsenates isolated in urine from exposed humans and animals are much less toxic than the inorganic forms. Wide species differences in methylation capability even among primates have raised the possibility that other detoxification pathways exist, and observations that the methylated forms are also found at low levels in the highly toxic trivalent state in animal tissues and in human urine (Aposhian *et al.*, 2000) have prompted re-evaluation of their roles. Identification of an AsIII-methyltransferase and exploration how it mediates toxic effects in cells where it is expresssed (Drobna *et al.*, 2005) promise to clarify this important issue. For the epidermis, where little methylation occurs, effects of the inorganic forms evidently dominate. As shown by many labs, effects of arsenate (the most common form in drinking water) in vivo or in culture are mediated by reduction to arsenite (Patterson *et al.*, 2003).

Arsenic is a weak mutagen at best in bacteria and mammalian cells, but it does induce DNA deletions and chromosomal aberrations and acts as a co-mutagen, possibly by interfering with DNA repair (Rossman *et al.*, 2004). Arsenic was recently found to be a transplacental carcinogen in mice, leading to an increase in tumors of the liver, adrenal gland, lung, and ovary in adulthood among animals exposed in utero (Waalkes *et al.*, 2004). A lack of epidermal tumors in these mice suggests species specificity in tissue response, and finding tumors in tissues with a substantial background rate could suggest enhancement of an endogenous carcinogenic process (Rossman, 2003). In mice where the skin is irradiated with ultraviolet light, arsenic acts as a cocarcinogen (Rossman *et al.*, 2004), and in Tg.AC mice, expressing an activated ras oncogene in the epidermis, arsenic enhances phorbol ester tumor promotion (Germolec *et al.*, 1997). Although arsenic is thought to elicit cancer in regions of the skin not receiving high sun exposure (e.g., the palms and soles), careful examination of epidemiological data in Bangladesh indicate sun exposure is a risk factor for arsenical keratoses, precursors for cancer (Chen *et al.*, 2006). High arsenic exposure from drinking water also appears to promote skin lesions in users of betel nut (McCarty *et al.*, 2006), a source of genotoxic nitrosamines known to be activated by cytochrome P450 activities in keratinocytes of the oral cavity (Miyazaki *et al.*, 2005). Among the proposed mechanisms of arsenic action, generation of reactive oxygen in target cells is a likely contributor to such carcinogenic and other pathological effects. This phenomenon has been proposed to result from activation of NADPH oxygenases (Smith *et al.*, 2001), damage to mitochondria (Liu *et al.*, 2005) or, in the case of the methylated forms, (auto)oxidation (Kitchin and Ahmad, 2003). Consequent formation of 8-hydroxyguanine or -guanosine, consistent with low-level mutagenesis, has been detected in vivo and in culture. Reactive oxygen generation could also account for the hyperplastic response of mouse skin to arsenic (Rossman *et al.*, 2004) and the broad effects in target cells (Rea *et al.*, 2003), including central signaling molecules such as focal adhesion kinase (Yancy *et al.*, 2005).

REFERENCES

Ahmad N, Mukhtar H: Cytochrome P450: A target for drug development for skin diseases. *J Invest Dermatol* 123:417–425, 2004.

Alvarez-Roman R, Naik A, Kalia Y, *et al.*: Visualization of skin penetration using confocal laser scanning microscopy. *Eur J Pharm Biopharm* 58:301–316, 2004.

Amin S, Freeman S, Maibach HI: Systemic toxicity in man secondary to percutaneous absorption, in Roberts MS, Walters KA (eds.): *Dermal Absorption and Toxicity Assessment*. New York: Marcel Dekker, 1998, pp. 103–125.

Aposhian HV, Gurzau ES, Le XC, *et al.*: Occurrence of monomethylarsonous acid in urine of humans exposed to inorganic arsenic. *Chem Res Toxicol* 13:693–697, 2000.

Arts JHE, Mommers C, de Heer C: Dose-response relationships and threshold levels in skin and respiratory allergy. *Crit Rev Toxicol* 36:219–251, 2006.

Baccarelli A, Pesatori AC, Consonni D, *et al.*: Health status and plasma dioxin levels in chloracne cases 20 years after the Seveso, Italy accident. *Br J Dermatol* 152:459–465, 2005.

Barratt MD: Structure-activity relationships and prediction of the phototoxicity and phototoxic potential of new drugs. *Altern Lab Anim* 32:511–524, 2004.

Belsito DV: Occupational contact dermatitis: Etiology, prevalence, and resultant impairment/disability. *J Am Acad Dermatol* 53:303–313, 2005.

Betts CJ, Dearman RJ, Kimber I, *et al.*: Potency and risk assessment of a skin sensitizing disperse dye using the local lymph node assay. *Contact Dermatitis* 52:268–272, 2005.

Boukhman MP, Maibach HI: Thresholds in contact sensitization: Immunologic mechanisms and experimental evidence in humans—An overview. *Food ChemToxicol* 39:1125–1134, 2001.

Brown HS, Bishop DR, Rowan CA: The role of skin absorption as a route of exposure for volatile organic compounds (VOCs) in drinking water. *Am J Public Health* 74:479–484, 1984.

Buchholz BA, Fultz E, Haack KW, *et al.*: HPLC-accelerator MS measurement of atrazine metabolites in human urine after dermal exposure. *Analyt Chem* 71:3519–3525, 1999.

Chave TA, Mortimer NJ, Sladden MJ, *et al.*: Toxic epidermal necrolysis: Current evidence, practical management and future directions. *Br J Dermatol* 153:241–253, 2005.

Chen Y, Graziano JH, Parvez F, *et al.*: Modification of risk of arsenic-induced skin lesions by sunlight exposure, smoking, and occupational exposures in Bangladesh. *Epidemiology* 17:459–467, 2006.

Choi MJ, Maibach HI: Liposomes and niosomes as topical drug delivery systems. *Skin Pharmacol Physiol* 18:209–219, 2005.

Cohen DE: Contact dermatitis: A quarter century perspective. *J Am Acad Dermatol* 51:S60–S63, 2004.

Cook N, Freeman S: Report of 19 cases of photoallergic contact dermatitis to sunscreens seen at the Skin and Cancer Foundation. *Australas J Dermatol* 42:257–259, 2001.

Cross SE, Anderson C, Thompson MJ, *et al.*: Is there tissue penetration after application of topical salicylate formulations? *Lancet* 350:636, 1997.

Curtin GM, Hanausek M, Walaszek Z, *et al.*: Short-term biomarkers of cigarette smoke condensate tumor promoting potential in mouse skin. *Toxicol Sci* 89:66–74, 2006.

Davidson T, Kluz T, Burns FJ, *et al.*: Exposure to chromium (VI) in the drinking water increases the susceptibility to UV-induced skin tumors in hairless mice. *Toxicol Appl Pharmacol* 196:431–437, 2004.

del Giudice P, Yves P: The widespread use of skin lightening creams in Senegal: A persistent public health problem in West Africa. *Int J Dermatol* 41:69–72, 2002.

Del Rosario RN, Barr RJ, Graham BS, *et al.*: Exogenopus and endogenous cutaneous anomalies and curiosities. *Am J Dermatopathol* 27:259–2667, 2005.

DeLeo VA: Photocontact dermatitis. *Dermatol Ther* 17:279–288, 2004.

Doutre MS: Occupational contact urticaria and protein contact dermatitis. *Eur J Dermatol* 15:419–424, 2005.

Drobna Z, Waters SB, Devesa V, *et al.*: Metabolism and toxicity of arsenic in humnan urothelial cells expressing rat arsenic (+3 oxidation state)-methyltransferase. *Toxicol Appl Pharmacol* 207:147–159, 2005.

Du L, Neis MM, Ladd PA, *et al.*: Effects of the differentiated keratinocyte phenotype on expression levels of CYP1-4 family genes in human skin cells. *Toxicol Appl Pharmacol* 213:135–144, 2006.

Elias PM: Role of lipids in barrier function of the skin, in Mukhtar H (ed.): *Pharmacology of the Skin*. Boca Raton: CRC Press, 1992, pp. 29–38.

Emmett EA: Occupational contact dermatitis II: Risk assessment and prognosis. *Am J Contact Dermatitis* 14:21–30, 2003.

Epstein JH: Phototoxicity and photoallergy. *Sem Cutaneous Med Surgery* 18:274–284, 1999.

Fisher AA: Unique reactions of scrotal skin to topical agents. *Cutis* 44:445–447, 1989.

Fournier A, Murray MW: Application of phorbol ester to mouse skin causes a rapid and sustained loss of protein kinase C. *Nature* 330:767–769, 1987.

French LE, Trent JT, Kerdel FA: Use of intravenous immunoglobulin in toxic epidermal necrolysis and Stevens-Johnson syndrome: Our current understanding. *Int Immunopharmacol* 6:543–549, 2006.

Gawkrodger DJ: Occupational skin cancers. *Occupational Med* 54:458–463, 2004.

Germolec DR, Spalding J, Boorman GA, *et al.*: Arsenic can mediate skin neoplasia by chronic stimulation of keratinocyte-derived growth factors. *Mutation Res* 386:209–218, 1997.

Gerner I, Barratt MD, Zinke S, et al.: Development and validation of a list of structure-activity relationship rules to be used in expert systems for prediction of the skin-sensitizing properties of chemicals. *Altern Lab Anim* 32:487–509, 2004.

Geyer HJ, Schramm K-W, Feicht EA, et al.: Half lives of tetra-, penta-, hexa-, hepta- and octachlorodibenzo-p-dioxin in rats, monkeys and humans—A critical review. *Chemosphere* 48:631–644, 2002.

Goossens A: Photoallergic contact dermatitis. *Photodermatol Photoimmunol Photomed* 20:121–125, 2004.

Gruchalla RS, Pirmohamed M: Antibiotic allergy. *N Engl J Med* 354:601–609, 2006.

Holden CR, Gawkrodger DJ: 10 years' experience of patch testing with a shoe series in 230 patients: Which allergens are important? *Contact Dermatitis* 53:37–39, 2005.

Hotchkiss SAM: Dermal metabolism, in Roberts MS, Walters KA (eds.): *Dermal Absorption and Toxicity Assessment.* New York: Marcel Dekker, 1998, pp. 43–101.

Humble MC, Trempus CS, Spalding JW, et al.: Biological, cellular and molecular characterisitics of an inducible transgenic skin tumor model: A review. *Oncogene* 24:8217–8228, 2005.

Jacobs A: Prediction of 2-year carcinogenicity study results for pharmaceutical products: How are we doing? *Toxicol Sci* 88:18–23, 2005.

Jiang YJ, Kim P, Elias PM, et al.: LXR and PPAR activators stimulate cholesterol sulfotransferase type 2 isoform 1b in human keratinocytes. *J Lipid Res* 46:2657–2666, 2005.

Kao J, Hall J: Skin absorption and cutaneous first pass metabolism of topical steroids: In vitro studies with mouse skin in organ culture. *J Pharmacol Exper Therap* 241:482–487, 1987.

Khan WA, Das M, Stick S, et al.: Induction of epidermal NAD(P)H:quinone reductase by chemical carcinogens: A possible mechanism for the detoxification. *Biochem Biophys Res Commun* 146:126–133, 1987.

Kimbrough RD: Porphyrias and hepatotoxicity. *Annals NY Acad Sci* 514:289–296, 1987.

Kitchen KT, Wallace K: Arsenite binding to synthetic peptifdes based on the Zn finger region and the estrogen binding region of the human estrogen receptor-α. *Toxicol Appl Pharmacol* 206:66–72, 2005.

Kitchin KT, Ahmad S: Oxidative stress as a possible mode of action for arsenic carcinogenesis. *Toxicol Lett* 137:3–13, 2003.

Krueger GG, Pershing LK: Human skin xenografts to athymic rodents as a system to study toxins delivered to or through skin, in Wang RGM, Knaak JB, Maibach HI (eds.): *Health Risk Assessment Dermat and Inhalation Exposure and Absorption of Toxicants.* Boca Raton: CRC Press, 1993, pp. 413–452.

Kynemund Pedersen L, Agner T, Held E, et al.: Methyldibromoglutaronitrile in leave-on products elicits contact allergy at low concentration. *Br J Dermatol* 151:817–822, 2004.

Laughter D, Istvan JA, Tofte SJ, et al.: The prevalence of atopic dermatitis in Oregon school children. *J Am Acad Dermatol* 43:649–655, 2000.

Legros L, Cassuto J-P, Ortonne J-P: Imatinib mesilate (Glivec): A systemic depigmenting agent for extensive vitiligo. *Br J Dermatol* 153:691–692, 2005.

Lindelof B, Sigurgeirsson B, Tegner E, et al.: PUVA and cancer risk: The Swedish follow-up study. *Br J Dermatol* 141:108–112, 1999.

Lipozencic J, Wolfe R: Life-threatening severe allergic reactions: Urticaria, angioedema, and anaphylaxis. *Clin Dermatol* 23:193–205, 2005.

Liu S-X, Davidson MM, Tang X, et al.: Mitochondrial damage mediates genotoxicity of arsenic in mammalian cells. *Cancer Res* 65:3236–3242, 2005.

Mark BJ, Slavin RG: Allergic contact dermatitis. *Med Clin N Am* 90:169–185, 2006.

Martin-Bouyer G, Lebreton R, Toga M, et al.: Outbreak of accidental hexachlorophene poisoning in France. *Lancet* 1:91–95, 1982.

Mazumdur DNG, Haque R, Ghosh N, et al.: Arsenic levels in drinking water and prevalence of skin lesions in West Bengal, India. *Int J Epidemiol* 27:871–877, 1998.

Mazumdur DNG, Steinmaus C, Bhattacharya P, et al.: Bronchiectasis in persons with skin lesions resulting from arsenic in drinking water. *Epidemiol* 16:760–765, 2005.

McCarty KM, Houseman EA, Quamruzzaman Q, et al.: The impact of diet and betel nut use on skin lesions associated with drinking-water arsenic in Pabna, Bangladesh. *Environ Health Perspect* 114:334–340, 2006.

McKnight RH, Spiller HA: Green tobacco sickness in children and adolescents. *Pub Health Rep* 120:602–605, 2005.

McManus J, Huebner K: Vesicants. *Crit Care Clin* 21:707–718, 2005.

Melnikova VO, Ananthaswamy HN: Cellular and molecular events leading to the development of skin cancer. *Mutation Res* 571:91–106, 2005.

Merk HF, Abel J, Baron JM, et al.: Molecular pathways in dermatotoxicology. *Toxicol Appl Pharmacol* 195:267–277, 2004.

Miller J, Djabali K, Chen T, et al.: Atrichia caused by mutations in the vitamin D receptor gene is a phenocopy of generalized atrichia caused by mutations in the hairless gene. *J Invest Dermatol* 117:612–617, 2001.

Miyazaki M, Sugawara E, Yoshimura T, et al.: Mutagenic activation of betel quid-specific N-nitrosamines catalyzed by human cytochrome P450 coexpressed with NADH-cytochrome P450 reductase in *Salmonella typhimurium* YG7108. *Mutation Res* 581:165–171, 2005.

Moan J, Peng Q: An outline of the hundred-year history of PDT. *Anticancer Res* 23:3591–3600, 2004.

Mukhtar H, Bickers DR: Comparative activity of the mixed function oxidases, epoxide hydratase, and glutathione S-transferase in liver and skin of the neonatal rat. *Drug Metab Dispos* 9:311–314, 1981.

Netzlaff F, Lehr C-M, Wertz PW, et al.: The human epidermis models EpiSkin, SkinEthic and EpiDerm: An evaluation of morphology and their suitability for testing photoxicity, irritancy, corrosivity and substance transport. *Eur J Pharm Biopharm* 60:167–178, 2005.

Nishigori C: Cellular aspects of photocarcinogenesis. *Photochem Photobiol Sci* 5:208–214, 2006.

Okey AB, Franc MA, Moffat ID, et al.: Toxicological implications of polymorphisms in receptors for xenobiotic chemicals: The case of the aryl hydrocarbon receptor. *Toxicol Appl Pharmacol* 207:S43–S51, 2005.

Owens DM, Spalding JW, Tennant RW, et al.: Genetic alterations cooperate with v-Ha-ras to accelerate multistage carcinogenesis in TG.AC transgenic mouse skin. *Cancer Res* 55:3171–3178, 1995.

Owens DM, Wei S-JC, Smart RC: A multihit, multistage model of chemical carcinogenesis. *Carcinogenesis* 20:1837–1844, 1999.

Park J-H, Troxel AB, Harvey RG, et al.: Polycyclic aromatic hydrocarbon (PAH) o-quinones produced by the aldo-keto-reductases (AKRs) generate abasic sites, oxidized pyrimidines and 8-oxo-dGuo via reactive oxygen species. *Chem Res Toxicol* 19:719–728, 2006.

Patterson TJ, Ngo M, Aronov PA, et al.: Biological activity of inorganic arsenic and antimony reflects oxidation state in cultured keratinocytes. *Chem Res Toxicol* 16:1624–1631, 2003.

Poland A, Knutson JC: 2,3,7,8-Tetrachlorodibeno-p-dioxin and related halogenated aromatic hydrocarbons: Examination of the mechanism of toxicity. *Ann Rev Pharmacol Toxicol* 22:517–554, 1982.

Poland A, Palen D, Glover E: Tumor promotion by TCDD in skin of HRS/J hairless mice. *Nature* 300:271–273, 1982.

Potts RO, Guy RH: Predicting skin permeability. *Pharmacol Res* 9:663–669, 199.

Pratt MD, Belsito DV, Deleo VA, et al.: North American Contact Dermatitis Group patch-test results, 2001–2002 study period. *Dermatitis* 15:176–183, 2004.

Raza H, Agarwal R, Mukhtar H: Cutaneous glutathione S-transferases, in Mukhtar H (ed.): Pharmacology of the Skin. Boca Raton: CRC Press, 1992, pp. 131–137.

Rea MA, Gregg JP, Qin Q, et al.: Global alteration of gene expression in human keratinocytes by inorganic arsenic. *Carcinogenesis* 24:747–756, 2003.

Reines HD, Seifert PC: Patient safety: Latex allergy. *Surg Clin North Am* 85:1329–1340, 2005.

Riviere JE, Brooks JD: Predicting skin permeability from complex chemical mixtures. *Toxicol Appl Pharmacol* 208:99–110, 2005.

Rossman TG: Mechanism of arsenic carcinogenesis: An integrated approach. *Mutation Res* 533:37–65, 2003.

Rossman TG, Uddin AN, Burns FJ: Evidence that arsenite acts as a cocarcinogen in skin cancer. *Toxicol Appl Pharmacol* 198:394–404, 2004.

Roujeau J-C: Clinical heterogeneity of drup hypersensitivity. *Toxicol* 209:123–129, 2005.

Rubin H: Synergistic mechanisms in carcinogenesis by polycyclic aromatic hydrocarbons and by tobacco smoke: A bio-historical perspective with updates. *Carcinogenesis* 22:1903–1930, 2001.

Ryan CA, Gerberick GF, Gildea LA, *et al.*: Interactions of contact allergens with dendritic cells: Opportunities and challenges for the development of novel approaches to hazard assessment. *Toxicol Sci* 88:4–11, 2005.

Saarikoski ST, Rivera SP, Hankinson O, *et al.*: CYP2S1: A short review. *Toxicol Appl Pharmacol* 207:S62–S69, 2005

Saary J, Qureshi R, Palda V, *et al.*: A systematic review of contact dermatitis treatment and prevention. *J Am Acad Dermatol* 53:845–855, 2005.

Scheuplein RJ, Blank IH: Permeability of skin. *Physiol Rev* 51:702–747, 1971.

Schoen A, Beck B, Sharma R, *et al.*: Arsenic toxicity at low does: Epidemiological and mode of action considerations. *Toxicol Appl Pharmacol* 198:253–267, 2004.

Sheehan JM, Cragg N, Chadwick CA, *et al.*: Repeated ultraviolet exposure affords the same protection against DNA photodamage and erythema in human skin types II and IV but is associated with faster DNA repair in skin type IV. *J Invest Dermatol* 118:825–829, 2002.

Shimizu Y, Nakatsuru Y, Ichinose M, *et al.*: Benzo[a]pyrene carcinogenicity is lost in mice lacking the aryl hydrocarbon receptor. *Proc Natl Acad Sci USA* 97:779–782, 2000.

Smith KR, Klei LR, Barchowsky A: Arsenite stimulates plasma membrane NADPH oxidase in vascular endothelial cells. *Am J Lung Cell Molec Physiol* 280:L442–L449, 2001.

Spencer JM, Amonette R: Tanning beds and skin cancer: Artifical sun + Old Sol = real risk. *Clin Dermatol* 16:487–501, 1998.

Spritz RA: The gemntics of generalized vitiligo and associated autoimmunie diseases. *J Dermatol Sci* 41:3–10, 2006.

Stern RS, Nichols KT, Vakeva LH: Malignant melanoma in patients treated for psoriasis with methoxsalen (psoralen) and ultraviolet A radiation (PUVA). The PUVA follow-up study. *N Engl J Med* 336:1041–1045, 1997.

Storm JE, Collier SW, Stewart RF, *et al.*: Metabolism of xenobiotics during percutaneous penetration: Role of absorption rate and cutaneous enzyme activity. *Fund Appl Toxicol* 15:132–141, 1990.

Swanson HI: Cytochrome P450 expression in human keratinocytes: An aryl hydrocarbon receptor perspective. *Chem-Biol Interact* 149:69–79, 2004.

Tapio S, Grosche B: Arsenic in the etiology of cancer. *Mutation Res* 612:215–246, 2006.

Tauchi M, Hida A, Negishi T, *et al.*: Constitutive expression of aryl hydrocarbon receptor in keratinocytes causes inflammatory skin lesions. *Molec Cell Biol* 25:9360–9368, 2005.

Thami GP, Sarkar R: Coal tar: Past, present and future. *Clin Exp Dermatol* 27:99–103, 2004.

Tornier C, Rosdy M, Maibach HI: In vitro skin irritation testing on reconstituted human epidermis: Reproducibility for 50 chemicals tested with two proptocols. *Toxicol in Vitro* 20:401–416, 2006.

Toyoda M, Morohashi M: Pathogenesis of acne. *Med Electron Microsc* 34:29–40, 2001.

Uter W, Johansen JD, Orton DI, *et al.*: Clinical update on contact allergy. *Curr Opin Allergy Clin Immunol* 5:429–436, 2005.

van Birgelen APJM, Fase KM, van der Kolk J, *et al.*: Synergistic effect of 2,2′,4,4′,5,5′-hexachlorobiphenyl and 2,3,7,8-tetrachlorodibenzo-p-dioxin on hepatic porphyrin levels in the rat. *Environ Health Perspect* 104:550–557, 1996.

von Ehrenstein OS, Mazumdur DNG, Hira-Smith M, *et al.*: Pregnancy outcomes, infant mortality, and arsenic in drinking water in West Bengal, India. *Am J Epidemiol* 163:662–669, 2006.

von Ehrenstein OS, Mazumdur DNG, Yuan Y, *et al.*: Decrements in lung function related to arsenic in drinking water in West Bengal, India. *Am J Epidemiol* 162:533–541, 2005.

Waalkes MP, Liu J, Ward JM, *et al.*: Animal models for arsenic carcinogenesis: Inorganic arsenic is a transplacental carcinogen in mice. *Toxicol Appl Pharmacol* 198:377–384, 2004.

Walsh AA, deGraffenried LA, Rice RH: 2,3,7,8-Tetrachlorodibeno-p-dioxin sensitization of cultured human epidermal cells to carcinogenic heterocyclic amine toxicity. *Carcinogenesis* 16:2187–2191, 1995.

Wetter DA, Davis MDP, Yiannias JA, *et al.*: Patch test results from the Mayo Clinic Contact Dermatitis Group. *J Am Acad Dermatol* 53:416–421, 2005.

Wolf R, Orion E, Marcos B, *et al.*: Life-threatening acute adverse cutaneous drug reactions. *Clin Dermatol* 23:171–181, 2005.

Yancy SL, Shelden EA, Gilmont RR, *et al.*: Sodium arsenite exposure alters cell migration, focal adhesion localization, and decreases tyrosine phosphorylation of focal adhesion kinase in H9C2 myoblasts. *Toxicol Sci* 84:278–286, 2005.

Zeitouni NC, Oseroff AR, Shieh S: Photodynamic therapy for nonmelanoma skin cancers. Current review and update. *Molec Immunol* 39:1133–1136, 2003.

Zhai H, Fautz R, Fuchs A, *et al.*: Human scalp irritation compared to that of the arm and back. *Contact Dermatitis* 51:196–200, 2004.

CHAPTER 20

TOXIC RESPONSES OF THE REPRODUCTIVE SYSTEM

Paul M.D. Foster and L. Earl Gray Jr.

INTRODUCTION

Any evaluation of toxicity to reproduction will have as an important consideration that events may not only be on the adults having impact on their likelihood to have children, but also impact the viability and quality of life of their potential offspring and feasibly even affect later generations. That chemicals can adversely affect reproduction in males and females is not a new concept, one only has to look at the importance of drugs as contraceptives to realize how sensitive the reproductive system can be to external chemical influences to

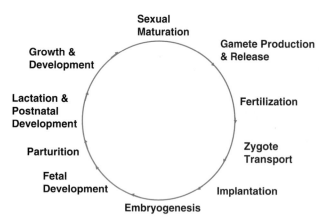

Figure 20-1. The Reproductive Cycle.

Table 20-1

Examples of reproductive physiology similarities among humans and rats

Steroid hormone control of reproductive function relies on testosterone, dihydrotestosterone, estradiol, and progesterone.

CNS-hypothalamic secretion of GnRH controls pituitary release and synthesis of FSH and LH.

FSH and LH regulate germ cell development after puberty, LH surges induce spontaneous ovulation in the female, LH regulates testis Leydig cell testosterone production.

Placental support of embryos. Placenta and fetal unit also produce hormones critical for pregnancy maintenance after the first week.

Hormonal regulation of uterine function and onset of delivery.

Androgens required to maintain male spermatogenesis and secondary sex characteristics.

Hormone-dependent mating and other sexually dimorphic behavior. "Rough and tumble" play behavior is sexually dimorphic behavior being imprinted by early androgens.

Lactation under complex hormonal regulation.

Dramatic endocrine changes resulting from CNS-HPG maturation responsible for puberty in males and females. Females generally attain puberty at an earlier age than males of the same species.

Key: CNS, central nervous system; GnRH, gonatropin-releasing hormone; FSH, follicle-stimulating hormone; LH, luteinizing hormone; HPG, hypothalamic-pituitary-gonadal.

disrupt this process. Of course in these cases, the failure of normal reproduction is a desired outcome in a contraceptive, but unfortunately we have had a number of catastrophes in which such failure has been unintentional. Many of the classic examples in chemical workers, or contamination of groundwater from chemical exposure such as dibromochloropropane (DBCP) or kepone (Chlordecone) have shown the sensitivity of human reproduction to these specific exposures (reviewed in (Cannon *et al.*, 1978; Faroon *et al.*, 1995; Winker and Rudiger, 2006). There have been significant improvements in our ability to test for effects on reproduction for chemicals, agrochemicals and drugs, but unfortunately such adverse episodes continue to occur in, for example, the more recent reports of the effects of 2-bromopropane in chemical workers (both male and female) in Korea (reviewed in Boekelheide *et al.*, 2004).

Recent trends in human fertility, fecundity—changing social influences (age at which women have their first child) and the knowledge that populations in many western countries are no longer self sustaining, coupled with the advent of assisted reproductive techniques (ARTs), where according to a recent paper 5.9% of all live births in Denmark used these ARTs (Andersen *et al.*, 2005), all point to the potential for declines in normal human reproduction. Underlying all these issues with human reproductive performance is the concept that exposure to environmental chemicals and drugs may be contributing to these declines.

The advent of the endocrine disruptor debate provided a major impetus to the examination of the methods used in screening and testing for reproductive (and other) toxicity, and highlighted a number of shortfalls, not least in how we should evaluate the latent effects on adults of in utero exposures. However, this Chapter will not specifically address the emerging issue of the fetal origins of adult disease as proposed by Barker (Barker, 1995, 1999; Barker *et al.*, 1993; Barker *et al.*, 1989).

This chapter will take the reproductive cycle (Fig. 20-1) as the biological basis for the description of toxicity to reproduction rather than an encyclopedic approach. The basic biology of the different lifestages and processes that are requisites for normal reproduction will be discussed and, where possible, the differences between experimental animals and humans highlighted (see Tables 20-1 and 20-2). These processes will then be placed into perspective by reference to a number of case studies of selected chemicals chosen to illustrate a range of modes of action and how they can perturb reproduction.

Special attention will be focused on endocrine disruption, methods proposed for screening and testing and the selection of chemicals with specific pharmacologies (e.g., estrogen or antiandrogen) to illustrate the types of toxicities produced at different lifestages.

The chapter will also provide basic information on testing methodologies for chemicals, pesticides and drugs, but placed into the reproductive cycle framework. Thus, it will examine the lifestages that are exposed and when specific evaluations are undertaken. Lastly, we have included a section on the evaluation of data and weight of evidence, specifically how one looks at concordance of end points with examples of the types of profiles observed (based on the examples used previously). We do not believe that we have seen this anywhere before, or in this context, and hopefully this will be a useful tool for students and professionals alike.

THE REPRODUCTIVE CYCLE

If one considers the purpose of the reproductive system as the production of good quality gametes, capable of fertilization and producing a viable offspring which in turn can successfully reproduce, then it is clear that a large number of complex processes need to be orchestrated in a precise, sequential order for optimal performance at different stages of the lifecycle of the animal, or human. Thus, following fertilization of an egg by a sperm, the resulting zygote must be transported along the oviduct while maturing into an early embryo. This embryo is then required to implant in the uterus successfully, such that the developing conceptus can differentiate, produce a placenta and normal embryogenesis and fetal development occur. Once the fetus has completed in utero growth and differentiation, parturition needs to occur at the correct time and the neonate be born and then proceed successfully through the lactation phase of development and be weaned.

When the male and female offspring enter puberty after infancy, they need to acquire sexual characteristics as young adults

Table 20-2

Examples in which the reproductive strategy of the rat differs from that of the human

1. The rat is a short (22.5 day) gestation species. Pregnancy in humans is 9 month.
2. The rat placenta lacks aromatase; estrogen is produced during pregnancy by the ovary. Human placental tissue expresses high levels of aromatase.
3. In the rat, sexual differentiation of the reproductive tract is perinatal, whereas central nervous system (CNS) sexual differentiation is a postnatal event, regulated to a great degree by aromatization of testosterone to estradiol (play behavior, an exception, is androgen dependent in both rats [Hotchkiss *et al.*, 2002, 2003] and humans [Hines, 2003]). In nonhuman primates and presumably humans, more CNS events are prenatal, and androgens are more important than in rats (Goy and Phoenix, 1972; Goy and Resko, 1972; Goy *et al.*, 1988; Hines, 2003).
4. The rat has a 4- to 5-day estrous cycle, with no functional corporus luteum. The estrous cycle can be monitored easily by examining daily cytology. The female rat displays sexual receptivity only during estrus after "lights out" after a proestrus vaginal smear. This behavior is exquisitely dependent on estrogen followed by progesterone. Humans have a menstrual cycle approximately 28 days in duration and do not display periods of peak behavioral estrus during the cycle. Corpora luteal function is sustained for approximately 10 days by mating-induced cervical stimulatory prolactin surges in rats, whereas the human menstrual cycle has a spontaneous luteal phase of 10 to 14 days after ovulation.
5. Male rat sex behavior can be induced by estrogens and involves multiple series of ejaculations in a single mating. Mating involves approximately 10 mounts, with intromission before each ejaculation, followed by a postejaculatory interval before the onset of the next series. In nonhuman primates and presumably humans, male sex behavior is androgen mediated.
6. Both ovaries spontaneously release several ova in response to a luteinizing hormone surge into separate uterine horns, each with a separate cervix in the rat; whereas in women, a single ovum is typically ovulated during each cycle.
7. Pregnancy is easily disrupted by estrogens in rats, but not in humans. Rats, unlike humans, are a litter-bearing species.
Most strains used for toxicology testing have litters of 10 to 12 pups. Spontaneous reproductive malformations are very rare in the rat, whereas in humans, some malformations such as cryptorchidism occur in 3% of newborn boys.
8. Spermatogenesis begins at approximately 5 days of age in the rat; the spermatogenic cycle is about 53 days of age, and sperm appear in the epididymis at about 55 days of age. In humans, spermatogenesis begins during puberty at 10 to 14 yr of age, and the entire spermatogenic cycle is approximately 75 days in duration.
9. Puberty in the rat (as measured by the age at vaginal opening and the onset of estrous cyclicity) occurs at about 32 days of age in females and 42 days of age (as measured by preputial separation an androgen-dependent event) in male SD and LE rat strains. In humans, puberty occurs at 9 to 12 yr of age in girls, and 10 to 14 yr of age in boys.
10. Fertility begins to decline in the female rat at about 6 mo of age, especially if never mated and allowed to cycle continuously. Fertility begins to decline in women at about 35 yr of age, and at 40 yr of age, approximately 50% of women are infertile.

For a review of reproductive physiology, see Knobil E, Neill JD, eds.: *The Physiology of Reproduction*, 2nd ed, Vol 1 and 2. New York: Raven Press, 1994.

with mature reproductive systems. Acquisition of sexual maturity involves the generation of gametes by the gonads which in turn can result in the production of the next generation. For the parental animals, once their reproductive lifespan has finished, the process of reproductive senescence then occurs. This myriad of processes all involve complex interplay between tissues and cells, the vast majority of these processes being under complex hormonal control that provides the critical signals and precise timing of these events.

Not surprisingly, it is possible to perturb this complex series of events and thus disturb the process and purpose of reproduction. Indeed, all these processes can be targets for the action of specific agents that can disturb these events leading to adverse effects on reproduction, such that the normal production of viable offspring cannot occur. It is thus important to consider in an evaluation of reproductive toxicity that while simple yes/no answers as to whether a particular agent can be a reproductive toxicant are possible, and indeed are used, any description of such toxicity has to be in the context of the lifestage of exposure and effect. There are examples of chemicals that can have different effects on reproduction, at different lifestages, via different modes of action/mechanisms. Indeed it might be useful for this particular aspect of toxicity to modify the adage of Paracelsus to "It is the **timing** of the dose that makes the poison." That is the dose of the toxic chemical and its resultant effects will be dependent on when in the lifestage of the organism that the chemical is administered and evaluated.

The next sections will examine some of the hormonal and other control mechanisms that have been deduced from careful physiological studies in experimental animals and humans (see Table 20-3) to provide more information as to where chemicals may produce their effects. Rather than provide a laundry list of chemicals that can produce effects on reproduction, one or two examples will be mentioned to illustrate the variety of processes that can be affected with referral to more detailed references. While reviewing the mammalian reproductive cycle one could start in any position, we have decided to begin with the development of the reproductive system in utero that occurs with the process of sexual differentiation of the embryo and the move forward around the cycle as depicted in Fig. 20-1.

REPRODUCTIVE DEVELOPMENT AND SEXUAL DIFFERENTIATION

During early human development there is a short period immediately prior to sexual differentiation when the gonad is sexually indifferent and it is not until the seventh week of gestation that male and female morphological characteristics begin to develop. In rodents, the embryo remains sexually indifferent and possesses both male and female reproductive tract primordia until embryonic day 13.5 regardless of its genetic sex.

Table 20-3
Reproductive Parameters for Various Species

SPECIES	AGE AT PUBERTY/ PERIOD	SEXUAL CYCLE DURATION (DAYS)	OVULATION		GESTATION	
			TIME	TYPE	IMPLANTATION (DAYS)	PARTURITION (DAYS)
Mouse	5–6 wk	4	2–3 hr	S	4–5	19 (19–21)
Rat	6–11 wk	4–6	8–11 hr	S	5–6	21–22
Rabbit	6–7 mo	Indefinite	10 hr	I	7–8	31 (30–35)
Hamster	5–8 wk	4	Early estrus	S	5+	16 (15–18)
Guinea Pig	8–10 wk	16–19	10 hr	S	6	67–68
Ferret	8–12 mo	Seasonal	30–36 hr	I	12–13	42
Cat	6–15 mo	Seasonal	24–56 hr	I	13–14	63 (52–69)
Dog	6–8 mo	9	1–3 days	S	13–14	61 (53–71)
Monkey	3 yr	28	9–20 days	S	9	168 (146–180)
Man	12–16 yr	27–28	13–15 days	S	7.5	267 (ovulation)

S = Spontaneous
I = Induced

Gonadogenesis begins with proliferation of the mesodermal (coelomic) epithelium which invades the underlying mesenchyme, resulting in a longitudinal thickening on the medial side of the mesonephros, known as the gonadal ridge (Byskov, 1986). The invading epithelium begins to form primitive sex cords in the gonadal ridge which are surrounded by undifferentiated mesenchyme (Pelliniemi, 1975). Primordial germ cells, or primitive sex cells, are first visible in the fourth week in the caudal region of the yolk sac near the origin of the allantois and migrate along the hindgut, up the dorsal mesentery and into the gonadal ridges (Eddy *et al.*, 1981). The primordial germ cells divide mitotically during migration and continue to proliferate as they migrate under the underlying mesenchyme and are incorporated into the primary sex cords (Moore, 1982). As the primitive cords begin to form, the mesenchyme is invaded by capillaries. The indifferent gonad now consists of an outer cortex and an inner medulla. In the rodent, formation of the gonadal cords is a rapid process that occurs at gestational day 13 via transitory epithelial cell aggregates along the length of the gonadal ridge (Paranko *et al.*, 1983).

Gonadal differentiation is dependent on signals from the Y chromosome which contains the genes necessary to induce testicular morphogenesis. One of these signals is the SRY gene which is the sex-determining region on the short arm of the Y chromosome (Koopman *et al.*, 1990) and acts as a "switch" to initiate transcription of other genes which contribute to testicular organogenesis. In the absence of the SRY protein, the gonad remains indifferent for a short period of time before differentiating into an ovary.

The first morphological sign of testis formation is the aggregation of primordial germ cells and somatic cells (primitive Sertoli cells). These aggregates develop from the gonadal blastema into plate-like structures which then develop into simple arches of elongated testicular cords (Paranko *et al.*, 1983). Throughout differentiation, the testicular cords remain connected to the basal portion of the mesonephric cell mass. The cords gradually transform and extend into the medulla of the gonad, where they branch and anastomose to form a network of cords, known as the rete testis (Moore, 1982). A characteristic and diagnostic feature of testicular development is development of a thick fibrous capsule, the tunica albuginea. As this capsule develops the connection of the prominent testicular (seminiferous) cords with the surface epithelium is disrupted. Gradually the testis separates from the regressing mesonephros, becoming

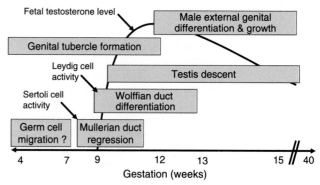

Figure 20-2. Male sexual differentiation in humans during gestation.

(Reproduced with permission from Klonisch T, Fowler PA, Hombach-Klonisch S: Molecular and genetic regulation of testis descent and external genitalia development. *Dev Biol* 270:1–18, 2004. Elsevier Science.)

suspended by its own mesentery. Concurrent with testicular cord formation, fetal Leydig cells differentiate from loosely packed, undifferentiated mesenchymal cells in the interstitium (Pelliniemi, 1975). These interstitial Leydig cells produce the male sex hormone testosterone, which induces masculine differentiation of the Wolffian duct and external genitalia. Intratesticular vasculature differentiates in the gonadal mesenchyme along with the growth of epithelial components. A testis-specific distribution of blood vessels is obvious from an early phase of testicular development (Pelliniemi, 1975). See Fig. 20-2 for a diagrammatic representation of sexual differentiation in the human male.

The fetal testis is composed of testicular cords containing supporting immature Sertoli cells and centrally placed spermatogonia, derived from the surface epithelium and primordial germ cells respectively. These cords are surrounded by a highly vascularized interstitium containing fetal Leydig cells and mesenchyme (Pelliniemi and Niei, 1969). The testicular cords remain without a lumen throughout the fetal period. The seminiferous cords turn into tubules when the Sertoli cells undergo terminal differentiation. This occurs after birth when they finish dividing (roughly at the onset of puberty). They develop tight junctions between adjacent cells, and apical secretion of fluid begins as these cells become highly

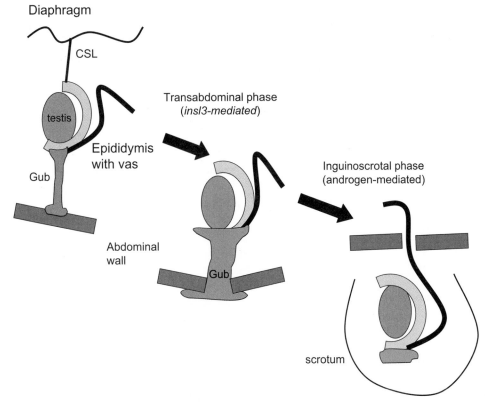

Figure 20-3. The two distinct phases of testicular descent in mammals.

The first (transabdominal phase) mediated by insl3 from the fetal testis involving the removal of the cranial suspensory ligament (CSL) and development of the gubernaculum (gub). The second (inguinoscrotal phase) being androgen mediated. (Reproduced with permission from Klonisch T, Fowler PA, Hombach-Klonisch S: Molecular and genetic regulation of testis descent and external genitalia development. *Dev Biol* 270:1–18, 2004. Elsevier Science.)

polarized. Thus, the lumen forms as Sertoli cells develop their mature phenotype.

In the rodent and human species, fetal testicular androgen production is not only necessary for proper testicular development and normal male sexual differentiation but also differentiation of the Wolffian ducts into the epididymides, vasa deferentia, and seminal vesicles (Barker *et al.*, 1993; Berman *et al.*, 1995; Imperato-McGinley *et al.*, 1992; Kassim *et al.*, 1997; Roy and Chatterjee, 1995; Silversides *et al.*, 1995; Veyssiere *et al.*, 1982; Wilson and Lasnitzki, 1971).

Androgens derived from the Leydig interstitial cells stimulate the mesonephric (or Wolffian) ducts to form the male genital ducts, while Sertoli cells produce Müllerian Inhibiting Substance (MIS or Anti Müllerian Hormone (AMH)) which suppresses development of the paramesonephric (Müllerian) ducts, or female genital ducts.

There is differential maturation of the mesonephric ducts depending on location. Near the testis, some tubules persisting and are transformed into efferent ductules, which open into the mesonephric duct, forming the ductus epididymis. Distal to the epididymis, the mesonephric ducts acquire a thickening of smooth muscle to become the ductus deferens, or vas deferens (Moore, 1982).

Development of the external genitalia is similar in the two sexes. In the human the external genitalia are indistinguishable until the ninth week of gestation, and not fully differentiated until the twelfth week of development. Development of the external genitalia coincides with gonadal differentiation. Early in the fourth week of

gestation, the sexually undifferentiated fetus develops a genital tubercle at the cranial end of the cloacal membrane. Labioscrotal (genital) swellings and urogenital (urethral) folds then develop on each side of the cloacal membrane. The genital tubercle then elongates forming a phallus. In response to testicular androgens the phallus enlarges and elongates forming the penis while the labioscrotal swellings ultimately form the scrotum. At the end of the sixth week of gestation, the urorectal septum fuses with the cloacal membrane dividing the membrane into a dorsal anal and a ventral urogenital membrane. Approximately a week following, these membranes rupture forming the anus and urogenital orifice, respectively (Moore, 1982).

Fetal testicular androgens are responsible for the induction of masculinization of the indifferent external genitalia. The testis remains caudally positioned during the tenth to fifteenth week until entry into the inguinal canal and transabdominal descent. Testicular descent through the inguinal canal begins in the twenty-eighth week and the testes enter the scrotum by the thirty-second week. At birth, the testes reach the bottom of the scrotum (Moore, 1982). There are two critical phases of testis descent, transabdominal and inguinoscrotal, essential to move the testes into the scrotum. Although the precise mechanisms of testicular descent, and causes of cryptorchidism, remain unclear the insulin-like peptide hormone INSL3 and fetal testicular androgens are known to play a critical role (Klonisch *et al.*, 2004)—see Fig. 20-3. Cryptorchidism or undescended testes occurs in about 3% of full-term and 30% of preterm males making it the most common human birth defect (Boisen *et al.*,

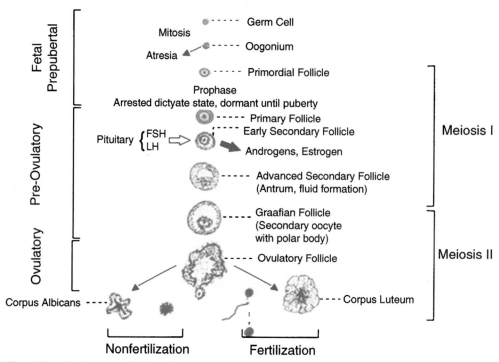

Figure 20-4. Development of the Oocyte.

2004). However, a comparative study of the prevalence of cryptorchidism in cohorts of children in Denmark and Finland, a higher prevalence of cryptorchidism was observed in Denmark, with a 9% incidence rate in full-term males reported at birth (Boisen *et al.*, 2004). These data add further evidence to the concept that there is a significant geographical difference in male reproductive health in two neighboring countries, and therefore potential exposure to similar environmental effects. As the major difference was found in the milder forms of cryptorchidism, an environmental rather than a genetic basis for effect is favored. If correct, there is a need to determine the nature of the environmental agents responsible, because similar agents may well be implicated in the trends noted in other geographically diverse countries where an increasing frequency of cryptorchidism and testicular cancer has been found (Boisen *et al.*, 2004).

Thus male, but not female, reproductive tract development is totally hormonally dependent and thus inherently more susceptible to endocrine disruption (see section "Endocrine Disruption" including "Screening and Puberty"). It is also of note to mention that the early development and triggers of the testis are mediated by direct hormone action before the establishment of the hypothalamic-pituitary-gonadal (HPG) axis.

GAMETOGENESIS

Formation and production of gametes in mammals begins in early embryonic life with the development of primordial germ cells in the genital ridge and movement of these cells into what will become the gonads (see section on sex differentiation). The critical feature in the production of gametes is the process of meiosis.

The basic features of meiosis—two cell divisions with no intervening DNA replication, results in a halving of the chromosome complement—is conserved throughout evolution. Thus, it is not surprising that the general outline applies to both mammalian males and females. However, the strategies employed are remarkably different between the sexes. The mammalian oocyte begins meiosis during fetal development but arrests partway through meiosis I and does not complete the first division until ovulation; the second division is completed only if the egg is fertilized (see Fig. 20-4). Oogenesis therefore requires several start and stop signals and, in some species (e.g., the human), may last for more than 10 years. In contrast, male meiosis begins at puberty and is a continuous process, with spermatocytes progressing from prophase through the meiotic second division in little more than a week. This difference in strategy has implications for the action of toxicants and critical time periods when these cells may be vulnerable to attack (see section on male and female reproductive system). Critical to this is the understanding that the complement of oocytes available to the mammalian female is complete at birth, whereas in the male there is significant stem cell (spermatogonial) renewal to maintain the significantly higher number of germ cells available in males.

NEONATAL DEVELOPMENT

At birth, or even late in gestation, male rats display longer anogenital distances (AGD) than do female rats with neonatal male AGD being more than twice as long as females (Gray *et al.*, 1999). There are homologous sex differences in humans (Longnecker *et al.*, 2007; Swan *et al.*, 2005). Administration of androgen receptor (AR) antagonists or inhibitors of testosterone synthesis can demasculinize male AGD whereas androgen administration during this period lengthens female AGD (Gray *et al.*, 1994, 1999; Hotchkiss *et al.*, 2007; Wolf *et al.*, 2002).

In addition, in many mammalian species, including humans and rats, males of the species engage in more aggressive play than do females (Hines, 2003; Hotchkiss *et al.*, 2003). In the rat, play behavior is displayed for a period of a few weeks around 35 days of age and males engage in more rough and tumble aggressive play than do females. This behavior differentiates during neonatal life and exposure to antiandrogens like flutamide or vinclozolin shortly after birth demasculinizes this behavior such that treated males engage in female-like play at about 35 days of age. In contrast, neonatal androgen treatments masculinize female rat play behavior such that they will engage in male-like levels of rough and tumble play. In humans, sexually dimorphic play behaviors are displayed fairly early in life. Congenital adrenal hyperplasia (CAH) daughters, exposed to high levels of adrenal androgens in utero display male-like play (Hines and Kaufman, 1994). Normally in the rat, the development of this behavior differentiates under the influence of a neonatal surge in testosterone in the first few days of pregnancy, after which fetal testis Leydig cells regress and testosterone production declines to very low levels for a few weeks until the emergence of the adult Leydig cells occurs in the testis prior to puberty (Huhtaniemi and Pelliniemi, 1992). In rodents but not humans, interestingly the first wave of spermatogenesis is initiated at about 4 days of age.

INFANTILE DEVELOPMENT

Later in lactation, during the infantile period of development, several key events occur in the reproductive system of rats including emergence of the nipple buds and areolae in females and maturation of the hypothalamic-pituitary axis. Emergence of the nipple buds is an event most visible around 13 days of age which is prevented in males by prenatal androgen-induced atrophy of the nipple anlagen. It is noteworthy that male rats with the shortest AGD and highest numbers of female-like nipples have a very high likelihood of displaying reproductive tract lesions like hypospadias or epididymal agenesis (Barlow et al., 2004; Hotchkiss et al., 2007). Similarly, prenatally androgen treated females with the longest AGDs and reduced infant nipple numbers are more likely to display reproductive tract malformations (retained male tissues or vaginal agenesis) than less affected females (Hotchkiss et al., 2007). In addition, the effects on AGD are permanent in both sexes (Barlow et al., 2004; Hotchkiss et al., 2004, 2007) with nipple buds being permanent in males.

PUBERTAL DEVELOPMENT

Scientific evidence increasingly supports the concerns about environmentally induced alterations of pubertal events in girls and boys. In addition, experimental animal data are consistent with a potential role of environmental factors in inducing altered pubertal maturation in humans. Puberty is the stage of life when an individual matures from a child, through adolescence to full maturity. The process is marked by dramatic development of hormone dependent sexual characteristics, somatic growth, and sexual and social behaviors eventually resulting in full sexual maturity and reproductive capacity. The stages of puberty in boys and girls are determined using approaches including the Tanner Stages (Marshall and Tanner 1969, 1970) for breast and pubic hair development in girls and gonadal and pubic hair development in boys. Puberty in girls is also assessed using the age at menarche as a marker. Alternatively, increasing levels of estradiol or androgens in the serum prior to some of the development of some of the early physical markers can be used to determine the onset of puberty in girls and boys respectively.

Puberty is initiated by activation of the HPG and hypothalamic-pituitary-adrenal (HPA) axes (Ojeda and Heger, 2001; Ojeda et al., 2003) (see Fig. 20-5). At the onset, the HPG axis releases gonadotropin releasing hormone (GnRH) pulses with increasing frequency and amplitude which induces complimentary pulsatile secretions of luteinizing hormone (LH) and follicle-stimulating hormone

(FSH) from the anterior pituitary (Ojeda et al., 2003). In turn, LH and FSH stimulate the gonads inducing gonadarche characterized by the onset of gonadal hormone production. In the female, secretion of androgens from theca cells and estradiol from granulosa cells of maturing follicles prior to ovulation, followed by secretion of progesterone from the corpus luteum after ovulation, whereas in the male, LH stimulates testicular synthesis and secretion of androgens and insulin-like 3 peptide hormone from the Leydig cells of males. Interestingly, in most mammals including humans and rodents, puberty in the female normally precedes the age of puberty in the male.

In humans, adrenarche, the maturation of adrenal endocrine function, occurs early in pubertal development resulting in the growth of pubic hair, acne, and other secondary sex traits (Auchus and Rainey, 2004). These physical changes result from increasing adrenal synthesis and secretion of steroids including dehydroepiandrosterone (DHEA), dehydroepiandrosterone sulfate (DHEAS), and androstenedione, steroids with weak androgenic activities. Adrenarche is independent of gonadarche and typically occurs between 6 and 8 years of age in both sexes. Adrenarche occurs only in primates and is not associated with puberty in all primate species.

Precocious puberty is defined as the onset of sexual traits before 8 and 9 years of age in girls and boys, respectively, whereas puberty is considered as delayed in girls if thelarche is not displayed by 13 years and at 14 years of age in boys when testicular volume of less than 4 mL (Becker and Epperson, 2006; Biro et al., 2006; Den Hond and Schoeters, 2006; Himes, 2006; Muir, 2006; Ojeda et al., 2006; Papathanasiou and Hadjiathanasiou, 2006; Tuvemo, 2006). Delays in boys can occur as a result of either primary hypothalamic–pituitary or gonadal failure, from head trauma or from infection. While the majority of these delays are transient, some cases are associated with gene mutations resulting in either hypogonadotropic hypogonadism or primary gonadal failure.

Of greatest concern current is the observation that in the United States and several other countries, the age of onset of puberty over the past 40 years has decreased from 0.5 and 1.0 years in girls and the age at menarche has declined by about 0.2 years (Kaplowitz, 2006). Northern European countries have not reported such a trend. Similar trends in male puberty have not been observed and similar trends have not been seen in boys.

Some scientists have attributed the trends in pubertal maturation of girls to obesity rates in children. Rapid early weight gain, obesity, and early development have been associated with the development of insulin resistance and an exaggerated adrenarche (Buck et al., 2007). These endocrine alterations, together with elevated leptin levels and enhancement of hormonal activity by conversion of steroids to estrogens by fat cells, could affect the onset and progression of puberty in young obese girls. In addition, the role of environmental factors including endocrine disrupting chemicals (EDCs) in the etiology of this trend is also being investigated. Alterations of puberty in boys and girls can also be of genetic origin. Precocious puberty may result from early onset of HPG function or via gonadotropin-independent alterations.

Premature thelarche and premature adrenarche are often referred to as pseudoprecocious puberty when the full spectrum of pubertal changes do not occur. Premature thelarche in girls and gynecomastia in boys is known to result from direct exposure estrogen-containing personal care and "natural" products (Henley et al., 2007; Hertz, 1958; Massart et al., 2006). Although these conditions are usually resolved after termination of exposure, untoward

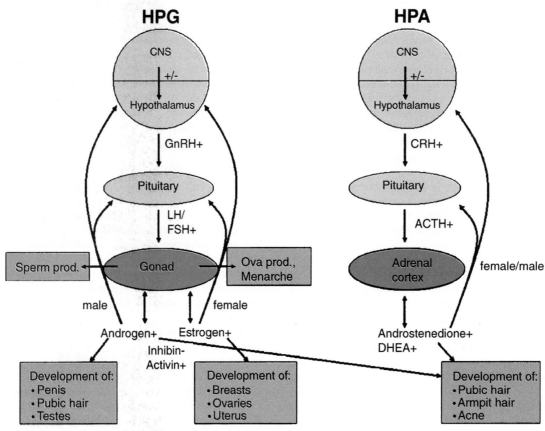

Figure 20-5. Endocrine control of puberty in males and females.

consequences of these conditions may occur with prolonged exposure including shortened stature due to effects of estrogens on the growth plates of the long bones and sexual–social behavior that is inappropriate for chronological age of the child (Wacharasindhu *et al.*, 2006). Concerns have also been expressed that premature thelarche may enhance the likelihood of developing diseases like breast cancer and endometriosis.

Numerous human studies have examined the relationships between environmental factors and human puberty. Many studies have shown a positive relation between body fat and onset of the growth spurt, breast development, or menarche (Battaglia *et al.*, 2005; Biro *et al.*, 2006; Dunger *et al.*, 2005; Himes, 2006; McCartney *et al.*, 2007). Environmental exposure to persistent halogenated organic chemicals such as polychlorinated biphenyls (PCBs) (Den Hond and Schoeters, 2006), DDT/DDE (Charlier, 2006; Gladen *et al.*, 2004; Krstevska-Konstantinova *et al.*, 2001; Ouyang *et al.*, 2005), brominated flame retardants (Blanck *et al.*, 2000), dioxin (Eskenazi *et al.*, 2000; Hauser *et al.*, 2005; Warner *et al.*, 2004; Wolff *et al.*, 2005), hexachlorobenzene (HCB) (Charlier, 2005, 2006), endosulfan (Saiyed *et al.*, 2003), and heavy metals also have been studied for associated with pubertal alterations but a consensus about the causative role of these chemicals in altering puberty has not been achieved.

Rodent Models of Puberty

Rodents provide important animal models in the study of the genetic and environmental factors that regulate puberty. In the rat, GnRH secretion is at low levels during juvenile development until GnRH release is activated by neuronal networks during puberty. During the

onset of puberty there is an increase in the excitatory amino acids and the peptide kisspeptin peptide (Tena-Sempere, 2006) along with decreases in inhibitory neurotransmitters gamma amino butyric acid (GABA), and opioid peptides. In addition, several growth factors like epidermal growth factor (EGF)-like ligands and members of the EGF receptor family contribute to glia-to-neuron communication (Ojeda *et al.*, 2006; Ojeda *et al.*, 2003). While the complete pathway triggering the onset of puberty in rodents has not yet been described, several early components have been identified including the kisspeptin-GPR-54 regulatory system. Mutations of the GPR54 receptor result in absence of puberty in humans and mice (Semple *et al.*, 2005). In addition, leptin (Vogel, 1996)and insulin-like growth factor 1 (IGF-1) Jaruratanasirikul *et al.*, 1999) appear to be in sustaining pubertal events once the process has been initiated.

In the laboratory rat the standard landmarks of puberty in the male are the age of male preputial separation (PPS), an androgen-mediated event, and the ages of vaginal opening (VO), an estrogen-mediated event, and first estrus, with VO normally coinciding with the first estrus and the onset of estrous cycles (Goldman *et al.*, 2000). In the laboratory mouse, VO is not a useful indicator of puberty because it is not associated with the ages at first estrus and the onset of estrous cyclicity.

The ages of VO in females and PPS in male rats were included as required endpoints in the 1998 USEPA multigenerational test guidelines (http://www.epa.gov/opptsfrs/publications/OPPTS_Harmonized/870_Health_Effects_Test_Guidelines/Series/870-3800.pdf). Furthermore, it is generally agreed among risk assessors that statistically significant alterations in pubertal maturation in the rat are adverse effects and these data have been used as a critical effect to establish reference doses in some cases (see the USEPA Vinclozolin risk assessment, 2002). Because EDCs share mechanisms of action in common with many of the drugs used to treat altered human pubertal development, it is biologically plausible that these EDCs would also alter pubertal onset in boys and girls, if children were exposed to sufficient levels of these chemicals during this critical stage of life.

Toxicants can alter puberty as a consequence of in utero, lactational, or pubertal exposures. In a multigenerational study, discerning the stage of life when exposure induced the alteration may be challenging, if possible at all, because dosing is not initiated in the parent (F_0) generation, the only generation with in utero and lactational exposure, until well after puberty. Some alternate reproductive test protocols (Gray et al., 1988a) can detect pubertal alterations in the F_0 generation since they initiate exposure right after weaning. In addition, short-term studies using the pubertal male and female rat assays (EDSTAC Final report, 1998) (Gray et al., 2004a) can help resolve this uncertainty since exposures are initiated directly to the weanling rat and continued for 20–30 days for females and males, respectively. Comprehensive reviews describing the toxicology of puberty in rodents are found elsewhere (Goldman et al., 2000; Stoker et al., 2000; Gray et al., 2004).

Studies using rats demonstrate that body weight at weaning is an important determinant of the age of VO in the female and PPS in the male. However, treatments that reduce growth by 10% or less have little effect on the attainment of the male and female pubertal landmarks. The onset of puberty can be altered in the male and female rat by disrupting the endocrine system at a variety of levels including the entire HPG axis. In addition to effects on the HPG axis, the landmarks of female rat puberty can be altered by the direct action of either estrogens or antiestrogens on VO and other components of the reproductive tract, whereas, androgens and antiandrogens can alter male rat pubertal landmarks by acting at the level of the male reproductive tract.

Because estrogen exposure in the peripubertal female rat can accelerate the onset of VO and at the age of the first estrus smear without accelerating the onset of regular estrous cycles it is useful to monitor all three landmarks of puberty in the female in order to discriminate pseudoprecocious puberty (accelerated age at VO but not the onset of estrous cyclicity) from true precocious puberty (both the ages at VO and the onset of estrous cyclicity are accelerated).

Selected Examples of Chemicals That Alter the Onset of Pubertal Landmarks in Rats After Acute in Utero and/or Lactational Exposures In utero exposure to 2, 3, 7, 8-tetrachlorodibenzo-p-dioxin (TCDD) (a single dose of 0.001 mg/kg on gestational day (GD) 15) delays the onset of pubertal landmarks in male and female rats (Gray et al., 1995; Gray and Ostby, 1995; Gray et al., 1997b; Gray et al., 1997c). The mode of action for these effects is not known but it likely involves permanent organizational effects of TCDD of the reproductive tract during sexual differentiation mediated via arylhydrocarbon receptor, AhR. In addition, the treated females display a persistent vaginal thread after puberty.

In utero exposure to the potent alkalating drug busulfan at (5 and 10 mg/kg sc on GD 15) destroys fetal germ cells resulting in gonadal atrophy and delayed puberty in both male and female rats (Gray and Ostby, 1998). Some females never displayed VO, or any other pubertal landmark likely due to a total absence of primary follicles in the ovary.

Prenatal androgen administration can induce agenesis of the lower vaginal canal in females, an effect that could be missed entirely of misconstrued as just a delay in VO unless the females are retained after weaning and thoroughly examined after the normal age at puberty (Hotchkiss et al., 2007). Conversely, prenatal antiandrogen-treatments can result in the formation of a lower vaginal "pouch" in treated male rats (Gray et al., 1994).

Administration of estrogens like ethinyl estradiol (EE) or methoxychlor (MXC) to the dam during gestation and lactation can accelerate VO in female rat offspring. In the higher dosage groups VO can be detected as early as 10–15 days of age, albeit a "pin-hole" like opening (Gray et al., 1989).

Peripubertal administration of EDCs can alter the onset of pubertal landmarks in male (Gray et al., 2004b; Monosson et al., 1999) and female rats (Goldman et al., 2000). Androgens play a key role in pubertal maturation in young males and antiandrogens like vinclozolin (Monosson et al., 1999), linuron (Gray et al., 1999), o,p' DDE (Kelce et al., 1995), prochloraz (Blystone et al., 2007), and the phthalates (Gray et al., 1999) produce measurable delays in this process. For example, vinclozolin treatment delayed pubertal maturation and retarded sex accessory gland and epididymal growth (at 30 and 100 mg/kg/d) (Monosson et al., 1999). Serum LH (significant at all dosage levels), testosterone and 5α-androstane, 3α,17β-diol (at 100 mg/kg/d) levels were increased. Testis size and sperm production, however, were unaffected. In contrast, reproductive toxicants like carbendazim that indirectly alter FSH levels without affecting serum testosterone fail to delay PPS even at dosage levels that cause profound alterations of testicular and hypothalamic-pituitary (FSH secretion) function (Gray et al., 1990).

The ease with which a delay in PPS, a landmark of puberty in the rat, can be measured enables us to use this endpoint to evaluate chemicals for this form of endocrine activity. A "pubertal male assay" including an assessment of PPS is being considered by the USEPA and others (Gray, 1998; Gray et al., 1997a; Stoker et al., 2000) for screening chemicals for endocrine activity, as mandated by 1996 U.S. legislation (the Food Quality Protection Act and Safe Drinking Water Act).

Selected Examples of Chemicals That Alter the Onset of Pubertal Landmarks in Rats After Peripubertal Exposures The "pubertal female rat assay" assay has been included in the proposed EDSTAC Tier 1 Screening (T1S) battery. In this assay, weanling female rats are dosed daily by gavage for 21 days and the age at VO (puberty) is monitored and the females are necropsied at about 42 days of age (reviewed by Goldman et al., 2000). Vaginal estrous cycles are also determined by daily observation by light microscopy of the cell types present in a vaginal lavage, taken from VO until necropsy. Necropsy measurements include serum thyroid hormones, and uterine and ovarian weight and histology. This assay detects alterations in thyroid hormone status, HPG function, and inhibition of steroidogenesis, estrogens and antiestrogens. Recently, in studies from different laboratories the pubertal female assay was found to be highly reproducible and very sensitive to certain endocrine activities including estrogenicity, inhibition of steroidogenesis, and antithyroid activity (Gray et al., 2004b) (see Table 20-4).

The "pubertal male assay rat" (Gray et al., 2004; Stoker et al., 2000; Monosson et al., 1999) detects alterations of thyroid function, HPG maturation, steroidogenesis, and altered steroid hormone function (androgen). Intact weanling males are exposed to the test substance for about 30 days, the age at puberty is determined and

Table 20-4

Chemicals evaluated by the U.S. Environmental Protection Agency (EPA) using the standardized pubertal female rat assay in two contract laboratories or key studies performed in other laboratories

STUDIES PERFORMED IN LABORATORY 1 FOR THE EPA

Ethinyl estradiol: Positive estrogenic control
Tamoxifen: Mixed estrogen agonist–antagonist; successfully identified mixed action
Ketoconazole: Inhibits steroidogenesis; caused ovarian histological changes
Methoxychlor: Estrogenic pesticide; successfully detected by accelerated puberty
Phenobarbital: Alters liver, hypothalamic, pituitary, and ovarian function; delays puberty
Studies performed in Laboratory 2 for the EPA
Methoxychlor: Estrogenic pesticide; successfully detected by accelerated puberty
Ketoconazole: Inhibits steroidogenesis; caused ovarian histological changes
Bisphenol A: Weakly estrogenic plastic monomer; negative for endocrine effects
Propylthiouracil: Antithyroid agent; lowered T4, increased thyroid-stimulating hormone, and caused thyroid histological
  changes at low doses that slightly delayed rat puberty
Fenarimol: Fungicide that weakly inhibits aromatase; slight delay in puberty, but lowered T4 and retarded growth
Atrazine: Herbicide that alters hypothalamic-pituitary function; delays puberty and growth
Key published studies performed in other laboratories
Methoxychlor: Estrogenic pesticide; accelerates puberty (Gray et al., 1989)b
Polybrominated diphenyl ether: DE71; antithyroid toxicant; affected thyroid endpoints and delayed puberty (Stoker
  et al., 2004b)b
Fadrazole: Potent aromatase inhibitor; delayed puberty (Marty et al., 1999)b
Antarelix: Gonadotropin-releasing hormone antagonist; delayed puberty (Ashby et al., 2002b)b
Octylphenol: Estrogenic surfactant; accelerates female rat puberty (Gray and Ostby, 1998)b
DES: Estrogenic pharmaceutical; accelerated puberty (Kim et al., 2002)b
Tamoxifen: A mixed agonist/antagonistic drug; accelerated puberty (Kim et al., 2002)b
ICI 182,780: Estrogen receptor (ER) antagonist; delayed puberty (Ashby et al., 2002a)b
ZM 189,154: ER antagonist; delayed puberty (Ashby et al., 2002a)b

Pubertal female assay data from contract laboratories (Summary available at http://www.epa.gov/scipoly/oscpendo/assayvalidation/meetings.htm.

reproductive tissues are evaluated and serum taken for optional hormonal analyses. This assay produced reproducible responses among different labs and was sensitive to androgens, antiandrogens, inhibitors of steroidogenesis and antithyroid activity. The chemicals studied to date in this assay are listed in Table 20-5.

When antiandrogenic chemicals are administered to juvenile male rats these chemicals do not induce malformations of the reproductive tract but pubertal development is delayed. Throughout puberty and into adulthood, the sex accessory glands and other androgen-dependent tissues (i.e., muscles, nervous system) continue to be dependent upon testosterone (T) and 5α-dihydrotestosterone (DHT) for maturation and maintenance of function (7). Several androgen dependent events occur during puberty, most notably the separation of the prepuce from the penis (PPS), followed 10 days to 2 weeks later by the appearance of mature sperm in the epididymis (Monosson et al., 1999). During pubertal maturation, there are gradual changes in serum concentrations of testosterone (T) and of its metabolite 5α-androstanediol. In very young rats, 5α-androstanediol is present in greater quantities than T. T concentrations begin to increase, however, as 5α-reductase activity decreases in the Leydig cells, resulting in higher serum T concentrations than androstanediol in older rats. Peak T concentrations generally occur around 50–60 days of age.

In addition to delaying PPS, some antiandrogens also alter serum LH and T, while others do not. In particular, peripubertal exposure to flutamide (from 23 to 38 days of age) or vinclozolin (from 23 to 55 days of age) causes reductions in prostate, seminal vesicle, and epididymis in rats whereas serum LH and testosterone are increased (Monosson et al., 1999).

SEXUAL MATURITY

Hypothalamo-Pituitary-Gonadal Axis

FSH and LH are glycoproteins synthesized and released from a subpopulation of the basophilic gonadotropic cells of the pituitary gland. Hypothalamic neuroendocrine neurons secrete specific releasing or release-inhibiting factors into the hypophyseal portal system, which carries them to the adenohypophysis, where they act to stimulate or inhibit the release of anterior pituitary hormones. GnRH acts on gonadotropic cells, thereby stimulating the release of FSH and LH. Native and synthetic forms of GnRH stimulate the release of both gonadotrophic hormones.

The neuroendocrine neurons have nerve terminals containing monoamines (norepinephrine, dopamine, serotonin) that impinge on them. Reserpine, chlorpromazine, and monoamine oxidase (MAO) inhibitors modify the content or actions of brain monoamines that affect gonadotrophin production.

In the female (see Fig. 20-6 for structure of the female reproductive tract of the rat and Fig. 20-7 for basic endocrine control), LH acts on thecal cells of the ovary to induce steroidogenesis, particularly the production of progesterone and androgens which are transferred to the granulosa cells which can be stimulated by FSH to produce estradiol. These steroids then feedback on the hypothalamus and

Table 20-5

Chemicals evaluated by the U.S. Environmental Protection Agency (EPA) using the standardized pubertal male rat assay in two contract laboratories or key studies performed in other laboratories

STUDIES PERFORMED IN LABORATORY 1 FOR THE EPA

Flutamide: Potent antiandrogenic drug; delayed puberty, among other effects
Ketoconazole: Inhibits steroidogenesis
Methyltestosterone: Androgenic drug; accelerated puberty
Phenobarbital: Alters liver, hypothalamic, pituitary, and testis function; delayed puberty, among other effects
Vinclozolin: Antiandrogenic fungicide; delayed puberty puberty, among other effects
Dibutyl Phthalate: Plasticizer that inhibits Leydig cell testosterone function; delayed puberty, among other effects

Studies performed in Laboratory 2 for the EPA
Vinclozolin: Antiandrogenic fungicide; delayed puberty puberty, among other effects
Linuron: Antiandrogenic herbicide; delayed puberty, among other effects
***p,p′*-DDE**: Antiandrogenic pesticide metabolite; delayed puberty, among other effects
Phenobarbital: Alters liver, hypothalamic, pituitary, and testis function; delayed puberty, among other effects
Methoxychlor: Estrogenic and antiandrogenic pesticide; reduced androgen-dependent tissues weights
Ketoconazole: Inhibits steroidogenesis
Atrazine: Herbicide, alters hypothalamic pituitary function; delays puberty and growth

Key published studies performed in other laboratories
Vinclozolin: Androgen receptor antagonistic fungicide; delayed puberty, increase serum T and luteinizing hormone
  (Monosson *et al.*, 1999)
Cyproterone acetate: Antiandrogenic drug; delayed puberty, among other effects
Polybrominated diphenyl ether, DE71; antithyroid toxicant; affected thyroid endpoints and delayed puberty (Stoker *et al.*, 2004a,b)
Finasteride: Potent inhibitor of enzyme 5 alpha reductase required for dihydrotesterone synthesis; reduced sex gland weight (Marty *et al.*, 2001)

Pubertal female and pubertal male assay data from contract laboratories (summary available at http://www.epa.gov/scipoly/oscpendo/assayvalidation/meetings.htm.)

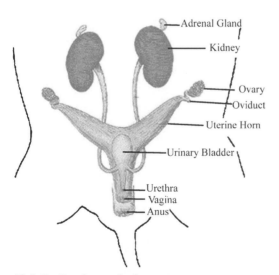

Figure 20-6. Rat Female reproductive system.

pituitary to regulate gonadotrophin production (see later sections on ovarian function).

Similarly in the male (see Fig. 20-8 for the basic structure of the male reproductive system and Fig. 20-9 for basic endocrine control), FSH acts primarily on the Sertoli cells, but it also appears to stimulate the mitotic activity of spermatogonia. LH stimulates steroidogenesis in the interstitial Leydig cells. A defect in the function of the testis (in the production of spermatozoa or testosterone)

will tend to be reflected in increased levels of FSH and LH in serum because of the lack of the "negative feedback" effect of testicular hormones.

The HPG feedback system is a very delicately modulated hormonal process. Several sites in the endocrine process can be perturbed by different chemicals.

Ovarian Function

Oogenesis Ovarian germ cells with their follicles have a dual origin; the theca or stromal cells arise from fetal connective tissues of the ovarian medulla, the granulosa cells from the cortical mesenchyme (Fig. 20-4). In women, about 400,000 follicles are present at birth in each human ovary. After birth, many undergo atresia, and those that survive are continuously reduced in number. Any chemical that damages the oocytes will accelerate the depletion of the pool and can lead to reduced fertility in females. About one-half of the numbers of oocytes present at birth remain at puberty; the number is reduced to about 25,000 by 30 years of age. About 400 primary follicles will yield mature ova during a woman's reproductive life span. During the approximately three decades of fecundity, follicles in various stages of growth can always be found. After menopause, follicles are no longer present in the ovary (Knobil and Neill, 1994).

Follicles remain in a primary follicle stage following birth until puberty, when a number of follicles start to grow during each ovarian cycle. However, most fail to achieve maturity. For the follicles that continue to grow, the first event is an increase in size of the primary oocytes. During this stage, fluid-filled spaces appear among the cells

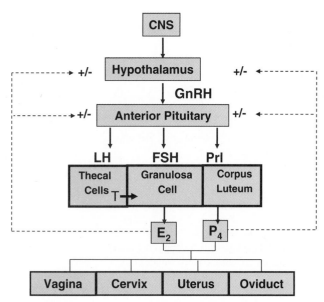

Figure 20-7. *Endocrine Control of the Female Reproductive cycle.*

CNS – Central Nervous system; GnRH – gonadotrophin releasing hormone; LH – luteinizing hormone; FSH – follicle stimulating hormone; Prl – Prolactin; T – testosterone; E_2 – estradiol; P_4 – progesterone.

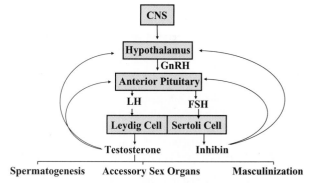

Figure 20-9. *Endocrine control of male reproduction.*

of the follicle, which unite to form a cavity or antrum, otherwise known as the Graafian follicle.

Primary oocytes undergo two specialized nuclear divisions, which result in the formation of four cells containing one-half the number of chromosomes (Fig. 20-4). The first meiotic division occurs within the ovary just before ovulation, and the second occurs just after the sperm fuses with the egg. In the first stage of meiosis, the primary oocyte is actively synthesizing DNA and protein in preparation for entering prophase. The DNA content doubles as each of the prophase chromosomes produces its mirror image. Each doubled chromosome is attracted to its homologous mate to form tetrads. The members of the tetrads synapse or come to lie side by side. Before separation, the homologous pairs of chromosomes exchange genetic material by a process known as crossing over. Thus, qualitative differences occur between the resulting gametes. Subsequent meiotic stages distribute the members of the tetrads to the daughter cells in such a way that each cell receives the haploid number of chromosomes. At telophase, one secondary oocyte and a polar body have been formed, which are no longer genetically identical.

The secondary oocyte enters the next cycle of division very rapidly; each chromosome splits longitudinally; the ovum and the three polar bodies now contain the haploid number of chromosomes and half the amount of genetic material. Although the nuclei of all four eggs are equivalent, the cytoplasm is divided unequally. The end products are one large ovum and three rudimentary ova (polar bodies), which subsequently degenerate. The ovum is released from the ovary at the secondary oocyte stage; the second stage of meiotic division is triggered in the oviduct by the entry of the sperm.

Although ovarian weight, unlike uterine weight, in the rat does not fluctuate during the estrous cycle, ovarian weight and histology can provide very useful information about the effects of toxicants on the female reproductive system. Ovarian weight can be reduced

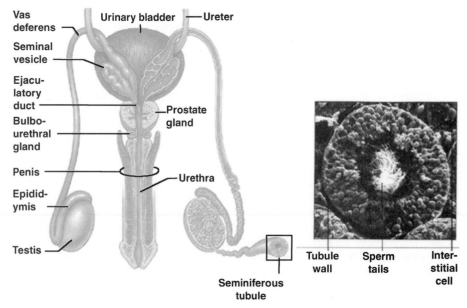

Figure 20-8. *Male reproductive system.*

by either depletion of oocytes or disruption of the HPG axis. Toxicants affect ovarian histology inducing a variety of lesions, including polyovular follicles, oocyte depletion, interstitial cell hyperplasia, corpora albanicans, and absence of corpora lutea, for example. In addition, ovarian tissue can be cultured ex vivo after in vivo treatment or in vitro at different stages of the estrous cycle or during pregnancy to assess their steroidogenic capacity (Berman and Laskey, 1993; Calafat et al., 2006; Gray et al., 1997a).

Case Study—Busulphan The drug busulfan is an alkylating agent used to treat several diseases in humans including chronic myelogenous leukemia, certain myeloproliferative disorders such as severe thrombocytosis and polycythemia vera and busulfan is also used in combination with other drugs to treat myelofibrosis. Busulfan has been used in very high doses and in combination with other drugs to destroy the bone marrow in preparation for a bone marrow transplant. Busulfan may interfere with the normal menstrual cycles in women and block sperm production in men. In addition, busulfan causes ovarian failure and prevents or delays the onset of puberty in girls (http://www.nlm.nih.gov/medlineplus/ druginfo/medmaster/a682248.html).

In the rat, busulfan produces a similar profile of reproductive effects, the most dramatic occuring in utero. In rodents, endocrine function during adulthood can be altered by prenatal exposure to fetal germ cell toxicants. The ovary of the treated female offspring, lacking oocytes, developing follicles (the source of most serum estradiol) or corpora lutea (the major source of progesterone) fails to produce sex hormones. Administration of busulfan (10 mg/kg ip 5–7 d before birth) specifically inhibits germ cell development (Hemsworth and Jackson, 1963) in rats. Offspring of rats dose with 2.5 and 5 mg busulfan/kg on gestational day 14 display permanent reproductive and CNS alterations (Gray and Ostby, 1998). The most severely affected females do not display estrous cycles or spontaneous sexual behavior as a consequence of this effect. Puberty was markedly delayed in females treated with 10 mg of busulfan. In male progeny, testicular (at 2.5 mg), epididymal (2.5 mg), and ejaculated sperm (5.0 mg) counts, fertility and fecundity (10 mg), measured under continuous breeding conditions, were reduced. In female progeny, fertility and fecundity (2.5 mg) and ovarian weight (5 mg) were reduced and the incidence of constant vaginal estrus was increased (10 mg). In addition to these reproductive effects, brain weight was reduced in both sexes all dosage groups, even though body and other nonreproductive organ weights were only affected in the high-dose group (10 mg). Even though the gonads of both sexes were affected at similar dosage levels, fertility and gonadal hormone production were much more easily disrupted in female than male offspring, because the steroid producing cells in the ovary fail to differentiate in the absence of the oocyte. In the male, Leydig cell numbers and steroidogenesis are not so dependent upon normal gametogenesis. Hence, the lack of oocytes in the female progeny results in a lack of estrous cyclicity and the spontaneous display of female mating behavior at proestrus. Technically, busulphan is not considered to be an EDC because the cells that it eliminates, the oocytes, do not display endocrine activity. However, this classification is of little import because in their absence, ovarian thecal and granulosa cell endocrine functions are severely impaired.

In addition to busulfan, several environmental chemicals have been shown to disrupt ovarian development and oocyte numbers in the rat or mouse. Oral administration of some of the benzidine-based dyes on days 8–12 of pregnancy in the mouse or rat produces reproductive effects in the female offspring similar to those seen with the lower dose levels of busulfan, albeit at much higher dose levels (1 g/kg/d) (Gray and Kelce, 1996).

4-Vinylcyclohexene (VCH) is a chemical intermediate used in the production of flame retardants, flavors and fragrances, in the manufacture of polyolefins, and as a solvent and in the manufacture of its diepoxide. Low levels of occupational exposure have been measured during the production and use of 1,3-butadiene. In the mouse, 4-VCH destroys the small preantral follicles in the ovaries (Hoyer and Sipes, 2007) and the monoepoxide metabolites, 1,2-VCH epoxide, 7,8-VCH epoxide, and the diepoxide, VCD, cause preantral follicle loss in rats as well as mice. Mice are more susceptible to VCH than rats because they are capable of its metabolic bioactivation. Follicle destruction by VCD is selective for primordial and primary follicles and results from upregulating the rate of atresia (apoptosis) through activation of proapoptotic signaling events selectively in the small preantral follicles.

MXC is an organochlorine pesticide and reproductive toxicant that also produces antral follicle atresia, in part by altering apoptotic regulators (Bcl-2 and Bax). MXC directly inhibits follicle growth partly by Bcl-2 and Bax pathways, and increases atresia partly through Bcl-2 pathways (Miller et a,., 2005) by inducing oxidative stress (Gupta et al., 2006a, 2006b). A diagrammatic representation of the sites of actions of female reproductive toxicants is presented in Fig. 20-10.

Ovarian Cycle

The cyclic release of pituitary gonadotropins involving the secretion of ovarian progesterone and estrogen is depicted in Fig. 20-11. These female sex steroids determine ovulation and prepare the female accessory sex organs to receive the male sperm. Sperm, ejaculated into the vagina, must make their way through the cervix into the uterus, where they are capacitated. Sperm then migrate into the oviducts, where fertilization takes place. The conceptus then returns from the oviducts to the uterus and implants into the endometrium. This axis can be disrupted, resulting in infertility at any level of the endocrine system. For example, chemicals that block the LH surge transiently can prevent or delay ovulation resulting in infertility or lower fecundity due to delayed fertilization of ova (Cooper et al., 1994, 2000; Goldman et al., 1997, 1994, 1993; Stoker et al., 1996, 1993, 2001, 2003, 2005).

Postovarian Processes

Female accessory sex organs function to bring together the ovulated ovum and the ejaculated sperm. The chemical composition and viscosity of reproductive tract fluids, as well as the epithelial morphology of these organs, are controlled by ovarian (and trophoblastic) hormones (see Fig. 20-6).

Oviducts The oviducts provide the taxis of the fimbria, which is under muscular control. The involvement of the autonomic nervous system in this process, as well as in oviductal transport of both the male and female gametes, raises the possibility that drugs known to alter the autonomic nervous system may alter function and therefore fertility. The progression of the fertilized eggs through the oviduct and uterus is under hormonal regulation and chemicals like the estrogens can stimulate oviductal transport and interfere with uterine endometrial function, precluding implantation (Cummings and Perreault, 1990).

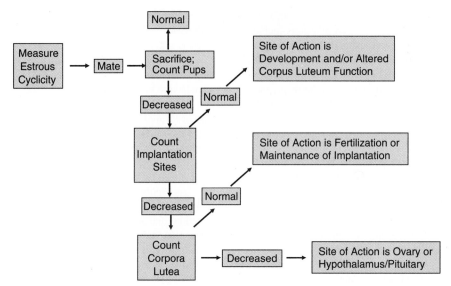

Figure 20-10. Sites of action for female reproductive toxicants.

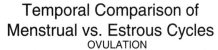

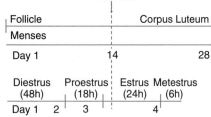

Figure 20-11. Comparison of the human menstrual cycle with the rat estrus cycle.

LH – luteinizing hormone; FSH – follicle stimulating hormone; PRL – Prolactin; E_2 – estradiol; P_4 – progesterone; hCG – human chorionic gonadotrophin; rCG – rat chorionic gonadotrophin.

Uterus Uterine endometrium reflects the cyclicity of the ovary as it is prepared to receive the conceptus. The myometrium's major role is contractile. In primates, at the end of menstruation, all but the deep layers of the endometrium are sloughed. Under the influence of estrogens from the developing follicle, the endometrium increases rapidly in thickness. The uterine glands increase in length but do not secrete to any degree. These endometrial changes are called proliferative. After ovulation, the endometrium becomes slightly edematous, and the actively secreting glands become tightly coiled and folded under the influence of estrogen and progesterone from the corpus luteum. These are secretory (progestational) changes (Fig. 20-11). When fertilization fails to occur, the endometrium is shed and a new cycle begins. Only primates menstruate (Knobil and Neill, 1994).

Other mammals have estrous cycles rather than menstrual cycles, see Figs. 20-12 and 20-13 for a diagrammatic comparison of the human menstrual and rat estrous cycles with regard to timing and endocrine control. In the young adult rat, the female has a 4–5 day estrous cycle which lacks a functional luteal phase (Knobil and Neill, 1994; Cooper *et al.*, 1984). During the estrous cycle the uterus and vagina display remarkable changes in morphology over

the brief cycle. Uterine weight and fluid content increase many folds during proestrus under the influence of estrogen. The vaginal cytology also changes daily throughout the estrous cycle and this can be monitored by examining the cytology of the cells sloughed from the vaginal epithelium into the lumen with daily vaginal lavages.

Uterine weight is a very useful index of estrogenicity in the immature or adult ovariectomized female rat. Since uterine weight and histology fluctuate greatly during the estrous cycle, studies which necropsy females at different stages of the cycle will often be too variable to detect anything but the most profound effects on these endpoints, but nonetheless it can still be a useful endpoint and should be measured. A single vaginal lavage, taken at necropsy could be used as a covariate to analyze for treatment effects. It is noteworthy that both uterine weight and ovarian histology provided useful information in a surprising number of cases in the assessment of chemicals in the Pubertal Female Rat Assay being validated by the USEPA, OSCP, EDSP (reports available at http://www.epa.gov/scipoly/oscpendo/).

TESTICULAR STRUCTURE AND FUNCTION

Targets for Toxicity

For the adult male, the overall objective of the reproductive process is the production of gametes capable of fertilization and the production of viable offspring. In considering these processes there are numerous potential targets for the action of chemicals upon the system (see Fig. 20-13). These would range from the action of dopamine analogues on the hypothalamus interrupting the normal secretion of GnRH, the action of estrogens on the pituitary (and hypothalamus) to interfere with gonadotropin (LH and FSH—see Fig. 20-7) production through direct effects on spermatogenesis—where the vast majority of toxicants have their site of action. However, there are specific examples of chemicals that may impair spermatogenesis via an indirect mechanism not specifically related to the HPG axis. So for example, there are a number of examples of nutritional deficits (and overexposures) of critical vitamins and minerals (e.g., vitamin A and zinc) that are essential for normal reproduction. Perturbing the homeostasis of these nutrients can lead to direct effects on spermatogenesis and subsequent issues with fertility. Similarly,

Comparative Endocrinology of Menstrual and Estrous Cycles and Early Pregnancy

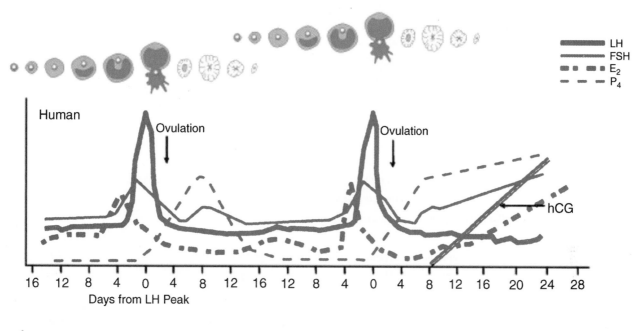

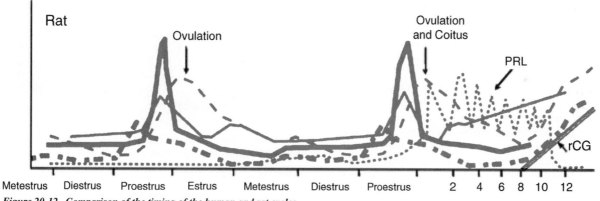

Figure 20-12. Comparison of the timing of the human and rat cycles.

chemicals that have direct effects on the liver (e.g., CCl₄) can disturb the normal metabolism of sex steroids leading to changes in clearance (predominantly of glucuronide and sulfate conjugates of hydroxytestosterones in the male), indirectly affecting the HPG axis and exerting effects on male reproduction.

While most experimental rodents normally employed in reproductive toxicity studies do not show marked seasonality in breeding performance, there are dramatic exceptions (for example, the hamster, where during the breeding season (or under lab conditions of 14-hours light and 10-hours dark) up to 10% of an adult male's body weight may be testicular tissue). In the hamster markedly changing the light dark cycle to reduce the hours of daylight can influence melatonin levels and through a cascade of signaling responses cause regression of the testes and concurrent decreases in testicular steroids and mating behavior. This is a normal circumstance in the wild, but care should be taken in laboratory situations to ensure appropriate housing for the conduct of reproduction studies with this species.

The testis also has a finely tuned circulatory system in mammals, termed the pampininform plexus, design to shunt the arterial venous blood supply and aid in scrotal cooling. Some chemicals can actually target this structure and the testis circulatory system to induce ischemic shock to the testis resulting in injury and reduced fertility, with cadmium being an example of a chemical that can induce testicular damage via this "indirect" mechanism (Setchell and Waites, 1970).

Testicular Structure and Spermatogenesis

The experimenter should be cognizant of these indirect mechanisms affecting male reproductive biology, however the overwhelming number of chemicals known to affect the male reproductive system appears to do so by a direct effect on the testis and an interference with the process of spermatogenesis. In rodents, there is a highly efficient process for the production of sperm in large numbers. A simple cross section of the testis from a rat (see Fig. 20-14), the

POTENTIAL TARGET SITES

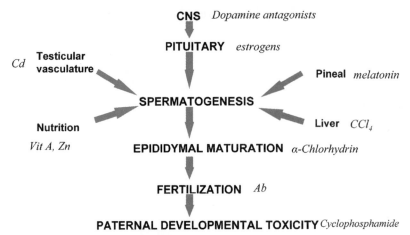

Figure 20-13. Potential target sites for male reproductive toxicants.

Examples of agents shown in italics.

most common species employed in reproductive toxicity studies, indicates that not all of the seminiferous tubules have an identical morphology. The generalized structure of the rat seminiferous tubule (see Figs 20-15 and 20-16) shows the organization of a number of different cell types comprising germ cells at different stages of differentiation supported by a somatic cell, the Sertoli cell, that provides structure to the epithelium and numerous support functions (e.g., hormonal signaling, nutrition, fluid provision, etc.) and serves to maintain the haploid germ cells in a protected environment (the so-called blood- tubule barrier) because these would be recognized as foreign by the host immune system. Thus, the seminiferous tubules can be divided into a number of physiological compartments (as indicated in Fig. 20-15) that facilitate the process of spermatogenesis. The boundary of the seminiferous tubule is surrounded by myoepithelial cells that aid in a peristaltic process in moving released spermatozoa present in the lumina of the tubules (at this time these sperm are both nonmotile and nonfertile) along the tubules through the rete testis (into which the seminiferous tubules open—these tubules have both ends attached to the rete) for further progression through the efferent ducts to the epididymis. It is here that a concentration of sperm and changes in their fluid environment occur as the sperm are ushered through the epididymis and acquire motility and fertilizing ability.

Spermatogenesis is an extremely ordered process in the rat (see Fig. 20-17). The spermatogonia have populations that act as the stem cells for the seminiferous tubules and a proportion of these cells then undergo a series of mitotic divisions to increase numbers, move into meiotic prophase and are then committed to becoming spermatozoa. These germ cells proceed through the various stages of prophase, preleptotene, leptotene, zygotene, and pachytene with increasingly larger cells that undertake DNA replication in preparation for the cells to enter meiosis. The germ cells enter diplotene and then diakinesis with two meiotic divisions, which eventually results in the production of the haploid spermatid population. These initially round cells then undergo an incredible metamorphosis to produce the elongated spermatozoa that mature and are then released into the seminiferous tubule lumen.

The spermatogonial stem cells undergo another round of mitotic division every approximately 13 days in the rat to produce

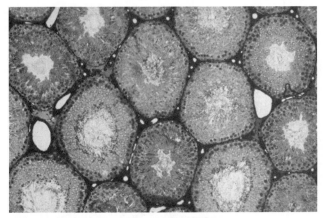

Figure 20-14. Control testis indicating different cellular associations noted in different seminiferous tubule cross-sections.

See also Fig. 20-19.

another wave of division and differentiation (see Fig. 20-18). For the rat, the time taken for a spermatogonial stem cell to become a mature spermatozoan takes approximately 8 weeks (and 10 weeks for humans) with an additional 10 days to 2 weeks for the released sperm to mature in the epididymis and be capable for ejaculation and fertilization of the ovum. One of the consequences of these successive longitudinal waves of differentiation is the highly ordered sequence of events reflected in seminiferous tubular morphology. The most primitive germ cells, the spermatogonia, reside at the periphery of the tubule and as they mature, they move toward the tubule lumen for eventual release (in a process termed spermiation). As can be seen from the Fig. 20-18, at any one time the tubule can contain cellular members from four and a half successive spermatogenic cycles, with the most primitive spermatogonia from the current cycle and the most mature, the late spermatids (about to become spermatozoa on release), generated up to 4.5 cycles earlier. Thus when we take a cross section through a seminiferous tubule, this is essentially taking a "snapshot" in time of the various spermatogenic cycles. This also explains why different tubular cross sections

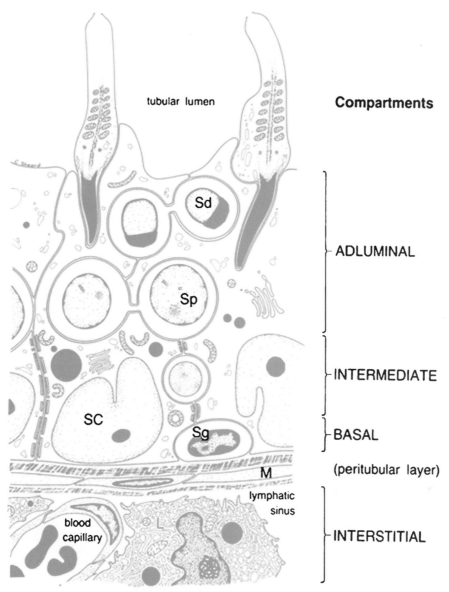

Figure 20-15. *Diagrammatic representation of a portion of a seminiferous tubule showing the cellular arragements and testicular compartments.*

Key: L – Leydig cell; M – myoepithelial peritubular cell; SC – Sertoli cell; Sd spermatid; Sg – spermatogonium and Sp – spermatocyte. (From Foster, 1988).

have different morphologies, depending on when this "snapshot" is taken because of different cellular associations resulting from different cycles. It is possible for the various species to construct a morphological diagram of the nature of these cellular associations (Fig. 20-19 illustrates this for the rat). The most common system employed for the rat was based on that published by Leblond and Clermont and describes 14 different patterns of cellular association (or stages—usually depicted by a roman numeral). We know that different biochemical events can go on during the different stages and indeed this can provide clues as to potential mode of action of chemicals that produce stage specific lesions. Such occurrences do occur regularly (e.g., certain phthalate esters, glycol ethers, antiandrogenic agents etc.). In the case of a phthalate ester given to an adult rat there is a marked stage specificity in response which coincides with those stages that have the highest concentrations of

FSH receptors (in the Sertoli cells of the tubule) (Creasy *et al.*, 1987). Other Sertoli cell in vitro data indicate that the phthalate ester metabolites responsible for in vivo damage could down regulate Sertoli cell responsiveness to FSH with regard to cAMP production (Lloyd and Foster, 1988) lending support to the establishment of a potential mode of action for this class of chemicals in adult rats.

At spermiation, when the step 19 spermatids are released into the seminiferous tubule lumen, the excess cytoplasm and cellular debris form a residual body that is then phagocytosed by the Sertoli cell. These bodies originate at the luminal surface of the tubule and then as they are resorbed, can be seen to move through the Sertoli cell toward the base of the tubule and eventually disappear. Delays in spermiation—that is step 19 late spermatids being retained beyond Stage VIII of the cycle are one of the more subtle yet commonly noted testicular lesions (e.g., boric acid, Chapin and Ku,

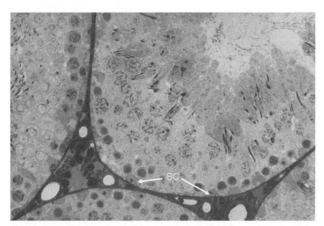

Figure 20-16. *Section of a rat seminiferous tubules showing the orientation of different germ cells and Sertoli cells (SC).*

Compare with Figs. 20-15 and 20-18.

1994; Gray *et al.*, 1990); dibromoacetic acid (Linder *et al.*, 1997; Melnick *et al.*, 2006); and hormonal withdrawal (Saito *et al.*, 2000) and are sometimes accompanied by abnormal residual body formation. Having this "extra" layer of germ cells is a lesion frequently missed by pathologists without a good knowledge and appreciation of the stages of the spermatogenic cycle.

Once sperm are released into the seminiferous tubule lumen and proceed to the epididymis, they can also be the target of toxi-

cant action. Chlorosugars and epichlohydrin have both been shown to inhibit energy metabolism in sperm that prevents them from functioning normally. The specificity of the response was noted, at least in part, from the specific isoform of lactate dehydrogenase found in testicular germs cells (LDH-X or C4) essential for energy production. We are now learning more about the molecular events that drive fertilization and it seems likely that here may be a potential target for the action of chemicals to disturb the process. We certainly know of the requirement for the expression of critical cell surface markers by the sperm that facilitate the normal binding of the sperm to the egg surface membrane. Lastly, there is the potential for effects in the male to induce paternally mediated developmental toxicity in the embryo/fetus. Whereas this is not a common occurrence it has been documented with one or two specific agents (e.g., cyclophosphamide, Trasler *et al.*, 1985).

The number of known environmental chemicals that produce adverse responses in human males is not large. All of these have been shown to induce effects in rodents and especially the rat, although there may be differences in sensitivity based on dose. Interestingly, a number of the classic human testicular toxicants (e.g., DBCP, gossypol) do not seem to produce infertility or testicular toxicity in the mouse, and so the rat is more commonly employed as a model for male reproductive toxicity studies. However, this does not imply that all chemicals known to produce injury in the rat would indeed show toxicity in man. The human does not employ a longitudinal wave for the production of sperm in the testis noted above for the rat, rather cellular associations are organized in a helical fashion that

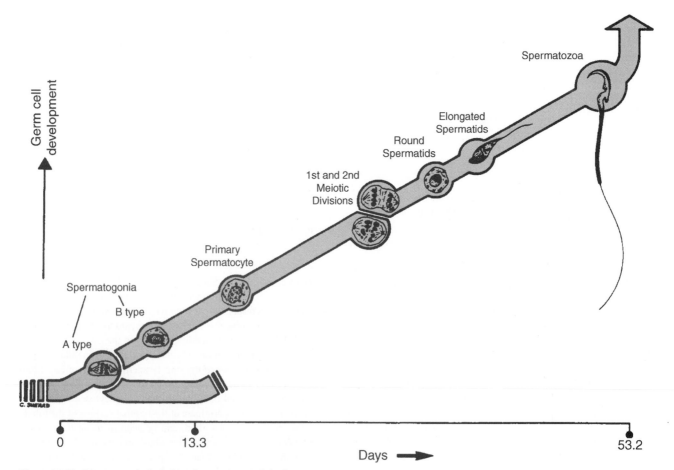

Figure 20-17. *Diagrammatic depiction of spermatogenesis in the rat.*

(From Foster, 1988).

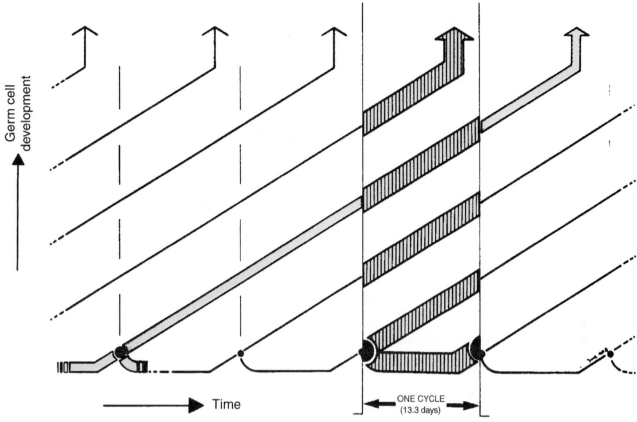

Figure 20-18. *The cyclicity of the seminiferous epithelium of the rat.*

The process whereby successive spermatogenic "waves" (see Fig. 20-18) are interrelated. A transverse section of a tubule covering one cycle of the epithelium will contain cellar representatives at different stages of maturity from successive waves. (From Foster, 1988).

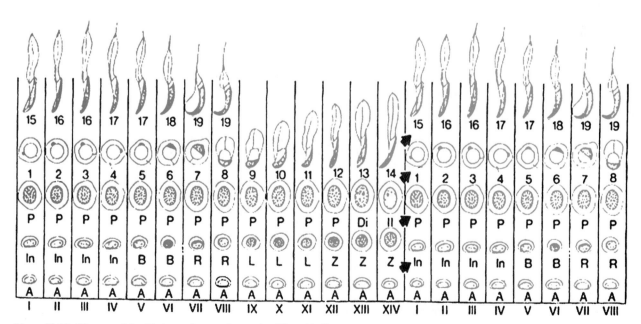

Figure 20-19. *Diagram of the 14 stages of spermatogenesis of the rat testis*

(After Leblond and Clermont, 1952). Each stage (Roman Numeral) contains different cellular associations of spermatogonia (A, IN or B), spermatocytes (R-resting/pre-leptotene; L – leptotene; Z – zygotene; P – pachytene; Di – diplotene, II – secondary), and spermatids (Arabic numerals 1-19). (From Foster, 1988).

is intrinsically less efficient for sperm production (when estimated on a sperm produced per gram of tissue basis) and thus humans are usually deemed more sensitive, from the risk assessment standpoint, because there are a greater range of values for semen parameters for the human population than the rat and a lesser decrement in sperm number or function is more likely to push larger numbers of men in the population into the infertile range.

Posttesticular Processes

Following the release of mature spermatids from the seminiferous epithelium, the extraneous cytoplasm and organelles form the residual body that is phagocytosed by the Sertoli cell and moves from the periphery of the tubule to its base. These nonmotile sperms are moved along the tubules by a peristaltic-like action of the myoepithelial cells of the tubule and eventually empty into the rete testis.

In rodents, but not humans, a large blood plexus forms over the rete (which is close to the surface and near the pole of the testis) where fluid exchange can take place. Sperm are then moved into the efferent ducts that exit in the testis. These ducts are rich in ER receptors (Oliveira et al., 2004) and the fluid from the seminiferous tubules contains steroid hormones, but is low in overall total protein.

The efferent ducts then empty into the caput (head) of the epididymis, which is a single highly coiled tube derived from the Wolffian duct in utero. The epididymis can be divided into three anatomical portions, the caput, corpus (body), and cauda (tail), which has a changing chemical environment and fluid composition from the efferent ducts through to the cauda. The sperm undergo maturation in the caput and corpus and begin to acquire motility, whereas the cauda is principally used for sperm storage, although expression of some critical surface markers does occur that are involved in the process of fertilization. In humans, the passage of sperm takes approximately 6 days and is longer in rats (~10 days). During the movement along the epididymal tubule, fluid is removed by active transport and this stage of the process is one that can be interfered with by toxicants resulting in an inappropriate environment for normal sperm development.

Most mammals possess seminal vesicles and a prostate (in experimental animals the exception is that dogs do not have seminal vesicles) and the accessory sex organs are depicted in Fig. 20-20. The physiology and anatomy of these organs varies widely among mammalian species with the rodent having a clear lobular pattern to the prostate that is not seen in humans. These organs are predominantly glandular/secretory in nature and produce much of the seminal plasma for the ejaculation of sperm to survive within the female reproductive tract. Other contributors to the seminal plasma are the epididymis and bulbourethral (Cowper's) glands. The seminal plasma contains many nutrients for sperm motion as well as distinct proteins and ion content. Any disturbance in these components may have an effect on subsequent fertility. For example, a diminution in energy substrates can affect sperm motion characteristics. These "accessory sex organs" are androgen dependent for their function and/or development and are frequently recorded in toxicity studies as indicators of androgen action. Indeed the Hershberger assay, used as part of the EPA's screening battery for endocrine disruptors (see section on Testing for Reproductive Toxicity), use changes in the weights of these organs as indicators of androgen or antiandrogen action in this pharmacological screen.

Semen volume varies considerably among species ranging from relatively small (1–10 mL: like humans) to much larger (~500 mL in boars).

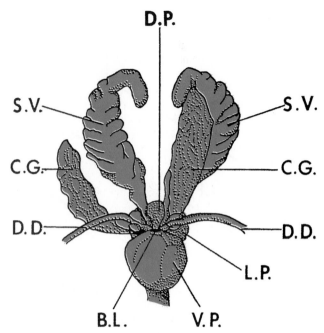

Figure 20-20. Anatomic relation of components of rodent sex accessory glands.

D.D. – ductus deferens; B.L. – bladder; V.P. – ventral prostate; L.P. – lateral prostate; C.G. – coagulating gland (also called the anterior prostate); S.V. – seminal vesicle; D.P. – dorsal prostate. (Reproduced with permission from Hayes AW: *Principles and Methods of Toxicology.* New York: Raven Press, 1982.)

Erection and Ejaculation

These physiologic processes are controlled by the CNS but are modulated by the autonomic nervous system. Parasympathetic nerve stimulation results in dilatation of the arterioles of the penis, which initiates an erection. Erectile tissue of the penis engorges with blood, veins are compressed to block outflow, and the turgor of the organ increases. In the human, afferent impulses from the genitalia and descending tracts, which mediate erections in response to erotic psychic stimuli, reach the integrating centers in the lumbar segments of the spinal cord. The efferent fibers are located in the pelvic splanchnic nerves (Andersson and Wagner, 1995).

Ejaculation is a two-stage spinal reflex involving emission and ejaculation. Emission is the movement of the semen into the urethra; ejaculation is the propulsion of the semen out of the urethra at the time of orgasm. Afferent pathways involve fibers from receptors in the glans penis that reach the spinal cord through the internal pudendal nerves. Emission is a sympathetic response affected by contraction of the smooth muscle of the vas deferens and seminal vesicles. Semen is ejaculated out of the urethra by contraction of the bulbocavernosus muscle. The spinal reflex centers for this portion of the reflex are in the upper sacral and lowest lumbar segments of the spinal cord; the motor pathways traverse the first to third sacral roots of the internal pudendal nerves.

Little is known concerning the effects of chemicals on erection or ejaculation (Woods, 1984). Pesticides, particularly the organophosphates, are known to affect neuroendocrine processes involved in erection and ejaculation. Many drugs act on the autonomic nervous system and affect potency (Table 20-5) (see also (Buchanan and Davis, 1984; Keene and Davies, 1999; Stevenson and Umstead, 1984). Impotence, the failure to obtain or sustain an erection, is rarely of endocrine origin; more often, the cause is psychological. The occurrence of nocturnal or early-morning erections implies that the neurologic and circulatory pathways involved in attaining an erection are intact and suggests the possibility of a psychological cause.

Normal penile erection depends upon the relaxation of smooth muscles in the corpora cavernosa. In response to sexual stimuli, cavernous nerves and endothelial cells release nitric oxide, which stimulates the formation of cyclic guanosine monophosphate (GMP) by guanylate cyclase. The drug sildenafil (Viagra) is used to treat erectile dysfunction; its mechanism of action resides in its ability to selectively inhibit cGMP-specific phosphodiesterase type 5. By selectively inhibiting cGMP catabolism in cavernosal smooth muscle cells, sildenafil restores the natural erectile response (Goldstein *et al.*, 1998; Uckert *et al.*, 2006). In the rat, prenatal exposure to the antiandrogenic fungicide vinclozolin induces a significant reduction of erections at all dose levels during the ex copula penile reflex tests in male offspring (Colbert *et al.*, 2005).

Case Studies for Effects on the Male

m-Dinitrobenzene *m*-Dinitrobenzene (*m*-DNB) has been extensively studied for its ability to produce a rapid deleterious effects on the rat testis since the mid-1980s. The earliest studies using a 10-week dosing regime (5 d/wk by gavage in corn oil) reported effects at 6 mg/kg/d (Linder *et al.*, 1986), while others have reported testicular injury after a single gavage oral dose of 25–50 mg/kg (Blackburn *et al.*, 1988). This paper also showed that the other isomers of DNB (*o*- and *p*-) were without testicular effects when given using the same dosing regime. Gray *et al.* (1988a) showed that the activity was via a direct mechanism and not secondary to changes in the HPG axis. Foster (1989) showed that 5-day dosing with 5 mg/kg/d produced a minimal to moderate testicular lesion within 2 weeks and 10 mg/kg/d a moderate to severe lesion. Testicular weight remained reduced for many weeks after the treatment period with significant dose-related effects on fertility (measured by pregnancy rate and implantation success). Similar studies have shown abnormal sperm function and failure of fertilization in rat in vitro fertilization (IVF) studies (Holloway *et al.*, 1990). Detailed electron microscopic evaluation has shown initial lesions to be present in the Sertoli cells of the testis, which results rapidly in germ cell apoptosis and death. The primary testicular effects on Sertoli cells (see Fig. 20-21) are consistent with the period of infertility noted in the breeding study (see Fig. 20-22) and could also be modeled in Sertoli-germ cell cultures where the *o*- and *p*-isomers were also without effect. A futile redox cycle has been proposed to explain the difference in isomer toxicity in which only *m*-DNB is metabolized to its nitroso metabolite and further to the hydroxylamine which is recycled back to the nitroso intermediate to reduce cellular reducing equivalents, such as reduced glutathione (GSH) (Cave and Foster, 1990; Ellis and Foster, 1992; Foster *et al.*, 1987; Reeve *et al.*, 2002).

Ethylene Glycol Monomethyl Ether (EGME) Since first published in 1979 (Nagano *et al.*, 1979) that EGME can elicit testicular toxicity in the mouse there has been significant effort expended on trying to understand the mode of action for the induction of these effects. Thus far, EGME has been shown to produce testicular toxicity in a wide variety of species, including nonmammals, the major toxicologically used species (rat, mouse, rabbit, dog) with reasonable evidence that it is likely to have effects in humans should exposure be high enough. A number of studies have described the pathogen-

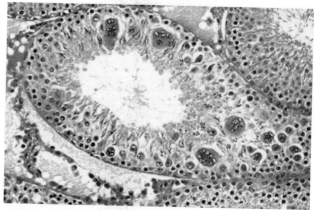

Figure 20-21. Seminiferous tubules 24 hours after m-Dinitrobenzene exposure (25 mg/kg).

Note multinucleate giant cells and germ cell debris sloughed into the tubular lumen.

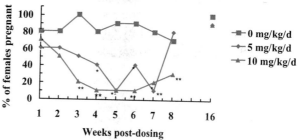

Figure 20-22. Effect of m-dinitrobenzene on percentage of females pregnant in a serial mating study design.

Note range of germ cell types affected consequent to the Sertoli cell injury produced by the compound. And the reversibility of the effects after 16 weeks (two spermatogenic waves – see Fig. 20-17). (Reproduced with permission from Foster PMD: Testicular organization and biochemical function, in Lamb JC, Foster PMD (eds.), *The Physiology and Toxicology of Male Reproduction*. New York: Academic Press, 1988, pp. 7–34.)

esis of the EGME lesion (predominantly in the rat) which seems to be common for the species thus far examined. The earliest features of these studies after a single dose (250 or 500 mg/kg/d) were that there are Sertoli cell vacuoles and swollen germ cell mitochondria, followed by (or concurrent with) a breakdown of the membrane between the Sertoli cell and the pachytene spermatocyte in a spermatogenic stage-specific manner. This is followed quickly (within hours) by the death of (probably those) pachytene spermatocytes (Creasy *et al.*, 1986; Creasy and Foster, 1984; Foster *et al.*, 1983). See Fig. 20-23.

EGME is metabolized to active intermediates; these are methoxyacetaldehyde and methoxyacetic acid (MAA). MAA has a longer half-life and is generally considered the more important of the two. Treating animals with MAA produces identical testicular lesions as that of the parent compound.

The spermatogenic stage specific effects are on the pachytene spermatocytes immediately before and during meiotic division (so, in Stages XII–XIV of the cycle in the rat (see Fig. 20-24), and also the early pachytene spermatocytes, at stages I–IV of the cycle). Dead germ cells can be seen as soon as 12 hours after an effective dose. Continued treatment at a low effective dose seems to affect just the vulnerable cell types so that a window of missing cells appears downstream from the stage of damage as time progresses (see

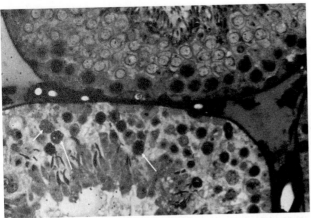

Figure 20-23. Effect of Ethylene glycol monomethyl ether (or its metabolite mehtoxyacetic acid) 24 hours after a single oral dose (100 mg/kg/d).

Note the damaged spermatocytes (arrows) in lower tubule compared to the upper normal tubule.

Fig. 20-24). As with other testis toxicants, higher dose levels produce a more widespread lesion involving other cell types (Foster *et al.*, 1987), producing immediate (<24 hours) and widespread damage and destruction within the tubules. The Sertoli cell vacuolization regresses after about 12 hours and is not a prominent feature of this lesion as it is with other agents like hexanedione, or some of the phthalate esters. Some weak evidence of involvement of this cell type also comes from some in vitro data with isolated seminiferous tubules. In this system molecules that inhibit transcellular calcium movement block the germ cell death from occurring, supporting a change in Sertoli cell communication to germ cells resulting in the rapid cell death after MAA treatment. Leydig cells do not seem to be pivotally involved in the pathogenesis. The lesion is not characteristic of a low-androgen testicular lesion, and reduced accessory sex organ weights are not a prominent feature associated with the early testicular pathology.

Decrements in fertility in the rat after acute treatment with EGME, are entirely consistent with the primary effect on pachytene spermatocyte germ cells, the prominent period of infertility being approximately 5–6 weeks after dosing when the pachytene spermatocytes should have matured to become mature sperm capable of fertilization based on the known kinetics of the process (Chapin *et al.*, 1985).

MATING BEHAVIOR IN THE RAT

Female rats are only sexually receptive on the day of proestrus, which is characterized by round nucleated and cornified epithelial cells in the vaginal lavage (Knobil and Neill, 1994) (Chap. 35). The period of receptivity begins at the onset of the dark phase of their light cycle, terminating later in the evening before the next stage of the cycle, defined as estrus which is typically characterized by the display of a vaginal lavage of mostly cornified epithelial cells. Serum estradiol rises during proestrus and this is followed by initiation of an LH surge shortly after onset of the dark phase of the light cycle which in turn induces ovulation and a brief increase in progesterone. This is normally the only time during which the female is receptive to the male and the display of this behavior can be induced in ovariectomized female rats by a sequence of injections of estradiol for a couple of days prior to mating followed by progesterone administration a few hours before the mating trial is

conducted, which must occur during the evening of the rat's diurnal cycle. Male and female rat mating behavior is sufficiently stereotyped that it can be easily quantified to assess the effects of toxicants on these behaviors (Gray and Ostby 1998; Gray *et al.*, 1988b).

During mating, the female rat displays proceptive behaviors like ear wiggling and darting to induce the male to mount, and when mounted the female is "receptive" displaying a lordosis posture characterized by a raised head and tail and fully arched back. The female maintains this posture for several seconds. In experienced male rats, the latency to the first mount is usually on a few seconds, but inexperienced males may take much longer. When the male rat mounts the lordosing female he will display a single pelvic thrust which may or may not result in intromission of the penis into the vagina. In rats, there is a rapid dismount after this single pelvic thrust. Within a few seconds, the male mounts again and this series continues until the male ejaculates. Ejaculation is usually identifiable by a slow dismount, after which the male retires for several minutes; a period termed the postejaculatory interval (PIE). During this period the male produces a 22 KHz vocalization, during which the female does not display proceptive behaviors (Porter *et al.*, 2005). Following the PIE, the series repeats itself several times throughout the evening. At the beginning of the second series, the male dislodges the copulatory plug, formed from the seminal secretions. The copulatory plug normally fits close to the cervix and it is necessary to facilitate sperm entry into the uterus. It is not unusual to find seven to eight copulatory plugs in the breeding cage the day after mating (Gray *et al.*, 1989). If mating does not occur, then the brief rise in serum progesterone declines by the next day.

In spontaneously ovulating species (e.g., rodents), the endocrine events are comparable with those in the menstrual cycle. In the rabbit, the LH surge and ovulation is a neural reflex produced by copulation (Knobil and Neill, 1994).

Cervix

The mucosa of the uterine cervix does not undergo cyclic desquamation, but there are regular changes in the cervical mucus. Estrogen, which makes the mucus thinner and more alkaline, promotes the survival and transport of sperm. Progesterone makes the mucus thick, tenacious, and cellular. The mucus is thinnest at the time of ovulation and dries in an arborizing, fernlike pattern on a slide. After ovulation and during pregnancy, it becomes thick and fails to form the fern pattern. Disruptions of the cervix may be expressed as disorders of differentiation (including neoplasia), disturbed secretion, and incompetence. Exfoliative cytologic (Papanicolaou's stain) and histologic techniques are currently used to assess disorders of differentiation. Various synthetic steroids (e.g., oral contraceptives) can affect the extent and pattern of cervical mucus.

Vagina

Estrogen produces a growth and proliferation of vaginal epithelium. The layers of cells become cornified and can be readily identified in vaginal smears. Vaginal cornification has been used as an index for estrogens. Progesterone stimulation produces a thick mucus and the epithelium proliferates, becoming infiltrated with leukocytes. The cyclic changes in the vaginal smear in rats are easily recognized. The changes in humans and other species are similar but less apparent. Analysis of vaginal fluid or cytologic studies of desquamated vaginal cells (quantitative cytochemistry) normally reflects ovarian function. However, administration of estrogenic toxicants can

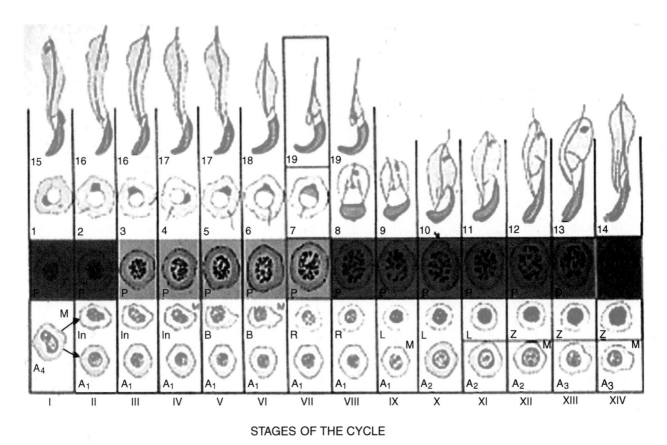

STAGES OF THE CYCLE

Figure 20-24. Stage specific lesions induced by methoxyacetic acid.

Intensity of shading indicates magnitude of effect on spermatocytes. (After Foster *et al.*, 1987).

induce persistent vaginal cornification in both immature and adult ovariectomized females by acting directly on the cellular dynamics and cell cycling of the vaginal epithelium (Gray *et al.*, 1988b, 1989). Vaginal sampling of cells and fluid might offer a reliable and easily available external monitor of internal function and dysfunction.

FERTILIZATION

Fertilization is the process whereby the genome from one generation is passed to the next to begin the development of a new organism. In mammals the oocyte is surrounded by two layers—an outer layer of cumulus cells and an inner layer of extracellular matrix termed the zona pellucida (see review by Hoodbhoy and Dean 2004). To reach the oocyte, the sperm must penetrate both layers that require high motility, the release of sperm enzymes and the presence of proteins that will facilitate binding of the sperm to the oocyte. Moreover, once fertilization has occurred, mechanisms must be in place to prevent the binding of further sperm to the fertilized oocyte (the zygote). To facilitate these activites, sperm must be capacitated (Hunter and Rodriguez-Martinez, 2004) and the secretion of enzymes (hyaluronidases) allows the sperm to penetrate through the cumulus cells to the zona pellucida. This special extracellular matrix is composed of three glycoproteins and cell surface factors then cause the sperm to release the secretory enzymes present in the acrosome via binding to the specific carbohydrates present in this matrix. The release of these enzymes enables the sperm to penetrate through the zona pellucida to then bind and fuse with the oocyte plasma membrane through specialized proteins to release

the genetic material into the oocyte as the male pronucleus which eventually combines with the genetic material from the female to form the zygote. Once sperm fusion has occurred, a "zona block" is initiated to prevent any further sperm entering through the zona pellucida and fusing with the oocyte membrane. The precise mechanisms of how this occurs have not been fully elucidated (Hoodbhoy and Dean, 2004).

IMPLANTATION

Implantation is an intricately timed event that allows mammals to nourish and protect their young during early development and results from an intimate relationship between the developing embryo and the differentiating uterus (see diagram in Fig. 20-25). Implantation can only occur when the embryo reaches the blastocyst stage and gains implantation competency, and the uterus, through steroid hormone dependent changes, attains a receptive state. This reciprocal interaction must occur between the blastocyst and uterus together with an increase in uterine vascular permeability at the site of blastocyst attachment. There are four stages that comprise early implantation in mammals: (1) apposition and adhesion of the blastocyst to the uterine lumen, (2) penetration of the epithelium, (3) decidualization of the stromal cells, and (4) trophoblastic invasion into the stromal vasculature. These four stages can vary in length and in precise order depending on the specific species studied and is further reviewed in (Aplin and Kimber, 2004; Lee and DeMayo, 2004; Schäfer-Somi, 2003; Tranguch *et al.*, 2005). The molecular understanding of these physiological events is far from complete,

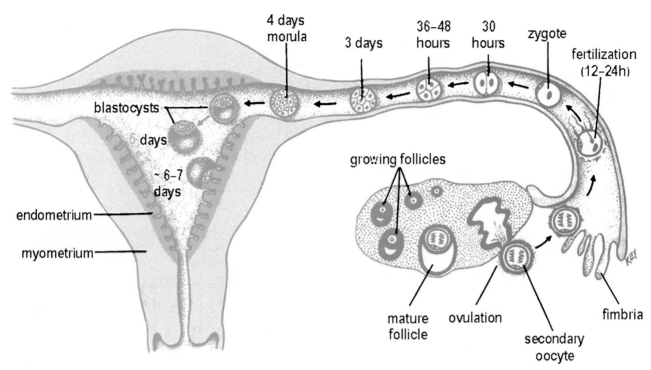

Figure 20-25. Fertilization and implantation in the female reproductive tract.

with data being generated mainly from studies in the mouse that have indicated through gene abalation in the uterus, a number of critical factors and cytokines and involved in implantation, however a number of these critical gene products (e.g., VEGF, BMP-2, wnt-4) have also been shown to produce early embryonic lethality when knocked out. Another important aspect of the implantation process common to many species (and offering an experimental tool to study implantation) is the embryonic diapause (or delayed implantation) evolved as a strategy to ensure proper implantation timing, depending on environmental conditions (see review by .Lopes *et al.*, 2004). The regulation of this phenomenon varies widely between species ranging from photoperiod through to hormonal or nutritional influences.

PLACENTA

The placenta plays a key role in pregnancy, mediating exchanges between the mother and fetus and maternal tolerance of antigens produced by the fetus. There are a huge number of different placental types exhibited by eutherian mammals that exhibit differences in both structure and endocrinology including significant difference between the major experimental animal species and humans (see reviews by Enders and Carter, 2004; Malassine *et al.*, 2003 and Fig. 20-26). Humans and monkeys possess a hemochorial placenta. Pigs, horses, and donkeys have an epitheliochorial type of placenta, whereas sheep, goats, and cows have a syndesmochorial type of placenta. In laboratory animals (e.g., rat, rabbit, and guinea pig),

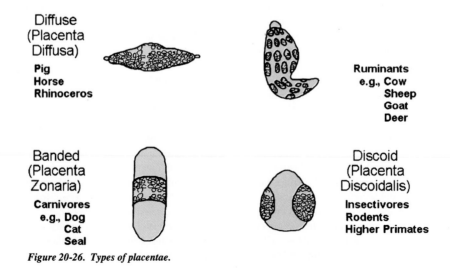

Figure 20-26. Types of placentae.

the placenta is termed a hemoendothelial type. Among the various species, the number of maternal and fetal cell layers ranges from six (e.g., pig, horse) to a single one (e.g., rat, rabbit). Primates, including humans, have three layers of cells in the placenta that a substance must pass across.

Early in implantation the blastocyst comes in contact with the endometrium and becomes surrounded by an outer layer or syncytiotrophoblast, a multinucleated mass of cells with no discernible boundaries, and an inner layer of individual cells, the cytotrophoblast. The syncytiotrophoblast erodes the endometrium, and the blastocyst implants. Placental circulation is then established and trophoblastic function continues. The blastocysts of most mammalian species implant about day 6 or 7 following fertilization. At this stage, the differentiation of the embryonic and extraembryonic (trophoblastic) tissues is apparent.

Trophoblastic tissue differentiates into cytotrophoblast and syncytiotrophoblast cells. The syncytiotrophoblast cells produce chorionic gonadotropin, chorionic growth hormones, placental lactogen, estrogen, and progesterone, which are needed to achieve independence from the ovary in maintaining the pregnancy. Rapid proliferation of the cytotrophoblast serves to anchor the growing placenta to the maternal tissue.

The developing placenta consists of proliferating trophoblasts, which expand rapidly and infiltrate the maternal vascular channels. Shortly after implantation, the syncytiotrophoblast is bathed by maternal venous blood, which supplies nutrients and permits an exchange of gases. Histotrophic nutrition involves yolk sac circulation; hemotrophic nutrition involves the placenta. Placental circulation is established quite early in women and primates and relatively much later in rodents and rabbits. One of the major differences in endocrine placental function between humans and rodents is in the production and regulation of progesterone necessary for the maintenance of pregnancy. In the rodent, the corpus luteum in the ovary has to produce progesterone throughout gestation and is regulated initially by pituitary prolactin secretion and then around midway through gestation by placental lactogens produced by the trophoblast. Thus, hypophysectomy (to remove pituitary influences) in a mouse does not terminate pregnancy after GD 11. In humans, the pituitary gland is not required for the initiation and maintenance of pregnancy, with maintenance of the corpus luteum to produce progesterone dependent on the secretion of human Chorionic Gonadotrophin (hCG) by the trophoblast. There is sufficient progesterone produced by the trophoblast after 8 weeks of gestation in humans to maintain pregnancy even in cases of ovariectomy.

Generally, the placenta is quite impermeable to chemicals/drugs with molecular weights of 1000 Da or more. Because most medications and xenobiotics have molecular weights of 500 Da or less, molecular size is rarely a factor in denying a drug's entrance across the placenta and into the embryo/fetus. Placental permeability to a chemical is affected by placental characteristics including thickness, surface area, carrier systems, and lipid-protein concentration of the membranes. The inherent characteristics of the chemical itself, such as its degree of ionization, lipid solubility, protein binding, and molecular size also affect its transport across the placenta.

PREGNANCY

In the female rat during mating, repeated cervical stimulation by the penis induces a surge of prolactin from the posterior pituitary within 20 minutes followed by the onset of twice-daily prolactin surges which persist for an 8- to 13-day period. During this pe-

riod, prolactin "rescues" the corpora lutea preventing regression. If sperm transport, fertilization or implantation are blocked, then the mated female is "pseudopregnant" for about 10–13 days (Swingle et al., 1951). During days 6–10 of pregnancy, sustained ovarian luteal function also requires pituitary LH. Pregnancy loss, i.e., full-litter resorption, can be induced at this stage of pregnancy by inhibition of pituitary LH secretion which in turn causes a reduction in serum progesterone levels (Bielmeier et al., 2004).

Midpregnancy of the rat is characterized by hypertrophic development of the corpus luteum which is dependent upon transition from the early LH and prolactin dependent phase of pregnancy to one that involves the secretion of hormones by the feto-placental unit (rCG and rPL) that induce rapid growth and differentiation of the corpora lutea, an increase in progesterone synthesis and a doubling in serum progesterone. Doody et al (1991) examined the levels of expression of mRNA species encoding cholesterol side-chain cleavage cytochrome P-450 (P-450scc), 17 α-hydroxylase cytochrome P-450 (P-450-17 α), aromatase cytochrome P-450 (P-450AROM) and 3 β-hydroxysteroid dehydrogenase (3 β-HSD) in rat ovaries during pregnancy. Expression of P-450scc mRNA is at low, but detectable, levels until day 14, thereafter expression increased to high levels (day 14–21 of gestation). Levels of P-450-17 α-mRNA on day 10 of gestation were low and decreased further on days 14 and 17. Expression of 3 β-HSD was decreased on day 10, but on days 14, 17, and 21 of gestation high mRNA levels were detectable. Ovarian expression of the three P-450AROM species is also dramatically increased between days 14 and 17 of pregnancy, but declines by day 21.

Because the transition from early to midpregnancy in the rat requires hormones from the feto-placental unit, if implantation or uterine decidualization are blocked by a chemical, then the female would resume her estrous cycles and the corpora lutea would regress (Knobil and Neill, 1994, Chap. 7). Chemicals that induce whole-litter loss at mid to late pregnancy may cause abortions in some of the females whereas others fail to deliver and appear pregnant for an unusually long period of time. Effects on female fertility due to disruption of hormones during pregnancy may be difficult to detect in standard testing studies if females are mated to similarly treated males if the chemical affects the reproductive system of both sexes. For example, with chronic di-n-butyl phthalate (DBP) administration at high dose levels induces whole litter loss at midpregnancy through reductions in ovarian progesterone production on GD 13. However, ovarian weight is not altered at GD 13 and the onset of female puberty, estrous cyclicity, and mating also were unaffected. This is in contrast to the robust reductions in testis size and histology, sex accessory gland size and sperm counts in pubertal males treated with DBP at 500 or 1000 mg/kg/d, treated F_0 females only display gross morphological reproductive alterations and reductions in uterine weights during midpregnancy. Hence, when female-mediated infertility is affected in this manner it may only be apparent when treated females are mated to untreated males. Chemicals that reduce serum progesterone production during pregnancy by inhibiting progesterone synthesis also may not alter the estrous cycles in the rat because the rat estrous cycle does not have a functional luteal phase, unlike humans.

Many abortifacients induce pregnancy loss by reducing progesterone levels in the rat. Generally, reducing midpregnancy progesterone levels by half or more are sufficient to terminate pregnancy (Carnathan et al., 1987). For example, treating pregnant rats with a prostaglandin F2alpha analogue ICI 81008, which reduces serum progesterone levels during pregnancy, induces full-litter loss in 40%

of 300 dams, while 25% had reduced litter sizes and 35% had normal litters (Warnock and Csapo, 1975). In comparison with the 107 control dams, all treated rats with full-litter loss had a drastic reduction in midpregnancy plasma progesterone levels. In contrast, those animals with only a partly resorbed litter only had a moderate reduction in progesterone until day 16. In contrast to progesterone, there was no correlation between plasma estradiol-17 beta levels and the consequences of treatment on pregnancy.

Corpora lutea function during pregnancy may also involve androgens and insulin-like 3 peptide hormone, in concert with lactogenic hormones. Whereas some of the androgenic actions are mediated by conversion of androgens to estrogens, pure androgenic effects also have been implicated (Goyeneche et al., 2002). Goyeneche et al. (2002) reported that AR mRNA and protein were expressed throughout gestation in the rat corpus luteum. In addition, they found that androstenedione, the main circulating androgen in pregnant rats, opposed luteal regression, reduced the number of cells undergoing apoptosis, and enhanced the levels of circulating progesterone.

PARTURITION

Parturition is a complex process involving fetal, placental, and maternal signals and the precise molecular events controlling this physiological process are not clear. Parturition is thought best to be thought of as a release from the inhibitory effects of pregnancy on the myometrium of the uterus rather than an active process, although the timing and order of the precise events is an active process. For most mammals the uterus is held in a quiescent state by high levels of progesterone and it is the decrease of progesterone that provides the trigger for parturition. In humans, this does not seem to be the case (i.e., levels of progesterone do not drop). Some authors have postulated that progesterone receptor inactivity does appear to be related to onset of labor and that local metabolism of progesterone in the cervix and uterus produces a localized decrease in progesterone that initiates labor. The fetus also directly contributes to the onset of parturition by activation of its HPA axis producing increased levels of cortisol. This in turn directly upregulates steroidogenic enzymes (especially CYP 17) in the fetus and placenta which in turn leads to changes in prostaglandin (particularly PGF2α) and oxytocin production to induce uterine contractions together with the increased activity of cytokines (including NF-κB and IL-1β). In humans there is no CYP 17 in the placenta which maybe related to the lack of change of progesterone (see recent reviews by Challis et al., 2005; Mendelson and Condon, 2005; Snegovskikh et al., 2006).

LACTATION

The endocrine control of lactation is one of the most complex physiologic mechanisms of human parturition. Mammogenesis, lactogenesis, galactopoiesis, and galactokinesis are all essential to assure proper lactation. Prolactin is the key hormone of lactation and seems to be the single most important galactopoietic (milk synthesis) hormone. Oxytocin, serotonin, opioids, histamine, substance P, and arginine-leucine modulate prolactin release by means of an autocrine/paracrine mechanism, whereas estrogen and progesterone hormones can act at the hypothalamic and adenohypophysial levels. Human placental lactogen and growth factors play an essential role to assure successful lactation during pregnancy with oxytocin being the most powerful galactokinetic (milk ejection) hormone (Buhimschi, 2004).

SENESCENCE

Reproductive senescence is usually preceded by a dysregulation of the HPG axis. This dysregulation leads to alterations in serum HPG hormones, accompanied an upregulation in GnRH, LH, and activin activities and a decrease in steroids in the brain. Receptors for these hormones in the brain are intimately involved in cell proliferation and differentiation in growth and development. In females, reproductive senescence is associated with a transition from regular to irregular estrus (menstrual) cycles leading to acyclicity and ultimately a loss of fertility. GnRH neurons in the brain are affected morphologically and it is the changes in GnRH neurosecretion with changes in pulsatility and preovulatory release that are causal in producing acyclicity. Perinatal exposure to toxicants with estrogenic activity can defeminize the HPG axis such that the females are acyclic and infertile while less affected females display the "delayed anovulatory syndrome" and become anovulatory and acyclic at an early age (Gray et al., 1989).

In males, a decrease in androgen is noted in around 20% of fit 60-year old men, but the value of androgen supplementation is not clear with regard to reproductive senescence. Dysregulation of the HPG axis is also found in aged male rats, with elevations in FSH and LH and decreased testosterone normally found. For reviews on reproductive senescence and possible associations with cognitive function see reviews by (Atwood et al., 2005; Keefe et al., 2006; Yin and Gore, 2006)

ENDOCRINE DISRUPTION (INCLUDING SCREENING AND PUBERTY)

Currently, the potential effects of "endocrine disrupting chemicals" (EDCs) on human health and the proven effects of EDCs on wildlife are a major focus among the scientific community. In 1996, the USEPA was given a mandate under the Food Quality Protection Act and Safe Drinking Water Act to develop test protocols to screen for endocrine effects. The initial impetus for these actions arose from a Work Session in 1991 on "Chemically Induced Alterations in Sexual Development: The Wildlife /Human Connection" (Colborn, 1994). Recent findings have contributed to these concerns; for example, it has been suggested that in utero exposure to environmental estrogens, antiandrogens or chemicals like phthalates or 2,3,7,8-TCDD could be responsible for the reported 50% decline in sperm counts in some areas and the apparent increase in cryptorchid testes (Toppari et al., 2001), testicular cancer (Skakkebaek, 2002), and hypospadias (Aho et al., 2000; Canning, 1999; Nassar et al., 2007; Paulozzi et al., 1997; Pierik et al., 2002; Porter et al., 2005; Toppari et al., 2001). The differences in sperm counts between regions are so large that they cannot be explained by methodological biases and "environmental effects are entirely plausible" (Giwercman et al., 2006; Jorgensen et al., 2001, 2002). Indeed, it has been proposed (Skakkebaek, 2002) that the secular deficits in these human reproductive end points could be plausibly linked and have an origin in fetal life as the testes are developing. These authors proposed the term Testicular Dysgenesis Syndrome (see Fig. 20-27) to explain the interrelationship of these findings.

Phthalate exposures have been associated with reduced AGD in boys and lower testosterone levels in men. In females, exposure to EDCs during development could contribute to earlier age at puberty and to increased incidences of endometriosis and breast cancer, for example. The original focus for the discussion of "endocrine disrupters" was research on toxicants reported to possess estrogenic

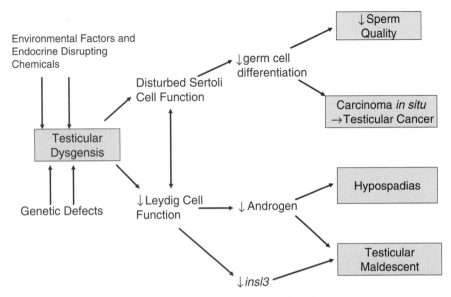

Figure 20-27. Testicular Dysgenesis Syndrome. The hypothesis (See Skakkebaek et al., 2002).

That events occurring during the development of the testis in fetal life can be related to the secular increases in a number of human reproductive disorders.

activity, with little consideration given to other mechanisms of endocrine toxicity; mechanisms that, in fact, may be of equal or greater concern. In addition, there has been a great deal of misinformation communicated on issues concerning endocrine disrupters; for example, nonestrogenic chemicals (i.e., phthalates and p,p'-DDE) are repeatedly reported to be estrogenic. There is a lack of appreciation for the fact that many endocrine disrupters (i.e., TCDD, EE) are very potent reproductive toxicants. In addition, there has been a tendency to dismiss the wildlife data as correlative, ignoring examples of clear, cause and effect relationships between chemical exposure and reproductive alterations (e.g., DDT metabolite effects in birds, PCB effects in fish, and environmental estrogen effects in domestic animals). There is a lack of recognition that subtle, low-dose reproductive effects seen in laboratory studies with endocrine disrupters will be difficult, if not impossible, to detect in typical epidemiological studies because of high variability normally seen in human reproductive function (e.g., time to fertility, fecundity, and sperm measures), the delayed appearance of the reproductive lesions and a lack of high quality exposure data. There is also a lack of appreciation for the complexity of the multiple mechanisms by which a single chemical can alter the endocrine milieu, to say nothing of the complex endocrine alterations induced by mixtures of chemicals.

We are now not only concerned about pesticides and other toxic substances in the environment, but the issue has broadened considerably due to the growing awareness that the list of EDCs present in the environment from human activities includes potent pharmaceutical products and phytosterols. Among these drugs are estrogens, antibiotics, beta-blockers, antiepileptics, and lipid regulating agents. One study reported that the pharmaceuticals found as contaminants of aquatic systems included 36 of 55 pharmaceuticals and five of nine metabolites measured including antiepileptic drugs (Kolpin *et al.*, 1998, 2002, 2004).

In the area of wildlife toxicology and ecosystem health, it is apparent that clear cut cause and effect relationships exist between exposure to EDCs and adverse effects in several vertebrate classes from fish to mammals. One challenge in interspecies extrapolation is

to link laboratory mechanistic studies with EDCs to both individual and population effects in the field.

Reports of U-shaped (nonmontonic), ultra-low-dose effects and nonthreshold effects for EDCs are challenging some of the basic assumptions of risk assessment for noncancer endpoints. While the focus of this debate has centered on the low-dose effects of bisphenol A (Ashby *et al.*, 1999; Nagel *et al.*, 1997; Owens and Chaney, 2005; vom Saal *et al.*, 1998, 2005; Welshons *et al.*, 2006), well documented U-shaped dose-response curves are known from many other in vitro and some in vivo studies. For example, administration of testosterone produces a well characterized and reproducible U-shaped dose response for spermatogenesis (Ewing *et al.*, 1977, 1979, 1981; Robaire *et al.*,1979) in the intact adult male rat. In vitro studies show that such responses do not always involve multiple mechanisms of action. Several AR ligands, antagonists at low to moderate concentrations, became AR agonists at high concentrations. Furthermore, the basic tenet of toxicology from Paracelceus (1564) that "dose alone determines the poison" is too limited for some EDCs because the timing of exposure dictates not only the effect but also whether the effects are adverse or beneficial. Even when administered during adult life, drugs with EDC-activity can simultaneously have a beneficial effect on one tissue and an adverse effect on another.

Known Effects of EDCs in Humans and Animals

The list of chemicals that are known to affect humans, domestic animals, and/or wildlife via functional developmental toxicity or endocrine mechanisms includes 2,3,7,8-TCDD, PCBs and polychlorinated dibenzofurans (PCDFs), methylmercury, EE, alkylphenols, plant sterols, fungal estrogens, androgens, chlordecone, DBCP, o,p'-DDD (Mitotane), o,p' DDT, and p,p'-DDE (Gray *et al.*, 2001) (Gray 2002). In addition to these xenobiotics, over 30 different drugs taken during pregnancy have been found to alter human development as a consequence of endocrine disruption. These drugs are not limited to estrogens, like diethylstilbestrol (DES). EDCs are known to alter human development via several mechanisms besides the estrogen receptor (ER): this includes binding to the AR, or retinoic acid (RAR, RXR) receptors, and by inhibition of steroidogenic enzymes or the synthesis of thyroid hormones. Findings on the effects of background levels of PCBs on the neurobehavioral development of the child have contributed to the concerns about the effects of EDCs on human health via alteration of hormone function including the thyroid (Brouwer et al., 1999; Tan and Zoeller, 2007). In summary, there are several hundred epidemiology studies showing associations among EDCs and adverse human health effects, however, none of these has been sufficiently studied to claim that "cause and effect" exists.

Known Effects of Drugs on Human Sexual Differentiation

In humans (Bardin and Catterall, 1981; Carmichael et al., 2005; Herbst, 1973; Ohyama, 2004) and laboratory rodents (Fisher, 2004; Foster et al., 2001; Gray et al., 2006), exposure to hormonally active chemicals during sex differentiation can produce pseudohermaphroditism. Androgenic drugs like Danazol and methyltestosterone can masculinize human females (i.e., "female pseudohermaphroditism") (Schardein, 2000; Kingsbury, 1985; Rosa, 1984). Laboratory studies demonstrate that these chemicals alter sex differentiation in rodents as well (Duck and Katayama, 1981). The drug aminoglutethimide, which alters steroid hormone synthesis in a manner identical to many fungicides, also masculinizes human females following in utero exposure (LeMaire et al., 1972; Schardein, 2000).

DES provides an unfortunate example of how in utero exposure to a potent endocrine disrupter with estrogenic activity can alter reproductive development in humans (Herbst, 1987; Shaffer, 2000; Veurink et al., 2005). Although a few cases of masculinized females were noted in the late 1950s, most of the effects of DES were not apparent until after the children attained puberty. Transplacental exposure of the developing fetus to DES causes clear cell adenocarcinoma of the vagina, as well as gross structural abnormalities of the cervix, uterus, and fallopian tube. These women are more likely to have an adverse pregnancy outcome, including spontaneous abortions, ectopic pregnancies, and premature delivery (DeCherney et al., 1981). Some of the pathological effects that develop in males following fetal DES exposure appear to result from an inhibition of androgen action or synthesis (underdevelopment or absence of the vas deferens, epididymis, and seminal vesicles) and anti- Mullerian duct factor (persistence of the Mullerian ducts) (Niculescu, 1985). DES may also have caused epididymal cysts, hypotrophic testes, and infertility in males.

Known Effects of Plant and Fungal Products in Animals and Humans

The phytoestrogens and fungal mycotoxins are naturally occurring and widespread in nature. Farnsworth et al. (1975) listed over 400 species of plants that contain potentially estrogenic isoflavonoids or coumestans or were suspected of being estrogenic based on biological grounds (Farnsworth, 1990). Plants contain many other compounds in addition to estrogens that can affect reproductive performance, such as the purported antiandrogenic activity in the oil from saw palmetto (Gordon and Shaughnessy, 2003).

Although most naturally occurring environmental estrogens are relatively inactive, when compared to steroidal estrogens or DES, the phytoestrogen miroestrol is almost as potent as estradiol in vitro and even more potent than estradiol when administered orally (Cain, 1960; Matsumura et al., 2005) . In addition, many plant estrogens occur in such high concentrations that they induce reproductive alterations in domestic animals (Adams 1990; Adams

and Sanders, 1988). "Clover disease," which is characterized by dystocia, prolapse of the uterus, and infertility, is observed in sheep grazed on highly estrogenic clover pastures. Permanent infertility (defeminization) can be produced in ewes by much lower amounts of estrogen over a longer time period than are needed to produce "clover disease." In domestic animals, feeds contaminated with the zearalenone-producing fungus (Fusarium sp.) induce adverse reproductive effects in a wide variety of domestic animals, including impaired fertility in cows and hyperestrogenism in swine and turkeys (Kuiper-Goodman et al., 1987).

Known Effects of Organochlorine Compounds in Humans

In addition to drugs and plant substances, several pesticides and toxic substances have been shown to alter human reproductive function (listed above). An accidental high dose in utero exposure to PCBs and PCDFs have been associated with reproductive alterations in boys, increased stillbirths, low birth weight, malformations, and IQ and behavioral deficits (58). In addition to the effects associated with this inadvertent exposure, relatively subtle adverse effects were seen in infants and children exposed to relatively low levels of PCBs and PCDFs (36). The authors reported that the lowest observed adverse effect levels (LOAELs) for developmental neurobehavioral and reproductive endpoints are currently within the range of current human body burdens based on Toxicity Equivalency Factors.

One metabolite of DDT was found to alter adrenal function with sufficient potency to be used as a drug to reduce adrenal androgen production (Knappe et al., 1997). o,p'-DDD (mitotane) is used to treat adrenal steroid hypersecretion associated with adrenal tumors. In addition to this usage, lower doses of mitotane restored menstruation in women with spanomenorrhea associated with hypertrichosis.

Occupational Exposures

Occupational exposure to pesticides and other toxic substances (i.e., chlordecone and DBCP) in the workplace have been associated with reduced fertility, lowered sperm counts, and/or endocrine alterations in male workers. Workers in Hopewell VA, exposed to high levels of chlordecone, an estrogenic (Hammond et al., 1979) and neurotoxic (Landrigan et al., 1980) organochlorine pesticide, displayed obvious signs of intoxication which included severe neurotoxicity and abnormal testicular function (Epstein, 1978; Reich and Spong, 1983). As this cohort was not followed, it is not known if the effects of chlordecone were completely reversible.

It is surprising to learn that occupational exposures to potential EDCs at effective concentrations apparently have not been entirely eliminated from the workplace. A series of publications from about 1990 to 1996 presented documentation of sexual impotence in chemical factory workers exposed to a DES-like stilbene derivative. National Institute of Occupation Safety and Health conducted two studies in response to complaints of impotence and decreased libido among male workers involved in the manufacture of 4,4'-diaminostilbene-2,2' disulfonic acid (DAS), a key ingredient in the synthesis of dyes and fluorescent whitening agents (Grajewski et al., 1996; Hammond et al., 1987; Quinn et al., 1990; Smith and Quinn, 1992; Whelan et al., 1996). Both current and former workers had lower serum testosterone levels (Grajewski et al., 1996) and reduced libido (Whelan et al., 1996) as compared to control workers. In addition, duration of employment was negatively correlated with testosterone levels. These studies replicated the observations reported by Quinn et al. (1990) who reported low levels of serum testosterone and problems with impotence in male workers. In a uterotropic assay, while DAS was only weakly to negligibly estrogenic (Smith and Quinn, 1992), a single sc 30 mg/kg dose of 4-nitrotoluene, a precursor of DAS, increased uterine weights without producing overt toxicity. Samples of DAS from the workplace displayed estrogenic activity.

Environmental Androgens

Androgenic activity has been detected in several complex environmental mixtures. Pulp and paper mill effluents (PME) from Florida, the Baltic Sea, the Great Lakes, and New Zealand (Ellis et al., 2003; Larsson and Forlin, 2002; Parks et al., 2001). PME effluents from sites on the Fenholloway River in Florida include a chemical mixture that binds AR and induces androgen-dependent gene expression in vitro. This mode of action is consistent with the masculinized female mosquitofish (Gambusia holbrooki) collected from contaminated sites on the river. Male-biased sex ratios of fish embryos have been reported near a pulp mill in broods of eelpout (Zoarces viviparus) in the vicinity of a large kraft pulp mill on the Swedish Baltic coast, suggesting that masculinizing compounds in the effluent were affecting gonadal differentiation and promoting skewed sex ratios. Efforts to date have not conclusively identified chemicals in PME responsible for androgenic activity (Durhan et al., 2002).

Effluents from beef-cattle concentrated animal feeding operations (CAFO) from Nebraska and Ohio have been shown to display androgenicity. Orlando et al. (2004) found that CAFO discharge at a site in Nebraska exhibited androgenic activity and found that fish (fathead minnow; Pimephales promelas) collected at the site displayed small gonads as compared to fish from a reference site. Durhan et al., (2005) detected the synthetic androgens 17α- and 17β-trenbolone in several water samples from a beef CAFO in Ohio where trenbolone acetate implants were used to stimulate weight gain and the samples collected from a direct discharge from the feedlot displayed significant androgenic activity in vitro. Complementary laboratory studies revealed both trenbolone isomers were androgenic in fathead minnows (Ankley et al., 2003) and the rats (Wilson et al., 2002). When administered in utero, 17β-trenbolone (TB) masculinized female rat offspring, increased AGD, nipple, and caused vaginal agenesis and induced male sex accessory tissues in females (Wolf et al., 2002). TB binds to ARs with high affinity and induces androgen-dependent gene expression in vitro at concentrations similar to those for DHT (Wilson et al., 2004).

In vivo androgenicity testing using the Hershberger assay shows that TB is as potent as testosterone propionate (TP) in inducing growth of the androgen-dependent levator ani-bulbocavernosus muscles (Wilson et al., 2002), being about 70 times more potent when administered sc versus orally.

Environmental Antiandrogens

Fungicides Vinclozolin and procymidone are two members of the dicarboximide fungicide class that act as AR antagonists (Kelce et al., 1994; Ostby et al., 1999). These pesticides, or their metabolites, competitively inhibit the binding of androgens to AR that leads to an inhibition of androgen-dependent gene expression in vitro and in vivo (Kelce et al., 1997). Peripubertal administration of antiandrogens can alter the onset of pubertal landmarks in the male rat (Monosson et al., 1999). Vinclozolin delays pubertal maturation and reduces sex accessory gland and epididymal growth and increases

serum LH, and testosterone and 5-androstane, 3,17-diol levels. In a Hershberger assay using castrated immature testosterone-treated male rats, vinclozolin and procymidone alone or in combination inhibited testosterone induced growth of androgen-dependent tissues (ventral prostate, seminal vesicles, and levator ani-bulbocavernosus muscles) in a dose-additive fashion (Gray et al., 2001).

Administration of vinclozolin during sexual differentiation demasculinizes and feminizes the male rat offspring such that treated males display female-like AGD at birth, retained nipples, hypospadias, suprainguinal ectopic testes, a blind vaginal pouch, and small to absent sex accessory glands (Gray et al., 1994). In contrast to the phthalates and linuron (see below), even at high dosages (200 mg/kg/d), epididymal hypoplasia was rare and no cases of gubernacular agenesis were noted. At low doses, vinclozolin reduces neonatal AGD and increases the incidence of retained nipples/areolae in infant male rats. In adult life, ventral prostate weight is permanently reduced and male offspring display permanent female-like nipples (Gray et al., 1999a). Treatment at 50 and 100 mg/kg/d induces hypospadias and other reproductive tract malformations. The most sensitive period of development to the disruptive effects of vinclozolin is GD 16–17 with less severe effects seen in males exposed to vinclozolin on GD 14–15 and GD 18–19. In addition, Hotchkiss et al. (2003) demonstrated that neonatal injection of vinclozolin at 200 mg/kg/d demasculinized aggressive play behavior in male rats at 35 days of age, indicating that CNS sexual differentiation was altered an anti-androgenic manner.

When procymidone is administered from day 14 of pregnancy to day 3 after birth, AGD is shortened in male pups, and the males display retained nipples, hypospadias, cryptorchidism, cleft phallus, a vaginal pouch, and reduced sex accessory gland size (Ostby et al., 1999). Procymidone also induces fibrosis, cellular infiltration, and epithelial hyperplasia in the dorsolateral and ventral prostatic and seminal vesicular tissues in the offspring when examined as adults.

Prochloraz is a fungicide that disrupts reproductive development and function by several modes of action (Noriega et al., 2005; Vinggaard et al., 2000, 2002). Prochloraz inhibits the steroidogenic enzymes 17, 20 lyase and aromatase and it is an AR antagonist. Wilson et al. (2004) found that prenatal prochloraz reduces fetal testis testosterone and increases progesterone production 10-fold on GD 18 without affecting Leydig cell insl3 mRNA levels. Prenatal prochloraz treatment delayed parturition and altered reproductive development in the male offspring in a dose-related manner (Noriega et al., 2005). Treated males displayed reduced AGD and female-like areolas and high-dose males displayed hypospadias but the epididymides and gubernacular ligaments were relatively unaffected.

Linuron (Herbicide) The herbicide linuron is a AR antagonist. It binds rat and human AR and inhibits DHT-hAR induced gene expression in vitro (Lambright et al., 2000; McIntyre et al., 2002a, 2002b). In vivo treatment with linuron elicits a positive response in the Hershberger assay for antiandrogens (Lambright et al., 2000). In utero linuron exposure produces dramatic effects in male rat offspring. More than half of the males exposed to 100 mg linuron/kg/d (GD14-18) display epididymal and testicular abnormalities (Gray et al., 1999b) with effects seen at dosage as low as 12.5 mg/kg/d (exposed from GD 10–22) (McIntyre et al., 2000). In contrast to the effects of vinclozolin and procymidone, malformed external genitalia and undescended testes were rarely displayed by linuron-exposed males. Interestingly, the syndrome of effects for linuron are atypical of an AR antagonist and more closely resembles those seen with in utero to phthalates which inhibit fetal Leydig cell insl3 hormone levels. Wilson *et al.* (2004) found that fetal testosterone production is significantly reduced in linuron treated fetal males, demonstrating that linuron is antiandrogenic via dual mechanisms of action.

***p,p′*-DDE (Pesticide Metabolite)** Kelce *et al.* (1995; 1997) found that *p,p′*-DDE displayed AR antagonism both in vivo and in vitro. In vitro, *p,p′*-DDE binds to the AR and inhibits androgen-dependent gene expression. In vivo, *p,p′*-DDE delays pubertal development in male rats by about 5 days at 100 mg/kg/d and inhibits androgen-stimulated tissue growth in the Hershberger assay which uses castrated immature androgen-treated male rats (Table 20-1). *p,p′*-DDE administered to Long Evans Hooded and Sprague-Dawley male rats in utero reducesAGD, induces nipples, and permanently reduces androgen-dependent organ weights (Gray *et al.*, 1999a).

Phthalates (Plasticizers) The phthalates represent a class of high production volume chemicals that alter reproductive development. While a few in vitro studies suggested that some of the phthalates are estrogenic, DBP injections do not induce a uterotropic response or estrogen-dependent sex behavior (lordosis) in the ovariectomized adult female rats (Gray, 1998). Likewise, oral DBP or diethylhexyl phthalate (DEHP) treatments fail to accelerate VO or induce constant estrus in the intact female rats. In addition, neither the phthalate diesters nor their monoester metabolites appear to compete significantly with androgens for binding to the AR at environmentally relevant concentrations (Foster *et al.*, 2001; Parks *et al.*, 2000; Stroheker *et al.*, 2005). In utero, some phthalate esters alter the development of the male rat reproductive tract at relatively low dosages. Prenatal exposure to DBP, benzyl-butyl phthalate (BBP), di-isononyl phthalate (DINP) and DEHP treatment cause a syndrome of effects, including underdevelopment and agenesis of the epididymis and other androgen-dependent tissues and testicular abnormalities (Foster *et al.*, 2001; Gray *et al.*, 2000). Among the antiandrogenic EDCs, the phthalates are unique in their ability to induce agenesis of the gubernacular cords, a tissue whose development is dependent upon the peptide hormone insulin-like peptide-3. Wilson *et al.* (2004) found that the phthalates reduced both insl3 mRNA and testosterone levels during sexual differentiation of the male rat.

When pregnant SD rats are dosed by gavage with DEHP from GD 8 to day 17 of lactation with 0, 11, 33, 100, or 300 mg/kg/d, in utero exposure induces a low incidence of abnormalities consistent with the aphthalate syndrome in the 11, 33, and 100 mg/kg/d dose groups along with subtle reductions in reproductive organ weights. In the high-dose group, more than 25% of the males display testicular and/or epididymal abnormalities. Pubertal DEHP treatment alone is sufficient to delay puberty in Long Evans (LE) and SD rats due to lowered testosterone levels.

Prenatal exposure to DBP from day 10 to 22 of gestation produces effects nearly identical to those seen with DEHP, with effects occurring at dosage levels of 50–100 mg/kg/d (Mylchreest *et al.*, 1999, 2000). When administered in 4-day periods of gestation (GD 8–11, 12–15 or 16–19), DBP at 500 mg/kg/d was most effective in altering sexual differentiation at GD 16–19 (Gray *et al.*, 1999b). When Carruthers and Foster (2005) exposed SD rats to DBP at 500 mg/kg/day for 2-day periods (GD 14 and 15, 15 and 16, 16 and

17, 17 and 18, 18, and 19, or 19 and 20) they also found that the critical window for abnormal development is GD 16–18.

DBP also disrupts reproductive function in the rabbit. In rabbits exposed to 400 mg DBP/kg/day in utero (GD 15–29), male offspring exhibit reduced numbers of ejaculated sperm, testis weight and accessory sex gland weight (Higuchi *et al.*, 2003). Additionally, DBP caused a slight increase in histological alterations of the testis, a doubling of abnormal sperm and hypospadias, hypoplastic prostate, and cryptorchid testes with carcinoma in situ-like cells were present in 1/17 DBP-treated male rabbits.

Environmental Estrogens

Methoxychlor is an estrogenic pesticide that produces variety of estrogen-like effects in the male and female rat. This pesticide requires metabolic activation in order to display full endocrine activity in vitro. The active metabolites of M bind ER and activate estrogen dependent gene expression in vitro (Wilson *et al.*, 2005) and in vivo in the female rat; M stimulates a uterotropic response, accelerates VO and induces constant estrus, reduces ovarian weight lacking corpora lutea and infertility in the female rat (Gray *et al.*, 1989; Chapin, 1997). Ovarian function is also altered by M exposure. In the ovariectomized female rat, M also induces estrogen-dependent reproductive and nonreproductive behaviors (Gray *et al.*, 1988) including female sex behaviors, running wheel activity, and food consumption. Unlike estradiol, M is as effective, or is more effective, when administered orally than when it is injected.

When given to the dam during pregnancy and lactation both male and female offspring are affected, with females being the more sensitive gender with effects ranging from VO at 5 mg/kg/d and above and infertility at 100 mg/kg/d and above. At 50 mg/kg/d F_1 females display irregular estrous cycles and reduced fecundity. F_1 male fertility is unaffected at doses up to 200 mg/kg/d, even though they display permanent reductions in testis and other reproductive organ weights at 50 mg/kg/d and above.

EE is a synthetic derivative of estradiol that is very bioactive orally. This estrogen is in almost all modern formulations of combined oral contraceptive pills. Over time, formulations have decreased the EE dose from as high as 100 μg/d to as low as 20 μg/d. EE is found in many aquatic systems contaminated by sewage effluents, originating principally from human excretion. Along with natural steroidal estrogens, EE plays a major role in causing widespread endocrine disruption in wild populations of fish species and other lower vertebrate species (Jobling and Tyler, 2006).

In the immature SD and Wistar female rat, 0.3 μg/kg/d of EE is effective in inducing uterine weight when given sc, whereas orally 1.0 μg EE/kg/d stimulates uterine weight (Kanno *et al.*, 2001).

Administration of 0.5 mg EE/kg/d accelerates VO by 5–7 days and induces vaginal cornification in LE and SD weanling rats. When administered to the dam during gestation and lactation over a broad dose response (0.05–50 μg/kg/d) range, F_1 female LE rats display a variety of reproductive tract lesions including cleft phallus, accelerated VO, and infertility at 5 and 50 μg/kg/d, whereas F_1 males are less severely affected. F_1 males did not display any reproductive tract malformations and seminal vesicle, ventral prostate and other androgen-dependent organ weights were not affected at any dose whereas testis and epididymal weights were reduced at 50 μg EE/kg/d. In a similar study with the SD rat, EE only affected F_1 females at 50 μg/kg/d and it was reported that they were not infertile and no effects were noted in the male offspring (Sawaki *et al.*, 2003).

EDC Screening Programs

In response to the 1996 legislative mandate for an endocrine screening and testing program, the EPA formed the Endocrine Disruptor Screening and Testing Advisory Committee (EDSTAC), which proposed a tiered screening and testing strategy for EDCs in its final report in 1998 (http://www.epa.gov/scipoly/oscpendo/history/finalrpt.htm). The EDSTAC proposal included the following: (1) a process to prioritize chemicals for evaluation and recommendations, for (2) screening (Tier 1), and for (3) testing (Tier 2) batteries. The recommended screening battery was designed to detect alterations of HPG function; estrogen, androgen, and thyroid hormone synthesis; and androgen receptor (AR) and ER-mediated effects in mammals and other taxa. Based on a "weight-of-evidence" analysis, chemicals positive in Tier 1 would be considered as potential EDCs and subjected to testing (Tier 2). Equivocal effects in Tier 1 could be replicated or evaluated further in additional short-term assays before more extensive Tier 2 testing was initiated. Tier 1 should include assays sensitive enough to detect EDCs, whereas issues of "dose-response, relevance of the route of exposure, sensitive life stages and adversity" would be resolved in the Tier 2 testing phase.

In Vivo Mammalian Assays   EDSTAC recommended the laboratory rat as the species of choice for the endocrine screening and testing assays. In vitro assays can produce false–positive responses at high concentrations due to a lack of specificity as assay conditions deteriorate. Although such false–positives can be eliminated by experimental measurement of Ki values, few in vitro screening strategies include Ki determinations to insure that the effects seen in binding and gene expression assays are the result of competitive inhibition of ER or AR. As a result, a high percentage of screened chemicals that are determined to be "positives" in vitro may not be true receptor ligands. Finally, because in vitro screening assays are unable to integrate the endocrine responses seen in the whole organism, the relationships between endocrine toxicity and other systemic effects cannot be simulated in vitro. To avoid the limitations described above, the EDSTAC proposed three short-term in vivo mammalian assays for the Tier 1 Screening Battery: the uterotropic, Hershberger, and pubertal female rat assays (Gray 1998; Gray *et al.*, 1997a; Gray *et al.*, 2002). Table 20-6 indicates the range of EDCs tested in validating these assays for use in the screening program.

Uterotropic Assay   Estrogen agonists and antagonists are detected in a 3-day uterotropic assay using subcutaneous administration of the test compound. Based on the evaluation of four variations of the uterotropic assay protocol in the OECD interlaboratory studies, all of the protocols have produced acceptable responses without regard to rat strain, diet, or housing conditions (Kanno *et al.*, 2001; 2003a,b; Owens and Ashby, 2002; Owens *et al.*, 2003, 2006; Owens and Koeter, 2003). The selected uterotropic assays for estrogens and antiestrogens use either the intact juvenile or the castrated ovariectomized adult/juvenile female rat.

Hershberger Assay   The second in vivo assay in T1S, the Hershberger assay, detects antiandrogenic activity simply by weighing androgen-dependent tissues in the castrated male rat (Gray, 1998; Gray *et al.*, 1997a, 2002; Hershberger *et al.*, 1953). In this assay, weights of the ventral prostate, Cowper's glands, seminal vesicle (with coagulating glands and fluids), glans penis, and levator ani/bulbocavernosus muscles are measured in castrated, testosterone-treated (or untreated) male rats after 10 days of oral treatment with the test compound. This assay is very sensitive for detection of androgens and antiandrogens. Other useful end-points that help reveal the mechanism of action and specificity of the response include weights of the adrenal, liver, and kidney, and measurements of serum (collected by cardiac puncture) levels of testosterone and LH. The Hershberger assay shows high sensitivity and specificity to chemicals with AR-mediated activity. Weakly antiandrogenic pesticides like *p,p'*-DDE and linuron are easily detected in the Hershberger assay (Lambright *et al.*, 2000; .Yamasaki *et al.*, 2003). Chemicals like finasteride, which inhibit 5-alpha reductase activity, are also active in this assay. They dramatically reduce male accessory sex gland weight with less effect on the levator ani/bulbocavernosus muscle, which has low levels of this enzyme. Chemicals that are positive in the Hershberger assay often produce adverse effects during puberty and after in utero exposure.

Pubertal Female Rat Assay   The third in vivo mammalian/rat assay included in the screening battery is the pubertal female rat assay has been in use for nearly two decades (Gray *et al.*, 1988a, 1989). In this assay, weanling female rats are dosed daily by gavage for 21 days while the age at VO (puberty) is monitored. The females are necropsied at about 42 days of age (reviewed by (Goldman *et al.*, 2000). Measurements include serum thyroid hormones, uterine and ovarian weight, and histology. This assay detects alterations in thyroid hormone status, HPG function, inhibition of steroidogenesis, estrogens, and antiestrogens, and has been found to be highly reproducible and very sensitive to certain endocrine activities including estrogenicity, inhibition of steroidogenesis, and antithyroid activity.

Alternative Screening Assays   Alternative in vivo assays were also discussed by EDSTAC and are being evaluated by the EPA. If they are of sufficient sensitivity, specificity, and relevance, they might replace or augment current T1S assays. However, whether they meet such criteria remains to be determined.

Pubertal Male Rat Assay   One promising alternative assay is the pubertal male rat assay (Stoker *et al.*, 2000), which detects alterations of thyroid function, HPG maturation, steroidogenesis, and altered steroid hormone function (androgen). Intact weanling males are exposed to the test substance for approximately 30 days. The age at puberty is determined by measuring the age at PPS, and reproductive tissues are evaluated and serum taken for optional hormonal analyses. The studies conducted on contract for EPA using the pubertal male assay are also presented on the EPA EDSP web site. This assay produced reproducible responses among different laboratories and was sensitive to androgens and antiandrogens.

In Utero-Lactational Assay   The EDSTAC recommended that the EPA develop and evaluate an in utero-lactational assay due to the unique sensitivity of the fetal reproductive system to disruption by some toxicants. For example, 2,3,7,8-TCDD (dioxin) alters sexual differentiation of male and female rats and hamsters at dosage levels approximately two orders of magnitude below those required to produce adverse effects in pubertal or adult rats (Gray *et al.*, 1997b, 1997c; Stoker *et al.*, 2000). One version of the proposed in utero-lactational assay now being evaluated by the EPA takes about 80 days and uses approximately 10 litters per group (120–150 pups). In this protocol, androgens and antiandrogens can be detected in approximately 2–3 weeks, and EDCs with antithyroid activity can be detected in infant or weanling offspring after 4–5 weeks of maternal treatment.

It is important to retain flexibility in the selection of new assays and endpoints for the screening and testing program so that new methods can be used as replacements or to augment the assays if they offer distinct advantages over the current battery of assays.

Table 20-6

Chemicals examined in protocols of the Organisation for Economic Cooperation and Development (OECD) and the U.S. Environmental Protection Agency (EPA), using standardized assays with oral or subcutaneous dosing

OECD UTEROTROPIC ASSAY (FOUR PROTOCOLS — ALL SUCCESSFULLY IDENTIFIED EACH CHEMICAL)

Ethinyl estradiol: Positive estrogenic control
Genistein: Phytoestrogen
Methoychlor: Estrogenic and antiandrogenic pesticide
Nonylphenol: Estrogenic "inert" ingredient and surfactant
o,p′-**DDT:** Estrogenic pesticide
Bisphenol A: Estrogenic plastic monomer
ZM 189,154: Antiestrogenic pharmaceutical
Dibutyl phthalate: Negative control; plasticizer that inhibits testis Leydig cells

OECD Hershberger assay (each chemical successfully identified)
Testosterone propionate: Androgenic positive control
Trenbolone: Androgenic veterinary pharmaceutical
Methyltestosterone: Potent androgenic pharmaceutical
Linuron: Antiandrogenic herbicide
p,p′-**DDE:** Antiandrogenic pesticide metabolite
Flutamide: Potent antiandrogenic pharmaceutical
Finasteride: Potent inhibitor of enzyme 5 alpha reductase required for DHT synthesis and full androgen-dependent growth of some sex accessory tissues
Vinclozolin: Antiandrogenic fungicide
Procymidone: Antiandrogenic fungicide

EPA in utero-lactational protocol (partially successful in identifying estrogenicity)
Methoxychlor: Estrogenic and antiandrogenic pesticide

EPA execution of adult intact male assay (did not successfully identify endocrine activity of either chemical)
Linuron: Antiandrogenic herbicide
Methoxychlor: Estrogenic and antiandrogenic pesticide

[a]Kanno *et al.*, 2001, 2002, 2003a,b; Owens and Koeter, 2003; Owens *et al.*, 2003 (see text).
[b]Yamasaki *et al.*, 2003 (see text).

Enhancements to current life cycle and multigenerational tests are also being considered in an effort to improve the quality of the data on EDCs that will be used for risk assessments. Scientists are attempting to minimize animal use by using as few animals as possible in the most precise and sensitive assays, by incorporating sensitive in vitro assays in T1S, and by using quantitative structure activity relationships (QSAR) models or high throughput prescreening assays in the prioritization of chemicals for use in vivo. It is also possible to avoid unwarranted animal use because chemicals negative in T1S are not subject to T2T. In addition, testing statistical "false positives" can be almost entirely eliminated by ensuring that T1S assay results are replicated in T1.5 before moving to T2T. Attempts to enhance T2T by adding more sensitive endpoints and a more thorough assessment of the animals already on study may also lead to additional reductions in animal use.

TESTING FOR REPRODUCTIVE TOXICITY

Screens and Multigeneration Studies

The testing of materials for reproductive toxicity has been refined over many decades to provide more comprehensive assessments of a test material's ability to affect the reproductive cycle in laboratory animal models and provide appropriate information to estimate potential risk of exposure to humans. The history and evolution of reproductive toxicity guidelines for pharmaceuticals has recently been reviewed (Collins, 2006). The types of protocols and guidelines employed depend on the type of chemical being tested and its intended use(s). For example, this would involve extensive and comprehensive testing of a food use pesticide, where all the population may be exposed, while much more limited information would be required for a specific drug (e.g., used to treat women for menopausal symptoms). In the specific drug case, the experimentation required would be directed at the "target" lifestage(s).

It should also be noted that comprehensive testing for reproductive toxicity normally involves the simultaneous exposures of both males and females. Only with specific protocol amendments will the affected sex(es) be determined (e.g., exposure of one sex, or a crossover mating study design in which treated males and females are mated with corresponding control animals). The details below apply to the rat, the most common species employed in reproductive toxicity studies. Suitable amendments can be made for other species (the mouse is sometimes used) and nonhuman primates occasionally employed—particularly for testing drugs.

A significant amount of attention has also been focused on the development of "screens" for reproductive toxicity as opposed to the more definitive protocols usually found in testing guidelines. Such a need has arisen primarily for the evaluation of the 80,000 chemicals used in commerce which have no reproductive toxicity testing information. Thus, the screens currently employed (and particularly the

OECD 421 and 422 guidelines) have been developed to prioritize chemicals for more comprehensive testing. Whereas such screening approaches can identify chemicals that have adverse effects on reproductive function, the dosing regimes, end points employed, number of dose levels used etc. serve only to provide a signal, albeit that the basic information is of a quality to set dose levels, or highlight potential areas of issue in more detailed studies. More problematic is what to do with negative data from these screens as these *do not* imply that the chemical tested is without reproductive toxicity, and may still present a risk to humans. Thus, the outcomes from such screens can be summarized as: "*a positive response is a positive, but a negative response is a maybe.*" More detailed information on the proposed screening battery for EDCs is provided in section "Endocrine Disruption" including "Screening and Puberty".

The most comprehensive assessment of reproductive toxicity would be provided by a protocol that exposes the animal model throughout the reproductive cycle (see Fig. 20-1) and involves the assessment of multiple end points at different lifestages during this continuous exposure. The protocol and guideline coming closest to this ideal is the multigeneration reproduction study used for the assessment of chemicals, pesticides, and some food additives (OECD 416, EPA OPPTS 870.3800, FDA "redbook" and the NTP Reproductive Assessment by Continuous Breeding [RACB]). These all represent variations on the general theme noted in Fig. 20-28 and Fig. 20-29 and the reader is pointed to the specific guidelines for more detailed explanation of the differences. In general, parental (F_0) animals are exposed for approximately 10 weeks prior to mating (based the duration of the spermatogenic wave of 8 weeks and the passage of sperm through the epididymis and the availability of mature sperm for fertilization) (see Fig. 20-16). Exposure continues through mating (and after the mating pairs are separated), continues through gestation, birth, and lactation. Litters maybe "standardized" to ensure equal lactational demand on the dams and normalize the growth of pups (litters are usually reduced to four males and four females per litter on PND 4). At weaning, F_1 litters are usually culled to one male and one female that are raised and exposed until adulthood and the exposure continues through the same processes in the second breeding generation which usually halts at weaning of the F_2 pups. These studies normally have at least 3 dose levels (with the highest dose level designed to induce some toxicity) and at least 20 litters produced per dose group. The RACB study is unusual in that two to three litters are produced in each generation and in its latest form, four males and females are retained from the last F_1 and F_2 litters to adulthood. These multigeneration studies normally encompass detailed measurements of reproductive performance (number of pregnant females from number of pairs mated, number of females producing a litter, litter size, number of live pups with their birth weights and sex). Measurement of growth and analysis of the reproductive organs in the F_0 parental generation is conducted (including specific evaluations of ovarian follicles, estrous cyclicity, and sperm parameters). Similar measurements to those undertaken for the F_0 are made on the F_1 parents, but in addition offspring are normally carefully examined at birth (and sexually dimorphic end points may be collected such asAGD), at weaning, and at puberty (particularly the assessment of VO and time of first estrus in females and belanopreputial separation in males) in addition to the adult measurements of reproductive performance, organ weights, histology etc. In the EPA multigeneration study design, only 10 adult animals per sex, per group, per generation are required to have their tissues evaluated histologically. For the OECD 416 design, this number will increase to 20 per sex per group (i.e., each male and female selected for breeding in the F_1 generation).

Multigeneration Reproduction Study

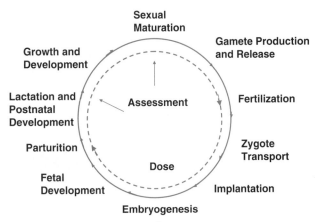

Figure 20-28. Multigeneration study.

Generally, only one mating is performed per generation, but in the presence of equivocal data, or clear indications that effects are becoming more adverse in succeeding generations, then extra litters or generations may be added to the standard designs to clarify potential reproductive toxicity.

Testing for Endocrine Disrupting Chemicals

In a tiered screening and testing approach, only chemicals that display positive reproducible responses in Tier 1 screening (T1S–see section "Endocrine Disruption" including "Screening and Puberty") or T1.5 would be evaluated further in full-life cycle or multigenerational tests. In Tier 2 testing (T2T), not T1S, issues of dose-response, relevance of the route of exposure, sensitive life stages, and adversity are resolved. For some endocrine activities, the number of sensitive endpoints and F_1 offspring examined in these assays should be expanded on a case-by-case basis.

AGD at birth and nipple/areola retention in infant female and male rats should be included in testing of androgens and antiandrogens, respectively, because they are sensitive, potentially permanent effects that are highly correlated with malformations and reproductive organ weight changes later in life (McIntyre *et al.*, 2001). These early alterations constitute part of the antiandrogen-induced developmental syndromes. The syndrome induced by the AR antagonists differs to some degree from that induced by the phthalates, which inhibit the synthesis of fetal testosterone and insulin-like 3 peptide (insl-31) hormones.

Developmental Syndromes and Tailored Testing   A careful evaluation of the male rat offspring allows one to distinguish the "phthalate syndrome," in which effects on reproductive development involve a decrease in fetal testicular testosterone and insl-3 peptide hormone biosynthesis (Gray *et al.*, 2002; Mylchreest and Foster, 2000; Mylchreest *et al.*, 1999; Parks *et al.*, 2001; Wilson *et al.*, 2004) from the "AR antagonist syndrome," induced by vinclozolin (Gray *et al.*, 1994, 1999b; Lim *et al.*, 2001) or flutamide (McIntyre *et al.*, 2001). The main distinction between the two syndromes is that the phthalate syndrome includes agenesis of the testis, epididymis, and gubernacular cord. These lesions are rarely seen in the AR antagonist syndrome, even when all of the males display hypospadias. In addition, of all chemicals that interfere with the

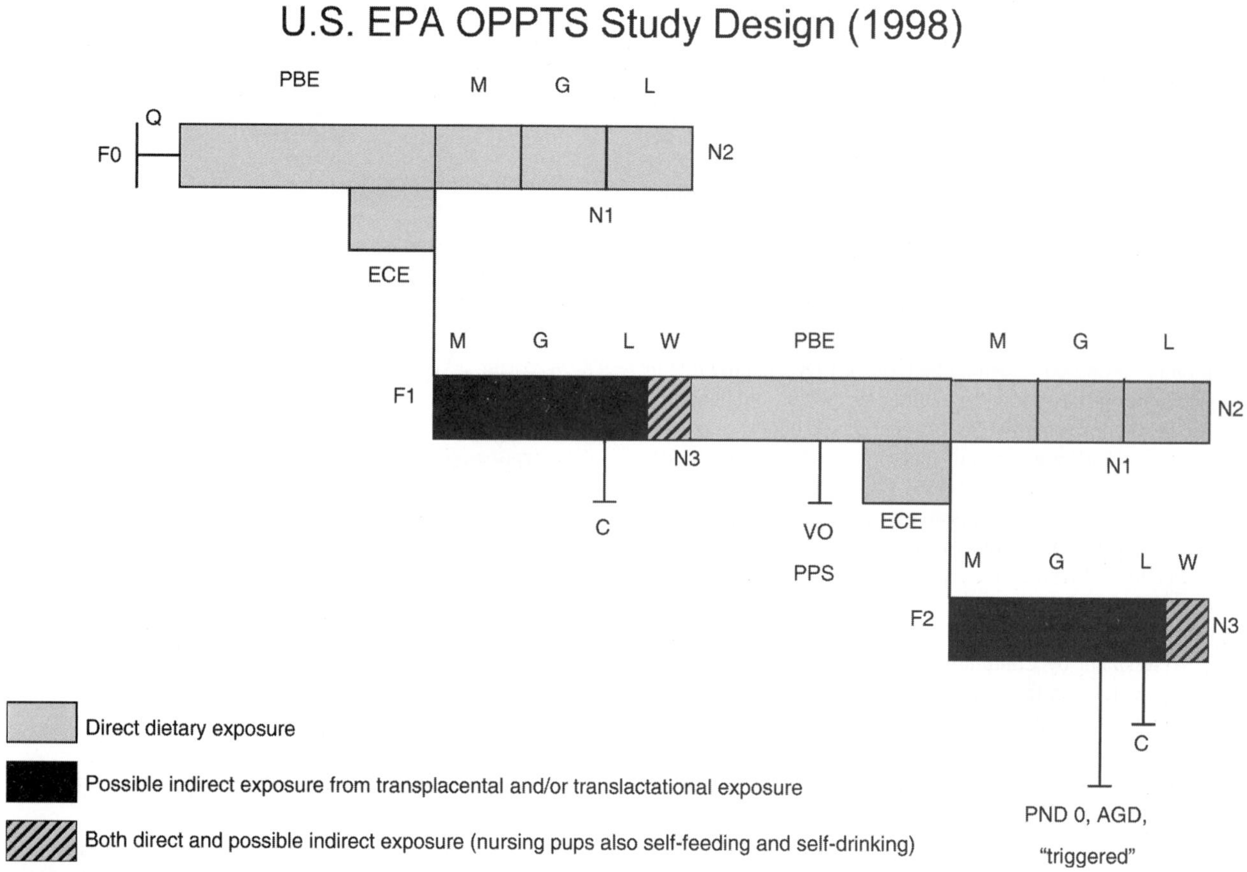

U.S. EPA OPPTS Study Design (1998)

Figure 20-29. Multigeneration reproduction study as recommended by EPA.

Key for the rat: Q – Quarantine (one week); PBE – Prebreed exposure (10 weeks); M – Mating (two weeks); G – Gestation (three weeks); L – Lactation (three weeks); VO – Vaginal opening (evaluated in F1 females on postnatal day 22 to acquisition); PPS – Preputial separation (evaluated in F1 males on postnatal day 35 to acquisition); W – Weaning (postnatal day 21); N1 – Necropsy of all paternal animals (organ weights, histology, andrological assessments); N2 – Necropsy of all maternal animals (organ weights, histology, ovarian follicle assessments); N3 – Necropsy of selected weanlings, three/sex/litter, if possible (organ weights); ECE – Estrous cyclicity evaluation (three weeks); C – Cull litters to ten pups (with equal sex ratio) on postnatal day 4; AGD – Anogenital distance measured in F2 pups on postnatal day 0 if triggered by effects on F1 reproductive development; N – Necropsy. Single generation reproduction study (e.g., OECD 415).

androgen signaling pathway in the fetal male rat, only the phthalates affect Leydig cell insl-3 hormone synthesis and cause undescended testes due to gubernacular agenesis (Wine *et al.*, 1997).

In contrast to the antiandrogens, which primarily affect the male offspring (see Table 20-7), in utero exposure to androgenic chemicals has more severe consequences for the female offspring (see Table 20-8). It is important to consider this information when tailoring T2T based on T1S results. For example, when the female rat fetus is exposed to testosterone (Hotchkiss *et al.*, 2007) or the veterinary pharmaceutical trenbolone, agenesis of the vagina and nipples is seen at a low rate in the lower dosage groups. In fact, most of the low-dose effects of androgens in the female offspring (retained prostatic and vesicular tissues, and nipple agenesis (Hotchkiss *et al.*, 2007; Wolf *et al.*, 2002) are effects that are likely to be missed in a standard necropsy.

When conducting a multigenerational study, it is important to summarize the data in a manner that clearly delineates the proportion of animals that are affected, indicating that they display any lesion (histological or gross pathology) consistent with the syndrome. In teratology studies, data are typically presented and analyzed in this manner, indicating the number of malformed/number observed on an individual and litter basis, whereas multigenerational studies are frequently presented and analyzed differently, even when clear teratogenic and other developmental responses are noted after birth. Multigenerational protocols are used in T2T because only these protocols expose the animals during all critical stages of development and examine reproductive function of offspring after they mature.

Although the new EPA multigenerational test provides for a comprehensive evaluation of the F_0 or parental generation, too few F_1 animals (offspring with developmental exposure) are examined after maturity to detect anything but the most profound reproductive teratogens (Gray and Foster, 2004). F_0 animals within a dose group typically respond in a similar fashion to the chemical exposure; however, the response to toxicants in utero can vary greatly even within a litter with only a few animals displaying severe reproductive malformations in the lower dosage groups. For example, dose-related adverse reproductive effects are seen in less than 10% of the F_1 offspring treated in utero with the phthalate DINP (male reproductive malformations, Gray *et al.*, 2000); 2,3,7,8-TCDD (permanent vaginal threads and ovarian atrophy, Gray *et al.*, 1997c); in utero busulfan (ovarian atrophy and delayed puberty, Gray and Ostby, 1998); DEHP (epididymal and testicular lesions, and linuron, McIntyre *et al.*, 2000); epididymal and testicular hypoplasia, and androgens (vaginal and nipple agenesis, Wolf *et al.*, 2002).

Table 20-7

Detecting developmental reproductive syndromes in male rat offspring. Multitude of effects of antiandrogens in male rat offspring that should be evaluated in Tier 2 testing studies displaying this activity in Tier 1 screening or other assays

Neonatal-infantile data

1   Anogenital distance at birth (1–3 days of age)
2   Areola/nipple retention in infant male rats at 13–14 days of age

External necropsy endpoints on all male rat offspring at maturity

1   Body weight any unusual malformations or anomalies, euthanize
2   Shave ventral surface from inguinal region to neck and count nipples and areolas (observer blind to treatment), record position of areolas and nipples.
3   Check animals for hypospadias, epispadias, cleft phallus, and measure AGD
4   Note if testes obviously undescended
5   Note if inguinal region soiled with urine
6   Note if prepuce partially or entirely detached from glans penis, especially if a persistent thread of tissue is present along frenulum.

Internal endpoints on all male rat offspring at maturity

1   Location of each testis (scrotal, abdominal, gubernaclum attached to abdominal wall)
2   Gubernacular cords, present or absent, and length in mm if abnormal
3   Note if present, cranial suspensory ligaments
4   Note if testes are small, absent, fluid filled, enlarged, appear infected or other
5   Note if epididymides are small, absent, or infected (record region of effects)
6   Note if ventral prostate is small, absent, or infected
7   Note if dorsolateral prostate is small, absent, or infected
8   Note if seminal vesicles are small, absent, infected, or one side larger than the other
9   Note if coagulating glands are small absent, infected, one side larger than the other or detached from seminal vesicles.
10 Note if kidneys display hydronephrosis, calcium deposits
11 Note presence of hydroureter
12 Note presence of bladder stones or bloody in bladder

Weigh the following organs on all male rat offspring at maturity

1   Each testis individually (examine histology of each testis)
2   Each corpus plus caput epididymis (examine histology of each segment)
3   Each cauda epididymis (examine histology of each segment)
4   Entire seminal vesicle, plus coagulating glands with fluid as a unit, if possible
5   Entire ventral prostate, if possible
6   Each kidney
7   Paired adrenals
8   Liver
9   Levator ani plus bulbocavernosus
10 Cowper's glands as a pair, if possible
11 Glans penis
12 Pituitary
13 Brain

Histology on all male F_1 offspring at maturity

1   Both testes
2   Both epididymides
3   Prostate glands
4   Any grossly abnormal reproductive tissues

Thus, a standard multigenerational protocol that examines only one F_1 animal per sex, per litter after maturity from 20 litters per dosage group, can detect statistically significant alterations only when they are displayed by 25% or more of the offspring. Histopathological alterations must be displayed by 50% or more of the offspring because a histological examination of the reproductive tract is required only in 10 F_1 animals per sex, per dose—far too few to detect anything but the most profound effects on reproductive development. Such an approach would also create uncertainty associated with lowest observed adverse effect levels (LOAELs) and no observed adverse effect levels (NOAELs) identified in multigenerational studies for chemicals that do not include either a complete assessment of all of the endpoints that constitute the syndrome, or those included in the EPA new Multigenerational Test Guidelines.

In "transgenerational" protocols (Gray, 1998a; Gray and Ostby, 1995; Gray et al., 1994, 1997c, 1999b,c, 2002; McIntyre et al., 1998,

Table 20-8

Detecting developmental reproductive syndromes in female rat offspring. Multitude of effects of androgens in female rat offspring that should be evaluated in Tier 2 testing studies

	Neonatal-infantile data in female rat offspring
1	Anogenital distance at birth (1–3 days of age)
2	Areola/nipple agenesis (complete or faint) in infant female rats at 13–14 days of age

	External necropsy endpoints on all female rat offspring at maturity
1	Body weight any unusual malformations or anomalies, euthanize
2	Shave ventral surface from inguinal region to neck and count nipples and areolas (observer blind to treatment), record position of areolas and nipples
3	Check animals for cleft phallus and measure AGD and position of vaginal opening
4	Note if inguinal region soiled with urine

	Internal endpoints on all female rat offspring at maturity
1	Location of ovaries in relationship to kidneys
2	Note if absent, cranial suspensory ligaments
3	Note if ovaries are small, cystic-fluid filled, enlarged, appear infected or other
4	Note if oviducts, uterus, or upper or lower vagina are small, absent, or infected (record region of effects) or fluid-filled
5	Note if ventral prostate tissue is present
6	Note if seminal vesicle tissue is present
7	Note if levator ani/bulbocavernosus muscle tissues are present
8	Note if other male tissues are present
9	Note if kidneys display hydronephrosis, calcium deposits
10	Note presence of hydroureter
11	Note presence of bladder stones or blood in bladder

	Weigh the following organs in all female offspring at maturity
1	Paired ovaries (histology)
2	Uterus with fluid (histology)
3	Vagina
4	Each kidney
5	Paired adrenals
6	Liver
7	Pituitary
8	Brain

	Histology on all female rat offspring at maturity
1	Both ovaries
2	Uterus
3	Vagina
4	Any suspected male reproductive tissues
5	Any grossly abnormal reproductive tissues

2000, 2001), we typically use fewer litters (7–10 per dose group) but examine all of the animals in each litter. These protocols actually use fewer animals but provide enhanced statistical power to detect reproductive effects in the F_1 generation. Additional factors, besides detection of adverse effects at necropsy or during data analysis and interpretation, limit interpretation of data from the standard multigenerational reproduction test. The life-long exposure of both males and females in the F_1 generation, which allows one to detect effects induced in utero, during lactation, or from direct exposure after puberty, can confound the identification of when the effect was induced (i.e., during adulthood vs. development) or even the affected sex. In studies, where the dosing period normally is terminated near birth or at weaning, precludes misinterpretation of the developmental origin of reproductive effects. Nevertheless, it is clear that transgenerational protocols would not be appropriate

for EDCs that induce low-dose alterations in the pubertal or adult animal in the F_0 generation.

Test Design and Numbers of F_1 Animals It is important to reiterate that the endpoints described above, which are sensitive to antiandrogens or androgens in utero (listed in detail in Gray and Foster, 2004), are not sensitive to xenoestrogens or some other EDCs. Thus, not all EDCs should be tested similarly to the androgens or antiandrogens. Testing should be tailored based on the pharmacological activity demonstrated in T1S. In addition, the developing fetus is not always the most sensitive life stage. Some EDCs disrupt pregnancy by altering maternal ovarian hormone production in F_0 dams at dosage levels that appear to be without direct effect on the offspring (Gray *et al.*, 1999b). In such cases, the standard EPA multigenerational protocol with minor enhancements would be

In Utero Lactational study Protocol

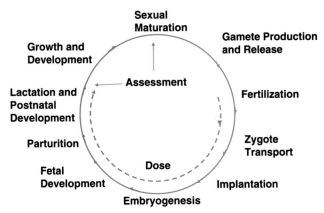

Figure 20-30. The in utero-lactational study design under review by EPA for the assessment of endocrine active agents.

recommended, or a transgenerational protocol with exposure continued after weaning. The transgenerational or in utero-lactational protocols (see Fig. 20-30) fill a gap in the testing program for EDCs that should be used only on a case-by-case basis, as indicated by the results of T1S and any Tier 1 repeat study.

Testing Pharmaceuticals

In the case of pharmaceuticals, it is rare for multigeneration studies to be conducted, because it is not common for all the population to use a specific drug and that exposure to the drug is not necessarily chronic and over many different lifestages. Typically three specific studies are undertaken based on the recommendations of the International Conference on Harmonization of Guidelines S5A: Detection of toxicity to reproduction for medicinal products (see Collins 2006 for specific study descriptions) although any permutation or specific design is open to the investigator to explore specific toxicity based on the pharmacology of the drug tested. The three "most likely" studies are as follows.

1. **A study of fertility and early embryonic development** (see Fig. 20-31). Parental adults are exposed to the test chemical for 2 weeks (females) or 4 weeks (males) prior to breeding and then during breeding. Females then continue their exposure through to implantation. Males can be necropsied for the end points noted above for the multigeneration studies after pregnancy has been confirmed, and for the pregnant females, necropsy takes place any time after midgestation. As with the multigeneration study, reproductive and target organs are weighed and examined histologically, sperm parameters are assessed in males and in females, the uterine implantation sites and ovarian *corpora lutea* are counted, as well as live and dead embryos.

   In this study design, the selection of the dosing regimen for males has been based on pragmatism in attempting to shorten the study, rather than the biology of spermatogenesis in the test species (as employed in the multigeneration study). It is thought that the majority of chemicals that might affect the male should be detectable (by histology) after 4 weeks exposure, however, there are a number of exceptions to this notion. One of the significant advantages of the pharmaceutical guideline approach is that the investigator is encouraged to tailor their testing proto-

Fertility and Early Embryonic Development Study

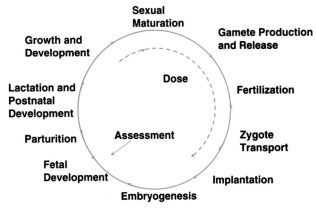

Figure 20-31. Fertility and Early embryonic study.

Pre-and Postnatal Development Study

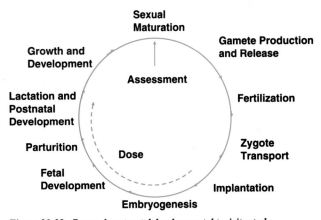

Figure 20-32. Pre-and post-natal developmental toxicity study.

Dosing is from implantation until the litters are weaned.

cols to reflect the best science and available knowledge. One potential disadvantage is that the basic approach does represent a theoretical "gap" as some chemicals may not manifest a testis histological lesion in 4 weeks and also there is a potential disassociation of structure (testis histology and sperm parameters) from function (male breeding performance).

2. **A study of effects on pre- and postnatal development including maternal function** (see Fig. 20-32). In this study, pregnant females are exposed from implantation until weaning of their offspring (usually PND 21 in the rat). After cessation of exposure, selected offspring (one male and one female per litter) are raised to adulthood and then mated to assess reproductive competence. These animals are observed for maturation and growth (but are not exposed). Puberty indices, as employed in the multigeneration study, are measured. In addition, sensory function, reflexes, motor activity, learning and memory are also evaluated.

3. **A study of embryo–fetal development** (see Fig. 20-33). This study tests for enhanced toxicity relative to that noted in pregnant females and unlike the previous two studies, is normally

Embryo–Fetal Development Study

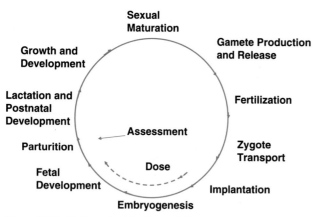

Figure 20-33. *Embryo–fetal developmental toxicity study as used by FDA guidelines.*

Dosing starts at implantations and continues to closure of the hard palate with an assessment of fetuses just prior to parturition.

EPA Prenatal Developmental Toxicity Study

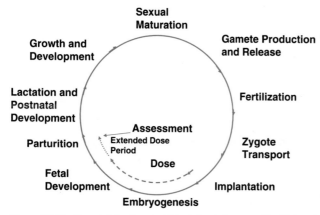

Figure 20-34. *Prenatal developmental toxicity study as used by EPA and OECD.*

Note the extended dose period compared with that used in Figure 20-33.

conducted in two species (typically the rat and rabbit). Exposure occurs between implantation and closure of the hard palate and females are killed just prior to parturition. At necropsy, dams are observed for any affected organs and *corpora lutea* are counted. Live and dead fetuses counted and examined for external, visceral, and skeletal abnormalities. In the evaluation of prenatal developmental toxicity for a chemical or pesticide (e.g., OPPTS 870.3700, OECD 414), exposure of the pregnant dams is usually longer and can be continuous throughout pregnancy or, more normally, from implantation until just prior to birth (see Fig. 20-34). Other end points measured in the dam and fetuses are identical between the pharmaceutical embryo-fetal toxicity study and that employed for evaluation of an industrial chemical or pesticide.

The FDA Center for Drug Evaluation and Research produced a draft guidance document in 2001 that explored how data should

Single Generation Reproduction Study

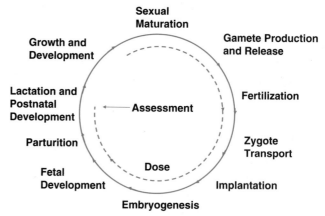

Figure 20-35. *Single generation reproduction study.*

be passed through an integrative process to assess a drug for reproductive toxicity. The tool is used in a tiered manner consisting of three sections (1) methods applicable to all datasets, (2) approaches applicable only to datasets without evidence of reproductive and developmental toxicity, and (3) approaches applicable to datasets with positive indications of reproductive and/or developmental toxicity. This integration would provide one of three summary risk conclusions that would be applied to the drug label namely (1) not anticipated to produce reproductive and/or developmental effects above the background incidence for humans when used in accordance with the dosing information on the product label; (2) the drug may increase the incidence of adverse reproductive and/or developmental events, or (3) that the drug is expected to increase the incidence of adverse reproductive and/or developmental effects in humans when used according to the product label.

An examination of the reproductive cycle in a comparison of these three most likely options for FDA studies indicates an obvious gap in the exposure regime for the complete reproductive cycle, namely exposure of weanlings through puberty to adulthood. This exposure period has become of increasing interest to many companies developing drugs for specific administration to infants and juveniles and as such "bridging type" protocols to be used in addition to the three "most likely" have been developed to specifically address toxicity that may occur after exposure during this specific lifestage (Hurtt *et al.*, 2004).

The single generation reproduction study (OECD 415) is used more frequently in Europe where specific testing guidelines for reproductive toxicity may be triggered by the tonnage production of a specific chemical. This design (see Fig. 20-35) has a common F_0 parental exposure period to that used in the multigeneration guideline (OECD multigeneration study—416). Estimates are made of the standard litter parameters and reproductive performance of the F_0 parents, but in this design the study halts at the weaning of the F_1 offspring and no estimate is made of effects on adult F_1 offspring, nor on the ability of this generation to reproduce. This study design provides critical information on parental reproductive effects but has very limited information on the offspring aside from pup number, growth and survival to weaning, and thus has limited utility in the estimation of transgenerational effects, or postnatal reproductive consequences.

Newer Guidelines and Approaches

The International Life Sciences Institute sponsored a new endeavor looking at how Agricultural Chemicals might be assessed for toxicity, including reproductive toxicity in a proposed lifestage approach (Cooper *et al.*, 2006) using an extended one-generation study (see Fig. 20-36) in the rat. This approach incorporated many of the changes made more recently to testing guidelines (including extra endocrine related end points) and attempted to streamline the testing of chemicals for toxicity. The lifestages protocol was one of a tiered set of proposed studies, such that all data available could be incorporated into the study design and interpretation of the data. The approach was very laudable in that it proposed (unfortunately only as an option) incorporation of toxicokinetic data generated during pregnancy and lactation into the study design, as has long been required in drug testing, to aid study design and data interpretation. In addition, end points evaluating (at least to some degree) developmental neurotoxicity and developmental immunotoxicity would be measured as a standard, rather than as a triggered option. Its major aim was to reduce the number of animals required and increase the information available on young animals. However, these compromises were not without some flaws compared to the current multigeneration study used for pesticides by EPA or OECD. The study would seek to be a substitute for the current multigeneration study in most instances. The proposal does offer the opportunity to undertake a classical multigeneration study in a second tier but only if adverse events were not found in the Tier 1 study. Thus, a negative in the extended one-generation study could mean a halt to testing for reproductive toxicity. In particular, the paper recommends the use of the shortened exposure period before breeding the parental animals, similar to that implied in the international conference on harmonization of guidelines (ICH) guideline for fertility and early embryonic development, but it is much harder to justify that pesticides and other agricultural chemicals, unlike drugs, will not have human exposure at least subchronically and moreover the divorce of reproductive structure (e.g., histopathology of the reproductive organs) from function (e.g., litter parameters) could have serious implications for classification and labeling in some parts of the world.

As noted above, the new NTP RACB study attempts to overcome some of the shortcomings noted in standard multigeneration studies and the ILSI/ACSA designs by maintaining at least four males and four females of each litter until PND 90 for a full examination of the animals at sexual maturity and the increased power associated with keeping extra animals to detect low incidence phenomena. A standard multigeneration study keeping only one male and female from each of 20 litters could only detect a 25% incidence of a reproductive tract malformation if the background incidence is typically 0—precisely the types of adverse responses noted in studies with endocrine disruptors. The RACB study also takes multiple litters per generation to ensure the detection of latent effects that might not be observable only on the first breeding.

EVALUATION OF TOXICITY TO REPRODUCTION

Concordance of End Points

As noted in the testing section R, our standard testing protocols do not allow for discrimination between male and female effects except by some method modification. However, there is built-in redundancy in the number and type of end points evaluated in these studies that could indicate male, female, or effects on both sexes during testing. The following examples give an outline of the types of end points evaluated typically in rat multigeneration studies (the species most commonly used for reproductive toxicity evaluations).

There are a number of general points that the investigator should note in any estimation of potential reproductive toxicity:

- Adequacy of experimental design and conduct. Was there sufficient statistical power in the evaluation(s)?
- Occurrence of common versus rare reproductive deficits. Biological versus statistical significance.
- Use of historical control data to place concurrent control data into perspective and to estimate population background incidence of various reproductive parameters and deficits.
- Known structure-activity relationships for inducing reproductive toxicity.
- Concordance of reproductive end points (e.g., did a decrease in litter size relate to ovarian histology and changes in vaginal cytology?).
- Did the reproductive deficits become more severe with increases in dose—for example, did histological changes at one dose level become decrements in litter size and then reductions in fertility at higher dose levels in any generation?
- Did the reproductive deficits increase in prevalence (more individuals and/or more litters) with dose level in any generation?
- Special care should be taken for decrements in reproductive parameters noted in the F_1 generation (and potentially later generations) that were not seen in the F_0 generation, which may suggest developmental, as well as reproductive, toxicity. Likewise, findings in an F_1 generation animal may (or may not) be reproduced in F_2 offspring. For example, effects in the F_1 generation on reproductive parameters may have resulted in the selection out of sensitive animals in the population, thus not producing F_2 offspring for subsequent evaluation.

The first primary indication of a decrement in reproduction is obtained from the inspection of litter parameters from a breeding and determination of any functional effects. Thus, it is normal to inspect for various treatment groups versus the control, the number of fertile pairings, the mean litter size, pup weight at birth (small litters tend to have higher pup weights), and the sex ratio (to determine if there is a selective effect on any one sex).

In the parental females there should also be an evaluation of potential maternal toxicity that may or may not impact on the reproductive performance of these animals; these measures are crude and usually restricted to body weight, food consumption, and clinical signs. Gestation length is normally recorded (and this maybe shortened or lengthened) together with any signs of dystocia. Chemicals with progestin-like activity may also produce midgestational bleeding observable on the fur/or in the cage. At weaning of the litter (usually PND 21 in the rat), the parental females are usually necropsied (if no further pairings are required) and the uteri examined for implantation sites (which can be compared to the number of offspring produced) and the ovaries examined for corpora lutea and corpora albicans. These data are not as definitive for pre- versus postimplantation loss as in the developmental toxicity study, because the female will begin to cycle around postnatal day 15 and have representative corpora lutea from both the pregnancy and the new ovarian cycle(s).

In immature females after weaning, measurements can be made of the onset of puberty (which may be accelerated or delayed)

ILSI/ ACSA F₁- extended one generation rat reproduction study

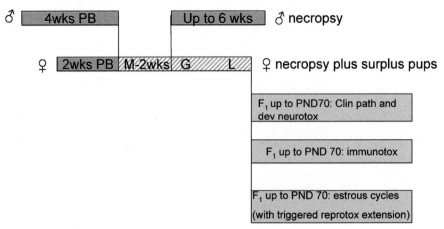

Figure 20-36. The ILSI/ACSA lifestages study for the evaluation of reproduction with developmental immunotoxicity and neurotoxicity.

through estimates of the date of VO and first estrus from vaginal smears. Some care needs to be used in the impact of other toxicity on these pubertal parameters and it is usual to normalize based on bodyweight. However, timing of puberty should not be normalized by body weight at acquisition of puberty (since a delay will invariably mean that the females are larger compared to controls and vice versa for acceleration). Instead, it is more likely that the investigator would employ weight at weaning as a covariate in the analysis of these pubertal end points.

As the female matures, estimates will be made of estrous cyclicity particularly if they are normal or abnormal (a rat normally has a 4–5 day cycle) and the duration of the cycles (for example, was persistent estrus or diestrus noted). Vaginal smears are also noted during mating and the presence of a sperm positive smear would indicate a successful mating that provides at least some surrogate of normal reproductive behavior from the breeding pair.

At necropsy of the adult F₁ female, weights and histopathology would be undertaken on critical organs (e.g., ovaries, uterus, pituitary and perhaps adrenal [as another steroidogenic organ]). Histopathology of the ovary is not straightforward and some guidelines require the evaluation of primordial follicle counts in step sections of the ovary. However, such an examination provides only limited information on one type of follicle and it is essential that the pathologists make their evaluation with regard to the normal expected patterns of the different follicular types (from primordial to antral), and when necessary undertake quantitative analysis to confirm an effect on ovarian follicular development.

In the parental males, similar types of evaluation are available to the investigator with regard to potential parental toxicity. Decreases in fertile pairings and litter size may be equally applicable for the detection of a male effect. The presence of a sperm positive smear in the female is indicative that the male has successfully mounted and mated with the female (note the presence of a copulatory plug is not the same because these may be formed from accessory sex organ fluids in the absence of sperm).

Males going through puberty can be estimated using the date of belanopreputial separation of the penis as an index. This androgen dependent end point in the male is also corrected for growth, but

the same caveats used in the female would apply to this male measurement. Decrements of ~10% body weight are normally without significant effect on male or female puberty indicies (Carney *et al.*, 2004). As the male matures and is bred with a female, observations of the precoital interval (the time between pairing and evidence of mating) can indicate treatment related effects on mating performance or behavior. However, it should be noted that if the female is at a random stage of estrus when introduced to the male, she may not allow mating until estrus is attained. Thus delays of more than 4–5 days in precoital interval should be carefully examined.

Once a pregnancy has been achieved and there is no requirement for further matings, the parental male is necropsied and organ weights and histological examination conducted usually of the testis, epididymis, prostate, seminal vesicles, and pituitary (and perhaps adrenal as for the female as another steroidogenic organ). Some studies also include other androgen-dependent organ weights such as the Levator ani-bulbocavernosus muscle, Cowper's gland, and penis. As with the ovary, histopathological examination of the testis requires some experience and the pathologist must be familiar with the different stages of the spermatogenic cycle. Although quantitative analysis of stage frequency is rarely required (and not useful in longer term studies) the noting of specific stages that may show a predilection for injury is most helpful, as is an appreciation of the different cellular associations affected within the seminiferous tubule. Such an analysis is essential in the detection of more subtle testicular effects.

At necropsy, a number of quantitative estimates can be made of sperm production and function. These can include testicular spermatid counts following homogenization (this end point entails destruction of one testis and has to be balanced with the information obtained from histopathology). A sperm sample is also taken from the vas or cauda epididymis for examination of sperm concentration, motility and morphology, which can be examined using manual methods. More often, computer assisted sperm analysis is used to evaluate these sperm end points and in addition further parameters can be collected, such as forward progressive motility, which is believed more closely related to fertility. Frequently, whole cauda epididymal sperm counts are also evaluated and normalized by weight.

Evaluation of male and female offspring follows the schema outline above for adults and for animals going through puberty. In addition, other useful end points may be included before weaning such as AGD, the presence of nipples and areolae (usually at postnatal day 13 before the pup fur has started to grow excessively to prevent examination), and the presence of certain reproductive tract malformations (see Tables 20-7 and 20-8). AGD and nipple retention are sexually dimorphic in the rat and under androgen control. Thus, normally AGD is twice the distance in males than females (this also seems to hold true for humans) and is dependent on levels of circulating DHT. In the normal male rat fetus, the presence of androgen around gestation day 17 causes the anlagen for the nipples to undergo apoptosis and thus males are born without nipples whereas females have the full complement of 12. The presence of an antiandrogen in males or an androgen in females would upset this balance to produce nipple retention in the males and a reduced number in the females reflective of the androgen status of these animals at critical periods of development. Some assessment must also be made of general growth of the offspring (usually bodyweight).

Consistency Across Generations

The F_0 reproductive parameters can differ markedly from those noted in the F_1 and similarly from the F_2 generation in a multigeneration study. Because exposure in a multigeneration study typically starts with the F_0 generation as young adults, critical periods of reproductive development have already taken place. The phthalates (e.g., DBP; Wine *et al.*, 1997) represent a classic example of weak effects noted in the F_0 generation (all the pairs were fertile but there was a small but significant effect on litter size and pup growth). In the F_1 generation where exposure is from conception to adulthood when these animals were bred at the same dose only 19/20 pairings resulted in a litter and thus the effects on reproduction were significantly enhanced in the F_1 generation and illustrate the importance of breeding the F_1 animals to detect functional effects on the offspring due to in utero exposure.

Differences between F_1 and F_2 generations can also arise. Here the exposure duration and critical windows of development are the same. However, because one normally only takes one male and female from each litter to generate the F_1 and F_2 parents it is distinctly possible that a selection bias can exist (e.g., if sensitive animals did not produce a litter, or the sensitive pups within a litter did not survive, then a pup from this pairing cannot be selected for further generations) and therefore potential effects may decrease in incidence or severity across generations. Other specific effects may increase severity in the F_2 versus the F_1. For example, a selective effect during in utero exposure of F_1 on the mammary gland would show the F_1 population as being normal with regard to reproduction, but when the F_1 animal becomes a parent, it cannot raise the F_2 adequately because of a mammary effect. In this instance there would be a more profound influence on the F_2 than the F_1 litters.

Graded Effects

In a similar fashion to developmental toxicity it is important to keep in mind the ability of changes in dose to alter the outcome of reproductive toxicity studies such that it is not just an increase in severity of a reproductive deficit that may be noted with increased dose but potentially an increased prevalence of a specific effect (on either an individual or litter basis). There may also be an increase in the severity of the type of lesion with the full constellation of the effects only noted at the highest dose level. Thus, for example, a single compound may produce a subtle effect on testis histology at low-dose levels. As the dose increases, this lesion may become more severe, with pathology noted in the epididymis, this in turn may affect semen parameters that result in a decrease in litter size and as the dose increases further, to a reduction in the number of fertile pairs—thus there is a continuum of effects that may be shown by a chemical producing reproductive toxicity that are interrelated and become important in selecting appropriate effect dose levels and therefore those exposures that maybe without effect.

REFERENCES

Adams NR: Permanent infertility in ewes exposed to plant oestrogens. *Aust Vet J* 67:197–201, 1990.

Adams NR, Sanders MR: Persistent infertility in ewes after prolonged exposure to oestradiol-17 beta. *J Reprod Fertil* 84:373–378, 1988.

Aho M, Koivisto AM, Tammela TL, Auvinen A: Is the incidence of hypospadias increasing? Analysis of Finnish hospital discharge data 1970–1994. *Environ Health Perspect* 108:463–465, 2000.

Andersen AN, Gianaroli L, Felberbaum R, de Mouzon J, Nygren K G: Assisted reproductive technology in Europe, 2001. Results generated from European registers by ESHRE. *Hum Reprod* 20:1158–1176, 2005.

Andersson KE, Wagner G: Physiology of penile erection. *Physiol Rev* 75:191–236, 1995.

Aplin JD, Kimber SJ: Trophoblast-uterine interactions at implantation. *Reprod Biol Endocrinol* 2:48, 2004.

Ashby J, Tinwell H, Haseman J: Lack of effects for low dose levels of bisphenol A and diethylstilbestrol on the prostate gland of CF1 mice exposed in utero. *Regul Toxicol Pharmacol* 30:156–166, 1999.

Atwood CS, Meethal SV, Liu T, *et al.*: Dysregulation of the hypothalamic-pituitary-gonadal axis with menopause and andropause promotes neurodegenerative senescence. *J Neuropathol Exp Neurol* 64:93–103, 2005.

Auchus RJ, Rainey WE: Adrenarche—physiology, biochemistry and human disease. *Clin Endocrinol (Oxf)* 60:288–296, 2004.

Bardin CW, Catterall JF: Testosterone: A major determinant of extragenital sexual dimorphism. *Science (New York)* 211:1285–1294, 1981.

Barker DJ: Fetal origins of coronary heart disease. *Bmj* 311:171–174, 1995.

Barker DJ: Fetal origins of cardiovascular disease. *Ann Med* 31 (Suppl 1):3–6, 1999.

Barker DJ, Hales CN, Fall CH, Osmond C, Phipps K, Clark PMl: Type 2 (non-insulin-dependent) diabetes mellitus, hypertension and hyperlipidaemia (syndrome X): Relation to reduced fetal growth. *Diabetologia* 36:62–67, 1993.

Barker DJ, Winter PD, Osmond C, Margetts B, Simmonds SJ: Weight in infancy and death from ischaemic heart disease. *Lancet* 2:577–580, 1989.

Barlow NJ, McIntyre BS, Foster PM: Male Reproductive Tract Lesions at 6, 12, and 18 Months of Age Following in Utero Exposure to Di(n-butyl) Phthalate. *Toxicol Pathol* 32:79–90, 2004.

Battaglia C, De Iaco P, Iughetti L, *et al.*: Female precocious puberty, obesity and polycystic-like ovaries. *Ultrasound Obstet Gynecol* 26:651–657, 2005.

Becker AL, Epperson CN: Female puberty: clinical implications for the use of prolactin-modulating psychotropics. *Child Adolesc Psychiatr Clin N Am* 15:207–220, 2006.

Berman DM, Tian H, Russell DW: Expression and regulation of steroid 5α-reductase in the urogenital tract of the fetal rat. *Mol Endo* 9:1561–1570, 1995.

Berman E, Laskey JW: Altered steroidogenesis in whole-ovary and adrenal culture in cycling rats. *Reprod Toxicol* 7:349–358, 1993.

Bielmeier SR, Best DS, Narotsky MG: Serum hormone characterization and exogeneous hormone rescue of bromodichloromethane-induced pregnancy loss in the F344 rat. *Toxicol Sci* 77:101–108, 2004.

Biro FM, Khoury P, Morrison JA: Influence of obesity on timing of puberty. *Int J Androl* 29:272–277, 2006; discussion 286-90.

Blackburn DM, Gray AJ, Lloyd SC, Sheard CM, Foster PMD: A comparison of the effects of the three isomers of dinitrobenzene on the testis in the rat. *Toxicol Appl Pharmacol* 92: 54–64, 1988.

Blanck HM, Marcus M, Tolbert PE, *et al.*: Age at menarche and tanner stage in girls exposed in utero and postnatally to polybrominated biphenyl. *Epidemiology* 11:641–647, 2000.

Blystone CR, Lambright CS, Howdeshell KL, *et al.*: Sensitivity of Fetal rat Testicular Steroidogenesis to Maternal Prochloraz Exposure and the Underlying Mechanism of Inhibition: Prochloraz reduced fetal testis testosterone. *Toxicol Sci* 97:512–519, 2007.

Boekelheide K, Darney SP, Daston GP, *et al.*: NTP-CERHR Expert Panel Report on the reproductive and developmental toxicity of 2-bromopropane. *Reprod Toxicol* 18:189–217, 2004.

Boisen KA, Kaleva M, Main KM, *et al.*: Difference in prevalence of congenital cryptorchidism in infants between two Nordic countries. *Lancet* 363:1264–1269, 2004.

Brouwer A, Longnecker MP, Birnbaum LS, *et al.*: Characterization of potential endocrine-related health effects at low-dose levels of exposure to PCBs. *EnvironHealth Perspect* 107 (Suppl 4): 639–649, 1999.

Buchanan JF, Davis LJ: Drug-induced infertility. *Drug Intell Clin Pharm* 18:122–132, 1984.

Buhimschi CS: Endocrinology of lactation. *Obstet Gynecol Clin North Am* 31:963–979, xii, 2004.

Byskov AG: Differentiation of mammalian embryonic gonad. *Physiol Rev* 66:71–117, 1986.

Cain JC: Miroestrol: An oestrogen from the plant *Pueraria mirifica*. *Nature* 188:774–777, 1960.

Calafat AM, Brock JW, Silva MJ, *et al.*: Urinary and amniotic fluid levels of phthalate monoesters in rats after the oral administration of di(2-ethylhexyl) phthalate and di-*n*-butyl phthalate. *Toxicology* 217:22–30, 2006.

Canning DA: Hypospadias trends in two US surveillance systems. Rise in prevalence of hypospadias. *J Urol* 161:366, 1999.

Cannon SSB, Veazey JJM, Jackson RRS, *et al.*: Epidemic kepone poisoning in chemical workers. *Am J Epidemiol* 107:529–537, 1978.

Carmichael SL, Shaw GM, Laurent C, Croughan MS, Olney RS, Lammer EJ: Maternal progestin intake and risk of hypospadias. *ArchPediatr Adolesc Med* 159:957–962, 2005.

Carnathan GW, Metcalf LE, Cochrane RL, Nutting EF, Black DL: Relationship between progesterone suppression and pregnancy in rats. *J Pharm Pharmacol* 39:401–404, 1987.

Carney EW, Zablotny CL, Marty MS, *et al.*: The effects of feed restriction during in utero and postnatal development in rats. *Toxicol Sci* 82:237–249, 2004.

Cave DA, Foster PMD: Modulation of m-dinitrobenzene and m-nitrosonitrobenzene toxicity in rat Sertoli—germ cell co-cultures. *Fund Appl Toxicol* 14:199–207, 1990.

Challis JR, Bloomfield FH, Bocking AD, *et al.*: Fetal signals and parturition. *J Obstet Gynaecol Res* 31:492–499, 2005.

Chapin R, Dutton S, Ross M, Lamb J: Effects of ethylene glycol monomethyl ether (EGME) on mating performance and epididymal sperm parameters in F344 rats. *Fundam Appl Toxicol* 5:182–189, 1985.

Chapin RE, Ku WW: The reproductive toxicity of boric acid. *Environ Health Perspect* 102 (Suppl 7): 87–91, 1994.

Charlier C: Endocrine effects of environmental pollutants. *Bull Mem Acad R Med Belg* 160:301–310, 2005.

Charlier C: Effects of environmental pollutants on hormone disturbances. *Bull Mem Acad R Med Belg* 161:116–124, 2006; discussion 124–6.

Colbert NK, Pelletier NC, Cote JM, *et al.*: Perinatal exposure to low levels of the environmental antiandrogen vinclozolin alters sex-differentiated social play and sexual behaviors in the rat. *Environ Health Perspect* 113:700–707, 2005.

Colborn T: The wildlife/human connection: Modernizing risk decisions. *Environ Health Perspect* 102 (Suppl 12): 55–59, 1994.

Cooper RL, Barrett MA, Goldman JM, *et al.*: Pregnancy alterations following xenobiotic-induced delays in ovulation in the female rat. *Fundam Appl Toxicol* 22:474–480, 1994.

Cooper RL, Lamb JC, Barlow SM, *et al.*: A tiered approach to life stages testing for agricultural chemical safety assessment. *Crit Rev Toxicol* 36:69–98, 2006.

Cooper RL, Roberts B, Rogers DC, Seay SG, Conn PM: Endocrine status versus chronologic age as predictors of altered luteinizing hormone secretion in the "aging" rat. *Endocrinology* 114:391–396, 1984.

Cooper RL, Stoker TE, Tyrey L, Goldman JM, McElroy WK: Atrazine disrupts the hypothalamic control of pituitary-ovarian function. *Toxicol Sci* 53:297–307, 2000.

Creasy DM, Beech LM, Gray TJ, Butler WH: An ultrastructural study of ethylene glycol monomethyl ether-induced spermatocyte injury in the rat. *Exp Mol Pathol* 45:311–322, 1986.

Creasy DM, Beech LM, Gray TJB, Butler WH: The ultrastructural effects of di-*n*-pentyl phthalate on the testis of the mature rat. *Exp Mol Pathol* 46:357–371, 1987.

Creasy DM, Foster PMD: The morphological development of glycol ether-induced testicular atrophy in the rat. *Exp Mol Path* 40:169–176, 1984.

Cummings AM, Perreault SD: Methoxychlor accelerates embryo transport through the rat reproductive tract. *Toxicol Appl Pharmacol* 102:110–116, 1990.

DeCherney AH, Cholst I, Naftolin F: Structure and function of the fallopian tubes following exposure to diethylstilbestrol (DES) during gestation. *Fertil Steril* 36: 741–745, 1981.

Den Hond E, Schoeters G: Endocrine disrupters and human puberty. *Int J Androl* 29:264–271, 2006; discussion 286–90.

Doody KJ, Lephart ED, Stirling D, *et al.*: Expression of mRNA species encoding steroidogenic enzymes in the rat ovary. *J Mol Endocrinol* 6:153–162, 1991.

Duck SC, Katayama KP: Danazol may cause female pseudo-hermaphroditism. *Fertil Steril* 35:230–231, 1981.

Dunger DB, Ahmed ML, Ong KK: Effects of obesity on growth and puberty. *Best Pract Res Clin Endocrinol Metab* 19:375–390, 2005.

Eddy E, Gong D, Fenderson A: Origin and migration of primoridal germ cells in mammals. *Gamete Research* 4:333–362, 1981.

Ellis MK, Foster PMD: The metabolism of 1,3-dinitrobenzene by rat testicular subcellular fractions. *Tox Letts* 62:201–208, 1992.

Enders AC, Carter AM: What can comparative studies of placental structure tell us?–A review. *Placenta* 25:S3–9, 2004.

Epstein SS: Kepone–hazard evaluation. *Sci Total Environ* 9:1–62, 1978.

Eskenazi B, Mocarelli P, Warner M, *et al.*: Seveso Women's Health Study: A study of the effects of 2,3,7,8-tetrachlorodibenzo-p-dioxin on reproductive health. *Chemosphere* 40:1247–1253, 2000.

Ewing LL, Desjardins C, Irby DC, Robaire B: Synergistic interaction of testosterone and oestradiol inhibits spermatogenesis in rats. *Nature* 269:409–411, 1977.

Ewing LL, Gorski RA, Sbordone RJ, Tyler JV, Desjardins C, Robaire B: Testosterone-estradiol filled polydimethylsiloxane subdermal implants: Effect on fertility and masculine sexual and aggressive behavior of male rats. *Biol Reprod* 21:765–772, 1979.

Ewing LL, Zirkin BR, Chubb C: Assessment of testicular testosterone production and Leydig cell structure. *Environ Health Perspect* 38:19–27, 1981.

Farnsworth NR: The role of ethnopharmacology in drug development. *Ciba Found Sympos* 154:2–11, 1990; discussion 11–21.

Faroon O, Kueberuwa S, Smith L, DeRosa C: ATSDR evaluation of health effects of chemicals. II. Mirex and chlordecone: Health effects, toxicokinetics, human exposure, and environmental fate. *Toxicol Ind Health* 11:1–203, 1995.

Fisher JS: Environmental anti-androgens and male reproductive health: Focus on phthalates and testicular dysgenesis syndrome. *Reproduction* 127:305–315, 2004.

Foster PM, Cook MW, Thomas LV, Walters DG, Gangolli SD: Differences in urinary metabolic profile from di-*n*-butyl phthalate-treated rats and hamsters. A possible explanation for species differences in susceptibility to testicular atrophy. *Drug Metab Dispos* 11:59–61, 1983.

Foster PM, Mylchreest E, Gaido KW, Sar M: Effects of phthalate esters on the developing reproductive tract of male rats. *Hum Reprod Update* 7:231–235, 2001.

Foster PMD: Testicular organization and biochemical function, in Lamb JC, Foster PMD (eds): *The Physiology and Toxicology of Male Reproduction*, New York: Academic Press, 1988, pp. 7–34.

Foster PMD: Studies on the toxicity of m-dinitrobenzene to the testicular Sertoli cell. *Arc. Tox Suppl* 13:3–17, 1989.

Foster PMD, Lloyd SC, Blackburn DM: Comparison of the in vivo and in vitro testicular effects produced by methoxy-, ethoxy- and *n*-butoxy acetic acids in the rat. *Toxicology* 43:17–30, 1987.

Giwercman A, Rylander L, Hagmar L, Giwercman YL: Ethnic differences in occurrence of TDS–genetics and/or environment? *IntJ Androl* 29:291–297, 2006; discussion 304–6.

Gladen BC, Klebanoff MA, Hediger ML, *et al.*: Prenatal DDT exposure in relation to anthropometric and pubertal measures in adolescent males. *Environ Health Perspect* 112:1761–1767, 2004.

Goldman JM, Laws SC, Balchak SK, Cooper RL, Kavlock RJ: Endocrine-disrupting chemicals: prepubertal exposures and effects on sexual maturation and thyroid activity in the female rat. A focus on the EDSTAC recommendations. *Crit Rev Toxicol* 30:135–196, 2000.

Goldman JM, Parrish MB, Cooper RL, McElroy WK: Blockade of ovulation in the rat by systemic and ovarian intrabursal administration of the fungicide sodium dimethyldithiocarbamate. *Reprod Toxicol* 11:185–190, 1997.

Goldman JM, Stoker TE, Cooper RL, McElroy WK, Hein JF: Blockade of ovulation in the rat by the fungicide sodium N-methyldithiocarbamate: relationship between effects on the luteinizing hormone surge and alterations in hypothalamic catecholamines. *Neurotoxicol Teratol* 16:257–268, 1994.

Goldman JM, Stoker TE, Perreault SD, Cooper RL, Crider MA: Influence of the formamidine pesticide chlordimeform on ovulation in the female hamster: Dissociable shifts in the luteinizing hormone surge and oocyte release. *Toxicol Appl Pharmacol* 121:279–290, 1993.

Goldstein I, Lue TF, Padma-Nathan H, Rosen RC, Steers WD, Wicker PA: Oral sildenafil in the treatment of erectile dysfunction. Sildenafil Study Group. *N Engl J Med* 338:1397–1404, 1998.

Gordon AE, Shaughnessy AF: Saw palmetto for prostate disorders. *Am Fam Physician* 67:1281–1283, 2003.

Goyeneche AA, Calvo V, Gibori G, Telleria CM: Androstenedione interferes in luteal regression by inhibiting apoptosis and stimulating progesterone production. *Biol Reprod* 66:1540–1547, 2002.

Grajewski B, Whelan EA, Schnorr TM, Mouradian R, Alderfer R, Wild DK: Evaluation of reproductive function among men occupationally exposed to a stilbene derivative: I. Hormonal and physical status. *Am J Ind Med* 29:49–57, 1996.

Gray L, Ostby J, Furr J, Lambright C, Hotchkiss A, Wilson V: Cumulative Effects of Endocrine Disrupters (EDCs): Synergy or Additivity? *The Toxicologist* 74:2004a.

Gray LE: Emerging issues related to endocrine disrupting chemicals and environmental androgens and antiandrogens, in Hutzinger O (ed.): *The Handbook of Environmental Chemistry*. Vol. 3, Heidelberg: Springer-Verlag, 2002, pp. 209–248.

Gray LE, Jr.: Tiered screening and testing strategy for xenoestrogens and antiandrogens. *Toxicol Lett* 102–103:677–680, 1998.

Gray LE, Jr., Kelce WR: Latent effects of pesticides and toxic substances on sexual differentiation of rodents. *Toxicol Ind Health* 12:515–531, 1996.

Gray LE, Jr., Kelce WR, Monosson E, Ostby JS, Birnbaum LS: Exposure to TCDD during development permanently alters reproductive function in male Long Evans rats and hamsters: Reduced ejaculated and epididymal sperm numbers and sex accessory gland weights in offspring

with normal androgenic status. *Toxicol Appl Pharmacol* 131:108–118, 1995.

Gray LE, Jr., Kelce WR, Wiese T, *et al.*: Endocrine Screening Methods Workshop report: detection of estrogenic and androgenic hormonal and antihormonal activity for chemicals that act via receptor or steroidogenic enzyme mechanisms. *Reprod Toxicol* 11:719–750, 1997a.

Gray LE, Jr., Ostby J: Effects of pesticides and toxic substances on behavioral and morphological reproductive development: Endocrine versus nonendocrine mechanisms. *Toxicol Ind Health* 14:159–184, 1998.

Gray LE, Jr., Ostby J, Ferrell J, *et al.*: A dose-response analysis of methoxychlor-induced alterations of reproductive development and function in the rat. *Fundam Appl Toxicol* 12:92–108, 1989.

Gray LE, Jr., Ostby J, Linder R, Goldman J, Rehnberg G, Cooper R: Carbendazim-induced alterations of reproductive development and function in the rat and hamster. *Fundam Appl Toxicol* 15:281–297, 1990.

Gray LE, Jr., Ostby J, Monosson E, Kelce WR: Environmental antiandrogens: Low doses of the fungicide vinclozolin alter sexual differentiation of the male rat. *Toxicol Ind Health* 15:48–64, 1999.

Gray LE, Jr., Ostby J, Sigmon R, *et al.*: The development of a protocol to assess reproductive effects of toxicants in the rat. *Reprod Toxicol* 2:281–287, 1988a.

Gray LE, Jr., Ostby J, Wilson V, *et al.*: Xenoendocrine disrupters-tiered screening and testing: filling key data gaps. *Toxicology* 181–182:371–382, 2002.

Gray LE, Jr., Ostby JS: In utero 2,3,7,8-tetrachlorodibenzo-*p*-dioxin (TCDD) alters reproductive morphology and function in female rat offspring. *Toxicol Appl Pharmacol* 133:285–294, 1995.

Gray LE, Jr., Ostby JS, Ferrell JM, Sigmon ER, Goldman JM: Methoxychlor induces estrogen-like alterations of behavior and the reproductive tract in the female rat and hamster: Effects on sex behavior, running wheel activity, and uterine morphology. *Toxicol Appl Pharmacol* 96:525–540, 1988b.

Gray LE, Jr., Ostby JS, Kelce WR: Developmental effects of an environmental antiandrogen: the fungicide vinclozolin alters sex differentiation of the male rat. *Toxicol Appl Pharmacol* 129:46–52, 1994.

Gray LE, Jr., Wilson V, Noriega N, *et al.*: Use of the laboratory rat as a model in endocrine disruptor screening and testing. *Ilar J* 45:425–437, 2004b.

Gray LE, Jr., Wilson VS, Stoker T, *et al.*: Adverse effects of environmental antiandrogens and androgens on reproductive development in mammals. *Int J Androl* 29:96–104, 2006; discussion 105–8.

Gray LE, Ostby J, Furr J, *et al.*: Effects of environmental antiandrogens on reproductive development in experimental animals. *Hum Reprod Update* 7:248–264, 2001.

Gray LE, Ostby JS, Kelce WR: A dose-response analysis of the reproductive effects of a single gestational dose of 2,3,7,8-tetrachlorodibenzo-*p*-dioxin in male Long Evans Hooded rat offspring. *Toxicol Appl Pharmacol* 146:11–20, 1997b.

Gray LE, Wolf C, Mann P, Ostby JS: In utero exposure to low doses of 2,3,7,8-tetrachlorodibenzo-*p*-dioxin alters reproductive development of female Long Evans hooded rat offspring. *Toxicol Appl Pharmacol* 146:237–244, 1997c.

Gupta RK, Miller KP, Babus JK, Flaws JA: Methoxychlor inhibits growth and induces atresia of antral follicles through an oxidative stress pathway. *Toxicol Sci* 93:382–389, 2006a.

Gupta RK, Schuh RA, Fiskum G, Flaws JA: Methoxychlor causes mitochondrial dysfunction and oxidative damage in the mouse ovary. *Toxicol Appl Pharmacol* 216:436–445, 2006b.

Hammond B, Katzenellenbogen BS, Krauthammer N, McConnell J: Estrogenic activity of the insecticide chlordecone (Kepone) and interaction with uterine estrogen receptors. *Proc Natl Acad Sci U S A* 76:6641–6645, 1979.

Hammond SK, Smith TJ, Ellenbecker MJ: Determination of occupational exposure to fabric brightener chemicals by HPLC. *Am Ind Hyg Assoc J* 48:117–121, 1987.

Hauser R, Williams P, Altshul L, *et al.*: Predictors of serum dioxin levels among adolescent boys in Chapaevsk, Russia: A cross-sectional pilot study. *Environ Health* 4:8, 2005.

Hemsworth BN, Jackson H: Effect of Busulphan on the Developing Ovary in the Rat. *J Reprod Fertil* 6:229–233, 1963.

Henley DV, Lipson N, Korach KS, Bloch CA: Prepubertal gynecomastia linked to lavender and tea tree oils. *N Engl J Med* 356:479–485, 2007.

Herbst AL: Exogenous hormones in pregnancy. *Clin Obstetr Gynecol* 16:37–50, 1973.

Herbst AL: The effects in the human of diethylstilbestrol (DES) use during pregnancy. *Princess Takamatsu Symp* 18:67–75, 1987.

Hershberger LG, Shipley EG, Meyer RK: Myotrophic activity of 19-nortestosterone and other steroids determined by modified levator ani muscle method. *Proceedings of the Society for Experimental Biology and Medicine. Society for Experimental Biology and Medicine. New York,* 83:175–180, 1953.

Hertz R: Accidental ingestion of estrogens by children. *Pediatrics* 21:203–206, 1958.

Himes JH: Examining the evidence for recent secular changes in the timing of puberty in US children in light of increases in the prevalence of obesity. *Mol Cell Endocrinol* 254–255:13–21, 2006.

Hines M: Sex steroids and human behavior: Prenatal androgen exposure and sex-typical play behavior in children. *Ann N Y Acad Sci* 1007:272–282, 2003.

Hines M, Kaufman FR: Androgen and the development of human sex-typical behavior: Rough-and-tumble play and sex of preferred playmates in children with congenital adrenal hyperplasia (CAH). *Child Dev* 65:1042–1053, 1994.

Holloway AJ, Moore HDM, Foster PMD: The use of in vitro fertilization to detect reductions in fertility of male rats exposed to 1,3-dinitrobenzene. *Fund Appl Toxicol* 14:113–122, 1990.

Hoodbhoy T, Dean J: Insights into the molecular basis of sperm-egg recognition in mammals. *Reproduction* 127:417–422, 2004.

Hotchkiss AK, Lambright CS, Ostby JS, Parks-Saldutti L, Vandenbergh JG, Gray LE, Jr.: Prenatal testosterone exposure permanently masculinizes anogenital distance, nipple development, and reproductive tract morphology in female Sprague-Dawley rats. *Toxicol Sci* 96:335–345, 2007.

Hotchkiss AK, Ostby JS, Vandenbergh JG, Gray LE Jr.: An environmental antiandrogen, vinclozolin, alters the organization of play behavior. *Physiol Behav* 79:151–156, 2003.

Hotchkiss AK, Parks-Saldutti LG, Ostby JS, *et al.*: A mixture of the "antiandrogens" linuron and butyl benzyl phthalate alters sexual differentiation of the male rat in a cumulative fashion. *Biol Reprod* 71:1852–1861, 2004.

Hoyer PB, Sipes IG: Development of an animal model for ovotoxicity using 4-vinylcyclohexene: a case study. *Birth Defects Res B Dev Reprod Toxicol* 80:113–125, 2007.

Huhtaniemi I, Pelliniemi LJ: Fetal Leydig cells: Cellular origin, morphology, life span, and special functional features. *Proc Soc Exp Biol Med* 201:125–140, 1992.

Hunter RH, Rodriguez-Martinez H: Capacitation of mammalian spermatozoa in vivo, with a specific focus on events in the Fallopian tubes. *Mol Reprod Dev* 67:243–250, 2004.

Hurtt ME, Daston G, Davis-Bruno K, *et al.*: Juvenile animal studies: Testing strategies and design. *Birth Defects Res B Dev Reprod Toxicol* 71:281–8, 2004.

Imperato-McGinley J, Sanchez RS, Spencer JR, Yee B, Vaughan ED: Comparison of the effects of the 5 alpha-reductase inhibitor finasteride and the antiandrogen flutamide on prostate and genital differentiation: Dose-response studies. *Endocrinology* 131:1149–1156, 1992.

Jaruratanasirikul S, Leethanaporn K, Pradutkanchana S, Sriplung H: Serum insulin-like growth factor-1 (IGF-1) and insulin-like growth factor binding protein-3 (IGFBP-3) in healthy Thai children and adolescents: Relation to age, sex, and stage of puberty. *J Med Assoc Thai* 82:275–283, 1999.

Jobling S, Tyler CR: Introduction: The ecological relevance of chemically induced endocrine disruption in wildlife. *Environ Health Perspect* 114(Suppl 1):7–8, 2006.

Jorgensen N, Andersen AG, Eustache F, *et al.*: Regional differences in semen quality in Europe. *Hum Reprod* 16:1012–1019, 2001.

Jorgensen N, Carlsen E, Nermoen I, *et al.*: East-West gradient in semen quality in the Nordic-Baltic area: A study of men from the general population in Denmark, Norway, Estonia and Finland. *Hum Reprod* 17:2199–2208, 2002.

Kanno J, Onyon L, Haseman J, Fenner-Crisp P, Ashby J, Owens W: The OECD program to validate the rat uterotrophic bioassay to screen compounds for in vivo estrogenic responses: Phase 1. *Environ Health Perspect* 109:785–794, 2001.

Kanno J, Onyon L, Peddada S, Ashby J, Jacob E, Owens W: The OECD program to validate the rat uterotrophic bioassay. Phase 2: Coded single-dose studies. *Environ Health Perspect* 111:1550–1558, 2003a.

Kanno J, Onyon L, Peddada S, Ashby J, Jacob E, Owens W: The OECD program to validate the rat uterotrophic bioassay. Phase 2: Dose-response studies. *Environ Health Perspect* 111:1530–1549, 2003b.

Kaplowitz P: Pubertal development in girls: Secular trends. *Curr Opin Obstet Gynecol* 18:487–491, 2006.

Kassim NM, McDonald SW, Reid O, Bennett NK, Gilmore DP, Payne AP: The effects of pre- and postnatal exposure to the nonsteroidal antiandrogen flutamide on testis descent and morphology in the Albino Swiss rat. *J Anat* 190:577–588, 1997.

Keefe DL, Marquard K, Liu L: The telomere theory of reproductive senescence in women. *Curr Opin Obstet Gynecol* 18:280–285, 2006.

Keene LC, Davies PH: Drug-related erectile dysfunction. *Adverse Drug React Toxicol Rev* 18:5–24, 1999.

Kelce WR, Monosson E, Gray LE, Jr.: An environmental antiandrogen. Recent *Prog Horm Res* 50:449–453, 1995.

Kingsbury AC: Danazol and fetal masculinization: A warning. *Med J Aust* 143:410–411, 1985.

Klonisch T, Fowler PA, Hombach-Klonisch S: Molecular and genetic regulation of testis descent and external genitalia development. *Dev Biol* 270:1–18, 2004.

Knappe G, Gerl H, Ventz M, Rohde W: The long-term therapy of hypothalamic-hypophyseal Cushing's syndrome with mitotane (o, p'-DDD). *Deutsche Medizinische Wochenschrift (1946)* 122:882–886, 1997.

Knobil E, Neill J: *The Physiology of Reproduction.* New York: Raven Press, 1994.

Kolpin DW, Furlong ET, Meyer MT, *et al.*: Pharmaceuticals, hormones, and other organic wastewater contaminants in U.S. streams, 1999–2000: A national reconnaissance. *Environ Sci Technol* 36:1202–1211, 2002.

Kolpin DW, Skopec M, Meyer MT, Furlong ET, Zaugg SD: Urban contribution of pharmaceuticals and other organic wastewater contaminants to streams during differing flow conditions. *Sci Total Environ* 328:119–130, 2004.

Kolpin DW, Thurman EM, Linhart SM: The environmental occurrence of herbicides: The importance of degradates in ground water. *Arch Environ Contam Toxicol* 35:385–390, 1998.

Koopman P, Munsterberg A, Capel B, Vivian N, Lovell-Badge R: Expression of a candidate sex-determining gene during mouse testis differentiation. *Nature* 348:450–452, 1990.

Krstevska-Konstantinova M, Charlier C, Craen M, *et al.*: Sexual precocity after immigration from developing countries to Belgium: Evidence of previous exposure to organochlorine pesticides. *Hum Reprod* 16:1020–1026, 2001.

Kuiper-Goodman T, Scott PM, Watanabe H: Risk assessment of the mycotoxin zearalenone. *Regul Toxicol Pharmacol* 7:253–306, 1987.

Lambright C, Ostby J, Bobseine K, *et al.*: Cellular and molecular mechanisms of action of linuron: An antiandrogenic herbicide that produces reproductive malformations in male rats. *Toxicol Sci* 56:389–399, 2000.

Landrigan PJ, Kreiss K, Xintaras C, Feldman RG, Heath CW, Jr.: Clinical epidemiology of occupational neurotoxic disease. *Neurobehav toxicol* 2:43–48, 1980.

Leblond CP, Clermont Y: Definition of the stages of the seminiferous epithelium in the rat. *Ann NY Acad Sci* 55:548–573, 1952.

Lee KY, DeMayo FJ: Animal models of implantation. *Reproduction* 128:679–695, 2004.

LeMaire WJ, Cleveland WW, Bejar RL, Marsh JM, Fishman L: Aminoglutethimide: A possible cause of pseudohermaphroiditism in females. *Am J Dis child (1960)* 124:421–423, 1972.

Linder RE, Hess RA, Strader LF: Testicular toxicity and infertility in male rats treated with 1,3-dinitrobenzene. *J Toxicol Environ Health* 19:477–489, 1986.

Linder RE, Klinefelter GR, Strader LF, Veeramachaneni DN, Roberts NL, Suarez JD: Histopathologic changes in the testes of rats exposed to dibromoacetic acid. *Reprod Toxicol* 11:47–56, 1997.

Lloyd SC, Foster PM: Effect of mono-(2-ethylhexyl)phthalate on follicle-stimulating hormone responsiveness of cultured rat Sertoli cells. *Toxicol Appl Pharmacol* 95:484–489, 1988.

Longnecker MP, Gladen BC, Cupul-Uicab LA, *et al.*: In Utero Exposure to the Antiandrogen 1,1-Dichloro-2,2-bis(p-chlorophenyl)ethylene (DDE) in Relation to Anogenital Distance in Male Newborns from Chiapas, Mexico. *Am J Epidemiol* 165:1015–1022, 2007.

Lopes FL, Desmarais JA, Murphy BD: Embryonic diapause and its regulation. *Reproduction* 128:669–678, 2004.

Malassine A, Frendo JL, Evain-Brion D: A comparison of placental development and endocrine functions between the human and mouse model. *Hum Reprod Update* 9:531–539, 2003.

Marshall WA, Tanner JM: Variations in pattern of pubertal changes in girls. *Arch Dis Child* 44:291–303, 1969.

Marshall WA, Tanner JM: Variations in the pattern of pubertal changes in boys. *Arch Dis Child* 45:13–23, 1970.

Massart F, Parrino R, Seppia P, Federico G, Saggese G: How do environmental estrogen disruptors induce precocious puberty? *Minerva Pediatr* 58:247–254, 2006.

Matsumura A, Ghosh A, Pope GS, Darbre PD: Comparative study of oestrogenic properties of eight phytoestrogens in MCF7 human breast cancer cells. *J steroid biochem mol bio* 94:431–443, 2005.

McCartney CR, Blank SK, Prendergast KA, *et al.*: Obesity and sex steroid changes across puberty: Evidence for marked hyperandrogenemia in pre- and early pubertal obese girls. *J Clin Endocrinol Metab* 92:430–436, 2007.

Melnick RL, Nyska A, Foster PM, Roycroft JH, Kissling GE: Toxicity and carcinogenicity of the water disinfection byproduct, dibromoacetic acid, in rats and mice. *Toxicology* 230:126–136, 2007.

Mendelson CR, Condon JC: New insights into the molecular endocrinology of parturition. *J Steroid Biochem Mol Biol* 93:113–119, 2005.

Miller KP, Gupta RK, Greenfeld CR, Babus JK, Flaws JA: Methoxychlor directly affects ovarian antral follicle growth and atresia through Bcl-2- and Bax-mediated pathways. *Toxicol Sci* 88:213–221, 2005.

Monosson E, Kelce WR, Lambright C, Ostby J, Gray LE, Jr.: Peripubertal exposure to the antiandrogenic fungicide, vinclozolin, delays puberty, inhibits the development of androgen-dependent tissues, and alters androgen receptor function in the male rat. *Toxicol Ind Health* 15:65–79, 1999.

Moore KL: *The Developing Human: Clinically Oriented Embryology.* Philadelphia: W. B. Saunders Company, 1982.

Muir A: Precocious puberty. *Pediatr Rev* 27:373–381, 2006.

Nagano K, Nakayama E, Koyano M, Oobayashi H, Adachi H, Yamada T: Testicular atrophy of mice induced by ethylene glycol mono alkyl ethers (author's transl). *Sangyo Igaku* 21:29–35, 1979.

Nagel SC, vom Saal FS, Thayer KA, Dhar MG, Boechler M, Welshons WV: Relative binding affinity-serum modified access (RBA-SMA) assay predicts the relative in vivo bioactivity of the xenoestrogens bisphenol A and octylphenol. *Environ Health Perspect* 105:70–76, 1997.

Nassar N, Bower C, Barker A: Increasing prevalence of hypospadias in Western Australia, 1980–2000. *Arch Dis Child* 92:580–584, 2007.

Niculescu AM: Effects of in utero exposure to DES on male progeny. *J Obstet Gynecol Neonatal Nurs* 14:468–470, 1985.

Ohyama K: Disorders of sex differentiation caused by exogenous hormones. *Nippon rinsho* 62:379–384, 2004.

Ojeda SR, Heger S: New thoughts on female precocious puberty. *J Pediatr Endocrinol Metab* 14:245–256, 2001.

Ojeda SR, Lomniczi A, Mastronardi C, *et al.*: Minireview: The neuroendocrine regulation of puberty: is the time ripe for a systems biology approach? *Endocrinology* 147:1166–1174, 2006.

Ojeda SR, Prevot V, Heger S, Lomniczi A, Dziedzic B, Mungenast A: The neurobiology of female puberty. *Horm Res* 60(Suppl 3):15–20, 2003.

Oliveira CA, Mahecha GA, Carnes K, *et al.*: Differential hormonal regulation of estrogen receptors ERalpha and ERbeta and androgen receptor expression in rat efferent ductules. *Reproduction* 128:73–86, 2004.

Ouyang F, Perry MJ, Venners SA, *et al.*: Serum DDT, age at menarche, and abnormal menstrual cycle length. *Occup Environ Med* 62:878–884, 2005.

Owens JW, Ashby J: Critical review and evaluation of the uterotrophic bioassay for the identification of possible estrogen agonists and antagonists: In support of the validation of the OECD uterotrophic protocols for the laboratory rodent. Organisation for Economic Co-operation and Development. *Crit Rev Toxicology* 32:445–520, 2002.

Owens JW, Chaney JG: Weighing the results of differing 'low dose' studies of the mouse prostate by Nagel, Cagen, and Ashby: Quantification of experimental power and statistical results. *Regul Toxicol Pharmacol* 43:194–202, 2005.

Owens W, Ashby J, Odum J, Onyon L: The OECD program to validate the rat uterotrophic bioassay. Phase 2: Dietary phytoestrogen analyses. *Environ Health Perspect* 111:1559–1567, 2003.

Owens W, Koeter HB: The OECD program to validate the rat uterotrophic bioassay: An overview. *Environ Health Perspect* 111:1527–1529, 2003.

Owens W, Zeiger E, Walker M, Ashby J, Onyon L, Gray LE, Jr.: The OECD program to validate the rat Hershberger bioassay to screen compounds for in vivo androgen and antiandrogen responses. Phase 1: Use of a potent agonist and a potent antagonist to test the standardized protocol. *Environ Health Perspect* 114:1259–1265, 2006.

Papathanasiou A, Hadjiathanasiou C: (2006). Precocious puberty. *Pediatr Endocrinol Rev* 3(Suppl 1):182–187, 2006.

Paranko J, Pelliniemi LJ, Vaheri A, Foidart JM, Lakkala-Paranko T: Morphogenesis and fibronectin in sexual differentiation of rat embryonic gonads. *Differentiation* 23(Suppl):S72–S81, 1983.

Paulozzi LJ, Erickson JD, Jackson RJ: Hypospadias trends in two US surveillance systems. *Pediatrics* 100:831–834, 1997.

Pelliniemi LJ: Ultrastructure of the early ovary and testis in pig embryos. *Am J Anat* 144:89–111, 1975.

Pelliniemi LJ, Niei M: Fine structure of the human foetal testis. I. The interstitial tissue. *Z Zellforsch Mikrosk Anat* 99, 507–522, 1969.

Pierik FH, Burdorf A, Nijman JM, de Muinck Keizer-Schrama SM, Juttmann RE, Weber RF: A high hypospadias rate in The Netherlands. *Hum Reprod* 17:1112–1115, 2002.

Porter MP, Faizan MK, Grady RW, Mueller BA: Hypospadias in Washington State: Maternal risk factors and prevalence trends. *Pediatrics* 115:e495–e499, 2005.

Quinn MM, Wegman DH, Greaves IA, *et al.*: Investigation of reports of sexual dysfunction among male chemical workers manufacturing stilbene derivatives. *Am J Ind Med* 18:55–68, 1990.

Reeve IT, Voss JC, Miller MG: 1,3-Dinitrobenzene metabolism and GSH depletion. *Chem Res Toxicol* 15:361–366, 2002.

Reich MR, Spong JK: Kepone: A chemical disaster in Hopewell, Virginia. *Int J Health Serv* 13:227–246, 1983.

Robaire B, Ewing LL, Irby DC, Desjardins C: Interactions of testosterone and estradiol-17 beta on the reproductive tract of the male rat. *Biol Reprod* 21:455–463, 1979.

Rosa FW: Virilization of the female fetus with maternal danazol exposure. *Am J Obstet Gynecol* 149:99–100, 1984.

Roy AK, Chatterjee B: Androgen action. *Crit Rev Eukaryot Gene Expr* 5:157–176, 1995.

Saito K, O'Donnell L, McLachlan RI, Robertson DM: Spermiation failure is a major contributor to early spermatogenic suppression caused by hormone withdrawal in adult rats. *Endocrinology* 141:2779–2785, 2000.

Saiyed H, Dewan A, Bhatnagar V, *et al.*: Effect of endosulfan on male reproductive development. *Environ Health Perspect* 111:1958–1962, 2003.

Schäfer-Somi S: Cytokines during early pregnancy of mammals: A review *Anim Reprod Sci* 75:73–94, 2003.

Schardein J: *Chemically induced birth defects*. New York: Marcel Dekker, 2000.

Semple RK, Achermann JC, Ellery J, *et al.*: Two novel missense mutations in g protein-coupled receptor 54 in a patient with hypogonadotropic hypogonadism. *J Clin Endocrinol Metab* 90:1849–1855, 2005.

Setchell BP, Waites GM: Changes in the permeability of the testicular capillaries and of the 'blood-testis barrier' after injection of cadmium chloride in the rat. *J Endocrinol* 47:81–86, 1970.

Shaffer NG: DES: A continuing health concern. *Pa med* 103:17, 2000.

Silversides DW, Price CA., Cooke GM: Effects of short-term exposure to hydroxyflutamide in utero on the development of the reproductive tract in male mice. *Can J Physiol Pharmacol* 73:1582–1588, 1995.

Skakkebaek NE: Endocrine disrupters and testicular dysgenesis syndrome. *Horm Res* 57(Suppl 2):43, 2002.

Smith ER, Quinn MM: Uterotropic action in rats of amsonic acid and three of its synthetic precursors. *J Toxicol Environ Health* 36:13–25, 1992.

Snegovskikh V, Park JS, Norwitz ER: Endocrinology of parturition. *Endocrinol Metab Clin North Am* 35:173–191, viii, 2006.

Stevenson JG, Umstead GS: Sexual dysfunction due to antihypertensive agents. *Drug Intell Clin Pharm* 18:113–121, 1984.

Stoker TE, Cooper RL, Goldman JM, Andrews JE: Characterization of pregnancy outcome following thiram-induced ovulatory delay in the female rat. *Neurotoxicol Teratol* 18:277–282, 1996.

Stoker TE, Goldman JM, Cooper RL: The dithiocarbamate fungicide thiram disrupts the hormonal control of ovulation in the female rat. *Reprod Toxicol* 7:211–218, 1993.

Stoker TE, Goldman JM, Cooper RL: Delayed ovulation and pregnancy outcome: effect of environmental toxicants on the neuroendocrine control of the ovary(1). *Environ Toxicol Pharmacol* 9:117–129, 2001.

Stoker TE, Jeffay SC, Zucker RM, Cooper RL, Perreault SD: Abnormal fertilization is responsible for reduced fecundity following thiram-induced ovulatory delay in the rat. *Biol Reprod* 68:2142–2149, 2003.

Stoker TE, Parks LG, Gray LE, Cooper RL: Endocrine-disrupting chemicals: Prepubertal exposures and effects on sexual maturation and thyroid function in the male rat. A focus on the EDSTAC recommendations. Endocrine Disrupter Screening and Testing Advisory Committee. *Crit Rev Toxicol* 30:197–252, 2000.

Stoker TE, Perreault SD, Bremser K, Marshall RS, Murr A, Cooper RL Acute exposure to molinate alters neuroendocrine control of ovulation in the rat. *Toxicol Sci* 84:38–48, 2005.

Swan SH, Main KM, Liu F, *et al.*: Decrease in anogenital distance among male infants with prenatal phthalate exposure. *Environ Health Perspect* 113:1056–1061, 2005.

Swingle WW, Seay P, Perlmutt J, Collins EJ, Barlow G, Jr., Fedor EJ: An experimental study of pseudopregnancy in rat. *Am J Physiol* 167:586–592, 1951.

Tan SW, Zoeller RT: Integrating basic research on thyroid hormone action into screening and testing programs for thyroid disruptors. *Crit Rev Toxicol* 37:5–10, 2007.

Tena-Sempere M: KiSS-1 and reproduction: focus on its role in the metabolic regulation of fertility. *Neuroendocrinology* 83:275–281, 2006.

Toppari J, Kaleva M, Virtanen HE: Trends in the incidence of cryptorchidism and hypospadias, and methodological limitations of registry-based data. *Hum Reprod Update* 7:282–286, 2001.

Tranguch S, Daikoku T, Guo Y, Wang H, Dey SK: Molecular complexity in establishing uterine receptivity and implantation. *Cell Mol Life Sci* 62:1964–1973, 2005.

Trasler JM, Hales BF, Robaire B: Paternal cyclophosphamide treatment of rats causes fetal loss and malformations without affecting male fertility. *Nature* 316:144–146, 1985.

Tuvemo T: Treatment of central precocious puberty. *Expert Opin Investig Drugs* 15:495–505, 2006.

Uckert S, Hedlund P, Andersson KE, Truss MC, Jonas U, Stief CG: Update on phosphodiesterase (PDE) isoenzymes as pharmacologic targets in urology: Present and future. *Eur Urol* 50:1194–1207, 2006; discussion 1207.

Veurink M, Koster M, Berg LT: The history of DES, lessons to be learned. *Pharm World Sci* 27:139–143, 2005.

Veyssiere G, Berger M, Jean-Faucher C, de Turckheim M, Jean C: Testosterone and dihydrotestosterone in sexual ducts and genital tubercle of rabbit fetuses during sexual organogenesis: Effects of fetal decapitation. *J Steroid Biochem* 17:149–154, 1982.

Vogel G: Leptin: A trigger for puberty? *Science* 274:1466–1467, 1996.

vom Saal FS, Cooke PS, Buchanan DL, *et al.*: A physiologically based approach to the study of bisphenol A and other estrogenic chemicals on the size of reproductive organs, daily sperm production, and behavior. *Toxicol Ind Health* 14:239–260, 1998.

vom Saal FS, Nagel SC, Timms BG, Welshons WV: Implications for human health of the extensive bisphenol A literature showing adverse effects at low doses: A response to attempts to mislead the public. *Toxicology* 212:244–252, 2005; author reply 253–4.

Wacharasindhu S, Petwijit T, Aroonparkmongkol S, Srivuthana S, Kingpetch K: Bone mineral density and body composition in Thai Precocious Puberty girls treated with GnRH agonist. *J Med Assoc Thai* 89:1194–1198, 2006.

Warner M, Samuels S, Mocarelli P, *et al.*: Serum dioxin concentrations and age at menarche. *Environ Health Perspect* 112:1289–1292, 2004.

Warnock DH, Csapo AI: Progesterone withdrawal induced by ICI 81008 in pregnant rats. *Prostaglandins* 10:715–724, 1975.

Welshons WV, Nagel SC, vom Saal FS: Large effects from small exposures. III. Endocrine mechanisms mediating effects of bisphenol A at levels of human exposure. *Endocrinology* 147:S56–69, 2006.

Whelan EA, Grajewski B, Wild DK, Schnorr TM, Alderfer R: Evaluation of reproductive function among men occupationally exposed to a stilbene derivative: II. Perceived libido and potency. *Am J Ind Med* 29:59–65, 1996.

Wilson JD, Lasnitzki I: Dihydrotestosterone formation in fetal tissues of the rabbit and rat. *Endocrinology* 89:659–668, 1971.

Wilson VS, Lambright C, Ostby J, Gray LE, Jr.: In vitro and in vivo effects of 17beta-trenbolone: a feedlot effluent contaminant. *Toxicol Sci* 70:202–211, 2002.

Wine RN, Li LH, Barnes LH, Gulati DK, Chapin RE: Reproductive toxicity of di-*n*-butylphthalate in a continuous breeding protocol in Sprague-Dawley rats. *Environ Health Perspect* 105:102–107, 1997.

Winker R, Rudiger HW: Reproductive toxicology in occupational settings: An update. *Int Arch Occup Environ Health* 79:1–10, 2006.

Wolf CJ, Hotchkiss A, Ostby JS, LeBlanc GA, Gray LE, Jr.: Effects of prenatal testosterone propionate on the sexual development of male and female rats: A dose-response study. *Toxicol Sci* 65:71–86, 2002.

Wolff MS, Britton JA, Russo JC: TCDD and puberty in girls. *Environ Health Perspect* 113:A17, 2005; author reply A18.

Yamasaki K, Sawaki M, Ohta R, *et al.*: OECD validation of the Hershberger assay in Japan: Phase 2 dose response of methyltestosterone, vinclozolin, and *p, p'*-DDE. *Environ Health Perspect* 111:1912–1919, 2003.

Yin W, Gore AC: Neuroendocrine control of reproductive aging: roles of GnRH neurons. *Reproduction* 131:403–414, 2006.

CHAPTER 21

TOXIC RESPONSES OF THE ENDOCRINE SYSTEM

Charles C. Capen

INTRODUCTION

Endocrine glands are collections of specialized cells that synthesize, store, and release their secretions directly into the bloodstream. They are sensing and signaling devices located in the extracellular fluid compartment and are capable of responding to changes in the internal and external environments to coordinate a multiplicity of activities that maintain homeostasis.

Endocrine cells that produce polypeptide hormones have a well-developed rough endoplasmic reticulum that assembles hormone and a prominent Golgi apparatus for packaging hormone into granules for intracellular storage and transport. Secretory granules are unique to polypeptide hormone- and catecholamine-secreting endocrine cells and provide a mechanism for intracellular storage of substantial amounts of preformed active hormone. When the cell receives a signal for hormone secretion, secretory granules are directed to the periphery of the endocrine cell, probably by the contraction of microfilaments.

Steroid hormone-secreting cells are characterized by prominent cytoplasmic lipid bodies that contain cholesterol and other precursor molecules. The lipid bodies are in close proximity to an extensive tubular network of smooth endoplasmic reticulum and large mitochondria which contain hydroxylase and dehydrogenase enzyme systems. These enzyme systems function to attach various side chains to the basic steroid nucleus. Steroid hormone-producing cells lack secretory granules and do not store significant amounts of preformed hormone. They are dependent on continued biosynthesis to maintain the normal secretory rate for a particular hormone.

Many diseases of the endocrine system are characterized by dramatic functional disturbances and characteristic clinicopathological alterations affecting one or several body systems. The affected animal or human patient may have clinical signs that primarily involve the skin (hair loss caused by hypothyroidism), nervous system (seizures caused by hyperinsulinism), urinary system (polyuria caused by diabetes mellitus, diabetes insipidus, and hyperadrenocorticism), or skeletal system (fractures induced by hyperparathyroidism) (Capen, 2006b).

The literature suggests that chemically induced lesions of the endocrine organs are most commonly encountered in the adrenal glands, followed in descending order by the thyroid, pancreas, pituitary, and parathyroid glands. In the adrenal glands, chemically induced lesions are most frequently found in the zona fasciculata/zona reticularis and to a lesser extent in either the zona glomerulosa or medulla. In a survey, conducted by the Pharmaceutical Manufacturers Association, of tumor types developing in carcinogenicity studies, endocrine tumors developed frequently in rats, with the thyroid gland third in frequency (behind the liver and mammary gland), followed by the pituitary gland (fourth), and adrenal gland (fifth). Selected examples of commonly encountered toxic endpoints involving endocrine organs in laboratory animals are discussed in this chapter. Mechanistic data is included whenever possible to aid in the interpretation of findings in animal toxicology studies and to determine their significance in risk assessment (Alison *et al.*, 1994).

PITUITARY GLAND

Normal Structure and Function

The pituitary gland (hypophysis) is divided into two major compartments: (1) the adenohypophysis (anterior lobe) of the human pituitary composed of the pars distalis, pars tuberalis, and pars intermedia; and (2) the neurohypophyseal system which includes the pars nervosa (posterior lobe), infundibular stalk, and nuclei (supraoptic and paraventricular) in hypothalamus that contain the neurosecretory neurons that synthesize and package into secretory granules the neurohypophyseal hormones. The pars intermedia forms the thin cellular zone between the adenohypophysis and neurohypophysis. The pituitary gland lies within the sella turcica of the sphenoid bone. The gland receives its blood supply via the posterior and anterior hypophyseal arteries which originate from the internal carotid arteries. Arteriolar branches penetrate the pituitary stalk near the median eminence, lose their muscular coat, and form a capillary plexus. These vessels drain into the hypophyseal portal veins which supply the adenohypophysis. The hypothalamic–hypophyseal portal system functionally is important as it transports the hypothalamic releasing- and release-inhibiting hormones directly to the adenohypophysis where they interact with their specific populations of trophic hormone-producing cells.

The adenohypophysis in many animal species completely surrounds the pars nervosa of the neurohypophyseal system in contrast to human beings where it is situated on the anterior surface. The pars distalis is the largest portion and is composed of the multiple populations of endocrine cells that secrete the pituitary trophic hormones. The secretory cells are surrounded by abundant capillaries derived from the hypothalamic–hypophyseal portal system (Capen, 1996a). The pars tuberalis consists of dorsal projections of supportive cells along the infundibular stalk. It functions primarily as a scaffold for

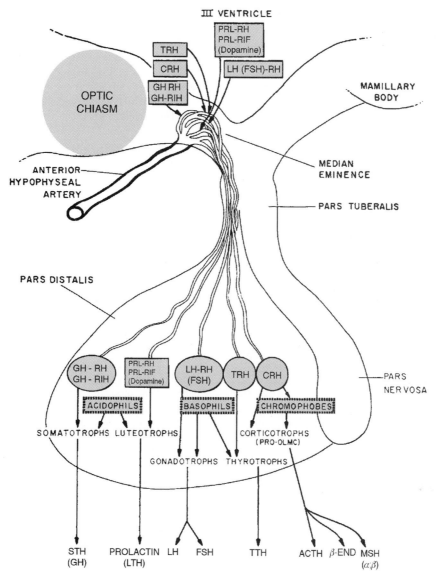

Figure 21-1. Control of trophic hormone secretion from the adenohypophysis by hypothalamic releasing hormones (RH) and release-inhibiting hormones (RIH).

The releasing and release-inhibiting hormones are synthesized by neurons in the hypothalamus, transported by axonal processes, and released into capillary plexus in the median eminence. They are transported to the adenohypophysis by the hypothalamic–hypophyseal portal system where they interact with specific populations of trophic hormone-secreting cells to govern the rate of release of preformed hormones, such as somatotropin (GH, STH), prolactin (LTH), prolactin (LTH), lutenizing hormone (LH), follicle-stimulating hormone (FSH), thyrotropic hormone (TTH), adrenocorticotropic hormone (ACTH), and melanocyte-stimulating hormone (MSH). There are RIH for those trophic hormones (e.g., prolactin and growth hormone) that do not directly influence the activity of target cells and result in production of a final endocrine product (hormone) that could exert negative feedback control.

the capillary network of the hypophyseal portal system during its course from the median eminence to the pars distalis. The pars intermedia is located between the pars distalis and pars nervosa and lines the residual lumen of Rathke's pouch. It contains two populations of endocrine cells in certain species. One of these cell types (B-cell) in the dog synthesizes and secretes adrenocorticotropic hormone (ACTH).

A specific population of endocrine cells is present in the pars distalis (and in the pars intermedia of dogs for ACTH) that synthesizes, processes, and secretes each of the pituitary trophic hor-

mones. Secretory cells in the adenohypophysis formerly were classified either as acidophils, basophils, or chromophobes based on the reactions of their secretory granules with pH-dependent histochemical stains. Based upon contemporary specific immunocytochemical procedures, acidophils can be further subclassified functionally into somatotrophs that secrete growth hormone (GH; somatotrophin) and luteotrophs that secrete luteotropic hormone (LTH; prolactin). Their granules contain simple protein hormones. Basophils include both gonadotrophs that secrete luteinizing hormone (LH) and follicle-stimulating hormone (FSH), and thyrotrophs that secrete thyrotropic hormone (thyroid-stimulating hormone [TSH]). Chromophobes are pituitary cells that by light microscopy do not have stainable cytoplasmic secretory granules. They include the pituitary cells involved with the synthesis of ACTH and melanocyte-stimulating hormone (MSH) in some species, nonsecretory follicular (stellate) cells, degranulated chromophils (acidophils and basophils) in the actively synthesizing phase of the secretory cycle, and undifferentiated stem cells of the adenohypophysis.

Each type of endocrine cell in the adenohypophysis is under the control of a specific releasing hormone from the hypothalamus (Fig. 21-1). These releasing hormones are small peptides synthesized and secreted by neurons of the hypothalamus. They are transported by short axonal processes to the median eminence where they are released into capillaries and are conveyed by the hypophyseal portal system to specific trophic hormone-secreting cells in the adenohypophysis. Each hormone stimulates the rapid release of preformed secretory granules containing a specific trophic hormone. Specific releasing hormones have been identified for TSH, FSH and LH, ACTH, and GH. Prolactin (PRL) secretion is stimulated by a number of factors, the most important of which appears to be thyrotropin-releasing hormone (TRH). Dopamine serves as the major prolactin-inhibitory factor and suppresses prolactin secretion and also inhibits cell division and DNA synthesis of luteotrophs (Parkening *et al.*, 1980). Dopamine also suppresses ACTH production by corticotrophs in the pars intermedia of some species. Another hypothalamic release-inhibiting hormone is somatostatin (somatotropin-release inhibiting hormone, SRIH). This tetradecapeptide inhibits the secretion of both growth hormone and TSH. Control of pituitary trophic hormone secretion also is affected by negative feedback by the circulating concentration of target organ (thyroid, adrenal cortex, and gonad) hormones.

The neurohypophysis is subdivided into three anatomic parts. The pars nervosa (posterior lobe of the human pituitary) represents the distal component of the neurohypophyseal system. The infundibular stalk joins the pars nervosa to the overlying hypothalamus and is composed of long axonal processes from neurosecretory neurons in the hypothalamus. It is composed of numerous capillaries, supported by modified glial cells (pituicytes), which are termination sites for the nonmyelinated axonal processes of neurosecretory neurons. The neurohypophyseal hormones (i.e., oxytocin and antidiuretic hormone) are synthesized in the cell body of hypothalamic neurons, packaged into secretory granules, transported by long axonal processes, and released into the bloodstream in the pars nervosa.

Antidiuretic hormone (ADH or vasopressin) and oxytocin are nonapeptides synthesized by neurons situated either in the supraoptic (primarily ADH) or paraventricular (primarily oxytocin) nuclei of the hypothalamus. ADH and its corresponding neurophysin are synthesized as part of a common larger biosynthetic precursor molecule, termed propressophysin. The hormones are packaged with a corresponding binding protein (i.e., neurophysin) into membrane-limited neurosecretory granules and transported by axons to the pars nervosa for release into the circulation. As the biosynthetic precursor molecules travel along the axons in secretion granules from the neurosecretory neurons, the precursors are cleaved into the active hormones and their respective neurophysins. These secretory products can be detected immunocytochemically. In Brattleboro rats with hereditary hypothalamic diabetes insipidus, nerve cells in the hypothalamus that normally produce ADH and neurophysin-I are negative immunocytochemically for both proteins whereas neurosecretory stain positive for cells that produce vasopressin and neurophysin-II are positive.

In addition to the specific trophic hormone-secreting cells, a population of supporting cells is also present in the adenohypophysis. These cells are referred to as stellate (follicular) cells and can be stained selectively with antibodies to S-100 protein. The stellate cells typically have elongate processes and prominent cytoplasmic filaments. These cells appear to provide a phagocytic or supportive function in addition to producing a colloid-like material that accumulates in follicles.

Mechanisms of Pituitary Toxicity

Pituitary tumors can be induced readily by sustained uncompensated hormonal derangements leading to increased synthesis and secretion of pituitary hormones. The absence of negative feedback inhibition of pituitary cells leads to unrestrained proliferation (hyperplasia initially, neoplasia later). This effect can be potentiated by the concurrent administration of ionizing radiation or chemical carcinogens.

In the pituitary–thyroid axis, thyroxine (T_4) and triiodothyronine (T_3) normally regulate the pituitary secretion of TSH by a classical negative feedback control system. Surgical removal or radiation-induced ablation of the thyroid or interference with the production of thyroid hormones by the use of specific chemical inhibitors of thyroid hormone synthesis leads to a stimulation of TSH synthesis and secretion with elevated blood levels. The thyrotrophic cells in the adenohypophysis undergo prominent hypertrophy. Subsequently, hyperplasia of the thyrotrophs occurs concurrently with hypertrophy as a consequence of the lack of normal negative feedback control. In rodents foci of hyperplasia may progress to the formation of adenomas in the pituitary gland. The role of gonadectomy in pituitary tumor induction has been studied most intensively in mice. The pituitary tumors induced by gonadectomy in mice are markedly strain-dependent and may contain FSH, LH, or both.

The administration of estrogens is a reproducible method for inducing pituitary tumors in certain experimental animals. The effect of exogenous estrogen on the rat pituitary includes stimulation of prolactin secretion and the induction of prolactin-secreting tumors (Hart, 1990). The administration of estrogens in susceptible strains results in elevated serum prolactin levels, increased numbers of prolactin cells within the pituitary, enhanced incorporation of tritiated thymidine within the gland, and increased mitotic activity (Osamura *et al.*, 1982). The pituitary of the ovariectomized F344 female rat is more responsive to the tumorigenic effect of diethylstilbestrol than the intact female; however, there is considerable variation in the induction of pituitary tumors by estrogens in different rat strains. For example, F344 and Holtzman rats respond to an initial estrogen stimulus by increasing the rate of DNA synthesis in the pituitary within 2–4 days. The rate of DNA synthesis declines after 7–10 days of treatment to unstimulated levels in the Holtzman strain but remains elevated in F344 rats.

Sarkar *et al.* (1982) have reported that estrogen-induced pituitary adenomas derived from prolactin-secreting cells are associated with loss of hypothalamic dopaminergic neurons, which normally inhibit the function of prolactin-secreting cells. Prolactin-producing tumors when transplanted subcutaneously were also associated with degenerative changes in hypothalamic dopaminergic neurons. The tumorigenic action of estrogen may not be due exclusively to its effect on the hypothalamus because estrogen can produce prolactinomas in pituitaries grafted beneath the renal capsule. The effects of estrogens on prolactin cells have been studied in hypophysectomized rats bearing transplanted pituitaries beneath the kidney capsule. The studies of El Etreby *et al.* (1988) using this model have shown

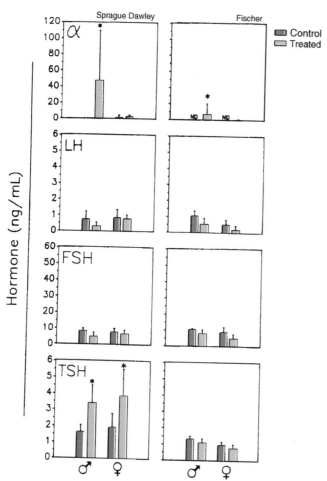

Figure 21-2. *Serum glycoprotein hormone levels in rats treated chronically with salmon calcitonin.*

Sprague–Dawley (left panels) or Fischer rats (right panels) were treated for 52 weeks with vehicle (open bars) or calcitonin (80 IU/kg/d) (black bars). Results are the mean ± SD; *P < 0.05. (From Jameson *et al.*, 1992).

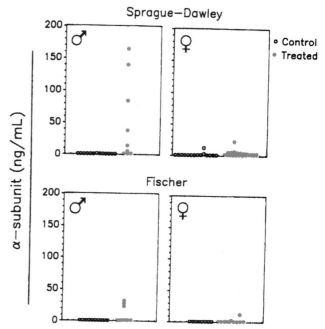

Figure 21-3. *Serum α-subunit levels in individual male rats treated chronically with calcitonin.*

The serum levels for individual animals are denoted as 0 = vehicle; ● = calcitonin-treated. (From Jameson *et al.*, 1992).

that dopamine agonists, including lisuride and bromocriptine, antagonize the direct stimulatory effects of estrogens on the prolactin cells. These dopamine agonists may act directly on dopaminergic receptors within the transplanted pituitaries.

Other chemicals, including caffeine, have been implicated in the development of pituitary adenomas in rats (Yamagami *et al.*, 1983). The administration of *N*-methylnitrosourea also is associated with the development of pituitary adenomas in Wistar rats. The neuroleptic agent sulpiride has been reported to cause the release of prolactin from the anterior pituitary in the rat and to stimulate DNA replication. The administration of clomiphene prevents the stimulation of DNA synthesis produced by sulpiride, but does not affect prolactin release from the gland. These findings suggest that the intracellular prolactin content of the pituitary plays a role in the regulation of DNA synthesis through a mechanism mediated by estrogens (Gunnison *et al.*, 1997).

Morphologic Alterations and Proliferative Lesions of Pituitary Cells

Jameson *et al.* (1992) reported that the administration of salmon calcitonin for one year to Sprague–Dawley and Fisher 344 rats was associated with an increased incidence of focal hyperplasia and adenomas in the pituitary. The association of calcitonin treatment and pituitary tumors was dose-dependent and was more pronounced with salmon calcitonin than with porcine calcitonin (Brown *et al.*, 1993). Using both immunohistochemical analysis and measurements of serum hormone levels, they provided evidence that prolonged administration of calcitonin resulted in pituitary tumors that produced the common α-subunit of the glycoprotein hormones (leutinizing hormone [LH], follicle-stimulating hormone [FSH] and thyroid-stimulating hormones [TSH]), a type of tumor that has been reported to comprise a significant fraction of pituitary tumors in humans. Immunohistochemistry and in situ hybridization demonstrated that most pituitary tumors associated with the chronic administration of high doses of calcitonin expressed a glycoprotein hormone α-subunit, whereas expression of the α-subunit was identified infrequently in hyperplastic lesions of control rats.

Serum levels of each of the major pituitary hormones were measured in both sexes of Sprague–Dawley and Fisher rats administered calcitonin. There were no significant alterations in the circulating levels of growth hormone, prolactin, or ACTH and the tumors were negative by immunohistochemical and in situ hybridization assessment for these hormones. Serum LH and FSH levels were unaffected by the treatment with calcitonin; however, TSH levels were elevated 2.1-fold after calcitonin treatment in Sprague–Dawley but not Fischer rats of both sexes (Fig. 21-2). Interestingly, thyroid weights were decreased by 43% in calcitonin-treated male rats and there was atrophy of thyroid follicular cells in some treated rats, suggesting that the immunoreactivity detected by the TSH assay was not biologically active. After treatment with calcitonin, serum α-subunit levels were increased at least 20-fold in Sprague–Dawley males and fourfold in male Fischer rats (Figs. 21-3 and 21-4). There was a good correlation between histopathologic evidence of α-subunit-producing pituitary tumors and elevated serum levels. In each of the calcitonin-treated rats that had adenomas, the tumors were positive

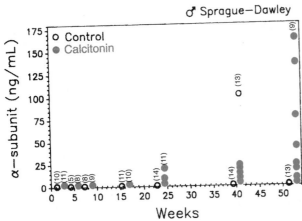

Figure 21-4. *Time course for the increase in serum α-subunit levels in male Sprague–Dawley rats.*

Symbols in the undetectable range represent values for more than one animal. The number of animals in each group is shown in parenthesis. 0 = control; ● = calcitonin-treated. (From Jameson *et al.*, 1992).

for α-subunit by immunohistochemistry and in situ hybridization for expression of α-subunit mRNA.

Serum levels of α-subunit were elevated in male Sprague–Dawley rats after 2, 5, 8, 16, 24, 40, and 52 weeks to determine the time course for hormone elevation. Elevated levels of α-subunit were detected as early as 24 weeks in rats treated with calcitonin and the majority of animals had increased α-subunit levels by 40 weeks of treatment (Fig. 21-4), suggesting that pituitary tumors developed only after several months of exposure to calcitonin. Levels of α-subunit in vehicle-treated rats were below the detection limits of the assay at each time point.

The studies reported by Jameson *et al.* (1992) did not determine whether the effects of calcitonin on the pituitary were direct or indirect. Calcitonin is known to be produced in large amounts in the posterior hypothalamus and median eminence where it may normally exert an effect on the hypothalamus–pituitary axis. Calcitonin receptors have been identified in the hypothalamus and lower numbers of receptors are found in the pituitary gland. A striking feature of the calcitonin-induced pituitary tumors and elevated serum α-subunit levels was the predilection for male compared with female rats. The basis for the sex- and species-specific effects of calcitonin was not determined. The relevance of the effects of calcitonin in the rat pituitary gland to human pathophysiology is uncertain at present. However, neither the treatment of patients with calcitonin nor patients with the multiple endocrine neoplasia syndrome II with medullary thyroid cancer and elevated serum calcitonin levels have resulted in the development of pituitary tumors. The doses of calcitonin used in rats were from 25- to 50-fold greater on a per-weight basis than doses administered to patients. In addition, several strains of rats are known to be highly predisposed to develop pituitary tumors compared to humans.

The high frequency of spontaneous pituitary adenomas in laboratory rats is a well-recognized phenomenon which must be considered in any long-term toxicological study (Attia, 1985). The incidence of pituitary tumors is determined by many factors including strain, age, sex, reproductive status, and diet (Berry, 1986). Studies from the National Toxicology Program (NTP) historical database of 2-year-old F344 rats have shown that the incidence of pituitary adenomas was 21.7% and 44% for males and females, respectively. Corresponding figures for carcinomas arising in the adenohypophysis

were 2.4% and 3.5% for males and females, respectively. Numerous hypotheses have been invoked to explain the high incidence of pituitary adenomas in certain inbred rat strains. Both hereditary factors and the levels of circulating sex steroids have been suggested as important etiological mechanisms. The hypothalamus has also been incriminated in the development of these tumors (Azad *et al.*, 1989). Age-related hypothalamic changes may result in diminished activity of dopamine, the major prolactin-inhibitory factor.

Numerous studies have demonstrated the striking degree of strain variation in the incidence of pituitary tumors in rats, which has been reported to range from 10% to more than 90% (van Putten *et al.*, 1988; van Putten and van Zwieten, 1988; Sher *et al.*, 1982; Haseman *et al.*, 1998; Pickering and Pickering, 1984). Particularly high incidences of pituitary adenomas have been reported in Wistar, WAG/Rij, Osborne–Mendel, Long–Evans, Amsterdam, and Columbia-Sherman rats. In the BN/Bi strain, pituitary adenomas have been found in 26% of females and 14% of males. Adenomas were identified in 95% of females and 96% of males in the WAG/Rij strain whereas (WAG/Rij 3 BN) F_1 rats had incidences of 83% for females and 64% for males. Rapid body growth rates and high levels of conversion of feed to body mass in early life or high protein intake in early adult life predispose any strain of rat to the development of pituitary adenomas (Keenan *et al.*, 1994, 1995). In rats fed a low protein diet (less than 12.7% crude protein), the overall tumor incidence, the numbers of multifocal tumors, and the degree of cellular atypia within tumors are significantly lower than in rats fed a standard diet.

Cystoid Degeneration   Cystoid degeneration has been used to describe foci of parenchymal cell loss in the adenohypophysis. Foci of cystoid degeneration (50–150 mm in diameter) have margins composed of normal secretory cells of the pars distalis. Cystoid degeneration also may occur in hyperplastic foci and in neoplasms of the pituitary. The frequency of cystoid degeneration is increased by feeding diets containing diethylstilbestrol to female C3H HeN (MTV+) mice.

Pituitary Hyperplasia and Neoplasia   The separation between focal hyperplasia, adenoma, and carcinoma utilizing histopathological techniques is difficult in the pituitary gland. However, criteria for their separation have been established and should be applied in a consistent manner in the evaluation of proliferative lesions of the pituitary gland (Barsoum *et al.*, 1985; Berkvens *et al.*, 1980). For the specific trophic hormone-secreting cells of the adenohypophysis there appears to be a continuous spectrum of proliferative lesions between diffuse or focal hyperplasia and adenomas derived from a specific population of secretory cells. It appears to be a common feature of endocrine glands that prolonged stimulation of a population of secretory cells predisposes to the subsequent development of a higher than expected incidence of focal hyperplasia and tumors. Long-continued stimulation may lead to the development of clones of cells within the hyperplastic foci that grow more rapidly than the rest and are more susceptible to neoplastic transformation when exposed to the right combination of promoting carcinogens.

Focal ("nodular") hyperplasia in the adenohypophysis appears as multiple small areas that are well demarcated but not encapsulated from adjacent normal cells. Cells in areas of focal hyperplasia closely resemble the cells of origin; however, the cytoplasmic area may be slightly enlarged and the nucleus more hyperchromatic than in the normal cells. Adenomas usually are solitary nodules that are larger than the often multiple areas of focal hyperplasia. They are sharply demarcated from the adjacent normal pituitary glandular parenchyma and there often is a thin, partial to complete, fibrous capsule. The adjacent parenchyma is compressed to varying degrees depending on the size of the adenoma. Cells composing an adenoma closely resemble the cells of origin morphologically and in their architectural pattern of arrangement.

Carcinomas usually are larger than adenomas in the pituitary and usually result in a macroscopically detectable enlargement. Histopathological features that are suggestive of malignancy include extensive intraglandular invasion, invasion into adjacent structures (e.g., dura mater, sphenoid bone), formation of tumor cell thrombi within vessels, and particularly the establishment of metastases at distant sites. The growth of neoplastic cells subendothelially in highly vascular benign tumors of the pituitary should not be mistaken for vascular invasion. Malignant cells often are more pleomorphic than normal, but nuclear and cellular pleomorphism are not a consistent criterion to distinguish adenoma from carcinoma in the adenohypophysis of rodents.

The vast majority of pituitary adenomas in humans and rodents have been described as chromophobic in type by light microscopy; however, many of these tumors have been found to stain for prolactin by immunohistochemistry. Of the prolactin-producing tumors, most are sparsely granulated with low levels of prolactin immunoreactivity by immunohistochemistry and having small numbers of secretory granules by electron microscopy (McComb *et al.*, 1984,1985; Sandusky *et al.*, 1988). Diffuse hyperplasia of the prolactin cells has been observed adjacent to some adenomas. The development of tumors and hyperplasia of prolactin-secreting cells often is accompanied by increasing serum levels of prolactin. Occasionally, prolactin cells within adenomas may be admixed with FSH/LH-, TSH-, or ACTH-positive cells in the rat pituitary.

ADRENAL CORTEX

Normal Structure and Function

The adrenal cortex is composed of three distinct zones. The outer zone is the zona glomerulosa and is composed of a thin region of columnar cells arranged in an arched or arcuate pattern. This zone is also called the zona multiformis in animals because of its different patterns of arrangement of secretory cells. The zona glomerulosa produces the steroid hormone, aldosterone, which is responsible for increasing sodium reabsorption and stimulating potassium excretion by the kidneys and thereby indirectly regulating extracellular fluid volume. Loss of this zone or the inability to secrete aldosterone may result in death due to retention of high levels of potassium with excess loss of sodium, chloride, and water. The zona fasciculata is the thickest zone (>70% of the cortex) and is composed of columns of secretory cells separated by prominent capillaries. The cells are polyhedral and have many intracellular lipid droplets. This zone produces glucocorticoids. The zona reticularis is also composed of polyhedral cells, whose arrangement is less linear and more as round nests or clumps of cells. The zona reticular produces glucocorticoids and in some species small amounts of sex steroids, namely, androgens, estrogens, and progestins. This zone is more distinct in rats compared to mice.

These are unique anatomical features of the adrenal gland blood supply that are important for its function and development of lesions. The gland is supplied by arterioles that penetrate the capsule, lose their muscular wall, and form a capillary bed that supplies the adrenal cortex. The arterioles that penetrate the capsule have a rapid reduction in lumen diameter and are a common site of emboliza-

tion of bacteria or tumor cells. The capillaries of the cortex supply blood to the medulla via the cortical–medullary portal blood system. This results in a high concentration of glucocorticoids in the blood supplied to the medulla. Some of the arterioles directly supply the medulla with blood, so the medulla has two sources of blood, namely, cortical capillaries and primary arterioles. Blood leaves the adrenal gland via medullary veins.

Ultrastructural features of the cortical cells can be very useful for their identification. All three zones have prominent mitochondria that can be distinguished by the shape of their cristae. Cells of the zona glomerulosa are characterized by prominent mitochondria and Golgi apparatus, whereas cells of the zona fasciculata have many cytoplasmic lipid droplets, mitochondria with vesicular cristae, and abundant smooth endoplasmic reticulum. The zona reticularis is distinguished by the presence of prominent lysosomes in the cytoplasm.

The adrenal cortex of animals is prone to develop degenerative and proliferative lesions, the etiology of which may be either spontaneous in nature or experimentally induced (Ribelin, 1984). Therefore, testing of xenobiotic chemicals using various laboratory animal species is a valid means of assessing the toxic potential for humans exposed to various xenobiotic chemicals. The choice of test animal species also is critical as a number of studies have demonstrated that there often is a variable species susceptibility to chemical toxicity. This suggests that interspecies differences in metabolism play a role in the development of adrenal cortical toxicity and in the inhibition of steroidogenesis. The age of the test animal, to a lesser degree, can be a factor in the development of chemically induced adrenal cortical lesions.

The adrenal (suprarenal) glands in mammals are flattened bilobed organs located in close proximity to the kidneys. The adrenal glands receive arterial blood from branches of the aorta or from the phrenic, renal, and lumbar arteries resulting in a subcapsular sinusoidal vascular plexus that drains through the cortex into the medulla. The ratio of cortex:medulla is approximately 2:1 in healthy laboratory-reared animals.

The cortex is histologically characterized by defined regions or zones. The cortical zones consist of the zona glomerulosa (multiformis), zona fasciculata, and zona reticularis. The zones are not always clearly delineated, as in the normal rat adrenal cortex. The mineralocorticoid-producing zona glomerulosa (multiformis) (approximately 15% of the cortex) contains cells aligned in a sigmoid pattern in relationship to the capsule. Degeneration of this zone or an interference in the ability to produce mineralocorticoids (namely, aldosterone) results in a life-threatening retention of potassium and hypovolemic shock associated with the excessive urinary loss of sodium, chloride, and water. The largest part of the cortex is the zona fasciculata comprising >70% of the cortical width. Cells in this zone are arranged in long anastomosing columns separated by vascular sinusoids and are responsible for the secretion of glucocorticoid hormones (e.g., corticosterone or cortisol). The innermost portion of the cortex is the zona reticularis (>15% of the cortex), which secretes minute quantities of adrenal sex hormones.

The adrenal cortical cells contain large cytoplasmic lipid droplets which consist of cholesterol and other steroid hormone precursors. The lipid droplets are in close proximity to the smooth endoplasmic reticulum and large mitochondria which contain the specific hydroxylase and dehydrogenase enzyme systems required to synthesize the different steroid hormones. Unlike polypeptide-hormone-secreting cells, there are no secretory granules in the cytoplasm because there is direct secretion without significant storage of preformed steroid hormones.

Steroid-hormone-producing cells of the adrenal cortex synthesize a major parent steroid with one to four additional carbon atoms added to the basic 17-carbon steroid nucleus. Because steroid hormones are not stored in any significant amount, a continued rate of synthesis is required to maintain a normal secretory rate. Once in the circulation, cortisol or corticosterone are bound reversibly to plasma proteins (such as transcortin, albumin). Under normal conditions 10% of the glucocorticoids are in a free unbound state.

Adrenal steroids are synthesized from cholesterol by specific enzyme-catalyzed reactions and involve a complex shuttling of steroid intermediates between mitochondria and endoplasmic reticulum. The specificity of mitochondrial hydroxylation reactions in terms of precursor acted upon and the position of the substrate which is hydroxylated is confined to a specific cytochrome P-450. The common biosynthetic pathway from cholesterol is the formation of pregnenolone, the basic precursor for the three major classes of adrenal steroids. Pregnenolone is formed after two hydroxylation reactions at the carbon 20 and 22 positions of cholesterol and a subsequent cleavage between these two carbon atoms. In the zona fasciculata, pregnenolone is first converted to progesterone by two microsomal enzymes. Three subsequent hydroxylation reactions occur involving, in order, carbon atoms at the 17, 21, and 11 positions. The resulting steroid is cortisol, which is the major glucocorticoid in teleosts, hamsters, dogs, nonhuman primates, and humans. Corticosterone is the major glucocorticoid produced in amphibians, reptiles, birds, rats, mice, and rabbits. It is produced in a manner similar to the production of cortisol, except that progesterone does not undergo 17α-hydroxylation and proceeds directly to 21-hydroxylation and 11β-hydroxylation.

In the zona glomerulosa, pregnenolone is converted to aldosterone by a series of enzyme-catalyzed reactions similar to those involved in cortisol formation; however, the cells of this zone lack the 17α-hydroxylase and thus cannot produce 17α-hydroxyprogesterone which is required to produce cortisol. Therefore, the initial hydroxylation product is corticosterone. Some of the corticosterone is acted on by 18-hydroxylase to form 18-hydroxycorticosterone, which in turn interacts with 18-hydroxysteroid dehydrogenase to form aldosterone. Since 18-hydroxysteroid dehydrogenase is found only in the zona glomerulosa, it is not surprising that only this zone has the capacity to produce aldosterone. In addition to the aforementioned steroid hormones, cells in the zona reticularis also produce small amounts of sex steroids including progesterone, estrogens, and androgens.

The mineralocorticoids (e.g., aldosterone) are the major steroids secreted from the zona glomerulosa under the control of the rennin-angiotensin II system. The mineralocorticoids have their effects on ion transport by epithelial cells, particularly renal cells, resulting in conservation of sodium (chloride and water) and loss of potassium. In the distal convoluted tubule of the mammalian nephron, a cation exchange exists which promotes the resorption of sodium from the glomerular filtrate and the secretion of potassium into the lumen.

Under conditions of decreased blood flow or volume, the enzyme renin is released into the circulation at an increased rate by cells of the juxtaglomerular apparatus of the kidney. Renin release has also been associated with potassium loading or sodium depletion. Renin in the peripheral circulation acts to cleave a plasma globulin precursor (angiotensinogen produced by the liver) to angiotensin-I. An angiotensin-converting enzyme (ACE) subsequently hydrolyzes angiotensin-I to angiotensin-II, which acts as a trophic hormone to stimulate the synthesis and secretion of aldosterone. Under normal conditions negative feedback control to inhibit further renin release is exerted by the elevated levels of angiotensin (principally angiotensin-II) as well as the expanded extracellular fluid volume resulting from the increased electrolyte (sodium and chloride) and water reabsorption by the kidney.

The principal control for the production of glucocorticoids by the zona fasciculata and zona reticularis is exerted by adrenocorticotropin (ACTH), a polypeptide hormone produced by corticotrophs in the adenohypophysis of the pituitary gland. ACTH release is largely controlled by the hypothalamus through the secretion of corticotropin-releasing hormone (CRH). An increase in ACTH production results in an increase in circulating levels of glucocorticoids and under certain conditions also can result in weak stimulation of aldosterone secretion. Negative feedback control normally occurs when the elevated blood levels of cortisol act either on the hypothalamus, anterior pituitary, or both to cause a suppression of ACTH secretion (Rothuizen *et al.*, 1991).

Fetal Adrenal Cortex A specialized fetal adrenal cortex exists in primates during late gestation (Mesiano and Jaffe, 1997). The cortex is composed of large polyhedral cells that produce abundant cortisol and estrogen precursors. The hormones secreted by the cortex are important for normal development of the fetus, and the steroid precursor dihydroepiandrosterone is converted to estrogen by the placenta. The cells of the fetal cortex are produced in the outer cortex and migrate medially, where they undergo hypertrophy and eventually apoptosis. After birth, there is a rapid regression, apoptosis, and lysis of the fetal cortex with dilatation of cortical capillaries and replacement by the typical three cortical zones. It is important not to misinterpret this as a lesion in neonatal primates since it represents physiological replacement of the fetal cortex with the definitive postnatal adrenal cortex.

X-Zone of Adrenal Gland The X-zone in the mouse adrenal cortex is a similar unique physiologic phenomenon as the fetal cortex in primates. In contrast to the fetal cortex of primates, the X-zone develops postnatally in the inner cortex of mice and is fully formed at weaning. Its function is unknown, but it may be similar to the fetal zone in primates. After weaning, the X-zone degenerates at variable rates, depending on the sex of the mouse. In male mice, the X-zone undergoes degeneration at puberty with accumulation of intracellular fat globules. In unbred females, the zone undergoes slow regression and degeneration during the first pregnancy. As with the fetal zone in primates, it is important not to misinterpret the degeneration associated with regression of the X-zone in mice as a lesion.

Mechanisms of Adrenal Cortical Toxicity

The reason the adrenal cortex is predisposed to the toxic effects of xenobiotic chemicals appears to be related to at least two factors. First, adrenal cortical cells of most animal species contain large stores of lipids used primarily as substrate for steroidogenesis. Many adrenal cortical toxic compounds are lipophilic and therefore can accumulate in these lipid-rich cells. Second, adrenal cortical cells have enzymes capable of metabolizing xenobiotic chemicals, including enzymes of the cytochrome P450 family. Many of these enzymes function in the biosynthesis of endogenous steroids and are localized in membranes of the endoplasmic reticulum or mitochondria. A number of toxic xenobiotic chemicals serve as

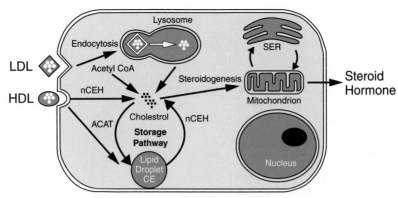

Figure 21-5. Cholesterol metabolism and steroid biosynthesis in adrenocortical and ovarian interstitial cells.

Cholesterol is the substrate for steroid biosynthesis. Conversion of cholesterol to pregnenolone occurs in the mitochondria and oxidative reactions catalyzed by P450 enzymes occur in the smooth endoplasmic reticulum and mitochondria. Sources of cholesterol include lipoprotein uptake from serum (LDL and HDL), de novo synthesis from acetate via the acetyl coenzyme A pathway, and hydrolysis of cholesteryl ester (CE) by neutral CE hydrolase (nCEH). The storage pool in the form of lipid droplets is derived principally from the conversion of free cholesterol to CE catalyzed by acyl coenzyme A:cholesterol acyltransferase (ACAT). Direct uptake of CE from serum to the storage pool is minimal in the rat. (From Latendresse *et al.*, 1993).

pseudosubstrates for these enzymes and can be metabolized to reactive toxic compounds. These reactive compounds result in direct toxic effects by covalent interactions with cellular macromolecules or through oxygen activation with the generation of free radicals (Colby, 1988; Hinson and Raven, 2006).

Impaired Steroidogenesis Impaired steroidogenesis is an important mechanism of toxicity in the adrenal cortex. It can occur by inhibition of cholesterol biosynthesis or metabolism and by disruption of cytochrome P-450 enzymes. Both these mechanisms will lead to the accumulation of increased cytoplasmic lipid in the form of discrete droplets.

Toxin Activation by CYP-450 Enzymes Toxins may be activated by many of the cytochrome P-450 enzymes in the cortical cells. Activation of toxins can result in the generation of reactive oxygen metabolites, membrane damage, and produce phospholipidosis in the cells.

Exogenous Steroids Exogenous steroids can disrupt normal function and structure of the adrenal cortex. Exogenous agonists will induce negative feedback inhibition of ACTH secretion by the pituitary and will result in atrophy of the zona fasciculata and reticularis. Some steroids, such as the sex steroids, can induce proliferative lesions in the adrenal cortex. Exogenous steroid antagonists will block steroid hormone action, lead to increased ACTH secretion, and diffuse hyperplasia of the cortex.

There is considerable species variation in the response of the adrenal cortex to exogenous chemicals. This is due to both inherent differences in the sensitivity to certain drugs and differences in the metabolic pathways of steroidogenesis. An interesting example is *o,p'*-DDD (Mitotane) which was originally developed to treat metastatic adrenal cortical cancer in humans; however, humans are relatively insensitive to the effects of *o,p'*-DDD, and the drug was not useful in the treatment of adrenal cancer. In contrast, dogs are more sensitive to the effects of *o,p'*-DDD, and it has been used effectively to treat pituitary-dependent hyperadrenocorticism due to autonomous secretion of ACTH by pituitary (corticotroph) tumors in a dose-dependent manner. *o,p'*-DDD is a selective toxin for the zona fasciculata and reticularis, thereby sparing the important functions of the zona glomerulosa (Vilar and Tullner, 1959).

The zonae reticularis and fasciculata appear to be the principal targets of xenobiotic chemicals in the adrenal cortex. Classes of chemicals known to be toxic for the adrenal cortex include short chain (3 or 4 carbon) aliphatic compounds, lipidosis-inducers, and amphiphilic compounds (Yarrington *et al.*, 1981, 1983, 1985). A variety of other compounds also may affect the medulla. The most potent aliphatic compounds are of 3-carbon length with electronegative groups at both ends. These compounds frequently produce necrosis, particularly in the zonae fasciculata and reticularis. Examples include acrylonitrile, 3-aminopropionitrile, 3-bromopropionitrile, 1-butanethiol, and 1,4-butanedithiol (Szabo *et al.*, 1980). By comparison, lipidosis inducers can cause the accumulations, often coalescing, of neutral fats which may be of sufficient quantity to cause a reduction or loss of organellar function and eventual cell destruction.

Lipidosis-Producing Compounds Cholesterol is the precursor substrate required to synthesize steroid hormones. Steroidogenic cells obtain cholesterol exogenously from serum lipoproteins and endogenously from *de novo* synthesis via the acetyl coenzyme A pathway (Fig. 21-5). The adrenal cortical cells and OI cells in the rat preferentially utilize serum high-density lipoproteins (HDLs) for their primary source of cholesterol and resort to *de novo* synthesis if HDL does not meet the demand of steroidogenesis. This is in contrast to Leydig cells of the testis, which preferentially utilizes *de novo* synthesis of cholesterol and uses an exogenous source only when intracellular synthesis does not meet the demand and the cholesterol pool has been depleted (Payne *et al.*, 1985). Examples of the compounds causing lipidosis include aminoglutethimide, amphenone, and anilines.

Tricresyl phosphate (TCP) and other triaryl phosphates cause a defect in cholesterol metabolism by blocking both the uptake from

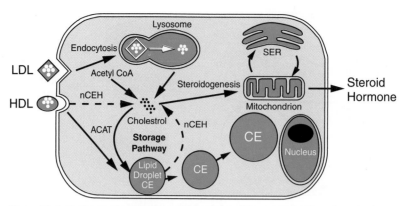

Figure 21-6. *Pathogenesis of cholesteryl lipidosis in adrenocortical cells and ovarian interstitial cells.*

The defect in cholesterol metabolism occurs in the uptake from serum and storage pathways. An inhibition of neutral cholesteryl ester hydrolase (nCEH) by a xenobiotic chemical results in the accumulation of CE in the form of lipid droplets in the cytoplasm. Acyl coenzyme A:cholesterol acyltransferase (ACAT) (catalyzes the formation of CE from cholesterol) activity remains near normal levels. (From Latendresse *et al.*, 1993).

serum and storage pathways. An inhibition of cytosolic neutral cholesteryl ester hydroxylase (nCEH) by triaryl phosphate (97% inhibition compared to controls) results in the progressive accumulation of cholesteryl ester in the form of lipid droplets in the cytoplasm of adrenal cortical and ovarian interstitial (OI) cells (Fig. 21-6) but not in testicular Leydig cells of rats (Latendresse *et al.*, 1993). Acyl coenzyme A: cholesterol acyl transferase (ACAT), an enzyme that esterifies cholesterol to make cholesteryl ester, was depressed only 27% (compared to controls) resulting in elevated intracellular storage of cholesterol in the form of lipid droplets (Fig. 21-7) (Latendresse *et al.*, 1994a,b, 1995).

Disruption of Membrane Organellar Membrane Turnover Biologically active cationic amphiphilic compounds produce a generalized phospholipidosis that involves primarily the zonae reticularis and fasciculata and produce microscopic phospholipid-rich inclusions. These compounds affect the functional integrity of lyso-somes, which appear ultrastructurally to be enlarged and filled with membranous lamellae or myelin figures. Examples of compounds known to induce phospholipidosis include chloroquine, triparanol, and chlorphentermine.

Selective Destruction of Mitochondria and Smooth Endoplasmic Reticulum In addition, there is a miscellaneous group of chemicals that affect hydroxylation and other functions of mitochondrial and microsomal fractions (e.g., smooth endoplasmic reticulum) in the adrenal cortex. Examples of these compounds include *o,p'*-DDD and α-(1,4-dioxido-3-methylquinoxalin-2-yl)-*N*-methylnitrone (DMNM). Other compounds in this miscellaneous category cause their effects by means of cytochrome P-450 metabolism and the production of toxic metabolites. A classic example is the activation of carbon tetrachloride, resulting in lipid peroxidation and covalent binding to cellular macromolecules of the adrenal cortex.

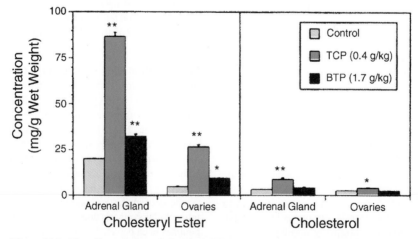

Figure 21-7. *The effects of tricresyl phosphate (TCP) and butylated triphenyl phosphate (BTH) on the concentration of cholesteryl ester (CE) and cholesterol in adrenal gland and ovary of rats.*

Mean ± SEM ($n = 8$–9) mg/g wet weight of adrenal organ and ovary. ***Different ($p \leq 0.01$, $p \leq 0.05$, respectively) from control. (From Latendresse *et al.*, 1993).

Studies with o,p'-DDD have shown a dose-dependent mitochondrial degeneration with vacuolization in the zonae fasciculata and reticularis (cortisol- and sex hormone-producing zone) with sparing of the aldosterone-producing zona glomerulosa (multiformis) (Hart *et al.*, 1971). The canine adrenal cortex is unusually sensitive to the cytotoxic effects of o,p'-DDD, which has led to the development of an effective drug (Lysodren or Mitotane) for the medical management of pituitary-dependent hypercortisolism (Cushing's disease). Cessation of weekly maintenance treatment with o,p'-DDD after regression of clinical signs often results in a recrudescence of functional disturbances of cortisol-excess due to chronic ACTH over-stimulation of the adrenal cortex leading to hypertrophy and hyperplasia of the cortisol-producing zones. The canine adrenal cortex is considerably more sensitive to the effects of o,p'-DDD than the adrenal cortices of humans.

Selective Inhibition of Angiotensin Converting Enzyme (ACE)
Drugs such as Captopril, used in the medical management of hypertension, selectively inhibit ACE and result in atrophy of the outer zona glomerulosa (multiformis) in the adrenal cortex. Inhibition of ACE decreases the synthesis of angiotensin II from angiotensin I leading to trophic atrophy of the zona glomerulosa. The decreased production of aldosterone results in decreased renal tubular reabsorption of sodium and chloride, increased serum potassium due to decreased tubular excretion, and decreased tubular reabsorption of water resulting in lower blood volume and pressure.

Selective Inhibition of ACYL-CoenzymeA: Cholesterol ACYL Transferase (ACAT) Compounds that inhibit ACAT often result in degeneration of the zonae fasciculata and reticularis in the adrenal cortex. There is a distinct species sensitivity with dogs > guinea pigs > rabbits > monkeys > rats. It is uncertain whether the mechanism of toxicity is due to a direct cytotoxic effect of the compound or the result of the selective ACAT inhibition (Dominick *et al.*, 1993a,b; Reindel *et al.*; 1994; Junquero *et al.*, 2001; Robertson *et al.*, 2001).

Many of the chemicals that cause morphological changes in the adrenal glands also affect cortical function. Chemically induced changes in adrenal function result either from blockage of the action of adrenocorticoids at peripheral sites or by inhibition of synthesis and/or secretion of hormone. In the first mechanism, many antisteroidal compounds (antagonists) act by competing with or binding to steroid hormone-receptor sites; thereby, either reducing the number of available receptor sites or by altering their binding affinity. Cortexolone (11α-deoxycortisol) an antiglucocorticoid and spironolactone, an antimineralocorticoid, are two examples of peripherally acting adrenal cortical hormone antagonists.

Xenobiotic chemicals affecting adrenal function often do so by altering steroidogenesis and result in histologic and ultrastructural changes in adrenal cortical cells. For example, chemicals causing increased lipid droplets often inhibit the utilization of steroid precursors, including the conversion of cholesterol to pregnenolone. Chemicals that affect the fine structure of mitochondria and smooth endoplasmic reticulum often impair the activity of 11α-, 17α-, and 21α-hydroxylases, respectively, and are associated with lesions primarily in the zonae reticularis and fasciculata. Atrophy of the zona glomerulosa may reflect specific inhibition of aldosterone synthesis or secretion, either directly (e.g., inhibition of 18α- hydroxylation) or indirectly (e.g., suppression of the rennin-angiotensin system II) by chemicals such as spironolactone and captopril.

It is well documented that synthetic and naturally occurring corticosteroids are potent teratogens in laboratory animals. The principal induced defect is cleft lip or palate; however, there is a paucity of information on the direct effect of xenobiotic chemicals on the development of the adrenal cortex. For example, adrenal aplasia occurred in 7.6 of 9.8% of white Danish rabbits when thalidomide was given to their dams.

Pathologic Alterations and Proliferative Lesions in Cortical Cells

Macroscopic lesions of chemically affected adrenal glands are characterized either by enlargement or reduction in size that often is bilateral. Cortical hypertrophy due to impaired steroidogenesis or hyperplasia due to long-term stimulation often is present when the adrenal cortex is increased in size. Small adrenal glands often are indicative of degenerative changes or trophic atrophy of the adrenal cortex. Midsagittal longitudinal sections of adrenal glands under the above conditions will reveal either a disproportionately wider cortex relative to the medulla or vice versa, resulting in an abnormal cortical:medullary ratio. Nodular lesions that distort and enlarge one or both adrenal glands suggest that a neoplasm is present. A single well-demarcated nodular lesion suggests a cortical adenoma whereas widespread incorporation of the entire adrenal gland by a proliferative mass is suggestive of cortical carcinoma, especially if there is evidence of local invasion into periadrenal connective tissues or into adjacent blood vessels and the kidney.

Non-neoplastic lesions of the adrenal cortex induced by xenobiotic chemicals are characterized by changes ranging from acute progressive degeneration to reparative processes such as multifocal hyperplasia. Early degenerative lesions characterized by enlarged cortical cells filled with cytoplasmic vacuoles (often lipid) may result in a diffuse hypertrophy of the cortex. A lesion of this type has been observed in rats treated with an antibacterial compound α-(1,4-dioxido-3-methylquinoxalin-2-yl)-N-methylnitrone (DMNM). This type of vacuolar degeneration is a reflection of impaired steroidogenesis resulting in an accumulation of steroid precursors. More destructive lesions such as hemorrhage and/or necrosis are associated with an inflammatory response in the cortex. If the zona glomerulosa remains functional there will be no life-threatening electrolyte disturbances and no signs of hypoadrenocorticism (Addison's disease). While many chemical agents that affect the adrenal cortex initially involve the zona reticularis and inner zona fasciculata, certain chemicals such as DMNM can cause a progressive degeneration of the entire adrenal cortex. Occasionally, a chemical's effect is limited to a specific zone of the adrenal cortex and may be species specific (Yarrington and Johnston, 1994).

Ultrastructural alterations of adrenal cortical cells associated with chemical injury are quite diverse in nature. The zonae reticularis and fasciculata typically are most severely affected, although eventually the lesions involve the zona glomerulosa. These lesions may be classified as follows: endothelial damage (e.g., acrylonitrile), mitochondrial damage (e.g., DMNM, o, p'-DDD, amphenone), endoplasmic reticulum disruption (e.g., triparanol), lipid aggregation (e.g., aniline), lysosomal phospholipid aggregation (e.g., chlorophentermine), and secondary effects due to embolization by medullary cells (e.g., acrylonitrile). Mitochondrial damage with vacuolization and accompanying changes in the endoplasmic reticulum and autophagocytic responses appear to be among the most common ultrastructural changes observed following chemical injury in the adrenal cortex. Because mitochondria and smooth endoplasmic reticulum form an intimate subcellular organellar network in cortical cells with important hydroxylases and dehydrogenase enzymes, it is not surprising that many chemical agents altering the ultrastructural morphology of cortical cells inhibit steroidogenesis.

Chemically induced proliferative lesions of the adrenal cortex are less frequently reported and include hyperplasia, adenoma, and carcinoma. Unlike the diffuse cortical hyperplasia/hypertrophy associated with excess ACTH stimulation, chemically induced hyperplasia usually is nodular in type, often multiple in distribution, and composed of increased numbers of normal or vacuolated cortical cells.

A variety of different chemicals are associated with an increased incidence of adrenal cortical neoplasia. Most of the reported tumors tend to be benign (adenomas) although an occasional tumor may be malignant (carcinomas). The zonae reticularis and fasciculata are more prone to develop tumors following chemical injury whereas the zona glomerulosa is spared unless invaded by an expanding tumor in the adjacent zones of the cortex. The tumorigenic agents of the adrenal cortex have a diverse chemical nature and use.

Spontaneous proliferative lesions may be found in all zones of the adrenal cortex but in adult rats are found most frequently in the zona fasciculata. Spontaneous nodular hyperplasia of the adrenal cortex is common in the rabbit, golden hamster, rat, mouse, dog, cat, horse, and baboon. Naturally occurring adrenal cortical tumors are found infrequently in domestic animals, except adult dogs and castrated male goats. However, cortical adenomas and (to a lesser extent) cortical carcinomas have been reported in moderately high incidence in certain strains of laboratory hamsters (e.g., BIO 4.24 and BIO 45.5 strains) and rat (e.g., Osborne–Mendel, WAG/Rij, BUF, and BN/Bi strains). The incidence often increases markedly in rats over 18 months of age. Adrenal cortical neoplasms in mice are uncommon but the incidence may be increased by gonadectomy.

Assessment of Function of the Adrenal Cortex

It may be useful to measure the function of the adrenal cortex. This can be accomplished by measuring glucocorticoid hormone concentrations in the blood or urine (expressed as a ratio to creatinine). It is important to remember the diurnal variations in secretion. Provocative testing is a useful tool to evaluate the functional capacity of the zonae fasciculata and reticularis by measuring the increase in secretion of glucocorticoids in response to exogenous ACTH. Light and electron microscopy and histomorphometry (cortico:medullary ratio and width of different cortical zones) are useful to characterize lesions that may disrupt the function of the cortical cells.

ADRENAL MEDULLA

Normal Structure and Function

The medulla constitutes approximately 10% of the volume of the adrenal gland. In the normal rodent adrenal gland and in most other laboratory animal species the medulla is sharply demarcated from the surrounding cortex. The bulk of the medulla is composed of chromaffin cells, which are the sites of synthesis and storage of the catecholamine hormones (Tischler et al., 1988a). In the rat and mouse, norepinephrine and epinephrine are stored in separate cell types that can be distinguished ultrastructurally after fixation in glutaraldehyde and postfixation in osmium tetroxide. The norepinephrine-containing core of the secretory granules appears electron-dense and is surrounded by a wide submembranous space

whereas epinephrine-containing granules are less dense, have a finely granular core, and a narrow space beneath the limiting membrane. Granules of varying densities may be found in the same cell types in the adrenal medulla of immature rats (Tischler and DeLellis, 1988a). Human adrenal medullary cells may contain both norepinephrine and epinephrine within a single chromaffin cell.

The adrenal medulla contains variable numbers of ganglion cells in addition to chromaffin cells (Reznik et al., 1980). A third cell type has been described in the medulla and designated the small granule-containing (SGC) cell or small intensely fluorescent (SIF) cell. These cells morphologically appear intermediate between chromaffin cells and ganglion cells, and may function as inter-neurons. The adrenal medullary cells also contain serotonin and histamine, but it has not been determined if these products are synthesized in situ or taken up from the circulation. A number of neuropeptides also are present in rat chromaffin cells including enkephalins, neurotensin, and neuropeptide Y.

In the catecholamine biosynthetic pathway, tyrosine is acted on by tyrosine hydroxylase to produce dopa, which is converted to dopamine by dopa decarboxylase. Dopamine in turn, is acted on by dopamine beta-hydroxylase to form norepinephrine, which is converted to epinephrine by phenylethanolamine-N-methyltransferase (PNMT). Tyrosine hydroxylase and PNMT are the principal rate limiting steps in catecholamine synthesis. The conversion of tyrosine into dopa and dopamine occurs within the cytosol of chromaffin cells. Dopamine then enters the chromaffin granule where it is converted to norepinephrine. Norepinephrine leaves the granule and is converted into epinephrine in the cytosol and epinephrine re-enters and is stored in the chromaffin granule. In contrast to the synthesis of catecholamines, which occurs in the cytosol, neuropeptides and chromogranin-A proteins are synthesized in the granular endoplasmic reticulum and are packaged into granules in the Golgi apparatus.

Innervation plays an important role in regulating the functions of chromaffin cells. During adult life, stresses such as insulin-induced hypoglycemia or reserpine-induced depletion of catecholamines produces a reflex increase in splanchnic nerve discharge, resulting both in catecholamine secretion and transsynaptic induction of catecholamine biosynthetic enzymes, including tyrosine hydroxylase. These effects become apparent during the first week of life, following an increase in the number of nerve terminals in the adrenal medulla. Other environmental influences including growth factors, extracellular matrix, and a variety of hormonal signals that generate cyclic AMP, may also regulate the function of chromaffin cells.

Mechanisms of Adrenal Medullary Toxicity

Proliferative lesions of the medulla, particularly in the rat, have been reported to develop as a result of a variety of different mechanisms (Rosol et al., 2001; Tischler et al., 1985, 1988b, 1991). Warren et al. (1966) studied over 700 pairs of rats with parabiosis and found that more than 50% of male irradiated rats developed adrenal medullary tumors. A relationship exists between adenohypophyseal (anterior pituitary) hormones and the development of adrenal medullary proliferative lesions (Manger et al., 1982). For example, the long-term administration of growth hormone is associated with an increased incidence of pheochromocytomas as well as the development of tumors at other sites. Prolactin-secreting pituitary tumors, which occur commonly in many rat strains, also play a role in the development of proliferative medullary lesions. In addition,

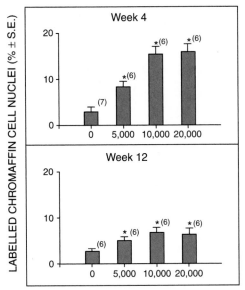
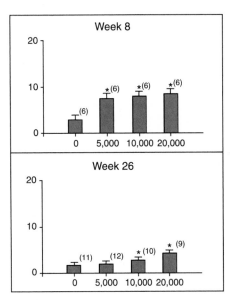

Figure 21-8. Effects of vitamin D_3 on percent of chromaffin cells labeled with BrdU during weeks 4, 8, 12, and 26 of dietary supplementation.

Asterisks indicate statistically significant increases over corn oil controls. Numbers in parenthesis indicate numbers of rats scored for each point. Premature deaths or euthanasia caused loss of three animals from the 20,000 IU/kg/day group, two from the 10,000 IU/kg/day group and one control. Histological examination of these animals' adrenal glands showed no detectable abnormalities. One extra animal at the start of the experiment was assigned to the control group at week 1. At least 2500 chromaffin cells were scored for each rat. (From Tischler *et al.*, 1999).

several neuroleptic compounds that increase prolactin secretion by inhibiting dopamine production have been associated with an increased incidence of proliferative lesions of medullary cells in chronic toxicity studies in rats.

Both nicotine and reserpine have been implicated in the development of adrenal medullary proliferative lesions in rats. Both chemicals act by a shared mechanism since nicotine directly stimulates nicotinic acetylcholine receptors whereas reserpine causes a reflex increase in the activity of cholinergic nerve endings in the adrenal (Tischler *et al.*, 1995). A short dosing regimen of reserpine administration in vivo stimulates proliferation of chromaffin cells in the adult rat and the mechanism may involve a reflex increase in neurogenic stimulation via the splanchnic nerve. Several other drugs have been reported to increase the incidence of adrenal medullary proliferative lesions. These include zomepirac sodium (a nonsteroidal inflammatory drug) (Mosher and Kircher, 1988), isoretinoin (a retinoid), and nafarelin (LHRH analog), atenolol (β-adrenergic blocker), terazosin (α-adrenergic blocker), ribavirin (antiviral), and pamidronate (bisphosphonate) (Davies and Monro, 1995).

Lynch *et al.* (1996) have reported that nutritional factors have an important modulating effect on the spontaneous incidence of adrenal medullary proliferative lesions in rats. Several sugars and sugar alcohols have produced adrenal medullary tumors at high dosages (concentrations of 10–20% in the diet), including xylitol, sorbitol, lacitol, and lactose (Baer, 1988). Although the exact mechanism involved is not completely understood, an important role for calcium has been suggested. High doses of slowly absorbed sugars and starches increase the intestinal absorption and urinary excretion of calcium. Hypercalcemia is known to increase catecholamine synthesis in response to stress, and low-calcium diets will reduce the incidence of adrenal medullary tumors in xylitol-treated rats. Other

compounds that may act by a similar mechanism of altered calcium homeostasis include the retinoids (which produce hypercalcemia) and conditions such as progressive nephrocalcinosis in aging male rats treated with nonsteroidal anti-inflammatory agents.

Roe and Bar (1985) have suggested that environmental and dietary factors may be more important than genetic factors as determinants of the incidence of adrenal medullary proliferative lesions in rats. The incidence of adrenal medullary lesions can be reduced by lowering the carbohydrate content of the diet. Several of the chemicals that increase the incidence of adrenal medullary lesions, including sugar alcohols, increase absorption of calcium from the gut. Calcium ions as well as cyclic nucleotides and prostaglandins may act as mediators capable of stimulating both hormonal secretion and cellular proliferation.

Tischler *et al.* (1996, 1999) presented data that vitamin D is the most potent in vivo stimulus yet identified for chromaffin cell proliferation in the adrenal medulla. Vitamin D_3 (5000, 10,000, or 20,000 IU/kg/day in corn oil) resulted in a four- to fivefold increase in bromodeoxyuridine (BrdU) labeling at week 4 that diminished to a twofold increase by week 26 (Fig. 21-8). An initial preponderance of epinephrine-labeled (PNMT-positive) cells subsequently gave way to norepinephrine-labeled cells. By week 26, 89% of rats receiving the two highest doses of vitamin D_3 had focal medullary proliferative lesions (BrdU-labeled focal hyperplasia, "hot spots") and pheochromocytomas in contrast to absence of proliferative lesions in controls. This increase in medullary cell proliferation was associated with a significant increase in circulating levels of both calcium and phosphorus after vitamin D administration (Fig. 21-9). The nuclei of hyperplastic chromaffin cells were labeled by BrdU but were phenylethanolamine-*N*-methyl transferase-negative indicating that they most likely were norepinephrine-producing cells

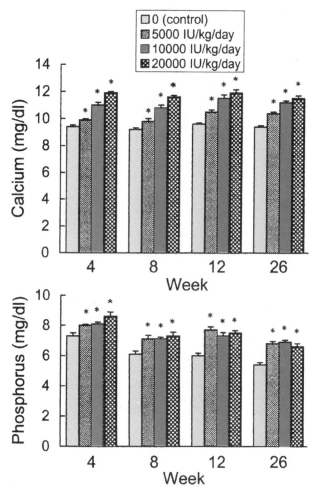

Figure 21-9. Effects of vitamin D₃ on serum calcium and phosphorus levels at weeks 4, 8, 12, and 26. Sustained perturbation of both Ca⁺⁺ and PO₄ concentrations persisted throughout the time course. (From Tischler et al., 1999).

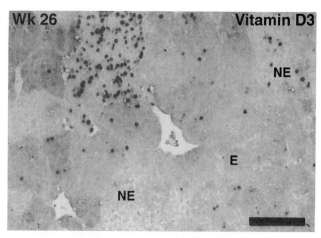

Figure 21-10. Photomicrographs of adrenal medullary sections stained for BrdU (dark nuclei) and PNMT (dark cytoplasm) to compare BrdU labeling of epinephrine (E) and norepinephrine (NE) cells.

Vitamin D₃ (20,000 IU/kg/day) caused a dramatic increase in BrdU labeling of predominantly E-cells at week 4. The response was greatly reduced at week 26 and there was no longer an E-cell predominance. A representative hyperplasic nodule in the vitamin D₃-stimulated adrenal medulla at week 26 (top left) is densely labeled with BrdU and is PNMT-negative (bar = 100 μm). (From Tischler et al., 1999).

Pathologic Alterations and Proliferative Lesions of Adrenal Medullary Cells

Adrenal Medullary Hyperplasia and Neoplasia   The adrenal medulla undergoes a series of proliferative changes ranging from diffuse hyperplasia to benign and malignant neoplasia. The latter neoplasms have the capacity to invade locally and to metastasize to distant sites. Diffuse hyperplasia is characterized by symmetrical expansion of the medulla with maintenance of the usual sharp demarcation between the cortex and the medulla. The medullary cell cords often are widened, but the ratio of norepinephrine to epinephrine cells is similar to that of normal glands. Focal hyperplastic lesions are often juxtacortical but may occur within any area of the medulla. The small nodules of hyperplasia in general are not associated with compression of the adjacent medulla; however, the larger foci may be associated with limited medullary compression. The foci of adrenal medullary hyperplasia are typically composed of small cells with round to ovoid nuclei and scanty cytoplasm. At the ultrastructural level, the cells composing these focal areas of hyperplasia contain small numbers of dense core secretory granules resembling the granules of SIF or SGC cells (Tischler and DeLellis, 1988b).

Larger benign adrenal medullary proliferative lesions are designated as pheochromocytomas. These lesions may be composed of relatively small cells similar to those found in smaller hyperplastic foci or larger chromaffin cells or a mixture of small and large cells. According to some authors, the lack of a positive chromaffin reaction in these focal proliferative lesions precludes the diagnosis of pheochromocytoma; however, the chromaffin reaction is quite insensitive and catecholamines (particularly norepinephrine) can be demonstrated in these proliferative lesions by biochemical extraction studies and by the formaldehyde- or glyoxylic-acid-induced fluorescence methods. Even in some of the larger medullary lesions, the chromaffin reaction is equivocal but catecholamines can be demonstrated both biochemically and histochemically.

of the rat medulla (Fig. 21-10). The proliferative lesions usually were multicentric, bilateral, peripheral in location in the medulla, nearly all were PNMT negative, and appeared to represent morphologic continuum rather than separate entities. Earlier studies reported by the same research group had demonstrated that the vitamin D₃ (20,000, 40,000 IU/kg/day) increase in chromaffin cell proliferation was observed as early as 1 week and had declined by 4 weeks. These findings support the hypothesis that altered calcium homeostasis is involved in the pathogenesis of pheochromocytomas in rodents, most likely through effects on increasing chromaffin cell proliferation (Fig. 21-11). Vitamin D₃, calcitrol (active metabolite of D₃), lactose, and xylitol all failed to stimulate directly the proliferation of rat chromaffin cells in vitro.

In summary, three dietary factors have been suggested to lead to an increased incidence of adrenal medullary proliferative lesions in chronic toxicity studies in rats (Roe and Bar, 1985). These are (1) excessive intake of food associated with feeding ad libitum; (2) excessive intake of calcium and phosphorus, since commercial diets contain 2–3 times more calcium and phosphorus than needed by young rats; and (3) excessive intake of other food components (e.g., vitamin D and poorly absorbable carbohydrates) which increase calcium absorption.

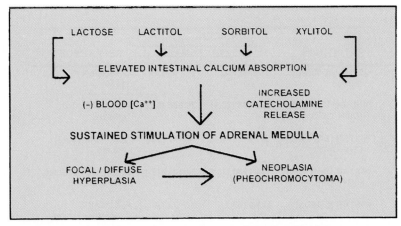

Figure 21-11. Pathogenesis of adrenal medullary proliferative lesions associated with ingestion of polyols resulting in elevation of the blood calcium concentration. (Modified from Lynch et al., 1996).

Malignant pheochromocytomas invade the adrenal capsule and often grow in the periadrenal connective tissues with or without distant metastases.

Proliferative lesions occur with high frequency in many strains of laboratory rats. The incidence of these lesions varies with strain, age, sex, diet, and exposure to drugs, and a variety of environmental agents (Nyska *et al.*, 1999; Roe *et al.*, 1995). Studies from the NTP historical database of two-year-old F344 rats have reported that the incidence of pheochromocytomas was 17.0% and 3.1% for males and females, respectively. Malignant pheochromocytomas were detected in 1% of males and 0.5% of females. In addition to F344 rats, other strains with a high incidence of pheochromocytomas include Wistar, NEDH (New England Deaconess Hospital), Long–Evans, and Sprague–Dawley. Pheochromocytomas are considerably less common in Osborne–Mendel, Charles River, Holtzman, and WAG/Rij rats. Most studies have revealed a higher incidence in males than in females (Figs. 21-12 and 21-13). Crossbreeding of animals with high and low frequencies of adrenal medullary proliferative lesions results in F_1 animals with an intermediate tumor frequency. Pheochromocytomas are less common in mice than in most strains of rats.

There is a conspicuous relationship between increasing age and the frequency, size, and bilateral occurrence of adrenal medullary proliferative lesions in the rat. In the Long–Evans strain, medullary nodules have been found in less than 1% of animals under 12 months of age. The frequency increases to almost 20% in 2-year-old animals and to 40% in animals between 2 and 3 years of age. The mean tumor size increases progressively with age as does the frequency of bilateral and multicentric occurrence.

A variety of techniques may be used for the demonstration of catecholamines in tissue sections. The chromaffin reaction is the oxidation of catecholamines by potassium dichromate solutions and results in the formation of a brown-to-yellow pigment in medullary tissue. The chromaffin reaction as traditionally performed possesses a low level of sensitivity and should not be used for the definitive demonstration of the presence of catecholamines in tissues. Similarly, both the argentaffin and argyrophil reactions, which have been used extensively in the past for the demonstration of chromaffin cells, also possess low sensitivity and specificity. Fluorescence techniques using formaldehyde or glyoxylic acid represent the methods of choice for the demonstration of catecholamines at the cellular level. These aldehydes form highly fluorescent derivatives

	INCIDENCE (%)		
RAT STRAIN	MALES (%)	FEMALES (%)	REFERENCE
CHARLES RIVER-CD	109/1211 (9.0)	24/1204 (2.0)	SHER *et al.* (1982)
F344 (NTP)	158/1794 (8.8)	55/1754 (3.1)	GOODMAN *et al* (1979)
HOLTZMAN	4/806 (0.5)	3/618 (0.5)	SCHARDIEN *et al* (1968)
F344	76/448 (17.0)	14/450 (3.1)	SHER *et al.* (1982)

Figure 21-12. Rat strains with a high incidence of pheochromocytomas. (Modified from Lynch et al., 1996).

| RAT STRAIN | INCIDENCE (%) | | REFERENCE |
	MALES (%)	FEMALES (%)	
OSBORNE-MENDEL (NTP)	21/975 (2.2)	9/970 (0.9)	GOODMAN et al. (1980)
SPRAGUE-DAWLEY (CIBA-GEIGY)	121/578 (20.9)	36/585 (6.2)	McMARTIN et al. (1992)
WISTAR (BOR:WISW [SPF Cpb])	131/445 (29.4)	16/447 (3.6)	BOMHARD (1992) (30 mo.)
WISTAR (BOR:WISW [SPF Cpb])	133/1230 (10.6)	27/1242 (2.1)	BOMHARD & RINKE (1994) (24 mo.)
WISTAR (LOBUND)	46/66 (69.2)	NO DATA	POLLARD & LUCKERT (1989)

Figure 21-13. Rat strains with a low incidence of pheochromocytomas. (Modified from Lynch et al., 1996).

with catecholamines, which can be visualized by ultraviolet microscopy. Immunohistochemistry provides an alternative approach for the localization of catecholamines in chromaffin cells and other cell types. Antibodies are available that permit epinephrine- and norepinephrine-containing cells to be distinguished in routinely fixed and embedded tissue samples. Several of the important enzymes involved in the biosynthesis of catecholamine hormones also may be demonstrated by immunohistochemical procedures. Antibodies to chromogranin-A can be used for the demonstration of this unique protein in chromaffin cells (Puchacz *et al.*, 1996; Tischer *et al.*, 1990, 1994).

Pheochromocytomas in rats and human beings are both composed of chromaffin cells with variable numbers of hormone-containing secretory granules (Fig. 21-14). The incidence is high in many strains of rats by comparison to human patients where pheochromocytomas are uncommon except in patients with inherited clinical syndromes of multiple endocrine neoplasia (MEN). These tumors in rats usually do not secrete excess amounts of catecholamines whereas human pheochromocytomas episodically secrete increased amounts of catecholamines leading to hypertension

and other clinical disturbances. There appears to be a striking species difference in the response of medullary chromaffin cells to mitogenic stimuli with rats being very sensitive compared to humans (Fig. 21-14).

Tischler and Riseberg (1993) reported that adult rat chromaffin cells had a marked (10–40%) increase in bromodeoxyuridine (BrdU) labeled nuclei in vitro following the addition of the following mitogens: nerve growth factor (NGF), fibroblast growth factor (FGF), forskolin, and phorbol myristate (PMA) whereas human chromaffin cells had a minimal (<0.1%) response to the same mitogens (Fig. 21-15). This striking difference in sensitivity to mitogenic stimuli may explain the lower frequency of adrenal medullary proliferative lesions in humans compared to many rat strains (Tischler and Riseberg, 1993). The mouse adrenal medulla, which like humans has a low spontaneous incidence of proliferative lesions of chromaffin cells, also failed to respond to a variety of mitogenic stimuli (Fig. 21-15). These findings and others suggest that chromaffin cells of the rat represent an inappropriate model to assess the potential effects of xenobiotic chemicals on chromaffin cells of the human adrenal medulla (Lynch *et al.*, 1996).

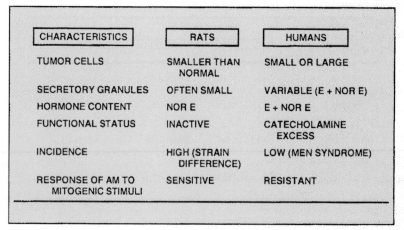

CHARACTERISTICS	RATS	HUMANS
TUMOR CELLS	SMALLER THAN NORMAL	SMALL OR LARGE
SECRETORY GRANULES	OFTEN SMALL	VARIABLE (E + NOR E)
HORMONE CONTENT	NOR E	E + NOR E
FUNCTIONAL STATUS	INACTIVE	CATECHOLAMINE EXCESS
INCIDENCE	HIGH (STRAIN DIFFERENCE)	LOW (MEN SYNDROME)
RESPONSE OF AM TO MITOGENIC STIMULI	SENSITIVE	RESISTANT

Figure 21-14. Characteristics of pheochromocytomas in rats compared to humans. (Modified from Lynch et al., 1996).

BrdU INCORPORATION *IN VITRO*

	CONTROL	NGF	FGF	FORSKOLIN	PMA
RAT	<1%	UP TO 40%	UP TO 40%	UP TO 40%	UP TO 10%
HUMAN	<0.1%	<0.1%	<0.1%	<0.1%	<0.1%
BOVINE	0	0	0	0	0
MOUSE	<0.1%	0	UP TO 5%	UP TO 1%	UP TO 1%

PM = PHORBOL MYRISTATE; NGF = NERVE GROWTH FACTOR; FGF = FIBROBLAST GROWTH FACTOR; BrdU = BROMODEOXYURIDINE

[1] RAT (3- TO 9-MONTH-OLD MALE AND FEMALE F344 OR CHARLES RIVER SPRAGUE-DAWLEY) BOVINE (ADULT FEMALE); [2] MOUSE (12/SVJ x C57 L/6J; 3-MONTH-OLD FEMALES)

FROM: TISCHLER AND RISEBERG. ENDOCRINE PATH 4:1993, 15-19

Figure 21-15. Species differences in mitogenic responses of chromaffin cells in vitro from adult rat, human, bovine, and mouse adrenals. (From Tischler and Riseberg (1993).

Chemically Induced Medullary Toxicity

Medullary chromaffin cells in rats are susceptible to acute necrosis and cytolysis by salinomycin, which occurs in less than 10 hours (Chen-Pan *et al.*, 1999). However, the adrenal medulla is capable of replenishing the chromaffin cells in as little as 24 hours by an unknown mechanism. It appears that the adrenal medulla recruits undifferentiated chromaffin cells to repopulate the medulla by a rapid and orderly process of differentiation. Repopulation is not dependent on mitosis. Therefore, chemically induced acute necrosis of the adrenal medulla may be easily overlooked if short experimental time points (<24 hours) were not examined.

Chen-Pan *et al.* (2002), in a subsequent study with salinonycin, found the rapid recovery to be based on differentiation of preexisting primitive undifferentiated chromaffin cells, rather than by mitosis, due to a lack of 5-bromo-2-deoxyuridine incorporation in the differentiating and/or differentiated chromaffin cells. Schwann cells actively functioned as phagocytes and appeared to indirectly stimulate the differentiation of undifferentiated chromaffin cells. Inflammatory cells were rare with only a few lymphocytes evident inside the clusters of necrotic medullary cells.

THYROID GLAND (FOLLICULAR CELLS)

Normal Structure and Function

The thyroid gland is the largest of the endocrine organs that functions exclusively as an endocrine gland (Capen 2000). The basic histologic structure of the thyroid is unique for endocrine glands, consisting of follicles of varying size (20–250 μm) that contain colloid produced by the follicular cells (thyrocytes). The follicular cells are cuboidal to low columnar (under conditions of normal iodine intake) and their secretory polarity is directed toward the lumen of the follicles. An extensive network of interfollicular capillaries provides the follicular cells with an abundant blood supply. Follicular cells have extensive profiles of rough endoplasmic reticulum and a large Golgi apparatus in their cytoplasm for synthesis and packaging substantial amounts of protein (e.g., thyroglobulin) that are then transported into the follicular lumen. The interface between the luminal side of follicular cells and the colloid is modified by numerous microvillous projections.

The synthesis of thyroid hormones is unique among endocrine glands because the final assembly of hormone occurs extracellularly within the follicular lumen. Essential raw materials, such as iodide ion (I^-), are trapped by follicular cells from plasma, transported rapidly against a concentration gradient to the lumen of the follicle, and oxidized by a peroxidase enzyme in the microvillar membranes to iodine (I_2).

Biosynthesis of Thyroid Hormones The assembly of thyroid hormones within the follicular lumen is made possible by a unique protein, thyroglobulin, synthesized by follicular cells (Fig. 21-16). Thyroglobulin is a high molecular-weight glycoprotein synthesized in successive subunits on the ribosomes of the endoplasmic reticulum in follicular cells. The constituent amino acids (tyrosine and others) and carbohydrates (mannose, fructose, galactose) are derived from the circulation. Recently synthesized thyroglobulin leaving the Golgi apparatus is packaged into apical vesicles which are extruded into the follicular lumen. The amino acid tyrosine, an essential component of thyroid hormones, is incorporated within the molecular structure of thyroglobulin. Iodine is bound to the tyrosyl residues in thyroglobulin at the apical surface of follicular cells to form successively monoiodotyrosine (MIT) and diiodotyrosine (DIT). These biologically inactive iodothyronines subsequently are coupled together under the influence of the thyroperoxidase to form the two biologically active iodothyronines (thyroxine-T4, triiodothyronine-T3) secreted by the thyroid gland.

The functionally important thyroperoxidase enzyme in the thyroid hormone synthetic pathway is present in the apical plasma membrane and microvilli as well as in other membranous structures of the follicular cells (Tice and Wollman, 1972, 1974). Thyroperoxidase is a membrane-bound, heme-containing glycoprotein composed of 933 amino acids with a transmembrane domain. This important enzyme oxidizes (in the presence of hydrogen peroxidase) iodide ion (I^-) taken up by follicular cells through the function of the sodium-iodide symporter into reactive iodine (I_2), which binds to the tyrosine residues in the thyroglobulin. Iodine is incorporated not

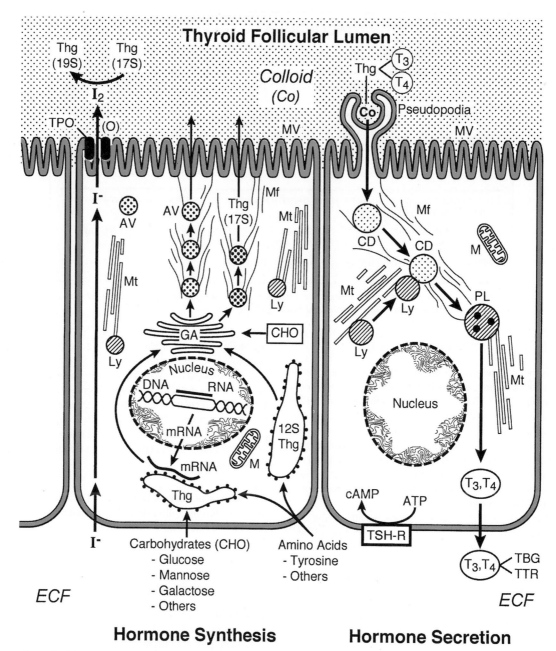

Figure 21-16. Normal thyroid follicular cells illustrating two-way traffic of materials from capillaries into the follicular lumen and from lumen back into interfollicular capillaries.

Raw materials, such as iodine, are concentrated by follicular cells and rapidly transported into the lumen (left). Amino acids (tyrosine and others) and sugars are assembled by follicular cells into thyroglobulin (thg), packaged into apical vesicles (AV), and released into the lumen. The iodination of tyrosyl residues occurs within the thyroglobulin molecule to form thyroid hormones in the follicular lumen. Elongation of microvilli and endocytosis of colloid by follicular cells occurs in response to thyroid-stimulating hormone (TSH) stimulation (right). The intracellular colloid droplets (Co) fuse with lysosomal bodies (Ly), active thyroid hormone is enzymatically cleaved from thyroglobulin, and free tetraiodothyronine (T4) and triiodothyronine (T3) are released into circulation. M, mitochondria; N, nucleus; CHO, carbohydrates; GA, Golgi apparatus; R, receptor; TgB, thyroid-binding globulin; PL, phagolysosome; TTR, transthyretin; ECF, extra cellular fluids; Mf, microfilaments; and Mt, microtubules. (From Capen, 2004).

only into newly synthesized thyroglobulin recently delivered to the follicular lumen but also into molecules already stored in the lumen. Thyroperoxidase also functions as a coupling enzyme to combine MIT and DIT to form triiodothyronine (T3) or two DITs to form thyroxine (T4).

The mechanism of active transport of iodide has been shown to be associated with a sodium-iodide (Na+-I−) symporter (NIS) present in the basolateral membrane of thyroid follicular cells (Fig. 21-17) (LaPerle and Jhiang, 2003). Transport of iodide ion across the thyroid cell membrane is linked to the transport of Na+.

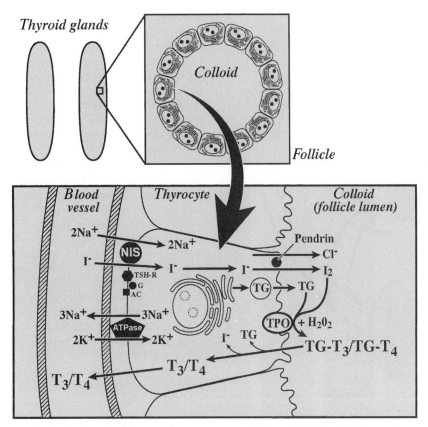

Figure 21-17. The sodium-iodide (NA+-I⁻) symporter (NIS) and thyroid hormone biosynthesis.

The NIS located in the basolateral membrane of thyroid follicular cells is responsible for the rapid uptake and concentration of iodide ion (I^-) from the circulation. The enzyme thyroperoxidase (TPO) in microvilli on the lumenal surface oxidizes I^- in the presence of hydrogen peroxide (H_2O_2) to reactivate iodine (I_2) that subsequently binds to tyrosyl residues in the thyroglobulin (TG) molecule of the colloid. Pendrin is a CI^-/I^- transport protein on the apical surface of thyrocytes. AC, adenylate cyclase; CD, colloid droplet; CI-, chlorine ion; G, G protein; I^-, iodide ion; R, receptor; T3, triiodothyronine; T4, tetraiodothyronine (thyroxine); and TSH, thyroid-stimulating hormone. (From La Perle *et al.*, 2003.)

The ion gradient generated by the Na^+–K^+ ATPase appears to be the driving force for the active co-transport of iodide. The transporter protein is present in the basolateral membrane of thyroid follicular cells and is a large protein containing 643 amino acids with 13 transmembrane domains.

Other tissues such as the salivary gland, gastric mucosa, choroid plexus, ciliary body of the eye, and lactating mammary gland also have the capacity to actively transport iodide, albeit at a much lower level than the thyroid (Lacroix *et al.*, 2001). In the salivary glands the NIS protein has been detected in ductal cells but not in acinar cells. Only the thyroid follicular cells accumulate iodide in a TSH-dependent manner.

The NIS gene is complex (15 exons, 14 introns) and its expression in the thyroid is upregulated by TSH. The functionally active iodine transport system in the thyroid gland has important pathophysiologic applications in the evaluation, diagnosis, and treatment of several thyroid disorders, including cancer. The NIS and active transport of iodide can be selectively inhibited by competitive anion inhibitors (e.g., perchlorate, thiocyanate); thereby, effectively blocking the ability of the gland to iodinate tyrosine residues in thyroglobulin and synthesize thyroid hormones.

The ability of NIS to concentrate iodide holds clinical relevance, in addition to its physiological importance, by providing the basis for using radioactive iodine in the treatment and management of various thyroid diseases. Radioactive iodine is commonly used to destroy hyperactive thyrocytes in patients with thyrotoxicosis, to ablate normal and malignant thyroid tissues in patients who have undergone total thyroidectomy for thyroid carcinoma, and to perform whole-body scans for the detection of recurrent and metastatic thyroid cancer.

Iodide ion once within the thyrocyte is passively transported via pendrin into the follicular lumen (Royaux *et al.* 2000; Kohn *et al.* 2001). Pendrin is a ~86 kDa chloride/iodide transport protein, is located at the apical membrane of thyrocytes, and is responsible for the transport of iodide ion into the follicular lumen (Fig. 21-17) (Scott *et al.*, 1999). It is the product of the gene responsible for Pendred syndrome, a genetic disorder in human patients characterized clinically by sensorineural hearing loss and goiter (Everett *et al.*, 1999, 2001; Kopp, 1999; Bidart *et al.*, 2000). Pendrin is characterized by 11 or 12 putative-transmembrane domains and is closely related to a family of sulfate transport proteins; however, pendrin does not transport sulfate and unlike NIS does not require sodium for its transport of iodide.

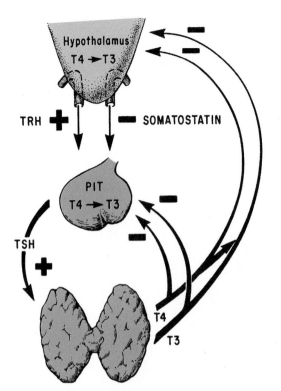

Figure 21-18. Hypothalamic–pituitary–thyroid axis.

Thyroid-stimulating hormone (TSH) from the pituitary stimulates the secretion of both the tetraiodothyronine (T_4) and triiodothyronine (T_3). These act at the pituitary (PIT) level to control secretion of TSH by a negative-feedback mechanism. In addition, T_4 is converted to T_3 within the pituitary by a monodeiodinase. TSH secretion is stimulated by thryotropin-releasing hormone (TRH) from the hypothalamus and inhibited by somatostatin and, to a lesser extent, by dopamine. Thyroid hormones act at the hypothalamus to stimulate the secretion of somatostatin. T_4 also is deiodinated to T_3 within the hypothalamus, and this conversion may play a role in feedback regulation. (From Reichlin, 1998.)

Thyroid Hormone Secretion   The secretion of thyroid hormones from stores within luminal colloid is initiated by elongation of microvilli on follicular cells and formation of pseudopodia. These elongated cytoplasmic projections are increased by pituitary TSH, extend into the follicular lumen, and indiscriminatingly phagocytize a portion of adjacent colloid (Fig. 21-16). Colloid droplets within follicular cells subsequently fuse with numerous lysosomal bodies that contain proteolytic enzymes (Wollman *et al.*, 1964; Sagartz *et al.*, 1995; Ozaki *et al.*, 1995; Nilsson *et al.*, 1986). Triiodothyronine (T_3) and thyroxine (T_4) are released from the thyroglobulin molecule and because of their hydrophobic nature diffuse out of follicular cells into the adjacent capillaries. The biologically inactive iodotyrosines (MIT, DIT) simultaneously released from the colloid droplets are deiodinated enzymatically and the iodide generated is either recycled to the follicular lumen to iodinate new tyrosyl residues or released into the circulation under normal conditions. Thyroxine is rapidly bound in plasma to albumin and several globulin fractions (especially high-affinity thyroxine-binding globulin [TBG]) produced by the liver, and triiodothyronine is bound to albumin (transthyretin) and one globulin fraction in dogs.

Negative feedback control of thyroid hormone secretion is accomplished by the coordinated response of the adenohypophysis and specific hypothalamic nuclei to circulating levels of thyroid hormones (especially T_3). A decrease in thyroid hormone concentration in plasma is sensed by groups of neurosecretory neurones in the hypothalamus that synthesize and secrete a small peptide (3 amino acids), thyrotropin-releasing hormone (TRH), into the hypophyseal portal circulation. Thyroid-stimulating hormone (TSH) or thyrotropin (TTH) is conveyed to thyroid follicular cells where it binds to the basilar aspect of the cell, activates adenyl cyclase, and increases the rate of biochemical reactions concerned with the synthesis and secretion of thyroid hormones (Wynford-Thomas *et al.*, 1987) (Fig. 21-18).

Biologic Effects of Thyroid Hormones   Thyroxine (T_4) and triiodothyronine (T_3) once released into the circulation act on many different target cells in the body. The overall functions of the hormones are similar though much of the biologic activity is the result of monodeiodination by 5′-deiodinase to 3,5,3′-triiodothyronine (active T_3) prior to interacting with target cells. Under certain conditions (protein starvation, neonatal animals, liver and kidney disease, febrile illness, etc.) or exposure to xenobiotic chemicals, thyroxine is preferentially monodeiodinated by 5′-deiodinase to 3,3′,5′-triiodothyronine ("reverse T3"). Because this form of T_3 is biologically inactive, monodeiodination to form reverse T3 provides a mechanism to attenuate the metabolic effects of thyroid hormones in peripheral tissues.

The overall physiologic effects of thyroid hormones are to: increase the basal metabolic rate; make more glucose available to meet the elevated metabolic demands by increasing glycolysis, gluconeogenesis, and glucose absorption from the intestine; stimulate new protein synthesis; increase lipid metabolism and conversion of cholesterol into bile acids and other substances; activate lipoprotein lipase and increase sensitivity of adipose tissue to lipolysis by other hormones; stimulate the heart rate, cardiac output, and blood flow; increase neural transmission, cerebration, and neuronal development in young animals (Lima *et al.*, 2001).

The subcellular mechanism of action of thyroid hormones resembles that for steroid hormones in that free hormone enters target cells and binds loosely to cytosol-binding proteins (Fig. 21-19). Free triiodothyronine initially binds to receptors on the inner mitochondrial membrane to activate mitochondrial energy metabolism, and subsequently binds to high-affinity nuclear receptors and increases transcription of the genetic message (mRNA) to facilitate new protein synthesis (e.g., structural, enzymatic, and binding proteins).

Thyroid hormone functions in target cells are mediated by three nuclear receptors: T_3R alpha$_1$, T_3R beta$_1$, and T_3R beta$_2$ that are encoded by two genes, namely T_3R alpha and T_3R beta. Thyroid hormones are essential for numerous postnatal developmental processes including growth and neurogenesis. The T_3R alpha gene is widely expressed from early development whereas the T_3R beta gene is highly restricted and expressed later in development (Fraichard *et al.*, 1997). Mice with targeted disruption of the T_3R alpha gene have markedly reduced production of both T_4 and T_3 associated with growth arrest and delayed development of bones and small intestine.

Species Differences in Thyroid Hormone Economy

Long-term perturbations of the pituitary–thyroid axis by various xenobiotics or physiological alterations (e.g., iodine deficiency, partial thyroidectomy, and natural goitrogens in food) are more likely to predispose the laboratory rat to a higher incidence of proliferative lesions (e.g., hyperplasia and benign tumors [adenomas] of follicular

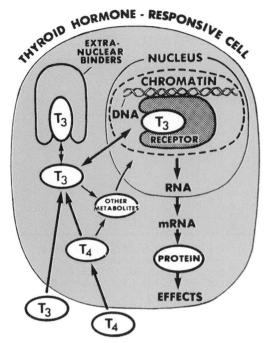

Figure 21-19. Subcellular mechanism of action of thyroid hormones in target cells.

Free triiodothyronine (T_3) primarily enters target cells because most of the tetraiodothyronine (T_4) undergoes monodeiodination in the liver or elsewhere in the periphery to form T_3. In the cell T_3 binds either to cytosolic-binding proteins (CBPs) or to high-affinity receptors on the inner mitochondrial (MT) membrane and activates oxidative phosphorylation in target cells. Binding to nuclear receptors by T_3 increases transcription of messenger RNA, which returns to the cytoplasm to direct the synthesis of new proteins. The increased synthesis of new proteins (structural or enzyme) carries out the multiple biological effects of the thyroid hormones.

cells) in response to chronic TSH stimulation than in the human thyroid (Capen and Martin, 1989; Curran and DeGroot, 1991; Capen, 1997; Zbinden *et al.*, 1988). This is particularly true in the male rat which has higher circulating levels of TSH than in females. The greater sensitivity of the rodent thyroid to derangement by drugs, chemicals, and physiological perturbations also is related to the shorter plasma half-life of thyroxine T_4 in rats than in humans due to the considerable differences in the transport proteins for thyroid hormones between these species (Döhler *et al.*, 1979).

The plasma T_4 half-life in rats is considerably shorter (12–24 hours) than in humans (5–9 days). In human beings and monkeys circulating T_4 is bound primarily to thyroxine-binding globulin (TBG), but this high-affinity binding protein is not present in rodents, birds, amphibians, or fish (Table 21-1).

The binding affinity of TBG for T_4 is approximately one thousand times higher than for prealbumin. The percent of unbound active T_4 is lower in species with high levels of TBG than in animals in which T_4 binding is limited to albumin and prealbumin. Therefore, a rat without a functional thyroid requires about 10 times more T_4 (20 μg/kg body weight) for full substitution than an adult human (2.2 μg/kg body weight). Triiodothyronine (T_3) is transported bound to TBG and albumin in human beings, monkey, and dog but only to albumin in mouse, rat, and chicken (Table 21-2). In general, T_3 is bound less avidly to transport proteins than T_4, resulting in a faster turnover and shorter plasma half-life in most species. These differences in plasma half-life of thyroid hormones and binding to

Table 21-1
Thyroxine (T_4) Binding to Serum Proteins in Selected Vertebrate Species

SPECIES	T_4-BINDING GLOBULIN	POSTALBUMIN	ALBUMIN	PREALBUMIN
Human being	++*	—	++	+
Monkey	++	—	++	+
Dog	++*	—	++	—
Mouse	—*	++	++	—
Rat	—	+	++	+
Chicken	—	—	++	—

+, ++, Degree of T_4 binding to serum proteins; —, absence of binding of T_4 to serum proteins. (From Döhler *et al.*, 1979).

Table 21-2
Triiodothyronine (T_3) Binding to Serum Proteins in Selected Vertebrate Species

SPECIES	T_4-BINDING GLOBULIN	POSTALBUMIN	ALBUMIN	PREALBUMIN
Human being	+*	—	+	—
Monkey	+	—	+	—
Dog	+	—	+	—
Mouse	—*	+	+	—
Rat	—	—	+	—
Chicken	—	—	+	—

+, ++, Degree of T_3 binding to serum proteins; —, absence of binding of T_3 to serum proteins. (From Döhler *et al.*, 1979).

transport proteins between rats and human beings may be one factor in the greater sensitivity of the rat thyroid to developing hyperplastic and/or neoplastic nodules in response to chronic TSH stimulation.

Thyroid-stimulating hormone levels are higher in male than female rats and castration decreases both the baseline serum TSH and response to thyrotropin-releasing hormone (TRH) injection. Follicular cell height often is higher in male than in female rats in response to the greater circulating TSH levels. The administration of exogenous testosterone to castrated male rats restores the TSH level to that of intact rats. Malignant thyroid tumors (carcinomas or "cancer") develop at a higher incidence following irradiation in males than females (2:1) and castration of irradiated male rats decreases the incidence to that of intact irradiated female rats. Testosterone replacement to castrated male rats restores the incidence of irradiation-induced thyroid carcinomas in proportion to the dose of testosterone and, similarly, serum TSH levels increase proportionally to the dose of replacement hormone. Likewise, higher incidence of follicular cell hyperplasia and neoplasia has been reported in males compared to female rats following the administration of a wide variety of drugs and chemicals in chronic toxicity/carcinogenicity testing.

There are also marked species differences in the sensitivity of the functionally important peroxidase enzyme to inhibition by xenobiotics. Thioamides (e.g., sulfonamides) and other chemicals can selectively inhibit the thyroperoxidase and significantly interfere with the iodination of tyrosyl residues incorporated in the thyroglobulin molecule, thereby, disrupting the orderly synthesis of T_4 and T_3. A number of studies have shown that the long-term administration of sulfonamides results in the development of thyroid nodules frequently in the sensitive species (such as the rat, dog, and mouse)

PROMOTING EFFECT OF IODINE DEFICIENCY (ID) ON THYROID

CARCINOGENESIS INDUCED BY N-NITROSOMETHYLUREA (NMU) AT 33 WEEKS

GROUP	THYROID WEIGHT ($\bar{x}$ mg + SD)	DIFFUSE FC HYPERPLASIA (%)	FOLLICULAR CELL (FC) ADENOMA (%)	FOLLICULAR CELL (FC) CARCINOMA (%)	TOTAL FOCAL FC LESIONS (no./cm^2)
NMU + ID DIET	632 ± 208*	100×	100××	100××××	11 ± 6
NMU + IODINE ADEQUATE (IA) DIET	46 ± 13**	0	70×××	10	14 ± 14
NMU + CONTROL DIET	29 ± 4***	0	50	0	17 ± 20
ID DIET	109 ± 12****	100×	0	0	0.4 ± 0.8
IODINE ADEQUATE DIET	40 ± 16	0	0	0	0
CONTROL DIET	36 ± 4	0	0	0	0

```
  *   P<0.01 vs. GROUPS 2, 3, 4, 5, or 6          x    P<0.001 vs. GROUPS 2, 3, 5 or 6
 **   P<0.05 vs. GROUPS 3 or 4                   xx    P<0.001 vs. GROUPS 4, 5, or 6
***   P<0.01 vs. GROUP 4                        xxx    P<0.01 vs. GROUPS 4, 5, or 6
****  P<0.01 vs. GROUPS 5 or 6                 xxxx    P<0.001 vs. GROUPS 2, 3, 4, 5, or 6
```

CONTROL DIET = STERILIZABLE WAYNE BLOX DIET; IODINE ADEQUATE = ID (REMINGTON)
DIET + 0.01 gm/kg K IODATE.
NMU 41 mg/kg IV AT 6 WK OF AGE (2 WK BEFORE DIETS STARTED).

Figure 21-20. The potent promoting effects of increased TSH secretion caused by iodine deficiency demonstrated in rats administered a single intravenous dose of a known initiator (N-nitrosomethylurea) of thyroid neoplasms. (Redrawn from Ohshima and Ward, 1984).

but not in species resistant (e.g., monkey, guinea pig, chicken, and human beings) to the inhibition of peroxidase in follicular cells.

Mechanisms of Thyroid Follicular Cell Toxicity

Numerous studies have reported that chronic treatment of rodents with goitrogenic compounds results in the development of follicular cell adenomas (Capen, 1996b, 1998, 1999, 2006a; Hard, 1988). Thiouracil and its derivatives have this effect in rats (Napalkov, 1976) and mice (Morris, 1955). This phenomenon has also been observed in rats that consumed brassica seeds (Kennedy and Purves, 1941), erythrosine (FD&C Red No. 3) (Borzelleca *et al.*, 1987; Capen and Martin, 1989), sulfonamides (Swarm *et al.*, 1973), and many other compounds (Paynter *et al.*, 1988; Hill *et al.*, 1989). The pathogenetic mechanism of this phenomenon has been understood for some time (Furth, 1954) and is widely accepted by the scientific community. These goitrogenic agents either directly interfere with thyroid hormone synthesis or secretion in the thyroid gland, increase thyroid hormone catabolism and subsequent excretion into the bile, or disrupt the peripheral conversion of thyroxine (T_4) to triiodothyronine (T_3). The ensuing decrease in circulating thyroid hormone levels results in a compensatory increased secretion of pituitary thyroid-stimulating hormone (TSH) (Hotz *et al.*, 1997). The receptor-mediated TSH stimulation of the thyroid gland leads to proliferative changes of follicular cells that include hypertrophy, hyperplasia, and ultimately, neoplasia in rodents (Hill *et al.*, 1998, 1999; Hurley *et al.*, 1998).

Excessive secretion of TSH alone (i.e., in the absence of any chemical exposure) has also been reported to produce a high incidence of thyroid tumors in rodents (Ohshima and Ward, 1984, 1986). This has been observed in rats fed an iodine-deficient diet (Axelrod and Leblond, 1955) and in mice that received TSH-secreting pituitary tumor transplants (Furth, 1954). The pathogenetic mechanism of thyroid follicular cell tumor development in rodents involves a sustained excessive stimulation of the thyroid gland by TSH. In addition, iodine deficiency is a potent promoter of the development

of thyroid tumors in rodents induced by intravenous injection of *N*-methyl-*N*-nitrosourea (Fig. 21-20) (Ohshima and Ward, 1984). The subsequent parts of thyroid section discuss specific mechanisms by which xenobiotic chemicals disrupt thyroid hormone synthesis and secretion, induce hepatic microsomal enzymes that enhance thyroid hormone catabolism or inhibit enzymes involved in monodeiodination in peripheral tissues that result in perturbations of thyroid hormone economy, which in rodents predisposes to the development of follicular cell tumors in chronic studies.

Xenobiotic Chemicals that Directly Inhibit Thyroid Hormone Synthesis

Blockage of Iodine Uptake The biosynthesis of thyroid hormones is unique among endocrine glands because the final assembly of the hormones occurs extracellularly within the follicular lumen. Essential raw materials, such as iodide, are trapped efficiently at the basilar aspect of follicular cells from interfollicular capillaries, transported rapidly against a concentration gradient to the lumen, and oxidized by a thyroid peroxidase in microvillar membranes to reactive iodine (I_2) (Fig. 21-21). The mechanism of active transport of iodide has been shown to be associated with a sodium-iodide (Na^+-I^-) symporter (NIS) present in the basolateral membrane of thyroid follicular cells. Transport of iodide ion across the thyroid cell membrane is linked to the transport of Na^+. The ion gradient generated by the Na^+-K^+ ATPase appears to be the driving force for the active co-transport of iodide. The transporter protein is present in the basolateral membrane of thyroid follicular cells (thyrocytes) and is a large protein containing 643 amino acids with 13 transmembrane domains.

Immunohistochemical staining using a polyclonal antibody against the human NIS fusion protein (hNIS) revealed that expression of the protein is heterogenous in the normal human thyroid and detected only in occasional thyrocytes of a follicle (Jhiang *et al.*, 1998b). The hNIS-positive thyrocytes usually were detected in small

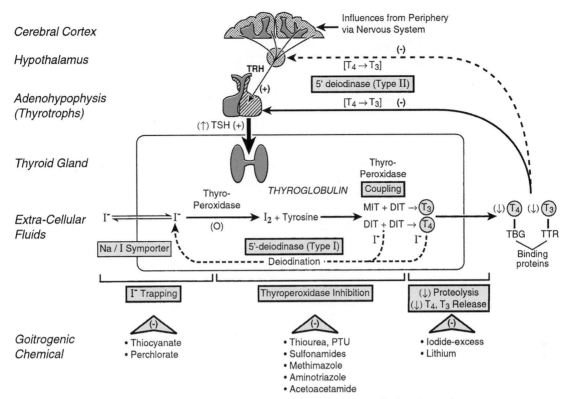

Figure 21-21. Mechanism of action of giotrogenic chemicals on thyroid hormone synthesis and secretion.

Chemicals can interfere with thyroid function either by (a) blocking iodide ion trapping, (b) inhibiting organic binding–coupling, or (c) disrupting proteolysis and release of T_4 and T_3 from colloid. DIT, diiodotyrosine; I_2, reactive iodine; MIT, monoiodotyrosine; PTU, propylthiouracil; T_3, triiodothyronine; T_4, tetraiodothyronine; TBG, thyroxine-binding globulin; TRH, thyrotropin-releasing hormone; and TSH, thyroid-stimulating hormone. (From Capen, 2004a.)

follicles composed of cuboidal to columnar cells but rarely were detected in large follicles composed of flattened thyrocytes. The heterogeneity of hNIS expression among thyroid follicles is consistent with the finding that iodide concentrating ability also varies between follicles in the thyroid gland (Spitzweg *et al.*, 2000).

Other tissues such as the salivary gland, gastric mucosa, choroid plexus, ciliary body of the eye, and lactating mammary gland also have the capacity to actively transport iodide, albeit at a much lower level than the thyroid. In the salivary glands the hNIS protein was detected in ductal cells but not in acinar cells. Only the thyroid follicular cells accumulate iodide in a TSH-dependent manner. The NIS gene is complex (15 exons, 14 introns) and its expression in the thyroid is upregulated by TSH. The functionally active iodine transport system in the thyroid gland has important clinical applications in the evaluation, diagnosis, and treatment of several thyroid disorders, including cancer. The NIS and active transport of iodide can be selectively inhibited by competitive anion inhibitors; thereby, effectively blocking the ability of the gland to iodinate tyrosine residues in thyroglobulin and synthesize thyroid hormones.

The initial step in the biosynthesis of thyroid hormones is the uptake of iodide from the circulation and transport against a gradient across follicular cells to the lumen of the follicle. A number of anions act as competitive inhibitors of iodide transport in the thyroid, including perchlorate (ClO_4^-), thiocyanate (SCN^-), and pertechnetate (Fig. 21-21) (Atterwill *et al.*, 1987). Thiocyanate is a potent inhibitor of iodide transport and is a competitive substrate for the thyroid peroxidase but it does not appear to be concentrated in the

thyroid. Blockage of the iodide trapping mechanism has a disruptive effect on the thyroid–pituitary axis, similar to iodine deficiency. The blood levels of T_4 and T_3 decrease, resulting in a compensatory increase in the secretion of TSH by the pituitary gland. The hypertrophy and hyperplasia of follicular cells following sustained exposure results in increased thyroid weights and the development of goiter.

Perchlorate from combustion of solid-propelled rocket engines and missiles, and other environmental sources (e.g., explosives, fireworks, road flares, commercial fertilizers, and airbag inflation systems) has contaminated water sources nationwide and more than 11 million people have perchlorate in their public drinking water at concentrations of 4 ppb (4 μg/L). Perchlorate is an ion that can affect thyroid function because it competitively inhibits the transport of iodine into thyroid follicular cells by inhibiting the action of the sodium-iodide symporter (Soldin *et al.*, 2001; Clewell *et al.*, 2004). Exposure to perchlorate in drinking water is a concern due to potential disruption of thyroid function with the development of hypothyroidism at various stages of life and subsequent effects on neuro-intellectual development (Li *et al.*, 2000; Lamm *et al.*, 1999; Lamm and Doemland, 1999). A normal secretion of thyroid hormones are required for the development and growth of neurones and supporting glial cells, the formation of synapses between neurones, the formation of myelin sheaths surrounding neuronal processes, and the development of neurotransmitters (National Research Council, 2005).

Review of the extensive scientific literature following perchlorate exposure or administration to humans and animals by a National Academy of Sciences committee concluded that the most

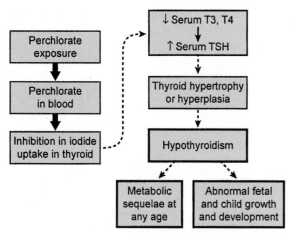

Figure 21-22. Suggested mode-of-action model for perchlorate toxicity in humans.

Solid arrows represent outcomes observed in humans during perchlorate exposure. Dashed arrows represent outcomes not clearly demonstrated in humans exposed to perchlorate but biologically plausible in absence of adequate compensation. The thyroid response to increased serum TSH concentrations and the independent increase in thyroid iodide uptake would act to raise T_3 and T_4 production to normal and thus prevent later steps of the model from occurring. (From Health Implications of Perchlorate Ingestion. National Research Council, The National Academic Press, Washington, DC, 2005).

reasonable mode of action pathway of events after perchlorate exposure would be changes in thyroid hormones and TSH secretion followed by thyroid follicular cell hypertrophy and hyperplasia. Hypothyroidism would develop only in people unable to compensate with an increased thyroid iodide uptake (National Research Council, 2005) (Fig. 21-22). Mechanisms exist that permit the body to compensate for decreases in T_4 and T_3 production. The compensatory increase in TSH secretion and thyroidal iodide uptake returns T_4 and T_3 production to normal without causing adverse affects (National Research Council, 2005). Any effects that follow and result from hypothyroidism (e.g., metabolic sequelae at any age such as decreased basal metabolic rate and slowing of function of many organ systems or abnormal growth and development of fetuses and children) clearly would be adverse. The Committee that investigated the health implications of perchlorate ingestion concluded that transient changes in serum thyroid hormones or TSH concentrations are not adverse effects but simply biochemical changes that might precede adverse effects. Based upon clinical studies, occupational and environmental epidemiologic studies, and investigations following the long-term administration of perchlorate to patients with hyperthyroidism, the committee recommended that a perchlorate reference dose (RfD) of 0.0007 µg/kg/day should protect the health of even the most sensitive populations (National Research Council, 2005). This is equivalent to 24.5 ppb concentration of perchlorate in drinking water assuming a body weight of 70 kg, daily water consumption of 2 L and drinking water as the only dietary source of perchlorate (DeGroef *et al.*, 2006). Recent studies in healthy volunteers have reported that 6 months of exposure to perchlorate at doses up to 3 mg/day had no effect on thyroid function including thyroidal iodide uptake as well as serum levels of thyroid hormones, TSH, and thyroglobulin (Braverman *et al.*, 2006).

Sodium chlorate ($NaClO_3$) is another xenobiotic chemical that results in perturbations of thyroid hormone economy, most likely by an inhibition of sodium-iodide symporter, and in chronic stud-

- THIOUREA
- PROPYLTHIOUREA (PTU)
- ANILINE DERIVATIVES: SULFONAMINDES
  – SULFAMETHAZINE
  – MANY OTHERS, NOT ALL
- METHIMAZOLE, CARBIMAZOLE
- AMINOTRIAZOLE
- ACETOACETAMIDE

Figure 21-23. Chemicals disrupting thyroid function (decreased synthesis of thyroid hormones) by inhibiting thyroperoxidase.

ies increased the incidence of thyroid follicular cell tumors when administered in drinking water to rats (Hooth *et al.*, 2001). The dose-dependent decrease in serum T4 was greater after 4 than 21 days but on day 90 T4 levels were similar to controls. The significant compensatory increases in serum TSH were greater after 4 and 21 days than at 90 days when only the high dose rats had a very modest increase in circulating levels. This increase in TSH is associated with the administration of $NaClO_3$ resulted in a 13% incidence of thyroid follicular cell adenoma plus carcinoma in males and a 9% incidence in females compared to 2% in controls of both sexes (Hooth *et al.*, 2001).

Inhibition of Thyroid Peroxidase Resulting in an Organification Defect A wide variety of chemicals, drugs, and other xenobiotics affect the second step in thyroid hormone biosynthesis (Fig. 21-21). The stepwise binding of iodide to the tyrosyl residues in thyroglobulin requires oxidation of inorganic iodide (I^2) to molecular (reactive) iodine (I_2) by the thyroid peroxidase present in the luminal aspect (microvillar membranes) of follicular cells and adjacent colloid. Classes of chemicals that inhibit the organification of thyroglobulin include (1) the thionamides (such as thiourea, thiouracil, propylthiouracil, methimazole, carbimazole, and goitrin); (2) aniline derivatives and related compounds (e.g., sulfonamides, paraaminobenzoic acid, paraaminosalicylic acid, and amphenone); (3) substituted phenols (such as resorcinol, phloroglucinol, and 2,4-dihydroxybenzoic acid); and (4) miscellaneous inhibitors (e.g., aminotriazole, tricyanoaminopropene, antipyrine, and its iodinated derivative [iodopyrine]) (Fig. 21-23).

Many of these chemicals exert their action by inhibiting the thyroid peroxidase which results in a disruption both of the iodination of tyrosyl residues in thyroglobulin and also the coupling reaction of iodotyrosines [(e.g., monoiodothyronine (MIT) and diiodothyronine (DIT)] to form iodothyronines (T_3 and T_4) (Fig. 21-24). Propylthiouracil (PTU) has been shown to affect each step in thyroid hormone synthesis beyond iodide transport in rats. The order of susceptibility to the inhibition by PTU is the coupling reaction (most susceptible), iodination of MIT to form DIT, and iodination of tyrosyl residues to form MIT (least susceptible). Thiourea differs from PTU and other thioamides in that it neither inhibits guaiacol oxidation (the standard assay for peroxidase) nor inactivates the thyroid peroxidase in the absence of iodine. Its ability to inhibit organic iodinations is due primarily to the reversible reduction of active I_2 to $2I^-$.

The goitrogenic effects of sulfonamides have been known for more than 50 years, since the reports of the action of sulfaguanidine on the rat thyroid. Sulfamethoxazole and trimethroprim exert a potent goitrogenic effect in rats, resulting in marked decreases in circulating T_3 and T_4, a substantial compensatory increase in TSH,

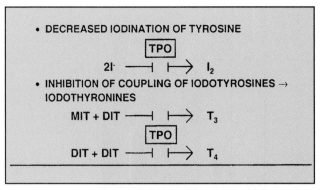

Figure 21-24. Mechanisms by which xenobiotic chemicals decrease thyroid hormone synthesis by inhibiting thyroperoxidase in follicular cells.

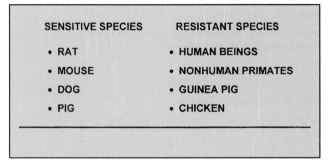

Figure 21-25. Variable species sensitivity of thyroperoxidase inhibition by sulfonamides. (From Takayama et al., 1986).

and increased thyroid weights due to follicular cell hyperplasia. The dog also is a species sensitive to the effects of sulfonamides, resulting in markedly decreased serum T_4 and T_3 levels, hyperplasia of thyrotrophic basophils in the pituitary gland, and increased thyroid weights.

By comparison, the thyroids of monkeys and human beings are resistant to the development of changes that sulfonamides produce in rodents (rats and mice) and the dog. Rhesus monkeys treated for 52 weeks with sulfamethoxazole (doses up to 300 mg/kg/day) with and without trimethroprim had no changes in thyroid weights and the thyroid histology was normal. Takayama *et al.* (1986) compared the effects of PTU and a goitrogenic sulfonamide (sulfamonomethoxine) on the activity of thyroid peroxidase in the rat and monkey using the guaiacol peroxidation assay. The concentration required for a 50% inhibition of the peroxidase enzyme was designated as the inhibition constant$_{50}$ (IC_{50}). When the IC_{50} for PTU was set at 1 for rats it took 50 times the concentration of PTU to produce a comparable inhibition in the monkey. Sulfamonomethoxine was almost as potent as PTU in inhibiting the peroxidase in rats. However, it required about 500 times the concentration of sulfonamide to inhibit the peroxidase in the monkey compared to the rat. Studies such as these with sulfonamides demonstrate distinct species differences between rodents and primates in the response of the thyroid to chemical inhibition of hormone synthesis. It is not surprising that the sensitive species (e.g., rats, mice, and dogs) are much more likely to develop follicular cell hyperplasia and thyroid nodules after long-term exposure to sulfonamides than the resistant species (e.g., subhuman primates, human beings, guinea pigs, and chickens) (Fig. 21-25).

Recent evidence suggests that propylthiouracil (PTU) or feeding a low iodine diet markedly increase thyroid follicular cell proliferation in rats by disrupting the movement of small molecular weight ions and molecules through gap junctions (Kolaja *et al.*, 2000). Inhibition of gap-junction intercellular communication (GJIC) prior to induction of cell proliferation has been reported with several tumor promoters and in proliferative diseases. After 14 days of either PTU or a low iodine diet (plus 1% $KClO_4$ in water) serum T_3 and T_4 were decreased to undetectable levels, serum TSH was increased significantly and thyroid follicular cell proliferation was increased nearly threefold. This was accompanied by a 30–35% decrease in GJIC (determined by an ex vivo method with Lucifer-yellow—a small molecular weight [457] fluorescent dye) and a twofold increase in apoptosis in both treated groups. Therefore, inhibition of GJIC by PTU or a low iodine diet may result in increased thyroid follicular cell proliferation, similar to other tissues, possibly by disrupting the passage of regulatory substance(s) through these highly permeable intercellular channels.

A contemporary example of a chemical acting as a thyroperoxidase inhibitor is sulfamethazine (Poirier *et al.*, 1999). This is a widely used antibacterial compound in food-producing animals with a current permissible tissue residue level of 100 ppb. Carcinogenicity studies at NCTR reported a significant increase of thyroid tumors in male Fischer 344 rats administered the high dose (2400 ppm) of sulfamethazine (McClain, 1995). The incidence of thyroid tumors was increased in both male and female $B_6C_3F_1$ mice after two years in the high-dose (4800 ppm) group but not in the lower dose groups. Quantitative risk assessment based upon these carcinogenicity findings, using low-dose linear extrapolation, yielded a 1×10^6 lifetime risk of 90 ppb in female rats and 40 ppb in male rats. A consideration of the ratio of intact drug to metabolites further reduced the tissue residue level to 0.4 ppb, which would be unachievable in practice (McClain, 1995).

A number of mechanistic studies have been performed in collaboration with Dr. McClain and others with the objective of developing a database that would support the hypothesis that the thyroid tumors observed in rats and mice from chronic studies were secondary to hormonal imbalances following the administration of high doses of sulfamethazine. In a 4-week mechanistic study, the effects of 10 dose levels (0–12,000 ppm) of sulfamethazine, spanning the range that induced thyroid tumors in rodents, were evaluated on thyroid hormone economy in Sprague–Dawley rats. There was a characteristic log–dose response relationship in all parameters of thyroid function evaluated. There were no significant changes at the six lower doses (20–800 ppm) of sulfamethazine, followed by sharp relatively linear changes at the four higher dose levels (1600–12,000 ppm) in percent decrease of serum T_3 and T_4, increase in serum TSH, and increase in thyroid weight. A similar, nonlinear dose response was present in the morphologic changes of thyroid follicular cells following the feeding of varying levels of sulfamethazine. Follicular cell hypertrophy was observed at lower doses of sulfamethazine than hyperplasia, which was increased only at dose levels of 3300 ppm and above (Fig. 21-26).

Other mode-of-action studies have demonstrated sulfamethazine to be a potent inhibitor of thyroperoxidase in rodents with an IC_{50} of 1.2×10^{-6} M. The morphologic effects on the thyroid were reversible after withdrawal of compound, and supplemental T_4 in the diet inhibited the development of the functional and morphologic changes in thyroid follicular cells (McClain, 1995). Hypophysectomized rats (with no TSH) administered sulfamethazine did not develop morphologic changes in the thyroid. Sulfamethazine

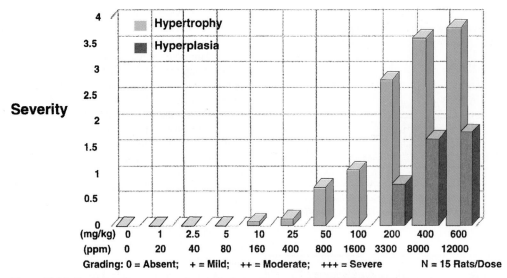

Figure 21-26. *Nonlinear dose–response in morphologic changes in thyroid follicular cells in response to 10 dose levels of sulfamethazine administered in the feed to male Sprague–Dawley rats. (From Capen, 1997).*

did not increase thyroid cell proliferation in vitro in the absence of TSH and there was no effect on thyroid structure/function in cynomologous monkeys administered sulfamethazine. Nonhuman primates and human beings are known to be more resistant than rodents to the inhibition of thyroperoxidase.

Xenobiotic Chemicals that Disrupt Thyroid Hormone Secretion

Blockage of Thyroid Hormone Secretion Relatively few chemicals selectively inhibit the secretion of thyroid hormone from the thyroid gland (Fig. 21-21). An excess of iodine has been known for years to inhibit secretion of thyroid hormone and occasionally can result in goiter and subnormal function (hypothyroidism) in animals and human patients. High doses of iodide have been used therapeutically in the treatment of patients with Grave's disease and hyperthyroidism to lower circulating levels of thyroid hormones. Several mechanisms have been suggested for this effect of high iodide levels on thyroid hormone secretion, including a decrease in lysosomal protease activity (in human glands), inhibition of colloid droplet formation (in mice and rats), and inhibition of TSH-mediated increase in cAMP (in dog thyroid slices). Rats fed an iodide-excessive diet had a hypertrophy of the cytoplasmic area of follicular cells with an accumulation of numerous colloid droplets and lysosomal bodies (Collins and Capen, 1980a; Kanno *et al.*, 1994; Many *et al.*, 1985). However, there was limited evidence ultrastructurally of the fusion of the membranes of these organelles and of the degradation of the colloid necessary for the release of active thyroid hormones (T_4 and T_3) from the thyroglobulin. Circulating levels of T_4, T_3, and rT_3 all would be decreased by an iodide-excess in rats.

Lithium has also been reported to have a striking inhibitory effect on thyroid hormone release (Fig. 21-21). The widespread use of lithium carbonate in the treatment of manic states occasionally results in the development of goiter with either euthyroidism or occasionally hypothyroidism in human patients. Lithium inhibits colloid droplet formation stimulated by cAMP in vitro and inhibits the release of thyroid hormones.

Xenobiotic-Induced Thyroid Pigmentation or Alterations in Colloid

The antibiotic minocycline produces a striking black discoloration of the thyroid lobes in laboratory animals and humans with the formation of brown pigment granules within follicular cells (Ambrogio *et al.*, 1999; Eisen and Hakim, 1998; Tajima *et al.*, 1985). The pigment granules stain similarly to melanin and are best visualized on thyroid sections stained with the Fontana–Masson procedure. Electron-dense material first accumulates in lysosome-like granules and in the rough endoplasmic reticulum. The pigment appears to be a metabolic derivative of minocycline and the administration of the antibiotic at high dose to rats for extended periods may result in a disruption of thyroid function and the development of goiter. The release of T_4 from perfused thyroids of minocycline-treated rats was significantly decreased but the follicular cells retained the ability to phagocytose colloid in response to TSH and had numerous colloid droplets in their cytoplasm.

Other xenobiotics [or metabolite(s)] selectively localize in the thyroid colloid of rodents resulting in abnormal clumping and increased basophilia to the colloid. Brown to black pigment granules may be present in follicular cells, colloid, and macrophages in the interthyroidal tissues resulting in a macroscopic darkening of both thyroid lobes. The physiochemically altered colloid in the lumen of thyroid follicles appears to be less able than normal colloid either of reacting with organic iodine in a step-wise manner to result in the orderly synthesis of iodothyronines or being phagocytized by follicular cells and enzymatically processed to release active thyroid hormones into the circulation. Serum T_4 and T_3 are decreased, serum TSH levels are increased by an expanded population of pituitary thyrotrophs, and thyroid follicular cells undergo hypertrophy and hyperplasia. As would be expected, the incidence of thyroid follicular cell tumors in 2-year carcinogenicity studies is increased at the higher dose levels usually with a greater effect in males than females. Autoradiographic studies often demonstrate tritiated material to be preferentially localized in the colloid and not within follicular cells. Tissue distribution studies with ^{14}C-labelled compound may reveal preferential uptake and persistence in the thyroid gland compared to other tissues. However, thyroperoxidase activity is normal

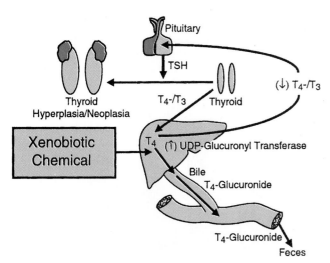

Figure 21-27. Hepatic microsomal enzyme induction by the chronic administration of xenobiotic chemicals leading to thyroid follicular cell hyperplasia and neoplasia.

and the thyroid's ability to take up radioactive iodine often is increased compared to controls in response to the greater circulating levels of TSH. Similar thyroid changes and/or functional alterations usually do not occur in dogs, monkeys, or humans.

Hepatic Microsomal Enzyme Induction

Hepatic microsomal enzymes play an important role in thyroid hormone economy because glucuronidation is the rate-limiting step in the biliary excretion of T_4 and sulfation primarily by phenol sulfotransferase for the excretion of T_3 (Vansell and Klaassen, 2001, 2002a; Shelby *et al.*, 2003; Dunn and Klaassen, 2000). Long-term exposure of rats to a wide variety of different chemicals may induce these enzyme pathways and result in chronic stimulation of the thyroid by disrupting the hypothalamic–pituitary–thyroid axis (Curran and DeGroot, 1991; Vansell and Klaassen, 2002b). The resulting chronic stimulation of the thyroid by increased circulating levels of TSH often results in a greater risk of developing tumors derived from follicular cells in 2-year or lifetime chronic toxicity/carcinogenicity studies with these compounds in rats (Fig. 21-27). Recent studies have suggested that glucuronidation and enhanced biliary excretion of T_3 may be the reason why serum TSH is increased in short-term (7 days) studies with some microsomal enzyme-inducing chemicals (e.g., phenobarbital, pregnenolone-16α-carbonitrile) but is less affected with others (3-methylcholanthrene, PCB). However, microsomal enzyme inducers are more effective in reducing serum T_4 than serum T_3 (Hood and Klaassen, 2000a). Outer-ring deiodinase (ORD) activity, an enzyme involved in the peripheral conversion of T_4 (major secretory product of the thyroid) to T_3, was reduced (not increased as would be expected if this was the mechanism) following the administration of four well-characterized enzyme inducers in rats. Type I ORD was measured in thyroid, kidney, and liver whereas type II ODR was quantified in brown adipose tissue, pituitary gland, and brain (Hood and Klaassen, 2000b).

Xenobiotics that induce liver microsomal enzymes and disrupt thyroid function in rats include CNS-acting drugs (e.g., phenobarbital, benzodiazepines); calcium channel blockers (e.g., nicardipine, bepridil); steroids (spironolactone); retinoids; chlorinated hydrocarbons (e.g., chlordane, DDT, TCDD), polyhalogenated biphenyls (PCB, PBB), among others (Waritz *et al.*, 1996). Most of the hep-

atic microsomal enzyme inducers have no apparent intrinsic carcinogenic activity and produce little or no mutagenicity or DNA damage. Their promoting effect on thyroid tumors usually is greater in rats than in mice, with males more often developing a higher incidence of tumors than females. In certain strains of mice these compounds alter liver cell turnover and promote the development of hepatic tumors from spontaneously initiated hepatocytes.

Phenobarbital has been studied extensively as the prototype for hepatic microsomal inducers that increase a spectrum of cytochrome P-450 isoenzymes (McClain *et al.*, 1988). McClain *et al.* (1989) reported that the activity of uridine diphosphate glucuronyltransferase (UDP-GT), the rate-limiting enzyme in T_4 metabolism, is increased in purified hepatic microsomes of male rats when expressed as picomoles/min/mg microsomal protein (1.3-fold) or as total hepatic activity (3-fold). This resulted in a significantly higher cumulative (4-hours) biliary excretion of ^{125}I-T_4 and bile flow than in controls.

Phenobarbital-treated rats develop a characteristic pattern of changes in circulating thyroid hormone levels (McClain *et al.*, 1988, 1989). Plasma T_3 and T_4 are markedly decreased after 1 week and remain decreased for 4 weeks. By 8 weeks T_3 levels return to near normal due to compensation by the hypothalamic–pituitary–thyroid axis. Serum TSH values are elevated significantly throughout the first month but often decline after a new steady state is attained. Thyroid weights increase significantly after 2–4 weeks of phenobarbital, reach a maximum increase of 40–50% by 8 weeks, and remain elevated throughout the period of treatment.

McClain *et al.* (1988) in a series of experiments have shown that supplemental administration of thyroxine (at doses that returned the plasma level of TSH to the normal range) blocked the thyroid tumor-promoting effects of phenobarbital and that the promoting effects were directly proportional to the level of plasma TSH in rats. The sustained increase in circulating TSH levels results initially in hypertrophy of follicular cells, followed by hyperplasia, and ultimately places the rat thyroid at greater risk to develop an increased incidence of benign tumors.

Phenobarbital has been reported to be a thyroid gland tumor promoter in a rat initiation–promotion model. Treatment with a nitrosamine followed by phenobarbital has been shown to increase serum TSH concentrations, thyroid gland weights, and the incidence of follicular cell tumors in the thyroid gland (McClain *et al.*, 1988, 1989). These effects could be decreased in a dose-related manner by simultaneous treatment with increasing doses of exogenous thyroxine. McClain *et al.* (1989) have demonstrated that rats treated with phenobarbital have a significantly higher cumulative biliary excretion of ^{125}I-thyroxine than controls (Fig. 21-28). Most of the increase in biliary excretion was accounted for by an increase in T_4-glucuronide due to an increased metabolism of thyroxine in phenobarbital-treated rats. This is consistent with enzymatic activity measurements which result in increased hepatic T_4-UDP-glucuronyl transferase activity in phenobarbital-treated rats (Fig. 21-29). Results from these experiments are consistent with the hypothesis that the promotion of thyroid tumors in rats was not a direct effect of phenobarbital on the thyroid gland but rather an indirect effect mediated by TSH secretion from the pituitary secondary to the hepatic microsomal enzyme-induced increase of T_4 excretion in the bile.

The activation of the thyroid gland during the treatment of rodents with substances that stimulate thyroxine catabolism is a well-known phenomenon and has been investigated extensively with phenobarbital and many other compounds (Curran and DeGroot, 1991). It occurs particularly with rodents, first because UDP-glucuronyl transferase can easily be induced in rodent species, and second

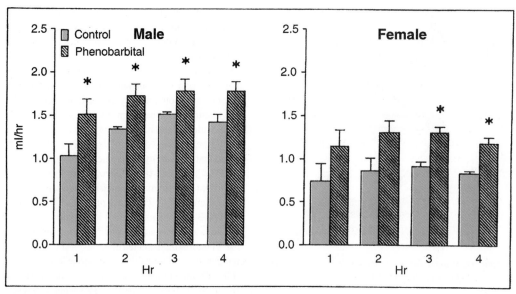

Figure 21-28. Cumulative biliary excretion of [125] ***I-thyroxine (percentage of administered dose) in control and pheno-barbital treated rats (100 mg/kg/day in the diet for 4–6 weeks).***

Phenobarbital treatment resulted in an increase in the cumulative excretion of thyroxine over a 4-hour period. Thin layer chromatography of bile samples indicated that most of the increase in biliary excretion was accounted for by an increase in the fraction corresponding to thyroxine-glucuronide. (From McClain, 1998).

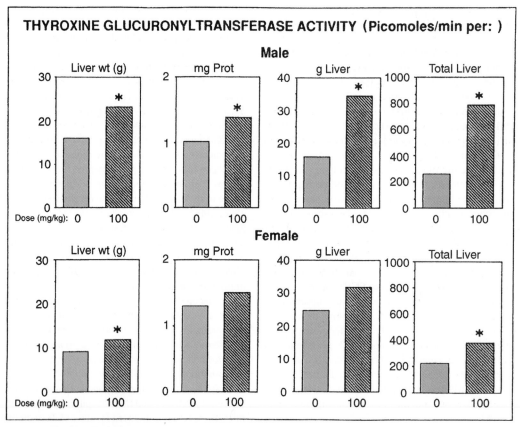

Figure 21-29. Hepatic thyroxine glucuronyltransferase activity in control and phenobarbital-treated rats (100 mg/kg/day in the diet for 4 weeks).

Glucuronyltransferase activity was measured in hepatic microsomes using thyroxine as a substrate. Phenobarbital treatment induced thyroxine-glucuronyltransferase in male and female rats; however, the effect in male rats was quantitatively larger. (From McClain, 1998).

because thyroxine metabolism takes place very rapidly in rats in the absence of thyroxine-binding globulin. In humans a lowering of the circulating T_4 level but no change in TSH and T_3 concentrations has been observed only with high doses of very powerful enzyme-inducing compounds, such as rifampicin with and without antipyrine.

Although phenobarbital is the only UDP-glucuronyl transferase (UDP-GT) inducer that has been investigated in detail to act as a thyroid tumor promoter, the effects of other well-known UDP-GT inducers on the disruption of serum T_4 TSH and thyroid gland have been investigated. For example, pregnenolone-16α-carbonitrile (PCN), 3-methylcholanthrene (3MC), and aroclor 1254 (PCB) induce hepatic microsomal UDP-GT activity toward T_4 (Barter and Klaassen, 1992a). These UDP-GT inducers reduce serum T_4 levels in both control as well as in thyroidectomized rats that are infused with T_4, indicating that reductions in serum T_4 levels are not due to a direct effect of the inducers on the thyroid gland (Barter and Klaassen, 1992b, 1994). However, serum TSH levels and the thyroid response to reductions in serum T_4 levels by UDP-GT inducers are not always predictable. While PCN increased serum TSH and resulted in thyroid follicular cell hyperplasia, similar to that observed with phenobarbital, 3MC and PCB in these short-duration experiments and at the dose levels used did not increase serum TSH levels or produce thyroid follicular cell hyperplasia (Hood et al., 1995; Liu et al., 1995). These findings support the overall hypothesis that UDP-GT inducers can adversely affect the thyroid gland by a secondary mechanism, but this applies only to those UDP-GT inducers that increase serum TSH in addition to reducing serum T_4 (Kolaja and Klaassen, 1998).

Additional investigations by this research group demonstrated that hepatic microsomal enzyme-inducing xenobiotic chemicals [e.g., phenobarbital and pregnenolone-16α-carbonitrile (PCN)] increased serum TSH (0–75%) much less than the thyroperoxidase inhibitor propylthiouracil (PTU) (830%) (Hood et al., 1999a,b). Phenobarbital and PCN administration increased thyroid weight approximately 80% compared to a 500% increase in PTU-treated rats. Thyroid follicular cell proliferation (determined by BrdU labeling) was increased 260, 330, and 850% in rats treated with phenobarbital, PCN, and PTU, respectively, for 7 days but the labeling index had returned to control levels by the 45th day of treatment. These findings demonstrate that certain hepatic microsomal enzyme-inducing chemicals that result in mild to modest elevations in serum TSH lead to dramatic increases in thyroid follicular cell proliferation which peaked after 7 days of treatment and then rapidly returned to control values (Klaassen and Hood, 2001). These findings are similar to those of Wynford-Thomas et al. (1982), who reported a maximal proliferative response (evaluated by mitotic index) after 7 days of treatment with aminotriazole (a thyroperoxidase inhibitor). The decline in thyroid follicular cell proliferation was suggested to be due to desensitization of the cells to the mitogenic actions of TSH (Wynford-Thomas et al., 1982a).

Hood et al. (1999) reported that moderate increases in serum TSH of between 10 and 20 ng/mL increased the number of proliferating thyroid follicular cells but had no effect on thyroid weight, emphasizing that small increases in serum TSH can be sufficient to stimulate proliferation. These important findings suggest that quantitation of follicular cell proliferation may be more useful than thyroid weights for assessing alterations in thyroid growth in rats administered xenobiotic chemicals that produce only small to moderate increases in serum TSH.

Another classic example of a chemical that induces hepatic microsomal enzymes and disrupts thyroid function are the polychlorinated biphenyls (Vansell et al., 2004). Polychlorinated biphenyls are commonly used industrial compounds that have been released into the environment and have caused widespread contamination. The disease-producing capability of these compounds includes alterations in reproduction, growth, and development. PCBs cause a significant reduction in serum levels of thyroid hormones due to alterations in thyroid structure, in addition to the well-known induction of hepatic UDP-glucuronyl transferase and increased secretion of thyroxine-glucuronide in the bile (Collins and Capen, 1980b).

Feeding of PCB produced a dose-dependent significant reduction in serum T_4 levels in rats. Following withdrawal of PCB from the diet, blood T_4 levels return to the normal range at 35 weeks but not at 12 weeks. These changes in circulating levels of T_4 were accompanied by a striking hypertrophy and hyperplasia of thyroid follicular cells compared with controls. The most consistent lesions in follicular cells following the feeding of PCB were the accumulation of numerous large colloid droplets and irregularly shaped lysosomal bodies in the expanded cytoplasmic area. Microvilli on the lumenal surface were shortened with abnormal branchings. The chronic administration (12-week) of PCB resulted in a striking distention of many follicular cells with large lysosomal bodies that were strongly acid phosphatase positive and with colloid droplets, blunt and abnormally branched microvilli, and mitochondrial vacuolation. The principal lesion produced by PCB in follicular cells that contributed to the altered thyroid function appeared to be an interference in the interaction between the numerous colloid droplets and lysosomal bodies that is necessary for the enzymatic release of thyroid hormones.

Another recently-investigated example of an inducer of hepatic microsomal enzymes that increase the incidence of thyroid follicular cell tumors in rats is pyrethrins. Pyrethrins comprise a mixture of natural products isolated from Pyrethrum flowers, which have been used for many years as an insecticide for household and other applications. Pyrethrins exhibit a low order of oral toxicity in mammals and are rapidly metabolized. Short-term tests for genotoxic potential have demonstrated that pyrethrins are not genotoxic agents. Pyrethrins were not carcinogenic to male and female CD-1 mice in an 18-month study when administered at dietary levels of 0, 100, 2500, and 5000 ppm (Schoenig, 1995). The treatment of male and female Sprague–Dawley (CD) rats for 2 years with 100 ppm pyrethrins had no effect on tumor incidence. However, higher doses of pyrethrins produced effects in the liver of female rats and in the thyroid glands of both sexes. A small increase in the incidence of hepatocellular adenoma was observed in female rats given 3000 ppm pyrethrins. Although treatment with 1000 ppm pyrethrins had no significant effect on the incidence of thyroid gland follicular cell tumors in female rats, the combined incidence of follicular cell adenomas and/or carcinomas was significantly increased in male rats given 1000 and 3000 ppm pyrethrins and in female rats fed 3000 ppm pyrethrins.

In a subsequent mechanistic study, male Sprague–Dawley (CD) rats were fed diets containing 0 and 8000 ppm pyrethrins and female rats diets containing 0, 100, 3000, and 8000 ppm pyrethrins for periods of 7, 14, and 42 days followed by 42 days reversal (Finch et al., 2006). Rats also were fed diets containing 1200–1558 ppm sodium phenobarbital (NaPb) for 7 and 14 days as a positive control. Treatment of male rats with 8000 ppm pyrethrins, female rats with 3000 and 8000 ppm pyrethrins, and both sexes with NaPb resulted in increased thyroid gland weights

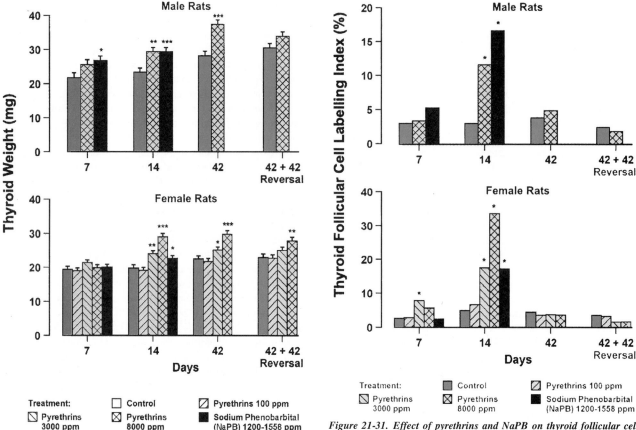

Figure 21-30. *Effect of pyrethrins and NaPB on thyroid weights of Sprague–Dawley rats. (From Finch et al., 2006).*

Figure 21-31. *Effect of pyrethrins and NaPB on thyroid follicular cell labelling index of Sprague–Dawley rats. (From Finch et al., 2006).*

(Fig. 21-30) associated with follicular cell hypertrophy. Thyroid follicular cell replicative DNA synthesis was increased by treatment of both males and females with pyrethrins and NaPb for 14 days (Fig. 21-31). Treatment with pyrethrins and NaPb increased serum TSH (Fig. 21-32) and reduced serum levels of T_4 (Fig. 21-33) (Finch et al., 2006).

The treatment of male and female rats with 8000 ppm pyrethrins for 7, 14, and 42 days and 1200–1558 ppm NaPb for 7 and 14 days produced increases in hepatic microsomal cytochrome P450 (CYP) content and a marked induction of CYP2B-dependent 7-pentoxyresorufin O-depentylase and testosterone 16β-hydroxylase activities (Price et al., 2007). Significant increases also were observed in CYP3A-dependent testosterone β-hydroxylase and thyroxine UDP-glucuronosyltransferase activities (Fig. 21-34). Relative potency calculations indicated that NaPb was 8.8 and 3.8X more potent than pyrethrins in inducing CYP2B and CYP3A enzymes in male and female rats, respectively. Hepatic effects of pyrethrins were dose-dependent in female rats (100 ppm being a no effect level) and after the cessation of treatment were reversible in both sexes. The mode of action of pyrethrins-induced rat liver and thyroid tumors appears to be similar to that of other nongenotoxic inducers of hepatic xenobiotic metabolism (Price et al., 2007).

In addition to disturbances in thyroid hormone economy associated with induction of hepatic microsomal enzymes and increased biliary excretion of conjugated thyroid hormones, recent studies have reported xenobiotic chemical-induced rapid hepatobiliary clearance of unconjugated T_4 (Wong et al., 2005). Serum T_4 levels were significantly lowered after 12 hours and were undetectable after 72 hours of administration of a selective corticotrophin-releasing factor (CRF) receptor-1 antagonist to male Sprague–Dawley rats. By comparison propylthiouracil (PTU) (used as a positive control) did not lower serum T4 levels until 72 hours. A significant compensatory increase in serum TSH also was detected after 12 hours with the CRF-1 receptor-1 antagonist compared to after 48 hours with PTU. A decreased mean ^{125}I–T_4 plasma concentration was detected after 1 hour when the first sample was collected and continued to rapidly decrease over a 24-hours period. Phenobarbital (used as a positive control) resulted only in a slight decrease of ^{125}I–T_4 in plasma compared to controls over a similar 24-hours experimental period (Wong et al., 2005). A single oral dose of the compound resulted in a rapid (at 3 hours) significant increase in mRNA for hepatic organic anion transporting protein (Oatp2) that persisted over the 24 hours of the experiment. Other studies have reported that microsomal enzyme inducers can increase the expression of these transporter proteins that mediate the uptake of xenobiotics from blood into the liver (Klaassen and Slitt, 2005). In addition, the CRF receptor-1 antagonist also induced the mRNA's of the multidrug resistance protein-2, a canalicular transporter, that mediates the efflux of compounds from liver into bile (Johnson and Klaassen, 2002a,b; Klaassen, 2002; Wong et al., 2005; Chen and Klaassen, 2004; Chen et al., 2003, 2005; Cheng et al., 2005; Cherrington et al., 2002, 2003; Guo et al., 2002; Maher et al., 2005; Slitt et al., 2006).

Xenobiotic chemical-induced perturbations in thyroid hormone economy are encountered more frequently in rats than in mice. Viollon-Badie et al. (1999) administered four classic hepatic microsomal enzyme-inducing chemicals (e.g., clofibrate [300 mg/kg],

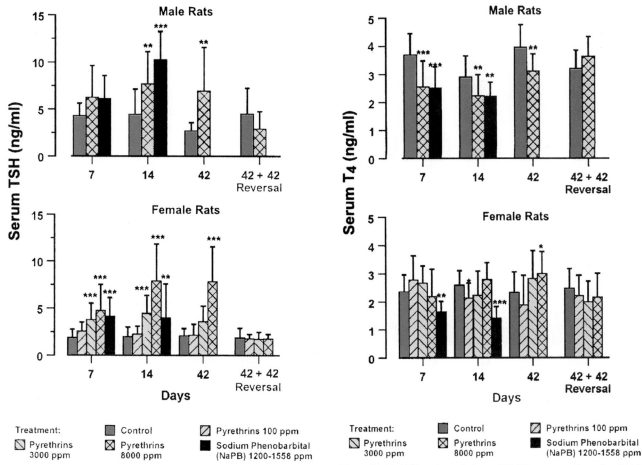

Figure 21-32. *Effect of pyrethins and NaPB on serum TSH in Sprague–Dawley rats. (From Finch et al., 2006).*

Figure 21-33. *Effect of pyrethrins and NaPB on serum thyroxine (T₄) in Sprague–Dawley rats. (From Finch et al., 2006).*

phenobarbital (PB) [80 mg/kg], pregnenolone-16α carbonitrile [PCN] [100 mg/kg], and β-naphthoflavone [80 mg/kg]) to rats and mice and compared the effects on hepatic T_4-UDP-glucuronyl transferase. Rats had a consistent and significant increase in enzyme activity whereas the modest increase in mice was not significant compared to controls. However, Hood *et al.* (2003) clearly demonstrated that B6C3F male mice respond to classic hepatic enzyme inducers (e.g., PB, PCB, PCN, and 3-methylcholanthrene (3-MC) by increasing liver weight, increased hepatic T4-UDP-glucuronyl transferase activity, decreased serum T_4 (only with PB and PCB), and increased serum TSH (markedly by PCN and 3-MC, only slight by PB and PCB). All four microsomal enzyme inducers dramatically increased thyroid follicular cell proliferation in mice as quantitated by the BrdU-labeling index.

There is no convincing evidence that humans treated with drugs or exposed to chemicals that induce hepatic microsomal enzymes are at increased risk for the development of thyroid cancer (Curran and DeGroot, 1991). In a study on the effects of microsomal enzyme-inducing compounds on thyroid hormone metabolism in normal healthy adults, phenobarbital (100 mg daily for 14 days) did not affect the serum T_4, T_3, or TSH levels (Ohnhaus *et al.*, 1981). A decrease in serum T_4 levels was observed after treatment with either a combination of phenobarbital plus rifampicin or a combination of phenobarbital plus antipyrine; however, these treatments had no effect on serum T_3 or TSH levels (Ohnhaus and Studer, 1983). Epidemiological studies of patients treated with therapeutic doses

of phenobarbital have reported no increase in risk for the development of thyroid neoplasia (Clemmesen *et al.*, 1974; Clemmesen and Hjalgrim-Jensen, 1977, 1978, 1981; White *et al.*, 1979; Friedman, 1981; Shirts *et al.*, 1986; Olsen *et al.*, 1989). Highly sensitive assays for thyroid and pituitary hormones are readily available in a clinical setting to monitor circulating hormone levels in patients exposed to chemicals potentially disruptive of pituitary–thyroid axis homeostasis.

Likewise, there is no substantive evidence that humans treated with drugs or exposed to chemicals that induce hepatic microsomal enzymes are at increased risk for the development of liver cancer. This is best exemplified by the extensive epidemiological information on the clinical use of phenobarbital. Phenobarbital has been used clinically as an anticonvulsant for more than 80 years. Relatively high microsomal enzyme-inducing doses have been used chronically, sometimes for lifetime exposures, to control seizure activity in human beings. A study of over 8000 patients admitted to a Danish epilepsy center from 1933 to 1962 revealed no evidence for an increased incidence of hepatic tumors in phenobarbital-treated humans when patients receiving thorotrast, a known human liver carcinogen, were excluded (Clemmesen and Hjalgrim-Jensen, 1978). A follow-up report on this patient population confirmed and extended this observation (Clemmesen and Hjalgrim-Jensen, 1981; Olsen *et al.*, 1989). The results of two other smaller studies (2099 epileptics and 959 epileptics) also revealed no hepatic tumors in patients treated with phenobarbital (White *et al.*, 1979).

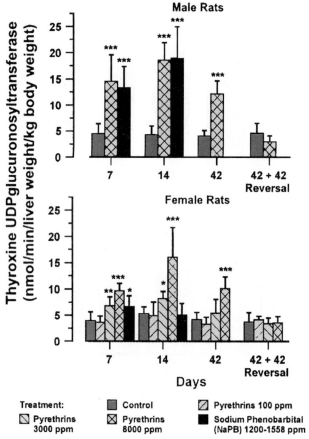

Figure 21-34. Effect of pyrethrins and NaPB on hepatic T₄-UDP-GT (nmol/min/liver wt./body wt.) in Sprague–Dawley rats. (From Finch et al., 2006).

Chemical Inhibition of 5'-Monodeiodinase

FD&C Red No. 3 (erythrosine) is an example of a well-characterized xenobiotic that results in perturbations of thyroid function in rodents and in long-term studies is associated with an increased incidence of benign thyroid tumors. Red No. 3 is a widely used color additive in foods, cosmetics, and pharmaceuticals. A chronic toxicity/carcinogenicity study revealed that male Sprague–Dawley rats

fed a 4% dietary concentration of Red No. 3 beginning in utero and extending over their lifetime (30 months) developed a 22% incidence of thyroid adenomas derived from follicular cells compared to 1.5% in control rats and a historical incidence of 1.8% for this strain (Borzelleca *et al.*, 1987; Capen, 1989) (Fig. 21-35). There was no significant increase in follicular cell adenomas in the lower dose groups of male rats or an increase in malignant thyroid follicular cell tumors. Female rats fed similar amounts of the color did not develop a significant increase in either benign or malignant thyroid tumors. Feeding of the color at the high dose (4%) level provided male rats with 2464 mg/kg of Red No. 3 daily; by comparison human consumption in the United States is estimated to be 0.023 mg/kg/day.

The results of mechanistic studies with FD&C Red No. 3 have suggested that a primary (direct) action on the thyroid is unlikely to result from: (1) failure of the color (^{14}C-labeled) to accumulate in the gland, (2) negative genotoxicity and mutagenicity assays, (3) lack of an oncogenic response in mice and gerbils, (4) a failure to promote thyroid tumor development at dietary concentrations of 1.0% or less in male and female rats (Capen, 1989), and (5) no increased tumor development in other organs. Investigations with radiolabeled compound have demonstrated that the color does not accumulate in the thyroid glands of rats following the feeding of either 0.5% or 4.0% FD&C Red No. 3 for 1 week prior to the oral dose of ^{14}C-labeled material.

Mechanistic investigations with FD&C Red No. 3 included, among others, a 60-day study of male Sprague–Dawley rats fed either 4% (high dose) or 0.25% (low dose) Red No. 3 compared to controls, whose food was without the color, in order to determine the effects of the color on thyroid hormone economy. The experimental design of the study was to sacrifice groups of rats ($n = 20$ rats/interval and dose) fed Red No. 3 and their control groups after 0, 3, 7, 10, 14, 21, 30, and 60 days.

A consistent effect of Red No. 3 on thyroid hormone economy was the striking increase in serum reverse T_3 (Fig. 21-36). In the rats fed high doses, reverse T_3 was increased at all intervals compared to controls and this also held for rats killed at 10, 14, and 21 days in the low-dose group. The mechanisms responsible for the increased serum reverse T_3 appear to be, first, substrate (T_4) accumulation due to 5'-monodeiodinase inhibition with subsequent conversion to reverse T_3 rather than active T_3; and, second, reverse T_3 accumulation due to 5'-monodeiodinase inhibition resulting in an inability to degrade reverse T_3 further to diiodothyronine (T_2).

Groups	Original Study					High-Dose Study	
	I_A	I_B	II	III	IV	I_C	V
Red No. 3 (%)	0	0	0.1	0.5	1.0	0	4.0
(mg/kg/day)	–	–	(49)	(251)	(507)	–	(2.464)
F.C. Adenoma (%)	0	0	0	2.9	1.5	1.5	21.8
F.C. Carcinoma (%)	0	0	4.5	1.5	4.4	2.9	4.4
Cystic follicular hyperplasia (%)	2.9	1.5	12	16.2	7.3	0	23.2
Diffuse or focal F.C. hyperplasia (%)	1.4	0	7.	7.4	26.1	5.8	87.0
Follicular cysts (%)	10	14.5	9.0	11.8	11.6	2.9	14.5

Figure 21-35. Thyroid lesions in male Sprague–Dawley rats fed varying doses of FD&C Red No. 3 beginning in utero and for a lifetime of 30 months. (From Borzelleca et al., 1987).

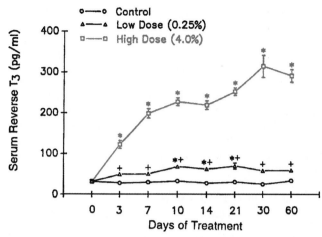

Figure 21-36. *Rapid and significant increase in serum reverse triiodothyronine (rT$_3$) levels in Sprague–Dawley rats (N = 20 per group and interval) administered a high (4%) and low (0.25%) dose of FD&C Red No. 3.*

The significant increase in rT$_3$ was detected at the initial interval of 3 days and persisted during the 60-day experiment in the high-dose group. (Courtesy of the Certified Color Manufacturers Association, Inc., and Dr. L.E. Braverman and Dr. W.J. DeVito, University of Massachusetts Medical School.)

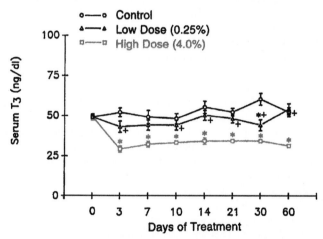

Figure 21-37. *Changes in serum triiodothyronine (T$_3$) following administration of a high (4%) and low (0.25%) dose of FD&C Red No. 3 in the diet to Sprague–Dawley rats. (Courtesy of the Certified Color Manufacturers, Inc., and Dr. L.E. Braverman and Dr. W.J. DeVito, University of Massachusetts Medical School.)*

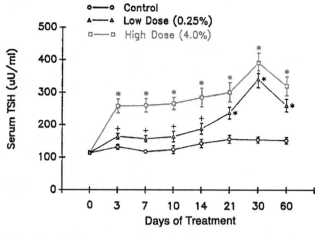

Figure 21-38. *Changes in serum thyroid-stimulating hormone (TSH) following administration of a high (4%) and low (0.25%) dose of FD&C Red No. 3 in the diet to Sprague–Dawley rats. (Courtesy of the Certified Color Manufacturers Association, Inc. and Dr. L.E. Braverman and Dr. W.J. DeVito, University of Massachusetts Medical School.)*

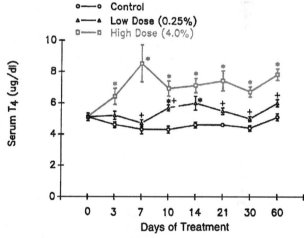

Figure 21-39. *Changes in serum thyroxine (T$_4$) following administration of a high (4%) and low (0.25%) dose of FD&C Red No. 3 in the diet to Sprague–Dawley rats. (Courtesy of the Certified Color Manufacturers Association, Inc., and Dr. L.E. Braverman and Dr. W.J. DeVito, University of Massachusetts Medical School.)*

Serum triiodothyronine (T$_3$) was decreased significantly at all intervals in rats of the high-dose group compared to interval controls (Fig. 21-37). The mechanism responsible for the reduced serum T$_3$ following feeding of Red No. 3 was decreased monodeiodination of T$_4$ due to an inhibition of the 5'-monodeiodinase by the color.

Serum TSH was increased significantly at all intervals in rats of the high-dose (4%) group compared to controls. Rats fed 0.25% Red No. 3 had increased serum TSH only at days 21, 30, and 60 (Fig. 21-38). The mechanism responsible for the increased serum TSH following ingestion of Red No. 3 was a compensatory response by the pituitary gland to the low circulating levels of T$_3$ that resulted from an inhibition of the 5'-monodeiodinase. Serum T$_4$ also was increased at all intervals in rats fed 4% Red No. 3 compared to controls (Fig. 21-39). The mechanism responsible for the increased serum T$_4$

was, first, accumulation due to an inability to monodeiodinate T$_4$ to T$_3$ in the liver and kidney from the inhibition of 5'-monodeiodinase by the color; and, second, TSH stimulation of increased T$_4$ production by the thyroid gland.

[125]I-labeled T$_4$ metabolism was altered in liver homogenates prepared from rats fed 4% FD&C Red No. 3. Degradation of labeled T$_4$ was decreased to approximately 40% of the values in control homogenates (Fig. 21-40). This was associated with a 75% decrease in percent generation of ^{125}I and an approximately 80% decrease in percent generation of ^{125}I-labeled T$_3$ from radiolabeled T$_4$ substrate. These mechanistic investigations suggested that the color results in a perturbation of thyroid hormone economy in rodents by inhibiting the 5'-monodeiodinase in the liver, resulting in long-term stimulation of follicular cells by TSH, which over their lifetime predisposed to an increased incidence of thyroid tumors (Borzelleca *et al.*, 1987; Capen and Martin, 1989). The color tested negative in

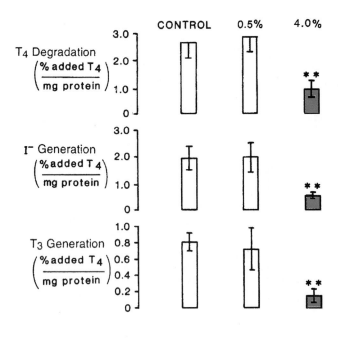

**P<0.001 4% vs. Control

Figure 21-40. Effects of dietary FD&C Red No. 3 on the hepatic metabolism of ^{125}I-labeled thyroxine in male Sprague–Dawley rats fed diets containing 0.5 and 4.0% color compared to controls. (Courtesy of the Certified Color Manufacturers Association, Inc. and the late Sidney H. Ingbar, M.D.)

standard genotoxic and mutagenic assays, and it did not increase the incidence of tumors in other organs.

Morphometric evaluation was performed on thyroid glands from all rats at each interval during the 60-day study. Four levels of exposure of rat thyroid to Red No. 3 were evaluated, with 25 measurements from each rat. The direct measurements included the diameter of thyroid follicles, area of follicular colloid, and height of follicular cells. Thyroid follicular diameter was decreased significantly in both low- and high-dose groups at 3, 7, 10, and 14 days compared to interval controls. The area of follicular colloid generally reflected the decrease in thyroid follicular diameter and was decreased significantly at days 3 and 10 in high-dose rats and days 7 and 10 in the low-dose group compared to interval controls. These reductions in thyroid follicular diameter and colloid area were consistent with morphological changes expected in response to an increased serum TSH concentration.

Thyroid follicular height was increased significantly only after feeding FD&C Red No. 3 for 60 days in both the high- and low-dose groups compared to interval controls. The absence of morphometric evidence of follicular cell hypertrophy at the shorter intervals was consistent with the modest increase (15.8%) in thyroid gland:body weight ratio after this relatively short exposure to the color. The lack of follicular cell hypertrophy at the shorter intervals of feeding Red No. 3 in rats with severalfold elevations in serum TSH levels may be related, in part, to the high iodine content (58% of molecular weight) interfering with the receptor-mediated response of thyroid follicular cells to TSH. The thyroid responsiveness to TSH is known to vary inversely with iodine content (Ingbar, 1972; Lamas and Ingbar, 1978). Thyroid glands of rats fed FD&C Red No. 3 would be exposed to an increased iodine concentration primarily from sodium iodide contamination of the color and, to a lesser extent, from metabolism of the compound and release of iodide.

Secondary Mechanisms of Thyroid Tumorigenesis and Risk Assessment

Understanding the mechanism of action of xenobiotics on the thyroid gland provides a rational basis for extrapolation findings from long-term rodent studies to the assessment of a particular compound's safety for humans (McClain, 1994). Many chemicals and drugs disrupt one or more steps in the synthesis and secretion of thyroid hormones, resulting in subnormal levels of T_4 and T_3, associated with a compensatory increased secretion of pituitary TSH (Fig. 21-41). When tested in highly sensitive species, such as rats and mice, early on these compounds resulted in follicular cell hypertrophy/hyperplasia and increased thyroid weights, and in long-term studies they produced an increased incidence of thyroid tumors by a secondary (indirect) mechanism associated with hormonal inbalances.

Review of the U.S. *Physicians' Desk Reference* (PDR) reveals a number of marketed drugs that result in a thyroid tumorigenic response when tested at high concentrations in rodents, primarily in rats. A broad spectrum of product classes are represented including antibiotics, calcium-channel blockers, antidepressants, hypolipidemic agents, amongst others (Fig. 21-42). Amiodarone (an antiarrhythmic drug) and iodinated glycerol (an expectorant) are highly iodinated molecules that disrupt thyroid hormone economy by mechanisms similar to the food color, FD&C Red No. 3 (Fig. 21-43).

In the secondary mechanism of thyroid oncogenesis in rodents, the specific xenobiotic chemical or physiological perturbation evokes another stimulus (e.g., chronic hypersecretion of TSH) that promotes the development of nodular proliferative lesions (initially hypertrophy, followed by hyperplasia, subsequently adenomas, infrequently carcinomas) derived from follicular cells (Hiasa *et al.*, 1987). Thresholds for "no effect" on the thyroid gland can be established by determining the dose of xenobiotic that fails to elicit an elevation in the circulating level of TSH. Compounds acting by this indirect (secondary) mechanism with hormonal imbalances usually show little or no evidence for mutagenicity or for producing DNA damage.

In human patients who have marked changes in thyroid function and elevated TSH levels, as is common in areas with a high incidence of endemic goiter due to iodine deficiency, there is little if any increase in the incidence of thyroid cancer (Doniach, 1970; Curran and DeGroot, 1991). The relative resistance to the development of thyroid cancer in humans with elevated plasma TSH levels is in marked contrast to the response of the thyroid gland to chronic TSH stimulation in rats and mice. The human thyroid is much less sensitive to this pathogenetic phenomenon than rodents (McClain *et al.*, 1989).

Human patients with congenital defects in thyroid hormone synthesis (dyshormonogenetic goiter) and markedly increased circulating TSH levels have been reported to have an increased incidence of thyroid carcinomas (McGirr *et al.*, 1959; Cooper *et al.*, 1981). Likewise, thyrotoxic patients with Grave's disease, in which follicular cells are autonomously stimulated by an immunoglobulin (long-acting thyroid stimulator, or LATS) also appear to be at greater risk of developing thyroid tumors (Clements, 1954; Pendergrast *et al.*, 1961). Therefore, the literature suggests that prolonged stimulation of the human thyroid by TSH will induce neoplasia only in exceptional circumstances, possibly by acting together with some other metabolic or immunologic abnormality (Curran and DeGroot, 1991).

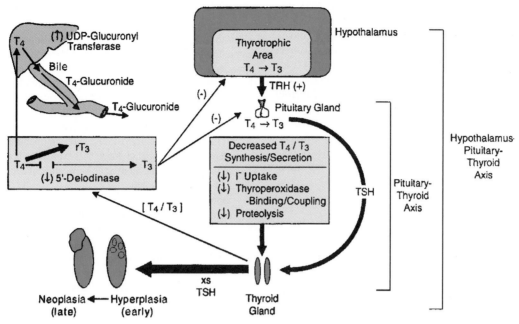

Figure 21-41. Multiple sites of disruption of the hypothalamic–pituitary–thyroid axis by xenobiotic chemicals.

Chemicals can exert direct effects by disrupting thyroid hormone synthesis or secretion and indirectly influence the thyroid through an inhibition of 5′-deiodinase or by inducing hepatic microsomal enzymes (e.g., T_4-UDP glucuronyltransferase). All of these mechanisms can lower circulating levels of thyroid hormones (T_4 and/or T_3), resulting in a release from negative-feedback inhibition and increased secretion of thyroid-stimulating hormone (TSH) by the pituitary gland. The chronic hypersecretion of TSH predisposes the sensitive rodent thyroid gland to develop an increased incidence of focal hyperplastic and neoplastic lesions (adenomas) by a secondary (epigenetic) mechanism.

DRUG	PRODUCT CLASS	SPECIES
● MINOCYCLINE	ANTIBIOTIC	R
● OXAZEPAM	ANTIANXIETY	R
● NICARDIPINE	Ca-CHANNEL BLOCKER	R
● SERTRALINE	ANTIDEPRESSANT	R
● SIMVASTATIN	HYPOLIPIDEMIC	R
● SPIRONOLACTONE	DIURETIC	R
● VIDARABINE	ANTIVIRAL	R

Figure 21-42. Examples of marketed drugs with a tumorigenic response in the thyroid gland of rats. (Modified from Davis and Monro, 1995).

DRUG	PRODUCT CLASS	SPECIES
● AMIODARONE	ANTIARRHYTHMIC	R
● ATENOLOL	β-ADRENERGIC BLOCKER	R
● BEPRIDIL	Ca-CHANNEL BLOCKER	R
● DAPSONE	ANTINEOPLASTIC	R
● GRISEOFULVIN	ANTIBIOTIC	R
● IODINATED GLYCEROL	EXPECTORANT	R
● METHINAZOLE	ANTI-THYROID	R
● MIDAZOLAM	SEDATIVE	R

Figure 21-43. Marketed drugs with a thyroid tumorigenic response. (Modified from Davis and Monro, 1995).

Initiating Chemicals in Thyroid Carcinogenesis

In contrast to the previous categories of indirect-acting thyrotoxic compounds, certain chemicals and irradiation appear to have a direct effect on the thyroid gland resulting in genetic damage that leads to cell transformation and tumor formation in animals (Doniach, 1963; Lee *et al.*, 1982; Capen *et al.*, 1999). Examples of thyroid initiators include 2-acetylaminofluorine (2-AAF), *N*-methyl-*N*-nitrosourea [MNU], *N*-bis(2-hydroxypropyl) nitrosamine [DHPN], methylcholanthrene, dichlorobenzidine, and polycyclic hydrocarbons. Chemicals in this group often increase the incidence of both benign and malignant thyroid tumors. Iodine deficiency is a strong promoter of MNU-initiated thyroid tumors in rats.

Thyroid Tumors in Humans

Thyroid carcinomas are the most common endocrine neoplasms in humans, affecting approximately 1% of the population (Sherman, 2003). Roughly 95% of all thyroid tumors are of thyroid follicular epithelial cell origin, including papillary, follicular, and anaplastic thyroid carcinomas. The remaining 5% are medullary thyroid carcinomas of C-cell origin (Cho *et al.*, 1999; Sherman, 2003). The subclassification of thyroid cancers into these four categories is clinically significant. Papillary thyroid carcinomas metastasize via lymphatics to local lymph nodes in an estimated 50% of cases but have the most favorable prognosis, with a 98% 10-year survival rate. Follicular carcinomas are associated with poorer prognoses. Follicular thyroid carcinomas are more prevalent in areas of dietary iodine deficiency, metastasize hematogenously, and are less likely than papillary thyroid carcinomas to take up radioactive iodide for imaging and therapeutic ablation. However, the 10-year survival rate for follicular thyroid carcinomas is still high at 92%. Anaplastic thyroid carcinomas are almost invariably fatal due to rapid invasion of critical structures in the neck, distant metastases, and a failure to take up radioactive iodide.

Medullary thyroid carcinomas, also commonly known as C-cell carcinomas, arise from calcitonin-secreting C-cells and are associated with inherited syndromes, such as multiple endocrine neoplasia (MEN), in approximately 20–25% of cases (Cho *et al.*, 1999; Sherman, 2003). Medullary carcinomas frequently metastasize via the bloodstream, in addition to lymphatic spread, and are treated with surgical resection and/or external beam radiation. In contrast to follicular origin thyroid tumors, C-cells and tumors arising from them do not have the ability to take up radioactive iodide. The five-year survival rate for medullary thyroid carcinomas is approximately 50%.

Genetic Events in Thyroid Tumors of Follicular Cell Origin

Thyroid follicular cells are responsible for iodide uptake and thyroid hormone synthesis and can undergo neoplastic transformation to carcinomas of three histotypes: papillary, follicular, and anaplastic. It is well known that papillary thyroid carcinomas can occur secondary to ionizing radiation exposure, particularly in children (Sherman, 2003; Boice, 2005). After the Chernobyl nuclear reactor accident in 1986, the incidence of thyroid carcinomas in children in affected areas of Belarus increased from less than one per million to more than 90 per million (Cardis *et al.*, 2005). The primary known molecular mechanism of radiation-induced papillary carcinoma development is through the Ret/PTC group of oncogenes. *Ret* proto-oncogene is a receptor tyrosine kinase normally involved in the glial-derived neurotropic factor signaling pathway in neuroendocrine and neural cells. In thyroid follicular cells, the alignment of chromosomes during interphase places the *ret* proto-oncogene in close proximity to several other constitutively expressed genes with which it can recombine during repair of ionizing radiation-induced double-stranded DNA breaks (Nikiforov, 2002, 2000). These Ret/PTC rearrangements allow for unregulated expression of chimeric oncoproteins with constitutive tyrosine kinase activity. Ret/PTC expression is found in roughly one-third of all papillary carcinomas, but in the majority of all radiation-induced papillary carcinomas (Klugbauer *et al.*, 1995). Whereas Ret/PTC1-expressing papillary carcinomas are often well differentiated, Ret/PTC3 expression is associated with a solid phenotype and a more aggressive clinical course (Nikiforov, 2002; Williams *et al.*, 2004).

Sporadic papillary thyroid carcinomas unrelated to radiation exposure make up more than two-thirds of all cases, and several genetic events have been identified as important in their tumorigenesis (Nikiforov, 2004). A form of the B-type Raf kinase, or BRAF, with a point mutation resulting in V600E has been identified in approximately 45% of sporadic papillary carcinomas, particularly the tall-cell variant (Xing, 2005). BRAF expression has been associated with dedifferentiation and disease progression. NTRK1 is a receptor tyrosine kinase normally involved in nerve growth factor signaling (Tallini, 2002). Like Ret/PTC rearrangements, NTRK1 can recombine with the 5′ end of other heterologous genes and form a constitutively active oncogene, such as TRK-T1, leading to papillary carcinomas. However, NTRK1 rearrangements are less frequent than Ret/PTC rearrangements and are not associated with radiation exposure.

Genetically Engineered Mouse Models of Thyroid Cancer

Genetically engineered mouse models of thyroid cancer facilitate analysis of the roles of specific genetic mutations in thyroid tumorigenesis (Jhiang *et al.*, 1996, 1998b; Sagartz *et al.*, 1997; Capen and Sagartz, 1998). Because thyroid cancer truly encompasses several diseases with different etiologies and relevant genetic mutations, no single transgenic mouse model of thyroid cancer can fully recapitulate the full spectrum of disease. However, several models have successfully reproduced various aspects and have offered insight into genetic mutations underlying thyroid tumorigenesis. These mouse models of thyroid cancer offer examples of positive genotype–phenotype correlation (Knostman *et al.*, 2007) (Table 21-3).

Over the past decade, several genetically engineered mouse models of thyroid cancer have been utilized to replicate variants of the human disease (Table 21-3). In most cases, transgenic mice have been produced using the highly active bovine thyroglobulin (Tg) promoter to specifically target transgene expression to thyroid follicular cells or using the human or rat calcitonin/calcitonin gene-related peptide (CGRP) promoter to target transgene expression to C-cells. In some cases, tumor suppressor gene knockout mice have been created and cross-bred with transgenic mice expressing thyroid-specific oncogenes, resulting in increased tumorigenesis and/or an aggressive phenotype. Transgenic mice expressing Ret/PTC1, Ret/PTC3 Trk-T1, BRAF or ras offer a reasonable approximation of the features of papillary thyroid carcinomas in humans. However, even with a p53 knock-out, no model has been able to demonstrate significant tumor dedifferentiation or metastasis (LaPerle *et al.*, 2000). One limitation has been the fact that p53 knockout mice develop extrathyroidal neoplasms at a high rate,

Table 21-3

Comparison of Human Thyroid Tumors and Genetically Engineered Mouse Models of Thyroid Cancer with Similar Genetic Mutations

GENETIC ALTERATION	TUMOR MORPHOLOGY		BIOLOGIC BEHAVIOR		HORMONAL DERANGEMENT	
	HUMAN	MOUSE	HUMAN	MOUSE	HUMAN	MOUSE
Ret/PTC1	Typical PTC	Typical PTC	Frequent local invasion, regional lymph node and less common distant metastases	Local invasion without any metastasis	None typical	Hypothyroidism
Ret/PTC3	Typical to solid PTC	Typical to solid PTC	Frequent local invasion, regional lymph node and less common distant metastases	Local invasion with rare lymph node metastases	None typical	NR
BRAF^{V600E}	Tall-cell variant or typical PTC with necrosis and anaplasia	Tall-cell variant or typical PTC with foci of anaplasia	Very frequent local invasion and anaplasia; loss of differentiation markers	Local invasion and anaplasia; maintenance of thyroglobulin expression	None typical	High TSH euthyroid
TRK	Typical PTC	PTC with absence of characteristic nuclear abnormalities	Local invasion, regional lymph node and less common distant metastases	Invasion not reported; absence of metastases	None typical	None
ras	FTC or follicular variant PTC	Typical PTC	Local invasion, regional lymph node, and/or hematogenous metastases	Local invasion with rare lung metastases	None typical	None
p53 inactivation/loss	ATC	Increased anaplasia, invasion and metastases in Ret/PTC models of PTC (p53 not examined alone)	Rapid local invasion and metastases with loss of differentiation markers	Local invasion with rare metastases and early death	None typical	Hypothyroidism (in combination with Ret/PTC transgene expression)
Ret	MTC	MTC +/− PTC	C-cell hyperplasia progressing to MTC*; distant spread common in advanced disease; tumors produce calcitonin	C-cell hyperplasia progressing to MTC; very rare metastases; tumors produce calcitonin	Hypercalcitonism	Hypercalcitonism

PTC, papillary thyroid carcinoma; FTC, follicular thyroid carcinoma; ATC, anaplastic thyroid carcinoma; MTC, medullary thyroid carcinoma; NR, not reported; *hereditary cases (e.g., MEN 2A) From Knostman *et al.*, 2007.

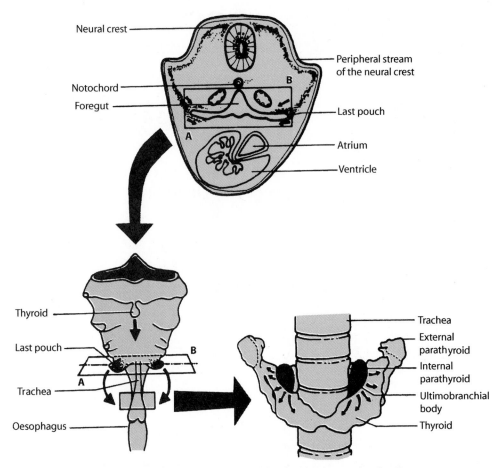

Figure 21-44. Schematic representation of neural crest origin of calcitonin-secreting C-cells.

Primordial cells arising from neural crest migrate ventrally during embryonic life to become incorporated in the last (ultimobranchial) pharyngeal pouch. The ultimobranchial body fuses with primordia of the thyroid and distributes C-cells to varying degrees throughout the mammalian thyroid gland. (From Foster *et al.*, 1972).

resulting in a shortened life span. A tissue-specific p53 knockout would help to eliminate this problem and allow the mice to live long enough to potentially develop more advanced thyroid cancer (Knostman *et al.*, 2007).

Follicular thyroid carcinoma has been primarily investigated using a single mouse model, $TR\beta^{PV/PV}$. The limitation of this model is the presence of hyperthyroidism and thyroid hormone resistance, which is not typical of the human disease. Because follicular thyroid carcinomas are more common in areas of dietary iodide deficiency, it is interesting that chronic TSH stimulation in the $TR\beta^{PV/PV}$ mice resulted in this type of neoplasm. However, rodents are notoriously susceptible to thyroid neoplasia due to perturbations of the pituitary–thyroid axis (Capen, 1997, 2001).

Many of the mouse models of thyroid follicular cell neoplasia fail to reproduce the normal hormonal milieu present in humans with thyroid cancer. For example, derangement of thyroid function in mouse models remains a problem. Rapid onset of dysplasia or neoplasia replacing the majority of the normal thyroid tissue, especially in neonatal and juvenile mice, often results in significant hypothyroidism unless thyroid hormone supplementation is instituted. In addition, human thyroid neoplasms are more than twofold more common in women than in men, suggesting that estrogen plays a role in tumorigenesis, while no sex predilection has been achieved in the current mouse models.

THYROID C-CELLS

Normal Structure and Function

Calcitonin (CT) has been shown to be secreted by a second population of endocrine cells in the mammalian thyroid gland that are much less numerous than follicular cells. C-cells (parafollicular or light cells) are distinct from follicular cells in the thyroid that secrete T_4 and T_3 (Nonidez, 1931–32; Kalina and Pearse, 1971). They are situated either within the follicular wall immediately beneath the basement membrane or between follicular cells and as small groups of cells between thyroid follicles. C-cells do not border the follicular colloid directly, and their secretory polarity is oriented toward the interfollicular capillaries. The distinctive feature of C-cells, compared to thyroid follicular cells, is the presence of numerous small membrane-limited secretory granules in the cytoplasm. Immunocytochemical techniques have localized the calcitonin activity of C-cells to these secretory granules (DeGrandi *et al.*, 1971).

Calcitonin-secreting thyroid C-cells have been shown to be derived embryologically from cells of the neural crest. Primordial cells from the neural crest migrate ventrally and become incorporated within the last (ultimobranchial) pharyngeal pouch (Foster *et al.*, 1972) (Fig. 21-44). They move caudally with the ultimobranchial body to the point of fusion with the midline thyroglossal duct

Thyroid C-Cell

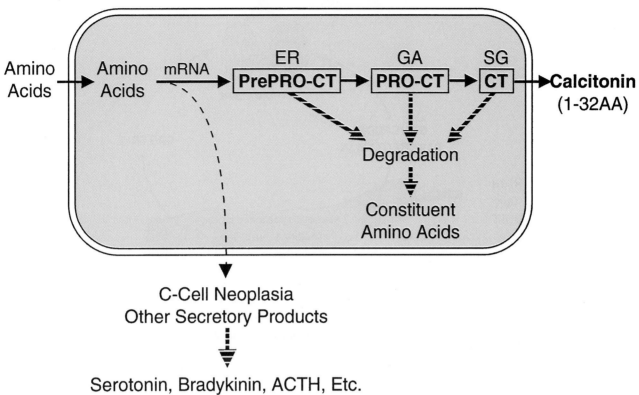

Figure 21-45. Biosynthesis of calcitonin in C-cells of the thyroid gland.

Preprocalcitonin (prePRO-CT) and procalcitonin (PRO-CT) are biosynthetic precursors that undergo posttranslational processing to form biologically active calcitonin (CT). Some of these precursor molecules and biologically active calcitonin may undergo enzymatic degradation to the constituent amino acids (AAs) prior to secretion from the C cell. Under certain disease conditions (e.g., neoplasms), C-cells may secrete other neuroendocrine products, including serotonin, bradykinin, and adrenocorticotropic hormone (ACTH). ER, endoplasmic reticulum; GA, Golgi apparatus; mRNA, messenger ribonucleic acid; and SG, secretory granule.

primordia that gives rise to the thyroid gland. The ultimobranchial body fuses with and is incorporated into the thyroid near the hilus in mammals and C-cells subsequently are distributed throughout the gland. Although C-cells are present throughout the thyroid gland of humans and most other mammals in postnatal life, they often remain more numerous near the hilus and point of fusion with the ultimobranchial body. Under certain conditions colloid-containing follicles lined by follicular cells also can differentiate from cells of ultimobranchial origin (Leblanc *et al.*, 1990; Teitelbaum *et al.*, 1970).

In contrast to the iodothyronines (T$_4$ and T$_3$) produced by follicular cells, calcitonin is a polypeptide hormone composed of 32 amino acid residues arranged in a straight chain (Copp, 1970). Calcitonin is synthesized as part of a larger biosynthetic precursor molecule (Wolfe, 1982) called pre-procalcitonin (Fig. 21-45). It is transported to the Golgi apparatus where it is converted to procalcitonin and then to calcitonin prior to packaging in membrane-limited secretory granules. Depending upon the need for calcitonin, a proportion of the precursors and active hormone undergo degradation prior to release from C-cells. The concentration of calcium ion in plasma and extracellular fluids is the principal physiological stimulus for the secretion of CT by C-cells. CT is secreted continuously under conditions of normocalcemia but the rate of secretion of CT is increased greatly in response to elevations in blood calcium. C-cells

store substantial amounts of CT in their cytoplasm in the form of membrane-limited secretory granules. In response to hypercalcemia there is a rapid discharge of stored hormone from C-cells into interfollicular capillaries. The hypercalcemic stimulus, if sustained, is followed by hypertrophy of C-cells and an increased development of cytoplasmic organelles concerned with the synthesis and secretion of CT. Hyperplasia of C-cells occurs in response to long-term hypercalcemia. When the blood calcium is lowered, the stimulus for CT secretion is diminished and numerous secretory granules accumulate in the cytoplasm of C-cells.

Calcitonin exerts its function by interacting with target cells, primarily in bone and kidney. The action of calcitonin is antagonistic to that of parathyroid hormone on mobilizing calcium from bone, but synergistic on decreasing the renal tubular reabsorption of phosphorus. The storage of large amounts of preformed hormone in C-cells and rapid release in response to moderate elevations of blood calcium are a reflection of the physiologic role of calcitonin as an "emergency" hormone to protect against the development of hypercalcemia. Calcitonin and parathyroid hormone, acting in concert, provide a dual negative feedback control mechanism to maintain the life-sustaining concentration of calcium ion in extracellular fluids within narrow limits. Calcitonin secretion is increased in response to a high-calcium meal often before a significant rise in plasma calcium can be detected. Gastrin, pancreozymin,

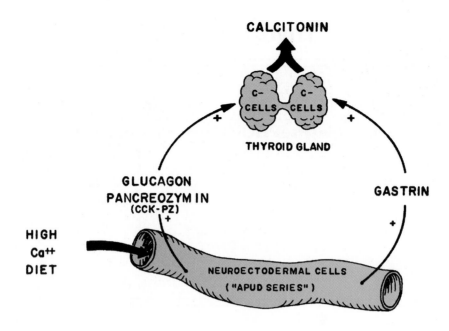

GASTROINTESTINAL- THYROID C CELL AXIS

Figure 21-46. The gastrointestinal hormone-thyroid C-cell axis.

This axis provides a mechanism for rapid release of calcitonin from the thyroid in response to a high-calcium diet before a significant elevation in blood calcium occurs. (From Rosol and Capen, 1997).

and intestinal glucagon are examples of gastrointestinal hormones whose secretion is stimulated by an oral calcium load which, in turn, act as secretagogues for calcitonin release from the thyroid gland (Fig. 21-46).

The calcitonin gene is expressed differently in thyroid (C-cells) than in neural tissues (Steenbergh *et al.*, 1984; Jacobs, 1985). In C-cells of the mammalian thyroid, the mRNA encodes primarily for pre-procalcitonin with a molecular weight of 17,400 Da, whereas in neural tissues there is alternative RNA processing and encoding for pre-procalcitonin gene-related peptide (CGRP). This CGRP is a neuropeptide composed of 37 amino acids with a molecular weight of 15,900 Da and participates in nociception, ingestive behavior, and modulation of the nervous and endocrine systems.

The structure of calcitonin differs considerably between species. The molecular structure of calcitonin for five selected species share only 9 of the 32 amino acid residues. However, the amino terminal portion of the calcitonin molecule is similar in all species. It consists of a seven-member ring enclosed by an intrachain (1–7) disulfide bridge. The complete sequence of 32 amino acids and the disulfide bond are essential for full biologic activity. It is surprising that on a weight basis, salmon calcitonin is more potent in lowering blood calcium than any of the other calcitonins when administered to mammals, including humans. The reason for the greater biologic potency of salmon calcitonin in mammals is uncertain but probably is related to an increased resistance to metabolic degradation and longer half-life or to a greater affinity for receptor sites in bone and other target tissues.

Serum levels of calcitonin are best measured by radioimmunoassay (RIA). Because of the low degree of homology of calcitonin between species there is poor cross reactivity of RIAs for calcitonin. There is comparatively limited need to measure calcitonin in clinical veterinary medicine due to the low incidence of

calcitonin-secreting neoplasms and metabolic disorders resulting from abnormal levels of calcitonin. Since the sequencing of canine calcitonin, a canine-specific RIA has been developed to measure serum calcitonin in dogs (Hazewinkel, 1991).

Mechanisms of Thyroid C-cell Toxicity

Nodular and/or diffuse hyperplasia of C-cells occurs with advancing age in many strains of laboratory rats and in response to long-term hypercalcemia in certain animal species and human beings. Focal aggregation of C-cells near the thyroid hilus are a normal anatomical finding in the thyroids of dogs and should not be over-interpreted as areas of C-cell hyperplasia. There is suggestive evidence that focal or diffuse hyperplasia precedes the development of C-cell neoplasms (DeLellis *et al.*, 1977, 1979, 1986) (Fig. 21-47). Other studies (Triggs and Williams, 1977) have demonstrated elevated circulating levels of immunoreactive calcitonin in rats with C-cell neoplasms compared to either young or old rats without C-cell tumors. Neither consistent changes in total blood calcium and phosphorus nor bone lesions have been reported in rats with calcitonin-secreting C-cell neoplasms.

Triggs and Williams (1977) reported that radiation (5 or 10 µCi ^{131}I) increased the incidence of C-cell (as well as follicular cell) thyroid tumors in Wistar rats but that high dietary calcium intake (2000 mg/100 g) did not further increase the incidence of C-cell tumors in irradiated rats. Further studies by Thurston and Williams (1982) found that irradiated rats receiving diets high in vitamin D that developed hypercalcemia had a higher incidence of C-cell tumors than rats fed diets adequate or deficient in vitamin D. Stoll *et al.* (1978) reported that the antithyroid drug, thiamazole, can result in proliferative lesions (hyperplasia and adenoma) in thyroid C-cells as well as in follicular cells in rats.

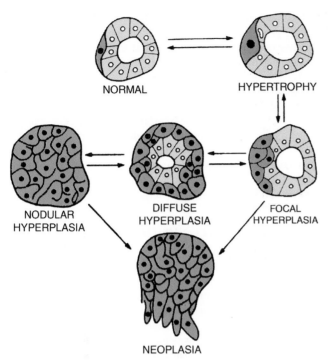

Figure 21-47. Focal and nodular hyperplasia of C-cells in the thyroid often precedes the development of C-cell neoplasms. (From DeLellis et al., 1977).

Thyroid C-cells are known to have receptors for certain gastrointestinal hormones that permit the release of calcitonin from the thyroid gland following a high-calcium meal prior to significant elevations in the blood calcium concentration. The link between the gastrointestinal tract and thyroid C-cells has been demonstrated following pharmacologically induced elevations of the gastrointestinal hormone, gastrin, during treatment with the gastric acid secretion inhibitor, omeprazole (Yeomans, 1994).

Another of the gastrointestinal hormones that can influence thyroid C-cell function glucagon-like peptide-1 (GLP-1), which is being developed for the treatment of diabetes mellitus either as monotherapy or with other glucose-lowering drugs. Glucagon-like peptide-1 is an incretin hormone secreted by L-cells in the lower intestine (Kieffer and Habener, 1999) and is a potent stimulus of insulin biosynthesis and release from beta cells of the pancreas (Drucker *et al.*, 1987; Holz *et al.*, 1993; Bulotta *et al.*, 2002, 2003). Circulating levels of calcitonin can serve as a specific and sensitive biomarker for drugs or chemicals that stimulate thyroid C-cells by a receptor-mediated mechanism. Preclinical studies for pharmacologic agents that altered homeostasis, such as recombinant human PTH 1-34 (Teriparatide, Forteo®), have reported stimulation of thyroid C-cells and an increased incidence of C-cell tumors in rats (FDA, 2005). Not surprisingly, an increased incidence of C-cell tumors was reported in a 2-year rat study with a GLP-1 receptor agonist (Exenatide), the first approved drug in this class for the treatment of type 2 diabetes mellitus (FDA, 2005a). However, C-cells in the thyroids of monkeys and humans have a much lower expression of GLP-1 receptors that would result in a much lower level of C-cell stimulation and calcitonin release in response to a GLP-1 agonist. The C-cell proliferative lesions observed in rats following chronic GLP-1 agonist administration are unlikely to be of relevance to humans.

Morphologic Alterations and Proliferative Lesions of Thyroid C-cells

C-cell proliferative lesions occur commonly in many rat strains but are uncommon in the mouse. Rat strains with high incidences of these lesions include WAG/Rij, Sprague–Dawley, Fisher, Wistar, Buffalo, and Osborne–Mendel. The incidence varies from 19% to 33% with no obvious sex differences. Burek (1978) reported that crossbreeding of high (WAG/Rij) and low (BN/Bi) incidence strains results in F_1 animals with intermediate tumor incidences. As with proliferative lesions of other endocrine organs there is a correlation between the age of the animal and the presence of the entire spectrum of C-cell proliferative lesions. For example, Long–Evans rats under 1 year of age rarely have C-cell neoplasms in the thyroid. Rats which were between 12 and 24 months of age had a 10% incidence whereas approximately 20% of 2- to 3-year-old rats had C-cell tumors. Similarly, the frequency of focal and diffuse C-cell hyperplasia increased progressively with age in this strain of rat. According to the NTP historical database of 2-year-old F344 rats, the incidence of C-cell neoplasms was 8.9% in males and 8.5% in females.

There are two types of C-cell hyperplasia, namely diffuse and focal (nodular) hyperplasia (Fig. 21-47). In diffuse hyperplasia, the numbers of C-cells are increased throughout the thyroid lobe to a point where they may be more numerous than follicular cells. In contrast to the predominantly central distribution of C-cells in thyroids from young rats, C-cells in the more severe forms of hyperplasia extend to the extreme upper and lower poles as well as the peripheral regions of the lobes. Focal (nodular) hyperplasia of C-cells often occurs concurrently with diffuse hyperplasia in the thyroid glands of rats. Follicular cells adjacent to the proliferating C-cells often are compressed and atrophic with prominent supranuclear accumulations of lipofuscin. In the later stages, follicles with intense C-cell hyperplasia often assume irregular, twisted, and elongate configurations. Occasional colloid-filled thyroid follicles are entrapped among the proliferating C-cells.

The histological distinction between focal hyperplasia and adenoma of C-cells is indistinct and somewhat arbitrary. The diagnosis of C-cell hyperplasia refers to a focal or diffuse increase of C-cells between thyroid follicles and/or within the follicular basement membrane. The C-cells appear normal with an abundant, lightly eosinophilic, granular cytoplasm and a round-to-oval nucleus with finely stippled chromatin. In focal C-cell hyperplasia the accumulations of proliferating C-cells are of a lesser diameter than five average colloid-containing thyroid follicles with minimal evidence of compression of adjacent follicles. Hyperplastic C-cells within the follicular basement membrane may compress individual thyroid follicles.

The ultimobranchial body (last, usually fifth, pharyngeal pouch) that delivers the neural crest-derived C-cells to the postnatal thyroid gland fuses with each thyroid lobe at the hilus during embryonic development and distributes C-cells throughout each lobe to varying degrees in different species (Fig. 21-44). In the dog, nodular aggregations of C-cells frequently persist along the course of the major vessels to the thyroid; therefore, C-cell hyperplasia in dogs should be diagnosed only when there is a definite increase in C-cells throughout each thyroid lobe compared to age-matched controls. Both thyroid lobes should be sectioned longitudinally in a consistent manner for microscopic evaluation. This will minimize the prominent regional differences of C-cells in the thyroid glands of normal dogs that can result in the over interpretation of these focal aggregations of C-cells as a significant lesion. There are occasional ultimobranchial-derived, colloid-containing follicles within the focal accumulations of microscopically normal C-cells along the course of vessels within the thyroid lobe or in the connective tissues of the thyroid hilus in dogs.

By comparison C-cell adenomas are discrete, expansive masses of C-cells larger than five average colloid-containing thyroid follicles. Adenomas either are well circumscribed or partially encapsulated from adjacent thyroid follicles that often are compressed to varying degrees. C-cells comprising an adenoma may be subdivided by fine connective tissue septae and capillaries into small neuroendocrine packets. Some C-cell adenomas are composed of larger pleomorphic cells with amphophilic cytoplasm, large nuclei with coarsely clumped chromatin, prominent nucleoli, and bear a histological resemblance to ganglion cells. Occasional amyloid deposits may be found both in nodular hyperplasia and in adenomas.

C-cell carcinomas often result in macroscopic enlargement of one or both thyroid lobes due to the extensive proliferation and infiltration of C-cells. There is evidence of intrathyroidal and/or capsular invasion by the malignant C-cells, often with areas of hemorrhage and necrosis within the neoplasm. The malignant C-cells are more pleomorphic than those comprising benign proliferative lesions. Immunoperoxidase reactions for calcitonin generally are more intense in diffuse or nodular hyperplasia; whereas, in adenomas and carcinomas calcitonin immunoreactivity is much more variable between tumors and in different regions of a tumor. Hyperplastic C-cells adjacent to adenomas and carcinomas usually are intensely positive for calcitonin. In addition to calcitonin, some of the tumor cells and adjacent hyperplastic C-cells have positive staining for somatostatin or bombesin.

Medullary thyroid carcinomas in humans, also commonly known as C-cell carcinomas, arise from calcitonin-secreting C-cells and are associated with inherited syndromes, such as multiple endocrine neoplasia (MEN), in approximately 20–25% of cases (Cho et al., 1999; Sherman, 2003). Medullary carcinomas frequently metastasize via the bloodstream, in addition to lymphatic spread, and are treated with surgical resection and/or external beam radiation. In contrast to follicular origin thyroid tumors, C-cells and tumors arising from them do not have the ability to take up radioactive iodide. The five-year survival rate for medullary thyroid carcinomas is approximately 50%.

Genetic Events in Tumors of Thyroid C-cells

Medullary thyroid carcinomas, or C-cell carcinomas, arise from the calcitonin-secreting parafollicular C-cells of the thyroid gland. These tumors can occur as part of an inherited syndrome, such as multiple endocrine neoplasia (MEN) type 2A or type 2B, or familial medullary thyroid carcinoma (FMTC), which together account for 20–25% of all medullary thyroid carcinomas (Cho et al., 1999; Sherman, 2003; Quayle and Moley, 2005). The ret proto-oncogene, which can undergo rearrangements in papillary carcinoma as previously described, is also important in initiating medullary carcinoma. In medullary carcinoma, the full-length ret proto-oncogene has gain-of-function point mutations involving one of several possible codons (Michiels et al., 1997; Cranston and Ponder, 2003; Quayle and Moley, 2005). As a result, Ret is constitutively active in the neuroendocrine tissues normally expressing this protein, such as thyroid C-cells and neuroendocrine cells of the adrenal medulla. All of the known hereditary forms of medullary carcinoma are autosomal dominant and involve ret mutations. While sporadic medullary

carcinomas comprise more than 75% of cases, little is known about specific genetic mutations initiating this form of thyroid cancer. However, somatic ret point mutations have been identified in up to 50% of sporadic cases (Gimm and Dralle, 1999; Knostman et al., 2007).

Reproduction of the MEN 2A syndrome using CGRP-Ret[C634R] has been quite successful. However, in this model, as well as the Rb[+/−] models, there appears to be a significant contribution of background strain to the development of medullary thyroid carcinomas. In addition, these models develop several extrathyroidal neoplasms common to the MEN 2A syndrome, whereas only the CGRP-v-Ha-ras model mimics the presence of medullary thyroid carcinoma alone, which is the most common form of the disease in humans.

PARATHYROID GLAND

Calcium Metabolism

Calcium plays a key role as an essential structural component of the skeleton and also in many fundamental biological processes. These processes include neuromuscular excitability, membrane permeability, muscle contraction, enzyme activity, hormone release, and blood coagulation, among others. The precise control of calcium in extracellular fluids is vital to health. To maintain a constant concentration of calcium, despite marked variations in intake and excretion, endocrine control mechanisms have evolved that primarily consist of the interactions of three major hormones—parathyroid hormone (PTH), calcitonin (CT), and cholecalciferol (vitamin D) (Fig. 21-48).

Disruption of the normal regulation of calcium balance in animals results in hypercalcemia or hypocalcemia and can lead to metabolic disease and death. Pathological effects associated with abnormal levels of calcium in the body include mineralization of vital organs and other soft tissues, rickets, osteoporosis, and metabolic disorders (Siesjo, 1989).

Approximately 99% of the calcium of the body is present in the inorganic matrix of bone as hydroxyapatite. Most of the remaining calcium is sequestered in the plasma membrane and endoplasmic reticulum of cells. Extracellular fluid contains 0.1% of the body's calcium mass with a total calcium concentration of about 2.5 mmol/L. Extracellular and serum calcium exists in three forms: (1) ionized, (2) complexed to anions such as citrate, bicarbonate, phosphate, or lactate (5% of total calcium), and (3) protein bound (Fig. 21-49). The protein-bound fraction of Ca^{2+} is dependent on the pH of the serum and is principally bound to negatively charged sites on albumin with smaller amounts bound to globulins. As the pH of serum becomes more acidic, the $[Ca^{2+}]$ will increase due to the competition of hydrogen ions $[H^+]$ for binding to the negatively charged sites on serum proteins. Approximately 50% of the extracellular calcium (1.2 mmol/L) is in the ionized form (Ca^{2+}), which is the biologically active form of calcium (Fig. 21-49). The ionized and complexed Ca^{2+} compose the ultrafilterable fraction of Ca^{2+} and represent the fraction that is present in the glomerular filtrate. Neonatal animals have slightly greater concentrations of extracellular calcium compared to adult animals. There is very little calcium in the cytosol, approximately 100 nM, which is predominantly in the ionized form.

Calcium serves two primary functions in the body: (1) structural integrity of bones and teeth, and (2) as a messenger or regulatory ion. There is a 10,000-fold concentration gradient of Ca^{2+} between the extracellular fluid (1.2 mmol/L) and the cytoplasm

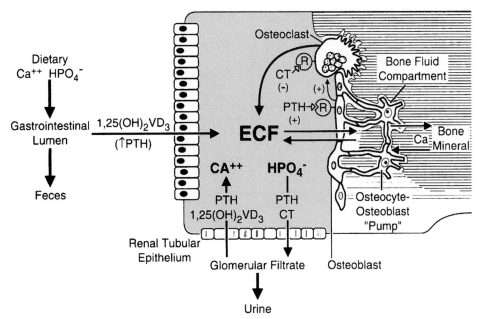

Figure 21-48. Interrelationship of parathyroid hormone (PTH), calcitonin (CT), and 1,25-dihydroxycholecalciferol (1,25(OH)₂VD₃) in the hormonal regulation of calcium (Ca) and phosphorus in extracellular fluids.

Receptors for PTH are on osteoblasts and for CT on osteoclasts in bone. PTH and CT are antagonistic in their action on bone but synergistic in stimulating the renal excretion of phosphorus. Vitamin D exerts its action primarily on the intestine to enhance the absorption of both calcium and phosphorus.

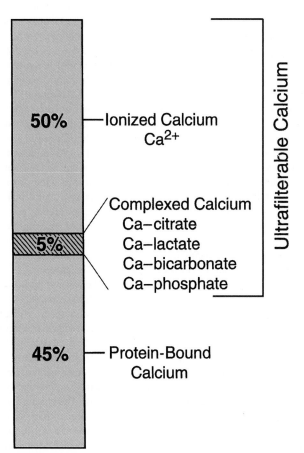

Figure 21-49. Fractions of extracellular calcium (Ca). (From Rosol et al., 1995.)

(100 nM). This gradient permits Ca^{2+} to function as a signaling ion to activate intracellular processes. The lipid bilayer of the cell membrane has a low permeability to Ca^{2+}; therefore, influx of Ca^{2+} into the cytoplasm is controlled by a heterogeneous group of calcium channels regulated by membrane potential, cell membrane receptors, or intracellular secondary messengers. Influx of Ca^{2+} into cells can: (1) regulate cellular function by interactions with intracellular calcium-binding proteins (e.g., calmodulin) and calcium-sensitive protein kinases, and (2) stimulate biologic responses such as neurotransmitter release, contraction, and secretion. Ionized calcium also plays an important role in cell adhesion and blood coagulation. In addition, Ca^{2+} may regulate cellular function by binding to a G-protein-linked Ca^{2+}-sensing receptor in the cell membrane, such as in parathyroid chief cells or renal epithelial cells (Brown *et al.*, 1995).

The kidney normally reabsorbs 98% or more of the filtered calcium. This high degree of reabsorption is an important mechanism to maintain the balance of calcium in the body. If necessary, the kidneys excrete large amounts of calcium in the urine. Ionized and complexed calcium enters the glomerular filtrate by convection and is reabsorbed by the renal tubules. The kidneys reabsorb approximately 40-fold more calcium than is absorbed by the intestinal tract due to the high degree of blood flow and ultrafiltration in the glomerulus. Reduction of glomerular filtration impairs the ability of the kidneys to excrete calcium. About 70% of filtered calcium is reabsorbed in the proximal convoluted tubules by diffusion and convection with water uptake between the epithelial cells. The thick ascending loop of Henle also absorbs about 20% of the filtered calcium, but the precise mechanism is unclear. Much of the calcium reabsorption appears to be passive, but an active component (Rouse and Suki, 1990) may also be present in the distal convoluted tubule, which reabsorbs approximately 10% of the

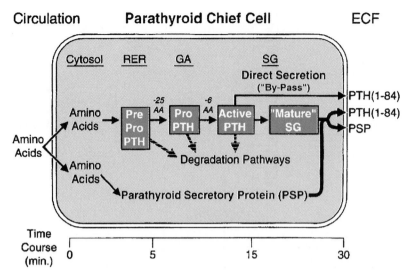

Figure 21-50.   Biosynthesis of parathyroid hormone (PTH) and parathyroid secretory protein (PSP) by parathyroid chief cells.

Active PTH is synthesized as a larger biosynthetic precursor molecule (preproPTH) that undergoes rapid posttranslational processing to proPTH prior to secretion from chief cells as active PTH (amino acids 1–84).

filtered calcium. The principal stimulator of calcium reabsorption in the distal convoluted tubule is parathyroid hormone. Reabsorption of calcium in the distal convoluted tubule is an active transcellular process requiring the presence of calcium channels in the luminal cell membrane, intracellular calcium-binding proteins, such as calbindins, a Ca^{2+}-ATPase, and Na^+/Ca^{2+} exchanger in the basolateral cell membranes. Renal epithelial cells express the Ca^{2+}-sensing receptor on their cell membranes and the distribution of the receptor overlaps with the localization of PTH receptors, so the kidneys may partially autoregulate the renal reabsorption of calcium based on concentration of Ca^{2+} in the blood.

Normal Structure and Function of Chief Cells

Biosynthesis of Parathyroid Hormone   Parathyroid glands are present in all air-breathing vertebrates. Phylogenetically, the parathyroids first appeared in amphibians, coincidentally with the transition of life from an aquatic to a terrestrial environment. It has been suggested that the appearance and development of parathyroid glands may have arisen from the need to protect against the development of hypocalcemia and the necessity to maintain skeletal integrity in terrestrial animals, which often are in a relatively low-calcium, high-phosphorus environment (Capen *et al.*, 1996).

The parathyroid glands in most animal species consist of two pairs of glands, the internal and the external parathyroids, usually situated in the anterior cervical region in close proximity to the thyroid gland. The laboratory rat is an exception to this general rule as they have a single pair of parathyroids closely associated with the thyroid lobes. Embryologically, both parathyroid glands are of entodermal origin. The external parathyroid is derived from the third (III) and the internal parathyroid is derived from the fourth (IV) pharyngeal pouches, in close association with the primordia of the thymus (Capen, 1996c).

Parathyroid chief cells in humans and many animal species store relatively small amounts of preformed hormone but they respond quickly to variations in the need for hormone by changing the rate of hormone synthesis. Parathyroid hormone, like many peptide hormones, is first synthesized as a larger biosynthetic precursor molecule that undergoes posttranslational processing in chief cells. Preproparathyroid hormone (preproPTH) is the initial translation product synthesized on ribosomes of the rough endoplasmic reticulum in chief cells. It is composed of 115 amino acids and contains a hydrophobic signal or leader sequence of 25 amino acid residues that facilitates the penetration and subsequent vectorial discharge of the nascent peptide into the cisternal space of the rough endoplasmic reticulum (Kronenberg *et al.*, 1986) (Fig. 21-50). PreproPTH is rapidly converted within 1 min or less of its synthesis to proparathyroid hormone (ProPTH) by the proteolytic cleavage of 25 amino acids from the NH_2-terminal end of the molecule (Habener, 1981). The intermediate precursor, proPTH, is composed of 90 amino acids and moves within membranous channels of the rough endoplasmic reticulum to the Golgi apparatus (Fig. 21-50). Enzymes within membranes of the Golgi apparatus cleave a hexapeptide from the NH_2-terminal (biologically active) end of the molecule forming active PTH. Active PTH is packaged into membrane-limited, macromolecular aggregates in the Golgi apparatus for subsequent storage in chief cells. Under certain conditions of increased demand (e.g., a low calcium ion concentration in the extracellular fluid compartment), PTH may be released directly from chief cells without being packaged into secretion granules by a process termed *bypass secretion*.

Although the principal form of active PTH secreted from chief cells is a straight chain peptide of 84 amino acids (molecular weight 9500), the molecule is rapidly cleaved into amino- and carboxyterminal fragments in the peripheral circulation and especially in the liver. The purpose of this fragmentation is uncertain because the biologically active amino-terminal fragment is no more active than the entire PTH molecule (amino acids 1–84). The plasma half-life of the N-terminal fragment is considerably shorter than that of the biologically inactive carboxy-terminal fragment of parathyroid hormone. The C-terminal and other portions of the PTH molecule are degraded primarily in the kidney and tend to accumulate with chronic renal disease (Goltzman *et al.*, 1986).

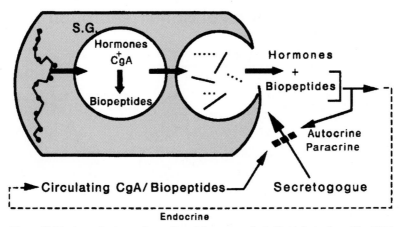

Figure 21-51. Autocrine/paracrine action of chromogranin A (CgA)-derived peptides. PTH and CgA are co-released from chief cells in response to a low calcium ion signal.

Pancreastatin (PST) is a 49 amino acid peptide derived from CgA that exerts local negative feedback on chief cells and decreases PTH secretion from chief cells. (Modified from Cohn *et al*,. 1993).

Control of Parathyroid Hormone Secretion Although secretory cells in the parathyroid gland store small amounts of preformed hormone, they are capable of responding to minor fluctuations in calcium concentration by rapidly altering the rate of hormonal secretion and more slowly by altering the rate of hormonal synthesis. In contrast to most endocrine organs that are under complex controls involving both long and short feedback loops, the parathyroids have a unique feedback controlled by the concentration of calcium (and to a lesser extent magnesium) ion in serum. The concentration of blood phosphorus has no direct regulatory influence on the synthesis and secretion of PTH; however, several disease conditions with hyperphosphatemia in both animals and humans are associated clinically with secondary hyperparathyroidism. An elevated blood phosphorus level may lead indirectly to parathyroid stimulation by virtue of its ability to lower blood calcium, primarily by suppressing the 1α-hydroxylase in the kidney and decreasing the production of the active form of vitamin D [1,25-$(OH)_2$-cholecalciferol], thereby diminishing the rate of intestinal calcium absorption. Magnesium ion has an effect on parathyroid secretion rate similar to that of calcium, but its effect is not equipotent to that of calcium.

The concentration of ionized calcium in serum and extracellular fluid can regulate cellular function by interacting with a recently identified Ca^{2+}-sensing receptor in the plasma membrane of various cells (Brown and Hebert, 1996; Chattopadhyay *et al*., 1996). The cell membrane Ca^{2+} receptor is coupled to G-protein and the 7-transmembrane domain of this receptor is unique because the ligand for the receptor is an ion. The Ca^{2+} receptor plays an important role in the regulation of extracellular Ca^{2+} homeostasis and is present on parathyroid chief cells, thyroid C-cells, renal epithelial cells, brain, and placenta amongst other tissues. The Ca^{2+} receptor is responsible for sensing serum Ca^{2+} concentration and modifying parathyroid hormone secretion, calcitonin secretion, and calcium transport by renal epithelial cells. Mutations in one or both of the Ca^{2+}-sensing receptor genes in humans results in familial hypocalciuric hypercalcemia or neonatal severe hypercalcemia, respectively, due to an inadequate ability to sense the extracellular Ca^{2+} concentration and coordinate the appropriate cellular response.

The serum $[Ca^{2+}]$ that results in half maximal PTH secretion is defined as the serum calcium "set-point" and is stable for an individual animal. The sigmoidal relationship between serum $[Ca^{2+}]$ and PTH secretion permits the chief cells to respond rapidly to a reduction in serum Ca^{2+}. The major inhibitors of PTH synthesis and secretion are increased serum $[Ca^{2+}]$ and 1,25-dihydroxyvitamin D. Inhibition of PTH synthesis by 1,25-dihydroxyvitamin D completes an important endocrine feedback loop between the parathyroid chief cells and the renal epithelial cells because PTH stimulates renal production of 1,25-dihydroxyvitamin D.

Chief cells synthesize and secrete another major protein termed "parathyroid secretory protein (I)" or chromogranin A (CG-A). It is a higher molecular weight molecule (70 kD) composed of 430–448 amino acids that is co-stored and secreted with PTH. A similar molecule has been found in secretory granules of a wide variety of peptide hormone-secreting cells and in neurotransmitter secretory vesicles (Doss *et al*., 1998). An internal region of the parathyroid secretory protein or chromogranin A molecule is identical in sequence to pancreastatin, a C-terminal amidated peptide, that inhibits glucose-stimulated insulin secretion. This 49 amino acid proteolytic cleavage product (amino acids number 240–280) of parathyroid secretory protein has been reported to inhibit low calcium-stimulated secretion of parathyroid hormone and chromogranin A from parathyroid cells. These findings suggest that chromogranin A-derived peptides may act locally in an autocrine manner to inhibit the secretion of active hormone by endocrine cells, such as chief cells of the parathyroid gland (Fasciotto *et al*., 1990; Barbosa *et al*., 1991; Cohn *et al*., 1993) (Fig. 21-51).

Although the functions of CGA are still under investigation, several roles have been postulated. Chromogranin A is suspected to play an important role in the maturation of secretory granules. Inside the Golgi apparatus, CGA is involved in the packaging of the contents of newly formed vesicles. Chromogranin A precipitates as it diffuses into the trans-Golgi network and secretory products such as parathyroid hormone become entrapped in the growing CGA conglomerate and are subsequently packaged into secretory granules. Chromogranin A has a large calcium-binding capacity which may enhance the stability of secretory vesicles. As granules mature, they accumulate up to 40 mM of calcium, which also may serve as a route of Ca^{2+} secretion. Chromogranin A-calcium complexes are important in maintaining the integrity of the secretory granules.

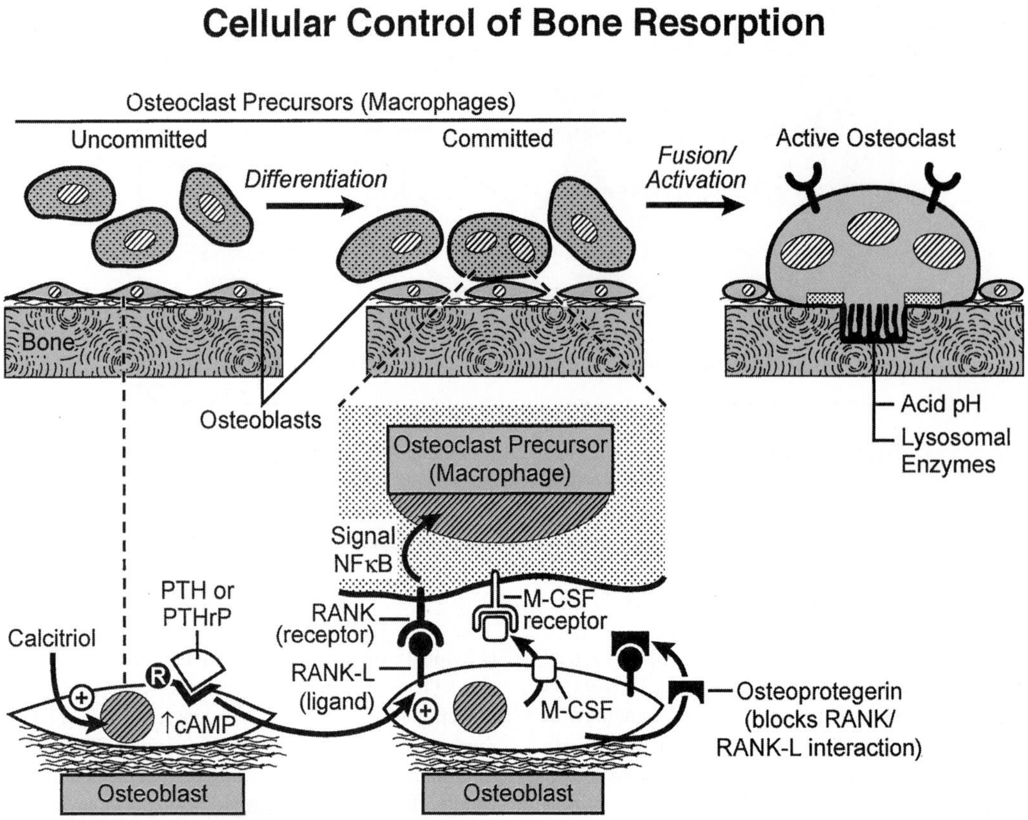

Cellular Control of Bone Resorption

Figure 21-52. Cellular control of bone resorption.

Specific receptors for parathyroid hormone (PTH and PTH-rP) are present on osteoblasts but not on osteoclasts. RANK L is a membrane-bound protein on osteoblasts that stimulates differentiation of cells of the osteoclast lineage. Expression of RANK L in osteoblasts is upregulated by osteotrophic factors such as PTH, calcitriol, and interleukin 11. M-CSF, macrophage colony-stimulating factor; PTH-rP, parathyroid hormone-related peptide; R, receptor for PTH or PTH-rP; R, receptor; and RANK L, receptor activator NF-κB ligand. (From Capen, 2004).

The absence of calcium causes dissociation of protein complexes and results in osmotic lysis of the vesicle.

The intragranular functions of CGA include hormone packaging, stabilization of the granule against osmotic gradients, and the excretion of intracellular calcium. During the process of secretion, the contents of secretory granules are extruded into the pericapillary space. The pH and calcium concentration of the extracellular fluid promote the dissociation of CGA complexes and solubilization of bound calcium and other contents of the granule. Once solubilized, extracellular peptidases cleave CGA into biologically active peptides, which act as paracrine or autocrine regulators of endocrine secretion (Deftos, 1991).

Biologic Effects of Parathyroid Hormone Parathyroid hormone is the principal hormone involved in the minute-to-minute, fine regulation of blood calcium in mammals. It exerts its biologic actions by directly influencing the function of target cells, primarily in the bone and kidney, and secondarily in the intestine to maintain plasma calcium at a level sufficient to ensure the optimal functioning of a wide variety of body cells. In general, the most important biologic effects of PTH are to: (1) elevate the blood concentration of calcium, (2) decrease the blood concentration of phosphorus, (3) increase the urinary excretion of phosphorus by a decreased rate of tubular reabsorption, (4) increase the renal tubular reabsorption of calcium, (5) increase the rate of skeletal remodeling and the net rate of bone resorption, (6) increase the numbers of osteoclasts on bone surfaces and the rate of osteolysis, (7) increase the urinary excretion of hydroxyproline, (8) activate adenylate cyclase in target cells, and (9) accelerate the formation of the principal active vitamin D metabolite (1,25-dihydroxycholecalciferol; 1,25-dihydroxy vitamin D) through a trophic effect of PTH on the 1α-hydroxylase in mitochondria on the epithelial cells lining the proximal convoluted tubules of the kidney.

Parathyroid hormone mobilizes calcium from skeletal reserves into the extracellular fluids. The response of bone to parathyroid hormone is biphasic. The immediate effects are the result of increasing the activity of existing osteocytes and osteoclasts. This rapid effect of PTH depends upon the continuous presence of hormone and results in an increased flow of calcium to the bone surface through the coordinated action of osteocytes and activation of endosteal lining cells (inactive osteoblasts). The later effects of parathyroid hormone on bone are of a greater magnitude of response and are not dependent upon the continuous presence of PTH. Osteoclasts are primarily responsible for the long-term actions of PTH on increasing bone resorption and overall bone remodeling. This is particularly interesting, in light of studies which have demonstrated the presence of receptors for PTH on osteoblasts but not on osteoclasts (Fig. 21-48).

Recombinant human PTH (1–34), the 34 amino acid N-terminal portion of the natural hormone, has been developed as a new treatment for osteoporosis. Teriparatide (Forteo®) administered by once-daily subcutaneous injection stimulated new bone formation by activating quiescent bone-lining cells, by stimulating osteoblast differentiation from precursor cells, and by inhibiting osteoblast apoptosis (Hock, 2001). This anabolic effect of PTH was distinct from its well-known catabolic effects on the skeleton through the activation of osteoclasts and increased bone resorption associated with chronic elevations of hormone in humans and animals from renal disease or nutritional imbalances. Teriparatide stimulates mineral apposition into trabecular, endocortical, and periosteal bone surfaces in rats, monkeys, and humans resulting in substantial increases in bone mass, improved architecture, and enhanced biomechanical strength (Sato *et al.*, 1997; Jerome *et al.*, 1999; Jiang *et al.*, 2003; Zanchetta *et al.*, 2003).

A 2-year rat carcinogenicity study reported that once-daily subcutaneous administration of Teriparatide resulted in large, dose-dependent increases in bone mass, as well as bone proliferative lesions, including osteosarcoma at all dose levels tested (Sato *et al.*, 2002; Vhale *et al.*, 2002). This study had several design features that differ from the intended short-term use of Teriparatide, making relevance of the rat findings difficult to assess in terms of safety for humans (Tashjian and Chabner, 2002). Rats were treated once daily for 24 months starting at approximately 2 months of age at initiation of treatment. The rats were treated for nearly their entire lifespan (70–80% of lifetime) and during the rapid phase of longitudinal skeletal growth (Vhale *et al.*, 2002). The intended clinical use of Teriparatide is up to 2 years of therapy in older patients with a mature skeleton, which corresponds to approximately 2–3% of the human lifespan.

A long-term study subsequently was conducted in female F344 rats to determine the relative importance of dose, treatment duration, and age at initiation of treatment on the incidence of bone proliferative lesions induced by Teriparatide (Vhale *et al.*, 2004). Treatment groups consisted of different combinations of dose (0, 5, or 30 μg/kg/day), treatment duration (6, 20, or 24 months) and age at initiation of treatment (2 or 6 months of age). Significant increases in the incidence of bone tumors (osteoma, osteoblastoma, and osteosarcoma) appeared in rats treated with 30 μg/kg for 20 or 24 months. No neoplasms were found when rats were administered 5 μg/kg at 6 months of age and continued for either 6 or 20 months (up to 70% of lifespan). These results demonstrated that treatment duration and administered dose are important factors in the induction of bone tumors in rats by Teriparatide (Vhale *et al.*, 2004; Sato *et al.*, 2002).

Bone resorption is a complex, multistep process that involves the activation of multiple genes and the action of multiple hormones (Teitelbaum, 2000). Most hormones and cytokines that are involved in the regulation of bone resorption (e.g., parathyroid hormone, calcitriol, interleukin-1 beta, tumor necrosis factor [TNF], interleukin-6, and prostaglandin E_2) act via receptors on osteoblasts. Three new family members of the TNF ligand and receptor signaling system have been identified and cloned recently that play a critical role in the regulation of bone resorption (Hofbauer, 1999; American Society for Bone and Mineral Research [ASBMR] Special Committee on Nomenclature, 2000; Hofbauer *et al.*, 2000). In the presence of permissive concentrations of macrophage colony-stimulating factor (M-CSF), the new TNF superfamily molecules constitute the common pathway for regulation of osteoclast formation and function by cells of the osteoblast lineage, thereby, mediating the biologic effects of many upstream hormones and cytokines (Suda *et al.*, 1999).

Control of Osteoclast Function by Products of Osteoblast Cell Lineage

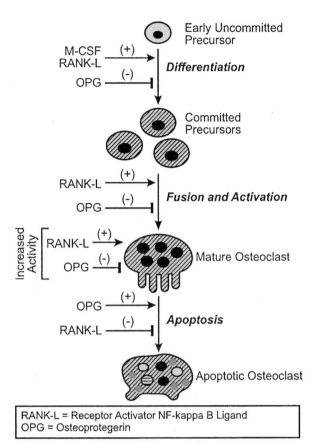

RANK-L = Receptor Activator NF-kappa B Ligand
OPG = Osteoprotegerin

Modified from Hofbauer et al. J.B.M.R. 15,2000

Figure 21-53. *Control of osteoclast functions by products of osteoblast cell lineage.*

Note that all steps of osteoclast formation and function are regulated by the OPG-L/OPG ratio, including initiation of differentiation, fusion of preosteoclasts to form active mature osteoclasts, regulation of osteoclast function, and osteoclast apoptosis. M-CSF is required only for the initiation of differentiation by uncommitted osteoclast precursors in bone marrow. M-CSF, macrophage colony-stimulating factor; OCIF, osteoclastogenesis inhibitory factor; ODF, osteoclast differentiation factor; OPG, osteoprotegerin; OPG L, osteoprotegerin ligand; and RANK L, receptor activator NF-κB ligand. (Modified and redrawn from Hofbauer *et al.*, 2000.)

RANK, RANK Ligand and Osteoprotegerin   The receptor ligand (RANK ligand or RANK L) is a membrane-bound protein on osteoblasts that serves as a common mediator for osteoclastic bone resorption (Takahashi *et al.*, 1999; Martin and Gillespie, 2001). This ligand (initially termed osteoclast differentiation factor [ODF]) and osteoprotegrin ligand [OPG L] is produced by osteoblast lineage cells and stimulates differentiation of cells of the osteoclast lineage, enhances the functional activity of mature osteoclasts, and prolongs osteoclast life by inhibiting apoptosis (ASBMR Special Committee on Nomenclature 2000; Hock *et al.*, 2001) (Figs. 21-52 and 21-53). Targeted deletion of the receptor ligand in mice leads to osteopetrosis, shortened bones, impaired tooth eruption, and immunologic abnormalities. Expression of RANK L in osteoblasts/stromal cells

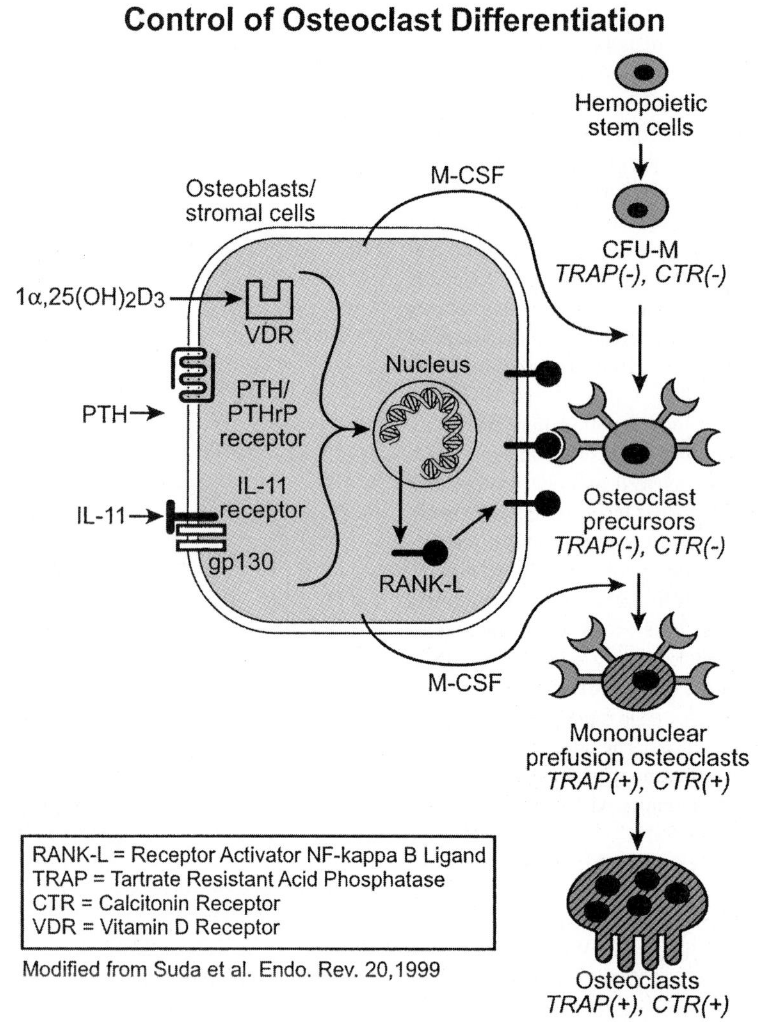

Control of Osteoclast Differentiation

RANK-L = Receptor Activator NF-kappa B Ligand
TRAP = Tartrate Resistant Acid Phosphatase
CTR = Calcitonin Receptor
VDR = Vitamin D Receptor

Modified from Suda et al. Endo. Rev. 20,1999

Figure 21-54. Concept of osteoclast differentiation.

Osteotropic factors such as $1\alpha,25(OH)_2D_3$ (dihydroxycholecalciferol), parathyroid hormone (PTH), and interleukin-11 (IL-11) stimulate osteoclast formation in co-cultures of osteoblasts/stromal cells and hemopoietic cells. Target cells for these factors are osteoblasts/stromal cells. Three different signaling pathways mediated by the vitamin D receptor (VDR), PTH/PTH-rP receptor, and gp130 similarly induce osteoclast differentiation factor (ODF) or stromal osteoclast-forming activity (SOFA) as a membrane-associated factor in osteoblasts/stromal cells. Osteoclast progenitors of the monocyte–macrophage lineage recognize ODF/SOFA in osteoblasts/stromal cells through cell-to-cell interaction and then differentiate into osteoclasts. Macrophage colony-stimulating factor (M-CSF) produced by osteoblasts/stromal cells is a prerequisite for both proliferation and differentiation of osteoclast progenitors. CFU-M, colony-forming unit-megakaryocyte; CTR, calcitonin receptor; PTH-rP, parathyroid hormone-related peptide; RANK L, receptor activator NF-κB ligand; and TRAP, tartrate-resistant acid phosphatase. (Modified and redrawn from Suda *et al.*, 1999.)

is upregulated by osteotrophic factors such as calcitriol, PTH, and interleukin-11 (Suda *et al.*, 1999). This molecule is identical to TNF-related activation-induced cytokine (TRANCE) or receptor activator of NF-kappa B ligand (RANK L) reported to stimulate T-cell growth and dendritic cell function in the immunology literature (ASBMR Special Committee on Nomenclature, 2000).

The membrane receptor (RANK) for the ligand (RANK L) on cells of the osteoclast lineage is identical with a receptor of similar name identified previously on immune cells (Suda *et al.*, 1999; ASBMR Special Committee on Nomenclature, 2000) (Fig. 21-51).

The receptor also has been referred to in the literature as osteoclast differentiation and activation receptor [ODAR]. Binding of the ligand to this receptor activates signaling pathways in osteoclasts that lead to increased functional activity. Osteoclast precursors express RANK, recognize RANK L through cell-to-cell interaction with osteoblasts/stromal cells, and differentiate into prefusion osteoclasts in the presence of M-CSF. Mice made deficient in RANK by targeted deletion of the gene develop severe osteopetrosis due to decreased osteoclast function and fail to develop peripheral lymph nodes (ASBMR Special Committee on Nomenclature, 2000).

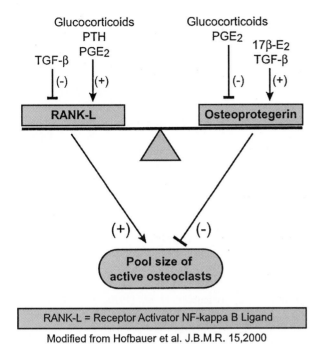

RANK-L = Receptor Activator NF-kappa B Ligand

Modified from Hofbauer et al. J.B.M.R. 15,2000

Figure 21-55.   Regulation of osteoclast functions by cytokines.

The convergence hypothesis proposes two levels of regulation of osteoclast funtions. A variety of upstream cytokines and hormones alter the pool size of active osteoclasts by converging at the level of OPG L/ODF and OPG/OCIF. These two downstream factors serve as the final effectors for osteoclastogenesis and also affect osteoclast activation and osteoclast apoptosis. At steady state, there is a balance of levels of OPG L/ODF and OPG/OCIF that maintain a pool size of active osteoclasts that supports normal levels of bone resorption. When a change in one or more upstream factors tilts the balance toward a functional excess of OPG L/ODF, the pool size decreases. 17β-E2, 17β-estradiol; PGE_2, prostaglandin E_2; PTH, parathyroid hormone; RANK-L, receptor activator of NF-κB ligand; and TGF-β, transforming growth factor β. (Modified and redrawn from Hofbauer *et al.*, 2000.)

Osteoprotegerin (OPG) ("decoy receptor") is a novel member of the TNF receptor superfamily produced by cells of the osteoblast lineage/stromal cells and a negative regulator of bone resorption (Hofbauer, 1999; Hofbauer *et al.*, 2000) (Figs. 21-52 and 21-53). When this soluble decoy receptor binds to the ligand (RANK L) it prevents the ligand from binding to its biological membrane receptor (RANK) thereby resulting in its inactivation. Overexpression of this decoy receptor in transgenic mice leads to osteopetrosis associated with decreased osteoclast formation and function. In contrast, targeted gene ablation in mice results in severe osteoporosis and arterial mineralization (ASBMR Special Committee on Nomenclature, 2000).

These recent findings clearly indicate that microenvironment in bone marrow provided by osteoblast lineage/stromal cells regulate osteoclast differentiation and function. Osteoclast formation appears to be determined by the ratio of RANK L:OPG, and alterations in this ratio may be a major cause of bone loss in certain metabolic disorders such as estrogen-deficiency and glucocorticoid-excess (Hofbauer *et al.*, 2000; Rodan and Martin, 2000) (Figs. 21-54 and 21-55). A long-term increase in the secretion of PTH also may result in the formation of greater numbers of osteoblasts and an increase in bone formation and resorption. However, because bone resorption by osteoclasts usually is greater than bone formation by osteoblasts, there is a net negative balance in skeletal mass.

The initial binding of PTH to osteoblasts lining bone surfaces causes the cells to contract, thereby exposing the underlying mineral to osteoclasts (Fig. 21-48). If the increase in PTH is sustained, the size of the active osteoclast pool in bone is increased by the activation of progenitor cells of the osteoclastic lineage. The plasma membrane of osteoclasts in intimate contact with the resorbing bone surface is modified to form a series of membranous projections referred to as the brush "ruffled" border. This area of active bone resorption is isolated from the extracellular fluids by adjacent transitional "sealing" zones, thereby localizing the lysosomal enzymes and acidic environment to the immediate area undergoing dissolution. The mineral and organic components such as hydroxyproline released from bone are phagocytized by osteoclasts and transported across the cell in transport vesicles to be released into the extracellular fluid compartment.

Parathyroid hormone also has a direct and rapid effect on renal tubular function. About 5–10 minutes after PTH administration, the reabsorption of phosphate is decreased, causing phosphaturia. The site of action of PTH on the tubular reabsorption of phosphate has been localized by micropuncture methods to the proximal convoluted tubule of the nephron. In addition, PTH leads to the increased urinary excretion of potassium, sodium bicarbonate, cyclic adenosine monophosphate, and amino acids. Although the effect of PTH on the tubular reabsorption of phosphate has been considered to be of importance, the capability of PTH to enhance the renal reabsorption of calcium is of more importance in the maintenance of calcium homeostasis. This effect of PTH upon tubular reabsorption of calcium appears to be due to a direct action on cells of the distal convoluted tubule of the kidney nephron. The other important effect of PTH on the kidney is the regulation of the conversion of 25-hydroxycholecalciferol to 1,25-dihydroxycholecalciferol and other metabolites of vitamin D.

Assay of Parathyroid Hormone

Under normal conditions, PTH is secreted continuously from chief cells. Biologically active parathyroid hormone is a linear peptide chain of 84 amino acids which is cleaved in the liver and possibly elsewhere, an amino-terminal fragment comprising approximately one-third of the PTH molecule, and a larger carboxy-terminal fragment which is biologically inactive. Parathyroid hormone is secreted in two forms by chief cells: *first*, an intact PTH peptide comprising amino acids 1 through 84 (PTH 1-84) and *second*, a C-terminal peptide (PTH 35–84). Intact PTH (1–84) is the principal circulating biologically active form of PTH, has a half-life of less than 5 minutes, and is rapidly removed from the circulation by endopeptidases in hepatic Kupffer cell membranes or by glomerular filtration (Arnaud and Pun, 1992). Some C-terminal peptide is released into the circulation by Kupffer cells and is then cleared by the kidney. The kidney is a major organ for the degradation of PTH. As a result the C-terminal PTH fragment has a biological half-life that is longer than that of intact PTH (1–84) and is present in the serum in higher concentrations (50–90% of total PTH), especially in cases of hyperparathyroidism associated with chronic renal disease.

The multiple forms of PTH and PTH fragments in the circulation made the development of specific and sensitive radioimmunoassays (RIAs) for this hormone difficult. Early assays for PTH were single-site radioimmunoassays for C-terminal peptides. These assays were suboptimal because both the biologically active and inactive forms of PTH were quantified; nevertheless, the assay was clinically useful to diagnose and monitor hyperparathyroidism in patients with normal renal function. Mid-region and C-terminal RIAs measure both intact PTH (active) and C-terminal PTH (inactive) which renders them less clinically relevant. In addition, conditions that reduce the glomerular filtration rate, such as renal failure, result in a large increase in the serum concentration of C-terminal PTH. Concentrations of intact PTH in the serum of animals are best measured by a two-site immunoradiometric assay (IRMA).

Xenobiotic Chemical-Induced Toxic Injury of Parathyroids

Ozone Inhalation of a single dose of ozone (0.75 ppm) for 4–8 hours has been reported to produce light and electron microscopic changes in parathyroid glands (Atwal and Wilson, 1974). Subsequent studies have utilized longer (48-hours) exposure to ozone in order to define the pathogenesis of the parathyroid lesions (Atwal et al., 1975; Atwal, 1979). Initially (1–5 days post-ozone exposure), many chief cells undergo compensatory hypertrophy and hyperplasia with areas of capillary endothelial cell proliferation, interstitial edema, degeneration of vascular endothelium, formation of platelet thrombi, leukocyte infiltration of the walls of larger vessels in the gland, and disruption of basement membranes. Chief cells had prominent Golgi complexes and endoplasmic reticulum, aggregations of free ribosomes, and swelling of mitochondria (Atwal and Pemsingh, 1981).

Inactive chief cells with few secretory granules predominate in the parathyroids in the later stages of exposure to ozone. There was evidence of parathyroid atrophy from 12 to 20 days post-ozone exposure with mononuclear cell infiltration and necrosis of chief cells. The reduced cytoplasmic area contained vacuolated endoplasmic reticulum, a small Golgi apparatus, and numerous lysosomal bodies. Plasma membranes of adjacent chief cells were disrupted resulting in coalescence of the cytoplasmic area. Fibroblasts with associated collagen bundles were prominent in the interstitium and the basal lamina of the numerous capillaries often was duplicated.

The parathyroid lesions in ozone-exposed animals are similar to isoimmune parathyroiditis in other species (Lupulescu et al., 1968). Antibody against parathyroid tissue was localized near the periphery of chief cells by indirect immunofluorescence, especially 14 days following ozone injury (Atwal et al., 1975).

Aluminum Evidence for a direct effect of aluminum on the parathyroid was suggested from studies of patients with chronic renal failure treated by hemodialysis with aluminum-containing fluids or orally administered drugs containing aluminum. These patients often had normal or minimal elevations of immunoreactive parathyroid hormone (iPTH), little histological evidence of osteitis fibrosa in bone, and a depressed response by the parathyroid gland to acute hypocalcemia (Bourdeau et al., 1987). Studies by Morrissey et al. (1983) have reported that an increase in aluminum concentration in vitro over a range of 0.5–2.0 mM in a low calcium medium (0.5 mM) progressively inhibited the secretion of PTH. At 2.0 mM aluminum, PTH secretion was inhibited by 68% while high calcium-containing medium (2.0 mM) without aluminum maximally inhibited PTH secretion only 39%. The inhibition of PTH secretion by aluminum does not appear to be related to an irreversible toxic effect because normal secretion was restored when parathyroid cells were returned to 0.5 mM calcium medium without aluminum. The incorporation of [^{3}H] leucine into total cell protein, parathyroid secretory protein, proparathyroid hormone, or PTH was not affected

by aluminum; however, the secretion of radiolabeled protein by dispersed parathyroid cells was inhibited by aluminum (Morrissey et al., 1983).

The molecular mechanism by which aluminum inhibits PTH secretion, reducing diglyceride levels in chief cells (Morrissey and Slatopolsky, 1986), appears to be similar to that of the calcium ion. Aluminum appears to decrease diglyceride synthesis, which is reflected in a corresponding decrease in synthesis of phosphatidylcholine and possible triglyceride; however, phosphatidylinositol synthesis was not affected by aluminum.

Calcium regulates PTH gene expression by a post-transcriptional mechanism plus parathyroid gland growth through activation of the calcium-sensory receptor. Aluminum impairs parathyroid function through a calcium-like mechanism due to a lack of specificity of the calcium-sensing receptor. In addition, aluminum decreases parathyroid calcium-sensing receptor mRNA levels and the regulatory mechanism was post-transcriptional (González-Suárez et al., 2005).

L-Asparaginase Tettenborn et al. (1970) and Chisari et al. (1972) reported that rabbits administered L-asparaginase develop severe hypocalcemia and tetany characterized by muscle tremors, opisthotonos, carpopedal spasms, paralysis, and coma. This drug was of interest in cancer chemotherapy because of the beneficial effects of guinea pig serum against lymphosarcoma in mice.

Parathyroid chief cells appeared to be selectively destroyed by L-asparaginase (Young et al., 1973). Chief cells were predominately inactive and degranulated, with large autophagic vacuoles present in the cytoplasm of degenerating cells. Cytoplasmic organelles concerned with synthesis and packaging of secretory products were poorly developed in chief cells. Rabbits developed hyperphosphatemia, hypomagnesemia, hyperkalemia, and azotemia in addition to acute hypocalcemia. Rabbits with clinical hypocalcemic tetany did not recover spontaneously; however, administration of parathyroid extract prior to or during treatment with L-asparaginase decreased the incidence of hypocalcemic tetany.

The development of hypocalcemia and tetany have not been observed in other experimental animals administered L-asparaginase (Oettgen et al., 1970). However, this response may not be limited to the rabbit because some human patients receiving the drug also have developed hypocalcemia (Jaffe et al., 1972). The L-asparaginase-induced hypoparathyroidism in rabbits is a valuable model for investigating drug-endocrine cell interactions, somewhat analogous to the selective destruction of pancreatic beta cells by alloxan with production of experimental diabetes mellitus.

Proliferative Lesions of Parathyroid Chief Cells

Chief Cell Tumors Parathyroid adenomas in adult-aged rats vary in size from microscopic to unilateral nodules several millimeters in diameter, located in the cervical region by the thyroids or infrequently in the thoracic cavity near the base of the heart. Parathyroid neoplasms in the precardiac mediastinum are derived from ectopic parathyroid tissue displaced into the thorax with the expanding thymus during embryonic development. Tumors of parathyroid chief cells do not appear to be a sequela of long-standing secondary hyperparathyroidism of either renal or nutritional origin (Capen, 1997b). The unaffected parathyroid glands may be atrophic if the adenoma is functional, normal if the adenoma is nonfunctional, or enlarged if there is concomitant hyperplasia. In functional adenomas the normal mechanism by which PTH secretion is regulated, changes in the concentration of blood calcium ion, is lost and hormone secretion is excessive in spite of an increased level of blood calcium.

Adenomas are solitary nodules that are sharply demarcated from adjacent parathyroid parenchyma. Because the adenoma compresses the rim of surrounding parathyroid to varying degrees depending upon its size, there may be a partial fibrous capsule, resulting either from compression of existing stroma or from proliferation of fibrous connective tissue.

Adenomas are usually nonfunctional (endocrinologically inactive) in adult-aged rats from chronic toxicity/carcinogenicity studies (Capen, 1997b; Arnold et al., 2003). Chief cells in nonfunctional adenomas are cuboidal or polyhedral and arranged either in a diffuse sheet, lobules, or acini with or without lumens. Chief cells from functional adenomas often are closely packed into small groups by fine connective tissue septae. The cytoplasmic area varies from normal size to an expanded area. There is a much lower density of cells in functional parathyroid adenoma compared to the adjacent rim with atrophic chief cells.

Larger parathyroid adenomas, such as those that are detected macroscopically, often nearly incorporate the entire affected gland. A narrow rim of compressed parenchyma may be detected at one side of the gland or the affected parathyroid may be completely incorporated by the adenoma. Chief cells in this rim often are compressed and atrophic due to pressure and the persistent hypercalcemia. Peripherally situated follicles in the adjacent thyroid lobe may be compressed to a limited extent by larger parathyroid adenomas. The parathyroid glands that do not contain a functional adenoma also undergo trophic atrophy in response to the hypercalcemia and become smaller.

Influence of Age on Development of Parathyroid Tumors   There are relatively few chemicals or experimental manipulations reported in the literature that increase the incidence of parathyroid tumors. Long-standing renal failure with intense diffuse hyperplasia does not appear to increase the development of chief cell tumors in rats. The historical incidence of parathyroid adenomas in untreated control male F344 rats in studies conducted by the NTP was 4/1315 (0.3%), and for female F344 rats it was 2/1330 (0.15%). However, parathyroid adenomas are an example of a neoplasm in F344 rats whose incidence increases dramatically when life span data are compared to 2-year studies. Solleveld et al. (1984) reported that the incidence of parathyroid adenomas increased in males from 0.1% at 2 years to 3.1% in lifetime studies. Corresponding data for female F344 rats was 0.1% at 2 years and 0.6% in lifetime studies.

Influence of Gonadectomy   Oslapas et al. (1982) reported an increased incidence of parathyroid adenomas in female (34%) and male (27%) rats of the Long–Evans strain administered 40 μCi sodium ^{131}I and saline at 8 weeks of age. There were no significant changes in serum calcium, phosphorus, and parathyroid hormone compared to controls. Gonadectomy performed at 7 weeks of age decreased the incidence of parathyroid adenomas in irradiated rats (7.4% in gonadectomy vs. 27% in intact controls) but there was little change in the incidence of parathyroid adenomas in irradiated females. X-irradiation of the thyroid–parathyroid region also increased the incidence of parathyroid adenomas. When female Sprague–Dawley rats received a single absorbed dose of X-rays at 4 weeks of age, they subsequently developed a 24% incidence of parathyroid adenomas after 14 months (Oslapas et al., 1981).

Influence of Xenobiotic Chemicals   Parathyroid adenomas have been encountered infrequently following the administration of a variety of chemicals in 2-year bioassay studies (Capen, 1997a,b). In a study with the pesticide Rotenone in F344 rats, there appeared to be an increased incidence of parathyroid adenomas in high-dose (75 ppm) males (4 of 44 rats) compared to either low-dose (38 ppm) males, control males (1 of 44 rats), or NTP historical controls (0.3%) (Abdo et al., 1988). It was uncertain whether the increased incidence of this uncommon tumor was a direct effect of Rotenone feeding or the increased survival in high-dose males. Chief cell hyperplasia was not present in parathyroids that developed adenomas.

Influence of Irradiation and Hypercalcemia Induced by Vitamin D   Wynford-Thomas et al. (1982) reported that irradiation significantly increases the incidence of parathyroid adenomas in inbred Wistar albino rats and that the incidence could be modified by feeding diets with variable amounts of vitamin D. Neonatal Wistar rats were given either 5 or 10 μCi radioiodine (^{131}I) within 24 h of birth. In rats 12 months of age and older, parathyroid adenomas were found in 33% of rats administered 5 μCi ^{131}I and in 37% of rats given 10 μCi ^{131}I compared to 0% in unirradiated controls. The incidence of parathyroid adenomas was highest (55%) in normocalcemic rats fed a low vitamin D diet and lowest (20%) in irradiated rats fed a high vitamin D diet (40,000 IU/kg) that had a significant elevation in plasma calcium.

Age-Related Changes in Parathyroid Function

Serum immunoreactive parathyroid hormone (iPTH) (as well as calcitonin [iCT]) have been reported to be different in young compared to aged Fischer 344 (F344) rats; however, the serum calcium concentration does not change with age (Wongsurawat and Armbrecht, 1987). This suggests that the regulation of iPTH (and iCT) secretion may be affected by the process of aging. The decreased responsiveness of chief cells to calcium may be due to age-related changes in the regulation of the secretory pathway. This could include age-related changes in the effect of calcium on release of stored PTH, intracellular degradation of PTH, or modification of adenylate cyclase activity as observed in other tissues that utilize calcium as an intermediary signal (Brown, 1982). Therefore, the sensitivity of parathyroid chief cells to circulating calcium ion concentration appears not to be fixed but may change during development, aging, and in response to certain disease processes.

The increased secretion of iPTH with advancing age in rats could be due to several factors (Capen, 1994): *first*, an increased number of parathyroid secretory cells with age or *second*, an altered regulation of chief cells in response to calcium ion associated with the process of aging. For example, a decreased sensitivity of chief cells to negative feedback by calcium ion could result in the higher blood levels of iPTH in aged F344 rats. Wada et al. (1992) reported that the early age-related rise in plasma PTH in F344 rats was neither a consequence of low plasma calcium nor of renal insufficiency. Age-related changes in the responsiveness of chief cells to circulating levels of other factors which modulate iPTH secretion, particularly 1,25-dihydroxycholecalciferol and alpha and beta adrenergic catecholamines, also could contribute to the variations in blood levels of iPTH in rats of different ages. In addition, target cell responsiveness to PTH also decreases with advancing age in rats. PTH does not increase the renal production of 1,25-dihydroxyvitamin D in adult (13-month-old) male F344 rats compared to young (2-month-old) rats where its production

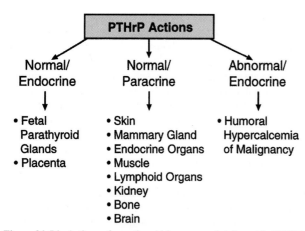

Figure 21-56. Actions of parathyroid hormone-related protein (PTHrP) under normal and abnormal conditions. (From Rosol and Capen, 1997.)

was increased 61% (Armbrecht *et al.*, 1982). Older rats have a decreased calcemic response and decreased renal production of 1,25-dihydroxycholecalciferol compared to young rats (Armbrecht *et al.*, 1982; Kalu *et al.*, 1982).

Parathyroid Hormone-Related Protein (PTHrP)

Relationship to Parathyroid Hormone   Parathyroid hormone-related protein (PTHrP) was first identified in 1982 as an important PTH-like factor that plays a central role in the pathogenesis of cancer-associated hypercalcemia (humoral hypercalcemia of malignancy). PTHrP is a 139, 141, or 173 amino acid peptide, originally isolated from human and animal tumors associated with humoral hypercalcemia of malignancy (Gröne *et al.*, 1997). Humoral hypercalcemia of malignancy (HHM) (pseudohyperparathyroidism) is a syndrome associated with diverse malignant neoplasms in animal and human patients (Rosol and Capen, 1992, 1997, 2000). Characteristic clinical findings in patients with HHM include hypercalcemia, hypophosphatemia, hypercalciuria (often with decreased fractional calcium excretion), increased fractional excretion of phosphorus, increased nephrogenous cAMP, and increased osteoclastic bone resorption. Hypercalcemia is induced by humoral effects on bone, kidney, and possibly the intestine. The PTHrP peptide shares 70% sequence homology with the first 13 amino acids of intact PTH. The N-terminal region of PTHrP (amino acids 1–34) binds to and activates PTH receptors in bone and kidney cells with equal affinity as PTH. However, PTHrP is not strictly a calcium-regulating hormone and it has been determined that PTHrP is widely produced in the body and acts as a paracrine factor in the tissues in which it is produced (Fig. 21-56).

Role in the Fetus   The fetus maintains higher concentrations of serum calcium compared to the dam (Care, 1991). Because the fetal parathyroid glands produce low levels of PTH, the mechanism of maintaining increased serum concentrations of calcium was unknown until the finding that PTHrP maintains calcium balance in the fetus (Care, 1991) and is the major hormone secreted by the chief cells of the fetal parathyroid glands. The PTHrP produced by the placenta also stimulates the uptake of calcium by the fetus. Parathyroid hormone-related peptide plays a role in the differentiation of many tissues during gestation and is especially important in the growth and development of bone. Growth of cartilage at the

epiphyseal plate is regulated by the actions or PTHrP which stimulates chondrocyte proliferation, inhibits apoptosis, and inhibits the maturation of chondrocytes from the proliferative zone to the hypertrophic zone (Vortkamp *et al.*, 1996), responses which are dependent on the translocation of PTHrP to the nucleus and nucleolus (Henderson *et al.*, 1995).

Role in Adults   Many tissues in adult animals including endocrine glands, smooth, skeletal, and cardiac muscles, brain, lymphocytes, lactating mammary gland, kidney, prostate gland, lung, skin, and bone produce PTHrP. The function of PTHrP in most of these tissues is incompletely understood, but likely is an autocrine or paracrine regulatory factor. Circulating concentrations of PTHrP in normal animals and humans are low (<1 pM) (Burtis, 1992; Rosol *et al.*, 1995) and the PTH/PTHrP receptor is often expressed on the same or adjacent cells in tissues that synthesize PTHrP.

Epidermal keratinocytes produce PTHrP which plays a role in their proliferation or differentiation. However, keratinocytes do not contain the classic PTH/PTHrP receptor, which suggests that keratinocytes have an alternate PTHrP receptor (Orloff *et al.*, 1992). The greatest concentration of PTHrP is found in milk (10–100 nmol/L) and is 10,000 to 100,000-fold greater than in the serum (Ratcliffe, 1992; Riond *et al.*, 1995). The function of PTHrP in the mammary gland and in milk is poorly understood at present. However, over-expression of PTHrP in the mammary gland during glandular development prior to lactation results in glandular hypoplasia due to a reduction in the morphogenesis and branching of the mammary ducts.

Biologically active PTHrP produced by alveolar epithelial cells during lactation results in the high concentration of PTHrP in milk and this PTHrP may play a role in stimulating the transport of calcium by alveolar epithelial cells from serum to milk (Parfitt, 1987; Barlet *et al.*, 1992). Synthesis of PTHrP by the mammary gland abruptly ceases when suckling stops and the gland undergoes involution. The PTHrP peptide is enzymatically cleaved in milk, but the N-terminal PTHrP fragment retains biologic activity. Although circulating concentrations of PTHrP may be minimally increased in lactating dams, no significant relationship has been demonstrated between PTHrP and the pathogenesis of parturient hypocalcemia and paresis in lactating dairy cattle (Riond *et al.*, 1996). Hence PTHrP from the mammary gland likely plays a minor role in the systemic calcium balance of lactating animals but may have physiological functions in suckling neonates, such as regulation of growth or differentiation of the gastrointestinal tract.

TESTIS

Structure and Endocrinologic Regulation of Leydig (Interstitial) Cells

Leydig (interstitial) cell tumors are one of the more frequently occurring endocrine tumors in rodents in chronic toxicity/carcinogenicity studies, and a great deal of research has been published in the literature investigating their pathogenesis and implications for safety assessment. Rodent testicular tumors are classified into five general categories including tumors derived from cells of the gonadal stroma, neoplasms of germ cell origin, tumors derived from adnexal structures or serous membranes, and, lastly, a group of tumors derived from the supporting connective tissues and vessels of the testis.

Neoplasms of the gonadal stroma include benign and malignant tumors derived from Leydig (interstitial) cells, Sertoli cells

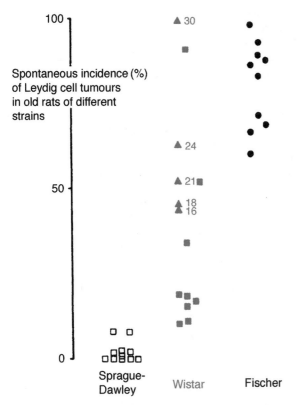

Figure 21-57. Spontaneous incidence of Leydig cell tumors of the testis in Sprague–Dawley, Wistar, and Fischer rats. (From Bär, 1992).

carcinogenicity studies, including the Fischer 344 and Wistar strains. The spontaneous incidence of Leydig cell tumors in three different strains of rats is illustrated in Fig. 21-57 (Bär, 1992). The actual incidence of Leydig cell tumors in old rats is lowest in Sprague–Dawley, highly variable in Wistar rats, and highest in Fischer rats (in which the incidence at 2 years of age often approaches 100%). The specific numerical incidence of benign Leydig cell tumors in rats also will vary considerably depending upon the histological criteria used by the pathologist in the separation of focal hyperplasia from adenomas.

In comparison to rodents, the incidence of Leydig cell tumors in human patients is extremely rare, something to the order of one in five million with age peaks at approximately 30 and 60 years. Ninety or more percent of Leydig cell tumors in humans are benign and some appear to be endocrinologically active and associated clinically with gynecomastia. The most common and clinically important testicular neoplasms in men are of germ cell origin (e.g., seminona). By comparison, germ cell tumors are rare in rodents either as a spontaneous lesion or following exposure to large doses of xenobiotic chemicals.

Although the numbers of Leydig cells vary somewhat among different animal species and humans, the basic structural arrangement is similar. In the rat, there are small groups of Leydig cells clustered around blood vessels in the interstitium, between seminiferous tubules with an incomplete layer of endothelial cells around the groups of Leydig cells. In humans, the Leydig cells are present as small groups in the interstitium near blood vessels or in loose connective tissue but without the surrounding layer of endothelial cells. Leydig cells are much more numerous in some animal species, such as the domestic pig. Microscopic evaluation of the normal rat testis reveals the inconspicuous clusters of Leydig cells in the interstitium between the much larger seminiferous tubules composed of spermatogonia and Sertoli cells. The close anatomic association of Leydig cells and interstitial blood vessels permits the rapid exchange of materials between this endocrine cell population and the systemic circulation.

The endocrinological regulation of Leydig cells involves the coordinated activity of the hypothalamus and adenohypophysis (anterior pituitary) with negative feedback control exerted by the blood concentration of gonadal steroids (Fig. 21-58). Hypothalamic

of the seminiferous tubules, as well as a rare mixed tumor with an admixture of both cell types. The Leydig cell tumor is the most common tumor developing in the rodent testis and frequently presents a problem in separating between focal hyperplasia and early neoplastic growth (i.e., adenoma formation).

The incidence of Leydig cell tumors in old rats varies considerably depending upon the strain. In general, Sprague–Dawley, Osborne–Mendel, and Brown–Norway strains have a much lower incidence than other strains frequently used in chronic toxicity/

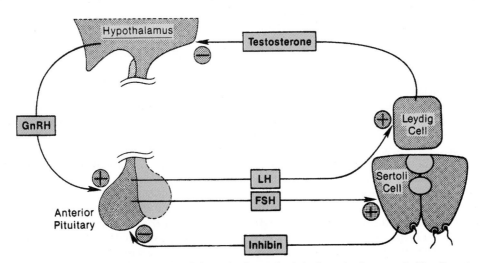

Figure 21-58. Hypothalamus–anterior pituitary gland–gonad axis in the endocrine control of Leydig and Sertoli cells by luteinizing hormone (LH) and follicle-stimulating hormone (FSH). (From Hedge et al., 1987).

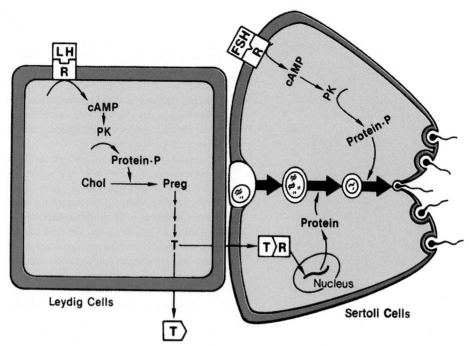

Figure 21-59. Hormonal control of testicular function.

Luteinizing hormone (LH) stimulates testosterone (T) release by binding to its receptor (R) and increasing the conversion of cholesterol (chol) to pregnenolone (preg) via a cAMP-protein kinase (PK) cascade. Spermatogenesis (bold arrows) is controlled by both FSH and testosterone acting via Sertoli cells. (From Hedge *et al.*, 1987.)

gonadotrophin-releasing hormone (GnRH) stimulates the pulsatile release of both luteinizing hormone (LH) and follicle-stimulating hormone (FSH) from gonadotrophs in the adenohypophysis. Luteinizing hormone is the major trophic factor controlling the activity of Leydig cells and the synthesis of testosterone. The blood levels of testosterone exert negative feedback on the hypothalamus and, to a lesser extent, on the adenohypophysis. Follicle-stimulating hormone binds to receptors on Sertoli cells in the seminiferous tubules and, along with the local concentration of testosterone, plays a critical role in spermatogenesis. Testosterone, by controlling GnRH release, is one important regulator of FSH secretion by the pituitary gland. The seminiferous tubules also produce a glycopeptide, designated as inhibin, that exerts negative feedback on the release of FSH by the gonadotrophs.

Leydig cells have a similar ultrastructural appearance as other endocrine cells that synthesize and release steroid hormones. The abundant cytoplasmic area contains numerous mitochondria, abundant profiles of smooth endoplasmic reticulum, prominent Golgi apparatuses associated with lysosomal bodies, and occasional lipofucsin inclusions. However, they lack the hormone-containing secretory granules that are found characteristically in peptide-hormone-secreting endocrine cells.

The hormonal control of testicular function is largely the result of the coordinated activities of LH and FSH from the pituitary gland. LH binds to high-affinity, low-capacity receptors on the surface of Leydig cells and activates adenylate cyclase in the plasma membrane resulting in the generation of an intracellular messenger, cyclic AMP (Fig. 21-59). The cyclic AMP binds to a protein kinase, resulting in the phosphorylation of a specific set of proteins in the cytosol, which increases the conversion of cholesterol to pregnenolone by making more substrate available and increasing the activity of an enzyme that cleaves the side chain of cholesterol. The pregnenolone in Leydig cells is rapidly converted to testosterone, which is released into interstitial blood vessels or taken up by adjacent Sertoli cells. Testosterone in Sertoli's cells binds to nuclear receptors where it increases genomic expression and transcription of mRNAs that direct the synthesis of proteins (e.g., androgen-binding protein and others) involved in spermatogenesis. In the rat, the mitotic phase of gametogenesis can occur without hormonal stimulation but testosterone is necessary for meiosis of spermatocytes to spermatids. FSH is required for the later stages for spermatid maturation to spermatazoa (Fig. 21-59). Once FSH and testosterone initiate spermatogenesis at puberty in the rat, testosterone alone is sufficient to maintain sperm production.

Pathology of Leydig (Interstitial) Cell Tumors

Before discussing the pathology of focal proliferative lesions of Leydig cells, a few points should be made about the importance of standardized sectioning methods for the complete evaluation of the rodent testis. It is not unusual to have less than optimal sections to evaluate, due either to a lack of a consistent plane of section or to inadequate fixation. The goal should be to include the largest testicular area containing all anatomic features on a mid-sagittal section along the long axis of the testis to include spermatic vessels, attachment sites of the epididymis, tubulus rectus, and intratesticular rete testis. It is also important to emphasize the need to cut the thick outer covering (tunica albuginea) of the testis at several points prior to immersion in the fixative, in order to permit more rapid penetration of the formalin or other fixing solution.

The major issue in the interpretation of focal proliferative lesions of Leydig cells in the rodent testis is the accurate and

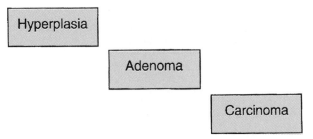

Figure 21-60. Multistage model of carcinogenesis of proliferative lesions in endocrine tissues of rodents.

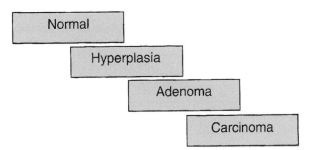

Figure 21-61. Morphological continuum of proliferative lesions in endocrine tissues of rodents.

consistent separation of focal hyperplasia from benign tumors (adenomas) that possess autonomous growth. The separation of focal hyperplasia from adenomas derived from Leydig cells is arbitrary based upon current methods of evaluation and often is based primarily on the size of the focal lesion, since cytologic features usually are similar between focal hyperplastic and benign neoplastic lesions derived from Leydig cells.

In the multistage model of carcinogenesis, proliferative lesions are designated as beginning with hyperplasia, often progressing to benign tumors (adenomas), and infrequently a few assume malignant potential and form carcinomas ("cancer") (Fig. 21-60). Although this terminology often is applied to focal proliferative lesions in rodent endocrine tissues for convenience and standardization, it is essential to understand that the separation, especially between focal hyperplasia and adenoma, is based primarily on size and morphologic changes in the proliferating Leydig cells. It is important to emphasize that focal proliferative lesions in rodent endocrine tissues also including Leydig cells, adrenal medullary cells, thyroid follicular and C-cells, among others, represent a morphologic continuum that begins with hyperplasia and progresses often but not always to the formation of adenomas that grow autonomously and only occasionally undergo a malignant transformation to form carcinomas ("cancer") (Fig. 21-61).

The National Toxicology Program (NTP), in an attempt to standardize the classification of focal proliferative lesions of Leydig cells between studies with different xenobiotic chemicals and different testing laboratories, established the following diagnostic criteria (Boorman *et al.*, 1987): (1) hyperplasia was defined as a focal collection of Leydig cells with little atypia and a diameter of less than one seminiferous tubule. (2) An adenoma was defined as a mass of Leydig cells larger in diameter than one seminiferous tubule with some cellular atypia and compression of adjacent tubules. (3) It was emphasized that the separation was arbitrary since at that time little was known about the biological behavior of these lesions in rodents.

A more contemporary set of diagnostic criteria for focal proliferative lesions of Leydig cells has been published recently by the Society of Toxicologic Pathologists (STP) (McConnell *et al.*, 1992). Recognizing that many small focal proliferative lesions of Leydig cells (i.e., between 1 and 3 tubule diameters) will regress following removal of the inciting stimulus, they recommend the diagnosis of Leydig cell adenoma be used for a mass of interstitial cells equal to or greater than the diameter of three adjacent seminiferous tubules plus one or more of the following criteria: symmetrical peripheral compression of adjacent tubules, evidence of cellular pleomorphism, or an increase in the nuclear:cytoplasmic ratio, an endocrine sinusoidal vascular network, increased mitotic activity, or coalescence of adjacent cell masses.

Leydig cell neoplasms in laboratory rats rarely undergo malignant transformation with progression to the development of carcinomas ("cancer"). Histological features of malignancy include invasion into the epididymus, spermatic cord, or tunica albuginea. The most definitive criteria of malignancy is the demonstration of metastases in extratesticular sites. Leydig cell carinomas are large and often distort the overall contour of the affected testis with extensive areas of both hemorrhage and necrosis. The cytology of Leydig cell carcinomas usually is more pleomorphic than with adenomas consisting of an admixture of poorly differentiated cells with an increased nuclear:cytoplasmic ratio and larger, more differentiated cells with an abundant vacuolated eosinophilic cytoplasmic area. The frequency of mitotic figures may be increased either in focal areas or throughout the Leydig cell carcinomas. The most convincing evidence of malignancy in carcinomas is the establishment of foci of growth outside of the testis, such as multiple foci of tumor cell emboli growing within and distending vessels of the lung.

Mechanisms of Leydig (Interstitial) Cell Tumor Development

Leydig (interstitial) cells of the testis frequently undergo proliferative changes with advancing age and following chronic exposure to large doses of xenobiotic chemicals. In addition, it should be emphasized that the "sensitivity" of rodent endocrine tissues, such as Leydig cells of the testis and other populations of endocrine cells, appears to be increasing over time particularly if one compares data generated in the 1970s to that gathered in the 1990s for the same compound (Table 21-4). This appears to be the result of several factors, including: (1) animal husbandry practices, such as specific pathogen-free conditions, that result in a greater survival for 2 years,

Table 21-4

Changes in Rodent Endocrine Sensitivity Over Time (1970s–1990s)

1. Animal husbandry practices
   - Specific pathogen-free (SPF) conditions
     —greater survival to 2 years+
   - High body weight (obesity)
   - Immobility
2. Genetic selection process
   - High productivity
     —Large litters
     —High lactation yield
   - Rapid growth

Table 21-5

Pathogenic Mechanisms for Development of Leydig (Interstitial) Cell Proliferative Lesions in Rodents

- Physiological perturbations
  Cryptorchidism
  Compromised blood supply
  Heterotransplantation (spleen)
- Hormonal imbalances
  Decreased testosterone
  Increased estrogens (mice, hamsters)
  Increased pituitatry gonadotropins (e.g., LH)
- Irradiation
- Species/strain differences
  Chemicals
  Cadmium salts
  2-Acetoaminofluorene

Table 21-6

Effect of Food Restriction on the Development of Interstitial (Leydig) Cell Adenomas in F344 Rats*

| FEEDING | RATS (NO.)* | INTERSTITIAL CELL ADENOMAS | |
		NO.	%
Ad libitum	49	24	49
Food restricted (40%)	52	10	19

*Lifetime study without periodic sacrifice removals (died from spontaneous disease) (From Thurman *et al.*, 1994).

Table 21-7

Effect of Food Restriction on the Development of Interstitial (Leydig) Cell Adenomas in F344 Rats*

| FEEDING | RATS (NO.)* | INTERSTITIAL CELL ADENOMAS | |
		NO.	%
Ad libitum	−98	59	60
Food restricted (40%)	112	26	23

*Lifetime study with periodic removal of serially sacrificed rats (died from spontaneous disease) (From Thurman *et al.*, 1994).

Table 21-8

Effects of Food Restriction on the Development of Interstitial (Leydig) Cell Adenoma (ICA) in F344 Rats at Different Ages

| AGE AT SACRIFICE (MOS.) | ICA [TUMORS/NO. RATS (%)] | |
	AD LIBITUM	FEED-RESTRICTED (40%)
12	0/12 (0)	0/12 (0)
18	5/12 (42)	0/12 (0)
24	10/12 (83)	1/12 (8)
30	9/9 (100)	2/12 (17)
36	—	4/9 (44)

(From Thurman *et al.*, 1994.)

high body weight related to over feeding, and immobility; and (2) the genetic selection process for high productivity and rapid growth.

Pathogenic mechanisms reported in the literature to be important in the development of proliferative lesions of Leydig cells include irradiation, the species and strain differences mentioned previously, and exposure to certain chemicals such as cadmium salts (Waalkes *et al.*, 1997) and 2-acetoaminofluorene (Prentice and Meikle, 1995) (Table 21-5). Other pathogenic mechanisms include physiological perturbations such as cryptorchidism, a compromised blood supply to the testis, or heterotransplantation into the spleen. Data from several studies in the recent literature emphasize the importance of several of these pathogenetic factors in the frequent development of Leydig cell tumors in rats. Thurman *et al.* (1994) reported the effects of food restriction on the development of Leydig cell adenomas in the high incidence strain of Fischer 344 rats (Table 21-6). Beginning at 13 weeks of age, rats were either continued on an ad libitum feeding or they were food-restricted 40% (NIH-31 diet with 1.673 fat soluble and B vitamins) over their lifetime until they died or became moribund due to spontaneous disease. The incidence of Leydig cell adenomas was decreased to 19% in food-restricted rats compared to 49% in the ad-libitum-fed group (Table 21-6). In another group from the food restriction study reported by Thurman *et al.* (1994), rats were periodically removed for serial sacrifice at 6-month intervals. Food restriction resulted in a similar marked reduction in Leydig cell adenomas (23% compared to 60% in ad-libitum-fed rats) (Table 21-7). Examination of the serially sacrificed F344 rats in this study also demonstrated that feed restriction delayed the onset of development, as well as decreasing the incidence of Leydig cell adenomas compared to the ad-libitum-fed group (Table 21-8). For example, at the 30-month sacrifice, only 17% of feed-restricted F344 rats had developed Leydig cell adenomas compared to 100% in the ad libitum group.

Disturbances of the Hypothalamic–Hypophyseal–Gonadal Axis
Hormonal imbalances also are important factors in the development of focal proliferative lesions of Leydig cells, including increased estrogenic steroids in mice and hamsters and elevated pituitary gonadotrophins resulting from the chronic administration of androgen receptor antagonists, 5α-reductase inhibitors, testosterone biosynthesis inhibitors, GnRH agonists, and aromatase inhibitors

(Fig. 21-62) (Clegg *et al.*, 1997; Cook *et al.*, 1992, 1999). Many xenobiotic chemicals when administered chronically to rats disrupt the hypothalamic–pituitary–testis axis at one of several possible sites interfering with negative feedback control, resulting in an over production of luteinizing hormone (LH) that causes the proliferative

- ANDROGEN RECEPTOR ANTAGONISTS (RATS)
- 5α-REDUCTASE INHIBITORS (RAT, MOUSE)
- TESTOSTERONE BIOSYNTHESIS INHIBITORS (RAT)
- AROMATASE INHIBITORS (DOG, RAT)
- DOPAmine AGONISTS (RAT)
- GnRH AGONISTS (RAT)
- ESTROGEN AGONISTS / ANTAGONISTS (MOUSE)

Figure 21-62. Model of action of nongenotoxic compounds that produce Leydig cell hyperplasia/adenoma in rodents.

Table 21-9

Effect of Aging and Testosterone on the Incidence of Interstitial Cell Adenomas (ICA) and Hyperplasia (ICH) in Fischer 344 Rats

TREATMENT (23 WEEKS)	TERMINAL AGE (WEEKS)	ICA % (NO./NO. TESTES)	ICH % TESTES	ICH* (NODULES/ TESTES)	SERUM LH (ng/ml)*
0	42	0 (0/20)	10	0.3 ± 0.8	20.9 ± 19.5
0	50	0 (0/20)	95	5.0 ± 2.3	N.D.
0	60	0 (0/10)	90	8.3 ± 7.0	48.7 ± 16.7
0	70	70 (14/20)	100	11.1 ± 6.2	22.1 ± 8.4
Testosterone[†]	70	0 (0/10)[‡]	0[‡]	0.0 ± 0.0[‡]	8.4 ± 8.8[‡]

*Mean ± S.D.

[†]Silastic tubes implanted subcutaneously at 42 weeks.

[‡] $P < 0.05$ compared to controls.

NTP Criteria: ICA greater and ICH less than one normal seminiferous tubule diameter (From Chatani *et al.*, 1990).

changes (hyperplasia, adenoma) in Leydig cells (Fig. 21-63). For example, chronic exposure to chemicals with antiandrogenic activity, such as procymidone due to binding to the androgen receptor, increases circulating levels of LH and results in stimulation of Leydig cells leading to an increased incidence of hyperplasia and adenomas in rats (Murakami *et al.*, 1995).

Investigations reported by Chatani *et al.* (1990) documented the importance of hormonal imbalances on the incidence of Leydig cell adenomas and hyperplasia in Fischer rats (Table 21-9). The incidence of adenomas was 70% and of hyperplasia 100% in control rats killed at 70 weeks of age. In rats administered testosterone for 28 weeks (by silastic tubes implanted subcutaneously at 42 weeks of age), the incidence of Leydig cell adenomas and hyperplasias was decreased to 0% for both at 70 weeks of age. This dramatic reduction in the incidence of focal proliferative lesions of Leydig cells was associated with a significant lowering in circulating levels of LH, through negative feedback exerted by testosterone on the pituitary gland.

The important studies reported by Chatani *et al.* (1990) also demonstrated that hormones other than testosterone could markedly decrease the development of Leydig cell adenomas in F344 rats (Table 21-9). The administration of estradiol-17β for 28 weeks (by silastic tubes implanted subcutaneously) decreased the incidence of Leydig cell adenomas to 0% (compared to 100% in controls) and significantly reduced serum LH, due to negative feedback control on the pituitary gland. An LH-releasing hormone agonist administered continuously for 28 weeks (injection of microcapsules every 4 weeks at a dose of 5 mg/2 mL/kg) also decreased the incidence of Leydig cell adenomas to 0% and significantly decreased circulating LH levels, most likely a result of the known downregulation of LH–RH receptors on pituitary gonadotrophs (Table 21-10).

The studies of Bartke *et al.* (1985) demonstrated that hyperprolactinemia also markedly decreased the incidence of Leydig cell adenomas in Fischer rats (Table 21-11). Pituitaries transplanted beneath the renal capsule (four per rat) resulted in a chronic elevation of circulating prolactin levels, owing, most likely, to the lack of dopamine inhibition of prolactin secretion, which occurs when the pituitary gland is in its normal anatomic location in close proximity to the hypothalamus. In this interesting experiment, 83% of sham-operated rats developed Leydig cell adenomas at 21–24 months of

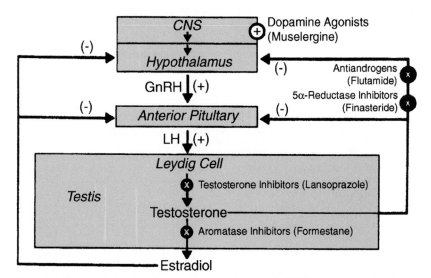

Figure 21-63. Regulation of the hypothalamic–pituitary–testis (HPT) axis and control points for potential disruption by xenobiotic chemicals.

Symbols: (+) feedback stimulation; (−) feedback inhibition; ⊕ receptor stimulation; ⊗ enzyme or receptor inhibition. (Modified from Cook *et al.*, 1999).

Table 21-10

Effect of Testosterone, Estradiol, and LH-RH Agonist on Incidence of Interstitial Cell Adenoma (ICA) in F344 Rats

TREATMENT (28 WEEKS)	TERMINAL AGE (WEEKS)	ICA % (NO./NO. TESTES)	SERUM LH (ng/mL)*
Control	88	100 (18/18)	12.9 ± 11.7
Testosterone[†]	88	0 (0/18)[‡]	1.7 ± 1.6[‡]
Estradiol-17β[†]	88	0 (0/18)[‡]	4.7 ± 2.4[‡]
LH-RH Agonist[‡]	88	0 (0/16)[‡]	4.9 ± 3.5[‡]

*Mean ± SD.

[†]Silastic tubes implanted subcutaneously.

[‡] $P < 0.05$ compared to controls.

[+]Injected subcutaneously at 60 weeks of age.

NTP criteria: ICA greater than one normal seminiferous tubule diameter (From Chatani *et al.*, 1990).

age, whereas 0% of rats developed tumors in animals with ectopic pituitaries and elevated serum prolactin levels.

The administration of a calcium-channel blocker (SVZ 200-110) at high doses (62.5 mg/kg/day for 2 years) significantly increased the incidence of Leydig cell adenomas in Sprague–Dawley rats. Endocrinological studies demonstrated that increased serum levels of LH and FSH were present only after 52 and 66 weeks, respectively, and persisted to week 104 for LH. This compound is unusual in that most xenobiotic chemicals that cause hormonal imbalances result in earlier significant changes in circulating hormone levels.

Inhibition of Testosterone Synthesis   Another important mechanism by which xenobiotic chemicals increase the incidence of Leydig cell tumors in rats is by inhibition of testosterone synthesis by cells in the testis. For example, lansoprazole is a substituted benzimidazole which inhibits the hydrogen-potassuim ATPase (proton pump) responsible for acid secretion by the parietal cells in the fundic mucosa of the stomach (Fort *et al.*, 1995). The presence of the imidazole moiety in lansoprazole was suggestive of an effect on testosterone synthesis because several imidazole compounds (e.g., ketoconazole and miconazole) are known to inhibit testosterone synthesis. Lansoprazole resulted in decreased circulating levels of testosterone, increased levels of LH, and an increased incidence of

Leydig cell hyperplasia and benign neoplasia (adenomas) in chronic studies in rats (Fort *et al.*, 1995). The most sensitive site for inhibition of testosterone synthesis by lansoprazole was the transport of cholesterol to the cholesterol side chain cleavage enzyme.

Leydig Cell Tumorigenesis in Rodents and Relevance for Human Risk Assessment   Although several hormonal imbalances result in an increased incidence of Leydig cell tumors in rodents, in human patients several disease conditions associated with chronic elevations in serum LH (including Klinefelter's syndrome and gonadotroph adenomas of the pituitary gland) have not been associated with an increased development of this type of rare testicular tumor.

There are a number of reports in the literature of xenobiotic chemicals (many of which are marketed drugs) that increase the incidence of proliferative lesions of Leydig cells in chronic toxicology/carcinogenicity in rats. These include indomethacin, lactitol, muselergine, cimetidine, gemfibrozil, and flutamide, among many others (Table 21-12).

Flutamide is a potent nonsteroidal, antiandrogen compound that displaces testosterone from specific receptors in target cells and decreases negative feedback on the hypothalamus–pituitary gland, resulting in elevated circulating levels of LH and FSH. The chronic administration of flutamide is known to result in a striking increase in the incidence of Leydig cell adenomas in rats. The Schering-Plough Research Institute's Department of Drug Safety and Metabolism completed an important reversibility study in which Sprague–Dawley rats were administered flutamide daily either for 1 year, 1 year followed by a 1-year recovery period, or continuously for 2 years (Table 21-13). This important study emphasizes the lack of autonomy of many focal proliferative lesions of Leydig cells in rats and their continued dependence upon compound administration for stimulation of growth. There was a reduction in the incidence of Leydig cell adenomas (using the conservative NTP criteria of greater than 1 tubule diameter) in rats administered 3 dose levels of flutamide daily for 1 year followed by a 1-year recovery prior to termination, compared to rats given flutamide for 1 year and immediately evaluated (Table 21-13). Conversely, in rats administered flutamide for 2 years the numbers of adenomas continued to increase until 95% of animals in the mid- and high-dose groups (30 and 50 μg/kg, respectively) had developed Leydig cell tumors. There also was a marked reduction in the incidence of focal hyperplasia (focus less than 1 tubule diameter) after 1 year of

Table 21-11

Effect of Hyperprolactinemia from Ectopic Pituitary Transplants on the Incidence of Interstitial Cell Adenoma (ICA) and Testicular/Seminal Vesicle Weights in Fischer 344 Rats

RAT GROUP	ICA % (NO./NO. RATS)	TESTES' WEIGHT (gm)*	SEMINAL VESICLES' WEIGHT (gm)*
Sham-operated			
With tumors	83 (20/24)	4.88 ± 0.22[‡]	0.55 ± 0.08[‡]
Without tumors	17 (4/24)	2.66 ± 0.48	1.35 ± 0.14
Pituitary-grafted[†]			
With tumors	0 (0/0)	—	—
Without tumors	100 (24/24)	2.79 ± 0.05	1.26 ± 0.07

*Mean ± SE.

[†]Pituitary transplants (4/rat) beneath renal capsule or sham-operated at 2–5 mos. of age; terminated at 21–24 mos. of age.

[‡] $P < 0.05$ compared to other two groups.

From Bartke *et al.* (1985).

Table 21-12

Selected Examples of Drugs that Increase the Incidence of Proliferative Lesions of Leydig Cells in Chronic Exposure Studies in Rats or Mice

NAME	SPECIES	CLINICAL INDICATION	REFERENCE
Indomethacin	R	Anti-inflammatory	Roberts *et al.* (1989)
Lactitol	R	Laxative	Bär (1992)
Metronidazole	R	Antibacterial	Rustia and Shubik (1979)
Muselergine	R	Parkinson's disease	Prentice *et al.* (1992)
Buserelin	R	Prostatic and breast carcinoma, endometriosis	Donaubauer *et al.* (1989)
Cimetidine	R	Reduction of gastric acid secretion	PDR (1992)
Flutamide	R	Prostatic carcinoma	PDR (1992)
Gemfibrozil	R	Hypolipidemia	Fitzgerald *et al.* (1981)
Spironolactone	R	Diuretic	PDR (1994)
Nararelin	R	LH-RH Analog	PDR (1994)
Tamoxifen	M	Antiestrogen	PDR (1994)
Vidarabine	R	Antiviral	PDR (1994)
Clofibrate	R	Hypolipidemia	PDR (1994)
Finasteride	M	Prostatic hyperplasia	Prahalada *et al.* (1994)

Table 21-13

Flutamide: Incidence of Interstitial Cell (IC) Adenoma in Sprague–Dawley Rats after Various Dosing Intervals

	1-YEAR DOSING+											
	1-YEAR DOSING				1-YEAR POSTDOSE				2-YEAR DOSING			
DOSE	0	10	30	50	0	10	30	50	0	10	30	50
Number/Group	58	57	57	57	52	53	53	53	55	55	55	55
IC adenoma (>1 tubule)	0	28	43	40	6	25	23	25	6	50	52	52
IC hyperplasia (<1 tubule)	6	39	44	48	8	7	10	17	5	12	9	12

Courtesy of Schering Plough Research Institute, Department of Drug Safety and Metabolism, Lafayette, New Jersey.

recovery, compared to rats terminated immediately following 1 year of flutamide administration, a finding that emphasizes the frequent reversibility of these small proliferative lesions of Leydig cells.

Although a number of xenobiotic chemicals have been reported to increase the incidence of Leydig cell adenomas in chronic studies in rats, similar compounds such as cimetidine, ketoconazole, and certain calcium channel-blocking drugs have not resulted in an increased incidence of Leydig cell neoplasia in man. In summary, Leydig cell tumors are a frequently occurring tumor in rats, often associated mechanistically with hormonal imbalances; however, they are not an appropriate model for assessing the potential risk to human males of developing this rare testicular tumor.

OVARY

Ovarian Tumors in Rodents

Ovarian tumors in rodents can be subdivided into five broad categories including epithelial tumors, sex cord-stromal tumors, germ cell tumors, tumors derived from nonspecialized soft tissues of the ovary, and tumors metastatic to the ovary from distant sites. The epithelial tumors of the ovary include cystadenomas and cystadenocarcinomas, tubulostromal adenomas, and mesothelioma. The tubular (or tubulostromal) adenomas are the most important of the ovarian tumors in mice, and they are the tumors whose incidence often is

increased by various endocrine perturbations associated with exposure to xenobiotics, senescence, or inherited genic deletion (Murphy and Beamer, 1973). Tubular adenomas are a unique lesion that develops frequently in the mouse ovary, accounting for approximately 25% of naturally occurring ovarian tumors in this species (Rehm *et al.*, 1984; Alison and Morgan, 1987). They are uncommon in rats, rare in other animal species, and not recognized in the ovaries of women. In some ovarian tumors of this type in mice, there is an intense proliferation of stromal (interstitial) cells of sex cord origin. These tumors often are designated tubulostromal adenomas or carcinomas to reflect the bimorphic appearance.

The tubulostromal adenomas in mice are composed of numerous tubular profiles derived from the surface epithelium, plus abundant large luteinized stromal cells from the ovarian interstitium (Capen, 2004; Capen *et al.*, 1995). The differences in histological appearance of this type of unique ovarian tumor in mice are interpreted to represent a morphological spectrum with variable contributions from the surface epithelium and sex cord-derived ovarian interstitium rather than being two distinct types of ovarian tumors. The histogenic origin of this unique ovarian tumor in mice has been a controversial topic in the literature but most investigators currently agree that it is derived from the ovarian surface epithelium, with varying contributions from stromal cells of the ovarian interstitium. However, some early reports suggested an origin from the rete ovarii or thecal/granulosal cells of the ovary.

Another important group of ovarian tumors are those derived from the sex cords and/or ovarian stroma. These include the granulosal cell tumors, luteoma, thecoma, Sertoli cell tumor, tubular adenoma (with contributions from ovarian stroma), and undifferentiated sex cord-stromal tumors. The granulosal cell tumor is the most common of this group which, according to Alison and Morgan (1987), accounts for 27% of naturally occurring ovarian tumors in mice. Granulosal cell tumors may develop within certain tubular or tubulostromal adenomas following a long-term perturbation of endocrine function associated with genic deletion, irradiation, oocytotoxic chemicals, and neonatal thymectomy (Li and Gardner, 1949; Hummel, 1954; Frith et al., 1981; Davis and Maronpot, 1996).

Mechanisms of Ovarian Tumorigenesis

Five model systems of ovarian tumorigenesis in mice have been reported in the literature. The first model system identified was the production of ovarian neoplasms by radiation (Furth and Boon, 1947; Gardner, 1950). After acute radiation exposure, the initial change was a rapid loss of oocytes and a destruction of graafian follicles. There was proliferation and down-growth of the ovarian epithelium into the stroma within 10 weeks after radiation exposure. The first ovarian tumors developed approximately 1 year after exposure. The tubular adenomas that develop following radiation often were bilateral, endocrinologically inactive, and not lethal unless they reached a very large size. Some irradiated mice also developed endocrinologically active granulosal cell tumors, which transplantation experiments have shown to be different from the tubular adenomas. Granulosal cell tumors were transplantable into the spleen and often grew rapidly, whereas tubular adenomas grew slowly after transplantation, most successfully in castrated animals.

The second model of ovarian tumorigenesis arose out of the work published by Biskind and Biskind (1944). They transplanted ovaries into the spleen of castrated rats to prevent negative feedback by circulating sex hormones on the hypothalamus and pituitary gland because estrogen is degraded as it circulates through the liver. Transplantation resulted in a rapid loss of ovarian follicles as well as an interference with estrogen feedback on the hypothalamus. Following the loss of graafian follicles, the epithelial covering of the ovary began to proliferate and invaginate into the ovary, with an accompanying increase in stromal tissue that ultimately resulted in the formation of tubular adenomas and, occasionally, granulosal cell tumors (Guthrie, 1957). The presence of a single functioning gonad prevented the development of the proliferative lesions in the ovary, suggesting that the lack of negative feedback from estrogen was necessary for the changes to develop. Administration of exogenous estrogen or testosterone after transplantation completely suppressed development of the proliferative changes in the ovarian cortex.

The third model of ovarian tumorigenesis was described by Marchant (1957, 1960), who reported that ovarian tumors developed in mice exposed to dimethylbenzanthracene. This chemical is a reproductive toxicant that is cytotoxic to oocytes, resulting in the loss of graafian follicles from the ovary. This was followed by a proliferation of the interstitial (stromal) tissue, invaginations of the surface epithelium, and subsequent development of tubular adenomas and occasionally granulosal cell tumors of the ovary (Taguchi et al., 1988). Support for an endocrinological mechanism of hormonal imbalance included the observation that the xenobiotic chemical first must cause sterility, because the presence of a single normal gonad prevented the development of the hyperplastic lesions and tumors of

the ovary. The administration of estrogen prevented tumor formation even in sterile mice, and hypophysectomy also prevented the development of ovarian tumors.

The fourth model of ovarian tumorigenesis was described by Nishizuki et al. (1979). They reported that removal of the thymus from neonatal mice resulted in ovarian dysgenesis and the development of ovarian tumors. Thymectomy prior to 7 days of age resulted in an immune-mediated destruction of follicles in the ovary. Because estrogen was not produced by the follicles, these mice also developed hormone-mediated proliferative lesions and ovarian tumors identical to those in the previously described models. After the immune-mediated destruction of follicles, there was a proliferation of the interstitial (stromal) and surface epithelial cells of the ovary, resulting in the formation of tubular adenomas. If the mice survived for longer periods, some animals developed granulosal cell tumors and luteomas in the ovary. Because this model also did not involve exposure to any carcinogen, it is another indication that the prerequisite for ovarian tumor response in mice is the production of sterility, which results in hormonal imbalances that lead to stimulation of the sensitive populations of target cells (Michael et al., 1981). The fifth model system of ovarian tumorigenesis in rodents is associated with administration of xenobiotic chemicals.

Ovarian Tumors Associated Xenobiotic Chemicals

Nitrofurantoin Nitrofurantoin is an example of a chemical that, when fed at high doses to mice for 2 years in an NTP study, increased the incidence of ovarian tumors of the tubular or tubulostromal type (Table 21-14). Nitrofurantoin fed at both low (1300 ppm) and high (2500 ppm) doses to B6C3F1 mice caused sterility due to the destruction of ovarian follicles, leading to hormonal imbalances, which resulted in the development of an increased incidence of this unique type of ovarian tumor.

Mice administered nitrofurantoin had a consistent change in the ovarian cortex, termed *ovarian atrophy*. This lesion was characterized by an absence of graafian follicles, developing ova, and corpora lutea; by focal or diffuse hyperplasia with localized or diffuse downgrowth of surface epithelium into the ovary; and by varying numbers of polygonal, often vacuolated, sex-cord-derived stromal (interstitial) cells between the tubular profiles. The ovaries were small, had irregular surfaces due to the tubular down-growths into the cortex, and had scattered eosinophilic stromal cells between tubular profiles. In addition, there was a lack of graafian follicles and corpora lutea throughout the ovarian cortex.

The benign ovarian tumors in this study were classified either as tubular adenomas (5 of 50 mice) or as tubulostromal tumors (4 of 50 mice) (Table 21-14). In tubulostromal adenomas, the proliferating stromal (interstitial) cells between the tubules were considered to represent a significant component of the lesion. However, the separation between these two types of proliferating ovarian lesions in mice was not distinct and both appeared to be part of a continuous morphological spectrum. Because all treated mice in the NTP nitrofurantoin feeding study were sterile due to ovarian atrophy, an indirect mechanism secondary to a disruption of endocrine function leading to hormonal imbalances was suggested to explain the development of the ovarian tubular adenomas.

The results of an investigative study demonstrated that nitrofurantoin had an effect on graafian follicles in the ovary of B6C3F1 mice. Female mice of the same strain were fed 350 or 500 mg/kg/day of nitrofurantoin beginning at 7 weeks of age. These levels approximate the low (1300 ppm) and high (2500 ppm) doses used in the

Table 21-14

NTP Nitrofurantoin Study of Treatment-Related Ovarian Lesions in B₆C₃F₁ Mice (50/Group Exposed for 2 Years in Feed)

LESION	CONTROL	LOW DOSE (0.13%)	HIGH DOSE (0.25%)
Tubular adenoma	0	0	5*
Tubulostromal adenoma	0	0	4†
Benign GCT	0	3	2
Malignant GCT	0	0	1
Cystadenoma	2	1	1
Cysts	14	15	10
Abscess	18	0	0
Ovarian atrophy	0	49	48
Survival at 2 years	19	37	37

NTP, National Toxicology Program; GCT, Granulosal cell tumor.
*Trend test positive ($P \leq 0.05$).
†Fischer exact test positive ($P \leq 0.05$).

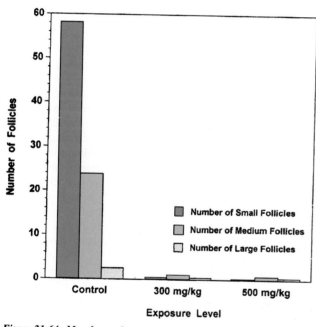

Figure 21-64. Morphometric evaluation of ovaries of mice following the administration of 350 and 500 mg/kg/day of nitrofurantoin.

The numbers of small, medium, and large ovarian follicles were numerically decreased after 17 weeks and significantly decreased after 43 and 64 weeks due to a direct action of the nitrofurantoin.

NTP study with nitrofurantoin. Ten female mice per group were sacrificed at 4, 8, 13, 17, 43, and 64 weeks of feeding nitrofurantoin. The numbers of follicles were quantified from nitrofurantoin-treated and control mice on serial sections of the ovary. The morphometric data revealed that the numbers of small, medium, and large follicles in nitrofurantoin-treated mice were numerically decreased at 17 weeks compared with controls and were significantly decreased in rats fed 350 and 500 mg/kg/day nitrofurantoin after 43 and 64 weeks (Fig. 21-64). All mice in the treated groups were sterile by 43 weeks of feeding nitrofurantoin.

Selective Estrogen Receptor Modulators Selective estrogen receptor modulators (SERMs) are compounds that have estrogen ago-

nist effects on some tissues and estrogen antagonist actions on other tissues (Cohen *et al.*, 2000). The triphenylethylene SERMs tamoxifen and toremifene have estrogen antagonist effects in the breast and currently are used in the medical management of breast cancer. The benzothiophene SERM raloxifene has estrogen agonist effects on bone and serum lipids but estrogen antagonist actions on the uterus and breast (Delmas *et al.*, 1997). This is in contrast to tamoxifen that has an estrogen agonist effect on bone and also may stimulate the uterine endometrium. These SERMs (e.g., tamoxifen, toremifene, and raloxifene) all have been reported to increase the incidence of ovarian tumors when administered chronically to mice. For example, CD₁, mice administered raloxifene (9, 50, 225 mg/kg) per day for 21 months developed an increased incidence of granulosa/theca cell tumors (benign and malignant) and tubular/papillary adenomas of the ovary. However, there is no evidence of an increased risk for ovarian cancer in women administered SERMs since tamoxifen has been used clinically since 1978 (Fisher *et al.*, 1994; Cook *et al.*, 1995).

Raloxifene binds to the estrogen receptor (Yang *et al.*, 1996) and appears to block the negative feedback of circulating levels of estrogen on the hypothalamus, resulting in a sustained increase in circulating levels of LH. Mice (CD₁) administered raloxifene (233 or 236 mg/kg) daily for 2 and 4 weeks had a dose-dependent significant elevation of serum LH levels (4- to 7-fold and 4.4-fold compared to controls, respectively) (Cohen *et al.*, 2000). Raloxifene-treated mice had sustained elevations in serum LH over a 24-hour period and did not have the preovulatory LH surge present in many control mice. Histomorphologic changes in the ovary were indicative of arrested follicular maturation including anovulatory hemorrhagic follicles, some developing follicles, and few corpora lutea. Following a recovery period of 3 weeks during which no raloxifene was administered, serum LH concentrations were indistinguishable from controls and follicular maturation and corpora lutea distribution were normal. Raloxifene binding to the estrogen receptor resulted in an elevation of serum LH and ovarian tumor development similar to those in estrogen receptor-α knock-out mice with genetic deletion of the estrogen receptor (Korach, 1994), suggesting that the tumors in both instances develop secondary to the hormonal imbalances.

Ovarian Tumors in Mutant Strains of Mice

Wˣ/Wᵛ Strain with Genetic Deletion of Germ Cells in Ovarian Cortex In an attempt to arrive at further mechanistic explanations for the development of tubular adenomas in B6C3F1 mice fed high doses of nitrofurantoin, ovaries were evaluated from several mutant mouse strains not exposed to any xenobiotic chemicals but that are known to develop ovarian tumors (Blaakaer *et al.*, 1995). In this mutant mouse strain, referred to as Wˣ/Wᵛ, few germ cells migrate into the ovary during development. Murphy (1972) reported that less than 1% of the normal complement of oocytes were present in the ovary at 1 day of age and the numbers of graafian follicles decrease progressively until none were present at 13 weeks of age. In this mutant mouse strain (Wˣ/Wᵛ), a mutant allele at the C-kit locus encodes for a defective protein kinase receptor, resulting in an inability to respond to stem cell growth factor encoded by the Steel locus (Majumder *et al.*, 1988; Witte, 1990). A failure of proliferation of primordial germ cells during gonadogenesis leads to the marked reduction of graafian follicles in the ovarian cortex.

Ovaries from mutant mice at age 13 weeks were small, had an irregular surface, were devoid of graafian follicles, and had numerous hyperplastic tubules growing into the cortex. These tubules were lined by a hyperplastic cuboidal epithelium similar to that on the surface of the ovary. Interspersed between the tubular profiles were luteinized stromal cells of the ovarian interstitium with a lightly eosinophilic, often vacuolated, cytoplasm. The proliferative changes observed in the ovary of these mutant (Wˣ/Wᵛ) mice at 13 weeks of age were similar morphologically to the ovarian atrophy lesions in the NTP nitrofurantoin study.

The ovaries of heterozygous controls (1/1) of this strain were larger than in the mutant mice and had a histological appearance similar to normal mouse ovaries. The ovarian cortex in control mice had plentiful graafian follicles with developing ova. The surface epithelium covering the ovary consisted of a single layer of cuboidal cells without the down-growth of tubules into the underlying cortex.

The ovaries of mutant (Wˣ/Wᵛ) mice at 22 weeks of age had a more intense proliferation of surface epithelium either with extensive down-growths of hyperplastic tubules into the cortex or the formation of small tubular adenomas. The tubular adenomas in the mutant (Wˣ/Wᵛ) mice with genetic deletion of graafian follicles but without any exposure to xenobiotic chemicals were composed of proliferating tubules of surface epithelium that replaced much of the ovary. They were similar microscopically to the smaller tubular adenomas in the B6C3F1 mice fed the high dose (2500 ppm) of nitrofurantoin in the 2-year NTP feeding study. Interspersed between the hyperplastic profiles of surface epithelium in the tubular adenomas were scattered luteinized stromal cells with varying degrees of vacuolation of the eosinophilic cytoplasm. In mutant (Wˣ/Wᵛ) mice, age 22 weeks, whose ovaries had been under long-term intense gonadotrophin stimulation, there appeared to be a morphological continuum between ovarian atrophy and tubular adenomas.

At age 20 months, ovaries of the mutant (Wˣ/Wᵛ) mice without any exposure to xenobiotic chemicals consistently had large tubular adenomas that incorporated all of the ovarian parenchyma and greatly enlarged the ovary. These neoplasms were similar histologically to the larger tubular adenomas in the high-dose (2500 ppm) mice of the NTP study. Several of the larger ovarian neoplasms of the 20-month-old mutant mice had evidence of malignancy with invasion of tumor cells through the ovarian capsule into the periovarian tissues, often accompanied by a localized desmoplastic response. Histopathologic evidence of malignancy was not observed in the ovarian tubular adenomas from the high-dose (2500 ppm) female mice in the NTP study. An occasional mutant mouse at 20 months of age also had developed focal areas of hyperplasia of granulosa cells or small granulosal cell tumors.

- **TUMORS DEVELOP ONLY IN STERILE MICE**

- **REQUIRES AN INTACT HYPOTHALAMUS-PITUITARY-OVARIAN AXIS**

- **EXOGENOUS ESTROGEN PREVENTS OVARIAN TUMOR DEVELOPMENT**

Figure 21-65. Secondary mechanisms of ovarian oncogenesis in mice.

Hypogonadal (hpg/hpg) Mice Unable to Synthesize Hypothalamic Gonadotrophin-Releasing Hormone (GnRH) Mutant hypogonadal mice, designated hpg/hpg, are unable to synthesize normal amounts of hypothalamic GnRH (Tennent and Beamer, 1986). They have low circulating levels of pituitary gonadotrophins, and boast FSH and LH; however, these hypogonadal mice have a normal complement of ovarian follicles (Cattanach *et al.*, 1977).

In the studies of Tennent and Beamer (1986), both genetically normal littermates and hypogonadal (hpg/hpg) mice were irradiated at age 30 days to destroy the oocytes. The irradiated control mice of this strain produced normal amounts of pituitary gonadotrophic hormones and developed ovarian tubular adenomas at age 10–15 months. The tumors that developed in the absence of any exposure to xenobiotic chemicals had similar histological characteristics as tubular adenomas in the high-dose (2500 ppm) females of the nitrofurantoin study. They either were small nodules involving only a portion of the ovary or large masses that completely incorporated the affected gonad. They were composed predominantly of tubular profiles, some of which were dilated, with interspersed stromal cells.

The irradiated hypogonadal (hpg/hpg) mice failed to develop tubular adenomas or to have intense hyperplasia of the ovarian surface epithelium and interstitial (stromal) cells, in the absence of GnRH and with low circulating levels of pituitary gonadotrophins. The ovaries of irradiated hypogonadal mice were small and had single- or multiple-layered follicles, without oocytes, scattered throughout the ovary. There also was an absence of stromal cell hypertrophy and hyperplasia, a change frequently observed in ovaries of the irradiated normal littermates.

The experiments reported by Tennent and Beamer (1986) demonstrated that a normal secretion of hypothalamic GnRH and pituitary gonadotrophins was necessary for the intense proliferation of ovarian surface epithelium and stromal cells, leading to the formation of tubular adenomas in mice, which develop subsequent to irradiation-induced loss of ovarian follicles and decreased ability to produce gonadal steroids (especially estradiol-17β).

Genetically Engineered Mouse Models of Ovarian Tumors Transgenic mice expressing a chimeric lutenizing hormone (LH) β submit (LHβ) in pituitary gonadotrophs have increased pituitary expression of LH mRNA and elevated circulating levels of LH (as well as estradiol and testosterone) but are infertile (Risma *et al.*, 1995, 1997). They ovulate infrequently, maintain a prolonged luteal phase, and develop a variety of ovarian lesions including cyst (blood and fluid filled) formation and ovarian tumors. A subset of LHβ transgenic mice developed ovarian granulosa and theca-interstitial cell tumors by 4–8 months of age as a result of the chronic stimulation

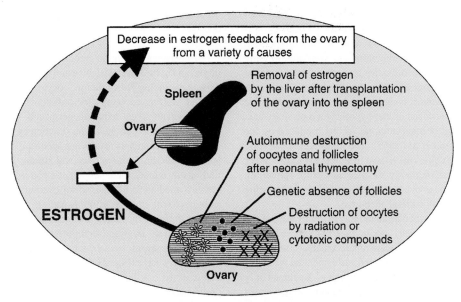

Figure 21-66. Multiple pathogenic mechanisms in ovarian tumorigenesis of mice resulting in decreased negative feedback by diminished levels of gonadal steroids, particularly estrogen.

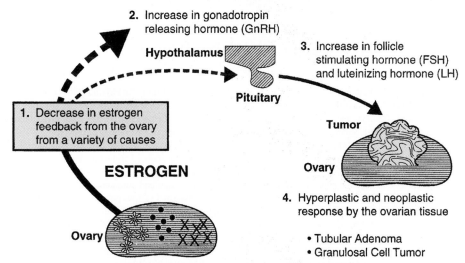

Figure 21-67. Decreased circulating estrogens release the hypothalamus–pituitary gland from negative feedback inhibition.

The increased gonadotrophin levels (LH and FSH) result in the mouse ovary being at greater risk of developing tubular adenomas in chronic studies.

by the elevated gonadotropin (LH) levels. The findings of granulosa and stromal cell tumors in transgenic mice whose only genetic alteration is the addition of a gene encoding a chimeric gonadotropin suggest that abnormal gonadotropin stimulation is tumorigenic to the ovary in mice. In addition, genetically altered mice deficient in inhibin (hormone which suppresses the secretion of follicle stimulating hormone [FSH]) have elevated blood concentrations of FSH (two- to threefold) and develop granulosa cell tumors and mixed or incompletely differentiated gonadal stromal tumors of the ovary (Matzuk *et al.*, 1992; Amsterdam and Selvaraj, 1997).

Another example of hormonal dysregulation leading to the induction of ovarian tumors are the estrogen receptor knockout (ERKO) mice that lack the alpha estrogen receptors and are unable to regulate gonadotropin secretion due to a lack of negative feedback control by the blood estrogen level (Lubahn *et al.*, 1993; Korach,

1994). Female mice are infertile with hypoplastic uteri and hyperemic ovaries with no detectable corpora lutea. There was no uterine stimulation (uterotropic response) when treated with tamoxifen (an estrogen agonist in mice). ERKO mice also develop ovarian granulosal cell tumors in response to the chronic elevations in circulating gonadotropin levels.

Secondary Mechanisms of Ovarian Tumoringenesis in Rodents

A review of studies on mutant mice and the NTP study of nitrofurantoin support an interpretation that the unique intense hyperplasia of ovarian surface epithelium and stromal cells, leading eventually to an increased incidence of tubular adenomas and occasionally granulosa cell tumors, develops secondary to chronic pituitary gonadotrophic hormone stimulation (Willemsen *et al.*, 1993). Factors that destroy or greatly diminish the numbers of ovarian follicles, such as senescence, genetic deletion of follicles, X-irradiation, drugs and chemicals such as nitrofurantoin, and early thymectomy with the development of autoantibodies to oocytes, are known to diminish sex steroid hormone secretion by the ovary. This results in elevated circulating levels of gonadotrophins, especially LH, due to decreased negative feedback on the hypothalamic-pituitary axis by estrogens and possibly other humoral factors produced by the graafian follicles (Carson *et al.*, 1989). The long-term stimulation of stromal (interstitial) cells, which have receptors for LH (Beamer and Tennent, 1986), and, indirectly, the ovarian surface epithelium appears to place the mouse ovary at increased risk for developing the unique tubular or tubulostromal adenomas.

The finding of similar tubular adenomas in the ovaries of the xenobiotic-treated and genetically sterile mice not exposed to exogenous chemicals supports the concept of a secondary (hormonally mediated) mechanism of ovarian oncogenesis associated with hormonal imbalances (Fig. 21-65). The ovarian tumors developed only in sterile mice in which the pituitary–hypothalamic axis was intact; administration of exogenous estrogen early in the course will prevent ovarian tumor development. The intense proliferation of ovarian surface epithelium and stromal (interstitial) cells with the development of unique tubular adenomas in response to sterility does not appear to have a counterpart in the ovaries of human adult females.

Experimental ovarian carcinogenesis has been investigated in inbred and hybrid strains of mice and induced by a diversity of mechanisms, including X-irradiation, oocytotoxic xenobiotic chemicals, ovarian grafting to ectopic or orthotopic sites, neonatal thymectomy, mutant genes reducing germ cell populations, and aging (Fig. 21-66). Disruptions in the function of graafian follicles by a variety of mechanisms results in a spectrum of ovarian proliferative lesions, including tumors (Hsu and Hsueh, 1997; Rao, 1981). The findings in mutant mice support the concept of a secondary (hormonally mediated) mechanism of ovarian carcinogenesis in mice, associated with sterility. Multiple pathogenetic factors that either destroy or diminish the numbers of graafian follicles in the ovary result in decreased sex hormone secretion (especially estradiol-17β), leading to a compensatory overproduction of pituitary gonadotrophins (particularly LH) (Fig. 21-66), which places the mouse ovary at an increased risk for developing tumors (Fig. 21-67). The intense proliferation of ovarian surface epithelium and stromal (interstitial) cells with the development of unique tubular adenomas in response to sterility does not appear to have a counterpart in the ovaries of human adult females.

REFERENCES

Abdo KM, Eustis SL, Haseman J, *et al.*: Toxicity and carcinogenicity of rotenone given in the feed to F344/N rats and B6C3F1 mice for up to two years. *Drug Chem Toxicol* 11:225–235, 1988.

Alison RH, Capen CC, Prentice DE: Neoplastic lesions of questionable significance to humans. *Toxicol Pathol* 22:179–186, 1994.

Alison RH, Morgan KT: Ovarian neoplasms in F344 rats and B6C3F1 mice. *Environ Health Perspect* 73:91–106, 1987.

Ambrogio SS, Connelly J, DiMaio D: Minocycline pigmentation of heart valves. *Cardiovas Pathol* 8:329–332, 1999.

Amsterdam A, Selvaraj N: Control of differentiation, transformation, and apoptosis in granulosa cells by oncogenes, oncoviruses, and tumor suppressor genes. *Endocr Rev* 18:435–461, 1997.

Armbrecht HJ, Wongsurawat N, Zenser TV, *et al.*: Differential effects of parathyroid hormone on the renal 125-dihydroxyvitamin D3 and 24,25-dihydroxyvitamin D3 production of young and adult rats. *Endocrinology* 111:1339–1344, 1982.

Arnaud CD, Pun K-K. Metabolism and assay of parathyroid hormone, in Coe FL, Favus MJ (eds.): *Disorders of Bone and Mineral Metabolism.* New York: Raven, 1992, pp. 107–122.

Arnold LL, Eldam M, van Gemert M, *et al.*: Chronic studies evaluating the carcinogenicity of monomethylarsonic acid in rats and mice. *Toxicology* 90:197–219, 2003.

Atterwill CK, Collins P, Brown CG, *et al.*: The perchlorate discharge test for examining thyroid function in rats. *J Pharmacol Meth* 18:199–203, 1987.

Attia MA: Neoplastic and non-neoplastic lesions in aging female rats with special reference to the functional morphology of the hyperplastic and neoplastic changes in the pituitary gland. *Arch Toxicol* 57:77–83, 1985.

Atwal OS: Ultrastructural pathology of ozone-induced experimental parathyroiditis. IV. Biphasic activity in the chief cells of regenerating parathyroid glands. *Am J Pathol* 95:611–632, 1979.

Atwal OS, Pemsingh RS: Morphology of microvascular changes and endothelial regeneration in experimental ozone-induced parathyroiditis. III. Some pathologic considerations. *Am J Pathol* 102:297–307, 1981.

Atwal OS, Samagh BS, Bhatnagar MK: A possible autoimmune parathyroiditis following ozone inhalation. II. A histopathologic, ultrastructural, and immunofluorescent study. *Am J Pathol* 80:53–68, 1975.

Atwal OS, Wilson T: Parathyroid gland changes following oxone inhalation. A morphologic study. *Arch Environ Health* 28:91–100, 1974.

Axelrod AA, Leblond CP: Induction of thyroid tumors in rats by low iodine diet. *Cancer* 8:339–367, 1955.

Azad N, Nayyar R, Tentler J, *et al.*: Anatomical and functional effects of estrogen-induced prolactinomas on the rat hypothalamus. *J Exp Pathol* 4:237–249, 1989.

Baer A: Sugars and adrenomedullary proliferative lesions: The effects of lactose and various polyalcohols. *J Am Coll Toxicol* 7:71–81, 1988.

Bär A: Significance of Leydig cell neoplasia in rats fed lactitol or lactose. *J Am Coll Toxicol* 11:189–207, 1992.

Barbosa JA, Gill BM, Takiyyuddin MA, *et al.*: Chromogranin A: Post-translational modifications in secretory granules. *Endocrinology* 128:174–190, 1991.

Barlet JP, Champredon C, Coxam V, *et al.*: Parathyroid hormone-related peptide might stimulate calcium secretion into the milk of goats. *J Endocrinol* 132:353–359, 1992.

Barsoum NJ, Moore JD, Gough AW, *et al.*: Morphofunctional investigations on spontaneous pituitary tumors in Wistar rats. *Toxicol Pathol* 13:200–208, 1985.

Barter RA, Klaassen CD: Rat liver microsomal UDP-glucuronosyltransferase activity toward thyroxine: Characterization, induction, and form specificity. *Toxicol Appl Pharmacol* 115:261–267, 1992a.

Barter RA, Klaassen CD: UDP-glucuronosyltransferase inducers reduce thyroid hormone levels in rats by an extrathyroidal mechanism. *Toxicol Appl Pharmacol* 113:36–42, 1992b.

Barter RA, Klaassen CD: Reduction of thyroid hormone levels and alteration of thyroid function by four representative UDP-glucuronosyltransferase inducers in rats. *Toxicol Appl Pharmacol* 128:9–17, 1994.

Bartke A, Sweeney CA, Johnson L, *et al.*: Hyperprolactinemia inhibits development of Leydig cell tumors in aging Fischer rats. *Exp Aging Res* 11:123–128, 1985.

Beamer WG, Tennent BJ: Gonadotropin uptake in genetic and irradiation models of ovarian tumorigenesis. *Biol Reprod* 34:761–770, 1986.

Berkvens JM, van Nesselrooy JHJ, Kroes R, *et al.*: Spontaneous tumours in the pituitary gland of old Wistar rats. A morphological and immunocytochemical study. *J Pathol* 130:179–191, 1980.

Berry PH: Effect of diet or reproductive status on the histology of spontaneous pituitary tumors in female Wistar rats. *Vet Pathol* 23:606–618, 1986.

Bidart J-M, Mian C, Lazar V, *et al.*: Expression of pendrin and the Pendred syndrome (PDS) gene in human thyroid tissues. *J Clin Endocrinol Metab* 85:2028–2033, 2000.

Biskind MS, Biskind JR: Development of tumors in the rat ovary after transplantation into the spleen. *Proc Soc Exp Biol Med* 55:176–179, 1944.

Blaakaer J, Baeksted M, Micic S, *et al.*: Gonadotrophin-releasing hormone agonist suppression of ovarian tumorigenesis in mice of the Wx/Wv genotype. *Biol Reprod* 53:775–779, 1995.

Boice JD Jr: Radiation-induced thyroid cancer—What's new? *J Natl Cancer Inst* 97:703–705, 2005.

Boorman GA, Hamlin MH, Eustis SL: Focal interstitial cell hyperplasia, testis, rat, in Jones TC, Möhr U, Hunt RD (eds.): *Monographs on Pathology of Laboratory Animals*. Berlin: Springer-Verlag, 1987, pp. 200–220.

Borzelleca JF, Capen CC, Hallagan JB: Lifetime toxicity carcinogenicity study of FC&C Red No. 3 (erythrosine) in rats. *Food Chem Toxicol* 25:723–733, 1987.

Bourdeau AM, Plachot JJ, Cournot-Witmer G, *et al.*: Parathyroid response to aluminum in vitro: Ultrastructural changes and PTH release. *Kidney Int* 31:15–24, 1987.

Braverman LE, He X, Pino S, *et al.*: The effect of perchlorate, thiocyanate, and nitrate on thyroid function in workers exposed to perchlorate long-term. *J Clin Endocrinol Metabol* 90(2):700–706, 2005.

Braverman LE, Pearce EN, HE X, *et al.*: Effects of six months of daily low-dose perchlorate exposure on thyroid function in healthy volunteers. *J Clin Endocrinol Metabol* 91(7):2721–2724, 2006.

Brown EM: PTH secretion in vivo and in vitro. Regulation by calcium and other secretagogues. *Miner Electrolyte Metab* 8:130–150, 1982.

Brown EM, Hebert SC: A cloned extracellular Ca^{2+}-sensing receptor: Molecular mediator of the actions of extracellular Ca^{2+} on parathyroid and kidney cells? *Kidney Int* 49:1042–1046, 1996.

Brown EM, Pollak M, Seidman CE, *et al.*: Calcium-ion-sensing cell-surface receptors. *N Engl J Med* 333:234–240, 1995.

Brown WR, Fetter AD, Van Ryzin RJ, *et al.*: Proliferative pituitary lesions in rats treated with salmon or porcine calcitonin. *Toxicol Pathol* 21:81–86, 1993.

Bulotta A, Hui H, Anastasi E, *et al.*: Cultured pancreatic ductal cells undergo cell cycle re-distribution and beta-cell-like differentiation in response to glucagon-like peptide I. *J Molecular Endocrinol* 29:347–360, 2002.

Burek JD: *Pathology of Aging Rats.* West Palm Beach, Florida: CRC Press, Inc., 1978.

Burns-Naas LA, Zorbas M, Jessen B, *et al.*: Increase in thyroid tumors in nelfinaver-treated rats is consistent with a rat-specific mechanism of thyroid neoplasia. *Hum Exp Toxicol* 24:643–654, 2005.

Burtis WJ: Parathyroid hormone-related protein: Structure, function, and measurement. *Clin Chem* 38:2171–2183, 1992.

Capen CC: Mechanistic considerations for thyroid gland neoplasia with FD&C Red No. 3 (erythrosine), in *The Toxicology Forum.* Proceedings of the 1989 Annual Winter Meeting, Washington, DC, 1989, pp. 113–130.

Capen CC: Age-related changes in structure and function of the parathyroid gland in laboratory rats, in Mohr U, Dungworth DL, Capen CC (eds.): *Pathobiology of the Aging Rat*, vol. II. Washington, DC: International Life Sciences Press (ILSI), 1994, pp. 199–226.

Capen CC: Functional and pathologic interrelationships of the pituitary gland and hypothalamus in animals, in Jones TC, Capen, CC, Mohr U (eds.): *Endocrine System. Series II. Monographs on Pathology of Laboratory Animals*, 2nd edn, International Life Sciences Institute Series. Berlin, Heidelberg, New York: Springer-Verlag, Inc., 1996a, pp. 3–32.

Capen CC: George Scott memorial lecture on mechanistic toxicology, in *The Toxicology Forum.* Proceedings of the 1996 Annual Summer Meeting, Aspen, CO, 7–12 July 1996b, pp. 441–465.

Capen CC: Pathobiology of parathyroid gland structure and function in animals, in Jones TC, Capen CC, Mohr U (eds.): *Endocrine System. Series II. Monographs on Pathology of Laboratory Animals*, 2nd edn, International Life Sciences Institute Series. Berlin, Heidelberg, New York: Springer-Verlag, Inc., 1996c, pp. 293–327.

Capen CC: Chemically induced injury of the parathyroid glands: Pathophysiology and mechanistic considerations, in Thomas JA, Colby H (eds.): *Endocrine Toxicology*, 2nd edn. Washington DC: Taylor and Francis, 1997a, pp. 1–42.

Capen, CC: Toxic responses of the parathyroid gland, in Sipes IG, McQueen CA, Gandolfi AJ (eds.): *Comprehensive Toxicology*, vol. 10, Chap. 51; Boekelheide K, *et al.* (eds.): *Reproductive and Endocrine Toxicology*. Oxford, New York, Tokyo: Elsevier Science/Pergamon, 1997b, pp. 679–689.

Capen CC: Mechanistic data and risk assessment of selected toxic end points of the thyroid gland. *Toxicol Pathol* 25:39–48, 1997.

Capen CC: Correlation of mechanistic data and histopathology in the evaluation of selected toxic endpoints of the endocrine system. *Toxicol Lett* 102–103:405–409, 1998.

Capen CC: Thyroid and parathyroid toxicology, in Harvey PW, Rush K, Cockburn A (eds.): *Endocrine and Hormonal Toxicology*. Sussex, England: John Wiley & Sons, Ltd., 1999, pp. 33–66.

Capen, CC: Comparative anatomy and physiology of the thyroid, in Braverman LE, Utiger RD (eds.): *Werner and Ingbar's The Thyroid: A Fundamental and Clinical Text*, 8th edn, Chap. 3. Philadelphia: Lippincott-Raven Publishers, 2000, pp. 20–44.

Capen CC: Overview of structural and functional lesions in endocrine organs of animals. *Toxicol Pathol* 29:8–33, 2001.

Capen CC: Tumors of the endocrine glands, in Meuten DJ (ed.): *Moulton's Tumors in Domestic Animals*, 4th edn. Ames, IA: Blackwell Science/Iowa State University Press, 2002, pp. 607–696.

Capen CC: Mechanisms of ovarian carcinogenesis. *Toxicol Pathol* 32:1–6, 2004.

Capen CC: Pathophysiology of the thyroid gland, in Dunlop RH, Malbert C, (eds.): *Veterinary Pathophysiology*. Ames, Iowa: Blackwell Publishing, 2004a, pp. 444–469.

Capen CC: Comparative toxicology of the thyroid gland. *Proceedings of the Midwest Regional Chapter of the Society of Toxicology*. Lincolnshire IL, 12 May 2006a.

Capen CC.: The endocrine glands, in Maxie MG (ed.): *Pathology of Domestic Animals*, 5th edn, vol. 3, Chap. 3. Amsterdam, New York: Elsevier, 2006b, pp. 325–428.

Capen CC, Beamer WG, Tennent BJ, *et al.*: Mechanisms of hormone-mediated carcinogenesis of the ovary in mice. *Mutat Res* 333:143–151, 1995.

Capen CC, De Lellis RA, Williams ED: Experimental thyroid carcinogenesis: Role of radiation and xenobiotic chemicals, in Karaoglou TG, Williams ED (eds.): *Radiation and Thyroid Cancer*. Singapore: World Scientific, 1999, pp. 167–176.

Capen CC, Gröne A, Bucci TJ, *et al.*: Changes in structure and function of the parathyroid gland, in Mohr U, Dungworth D, Capen C, Sundberg J (eds.): *Pathobiology of the Aging Mouse*. Washington, DC: International Life Sciences (ILSI) Press, 1996, pp. 109–124.

Capen CC, Martin SL: Endocrine system: Introduction, in Aiello SE (ed.): *The Merck Veterinary Manual*, 8th edn. New Jersey: Merck & Co., 1998, pp. 380–386.

Capen CC, Martin SL: The effects of xenobiotics on the structure and function of thyroid follicles and C-cells. *Toxicol Pathol* 17:266–293, 1989.

Capen CC, Sagartz J: A Ret transgenic mouse model of thyroid carcinogenesis. *Lab Anim Sci* 48:580–583, 1998.

Cardis E, Kesminiene A, Ivanov V, *et al*: Risk of thyroid cancer after exposure to ^{131}I in childhood. *J Natl Cancer Inst* 97:724–732, 2005.

Care AD: The placental transfer of calcium. *J Dev Physiol* 15:253–257, 1991.

Carson RS, Zhang Z, Hutchinson LA, *et al.*: Growth factors in ovarian function. *J Reprod Fert* 85:735–746, 1989.

Cattanach BM, Iddon A, Charlton HM, *et al.*: Gonadotropin releasing hormone deficiency in a mutant mouse with hypogonadism. *Nature* 269:238–240, 1977.

Chatani F, Nonoyama T, Katsuichi S, et al.: Stimulatory effect of luteinizing hormone on the development and maintenance of 5a-reduced steroid-producing testicular interstitial cell tumors in Fischer 344 rats. Anticancer Res 10:337–342, 1990.

Chattopadhyay N, Mithal A, Brown EM: The calcium-sensing receptor: A window into the physiology and pathophysiology of mineral ion metabolism. Endocr Rev 17:289–307, 1996.

Chen C, Klaassen CD: Rat multidrug resistance protein 4 (Mrp4, Abcc4): molecular cloning, organ distribution, postnatal renal expression, and chemical inducibility. Biochem Biophys Res Comm 317:46–53, 2004.

Chen C, Slitt AL, Dieter MZ, et al.: Up-regulation of Mrp4 expression in kidney of Mrp2-deficient TR− rats. Biochem Pharmacol 70:1088–1095, 2005.

Chen C, Staudingere JL, Klaassen CD: Nuclear receptor, pregnane X receptor, is required for induction of UDP-glucurononsyltransferases in mouse liver by pregnenolone-16α-carbonitrile. Drug Metab Disp 31:908–915, 2003.

Cheng X, Maher J, Dieter MZ, et al.: Regulation of mouse organic anion-transporting polypeptides (OATPS) in liver by prototypical microsomal enzyme inducers that activate distinct transcription factor pathways. Drug Metabol Disposition 33:1276–1282, 2005.

Chen-Pan C, Pan IJ, Yamamoto, Y, et al.: Prompt recovery of damaged adrenal medullae induced by salinomycin. Toxicol Pathol 27:563–572, 1999.

Chen-Pan C, Pan IJ, Yamamoto, Y, et al.: Recovery of injured adrenal medulla by differentiation of pre-existing undifferentiated chromaffin cells. Toxicol Pathol 30:165–172, 2002.

Cherrington NJ, Haartley DP, Li N, et al.: Organ distribution of multidrug resistance proteins 1, 2, and 3 (Mrp1, 2, and 3) mRNA and hepatic induction of Mrp3 by constitutive androstane receptor activators in rats. J Pharm Exp Toxicol 300:97–104, 2002.

Cherrington NJ, Slitt AL, Maher JM, et al.: Induction of multidrug resistance protein 3 (MRP3) in vivo is independent of constitutive androstane receptor. Drug Metabol Disp 31:1315–1319, 2003.

Chisari FV, Hochstein HD, Kirschstein RL: Parathyroid necrosis and hypocalcemic tetany induced in rabbits by L-asparaginase. Am J Pathol 69:461–476, 1972.

Cho J-Y, Sagartz JE, Capen CC, et al.: Early cellular abnormalities induced by Ret/PTC1 oncogene in thyroid-targeted transgenic mice. Oncogene 18:3659–3665, 1999.

Cho J-Y, Sagartz JE, Capen CC, et al: Early cellular abnormalities induced by Ret/PTC1 oncogene in thyroid-targeted transgenic mice. Oncogene 18:3659–3665, 1999.

Clegg ED, Cook JC, Chapin RE, et al.: Leydig cell hyperplasia and adenoma formation: Mechanisms and relevance to humans. Reprod Toxicol 11:107–121, 1997.

Clements FW: Relationship of thyrotoxicosis and carcinoma of thyroid to endemic goiter. Med J Aust 2:894–899, 1954.

Clemmesen J, Fuglsang-Frederiksen V, Plum CM: Are anticonvulsants oncogenic? Lancet 1:705–707, 1974.

Clemmesen J, Hjalgrim-Jensen S: On the absence of carcinogenicity to man of phenobarbital, in: Statistical Studies in the Aetiology of Malignant Neoplasms. Acta Pathol Microb Scand 261(Suppl):38–50, 1977.

Clemmesen J, Hjalgrim-Jensen S: Is phenobarbital carcinogenic? A follow-up of 8078 epileptics. Ecotoxicol Environ Safety 1:255–260, 1978.

Clemmesen J, Hjalgrim-Jensen S: Does phenobarbital cause intracranial tumors? A follow-up through 35 years. Ecotoxicol Environ Safety 5:255–260, 1981.

Clewell RA, Merill EA, Narayanan L, et al.: Evidence for competitive inhibition of iodide uptake by perchlorate and translocation of perchlorate into the thyroid. Intl J Toxicol 23:17–23, 2004.

Cohen IR, Sims ML, Robbins MR, et al.: The reversible effects of raloxifene on luteinizing hormone levels and ovarian morphology in mice. Reprod Toxicol 14:37–44, 2000.

Cohn DV, Fasciotto BH, Zhang J-X, et al.: Chemistry and biology of chromogranin A (secretory protein-I) of the parathyroid and other endocrine glands, in Bilezikian JP, Marcus R, Levine MA (eds.): The Parathyroids: Basic and Clinical Concepts. New York: Raven Press, 1993, pp. 107–119.

Colby HD: Adrenal gland toxicity: Chemically induced dysfunction. J Am Col Toxicol 7:45–69, 1988.

Collins WT Jr, Capen CC: Ultrastructural and functional alterations in thyroid glands of rats produced by polychlorinated biphenyls compared with the effects of iodide excess and deficiency, and thyrotropin and thyroxine administration. Virchows Arch B Cell Pathol 33:213–231, 1980a.

Collins WT Jr, Capen CC: Biliary expression of ^{125}I-thyroxine and fine structural alterations in the thyroid glands of Gunn rats fed polychlorinated biphenyls. Lab Invest 43:158–164, 1980b.

Cook JC, Klinefelter GR, Hardisty JF, et al.: Rodent Leydig cell tumorigenesis: A review of the physiology, pathology, mechanisms, and relevance to humans. Crit Rev Toxicol 29:169–261, 1999.

Cook JC, Murray SM, Frame SR, et al.: Induction of Leydig cell adenomas by ammonium perfluorooctanoate: A possible endocrine-related mechanism. Toxicol Appl Pharmacol 113:209–217, 1992.

Cook LS, Weiss NS, Schwartz SM, et al.: Population-based study of tamoxifen therapy and subsequent ovarian, endometrial, and breast cancers. J Natl Cancer Inst 87:1359–1364, 1995.

Cooper DS, Axelrod L, DeGroot LJ, et al.: Congenital goiter and the development of metastatic follicular carcinoma with evidence for a leak of non-hormonal iodide: Clinical, pathological, kinetic, and biochemical studies and a review of the literature. J Clin Endocrinol Metab 52:294–306, 1981.

Copp DH: Endocrine regulation of calcium metabolism. Annu Rev Physiol 32:61–86, 1970.

Cranston AN, Ponder BAJ: Modulation of medullary thyroid carcinoma penetrance suggests the presence of modifier genes in a RET transgenic mouse model. Cancer Res 63:4777–4780, 2003.

Curran PG, DeGroot LJ: The effect of hepatic enzyme-inducing drugs on thyroid hormones and the thyroid gland. Endocr Rev 12:135–150, 1991.

Davies TS, Monro A: Marketed human pharmaceuticals reported to be tumorigenic in rodents. J Am Coll Toxicol 14:90–107, 1995.

Davis BJ, Maronpot RR: Chemically associated toxicity and carcinogenicity of the ovary, in Huff J, Boyd J, Barrett J (eds.): Cellular and Molecular Mechanisms of Hormonal Carcinogenesis: Environmental Influences. New York: Wiley-Liss, 1996, pp. 285–309.

Deftos L: Chromogranin A: Its role in endocrine function and as an endocrine and neuroendocrine tumor marker. Endocr Rev 12:181–197, 1991.

DeGrandi PB, Kraehenbuhl JP, Campiche MA: Ultrastructural localization of calcitonin in the parafollicular cells of the pig thyroid gland with cytochrome c-labeled antibody fragments. J Cell Biol 50:446–456, 1971.

DeGroef B, Decallonne BR, Van der Geyten S, et al.: Perchlorate versus other environmental sodium/iodide symporter inhibitors: Potential thyroid-related health effects. Euro J Endocrinol 155:17–25, 2006.

DeLellis RA, Dayal Y, Tischler AS, et al.: Multiple endocrine neoplasia syndromes. Cellular origins and interrelationships. Int Rev Exp Pathol 28:163–215, 1986.

DeLellis RA, Nunnemacher G, Bitman WR, et al.: C-cell hyperplasia and medullary thyroid carcinoma in the rat: An immunohistochemical and ultrastructural analysis. Lab Invest 40:140–154, 1979.

DeLellis RA, Nunnemacher G, Wolfe HJ: C cell hyperplasia, an ultrastructural analysis. Lab Invest 36:237–248, 1977.

Delmas PD, Bjarnason NH, Mitlak BH, et al.: Effects of raloxifene on bone mineral density, serum cholesterol concentrations, and uterine endometrium in postmenopausal women. N Engl J Med 337:23:1641–1647, 1997.

Dieter MZ, Maher JM, Cheng X, et al.: Expression and regulation of the sterol half-transporter genes ABCG5 and ABCG8 in rats. Comp Biochem Physiol 139:209–218, 2004.

Döhler K-D, Wong CC, von zut Mühlen A: The rat as model for the study of drug effects on thyroid function: consideration of methodological problems. Pharmacol Ther 5:305–313, 1979.

Dominick MA, Bobrowski WA, MacDonald JR, *et al.*: Morphogenesis of a zone-specific adrenocortical cytotoxicity in guinea pigs administered PD 132301-2, an inhibitor of acyl-CoA; cholesterol acyltransferase. *Toxicol Pathol* 21:54–62, 1993.

Dominick MA, McGuire EJ, Reindel JF, *et al.*: Subacute toxicity of a novel inhibitor of acyl-CoA: Cholesterol acyltransferase in beagle dogs. *Fundam Appl Toxicol* 20:217–224, 1993.

Donaubauer HH, Kramer M, Krieg K, *et al.*: Investigations of the carcinogenicity of the LH-RH analog buserelin (HOE 766) in rats using the subcutaneous route of administration. *Fundam Appl Toxical* 9:738–752, 1987.

Doniach I: Effects including carcinogenesis of ^{131}I and X ray on the thyroid of experimental animals: A review. *Health Phys* 9:1357–1362, 1963.

Doniach I: Aetiological consideration of thyroid carcinoma, in Smithers D (ed.): *Tumors of the Thyroid Gland*. London: E & S Livingstone, 1970, pp. 55–72.

Doss JC, Gröne A, Capen CC, *et al.*: Immunohistochemical localization of chromogranin A in endocrine tissues and endocrine tumors of dogs. *Vet Pathol* 35:312–315, 1998.

Drucker DJ, Philippe J, Mojsov S, *et al.*: Glucagon-like peptide I stimulates insulin gene expression and increases cyclic AMP levels in a rat islet cell line. *Proc Natl Acad Sci USA* 84:3434–3438, 1987.

Dunn RT, Klaassen CD: Thyroid hormone modulation of rat sulphotransferase mRNA expression. *Xenobiotica* 30:345–357, 2000.

Eisen D, Hakim MD: Minocycline-induced pigmentation. Incidence, prevention and management. *Drug Safety* 18:431–440, 1998.

El Etreby MF, Lorenz B. Habenicht UF: Immunocytochemical studies on the pituitary gland and spontaneous pituitary tumors of Sprague-Dawley rats. *Pathol Res Pract* 183:645–650, 1988.

Everett LA, Belyantseva IA, Noben-Trauth K, *et al.*: Targeted disruption of mouse *PDS* provides insight about the inner-ear defects encountered in Pendred Syndrome. *Hum Mol Genet* 10:153–161, 2001.

Everett LA, Morsli H, Wu DK, *et al.*: Expression pattern of the mouse ortholog of the Pendred's syndrome gene (*Pds*) suggests a key role for pendrin in the inner ear. *Proc Natl Acad Sci U S A* 96:9727–9732, 1999.

Evista Package Insert. Indianapolis, IN: Eli Lilly, 1997.

Fasciotto BH, Gorr S-U, Bourdeau AM, *et al.*: Autocrine regulation of parathyroid secretion: Inhibition of secretion by chromogranin-A (secretory protein-I) and potentiation of secretion by chromogranin-A and pancreastatin antibodies. *Endocrinology* 127:1329–1335, 1990.

Federal Drug Administration, USA. Byetta (Exenatide), *FDA Pharmacology Review.* [http://www.fda.gov/cder/foi/nda/2005/021773 Byetta_pharmr.pdf, 2005b]

Federal Drug Administration, USA. Forteo (Teriparatide), *FDA Medical Review, Part 3.* [http://www.fda.gov/cder/foi/nda/2002/21-31 Forteo Mmedr P3.pdf, 2005a]

Finch JM, Osimtz TG, Gabriel KL, *et al.*: A mode of action for the induction of thyroid gland tumors by pyrethrins in the rat. *Toxicol Appl Pharmacol* 214:253–262, 2006.

Fisher B, Costantino JP, Redmond CK, *et al.*: Endometrial cancer in tamoxifen-treated breast cancer patients: Findings from the National Surgical Adjuvant Breast and Bowel Project (NSABP) B-14. *J Natl Cancer Inst* 86:527–537, 1994.

Fort FL, Miyajima H, Ando T, *et al.*: Mechanism for species-specific induction of Leydig cell tumors in rats by lansoprazole. *Fundam Appl Toxicol* 26:191–202, 1995.

Foster GV, Byfield PGH, Gudmundsson TV: Calcitonin, in MacIntyre I (ed.): *Clinics in Endocrinology and Metabolism*, vol. 1. Philadelphia: WB Saunders, 1972, pp. 93–124.

Fraichard A, Chassande O, Plateroti M, *et al*: The T_3R gene encoding a thyroid hormone receptor is essential for post-natal development and thyroid hormone production. *Embo J* 16:4412–4420, 1997.

Friedman GD: Barbiturates and lung cancer in humans. *JNCI* 67:291–295, 1981.

Frith CH, Botts S, Jokinen MP, *et al.*: Non-proliferative lesions of the endocrine system in rats, in *Guides for Toxicologic Pathology*. Washington DC: STP/ARP/AFIP, 2000, pp. 1–22.

Frith CH, Zuna RF, Morgan K: A morphologic classification and incidence of spontaneous ovarian neoplasms in three strains of mice. *J Natl Cancer Inst* 67:693–702, 1981.

Furth J, Boon MC: Induction of ovarian tumors in mice by X-rays. *Cancer Res* 7:241–245, 1947.

Furth J: Morphologic changes associated with thyrotropin-secreting pituitary tumors. *Am J Pathol* 30:421–463, 1954.

Gardner WU: Ovarian and lymphoid tumors in female mice subsequent to Roentgen-Ray irradiation and hormone treatment. *Proc Soc Exper Biol Med* 75:434–436, 1950.

Gimm O, Dralle H: C-cell cancer-prevention and treatment. *Langenbecks Arch Surg* 384:16–23, 1999.

Goltzman D, Bennett HPJ, Koutsilieris M, *et al.*: Studies of the multiple molecular forms of bioactive parathyroid hormone and parathyroid hormone2Dlike substances. *Recent Prog Horm Res* 42:665–703, 1986.

González-Suárez I, Álverez-Hernández D, Córrillo-Lopez N, *et al.*: Aluminum post-transcription regulation of parathyroid hormone synthesis: A role for the calcium-sensing receptor. *Kidney Intl* 68:2484–2496, 2005.

Gröne A, Rosol TJ, McCauley K, *et al.*: Cancer-associated hypercalcemia: parathyroid hormone-related protein (PTHrP) expression in low and high serum calcium variants of the canine apocrine adenocarcinoma (CAC-8) model of humoral hypercalcemia in nude mice, in Norman AW, Bouillonn R, Thomasset M (eds.): *Abstracts (No. 80) of Tenth Workshop on Vitamin D.* Strasbourg, France, 24–29 May 1997, p. 45; and published *Vitamin D - Chemistry, Biology, and Clinical Applications of the Steroid Hormone.* University of California Printing and Reprographics, 1997, pp. 497–498.

Gunnison AF, Bowers A, Nadziejko C, *et al.*: Modulation of the inflammatory effects of inhaled ozone in rats by subcutaneous prolactin-secreting, pituitary-derived tumors. *Fundam Appl Toxicol* 37:88–94, 1997.

Guo GL, Choudhuri S, Klaassen: Induction profile of rat organic anion transporting polypeptide 2 (oatp2) by prototypical drug-metabolizing enzyme inducers that activate gene expression through ligand-activated transcription factor pathways. *J Pharmacol Exp Ther* 300:206–212, 2002.

Guthrie MJ: Tumorigenesis in intrasplenic ovaries in mice. *Cancer* 10:190–203, 1957.

Habener JF: Recent advances in parathyroid hormone research. *Clin Biochem* 14:223–229, 1981.

Hard GC: Recent developments in the investigation of thyroid regulation and thyroid carcinogenesis. *Environ Health Perspect* 106:427–436, 1998.

Hart JE: Endocrine pathology of estrogens: Species differences. *Pharmac Ther* 47:203–218, 1990.

Hart MM, Swackhamer ES, Straw JA: Studies on the site of action of *o,p'*-DDD in the dog adrenal cortex. II. TPNH- and corticosteroid precursor-stimulation of *o,p'*-DDD inhibited steroidogenesis. *Steroids* 17:575–586, 1971.

Haseman JK, Hailey JR, Morris RW: Spontaneous neoplasm incidences in Fischer 344 rats and B6C3F$_1$ mice in two-year carcinogenicity studies: A national toxicology program update. *Toxicol Pathol* 26:428–441, 1998.

Hazewinkel HAW: Dietary influences on calcium homeostasis and the skeleton, in *Proceedings of the First Purina International Nutrition Symposium.* Orlando FL: Eastern States Veterinary Conference, 1991, pp. 51–61.

Henderson JE, Amizuka N, Warshawsky H, *et al*: Nucleolar localization of parathyroid hormone-related peptide enhances survival of chondrocytes under conditions that promote apoptotic cell death. *Mol Cell Biol* 15:4064–4075, 1995.

Hiasa Y, Kitahori Y, Kato Y, *et al.*: Potassium perchlorate, potassium iodide, and propylthiouracil: Promoting effect on the development of thyroid tumors in rats treated with N-Bis(2-hydroxypropyl)-nitrosamine. *Jpn J Cancer Res* 78:1335–1340, 1987.

Hill RN, Crisp TM, Hurley PM, *et al.*: Risk assessment of thyroid follicular cell tumors. *Environ Health Perspect* 106:447–457, 1998.

Hill RN, Erdreich LS, Paynter O, *et al.*: Thyroid follicular cell carcinogenesis. *Fundam Appl Toxicol* 12:629–697, 1989.

Hill RN, Erdreich LS, Paynter O, *et al.*: Assessment of thyroid follicular cell tumors. Risk Assessment Forum, U.S. Environmental Protection Agency, Washington, DC, March 1999, pp. 1–43.

Hinson JP, Raven PW: Effects of endocrine-disrupting chemicals on adrenal function. *Best Pract Clin Endocrinol Metabol* 20:111–120, 2006.

Hock JM: Anabolic actions of PTH in the skeleton of animals. *J Musculoskeletal Neurol Interactions* 2:33–47, 2001.

Hock JM, Krishnan V, Onyia JE, *et al.*:Osteoblast apoptosis and bone turnover. *J Bone Miner Res* 16:975–984, 2001.

Hofbauer LC: Osteoprotegerin ligand and osteoprotegerin: Novel implications for osteoclast biology and bone metabolism. *Eur J Endocrinol* 141:195–210, 1999.

Hofbauer LC, Khosla S, Dunstan CR, *et al*: The roles of osteoprotegerin and osteoprotegerin ligand in the paracrine regulation of bone resorption. *J Bone Miner Res* 15:2–12, 2000.

Holz GG, Kühtreiber WM, Habener JF: Pancreatic beta cells are rendered glucose-competent by the insulinotrophic hormone, glucagon-like peptide-1 (7-37). *Nature* 361:362–365, 1993.

Hood A, Allen ML, Liu Y, *et al.*: Induction of T4 UDP-GT activity, serum thyroid stimulating hormone and thyroid follicular cell proliferation in mice treated with microsomal enzyme inducers. *Toxicol Appl Pharmacol* 188:6–13, 2003.

Hood A, Harstad E, Klaassen CD: Effects of UDP-glucuronosyltransferase (UDP-GT) inducers on thyroid cell proliferation. *Toxicologist* 15:229, 1995.

Hood A, Hashmi R, Klaassen CD: Effects of microsomal enzyme inducers on thyroid-follicular cell proliferation, hyperplasia, and hypertrophy. *Toxicol Appl Pharmacol* 160:163–170, 1999a.

Hood A, Klaassen CD: Differential effects of microsomal enzyme inducers on *in vitro* thyroxine (T_4) and triiodothyronine (T_3) glucuronidation. *Toxicol Sci* 55:78–84, 2000a.

Hood A, Klaassen CD: Effects of microsomal enzyme inducers on outer-ring deiodinase activity toward thyroid hormones in various rat tissues. *Toxicol Appl Pharmacol* 163:240–248, 2000b.

Hood A, Liu YP, Gattone VH II, *et al.*: Sensitivity of thyroid gland growth to thyroid stimulating hormone (TSH) in rats treated with antithyroid drugs. *Toxicol Sci* 49:263–271, 1999b.

Hood A, Liu YP, Klaassen CD: Effects of phenobarbital, pregnenolone-16α-carbonitrile, and propylthiouracil on thyroid follicular cell proliferation. *Toxicol Sci* 50:45–53, 1999a.

Hooth MJ, DeAngelo AV, George MH, *et al.*: Subchronic sodium chlorate exposure in drinking water results in a concentration-dependent increase in rat thyroid follicular cell hyperplasia. *Toxicol Pathol* 29:250–259, 2001.

Hotz KJ, Wilson AGE, Thake DC, *et al.*: Mechanism of thiazopyr-induced effects on thyroid hormone homeostasis in male Sprague-Dawley rats. *Toxicol Appl Pharmacol* 142:133–142, 1997.

Hsu SY, Hsueh AJW: Hormonal regulation of apoptosis: An ovarian perspective. *Trends Endocrinol Metab* 8:207–213, 1997.

Hummel KP: Induced ovarian tumors. *JNCI* 15:711–715, 1954.

Hurley PM, Hill RN, Whiting RJ: Mode of carcinogenic action of pesticides inducing thyroid follicular cell tumors in rodents. *Environ Health Perspect* 106:437–445, 1998.

Ingbar SH: Autoregulation of the thyroid. Response to iodide excess and depletion. *Mayo Clin Proc* 47:814, 1972.

Jacobs JW: Calcitonin gene expression. *J Bone Miner Res* 3:151, 1985.

Jaffe N, Traggis D, Lakshmi D, *et al.*: Comparison of daily and twice-weekly schedule of L-asparaginase in childhood leukemia. *Pediatrics* 49:590–595, 1972.

Jameson JL, Weiss J, Polak JM, *et al.*: Glycoprotein hormone alpha-subunit-producing pituitary adenomas in rats treated for one year with calcitonin. *Am J Pathol* 140:75–84, 1992.

Jerome CP, Johnson CS, Vafai HT, *et al.*: Effect of treatment for 6 months with human parathyroid hormone (1-34) peptide in ovariectomized cynamolgus monkeys (*Macaca fascicularis*). *Bone* 25:301–309, 1999.

Jhiang SM, Cho J-Y, Furminger TL, *et al.*: Thyroid carcinomas in RET/PTC transgenic mice, in Schwab M, Rabes H, Munk K, Hofschneider PH (eds.): *Genes and Environment in Cancer. Recent Results in Cancer Research*, 1998b, pp. 265–270.

Jhiang SM, Cho J-Y, Ryu K-Y, *et al.*: An immunohistochemical study of Na+/I⁻ symporter in human thyroid tissues and salivary gland tissues. *Endocrinology* 139:4416, 1998.

Jhiang SM, Sagartz JE, Tong Q, *et al.*: Targeted expression of the *ret*/PTC1 oncogene induces papillary thyroid carcinomas. *Endocrinology* 137:375–378, 1996.

Jiang Y, Zhao JJ, Mitlak BH, *et al.*: Teriparatide [recombinant human parathyroid hormone (1-34)] improved both cortical and cancellous bone structure. *J Bone Min Res* 18:1932–1941, 2003.

Johnson DR, Klaassen CD: Regulation of rat multidrug resistance protein 2 by classes of prototypical microsomal enzyme inducers that activate distinct transcription pathways. *Toxicol Sci* 67:182–189, 2002a.

Johnson DR, Klaassen CD: Role of rat multidrug resistance protein 2 in plasma and biliary disposition of dibromosulfophthalein after microsomal enzyme induction. *Toxicol Appl Pharmacol* 180:56–63, 2002b.

Junquero P, Pilon A, Carilla-Durand E, *et al.*: Lack of toxic effects of F12511, a novel potent inhibitor of ACYL-co-enzymeA:cholesterol O-ACYL transferase, on human adrenal cortical cells in culture. *Biochem Pharmacol* 61:387–398, 2001.

Kalina M, Pearse AGE: Ultrastructural localization of calcitonin in C-cells of dog thyroid: An immunocytochemical study. *Histochemie* 26:1–8, 1971.

Kalu DN, Hardin RR, Murata I, *et al.*: Age-dependent modulation of parathyroid hormone action. *Age* 5:25–29, 1982.

Kanno J, Nemoto T, Kasuga T, *et al.*: Effects of a six-week exposure to excess iodide on thyroid glands of growing and nongrowing male Fischer-344 rats. *Toxicol Pathol* 22:23–28, 1994.

Keenan KP, Smith PF, Hertzog P, *et al.*: The effects of overfeeding and dietary restriction on Sprague-Dawley rat survival and early pathology biomarkers of aging. *Toxicol Pathol* 22:300–315, 1994.

Keenan KP, Soper KA, Smith PF: Diet, overfeeding, and moderate dietary restriction in control Sprague-Dawley rats: I. Effects on spontaneous neoplasms. *Toxicol Pathol* 23:269–286, 1995.

Kennedy TH, Purves HD: Studies on experimental goiter: Effect of *Brassica* seed diets on rats. *Br J Exp Pathol* 22:241–244, 1941.

Klaassen CD: Xenobiotic transporters: Another protective mechanism for chemicals. *Intl J Toxicol* 21:7–12, 2002.

Klaassen CD, Hood AM: Effects of microsomal enzyme inducers on thyroid follicular cell proliferation and thyroid hormone metabolism. *Toxicol Pathol* 29:34–40, 2001.

Klaassen CD, Slitt AL: Regulation of hepatic transporters by xenobiotic receptors. *Current Drug Metabol* 6:309–328, 2005.

Klugbauer S, Lengfelder E, Demidchik EP, *et al.*: High prevalence of RET rearrangement in thyroid tumors of children from Belarus after the Chernobyl reactor accident. *Oncogene* 11:2459–2467, 1995.

Knostman KAB, Jhiang SM, Capen CC: Genetic models in thyroid cancer: The role of mouse models. *Vet Pathol* 44:1–14, 2007.

Kohn LD, Suzuki K, Nakazato M, *et al*: Effects of thyroglobulin and pendrin on iodide flux through the thyrocyte. *Trends Endocrinol Metab* 12:10–16, 2001.

Kolaja KL, Klaassen CD: Dose-response examination of UDP-glucuronosyltransferase inducers and their ability to increase both TGF-β expression and thyroid follicular cell apoptosis. *Toxicol Sci* 46:31–37, 1998.

Kolaja KL, Petrick JS, Klaassen CD: Inhibition of gap-junctional-intercellular communication in thyroid-follicular cells by propylthiouracil and low iodine diet. *Toxicology* 143:195–202, 2000.

Kopp P: Pendred's syndrome: Identification of the genetic defect a century after its recognition. *Thyroid* 9:65–69, 1999.

Korach KS: Insights from the study of animals lacking functional estrogen receptor. *Science* 266:1524–1527, 1994.

Kronenberg HM, Igarashi T, Freeman MW, *et al.*: Structure and expression of the human parathyroid hormone gene. *Recent Prog Horm Res* 42:641–663, 1986.

Lacroix L, Mian C, Caillou B, *et al*: Na$^+$/I$^-$ symporter and Pendred syndrome gene and protein expressions in human extra-thyroidal tissues. *Eur J Endocrinol* 144:297–302, 2001.

Lamas L, Ingbar SH: The effect of varying iodine content on the susceptibility of thyroglobulin to hydrolysis by thyroid acid protease. *Endocrinology* 102:188–197, 1978.

Lamm SH, Braverman LE, Li FX, *et al*.: Thyroid health status of ammonium perchlorate workers: A cross-sectional occupational health study. *J Occup Environ Med* 41:248–260, 1999.

Lamm SH, Doemland M: Has perchlorate in drinking water increased the rate of congenital hypothyroidism? *J Occup Environ Med* 41:409–411, 1999.

LaPerle KMD, Jhiang SM: Iodine: Symporter and oxidation, thyroid hormone biosynthesis, in Henry HL, Norman AW (eds.): *Encyclopedia of Hormones*, Amsterdam: Academic Press, 2003, 2:519–522.

LaPerle KMD, Jhiang SM, Capen, CC: Loss of p53 promotes anaplasia and local invation in ret/PTC1-induced thyroid carcinomas. *Am J Pathol* 157:671–677, 2000.

Latendresse JR, Azhar S, Brooks CL, *et al*.: Pathogenesis of cholesteryl lipidosis of adrenocortical and ovarian interstitial cells in F344 rats caused by tricresyl phosphate and butylated triphenyl phosphate. *Toxicol Appl Pharmacol* 122:281–289, 1993.

Latendresse JR, Brooks CL, Capen CC: Pathologic effects of butylated triphenyl phosphate-based hydraulic fluid and tricresyl phosphate on the adrenal gland, ovary and testis in the F344 rat. *Toxicol Pathol* 22:341–352, 1994a.

Latendresse JR, Brooks CL, Capen CC: Toxic effects of butylated triphenyl phosphate-based hydraulic fluid and tricresyl phosphate in female F344 rats. *Vet Pathol* 32:394–402, 1995.

Latendresse JR, Brooks CL, Fleming CD, *et al*.: Reproductive toxicity of butylated triphenyl phosphate (BTP) and tricresyl phosphate (TCP) fluids in F344 rats. *Fundam Applied Toxicol* 22:392–399, 1994b.

Leblanc B, Paulus G, Andreu M, *et al*.: Immunocytochemistry of thyroid C-cell complexes in dogs. *Vet Pathol* 27:445–452, 1990.

Lee W, Chiacchierini RP, Shleien B, *et al*: Thyroid tumors following ^{131}I or localized X irradiation to the thyroid and pituitary glands in rats. *Radiat Res* 92:307–319, 1982.

Li MH, Gardner WU: Further studies on the pathogenesis of ovarian tumors in mice. *Cancer Res* 9:35–44, 1949.

Li Z, Li FX, Byrd D, *et al*.: Neonatal thyroxine level and perchlorate in drinking water. *J Occup Environ Med* 42:200–205, 2000.

Lima FRS, Gervais A, Colin C, *et al*.: Regulation of microglial development: A novel role for thyroid hormone. *J Neurosci* 21:2028–2038, 2001.

Liu J, Liu Y, Barter RA, *et al*.: Alteration of thyroid homeostais by UDP-glucuronosyltransferase inducers in rats: A dose-response study. *J Pharmacol Exp Ther* 273:977–985, 1995.

Lubahn DB, Moyer JS, Golding TS, *et al*.: Alteration of reproductive function but not prenatal sexual development after insertional disruption of the mouse estrogen receptor gene. *Proc Natl Acad Sci U S A* 90:11162–11166, 1993.

Lupulescu A, Potorac E, Pop A: Experimental investigation on immunology of the parathyroid gland. *Immunology* 14:475–482, 1968.

Lynch BS, Capen CC, Nestmann ER, *et al*.: Review of subchronic/chronic toxicity of antimony potassium tartrate. *Reg Toxicol Pharmacol* 30:9–17, 1999.

Lynch BS, Tischler AS, Capen C, *et al*.: Low digestible carbohydrates (polyols and lactose): Significance of adrenal medullary proliferative lesions in the rat. *Regul Toxicol Pharmacol* 23:256–297, 1996.

Maher JM, Cherrington NJ, Slitt AL, *et al*.: Tissue distribution and induction of the rat multidrug resistance-associated proteins 5 and 6. *Life Sci* 78:2219–2225, 2005.

Majumder S, Brown K, Qiu F-H, *et al*.: c-kit Protein, a transmembrane kinase: Identification in tissues and characterization. *Mol Cell Biol* 8:4896–4903, 1988.

Manger WM, Hulse MC, Forsyth MS, *et al*.: Effect of pheochromocytoma and hypophysectomy on blood pressure and catecholamines in NEDH rats. *Hypertension* 4(Suppl 2):200–202, 1982.

Many M-C, Denef J-F, Haumont S, *et al*.: Morphological and functional changes during thyroid hyperplasia and involution in C3H mice: Effects of iodine and 3,5,3′-triiodothyronine during involution. *Endocrinology* 116:798, 1985.

Marchant J: The chemical induction of ovarian tumours in mice. *Br J Cancer* 11:452–464, 1957.

Marchant J: The development of ovarian tumors in ovaries grafted from mice treated with dimethylbenzanthracene. Inhibition by the presence of normal ovarian tissue. *Br J Cancer* 14:514–519, 1960.

Martin TJ, Gillespie MT: Receptor activator of nuclear factor kappa B ligand (RANK L): Another link between breast and bone. *Trends Endocrinol Metab* 12:2–4, 2001.

Matzuk MM, Finegold MJ, Su JG, *et al*.: Alpha-inhibin is a tumour-suppressor gene with gonadal specificity in mice. *Nature* 360:313–319, 1992.

McClain RM: Mechanistic considerations in the regulation and classification of chemical carcinogens, in Kotsonis FN, Mackey M, Hjelle J (eds.): *Nutritional Toxicology*. New York: Raven Press, 1994, pp. 273–304.

McClain RM: The use of mechanistic data in cancer risk assessment: Case example—Sulfonamides, in *Low-Dose Extrapolation of Cancer Risks: Issues and Perspectives*, International Life Sciences Institute Series. Washington DC: ILSI Press, 1995, pp. 163–173.

McClain RM, Levin AA, Posch R, Downing JC: The effects of phenobarbital on the metabolism and excretion of thyroxine in rats. *Toxicol Appl Pharmacol* 99:216–228, 1989.

McClain RM, Posch RC, Bosakowski T, *et al*.: Studies on the mode of action for thyroid gland tumor promotion in rats by phenobarbital. *Toxicol Appl Pharmacol* 94:254–265, 1988.

McComb DJ, Kovacs K, Beri J, *et al*.: Pituitary adenomas in old Sprague-Dawley rats: A histologic, ultrastructural, and immunocytochemical study. *J Natl Cancer Inst* 73:1143–1166, 1984.

McComb DJ, Kovacs K, Beri J, *et al*.: Pituitary gonadotroph adenomas in old Sprague-Dawley rats. *J Submicrosc Cytol* 17:517–530, 1985.

McConnell RF, Westen HH, Ulland BM, *et al*.: Proliferative lesions of the testes in rats with selected examples from mice. *Guides for Toxicologic Pathology*, STP/ARP/AFIP, Washington, DC, 1992, pp. 1–32.

McGirr EM, Clement WE, Currie AR, Kennedy JS: Impaired dehalogenase activity as a cause of goiter with malignant changes. *Scott Med J* 4:232–242, 1959.

Mesiano S, Jaffe RB: Developmental and functional biology of the primate fetal adrenal cortex. *Endocr Rev* 18:378–403, 1997.

Michael SD, Taguchi O, Nishizuka Y: Changes in hypophyseal hormones associated with accelerated aging and tumorigenesis of the ovaries in neonatally thymectomized mice. *Endocrinology* 108:2375–2380, 1981.

Michiels F-M, Chappuis S, Caillou B, *et al*.: Development of medullary thyroid carcinoma in transgenic mice expressing the RET protooncogene altered by a multiple endocrine neoplasia type 2A mutation. *Proc Natl Acad Sci* USA 94:3330–3334, 1997.

Morris HP: The experimental development and metabolism of thyroid gland tumors. *Adv Cancer Res* 3:51–115, 1955.

Morrissey J, Rothstein M, Mayor G, Slatopolsky E: Suppression of parathyroid hormone secretion by aluminum. *Kidney Int* 23:699–704, 1983.

Morrissey J, Slatopolsky E: Effect of aluminum on parathyroid hormone secretion. *Kidney Int* 29:S41–S44, 1986.

Mosher AH, Kircher CH: Proliferative lesions of the adrenal medulla in rats treated with Zomepirac sodium. *J Am Coll Toxicol* 7:83–93, 1988.

Murakami M, Hosokawa S, Yamada T, *et al*.: Species-specific mechanism in rat Leydig cell tumorigenesis by procymidone. *Toxicol Appl Pharmacol* 131:244–252, 1995.

Murphy ED, Beamer WG: Plasma gonadotrophin levels during early stages of ovarian tumorigenesis in mice of the Wx/Wv genotype. *Cancer Res* 33:721–723, 1973.

Murphy ED: Hyperplastic and early neoplastic changes in the ovaries of mice after genic deletion of germ cells. *J Natl Cancer Inst* 48:1283–1295, 1972.

Napalkov NP: Tumours of the thyroid gland, in Turusov VS (ed.): *Pathology of Tumors in Laboratory Animals. Part 2. Tumors of the Rat*, No. 6, vol. 1. Lyon, France: IARC Scientific Publication, 1976, pp. 239–272.

National Research Council: *Health Implications of Perchlorate Ingestion.* Washington, DC: National Academic Press, 2005, pp. 1–260.

Nikiforova MN, Stringer JR, Blough R, et al.: Proximity of chromosomal loci that participate in radiation-induced rearrangements in human cells. *Science* 290:138–41, 2000.

Nikiforov YE: RET/PTC rearrangement in thyroid tumors. *Endocr Pathol* 13:3–16, 2002.

Nikiforov YE: Genetic alterations involved in the transition from well-differentiated to poorly differentiated and anaplastic thyroid carcinomas. *Endocr Pathol* 15:319–328, 2004.

Nilsson M, Engström G, Ericson LE: Graded response in the individual thyroid follicle cell to increasing doses of TSH. *Mol Cell Endocrinol* 44:165, 1986.

Nishizuki Y, Sakakura T, Taguchi O: Mechanism of ovarian tumorigenesis in mice after neonatal thymectomy. *J Natl Cancer Inst Monogr* 51:89–96, 1979.

Nonidez José F: The origin of the 'parafollicular' cell, a second epithelial component of the thyroid gland of the dog. *Am J Anat* 49:479–505, 1931–32.

Nyska A, Haseman JK, Hailey JR, et al.: The association between severe nephropathy and pheochromocytoma in the male F344 rat—The national toxicology program experience. *Toxicol Pathol* 27:456–462, 1999.

Oettgen HF, Old LJ, Boyse EA, et al.: Toxicity of E. coli L-asparaginase in man. *Cancer* 25:253–278, 1970.

Ohnhaus EE, Burgi H, Burger A, Studer H: The effect of antipyrine, phenobarbital, and rifampicin on the thyroid hormone metabolism in man. *Eur J Clin Invest* 11:381–387, 1981.

Ohnhaus EE, Studer H: A link between liver microsomal enzyme activity and thyroid hormone metabolism in man. *Br J Clin Pharmacol* 15:71–76, 1983.

Ohshima M, Ward JM: Dietary iodine deficiency as a tumor promoter and carcinogen in male F344/NCr rats. *Cancer Res* 46:877–883, 1986.

Ohshima M, Ward JM: Promotion of N-methyl-N-nitrosourea-induced thyroid tumors by iodine deficiency in F344/NCr rats. *JNCI* 73:289–296, 1984.

Olsen JH, Boice JD, Jensen JP, Fraumeni JF Jr: Cancer among epileptic patients exposed to anticonvulsant drugs. *J Natl Cancer Inst* 81:803–808, 1989.

Orloff JJ, Ganz MB, Ribaudo AE, et al.: Analysis of PTHrP binding and signal transduction mechanisms in benign and malignant squamous cells. *Am J Physiol* 262:E599–E607, 1992.

Osamura RY, Komatsu N, Izumi S, et al.: Ultrastructural localization of prolactin in the rat anterior pituitary glands by pre-embedding peroxidase-labeled antibody method: Observations in normal, castrated, or estrogen-stimulated specimen. *J Histochem Cytochem* 30:919–925, 1982.

Oslapas R, Prinz R, Ernst K, et al.: Incidence of radiation-induced parathyroid tumors in male and female rats. *Clin Res* 29:734A, 1981.

Oslapas R, Shah KH, Hoffman, et al.: Effect of gonadectomy on the incidence of radiation-induced parathyroid tumors in male and female rats. *Clin Res* 30:401A, 1982.

Ozaki A, Sagartz JE, Capen CC: Phagocytic activity of FRTL-5 rat thyroid follicular cells as measured by ingestion of fluorescent latex beads. *Exp Cell Res* 219:547–554, 1995.

Parfitt AM: Bone and plasma calcium homeostasis. *Bone* 8(Suppl 1):S1–S8l, 1987.

Parkening TA, Collins TJ, Smith ER: A comparative study of prolactin levels in five species of aged female laboratory rodents. *Biol Reprod* 22:513–518, 1980.

Payne AH, Quinn PG, Stalvey JRD: The stimulation of steroid biosynthesis by luteinizing hormone, in Ascoli M (ed.): *Luteinizing Hormone Action and Receptors*. Boca Raton, Florida: CRC Press, 1985, pp. 136–173.

Paynter OH, Burin GJ, Jaeger RB, Gregorio CA: Goitrogens and thyroid follicular cell neoplasia: Evidence for a threshold process. *Reg Toxicol Pharmacol* 8:102–119, 1988.

Pendergrast WJ, Milmore BK, Marcus SC: Thyroid cancer and toxicosis in the United States: Their relation to endemic goiter. *J Chronic Dis* 13:22–38, 1961.

Pickering CE, Pickering RG: The effect of repeated reproduction on the incidence of pituitary tumours in Wistar rats. *Lab Anim* 18:371–378, 1984.

Poirier LA, Doerge DR, Gaylor DW, et al.: An FDA review of sulfamethazine toxicity. *Regul Toxicol Pharmacol* 30:217–222, 1999.

Prahalada S, Majka JA, Soper KA, et al.: Leydig cell hyperplasia and adenomas in mice treated with finasteride, a 5 α-reductase inhibitor: A possible mechanism. *Fundam Appl Toxicol* 22:211–219, 1994.

Prentice DE, Meikle AW: A review of drug-induced Leydig cell hyperplasia and neoplasia in the rat and some comparisons with man. *Hum Exp Toxicol* 14:562–572, 1995.

Prentice DE, Siegel RA, Donatsch P, Qureshi S, Ettlin RA: Mesulergine induced Leydig cell tumours, a syndrome involving the pituitary-testicular axis of the rat. *Arch Toxicol* 15(Suppl.):197–204, 1992.

Price RJ, Walters DG, Finch JM, et al.: Mode of action of pyrethrins: Induction of rat hepatic xenobiotic metabolizing enzyme activities. *Toxicol Appl Pharmacol* 218:186–195, 2007.

Puchacz E, Stumpf WE, Stachowiak EK, et al.: Vitamin D increases expression of the tyrosine hydroxylase gene in adrenal medullary cells. *Mol Brain Res* 36:193–196, 1996.

Quayle FJ, Moley JF: Medullary thyroid carcinoma: Including MEN 2A and MEN 2B syndromes. *J Surg Oncol* 89:122–129, 2005.

Rao AR: Effects of carcinogen and/or mutagen on normal and gonadotrophin-primed ovaries of mice. *Int J Cancer* 28:105–110, 1981.

Ratcliffe WA: Role of parathyroid hormone-related protein in lactation. *Clin Endocrinol* 37:402–404, 1992.

Rehm S, Dierksen D, Deerberg F: Spontaneous ovarian tumors in Han:NMRI mice: Histologic classification, incidence, and influence of food restriction. *J Natl Cancer Inst* 72:1383–1395, 1984.

Reindel JF, Dominick MA, Bocan TM, et al.: Toxicologic effects of a novel acyl-CoA: Cholesterol acyltransferase (ACAT) inhibitor in cynomolgus monkeys. *Toxicol Pathol* 22:510–518, 1994.

Reznik G, Ward JM, Reznik-Shuller H: Ganglioneuromas in the adrenal medulla of F344 rats. *Vet Pathol* 17:614–621, 1980.

Ribelin WE: The effects of drugs and chemicals upon the structure of the adrenal gland. *Fundam Appl Toxicol* 4:105–119, 1984.

Riond J-L, Kocabagli N, Cloux F, et al.: Parathyroid hormone-related protein in the colostrum of paretic post parturient dairy cows. *Vet Rec* 138:333–334, 1996.

Riond J-L, Kocabagli N, Forrer R, et al.: Repeated daytime measurements of the concentrations of PTHrP and other components of bovine milk. *J Anim Physiol Anim Nutr* 74:194–204, 1995.

Risma KA, Clay CM, Nett TM, et al.: Targeted overexpression of luteinizing hormone in transgenic mice leads to infertility, polycystic ovaries, and ovarian tumors. *Proc Natl Acad Sci U S A* 92:1322–1326, 1995.

Risma KA, Hirshfield AN, Nilson JH: Elevated luteinizing hormone in prepubertal transgenic mice causes hyperandrogenemia, precocious puberty, and substantial ovarian pathology. *Endocrinology* 138:3540–3547, 1997.

Roberts SA, Nett TM, Hartman HA, Adams TE, Stoll RE: SDZ 2000-110 induces Leyding cell tumors by increasing gonadotropins in rats. *J Am Coll Toxicol* 8:487–505, 1989.

Robertson DG, Breider MA, Milad MA: Preclinical safety evaluation of Avasimide in Beagle dogs: An ACAT inhibitor with minimal adrenal effects. *Toxicol Sci* 59:324–334, 2001.

Rodan GA, Martin TJ: Therapeutic approaches to bone diseases. *Science* 289:1508–1514, 2000.

Roe FJC, Bar A: Enzootic and epizootic adrenal medullary proliferative disease of rats: Influence of dietary factors which affect calcium absorption. *Human Toxicol* 4:27–52, 1985.

Roe FJC, Lee PN, Conybeare G, et al.: The biosure study: Influence of composition of diet and food consumption on longevity, degenerative diseases and neoplasia in Wistar rats studied for up to 30 months post weaning. *Fd Chem Toxic* 33(Suppl 1):1S–100S, 1995.

Rosol TJ, Capen CC: Biology of disease: Mechanisms of cancer-induced hypercalcemia. *Lab Invest* 67:680–702, 1992.

Rosol TJ, Capen CC: Calcium-regulating hormones and diseases of abnormal mineral (calcium, phosphorus, magnesium) metabolism, in Kaneko JJ, Harvey JW, Bruss ML (eds.): *Clinical Biochemistry of Domestic animals*, 5th edn. New York: Academic Press, 1997, pp. 619–702.

Rosol TJ, Capen CC: Humoral hypercalcemia of malignancy, in Feldman B, Zinkl J, Jain N (eds.): *Schalm's Veterinary Hematology. Section: Lymphoid Neoplasia*, 5th edn, Chap. 98. Baltimore MD: Williams and Wilkins, 2000, pp. 660–666.

Rosol TJ, Chew DJ, Nagode LA, et al.: Pathophysiology of calcium metabolism. *Vet Clin Pathol* 24:49–63, 1995.

Rosol TJ, Yarrington JT, Latendresse J, et al.: Adrenal gland: Structure, function, and mechanisms of toxicity. *Toxicol Pathol* 29:41–48, 2001.

Rothuizen J, Reul JM, Rijnberk A, et al.: Aging and the hypothalamus-pituitary-adrenocortical axis, with special reference to the dog. *Acta Endocrinol* 125(Suppl.):73–76, 1991.

Rouse D, Suki WN: Renal control of extracellular calcium. *Kidney Int* 38:700–708, 1990.

Royaux IE, Suzuki K, Mori A, et al.: Pendrin, the protein encoded by the Pendred syndrome gene (*PDS*), is an apical porter of iodide in the thyroid and is regulated by thyroglobulin in FRTL-5 cells. *Endocrinology* 141:839–845, 2000.

Sagartz JE, Jhiang SM, Tong Q, Capen CC: Thyroid stimulating hormone promotes growth of thyroid carcinomas in transgenic mice with targeted expression of ret/PTC$_1$ oncogene. *Lab Invest* 76:307–318, 1997.

Sagartz JE, Ozaki A, Capen CC: Phagocytosis of fluorescent beads by rat thyroid follicular (FRTL-5) cells: Comparison with iodine uptake as an index of functional activity of thyrocytes *in vitro*. *Toxicol Pathol* 23:635–643, 1995.

Sandusky GE, Van Pelt CS, Todd GC, et al.: An immunocytochemical study of pituitary adenomas and focal hyperplasia in old Sprague-Dawley and Fischer 344 rats. *Toxicol Pathol* 16:376–380, 1988.

Sarkar DK, Gottschall PE, Meites J: Damage to hypothalamic dopaminergic neurons is associated with development of prolactin-secreting pituitary tumors. *Science* 218:684–686, 1982.

Sato M, Vhale J, Schmidt A, et al.: Abnormal bone architecture and biomechanical properties with near-lifetime treatment of rats with PTH. *Endocrinology* 143:3230–3242, 2002.

Sato M, Zeng GQ, Turner CH: Biosynthetic human parathyroid hormone (1-34) effects on bone quality in aged ovariectomized rats. *Endocrinology* 138:4330–4337, 1997.

Satoh H, Kajimura T, Chen C-J, et al.: Invasive pituitary tumors in female F344 rats induced by estradiol dipropionate. *Toxicol Pathol* 25:462–469, 1997.

Schoenig GP: Mammalian toxicology of pyrethrum extract, in Casida JE, Quistad JD (eds.): *Pyrethrum Flowers Production, Chemistry, Toxicology, and Uses*. New York: Oxford University Press, 1995, pp. 249–257.

Scott DA, Wang R, Kreman TM, et al.: The Pendred syndrome gene encodes a chloride-iodide transport protein. *Nat Genet* 21:440–443, 1999.

Shelby MK, Cherrington NJ, Vansell, et al.: Tissue mRNA expression of the rat UDP-glucuronosyltransferase gene family. *Drug Metab Disp* 31:326–333, 2003.

Sher SP, Jensen RD, Bokelman DL: Spontaneous tumors in control F344 and Charles River-CD rats and Charles River CD-1 and B6C3HF1 mice. *Toxicol Lett* 11:103–110, 1982.

Sherman SI: Thyroid Carcinoma. *Lancet* 361:501–511, 2003.

Shirts SB, Annegers JF, Hauser WA, Kurland LT: Cancer incidence in a cohort of patients with seizure disorders. *JNCI* 77:83–87, 1986.

Siesjo BK: Calcium and cell death. *Magnesium* 8:223–237, 1989.

Slitt AL, Cherrington NJ, Fisher CD, et al.: Induction of genes for metabolism and transport by trans-stilbene oxide in livers of Sprague-Dawley and Wistar-Kyoto rats. *Drug Metabol Disposition* 34:1190–1197, 2006.

Soldin OP, Braverman LE, Lamm: Perchlorate clinical pharmacology and human health: A review. *Therap Drug Monit* 23:316–331, 2001.

Solleveld HA, Haseman JK, McConnell EE: National history of body weight gain, survival and neoplasia in the F344 rat. *JNCI* 72:929–940, 1984.

Spitzweg C, Heufelder AE, Morris JC: Review: Thyroid iodine transport. *Thyroid* 10:321–330, 2000.

Steenbergh PH, Hoppener JWM, Zandberg J, et al.: Calcitonin gene related peptide coding sequence is conserved in the human genome and is expressed in medullary thyroid carcinoma. *J Clin Endocrinol Metab* 59:358–360, 1984.

Stoll R, Faucounau N, Maraud R: Les adenomes a cellules folliculaires et parafolliculaires de la thyroide du rat soumis au thiamazole. [Development of follicular and parafollicular adenomas in the thyroid of rats treated with thiamazole.] *Ann Endocrinol (Paris)*, 39:179–189, 1978.

Suda T, Takahashi N, Udagawa N, et al.: Modulation of osteoclast differentiation and function by the new members of the tumor necrosis factor receptor and ligand families. *Endocr Rev* 20:345–357, 1999.

Swarm RL, Roberts GKS, Levy AC: Observations on the thyroid gland in rats following the administration of sulfamethoxazole and trimethoprim. *Toxicol Appl Pharmacol* 24:351–363, 1973.

Szabo S, Huttner I, Kovacs K, et al.: Pathogenesis of experimental adrenal hemorrhagic necrosis ("apoplexy"). Ultrastructural, biochemical, neuropharmacologic, and blood coagulation studies with acrylonitrate in the rat. *Lab Invest* 42:533–546, 1980.

Taguchi O, Michael SD, Nishizuka Y: Rapid induction of ovarian granulosa cell tumors by 7,12-dimethylbenz[a]anthracene in neonatally estrogenized mice. *Cancer Res* 48:425–429, 1988.

Tajima K, Miyagawa J-I, Nakajima H, et al.: Morphological and biochemical studies on minocycline-induced black thyroid in rats. *Toxicol Appl Pharmacol* 81:393–400, 1985.

Takahashi N, Udagawa N, Suda T: A new member of tumor necrosis factor ligand family, ODF/OPGL/TRANCE/RANKL, regulates osteoclast differentiation and function. *Biochem Biophys Res Commun* 256:449–455, 1999.

Takayama S, Aihara K, Onodera T, et al., Antithyroid effects of propylthiouracil and sulfamonomethoxine in rats and monkeys. *Toxicol Appl Pharmacol* 82:191–199, 1986.

Tallini G: Molecular pathobiology of thyroid neoplasms. *Endocr Path* 13:271–288, 2002.

Tashjian AH, Chabner BA: Clinical safety of recombinant human parathyroid hormone (1-34) in the treatment of osteoporosis in postmenopausal women and men. *J Bone Min Res* 17:1151–1161, 2002.

Teitelbaum SL, Moore KE, Shieber W: C cell follicles in the dog thyroid: Demonstration by in vivo perfusion. *Anat Rec* 168:69–78, 1970.

Teitelbaum SL: Bone resorption by osteoclasts. *Science* 289:1504–1508, 2000.

Tennent BJ, Beamer WG: Ovarian tumors not induced by irradiation and gonadotropins in hypogonadal (*hpg*) mice. *Biol Reprod* 34:751–760, 1986.

Tettenborn D, Hobik HP, Luckhaus G: Hypoparathyroidismus beim Kaninchen nach Verabreichung von L-asparaginase. *Arzneimittelforschung* 20:1753–1755, 1970.

Thurman JD, Bucci TJ, Hart RW, Turturro A: Survival, body weight, and spontaneous neoplasms in ad libitum-fed and food-restricted Fischer-344 rats. *Toxicol Pathol* 22:1–9, 1994.

Thurston V, Williams ED: Experimental induction of C-cell tumours in thyroid by increased dietary content of vitamin D2. *Acta Endocrinol* 100:41–45, 1982.

Tice LW, Wollman SH: Ultrastructural localization of peroxidase activity on some membranes of the typical thyroid epithelial cell. *Lab Invest* 26:23–34, 1972.

Tice LW, Wollman SH: Ultrastructural localization of peroxidase on pseudopods and other structures of the typical thyroid epithelial cell. *Endocrinology* 94:1555–1567, 1974.

Tischler AS, DeLellis RA, Nunnemacher G, et al.: Acute stimulation of chromaffin cell proliferation in the adult rat adrenal medulla. *Lab Invest* 58:733–735, 1988.

Tischler AS, DeLellis RA, Perlman RL, et al.: Spontaneous proliferative lesions of the adrenal medulla in aging Long-Evans rats: Comparison to PC12 cells, small granule-containing cells, and human adrenal medullary hyperplasia. *Lab Invest* 53:486–498, 1985.

Tischler AS, DeLellis RA: The rat adrenal medulla. I. The normal adrenal. *J Am Coll Toxicol* 7:1–21, 1988a.

Tischler AS, DeLellis RA: The rat adrenal medulla. II. Proliferative lesions. *J Am Coll Toxicol* 7:23–44, 1988b.

Tischler AS, McClain RM, Childers H, *et al.*: Neurogenic signals regulate chromaffin cell proliferation and mediate the mitogenic effect of reserpine in the adult rat adrenal medulla. *Lab Invest* 65:374–376, 1991.

Tischler AS, Powers JF, Downing JC, *et al.*: Vitamin D₃, lactose, and xylitol stimulate chromaffin cell proliferation in the rat adrenal medulla. *Toxicol Appl Pharmacol* 140:115–123, 1996.

Tischler AS, Powers JF, Pignatello M, *et al.*: Vitamin D₃-induced proliferative lesions in the rat adrenal medulla. *Toxicol Sci* 51:9–18, 1999.

Tischler AS, Riseberg J, Cherington V: Multiple mitogenic signaling pathways in chromaffin cells: A model for cell cycle regulation in the nervous system. *Neurosci Lett* 168:181–184, 1994.

Tischler AS, Riseberg J: Different responses to mitogenic agents by adult rat and human chromaffin cells in vitro. *Endocrine Pathol* 4:15–19, 1993.

Tischler AS, Ruzicka LA, Van Pelt CS, *et al.*: Catecholamine-synthesizing enzymes and chromogranin proteins in drug-induced proliferative lesions of the rat adrenal medulla. *Lab Invest* 63:44–51, 1990.

Tischler AS, Ziar J, Downing JC, *et al.*: Sustained stimulation of rat adrenal chromaffin cell proliferation by reserpine. *Toxicol Appl Pharmacol* 135:254–257, 1995.

Triggs SM, Williams ED: Experimental carcinogenesis in the rat thyroid follicular and C-cells. *Acta Endocrinol* 85:84–92, 1977.

van Putten LJA, van Zwieten MJ, Mattheij JAM, *et al.*: Studies on prolactin-secreting cells in aging rats of different strains. I. Alterations in pituitary histology and serum prolactin levels as related to aging. *Mech Ageing Dev* 42:75–90, 1988.

van Putten LJA, van Zwieten MJ: Studies on prolactin-secreting cells in aging rats of different strains. II. Selected morphological and immunocytochemical features of pituitary tumors correlated with serum prolactin levels. *Mech Ageing Dev* 42:115–127, 1988.

Vansell NR, Klaassen CD: Increased biliary excretion of thyroxine by microsomal enzyme inducers. *Toxicol Appl Pharmacol* 176:187–194, 2001.

Vansell NR, Klaassen CD: Effect of microsomal enzyme inducers on the biliary excretion of triiodothyronine (T3) and its metabolites. *Toxicol Sci* 65:184–191, 2002a.

Vansell NR, Klaassen CD: Increase in rat liver UDP-glucuronosyltransferase mRNA by microsomal enzyme inducers that enhance thyroid hormone glucuronidation. *Drug Metabol Disp* 30:240–246, 2002b.

Vansell NR, Muppidi JR, Habeebu SM, *et al.*: Promotion of thyroid tumors in rats by pregnenolone-16a-carbonitrile (PCN) and polychlorinated biphenyl (PCB). *Toxicol Sci* 81:50–59, 2004.

Vhale JL, Long GG, Sandusky G, *et al.*: Bone neoplasms in F344 rats given Teriparatide [rhPTH(1–34)] are dependent on duration of treatment and dose. *Toxicol Pathol* 32:426–438, 2004.

Vhale JL, Sato M, Long GG, *et al.*: Skeletal changes in rats given daily subcutaneous injections of recombinant human parathyroid hormone (1–34) for 2 years and relevance to human safety. *Toxicol Pathol* 30:312–321, 2002.

Vilar O, Tullner WW: Effects of o,p′-DDD on histology and 17-hydroxycorticosteroid output of the dog adrenal cortex. *Endocrinology* 65:80–86, 1959.

Viollon-Badie C, Lassere D, Debruyne E, *et al.*: Phenobarbitol, β-naphthoflavone, clofibrate, and pregnenolone-16α-carbonitrile do not affect hepatic thyroid hormone UDP-Glucuronosyltransferase activity, and thyroid gland function in mice. *Toxicol Appl Pharmacol* 155:1–12, 1999.

Vortkamp A, Lee K, Lanske B, *et al.*: Regulation of rate of cartilage differentiation by Indian hedgehog and PTH-related protein. *Science* 273:613–622, 1996.

Waalkes MP, Rehm S, Devor DE: The effects of continuous testosterone exposure on spontaneous and cadmium-induced tumors in the male Fischer (F344/NCr) rat: Loss of testicular response. *Toxicol Appl Pharmacol* 142:40–46, 1997.

Wada L, Daly R, Kern D, *et al.*: Kinetics of 1,25-dihydroxyvitamin D metabolism in the aging rat. *Am J Physiol* 262 (*Endocrinol Metab*, 25): E906–E910, 1992.

Waritz RS, Steinberg M, Kinoshita FK, *et al.*: Thyroid function and thyroid tumors in toxaphene-treated rats. *Regul Toxicol Pharmacol* 24:184–192, 1996.

Warren S, Gruzdev L, Gates O, *et al.*: Radiation induced adrenal medullary tumors in the rat. *Arch Pathol* 82:115–118, 1966.

White SJ, McLean AEM, Howland C: Anticonvulsant drugs and cancer. A cohort study in patients with severe epilepsy. *Lancet* 2:458–461, 1979.

Willemsen W, Kruitwagen R, Bastiaans B, *et al.*: Ovarian stimulation and granulosa-cell tumour. *Lancet* 341:986–988, 1993.

Williams ED, Abrosimov A, Bogdanova T, *et al.*: Thyroid carcinoma after Chernobyl latent period, morphology and aggressiveness. *Br J Cancer* 90:2219–2224, 2004.

Witte ON: Steel locus defines new multipotent growth factor. *Cell* 63:5–6, 1990.

Wolfe HJ: Calcitonin: Perspectives and current concepts. *J Endocrinol Invest* 5:423–432, 1982.

Wollman SH, Spicer SS, Burstone MS: Localization of esterase and acid phosphatase in granules and colloid droplets in rat thyroid epithelium. *J Cell Biol* 21:191–201, 1964.

Wong H, Lehman-McKeeman LD, Grubb MF, *et al.*: Increase hepatobiliary clearance of unconjugated thyroxine determines DMP 904-induced alterations in thyroid hormone homeostasis in rats. *Toxico Sci* 84:232–242, 2005.

Wongsurawat N, Armbrecht HJ: Comparison of calcium effect on in vitro calcitonin and parathyroid hormone release by young and aged thyroparathyroid glands. *Exp Gerontol* 22:263–269, 1987.

Wynford-Thomas D, Smith P, Williams ED: Proliferative response to cyclic AMP elevation of thyroid epithelium in suspension culture. *Mol Cell Endocrinol* 51:163, 1987.

Wynford-Thomas D, Stringer BM, Williams ED: Desensitisation of rat thyroid to the growth-stimulating action of TSH during prolonged goitrogen administration. Persistence of refractoriness following withdrawal of stimulation. *Acta Endocrinol Copenh* 101:562–569, 1982a.

Wynford-Thomas D, Stringer BM, Williams ED: Dissociation of growth and function in the rat thyroid during prolonged goitrogen administration. *Acta Endocrinol Copenh* 101:210–216, 1982b.

Wynford-Thomas V, Wynford-Thomas D, Williams ED: Experimental induction of parathyroid adenomas in the rat. *JNCI* 70:127–134, 1982.

Xing M: BRAF mutation in thyroid cancer. *Endocr Relat Cancer* 12:245–262, 2005.

Yamagami T, Handa H, Takeuchi J, *et al.*: Rat pituitary adenoma and hyperplasia induced by caffeine administration. *Surg Neurol* 20:323–331, 1983.

Yang NN, Venugopalan M, Hardikar S, *et al.*: Identification of an estrogen response element activated by metabolites of 17β-estradiol and raloxifene. *Science* 273:1222–1225, 1996.

Yarrington JT, Huffman KW, Gibson JP: Adrenocortical degeneration in dogs, monkeys, and rats treated with i-(1,4-dioxido-3-methylquinoxalin-2-yl)-*N*-methylnitrone. *Toxicol Lett* 8:229–234, 1981.

Yarrington JT, Huffman KW, Leeson GA, *et al.*: Comparative toxicity of the hematinic MDL 80,478- effects on the liver and adrenal cortex of the dog, rat and monkey. *Fundam Appl Toxicol* 3:86–94, 1983.

Yarrington JT, Johnston JO: Aging in the adrenal cortex, in Mohr U, Dungworth DL, Capen CC (eds.): *Pathobiology of the Aging Rat.* Washington, DC: ILSI Press, 1994, pp. 227–244.

Yarrington JT, Latendresse JR, Capen CC: Toxic responses of the adrenal cortex, in Sipes IG, McQueen CA, Gandolfi AJ (eds.): *Comprehensive Toxicology*, vol. 10, Chap. 49; Boekelheide K, *et al.* (eds.): *Reproductive and Endocrine Toxicology.* Oxford, New York, Tokyo: Elsevier Science/Pergamon, 1997, pp. 647–658.

Yarrington JT, Loudy DE, Sprinkle DJ, *et al.*: Degeneration of the rat and canine adrenal cortex caused by i-(1,4-dioxido-3-methylquinoxalin-2-yl)-*N*-methylnitrone (DMNM). *Fundam Appl Toxicol* 5:370, 1985.

Yeomans ND, Omeprazole: Short and long-term safety. *Adverse Drug Reac Toxicol Rev* 13:145–156, 1994.

Young DM, Olson HM, Prieur DJ, *et al*.: Clinicopathologic and ultrastructural studies of L-asparaginase-induced hypocalcemia in rabbits. An experimental animal model of acute hypoparathyroidism. *Lab Invest* 29:374–386, 1973.

Zanchetta JR, Bodago CE, Ferretti JL, *et al*.: Effects of Teriparatide [recombinant human parathyroid hormone (1–34)] on cortical bone in postmenopausal women with osteoporosis. *J Bone Min Res* 18:539–543, 2003.

Zbinden G: Hyperplastic and neoplastic responses of the thyroid gland in toxicological studies. *Arch Toxicol* Suppl 12:98–106, 1988.

UNIT 5

TOXIC AGENTS

CHAPTER 22

TOXIC EFFECTS OF PESTICIDES

Lucio G. Costa

INTRODUCTION

Pesticides can be defined as any substance or mixture of substances intended for preventing, destroying, repelling, or mitigating pests. Pests can be insects, rodents, weeds, and a host of other unwanted organisms (Ecobichon, 2001a). Thus, pesticides occupy a rather unique position among the many chemicals that we encounter daily, in that they are deliberately added to the environment for the purpose of killing or injuring some form of life. Ideally, their injurious action would be highly specific for undesirable targets; in fact, however, most pesticides are not highly selective, but are generally toxic to many nontarget species, including humans. Thus, the use of pesticides must minimize the possibility of exposure of nontarget organisms to injurious quantities of these chemicals (Murphy, 1986).

It is not uncommon for people to refer to pesticides as a single unitary class of chemicals, while in fact the term pesticide should be equated to that of pharmaceutical drugs. As there are dozens of drugs with different therapeutical indications and different mechanisms of action, several different classes of pesticides exist, with different uses, mechanisms and, hence, toxic effects in nontarget organisms. The most common classification of pesticides relies on the target species they act on. The four major classes (and their target pests) are those of insecticides (insects), herbicides (weeds), fungicides (fungi, molds), and rodenticides (rodents), but there are also acaricides (mites), molluscides (snails, other mollusks), miticides (mites), larvicides (larvae), and pediculocides (lice). In addition, for regulatory purposes, plant growth regulators, repellants, and attractants (pheromones) often also fall in this broad classification of chemicals. Furthermore, within each class, several subclasses exist, with substantially different chemical and toxicological characteristics. For example, among insecticides, one can find organophosphorus compounds, carbamates, organochlorines, pyrethroids, and many other chemicals. Even within each of these subclasses, significant differences can exist, as is the case, for example, of organochlorine compounds such as DDT, aldrin, or chlordecone. Thus, detailed knowledge of the toxicological characteristics of each chemical is needed to properly evaluate their potential risks for nontarget species.

The literature pertaining to the chemistry, development, nomenclature, biotransformation and degradation, environmental effects, toxicity in target and nontarget species, and mode of action of pesticides over the past 60 years is very extensive, and the reader is referred to the monographs of O'Brien (1967), Ecobichon and Joy (1982), Hayes (1982), Wagner (1983), Matsumura (1985), Costa *et al.* (1987), Baker and Wilkinson (1990), Dikshith (1991), Hayes and Laws (1991), Chambers and Levi (1992), and Krieger (2001), for more indepth discussions.

HISTORICAL DEVELOPMENTS

Pesticides have been used to a limited degree since ancient times. The Ebers Papyrus, written about 1500 B.C., lists preparations to expel fleas from the house. The oldest available record is Homer's mention (about 1000 B.C.) that Odysseus burned sulfur "... to purge the hall and the house and the court" (Odyssey XXII, 493–494). Pliny the Elder (A.D. 23–79) collected in his Natural History many anecdotes on the use of pesticides in the previous three to four centuries (Shepard, 1939). Dioscorides, a Greek physician (A.D. 40–90), knew of toxic properties of sulfur and arsenic. There are records showing that by A.D. 900 the Chinese were using arsenic sulfides to control garden insects. *Veratrum album* and *Veratrum nigrum,* two species of false hellebore, were used by the Romans as rodenticides (Shepard, 1939). In 1669, the earliest known record of arsenic as an insecticide in the Western world mentioned its use with honey as an ant bait. Use of tobacco as contact insecticide for plant lice was mentioned later in the same century. Copper compounds were known since the early 1800s to have fungicidal value, and the Bordeaux mixture (hydrated lime and copper sulfate) was first used in France in 1883. Hydrocyanic acid, known to the Egyptians and the Romans as a poison, was used as a fumigant in 1877 to kill museum pests in insect collections, and carbon disulfide has been used as a fumigant since 1854 (Costa, 1987). Even in this century, until the 1930s, pesticides were mainly of natural origins or inorganic compounds. Arsenicals have played a major role in pest control, first as insecticides, then as herbicides. Sulfur has been widely used as a fumigant since the early 1800s, and remains one of the most widely used fungicides as of today. Nicotine has been widely used as an insecticide all over the world, as has been rotenone, used as a fish poison in South America since 1725 (Costa, 1987). Mercuric chloride was used as a fungicide since 1891, slowly replaced by phenylmercury and alkylmercury. Outbreaks of poisoning with the latter compounds (Bakir *et al.*, 1973) have led to a ban on these chemicals.

The period between 1935 and 1950 was characterized by the development of major classes of pesticides, particularly insecticides. In 1939 Paul Müller found that DDT (dichlorodiphenyltrichloroethane), which had been first synthesized in 1874, acted as a poison on flies, mosquitoes, and other insects. DDT was commercialized in 1942 and was used extensively and successfully for the control of typhus epidemics and particularly of malaria. Together with DDT, other chlorinated hydrocarbon insecticides were developed. In the early 1940s, scientists in England and France recognized the gamma isomer of hexachlorocyclohexane, commonly known as lindane, which had been first synthesized in 1825 by Faraday, as a highly potent insecticide (Ecobichon, 1992). Starting in the mid-1940s several other chlorinated insecticides were commercialized, including chlordane, heptachlor, aldrin, and dieldrin. The organophosphorus insecticides were first synthesized in Germany in the late 1930s. Gerhard Schrader, a chemist at the I. G. FarbenIndustrie in Germany, is considered the "father" of organophosphorus insecticides. The first one, tetraethylpyrophosphate (TEPP), was brought to the market in 1944, but had little success because of its instability in aqueous solution. Several thousand molecules were synthesized by Schrader, and one (code name E605) was eventually introduced into the agricultural market under the trade name parathion, to become one of the most widely employed insecticides in this class. During those years, compounds of much greater toxicity than parathion, such as sarin, soman, and tabun, were also synthesized as potential chemical warfare agents. The mechanisms of action of organophosphates, i.e., inhibition of acetylcholinesterase, was soon discovered, primarily by knowledge of the effects and mechanism of action of physostigmine. This alkaloid had been isolated in 1864 from Calabar beans, the seeds of *Physostigma venenosum,* a perennial plant in tropical West Africa, and its mode of action as a cholinesterase inhibitor was identified in 1926 (Casida, 1964). Despite the early studies on physostigmine, the carbamates were introduced as insecticides only in the early 1950s. Though pyrethrum flower and extracts had been used for several centuries, pyrethrins were characterized only between 1910 and 1924 (Casida, 1980). This led then to the development of synthetic pyrethroids, the first of which, allethrin, was followed by several others in the early 1970s, particularly because of the work of Michael Elliott in England and of scientists at Sumitomo Chemical Company in Japan. Several other classes of insecticides (e.g., avermectins, neonicotinoids, N-phenylpyrazoles) have also been developed in the past few decades.

The past 60 years have also seen the development of hundreds of other chemicals used as herbicides, fungicides, and rodenticides. The development of thioureas, such as ANTU, and of anticoagulants such as warfarin, as rodenticides, dates back to the mid to late 1940s. A few years later, two important fumigants were introduced, 1,2-dichloropropene and methyl bromide. In the 1950s, phenylureas and chlorophenoxy compounds were developed as herbicides, together with the fungicides captan and folpet. Triazines, chloroacetanilides and paraquat, all widely used herbicides, came to the market in the 1960s, and so did the important class of dithiocarbamate fungicides, while the herbicide glyphosate was introduced in the mid-1970s.

ECONOMICS AND PUBLIC HEALTH

As with all chemicals, including therapeutic drugs, the use of pesticides must take into consideration the balance of the benefits that may be expected versus the possible risks of injury to human health or degradation of environmental quality. Pesticides play a major role in the control of vector-borne diseases, which represent a major threat to the health of large human populations. Pesticides of various types are used in the control of insects, rodents, and other pests that are involved in the life cycle of vector-borne diseases such as malaria, filariasis, yellow fever, viral encephalitis, typhus, and many others (Novak and Lampman, 2001). The case of DDT exemplifies the difficulty in striking a balance between benefits of its use and risks, in this case mainly to the environment. When introduced in 1942, DDT appeared to hold immense promise of benefit to agricultural economics and protection of public health against vector-borne diseases. For example, in the Italian province of Latina there were 175 new cases of malaria in 1944, but after a DDT spray control program was initiated, no new cases of malaria appeared by 1949 (Murphy, 1986). Indeed, at the time, the public health benefits of DDT were viewed so great that Mueller was awarded the Nobel prize in Medicine in 1948. However, because of its bioaccumulation in the environment and its effects on bird reproduction, DDT was eventually banned in most countries by the mid-1970s. In South Africa, DDT was only banned in 1996, and at the time <10,000 cases of malaria were registered in that country. By the year 2000, cases of malaria had increased to 62,000, but with the reintroduction of DDT at the end of that year, cases were down to 12,500 (Maharaj et al., 2005). There are still hundreds of millions of people in the world who are at risk from schistosomiasis, filariasis, and intestinal worm infestations, particularly in Africa and some Asian countries, and these major health problems require a continuous judicious use of pesticides (Novak and Lampman, 2001).

In many parts of the world, excessive loss of food crops to insects or other pests may contribute to possible starvation, and use of pesticides seems to have a favorable cost-benefit relationship (Murphy, 1986). In developed countries, pesticides allow production of abundant, inexpensive, and attractive fruits and vegetables, as well as grains. In this case, cost-benefit considerations are based on economic considerations, particularly with regard to labor costs. Along with insecticides, herbicides and fungicides play a major role in this endeavor. Loss of harvested crops by postharvest infestation by insects, fungi, and rodents is also a major problem (Ecobichon, 2001a,b), that is dealt with by the use of fumigants and other pesticides. Pesticides, particularly herbicides, also find useful application in forestry, during reforestation, as well as the clearing of roadways, train tracks and utilities' rights of way. In the urban setting, pesticides find multiple uses in the home and garden area, to control insects, weeds and other pests (Rust, 2001; Marsh, 2001). It is estimated that 75% of households in the United States utilize some form of pesticides (Table 22-1). These could include, for example, chemicals to control termite, cockroach or rodent infestations, herbicides to control weeds in the garden, or insect repellents.

Use of Pesticides

It is commonly believed that there is a continuous increase in the use of pesticides. While this is certainly true for the period 1950–1980, in the past twenty years or so, use of pesticides (as amount of active ingredient) has actually reached a plateau (Table 22-2). This is due in part to the utilization of more efficacious compounds, that require less active ingredients to be applied to obtain the same degree of pest control, and in part to the introduction of integrated pest management approaches and organic farming, at least in the developed countries. Expenditures on pesticides, however, have increased (Table 22-2), as new chemicals are more expensive than older ones.

Table 22-1

Number of U.S. Households Using Pesticides (2000)

PESTICIDE TYPE	US HOUSEHOLDS (MILLIONS)	% OF TOTAL HOUSEHOLDS[1]
Insecticides	59	56
Herbicides	41	39
Fungicides	14	13
Repellents	53	50
Disinfectants	59	56
Any pesticide	78	74

[1] Based on 105.5 million households and a population of 281.4 million (U.S. Census Bureau, 2000).
SOURCE: Kiely et al., 2004.

Table 22-2

Use and Expenditure on Pesticides in the United States in All Market Sectors: 1985–2000

YEAR	USE[1]	EXPENDITURE[2]
1985	1,304	6,706
1990	1,201	7,727
1995	1,210	10,781
2000	1,234	11,165

[1] Millions of pounds of active ingredients. Excludes preservatives, specialty biocides and chlorine/hypochlorites.
[2] Millions of dollars.
SOURCE: Kiely et al., 2004.

Table 22-3

U.S. and World Use of Pesticides: 2001

Pesticide	UNITED STATES mil. lbs of a.i.	%	WORLD mil. lbs of a.i.	%
Herbicides[1]	553	46	1,870	37
Insecticides	105	9	1,232	24
Fungicides	73	6	475	9
Other[2]	472	39	1,469	29
TOTAL	1,203	100	5,046	100

[1] Includes herbicides and plant growth regulators.
[2] Other = rodenticides, fumigants, nematocides, molluscicides, and other chemicals. a.i. = active ingredient.
SOURCE: Kiely et al., 2004.

In the United Stastes, almost half of the pesticides used are herbicides, while in other countries, particularly Africa, Asia, and Central America, there is also a substantial use of insecticides (Table 22-3). Because the latter compounds are generally more acutely toxic, they contribute to the still large number of yearly pesticide poisonings (see below). Tables 22-4 and 22-5 show the main pesticides used in the agricultural, and home and garden sectors in the United States

Pesticides are often, if not always, used as multiagent formulations, in which the active ingredient is present together with other ingredients to allow mixing, dilution, application, and stability. These other ingredients are lumped under the term "inert" or "other" (Tominack, 2000). Though they do not have pesticidal action, such inert ingredients may not always be devoid of toxicity; thus, an ongoing task of manufacturers and regulatory agencies is

Table 22-4

Most Commonly Used Conventional Pesticide Active Ingredients in the United States in the Agricultural Market Sector: 2001[1]

ACTIVE INGREDIENT	TYPE	MILLIONS OF POUNDS
Glyphosate	H	85–90
Atrazine	H	74–80
Metam sodium	Fum	57–62
Acetochlor	H	30–35
2,4-D	H	28–33
Malathion	I	20–25
Methyl bromide	Fum	20–25
Dichloropropene	Fum	20–25
Metolachlor-s	H	20–24
Metolachlor	H	15–22
Pendimethalin	H	15–19
Trifluralin	H	12–16
Chlorothalonil	F	8–11
Copper salts	F	8–10
Chlorpyrifos	I	8–10

[1]Does not include sulfur (172 mil. lb) and petroleum oil (60 mil. lb). H = herbicide; I = insecticide; F = fungicide; Fum = fumigant.
SOURCE: Kiely *et al.*, 2004.

Table 22-5

Most Commonly Used Conventional Pesticide Active Ingredients, House and Garden Market Sector: 2001[1]

ACTIVE INGREDIENT	TYPE	MILLIONS OF POUNDS
2,4-D	H	8–11
Glyphosate	H	5–8
Pendimethalin	H	3–6
Diazinon	I	4–6
MCPP	H	4–6
Carbaryl	I	2–4
Dicamba	H	2–4
Malathion	I	2–4
DCPA	H	1–3
Benefin	H	1–3

[1]Does not include compounds used for moth control (paradiclorobenzene, 30–35 mil. lb; naphtalene, 2–4 mil. lb) and insect repellents (DEET, 5–7 mil. lb).
H = herbicide; I = insecticide
SOURCE: Kiely *et al.*, 2004.

to assure that inert ingredients do not pose any unreasonable risk of adverse health effects (Tominack, 2000).

Exposure

Exposure to pesticides can occur via the oral or dermal routes or by inhalation. From a quantitative perspective, oral exposure lies on the extremes of a hypothetical dose–response curve. High oral doses, leading to severe poisoning and death, are achieved as a result of pesticide ingestion for suicidal intents, or of accidental ingestion, commonly due to storage of pesticides in improper containers. Chronic low doses on the other hand, are consumed by the general population as pesticide residues in food, or as contaminants in drinking

water. Regulations exist to ensure that pesticide residues are maintained at levels below those that would cause any adverse effects (see below). Workers involved in the production, transport, mixing and loading, and application of pesticides, as well as in harvesting of pesticide-sprayed crops, are at highest risk for pesticide exposure. The dermal route is thought in this case to offer the greatest potential for exposure, with a minor contribution of the respiratory route when aerosols or aerial spraying are used. In these latter cases, bystanders or individuals living in proximity of the spraying may also be exposed because of off-target drifts. In the occupational setting, dermal exposure during normal handling or application of pesticides, or in case of accidental spillings, occurs in body areas not covered by protective clothing, such as the face or the hands. Furthermore, deposition of pesticides on clothing may lead to slow penetration through the tissue and/or to potential exposure of others, if clothes are not changed and washed upon termination of exposure. Several methodologies exist to assess exposure by passive dosimetry, such as the use of absorbent cloth or paper patches, of biosensors, or of tracers followed by video imaging (USEPA 1999; Fenske *et al.*, 1986). Biological monitoring is also used, to measure the absorbed dose of pesticides. Analysis of body fluids and excreta, usually urine, for parent compound or metabolites, can provide both a quantitative and a qualitative measurement of absorbed dose. The advantage of such approach over passive dosimetry is that it evaluates actual, rather than potential absorption, and integrates absorption from all routes of exposure. In some cases, modifications of biochemical parameters or a consequence of exposure can be measured as an indication of both exposure and of a biological effect. This is the case, for example, of measurements of plasma or erythrocyte cholinesterases upon exposure to organophosphorus insecticides (Storm *et al.*, 2000).

Human Poisoning

Pesticides are not always selective for their intended target species, and adverse health effects can occur in nontarget species, including humans. In the general population and in occupationally exposed workers, a primary concern relates to a possible association between pesticide exposure and increased risk of cancer (Alavanja *et al.*, 2004; Pearce and McLean, 2005; Jaga and Dharmani, 2005). More recently, the acknowledgment that pesticide standards are based on healthy adults, and thus may not be sufficiently protective of susceptible populations, such as children, has led to new concerns, research, and regulations (NRC, 1993; Colborn, 2006). Evidence that some pesticides may act as endocrine disruptors, possibly contributing to various adverse effects in humans, including cancer and reproductive and developmental toxicity, has also prompted additional concerns and initiatives (Porterfield, 2000; Safe, 2005). Yet, from a global perspective, the major problem with pesticides remains that of acute human poisoning. The World Health Organization (WHO) estimated that there are around three million hospital admissions for pesticide poisoning each year, that result in around 220,000 deaths (WHO, 1990). Most occur in developing countries, particularly in Southeast Asia, and a large percentage is due to intentional ingestion for suicide purposes (Gunnell and Eddleston, 2003). The WHO has recommended a classification of pesticides by hazard, where acute oral or dermal toxicities in rats were considered (Table 22-6; IPCS, 2005). An analysis of commercially available pesticides indicates that, as a class, insecticides are the most acutely toxic. Indeed, among the 74 active ingredients listed in Class 1A (Extremely hazardous) and Class 1B (Highly hazardous), 48 (65%) are insecticides, in particular organophosphates

Table 22-6
WHO-Recommended Classification of Pesticides by Hazard

| | | LD$_{50}$ IN RAT (mg/kg body weight) | | | |
| | | ORAL | | DERMAL | |
CLASS		SOLIDS	LIQUIDS	SOLIDS	LIQUIDS
Ia	Extremely hazardous	5 or less	20 or less	10 or less	40 or less
Ib	Highly hazardous	5–50	20–200	10–100	40–400
II	Moderately hazardous	50–500	200–2000	100–1000	400–4000
III	Slightly hazardous	Over 500	Over 2000	Over 1000	Over 4000
IV+	Unlikely to present hazard in normal use	Over 2000	Over 3000	Over 4000	Over 6000

SOURCE: IPCS, 2005.

(IPCS, 2005). Rodenticides are also highly toxic to rats, but do not present the same hazard to humans. Indeed, warfarin, one of the most widely used rodenticides, is the same chemical used as an effective "blood thinner" (anticoagulant) for prevention of stroke and other blood clot related conditions. Herbicides, again as a class, have generally moderate to low acute toxicity, one exception being paraquat (which has a low dermal toxicity but causes fatal effects when ingested). Fungicides vary in their acute toxicity, but this is usually low.

Reports of human poisonings worldwide confirm this analysis. In Costa Rica between 1980 and 1986, 3330 individuals were hospitalized for pesticide poisoning, and 429 died. Cholinesterase inhibitors (organophosphates and carbamates) caused 63% of hospitalizations and 36% of deaths, while paraquat accounted for 24% of hospitalizations and 60% of deaths. Cholinesterase inhibitors also caused more than 70% of occupational accidents (Wesseling et al., 1993). Of 335 poisoning deaths in Manipal, India, in the 1990s, 70% were due to cholinesterase inhibitors (Mohanty et al., 2004). In Sri Lanka between 1986 and 2000, hospital admissions for pesticide poisoning were 12–20 thousand/year, with approximately a 10% fatality rate (Roberts et al., 2003). Organophosphates and the organochlorine insecticide endosulfan (which was banned in 1998), were the compounds most commonly involved. The same pattern of poisoning can also be seen in developed countries. For example, in Greece, the number of poisonings ranged between 1200 and 1700/year during the periods 1988–1999. Of these, 40% were due to occupational exposure and 45% to accidental exposure. Organophosphates, carbamates and paraquat were again involved in the majority of cases (Bertsias et al., 2004). In a four year period in Japan, 346 cases of pesticide poisoning were reported; in this case 70% were due to suicide attempts. Again, cholinesterase inhibitors and paraquat were involved in more than 60% of poisonings. Death rate from poisoning with paraquat was over 70%, whereas it was <10% with the herbicides glyphosate or glufosinate (Nagami et al., 2005).

Regulatory Mandate

The awareness that the misuse of pesticides may pose potential health hazards has led to a realm of regulatory measures to ensure their safe use and the protection of the population. In the United States, the primary authority for pesticide regulation resides with the U.S. Environmental Protection Agency (EPA), under the Federal Insecticide, Fungicide and Rodenticide Act (FIFRA) and the Federal Food, Drug and Cosmetic Act (FFDCA). Under FIFRA,

EPA registers pesticides for use, whereas under FFDCA, EPA establishes maximum allowable levels of pesticide residues (tolerances) in foods and animal feeds, which are enforced by other federal agencies (Fenner-Crisp, 2001).

The first legislation passed in the United States was the Federal Insecticide Act of 1910, which only prohibited the manufacture of any insecticide or fungicide that was adulterated or misbranded. FIFRA was originally passed by Congress in 1947, adding the requirement of registration by the Secretary of Agriculture before sale of insecticides, rodenticides, fungicides, and herbicides. Amendments in subsequent years added other pesticides to FIFRA jurisdiction, and provided the U.S. Department of Agriculture (USDA) with the authority to deny, suspend or cancel registrations of products. In 1954, Congress amended the FFDCA to require the Food and Drug Administration (FDA) to establish tolerances for pesticides in raw agricultural commodities. This was extended four years later to processed foods. In 1970, the primary federal authority for the regulation of pesticides was transferred from USDA and FDA to the newly formed EPA. Between 1970 and 1990, FIFRA was amended several times, to address various issues related to pesticide safety and registration processes.

In 1996, the Food Quality and Protection Act (FQPA) brought important changes to pesticide regulations in the United States, that affected both FIFRA and FFDCA. For example, FQPA provided the statutory mandate, under FIFRA, for continuing the expedited consideration of applications for pesticides that may provide reduced risks for human health, nontarget species, and the environment (Fenner-Crisp, 2001). Perhaps more significant were the changes to the FFDCA mandate. In 1958, an amendment of the FFDCA, the Delaney clause (Section 409), stated that "...no additive shall be deemed safe if it is found to induce cancer when ingested by man or animal or if it is found, after tests which are appropriate for the evaluation of the safety of food additives, to induce cancer in man or animal..." Pesticides were included in this "additive" legislation. Under FQPA, however, pesticide residues are excluded from the definition of food additive, and the Delaney clause no longer applies to residues in food. Thus, tolerances can be set also for carcinogens. FQPA also directs EPA to consider aggregate exposure in the risk assessment process, i.e., exposure which occurs from all food uses for a pesticide, as well as from exposures that occur from nonoccupational sources (e.g., drinking water, indoor residential or school use, etc.). Additionally, EPA must consider whether certain pesticides, as well as other substances, may have the same mechanism of toxicity, and if so, carry out a cumulative risk assessment.

Table 22-7

Basic Toxicology Testing Requirements for Pesticide Registration

TEST	ANIMAL SPECIES*
Acute lethality (oral, dermal, inhalation)	Rat, mouse, guinea pig, rabbit
Dermal irritation	Rabbit, rat, guinea pig
Dermal sensitization	Guinea pig
Eye irritation	Rabbit
Acute delayed neurotoxicity	Hen
Genotoxicity studies (in vitro, in vivo)	Bacteria, mammalian cells, mouse, rat, drosophila
Teratogenicity	Rabbit, rodent (mouse, rat, hamster)
Two–four week toxicity study (oral, dermal, inhalation)	Rat, mouse
90-Day toxicity study (oral)	Rat
Chronic toxicity study (oral; 6 months–2 years)	Rat, dog
Oncogenicity study	Rat, mouse
Reproductive/fertility study	Rat
Developmental neurotoxicity study	Rat

*Substantial efforts are being devoted to develop alternative nonanimal test systems. As of 2006, only one in vitro test (for primary irritation) has been validated and accepted by EU regulatory bodies (OECD).

Another change introduced by FQPA gives EPA the mandate to assess special risks of pesticides to infants and children. The Agency must assess aggregate risks based on dietary consumption patterns of children, possible susceptibility of infants and children to pesticides, and cumulative effects of compounds that share the same mechanism of toxicity. In the absence of adequate data, an additional default 10-fold safety factor should be applied to ensure children's safety. Finally, provisions are included for EPA to determine whether certain substances may have endocrine disrupting effects in humans. Additional regulations concerning pesticides are present in other laws, such as the Safe Drinking Water Act or the Clean Air Act.

Under FIFRA, all pesticides sold or distributed in the United States must be registered by the EPA. Older products, registered before 1984, must undergo a re-registration process. To register a pesticide or a formulated product, a large number of studies (over 140) are required, a process that takes several years and anywhere between $50 and $100 million. The data base should include information on product and residue chemistry, environmental fate, toxicology, biotransformation/degradation, occupational exposure and reentry protection, spray drift, environmental impact on nontarget species (birds, mammals, aquatic organisms, plants, soil), environmental persistence and bioaccumulation, as well as product performance and efficacy. Table 22-7 lists the basic requirements regarding toxicology data needed for new pesticide registration (see also Chap. 2). New tiered approaches to toxicity testing for agricultural chemicals, that would reduce the use of animals and improve the risk assessment process, have been recently proposed (Doe et al., 2006; Cooper et al., 2006).

Other nations, such as Canada, Japan, and most European countries have promulgated legislation similar to that of the United States for registration of pesticides. In 1991, the European Union (EU) passed a directive that created a harmonized Union-wide framework for pesticide regulation. Applications for registration can be directed to the EU, or at the level of individual member states. Some developing nations, with a shortage of trained technical, scientific, and legal professionals to develop their own legislation, have adopted the regulatory framework of one or another industrialized nation. The World Health Organization provides guidance, particularly with the setting of acceptabe daily intake (ADI) values for pesticides, through its Joint FAO/WHO Meeting on Pesticide Residues

(JMPR). In a few countries, still no legislation has been introduced to curb adverse effects of pesticides on the environment and human health.

INSECTICIDES

Insecticides play a most relevant role in the control of insect pests, particularly in developing countries. All of the chemical insecticides in use today are neurotoxicants, and act by poisoning the nervous systems of the target organisms (Table 22-8). The central nervous system of insects is highly developed and not unlike that of mammals, and the peripheral nervous system, though less complex, also presents striking similarities (Ecobichon, 2001a). Thus, insecticides are mostly not species-selective with regard to targets of toxicity, and mammals, including humans, are highly sensitive to their toxicity. When selectivity exists, this is often due to differences in detoxication pathways between insects and mammals, or to differential interactions with their target. As a class, insecticides have higher acute toxicity toward nontarget species compared to other pesticides. Some of them, most notably the organophosphates, are involved in a great number of human poisonings and deaths each year. The literature pertaining to the chemistry, development, biotransformation, environmental effects, and toxicity in target and nontarget species of insecticides is extensive, and the reader should refer to the monographs of O'Brien (1967), Hayes (1982), Ecobichon and Roy (1982), Matsumura (1985), Ford et al. (1986), Clark and Matsumura (1986), Costa et al. (1987), Hayes and Laws (1991), Chambers and Levi (1992), Krieger (2001), and Gupta (2006).

Organophosphorus Compounds

Although a number of organic phosphorus (OP) compounds were synthesized in the 1800s, their development as insecticides only occurred in the late 1930s and early 1940s (Gallo and Lawryk, 1991; Costa, 1988). The German chemist Gerhard Schrader is credited for the discovery of the general chemical structure of anticholinesterase OP compounds, and for the synthesis of the first commercialized OP insecticide [Bladan, containing TEPP (tetraethyl pyrophosphate) as the active ingredient], and for one of the most known, parathion, in

Table 22-8
Molecular Targets of the Major Classes of Insecticides

TARGET	INSECTICIDE	EFFECT
Acetylcholinesterase	Organophosphates	Inhibition
	Carbamates	Inhibition
Sodium channels	Pyrethroids (Type I and II)	Activation
	DDT	Activation
	Dihydropyrazoles	Inhibition
Nicotinic acetylcholine receptors	Nicotine	Activation
	Neonicotinoids	Activation
GABA receptors-gated chloride channels	Cyclodienes	Inhibition
	Phenylpyrazoles	Inhibition
	Pyrethroids (Type II)	Inhibition
Glutamate-gated chloride channels[1]	Avermectins	Activation
Octopamine receptors[2]	Formamidines	Activation
Mitochondrial complex I	Rotenoids	Inhibition

[1]Found only in insects. In mammals avermectins activate $GABA_A$ receptors.

[2]In mammals, formamidines activate $alpha_2$-adrenoceptors.

1944. Since then, hundreds of OP compounds have been made and commercialized worldwide in a variety of formulations. More than half of the insecticides used are OPs, and some OPs are among the most extensively used pesticides.

The chemistry of OPs has been thoroughly investigated (Chambers *et al.*, 2001). The general structure of OP insecticides can be represented by

$$R_1 \diagdown \quad \diagup O\ (or\ S)$$
$$P$$
$$R_2 \diagup \quad \diagdown X$$

Where X is the so-called "leaving group," that is displaced when the OP phosphorylates acetylcholinesterase (AChE), and is the most sensitive to hydrolysis; R_1 and R_2 are most commonly alkoxy groups (i.e., OCH_3 or OC_2H_5), though other chemical substitutes are also possible; either an oxygen or a sulfur (in this case the compound should be defined as a phosphorothioate) are also attached to the phosphorus with a double bond. Based on chemical differences, OPs can be divided into several subclasses, which include phosphates, phosphorothioates, phosphoramidates, phosphonates, and others (Chambers *et al.*, 2001). Figure 22-1 shows the chemical structures of some commonly used OPs. Most are phosphorothioates, and need to be bioactivated in vivo to their oxygen analogs to exert their toxic action, but some (e.g., dichlorvos or the nerve agent sarin) have P=O bonds. Most OPs used as insecticides have two methoxy or ethoxy side chains (Fig. 22-1).

Biotransformation   The complex array of reactions involved in the biotransformation of OPs in target and nontarget species has been the subject of extensive investigations (Tang *et al.*, 2006). For all compounds that contain a sulfur bound to the phosphorus, a metabolic bioactivation is necessary for their biological activity to be manifest, as only compounds with a P=O moiety are effective inhibitors of AChE. This bioactivation consists in an oxidative desulfuration mediated, mostly but not exclusively in the liver, by cytochrome P450 enzymes (CYPs), and leading to the formation of an "oxon," or oxygen analog of the parent insecticide (Fig. 22-2). Though this reaction has been known for several decades, the exact CYP isoforms involved have only been recently investigated, and available data suggest that the overall picture is quite complex. Multiple CYPs have been shown to activate organophosphorothioates to their oxons, with different substrate specificities. For example, diazinon is activated by human hepatic CYP2C19, whereas parathion is activated primarily by CYP3A4/5 and CYP2C8, and chlorpyrifos by CYP2B6 (Kappers *et al.*, 2001; Tang *et al.*, 2001; Mutch *et al.*, 2003). In addition to oxidative desulfuration, other reactions can activate OPs (Costa, 1988). Of relevance to insecticidal OPs is thioether oxidation (formation of a sulfoxide, S=O, followed by the formation of a sulfone, O=S=O) which occurs in the leaving group moiety, and is also catalyzed by CYPs. For example, in case of the OP disulfoton, the sulfoxide and the sulfone are more potent inhibitors of AChE than the parent compound. Many other biochemical reactions are detoxication reactions, as they lead to metabolites of lesser or no toxicity (Fig. 22-2). Some, e.g., oxidative dearylation or *O*-dealkylation, are mediated by CYPs, and differences between CYPs exist also in the detoxication process. For example, dearylation of chlorpyrifos is catalyzed primarily by CYP2C19, whereas that of parathion by CYP2B6 (Tang *et al.*, 2001; Hodgson, 2003). Catalytic hydrolysis by phosphotriesterases, known as A-exterases (which are not inhibited by OPs), also plays an important role in the detoxication of certain OPs. One example is the enzyme paraoxonase (PON1) which hydrolyzes the oxons of chlorpyrifos and diazinon, and at least in vitro, also of parathion (Costa *et al.*, 2002; Li *et al.*, 2000). Noncatalytic hydrolysis of OPs also occurs when these compounds phosphorylate serine esterases classified as B-esterases, that are inhibited by OPs but cannot catalytically hydrolyze them. Examples are the carboxylesterases (CarE) and butyrylcholinesterase (BuChE), in addition to the OP target, AChE. CarE also performs a catalytic hydrolysis of the carboxylic esters of malathion, and is believed to be a major determinant of its low toxicity in mammals. Indeed, insects have low CarE activity, and inhibition of CarE by other OPs greatly potentiates the toxicity of malathion in mammals (Murphy, 1986). Glutathione *S*-transferases may also contribute to the detoxication of OPs, particularly the methoxy compounds (Abel *et al.*, 2004).

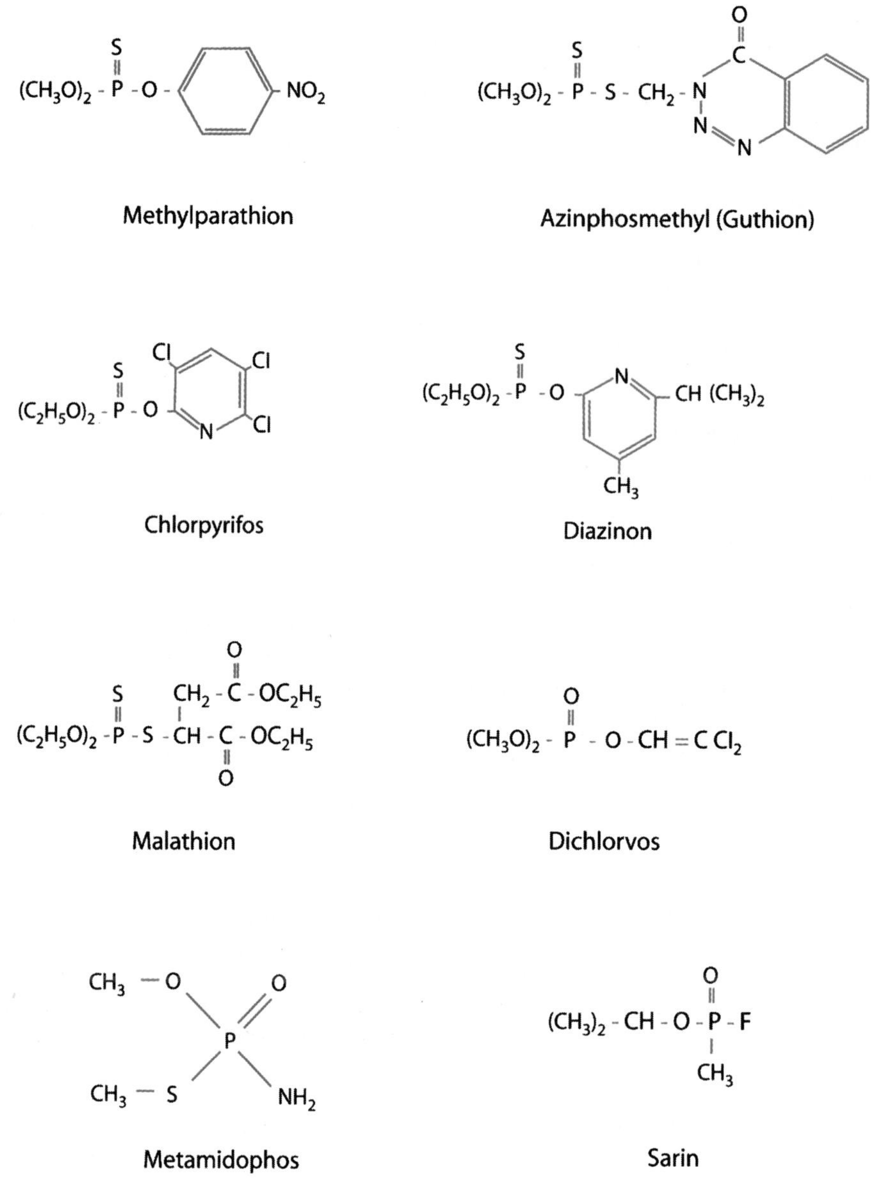

Figure 22-1. Structures of some organophosphorus insecticides and of the nerve agent sarin.

Note that most commonly used compounds are organophosphorothioates (i.e., have a P=S bond) but some, including sarin, have a P=O bond and do not require metabolic activation.

Signs and Symptoms of Toxicity and Mechanism of Action OP insecticides have high acute toxicity, with oral LD_{50} values in rat often below 50 mg/kg, though for some widely used compounds (e.g., chlorpyrifos, diazinon) toxicity is somewhat lower, due to effective detoxication. One exception is malathion, which has an oral LD_{50} in rat of >1 g/kg, due, as said, to rapid detoxication by CarE. For several OPs acute dermal toxicity is also high, with some exceptions being azinphosmethyl and malathion (Murphy, 1986). The primary target for OPs is AChE, a B-esterase whose physiological role is that of hydrolyzing acetylcholine, a major neurotransmitter in the central and peripheral (autonomic and motor-somatic) nervous systems. Acetylcholine released from cholinergic nerve terminals is disposed of solely through hydrolysis by AChE. In fact, in contrast to other neurotransmitters (e.g., norepinephrine), it is choline, the product of acetylcholine hydrolysis by AChE, that is taken up by the presynaptic terminal. Hence, inhibition of AChE by OPs causes accumulation of acetylcholine at cholinergic synapses, with overstimulation of cholinergic receptors of the muscarinic and nicotinic type. As these receptors are localized in most organs of the body, a "cholinergic syndrome" ensues, which includes increased sweating and salivation, profound bronchial secretion, bronchoconstriction, miosis, increased gastrointestinal motility, diarrhea, tremors, muscular twitching, and various central nervous system effects (Table 22-9). When death occurs, this is believed to be due to respiratory failure due to inhibition of respiratory centers in the brain stem, bronchoconstriction and increased bronchial secretion, and flaccid paralysis of respiratory muscles (Gallo and Lawryk, 1991; Lotti, 2000, 2001). The time interval between exposure and onset of symptoms varies with the route and degree of exposure, and the chemical nature of the OP. The first signs to appear are usually muscarinic,

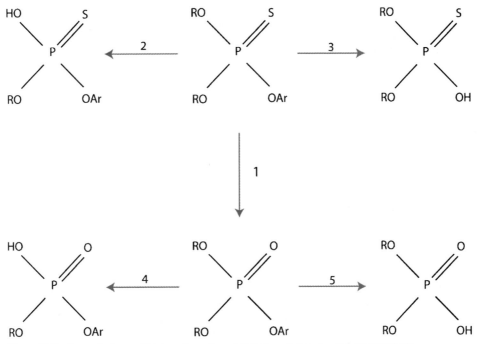

Figure 22-2. General scheme of biotransformation of dialkyl, aryl phosphorothioate insecticides.

Reaction 1 is the bioactivation, by oxidative desulfuration, of the parent compound to the active metabolite, the oxon. The other reactions are enzymatic detoxication reactions that yield products that do not inhibit acetylcholinesterase. Reaction 2 and 4 are dealkylation reactions, while reaction 3 is a dearylation. All are mediated by various cytochromes P450. Reaction 5 is a hydrolytic reaction, catalyzed by paraoxonase (PON1). Note that not all reactions occur with every organophosphorus insecticide.

which may or may not be in combination with nicotinic signs. While respiratory failure is a hallmark of severe OP poisoning, mild poisoning and/or early stages of an otherwise severe poisoning may display no clear-cut signs and symptoms (Lotti, 2001). Therefore, diagnosis is made through symptom recognition; miosis is observed most often, followed by gastrointestinal symptoms (nausea, vomiting, abdominal pain) and hypersalivation.

The interaction of OPs with AChE has been studied in much detail. OPs with a P=O moiety phosphorylate an hydroxyl group on serine in the active (esteratic) site of the enzyme, thus impeding its action on the physiological substrate (Fig. 22-3). The first reaction leads to the formation of a Michaelis complex, while a subsequent reaction leads to phosphorylated AChE (Table 22-10). Rates of these two reactions, that are usually very rapid, indicate the affinity of the enzyme for a given OP. The bond between the phosphorus atom and the esteratic site of the enzyme is much more stable than the bond between the carbonyl carbon of acetate (in acetylcholine) at the same enzyme site. While breaking of the carbon–enzyme bond is complete in a few microseconds, breaking of the phosphorus-enzyme bond can take from a few hours to several days, depending on the chemical structure of the OP. Phosphorylated AChE is hydrolyzed by water at a very slow rate (Fig. 22-3; Table 22-10), and the rate of "spontaneous reactivation" depends on the chemical nature of the R substituents. Reactivation decreases in the order demethoxy > diethoxy ≫ diisopropoxy (Gallo and Lawryk, 1991). Whereas water is a weak nucleophilic agent, certain hydroxylamine derivatives, known as oximes, can facilitate dephosphorylation of AChE, and are utilized in the therapy of OP poisoning (see below). Reactivation of phosphorylated AChE does not occur once the enzyme-inhibitor complex has "aged" (Fig. 22-3). Aging consists of the loss

(by nonenzymatic hydrolysis) of one of the two alkyl (R) groups, and the rate of aging depends on the nature of the alkyl group. When phosphorylated AChE has aged, the enzyme can be considered to be irreversibly inhibited, and the only means of replacing its activity is through synthesis of new enzyme, a process that may take days.

Treatment of Poisoning   Upon OP poisoning, prompt treatment is essential. Procedures aimed at decontamination and/or at minimizing absorption depend on the route of exposure. In case of dermal exposure, contaminated clothing should be removed, and the skin washed with alkaline soap (Lotti, 2001). Special attention should be exercised by medical personnel, because passive contamination may occur. In case of ingestion, procedures to reduce absorption from the gastrointestinal tract do not appear to be very effective (Lotti, 2001). Atropine represents the cornerstone of the treatment for OP poisoning; it is a muscarinic receptor antagonist, and thus prevents the action of accumulating acetylcholine on these receptors. Atropine is preferably given intravenously, though the intramuscular route is also effective. The best clinical approach is to administer doses of atropine large enough to achieve evidence of atropinization, i.e., flushing, dry mouth, changes in pupil size, bronchodilation, and increased heart rate; atropinization should be maintained for at least 48 hours (Lotti, 2001). Indicative doses of atropine are 1 mg or 2–5 mg in case of mild or moderate poisoning, respectively. Higher doses by continuous infusion may be required in severe cases. Overdosage with atropine is rarely serious in OP poisoned patients (Lotti, 2001).

Oximes, such as pralidoxime (2-PAM) are also used in the therapy of OP poisoning. 2-PAM contains a positively charged atom capable of attaching to the anionic site of AChE, and facilitate

Table 22-9
Signs and Symptoms of Acute Poisoning with Anticholinesterase Compounds

SITE AND RECEPTOR AFFECTED	MANIFESTATIONS
Exocrine glands (M)	Increased salivation, lacrimation, perspiration
Eyes (M)	Miosis, blurred vision
Gastrointestinal tract (M)	Abdominal cramps, vomiting, diarrhea
Respiratory tract (M)	Increased bronchial secretion, bronchoconstriction
Bladder (M)	Urinary frequency, incontinence
Cardiovascular system (M)	Bradycardia, hypotension
Cardiovascular system (N)	Tachycardia, transient hypertension
Skeletal muscles (N)	Muscle fasciculations, twitching, cramps, generalized weakness, flaccid paralysis
Central nervous system (M,N)	Dizziness, lethargy, fatigue, headache, mental confusion, depression of respiratory centers, convulsions, coma

M = muscarinic receptors; N = nicotinic receptors.

dephosphorylation of the enzyme (Fig. 22-4), thus restoring the catalytic site of AChE to its function. However, this chemical reaction occurs only when the phosphorylated AChE has not undergone aging. Dosing regimens for various oximes depend on the specific compound and the severity of OP poisoning. For example, for pralidoxime chloride, an initial 1 g dose given intravenously is recommended, followed after 15–30 minutes by another 1 g if no improvement is seen. If still no improvement is seen, an infusion of 0.5 g/h can be started (Lotti, 2001). The recommended dosage schedule is aimed at achieving a plasma oxime concentration of 4 mg/L, which was shown to be effective for pralidoxime methanesulfonate in cats poisoned with a quaternary analogue of sarin (Sundwall, 1961). While animal data consistently show a marked positive effect of oximes, several authors reported limited or no efficacy of oximes in the treatment of OP poisoning (Bismuth et al., 1992; Singh et al., 1995; Buckley et al., 2005). A recent meta-analysis of several studies of OP-poisoned patients concluded that use of oximes was associated "with either a null effect or possible harm" (Peter et al., 2006). On the other hand, inadequate dosing has been held as a major factor for lack of response to oxime therapy (Johnson et al., 2000; Eddleston et al., 2002). Furthermore, poisoning by OPs bearing two methoxy groups (malathion, methylparathion, dimethoate) is considered to be rather resistant to oxime therapy (Worek et al., 1999a). Additionally, time of oxime administration following OP poisoning is crucial, as their therapeutic window is determined by the rate of aging. For example, 1 day after intoxication with a dimethyl phosphoryl compound, virtually all phosphorylated AChE would be expected to be in the aged form, so that oxime therapy will be useless by that time (Johnson et al., 2000). Oximes also have the potential to form stable phosphoryl oximes that have themselves anticholinesterases activity; for this reason, and because of rapid reactivation of carbamylated AChE, oximes are not indicated in case of poisoning with carbamate insecticides.

In addition to oximes, diazepam (10–20 mg) is also used in the treatment of acute OP poisoning to relieve anxiety in mild cases, and to reduce muscle fasciculations and antagonize convulsions in the more severe cases (Lotti, 2001).

Biochemical Measurements   In addition to synapses, AChE is also present in red blood cells (RBC). Additionally, BuChE, also known as pseudo-cholinesterase, is found in plasma. The physiological functions of these enzymes are yet to be discovered. Never-

theless, because activity of both enzymes is usually inhibited upon exposure to OPs, their measurement is widely used as an indication of exposure, and/or biological effect of OPs. The specificity and usefulness of measurements of RBC AChE and of plasma BuChE in case of OP exposure have been debated for some time (Lotti, 1995). The main issues can be summarized as follows (Costa et al., 2005): (1) Different OPs may inhibit AChE or BuChE to a different degree. For example, the oxygen analogs of malathion, diazinon and chlorpyrifos, and dichlorvos, are stronger inhibitors of plasma BuChE than of RBC AChE. (2) There is a high degree of variability of enzyme activity (particularly of BuChE) among individuals, in part due to genetic differences (see below). This requires establishment of a baseline value for each individual, or in case this is not available, of repeated postexposure measurements to determine possible changes back toward baseline values. (3) RBC AChE activity is better correlated with target tissue (e.g., brain, diaphragm) AChE, than is plasma BuChE activity, as indicated by animal studies (Padilla et al., 1994). There is also a good correlation between the severity of signs and symptoms of poisoning and the degree of inhibition of RBC AChE (Lotti, 2001). (4) Neither measurement is specific for a certain OP, and indeed, other insecticides, such as carbamates, also inhibit AChE and BuChE. (5) A 30% or greater decrease of plasma BuChE from pre-exposure baseline raises a red flag, and requires health and workplace surveillance, and removal of the worker from the exposure; however, the toxicological significance of such decrease is still much debated (Carlock et al., 1999; USEPA, 2000). Despite these caveats, measurements of plasma BuChE, and particularly of RBC AChE, remain a very valid way to determine exposure to OPs, and early biological effects of OP exposure, to be used as confirmation of diagnosis of OP poisoning, or to monitor occupationally exposed workers. Several methods exist to measure activity of these two enzymes (Reiner and Simeon-Rudolf, 2006). Whole blood AChE may also be measured, considering that only about 10% of the activity is due to the plasma enzyme (Worek et al., 1999b).

Several analytical methods are available to measure OPs and their metabolites in body fluids; the parent compound is measured in blood, whereas metabolites are measured in urine (Lotti, 2001). These measurements are rarely carried out in the clinical setting, but are extensively utilized in epidemiological studies; indeed, determination of metabolite levels in urine is the most practical method to estimate exposure to OPs (Maroni et al., 2000). Such metabolites

Table 22-10

Rates of Cholinesterase Inhibition by Carbamate and Organophosphorus Esters

$$EH + AB \underset{k_{-1}}{\overset{k_1}{\rightleftharpoons}} EHAB \overset{k_2}{\to} EA + BH \overset{k_3}{\to} EH + AOH$$

		REACTION RATES	
PARAMETER	KINETIC CONSTANT	CARBAMATE	ORGANOPHOSPHORUS
Complex formation	k_{-1}/k_1	Rapid	Rapid
Inhibition rate	k_2	Variable	Rapid to moderately rapid
Reactivation rate	k_3	Relatively rapid	Slow to extremely slow

SOURCE: Ecobichon (2001a; 2001b).

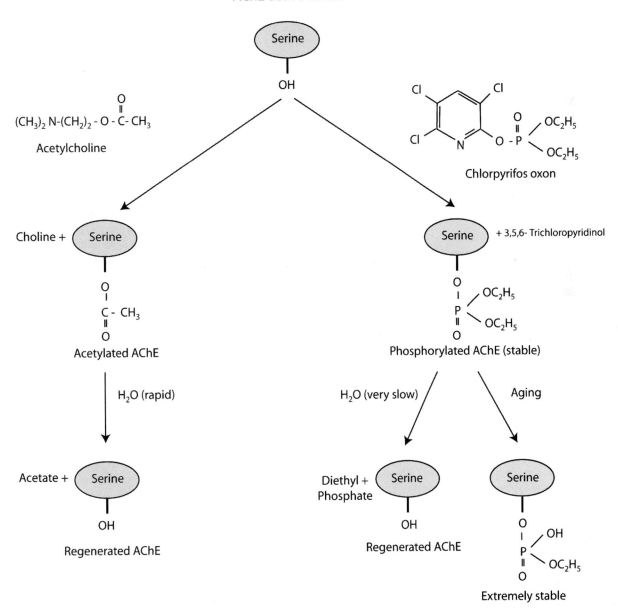

Figure 22-3. *Scheme of hydrolysis of acetylcholine by acetylcholinesterase (AChE) and reaction of chlorpyrifos oxon with AChE.*

(See text for details).

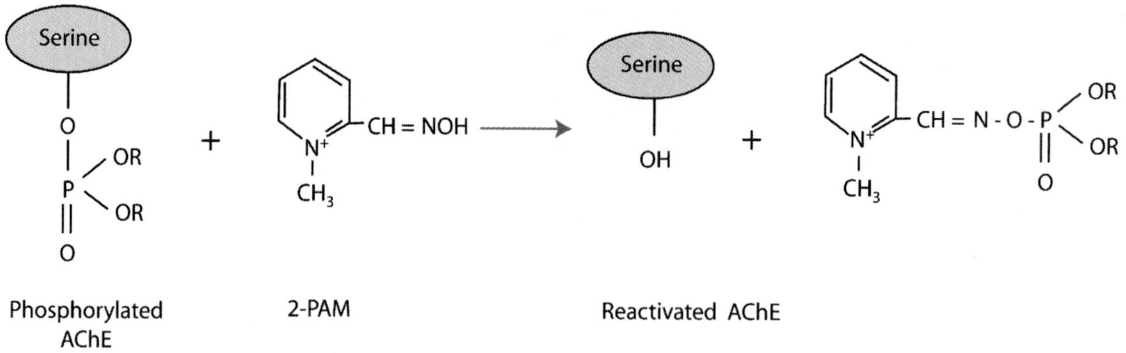

Figure 22-4. Reactivation of phosphorylated acetylcholinesterase by pralidoxime (2-PAM).

Note that 2-PAM is only effective before the phosphorylated enzyme has undergone the aging reaction.

Table 22-11

Examples of Alkylphosphates in Urine

METABOLITE	ORGANOPHOSPHATE
DMP (Dimethylphosphate)	Methylparathion, methylchlorpyrifos, dichlorvos, trichlorfon
DEP (Diethylphosphate)	Parathion, diazinon, chlorpyrifos
DMTP (Dimethylthiophosphate)	Azinphos-methyl (Guthion), fenitrothion
DETP (Diethylthiophosphate)	Diazinon, parathion, chlorpyrifos

SOURCE: Maroni *et al.* (2000).

include alkylphosphate derivatives, as well as chemical residues (the "leaving group") specific for each compound. The alkylphosphates or alkyl-(di)-thiophosphates are the result of metabolism of parent compounds or their oxygen analogs by CYPs or esterases. They are not specific for a certain OP, but are useful to assess exposure to (or internal dose of) several OPs. Some alkylphosphate metabolites of commonly used OPs are shown in Table 22-11. Other metabolites are specific for certain OP compounds; for example, p-nitrophenol in urine is an indicator of exposure to parathion or methyl parathion, whereas 3,5,6–trichloropyridinol is useful to assess exposure to chlorpyrifos or methyl chlorpyrifos. While measurements of urinary metabolites of OPs have been widely used to assess exposure to OP from occupational, environmental, and dietary sources, caution should be exercised when interpreting results, as dialkylphosphates, and also leaving groups, can be found in the environment, including food and drinks, as a result of OP degradation. This would lead to an overestimate of OP exposure (Lu *et al.*, 2005).

The Intermediate Syndrome A second distinct manifestation of exposure to OPs is the so-called intermediate syndrome, which was first conceptualized by clinicians in Sri Lanka involved in the treatment of suicide attempts (Senanayake and Karalliedde, 1987). The intermediate syndrome is seen in 20–50% of acute OP poisoning cases, and has been observed following exposure to a large variety of OPs. The syndrome develops one to several days after the poisoning, during recovery from cholinergic manifestations, or in some cases, when patients are completely recovered from the initial cholinergic crisis. Prominent features of the intermediate syndrome

are a marked weakness of respiratory, neck, and proximal limb muscles. Mortality due to respiratory paralysis and complications ranges from 15–40%, and recovery in surviving patients usually takes up to 15 days. The intermediate syndrome is not a direct effect of AChE inhibition, and its precise underlying mechanisms are unknown. One hypothesis is that muscle weakness may result from nicotinic receptor desensitization due to prolonged cholinergic stimulation (Lotti, 2001). There is no specific treatment for the intermediate syndrome and intervention is exclusively supportive.

Organophosphate-Induced Delayed Polyneuropathy A few OPs may also cause another type of toxicity, known as organophosphate-induced delayed polyneuropathy (OPIDP). Signs and symptoms include tingling of the hands and feet, followed by sensory loss, progressive muscle weakness and flaccidity of the distal skeletal muscles of the lower and upper extremities, and ataxia (Lotti, 1992; Ehrich and Jortner, 2001; Lotti and Moretto, 2005). These may occur 2–3 weeks after a single exposure, when signs of both the acute cholinergic and the intermediate syndromes have subsided. OPIDP can be classified as a distal sensorimotor axonopathy. Neuropathological studies in experimental OPIDP have evidenced that the primary lesion is a bilateral degenerative change in distal levels of axons and their terminals, primarily affecting larger/longer myelinated central and peripheral nerve fibers, leading to breakdown of neuritic segments and the myelin sheaths (Ehrich and Jortner, 2001). OPIDP is not related to AChE inhibition. Indeed, one of the compounds involved in several epidemics of this neuropathy, including the so-called Ginger-Jake paralysis in the 1930s in the United States, is TOCP (tri-ortho-cresyl phosphate), which is a very poor AChE inhibitor. Extensive studies carried out in the past 30 years (Johnson, 1982; Johnson and Glynn, 2001; Lotti, 1992) have identified the target for OPIDP as an esterase, present in nerve tissues as well as other tissues (e.g., lymphocytes), named neuropathy target esterase (NTE). Several OPs, depending on their chemical structure, can inhibit NTE, as do some non-OPs, such as certain carbamates and sulfonyl fluorides. Phosphorylation of NTE by OPs is similar to that observed for AChE. However, only OPs whose chemical structure leads to aging of phosphorylated NTE (by a process analogous to that described for AChE) can cause OPIDP. Other compounds that inhibit NTE but cannot undergo the aging reaction, are not neuropathic, indicating that inhibition of NTE catalytic activity is not the mechanism of axonal degeneration. For OPIDP to be initiated, phosphorylation and subsequent aging of at least 70% of NTE is necessary, and this two-step process occurs within hours of

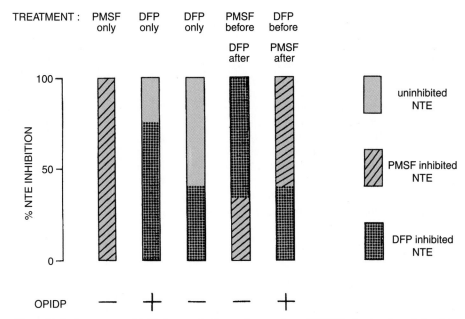

Figure 22-5. *A summary of initiation, protection and promotion of OPIDP, showing the relationships among dosing, NTE inhibition and clinical response, when DFP (diisopropylfluorophosphate) and PMSF (phenylmethanesulfonyl fluoride) are given alone or in combination.*

With permission from Lotti M, Caroldi S, Capodicasa E *et al.*: Promotion of organophosphate-induced delayed polyneuropathy by phenylmethanesulfonyl fluoride. *Toxicol Appl Pharmacol* 108:234–241, 1991.

poisoning. When the first clinical signs of OPIDP are evident some weeks later, NTE activity has recovered. Hypotheses to explain the consequences of OP-NTE interactions include a loss of nonesterase functions of NTE, that would be essential for the axon, or a gain of toxic function of phosphorylated/aged NTE (Lotti and Moretto, 2005). Though reductions in axonal transport have been found to precede overt clinical signs, the exact chain of events occurring between phosphorylation and aging of NTE and axonal degeneration remain obscure. The physiological functions(s) of NTE are also unknown. Recent studies have shown that NTE has a 41% identity with the Swiss Cheese Protein (SWS) in neurons of *Drosophila*. Studies in genetically modified mice have indicated that NTE is required for normal blood vessel and placental development, and that absence of brain NTE results in neuronal degeneration and loss of endoplasmic reticulum in various brain areas (Moser *et al.*, 2004; Akossoglou *et al.*, 2004). Interestingly, in *Drosophila* SWS mutants, extensive vacuolation is seen in the brain (Kretzschmar *et al.*, 1997). NTE also appears to play a role in membrane lipid metabolism, and may be involved in intra-neuronal membrane trafficking and lipid homeostasis (Zaccheo *et al.*, 2004; Glynn, 2006). However, the most crucial issues in the mechanisms of OPIDP development and progression remain obscure.

Though several epidemics of OPIDP have occurred in the past, its occurrence in humans is now rare. Before commercialization, OPs must undergo specific neurotoxicity testing in the hen (one of the most sensitive species) to determine whether OPIDP is produced (Moretto, 1999). High doses of OPs are used, and animals are protected from acute cholinergic toxicity with atropine, and clinical, morphological, and biochemical measurements are carried out. In vitro tests can provide the ratio of relative inhibitory potency toward AChE and NTE, but these have not been accepted by regulatory agencies (Ehrich *et al.*, 1997). Despite these tests, a few commercialized OPs (metamidophos, trichlorfon, chlorpyrifos) have caused

OPIDP in humans, mostly as a result of extremely high exposures in suicide attempts (Lotti and Moretto, 2005). Though it was once thought that some animal species (e.g., rodents) were insensitive to OPIDP, only mice appear to be somewhat resistant (Veronesi *et al.*, 1991). On the other hand, age is an important determinant of susceptibility, with young animals displaying more resistance; in young chicks the threshold for NTE inhibition and aging is >90% vs. 70% in adult hens (Peraica *et al.*, 1993). Children are also more resistant to OPIDP.

As noted earlier, compounds that inhibit NTE but do not age, do not cause OPIDP. When given to experimental animals *before* a neuropathic OP, these compounds exert a protective role, by occupying the NTE active site. However, when given *after* a neuropathic OP, these compounds have been shown to promote OPIDP (Fig. 22-5; Lotti *et al.*, 1991; Lotti, 2002a,b). By borrowing a terminology used for carcinogenic compounds, agents that phosphorylate NTE and age have been named initiators, whereas NTE inhibitors that do not initiate NTE but can promote it, have been named promoters (Lotti, 2002a,b). It is easy to understand why these latter compounds would be protective when given before an OP initiator; however, how they are able to promote OPIDP is still unknown. Promoters can also potentiate axonal degeneration caused by means other than OPs, such as traumatic nerve lesion, or 2,5-hexanedione (Moretto, 2000). Furthermore, promotion has also been shown to occur, in some cases, even when the promoter is given at doses that do not inhibit NTE, suggesting that another protein, rather than NTE, may be the target for the promoting effect. Because promotion is less efficient in chicks, where the compensation/repair mechanisms are thought to be more efficient, an hypothesis is that promotion may directly affect compensation/repair mechanism(s) of the nervous system (Lotti, 2002a,b). The issue of promotion may have a bearing on risk assessment of potential insecticide mixtures. Indeed, exposure to an initiator at a dose lower than that required to elicit OPIDP, would nevertheless result in OPIDP if followed by exposure to a promoter.

Genetic Susceptibility   Genetically determined variations in biotransformation enzymes or target molecules can modify the response to OPs (Costa, 2001). As discussed earlier, CYPs are important for the activation and detoxication of OPs. Variant forms of several CYPs have been identified, and these polymorphisms confer differences in catalytic activity or levels of expression which may result in varying rates of oxidation of OPs. Limited in vitro studies have indeed shown that polymorphic forms of some CYPs (e.g., CYP2C19 or CYP3A4) cause differential desulfuration and dearylation of chlorpyrifos (Hodgson, 2003), but their overall influence on OP toxicity in vivo has not been investigated. The liver and plasma A-esterase paraoxonase (PON1), which detoxifies chlorpyrifos oxon and diazoxon, also presents several polymorphisms in the coding and promoter regions, that affect the catalytic efficiency of the enzyme toward different substrates (the Q192R polymorphism), and its level of expression (e.g., the C-108T polymorphism) (Costa et al., 2002, 2003). Studies in transgenic animal models have clearly indicated that PON1 "status," encompassing both the Q192R polymorphism and the level of PON1 activity, plays a most relevant role in modulating the acute toxicity of some OPs (Fig. 22-6; Li et al., 2000; Cole et al., 2005).

High levels of BuChE are present in plasma, and OPs can inhibit its activity. Though its physiological function is unclear, BuChE, by scavenging OPs, can guard against their toxicity, as the OP would be unavailable for reaction with its primary target AChE (Costa, 2001). At least 39 genetic variants of BuChE have been identified, with nucleotide alterations in the coding region. Several of these variants are silent, but they are rare; most common variants have a reduced activity and are far less efficient scavengers of cholinesterase inhibitors (Lockridge and Masson, 2000; Goodal, 2006). Individuals with such BuChE variants would be predicted to be more susceptible to OP toxicity, as suggested by a study in Brazilian farmers (Fontoura-da-Silva and Chautard-Friere-Maira, 1996). To date, only a few genetic variants of human AChE have been described (Goodal, 2006). One resulted in an amino acid change but had no effect on the catalytic properties of the enzyme (Masson et al., 1994), whereas a polymorphism in the distal promoter region was associated with an enhanced response to pyridostigmine (Shapira et al., 2000). A third study identified several polymorphisms in the coding region, that also did not appear to alter the catalytic action of AChE (Hasin et al., 2004). Transgenic mice carrying one deficient AChE allele (AChE $^{+/-}$) are healthy, and display supersensitivity to OPs (Lockridge et al., 2005). Genetic polymorphisms of AChE in humans that would cause partial AChE deficiency have been hypothesized, but not yet demonstrated; such individuals would be expected to display increased susceptibility to OP toxicity.

Long-Term Toxicity   Whereas the effects of acute exposure to OPs have been clearly identified and characterized by thousands of animal studies and cases of human poisonings, there is still controversy on possible long-term effects of OPs. That acute exposure to high doses of OPs may result, in some cases, in long-lasting adverse health effects (particularly in the CNS) has been shown in animals, as well as humans (Sanchez-Santed et al., 2004; Rosenstock et al., 1991). More controversial is the possibility that low exposure to OPs, at doses that produce no cholinergic signs, may lead to long-term adverse health effects, particularly in the central and peripheral

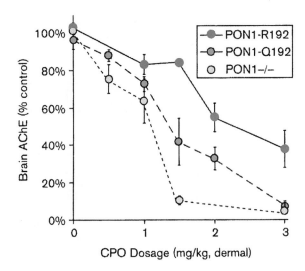

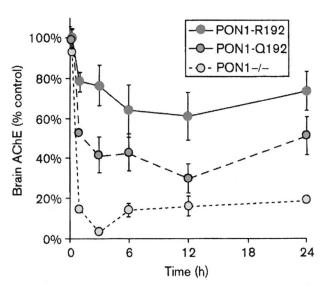

Figure 22-6. Dose–response (top panel) and time-course (bottom panel) of brain acetylcholinesterase (AChE) inhibition by chlorpyrifos oxon (CPO) in PON1 knockout mice (PON1 -/-) or in mice expressing either of the two human PON1 $_{R192}$ or PON1 $_{Q192}$ transgenes in place of endogenous mouse PON1.

Note that mice lacking PON1 are most sensitive to CPO toxicity, while those expressing human PON1 $_{R192}$ are most resistant. Mice expressing human PON1 $_{Q192}$ show intermediate sensitivity, despite expressing similar levels of PON1. The experiments indicate the role of PON1 "status" in modulating the toxicity of CPO. Modified with permission from Cole TB, Walter BJ, Shih DM et al.: Toxicity of chlorpyrifos and chlorpyrifos oxon in a transgenic mouse model of the human paraoxonase (PON1) Q192R polymorphism. *Pharmacogenet Genomics* 15:589–598, Lippincott Williams & Wilkins (http://lww.com), 2005.

nervous systems. Chronic exposure of animals to OPs, at doses that significantly inhibit AChE, but may not be associated with clinical signs, results in the development of tolerance to their cholinergic effects (which is mediated, at least in part, by down-regulation of cholinergic receptors), and has been associated with neurobehavioral abnormalities, particularly at the cognitive level (Costa et al., 1982; Prendergast et al., 1998). Evidence describing long-term

Figure 22-7. Structures of some carbamate insecticides, with indication of acute oral and dermal toxicity in the rat, and of water solubility.

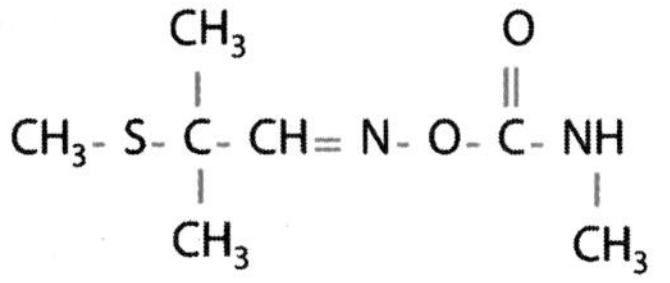

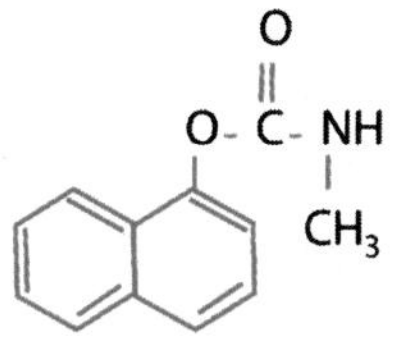

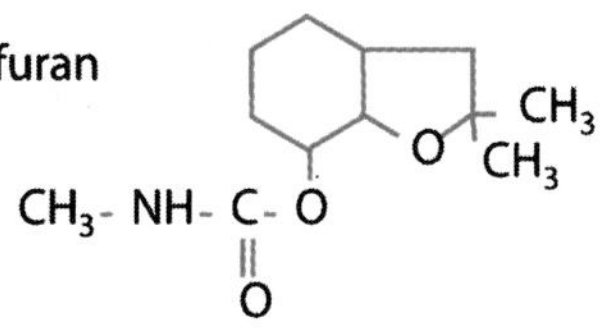

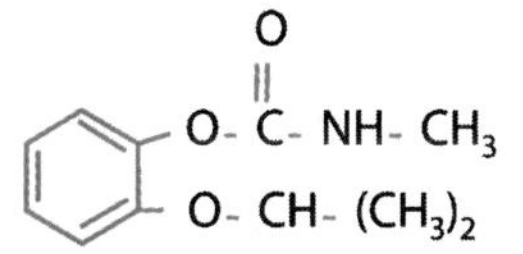

neuropsychological or neuropsychiatric alterations in humans upon low chronic exposure is contradictory (Daniell *et al.*, 1992; Jamal and Julu, 2002), and most recent expert reviews tend to conclude that the balance of evidence does not support the existence of clinically significant neuropsychological effects, neuropsychiatric abnormalities, or peripheral nerve dysfunction in humans chronically exposed to low levels of OPs (Ray, 1998; Lotti 2002a,b; Colosio *et al.*, 2003; IOM, 2000). Yet, research in this area, and the ensuing debate, will undoubtedly continue.

OPs as a class are not considered to be mutagenic, and there is little evidence that they may be carcinogenic. Immunotoxicity of OPs has been suggested from in vitro or high dose animal studies, but evidence in humans is lacking. Some OPs have also endocrine disrupting activities in vitro (Tamura *et al.*, 2003), but in vivo studies, even at dose levels that inhibit brain AChE activity, have not substantiated these findings (Okahashi *et al.*, 2005).

Developmental Toxicity and Neurotoxicity   In the past decade, a report from the National Academy of Sciences has highlighted the potential higher exposure of children to pesticides (NRC, 1993), and FQPA indicates that in the risk assessment process, an additional safety factor should be included to ensure protection of children who are presumed to be more sensitive to the effects of toxicants (FQPA, 1996). Experimental data indicate that young animals are more sensitive to the acute toxicity of OPs (Costa, 2006). This increased sensitivity does not appear to be due to intrinsic differences in AChE, but rather to lower detoxication abilities of young animals.

For example, low detoxication by CYPs or PON1 accounts for the age-dependent susceptibility of parathion and chlorpyrifos, respectively (Benke and Murphy, 1975; Mortensen *et al.*, 1996). In contrast, as discussed earlier, the young appear to be more resistant to OPIDP. In recent years, accumulating evidence suggests perinatal exposure to OPs may cause developmental neurotoxicity. Studies in rodents indicate that OPs can affect various cellular processes (e.g., DNA replication, neuronal survival, neurite outgrowth), noncholinergic pathways (e.g., serotoninergic synaptic functions, the adenylate cylase system), and cause various behavioral abnormalities (Song *et al.,* 1997; Dam *et al.,* 1998; Jett *et al.,* 2001; Aldridge *et al.,* 2003; Ricceri *et al.,* 2003; Garcia *et al.,* 2005). Such effects were often seen at dose levels that produced no cholinergic signs of toxicity. These findings, together with results of biomonitoring studies that indicate exposure of children, particularly in inner cities and farming communities, to OPs, have led to regulatory restrictions on the use of certain OPs, and to heightened concern for their potential neurotoxic effects in children (Eskenazi *et al.,* 1999; Weiss *et al.,* 2004). Furthermore, specific guidelines for developmental neurotoxicity have been implemented (Tilson, 2000).

Carbamates

Carbamate insecticides have a variety of chemical structures (Fig. 22-7), but all derive from carbamic acid, the majority being *N*-methylcarbamates. They present different degrees of acute oral toxicity, ranging from moderate to low toxicity such as carbaryl, to

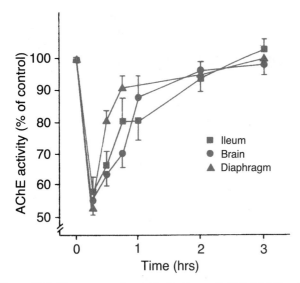

Figure 22-8. Time-course of acetylcholinesterase (AChE) inhibition in different tissues of mice following administration of a single dose of the carbamate insecticide propoxur (10 mg/kg, i.p.).

Note the near complete recovery of AChE activity two hours after propoxur administration. With permission from Costa LG, Hand H, Schwab BW *et al.*: Tolerance to the carbamate insecticide propoxur. *Toxicology* 21:267–278, Elsevier, 1981.

extremely high toxicity, such as aldicarb (Fig. 22-7). Dermal toxicity is lower, but skin penetration is increased by organic solvents and emulsifiers present in most formulations (Ecobichon, 2001b). Carbamates are susceptible to a variety of enzyme-catalyzed biotransformation reactions, and the principal pathways involve oxidation and hydrolysis (Fukuto, 1972; Tang *et al.*, 2006). For the most part, the metabolites are devoid of biological activity, but this is not always the case. For example, two metabolites of aldicarb, the sulfoxide and the sulfone, are more potent anticholinesterases than the parent compound (Risher *et al.*, 1987). The mechanism of toxicity of carbamates is analogous to that of OPs, in that they inhibit AChE. However, inhibition is transient and rapidly reversible, because there is rapid reactivation of the carbamylated enzyme in the presence of water (Table 22-10). Additionally, carbamylated AChE does not undergo the aging reaction. The sign and symptoms of carbamate poisoning are the same as observed following intoxication with OPs, and include miosis, urination, diarrhea, salivation, muscle fasciculation, and CNS effects (Table 22-9). However, differently from OPs, acute intoxication by carbamates is generally resolved within a few hours. Figure 22-8 shows experimental data on AChE inhibition by propoxur in mice; maximal inhibition is achieved very rapidly, as carbamates are direct AChE inhibitors and do not require metabolic bioactivation, and enzyme activity returns to control levels within two hours. Carbamates also inhibit BuChE; the degree of such inhibition varies depending on the specific compound, but is generally modest after moderate exposure (when, however, inhibition of red blood cells and nervous tissue AChE can be substantial), and equivalent to that of AChE after severe exposure (Ecobichon, 2001b).

The transient nature of AChE inhibition following carbamate exposure poses several problems in measurements of its activity. First, measurements should be made shortly (a few hours at most) following exposure; otherwise, even if severe inhibition and symptoms of toxicity were present, the latter would be resolved, and

no enzyme inhibition would be detected. Secondly, particular care should be taken even if blood samples are drawn shortly after exposure, as temperature and time elapsed before the assay would cause reversal of inhibition. The treatment of carbamate intoxication relies on the use of the muscarinic antagonist atropine. Use of oximes is generally not recommended, as 2-PAM has been shown to aggravate the toxicity of carbaryl (Murphy, 1986). Yet, oximes may have beneficial effects in case of other carbamates such as aldicarb (Ecobichon, 2001b). There are several cases of human poisoning associated with exposure to various carbamates, in particular carbaryl (Cranmer, 1986) and propoxur (Hayes, 1982). Most cases, however, involved aldicarb. This compound, which has a very high acute toxicity, is also highly water soluble (Fig. 22-7). Though, because of this characteristic, it is not registered for use on any fruit or vegetable having a high water content, its illegal use in hydroponically grown cucumbers, and in watermelons have led to outbreaks of poisoning (Goes *et al.*, 1980; Goldman *et al.*, 1990). Contamination of drinking water has also been reported (Zaki *et al.*, 1982). Carbamates can inhibit NTE, but because carbamylated NTE cannot age, they are thought to be unable to initiate OPIDP. Additionally, when given before a neuropathic organophosphate, carbamates offer protection against OPIDP (Johnson and Lawerys, 1969), but when given after, they can promote OPIDP (Lotti, 2002b). A few case reports indicate that exposure to very high dosages of methylcarbamates (e.g., carbaryl, carbofuran), may result in a peripheral polyneuropathy similar to OPIDP (Dickoff *et al.*, 1987; Yang *et al.*, 2000). This would imply that aging is not required for OPIDP to develop, or, alternatively, that in these cases, carbamates may have amplified a pre-existing subclinical neuropathy. Carefully conducted animal studies would be needed to substantiate this hypothesis.

Subchronic and chronic toxicity studies on carbamate insecticides have been carried out mostly for registration purposes, and their main findings (inhibition of cholinesterases, effects on organ weight and hematological parameters, histopathological changes) are described in detail by Baron (1991). Development of tolerance to some carbamates (propoxur, carbaryl) upon repeated exposure has been observed, and this appears to be due to an induction of microsomal enzymes (Costa *et al.*, 1981). As a class, methylcarbamates are not mutagenic, and there is also no evidence of carcinogenicity. Embryotoxicity or fetotoxicity are observed only at maternally toxic doses (Baron, 1991). Limited evidence suggests that carbamates (e.g., aldicarb) may be more acutely toxic to young animals than to adults (Moser, 1999), possibly because of lower detoxication, but this aspect has not been investigated in the same detail as for OPs.

Pyrethroids

Pyrethrins were first developed as insecticides from extracts of the flower heads of *Chrisanthenum cinerariaefolium*, whose insecticidal potential was appreciated in ancient China and Persia. However, because pyrethrins were decomposed rapidly by light, synthetic analogs, the pyrethroids, were developed. Because of their high insecticidal potency, relatively low mammalian toxicity, lack of environmental persistence, and low tendency to induce insect resistance, pyrethroids have encountered much success in the past thirty years, and now account for more than 25% of the global insecticide market (Soderlund *et al.*, 2002). Pyrethroids are used widely as insecticides both in the house and in agriculture, in medicine for the topical treatment of scabies and head lice, and in tropical countries in soaked bed nets to prevent mosquito bites. Pyrethroids are known to alter the normal function of insect nerves by modifying the kinetics of voltage-sensitive sodium channels, which mediate the transient increase in the sodium permeability of the nerve membrane that underlies the nerve action potential (Soderlund *et al.*, 2002). All pyrethroid insecticides contain an acid moiety, a central ester bond, and an alcohol moiety (Fig. 22-9). The acid moiety contains two chiral carbons, thus pyrethroid typically exist as stereoisomeric compounds (*trans* and *cis*). Additionally, some pyrethroids also have a chiral carbon on the alcohol moiety, allowing for a total of eight different stereoenantiomers. These chemical considerations are relevant, as pyrethroids' effects on sodium channels, their insecticidal activity, and their mammalian toxicity, are stereospecific. The *cis* isomers are generally more toxic than the corresponding *trans* isomers (Casida *et al.*, 1983). The acute oral mammalian toxicity of pyrethroids is generally low. Values of LD_{50} range, for example, from 100 mg/kg (deltamethrin) to 10,000 mg/kg (phenothrin). To underline the relevance of stereospecificity, the LD_{50} for 1R, *trans*-resmethrin is 8,000 mg/kg, but that of 1R, *cis*-resmethrin is 100 mg/kg (Casida *et al.*, 1983). The low mammalian toxicity of pyrethroids is confirmed by the fact that despite their extensive worldwide use, there are relatively few reports of human poisonings, and only a dozen deaths (Bradberry *et al.*, 2005). Most deaths occurred following accidental or intentional exposure to pyrethroids. For example, a 45-year-old man died three hours after eating beans and cheese prepared using a 10% cypermethrin solution instead of oil (Poulos *et al.*, 1982). The dermal toxicity of pyrethroid is even lower, because of limited absorption through the skin.

Upon absorption, pyrethroids are very rapidly metabolized through two major biotransformation routes: hydrolysis of the ester linkage, which is catalyzed by hepatic and plasma carboxylesterases, and oxidation of the alcohol moiety by cytochromes P450 (Miyamoto, 1976; Soderlund and Casida, 1977). These initial reactions are followed by further oxidations, hydrolysis and conjugation with sulfate or glucuronide. The relative importance of the hydrolytic or oxidative biotransformation varies from compound to compound, and from isomer to isomer for each pyrethroid. For example, the *trans* isomer of permethrin is more susceptible to hydrolysis by carboxylesterase than the *cis* isomer (Soderlund and Casida, 1977; Ross *et al.*, 2006). Type II pyrethroids (see below) are less sensitive to hydrolysis. For instance, deltamethrin, a type II pyrethroid containing a cyano group (Fig. 22-9), and present solely as the *cis* isomer, is more extensively metabolized by hepatic cytochromes P450, particularly CYP1A2 and CYP1A1 (Vmax/Km = 34.9), than by liver carboxylesterase (Vmax/Km = 11.5) (Anand *et al.*, 2006a). Though it has been suggested that oxidative metabolism may lead in some cases, to bioactivation of certain pyrethroids (Dayal *et al.*, 2003; Ray and Fry, 2006), the current line of evidence would suggest that hydrolytic and oxidative metabolism achieve detoxication of the parent, active compound (Soderlund *et al.*, 2002). Inhibition of cytochromes P450 by piperonyl butoxide indeed increases pyrethroid toxicity, and so does inhibition of carboxylesterase (Casida *et al.*, 1983). Piperonyl butoxide is added to most pyrethroid formulations as a synergist. Inhibition of carboxylesterase may be of significance, if unauthorized pyrethroid/organophosphate mixtures are utilized (Ray and Forshaw, 2000). In fact, several organophosphates inhibit carboxylesterase activity, and may thus be expected to potentiate pyrethroid toxicity (Choi *et al.*, 2004).

Signs and Symptoms of Toxicity and Mechanism of Action
The acute mammalian toxicity of pyrethroids is well character-

Table 22-12

Classification of Pyrethroid Insecticides Based on Toxic Signs in Rats

SYNDROME	SIGNS AND SYMPTOMS	EXAMPLES
Type I (T syndrome)	Aggressive sparring Increased sensitivity to external stimuli Whole body tremors Prostration	Allethrin Bioallethrin Resmethrin Phenothrin
Type 2 (CS syndrome)	Pawing and burrowing Profuse salivation Coarse Tremor Choreoatetosis Clonic seizures	Deltamethrin Fenvalerate Cypermethrin Cyhalothrin

ized. Based on toxic signs in rats, pyrethroids have been divided into two types (Table 22-12; Verschoyle and Aldridge, 1980). Type I compounds produce a syndrome consisting in marked behavioral arousal, aggressive sparring, increased startle response, and fine body tremor progressing to whole-body tremor and prostration (Type I or T syndrome). Type II compounds produce profuse salivation, coarse tremor progressing to choreoatetosis and clonic seizures (Type II or CS syndrome) (Soderlund *et al.*, 2002; Ray and Fry, 2006). A key structural difference between type I and type II pyrethroids is the presence only in the latter of a cyano group at the α carbon of the alcohol moiety of the compound (Fig. 22-9). However, certain pyrethroids (e.g., cyphenothrin, flucythrinate) elude such classification, as they produce a combination of the two syndromes (Soderlund *et al.*, 2002; Ray and Fry, 2006).

The mode of action of pyrethroids in mammals is the same as in insects, disruption of the voltage-gated sodium channels (Narahashi, 1996). Pyrethroids bind to the α subunit of the sodium channel and slow the activation (opening), as well as the rate of inactivation (closing) of the sodium channel, leading to a stable hyperexcitable state. Sodium channels then open at more hyperpolarized potentials, and are held open longer, allowing more sodium ions to cross and depolarize the neuronal membrane (Shafer *et al.*, 2005). In general, type II compounds delay the inactivation of sodium channels substantially longer (>10 ms) than do type I compounds (<10 ms) (Ray and Fry, 2006). Type I compounds prolong channel opening only long enough to cause repetitive firing of action potential (repetitive discharge), analogously to DDT (Vijveberg *et al.*, 1982); type II compounds hold the channels open for such long periods that the membrane potential ultimately becomes depolarized to the point at which generation of action potential is not possible (depolarization-dependent block) (Fig. 22-10; Shafer *et al.*, 2005). These differences in the time of opening of sodium channels are believed to be at the basis of the differences observed between the T and CS syndromes (Ray and Fry, 2006). The higher sensitivity of insects to pyrethroid toxicity, compared to mammals, is believed to result from a combination of higher sensitivity of insect sodium channels, lower body temperature (as pyrethroids show a negative temperature coefficient of action), and slower biotransformation (Ray and Fry, 2006). Type II pyrethroids, but not type I compounds, also bind to, and inhibit $GABA_A$-gated chloride channels (Lawrence and Casida, 1983), albeit at higher concentrations than those sufficient to affect

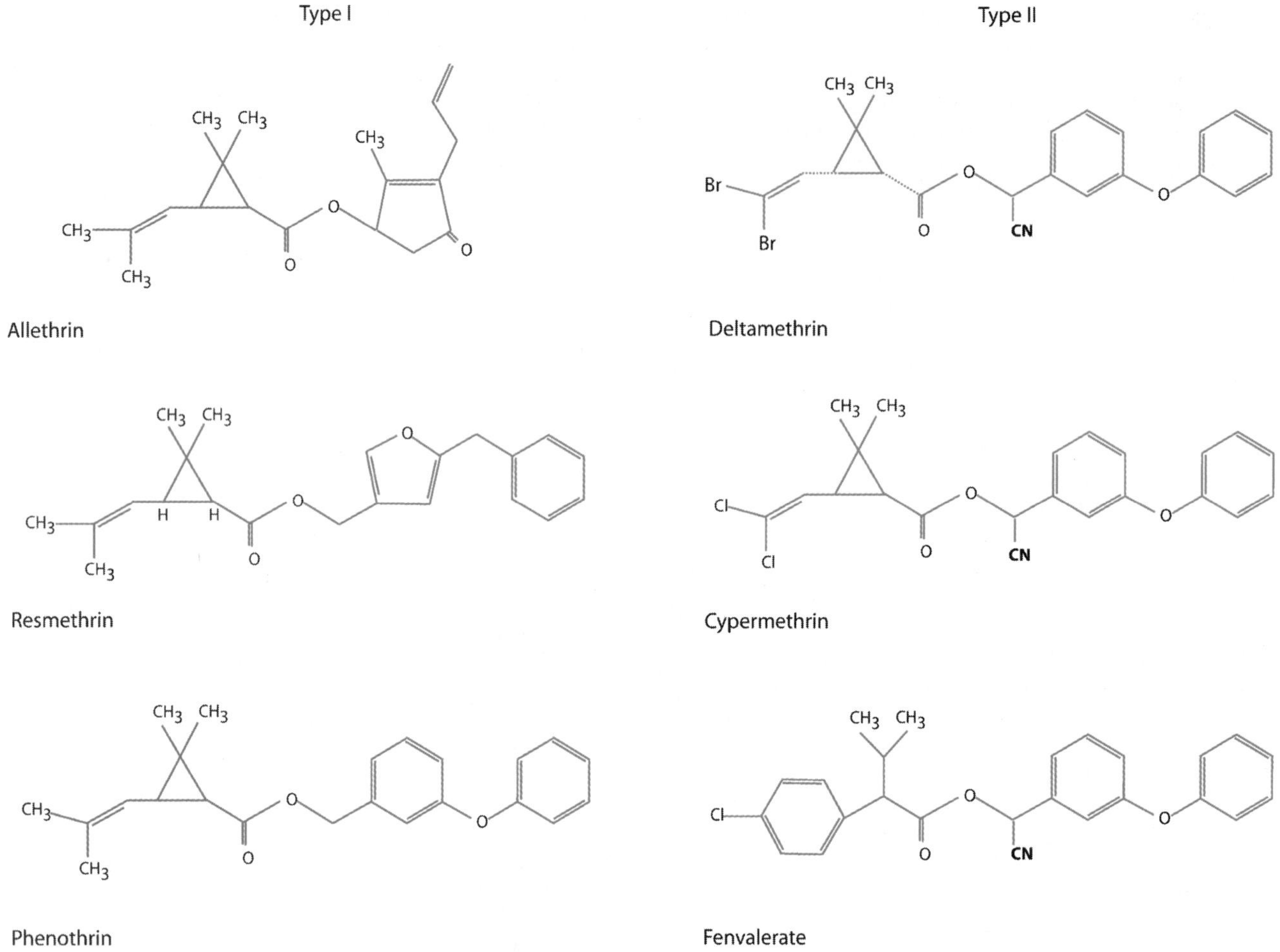

Figure 22-9. *Structures of Type I (left) and Type II (right) pyrethroid insecticides. Note that all Type II pyrethroids display a cyano (CN) group.*

sodium channels (10^{-7}M vs 10^{-10}M). This effect is believed to contribute to the seizures that accompany severe type II pyrethroid poisoning. However, drugs that enhance GABAergic transmission (e.g., diazepam), have modest effects toward deltamethrin-induced choreoatetosis or seizures. Type II pyrethroids, such as deltamethrin, also inhibit at low concentration (10^{-10}M) voltage-dependent chloride channels (Forshaw *et al.*, 1993). Because chemicals that open these chloride channels, such as ivermectin and pentobarbital, antagonize pyrethroid-induced choreoatetosis and salivation, inhibition of maxi voltage-dependent chloride channels by pyrethroid may contribute to the type II poisoning syndrome (Forshaw *et al.*, 2000). Other reported targets for pyrethroids include calcium ATPase and voltage-gated calcium channels, which are however, affected at higher concentrations (10^{-5} M and 10^{-6}M, respectively). Of potential interest was the observation that several pyrethroids could stimulate protein kinase C-dependent protein phosphorylation at very low concentrations (10^{-13}M), (Enan and Matsumura, 1993), but whether this interaction is involved in the modulation of sodium and/or chloride channels remains to be determined.

Young animals are more sensitive to the acute toxicity of certain pyrethroids, such as deltramethrin and cypermethrin (Sheets, 2000), most likely because of a lesser capacity for metabolic detoxification (Anand *et al.*, 2006b); however, only minor age-related differences were found for other compounds (Sheets, 2000). Some studies have suggested that certain pyrethroids may cause devel-

opmental neurotoxicity, but current evidence has been judged inadequate (Shafer *et al.*, 2005). Furthermore, levels of background pyrethroid exposure (presumably through residues in the diet) in children has been found to be of orders of magnitude lower than the corresponding acceptable daily intake (Heudorf *et al.*, 2004). Also, the use of deltamethrin-impregnated bed nets does not appear to pose any health risk in children and neonates (Barlow *et al.*, 2001), while substantially reducing infant mortality from malaria (Alonso *et al.*, 1991).

Upon occupational exposure, the primary adverse effect resulting from dermal contact with pyrethroids is paresthesia (Flannigan *et al.*, 1985; He *et al.*, 1989). Symptoms include continuous tingling or pricking or, when more severe, burning. The condition reverses in about 24 hours, and topical application of vitamin E has been shown to be an effective treatment. Paresthesia is presumably due to abnormal pyrethroid-induced repetitive activity in skin nerve terminals (Ray and Fry, 2006).

Chronic studies with pyrethroids indicate that at high dose levels they cause slight liver enlargement often accompanied by some histopathological changes. There is little evidence of teratogenicity and mutagenicity (Miyamoto, 1976; Ray, 1991). An increased rate of lymphoma incidence in rodents has been reported for deltamethrin, but the effect was not dose-dependent (Cabral *et al.*, 1990). There is no compelling evidence that pyrethroids may act as endocrine disruptors (Kim *et al.*, 2004). Pyrethroids are particularly toxic to fish, but not to birds (Miyamoto, 1976).

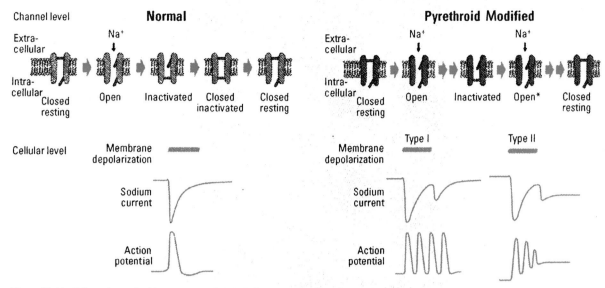

Figure 22-10. Effect of pyrethroids on neuronal excitability.

Depolarization opens voltage sensitive sodium channels (VSSCs) allowing Na^+ to enter the cell. To limit Na^+ entry and depolarization length, VSSCs inactivate and return to a "resting" state before reopening (top left). Pyrethroids delay inactivation (double arrows between states) of the channel and allow continued Na+ flux (Open *) (top right). Under normal circumstances, depolarization leads to a rapidly inactivating current, and generates a single action potential (bottom left). Pyrethroid-modified VSSCs remain open when depolarization ends, resulting in a "tail" current. Type I compounds depolarize the cell membrane above the threshold for action potential generation, resulting in a series of action potential (repetitive firing). Type II compounds cause greater membrane depolarization, diminishing the Na^+ electrochemical gradient and subsequent action potential amplitude, eventually leading to depolarization-dependent block (bottom right). From Shafer *et al.* (2005) with permission.

Organochlorine Compounds

The organochlorine insecticides include the chlorinated ethane derivatives, such as DDT and its analogues; the cyclodienes, such as chlordane, aldrin, dieldrin, heptachlor, endrin, and toxaphene; the hexachlorocyclohexanes, such as lindane; and the caged structures mirex and chlordecone (Figs. 22-11 and 22-12). From the 1940s to the 1970s and 1980s, the organochlorine insecticides enjoyed wide use in agriculture, structure insect control, and malaria control programs. Their acute toxicity is moderate (less than that of organophosphates), but chronic exposure may be associated with adverse health effects particularly in the liver and the reproductive system. Primarily because of ecological considerations, these compounds have been banned in most countries in the past thirty years. Yet, because of their environmental persistence and high lipophilicity, exposure to these compounds continues, most notably through the diet. Furthermore, some, such as DDT, are being reintroduced in part of the world for malaria control; hence, a discussion of their toxicity has more than historical value.

DDT and Its Analogues   DDT [1,1,1-trichloro-2, 2-bis (4-chlorophenyl) ethane] was first synthesized by O. Zeidler in 1874, but its insecticidal activity was discovered only in 1939 by Paul Mueller in Switzerland. Early experiments showed that DDT was effective against a wide variety of agricultural pests, as well as against insects that transmit some of the world's most serious diseases, such as typhus, malaria, and yellow fever. In the United States, annual use of DDT rose until 1959 to about 36,000 tons, after which it declined gradually until its ban in 1972 (Rogan and Chen, 2005). However, as said, because of its high persistence, global redistribution, and its current use in many parts of the world, a discussion of the toxicology of DDT is still of relevance (Longnecker, 2005). While

DDT is the universally accepted common name of the insecticide, technical-trade DDT is a mixture of several isomers (Fig. 22-11), with p,p'-DDT being responsible for the insecticidal activity.

DDT has a moderate acute toxicity when given by the oral route, with an LD_{50} of about 250 mg/kg; p,p'-DDT is at least 10-fold more toxic than o, p'-DDT (Smith, 2001). Dermal absorption of DDT is very limited, resulting in dermal LD_{50} values of >1000 mg/kg. In humans, oral doses of 10–20 mg/kg produce illness, but doses as high as 285 mg/kg have been ingested accidentally without fatal results. Toxicity from dermal exposure in humans is also low, as evidenced by the lack of significant adverse health effects when thousands of people were liberally dusted with this compound. Upon absorption, DDT distributes in all tissues, and the highest concentrations are found in adipose tissue. DDT is also extensively but slowly metabolized, with DDE, DDD and DDA (in each case both the p,p' and the o,p' isomers) being the primary metabolites in humans (Smith, 2001). DDE is also stored in adipose tissue. Excretion is through the bile, urine, and the milk.

Acute exposure to high doses of DDT causes motor unrest, increased frequency of spontaneous movements, abnormal susceptibility to fear and hypersusceptibility to external stimuli (light, touch, sound). This is followed by the development of fine tremors, progressing to coarse tremors, and eventually tonic-clonic convulsions. Symptoms usually appear several hours after exposure, and death, usually due to respiratory failure, may follow after 24–72 hours (Ecobichon and Joy, 1982). Signs and symptoms of poisoning are similar in most animals species, with dogs displaying prominent convulsions. There is no evidence that young animals may be more sensitive than adults to the acute toxicity of DDT, and they may actually be less sensitive (Smith, 2001). In humans, the earliest symptom of poisoning by DDT is hyperesthesia of the mouth and lower part of the face, followed by paresthesia of the same area and of the tongue.

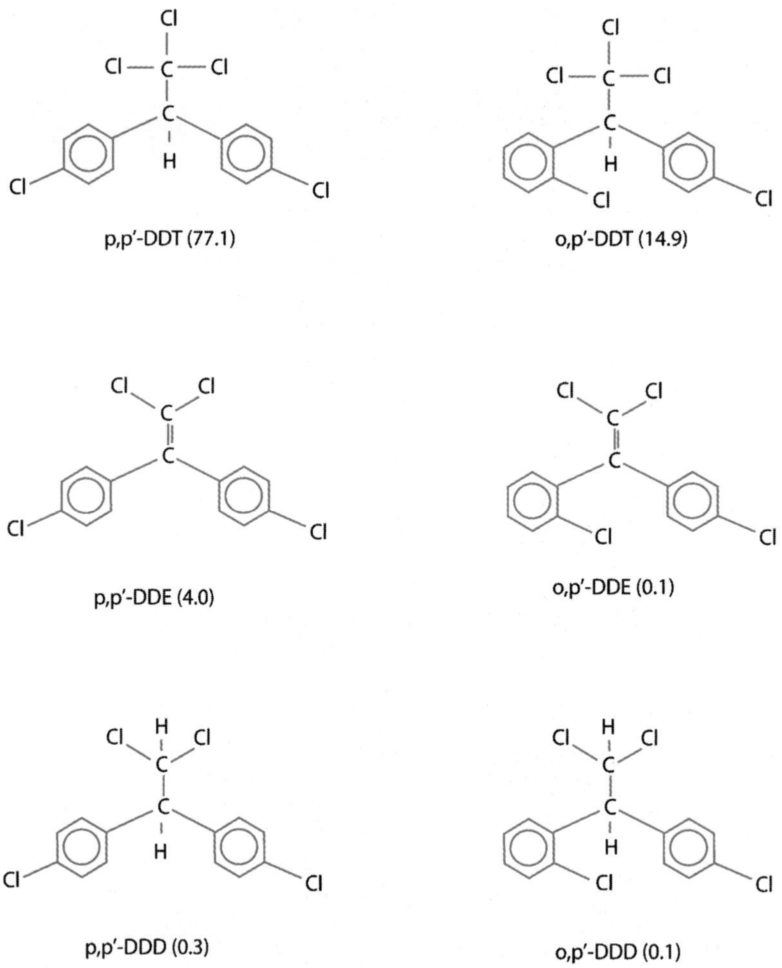

Figure 22-11. Structures of the organochlorine insecticide p,p'-DDT and its isomers.

The percentage of each isomer present in technical grade DDT is indicated in parenthesis. DDE and DDD also result from biotransformation of DDT.

Dizziness, tremor of the extremities, confusion and vomiting follow, while convulsions occur only in severe poisoning.

Signs and symptoms of acute poisoning clearly point at the nervous system as the primary target for DDT toxicity (Woolley, 1982). Both in insects and in mammals, DDT interferes with the sodium channels in the axonal membrane by a mechanism similar to that of Type I pyrethroids (Vijverberg et al., 1982). DDT has little or no effect on the resting potential or the rising phase and peak amplitude of the action potential. However, it greatly prolongs the depolarizing (negative) afterpotential of the action potential, and this produces a period of increased neuronal excitability immediately after the spike phase. This, in turn, enhances the probability of repetitive firing, and the insurgence of a "train" of action potentials (Fig. 22-13). Voltage clamp studies have shown that the principal effect of DDT is to slow down the closing of sodium channels once they have opened, while having little or no effect on closed gates. In addition to this effect on sodium channels, DDT also affects ATPases. Though DDT inhibits Na^+, K^+-ATPase, this action would not contribute to its neurotoxic effect (Matsumura and Patil, 1969). Rather, inhibition of a Ca^{2+}-ATPase (an ecto-ATPase, located on the outside of the cell membrane) may be involved in the effects of DDT. As the function of this Ca^{2+}-ATPase is believed to be that of maintaining high external calcium concentrations, its inhibition would lower external calcium and contribute to membrane instability and repetitive firing (Matsumura and Ghiasuddin, 1979). Several neurochemical studies have also shown that DDT exposure alters the levels of some neurotransmitters such as acetylcholine, norepinephrine, and serotonin, as well as of cyclic GMP, but these effects appear to be the results, rather than the cause, of DDT-induced neurotoxicity (Woolley, 1982). Treatment for DDT poisoning focuses on the nervous system. In animals, phenytoin and calcium gluconate have been found to reduce DDT-induced tremors and mortality, respectively. In humans, in addition to decontamination and supportive treatment, diazepam or phenobarbital may be beneficial to control convulsions, if present.

While acute exposure to DDT is a rare event, chronic exposure has been, and still is, a primary concern. In this regard, an important target for DDT is the liver. DDT and DDE increase liver weight and cause hepatic cell hypertrophy and necrosis, and are potent inducers of cytochromes P450, particularly CYP2B and CYP3A (Smith, 1991, 2001). DDT has been shown to be hepatocarcinogenic in mice and rats, but results in other species are inconclusive. DDT also increased incidence of lung tumors and adenomas in mice. Both DDE and DDD were also shown to be carcinogenic, causing primarily an increase in liver tumors. DDT is not genotoxic in in vitro and in vivo tests. Based on animal data, DDT is classified as a possible human carcinogen by IARC; however, evidence of human carcinogenicity

Approx. LD$_{50}$ (mg/kg)

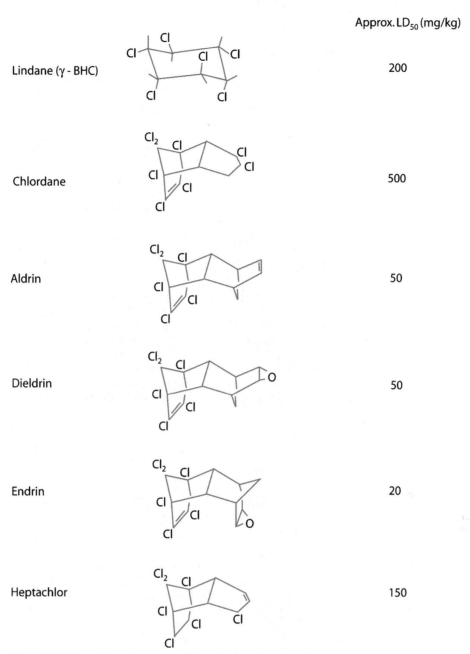

Lindane (γ - BHC)	200
Chlordane	500
Aldrin	50
Dieldrin	50
Endrin	20
Heptachlor	150

Figure 22-12. Structure and acute toxicity (oral LD$_{50}$ in rat) of selected organochlorine insecticides of different chemical classes

(See text for details).

is still inconclusive. Along with many negative studies, there is some, albeit contradictory, evidence of increased risks for pancreatic cancer, liver cancer, and multiple myeloma, associated with exposure to DDT (Turosov *et al.*, 2002; Beard, 2006). Given the endocrine disrupting actions of DDT and DDE (see below), particular attention has been devoted to possible associations between exposure to these compounds and hormonally sensitive cancers, such as those of the breast, the endometrium and the prostate, but the results have been inconclusive (Safe, 2005; Beard, 2006).

Methoxychlor [2,2-bis (p-methoxyphenyl) −1, 1, 1-trichloroethane) is the p,p′-dimethoxy analog of p,p′-DDT. Because of its low acute toxicity (LD$_{50}$ in rat = 5000 mg/kg) and short

biological half-life, its use has greatly expanded following the ban of DDT. Furthermore, methoxychlor is rapidly metabolized, and does not accumulate in tissues. Though convulsions have been reported in dogs after high doses, in the rat depression of the central nervous system, mild tremors, diarrhea and anorexia were observed (Smith, 2001). Upon chronic exposure, methoxychlor has been found to be a modest inducer of liver microsomal enzymes, and to cause chronic nephritis, and hypertrophy of kidneys, mammary glands, and uterus. Testicular atrophy and decreased spermatogenesis were also observed. Evidences of mutagenicity and carcinogenicity are inconclusive. Methoxychlor is metabolized by CYP2C19 and CYP1A2 to demethylated compounds, which

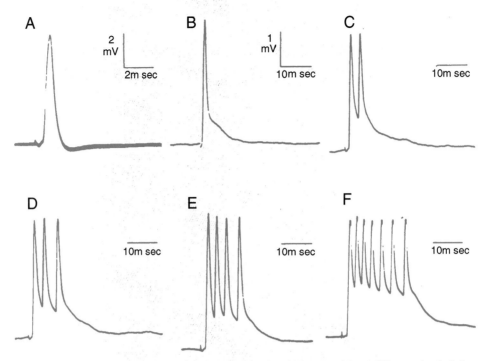

Figure 22-13. Action potential of a single nerve fiber from the sciatic nerve of the toad Xenopus laevis, before (A), and 65, 85, 90, 105, and 135 min (B–F) after in vitro exposure to 10^{-4} M DDT. Note the difference in time-scale between A and B. The first observable effect is the development of a negative after-potential (B). With time of exposure, repetitive spike discharge is initiated and increased in proportion to the amplitude of the negative after-potential (C-F).

With permission from Van den Bercken J: The effect of DDT and dieldrin on myelinated nerve fibers. *Eur J Pharmacol* 20:205–214, Elsevier, 1972.

have estrogenic activity (Smith, 2001); these are likely responsible for the effects caused by methoxychlor on the reproductive system in both male and female animals.

Hexachlorocyclohexanes and Cyclodienes   These two families of organochlorine insecticides comprise a large number of compounds that share a similar mechanism of neurotoxic action. Lindane is the γ isomer of benzene hexachloride (BHC; 1,2,3,4,5,6- hexachlorocyclohexane) (Fig. 22-12). BHC is composed of eight stereoisomers, and the γ isomer is the one with insecticidal activity (Smith, 1991). Cyclodiene compounds include chlordane, dieldrin, aldrin (which is rapidly metabolized to dieldrin), heptachlor, and endrin (Fig. 22-12). Toxaphene, a complex mixture of chlorinated bornanes and camphenes, is also classified as an organochlorine insecticide. All of these compounds were introduced in the late 1940s to early 1950s, and have experienced wide use before being banned in most countries due to their persistence and environmental and human health effects, one exception being lindane. Lindane has been used as an insecticide in agriculture and has found many uses as a scabicide and pediculocide in lotions and shampoos. The primary use of chlordane has been for termite control, while other compounds were primarily used in agriculture. Endrin was registered for use as a rodenticide to control voles in orchards, a testament to its rather high acute toxicity, compared to most other organochlorines (Fig. 22-12).

Lindane and cyclodienes have moderate to high acute oral toxicity (Fig. 22-12). However, in contrast to DDT, these compounds are readily absorbed through the skin. The primary target for their toxicity is the central nervous system. Unlike DDT, tremor is essentially absent, but convulsions are a prominent aspect of poisoning. These are due to the ability of these compounds to interfere with γ-aminobutyric acid (GABA)–mediated neurotransmission. GABA is an important neurotransmitter in the mammalian and insect CNS and in the insect neuromuscular junction. GABA receptors are members of the superfamily of ligand-gated ion channels that contain a chloride ionophore; by binding to these receptors, endogenous GABA causes the opening of chloride channels resulting in hyperpolarization of the membrane. Lindane and cyclodienes bind to a specific site (the picrotoxin site) on the chloride channel, thereby blocking its opening and thus antagonizing the "inhibitory" action of GABA (Cole and Casida, 1986; Eldefrawi and Eldefrawi, 1987; Narahashi, 1996). Treatment of acute poisoning is symptomatic; phenobarbital and diazepam can be used as anticonvulsants. Additional reported neurochemical effects of organochlorine insecticides include inhibition of Na^+- K^+, Ca^{2+}, and Mg^{2+} -ATPases, and changes in neurotransmitter levels.

As with DDT, these compounds are slowly metabolized, and have a tendency to bioaccumulate in adipose tissue; they are also excreted in milk. Cyclodienes are inducers of microsomal biotransformation enzymes and cause liver enlargement upon chronic exposure (Smith, 1991). They are not genotoxic, but have been shown to act as tumor promoters and cause liver tumors in mice. As with DDT, they are extremely persistent in the environment, and some have endocrine disrupting properties.

Mirex and Chlordecone   These two organochlorine insecticides have a cage-like structure and were introduced in the late 1950s for

Table 22-13

Concentration of DDT in a Lake Michigan Food Chain

	DDT (ppm)
Water	0.000002
Bottom mud	0.014
Fairy shrimp	0.410
Coho salmon, lake trout	3–6
Herring gull	99

SOURCE: Harrison *et al.* (1970).

use against fire ants and leaf-eating insects, respectively. Chlordecone (Kepone) has been the most studied because of one episode which involved 148 workers in a chlordecone producing factory in Hopewell, Virginia, between 1973 and 1975 (Taylor *et al.*, 1978). The primary manifestation of chlordecone toxicity is the presence of tremors, which are observed in animals as well as in humans (Guzelian, 1982). The exact mechanism of chlordecone neurotoxicity has not been elucidated, but it is believed to involve inhibition of ATPases (both Na^+-K^+ and Mg^{++} ATPases), and ensuing inhibition of the uptake of catecholamines (Desaiah, 1982). In contrast to cyclodienes, chlordecone does not cause seizures.

Chlordecone induces hepatic drug metabolizing enzymes, and causes hepatosplenomegaly in rats and humans. It is not mutagenic, but can induce liver tumors in rodents (Smith, 1991). Chlordecone also causes reproductive toxicity in animals, likely by mimicking the effects of excessive estrogens. Low or absent sperm count was found in chlordecone-exposed workers (Taylor *et al.*, 1978; Guzelian, 1982). Cholestyramine, an anion-exchange resin, has been shown effective both in animals and humans as a means to increase fecal excretion of chlordecone, probably by sequestering the unmetabolized compound that is secreted into the intestinal lumen via biliary excretion; this interrupts enterohepatic circulation and shortens the biological half-life (Guzelian, 1982).

Environmental Ubiquity and Persistence The properties (low volatility, chemical stability, lipid solubility, slow rate of biotransformation, and degradation) that made organochlorine compounds such effective insecticides, also brought about their demise because of their persistence in the environment, bioconcentration and biomagnification in food chains, and the acquisition of biologically active body burdens at higher trophic levels (Ecobichon, 2001a). Sweden banned DDT in 1970, the United States in 1972, and the UK in 1986. Most other organochlorine insecticides were also banned in the United States during this period; for example, aldrin and dieldrin in 1975, toxaphene in 1982, and chlordane in 1988. These bans occurred largely on the basis of ecological considerations. Their extensive use and their environmental persistence made them widespread pollutants. Studies carried out in the Great Lakes region in the United States exemplify the nature and the extent of the problem. Table 22-13 shows the tendency of DDT to bioaccumulate in the food chain. Adverse effects on bird reproduction (e.g., eggshell thinning) were among the first ecological effects to be identified and denounced (Carson, 1962; Peakall, 1970), and played an important role in the decision to ban DDT (USEPA, 1975). Monitoring of organochlorine insecticides in fish in the Great Lakes shows extreme high levels in 1970 (e.g., 20,000 ng/g of total DDT, which also includes DDE and DDD), and a progressive decline after the use of these compounds was restricted or banned (Hickey *et al.*, 2006).

Because of their stability and high lipophilicity, organochlorines are present in adipose tissues of most individuals. For example, DDE, the breakdown product of DDT in the environment and the result of its biotransformation, is an extremely stable compound ($t_{1/2} = 7$–11 years), which accumulates in fat, and is usually found in human tissue at the highest concentration. Studies in populations from different countries in the 1960s showed that all adipose tissue samples contained DDT at concentrations ranging from 5–20 mg/kg (ppm), with DDE accounting for about 60% of total DDT (WHO, 1979). Though concentrations of DDT in humans show a decreasing trend, those of DDE, which is ingested with food, particularly meat and fish, remain more constant or decrease only slightly. Organochlorine insecticides are also excreted in the milk. Though levels have decreased in most countries in the last decades (Smith, 1999), elevated levels remain in several developing countries (Table 22-14; Chao *et al.*, 2006). Data presented in Table 22-14 also indicate a differential DDE/DDT ratio among milk samples from different populations; a higher ratio is an indication of high environmental persistence and continuous bioaccumulation, while a low DDE/DDT ratio indicates recent exposure to DDT, as the biological half-life of DDT is shorter than DDE (Jaga and Dharmani, 2003).

Endocrine Disruption An endocrine, or hormone, disruptor can be defined as an exogenous chemical that interferes with the synthesis, secretion, transport, binding, action or elimination of natural hormones in the body, that are responsible for the maintenance of homeostasis, reproduction, development and behavior (Crisp *et al.*, 1998). Several pesticides may fall into this category, and among these, a large number are organochlorine insecticides. The o,p'-isomer of DDT, which comprise approximately 15% of the technical grade product (Fig. 22-11), has estrogenic properties, in that it can act as an agonist at estrogen receptors (ER) α and β (Table 22-15). A metabolite of DDT, p,p'-DDE, in contrast, inhibits androgen binding to androgen receptor (Table 22-15; Kelce *et al.*, 1995). Metabolites of the DDT analog, methoxychlor, are active as ERα agonists, ERβ antagonists and are antiandrogenic. Chlordecone also has estrogenic properties (Table 22-15; Guzelian, 1982). Other organochlorine compounds with weak estrogenic activity are dieldrin, endosulfan, toxaphene, lindane and the β isomer of hexachlorocyclohexane (βBHC). In all cases, the potency of the insecticides or their metabolites were several orders of magnitude less then those of the hormones. Experimental studies have shown that administration of these compounds to animals can cause hormonally-mediated adverse health effects. For example, p,p'-DDE had clear antiandrogenic effect when given to fetal, pubertal, and adult male rats (Kelce *et al.*, 1995). Several studies have shown that chlordecone and methoxychlor affect the male reproductive system (Guzelian, 1982; Kavlock, 2001). Of possible relevance is the recent finding that exposure to methoxychlor during gestation (E8–E15) induced transgenerational defects in spermatogenic capacity and sperm viability, i.e., these abnormalities were also observed in F2 generation animals (Anway *et al.*, 2005). All these findings, though provocative, were obtained at dosage levels that far exceed anticipated environmental exposure. It has been suggested that estrogen equivalents from phytoestrogens present in foods and beverages are several orders of magnitude higher than estrogen equivalents resulting from estrogenic organochlorine insecticide contaminants in food (Safe, 2000). More importantly, the association between exposure to organochlorine compounds and possible related diseases in humans (breast cancer, decreased sperm count, cryptorchidism, testicular cancer,

Table 22-14

Levels of p,p'-DDT and p,p'-DDE (ng/g lipid) in Human Milk from Selected Countries

COUNTRY	SAMPLING YEAR	N	p,p'-DDT	p,p'-DDE	DDE/DDT	REFERENCE
Sweden	1997	40	14	129	9.2	1
Japan	1998	49	18	270	15.0	2
New Zealand	1998	53	26	626	24.1	3
United Kingdom	2001–03	54	6.2	150	24.2	4
Taiwan	2000–01	30	22	301	13.7	5
Mexico	1997–98	60	651	3997	6.1	6
Thailand	1998	25	2600	8210	3.2	7
China (Guangzhou)	2000	54	700	2850	4.1	8
Vietnam	2000–01	96	223	1956	8.8	9
Turkey	2003	37	65	1522	28.0	10

References: 1. Noren and Meironyte, 2000; 2. Konishi *et al.*, 2001; 3. Bate *et al.*, 2002; 4. Kalantzi *et al.*, 2004; 5. Chao *et al.*, 2006; 6. Waliszewski *et al.*, 1999; 7. Stuetz *et al.*, 2001; 8. Wong *et al.*, 2002; 9. Minh *et al.*, 2004; 10. Erdogrul *et al.*, 2004.

Table 22-15

Potency of DDT and its Metabolites, and of Chlordecone at Androgen and Estrogen Receptors

COMPOUND	ANDROGEN RECEPTOR	ESTROGEN RECEPTOR
	IC$_{50}$ (μM)	
p,p'-DDT	75	>1000
p,p'-DDE	5	>1000
o,p'-DDT	95	5
p,p'-DDD	90	>1000
Chlordecone	125	3
17β-estradiol	0.5	0.002

SOURCE: Kelce *et al.* (1995).

etc.) is weak at best, and inconclusive (Golden *et al.*, 1998; Safe, 2005). Nevertheless, the possibility that these chemicals, as well as several other endocrine disruptors, may contribute to hormonally mediated cancers, reproductive effects, and developmental abnormalities, should not be discounted, and additional research in this area is warranted.

DDT and Public Health: Risk-Benefit Considerations The Stockholm Convention on Persistent Organic Pollutants, ratified in 2004 by 50 states, outlawed the use of 12 industrial chemicals (the "Dirty Dozen"), including DDT. Yet, an exemption clause allows malaria-endemic nations to continue utilizing DDT for indoor residual wall spraying. The United Nations Environment Program estimates that about 25 countries would use DDT under this exemption from its ban. This situation is keeping the debate on the risks and benefits of DDT usage very much alive. On one hand, the environmental and human health effects of DDT are evident; on the other, one has to come to grips with the burden of mortality from malaria worldwide. Indeed, each year up to three million deaths due to malaria occur throughout the world, with 90% occurring in Africa (Breman *et al.*, 2004). Most such mortality occurs in the first five years of life (Rogan and Chen, 2005). Thus, use of DDT might reduce mortality from malaria and overall infant mortality, if spraying is carried out according to planned schedule, which is not always the case, and if malaria-transmitting mosquitoes do not become resistant to DDT, a problem that in the past has forced switching to other insecticides. The successful results obtained in South Africa in recent years (see earlier section "Economics and Public Health"), would support a continuous use of DDT. Indoor residual spraying might not cause the ecological effects that caused the ban of DDT, but could expose humans to amounts of DDT that may cause adverse health effects. In this regard, reproductive outcomes are of most concern. In particular, preterm births and early weaning (decreased duration of lactation), which can lead to increased infant mortality, have been associated with DDT exposure (Chen and Rogan, 2003; Rogan and Chen, 2005), though findings are controversial (Roberts *et al.*, 2004). DDT remains, however, a public health intervention that is cheap, long lasting, and effective. Its judicious use should be combined with that of insecticide-treated bed nets, to prevent mosquito biting, and with a better availability of therapeutic interventions in affected populations.

Other Old and New Insecticides

Rotenoids The roots of the East Asian Derris plants, particularly *Derris Elliptica,* and those of *Lonchocarpus utilis* and *Lonchocarpus urucu* in South America contain at least six rotenoid esters, among which the most abundant is rotenone. Rotenone is used as an agricultural insecticide/acaricide, particularly in organic farming (Isman, 2006). It is rather persistent in food crops after treatment, as indicated by half-life of 4 days in olives (Cabras *et al.*, 2002). Rotenone is very toxic to fish; root extracts were used to paralyze fish for capture and consumption, and rotenone is still used in fishery management. Toxicity of rotenone in target and nontarget species is due to its ability to inhibit, at nanomolar concentrations, the mitochondrial respiratory chain, by blocking electron transport at NADH-ubiquinone reductase, the energy conserving enzyme complex commonly known as Complex I. Insect and fish mitochondria are particularly sensitive to Complex I inhibition (Degli Esposti, 1998). Purified rotenone has a high acute toxicity in rodents and dogs, and is less toxic to rabbits and birds (Ujvary, 2001). Poisoning symptoms include initial increased respiratory and cardiac rates, clonic and tonic spasms, and muscular depression, followed by respiratory depression. Acute intoxication in humans is rare, and the lethal dose in adults has been estimated at >140 mg/kg. However, a case report describes a fatal case in a 3.5-year-old girl who ingested an estimated 40 mg/kg of rotenone. Of note is that the label on the insecticide, which was manufactured in France and recommended for external use on animals, had stated "Natural Product – Non Toxic" (De Wilde *et al.*, 1986).

In recent years, rotenone has received much attention because of its potential role in the etiology of Parkinson's disease. An earlier study by Heikkila *et al.* (1985) showed that stereotaxic administration to rats of rotenone damaged the dopaminergic nigrostriatal pathway, same as what observed with MPP$^+$ (1-methyl-4-phenyl pyridinium, the active metabolite of 1-methyl-4-phenyl- 1,2,3,6-tetrahydropyridine, MPTP), a known parkinsonism-causing chemical, which is also a Complex I inhibitor (Degli Esposti, 1998). More recent studies have shown that administration of rotenone to rats (2–3 mg/kg/d for 1–5 weeks) caused selective nigrostriatal degeneration, though inhibition of Complex I was observed uniformly in brain (Betarbet *et al.*, 2000; Sherer *et al.*, 2003). The finding that rotenone also produced protein inclusions, similar to Lewy bodies, that stained positively for ubiquitin and alpha-synuclein, suggests that the rotenone model for Parkinson's disease would be even better than the MPTP model (Betarbet *et al.*, 2002). However, the severe systemic toxicity of rotenone, the high variability across and within strains, and reports on nonspecific CNS effects (LaPointe *et al.*, 2004), have also pointed out the limitations of the rotenone model (Li *et al.*, 2005). There is no evidence of Parkinson's disease-like clinical signs or neurodegenerative pathology in chronic dietary studies (Hollingworth, 2001). Thus, although rotenone may represent an useful experimental model, its primary role, if any, in the etiology of Parkinson's disease in the general population is still unproven (Hollingworth, 2001; Li *et al.*, 2005).

Nicotine The tobacco plant (*Nicotiana tabacum, Nicotiana rustica*) was introduced in Europe in 1559 from the Americas where it had long been cultivated primarily for smoking. Tobacco extracts have been used to repel and kill insects since 1690, and tobacco smoke was also used for fumigation (Ujvary, 2001). Nicotine is an alkaloid extracted from the leaves of tobacco plants, and is used as a free base or as the sulfate salt. The most notorious commercial preparation, Black Leaf 40, has been discontinued. Very little nicotine is used currently in the United States, but nicotine is still used as a minor insecticide in some Asian countries. It is a systemic insecticide effective toward a wide range of insects, including aphids, thrips, and whiteflies (Ujvary, 1999). As the primary component of tobacco used for smoking or chewing, nicotine's pharmacology and toxicology have been thoroughly investigated (Benowitz, 1996; Taylor, 1996). Nicotine exerts its pharmacological and toxic effects in mammals and insects by activating nicotinic acetylcholine receptors (nAChRs). In vertebrates, nAChRs are expressed at neuromuscular junctions, in the PNS and in the CNS; in insects, nAChRs are confined to the nervous system (Eldefrawi and Eldefrawi, 1997). Interaction of nicotine with nAChRs produces initial stimulation followed by protracted depolarization, which results in receptor paralysis. The overall effect is the summation of stimulatory and inhibitory effects of nicotine at all sites expressing nAChRs. At high doses, parasympathetic stimulation and ganglionic and neuromuscular blockade predominate (Matyunas and Rodgers, 2001). Nicotine has a high acute toxicity in vertebrates, with LD$_{50}$s usually below 50 mg/kg (Ujvary, 2001). Signs and symptoms of poisoning include nausea, vomiting, muscle weakness, respiratory effects, headache, lethargy, and tachycardia. Most cases of poisoning with nicotine occur after exposure to tobacco products, or gum or patches.

Workers who cultivate, harvest, or handle tobacco may experience green tobacco sickness, caused by dermal absorption of nicotine.

Neonicotinoids By various chemical modifications of nicotine and other nAChRs agonists, new classes of insecticides have been developed that contain a nitromethylene, nitroimine or cyanoimine group, and are referred to as neonicotinoids. One of the first compounds synthesized was nithiazine, a nitromethylenyl heterocyclic compound highly toxic toward insects but with low mammalian toxicity. Nithiazine was not developed commercially because of its photo-instability. Further structure-activity studies led to the development of imidacloprid, nitenpyram, acetamiprid, and other neonicotinoid compounds (Fig. 22-14; Matsuda *et al.*, 2001). The insecticidal activity of neonicotinoids is attributed to activation of nAChRs. They are used primarily for crop protection as systemic insecticides, but are also effective against fleas in cats and dogs (Schenker *et al.*, 2003). The mammalian toxicity of neonicotinoids is similar to that of nicotine, and correlates with agonist action and binding affinity at the nAChRs. Acute oral toxicity (LD50) in rats ranges from 180 to >2000 mg/kg (Fig. 22-14), while dermal toxicity is much lower (2000–5000 mg/kg), likely because of the low lipophilicity (Tomizawa and Casida, 2005). Signs and symptoms of toxicity are attributable to stimulation of nAChRs. Some neonicotinoids (imidocloprid, thiacloprid) are particularly toxic to birds, others (thiacloprid) to fish. Most neonicotinoids are not mutagenic or carcinogenic, nor teratogenic. Neonicotinoids undergo limited biotransformation in mammals, involving mostly cytochrome P450-mediated oxidative reactions (Sheets, 2001; Tomizawa and Casida, 2005). Neonicotinoids account for 10–15% of the total insecticide market, and their use is increasing faster than other insecticides (Matsuda *et al.*, 2001; Tomizawa and Casida, 2005). The main reason for their success lies in their selectivity profile, which is largely attributable to their specificity toward insect vs. mammalian nAChRs. The nAChR consists of diverse subtypes assembled in combination from ten α and four β, γ, δ, ε subunits. The most abundant subtypes in the vertebrate nervous system are $\alpha 4\beta 2$ and $\alpha 7$, which are insensitive and sensitive, respectively, to α-bungarotoxin. In insects, neonicotinoids have been shown to bind to at least three pharmacologically distinct nAChRs (Sheets, 2001; Matsuda *et al.*, 2001). Table 22-16 shows the in vitro effects of some neonicotinoids toward insect nAChRs and mammalian $\alpha 4\beta 2$ nAChRs, and compares them to nicotine. Structural features of neonicotinoids that contribute to their selective actions at insect nAChRs have been described (Nakayama and Sukekawa, 1998; Matsuda *et al.*, 2001; Tomizawa and Casida, 2005).

Formamidines Formamidines, such as chlordimeform [(N'-(4-chloro-o-tolyl)-N, N-dimethylformamidine] or amitraz [N'-2,4-(dimethyl-phenyl)-N-N ((2,4-dimethylphenyl) imino) methyl-N-methanimidamide] are used in agriculture and in veterinary medicine as insecticides/acaricides (Hollingworth, 1976). Their structures are closely related to the neurotransmitter norepinephrine (Fig. 22-15). In invertebrates, these compounds exert their toxicity by activating an octopamine-dependent adenylate cyclase (Nathanson, 1985). In mammals, symptoms of formamidines poisoning are sympathomimetic in nature (Beeman and Matsumura, 1973). The similarity between insect octopamine receptors and mammalian α_2-adrenergic receptors had suggested the latter as a possible target for formamidines. In vivo and in vitro studies have indeed shown that formamidines act as rather selective

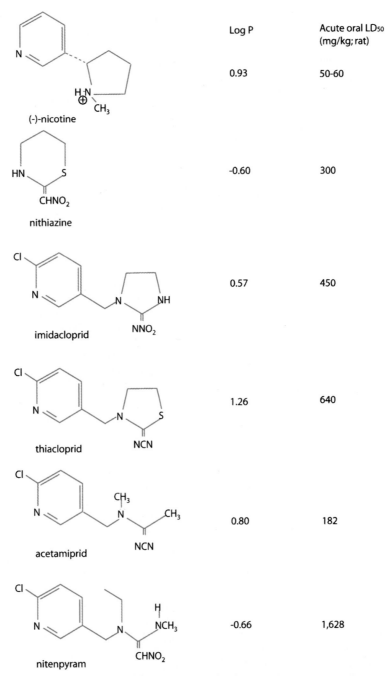

	Log P	Acute oral LD$_{50}$ (mg/kg; rat)
(-)-nicotine	0.93	50-60
nithiazine	-0.60	300
imidacloprid	0.57	450
thiacloprid	1.26	640
acetamiprid	0.80	182
nitenpyram	-0.66	1,628

Figure 22-14. Structures of nicotine and of neonicotinoid insecticides with indication of their acute oral toxicity in rat and their octanol/water partition (P).

Data are derived from Tomizawa and Casida (2005).

agonists at α_2–adrenergic receptors (Hsu and Lu, 1984; Hsu and Kakuk, 1984; Costa et al., 1988; Altobelli et al., 2001). Chlordimeform's metabolism plays a most relevant role in its toxicity. The N-demethylated metabolite (desmethylchlordimeform) is more acutely toxic than chlordimeform, and displays a >400-fold higher potency toward α_2–adrenoceptors (Ghali and Hollingsworth, 1985; Costa and Murphy, 1987). Two other metabolites of chlordimeform, 4-chloro-toluidine and N-formyl-4-chloro-o-toluidine, are believed to be responsible for the observed haemangioendotheliomas in mice observed in carcinogenicity studies (IPCS, 1998). Chlordimeform was classified as a probable human carcinogen (Group 2A) by IARC

in 1990. Given the increasing evidence of an association between exposure to chlordimeform and 4-chloro-o-toluidine and bladder cancer (Popp et al., 1992), chlordimeform was withdrawn form the market in 1992. Amitraz, in contrast, remains on the market and is still used worldwide for the control of ectoparasites in farm animals and crops. In recent years several cases of acute amitraz poisoning have been reported, particularly in Turkey, and most involved children (Yaramis et al., 2000; Caksen et al., 2003; Elinav et al., 2005; Proudfoot, 2003). Signs and symptoms of poisoning mimicked those of α_2-adrenergic receptor agonists such as clonidine, and included nausea, hypotension, hyperglycemia, bradycardia, and

Table 22-16

Specificity of Neonicotinoids for Insect and Vertebrate nAChRs

INSECTICIDE	IC50 (nM)		SELECTIVITY RATIO
	INSECT	VERTEBRATE $\alpha 4\beta 2$	
Imidacloprid	4.6	2,600	565
Acetamiprid	8.3	700	84
Thiacloprid	2.7	860	319
Nitenpyram	14.0	49,000	3,500
(-)Nicotine	4000	7	0.002

SOURCE: Tomizawa and Casida, 2005.

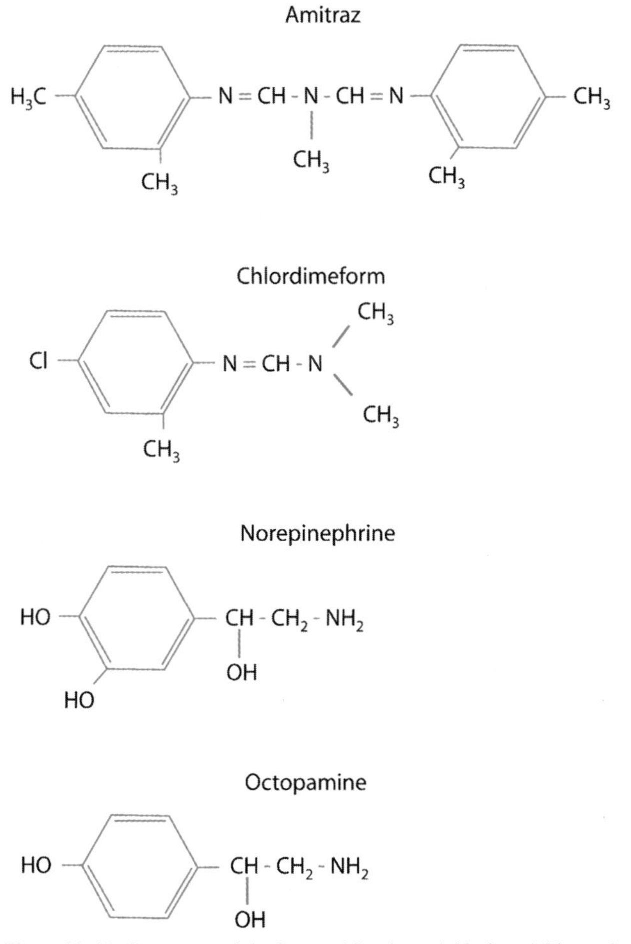

Figure 22-15. *Structures of the formamidine insecticides/acaricides ami-traz and chlordimeform. Structures of the mammalian neurotransmitter norepinephrine and of the insect neurotransmitter octopamine are also shown.*

miosis. No deaths occurred. Though α_2-adrenoceptor antagonists such as yohimbine have proven useful as antidotes in animals (Andrade and Sakate, 2003), their usefulness in managing amitraz poisoning in humans has not been evaluated.

Avermectins The avermectins are macrocyclic lactones, first iso-lated in 1975 from the fermentation broth of the actinomycete *Streptomyces avermitilis,* which originated from a Japanese soil

sample (Campbell, 1989; Fisher and Mrozik, 1992). This fungus synthesizes eight individual avermectins, of which avermectin B_{1a} displays the highest antiparasitic activity. Currently, abamectin (a mixture of 80% avermectin B_{1a} and 20% avermectin B_{1b}) is used as an insecticide, whereas the semisynthetic derivatives of avermectin B_{1a}, emamectin benzoate, and ivermectin, are used as insecticides, and for parasite control in human and veterinary medicine, respec-tively (Stevens and Breckenridge, 2001). Abamectin is used primar-ily to control mites, whereas emamectin benzoate is effective at con-trolling lepidopterian species in various crops. Ivermectin is used as an antihelmintic and antiparasitic drug in veterinary medicine, and in humans it has proven to be an effective treatment for in-fection of intestinal threadworms, onchocerciasis (river blindness), and lymphatic filariasis (Stevens and Breckenridge, 2001). In insects and nematodes, avermectins exert their toxic effects by binding to, and activating, glutamate-dependent chloride channels (Arena *et al.*, 1995). Avermectins have a high acute toxicity, with oral LD_{50}s in rats of 11 (abamectin) to 80 (emamectin) mg/kg. Toxicity is higher in neonate animals, possibly because of a deficient blood-brain barrier (Stevens and Breckenridge, 2001). Signs and symptoms of intoxica-tion include hyperexcitability, tremors, and incoordination, followed by ataxia and coma-like sedation. These effects are due to the ability of avermectins to activate $GABA_A$ receptor-gated chloride channels in the vertebrate CNS (Pong *et al.*, 1982; Fisher and Mrozik, 1992). Activity at $GABA_A$ receptors also mediates the anticonvulsant ef-fects of avermectins, but because the same target seems to mediate both pharmacological and toxic effects, the potential of avermectins as anticonvulsants is limited (Dawson *et al.*, 2000). Avermectins are also strong inhibitors of P-glycoprotein, a plasma membrane protein whose main function is the ATPase-dependent transport of foreign substances from the cell (Didier and Loor, 1996). As such, avermectins are being investigated for their potential ability to in-hibit multidrug resistance of tumor cells (Korystov *et al.*, 2004). In this respect, the complete sequencing of the *S. avermitilis* genome would allow the definition of the precise biosynthetic pathways and regulatory mechanisms for avermectins, which in turn may lead to engineering of this fungus to produce pharmacological compounds of interest (Yoon *et al.*, 2004). Given the wide use of avermectins, and particularly that of ivermectin in Africa, there is little evidence of adverse health effects in humans. The major effect following ad-ministration of active doses of ivermectin (0.1–0.2 mg/kg) is a se-vere inflammatory response (the Mazzotti reaction), characterized by pruritis, erithema, vesicle and papulae formation, and attributable to the killing of microfiliae which dislodge from their site of infes-tation and are transported in the blood and body fluids (Ackerman *et al.*, 1990).

Phenylpyrazoles A relatively new class of insecticides is that of phenylpyrazole derivatives, of which fipronil, commercialized in the mid-1990s, was the first one brought to market. Fipronil is a broad-spectrum insecticide with moderate mammalian toxicity (LD_{50} in rat: oral, 97 mg/kg; dermal, >2000 mg/kg), and a high selectivity for target species. Fipronil acts as a blocker of the $GABA_A$-gated chlo-ride channel, but binds to a site different from the picrotoxin binding site used by organochlorine insecticides. It also has a much higher specificity for insect receptors over mammalian receptors (Hainzl *et al.*, 1998). There is no evidence that fipronil is an eye or skin ir-ritant, or has any mutagenic, carcinogenic, or teratogenic effects. A number of human poisonings with fipronil have been reported that resulted from accidental or intentional ingestion. Less than 20% of the patients developed seizures, and all recovered (Mohamed *et al.*, 2004).

Bacillus Thuringiensis   The past decade has seen increasing research and development in the area of biopesticides, that is pesticides derived from natural materials such as plants, bacteria, and fungi. As of 2001, there were 195 registered biopesticide active ingredients in the United States, and 780 products. Biopesticides fall into three major classes: (1) Microbial pesticides, which consist of a microorganism (e.g., a bacterium, fungus or protozoan) as the active ingredient. The most widely used microbial pesticides are subspecies and strains of *B. thuringiensis* (Bt) which act as insecticides. Other microbial pesticides can control different kinds of pests; for example there are fungi that can control certain weeds, and others that can kill specific insects. (2) Plant-incorporated-protectants, which are pesticidal substances that plants produce from genetic material that has been added to the plant. For example, a plant can be genetically manipulated to produce the Bt pesticidal protein. (3) Biochemical pesticides, that are naturally occurring substances that control pests by nontoxic mechanisms. Examples are sex pheromones, that interfere with mating of insects, or various scented plant extracts that attract insect pests to traps (Sudakin, 2003). Biopesticides represent a little more than 1% of the world pesticide market, but Bt products represent 80% of all biopesticides sold (Whalon and Wingend, 2003). Bt is a soil microorganism that produces proteins that are selectively toxic to certain insects. Its name comes from the German region of Thuringia, where this strain was found in 1915. Bt-based microbial insecticides were commercialized in France in 1938 and in the United States in 1961. Over 150 insecticidal crystal proteins (Cry) have been identified in Bt and in the closely related *Bacillus cereus* (Schnepf *et al.*, 1998). After ingestion of Bt by an insect, the crystal proteins are solubilized, and proteolytically processed to active toxins (δ-endotoxin) in the insect's midgut. Here they bind to specific receptors in the epithelial cells and insert into the cellular membrane. Next, aggregation of inserted crystal protein occurs, resulting in the formation of pores, which lead to changes in K^+ fluxes across the epithelial cells, and to changes in pH. Ultimately, cells of the midgut epithelium are destroyed by the high pH and by osmotic lysis. Insects eventually die as a result of gut paralysis and feeding inhibition, and subsequent starvation and septicemia (Gringorten, 2001). Bt targets primarily leaf-feeding lepidoptera, breaks down rapidly in UV light, and exhibits low mammalian toxicity. The basis for the selective toxicity of Bt is attributed to the fact that crystalline Bt endotoxins require activation by alkalis and/or digestion, conditions absent in the mammalian stomach (Ujvary, 2001). A summary of the toxicology studies in mammals of Bt-based insecticides is provided by McClintock *et al.* (1995). Adverse health effects in humans are infrequent and include allergic reactions and infections (Ujvary, 2001). Bt genes are also expressed in a variety of crop plants, most notably cotton and corn. Thus, the plant, instead of the Bt bacterium, produces the substance that affects the insect upon feeding. Resistance can develop to Bt toxins that involves alterations in the processing of Cry toxin in the insect's gut or in its binding to receptors (Whalon and Wingerd, 2003).

INSECT REPELLENTS

Insect-transmitted diseases remain a major source of illness and death worldwide, as mosquitoes alone transmit disease to more than 700 million persons annually (Fradin and Day, 2002). Though insect-borne diseases represent a greater health problem in tropical and subtropical climates, no part of the world is immune to their risks. For example, in 1999, the West Nile virus, transmitted by mosquitoes, was detected for the first time in the western hemisphere. In the New York City area, 62 persons infected with the West Nile virus were hospitalized and seven died (Nash *et al.*, 2001). Other arthropod-borne viral diseases (e.g., equine encephalitis) and tick-borne diseases (e.g., Lyme disease) are also of concern; additionally, other insect bites can be associated with variable adverse health effects, from mild irritation and discomfort to possible allergic reactions. Insect repellents are thus widely used to provide protection toward insect bites. The best known and most widely used insect repellent is DEET. Botanical insect repellents based on citronella or oil of eucalyptus, and a biopesticide structurally similar to the aminoacid alanine are also commercialized in Europe and the United States (Fradin and Day, 2002). A new compound, picaridin, has been recently approved for use as an insect repellent; it is effective against biting flies, mosquitoes, ticks and fleas, and has a very favorable toxicological profile (USEPA, 2005).

DEET

DEET (*N*, *N*-diethyl-m-toluamide or *N*, *N*-diethyl-3-methyl-benzamide) was first developed by the USDA in 1946 for use in the military, and was registered as an insect repellent for the general public in 1957. The USEPA estimates that 30% of the U.S. population uses DEET every year. More than 200 formulations exist with varying concentrations of DEET (commonly 4.75–40%) which are applied directly to the skin or on clothing. DEET is very effective at repelling insects, flies, fleas, and ticks, and protection time increases with increasing concentrations (Fradin and Day, 2002). Percutaneous absorption of DEET varies from 7.9 to 59%, depending on the species tested and the conditions of the study (Osimitz and Murphy, 1997). DEET undergoes oxidative biotransformation catalyzed by various cytochromes P450, and is excreted mostly in the urine (Sudakin and Trevathan, 2003). DEET has low acute toxicity, with LD_{50} values in the rat of 1892 mg/kg (oral) and >5,000 mg/kg (dermal) (Schoenig and Osimitz, 2001). From 1961 to 2002, eight deaths were reported related to DEET: three resulted from deliberate ingestion, while two were reported following dermal exposure (Tenenbein, 1987; Bell *et al.*, 2002). The remaining three cases were children, age 17 months to 6 years (Zadikoff, 1979). Subchronic toxicity studies in various species did not reveal major toxic effects, with the exception of renal lesions in male rats; these were considered to be reflective of α_{2u}-globulin induced nephropathy, a condition unique to male rats and not occurring in humans (Schoenig and Osimitz, 2001). No significant effects of DEET were seen in mutagenicity, reproductive toxicity, and carcinogenicity studies. Acute and chronic neurotoxicity studies also provided negative results (Schoenig *et al.*, 1993). Yet, several case reports over the past 40 years have indicated neurological effects of DEET, and most of these were in children (Petrucci and Sardini, 2000; Osimitz and Murphy, 1997; Hampers *et al.*, 1999; Sudakin and Trevathan, 2003; Briassoulis *et al.*, 2001; MMWR, 1989; Gryboski *et al.*, 1961). The most common symptoms reported were seizures. Given that seizure disorders occur in 3–5% of children, and almost 30% of children in the United States are utilizing DEET, an association just by chance is certainly possible. Possible mechanism(s) responsible for neurotoxic effects of DEET are unknown, though it has been suggested that DEET's structure is similar to that of nikethamide, a convulsant (Briassoulis *et al.*, 2001). It has also been suggested that DEET may disrupt the permeability of the blood–brain barrier,

Table 22-17
Some Mechanisms of Action of Herbicides

MECHANISM	CHEMICAL CLASSES (EXAMPLE)
Inhibition of photosynthesis	Triazines (atrazine), Substitued ureas (diuron), Uracils (bromacil)
Inhibition of respiration	Dinitrophenols
Auxin growth regulators	Phenoxy acids (2,4-D), Benzoic Acids (dicamba), Pyridine acids (picloram)
Inhibition of protein synthesis	Dinitroanilines
Inhibition of lipid synthesis	Aryloxyphenoxyproprionates (diclofop)
Inhibition of specific enzymes	
• Glutamine synthetase	Glufosinate
• Enolpyruvylshikimate -3- phosphate synthetase	Glyphosate
• Acetalase synthase	Sulfonylureas
Cell membrane disruptors	Bipyridyl derivatives (Paraquat)

but results are inconclusive (Abdel-Rahman *et al.*, 2002). Overall, given its long-standing and widespread use, DEET appears to be relatively safe when used as recommended (Osimitz and Murphy, 1997; Koren *et al.*, 2003). A risk assessment by the Canadian Pest Management Regulatory agency has recommended, however, that toddlers and children, up to 12 years old, should only be exposed to products with up to 10% DEET (Sudakin and Trevathan, 2003). For all other individuals, products with up to 30% DEET can be used, as they appear safe and effective (Fradin and Day, 2002).

HERBICIDES

Herbicides are chemicals that are capable of either killing or severely injuring plants. They represent a very broad array of chemical classes and act at a large number of sites of metabolic functions and energy transfer in plant cells (Duke, 1990). Some of the various mechanisms by which herbicides exert their biological effects are shown in Table 22-17, together with examples for each class. Another method of classification pertains to how and when herbicides are applied. Thus, *preplanting* herbicides are applied to the soil before a crop is seeded; *preemergent* herbicides are applied to the soil before the time of appearance of unwanted vegetation; and *postemergent* herbicides are applied to the soil or foliage after the germination of the crop and/or weeds (Ecobichon, 2001a). Herbicides are also divided according to the manner they are applied to plants. *Contact* herbicides are those that affect the plant that was treated, while *translocated* herbicides are applied to the soil or to above-ground parts of the plant, and are absorbed and circulated to distant tissues. Nonselective herbicides will kill all vegetation, while selective compounds are those used to kill weeds without harming the crops. In the past decade, the development of herbicide-resistant crops through transgenic technology has allowed the use of nonselective compounds as selective herbicides (Duke, 2005). A final classification, of relevance to adverse health effects in nontarget species, relies, on the other hand, on chemical structures, as indicated below.

For the past several decades, herbicides have represented the most rapidly growing sector of the agrochemical market, and these compounds now represent almost half of the pesticides used in the

United States, and more than one-third of those utilized worldwide (Table 22-3). This can be ascribed in part to movement to monocultural practices, where the risk of weed infestation has increased, and to mechanization of agricultural practices because of increased labor costs. In addition to agriculture and home and garden uses, herbicides are also widely utilized in forestry management and to clear roadsides, utilities' rights of way, and industrial areas.

In terms of general toxicity, herbicides, as a class, display relatively low acute toxicity, compared for example to most insecticides. There are exceptions, however, such as paraquat. A number of herbicides can cause dermal irritation and contact dermatitis, particularly in individuals prone to allergic reactions. Other compounds have generated much debate for their suspected carcinogenicity or neurotoxicity. The principal classes of herbicides associated with reported adverse health effects in humans are discussed below.

Chlorophenoxy Compounds

Chlorophenoxy herbicides are characterized by an aliphatic carboxylic acid moiety attached to a chlorine-or-methyl-substituted aromatic ring. The most commonly used compound of this class is 2,4-dichlorophenoxyacetic acid (2,4-D), while others are 2,4,5-trichlorophenoxyacetic acid (2,4,5-T) and 4-chloro-2-methylphenoxyacetic acid (MCPA) (Fig. 22-16). Chlorophenoxy herbicides are chemical analogues of auxin, a plant growth hormone, and produce uncontrolled and lethal growth in target plants. Because the auxin hormone is critical to the growth of many broad-leaved plants, but is not used by grasses, chlorophenoxy compounds can suppress the growth of weeds (e.g., dandelions) without affecting the grass. Once absorbed, they selectively eliminate broad-leaved plants, due to their larger leaf area and greater absorption. 2,4-D is one of the most widely used herbicides throughout the world, and is primarily used in agriculture to control weeds in corn and grain, in forestry, and in lawn care practices. 2,4,5-T has been largely withdrawn from use because of concerns that arose from contamination of some formulations with 2,3,7,8-tetrachlorodibenzo-*p*-dioxin (TCDD), which can derive from the reaction of two molecules of 2,4,5-trichlorophenol (Fig. 22-17). A 50:50 mixture of the n-butyl esters of 2,4,-D and 2,3,5-T, known as Agent Orange (from the color of the barrels which contained it), was extensively used as a defoliant during the Vietnam War, and was found to be contaminated with TCDD to a maximum of 47 μg/g. Exposure of military personnel and Vietnamese population to Agent Orange has raised concerns on possible long-term health effects, particularly carcinogenicity and reproductive toxicity (IOM, 1996), which are ascribed to the presence of TCDD.

2,4-D is a compound of low to moderate acute toxicity, with oral LD_{50}s in rodents of 300–2000 mg/kg. The dog is more sensitive, possibly because of its lower ability to eliminate organic acids via the kidney. Upon oral exposure, 2,4-D is rapidly absorbed, and its salts and esters rapidly dissociate or hydrolyze in vivo, so that toxicity depends primarily on the acid form. It binds extensively to serum albumin, but does not accumulate in tissue, and is excreted almost exclusively through the urine. Ingestion of 2,4-D has caused several cases of acute poisoning in humans, usually at doses above 300 mg/kg, though lower doses have been reported to elicit symptoms. Vomiting, burning of the mouth, abdominal pain, hypotension, myotonia and CNS involvement including coma, are among the clinical signs observed (Bradberry *et al.*, 2000; 2004a). Management of 2,4-D poisoning appears to be aided by urine alkalinization, through intravenous administration of bicarbonate (Proudfoot *et al.*, 2004;

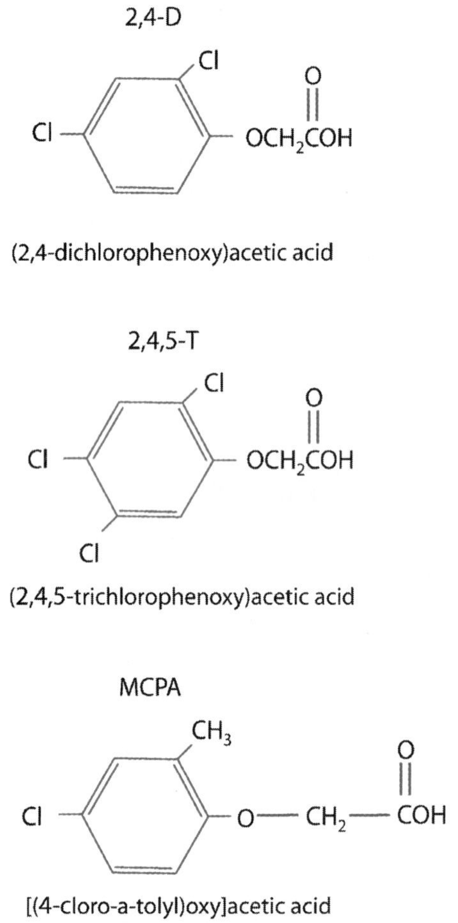

2,4-D

(2,4-dichlorophenoxy)acetic acid

2,4,5-T

(2,4,5-trichlorophenoxy)acetic acid

MCPA

[(4-cloro-a-tolyl)oxy]acetic acid

Figure 22-16. Structures of three chlorophenoxy acid herbicides.

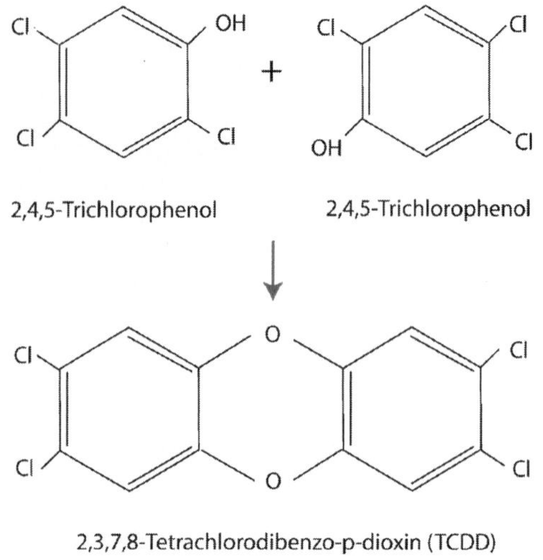

2,4,5-Trichlorophenol   2,4,5-Trichlorophenol

2,3,7,8-Tetrachlorodibenzo-p-dioxin (TCDD)

Figure 22-17. Formation of 2,3,7,8-tetrachlorodibenzo-p-dioxin (TCDD) during the synthesis of 2,4,5-T because of reaction between two molecules of 2,4,5-trichlorophenol.

Table 22-18

Effect of Urine Alkalinization on Renal Clearance and Plasma Half-Life of 2,4-D

URINE pH	RENAL CLEARANCE (mL/min)	HALF-LIFE (h)
5.10–6.5	0.28	219
6.55–7.5	1.14	42
7.55–8.8	9.60	4.7

SOURCE: Park *et al.*, (1977).

Bradberry *et al.*, 2004a). Ionization of an acid, such as 2,4-D, is increased in an alkaline environment. Though, at pH 5.0, practically all 2,4-D would already be ionized, further alkalinization of urine, to pH 7.5 or above, would reduce the non-ionized fraction from approximately 0.53 to 0.0017%. As a result, the fraction prone to reabsorption would be >300-times lower (Bradberry *et al.*, 2004a). This explains why alkalinization of the urine diminishes reabsorption and increases 2,4-D elimination. An example of the effect of urine alkalinization on 2,4-D renal clearance and plasma half-life is given in Table 22-18. Dermal exposure is by far the major route of unintentional exposure to 2,4-D in humans. Dermal absorption studies in rats, mice and rabbit, indicate an absorption of 12–36%; the absorption in humans, however, is lower (2–10%), and is usually less than 6% (Ross *et al.*, 2005). Acute poisoning by 2,4-D via the dermal route is thus uncommon; no reports of systemic toxicity following dermal exposure have been reported for over 20 years, and no fatalities have ever occurred (Bradberry *et al.*, 2004a).

The precise mechanisms of toxicity of chlorophenoxy herbicides have not been completely elucidated, but experimental studies indicate the possible involvement of three actions: (1) Cell membrane damage; (2) Interference with metabolic pathways involving acetyl-coenzyme A; (3) Uncoupling of oxidative phosphorylation (Bradberry *et al.*, 2000). The toxicity of chlorophenoxy herbicides has been summarized in several reviews (Sterling and Arundel, 1986; Munro *et al.*, 1992; Garebrant and Philbert, 2002). 2,4-D and its salts and esters are not teratogenic in mice, rats, or rabbits,

unless the ability of the dam to excrete the chemical is exceeded. There is also no convincing evidence that 2,4-D is associated with human reproductive toxicity (Garabrant and Philbert, 2002). Subchronic and chronic toxicity studies have not provided evidence of immunotoxicity, and there is very limited evidence that 2,4-D may affect the nervous system (Mattsson *et al.*, 1997). There are, however, several case reports suggesting an association between exposure to 2,4-D and neurologic effects like peripheral neuropathy, demyelination and ganglion degeneration in the CNS, reduced nerve conduction velocity, mytonia and behavioral alterations (Garabrant and Philbert, 2002).

Numerous in vitro and in vivo studies with 2,4-D indicate that it has very little genotoxic potential (Munro *et al.*, 1992). Long-term bioassays in rats, mice and dogs provided no evidence to suggest that 2,4-D is a carcinogen in any of these species. An earlier study in rat reported an increase in the incidence of brain astrocytomas in male animals, only at the highest dose tested (45 mg/kg/d) (Serota *et al.*, 1986). However, a review of this study concluded that the observed tumors were not treatment-related (Munro *et al.*, 1992), and more recent studies did not replicate the original finding (Charles *et al.*, 1996). Nevertheless, the chlorophenoxy herbicides have attracted much attention because of the association between exposure and non-Hodgkin's lymphoma or soft-tissue sarcoma, found in a small number of epidemiological studies (Hoar *et al.*, 1986; Hardell *et al.*, 1994). In a recent review that follows several previous ones discussing this topic (Woods *et al.*, 1987; Munro *et al.*, 1992; USEPA, 1994), Garabrant and Philbert (2002) evaluated all cohort and case-control studies available to date, and concluded that the evidence from epidemiological studies was not adequate

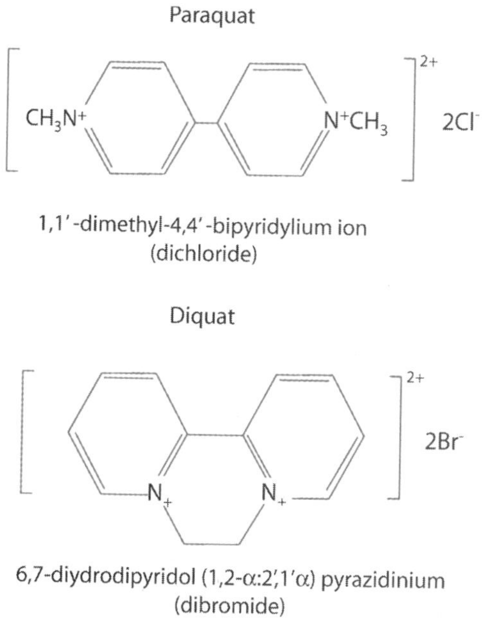

Paraquat

1,1'-dimethyl-4,4'-bipyridylium ion
(dichloride)

Diquat

6,7-diydrodipyridol (1,2-α:2',1'α) pyrazidinium
(dibromide)

Figure 22-18. Structures of the bipyridyl herbicides paraquat and diquat, marketed as the dichloride and dibromide salts, respectively.

to conclude that exposure to 2,4-D is associated with soft-tissue sarcoma, non-Hodgkin's lymphoma or Hodgkin's disease. 2,4-D is classified as a Group D agent (not classifiable as to human carcinogenicity) (USEPA, 1997).

Bipyridil Compounds

This class of herbicides comprises paraquat and diquat (Fig. 22-18). Of these, paraquat (1,1'-dimethyl-4,4'-bipyridilium dichloride) is of most toxicological concern, and will be discussed in more detail. First described in 1882, paraquat's redox properties were discovered in 1933, when the compound was called methyl viologen. Paraquat, introduced as a herbicide in 1962, is formulated as an aqueous solution or as a granular formulation. Paraquat is a fast-acting, nonselective contact herbicide, used to control broad-leaved weeds and grasses in plantations and fruit orchards, and for general weed control (Lock and Wilks, 2001a).

Paraquat has one of the highest acute toxicity among herbicides; its oral LD_{50} in rat is approximately 100 mg/kg, while guinea pigs, rabbits, and monkeys are more sensitive. Paraquat is more toxic when given by the i.p. route (LD_{50} in rats = 10–20 mg/kg), suggesting that it is poorly absorbed from the gastrointestinal tract. Paraquat is also poorly absorbed through the skin. Upon absorption, independent of the route of exposure, paraquat accumulates in the lung and the kidney, and these two organs are the most susceptible to paraquat-induced injury. Paraquat is very poorly metabolized, and is excreted almost unchanged in the urine. Paraquat has minimal to no genotoxic activity, is not carcinogenic in rodents, has no effect on fertility, is not teratogenic, and only produces fetotoxicity at maternally toxic doses (Lock and Wilks, 2001a). Thus, the major toxicological concerns for paraquat are related to its acute systemic effects, particularly in the lung, and secondarily, the kidney. Rose *et al.* (1974) first described an energy-dependent accumulation of paraquat in lung tissue, particularly, but not exclusively, in type II alveolar epithelial cells. The loss of paraquat from lung tissue following in vivo administration is slow. Thus, the basis for the selective

toxicity of paraquat to the lung resides in its ability to concentrate in alveolar type II and I cells and Clara cells.

The mechanism(s) by which paraquat is toxic to living cells have been extensively investigated (Autor, 1974; Bus and Gibson, 1984; Smith, 1987). Paraquat can be reduced to form a free radical, which in the presence of oxygen, rapidly reoxidizes to the cation, with a concomitant production of superoxide anion ($O2^-$). Thus, once paraquat enters a cell, it undergoes alternate reduction followed by reoxidation, a process known as redox cycling (Adam *et al.*, 1990). Superoxide dismutases (SOD) are a family of metalloenzymes that can dismutate superoxide anions to hydrogen peroxide and oxygen. The finding that transgenic mice lacking copper/zinc SOD show marked increase in sensitivity to paraquat (Ho *et al.*, 1998), supports a role for superoxide anions in paraquat's cellular toxicity. Nevertheless, superoxide anion itself is unlikely to be the ultimate toxic species (Lock and Wilks, 2001a). Three hypotheses have been proposed to account for the ensuing cytotoxicity, which are not mutually exclusive. The generation of superoxide anion and subsequently of hydroxy radicals, would initiate lipid peroxidation, ultimately leading to cell death (Bus and Gibson, 1984). Intracellular redox cycling of paraquat would also result in the oxidation of NADPH, leading to its cellular depletion, which is augmented by the detoxification of hydrogen peroxide formed in the glutathione peroxidase/reductase enzyme system to regenerate GSH (Fig. 22-19). A third hypothesis is that paraquat toxicity is due to mitochondrial damage; however, paraquat does not affect complex I in isolated brain mitochondria (Richardson *et al.*, 2005).

Upon acute exposure to lethal doses of paraquat, mortality may occur 2–5 days after dosing, though death can also occur after longer periods (Clark *et al.*, 1966). Damage to alveolar epithelial cells is seen within 24 hours after exposure. Damage progresses in the following 2–4 days with large areas of the alveolar epithelium completely lost. This is followed by alveolar edema, extensive infiltration of inflammatory cells into the alveolar interstitium, and finally death due to severe anoxia (Smith and Heath, 1976). Survivors of this first phase, called the destructive phase, show extensive proliferation of fibroblasts in the lung. The second phase, called the proliferative phase, is characterized by attempts by the alveolar epithelium to regenerate and restore normal architecture, and presents itself as an intensive fibrosis (Smith and Heath, 1976). Some individuals who survive the first phase may still die from the progressive loss of lung function several weeks after exposure.

Attempts to develop treatments for paraquat poisoning have focused on prevention of absorption from the gastrointestinal tract, removal from the bloodstream, prevention of its accumulation in the lung, use of free radical scavengers, and prevention of lung fibrosis (Lock and Wilks, 2001a). Though some approaches have shown promises in vitro or in isolated lung tissue preparations, only the first one, removal of the ingested material by emesis or purgation of the gastrointestinal tract, has been shown to be effective in vivo in animals.

Since its introduction as a herbicide, there have been thousands of episodes of acute poisoning with paraquat in humans, a large percentage of which results in death (Malone *et al.*, 1971; Casey and Vale, 1994; Wesseling *et al.*, 2001). Most cases involved ingestion of a 20% paraquat concentrate solution for suicidal purposes, or as a result of accidental poisoning due to decanting in unlabeled drink bottles or containers. To avoid the latter, in the 1980s, the manufacturers added a blue pigment, a stenching compound, and an emetic substance to the formulation, to make severe unintentional poisoning due to oral intake virtually impossible (Sabapathy, 1995). As

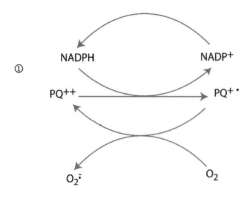

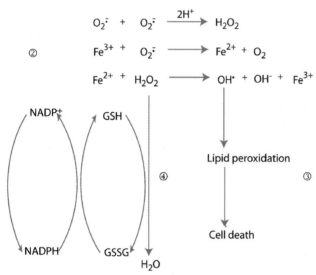

Figure 22-19. Mechanism of toxicity of paraquat.

(1) Redox cycling of paraquat utilizing NADPH; (2) formation of hydroxy radicals leading to lipid peroxidation (3); (4) detoxication of H_2O_2 via glutathione reductase/peroxidase couple, utilizing NADPH. Modified from Smith (1987), with permission from Palgrave Macmillan.

said, absorption of paraquat across the human skin is very low (but is increased by damage to skin, and paraquat is a skin irritant), and inhalation exposure is even lower. Few cases of paraquat poisoning have been reported following dermal exposure. Signs and symptoms of paraquat poisoning in humans reflect those previously described. A dose of 20–30 mg/kg can cause mild poisoning, while 30–50 mg/kg can cause delayed development of pulmonary fibrosis, which can be lethal. Higher doses usually cause death within a few days due to pulmonary edema, and renal and hepatic failure (Smith and Heath, 1976). No single therapeutic intervention, among those outlined earlier, has proven efficacious in case of severe acute paraquat poisoning (Bismuth et al., 1982). In rare instances, heart/lung transplant has been used to treat severely paraquat-poisoned patients.

Chronic exposure of experimental animals to paraquat affects the same target organs of acute toxicity, i.e., the lung and the kidney, and no-effect levels have been established. Under normal use conditions, exposure to paraquat is very low and can be monitored by measuring paraquat levels in urine, as the compound is excreted unchanged. In the late 1970s concern was raised about possible exposure of marijuana smokers to paraquat by inhalation. Paraquat was indeed used to destroy marijuana fields, and residues were still present in the final products (Landrigan et al., 1983). However, no clinical cases were identified.

Chronic paraquat exposure has also been suggested as a possible etiological factor in the development of Parkinson's disease, and the first suggestion came from a study in the Canadian province of Quebec (Barbeau et al., 1986). The hypothesis arose by the structural similarity of paraquat to MPP^+ (1-methyl-4-phenylpyridinium ion), the toxic metabolite of MPTP (1-methyl-4-phenyl-1,2,3,5-tetrahydropyridine). MPP^+ itself was initially developed as a possible herbicide, but was never commercialized. It has been argued that paraquat, being positively charged, cannot easily pass the blood–brain barrier. Yet, animal studies have shown that paraquat can cause CNS effects, most notably a neurodegeneration of dopaminergic neurons (McCormack et al., 2002). Paraquat may be transported into the brain by a neutral amino acid transporter, such as the system L carrier (LAT-1) (Shimizu et al., 2001). The ability of paraquat to cause oxidative damage through a free radical mechanism may explain the selective vulnerability of dopaminergic neurons, which are per se more susceptible to oxidative damage (McCormack et al., 2005). Paraquat neurotoxicity is, however, distinct from that of MPTP or rotenone (Richardson et al., 2005). Whereas these animal studies are of interest, there is still no solid evidence that paraquat may be associated with Parkinson's disease in humans (Li et al., 2005). Furthermore, a 5–10 years follow-up of individuals who survived paraquat poisoning did not provide any evidence of parkinsonism (Zilker et al., 1988).

Despite the chemical similarity to paraquat (Fig. 22-18), the herbicide diquat presents a different toxicological profile. Acute toxicity is somewhat lower, with oral LD_{50} in rats of approximately 200 mg/kg (Lock and Wilks, 2001b). Diquat is not a skin sensitizer, has minimal or no genotoxic activity, is not carcinogenic in rodents, has no effect on fertility, and is not teratogenic. In contrast to paraquat, it does not accumulate in the lung, and no lung toxicity is seen upon acute or chronic exposure. Upon chronic exposure, target organs for toxicity are the gastrointestinal tract, the kidney, and particularly the eye. Diquat indeed causes a dose- and time-dependent appearance of cataracts in both rats and dogs (Lock and Wilks, 2001b). Like paraquat, diquat can be reduced to form a free radical and then reoxidized in the presence of oxygen, with the concomitant production of superoxide anion. This process of redox cycling occurs in the eye and is believed to be the likely mechanism of cataract formation (Lock and Wilks, 2001b). A limited number of cases of human poisoning with diquat have occurred. Clinical symptoms include nausea, vomiting, diarrhea, ulceration of mouth and esophagus, decline of renal functions and neurologic effects, but no pulmonary fibrosis. As for paraquat, therapy for intoxication is directed at preventing absorption and enhancing elimination (Vanholder et al., 1981; Lock and Wilks, 2001b).

Chloroacetanilides

Representative compounds of this class of herbicides are alachlor, acetochlor, and metolachlor (Fig. 22-20), which are used to control herbal grasses and broad-leaved weeds in a number of crops (corn, soybeans, peanuts). Chloroacetanilides display moderate to low acute toxicity, with oral LD_{50} in rat ranging from about 600 mg/kg (propachlor) to 2800 mg/kg (metolachlor). Dermal LD_{50} values are higher, indicating poor absorption of these compounds across the skin (Heydens et al., 2001). Subchronic and chronic toxicity studies, carried out in multiple species, have identified the liver and kidney as principal target organs, and no-adverse-effect

Alachlor

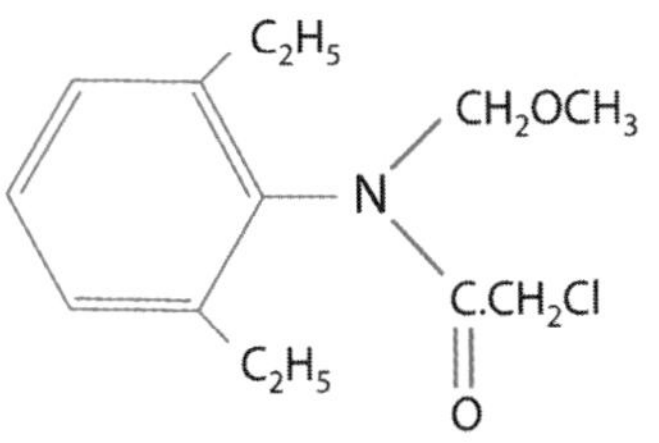

2-chloro-2',6'-diethyl-N-(methoxymethyl)
acetanilide

Metolachlor

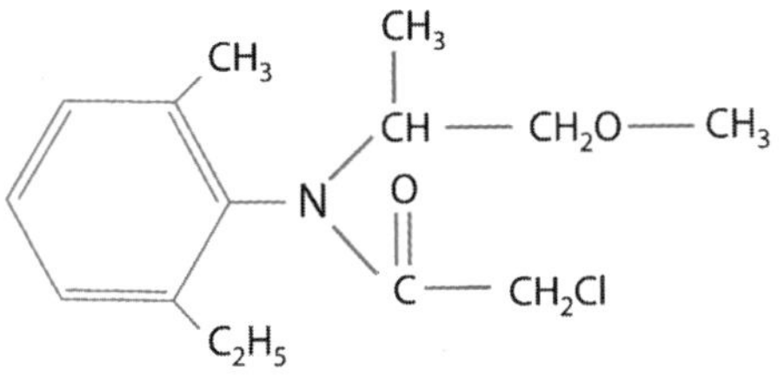

2-chloro-N-(2-ethyl-6-methylpheynyl)-N-
(2-methoxy-1-methylethyl)-acetamide

Acetochlor

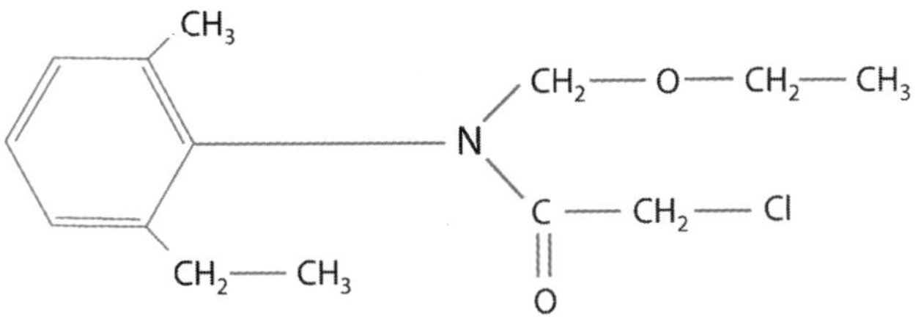

2-chloro-N-(ethoxymethyl)-N-
2-ethyl-6-methylphenyl)-acetamide

Figure 22-20. Structures of chloroacetanilide herbicides.

levels have been established. Alachlor was found to produce an ocular lesion, termed "progressive uveal degeneration syndrome," in rats (Heydens, 1998). However, an investigation of similar eye abnormalities in alachlor production workers considered to have the highest alachlor exposure, provided no evidence of ocular disease (Ireland *et al.*, 1994). None of the chloroacetanilides appears to be teratogenic or cause reproductive or developmental toxicity (Heydens *et al.*, 2001).

Chloroacetanilides have been extensively tested for genotoxicity in vitro and in vivo, and these studies indicate, on the basis of a weight-of-evidence approach, that these compounds are not genotoxic (Ashby *et al.*, 1996; Heydens *et al.*, 1999, 2001). Yet these compounds have been shown to induce tumors at various sites in rats. Tumors in mice (lung adenomas), found with alachlor and acetochlor, were considered not to be treatment-related (Ashby *et al.*, 1996; Heydens *et al.*, 1999). In rats, nasal epithelial (olfactory) tumors and thyroid follicular tumors were observed in carcinogenic-

ity studies with alachlor, acetochlor, and butachlor, while glandular stomach tumors were found with alachlor and butachlor. These findings led to the classification of alachlor, acetochlor, and butachlor as probable human carcinogens (Group B2). The discovery of alachlor in well water led to cancellation of its registration in some countries, and to its restriction in others. A series of mechanistic studies in the past decade has provided evidence that tumors observed in rats may be species-specific, show a threshold, and are not due to genotoxic mechanisms, and hence may not be relevant to humans (Ashby *et al.*, 1996; Heydens *et al.*, 1999, 2001). Alachlor and other chloroacetanilides are extensively metabolized in rats; more than 30 metabolites have been identified in this species, whereas in primates alachlor is metabolized to a limited number of glutathione and glucuronide metabolites. Furthermore, in rats, biliary excretion and enterohepatic recirculation of metabolites is observed, whereas in primates excretion is primarily via the kidneys. Thus, in rats, alachlor and butachlor are initially metabolized in the liver via the cytochrome P450 pathway and by glutathione conjugation, and the metabolites undergo enterohepatic circulation and further metabolism in liver and nasal tissue, to form the putative carcinogenic metabolite diethyl quinoneimine (DEIQ) (Feng *et al.*, 1990). In the case of acetochlor, the carcinogenic metabolite is EMIQ, an acetochlor quinoneimine compound analogous to DEIQ. Quinoneimines are electrophilic, deplete glutathione and exert cellular toxicity, which is followed by regenerative cell proliferation. Whole-body autoradiography studies have shown that alachlor-derived radioactivity specifically localizes in the nasal mucosa of rats, but not mice or monkeys. Furthermore, the ability of rat nasal tissue to form DEIQ is much higher than human nasal tissue (Wilson *et al.*, 1995). With regard to stomach and thyroid tumors, it is suggested that these result from tissue-specific toxicity, leading to compensatory cell proliferation in the fundic mucosa, and to alterations of thyroid stimulating hormone homeostasis. Both are believed to be threshold-sensitive phenomena. Epidemiological investigations in workers involved in the manufacturing of alachlor have not demonstrated any evidence of increased mortality or cancer incidence (Leet *et al.*, 1996).

Triazines

The family of triazine herbicides comprises several compounds (atrazine, simazine, propazine; Fig. 22-21), that are extensively used for the preemergent control of broad-leaved weeds (Stevens *et al.*, 2001). Triazines have low acute oral and dermal toxicity, and chronic toxicity studies indicate primarily decreased body weight gain. In dogs, cardiotoxicity is seen with atrazine, and was used to derive the NOEL for this compound (0.5 mg/kg/d) (Gammon *et al.*, 2005). There is no evidence that triazines are teratogenic, nor developmental or reproductive toxicants. Evidence from in vitro and in vivo studies indicate that atrazine is not genotoxic (Brusick, 1994), although a more recent study has suggested a possible clastogenic effect (Taets *et al.*, 1998). Oncogenicity studies found that triazines cause an increased incidence of mammary carcinomas in female Sprague–Dawley rats (Stevens *et al.*, 2001; Gammon *et al.*, 2005). Such tumors were not observed in male Sprague–Dawley rats, or in Fischer 344 rats or CD-1 mice of either sex (IARC, 1999; Stevens *et al.*, 2001). It is believed that such mammary tumors arise from an endocrine effect that might be expected to show a threshold. In contrast to most rodent species, female Sprague–Dawley rats have a high degree of spontaneous mammary tumors, due to their reproductive aging; they display prolonged or persistent estrus associated with high estrogen levels (Eldridge *et al.*, 1996). This is supported by the

Atrazine

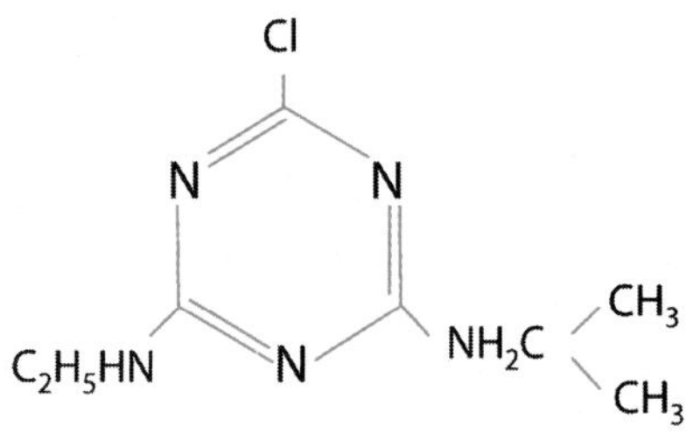

2-chloro-4(ethylamino)-6-
(isopropylamino)-s-triazine

Simazine

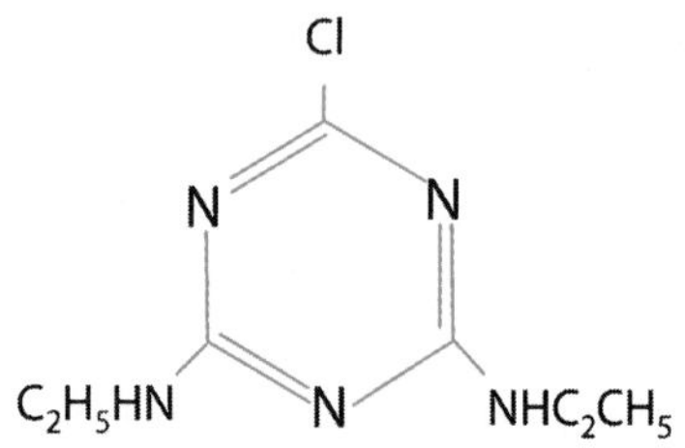

2-chloro-4,6(ethylamino)-
s-triazine

Propazine

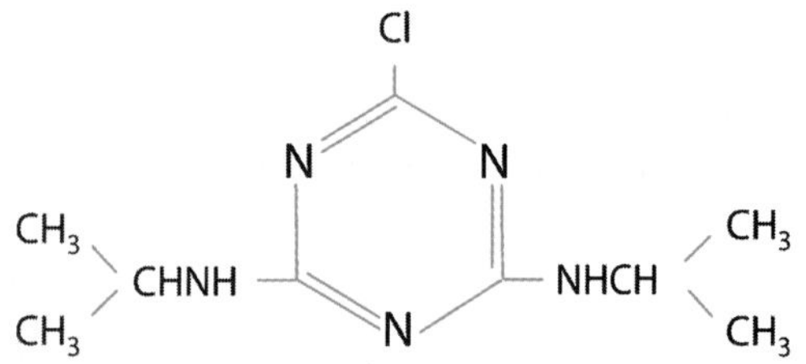

2-chloro-4,6 bis(isopropylamino)-
s-triazine

Figure 22-21. *Structures of triazine herbicides.*

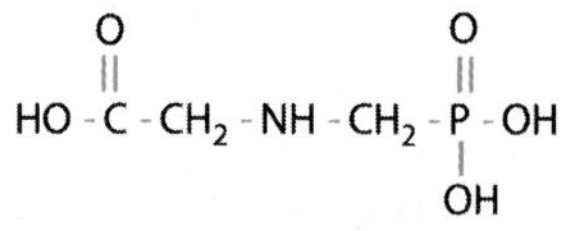

Glyphosate

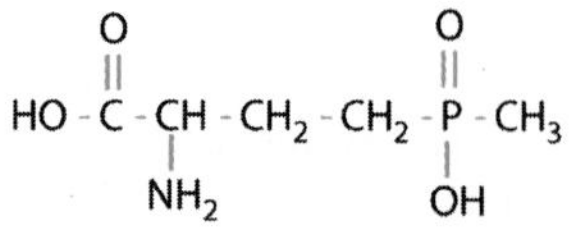

Glufosinate

Figure 22-22. *Structures of the phosphomethyl amino acids glyphosate and glufosinate. Note that though having a P=O moiety like organophosphates, these compounds are not acetylcholinesterase inhibitors.*

et al., 2003). Both atrazine and simazine are classified as Group 3 carcinogens (not classifiable as to its carcinogenicity to humans) by IARC.

Though exposure to atrazine through residues in food commodities is very low, contamination of ground water and drinking water is common (Villanueva *et al.*, 2005). Several European countries have banned the use of atrazine in recent years, mainly because it was often detected at levels exceeding the 0.1 mg/L standard for drinking water. Recent publications have reported a possible feminization of frogs, measured in laboratory and field studies, by atrazine levels around 0.1 mg/L (Hayes *et al.*, 2002). However, other investigators failed to reproduce these findings (Carr *et al.*, 2003). The USEPA has concluded that the conflicting results do not allow any firm conclusion in this regard, and that further studies are needed (USEPA, 2003). Nevertheless, the known hormonal effects of triazines call for careful evaluation of endocrine disrupting effects of these herbicides.

Phosphonomethyl Amino Acids

The two compounds of this class are glyphosate (N-phosphonomethyl glycine) and glufosinate (N-phosphonomethyl homoalanine). Both are broad-spectrum nonselective systemic herbicides used for postemergent control of annual and perennial plants, and are marketed primarily as the isopropylamine salt (glyphosate) or ammonium salt (glufosinate). Though both compounds contain a P=O moiety (Fig. 22-22), they are not organophosphates, but rather organophosphonates, and do not inhibit AChE (Farmer, 2001).

Glyphosate   Glyphosate exerts its herbicidal action by inhibiting the enzyme 5-enolpyruvylshikimate-3-phosphate synthase, responsible for the synthesis of an intermediate in the biosynthesis of various amino acids. Although important in plant growth, this metabolic pathway is not present in mammals. The toxicity profile of technical grade glyphosate is unremarkable (Williams *et al.*, 2000; Farmer, 2001). Oral and dermal LD_{50} are >5000 mg/kg, and chronic toxicity studies show only nonspecific effects, such as failure to gain weight. It has no teratogenic, developmental or reproductive effects. Genotoxicity and carcinogenicity studies in animals were negative; on the basis of all available evidence glyphosate has been classified as a Group E compound (evidence of noncarcinogenicity in humans) by the USEPA (Farmer, 2001).

finding that ovariectomy eliminates mammary tumors in Sprague–Dawley rats that arise both spontaneously and as a result of atrazine administration (Stevens *et al.*, 1999). The possible mechanisms for the effect of atrazine involve an action on pituitary luteinizing hormone, regulated by hypothalamic gonadothropin-releasing hormone, in turn controlled by hypothalamic norepinephrine (Cooper *et al.*, 2000). Some regulatory agencies have thus concluded that mammary tumors in female Sprague–Dawley rats are formed via a secondary, hormone-mediated mechanism, of little or no toxicological relevance to humans. Epidemiological studies of triazine herbicides and cancer have provided inconclusive results (Sathiakumar and Delzell, 1997). More recent studies have suggested an increased risk of prostate cancer associated with triazine herbicides (Mills and Yang, 2003), but this has not been substantiated by others (Alavanja

Glyphosate is one of the most widely used herbicides in the United States and worldwide (Table 22-4), and the development of transgenic crops that can tolerate glyphosate treatment have expanded its utilization. Given its widespread use, including the home and garden market, accidental or intentional exposure to glyphosate is inevitable. For example, in the period 2001–2003, there were over 13,000 reports to the American Association of Poisons Control Centers' Toxic Exposure Surveillance System relating to glyphosate exposure (Bradberry et al., 2004b). There was a major adverse outcome in 18 patients, and five died. Several other cases of glyphosate ingestions have been published, with a 10–15% mortality rate (Sawada et al., 1988; Talbot et al., 1991; Lee et al., 2000; Stella and Ryan, 2004; Bradberry et al., 2004b). Given the low acute toxicity of glyphosate itself, the attention has been focused on its formulation, which contains surfactants to aid its penetration. The most widely used glyphosate product is Roundup® which is formulated as a concentrate containing water, 41% glyphosate (as isopropylamine salt) and 15% polyoxethyleneamine (POEA). Animal studies suggest that the acute toxicity of this glyphosate formulation is due to the surfactant POEA, which has an oral LD in rat of 1200 mg/kg (Bradberry et al., 2004b). Mild intoxication results mainly in transient gastrointestinal symptoms, while moderate or severe poisoning presents with gastrointestinal bleeding, hypotension, pulmonary dysfunction and renal damage (Talbot et al., 1991).

Glufosinate Glufosinate is a nonselective contact herbicide that acts by irreversibly inhibiting glutamine synthetase (Ebert et al., 1990). Plants die as a consequence of the increased levels of ammonia. Mammals have other metabolizing systems that can cope with the effects on glutamine synthetase activity to a certain limit. In brain, however, inhibition of >10% of this enzyme activity is considered an adverse effect (EFSA, 2005). Glufosinate has relatively low acute toxicity, and chronic toxicity studies provided a NOAEL of 4.5 mg/kg/d, based on decreased glutamine synthetase activity. There is no evidence of genotoxicity or carcinogenicity, or direct effects on reproductive performance and fertility. Developmental toxic effects were found in rabbits (premature deliveries, abortions, dead fetuses). The most commonly used form of glufosinate is as ammonium salt, which is formulated with an anionic surfactant. Several cases of acute human poisoning from glufosinate ammonium-containing products have been reported, particularly in Japan, due to suicidal intent or accidental misuse. Symptoms include gastrointestinal effects, impaired respiration, neurological disturbance, and cardiovascular effects (Koyama et al., 1994; Watanabe and Sano, 1998; Ujvary, 2001). Though glufosinate does not inhibit cholinesterase, a reduction of red blood cell and plasma cholinesterase was found in poisoned patients. As is the case for glyphosate, a role for the surfactant in the acute toxicity has been proposed, particularly with regard to the cardiovascular effects (Ujvary, 2001).

FUNGICIDES

Fungal diseases are virtually impossible to control without chemical application. Fungicidal chemicals are derived from a variety of structures, from simple inorganic compounds, such as copper sulfate, to complex organic compounds. The majority of fungicides are surface or plant protectants, and are applied prior to potential infection by fungal spores, either to plants or to postharvest crops. Other fungicides can be used therapeutically, to cure plants when

an infestation has already begun. Still others are used as systemic fungicides, that are absorbed and distributed throughout the plant.

With few exceptions, fungicides have low acute toxicity in mammals. However, several produce positive results in genotoxicity tests and some have carcinogenic potentials. The effects are often associated with the mechanisms by which these compounds act on their targets, the fungi. A 1987 evaluation by the National Research Council concluded that fungicides, though accounting for only 7% of all pesticide sales, and less than 10% of all pounds of pesticides applied, accounted for about 60% of estimated dietary oncogenic risk (NRC, 1987). Some fungicides have been associated with severe epidemics of poisoning, and have thus been banned. Methylmercury was associated with poisoning in Iraq, when treated grains were consumed (Bakir et al., 1973). Hexachlorobenzene (HCB), used in the 1940–1950s to treat seed grains, was associated with an epidemic of poisoning in Turkey from 1955 to 1959 (Cam and Nigogosyan, 1963). HCB has a high cumulative toxicity and caused a syndrome called black sore, characterized by blistering and epidermolysis of the skin, pigmentation and scarring. HCB also causes porphyria as well as hepatomegaly and immunosuppression (Ecobichon, 2001a). The main classes of fungicides currently in use are discussed below; additional discussions of fungicide use and toxicity can be found in Hayes (1982) and in Edwards et al. (1991).

Captan and Folpet

Captan and folpet are broad-spectrum protectant fungicides; together with captafol, which was taken off the market in 1988, they are called chloroalkylthio fungicides, due to the presence of side chains containing chlorine, carbon, and sulfur (Fig. 22-23). Captan was first registered in the United States in 1949, and folpet followed a few years later. As for most fungicides, captan and folpet have low acute oral and dermal toxicity (LD$_{50}$ = ~5g/kg). They are potent eye irritants, but only mild skin irritants. Dermal absorption is low. Both are extensively and rapidly metabolized in mammals, through hydrolysis and thiol interactions, with thiophosgene being a common metabolite (Gordon, 2001). Captan and folpet, as well as thiophosgene, are mutagenic in in vitro tests; however, in vivo mutagenicity tests are mostly negative, possibly because of the rapid degradation of these compounds. Both fungicides induce the development of duodenal tumors in mice, and on this basis, they are classified by the USEPA as probable human carcinogens. The mode of action for these tumors is thought to be dependent on irritation and cell loss in the intestinal villi, followed by a compensatory increase in proliferation in the crypt compartment (Gordon, 2001). Captan and folpet share a common mechanism of toxicity with regard to the development of duodenal tumors in mice, as well as other toxicity end points, and are considered for cumulative risk assessment under the FQPA (Bernard and Gordon, 2000). Tumors observed in rats (renal adenomas and uterine sarcomas) are suggested not to be treatment-related (Gordon, 2001), but are considered in the carcinogenicity classification of these fungicides. Because of their structural similarity to the potent teratogen thalidomide (Fig. 22-23), chloroalkylthio fungicides have been extensively tested in reproductive/developmental studies in multiple species, but no evidence of teratogenicity has been found (McLaughlin et al., 1969).

Dithiocarbamates

Dithiocarbamates are a group of fungicides that have been widely used since the 1940s to control about 400 fungal pathogens in a

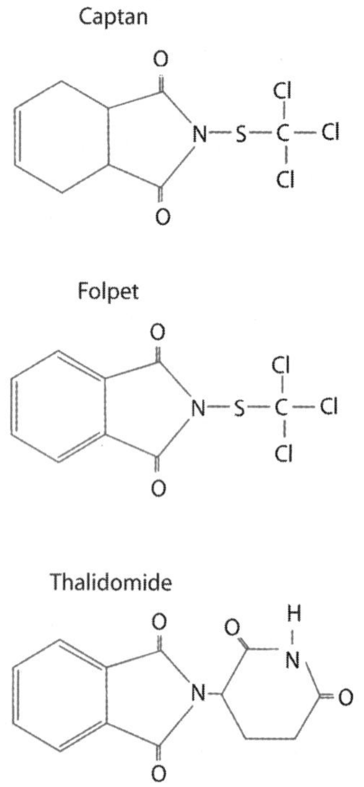

Captan

Folpet

Thalidomide

Figure 22-23. Structures of the phthalimide fungicides captan and folpet. The structure of thalidomide is also shown, though phthalimides have been shown not to be teratogenic, despite structural similarities.

Maneb

manganese ethylenebisdithiocarbamate

Zineb

zinc ethylenebisdithiocarbamate

Thiram

bis(diethylthio-carbamoyl)disulfide

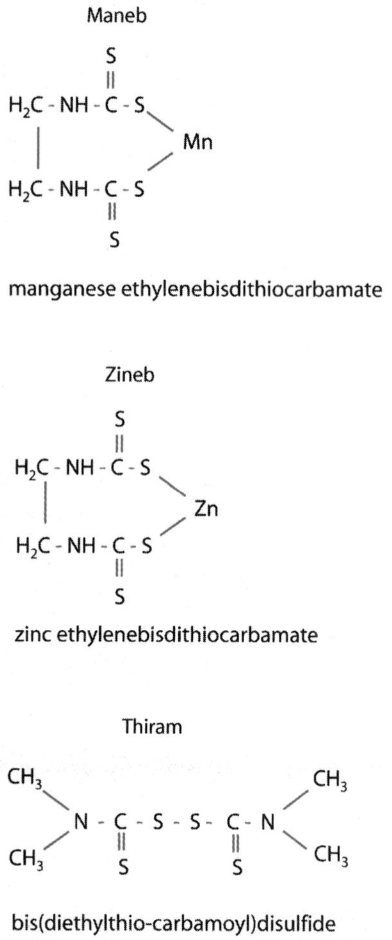

Figure 22-24. Structures of three dithiocarbamate fungicides.

variety of crops. The nomenclature of many of these compounds arises from the metal cations with which they are associated; thus, there are for example Maneb (Mn), Ziram and Zineb (Zn), and Mancozeb (Mn and Zn) (Fig. 22-24). Thiram is an example of dithiocarbamate without a metal moiety (Fig. 22-24). The dithiocarbamates have low acute toxicity by the oral, dermal, and respiratory route (Hurt *et al.*, 2001). However, chronic exposure is associated with adverse effects that may be due to the dithiocarbamate acid or the metal moiety. These compounds are metabolized to a common metabolite, ethylenethiourea (ETU), which is responsible for the effects of dithiocarbamates on the thyroid. ETU produced thyroid tumors in rats and mice, that result from the inhibition of the synthesis of the thyroid hormones thyroxine (T4) and triiodothyronine (T3). This leads to elevated serum levels of thyroid stimulating hormone (TSH), via feedback stimulation of the hypothalamus and the pituitary, and subsequent hypertrophy and hyperplasia of thyroid follicular cells, that progresses to adenomas and carcinomas (Chhabra *et al.*, 1992). Similarly, dithiocarbamates alter thyroid hormone levels, and cause thyroid hypertrophy. The hormonal mechanism of thyroid tumors would imply a threshold model for hazard assessment. ETU also causes liver tumors in mice, by yet unknown mechanisms, although levels of ETU resulting from fungicide metabolism at maximum tolerated doses are believed to be insufficient to produce hepatic tumors (Hurt *et al.*, 2001). Neither dithiocarbamates nor ETU are genotoxic in in vitro and in vivo tests.

Developmental toxicity and teratogenicity is observed with dithiocarbamates and ETU at maternally toxic doses. These effects are ascribed to an effect of ETU on the thyroid. A key concern with chemicals affecting thyroid functions, is their potential developmental neurotoxicity, given the essential role of thyroid hormones in brain development (Chan and Kilby, 2000), and this deserves further investigation. There is also some evidence that dithiocarbamates may cause neurotoxicity by mechanisms not involving ETU.

High doses of several of these compounds cause hind limb paralysis, which is possibly related to the release of the carbon disulfide moiety (Johnson *et al.*, 1998). Chronic exposure to Maneb has been associated with parkinsonism, which is likely ascribed to exposure to the manganese moiety, rather than the dithiocarbamate (Ferraz *et al.*, 1988; Meco *et al.*, 1994). Maneb has also been shown to produce nigrostriatal degeneration when given in combination with paraquat (Thiruchelvam *et al.*, 2000), and to potentiate the neurotoxicity of MPTP (McGrew *et al.*, 2000). It has been shown that Maneb affects dopaminergic neurons by inhibiting mitochondrial functions (Zhang *et al.*, 2003).

The structure of dithiocarbamate fungicides resembles that of disulfiram, a compound used therapeutically to produce intolerance to alcohol, by virtue of its ability to inhibit aldehyde dehydrogenase. Interactions of dithiocarbamates with alcohol, leading to elevation in acetaldehyde levels, have been reported (Edwards *et al.*, 1991).

Chlorothalonil

Chlorothalonil (Bravo[®]) is a halogenated benzonitrile fungicide (Fig. 22-25), widely used to treat vegetable, ornamental, and orchard diseases (Table 22-4). Whereas oral and dermal toxicities are low (LD$_{50}$s = 5–10 g/kg), it is highly toxic by the intraperitoneal and inhalation routes. It also causes severe irreversible eye lesions in the rabbit, because of its irritant properties. Dermal absorption is low, but following oral administration, chlorothalonil is rapidly

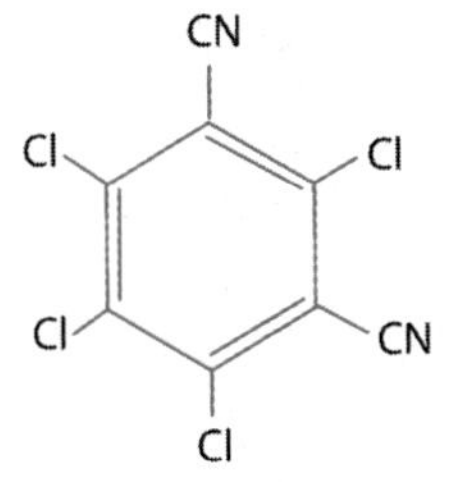

CN

Cl | Cl

Cl | CN

Cl

Chlorothalonil

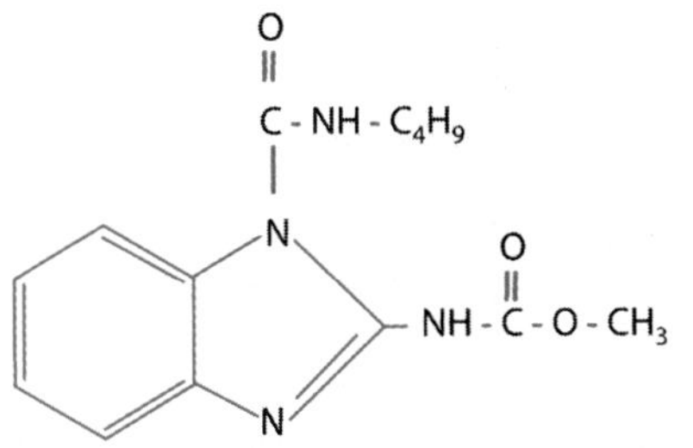

O
‖
C - NH - C₄H₉
|
N

O
‖
NH - C - O - CH₃

N

Benomyl

Figure 22-25. Structures of the fungicides choroathalonil and benomyl.

absorbed and metabolized through glutathione conjugation. Chlorathalonil is not mutagenic in in vitro and in vivo tests (Parsons, 2001). Tumors in the forestomach and the kidney have been found in chronic toxicity studies in both rats and mice, but not in dogs. Tumors are believed to be due to regenerative hyperplasia, and it is assumed that a threshold can be established for carcinogenicity (Parsons, 2001). Chlorothalonil is not a reproductive or developmental toxicant. Known adverse effects in humans are limited to its irritant effects on the eye and the skin.

Benzimidazoles

Benomyl is the main representative of this class of fungicides (Fig. 22-25). It inhibits fungal growth by binding to tubulin, and this mechanism also accounts for its toxic effects in mammals. Acute toxicity is low, whereas chronic studies have found effects in the liver, testes, bone marrow and gastrointestinal tract (Mull and Hershberger, 2001). Because of its ability to disrupt microtubule assembly during cell division, Benonyl causes chromosomal aberrations (aneuploidy) both in vitro and in vivo, but does not interact directly with DNA. Liver tumors have been observed in chronic oncogenicity studies in mice. The action on dividing cells has also raised concern for Benomyl's potential teratogenicity and developmental toxicity. Teratogenic effects were observed following administration of high doses of Benomyl and Carbendazim (a metabolite of Benomyl, which is commercialized as a fungicide but not in the United States) to rats (Mull and Hershberger, 2001). However, such effects were not seen in feeding studies in rats or rabbits. Anecdotal evidence suggests that maternal exposure to Benomyl may result in anophthalmia in humans, but epidemiological studies did not demonstrate any convincing association (Spagnolo *et al.*, 1994).

Inorganic and Organometal Fungicides

Several inorganic and organic metal compounds are, or have been, used as fungicides (Clarkson, 2001). The fungicidal activity of

soluble copper salts was discovered as early as 1807, and by 1890 copper sulfate found extensive use, particularly in the formulation known as Bordeaux mixture (copper sulfate and calcium hydroxide). Copper sulfate has overall low toxicity and remains one of the most widely used fungicides (Table 22-4). Among organotin compounds, triphenyltin acetate is used as a fungicide, while tributyltin is utilized as an antifouling agent. Triphenyltin has moderate to high acute toxicity, but may cause reproductive toxicity and endocrine disruption (Golub and Doherty, 2004). Organic mercury compounds, such as methylmercury, were used extensively as fungicides in the past for the prevention of seed-borne diseases in grains and cereals. Given their high toxicity, particularly neurotoxicity, and large episodes of human poisoning (Bakir *et al.*, 1973), their use has since been banned. A discussion of organometal compounds is found in Chap. 23.

RODENTICIDES

Rats and mice can cause health and economic damages to humans. Rodents are vectors for several human diseases, including plague, endemic rickettsiosis, spirochetosis, and several others; they can occasionally bite people; they can consume large quantities of postharvest stored foods, and can contaminate foodstuff with urine, feces, and hair, that may cause diseases. Hence, there is a need to control rodent population. Limiting their access to feed and harborage, and trapping, are two approaches; however, rodenticides still play and will likely continue to play an important role in rodent control. To be effective, yet safe, rodenticides must satisfy several criteria: (1) the poison must be very effective in the target species once incorporated into bait in small quantity; (2) baits containing the poison must not excite bait shyness, so that the animal will continue to eat it; (3) the manner of death must be such that survivors do not become suspicious of its cause; and (4) it should be species-specific, with considerable lower toxicity to other animals (Murphy, 1986; Ecobichon, 2001a).

The compounds used as rodenticides comprise a diverse range of chemical structures having a variety of mechanisms of action. The ultimate goal is to obtain the highest species selectivity; in some cases (e.g., norbormide) advantage has been taken of the physiology and biochemistry unique to rodents. With other rodenticides, the sites of action are common to most mammals, but advantage is taken of the habits of the pest animal and/or the usage, thereby minimizing toxicity for nontarget species. Because rodenticides are used in baits which are often placed in inaccessible places, widespread exposures or contaminations are unlikely. However, toxicologic problems can arise from acute accidental ingestions or from suicidal/homicidal attempts. In particular, poison centers receive thousands of calls every year related to accidental ingestions of rodenticide baits by children, most of which are resolved without serious consequences.

Fluoroacetic Acid and Its Derivatives

Sodium fluoroacetate (Compound 1080) and fluoroacetamide are the main representatives of this class of rodenticides. They are white in color and odorless, and due to their high mammalian toxicity, their use is restricted to trained personnel. Both compounds have indeed high acute toxicity (oral LD_{50}s in the rat = 2 and 13 mg/kg, respectively). The main targets of toxicity are the central nervous system and the heart. Fluoroacetate is incorporated into fluoracetyl-coenzyme A, which condenses with oxolacetate to form fluorocitrate, which inhibits mitochondrial aconitase. This results in inhibition of the Krebs cycle, leading to lowered energy production, reduced oxygen consumption, and reduced cellular concentration of ATP. Blockage of energy metabolism is believed to account for most signs of toxicity, though some may be due to accumulation of citrate, which is a potent chelator of calcium ions (Pelfrene, 2001). Since 1946, when sodium fluoroacetate was introduced in the United States, several cases of human poisoning have been reported. Initial gastrointestinal symptoms are followed by severe cardiovascular effects (ventricular tachycardia, fibrillation, hypotension), as well as CNS effects (agitation, convulsions, coma). The estimated lethal dose in humans ranges from 2–10 mg/kg. There is no specific antidote for sodium fluoroacetate. Monacetin (60% glycerol monoacetate) has proved beneficial in the treatment of poisoned primates. Use of procainamide (for cardiac arrhythmia) and barbiturates (to control seizures) are also indicated. Use of Compound 1080 in the United States is severely restricted primarily because of toxicity to nontarget animals, such as dogs.

Thioureas

The discovery of α-naphtyl thiourea (ANTU) occurred fortuitously in the mid-1940s in the Psychobiological Laboratory of Curt Richter in Baltimore. While studying thioureas, favored by geneticists for taste tests, because they are so bitter to some people and tasteless to others, he discovered that ANTU was lethal yet tasteless to rodents, while being of low toxicity to humans (Keiner, 2005). A wide range of acute oral LD_{50} values has been reported for different species, the rat being the most sensitive at 6 mg/kg, and the monkey the least susceptible at 4 g/kg. The main target of toxicity is the lung, where ANTU causes marked edema of the subepithelial spaces of the alveolar walls. ANTU is believed to be biotransformed to a reactive intermediate which binds to lung macromolecules; however, the exact mechanism of its toxicity is unknown. Young rats are resistant to the chemical, whereas older rats become tolerant to it; both situations have been ascribed to developmentally low, or to ANTU-induced inhibition of, microsomal enzymes involved in its bioactivation (Boyd and Neal, 1976). There are no reports of human poisonings with ANTU. However, several cases involving a combination of chloralose and ANTU were reported in France; symptoms included motor agitation and coma, both characteristic of chloralose poisonings, and pulmonary effects, due to ANTU, but all patients recovered (Pelfrene, 2001). Suggestions that the presence of an impurity in ANTU, β-naphthylamine, may increase risk of bladder cancer, remain unsubstantiated (Case, 1966; Pelfrene, 2001).

Anticoagulants

Following the report of an hemorrhagic disorder in cattle that resulted from the ingestion of spoiled sweet clover silage, the hemorrhagic agent was identified in 1939 as bishydroxycoumarin (dicoumarol). In 1948, a more potent synthetic congener was introduced as an extremely effective rodenticide; the compound was named warfarin, as an acronym derived from the name of the patent holder, Wisconsin Alumni Research Foundation (Majerus and Tollefsen, 2006). In addition to their use as rodenticides, coumarin derivatives, including warfarin itself, are used as anticoagulant drugs and have become a mainstay for prevention of thromboembolic disease (Majerus and Tollefsen, 2006). Coumarins antagonizes the action of vitamin K in the synthesis of clotting factors (factors II, VII, IX, and X). Their specific mechanism involves inhibition of the enzyme vitamin K epoxide reductase, which regenerates reduced vitamin K necessary for sustained carboxylation and synthesis of relevant clotting factors (Fig. 22-26). The acute oral toxicity of warfarin in rats is approx. 50–100 mg/kg, whereas the 90-day dose LD_{50} has been reported as 0.077 mg/kg, indicating that multiple doses are required before toxicity develops.

Human poisonings by these rodenticides are rare because they are dispersed in grain-based baits. However, there is a significant number of suicide or homicide attempts or of accidental consumption of warfarin. One often reported case involved a Korean family that consumed a diet of corn containing warfarin over a two-week period. Symptoms (massive bruises, hematomata, gum and nasal hemorrhage) appeared about 10 days after the beginning of the warfarin consumption. Consumption of warfarin in this episode was estimated to be in the order of 1–2 mg/kg/d (Lange and Terveer, 1954). Monitoring of anticoagulant therapy is done by measuring prothrombin time (PT) in comparison to normal pooled plasma. Values of INR (International Normatized Ratio) are then derived, with a target value of 2–3. In case of poisoning, PT is significantly longer, and leads to severe internal bleeding. When INR is above 5, vitamin K can be given as an antidote.

The appearance of rats resistant to warfarin and to other early anticoagulant rodenticides, led to the development of "second generation" anticoagulants. Some are coumarins, such as the "super-warfarins" brodifacoum or difenacoum, whereas others are indan-1,3 -dione derivatives (diphacinone, chlorophacinone). These compounds essentially act like warfarin, but have prolonged half-lives (e.g., brodifacoum 156 hours vs. warfarin 37 hours), and cause very long-lasting inhibition of coagulation. Some are extremely toxic to most mammalian species; for example the oral LD_{50} of brodifacoum is about 0.3 mg/kg in rat, rabbit, and dog (Pelfrene, 2001).

Other Compounds

Norbormide This compound shows a remarkable selectivity in both toxicity and pharmacological effects. Oral LD_{50} in rat is about 5–10 mg/kg, whereas in dog and monkey 1000 mg/kg produces no effect. Such species difference in toxicity seems to be accounted for by differences in response of the peripheral blood vessels to norbormide-induced vasoconstriction. The exact mechanisms of this effect are not known.

Zinc Phosphide The toxicity of this chemical can be accounted for by the phosphine gas (PH_3) formed on ingestion following a hydrolytic reaction with water in the stomach. Phosphine causes widespread cellular toxicity with necrosis of the gastrointestinal tract and injury to liver and kidney. Cases of human poisoning have been reported (Ecobichon, 2001a). Additional inorganic compounds that have been used as rodenticides include aluminum phosphide, thallium sulfate, and arsenic salts. Thallium sulfate has the unusual feature of causing extensive alopecia (hair loss); because of its high acute toxicity in nontarget species, it was banned in the United States in 1972 (Clarkson, 2001).

Other Some rodenticides used in the past that have become obsolete include strychnine, an extremely poisonous alkaloid derived from the seeds of *Strychnos nux-vomica,* which is a potent convulsant; red squill (sea onion) and its bioactive principle, scilliroside, which affect the cardiovascular and central nervous systems and cause emesis; the inability of rodents to vomit explains the rather selective action in these species; and pyriminyl, a substituted urea

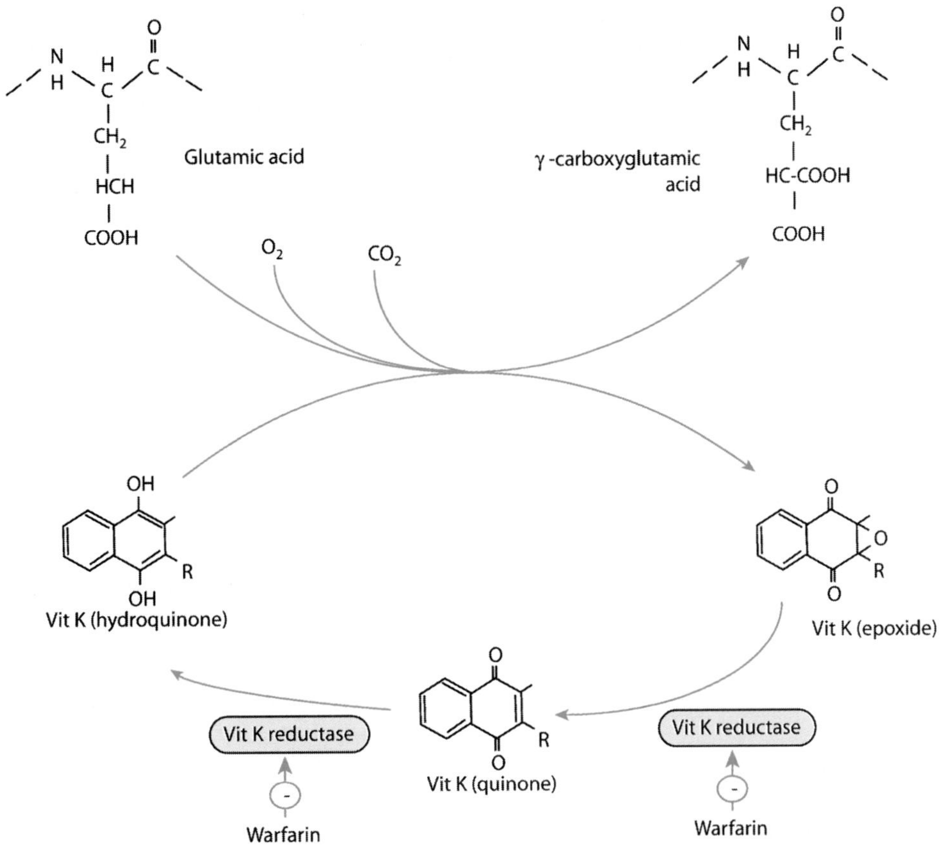

Figure 22-26. Site of action of the anticoagulant rodenticide warfarin.

Reduced vitamin K (hydroquinone) serves as cofactor for the conversion of glutamic acid to γ-carboxyglutamic acid in the peptide chains of coagulation factors II, VII, IX, and X. During this reaction, vitamin K is oxidized to an epoxide that is then reduced to quinone and hydroquinone by vitamin K reductase, which is inhibited by warfarin.

introduced in 1975 but withdrawn in the United States a few years later. This compound targets complex I in the mitochondria, and there are many reports of human poisoning in the short period of its use (Pelfrene, 2001). As many other ureas, it has diabetogenic properties.

FUMIGANTS

A large number of compounds are used for soil fumigation or for fumigating postharvest commodities. They are active toward insects, mites, nematodes, weed seeds, fungi or rodents, and have in common the property of being in the gaseous form at the time they exert their pesticidal action. They can be liquids that readily vaporize (e.g., ethylene dibromide), solids that can release a toxic gas on reaction with water (e.g., phosphine released by aluminum phosphide), or gases (e.g., methyl bromide). For soil fumigation, the compound is injected directly into the soil, which is then covered with plastic sheeting, which is sealed. By eliminating unwanted pests, this treatment enhances the quality of the crops and increases yield. Fumigation of postharvest commodities, such as wheat, cereals, and fruits to eradicate pest infestations, typically occurs where the commodities are stored (e.g., warehouses, grain elevators, ship holds). Compounds used as fumigants are usually nonselective, highly reactive, and cytotoxic. They provide a potential hazard from the standpoint of inhalation exposure, and to a minor degree for dermal exposure or ingestion, in case of solids or liquids. Several fumigants used in the past are no longer marketed

because of toxicological concerns. These include, for example, carbon disulfide, which is neurotoxic; carbon tetrachloride, a potent hepatotoxicant; 1,2-dibromo-3-chloropropane, a male reproductive toxicant; and ethylene dibromide, a carcinogen. Their toxicity is discussed in other sections of the book. Some of the most commonly used fumigants are discussed below.

Methyl Bromide

Methyl bromide is a broad-spectrum pesticide, used for soil fumigation, commodity treatment, and structural fumigation. It has been used as a fumigant for over 50 years, and its use is strictly controlled and restricted to certified applicators. Since the mid-1990s, use of methyl bromide has substantially decreased, because of environmental and toxicological concerns (Ruzo, 2006). Methyl bromide is thought to contribute to ozone depletion in the stratosphere. In 1987, with the signing of the Montreal Protocol on Substances that Deplete the Ozone Layer, the international community initiated a series of steps to reduce emissions of ozone-depleting products, including methyl bromide. Concerns on certain toxicological aspects of methyl bromide, have also contributed to its decreasing use, and to the search of viable alternatives (Ruzo, 2006; Schneider *et al.*, 2003). Yet, while several countries are substantially curtailing the use of methyl bromide, this compound still remains one of the most extensively used pesticides in the United States (Table 22-4; Ruzo, 2006), likely for convenience and economic reasons (Norman, 2005; McCook, 2006).

The acute toxicity of methyl bromide relates to both its concentration and the duration of exposure. For example, LC_{50} values in rats were 2833 ppm for a 30 minute exposure, and 302 ppm for an 8 hour exposure (Piccirillo, 2001). Between 1953 and 1981, 301 cases of systemic poisoning and 60 fatalities resulted from use of methyl bromide as a fumigant (Alexeef and Kilgore, 1983). Additional cases of human intoxication have since been reported (Herzstein and Cullen, 1990). Acute exposure results in respiratory, gastrointestinal and neurologic symptoms; the latter include lethargy, headache, seizures, paresthesias, peripheral neuropathy, and ataxia, and are considered to be more relevant than other toxic effects for human risk assessment (Alexeef and Kilgore, 1983; Lifshitz and Gavrilov, 2000; Piccirillo, 2001). Acute and chronic neurotoxicity studies in rats have demonstrated behavioral effects and morphological lesions, which were concentration- and time-dependent (Piccirillo, 2001). Long-lasting behavioral and neuropsychiatric effects are also seen in humans (De Haro et al., 1997; Lifshitz and Gavrilov, 2000). The mechanism(s) underlying methyl bromide neurotoxicity are not known. Depletion of GSH in brain areas was observed following exposure of rats to methyl bromide (140 ppm for 6 h/d, for 5 days) (Davenport et al., 1992). This may be due to conjugation of methyl bromide with GSH. The role of GSH and the possible ensuing increase in oxidative stress in methyl bromide neurotoxicity remains, however, uncertain. In various subchronic toxicity studies, the NOEL for neurotoxicity ranges between 18 and 200 ppm (Piccirillo, 2001).

Methyl bromide is positive in several genotoxicity tests in vitro and in vivo. Carcinogenicity studies produced carcinomas in the forestomach of rats following oral ingestion, and increased incidence of adenomas of the pituitary gland in male rats in an inhalation study. Other studies in rats and mice, however, provided no evidence of carcinogenicity. Methyl bromide is classified by IARC in Group 3 (not classifiable as to its carcinogenicity to humans), given the limited evidence in animals and the inadequate evidence in humans. As methyl bromide is an odorless and colorless gas, another fumigant, chloropicrin, which has a pungent odor and causes irritation of the eyes, is often used in conjunction with methyl bromide and other fumigant mixtures, to warn against potentially harmful exposures.

1,3–Dichloropropene

1,3–Dichloropropene, first introduced over fifty years ago, is a soil fumigant, extensively utilized (see Table 22-4) for its ability to control soil nematodes. It has a moderate to high acute toxicity in animals (oral LD_{50} in rats: 130–713 mg/kg; dermal LD_{50}: >1200 mg/kg; inhalation LD_{50}: ~ 1000 ppm). Human fatalities following oral exposure have been reported (Hernandez et al., 1994). 1,3–Dichloropropene is an irritant, and can cause redness and necrosis of the skin. It is extensively metabolized, with the mercapturic acid conjugate being the major urinary metabolite. Data on genotoxicity are contradictory, and carcinogenicity studies in rodents have found an increase in benign liver tumors in rats but not in mice, after oral administration (Stebbins et al., 2000), and of benign lung adenomas in mice following inhalation exposure (Lomax et al., 1989). The toxicology of 1,3 - dichloropropene has been recently reviewed (Stott et al., 2001).

Metam Sodium

Metam sodium ($C_2H_4NNaS_2$) is a widely used soil fumigant (Table 22-4), whose toxic action toward soil nematodes, fungi, and weed seeds is due to its hydrolysis product, methyl isothiocyanate (MITC). In mammals, metam sodium is metabolized in vivo to carbon disulfide and MITC (Pruett et al., 2001). In humans, metam sodium can act as a contact sensitizer, inducing allergic dermatitis, possibly due to MITC. Immunotoxicity is observed in rodents. In 1991, because of the derailment of a train car, approximately 19,000 gallons of metam sodium was spilled into the Sacramento River in California, causing a large kill of aquatic organisms. Symptoms reported by exposed individuals included headache, eye irritation, nausea, shortness of breath and dermatitis (Pruett et al., 2001). Metam sodium is increasingly being used as an alternative to methyl bromide (Ruzo, 2006).

Sulfur

Elemental sulfur is considered the oldest of all pesticides, and its pesticidal properties were known to the ancient Greeks as early as 1000 B.C. (Tweedy, 1981). It is very effective as a fumigant for the control of many plant diseases, particularly fungal diseases, and still represents the most heavily used crop protection chemical in the United States (Table 22-4). Sulfur finds its major uses in grapes and tomatoes, and can be used in organic farming (Gammon et al., 2001). Though it is generally considered an environmentally and toxicologically safe compound, elemental sulfur used as a fungicide can make the soil too acidic for the continuous optimal growth of a particular crop (Gammon et al., 2001). The primary health effect in humans associated with the agricultural use of elemental sulfur is dermatitis (Gammon et al., 2001). In ruminants, excessive sulfur ingestion can cause cerebrocortical necrosis (polioencephalomalacia), possibly due to its conversion by microorganisms in the rumen to hydrogen sulfide (Gammon et al., 2001).

REFERENCES

Abdel-Rhaman A, Shetty AK, Abou-Donia MB: Disruption of the blood-brain barrier and neuronal cell death in cingulate cortex, dentate gyrus, thalamus, and hypothalamus in a rat model of Gulf War syndrome. *Neurobiol Dis* 10:306–326, 2002.

Abel EL, Bammler TK, Eaton DL: Biotransformation of methyl parathion by glutathione S-transferases. *Toxicol Sci* 79:224–232, 2004.

Ackerman SJ, Kephart GM, Francis H, et al.: Eosinophil degranulation: An immunologic determinant in the pathogenesis of the Mazzotti reaction in human onchocerciasis. *J Immunol* 144:3961–3969, 1990.

Adam A, Smith LL, Cohen GM: An evaluation of the redox cycling potencies of paraquat and nitrofurantoin in microsomal and lung slice systems. *Biochem Pharmacol* 40:1533–1539, 1990.

Akossoglou K, Malester B, Xu J, et al.: Brain-specific deletion of neuropathy target esterase/Swiss cheese results in neurodegeneration. *Proc Natl Acad Sci USA* 101:5075–5080, 2004.

Alavanja MCR, Dosemeci M, Samanic C, et al.: Pesticides and lung cancer risk in the agricultural health study cohort. *Am J Epidemiol* 160:876–885, 2004.

Alavanja MCR, Samanic C, Dosemeci M, et al.: Use of agricultural pesticides and prostate cancer risk in the agricultural health study cohort. *Am J Epidemiol* 157:800–814, 2003.

Aldridge JE, Seidler FJ, Meyer A, et al.: Serotoninergic systems targeted by developmental exposure to chlorypyrifos: Effects during different critical periods. *Environ Health Perspect* 111:1736–1743, 2003.

Alexeef GV, Kilgore WW: Methyl bromide. *Residue Rev* 88:101–153, 1983.

Alonso L, Lindsay SW, Armstrong JRM, et al.: The effect of insecticide-treated bed nets on mortality of Gambian children. *Lancet* 337:1499–1502, 1991.

Altobelli D, Martire M, Maurizi S, et al.: Interaction of formamidine pesticides with the presynaptic α_2-adrenoceptor regulating [^{3}H] noradrenaline release from rat hypothalamic synaptosomes. *Toxicol Appl Pharmacol* 172:179–185, 2001.

Anand SS, Bim KB, Padilla S, et al.: Ontogeny of hepatic and plasma metabolism of deltamethrin in vitro: Role in age-dependent acute neurotoxicity. *Drug Metab Dispos* 34:389–397, 2006b.

Anand SS, Bruckner JV, Haines WT, et al.: Characterization of deltamethrin metabolism by rat plasma and liver microsomes. *Toxicol Appl Pharmacol* 212:156–166, 2006a.

Andrade SF, Sakate M: The comparative efficacy of yohimbine and atipamezole to treat amitraz intoxication in dogs. *Vet Hum Toxicol* 45:124–127, 2003.

Anway MD, Cupp AS, Uzumcu M, et al.: Epigenetic transgenerational actions of endocrine disruptors and male fertility. *Science* 306:1466–1468, 2005.

Arena JP, Liu KK, Paress PS, et al.: The mechanism of action of avermectins in *Caenorhabditis elegans:* Correlation between activation of glutamate-sensitive chloride current, membrane binding and biological activity. *J Parasitol* 81:286–294, 1995.

Ashby J, Kier L, Wilson AGE: Evaluation of the potential carcinogenicity and genetic toxicity to humans of the herbicide acetochlor. *Hum Exp Toxicol* 15:702–735, 1996.

Autor AP: *Biochemical Mechanisms of Paraquat Toxicity.* New York: Academic Press, 1974.

Baker SR, Wilkinson DF (eds): *The Effects of Pesticides on Human Health.* Princeton: Princeton Scientific Publishing, 1990, pp. 438.

Bakir F, Damluji SF, Amin-Zaki L, et al.: Methylmercury poisoning in Iraq. *Science* 181:230–241, 1973.

Barbeau A, Roy M, Clourier L, et al.: Environmental and genetic factors in the etiology of Parkinson's disease. *Adv Neurol* 45:299–306, 1986.

Barlow SM, Sullivan FM, Lines J: Risk assessment of the use of deltamethrin on bed nets for the prevention of malaria. *Food Chem Toxicol* 39:407–422, 2001.

Baron RL: Carbamate insecticides, in Hayes WJ, Laws ER (eds): *Handbook of Pesticide Toxicology.* San Diego: Academic Press, 1991, pp. 1125–1189.

Barr DB, Allen R, Olsson AO, et al.: Considerations of selective metabolites of organophosphorus pesticides in the United States population. *Environ Res* 99:314–326, 2005.

Bate MN, Thomson B, Garrett N: Reduction in organochlorine levels in the milk of New Zealand. *Arch Environ Health* 57:591–597, 2002.

Beard J: DDT and human health. *Science Total Environ* 355:78–89, 2006.

Beeman RW, Matsumura F: Chlordimeform: A pesticide acting upon amine regulatory mechanisms. *Nature* 242:273–274, 1973.

Bell JW, Veltri JC, Page BC: Human exposures to N, N-diethyl-m-toluamide insect repellents reported to the American Association of Poison Control Centers 1993–1997. *Int J Toxicol* 21:341–352, 2002.

Benke G, Murphy SD: The influence of age on the toxicity and metabolism of methylparathion and parathion in male and female rats. *Toxicol Appl Pharmacol* 31:254–269, 1975.

Benowitz NL: Pharmacology of nicotine: Addiction and therapeutics. *Annu Rev Pharmacol Toxicol* 36:597–613, 1996.

Bernand BK, Gordon EB: An evaluation of the common mechanism approach to the Food Quality Protection Act: Captan and four related fungicides, a practical example. *Int J Toxicol* 19:43–61, 2000.

Bertsias GJ, Katonis P, Tzanakakis G, et al.: Review of clinical and toxicological features of acute pesticide poisoning in Crete (Greece) during the period 1991–2001. *Med Sci Monit* 10:CR622–627, 2004.

Betarbet R, Sherer TB, Greenamyre JT: Animal models of Parkinson's disease. *Bioessays* 24:308–318, 2002.

Betarbet R, Sherer TB, MacKenzie G, et al.: Chronic systemic pesticide exposure reproduces features of Parkinson's disease. *Nature Neurosci* 3:1301–1306, 2000.

Bismuth C, Garnier R, Dolly S, et al.: Prognosis and treatment of paraquat poisoning: A review of 28 cases. *Clin Toxicol* 19:461–474, 1982.

Bismuth C, Inns RH, Marrs TC: Efficacy, toxicity and clinical use of oximes in anticholinesterases poisoning, in Ballantyne B, Marrs TC (eds): *Clinical and Experimental Toxicology of Organophosphates and Carbamates.* Oxford: Butterworth-Heinemann, 1992, pp. 555–577.

Boyd MR, Neal RA: Studies on the mechanism of toxicity and of development of tolerance to the pulmonary toxic α-naphthylthiourea (ANTU). *Drub Metab Dispos* 4:314–322, 1976.

Bradberry SM, Cage SA, Proudfoot AT, et al.: Poisoning due to pyrethroids. *Toxicol Rev* 24:93–106, 2005.

Bradberry SM, Proudfoot AT, Vale JA: Poisoning due to chlorophenoxy herbicides. *Toxicol Rev* 23:65–73, 2004a.

Bradberry SM, Proudfoot AT, Vale JA: Glyphosate poisoning. *Toxicol Rev* 23:159–167, 2004b.

Bradberry SM, Watt BE, Proudfoot AT, et al.: Mechanisms of toxicity, clinical features, and management of acute chlorophenoxy herbicide poisoning: A review. *Clin Toxicol* 39:111–122, 2000.

Breman JG, Alilio MS, Mills A: Conquering the intolerable burden of malaria: What's new, what's needed: A summary. *Am J Trop Med Hyg* 71 (suppl 2):1–15, 2004.

Briassulis G, Niarloglou M, Hatzis T: Toxic encephalopathy associated with use of DEET insect repellents: A case analysis of its toxicity in children. *Hum Exp Toxicol* 20:8–14, 2001.

Brooks GT: *Chlorinated Insecticides. Vol I. Technology and Application; Vol. II. Biological and Environmental Aspects.* Cleveland: CRC Press, 1974, pp. 249, 197 (Vol. I and II, resp.).

Brusick DJ: An assessment of the genetic toxicity of atrazine: Relevance to human health and environmental effects. *Mutat Res* 317:133–144, 1994.

Buckley NA, Eddleston M, Szinicz L: Oximes for acute organophosphate pesticide poisoning. *Cochrane Database Syst Rev* Issue 1. Art No. CD005085, 2005.

Burkhart KK: Anticoagulant rodenticides, in Ford MD, Delaney KA, Ling LJ, Erickson T (eds): *Clinical Toxicology.* Philadelphia: WB Saunders, 2001, pp. 848–853.

Bus JS, Gibson JE: Paraquat: Model for oxidant-initiated toxicity. *Environ Health Perspect* 55:37–46, 1984.

Cabras P, Caboni P, Cabras M, et al.: Rotenone residues in olives and in olive oil. *J Agric Food Chem* 50:2576–2580, 2002.

Cabral JR, Galendo D, Laval M, et al.: Carcinogenicity studies with deltamethrin in mice and rats. *Cancer Lett* 49:147–152, 1990.

Caksen H, Odabas D, Arslan S, et al.: Report of eight children with amitraz intoxication. *Hum Exp Toxicol* 22:95–97, 2003.

Cam C, Nigogosyan G: Acquired toxic porphyria cutanea tarda due to hexachlorobenzene. *J Am Med Assoc* 183:88–91, 1963.

Campbell WC (ed): *Ivermectin and Abamectin.* New York: Springer-Verlag, 1989, pp. 363.

Carlock LL, Chen WL, Gordon EB, et al.: Regulating and assessing risks of cholinesterase-inhibiting pesticides: Divergent approaches and interpretations. *J Toxicol Environ Health B Crit Rev* 2:105–160, 1999.

Carlock LL, Dotson TA: Metam-sodium, in Krieger R (ed): *Handbook of Pesticide Toxicology.* San Diego: Academic Press, 2001, pp. 1867–1879.

Carr JA, Gentles A, Smith EE, et al.: Response of larval *Xenopus laevis* to atrazine: Assessment of growth, metamorphosis, and gonadal and laryngeal morphology. *Environ Toxicol Chem* 22:396–405, 2003.

Carson R: *Silent Spring.* Boston: Houghton Mifflin, 1962.

Case RAM: Tumours of the urinary tract as an occupational disease in several industries. *Ann R Coll Surg Engl* 39:213–235, 1966.

Casey P, Vale JA: Deaths from pesticide poisoning in England and Wales: 1945–1989. *Hum Exp Toxicol* 13:95–101, 1994.

Casida JE: Esterase inhibitors as pesticides. *Science* 146:1011–1017, 1964.

Casida JE: Pyrethrum flowers and pyrethroid insecticides. *Environ Health Perspect* 34:189–202, 1980.

Casida JE, Gammon DW, Glickman AH, *et al.*: Mechanisms of selective action of pyrethroid insecticides. *Annu Rev Pharmacol Toxicol* 23:413–438, 1983.

Chambers HW, Boone JS, Carr RL, *et al.*: Chemistry of organophosphorus insecticides, in Krieger R (ed): *Handbook of Pesticide Toxicology.* San Diego: Academic Press, 2001, pp. 913–917.

Chambers JE, Levi PE (eds): *Organophosphates: Chemistry, Fate and Effects.* San Diego: Academic Press, 1992, pp. 443.

Chan S, Kilby MD: Thyroid hormone and fetal central nervous system development. *J Endocrinol* 165:1–8, 2000.

Chao HR, Wang SL, Lin TC, *et al.*: Levels of organochlorine pesticides in human milk from central Taiwan. *Chemosphere* 62:1776–1785, 2006.

Charles JM, Bond DM, Jeffries TK, *et al.*: Chronic dietary toxicity/oncogenicity studies on 2,4- dichlorophenoxyacetic acid in rodents. *Fundam Appl Toxicol* 33:166–172, 1996.

Chen A, Rogan WJ: Nonmalarial infant deaths and DDT use for malaria control. *Emerg Infect Dis* 9:960–964, 2003.

Chhabra RS, Eustis S, Haseman JK, *et al.*: Comparative carcinogenicity of ethylene thiourea with or without perinatal exposure in rats and mice. *Fundam Appl Toxicol* 18:405–417, 1992.

Choi J, Hodgson E, Rose RL: Inhibitions of trans-permethrin hydrolysis in human liver fractions by chlorpyrifos oxon and carbaryl. *Drug Metabol Drug Interact* 20:233–246, 2004.

Clark DG, McElligott TF, Hurst EW: The toxicity of paraquat. *Br J Ind Med* 23:126–132, 1966.

Clark JM, Matsumura F (eds): *Membrane Receptors and Enzymes as Targets of Insecticidal Action.* New York: Plenum Press, 1986, pp. 256.

Clarkson TW: Inorganic and organometal pesticides, in Krieger R (ed): *Handbook of Pesticide Toxicology.* San Diego: Academic Press, 2001, pp. 1357–1428.

Colborn T: A case for revisiting the safety of pesticides: A closer look at neurodevelopment. *Environ Health Perspect* 114:10–17, 2006.

Cole LM, Casida JE: Polychlorocycloalkane insecticide-induced convulsions in mice in relation to disruption of the GABA-regulated chloride ionophore. *Life Sci* 39:1855–1862, 1986.

Cole TB, Walter BJ, Shih DM, *et al.*: Toxicity of chlorpyrifos and chlorpyrifos oxon in a transgenic mouse model of the human paraoxonase (PON1) Q192R polymorphism. *Pharmacogenet Genomics* 15:589–598, 2005.

Colosio C, Tiramani M, Maroni M: Neurobehavioral effects of pesticides: State of the art. *Neurotoxicology* 24:577–591, 2003.

Cooper RL, Lamb JC, Barlow SM, *et al.*: A tiered approach to life testing for agricultural risk assessment. *Crit Rev Toxicol* 36:69–98, 2006.

Cooper RL, Stoker TE, Tyrey L, *et al.*: Atrazine disrupts the hypothalamic control of pituitary-ovarian function. *Toxicol Sci* 53:297–307, 2000.

Costa LG: Toxicology of pesticides: A brief history, in Costa LG, Galli CL, Murphy SD (eds): *Toxicology of Pesticides: Experimental, Clinical and Regulatory Perspectives.* Heidelberg: Springer-Verlag, 1987, pp. 1–10.

Costa LG: Organophosphorus compounds, in Galli CL, Manzo L, Spencer PS (eds): *Recent Advances in Nervous System Toxicology.* New York: Plenum Press, 1988, pp. 203–246.

Costa LG: Pesticide exposure. Differential risk for neurotoxic outcomes due to enzyme polymorphisms. *Clin Occup Environ Med* 1:511–523, 2001.

Costa LG: Current issues in organophosphate toxicology. *Clin Chim Acta* 366:1–13, 2006.

Costa LG, Cole TB, Jarvik GP, *et al.*: Functional genomics of the paraoxonase (PON1) polymorphisms: Effect on pesticide sensitivity, cardiovascular disease and drug metabolism. *Annu Rev Med* 54:371–392, 2003.

Costa LG, Cole TB, Vitalone A, *et al.*: Measurement of paraoxonase (PON1) status as a potential biomarker of susceptibility to organophosphate toxicity. *Clin Chim Acta* 352:37–47, 2005.

Costa LG, Galli CL, Murphy SD (eds): *Toxicology of Pesticides: Experimental, Clinical and Regulatory Perspectives.* Heidelberg: Springer-Verlag, 1987, pp. 320.

Costa LG, Hand H, Schwab BW, *et al.*: Tolerance to the carbamate insecticide propoxur. *Toxicology* 21:267–278, 1981.

Costa LG, Li WF, Richter RJ *et al.*: PON1 and organophosphate toxicity, in Costa LG, Furlong CE (eds): *Paraoxonase (PON1) in Health and Disease: Basic and Clinical Aspects.* Norwell, MA: Kluwer Academic Publishers, 2002, pp. 165–183.

Costa LG, Murphy SD: Interaction of the pesticide chlordimeform with adrenergic receptors in mouse brain: An in vitro study. *Arch Toxicol* 59:323–327, 1987.

Costa LG, Olibet G, Murphy SD: Alpha$_2$-adrenoceptors as a target for formamidine pesticides: In vitro and in vivo studies in mice. *Toxicol Appl Pharmacol* 93:319–328, 1988.

Costa LG, Schwab BW, Murphy SD: Tolerance to anticholinesterase compounds in mammals. *Toxicology* 25:79–97, 1982.

Cranmer MF: Carbaryl. A toxicological review and risk analysis. *Neurotoxicology* 7:247–332, 1986.

Crisp TM, Clegg ED, Cooper RL, *et al.*: Environmental endocrine disruption: An effects assessment and analysis. *Environ Health Perspect* 106 (suppl 1):11–56, 1998.

Dam K, Seidler FJ, Slotkin TA: Developmental neurotoxicity of chlorpyrifos: Delayed targeting of DNA synthesis after repeated administration. *Dev Brain Res* 108:39–45, 1998.

Daniell WE, Barnhart S, Demers P, *et al.*: Neuropsychological performance among pesticide applicators. *Environ Res* 59:217–228, 1992.

Davenport CJ, Ali SF, Miller FJ, *et al.*: Effect of methylbromide on regional brain glutathione, glutathione S-transferases, monoamines, and amino acids in F344 rats. *Toxicol Appl Pharmacol* 112:120–127, 1992.

Dawson GR, Wafford KA, Smith A, *et al.*: Anticonvulsant and adverse effects of avermectin analogs in mice are mediated through the γ-aminobutyric acid$_A$ receptor. *J Pharmacol Exp Ther* 295:1051–1060, 2000.

Dayal M, Parmar D, Dhawan A, *et al.*: Effect of pretreatment of cytochrome P450 (P450) modifiers on neurobehavioral toxicity induced by deltamethrin. *Food Chem Toxicol* 41:431–437, 2003.

Degli Esposti M: Inhibitors of NADH-ubiquinone reductase: An overview. *Biochim Biophys Acta* 1364:222–235, 1998.

De Haro L, Gastaut JL, Jouglard J, *et al.*: Central and peripheral neurotoxic effects of chronic methyl bromide intoxication. *J Toxicol Clin Toxicol* 35:29–34, 1997.

Desaiah D: Biochemical mechanisms of chlordecone neurotoxicity: A review. *Neurotoxicology* 3:103–110, 1982.

DeWilde AR, Heyndrickx A, Carton D: A case of fatal rotenone poisoning in a child. *J Forensic Sci* 31:1492–1498, 1986.

Dickoff DJ, Gerber O, Turovsky Z: Delayed neurotoxicity after ingestion of carbamate pesticide. *Neurology* 37:1229–1231, 1987.

Didier A, Loor F: The abamectin derivative invermectin is a potent P-glycoprotein inhibitor. *Anticancer Drugs* 7:745–757, 1996.

Dikshith TSS (ed): *Toxicology of Pesticide in Animals.* Boca Raton: CRC Press, 1991, pp. 255.

Doe JE, Boobis AR, Blacker A, *et al.*: A tiered approach to systemic toxicity testing for agricultural risk assessment. *Crit Rev Toxicol* 36:37–68, 2006.

Duke SO: Overview of herbicide mechanisms of action. *Environ Health Perspect* 87:263–271, 1990.

Duke SO: Taking stock of herbicide-resistant crops ten years after introduction. *Pest Manag Sci* 61:211–218, 2005.

Ebert E, Leist KH, Mayer D: Summary of safety evaluation of toxicity studies of glufosinate ammonium. *Food Chem Toxicol* 28:339–349, 1990.

Ecobichon DJ: Introduction, in Ecobichon DJ, Roy RM (eds): *Pesticides and Neurological Diseases.* Boca Raton: CRC Press, 1992, pp. 1–14.

Ecobichon DJ: Toxic effect of pesticides, in Klaassen CD (ed): *Casarett and Doull's Toxicology. The Basic Science of Poisons.* New York: McGraw-Hill, 2001a, pp. 763–810.

Ecobichon DJ: Carbamate insecticides, in Krieger R (ed): *Handbook of Pesticide Toxicology.* San Diego: Academic Press, 2001b, pp. 1087–1106.

Ecobichon DJ, Joy RM: *Pesticides and Neurological Diseases.* Boca Raton: CRC Press, 1982, pp. 281.

Eddleston M, Szinicz L, Eyer P, *et al.*: Oximes in acute organophosphorus pesticide poisoning: A systematic review of clinical trials. *QJ Med* 95:275–283, 2002.

Edwards IR, Ferry DG, Temple WA: Fungicides and related compounds, in Hayes WJ, Laws ER (eds): *Handbook of Pesticide Toxicology.* Vol. 3. San Diego: Academic Press, 1991, pp. 1409–1470.

EFSA (European Food Safety Agency): Conclusion regarding the peer-review of the pesticide risk assessment of the active substance glufosinate. *EFSA Scientific Report* 27:1–81, 2005.

Ehrich M, Correll L, Veronesi B: Acetylcholinesterase and neuropathy target esterase inhibitions in neuroblastoma cells to distinguish organophosphorus compounds causing acute and delayed neurotoxicity. *Fundam Appl Toxicol* 38:55–63, 1997.

Ehrich M, Jortner BS: Organophosphorus-induced delayed neuropathy, in Krieger R (ed): *Handbook of Pesticide Toxicology.* San Diego: Academic Press, 2001, pp. 987–1012.

Eldefrawi AT, Eldefrawi ME: Receptors for γ-aminobutyric acid and voltage-dependent chloride channels as targets for drugs and toxicants. *FASEB J* 1:262–271, 1987.

Eldefrawi ME, Eldefrawi AT: Comparative molecular and pharmacological properties of cholinergic receptors in insects and mammals, in Hedin PA, Hollingworth RM, Masler EP, Miyamoto J, Thompson DG (eds): *Phytochemicals in Pest Control.* Washington, DC: American Chemical Society, 1997, pp. 327–338.

Eldridge JC, Stevens JT, Wetzel LT, *et al.*: Atrazine: Mechanisms of hormonal imbalance in female SD rats. *Fundam Appl Toxicol* 42:2–5, 1996.

Elinav E, Shapira Y, Ofran Y, *et al.*: Near-fatal amitraz intoxication: The overlooked pesticide. *Basic Clin Pharmacol Toxicol* 97:185–187, 2005.

Enan E, Matsumura F: Activation of phosphoinositide protein kinase C pathway in rat brain tissue by pyrethroids. *Biochem Pharmacol* 45:703–710, 1993.

Erdogrul O, Covaci A, Kurtul N, *et al.*: Levels of organohalogenated persistent pollutants in human milk from Kahramanmaras region, Turkey. *Environ Int* 30:659–666, 2004.

Eskenazi B, Bradman A, Castorina R: Exposures to children to organophosphate pesticides and their potential health effects. *Environ Health Perspect* 107 (suppl 3):409–419, 1999.

Farmer D:Inhibitors of aromatic acid biosynthesis, in Krieger R (ed): *Handbook of Pesticide Toxicology.* San Diego: Academic Press, 2001, pp. 1667–1671.

Feng P, Wilson AGE, McClanahan R, *et al.*: Metabolism of alachlor by rat and mouse liver and nasal turbinate tissues. *Drug Metab Dispos* 18:373–377, 1990.

Fenner-Crisp PA: Risk assessment and risk management: The regulatory process, in Krieger R (ed): *Handbook of Pesticide Toxicology.* San Diego: Academic Press, 2001, pp. 681–689.

Fenske RA, Wong SM, Leffingwell JT, *et al.*: A video imaging technique for assessing dermal exposure. II. Fluorescent tracer testing. *Am Ind Hyg Assoc J* 47:771–775, 1986.

Ferraz HB, Bertolucci PH, Pereira JS, *et al.*: Chronic exposure to the fungicide maneb may produce symptoms and signs of CNS manganese intoxication. *Neurology* 38:550–553, 1988.

Fisher MH, Mrozik H: The chemistry and pharmacology of avermectins. *Annu Rev Pharmacol Toxicol* 32:537–553, 1992.

Flannigan SA, Tucker SB, Key MM, *et al.*: Synthetic pyrethroid insecticides: A dermatological evaluation. *Br J Ind Med* 42:363–372, 1985.

Fontoura-da-Silva SE, Chautard-Friere-Maira EA: Butyrylcholinesterase variants (BChE and ChE1 loci) associated with erythrocyte acetylcholinesterase inhibition in farmers exposed to pesticides. *Hum Hered* 46:142–147, 1996.

Ford MG, Lunt GG, Reay RC, *et al.* (eds): *Neuropharmacology and Pesticide Action.* Chichester: Ellis Norwood, 1986, pp. 512.

Forshaw PJ, Lister T, Ray DE: Inhibition of a neuronal voltage-dependent chloride channel by the type II pyrethroid, deltamethrin. *Neuropharmacology* 32:105–111, 1993.

Forshaw PJ, Lister T, Ray DE: The role of voltage-gated chloride channels in Type II pyrethroid insecticide poisoning. *Toxicol Appl Pharmacol* 163:1–8, 2000.

FQPA (Food Quality Protection Act). Public Law 1996, 104–170.

Fradin MS, Day JF: Comparative efficacy of insect repellents against mosquito bites. *New Engl J Med* 347:13–18, 2002.

Fukuto TR: Metabolism of carbamate insecticides. *Drug Metab Rev* 1:117–152, 1972.

Gallo MA, Lawryk NJ: Organic phosphorus pesticides, in Hayes WJ, Laws ER (eds): *Handbook of Pesticide Toxicology.* San Diego: Academic Press,1991, pp. 917–1123.

Gammon DW, Aldous CN, Carr WC, *et al.*: A risk assessment of atrazine use in California: Human health and ecological aspects. *Pest Manag Sci* 61:331–355, 2005.

Gammon DW, Moore TB, O'Malley MA: A toxicological assessment of sulfur as a pesticide, in Krieger R (ed): *Handbook of Pesticide Toxicology.* San Diego: Academic Press, 2001, pp. 1781–1791.

Garabrandt DH, Philbert MA: Review of 2,4- dichloropheynoxyacetic acid (2,4-D) epidemiology and toxicology. *Crit Rev Toxicol* 34:233–257, 2002.

Garcia SJ, Seidler FJ, Slotkin TA: Developmental neurotoxicity of chlorypyrifos: Targeting glial cells. *Environ Toxicol Pharmacol* 19:455–461, 2005.

Ghali TG, Hollingworth RM: Influence of mixed function oxygenase metabolism on the acute neurotoxicity of the pesticide chlordimeform in mice. *Neurotoxicology* 6:215–238, 1985.

Glynn P: A mechanism for organophosphate-induced delayed neuropathy. *Toxicol Lett* 162:94–97, 2006.

Goes AE, Savage EP, Gibbons G, *et al.*: Suspected foodborne carbamate pesticide intoxications with the ingestion of hydroponic cucumbers. *Am J Epidemiol* 111:254–259, 1980.

Golden RJ, Noller KL, Titus-Enrstoff L, *et al.*: Environmental endocrine modulators and human health: An assessment of biological evidence. *Crit Rev Toxicol* 28:109–227, 1998.

Goldman LR, Smith DF, Neutra RR, *et al.*: Pesticide food poisoning from contaminated watermelons in California, 1985. *Arch Environ Health* 45:229–236, 1990.

Golub M, Doherty J: Triphenyltin as a potential human endocrine disruptor. *J Toxicol Environ Health B Crit Rev* 7:281–295, 2004.

Goodal R: Cholinesterase pharmacogenetics, in Gupta RC (ed): *Toxicology of Organophosphate and Carbamate Compounds.* Amsterdam: Elsevier, 2006, pp. 187–198.

Gordon EB: Captan and Folpet, in Krieger R (ed): *Handbook of Pesticide Toxicology.* San Diego: Academic Press, 2001, pp. 1711–1742.

Gringorten JL: Ion balance in the Lepidopteran midgut and insecticidal action of *Bacillus thuringiensis*, in Isheaya I (ed): *Biochemical Sites of Insecticide Action and Resistance.* Heidelberg: Springer, 2001, 167–207.

Gryboski J, Weinstein D, Ordway NK: Toxic encephalopathy apparently related to the use of an insect repellent. *New Engl J Med* 264:289–290, 1961.

Gunnell D, Eddleston M: Suicide by intentional ingestion of pesticides: A continuing tragedy in developing countries. *Int J Epidemiol* 32:902–909, 2003.

Gupta RC (ed): *Toxicology of Organophosphate and Carbamate Compounds.* Amsterdam: Elsevier, 2006, pp. 763.

Guzelian PS: Comparative toxicology of chlordecone (Kepone) in humans and experimental animals. *Annu Rev Pharmacol Toxicol* 22:89–113, 1982.

Hainzl D, Cole LM, Casida JE: Mechanisms for selective toxicity of fipronil insecticide and its sulfone metabolite and desulfinyl photoproduct. *Chem Res Toxicol* 11:1529–1535, 1998.

Hampers LC, Oker E, Leikin JB: Topical use of DEET insect repellent as a cause of severe encepholopathy in a healthy adult male. *Acad Emerg Med* 6:1295–1297, 1999.

Hardell L, Eriksson M, Degerman A: Exposure to phenoxyacetic acids, chlorophenols or organic solvents in relation to histopathology, stage, and anatomical localization of non-Hodgkin's lymphoma. *Cancer Res* 54:2386–2389, 1994.

Harrison ML, Loucks OL, Mitchell JW, *et al.*: Systems studies of DDT transport. *Science* 170:503–508, 1970.

Hasin Y, Avidan N, Bercovich D, *et al.*: A paradigm for single nucleotide polymorphism anlysis: The case of the acetylcholinesterase gene. *Hum Mutat* 24:408–416, 2004.

Hayes, WJ: *Pesticides Studied in Man*. Baltimore: Williams & Wilkins, 1982, pp. 672.

Hayes TB, Collins A, Lee M, *et al.*: Hermaphroditic, demasculinized frogs after exposure to the herbicide atrazine at low ecologically relevant doses. *Proc Natl Acad Sci USA* 99:5476–5480, 2002.

Hayes WJ, Laws ER (eds): *Handbook of Pesticide Toxicology.* San Diego: Academic Press, 1991 pp. 1576.

He F, Wang S, Liu L, *et al.*: Clinical manifestations and diagnosis of acute pyrethroid poisoning. *Arch Toxicol* 63:54–58, 1989.

Heikkila RE, Nicklas WJ, Vyas I, *et al.*: Dopaminergix toxicity of rotenone and the 1-methyl-4-phenylpyridinium ion after their stereotaxic administration to rats: Implication for the mechanism of 1-methyl-4-phenyl-1,2,3,6-tetrahydropyridine toxicity. *Neurosci Lett* 62:389–394, 1985.

Hernandez AF, Martin-Rubi JC, Ballesteros JL, *et al.*: Clinical and pathological findings in fatal 1, 3-dichloropropene intoxication. *Hum Exp Toxicol* 13:303–306, 1994.

Hertzstein J, Cullen MR: Methyl bromide intoxication in four field workers during removal of soil fumigation sheets. *Am J Ind Med* 17:321–326, 1990.

Heudorf U, Angerer J, Drexler H: Current internal exposure to pesticides in children and adolescents in Germany: Urinary levels of metabolites of pyrethroid and organophosphorus insecticides. *Int Arch Occup Environ Health* 77:67–72, 2004.

Heydens WF: Summary of toxicology studies with alachlor. *J Pest Sci* 24:75–82, 1998.

Heydens WF, Lamb IC, Wilson AGE: Chloroacetanilides, in Krieger R (ed): *Handbook of Pesticide Toxicology.* San Diego: Academic Press, 2001, pp. 1543–1558.

Heydens WF, Wilson AGE, Kier LD, *et al.*: An evaluation of the carcinogenic potential of the herbicide alachlor to man. *Human Exp Toxicol* 18:363–391, 1999.

Hickey JP, Batterman SA, Chernyak SM: Trends of chlorinated organic contaminants in Great Lakes trout and walleye from 1970 to 1998. *Arch Environ Contam Toxicol* 50:97–110, 2006.

Ho YS, Magnenat JL, Gargano M, *et al.*: The nature of antioxidant defense mechanisms: A lesson from transgenic mice. *Environ Health Perspect* 106:1219–1228, 1998.

Hoar SK, Blair A, Holmes FF, *et al.*: Agricultural herbicide use and risk of lymphoma and soft-tissue sarcoma. *JAMA* 256:1141–1147, 1986.

Hodgson E: In vitro human phase I metabolism of xenobiotics I: Pesticides and related compounds used in agriculture and public health, May 2003. *J Biochem Mol Toxicol* 17:201–206, 2003.

Hollingworth RM: Chemistry, biological activity and uses of formamidine pesticides. *Environ Health Perspect* 14:57–69, 1976.

Hollingworth RM: Inhibitors and uncouplers of mitochondrial oxidative phosphorylation, in Krieger R (ed): *Handbook of Pesticide Toxicology.* San Diego: Academic Press, 2001, pp. 1169–1261.

Hsu WH, Kakuk TJ: Effects of amitraz and chlordimeform on heart rate and pupil diameter in rats: Mediated by alpha$_2$-adrenoceptors. *Toxicol Appl Pharmacol* 73:411–415, 1984.

Hsu WH, Lu ZH: Amitraz-induced delay of gastrointestinal transit in mice: Mediated by alpha$_2$-adrenergic receptors. *Drug Dev Res* 4:655–660, 1984.

Hurt S, Ollinger J, Arce G, *et al.*: Dialkyldithiocarbamates (EBDCs), in Krieger R (ed): *Handbook of Pesticide Toxicology.* San Diego: Academic Press, 2001, pp. 1759–1779.

IARC (International Agency for Research on Cancer): Atrazine. *IARC Monogr Eval Carcinog Risks Hum* 73:59–113, 1999.

IOM (Institute of Medicine): *Veterans and Agent Orange. Update 1996.* Washington DC: National Academy Press, 1996, pp. 365.

IOM (Institute of Medicine): *Gulf War and Health. Vol. I.* Washington DC: National Academy Press, 2000, pp. 408.

IPCS (International Programme on Chemical Safety): *Chlordimeform.* Environmental Health Criteria 1999. Geneva: World Health Organization, 1998, pp. 159.

IPCS (International Programme on Chemical Safety): *The WHO Recommended Classification of Pesticides by Hazard and Guidelines to Classification: 2004*. Geneva: World Health Organization, 2005, pp. 58.

Ireland B, Acquarella, J, Farrell T, *et al.*: Evaluation of ocular health among alachlor manufacturing workers. *J Occup Med* 36:738–742, 1994.

Isman MB: Botanical insecticides, deterrents and repellents in modern agriculture and an increasingly regulated world. *Annu Rev Entomol* 51:45–66, 2006.

Jaga K, Dharmani C: Global surveillance of DDT and DDE levels in human tissues. *Int J Occup Med Environ Health* 16:7–20, 2003.

Jaga K, Dharmani C: The epidemiology of pesticide exposure and cancer: A review. *Rev Environ Health* 20:15–38, 2005.

Jamal GA, Julu POO: Low level exposure to organophosphate esters may cause neurotoxicity. *Toxicology* 181:22–33, 2002.

Jett DA, Navoa RV, Beckles RA, *et al.*: Cognitive function and cholinergic neurochemistry in weanling rats exposed to chlorpyrifos. *Toxicol Appl Pharmacol* 174:89–98, 2001.

Johnson DJ, Graham DG, Amarnath V, *et al.*: Release of carbon disulfide is a contributing mechanism in the axonopathy produced by N, N – diethyldithiocarbamate. *Toxicol Appl Pharmacol* 148:288–296, 1998.

Johnson MK: The target for initiation of delayed neurotoxicity by organophosphorus esters: Biochemical studies and toxicological applications. *Rev Biochem Toxicol* 4:141–212, 1982.

Johnson MK, Glynn P: Neuropathy target esterase, in Krieger R (ed): *Handbook of Pesticide Toxicology.* San Diego: Academic Press, 2001, pp. 953–965.

Johnson MK, Jacobsen D, Meredith TJ, *et al.*: Evaluation of antidotes for poisoning by organophosphorus pesticides. *Emerg Med* 12:22–37, 2000.

Johnson MK, Lauwerys R: Protection by some carbamates against the delayed neurotoxic effects of diisopropyl phosphorofluoridate. *Nature* 222:1066–1067, 1969.

Kalantzi OI, Martin FL, Thomas GO, *et al.*: Different levels of polybrominated diphenyl ethers (PBDEs) and chlorinated compounds in breast milk from two UK regions. *Environ Health Perspect* 112:1086–1091, 2004.

Kappers WA, Edwards RJ, Murray S, *et al.*: Diazinon is activated by CYP2C19 in human liver. *Toxicol Appl Pharmacol* 177:68–76, 2001.

Kavlock RJ: Pesticides as endocrine-disrupting chemicals, in Krieger R (ed): *Handbook of Pesticide Toxicology.* San Diego: Academic Press, 2001, pp. 727–746.

Keiner C: Wartime rat control, rodent ecology, and the rise and fall of chemical rodenticides. *Endeavour* 29:119–125, 2005.

Kelce WR, Stone CR, Laws SC, *et al.*: Persistent DDT metabolite p,p′–DDE is a potent androgen receptor antagonist. *Nature* 375:581–585, 1995.

Kiely T, Donaldson D, Grube A: Pesticide Industry Sales and Usage. 2000 and 2001 Market Estimates. Washington DC: USEPA, 2004, pp. 33.

Kim IY, Shin JH, Kim HS, *et al.*: Assessing estrogenic activity of pyrethroid insecticides using in vitro combination assays. *J Reprod Develop* 50:245–255, 2004.

Konishi Y, Kuwabara K, Hori S: Continuous surveillance of organochlorine compounds in human breast milk from 1972 to 1998 in Osaka, Japan. *Arch Environ Contam Toxicol* 40:571–578, 2001.

Koren G. Matsui D, Bailey B: DEET-based insect repellents: Safety implications for children and pregnant and lactating women. *Can Med Assoc J* 169:209–212, 2003.

Korystov YN, Ermakova NV, Kublik LN, *et al.*: Avermectins inhibit multidrug resistance of tumor cells. *Eur J Pharmacol* 493:57–64, 2004.

Koyama K, Andou Y, Saruki K, *et al.*: Delayed and severe toxicity of a herbicide containing glufosinate and a surfactant. *Vet Hum Toxicol* 36:17–18, 1994.

Kretzschmar D, Mason G, Sharma S, *et al.*: The Swiss cheese mutant causes glial hyperwrapping and brain degeneration in Drosophila. *J Neurosci* 17:7425–7432, 1997.

Krieger R (ed): *Handbook of Pesticide Toxicology.* San Diego: Academic Press, 2001, pp. 1908.

Landrigan PJ, Powell KE, James LE, *et al.*: Paraquat and marijuana-epidemiologic risk assessment. *Am J Public Health* 73:784–788, 1983.

Lange PF, Terveer J: Warfarin poisoning; report of fourteen cases. *US Armed Forces J* 5:872–877, 1954.

Lapointe N, St-Hilaire M, Martinoli MG, *et al.*: Rotenone induces non-specific central nervous system and systemic toxicity. *FASEB J* 18:717–719, 2004.

Lawrence LJ, Casida JE: Stereospecific action of pyrethroid insecticides on the γ-aminobutyric acid receptor-ionophore complex. *Science* 221:1399–1401, 1983.

Lee HL, Chen KW, Chi CH, *et al.*: Clinical presentations and prognostic factors of a glyphosate-surfactant herbicide intoxication: A review of 131 cases. *Acad Emerg Med* 7:906–910, 2000.

Leet T, Acquavella J, Lynch C, *et al.*: Cancer incidence among alachlor manufacturing workers. *Am J Ind Med* 30:300–306, 1996.

Li AA, Mink PJ, McIntosh LJ, *et al.*: Evaluation of epidemiologic and animal data associating pesticides with Parkinson's disease. *J Occup Environ Med* 47:1059–1087, 2005.

Li WF, Costa LG, Richter RJ, *et al.*: Catalytic efficiency determines the in vivo efficacy of PON1 for detoxifying organophosphates. *Pharmacogenetics* 10:767–779, 2000.

Lifshitz M, Gavrilov V: Central nervous system toxicity and early peripheral neuropathy following dermal exposure to methyl bromide. *Clin Toxicol* 38:799–801, 2000.

Lock EA, Wilks MF: Paraquat, in Krieger R (ed): *Handbook of Pesticide Toxicology.* San Diego: Academic Press, 2001a, pp. 1559–1603.

Lock EA, Wilks MF: Diquat, in Krieger R (ed): *Handbook of Pesticide Toxicology.* San Diego: Academic Press, 2001b, pp. 1605–1621.

Lockridge O, Duysen EG, Voelker T, *et al.*: Life without acetylcholinesterase: The implications of cholinesterase inhibition toxicity in AChE-knockout mice. *Environ Toxicol Pharmacol* 19:463–469, 2005.

Lockridge O, Masson P: Pesticides and susceptible populations: People with butyrylcholinesterase genetic variants may be at risk. *Neurotoxicology* 21:113–126, 2000.

Lomax LG, Stott WT, Johnson KA, *et al.*: The chronic toxicity and oncogenicity of inhaled technical grade 1, 3-dichloropropene in rats and mice. *Fundam Appl Toxicol* 12:418–431, 1989.

Longnecker MP: Invited commentary: Why DDT matters now. *Am J Epidemiol* 162:726–728, 2005.

Lotti M: The pathogenesis of organophosphate neuropathy. *Crit Rev Toxicol* 21:465–487, 1992.

Lotti M: Cholinesterase inhibition: Complexities in interpretation. *Clin Chem* 41:1814–1818, 1995.

Lotti M: Organophosphorus compounds, in Spencer PS, Schaumburg HH, Ludolph AC (eds): *Experimental and Clinical Neurotoxicology.* Oxford: Oxford University Press, 2000, pp. 898–925.

Lotti M: Clinical toxicology of anticholinesterases in humans, in Krieger R (ed): *Handbook of Pesticide Toxicology.* San Diego: Academic Press, 2001, pp. 1043–1085.

Lotti M: Low level exposures to organophosphorus esters and peripheral nerve functions. *Muscle Nerve* 25:492–504, 2002a.

Lotti M: Promotion of organophosphate-induced delayed polyneuropathy by certain esterase inhibitors. *Toxicology* 181–182:245–248, 2002b.

Lotti M, Caroldi S, Capodicasa E, *et al.*: Promotion of organophosphate-induced delayed polyneuropathy by phenylmethanesulfonyl fluoride. *Toxicol Appl Pharmacol* 108:234–241, 1991.

Lotti M, Moretto A: Organophosphate-induced delayed polyneuropathy. *Toxicol Rev* 24:37–49, 2005.

Lu C, Bravo R, Caltabiano LM, *et al.*: The presence of dialkylphosphates in fresh fruit juices: Implications for organophosphorus pesticide exposure and risk assessments. *J Toxicol Environ Health Part A* 68:209–227, 2005.

Maharaj R, Mthembu DJ, Sharp BL: Impact of DDT re-introduction on malaria transmission in KwaZulu-Natal. *S Afr Med J* 95:871–874, 2005.

Majerus PW, Tollefsen DM: Blood coagulation and anticoagulants, thrombolytic, and antiplatelet drugs, in Brunton LL (ed): *Goodman and Gilman's The Pharmacological Basis of Therapeutics.* New York: McGraw-Hill, 2006, pp. 1467–1488.

Malone JDG, Carmody M, Keogh B, *et al.*: Paraquat poisoning – A review of nineteen cases. *J Ir Med Assoc* 64:59–68, 1971.

Maroni M, Colosio C, Ferioli A, *et al.*: Biological monitoring of pesticide exposure: A review. *Toxicology* 143:5–118, 2000.

Marsh RE: Vertebrate pest control chemicals and their use in urban and rural environments, in Keirger R (ed): *Handbook of Pesticide Toxicology.* San Diego: Academic Press, 2001, pp. 251–262.

Masson P, Froment MT, Sorenson RC, *et al.*: Mutation His322Asn in human acetylcholinesterase does not alter electrophoretic and catalytic properties of the erythrocyte enzyme. *Blood* 83:3003–3005, 1994.

Matsuda K, Buckingam SD, Kleier D, *et al.*: Neonicotinoids: Insecticides acting on insect nicotinic acetylcholine receptors. *Trends Pharmacol Sci* 22:573–580, 2001.

Matsumura F: *Toxicology of Insecticides.* New York: Plenum Press, 1985, pp. 598.

Matsumura F, Ghiasuddin SM: Characteristics of DDT-sensitive Ca-ATPase in the axonic membrane, in Narahashi T (ed): *Neurotoxicology of Insecticides and Pheromones.* New York: Plenum Press, 1979, pp. 245–257.

Matsumura F, Patil KC: Adenosin triphosphatase sensitive to DDT in synapses of rat brain. *Science* 166:121–122, 1969.

Mattsson JL, Charles JM, Yano BL, *et al.*: Single-dose and chronic dietary neurotoxicity screening studies on 2,4-dichlorophenoxyacetic acid in rats. *Fundam Appl Toxicol* 40:11–119, 1997.

Matyunas NG, Rodgers GC: Nicotine poisoning, in Ford MD, Delaney KA, Ling LJ, Erickson T (eds): *Clinical Toxicology.* Philadelphia: WB Saunders, 2001, pp. 985–989.

McClintock JT, Schaffer CR, Sjobald RD: A comparative review of the mammalian toxicity of *Bacillus thuringiensis*–based pesticides. *Pestic Sci* 45:95–106, 1995.

McCook A: The banned pesticide in our soil. *Scientist* 20:40–45, 2006.

McCormack AL, Atienza JG, Johnston LC, *et al.*: Role of oxidative stress in paraquat-induced dopaminergic cell degeneration. *J Neurochem* 93:1030–1037, 2005.

McCormack AL, Thiruchelvam M, Manning-Bog AB, *et al.*: Environmental risk factors and Parkinson's disease: Selective degeneration of nigral dopaminergic neurons caused by the nerbicide paraquat. *Neurobiol Dis* 10:119–127, 2002.

McGrew DM, Irwin I, Langston JW: Ehtylene-bisdithiocarbamate enhances MPTP-induced striatal dopamine depletion in mice. *Neurotoxicology* 21:309–312, 2000.

McLaughlin J, Reynaldo EF, Lamar JK, *et al.*: Teratology studies in rabbits with captan, folpet and thalidomide. *Toxicol Appl Pharmacol* 14:641, 1969.

Meco G, Bonifati V, Vanacore N, *et al.*: Parkinsonism after chronic exposure to the fungicide maneb (manganese ethylene-bis-dithiocarbamate). *Scand J Work Environ Health* 20:301–305, 1994.

Mills PK, Yang R: Prostate cancer risk in California farm workers. *J Occup Environ Med* 45:249–258, 2003.

Minh NH, Somaya M, Minh TB, *et al.*: Persistent organochlorine residue in human breast milk from Hanoi and Hochiminh City, Vietnam: Contamination, accumulation kinetics and risk assessment for infants. *Environ Pollut* 129:431–441, 2004.

Miyamoto J: Degradation, metabolism and toxicity of synthetic pyrethroids. *Environ Health Perspect* 14:15–28, 1976.

MMWR (Morbidity and Mortality Weekly Reports): Seizures temporarily associated with use of DEET insect repellents – New York and Connecticut. *MMWR* 38:678–680, 1989.

Mohamed F, Senarathna L, Percy A, *et al.*: Acute human self-poisoning with the N- phenylpyrazole insecticide fipronil—a GABA$_A$ -gated chloride channel blocker. *J Toxicol Clin Toxicol* 42:955–963, 2004.

Mohanty MK, Kumar V, Pastia BK, *et al.*: An analysis of poisoning deaths in Manipal, India. *Vet Hum Toxicol* 46:208–209, 2004.

Moretto A: Testing for organophosphate delayed neuropathy, in Maines MD, Costa LG, Reed DJ, *et al.* (eds): *Current Protocols in Toxicology.* New York: John Wiley & Sons, 1999, pp. 11.5.1–11.5.14.

Moretto A: Promoters and promotion of axonopathies. *Toxicol Lett* 112–113:17–21, 2000.

Mortensen S, Chandra S, Hooper M, et al.: Maturational differences in chlorpyrifos-oxonase activity may contribute to age-related sensitivity to chlorpyrifos. J Biochem Toxicol 1:279–287, 1996.

Moser M, Li Y, Varpel K, et al.: Placental failure and impaired vasculogenesis result in embryonic lethality for neuropathy target esterase-deficient mice. Mol Cell Biol 24:1667–1679, 2004.

Moser V: Companion of aldicarb and metamidophos neurotoxicity at different ages in the rat: Behavioral and biochemical parameters. Toxicol Appl Pharmacol 157:94–106, 1999.

Mull RL, Hershberger LW: Inhibitors of DNA biosynthesis – mitosis: benzimidazoles. The Benzimidazole fungicides Benomyl and Carbendazim, in Krieger R (ed): Handbook of Pesticide Toxicology. San Diego: Academic Press, 2001, pp. 1673–1699.

Munro IC, Carlo GL, Orr JC, et al.: A comprehensive, integrated review and evaluation of the scientific evidence relating to the safety of the herbicide 2,4-D. J Am Coll Toxicol 11:559–664, 1992.

Murphy SD: Toxic effects of pesticides, in Klaassen CD, Amdur MO, Doull J (eds): Casarett and Doull's Toxicology. The Basic Science of Poisons. New York: Macmillan, 1986, pp. 519–581.

Mutch E, Daly AK, Leathart JBS, et al.: Do multiple cytochrome P450 isoforms contribute to parathion metabolism in man? Arch Toxicol 77:313–320, 2003.

Nagami H, Nishigaki Y, Matsushima S, et al.: Hospital-based survey of pesticide poisoning in Japan, 1998–2002. Int J Occup Environ Health 11:180–184, 2005.

Nakayama A, Sukekawa M: Quantitative correlation between molecular similarity and receptor-binding activity of neonicotinoid insecticides. Pestic Sci 52:104–110, 1998.

Narahashi T: Neuronal ion channels as the target sites of insecticides. Pharmacol Toxicol 78:1–14, 1996.

Nash D, Mostashari F, Fine A, et al.: The outbreak of West Nile virus infection in the New York City area in 1999. New Eng J Med 344:1807–1814, 2001.

Nathanson JA: Characterization of octopamine-sensitive adenylate cyclase: Elucidation of a class of potent and selective octopamine-2 receptor agonists with toxic effects in insects. Proc Natl Acad Sci USA 82:599–603, 1985.

Noren K, Meironyte D: Certain organochlorine and organobromine contaminants in Swedish human milk in perspective of past 20–30 years. Chemosphere 40:1111–1123, 2000.

Norman CS: Potential impact of imposing methylbromide phaseout on US strawberry growers: A case study of nomination for a critical use exemption under the Montreal Protocol. J Environ Manag 75:167–176, 2005.

NRC (National Research Council): Regulating Pesticides in Food: The Delaney Paradox. Washington DC: National Academy Press, 1987, pp. 288.

NRC (National Research Council): Pesticides in the Diets of Infants and Children. Washington DC: National Academy Press, 1993, pp. 386.

Novak RJ, Lampman RL: Public health pesticides, in Krieger R (ed): Handbook of Pesticide Toxicology. San Diego: Academic Press, 2001, pp. 181–201.

O'Brien RD: Insecticides: Action and Metabolism. New York: Academic Press, 1967, pp. 332.

Okahashi N, Sano M, Miyata K, et al.: Lack of evidence for endocrine disrupting effects in rats exposed to fenitrothion in utero and from weaning to maturation. Toxicology 206:17–31, 2005.

Osimitz TG, Murphy JV: Neurological effects associated with use of the insect repellent N, N-diethyl-m-toluamide (DEET). Clin Toxicol 35:435–441, 1997.

Padilla S, Wilson VA, Bushnell PJ: Studies on the correlation between blood cholinesterase inhibition and target tissue inhibition in pesticide-treated rats. Toxicology 92:11–25, 1994.

Park J, Darrien I, Prescott LF: Pharmacokinetic studies in severe intoxication with 2,4-D and mecoprop. Proc Eur Soc Toxicol 18:154–155, 1977.

Parsons PP: Mammalian toxicokinetics and toxicity of chlorothalonie, in Krieger R (ed): Handbook of Pesticide Toxicology. San Diego: Academic press, 2001, pp. 1743–1757.

Peakall DB: Pesticides and the reproduction of birds. Sci Am 222:72–78, 1970.

Pearce N, McLean D: Agricultural exposures and non-Hodgkin's lymphoma. Scand J Work Environ Health 31 (Suppl 1):18–25, 2005.

Pelfrene AF: Rodenticides, in Krieger R (ed): Handbook of Pesticide Toxicology. San Diego: Academic Press, 2001, pp. 1793–1836.

Peraica M, Capodicasa E, Moretto A, et al.: Organophosphate polyneuropathy in chicks. Biochem Pharmacol 45:131–135, 1993.

Peter JV, Moran JL, Graham P: Oxime therapy and outcomes in human organophosphate poisoning: An evaluation using meta-analytic techniques. Crit Care Med 34:502–510, 2006.

Petrucci N, Sardini S: Severe neurotoxic reaction associated with oral ingestion of low-dose diethyltoluamide-containing insect repellent in a child. Pediatr Emerg Care 16:341–342, 2000.

Piccirillo VJ: Methyl bromide, in Krieger R (ed): Handbook of Pesticide Toxicology. San Diego: Academic Press, 2001, pp. 1837–1845.

Pong SS, DeHaven R, Wang CC: A comparative study of avermectin B_{1A} and other modulators of the γ-aminobutyric acid receptor-chloride ion channel complex. J Neurosci 2:966–971, 1982.

Popp W, Schmieding W, Speck M et al.: Incidence of bladder cancer is a cohort of workers exposed to 4-chloro-o-toluidine while synthesizing chlordimeform. Br J Ind Med 49:529–531, 1992.

Porterfield SP: Thyroidal dysfunction and environmental chemicals. Potential impact on brain development. Environ Health Perspect 108 (suppl 3):433–438, 2000.

Poulos L, Athanaselis S, Coutselinis A: Acute intoxication with cypermethrin (NRDC 149). J Toxicol Clin Toxicol 19:519–520, 1982.

Prendergast MA, Terry AV, Buccafusco JJ: Effects of chronic, low-level organophosphate exposure on delayed recall, discrimination, and spatial learning in monkeys and rats. Neurotoxicol Teratol 20:115–122, 1998.

Proudfoot AT: Poisoning with amitraz. Toxicol Rev 22:71–74, 2003.

Proudfoot AT, Krenzelak EP, Vale JA: Position paper on urine alkalinization. J Toxicol Clin Toxicol 42:1–26, 2004.

Pruett SB, Myers LP, Keil DE: Toxicology of metam sodium. J Toxicol Environ Health Part B 4:207–222, 2001.

Ray DE: Pesticides derived from plants and other organisms in Hayes WJ, Lawd ER (eds): Handbook of Pesticide Toxicology. San Diego: Academic Press, 1991, pp. 585–636.

Ray DE: Chronic effects of low level exposure to anticholinesterases – a mechanistic review. Toxicol Lett 103:527–533, 1998.

Ray DE, Forshaw PJ: Pyrethroid insecticides: Poisoning, syndromes, synergies and therapy. Clin Toxicol 38:95–101, 2000.

Ray DE, Fry JR: A reassessment of the neurotoxicity of pyrethroid insecticides. Pharmacol Therap 111:174–193, 2006.

Reiner E, Simeon-Rudolf V: Methods for measuring cholinesterase activities in human blood, in Gupta RC (ed): Toxicology of Organophosphate and Carbamate Compounds. Amsterdam: Elsevier, 2006, pp. 199–208.

Ricceri L, Markina N, Valanzano A, et al.: Developmental exposure to chlorpyrifos alters reactivity to environmental and social cues in adolescent mice. Toxicol Appl Pharmacol 191:189–201, 2003.

Richardson JR, Quan Y, Sherer TB, et al.: Paraquat neurotoxicity is distinct from that of MPTP and rotenone. Toxicol Sci 88:193–201, 2005.

Risher JF, Miuk FL, Stara JF: The toxicologic effects of the carbamate insecticide aldicarb in mammals: A review. Environ Health Perspect 72:267–281, 1987.

Roberts D, Curtis C, Tren R, et al.: Malaria control and public health. Emerg Infect Dis 10:1170–1171, 2004.

Roberts DM, Karunarathna A, Buckley NA, et al.: Influence of pesticide regulation on acute poisoning deaths in Sri Lanka. Bull World Health Organ 81:789–798, 2003.

Rogan WJ, Chen A: Health risks and benefits of bis (4-chlorophenyl) -1, 1,1 –trichloroethane (DDT). Lancet 366:763–773, 2005.

Rose MS, Smith LL, Wyatt I: Evidence for the energy-dependant accumulation of paraquat into rat lung. Nature 252:314–315, 1974.

Rosenstock L, Keifer M, Daniell WE, et al.: Chronic central nervous system effects of acute organophosphate pesticide intoxication. Lancet 338:223–227, 1991.

Ross JH, Driver JH, Harris SA, *et al.*: Dermal absorption of 2,4-D: A review of species differences. *Regul Toxicol Pharmacol* 41:82–91, 2005.

Ross MK, Borazjani A, Edward CC, *et al.*: Hydrolytic metabolism of pyrethroids by human and other mammalian carboxylesterase. *Biochem Pharmacol* 71:657–669, 2006.

Rust MK: Insecticides and their use in urban structural pest control, in Krieger R (ed): *Handbook of Pesticide Toxicology.* San Diego: Academic Press, 2001, pp. 243–250.

Ruzo LO: Physical, chemical and environmental properties of selected chemical alternatives for the pre-plant use of methyl bromide as soil fumigant. *Pest Manag Sci* 62:99–113, 2006.

Sabapathy NN: Paraquat formulation and safety management, in Bismuth C, Hall AH (eds): *Paraquat Poisoning.* New York: Dekker, 1995, pp. 335–347.

Safe S: Endocrine disruptors and human health – is there a problem? An update. *Environ Health Perspect* 108:487–493, 2000.

Safe S: Clinical correlates of environmental endocrine disruptors. *Trends Endocrinol Metab* 16:139–144, 2005.

Sanchez-Santed F, Canadas F, Flores P, *et al.*: Long-term functional neurotoxicity of paraoxon and chlorpyrifos oxon: Behavioral and pharmacological evidence. *Neurotoxicol Teratol* 26:304–317, 2004.

Sathiakumar N, Delzell E: A review of epidemiologic studies of triazine herbicides and cancer. *Crit Rev Toxicol* 27:599–612, 1997.

Sawada Y, Nagai Y, Ueyama M, *et al.*: Probable toxicity of surface-active agent in commercial herbicide containing glyphosate. *Lancet* Feb. 6:299, 1988.

Schenker R, Tinembart O, Humbert-Droz E, *et al.*: Comparative speed of kill between nitenpyram, fipronil, imidacloprid, selamectin and cythioate against adult *ctenocephalides felis* (Bouché) on cats and dogs. *Vet Parasitol* 112:249–254, 2003.

Schneider SM, Rosskopf EN, Leesch JG, *et al.*: United States Department of Agriculture – Agricultural Research Service research on alternatives to methyl bromide: Pre-plant and post-harvest. *Pestic Manag Sci* 59:814–826, 2003.

Schnepf E, Crickmore N, Van Rie J, *et al.*: *Bacillus thuringiensis* and its pesticidal crystal proteins. *Microbiol Mol Biol Rev* 62:775–806, 1998.

Schoenig GP, Hartnagel RE, Schardein JL, *et al.*: Neurotoxicity evaluation of N, N-diethyl-m-toluamide (DEET) in rats. *Fund Appl Toxicol* 21:355–365, 1993.

Schoenig GP, Osimitz TH: DEET, in Krieger R (ed): *Handbook of Pesticide Toxicology.* San Diego: Academic Press, 2001, pp. 1439–1459.

Senanayake N, Karalliedde L: Neurotoxic effects of organophosphate insecticides. An intermediate syndrome. *New Engl J Med* 316:761–763, 1987.

Serota DG.: *Combined chronic toxicity and oncogenicity study in rats with 2,4-D acid,* Unpublished Report 2184-102, Hazleton Laboratories, Inc., Vienna, VA 1986.

Shafer TJ, Meyer DA, Crofton KM: Developmental neurotoxicity of pyrethroid insecticides: Critical review and future research needs. *Environ Health Perspect* 113:123–136, 2005.

Shapira M, Tur-Kaspa I, Bosgraaf L, *et al.*: A trancription-activating polymorphism in the AChE promoter associated with acute sensitivity to anti-acetylcholinesterases. *Hum Mol Genet* 9:1273–1281, 2000.

Sheets LP: A consideration of age dependent differences in susceptibility to organophosphorus and pyrethroid insecticides. *Neurotoxicology* 21:57–64, 2000.

Sheets LP: Imidacloprid: A neonicotinoid insecticide, in Krieger R (ed): *Handbook of Pesticide Toxicology.* San Diego: Academic Press, 2001, pp. 1123–1130.

Shepard HH: *The Chemistry and Toxicology of Insecticides.* Minneapolis: Burgess Publishing Company, 1939, pp. 383.

Sherer TB, Kim JH, Betarbet R, *et al.*: Subcutaneous rotenone exposure causes highly selective dopaminergic degeneration and α-synuclein aggregation. *Exp Neurol* 179:6–16, 2003.

Shimizu K, Ohtaki K, Matsubara K, *et al.*: Carrier-mediated processes in blood-brain barrier penetration and neural uptake of paraquat. *Brain Res* 906:135–142, 2001.

Singh S, Batra YK, Singh SM, *et al.*: Is atropine alone sufficient in acute severe organophosphorus poisoning? Experience of a North West Indian Hospital. *Int J Clin Pharmacol Ther* 33:628–630, 1995.

Smith AG: Chlorinated hydrocarbon insecticides, in Hayes WJ, Laws ER (eds): *Handbook of Pesticide Toxicology.* San Diego: Academic Press, 1991, pp. 731–915.

Smith AG: DDT and its analogs, in Krieger R (ed): *Handbook of Pesticide Toxicology.* San Diego: Academic Press, 2001, pp. 1305–1355.

Smith D: Worldwide trends in DDT levels in human breast milk. *Int J Epidemiol* 28:179–188, 1999.

Smith LL: Mechanism of paraquat toxicity in the lung and its relevance to treatment. *Hum Toxicol* 6:31–36, 1987.

Smith LL, Heath D: Paraquat. *CRC Crit Rev Toxicol* 4:411–445, 1976.

Soderlund DM, Casida JE: Effects of pyrethroid structure on rates of hydrolysis and oxidation by mouse liver microsomal enzymes. *Pestic Biochem Physiol* 7:391–401, 1977.

Soderlund DM, Clark JM, Sheets LP, *et al.*: Mechanisms of pyrethroid neurotoxicity: Implications for cumulative risk assessment. *Toxicology* 171: 3–59, 2002.

Song X, Seidler FJ, Saleh JL, *et al.*: Cellular mechanisms for developmental toxicity of chlorpyrifos: Targeting the adenylate cyclase signaling cascade. *Toxicol Appl Pharmacol* 145:158–174, 1997.

Spagnolo A, Bianchi F, Calabro A, *et al.*: Anophthalmia and benomyl in Italy: A multicenter study based on 940,615 newborns. *Reprod Toxicol* 8:397–403, 1994.

Stebbins KE, Johnson KA, Jeffries TK, *et al.*: Chronic toxicity and oncogenicity studies of ingested 1, 3-dichloropropene in rats and mice. *Reg Toxicol Pharmacol* 32:1–13, 2000.

Stella J, Ryan M: Glyphosate herbicide formulation: A potentially lethal ingestion. *Emerg Med Australia* 16:235–239, 2004.

Sterling TD, Arundel AV: Health effects of phenoxy herbicides. *Scand J Work Environ Health* 12:161–173, 1986.

Stevens JT, Breckenridge CB: The avermectins: Insecticidal and antiparasitic agents, in Krieger R (ed): *Handbook of Pesticide Toxicology.* San Diego: Academic Press, 2001, pp. 1157–1167.

Stevens JT, Breckenridge CB, Simpkins J, *et al.*: Symmetrical and asymmetrical triazine herbicides, in Krieger R (ed): *Handbook of Pesticide Toxicology.* San Diego: Academic Press, 2001, pp. 1511–1519.

Stevens JT, Breckenridge CB, Wetzel LT, *et al.*: A risk characterization for atrazine: Oncogenicity profile. *J Toxicol Environ Health* 56:69–109, 1999.

Storm E, Rozman KK, Doull J: Occupational exposure limits for organophosphate pesticides based on inhibition of red blood cell acetylcholinesterase. *Toxicology* 150:1–29, 2000.

Stott WT, Gollapudi BB, Rao KS: Mammalian toxicity of 1,3 – Dichloropropene. *Rev Environ Contam Toxicol* 168:1–42, 2001.

Stuetz W, Propamontol T, Erhardt JG, *et al.*: Organochlorine pesticide residues in human milk of a Hmong hill tribe living in Northern Thailand. *Sci Total Environ* 273:53–60, 2001.

Sudakin DK: Biopesticides. *Toxicol Rev* 22:83–90, 2003.

Sudakin DL, Trevathan WR: DEET: A review and update of safety and risk in the general population. *J Toxicol Clin Toxicol* 41:831–830, 2003.

Sundwall A: Minimum concentrations of N-methylpyridinium -2-aldoxime methane sulphonate (P2S) which reverse neuromuscular block. *Biochem Pharmacol* 8:413–417, 1961.

Taets C, Aref S, Rayburn AL: The clastogenic potential of triazine herbicide combinations found in potable water supplies. *Environ Health Perspect* 106:197–201, 1998.

Talbot AR, Shiaw MH, Huang JS, *et al.*: Acute poisoning with a glyphosate surfactant herbicide (Round-up): A review of 93 cases. *Hum Exp Toxicol* 10:1–8, 1991.

Tamura H, Yoshikawa H, Gaido KW, *et al.*: Interaction of organophosphate pesticides and related compounds with the androgen receptor. *Environ Health Perspect* 111:545–552, 2003.

Tang J, Cao Y, Rose RL, *et al.*: Metabolism of chlorpyrifos by human cytochrome P450 isoforms and human, mouse and rat liver microsomes. *Drug Metab Dispos* 29:1201–1204, 2001.

Tang J, Rose RL, Chambers JE: Metabolism of organophosphorus and carbamate pesticides, in Gupta RC (ed): *Toxicology of Organophosphate and Carbamate Compounds.* Amsterdam: Elsevier, 2006, pp. 127–143.

Taylor JR, Selhorst JB, Houff SA, *et al.*: Chlordecone intoxication in man. I. Clinical observations. *Neurology* 28:626–630, 1978.

Taylor P: Agents acting at the neuromuscular junction and autonomic ganglia, in Hardman JG, Limbird LE (ed): *Goodman & Gilman's The Pharmacological Basis of Therapeutics.* New York: McGraw-Hill, 1996, pp. 177–197.

Tenenbein M: Severe toxic reactions and death following the ingestion of diethyltoluamide-containing insect repellents. *J Am Med Assoc* 258:1509–1511, 1987.

Thiruchelvam M, Richfield EK, Baggs RB, *et al.*: The nigrostriatal dopaminergic system as a preferential target of repeated exposures to combined paraquat and maneb: Implications for Parkinson's disease. *J Neurosci* 20:9207–9214, 2000.

Tilson HA: Neurotoxicology risk assessment guidelines: Developmental neurotoxicology. *Neurotoxicology* 21:189–194, 2000.

Tominack RL: Herbicide formulations. *Clin Toxicol* 38:129–135, 2000.

Tomizawa M, Casida JE: Neonicotinoid insecticide toxicology: Mechanisms of selective action. *Annu Rev Pharmacol Toxicol* 45:247–268, 2005.

Turosov V, Rakitsky V, Tomatis L: Dichlorodiphenyltrichloroethane (DDT): Ubiquity, persistence, and risks. *Environ Health Perspect* 110:125–128, 2002.

Tweedy BW: Inorganic sulfur as a fungicide. *Residue Rev* 78:43–68, 1981.

Ujvary I: Nicotine and other insecticidal alkaloids, in Yamamoto I, Casida JE (eds): *Nicotinoid Insecticides and the Nicotinic Acetylcholine Receptor.* Tokyo: Springer Verlag, 1999, pp. 29–69.

Ujvary I: Pest control agents from natural products, in Krieger R (ed): *Handbook of Pesticide Toxicology.* San Diego: Academic Press, 2001, pp. 109–179.

USEPA (U.S. Environmental Protection Agency): *DDT: A review of Scientific and Economic Aspects of the Decision to Ban its Use as a Pesticide.* Washington DC: USEPA, 1975, pp. 300.

USEPA (U.S. Environmental Protection Agency): A SAB report: Assessment of potential 2,4-D carcinogenicity. Review of epidemiological and other data on potential carcinogenicity of 2,4-D. U.S. Environmental Protection Agency, Science Advisory Board, Washington, DC, 1994.

USEPA (U.S. Environmental Protection Agency): Carcinogenicity peer review (4th) of 2, 4- dichlorophenoxyacetic acid (2,4-D). 1-29-1997.

USEPA (U.S. Environmental Protection Agency): Exposure Factors Handbook, EPA/600/C-99/001, February. Washington DC: US EPA, Office of Research and Development, 1999.

USEPA (U.S. Environmental Protection Agency): The use of data on cholinesterase inhibition for risk assessments of organophosphorus and carbamate pesticides. Washington, DC: USEPA, 2000, pp. 50 (accessible online at http://www.epa.gov/pesticides/trac/science/cholin.pdf).

USEPA (U.S. Environmental Protection Agency): Potential developmental effects of atrazine in amphibians (www.epa.gov/oscpmont/sap/2003/june/junemeetingreport.pdf).

USEPA (U.S. Environmental Protection Agency): Picaridin, 2005 (http://www.epa. gov/opprd001/factsheets/picaridin.pdf).

Van den Bercken J: The effect of DDT and dieldrin on myelinated nerve fibers. *Eur J Pharmacol* 20:205–214, 1972.

Vanholder R, Colardyn F, De Reuck J, *et al.*: Diquat intoxication—Report of two cases and review of the literature. *Am J Med* 70:1267–1271, 1981.

Veronesi B, Padilla S, Blackmon K, *et al.*: Murine susceptibility to organophosphorus-induced delayed neuropathy (OPIDN). *Toxicol Appl Pharmacol* 107:311–324, 1991.

Verschoyle RD, Aldridge WN: Structure-activity relationships of some pyrethroids in rats. *Arch Toxicol* 45:325–329, 1980.

Vijverberg HPM, van der Zalm JM, van den Bercken J: Similar mode of action of pyrethroids and DDT on sodium channel gating in myelinated nerves. *Nature* 295:601–603, 1982.

Villanueva CM, Durand G, Coutté MB, *et al.*: Atrazine in municipal drinking water and risk of low birth weight, pre-term delivery, and small-for-gestational-age status. *Occup Environ Med* 62:400–405, 2005.

Wagner SL: *Clinical Toxicology of Agricultural Chemicals.* Park Ridge, NJ: Noyes Data Corporation, 1983, pp. 306.

Waliszewski SM, Aguirre AA, Infanzon RM, *et al.*: Comparison of organochlorine pesticide levels in adipose tissue and human milk of mothers living in Veracruz, Mexico. *Bull Environ Contem Toxicol* 62:685–690, 1999.

Watanabe T, Sano T: Neurological effects of glufosinate poisoning with a brief review. *Hum Exp Toxicol* 17:35–39, 1998.

Weiss B, Amler S, Amler SW: Pesticides. *Pediatrics* 113:1030–1036, 2004.

Wesseling C, Castillo L, Elinder CG: Pesticide poisonings in Costa Rica. *Scand J Work Environ Health* 19:227–235, 1993.

Wesseling C, van Wendel De Joode B, Ruepert C, *et al.*: Paraquat in developing countries. *Int J Occup Environ Health* 7:275–286, 2001.

Whalon ME, Wingend BA: Bt: Mode of action and use. *Arch Insect Biochem Physiol* 54:200–211, 2003.

WHO (World Health Organization): DDT and its derivatives. *Environmental Health Criteria 9.* Geneva: WHO, 1979, pp. 194.

WHO (World Health Organization): *Public Health Impact of Pesticides Used in Agriculture.* Geneva: WHO, 1990.

Williams GM, Kroes R, Munro IC: Safety evaluation and risk assessment of the herbicide Roundup and its active ingredient, glyphosate, for humans. *Reg Pharmacol Toxicol* 31:117–165, 2000.

Wilson AGE, Lau H, Asbury KJ, *et al.*: Metabolism of alachlor by human nasal tissue. *Fundam Appl Toxicol* 15:1398, 1995.

Wong CK, Leung KM, Poon BH, *et al.*: Organochlorine hydrocarbons in human breast milk collected in Hong Kong and Guangzhou. *Arch Environ Contam Toxicol* 43:364–372, 2002.

Woods JS, Polissar L, Severson RK, *et al.*: Soft tissue sarcoma and non-Hodgkin's lymphoma in relation to phenoxyherbicide and chlorinated phenol exposure in western Washington. *J Natl Cancer Inst* 78:899–910, 1987.

Woolley DE: Neurotoxicity of DDT and possible mechanisms of action, in Prasad KN, Vernadakis A (eds): *Mechanisms of Action of Neurotoxic Substances.* New York: Raven Press, 1982, pp. 95–141.

Worek F, Diebold C, Eyer P: Dimethylphosphoryl-inhibited human cholinesterases: Inhibition, reactivation and aging kinetics. *Arch Toxicol* 73:7–14, 1999a.

Worek F, Mast U, Kiderlen D, *et al.*: Improved determination of acetylcholinesterase activity in human whole blood. *Clin Chim Acta* 288:73–90, 1999b.

Yang PY, Taso TC, Lin JL, *et al.*: Carbofuran-induced delayed neuropathy. *J Toxicol Clin Toxicol* 38:43–46, 2000.

Yaramis A, Soker M, Bilici M: Amitraz poisoning in children. *Hum Exp Toxicol* 19:1–3, 2000.

Yoon YJ, Kim ES, Hwang YS, *et al.*: Avermectin: Biochemical and molecular basis of its synthesis and regulation. *Appl Microbiol Biotechnol* 63:626–634, 2004.

Zaccheo O, Dinsdale D, Meacock PA, *et al.*: Neuropathy target esterase and its yeast homologue degrade phosphatidylcholine to glycerophosphocholine in living cells. *J Biol Chem* 279:24024–24033, 2004.

Zadikoff CM: Toxic encephalopathy associated with use of insect repellents. *J Pediatr* 95:140–142, 1979.

Zaki MM, Moran D, Harris D: Pesticide in ground-water: The aldicarb story in Suffolk County, New York. *Am J Public Health* 72:1391–1395, 1982.

Zhang J, Fitsanakis VA, Gu G, *et al.*: Manganese ethylene-bis-dithiocarbamate and selective dopaminergic neurodegeneration in rat: A link through mitochondrial dysfunction. *J Neurochem* 84:336–346, 2003.

Zilker T, Fogt F, von Clarmann M: Kein Parkinsonsyndrom nach akuter paraquat intoxikation. *Klin Wochenschr* 66:1138–1141, 1988.

CHAPTER 23

TOXIC EFFECTS OF METALS

Jie Liu, Robert A. Goyer, and Michael P. Waalkes

INTRODUCTION

What is a Metal?

The definition of a metal is not inherently obvious and the differences between metallic and nonmetallic elements can be subtle (Vouk, 1986a). Metals are typically defined by physical properties of the element in the solid state, but they vary widely with the metallic element. General metal properties include high reflectivity (luster); high electrical conductivity; high thermal conductivity; and mechanical ductility and strength. A toxicologically important characteristic of metals is that they may react in biological systems by losing one or more electrons to form cations (Vouk, 1986a). In the periodic table, within a group there is often a gradual transition from nonmetallic to metallic properties going from lighter to heavier atoms (e.g., Group IVa transitions from carbon to lead). Many metals exhibit variable oxidation states. Various names are applied to subsets of metallic elements including alkali metals (e.g., lithium and sodium), the alkaline earth metals (e.g., beryllium and magnesium), the transition (or heavy) metals (e.g., cadmium and zinc), and the metalloids (e.g., arsenic and antimony), which have characteristics between metal and nonmetals.

In the periodic table, over 75% of the elements are regarded as metals and eight are considered metalloids. This chapter discusses metals that have been reported to produce significant toxicity in humans. This discussion will include major toxic metals (e.g., lead, cadmium), essential metals (e.g., zinc, copper), medicinal metals (e.g., platinum, bismuth), and minor toxic metals including metals in emerging technology (e.g., indium, uranium). *Metal Toxicology* will also discuss toxic metalloids (e.g., arsenic, antimony) and certain nonmetallic elemental toxicants (e.g., selenium, fluoride). An overview of *Metal Toxicology* is shown in Fig. 23-1.

Metals as Toxicants

The use of metals has been critical to the progress and success of human civilization. It would be difficult to image an advanced society without extensive utilization of metallic compounds. Metals are unique among pollutant toxicants in that they are all naturally occurring and, in many cases, are ubiquitous within the human environment. Thus, regardless of how safely metals are used in industrial processes or consumer products, some level of human exposure is inevitable. In addition, all life has evolved in the presence of metals and organisms have been forced to deal with these potentially toxic, yet omnipresent, elements. In fact, many metals have become essential to various biological processes. Essentiality goes hand-in-hand with intentional accumulation and safe transport, storage, and usage mechanisms. Nonetheless, even essential metals will become toxic with increasing exposure. It is often the case that the nonessential toxicant metals mimic essential metals and thereby gain access to, and potentially disrupt, key cellular functions. This can also account for bioaccumulation of toxic metals.

Metals differ from other toxic substances because, as elements, they are neither created nor destroyed by human endeavors. What human industry has accomplished is to concentrate metals in the biosphere. The anthropogenic contribution to the levels of metals in air, water, soil, and food is well recognized (Beijer and Jernelov, 1986). Human use of metals can also alter the chemical form or speciation of an element and thereby impact toxic potential. With a few notable exceptions, most metals are only sparingly recycled once used. These factors combine to make metals very persistent in the human environment.

Metals are certainly one of the oldest toxicants known to humans due to their very early use. For instance, human use of lead

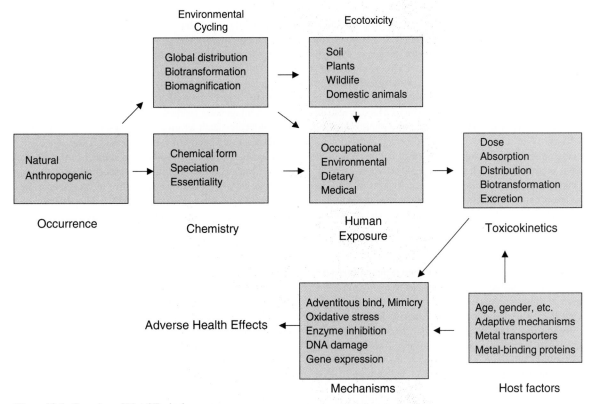

Figure 23-1. Overview of Metal Toxicology.

probably started prior to 2000 BC, when abundant supplies were obtained from ores as a byproduct of smelting silver. The first description of abdominal colic in a man who extracted metals is credited to Hippocrates in 370 BC. Arsenic and mercury are discussed by Theophrastus of Erebus (370–287 BC), and Pliny and Elder (AD 23–79). Arsenic was used early on for decoration in Egyptian tombs and as a "secret poison," whereas mercury assumed almost a mystical stature in early science and was a large focus of alchemy. However, most of the use of the metals has occurred since the onset of the industrial revolution. In this regard, many of the metals of toxicological concern today were only relatively recently discovered. For instance, cadmium was first recognized in the early 1800s, and it was much later before the metal was widely used. The toxicological importance of some of the rarer or lesser used metals might well increase with new applications, such as chemotherapy and microelectronics, or other emerging technologies.

Historically, metal toxicology largely concerned acute or overt, high-dose effects, such as abdominal colic from lead or the bloody diarrhea and uropenia after mercury ingestion. Because of advances in our understanding of potential toxicity of metals, and consequent improvements in industrial hygiene and stricter environmental standards, such acute high-dose effects are now uncommon. Focus has shifted to subtle, chronic, low-dose effects, in which cause-and-effect relationships may not be immediately clear. These might include a level of effect that causes a change in an important, but highly complex index of affected individual's performance, such as lower than expected IQs due to childhood lead exposure. Other important chronic toxic effects include carcinogenesis, and several metals have emerged as human carcinogens. Assigning responsibility for such toxicological effects can often be difficult, particularly when the endpoint in question lacks specificity, in that it may be a

complex disease caused by a number of different chemicals or even combinations of chemicals. In addition, humans are never exposed to only a single metal, but rather to complex mixtures. The metals as a class of toxicants clearly present many challenges in toxicological research.

The elemental nature of metals impacts their biotransformation and toxicity, as detoxification by destructive metabolism to subcomponents of lesser toxicity cannot occur with these atomic species. In essence, as elemental species metals are non-biodegradable. This indestructibility combined with bioaccumulation contributes to the high concern for metals as toxicants. Most elemental metals tend to form ionic bonds. However, biological conjugation to form organometallic compounds can occur for various metals (Dopp *et al.*, 2004), particularly with metalloids, like arsenic, that show mixed carbonaceous and metallic qualities. The redox capacity of a given metal or metallic compound should also be considered as part of its metabolism. The metabolism of metals is intricate and subtle but can directly impact toxic potential.

Movement of Metals in the Environment

Metals are redistributed naturally in the environment by both geologic and biologic cycles. Rainwater dissolves rocks and ores and transports materials, including metals, to rivers and underground water (e.g., arsenic), depositing and stripping materials from adjacent soil and eventually transporting these substances to the ocean to be precipitated as sediment or taken up into forming rainwater to be relocated elsewhere. Biological cycles moving metals include biomagnification by plants and animals resulting in incorporation into food cycles. In comparison, human activity often intentionally shortens the residence time of metals in ore deposits, and can result in the formation of new, non-naturally occurring metallic compounds. For instance, cadmium distribution mainly comes from human activities. Human industry greatly enhances metal distribution in the global environment by discharge to soil, water, and air, as exemplified by the 200-fold increase in lead content of Greenland ice since the onset of the industrial revolution. Mercury undergoes global cycling with elevated levels being found far from points of discharge, as, for example, with mercury in the Arctic Ocean. Mercury also undergoes biomethylation and biomagnification by aquatic organisms (see Fig. 23-6).

Increased distribution of metals and metal compounds in the environment, especially through anthropogenic activities, raises increasing concern for ecotoxicological effects. Reports of metal intoxication are common in plants, aquatic organisms, invertebrates, fish, sea mammals, birds, and domestic animals. The ecotoxicity of various metals is discussed under each individual section. Mercury poisoning from consumption of fish containing high levels of methylmercury and cadmium poisoning from consumption of rice grown in soils contaminated with cadmium from industrial discharges are examples of human consequences from environmental pollution.

Not all human toxicity occurs from metals deposited in the biosphere by human activity. For example, chronic arsenic poisoning from high levels of naturally occurring inorganic arsenic in drinking water is a major health issue in many parts of the world. Endemic intoxication from excess fluoride, selenium, or thallium can all occur from natural high environmental levels.

Chemical Mechanisms of Metal Toxicology

The precise chemical basis of metal toxicology is inadequately understood but a uniform mechanism for all toxic metals is implausible because of the great variation in chemical properties and toxic endpoints. Chemically, metals in their ionic form can be very reactive and can interact with biological systems in a large variety of ways. In this regard, a cell presents numerous potential metal-binding ligands. For instance, metals like cadmium and mercury readily attach to sulfur in proteins as a preferred bio-ligand. Such adventitious binding is an important chemical mechanism by which exogenous metals exert toxic effects that can result in steric re-arrangement that impairs the function of biomolecules (Kasprzak, 2002). An example would be the inhibition of enzyme activity by metal interaction at sites other than the active center, such as the inhibition of heme synthesis enzymes by lead. The inhibition of biologically critical enzymes is an important molecular mechanism of metal toxicology.

The metals can show more specific forms of chemical attack through mimicry. In this regard the toxic metals may act as mimics of essential metals, binding to physiological sites that normally are reserved for an essential element. Owing to their rich chemistry, essential metals control, or are involved in, a variety of key metabolic and signaling functions (Kasprzak, 2002; Cousins et al., 2006). Through mimicry, the toxic metals may gain access to, and potentially disrupt a variety of important or even critical metal-mediated cellular functions. For example, mimicry for, and replacement of zinc, is a mechanism of toxicity for cadmium, copper, and nickel. Thallium mimics potassium and manganese mimics iron as a critical factor in their toxicity. Mimicry of arsenate and vanadate for phosphate allows for cellular transport of these toxic elements whereas selenate, molybdate, and chromate mimic sulfate and can compete for sulfate carriers and in chemical sulfation reactions (Bridges and Zalpus, 2005). Organometallic compounds can also act as mimics of

biological chemicals, as, for example, with methylmercury, which is transported by amino acid or organic anion transporters (Bridges and Zalpus, 2005). Indeed, molecular or ionic mimicry at the level of transport is often a key event in metal toxicity.

Another key chemical reaction in metal toxicology is metal-mediated oxidative damage. Many metals can directly act as catalytic centers for redox reactions with molecular oxygen or other endogenous oxidants, producing oxidative modification of biomolecules such as proteins or DNA. This may be a key step in the carcinogenicity of certain metals (Kasprzak, 2002). Besides oxygen-based radicals, carbon- and sulfur-based radicals may also occur. Nickel and chromium are two examples of metals that act, at least in part, by generation of reactive oxygen species or other reactive intermediates (Kasprazak, 2002). Alternatively, metals may displace redox active essential elements from their normal cellular ligands, which, in turn, may result in oxidative cellular damage. For instance, cadmium, which is not redox active, may well cause oxidative stress through the release of endogenous iron, an element with high redox activity (Valko et al., 2006).

Metals in their ionic form can be very reactive and form DNA and protein adducts in biological systems. For example, once hexavalent chromium enters the cell it is reduced by various intracellular reductants to give reactive trivalent chromium species that form DNA adducts or DNA-protein cross-links, events likely to be important in chromium genotoxicity (Zhitkovich, 2005). Metals can also induce an array of aberrant gene expression, which, in turn, produces adverse effects. For example, nickel can induce the expression of Cap43/NDRG1, under the control of the hypoxia-inducible transcription factor (HIF-1), which is thought to play a key role in nickel carcinogenesis (Costa et al., 2005). An array of aberrant hepatic gene expressions occurs in adult mice after in utero arsenic exposure, which could be an important molecular event in arsenic hepatocarcinogenesis (Liu et al., 2006).

Factors Impacting Metal Toxicity

The standard factors that impact the toxic potential of all chemicals apply to the metals as well. Exposure-related factors include dose, route of exposure, duration, and frequency of exposure. Because metals can be quite reactive, and the portal of entry is often initially the organ most affected, as with the lung after inhalation.

Host-based factors that can impact metal toxicity include age at exposure, gender, and capacity for biotransformation. For instance, it is quite clear that younger subjects are often more sensitive to metal intoxication, as, for example, with the neurotoxicity of lead in children. The major pathway of exposure to many toxic metals in children is food, and children consume more calories per pound of body weight than adults. Moreover, children have higher gastrointestinal absorption of metals, particularly lead. The rapid growth and proliferation in the perinate represent opportunities for toxic effects, including potentially carcinogenesis, of metallic agents, and several metals (e.g., arsenic, nickel, lead, and chromium) are transplacental carcinogens in rodents. Fetal-stage toxicity of metals is well documented, as with methylmercury, and many metals are teratogenic. For many inorganics there is no impediment to transplacental transport, as with lead or arsenic, and human fetal blood lead levels are similar to maternal levels. Elderly persons are also believed to be generally more susceptible to metal toxicity than younger adults. Recognition of factors that influence toxicity of a metal is important in determining risk, particularly in susceptible subpopulations.

Chemical-related factors directly impact the toxic potential of metals. This would include the precise metal compound and its valence state or speciation. For instance, methylmercury is a potent neurotoxin, whereas the inorganic mercurials primarily attack the kidney. Similarly, the oxidation state of chromium can differentiate the essential (naturally occurring trivalent chromium) from toxic species (hexavalent chromium).

Lifestyle factors such as smoking or alcohol ingestion may have direct or indirect impacts on the level of metal intoxication. For instance, cigarette smoke by itself contains many toxic metals, such as cadmium, and it is thought that smoking will double the life-time burden of cadmium in nonoccupationally exposed individuals. Other components of cigarette smoke may also influence pulmonary effects, as, for instance, with metals that are lung carcinogens. Alcohol ingestion may influence toxicity by altering diet, reducing essential mineral intake, and altering hepatic iron deposition. The composition of the diet can significantly alter gastrointestinal absorption of various dietary metals.

The essentiality of metals has direct bearing on the toxic potential of a metal. Any "free" ionic metal would be potentially toxic due to reactive potential. The need to accumulate essential metals dictates the evolution of systems for the safe transport, storage, and utilization as well as, within limits, elimination of excess. For example, metallothionein is a metal-binding protein that may function in the homeostatic control of zinc (Cousins et al., 2006), and may represent a storage or transport form of this metal. Such factors imply that a threshold would exist for toxicity due to essential metal exposure. In this regard, the essential metallic elements would be expected to show a "U"-shaped dose–response curve in that, at very low exposure levels, toxic adverse effects would occur from deficiency, but at high exposure levels toxicity also occurs. The nonessential toxic metals can mimic essential elements and disrupt homeostasis, as with cadmium which will potentially displace zinc to bind to zinc-dependent transcription factors and enzymes (Waalkes, 2003).

Adaptive mechanisms can be critical to the toxic effects of metals, and organisms have a variety of ways in which they can adapt to otherwise toxic metal insults. Typically, adaptation is acquired after the first few exposures and can be long lasting or transient after exposure ceases. Adaptation can be at the level of uptake or excretion, or with some metals, through long-term storage in a toxicological inert form. For instance, it appears enhanced arsenic efflux is involved in acquired tolerance to the metalloid on the cellular level (Liu et al., 2001). Conversely, intentional sequestration of toxic metals is another adaptive tactic and examples of such long-term storage include lead-inclusion bodies, which form in various organs and contain protein-immobilized lead in a distinct cellular aggresome. These bodies are thought to be protective by limiting the level of free, and therefore toxic, lead within the cell, and the inability to form such bodies clearly increases the chronic toxic effects of lead, including carcinogenesis (Waalkes et al., 2004c). Similarly, cadmium exposure causes the overexpression of metallothionein which will sequester cadmium and reduce its toxicity as an adaptive mechanism (Klaassen and Liu, 1998). Metal exposure can also induce a cascade of molecular/genetic responses that may, in turn, reduce toxicity, such as with metal-induced oxidative stress responses (Valko et al., 2006). It is clear that acquired metal adaptation, although allowing immediate cellular survival, may in fact be a potential contributing factor in long-term toxicity (Waalkes et al., 2000). For instance, acquired self-tolerance to cadmium- or arsenic-induced apoptosis may actually contribute to eventual carcinogenesis by allowing survival of damaged cells that would otherwise have been eliminated (Hart et al., 2001; Pi et al., 2005).

Biomarkers of Metal Exposure

Biomarkers of exposure, toxicity, and susceptibility are important in assessing the level of concern with metal intoxication. Exposure biomarkers, such as concentrations in blood or urine, have long been used with metals. Techniques in molecular toxicology have greatly expanded the possibilities for biomarkers. Thus, in the case of chromium, DNA–protein complexes may serve as a biomarker of both exposure and carcinogenic potential. The capacity for expression of genes that potentially play protective roles against metal toxicity, as, for example, with metallothionein and heme oxygenase, show promise as markers of both effect and susceptibility. The use of such biomarkers may well allow identification of particularly sensitive subpopulations.

Estimates of the relationship of exposure level to toxic effects for a particular metal are in many ways a measure of the dose–response relationships discussed in great detail earlier in this book. The dose of a metal is a multidimensional concept and is a function of time as well as concentration. The most toxicologically relevant definition of dose is the amount of active metal within cells of target organs. The active form is often presumed to be the free metal, but it is technically difficult or impossible to precisely determine.

A critical indicator of retention of a metal is its biological half-life, or the time it takes for the body or organ to excrete half of an accumulated amount. The biological half-life varies according to the metal as well as the organ or tissue. For example, the biological half-lives of cadmium in kidney and lead in bone are 20–30 years, whereas for some metals, such as arsenic or lithium, they are only a few hours to days. For many metals, more than one half-life is needed to fully describe the retention. The half-life of lead in blood is only a few weeks, as compared to the much longer half-life in bone. After inhalation of mercury vapor, at least two half-lives describe the retention in brain, one on the order of a few weeks and the other measured in years. Continued metal exposure clearly complicates retention kinetics.

Blood, urine, and hair are the most accessible tissues for quantifying metal exposure. Results from single measurements may reflect recent exposure or long-term or past exposure, depending on retention time in the particular tissue. Blood and urine concentrations usually, but not always, are reflective of more recent exposures and correlate with acute adverse effects. An exception is urinary cadmium, which may reflect kidney damage related to a renal cadmium accumulation over several decades. Hair can be useful in assessing variations in exposure to metals over the period of its growth. Analyses can be performed on segments of the hair, so that metal content of the newest growth can be compared with past exposures. Hair levels of mercury have been found to be a reliable measure of exposure to methylmercury. For most other metals, however, hair is not a reliable tissue for measuring exposure because of metal deposits from external contamination that may complicate analysis.

Metal-binding Proteins and Metal Transporters

Protein binding of metals is a critical aspect of essential and toxic metal metabolism (Zalpus and Koropatnick, 2000). Many different types of proteins play roles in the disposition of metals in the body. Nonspecific binding to proteins, like serum albumin or hemoglobin, act in metal transport and tissue distribution. Metals vary in their preferred site of proteinaceous binding, and can attack a variety of amino acid residues. For instance, cysteine sulfurs are preferred by cadmium and mercury, and these residues are commonly involved with overall protein structure. In addition, proteins with specific metal-binding properties play special roles in the trafficking of specific essential metals, and toxic metals may interact with these proteins through mimicry. Metal-binding proteins are an important, emerging issue in the physiology and toxicology of metals and only a few examples are highlighted here.

The *metallothioneins* are a very important class of metal-binding proteins that function in essential metal homeostasis and metal detoxification (Klaassen *et al.*, 1999). They are small (6000 Da), soluble, and rich in internally oriented thiol ligands. These thiol ligands provide the basis for high-affinity binding of several essential and toxic metals including zinc, cadmium, copper, and mercury. The metallothioneins are highly inducible by a variety of metals or other stimulants. Metallothioneins clearly play an important role in metal toxicity, as illustrated in the discussion of cadmium below.

Transferrin is a glycoprotein that binds most of the ferric iron in plasma and helps transport iron across cell membranes. The protein also transports aluminum and manganese. *Ferritin* is primarily a storage protein for iron. It has been suggested that ferrin may serve as a general metal detoxicant protein, because it binds a variety of toxic metals including cadmium, zinc, beryllium, and aluminum.

Ceruloplasmin is a copper-containing glycoprotein oxidase in plasma that converts ferrous iron to ferric iron, which then binds to transferrin. This protein also stimulates iron uptake by a transferrin-independent mechanism.

In all cells there are mechanisms for metal ion homeostasis that frequently involve a balance between uptake and efflux systems. A rapidly increasing number of metal transport proteins are being discovered that transport metals across cell membranes and organelles inside the cells. Metal transporters are important for cellular resistance to metals or metalloids (Rosen, 2002). For instance, enhanced efflux via multidrug resistance protein pumps is involved in acquired tolerance to arsenic (Liu *et al.*, 2001), wheraes decreased influx via reduced calcium G-type channels is involved in acquired tolerance to cadmium (Leslie *et al.*, 2006). Over ten zinc transporters and four Zip family proteins are involved in cellular zinc transport, trafficking, and signaling (Cousins *et al.*, 2006). The importance of metal transporters in human diseases is well illustrated by Menkes disease and Wilson disease, which are caused by genetic mutations in the copper-transport protein gene *ATP7A*, resulting in copper deficiency (Menkes disease), or *ATP7B*, resulting in copper overload (Wilson disease) (see Fig. 23-7).

Pharmacology of Metals

Metal and metal compounds have a long history of pharmacological use. Metallic agents, largely because of their potential toxicity, have been often used in chemotherapeutic settings. For instance, mercury was used in the treatment of syphilis as early as the 16th century. Similarly, Ehrlich's *magic bullet* (arsphenamine) was an organoarsenical. Today, many metallic chemicals remain valuable pharmacological tools in the treatment of human disease, as exemplified by the highly effective use of platinum compounds in cancer chemotherapy. In addition, gallium and titanium complexes are promising metal compounds in cancer chemotherapy. Other medicinal metals used today include aluminum (antacids and buffered analgesics), bismuth (peptic ulcer and *Helicobacter pylori* asso-

ciated gastritis), lithium (mania and bipolar disorders), and gold (arthritis).

Treatment of metal poisoning is sometimes used to prevent, or even attempt to reverse, toxicity. The typical strategy is to give metal chelators that will complex the metal and enhance its excretion (Klaassen, 2001). Most chelators are not specific and will interact with a number of metals, eliminating more than the metal of concern. In addition, the vast array of biological metal ligands is a formidable barrier to chelator efficacy (Klaassen, 2001). Metal chelation therapy should be considered a secondary alternative to reduction or prevention of toxic metal exposures. Such therapy can be used for many different metals including lead, mercury, iron, and arsenic. For detailed discussion on the pharmacology of chelation therapy, see Klaassen (2001).

MAJOR TOXIC METALS

Arsenic

Arsenic (As) is a toxic and carcinogenic metalloid. The word *arsenic* is from the Persian word *Zarnikh*, as translated to the Greek *arsenikon*, meaning "yellow orpiment." Arsenic has been known and used since ancient times as the *Poison of Kings and the King of Poisons*. The element was first isolated in about 1250. Arsenicals have been used since ancient times as drugs and even today are very effective against acute promyelocytic leukemia (Soignet *et al.*, 2001). Arsenic exists in the trivalent and pentavalent forms and is widely distributed in nature. The most common inorganic trivalent arsenic compounds are arsenic trioxide and sodium arsenite, while common pentavalent inorganic compounds are sodium arsenate, arsenic pentoxide, and arsenic acid. Important organo-arsenicals include arsenilic acid, arsenosugars, and several methylated forms produced as a consequence of inorganic arsenic biotransformation in various organisms, including humans. Arsine (AsH_3) is an important gaseous arsenical.

Occupational exposure to arsenic occurs in the manufacture of pesticides, herbicides, and other agricultural products. High exposure to arsenic fumes and dusts may occur in smelting industries (ATSDR, 2005a). Environmental arsenic exposure mainly occurs from arsenic-contaminated drinking water. Arsenic in drinking water is often from natural sources. Although most U.S. drinking water contains arsenic at levels lower than 5 μg/L (ppb), it has been estimated that about 25 million people in Bangladesh alone drink water with arsenic levels above 50 ppb (IARC, 2004). Environmental exposure to arsenic also occurs from burning of coal containing naturally high levels of arsenic (Liu *et al.*, 2002), and perhaps from wood treated with arsenical preservatives (Khan *et al.*, 2006). It is not known, however, to what extent arsenic-treated wood products contribute to human exposure. Food, especially seafood, may contribute significantly to daily arsenic intake. Arsenic in seafood is largely in an organic form called arsenobetaine that is much less toxic than the inorganic forms (ATSDR, 2005a).

Toxicokinetics Inorganic arsenic is well absorbed (80–90%) from the gastrointestinal tract, distributed throughout the body, often metabolized by methylation, and then excreted primarily in urine (NRC, 2001). Arsenic compounds of low solubility (e.g., arsenic trioxide, arsenic selenide, lead arsenide, and gallium arsenide) are absorbed less efficiently after oral exposure. Skin is a potential route of exposure to arsenic, and systemic toxicity has been reported in persons having dermal contact with solutions of inorganic arsenic

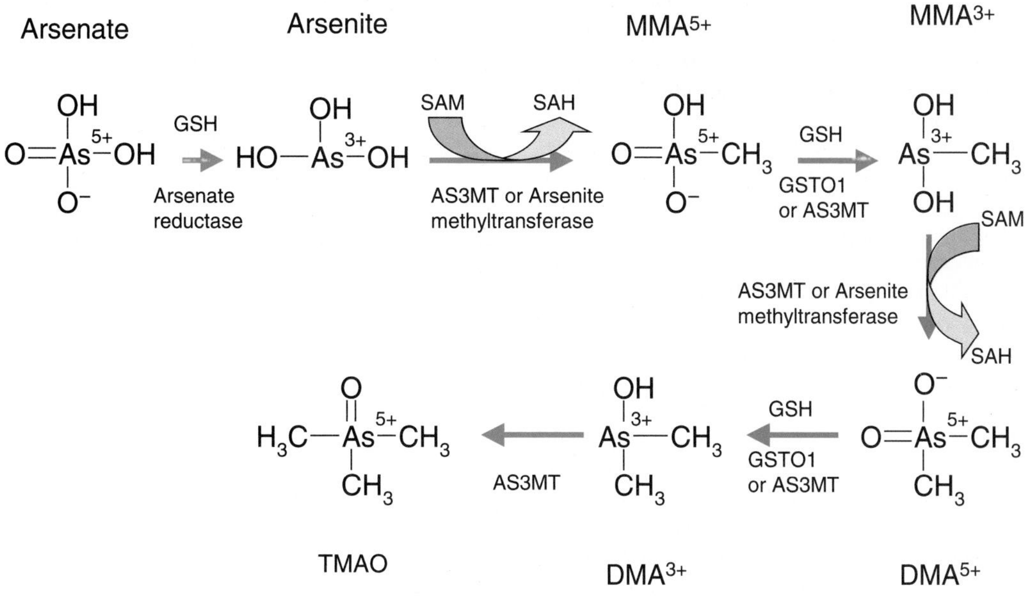

Figure 23-2. Arsenic Metabolism.

GSH, reduced glutathione; GSTO1, glutathione S-transferase omega-1; SAM, S-adenosylmethionine; SAH, S-adenosyl-homocysteine; AS3MT, arsenic methyltransferase (Cyt19); MMA^{5+}, monomethylarsonic acid; MMA^{3+}, monomethylarsonous acid; DMA^{5+}, dimethylarsinic acid; DMA^{3+}, dimethylarsinous acid; TMAO, trimethylarsenic oxide.

(Hostynek *et al.*, 1993). Airborne arsenic is largely trivalent arsenic oxide. Deposition in airways and absorption of arsenicals from lungs is dependent on particle size and chemical form. Excretion of absorbed arsenic is mainly via the urine. The whole-body biological half-life of ingested arsenic is about 10 hours, and 50–80% is excreted over 3 days. The biological half-life of methylated arsenicals is in the range of 30 hours. Arsenic has a predilection for skin and is excreted by desquamation of skin and in sweat, particularly during periods of profuse sweating. It also concentrates in forming fingernails and hair. Arsenic exposure produces characteristic transverse white bands across fingernails (Mees' line), which appear about 6 weeks after the onset of symptoms of arsenic toxicity. Arsenic in the fingernails and hair has been used as a biomarker for exposure, including both current and past exposures, while urinary arsenic is a good indicator for current exposure.

Methylation of inorganic arsenic species is no longer considered as a detoxication process, as recent work has identified the highly toxic trivalent methylated arsenicals. Some animal species even lack arsenic methylation capacity, perhaps as an adaptation mechanism. Figure 23-2 illustrates the biotransformation of arsenic. Arsenate (As^{5+}) is rapidly reduced to arsenite (As^{3+}) by arsenate reductase (presumably purine nucleoside phosphorylase). Arsenite is then sequentially methylated to form methylarsonate (MMA^{5+}) and dimethylarsinic acid (DMA^{5+}) by arsenic methyltransferase (AS3MT or Cyt19) or arsenite methyltransferase using S-adenosylmethionine (SAM) as a methyl group donor. The intermediate metabolites, methylarsonous acid (MMA^{3+}) and dimethylarsinous acid (DMA^{3+}), are generated during this process, and these trivalent methylated arsenicals are now thought to be more toxic than even the inorganic arsenic species (Aposhian and Aposhian, 2006; Thomas *et al.*, 2007). In humans, urinary arsenicals are composed of 10–30% inorganic arsenicals, 10–20% MMA, and 55–76% DMA (NRC, 2001). However, large variations in arsenic methylation occur due to factors such as age and sex, and it is suspected that ge-

netic polymorphisms may exist. Arsenic metabolism also changes through the course of pregnancy, reflected in higher urinary excretion of DMA and lower urinary levels of inorganic arsenic and MMA, which may have toxicologic impact on the developing fetus (Hopenhayn *et al.*, 2003).

Toxicity

Acute Poisoning Ingestion of large doses (70–180 mg) of inorganic arsenic can be fatal. Symptoms of acute intoxication include fever, anorexia, hepatomegaly, melanosis, cardiac arrhythmia and, in fatal cases, eventual cardiac failure. Acute arsenic ingestion can damage mucous membranes of the gastrointestinal tract, causing irritation, vesicle formation, and even sloughing. Sensory loss in the peripheral nervous system is the most common neurologic effect, appearing at 1–2 weeks after large doses and consisting of Wallerian degeneration of axons, a condition that is reversible if exposure is stopped. Anemia and leucopenia, particularly granulocytopenia, occur a few days following high-dose arsenic exposure and are reversible. Intravenous arsenic infusion at clinical doses in the treatment of acute promyelocytic leukemia may be significantly or even fatally toxic in susceptible patients, and at least three sudden deaths have been reported (Westervelt *et al.*, 2001). Acute exposure to a single high dose can produce encephalopathy, with signs and symptoms of headache, lethargy, mental confusion, hallucination, seizures, and even coma (ATSDR, 2005a).

Arsine gas, generated by electrolytic or metallic reduction of arsenic in nonferrous metal production, is a potent hemolytic agent, producing acute symptoms of nausea, vomiting, shortness of breath, and headache accompanying the hemolytic reaction. Exposure to arsine is fatal in up to 25% of the reported human cases and may be accompanied by hemoglobinuria, renal failure, jaundice, and anemia in nonfatal cases when exposure persists (ATSDR, 2005a).

Chronic Toxicity   The skin is a major target organ in chronic inorganic arsenic exposure. In humans, chronic exposure to arsenic induces a series of characteristic changes in skin epithelium. Diffuse or spotted hyperpigmentation and, alternatively, hypopigmentation can first appear between 6 months to 3 years with chronic exposure to inorganic arsenic. Palmar-plantar hyperkeratosis usually follows the initial appearance of arsenic-induced pigmentation changes within a period of years (NRC, 2001). Skin cancer is common with protracted high-level arsenical exposure (see below).

Liver injury, characteristic of long-term or chronic arsenic exposure, manifests itself initially as jaundice, abdominal pain, and hepatomegaly (NRC, 2001; Mazumder, 2005). Liver injury may progress to cirrhosis and ascites, even to hepatocellular carcinoma (Centeno *et al.*, 2002; Liu *et al.*, 2002).

Repeated exposure to low levels of inorganic arsenic can produce peripheral neuropathy. This neuropathy usually begins with sensory changes, such as numbness in the hands and feet but later may develop into a painful "pins and needles" sensation. Both sensory and motor nerves can be affected, and muscle tenderness often develops, followed by weakness, progressing from proximal to distal muscle groups. Histological examination reveals a dying-back axonopathy with demyelination, and effects are dose-related (ATSDR, 2005a).

An association between ingestion of inorganic arsenic in drinking water and cardiovascular disease has been shown (NRC, 2001; Chen *et al.*, 2005; Navas-Acien *et al.*, 2005). Peripheral vascular disease has been observed in persons with chronic exposure to inorganic arsenic in the drinking water in Taiwan. It is manifested by acrocyanosis and Raynaud's phenomenon and may progress to endarteritis and gangrene of the lower extremities (Blackfoot disease). Arsenic-induced vascular effects have been reported in Chile, Mexico, India, and China, but these effects do not compare in magnitude or severity to Blackfoot disease in Taiwanese populations, indicating other environmental or dietary factors may be involved (Yu *et al.*, 2002).

Some studies have shown an association between high arsenic exposure in Taiwan and Bangladesh and an increased risk of diabetes mellitus, but the data for occupational exposure is inconsistent (Navas-Acien *et al.*, 2006). Additional research is required to verify a link between inorganic arsenic exposure and diabetes.

Immunotoxic effects of arsenic have been suggested (ATSDR, 2005a). The hematologic consequences of chronic exposure to arsenic may include interference with heme synthesis, with an increase in urinary porphyrin excretion, which has been proposed as a biomarker for arsenic exposure (Ng *et al.*, 2005).

Mechanisms of Toxicity   The trivalent compounds of arsenic are thiol-reactive, and thereby inhibit enzymes or alter proteins by reacting with proteinaceous thiol groups. Pentavalent arsenate is an uncoupler of mitochondrial oxidative phosphorylation, by a mechanism likely related to competitive substitution (mimicry) of arsenate for inorganic phosphate in the formation of adenosine triphosphate. Arsine gas is formed by the reaction of hydrogen with arsenic, and is a potent hemolytic agent (NRC, 2001).

In addition to these basic modes of action, several mechanisms have been proposed for arsenic toxicity and carcinogenicity. Arsenic and its metabolites have been shown to produce oxidants and oxidative DNA damage, alteration in DNA methylation status and genomic instability, impaired DNA damage repair, and enhanced cell proliferation (NRC, 2001; Rossman, 2003). Unlike many carcinogens, arsenic is not a mutagen in bacteria and acts weakly in mammalian cells, but can induce chromosomal abnormalities, aneuploidy, and micronuclei formation. Arsenic can also act as a co-mutagen and/or co-carcinogen (Rossman, 2003; Chen *et al.*, 2005). These mechanisms are not mutually exclusive and multiple mechanisms likely account for arsenic toxicity and carcinogenesis. Some mechanisms, however, may be organ specific.

Carcinogenicity   The carcinogenic potential of arsenic was recognized over 110 years ago by Hutchinson, who observed an unusual number of skin cancers occurring in patients treated for various diseases with medicinal arsenicals. IARC (2004) has classified arsenic as a known human carcinogen, associated with tumors of the skin, lung, and urinary bladder, and possibly kidney, liver, and prostate (NRC, 2001; IARC, 2004).

Arsenic-induced skin cancers include basal cell carcinomas and squamous cell carcinomas, both arising in areas of arsenic-induced hyperkeratosis. The basal cell cancers are usually only locally invasive, but squamous cell carcinomas may have distant metastases. In humans, the skin cancers often, but not exclusively, occur on areas of the body not exposed to sunlight (e.g., on palms of hands and soles of feet). They also often occur as multiple malignant lesions. Animal models have shown that arsenic acts as a rodent skin tumor copromoter with 12-*O*-teradecanoyl phorbol-13-acetate in v-Ha-*ras* mutant Tg.AC mice (Germolec *et al.*, 1998) or as a co-carcinogen with UV irradiation in hairless mice (Rossman *et al.*, 2001).

The association of internal tumors in humans with arsenic exposure is well recognized (NRC, 2001). This includes arsenic-induced tumors of the urinary bladder, and lung, and potentially the liver, kidney, and prostate. In rats, the methylated arsenic species, DMA^{5+}, is a urinary bladder tumor initiator and promoter (Wei *et al.*, 2002) and produces urothelial cytotoxicity and proliferative regeneration with continuous exposure (Cohen *et al.*, 2001). However, the relevance of this finding to inorganic arsenic carcinogenesis must be extrapolated cautiously, due to the high dose of DMA required to produce these changes in rats (NRC, 2001).

In contrast to most other human carcinogens, it has been difficult to confirm the carcinogenicity of inorganic arsenic in experimental animals. Recently, a transplacental arsenic carcinogenesis model has been established in mice. Short-term exposure of the pregnant rodents from gestation day 8 to day 18, a period of general sensitivity to chemical carcinogenesis, produces tumors in the liver, adrenal, ovary, and lung of offspring as adults (Waalkes *et al.*, 2003, 2004a). The tumor spectrum after in utero arsenic exposure resembles estrogenic carcinogens and is associated with overexpression of estrogen-linked genes (Liu *et al.*, 2006), and thus a hypothesis that arsenic may somehow act on estrogen signaling to produce hepatocarcinogenic effects has been proposed (Waalkes *et al.*, 2004b). Indeed, when in utero arsenic exposure is combined with postnatal treatment with the synthetic estrogen diethylstilbestrol, synergistic increases in malignant urogenital system tumors, including urinary bladder tumors and liver tumors, are observed (Waalkes *et al.*, 2006a,b). As a corollary in humans, increased mortality occurs from lung cancer in young adults following in utero exposure to arsenic (Smith *et al.*, 2006). Thus, the developing fetus appears to be hypersensitive to arsenic carcinogenesis.

Treatment   For acute arsenic poisoning, treatment is symptomatic, with particular attention to fluid volume replacement and support of blood pressure. The oral chelator penicillamine or succimer

(2,3-dimercaptosuccinic acid, DMSA) is effective in removing arsenic from the body. Dimercaptopropanesulfonic acid (DMPS) has also been used for acute arsenic poisoning with fewer side effects (Aposhian and Aposhain, 2006). However, for chronic poisoning, chelator therapy has not proven effective in relieving symptoms (Rahman *et al.*, 2001; Liu *et al.*, 2002) except for a limited preliminary trial with DMPS (Mazumder, 2005). The best strategy for preventing chronic arsenic poisoning is by reducing exposure.

Beryllium

Beryllium (Be), an alkaline earth metal, was discovered in 1798. The name beryllium comes from the Greek *beryllos*, a term used for the mineral beryl. Beryllium compounds are divalent. Beryllium alloys are used in automobiles, computers, sports equipment, and dental bridges. Pure beryllium metal is used in nuclear weapons, aircraft, X-ray machines, and mirrors. Human exposure to beryllium and its compounds occur primarily in beryllium manufacturing, fabricating, or reclaiming industries. Individuals may also be exposed to beryllium from implanted dental prostheses. The general population is exposed to trace amounts of beryllium through the air, food, and water, as well as from cigarette smoke (WHO, 1990; ATSDR, 2002).

Toxicokinetics The primary route of exposure to beryllium compounds is through the lungs. After being deposited in the lung, beryllium is slowly absorbed into the blood. In patients accidentally exposed to beryllium dust, serum beryllium levels peak about 10 days after exposure with a biological half-life of 2–8 weeks (ATSDR, 2002). Gastrointestinal and dermal absorption of beryllium is low (<1%), but incidental oral exposure to soluble beryllium compounds or exposure through damaged skin may significantly contribute to total body burden (Deubner *et al.*, 2001). Most of the beryllium circulating in the blood is bound to serum proteins, such as prealbumins and globulins. A significant part of the inhaled beryllium is stored in the bone and lungs. More soluble beryllium compounds are distributed to the liver, lymph nodes, spleen, heart, muscle, skin, and kidney. Elimination of absorbed beryllium occurs mainly in the urine and only to a minor degree in the feces. Because of the long residence time of beryllium in the skeleton and lungs, its biological half-life is over one year (WHO, 1990; ATSDR, 2002).

Toxicity

Skin Effects Effects in the skin are the most common beryllium-related toxicity. Exposure to soluble beryllium compounds may result in conjunctivitis and papulovesicular dermatitis of the skin, which is likely an inflammatory response to beryllium. Beryllium exposure may also cause a delayed-type hypersensitivity reaction in skin, which is a cell-mediated immune response. If insoluble beryllium-containing materials become embedded under the skin, a chronic granulomatous lesion develops, which may be necrotizing and ulcerative. Skin is a route of beryllium exposure and sensitization, and the beryllium sulfate skin test and the beryllium lymphocyte proliferation test have been used to identify beryllium-sensitive individuals (Fontenot *et al.*, 2002; Tinkle *et al.*, 2003). Beryllium fluoride patch test may in itself be sensitizing, which has been replaced by the use of 1% beryllium sulfate (ATSDR, 2002; Fontenot *et al.*, 2002).

Acute Chemical Pneumonitis Inhalation of beryllium can cause a fulminating inflammatory reaction of the entire respiratory tract, involving the nasal passages, pharynx, tracheobronchial airways, and the alveoli. In the most severe cases, it produces acute fulminating pneumonitis. This occurs almost immediately following inhalation of aerosols of soluble beryllium compounds, particularly the fluoride, during the ore extraction process. Fatalities have occurred, although recovery is generally complete after a period of several weeks or even months.

Chronic Granulomatous Disease Berylliosis, or chronic beryllium disease (CBD), was first described among fluorescent lamp workers exposed to insoluble beryllium compounds, particularly beryllium oxide. Granulomatous inflammation of the lung, along with dyspnea on exertion, cough, chest pain, weight loss, fatigue, and general weakness, are the most typical features. Impaired lung function and hypertrophy of the right heart are also common. Chest X-ray shows miliary mottling. Histologically, the alveoli contain small interstitial granulomas resembling those seen in sarcoidosis. In severe cases, CBD may be accompanied by cyanosis and hypertrophic osteoarthropathy (WHO, 1990; ATSDR, 2002). Beryllium sensitization following initial exposure can progress to CBD (Newman *et al.*, 2005). As the lesions progress, interstitial fibrosis increases, with loss of functioning alveoli, impairment of effective air-capillary gas exchange, and increasing respiratory dysfunction. CBD involves an antigen-stimulated, cell-mediated immune response. Human leukocyte antigen, T cells, and proinflammatory cytokines (TNF-α and IL-6) are believed to be involved in the pathogenesis of CBD (Fontenot *et al.*, 2002; Day *et al.*, 2006).

Carcinogenicity A number of epidemiology studies in U.S. beryllium workers found that death due to lung cancer was increased, along with increased incidence of respiratory diseases. The increase in lung cancers are linked to high exposure levels which occurred prior to stricter exposure regulations introduced in the 1950s. The likelihood of lung cancer was greater in workers with acute beryllium disease than CBD (ATSDR, 2002; Gordon and Bowser, 2003). Beryllium has been classified as a human carcinogen (IARC, 1993).

Experimental studies confirmed carcinogenic potential of beryllium compounds by inhalation. For example, a single, short (<48 min) exposure to 410–980 mg/m^3 beryllium metal aerosol induced lung tumors in rats 14 months after exposure. Chronic beryllium sulfate inhalation (13 months, 0.034 mg Be/m^3) resulted in 100% lung tumor incidence in rats (Gordon and Bowser, 2003). Injection of beryllium compounds also induced osteosarcomas in rabbits (WHO, 1990). Beryllium compounds are negative in bacterial mutation assays. In mammalian cells, soluble beryllium compounds show weak mutagenic potential, but can induce malignant transformation. The ability of beryllium compounds to produce chromosomal aberrations is controversial, and appears to depend on the compound, dose, and experimental conditions (Gordon and Bowser, 2003). The carcinogenic mechanism of beryllium is not yet clear. Several molecular events can occur including oncogene activation (K-*ras*, c-*myc*, c-*fos*, c-*jun*, and c-*sis*), and tumor suppressor gene dysregulation (p53, p16), but mutations in *p53* or K-*ras* are not evident. Beryllium-induced lung tumors show hypermethylation of p16 leading to loss of expression, and have decreased expression of genes associated with DNA repair (Gordon and Bowser, 2003).

Cadmium

Cadmium (Cd) is a toxic transition metal that was discovered in 1817 as an impurity of "calamine" (zinc carbonate) for which it is named (from the Latin *cadmia*). Until recently the industrial use of cadmium was quite limited, but now it has become an important metal with many uses. About 75% of cadmium produced is used in batteries, especially nickel–cadmium batteries. Because of its noncorrosive properties, cadmium has been used in electroplating or galvanizing alloys for corrosion resistance. It is also used as a color pigment for paints and plastics, in solders, as a barrier to control nuclear fission, as a plastic stabilizer and in some special application alloys. This metal is typically found in ores with other metals, and is commercially produced as a byproduct of zinc and lead smelting, which are sources of environmental cadmium. Cadmium ranks close to lead and mercury as one of the top toxic substances (Jarup *et al.*, 1998; ATSDR, 1999).

Exposure   Food is the major source of cadmium for the general population. Many plants readily accumulate cadmium from soil. Both natural and anthropogenic sources of cadmium contamination occur for soil, including fallout of industrial emissions, some fertilizers, soil amendments, and use of cadmium-containing water for irrigation, all resulting in a slow but steady increase in the cadmium content in vegetables over the years (Jarup *et al.*, 1998). Shellfish accumulate relatively high levels of cadmium (1–2 mg/kg), and animal liver and kidney can have levels higher than 50 μg Cd/kg. Cereal grains such as rice and wheat, and tobacco concentrate cadmium to levels of 10–150 μg Cd/kg. With nearby industrial emission, air can be a significant source of direct exposure or environmental contamination. Total daily cadmium intake from all sources in North America and Europe ranges from 10 to 30 μg Cd/day. Of this about 10% or less is retained (Jarup *et al.*, 1998). Cigarette smoking is a major nonoccupational source of cadmium exposure, because of cadmium in the tobacco. Smoking is thought to roughly double the life-time body burden of cadmium (Satarug and Moore, 2004).

Historically, levels of cadmium in the workplace have dramatically improved with the appreciation of its potential toxicity in humans, development of safety restrictions, and improved industrial hygiene. Inhalation is the dominant route of exposure in occupational settings. Airborne cadmium in the present-day workplace environment is generally 5 μg/m^3 or less and occupational standards range from 2 to 50 μg/m^3. Occupations potentially at risk from cadmium exposure include those involved with refining zinc and lead ores, iron production, cement manufacture, and industries involving fossil fuel combustion, all of which can release airborne cadmium. Other occupations include the manufacture of paint pigments, cadmium-nickel batteries, and electroplating (WHO, 1992; ATSDR, 1999).

Toxicokinetics   Gastrointestinal absorption of cadmium is limited to 5–10% of a given dose. Cadmium absorption can be increased by dietary deficiencies of calcium or iron and by diets low in protein. In the general population, women have higher blood cadmium levels than men, possibly due to increased oral cadmium absorption because of relatively low iron stores in women of childbearing age. Indeed, women showing low serum ferritin levels have twice the normal rate of oral cadmium absorption (Berglund *et al.*, 1994). It has recently been shown that rats on an iron-deficient diet have an increased absorption of cadmium, which correlated with the upreg-ulation of the iron transporter, DMT, which transports both iron and cadmium (Ryu *et al.*, 2004). Absorption of cadmium after inhalation is generally greater, ranging from 5 to 35%, depending on the specific compound, site of deposition, and particle size. For instance, 50% of cadmium fumes, as generated in cigarette smoke, may be absorbed. It is thought that as much as 100% of cadmium eventually reaching the alveoli can be transferred to blood (Satarug and Moore, 2004).

Once absorbed, cadmium is very poorly excreted and only about 0.001% of the body burden is excreted per day. Both urinary and fecal excretory routes are operative (ATSDR, 1999; Satarug and Moore, 2004). Cadmium transport into cells is mediated through calcium channels (Leslie *et al.*, 2006) and through molecular mimicry (Zalpus and Ahmad, 2003). Gastrointestinal excretion occurs through the bile as a glutathione complex. Cadmium excretion in urine increases relative to body burden (Friberg *et al.*, 1986; ATSDR, 1999). Cadmium is nephrotoxic, and when renal pathology is present the urinary excretion of cadmium is increased due to decreased renal absorption of filtered cadmium (Zalpus and Ahmad, 2003).

The relationship of cadmium metabolism and toxicity is shown in Fig. 23-3. Cadmium is transported in blood by binding to albumin and other larger molecular-weight proteins. It is rapidly taken up by tissues and is primarily deposited in the liver and to a lesser extent in the kidney. In the liver, kidney, and other tissues, cadmium induces the synthesis of metallothionein (MT), a low-molecular-weight, high affinity metal-binding protein (Klaassen *et al.*, 1999). Cadmium is stored in the liver primarily as cadmium–MT. Cadmium–MT may be released from the liver and transported via blood to the kidney, where it is reabsorbed and degraded in the lysosomes of the renal tubules. This releases cadmium to induce more cadmium–MT complex or cause renal toxicity.

Blood cadmium levels in nonoccupationally exposed, nonsmokers are usually less than 1 μg/L. Cadmium does not readily cross the placenta. Breast milk is not a major source of early life exposure. About 50–75% of the retained cadmium is found in the liver and kidneys. The biological half-life of cadmium in humans is not known exactly, but is probably in the range of 10–30 years.

Toxicity   Acute, high-dose cadmium toxicity in humans is now a rare event. Acute cadmium toxicity from the ingestion of high concentrations of cadmium in the form of heavily contaminated beverages or food causes severe irritation to the gastrointestinal epithelium. Symptoms include nausea, vomiting, and abdominal pain. Inhalation of cadmium fumes or other heated cadmium-containing materials may produce acute pneumonitis with pulmonary edema. Inhalation of large doses of cadmium can be lethal for humans (ATSDR, 1999). Acute cadmium toxicity depends on solubility of cadmium compounds (ATSDR, 1999). For instance, with acute inhalation exposures, the more soluble cadmium chloride, oxide fume, and carbonate are more toxic than the relatively less soluble sulfide (Klimisch, 1993). The major long-term toxic effects of low-level cadmium exposure are renal injury, obstructive pulmonary disease, osteoporosis, and cardiovascular disease. Cancer is primarily a concern in occupationally exposed groups. The chronic toxic effects of cadmium are clearly a much greater concern than the rare acute toxic exposures.

Nephrotoxicity   Cadmium is toxic to tubular cells and glomeruli, markedly impairing renal function. Pathologically, these lesions

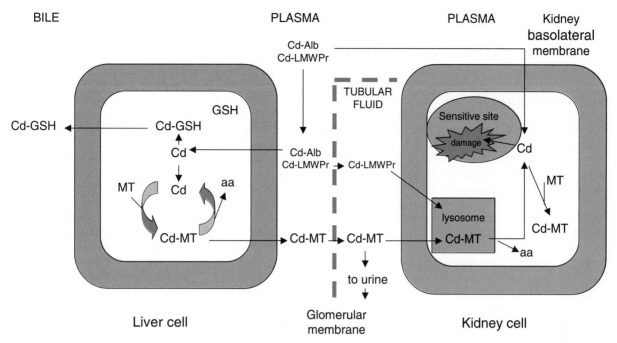

Figure 23-3. *Cadmium Transport, Protein-Binding, and Toxicity.*

GSH, glutathione; MT, metallothionein; aa, amino acids; Cd-Alb, Cd-albumin; Cd-LMWPr, Cd associated with low molecular weight proteins.

consist of initial tubular cell necrosis and degeneration, progressing to an interstitial inflammation and fibrosis. There appears to be a critical concentration of cadmium in the renal cortex that, once exceeded, is associated with tubular dysfunction. This concentration depends on the individual, and chronic cadmium nephropathy is seen in about 10% of the population at renal concentrations of ~200 μg/g and in about 50% of the population at about 300 μg/g. Because of the potential for renal toxicity, there is considerable concern about the levels of dietary cadmium intake for the general population. In fact, it is thought that upwards of 7% of the general population may have significant cadmium-induced kidney alterations due to chronic exposure with kidney cadmium levels as low as 50 μg/g (Jarup *et al.*, 1998).

Cadmium-induced renal toxicity is reflected by proteinuria as a result of renal tubular dysfunction. The predominant proteins include β_2-microglobulin, *N*-acetyl-β-D-glucosaminidase (NAG), and MT, as well as retinol-binding protein, lysozyme, ribonuclease, α_1-microglobulin, and immunoglobulin light chains (Bernard, 2004; Chen *et al.*, 2006). The presence of larger proteins, like albumin and transferrin, in the urine after occupational cadmium exposure suggests a glomerular effect as well. The pathogenesis of the glomerular lesion in cadmium nephropathy is not well understood (Bernard, 2004). Urinary excretions of proteins and cadmium have been used as biomarkers for cadmium exposure.

The induction of MT by cadmium and the subsequent sequestration of cadmium as the cadmium–MT complex likely protect tissues from cadmium toxicity. However, if cadmium–MT complex is injected it is acutely nephrotoxic (Nordberg, 2004). This led to the hypothesis that the cadmium–MT complex was responsible for chronic cadmium nephropathy. In this scenario, cadmium–MT released from the liver would be filtered by the kidney and reabsorbed in proximal tubule cells, where it is degraded releasing locally high levels of "free" cadmium (Fig. 23-3). Nephrotoxicity in normal rats following liver transplantation from cadmium-exposed

rats supported this hypothesis (Chan *et al.*, 1993). However, MT-null mice, which are unable to produce the major forms of MT, are hypersensitive to chronic cadmium nephropathy (Liu *et al.*, 1998a), suggesting that cadmium nephropathy is not necessarily mediated through the cadmium–MT complex. Kidney pathology from a single injection of cadmium–MT also differs greatly from that induced by chronic oral inorganic cadmium exposure (Liu *et al.*, 1998b). Inorganic cadmium can be taken into the kidney from the basolateral membrane, and is more toxic than cadmium–MT to cultured renal cells (Prozialeck *et al.*, 1993; Liu *et al.*, 1994; Zalpus and Ahmad, 2003). It is likely that inorganic cadmium can bind to other low-molecular proteins or other complexes for renal uptake, and these complexes can contribute to chronic cadmium nephropathy (Zalpus and Ahmad, 2003).

Chronic Pulmonary Disease   Cadmium inhalation is toxic to the respiratory system in a fashion related to the dose and duration of exposure. Cadmium-induced obstructive lung disease in humans can be slow in onset, and results from chronic bronchitis, progressive fibrosis of the lower airways, and accompanying alveolar damage leading to emphysema. Pulmonary function is reduced with dyspnea, reduced vital capacity, and increased residual volume. The pathogenesis of these lung lesions is not completely understood, but can be duplicated in rodents (WHO, 1992; ATSDR, 1999). The chronic effects of cadmium on the lung clearly increased the mortality of cadmium workers with high exposure.

Skeletal Effects   Occupational cadmium exposure is a well recognized cause for renal tubular dysfunction associated with hypercalciuria, renal stone formation, osteomalacia, and osteoporosis (Kazantzis, 2004). The long-term consumption of cadmium-contaminated rice caused *Itai-Itai* disease, which occurred mostly in multiparous elderly women and was characterized by severe osteomalacia and osteoporosis, resulting in bone deformities and concomitant renal dysfunction. Vitamin D deficiency and perhaps other nutritional deficiencies are thought to be cofactors in *Itai-Itai* disease. Issues with loss of bone density, height loss, and increased bone fractures have now been reported in populations exposed to far lower levels of environmental cadmium than *Itai-Itai* victims (Kazantzis, 2004). Cadmium affects calcium metabolism, at least partially through renal dysfunction, and excess excretion of calcium often occurs in the urine. The skeletal changes are probably related to calcium loss and interference with the actions of parathyroid hormone and vitamin D. Cadmium may also act directly on bone and animal studies have shown the metal stimulates osteoclast activity, resulting in the breakdown of bone matrix. Cadmium in bone interferes with calcification and bone remodeling (Wang and Bhattacharyya, 1993). In accord with human victims of *Itai-Itai*, multiparity in mice enhances the osteotoxicity of cadmium (Bhattacharyya *et al.*, 1988).

Cardiovascular Effects   Some epidemiologic evidence suggests cadmium may be an etiologic agent for cardiovascular disease including hypertension, although these associations are not observed in all studies (Jarup *et al.*, 1998). The population-based U.S. NHANES II study and studies in Belgium (Staessen *et al.*, 1996) have not supported a role for cadmium in the etiology of hypertension or cardiovascular disease in humans. Animal studies indicate that cadmium may be toxic to myocardium (Kopp *et al.*, 1982), although the relevance of these results to humans is not clear.

Neurotoxicity   There is only limited data from animals and humans that cadmium can be neurotoxic (Jarup *et al.*, 1998; ATSDR, 1999). Studies in humans have suggested a relationship between abnormal behavior and/or decreased intelligence in children and adults exposed to cadmium, but are typically complicated by exposure to other toxic metals. Furthermore, the blood–brain barrier severely limits cadmium access to the central nervous system, and a direct toxic effect appears to occur only with cadmium exposure prior to blood–brain barrier formation (young children), or with blood–brain barrier dysfunction under certain pathological conditions. Additionally, the choroid plexus epithelium may accumulate high levels of cadmium reducing access to other areas (Zheng, 2001). Although a special form of MT (MT-3) occurs in the brain, the role of MT in cadmium neurotoxicity is incompletely defined (Klaassen *et al.*, 1999).

Carcinogenicity   Cadmium compounds are considered to be human carcinogens (IARC, 1993; NTP, 2004). In humans, occupational respiratory exposure to cadmium has been most clearly associated with lung cancer (IARC, 1993; NTP, 2004). Early human studies also indicated a possible link to cancer of the prostate, which has not been confirmed by more recent work (Sahmoun *et al.*, 2005), despite evidence that the prostate can be a target of cadmium carcinogenesis in rats (Waalkes, 2003). Both the kidney and pancreas accumulate high concentrations of cadmium and exposure to cadmium may also be associated with human renal (Il'yasora and Schwartz, 2005) and pancreatic cancer (Schwartz and Reis, 2000; Kriegel *et al.*, 2006).

Multiple rodent studies have confirmed that inhalation of various cadmium compounds will lead to lung cancer (IARC, 1993; Waalkes, 2003; NTP, 2004). Lung tumors can also be produced by systemic cadmium exposure in mice (Waalkes, 2003). Beyond the lung, in rodents cadmium can produce a variety of tumors, including malignant tumors at the site of repository injection (subcutaneous, etc.). Compounds such as cadmium chloride, oxide, sulfate, sulfide, and cadmium powder produce local sarcomas in rodents after subcutaneous or intramuscular injections. A single injection can be effective, but multiple injections of cadmium at the same site cause more aggressive sarcomas that show a higher rate of local invasion and distant metastasis. The relevance of injection site sarcoma production to human cancer is unclear. Cadmium also induces tumors of the testes, specifically benign Leydig cell tumors, but this is likely due to a high-dose mechanism involving acute testicular necrosis, degenerative testicular atrophy, and subsequent over-stimulation by luteinizing hormone, factors very likely of limited relevance in humans (Waalkes, 2003). Other studies have found that cadmium exposure can induce tumors of the pancreas, adrenals, liver, kidney, pituitary, and hematopoietic system in mice, rats, or hamsters. Cadmium can be carcinogenic in animals after inhalation or oral administration or by various injection routes (Waalkes, 2003). Various studies indicate zinc administration will generally block cadmium carcinogenesis, whereas dietary zinc deficiency can enhance the response (IARC, 1993; Waalkes, 2003; NTP, 2004). The mechanism of cadmium carcinogenesis is poorly understood (Waalkes, 2003).

Treatment   At the present time, there is no effective clinical treatment for cadmium intoxication. In experimental systems some chelators can reduce acute cadmium-induced mortality (Klaassen *et al.*, 1984), but chelation therapy for cadmium generally results in significant adverse effects.

Chromium

Chromium (Cr) was named from the Greek word "*chroma*" meaning color, because of the many colorful compounds made from it. Chromium is part of the mineral crocoite (lead chromate), and the element was first isolated in 1798. Hexavalent chromium (Cr^{6+}) is a by-product of various industrial processes. Hexavalent chromium is a human carcinogen and produces a variety of toxic effects (ATSDR, 2000). The major industrial source of chromium is from chromite ore. Chromates are produced by smelting, roasting, and extraction processes. Ferrochrome is used for the production of stainless steel and alloys. Sodium chromate and dichromate are the principal substances for the production of chromium chemicals. Chromium compounds are used for plating, leather tanning, and the manufacture of dyes and pigments, cooking utensils and as wood preservatives (ATSDR, 2000). Chromium in ambient air originates primarily from industrial sources, particularly ferrochrome production, ore refining, and chemical processing. Chromium fallout is deposited on land and water, and eventually, in sediments. Widespread industrial uses have increased chromium levels in the environment. The hexavalent chromium compounds are also toxic to the ecosystems, and microbial and plant variants occur that adapt to high chromium levels in the eco-environment (Cervantes *et al.*, 2001). Up to 38% of drinking water supplies in California have detectable levels of hexavalent chromium, but little is known about the health effects from environmental exposures (Costa and Klein, 2006; Sedman *et al.*, 2006). Cobalt-chromium alloy hip replacement can increase blood levels of chromium (Bhamra and Case, 2006).

Trivalent chromium (Cr^{3+}) is a naturally occurring essential trace nutrient important for glucose metabolism and will be discussed separately in the "Essential Metal" section.

Toxicokinetics Absorption of hexavalent chromium compounds is higher (2–10%) than that of trivalent chromium compounds (0.5–2%). Hexavalent chromium readily crosses cell membranes on carriers for sulfate and phosphate, whereas the less insoluble trivalent chromium compounds are absorbed via passive diffusion and phagocytosis. Absorption of inhaled chromium compounds takes place in the lung via transfer across alveolar cell membranes. Dermal absorption depends on the chemical form, the vehicle, and the integrity of the skin. Concentrated potassium chromate may cause chemical burns in the skin that facilitate absorption. Once in the blood, hexavalent chromium is taken up by erythrocytes, whereas trivalent chromium is only loosely associated with erythrocytes. Chromium compounds are distributed to all organs of the body, with high levels in liver, spleen, and kidney. Particles containing chromium can be retained in the lungs for years. Absorbed chromium is excreted primarily in urine. The half-life for excretion of potassium chromium is about 35–40 hours (ATSDR, 2000; Sedman *et al.*, 2006).

Once hexavalent chromium enters cells, it is reduced intracellularly by ascorbic acid, glutathione, and/or cysteine, ultimately to trivalent chromium. It is thought that the toxicity of hexavalent chromium compounds results from damage to cellular components during this process, including the generation of free radicals and the formation of DNA adducts (Zhitkovich, 2005).

Toxicity Toxic effects have been attributed primarily to airborne hexavalent chromium compounds in industrial settings. Hexavalent chromium is corrosive and may cause chronic ulceration and perforation of the nasal septum, as well as chronic ulceration of other skin surfaces (ATSDR, 2000). Hexavalent chromium elicits allergic contact dermatitis among previously sensitized individuals, which is a type-IV allergic reaction inducing skin erythema, pruritus, edema, papule, and scars. The prevalence of chromium sensitivity is less than 1% among the general population (Proctor *et al.*, 1998). Occupational exposure to chromium may be a cause of asthma (Bright *et al.*, 1997). Accidental ingestion of high doses of hexavalent chromium compounds may cause acute renal failure characterized by proteinuria, hematuria, and anuria, but kidney damage from lower-level chronic exposure is equivocal (ATSDR, 2000).

Carcinogenicity Occupational exposure to hexavalent chromium compounds, particularly in the chrome production and pigment industries, is associated with increased risk of lung caner, and hexavalent chromium-containing compounds are considered to be human carcinogens (IARC, 1990). Hexavalent chromium compounds are genotoxic. A review of more than 700 sets of short-term genotoxicity test results with 32 chromium compounds revealed 88% of hexavalent chromium compounds were positive, as a function of solubility and bioavailability to target cells (De Flora, 2000). Trivalent chromium compounds were generally nongenotoxic, probably because trivalent chromium is not readily taken up by cells (De Flora, 2000). Once hexavalent chromium enters the cell, it is reduced by various intracellular reductants to give reactive trivalent chromium species. During the reduction process, various genetic lesions can be generated, including chromium–DNA adducts, DNA protein cross-links, DNA–chromium intrastrand cross-links, DNA strand breaks, and oxidized DNA bases (O'Brien *et al.*, 2003; Zhitkovich, 2005). Hexavalent chromium compounds are mutagenic, causing base substitutions, deletions, and transversions in bacterial systems, and hypoxanthine guanine phosphoribosyl transferase, *supF* muta-

tions, etc., in mammalian mutagenesis systems (Cohen *et al.*, 1993; O'Brien *et al.*, 2003).

Hexavalent chromium compounds also react with other cellular constituents during the intracellular reduction process. They can cause the generation of reactive oxygen radicals, inhibit protein synthesis and arrest DNA replication. Hexavalent chromium can also cause disturbances of the p53 signaling pathway, cell cycle arrest, apoptosis, interference of DNA damage repair, and neoplastic transformation. All these effects could well play an integrated role in chromium carcinogenesis (O'Brien *et al.*, 2003; Costa and Klein, 2006).

Inhaled chromium compounds can penetrate to many tissues in the body, and thus have the potential to cause cancer at sites other than the lung. Accumulating evidence indicates an association between cancers of the bone, prostate, hematopoietic system, stomach, kidney, and urinary bladder and hexavalent chromium exposure (Costa, 1997). Furthermore, exposure of hexavalent chromium compounds through the drinking water enhances UV-induced skin cancer in the hairless mouse model (Costa and Klein, 2006). An association of hexavalent chromium in the drinking water with stomach cancer has also been reported (Sedman *et al.*, 2006).

Lead

Lead (Pb) has been used by humans for at least 7000 years, because it is widespread, easy to extract, and easy to work with. It is highly malleable and ductile as well as easy to smelt. In the early Bronze Age, lead was used with antimony and arsenic. Lead's elemental symbol Pb, is an abbreviation of its Latin name *plumbum*. Lead in lead compounds primarily exists in the divalent form. Metallic lead (Pb^0) is resistant to corrosion and can combine other metals to form various alloys. Organolead compounds are dominated by Pb^{4+}. Inorganic lead compounds are used as pigments in paints, dyes, and ceramic glazes. Organolead compounds were used as gasoline additives. Lead alloys are used in batteries, shields from radiation, water pipes, and ammunition. Environmental lead comes mainly from human activity and is listed as a top toxic substance (ATSDR, 2005c). The phasing out of leaded gasoline, the removal of lead from paint, solder, and water supply pipes have significantly lowered blood lead levels (BLL) in the general population. Lead exposure in children still remains a major health concern. Lead is not biodegradable and the concerns for ecotoxicity of lead are increasing. For instance, the leaded fish sinkers or pellets lost in the bottom of lakes and river banks can be mistaken for stone and ingested by birds causing adverse effects including death (De Francisco *et al.*, 2003).

Exposure Lead-containing paint is a primary source of lead exposure in children. Major environmental sources of lead for infants and toddlers up to 4 years of age is hand-to-mouth transfer of lead-containing paint chips or dust from floors of older housing (Manton *et al.*, 2000). Lead in household dust can also come from outside of the home and may be related to lead in neighborhood soil (von Lindren *et al.*, 2003). A major route of exposure for the general population is from food and water. Dietary intake of lead has decreased dramatically in recent years, and for infants, toddlers, and young children is <5 μg/day (Manton *et al.*, 2005). A review by the EPA in 2004 found lead levels in 71% of the water systems in the US showed <5 μg Pb/L (ppb). Only 3.6% exceeded the action level of 15 ppb. Lead in urban air is generally higher than rural air. Air lead in rural areas of eastern United States is typically 6–10 ng/m³ (ATSDR, 2005c).

Other potential sources of lead exposure are recreational shooting, hand-loading ammunition, soldering, jewelry making, pottery making, gun smithing, glass polishing, painting, and stained glass crafting. Workplace exposure is gradually being reduced. Herbal medicines could be potential sources of lead exposure. Certain Ayurvedic herbal products were found to be contaminated with lead ranging up to 37 mg/g and over 55 cases of lead poisoning have been related to the ingestion of herbal medicines (Patrick, 2006).

Blood lead levels (BLL) are commonly used for monitoring human exposure to lead. The uses of other biomarkers for lead exposure have been critically reviewed (Barbosa *et al.*, 2005).

Toxicokinetics   Adults absorb 5–15% of ingested lead and usually retain less than 5% of what is absorbed. Children absorb 42% of ingested lead with 32% retention (Ziegler *et al.*, 1978). Lead absorption can be enhanced by low dietary iron and calcium, especially in children (Mahaffey, 1985). Airborne lead is a minor component of exposure. Lead absorption by the lungs depends on the form (vapor versus particle), particle size, and concentration. About 90% of lead particles in ambient air that are inhaled are small enough to be retained. Absorption of retained lead through alveoli is relatively efficient.

Lead in blood is primarily (99%) in erythrocytes bound to hemoglobin, only 1% of circulating lead in serum is available for tissue distribution (ATSDR, 2005c). Lead is initially distributed to soft tissues such as kidney and liver, and then redistributed to skeleton and hair. The half-life of lead in blood is about 30 days. The fraction of lead in bone increases with age from 70% of body burden in childhood to as much as 95% in adulthood, with a half-life of about 20 years. Lead in trabecular bone is more labile and has a shorter turnover time than cortical bone. Lead released from bones may contribute up to 50% of the lead in blood, and is a significant source of endogenous exposure. Bone lead release may be important in adults with accumulated occupational exposure and in women due to bone resorption during pregnancy, lactation, menopause, and from osteoporosis (Silbergeld *et al.*, 1988; Gulson, *et al.*, 2003). Lead crosses the placenta, so that cord blood generally correlates with maternal BLL but is often slightly lower. Lead accumulation in fetal tissues, including brain, is proportional to maternal BLL (Goyer, 1996).

The major route of excretion of absorbed lead is the kidney. Renal excretion of lead is usually through glomerular filtrate with some renal tubular resorption. Fecal excretion via biliary tract accounts for one-third of total excretion of absorbed lead (ATSDR, 2005c).

Physiological-based pharmacokinetic (PBPK) models have been developed for lead risk assessment. The O'Flaherty model is a model for children and adults; The integrated exposure uptake (IEUBK) model is developed by EPA for predicting BLL in children. The Leggett model allows simulation of lifetime exposures and can be used to predict blood lead in both children and adults (ATSDR, 2005c).

Toxicity   Lead can induce a wide range of adverse effects in humans depending on the dose and duration of exposure. The toxic effects range from inhibition of enzymes to the production of severe pathology or death (Goyer, 1990). Children are most sensitive to effects in the central nervous system, while in adults peripheral neuropathy, chronic nephropathy, and hypertension are concerns. Other target tissues include the gastrointestinal, immune, skeletal,

and reproductive systems. Effects on the heme biosynthesis provide a sensitive biochemical indicator even in the absence of other detectable effects.

Neurological, Neurobehavioral, and Developmental Effects in Children   Clinically overt lead encephalopathy may occur in children with high exposure to lead, probably at BLL of 70 μg/dL or higher. Symptoms of lead encephalopathy begin with lethargy, vomiting, irritability, loss of appetite, and dizziness, progressing to obvious ataxia, and a reduced level of consciousness, which may progress to coma and death. The pathological findings at autopsy are severe edema of the brain due to extravasations of fluid from capillaries in the brain. This is accompanied by the loss of neuronal cells and an increase in glial cells. Recovery is often accompanied by sequelae including epilepsy, mental retardation, and, in some cases, optic neuropathy and blindness (Goyer, 1990; Bellinger, 2004; ATSDR, 2005c; Laraque and Trasande, 2005).

The most sensitive indicators of adverse neurological outcomes are psychomotor tests or mental development indices, and broad measures of IQ. Most studies report a 2- to 4-point IQ deficit for each μg/dL increase in BLL within the range of 5–35 μg/dL. The Centers for Disease Control and Prevention set the goal of eliminating ≥ 10 μg/dL BLL in children by 2010 (CDC, 2005). However, effects of lead on IQ may occur below this level (Bellinger, 2004). Recent studies found that deficits in cognitive and academic skills could occur with BLL < 5.0 μg/dL (Lamphear *et al.*, 2000). A study of a cohort of children from pregnancy through 10 years of age found that lead exposure around 28 weeks of gestation is a critical period for later child intellectual development, and lead's effect on IQ occurs with first few μgs of BLL (Schnaas *et al.*, 2006).

Lead can affect the brain by multiple mechanisms (Goyer, 1996; ATSDR, 2005c). Lead may act as a surrogate for calcium and/or disrupt calcium homeostasis. The stimulation of protein kinase C may result in alteration of blood–brain barrier and inhibition of cholinergic modulation of glutamate-related synaptic transmissions. Lead affects virtually every neurotransmitter system in the brain, including glutamatergic, dopaminergic, and cholinergic systems. All these systems play a critical role in synaptic plasticity and cellular mechanisms for cognitive function, learning, and memory.

Neurotoxic Effects in Adults   Adults with occupational exposure may demonstrate abnormalities in a number of measures in neurobehavior with cumulative exposures resulting from BLL > 40 μg/dL (Lindgren *et al.*, 1996). Peripheral neuropathy is a classic manifestation of lead toxicity in adults. More than a half-century ago, footdrop and wristdrop characterized the house painter and other workers with excessive occupational exposure to lead but are rare today. Peripheral neuropathy is characterized by segmental demyelination and possibly axonal degeneration. Motor nerve dysfunction, assessed clinically by electrophysiological measurement of nerve conduction velocities, occurred with BLL as low as 40 μg/dL (Goyer, 1990).

Hematologic Effects   Lead has multiple hematologic effects, ranging from increased urinary porphyrins, coproporphyrins, δ-aminolevulinic acid (ALA), and zinc-protoporphyrin to anemia. The heme biosynthesis pathway and the sites of lead interference are shown in Fig. 23-4. The most sensitive effects of lead are the inhibition of δ-aminolevulinic acid dehydratase (ALAD) and ferrochelatase. ALAD catalyzes the condensation of two units of ALA to form phorphobilinogen (PBG). Inhibition of ALAD results in

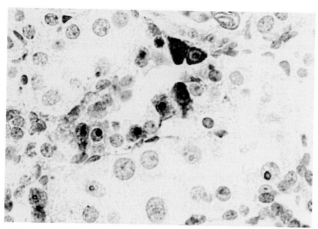

Figure 23-4. Metallothionein Intensity and Localization in Lead-Induced Nuclear Inclusion Bodies from the Kidneys of Wild-type Mice.

Immunohistochemical assessment of a representative section including inclusion bodies showing intense surface staining for metallothionein (*dark brown*; x400) (From Waalkes *et al.*, 2004c, with permission).

accumulation of ALA. Ferrochelatase catalyzes the insertion of iron into the protoporphyrin ring to form heme. Inhibition of ferrochelatase results in accumulation of protophorphyrin IX, which takes the place of heme in the hemoglobin molecule and, as the erythrocytes containing protoporphyrin IX circulate, zinc is chelated at the site usually occupied by iron. Erythrocytes containing zinc-protoporphyrin are intensely fluorescent and may be used to diagnose lead exposure. Feeding lead to experimental animals also raises

heme oxygenase activity, resulting in increases in bilirubin formation. Anemia only occurs in very marked cases of lead toxicity, and is microcytic and hypochromic, as in iron deficiency. The changes in ALAD in peripheral blood and excretion of ALA in urine correlate with BLL and serve as early biochemical indices of lead exposure (ATSDR, 2005c).

Genetic polymorphisms have been identified for alleles of the *ALAD* gene which may affect the toxicokinetics of lead. However, no firm evidence exists for an association between *ALAD* genotype and susceptibility to lead toxicity at background exposures, and thus, population testing for *ALAD* polymorphism is not justified (Kelada *et al.*, 2001).

Renal Toxicity   Acute lead nephrotoxicity consists of proximal tubular dysfunction and can be reversed by treatment with chelating agents. Chronic lead nephrotoxicity consists of interstitial fibrosis and progressive nephron loss, azotaemia and renal failure (Goyer, 1989). A characteristic microscopic change is the presence of intranuclear inclusion bodies (Fig. 23-5). By light microscopy the inclusions are dense, homogeneous, and are eosinophilic with hematoxylin and eosin staining. The bodies are composed of a lead–protein complex. The protein is acidic and contains large amounts of aspartic and glutamic acids with little cystine. The inclusion bodies are a form of aggresome accumulating large amounts of lead in a relatively inert, nontoxic state. Metallothionein-null mice cannot form inclusion bodies following lead treatment and are hyper-sensitive to lead-induced nephropathy and carcinogenesis, suggesting that lead inclusion body formation requires metallothionein as a participant (Qu *et al.*, 2002; Waalkes *et al.*, 2004c). In fact, metallothionein is found on the outer surface of lead inclusion bodies, indicating

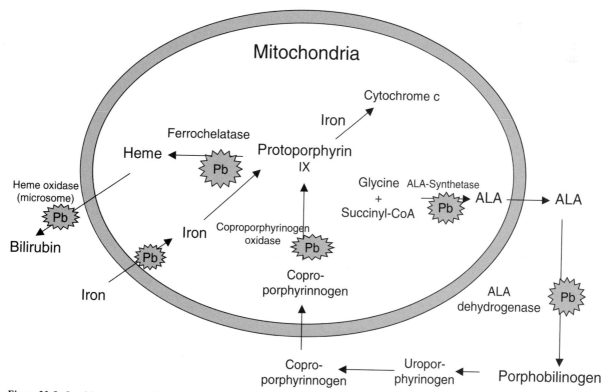

Figure 23-5. Lead Interruption of Heme Biosynthesis.

ALA, δ-aminolevulinate; Pb, sites for lead effects. The major lead inhibition sites are ALA dehydrogenase and ferrochelatase.

that it may transport the metal to the forming inclusion (Waalkes *et al.*, 2004c). Lead nephrotoxicity impairs the renal synthesis of heme-containing enzymes in the kidney, such as heme-containing hydroxylase involved in vitamin D metabolism causing bone effects (ATSDR, 2005c). Hyperuricemia with gout occur more frequently in the presence of lead nephropathy (Batuman, 1993). Lead nephropathy is also a cause of hypertension (Gonick and Behari, 2002).

Effects on Cardiovascular System   There is evidence of a causal relationship between lead exposure and hypertension (Gonick and Behari, 2002; ATSDR, 2005c). A study related bone lead with blood pressure in a cohort of 590 men that indicated an increase in hypertension for individuals with elevated bone lead (Hu *et al.*, 1996). Analysis of data from the National Health and Nutrition Examination Survey (NHANES II) for the U.S. population, including BLL and blood pressure measurements in a general population (5803 people aged 12–74), found a correlation between BLL at relatively low levels and blood pressure (Harlan, 1988). An epidemiology reappraisal using meta-analysis of 58,518 subjects from both the general population and occupationally exposed groups from 1980 to 2001 suggested a weak, but significant association between BLL and blood pressure (Nawrot *et al.*, 2002). Elevated blood pressure is more pronounced in middle age than at young age (ATSDR, 2005c).

A review of chronic lead exposure on blood pressure in experimental animals indicated that at lower doses, lead consistently produced hypertension effects, whereas at higher doses results are inconsistent (Victery, 1988). The pathogenesis of lead-induced hypertension is multifactorial including: (1) inactivation of endogenous nitric oxide and cGMP, possibly through lead-induced reactive oxygen species; (2) changes in the rennin–angiotensin–aldosterone system, and increases in sympathetic activity, important humoral components of hypertension; (3) alterations in calcium-activated functions of vascular smooth muscle cells including contractility by decreasing Na^+/K^+-ATPase activity and stimulation of the Na^+/Ca^{++} exchange pump; and (4) a possible rise in endothelin and thromboxane (Gonick and Behari, 2002; Vaziri and Sica, 2004).

Immunotoxicity   The developing immune system is sensitive to toxic effects of lead (Dietert *et al.*, 2004). A hallmark of lead-induced immunotoxicity is a pronounced shift in the balance in T helper cell function toward Th2 responses at the expense of Th1 functions, resulting in elevated IgE levels. Increased IgE levels and inflammatory cytokines were found in lead-exposed neonatal rodents, and there is an association between BLL and elevated IgE levels in children (Karmaus *et al.*, 2005; Luebke *et al.*, 2006). Thus, lead immunotoxicity might be a risk factor for childhood asthma (Dietert *et al.*, 2004). In experimental animals, lead has been shown to target macrophages and T cells, especially CD4+ T cells. In occupational exposure, lead-associated changes include altered T-cell subpopulations, reduced immunoglobin levels, and reduced polymorphonuclear leukocyte chemotactic activity (Dietert *et al.*, 2004; Luebke *et al.*, 2006).

Bone Effects   Lead has an extremely long half-life in bone, accounting for over 90% of the body lead in adults. Lead can affect bone by interfering with metabolic and homeostatic mechanisms including parathyroid hormone, calcitonin, vitamin D, and other hormones that influence calcium metabolism. Lead substitutes for calcium in bone (Pounds *et al.*, 1991). Lead is known to affect osteoblasts, osteoclasts, and chrondrocytes and has been associated with osteoporosis and delays in fracture repair (Carmouche *et al.*,

2005). In children exposed to lead, a higher bone mineral density (BMD) was observed. This may be due to accelerated bone maturation through inhibition of parathyroid hormone-related peptide, may ultimately result in lower peak BMD in young adulthood, and might predispose subjects to osteoporosis later in life (Campbell *et al.*, 2004). A positive association between lead exposure and dental caries in children has been shown in a number of studies. Lead is deposited in teeth, inhibits mineralization of enamel and dentine, and affects metabolism of the cells in the dental pulp (ATSDR, 2005c).

Other Effects   Lead colic is a major gastrointestinal symptom of severe lead poisoning, and is characterized by abdominal pain, nausea, vomiting, constipation, and cramps (ATSDR, 2005c). It is rarely seen today.

Lead-induced gametotoxic effects have been demonstrated in both male and female animals (Goyer, 1990). There is also evidence that lead may disrupt the hypothalamic–pituitary–gonadal axis. An increase in the maternal BLL may also contribute to premature birth and reduced birth weight (ATSDR, 2005c).

Carcinogenicity   The association of lead exposure with increased human cancer risk was strengthened by recent studies (ATSDR, 2005c), and inorganic lead compounds were recently reclassified as probably carcinogenic to humans (IARC, 2004). A study of a cohort of 20,700 workers coexposed to lead and engine exhaust found a 1.4 fold increase in the overall cancer incidence and a 1.8 fold increase in lung cancer among those who ever had elevated BLLs (Anttila *et al.*, 1995). Another epidemiological study of 27,060 brain cancer cases and 108,240 controls that died of nonmalignant disease in US from 1984 to 1992 provides evidence for a potential link between occupational exposure to lead and brain cancer (Cocco *et al.*, 1998). A meta-analysis of published data on cancer incidence among workers in various industries with lead exposure indicates a significant excess of cancer deaths from stomach cancer, lung cancer, and bladder cancer (Fu and Boffetta, 1995). Analysis of eight principal studies with well-documented lead exposures suggests associations of lead exposure with increased lung and stomach cancers (Steenland and Boffetta, 2000). However, workers were not only exposed to lead alone, and exposures to other potential carcinogens such as arsenic, cadmium, and engine exhausts could confound these interpretations. Lead does not appear to be directly genotoxic in vivo or in vitro, and lead may interact with other toxicants to facilitate chemical carcinogenesis (Silbergeld, 2003).

Lead is a nephrocarcinogen in adult rodents (Waalkes *et al.*, 1995, 2004c; IARC, 2006). Lead-induced renal tumors also occur after perinatal exposure in the absence of the extensive chronic nephropathy (Waalkes *et al.*, 1995). Metallothionein-null mice, which do not form lead inclusion bodies, are hypersensitive to lead-induced proliferative lesions of the kidney (Waalkes *et al.*, 2004c).

Several mechanisms have been proposed for lead-induced carcinogenesis, including regenerative repair, inhibition of DNA synthesis or repair, generation of reactive oxygen species with oxidative damage to DNA, substitution of lead for zinc in transcriptional regulators, interaction with DNA-binding proteins, and aberrant gene expression (Silbergeld *et al.*, 2000; Qu *et al.*, 2002; Silbergeld, 2003).

Treatment   Chelation therapy is warranted in workmen with BLL > 60 μg/dL. For children, criteria have been established (Laraque and

Table 23-1

Blood Lead Levels (BLL) in Children as an Indicator for Risk Assessment

BLL (μG/DL)	RISK LEVEL	POTENTIAL EFFECT WITH BLL (μG/DL)
<10	I	
10–14	II, moderate	IQ Deficits (10–15), ALA-D inhibition (10)
15–19	II, moderate	Developmental effects (10–15)
20–44	III, high	Increased U-ALA (40), decrease nerve, conduction velocity, hearing, vitamin D metabolism
45–69	IV, urgent	Nephropathy, colic (40–60)
>70	V, emergency	Encephalopathy, anemia (80–100)

Trasande, 2005) that may serve as guidelines to assist in evaluating the individual case with potential health effects (Table 23-1). The oral chelating agent dimercaptosuccinic acid (DMSA, also called Succimer) has advantages over EDTA in that it can be given orally and is effective in temporarily reducing BLL. However, DMSA does not improve long-term BLL in children, nor reduce brain lead levels beyond the cessation of lead exposure alone (Cremin et al., 1999; O'Connor and Rich, 1999). A recent study shows that DMAS lowered BLL in children, but had no detectable benefit on learning and behavior (Dietrich et al., 2004).

Mercury

Mercury (Hg) was named after the Greco-Roman god known for swift flight. Also called quicksilver, metallic mercury is in liquid state at room temperature. The symbol Hg was derived from the Latinized Greek *hydrargyrum*, meaning "water" and "silver." Mercury was known in ancient times from ~1500 BC. By 500 BC mercury was used to make amalgams with other metals. Mercury vapor (Hg^0) is much more hazardous than the liquid form. Mercury binds to other elements (such as chlorine, sulfur, or oxygen) to form inorganic mercurous (Hg^{1+}) or mercuric (Hg^{2+}) salts. This metal can form a number of stable organometallic compounds by attaching to one or two carbon atoms. Methylmercury (CH_3Hg^+, or MeHg) is the toxicologically most important organic form (ATSDR, 1999). Mercurial compounds have characteristic toxicokinetics and health effects that depend on oxidation state and associated organic species.

Global Cycling and Ecotoxicology Mercury exemplifies movement of metals in the environment (Fig. 23-6). Atmospheric mercury, in the form of mercury vapor (Hg^0), is derived from natural degassing of the earth's crust and through volcanic eruptions as well as from evaporation from oceans and soils. Anthropogenic sources have become a significant contributor to atmospheric mercury. These include emissions from metal mining and smelting (mercury, gold, copper, and zinc), coal-combustion, municipal incinerators, and chloralkali industries. Mercury vapor is a chemically stable monatomic gas and its residence time in atmosphere is about one year. Thus, mercury is globally distributed even from point resources. Eventually, it is oxidized to a water-soluble inorganic form (Hg^{2+}) and returned to the earth's surface in rainwater. At this stage, the metal may be reduced back to mercury vapor and returned to the atmosphere, or it may be methylated by microorganisms present in sediments of bodies of fresh and ocean water. This natural biomethylation reaction produces methylmercury (MeHg). Methylmercury enters the aquatic food chain starting with plankton, then herbivorous fish, and finally ascending to carnivorous fish and sea mammals. On the top of the food chain, tissue mercury can rise to levels 1800 to 80,000 times higher than levels in the surrounding water. This biomethylation and bioconcentration result in human exposure to methylmercury through consumption of fish (Clarkson, 2002; Risher et al., 2002). Organomercurial compounds are generally more toxic than inorganic mercury to aquatic organisms, aquatic invertebrates, fish, plants, and birds. Organisms in the larval stages are generally more sensitive to toxic effects of mercury (Boening, 2000).

Exposure

Dietary Exposure Consumption of fish is the major route of exposure to methylmercury. Unlike the case of polychlorinated biphenyls, which are also deposited in fat, cooking the fish does not lower the methylmercury content. Inorganic mercury compounds are also found in food. The source of inorganic mercurial is unknown but the amounts ingested are far below known toxic levels. Mercury in the atmosphere and in drinking water is generally so low that they do not constitute an important source of exposure to the general population (ATSDR, 1999; Clarkson, 2002).

Occupational Exposure Inhalation of mercury vapor can occur from the working environment, as in the chloralkali industry, where mercury is used as a cathode in the electrolysis of brine. Occupational exposure may also occur during manufacture of a variety of scientific instruments and electrical control devices, and in dentistry where mercury amalgams are used in tooth restoration. In the processing of and extraction of gold, especially in developing countries, large quantities of metallic mercury are used to form an amalgam with gold. The amalgam is then heated to drive off the mercury, resulting in a substantial atmospheric release (ATSDR, 1999; Eisler, 2003).

Medicinal Exposure Mercury was an important constituent of drugs for centuries and was used as an ingredient in diuretics, antiseptics, skin ointments, and laxatives. These uses have largely been replaced by safer drugs. Thimerosal contains the ethylmercury radical attached to the sulfur group of thiosalicylate (49.6% mercury by weight as ethylmercury), and has been used as a preservative in many vaccines since 1930s. The use of mercury amalgam in dental restoration releases mercury vapor in the oral cavity and can result in increased mercury body burden. However, the amounts are low compared to occupational exposure (Clarkson et al., 2003).

Accidental Exposure Fatal mercury poisonings come mainly from accidental exposure. Elemental mercury spills can occur in many ways, such as from broken elemental mercury containers, medicinal devices, barometers, and from melting tooth amalgam fillings to recover silver. Inhalation of large amount of mercury vapor can be deadly (Baughman, 2006). Oral ingestion of large amounts of inorganic mercury chloride has also been lethal in suicide cases (ATSDR, 1999). A well-known organomercurial poisoning episode was from consumption of fish contaminated with methylmercury from industrial waste in Minamata, Japan. Consumption of grains and rice treated with methylmercury or ethylmercury as fungicides

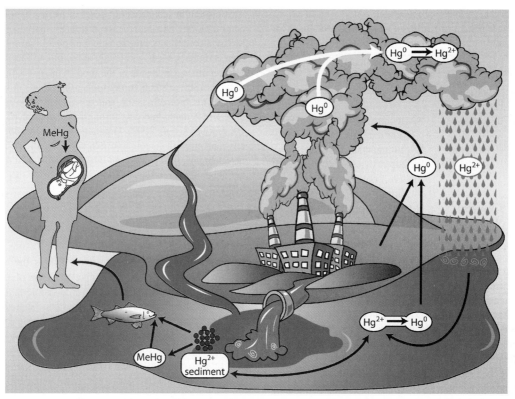

Figure 23-6. The Movement of Mercury in the Environment.

In nature, mercury vapor (Hg^0), a stable monoatomic gas, evaporates from the earth's surface (both soil and water) and is emitted by volcanoes. Anthropogenic sources include emissions from coal-burning power stations and municipal incinerators. After $\sim$1 year, mercury vapor is converted to soluble form (Hg^{2+}) and returned to the earth by rainwater. It may be converted back to the vapor by microorganisms and reemitted into the atmosphere. Thus, mercury may recirculate for long periods. Mercury attached to aquatic sediments is subjected to microbial conversion to methylmercury, starting with plankton, then herbivorous fish, and finally ascending to carnivorous fish and sea mammals. This biomethylation and biomagnification result in human exposure to methylmercury through consumption of fish, and poses the health risk to humans, especially the developing fetus.

to prevent plant root diseases in Iraq and China also led to a significant number of poisonings (Clarkson, 2002; Risher *et al.*, 2002). Contact with even a small amount of dimethylmercury (CH_3CH_3Hg) can penetrate laboratory gloves resulting in rapid transdermal absorption, delayed cerebellar damage and death (Nierenberg *et al.*, 1998).

Toxicokinetics

Mercury Vapor   Mercury vapor is readily absorbed (about 80%) in the lungs, rapidly diffuses across alveolar membranes into the blood, and distributes to all tissues in the body due to its high lipid solubility. Once the vapor has entered the cell, it is oxidized to divalent inorganic mercury by tissue and erythrocyte catalase. A significant portion of mercury vapor crosses the blood–brain barrier and placenta before it is oxidized by erythrocytes, and thus shows more neurotoxicity and developmental toxicity compared to administration of inorganic mercury salts which cross membranes less rapidly. After mercury vapor undergoes oxidation, its deposition resembles inorganic mercury. Approximately 10% of mercury vapor is exhaled within a week of exposure, and that converted to inorganic mercury is excreted mainly in urine and feces, with a half-life of 1–2 months (ATSDR, 1999; Clarkson *et al.*, 2003). Liquid metallic mercury,

such as that swallowed from a broken thermometer, is only poorly absorbed by the gastrointestinal tract (0.01%), is not biologically reactive, and is generally thought to be of little or no toxicological consequence.

Inorganic Mercury   Inorganic mercury is poorly absorbed from the gastrointestinal tract. Absorption ranges 7% to 15% of ingested dose, depending on the inorganic compound. A small portion of absorbed inorganic mercury is formed by reduction in tissues and exhaled as mercury vapor. The highest concentration of inorganic mercury is found in kidney, a major target. Renal uptake of mercury salts occurs through two routes: from luminal membranes in renal proximal tubule in the form of the cysteine S-conjugates (Cys-S-Hg-S-Cys) or from the basolateral membrane through organic anion transporters (Bridges and Zalpus, 2005). Inorganic mercury salts do not readily pass blood–brain barrier or placenta and are mainly excreted in urine and feces, with a half-life of about 2 months.

Methylmercury   Methylmercury is well absorbed from the gastrointestinal tract. About 95% of methylmercury ingested from fish is absorbed. It is distributed to all tissues in about 30 hours. About 10% of absorbed methylmercury is distributed to the brain and 5% remains in blood. The concentration in erythrocytes is 20 times that in plasma. Methylmercury is bound to thiol-containing molecules such as cysteine (CH₃Hg-*S*-Cys), which mimic methionine to cross the blood–brain barrier and placenta through the neutral amino acid carrier. Methylmercury avidly accumulates in hair, and although concentrations are proportional to that in blood, they are about 250-fold higher. Thus, hair mercury is often used as an indicator of exposure. Methylmercury undergoes extensive enterohepatic recycling, which can be interrupted to enhance fecal excretion. Methylmercury is slowly metabolized to inorganic mercury by microflora in intestine (about 1% of the body burden per day). In contrast to inorganic mercury, 90% of the methylmercury is eliminated from the body in the feces, and less than 10% is in the urine, with a half-life of 45–70 days (Clarkson, 2002; Risher *et al.*, 2002; Bridges and Zalpus, 2005).

The disposition of ethylmercury is similar to methylmercury. The major differences include that the conversion to inorganic mercury in the body is much faster for ethylmercury, which can result in renal injury. The mercury concentrations in brain are lower for ethylmercury than methylmercury. The half-life for ethylmercury is only 15–20% of that for methylmercury (Clarkson *et al.*, 2003).

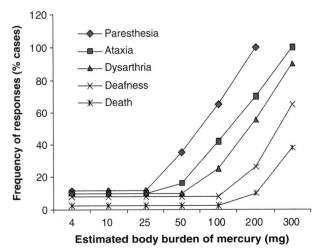

Figure 23-7. A Dose–Response Simulation of Estimated Methylmercury Body Burden and the Onset and Frequency of Symptoms from Iraq Epidemic Poisoning in 1970s.

Toxicity

Mercury Vapor   Inhalation of mercury vapor at extremely high concentrations may produce an acute, corrosive bronchitis and interstitial pneumonitis and, if not fatal, may be associated with central nervous system effects such as tremor or increased excitability. With chronic exposure to mercury vapor, the major effects are on the central nervous system. Early signs are nonspecific, and this condition has been termed the *asthenic-vegetative syndrome* or *micromercurialism*. Identification of the syndrome requires neurasthenic symptoms and three or more of the following clinical findings: tremor, enlargement of the thyroid, increased uptake of radioiodine in the thyroid, labile pulse, tachycardia, dermographism, gingivitis, hematologic changes, or increased excretion of mercury in urine. The triad of tremors, gingivitis, and erethism (memory loss, increased excitability, insomnia, depression, and shyness) has been recognized historically as the major manifestation of mercury poisoning from inhalation of mercury vapor. Sporadic instances of proteinuria and even nephrotic syndrome may occur in persons with exposure to mercury vapor, particularly with chronic occupational exposure. The pathogenesis is probably immunologically similar to that occuring after exposure to inorganic mercury (ATSDR, 1999; Clarkson, 2002). Mercury vapor release from amalgam is in general too low to cause significant toxicity (Clarkson *et al.*, 2003; Factor-Litvak *et al.*, 2003; Horsted-Bindslev, 2004).

Inorganic Mercury   Kidney is the major target organ for inorganic mercury (ATSDR, 1999). Although a high dose of mercuric chloride is directly toxic to renal tubular cells, chronic low-dose exposure to mercury salts may induce an immunologic glomerular disease (Bigazzi, 1999). Exposed persons may develop proteinuria that is reversible after they are removed from exposure. Experimental studies have shown that the pathogenesis has two phases including an early phase characterized by an anti-basement membrane glomerulonephritis, followed by a superimposed immune-complex glomerulonephritis with transiently raised concentrations of circulating immune complexes (Henry *et al.*, 1988). The pathogenesis of the nephropathy in humans appears similar, although antigens have not been characterized. In humans, the early glomerular nephritis

may progress to interstitial immune-complex nephritis (Pelletier and Druet, 1995; Bigazzi, 1999).

Methylmercury   The major human health effect from exposure to methylmercury is neurotoxicity. Clinical manifestations of neurotoxicity include paresthesia (a numbness and tingling sensation around the mouth, lips) and ataxia, manifested as a clumsy, stumbling gait, and difficulty in swallowing and articulating words. Other signs include neurasthenia (a generalized sensation of weakness), vision and hearing loss, and spasticity and tremor. These may finally progress to coma and death. Neuropathological observations have shown that the cortex of the cerebrum and cerebellum are selectively involved with focal necrosis of neurons, lysis, and phagocytosis, and replacement by glial cells. These changes are most prominent in the deeper fissures (sulci), as in the visual cortex and insula. The overall acute effect is cerebral edema, but with prolonged destruction of gray matter and subsequent gliosis, cerebral atrophy results (Takeuchi, 1977). A study of the Iraq epidemic of methylmercury exposure (Bakir *et al.*, 1973) has provided dose–response estimates of the body burden of mercury required for the onset and frequency of symptoms (Fig. 23-7).

Mechanism of Toxicity   High-affinity binding of divalent mercury to sulfhydryl groups of proteins in the cells is an important mechanism for producing nonspecific cell injury or even cell death. Other general mechanisms, such as the interruption of microtubule formation, inhibition of enzymes, oxidative stress, interruption of protein and DNA synthesis, and autoimmune responses, have also been proposed (ATSDR, 1999; Clarkson, 2002). Mercury causes overexpression of metallothionein and glutathione system-related genes in rat tissues (Brambila *et al.*, 2002; Liu *et al*, 2003), probably as an adaptive mechanism.

Sensitive Sub-populations

Early life stages are particularly vulnerable to mercury intoxication (Counter and Buchanan, 2004). In Minamata, Japan, pregnant women who consumed fish contaminated with methylmercury, manifested mild or minimal symptoms, but gave birth to infants with severe developmental disabilities, raising initial concerns for mercury as a developmental toxicant.

Methylmercury crosses the placenta and reaches the fetus, and is concentrated to a level in fetal brain at least 5–7 times that of maternal blood (Clarkson, 2002). Prenatal methylmercury exposure at high levels can induce widespread damage to the fetal brain. However, the observed effects from low-level exposures are inconsistent (Counter and Buchanan, 2004; Davidson *et al.*, 2004). In the Seychelles Children Development Study, a group with significant methylmercury exposure from a diet predominantly of fish was studied for adverse developmental effects. These children were examined six times over 11 years using extensive batteries of age-appropriate developmental end-points, but no convincing associations were found except for delayed walking (Davidson *et al.*, 2006). The National Research Council reviewed the epidemiologic studies relating in utero methylmercury exposure and fetal neurological development. It concluded that the current EPA reference dose (RfD) for methylmercury of 0.1 μg/kg per day or 5.8 μg/L cord blood is scientifically justifiable for protection of human health (NRC, 2000). The RfD is equivalent to 12 ppm methylmercury in maternal hair.

The safety of thimerosal (ethylmercury) used in childhood vaccines has also received extensive attention. A recent review indicates that thimerosal is safe at the doses used in vaccines, except for a potential for local hypersensitivity (Clarkson *et al.*, 2003). However, some infants may be exposed to cumulative levels of mercury during the first six months of life that may exceed EPA recommendations (Ball *et al.*, 2001). Steps have been rapidly taken to remove thimerosal from vaccines in the US by switching to single-dose vials that do not require preservatives. Nonetheless, the World Health Organization concluded that it is safe to continue using thimerosal in vaccines, which is important for developing countries where it is essential to use multidose vials (Clarkson *et al.*, 2003).

Although the use of mercury amalgam in children can contribute to mercury exposure, the exposure is too low to cause significant toxicological effects (DeRouen *et al.*, 2006).

Acrodynia occurred in children chronically exposed to inorganic mercury compounds in teething powder and diaper disinfectants, as well as to organomercurials. Acrodynia is characterized by pink hands and feet (also called Pink Disease). These subjects are photophobic and suffer from joint pains (Clarkson, 2002).

Treatment   Therapy for mercury poisoning should be directed toward lowering the concentration of mercury at the critical organ or site of injury. For the most severe cases, particularly with acute renal failure, hemodialysis may be the first measure, along with administration of chelating agents for mercury, such as cysteine, EDTA, BAL, or penicillamine. Caution should be taken to avoid inappropriate use of chelating agents in putative mercury poisoning patients (Risher and Amler, 2005).

Chelation therapy is not very helpful for alkyl mercury exposure. Biliary excretion and reabsorption by the intestine can be interrupted by oral administration of a nonabsorbable thiol resin, which can bind mercury and enhance fecal excretion (Clarkson, 2002).

Nickel

Nickel (Ni) has been in use since ancient times. However, because the ores of nickel were easily mistaken for ores of silver, a more complete understanding of this metal and its specific use dates to more contemporary times. In 1751, nickel was first isolated from the ore kupfernickel (niccolite) for which it is named. Metallic nickel is produced from sulfide and silicate-oxide ores. In the US ~200,000 metric tons of nickel are used each year. Nickel is used in various metal alloys, including stainless steels and in electroplating. Major properties of nickel alloys include strength, corrosion resistance, and good thermal and electrical conductivity. Occupational exposure to nickel occurs by inhalation of nickel-containing aerosols, dusts, or fumes, or dermal contact in workers engaged in nickel production (mining, milling, refinery, etc.) and nickel-using operations (melting, electroplating, welding, nickel–cadmium batteries, etc.) (ATSDR, 2005d). Nickel is ubiquitous in nature, and the general population is exposed to low levels of nickel in air, cigarette smoke, water, and food. These exposures are generally too low to be of toxicological concern (Kasprzak *et al.*, 2003). Nickel has various oxidation states but the 2+ oxidation state is the most prevalent form in biosystems. The major soluble nickel compounds are nickel acetate, nickel chloride, nickel sulfate, and nickel nitrate. The important water-insoluble nickel compounds include nickel sulfide, nickel subsulfide, nickel oxide, nickel carbonyl, and nickel carbonate (ATSDR, 2005d).

Toxicokinetics   Inhaled nickel particles are deposited in the respiratory tract and, as with all inhaled particles, the site of deposition depends on the particle size. Large particles (5–30 μm) deposit in the nasopharyngeal area via impaction, smaller particles (1–5 μm) enter the trachea and bronchiolar region by sedimentation, and particles smaller than 1 μm enter the alveolar space. About 25–35% of the inhaled nickel that is retained in the lungs is absorbed into the blood. The insoluble nickel particles can be taken up into cells by phagocytosis. In the skin the rate of absorption depends on the rate of penetration into the epidermis, which differs for different chemical forms of nickel. In humans, about 27% of a single oral dose of nickel in drinking water is absorbed, whereas only about 1% is absorbed when nickel is given with food. Intestinal nickel absorption occurs through calcium or iron channels, or by the divalent metal transport protein-1 (ATSDR, 2005d).

The main transport proteins of nickel in blood are albumin, histidine, and α_2-microglobulin. Nickelplasmin and metallothionein also bind and transport nickel. Following inhalation exposure, nickel is distributed to the lungs, skin, kidneys, liver, pituitary, and adrenals. The half-life of nickel is 1–3 days for nickel sulfate, 5 days for nickel subsulfide, and more than 100 days for nickel oxide (ATSDR, 2005d). Absorbed nickel is excreted into urine. Urinary nickel correlates closely with exposure to airborne levels of insoluble nickel compounds. Thus, urinary nickel may serve as a suitable measure of current nickel exposure.

The marked differences in carcinogenic activities of various nickel compounds may be due to differences in delivery of nickel to specific cells and subcellular target molecules. For example, injection of animals with crystalline nickel subsulfide or crystalline nickel sulfide results in a high incidence of tumors at the site of injection sites, although tumors are not observed in animals similarly injected with soluble nickel sulfate. The crystalline nickel particles can be actively phagocytized and deliver larger quantities of nickel ions into the nucleus than water-soluble nickel compounds (Kasprzak *et al.*, 2003; Costa *et al.*, 2005).

Essentiality of nickel in higher organisms is questionable, although nickel may be nutritionally essential for some plants, bacteria, and invertebrates. Nickel deficiency syndromes have not been reported in humans and nickel-dependent enzymes or cofactors are unknown (Denkhaus and Kalnikow, 2002).

Toxicity

Contact Dermatitis   Nickel-induced contact dermatitis is the most common adverse health effect from nickel exposure and is found in 10–20% of the general population. It can result from exposure to airborne nickel, liquid nickel solutions, or prolonged skin contact with metal items containing nickel, such as coins and jewelry. Nickel sensitization usually arises from prolonged contact with nickel or exposure to a large dose of nickel. The resulting dermatitis is an inflammatory reaction mediated by type IV delayed hypersensitivity (ATSDR, 2005d).

Nickel Carbonyl Poisoning   Metallic nickel combines with carbon monoxide to form nickel carbonyl ($Ni[CO]_4$), which decomposes to nickel and carbon monoxide on heating to 200°C (the Mond process). This reaction provides a convenient and efficient method for nickel refining. However, nickel carbonyl is extremely toxic, and many cases of acute toxicity have been reported. Intoxication begins with headache, nausea, vomiting, and epigastric or chest pain, followed by cough, hyperpnea, cyanosis, gastrointestinal symptoms, and weakness. The symptoms may be accompanied by fever and leukocytosis. The more severe cases can progress to pneumonia, respiratory failure, and eventually to cerebral edema and death.

Carcinogenicity   Nickel is a respiratory tract carcinogen in nickel-refining industry workers (IARC, 1990). Risks are highest for lung and nasal cancers among workers heavily exposed to nickel sulfide, nickel oxide, and metallic nickel. A cohort of 418 workers employed in a Finnish refinery reported a twofold increased incidence of lung cancer and a large increase in sinonasal cancers (Karjalainen *et al.*, 1992). A follow-up of this study, including a total of 1155 workers, confirmed an elevated risk of lung and nasal cancers among refinery workers, with a greater risk among workers with a longer latency (greater than 20 years) (Anttila *et al.*, 1998). Because the refining of nickel in the plants that were studied involved the Mond process, with the formation of nickel carbonyl, it was believed for some time that nickel carbonyl was the principal carcinogen. However, additional epidemiologic studies of workers in refineries that do not use the Mond process also showed an increased risk of respiratory cancer, suggesting that the source of the increased risk is the mixture of nickel sulfides present in molten ore. Studies with experimental animals have shown that the nickel subsulfite produces local tumors at injection sites and lung tumors by inhalation in rats. Differences in the carcinogenic activities of nickel compounds may be attributed to variations in their solubility and capacities to provide nickel ions at critical sites within target cells (Sunderman, 1989; Costa, 2005). However, nickel compounds lose their original chemical identity upon entering the blood, so that it is not possible to identify the original source of exposure (Grant and Mushak, 1989). Carcinogenesis studies of soluble nickel compounds have also yielded positive results in rodents (Kasprzak *et al.*, 2003). For instance, nickel acetate is a complete transplacental carcinogen for the rat pituitary and initiator of kidney tumors in the rat (Diwan *et al.*, 1992). However, many rodent studies using soluble nickel compounds or metallic nickel have yielded negative results (Oller, 2002; Sivulka, 2005).

Mechanism for Nickel Carcinogenesis   The carcinogenicity of nickel was thought to be due to the ionic nickel species, but on this basis alone it is difficult to explain the differences in carcinogenic potency between different nickel compounds. Some studies suggest that water-insoluble crystalline nickel compounds were responsible for lung and nasal cancers (IARC, 1990). However, not all water-insoluble crystalline nickel compounds induce tumors, so factors other than solubility are probably involved.

Carcinogenic nickel particles that are phagocytized and deliver large quantities of nickel ions into the nucleus are generally not mutagenic but are clastogenic (Costa *et al.*, 2005). Crystalline nickel sulfide compounds produce specific chromosomal damage, notable in the heterochromatic long arm of the X chromosome which suffers regional decondensation, frequent deletions, and other aberrations (Costa *et al.*, 2005). Nickel compounds also produce chromosomal abnormalities such as sister chromatid exchange, especially in hetrochromatin, micronuclei formation in human lymphocytes, microsatellite mutations in human lung cancer cells, and mutations in renal cells (Kasprzak *et al.*, 2003).

Epigenetic Effects   A broad spectrum of epigenetic effects occurs with nickel and include alterations in gene expression resulting from DNA hypermethylation and histone hypoacetylation. A notable nickel-inducible gene is Cap43/NDRG1, under the control of the hypoxia-inducible transcription factor (HIF-1). During tumor development, HIF-1 facilitates angiogenesis and regulates numerous genes including glucose transport and glycolysis, which are essential for tumor growth. A correlation of overexpression of Cap43 with the neoplastic state of the cells was noted (Costa *et al.*, 2005). Another nickel-induced gene amplification is the Ect2 gene. The Ect2 protein is overexpressed in nickel-transformed cells, which can cause microtubule disassembly and cytokinesis, and may contribute to morphological changes in cells (Clemens *et al.*, 2005). Nickel produces rather low, but measurable reactive oxygen species in cells and depletes cellular glutathione. Oxidative DNA damage (including the formation of 8-hydroxyguanine and DNA strand breaks), oxidative protein damage and lipid peroxidation, as well as inhibition of DNA repair enzymes, can be observed following nickel exposure (Kasprzak *et al.*, 2003; Valko *et al.*, 2005).

Sunderman and Barber (1988) proposed that nickel interacts with DNA by replacement of zinc in zinc-binding sites of DNA-binding proteins. DNA-binding proteins with finger loop domains have been identified on some proto-oncogenes and are thought to be likely targets for metal toxicity. In addition, nickel may interfere with the metabolism of iron, calcium, magnesium, or manganese to produce its toxic or carcinogenic effects (Kasprzak *et al.*, 2003).

Treatment of Nickel Toxicity   Blood nickel levels immediately following exposure to nickel carbonyl provide a guideline as to the severity of exposure and are an indication for chelation therapy (Sunderman, 1979). Sodium diethylcarbodithioate (DDTC) is the preferred drug. Disulfiram, another nickel-chelating agent, has been used in nickel dermatitis and in nickel carbonyl poisoning. Other chelating agents, such as D-penicillamine and DMPS, provide some degree of protection from clinical effects (Blanusa *et al.*, 2005).

ESSENTIAL METALS WITH POTENTIAL FOR TOXICITY

Cobalt

Cobalt (Co) is a relatively rare, ferromagnetic transition metal first isolated in the 1730s. The name cobalt comes from the German word *kobalt*, which is derived from *kobold* meaning "goblin," a name applied by miners of the time to cobalt ore, which was thought to be worthless and poisonous. Cobalt is usually not mined alone and tends to be produced primarily as a byproduct of copper and nickel mining. Cobalt is useful in various alloys, where it provides corrosion- and wear-resistance, and in cemented carbides ("hard" metals). It is used in permanent magnets, as a paint or varnish dryer, in catalysts, and in pigments production.

Toxicokinetics The toxicokinetics and possible adverse health effects of inorganic cobalt compounds have been reviewed (Elinder and Friberg, 1986; De Boeck *et al.*, 2003). Cobalt absorption depends on the compound. Less than 5% of an oral dose of cobalt oxide is absorbed whereas about 30% of an oral dose of cobalt chloride is absorbed in rodents (Elinder and Friberg, 1986). Oral absorption of cobalt varies widely in humans, and it is estimated to be between 5% and 45% (Elinder and Friberg, 1986). Increasing doses of cobalt results in a decreasing proportional absorption so increased cobalt levels tend not to cause significant accumulation. Absorption of inhaled cobalt compounds appears to be relatively effective in humans and animals (Elinder and Friberg, 1986). About 80% of absorbed cobalt is excreted in urine, and about 15% is excreted in feces. The liver, kidneys, adrenals, and thyroid have relatively high concentrations. The normal levels in human urine and blood are about 1.0 and 0.18 μg/L, respectively. Cobalt in blood is largely associated with red blood cells.

Essentiality Cobalt is an essential nutrient, in small amounts, to mammals, including humans. The essential form of cobalt is cobalamin, a cobalt-containing tetrapyrrolic ring and critical component of Vitamin B_{12}. Vitamin B_{12} is required for the production of red blood cells and in the prevention of pernicious anemia. Insufficient natural levels of cobalt in the diet of sheep and cattle result in cobalt deficiency disease, characterized by anemia and loss of weight or retarded growth. If other requirements for cobalt exist, they are not well defined (Herbert, 1996).

Toxicity Occupational inhalation of cobalt-containing dust in industrial settings may cause respiratory irritation at air concentrations between 0.002 to 0.01 mg/m^3. Higher concentrations may be a cause of "hard metal" pneumoconiosis, a progressive form of pulmonary interstitial fibrosis. Occupational dermal exposure is sometimes associated with an allergic dermatitis.

Although the data linking cobalt exposure to cancer in humans is considered inadequate (IARC, 1991; NTP, 2004), in rodents, inhalation of cobalt sulfate induces lung tumors, including carcinoma, in rats and mice (Bucher *et al.*, 1999). Repository injections or implantation of various cobalt compounds can produce local sarcomas in rodents (IARC, 1991). The mechanism by which cobalt produces cancer is not defined.

Cobalt can be erythropoietic when excessive amounts are ingested by most mammals, including humans (Elinder and Friberg, 1986). Chronic oral administration of high levels of cobalt for the treatment of anemia can cause goiter, and epidemiologic studies suggest that the incidence of goiter is higher in regions containing increased levels of cobalt in water and soil. The goitrogenic effect has been elicited by the oral administration of 3–4 mg/kg to children in the course of treatment of sickle cell anemia. Intravenous exposure to cobalt can cause increased blood pressure, slowed respiration, tinnitus, and deafness due to nerve damage. Cardiomyopathy with signs of congestive heart failure has been associated with excessive cobalt intake (>10 mg/day), particularly from drinking beer

to which cobalt was added as a foaming agent. Autopsy findings in such cases have found a tenfold increase in the cardiac levels of cobalt. In animals, myocardial degeneration can be produced by cobalt injection. In rats cobalt injection will produce hyperglycemia due to pancreatic β-cell damage (Seghizzi *et al.*, 1994).

Copper

Copper (Cu) has been used for many centuries. By 2000 BC, copper–tin alloys or 'bronze' were in wide use in Europe. In Roman times, copper became known as *cyprium* because so much of it was mined in Cyprus, and eventually Anglicized into *copper*. Copper is an essential element widely distributed in nature. Food, beverages, and drinking water are major sources of exposure in the general population. Daily intake of copper in adults varies between 0.9 and 2.2 mg, and in children between 0.6 to 0.8 mg (WHO, 1998). The Recommended Dietary Allowance (RDA) of copper varies according to age, pregnancy, and lactation, and for adults is 0.9 mg/day (IOM, 2001).

Copper exposure in industry is primarily from inhaled particulates in mining or metal fumes in smelting operations, welding, or related activities. Excess copper in the water represents a risk factor to the aquatic environment, producing endocrine disruption and other toxic effects in fish (Handy, 2003).

Toxicokinetics Approximately 55% to 75% of an oral dose of copper is absorbed from the gastrointestinal tract, primarily in the duodenum. Intestinal copper absorption can be reduced by zinc, iron, molybdate, and fructose (IOM, 2001). The cellular transport and metabolism of copper comprises a series of copper-binding proteins and small peptides, such as albumin, ceruloplasmin, glutathione, metallothionein, and cytosolic copper chaperons, which work in conjunction with copper-ATPases to maintain copper homeostasis (Harris, 2000; Mercer, 2001). Copper levels are maintained mainly through control of excretion, although copper binding to hepatic metallothionein may act as a form of copper storage. In mammals, little copper is excreted into the urine, and the bile is the major route of excretion. Bile secretion, enterohepatic recirculation, and intestinal absorption all help to control copper status.

Essentiality Copper is an essential component of several metalloenzymes, including type A oxidases and type B monoamine oxidases. Of the type B oxidases, cytochrome *c*-oxidase is probably the most important because it catalyzes a key reaction in energy metabolism, and inherited mutational defects can result in severe pathology in humans (Hamza and Gitlin, 2002). Of the type A oxidases, lysyl oxidase plays a major role in the formation and repair of extracellular matrix by oxidizing lysine residues in elastin and collagen, thereby initiating the covalent crosslinkage (Kagan and Li, 2003). Copper/zinc superoxide dismutase is present in most cells, particularly of the brain, thyroid, liver, lung, and blood, and helps protect from oxygen toxicity by reducing superoxide radicals to hydrogen peroxide (Valko *et al.*, 2005).

Copper deficiency is uncommon in humans. Copper deficiency can occur as a result of malnutrition, overdose of molybdenum, or excessive consumption of zinc (Maret and Standstead, 2006). Copper deficiency manifests clinically by hypochromic, microcytic anemia that is refractory to iron supplementation and predisposes to infection. This deficiency is sometimes accompanied by bone abnormalities. Less frequent manifestations are hypopigmentation of the hair and hypotonia. Biomarkers of copper deficiency include serum and urine copper levels, ceruloplasmin concentration, and copper-dependent enzyme activities (IOM, 2001).

Toxicity The most commonly reported adverse heath effects of excess oral copper intake are gastrointestinal distress. Nausea, vomiting, and abdominal pain have been reported shortly after drinking solutions of copper sulfate or beverages stored in containers that readily release copper (Pizarro *et al.*, 1999). Ingestion of drinking water with >3 mg Cu/L will produce gastrointestinal symptoms. Ingestion of large amounts of copper salts, most frequently copper sulfate, may produce hepatic necrosis and death. Epidemiological studies have not found any relation between copper exposure and cancer (WHO, 1998).

Hereditary Disease of Copper Metabolism

Menkes Disease This is a rare sex-linked genetic defect in copper metabolism resulting in copper deficiency in male infants. It is characterized by peculiar hair, failure to thrive, severe metal retardation, neurologic impairment, and death usually by 5 years of age. Bones are osteoporotic with flared metaphases of the long bones and bones of the skull. There is extensive degeneration of the cerebral cortex and of white matter. The gene responsible for Menkes disease, *ATP7A*, belongs to the family of ATPases and is a copper transporter (Fig. 23-8). Deficiency in this copper transporter in Menkes disease blocks copper transport across the basolateral membrane of intestinal cells into the portal circulation, resulting in accumulation of copper in the entrocytes and systemic copper deficiency in the body. The transport of copper to the brain is also blocked, causing severe neurological abnormalities (Mercer, 2001). Animal models for copper deficiency support the importance of adequate copper intake during embyrogenesis and early development (Shim and Harris, 2003).

Wilson Disease This is an autosomal recessive genetic disorder of copper metabolism characterized by the excessive accumulation of copper in liver, brain, kidneys, and cornea. Serum ceruloplasmin is low and serum copper not bound to ceruloplasmin is elevated. Urinary excretion of copper is high. Clinical abnormalities of the nervous system, liver, kidneys, and cornea are related to copper accumulation. Patients with Wilson disease have impaired biliary excretion of copper, which is believed to be the fundamental cause of the copper overload. Genetic studies have identified the defect in copper transport as mutations of the Wilson disease locus (WND) on chromosome 13, encoding P-type ATPase (*ATP7B*) (WHO, 1998; Harris, 2000). There appears to be several polymorphisms of the defect, which may explain the clinical variability in the disorder. Diagnosis may be suspected with elevated serum copper but must be confirmed by liver biopsy and elevated liver copper (normally 15–55 μg/g versus > 250 μg/g in Wilson disease). Animal models of Wilson disease include the toxic milk (Tx) mouse and the Long–Evans Cinnamon (LEC) rats. Both rodent models develop hepatocellular damage from abnormal copper accumulation associated with mutations in *ATP7B*, but do not exhibit the neurological symptoms associated with the human disease (Shim and Harris, 2003).

Hereditary Aceruloplasnaemia This is the autosomal recessive genetic disorder of copper-binding protein ceruloplasmin, associ-

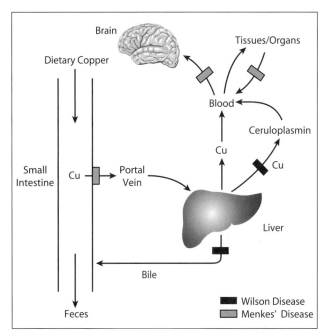

Figure 23-8. Pathways of Copper in the Body and Defects in Menkes' and Wilson Diseases.

Copper is absorbed by the enterocytes of the small intestine and transported across the basolateral membrane of enterocytes into the portal circulation. This later process is defective in Menkes' disease patients and results in accumulation of copper in the enterocytes and overall copper deficiency in the body. Most of the newly absorbed copper is normally taken up by the liver. In cases of copper overload, excess copper is excreted in the bile and this process is blocked in Wilson disease, as is the delivery of copper to ceruloplasmin, the principal copper carrier in the blood. Other low molecular weight proteins such as Cu–metallothionein and Cu–histine are also proposed to be important sources of copper to tissues. The transport of copper to the brain is blocked in patients with Menkes' disease, leading to the severe neurological abnormalities (Adapted from Mercer, 2001, with permission from Elsevier).

ated with the iron-overload syndrome. Clinical signs and symptoms include mental confusion, memory loss, dementia, cerebellar ataxia, altered motor function, retinal degeneration, and diabetes (WHO, 1998). Ceruloplasmin-null mice accumulate iron predominantly in organs of reticuloendothelial system. In these mice, hematologic indices and serum iron are abnormal by 10 weeks of age, with profound iron overload in the spleen and liver. Hepatic copper deposition is also approximately doubled in these mice. However, neurodegeneration and diabetes are not observed in these mice (Shim and Harris, 2003).

Indian Childhood Cirrhosis (ICC) This is a disorder occurring in young children characterized by jaundice due to an insidious and progressive liver disease. Two distinguishing features are a widespread brown orcein staining (indicating copper) and intralobular hepatic fibrosis progressing to portal cirrhosis and chronic inflammation. The etiology is not known but it is suspected that bottle feeding of milk contaminated with copper from storage in brass vessels may be important. However, epidemiological studies also suggest an autosomal recessive genetic component because of strong familial occurrence and high consanguinity among affected children (WHO, 1998).

Idopathic Copper Toxicosis or Non-Indian Childhood Cirrhosis
This is a rare disorder in children similar to ICC occurring in some
Western countries. The largest series of cases are reported from the
Tyrol region of Austria. This population also used copper vessels
to store milk, and the incidence of the disorder has declined since
replacement of the copper vessels. A number of other cases have
been reported from other parts of the world, some from increased
amounts of copper in drinking water (WHO, 1998).

Treatment   Clinical improvement can be achieved by chelation of copper with D-penicillamine, Trien [triethylene tetramine
2HCl)], zinc acetate, and tetrathiomolybdate. The combination
of tetrathiomolybdate and zinc acetate is more effective (Brewer,
2005). *N*-Acetylcystein amide can cross the blood–brain barrier
and was developed to help prevent neurodegenerative disorders (Cai
et al., 2005).

Iron

Iron (Fe) is a very abundant transition metal. Iron came into use
around 4000 BC. An early source of iron was from fallen meteorites
and the name may derive from the Ethruscan word *aisar* which
means "the gods." Iron is an essential metal for erythropoiesis and
a key component of hemoglobin, myoglobin, heme enzymes, met-
alloflavoprotein enzymes, and mitochondrial enzymes. In biological
systems, iron mainly exists as the ferrous (2+) and ferric (3+) forms.
Toxicologic considerations are important in terms of iron deficiency,
accidental acute exposures, and chronic iron overload due to idiopathic hemochromatosis or as a consequence of excess dietary iron
or frequent blood transfusions (Yip and Dallman, 1996; IOM, 2001;
Papanikolaou and Pantopoulos, 2005).

Toxicokinetics   Iron metabolism is regulated by a complex series
of events that maintain homeostasis, mainly involving absorption,
storage, and excretion. Heme iron from meat, poultry, and fish is
highly bioavailable. Nonheme iron absorption is influenced by its
solubility and by other dietary factors, such as vitamin C (ascorbic acid) which enhances uptake. Absorption involves movement of
ferrous ions from the intestinal lumen into the mucosal cells via the
divalent metal transporter protein-1 (DMT-1) and then transfer from
the mucosal cell to the plasma, where iron is bound to transferrin
for transport and distribution. Transferrin is a β1-globulin with a
molecular weight of 75,000 and is produced in the liver. Transferrin
delivers iron to tissues by binding to transferrin receptor-1(TfR1) on
the cell membrane, followed by endocytosis. Iron is then released in
the acidic endosomal vesicle. The human body contains $\sim$3–5 g of
iron. About two-thirds of body iron is in hemoglobin, 10% is in myoglobin and iron-containing enzymes, and the remainder is bound to
the iron storage proteins like ferritin and hemosiderin, stored in
liver and reticuloendothelial cells in the spleen and bone marrow.
Iron stores serve as a reservoir to supply cellular iron needs, mainly
for hemoglobin production. Erythrocyte destruction and production
are responsible for most iron turnover. Hepcidin, a small peptide
of liver origin, modulates iron absorption in response to erythropoiesis (Papanikolaou and Pantopoulos, 2005). The major route of
excretion of iron is into the gastrointestinal tract and eventually the
feces. Daily iron losses from urine, gastrointestinal tract, and skin
are $\sim$0.08, 0.6, and 0.2 mg/day, respectively.

Essentiality and Deficiency   Iron deficiency is the most common
nutritional deficiency worldwide, affecting infants, young children,
and women of child-bearing age. The critical period for iron deficiency in children is between the ages of 6 months and 2 years. The
major manifestation of iron deficiency is anemia with microcytic
hypochromic red blood cells. Other effects of iron deficiency include
impaired psychomotor development and intellectual performance,
decreased resistance to infection, adverse pregnancy outcomes, and
possibly increased susceptibility to lead and cadmium toxicity. Oral
ferrous sulfate is the treatment of choice for iron deficiency.

Toxicity   Acute iron poisoning from accidental ingestion of iron-
containing dietary supplements is the most common cause of acute
toxicity. It most often occurs in children. A decrease in occurrence
of this type of poisoning followed the introduction of childproof lids
on prescription medicines and vitamin supplements. Severe toxicity occurs after the ingestion of more than 0.5 g of iron or 2.5 g
of ferrous sulfate. Toxicity occurs about 1–6 hours after ingestion.
Symptoms include abdominal pain, diarrhea, and vomiting. Of particular concern are pallor or cyanosis, metabolic acidosis, and cardiac collapse. Death may occur in severely poisoned children within
24 hours. Supportive therapy and iron chelation with deferoxamine
should be used as soon as possible. Inhalation of iron oxide fumes or
dust may cause pneumoconiosis in occupational settings (Dotherty
et al., 2004).

   Chronic iron toxicity from iron overload in adults is a relatively
common problem. There are three basic ways in which excessive
amounts of iron can accumulate in the body. The first is hereditary hemochromatosis due to abnormal absorption of iron from the
intestinal tract. Hereditary hemochromatosis is an autosomal recessive disorder attributed to mutation in the hemochromatosis gene.
About 90% of patients are homozygous for C282Y mutation, while
a few patients are heterozygotes for C282Y with a second mutation
for H63D. The frequency of homozygosity is $\sim$0.3–0.4% in populations of European ancestry. The second possible cause of iron
overload is excess intake via the diet or from oral iron preparations.
The third circumstance in which iron overload can occur is repeated
blood transfusions for some form of refractory anemia and is referred to as *transfusional siderosis*. The pathologic consequences
of iron overload are similar regardless of the basis. *Hemosiderosis*
refers to increased iron stores in the form of hemosiderin. The body
iron content can increase 20–40 g, up to 10 times higher than normal
levels. *Hemochromatosis* refers to excessive deposition of iron that
causes organ damage, often resulting in fibrosis. Inhalation of iron
oxide fumes or dust by workers in hematic mines (mainly Fe_2O_3),
steel workers, and welders may produce siderosis (nonfibrotic), and
in some cases silicosis (fibrotic) in the lung, with increases in total
body iron (Doherty *et al.*, 2006). Liver iron overload from hereditary
hemochromatosis is associated with a high risk for hepatocellular
carcinoma, as well as with other malignancies (Papanikolaou and
Pantopoulos, 2005).

   Increased body iron may play a role in the development
of cardiovascular disease. It is suspected that iron may act as a
catalyst to produce free radical damage resulting in artherosclero-
sis and ischemic heart disease (Alpert, 2004). This iron hypothesis is controversial, but it is clear that mortality from cardiovascular disease is correlated with liver iron overload (Yuan and
Li, 2003). Several neurodegenerative disorders are associated with
aberrant iron metabolism in the brain, such as neuroferritinopathy,

aceruloplasminemia, and manganism (Aschner *et al.*, 2005; Papanikolaou and Pantopoulos, 2005).

Treatment   Desferrioxamine is the chelator of choice for the treatment of acute iron intoxication and chronic iron overload. Iron chelators have also been proposed for the treatment of cancers with iron overload (Buss *et al.*, 2004).

Magnesium

Magnesium (Mg) was recognized as an element in 1755. The name originates from the Greek word for a district in Thessaly called *Magnesia*. Magnesium is a nutritionally essential metal that plays a key role in a wide range of important fundamental cellular reactions (Shils, 1996). Nuts, cereals, seafood, and meats are good dietary sources of magnesium. The drinking water content of magnesium increases with hardness of the water. Magnesium citrate, oxide, sulfate, hydroxide, and carbonate are widely taken as antacids or cathartics. Magnesium hydroxide, or milk of magnesia, is one of the universal antidotes for poisoning. Topically, the sulfate is also used to relieve inflammation. Parenteral administration of magnesium sulfate has been used in the treatment of seizures associated with eclampsia of pregnancy and acute nephritis.

Toxicokinetics   Oral magnesium is absorbed mainly in the small intestine. The colon also absorbs some magnesium. Calcium and magnesium are competitive with respect to absorption, and excess calcium will partially inhibit magnesium absorption. Serum magnesium levels are remarkably constant. Magnesium is excreted into the digestive tract by the bile and in pancreatic and intestinal juices. Approximately 60–65% of the total body magnesium is in the bone, 27% in muscle, 6–7% in other organs, and only 1% is in extracellular fluid. Of the magnesium filtered by the glomeruli about 95% is reabsorbed, an important factor in maintaining homeostasis.

Essentiality and Deficiency   Magnesium is a cofactor of many enzymes. In the glycolytic cycle, there are seven key enzymes that require divalent magnesium. Magnesium-containing enzymes are also involved in the citric acid cycle and in beta oxidation of fatty acids. Deficiency may occur as a complication of various disease states such as malabsorption syndromes, renal dysfunction, and endocrine disorders. Magnesium deficiency in humans causes neuromuscular irritability, frank tetany, and even convulsions. Magnesium deficiency induces an inflammatory syndrome (Mazur *et al.*, 2007), and is a risk factor for diabetes mellitus, hypertension, hyperlipidemia, and ischemic heart diseases (Ueshima, 2005). Supplementation of magnesium, either by intravenous or oral administration, is beneficial.

Toxicity   In industrial exposures, no ill effects are produced with a twofold increase in serum magnesium, although concurrent increases occur in serum calcium. Inhaled freshly generated magnesium oxide can cause metal fume fever, similar to that caused by zinc oxide. In nonoccupationally exposed individuals, toxicity can occur when magnesium-containing drugs, usually antacids, are ingested chronically by persons with serious renal failure. The toxic effects may progress from nausea and vomiting to hypotension, electrocardiograph abnormalities, central nervous system effects, coma, and systolic cardiac arrest (Shils, 1996). Magnesium toxicity can sometimes be counteracted with calcium infusion.

Manganese

Manganese (Mn) was in use in prehistoric times. Paints that were pigmented with manganese dioxide can be traced back to ancient times. The pure element was isolated in 1774 and named after the Latin *magnes*, meaning "magnet." Manganese is an essential metal required for many metabolic and cellular functions. Manganese metalloenzymes include arginase, glutamine synthetase, phosphoenolpyruvate decarboxylase, and manganese superoxide dismutase (Aschner and Aschner, 2005). Manganese is also a cofactor for a number of enzymatic reactions. Manganese exists in many valences but the divalent cation is by far the predominant species within cells. Divalent manganese may be oxidized to the more reactive and toxic trivalent form. The major source of manganese intake is from the food. Vegetables, grains, fruits, nuts, and tea are rich in manganese. Daily manganese intake ranges from 2 to 9 mg (ATSDR, 2000). The Adequate Intake is 2.3 and 1.8 mg/day for adult men and women, respectively (IOM, 2002).

Occupational exposures to high concentrations of manganese can occur in a number of settings, including manganese dioxide mines and smelters. Significant exposure can also occur in factories making manganese steel alloys, electrical coils, batteries, glass, welding rods, and during production of potassium permanganate ($KMnO_4$). The industrial use of manganese has expanded in recent years as a ferroalloy in the iron industry and as a component of alloys used in welding (Crossgrove and Zheng, 2004).

Environmental exposures are often associated with manganese-based organometallic pesticides, maneb and mancozeb. Manganese intoxication has also been reported after ingestion of contaminated water (ATSDR, 2000; Crossgrove and Zheng, 2004). There is current interest in the toxicology of manganese-containing fuel additive methylcyclopentadienyl manganese tricarbonyl (MMT). In addition, manganese compounds, such as mangafodipir are increasingly used as MRI enhancers in clinical imaging techniques.

Toxicokinetics   Approximately 1–5% of ingested manganese is normally absorbed. Interactions between manganese, and iron, as well as other divalent elements, occur and impact the toxicokinetics of manganese especially following oral exposure (Roth and Garrick, 2003). Iron and manganese can compete for the same binding protein in serum (transferrin) and the same transport systems (divalent metal transporter, DMT1). Inhalation of particulate manganese may result in direct transfer to brain tissue via the olfactory system (Tjalve and Henriksson, 1999). Within the plasma, manganese is largely bound to gamma globulin and albumin, with a small fraction bound to transferrin. Manganese concentrates in mitochondria, so that tissues rich in these organelles, like pancreas, liver, kidneys, and intestines, have the highest concentrations of manganese. Manganese readily crosses the blood–brain barrier and accumulates in specific brain regions (Crossgrove and Zheng, 2004). Manganese is eliminated in the bile and reabsorbed in the intestine. The principal route of manganese excretion is with the feces. Biliary excretion is poorly developed in neonates and exposure during this period may result in increased delivery of manganese to the brain and other tissues (Aschner and Aschner, 2005).

Essentiality and Deficiency   Manganese deficiency has been produced in many species of animals, but questions remain about whether deficiency has actually been demonstrated in humans

(WHO, 1996). Deficiency in animals results in impaired growth, skeletal abnormalities, and disturbed reproductive function.

Toxicity Chronic manganese-induced neurotoxicity (manganism) is of great concern and the brain is considered the most sensitive organ to manganese. Neurotoxicity due to inhalation of airbone manganese ranging from 0.027 to 1 mg Mn/m^3 has been reported in a number of occupational settings. Overt manganism occurs in workers exposed to aerosols containing extremely high levels ($>1-5$ mg Mn/m^3). Neurotoxicity also occurs following ingestion of manganese contaminated water (1.8 to 14 ppm; Aschner et al., 2005). Manganism is associated with elevated brain levels of manganese, primarily in those areas known to contain high concentrations of nonheme iron, such as the substantia nigra, basal ganglia, caudate-putamen, globus pallidus, and subthalamic nuclei. Early manifestations of manganese neurotoxicity include headache, insomnia, memory loss, muscle cramps, and emotional instability. Initial outward symptoms progress gradually and are mainly psychiatric. As exposure continues and the disease progresses, patients may develop prolonged muscle contractions (dystonia), decreased muscle movement (hypokinesia), rigidity, hand tremor, speech disturbances, and festinating "cock-walk" gait. These signs are associated with damage to dopaminergic neurons that control muscle movement (Crossgrove and Zheng, 2004; Aschner et al., 2005). Specialized T1-weighted magnetic resonance brain imaging of manganism patients indicates high levels in the basal ganglia and especially in the globus pallidus.

Inhalation of manganese-containing dust in certain occupational settings can lead to an inflammatory response in the lung. Symptoms of lung irritation and injury may include cough, bronchitis, pneumonitis, and occasionally, pneumonia (ATSDR, 2000). Men working in plants with high concentrations of manganese dust show an incidence of respiratory disease that is 30 times greater than normal. Manganese exposure also alters cardiovascular function in animals and humans, as evidenced by abnormal electrocardiogram and the inhibition of myocardial contraction. Manganese dilates blood vessels and induces hypotension (Jiang and Zheng, 2005). When manganese is combined with bilirubin, it produces intrahepatic cholestasis by acting on the synthesis and degradation of cholesterol and the inhibition of the transport pump Mrp2 (Akoume et al., 2003). Liver cirrhosis is a major contributing factor for hepatic encephalopathy, often associated with increased manganese levels in the brain (Mas, 2006).

Interactions between manganese and iron play a role in manganese toxicity. The coaccumulation of iron with manganese in the globus pallidus raises the concern that iron may be a contributing factor facilitating neuronal cell loss during manganese intoxication. Chronic exposure to manganese alters iron concentrations in blood and cerebrospinal fluid, presumably due to manganese–iron interaction at certain iron–sulfur containing proteins, which regulate iron homeostasis. Manganese intoxication in monkeys causes elevated iron deposition in the globus pallidus and substantia nigra. The excess iron may produce oxidative stress via the Fenton reaction, leading to neuronal damage. Dysfunctional iron metabolism has also been seen in manganism patients. Serum parameters associated with iron metabolism, such as ferritin, transferrin, and total-iron-binding capacity are significantly altered (Roth and Garrick, 2003; Crossgrove and Zheng, 2004). High levels of total iron and iron-associated oxidative stress, decreased ferritin, and abnormal mitochondrial complex-1 have been repeatedly reported in postmortem samples of substantia nigra from manganism patients.

Available data indicate that inorganic manganese is not carcinogenic in humans or rodents, and negative in Ames test, but may cause DNA damage and chromosome aberrations in vitro in mammalian cells (Gerber et al., 2002).

Molybdenum

Molybdenum (Mo) was first separated from lead and graphite in 1778. Molybdenum was derived from Greek molybdos meaning "lead-like." As an essential element, molybdenum acts as a cofactor for at least three enzymes in humans: sulfite oxidase, xanthine oxidase, and aldehyde oxidase. Molybdenum exists in five oxidation states but the predominant species are Mo^{4+} and Mo^{6+}. Molybdenum concentration in food varies considerably depending on the local environment. Molybdenum is added in trace amounts to fertilizers to stimulate plant growth. The human requirement for molybdenum is low and easily provided by a common US diet. The RDA for molybdenum is 45 μg/day (IOM, 2001).

The most important mineral source of molybdenum is molybdenite (MoS$_2$). The industrial uses of this metal include the manufacture of high temperature-resistant steel alloys for gas turbines and jet aircraft engines and in the production of catalysts, lubricants, and dyes. Ammonium tetrathiomolybdate is used as a molybdenum-donating copper chelator in treatment of Wilson disease (Brewer, 2003).

Toxicokinetics Water-soluble molybdenum compounds are readily absorbed when ingested. In laboratory animals, gastrointestinal absorption varies between 75% and 95%. In humans, absorption of molybdenum after oral intake varies from 28% to 77% (Vyskocil and Viau, 1999). Once absorbed, molybdenum rapidly appears in blood and most tissues. The highest molybdenum concentrations are found in kidneys, liver, and bones. Very little molybdenum appears to cross the placenta. When elevated exposure is ceased, tissue concentrations quickly return to normal levels. Molybdenum metabolism is related to copper and sulfur. Exposure to molybdenum decreases intestinal absorption of copper and sulfate, and impairs the sulfation of chemicals (Boles and Klaassen, 2000). Excretion, primarily via the urine, is rapid and 36–90% of a dose of molybdenum is excreted in urine in experimental animals. In humans, the urinary excretion ranges from 17% to 80% of the total dose. Very little ($<1\%$) of molybdenum excretion is via bile (Vyskocil and Viau, 1999). When consuming a low-molybdenum diet, the intestinal molybdenum absorption and tissue uptake are increased, while urinary excretion is decreased to reduce the molybdenum loss. With high dietary intake, urinary excretion can be dramatically increased to help eliminate excess molybdenum (Novotny and Turnlund, 2006).

Essentiality and Deficiency Molybdenum deficiency has been described in various animal species and consists of disturbances in uric acid metabolism and sulfite metabolism. Molybdenum cofactor (Moco) deficiency is a pleiotropic genetic disorder characterized by the loss of the molybdenum-dependent enzymes sulfite oxidase, xanthine oxidoreductase, and aldehyde oxidase, due to mutations in the genes involved with Moco biosynthesis. This rare human genetic metabolic disorder is characterized by severe neurodegeneration resulting in early childhood death (Schwarz, 2005).

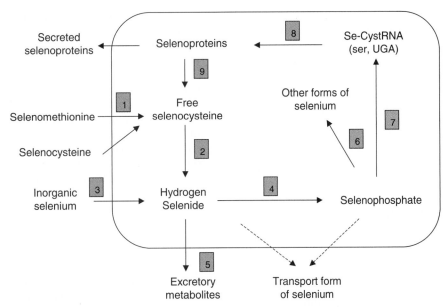

Figure 23-9. Selenium Metabolism Pathways.

(1) The transulfuration pathway; (2) seleno-cysteine β-lyase; (3) reduction by glutathione; (4) selenophosphate synthetase; (5) methylation; (6) replacement of sulfur in tRNA by selenium; (7) replacement of oxygen in serine to produce selenocysteine; (8) decoding of UGA in mRNA with insertion of selenocysteine into primary structure of protein; and (9) proteolytic breakdown of proteins. The origin and identity of the transport form for selenium is unknown, as indicated by the broken lines.

Toxicity Molybdenum is of low toxicity. Chronic exposure to excess molybdenum in humans is characterized by high uric acid levels in serum and urine. A gout-like syndrome has been observed in inhabitants exposed to high levels of environmental molybdenum or among workers exposed to molybdenum in a copper–molybdenum plant (Vyskocil and Viau, 1999). When inhaled, both metallic molybdenum and sparingly soluble molybdenum trioxide have been reported to cause pneumoconiosis. Molybdenosis (teart) is a form of molybdenum poisoning that produces a disease in ruminants similar to copper-deficiency (Barceloux, 1999). Generally, soluble molybdenum compounds are more toxic than insoluble compounds. In many ways molybdenum toxicity resembles copper deficiency. Treatment with supplemental copper can often reverse the adverse effects of excess molybdenum (Vyskocil and Viau, 1999). Conversely, treatment of Wilson disease with molybdenum compounds is used to reduce copper burden. Molybdenum treatment may also be beneficial for angiogenesis, inflammation, and other disorders associated with excess copper (Brewer, 2003).

Selenium

Selenium (Se) was discovered in 1817, and named after the Greek word *selene* meaning moon. Although technically a nonmetal, certain forms have metal-like properties. Selenium is an essential element found in selenoproteins and deficiency is recognized in humans and animals (Ziegler and Filer, 1996). Selenium is also toxic and high doses cause overt selenium poisoning (*selenosis*). The availability and the toxic potential of selenium compounds are related to their chemical forms and, most importantly, to solubility. Selenium occurs in nature and biological systems as selenate (Se^{6+}), selenite (Se^{4+}), selenide (Se^{2+}), and elemental selenium (Se^{0}) (ATSDR, 2003).

Foods are a good source of selenium. Seafood (especially shrimp), meat, milk products, and grains provide the largest amounts in the diet. Levels of selenium in river water vary, depending on environmental and geological factors. Combustion of coal and other fossil fuels are the primary sources of airborne selenium compounds. Occupational exposure come from selenium refining operations, metal smelting, and milling operations, incineration of rubber tires and municipal waste (ATSDR, 2003).

Toxicokinetics Orally administered selenite, selenate, and selenomethione are readily absorbed, often greater than 80%, whereas elemental selenium and selenides are virtually insoluble and poorly absorbed. Because of their insolubility, these forms may be regarded as an inert selenium sink. Monogastric animals have higher intestinal absorption than ruminants, probably because selenite is reduced to an insoluble form in rumen. Selenium accumulates in many tissues, with the highest accumulation in the liver and kidney. Selenium is transferred through the placenta to the fetus, and it also appears in milk. Levels in milk are dependent on dietary intake. Selenium in red blood cells is associated with glutathione peroxidase and is about three times more concentrated than in plasma. Selenium is primarily eliminated in urine and feces. In cases of acute exposure to toxic concentrations of selenium, significant amounts are eliminated in expired air, causing the characteristic "garlic breath" (ATSDR, 2003).

Selenium metabolism is well regulated in order to meet several metabolic needs (Fig. 23-9). Inorganic selenium and selenocysteine undergo stepwise reduction to the key intermediate hydrogen selenide, which is either transformed to selenophosphate for selenoprotein synthesis or excreted into breath or urine after being transformed into methylated metabolites of selenide (ATSDR, 2003). Selenophosphate is involved in the synthesis of selenocystein tRNA according to the UGA code for the selenocysteine residue. The translation of selenoprotein mRNA requires *cis*-acting sequences in the mRNA and transacting factors dedicated to selenocysteine incorporation (Driscoll and Copeland, 2003). Selenoprotein synthesis is highly dependent on selenium availability.

Essentiality and Deficiency Selenium is notable for its actions in antioxidant systems through involvement in over 20 selenoproteins (Tapiero *et al.*, 2003). For instance, glutathione peroxidase is the selenium-dependent enzyme that reduces peroxides using glutathione, and thereby protects membrane lipids, proteins, and nucleic acids from damage by oxidants or free radicals. The enzyme thioredoxin reductase is another selenium-dependent enzyme that has an important role in body's defense against oxidative damage. Selenoprotein P is the major plasma selenoprotein, and serves as an antioxidant in the extracellular space and transports selenium from the liver to other tissues. Selenium W is a low-molecular-weight selenoprotein and may have redox functions. Iodothreonine deiodinases are selenoproteins contributing to systemic or local thyroid hormone homeostasis. Selenium content in endocrine tissues (thyroid, adrenals, pituitary, testes, and ovary) is higher than many other organs. Hormones and growth factors also regulate expression of selenoproteins (Kohrle *et al.*, 2005).

The most extensively documented deficiency of selenium in humans is Keshan disease. This is an endemic cardiomyopathy first discovered in Keshan County in China where there are very low concentrations of selenium in the soil and food, and Keshan disease patients show very low plasma selenium levels. This deficiency occurs most frequently in children under 15 years of age and in women of child-bearing age and is characterized by various degrees of cardiomegaly and cardiac decompensation. Deficiency of selenium also occurs in domestic animals and rodents. Selenium supplement reduces these adverse effects (WHO, 1987; Tinggi, 2003).

Kashin-Beck disease is an osteoarthropathy found in areas where combined deficiency of selenium and iodine occur with elevated exposure to mycotoxin and fulvic acids (Sudre and Mathieu, 2001). Selenium deficiency is a major contributing factor in this disease. Other potential effects of selenium deficiency include immune dysfunction, and susceptibility to cancer or infectious/inflammatory diseases (Tapiero *et al.*, 2003; Ryan-Harshman and Aldoori, 2005).

The National Research Council's Food and Nutrition Board recommends 200 μg/day as the safe upper limit in adults (Duffield-Lillico *et al.*, 2002). Metabolic balance studies in adults indicate about 70 μg/day is required to maintain selenium balance and presumably to satisfy selenium requirement. Data indicate that daily intake less than 20 μg can cause Keshan disease.

Toxicity Acute selenium toxicity in humans is rare. Intentional or accidental ingestion of a large dose of sodium selenate or sodium selenite can be life-threatening. Symptoms of fatal selenium intoxication include nausea and vomiting, followed by pulmonary edema and rapid cardiovascular collapse (Hunsaker *et al.*, 2005).

Chronic selenium toxicity (*selenosis*) can occur with environmental exposure when the intake exceeds the excretory capacity. Effects are mainly dermal and neurological including hair and finger nail loss, tooth discoloration, numbness, paralysis, and occasional hemiplegia. Selenosis occurred in several villages in China where people were exposed to very high selenium in food (ATSDR, 2003). Intoxication from environmental selenium has also been noted in

people residing in Venezuela and South Dakota. Selenium toxicity in animals was recognized in South Dakota when the livestock that had been grazed in areas with high soil selenium developed *alkali disease* and *blind staggers*. In a study of people living in this area, poor dentition, a yellowish discoloration of the skin, skin eruptions, and diseased fingernails and toe nails were found (WHO, 1987).

Plants vary in their ability to accumulate selenium. Grasses, grains, and most weeds do not accumulate selenium even when grown in high selenium areas, so that these plants add little to the selenium content of livestock feed. But there are several plant species that are classified as "selenium accumulators" and they may contain selenium at very high concentrations (100–10,000 mg/kg). These plants usually grow in nonagricultural areas and when consumed by livestock may cause selenium intoxication. Selenium has produced loss of fertility and congenital defects and is considered embryotoxic and teratogenic in animals (WHO, 1987).

Selenium has various bioinorganic interactions, which may affect the toxicity of selenium or other metals. Selenium forms insoluble complexes with various metals, as for example, with arsenic. Selenium complexation can increase the biliary excretion of various metals. Selenium forms complexes with copper, and toxicity of either selenium or copper is influenced by the intake of the other elements. The methylation of selenium can influence other methylation reactions, and can alter arsenic metabolism and toxicity (Zeng *et al.*, 2005). Selenium prevents the toxic effects of cadmium and can reduce the toxic effects of methylmercury. The mechanisms for these interactions are only partially understood, but their occurrence influences the determination of safe and toxic levels of selenium for the general population (WHO, 1987, 1996).

Some epidemiologic data have linked low blood selenium levels and increased cancer risk in various populations (ATSDR, 2003). Selenium supplementations appear to decrease human cancer rates, especially for prostate cancer (Duffield-Lillico *et al.*, 2002). Increasing selenium content of forage crops has been shown to be beneficial in reducing cancer risk. Some experimental evidence supports a role for selenium in reduction of spontaneous tumors or tumors formed by organic carcinogens in rats and mice. Synthetic organoselenium compounds have been under trial as chemotherapeutics (Tapiero *et al.*, 2003).

Trivalent Chromium

Essentiality Trivalent chromium (Cr^{3+}) is a naturally occurring essential trace nutrient serving an important role in glucose metabolism by enhancing insulin signaling (IOM, 2001). The glucose tolerance factor is a complex of trivalent chromium, nicotinic acid, and amino acids, and physiologically potentiates the action of insulin in glucose, lipid, and protein metabolism (IOM, 2001). Other effects of trivalent chromium include the beneficial roles in growth, immune response, and stress (Ziegler and Filer, 1996). The tissue levels of chromium are reduced among diabetic individuals, but the effects of chromium supplementation in type-2 diabetes are still controversial (Cefalu and Hu, 2004). The adequate intake of chromium is now proposed as 35 and 25 μg/kg/day for men and women, respectively, which is lower than previous 50–200 μg/day. Chromium picolinate, the best-selling nutritional supplement was thought to have adverse effects and might have potential to cause cancer (Vincent, 2004), but more evidence is needed to make conclusions.

Zinc

Zinc (Zn) was named after the German word *zink* meaning tin. Zinc has been used since ancient times, including uses in alloys and medicines. An essential metal, zinc deficiency results in severe health consequences. However, zinc toxicity is relatively uncommon and occurs only at very high exposure levels. Zinc is ubiquitous in the environment so that it is present in most foodstuffs, water, and air. The major route of zinc intake is through the diet, the contents of which vary from 5.2 to 16.2 mg Zn/day (ATSDR, 2005f). Recommend Dietary Allowance for zinc is 11 and 8 mg/day for men and women, respectively (IOM, 2001).

Occupational exposure to dusts and fumes of metallic zinc occurs in zinc mining and smelting. The zinc content of substances in contact with galvanized copper or plastic pipes may be high. Many countries regulate workplace levels of zinc oxide fume and dust at levels between 5 and 10 mg/m^3 (WHO, 1998).

Toxicokinetics The absorption of zinc from the gastrointestinal tract is homeostatically regulated. About 20–30% of ingested zinc is absorbed. Zinc uptake from the intestinal lumen involves passive diffusion and a carrier-mediated process through specific zinc transporters such as ZnT-1. Intestinal absorption of zinc can be reduced by dietary fiber, phytates, calcium and phosphorus, while amino acids, picolinic acid, and prostaglandin E2 can enhance zinc absorption. Once absorbed, zinc is widely distributed throughout the body. The total zinc content of the human body is in the range of 1.5–3 g. Most of this is found in muscle (60%), bone (30%), skin/hair (8%), liver (5%), and pancreas (3%). The highest concentrations of zinc are found in prostate, pancreas, liver, and kidney. In plasma, zinc concentration is about 1 mg/L, and is bound to albumin (60–80%), which represents the metabolically active pool of zinc. The remainder is bound to α_2-macroglobulin and trasferrin. Zinc is excreted in both urine and feces. The concentration of zinc in the plasma is not a sensitive indicator of zinc status and does not reflect the dose–response relationship between zinc levels in the body and effects at various target sites. Zinc ions are involved as inter- and intracellular messengers and the homeostasis of zinc has to be tightly controlled. The most reliable index of zinc status is the determination of zinc balance, using a U-shaped homeostatic model to analyze the relationship between intake and excretion (WHO, 1998).

Zinc is an effective inducer of metallothionein synthesis and, when metallothionein is saturated in intestinal cells, zinc absorption is decreased. Metallothionein is also an important storage depot for cellular zinc. Liver metallothionein concentration is influenced by hormonal factors, including adrenocorticotropic hormone and parathyroid hormone, and various stimuli that impact zinc metabolism. The high concentration of zinc in the prostate is probably related to the rich content of zinc-containing enzyme acid phosphatase.

Essentiality and Deficiency More than 300 catalytically active zinc metalloenzymes and 2000 zinc-dependent transcription factors exist (Ziegler and Filer, 1996; Cai *et al.*, 2005). Zinc participates in a wide variety of metabolic processes, supports a healthy immune system, and is essential for normal growth and development during pregnancy, childhood, and adolescence. Zinc deficiency is related to poor dietary zinc intake, dietary phytate intake, chronic illness, or over-supplementation with iron or copper (Prasad, 2004). Symptoms of zinc deficiency include growth retardation, appetite loss, alopecia, diarrhea, impaired immune function, cognitive impairments, dermatitis, delayed healing of wounds, taste abnormalities, and impaired sexual function (Prasad, 2004; Cai *et al.*, 2005; Cousins, 2006). *Acrodermatitis enteropathica* is a rare genetically based, heredity disorder involving zinc deficiency due to poor intestinal absorption (Perafan-Riveros *et al.*, 2002). Zinc supplementation, alone or with other micronutrients, is recommended for zinc-deficient children, especially in developing countries.

Therapeutic uses of zinc include the treatment of acute diarrhea in infants with severe zinc deficiency, the treatment of common cold by its antiviral and immunomodulatory effects, therapy for Wilson disease to help reduce copper burden and to induce metallothionein, and in the prevention of blindness in age-related macular degeneration (Prasad, 2004).

Toxicity Acute zinc toxicity from excessive ingestion is uncommon, but gastrointestinal distress and diarrhea have been reported following ingestion of beverages standing in galvanized cans. Following inhalation of zinc oxide, and to a lesser extent other zinc compounds, the most common effect is "metal-fume fever" characterized by fever, chest pain, chills, cough, dyspnea, nausea, muscle soreness, fatigue, and leukocytosis. Acute inhalation of high levels of zinc chloride as in the military use of "smoke bombs" results in more pronounced damage to the mucous membrane including interstitial edema, fibrosis, pneumonitis, bronchial mucosal edema, and ulceration. Following long-term exposure to lower doses of zinc, symptoms generally result from a decreased dietary copper absorption, leading to early symptoms of copper deficiency, such as decreased erythrocyte number or decreased hematocrit.

Neuronal Toxicity Zinc has dual effects in the brain. As an essential cofactor for numerous enzymes and proteins, zinc deficiency may alter activity of the antioxidant enzyme Cu–Zn–superoxide dismutase (SOD), resulting in excess free radicals that are damaging to cell membranes (Valko *et al.*, 2005). A genetic abnormality of Cu–Zn–SOD may be the basis of a familial form of amyotrophic lateral sclerosis (Selverstone Valentine *et al.*, 2005). Zinc can also act as a neurotransmitter for normal brain functions (Frederickson *et al.*, 2005; Cousins *et al.*, 2006). Zinc modulates the solubility of β-amyloid in the brain and protects against β-amyloid toxicity, but excess zinc may trigger neuronal death that is independent or synergistic with the toxic effect of β-amyloid (Valko *et al.*, 2005). In addition, excess zinc released by oxidants can act as a potent neurotoxin (Frederickson *et al.*, 2005). Synaptically released zinc might contribute to excitotoxic brain injury, and the release of excess, toxic free zinc into the brain that occurs during excitotoxic brain injury could be a factor that sets the stage for the later development of Alzheimer's disease.

Pancreatic Toxicity Because large amounts of zinc accumulate in secretory granules of pancreatic islet beta-cells, zinc released under certain conditions can affect the function or survival of islet cells and cause beta-cell death. Excess dietary zinc is associated with damage to exocrine pancreas. A single, high-dose injection of zinc increases plasma α-amylase activity and can produce fibrosis and necrosis of pancreatic exocrine cells, but does not affect the islets of Langerhans cells (Cai *et al.*, 2005).

Zinc and Carcinogenicity Epidemiological studies of workers in electrolytic zinc and copper refining industries have not found an increased incidence of cancer associated with occupational zinc inhalation. Oral zinc supplementation does not appear to have a significant effect on cancer incidence (ATSDR, 2005f). In addition, zinc deficiency may be associated with increased risk of cancer in humans (Prasad and Kucuk, 2002). Zinc supplementation could decrease oxidative stress and improve immune function, which may be a possible mechanism for its cancer preventive activity (Prasad and Kucuk, 2002). In experimental animals, zinc prevents cadmium-induced testicular cancer, but facilitates cadmium-induced prostate tumors (Waalkes, 2003).

METALS RELATED TO MEDICAL THERAPY

Aluminum

Aluminum (Al) is the third most abundant metal in the earth's crust after oxygen and silicon. Elemental aluminum was first identified in 1827. Due to its high reactivity, aluminum is not found in the free-state in nature. Chemical compounds of aluminum occur typically in the trivalent valence state (Al^{3+}). As a hard trivalent ion, aluminum binds strongly to oxygen-donor ligands such as citrate and phosphate. The chemistry of aluminum compounds is complicated by a tendency to hydrolyze and form polynuclear species, many of which are sparingly soluble (Harris et al., 1996).

Aluminum has many uses, mainly in the form of alloys, and finds use in packing, construction, transportation, electrical applications, and beverage cans. Aluminum compounds are also used as food additives. Human exposure to aluminum comes primarily from food and secondarily from drinking water. The amount of aluminum in the food supply is small compared to pharmaceutical use of aluminum in antacids and buffered analgesics (Soni et al., 2001). Occupational exposures to aluminum occur during mining and processing, as well as in aluminum welding. The levels of exposure can vary greatly according to the type of industry and hygiene conditions. Inhalation of aluminum-containing dust particles is of health concern (WHO, 1997).

Aluminum exists predominantly in forms that are innocuous to humans and most species. However, acid conditions, such as acid rain or dry acid deposition, can dramatically increase the amount of aluminum in ecosystems, resulting in well-described destructive effects on plants, fish, and other wildlife. However, aluminum is not bioaccumulated to any significant extent except in the tea plant (Sparling and Lowe, 1996).

Toxicokinetics Aluminum is poorly absorbed following either oral or inhalation exposure and is essentially not absorbed dermally. Inhalation of particulate aluminum may result in direct transfer to brain tissue via the olfactory system (Tjalve and Henriksson, 1999). Less than 1% of aluminum in the diet is absorbed. Absorption from the gut depends largely on pH and the presence of complexing ligands, particularly carboxylic acids, through which aluminum becomes absorbable. For example, intestinal absorption is enhanced in the presence of citrate. Biological speciation is also of major importance in distribution and excretion of aluminum in mammals (Harris et al., 1996). In plasma, 80–90% of aluminum binds to transferrin, an iron-transport protein with receptors in many tissues. The transferrin pathway is also considered a mechanism for aluminum transport across the blood–brain barrier (Van Landeghem et al., 1998). Lung, liver, and bone have the highest concentrations of aluminum (WHO, 1997). Aluminum is removed from blood by the kidneys and excreted in urine. In patients with impaired renal function, tis-

sue aluminum concentrations can increase and are associated with encephalopathy and osteomalacia.

Aluminum compounds can alter absorption of other elements in the gastrointestinal tract. For instance, aluminum inhibits fluoride absorption and may decrease the absorption of calcium and iron compounds and salicylic acid, which, in turn, may affect the absorption of aluminum (Exley et al., 1996). The binding of phosphorus by aluminum in the intestinal tract can lead to phosphate depletion and potentially, osteomalacia. Aluminum interacts with calcium in bone and kidney, resulting in aluminum osteodystrophy (Goyer, 1997). Aluminum may also alter gastrointestinal tract motility by inhibition of acetylcholine-induced contractions, which is probably why aluminum-containing antacids often cause constipation.

Toxicity Acute aluminum toxicity is rare. Most cases of aluminum toxicity in humans are observed in patients with chronic renal failure, or in persons exposed to aluminum in the workplace, with the lung, bone, and central nervous system as major target organs. Aluminum affects similar target organs in animals and can produce developmental effects.

Lung and Bone Toxicity Occupational exposure to aluminum dust can produce lung fibrosis in humans, but this effect is probably due to lung overload caused by excessive deposition of dust (Morrow, 1992). Osteomalacia has been associated with excessive intake of aluminum-containing antacids in otherwise healthy individuals. This is assumed to be due to interference with intestinal phosphate absorption. Osteomalacia also can occur in uremic patients exposed to aluminum in the dialysis fluid. In these patients, osteomalacia may be a direct effect of aluminum on bone mineralization as bone levels are high (Soni et al., 2001).

Neurotoxicity Aluminum is neurotoxic to experimental animals, with wide species- and age-variations. In susceptible animals, such as rabbits and cats, aluminum toxicity is characterized by progressive neurological impairment resulting in death associated with status epilepticus (WHO, 1997). The most prominent early pathologic change is the accumulation of neurofibrillary tangles (NFTs) in large neurons, proximal axons, and dentrites of neurons of many brain regions. This is associated with loss of synapses and atrophy of the dendritic tree. Not all species show this reaction to aluminum. For instance, rats fail to develop NFTs or encephalopathy and monkeys develop NFTs only after more than a year of aluminum infusion. Impairment of cognitive and motor function and behavioral abnormalities are often observed. Whereas studies in animals have provided some insights into the mechanisms of the neurotoxicity of aluminum in experimental models, the relationship to any human disease is still uncertain.

Dialysis Dementia This is a progressive, neurologic syndrome reported in patients on long-term intermittent hemodialysis for chronic renal failure (Alfrey, 1993). The first symptom in these patients is a speech disorder followed by dementia, convulsions, and myoclonus. The disorder, which typically arises after 3–7 years of dialysis treatment, may be due to aluminum intoxication. The aluminum content of brain, muscle, and bone increases in these patients. Sources of the excess aluminum may be from oral aluminum hydroxide commonly given to these patients or from aluminum in dialysis fluid derived from the tap water used to prepare the dialysate fluid. The high serum aluminum concentrations may be related to increased parathyroid hormone levels which are due to low blood calcium and osteodystrophy common in patients with chronic renal disease. The syndrome may be prevented by avoiding the use of aluminum-containing oral phosphate binders and by monitoring of aluminum in the dialysate.

The Chamorro people of the Marina Islands in the Western Pacific Ocean, particularly Guam and Rota, have an unusually high incidence of neurodegeneration of the Alzheimer's type. Garruto *et al.* (1984, 1985) noted that the volcanic soils of the regions of Guam with a high incidence of Amyotrophic Lateral Sclerosis and Parkinsonism-Dementia Syndromes (ALS-PD) contained high concentrations of aluminum and manganese and were low in calcium and magnesium. They postulated that a low intake of calcium and magnesium induced secondary hyperparathyroidism, resulting in an increase in the deposition of calcium, aluminum, and other toxic metals, and eventually in neuronal injury and death. How and why aluminum enters the brain of these people is unclear. The incidence of these disorders dramatically decreased or disappeared during the past 60 years, possibly as the result of radical socioeconomic, ethnographic, and ecologic changes brought about by the rapid westernization of Guam, rather than genetic factors (Garruto *et al.*, 1985; Plato *et al.*, 2003).

Alzheimer's Disease A possible relationship between aluminum and Alzheimer's disease has been a matter of speculation for decades. The basis for this relationship is the finding of increased aluminum levels in Alzheimer brains, neurofibrillary lesions in experimental animals, and the fact that aluminum is associated with various components of the pathologic lesions in Alzheimer brain tissue. However, elevated aluminum levels in Alzheimer brains may be a consequence and not a cause of the disease. The reduced effectiveness of the blood–brain barrier in Alzheimer's might allow more aluminum into the brain. Also, recent studies have raised the possibility that the staining methods in earlier studies may have lead to aluminum contamination (Makjanic *et al.*, 1998). Furthermore, the neurofibrillary tangles seen in aluminum encephalopathy differ structurally and chemically from those in Alzheimer's (WHO, 1997). Epidemiological studies examining the role of aluminum exposure in Alzheimer's disease arrive at conflicting conclusions. An examination of 20 epidemiological studies concluded that there is not enough evidence to support a primary causative role of aluminum in Alzheimer's disease, and aluminum does not induce Alzheimer's pathology in vivo in any species, including humans (WHO, 1997). However, there is increasing evidence suggesting a link between aluminum in the brain and other neurodegenerative diseases (Kawahara, 2005).

Treatment Chelation therapy for aluminum, mostly in dialyzed and/or uremic patients, resembles that for iron overload, with deferoxamine and deferiprone (Blanusa *et al.*, 2005).

Bismuth

Bismuth (Bi) is a metal with a stable valence of 3+. The name *bisemutum* is from German *Wismuth*, perhaps from the term *weiße Masse*, for "white mass." It was confused in early times with tin and lead due to its resemblance to those elements. Bismuth was shown to be distinct from lead in 1753. The solubility of most bismuth salts is low but can be affected by pH and the presence of sulfhydryl- or hydroxy-containing ligands. The significance of environmental

and occupational bismuth exposure is unknown. Human exposure to bismuth generally is due to medicinal use.

Trivalent insoluble bismuth salts such as bismuth subnitrate, subcarbonate, and subgallate, are used for various gastrointestinal disorders including diarrhea, flatulence, constipation, cramps, and dyspepsia. Colloidal bismuth subcitrate, bismuth subsalicylate, and the more recently developed ranitidine bismuth citrate, are widely used to treat peptic ulcer and *Helicobacter pylori* associated gastritis. Outdated medicinal applications include the use of bismuth salts for treatment of syphilis, malaria, warts, stomatitis, and infections of the upper respiratory tract (Slikkerveer and de Wolf, 1996). A new potential application includes the use of bismuth subnitrate to prevent cisplatin nephrotoxicity, probably due to a specific induction of renal metallothionein (Kondo *et al.*, 2004). The use of alpha-particle emitting bismuth compounds as radio-therapeutic agents, and the use of certain bismuth compounds as antitumor agents show some promise (Tiekink, 2002).

Toxicokinetics Most bismuth compounds are insoluble and poorly absorbed from the gastrointestinal tract or when applied to the skin. The three widely used compounds, colloidal tripotassium dicitrato bismuthate, bismuth subsalicylate, and ranitidine bismuth citrate are all poorly absorbed (<1%) (Tillman *et al.*, 1996). The highest concentrations of bismuth are found in kidneys, and to a lesser extent in the brain, liver, and bone (Slikkerveer and de Wolf, 1996; Larsen *et al.*, 2005). Passage of bismuth into the amniotic fluid and fetus has been demonstrated. Bismuth is cleared from the body through urine and feces (Gregus and Klaassen, 1986). Traces of bismuth can be found in milk and saliva. The elimination half-life is reported to be about 21 days, depending on bismuth compounds.

Toxicity Bismuth-containing medications are consumed worldwide and the risk of bismuth-related toxicity in the general population is relatively low. The main target organs for bismuth toxicity are kidney, brain, and bone (Slikkerveer and de Wolf, 1996; Tillman *et al.*, 1996; Larsen *et al.*, 2005). Acute renal injury is related to very high doses of bismuth, or to oral intake of organic bismuth compounds such as bismuth sodium triglycocollamate or thioglycollate, particularly in children. The tubular epithelium is the primary site of toxicity, where bismuth produces degeneration of renal tubular cells and nuclear inclusion bodies composed of bismuth–protein complex analogous to those found with lead exposure (Fowler and Goyer, 1975). A large single oral dose of colloidal bismuth subcitrate damages the proximal tubes, but the damage is reversible in both humans and animals (Leussink *et al.*, 2001).

An episode of bismuth-associated encephalopathy in France in the 1970s revealed a potential neurotoxic effect of bismuth, although it cannot be exclusively attributed to bismuth alone (Slikkerveer and de Wolf, 1996). Using autometallography, high amounts of bismuth were found in the reticular and hypothalamic nuclei, in the oculomotor and hypoglossal nuclei and in Purkinje cells following 8-month exposure to bismuth. Axonal transport seems to influence the distribution of bismuth. Ultrastructurally, accumulation of bismuth was seen in lysosomes (Larsen *et al.*, 2005).

Treatment The most effective treatment of bismuth toxicity is to discontinue bismuth intake. Chelation therapy using dimercaprol (BAL), 2,3-dimercaptoduccinic acid (DMSA), and 2,3-dimercapto-propane-1-sulfonic acid (DMPS) reduces the bismuth concentration in most organs (especially kidney and liver) and increase elimination of bismuth in urine. BAL was the only chelator effective in lowering brain bismuth concentrations (Slikkerveer and de Wolf, 1996).

Gallium

Gallium (Ga) has a very low melting point with the main valence state of 3+ (gallic), although the 2+ (gallous) form can also form stable gallium compounds. Gallium, stemming from *Gallia* meaning Gaul or France, was predicted to exist prior to being discovered in 1875 by its characteristic spectrum. Gallium is of interest because of the use of radiogallium as a diagnostic tool for the localization of bone lesions. Nonradioactive gallium nitrate has been used as an antitumor agent and in the treatment of hypercalcemia. Gallium is obtained as a by-product of copper, zinc, lead, and aluminum refining and is used in high-temperature thermometers, as a substitute for mercury in arc lamps, as a component of metal alloys, and as a seal for vacuum equipment. Gallium arsenide is a widely used semiconductor material. Gallium is the only metal other than mercury that is liquid at, or near room temperature.

Toxicokinetics Gallium salts are sparingly absorbed from the gastrointestinal tract, but accumulation in tissues can be observed after repeated administrations. The oral bioavailability is improved with gallium complexes such as gallium maltolate. Gallium accumulates mainly in bone, inflammatory lesions, and tumors, as well as in the liver, spleen, and kidney. Gallium binds to plasma transferrin and enters cells by iron transport mechanisms. Urine is the major route of gallium excretion (Bernstein, 1998; Jakupec and Keppler, 2004).

Toxicity The trivalent gallium cation biologically resembles ferric iron. It affects cellular acquisition of iron by binding to transferrin and interacts with the iron-dependent enzyme ribonucleotide reductase, resulting in decreased dNTP pools and inhibition of DNA synthesis (Bernstein, 1998). The abundance of transferrin receptors and ribonucleotide reductase renders tumor cells susceptible to the cytotoxicity of gallium. Use of bolus intravenous injection of gallium nitrate in the treatment of lymphoma and bladder cancer is limited by potential nephrotoxicity, which can be reduced by slow continuous infusion over several days (Jakupec and Keppler, 2004). Gallium nitrate is an effective treatment for cancer-related hypercalcemia and diseases associated with accelerated bone loss including myeloma, bone metastasis, Paget's disease, and osteoporosis. It accumulates in metabolically active regions of bone and favorably alters the mineral properties to enhance hydroxyapatite crystallization and reduce mineral solubility. Gallium inhibits osteoclastic bone resorption without poisoning the osteoclast cells, yielding a skeletal system with increased calcium and phosphate content and improved strength (Bockman, 2003). Adverse effects may include nausea, vomiting, and anemia. Less frequent are gallium-induced neurologic, pulmonary, and dermatologic effects.

Acute and chronic toxicity to lung, testes, and kidney are associated with exposures of gallium arsenide in animals, although the role of the individual metals in this response is unclear (Tanaka, 2004). There is little information regarding adverse effects of gallium compounds following occupational exposure.

Gold

Gold (Au) was well known and highly valued since prehistoric times. Gold is widely distributed but usually in small quantities. The metal has a number of industrial uses because of its electrical and thermal conductivity. Monovalent organogold salts (e.g., auranofin, aurothioglucose, gold sodium thiomalate) are used for the treatment of rheumatoid arthritis. Mono- and trivalent coordinated gold complexes have antitumor potential (Kostova, 2006). The health risks associated with gold mining, especially miners who used elemental mercury to amalgamate and extract gold, have been recently reviewed (Eisler, 2003).

Toxicokinetics Gold salts are poorly absorbed from the gastrointestinal tract. The more water-soluble, therapeutic gold compounds are absorbed after intramuscular injection, and peak concentration in blood is reached in 2–6 hours. Gold is initially bound to serum albumin, and then distributes to various tissues. With continued therapy, the concentration of gold in synovium of affected joints is 10 times that of muscle, bone, or fat. Gold deposits are also found in macrophages, kidney, liver, testes, and skin. About 60–90% of gold is excreted via the kidney while 10–40% occurs via biliary excretion into feces. Chelators such as dimercaprol may increase the excretion of gold. Gold has a long biological half-life, and elevated tissue and blood levels can be demonstrated for months after cessation of treatment.

Toxicity Contact dermatitis is the most frequently reported toxic reaction to gold and is sometimes accompanied by stomatitis, probably involving an allergic mechanism. Gold-induced allergic responses include delayed hypersensitivity, formation of intracutaneous nodules and immunogenic granuloma, as well as the occurrence of eczema (Hostynek, 1997).

The use of gold in the form of organic salts to treat rheumatoid arthritis may be complicated by the development of proteinuria and the nephrotic syndrome, which morphologically consists of immune-complex glomerulonephritis, with granular deposits along the glomerular basement membrane and in the mesangium (Hostynek, 1997; Bigazzi, 1999). The pathogenesis of the immune-complex disease is not certain, but gold may behave as a hapten and generate the production of antibody complexes for the glomerular deposits (Voil *et al.*, 1977).

Gold miners have increased frequency of pulmonary diseases, including tumors, and increased prevalence of infectious diseases. Mercury intoxication associated with gold mining activities is well documented (Eisler, 2003).

Lithium

Lithium (Li) is one of the lightest metallic elements. Lithium was discovered in 1817, and the name was derived from the Greek *lithos* for stone. Lithium shares its group with sodium and potassium, and is widely distributed in nature. Lithium is used in batteries, alloys, catalysts, photographic materials, and in the space industry. Lithium hydride produces hydrogen on contact with water and is used in manufacturing electronic tubes, in ceramics, and in chemical analysis. Groundwater contamination with lithium from man-made waste disposal could be a risk factor for the aquatic environment (Kszos and Stewart, 2003). Lithium carbonate and lithium citrate are widely used for mania and bipolar disorders. In this regard, lithium is active possibly through its effects on signal transduction, such as phosphoinositide hydrolysis, glycogen synthase kinase-3, and neurotropic cascades (Lenox and Hahn, 2000; Quiroz *et al.*, 2004). Topical applications of lithium succinate are still used in the treatment of seborrhoic dermatitis (Sparsa and Bonnetblane, 2004).

Toxicokinetics Lithium is readily absorbed from the gastrointestinal tract, with peak therapeutic levels at 30 minutes to 3 hours post-ingestion. Lithium is not bound to plasma proteins but is associated with red blood cells. Lithium is distributed to total body water with higher levels in kidney, thyroid, and bone as compared to other tissues. Excretion is chiefly through the kidneys with 80% of the filtered lithium reabsorbed. The usual elimination half-life is 12–27 hours, but it may rise to nearly 60 hours if renal function is compromised. Lithium can substitute for sodium or potassium on several transport proteins. It enters cells via the amiloride-sensitive sodium channel or the Na/H$^+$ exchanger. The greater part of lithium is retained in the cells, perhaps at the expense of potassium. In general it may be competing with sodium at certain sites, such as in renal tubular reabsorption (Timmer and Sands, 1999).

Toxicity From the industrial point of view, except for lithium hydride, none of the other salts is considered hazardous, nor is the metal very toxic itself. Lithium hydride is intensely corrosive and may produce burns on the skin because of the formation of hydroxides (Cox and Singer, 1981). Intoxications related to lithium exposure are mainly related to its medicinal uses (Timmer and Sands, 1999), as the therapeutic index of lithium is very narrow. In this regard, 0.7–1.2 mmol/L is considered an adequate therapeutic blood level, while blood levels only threefold higher commonly result in severe symptoms such as seizures and coma. The toxic responses to lithium include neuromuscular changes (tremor, muscle hyper-irritability, and ataxia), central nervous system disorders (blackout spells, epileptic seizures, slurred speech, coma, psychosomatic retardation, and increased thirst), cardiovascular disturbances (cardiac arrhythmia, hypertension, and circulatory collapse), gastrointestinal symptoms (anorexia, nausea, and vomiting), and renal damage (albuminuria and glycosuria). The renal lesions are believed to be due to temporary hypokalemic nephritis. Long-term sequelae from acute lithium poisoning include cognitive losses such as impaired memory, attention and executive functions, and visuospatial deficits (Brumm et al., 1998).

Chronic lithium nephrotoxicity and interstitial nephritis may occur with long-term exposure even when lithium levels remain within the therapeutic range. Lithium nephrotoxicity primarily targets distal and collecting tubes, with a higher incidence of proteinuria and associated glomerular pathology (Markowitz et al., 2000). Chronic lithium-induced neurotoxicity, nephritis and thyroid dysfunction may occur, especially in susceptible patients with identifiable clinical risk factors such as nephrogenic diabetes insipididus, older age, abnormal thyroid function, and impaired renal function (Oakley et al., 2001).

Lithium overdose and toxicity may be treated by the administration of diuretics (amiloride) and lowering of blood levels via hemodialysis. Treatment with diuretics must be accompanied by replacement of water and electrolytes (Timmer and Sands, 1999).

Platinum

Platinum (Pt) is a malleable, ductile, silvery-white noble metal. Naturally occurring platinum and platinum-rich alloys have been known for a long time. The first European reference to platinum appeared in 1557 and the element was isolated in 1741. In platinum compounds, the maximum oxidation state is 6+, while the 2+ and 4+ valences are most stable. Platinum is found in nature either in the metallic form or in a number of mineral forms in various ores. Environmental platinum levels are very low. Platinum compounds are used as automobile catalysts, in jewelry, in electronics, and in dental alloys. Platinum coordination complexes are very important antitumor agents. Occupational exposure can be higher than the exposure limit of 2 μg/m^3 in some settings (WHO, 1991).

Toxicokinetics Following a single inhalation exposure, most of the inhaled platinum is rapidly cleared from the lungs by mucociliary action, swallowed, and excreted in the feces, with half-life of about 24 hours. A small portion is detected in the urine, indicating very little platinum is absorbed. After intravenous administration of clinical doses, the drug has an initial elimination half-life in plasma of 25–50 min. More than 90% of the platinum in the blood is covalently bound to plasma proteins. After administration of the main metallochemotherapeutic form, cis-dichlorodiammine platinum(II) (cisplatin), high concentrations are found in the kidney, liver, intestine, spleen, and testes, but there is poor penetration into the brain. Only a small portion of the drug is excreted by the kidney during the first 6 hours. By 24 hours up to 25% is excreted, while by 5 days up to 43% of the administered dose is recovered in the urine (WHO, 1991; Hardman et al., 2001).

Toxicity Platinum can produce profound hypersensitivity reactions in susceptible individuals (WHO, 1991). The signs of hypersensitivity include urticaria, contact dermatitis of skin, and respiratory distress, ranging from irritation to an asthmatic syndrome, following exposure to platinum dust. The skin and respiratory changes are termed *platinosis*. They are mainly confined to persons with a history of industrial exposure to soluble compounds such as sodium chloroplatinate, although cases resulting from the wearing of platinum jewelry have been reported (WHO, 1991). The complex salts of platinum may act as powerful allergens, particularly ammonium hexachloroplatinate and hexachloroplatinic acid. Platinum salt sensitization may persist for years after cessation of exposure (Brooks et al., 1990). Halogeno complex salts of platinum are potent allergens provoking Type I allergic symptoms in platinum refining workers. Skin prick tests can detect sensitization at an early stage and is the mainstay of surveillance programs (WHO, 1991; Linnett, 2005).

Antitumor Effects of Platinum Complexes The platinum-coordinated complexes are important antitumor agents, including cisplatin, carboplatin, and oxaliplatin (Hardman et al., 2001). They are routinely administered, often in combination with other anti-cancer drugs, in the treatment of a wide spectrum of malignancies, especially epithelial cancers. They have become the foundation for curative regimens for advanced testicular cancer and have notable activity against cancers of head and neck, bladder, esophagus, lung, and ovary (Hardman et al., 2001). Platinum complexes are neutral and have a pair of cis-leaving groups. Low intracellular chloride concentrations favor hydrolysis of chloride-leaving groups in cisplatin to yield a positively charged molecule, which then reacts with DNA and proteins, forming both intrastrand and interstrand DNA cross-links with guanine and/or adenine. In tumor cells, the replication of DNA is impaired due to cisplatin-induced DNA cross-links, while in normal cells, guanine is repaired before replication. The formation of DNA-adducts with platinum is also responsible for cytotoxicity (WHO, 1991; Hardman et al., 2001).

Carcinogenic Effects of Platinum Complexes Although cisplatin has antitumor activity in humans, it is considered to be a probable carcinogen in humans (IARC, 1987) and is clearly carcinogenic in rodents. In fact, in mice deficient in metallothionein, cisplatin can induce tumors at clinically relevant doses (Waalkes *et al.*, 2006c). Cisplatin is a strong mutagen in bacterial systems and causes chromosomal aberrations in cultured hamster cells and a dose-dependent increase in sister chromatid exchanges.

Toxicities of Platinum Antitumor Complexes   Cisplatin is a nephrotoxin, which often compromises its usefulness as a therapeutic agent. Platinum compounds with antitumor activity produce proximal and distal tubular cell injury, mainly in the corticomedullary region, where the concentration of platinum is highest (Madias and Harrington, 1978). Associated with cisplatin nephrotoxicity is the risk for electrolyte abnormalities. In comparison, carboplatinum and oxaliplatinum, given at standard chemotherapeutic doses, are not considered as highly nephrotoxic (Markman, 2003).

Neurotoxicity is another dose-limiting factor, particular when platinum complexes are combined with other potential neurotoxic drugs such as paclitaxel. Hearing loss can occur and can be unilateral or bilateral but tends to be more frequent and severe with repeated doses. Marked nausea and vomiting occur in most patients receiving the platinum complexes but can be controlled with ondanserton or high-dose of corticosteroids. Bone marrow suppression, manifested as anemia, neutropenia, and thrombocytopenia are relatively common during treatment with platinum complexes, especially when given in combination with fluorouracil. Carboplatin treatment has a higher myelotoxic risk than cisplatin and oxaliplatin (Hardman *et al.*, 2001; Markman, 2003).

MINOR TOXIC METALS

Antimony

Antimony (Sb) is a metalloid that belongs to the same periodic group as arsenic. Antimony was recognized in antiquity (3000 BC or earlier) in various compounds for its fine casting qualities, and the description of its isolation appeared in 1540. The name antimony may come from the Greek words "anti" and "monos," which means "opposed to solitude" as it was thought never to exist in its pure form. Most antimony compounds are of tri- and pentavalent states. Antimony has many uses including in alloys, and in production of fireproofing chemicals, ceramics, glassware, and pigments. Antimony potassium tartrate has been used medically in the treatment of schistosomiasis, and pentavalent antimony compounds are preferred drugs for leishmaniasis (DeBoeck *et al.*, 2003). Similar to arsenic trioxide, trivalent antimony compounds also show some antitumor potential (Tiekink, 2002). Occupational antinomy exposure comes from industrial emissions. Food is the major route for environmental exposure, but the exposure levels are generally low. The average daily intake from food and water is estimated at about 5 μg (ATSDR, 1992).

The disposition of antimony in the body resembles that of arsenic (Gebel, 1997). Most antimony compounds are absorbed from the lung and the gastrointestinal tract. The major sites of antimony accumulation are the liver, kidney, lung, spleen, and blood. The accumulation of antimony in blood may be due to high affinity of trivalent antimony for erythrocytes (ATSDR, 1992). In humans and rodents, pentavalent antimony is only sparingly reduced to the trivalent form, and evidence of antimony methylation in mammals is low (Gebel, 1997). The pentavalent form is predominantly excreted in urine, whereas trivalent antimony is conjugated to GSH and is excreted via the bile and found mainly in feces.

Toxicity   Most information about antimony toxicity has been obtained from industrial experiences. Occupational exposures are usually by inhalation of dust containing antimony compounds, such as the pentachloride, trichloride, trioxide, and trisulfide. Acute toxicity from the pentachloride and trichloride exposures include rhinitis and, in severe exposures, even acute pulmonary edema. Chronic exposure by inhalation of other antimony compounds results in rhinitis, pharyngitis, trachitis, and, over the longer term, bronchitis and eventually pneumoconiosis with obstructive lung disease and emphysema. Transient skin eruptions (antimony spots) may occur in workers with chronic exposure (Elinder and Fridberg, 1986). Trivalent forms of antimony appear more toxic and may produce cardiotoxicity involving arrhythmias, myocardial damage, and cardiac arrest (Winship, 1987). In rodent subchronic/chronic studies with antimony potassium tartrate, relatively low toxicity was reported (Lynch *et al.*, 1999).

The chemico-toxicological similarity between arsenic and antimony has prompted research on mutagenic and carcinogenic potential of antimony compounds. Antimony trioxide is considered an animal carcinogen (IARC, 1987), but human data is difficult to evaluate given frequent co-exposure to arsenic (Leonard and Garber, 1996; DeBoeck *et al.*, 2003). Antimony compounds are generally negative in nonmammalian genotoxicity tests, while mammalian tests usually give positive results for trivalent but negative results for pentavalent antimony compounds. The in vivo potential of antimony to induce chromosome aberrations appears inconsistent (Leonard and Gerber, 1996; DeBoeck *et al.*, 2003).

The metal hydride of antimony, stibine (SbH_3), is a highly toxic gas that can be generated when antimony is exposed to reducing acids or when certain batteries are overcharged. High-purity stibine is also used in the production of semiconductors and, like arsine (AsH_3), causes hemolysis.

Barium

Barium (Ba) is an alkaline earth metal found in environment in the 2+ oxidation state. Barium was first identified in 1774, and named after the Greek word *barys* meaning "heavy." Barium and barium compounds are used in electronics (barium alloys), as rodenticides (barium carbonate), as pigments (barium carbonate and sulfate), and as X-ray contrast media (barium sulfate). Barium is relatively abundant in nature and is found in plants and animal tissue. Some foods, such as Brazil nuts, pecans, and seafood, may contain high amounts of barium. Barium from natural sources may exceed Federal government standards in some freshwater, although the amount of barium found in food and water usually is not high enough to be a health concern. Occupational exposure to barium primarily occurs in workers who inhale barium sulfate from working with the ore, barite, and barium carbonate dust during the mining and manufacturing (ATSDR, 2005b).

Insoluble barium sulfate is not absorbed from the gastrointestinal tract, and is nontoxic to humans. Ingested soluble compounds are absorbed, but vary greatly and are affected by many factors such as age, duration, dose, and amounts of other elements in the intestine. Aerosols of soluble barium compounds are well absorbed in the lung. Bone and teeth are the major sites of barium deposition, containing up to 90% of the body burden. The remainder of barium in the body is found in soft tissues, such as the lung, aorta, brain, heart, spleen, liver, and pancreas (Dallas and Williams, 2001). Once filtered by the glomeruli, barium is reabsorbed by the renal tubules with only small amounts appearing in the urine. The major route of barium excretion is the feces. The elimination half-life is about 3 to 4 days.

Toxicity Occupational poisoning by barium is uncommon, but a benign pneumoconiosis (*baritosis*) may result from inhalation of barium sulfate (barite) dust or barium carbonate. This is not incapacitating and is usually reversible with cessation of exposure. Accidental poisoning from ingestion of an acute toxic dose (over 200 mg) of soluble barium salt results in intractable vomiting, severe diarrhea, and gastrointestinal hemorrhage. Cardiac arrest is often the cause of death (ATSDR, 2005f). Profound hypokalemia and muscle weakness progressing to flaccid paralysis are the hallmarks of barium poisoning (Johnson and VanTassell, 1991). The mechanism of toxicity probably involves the blocking of calcium activated potassium channels responsible for cellular efflux of potassium. As a result, intracellular potassium rises and extracellular levels fall leading to hypokalemia. The progressive muscle weakness seen in barium intoxication in humans could be due to barium-induced hypokalemia rather than a direct effect on muscles, which is not observed in experimental animals. Treatment with intravenous potassium appears beneficial.

Following long-term exposure to barium, nephrotoxicity has been observed in rats and mice. Animal studies designed to assess cardiovascular function have not found significant alterations. Barium compounds are not considered carcinogenic in rodents and there is no evidence in humans (ATSDR, 2005f; Dallas and Williams, 2001).

Cesium

Cesium (Cs) is a soft silvery-gold alkali metal discovered in 1860, and named after the Latin word *caesius* meaning "sky blue." Similar to mercury and gallium, metallic cesium exists in the liquid state at slightly above room temperature, and is used in vacuum tubes and in atomic clocks. Cesium compounds only have the 1+ oxidation state, and are used as catalysts in inorganic chemistry, in pharmaceuticals, as well as in scintillation counters. ^{137}Cesium is a by-product of nuclear reactions and is used in radiation therapy (ATSDR, 2004).

The Chernobyl nuclear plant accident in 1986 resulted in a large release of cesium into atmosphere, which then spread as radioactive fallout into the soil, rivers, and lakes, causing serious ecological problems in the Northern Europe. The transfer of radio-cesium into the food chain and into sheep and reindeer may contribute to human cesium exposure (Howard and Howard, 1997). These ecological issues remain in some areas even decades after the original accident (Bell and Shaw, 2005).

Most cesium compounds are water soluble and are well absorbed through inhalation, ingestion, or skin contact. Once in the blood, cesium is rapidly distributed throughout the body, with higher concentrations in muscles. Cesium can cross the placenta and appears in milk. Cesium mimics potassium for cellular transport. Urinary excretion is the primary route of elimination of cesium from the body. The biological half-life of cesium is variable, ranging from 50 to 150 days (ATSDR, 2004). A physiologically based kinetic model has been developed to describe the distribution and retention of cesium in humans (Leggett *et al.*, 2003).

Toxicity

Radioactive Cesium Exposure to radioactive cesium (^{134}Cs and ^{137}Cs) is of much greater human health concern than nonradioactive cesium. The initial symptoms following radioactive cesium exposure include nausea, vomiting, and diarrhea. Local skin blistering is common when there is significant dermal contact. With continued exposure to radioactive cesium, adverse neurological and developmental effects can be observed. Symptoms can eventually progress to bone morrow suppression, infection, hemorrhage, and even death (ATSDR, 2004).

Non-radioactive Cesium Compounds Stable (nonradioactive) cesium compounds are relatively less toxic. High-dose exposure can cause irritation to the gastrointestinal tract and to the eye (ATSDR, 2004). Cardiac arrhythmia and QT wave prolongation have been observed in several case reports following ingestion of cesium salts as homeopathic remedies for cancer treatment (ATSDR, 2004; Dalal *et al.*, 2004). Adverse developmental effects of cesium chloride have been observed in rodents (Messiha, 1994). Prussian blue has been approved in the treatment of cesium poisoning (Thompson and Callen, 2004).

Fluorine

Fluorine (F) was isolated in 1886 by Henri Moissan for which he was awarded the 1906 Nobel Prize in Chemistry. Fluorides are organic and inorganic compounds containing the nonmetallic element fluorine. Fluoride is an essential component for normal mineralization of bones and dental enamel, and it has been widely used to reduce the prevalence and severity of dental caries in children and adults. Flurosilicic acid and sodium fluorosilicate have been used in water fluoridation since 1940s. Adequate intake level is about 0.05 mg/kg/day in adults but is much lower for infants (Ziegler and Filer, 1996; ATSDR, 2003). Toxicologically important fluoride compounds include hydrogen fluoride and sodium fluoride. The major sources of fluorides intake in the general population are water, food, and fluoride-containing dental products. However, excessive intake of fluorides has been observed from environmental sources, including from drinking water with naturally high fluoride (Meenakshi and Masheshwari, 2006), or from exposure to indoor fluoride air pollution from the use of high fluoride-containing coal (Ando *et al.*, 1998; Liu *et al.*, 2002).

Fluorides are readily absorbed (75–90%) from the gastrointestinal tract. Once absorbed, fluorides are rapidly distributed throughout the body. Approximately 99% of the fluoride in the body is found in bones and teeth. Fluoride is incorporated into bone by replacing the hydroxyl ion in hydroxyapatite to form hydroxyfluoapatite. Fluoride in bone can be remobilized slowly as a result of the ongoing process of bone remodeling, especially in the young children. Fluoride is readily transferred across the placenta but poorly transferred to breast milk. Fluorides are mainly excreted in urine. Plasma and urine fluoride levels are related to fluoride intake and are a biomarker for excess exposure, while hair, fingernails, and tooth enamel are indicators of long-term response (ATSDR, 2003).

Toxicity

Dental Fluorosis Excessive fluoride intake from water during the period of enamel formation in children can cause dental fluorosis. In its mild form, dental fluorosis is characterized by white, opaque areas on the tooth surface. In its severe form, it is manifested as yellowish brown to black stains and severe pitting of the teeth. Dental fluorosis incidence and severity in some instances can be decreased by the cessation of water fluoridation (Clark *et al.*, 2006). Inappropriate use of fluoride toothpaste and fluoride supplements in young children is a risk factor for dental fluorosis (Browne *et al.*, 2005). Dental fluorosis is more common and severe in areas of endemic environmental fluorosis (Ando *et al.*, 1998; Meenakshi and Masheshwari, 2006).

Skeletal Fluorosis Long-term exposure to very high oral doses of fluoride or occupational exposure to cryolite dusts can result in skeletal fluorosis. Cases of skeletal fluorosis are predominantly found in developing countries, particularly in India and China, and are associated with high fluoride intake coupled with malnutrition (Ando *et al.*, 1998; ATSDR, 2003; Meenakshi and Masheshwari, 2006). Skeletal fluorosis does not usually manifest symptomatically until the disease attains an advanced stage. Fluoride is mainly deposited in the neck, knee, pelvic, and shoulder joints and/or bones, which makes it difficult to move or walk. The symptoms of skeletal fluorosis are similar to arthritis, and early on include sporadic pain, back stiffness, burning-like sensation, pricking and tingling in the limbs, muscle weakness, and chronic fatigue. These symptoms are associated with abnormal calcium deposits in bones and ligaments. In the advanced stage, symptoms include osteoporosis in long bones, and bone outgrowth. The vertebrae may fuse together and eventually the victim may be crippled (crippling skeletal fluorosis), a disability often accompanied by kyphosis (humbacked) or lordosis (arched back).

There are conflicting data regarding the association between fluoride exposure and the incidence of osteosarcoma, a rare bone malignancy (ATSDR, 2003). A recent case-control study in the United States found an association between fluoride exposure in drinking water during childhood and the incidence of osteosarcoma among males but not among females (Bassin *et al.*, 2006). This pattern is similar to the findings from the National Toxicology Program rodent study in which osteosarcoma occurred in male rats exposed to sodium fluoride in the drinking water, with a weak but statistically significant dose–response trend (NTP, 1990). However, caution should be taken to make conclusions and more studies are needed in this regard (Douglass and Joshipura, 2006).

Other health effects include respiratory tract, skin, and eye irritation following inhalation exposure to hydrogen fluoride or fluorine gas. Gastrointestinal symptoms occur with excess ingestion of fluoride (ATSDR, 2003). Chronic endemic fluorosis may also lead to muscle fiber degeneration, low hemoglobin levels, skin ruches, neurological manifestations, compromised immunity, and endocrine effects (Meenakshi and Masheshwari, 2006). Endemic fluorosis from coal burning in China often occurs concurrently with arsenicosis (Liu *et al.*, 2002).

Germanium

Germanium (Ge) is a metalloid-like antimony and arsenic. The discovery of germanium as a predicted analog of silicon in the 1880s was a key confirmation of the developing theory of elemental periodicity. Chemically similar to tin, germanium can form a large number of organometallic compounds such as dimethyl germanium and germanium tetrahydride. Stable oxidation states include divalent and tetravalent germanium. In the semiconductor industry, germanium transistors found countless uses in solid-state electronics up to the mid-1970s, but then were largely replaced by silicon. Currently it is used in infrared night vision systems, fiber optics, as a polymerization catalyst, and in alloys with other metals. Silicon germanide (SiGe) is emerging as an important semiconductor metal for use in high speed integrated circuits. Germanium is commercially derived from zinc ore processing or as a combustion by-product of certain coals. Ultra pure germanium can be obtained from other metals by fractional distillation of the volatile germanium tetrachloride.

The diet is the dominant source of germanium exposure in the general population while occupational exposure is predominantly by inhalation. Germanium concentrations in most foods are similar to the natural abundance level of about 0.6 to 1.0 ppm in soils, although higher levels have been reported in some canned foods (Vouk, 1986b). Daily germanium intake from food in humans is reported to be about 1.5 mg of which 96% is absorbed (Vouk, 1986b). Intake of germanium from drinking water appears negligible. Considerable amounts of germanium are emitted into the air by coal combustion although exposure from air is limited in the general population. There is no evidence of any essential function of germanium.

Inorganic germanium compounds are rapidly and effectively absorbed after oral exposure. Elemental germanium particles are likewise rapidly cleared from the lung and soon appear in distant tissues (Vouk, 1986b). Absorbed germanium is widely distributed throughout the body with the highest concentrations occurring in many tissues including the liver, kidney, and spleen. Absorption and distribution appears to be largely independent of the germanium compound, as both sodium germanate and tetraethylgermanium are widely distributed without evidence of selective retention or storage after oral exposure in mice (Vouk, 1986b). In both humans and laboratory animals, germanium is excreted mainly via the kidneys with whole-body half-life of 1 to 4 days. Hair and nails may be useful media for biological monitoring.

There appear to be no reports on systemic toxicity of germanium after occupational exposure. There are, however, at least 31 case reports of renal failure in humans after ingestion of inorganic or organometallic germanium compounds mainly through consumption of germanium-containing dietary supplements or elixirs for various diseases (Takeuchi *et al.*, 1992; Tao and Bolger, 1997). Among these cases nine deaths were reported (Tao and Bolger, 1997). Levels of germanium consumed were ~15 to 300 g and were ingested over a period of 2 to 36 months (Tao and Bolger, 1997). Excessive germanium consumption from such sources induces various symptoms including renal dysfunction involving tubular degeneration, anemia, muscle weakness, and peripheral neuropathy. Recovery of renal function is slow and incomplete (Tao and Bolger, 1997). Although reports on the efficacy of germanium supplementation against diseases like cancer and AIDS persist, germanium supplementation has not been clearly shown to be of value and the USFDA considers such germanium products to present a potential human health risk (Tao and Bolger, 1997).

Spirogermanium (2-aza-8-germanspiro[4,5] decane-2-propamine-8,8-diethyl-*N*,*N*-dimethyl dichloride) was neurotoxic to humans after intravenous injection for the treatment of cancer (Vouk, 1986b). The effects were reversible and included ataxia and seizures. Neurotoxic effects are also observed in dogs (Vouk, 1986).

There is no evidence of germanium carcinogenicity in humans. In rodents limited testing indicates germanium is not carcinogenic in rats and it has no mutagenic activity (Gerber and Leonard, 1997). Dimethyl germanium oxide can produce embryonic resorption and fetal malformations in animals.

Indium

Indium (In) is a posttransitional metal, named after the indigo line in its atomic spectrum, which was discovered and isolated in the 1860s. Indium is a rare metal with a principal valence state of 3+ and is recovered as a by-product of zinc smelting. In its metallic forms, indium is used in liquid displays, semiconductors, alloys, solders, and as a hardening agent for bearings. Indium arsenide and indium phosphide are chemical forms commonly used in semiconductors (Tanaka, 2004). The most common isotope of indium is slightly radioactive, a characteristic exploited in medical imaging and nuclear medicine. Indium is considered to be a nonessential metal.

The human daily intake of indium has been estimated in the range of 8 to 10 μg. The most common routes of exposure for the general population are inhalation and ingestion while in occupational exposure inhalation predominates. Indium compounds are poorly absorbed when ingested or after intratracheal instillation but may show moderate absorption after inhalation (Fowler, 1986; Zheng et al., 1994). Indium derived from oral or intratracheal instillation of indium phosphide is uniformly distributed between major organs and is excreted in the urine and feces (Zheng et al., 1994). Ionic indium is transported bound to transferrin and is cleared from the blood within 3 days of an intravenous injection in mice (Fowler, 1986).

Toxicity There appear to be no meaningful reports of local or systemic indium toxicity in humans after oral or inhalation exposure. Animal data on indium indicate that toxicity is related to the chemical form and route of exposure (NTP, 2001). Acute toxicity in animals is generally greatest after inhalation or intravenous injection, and limited after oral exposure (NTP, 2001). In this regard, intravenous injection of indium chloride in mice or rats produces extensive renal and liver necrosis (Fowler, 1986). Intratracheal instillation of the indium chloride produces severe inflammation and pulmonary damage with fibrosis in mice (Blazka et al., 1994). Lung instillation of indium phosphide can produce alveolar or bronchiolar cell hyperplasia in hamsters (Tanaka et al., 1996). The intratracheal instillation of indium phosphide produces little systemic toxicity (Oda, 1997). Indium trichloride showed no evidence of reproductive toxicity in mice, although it did adversely affect fetal survival (Chapin et al., 1995). Teratogenic effects have been observed with intravenously injected indium compounds in rats and hamsters (Ferm and Carpenter, 1970; Nakajima et al., 1998, 2000), but not in mice (Nakajima et al., 2000). Oral indium is teratogenic only at doses that induce maternal toxicity (Ungvary et al., 2000). Inhalation of indium phosphide or oral exposure to indium chloride by pregnant rats results in fetal indium concentrations that are similar to maternal blood levels (Ungvary et al., 2000; NTP, 2001) indicating the placenta does not perturb indium.

Because of its use in the microelectronics industry, indium phosphide was tested recently by the National Toxicology Program (NTP, 2001). After inhalation of indium phosphide for up to 2 years there was clear evidence of pulmonary carcinogenic activity in both male and female rats and mice. This included production of lung adenoma and carcinoma after inhalation of indium phosphide. Concurrent genetic toxicity testing, specifically micronucleated erythrocytes in peripheral mouse blood, was negative (NTP, 2001). Further study indicated inhaled indium phosphide particles likely acted through chronic inflammation in conjunction with production of reactive oxygen species and epithelial cell proliferation (Gottschling et al., 2001).

Palladium

Palladium (Pd) belongs to the platinum group metals. Palladium was discovered in 1803, and named after the asteroid Pallas. Palladium occurs together with other platinum group metals (platinum, rhodium, ruthenium, iridium, and osmium) at very low concentrations in earth crust, and is recovered as a by-product of refining nickel, platinum, and other base metals. Palladium compounds commonly exhibit oxidation state of 2+, although compounds with the oxidation state 4+ are observed. Organopalladium compounds also exist. Palladium is used in automobile catalysts, in dentistry (for crowns and bridges), in electrical appliances, and in jewelry. Environmental palladium levels are increasing, but exposure in the general population is low. Dental alloys and work in metal refining or catalyst manufacture can be major sources of palladium exposure (WHO, 2002; Kielhorn et al., 2002).

Palladium chloride is poorly absorbed from the gastrointestinal tract or from subcutaneous injection sites. After intravenous administration of palladium compounds, palladium is distributed to kidney, liver, spleen, lung, and bone. In cells, palladium compounds likely complex with amino acids, proteins, DNA, and other macromolecules. Orally administered palladium is poorly absorbed and eliminated in feces, whereas intravenous palladium is mainly eliminated in the urine. Half-lives range from 5 to 12 days (WHO, 2002).

Toxicity Palladium sensitization is a major health concern, as very low doses are sufficient to cause allergic reactions in susceptible individuals. Persons with known nickel allergy may be especially susceptible (Kielhorn et al., 2002). Contact dermatitis is a main manifestation of palladium sensitivity, unlike that with platinum. Immediate hypersensitivity (type I) reactions to palladium have been reported in refinery workers sensitized to platinum (Ravindra et al., 2004). Palladium sensitization is often from dental alloys or jewelry. Occupational exposure to palladium salts may cause skin and eye irritation, and occasionally asthma (Kielhorn et al., 2002; WHO, 2002).

There is some evidence that palladium chloride is carcinogenic after oral exposure in rodents, but the validity of this study was questioned due to methodology deficiencies (Ravindra et al., 2004). Palladium compounds are negative in bacterial mutagenicity tests and in micronucleus test in human peripheral lymphocytes. Tetraammine palladium hydrogen carbonate induced a clastogenic response to lymphocytes in vitro but did not produce positive results in the micronucleus test (WHO, 2002). Some organopalladium complexes have been shown to have antitumor potential similar to that of cisplatin (WHO, 2002; Abu-Surrah and Kettunen, 2006).

Silver

Sliver (Ag) is a rare, naturally occurring element found as a soft, "silver" colored metal. Silver was known since ancient times and was separated from lead as early as the 4000 BC. The chemical symbol for silver is Ag, and is from its Latin name *argentum*. Metallic silver and 1+ oxidation forms are common. Silver metal is used for jewelry, silverware, electronic equipment, and dental filling. Soluble silver salts (e.g., silver nitrate and silver sulfide) have been used to treat bacteria infection. Silver halide is used in the manufacture of photographic plates, while silver sulfadiazine is used in the treatment of burns. Occupational exposure occurs mainly from inhalation of silver fumes and dusts in a number of settings (ATSDR,

1990; Drake and Hazelwood, 2005). Dietary intake is in the range of 70 to 90 μg/day, which is much less than the silver intake from medicinal uses. For drinking water disinfection, WHO permissible level is 0.1 mg silver/L (Pelkonen *et al.*, 2003)

Sliver compounds can be absorbed orally, by inhalation, and through damaged skin. Ingested silver compounds are absorbed at a level of less than 10%, and only 2–4% is retained in tissues. Metallic silver and insoluble silver compounds are not readily taken up by the body, and pose minimal health risk (Drake and Hazelwood, 2005). In mice given drinking water containing silver nitrate (0.03 mg/L for 2 weeks), silver was widely distributed to most tissues including muscle, cerebellum, spleen, duodenum, heart, lung, liver, and kidney (Pelkonen *et al.*, 2003). Silver can cross the blood–brain barrier and produce long-lasting deposits in many structures of the nervous system (Rungby, 1990) and is located almost exclusively in lysosomes of neuronal cells (Stoltenberg *et al.*, 1994). Uptake of silver into lysosomes probably occurs through a carrier-mediated process (Havelaar *et al.*, 1998). Autopsy findings after silver treatment of burn victims indicate the highest levels occur in skin, gingiva, cornea, liver, and kidneys. Urine silver analysis as a biomarker is useful only following a high degree of exposure because little silver is excreted in urine.

Toxicity   The most common health effects associated with prolonged exposure to silver compounds are the development of a characteristic, irreversible pigmentation of the skin (argyria) and/or the eyes (argyrosis). The affected area becomes bluish-gray or ash gray. This is most prominent in the areas of the body exposed to sunlight, as light acts as a catalyst by triggering the photoreduction of these compounds to form metallic silver, similar to the process of developing a photographic negative. Metallic silver is subsequently oxidized by tissue and is bound as silver sulfide. Black silver sulfide and silver selenide complexes bound to tissue are identified as silver particle deposits. Argyria has two forms, local and general. Localized argyria is caused by direct, local contact with silver such as through jewelry, and involves the formation of gray-blue patches on the skin or may manifest itself in the conjunctiva of the eye. In generalized argyria, the skin shows widespread pigmentation, often spreading from the face to most uncovered parts of the body.

Chelating therapy and dermal abrasion are ineffective in removing silver deposits from the body and there is no effective treatment for argyria. Argyria can be considered a mechanism for detoxication of silver by sequestering it in the tissues as nontoxic silver–protein complexes or silver sulfide (ATSDR, 1990; Drake and Hazelwood, 2005).

The respiratory tract may be affected in severe cases of silver intoxication. Chronic bronchitis has also been reported to result from medicinal use of colloidal silver (ATSDR, 1990). Large oral doses of silver nitrate may cause severe gastrointestinal irritation due to its caustic action. Lesions of the kidneys and lungs and arteriosclerosis have been attributed to both industrial and medicinal exposures. Animal experiments indicate that silver may disturb copper metabolism (Hirasawa *et al.*, 1994) and that metallothionein may protect against the toxic action of silver (Shinogi and Maezumi, 1993).

Tellurium

Tellurium (Te) is a metalloid chemically related to selenium and sulfur. Discovered in the 1780s, tellurium is named after the Latin

word for earth (*tellus*). It is naturally found as the telluride of gold or combined with various other metals. Produced most often as a by-product of electrolytic copper refining, tellurium is used as an additive to improve metallurgic characteristics of copper, steel, and lead alloys (Gerhardsson *et al.*, 1986). Tellurium vapor is used in "daylight" lamps and as a semiconductor in combination with other metals. It is also used in explosives, specialized glass, and in thermoelectric and electronic devices.

Tellurium in food is probably in the form of tellurates. The estimated human daily intake is about 100 μg. Condiments, dairy products, nuts, and fish have relatively high concentrations of tellurium. Some plants, such as cactus, accumulate tellurium from the soil. The average body burden in humans is about 600 mg, mainly in bone.

The biochemistry and toxicity of inorganic and organometallic tellurium compounds have been reviewed (Taylor, 1996; Nogueira *et al.*, 2004). Soluble tetravalent tellurates, absorbed into the body after oral administration, are reduced to tellurides, partly methylated, and then exhaled as dimethyl telluride. The dimethylated form is responsible for the characteristic garlic odor in persons intoxicated by tellurium compounds. Food is the main source of tellurium for the general population, while in industrial exposure inhalation would predominate. Some organometallic tellurium compounds are absorbed through the skin. Respiratory absorption data are limited, but inhaled tellurium compounds are likely well absorbed. After oral exposure of tellurides 10–20% of the ingested dose is absorbed (Gerhardsson *et al.*, 1986). The kidney, bone, and liver accumulate tellurium and it is estimated that bone stores may have a half-life of up to 2 years or more (Gerhardsson *et al.*, 1986). The urine and bile are the principal routes of excretion. Tellurium crosses the blood–brain barrier and the placenta.

Toxicity   Of toxicological importance are elemental tellurium, the gases hydrogen telluride and tellurium hexafluoride, and the water-soluble sodium or potassium tellurites and tellurates (Gerhardsson *et al.*, 1986). Many organometallic forms of tellurium exist. Tellurates and tellurium are of generally low toxicity, but tellurites are typically more toxic. Acute intoxication by inhalation results in sweating, nausea, a metallic taste, and garlic smelling breath. In fact, garlic breath is an indicator of exposure to tellurium by dermal, inhalation, or oral routes. The cases of tellurium intoxication reported from industrial exposure do not appear to have been life threatening. Two deaths occurred within 6 hours of accidental poisoning by mistaken injection of sodium tellurite (instead of sodium iodine) into the ureters during retrograde pyelography (Gerhardsson *et al.*, 1986). The victims had garlic breath, renal pain, cyanosis, vomiting, stupor, and loss of consciousness. The amount of sodium telluride injected was about 2 g.

In rats, chronic exposure to high doses of tellurium dioxide produces renal and hepatic injury (Gerhardsson *et al.*, 1986). Rats fed metallic tellurium at 1% of the diet develop demyelination of peripheral nerves (Goodrum, 1998), probably due to the inhibition of cholesterol biosynthesis (Laden and Porter, 2001). Remyelination occurs after cessation of tellurium exposure (Morell *et al.*, 1994).

There are no data on human carcinogenicity of tellurium. Lifetime exposure to sodium tellurite at 2 mg Te/L drinking water had no effect on tumor incidence in rats. Some tellurium compounds show mutagenic potential (Gerhardsson *et al.*, 1986). Tellurium compounds produce hydrocephalus in rats after gestational exposure between day 9 and 15.

Thallium

Thallium (Tl) is one of the most toxic metals. Thallium (from the Greek word *thallos* meaning "a green shoot or twig") was discovered in 1861. The thallium ion has a similar charge and ion radius as the potassium ion, and its toxic effects may result from interference with the biological functions of potassium. Thallium is obtained as a by-product of the refining of iron, cadmium, and zinc, and is used as a catalyst in alloys, and in optical lenses, jewelry, low-temperature thermometers, semiconductors, dyes, pigments, and scintillation counters. It has been used medicinally as a depilatory. Thallium compounds, chiefly thallous sulfate, were used as rat poisons and insecticides. Once the commonest sources of human thallium poisoning, the use of thallium as rodenticides or insecticides is now banned (WHO, 1996; Peter and Viraraghavan, 2005). Industrial poisoning is a risk in the manufacture of fused halides for the production of lenses and windows. Naturally high thallium concentration in soils and consequent uptake into edible plants in Southwest Guizhou, China caused locally chronic thallium poisoning (Xiao *et al.*, 2004).

Thallium is absorbed through the skin and gastrointestinal tract. The highest concentrations of thallium poisoning are in the kidney. Following the initial exposure, large amounts are excreted in urine during the first 24 hours, but after that urinary excretion becomes slow and the feces becomes an important route of excretion. The half-life of thallium in humans has been reported to range from 1 to 30 days and depends on the initial dose. Thallium undergoes enterohepatic recirculation. Prussian blue, the most commonly used antidote, is given orally to break the enterohepatic recycling by trapping thallium secreted into bile and carried it into the feces (WHO, 1996). Thallium can transfer across the placenta and is found in breast milk, and may cause toxicity in the offspring (Hoffman, 2000).

Toxicity   The triad of gastroenteritis, polyneuropathy, and alopecia is regarded as the classic syndrome of thallium poisoning (WHO, 1996). Other signs and symptoms also occur depending on the dose and duration of exposure. The estimated acute lethal dose in humans is 10 to 15 mg/kg. Death is due mainly to renal, central nervous system, and cardiac failure within a few days to two weeks (WHO, 1996; Galvan-Arzate and Santamaria, 1998; Peter and Viraraghavan, 2005).

Alopecia is the best-known effect of thallium poisoning. Depilation begins about 10 days after ingestion and complete hair loss can occur in about 1 month. Other dermal signs may include palmar erythema, acne, anhydrosis, and dry scaly skin due to the toxic effects of thallium on sweat and sebaceous glands. After oral ingestion of thallium, gastrointestinal symptoms occur, including nausea, vomiting, gastroenteritis, abdominal pain, and gastrointestinal hemorrhage. Neurological symptoms usually appear 2–5 days after acute exposure, depending on the age and the level of exposure. A consistent and characteristic feature of thallium intoxication in humans is the extreme sensitivity of the legs, followed by the "burning feet syndrome" and paresthesia. Central nervous system toxicity is manifest by hallucinations, lethargy, delirium, convulsions, and coma. The acute cardiovascular effects of thallium initially manifested by hypotension and bradycardia due to direct effects of thallium on sinus node and cardiac muscle. This is followed by hypertension and tachycardia due to vagal nerve degeneration. In severe cases, cardiac failure occurs (Milkey and Oehme, 1993).

Major symptoms of chronic thallium poisoning include anorexia, headache, and abnormal pain. Other toxic effects of thal-

lium include fatty infiltration and necrosis of the liver, nephritis, pulmonary edema, degenerative changes in the adrenals, and degeneration of the peripheral and central nervous system. In severe cases, alopecia, blindness, and even death have been reported as a result of long-term systemic thallium intake.

A recent review on thallium poisoning during pregnancy in humans gives a range of fetal effects from severe toxicity to normal development. The only consistent effect identified is a trend toward prematurity and low birth weight in children exposed to thallium during early gestation (Hoffman, 2000). Evidence that thallium is mutagenic or carcinogenic is scanty (Leonard and Gerber, 1997). However, it may be teratogenic, especially with regard to cartilage and bone formation, but most of the evidence comes from birds and not mammals.

Treatment   Therapy for thallium intoxication combines forced diuresis, use of activated charcoal, prevention of reabsorption by administration of Prussian blue, and administration of potassium ferric hexacyanoferrate (WHO, 1996). Prussian blue is the recommended drug of choice in acute thallium poisoning (Hoffman, 2003).

Tin (Sn)

Tin (Sn) is a silver–white metal. The name tin derives from the Anglo-Saxon, *tin*, through the Latin, *stannum*. Tin is one of the earliest metals known and was used as a component of bronze from antiquity. Because of its hardening effect on copper, tin was used in bronze implements as early as 3500 BC. However, the pure metal was not used until 600 BC. Metallic tin can combine with chloride, sulfur, or oxygen to form inorganic tin compounds (stannous, Sn^{2+} and stannic, Sn^{4+}). Tin can also bind with carbon to form a number of toxicologically important organotin compounds including dimethyltin, dibutyltin, dioctyltin, triphenyltin, and tricyclohexyltin (ATSDR, 2005e). Currently, tin is used in the manufacture of various alloys, such as bronze and brass, for fabricating window glass and in solders, but was previously widely used in food packaging. Stannic chlorides are used in dyeing textiles. Organic tin compounds have been used in fungicides, bactericides, and slimicides, as well as in plastics as stabilizers. The average daily intake of tin from all sources is about 4.0 mg, considerably lower than the 17 mg estimated in previous decades, thanks to better food packaging technology (Winship, 1988; Blunden and Wallace, 2003). Organotin compounds are ubiquitous contaminants in the environment. Bioconcentration in aquatic organisms and ecotoxicity are dependent on the bioavailability of the particular compounds. Some tin compounds, especially organotins, show high bioavailability and may pose adverse effects toward aquatic ecosystems (Fent, 1996).

Inorganic tin compounds are poorly absorbed after oral, inhalation, or dermal exposures. For example, only 3% of stannous and <1% of stannic compounds are absorbed from the gastrointestinal tract (Rudel, 2003). The majority of an oral dose of inorganic tin ends up in the feces, while only a small portion of absorbed tin is eliminated via urine (Rudel, 2003). Studies on animals reveal that administration of inorganic tin compounds reduces copper absorption (Yu and Beynen, 1995). The organotin compounds, particularly trimethyltin and triethyltin compounds are better absorbed than inorganic tins. The tissue distribution of tin from these organometallic compounds shows the highest concentration in the bone, liver, kidney, and lung, with smaller amounts in the muscle, spleen, heart, or brain. Tetra-, tri-, and diethyltin undergo dealkylation to ethyltin compounds, whereas tributyltin is dealkylated to di- and mono-butyltin compounds. Phenyltin compounds undergo dearylation, mainly by microsome monooxygenase and P450 enzymes (Winship, 1988; ATSDR, 2005e).

Toxicity Metallic tin and inorganic tin compounds are relatively nontoxic. Ingestion of food items contaminated with high levels of inorganic tins may cause acute gastroenteritis, while chronic inhalation of inorganic tins (e.g., stannic oxide dust or fumes) may lead to benign nonfibrotic pneumoconiosis called *stannosis* (Blunden and Wallace, 2003; ATSDR, 2005e).

Some organic tin compounds are highly neurotoxic, particularly triethyltin and trimethyltin, and cause encephalopathy and cerebral edema. Toxicity declines as the number of carbon atoms in the chain increases. An outbreak of neurotoxicity of almost epidemic nature took place in France in the 1950s due to the oral ingestion of a preparation (Stalinon) containing diethyltin diodide for the treatment of skin disorders (WHO, 1980). Trimethyltin produces degenerative lesions in the hippocampus and associated structure of the limbic system in primates and rodents. The lesions are characterized by neuron cell apoptosis with astrocyte swelling and gliosis. Microglia and astrocyte activation with the production of proinflammatory cytokines may well contribute to the lesion. Triethyltin produces cerebral edema in experimental animals (Rohl and Sievers, 2005; ATSDR, 2005e).

Triphenyltin, tributyltin, dibutyltin, and dioctyltin compounds produce immunotoxicity in experimental animals, characterized by thymic atrophy, and suppression of T-cell-mediated immune response (ATDSR, 2005e). Acute burns or subacute dermal irritation has been reported among workers as a result of dermal tributyltin exposure (Winship, 1988). Exposure of pregnant animals to organotin compounds such as tributyltin may induce developmental and endocrine disrupting effects (Adeeko *et al.*, 2003; ATSDR, 2005e).

Experimental studies have failed to find convincing evidence of carcinogenicity, mutagenicity, or teratogenicity of inorganic tin compounds (Winship, 1988). There is inadequate information to assess carcinogenic potential of organotin compounds in animals, and they are considered not classifiable as to human carcinogenicity (ATSDR, 2005). Studies of genotoxicity of organotin compounds have give mixed results depending on the specific compound and test system. Triphenyltin compounds are positive for induction of micronuclei and sister chromatid exchange in Chinese hamster cells.

Titanium

Titanium (Ti) was discovered in 1791. Titanium is named for the *Titans* of Greek mythology. Most titanium compounds are in the 4+ oxidation state (titanic), but the 3+ oxidation state (titanous) and 2+ compounds can occur. Titanium can form organometallic compounds. Because of its resistance to corrosion, inertness, and tensile strength, titanium has many metallurgic applications, and finds use in aircraft, armor plating, naval ships, missiles, and as a component of surgical implants and prostheses. Titanium dioxide, the most widely used titanium compound, is used as a white pigment in paints, paper, toothpaste, and plastics, as a food additive to whiten flour, in dietary products, and confections, and as a whitener in cosmetics. Titanium complexes (such as titanium diketonate and budotitane) and titanocene complexes (such as titanocene dichloride) have undergone clinical trials as cancer chemotherapeutics (Melendez, 2002; Caruso and Rossi, 2004). Titanium tetrachloride is used to make titanium metal and other titanium-containing compounds. Occupation exposures to titanium tetrachloride can be of toxicological concern (ATSDR, 1997).

Approximately 3% of an oral dose of inorganic titanium is absorbed. The majority of the absorbed dose is excreted in the urine. The normal urinary concentration of titanium has been estimated at 10 μg/L (Kazantzis, 1981), and the estimated total body burden of titanium is about 15 mg. As a result of inhalation exposure, the lungs accumulate titanium where it remains for long periods. Lung burdens increase with age and vary according to geographic location. Concentration in liver (8 μg/g) and kidney (6 μg/g) are similar. Titanium may circulate in plasma bound to transferrin (Messori *et al.*, 1999), which is thought to be a mediator for delivery of titanium to tumor cells (Desoize, 2004).

Toxicity Occupational inhalation exposure to titanium tetrachloride ($TiCl_4$) can produce mild to severe pulmonary injury because it undergoes rapid hydrolysis upon contact with water to form hydrochloric acid, titanium oxychloride, and titanium dioxide (TiO_2). Occupational exposure to titanium dioxide occurs during production. Titanium dioxide is classified as a nuisance particulate with a threshold limit value of 10 mg/m^3 (ATSDR, 1997). Inhalation and instillation of titanium particles coated with alumina and/or amorphous silica produce mild and reversible pulmonary effects. The base pigment-grade and/or nanoscale titanium dioxide particles produce minimal pulmonary toxicity, regardless of particle size and surface area (Warheit *et al.*, 2005, 2006). In general, titanium dioxide has been considered toxicologically inert regardless of route of exposure.

Epidemiological studies have not found the association of titanium exposure with increased risk of lung cancer and chronic respiratory diseases (Fayerweather *et al.*, 1992; Fryzek *et al.*, 2003). Titanium dioxide is not carcinogenic in rats or mice (NCI, 1979; Bernard *et al.*, 1990).

Titanium compounds and related metallocenes have recently shown chemotherapeutic activity toward gastrointestinal, breast, lung, and skin cancer (Melendez, 2002; Caruso and Rossi, 2004; Desoize, 2004). The mechanism of action of titanium compounds appears different from platinum compounds, and nephrotoxicity and myelotoxicity are not prominent.

Uranium

Uranium (U) is a heavy metal and its use dates at least back to AD 79. Uranium was discovered by the German chemist Martin Kloproth in 1789 in a mineral called pitchblende, and was named after Uranus, the planet, which had been discovered 8 years earlier. Uranium naturally occurs in three radioisotopes: ^{234}U, ^{235}U, and ^{238}U. ^{235}U is of particular interest in nuclear weapons and nuclear reactions. Thus, uranium ore is chemically enriched to increase ^{235}U content from 0.72% to 2–4%. The by-product of this process is called depleted uranium, which has decreased ^{235}U and has 40% less radioactivity than natural uranium (ATSDR, 1999). Depleted uranium has been used in military applications as warheads and tank armor. Nonmilitary uses include counterweights in airplanes and shields against radiation in hospitals (Craft *et al.*, 2004). The chemical toxicity of uranium compounds is a health concern, rather than their radiation. Depleted uranium has the same chemical toxicity potential as natural uranium (ATSDR, 1999; Craft *et al.*, 2004).

Uranium has five oxidation states but only the 4+ and 6+ forms are stable enough to be of practical importance. The 6+ oxidation state forms the uranyl ion (UO_2^{2+}), which further forms water-soluble compounds and is an important species of uranium in body fluids. The uranyl ion is also the most prevalent form in the environment (Sheppard *et al.*, 2005). The ecotoxicity of uranium and uranyl carbonate complexes to plants, aquatic life, and birds has been recently reviewed (Sheppard *et al.*, 2005).

Absorption of uranium compounds is low by all exposure routes. Absorption of inhaled uranium compounds occurs in respiratory tract via transfer across cell membranes, and is dependent on the particle size and solubility. Absorption from the gastrointestinal tract can vary from 0.1% to 6%, depending on the specific uranium compound. Once in the blood, uranium is distributed to the organs of the body. Uranium in body fluids generally exists as uranyl ion complexed with citrate and bicarbonate. Uranium preferentially distributes to bone (66%), liver (16%), kidney (8%), and then other tissues (10%). Two-thirds of the uranium in the blood is excreted in urine over the first 24 hours, but bone deposits of uranium last for about 1.5 years (ATSDR, 1999; Craft *et al.*, 2004).

Toxicity   The kidney is the most sensitive organ for uranium toxicity. The primary target is the renal proximal tubule, but the glomeruli may also be affected. Biomarkers of tubular effects include enzymuria, and increased excretion of low molecular weight proteins, amino acids, and glucose. Glucosuria is the most persistent biomarker for uranium-induced tubular dysfunction. Biomarkers for glomerular toxicity include urinary albuminuria, and elevated blood creatinine and urea nitrogen. Pathological and functional changes occur within days following acute exposure and are manifested by injury to renal tubular epithelial cells. Renal effects from acute exposure to uranium appear to have some relationship to peak kidney concentrations regardless of chemical form and route of exposure and are usually transient or reversible (Diamond *et al.*, 2005). Overt renal effects are observed with peak kidney uranium concentrations above 2 μg U/g, but mild renal tubular dysfunction from chronic exposure may occur at even lower renal concentrations. There appears to be a trend toward increase in severity of renal toxicity with increase in length exposure and urinary uranium levels (Thun *et al.*, 1985; Squibb *et al.*, 2005).

Challenges remain for establishing any causal relationship between human uranium exposure and birth defects and/or gonadal endocrine dysfunction, since these studies are confounded by co-exposure to other toxicants and inadequate exposure assessments (Craft *et al.*, 2004; Hindin *et al.*, 2005). However, uranium and depleted uranium can be developmental toxicants when given orally or subcutaneously to mice. Decreased fertility, embryo/fetal toxicity, teratogenicity, and reduced growth of the offspring have been observed in rodents following uranium exposure during different periods of gestation. Bone is a major site of uranium accumulation, and chronic uranium intoxication may result in diminished bone growth and osteoporosis. There is also increasing concern of potential neurotoxicity of uranium (Craft *et al.*, 2004; Jiang and Aschner, 2006).

A higher incidence of lung cancer has been found in uranium miners and is probably due to radon and its daughter products, but not to uranium itself (ATSDR, 1999). Gulf war veterans who were wounded subsequent to the explosion of armor-piercing shells containing depleted uranium often retain small fragments of the metal. This has created concern for the potential long-term effects of such embedded uranium fragments. Although there are no human data, a recent study in rats indicates that embedded depleted uranium fragments can cause localized proliferative reactions and soft tissue

sarcomas in rats (Hahn *et al.*, 2002). Embedded tungsten alloy containing depleted uranium rapidly induced malignant rhabdomyosarcomas as early as one month postimplantation in rats (Kalinich *et al.*, 2005).

Vanadium

Vanadium (V) is a transition metal discovered in the early 1800s and is named after the goddess of beauty in Scandinavian mythology, *Vanadis*, because of its beautiful multicolored chemical compounds. Vanadium may be an essential trace element, but definitive evidence that a vanadium-deficiency disease occurs in humans is lacking (Mukherjee *et al.*, 2004). It does appear to be an essential nutrient metal for ascidians, chickens, and rats (Lagerkvist *et al.* 1986). It has several oxidation states, the most common being 3+, 4+, and 5+. The metal can be found as halides, such as the tetrachloride, and oxides, such as vanadium pentoxide. Organometallic vanadium compounds are generally unstable. Vanadium is recovered from vanadium containing ores and from fossil fuels. Vanadium compounds are used in the hardening of steel, in the manufacture of pigments, in photography, and as catalysts.

Food is the major source of human exposure. Significant amounts of vanadium are found in seafood, mushrooms, dill seed, milk, meat, cereals, and vegetables (Lagerkvist *et al.* 1986; Mukherjee *et al.*, 2004). Concentrations in the drinking water largely depend on geographic location. Concentrations in rural air are much lower than in urban air, largely due to fossil fuel combustion (Lagerkvist *et al.*, 1986). The daily intake is estimated in the US population to range from 10 to 60 μg. The normal blood and urine levels are estimated to be around 1 and 10 nmol/L, respectively (Sabbioni *et al.*, 1993).

The lungs absorb about 25% of soluble vanadium compounds, but the absorption of vanadium salts from the gastrointestinal tract is generally poor (Lagerkvist *et al.*, 1986). Some dermal absorption of soluble compounds is possible but probably represents a minor route for humans. Once absorbed, extracellular vanadium will be in the form of vanadate (5+) and most likely in the vanadyl (4+) form after entering cells. After experimental exposure by various routes in rodents, the highest amounts of vanadium are found in the bone, kidney, liver, and spleen (Lagerkvist *et al.*, 1986). Brain levels are considerably lower than other tissues indicating limited transport across the blood–brain barrier. After parenteral exposure, vanadium is rapidly excreted in the urine with a biological half-life of 20 to 40 hours.

Toxicity   The toxicity of vanadium compounds usually increases as the valence increases and the pentavalent compounds are the most toxic. After occupational exposure to airborne vanadium, its toxic actions are largely confined to irritation of the respiratory tract, eyes, and skin (Lagerkvist *et al.*, 1986). Interestingly, there is usually a latent period of 1 to 6 days before the adverse effects of vanadium appear, although the effects are usually reversible. Bronchitis and bronchopneumonia are more frequent in workers exposed to vanadium compounds. In industrial exposures to vanadium pentoxide dust, a characteristic greenish-black discoloration of the tongue occurs due to deposition of vanadium. There is some evidence that a sensitization reaction may occur with repeated exposures (Lagerkvist *et al.*, 1986). Gastrointestinal distress, nausea, vomiting, abdominal pain, cardiac palpitation, tremor, nervous depression, and kidney damage have also been linked with industrial vanadium exposure (Lagerkvist *et al.*, 1986; Barceloux, 1999).

There are a variety of proposed pharmacological uses for vanadium compounds, including lowering cholesterol, triglycerides, and glucose levels, and some evidence indicates it can prevent tumor growth or formation in rodents (Mukherjee *et al.*, 2004). There are no data indicating a carcinogenic potential for vanadium compounds in animals or man, and vanadium compounds are only weakly mutagenic (Leonard and Gerber, 1994). Reproductive toxicology data are sparse but may indicate some potential (Domingo, 1994), and there is some evidence of teratogenic potential in hamsters or mice (Lagerkvist *et al.*, 1986).

ACKNOWLEDGMENT

The authors thank Drs. Erick Tokar, Jean-Francois Coppin, Wei Qu, Lamia Benbrahim-Tallaa, and Larry Keefer for their critical review of this manuscript. This work was supported by the Intramural Research Program of the NIH, National Cancer Institute, Center for Cancer Research. The authors have no compelling financial interest and the content of this publication does not necessarily reflect the views or policies of the Department of Health and Human Services.

REFERENCES

Abu-Surrah AS, Kettunen M: Platinum group antitumor chemistry: Design and development of new anticancer drugs complementary to cisplatin. *Curr Med Chem* 13:1337–1357, 2006.

Adeeko A, Li D, Forsyth DS: Effects of in utero tributyltin chloride exposure in the rat on pregnancy outcome. *Toxicol Sci* 74:407–415, 2003.

Akoume MY, Tuchweber B, Plaa GL, *et al.*: The role of mdr2 in manganese-bilirubin induced cholestasis in mice. *Toxicol Lett* 148:41–51, 2004.

Alfrey AC: Aluminum toxicity in patients with chronic renal failure. *Ther Drug Monit* 15:593–597, 1993.

Alpert PT: New and emerging theories of cardiovascular disease: Infection and elevated iron. *Biol Res Nurs* 6:3–10, 2004.

Ando M, Tadano M, Asanuma S, *et al.*: Health effects of indoor fluoride pollution from coal burning in China. *Environ Health Perspect* 106:239–244, 1998.

Anttila A, Heikkila P, Pukkala E, *et al.*: Excess lung cancer among workers exposed to lead. *Scand J Work Environ Health* 21:460–469, 1995.

Anttila A, Pukkala E, Aitio A, *et al.*: Update of cancer incidence among workers at a copper/nickel smelter and nickel refinery. *Int Arch Occup Environ Health* 71:245–250, 1998.

Aposhian HV, Aposhian MM. Arsenic toxicology: Five questions. *Chem Res Toxicol* 19:1–15, 2006.

Aschner M, Erikson KM, Dorman DC: Manganese dosimetry: Species differences and implications for neurotoxicity. *Crit Rev Toxicol* 35:1–32, 2005.

Aschner JL, Aschner M. Nutritional aspects of manganese homeostasis. *Mol Aspects Med* 26:353–362, 2005.

ATSDR: *Toxicological Profile for Silver.* Agency for Toxic Substances and Disease Registry, Atlanta, Georgia, 1990, pp. 1–145.

ATSDR: *Toxicological Profile for Antimony.* Agency for Toxic Substances and Disease Registry, 1992, pp. 1–207.

ATSDR: *Toxicological Profile for Titanium Tetrachloride.* Agency for Toxic Substances and Disease Registry, Atlanta, Georgia, 1997, pp. 1–109.

ATSDR: *Toxicological Profile for Cadmium (update).* Agency for Toxic Substances and Disease Registry, 1999a, pp. 1–397.

ATSDR: *Toxicological Profile for Mercury (update).* Agency for Toxic Substances and Disease Registry, Atlanta, Georgia, 1999b, pp. 1–485.

ATSDR: *Toxicological Profile for Uranium (update).* Agency for Toxic Substances and Disease Registry, Atlanta, Georgia, 1999c, pp. 1–398.

ATSDR: *Toxicological Profile for Chromium (update).* Agency for Toxic Substances and Disease Registry, Atlanta, Georgia, 2000a, pp. 1–419.

ATSDR: *Toxicological Profile for Manganese (update).* Agency for Toxic Substances and Disease Registry, Atlanta, Georgia, 2000b, pp. 1–398.

ATSDR: *Toxicological Profile for Beryllium (update).* Agency for Toxic Substances and Disease Registry, Atlanta, Georgia, 2002, pp. 1–247.

ATSDR: *Toxicological Profile for Fluorides, Hydrogen Fluoride, and Fluorine (Update).* Agency for Toxic Substances and Disease Registry, Atlanta, Georgia, 2003a, pp. 1–356.

ATSDR: *Toxicological Profile for Selenium (update).* Agency for Toxic Substances and Disease Registry, Atlanta, Georgia, 2003b, pp. 1–418.

ATSDR: *Toxicological Profile for Cesium.* Agency for Toxic Substances and Disease Registry, Atlanta, Georgia, 2004, pp. 1–244.

ATSDR: *Toxicological Profile for Arsenic (update).* Agency for Toxic Substances and Disease Registry, Atlanta, Georgia, 2005a, pp. 1–357.

ATSDR: *Toxicological Profile for Barium (update).* Agency for Toxic Substances and Disease Registry, Atlanta, Georgia, 2005b, pp. 1–197.

ATSDR: *Toxicological Profile for Lead (update).* Agency for Toxic Substances and Disease Registry, Atlanta, Georgia, 2005c, pp. 1–577.

ATSDR: *Toxicological Profile for Nickel (update).* Agency for Toxic Substances and Disease Registry, Atlanta, Georgia, 2005d, pp. 1–351.

ATSDR: *Toxicological Profile for Tin (update).* Agency for Toxic Substances and Disease Registry, Atlanta, Georgia, 2005e, pp. 1–376.

ATSDR: *Toxicological Profile for Zinc (update).* Agency for Toxic Substances and Disease Registry, Atlanta, Georgia, 2005f, pp. 1–307.

Ball LK, Ball R, Pratt RD: An assessment of thimerosal use in childhood vaccines. *Pediatrics* 107:1147–1154, 2001.

Bakir F, Damluji SF, Amin-Zaki L, *et al.*: Methylmercury poisoning in Iraq. *Science* 181:230–241, 1973.

Barbosa F Jr, Tanus-Santos JE, Gerlach RF, *et al.*: A critical review of biomarkers used for monitoring human exposure to lead: Advantages, limitations, and future needs. *Environ Health Perspect* 113:1669–1674, 2005.

Barceloux DG: Molybdenum. *J Toxicol Clin Toxicol* 37:231–137, 1999.

Barceloux DG: Vanadium. *J Toxicol Clin Toxicol* 37:265–278, 1999.

Bassin EB, Wypij D, Davis RB, *et al.*: Age-specific fluoride exposure in drinking water and osteosarcoma (United States). *Cancer Causes Control* 17:421–428, 2006.

Batuman V: Lead nephropathy, gout, and hypertension. *Am J Med Sci* 305:241–247, 1993.

Baughman TA: Elemental mercury spills. *Environ Health Perspect* 114:147–152, 2006.

Bellinger DC: Lead. *Pediatrics* 113:1016–1022, 2005.

Beijer K, Jernelov A: General chemistry of metals, in Friberg L, Nordberg GF, Voul VB (eds.): *Handbook of The Toxicology of Metals.* New York: Elsevier, 1986, pp. 68–84.

Bell JN, Shaw: Ecological lessons from the Chernobyl accident. *Environ Int* 31:771–777, 2005.

Berglund M, Akesson A, Nermell B, *et al.*: Intestinal absorption of dietary cadmium in women depends on body iron stores and fiber intake. *Environ Health Perspect* 102:1058–1066, 1994.

Bernard A: Renal dysfunction induced by cadmium: Biomarkers of critical effects. *Biometals* 17:519–523, 2004.

Bernard BK, Osheroff MR, Hofmann A, *et al.*: Toxicology and carcinogenesis studies of dietary titanium dioxide-coated mica in male and female Fischer 344 rats. *J Toxicol Environ Health* 29:417–429, 1990.

Bernstein LR: Mechanisms of therapeutic activity for gallium. *Pharmacol Rev* 50:665–681, 1998.

Bhamra MS, Case CP: Biological effects of metal-on-metal hip replacements. *Proc Inst Mech Eng* 220:379–384, 2006.

Bhattacharyya MH, Whelton BD, Peterson DP, *et al.*: Skeletal changes in multiparous mice fed a nutrient-sufficient diet containing cadmium. *Toxicology* 50:193–204, 1988.

Bigazzi PE: Metals and kidney autoimmunity. *Environ Health Perspect* 107(Suppl 5):753–565, 1999.

Blanusa M, Varnai VM, Piasek M, *et al.*: Chelators as antidotes of metal toxicity: Therapeutic and experimental aspects. *Curr Med Chem* 12:2771–2294, 2005.

Blazka ME, Tepper JS, Dixon D, *et al.*: Pulmonary response of Fischer 344 rats to acute nose-only inhalation of indium trichloride. *Environ Res* 67:68–83, 1994.

Blunden S, Wallace T: Tin in canned food: A review and understanding of occurrence and effect. *Food Chem Toxicol* 41:1651–62, 2003.

Bockman R: The effects of gallium nitrate on bone resorption. *Semin Oncol* 30(2 Suppl 5):5–12, 2003.

Boening DW: Ecological effects, transport, and fate of mercury: A general review. *Chemosphere* 40:1335–1351, 2000.

Boles JW, Klaassen CD: Effects of molybdate and pentachlorophenol on the sulfation of acetaminophen. *Toxicology* 146:23–35, 2000.

Brambila E, Liu J, Morgan DL, *et al.*: Effect of mercury vapor exposure on metallothionein and glutathione s-transferase gene expression in the kidney of nonpregnant, pregnant, and neonatal rats. *J Toxicol Environ Health A* 65:1273–1288, 2002.

Brewer GJ: Tetrathiomolybdate anticopper therapy for Wilson's disease inhibits angiogenesis, fibrosis and inflammation. *J Cell Mol Med* 7:11–20, 2003.

Brewer GJ: Neurologically presenting Wilson's disease: Epidemiology, pathophysiology and treatment. *CNS Drugs* 19:185–192, 2005.

Bridges CC, Zalpus RK: Molecular and ionic mimicry and the transport of toxic metals. *Toxicol Appl Pharmacol* 204:274–308, 2005.

Bright P, Burge PS, O'Hickey SP: Occupational asthma due to chrome and nickel electroplating. *Thorax* 52:28–32, 1997.

Browne D, Whelton H, O'Mullane D: Fluoride metabolism and fluorosis. *J Dent* 33:177–186, 2005.

Brooks SM, Baker DB, Gann PH, *et al.*: Cold air challenge and platinum skin reactivity in platinum refinery workers. Bronchial reactivity precedes skin prick response. *Chest* 97:1401–1407, 1990.

Brumm VL, van Gorp WG, Wirshing W: Chronic Neuropsychological sequelae in a case of severe lithium intoxication. *Neuropsychiatr Neuropsychol Behav Neurol* 11:245–249, 1998.

Bucher JR, Hailey JR, Roycroft JR, *et al.*: Inhalation toxicity and carcinogenicity studies of cobalt sulfate. *Toxicol Sci* 49:56–67, 1999.

Buss JL, Greene BT, Turner J, *et al.*: Iron chelators in cancer chemotherapy. *Curr Top Med Chem* 4:1623–635, 2004.

Cai L, Li XK, Song Y, *et al.*: Essentiality, toxicology and chelation therapy of zinc and copper. *Curr Med Chem* 12:2753–2763, 2005.

Campbell JR, Rosier RN, Novotny L, *et al.*: The association between environmental lead exposure and bone density in children. *Environ Health Perspect* 112:1200–1203, 2004.

Carmouche JJ, Puzas JE, Zhang X, *et al.*: Lead exposure inhibits fracture healing and is associated with increased chondrogenesis, delay in cartilage mineralization, and a decrease in osteoprogenitor frequency. *Environ Health Perspect* 113:749–755, 2005.

Caruso F, Rossi M: Antitumor titanium compounds. *Mini Rev Med Chem* 4:49–60, 2004.

CDC: Blood lead levels—United States, 1999–2002. *Morb Mortal Wkly Rep (MMWR)* 54:513–516, 2005.

Cefalu WT, Hu FB: Role of chromium in human health and in diabetes. *Diabetes Care* 27:2741–2751, 2004.

Centeno JA, Mullick FG, Martinez L, *et al.*: Pathology related to chronic arsenic exposure. *Environ Health Perspect* 110(Suppl 5):883–886, 2002.

Cervantes C, Campos-Garcia J, Devars S, *et al.*: Interactions of chromium with microorganisms and plants. *FEMS Microbiol Rev* 25:335–347, 2001.

Chan HM, Zhu LF, Zhong R, *et al.*: Nephrotoxicity in rats following liver transplantation from cadmium-exposed rats. *Toxicol Appl Pharmacol* 123:89–96, 1993.

Chapin RE, Harris MW, Hunter ES III, *et al.*: The reproductive and developmental toxicity of indium in the Swiss mouse. *Fundam Appl Toxicol* 27:140–148, 1995.

Chen CJ, Hsu LI, Wang CH, *et al.*: Biomarkers of exposure, effect, and susceptibility of arsenic-induced health hazards in Taiwan. *Toxicol Appl Pharmacol* 206:198–206, 2005.

Chen L, Jin T, Huang B, *et al.*: Critical exposure level of cadmium for elevated urinary metallothionein—An occupational population study in China. *Toxicol Appl Pharmacol.* 215:93–99, 2006.

Clark DC, Shulman JD, Maupome G, *et al.*: Changes in dental fluorosis following the cessation of water fluoridation. *Community Dent Oral Epidemiol* 34:197–204, 2006.

Clarkson TW: The three modern faces of mercury. *Environ Health Perspect* 110(Suppl 1):11–23, 2002.

Clarkson TW, Magos L, Myers GJ: The toxicology of mercury—Current exposures and clinical manifestations. *N Engl J Med* 349:1731–1737, 2003.

Clemens F, Verma R, Ramnath J, *et al.*: Amplification of the Ect2 protooncogene and over-expression of Ect2 mRNA and protein in nickel compound and methylcholanthrene-transformed 10T1/2 mouse fibroblast cell lines. *Toxicol Appl Pharmacol.* 206:138–149, 2005.

Cocco P, Dosemeci M, Heineman EF: Brain cancer and occupational exposure to lead. *J Occup Environ Med* 40:937–942, 1998.

Cohen MD, Kargacin B, Klein CB, *et al.*: Mechanisms of chromium carcinogenicity and toxicity. *Crit Rev Toxicol* 23:255–281, 1993.

Cohen SM, Yamamoto S, Cano M, Arnold L: Urothelial cytotoxicity and regeneration induced by dimethylarsinic acid in rats. *Toxicol Sci* 59:68–74, 2001.

Costa M: Toxicity and carcinogenicity of Cr(VI) in animal models and humans. *Crit Rev Toxicol* 27:431–442, 1997.

Costa M, Klein CB: Toxicity and carcinogenicity of chromium compounds in humans. *Crit Rev Toxicol* 36:155–163, 2006.

Costa M, Davidson TL, Chen H, *et al.*: Nickel carcinogenesis: Epigenetics and hypoxia signaling. *Mutat Res* 592:79–88, 2005.

Counter SA, Buchanan LH: Mercury exposure in children: A review. *Toxicol Appl Pharmacol* 198:209–230, 2004.

Cousins RJ, Liuzzi JP, Lichten L: Mammalian zinc transport, trafficking, and signals. *J Biol Chem* 281:24085–24089, 2006.

Cox M, Singer I: Lithium, in Bronner F, Coburn JW (eds.): *Disorders of Mineral Metabolism*. New York: Academic Press, 1981, pp. 369–438.

Craft E, Abu-Qare A, Flaherty M, *et al.*: Depleted and natural uranium: Chemistry and toxicological effects. *J Toxicol Environ Health B Crit Rev* 7:297–317, 2004.

Cremin JD Jr, Luck ML, Laughlin NK, *et al.*: Efficacy of succimer chelation for reducing brain lead in a primate model of human lead exposure. *Toxicol Appl Pharmacol* 161:283–293, 1999.

Crossgrove J, Zheng W. Manganese toxicity upon overexposure. *NMR Biomed* 17:544–553, 2004.

Dalal AK, Harding JD, Verdino RJ: Acquired long QT syndrome and monomorphic ventricular tachycardia after alternative treatment with cesium chloride for brain cancer. *Mayo Clin Proc* 79:1065–1069, 2004.

Dallas CE, Williams PL: Barium: Rationale for a new oral reference dose. *J Toxicol Environ Health B Crit Rev* 4:395–429, 2001.

Day GA, Stefaniak AB, Weston A, *et al.*: Beryllium exposure: Dermal and immunological considerations. *Int Arch Occup Environ Health* 79:161–164, 2006.

Davidson PW, Myers GJ, Weiss B, *et al.*: Prenatal methyl mercury exposure from fish consumption and child development: A review of evidence and perspectives from the Seychelles Child Development Study. *Neurotoxicology* 27:1106–1109, 2006.

Davidson PW, Myers GJ, Weiss B: Mercury exposure and child development outcomes. *Pediatrics* 113(4 Suppl):1023–1029, 2004.

De Boeck M, Kirsch-Volders M, Lison D: Cobalt and antimony: Genotoxicity and carcinogenicity. *Mutat Res* 533:135–152, 2003.

De Flora S: Threshold mechanisms and site specificity in chromium(VI) carcinogenesis. *Carcinogenesis* 21:533–541, 2000.

De Francisco N, Ruiz Troya JD, Aguera EI: Lead and lead toxicity in domestic and free living birds. *Avian Pathol* 32:3–13, 2003.

Denkhaus E, Salnikow K. Nickel essentiality, toxicity, and carcinogenicity. *Crit Rev Oncol Hematol* 42:35–56, 2002.

DeRouen TA, Martin MD, Leroux BG, *et al.*: Neurobehavioral effects of dental amalgam in children: A randomized clinical trial. *JAMA* 295:1784–1792, 2006.

Desoize B: Metals and metal compounds in cancer treatment. *Anticancer Res.* 24:1529–1544, 2004.

Deubner DC, Lowney YW, Paustenbach DJ, *et al.*: Contribution of incidental exposure pathways to total beryllium exposures. *Appl Occup Environ Hyg* 16:568–578, 2001.

Diamond GL, Zalpus R: Nephrotoxicity of Metals, in Tarloff JB, Lash LH (eds.): *Toxicology of the Kidney*, 3rd edn, Chap. 22. Boca Raton: CRC Press, 2005, pp. 971–979.

Diwan BA, Kasprzak KS, Rice JM: Transplacental carcinogenic effects of nickel(II) acetate in the renal cortex, renal pelvis and adenohypophysis in F344/NCr rats. *Carcinogenesis* 13:1351–1377, 1992.

Dietert RR, Lee JE, Hussain I, *et al.*: Developmental immunotoxicology of lead. *Toxicol Appl Pharmacol* 198:86–94, 2004.

Doherty MJ, Healy M, Richardson SG, *et al.*: Total body iron overload in welder's siderosis. *Occup Environ Med* 61:82–85, 2006.

Domingo JL: Metal-induced developmental toxicity in mammals: A review. *J Toxicol Environ Health* 42:123–141, 1994.

Dopp E, Hartmann LM, Florea AM, *et al.*: Environmental distribution, analysis, and toxicity of organometal(loid) compounds. *Crit Rev Toxicol* 34:301–333, 2004.

Douglass CW, Joshipura K: Caution needed in fluoride and osteosarcoma study. *Cancer Causes Control* 17:481–482, 2006.

Drake PL, Hazelwood KJ: Exposure-related health effects of silver and silver compounds: A review. *Ann Occup Hyg* 49:575–585, 2005.

Driscoll DM, Copeland PR: Mechanism and regulation of selenoprotein synthesis. *Annu Rev Nutr* 23:17–40, 2003.

Duffield-Lillico AJ, Reid ME, Turnbull BW, *et al.*: Baseline characteristics and the effect of selenium supplementation on cancer incidence in a randomized clinical trial: A summary report of the Nutritional Prevention of Cancer Trial. *Cancer Epidemiol Biomarkers Prev* 11:630–639, 2002.

Elinder C-G, Friberg L: Antimony, in Friberg L, *et al.* (eds.): *Handbook on the Toxicology of Metals*. Amsterdam: Elsevier, 1986, pp. 26–42.

Eisler R: Health risks of gold miners: A synoptic review. *Environ Geochem Health* 25:325–345, 2003.

Exley C, Burgess E, Day JP, *et al.*: Aluminum toxicokinetics. *J Toxicol Environ Health* 48:569–584, 1996.

Factor-Litvak P, Hasselgren G, Jacobs D, *et al.*: Mercury derived from dental amalgams and neuropsychologic function. *Environ Health Perspect* 111:719–723, 2003.

Fayerweather WE, Karns ME, Gilby PG, *et al.*: Epidemiologic study of lung cancer mortality in workers exposed to titanium tetrachloride. *J Occup Med* 34:164–169, 1992.

Fent K: Ecotoxicology of organotin compounds. *Crit Rev Toxicol* 26:1–117, 1996.

Ferm VH, Carpenter SJ: Teratogenic and embryopathic effects of indium, gallium, and germanium. *Toxicol Appl Pharmacol* 16:166–170, 1970.

Fontenot AP, Maier LA, Canavera SJ, *et al.*: Beryllium skin patch testing to analyze T cell stimulation and granulomatous inflammation in the lung. *J Immunol* 168:3627–3634, 2002.

Fowler BA: Indium, in Friberg L, Nordberg GF, Voul VB (eds.): *Handbook of The Toxicology of Metals*. New York: Elsevier, 1986, pp. 267–275.

Fowler BA, Goyer RA: Bismuth localization within nuclear inclusions by x-ray microanalysis. Effects of accelerating voltage. *J Histochem Cytochem* 23:722–726, 1975.

Friberg L, Elinder C-G, Kjellstrom T, Nordberg GF (eds.):*Cadmium and Health: A Toxicological and Epidemiological Appraisal*, vol. 1. Boca Raton: CRC Press, 1986, pp. 1–307.

Frederickson CJ, Koh JY, Bush AI: The neurobiology of zinc in health and disease. *Nat Rev Neurosci* 6:449–462, 2005.

Fryzek JP, Chadda B, Marano D, *et al.*: A cohort mortality study among titanium dioxide manufacturing workers in the United States. *J Occup Environ Med* 45:400–409, 2003.

Fu H, Boffetta P: Cancer and occuparional exposure to inorganic lead compounds: A meta-analysis of published data. *Occup Environ Med* 52:73–81, 1995.

Galvan-Arzate S, Santamaria A: Thallium toxicity. *Toxicol Lett* 99:1–13, 1998.

Grandjean P, Weihe P, White RF, *et al.*: Cognitive deficit in 7-year old children with prenatal exposure to methylmercury. *Neurotoxicol Teratol* 19:417–428, 1997.

Garruto RM, Fukatsu R, Yanagihara R, *et al.*: Imaging of calcium and aluminum in neurofibrillary tangle-bearing neurons in parkinsonism-dementia of Guam. *Proc Natl Acad Sci U S A* 81:1875–1879, 1984.

Garruto RM, Yanagihara R, Gajdusek DC: Disappearance of high-incidence amyotrophic lateral sclerosis and parkinsonism-dementia on Guam. *Neurology* 35:193–198, 1985.

Gebel T: Arsenic and antimony: comparative approach on mechanistic toxicology. *Chem Biol Interact* 107:131–144, 1997.

Gerber GB, Leonard A, Hantson P: Carcinogenicity, mutagenicity and teratogenicity of manganese compounds. *Crit Rev Oncol Hematol* 42:25–34, 2002.

Gerber GB, Leonard A: Mutagenicity, carcinogenicity and teratogenicity of germanium compounds. *Mutat Res* 387:141–146, 1997.

Gerhardsson L, Glover JR, Nordberg GF, Vouk V: Tellurium, in Friberg L, Nordberg GF, Voul VB (eds.): *Handbook of The Toxicology of Metals*. New York: Elsevier, 1986, pp. 255–266.

Germolec DR, Spalding J, Yu HS, *et al.*: Arsenic enhancement of skin neoplasia by chronic stimulation of growth factors. *Am J Pathol* 153:1775–1785, 1998.

Gonick HC, Behari JR: Is lead exposure the principal cause of essential hypertension? *Med Hypotheses* 59:239–246, 2002.

Goodrum JF: Role of organotellurium species in tellurium neuropathy. *Neurochem Res* 23:1313–1319, 1998.

Gordon T, Bowser D: Beryllium: genotoxicity and carcinogenicity. *Mutat Res.* 533:99–105, 2003.

Gottschling BC, Maronpot RR, Hailey JR, *et al.*: The role of oxidative stress in indium phosphide-induced lung carcinogenesis in rats. *Toxicol Sci* 64:28–40, 2001.

Goyer RA: Mechanisms of lead and cadmium nephrotoxicity. *Toxicol Lett* 46:153–162, 1989.

Goyer RA: Lead toxicity: From overt to subclinical to subtle health effects. *Environ Health Perspect* 86:177–181, 1990.

Goyer RA: Results of lead research: prenatal exposure and neurological consequences. *Environ Health Perspect* 104:1050–1054, 1996.

Goyer RA: Toxic and essential metal interactions. *Annu Rev Nutr* 17:37–50, 1997.

Grant LD, Mushak P: Specification of metals and metal compounds: implications for biological monitoring and development of regulatory approaches. *Toxicol Ind Health* 5:891–908, 1989.

Gregus Z, Klaassen CD: Disposition of metals in rats: A comparative study of fecal, urinary, and biliary excretion and tissue distribution of eighteen metals. *Toxicol Appl Pharmacol* 85:24–38, 1986.

Gulson BL, Mizon KJ, Korsch MJ, *et al.*: Mobilization of lead from human bone tissue during pregnancy and lactation—A summary of long-term research. *Sci Total Environ* 303:79–104, 2003.

Hahn FF, Guilmette RA, Hoover MD: Implanted depleted uranium fragments cause soft tissue sarcomas in the muscles of rats. *Environ Health Perspect* 110:51–59, 2002.

Handy RD: Chronic effects of copper exposure versus endocrine toxicity: Two sides of the same toxicological process? *Comp Biochem Physiol Part A* 135:25–38, 2003.

Hamza I, Gitlin JD: Copper chaperones for cytochrome c oxidase and human disease. *J Bioenerg Biomembr* 34:381–388, 2002.

Hardman JG, Limbird LE, Gilman AG (eds.). The *Pharmacological Basis of Therapeutics*.New York: McGraw-Hill, 2001, pp. 1432–1435.

Harlan WR: The relationship of blood lead levels to blood pressure in the US population. *Environ Health Perspect* 78:9–13, 1988.

Harris ED: Cellular copper transport and metabolism. *Annu Rev Nutr* 20:291–310, 2000.

Harris WR, Berthon G, Day JP, *et al.*: Speciation of aluminum in biological systems. *J Toxicol Environ Health* 48:543–568, 1996.

Hart BA, Potts RJ, Watkin RD: Cadmium adaptation in the lung—A double-edged sword? *Toxicology* 160:65–70, 2001.

Howard BJ, Howard DC: Health impacts of large releases of radionuclides. The radioecological significance of semi-natural ecosystems. *Ciba Found Symp* 203:21–45, 1997.

Havelaar AC, de Gast IL, Snijders S: Characterization of a heavy metal ion transporter in the lysosomal membrane. *FEBS Lett* 436:223–227, 1998.

Henry GA, Jarnot BM, Steinhoff MM, *et al.*: Mercury-induced renal autoimmunity in the MAXX rat. *Clin Immunol Immunopathol* 49:187–203, 1988.

Herbert V: Vitamin B-12, in Ziegler EE, Filer LJ (eds.): *Present Knowledge in Nutrition*. Washington, DC: ILSI, 1996, pp. 191–205.

Hindin R, Brugge D, Panikkar B: Teratogenicity of depleted uranium aerosols: A review from an epidemiological perspective. *Environ Health* 26:4–17, 2005.

Hirasawa F, Sato M, Takizawa Y: Organ distribution of silver and the effect of silver on copper status in rats. *Toxicol Lett* 70:193–201, 1994.

Hunsaker DM, Spiller HA, Williams D: Acute selenium poisoning: Suicide by ingestion. *J Forensic Sci* 50:942–946, 2005.

Hoffman RS: Thallium poisoning during pregnancy: A case report and comprehensive literature review. *J Toxicol Clin Toxicol* 38:767–775, 2000.

Hoffman RS: Thallium toxicity and the role of Prussian blue in therapy. *Toxicol Rev* 22:29–40, 2003.

Horsted-Bindslev P: Amalgam toxicity—Environmental and occupational hazards. *J Dent* 32:359–365, 2004.

Hopenhayn C, Huang B, Christian J, *et al.*: Profile of urinary arsenic metabolites during pregnancy. *Environ Health Perspect* 111:1888–1891, 2003.

Hostynek JJ, Hinz RS, Lorence CR, *et al.*: Metals and the skin. *Crit Rev Toxicol* 23:171–235, 1993.

Hostynek JJ: Gold: An allergen of growing significance. *Food Chem Toxicol* 35:839–844, 1997.

Hu H, Aro A, Payton M, *et al.*: The relationship of bone and blood lead to hypertension. *JAMA* 275:1171–1176, 1996.

IARC: IARC monographs on the evaluation of carcinogenic risks to humans. *Overall Evaluations of Carcinogenicity: An Updating of IARC Monographa*, vols. 1 to 42. Lyon, France: IARC, 1987.

IARC: IARC monographs on the evaluation of carcinogenic risks to humans. *Chromium, Nickel and Welding*, vol. 49. Lyon, France: IARC, 1990, pp. 1–677.

IARC: IARC Monographs on the evaluation of carcinogenic risks to humans. *Chlorinated Drinking Water Chlorination by-Products Some Other Halogenated Compounds Cobalt and Cobalt Compounds*, vol. 52. Lyon, France: IARC, 1991, pp. 1–544.

IARC: IARC Monographs on the evaluation of carcinogenic risks to humans. *Beryllium, Cadmium, Mercury and Exposures in the Glass Manufacturing Industry*, vol. 58. Lyon, France: IARC, 1993, pp. 41–117.

IARC: IARC Monographs on the evaluation of carcinogenic risks to humans. *Arsenic in Drinking Water: Some Drinking Water Disinfectants and Contaminants, including Arsenic*, vol. 84. Lyon, France: IARC, 2004, pp. 269–477.

IARC: IARC monographs on the evaluation of carcinogenic risks to humans. *Inorganic Lead and Organic Lead Compounds*, vol. 87.Lyon, France: IARC, 2006.

IOM: Institute of Medicine, Food and Nutrition Boards (eds.): *Dietary Reference Intakes*. Washington, DC: National Academic Press, 2001, pp. 1–769.

Il'yasova D, Schwartz GG: Cadmium and renal cancer. *Toxicol Appl Pharmacol* 207:179–186, 2005.

Jakupec MA, Keppler BK: Gallium in cancer treatment. *Curr Top Med Chem* 4:1575–1583, 2004.

Jarup L, Berglund M, Elinder CG, *et al.*: Health effects of cadmium exposure—A review of the literature and a risk estimate. *Scand J Work Environ Health* 24(Suppl 1):1–51, 1998.

Jiang GC, Aschner M: Neurotoxicity of depleted uranium: reasons for increased concern. *Biol Trace Elem Res* 110:1–18, 2006.

Jiang Y, Zheng W: Cardiovascular toxicities upon manganese exposure. *Cardiovasc Toxicol* 5:345–354, 2005.

Johnson CH, VanTassell VJ: Acute barium poisoning with respiratory failure and rhabdomyolysis. *Ann Emerg Med* 20:1138–1142, 1991.

Kagan HM, Li W: Lysyl oxidase: properties, specificity, and biological roles inside and outside of the cell. *J Cell Biochem* 88:660–672, 2003.

Kalinich JF, Emond CA, Dalton TK, *et al.*: Embedded weapons-grade tungsten alloy shrapnel rapidly induces metastatic high-grade rhabdomyosarcomas in F344 rats. *Environ Health Perspect* 113:729–734, 2005.

Karjalainen S, Kerttula R, Pukkala E: Cancer risk among workers at a copper/nickel smelter and nickel refinery in Finland. *Int Arch Occup Environ Health* 63:547–551, 1992.

Karmaus W, Brooks KR, Nebe T, *et al.*: Immune function biomarkers in children exposed to lead and organochlorine compounds: A cross-sectional study. *Environ Health* 4:1–10, 2005.

Kawahara M: Effects of aluminum on the nervous system and its possible link with neurodegenerative diseases. *J Alzheimers Dis* 8:171–82; discussion 209–15, 2005.

Kasprzak KS: Oxidative DNA and protein damage in metal-induced toxicity and carcinogenesis. *Free Radic Biol Med* 32:958–967, 2002.

Kasprzak KS, Sunderman FW Jr, Salnikow K: Nickel carcinogenesis. *Mutat Res* 533:67–97, 2003.

Kazantzis G: Role of cobalt, iron, lead, manganese, mercury, platinum, selenium, and titanium in carcinogenesis. *Environ Health Perspect* 40:143–161, 1981.

Kazantzis G: Cadmium, osteoporosis and calcium metabolism. *Biometals* 17:493–498, 2004.

Kelada SN, Shelton E, Kaufmann RB, *et al.*: Delta-aminolevulinic acid dehydratase and lead toxicity, a HuGE review. *Am J Epidemiol* 154:1–13, 2001.

Khan BI, Solo-Gabriele HM, Townsend TG, *et al.*: Release of arsenic to the environment from CCA-treated wood. 1. Leaching and speciation during service. *Environ Sci Technol* 40:988–993, 2006.

Kielhorn J, Melber C, Keller D, *et al.*: Palladium—A review of exposure and effects to human health. *Int J Hyg Environ Health* 205:417–432, 2002.

Klaassen CD: Heavy metals and heavy-metal antagonists, in Hardman JG, Limbird LE, Gilman AG (eds.): The *Pharmacological Basis of Therapeutics*. New York: McGraw-Hill, 2001, pp. 1851–1876.

Klaassen CD, Liu J: Induction of metallothionein as an adaptive mechanism affecting the magnitude and progression of toxicological injury. *Environ Health Perspect* 106(Suppl 1):297–300, 1998.

Klaassen CD, Liu J, Choudhuri S: Metallothionein: An intracellular protein to protect against cadmium toxicity. *Annu Rev Pharmacol Toxicol* 39:267–294, 1999.

Klaassen CD, Waalkes MP, Cantilena LR Jr: Alteration of tissue disposition of cadmium by chelating agents. *Environ Health Perspect* 54:233–242, 1984.

Klimisch HJ: Lung deposition, lung clearance and renal accumulation of inhaled cadmium chloride and cadmium sulphide in rats. *Toxicology* 84:103–124, 1993.

Kohrle J, Jakob F, Contempre B, *et al.*: Selenium, the thyroid, and the endocrine system. *Endocr Rev* 26:944–984, 2005.

Kondo Y, Himeno S, Satoh M, *et al.*: Citrate enhances the protective effect of orally administered bismuth subnitrate against the nephrotoxicity of cis-diamminedichloroplatinum. *Cancer Chemother Pharmacol* 53:33–38, 2004.

Kopp SJ, Glonek T, Perry HM Jr, *et al.*: Cardiovascular actions of cadmium at environmental exposure levels. *Science* 217:837–839, 1982.

Kostova I: Gold coordination complexes as anticancer agents. *Anticancer Agents Med Chem* 6:19–32, 2006.

Kriegel AM, Soliman AS, Zhang Q, *et al.*: Serum cadmium levels in pancreatic cancer patients from the East Nile Delta region of Egypt. *Environ Health Perspect* 114:113–119, 2006.

Kszos LA, Stewart AJ: Review of lithium in the aquatic environment: Distribution in the United States, toxicity and case example of groundwater contamination. *Ecotoxicology* 12:439–447, 2003.

Laden BP, Porter TD: Inhibition of human squalene monooxygenase by tellurium compounds: Evidence of interaction with vicinal sulfhydryls. *J Lipid Res* 42:235–240, 2001.

Lagerkvist B, Nordberg GF, Vouk V: Vanadium, in Friberg L, Nordberg GF, Voul VB (eds.): *Handbook of The Toxicology of Metals.* New York: Elsevier, 1986, pp. 638–663.

Lamphear BP, Dietrich K, Auinger P, *et al.*: Cognitive deficits associated with blood lead concentrations <10 μg/dL in US children and adolescents. *Public Health Rep* 115:521–529, 2000.

Laraque D, Trasande L: Lead poisoning: successes and 21st century challenges. *Pediatr Rev* 26:435–443, 2005.

Larsen A, Stoltenberg M, Sondergaard C, *et al.*: In vivo distribution of bismuth in the mouse brain: influence of long-term survival and intracranial placement on the uptake and transport of bismuth in neuronal tissue. *Basic Clin Pharmacol Toxicol* 97:188–196, 2005.

Leggett RW, Williams LR, Melo DR, *et al.*: A physiologically based biokinetic model for cesium in the human body. *Sci Total Environ* 317:235–255, 2003.

Leonard A, Gerber GB: Mutagenicity, carcinogenicity and teratogenicity of vanadium compounds. *Mutat Res* 317:81–88, 1994.

Leonard A, Gerber GB: Mutagenicity, carcinogenicity and teratogenicity of antimony compounds. *Mutat Res* 366:1–8, 1996.

Leonard A, Gerber GB: Mutagenicity, carcinogenicity and teratogenicity of thallium compounds. *Mutat Res* 387:47–53, 1997.

Lenox RH, Hahn CG: Overview of the mechanism of action of lithium in the brain: Fifty-year update. *J Clin Psychiatry* 61(Suppl 9):5–15, 2000.

Leussink BT, Slikkerveer A, Engelbrecht MR, *et al.*: Bismuth overdosing-induced reversible nephropathy in rats. *Arch Toxicol* 74:745–754, 2001.

Leslie EM, Liu J, Klaassen CD, *et al.*: Acquired cadmium resistance in metallothionein-I/II(-/-) knockout cells: Role of the T-type calcium channel Cacnalpha1G in cadmium uptake. *Mol Pharmacol* 69:629–639, 2006.

Lindgren KN, Masten VL, Ford DP: Relation of cumulative exposure to inorganic and neuropsychological test performance. *Occup Environ Med* 53:472–477, 1996.

Linnett PJ: Concerns for asthma at pre-placement assessment and health surveillance in platinum refining—A personal approach. *Occup Med (Lond)* 55:595–599, 2005.

Liu J, Liu Y, Klaassen CD: Nephrotoxicity of CdCl2 and Cd-metallothionein in cultured rat kidney proximal tubules and LLC-PK1 cells. *Toxicol Appl Pharmacol* 128:264–270, 1994.

Liu J, Liu Y, Habeebu SS, *et al.*: Susceptibility of MT-null mice to chronic CdCl2-induced nephrotoxicity indicates that renal injury is not mediated by the CdMT complex. *Toxicol Sci* 46:197–203, 1998a.

Liu J, Habeebu SS, Liu Y, *et al.*: Acute CdMT injection is not a good model to study chronic Cd nephropathy: Comparison of chronic CdCl2 and CdMT exposure with acute CdMT injection in rats. *Toxicol Appl Pharmacol* 153:48–58, 1998b.

Liu J, Chen H, Miller DS, *et al.*: Overexpression of glutathione S-transferase pi and multidrug resistance transport proteins is associated with acquired tolerance to inorganic arsenic. *Mol Pharmacol* 60:302–309, 2001.

Liu J, Lei D, Waalkes MP, *et al.*: Genomic analysis of the rat lung following elemental mercury vapor exposure. *Toxicol Sci* 74:174–181, 2003.

Liu J, Zheng B, Aposhian HV, *et al.*: Chronic arsenic poisoning from burning high-arsenic-containing coal in Guizhou, China. *Environ Health Perspect* 110:119–122, 2002.

Liu J, Xie Y, Ducharme DM, *et al.*: Global gene expression associated with hepatocarcinogenesis in adult male mice induced by in utero arsenic exposure. *Environ Health Perspect* 114:404–411, 2006.

Luebke RW, Chen DH, Dietert R: The comparative immunotoxicity of five selected compounds following developmental or adult exposure. *J Toxicol Environ Health B Crit Rev* 9:1–26, 2006.

Lynch BS, Capen CC, Nestmann ER, *et al.*: Review of subchronic/chronic toxicity of antimony potassium tartrate. *Regul Toxicol Pharmacol* 30:9–17, 1999.

Madias NE, Harrington JT: Platinum nephrotoxicity. *Am J Med* 65:307–314, 1978.

Mahaffey KR: Factors modifying susceptibility to lead toxicity, in Mahaffey KR (ed.): *Dietary and Environmental Lead: Human Health Effects.* New York: Elsevier, 1985, pp. 373–420.

Makjanic J, McDonald B, Chen LHCP, *et al.*: Absence of aluminium in neurofibrillary tangles in Alzheimer's disease. *Neurosci Lett* 240:123–126, 1998.

Manton WI, Angle CR, Stanek KL, *et al.*: Acquisition and retention of lead by young children. *Environ Res* 82:60–80, 2000.

Manton WI, Angle CR, Krogstrand KL: Origin of lead in the United States diet. *Environ Sci Technol* 15:8995–9000. 2005

Maret W, Standstead HH: Zinc requirements and the risks and benefits of zinc supplementation. *J Trace Elem Med Biol* 20:3–18, 2006.

Markman M: Toxicities of the platinum antineoplastic agents. *Expert Opin Drug Saf* 2:597–607, 2003.

Markowitz GS, Radhakrishnan J, Kambham N, *et al.*: Lithium nephrotoxicity: A progressive combined glomerular and tubulointerstitial nephropathy. *J Am Soc Nephrol* 11:1439–448, 2000.

Mas A: Hepatic encephalopathy: From pathophysiology to treatment. *Digestion* 73(Suppl 1):86–93, 2006.

Mazumder DN: Effect of chronic intake of arsenic-contaminated water on liver. *Toxicol Appl Pharmacol* 206:169–175, 2005.

Mazur A, Maier JA, Rock E: Magnesium and the inflammatory response: Potential physiopathological implications. *Arch Biochem Biophys* 458:48–56, 2007.

Meenakshi RC, Maheshwari SK: Fluoride in drinking water and its removal. *J Hazard Mater* 137: 456–463, 2006.

Melendez E: Titanium complexes in cancer treatment. *Crit Rev Oncol Hematol* 42:309–315, 2002.

Mercer JF: The molecular basis of copper-transport diseases. *Trends Mol Med* 7:64–69, 2001.

Messiha FS: Developmental toxicity of cesium in the mouse. *Gen Pharmacol* 25:395–400, 1994.

Messori L, Orioli P, Banholzer V, *et al.*: Formation of titanium(IV) transferrin by reaction of human serum apotransferrin with titanium complexes. *FEBS Lett* 442:157–161, 1999.

Morell P, Toews AD, Wagner M, *et al.*: Gene expression during tellurium-induced primary demyelination. *Neurotoxicology* 15:171–180, 1994.

Morrow PE: Dust overloading of the lungs: Update and appraisal. *Toxicol Appl Pharmacol* 113:1–12, 1992.

Mukherjee B, Patra B, Mahapatra S, *et al.*: Vanadium—An element of atypical biological significance. *Toxicol Lett* 150:135–143, 2004.

Mulkey JP, Oehme FW: A review of thallium toxicity. *Vet Hum Toxicol* 35:445–453, 1993.

Nakajima M, Takahashi H, Sasaki M, *et al.*: Developmental toxicity of indium chloride by intravenous or oral administration in rats. *Teratog Carcinog Mutagen* 18:231–238, 1998.

Nakajima M, Takahashi H, Sasaki M, *et al.*: Comparative developmental toxicity study of indium in rats and mice. *Teratog Carcinog Mutagen* 20:219–227, 2000.

Navas-Acien A, Sharrett AR, Silbergeld EK, *et al.*: Arsenic exposure and cardiovascular disease: A systematic review of the epidemiologic evidence. *Am J Epidemiol* 162:1037–1049, 2005.

Navas-Acien A, Silbergeld EK, Streeter RA, *et al.*: Arsenic exposure and type 2 diabetes: A systematic review of the experimental and epidemiological evidence. *Environ Health Perspect* 114:641–648, 2006.

Nawrot TS, Thijs L, Den Hond EM, *et al.*: An epidemiological re-appraisal of the association between blood pressure and blood lead: A meta-analysis. *J Hum Hypertens* 16:123–131, 2002.

Nierenberg DW, Nordgren RE, Chang MB, *et al.*: Delayed cerebellar disease and death after accidental exposure to dimethylmercury. *N Engl J Med* 338:1672–1676, 1998.

NCI: *Bioassay of Titanium Dioxide for Possible Carcinogenesity.* National Cancer Institute Carcinogenesis Technical Report No. 97, d79-1347. Washington, DC: NCI/DHEW, 1979.

Newman LS, Mroz MM, Balkissoon R, *et al.*: Beryllium sensitization progresses to chronic beryllium disease: A longitudinal study of disease risk. *Am J Respir Crit Care Med* 171:54–60, 2005.

Ng JC, Wang JP, Zheng B, *et al.*: Urinary porphyrins as biomarkers for arsenic exposure among susceptible populations in Guizhou province, China. *Toxicol Appl Pharmacol* 206:176–184, 2005.

NRC: *Toxicological Effects of Methylmercury/Committee on the Toxicological Effects of Methylmercury, Board on Environmental Studies and Toxicology, Commission on Life Sciences.* Washington, DC: National Research Council, National Academy. 2000, pp. 1–344.

NRC: *Arsenic in the Drinking Water (update).* Washington, DC: National Research Council, National Academy, 2001, pp. 1–225.

Nogueira CW, Zeni G, Rocha JB: Organoselenium and organotellurium compounds: Toxicology and pharmacology. *Chem Rev* 104:6255–6285, 2004.

Nordberg GF: Cadmium and health in the 21st century—Historical remarks and trends for the future. *Biometals* 17:485–489, 2004.

Novotny JA, Turnlund JR: Molybdenum kinetics in men differ during molybdenum depletion and repletion. *J Nutr* 136:953–977, 2006.

NTP: NTP toxicology and carcinogenesis studies of sodium fluoride (CAS No. 7681-49-4) in F344/N rats and B6C3F1 mice (drinking water studies). *Natl Toxicol Program Tech Rep Ser* 393:1–448, 1990.

NTP: Toxicology and carcinogenesis studies of indium phosphide (CAS No. 22398-90-7) in F344/N rats and B6C3F1 mice (inhalation studies). *Natl Toxicol Program Tech Ser* 499:7–340, 2001.

NTP: Cadmium and cadmium compounds. *National Toxicology Program Report on Carcinogens,* 11th edn, 2004, pp. III42–III44.

NTP: Cobalt sulfate CAS No. 10124-43-3. *Report on Carcinogens,* 11th edn, 2004, pp. 70–72.

Oakley PW, Whyte IM, Carter GL: Lithium toxicity: An iatrogenic problem in susceptible individuals. *Aust N Z J Psychiatry* 35:833–840, 2001.

O'Brien TJ, Ceryak S, Patierno SR: Complexities of chromium carcinogenesis: Role of cellular response, repair and recovery mechanisms. *Mutat Res* 533:3–36, 2003.

O'Connor ME, Rich D: Children with moderately elevated lead levels: Is chelation with DMSA helpful? *Clin Ped* 38:325–331, 1999.

Oda K: Toxicity of a low level of indium phosphide (InP) in rats after intratracheal instillation. *Ind Health* 35:61–68, 1997.

Oller AR: Respiratory carcinogenicity assessment of soluble nickel compounds. *Environ Health Perspect* 110(Suppl 5):841–844, 2002.

Papanikolaou G, Pantopoulos K: Iron metabolism and toxicity. *Toxicol Appl Pharmacol* 202:199–211, 2005.

Patrick L: Lead toxicity, a review of the literature. Part 1: Exposure, evaluation, and treatment. *Altern Med Rev* 11:2–22, 2006.

Pelkonen KH, Heinonen-Tanski H, Hanninen OO: Accumulation of silver from drinking water into cerebellum and musculus soleus in mice. *Toxicology* 186:151–157, 2003.

Pelletier L., Druet P: Immunotoxicology of metals, in Goyer RA, Cherian MG (eds.): *Handbook of Experimental Pharmacology,* vol. 115. Heidelberg, Germany: Springer-Verlag, 1995, pp. 77–92.

Perafan-Riveros C, Franca LF, Alves AC, *et al.*: Acrodermatitis enteropathica: case report and review of the literature. *Pediatr Dermatol* 19:426–431, 2002.

Peter AL, Viraraghavan T: Thallium: a review of public health and environmental concerns. *Environ Int* 31:493–501, 2005.

Pi J, He Y, Bortner C, *et al*: Low level, long-term inorganic arsenite exposure causes generalized resistance to apoptosis in cultured human keratinocytes: potential role in skin co-carcinogenesis. *Int J Cancer* 116:20–26, 2005.

Pizarro F, Olivares M, Gidi V, Araya M: The gastrointestinal tract and acute effects of copper in drinking water and beverages. *Rev Environ Health* 14:231–238, 1999.

Plato CC, Garruto RM, Galasko D, *et al*: Amyotrophic lateral sclerosis and parkinsonism-dementia complex of Guam: changing incidence rates during the past 60 years. *Am J Epidemiol* 157:149–157, 2003.

Pounds JG, Long GJ, Rosen JF: Cellular and molecular toxicity of lead in bone. *Environ Health Perspect* 91:17–32, 1991.

Prasad AS, Kucuk O: Zinc in cancer prevention. *Cancer Metastasis Rev* 21:291–295, 2002.

Prasad AS: Zinc deficiency: Its characterization and treatment. *Met Ions Biol Syst* 41:103–137, 2004.

Proctor DM, Fredrick MM, Scott PK, *et al.*: The prevalence of chromium allergy in the United States and its implications for setting soil cleanup: A cost-effectiveness case study. *Regul Toxicol Pharmacol* 28:27–37, 1998.

Prozialeck WC, Wellington DR, Lamar PC: Comparison of the cytotoxic effects of cadmium chloride and cadmium-metallothionein in LLC-PK1 cells. *Life Sci* 53:PL337–PL342, 1993.

Qu W, Diwan BA, Liu J, *et al.*: The metallothionein-null phenotype is associated with heightened sensitivity to lead toxicity and an inability to form inclusion bodies. *Am J Pathol* 160:1047–1056, 2002.

Quiroz JA, Gould TD, Manji HK: Molecular effects of lithium. *Mol Interv* 4:259–272, 2004.

Rahman MM, Chowdhury UK, Mukherjee SC, *et al*: Chronic arsenic toxicity in Bangladesh and West Bengal, India—A review and commentary. *J Toxicol Clin Toxicol* 39:683–700, 2001.

Ravindra K, Bencs L, Van Grieken R: Platinum group elements in the environment and their health risk. *Sci Total Environ* 318:1–43, 2004.

Risher JF, Murray HE, Prince GR: Organic mercury compounds: Human exposure and its relevance to public health. *Toxicol Ind Health* 18:109–160, 2002.

Risher JF, Amler SN: Mercury exposure: evaluation and intervention the inappropriate use of chelating agents in the diagnosis and treatment of putative mercury poisoning. *Neurotoxicology* 26:691–699, 2005.

Rohl C, Sievers J: Microglia is activated by astrocytes in trimethyltin intoxication. *Toxicol Appl Pharmacol* 204:36–45, 2005.

Rosen BP: Transport and detoxification systems for transition metals, heavy metals and metalloids in eukaryotic and prokaryotic microbes. *Comp Biochem Physiol A Mol Integr Physiol* 133:689–693, 2002.

Rossman TG: Mechanism of arsenic carcinogenesis: An integrated approach. *Mutat Res* 533:37–65, 2003.

Rossman TG, Uddin AN, Burns FJ, *et al.*: Arsenite is a cocarcinogen with solar ultraviolet radiation for mouse skin: An animal model for arsenic carcinogenesis. *Toxicol Appl Pharmacol* 176:64–71, 2001.

Roth JA, Garrick MD: Iron interactions and other biological reactions mediating the physiological and toxic actions of manganese. *Biochem Pharmacol* 66:1–13, 2003.

Rudel H: Case study: Bioavailability of tin and tin compounds. *Ecotoxicol Environ Saf* 56:180–189, 2003.

Rungby J: An experimental study on silver in the nervous system and on aspects of its general cellular toxicity. *Dan Med Bull* 37:442–449, 1990.

Ryan-Harshman M, Aldoori W: The relevance of selenium to immunity, cancer, and infectious/inflammatory diseases. *Can J Diet Pract Res* 66:98–102, 2005.

Ryu DY, Lee S-J, Park DW, Choi B-S, Klaassen CD, Park J-D: Dietary iron regulates intestinal cadmium absorption thorugh iron transporters in rats. *Toxicol Lett* 152: 19–25, 2004.

Sabbioni E, Pozzi G, Devos S, *et al.*: The intensity of vanadium(V)-induced cytotoxicity and morphological transformation in BALB/3T3 cells is dependent on glutathione-mediated bioreduction to vanadium(IV). *Carcinogenesis* 14:2565–2568, 1993.

Sahmoun AE, Case LD, Jackson SA, *et al.*: Cadmium and prostate cancer: A critical epidemiologic analysis. *Cancer Invest* 23:256–263, 2005.

Satarug S, Moore MR: Adverse health effects of chronic exposure to low-level cadmium in foodstuffs and cigarette smoke. *Environ Health Perspect* 112:1099–1103, 2004.

Schnaas L, Rothenberg SJ, Flores M-F, *et al*: Reduced intellectual development I children with prenatal lead exposure. *Environ Health Perspect* 114:791–797, 2006.

Schwarz G: Molybdenum cofactor biosynthesis and deficiency. *Cell Mol Life Sci* 62:2792–2810, 2005

Schwartz GG, Reis IM: Is cadmium a cause of human pancreatic cancer? *Cancer Epidemiol Biomarkers Prev* 9:139–145, 2000.

Sedman RM, Beaumont J, McDonald TA, *et al.*: Review of the evidence regarding the carcinogenicity of hexavalent chromium in drinking water. *J Environ Sci Health C Environ Carcinog Ecotoxicol Rev* 24:155–182, 2006.

Seghizzi P, D'Adda F, Borleri, *et al.*: Cobalt myocardiopathy. A critical review of literature. *Sci Total Environ* 150:105–109, 1994.

Selverstone Valentine J, Doucette PA, Zittin Potter S: Copper-zinc superoxide dismutase and amyotrophic lateral sclerosis. *Annu Rev Biochem* 74:563–593, 2005.

Sheppard SC, Sheppard MI, Gallerand MO, *et al.*: Derivation of ecotoxicity thresholds for uranium. *J Environ Radioact* 79:55–83, 2005.

Shils ME: Magnesium, in Ziegler EE, Filer LJ (eds.): *Present Knowledge in Nutrition*. Washington, DC: ILSI, 1996, pp 256–264.

Shim H, Harris ZL: Genetic defects in copper metabolism. *J Nutr* 133(5 Suppl 1):1527S–1531S, 2003.

Shinogi M, Maeizumi S: Effect of preinduction of metallothionein on tissue distribution of silver and hepatic lipid peroxidation. *Biol Pharm Bull* 16:372–374, 1993.

Silbergeld EK, Schwartz J, Mahaffey K: Lead and osteoporosis: Mobilization of lead from bone in postmenopausal women. *Environ Res* 47:79–94, 1988.

Silbergeld EK, Waalkes M, Rice JM: Lead as a carcinogen: Experimental evidence and mechanisms of action. *Am J Ind Med* 38:316–323, 2000.

Silbergeld EK: Facilitative mechanisms of lead as a carcinogen. *Mutat Res* 533:121–133, 2003.

Sivulka DJ: Assessment of respiratory carcinogenicity associated with exposure to metallic nickel: A review. *Regul Toxicol Pharmacol* 43:117–133, 2005.

Slikkerveer A, de Wolff FA: Toxicity of bismuth and its compounds, in Chang LW, Magos L, Suzuki T (eds.): *Toxicology of Metals* 1996. New York: CRC Press, pp. 439–454.

Smith AH, Marshall G, Yuan Y, *et al.*: Increased mortality from lung cancer and bronchiectasis in young adults after exposure to arsenic in utero and in early childhood. *Environ Health Perspect* 114:1293–1296, 2006.

Soignet SL, Frankel SR, Douer D, *et al.*: United States multicenter study of arsenic trioxide in relapsed acute promyelocytic leukemia. *J Clin Oncol* 19:3852–3860, 2001.

Soni MG, White SM, Flamm WG, *et al.*: Safety evaluation of dietary aluminum. *Regul Toxicol Pharmacol* 33:66–79, 2001.

Sparling DW, Lowe TP: Environmental hazards of aluminum to plants, invertebrates, fish, and wildlife. *Rev Environ Contam Toxicol* 145:1–127, 1996.

Sparsa A, Bonnetblanc JM: [Lithium] *Ann Dermatol Venereol* 131:255–261, 2004.

Squibb KS, Leggett RW, McDiarmid MA: Prediction of renal concentrations of depleted uranium and radiation dose in Gulf War veterans with embedded shrapnel. *Health Physics* 89: 267–273, 2005.

Staessen JA, Buchet JP, Ginucchio G, *et al.*: Public health implications of environmental exposure to cadmium and lead: An overview of epidemiological studies in Belgium. Working Groups. *J Cardiovasc Risk* 3:26–41, 1996.

Steenland K, Boffetta P: Lead and cancer in humans: Where are we now? *Am J Ind Med* 38:295–299, 2000.

Stoltenberg M, Juhl S, Poulsen EH: Autometallographic detection of silver in hypothalamic neurons of rats exposed to silver nitrate. *J Appl Toxicol* 14:275–280, 1994.

Sudre P, Mathieu F: Kashin-Beck disease: From etiology to prevention or from prevention to etiology? *Int Orthop* 25:175–179, 2001.

Sunderman FW Jr, Morgan LG, Andersen A, *et al.*: Histopathology of sinonasal and lung cancers in nickel refinery workers. *Ann Clin Lab Sci* 19:44–50, 1989.

Takeuchi A, Yoshizawa N, Oshima S, *et al.*: Nephrotoxicity of germanium compounds: Report of a case and review of the literature. *Nephron* 60:436–442, 1992.

Takeuchi T: Neuropathology of Minamata disease in Kumamoto: Especially at the chronic stage, in Roisin L, Shiaki H, Greevic N (eds.): *Neurotoxicology*. New York: Raven Press, 1977, pp 235–246.

Tanaka A, Hisanaga A, Hirata M, *et al.*: Chronic toxicity of indium arsenide and indium phosphide to the lungs of hamsters. *Fukuoka Igaku Zasshi* 87:108–15, 1996.

Tanaka A: Toxicity of indium arsenide, gallium arsenide, and aluminium gallium arsenide. *Toxicol Appl Pharmacol* 198:405–411, 2004.

Tao SH, Bolger PM: Hazard assessment of germanium supplements. *Regul Toxicol Pharmacol* 25:211–219, 1997.

Tapiero H, Townsend DM, Tew KD: The antioxidant role of selenium and seleno-compounds. *Biomed Pharmacother* 57:134–144, 2003.

Taylor A: Biochemistry of tellurium. *Biol Trace Elem Res* 55:231–239, 1996.

Thomas DJ, Styblo M, Lin S: The cellular metabolism and systemic toxicity of arsenic. *Toxicol Appl Pharmacol* 176:127–144, 2001.

Thomas DJ, Li J, Waters SB, *et al.*: Arsenic (+3 oxidation state) methyltransferase and the methylation of arsenicals. *Exp Biol Med* 232: 3–13, 2007.

Thompson DF, Callen ED: Soluble or insoluble prussian blue for radiocesium and thallium poisoning? *Ann Pharmacother* 38:1509–1514, 2004.

Thun MJ, Baker DB, Steenland K, *et al.*: Renal toxicity in uranium mill workers. *Scand J Work Environ Health* 11:83–90, 1985.

Tinggi U: Essentiality and toxicity of selenium and its status in Australia: A review. *Toxicol Lett* 137:103–110, 2003.

Tjalve J, Henriksson H: Uptake of metals in the brain via olfactory pathways. *Neurotoxicology* 20:181–195, 1999.

Tiekink ER: Antimony and bismuth compounds in oncology. *Crit Rev Oncol Hematol* 42:217–224, 2002.

Tillman LA, Drake FM, Dixon JS, *et al.*: Review article: Safety of bismuth in the treatment of gastrointestinal diseases. *Aliment Pharmacol Ther* 10:459–467, 1996.

Timmer RT, Sands JM: Lithium intoxication. *J Am Soc Nephrol* 10:666–674, 1999.

Tinkle SS, Antonini JM, Rich BA: Skin as a route of exposure and sensitization in chronic beryllium disease. *Environ Health Perspect* 111:1202–1208, 2003.

Tjalve H, Henriksson J: Uptake of metals in the brain via olfactory pathways. *Neurotoxicology* 20:181–195, 1999.

Ueshima K: Magnesium and ischemic heart disease: a review of epidemiological, experimental, and clinical evidences. *Magnes Res* 18:275–284, 2005.

Ungvary G, Szakmary E, Tatrai E, *et al.*: Embryotoxic and teratogenic effects of indium chloride in rats and rabbits. *J Toxicol Environ Health A.* 59:27–42, 2000.

Valko M, Morris H, Cronin MT: Metals, toxicity and oxidative stress. *Curr Med Chem* 12:1161–1208, 2005.

Valko M, Rhodes CJ, Moncol J, *et al.*: Free radicals, metals and antioxidants in oxidative stress-induced cancer. *Chem Biol Interact* 160:1–40, 2006.

Van Landeghem GF, de Broe ME, D'Haese PC: Al and Si: their speciation, distribution, and toxicity. *Clin Biochem* 31:385–397, 1998.

Vaziri ND, Sica DA: Lead-induced hypertension: role of oxidative stress. *Curr Hypertens Rep* 6:314–320, 2004.

Victery W: Evidence for effects of chronic lead exposure on blood pressure in experimental animals: An overview. *Environ Health Perspect* 78:71–76, 1988.

Vincent JB: Recent developments in the biochemistry of chromium(III). *Biol Trace Elem Res* 99:1–16, 2004.

Viol GW, Minielly JA, Bistricki T: Gold nephropathy: Tissue analysis by X-ray fluorescent spectroscopy. *Arch Pathol Lab Med* 101:635–640, 1977.

von Lindren IH, Spalinger SM, Bero BN, *et al.*: The influence of soil remediation on lead in house dust. *Sci Total Environ* 303:59–78, 2003.

Vouk VB: General chemistry of metals, in Friberg L, Nordberg GF, Vouk VB (eds.): *Handbook of The Toxicology of Metals*. New York: Elsevier, 1986a, pp. 14–35.

Vouk VB: Germanium, in Friberg L, Nordberg GF, Vouk VB (eds.): *Handbook of The Toxicology of Metals*. New York: Elsevier, 1986b, pp. 255–266.

Vyskocil A, Viau C: Assessment of molybdenum toxicity in humans. *J Appl Toxicol* 19:185–192, 1999.

Waalkes MP, Diwan BA, Ward JM, *et al.*: Renal tubular tumors and atypical hyperplasias in B6C3F1 mice exposed to lead acetate during gestation and lactation occur with minimal chronic nephropathy. *Cancer Res* 55:5265–5271, 1995.

Waalkes MP, Fox DA, States JC, *et al.*: Metals and disorders of cell accumulation: Modulation of apoptosis and cell proliferation. *Toxicol Sci* 56:255–261, 2000.

Waalkes M: Cadmium carcinogenesis. *Mutat Res* 533:107–120, 2003.

Waalkes MP, Ward JM, Liu J: Transplacental carcinogenicity of inorganic arsenic in the drinking water: Induction of hepatic, ovarian, pulmonary, and adrenal tumors in mice. *Toxicol Appl Pharmacol* 186:7–17, 2003.

Waalkes MP, Ward JM, Diwan BA: Induction of tumors of the liver, lung, ovary and adrenal in adult mice after brief maternal gestational exposure to inorganic arsenic: Promotional effects of postnatal phorbol ester exposure on hepatic and pulmonary, but not dermal cancers. *Carcinogenesis* 25:133–141, 2004a.

Waalkes MP, Liu J, Chen H, *et al.*: Estrogen signaling in livers of male mice with hepatocellular carcinoma induced by exposure to arsenic in utero. *J Natl Cancer Inst* 96:466–474, 2004b.

Waalkes MP, Liu J, Goyer RA, Diwan BA: Metallothionein-I/II double knockout mice are hypersensitive to lead-induced kidney carcinogenesis: Role of inclusion body formation. *Cancer Res.* 64:7766–7772, 2004c.

Waalkes MP, Liu J, Ward JM, Urogenital carcinogenesis in female CD1 mice induced by in utero arsenic exposure is exacerbated by postnatal diethylstilbestrol treatment. *Cancer Res* 66:1337–1345, 2006a.

Waalkes MP, Liu J, Ward JM, Enhanced urinary bladder and liver carcinogenesis in male CD1 mice exposed to transplacental inorganic arsenic and postnatal diethylstilbestrol or tamoxifen. *Toxicol Appl Pharmacol.* 215:295–305, 2006b.

Waalkes MP, Liu J, Kasprzak KS, *et al.*: Hypersusceptibility to cisplatin carcinogenicity in metallothionein-I/II double knockout mice: Production of hepatocellular carcinoma at clinically relevant doses. *Int J Cancer* 119:28–32, 2006c.

Wang C, Bhattacharyya MH: Effect of cadmium on bone calcium and 45Ca in nonpregnant mice on a calcium-deficient diet: Evidence of direct effect of cadmium on bone. *Toxicol Appl Pharmacol* 120:228–239, 1993.

Warheit DB, Brock WJ, Lee KP, *et al.*: Comparative pulmonary toxicity inhalation and instillation studies with different TiO2 particle formulations: Impact of surface treatments on particle toxicity. *Toxicol Sci* 88:514–524, 2005.

Warheit DB, Webb TR, Sayes CM, *et al.*: Pulmonary instillation studies with nanoscale TiO2 rods and dots in rats: Toxicity is not dependent upon particle size and surface area. *Toxicol Sci* 91:227–236, 2006.

Wei M, Wanibuchi H, Morimura K, *et al.*: Carcinogenicity of dimethylarsinic acid in male F344 rats and genetic alterations in induced urinary bladder tumors. *Carcinogenesis* 23:1387–1397, 2002.

Westervelt P, Brown RA, Adkins DR, *et al.*: Sudden death among patients with acute promyelocytic leukemia treated with arsenic trioxide. *Blood* 98:266–271, 2001.

WHO: IPCS Environmental Health Creteria. *Aluminum*, vol. 194. Geneva: World Health Organization, 1997, pp. 1–282.

WHO: IPCS Environmental Health Creteria. *Beryllium*, vol. 106. Geneva: World Health Organization, 1990, pp. 1–210.

WHO: IPCS Environmental Health Creteria. *Cadmium*, vol. 134. Geneva: World Health Organization, 1990, pp. 1–220.

WHO: IPCS Environmental Criteria. *Copper*, vol. 200. Geneva: World Health Organization, 1998, pp. 1–360.

WHO: IPCS Environmental Health Creteria. *Platinum*, vol. 125. Geneva: World Health Organization, 1991, pp. 1–167.

WHO: IPCS Environmental Health Creteria. *Palladium*, vol. 226. Geneva: World Health Organization, 2002, pp. 1–201.

WHO: IPCS Environmental Health Criteria. *Selenium*, vol. 58. Geneva: World Health Organization, 1987, pp. 1–238.

WHO: IPCS Environmental Health Criteria. *Thallium*, vol. 182. Geneva: World Health Organization, 1996.

WHO: IPCS Environmental Health Criteria. *Tin and Organotin Compounds: A Preliminary Review*, vol. 15. Geneva: World Health Organization, 1980.

WHO: IPCS Environmental Health Criteria. *Zinc*, vol. 221. Geneva: World Health Organization, 1998, pp. 1–360.

Winship KA: Toxicity of antimony and its compounds. *Adverse Drug React Acute Poisoning Rev* 6:67–90, 1987.

Winship KA: Toxicity of tin and its compounds. *Adverse Drug React Acute Poisoning Rev* 7:19–38, 1988.

Xiao T, Guha J, Boyle D, *et al.*: Environmental concerns related to high thallium levels in soils and thallium uptake by plants in southwest Guizhou, China. *Sci Total Environ* 318:223–244, 2004.

Yip R, Dallman PR: Iron, in Ziegler EE, Filer LJ (eds.): *Present Knowledge in Nutrition.* Washington, DC: ILSI, 1996, pp. 277–292.

Yu HS, Lee CH, Chen GS: Peripheral vascular diseases resulting from chronic arsenical poisoning. *J Dermatol* 29:123–130, 2002.

Yu S, Beynen AC: High tin intake reduces copper status in rats through inhibition of copper absorption. *Br J Nutr* 73:863–869, 1995.

Yuan XM, Li W: The iron hypothesis of atherosclerosis and its clinical impact. *Ann Med* 35:578–591, 2003.

Zalpus RK, Koropatnick J: *Molecular Biology and Toxicology of Metals.* New York: Taylor & Francis, 2000.

Zalpus RK, Ahmad S: Molecular handling of cadmium in transporting epithelia. *Toxicol Appl Pharmacol* 186:163–188, 2003.

Zheng W: Toxicology of choroid plexus: Special reference to metal-induced neurotoxicities. *Microsc Res Tech* 52:89–103, 2001.

Zheng W, Winter SM, Kattnig MJ, *et al.*: Tissue distribution and elimination of indium in male Fischer 344 rats following oral and intratracheal administration of indium phosphide. *J Toxicol Environ Health* 43:483–494, 1994.

Ziegler EE, Edwards BB, Jensen RL, *et al.*: Absorption and retention of lead by infants. *Pediatr Res* 12:29–34, 1978.

Ziegler EE, Filer LJ (eds.): *Present Knowledge in Nutrition.* Washington, DC: ILSI, 1996, pp. 1–684.

Zhitkovich A: Importance of chromium-DNA adducts in mutagenicity and toxicity of chromium(VI). *Chem Res Toxicol* 18:3–11, 2005.

CHAPTER 24

TOXIC EFFECTS OF SOLVENTS AND VAPORS

James V. Bruckner, S. Satheesh Anand, and D. Alan Warren

INTRODUCTION

The term *solvent* refers to a class of liquid organic chemicals of variable lipophilicity and volatility. These properties, coupled with small molecular size and lack of charge, make inhalation the major route of solvent exposure and provide for ready absorption across the lung, gastrointestinal (GI) tract, and skin. In general, the lipophilicity of solvents increases with increasing numbers of carbon and/or halogen atoms, while volatility decreases. Organic solvents are frequently used to dissolve, dilute, or disperse materials that are insoluble in water. As such they are widely employed as degreasers and as constituents of paints, varnishes, lacquers, inks, aerosol spray products, dyes, and adhesives. Other uses are as intermediates in

chemical synthesis, and as fuels and fuel additives. Most organic solvents are refined from petroleum. Many such as naphthas and gasoline are complex mixtures, often consisting of hundreds of compounds. Early in the twentieth century, there were perhaps a dozen or so known and commonly used solvents. By 1981, this number had climbed to approximately 350 (OSHA, 2006).

Solvents are classified largely according to molecular structure or functional group. Classes of solvents include aliphatic hydrocarbons, many of which are chlorinated (i.e., halocarbons); aromatic hydrocarbons; alcohols; ethers; esters/acetates; amides/amines; aldehydes; ketones; and complex mixtures that defy classification. The main determinants of a solvent's inherent toxicity are: (1) its number of carbon atoms; (2) whether it is saturated or has double

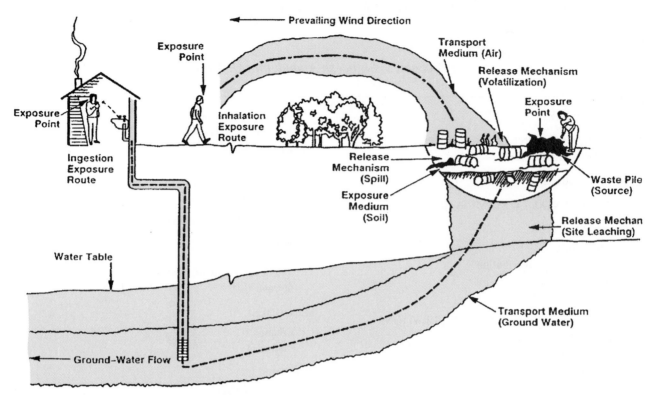

Figure 24-1. Solvent exposure pathways and media.

Adapted from EPA Risk Assessment Guidance for Superfund. *Human Health Evaluation Manual Part A, Interim Final*. Washington, DC: Office of Emergency and Remedial Response, 1989.

or triple bonds between adjacent carbon atoms; (3) its configuration (i.e., straight chain, branched chain, or cyclic); and (4) the presence of functional groups. Some class-wide generalizations regarding toxicity can be made. For example, the more lipophilic a hydrocarbon, the more potent a central nervous system (CNS) depressant it is; amides/amines tend to be potent sensitizers; aldehydes are particularly irritating; hydrocarbons that are extensively metabolized tend to be more cytotoxic/mutagenic; and many unsaturated, short-chain halocarbons are animal carcinogens. The toxicity of solvents within the same class can vary dramatically. For example, 1,1,1-trichloroethane (TRI) and 1,1,2-trichloroethylene (TCE) are both halocarbons with three chlorine atoms, yet the unsaturated TCE is carcinogenic in the rat and mouse, but TRI is not. Similar results have been reported for 2,4- and 2,6-diaminotoluene in rodents, as only the 2,4 isomer is capable of inducing significant hepatocyte proliferation and liver tumors. Slight structural differences in solvent metabolites are also of toxicological consequence. The peripheral neuropathy induced by *n*-hexane and 2-hexanone is dependent on the production of the γ-diketone metabolite, 2,5-hexanedione. Diketones lacking the gamma structure are not neurotoxic. Thus, subtle differences in chemical structure can translate into dramatic differences in toxicity.

Nearly everyone is exposed to solvents in the conduct of their normal activities. Consider, for example, a person who works in an aircraft factory as a metal degreaser (TCE exposure); drives to the neighborhood bar after work and has a few drinks (ethanol exposure) and cigarettes (benzene and styrene exposure); stops on the way home at a self-service filling station for gasoline (benzene, toluene, 1,3-butadiene exposure) and the dry cleaner's for laundry [tetrachloroethylene (PERC) exposure]; and after dinner enjoys his

hobby of model shipbuilding that requires the use of glue (toluene exposure). While everyone may not identify with the above scenario, detailed surveys of indoor and outdoor air, such as the EPA's Total Exposure Assessment Methodology (TEAM) and National Human Exposure Assessment Survey (NHEXAS) studies, indicate that airborne solvent exposure is unavoidable (Wallace, 1990; Clayton *et al.*, 1999). Drinking water is also a common source of solvent exposure due to discharge of solvents into surface and groundwaters and the presence of disinfection by-products, including the animal carcinogen chloroform ($CHCl_3$). Trichloroacetic acid (TCA), and dichloroacetic acid (DCA), metabolites of TCE and PERC, are also common disinfection by products.

Environmental exposures to solvents in air and groundwater are frequent subjects of toxic tort litigation, despite concentrations that are typically in the low parts per billion (ppb) range. Multiple exposure pathways frequently exist (Fig. 24-1). Although not represented in Fig. 24-1, household use of solvent-contaminated water may result in solvent intake from inhalation and dermal absorption as well as ingestion (Weisel and Jo, 1996; Nuckols *et al.*, 2005). In many cases, environmental risk assessments require that risks be determined for physiologically diverse individuals who are exposed to several solvents by multiple exposure pathways. As an aid to the risk assessment process, the U.S. EPA has derived toxicity factors for many of the most toxic solvents. These toxicity factors are referred to as reference concentrations (RfCs), reference doses (RfDs), and cancer slope factors (CSFs). Values for a number of these are available from the EPA's online Integrated Risk Information System (IRIS). Additional sources of exposure guidelines for noncancer end points are found in the *Toxicologic Profiles* of the U.S. Agency for Toxic Substances and Disease Registry (ATSDR).

These profiles often contain minimal risk levels that are derived in a similar manner to EPA's RfCs and RfDs, but are frequently based on different critical studies or derived with different uncertainty factors.

Occupational solvent exposures involve situations ranging from a secretary using typewriter correction fluid to the loading and off-loading of tanker trucks with thousands of gallons of gasoline. The greatest industrial use of solvents is as metal degreasers. This work environment is typically where the highest exposures occur, mainly via inhalation and secondarily via dermal contact. An estimated 10 million people are potentially exposed to organic solvents in the workplace (OSHA, 2006). Many of the most severe exposures to solvents have occurred as a result of their use in confined spaces with inadequate ventilation. While the U.S. Occupational Safety and Health Administration (OSHA) has established legally enforceable permissible exposure limits (PELs) for over 100 solvents, most PELs are outdated. The majority of existing PELs were adopted from the list of threshold limit values (TLVs) published some years ago by the American Conference of Governmental Industrial Hygienists (ACGIH). Many current TLVs are more stringent than the PELs but do not carry the weight of law. Whereas the ACGIH's TLVs for an 8-hour workday, 40-hour workweek are designed to be protective for a working lifetime, its short-term exposure limits (STELs) and ceiling values are designed to protect against the acute effects of high-level, short-term solvent exposure. If warranted, ACGIH will assign a skin notation to a solvent, indicating that a significant contribution to overall exposure is possible by the dermal route, either by contact with vapors or direct skin contact with the liquid. Biological monitoring in the workplace should find increasing use as technologic advances are made, because it often provides a better measure of exposure than classic industrial hygiene monitoring. The ACGIH has published over 50 Biological Exposure Indices (BEIs), on which bases the safety of internal measures of exposure can be judged (ACGIH, 2006).

Most solvent exposures involve a mixture of chemicals, rather than a single compound. Our knowledge of the toxicity of solvent mixtures is rudimentary relative to the toxicology of individual solvents. While the assumption is frequently made that the toxic effects of multiple solvents are additive, solvents may also interact synergistically or antagonistically. For example, repetitive alcohol consumption induces certain cytochrome P450s (CYPs), and may therefore enhance the metabolic activation of other solvents to cytotoxic metabolites. Ethanol intake near the time of exposure to such solvents, in contrast, may competitively inhibit their metabolism and be protective. Another well-characterized example of solvent antagonism is the competitive metabolic interaction between benzene and toluene (Medinsky et al., 1994). Coexposure to these chemicals results in diminished benzene metabolism, genotoxicity, and erythropoietic toxicity relative to that which follows benzene exposure alone. It is now recognized that significant data gaps exist in the area of mixtures toxicology, and that these can be significant sources of uncertainty in risk assessments. Physiologically based toxicokinetic (PBTK) models are being developed by different research groups to predict the impact of metabolic induction and inhibition on the kinetics of individual components of specific mixtures (Barton et al., 1995; Haddad et al., 2000; Dobrev et al., 2001).

Although some solvents are less hazardous than others, virtually all can cause adverse effects. Provided that the dose or concentration is sufficient, most have the potential to induce some level of narcosis and cause respiratory and mucous membrane irritation. A number of solvents are animal carcinogens, but only a handful have been classified as known human carcinogens. Herein lies a major challenge for toxicology—determining the human relevance of tumors observed in chronic, high-dose rodent studies. As with other chemicals, whether adverse health effects occur from solvent exposure is dependent on several factors: (1) toxicity of the solvent; (2) exposure route; (3) amount or rate of exposure; (4) duration of exposure; (5) individual susceptibility; and (6) interactions with other chemicals. Adverse health effects may occur acutely and be readily discernible, or they may be the result of chronic exposure and have insidious onset. Numerous epidemiologic studies of environmentally- and occupationally-exposed populations have been conducted for some solvents, but most human risk assessments remain heavily reliant upon extrapolation from high-dose animal studies. One must bear in mind that the toxic effects and their underlying mechanisms discussed herein may be operative only in certain animal species or strains and under certain exposure conditions. Care must therefore be taken in generalizing beyond the experimental conditions under which data are collected. While a relatively small number of commercially available solvents is discussed in this chapter, those selected for discussion are thought to best demonstrate principles of solvent toxicology, are of particular commercial importance, and/or are currently garnering significant attention from the toxicological and regulatory communities. A book chapter that examines solvents from an organ systems standpoint, in contrast to the discussion of individual solvents herein, is that of Gerr and Letz (1998).

IS THERE A SOLVENT-INDUCED CHRONIC ENCEPHALOPATHY?

The CNS-depressant effects of acute, high-level exposures and the potential for permanent neurologic damage in chronic solvent abusers are not a matter of debate. It is also clear that chronic, moderate-to-high-level exposure to a few solvents such as n-hexane and carbon disulfide can cause specific degenerative changes in the CNS or the peripheral nervous system (PNS). Far less clear is whether chronic, low-level exposure to virtually any solvent or solvent mixture can produce a pattern of neurologic dysfunction referred to as painters' syndrome, organic solvent syndrome, psychoorganic syndrome, and chronic solvent encephalopathy (CSE). CSE is characterized by nonspecific symptoms (e.g., headache, fatigue, mood disturbances, and sleep disorders) with or without changes in neuropsychological function. There is a reversible form of CSE referred to as neuroasthenic syndrome that consists of symptoms only, and both "mild" and "severe" forms accompanied by objective signs of neuropsychological dysfunction that may or may not be fully reversible. This syndrome was first described in the Scandinavian occupational literature in the late 1970s in solvent-exposed painters (Axelson et al., 1976; Arlien-Soborg et al., 1979). Since that time, numerous studies from Scandinavia have been published purporting that solvents as a class have chronic neurotoxic properties. These countries, as well as few others in Europe (i.e., Germany, Austria, and Belgium) have passed legislation recognizing CSE as a compensable occupational disability (Triebig and Hallermann, 2001). Scientists outside of Scandinavia, including many in the United States, have generally been less willing to recognize CSE as a legitimate disease state and have published studies to the contrary (Triebig et al., 1988; Bleecker et al., 1991; Spurgeon et al., 1994).

In response to the numerous reports of CSE, two conferences were convened in 1985. The first was held in Copenhagen by the Nordic Council of the World Health Organization (WHO, 1985).

Table 24-1

Proposed Categories of Solvent-Induced Encephalopathy

CATEGORY	CLINICAL MANIFESTATIONS
Type 1	*Symptoms only*: The patient complains of nonspecific symptoms such as fatigability, memory impairment, difficulty in concentration, and loss of initiative. These symptoms are reversible if exposure is discontinued, and there is no objective evidence of neuropsychiatric dysfunction.
Type 2A	*Sustained personality or mood change*: There is a marked and sustained change in personality involving fatigue, emotional lability, impulse control, and general mood and motivation.
Type 2B	*Impairment in intellectual function*: There is difficulty in concentration, impairment of memory, and a decrease in learning capacity. These symptoms are accompanied by objective evidence of impairment. There may also be minor neurologic signs. The complete reversibility of type 2B is questionable.
Type 3	*Dementia*: In this condition, marked global deterioration in intellect and memory is often accompanied by neurologic signs and/or neuroradiologic findings. This condition is, at best, poorly reversible, but is generally nonprogressive once exposure has ceased.

SOURCE: Reproduced from Cranmer (1986), with permission from Elsevier.

The second, in Raleigh, NC, was attended by an international group of scientists from academia, industry, and government (Cranmer, 1986). The categorization scheme that resulted from the Raleigh meeting is presented in Table 24-1. The WHO scheme is similar. Among those who utilize the categorization scheme, it is generally believed that the most severe CSE category, type 3, results from repeated, severe intoxications like those experienced by solvent abusers. CSE types 1 and 2, on the other hand, are thought to be associated with prolonged, low-to-moderate-level exposure common to work environments. A major criticism of the categorization scheme is the lack of consideration of inhaled solvent concentration and exposure duration. While no consensus exists, even most CSE proponents believe that solvent exposure must occur for some 10 years before clinical symptoms are manifest. Citing growing acceptance of CSE outside of Scandinavia, some scientists and physicians advocate for refinement of existing diagnostic criteria and a unified categorization scheme (van der Hoek *et al.*, 2000, 2001).

Table 24-2

Functions that May Be Assessed in a Neuropsychological Evaluation

Psychomotor functions
   Reaction time
   Motor speed and dexterity
   Eye-hand coordination
Sustained attention/concentration and perceptual speed
Verbal and nonverbal memory
   Immediate memory
   Delayed memory
Learning
Visual constructive ability
Conceptual ability
Evaluation of personality and affect

SOURCE: Reproduced from Cranmer (1986), with permission from Elsevier.

CSE researchers typically rely upon self-reported symptoms and a clinical neuropsychological evaluation (Table 24-2), and to a much lesser extent on diagnostic tests such as electroencephalography and computerized brain tomography. It has been argued that the neuropsychological tests are of questionable validity, sensitivity, specificity, and predictive value. It has also been noted that many investigations of CSE are fraught with methodologic flaws. For example, CSE investigators frequently fail to measure premorbid function or intellect; employ a reference population; control adequately for the potential confounders of age, alcohol use, other CNS diseases, and other chemicals; corroborate functional deficits with objective evidence of brain disease; and/or examine exposure–response relationships. The importance of doing so is best exemplified by the reanalysis of individuals originally reported in the seminal study by Arlien-Soborg *et al.* (1979) to have "painters' syndrome." When the influences of age, education, and intelligence were considered, the previously reported reduction in neuropsychological test scores disappeared (Gade *et al.*, 1988). Another example is that of Cherry *et al.* (1985), who demonstrated the importance of matching solvent-exposed and control groups for preexposure intellect before making a diagnosis of CSE. More recently, Albers *et al.* (2000) reportedly found no objective evidence of toxic encephalopathy among 52 railroad workers with long-term solvent exposure and diagnosis of CSE.

It is evident that resolution of the controversial issue of CSE will come only through the conduct of well-designed and controlled epidemiological studies, especially considering the absence of an appropriate animal model. Brief, but insightful reviews of CSE by Rosenberg (1995) and Schaumburg and Spencer (2000) have been published. These reviews conclude that the current literature, including the "landmark" North American study of 187 paint-manufacturing workers (Bleecker *et al.*, 1991), does not support chronic low-level solvent exposure as a cause of *symptomatic* CNS or PNS dysfunction. This does not preclude, however, the possibility that such exposure can be associated with *subclinical* cognitive dysfunction in the form of slight psychomotor and attentional deficit disorders. For the viewpoint of CSE proponents, readers are directed to texts by Arlien-Soborg (1992) and Kilburn (1998).

SOLVENT ABUSE

Inhalants are volatile substances that can be inhaled to induce a psychoactive or mind-altering effect. Their abuse has become a major drug problem worldwide, particularly in disadvantaged populations and among adolescents (Dinwiddie, 1994; Marelich, 1997). The epidemiology of inhalant abuse in the United States is receiving considerable attention (Spiller, 2004; Wu *et al.*, 2004), with almost one in five 8th graders claiming to have used inhalants according to the most recent National Institute on Drug Abuse (NIDA)-sponsored survey (Johnston *et al.*, 2006). Solvents are among the most popular classes of drugs of abuse, given their presence in a multitude of inexpensive, readily available products that are legal to buy and possess. These products are used for common household and industrial purposes and include paint thinners and removers, dry-cleaning fluids, degreasers, gasoline, glues, typewriter fluid, nail polish remover, felt-tip marker fluids, and aerosols such as fabric protector sprays and spray paints. Solvents are often among the first drugs used by children and adolescents. Early use of inhalants is often a precursor to abuse of multiple illegal substances (Wu *et al.*, 2004). Research suggests that adverse socioeconomic conditions, a history of child abuse, poor grades, and dropping out of school are all factors contributing to inhalant abuse (NIDA, 2005).

Solvent abuse is a unique exposure situation in that participants repeatedly subject themselves to vapor concentrations high enough to produce effects that resemble alcohol intoxication. Solvents can be breathed in through the nose or the mouth by "sniffing" or "snorting" vapors from containers; spraying aerosols directly into the nose or mouth; "bagging" by inhaling vapors from substances sprayed or deposited inside a plastic or paper bag; or "huffing" from a solvent-soaked rag stuffed into the mouth (NIDA, 2005). Although dependent on the pattern of inhalation, blood levels of solvents typically peak minutes after inhalation begins, and the abuser can begin to experience intoxication after a matter of seconds. While intoxication may last only a few minutes, abusers frequently seek to prolong the "high" by inhaling repeatedly over the course of several hours. In extreme circumstances, death may be a consequence of cardiac arrhythmias, asphyxiation, and/or cachexia.

Relatively little is known about the neuropharmacology of abused solvents, although they appear to have much in common with the classical CNS-depressant drugs like ethanol and barbiturates, including the potential for tolerance and dependence (Balster, 1998). Commonly used solvents have been shown to alter the function of a variety of ligand-gated ion channels, including those activated by glycine, gamma-aminobutyric acid (GABA) and *N*-methyl-D-aspartate (NMDA) (Beckstead *et al.*, 2000; Cruz *et al.*, 2000). Recent evidence links high-level toluene exposure in rats to increased dopaminergic neurotransmission within the mesolimbic reward pathway, an effect thought to underlie the abuse potential of numerous drugs (Reigel and French, 2002; Reigel *et al.*, 2004). Toluene, as well as TCE and TRI, have been shown to enhance serotonin-3 receptor function, which has also been implicated in the reinforcing properties of abused drugs (Lopreato *et al.*, 2003).

Whereas the intoxicating effects achieved through acute solvent abuse are reversible, abuse may be continued for years and result in residual organ damage. For example, chronic abuse of products containing *n*-hexane and methyl-*n*-butyl ketone can cause peripheral neuropathies. Blood dyscrasias, liver damage, kidney injury, and hearing impairment are seen in patients who have abused solvents injurious to these organs. It has been known for some time that the brain is not spared residual damage, with long-term

neurologic and psychological sequelae (Ron, 1986; Caldemeyer *et al.*, 1996). More recently, Rosenberg *et al.* (2002) reported increased incidences of neurologic and neuropsychological effects in chronic solvent abusers compared to a control group of chronic drug abusers. Solvent abusers did significantly worse on tests of working memory and executive cognitive function, and a much higher percentage of the patients (44 vs. 25.5%) had structural abnormalities in subcortical regions of the brain (i.e., basal ganglia, cerebellum, pons, and thalamus) as visualized by MRI (Fig. 2). Solvent abusers also showed moderate to severe, diffuse abnormality of the cerebral white matter, consistent with that seen in earlier studies of neuropsychologically impaired toluene abusers (Rosenberg *et al.*, 1988a,b; Filley *et al.*, 1990). Nearly two decades ago, Rosenberg and colleagues termed this condition "white matter dementia" (myelinated neurons are white in appearance) that was characterized primarily by diffuse cerebral, cerebellar and brainstem atrophy, and ventricular enlargement (Fig. 24-2). More recently, dementia in toluene abusers has been referred to as "toluene leukoencephalopathy" (Filley and Kleinschmidt-DeMasters, 2001; Filley *et al.*, 2004). Leukoencephalopathy, also known as multifocal demyelinating disease, involves structural alteration of cerebral white matter, in which the myelin sheaths that cover nerve fibers are destroyed but axons are largely spared. Thus, toluene is among the long list of white matter toxins identified to date.

ENVIRONMENTAL CONTAMINATION

Widespread use of solvents has resulted in their dissemination throughout the environment (Fig. 24-1). Everyone is exposed daily to solvents, albeit in minute amounts (Ashley *et al.*, 1994; Churchill *et al.*, 2001; Blount *et al.*, 2006). Because solvents as a chemical class are volatile, the preponderance of solvents entering the environment do so by evaporation. The majority of the more volatile organic chemicals (VOCs) volatilize when products containing them (e.g., aerosol propellants, paint thinners, cleaners, and soil fumigants) are used as intended. Solvent loss into the atmosphere also occurs during production, processing, storage, and transport activities, resulting in elevated concentrations in air in the proximity of point sources. Winds dilute and disperse solvent vapors across the world. Atmospheric concentrations of most VOCs are usually extremely low [i.e., nondetectable to nanograms or a few micrograms per cubic meter (m^3) of air]. Relatively high concentrations of certain solvents (e.g., 10–520 $\mu g/m^3$, or 3–163 ppb of benzene) have been measured in urban areas, around petrochemical plants, and in the immediate vicinity of hazardous waste sites (Bennett, 1987). Motor vehicle exhaust is a major contributor to hydrocarbon emissions (Mohamed *et al.*, 2002). Fraser *et al.* (1998) measured extremely high levels of benzene, toluene, ethylbenzene, and xylenes in a Los Angeles roadway tunnel.

Solvent contamination of drinking water supplies is of major health concern. Although the majority of a solvent spilled onto the ground evaporates, some may permeate the soil and migrate through it until reaching groundwater or an impermeable material. In years past, the more lipophilic solvents were generally regarded as water insoluble. It is now recognized that all solvents are soluble in water to some extent. Some (e.g., alcohols, ketones, glycols, and glycol ethers) are freely water soluble. Maximum solubilities of some common hydrocarbon solvents range from 10 mg/L (ppm) for *n*-hexane to 24,000 mg/L for bromochloromethane. High concentrations of VOCs are sometimes found in the effluent of facilities of rubber producers, chemical companies, petrochemical plants, and

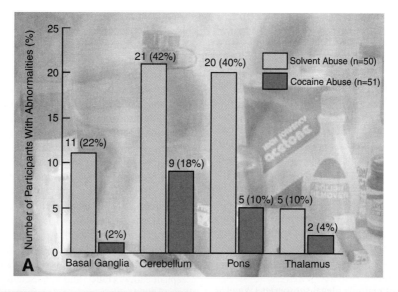

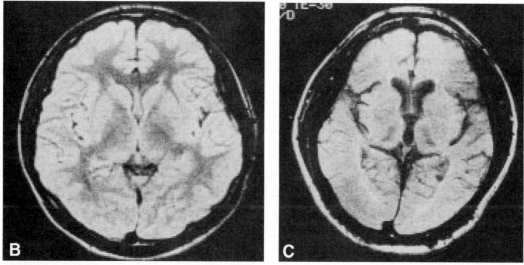

Figure 24-2. (A): Inhalant and cocaine abusers with subcortical abnormalities, by brain region affected. (B–C): Brain damage in a toluene abuser.

(A) Magnetic resonance imaging (MRI) scans of chronic inhalant abusers and chronic cocaine abusers showed more frequent occurrence of abnormalities in the basal ganglia, cerebellum, pons, and thalamus for those who abused solvents. (Available at http://www.drugabuse.gov/NIDA_notes/NNVol17N4/Chronic.html): [From NIDA Notes, 2002]. MRI shows marked atrophy (shrinkage) of brain tissue in a toluene abuser (C) compared to a nonabusing individual (B). Note the smaller size and the larger empty (dark) space within the toluene abuser's brain. The white outer circle in each image is the skull. (Available electronically at http://www.drugabuse.gov/PDF/RRInhalants.pdf): (Courtesy of Neil Rosenberg, M.D., as published in NIDA Research Report Series, March 2005).

paper mills. Concentrations diminish rapidly after VOCs enter bodies of water, primarily due to dilution and evaporation. VOCs in waters rise to the surface or sink to the bottom, according to their density. VOCs on the surface will largely evaporate. VOCs on the bottom must depend on solubilization in the water or upon mixing by current or wave action to reach the surface. VOCs in groundwater tend to remain trapped until the water reaches the surface, although some are subject to microbial modification. Concentrations in well water are rarely high enough for acute or subacute toxicity to be of concern. The very low levels of some solvents typically found in water have, however, caused a great deal of concern and debate about their carcinogenic potential.

Potential health effects of solvent contaminants of water have received considerable attention over the past 30+ years. A report by Mason and McKay (1974), of an increased incidence of cancer in persons who drank water from the Mississippi River, prompted the EPA to analyze the water supply of New Orleans. The finding of some 76 synthetic organic chemicals, many of which were solvents, prompted passage of the Safe Drinking Water Act in 1974. $CHCl_3$ is the most frequently found VOC in finished drinking water supplies in the United States (ATSDR, 1997a). It and certain other trihalomethanes are formed by reaction of the chlorine added as a disinfectant with natural organic compounds present in the water. Levels of solvents found in drinking water in the United States are typically in the nanogram per liter (ppt) to microgram per liter (ppb) range, though concentrations in the low milligram per liter (ppm) range are found in water from wells situated in solvent plumes from hazardous waste sites and other point discharges. Of the thousands of chemicals found at hazardous waste sites, six of the ten most commonly present in groundwater are solvents (Fay and Mumtaz, 1996; Fay, 2006).

People are subjected to solvents in environmental media by inhalation, ingestion, and skin contact. Considerable effort was devoted by the EPA, from 1979 to 1985, to assess personal exposure to solvents in different locales of the United States. TRI, PERC, benzene, xylenes, and ethylbenzene were most frequently found in highest concentrations ($\sim$1–32 μg/m^3) in air (Wallace *et al.*, 1987). Exhaled breath levels of some chemicals (e.g., CHCl$_3$, ethylbenzene) corresponded to indoor air levels. Personal activities (e.g., smoking, visiting a dry cleaner and service station) and occupational exposures were believed to be largely responsible for relatively high exposures to other VOCs (e.g., benzene, toluene, xylenes, and PERC) (Ashley *et al.*, 1994). Subsequent studies, accounting for all pertinent exposure pathways, were conducted by the EPA in the mid-1990s (Gordon *et al.*, 1999). Elliott *et al.* (2006) recently reported indoor exposures to VOCs did not have adverse effects on the respiratory function of 953 adults surveyed, with the exception of 1,4-dichlorobenzene, a component of air fresheners, toilet bowl deodorants, and mothballs. CHCl$_3$ was found to be the most prevalent VOC in drinking water. It should be recognized that CHCl$_3$ and other VOCs volatilize to some degree during home water usage, particularly when the water is heated. Thus, a significant proportion of one's total exposure to VOCs in tap water can occur via inhalation (Weisel and Jo, 1996), though the contribution of dermal exposure is relatively modest (Thrall *et al.*, 2002).

TOXICOKINETICS

Toxicokinetic (TK) studies are playing an increasingly important role in reducing uncertainties in risk assessments of solvents (Leung and Paustenbach, 1995; Andersen, 2003; Clewell and Andersen, 2004). The fundamental goal of TK studies is to delineate the uptake and disposition of chemicals and certain of their metabolites in the body. It is now recognized that toxicity is a dynamic process, in which the degree and duration of injury of a target tissue are dependent on the net effect of toxicodynamic (TD) and TK processes including systemic absorption, tissue deposition, metabolism, interaction with cellular components, elimination, and tissue repair. Estimation of risk of toxicity from TK data is based on the fundamental concept that the intensity of response from an administered dose is dependent on the amount(s) of biologically active chemical moiety(ies) present in a target tissue (i.e., the tissue dose). A related concept is that the tissue dose in a given target organ in one species will have the same degree of effect as an equivalent target organ dose in a second species. This concept of tissue dose equivalence appears to be applicable in many cases to solvents (Andersen, 1987), although TD differences are possible. Gaining an understanding of how the processes that govern solvent kinetics vary with dose, route of exposure, species, and even different individuals greatly reduces the number of assumptions that have to be made in assessment of health risks from exposure and toxicity/carcinogenicity data.

Volatility and lipophilicity are two of the most important properties of solvents that govern their absorption and deposition in the body. Most solvents are volatile under normal usage conditions, though volatility varies from compound to compound. Lipophilicity

can also vary substantially, from quite water soluble (e.g., glycols, esters, and alcohols) to quite lipid soluble (e.g., halocarbons and aromatic hydrocarbons). Many solvents of particular concern at present are relatively lipid soluble and volatile, hence their designation as VOCs. These compounds have a relatively low molecular weight and are uncharged. Thus, they pass freely through membranes from areas of high-to-low concentration by passive diffusion.

Absorption

The majority of systemic absorption of inhaled VOCs occurs in the alveoli, although limited absorption has been demonstrated to occur in the upper respiratory tract (Stott and McKenna, 1984). Gases in the alveoli are thought to equilibrate almost instantaneously with blood in the pulmonary capillaries (Goldstein *et al.*, 1974). Blood:air partition coefficients (PCs) of VOCs are important determinants of the extent of their uptake. A PC is defined by Gargas *et al.* (1989) as the ratio of concentration of VOC achieved between two different media at equilibrium. As blood is largely aqueous, the more hydrophilic solvents have relatively high blood:air PCs, which favor extensive uptake. Gargas *et al.* (1989) determined in vitro PCs for 55 VOCs in F-344 rats. Human blood:air values were measured for 36 of the compounds. Because VOCs diffuse from areas of high-to-low concentration, increases in respiratory rate (to maintain a high alveolar concentration) and in cardiac output/pulmonary blood flow (to maintain a large concentration gradient by removing capillary blood containing the VOC) enhance systemic absorption.

Systemic uptake of solvents during ongoing inhalation exposures is dependent on tissue loading and metabolism, in addition to the factors noted above. Percent uptake is initially high, but progressively declines as the chemical accumulates in tissues, and the level of chemical in venous blood returning to the pulmonary circulation increases. A near steady state, or equilibrium will soon be reached upon inhalation of a fixed concentration of lipophilic solvents. The approach to equilibrium is asymptotic. Despite continued inhalation of lipophilic solvents, levels in the blood and tissues (other than fat) generally only increase modestly. Percent uptake remains relatively constant for the duration of exposure, with metabolism and accumulation in adipose tissue largely responsible for the continuing absorption. Hydrophilic solvents take considerably longer to reach steady-state, due to the extended time required for equilibration of chemical in the inspired air with that in the total body water (Goldstein *et al.*, 1974).

Solvents are well absorbed from the GI tract. Peak blood levels are observed within a few minutes of dosing fasted subjects, although the presence of fatty food in the GI tract can significantly delay absorption. It is now usually assumed that 100% of an oral dose of most solvents is absorbed systemically. The vehicle or diluent in which a solvent is ingested can affect its absorption and TK. Kim *et al.* (1990a,b), for example, found that a corn oil vehicle served as a reservoir in the gut to delay GI absorption of carbon tetrachloride (CC1$_4$) in rats. Although bioavailability of CC1$_4$ given in corn oil and in an aqueous emulsion was the same, peak blood CC1$_4$ levels and acute hepatotoxicity were much lower in the corn oil group. Other factors that can influence the oral absorption of other classes of chemicals have relatively little influence on most lipophilic solvents, due to their rapid passive diffusion throughout the GI tract.

Absorption of solvents through the skin can result in both local and systemic effects. Skin contact with vapors and concentrated solutions of solvents is a common occurrence in the workplace. Dermal contact with solvent contaminants of water can also occur in the home and in recreational settings (Weisel and Jo, 1996). Lipophilic solvents penetrate the stratum corneum, the skin's barrier to absorption, by passive diffusion. Important determinants of the rate of dermal absorption of solvents include the chemical concentration, surface area exposed, exposure duration, integrity and thickness of the stratum corneum, and lipophilicity and molecular weight of the solvent (EPA, 1998). Skin penetration can be quantified in laboratory animals and humans by a variety of in vitro and in vivo techniques (Morgan et al., 1991; Nakai et al., 1999). Although absorption rates measured by these methods may vary numerically, there is often good agreement in their relative ranking of chemicals' ability to penetrate the skin. Dermal permeability constants are typically two to four times lower for human than for rodent skin (McDougal et al., 1990). The extent of dermal absorption in occupational and environmental exposure settings should be taken into account when conducting risk assessments of solvents.

Transport and Distribution

Chemicals and nutrients absorbed into portal venous blood from the GI tract can be removed from the bloodstream by first-pass, or presystemic elimination. As VOCs are rapidly absorbed and human intestinal epithelium apparently does not contain cytochrome $P450$ 2E1 (Paine et al., 2006), the primary CYP isoform that metabolizes low doses of many VOCs, their first-pass GI metabolism should be negligible. Blood in the portal venous circulation passes through the liver before reentering the venous circulation. Solvents are also subject to exhalation by the lungs during their first pass through the pulmonary circulation. Those solvents that are well metabolized and quite volatile are most efficiently eliminated before they enter the arterial blood. The efficiency of the hepatic first-pass elimination is thus dependent on the chemical, as well as the rate at which it arrives in the liver. Pulmonary first-pass elimination, in contrast, is believed to be a zero-order process, as a fixed percentage of the chemical was hypothesized to exit the pulmonary blood at each pass through the pulmonary circulation (NAS, 1986). Indeed, Lee et al. (1996) demonstrated in rats that pulmonary first-pass elimination of TCE was relatively constant over a range of doses, but that hepatic elimination was inversely related to dose. Andersen (1981) concludes that the liver is capable of removing "virtually all" of an orally administered VOC, if the amount in the portal blood is not great enough to saturate metabolism. This hypothesis, if demonstrated experimentally, could have a profound effect on extrahepatic cancer and noncancer risk estimates of environmentally encountered levels of solvents in ingested media.

Solvents are transported by the arterial blood and taken up according to tissue blood flow and mass and tissue:blood PCs (Astrand, 1983). Relatively hydrophilic solvents solubilize to different extents in plasma. Nevertheless, as much as 50% of such compounds may still be carried by erythrocytes (Lam et al., 1990). These researchers found that lipophilic solvents do not bind appreciably to plasma proteins or hemoglobin, but partition into hydrophobic sites in these molecules. Lipophilic solvents also partition into phospholipids, lipoproteins, and cholesterol present in the blood. The brain is an example of a rapidly perfused tissue with a relatively high lipid content. Lipophilic solvents therefore quickly accumulate in the brain after the initiation of exposures (Warren et al., 2000). Inhalation of halothane, TCE, and CHCl$_3$ can produce CNS effects as profound as surgical anesthesia within as little as 1–2 minutes. Redistribution to poorly perfused, lipoidal tissues will subsequently occur. Adipose

tissue gradually accumulates relatively large amounts of VOCs, and slowly releases them back into the blood due to high fat:blood PCs and low blood perfusion rates.

Route of exposure can significantly influence target organ deposition and toxicity of solvents. Much of the pre-1980s toxicology database for solvents comprised results of inhalation studies. Inhalation is the major route of occupational exposure to these chemicals. Since then, much attention has been focused on potential health effects of VOC contaminants of food and drinking water. Due to the initial paucity of oral data, regulatory agencies sometimes extrapolated directly from inhalation data to predict risks of ingested VOCs. Such a practice is obviously not scientifically valid, when physiological differences in the absorption pathways are taken into account. All the cardiac output passes through the pulmonary circulation versus $\sim$20% for the GI tract. Also, the alveolar surface area for absorption is approximately 20 times that of the entire GI tract in humans. VOCs absorbed in the lungs directly enter the arterial circulation and are transported throughout the body. In contrast, VOCs absorbed from the GI tract largely enter the portal circulation and are subject to first-pass elimination by both the liver and the lungs. The human GI epithelium contains certain monooxygenases, such as CYP3A4 (Ding and Kaminsky, 2003), though they do not participate to a significant extent in metabolism of most solvents. It is not surprising then that extrahepatic organs receive a greater dose following inhalation of VOCs. The liver should take up and metabolize a portion of many VOCs following ingestion. This has been demonstrated in rats receiving the same systemic dose of CC1$_4$ over the same time frame by inhalation and gastric infusion (Sanzgiri et al., 1997).

The pattern of ingestion of solvents can significantly influence their TK and health effects. For convenience, test chemicals are typically given daily to animals as a single bolus by gavage in short- and long-term oral toxicity and carcinogenicity studies. Actual human exposures to solvents in drinking water are quite different, in that people typically ingest water in divided doses. High, daily gavage doses of CHCl$_3$ and other halocarbons have produced hepatocellular carcinoma in B6C3F1 mice. No evidence of hepatic tumorigenesis was seen, however, when these mice were given the same doses of the chemical in their drinking water (Jorgenson et al., 1985; Klaunig et al., 1986). Female B6C3F1 mice exhibited hepatocellular necrosis and regenerative hyperplasia when gavaged with CHCl$_3$. Consumptions of the same doses in water were without ill effect (Larson et al., 1994). Similarly, the maximum blood level of CC1$_4$ was found to be 35 times higher and hepatotoxicity more severe in rats dosed with CC1$_4$ by gavage, than in those given the same dose over 2 hours by gastric infusion (Sanzgiri et al., 1995). Oral bolus doses of solvents can cause damage by exceeding the capacity of hepatic and pulmonary first-pass elimination, as well as protection and repair processes of cells.

The rate of systemic elimination of different solvents varies considerably. The two major routes of systemic elimination of VOCs are metabolism and exhalation. The rate and extent of metabolic clearance are dose- and compound-dependent. Exhalation is determined largely by the rate of pulmonary blood flow, the chemical's air:blood PC, and the alveolar ventilation rate. The more volatile, lipophilic VOCs are exhaled the most readily, because they have the higher air:blood PCs (Gargas et al., 1989). A good "case in point" is the comparison of toluene with acetone. The extent of CNS depression caused by each chemical is dependent on the concentration of the parent compound present in the brain (Bruckner and Peterson, 1981). As can be seen in Fig. 24-3, recovery of rats from toluene

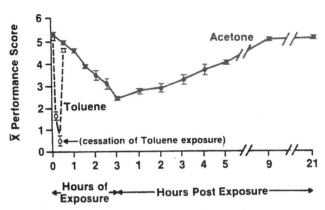

Figure 24-3. Comparison of the induction of and recovery from toluene and acetone narcosis.

Rats inhaled 45 mg/L of toluene or acetone for 20 minutes or 3 h, respectively. Animal performance/reflexes were monitored periodically as measures of the degree of CNS depression. [Reproduced from Bruckner and Peterson (1981), with permission from Elsevier.]

anesthesia occurs within minutes of exposure cessation. This can be attributed to redistribution of toluene from the brain to body fat and other tissues, as well as to relatively rapid metabolism and exhalation. In contrast, recovery from acetone narcosis does not occur for at least 9 hours post exposure. As acetone is water soluble, limited amounts are deposited in the brain. It is instead distributed in the considerable volume of the blood and other body water. Clearance of acetone is slow due to its large volume of distribution and its relatively slow metabolism and exhalation. Acetone's water solubility is responsible for its relatively low air:blood PC and retention in the pulmonary blood. Thus, acetone is available for diffusion into the brain and induction of a modest degree of CNS depression for a prolonged time.

Body fat plays an important role in the elimination of lipophilic solvents. Blood levels of such solvents drop very rapidly during the initial elimination phase following cessation of exposure. This so-called redistribution phase is characterized by rapid diffusion of solvents from the blood into tissues. Equilibration of adipose tissue is prolonged due to the small fraction of cardiac output (~3%) supplying fat depots (Goldstein *et al.*, 1974). Body fat increases the volume of distribution and total body burden of lipophilic solvents. Deequilibration from adipose tissue during the terminal elimination phase is prolonged, due to slow blood flow and high fat:blood PCs. Sato *et al.* (1975) demonstrated slower elimination of benzene from females than from male rats and humans, due to the female's higher body fat content. Rats with more body fat exhibited leukopenia during chronic benzene exposure.

Metabolism

Biotransformation plays a key role in modulating the toxicities of many solvents. Many solvents are poorly soluble in water. Certain cellular enzymes can convert them to relatively water-soluble derivatives, which may be more readily eliminated in the largely aqueous urine and/or bile. Conversion of a bioactive parent compound to a less bioactive or inactive metabolite(s) that (is/are) efficiently eliminated is termed *metabolic inactivation*, or *detoxification*. Toluene, for example, accumulates in neuronal membranes and inhibits their functions. Toluene is metabolized to hydroxyl and carboxyl metabo-

lites, which are too polar to accumulate or remain in substantial quantities in neuronal membranes. Thus, metabolism serves to detoxify and to accelerate the elimination of toluene. Metabolism of other solvents can produce reactive metabolites that are cytotoxic and/or mutagenic. This phenomenon is known as *metabolic activation*, or *bioactivation*. Benzene, for example, is oxidized to a variety of quinones and semiquinones that can produce hematopoietic toxicities and leukemia (Snyder, 2004). Benzene and many other VOCs are converted via multiple metabolic pathways to products of varying toxicity. Some of these competing pathways are considered bioactivation, others detoxification pathways. A variety of factors can influence the prominence of the different pathways and hence alter toxicity outcomes.

The initial step in biotransformation of relatively lipophilic solvents is catalyzed primarily by microsomal CYPs. They are a "superfamily" of hemoproteins that act as terminal oxidases of the mixed-function oxidase system. Their mode of action is described in Chap. 6. CYPs can catalyze a number of oxidative reactions, as well as certain reductive reactions (Omiecinski *et al.*, 1999). Some 40 different human CYP isoforms have been identified to date, but six of them (CYPs 2D6, 2C9, 3A4, 1A2, 2C19, and 2E1) account for the majority of xenobiotic metabolism (Smith *et al.*, 1998; Rendic, 2002). CYPs are generally thought to have broad, overlapping substrate specificities, as demonstrated by Kobayashi *et al.* (2002) in rats. It is believed by some authorities that enzyme kinetics under physiological conditions may favor one or two isoforms as the primary catalysts for a given chemical (Wrighton and Stevens, 1992). Different isoforms can predominate at different concentrations of a chemical.

The outcome of exposure to a potentially toxic solvent can depend on the relative abundance of CYP isoforms. Expression of CYPs can differ considerably as a result of genetic polymorphisms and exposure to chemicals that induce or inhibit specific isoforms. A number of factors have been found to be sources of individual variability in CYP induction (Tang *et al.*, 2005). Inheritable gene alterations, such as base changes and deletions, can result not only in functionally deficient enzymes, but also in the absence of certain P450s (Daly *et al.*, 1993). As CYPs have different modes of regulatory control, their expression in response to various inducers and inhibitors varies. It should also be recognized that frequently there are interspecies differences in the presence, regulation, and catalytic activities of P450s (Lewis *et al.*, 1998).

There has been a focus on identification of CYPs that participate in the metabolism of individual solvents. Nakajima *et al.* (1992a) found that low concentrations of TCE in rat liver were metabolized primarily by CYP2E1, a constitutive, high-affinity, low-capacity isoform. CYP2B1/2, a low-affinity, high-capacity form predominated under high-dose (substrate) conditions. CYP2E1 was observed to be a major contributor to the metabolism of TCE and benzene, but not toluene. CYP1A1 catalyzed the formation of *o*-cresol, but not benzyl alcohol from toluene. CYP1A1 oxidized TCE in mice but not in rats. Thus, CYP isoforms exhibit species selectivity, substrate selectivity, and regioselectivity for solvents (Nakajima, 1997).

CYP2E1 is a major catalyst of the oxidation of a variety of low-molecular-weight xenobiotics, including many solvents. CYP2E1 is found predominantly in liver, with lower levels present in kidneys, lungs, brain, testes, and other extrahepatic tissues of rodents and humans (Lieber, 1997). Guengerich *et al.* (1991) reported that human CYP2E1 is primarily responsible for oxidation of some 16 halogenated and aromatic hydrocarbons, including benzene, styrene, $CHCl_3$, TCE, and vinyl chloride. These compounds are oxidized to electrophilic metabolites, capable of causing cytotoxicity and/or mutagenicity (Raucy et al., 1993). The isozyme is also responsible for reduction of CCl_4 to free radicals (see the discussion of CCl_4 in this chapter). CYP2E1 activity is associated with the pathogenesis of alcoholic cirrhosis, through formation of highly reactive oxygen radicals and acetaldehyde from ethanol (Lieber, 1997; Caro and Cederbaum, 2004). CYP2E1 is inducible by ethanol, acetone, pyridazine, chlorzoxazone, isoniazid, and other of its substrates. Activity of the isoform varies from species to species (Nakajima, 1997) and from human to human (Lipscomb et al., 1997). Overnight fasting is widely recognized to induce CYP2E1, due in part to release of acetone during lipolysis (Bruckner et al., 2002). Starving rats, however, apparently must engage in coprophagy for induction to occur (Chung et al., 2001). Such differences in CYP2E1 activity/levels may play a major role in susceptibility to the toxicity and carcinogenicity of ethanol and a number of other solvents.

A variety of environmental factors can predispose people to harmful effects of solvents by altering P450s (Lof and Johanson, 1998). Ethanol is an effective CYP2E1 inducer when ingested repeatedly in substantial amounts. The person who drinks in such a manner may be subject to potentiation of solvent toxicity, due to increased solvent metabolic activation (Manno et al., 1996). Conversely, ethanol consumed at about the same time as a solvent exposure can be protective by competitively inhibiting metabolic activation of the solvent (Lieber, 1997). Thus, the timing of exposures is important. Folland et al. (1976) reported severe CCl_4-induced hepatorenal injury in workers at an isopropyl alcohol bottling plant. These subjects' preexposure to the alcohol, which is metabolized to acetone, had markedly induced CYP2E1. Their induced condition resulted in a substantial increase in the metabolic activation and cytotoxicity of CCl_4, upon inhalation of normally nontoxic concentrations of the halocarbon.

The metabolic basis of solvent interactions receives considerable attention. The consequence of CYP2E1 induction by one solvent or drug depends on the nature of the second solvent. Kaneko et al. (1994) reported that ethanol pretreatment of rats has a more profound effect on the TK of TRI (poorly metabolized) than TCE (well metabolized). Similarly, ethanol pretreatment of rats results in a greater increase in metabolism and hepatotoxicity of CCl_4 (relatively poorly metabolized) than $CHCl_3$ (well metabolized) (Wang et al., 1997). As capacity- (i.e., metabolic capacity of the liver) limited metabolism prevails for poorly metabolized solvents, irrespective of dose, induction of their metabolism could be toxicologically significant in high (occupational) or low (environmental) exposure settings. In contrast, alterations of the bioactivation of low doses of well-metabolized solvents should be of little consequence, as their biotransformation is perfusion (i.e., hepatic blood flow) limited. Lipscomb et al. (2003) utilized a PBTK model to calculate that a six-fold interindividual difference in TCE metabolism resulted in <2% change in the total amount of TCE oxidized by persons inhaling 50 ppm for 8 hours or drinking 2 L of water containing 5-ppb TCE. Under such circumstances, interindividual metabolic differences would have little influence on cancer risks posed by trace levels of such solvents.

Physiological Modeling

PBTK models have been developed to provide predictions of chemical concentrations in blood and tissues as a function of time. PBTK models are thus used to relate the administered dose to the blood and/or tissue dose of parent compound and/or bioactive moiety. If there is, sufficient knowledge of the physiology of the test animal/tissue and interactions of the bioactive moiety with cellular components and ensuing responses, physiologically based toxicodynamic (PBTD) models can be developed (Conolly and Andersen, 1991). Few PBTD models have been published to date. Tan et al. (2003) linked an existing PBTK model for $CHCl_3$ with data for hepatocellular death and regenerative hyperplasia to predict liver tumor response in mice. Development of PBTK models for anesthetic gases and other pharmaceutical agents was initially undertaken in the 1920s and 1930s. Modeling enjoyed widespread use in the design of experiments and dosage regimens for drugs, but the practice was not extended to industrial chemicals until the 1970s and 1980s. A "benchmark" paper by Ramsey and Andersen (1984) described the development of a PBTK model for styrene. By 1995, PBTK models had been developed for ~50 chemical environmental contaminants (Leung and Paustenbach, 1995). Some 28 of these 50 chemicals were solvents. Andersen (2003) more recently identified some 700 papers that dealt with PBTK models and/or their applications to toxicology and risk assessment. Thus, it is clear that physiological models are being developed and used with increasing frequency to incorporate dosimetry and mechanistic data into noncancer and cancer risk assessments (Krishnan and Johanson, 2005).

Physiological modeling accounts for species- and dose-dependent shifts from linear to nonlinear kinetics, which impact tissue doses of bioactive moiety or moieties. The models are well suited for species-to-species extrapolations, because human physiological and metabolic parameter values can be inputted into animal models, and simulations of target tissue doses and effects in humans generated. Thus, solvent exposures necessary to produce the same target organ dose in humans, as those found experimentally to cause unacceptable cancer or noncancer risks in test animals, can be determined in some cases with reasonable certainty. In the limited number of cases where there may be species differences in tissue sensitivity, PBTD models can be used to forecast toxicologically effective target organ doses. The influence of interindividual variability in model parameters is now receiving considerable attention (Price et al., 2003a). Several groups of investigators are performing model fitting in a Bayesian framework using Markov chain Monte Carlo simulation to reduce parameter uncertainty (Jonsson and Johanson, 2001, 2002).

POTENTIALLY SENSITIVE SUBPOPULATIONS

There is considerable variability in responses of humans to solvents and other xenobiotics (Hattis et al., 1987). Although information on interindividual differences in the kinetics and toxicity of solvents is usually limited, some significant differences are reported and should be taken into account in risk assessments (Grassman et al., 1998; Hattis et al., 1999). Children within specific age groups appear to be even more variable than adults (Hattis et al., 2003). Current EPA cancer and noncancer risk assessment practices are generally considered to be quite protective of potentially vulnerable subgroups, due to the use of multiple uncertainty factors and conservative default assumptions.

Endogenous Factors

Children Currently, there is considerable interest in regulatory and scientific issues related to protection of children's health. The potential sensitivity of infants and children to pesticides and other chemicals was brought to the public's attention by a National Academy of Sciences' report (NAS, 1993; Bruckner, 2000). The ensuing Presidential Executive Order 13045 in 1997, directed all federal agencies to make protection of children a high priority and to consider risks to children when making policies and setting standards. The Food Quality and Protection Act of 1996, dictated that an additional 10-fold safety/uncertainty factor be used in pesticide risk assessments when pediatric toxicity and TK data are unavailable. This is almost always the case for insecticides, solvents, and other chemical contaminants. Application of the 10-fold children's safety factor to non-pesticides has been considered. The Pediatric Research Equity Act of 2003 requires pharmaceutical companies seeking FDA's approval of new drugs to frequently assess a compound's safety and efficacy at different doses in pediatric patients.

Very little information is available on the toxic potential of solvents and most other chemicals in infants and children. There are several well-known examples of compounds (e.g., lead, thalidomide, chloromycetin, and valium) to which fetuses or neonates are particularly susceptible. Results of experiments with chlorpyrifos in immature rats raised enough concern about possible neurodevelopmental disorders in children that use of a number of organophosphates was severely restricted, and they have largely been removed from the market (Colborn, 2006). Compilations of maximally tolerated doses (MTDs) of chemotherapeutic drugs are among our most definitive data on age-dependent toxicity in humans. Clinical trials of diverse groups of antineoplastic drugs revealed that their toxic effects are often similar qualitatively, and usually differ quantitatively by a factor of ≤ 2 (NAS, 1993). MTDs for children are frequently higher than that for adults (Bruckner, 2000). Ginsberg et al. (2002) assembled a database with which TK parameters for adults and children can be compared for 45 drugs. These developmental metabolic profiles are relevant to some solvents and other environmental chemicals.

Increasing numbers of toxicology studies are being carried out in immature laboratory animals. The most comprehensive data sets available are still compilations of LD_{50} values from experiments with immature rodents (Done, 1964; Goldenthal, 1971). These data, like the aforementioned MTD compilations, reveal that immature animals are more sensitive to some but not to all chemicals. Variances are usually no more than two- to three-fold, but can be as much as 10-fold. The younger and more immature a subject, the more different its response from that of the adult. The newborn mouse and rat more nearly resemble the human fetus during the third trimester than during the neonate's initial weeks and months of life. Thus, it is not surprising that newborn rodents are usually much more sensitive to many toxicants than are human newborns. Growth and maturation are, of course, much more rapid in rodents. A few days growth of mice and rats can result in substantial changes in metabolism, disposition, and toxicity (Ginsberg et al., 2004). It is generally accepted that there are "windows of vulnerability," or periods during the development of the nervous, audiovisual, immune, endocrine, and other organ systems when the intricate, fragile maturational processes may be particularly sensitive to xenobiotics (Faustman et al., 2000; Dorman et al., 2001; Scheuplein et al., 2002). These windows occur at different ages and last for different periods of time in different species. This makes the choice of an appropriate animal model for children complex and cross-species comparisons more difficult than usual with adult risk assessments (Ginsberg et al., 2004; Morford et al., 2004).

Despite a paucity of data, some logical assumptions can be made about age-dependent changes in the TK and toxicity of solvents. GI absorption of solvents would not be expected to vary with age, as most solvents are absorbed rapidly and completely by passive diffusion from the entire GI tract. Systemic absorption of inhaled solvents may be greater in infants and children. Their cardiac output and respiratory rates are relatively high, although their alveolar surface area is lower than that of adults (Sarangapani et al., 2003). Reduced plasma protein binding in neonates and infants may be of consequence for certain solvent metabolites. Low-binding capacity for TCA, for example, could result in more of the mouse hepatocarcinogen being available for hepatic uptake, as well as for renal clearance. Extracellular water, expressed as percent of body weight, is highest in newborns and diminishes through childhood. The larger volume of distribution for water-soluble solvents results in their slower clearance and longer duration of action. Body fat is high from ~6 months to 3 years of age, then steadily decreases until adolescence, when it increases again in females. As lipophilic solvents accumulate in adipose tissue, more body fat would result in higher body burdens, slower clearance, and longer duration of action (NAS, 1993).

Changes in xenobiotic biotransformation during maturation may have the greatest impact on susceptibility to chemical toxicity and carcinogenicity. Low liver P450-mediated and liver and plasma carboxylesterase-mediated detoxification of deltamethrin, a pyrethroid insecticide, results in elevated blood and brain levels of the neurotoxic parent compound and severe acute poisoning of neonatal and preweanling rats (Anand et al., 2006a). Poisonings of premature and term human newborns by benzyl alcohol, hexachlorophene, valium, chloramphenicol, and certain other compounds are primarily attributable to deficits in hepatic Phase II metabolic (i.e., conjugative) capacity. Maturational studies of human liver reveal that CYP isoforms are expressed asynchronously (Cresteil, 1998). More recently there have been comprehensive efforts to characterize the ontogeny of human hepatic Phase I (Hines and McCarver, 2002; Stevens et al., 2003; Johnsrud et al., 2003) and Phase II (McCarver and Hines, 2002) enzymes from gestation through adolescence. Levels of CYP2E1, the primary catalyst of oxidation of a variety of solvents, are very low in fetal liver, increase steadily for the first year, and remain relatively constant through adolescence (Cresteil, 1998; Johnsrud et al., 2003). Blanco et al. (2000) failed to find an age-related difference in the maximal in vitro activity of CYP2E1 or other CYP isoforms in liver microsomes from donors 0.5 to– 93 years old. More rapid systemic clearance of many compounds by young children than by adults (Ginsberg et al., 2002) is generally believed to result from the child's liver's larger volume and more rapid perfusion rate (Murry et al., 1995; Noda et al., 1997; Sarangapani et al., 2003). Glomerular filtration and renal tubular secretion are quite low at birth, but increase substantially during the first 6 months to 1 year (Scheuplein et al., 2002). The half-life of creatinine, a substance eliminated entirely by glomerular filtration, is about half the adult value at 1 year. The net result of multiple age-related TK changes, some with offsetting effects, is usually difficult to predict.

A number of authorities have advocated the use of PBTK/TD models to collectively account for the unique and changing characteristics of children (Clewell et al., 2004; Daston et al., 2004; Landrigan et al., 2004). Considerable attention is being devoted to this pursuit, but the number of models published to date for solvents and other chemicals is quite limited. Pelekis et al. (2001) used simplified PBTK model-based algebraic equations and ranges of physiological and biochemical parameters (in lieu of measured values) to simulate tissue doses of a series of solvents in children and adults. The authors concluded that the child–adult differences of parent compounds were modest for inhalation exposures. Sarangapani et al. (2003) developed a PBTK model that integrated key age-specific respiratory tract parameters, such that the disposition of four VOCs (styrene, vinyl chloride, isopropanol, and PERC) could be forecast in children and adults. Differences in blood levels of parent compounds in infants and adults were comparable or varied <2-fold during the first year of life. Blood metabolite concentrations or the amounts metabolized in the liver or lung, microsomes, however, often varied substantially with age. Price et al. (2003b) utilized some age-specific physiological and biochemical data to model the kinetics of inhaled furan in blood of children and adults. Physiological parameter values (e.g., metabolic and alveolar ventilation rates) for some or all age groups were unavailable and had to be estimated. Nong et al. (2006) incorporated measured age-specific liver volumes and CYP2E1 content into a PBPK model for toluene to predict internal doses (blood levels) of the parent compound in adults and in children of different age groups. CYP2E1 content was the key model input parameter for neonates, whereas liver blood-flow rate was predominant after a few months of age. Combined interindividual and interage variability in blood level versus time curves was within a factor of 2, except for the neonates, which had somewhat higher AUCs.

Clewell et al. (2004) recently developed what they termed a life-stage model to simulate blood levels of four solvents [isopropanol, vinyl chloride, methylene chloride (MC), and PERC] and their primary metabolite in different life stages. This was intended to be a preliminary model, in view of the lack of validated models for the younger groups and the required number of simplifying assumptions in the face of uncertainties about many age-specific parameters. In general, dose metrics for the chemicals across life stages were within a factor of 2, except during the early postnatal period when the largest TK differences occurred. These and the observations of Pelekis et al. (2001) and Nong et al. (2006) are well within the TK component of 3.2 of the classical 10-fold interspecies factor. Potential PD differences, of course, are not taken into account here. Gentry et al. (2003) took a similar approach to forecast internal dosimetry of vinyl chloride, isopropanol, MC, and PERC in human offspring during pregnancy and lactation. In general, blood concentrations of the VOCs were lower in neonates during lactation than in the fetus during gestation. Fetal/neonatal VOC exposures were generally several orders of magnitude lower than maternal exposures. The relatively low systemic exposures and low metabolic capacity should reduce the risks from reactive metabolites of these solvents during these periods.

Elderly   The elderly, like infants and children, may be more or less sensitive to the toxicity of solvents than younger adults. Data are sorely lacking on the relative susceptibility of geriatric populations to solvents and other industrial chemicals. The aging CNS undergoes changes (e.g., neuronal loss, altered neurotransmitter and receptor levels, and reduced adaptability to effects of toxicants) (Ginsberg et al., 2005), that may predispose to more pronounced neurologic effects by solvents. Older people do appear to be more sensitive to the CNS-depressant effects of ethanol, due in part to lower gastric alcohol dehydrogenase (ADH) activity (Seitz et al., 1993). Kiesswetter et al. (1997) observed the most pronounced neurobehavorial effects in older workers with the highest single or mixed organic solvent exposures. Memory, attention, visual perception, and motor skills diminish with aging, even in the absence of chemical exposure. The aforementioned experimental findings could be interpreted as merely additive, or as exacerbation during a vulnerable life stage. Paradoxically, a subsequent investigation by Kiesswetter et al. (2000), this time of toluene-exposed rotogravure printers, revealed fewer symptoms and better psychometric performance in older workers with higher exposure levels. A limited number of studies of this phenomenon by other investigators are no more definitive.

Investigations of adverse effects of solvents on old animals have been quite limited. Attention has been primarily focused on age-related susceptibility of rodents to liver damage. Susceptibility varies dramatically from one chemical to another. Rikans and Hornbrook (1997) reviewed studies showing increased susceptibility of geriatric F-344 rats to allyl alcohol, but there was no apparent age dependency with bromobenzene. Results varied with species, strain, and gender. CCl_4 hepatotoxicity was less severe in 28-month-old female F-344 rats than in young adults (Rikans et al., 1999), but more severe in 28-month-old male F-344 rats (Schoeffner et al., 1996). No effects of aging on hepatic CYP2E1 levels, CCl_4 metabolic activation, glutathione (GSH) levels, antioxidants, or ability to suppress oxidative damage were found. Wauthier et al. (2004) saw no changes in CYP2E1 protein or mRNA in 18-month-old male Wistar rats, but did observe decreased CYP2E1 activity. The investigators attributed this phenomenon to oxidative stress on the isoform. More severe CCl_4-induced DNA damage in hepatocytes from older mice was shown to be due to preexisting oxidative DNA damage and a higher incidence of DNA strand breaks in the older animals (Lopez-Diazguerrero et al., 2005). Thus, normal aging processes can be accentuated by chemical stressors.

TK changes during aging have primarily been of interest in the field of drug therapeutics (Bressler and Bahl, 2003; McLean and LeCouteur, 2004). Federal agencies including the EPA are now focusing more attention on exposures and potential vulnerabilities of the elderly to toxic chemicals (Geller and Zenick, 2005). As there are few pertinent geriatric animal or human toxicology studies, it would be worthwhile to consider information on age-specific factors that govern the TK of solvents. Data for a substantial number of geriatric TK indices are inadequate. Clewell et al. (2002) and Sarangapani et al. (2003) have compiled comprehensive reviews and evaluations of the age-specific TK parameters that are available. Splanchnic blood flow decreases with age more rapidly than cardiac output. This seems unlikely to affect the GI absorption of solvents, as they are readily absorbed by passive diffusion. Dermal absorption could be influenced by loss of integrity of the stratum corneum, reduction in skin surface lipids and atrophy of the dermal capillary network (Roskos et al., 1989). Total lung capacity does not change with age, but vital capacity (mobile volume) diminishes progressively due to loss of lung elasticity and strength of the respiratory muscles. Residual capacity (fixed volume) increases with progressive narrowing and closure of small airways (Ritschel, 1988). Other alterations contributing to lower pulmonary absorption include decreases in alveolar surface area, membrane permeability and capillary blood volume, and thicker alveolar cell membranes (Clewell et al., 2002). Nevertheless, inhalation PBPK model predictions of steady-state blood concentrations of isopropanol, styrene, vinyl chloride, and PERC differed very little among 10-, 15-, 25-, 50-, and 75-year-old humans (Sarangapani et al., 2003).

Age influences the distribution of xenobiotics in the body, as well as their metabolism and elimination (Bressler and Bahl, 2003). With aging, body fat content usually increases substantially at the expense of the lean mass (i.e., skeletal muscle) and body water. Thus, polar solvents tend to reach higher blood levels during exposures. Relatively lipid-soluble solvents accumulate in adipose tissue and are released slowly to sites of action, metabolism, and elimination. Ginsberg et al. (2005) assembled clearance and half-life ($t^1/_2$) data for 46 drugs in 4500 subjects. Clearance was typically slower and half-life longer after the age of 60 years, particularly in those 80–84 years old. Cardiac output diminishes 30–40% between the ages of 25 and 65 years, as do renal and hepatic blood flows (Woodhouse and Wynne, 1992; Cody, 1993; McLean and Le Couteur, 2004). The latter two research groups and Clewell et al. (2002) concluded that reduced hepatic clearance of flow- and capacity-limited xenobiotics in the elderly was due primarily to reductions in liver blood flow and liver size. McLean and Le Couteur (2004) presented evidence that aging of the sinusoidal endothelium reduced oxygen delivery and drug transfer from blood to hepatocytes. Schmucker (2005) and Herrlinger and Klotz (2001) did not find significant relationships between aging and P450 activities in human liver. Cotreau et al. (2005) did describe some reports of age-related decreases in CYP3A4, an isoform of limited relevance to solvent metabolism. Kinirons and O'Mahony (2004) reviewed reports of declining drug metabolism in frail versus healthy elderly. With the exception of an ~70% decline in male-specific CYP2C11, senescence had little effect on pre- or post-phenobarbital induction of expression of some 12 constitutive and inducible P450s in Sprague–Dawley rats (Agrawal and Shapiro, 2003).

Information is available on certain age-related aspects of xenobiotic clearance other than metabolism. Plasma protein binding of drugs generally remains unaltered or diminishes modestly with age (Grandison and Boudinot, 2000). Hepatic and/or renal dysfunction more often account for altered protein binding. No information apparently exists on effects of aging on most transporters (Kinirons and O'Mahony, 2004). Renal clearance diminishes with advancing age, due to parallel annual decreases of ~0 .65% in glomerular filtration and maximal tubular secretory capacity beyond the age of 30 years. The foregoing TK factors may significantly influence tissue dosimetry and in turn responses of geriatric populations to solvents and other chemicals.

PBTK models should be useful for integrating the age-related physiological and metabolic changes into a quantitative framework to forecast their net effect on blood and tissue time courses of parent compounds and metabolites. Very few such "geriatric" models have been published. McMahon et al. (1994) employed a PBTK model to demonstrate that reduced urinary elimination of benzene metabolites by geriatric mice was due to decreased renal blood flow rather than altered formation of metabolites. Corley et al. (2005c) incorporated a number of age-, gender-, and species-specific physiological and biochemical parameters into a preexisting PBTK model for 2-butoxyethanol (BE), in order to predict the kinetics of BE and butoxyacetic acid (BAA), BE's major metabolite, in male and female mice and rats of different ages. The life-stage PBTK model of Clewell and colleagues was used to simulate human blood concentrations of several VOCs and their major metabolite (or metabolic rate) from infancy through the age of 75 years. Blood levels of the parent compounds remained relatively constant during adulthood, but metabolite levels or amounts metabolized frequently varied during the pediatric and geriatric years (Sarangapani et al., 2003). In a subsequent publication, blood levels of PERC and its major metabolite, TCA, were predicted to progressively rise during adulthood and old age by a PBTK model. Clewell et al. (2004) attributed this phenomenon to relatively low pulmonary and metabolic clear-

ance, coupled with accumulation of the lipophilic solvent in ample amounts of adipose tissue. Much work remains to be done to refine these generic PBTK models and to integrate them with significant geriatric PD changes (Burton et al., 2005).

Gender Some of the physiological and biochemical differences between men and women have the potential to alter tissue dosimetry and health effects of certain solvents. Clewell et al. (2002) have provided one of the most recent and comprehensive reviews of the potential impact of gender differences on chemicals' TK. There was no convincing evidence of sex differences in GI absorption rate constants. The investigators located few data on gender-dependent dermal or pulmonary absorption of solvents or other chemicals. Sarangapani et al. (2003) published tables of a number of age-specific factors (e.g., cardiac output, pulmonary ventilation rate, and pulmonary surface area) that dictate pulmonary absorption of VOCs. These rates and values were generally higher for males, but a PBPK model's predictions of steady-state blood concentrations for inhaled isopropanol, styrene, vinyl chloride, and PERC were largely sex independent (Sarangapani et al., 2003).

Distribution of water- and lipid-soluble solvents can vary substantially between men and women (Schwartz, 2003). Most men have more lean body mass and larger body size. Women typically have smaller volumes of distribution for polar solvents, but larger volumes of distribution for lipophilic solvents (Gandhi et al., 2004). Lean body mass decreases from 76 to 52%, and body fat increases from 33 to 49% in females between the ages of 25 years and 65–70 years. Nomiyama and Nomiyama (1974) found that women retain less inhaled acetone and ethyl acetate than similarly exposed men. Levels of toluene and TCE in expired air of females are lower, reflecting greater fat deposition and retention of these lipophilic chemicals. Similarly, women exhibit significantly higher respiratory uptake of 1,3-butadiene, another lipophilic VOC (Lin et al., 2001b). Clewell et al. (2004) utilized their life-stage PBPK model to predict blood levels of PERC and TCA, its major metabolite, in men and women over a lifetime of daily ingestion of 1 μg PERC/kg. The women were predicted to attain significantly higher blood PERC and TCA concentrations, ostensibly due to PERC's greater storage in fat and relatively low pulmonary and metabolic clearance.

The major sex differences in P450-mediated hepatic metabolism in rats are not seen in humans or most other mammals (Nakajima, 1997). Rinn et al. (2004) did recently find many significant differences in gene expression in the liver, kidney, and reproductive tissues of male and female mice. Some of the differentially expressed genes involve drug and steroid metabolism, but the biological significance of these variances is unknown. No marked gender differences in P450-catalyzed oxidation reactions have been identified in humans (Schmucker et al., 1990; Mugford and Kedderis, 1998). Other investigators have described modestly higher levels and activities of certain liver P450s in males, including CYP2E1, CYP1A2, and CYP2D6 (Schwartz, 2003). Many CYP3A substrates do not exhibit sex-dependent differences in clearance, though some researchers reported differences for certain substrates (Cotreau et al., 2005). Gender-specific metabolism data for most hydrocarbon solvents are lacking. Men exhibit somewhat lower blood ethanol levels than women upon ingestion of equal doses, due in part to more extensive ADH-catalyzed metabolism of the alcohol by the male gastric mucosa (Frezza et al., 1990). UDP glucuronyl transferase activity appears to be somewhat higher in males. Women seem to have modestly lower glomerular filtration rates, though information on renal tubular secretion and reabsorption processes is lacking.

A gender-specific PBTK model was developed to assess the relative risks (RRs) of benzene exposures (Brown *et al.*, 1998). Women were found to have a higher blood:air partition coefficient, a higher percent of body fat and higher maximum rate of benzene metabolism than men. Women exhibited higher blood benzene levels and a 23–26% increase in benzene metabolism, potentially placing them at greater risk than men with equivalent exposures.

Relatively little is known about potential influences of contraceptives, hormone replacement therapy, or pregnancy on the metabolism and disposition of xenobiotics (Gleiter and Gundert-Remy, 1996). The menstrual cycle with its hormone changes may influence the metabolism of some xenobiotics (Fletcher *et al.*, 1994). Watanabe *et al.* (1997) found that estradiol changes during the estrous cycle of rats affected both UDP-glucuronyl transferase and NADPH-cytochrome *c* reductase activities. Experiments by Nakajima *et al.* (1992b) demonstrated that pregnancy of rats resulted in significant reductions in hepatic P450 content, as well as the metabolism of both toluene and TCE. Pregnancy results in a 40% increase in tidal volume, which may increase the absorption of inhaled VOCs. Plasma volume increases ~50% in pregnant women, resulting in a decrease in albumin concentration and plasma protein binding of many drugs (Fletcher *et al.*, 1994). Cardiac output increases ~50%, due to increases in stroke volume and heart rate (Silvaggio and Mattison, 1994). Uterine blood flow, renal plasma flow, and glomerular filtration rise substantially, though no information on hepatic blood flow is apparently available. These TK factors need to be considered when assessing risks and setting occupational exposure limits for this subpopulation.

Gentry *et al.* (2003) described an approach for use of PBTK modeling to compare maternal and fetal/neonatal blood and tissue dosimetry during pregnancy and lactation. In general, blood levels of isopropanol, vinyl chloride, MC, and PERC were predicted to be lower in the human neonate during lactation than in the fetus during gestation. Simulated vinyl chloride levels, for example, were 4 orders of magnitude lower in the neonates. Fetal/neonatal isopropanol levels were forecast to be orders of magnitude lower than maternal levels. Corley *et al.* (2003) evaluated the state-of-the-science in PBTK/TD modeling of the developing embryo, fetus, and neonate.

Genetics A variety of genetic polymorphisms for biotransformation have been found to occur at different frequencies in different ethnic groups (Daly *et al.*, 1993). Polymorphisms for xenobiotic-metabolizing enzymes may affect the quantity and quality of enzymes and the outcomes of exposures to solvents (Ingelman-Sundberg *et al.*, 1994). It is important to note that culturally linked environmental factors also contribute to ethnic differences in metabolism and disposition of solvents and other chemicals. It is often difficult to disentangle the influences of genetic traits from those of different lifestyles, socioeconomic status, and geographic settings.

Ethnic differences in regulating the expression of CYP isozymes and other enzymes are associated with some variations in drug and solvent metabolism (Ingelman-Sundberg *et al.*, 1994; Weber, 1999). Shimada *et al.* (1994) found that Caucasians had higher total hepatic CYP levels than Japanese. Caucasians exhibited higher CYP2E1 activities, as reflected by aniline *p*-hydroxylation and 7-ethoxycoumarin *O*-deethylation. Individuals with two linked

polymorphisms in the transcription regulatory region of the CYP2E1 gene exhibited greater expression of the isoform. Reported frequencies of these rare alleles were 2% in Caucasians, 2–5% in African Americans, and 24–27% in Japanese (Kato *et al.*, 1992). Kawamoto *et al.* (1995) found that a CYP2E1 polymorphism in Japanese workers did not affect metabolism of toluene to benzoic acid, but that CYP1A1 and aldehyde dehydrogenase (ALDH2) polymorphisms did. ALDH2 deficiency can result in elevated CNS levels of toluene and benzaldehyde (Wilkins-Haug, 1997) in toluene-exposed individuals. About half of the Japanese population lacks ALDH2, due to a structural point mutation in the ALDH2 gene. Pronounced interethnic differences in rates of ethanol metabolism have been associated with a number of ADH and ALDH polymorphisms (Pastino *et al.*, 2000).

Ethnic differences have been demonstrated for some phase II biotransformation reactions. Glutathione *S*-transferases (GSTs) are a family of enzymes, some of which promote the detoxification of electrophilic metabolites by catalyzing their conjugation with reduced glutathione (GSH). GST theta-mediated conjugation with GSH is the first step in metabolic activation of MC to formaldehyde, a putative carcinogen. Individuals with a null/null genotype for GST theta are thus at a lower risk of developing cancer from MC (El-Masri *et al.*, 1999). The prevalence of this genotype ranges from 10% in Mexican Americans to 60–65% in Chinese and Koreans (Nelson *et al.*, 1995). GSTs participate in conjugating relatively small percentages of doses of TCE (Lash *et al.*, 2000b) and PERC (Lash and Parker, 2001). These pathways, however, can lead to production of cytotoxic, mutagenic metabolites in the kidney. No information was located on the influence of GST polymorphisms on TCE kidney cancer risks.

Increased susceptibility to different cancers has been reported to be associated with certain genetic polymorphisms, which occur with different frequencies in different ethnic groups (Daly *et al.*, 1993; Raunio *et al.*, 1995). Significant variations in allelic distributions for isoforms including CYP2E1, CYP2D6, CYP1A1, and GSTM1 have been observed in different racial groups. Results of investigations of relationships between occurrence of defective alleles for CYP2E1 and cancer incidence have been contradictory. Studies with more statistical power of selected ethnic groups need to be conducted to clarify the roles of CYP polymorphisms in cancers. Although molecular markers clearly indicate variances in CYP genes, biologically plausible mechanisms linking specific genotypes with specific outcomes are lacking at present.

Genetic polymorphisms, variable transporter activities, genetic variants of receptors and regulatory proteins, and environmental factors can play roles in individual variability in P450 induction (Tang *et al.*, 2005). Lipscomb *et al.* (1997) described substantial differences in activity and/or content of CYP2E1 within the U.S. population. Lipscomb (2004) incorporated extremes in CYP2E1-mediated metabolism into a PBTK model for TCE and learned there was very little impact on TCA dosimetry. Intersubject differences in hepatic blood flow did have a pronounced effect on TCE biotransformation, as TCE is an extensively metabolized (liver blood flow limited) compound. Wenker *et al.* (2001) similarly reported that interindividual genetic polymorphisms in CYP2E1 and several other CYPs did not affect the metabolism of styrene, another flow-limited compound. Kedderis (1997) utilized a PBTK-modeling approach to confirm this phenomenon, but found the opposite to be true for poorly metabolized (capacity limited) VOCs such as PERC and CCl$_4$ (i.e., interindividual differences in metabolic capacity may significantly affect their biotransformation). Haber *et al.* (2002) integrated human data on the incidence of a GST null polymorphism with a PBTK model for MC to forecast an ~30% decrease in the mean population cancer risk.

Exogenous Factors

P450 Inducers   Considerable effort has been devoted to investigation of effects of enzyme inducers on solvent metabolism and toxicity. Preexposure to drugs and other chemicals, which induce CYP isoforms that metabolically activate particular solvents, can markedly potentiate the solvents' toxicity. As described in the subsection on Metabolism, CYP2E1 is a high-affinity, low-capacity isoform responsible for activation of a wide variety of low-molecular-weight hydrocarbon and halocarbon solvents to cytotoxins and mutagens (Guengerich *et al.*, 1991). A number of CYP2E1 substrates (e.g., ethanol and other alcohols, acetone and other ketones, pyridine and pyridazine, isoniazid, acetaminophen, and chlorzoxazone) can act as inducers of the isoform. Preexposure to many of these can thus markedly increase the metabolic activation and adverse effects of certain solvents. The minimal hepatocytotoxicity caused by CCl_4 alone (Panel B, Fig. 24-4) can be contrasted with the centrilobular necrosis (Panel C, Fig. 24-4) in rats pretreated with 2-butanol before the same CCl_4 dose (Traiger and Bruckner, 1976). CYP2E1 is present in many organs and tissues, as are other CYPs that metabolize solvents. Although levels/activities are highest in liver, induction in extrahepatic tissues can result in increased metabolic activation in situ that may be toxicologically significant. It is worthy of note that many chemicals that induce P450s also induce detoxifying enzymes (e.g., epoxide hydrolase, glucuronyl- and sulfotransferases). A number of naturally occurring organosulfur compounds in allium vegetables have been demonstrated to induce these enzymes in the liver, kidney, intestines, and lungs of Wistar rats (Guyonnet *et al.*, 1999).

It should be recognized that timing of exposures to ≥ 2 P450 inducers is important. Sato *et al.* (1991) demonstrated that alcohol competitively inhibited the biotransformation of TCE when the exposures were concurrent. Alternatively, preexposure to ethanol stimulated TCE metabolism. As described previously in the Metabolism subsection, increased metabolic capacity in an individual is of little consequence for environmentally encountered levels of blood-flow-limited (i.e., extensively metabolized) solvents (e.g., TCE, vinyl chloride, MC, and $CHCl_3$). Thus, genetically predisposed or induced individuals should be at no greater cancer risk from these solvents than the average person.

P450 Inhibitors   An increasing number of drugs and other chemicals, dietary supplements, fruit juices, and vegetable constituents are being identified as inhibitors and/or inducers of P450s, Phase II enzymes, and efflux transporters (Halpert *et al.*, 1994; Lin and Lu, 2001; Huang and Lesko, 2004). It should be recalled that mechanisms of P450 inhibition can be categorized as reversible, quasi-reversible, and irreversible. Reversible inhibition is transient, with the normal function of the CYP continuing after elimination of the inhibitor. Both quasi- and irreversible inhibitions result from the enzyme's formation of a reactive metabolite. With quasi-reversible inhibition, the metabolite and enzyme form a complex that is so stable that the intact enzyme may be unavailable for further metabolism. With mechanism based or suicide inhibition, the reactive metabolite irreversibly inhibits the enzyme by binding to its active site. Experiments by Lilly *et al.* (1998) indicate that this is the mechanism by which epoxide metabolites of *trans*- and *cis*-1,2-dichloroethylene

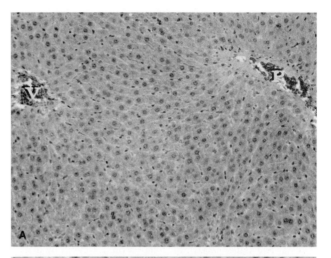

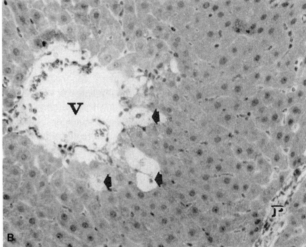

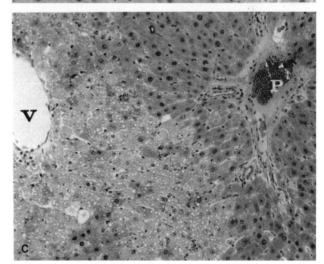

Figure 24-4. Potentiation of CCl_4 hepatotoxicity by 2-butanol.

Rats were (A) untreated; (B) given 0.1 mL/kg CCl_4/kg IP; or (C) pretreated with 2-butanol (2.2 mL/kg PO) 16 hours before 0.1 mL/kg CCl_4 IP. Cenral veins and portal triads are designated V and P, respectively. Occasional hepatocytes adjacent to the central vein are vacuolated in (B). Note the demarcation between vacuolated/necrotic centrilobular and midzonal cells, and normally appearing periportal cells in (C). Hematoxylin and eosin stain. (A) and (C) ×315; (B) ×480. [Reproduced from Traiger and Bruckner, 1976, with permission from ASPET.]

inhibit CYP2E1. Fisher *et al.* (2004) subsequently reported that metabolites generated from a single oral dose of CC1$_4$ as low as 1 mg/kg are suicide inhibitors of CYP2E1 and CYP2B2 in B6C3F1 mice. The net result of this action by CC1$_4$ is reduced formation of TCA from coadministered PERC. However, Blobaum (2006) recently described reversible inactivation of CYP2E and CYP2B isoforms during their mechanism-based inactivation by small *tert*-butyl terminal alkynes.

Flavanoids in grapefruit juice were one of the first classes of naturally occurring compounds to be documented to produce clinically significant increases in levels of therapeutic agents metabolized by CYP3A4 (Chan *et al.*, 1998). Flavanoids in red wine exerted a similar effect on intestinal CYP3A4, but white wine had little influence. Bergamottin, a furanocoumarin in grapefruit and lime juice, was subsequently found to inhibit human CYP3A4 activity (Bailey *et al.*, 2003) as well as intestinal P-glycoprotein efflux transporters (Dresser and Bailey, 2003). St. John's wort, a top-selling dietary supplement taken for depression, selectively induced CYP3A4 in the small intestine (Huang and Lesko, 2004). Echinacea inhibited human intestinal CYP3A, but induced hepatic CYP3A. Ginsenosides exhibited no or weak inhibition of several human CYPs, but some of the compounds' major intestinal metabolites inhibited a wide range of CYPs (Liu *et al.*, 2006). Certain components of ginko biloba, frequently used for memory impairment, were potent inhibitors of human recombinant CYP1B1, CYP1A1, and CYP1A2 (Chang *et al.*, 2006). Identification of isoform-selective, nontoxic inhibitors may eventually lead to modulation of human xenobiotic metabolism for therapeutic purposes (Halpert *et al.*, 1994). There are large interindividual responses to CYP enzyme inducers and inhibitors (Lin and Lu, 2001).

Physical Activity Exercise can significantly affect the kinetics of xenobiotics (van Baak, 1990), but is often not considered in occupational risk assessments of solvents. Exercise increases two of the major determinants of VOC uptake, alveolar ventilation rate, and cardiac output/pulmonary blood flow. Polar solvents with relatively high blood:air PCs (e.g., acetone, ethanol, and ethylene glycol) are very rapidly absorbed into the pulmonary circulation. Alveolar ventilation is rate limiting for these chemicals. In contrast, pulmonary blood flow and metabolism are rate limiting for uptake of the more lipophilic solvents (Johanson and Filser, 1992). Heavy exercise can increase pulmonary uptake of relatively polar solvents as much as five-fold in human subjects (Astrand, 1983). Light exercise doubles uptake of relatively lipid-soluble solvents, but no further increases occur at higher workloads. Blood flow to the liver and kidneys diminishes with exercise, so biotransformation of well-metabolized solvents and urinary elimination of polar metabolites may be diminished (Lof and Johanson, 1998). Dankovic and Bailer (1994) modified the human PBTK model of Reitz *et al.* (1989) for MC to reflect light work conditions. The modified model predicted that light exercise would result in a two-fold increase in hepatic MC deposition and in metabolite formation via P450- and GSH-dependent pathways. Jonsson *et al.* (2001) developed a population PBTK model for humans inhaling MC during moderate-to-heavy exercise. The focus of the study was on interindividual variability in MC metabolism and TK introduced by increased hepatic perfusion rates.

Diet Dietary habits can influence the absorption, metabolism, and toxicity of solvents in several ways. Factors that influence gastric emptying would not be expected to influence systemic absorption of VOCs, as they are so rapidly absorbed by passive diffusion throughout the GI tract. The mere bulk of food in the GI lumen, however, can inhibit absorption by preventing contact of the chemical with the GI epithelium. VOCs in the GI tract partition into dietary lipids, largely remaining there until the lipids are emulsified and absorbed. This serves to substantially delay uptake of lipophilic solvents such as CC1$_4$, resulting in lower, prolonged blood CC1$_4$ levels and diminished hepatotoxicity in rats (Kim *et al.*, 1990a). Food intake increases splanchnic blood flow, which favors GI absorption. The elevation in liver blood flow would be expected to enhance the biotransformation of low doses of well-metabolized solvents, but to have little effect on first-pass metabolism of relatively high (i.e., saturating) doses (Tam, 1993). Consumption of a high-fat diet results in a selective increase in hepatic CYP2E1 activity and protein levels in male Sprague–Dawley rats (Raucy *et al.*, 1991). Elevation of plasma ketone bodies appears to be implicated in this process, because acetone is a potent CYP2E1 inducer. Carbohydrate deficiency has been recognized for many years to enhance the metabolism of a series of VOCs in rats, but not to alter their conjugation (Sato and Nakajima, 1985). High protein diets and diets low in protein and high in carbohydrates lead to CYP1A2 increases and decreases, respectively (Glue and Clement, 1999). Psoralens (found in parsley, parsnip, and celery) reduce CYP1A2 activity, whereas food cooked over charcoal enhances it. Effects of other foods, fruit juices, and food supplements are addressed in the preceding subsections on P450 Inducers and Inhibitors.

Fasting results in decreased liver GSH levels due to interrupted intake of amino acids required for its synthesis. GSH plays a key role in the detoxification of electrophilic metabolites of a number of solvents. Short-term fasting ($\sim$8–24 hours) results in induction of liver CYP2E1 and increase in metabolism of a number of aromatic hydrocarbons and halocarbons (Nakajima *et al.*, 1982). The hepatotoxicity of CC1$_4$, which requires CYP2E1-catalyzed metabolic activation, is more severe in fasted animals. In contrast, long-term food deprivation (i.e., starvation) results in decreased synthesis and activity of P450s.

Clock Time Many physiological and biochemical processes that impact solvent TK exhibit circadian, or diurnal rhythms. A series of investigations have been conducted to delineate molecular control mechanisms of diurnal oscillation in mammals. The phenomenon appears to be controlled by a "master pacemaker" in the suprachiasmatic nuclei (SCN) of the hypothalamus of mice (Panda *et al.*, 2002). Genetic and genomic analyses of the SCN and liver indicate that a relatively small number of output genes are directly regulated by core oscillator components. Rate-limiting steps in major cellular pathways/processes are being identified as key sites of circadian regulation. Recent experiments reveal that transcriptional feedback is required for maintenance of circadian rhythmicity (Sato *et al.*, 2006).

Several research groups have discovered circadian rhythms in susceptibility of rats to liver damage by various VOCs, including CC1$_4$, CHC1$_3$, 1,1-dichloroethylene (1,1-DCE), ethanol, and styrene (Labrecque and Belanger, 1991). In each instance, the chemicals were most toxic when given during the initial part of the rodents' dark/active cycle. Low hepatic GSH levels at this time were an important contributing factor to the increased liver injury by 1,1-DCE and CHC1$_3$. Restricted food intake during sleep resulted in lipolysis and formation of acetone, which contributed to the diurnal induction of CYP2E1 and the ensuing increases in hepatic metabolic activation and cytotoxicity of CCl_4 in male rats during the early part of the animals' active cycle (Bruckner *et al.*, 2002). Skrzypinska-Gawrysiak *et al.* (2000) also observed that male mice were most susceptible to CCl_4 hepatotoxicity when dosed at a similar time. Furukawa *et al.* (1999) attributed high hepatic microsomal 7-alkoxycoumarin *O*-dealkylase activity during male rats' active cycle to diurnal secretion of growth hormone. Clearance rates for a number of well-metabolized compounds, including ethanol (Sturtevant *et al.*, 1978) and nicotine (Gries *et al.*, 1996), are maximal in human subjects during the first part of their active/wake cycle. Hepatic blood flow and acetone levels in expired air of humans peak before breakfast. Thus, humans may also be more susceptible during this time to the toxicity of solvents that undergo metabolic activation.

Diseases Illness can be a major source of variability in response to solvents. Impaired drug metabolism and clearance are commonly seen in patients with cirrhosis and hepatitis (Welling and Pool, 1996). Reduced metabolism of solvents may result from decrease in hepatic parenchymal mass, diminished enzymatic activity, and/or decreased portal blood flow (McLean and Morgan, 1991). Lower levels of CYP2E1, CYP1A2 and GSH are seen in livers of patients with cirrhosis (Murray, 1992). Reduced P450-catalyzed metabolic activation of certain solvents can be protective, but diminished capacity to conjugate electrophilic metabolites with GSH would have the opposite effect. Plasma levels of albumin and a_1-acid glycoprotein fall in cirrhotic patients. Thus, plasma protein binding of many xenobiotic metabolites decreases and their rate of elimination increases (McLean and Morgan, 1991). Definitive information is lacking, however, on the net effect of common liver diseases on solvents.

Chronic kidney disease is becoming increasingly prevalent in the United States over the past decade (Dowling, 2002). Progressive loss of kidney function leads to impaired renal excretion of numerous chemicals and metabolites that may be toxic or pharmacologically active. Renal failure can result in downregulation of the expression of some liver P450s, but have no effect on others (Leblond *et al.*, 2001). Effects on hepatic clearance of therapeutic chemicals can thus vary widely. The mechanisms of these effects on gene expression are unclear, as is their applicability to solvents. The plasma protein binding of many xenobiotics is reduced in patients with compromised renal function, apparently due to retention of substances that compete for protein-binding sites, as well as reduced albumin synthesis. Clearance of highly metabolized xenobiotics thus appears to depend on potentially offsetting influences of altered metabolism, decreased plasma protein binding, and decreased renal excretion (Yuan and Venitz, 2000). Impairment of renal metabolic activation via oxidation or β-lyase-mediated conversion of GSH metabolic intermediates of TCE and PERC (see subsections on these chemicals for details) to reactive, mutagenic metabolites would be protective.

Diabetes mellitus is a metabolic disease characterized by hyperglycemia as a result of insulin deficiency (Type I) or insulin resistance (Type II). Type II accounts for 90% of cases. Approximately 21 million people suffer from diabetes in the United States. A prominent effect of chemically induced Type I diabetes in rats is induction of CYP2E1. Elevation of acetone, but apparently not the other ketone bodies is responsible for the CYP2E1 increase. Hypoinsulinemia may play a role, in that insulin downregulates CYP2E1 mRNA in rat hepatoma cells and primary cultures of rat hepatocytes (Cheng and Morgan, 2001). In contrast, CYP2E1 is not affected in Type II diabetic animals (Sawant *et al.*, 2004). Neither Type I nor Type II diabetes influences CYP2E1 activity in humans (Lucas *et al.*, 1998; Cheng and Morgan, 2001). Nevertheless, animal studies show that Type II diabetes increases susceptibility to hepatotoxicants including allyl alcohol and CCl_4 (Sawant *et al.*, 2004), apparently due to inhibition of tissue repair. Devi and Mehendale (2005, 2006) subsequently demonstrated inhibition of expression of genes involved in cell division and protease inhibitors, as well as enhanced gene expression of proteases in Type I diabetic rats. These events may be important in delayed tissue repair following chemical cytotoxicity in diabetics.

Persons with bacterial infections may be more sensitive to cytotoxic actions of solvents. Endotoxin, which includes a lipopolysaccharide, is released from the cell wall of gram-negative organisms. The lipopolysaccharide causes the release of inflammatory mediators, which alter cell membranes, intercellular signaling, and gene expression (Roth *et al.*, 1997). These effects may render cells more susceptible to damage by solvents and other chemicals. Exposure of animals to small amounts of endotoxin potentiates liver injury by CCl_4, halothane, allyl alcohol, ethanol, and other solvents (Roth *et al.*, 1997). Endotoxin apparently activates Kupffer cells to release inflammatory mediators and cytotoxic moieties to hepatocytes (Thurman, 1998).

CHLORINATED HYDROCARBONS

Trichloroethylene

TCE is a widely used solvent identified at over one-half of the nearly 1300 hazardous waste sites that make up the EPA's National Priorities List (ATSDR, 2006a). TCE is released into the atmosphere from vapor degreasing operations; however, direct discharges to surface waters and groundwater from disposal operations have been frequent occurrences. As a result, TCE can be released to indoor air by vapor intrusion through underground walls and floors and by volatilization from the water supply. TCE has recently received a great deal of attention from the scientific and regulatory communities, due in large part to the EPA's efforts to update the chemical's two-decade-old risk assessment.

Moderate-to-high doses of TCE, as with other halocarbons, are associated with a number of noncancer toxicities (Barton and Das, 1996). TCE has been implicated in the development of autoimmune disorders and immune system dysfunction (Gilbert *et al.*, 1999; Blossom and Gilbert, 2006), and has been investigated for its potential as a male reproductive toxicant (Forkert *et al.*, 2003; Xu *et al.*, 2004). The effect of gestational exposure to TCE or its oxidative metabolites on cardiac development is a subject that has invoked considerable debate, as conflicting results exist (Fisher *et al.*, 2001; Johnson *et al.*, 2003; Watson *et al.*, 2006). The issue of TCE's effect on ocular development has also recently reemerged (Warren *et al.*, 2006). Cancer remains the dominant issue for TCE, however. Attempts to understand the mechanistic underpinnings of TCE's carcinogenicity in rodent models and their relevance to humans have resulted in a massive body of published data. Nonetheless, uncertainties remain that plague the risk-assessment process. Even so, TCE provides a stellar example of how research can be utilized to generate experimental and epidemiological data for use in a regulatory context. A 16-article series of state-of-the-science papers, upon which the EPA relied heavily for its 2001 draft risk assessment, was published (Scott and Cogliano, 2000).

Cancer Epidemiology   There are many published studies of cancer incidence and mortality among TCE-exposed populations including Morgan *et al.* (1998), Blair *et al.* (1998), Boice *et al.* (1999), and Ritz (1999), of whom all but the latter examined cancer mortality or incidence among aircraft-manufacturing or maintenance workers. In addition to these U.S. studies, the mortality/incidence experiences of Swedish, Finnish, German, and Danish worker cohorts have been examined (Axelson *et al.*, 1994; Anttila *et al.*, 1995; Henschler *et al.*, 1995; Hansen *et al.*, 2001; Raaschou-Nielsen *et al.*, 2003). Most of the studies mentioned above constitute what the meta-like analysis of Wartenberg *et al.* (2000) referred to as Tier I studies, meaning TCE exposure was better characterized than in cohort studies in lower tiers. Thus, Tier I studies received a greater weighting from Wartenberg and colleagues when making causal inferences than lower-tier cohort studies, case–control studies, and community-based studies. Among the Tier I studies, evidence for an excess incidence of cancer was strongest for the kidney (RR = 1.7, 95% confidence interval (CI) = 1.1–2.7), liver (RR = 1.9, 95% CI = 1.0–3.4), and non-Hodgkin's lymphoma (NHL) (RR = 1.5, 95% CI = 0.9–2.3). These investigators also contend that the data support weak associations between TCE exposure and multiple myeloma, Hodgkin's disease, and cancers of the prostate, skin, and cervix.

While not as comprehensive as that of Wartenberg *et al.* (2000), other reviews of epidemiological studies have been conducted. Weiss (1996) concluded that the evidence for the carcinogenicity of TCE was "quite limited." He acknowledged that there was some suggestive evidence that TCE could possibly be associated with NHL and cancers of the liver, biliary tract, and kidney. Another review of cohort and case–control studies concluded that the totality of the evidence did not support a role for TCE in renal cell cancer (RCC) (McLaughlin and Blot, 1997). Morgan *et al.* (1998) combined their data with that of others in a meta-analysis-like approach that resulted in slight, statistically insignificant elevations in meta-standardized mortality ratios for cancers of the liver, prostate, kidney, bladder, and NHL. More recent reviews of the epidemiological literature have reported either no significant increases in cancer risk (Wong, 2004; Alexander *et al.*, 2006), or a modest positive association in the case of TCE exposure and NHL (Mandel *et al.*, 2006).

The report of Henschler *et al.* (1995) was the first in a series of German studies that has provided the strongest evidence to date for an association between TCE and RCC. These authors reported on a cohort of male cardboard factory workers who were exposed to moderate to extremely high concentrations of TCE. By the closing date of the study, five of the 169 exposed workers had been diagnosed with kidney cancer versus none of the 190 controls. This resulted in standardized incidence ratios (SIRs) of 7.97 (95% CI = 2.59–18.59) and 9.66 (95% CI = 3.14–22.55), using Danish and German Cancer Registry data for comparison, respectively. A single U.S. study had previously reported a weaker, but significantly elevated SIR for RCC (SIR = 3.7, 95% CI = 1.4–8.1) among paperboard workers exposed to TCE (Sinks *et al.*, 1992). German researchers also conducted a hospital-based case–control study with 58 RCC patients and 84 patients from accident wards who served as controls. Of the 58 RCC patients, 19 had histories of occupational TCE exposure for at least 2 years, compared to only five of the controls. After adjustment for potential confounders, an association between RCC and long-term exposure to TCE was reported [odds ratio (OR) = 10.80, 95% CI = 3.36–34.75] (Vamvakas *et al.*, 1998). These studies find some support in a recently published case–control study of TCE exposure and RCC risk conducted in France (Charbotel *et al.*, 2006).

The studies detailed above provide some evidence of a link between kidney cancer and TCE, although the link may be operative only under very high exposure conditions. As will be discussed later, the application of molecular biology techniques to the issue of TCE and kidney cancer has strengthened the argument for a causal association. Controversy surrounds the German studies, as indicated in a critical review by Green and Lash (1999) to which the researchers responded (Vamvakas *et al.*, 2000).

Metabolism   With rare exception, the toxicities associated with TCE are thought to be mediated by metabolites rather than parent compound. Even the CNS-depressant effects of TCE are due in part to the sedative properties of the metabolites, trichloroethanol (TCOH) and chloroform. Understanding TCE's metabolism is thus a prerequisite to elucidating its mechanisms of action and accurately assessing human risks. Much experimental effort has been expended to this end.

TCE is rapidly absorbed into the systemic circulation via the oral and inhalation routes. The majority of TCE undergoes oxidation in the liver by CYPs, with a small proportion being conjugated with GSH via GSTs. Thus, two distinct metabolic pathways exist for TCE. The oxidative pathway is shown to the left in Fig. 24-5, and the GSH pathway is shown to the right (Lash *et al.*, 2005). This schematic represents a simplification of what is a complex metabolic scheme, as detailed in the state-of-the-science paper by Lash *et al.* (2000a). As shown, TCE may be oxidized to yield one of three initial metabolites: chloral, TCE-epoxide, and dichloroacetylchloride. These metabolites rapidly undergo oxidation and/or reduction to yield trichloroacetate (TCA) and TCOH, the major end products of the oxidative pathway. TCOH is either oxidized to TCA or glucuronidated. TCOH glucuronide is excreted via the urine and bile. That in the bile may undergo enterohepatic recirculation by hydrolysis to TCOH in the gut, with reabsorption and the possibility of conversion to TCA. TCA accumulates in the body due to strong plasma protein binding and slow excretion. In contrast, blood levels of DCA, formed by TCA dechlorination or from TCOH, are very low or nondetectable in humans.

Relatively small amounts of TCE can be conjugated in the liver with GSH to form *S*-(1,2-dichlorovinyl)glutathione (DCVG). DCVG is then effluxed from the hepatocyte into plasma and bile for translocation to the kidney and small intestine, respectively. The plasma DCVG is intrarenally converted by γ-glutamyltransferase and dipeptidases to the cysteine conjugate *S*-(1,2-dichlorovinyl)-L-cysteine (DCVC). The DCVG secreted into bile can undergo extrarenal processing to DCVC, that is subsequently delivered to the kidney by enterohepatic recirculation. DCVC represents a branch point in the pathway. It may be detoxified through *N*-acetylation or bioactivated to reactive thiols via renal β-lyase located in renal proximal tubular cells (or to a lesser extent, bioactivated to DCVC sulfoxide via flavin-containing monooxygenases).

Modes of Action in Target Tissues   Both metabolic pathways are implicated in the carcinogenicity of TCE: reactive metabolite(s) of the GSH pathway in kidney tumors in rats, and oxidative metabolites in liver and lung tumors of mice. That tumor formation in many cases is species-, strain-, sex-, and route of exposure –dependent has provided clues as to TCE's modes of carcinogenic action. Whereas substantial progress has been made on the mechanistic front, the reader should not infer from the text that follows that all modes of action are known with absolute certainty. Rather, they should

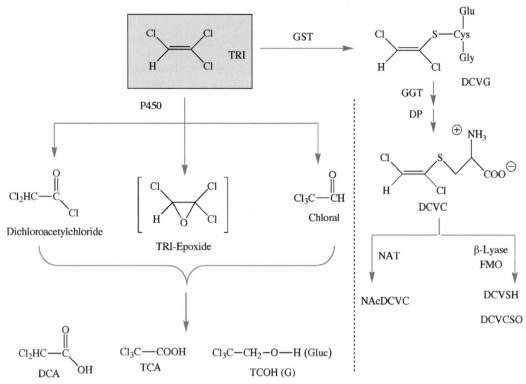

Figure 24-5. General scheme of metabolism for TCE.

Abbreviations: β-lyase, cysteine conjugate β-lyase; DCA, dichloroacetate; DCVC, S-(1,2-dichlorovinyl)-L-cysteine; DCVSH, 1,2-dichlorovinylthiol; DCVCSO, DCVC sulfoxide; DCVG, S-(1,2-dichlorovinyl)glutathione; DP, dipeptidase; FMO, flavin-containing monooxygenase; GGT, γ-glutamyltransferase; GST, GSH S-transferase; P450, cytochrome P450; TCA, trichloroacetate; TCOH, trichloroethanol; TCOG, TCOH glucuronide.
[Reproduced from Lash *et al.* (2005), with permission from Elsevier.]

be considered working hypotheses that await further experimental confirmation.

Liver Cancer   TCE induces malignant liver cancer in B6C3F1 mice but not in other strains of mice or in rats. This differential susceptibility can be explained by the greater capacity of the mouse to metabolize TCE via the oxidative pathway. B6C3F1 mice also develop liver tumors when chloral hydrate (CH), TCA, and DCA are administered in high doses, suggesting that one or more of these metabolites are ultimately responsible for TCE-induced liver cancer. Of the three, TCA and/or DCA are/is most likely responsible, as TCE metabolism results in extremely low blood levels of CH due to its rapid oxidation to TCA or reduction to TCOH. The sensitivity of B6C3F1 mice to TCE further suggests that liver tumor formation might be related to the abnormally high frequency of spontaneously initiated cells in this mouse strain, which manifests itself as an unusually high background liver tumor incidence. While TCA and/or DCA might induce liver tumors in B6C3F1 mice by simply promoting preexisting initiated cells, the finding that DCA (but not TCA) also induces liver tumors in F-344 rats suggests that another mechanism might also be operable.

As for a promotional mechanism for TCE, peroxisome proliferation represents a more viable mechanism than does overt cytotoxicity and reparative cell proliferation. As peroxisomes contain a variety of oxidative enzymes, peroxisome proliferation results in an increased potential for oxidative DNA damage and decreased gap junctional intercellular communication, both of which have been im-

plicated in neoplastic transformation. At tumorigenic doses, TCA induces sustained peroxisome proliferation in B6C3F1 mice. The peroxisome-proliferative response to DCA is transient, however, and requires a dose higher than that capable of inducing tumors. Therefore, a primary role for TCA is likely if liver tumor promotion occurs via peroxisome proliferation. Research supports a dominant role for the peroxisome proliferator-activated receptor alpha (PPAR-α) in mediating the effects associated with hepatocarcinogenesis upon TCE exposure of mice, including hepatocellular proliferation and most gene expression changes in the liver (Laughter *et al.*, 2004).

An alternative promotional mechanism is suggested by evidence that TCA and DCA depress replication rates of normal hepatocytes, conferring a selective growth advantage to initiated tumorigenic cells. This is referred to as *negative selection*. At high tumorigenic doses, DCA (but not TCA) is thought to stimulate cell replication within tumors. Interestingly, DCA tumors overexpress the insulin receptor relative to surrounding normal tissue. As overexpression of the insulin receptor is associated with the suppression of transforming growth factor-β 1 (TGF-β1)-induced apoptosis in human liver cells, it is conceivable that DCA could promote cancer by a dual mechanism: enhanced mitotic activity and decreased apoptotic activity of preneoplastic cells.

Experimental efforts continue to discern the contributions of TCA and DCA to the induction of liver tumors in mice by TCE (Bull *et al.*, 2002). Data suggest that if both contribute, they do so by distinct mechanisms, because DCA-promoted liver tumors differ phenotypically from those of TCA. DCA- and TCA-induced tumors also differ as to whether their depression of cytosine methylation is reversible upon cessation of treatment (Tao *et al.*, 1998). This is particularly important as DNA hypomethylation, including that of the proto-oncogenes c-jun and c-myc, may be an epigenetic mechanism for the tumorigenicity of DCA and TCA (Tao *et al.*, 2004). It appears that hypomethylation due to TCA and DCA induces DNA replication and prevents the methylation of newly synthesized strands of DNA (Ge *et al.*, 2001). Tao *et al.* (2000) have reported that DCA and TCA do so by virtue of their depletion of *S*-adenosylmethionine (SAM), which normally supplies the methyl group for the methylation process. A comprehensive review of mechanisms by which TCE may induce liver cancer can be found in the state-of-the-science paper by Bull (2000).

Kidney Cancer TCE exposure by inhalation or ingestion results in kidney tumors in male but not female rats. The susceptibility of the male rat can be explained by its greater capacity for TCE metabolism via the GSH pathway. TCE-induced kidney tumors are believed to result from reactive metabolite(s) of this pathway, particularly DCVC. DCVC is bioactivated in proximal tubular cells to a reactive thiol, *S*-(1,2-dichlorovinyl)thiol, which is chemically unstable and rearranges to reactive species capable of alkylating cellular nucleophiles, including DNA. The resulting DNA mutations can lead to alterations in gene expression, which in turn apparently lead to neoplastic transformation and tumorigenesis via a genotoxic mode of action.

Alternatively, there are many processes that can lead to proximal tubular cytotoxicity and subsequent tumor formation via a nongenotoxic mode of action. Reactive metabolites formed within proximal tubular cells exposed to high doses of DCVC result in oxidative stress, alkylation of cytosolic and mitochondrial proteins, marked ATP depletion, and perturbations of Ca^{2+} homeostasis. Tubular necrosis ensues, with subsequent reparative proliferation that can alter gene expression and, in turn, alter the regulation of cell growth and differentiation. Modes of action for TCE-induced kidney tumor formation are discussed in greater detail by Lash *et al.* (2000b) in their state-of-the-science paper, and more recently by Lock and Reed (2006).

Animal studies typically provide insight into mode of action, but in the case of TCE-induced RCC, human studies have been of significant value. Bruning *et al.* (1997a) analyzed tumor tissues from 23 RCC patients with occupational histories of long-term, high-level TCE exposure. Tumor cell DNA was isolated and analyzed for somatic mutations of the von-Hippel Lindau (VHL) tumor suppressor gene. Compared to VHL gene mutation rates of 33–55% in TCE-unexposed RCC patients, all 23 TCE-exposed RCC patients exhibited aberrations of the VHL gene. In a follow-up study, Brauch *et al.* (1999) sought to determine whether TCE produced a specific mutational effect in the VHL gene. These investigators analyzed VHL gene sequences in DNA isolated from renal cell tumors from patients exposed to high levels of TCE in metal-processing factories. Renal cell tumors of TCE-exposed patients showed somatic VHL mutations in 33 of 44 cases (75%). Of the 33 cases with VHL mutations, a specific mutational hot spot at VHL nucleotide 454 was observed in 13 cases. The nucleotide 454 mutation was not found in any of the 107 RCC patients without TCE exposure or among 97 healthy subjects, 47 of whom had a history of TCE exposure. These data suggest that the VHL gene might be a specific and susceptible target of TCE, a concept strengthened by a more recent study reporting the VHL mutation frequency among TCE-exposed versus nonexposed RCC patients (Brauch *et al.*, 2004).

Bruning and Bolt (2000) suggest that reactive metabolite(s) of the GSH pathway may have a genotoxic effect on the proximal tubule of the human kidney, but that full development of a malignant tumor requires a promotional effect such as cell proliferation in response to tubular damage. If this is true, then RCC secondary to TCE exposure would be a threshold response. The question of whether chronic tubular damage occurs in renal tumor formation is thus an important one. Answers have come from the use of electrophoresis to examine protein excretion patterns in the urine of RCC patients with and without a history of chronic, high-level TCE exposure (Bruning *et al.*, 1996). Protein excretion patterns indicative of tubular damage were identified in all 17 TCE-exposed cases, but in only about one-half of the 35 controls. This observation suggests that chronic tubular damage may be a prerequisite to TCE-induced RCC. Bruning *et al.* (1999) subsequently published a larger study supportive of this concept.

That TCE induces kidney tumors via a threshold-dependent process is supported by the occurrence of human RCC only among cases with unusually high and prolonged TCE exposure. However, factors other than the intensity and duration of exposure may determine one's susceptibility to TCE-induced RCC. Bruning *et al.* (1997b) have investigated the influence of GST isozyme polymorphisms on RCC risk using long-term, highly exposed workers with or without RCC. These investigators reported an unequal distribution of GSTμ1 and GSTθ1 polymorphisms among RCC cases and controls, which suggested a higher risk for RCC in TCE-exposed persons carrying either the GSTθ1 or GSTμ1 polymorphic gene. GSTμ is thought to function to detoxify reactive electrophiles, while GSTθ is primarily involved in conjugation reactions.

Harth *et al.* (2005) have published a recent review that concludes that TCE can be considered a renal carcinogen for which a practical threshold exists. Further support for a threshold comes from the use of the Eker rat model that carries a germline alteration of the tuberous sclerosis 2 (Tsc-2) tumor suppressor gene. This mutation results in an increased susceptibility to spontaneous and carcinogen-induced RCC, as tumors arise after inactivation of the remaining normal allele of the Tsc-2 gene. Mally *et al.* (2006) exposed Eker rats to TCE and rat kidney epithelial cells carrying the Tsc-2 mutation to DCVC. TCE did not initiate malignant transformation of renal epithelial cells in vivo, whereas DCVC reduced cell survival by 50% and transformed rat kidney epithelial cells in vitro to a neoplastic phenotype. Importantly, DCVC's transformation did not involve mutations in the VHL or Tsc-2 tumor suppressor genes, suggesting that renal tumor formation by DCVC is not the result of altered genes critical for renal tumor development, but rather toxic injury and regenerative repair. While the above study was conducted with rat kidney epithelial cells, efforts to understand the action of DCVC at the molecular level are being explored in cultured human renal proximal tubular cells (HRPTC) (Lash *et al.*, 2005). Such efforts include that of Lock *et al.* (2006), who have reported gene expression changes in HRPTC following DCVC treatment. Interestingly, DCVC has been a model nephrotoxicant in a series of recent studies to investigate the circumstances under which renal tissue repair might occur after exposure rather than a progression to renal failure (Vaidya *et al.*, 2003; Korrapati *et al.*, 2006; Dnyanmote *et al.*, 2006).

Lung Cancer As discussed in the state-of-the science paper by Green (2000), inhaled TCE is carcinogenic to the mouse lung but not to that of the rat. Oral TCE is not carcinogenic to the lung, probably due to first-pass hepatic metabolism that limits the amount of TCE reaching the organ. The primary target of TCE in the mouse lung is the nonciliated Clara cell. Cytotoxicity is characterized by vacuolization and increased replication of these cells in the bronchiolar epithelium. A dose-dependent reduction in the CYP activity in Clara cells is observed as well. This loss of metabolic activation capacity can be thought of as an adaptive response. Clara cells recover morphologically during repeated daily inhalation exposures to TCE.

Chloral is the putative toxicant responsible for pulmonary tumor formation. Clara cells of the mouse efficiently metabolize TCE to TCA and chloral. Chloral accumulates, due to its efficient production and the low activity of ADH, the enzyme responsible for its reduction to TCOH. The Clara cells' lack of glucuronosyltransferase, the enzyme that normally catalyzes the formation of TCOH glucuronide, has also been implicated in chloral accumulation. Species differences in susceptibility of the lung to TCE are due in part to mouse lung Clara cells having a much higher level of CYP2E1 than those of the rat, and thus a much higher capacity to metabolize TCE to chloral. Also, Clara cells in mice are much more numerous than in rats. A critical role for chloral is supported by the findings that its administration to mice, but not that of TCA or TCOH, causes Clara cell toxicity identical to that of TCE. Chloral does appear to have some genotoxic potential, especially in regard to inducing aneuploidy. However, the fact that tumors are not seen in species where cytotoxicity does not occur strongly implicates cytotoxicity and reparative proliferation in tumor formation. In an effort to test the hypothesis that bronchiolar damage by TCE is associated with bioactivation within Clara cells, Forkert *et al.* (2006) administered TCE i.p. to CD-1 mice. The result was dose-dependent production of dichloroacetyl lysine adducts in Clara cells (used as an in vivo marker of TCE metabolism) that correlated with bronchiolar damage. The study also suggested that CYP2F2 may play a more important role than CYP2E1 in TCE metabolism and cytotoxicity within the lung.

Risk Assessment   The human relevance of TCE-induced rodent tumors is an unresolved issue. For liver tumors, humans appear to be more similar to rats than mice in their capacity for oxidative TCE metabolism. For kidney tumors, evidence exists that TCE bioactivation via the GSH pathway is greater in rats than in humans. As for promotional mechanisms, rodent liver is much more responsive to the action of peroxisome proliferators than human liver, and α_{2u}-globulin nephropathy is thought to be specific to the male rat. With regard to lung cancer, the CYP content and the number of Clara cells in the human lung are fraction of those in the mouse. This suggests that the risk for chloral accumulation in humans is minimal. It thus appears as though direct extrapolation from rodent data would substantially overstate human TCE cancer risk.

Numerous hypotheses are available concerning carcinogenic modes of action in the liver, lung, and kidney of rodents, in particular. Just how compelling these hypotheses are is still the subject of debate, as exemplified by the critical response of EPA scientists (Caldwell *et al.*, 2006) to a recent attempt to apply a margin of exposure approach (i.e., a nonlinear dose–response extrapolation) in TCE risk assessment (Clewell and Andersen, 2004, 2006). In 2001, EPA issued its draft risk assessment on TCE (EPA, 2001). The document elicited much debate, which prompted the EPA and other federal agencies to request a scientific review of TCE by a NAS expert panel. Their report was released in 2006. It recommended,

among other things, a new meta-analysis of the epidemiological data and the precautionary extrapolation of cancer risk using a linear model, because modes of action are not known with certainty.

Tetrachloroethylene

Tetrachloroethylene (perchloroethylene, PERC) is commonly used as a dry cleaner, fabric finisher, degreaser, rug and upholstery cleaner, paint and stain remover, solvent, and chemical intermediate. The highest exposures usually occur in occupational settings via inhalation. Much attention is now focused on adverse health effects that may be experienced by dry cleaners and other persons living in the proximity of such facilities (Garetano and Gochfeld, 2000). Echeverria *et al.* (1995), for example, reported adverse effects on visuospatial functions of dry cleaners. PERC is frequently detected in the low ppt range in the breath and blood of the general populace (Ashley *et al.*, 1994; Churchill *et al.*, 2001; Blount *et al.*, 2006). Although releases are primarily to the atmosphere, PERC enters surface and groundwaters by accidental and intentional discharges (ATSDR, 1997c). Levels in the ppb range are reported in municipal water in areas of New England, where PERC was used in a process to treat plastic water pipe (Paulu *et al.*, 1999). Fay (2006) reports that PERC is the third most frequently found chemical contaminant in groundwater at hazardous waste sites in the United States.

The systemic disposition and metabolism of PERC and trichloroethylene (TCE) are similar in many respects. Both chemicals are well absorbed from the lungs and GI tract, distributed to tissues according to their lipid content, partially exhaled unchanged, and metabolized by hepatic CYPs, primarily CYP2E1. PERC is initially oxidized by the CYPs to PERC oxide. PERC is oxidized to a much lesser degree than TCE, though the two have a common major metabolite, TCA. Some of the TCA may be converted to DCA (Lash and Parker, 2001). GSH conjugation is a minor metabolic pathway, quantitatively for TCE and PERC. The resulting conjugates of TCE and PERC are S-(dichlorovinyl)glutathione (DCVG) and S-(trichlorovinyl)glutathione (TCVG), respectively. These are excreted into the bile, where they are cleaved to S-(dichlorovinyl)-L-cysteine (DCVC) and S-(trichlorovinyl)-L-cysteine (TCVC) (Birner *et al.*, 1994). TCVC can be detoxified by acetylation in the liver and excreted in the urine, or metabolically activated by cleavage by a β-lyase in the kidney to dichlorothioketene and other reactive metabolites. These can covalently bind to proteins and other macromolecules, or react with water to form DCA. DCA is also believed to be formed in small amounts from TCE (see previous subsection on TCE). Dichlorothioketene is purported to be the ultimate PERC metabolite responsible for nephrotoxicity and mutagenicity by Volkel *et al.* (1998). Other reactive metabolites include 1,2,2-trichlorovinylthiol and mercapturate sulfoxide (Lash and Parker, 2001).

PERC's capacity to produce acute or chronic hepatorenal toxicity in laboratory animals and humans is quite limited. Near-lethal i.p. doses of PERC were required to cause acute liver or kidney injury in mice (Klaassen and Plaa, 1966). Liver injury was not seen in B6C3F1 mice or Osborne–Mendel rats gavaged with up to ~1000 mg/kg daily for 78 weeks (NCI, 1977). Dose-dependent karyomegaly was observed in the renal proximal tubular epithelium of mice and rats inhaling PERC for 103 weeks (NTP, 1986). This change was most prominent in the male rats. Green *et al.* (1990) found increases in protein droplets and cell proliferation in the proximal tubular epithelium of male F-344 rats gavaged with 1500 mg PERC/kg daily for up to 42 days. These alterations are

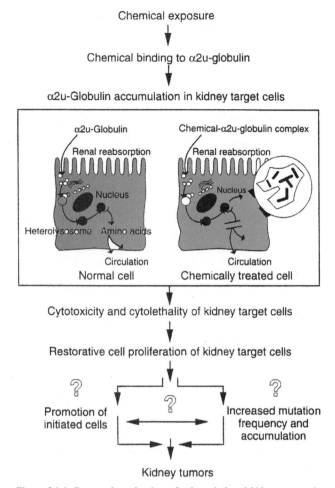

Chemical exposure

Chemical binding to α2u-globulin

α2u-Globulin accumulation in kidney target cells

α2u-Globulin   Chemical-α2u-globulin complex

Renal reabsorption   Renal reabsorption

Nucleus   Nucleus

Heterolysosome   Amino acids

Circulation   Circulation
Normal cell   Chemically treated cell

Cytotoxicity and cytolethality of kidney target cells

Restorative cell proliferation of kidney target cells

Promotion of   Increased mutation
initiated cells   frequency and
          accumulation

Kidney tumors

Figure 24-6. Proposed mechanism of solvent-induced kidney cancer in male rats involving α_{2u}-globulin.

[Used with permission of Borghoff *et al.*: *CIIT Activities* 16(10): 1–8, 1996.]

accompanied by an increase in α_{2u}-globulin, a male rat-specific protein (Fig. 24-6). Modest changes in a few indices of liver or kidney cell function in dry-cleaning workers (Gennari *et al.*, 1992; Brodkin *et al.*, 1995; Verplanke *et al.*, 1999) suggest that relatively minor effects may occur in humans with relatively high, chronic exposures. Philip *et al.* (2007) recently found that aqueous gavage of mice with 150, 500 or 1000 mg PERC/kg/day produced mild to moderate liver injury that regressed over a 30-day dosing period. No evidence of kidney damage was seen.

PERC's potential to cause cancer in humans continues to be a subject of considerable controversy. Male and female B6C3F1 mice, gavaged with very high doses of PERC for up to 78 weeks, exhibited an increase in hepatocellular carcinoma (NCI, 1977). No increase in tumor incidence was seen in Osborne–Mendel rats. Hepatocellular carcinoma was seen again in B6C3F1 mice inhaling 100 or 200 ppm PERC over a 2-year period (NTP, 1986). There was a low incidence of renal adenomas and carcinomas in male F-344 rats exposed to 200 or 400 ppm PERC. Such tumors are *rare* in this species. There was also a significant increase over controls in mononuclear-cell leukemia in the male and female rats, but ∼50% of the controls had this disease.

There have been many epidemiological studies of cancer incidence and mortality in groups of dry cleaners and other persons occupationally exposed to PERC (ATSDR, 1997c). Some researchers

have reported findings of excess incidences of different cancers, while others have not. Frequently, there was not a determination of the degree or duration of PERC exposure, or consideration of major confounding factors (e.g., exposure to other solvents/chemicals, smoking, alcohol consumption, and socioeconomic status). Nevertheless, there was sufficient information for Weiss (1995) to conclude that cigarette smoking and alcohol consumption could only partially account for an increased rate of esophageal cancer in dry cleaners. Kidney cancer incidences did not appear to be elevated. McLaughlin and Blot (1997) reevaluated available epidemiological data, and concluded that they did not support a cause-and-effect relationship between either PERC or TCE and kidney cancer. Boice *et al.* (1999) and Mundt *et al.* (2003) similarly concluded that there did not appear to be a relationship between occupational PERC exposure and cancer at any specific site.

The relevance of the male rat kidney tumor findings to humans has received considerable attention. Several mechanisms have been proposed for the development of renal cell carcinoma in PERC-exposed male rats. Some oxidative metabolites (TCA and DCA) modify cell signaling pathways, while reactive metabolites of the GSH pathway are cytotoxic and mutagenic (Lash and Parker, 2001). Chronic exposure to high doses of PERC can cause ongoing cell death, regenerative hyperplasia, and the opportunity for fixation of DNA damage and spontaneous errors in replication during repair. Increased cell replication, protein droplet accumulation, and enhanced α_{2u}-globulin levels in the P2 segment of renal proximal tubules appear to be unique to male rats (Green *et al.*, 1990). Melnick and Kohn (1999), however, have pointed out that mechanism(s) of interaction between α_{2u}-globulin accumulation and kidney cancer is(are) unknown, and that quantitative relationships between key biological processes have yet to be demonstrated. They offered an alternative hypothesis, namely the α_{2u}-globulin may bind to and thereby increase the renal concentration and action of a proximate carcinogen. As described above, a limited amount of PERC can be metabolized to TCVC, which in turn is detoxified or cleaved in the kidneys to cytotoxic and mutagenic products such as dichlorothioketene. Upon equivalent inhalation exposures of Wistar rats and humans to PERC, the rats excreted substantially larger amounts of DCA and acetylated TCVC (Volkel *et al.*, 1998). These observations were consistent with in vitro findings of greater conversion of PERC to TCVC by rat liver cytosol and of a 10-fold higher β-lyase-mediated metabolism of TCVC by rat than by human kidney (Green *et al.*, 1990; Cooper, 1994). These data indicate that human kidney has limited capacity to generate reactive metabolites from PERC by the GSH and β-lyase pathways.

Such metabolic and physiological differences between species (Lash *et al.*, 1998) can be input into PBTK models and used to predict inter- and intraspecies differences in metabolite dosimetry and cancer risks. Clewell *et al.* (2005) reviewed published PBTK PERC models and found just one, that by Gearhart *et al.* (1993), included a description of TCA kinetics. A second model with a TCA pathway (Jang and Droz, 1997) was subsequently located in the literature. Their data and model predictions showed that Asians exhibited higher PERC blood and breath levels and lower urinary TCA levels than Caucasians, consistent with slower PERC metabolism by the Asians. Quite recently, Covington *et al.* (2006) published a human model that provided for metabolism of PERC to TCA in the liver and kidney. A hierarchial Bayesian analysis was conducted to characterize the variability of estimates of the fractional metabolism of PERC in a population. Lash and Parker (2001) recommended that future PBTK models for PERC include a submodel for the GSH pathway.

1,1,1-Trichloroethane

1,1,1-Trichloroethane (methyl chloroform, TRI) is a widely used organic solvent. Its popularity as a metal degreaser, general purpose solvent, spot cleaner, and component of aerosols and a variety of household products increased substantially with the decline in manufacture of other halocarbons found to be high-dose rodent carcinogens and potential human carcinogens. TRI has not been shown to be carcinogenic in mice, rats, or humans (ATSDR, 2006b). Utilization of TRI declined during the 1990s, however, due to its ozone-depleting properties (Doherty, 2000). The VOC was to be phased out of use under the Montreal Protocol by 2002, but it continues to be manufactured and sold in large quantities in the United States and other countries.

The highest exposures to TRI occur via inhalation in occupational settings, but many persons encounter the VOC at home by use of commercial products and tap water containing it. Ashley *et al.* (1994) reported TRI and other VOCs in the blood of >75% of 600+ nonoccupationally exposed individuals. TRI and trichloroethylene (TCE) were also frequently detected in a subset of 982 adults examined in the NHANES III survey (Churchill *et al.*, 2001), and more recently in 951 other members of the general population (Blount *et al.*, 2006). TRI, TCE, and PCE comprise the most common ternary chemical mixture in groundwater at hazardous waste sites in the United States (Fay, 2006). TRI and other VOCs in groundwater can remain trapped for years and serve as a source of low-level exposure for large populations.

The primary pharmacological manifestation of acute or chronic inhalation of TRI is CNS depression, ranging in severity from slight headache or dizziness to anesthesia and death (ATSDR, 2006b). The current threshold limit value (TLV) of 350 ppm was established to prevent decrements in workers' mental and physical functions, though slight sedative effects have been reported by one group of investigators at 200 ppm (Muttray *et al.*, 2000). TRI has a very limited cytotoxic potential, ostensibly due to its quite limited biotransformation to relatively nontoxic metabolites (e.g., TCA and TCOH). Male rats gavaged five times weekly for as long as 12 days with up to 5 g TRI/kg died from effects of repeated, protracted CNS depression, but exhibited only slight hepatotoxicity (Bruckner *et al.*, 2001). Quast *et al.* (1988) saw only minimal histological changes in the liver of F-344 rats inhaling 1500-ppm TRI 6 h/d, 5 d/week for up to 2 years. It is worthy of note that even higher inhaled concentrations of TRI, particularly when accompanied by hypoxia and stress, can sensitize the myocardium to catecholamines, producing cardiac arrhythmias (Reinhardt *et al.*, 1973).

There is a relatively large rodent and human kinetic database for inhaled TRI. Inhalation experiments with human volunteers have been limited to monitoring blood and exhaled breath levels. The EPA has recently evaluated a number of TRI PBTK models for use in derivation of RfDs for its IRIS database. The model of Reitz *et al.* (1988) proved satisfactory, in that it accurately predicted the time–course of TRI in human, rat, and mouse blood for different inhalation scenarios. No brain deposition data were available then, so it was necessary to assume that blood TRI levels accurately reflect brain levels. Warren *et al.* (1998, 2000) demonstrated a high degree of correlation between brain and blood TRI levels in TRI-exposed mice and rats, as well as reasonable correlation between brain levels and CNS effects.

Methylene Chloride

Methylene chloride (dichloromethane, MC) enjoys widespread use as a solvent in industrial processes, food preparation, degreasing

agents, aerosol propellants, and agriculture. Thus, large numbers of people are exposed occupationally and in the home. The primary route of exposure to this very volatile solvent is inhalation. The preponderance of MC escaping into the environment does so by volatilization (ATSDR, 1998b). The VOC is also frequently found in wastewater discharges and in air and water at hazardous waste sites (Fay and Mumtaz, 1996).

The TK of MC have been well characterized in humans and rodents. Inhaled MC was extensively absorbed and reached a near steady state in the blood of human subjects with 1–2 hours of continuous exposure (DiVincenzo and Kaplan, 1981). Less than 5% of the absorbed dose was exhaled unchanged. Some 25–34% was exhaled as carbon monoxide, the major end metabolite of MC. Exposure of the volunteers to 50, 100, 150, and 200 ppm for 7.5 hours produced peak blood carboxyhemoglobin saturations of 1.9, 3.4, 5.3, and 6.8%, respectively. MC was very rapidly eliminated from the body and did not accumulate over a 5-day-exposure regimen. Metabolism of MC in humans and rodents is believed to occur via three pathways (Andersen *et al.*, 1987). One entails CYP2E1-catalyzed oxidation to carbon monoxide via formyl chloride, a reactive intermediate. The second, a GSH-mediated pathway, involves a theta-class GST, GSTT1-1. The P450 pathway is a high-affinity, low-capacity pathway that predominates at MC concentrations present in occupational and environmental settings. The GST pathway is a low-affinity, high-capacity pathway operative at the high exposure levels used in cancer bioassays (Green, 1997). With the third pathway, it is postulated that CO_2 is also formed via the oxidative pathway by reaction of formyl chloride with a nucleophile such as GSH (Fig. 24-7).

MC has only a limited systemic toxicity potential. High, repeated inhalation exposures are required to produce slight, reversible changes in the liver of rodents. Centrilobular vacuolization and focal necrosis occur in the livers of rats exposed 6 h/d, 5 d/week for 2 years to 500–4000-ppm MC (Burek *et al.*, 1984; Mennear *et al.*, 1988). Manifestations of kidney injury are infrequent in laboratory animals, but are occasionally reported in persons subjected to high vapor levels. As described above, the carbon monoxide that is formed from MC binds to hemoglobin to produce dose-dependent increases in carboxyhemoglobin. It is generally accepted that tissue hypoxia can contribute to acute CNS effects of MC. There are few reports of residual neurologic dysfunction in MC-exposed employees (Lash *et al.*, 1991; ATSDR, 1998b).

Occupational and environmental MC exposures are of concern primarily because of MC's carcinogenicity in rodents and its potential as a human carcinogen. Burek *et al.* (1984) saw increased numbers of salivary gland sarcomas in male rats and benign mammary tumors in female rats exposed to very high MC vapor levels 5 times weekly over 2 years. Hamsters were not affected. Benign mammary tumors in female rats were also seen in subsequent inhalation bioassays (Nitschke *et al.*, 1988; Mennear *et al.*, 1988). Dose-dependent increases in lung and liver tumors in male and female B6C3F1 mice were also found in the latter investigation. Epidemiology studies of workers exposed to MC have not revealed increases in mortality from lung or liver tumors (ATSDR, 1998b). There have been occasional reports of cancer excess in other organs, including the pancreas (Hearne *et al.*, 1990) and the prostate and cervix (Gibbs *et al.*, 1996). Upon a comprehensive review of the epidemiology literature, Dell *et al.* (1999) and Starr *et al.* (2006) concluded that occupational studies to date provide little evidence of MC carcinogenicity in humans.

There has been a great deal of research to define mechanisms of MC carcinogenicity, in order to more clearly understand the relevance of the murine tumors to humans (Green, 1997). Liver and lung

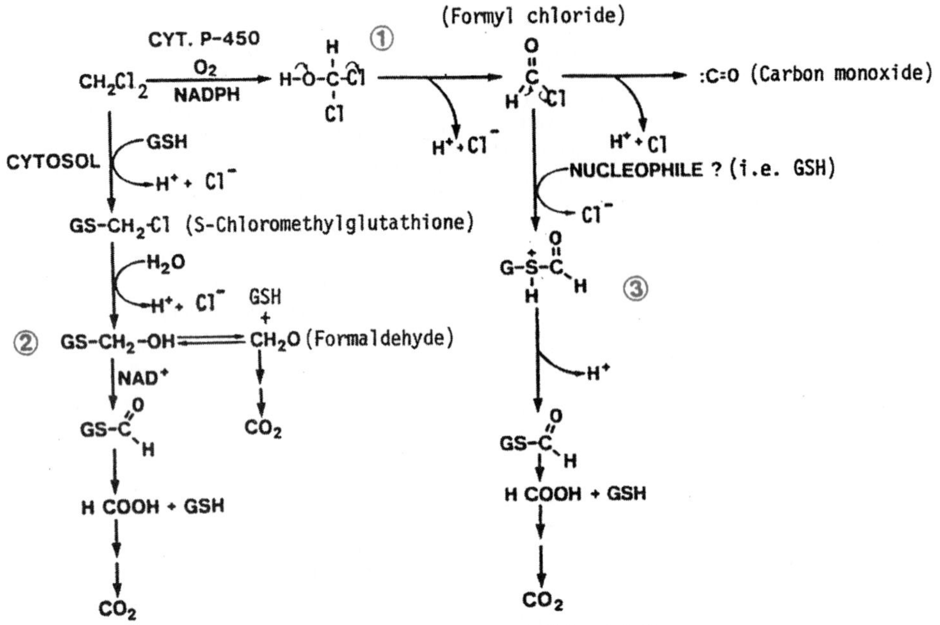

Figure 24-7. Proposed pathways for methylene chloride (CH_2Cl_2) metabolism.

(1) Mixed function oxidase pathway; (2) glutathione transferase pathway; and (3) nucleotide pathway.
[Modified from Andersen et al. (1987), with permission from Elsevier.]

tumors in mice do not seem to be associated with overt cytotoxicity or increased replicative DNA synthesis (Maronpot et al., 1995). Induction of the tumors in mice is generally believed to be due to a reactive intermediate generated via the GST pathway (Andersen et al., 1987). GSTT1-1 in liver and lung catalyzes conversion of MC to S-chloromethylglutathione ($GSCH_2Cl$), which apparently breaks down rapidly to GSH and formaldehyde. $GSCH_2Cl$ has yet to be isolated and quantified. Metabolism of MC via the GST pathway is an order of magnitude greater in mouse than in rat liver. Metabolic rates in hamster and human liver are even lower (Reitz et al., 1989; Thier et al., 1998). High GSTT1-1 activity was measured in the nuclei of mouse centrilobular hepatocytes. Mice may be unique in that extensive metabolic activation of MC to an unstable intermediate occurs in the proximity of the DNA. It would be useful in future PBTK models to include subcompartments for cytosolic and nuclear GST activities (Starr et al., 2006). GSTT1-1 was also detected in relatively high levels in mouse lung Clara cells and ciliated cells at alveolar/bronchiolar junctions. $GSCH_2Cl$ apparently causes single-strand breaks in vivo and in vitro in DNA of mouse liver and lung (Graves et al., 1995). No DNA breaks were detected in hamster or human hepatocytes in vitro. Casanova and coworkers have proposed an alternate mechanism of MC carcinogenicity, namely formation of DNA–protein cross-links (DPX) by formaldehyde. Upon incubation of MC with hepatocytes from mice, rats, hamsters, and humans, DPX were found only in the mouse samples (Casanova et al., 1996). Formaldehyde–RNA adducts, a more sensitive marker than DPX, were subsequently found in human hepatocytes incubated with MC, although the adducts were seven times more prevalent in mouse hepatocytes (Casanova et al., 1997).

We now have a substantial amount of information on the TK and mechanism(s) of carcinogenicity of MC. Considerable time and money have been spent on MC research by federal agencies, academia, and industry. MC was one of the first chemicals for which PBTK modeling was employed by the EPA in cancer risk estimation. Although uncertainties remain, species differences appear to

be largely quantitative rather than qualitative. Flux through both the P450 and GST pathways is substantially greater in mice than in rats or humans. Interindividual variability in the rate of MC oxidation by 13 human subjects is reported to be quite small (Sweeney et al., 2004). Persons with a GSTT1-1 null genotype (Nelson et al., 1995; Haber et al., 2002) may not be at risk from certain MC-induced tumors. This concept has been incorporated into cancer risk assessments based upon PBTK estimation of DPX formation in humans (El-Masri et al., 1999; Jonsson and Johanson, 2001).

Carbon Tetrachloride

CCl_4 previously enjoyed widespread use as a solvent, cleaning agent, fire extinguisher, synthetic intermediate, grain fumigant, and human anthelmintic. Its use has steadily declined since the 1970s, due to its hepatorenal toxicity, carcinogenicity, and contribution to atmospheric ozone depletion (ATSDR, 2005). Nevertheless, CCl_4 appears to be ubiquitous in ambient air in the United States, and it is still found in groundwater from some wells and waste sites. CCl_4 is a classic hepatotoxin, but kidney injury is often more severe in humans. There does not appear to be a good animal model for CCl_4-induced kidney toxicity.

The time–course of CCl_4-induced acute liver injury has been well characterized (ATSDR, 2005). Early signs of hepatocellular injury in rats include dissociation of polysomes and ribosomes from rough endoplasmic reticulum, disarray of smooth endoplasmic reticulum, inhibition of protein synthesis, and triglyceride accumulation. Hypomethylation of RNA is thought to contribute to inhibition of lipoprotein synthesis, thereby playing a role in steatosis (Clawson et al., 1987). Ingested CCl_4 reaches the liver, undergoes metabolic activation, produces lipid peroxidation, covalently binds, and inhibits microsomal ATPase activity within minutes in rats. Single cell necrosis, evident 5–6 hours post dosing, progresses to maximal centrilobular necrosis within 24–48 hours. Most microsomal enzyme activities are significantly depressed (Recknagel et al., 1989).

A variety of cytoplasmic enzymes are released from dead and dying hepatocytes into the bloodstream. The activity of these enzymes in serum generally parallels the extent of necrosis in the liver. Cellular regeneration, manifest by increased DNA synthesis and cell cycle progression, is maximal 36–48 hours post dosing (Rao *et al.*, 1997).

Development of cellular resistance and tissue repair are important in limiting CCl_4 hepatotoxicity, and in recovery (Mehendale, 2005). Alterations in transmembrane carrier proteins have been discovered in hepatocytes of CCl_4-treated mice. CCl_4 results in reduced expression of genes associated with extraction of bile acids and organic ions from sinusoidal blood, as well as upregulation of certain detoxification genes (Aleksunes *et al.*, 2005). CCl_4 also produces differential upregulation in multidrug resistance proteins that are involved in export of oxidative stress products and metabolites. Hepatocellular regeneration has been shown to begin within 6 hours of a small dose of CCl_4, just as centrilobular necrosis is becoming evident (Lockard *et al.*, 1983). This early-phase regeneration (arrested G_2 hepatocytes activated to proceed through mitosis) is followed at $\sim$24 hours by the secondary phase of regeneration (hepatocytes mobilized from G_o/G_1 to proceed through mitosis (Bell *et al.*, 1988).

It is likely that the mechanism of liver injury by CCl_4 has received more attention than that of any other chemical. Nevertheless, there is still considerable debate about the relative importance of different actions of CCl_4, notably covalent binding and lipid peroxidation. CCl_4 is known to be metabolized by P450-dependent reductive dehalogenation to a trichloromethyl radical ($CCl_3\cdot$). This radical can bind covalently to nucleic acids to initiate liver cancer, and bind to lipids and proteins, causing structural damage of membranes and inhibition of a variety of enzymes. $CCl_3\cdot$ may also react with oxygen to produce Cl_3OO, the highly reactive trichloromethyl peroxy radical. $CCl_3\cdot$ can also attack enoic fatty acids, leading to organic free radicals, which may in turn react with oxygen to form peroxides and other cytotoxic metabolites (Recknagel *et al.*, 1989; Plaa, 2000; Weber *et al.*, 2003). This self-perpetuating process is known as lipid peroxidation. It destroys polyunsaturated fatty acids, especially those associated with phospholipids, altering permeabilities of organelles, and resulting in a loss of calcium homeostasis. Numerous studies have shown various antioxidants to ameliorate CCl_4 cytotoxicity in vitro and in vivo. Chemicals that inhibit CCl_4 covalent binding are also protective. In vivo experiments in rats by Padron *et al.* (1996) demonstrated that both of these degenerative processes (i.e., covalent binding and lipid peroxidation) were necessary for CCl_4 cytotoxicity. Liu *et al.* (1995) have proposed that CCl_4 oxidative stress in the liver enhances nuclear factor kappa B activity, which in turn promotes expression of proinflammatory cytotoxic cytokines. Shi *et al.* (1998) proposed apoptosis as an additional/alternate mechanism of CCl_4-induced cell death.

Perturbation of intracellular calcium (Ca^{2+}) homeostasis appears to be an integral part of CCl_4 cytotoxicity (Stoyanovsky and Cederbaum, 1996). Increased cytosolic Ca^{2+} levels may result from influx of extracellular Ca^{2+} due to plasma membrane damage and from decreased intracellular Ca^{2+} sequestration. Elevation of intracellular Ca^{2+} in hepatocytes can cause activation of phospholipase A_2 and exacerbation of membrane damage (Glende and Recknagel, 1992). Elevated Ca^{2+} may also be involved in alterations in calmodulin and phosphorylase activity, as well as changes in nuclear protein kinase C activity (Omura *et al.*, 1999). High intracellular Ca^{2+} levels activate a number of catabolic enzymes including proteases, endonucleases, and phospholipases, which kill cells via apoptosis or necrosis (Weber *et al.*, 2003). The hydrolytic enzyme calpain mediates progression of acute CCl_4-induced liver injury by leaking from dying hepatocytes and attacking neighboring cells (Limaye *et al.*, 2003). Ca^{2+} may stimulate the release of cytokines and eicosanoids from Kupffer cells. Edwards *et al.* (1993) demonstrated that destruction of Kupffer cells prior to CCl_4 dosing of rats resulted in significant reductions in neutrophil infiltration and hepatocellular injury. Macrophages are known to release a number of inflammatory mediators, such as tumor necrosis factor alpha (TNF-α), that are cytotoxic (Morio *et al.*, 2001). CCl_4 hepatocytotoxicity is obviously a complex, multifactorial process that is likely to continue to receive considerable attention.

CCl_4 has frequently been used as a model hepatotoxic compound with which to examine the influence of various factors that alter P450s. CYP2E1 is primarily responsible for catalyzing the bioactivation of low doses of CCl_4 in humans. CYP3A contributes to the metabolism of higher doses (Zangar *et al.*, 2000). The preeminent role of CYP2E1 in animals is clearly demonstrated by the protection-afforded CCl_4-treated rodents by CYP2E1 antibody (Castillo *et al.*, 1992), the CYP2E1 inhibitor 3-amino-1,2,4-triazole (Padron *et al.*, 1996), and the absence of CYP2E1 expression (Wong *et al.*, 1998). As discussed previously, a variety of conditions that induce CYP2E1 potentiate CCl_4 hepatotoxicity in test animals and humans. Sufficient doses of CYP2E1 inhibitors, including natural constituents of foods (described in the subsection on P450 inhibitors), can inhibit CCl_4 toxicity (Lieber, 1997). Taieb *et al.* (2005) recently discovered protein 8, a transcription factor that regulates the expression of genes that protect cells from stress, rapidly triggered CYP2E1 downregulation in CCl_4-dosed mice, thereby minimizing CCl_4 bioactivation.

Chloroform

The primary use of chloroform ($CHCl_3$, trichloromethane) is in the production of the refrigerant chlorodifluoromethane (Freon 22), but this use is expected to diminish as chlorine-containing fluorocarbons are phased out under the Montreal Protocol. $CHCl_3$ was among the first inhalation anesthetics, but it was replaced by safer compounds after about 1940. $CHCl_3$ is a by-product of drinking water chlorination and has been measured in municipal drinking water supplies in concentrations as high as several hundred ppb, although levels are usually <25 ppb (ATSDR, 1997a). $CHCl_3$ has also been found in ppb concentrations in swimming pool water and surrounding air (Aggazzotti *et al.*, 1995). Like many other halocarbons, $CHCl_3$ can invoke CNS symptoms at subanesthetic concentrations similar to those of alcohol intoxication and can sensitize the myocardium to catecholamines, possibly resulting in cardiac arrhythmias.

The reproductive and developmental toxicities of $CHCl_3$ are rather unremarkable. Schwetz *et al.* (1974) found that inhalation of 100–300-ppm $CHCl_3$ by pregnant rats caused a high incidence of fetal resorption, retardation of fetal development, and a low incidence of fetal anomalies. Murray *et al.* (1979) reported that gestational exposure to 100-ppm $CHCl_3$ resulted in the decreased ability of mice to maintain pregnancy, as well as cleft palate, decreased fetal weight and length, and decreased ossification in pups. Very high $CHCl_3$ concentrations retarded development and induced diffuse cell death in cultured rat embryos (Brown-Woodman *et al.*, 1998). These studies support $CHCl_3$ as a weak teratogen, but negative studies employing maternally toxic doses argue against this characterization (Thompson *et al.*, 1974; NTP, 1997a). The EPA's IRIS profile for $CHCl_3$ notes that in reproductive/developmental studies, maternal toxicity and fetal effects occurred at doses higher than those that produced liver toxicity in the dog study by Heywood *et al.* (1979).

The latter study serves as the basis for EPA's benchmark dose-based RfD (EPA, 2006a).

Under certain conditions $CHCl_3$ is hepatotoxic and nephrotoxic. These toxicities are potentiated by aliphatic alcohols, ketones, and DCA and TCA (Davis, 1992). Albeit at low doses, numerous disinfection by-products such as the rodent carcinogens TCA and DCA are routinely consumed with $CHCl_3$ in finished drinking water. For this reason, mixture studies are particularly relevant. Consider, for example, the studies of Pereira *et al.* (2001) in which *N*-methyl-*N*-nitrosourea-initiated B6C3F1 mice were exposed to DCA with or without $CHCl_3$. $CHCl_3$ prevented the hypomethylation and increased mRNA expression of the proto-oncogene c-myc and the promotion of liver tumors by DCA. Conversely, $CHCl_3$ increased DCA-induced DNA hypomethylation and enhanced the DCA promotion of kidney tumors. Thus, concurrent exposure to two rodent carcinogens, $CHCl_3$ and DCA, resulted in less than additive activity in one organ and synergism in another (Pereira *et al.*, 2001; Tao *et al.*, 2005). This exemplifies the difficulty in assessing the risks posed by solvent mixtures.

Tolerance or adaptation to $CHCl_3$'s hepatorenal toxicity and carcinogenicity has been observed in some mouse strains after repeated exposure. This phenomenon was first investigated by Pereira and Grothaus (1997), who reported preexposure of mice to low doses of $CHCl_3$ in drinking water-induced resistance to hepatotoxicity and cell proliferation following a higher gavage dose. This was presumed at the time to result from suicidal inhibition of the P450s responsible for $CHCl_3$'s activation. More recently, mice exposed daily for 7, 14, and 30 days were found to have a robust regenerative response in target tissues, which prevented the progression of injury (Anand *et al.*, 2006b). Blood and tissue levels of $CHCl_3$ after repeated exposure were substantially lower than those following a single exposure, owing to increased elimination of $CHCl_3$ via exhalation. These same researchers also reported that priming mice with $CHCl_3$ prior to a lethal dose stimulated compensatory hepato- and nephrogenic repair, limiting the progression of injury and resulting in 100% survival. Relative to unprimed mice, there was no difference in hepatic or renal CYP2E1 activity, though GSH and GSH reductase activity were upregulated in the kidney (but not in the liver), with a consequent decrease in renal covalent binding. The area under the blood $CHCl_3$ versus time curve (AUC) was 40% lower in primed versus unprimed mice, but increased elimination via exhalation was not responsible for the reduction in internal exposure in this particular case (Philip *et al.*, 2006). Taken together, these studies suggest that TK and TD factors contribute to the tolerance observed to $CHCl_3$ toxicity. Mehendele and colleagues have conducted a series of studies with $CHCl_3$, alone or in combination with other hepatotoxicants, to further discern the role of tissue repair in toxicant-induced injury. These studies have provided valuable insight into the importance of both the timing of the tissue repair response and its magnitude as pivotal determinants of the outcome of toxicant-induced injury and emphasize the need to consider repair processes in predictive toxicology (Anand *et al.*, 2003, 2005; Mehendale, 2005).

The status of $CHCl_3$ as a rodent carcinogen is indisputable. It causes liver and kidney tumors that are species-, strain-, sex-, and route of exposure-dependent. $CHCl_3$-induced liver tumors in mice and their dependence on ongoing liver necrosis were reported near the end of World War II (Eschenbrenner and Miller, 1945). These same authors observed that male but not female mice suffered kidney necrosis. This observation was supported by the report of Roe *et al.* (1979) that $CHCl_3$ ingested in a toothpaste base resulted in

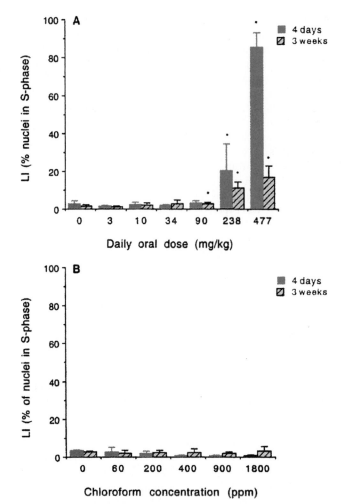

Figure 24-8. *Hepatocyte liver LI in female B6C3F1 mice given $CHCl_3$ orally in corn oil (A) or drinking water (B) for 4 days or 3 weeks.*

The LI is defined as the percent of hepatocyte nuclei positive for 5-bromo-2'-deoxyuridine immunohistochemical staining (i.e., percent of cells in the S phase, the period of DNA synthesis during the cell cycle). Values represent the mean ± SD for five mice. Asterisks (∗) denote a significant difference from similarly treated control mice (<0.05). Note that 1800-ppm $CHCl_3$ in water corresponds to a cumulative uptake of 329 mg/kg/d. [Reproduced with permission of Larson *et al.* (1994).]

renal tumors in male but not female mice. This sex difference is thought to be attributable to testosterone-mediated differences in renal CYP activity (Smith *et al.*, 1984). The NCI (1976) cancer bioassay demonstrated renal tumors in male rats and an extremely high incidence of liver tumors in both sexes of B6C3F1 mice gavaged with $CHCl_3$ in corn oil. In 1985, Jorgenson and colleagues reported that daily doses of $CHCl_3$ in drinking water comparable to those in the NCI gavage assay also produced renal tumors in rats, but failed to cause liver tumors in B6C3F1 mice. This finding provided evidence that the dose rate of $CHCl_3$ was a determinant of liver tumor formation, supporting the existence of a threshold mechanism. Hard *et al.* (2000) have reevaluated the kidneys from the Jorgenson *et al.* (1985) study and have confirmed the presence of chronic renal tubule injury, indicative of renal tumor formation via an epigenetic mechanism. In what may be a landmark study, Larson *et al.* (1994) compared cytotoxicity and cell proliferation in female B6C3F1 mice given $CHCl_3$ by gavage in corn oil versus ad libitum ingestion in drinking water. As seen in Fig. 24-8, the hepatocyte-labeling index, a measure of the proliferative response, differed between the two dosage regimens at comparable doses. Pereira (1994) reported essentially the same observation. This suggests that ingestion of $CHCl_3$ in small increments, similar to drinking water patterns of humans, fails to produce a sufficient amount of cytotoxic metabolite(s) per unit time to overwhelm detoxification and other protective mechanisms.

Potentiation of $CHCl_3$'s toxicity by CYP inducers and protection by GSH and P450 inhibitors suggest that a metabolite, presumably phosgene, is responsible for $CHCl_3$'s hepatorenal toxicity. Both target organs metabolize $CHCl_3$ to phosgene. There is evidence that CYP2E1 and CYP2B1/2 metabolically activate $CHCl_3$, but the former isoform is thought to catalyze $CHCl_3$ metabolism at a lower concentration than the latter (Nakajima *et al.*, 1995). By using an irreversible CYP2E1 inhibitor and CYP2E1-knockout mice, Constan *et al.* (1999) have demonstrated that metabolism of $CHCl_3$ by CYP2E1 is required for liver and kidney necrosis and cell proliferation. The electrophilic intermediate generated by $CHCl_3$'s metabolism (i.e., phosgene) is initially detoxified by covalently binding to cytosolic GSH. Once GSH is depleted, phosgene is free to covalently bind hepatic and renal proteins and lipids. Such binding damages membranes and other intracellular structures, leading to necrosis and subsequent reparative cellular proliferation. Sustained proliferation with repeated exposures promotes tumor formation in rodents by irreversibly "fixing" spontaneously altered DNA and clonally expanding initiated cells. The expression of certain genes, including *myc* and *fos*, is altered during regenerative cell proliferation in response to $CHCl_3$-induced cytotoxicity (Sprankle *et al.*, 1996; Kegelmeyer *et al.*, 1997). While the identity of phosgene's intracellular targets is largely unknown, Guastadisegni *et al.* (1999) have reported that phosgene reacts with phosphatidylethanolamine (PE). The adduct formed appears to consist of two PE moieties cross-linked at the amino head groups by the carbonyl moiety of phosgene. $CHCl_3$-modified PE preferentially accumulates on inner mitochondrial membranes, inducing ultrastructural modifications and inhibiting functions of the organelle. These researchers observed the induction of hepatic apoptosis and necrosis in $CHCl_3$-treated Sprague–Dawley rats and pointed out that apoptosis may be initiated by the release of regulatory factors normally sequestered in mitochondria, in particular Ca^{2+}. Evidence that Ca^{2+} perturbation plays a role in $CHCl_3$ toxicity comes from a report of Ca^{2+} mobilization in Madin–Darby canine kidney cells using Fura-2 as a Ca^{2+} probe. $CHCl_3$, albeit in millimolar concentrations, increased the cytosolic Ca^{2+} levels by releasing Ca^{2+} from multiple sites within the cell (Jan *et al.*, 2000).

There is no evidence of covalent binding of $CHCl_3$ metabolites to nucleic acids. There is binding to nuclear histone, which plays a key role in controlling DNA expression and might be a mechanism of $CHCl_3$'s carcinogenicity (Diaz and Castro, 1980; Fabrizi *et al.*, 2003). It has been hypothesized that the induction of oxidative stress and depletion of GSH by $CHCl_3$ may lead to indirect genotoxicity that could contribute to carcinogenicity. This hypothesis is supported by the small dose-dependent increase in M(1)dG adducts (malondialdehyde reacts with DNA to form adducts to deoxyguanosine), DNA strand breakage, and lipid peroxidation in $CHCl_3$-treated rat hepatocytes in the absence of any increase in DNA oxidation (Beddowes *et al.*, 2003). Such a mechanism would still be threshold dependent, given its reliance on the initial depletion of antioxidants.

Currently, the EPA classifies $CHCl_3$ as a probable human carcinogen (group B2), meaning there is sufficient evidence for carcinogenicity in animals and inadequate or no evidence in humans.

Experimental evidence and the prevailing opinion that $CHCl_3$ is nongenotoxic, indicates that the relationship between $CHCl_3$ dose and tumor formation is nonlinear. The EPA has, as is called for in its new *Guidelines for Carcinogen Risk Assessment* (EPA, 2005), considered mode of action in the determination of $CHCl_3$'s cancer risk and relied on a nonlinear dose–response approach and the use of margin-of-exposure analysis. In doing so, the Agency concluded that the RfD for noncancer effects, based on the dog study of Heywood *et al.* (1979), was adequately protective for cancer by the oral route on the basis of cancer and noncancer effects having a common link through cytotoxicity. The wealth of mechanistic data available continues to inform the risk assessment for $CHCl_3$. For example, Constan *et al.* (2002) exercised a PBTK dosimetry model to compare hepatic responses in mice and humans to inhaled $CHCl_3$. They concluded that no safety factor was needed to account for interspecies differences in inhalation cancer risk. Additionally, Tan *et al.* (2003) have published a PBTK/TD model for $CHCl_3$ to describe the plausible mechanism linking the hepatic metabolism of $CHCl_3$ to hepatocellular killing and regenerative proliferation, thereby creating a predictive model that most accurately reflects the current science.

AROMATIC HYDROCARBONS

Benzene

Benzene produced commercially in the United States is derived primarily from petroleum. Benzene has been utilized as a general purpose solvent, but it is now used principally in the synthesis of other chemicals (ATSDR, 2006c). The percentage by volume of benzene in gasoline is 1–2%. Benzene plays an important role in unleaded gasoline due to its antiknock properties. Inhalation is the primary route of exposure in industrial and in everyday settings. Cigarette smoke is the major source of benzene in the home (Wallace, 1996). Smokers have benzene body burdens that are six to 10 times greater than those of nonsmokers. Passive smoke can be a significant source of benzene exposure to nonsmokers. Gasoline vapor emission and auto exhaust are the other key contributors to exposures of the general populace.

The most important adverse effect of benzene is hematopoietic toxicity. Chronic exposure to benzene can lead to bone marrow damage, which may be manifest initially as anemia, leukopenia, thrombocytopenia, or a combination of these. Bone marrow depression appears to be dose dependent in both laboratory animals and humans. Continued exposure may result in marrow aplasia and pancytopenia, an often fatal outcome. Survivors of aplastic anemia frequently exhibit a preneoplastic state, termed myelodysplasia, which may progress to myelogenous leukemia (Snyder, 2002; Bird *et al.*, 2005).

There is strong evidence from epidemiological studies that high-level benzene exposures result in an increased risk of acute myelogenous leukemia (AML) in humans (Bergsagel *et al.*, 1999; ATSDR, 2006a). Evidence of increased risks of other cancers in such populations is less compelling. Only AML incidence was significantly elevated in the largest cohort study to date, in which ~75,000 benzene-exposed workers in 12 cities in China were evaluated (Yin *et al.*, 1996). Marginal, nonsignificant increases were seen for lung cancer and chronic myelogenous leukemia. A subsequent study of some 250 Chinese shoe workers who inhaled low (≤ 1 to ≥ 10 ppm) levels of benzene revealed dose-dependent hematotoxicity (Lan *et al.*, 2004). Exposures of 100 of these employees

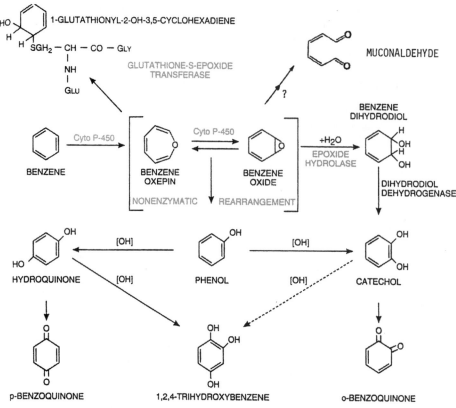

Figure 24-9. Biotransformation of benzene.

A question mark leads from the oxepin-oxide compartment to muconaldehyde because the substrate for the ring opening has yet to be identified. The dotted line leading to 1,2,4-trihydroxybenzene (1,2,4-T) indicates that it is not clear what the relative contributions of hydroquinone and catechol are to 1,2,4-T. [Modified and used with permission of Rangan and Snyder (1997).]

to ≤1 ppm reduced mature white cell and platelet counts, as well as myeloid progenitor cell colony formation. The progenitors were more sensitive to benzene than mature white cells. Polymorphisms in myeloperoxidase (an enzyme that metabolizes benzene to toxic quinones and free radicals) and NAD(P)H:quinone oxidoreductase (an enzyme that protects against these moieties) conferred increased susceptibility to white cell decreases. Turtletaub and Mani (2003) found that formation of DNA and protein adducts in mouse liver and bone marrow was dose dependent over a range of benzene doses, the lowest of which was 5 μg/kg.

Types of cancer other than AML have been tentatively attributed to benzene. Some investigations of persons exposed to engine exhausts have reported a significant association with multiple myeloma. Bezabeth *et al.* (1996) and Bergsagel *et al.* (1999) have concluded, however, that there is no scientific evidence to support a causal relationship between benzene exposure and multiple myeloma. Increased incidences of malignant lymphomas and a variety of solid tumors were found in male and female B6C3F1 mice dosed orally with high doses of benzene for up to 103 weeks (Huff *et al.*, 1989). Male and female F-344 rats in this bioassay exhibited excesses of Zymbal gland, skin, and oral cavity carcinomas. Thus, benzene is clearly an animal and human carcinogen, but major species differences exist.

It is essential to understand the metabolism of benzene in order to address its mechanisms of toxicity. The initial metabolic step (Fig. 24-9), oxidation of benzene to an epoxide (i.e., benzene oxide),

is catalyzed primarily by hepatic CYP2E1. Valentine *et al.* (1996) demonstrated that benzene-treated transgenic CYP2E1 knockout mice had relatively low levels of all benzene metabolites in their urine. A 5-day, 200-ppm benzene inhalation regimen produced severe genotoxicity and cytotoxicity in wild-type B6C3F1 mice, but no adverse effects in the knockout mice. Benzene oxide, which is in equilibrium with its oxepin form, is further metabolized by three pathways: (1) conjugation with GSH to form a premercapturic acid, which is converted to phenyl-mercapturic acid; (2) rearrangement nonenzymatically to form phenol; and (3) hydration by epoxide hydrolase to benzene dihydrodiol, which in turn can be oxidized by dihydrodiol dehydrogenase to catechol. If phenol is hydroxylated in the *ortho* position, more catechol will be formed. Catechol can be converted to *o*-benzoquinone. If benzene is hydroxylated in the *para* position, *p*-hydroquinone is formed. It can be oxidized to *p*-benzoquinone. The *o*- and *p*-benzoquinones are believed to be among the ultimate toxic metabolites of benzene. Another potentially toxic metabolite, muconaldehyde, may arise from ring opening of benzene oxide. Muconaldehyde undergoes a series of reactions that ultimately lead to *t,t*-muconic acid, an end metabolite found in the urine (Golding and Watson, 1999; Snyder, 2004).

Metabolism of benzene occurs primarily in the liver, though metabolism in bone marrow is believed by many authorities to play the key role in myelotoxicity. Levels of DNA and protein adducts were significantly higher in bone marrow than liver of benzene-dosed mice (Turtletaub and Mani, 2003). It has been generally accepted that phenolic conjugates are formed in the liver and transported via the blood to the bone marrow, where they are hydrolyzed and oxidized to quinones. Researchers have been unable to reproduce benzene toxicity, however, by giving individual phenolic metabolites to animals. The quinones are believed to be too reactive to be transported in the bloodstream. Lindstrom et al. (1997) have reported that benzene oxide has an estimated half-life of 7.9 minutes in rat blood, and thus may be able to travel from the liver to the bone marrow. Ring-opened metabolites of muconaldehyde, which are less reactive, could be transported to bone marrow and reoxidized. Bernauer et al. (1999) measured activity and levels of CYP2E1 in the liver and bone marrow of five strains of mice of varying sensitivity to benzene. CYP2E1 amounts and activities were considerably greater in the liver than the marrow, but no interstrain differences were seen in either tissue. It is likely that non-CYP enzymes (e.g., peroxidase, myeloperoxidase, and cyclooxygenase) play an important role in generation of semiquinones and quinones in bone marrow (Ross et al., 1996). Snyder (2004) concluded that benzene hematopoietic toxicity and leukemogenesis are primarily a function of the bone marrow, a site remote from the liver where most benzene metabolism occurs.

Benzene's metabolic pathways appear to be qualitatively, though not quantitatively similar in species studied to date (Henderson, 1996). Mice have a greater overall capacity to metabolize benzene than do rats or primates. Mani et al. (1999) reported good correlation between protein–DNA adduct levels in bone marrow and susceptibility to benzene genotoxicity and carcinogenesis in F-344 rats and three strains of mice. The B6C3F1 mouse shows the highest adduct levels and is the most sensitive of the animals tested. Powley and Carlson (1999) reported similar findings upon measurement of benzene metabolism in mouse, rat, rabbit, and human lung and liver microsomes. A paucity of information is available on the ability of human bone marrow to metabolically activate benzene.

Factors that alter the metabolism of benzene have the potential to influence the hematopoietic toxicity and carcinogenicity of the VOC. Pretreatment of rats with ethanol, a CYP2E1 inducer, enhanced metabolism of benzene and potentiated its acute and subacute myelotoxicity in rats (Nakajima et al., 1985) and mice (Marrubini et al., 2003). Phenobarbital had a negligible effect. Pretreatment of male B6C3F1 mice with acetone, another CYP2E1 inducer, increased benzene oxidation by about five-fold (Kenyon et al., 1996). Pretreatment with diethyldithiocarbamate, a CYP2E1 inhibitor, completely abolished benzene oxidation. Co-exposure of F-344 rats to gasoline and benzene resulted in competitive metabolic inhibition (Travis et al., 1992). Metabolism of benzene by hepatic microsomes from 10 human donors was directly proportional to CYP2E1 activity in the samples (Seaton et al., 1994). Thus, it would be anticipated that CYP2E1 polymorphisms may influence susceptibility to benzene toxicity. Male mice have consistently been found to be more sensitive than females to genotoxic effects of benzene. PBTK analysis of data from gas uptake experiments with B6C3F1 mice of both sexes revealed that the optimized maximum rate of benzene metabolism was twice as high in males (Kenyon et al., 1996). It is not known whether there is a sex-dependent difference in benzene metabolism in humans. Sato et al. (1975) saw a more rapid rate of pulmonary elimination of benzene in men than in women following inhalation of 25 ppm for 2 hours. Benzene was retained longer in the females due to their higher body fat content. Unfortunately, most epidemiology studies of benzene-exposed workers have not provided a gender comparison. Li et al. (1994) did not see a statistically significant difference in cancer mortality between

male and female workers exposed to benzene, though risks tended to be somewhat higher for males.

There are a number of cell populations in the bone marrow that may serve as targets for benzene metabolites. Benzene exposure in vivo results in inhibited growth and development of pluripotential bone marrow stem cells. More mature precursors, such as stromal cells and erythroid and myeloid colony-forming units, are also affected. Trush et al. (1996) point out that hydroquinone-induced inhibition of interleukin (IL)-1 synthesis by stromal macrophages results in altered differentiation of myeloid and lymphoid cells that are normally active in immune responses. These investigators also note that killing of stromal macrophages and fibroblasts could result in such a pronounced reduction of cytokines and growth factors that immature and committed hematopoietic progenitors would die from apoptosis. The erythroid series is more susceptible than the myeloid series to benzene-induced cytotoxicity. Immature myeloid cells can proliferate when the development of erythroid cells is restricted and acquire neoplastic characteristics upon dedifferentiation. The end result is AML (Golding and Watson, 1999).

Investigations of benzene toxicity/leukemogenesis have uncovered a variety of potential mechanisms (Golding and Watson, 1999; Snyder, 2002; Bird et al., 2005). As mentioned before, experimental evidence indicates that the complementary actions of benzene and several of its metabolites are required for myelotoxicity. It has been recognized for 20 years that a number of benzene metabolites can bind covalently to GSH, proteins, DNA, and RNA. This can result in disruption of the functional hematopoietic microenvironment by inhibition of enzymes, destruction of certain cell populations, and alteration of the growth of other cell types. Covalent binding of hydroquinones to spindle-fiber proteins will inhibit cell replication (Smith, 1996). In vitro studies have established that reactive benzene metabolites bind covalently to DNA of several tissues of different species. Through the use of accelerator mass spectrophotometry, Creek et al. (1997) have demonstrated DNA binding in mice exposed to extremely low ^{14}C-benzene levels. The binding was dose dependent over a wide range of doses. DNA adduct levels were so low, however, that this mechanism alone may be insufficient to fully account for leukemogenic effects.

It appears likely that oxidative stress contributes to benzene toxicity. As the bone marrow is rich in peroxidase activity, phenolic metabolites of benzene can be activated there to reactive quinone derivatives. Ross et al. (1996) discovered that myeloperoxidase present in murine and human progenitor cells could bioactivate hydroquinone to p-benzoquinone. Electron spin resonance experiments by Hiraku and Kawanishi (1996) revealed the formation of a semiquinone radical in p-benzoquinone-treated HL-60 cells (a human myeloid cell line). This suggested that reactive oxygen moieties (e.g., O_2^- and H_2O_2) are produced via the formation of the semiquinone radicals. These active oxygen species can cause DNA strand breaks or fragmentation, leading to cell mutation or apoptosis, respectively. Ross et al. (1996), however, pointed out that quinones can also inhibit proteases involved in induction of apoptosis. These authors noted that modulation of apoptosis may lead to aberrant hematopoiesis and neoplastic progression.

A number of biomarkers of exposure to benzene have been developed and carefully evaluated. Concentrations of the parent compound in exhaled breath parallel blood concentrations. Clayton et al. (1999) reported a high correlation between the extent of smoking-related activities and levels of benzene in exhaled breath of humans. Urinary excretion of a variety of benzene metabolites (i.e., phenol, catechol, hydroquinone, 1,2,4-trihydroxybenzene,

S-phenylmercapturic acid, and *t*,*t*-muconic acid) have been shown to be correlated with benzene exposure in occupational settings. Phenol, catechol, and hydroquinone, however, are neither sensitive nor specific biomarkers, because relatively high levels are found in nonexposed individuals (Medeiros *et al.*, 1997). Similarly, *t*,*t*-muconic acid is not specific, because it is a metabolite of sorbic acid, a common food additive. Boogaard and van Sittert (1996) conclude that *S*-phenylmercapturic acid, an end product of the conjugation of benzene oxide and GSH, is a suitable urinary biomarker for low-level benzene exposure because of its specificity and relatively long half-life. Adducts to hemoglobin and cysteine groups of proteins have been demonstrated in rodents, but not in humans. DNA damage has been detected in benzene-exposed workers (Liu *et al.*, 1996; Andreoli *et al.*, 1997), though such measures have not yet found widespread acceptance as biomarkers of effect.

A number of PBTK models have been developed to aid in predicting risks of myelotoxicity and leukemia posed to humans by benzene. Medinsky *et al.* (1989) published one of the first such models for benzene. They assumed that benzene metabolism followed Michaelis–Menten kinetics and occurred via benzene oxide. B6C3F1 mice, which are more sensitive than F-344 rats to benzene myelotoxicity, were predicted to metabolize two to three times more inhaled benzene. This and other PBTK models do not accurately simulate some laboratory data sets. Modeling benzene metabolism and disposition is difficult because of its inherent complexity and variability. In light of intricate dose–response relationships, Medinsky *et al.* (1996) emphasized the importance of considering competitive metabolic interactions between benzene and its metabolites, as well as the balance between enzymatic activation and inactivation processes. Cole *et al.* (2001) employed in vitro metabolic parameters for several pathways to construct a PBTK model that simulated most tissue dosimetry data sets for benzene-exposed mice quite well. Recently, Yokley *et al.* (2006) described a PBTK model that simulated tissue doses of benzene, benzene oxide, phenol, and hydroquinone in humans exposed orally and by inhalation. A Markov Chain Monte Carlo statistical technique was used to assess dissimilarities in population distributions of key model parameters. Variability in metabolic parameters and certain physiological parameters (e.g., organ weight) had to be inputed to accurately predict the range of human values.

Toluene

Toluene is present in paints, lacquers, thinners, cleaning agents, glues, and many other products. Toluene is also used in the production of other chemicals. Gasoline, which contains 5–7% toluene by weight, is the largest source of atmospheric emissions and exposure of the general populace (ATSDR, 2000). Inhalation is the primary route of exposure, though skin contact occurs frequently. Toluene is a favorite of solvent abusers, who intentionally inhale high concentrations to achieve a euphoric effect (Filley *et al.*, 2004). Large amounts of toluene enter the environment each year by volatilization. Relatively small amounts are released in industrial wastewater. Toluene is frequently found in water, soil, and air at hazardous waste sites (Fay and Mumtaz, 1996).

Toluene TK has been thoroughly characterized in humans and laboratory animals. Toluene is well absorbed from the lungs and GI tract. It rapidly accumulates in and affects the brain, due to that organ's high rate of blood perfusion and relatively high lipid content. Toluene subsequently is deposited in other tissues according to their lipid content, with adipose tissue attaining the highest levels.

Toluene is well metabolized, but a portion is exhaled unchanged. Hepatic P450s catalyze metabolism of toluene primarily to benzyl alcohol and lesser amounts of cresols. Benzyl alcohol is converted by ADH and aldehyde dehydrogenase (ALDH) to benzoic acid, which is primarily conjugated with glycine and eliminated in the urine as hippuric acid. Nakajima *et al.* (1992a) reported that CYP2E1 and CYP2C11 are primarily responsible for catalyzing the initial hydroxylation step in rat liver at low and high toluene levels, respectively. CYP2E1 is most active at low doses in humans (Nakajima *et al.*, 1997). Benignus *et al.* (1998) attempted to use a PBTK model to relate toluene blood levels to behavioral effects in rats and humans. It appeared that humans were more sensitive to increases in blood levels, but more rat data and much more human data are needed for model validation.

The CNS is the primary target organ of toluene and other alkylbenzenes. Manifestations of acute exposure range from slight dizziness and headache to unconsciousness, respiratory depression, and death. Occupational inhalation exposure guidelines are established to prevent significant decrements in psychomotor functions. Acute encephalopathic effects are rapidly reversible upon cessation of exposure (Fig. 24-3), and are not associated with neuroimaging changes (Filley *et al.*, 2004). Subtle neurologic effects have been described in some groups of occupationally exposed individuals. Exposure to ~100-ppm toluene for years may result in subclinical effects, as evidenced by altered brainstem auditory-evoked potentials (Abbate *et al.*, 1993) and changes in visual-evoked potentials (Vrca *et al.*, 1995). Foo *et al.* (1990) reported good correlation between toluene exposure and poor scores on neurobehavioral tests of 30 female rotogravure workers. Severe neurotoxicity is often diagnosed in persons who have abused toluene for a prolonged period. A relatively specific neurobehavioral profile is manifest including inattention, apathy, memory dysfunction, diminished visuospatial skills, frontal lobe dysfunction, and psychiatric status (Ron, 1986; Filley *et al.*, 2004). Magnetic resonance imaging reveals ventricular enlargement, cerebral atrophy and white matter hyperintensity, a characteristic profile termed toluene leukoencephalopathy. Such changes represent severe, chronic myelintoxicity. More advanced neuroimaging techniques may be able to reveal mild, subtle changes associated with early alterations in myelin of workers as well as toluene abusers (Caldemeyer *et al.*, 1996; Filley *et al.*, 2004). Rat pups subjected to high doses of toluene on days 6–19 of gestation exhibited a significant reduction in myelination per forebrain cell when they were 21 days old (Gospe and Zhou, 1998).

There is limited information on mechanisms by which toluene and similar solvents produced acute or residual CNS effects (Balster, 1998). The Meyer–Overton theory of partitioning of the lipophilic parent compounds into membrane lipids has been widely accepted for a century. It has been proposed that the presence of solvent molecules in cholesterol-filled interstices between phospholipids and sphingolipids changes membrane fluidity, thereby altering intercellular communication and normal ion movements (Engelke *et al.*, 1996). Such a process is reversible. An alternate hypothesis is that toluene partitions into hydrophobic regions of proteins and interacts with them, thereby altering membrane-bound enzyme activity and/or receptor specificity in a reversible manner (Balster, 1998). Other evidence suggests that toluene and other VOCs may act acutely by enhancing $GABA_A$ receptor function (Mihic *et al.*, 1994), attenuating NMDA receptor-stimulated calcium flux (Cruz *et al.*, 1998), and/or activating dopamingeric systems (von Euler, 1994). The mechanism of chronic toluene neurotoxicity is unknown. Toluene is known to be deposited in brain areas with the highest myelin content. Astrocytosis frequently accompanies myelin disruption (Gotohda *et al.*, 2000; Filley *et al.*, 2004).

As toluene is metabolized by CYPs, ADH, and ALDH, the chemical can interact with other xenobiotics metabolized by these enzymes. Concurrent exposure to solvents metabolized by the same CYP isoforms can result in competitive metabolic inhibition. Inoue *et al.* (1988) observed that benzene and toluene suppressed one another's metabolism in humans. Thus, the risk of leukopenia in workers exposed to benzene and toluene should be less than that in workers exposed to benzene alone. Pryor and Rebert (1992) found that toluene greatly reduced manifestations of peripheral neuropathy caused by *n*-hexane in rats. Although no interaction between toluene and xylenes was seen in humans inhaling low levels of each, simultaneous exposure to higher levels results in mutual metabolic suppression (Tardif *et al.*, 1991). Prior exposure to P450 inducers can result in increased rates of toluene metabolism/elimination and more rapid recovery from toluene-induced CNS depression. Nakajima and Wang (1994) observed that high concentrations of inhaled toluene moderately induced four of the six P450 isoforms that metabolize it, but inhibited the other two in rat liver.

High-level prenatal toluene exposures have produced growth and skeletal retardations in offspring of rodents and humans. The term "fetal solvent syndrome" was used to describe toluene-abusing women's children who exhibit microcephaly and cranial facial features similar to those with fetal alcohol syndrome (FAS) (Wilkins-Haug, 1997). The reproductive and developmental toxic potential of toluene was evaluated in a two-generation study of Sprague–Dawley rats (Roberts *et al.*, 2003). Both sexes of each generation were essentially exposed to 0, 100, 500, or 2,000 ppm toluene vapor 6 h/d, 7 d/week for 80 days premating and for 15 days of mating. Pregnant animals were also exposed from gestation days 1–20 and lactation days 5–21. No adverse effects were seen at any dose on fertility, reproductive performance, or maternal or pup behavior. Reduced fetal body weight and skeletal anomalies associated with growth retardation were manifest in the offspring of both generations subjected to 2000 ppm, but not to lower vapor levels (Roberts *et al.*, 2003).

Xylenes and Ethylbenzene

Large numbers of people are exposed to xylenes and ethylbenzene occupationally and environmentally (Wallace *et al.*, 1987). Xylenes (ATSDR, 2006d) and ethylbenzene (ATSDR, 1999), like benzene and toluene, are major components of gasoline and fuel oil. The primary uses of xylenes industrially are as solvents and synthetic intermediates. Most of these aromatics that are released into the environment evaporate into the atmosphere. They may also enter groundwater from oil and gasoline spills, leakage of storage tanks, and migration from waste sites.

The TK and acute toxicity of toluene, xylenes, and other aromatic solvents are quite similar. Xylenes and the others are well absorbed from the lungs and GI tract, distributed to tissues according to tissue blood flow and lipid content, exhaled unchanged to some extent, well metabolized by hepatic P450s, and largely excreted as urinary metabolites (Lof and Johanson, 1998). Nielsen and Alarie (1982) state that the potency of benzene and a series of alkylbenzenes, as sensory irritants of the upper respiratory tract of mice, increases with increasing lipophilicity. Acute lethality of hydrocarbons (i.e., CNS-depressant potency) also varies directly with lipophilicity (Swann *et al.*, 1974). There is limited evidence that chronic occupational exposure to xylenes is associated with residual neurologic effects (ATSDR, 2006c). Exposure con-

ditions, including the presence of other solvents, have usually not been characterized in such reports. Uchida *et al.* (1993), for example, reported increased subjective CNS symptoms in workers exposed for ~7 years to a mean of 21 ppm xylenes. The prevalence of symptoms was not dose dependent, nor were other solvent exposures characterized. This vapor concentration is significantly lower than current occupational exposure standards in the United States, which are established on the basis of acute irritancy or CNS effects. Savolainen *et al.* (1981) observed improved performance on a series of psychophysiological tests by humans inhaling 200 ppm *m*-xylene for 4 hours. An excitatory stage is often initially manifest in subjects, followed by functional inhibition with higher vapor concentrations and/or longer exposure periods. The current permissible exposure limit in the United States is 100 ppm.

Xylenes and ethylbenzene appear to have very limited capacity to adversely affect organs other than the CNS. Mild, transient liver and/or kidney toxicity have/has occasionally been reported in humans exposed to high vapor concentrations of xylenes. Little evidence of hepatorenal injury is typically manifest in laboratory animals (ATSDR, 2006c). Generally, hepatic P450s are moderately induced by alkylbenzenes (Gut *et al.*, 1993). Many investigators have reported xylenes to increase liver weight and to induce liver P450s in rats and other rodents. The *o*, *p*, and *m* isomers of xylene vary somewhat in their capacity to induce different P450 isoforms in different organs of rats (Backes *et al.*, 1993). Concurrent exposure to an alkylbenzene and another compound metabolized by P450s generally results in their competitive metabolic inhibition. Preexposure to an alkylbenzene, conversely, can result in increased metabolism of the other chemical.

The majority of alkylbenzenes do not appear to be genotoxic or carcinogenic. Ethylbenzene and styrene are two exceptions. Kidney injury and an increased incidence of renal adenoma and carcinoma (combined) were found in male F-344 rats exposed to 750 ppm ethylbenzene for up to 2 years (NTP, 1997b). Styrene's carcinogenic potential is discussed below.

Styrene

Styrene is primarily used in the manufacture of polystyrene items and in copolymers with acrylonitrile or 1,3-butadiene to produce synthetic rubber, latex, and reinforced plastics (Gibbs and Mulligan, 1997). Worker exposures in the rubber industry are of greatest concern toxicologically. Styrene is also often detected in the blood of nonoccupationally exposed populations (Churchill *et al.*, 2001; Blount *et al.*, 2006). Sources include tobacco smoke, auto exhaust, and emissions from building materials. Discharges from industry are the major source of environmental pollution (ATSDR, 1992).

There is considerable debate as to whether styrene is a human carcinogen. Styrene is toxic to the nasal epithelium of rats and mice, and hepatotoxic and pneumotoxic in mice. Workers exposed to ~25 ppm exhibit signs of mild hepatic injury and cholestasis (Brodkin *et al.*, 2001). Styrene is metabolized principally by CYP2E1- and CYP2F2-catalyzed side-chain oxidation to styrene-7,8-oxide (SO) in mouse lung and liver (Linhart *et al.*, 2000; Carlson, 2003). This epoxide is detoxified by the actions of epoxide hydrolase and GST. SO is detoxified much more efficiently by epoxide hydrolase in humans than in mice. SO can bind covalently to proteins and nucleic acids. It is carcinogenic to the forestomach of orally dosed mice and rats (Roe, 1994). Results of in vitro and in vivo mutagenicity and genotoxicity studies of styrene have been mixed

(ATSDR, 1992). Chromosomal aberrations, micronuclei, and/or sister chromatid exchange have been reported in employees in some high-exposure occupational settings, but not in others. Increased rates of different cancers have been reported in workers exposed to 1,3-butadiene and styrene in the synthetic rubber industry. The excesses of cancers have largely been attributed to 1,3-butadiene, though styrene may modify the actions of 1,3-butadiene and/or be implicated itself (Matonoski et al., 1997). Occasional findings of small increases in incidences of lymphatic and hematopoietic neoplasms in workers exposed primarily to styrene are not very robust (IARC, 2002). An inhalation cancer bioassay revealed increases in pulmonary adenomas and/or carcinomas in male and female mice, but four gavage studies were negative. (No reliable evidence of increased cancer incidence was seen in the four gavage, two other inhalation or one drinking water bioassay in rats (IARC, 2002).)

Workers in the reinforced plastics industry are exposed to styrene and SO. Tornero-Velez and Rappaport (2001) used a modified PBTK model to predict the relative contributions of inhaled styrene and SO to systemic levels of SO in humans. SO was forecast to present the greater cytogenetic hazard. Sarangapani et al. (2002) created a PBTK model with a multicompartment representation of the respiratory tract that included species-specific quantitative information on physiology, cellular composition, and metabolic capacity. The model-based analysis indicated that humans would be 100-fold less susceptible than mice to pulmonary tumors, based on predictions of SO concentrations in terminal bronchioles. Wenker et al. (2002) attempted to correlate key P450 metabolic capacities of 20 male volunteers with styrene clearance. The lack of correlation was attributed to the low inhaled vapor concentrations and styrene's blood flow-limited metabolism.

ALCOHOLS

Ethanol

Many humans experience greater exposure to ethanol (ethyl alcohol and alcohol) than to any other solvent. Not only is ethyl alcohol used as an additive in gasoline, as a solvent in industry, in many household products, and in pharmaceuticals, but it is also heavily consumed in intoxicating beverages. Frank toxic effects are less important occupationally than injuries resulting from psychomotor impairment. Driving under the influence of alcohol is, of course, the major cause of fatal auto accidents. In many states in the United States, a blood alcohol level of 80 mg/100 mL blood (80 mg%) is prima facie evidence of "driving while intoxicated." One's blood alcohol level and the time necessary to achieve it are controlled largely by the rapidity and extent of consumption of the chemical. Ethanol is distributed in body water and to some degree in adipose tissue. Alcohol is eliminated by urinary excretion, exhalation, and metabolism. The blood level in an average adult decreases by ≈ 16 mg% per hour. Thus, a person with a blood alcohol level of 120 mg% would require ≈ 8 hours to reach negligible levels.

Ethanol is metabolized to acetaldehyde by three enzymes: (1) The major pathway involves ADH-catalyzed oxidation to acetaldehyde. ADHs are present in various tissues including stomach, lung, eye, and liver, but the highest concentrations are found in the cytoplasm of hepatocytes (Yin et al., 1999). While hepatic ADH largely contributes to ethanol oxidation in humans (Lee et al., 2006), a PBTK model indicates both hepatic and gastric ADH contribute to first-pass metabolism of ethanol in rats, with gastric ADH playing a greater role at lower ethanol doses (Pastino and Conolly, 2000).

The oxidation they catalyze is reversible, but the acetaldehyde that is formed is rapidly oxidized by acetaldehyde dehydrogenase (ALDH) to acetate. Liver mitochondrial ALDH is the major enzyme responsible for acetaldehyde clearance. However, a recent PBTK model predicted the reversible conversion of acetaldehyde to alcohol by ADH to be an essential step in the systemic clearance of acetaldehyde (Umulis et al., 2005). (2) A second enzyme, catalase, utilizes H_2O_2 supplied by the actions of NADPH oxidase and xanthine oxidase. There is usually little H_2O_2 available in hepatocytes to support the reaction, so it is unlikely that catalase will normally account for more than 10% of ethyl alcohol metabolism. (3) The third enzyme, CYP2E1, is the principal isoform of the hepatic microsomal ethanol-oxidizing system.

Ethanol interacts with other solvents that are also metabolized by ADH and CYP2E1. Ethanol can be an effective antidote for poisoning by methanol, ethylene glycol, and diethylene glycol. As ethyl alcohol has a relatively high affinity for ADH, it competitively inhibits the metabolic activation of other alcohols and glycols. Pre-exposure to a single high dose or multiple doses of ethanol can induce CYP2E1, thereby enhancing the metabolic activation and potentiating the toxicity of a considerable number of other solvents and drugs such as acetaminophen (Lieber, 1997; Klotz and Ammon, 1998). Manno et al. (1996), for example, describe heavy drinkers who developed severe hepatorenal toxicity from CCl4 exposures, which caused no ill effects in nondrinkers. Other alcohols, such as 2-butanol (Fig. 24-4), can have analogous effects (Traiger and Bruckner, 1976). Chronic heavy drinkers may develop more severe hepatotoxicity associated with acetaminophen overdosing than non-alcoholics, due to increased formation and reduced detoxification of toxic metabolites (Riordan and Williams, 2002; Rumack, 2004). Such interactions are also described under the Metabolism and Exogenous Factors subsections in this chapter.

A variety of factors that modulate ADH, CYP2E1, and ALDH can influence adverse effects experienced by drinkers. Relatively low ADH and CYP2E1 activities increase systemic alcohol levels and prolong its effects, while low ALDH results in elevated acetaldehyde levels. Long-term ingestion of high alcohol doses can lead to alcohol dependency and cirrhosis, whereas high acetaldehyde levels may result in acute toxicity due to covalent binding to proteins and other macromolecules (Niemela, 1999). Ethanol-metabolizing enzymes exist in multiple molecular forms that are genetically controlled. Genetic polymorphisms of these enzymes contribute to different disease outcomes in different ethnic and racial populations (Crabb et al., 2004; Russo et al., 2004). Asians have higher frequencies of an ADH1*2 variant, which encodes for a rapidly metabolizing form of ADH, preventing alcoholism. White and black populations in the United States predominantly have an ADH1*1 allele (Russo et al., 2004), which encodes for a relatively inactive ADH (Lee et al., 2006), leading to increased risk of alcohol dependency. As for ALDH, some 50% of Asians have high levels of the inactive allele, ALDH2*2. Hence, this population experiences acetaldehyde-induced flushing, tachycardia, nausea, vomiting, and hyperventilation upon alcohol consumption. Whereas this syndrome offers protection against developing alcoholism, it increases the risk of acetaldehyde-related cancers, including esophageal, stomach, colon, lung, head, and neck tumors (Vasiliou et al., 2004). Hispanics, on the other hand, have very low levels of ADH1*2 and ALDH2*2, predisposing them to alcoholism and their offspring to fetal alcohol syndrome (FAS). Disulfiram, an ALDH inhibitor, is used to treat alcoholism, by enhancing acetaldehyde levels when alcohol is consumed. Whereas CYP2E1 polymorphism is reported in humans (Zintzaras *et al.*, 2006), its role in the pathogenicity of alcoholism is still unclear.

Gender differences in responses to ethanol are well recognized. Women are more sensitive to alcohol, and exhibit higher mortality at lower levels of consumption than men (Sato *et al.*, 2001; Brienza and Stein, 2002). Women exhibit somewhat higher blood levels than men following ingestion of equivalent doses of ethanol (Pikaar *et al.*, 1988). This phenomenon appears to be due in part to more extensive ADH-catalyzed metabolism of ethanol by the male gastric mucosa (Frezza *et al.*, 1990; Seitz *et al.*, 1993). Kinetic data indicate that hepatic ADH does not play a role in the sex difference in first-pass elimination of ethanol, though Chrostek *et al.* (2003) did report higher activities of ADH isoforms that efficiently oxidize ethanol in the liver of male subjects. Sex differences in ethanol metabolism in the remainder of the body appear to be small or nonexistent. A second factor contributing to the higher blood ethanol levels and greater CNS effects in women is their smaller volume of distribution for relatively polar solvents such as alcohols. It is well known that women are more susceptible to alcohol-induced hepatitis and cirrhosis (Thurman, 2000). A postulated mechanism for this sex difference is described below.

FAS is the most common, preventable cause of mental retardation. Diagnostic criteria for FAS include: (1) heavy maternal alcohol consumption during gestation; (2) pre- and postnatal growth retardation; (3) craniofacial malformations including microcephaly; and (4) mental retardation. Less complete manifestations of gestational ethanol exposure also occur and are referred to as fetal alcohol effects or alcohol-related neurodevelopmental disorder. The prevalence of FAS in the United States ranges from 0.5–2 cases per 1000 live births (May and Gossage, 2001; CDC, 2002). Although the total amount of alcohol consumed and the pattern of drinking are both important factors, peak maternal blood alcohol level is apparently the most important determinant of the likelihood of FAS and the severity of its effects. Overconsumption during all three trimesters of pregnancy can result in certain manifestations, dependent on the period of gestation during which ingestion occurs.

Despite an intensive research effort for three decades, the mechanisms underlying FAS remain unclear. Exposure of embryonic tissue to ethanol adversely affects many cellular functions critical to development, including protein and DNA synthesis, uptake of critical nutrients such as glucose and amino acids, and changes in several kinase-mediated signal transduction pathways (Shibley and Pennington, 1997). Alcohol may also harm the fetus indirectly as a result of the mother's malnutrition. Numerous mechanisms have been suggested as contributing to alcohol-induced fetal damage, although none has been established with certainty (Goodlett and Horn, 2001). Some studies have suggested that oxidative stress on fetal tissues is responsible (Henderson *et al.*, 1999), while others have implicated ethanol's effects on neurotransmitter-gated ion channels, particularly the NMDA receptor (Costa *et al.*, 2000), and its ability to trigger cell death via necrosis and apoptosis (Ikonomidou *et al.*, 2000; Goodlett and Horn, 2001). Others have reported that ethanol produces a long-lasting reduction in synaptic efficacy (Bellinger *et al.*, 1999) and alters the fetal expression of developmentally important genes such as msx2 and insulin-like growth factors (Singh *et al.*, 1996; Rifas *et al.*, 1997). Recent studies suggest that NMDA and GABA receptor-mediated apoptosis play critical roles in learning impairment (Ikonomidou *et al.*, 2000; Olney *et al.*, 2002; Toso *et al.*, 2006). Acetaldehyde may also contribute to the development of FAS, as it is shown to accumulate in the fetal brain after prenatal alcohol exposure (Hamby-Mason *et al.*, 1997)

and to be cytotoxic to cultured embryonic brain cells (Lee *et al.*, 2005).

A role for CYP2E1 in the induction of FAS has been hypothesized, given its expression in human cephalic tissues during embryogenesis (Boutelet-Bochan *et al.*, 1997). Results of in vitro experiments indicate that human CYP2E1 is effective in production of reactive oxygen intermediates (e.g., hydroxy radicals, superoxide anion, and H_2O_2) and in causation of lipid peroxidation (Dai *et al.*, 1993). Membrane lipids and a variety of enzymes are targets for free radical attack. Albano *et al.* (1999) have demonstrated a marked increase in covalent binding of hydroxyethyl radicals to hepatic microsomal proteins from rats following chronic ethanol administration. There is not yet direct evidence that hydroxyethyl radicals contribute to lipid peroxidation, but they do readily react with α-tocopherol, GSH, and ascorbic acid, thereby potentially lowering liver antioxidant levels in vivo. Albano *et al.* (1999) also describe evidence that hydroxyethyl radical-protein adducts in hepatocytes induce immune responses, which may contribute to chronic ethanol hepatotoxicity.

Alcohol-induced hepatotoxicity is postulated to be caused by elevation of endotoxin in the bloodstream. Endotoxin, released by the action of ethanol on gram-negative bacteria in the gut, is believed to be taken up by Kupffer cells, causing the release of inflammatory mediators that are cytotoxic to hepatocytes and chemoattractants for neutrophils (Bautista, 2000; Diehl, 2000). These mediators include interleukins, prostaglandins, free radicals, and TNF-α. Proinflammatory cytokines and oxidative stress stimulate collagen synthesis by hepatic stellate cells, leading to alcoholic fibrosis (Lieber, 2004). Acetaldehyde is also capable of upregulating collagen synthesis either directly or indirectly by inducing TGF-β1. Hence, polymorphisms of ALDH can increase the risk of fibrosis (Purohit and Brenner, 2006). Kupffer cells of female rats are more sensitive to endotoxin than those of males. Estrogen increases the sensitivity of Kupffer cells of rats to endotoxin, leading to increased production of TNF-α and death of hepatocytes (Thurman, 2000; Yin *et al.*, 2000; Colantoni *et al.*, 2003). This phenomenon is believed to account in part for the more severe hepatitis and cirrhosis commonly seen in female alcoholics (Thurman, 2000).

Alcohol-induced damage of the liver and other tissues is believed to result in part from nutritional disturbances, as well as toxic effects (Lieber, 2004; DiCecco and Francisco-Ziller, 2006). Lack of money, poor judgment, prolonged inebriation, and appetite loss contribute to poor nutrition and weight loss in alcoholics. A high percentage of calories in the alcoholic's diet is furnished by alcohol. Malabsorption of thiamine, diminished enterohepatic circulation of folate, degradation of pyridoxal phosphate, and disturbances in the metabolism of vitamins A and D can occur (Mezey, 1985). Prostaglandins released from endotoxin-activated Kupffer cells may be responsible for a hypermetabolic state in the liver. With the increase in oxygen demand, the viability of centrilobular hepatocytes would be most compromised, due to their relatively poor oxygen supply (Thurman, 1998). Metabolism of ethanol via ADH and ALDH results in a shift in the redox state of the cell. The metabolites and the more reduced state can result in hyperlactacidemia, hyperlipidemia, hyperuricemia, and hyperglycemia, leading to increased steatosis and collagen synthesis (Lieber, 2004).

Alcoholism can result in damage of extrahepatic tissues. Alcoholic myopathy is one of the more common consequences, occurring in 50% of alcohol abusers. The condition is characterized by reductions in skeletal muscle mass and strength (Adachi *et al.*, 2003; Preedy *et al.*, 2003). Alcoholic cardiomyopathy is a complex process that occurs in 20–25% of alcoholics. It results from decreased synthesis of cardiac contractile proteins, attack of oxygen radicals, increases in endoplasmic reticulum Ca^{2+}-ATPase and an antibody response to acetaldehyde–protein adducts (Richardson et al., 1998; Preedy et al., 2003). Interestingly, light-to-moderate drinking is reported to protect against atherosclerosis in the carotid artery, a major cause of ischemic stroke (Hillbom, 1999). Alcohol increases high-density lipoprotein (HDL) cholesterol by inducing the constituents, apo I and II, by increasing catabolism of very low-density lipoproteins and chylomicrons, and by delaying HDL catabolism (Kolovou et al., 2006). It is also hypothesized that ethanol metabolism in the vascular wall may inhibit oxidation of low-density lipoproteins (LDL), a requisite for atherogenesis. Phenolic antioxidants in wines may also inhibit LDL oxidation as well as reduce platelet aggregation. Conversely, heavy drinking appears to deplete antioxidants and have the opposite effects (Hillbom, 1999; Kolovou et al., 2006). Recent heavy drinking increases the risk of both hemorrhagic and ischemic strokes. Other organ systems can be adversely affected in alcoholics including the brain and GI tract (Kril et al., 1997; Rajendram and Preedy, 2005).

There is concern about the role of ethyl alcohol in carcinogenesis, due to the frequent consumption of alcoholic beverages by millions of people. IARC (1988) concluded that there was "sufficient evidence" for causation of tumors of the oral cavity, pharynx and larynx, esophagus, and liver of humans. Use of alcohol is also linked to a moderate increase in risk of lobular and hormone receptor-positive breast cancer in women (Li et al., 2003). Genotoxic effects by acetaldehyde and elevated estrogen levels are likely mechanisms (Boffetta and Hashibe, 2006). The original associations between alcohol and cancers came primarily from epidemiological case–control and cohort studies. One such cohort study of 276,000 American men showed increase in total cancer risk with increasing ethanol consumption (Boffeta and Garfinkel, 1990). In support of epidemiological studies, a rat study showed that ethanol induces tumors in various organs including oral cavity, tongue, and lips (Soffritti et al., 2002). Evidence suggests that the risk of alcohol-induced cancer in humans is modulated by genetic polymorphisms in enzymes responsible for alcohol metabolism, folate metabolism, and DNA repair (Boffetta and Hashibe, 2006). Ethanol and smoking act synergistically to cause oral, pharyngeal, and laryngeal cancers. It is generally believed that alcohol induces liver cancer by causing cirrhosis or other chronic liver damage and/or by enhancing the bioactivation of other carcinogens (Table 24-3).

Table 24-3
Possible Mechanisms of Ethanol Carcinogenicity

Congeners: additives and contaminants in alcoholic beverages influence carcinogenicity.
CYP2E1 induction by ethanol increases metabolic activation of procarcinogens.
Ethanol acts as a solvent for carcinogens, enhancing their absorption into tissues of the upper GI tract.
Ethanol affects the actions of certain hormones on hormone-sensitive tissues.
Immune function is suppressed by alcohol.
Absorption and bioavailability of nutrients are reduced by alcohol.

SOURCE: Adapted with permission of Ahmed (1995).

An international symposium (Purohit et al., 2005), sponsored by the National Institute on Alcohol Abuse and Alcoholism in 2004, concluded that chronic ethanol consumption may promote carcinogenesis by: (1) production of acetaldehyde, a weak mutagen and carcinogen; (2) induction of CYP2E1 and its associated oxidative stressors and conversion of procarcinogens to carcinogens; (3) depletion of SAM and, consequently, induction of global DNA hypomethylation; (4) increased production of inhibitory guanine nucleotide regulatory proteins and components of extracellular signal-regulated kinase-mitogen-activated protein kinase signaling; (5) accumulation of iron and associated oxidative stress; (6) inactivation of the tumor suppressor gene BRCA1 and increased estrogen responsiveness (primarily in the breast); and (7) impairment of retinoic acid metabolism.

Methanol

Methanol (methyl alcohol, wood alcohol, and CH_3OH) is primarily used as a starting material for the synthesis of chemicals such as formaldehyde, acetic acid, methacrylates, ethylene glycol, and methyl tertiary-butyl ether (MTBE). CH_3OH is found in windshield washer fluid, carburetor cleaners, antifreeze, and copy machine toner, and serves as fuel for Sterno™ heaters, model airplanes, and Indianapolis 500 racecars. It also functions as a denaturant for some ethyl and isopropyl alcohols, rendering them unfit for consumption. It is used to a limited extent as an alternative fuel for fleet vehicles (usually in a mixture of 85% CH_3OH and 15% gasoline) and is being explored as a gasoline additive and hydrogen source for fuel cell vehicles. Exposure of the general population also occurs via the consumption of fruits, fruit juices, vegetables, and alcoholic beverages that contain free CH_3OH or CH_3OH precursors. Indirect exposure occurs via the hydrolysis of the artificial sweetener, aspartame, and subsequent CH_3OH absorption from the gut. Very low-level exposures may occur via ambient air and drinking water. Of all chemicals reported, CH_3OH was ranked No. 1 for fugitive air emissions, No. 3 for point source air emissions, and No. 2 for surface water discharges according to the 2004 Toxic Release Inventory (EPA, 2006b). Persistence and bioaccumulation in the environment are not expected. The consumption of adulterated "bootleg" whiskey is a major cause of CH_3OH poisoning. Serious CH_3OH toxicity is most commonly associated with ingestion. Left untreated, acute CH_3OH poisoning in humans is characterized by an asymptomatic latent period of 12–24 hours followed by formic acidemia, ocular toxicity, coma, and in extreme cases death (Lanigan, 2001). Visual disturbances generally develop between 18 and 48 hours after ingestion and range from mild photophobia and misty or blurred vision to markedly reduced visual acuity and complete blindness (Eells et al., 1996). Although there is considerable variability among individuals in susceptibility to CH_3OH, a frequently cited lethal oral dosage is 1 mL/kg. Blindness and death have been reported with dosages as low as 0.1 mL/kg (ATSDR, 1993). CH_3OH's target within the eye is the retina, specifically the optic disk and optic nerve. Optic disk edema and hyperemia are seen, along with morphological alterations in the optic nerve head and the intraorbital portion of the optic nerve. Both axons and glial cells exhibit altered morphologies (Kavet and Nauss, 1990). Rods and cones, the photoreceptors of the retina, are also altered functionally and structurally (Seme et al., 1999). Evidence is accumulating that Müller cells, neuroglia that function in the maintenance of retinal structure and in intra- and intercellular transport, are early targets of CH_3OH (Garner et al., 1995a). There are indications of mitochondrial disruption in Müller and photoreceptor cells, which is consistent with the long-held view that formate inhibits the energy-generating mitochondrial enzyme, cytochrome *c* oxidase, which is critical for the proper functioning of highly oxidative organs like the retina. This mechanism might explain, at least in part, CH_3OH's selective toxicity to photoreceptors and other highly metabolically active cells (Eells *et al.*, 1996). Interestingly, exposure of rats to monochromatic red radiation from light-emitting diode arrays can aid in the recovery of rod and cone function in CH_3OH-treated rats and protect the retina from histopathological changes characteristic of formate toxicity (Eells *et al.*, 2003). This "photobiomodulation" is thought to be mediated by the ability of monochromatic red to near-IR light to improve mitochondrial respiratory chain function (i.e., increase cytochrome *c* oxidase activity), thereby initiating a signaling cascade that promotes cellular proliferation and cytoprotection.

As with CH_3OH's chronic toxicity, elucidation of the mechanism of CH_3OH's acute toxicity was hampered for years by species differences in susceptibility and the lack of appropriate animal models. Largely based on the work of Gilger and Potts (1955), it became apparent that only non-human primates respond to CH_3OH similarly to humans. The severe metabolic acidosis frequently seen in humans does not occur in rodents. In all mammalian species studied, CH_3OH is metabolized in the liver by ADH to formaldehyde (HCOH), which in turn is very rapidly converted via ALDH to formate. The conversion of formate to CO_2 then occurs via a two-step, tetrahydrofolate (THF)-dependent pathway. First, formate is converted to 10-formyl-THF by formyl-THF synthetase, after which 10-formyl-THF is oxidized to CO_2 by formyl-THF dehydrogenase (F-THF-DH). The species differences in susceptibility to CH_3OH are thought to result primarily from differences in the rate of THF-dependent oxidation of formate to CO_2. Because rodents have much higher hepatic THF levels than primates, formate does not accumulate as it does in humans and monkeys (Medinsky and Dorman, 1995; Martinasevic *et al.*, 1996). Another possible explanation is the lower F-THF-DH activity in primate liver (Johlin *et al.*, 1989). It is further speculated that primates are more susceptible to CH_3OH and formate toxicity due to their relative inability to excrete excess formate via the kidneys (Smith and Taylor, 1982). Regardless, susceptibility to CH_3OH-induced ocular toxicity is dependent on the relative rate of formate clearance. Dietary and chemical depletion of endogenous folate cofactors in rats have been shown to increase formate accumulation following CH_3OH, resulting in the development of metabolic acidosis and ocular toxicity similar to that observed in humans (Eells *et al.*, 1996, 2000). A simplified scheme of CH_3OH metabolism is presented in Fig. 24-10.

For years there was considerable debate whether HCOH or formate was responsible for CH_3OH's ocular toxicity. The finding that HCOH does not accumulate following CH_3OH treatment, even in folate-deficient monkeys that are profoundly sensitive to CH_3OH, argues against a role for HCOH. Also, species of differing susceptibility exhibit comparable blood HCOH half-lives. In contrast, formate has been shown to accumulate in the human and monkey following CH_3OH treatment. CH_3OH-derived formate has also been quantified in the vitreous humor, retina, and to a lesser extent the optic nerve (Eells *et al.*, 1996). Moreover, CH_3OH-induced retinal dysfunction, as indicated by diminution of the amplitude of electroretinogram (ERG) *a* and *b* waves, is negatively correlated in a linear fashion with blood formate concentrations (Eells *et al.*, 1996). Others have reported similar relationships between blood formate and ERG responses indicative of photoreceptor dysfunction (Seme *et al.*, 1999). Formate has also been shown to induce ocular toxicity

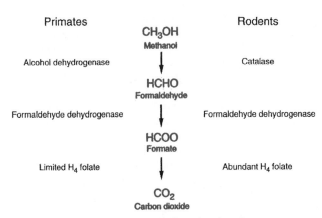

Figure 24-10. Scheme for the metabolism of methanol.

Major enzymes are listed for primates (*left*) and rodents (*right*). Conversion of formate to CO_2 is rapid in rodents, but relatively slow in primates. [Used with permission of Dorman DC, Welsch F: *CIIT Activities* 16:1–7, 1996.]

in monkeys and formate oxidation-inhibited rats in the absence of metabolic acidosis or a reduction in blood pH (Martin-Amat *et al.*, 1978; Eells *et al.*, 1996). Direct incubation of formate with cultured ocular cells caused ATP depletion and cytotoxicity (Treichel *et al.*, 2003). Thus, formate appears to act as a direct ocular toxin and not indirectly through the induction of an acidotic state, though acidosis may potentiate formate toxicity (since the inhibition of cytochrome oxidase increases as pH decreases and acidosis allows for greater diffusion of formic acid into cells).

The question has been raised whether ocular toxicity is simply a function of circulating formate reaching the visual tract, or whether metabolism in retinal or optic nerve tissues generates toxic metabolites locally. This is a legitimate question considering that metabolism of CH_3OH to HCOH via peroxisomal enzymes (catalase) has been demonstrated in rat retina in vitro (Garner *et al.*, 1995a), and the presence of cytoplasmic ALDH activity has been demonstrated in several regions of the rat and mouse eye, including the retina (Messiha and Price, 1983; McCaffery *et al.*, 1991). By use of a folate-deficient rat model, Garner *et al.* (1995b) showed that a level of blood formate generated by i.v. infusion of pH-buffered formate did not diminish the ERG *b*-wave amplitude generated by Müller cells of the retina, as did a comparable blood level of formate derived from CH_3OH. This suggests that the intraretinal metabolism of CH_3OH is necessary for the initiation of retinal toxicity by formate. Not only are the enzymes necessary to produce formate present in the retina, but so too are folate and F-THF-DH. F-THF-DH was found to be localized in the mitochondria of Müller cells, prompting the suggestion that F-THF-DH may serve a dual role, one protective of the Müller cell and the other toxic. Protection would come in the form of formate oxidation; toxicity from the overconsumption or depletion of ATP required for formate metabolism via the folate pathway (Martinasevic *et al.*, 1996).

The aforementioned findings raise concerns about the safety of CH_3OH exposure. Chamber studies of human volunteers exposed to 200 ppm CH_3OH for 4 or 6 hours showed no blood formate accumulation above background (Lee *et al.*, 1992; d'Alessandro *et al.*, 1994). Whereas this might be considered evidence that exposure at the current ACGIH TLV and OSHA PEL of 200 ppm poses no risk of ocular toxicity, such an interpretation may not be valid given that ocular toxicity may be a function of intraretinal CH_3OH metabolism rather than circulating formate levels.

The effects of acute, high CH_3OH exposures are well characterized compared to those of chronic, low-level exposures. Few reproductive/developmental studies and even fewer cancer bioassays have been conducted, due to the fact that rodents are not an ideal animal model for CH_3OH. Nonetheless, Soffritti *et al.* (2002) conducted a bioassay in which Sprague–Dawley rats received CH_3OH in their drinking water (0, 500, 5000, or 20,000 ppm) ad libitum for 104 weeks. The investigators concluded that CH_3OH was a multipotent carcinogen. However, they did reference two Japanese bioassays that found no evidence of carcinogenicity in B6C3F1 mice or F-344 rats exposed 20 h/d to 10-, 100-, or 1000-ppm CH_3OH by inhalation for 18 and 24 months, respectively (NEDO, 1987; Katoh, 1989).

The NTP Center for the Evaluation of Risks to Human Reproduction released a monograph on CH_3OH's reproductive/developmental toxicity, largely based on an expert panel report (NTP, 2003, 2004b). Among the conclusions was that CH_3OH is a potential developmental toxicant in humans, provided a high enough blood concentration of the parent compound (assumed to be the proximate teratogen) is achieved. As this conclusion was largely based on data in rodents that metabolize CH_3OH much differently than humans, its validity has been called into question (Clary, 2003). As such, the few reproductive/developmental studies in non-human primates are particularly informative. These studies reported that maternal exposure of monkeys to inhaled CH_3OH (200, 600, or 1800 ppm, 2.5 h/d, 7 d/week prior to breeding and throughout pregnancy) was not associated with maternal toxicity, reproductive loss, or congenital malformations in offspring, but was associated with a 6–8-day reduction in the mean length of pregnancy (Burbacher *et al.*, 2004a,b). Studies in rodents and rodent whole embryo cultures have implicated dysregulated cell death in the pathogenesis of CH_3OH-induced malformations, examined GSH status in the developing conceptus as it relates to vulnerability, and explored the basis for the increased sensitivity of the mouse embryo compared to the rat (Harris *et al.*, 2003, 2004; Degitz *et al.*, 2004; Hansen *et al.*, 2005).

Whereas there is still much to be learned about the mechanisms of CH_3OH toxicity, what is known allows for effective therapies if they are applied in a timely manner. The American Academy of Clinical Toxicology has published practice guidelines for the treatment of CH_3OH poisoning (Barceloux *et al.*, 2002). In cases of severe CH_3OH poisoning, there is a direct correlation between the formic acid concentration and increased morbidity and mortality. Sodium bicarbonate is usually given i.v. to correct severe acidosis, and case reports suggest that it may enhance renal formate excretion. Metabolic blockade is usually achieved with ethanol or 4-methylpyrazole (fomepizole), both acting as effective competitive inhibitors of ADH. Folate or folinic acid (activated folate) therapy is also indicated to increase the efficiency of formate oxidation. Hemodialysis is generally indicated when acidemia, high CH_3OH concentrations, or visual symptoms are present, although there is conflicting data on whether it appreciably shortens the elimination half-life of formate (Kerns *et al.*, 2002; Hantson *et al.*, 2005). Lastly, the treatment threshold of 20 mg CH_3OH/dL in a nonacidotic patient arriving early for care has been questioned as being overly conservative. This stems from a comprehensive review of worldwide CH_3OH poisonings that identified 126 mg/dL as the lowest early blood CH_3OH level ever clearly associated with acidosis (Kostic and Dart, 2003). CH_3OH exemplifies the benefits of knowing a chemical's mode of action when treating the poisoned patient. This knowledge also aids in identifying potentially sensitive subpopulations, such as those suffering from dietary folate deficiency. Research suggests, however, that even in a state of folate deficiency, the body probably contains sufficient folate stores to effectively detoxify small doses of CH_3OH-derived formate from exogenous sources (Medinsky *et al.*, 1997).

GLYCOLS

Ethylene Glycol

Ethylene glycol (1,2-dihydroxyethane, EG) is a constituent of antifreeze, deicers, hydraulic fluids, drying agents, and inks, and is used to make plastics and polyester fibers. Workers may be exposed dermally or by inhalation when solutions containing EG are heated or sprayed. The most important exposure route is ingestion, as EG may be accidentally swallowed, taken deliberately in suicide attempts, or used as a cheap substitute for ethanol. "Antifreeze" poisoning occurs frequently in cats and dogs that find its taste appealing. In 2004, there were 5562 human cases of EG exposure reported by the American Association of Poison Control Centers (23 fatal), nearly 40% of which were treated in a health-care facility (Watson *et al.*, 2005). EG enters the environment as a result of disposal of industrial and consumer products containing the chemical. It partitions into surface water and groundwater, but does not persist in any environmental medium and is practically nontoxic to aquatic organisms (Staples *et al.*, 2001).

The TK profile of EG is well characterized. All laboratory mammals and humans metabolize EG similarly. A series of papers has been published describing the TK of EG in Sprague–Dawley rats and CD-1 mice after administration of a single dose by the i.v., oral, or percutaneous routes (Frantz *et al.*, 1996a–c). Absorption from the GI tract of rodents and humans is very rapid and virtually complete, with cutaneous and pulmonary absorption are relatively slow and less extensive. Once absorbed, EG is distributed throughout the total body water. As illustrated in Fig. 24-11, EG is metabolized by NAD^+-dependent ADH to glycolaldehyde and on to glycolic acid (GA). GA is oxidized to glyoxylic acid by GA oxidase and lactic dehydrogenase. Glyoxylic acid may be converted to formate and CO_2, or oxidized by glyoxylic acid oxidase to oxalic acid (OA) (Wiener and Richardson, 1988; Frantz *et al.*, 1996b). The rate-limiting step in the metabolism of EG is the conversion of GA to glyoxylic acid, which results in accumulation of GA in the blood. EG has a half-life in humans of 3–8.6 hours (Leth and Gregersen, 2005). Under conditions of repetitive, low-dose exposure, EG is not expected to bioaccumulate given its rapid metabolism and elimination. Pregnancy status has no bearing on the TK of EG, GA, or OA, as demonstrated by comparisons of pregnant and nonpregnant Sprague–Dawley rats (Pottenger *et al.*, 2001).

The minimum acute lethal dose of EG in humans is estimated at ~1.4 mL/kg, which equates to 100 mL for a 70-kg adult (LaKind *et al.*, 1999; Hess *et al.*, 2004). Acute poisoning entails three clinical stages after an asymptomatic period, during which EG is metabolized: (1) a period of inebriation, the duration and degree depending on dose; (2) the cardiopulmonary stage 12–24 hours after exposure, characterized by tachycardia and tachypnea, which may progress to cardiac failure and pulmonary edema; and (3) the renal toxicity stage 24–72 hours postexposure. Metabolic acidosis, due largely to GA accumulation, can develop and become progressively more severe during stages 2 and 3 (Jacobsen *et al.*, 1984; Moreau *et al.*, 1998; Egbert and Abraham, 1999). Hypocalcemia can result from Ca^{2+} chelation by OA to form Ca^{2+} oxalate monohydrate (COM) crystals. Deposition of these crystals in kidney tubules is associated with

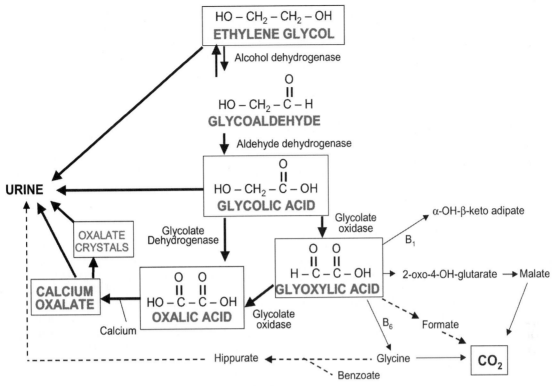

Figure 24-11. Metabolic scheme for ethylene glycol in animals.

Key metabolites that have been observed in vivo are highlighted in boxes. Dashed lines are theoretical pathways that have not been verified in vivo or in vitro. [Used with permission of Corley *et al.* (2005a).]

organ damage and potentially acute renal failure. Nephrotoxicity appears to be an acute, high-dose phenomenon, as no demonstrable kidney damage has been reported in occupational studies of groups such as airport deicing workers or Finnish auto mechanics (Laitinen *et al.*, 1995; Gerin *et al.*, 1997). COM crystal deposition has been reported in the walls of CNS blood vessels, with associated inflammation, edema, and sometimes neuropathy (Froberg *et al.*, 2006).

Based on high-dose rodent studies, including two lifetime dietary studies, EG has very limited chronic toxicity potential, exhibits no evidence of carcinogenicity, and does not appear to be a reproductive toxicant (DePass *et al.*, 1986; NTP, 1993). However, it can cause adverse developmental effects such as skeletal and soft tissue malformations and delayed ossification when administered during gestation at high doses (≥500 mg/kg/d) (ATSDR, 1997c). GA appears to be the proximate developmental toxicant, with metabolic acidosis playing an exacerbating, but not obligatory role (Carney *et al.*, 1996, 1999). Pottenger *et al.* (2001) have demonstrated that at teratogenic doses of EG, blood levels of GA are disproportionately high relative to the EG dose, further supporting GA as the proximate teratogen and implying a role for metabolic saturation. Corley *et al.* (2005d) have detailed the key events in EG-induced developmental toxicity and suggest the disruption of *hox* gene expression, fluid imbalance, and dysregulation of cell death in the embryo as mechanistic possibilities. The mechanism of GA's teratogenic action remains largely unknown, however, as does the relevance of defects in rodents given the absence of reported developmental effects in humans. The NTP Center for the Evaluation of Risks to Human Reproduction has released a monograph on EG's reproductive/developmental toxicity largely based on an expert panel report (NTP, 2004d,f). The over-

all conclusion was that EG exposures below the level of metabolic saturation should not result in developmental toxicity in humans. Further, because environmental and occupational exposures to humans are 2 to 3 orders of magnitude lower than those expected to result in metabolic saturation, such exposures are of negligible concern. Corley *et al.* (2005a) have developed a PBTK model of EG and GA and compared internal dose surrogates in rats and humans. Based on the comparisons, they also concluded that occupationally- or environmentally-exposed humans are unlikely to achieve blood levels of GA that have been associated with developmental toxicity in rats.

The chief concern about EG is renal toxicity after high dose, acute exposure. Although EG must be metabolized to toxic intermediates to induce kidney damage, the specific metabolite(s) and underlying mechanism(s) responsible remain to be fully elucidated. There is agreement, however, that the process involves a toxicant-induced proximal tubular necrosis leading to loss of renal function. Poldelski *et al.* (2001) exposed isolated mouse proximal tubule segments and human proximal tubular epithelial cells (HK-2) to GA, glycoaldehyde, glyoxylate, or OA for 15–60 minutes, on which basis they concluded glycoaldehyde and glyoxylate are the principal metabolites responsible for EG nephrotoxicity. This is contrary to the prevailing opinion that renal toxicity is due to the terminal metabolite, OA, which precipitates in the kidney in the form of COM crystals (Guo and McMartin, 2005). Corley *et al.* (2005d) have listed the key mechanistic events in the renal toxicity of EG: (1) metabolism of EG to OA via GA; (2) concentration of OA in tubular urine → precipitation of OA with Ca^{2+} → buildup of COM crystals in renal tubular epithelium → adherence of COM crystals to the plasma membrane of proximal tubular cells → subsequent intracellular uptake of COM crystals by endocytosis; and (3) physical trauma by COM crystals and/or production of free radicals and lipid peroxidation leading to cell necrosis, apoptosis and renal tubular degeneration. Clearly, the weight of evidence implicates OA is critical in the induction of renal damage, but a possible role for less frequently observed hippuric acid crystals and direct cytotoxicity by other metabolites cannot be ruled out. In vitro assays have indicated that both oxalate and COM crystals are injurious to renal epithelial cells (Thamilselvan and Khan, 1998). Also, renal damage has been observed occasionally following exposure to EG, without documentation of crystals in the kidney.

The intracellular target(s) of COM crystals is(are) not known with certainty, but it is well established that mitochondrial damage is a major mechanism for chemically mediated renal tubular necrosis. As such, COM crystals in the cytoplasm could directly affect mitochondria or be metabolized to release the oxalate ion that could do so. McMartin and Wallace (2005) hypothesized as much and demonstrated that COM produced a dose-dependent decrease in State 3 respiration in isolated rat kidney mitochondria, which they believe may be responsible for induction of a phenomenon known as mitochondrial permeability transition (MPT). MPT is characterized by an otherwise inpenetrant inner mitochondrial membrane undergoing transformation, whereby it becomes penetrable to solutes or large molecules. As a result of MPT induction, mitochondria undergo a rapid and progressive osmotic swelling, depolarization of mitochondrial membrane potential, and inhibition of oxidative phosphorylation/ATP synthesis, all of which can lead to either oncotic/ischemic cell death or apoptotic cell death. Additional insight into the pathogenesis of EG-induced renal damage has been provided by Chen et al. (2004), who provided male rats with 0.75% EG in their drinking water for 2, 4, and 8 weeks, after which the kidneys were processed for RNA isolation and microarray analysis using a rat-based chip. Changes in the expression of genes associated with tubular structure and function, oxidative damage, and inflammation were common. Increased expression of mitochondrial uncoupling protein was also observed, providing additional evidence of a mitochondrial target. EG has also been used as a model crystal-forming renal toxicant to determine the basis for COM crystal retention in the kidney. Studies with EG suggest that crystal retention in the kidney may depend on the expression of the proteins hyaluronan, osteopontin, and their mutual cell surface receptor CD44, all of which are upregulated in response to renal injury/inflammation, and under normal circumstances play a role in reestablishment of epithelial barrier integrity and restoration of renal function. However, their upregulation could turn a non-crystal-binding epithelium into a crystal-binding one, thereby setting the stage for crystal retention and renal injury (Asselman et al., 2003; Verhulst et al., 2003).

In cases of severe EG poisoning, early diagnosis and aggressive therapeutic intervention are essential for a favorable clinical outcome. A plasma EG level of 20 mg/dL is considered the threshold for kidney toxicity, if therapeutic strategy is based on EG concentration alone (Hess et al., 2004). However, no signs of renal injury have developed in patients at initial plasma GA concentrations of up to 10.1 mM or 76.7 mg/dL (Brent et al., 1999; Hess et al., 2004). In any case, treatment of EG poisoning involves three primary goals: (1) correction of the patient's metabolic acidosis; (2) inhibition of EG metabolism to its toxic metabolites; and (3) removal of EG and its toxic metabolites by hemodialysis, if necessary. As Guo and McMartin (2005) demonstrated that the renal cytotoxicity of COM crystals is potentiated by severe acidosis, its correction with bicarbonate should help ameliorate the development of renal toxicity. As with

CH_3OH, ethanol and 4-methylpyrazole (fomepizole) are frequently given as antidotes for EG poisoning and can prevent renal injury if given early in the course of intoxication. These ADH inhibitors block EG's metabolic bioactivation, thus minimizing the formation of toxic metabolites and allowing EG to be eliminated unchanged by the kidneys. There is increasing evidence that i.v. fomepizole may be more efficacious than ethanol as an antidote and obviate the need for hemodialysis in most EG-poisoned patients with normal renal function (Moreau et al., 1998; Brent et al., 1999; Sivilotti et al., 2000; Scalley et al., 2002). Watson (2000) has even stated that the results of fomepizole therapy support the recommendation that ethanol's use should be limited to settings where fomepizole is not available or contraindicated. The same editorial by Watson also supports the use of hemodialysis for renal insufficiency or metabolic acidosis rather than the traditional criterion of serum EG concentrations > 50 mg/dL. Interestingly, Corley and McMartin (2005) have refined a previously published PBTK model for EG and its GA metabolite in rats and humans to include hemodialysis, ethanol, and fomepizole as therapeutic interventions. This enabled the model to describe data from several human case reports of EG poisoning and demonstrated that fomepizole, if administered early enough, can indeed be more effective than ethanol or hemodialysis in inhibiting EG metabolism.

From a regulatory standpoint, EPA has established a RfD of 2 mg/kg/d based on kidney toxicity in the chronic rat feeding study by DePass et al. (1986) (EPA, 2006b). Palmer and Brent (2005) have recently derived a "chemical-specific adjustment factor" of 43.7 mg/kg/d based on a NOAEL for acute renal toxicity in humans. Although considerably higher than EPA's RfD, it is comparable to the Benchmark Dose 0.5 ($BMD_{0.5}$) for EG-induced nephrotoxicity of 49 mg/kg/d derived by Health Canada (2000).

Diethylene Glycol

Diethylene glycol (DEG) is similar in physicochemical properties to EG, but has a higher boiling point, viscosity, and specific gravity. DEG serves as a chemical intermediate in the production of polyester resins and polyurethanes, and as a solvent for shellacs and printing ink. It is hygroscopic, which leads to applications as a drying agent for natural and industrial gases, a humectant for cork and paper, and an additive in cosmetics.

DEG's use as an excipient in a liquid sulfanilamide preparation resulted in 105 deaths in the United States in 1937. This incident prompted passage of the Food, Drug and Cosmetic Act of 1938 (Wax, 1995). Use of DEG-contaminated propylene glycol or glycerin in various pharmaceuticals has caused multiple fatalities from renal failure in Nigeria, Bangladesh, India, and Haiti. In the Haitian incident, 109 cases of acute renal failure (with 88 deaths) were identified in children who received a locally manufactured acetaminophen syrup containing DEG-contaminated glycerin (O'Brien et al., 1998). The median lethal dose of DEG was estimated at 1.34 mL/kg. Renal failure was the "hallmark" finding in these cases, but hepatitis, pancreatitis, and severe neurologic manifestations (e.g., encephalopathy, optic neuritis with retinal edema, and unilateral facial paralysis) were frequently seen. Alfred et al. (2005) have presented seven cases of DEG poisoning characterized by metabolic acidosis, renal failure, and in three patients, neurotoxicity.

Compared to EG, toxicological data for DEG in animals are quite limited. Consistent with observations in human poisonings, Fitzhugh and Nelson (1946) reported dose-dependent hepatorenal injury in rats that consumed diets containing DEG. Kraul et al.

(1991) reported oliguria or polyuria, proteinuria, and other manifestations indicative of renal tubule injury in rats given a single i.p. dose of DEG. Similar to EG, renal tubular necrosis and COM crystal deposition in tubules have been observed following acute exposure of male rats (Hebert *et al.*, 1978). As for reproductive/developmental effects, high-dose gavage and dietary studies during gestation in mice, rats, and rabbits have largely been negative for embryotoxicity and teratogenicity (Ballantyne and Snellings, 2005). One study in mice employing a continuous breeding protocol has revealed diminished reproductive performance and fertility, as well as limited data on craniofacial malformations in live born and dead pups at drinking water exposures equivalent to 6.1 g/kg/d (Williams *et al.*, 1990). Citing this lone positive result and the developmental toxicity profile of EG, Ballantyne and Snellings (2005) gavaged CD-1 mice and CD rats with a range of DEG doses (559–11,180 mg/kg/d) on gestation days 6–15. They reported no embryotoxic or teratogenic effects at any dose in either species, except for delayed ossification consistent with reduced fetal body weight in rats.

Like EG, DEG is well absorbed from the GI tract, distributed throughout total body water and organs on the basis of blood flow, and initially metabolized by ADH and subsequently by ALDH (Heilmair *et al.*, 1993). The ether linkage of DEG is not cleaved and no appreciable amounts of EG or EG metabolites are formed from DEG, although small amounts of OA have occasionally been reported (Hebert *et al.*, 1978; Winek *et al.*, 1978). Based on studies in rats and dogs, unchanged DEG recovered in urine constitutes the majority of oral doses, with a single urinary metabolite, (2-hydroxyethoxy) acetic acid, accounting for most of the remainder (Lenk *et al.*, 1989; Wiener and Richardson, 1989; Mathews *et al.*, 1991). Differences in the toxicity/potency of DEG and EG can thus be explained by differences in their TK profiles. DEG's nephrotoxic moiety(ies) has (have) not been positively identified. As with EG, ADH inhibitors can be effective antidotes for DEG, as demonstrated by the use of fomezipole and hemodialysis to successfully treat a 17-month-old girl who ingested DEG (Brophy *et al.*, 2000).

Propylene Glycol

Propylene glycol (PG) is used as an intermediate in the synthesis of polyester fibers and resins, as a component of automotive antifreeze/coolants, and as a deicing fluid for aircraft. As PG is "generally recognized as safe" by the FDA, it is a constituent of many cosmetics, processed foods, and tobacco products, and serves as a diluent for oral, dermal, and i.v. drug preparations (ATSDR, 1997b). The most important routes of exposure in the general population are ingestion and dermal contact with products containing the compound. The use and disposal of deicing solutions is the major means by which PG is released to the environment. PG has a high mobility in soil and the potential to leach into groundwater, but is neither persistent nor bioaccumulative. Its soil and water half-lives are a few days under aerobic or anaerobic conditions. Workers in industries involved in manufacturing or use of products containing PG may be exposed to concentrations higher than the general population, particularly when these materials are heated or sprayed.

PG has a very low order of acute and chronic toxicity (ATSDR, 1997b; LaKind *et al.*, 1999). No organ system has been identified as a target for acute or chronic injury by PG, and there have been no accounts of human fatalities. Glover and Reed (1996) reported a typical clinical case in which a 2-year-old child experienced CNS depression and anion-gap acidosis after ingesting a hair gel containing PG. Clinical studies and case reports speak of individuals

with reactions to PG-containing drug preparations where preexisting conditions exist. For example, a patient with renal insufficiency secondary to chronic cocaine use developed metabolic acidosis after receiving lorazepam for sedation in which PG was a component of the i.v. formulation (Cawley, 2001). Wilson *et al.* (2000) reported a case of nearly fatal PG toxicity after i.v. diazepam in high doses for alcohol withdrawal. These same authors report on a case series detailing the risk of PG toxicity from i.v. benzodiazepine therapy (Wilson *et al.*, 2005).

Toxicity studies of PG in lab animals can be found in the literature, but findings of adverse effects are rare. Christopher *et al.* (1990) noted increases in anion-gap acidosis, CNS depression, and ataxia in cats ingesting high doses of PG, consistent with progressively elevated plasma lactate levels. PG has not been shown to be mutagenic and was negative for carcinogenicity in a chronic feeding study of male and female rats (Gaunt *et al.*, 1972). As for PG's reproductive/developmental toxicity, the NTP Center for the Evaluation of Risks to Human Reproduction released a monograph on the subject largely based on an expert panel report (NTP, 2004e,g). The overall conclusion was that there is negligible concern for adverse developmental/reproductive toxicity from PG exposures in humans, since animal studies have shown no such effect even at the highest doses tested.

PG's TK profile explains its relative lack of toxicity. As with other glycols, PG is readily absorbed from the GI tract and distributed throughout total body water and to organs on the basis of blood flow. Approximately 55% of PG is metabolized by ADH to lactaldehyde, while a significant percentage (~45%) is excreted unchanged by the kidneys (Morshed *et al.*, 1988). PG has a mean serum half-life in humans of 2–4 hours. Whereas excessive lactic acid from lactaldehyde metabolism is primarily responsible for metabolic acidosis observed in extreme exposures, lactate is a good substrate for gluconeogenesis, an efficient detoxification mechanism (NTP, 2004e,g). This detoxification mechanism typically does not allow lactic acid to accumulate to toxic levels, even under saturable metabolic conditions. The rate-limiting step in PG metabolism is its conversion to lactaldehyde. Saturation of this metabolic step in humans occurs at doses 8- to 10-fold lower than observed in laboratory animals. This is protective, because PG has a lower general toxicity than its metabolites (NTP, 2004e,g). As for EG and DEG, ADH inhibitors may competitively inhibit PG metabolism and thus be beneficial in the PG-poisoned patient. This is exemplified by a case of co-ingestion of ethanol and PG-containing antifreeze by a 61-year-old man absent of significant acid–base disturbance and minimal lactate elevation (Brooks and Wallace, 2002).

Two structural analogues of PG also have low hazard profiles. DPG (dipropylene glycol) and tripropylene glycol (TPG) are both widely used in personal care products such as perfumes, facial makeup, stick deodorants, and shaving and skin-care preparations. Their low hazard profiles are predictable, given that DPG is rapidly converted to PG, and TPG is rapidly hydrolyzed to DPG, which is further hydrolyzed to PG. The toxicity of these compounds has been summarized (UNEP, 1994, 2001). A negative DPG cancer bioassay was conducted in F-344 rats and B6C3F1 mice receiving the chemical via drinking water (Hooth *et al.*, 2004; NTP, 2004c).

GLYCOL ETHERS

If one alcohol residue of ethylene glycol (HO—CH$_2$—CH$_2$—OH) is replaced by an ether, the resulting compound is a monoalkyl glycol ether such as ethylene glycol monomethyl ether, also

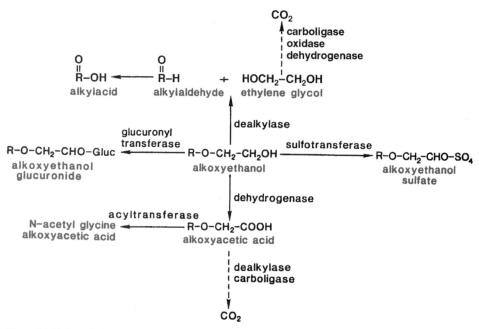

Figure 24-12. Metabolism of glycol ethers.

R denotes alkyl group of —CH₃,—CH₂—CH₃, or—CH₂—CH₂—CH₂—CH₃ for methoxy-, ethoxy-, or butoxyethanol, respectively. The formation of alkoxy glucuronide or sulfate conjugates has been identified only
for butoxyethanol. [Reproduced from Medinsky *et al.* (1990), with permission from Elsevier.]

called 2-methoxyethanol (2-ME; CH_3—O—CH_2—CH_2—OH).
If both alcohols are replaced by ethers, the result is a dialkyl glycol ether such as ethylene glycol dimethyl ether
(CH_3—O—CH_2—CH_2—O—CH_3). The alkyl group at the end
of the ether linkage may be a straight or branched short-chain
moiety (e.g., methyl, ethyl, n-propyl, isopropyl, or butyl). The
butyl moiety results in one of the most widely used glycol
ethers, 2-BE (CH_3—CH_2—CH_2—CH_2—O—CH_2—CH_2—OH).
Acetates of monoalkyl ethers such as 2-ME acetate
(CH_3—CO—O—CH_2—CH_2—O—CH_3) are also common solvents that undergo rapid ester hydrolysis to their parent glycol
ethers in vivo, and thus tend to exhibit the same toxicity profiles
as unesterified glycols. Glycol ethers exhibit properties of both
alcohols and ethers and are thus soluble in water and most organic
solvents. This dual solubility and a favorable evaporation rate,
make glycol ethers very popular solvents for surface coatings such
as varnishes and latex paints. Glycol ethers also find use as solvents
in paint thinners and strippers, inks, metal cleaning products, liquid
soaps, and household cleaners, and are used as jet fuel anti-icing
additives and in semiconductor fabrication. Human exposure
occurs mainly via inhalation, but also by dermal absorption.

Although glycol ether metabolism varies with chemical
structure, some generalizations are possible (Fig. 24-12). For
ethylene glycol monoalkyl ethers, the major metabolic pathway is oxidation via ADH and ALDH to alkoxyacetic acids.
For example, 2-ME and 2-BE are metabolized to methoxyacetic acid (MAA; CH_3—CO—O—CH_2—O—CH_3) and BAA
(CH_3—CO—O—CH_2—O—CH_2—CH_2—CH_2—CH_3), respectively.
The competing O-dealkylase pathway results in the cleavage of
the ether linkage to form ethylene glycol and an alkyl aldehyde.
Medinsky et al. (1990) reported that the relative contribution of
the oxidative pathway to metabolism of ethylene glycol ethers
increases with increasing alkyl chain length, whereas that of the

O-dealkylase pathway decreases. In contrast, the propylene series
of glycol ethers [e.g., propylene glycol monomethyl ether (PGME)]
is predominantly biotransformed to PG via O-dealkylation. Glycol
ethers may also be conjugated with glucuronide or sulfate, but
this is thought to occur mainly after saturation of other metabolic
pathways.

In vitro and in vivo toxicity studies demonstrate that some glycol ethers and their oxidative metabolites are reproductive, developmental, hematologic, and immunologic toxicants by all exposure
routes. A few have also tested positive in rodent cancer bioassays.
The metabolism of glycol ethers is considered a prerequisite to their
toxicity, as the alkoxyacetic acids are usually regarded as the ultimate toxicants. Their acetaldehyde precursors have also been implicated on occasion. A critical role for metabolism is supported by
the differential toxicities of glycol ethers metabolized via the oxidative and O-dealkylase pathways (Miller *et al.*, 1984; Ghanayem
et al., 1987). This differential toxicity has resulted in a dramatic
shift away from the production and use of certain low-molecular-
weight ethylene glycol ethers and their acetate esters (e.g., 2-ME
and 2-ethylene glycol monoethyl ether or 2-EE) toward those with
more favorable toxicity profiles such as ethylene, diethylene, and triethylene glycol butyl ethers and those in the low-molecular-weight
propylene series like PGME (de Ketttenis, 2005; Spencer, 2005).
Like several glycol ethers of the ethylene series, PBTK models
have been developed for PGME and its acetate in rats and humans
and exercised for risk assessment, including derivation of a RfC
and a RfD (Corley *et al.*, 2005b; Kirman *et al.*, 2005; Lemazurier
et al., 2005). Structure-activity relationships have been discerned in
studies of glycol ethers with various chemical substitution patterns
(Hardin *et al.*, 1984; Rawlings *et al.*, 1985; Hardin and Eisenmann,
1987; Ghanayem *et al.*, 1989). The reproductive and developmental toxicities of the monoalkyl glycol ethers, for example, tend to
decrease with increasing alkyl chain length, whereas hematotoxicity

increases. Thus, structure-activity relationships may not be universally applicable across multiple toxicological end points.

Reproductive Toxicity

Epidemiological studies have reported associations between glycol ether exposure and increased risk for spontaneous abortion, menstrual disturbances, and subfertility among women employed in the semiconductor industry (Schenker et al., 1995; Correa et al., 1996; Chen et al., 2002; Hsieh et al., 2005). These associations appear biologically plausible, given the reproductive toxicity of 2-ME and its active metabolite, MAA, is manifested as ovarian luteal cell hypertrophy and increased progesterone production in the female rat. Furthermore, MAA increased progesterone production in cultured human luteal cells at the same concentration it did in rat luteal cells, implying that it has the potential to alter ovarian luteal function in women (Almekinder et al., 1997; Davis et al., 1997). Reproductive effects, primarily reversible spermatotoxicity, have also been described for men exposed to glycol ethers, in some cases at concentrations well below current OSHA PELs for 2-ME (25 ppm) and 2-EE (200 ppm). For instance, Welch et al. (1988) found that painters exhibited oligospermia and azoospermia following average exposure to 2-EE and 2-ME at 2.7 and 0.8 ppm, respectively. In addition, men exposed to a mean level of 6.6-ppm 2-EE in a foundry had decreased numbers of sperm per ejaculate (Ratcliffe et al., 1989). Lastly, a large case–control study of male fertility clinic patients revealed a highly significant association between a diagnosis of impaired fertility and the detection of ethoxyacetic acid in urine (Veulemans et al., 1993).

Testicular effects in men are supported by experimental observations in animals including seminiferous tubule atrophy, abnormal sperm head morphology, necrotic spermatocytes, decreased sperm motility and count, and infertility (Lamb et al., 1984; Foote et al., 1995; Watanabe et al., 2000). Spermatocytes are among the first cells to be visibly affected following glycol ether exposure and their death involves apoptosis (Chapin et al., 1984; Brinkworth et al., 1995; Ku et al., 1995). Creasy and Foster (1984) noted a consistent order of spermatocyte susceptibility following oral administration of 2-ME or 2-EE to rats: dividing spermatocytes > early-pachytene spermatocytes > late-pachytene spermatocytes > mid-pachytene spermatocytes. Spermatocytes in the leptotene/zygotene stages of cell division, late-stage spermatids, and spermatogonia can be affected if the dose is increased and exposure prolonged.

As for mechanism of action, studies suggest several possibilities. Beattie et al. (1984) reported that rates of lactate accumulation in cultured rat Sertoli cells were significantly decreased by MAA. Lactate is the preferred metabolic substrate of spermatocytes. Also, 2-EE has been shown to increase oxygen consumption and decrease ATP levels in pachytene spermatocytes in a manner consistent with an uncoupled oxidative state (Oudiz and Zenick, 1986). Mebus et al. (1989) have, in addition, demonstrated that serine, acetate, sarcosine, and glycine attenuated the spermatotoxicity of 2-ME in the rat, suggesting MAA may interfere with the availability of one-carbon units for incorporation into purine and pyrimidine bases necessary for nucleic acid synthesis in pachytene spermatocytes. A mechanistic role for Ca^{2+} has been hypothesized and investigated in a series of studies by Chapin and colleagues. Ghanayem and Chapin (1990) observed that a Ca^{2+} channel blocker afforded protection against 2-ME-induced pachytene spermatocyte cell death. These authors reasoned that 2-ME perturbed Ca^{2+} homeostasis, which is consistent with observations of spermatocyte mitochondrial dis-

ruption. Involvement of Ca^{2+} was further suggested by observations that 2-ME activates a Ca^{2+}-dependent nuclease, cyclophilin A, found in pachytene spermatocytes and associated with spermatocyte apoptosis (Wine et al., 1997). Whereas an increase in intracellular Ca^{2+} is thought to trigger endonuclease activation, the protection afforded by Ca^{2+} channel blockers against MAA-induced spermatocyte apoptosis is apparently not mediated by preventing a rise in intracellular free Ca^{2+} (Li et al., 1997). Rather, because an intact relationship between Sertoli and germ cells is necessary for the morphological expression of MAA-induced spermatocyte apoptosis, it was reasoned that spermatocyte apoptosis is mediated by Sertoli cell-generated factor(s). This hypothesis proposes that transfer of this factor(s) from Sertoli cells into germ cells (or initiation of spermatocyte apoptosis by 2-ME-damaged Sertoli cells through direct Sertoli cell to germ cell communication), can be inhibited by Ca^{2+} channel blockers through their membrane-stabilizing effects and/or interaction with protein kinase C and/or calmodulin, both of which have demonstrated roles in apoptosis. The inhibition of protein kinase C and calmodulin has been shown to block MAA-induced spermatocyte cell death (Li et al., 1997).

Jindo et al. (2001) advanced the research of their predecessors by using cultured seminiferous tubules of juvenile rats to demonstrate that MAA-induced spermatocyte apoptosis could be blocked with protein kinase inhibitors. Several kinases (e.g., Src) increased immediately *around* dying spermatocytes in the immediate proximity of Sertoli cells. An increase was also noted in the phosphorylation of the endoplasmic reticulum chaperone glucose-regulated protein 94, known also as endoplasmin, that was located *inside* dying spermatocytes. This work implicates a role for kinase activity in the pathogenesis of MAA-induced spermatocyte apoptosis and suggests the involvement of Sertoli cells. Yet another investigation examined the role of tyrosine kinase pp60 (rat testicular Src), a tyrosine kinase encoded by the Src gene and involved in an array of cell signaling pathways, for its involvement in 2-ME-induced spermatocyte apoptosis. Sertoli cell cytoplasm was observed to be the principal site of Src immunoreactivity in control testis, while 2-ME treatment significantly induced Src expression in dying spermatocytes. In addition, MAA-induced apoptosis was blocked using Src inhibitors, further supporting a role for rat testicular Src in Sertoli-germ cell communication and spermatocyte toxicity of 2-ME (Wang et al., 2000). Furthermore, a suppression subtractive hybridization technique using whole testes from 2-ME-treated mice was employed to create mouse testis cDNA libraries enriched for gene populations either upregulated or downregulated by 2-ME (Wang and Chapin, 2000). A total of 70 clones was screened, and six of them were shown to be differentially expressed in the 2-ME lesion, three with increased expression, and three were suppressed. Interestingly, predicted peptide sequences of the six genes revealed several conserved motifs such as phosphorylation sites for protein kinase C and tyrosine kinase. Importantly, these gene changes were apparent at multiple germ cell stages and were localized in multiple germ cell types (Sertoli, interstitial, and peritubular cells). This further suggests the involvement of cell types other than the dying spermatocyte in the pathogenesis of 2-ME-induced spermatocyte death and helps explain the requirement for *intact* seminiferous tubules for in vitro replication of the pathology observed in vivo.

Developmental Toxicity

Exposure to certain glycol ethers during organogenesis (e.g., 2-ME and 2-EE) is toxic to the developing embryo, with effects seen in several animal models including non-human primates (Hardin *et al.*, 1986; Scott *et al.*, 1989). Others such as ethylene glycol butyl, propyl, and monohexyl ethers, and most PG ethers have either not induced fetal malformations or have a lower potential for developmental toxicity (Tyl *et al.*, 1989; Spencer, 2005). Structural anomalies in rodents have included a variety of minor skeletal variations, hydrocephalus, exencephaly, cardiovascular malformations, dilatation of the renal pelvis, craniofacial anomalies, and digit malformations. In the absence of structural defects, electrocardiograms of fetal rats from dams treated with 2-ME during gestation showed persistent, aberrant QRS waves, suggestive of an intraventricular conduction delay (Toraason and Breitenstein, 1988). Neurobehavioral changes and regional brain alterations of several neurotransmitters in offspring of rats treated with 2-ME or 2-EE have been reported (Nelson and Brightwell, 1984).

Little is known about the mechanism by which glycol ethers exert their developmental effects. 2-ME has served as a model toxicant to investigate the disposition of weak acids in the maternal–fetal unit and the hypothesis that weak acids such as MAA exert their effects by altering embryonic pH at critical stages of organogenesis (Nelson *et al.*, 1989; Clarke *et al.*, 1992; O'Flaherty *et al.*, 1995; Terry *et al.*, 1995). Ambroso *et al.* (1998) have applied confocal laser scanning microscopy, classical histopathology, and in situ immunohistochemistry to demonstrate that 2-ME caused a dose-dependent increase and expansion of apoptosis in gestation day 8 mouse embryos that could underlie 2-ME-induced neural tube defects. Such a mechanism has also been hypothesized for malformations induced by several prototypical teratogens like retinoic acid and ethanol.

Few epidemiological studies have addressed developmental effects of glycol ethers. Saavedra *et al.* (1997) described facial malformations and varying degrees of mental retardation in 44 offspring of mothers who were exposed occupationally to 2-ME and ethylene glycol at a factory producing capacitors in Mexico. There are a few reports published from a multicenter case–control study in Europe designed to investigate the role of maternal exposures at work and congenital malformations (Ha *et al.*, 1996; Cordier *et al.*, 1997; Lorente *et al.*, 2000). Preliminary results (Ha *et al.*, 1996) among mothers who were exposed to glycol ethers at work during pregnancy found excesses of oral clefts (OR = 2.0; 95% CI = 1.1–4.1) and CNS malformations (OR = 1.8; 95% CI = 1.1–3.3). In a study of 984 cases of major congenital malformations, Cordier *et al.* (1997) reported an overall OR of congenital malformations associated with glycol ether exposure of 1.44 (95% CI = 1.10–1.90), with significant associations for glycol ether exposure with cleft lip, multiple anomalies, and neural tube defects. Lorente *et al.* (2000) studied 100 mothers of babies with oral clefts and 751 mothers of healthy babies and reported a nonsignificant OR of 1.7 (95% CI = 0.9–3.3) for maternal occupational exposure to glycol ethers and cleft lip, with or without cleft palate. Maldonado *et al.* (2003) have reviewed the epidemiological evidence and determined that it is insufficient to determine whether occupational exposure to glycol ethers causes human congenital malformations.

Out of concern for the potential of ethylene glycol monoalkyl ethers as developmental toxicants, several PBTK models have been developed. Hays *et al.* (2000) developed a PBTK model for 2-ME and MAA in the pregnant rat that was capable of predicting embryonic concentrations. Gargas *et al.* (2000a,b) applied a PBTK model to estimate inhaled concentrations of 2-EE, its acetate ester, and 2-ME in humans that would result in blood levels equivalent to those observed at the rat NOAELs and LOAELs for developmental effects. Sweeney *et al.* (2001) applied Monte Carlo simulations to the models of Gargas and coworkers to account for the variability in TK and TD factors among humans and animals and derived occupational exposure limits to protect workers from developmental effects of 2-ME and 2-EE that were 1 to 2 orders of magnitude lower than current OSHA PELs. It is worthy of note that 2-ME has been largely removed from commerce due to its teratogenic potency.

Hematotoxicity

Some glycol ethers are hemolytic to red blood cells (RBCs). Typically, the osmotic balance of cells is disrupted, they imbibe water and swell, their ATP concentration decreases, and hemolysis occurs (Ghanayem, 1989). Nyska *et al.* (1999) reported that subchronic exposure to 2-BE causes disseminated thrombosis and bone infarctions in female, but not male rats, likely due to impedance of blood flow by intravascular hemolysis. It is thought that females might be susceptible, because they are less efficient in eliminating BAA, the hemolytic metabolite of 2-BE, and exhibit higher peak blood BAA levels. Young adult rats are more resistant to the hematologic effects of 2-BE than older rats, an observation attributed to depressed degradation and renal clearance of BAA in the older rats.

Species differ dramatically in their sensitivities to glycol ether-induced RBC deformity and hemolysis. Humans are less susceptible than rodents. This lower susceptibility even applies to RBCs from potentially sensitive subpopulations, such as the elderly and persons with hereditary blood disorders (Udden, 1994; Udden and Patton, 1994). A good example of using PBTK models in human risk assessment has been published by Corley *et al.* (1994). Based on comparisons of model output with data collected by Udden and colleagues on levels of 2-BE required to affect osmotic fragility of human RBCs, Corley and coworkers concluded that humans are unlikely to achieve hemolytic blood levels of BAA unless very large volumes of 2-BE are intentionally ingested. Udden (2005) has recently reported on the hemolytic effects of diethylene glycol butyl ether (DGBE) and its principal metabolite, butoxyethoxyacetic acid (BEAA), using rat and human RBCs in vitro. BEAA had weak hemolytic activity on rat erythrocytes, which is consistent with the finding of mild hemolysis when DGBE is administered to rats by gavage. However, such effects were absent in human RBCs exposed to DGBE or BEAA, indicating that it is unlikely hemolysis will occur in humans exposed to DGBE. Johnson *et al.* (2005) recently confirmed DGBE's low order of hematotoxicity in a 13-week drinking water study in F-344 rats that identified a NOAEL of 250 mg/kg/d, with minimal but statistically significant decreases in RBC count, hemoglobin, and hematocrit at 1000 mg/kg/d.

Hoflack *et al.* (1997) have shown 2-BE capable of inducing apoptosis in a human leukemia cell line and have hypothesized that the hematopoietic toxicity of 2-BE may be the result of its ability to induce apoptotic cell death. However, once inside the cell it is not entirely clear how hemolysis is accomplished, although the RBC membrane has long been the suspected target. Udden and Patton (2005) have utilized BAA to examine the mechanism of glycol ether hemolysis in rat RBCs in vitro. They concluded that the mode of action of BAA is to cause a colloid osmotic lysis of the RBC and speculated the following scenario: BAA causes Na^+ and Ca^{2+} to enter the cell $\rightarrow$ Ca^{2+} initially has a protective effect via the Ca^{2+}-activated potassium channel, which facilitates the loss of potassium, thereby compensating for the osmotic effect of increased cell Na^+ $\rightarrow$ Ca^{2+} subsequently has deleterious effects through activation of proteases and the loss of the normal asymmetric distribution of phospholipids (e.g., phosphatidylserine) in the membrane bilayer. These authors noted that preliminary studies in their laboratory have shown the movement of phosphatidylserine from the inner to the outer leaflet of the lipid bilayer of rat RBCs incubated with BAA. This "externalization" of phospatidylserine is associated with adhesion of RBCs to endothelial cells and the generation of thrombin, which is most interesting given reports of disseminated thrombosis and infarction in 2-BE-treated rats (Nyska *et al.*, 1999; Ghanayem *et al.*, 2001).

Immunotoxicity/Carcinogenicity

Based on changes in thymus and splenic weights/cellularities and a variety of in vitro and in vivo immune function assays, the immune system is a potential target for the oxidative metabolites of some glycol ethers. 2-ME and MAA have been employed almost exclusively in immunotoxicity investigations of glycol ethers. Not only have adult animals proven susceptible, but 2-ME exposure of pregnant mice induces fetal thymic atrophy/hypocellularity and a reduction in fetal liver prolymphocytes with potential implications for fetal immunity (Holladay *et al.*, 1994). Using B6C3F1 mice and gavage exposure, House *et al.* (1985) were among the first to report that 2-ME and MAA reduced thymus weight. Kayama *et al.* (1991) subsequently reported that 2-ME selectively depleted immature thymocytes in mice. Exon *et al.* (1991) not only reported thymic atrophy in rats exposed to 2-ME in drinking water, but also decreased antibody production, decreased splenocyte production of interferon-γ, and a reduction in spleen cellularity. Around the same time, the first in a lengthy series of studies by Smialowicz and colleagues was published (Smialowicz *et al.*, 1991a,b, 1992, 1994; Williams *et al.*, 1995; Kim and Smialowicz, 1997). This series has reported decreased thymus weights, reduced lymphoproliferative responses to mitogens, and reduced IL-2 production in splenocytes of F-344 rats exposed to 2-ME by gavage. It has also generated data indicating that not all glycol ethers are immunosuppressive, that mice are relatively insensitive to glycol ether immuosuppression compared to rats, and that rats of various strains show differential sensitivities. The Smialowicz series has further demonstrated that the relative insensitivity of mice is not a function of their more rapid clearance of MAA; that 2-ME is immunotoxic when applied dermally to F-344 rats; and that questions remain as to 2-ME's proximate immunotoxicant, as 2-methoxyacetaldehyde is more immunotoxic than MAA based on the ability to suppress IgM and IgG production by lymphocytes in F-344 rats.

As for cancer, only a few chronic bioassays have been conducted with glycol ethers. Two-year inhalation bioassays of 2-BE in F-344 rats and B6C3F1 mice revealed some evidence of carcinogenicity in male mice, based on increased incidences of hemangiosarcoma of the liver, as well as some evidence of carcinogenic activity in female mice, based on increased incidences of forestomach squamous cell papilloma or carcinoma (mainly papilloma) (NTP, 2000). In June 2004, an IARC working group evaluated the cancer risk of 2-BE and concluded that it is not classifiable as to its human carcinogenicity (Cogliano *et al.*, 2005). Likewise, EPA's IRIS profile for 2-BE currently indicates that the human carcinogenic potential of 2-BE cannot be determined at this time (EPA, 2006c). Since NTP's bioassays were completed, numerous studies have shed light on 2-BE's possible modes of action related to liver hemangiosarcomas and forestomach tumors and their implications for risk assessment (Park *et al.*, 2002; Siesky *et al.*, 2002; Poet *et al.*, 2003; Boatman *et al.*, 2004; Klaunig and Kamendulis, 2005; Corthals *et al.*, 2006). As discussed by Gift (2005), these studies suggest the following scenario: 2-BE consumed while grooming is metabolized to irritant

metabolites in the forestomach and/or irritant metabolites are formed in the upper respiratory tract and swallowed → chronic irritation → inflammation → hyperplastic effects → forestomach tumors. As for liver hemangiosarcomas, the following is suggested: 2-BE is metabolized to BAA → BAA causes hemolysis of RBCs → hemosiderin (iron) derived from released hemoglobin is taken up by and stored in phagocytic cells (e.g., Kupffer cells) of the spleen and liver → oxidative damage and increased synthesis of endothelial DNA are initiated by reactive oxygen species from excess iron or Kupffer cells, producing cytokines/growth factors that suppress apoptosis and promote cell proliferation → endothelial DNA mutations → potentiation and promotion of hepatic neoplastic cell populations. As further discussed by Gift (2005), the evidence suggests nonlinear modes of action in both cases and questionable human relevance of both tumor types. Several PBTK models have been developed and subsequently refined for 2-BE and BAA to aid in risk assessments (Corley *et al.*, 1994, 2005c; Lee *et al.*, 1998; Franks *et al.*, 2006).

Spencer *et al.* (2002) have reported a 2-year inhalation bioassay of PGME in F-344 rats and B6C3F1 mice that did not result in increases in neoplasia in either species except for kidney adenomas in male rats related to α_{2u}-globulin nephropathy. In contrast, a 2-year inhalation bioassay with propylene glycol mono-*t*-butyl ether (PGMBE) in F-344 rats and B6C3F1 mice also resulted in α_{2u}-globulin nephropathy in male rats, as well as liver tumors in male and female B6C3F1 mice at the highest concentration tested (1200 ppm) (NTP, 2004a; Doi *et al.*, 2004). Dill *et al.* (2004) have published information on PGMBE TK in rats and mice that demonstrate saturation of PGMBE metabolism/elimination at this tumor-producing concentration. The genotoxicity of some glycol ethers and their metabolites has been evaluated, with most exhibiting a lack of genotoxic potential and others yielding weakly positive responses in certain tests. Therefore, the role of genetic toxicology in the toxicities discussed above cannot be summarily dismissed, but is of unknown significance (Elliot and Ashby, 1997; NTP, 2000; Ballantyne and Vergnes, 2001).

FUELS AND FUEL ADDITIVES

Automotive Gasoline

Automotive gasoline is a complex mixture of hundreds of hydrocarbons predominantly in the C_4 to C_{12} range. The sheer number of people exposed in the manufacture, distribution, and use of gasoline make characterization of its acute and chronic toxicities important. Generalizations regarding gasoline toxicity must be made with care, because its composition varies with the crude oil from which it is refined, the refining process, and the use of specific additives. Experiments conducted with fully vaporized gasoline may not be predictive of actual risk, because humans are exposed primarily to the more volatile components in the range of C_4 to C_5. These hydrocarbons are generally regarded as less toxic than their higher-molecular-weight counterparts. Concern about gasoline exposure is fueled in part by the toxicities of certain components, some of which are classified by EPA as known or probable human carcinogens (e.g., benzene and 1,3-butadiene). The ACGIH has established a TLV for gasoline of 300 ppm to prevent ocular and upper respiratory tract irritation and a STEL of 500 ppm to avoid acute CNS depression.

Inhalation exposure to gasoline has been measured for service station attendants, self-service customers, truck drivers, distribution workers, and workmen removing leaking underground storage tanks (Kearney and Dunham, 1986; Shamsky and Samimi, 1987). In one survey, short-term exposures of self-service customers averaged about 6 ppm. The TLV is rarely exceeded in occupationally exposed individuals, due in part to the use of vapor scavenging systems. Brief exposures in excess of the STEL have, however, been documented for workers engaged in bulk handling operations (Phillips and Jones, 1978). The most extreme exposures occur to those intentionally sniffing gasoline for its euphoric effects. Several case reports of acute and chronic encephalopathies are testament to the dangers of this habit (Valpey et al., 1978; Fortenberry, 1985). In these cases, the identity of the offending agent(s) is often unclear. Gasoline is one of the most popular and lethal inhalants (Spiller, 2004; Wu et al., 2004), with deaths reported even among Aboriginal people in South Australia (Byard et al., 2003). An all too common occurrence is the ingestion of gasoline during siphoning events. This is typically followed by a burning sensation in the mouth and pharynx, as well as nausea, vomiting, and diarrhea resulting from GI irritation. If aspirated into the lungs, gasoline may produce pulmonary epithelial damage, edema, and pneumonitis. Thus, emetic therapy for gasoline ingestion is usually contraindicated.

Between 1986 and 2004, EPA identified 447,233 releases from underground petroleum storage tanks, many of which threaten groundwater that serves as the primary drinking water source for nearly one-half the U.S. population. Despite the number of releases, few community health studies have been conducted, and those that have are typically driven by concerns over leukemia risk owing to gasoline's benzene content. Consider for example the retrospective cohort study of the "Tranguch Gasoline Spill" in northeastern Pennsylvania (Patel et al., 2004). The standard incidence ratio for leukemia of all types was significantly elevated (4.40; 95% CI = 1.09–10.24), consistent with that reported by the Pennsylvania Department of Health. However, the excess was based on only four cases, two of whom had a history of smoking, a potential confounder. In addition, exposure was not well characterized, and only two of the subjects had acute myelogenous leukemia (AML), the leukemia type most strongly associated with benzene. Such a study exemplifies the problem with inferring causation for environmentally-exposed populations based on limited data.

Reese and Kimbrough (1993) and Caprino and Togna (1998) have reviewed the acute toxicity of gasoline and its additives. Like some other solvents, gasoline can sensitize the heart to catecholamines, defat the skin upon repeated contact, and induce hepatic P450s and UDP-glucuronyltransferase activities (Poon et al., 1995). The question of whether there is a "fetal gasoline syndrome" has been raised, although case reports are confounded by tetraethyl lead, alcohol abuse, and the possibility that an aberrant gene is distributed within the small Amerindian population where the cases reside (Hunter et al., 1979). There is a paucity of data on the reproductive toxicity of gasoline, but reports of enhanced estrogen metabolism and uterine atrophy among unleaded gasoline (UG)-treated mice suggest that this end point warrants investigation (Standeven et al., 1994a). Although dated, the study of Lykke and Stewart (1978) is of interest, because rats exposed to leaded gasoline at one-third the ACGIH TLV (i.e., 100 ppm) for 40 h/week for 6–12 weeks were observed to have a progressive interstitial fibrosis of the lungs associated with irregular alveolar collapse.

Prior to the identification of α_{2u}-globulin as the principal accumulating protein in the syndrome referred to as α_{2u}-globulin nephropathy, Kuna and Ulrich (1984) reported regenerative epithelium and dilated tubules in the kidneys of male rats exposed to 1552 ppm UG for 90 days. At about the same time, a chronic inhalation study revealed not only nephropathy, but also increased renal tumors in male rats (MacFarland et al., 1984). Subsequent studies by Halder et al. (1986) and Aranyi et al. (1986) showed that such nephropathy could not be produced by exposure of rats to a mixture of the butane and pentane components of gasoline or the 0°F to 145°F gasoline distillation fraction. These are thought to be more representative of human occupational exposures than wholly vaporized gasoline. In addition, the authors of a gavage screening study of 15 pure hydrocarbons and gasoline fractions concluded that branched aliphatic alkane components were primarily responsible for the nephropathy (Halder et al., 1985).

Investigations of mechanisms of the nephropathy and renal tumors included an assessment of unscheduled (a measure of genotoxicity) and replicative DNA synthesis (a measure of cell proliferation) in rat kidney cells exposed in vitro and in vivo to UG. No unscheduled DNA synthesis occurred, even at a tumorigenic dose, while a five- to eightfold increase in cell proliferation was observed (Loury et al., 1987). In a publication the same year by Olson et al. (1987), UG was reported to result in an increase in hyaline droplets harboring large accumulations of α_{2u}-globulin within proximal convoluted tubule epithelial cells. It was hypothesized that α_{2u}-globulin accumulated secondary to a defect in renal lysosomal degradation of the protein (Fig. 24-6). Supportive evidence for this hypothesis came from the demonstration that inhibition of the lysosomal peptidase, cathepsin B, caused a rapid accumulation of phagolysosomes and α_{2u}-globulin in the kidney similar to that of UG (Olson et al., 1988).

Further progress in elucidating the mechanism of α_{2u}-globulin nephropathy came from the demonstration that the UG component, 2,2,4-trimethylpentane (TMP), itself an inducer of α_{2u}-globulin nephropathy, was metabolized to 2,4,4-trimethyl-2-pentanol (TMPOH), which was selectively retained by the kidney of male rats. Subsequently, it was demonstrated that the sex-specific retention of TMPOH in the kidney was due to reversible binding with α_{2u}-globulin. This binding rendered the protein less digestible by lysosomal enzymes, which accounted for its accumulation (Charbonneau and Swenberg, 1988). This accumulation, in turn, led to cellular degeneration and necrosis, primarily in the P_2 segment of the proximal tubule. In response, regenerative proliferation occurs and promotes formation of renal cell tumors by irreversibly "fixing" spontaneously altered DNA and clonally expanding initiated cells. The promotional effects of gasoline and TMP on atypical cell foci and renal cell tumors have been demonstrated in male rats following initiation with N-ethyl-N-hydroxyethylnitrosamine (Short et al., 1989). NCI–Black–Reiter male rats, the only rat strain not to synthesize α_{2u}-globulin, are resistant to gasoline- and TMP-induced nephropathy (Dietrich and Swenberg, 1991). Thus, gasoline and TMP have been of great value in elucidating the mechanism of α_{2u}-globulin nephropathy and shedding light on its implications for renal tumorigenesis. Most toxicologists, and indeed the EPA, have concluded that renal tumors secondary to α_{2u}-globulin nephropathy are of little relevance, because humans do not synthesize α_{2u}-globulin.

Chronic inhalation of gasoline at high concentrations has also resulted in increased hepatocellular adenomas and carcinomas in female B6C3F1 mice, possibly due to the promotion of spontaneously initiated cells that occur with unusually high frequency in this mouse strain (MacFarland et al., 1984). This possibility is supported by reports that UG is a CYP inducer, mitogen, and liver tumor promoter in N-nitrosodiethylamine (DEN)-initiated female B6C3F1 mice (Standeven and Goldsworthy, 1993; Standeven et al., 1995; Moser et al., 1996a). CYP induction by UG has been attributed to "heavy UG" (components with boiling points > 100°C), whereas mitogenic activity is highly concentrated in UG components boiling from 100 to 132°C, for which the 2,2,3-, 2,2,4-, and 2,3,4-trimethylpentane isomers appear at least partially responsible (Standeven and Goldsworthy, 1994). It has been hypothesized that the liver tumor-promoting activity of UG is secondary to its estrogen antagonism, given that (1) UG is not a hepatocarcinogen in male mice; (2) estrogen inhibits liver tumor development initiated in mice but potentiates hepatic tumor promotion by UG; and (3) UG induces hepatic estrogen metabolism (Standeven et al., 1994b). The hypothesis that liver tumor promotion by UG depends on its interaction with estrogen is supported by the demonstration that tumor-promoting activity of UG was greatly attenuated in ovariectomized mice relative to intact mice (Moser et al., 1997). Further, the addition of estrogen to DEN-treated mice substantially reduces the percentage of hepatic foci with decreased levels of TGF-β1 compared to DEN-treated control mice or DEN + UG-treated mice, suggesting a promotional mechanism involving estrogen and the dysregulation of tumor growth factor(s) (Moser et al., 1996c). Whereas much attention has been given to its promotional potential, UG may also damage DNA, as it reportedly induces unscheduled DNA synthesis in hepatocytes from male and female mice treated in vivo and in cultured mouse, rat, and human hepatocytes (IARC, 1989b). The epidemiological evidence for an association between gasoline exposure and cancer in humans is inconclusive. Raabe (1993) has reviewed the carcinogenic potential of gasoline. IARC (1989b) classifies it as possibly carcinogenic to humans (Group 2B) primarily due to its benzene content. A comprehensive review of gasoline toxicity is provided in ATSDR's (1995) *Toxicological Profile for Gasoline.*

Vehicle emissions from gasoline combustion are a major contributor to urban air pollution, which is at unhealthy levels in numerous cities. In response, the Clean Air Act Amendments of 1990 require the use of oxygenated gasoline in such areas. Oxygenated gasoline contains additives that add oxygen to gasoline, thereby boosting its octane quality, enhancing combustion, and reducing exhaust emissions. MTBE and ethanol are the two most common oxygenates, although use of the former is being rapidly phased out due to widespread groundwater contamination and health concerns. As a result, the demand for ethanol–gasoline blends is increasing dramatically, raising concerns about how the two components might interact toxicologically. There is a dearth of information on this issue, but a 4-week inhalation study of an ethanol–gasoline mixture (6130-ppm ethanol and 500-ppm gasoline) in rats concluded that co-exposure showed additive and possibly some synergistic effects on growth, neurochemistry, and histopathology of the adrenal gland and respiratory tract. Effects were described as generally mild and adaptive in nature, and returned to normal after exposure cessation (Chu et al., 2005). The risks and benefits of ethanol as an oxygenate are discussed in detail by Williams et al. (2003), who point out several reasons why ethanol in gasoline can increase groundwater plume lengths and persistence of gasoline constituents in groundwater if ethanol blends are released into the environment. The most obvious concern is that longer or more persistent gasoline plumes could lead to a higher probability of gasoline constituents affecting public water wells. Meanwhile, another fuel additive, methylcyclopentadienyl manganese tricarbonyl (MMT), is receiving attention due to concerns that it could increase manganese inhalation exposures and pose a risk for neurotoxicity. The combustion of MMT gasoline results in the emission of fine Mn particulates mainly as Mn sulfate and Mn phosphate and smaller amounts of oxides. Several studies characterizing vehicular exhaust using MMT gasoline and describing the pharmacokinetics and neurobehavioral toxicity of Mn have

been recently published, some of which were mandated by EPA (Normandin et al., 2004; Dorman et al., 2006; Reaney et al., 2006; Tapin et al., 2006). Gasoline engine exhaust has been classified as possibly carcinogenic to humans (Group 2B), based largely on sufficient evidence in animals when condensates and exhaust extracts are tested (IARC, 1989a).

Methyl Tertiary-Butyl Ether

MTBE's high octane rating made it a logical replacement for tetraethyl lead as an octane booster for gasoline, and later as a gasoline oxygenator. As an oxygenator, MTBE makes fuel combustion more complete, thereby reducing pollutant emissions from automobile exhaust. MTBE may be added to gasoline at levels up to 15% by volume in order to comply with the 1990 Amendments to the Clean Air Act. By 1997, it was being used at the rate of 10 million gal/d, with more than one-third of the usage in California. While routine, low-level exposure of customers occurs at self-service stations, heightened concern about MTBE has resulted primarily from its contamination of groundwater by leaking underground gasoline tanks. It is highly water soluble, travels faster and farther in water than other gasoline components, and is resistant to degradation.

MTBE is well absorbed following oral, inhalation, and dermal exposure of humans and rats (Dekant et al., 2001; Prah et al., 2004; McGregor, 2006). The majority of absorbed MTBE is exhaled unchanged. Some MTBE is oxidized to *tert*-butyl alcohol (TBA) and HCOH. Whereas this oxidation is primarily CYP2A6 mediated in humans (Hong et al., 1999), it is largely CYP2B1 mediated in rats (Turini et al., 1998). TBA is relatively water soluble, so it tends to remain in the blood and extracellular fluid, and is slowly exhaled. TBA is further metabolized, first to 2-methyl-1,2-propanediol and then to 2-hydroxyisobutyrate, the major urinary metabolites of MTBE. In addition, glucuronide and sulfate conjugates of TBA are found in trace amounts in urine. Although HCOH is one of the oxidative metabolites of MTBE, it is undetectable after MTBE exposure in humans and rats, presumably due to its rapid metabolism. PBTK models have been developed to describe the dosimetry of MTBE and TBA following inhalation and oral exposures in rats and humans (Borghoff et al., 1996; Licata et al., 2001).

Concern about MTBE has led to numerous toxicity studies in humans and rodents, and a number of reviews of MTBE's toxicity are available (ATSDR, 1996b; EPA, 1997; Borak et al., 1998; McGregor, 2006). The review of Borak et al. (1998) focuses upon the acute human health effects of MTBE. It concludes, based on 19 reports of inhalation exposure to MTBE alone or in gasoline and 12 reports of parenteral MTBE administration to dissolve cholesterol gallstones, that no significant association exists between MTBE exposure and the acute symptoms commonly attributed to it. These symptoms include headache, eye, nose and throat irritation, cough, nausea, dizziness, and disorientation. The more recent review of McGregor (2006) is supportive of this conclusion.

In 1988, the EPA and industry developed a Testing Consent Order for MTBE under the Toxic Substances Control Act that precipitated investigations of MTBE's potential two-generation reproductive toxicity, developmental toxicity, in vivo mutagenicity, subchronic inhalation toxicity, oncogenicity, and neurotoxicity. Results of these studies are a major addition to the toxicity literature on MTBE and define several NOAELs (Bevan et al., 1997a,b; Bird et al., 1997; Daughtrey et al., 1997; Lington et al., 1997; McKee et al., 1997). The publication of Bird and colleagues is actually a recapitulation of reports by Chun et al. (1992) and Burleigh-Flayer

Table 24-4
Summary Results of MTBE Cancer Bioassays

AUTHORS	ANIMAL STRAIN/SPECIES	EXPOSURE ROUTE	POSITIVE RESULTS
Chun *et al.* (1992)	Fischer 344 rats	Inhalation	Kidney and testicular tumors (males)
Burleigh-Flayer *et al.* (1992)	CD-1 mice	Inhalation	Liver adenomas (females)
Belpoggi *et al.* (1995)	Sprague–Dawley rats	Oral	Testicular tumors (males)
			Leukemia + lymphoma (females)

et al. (1992), both of which are of particular value, as they represent two of only three MTBE cancer bioassays. In the Chun *et al.* study, male and female F-344 rats were exposed to 0-, 400-, 3000-, or 8000-ppm MTBE vapor 6 h/d, 5 d/week for 24 months. In the other inhalation study, Burleigh-Flayer *et al.* (1992) subjected male and female CD-1 mice to the same exposure regimen for 18 months. The only oral chronic bioassay is that by Belpoggi *et al.* (1995, 1997), who subjected male and female Sprague–Dawley rats by olive oil gavage to 0, 250, or 1000 mg/kg MTBE 4 d/week for 2 years. The results of the three MTBE animal cancer bioassays are presented in Table 24-4. In addition, Cirvello *et al.* (1995) and NTP (1995) have reported some evidence for the carcinogenicity of TBA in the kidney and thyroid after long-term drinking water exposure.

Taken at face value, one might interpret these cancer bioassay findings as ample evidence of carcinogenicity in animals and suggestive of a cancer risk for humans. The relevance of these findings to humans, however, has been a source of debate among toxicologists. Critics have questioned these studies on the basis of (1) the appropriateness of a combined incidence category for leukemias and lymphomas; (2) the possibility that renal tumors were secondary to male rat-specific α_{2u}-globulin nephropathy; (3) the possibility that Leydig cell tumors were a function of abnormally low testicular tumor rates in control animals or increased survival time of treated rats; (4) the questionable relevance of testicular tumors in rats to humans, given the species' differential responses of Leydig cells to proliferative stimuli; (5) the possibility that liver and kidney tumors are the result of high dose-induced chronic cytotoxicity, cell death, and reparative cell proliferation; (6) the questionable relevance of inhalation bioassays to prediction of drinking water risks; and (7) the use of an oil rather than a water-dosing vehicle, which could unduly influence MTBE's oral TK. Mennear (1997) and McGregor (2006) have discussed a number of these issues.

As an outgrowth of the uncertainties surrounding MTBE's human carcinogenicity risk, several mechanistic studies have been published. For example, after only 10 days of MTBE inhalation exposure, a strong positive linear relationship between renal α_{2u}-globulin concentration and cell proliferation was seen in the male F-344 rat (Prescott-Matthews *et al.*, 1997). This study, unlike the chronic bioassay of Chun *et al.* (1992), definitively identified the accumulating protein as α_{2u}-globulin. Williams and Borghoff (2001) have shown that TBA interacts with α_{2u}-globulin, which explains its accumulation in the male rat kidney following MTBE or TBA exposure. MTBE has been shown to be a hepatic mitogen in the female mouse, but not a promoter of tumor formation in DEN-initiated female mouse liver (Moser *et al.*, 1996b). It has been suggested in light of these findings, that MTBE may promote the growth of spontaneously initiated cell populations having genetic lesions different from those produced by DEN. Casanova and Heck (1997)

have reported a lack of concentration-, species-, and sex dependence in the formation of HCOH-induced DNA–protein cross-links and RNA–HCOH adducts in isolated female CD-1 mouse hepatocytes incubated with MTBE. As the cancer bioassay data suggest that hepatocarcinogenicity varies with all of these factors, these results do not support a role for HCOH in MTBE-induced liver tumor formation. Studies also indicate that MTBE causes endocrine dysregulation in rodents at high doses, suggesting the possibility that MTBE-induced tumor formation is hormonally mediated (Moser *et al.*, 1998; Williams *et al.*, 2000b). Changes in triiodothyronine, luteinizing hormone, testosterone, and estradiol levels have been discussed as possible mechanisms of MTBE-induced Leydig cell cancer (Williams and Borghoff, 2000; Williams *et al.*, 2000b; de Peyster *et al.*, 2003). Although it is generally accepted that MTBE induces certain tumors in animals through non-genotoxic mechanisms, experiments indicate that MTBE is mutagenic in some in a few in vitro test systems (Williams-Hill *et al.*, 1999; Zhou *et al.*, 2000).

Several mechanistic issues surrounding MTBE's toxicity, particularly its carcinogenicity, have yet to be resolved. Nonetheless, citing widespread groundwater contamination and health concerns, numerous states have instituted phased-in partial or complete bans of MTBE. This is in keeping with the opinion of EPA's *Blue Ribbon Panel on Oxygenates in Gasoline* that, in 1999, agreed that the use of MTBE and other gasoline additives that threaten drinking water supplies should be substantially reduced. To date, independent expert review groups who have assessed MTBE inhalation health risks (e.g., "Interagency Assessment of Oxygenated Fuels") have not concluded that the use of MTBE-oxygenated gasoline poses an imminent threat to public health. EPA's Office of Water has concluded that available data are not adequate to estimate potential health risks of MTBE at low exposure levels in drinking water, but that the data support the conclusion that MTBE is a potential human carcinogen at high doses. Fortunately, water-containing MTBE has an unpleasant taste and odor, which may alert consumers to the fact that their water is contaminated. Based on the results of studies of taste and odor thresholds for humans, an advisory guidance range of 20–40 μg/L has been set by the EPA to assure consumer acceptance and provide a large margin of safety from toxicity and carcinogenicity. California has derived both a cancer potency estimate and adopted a Public Health Goal of 13 ppb for MTBE in drinking water (Wang *et al.*, 1997). While many advocate for the suspension of MTBE's use in reformulated gasoline, such a decision should weigh the benefits against the risks associated with increased auto emissions of carcinogenic VOCs and the public health impact of increased CO_2 emissions and ozone formation. Two articles that discuss this subject in considerable detail are those of Spitzer (1997) and Erdal *et al.* (1997).

Jet Fuel

Jet A, jet propellant-8 (JP-8), and JP-8+100 are the predominant jet fuels in use today. All are kerosene-like mixtures of hundreds of aliphatic and aromatic hydrocarbons. Jet A is commercial aviation fuel, whereas JP-8 and JP-8+100 are military fuels. JP-8 is a mixture of Jet A plus three additives, whereas JP-8+100 contains JP-8 and an additional additive package. JP-8 is now the recognized battlefield fuel for all NATO forces and is used not only for aircraft, but also for ground vehicles and other equipment such as generators, cooking stoves, and tent heaters (NRC, 2003). Owing to slight differences in hydrocarbon composition and additives, JP-8 differs from its predecessor fuels (e.g., JP-4 and JP-5) in ways that impart added safety, enhance combat aircraft survivability, simplify battlefield logistics, and promote standardization with commercial jet fuel.

Civilian and military personnel are exposed to jet fuel by inhalation and dermal contact. Exposure can occur to liquid, vapor, or aerosol, each phase having a distinct composition and toxicity profile. Exposure is prevalent in aircraft refueling and maintenance operations and ground crews positioned behind jet aircraft during "cold starts" can become "drenched" in aerosol emissions. Jet fuel can be released into the environment by in-flight jettisoning and spills or leaks to soil or water during use, storage, or transportation. In many cases, the U.S. Department of Defense (DoD) is responsible for the cost of remediating contaminated military sites and contractor facilities, not to mention its responsibility to safeguard the health of military personnel. It is thus in DoD's interest to accurately characterize the toxicity of jet fuel. Much of the research conducted to date has been funded by the military. The Navy's Occupational Safety and Health Standards Board has proposed an 8-hour time-weighted average (TWA) PEL of 350 mg/m^3 and a 15-minute STEL of 1800 mg/m^3 for jet fuel vapors, but notes that exposure to aerosols that are much more toxic may necessitate reevaluation. The National Research Council (NRC) Subcommittee on Jet Propulsion Fuel 8 recommended that the 8-hour TWA be considered interim until further research is completed, and that the STEL be lowered to 1000 mg/m^3 to avoid acute CNS effects (NRC, 2003).

The complexity of jet fuel mixtures presents multiple challenges to toxicologists and risk assessors alike. One such challenge is to generate experimental exposures to jet fuel that accurately reflect those occurring in humans. The NRC Subcommittee on JP8 has reviewed the methods used to generate exposure atmospheres in several published studies using aerosol/vapor mixtures and suspects that the JP-8 concentrations may have been underreported, particularly in studies by Witten and colleagues (NRC, 2003). Therefore, it seems prudent at this time to discuss aerosol/vapor exposures in qualitative terms only. Because of concerns surrounding the quantitative accuracy of the exposure atmospheres, the NRC Subcommittee recommended an examination of the methods used for their characterization. To this end, Dietzel et al. (2005) have developed and validated a GC/MS method for JP-8, which was subsequently used to characterize the aerosol and vapor fractions of aerosolized fuel in one of the University of Arizona-based inhalation chambers previously utilized by Witten and colleagues.

Jet A, JP-8, and JP-8+100 have similar toxicity profiles, which suggests their toxicities are largely a function of hydrocarbon content rather than additives. Toxicity data on jet fuels have been well summarized (ATSDR, 1998a; NRC, 2003; Ritchie et al., 2003), but there remain several data gaps including genotoxicity. Most toxicity studies of jet fuels have focused on the two main portals of entry

(i.e., lung and skin) and the immune system. In subchronic and chronic rodent inhalation studies of jet fuel vapor, the chief finding has been renal toxicity and neoplasia in male rats consistent with α_{2u}-globulin nephropathy (Mattie et al., 1991; Bruner et al., 1993). Whereas the liver, kidneys, and testes in humans are not considered particularly sensitive targets of jet fuels, proteomic analyses of these tissues have been conducted in male rats subchronically exposed to JP-8 vapor (Witzmann et al., 2000a,b, 2003). Similarly, gene expression in the whole brain of rats repeatedly exposed to JP-8 vapor has been examined (Lin et al., 2001a, 2004), driven largely by reports of cognitive and motor deficits and neurochemical changes in jet fuel-exposed workers and experimental animals (Baldwin et al., 2001; Ritchie et al., 2001; Rossi et al., 2001; Bell et al., 2005).

Pulmonary Effects   The pulmonary effects of an aerosol/vapor mixture of JP-8 were initially investigated in rats with nose-only exposures designed to simulate military flightline exposures (Hays et al., 1995; Pfaff et al., 1995, 1996). Functional changes in the form of increases in pulmonary resistance and alveolar permeability were accompanied by a decrease in the concentration of the tachykinin Substance P (SP) in bronchoalveolar lavage fluid. Pathological changes were observed in lower pulmonary structures including inflammation of the terminal bronchioles, degeneration of alveolar type II epithelial (AIIE) cells and disruption of terminal bronchial airway epithelium. Most interestingly, the activity of neutral endopeptidase (NEP), an enzyme responsible for the metabolism of SP in the lung, was increased by exposure and a significant inverse relationship between SP and NEP activity demonstrated. Thus, JP-8 appears to exhibit a rather novel mechanism of lung injury that involves the reduction or depletion of SP due to its enhanced metabolism by NEP.

Because SP participates in the maintenance of airway epithelial cell competency, the effect of JP-8 and n-tetradecane (C$_{14}$), a primary constituent of JP-8, on epithelial barrier integrity was examined in vitro using paracellular mannitol flux in BEAS-2B human bronchial epithelial cells (Robledo et al., 1999). Noncytotoxic concentrations of JP-8 and C$_{14}$ produced dose-dependent increases in transepithelial mannitol flux that spontaneously reversed to control values over a 48-hour recovery period. This suggests that JP-8 and C$_{14}$ compromise the integrity of intercellular tight junctions that may precede and initiate the pathological alterations observed in whole animal studies. Evidence was also collected that SP's protective effect on the lung is largely mediated through the plasma membrane-bound neurokinin receptor, NK$_1$, present on airway epithelium from the trachea to the respiratory bronchioles (Robledo and Witten, 1999).

Among the most affected alveolar cells in rodent studies are AIIE cells. In support of the hypothesis that apoptotic cell death is responsible at least partially for JP-8's cytotoxicity in the lung, Stoica et al. (2001) reported that JP-8 results in morphological and biochemical changes characteristic of apoptosis in the rat AIIE cell line, RLE-6TN. Further, Boulares et al. (2002) have collected data that strongly suggest JP-8 triggers apoptosis in rat lung epithelial cells by inducing the generation of reactive oxygen species, depleting/reducing intracellular GSH, and markedly decreasing mitochondrial membrane potential, thereby initiating the apoptotic cascade (i.e., caspase-3 activation and DNA fragmentation).

A characteristic feature of the lung inflammatory response to JP-8 in rodents is vacuolization of AIIE cells and accumulation of pulmonary alveolar macrophages (PAM). The findings of Wang *et al.* (2002) suggest that JP-8 causes proinflammatory cytokine secretion not only by PAM, but also AIIE cells. The prolonged production of proinflammatory cytokines, together with the proteases produced by activated macrophages and neutrophils, are capable of producing a sustained immune response with increased risk for lung damage. Moreover, cocultures of AIIE cells and primary PAM indicate that the balance of cytokines released in response to JP-8 could possibly be regulated in vivo by cross-communication between the two cell types. Most recently, Espinoza *et al.* (2005) showed that the JP-8-induced expression of proinflammatory cytokine genes in AEII cells was mediated by the activation of PARP-1 (an enzyme coactivator of NF-kappaB) and NF-kappaB (a transcription factor that controls the expression of a variety of genes involved in inflammatory responses). The release of cytokines in the lung in response to JP-8 is similar to cytokine release from epidermal cells, which is thought to mediate, at least in part, the dermal and immune toxicities of JP-8 (see below). Further insight into the pulmonary effects of jet fuel has come from examinations of aerosolized JP-8's effect on gene and protein expression in lung cytosol and lung tissue of rats and mice (Witzmann *et al.*, 1999; Drake *et al.*, 2003; Espinoza *et al.*, 2005).

Immune Effects The immune system appears to be as susceptible to jet fuel as the lung, if not more so. Detrimental effects on the immune system of mice have been reported for aerosolized Jet A, JP-8, and JP-8+100 (Harris *et al.*, 2001a). Some effects were apparent just 1 hour after a single inhalation exposure with continued deterioration with each successive exposure (Harris *et al.*, 2002). As first reported by Harris *et al.* (1997a), mice exposed nose-only to a JP-8 aerosol/vapor mix exhibited decreased spleen and thymus weights and cellularities and an altered number of viable immune cells in lymph nodes, bone marrow, and peripheral blood. Depending on the immune tissue examined, different immune cell subpopulations were lost, including T and B cells and macrophages. In addition, JP-8 affected immune function as demonstrated by a concentration-dependent suppression of T-cell proliferation upon stimulation with the mitogen concanavalin A. In a short-term exposure study, Harris *et al.* (1997b) determined that JP-8-induced immunotoxicity persisted for at least 1 month after insult. These same authors later expanded the number of immune parameters examined and reported that aerosolized JP-8 exposure of mice nearly completely ablated natural killer cell function, suppressed the generation of lymphokine-activated killer cell activity, suppressed the generation of cytotoxic T lymphocytes from precursor T cells and inhibited helper T-cell activity (Harris *et al.*, 2000).

Ullrich (1999) has demonstrated that dermal application of JP-8 to mice can induce immune suppression. Ullrich found IL-10, a cytokine with potent immunosuppressive activity, in the serum of JP-8 dermally treated mice. He interpreted this as suggestive of an immune suppressive mechanism involving the upregulation of cytokine release. In a follow-up study, Ullrich and Lyons (2000) demonstrated that the immunosuppressive effect of dermally applied JP-8 appears to be specific to cell-mediated immune reactions (i.e., T-helper cell-driven cell-mediated immunity), as JP-8 had no effect on antibody production in immunized mice. Further, their study again implicated the release of cytokines from epidermal cells in immunosuppression, particularly prostaglandin E2 (PGE2) and IL-10. Ramos *et al.* (2004) have subsequently used platelet-activating factor (PAF) receptor antagonists to show that the PAF receptor, a signaling phospholipid which upregulates PGE2 synthe-

sis by keratinocytes, plays a critical role in jet fuel-induced immune suppression. Ramos *et al.* (2002) have also demonstrated that the dermal application of JP-8 and Jet A suppresses delayed-type hypersensitivity and immunologic memory upon rechallenge with a fungal pathogen, suggesting that jet fuel exposure may depress the protective effect of prior vaccination. Similar to that seen for pulmonary toxicity, aerosolized SP can both prevent and reverse some facets of JP-8-induced immunotoxicity, suggesting a key mechanistic role for the neuropeptide (Harris *et al.*, 1997c, 2001b). As reported for AIIE cells, JP-8 also induces apoptosis in primary mouse thymocytes (Stoica *et al.*, 2001). Exposure of mice to JP-8 in utero reportedly has implications for the immune system (Keil *et al.*, 2003).

Dermal Effects Owing to reports of severe contact dermatitis among military personnel, the dermal toxicity of jet fuel has been the subject of intensive investigation. A recent examination of dermal exposure in 124 U.S. Air Force fuel-cell maintenance workers, using a noninvasive tape-strip technique and naphthalene as a surrogate, confirmed that the skin provides a significant exposure route for JP-8 (Chao *et al.*, 2005). Dermal absorption and penetration of JP-8 and its component hydrocarbons have been examined in vitro using dermatomed rat skin and static diffusion cells and in vivo in weanling pigs (McDougal *et al.*, 2000; Singh *et al.*, 2003). Their cutaneous toxicity has been explored in pigs, rats, rabbits, and in vitro using human epidermal keratinocytes (HEK) (Kabbur *et al.*, 2001; Monteiro-Riviere *et al.*, 2001; Chou *et al.*, 2003; Singh and Singh, 2004). Dermal exposure to jet fuel can lead to skin irritation and sensitization and the disruption of skin barrier function. Research implicates cytokine release, oxidative stress and DNA damage/fragmentation as mechanistic underpinnings (Allen *et al.*, 2000; Rogers *et al.*, 2001; Gallucci *et al.*, 2004). Chronic dermal application of middle distillate fuels such as jet fuel can be weakly carcinogenic, though it has been effectively argued that such tumorigenicity is secondary to chronic irritation (Nessel, 1999; Nessel *et al.*, 1999).

The ultrastructural analysis of pig skin exposed to cotton fabric saturated with jet fuel suggests that the primary effect of exposure is damage of the stratum corneum barrier (Monteiro-Riviere *et al.*, 2004). This same publication reported that IL-8 release from HEK after JP-8 exposure was decreased by SP, which is an agonist for the NK₁ receptor present in keratinocytes and mechanistically linked to IL release. The attenuation of IL release in keratinocytes by SP and the protection SP affords against pulmonary and immunotoxicity suggests that there may be a common mechanistic linkage to these toxicities. However, studies suggest that jet fuel-induced cell death in skin is via necrosis, not apoptosis as observed in some other cell types such as AIIE cells and T lymphocytes (Stoica *et al.*, 2001). This was also demonstrated by Rosenthal *et al.* (2001), who observed JP-8-induced necrotic rather than apoptotic cell death in mouse skin fibroblasts and HEK in culture or grafted onto nude mice. These authors used immunoblot analysis to determine that necrosis of HEK appeared to be associated with the perturbation of the ratio between anti- and pro-survival members of the Bcl-2 family of proteins (i.e., the toxic, higher level of JP-8 decreased levels of the pro-survival proteins Bcl-2 and Bcl-x_L, while simultaneously elevating levels of the anti-survival proteins Bad and Bak). This has led to the suggestion that high intrinsic levels of Bcl-2 and Bcl-x_L may prevent apoptotic death of keratinocytes at low concentrations of JP-8, whereas modulation of Bcl-2 family members by high doses may lead to necrotic cell death.

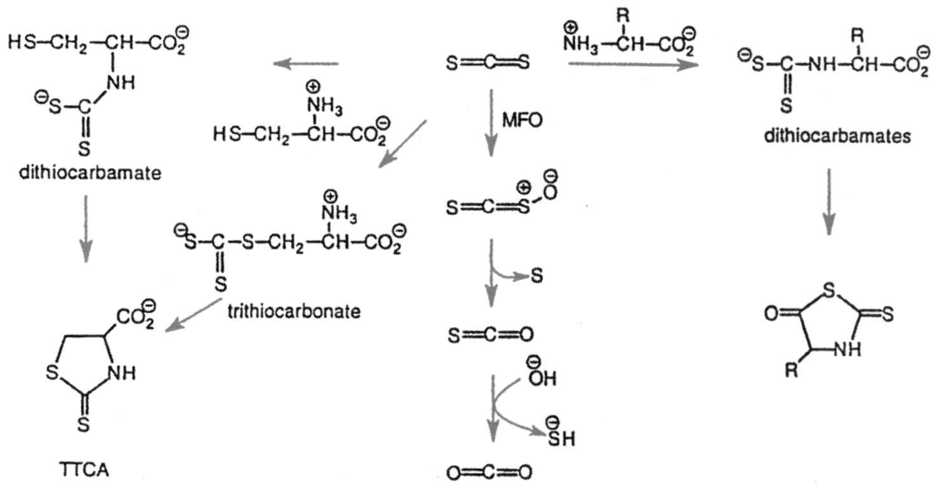

Figure 24-13. *Metabolism of carbon disulfide (CS$_2$).*

CS$_2$ is metabolized by the mixed-function oxidase (MFO) system to carbonyl sulfide, atomic sulfur and HS$^-$. Reaction of CS$_2$ with sulfhydryls of cysteine or GSH yields trithiocarbonates, which can cyclize to form thiazolidine-2-thione-4-carboxylic acid (TTCA). Reaction of CS$_2$ with amino groups of amino acids results in dithiocarbamate derivatives, which can cyclize to yield 2-thio-5-thiazolidinones; reaction of cysteine amine could also produce TTCA. CS$_2$ is also metabolized in the liver by P450s to an unstable oxygen intermediate, which spontaneously generates atomic sulfur, carbonyl sulfide (COS), and CO$_2$. [Reproduced with permission of Graham *et al.* (1995).]

As the skin allows for the selective absorption and penetration of various jet fuel components, one cannot assume that the internal or target tissue dose of chemical is qualitatively or quantitatively the same as that of the external dose (McDougal and Robinson, 2002). This has led to efforts to identify the offending components of jet fuel mixtures. Using static diffusion cells, McDougal *et al.* (2000) identified 12 components of JP-8 that fully penetrated rat skin and six components, all aliphatic hydrocarbons, which were partially absorbed or retained by the skin. This led these researchers to speculate that the aliphatic components of jet fuel may be the cause of skin irritation. Allen *et al.* (2001) exposed HEK to micromolar concentrations of four aliphatic hydrocarbon components of jet fuel and found that they all induced IL-8 release at subtoxic doses, further implicating aliphatic components. However, Chou *et al.* (2002) exposed HEK to 10 aliphatic jet fuel hydrocarbons (C6–C16) and found that the higher cytotoxicity of the shorter chain aliphatics did not correlate with their ability to induce IL-8 release, which peaked at mid-chain lengths (i.e., C9–C13). The toxicological interactions of jet fuel's aromatic and aliphatic components on HEK cells have also been explored (Yang *et al.*, 2006). The cytotoxicity and IL-8 release from these "mixed" hydrocarbon exposures were not always predictable based on the cytotoxic and IL-8 profiles of individual components. Muhammad *et al.* (2005) have exposed pigs topically to cotton fabric soaked with one of eight aliphatic hydrocarbons or one of six aromatic hydrocarbons and monitored skin irritation. Based on these data, coupled with data on IL-8 release, in vitro absorption and cytotoxicity, they postulate that tridecane and tetradecane may be the two most important hydrocarbons responsible for jet fuel-induced skin irritation. Jet fuel exemplifies well the difficulty in accurately predicting the dermal risk posed by a complex mixture based on limited knowledge of a few individual components. Progress toward this end has recently been made, as Kim *et al.* (2006) have published a dermatotoxicokinetic model of the skin that quantitatively characterizes the TK of three aromatic and three aliphatic jet fuel components following application

of a single dose of JP-8 to the forearm of human volunteers. As in lung tissue and lung cytosol of rodents, the capacity of JP-8 to alter gene or protein expression in HEK has been thoroughly examined (Espinoza *et al.*, 2004; Witzmann *et al.*, 2005; Chou *et al.*, 2006).

CARBON DISULFIDE

The major uses of carbon disulfide (CS$_2$) are in the production of rayon fiber, cellophane, and CCl$_4$ and as a solubilizer for waxes and oils (ATSDR, 1996a). Historically, exposures were particularly high during the early period of rayon production, and studies of these workers have been very informative as to CS$_2$'s toxicity. Human exposure is predominantly occupational, although CS$_2$ has been identified in at least 200 current or former EPA National Priority List hazardous waste sites (ATSDR, 1996a). Most industrial releases are to the atmosphere. The general public may be subjected to low vapor levels as demonstrated by detection of CS$_2$ in samples of breath and indoor and outdoor air surveyed in and around New York City (Phillips, 1992). Exposure to dithiocarbamate pesticides and drugs (e.g., the alcohol aversion drug, disulfiram) can result in indirect exposure to CS$_2$, as it is a product of their metabolism. However, there is evidence that the metabolic production of CS$_2$ is not unifying explanation for the neuropathies frequently associated with dithiocarbamate exposure (Tonkin *et al.*, 2000; Mulkey, 2001).

The relative contributions of parent compound and metabolites to most CS$_2$-induced toxicities are unknown. Two distinct metabolic pathways for CS$_2$ exist: (1) the direct interaction of CS$_2$ with free amine and sulfhydryl groups of amino acids and polypeptides to form dithiocarbamates and trithiocarbonates; and (2) microsomal metabolism of CS$_2$ to reactive sulfur intermediates capable of covalently binding tissue macromolecules (Graham *et al.*, 1995) (Fig. 24-13). The conjugation of CS$_2$ with sulfhydryls of cysteine or GSH results in the formation of 2-thiothiazolidine-4-carboxylic acid (TTCA), which is excreted in urine and has been frequently used as a biomarker of CS$_2$ exposure, especially among viscose rayon workers (Riihimaki *et al.*, 1992; Lee *et al.*, 1995). Several limitations of TTCA as a biomarker have been noted, and covalently cross-linked erythrocyte spectrin and hemoglobin have been discussed as potential alternatives (Valentine *et al.*, 1993, 1998). Nonetheless, the current ACGIH Biological Exposure Index (BEI) for CS_2 is 5 mg of TTCA per g of creatinine for a urine sample collected at the end of a workshift. Commentary on the derivation of this BEI has been published by Cox *et al.* (1992).

A few comprehensive reviews of CS_2's toxicity have been published (Beauchamp *et al.*, 1983; ATSDR, 1996a; WHO, 2002). CS_2 is capable of targeting multiple organ systems. There are numerous reports of enhanced noise-induced hearing loss and ophthalmological changes among workers exposed in the United States and abroad (Morata, 1989; Vanhoorne *et al.*, 1996; Chang *et al.*, 2003). The nervous and cardiovascular systems have garnered the most attention. The most common chronic effect is a distal sensorimotor neuropathy that preferentially affects long axons in the PNS and CNS (particularly the ascending and descending tracks of the spinal cord and the visual pathways). Encephalopathy with motor and congnitive impairment has also been reported following chronic, low-level exposure to CS_2 (Graham *et al.*, 1995). Several MRI studies report diffuse white matter lesions in chronically exposed workers similar to that described for "toluene leukoencephalopathy" among solvent abusers (Cho *et al.*, 2002; Ku *et al.*, 2003). For those particularly interested in the nervous system, the classic paper by Richter (1945) detailing his observations of chronic CS_2 poisoning in monkeys is recommended. Aftre 50 years, Rosenberg (1995) described the following clinical syndromes associated with CS_2:

(1) acute and chronic encephalopathy (often with prominent psychiatric manifestations); (2) polyneuropathy (both peripheral and cranial); (3) Parkinsonism; and (4) asymptomatic CNS and PNS dysfunction…. Pathologic changes occur in both the CNS and PNS…. CNS pathology consists of neuronal degeneration throughout the cerebral hemispheres, with maximal diffuse involvement in the frontal regions. Cell loss is also noted in the globus pallidus, putamen and cerebellar cortex, with loss of Purkinje cells. Vascular abnormalities with endothelial proliferation of arterioles may be seen, sometimes associated with focal necrosis or demyelination. PNS changes consist primarily of myelin swelling and fragmentation and large focal axonal swellings, characteristic of distal axonopathy.

Significant contributions to the understanding of CS_2's neurotoxicity have come from collaborative research by the NIEHS, EPA, and several universities (Harry *et al.*, 1998; Sills *et al.*, 1998, 2005). Studies were conducted with F-344 rats subchronically exposed to a range of CS_2 concentrations, in order to define the onset and temporal progression of neurotoxicity as manifest by multiple end points. These specific end points included TK changes in blood CS_2 levels and urinary TTCA, covalent cross-linking of blood and spinal cord proteins, alterations in axon/Schwann cell interactions as indicated by nerve growth factor mRNA expression, morphology of distal axonopathy, nerve conduction velocity and compound nerve action potential, and behavioral assessment using a Functional Observational Battery. This research showed sensitive end points at the cellular level that progressed to alterations in hindlimb and forelimb function, followed by electrophysiological and morphological changes. It supports the theory that the axonal degeneration that underlies CS_2's central–peripheral neuropathy results from the reaction of CS_2 [and perhaps carbonyl sulfide (COS)] with protein amino groups to yield initial adducts (dithiocarbamate derivatives). The adducts decompose to an electrophile (isothiocyanate for CS_2

and isocyanate for COS), which in turn reacts with protein nucleophiles on neurofilaments to cause covalent protein cross-linking. Progressive cross-linking of neurofilaments occurs during neurofilament transport along the axon, and covalently cross-linked masses of neurofilaments are thought to occlude axonal transport at the nodes of Ranvier, ultimately resulting in axonal swelling and degeneration (similar to that seen with 2,5-hexanedione). It should be noted that several other mechanisms for the disruption of neurofilament transport that underlie CS_2's axonopathy have been proposed including impaired energy metabolism, metal ion chelation by CS_2's dithiocarbamate derivatives, induction of vitamin deficiency, and disruption of cytoskeletal protein association by the increased phosphorylation of neurofilaments (Wilmarth *et al.*, 1993; Graham *et al.*, 1995).

One of the potentially more important outcomes of the collaborative research effort described above was the identification of thiourea cross-linking structures on erythrocyte spectrin and hemoglobin. This cross-linking exhibited a linear dose–response over the range of inhaled CS_2 concentrations examined, was detectable at subneurotoxic exposure levels, preceded axonal structural damage, and was positively correlated with neurofilament cross-linking (i.e., spectrin and hemoglobin cross-linking reflects neurofilament cross-linking). These findings suggest the utility of spectrin and hemoglobin cross-linking as sensitive biomarkers of exposure and effect, and potential alternatives or supplements to TTCA that was found to lack dose proportionality in the same studies (Valentine *et al.*, 1997, 1998; Moorman *et al.*, 1998).

Numerous worker studies support an association between CS_2 exposure and cardiovascular disease and related mortality. Elevated mortality from cardiovascular disease has been reported among viscose rayon workers in Finland, the United Kingdom, the United States, Scandinavia, and Poland (WHO, 2002). Viscose rayon worker studies reporting excess cardiovascular morbidity expand the range to Germany (Drexler *et al.*, 1996) and Japan (Takebayashi *et al.*, 2004). Further support for a CS_2–cardiovascular disease link comes from the examination of cardiovascular disease risk factors in workers, and to a lesser extent, experimental rodent studies. In workers, CS_2 exposure has been associated with elevations in blood pressure, total and LDL cholesterol, triglycerides, apolipoproteins, and lipid peroxidation in plasma, as well as reductions in HDL and antioxidant status (Egeland *et al.*, 1992; Vanhoorne *et al.*, 1992; Wronska-Nofer *et al.*, 2002; Luo *et al.*, 2003). Wronska-Nofer (1979) conducted studies in rats supporting a role for CS_2 in the elevation of blood cholesterol, whereas Lewis *et al.* (1999) found that exposure to as little as 50 ppm CS_2 significantly enhanced the rate of arterial fat deposition in mice placed on a western style, high-fat diet. Sulsky *et al.* (2002) have reviewed 37 studies addressing the CS_2–cardiovascular disease association and concluded that epidemiological evidence for an association was "mixed", with an effect on total and/or LDL cholesterol being the most consistent finding but of limited magnitude and uncertain clinical significance. Tan *et al.* (2002) conducted a meta-analysis of 11 cohort studies on CS_2's cardiovascular effects, that showed a small but significant correlation between CS_2 exposure and cardiovascular disease prevalence (pooled RR = 1.56; 95% CI = 1.12–2.1).

Taken together, studies suggest that CS_2 has the ability to accelerate atherosclerosis. Further, some have speculated that like neurotoxicity, protein cross-linking may also be involved in CS_2's promotion of the atherosclerotic process (Lewis *et al.*, 1999). As Price *et al.* (1997) point out, the cardiovascular mortality excesses seen in most published studies are among workers chronically exposed to high concentrations that no longer are observed in the workplace. These authors reviewed historical exposure and mortality data in the viscose rayon industry and estimated that chronic exposures of 15–20 ppm would not be associated with an increased risk of mortality due to ischemic heart disease. They were also instrumental in applying the benchmark dose method toward the establishment of EPA's RfC for CS_2 of 0.7 mg/m^3 (~0.22 ppm), that is based on reduced maximum motor conduction velocity in the peroneal

nerves of the NIOSH cohort of viscose rayon workers reported by Johnson *et al.* (1983) (Price *et al.*, 1996; EPA, 2006d). For the protection of workers, OSHA has established a PEL of 20 ppm as an 8-hour TWA and an acceptable ceiling concentration of 30 ppm. The ACGIH TLV was reduced from 10 to 1 ppm in 2006, as an 8-hour TWA based on neurologic end points. As a result, the ACGIH has placed CS_2's BEI under study and may move forward with a "notice of intended change" proposal in 2007.

REFERENCES

Abbate C, Giorgianni C, Munao F, Brecciaroli R: Neurotoxicity induced by exposure to toluene. An electropyhysiologic study. *Int Arch Occup Environ Health* 64:389–392, 1993.

ACGIH (American Conference of Governmental Industrial Hygienists): *2006 Threshold Limit Values (TLVs) and Biological Exposure Indices (BEIs)*. Cincinnati, OH, 2006.

Adachi J, Asano M, Ueno Y, et al.: Alcoholic muscle disease and biomembrane perturbations. *Nutr Biochem* 14:616–625, 2003.

Aggazzotti G, Fantuzzi G, Righi E, Predieri G: Environmental and biological monitoring of chloroform in indoor swimming pools. *J Chromatogr A* 710:181–190, 1995.

Agrawal AK, Shapiro BH: Constitutive and inducible hepatic cytochrome P450 isoforms in senescent male and female rats and response to low-dose phenobarbital. *Drug Metab Dispos* 31:612–619, 2003.

Ahmed FE: Toxicologycal effects of ethanol or human health. *Crit Rev Toxicol* 25: 347–367, 1995.

Albano E, French SW, Ingelman-Sundberg M: Hydroxyethyl radicals in ethanol hepatotoxicity. *Front Biosci* 4:533–540, 1999.

Albers JW, Wald JJ, Garabrant DH, et al.: Neurologic evaluation of workers previously diagnosed with solvent-induced toxic encephalopathy. *JOEM* 42:410–423, 2000.

Aleksunes LM, Slitt AM, Cherrington NJ, et al.: Differential expression of mouse hepatic transporter genes in response to acetaminophen and carbon tetrachloride. *Toxicol Sci* 83:44–52, 2005.

Alexander DD, Mink PJ, Mandel JH, Kelsh MA: A meta-analysis of occupational trichloroethylene exposure and multiple myeloma or leukemia. *Occup Med* 56:485–493, 2006.

Alfred S, Coleman P, Harris D, et al.: Delayed neurologic sequelae resulting from epidemic diethylene glycol poisoning. *Clin Toxicol* 43:155–159, 2005.

Allen DG, Riviere JE, Monteiro-Riviere NA: Identification of early biomarkers of inflammation produced by keratinocytes exposed to jet fuels jet A, JP-8, and JP-8 (100). *J Biochem Mol Toxicol* 14:231–237, 2000.

Allen DG, Riviere JE, Monteiro-Riviere NA: Analysis of interleukin-8 release from normal human epidermal keratinocytes exposed to aliphatic hydrocarbons: Delivery of hydrocarbons to cell cultures via complexation with α-cyclodextrin. *Toxicol in Vitro* 15:663–669, 2001.

Almekinder JL, Lennard DE, Walmer DK, et al.: Toxicity of methoxyacetic acid in cultured human luteal cells. *Fundam Appl Toxicol* 38:191–194, 1997.

Ambroso JL, Stedman DB, Elswick BA, Welsch F: Characterization of cell death induced by 2-methoxyethanol in CD-1 mouse embryos on gestation day 8. *Teratology* 58:231–240, 1998.

Anand SS, Kim K-B, Padilla S, et al.: Ontogeny of hepatic and plasma metabolism of deltamethrin in vitro: Role in age-dependent acute neurotoxicity. *Drug Metab Dispos* 34:389–397, 2006a.

Anand SS, Mumtaz MM, Mehendale HM: Dose-dependent liver regeneration in chloroform, trichloroethylene and allyl alcohol ternary mixture hepatotoxicity in rats. *Arch Toxicol* 79:671–682, 2005.

Anand SS, Philip BK, Palkar PS, et al.: Adaptive tolerance in mice upon subchronic exposure to chloroform: Increased exhalation and target tissue regeneration. *Toxicol Appl Pharmacol* 213:267–281, 2006b.

Anand SS, Soni MG, Vaidya VS, et al.: Extent and timeliness of tissue repair determines the dose-related hepatotoxicity of chloroform. *Int J Toxicol* 22:25–33, 2003.

Andersen ME: A physiologically based toxicokinetic description of the metabolism of inhaled gases and vapors: Analysis at steady state. *Toxicol Appl Pharmacol* 60:509–526, 1981.

Andersen, ME: Tissue dosimetry in risk assessment, or What's the problem here anyway? in Gillette JR, Jollow P (Chairs): *Drinking Water and Health*. Washington, DC: National Academy Press, 1987, Vol. 8, pp. 8–26.

Andersen ME: Toxicokinetic modeling and its applications in chemical risk assessment. *Toxicol Lett* 138:9–27, 2003.

Andersen ME, Clewell HJ, III, Gargas ML, et al.: Physiologically based pharmacokinetics and the risk assessment process for methylene chloride. *Toxicol Appl Pharmacol* 87:185–205, 1987.

Andreoli C, Leopardi P, Crebelli R: Detection of DNA damage in human lymphocytes by alkaline single cell gel electrophoresis after exposure to benzene or benzene metabolites. *Mutat Res* 377:95–104, 1997.

Anttila A, Pukkala E, Sallmen M, et al.: Cancer incidence among Finnish workers exposed to halogenated hydrocarbons. *J Occup Environ Med* 37:797–806, 1995.

Aranyi C, O'Shea WJ, Halder CA, et al.: Absence of hydrocarbon-induced nephropathy in rats exposed subchronically to volatile hydrocarbon mixtures pertinent to gasoline. *Toxicol Ind Health* 2:85–98, 1986.

Arlien-Soborg P: *Solvent Neurotoxicity*. Boca Raton, FL: CRC Press, 1992.

Arlien-Soborg P, Bruhn P, Gyldensted P, Melgaard, B: Chronic painters' syndrome: Chronic toxic encephalopathy in house painters. *Acta Neurol Scand* 60:149–156, 1979.

Ashley DL, Bonin MA, Cardinali FL, et al.: Blood concentrations of volatile organic compounds in a nonoccupationally exposed US population and in groups with suspected exposure. *Clin Chem* 40:1401–1404, 1994.

Asselman M, Verhulst A, de Broe ME, Verkoelen CF: Calcium oxalate crystal adherence to hyaluronan-, osteopontin-, and CD44-expressing injured/regenerating tubular epithelial cells in rat kidneys. *J Am Soc Nephrol* 14:3155–3166, 2003.

Astrand I: Effect of physical exercise on uptake, distribution and elimination of vapors in man, in Fiserova-Bergerova V (ed.): *Modeling of Inhalation Exposure to Vapors: Uptake, Distribution, and Elimination*. Boca Raton, FL: CRC Press, 1983, Vol. 2, pp. 107–130.

ATSDR (Agency for Toxic Substances and Disease Registry): *Toxicological Profile for Styrene*. Atlanta, GA: Public Health Service, 1992.

ATSDR (Agency for Toxic Substances and Disease Registry). Methanol toxicity. *Am Fam Physician* 47:163–171, 1993.

ATSDR (Agency for Toxic Substances and Disease Registry): *Toxicological Profile for Gasoline*. Atlanta, GA: Public Health Service, 1995.

ATSDR (Agency for Toxic Substances and Disease Registry): *Toxicological Profile for Carbon Disulfide*. Atlanta, GA: Public Health Service, 1996a.

ATSDR (Agency for Toxic Substances and Disease Registry): *Toxicological Profile For Methyl T-Butyl Ether*. Atlanta, GA: Public Health Service, 1996b.

ATSDR (Agency for Toxic Substances and Disease Registry): *Toxicological Profile for Chloroform.* Atlanta, GA: Public Health Service, 1997a.

ATSDR (Agency for Toxic Substances and Disease Registry): *Toxicological Profile for Ethylene Glycol and Propylene Glycol.* Atlanta, GA: Public Health Service, 1997b.

ATSDR (Agency for Toxic Substances and Disease Registry): *Toxicological Profile for Tetrachloroethylene.* Atlanta, GA: Public Health Service, 1997c.

ATSDR (Agency for Toxic Substances and Disease Registry): *Toxicological Profile for Jet Fuels (JP-5 and JP-8).* Atlanta, GA: Public Health Service, 1998a.

ATSDR (Agency for Toxic Substances and Disease Registry): *Toxicological Profile for Methylene Chloride.* Atlanta, GA: Public Health Service, 1998b.

ATSDR (Agency for Toxic Substances and Disease Registry): *Toxicological Profile for Ethylbenzene.* Atlanta, GA: Public Health Service, 1999.

ATSDR (Agency for Toxic Substances and Disease Registry): *Toxicological Profile for Toluene.* Atlanta, GA: Public Health Service, 2000.

ATSDR (Agency for Toxic Substances and Disease Registry): *Toxicological Profile for Carbon Tetrachloride.* Atlanta, GA: Public Health Service, 2005.

ATSDR (Agency for Toxic Substances and Disease Registry): *ToxFAQs for Trichloroethylene (TCE).* Atlanta, GA: Public Health Service, 2006a. http://www.atsdr.ege.gov/tfacts19.html.

ATSDR (Agency for Toxic Substances and Disease Registry): *Toxicological Profile for 1,1,1-Trichloroethane (Update).* Atlanta, GA: Public Health Service, 2006b.

ATSDR (Agency for Toxic Substances and Disease Registry): *Toxicological Profile Benzene.* Atlanta, GA: Public Health Service, 2006c.

ATSDR (Agency for Toxic Substances and Disease Registry): *Toxicological Profile for Xylenes.* Atlanta, GA: Public Health Service, 2006d.

Axelson O, Hane M, Hogstedt C: A case-referent study of neuropsychiatric disorders among workers exposed to solvents. *Scand J Work Environ Health* 2:14–20, 1976.

Axelson O, Selden A, Andersson K, *et al.*: Updated and expanded Swedish cohort study of trichloroethylene and cancer risk. *J Occup Med* 36:556–562, 1994.

Backes WL, Sequeira DJ, Cawley GF, Eyer CS: Relationship between hydrocarbon structure and induction of P450: Effects on protein levels and enzyme activities. *Xenobiotica* 23:1353–1366, 1993.

Bailey DG, Dresser GK, Bend JR: Bergamottin, lime juice, and red wine as inhibitors of cytochrome P450 3A4 activity: Comparison with grapefruit juice. *Clin Pharmacol Therap* 73:529–537, 2003.

Baldwin CM, Houston FP, Podgornik MN, *et al.*: Effects of aerosol-vapor JP-8 jet fuel on the functional observational battery, and learning and memory in the rat. *Arch Environ Health* 56:216–226, 2001.

Ballantyne B, Snellings WM: Developmental toxicity study with diethylene glycol dosed by gavage to CD rats and CD-1 mice. *Food Chem Toxicol* 43:1637–1646, 2005.

Ballantyne B, Vergnes JS: In vitro and in vivo genetic toxicology studies with diethylene glycol monohexyl ether. *J Appl Toxicol* 21:449–460, 2001.

Balster, RL: Neural basis of inhalant abuse. *Drug Alcohol Dep* 512:207–214, 1998.

Barceloux DG, Bond GR, Krenzelok EP, *et al.*: American Academy of Clinical Toxicology practice guidelines on the treatment of methanol poisoning. *J Toxicol Clin Toxicol* 40:415–446, 2002.

Barton HA, Creech JR, Godin CS, *et al.*: Chloroethylene mixtures: Pharmacokinetic modeling and in vitro metabolism of vinyl chloride, trichloroethylene, and trans-1,2-dichloroethylene in rat. *Toxicol Appl Pharmacol* 130:237–247, 1995.

Barton HA, Das S: Alternative for a risk assessment on chronic non-cancer effects from oral exposure to trichloroethylene. *Regul Toxicol Pharmacol* 24:269–285, 1996.

Bautista AP: Impact of alcohol on the ability of Kupffer cells to produce chemokines and its role in alcoholic liver disease. *J Gastroenterol Hepatol* 15:349–356, 2000.

Beattie PJ, Welsh MJ, Brabec MJ: The effect of 2-methoxyethanol and methoxyacetic acid on Sertoli cell lactate production and protein synthesis in vitro. *Toxicol Appl Pharmacol* 76:56–61, 1984.

Beauchamp RO, Bus JS, Popp JA, *et al.*: A critical review of the literature on carbon disulfide toxicity. *Crit Rev Toxicol* 11:169–278, 1983.

Beckstead MJ, Weiner JL, Eger EI, *et al.*: Glycine and gamma-aminobutyric acid (A) receptor function is enhanced by inhaled drugs of abuse. *Mol Pharmacol* 57:1199–1205, 2000.

Beddowes EJ, Faux SP, Chipman JK: Chloroform, carbon tetrachloride and glutathione depletion induce secondary genotoxicity in liver cells via oxidative stress. *Toxicology* 187:101–115, 2003.

Bell AN, Young RA, Lockard VG, Mehendale HM: Protection of chlordecone-potentiated carbon tetrachloride hepatotoxicity and lethality by partial hepatectomy. *Arch Toxicol* 61:392–405, 1988.

Bell IR, Brooks AJ, Baldwin CM, *et al.*: JP-8 jet fuel exposure and divided attention test performance in 1991 Gulf War veterans. *Aviat Space Environ Med* 76:1136–1144, 2005.

Belligner FP, Bedi KS, Wilson P, Wilce PA: Ethanol exposure during the third trimester equivalent results in long-lasting decreased synaptic efficacy but not plasticity in the CA1 region of the rat hippocampus. *Synapse* 31:51–58, 1999.

Belpoggi F, Soffritti M, Filippini F, Maltoni C: Results of long-term experimental studies on the carcinogenicity of methyl *tert*-butyl ether. *Ann NY Acad Sci* 837:77–95, 1997.

Belpoggi F, Soffritti M, Maltoni C: Methyl-tertiary-butyl ether (MTBE)-a gasoline additive-causes testicular and lymphophaematopoietic cancers in rats. *Toxicol Ind Health* 11:119–149, 1995.

Benignus VA, Boyes WK, Bushnell PG: A dosimetric analysis of behavioral effects of acute toluene exposure in rats and humans. *Toxicol Sci* 43:186–195, 1998.

Bennett GF: Air quality aspects of hazardous waste landfills. *Haz Waste Haz Mater* 4:119–138, 1987.

Bergsagel DE, Wong O, Bergsagel PL, *et al.*: Benzene and multiple myeloma: Appraisal of the scientific evidence. *Blood* 94:1174–1182, 1999.

Bernauer U, Vieth B, Ellrich R, *et al.*: CYP2E1-dependent benzene toxicity: The role of extrahepatic benzene metabolism. *Arch Toxicol* 73:189–196, 1999.

Bevan C, Neeper-Bradley TL, Tyl RW, *et al.*: Two-generation reproductive toxicity study of methyl tertiary-butyl ether (MTBE) in rats. *J Appl Toxicol* 17(S1):S13–S19, 1997a.

Bevan C, Tyl RW, Neeper-Bradley TL, *et al.*: Developmental toxicity evaluation of methyl tertiary-butyl ether (MTBE) by inhalation in mice and rabbits. *J Appl Toxicol* 17(S1) S21–S29, 1997b.

Bezabeth S, Engel A, Morris CB, Lamm SH: Does benzene cause multiple myeloma? An analysis of the published case–control literature. *Environ Health Perspect* 104(Suppl 6):1393–1398, 1996.

Bird MG, Burleigh-Flayer HD, Chun JS, *et al.*: Oncogenicity studies of inhaled methyl tertiary-butyl ether (MTBE) in CD-1 mice and F-344 rats. *J Appl Toxicol* 17:S45–S55, 1997.

Bird MG, Greim H, Snyder R, Rice JM: International symposium: Recent advances in benzene toxicity. *Chem-Biol Interact* 153–154:1–5, 2005.

Birner G, Richling C, Henschler D, *et al.*: Metabolism of tetrachloroethylene in rats: Identification of *N*-(dichloroacetyl)-L-cysteine and *N*-(trichloroacetyl)-L-lysine as protein adducts. *Chem Res Toxicol* 7:724–732, 1994.

Blair A, Hartge P, Stewart PA, *et al.*: Mortality and cancer incidence of aircraft maintenance workers exposed to trichloroethylene and other organic solvents and chemicals: Extended follow-up. *Occup Environ Med* 55:161–171, 1998.

Blanco JG, Harrison PL, Evans WE, Relling MV: Human cytochrome P450 maximal activities in pediatric versus adult liver. *Drug Metab Dispos* 28:379–382, 2000.

Bleecker ML, Bolla KI, Agnew J, *et al.*: Dose-related subclinical neurobehavioral effects of chronic exposure to low levels of organic solvents. *Am J Ind Med* 19:715–728, 1991.

Blobaum AL: Mechanism-based inactivation and reversibility: Is there a new trend in the inactivation of cytochrome P450 enzymes? *Drug Metab Dispos* 34:1–7, 2006.

Blossom SJ, Gilbert KM: Exposure to a metabolite of the environmental toxicant, trichloroethylene, attenuates CD4+ T cell activation-induced cell death by metalloproteinase-dependent FasL shedding. *Toxicol Sci* 92:103–114, 2006.

Blount BC, Kobelski RJ, McElprang DO, et al.: Quantification of 31 volatile organic compounds in whole blood using solid-phase microextraction and gas chromatography-mass spectrometry. *J Chromatogr B* 832:292–301, 2006.

Boatman R, Corley R, Green T, et al.: Review of studies concerning the tumorigenicity of 2-butoxyethanol in B6C3F1 mice and its relevance for human risk assessment. *J Toxicol Environ Health B Crit Rev* 7:385–398, 2004.

Boffeta P, Garfinkel L: Alcohol drinking and mortality among men enrolled in an American Cancer Society prospective study. *Epidemiology* 1:342–348, 1990.

Boffetta P, Hashibe M: Alcohol and cancer. *Lancet Oncol* 7:149–156, 2006.

Boice JD, Marano DE, Fryzek JP, et al.: Mortality among aircraft manufacturing workers. *Occup Environ Med* 56:581–597, 1999.

Boogaard PJ, van Sittert NJ: Suitability of S-phenylmercapturic acid and trans-trans-muconic acid as biomarkers for exposure to low concentrations of benzene. *Environ Health Perspect* 104(Suppl 6):1151–1157, 1996.

Borak J, Pastides H, Van Ert M, et al.: Exposure to MTBE and acute human health effects: A critical literature review. *Hum Ecol Assess* 4:177–200, 1998.

Borghoff SJ, Murphy JE, Medinsky MA: Development of physiologically based pharmacokinetic model for methyl tertiary-butyl ether and tertiary-butanol in male Fischer-344 rats. *Fundam Appl Toxicol* 30:264–275, 1996.

Boulares AH, Contreras FJ, Espinoza LA, Smulson ME: Roles of oxidative stress and glutathione depletion in JP-8 jet fuel-induced apoptosis in rat lung epithelial cells. *Toxicol Appl Pharmacol* 180:92–99, 2002.

Boutelet-Bochan H, Huang Y, Juchau MR: Expression of CYP2E1 during embryogenesis and fetogenesis in human cephalic tissues: Implications for the fetal alcohol syndrome. *Biochem Biophys Res Commun* 238:443–447, 1997.

Brauch H, Weirich G, Hornauer MA, et al.: Trichloroethylene exposure and specific somatic mutations in patients with renal cell carcinoma. *J Natl Cancer Inst* 91:854–861, 1999.

Brauch H, Weirich G, Klein B, et al.: VHL mutations in renal cell cancer: Does occupational exposure to trichloroethylene make a difference? *Toxicol Lett* 151:301–310, 2004.

Brent J, McMartin K, Phillips S, et al.: Fomepizole for the treatment of ethylene glycol poisoning. Methylpyrazole for Toxic Alcohols Study Group. *N Engl J Med* 340:832–838, 1999.

Bressler R, Bahl JJ: Principles of drug therapy for the elderly patient. *Mayo Clin Proc* 78:1564–1577, 2003.

Brienza RS, Stein MD: Alcohol use disorders in primary care: Do gender-specific differences exist? *J Gen Intern Med* 17:387–397, 2002.

Brinkworth MH, Weinbauer GF, Schlatt S, Nieschlag E: Identification of male germ cells undergoing apoptosis in adult rats. *J Reprod Fertil* 105:25–33, 1995.

Brodkin CA, Daniell W, Checkoway H, et al.: Hepatic ultrasonic changes in workers exposed to perchloroethylene. *Occup Environ Med* 52:679–685, 1995.

Brodkin CA, Moon J-D, Camp J, et al.: Serum hepatic biochemical activity in two populations of workers exposed to styrene. *Occup Environ Med* 58:95–102, 2001.

Brooks DE, Wallace KL: Acute propylene glycol ingestion. *J Toxicol Clin Toxicol* 40:513–516, 2002.

Brophy PD, Tenebein M, Gardner J, et al.: Childhood diethylene glycol poisoning treated with alcohol dehydrogenase inhibitor Fomepizole and hemodialysis. *Am J Kidney Dis* 35:958–962, 2000.

Brown EA, Shelley ML, Fisher JW: A pharmacokinetic study of occupational and environmental exposure with regard to gender. *Risk Anal* 18:205–213, 1998.

Brown-Woodman, PDC, Hayes LC, Huq F, et al.: In vitro assessment of the effect of halogenated hydrocarbons: Chloroform, dichloromethane, and dibromomethane on embryonic development of the rat. *Teratology* 57:321–333, 1998.

Bruckner, JV: Differences in sensitivity of children and adults to chemical toxicity: The NAS panel report. *Regul Toxicol Pharmacol* 31:280–285, 2000.

Bruckner JV, Kyle GM, Luthra R, et al.: Acute, short-term and subchronic oral toxicity of 1,1,1-trichloroethane in rats. *Toxicol Sci* 60:363–372, 2001.

Bruckner JV, Peterson RG: Evaluation of toluene and acetone inhalant abuse. I. Pharmacology and pharmacodynamics. *Toxicol Appl Pharmacol* 61:27–38, 1981.

Bruckner JV, Ramanathan R, Lee KM, Muralidhara S: Mechanisms of circadian rhythmicity of carbon tetrachloride hepatotoxicity. *J Pharmacol Exp Therap* 300:273–281, 2002.

Bruner RH, Kinkead ER, O'Neill TP, et al.: The toxicologic and oncogenic potential of JP-4 jet fuel vapors in rats and mice: 12-Month intermittent inhalation exposures. *Fundam Appl Toxicol* 20:97–110, 1993.

Bruning T, Bolt HM: Renal toxicity and carcinogenicity of trichloroethylene: Key results, mechanisms, and controversies. *Crit Rev Toxicol* 30:253–285, 2000.

Bruning T, Golka K, Makropoulos V, Bolt HM: Preexistence of chronic tubular damage in cases of renal cell cancer after long and high exposure to trichloroethylene. *Arch Toxicol* 70:259–260, 1996.

Bruning T, Weirich G, Hornauer MA, et al.: Renal cell carcinomas in trichloroethene (TRI) exposed persons are associated with somatic mutations in the von Hippel–Lindau (VHL) tumour suppressor gene. *Arch Toxicol* 71:332–335, 1997a.

Bruning T, Lammert M, Kempkes M, et al.: Influence of polymorphisms of GSTM1 and GSTT1 for risk of renal cell cancer in workers with long-term high occupational exposure to trichloroethene. *Arch Toxicol* 71:596–599, 1997b.

Bruning T, Mann H, Melzer H, et al.: Pathological excretion patterns of urinary proteins in renal cell cancer patients exposed to trichloroethylene. *Occup Med* 49:299–305, 1999.

Bull RJ: Mode of action of liver tumor induction by trichloroethylene and its metabolites, trichloroacetate and dichloroacetate. *Environ Health Perspect* 108(Suppl 2):241–259, 2000.

Bull RJ, Orner GA, Cheng RS, et al.: Contribution of dichloroacetate and trichloroacetate to liver tumor induction in mice by trichloroethylene. *Toxicol Appl Pharmacol* 182:55–65, 2002.

Burbacher TM, Grant KS, Shen DD, et al.: Chronic maternal methanol inhalation in nonhuman primates (*Macaca fascicularis*): Reproductive performance and birth outcome. *Neurotoxicol Teratol* 26:639–650, 2004a.

Burbacher TM, Shen DD, Lalovic B, et al.: Chronic maternal methanol inhalation in nonhuman primates (*Macaca fascicularis*): Exposure and toxicokinetics prior to and during pregnancy. *Neurotoxicol Teratol* 26:201–221, 2004b.

Burek JD, Nitschke KD, Bell TJ, et al.: Methylene chloride: A two-year inhalation toxicity and oncogenicity study in rats and hamsters. *Fundam Appl Toxicol* 4:30–47, 1984.

Burleigh-Flayer HD, Chun JS, Kintigh WJ: *Methyl Tertiary Butyl Ether: Vapor Inhalation Oncogenicity Study in CD Mice.* Export, PA: Bushy Run Research Center, 1992.

Burton DA, Allen MC, Bird JL, Faragher RA: Bridging the gap: Ageing, pharmacokinetics and pharmacodynamics. *J Pharm Pharmacol* 57:671–679, 2005.

Byard RW, Chivell WC, Gilbert JD: Unusual facial markings and lethal mechanisms in a series of gasoline inhalation deaths. *Am J Foren Med Path* 24:298–302, 2003.

Caldemeyer KS, Armstrong SW, George KK, et al.: The spectrum of neuroimaging abnormalities in solvent abuse and their clinical correlation. J Neuroimag 6:167–173, 1996.

Caldwell JC, Evans MV, Marcus AH, et al.: Comments on article "Applying mode-of-action and pharmacokinetic considerations in contemporary cancer risk assessments: An example with trichloroethylene" by Clewell and Andersen. Crit Rev Toxicol 36:291–294, 2006.

Caprino L, Togna GI: Potential health effects of gasoline and its constituents: A review of current literature (1990–1997) on toxicological data. Environ Health Perspect 106:115–125, 1998.

Carlson GP: In vitro metabolism of styrene to styrene oxide in liver and lung of CYP2E1 knockout mice. J Toxicol Environ Health A 66:861–869, 2003.

Carney EW, Freshour NL, Dittenber DA, Dryzga MD: Ethylene glycol developmental toxicity: Unraveling the roles of glycolic acid and metabolic acidosis. Toxicol Sci 50:117–126, 1999.

Carney EW, Liberacki AB, Bartels MJ, Breslin WJ: Identification of proximate toxicant for ethylene glycol developmental toxicity using rat whole embryo culture. Teratology 53:38–46, 1996.

Caro AA, Cederbaum, AI: Oxidative stress, toxicology, and pharmacology of CYP2E1. Annu Rev Pharmacol Toxicol 44:27–42, 2004.

Casanova M, Bell DA, Heck H d'A: Dichloromethane metabolism to formaldehyde and reaction of formaldehyde with nucleic acids in hepatocytes of rodents and humans with and without glutathione S-transferase T1 and M1 genes. Fundam Appl Toxicol 37:168–180, 1997.

Casanova M, Conolly RB, Heck H d'A: DNA–protein cross-links (DPX) and cell proliferation in B6C3F1 mice but not Syrian golden hamsters exposed to dichloromethane: Pharmacokinetics and risk assessment with DPX as dosimeter. Fundam Appl Toxicol 31:103–116, 1996.

Casanova M, Heck H d'A: Lack of evidence for the involvement of formaldehyde in the hepatocarcinogenicity of methyl tertiary-butyl ether in CD-1 mice. Chem-Biol Interact 105:131–143, 1997.

Castillo T, Koop DR, Kamimura S, et al.: Role of cytochrome P-450 2E1 in ethanol-, carbon tetrachloride- and iron-dependent microsomal lipid peroxidation. Hepatology 16:992–996, 1992.

Cawley MJ: Short-term lorazepam infusion and concern for propylene glycol toxicity: Case report and review. Pharmacotherapy 21:1140–1144, 2001.

CDC (Centers for Disease Control and Prevention). Fetal alcohol syndrome-Alaska, Arizona, Colorado, and New York, 1995–1997. Morbid Mortal Week Rep 51:433–435, 2002.

Chan WK, Nguyen LT, Miller VP, Harris RZ: Mechanism-based inactivation of human cytochrome P450 3A4 by grapefruit juice and red wine. Life Sci 62:135–142, 1998.

Chang S-J, Shih T-S, Chou T-C, et al.: Hearing loss in workers exposed to carbon disulfide and noise. Environ Health Perspect 111:1620–1624, 2003.

Chang TKH, Chen J, Yeung EYH: Effect of Ginkgo biloba extract on procarcinogen-bioactivating human CYP enzymes: Identification of isorhamnetin, kaempferol, and quercetin as potent inhibitors of CYP1B1. Toxicol Appl Pharmacol 213:18–26, 2006.

Chao YC, Gibson RL, Nylander-French LA: Dermal exposure to jet fuel (JP-8) in US Air Force personnel. Ann Occup Hyg 49:639–645, 2005.

Chapin RE, Dutton SD, Ross MD, et al.: The effects of ethylene glycol monomethyl ether on testicular histology in F344 rats. J Androl 5:369–380, 1984.

Charbonneau M, Swenberg JA: Studies on the biochemical mechanism of α_u-globulin nephropathy in rats. CIIT Activities 8:1–5, 1988.

Charbotel B, Fevotte J, Hours M, et al.: Case–control study on renal cell cancer and occupational exposure to trichloroethylene. Part II: Epidemiological aspects. Ann Occup Hyg 50:777–787, 2006.

Chen DH, Kaung HL, Miller CM, et al.: Microarray analysis of changes in renal phenotype in the ethylene glycol rat model of urolithiasis: Potential and pitfalls. BJU Int 94:637–650, 2004.

Chen PC, Hsieh GY, Wang JD, Cheng TJ: Prolonged time to pregnancy in female workers exposed to ethylene glycol ethers in semiconductor manufacturing. Epidemiology 13:191–196, 2002.

Cheng P-Y, Morgan ET: Hepatic cytochrome P450 regulation in disease states. Curr Drug Metab 2:165–183, 2001.

Cherry NH, Hutchins H, Pace T, Waldron JA: Neurobehavioral effects of repeated occupational exposure to toluene and paint solvents. Br J Ind Med 42:291–300, 1985.

Cho SK, Kim RH, Yim SH, et al.: Long-term neuropsychological effects and MRI findings in patients with CS$_2$ poisoning. Acta Neurol Scand 106:269–275, 2002.

Chou CC, Riviere JE, Monteiro-Riviere NA: Differential relationship between the carbon chain length of jet fuel aliphatic hydrocarbons and their ability to induce cytotoxicity vs. interleukin-8 release in human epidermal keratinocytes. Toxicol Sci 69:226–233, 2002.

Chou CC, Riviere JE, Monteiro-Riviere NA: The cytotoxicity of jet fuel aromatic hydrocarbons and dose-related interleukin-8 release from human epidermal keratinocytes. Arch Toxicol 77:384–391, 2003.

Chou CC, Yang JH, Chen SD, et al.: Expression profiling of human epidermal keratinocyte response following 1-minute JP-8 exposure. Cutan Ocul Toxicol 25:141–153, 2006.

Christopher MM, Eckfeldt JH, Eaton JW: Propylene glycol ingestion causes D-lactic acidosis. Lab Invest 62:114–118, 1990.

Chrostek L, Jelski W, Szmitkowski M, Puchalski Z: Gender-related differences in hepatic activity of alcohol dehydrogenase isoenzymes and aldehyde dehydrogenase in humans. J Clin Lab Anal 17:93–96, 2003.

Chu I, Poon R, Valli V, et al.: Effects of an ethanol-gasoline mixture: Results of a 4-week inhalation study in rats. J Appl Toxicol 25:193–199, 2005.

Chun JS, Burleigh-Flayer HD, Kintigh WJ: Methyl Tertiary Butyl Ether: Vapor Inhalation Oncogenicity Study in Fisher 344 Rats. Export, PA: Bushy Run Research Center, 1992.

Chung HC, Sung SH, Kim JS, et al.: Lack of cytochrome P450 2E1 (CYP2E1) induction in the rat liver by starvation without coprophogy. Drug Metab Dispos 29:213–216, 2001.

Churchill JE, Ashley DL, Kaye WE: Recent chemical exposures and blood volatile organic compound levels in a large population-based sample. Arch Environ Health 56:157–166, 2001.

Cirvello JD, Radovsky A, Heath JE, et al.: Toxicity and carcinogenicity of t-butyl alcohol in rats and mice following chronic exposure in drinking water. Toxicol Ind Health 11:151–165, 1995.

Clarke DO, Duignan JM, Welsch F: 2-Methoxyacetic acid dosimetry-teratogenicity relationships in CD-1 mice exposed to 2-methoxyethanol. Toxicol Appl Pharmacol 114:77–87, 1992.

Clary JJ: Methanol, is it a developmental risk to humans? Reg Toxicol Pharmacol 37:83–91, 2003.

Clawson GA, MacDonald J, Woo C: Early hypomethylation of 2′-0-ribose moieties in hepatocytes cytoplasmic ribosomal RNA underlies the protein synthesis defect produced by CC1$_4$. J Cell Biol 105:705–711, 1987.

Clayton CA, Pellizzari ED, Whitmore RW, et al.: National Human Exposure Assessment Survey (NHEXAS): Distributions and associations of lead, arsenic and volatile organic compounds in EPA Region 5. J Expos Anal Environ Epidemiol 9:381–392, 1999.

Clewell HJ, Teeguarden J, McDonald T, et al.: Review and evaluation of the potential impact of age- and gender-specific pharmacokinetic differences on tissue dosimetry. Crit Rev Toxicol 32(5):329–389, 2002.

Clewell HJ, Andersen ME: Applying mode-of-action and pharmacokinetic considerations in contemporary cancer risk assessments: An example with trichloroethylene. Crit Rev Toxicol 34:385–445, 2004.

Clewell HJ, Gentry PR, Kester JE, Andersen ME: Evaluation of physiologically based pharmacokinetic models in risk assessment: an example with perchloroethylene. Crit Rev Toxicol 35(5):413–433, 2005.

Clewell HJ, Andersen ME: Response to comments by Caldwell et al. on article "Applying mode-of-action and pharmacokinetic considerations in contemporary cancer risk assessments: An example with trichloroethylene." Crit Rev Toxicol 36:295–298, 2006.

Clewell HJ, Gentry PR, Covington TR, et al.: Evaluation of the potential impact of age- and gender-specific pharmacokinetic differences on tissue dosimetry. Toxicol Sci 79:381–393, 2004.

Cody RJ: Physiological changes due to age. Implications for drug therapy of congestive heart failure. Drugs Aging 3:320–334, 1993.

Cogliano VJ, Grosse Y, Baan RA, *et al.*: Meeting report: Summary of IARC monographs on formaldehyde, 2-butoxyethanol, and 1-tert-butoxy-2-propanol. *Environ Health Perspect* 113:1205–1208, 2005.

Colantoni A, Idilman R, De Maria N, *et al.*: Hepatic apoptosis and proliferation in male and female rats fed alcohol: Role of cytokines. *Alcohol Clin Exp Res* 27:1184–1189, 2003.

Colborn T: A case for revisiting the safety of pesticides: A closer look at neurodevelopment. *Environ Health Perspect* 114:10–17, 2006.

Cole CE, Tran HT, Schlosser PM: Physiologically based pharmacokinetic modeling of benzene metabolism in mice through extrapolation from in vitro to in vivo. *J Toxicol Environ Health A* 62:439–465, 2001.

Conolly RB, Andersen ME: Biologically based pharmacodynamic models: Tools for toxicological research and risk assessment. *Annu Rev Pharmacol Toxicol* 31:503–523, 1991.

Constan AA, Sprankle CS, Peters JM, *et al.*: Metabolism of chloroform by cytochrome P4502E1 is required for induction of toxicity in the liver, kidney, and nose of male mice. *Toxicol Appl Pharmacol* 160:120–126, 1999.

Constan AA, Wong BA, Everitt JI, Butterworth BE: Chloroform inhalation exposure conditions necessary to initiate liver toxicity in female B6C3F1 mice. *Toxicol Sci* 66:201–208, 2002.

Cooper AJL: Enzymology of cysteine S-conjugate β-lyases. *Adv Pharmacol* 27:71–113, 1994.

Cordier S, Bergeret A, Goujard J, *et al.*: Congenital malformations and maternal occupational exposure to glycol ethers. *Epidemiology* 8:355–363, 1997.

Corley RA, Bormett GA, Ghanayem BI: Physiologically based pharmacokinetics of 2-butoxyethanol and its major metabolite, 2-butoxyacetic acid, in rats and humans. *Toxicol Appl Pharmacol* 129:61–79, 1994.

Corley RA, Bartels MJ, Carney EW, *et al.*: Development of a physiologically based pharmacokinetic model for ethylene glycol and its metabolite, glycolic acid, in rats and humans. *Toxicol Sci* 85:476–490, 2005a.

Corley RA, Gies RA, Wu H, Weitz KK. Development of a physiologically based pharmacokinetic model for propylene glycol monomethyl ether and its acetate in rats and humans. *Toxicol Lett* 156:193–213, 2005b.

Corley RA, Grant DM, Farris E, *et al.*: Determination of age and gender differences in biochemical processes affecting the disposition of 2-butoxyethanol and its metabolites in mice and rats to improve PBPK modeling. *Toxicol Lett* 156:127–161, 2005c.

Corley RA, Meek ME, Carney EW: Mode of action: Oxalate crystal-induced renal tubule degeneration and glycolic acid-induced dysmorphogenesis – renal and developmental effects of ethylene glycol. *Crit Rev Toxicol* 35:691–702, 2005d.

Corley RA, Mast TJ, Carney EW, *et al.*: Evaluation of physiologically based models of pregnancy and lactation for their application in children's health risk assessments. *Crit Rev Toxicol* 33:137–211, 2003.

Corley RA, McMartin KE: Incorporation of therapeutic interventions in physiologically based pharmacokinetic modeling of human clinical case reports of accidental or intentional overdosing with ethylene glycol. *Toxicol Sci* 85:491–501, 2005.

Correa A, Gray R, Cohen R, *et al.*: Ethylene glycol ethers and risks of spontaneous abortion and subfertility. *Am J Epidemiol* 143:707–717, 1996.

Corthals SM, Kamendulis LM, Klaunig JE: Mechanism of 2-butoxyethanol-induced hemangiosarcomas. *Toxicol Sci* 92:378–386, 2006.

Costa ET, Savage DD, Valenzuela CF: A review of the effects of prenatal or early postnatal ethanol exposure on brain ligand-gated ion channels. *Alcohol Clin Exp Res* 24:706–715, 2000.

Cotreau MM, von Moltke LL, Greenblatt DJ: The influence of age and sex on the clearance of cytochrome P450 3A substrates. *Clin Pharmacokinet* 44:33–60, 2005.

Covington TR, Gentry PR, Van Landingham CB, *et al.*: The use of Markov chain Monte Carlo uncertainty analysis to support a public health goal for perchloroethylene. *Regul Toxicol Pharmacol* 2006. (in press)

Cox C, Lowry LK, Que Hee SS: Urinary 2-thiothiazolidine-4-carboxylic acid as a biological indicator of exposure to carbon disulfide: Derivation of a biological exposure index. *Appl Occup Environ Hyg* 7:672–676, 1992.

Crabb DW, Matsumoto M, Chang D, You M: Overview of the role of alcohol dehydrogenase and aldehyde dehydrogenase and their variants in the genesis of alcohol-related pathology. *Proc Nutr Soc* 63:49–63, 2004.

Cranmer JM: Proceedings of the workshop on neurobehavioral effects of solvents. *Neurotoxicology* 7:1–95, 1986.

Creasy DM, Foster PMD: The morphological development of glycol ether-induced testicular atrophy in the rat. *Exp Mol Pathol* 40:169–176, 1984.

Creek MR, Mani C, Vogel JS, Turteltaub KW: Tissue distribution and macromolecular binding of extremely low doses of [^{14}C]-benzene in B6C3F1 mice. *Carcinogenesis* 18:2421–2427, 1997.

Cresteil T: Onset of xenobiotic metabolism in children: Toxicological implications. *Food Add Contam* 15(Suppl):45–51, 1998.

Cruz SL, Balster RL, Woodward, JJ: Effects of volatile solvents on recombinant N-methyl-D-aspartate receptors expressed in *Xenopus* oocytes. *Br J Pharmacol* 131:1303–1308, 2000.

Cruz SL, Mirshahi T, Thomas B, *et al.*: Effects of the abused solvent toluene on recombinant N-methyl-D-aspartate and non-N-methyl-D-aspartate receptors expressed in Xenopus oocytes. *J Pharmacol Exp Therap* 286:334–340, 1998.

d'Alessandro A, Osterloh JD, Chuwers P, *et al.*: Formate in serum and urine after controlled methanol exposure at the threshold limit value. *Environ Health Perspect* 102:178–181, 1994.

Dai Y, Rashba-Step J, Cederbaum AI: Stable expression of human cytochrome P4502E1 in HepG2 cells: Characterization of catalytic activities and production of reactive oxygen intermediates. *Biochemistry* 32:6928–6937, 1993.

Daly AK, Cholerton S, Gregory W, Idle JR: Metabolic polymorphisms. *Pharmacol Therap* 57:129–160, 1993.

Dankovic, DA, Bailer AJ: The impact of exercise and intersubject variability on dose estimates for dichloromethane derived from a physiologically based pharmacokinetic model. *Fundam Appl Toxicol* 22:20–25, 1994.

Daston G, Faustman E, Ginsberg G, *et al.*: A framework for assessing risks to children from exposure to environmental agents. *Environ Health Perspect* 112:238–256, 2004.

Daughtrey WC, Gill MW, Pritts IM, *et al.*: Neurotoxicological evaluation of methyl tertiary-butyl ether in rats. *J Appl Toxicol* 17(S1):S57–S64, 1997.

Davis ME: Dichloroacetic acid and trichloroacetic acid increase chloroform toxicity. *J Toxicol Environ Health* 37:139–148, 1992.

Davis BJ, Almekinder JL, Flagler N, *et al.*: Ovarian luteal cell toxicity of ethylene glycol monomethyl ether and methoxy acetic acid in vivo and in vitro. *Toxicol Appl Pharmacol* 142:328–337, 1997.

de Ketttenis P: The historic and current use of glycol ethers: A picture of change. *Toxicol Lett* 156:5–11, 2005.

de Peyster A, MacLean KJ, Stephens BA, *et al.*: Subchronic studies in Sprague–Dawley rats to investigate mechanisms of MTBE-induced Leydig cell cancer. *Toxicol Sci* 72:31–42, 2003.

Degitz SJ, Rogers JM, Zucker RM, Hunter ES III: Developmental toxicity of methanol: Pathogenesis in CD-1 and C57BL/6J mice exposed in whole embryo culture. *Birth Defects Res A Clin Mol Teratol* 70:179–184, 2004.

Dekant W, Bernauer U, Rosner E, Amberg A: Biotransformation of MTBE, ETBE, and TAME after inhalation or ingestion in rats and humans. *Health Effects Inst Res Report* 102:29–71, 2001.

Dell LD, Mundt KA, McDonald M, *et al.*: Critical review of the epidemiology literature on the potential cancer risks of methylene chloride. *Int Arch Occup Environ Health* 72:429–442, 1999.

DePass LR, Garman RH, Woodside MD, *et al.*: Chronic toxicity and oncogenicity studies of ethylene glycol in rats and mice. *Fund Appl Toxicol* 7:547–565, 1986.

Devi SS, Mehendale HM: Disrupted G1 to S phase clearance via cyclin signaling impairs liver tissue repair in thioacetamide-treated type I diabetic rats. *Toxicol Appl Pharmacol* 207:89–102, 2005.

Devi SS, Mehendale HM: Microarray analysis of thioacetamide-treated type I diabetic rats. *Toxicol Appl Pharmacol* 212:69–78, 2006.

Diaz G, Castro JA: Covalent binding of chloroform metabolites to nuclear proteins—No evidence for binding to nucleic acids. *Cancer Lett* 9:213–218, 1980.

DiCecco SR, Francisco-Ziller N: Nutrition in alcoholic liver disease. *Nutr Clin Pract* 21:245–254, 2006.

Diehl AM: Cytokine regulation of liver injury and repair. *Immunol Rev* 174:160–171, 2000.

Dietrich DR, Swenberg JA: NCI–Black–Reiter (NBR) male rats fail to develop renal disease following exposure to agents that induce α-2u-globulin (α2u) nephropathy. *Fundam Appl Toxicol* 16:749–762, 1991.

Dietzel KD, Campbell JL, Bartlett MG, *et al.*: Validation of a gas chromatography/mass spectrometry method for quantification of aerosolized Jet Propellant 8. *J Chromatogr A* 1093:11–20, 2005.

Dill J, Fuciarelli A, Lee K, *et al.*: Toxicokinetics of propylene glycol mono-*t*-butyl ether following intravenous or inhalation exposure in rats and mice. *Inhal Toxicol* 16:271–290, 2004.

Ding X, Kaminsky LS: Human extrahepatic cytochromes P450: function in xenobiotic metabolism and tissue-selective chemical toxicity in the respiratory and gastrointestinal tracts. *Annu Rev Pharmacol Toxicol* 43:149–173, 2003.

Dinwiddie SH: Abuse of inhalants: A review. *Addiction* 89:925–939, 1994.

DiVincenzo GD, Kaplan CJ: Uptake, metabolism, and elimination of methylene chloride vapor by humans. *Toxicol Appl Pharmacol* 59:130–140, 1981.

Dnyanmote AV, Sawant SP, Lock EA, *et al.*: Calpastatin overexpression prevents progression of S-1,2-dichlorovinyl-L-cysteine (DCVC)-initiated acute renal injury and renal failure (ARF) in diabetes. *Toxicol Appl Pharmacol* 215:146–157, 2006.

Dobrev ID, Andersen ME, Yang RSH: Assessing interaction thresholds for trichloroethylene in combination with tetrachloroethylene and 1,1,1-trichloroethane using gas uptake studies and PBPK modeling. *Arch Toxicol* 75:134–144, 2001.

Doherty RE: A history of the production and use of carbon tetrachloride, tetrachloroethylene, trichloroethylene and 1,1,1-trichloroethane in the United States: Part 2-Trichloroethylene and 1,1,1-trichloroethane. *J Environ Forensics* 1:83–93, 2000.

Doi AM, Roycroft JH, Herbert RA, *et al.*: Inhalation toxicology and carcinogenesis studies of propylene glycol mono-t-butyl ether in rats and mice. *Toxicology* 199:1–22, 2004.

Done AK: Developmental pharmacology. *Clin Pharmacol Ther* 5:432–479, 1964.

Dorman DC, Allen SL, Byczkowski JZ, *et al.*: Methods to identify and characterize developmental neurotoxicity for human health risk assessment. III. Pharmacokinetics and pharmacodynamic considerations. *Environ Health Perspect* 109(Suppl 1):101–111, 2001.

Dorman DC, Struve MF, Clewell HJ III, Andersen ME: Application of pharmacokinetic data to the risk assessment of inhaled manganese. *Neurotoxicology* [E-pub ahead of print], 2006.

Dowling TC: Drug metabolism considerations in patients with chronic kidney disease. *J Pharm Practice* 15:419–427, 2002.

Drake MG, Witzmann FA, Hyde J, Witten ML: JP-8 jet fuel exposure alters protein expression in the lung. *Toxicology* 191:199–210, 2003.

Dresser GK, Bailey DG: The effects of fruit juices on drug disposition: A new model for drug interactions. *Eur J Clin Invest* 33(Suppl 2):10–16, 2003.

Drexler H, Ulm K, Hardt R, *et al.*: Carbon disulphide: IV. Cardiovascular function in workers in the viscose industry. *Int Arch Occup Environ Health* 69:27–32, 1996.

Echeverria D, White RF, Sampaio C: A behavioral evaluation of PCE exposure in patients and dry cleaners: A possible relationship between clinical and preclinical effects. *J Occup Environ Med* 37:667–680, 1995.

Edwards MJ, Keller BJ, Kauffman FC, Thurman RG: The involvement of Kupffer cells in carbon tetrachloride toxicity. *Toxicol Appl Pharmacol* 119:275–279, 1993.

Eells JT, Henry MM, Lewandowski MF, *et al.*: Development and characterization of a rodent model of methanol-induced retinal and optic nerve toxicity. *Neurotoxicology* 21:321–330, 2000.

Eells JT, Henry MM, Summerfelt P: Therapeutic photobiomodulation for methanol-induced retinal toxicity. *Proc Natl Acad Sci* 100:3439–3444, 2003.

Eells JT, Salzman MM, Lewandowski MR, Murray TG: Formate-induced alterations in retinal function in methanol-intoxicated rats. *Toxicol Appl Pharmacol* 140:58–69, 1996.

Egbert PA, Abraham K: Ethylene glycol intoxication: Pathophysiology, diagnosis, and emergency management. *ANNA J* 26:295–302, 1999.

Egeland GM, Burkhart GA, Schnorr TM, *et al.*: Effects of exposure to carbon disulphide on low density lipoprotein cholesterol concentration and diastolic blood pressure. *Br J Ind Med* 49:287–293, 1992.

Elliot BM, Ashby J: Review of the genotoxicity of 2-butoxyethanol. *Mutat Res* 387:89–96, 1997.

Elliott L, Longnecker MP, Kissling GE, London SJ: Volatile organic compounds and pulmonary function in the Third National Examination Survey. *Environ Health Perspect* 114:1210–1214, 2006.

El-Masri HA, Bell DA, Portier CJ: Effects of glutathione transferase theta polymorphism on the risk estimates of dichloromethane to humans. *Toxicol Appl Pharmacol* 158:221–230, 1999.

Engelke M, Tahti H, Vaalavirta L: Perturbation of artificial and biological membranes by organic compounds of aliphatic, alicyclic and aromatic structure. *Toxicol In Vitro* 10:111–115, 1996.

EPA (U.S. Environmental Protection Agency): *Drinking Water Advisory: Consumer Acceptability Advice and Health Effects Analysis on Methyl Tertiary-Butyl Ether (MtBE)*. Washington, DC: Office of Water, December 1997.

EPA (U.S. Environmental Protection Agency): *Risk Assessment Guidance for Superfund. Human Health Evaluation Manual Supplemental Guidance*, Dermal Risk Assessment, Interim Guidance. Washington, DC: Office of Emergency and Remedial Response, 1998, Vol. I.

EPA (U.S. Environmental Protection Agency): *Trichloroethylene health risk assessment: Synthesis and characterization. External review draft*. EPA/600/P-01/002A. National Center for Environmental Assessment, Washington, DC, 2001.

EPA (U.S. Environmental Protection Agency): *Guidelines for Carcinogen Risk Assessment*. Washington, DC: Risk Assessment Forum, EPA/630/P-03/001F, 2005.

EPA (U.S. Environmental Protection Agency). On-line Integrated Risk Information System (IRIS) Substance Profile—Chloroform. July 8, 2006a. http://www.epa.gov/iris/subst/0025.htm

EPA (U.S. Environmental Protection Agency): On-line integrated risk information system (IRIS) substance file—ethylene glycol. Washington, DC: July 30, 2006b. http://www.epa.gov/iris/subst/0238.htm

EPA (U.S. Environmental Protection Agency): On-line integrated risk information system (IRIS) substance file—ethylene glycol monobutyl ether (EGBE) (2-Butoxyethanol). Washington, DC: August 1, 2006c. http://www.epa.gov/iris/subst/0500.htm

EPA (U.S. Environmental Protection Agency): On-line integrated risk information system (IRIS) substance file—carbon disulfide. Washington, DC: July 17, 2006d. http://www.epa.gov/iris/subst/0217.htm

Erdal S, Gong H, Jr., Linn WS, Rykowski R: Projection of health benefits from ambient ozone reduction related to the use of methyl tertiary butyl ether (MTBE) in the reformulated gasoline program. *Risk Anal* 17:693–704, 1997.

Eschenbrenner AB, Miller E: Induction of hepatomas in mice by repeated oral administration of chloroform, with observations on sex differences. *J Natl Cancer Inst* 5:251–255, 1945.

Espinoza LA, Li P, Lee RY, *et al.*: Evaluation of gene expression profile of keratinocytes in response to JP-8 jet fuel. *Toxicol Appl Pharmacol* 200:93–102, 2004.

Espinoza LA, Valikhani M, Cossio MJ, *et al.*: Altered expression of γ-Synuclein and detoxification-related genes in lungs of rats exposed to JP-8. *Am J Resp Cell Mol* 32:192–200, 2005.

Exon JH, Mather GG, Bussiere JL: Effects of subchronic exposure of rats to 2-methoxyethanol or 2-butoxyethanol: Thymic atrophy and immunotoxicity. *Fundam Appl Toxicol* 16:830–840, 1991.

Fabrizi L, Taylor GW, Canas B, *et al.*: Adduction of the chloroform metabolite phosgene to lysine residues of human histone H2B. *Chem Res Toxicol* 16:266–275, 2003.

Faustman EM, Silbernagel SM, Fenske RA, *et al.*: Mechanisms underlying children's susceptibility to environmental toxicants. *Environ Health Perspect* 108(Suppl 1): 13–21, 2000.

Fay RM: Environmental pollutant mixtures in completed exposure pathways at hazardous waste sites. *Environ Toxicol Pharmacol*, 2006. (in press).

Fay RM, Mumtaz MM: Development of a priority list of chemical mixtures occurring at 1188 hazardous waste sites, using the HazDat database. *Food Chem Toxicol* 34:1163–1165, 1996.

Filley CM, Halliday W, Kleinschmidt-DeMasters BK: The effects of toluene on the central nervous system. *J Neuropathol Exp Neurol* 63:1–12, 2004.

Filley CM, Heaton RK, Rosenberg NL: White matter dementia in chronic toluene abuse. *Neurology* 40:532–534, 1990.

Filley CM, Kleinschmidt-DeMasters BK: Toxic leukoencephalopathy. *N Engl J Med* 345:425–432, 2001.

Fisher JW, Channel SR, Eggers JS, *et al.*: Trichloroethylene, trichloroacetic acid, and dichloroacetic acid: Do they affect fetal rat heart development? *Int J Toxicol* 20:257–67, 2001.

Fisher J, Lumpkin M, Boyd J, *et al.*: PBPK modeling of the interaction between carbon tetrachloride and tetrachloroethylene in mice. *Environ Toxicol Pharmacol* 16:93–105, 2004.

Fitzhugh OG, Nelson AA, *et al.*: Comparison of the chronic toxicity of triethylene glycol with that of diethylene glycol. *J Ind Hyg Toxicol* 28:40–43, 1946.

Fletcher CV, Acosta CP, Strykowski JM: Gender differences in human pharmacokinetics and pharmacodynamics. *J Adoles Health* 15:619–629, 1994.

Folland DS, Schaffner W, Ginn EH, *et al.*: Carbon tetrachloride toxicity potentiated by isopropyl alcohol. *JAMA* 236:1853–1856, 1976.

Foo SC, Jeyaratnam J, Koh D: Chronic neurobehavioral effects of toluene. *Br J Ind Med* 47:480–484, 1990.

Foote RH, Farrell PB, Schlafer DH, *et al.*: Ethylene glycol monomethyl ether effects on health and reproduction in male rabbits. *Reprod Toxicol* 9:527–539, 1995.

Forkert P-G, Lash L, Tardif R, *et al.*: Identification of trichloroethylene and its metabolites in human seminal fluid of workers exposed to trichloroethylene. *Drug Metab Dispos* 31:306–311, 2003.

Forkert P-G, Millen B, Lash LH, *et al.*: Pulmonary bronchiolar cytotoxicity and formation of dichloroacetyl lysine protein adducts in mice treated with trichloroethylene. *J Pharmacol Exp Ther* 316:520–529, 2006.

Fortenberry JD: Gasoline sniffing. *Am J Med* 79:740–744, 1985.

Franks SJ, Spendiff MK, Cocker J, Loizou GD: Physiologically based pharmacokinetic modeling of human exposure to 2-butoxyethanol. *Toxicol Lett* 162:164–173, 2006.

Frantz SW, Beskitt JL, Grosse CM, *et al.*: Pharmacokinetics of ethylene glycol. I. Plasma disposition after single intravenous, peroral, or percutaneous doses in female Sprague–Dawley rats and CD-1 mice. *Drug Metab Dispos* 24:911–921, 1996a.

Frantz SW, Beskitt JL, Grosse CM, *et al.*: Pharmacokinetics of ethylene glycol II. Tissue distribution, dose-dependent elimination, and identification of urinary metabolites following single intravenous, peroral or percutaneous doses in female Sprague–Dawley rats and CD-1 mice. *Xenobiotica* 26:1195–1220, 1996b.

Frantz SW, Beskitt JL, Tallant MJ, *et al.*: Pharmacokinetics of ethylene glycol. III. Plasma disposition and metabolic fate after single increasing intravenous, peroral, or percutaneous doses in the male Sprague–Dawley rat. *Xenobiotica* 26:515–539, 1996c.

Fraser MP, Cass GR, Simoneit BRT: Gas-phase and particle-phase organic compounds emitted from motor vehicle traffic in a Los Angeles roadway tunnel. *Environ Sci Technol* 32:2051–2060, 1998.

Frezza M, di Padova C, Pozzato G, *et al.*: High blood alcohol levels in women. The role of decreased gastric alcohol dehydrogenase activity and first-pass metabolism. *N Engl J Med* 322:95–99, 1990.

Froberg K, Dorion RP, McMartin KE: The role of calcium oxalate crystal deposition in cerebral vessels during ethylene glycol poisoning. *Clin Toxicol* 44:315-318, 2006.

Furukawa T, Manabe S, Watanabe T, *et al.*: Sex differences in the daily rhythm of hepatic P450 monooxygenase activities in rats is regulated by growth hormone release. *Toxicol Appl Pharmacol* 161:219–224, 1999.

Gade A, Mortensen EL, Bruhn P: "Chronic painter's syndrome." A reanalysis of psychological test data in a group of diagnosed cases, based on comparisons with matched controls. *Acta Neurol Scand* 77:293–306, 1988.

Gallucci RM, O'Dell SK, Rabe D, Fechter LD: JP-8 jet fuel exposure induces inflammatory cytokines in rat skin. *Int Immunopharmacol* 4:1159–1169, 2004.

Gandhi M, Aweeka F, Greenblatt, RM, Blaschke, TF: Sex differences in pharmacokinetics and pharmacodynamics. *Ann Rev Pharmacol Toxicol* 44:499–523, 2004.

Garetano G, Gochfeld M: Factors affecting tetrachloroethylene concentrations in residences above dry cleaning establishments. *Arch Environ Health* 55:59–68, 2000.

Gargas ML, Burgess RJ, Voisard, DE, *et al.*: Partition coefficients of low-molecular-weight volatile chemicals in various liquids and tissues. *Toxicol Appl Pharmacol* 98:87–99, 1989.

Gargas ML, Tyler TR, Sweeney LM, *et al.*: A toxicokinetic study of inhaled ethylene glycol monomethyl ether (2-ME) and validation of a physiologically based pharmacokinetic model for the pregnant rat and human. *Toxicol Appl Pharmacol* 165:53–62, 2000a.

Gargas ML, Tyler TR, Sweeney LM, *et al.*: A toxicokinetic study of inhaled ethylene glycol ethyl ether acetate and validation of a physiologically based pharmacokinetic model for rat and human. *Toxicol Appl Pharmacol* 165:63–73, 2000b.

Garner CD, Lee EW, Louis-Ferdinand RT: Muller cell involvement in methanol-induced retinal toxicity. *Toxicol Appl Pharmacol* 130:101–107, 1995a.

Garner CD, Lee EW, Terzo TS, Louis-Ferdinand RT: Role of retinal metabolism in methanol-induced retinal toxicity. *J Toxicol Environ Health* 44:43–56, 1995b.

Gaunt IF, Carpanini FM, Grasso P, Lansdown AB: Long-term toxicity of propylene glycol in rats. *Food Cosmet Toxicol* 10:151–162, 1972.

Ge R, Yang S, Kramer PM, *et al.*: The effect of dichloroacetic acid and trichloroacetic acid on DNA hypomethylation and cell proliferation in B6C3F1 mice. *J Biochem Mol Toxicol* 15:100–106, 2001.

Gearhart JM, Mahle DA, Greene RJ, *et al.*: Variability of physiologically-based pharmacokinetic (PBPK) model parameters and their effects on PBPK model predictions in a risk assessment for perchloroethylene (PCE). *Toxicol Lett* 68:131–144, 1993.

Geller AM, Zenick H: Aging and the environment: A research framework. *Environ Health Perspect* 113:1257–1262, 2005.

Gennari P, Naldi M, Motta R, *et al.*: γ-Glutamyltransferase isozyme pattern in workers exposed to tetrachloroethylene. *Am J Ind Med* 21:661–671, 1992.

Gentry PR, Covington TR, Clewell HJ III: Evaluation of the potential impact of pharmacokinetic differences on tissue dosimetry in offspring during pregnancy and lactation. *Regul Toxicol Pharmacol* 38:1–16, 2003.

Gerin M, Patrice S, Begin D, *et al.*: A study of ethylene glycol exposure and kidney function of aircraft de-icing workers. *Int Arch Occup Environ Health* 69:255–265, 1997.

Gerr F, Letz R: Organic solvents, in Rom WD (ed.): *Environmental and Occupational Medicine*, 3rd ed. Philadelphia: Lippincott-Raven, 1998, pp. 1091–1108.

Ghanayem BI: Metabolic and cellular basis of 2-butoxyethanol-induced hemolytic anemia in rats and assessment of human risk in vitro. *Biochem Pharmacol* 38:1679–1684, 1989.

Ghanayem BI, Burka LT, Matthews HB: Metabolic basis of ethylene glycol monobutyl ether (2-butoxyethanol) toxicity: Role of alcohol and aldehyde dehydrogenases. *J Pharmacol Exp Therap* 242:222–231, 1987.

Ghanayem BI, Burka LT, Matthews HB: Structure–activity relationships for the in vitro hematotoxicity of n-alkoxyacetic acids, toxic metabolites of glycol ethers. *Chem-Biol Interact* 70:339–352, 1989.

Ghanayem BI, Chapin RE: Calcium channel blockers protect against ethylene glycol monomethyl ether (2-methoxyethanol)-induced testicular toxicity. *Exp Mol Pathol* 52:279–290, 1990.

Ghanayem BI, Long PH, Ward SM, *et al.*: Hemolytic anemia, thrombosis, and infarction in male and female F344 rats following gavage exposure to 2-butoxyethanol. *Exp Toxicol Pathol* 53:97–105, 2001.

Gibbs BF, Mulligan CN: Styrene toxicity: An ecotoxicological assessment. *Ecotoxicol Environ Safety* 38:181–194, 1997.

Gibbs GW, Amsel J, Soden K: A cohort mortality study of cellulose triacetate-fiber workers exposed to methylene chloride. *J Occup Environ Med* 38:693–697, 1996.

Gift JS: U.S. EPA's IRIS assessment of 2-butoxyethanol: The relationship of noncancer to cancer effects. *Toxicol Lett* 156:163–178, 2005.

Gilbert KM, Griffin JM, Pumford NR: Trichloroethylene activates CD4+ T cells: Potential role in an autoimmune response. *Drug Metab Rev* 31:901–916, 1999.

Gilger AP, Potts AM: Studies on the visual toxicity of methanol: V. The role of acidosis in experimental methanol poisoning. *Am J Ophthalmol* 39:63–86, 1955.

Ginsberg G, Hattis D, Russ A, Sonawane B: Pharmacokinetic and pharmacodynamic factors that can affect sensitivity to neurotoxic sequelae in elderly individuals. *Environ Health Perspect* 113:1243–1249, 2005.

Ginsberg G, Hattis D, Sonawane B, *et al.*: Evaluation of child/adult pharmacokinetic differences from a database derived from the therapeutic drug literature. *Toxicol Sci* 66:185–200, 2002.

Ginsberg G, Slikker W, Jr, Bruckner JV, Sonawane B: Incorporating children's toxicokinetics into a risk framework. *Environ Health Perspect* 112:272–283, 2004.

Gleiter CH, Gundert-Remy U: Gender differences in pharmacokinetics. *Eur J Drug Metab Pharmacokinet* 21:123–128, 1996.

Glende EA Jr, Recknagel RO: Phospholipase A2 activation and cell injury in isolated rat hepatocytes exposed to bromotrichloromethane, chloroform and 1,1-dichloroethylene as compared to effects of carbon tetrachloride. *Toxicol Appl Pharmacol* 113:159–162, 1991.

Glover ML, Reed MD: Propylene glycol: The safe diluent that continues to cause harm. *Pharmacotherapy* 16:690–693, 1996.

Glue P, Clement RP: Cytochrome P450 enzymes and drug metabolism— Basic concepts and methods and assessment. *Cell Mol Neurobiol* 19:309–323, 1999.

Goldenthal EI: A compilation of LD50 values in newborn and adult animals. *Toxicol Appl Pharmacol* 18:185–207, 1971.

Golding BT, Watson WP: Possible mechanisms of carcinogenesis after exposure to benzene, in Singer B, Bartsch H (eds.): *Exocyclic DNA Adducts in Mutagenesis and Carcinogenesis*. Lyons, France: ARC, 1999, pp. 75–88, IARC Publ No. 150.

Goldstein A, Aronow L, Kalman, SM: Kinetics of the uptake and distribution of drugs administered by inhalation, in Pratt WB, Taylor P (eds.): *Principles of Drug Action. The Basis of Pharmacology*, 2nd ed. New York: Wiley, 1974, pp. 338–355.

Goodlett CR, Horn KH: Mechanisms of alcohol-induced damage to the developing nervous system. *Alcohol Res Health* 25:175–184, 2001.

Gordon SM, Callahan PJ, Nishioka MG, *et al.*: Residential environmental measurements in the National Human Exposure Assessment Survey (NHEXAS) pilot study in Arizona: Preliminary results for pesticides and VOCs. *J Expos Anal Environ Epidemiol* 9:456–470, 1999.

Gospe SM, Jr, Zhou SS: Toluene abuse embryopathy: Longitudinal neurodevelopmental effects of prenatal exposure to toluene in rats. *Reprod Toxicol* 12:119–126, 1998.

Gotohda T, Takunaga I, Kubo S-i, *et al.*: Effect of toluene inhalation on astrocytes and neutrotrophic factor in rat brain. *Forensic Sci Internat* 113:233–238, 2000.

Graham DG, Amarnath V, Valentine WM, *et al.*: Pathogenetic studies of hexane and carbon disulfide neurotoxicity. *Crit Rev Toxicol* 25:91–112, 1995.

Grandison MK, Boudinot FD: Age-related changes in protein binding of drugs: Implications for therapy. *Clin Pharmacokinet* 38:271–290, 2000.

Grassman JA, Kimmel CA, Neumann DA: Accounting for variability in responsiveness in human risk assessment, in Neumann DA, Kimmel CA (eds.): *Human Variability in Response to Chemical Exposures*. Washington, DC: International Life Sciences Institute, 1998, pp. 1–26.

Graves RJ, Coutts C, Green T: Methylene chloride-induced DNA damage: An interspecies comparison. *Carcinogenesis* 16:1919–1926, 1995.

Green LC, Lash TL: Renal cell cancer correlated with occupational exposure to trichloroethylene. *J Cancer Res Clin Oncol* 125:430–432, 1999.

Green T, Odum J, Nash JA, *et al.*: Perchloroethylene-induced rat kidney tumors: An investigation of the mechanisms involved and their relevance to humans. *Toxicol Appl Pharmacol* 103:77–89, 1990.

Green T: Methylene chloride induced mouse liver and lung tumors: An overview of the role of mechanistic studies in human safety assessment. *Hum Exp Toxicol* 16:3–13, 1997.

Green T: Pulmonary toxicity and carcinogenicity of trichloroethylene: Species differences and modes of action. *Environ Health Perspect* 108(Suppl 2):261–264, 2000.

Gries J-M, Benowitz N, Verotta D: Chronopharmacokinetics of nicotine. *Clin Pharmacol Ther* 60:385–395, 1996.

Guastadisegni C, Balduzzi M, Mancuso MT, Di Consiglio E: Liver mitochondria alterations in chloroform-treated Sprague–Dawley rats. *J Toxicol Environ Health* 57:415–429, 1999.

Guengerich FP, Kim DH, Iwasaki M: Role of human cytochrome P-450 IIE1 in the oxidation of many low molecular weight cancer suspects. *Chem Res Toxicol* 4:168–179, 1991.

Guo C, McMartin KE: The cytotoxicity of oxalate, metabolite of ethylene glycol, is due to calcium oxalate monohydrate formation. *Toxicology* 208:347–355, 2005.

Gut I, Terelius Y, Frantik E, *et al.*: Exposure to various benzene derivatives differently induces cytochromes P450 2B1 and P450 2E1 in rat liver. *Arch Toxicol* 67:237–243, 1993.

Guyonnet D, Siess M-H, Le Bon A-M, Suschetet M: Modulation of Phase II enzymes by organosulfur compounds from allium vegetables in rat tissues. *Toxicol Appl Pharmacol* 154:50–58, 1999.

Ha M-C, Cordier S, Dananche B, *et al.*: Congenital malformations and occupational exposure to glycol ethers: A European collaborative case–control study. *Occup Hyg* 2:417–421, 1996.

Haber LT, Maier A, Gentry PR, *et al.*: Genetic polymorphisms in assessing interindividual variability in delivered dose. *Regul Toxicol Pharmacol* 35:177–197, 2002.

Haddad S, Charest-Tardif G, Krishnan, K: Physiologically based modeling of the maximal effect of metabolic interactions on the kinetics of components of complex chemical mixtures. *J Toxicol Environ Health A* 61:209–223, 2000.

Halder CA, Holdsworth CE, Cockrell BY, Piccirillo VJ: Hydrocarbon nephropathy in male rats: Identification of the nephrotoxic components of unleaded gasoline. *Toxicol Ind Health* 1:67–87, 1985.

Halder CA, Van Gorp GS, Hatoum NS, Warne TM: Gasoline vapor exposures. Part II. Evaluation of the nephrotoxicity of the major C4/C5 hydrocarbon components. *Am Ind Hyg Assoc J* 47:173–175, 1986.

Halpert JR, Guengerich FP, Bend JR, Correia MA: Selective inhibitors of cytochromes P450. *Toxicol Appl Pharmacol* 125:163–175, 1994.

Hamby-Mason R, Chen JJ, Schenker S, *et al.*: Catalase mediates acetaldehyde formation from ethanol in fetal and neonatal rat brain. *Alcoholism: Clin Exper Res* 21:1063–1072, 1997.

Hansen J, Raaschou-Nielson O, Christensen JM, *et al.*: Cancer incidence among Danish workers exposed to trichloroethylene. *J Occup Environ Med* 43:133–139, 2001.

Hansen JM, Contreras KM, Harris C: Methanol, formaldehyde, and sodium formate exposure in rat and mouse conceptuses: A potential role of the visceral yolk sac in embryotoxicity. *Birth Defects Res A Clin Mol Teratol* 73:72–82, 2005.

Hantson P, Haufroid V, Wallemacq P: Formate kinetics in methanol poisoning. *Human Exp Toxicol* 24:55–59, 2005.

Hard GC, Boorman GA, Wolf DC: Re-evaluation of the 2-year chloroform drinking water carcinogenicity bioassay in Osborne–Mendel rats supports chronic renal tubule injury as the mode of action underlying the renal tumor response. *Toxicol Sci* 53:237–244, 2000.

Hardin BD, Eisenmann CJ: Relative potency of four ethylene glycol ethers for induction of paw malformations in the CD-1 mouse. *Teratology* 35:321–328, 1987.

Hardin BD, Goad PT, Burg JR: Developmental toxicity of four glycol ethers applied cutaneously to rats. *Environ Health Perspect* 57:69–74, 1984.

Hardin BD, Goad PT, Burg JR: Developmental toxicity of diethylene glycol monomethyl ether (diEGME). *Fundam Appl Toxicol* 6:430–439, 1986.

Harris C, Dixon M, Hansen JM: Glutathione depletion modulates methanol, formaldehyde and formate toxicity in cultured rat conceptuses. *Cell Biol Toxicol* 20:133–145, 2004.

Harris C, Wang SW, Lauchu JJ, Hansen JM: Methanol metabolism and embryotoxicity in rat and mouse conceptuses: Comparisons of alcohol dehydrogenase (ADH1), formaldehyde dehydrogenase (ADH3), and catalase. *Reprod Toxicol* 17:349–357, 2003.

Harris DT, Sakiestewa D, Robledo RF, *et al.*: Effects of short-term JP-8 jet fuel exposure on cell-mediated immunity. *Toxicol Ind Health* 16:78–84, 2000.

Harris DT, Sakiestewa D, Robledo RF, Witten M: Immunotoxicological effects of JP-8 jet fuel exposure. *Toxicol Ind Health* 13:43–55, 1997a.

Harris DT, Sakiestewa D, Robledo RF, Witten M: Short-term exposure to JP-8 jet fuel results in long-term immunotoxicity. *Toxicol Ind Health* 13:559–570, 1997b.

Harris DT, Sakiestewa D, Robledo RF, Witten M: Protection from JP-8 jet fuel induced immunotoxicity by administration of aerosolized substance P. *Toxicol Ind Health* 13:571–588, 1997c.

Harris DT, Sakiestewa D, Titone D, *et al.*: Jet fuel-induced immunotoxicity. *Toxicol Ind Health* 16:261–265, 2001a.

Harris DT, Sakiestewa D, Titone D, *et al.*: Substance P as prophylaxis for JP-8 jet fuel-induced immunotoxicity. *Toxicol Ind Health* 16:253–259, 2001b.

Harris DT, Sakiestewa D, Titone D, *et al.*: JP-8 jet fuel exposure results in immediate immunotoxicity, which is cumulative over time. *Toxicol Ind Health* 18:77–83, 2002.

Harry GJ, Graham DG, Valentine WM, *et al.*: Carbon disulfide neurotoxicity in rats: VIII. Summary. *Neurotoxicology* 19:159–162, 1998.

Harth V, Bruning T, Bolt HM: Renal carcinogenicity of trichloroethylene: Update, mode of action, and fundamentals for occupational standard setting. *Rev Environ Health* 20:103–118, 2005.

Hattis D, Banati P, Goble R, Burmaster DE: Human interindividual variability in parameters related to health risks. *Risk Anal* 19:711–726, 1999.

Hattis D, Erdreich L, Ballew M: Human variability in susceptibility to toxic chemicals—A preliminary analysis of pharmacokinetic data from normal volunteers. *Risk Anal* 7:415–426, 1987.

Hattis D, Ginsberg G, Sonawane B, *et al.*: Differences in pharmacokinetics between children and adults-II. Children's variability in drug elimination half-lives and in some parameters needed for physiologically-based pharmacokinetic modeling. *Risk Anal* 23:117–142, 2003.

Hays SM, Elswick BA, Blumenthal GM, *et al.*: Development of a physiologically based pharmacokinetic model of 2-methoxyethanol and 2-methoxyacetic acid disposition in pregnant rats. *Toxicol Appl Pharmacol* 163:67–74, 2000.

Hays Am, Parliman G, Pfaff JK, *et al.*: Changes in lung permeability correlate with lung histology in a chronic exposure model. *Toxicol Ind Health*, 11(3):325–36, 1995.

Health Canada: Priority substances list. *State-of-the-Science Report for Ethylene Glycol.* Health Canada and Environment Canada, 2000. http://www.ec.gc.ca/substances/ese/eng/psap/final/ethyleneglycol.cfm

Hearne FT, Pifer JW, Grose F: Absence of adverse mortality effects in workers exposed to methylene chloride: An update. *J Occup Med* 32:234–240, 1990.

Hebert JL, Fabre M, Auzepy P, Paillas J: Acute experimental poisoning by diethylene glycol: Acid base balance and histological data in male rats. *Toxicol Eur Res* 1:2890–2894, 1978.

Heilmair R, Lenk W, Lohr D: Toxicokinetics of diethylene glycol (DEG) in the rat. *Arch Toxicol* 67:655–666, 1993.

Henderson GI, Chen JJ, Schenker S: Ethanol, oxidative stress, reactive aldehydes, and the fetus. *Front Biosci* 4:D541–D550, 1999.

Henderson RF: Species differences in the metabolism of benzene. *Environ Health Perspect* 104(Suppl 6):1173–1175, 1996.

Henschler D, Vamvakas S, Lammert M, *et al.*: Increased incidence of renal cell tumors in a cohort of cardboard workers exposed to trichloroethene. *Arch Toxicol* 69:291–299, 1995.

Herrlinger C, Klotz U: Drug metabolism and drug interactions in the elderly. *Best Pract Res Clin Gastroenterol* 15:897–918, 2001.

Hess R, Bartels MJ, Pottenger LH: Ethylene glycol: An estimate of tolerable levels of exposure based on a review of animal and human data. *Arch Toxicol* 78:671–680, 2004.

Heywood R, Sortwell RJ, Noel PRB, *et al.*: Safety evaluation of toothpaste containing chloroform: III. Long-term study in beagle dogs. *J Environ Pathol Toxicol* 2:835–851, 1979.

Hillbom M: Oxidants, antioxidants, alcohol and stroke. *Front Biosci* 4:67–71, 1999.

Hines RN, McCarver DG: The ontogeny of human drug-metabolizing enzymes: Phase I oxidative enzymes. *J Pharmacol Exp Therap* 300:355–360, 2002.

Hiraku Y, Kawanishi S: Oxidative DNA damage and apoptosis induced by benzene metabolites. *Cancer Res* 56:5172–5178, 1996.

Hoflack J-C, Vasseur P, Poirier GG: Glycol ethers induce death and necrosis in human leukemia cells. *Biochem Cell Biol* 75:415–425, 1997.

Holladay SD, Comment CE, Kwon J, Luster MI: Fetal hematopoietic alterations after maternal exposure to ethylene glycol monomethyl ether: Prolymphoid cell targeting. *Toxicol Appl Pharmacol* 129:53–60, 1994.

Hong J-Y, Wang Y-Y, Bondoc FY, *et al.*: Metabolism of methyl *tert*-butyl ether and other gasoline ethers by human liver microsomes and heterologously expressed human cytochromes P450: Identification of CYP2A6 as a major catalyst. *Toxicol Appl Pharmacol* 160:43–48, 1999.

Hooth MJ, Herbert RA, Haseman JK, *et al.*: Toxicology and carcinogenesis studies of dipropylene glycol in rats and mice. *Toxicology* 204:123–140, 2004.

House RV, Lauer LD, Murray MJ, *et al.*: Immunological studies in B6C3F1 mice following exposure to ethylene glycol monomethyl ether and its principal metabolite methoxyacetic acid. *Toxicol Appl Pharmacol* 77:358–362, 1985.

Hsieh GY, Wang JD, Cheng TJ, Chen PC: Prolonged menstrual cycles in female workers exposed to ethylene glycol ethers in the semiconductor manufacturing industry. *Occup Environ Med* 62:510–516, 2005.

Huang S-M, Lesko LJL: Drug–drug, drug–dietary supplement, and drug–citrus fruit and other food interactions: What have we learned? *J Clin Pharmacol* 44:559–569, 2004.

Huff JE, Haseman JK, DeMarini DM, *et al.*: Multiple-site carcinogenicity of benzene in Fischer 344 rats and B6C3F1 mice. *Environ Health Perspect* 82:125–163, 1989.

Hunter AGW, Thompson D, Evans JA: Is there a fetal gasoline syndrome? *Teratology* 20:75–80, 1979.

IARC (International Agency for Research on Cancer): *IARC Monographs on the Evaluation of Carcinogenic Risks to Humans: Alcohol Drinking.* Lyons, France: World Health Organization, 1988, Vol. 44, pp. 251–259.

IARC (International Agency for Research on Cancer): *IARC Monographs on the Evaluation of Carcinogenic Risks to Humans. Diesel and Gasoline Engine Exhausts and Some Nitroarenes.* Lyons, France: World Health Organization, 1989a, Vol. 46.

IARC (International Agency for Research on Cancer): *IARC Monographs on the Evaluation of Carcinogenic Risks to Humans. Occupational Exposures in Petroleum Refining: Crude Oil and Major Petroleum Fuels.* Lyons, France: World Health Organization, 1989b, Vol. 45.

IARC (International Agency for Research on Cancer): *Summaries and Evaluations—Styrene (Group 2B).* Lyons, France: World Health Organization, 2002, Vol. 82, p. 437.

Ikonomidou C, Bittigau P, Ishimaru MJ, *et al.*: Ethanol-induced apoptotic neurodegeneration and fetal alcohol syndrome. *Science* 287:1056–1060, 2000.

Ingelman-Sundberg M, Johansson I, Persson I, *et al.*: Genetic polymorphism of cytochrome P450. Functional consequences and possible relationship to disease and alcohol toxicity, in Jansson B, Jornvall H, Rydberg U, *et al* (eds.): *Toward a Molecular Basis of Alcohol Use and Abuse.* Basel, Switzerland: Birkhauser Verlag, 1994, pp. 197–207.

Inoue O, Seiji K, Watanabe T, *et al.*: Mutual metabolic suppression between benzene and toluene in man. *Int Arch Occup Environ Health* 60:15–20, 1988.

Jacobsen D, Ovrebo S, Ostborg J, Sejersted OM: Glycolate causes the acidosis in ethylene glycol poisoning and is effectively removed by hemodialysis. *Acta Med Scand* 216:409–416, 1984.

Jan CR, Chen LW, Lin MW: Ca($^{2+}$) mobilization evoked by chloroform in Madin–Darby canine kidney cells. *J Pharmacol Exp Ther* 292:995–1001, 2000.

Jang J-Y, Droz PO: Ethnic differences in biological monitoring of several organic solvents II. A simulation study with a physiologically based pharmacokinetic model. *Int Arch Occup Environ Health* 70:41–50, 1997.

Jindo T, Wine RN, Li L-H, Chapin RE: Protein kinase activity is central to rat germ cell apoptosis induced by methoxyacetic acid. *Toxicol Pathol* 29:607–616, 2001.

Johanson G, Filser JG: Experimental data from closed chamber gas uptake studies in rodents suggest lower uptake rate of chemical than calculated from literature values on alveolar ventilation. *Arch Toxicol* 66:291–295, 1992.

Johlin FC, Swain E, Smith C, Tephly TR: Studies on the mechanism of methanol poisoning: Purification and comparison of rat and human liver 10-formyltetrahydrofolate dehydrogenase. *Mol Pharmacol* 35:745–750, 1989.

Johnson KA, Baker PC, Kan HL, *et al.*: Diethylene glycol monobutyl ether (DGBE): Two- and thirteen-week oral toxicity studies in Fischer 344 rats. *Food Chem Toxicol* 43:467–481, 2005.

Johnson BL, Boyd J, Burg JR, *et al.*: Effects on the peripheral nervous system of workers' exposure to carbon disulfide. *Neurotoxicology* 4:53–65, 1983.

Johnson PD, Goldberg SJ, Mays MZ, Dawson, BV, *et al.*: Threshold of trichloroethylene contamination in maternal drinking waters affecting fetal heart development in the rat. *Environ Health Perspect* 111:289–292, 2003.

Johnsrud EK, Koukouritaki SB, Divakaran K, *et al.*: Human hepatic CYP2E1 expression during development. *J Pharmacol Exp Therap* 307: 402–407, 2003.

Johnston LD, O'Malley PM, Bachman JG, Schulenberg, JE: *Monitoring the Future National Results on Adolescent Drug Use: Overview of Key Findings, 2005.* Bethesda, MD: National Institute on Drug Abuse, 2006, NIH Publication No. 06-5882, pp. 1–67.

Jonsson F, Bois F, Johanson G: Physiologically based pharmacokinetic modeling of inhalation exposure of humans to dichloromethane during moderate to heavy exercise. *Toxicol Sci* 59:209–218, 2001.

Jonsson F, Johanson G: A Bayesian analysis of the influence of GSTT1 polymorphism on the cancer risk estimate for dichloromethane. *Toxicol Appl Pharmacol* 174:99–112, 2001.

Jonsson F, Johanson G: Physiologically based modeling of the inhalation kinetics of styrene in humans using a Bayesian population approach. *Toxicol Appl Pharmacol* 179:35–49, 2002.

Jorgenson TA, Meierhenry EF, Rushbrook CJ, *et al.*: Carcinogenicity of chloroform in drinking water to male Osborne–Mendel rats and female B6C3F1 mice. *Fundam Appl Toxicol* 5:760–769, 1985.

Kabbur MB, Rogers JV, Gunasekar PG, *et al.*: Effect of JP-8 jet fuel on molecular and histological parameters related to acute skin irritation. *Toxicol Appl Pharmacol* 175:83–88, 2001.

Kaneko T, Wang P-Y, Sato A: Enzymes induced by ethanol differently affect the pharmacokinetics of trichloroethylene and 1,1,1-trichloroethane. *Occup Environ Med* 51:113–119, 1994.

Kato S, Shields PG, Caparoso NE, *et al.*: Cytochrome P450IIE1 genetic polymorphisms, racial variation, and lung cancer risk. *Cancer Res* 52:6712–6715, 1992.

Katoh M: New Energy Development Organization data. Presented at the Methanol Vapors and Health Effects Workshop: What we know and what we need to know—Summary Report. Washington, DC, ILSI Risk Science Institute/U.S. Environmental Protection Agency/Health Effects Institute/American Petroleum Institute, A-7, 1989.

Kavet R, Nauss KM: The toxicity of inhaled methanol vapors. *Crit Rev Toxicol* 21:21–50, 1990.

Kawamoto T, Koga M, Murata K, *et al.*: Effects of ALDH2, CYP1A1, and CYP2E1 genetic polymorphisms and smoking and drinking habits on toluene metabolism in humans. *Toxicol Appl Pharmacol* 133:295–304, 1995.

Kayama F, Yamashita U, Kawamoto T, Kodama Y: Selective depletion of immature thymocytes by oral administration of ethylene glycol monomethyl ether. *Int J Immunopharmacol* 13:531–540, 1991.

Kearney CA, Dunham DB: Gasoline vapor exposures at a high volume service station. *Am Ind Hyg Assoc J* 47:535–539, 1986.

Kedderis GL: Extrapolation of in vitro enzyme induction data to humans in vivo. *Chem-Biol Interact* 107:109–121, 1997.

Kegelmeyer AE, Sprankle CS, Horesovsky GJ, Butterworth BE: Differential display identified changes in mRNA levels in regenerating livers from chloroform-treated mice. *Mol Carcinogen* 20:288–297, 1997.

Keil DE, Warren DA, Jenny MJ, *et al.*: Immunological function in mice exposed to JP-8 jet fuel in utero. *Toxicol Sci* 76:347–356, 2003.

Kenyon EM, Kraichely RE, Hudson KT, Medinsky MA: Differences in rates of benzene metabolism correlate with observed genotoxicity. *Toxicol Appl Pharmacol* 136:49–56, 1996.

Kerns W, Tomaszewski C, McMartin K, *et al.*: Formate kinetics in methanol poisoning. *Clin Toxicol* 40:137–143, 2002.

Kiesswetter E, Sietmann B, Seeber A: Standardization of a questionnaire for neurotoxic symptoms. *Environ Res* 73:73–80, 1997.

Kiesswetter E, Sietmann B, Zupanic M, Seeber A: Neurobehavioral study on the interactive effects of age and solvent exposure. *Neurotoxicology* 21:685–696, 2000.

Kilburn KH: *Chemical Brain Injury*. New York: Van Nostrand Reinhold, 1998.

Kim B-S, Smialowicz RJ: The role of metabolism in 2-methoxyethanol induced suppression of in vitro polyclonal antibody responses by rat and mouse lymphocytes. *Toxicology* 123:227–239, 1997.

Kim D, Andersen ME, Nylander-French LA: A dermatotoxicokinetic model of human exposures to jet fuel. *Toxicol Sci* 93:22–33, 2006.

Kim HJ, Oden'hal S, Bruckner JV: Effect of oral dosing vehicles on the acute hepatotoxicity of carbon tetrachloride in rats. *Toxicol Appl Pharmacol* 102:34–49, 1990a.

Kim HJ, Bruckner JV, Dallas CE, Gallo JM: Effect of dosing vehicles on the pharmacokinetics of orally administered carbon tetrachloride in rats. *Toxicol Appl Pharmacol* 102:50–60, 1990b.

Kinirons MT, O'Mahony MS: Drug metabolism and aging. *Br J Clin Pharmacol* 57:540–544, 2004.

Kirman CR, Sweeney LM, Corley R, Gargas ML: Using physiologically-based pharmacokinetic modeling to address nonlinear kinetics and changes in rodent physiology and metabolism due to aging and adaptation in deriving reference values for propylene glycol methyl ether and propylene glycol methyl ether acetate. *Risk Anal* 25:271–284, 2005.

Klaassen CD, Plaa GL: Relative effects of various chlorinated hydrocarbons on liver and kidney function in mice. *Toxicol Appl Pharmacol* 9:139–151, 1966.

Klaunig JE, Kamendulis LM: Mode of action of butoxyethanol-induced mouse liver hemangiosarcomas and hepatocellular carcinomas. *Toxicol Lett* 156:107–115, 2005.

Klaunig JE, Ruch RJ, Pereira MA: Carcinogenicity of chlorinated methane and ethane compounds administered in drinking water to mice. *Environ Health Perspect* 69:89–95, 1986.

Klotz U, Ammon E: Clinical and toxicological consequences of the inductive potential of ethanol. *Eur J Clin Pharmacol* 54:7–12, 1998.

Kobayashi K, Urashima K, Shimada N, Chiba K: Substrate specificity for rat cytochrome P450 (CYP) isoforms: Screening with cDNA-expressed systems in rats. *Biochem Pharmacol* 63:889–896, 2002.

Kolovou GD, Salpea KD, Anagnostopoulou KK, Mikhailidis DP: Alcohol use, vascular disease, and lipid-lowering drugs. *J Pharmacol Exp Ther* 318:1–7, 2006.

Korrapati MC, Chilakapati J, Lock EA, *et al.*: Preplaced cell division— A critical mechanism of autoprotection against S-1,2-dichlorovinyl-L-cysteine-induced acute renal failure and death in mice. *Am J Physiol Renal Physiol* 291:F439–F455, 2006.

Kostic MA, Dart RC: Rethinking the toxic methanol level. *J Toxicol Clin Toxicol* 41:793–800, 2003.

Kraul H, Jahn F, Braunlich H: Nephrotoxic effects of diethylene glycol (DEG) in rats. *Exp Pathol* 42:27–32, 1991.

Kril JJ, Halliday GM, Svoboda MD, Cartwright H: The cerebral cortex is damaged in chronic alcoholics. *Neuroscience* 79:983–998, 1997.

Krishnan K, Johanson G: Physiologically-based pharmacokinetic and toxicokinetic models in cancer risk assessment. *J Environ Sci Health* 23:31–53, 2005.

Ku MC, Huang CC, Kuo HC, et al.: Diffuse white matter lesions in carbon disulfide intoxication: Microangiopathy or demyelination. *Eur Neurol* 50:220–224, 2003.

Ku WW, Wine RN, Chae BY, et al.: Spermatocyte toxicity of 2-methoxyethanol (ME) in rats and guinea pigs: Evidence for the induction of apoptosis. *Toxicol Appl Pharmacol* 134:100–110, 1995.

Kuna RA, Ulrich CE: Subchronic inhalation toxicity of two motor fuels. *J Am Col Toxicol* 3:217–229, 1984.

Labrecque G, Belanger PM: Biological rhythms in the absorption, distribution, metabolism and excretion of drugs. *Pharmacol Ther* 52:95–107, 1991.

Laitinen J, Liesivuori J, Savolainen H: Exposure to glycols and their renal effects in motor servicing workers. *Occup Med* 45:259–262, 1995.

LaKind JS, McKenna EA, Hubner RP, Tardiff RG: A review of the comparative mammalian toxicity of ethylene glycol and propylene glycol. *Crit Rev Toxicol* 29:331–365, 1999.

Lam C-W, Galen TJ, Boyd JF, Pierson DL: Mechanism of transport and distribution of organic solvents in blood. *Toxicol Appl Pharmacol* 104:117–129, 1990.

Lamb JC, IV, Gulati DK, Russell VS, et al.: Reproductive toxicity of ethylene glycol monoethyl ether tested by continuous breeding of CD-1 mice. *Environ Health Perspect* 57:85–90, 1984.

Lan O, Zhang L, Li G, et al.: Hematotoxicity in workers exposed to low levels of benzene. *Science* 306: 1774–1776, 2004.

Landrigan PG, Kimmel CA, Correa A, Esknazi B: Children's health and the environment: Public health issues and challenges for risk assessment. *Environ Health Perspect* 112:257–265, 2004.

Lanigan S: Final report on the safety assessment of methyl alcohol. *Int J Toxicol* 20(Suppl 1):57–85, 2001.

Larson JL, Wolf DC, Butterworth BE: Induced cytotoxicity and cell proliferation in the hepatocarcinogenicity of chloroform in female B6C3F1 mice: Comparison of administration by gavage in corn oil vs ad libitum in drinking water. *Fundam Appl Toxicol* 22:90–102, 1994.

Lash AA, Becker CE, So Y, Shore M: Neurotoxic effects of methylene chloride: Are they long lasting in humans? *Br J Ind Med* 48:418–426, 1991.

Lash LH, Fisher JW, Lipscomb JC, Parker JC: Metabolism of trichloroethylene. *Environ Health Perspect* 108(Suppl 2):177–200, 2000a.

Lash LH, Parker JC: Hepatic and renal toxicities associated with perchloroethylene. *Pharmacol Rev* 53:177–208, 2001.

Lash LH, Parker JC, Scott CS: Modes of action of trichloroethylene for kidney tumorigenesis. *Environ Health Perspect* 108(Suppl 2):225–240, 2000b.

Lash LH, Putt DA, Hueni SE, Horwitz BP: Molecular markers of trichloroethylene-induced toxicity in human kidney cells. *Toxicol Appl Pharmacol* 206:157–168, 2005.

Lash LH, Qian W, Putt DA, et al.: Glutathione conjugation of perchloroethylene in rats and mice in vitro: Sex-, species-, and tissue-dependent differences. *Toxicol Appl Pharmacol* 150:49–57, 1998.

Laughter AR, Dunn CS, Swanson CL, et al.: Role of the peroxisome proliferators-activated receptor alpha (PPARalpha) in responses to trichloroethylene and metabolites, trichloroacetate and dichloroacetate in mouse liver. *Toxicology* 203:83–98, 2004.

Leblond F, Guevin C, Demers C, et al.: Downregulation of hepatic cytochrome P450 in chronic renal failure. *J Am Soc Nephrol* 12:326–332, 2001.

Lee BL, Yang XF, New AL, Ong CN: Liquid chromatographic determination of urinary 2-thiothiazlidine-4-carboxylic acid, a biomarker of carbon disulphide exposure. *J Chromatogr B* 668:265–272, 1995.

Lee EW, Terzo TS, D'Arcy JB, et al.: Lack of blood formate accumulation in humans following exposure to methanol vapor at the current permissible exposure limit of 200 ppm. *Am Ind Hyg Assoc J* 53:99–104, 1992.

Lee KM, Bruckner JV, Muralidhara S, Gallo JM: Characterization of presystemic elimination of trichloroethylene and its nonlinear kinetics in rats. *Toxicol Appl Pharmacol* 139:262–271, 1996.

Lee KM, Bruckner JV, Muralidhara S, Gallo JM: Characterization of presystemic elimination of trichloroethylene and its nonlinear kinetics in rats. *Toxicol Appl Pharmacol* 139:262–271, 1996.

Lee KM, Dill JA, Chou BJ, Roycroft JH: Physiologically based pharmacokinetic model for chronic inhalation of 2-butoxyethanol. *Toxicol Appl Pharmacol* 153:211–226, 1998.

Lee RD, An SM, Kim SS, et al.: Neurotoxic effects of alcohol and acetaldehyde during embryonic development. *J Toxicol Environ Health A* 68:2147–2162, 2005.

Lee SL, Chau GY, Yao CT, et al.: Functional assessment of human alcohol dehydrogenase family in ethanol metabolism: Significance of first-pass metabolism. *Alcohol Clin Exp Res* 30:1132–1142, 2006.

Lemazurier E, Lecomte A, Robidel F, Bois FY: Propylene glycol monomethyl ether. A three-generation study of isomer beta effects on reproduction and developmental parameters in rats. *Toxicol Ind Health* 21:33–40, 2005.

Lenk W, Lohr D, Sonnenbichler J: Pharmacokinetics and biotransformation of diethylene glycol and ethylene glycol in the rat. *Xenobiotica* 19:961–979, 1989.

Leth PM, Gregersen M: Ethylene glycol poisoning. *Forensic Sci Int* 155:179–184, 2005.

Leung H-W, Paustenbach DJ: Physiologically based pharmacokinetic and pharmacodynamic modeling in health risk assessment and characterization of hazardous substances. *Toxicol Lett* 79:55–65, 1995.

Lewis DFV, Ioannides C, Parke DV: Cytochrome P450 and species differences in xenobiotic metabolism and activation of carcinogen. *Environ Health Perspect* 106:633–641, 1998.

Lewis JG, Graham DG, Valentine WM, et al.: Exposure of C57BL/6 mice to carbon disulfide induces early lesions of atherosclerosis and enhances arterial fatty deposits induced by a high fat diet. *Toxicol Sci* 49:124–132, 1999.

Li CI, Malone KE, Porter PL, et al.: The relationship between alcohol use and risk of breast cancer by histology and hormone receptor status among women 65–79 years of age. *Cancer Epidemiol Biomark Prev* 12:1061–1066, 2003.

Li G-L, Linet MS, Hayes RB, et al.: Gender differences in hematopoietic and lymphoproliferative disorders and other cancer risks by major occupational group among workers exposed to benzene in China. *J Occup Med* 36:875–881, 1994.

Li L-H, Wine RN, Miller DS, et al.: Protection against methoxyacetic-acid-induced spermatocyte apoptosis with calcium channel blockers in cultured rat seminiferous tubules: Possible mechanisms. *Toxicol Appl Pharmacol* 144:105–119, 1997.

Licata AC, Dekant W, Smith CE, Borghoff SJ: A physiologically based pharmacokinetic model for methyl tert-butyl ether in humans: Implementing sensitivity and variability analyses. *Toxicol Sci* 62:191–204, 2001.

Lieber CS: Alcoholic fatty liver: Its pathogenesis and mechanism of progression to inflammation and fibrosis. *Alcohol* 34:9–19, 2004.

Lieber CS: Cytochrome P4502E1: Its physiological and pathological role. *Physiol Rev* 77:517–544, 1997.

Lilly PD, Thorton-Manning JR, Gargas ML, et al.: Kinetic characterization of CYP2E1 inhibition in vivo and in vitro by the chloroethylenes. *Arch Toxicol* 72:609–621, 1998.

Limaye PB, Apte UM, Shankar K, et al.: Calpain release from dying hepatocytes mediates progression of acute liver injury induced by model hepatotoxicants. *Toxicol Appl Pharmacol* 191:211–226, 2003.

Lin B, Ritchie GD, Rossi J III, Pancrazio JJ: Gene expression profiles in the rat central nervous system induced by JP-8 jet fuel vapor exposure. *Neurosci Lett* 363:233–238, 2004.

Lin Y-S, Smith TJ, Kelsey KT, Wypij D: Human physiological factors in respiratory uptake of 1,3-butadiene. *Environ Health Perspect* 109:921–926, 2001a.

Lin B, Ritchie GD, Rossi J III, Pancrazio JJ: Identification of target genes responsive to JP-8 exposure in the rat central nervous system. *Toxicol Ind Health* 17:262–269, 2001a.

Lin JH, Lu AYH: Interindividual variability in inhibition and induction of cytochrome P450 enzymes. *Ann Rev Pharmacol Toxicol* 41:535–567, 2001.

Lindstrom AB, Yeowell-O'Connell K, Waidyanatha S, *et al.*: Measurement of benzene oxide in the blood of rats following administration of benzene. *Carcinogenesis* 18:1637–1641, 1997.

Lington AW, Dodd DE, Ridlon SA, *et al.*: Evaluation of 13-week inhalation toxicity study on methyl *t*-butyl ether (MTBE) in Fischer 344 rats. *J Appl Toxicol* 17(S1):S37–S44, 1997.

Linhart I, Gut I, Smejkal J, Novak J: Biotransformation of styrene in mice. Stereochemical aspects. *Chem Res Toxicol* 13:36–44, 2000.

Lipscomb JC: Evaluating the relationship between variance in enzyme expression and toxicant concentration in health risk assessment. *Human Ecol Risk Assess* 10:39–55, 2004.

Lipscomb JC, Garrett CM, Snawder JE: Cytochrome P450-dependent metabolism of trichloroethylene: Interindividual differences in humans. *Toxicol Appl Pharmacol* 142:311–318, 1997.

Lipscomb JC, Teuschler LK, Swartout J, *et al.*: The impact of cytochrome P450 2E1-dependent metabolic variance on a risk-relevant pharmacokinetic outcome in humans. *Risk Anal* 23:1221–1238, 2003.

Liu L, Zhang Q, Feng J, *et al.*: The study of DNA oxidative damage in benzene-exposed workers. *Mutation Res* 370:145–150, 1996.

Liu S-L, Esposti SD, Yao T, *et al.*: Vitamin E therapy of acute CCl₄-induced hepatic injury in mice is associated with inhibition of nuclear factor kappa B binding. *Hepatology* 22:1474–1481, 1995.

Liu Y, Zhang J-W, Li W, *et al.*: Ginsenoside metabolites, rather than naturally occurring ginsenosides, lead to inhibition of human cytochrome P450 enzymes. *Toxicol Sci* 91:356–364, 2006.

Lock EA, Barth JL, Argraves SW, Schnellmann RG: Changes in gene expression in human renal proximal tubule cells exposed to low concentrations of S-(1,2-dichlorovinyl)-L-cysteine, a metabolite of trichloroethylene. *Toxicol Appl Pharmacol* 216:319–330, 2006.

Lock EA, Reed CJ: Trichloroethylene: Mechanisms of renal toxicity and renal cancer and relevance to risk assessment. *Toxicol Sci* 91:313–331, 2006.

Lockard VG, Mehendale HM, O'Neal RM: Chlordecone-induced potentiation of carbon tetrachloride hepatotoxicity: A morphometric and biochemical study. *Exp Mol Pathol* 39:246–256, 1983.

Lof A, Johanson G: Toxicokinetics of organic solvents: A review of modifying factors. *Crit Rev Toxicol* 28:571–650, 1998.

Lopez-Diazguerrero NE, Luna-Lopez A, Gutierrez-Ruiz MC, *et al.*: Susceptibility of DNA to oxidative stressors in young and aging mice. *Life Sci* 77:2840–2854, 2005.

Lopreato GF, Phelan R, Borghese CM, *et al.*: Inhaled drugs of abuse enhance serotonin-3 receptor function. *Drug Alcohol Depend* 70:11–15, 2003.

Lorente C, Cordier S, Bergeret A, *et al.*: Maternal occupational risk factors for oral clefts. Occupational exposure and congenital malformation working group. *Scand J Work Environ Health* 26:137–145, 2000.

Loury DJ, Smith-Oliver T, Butterworth BE: Assessment of unscheduled DNA and replicative DNA synthesis in rat kidney cells exposed in vitro or in vivo to unleaded gasoline. *Toxicol Appl Pharmacol* 87:127–140, 1987.

Lucas D, Farez C, Bardou LG, *et al.*: Cytochrome P450 2E1 activity in diabetic and obese patients as assessed by chlorzoxazone hydroxylation. *Fundam Clin Pharmacol* 12:553–558, 1998.

Luo JC, Chang HY, Chang SJ, *et al.*: Elevated triglyceride and decreased high density lipoprotein level in carbon disulfide workers in Taiwan. *J Occup Environ Med* 45:73–78, 2003.

Lykke AWJ, Stewart BW: Fibrosing alveolitis (pulmonary interstitial fibrosis) evoked by experimental inhalation of gasoline vapours. *Experientia* 34:498, 1978.

MacFarland HN, Ulrich CE, Holdsworth CE, *et al.*: A chronic inhalation study with unleaded gasoline vapor. *J Am Col Toxicol* 3:231–248, 1984.

Maldonado G, Delzell E, Tyl RW, Sever LE: Occupational exposure to glycol ethers and human congenital malformations. *Int Arch Occup Environ Health* 76:405–423, 2003.

Mally A, Walker CL, Everitt JI, *et al.*: Analysis of renal cell transformation following exposure to trichloroethene in vivo and its metabolite S-(dichlorovinyl)-L-cysteine in vitro. *Toxicology* 224:108–118, 2006.

Mandel JH, Kelsh MA, Mink PJ, *et al.*: Occupational trichloroethylene exposure and non-Hodgkin's lymphoma: A meta-analysis and review. *Occup Environ Med* 63:597–607, 2006.

Mani C, Freeman S, Nelson DO, *et al.*: Species and strain comparisons in the macromolecular binding of extremely low doses of [¹⁴C] benzene in rodents using accelerator mass spectrophotometry. *Toxicol Appl Pharmacol* 159:83–90, 1999.

Manno M, Rezzadore M, Grossi M, Sbrana C: Potentiation of occupational carbon tetrachloride toxicity by ethanol abuse. *Hum Exp Toxicol* 15:294–300, 1996.

Marelich GP: Volatile substance abuse. *Crit Rev Allergy Immunol* 15:271–289, 1997.

Maronpot RR, Devereux TR, Hegi M, *et al.* Hepatic and pulmonary carcinogenicity of methylene chloride in mice: A search for mechanisms. *Toxicology* 102:73–81, 1995.

Marrubini G, Castoldi AF, Coccini T, Manzo L: Prolonged ethanol ingestion enhances benzene myelotoxicity and lowers urinary concentrations of benzene metabolite levels in CD-1 mice. *Toxicol Sci* 75:16–24, 2003.

Martin-Amat G, McMartin KE, Hayreh SS, *et al.*: Methanol poisoning: Ocular toxicity produced by formate. *Toxicol Appl Pharmacol* 45:201–208, 1978.

Martinasevic K, Green MD, Baron J, Tephly TR: Folate and 10-formyltetrahydrofolate dehydrogenase in human and rat retina: Relation to methanol toxicity. *Toxicol Appl Pharmacol* 141:373–381, 1996.

Mason TJ, McKay FW: *U.S. Cancer Mortality by County: 1950–1969*. Bethesda, MD: National Institutes of Health, 1974, DHEW Publ No NIH 74-615.

Mathews JM, Parker MK, Matthews HB: Metabolism and disposition of diethylene glycol in rat and dog. *Drug Metab Dispos* 19:1066–1070, 1991.

Matonoski G, Elliott E, Tao X, *et al.*: Lymphohematopoietic cancers and butadiene and styrene exposure in synthetic rubber manufacture. *Ann NY Acad Sci* 837:157–169, 1997.

Mattie DR, Alden CL, Newell TK, *et al.*: A 90-day continuous vapor inhalation toxicity study of JP-8 jet fuel followed by 20–21 months of recovery in Fischer 344 rats and C57BL/6 mice. *Toxicol Pathol* 19:77–87, 1991.

May PA, Gossage JP: Estimating the prevalence of fetal alcohol syndrome: A summary. *Alcohol Res Health* 25:159–167, 2001.

McCaffery P, Tempst P, Lara G, Drager U: Aldehyde dehydrogenase as a positional marker in the retina. *Development* 112:693–702, 1991.

McCarver DG, Hines RH: The ontogeny of human drug-metabolizing enzymes: Phase II conjugative enzymes and regulatory mechanisms. *J Pharmacol Exp Therap* 300:361–366, 2002.

McDougal JN, Jepson GW, Clewell HJ III, *et al.*: Dermal absorption of organic chemical vapors in rats and humans. *Fundam Appl Toxicol* 14:299–308, 1990.

McDougal JN, Pollard DL, Weisman W, *et al.*: Assessment of skin absorption and penetration of JP-8 jet fuel and its components. *Toxicol Sci* 55:247–255, 2000.

McDougal JN, Robinson PJ: Assessment of dermal absorption and penetration of components of a fuel mixture (JP-8). *Sci Total Environ* 288:23–30, 2002.

McGregor D: Methyl tertiary-butyl ether: Studies for potential human health hazards. *Crit Rev Toxicol* 36:319–358, 2006.

McKee RH, Vergnes JS, Galvin JB, *et al.*: Assessment of the in vivo mutagenic potential of methyl tertiary-butyl ether. *J Appl Toxicol* 17(S1):S31–S36, 1997.

McLaughlin JK, Blot WJ: A critical review of epidemiology studies of trichloroethylene and perchloroethylene and risk of renal-cell cancer. *Int Arch Occup Environ Health* 70:222–231, 1997.

McLean AJ, Le Couteur DG: Again biology and geriatric clinical pharmacology. *Pharmacol Rev* 56:163–184, 2004.

McLean AJ, Morgan DJ: Clinical pharmacokinetics in patients with liver disease. *Clin Pharmacokinetics* 21:42–69, 1991.

McMahon TF, Medinsky MA, Birnbaum LS: Age-related changes in benzene disposition in male C57BL/6N mice described by a physiologically based model. *Toxicol Lett* 74:241–253, 1994.

McMartin KE, Wallace KB: Calcium oxalate monohydrate, a metabolite of ethylene glycol, is toxic for rat renal mitochondrial function. *Toxicol Sci* 84:195–200, 2005.

Mebus CA, Welsch F, Working PK: Attenuation of 2-methoxyethanol induced testicular toxicity in the rat by simple physiological compounds. *Toxicol Appl Pharmacol* 99:110–121, 1989.

Medeiros AM, Bird MG, Witz G: Potential biomarkers of benzene exposure. *J Toxicol Environ Health* 51:519–539, 1997.

Medinsky MA, Dorman DC: Recent developments in methanol toxicity. *Toxicol Lett* 82/83:707–711, 1995.

Medinsky MA, Dorman DC, Bond JA, et al.: Pharmacokinetics of methanol and formate in female cynomolgus monkeys exposed to methanol vapors. *Res Rep Health Effects Inst* 77:1–38, 1997.

Medinsky MA, Kenyon EM, Seaton MJ, Schlosser PM: Mechanistic considerations in benzene physiological model development. *Environ Health Perspect* 104(Suppl 6):1399–1404, 1996.

Medinsky MA, Sabourin PJ, Lucier G, et al.: A physiological model for simulation of benzene metabolism by rats and mice. *Toxicol Appl Pharmacol* 99:193–206, 1989.

Medinsky MA, Schlosser PM, Bond JA: Critical issues in benzene toxicity and metabolism: The effect of interactions with other organic chemicals on risk assessment. *Environ Health Perspect* 102(Suppl 9):119–124, 1994.

Medinsky MA, Singh G, Bechtold WE, et al.: Disposition of three glycol ethers administered in drinking water to male F344/N rats. *Toxicol Appl Pharmacol* 102:443–455, 1990.

Mehendale HM: Tissue repair: An important determinant of final outcome of toxicant-induced injury. *Toxicol Pathol* 33:41–51, 2005.

Melnick RL, Kohn MC: Possible mechanisms of induction of renal tubule cell neoplasms in rats associated with α24-globulin: Role of protein accumulation versus ligand delivery to the kidney, in Cappen CC, Dybing E, Rice JM, Wilbourn JD (eds.): *Species Differences in Thyroid, Kidney and Urinary Bladder Carcinogenesis.* Lyons, France, 1999, IARC Publ No 147, pp 119–137.

Mennear JH: Carcinogenicity studies on MTBE: Critical review and interpretation. *Risk Anal* 17:673–681, 1997.

Mennear JH, McConnell EE, Huff JE, et al.: Inhalation and carcinogenesis studies of methylene chloride (dichloromethane) in F344/N rats and B6C3F1 mice. *Ann NY Acad Sci* 534:343–351, 1988.

Messiha FS, Price J: Properties and regional distribution of ocular aldehyde dehydrogenase in the rat. *Neurobehav Toxicol Teratol* 5:251–254, 1983.

Mezey E: Metabolic effects of ethanol. *Fed Proc* 44:134–138, 1985.

Mihic SJ, McQuilkin SJ, Eger EI, et al.: Potentiation of γ-aminobutyric acid type A receptor-mediated chloride currents by novel halogenated compounds correlated with their abilities to induce general anesthesia. *Mol Pharmacol* 46:851–857, 1994.

Miller RR, Hermann EA, Young JT, et al.: Ethylene glycol monomethyl ether and propylene glycol monomethyl ether: Metabolism, disposition, and subchronic inhalation toxicity studies. *Environ Health Perspect* 57:233–239, 1984.

Mohamed MF, Kang D, Aneja VP: Volatile organic compounds in some urban locations in United States. *Chemosphere* 47:863–882, 2002.

Monteiro-Riviere N, Inman A, Riviere J: Effects of short-term high-dose and low-dose exposure to Jet A, JP-8 and JP-8 + 100 jet fuels. *J Appl Toxicol* 21:485–494, 2001.

Monteiro-Riviere NA, Inman AO, Riviere JE: Skin toxicity of jet fuels: Ultra-structural studies and the effects of substance P. *Toxicol Appl Pharmacol* 195:339–347, 2004.

Moorman MP, Sills RC, Collins BJ, Morgan DL: Carbon disulfide neurotoxicity in rats: II. Toxicokinetics. *Neurotoxicology* 19:89–97, 1998.

Morata TC: Study of the effects of simultaneous exposure to noise and carbon disulfide on workers' hearing. *Scand Audiol* 18:53–58, 1989.

Moreau CL, Kerns W II, Tomaszewski CA, et al.: Glycolate kinetics and hemodialysis clearance in ethylene glycol poisoning. META Study Group. *J Toxicol Clin Toxicol* 36:659–666, 1998.

Morford LL, Henck JW, Breslin WJ, DeSesso JM: Hazard identification and predictability of children's health risk from animal data. *Environ Health Perspect* 112: 266–271, 2004.

Morgan DL, Cooper SW, Carlock DL, et al.: Dermal absorption of neat and aqueous volatile organic chemicals in the Fischer 344 rat. *Environ Res* 55:51–63, 1991.

Morgan RW, Kelsh MA, Zhao K, Heringer S: Mortality of aerospace workers exposed to trichloroethylene. *Epidemiology* 9:424–431, 1998.

Morio LA, Chiu H, Sprowles KA, et al.: Distinct roles of tumor necrosis factor-α and nitric oxide in acute liver injury induced by carbon tetrachloride in mice. *Toxicol Appl Pharmacol* 172:44–51, 2001.

Morshed KM, Nagpaul JP, Majumdar S, et al.: Kinetics of propylene glycol elimination and metabolism in the rat. *Biochem Med Metab Biol* 39:90–97, 1988.

Moser GJ, Wong BA, Wolf DC, et al.: Comparative short-term effects of methyl tertiary butyl ether and unleaded gasoline vapor in B6C3F1 mice. *Fundam Appl Toxicol* 31:173–183, 1996a.

Moser GJ, Wong BA, Wolf DC, et al.: Methyl tertiary butyl ether lacks tumor-promoting activity in *N*-nitrosodiethylamine-initiated B6C3F1 female mouse liver. *Carcinogenesis* 17:2753–2761, 1996b.

Moser GJ, Wolf DC, Harden R, et al.: Cell proliferation and regulation of negative growth factors in mouse liver foci. *Carcinogenesis* 17:1835–1840, 1996c.

Moser GJ, Wolf DC, Sar M, et al.: Methyl tertiary butyl ether-induced endocrine alterations in mice are not mediated through the estrogen receptor. *Toxicol Sci* 41:77–87, 1998.

Moser GJ, Wolf DC, Wong BA, Goldsworthy TL: Loss of tumor-promoting activity of unleaded gasoline in *N*-nitrosodiethylamine-initiated ovariectomized B6C3F1 mouse liver. *Carcinogenesis* 18:1075–1083, 1997.

Mugford CA, Kedderis GL: Sex-dependent metabolism of xenobiotics. *Drug Metab Rev* 30:441–498, 1998.

Muhammad F, Monteiro-Riviere NA, Riviere JE: Comparative in vivo toxicity of topical JP-8 jet fuel and its individual hydrocarbon components: Identification of tridecane and tetradecane as key constituents responsible for dermal irritation. *Toxicol Pathol* 33:258–266, 2005.

Mulkey ME: The determination of whether dithiocarbamate pesticides share a common mechanism of toxicity. Internal memorandum, U.S. EPA Office of Pesticide Programs, December 19, 2001, pp. 1–38. http//www.epa.gov/oppsrrdl/cummulative/dithiocarb.pdf

Mundt KA, Birk T, Burch MT: Critical review of the epidemiological literature on occupational exposure to perchloroethylene and cancer. *Int Arch Occup Environ Health* 76:473–491, 2003.

Murray FJ, Schwetz BA, McBride JG, Staples RE: Toxicity of inhaled chloroform in pregnant mice and their offspring. *Toxicol Appl Pharmacol* 50:515–522, 1979.

Murray M: P450 enzymes. Inhibition mechanisms, genetic regulation and effects of liver disease. *Clin Pharmacokinet* 23:132–146, 1992.

Murry DJ, Crom WR, Reddick WE, et al.: Liver volume as a determinant of drug clearance in children and adolescents. *Drug Metab Dispos* 23:1110–1116, 1995.

Muttray A, Kurten R, Jung D, et al.: Acute effects of 200 ppm 1,1,1-trichloroethane on the human EEG. *Eur J Med Res* 5:375–384, 2000.

Nakai JS, Stathopulos PB, Campbell GL, et al.: Penetration of chloroform, trichloroethylene, and tetrachloroethylene through human skin. *J Toxicol Environ Health* 58:157–170, 1999.

Nakajima T: Cytochrome P450 isoforms and the metabolism of volatile hydrocarbons of low relative molecular mass. *J Occup Health* 39:83–91, 1997.

Nakajima T, Elovaara E, Okino T, et al.: Different contributions of cytochrome P450 2E1 and P450 2B1/2 to chloroform hepatotoxicity in rat. *Toxicol Appl Pharmacol* 133:215–222, 1995.

Nakajima T, Koyama Y, Sato A: Dietary modification of metabolism and toxicity of chemical substances—with special reference to carbohydrate. *Biochem Pharmacol* 31:1005–1011, 1982.

Nakajima T, Okuyama S, Yonekura I, Sato A: Effects of ethanol and phenobarbital administration on the metabolism and toxicity of benzene. *Chem-Biol Interact* 55:23–38, 1985.

Nakajima T, Wang R-S, Elovaara E, *et al.*: A comparative study on the contribution of cytochrome P450 isozymes to metabolism of benzene, toluene and trichloroethylene in rat liver. *Biochem Pharmacol* 43:251–257, 1992a.

Nakajima T, Wang R-S, Katakura Y, *et al.*: Sex-, age- and pregnancy-induced changes in the metabolism of toluene and trichloroethylene in rat liver in relation to the regulation of cytochrome P450IIE1 and P450IIC11 content. *J Pharmacol Exp Therap* 261:869–874, 1992b.

Nakajima T, Wang R-S: Induction of cytochrome P450 by toluene. *Int J Biochem* 26:1333–1340, 1994.

Nakajima T, Wang R-S, Elovaara E, *et al.*: Toluene metabolism by cDNA-expressed human hepatic cytochrome P450. *Biochem Pharmacol* 53:271–277, 1997.

NAS (National Academy of Sciences): *Drinking Water and Health.* National Research Council. Washington, DC: National Academy Press, 1986, pp. 171–172.

NAS (National Academy of Sciences): *Pesticides in the Diets of Infants and Children.* National Research Council. Washington, DC: National Academy Press, 1993, pp. 1–12.

NAS (National Academy of Sciences): *Assessing the Human Health Risks of Trichloroethylene: Key Scientific Issues.* Committee on Human Health Risks of Trichloroethylene, National Research Council. Washington, DC: National Academies Press, 2006.

NCI (National Cancer Institute): *Carcinogenesis Bioassay of Chloroform.* National Technical Information Service No. PB264018/AS. Bethesda, MD: NCI, 1976.

NCI (National Cancer Institute): *Bioassay of Tetrachloroethylene for Possible Carcinogenicity.* NCI: DHEW Publ. No. NIH 77-813, Bethesda, MD: NCI, 1977.

NEDO (New Energy Development Organization): Toxicological research of methanol as a fuel for power station: Summary report on test with monkeys, rats and mice. *Tokyo*: 1–296, 1987.

Nelson BK, Brightwell WS: Behavioral teratology of ethylene glycol monomethyl and monoethyl ethers. *Environ Health Perspect* 57:43–46, 1984.

Nelson BK, Vorhees CV, Scott WJ, Hastings L: Effects of 2-methoxyethanol on fetal development, postnatal behavior, and embryonic intracellular pH of rats. *Neurotoxicol Teratol* 11:273–284, 1989.

Nelson HH, Wiencke JK, Christiani DC, *et al.*: Ethnic differences in the prevalence of the homozygous deleted genotype of glutathione *S*-transferase theta. *Carcinogenesis* 16:1243–1245, 1995.

Nessel CS: A comprehensive evaluation of the carcinogenic potential of middle distillate fuels. *Drug Chem Toxicol* 22:165–180, 1999.

Nessel CS, Freeman JJ, Forgash RC, McKee RH: The role of dermal irritation in the skin tumor promoting activity of petroleum middle distillates. *Toxicol Sci* 49:48–55, 1999.

NIDA (National Institute of Drug Abuse): *National Institute on Drug Abuse Research Report Series: Inhalant Abuse.* (NIH Publication No. 05-3818). Bethesda, MD, 2005, pp. 1–8.

Nielsen GD, Alarie Y: Sensory irritation, pulmonary irritation, and respiratory stimulation by airborne benzene and alkylbenzenes: Prediction of safe industrial exposure levels and correlation with their thermodynamic properties. *Toxicol Appl Pharmacol* 65:459–477, 1982.

Niemela O: Aldehyde–protein adducts in the liver as a result of ETH induced oxidative stress. *Front Biosci* 4:506–513, 1999.

Nitschke KD, Burek JD, Bell TJ, *et al.*: Methylene chloride: A 2-year inhalation toxicity and oncogenicity study in rats. *Fundam Appl Toxicol* 11:48–59, 1988.

Noda T, Todani T, Watanabe Y, Yamamoto S: Liver volume in children measured by computed tomography. *Pediatr Radiol* 27:250–252, 1997.

Nomiyama K, Nomiyama H: Respiratory retention, uptake and excretion of organic solvents in man. *Int Arch Arbeitsmed* 32:75–83, 1974.

Nong A, McCarver DG, Hines RN, Krishnan K: Modeling interchild differences in pharmacokinetics on the basis of subject-specific data on physiology and hepatic CYP2E1 levels: A case study with toluene. *Toxicol Appl Pharmacol* 214:78–87, 2006.

Normandin L, Ann Beaupre L, Salehi F, *et al.*: Manganese distribution in the brain and neurobehavioral changes following inhalation exposure of rats to three chemical forms of manganese. *Neurotoxicology* 25:433–441, 2004.

NRC (National Research Council): *Toxicologic Assessment of Jet-Propulsion Fuel 8.* Subcommittee on Jet-Propulsion Fuel 8, Committee on Toxicology. Washington, DC: National Academies Press, 2003.

NTP (National Toxicology Program): *Toxicology and Carcinogenesis Studies of Tetrachloroethylene (Perchloroethylene) in F344/N Rats and B6C3F1 Mice.* Research Triangle Park, NC, 1986.

NTP (National Toxicology Program): *Toxicology and Carcinogenesis Studies of Ethylene Glycol in B6C3F1 Mice (Feed Studies).* NIH Publ. No 93-3144. Research Triangle Park, NC, 1993.

NTP (National Toxicology Program): *Toxicology and Carcinogenesis Studies of t-Butyl Alcohol in F344/N Rats and B6C3F1 Mice* (Tech. Rep. Ser. No. 436; NIH Publ. No. 95-3167). Research Triangle Park, NC, 1995.

NTP (National Toxicology Program): Chloroform. NTP reproductive assessment by continuous breeding study. *Environ Health Perspect* 105(Suppl 1):285–286, 1997a.

NTP (National Toxicology Program): *Toxicology and Carcinogenesis Studies of Ethylbenzene in F344/N Rats and B6C3F1 Mice. (Inhalation Studies).* Research Triangle Park, NC, 1997b.

NTP (National Toxicology Program): NTP Toxicology and Carcinogenesis Studies 2-Butoxyethanol (CAS No. 111-76-2) in F344/N Rats and B6C3F1 Mice (Inhalation Studies). *Natl Toxicol Program Tech Rep Ser* 484:1–290, 2000.

NTP (National Toxicology Program): *NTP-CERHR Monograph on the Potential Human and Reproductive and Developmental Effects of Methanol.* NTP-Center for the Evaluation of Risks to Human Reproduction, U.S. DHHS, NIH Publication No. 03-4478, September 2003.

NTP (National Toxicology Program): NTP technical report on the toxicology and carcinogenesis studies of propylene glycol mono-t-butyl ether (CAS No. 57018-52-7) in F344/N rats and B6C3F1 mice and a toxicology study of propylene glycol mono-*t*-butyl ether in male NBR rats (inhalation studies). *Natl Toxicol Program Tech Rep Ser* 515:1–306, 2004a.

NTP (National Toxicology Program): NTP-CERHR expert panel on the reproductive and developmental toxicity of methanol. *Reprod Toxicol* 18:303–390, 2004b.

NTP (National Toxicology Program): NTP toxicology and carcinogenesis studies of dipropylene glycol (CAS No. 25265-71-8) in F344/N rats and B6C3F1 mice (drinking water studies). *Natl Toxicol Program Tech Rep Ser* 511:6–260, 2004c.

NTP (National Toxicology Program): NTP-CERHR expert panel report on the reproductive and developmental toxicity of ethylene glycol. *Repro Toxicol* 18:457–532 2004d.

NTP (National Toxicology Program): NTP-CERHR expert panel report on the reproductive and developmental toxicity of propylene glycol. *Repro Toxicol* 18:533–579, 2004e.

NTP (National Toxicology Program): NTP-CERHR *Monograph on the Potential Human Reproductive and Developmental Effects of Ethylene Glycol. NTP CERHR MON* 11:1-III36, 2004f.

NTP (National Toxicology Program): NTP-CERHR *Monograph on the Potential Human Reproductive and Developmental Effects of Propylene Glycol (PG). NTP CERHR MON* 12:i-III6, 2004g.

Nuckols JR, Ashley DL, Lyu C, *et al.*: Influence of tap water quality and household water use activities on indoor air and internal dose levels of trihalomethanes. *Environ Health Perspect* 113:863–870, 2005.

Nyska A, Maronpot RR, Long PH, *et al.*: Disseminated thrombosis and bone infarction in female rats following inhalation exposure to 2-butoxyethanol. *Toxicol Pathol* 27:287–294, 1999.

O'Brien KL, Selanikio JD, Hecdivert C, *et al.*: Epidemic of pediatric deaths from acute renal failure caused by diethylene glycol poisoning. *JAMA* 279:1175–1180, 1998.

O'Flaherty EJ, Nau H, McCandless D, *et al.*: Physiologically based pharmacokinetics of methoxyacetic acid: Dose-effect considerations in C57BL/6 mice. *Teratology* 52:78–89, 1995.

Olney JW, Wozniak DF, Farber NB, *et al.*: The enigma of fetal alcohol neurotoxicity. *Ann Med* 34:109–119, 2002.

Olson MJ, Garg BD, Murty CVR, Roy AK: Accumulation of α2u-globulin in the renal proximal tubules of male rats exposed to unleaded gasoline. *Toxicol Appl Pharmacol* 90:43–51, 1987.

Olson MJ, Mancini MA, Garg BD, Roy AK: Leupeptin-mediated alteration of renal phagolysosomes: Similarity to hyaline droplet nephropathy of male rats exposed to unleaded gasoline. *Toxicol Lett* 41:245–254, 1988.

Omiecinski CJ, Remmel RP, Hosagrahara VP: Concise review of the cytochrome P450s and their roles in toxicology. *Toxicol Sci* 4:151–156, 1999.

Omura M, Katsumata T, Misawa H, Yamaguchi M: Decreases in protein kinase and phosphatase activities in the liver nuclei of rats exposed to carbon tetrachloride. *Toxicol Appl Pharmacol* 160:192–197, 1999.

OSHA (Occupational Safety and Health Administration): Solvents. July 3, 2006. http://www.osha.gov/archive/oshinfo/priorities/solvents.html

Oudiz D, Zenick H: In vivo and in vitro evaluations of spermatotoxicity induced by 2-ethoxyethanol treatment. *Toxicol Appl Pharmacol* 84:576–583, 1986.

Padron AG, de Toranzo EGD, Castro JA: Depression of liver microsomal glucose 6-phosphatase activity in carbon tetrachloride-poisoned rats. Potential synergistic effects of lipid peroxidation and of covalent binding of haloalkane-derived free radicals to cellular components in the process. *Free Radic Biol Med* 21:81–87, 1996.

Paine MF, Hart HL, Ludington SS, *et al.*: The human intestinal cytochrome P450 "pie". *Drug Metab Dispos* 34:880–886, 2006.

Palmer RB, Brent J: Derivation of a chemical-specific adjustment factor (CSAF) for use in the assessment of risk from chronic exposure to ethylene glycol: Application of international programme for chemical safety guidelines. *Toxicol Appl Pharmacol* 207:576–584, 2005.

Panda S, Antoch MP, Miller BH, *et al.*: Coordinator transcription of key pathways in the mouse by the circadian clock. *Cell* 109:307–320, 2002.

Park J, Kamendulis LM, Klaunig JE. Effects of 2-butoxyethanol on hepatic oxidative damage. *Toxicol Lett* 126:19–29, 2002.

Pastino GM, Conolly RB: Application of a physiologically based pharmacokinetic model to estimate the bioavailability of ethanol in male rats: Distinction between gastric and hepatic pathways of metabolic clearance. *Toxicol Sci* 55:256–265, 2000.

Pastino GM, Flynn EJ, Sultatos LG: Genetic polymorphisms in ethanol metabolism: Issues and goals for physiologically based pharmacokinetic modeling. *Drug Chem Toxicol* 23:179–201, 2000.

Patel AS, Talbott EO, Zborowski JV, *et al.*: Risk of cancer as a result of community exposure to gasoline vapors. *Arch Environ Health* 59:497–503, 2004.

Paulu C, Aschengrau A, Ozonoff D: Tetrachloroethylene-contaminated drinking water in Massachusetts and the risk of colon-rectum, lung, and other cancers. *Environ Health Perspect* 107:265–271, 1999.

Pelekis M, Gephart LA, Lerman SE: Physiological-model-based derivation of the adult and child pharmacokinetic intraspecies uncertainty factors for volatile organic compounds. *Regul Toxicol Pharmacol* 33:12–20, 2001.

Pereira MA: Route of administration determines whether chloroform enhances or inhibits cell proliferation in the liver of B6C3F1 mice. *Fundam Appl Toxicol* 23:87–92, 1994.

Pereira MA, Grothaus M: Chloroform in drinking water prevents hepatic cell proliferation induced by chloroform administered by gavage in corn oil to mice. *Fundam Appl Toxicol* 37:82–87, 1997.

Pereira MA, Kramer PM, Conran PB, Tao L: Effect of chloroform on dichloroacetic acid and trichloroacetic acid-induced hypomethylation and expression of c-myc gene and on their promotion of liver and kidney tumors in mice. *Carcinogenesis* 22:1511–1519, 2001.

Pfaff J, Parton K, Lantz RC, *et al.*: Inhalation exposure to JP-8 jet fuel alters pulmonary function and substance P levels in Fischer 344 rats. *J Appl Toxicol* 15:249–256, 1995.

Pfaff JK, Tollinger BJ, Lantz RC, *et al.*: Neutral endopeptidase (NEP) and its role in pathological pulmonary change with inhalation exposure to JP-8 jet fuel. *Toxicol Ind Health* 12:93–103, 1996.

Philip BK, Anand SS, Palkar PS, *et al.*: Subchronic chloroform priming protects mice from a subsequently administered lethal dose of chloroform. *Toxicol Appl Pharmacol* 216:108–121, 2006.

Phillips CF, Jones RK: Gasoline vapor exposures during bulk handling operations. *Am Ind Hyg Assoc J* 39:118–128, 1978.

Phillips M: Detection of carbon disulfide in breath and air: A possible new risk factor for coronary artery disease. *Int Arch Occup Environ Health* 64:119–123, 1992.

Pikaar NA, Wedel M, Hermus RJJ: Influence of several factors on blood alcohol concentrations after drinking alcohol. *Alcohol Alcoholism* 23:289–297, 1988.

Plaa GL: Chlorinated methanes and liver injury: Highlights of the past 50 years. *Annu Rev Pharmacol Toxicol* 40:43–65, 2000.

Poet TS, Soelberg JJ, Weitz KK, *et al.*: Mode of action and pharmacokinetic studies of 2-butoxyethanol in the mouse with an emphasis on forestomach dosimetry. *Toxicol Sci* 71:176–189, 2003.

Poldelski V, Johnson A, Wright S, *et al.*: Ethylene glycol-mediated tubular injury: Identification of critical metabolites and injury pathways. *Am J Kidney Dis* 38:339–348, 2001.

Poon R, Chu IH, Bjarnason S, *et al.*: Short-term inhalation toxicity of methanol, gasoline, and methanol/gasoline in the rat. *Toxicol Ind Health* 11:343–361, 1995.

Pottenger LH, Carney EW, Bartels MJ: Dose-dependent nonlinear pharmacokinetics of ethylene glycol metabolites in pregnant (GD 10) and nonpregnant Sprague–Dawley rats following oral administration of ethylene glycol. *Toxicol Sci* 62:10–19, 2001.

Powley MW, Carlson GP: Species comparison of hepatic and pulmonary metabolism of benzene. *Toxicology* 139:207–217, 1999.

Prah J, Ashley D, Blount B, *et al.*: Dermal, oral, and inhalation pharmacokinetics of methyl tertiary butyl ether (MTBE) in human volunteers. *Toxicol Sci* 77:195–205, 2004.

Preedy VR, Ohlendieck K, Adachi J, *et al.*: The importance of alcohol-induced muscle disease. *Clin Sci* 104:287–294, 2003.

Prescott-Matthews JS, Wolf DC, Wong BA, Borghoff SJ: Methyl *tert*-butyl ether causes α2u-globulin nephropathy and enhanced renal cell proliferation in male Fischer-344 rats. *Toxicol Appl Pharmacol* 143:301–314, 1997.

Price B, Bergman TS, Rodriguez M, *et al.*: A review of carbon disulphide exposure data and the association between carbon disulfide exposure and ischemic heart disease mortality. *Regul Toxicol Pharmacol* 26:119–128, 1997.

Price B, Berner T, Henrich RT, *et al.*: A benchmark concentration for carbon disulfide: Analysis of the NIOSH carbon disulfide exposure database. *Regul Toxicol Pharmacol* 24:171–176, 1996.

Price PS, Conolly RB, Chaisson CF, *et al.*: Modeling interindividual variation in physiological factors used in PBPK models in humans. *Crit Rev Toxicol* 33:469–503, 2003a.

Price K, Haddad S, Krishnan K: Physiological modeling of age-specific changes in the pharmacokinetics of organic chemicals in children. *J Toxicol Environ Health A* 66:417–433, 2003b.

Pryor GT, Rebert CS: Interactive effects of toluene and hexane on behavior and neurophysiologic responses in Fischer-344 rats. *Neurotoxicology* 13:225–234, 1992.

Purohit V, Brenner DA: Mechanisms of alcohol-induced hepatic fibrosis: A summary of the Ron Thurman Symposium. *Hepatology* 43:872–878, 2006.

Purohit V, Khalsa J, Serrano J: Mechanisms of alcohol-associated cancers: Introduction and summary of the symposium. *Alcohol* 35:155–160, 2005.

Quast JF, Calhoun LL, Frauson LE: 1,1,1-Trichlorooethane formulation: A chronic inhalation toxicity and oncogenicity study in Fischer 344 rats and B6C3F1 mice. *Fund Appl Toxicol* 11:611–625, 1988.

Raabe GK: Review of the carcinogenic potential of gasoline. *Environ Health Perspect* 101:35–38, 1993.

Raaschou-Nielsen O, Hansen J, McLaughlin JK, *et al.*: Cancer risk among workers at Danish companies using trichloroethylene: A cohort study. *Am J Epidemiol* 158:1182–1192, 2003.

Rajendram R, Preedy VR: Effect of alcohol consumption on the gut. *Dig Dis* 23:214–221, 2005.

Ramos G, Kazimi N, Nghiem DX, *et al.*: Platelet activating factor receptor binding plays a critical role in jet fuel-induced immune suppression. *Toxicol Appl Pharmacol* 195:331–338, 2004.

Ramos G, Nghiem DX, Walterscheid JP, Ullrich SE: Dermal application of jet fuel suppresses secondary immune reactions. *Toxicol Appl Pharmacol* 180:136–144, 2002.

Ramsey JC, Andersen ME: A physiologically based description of the inhalation pharmacokinetics of styrene in rats and humans. *Toxicol Appl Pharmacol* 73:159–175, 1984.

Rao PS, Mangipudy RS, Mehendale HM: Tissue injury and repair as parallel and opposing responses to CCl4 hepatotoxicity: A novel dose–response. *Toxicology* 118:181–193, 1997.

Ratcliffe JM, Schrader SM, Clapp DE, *et al.*: Semen quality in workers exposed to 2-ethoxyethanol. *Br J Ind Med* 46:399–406, 1989.

Raucy JL, Kraner JC, Lasker JM: Bioactivation of halogenated hydrocarbons by cytochrome P4502E1. *Crit Rev Toxicol* 23:1–20, 1993.

Raucy JL, Lasker JM, Kraner JC, *et al.*: Induction of cytochrome P450IIE1 in the obese overfed rat. *Mol Pharmacol* 39:275–280, 1991.

Raunio H, Husgafvel-Pursianinen K, Anttila S, *et al.*: Diagnosis of polymorphisms in carcinogen-activating and inactivating enzymes and cancer susceptibility: A review. *Gene* 159:113–121, 1995.

Rawlings SJ, Shuker DE, Webb M, Brown NA: The teratogenic potential of alkoxy acids in post-implantation rat embryo culture: Structure–activity relationships. *Toxicol Lett* 28:49–58, 1985.

Reaney SH, Bench G, Smith DR: Brain accumulation and toxicity of Mn(II) and Mn(III) exposures. *Toxicol Sci* [E-pub ahead of print], 2006.

Recknagel RO, Glende EA Jr, Dolak JA, Waller RL: Mechanisms of carbon tetrachloride toxicity. *Pharmacol Therap* 43:139–154, 1989.

Reese E, Kimbrough RD: Acute toxicity of gasoline and some additives. *Environ Health Perspect* 101(Suppl 6):115–131, 1993.

Reigel AC, Ali SF, Torinese S, French ED: Repeated exposure to the abused inhalant toluene alters levels of neurotransmitters and generates peroxynitrite in nigrostriatal and mesolimbic nuclei in rat. *Ann NY Acad Sci* 1025:543–551, 2004.

Reigel AC, French ED: Abused inhalants and central reward pathways: Electrophysiological and behavioral studies in the rat. *Ann NY Acad Sci* 965:281–291, 2002.

Reinhardt CT, Mulllin LS, Maxfield ME: Epinephrine-induced cardiac arrhythmia potential of some common industrial solvents. *J Occup Med* 15:953–955, 1973.

Reitz RH, McDougal JN, Himmelstein MW, *et al.*: Physiologically-based pharmacokinetic modeling with methylchloroform: Implications for interspecies, high dose/low dose, and dose route extrapolations. *Toxicol Appl Pharmacol* 95:185–199, 1988.

Reitz RH, Mendrala AL, Guengerich FP: In vitro metabolism of methylene chloride in human and animal tissues: Use in physiologically based pharmacokinetic models. *Toxicol Appl Pharmacol* 97:220–246, 1989.

Rendic S: Summary of information on human CYP enzymes: Human P450 metabolism data. *Drug Metab Rev* 34:83–448, 2002.

Richardson PJ, Patel VB, Preedy VR: Alcohol and the myocardium. *Novartis Found Symp* 216:35–45, 1998.

Richter R: Degeneration of the basal ganglia in monkeys from chronic carbon disulfide poisoning. *J Neuropathol Exp Neurol* 4:324–353, 1945.

Rifas L, Towler DA, Avioli LV: Gestational exposure to ethanol suppresses msx2 expression in developing mouse embryos. *Proc Natl Acad Sci* 94:7549–7554, 1997.

Riihimaki V, Kivisto H, Peltonen K, *et al.*: Assessment of exposure to carbon disulfide in viscose production workers from urinary 2-thiothiazolidine-4-carboxylic acid determinations. *Am J Ind Med* 22:85–97, 1992.

Rikans LE, DeCicco LA, Hornbrook KR, Yamano T: Effect of age and carbon tetrachloride on cytokine concentrations in rat liver. *Mech Aging Develop* 108:173–182, 1999.

Rikans LE, Hornbrook KR: Age-related susceptibility to hepatotoxicants. *Environ Toxicol Pharmacol* 4:339–344, 1997.

Rinn JL, Rozowsky JS, Laurenzi IJ, *et al.*: Major molecular differences between mammalian sexes are involved in drug metabolism and renal function. *Dev Cell* 6:791–800, 2004.

Riordan SM, Williams R: Alcohol exposure and paracetamol-induced hepatotoxicity. *Addict Biol* 7:191–206, 2002.

Ritchie GD, Rossi J III, Nordholm AF, *et al.*: Effects of repeated exposure to JP-8 jet fuel vapor on learning of simple and difficult operant tasks by rats. *J Toxicol Environ Health* 64:385–415, 2001.

Ritchie GD, Still KR, Rossi J, *et al.*: Biological and health effects of exposure to kerosene-based jet fuels and performance additives. *J Toxicol Environ Health B* 6:357–451, 2003.

Ritschel WA: Physiology of the aged respiratory system, in Ritschel WA (ed.): *Gerontokinetics: The Pharmacokinetics of Drugs in the Elderly.* Caldwell, NJ: The Telford Press, 1988, p. 7.

Ritz B: Cancer mortality among workers exposed to chemicals during uranium processing. *J Occup Environ Med* 41:556–566, 1999.

Roberts LG, Bevans AC, Schreiner CA: Development and reproductive toxicity evaluation of toluene vapor in the rat. I. Reproductivity toxicity. *Repro Toxicol* 17:649–658, 2003.

Robledo RF, Barber DS, Witten ML: Modulation of bronchial epithelial cell barrier function by in vitro jet propulsion fuel 8 exposure. *Toxicol Sci* 51:119–125, 1999.

Robledo RF, Witten ML: NK1-receptor activation prevents hydrocarbon-induced lung injury in mice. *Am J Physiol* 276:L229–L238, 1999.

Roe FJ: Styrene: Toxicity studies–What do they show? *Crit Rev Toxicol* 24(Suppl 1):S117–S125, 1994.

Roe FJC, Palmer AK, Worden AN, Van Abbe NJ: Safety evaluation of toothpaste containing chloroform. I. Long-term studies in mice. *J Environ Pathol Toxicol* 2:799–819, 1979.

Rogers JV, Gunasekar PG, Garrett CM, *et al.*: Detection of oxidative species and low-molecular weight DNA in skin following dermal exposure with JP-8 jet fuel. *J Appl Toxicol* 21:521–525, 2001.

Ron MA: Volatile substance abuse: A review of possible long-term neurological, intellectual and psychiatric sequelae. *Br J Psychiatr* 148:235–246, 1986.

Rosenberg NL: Neurotoxicity of organic solvents, in Rosenberg NL (ed.): *Occupational and Environmental Neurology.* Newton, MA: Butterworth-Heinemann, 1995, pp. 71–113.

Rosenberg NL, Grigsby J, Dreisbach J, *et al.*: Neuropsychologic and MRI abnormalities associated with chronic solvent abuse. *J Toxicol Clin Toxicol* 40:21–34, 2002.

Rosenberg NL, Kleinschmidt-DeMasters BK, Davis KA, *et al.*: Toluene abuse causes central nervous system white matter changes. *Ann Neurol* 23:611–614, 1988a.

Rosenberg NL, Spitz MC, Filley CM, *et al.*: Central nervous system effects of chronic toluene abuse—Clinical, brainstem evoked response and magnetic resonance imaging studies. *Neurotoxicol Teratol* 10:489–495, 1988b.

Rosenthal DS, Simbulan-Rosenthal CMG, Liu WF, *et al.*: Mechanisms of JP-8 jet fuel cell toxicity. II. Induction of necrosis in skin fibroblasts and keratinocytes and modulation of levels of Bcl-2 family members. *Toxicol Appl Pharmacol* 171:107–116, 2001.

Roskos KV, Maibach HI, Guy RH: The effect of aging on percutaneous absorption in man. *J Pharmacokin Biopharmaceut* 17:617–630, 1989.

Ross D, Siegel D, Schattenberg DG, *et al.*: Cell-specific activation and detoxification of benzene metabolites in mouse and human bone marrow: Identification of target cells and potential role for modulation of apoptosis in benzene toxicity. *Environ Health Perspect* 104(Suppl 6):1177–1182, 1996.

Rossi J III, Nordholm AF, Carpenter RL, *et al.*: Effects of repeated exposure of rats to JP-5 or JP-8 jet fuel vapor on neurobehavioral capacity and neurotransmitter levels. *J Toxicol Environ Health A* 63:397–428, 2001.

Roth, RA, Harkema JR, Pestka JP, Ganey PE: Is exposure to bacterial endotoxin a determinant of susceptibility to intoxication from xenobiotic agents? *Toxicol Appl Pharmacol* 147:300–311, 1997.

Rumack BH: Acetaminophen misconceptions. *Hepatology* 40:10–15, 2004.

Russo D, Purohit V, Foudin L, Salin M: Workshop on alcohol use and health disparities 2002: A call to arms. *Alcohol* 32:37–43, 2004.

Saavedra D, Arteaga M, Tena M: Industrial contamination with glycol ethers resulting in teratogenic damage. *Ann NY Acad Sci* 837:126–137, 1997.

Sanzgiri UY, Kim HJ, Muralidhara S, *et al*.: Effect of route and pattern of exposure on the pharmacokinetics and acute hepatotoxicity of carbon tetrachloride. *Toxicol Appl Pharmacol* 134:148–154, 1995.

Sanzgiri UY, Srivatsan V, Muralidhara S, *et al*.: Uptake, distribution, and elimination of carbon tetrachloride in rat tissues following inhalation and ingestion exposures. *Toxicol Appl Pharmacol* 143:120–129, 1997.

Sarangapani R, Gentry PR, Covington TR, *et al*.: Evaluation of the potential impact of age- and gender-specific lung morphology and ventilation rate on the dosimetry of vapors. *Inhal Toxicol* 15:987–1016, 2003.

Sarangapani R, Teeguarden JG, Cruzan G, *et al*.: Physiologically based pharmacokinetic modeling of styrene and styrene oxide respiratory-tract dosimetry in rodents and humans. *Inhal Toxicol* 14:789–834, 2001.

Sato A, Endoh K, Kaneko T, Johanson G: Effects of consumption of ethanol on the biological monitoring of exposure to organic solvent vapors: A simulation study with trichloroethylene. *Br J Ind Med* 48:548–556, 1991.

Sato A, Nakajima T: Enhanced metabolism of volatile hydrocarbons in rat liver following food deprivation, restricted carbohydrate intake, and administration of ethanol, phenobarbital, polychlorinated biphenyl and 3-methylcholanthrene: A comparative study. *Xenobiotica* 15:67–75, 1985.

Sato A, Nakajima T, Fujiwara Y, Murayama N: Kinetic studies on sex difference in susceptibility to chronic benzene intoxication with special reference to body fat content. *Br J Ind Med* 32:321–328, 1975.

Sato N, Lindros KO, Baraona E, *et al*.: Sex difference in alcohol-related organ injury. *Alcohol Clin Exp Res* 25:40S–45S, 2001.

Sato TK, Yamada RG, Ukai H, *et al*.: Feedback repression is required for mammalian clock function. *Nat Genet* 38:312–319, 2006.

Savolainen K, Riihimaki V, Laine R, Kekoni J: Short-term exposure of human subjects to *m*-xylene and 1,1,1-trichloroethane. *Int Arch Occup Environ Health* 49:89–98, 1981.

Sawant SP, Dnyanmote AV, Shankar K, *et al*.: Potentiation of carbon tetrachloride hepatotoxicity and lethality in Type 2 diabetic rats. *J Pharmacol Exp Therap* 308:694–704, 2004.

Scalley RD, Ferguson DR, Piccaro JC, *et al*.: Treatment of ethylene glycol poisoning. *Am Fam Physician* 66:807–812, 2002.

Schaumburg HH, Spencer PS: Organic solvent mixtures, in Spencer PS, Schaumburg HH (eds.): *Experimental and Clinical Neurotoxicology*, 2nd ed. New York: Oxford University Press, 2000, pp. 894–897.

Schenker MB, Gold EB, Beaumont JJ, *et al*.: Association of spontaneous abortion and other reproductive effects with work in the semiconductor industry. *Am J Ind Med* 28:639–59, 1995.

Scheuplein R, Charnley G, Dourson M: Differential sensitivity of children and adults to chemical toxicity. I. Biological basis. *Regul Toxicol Pharmacol* 35:429–447, 2002.

Schmucker DL: Age-related changes in liver structure and function: Implications for disease? *Exper Gerontol* 40:650–659, 2005.

Schmucker DL, Woodhouse KW, Wang RK, *et al*.: Effects of age and gender on in vitro properties of human liver microsomal monooxygenases. *Clin Pharmacol Ther* 48:365–374, 1990.

Schoeffner DJ, Bruckner JV, Hatch GE, *et al*.: Age-dependent differences in carbon tetrachloride (CC1$_4$) hepatotoxicity in Fischer-344 rats. *Toxicologist* 30:289, 1996.

Schwartz JB: The influence of sex on pharmacokinetics. *Clin Pharmacokinet* 42:107–121, 2003.

Schwetz BA, Leong BK, Gehring PJ: Embryo- and fetotoxicity of inhaled chloroform in rats. *Toxicol Appl Pharmacol* 28:442–451, 1974.

Scott CS, Cogliano VJ: Trichloroethylene health risks—State of the science. *Environ Health Perspect* 108(Suppl 2):159–160, 2000.

Scott WJ, Fradkin R, Wittfoht W, Nau H: Teratologic potential of 2-methoxyethanol and transplacental distribution of its metabolite, 2-methoxyacetic acid, in non-human primates. *Teratology* 39:363–373, 1989.

Seaton MJ, Schlosser PM, Bond JA, Medinsky MA: Benzene metabolism by human liver microsomes in relation to cytochrome P450 2E1 activity. *Carcinogenesis* 15:1799–1806, 1994.

Seitz HK, Egerer G, Simanowski UA, *et al*.: Human gastric alcohol dehydrogenase activity: Effect of age, sex, and alcoholism. *Gut* 34:1433–1437, 1993.

Seme MT, Summerfelt P, Henry MM, *et al*.: Formate-induced inhibition of photoreceptor function in methanol intoxication. *J Pharmacol Exp Therap* 289:361–370, 1999.

Shamsky S, Samimi B: Organic vapors at underground gasoline tank removal sites. *Appl Ind Hyg* 2:242–245, 1987.

Shi J, Aisaki K, Ikawa Y, Wake K: Evidence of hepatocyte apoptosis in rat liver after the administration of carbon tetrachloride. *Am J Pathol* 153:515–525, 1998.

Shibley IA, Pennington SN: Metabolic and mitotic changes associated with the fetal alcohol syndrome. *Alcohol Alcoholism* 32:423–434, 1997.

Shimada T, Yamazaki H, Mimura M, *et al*.: Interindividual variations in human liver P-450 enzymes involved in the oxidation of drugs, carcinogens and toxic chemicals: Studies with liver microsomes of 30 Japanese and 30 Caucasians. *J Pharmacol Exp Therap* 270:414–423, 1994.

Short BG, Steinhagen WH, Swenberg JA: Promoting effects of unleaded gasoline and 2,2,4-trimethylpentane on the development of atypical cell foci and renal tubular cell tumors in rats exposed to *N*-ethyl-*N*-hydroxyethylnitrosamine. *Cancer Res* 49:369–378, 1989.

Siesky AM, Kamendulis LM, Klaunig JE: Hepatic effects of 2-butoxyethanol in rodents. *Toxicol Sci* 70:252–260, 2002.

Sills RC, Harry GJ, Valentine WM, Morgan DL: Interdisciplinary neurotoxicity inhalation studies: Carbon disulfide and carbonyl sulfide research in F344 rats. *Toxicol Appl Pharmacol* 207:S245–S250, 2005.

Sills RC, Morgan DL, Harry GJ: Carbon disulfide neurotoxicity in rats: I. Introduction and study design. *Neurotoxicology* 19:83–88, 1998.

Silvaggio T, Mattison DR: Setting occupational health standards: Toxicokinetic differences among and between men and women. *J Occup Med* 36:849–854, 1994.

Singh S, Singh J: Dermal toxicity and microscopic alteration by JP-8 jet fuel components in vivo in rabbit. *Environ Toxicol Phar* 16:153–161, 2004.

Singh S, Zhao K, Singh J: In vivo percutaneous absorption, skin barrier perturbation, and irritation from JP-8 jet fuel components. *Drug Chem Toxicol* 26:135–146, 2003.

Singh SP, Ehmann S, Snyder AK: Ethanol-induced changes in insulin-like growth factors and IGF gene expression in the fetal brain. *Proc Soc Exp Biol Med* 212:349–354, 1996.

Sinks T, Lushniak B, Haussler BJ, *et al*.: Renal cell cancer among paperboard printing workers. *Epidemiology* 3:483–489, 1992.

Sivilotti ML, Burns MJ, McMartin KE, Brent J: Toxicokinetics of ethylene glycol during fomepizole therapy: Implications for management. For the Methylpyrazole for Toxic Alcohols Study Group. *Ann Emerg Med* 36:114–125, 2000.

Skrzypinska-Gawrysiak M, Piotrowski JK, Sporny S: Circadian variations in hepatotoxicity of carbon tetrachloride in mice. *Internat J Occup Med Environ Health* 13:165–173, 2000.

Smialowicz RJ, Riddle MM, Luebke RW, *et al*.: Immunotoxicity of 2-methoxyethanol following oral administration in Fischer 344 rats. *Toxicol Appl Pharmacol* 109:494–506, 1991a.

Smialowicz RJ, Riddle MM, Rogers RR, *et al*.: Evaluation of the immunotoxicity of orally administered 2-methoxyacetic acid in Fischer 344 rats. *Fundam Appl Toxicol* 17:771–781, 1991b.

Smialowicz RJ, Riddle MM, Williams WC, *et al*.: Species and strain comparisons of immunosuppression by 2-methoxyethanol and 2-methoxyacetic acid. *Int J Immunopharmacol* 16:695–702, 1994.

Smialowicz RJ, Williams WC, Riddle MM, *et al.*: Comparative immuno-suppression of various glycol ethers orally administered to Fischer 344 rats. *Fundam Appl Toxicol* 18:621–627, 1992.

Smith DA, Abel SM, Hyland R, Jones BC: Human cytochromes P450s: Selectivity and measurement in vivo. *Xenobiotica* 28:1095–1128, 1998.

Smith EN, Taylor RT: Acute toxicity of methanol in the folate-deficient acatalasemic mouse. *Toxicology* 25:271–287, 1982.

Smith JH, Maita K, Sleight SD, Hook JB: Effect of sex hormone status on chloroform nephrotoxicity and renal mixed function oxidases in mice. *Toxicology* 30:305–316, 1984.

Smith MT: The mechanism of benzene-induced leukemia: A hypothesis and speculations on the causes of leukemia. *Environ Health Perspect* 104(Suppl 6):1219–1225, 1996.

Snyder R: Benzene and leukemia. *Crit Rev Toxicol* 32:155–210, 2002.

Snyder R: Xenobiotic metabolism and the mechanism(s) of benzene toxicity. *Drug Metab Rev* 36:531–547, 2004.

Soffritti M, Belpoggi F, Cevolani D, *et al.*: Results of long-term experimental studies on the carcinogenicity of methyl alcohol and ethyl alcohol in rats. *Ann NY Acad Sci* 982:46–69, 2002.

Spencer PJ: New toxicity data for the propylene glycol ethers—A commitment to public health and safety. *Toxicol Lett* 156:181–188, 2005.

Spencer PJ, Crissman JW, Stott WT, *et al.*: Propylene glycol monomethyl ether (PGME): Inhalation toxicity and carcinogenicity in Fischer 344 rats and B6C3F1 mice. *Toxicol Pathol* 30:570–579, 2002.

Spiller HA: Epidemiology of volatile substance abuse (VSA) cases reported to US poison control centers. *Am J Drug Alcohol Abuse* 30:155–165, 2004.

Spitzer HL: An analysis of the health benefits associated with the use of MTBE reformulated gasoline oxygenated fuels in reducing atmospheric concentrations of selected volatile organic compounds. *Risk Anal* 17:683–691, 1997.

Sprankle CS, Larson JL, Goldsworthy SM, Butterworth BE: Levels of *myc, fos,* Ha-*ras, met* and hepatocyte growth factor mRNA during regenerative cell proliferation in female mouse liver and male rat kidney after a cytotoxic dose of chloroform. *Cancer Lett* 101:97–106, 1996.

Spurgeon A, Glass DC, Calvert IA, *et al.*: Investigation of dose related neurobehavioral effects in paintmakers exposed to low levels of solvents. *Occup Environ Med* 51:626–630, 1994.

Standeven AM, Goldsworthy TL: Promotion of preneoplastic lesions and induction of CYP2B by unleaded gasoline vapor in female B6C3F1 mouse liver. *Carcinogenesis* 14:2137–2141, 1993.

Standeven AM, Blazer DG, Goldsworthy TL: Investigation of antiestrogenic properties of unleaded gasoline in female mice. *Toxicol Appl Pharmacol* 127:233–240, 1994a.

Standeven AM, Wolf DC, Goldsworthy TL: Interactive effects of unleaded gasoline and estrogen on liver tumor promotion in female B6C3F1 mice. *Cancer Res* 54:1198–1204, 1994b.

Standeven AM, Goldsworthy TL: Identification of hepatic mitogenic and cytochrome P-450-inducing fractions of unleaded gasoline in B6C3F1 mice. *J Toxicol Environ Health* 43:213–224, 1994.

Standeven AM, Wolf DC, Goldsworthy TL: Promotion of hepatic preneoplastic lesions in male B6C3F1 mice by unleaded gasoline. *Environ Health Perspect* 103:696–700, 1995.

Staples CA, Williams JB, Craig GR, Roberts KM: Fate, effects and potential environmental risks of ethylene glycol: A review. *Chemosphere* 43:377–383, 2001.

Starr TB, Matanoski G, Anders MW, Andersen ME: Workshop overview: Reassessment of the cancer risk of dichloromethane in humans. *Toxicol Sci* 91:20–28, 2006.

Stevens JC, Hines RN, Gu C, *et al.*: Developmental expression of the major human hepatic CYP3A enzymes. *J Pharmacol Exp Therap* 307:573–582, 2003.

Stoica BA, Boulares AH, Rosenthal DS, *et al.*: Mechanisms of JP-8 jet fuel toxicity. I. Induction of apoptosis in rat lung epithelial cells. *Toxicol Appl Pharmacol* 171:94–106, 2001.

Stott WT, McKenna MJ: The comparative absorption and excretion of chemical vapors by the upper, lower and intact respiratory tract of rats. *Fundam Appl Toxicol* 4:594–602, 1984.

Stoyanovsky DA, Cederbaum AI: Thiol oxidation and cytochrome P450-dependent metabolism of CCl4 triggers Ca^{+2} release from liver microsomes. *Biochemistry* 35:15839–15845, 1996.

Sturtevant RP, Sturtevant FM, Pauly JE, Scheving LE: Chronopharmacokinetics of ethanol. *Int J Clin Pharmacol* 16:594–599, 1978.

Sulsky SI, Hooven FH, Burch MT, Mundt KA: Critical review of the epidemiological literature on the potential cardiovascular effects of occupational carbon disulfide exposure. *Int Arch Occup Environ Health* 75:365–380, 2002.

Swann HE Jr, Kwon BK, Hogan GK, Snellings WM: Acute inhalation toxicology of volatile hydrocarbons. *Am Ind Hyg Assoc J* 35:511–518, 1974.

Sweeney LM, Kirman CR, Morgott DA, Gargas ML: Estimation of individual variation in oxidative metabolism of dichloromethane in human volunteers. *Toxicol Lett* 154:201–206, 2004.

Sweeney LM, Tyler TR, Kirman CR, *et al.*: Proposed occupational exposure limits for select ethylene glycol ethers using PBPK models and Monte Carlo simulations. *Toxicol Sci* 62:124–139, 2001.

Taieb D, Malicet C, Garcia S, *et al.*: Inactivation of stress protein 8 increases murine carbon tetrachloride hepatotoxicity via preserved CYP2E1 activity. *Hepatology* 42:176–182, 2005.

Takebayashi T, Nishiwaki Y, Uemura T, *et al.*: A six year follow up study of the subclinical effects of carbon disulphide exposure on the cardiovascular system. *Occup Environ Med* 61:127–134, 2004.

Tam YK: Individual variation in first-pass metabolism. *Clin Pharmacokinet* 25:300–328, 1993.

Tan X, Peng X, Wang F, *et al.*: Cardiovascular effects of carbon disulfide: Meta-analysis of cohort studies. *Int J Hyg Environ Health* 205:473–477, 2002.

Tan Y-M, Butterworth BE, Gargas ML, Conolly RB: Biologically motivated modeling of chloroform cytolethality and regenerative cellular proliferation. *Toxicol Sci* 75:192–200, 2003.

Tang C, Lin JH, Lu AYH: Metabolism-based drug-drug interactions: What determines individual variability in cytochrome P450 induction? *Drug Metab Dispos* 33:603–613, 2005.

Tao L, Kramer PM, Ge R, Pereira MA: Effect of dichloroacetic acid and trichloroacetic acid on DNA methylation in liver and tumors of female B6C3F1 mice. *Toxicol Sci* 43:139–144, 1998.

Tao L, Li Y, Kramer PM, *et al.*: Hypomethylation of DNA and the insulin-like growth factor-II gene in dichloroacetic and trichloroacetic acid-promoted mouse liver tumors. *Toxicology* 196:127–136, 2004.

Tao L, Wang W, Li L, *et al.*: DNA hypomethylation induced by drinking water disinfection by-products in mouse and rat kidney. *Toxicol Sci* 87:344–352, 2005.

Tao L, Yang S, Xie M, *et al.*: Effect of trichloroethylene and its metabolites, dichloroacetic acid and trichloroacetic acid, on the methylation and expression of c-Jun and c-Myc protooncogenes in mouse liver: Prevention by methionine. *Toxicol Sci* 54:399–407, 2000.

Tapin D, Kennedy G, Lambert J, Zayed J: Bioaccumulation and locomotor effects of manganese sulfate in Sprague–Dawley rats following subchronic (90 days) inhalation exposure. *Toxicol Appl Pharmacol* 211:166–174, 2006.

Tardif R, Lapare S, Plaa GL, Brodeur J: Effect of simultaneous exposure to toluene and xylene on their respective biological exposure indices in humans. *Int Arch Occup Environ Health* 63:279–284, 1991.

Terry KK, Elswick BA, Welsch F, Conolly RB: Development of a physiologically based pharmacokinetic model describing 2-methoxyacetic acid disposition in the pregnant mouse. *Toxicol Appl Pharmacol* 132:103–114, 1995.

Thamilselvan S, Khan SR: Oxalate and calcium oxalate crystals are injurious to renal epithelial cells: Results of in vivo and in vitro studies. *J Nephrol* 11:66–69, 1998.

Thier R, Wiebel FA, Hinkel A, *et al.*: Species differences in the glutathione transferase GSTT1-1 activity towards the model substrates methyl chloride and dichloromethane in liver and kidney. *Arch Toxicol* 72:622–629, 1998.

Thompson DJ, Warner SD, Robinson VB: Teratology studies on orally administered chloroform in the rat and rabbit. *Toxicol Appl Pharmacol* 29:348–357, 1974.

Thrall KD, Weitz KK, Woodstock AD: Use of real-time breath analysis and physiologically based pharmacokinetic modeling to evaluate dermal absorption of aqueous toluene in human volunteers. *Toxicol Sci* 68: 280–287, 2002.

Thurman RG: Mechanisms of hepatic toxicity II. Alcoholic liver injury involves activation of Kupffer cells by endotoxin. *Am J Physiol* 275:G605–G611, 1998.

Thurman RG: Sex-related liver injury due to alcohol involves activation of Kupffer cells by endotoxin. *Can J Gastroenterol* 14:129D–135D, 2000.

Tonkin EG, Erve JC, Valentine WM: Disulfiram produces a non-carbon disulfide-dependent schwannopathy in the rat. *J Neuropathol Exp Neurol* 59:786–797, 2000.

Toraason M, Breitenstein M: Prenatal ethylene glycol ether (EGME) exposure produces electrocardiographic changes in the rat. *Toxicol Appl Pharmacol* 95:321–327, 1988.

Tornero-Velez R, Rappaport SM: Physiological modeling of the relative contributions of styrene-7,8-oxide derived from direct inhalation and from styrene metabolism to the systemic dose in humans. *Toxicol Sci* 64:151–161, 2001.

Toso L, Roberson R, Woodard J, *et al.*: Prenatal alcohol exposure alters GABA(A)alpha(5) expression: A mechanism of alcohol-induced learning dysfunction. *Am J Obstet Gynecol* 195:1038–1044, 2006.

Traiger GJ, Bruckner JV: The participation of 2-butanone in 2-butanol-induced potentiation of carbon tetrachloride hepatotoxicity. *J Pharmacol Exp Therap* 196:493–500, 1976.

Travis CC, Fox MT, Simmons WM, Lyon BF: Co-exposure to gasoline vapor decreases benzene metabolism in Fischer-344 rats. *Toxicol Lett* 62:231–240, 1992.

Treichel JL, Henry MM, Skumatz CM, Eells JT, Burke JM: Formate, the toxic metabolite of methanol, in cultured ocular cells. *Neurotoxicology* 24:825–834, 2003.

Triebig G, Claus D, Csuzda I, *et al.*: Cross-sectional epidemiological study on neurotoxicity of solvents in paints and lacquers. *Int Arch Occup Environ Health* 60:233–241, 1988.

Triebig G, Hallermann J: Survey of solvent related chronic encephalopathy as an occupational disease in European countries. *Occup Environ Med* 58:575–581, 2001.

Trush MA, Twerdok LE, Rembish SJ, *et al.*: Analysis of target cell susceptibility as a basis for the development of a chemoprotective strategy against benzene-induced hematotoxicities. *Environ Health Perspect* 104(Suppl 6):1227–1234, 1996.

Turini A, Amato G, Longo V, Gervasi PG: Oxidation of methyl- and ethyl-tertiary-butyl ethers in rat liver microsomes: Role of the cytochrome P450 isoforms. *Arch Toxicol* 72:207–214, 1998.

Turtletaub KW, Mani C: Benzene metabolism in rodents at doses relevant to human exposure from urban air. *Res Report Health Effects Inst* 113:1–26, 2003.

Tyl RW, Ballantyne B, France KA, *et al.*: Evaluation of the developmental toxicity of ethylene glycol monohexyl ether vapor in Fischer 344 rats and New Zealand white rabbits. *Fundam Appl Toxicol* 12:269–280, 1989.

Uchida Y, Nakatsuka H, Ukai H, *et al.*: Symptoms and signs in workers exposed predominantly to xylenes. *Int Arch Occup Environ Health* 64:597–605, 1993.

Udden MM: Hemolysis and deformability of erythrocytes exposed to butoxyacetic acid, a metabolite of 2-butoxyethanol: II. Resistance in red blood cells from humans with potential susceptibility. *J Appl Toxicol* 14:97–102, 1994.

Udden MM: Effects of diethylene glycol butyl ether and butoxyethoxyacetic acid on rat and human erythrocytes. *Toxicol Lett* 156:95–101, 2005.

Udden MM, Patton CS: Hemolysis and deformability of erythrocytes exposed to butoxyacetic acid, a metabolite of 2-butoxyethanol: I. Sensitivity in rats and resistance in normal humans. *J Appl Toxicol* 14:91–96, 1994.

Udden MM, Patton CS: Butoxyacetic acid-induced hemolysis of rat red blood cells: Effect of external osmolarity and cations. *Toxicol Lett* 156:81–93, 2005.

Ullrich SE: Dermal application of JP-8 jet fuel induces immune suppression. *Toxicol Sci* 52:61–67, 1999.

Ullrich SE, Lyons HJ: Mechanisms involved in the immunotoxicity induced by dermal application of JP-8 jet fuel. *Toxicol Sci* 58:290–298, 2000.

Umulis DM, Gurmen NM, Singh P, Fogler HS: A physiologically based model for ethanol and acetaldehyde metabolism in human beings. *Alcohol* 35:3–12, 2005.

UNEP (United Nations Environment Programme): *SIDS Initial Assessment Report for SIAM 2 - Tripropylene Glycol*, July, 1994. http://www.inchem.org/documents/sids/sids/24800-44-0.pdf

UNEP (United Nations Environment Programme): *SIDS Initial Assessment Report for 11th SIAM—Dipropylene Glycol (Mixed Isomers and Dominant Isomer)*, January, 2001. http://www.inchem.org/documents/sids/sids/25265-71-8.pdf

Vaidya VS, Shankar K, Lock EA, *et al.*: Role of tissue repair in survival from *S*-(1,2-dichlorovinyl)-L-cysteine-induced acute renal tubular necrosis in the mouse. *Toxicol Sci* 74:215–227, 2003.

Valentine JL, Lee SS-T, Seaton MJ, *et al.*: Reduction of benzene metabolism and toxicity in mice that lack CYP2E1 expression. *Toxicol Appl Pharmacol* 141:205–213, 1996.

Valentine WM, Amarnath V, Amarnath K, *et al.*: Covalent modification of hemoglobin by carbon disulfide: III. A potential biomarker of effect. *Neurotoxicology* 19:99–108, 1998.

Valentine WM, Amarnath V, Graham DG, *et al.*: CS2-mediated cross-linking of erythrocyte spectrin and neurofilament protein: Dose response and temporal relationship to the formation of axonal swellings. *Toxicol Appl Pharmacol* 142:95–105, 1997.

Valentine WM, Graham DG, Anthony DC: Covalent cross-linking of erythrocyte spectrin by carbon disulfide in vivo. *Toxicol Appl Pharmacol* 121:71–77, 1993.

Valpey R, Sumi SM, Copass MK, Goble GJ: Acute and chronic progressive encephalopathy due to gasoline sniffing. *Neurology* 28:507–510, 1978.

Vamvakas S, Bruning T, Bolt HM, *et al.*: Renal cell cancer correlated with occupational exposure to trichloroethylene. *J Cancer Res Clin Oncol* 126:178–180, 2000.

Vamvakas S, Bruning T, Thomasson B, *et al.*: Renal cell cancer correlated with occupational exposure to trichloroethene. *J Cancer Res Clin Oncol* 124:374–382, 1998.

van Baak MA: Influence of exercise on the pharmacokinetics of drugs. *Clin Pharmacokinet* 19:32–43, 1990.

van der Hoek JAF, Verberk MM, Hageman G: Criteria for solvent-induced chronic toxic encephalopathy: A systematic review. *Int Arch Occup Environ Health* 73:362–368, 2000.

van der Hoek JAF, Verberk MM, van der Laan G, Hageman G: Routine diagnostic procedures for chronic encephalopathy induced by solvents: Survey of experts. *Occup Environ Med* 58:382–385, 2001.

Vanhoorne MH, De Bacquer D, De Backer G: Epidemiological study of the cardiovascular effects of carbon disulphide. *Int J Epidemiol* 21:745–752, 1992.

Vanhoorne M, De Rouck A, Bacquer D: Epidemiological study of the systemic ophthalmological effects of carbon disulfide. *Arch Environ Health* 51:181–188, 1996.

Vasiliou V, Pappa A, Estey T: Role of human aldehyde dehydrogenases in endobiotic and xenobiotic metabolism. *Drug Metab Rev* 36:279–299, 2004.

Verhulst A, Asselman M, Persy VP, *et al.*: Crystal retention capacity of cells in the human nephron: Involvement of CD44 and its ligands hyaluronic acid and osteopontin in the transition of a crystal binding—into a nonadherent epithelium. *J Am Soc Nephrol* 14:107–115, 2003.

Verplanke AJ, Leummens MH, Herber RF: Occupational exposure to tetrachloroethylene and its effects on the kidneys. *J Occup Environ Med* 41:11–16, 1999.

Veulemans H, Steeno O, Maschelein R, Groeseneken D: Exposure to ethylene glycol ethers and spermatogenic disorders in man: A case–control study. *Br J Ind Med* 50:71–78, 1993.

Volkel W, Friedewald M, Lederer E, *et al.*: Biotransformation of perchloroethene: Dose-dependent excretion of trichloroacetic acid, dichloroacetic acid, and *N*-acetyl-*S*-(trichlorovinyl)-L-cysteine in rats and humans after inhalation. *Toxicol Appl Pharmacol* 153:20–27, 1998.

von Euler G: Toluene and dopaminergic transmission, in Isaacon RL, Jensen KF (eds.): *The Vulnerable Brain and Environmental Risk. Toxins in Air and Water*. New York: Plenum Press, 1994, Vol. 3, pp. 301–321.

Vrca A, Bozicevic D, Karacic V, *et al.*: Visual evoked potentials in individuals exposed to long-term low concentrations of toluene. *Arch Toxicol* 69:337–340, 1995.

Wallace L: Major sources of exposure to benzene and other volatile organic chemicals. *Risk Anal* 10:59–64, 1990.

Wallace L: Environmental exposure to benzene: An update. *Environ Health Perspect* 104(Suppl 6):1129–1136, 1996.

Wallace LA, Pellizzari ED, Hartwell TD, *et al.*: A TEAM study: Personal exposures to toxic substances in air, drinking water, and breath of 400 residents of New Jersey, North Carolina, and North Dakota. *Environ Res* 43:290–307, 1987.

Wang PY, Kaneko T, Tsukada H, *et al.*: Dose- and route-dependent alterations in metabolism and toxicity of chemical compounds in ethanol-treated rats: Difference between highly (chloroform) and poorly (carbon tetrachloride) metabolized hepatotoxic compounds. *Toxicol Appl Pharmacol* 142:13–21, 1997.

Wang S, Young RS, Sun NN, Witten ML: In vitro cytokine release from rat type II pneumocytes and alveolar macrophages following exposure to JP-8 jet fuel in co-culture. *Toxicology* 173:211–219, 2002.

Wang W, Chapin RE: Differential gene expression detected by suppression subtractive hybridization in the ethylene glycol monomethyl ether-induced testicular lesion. *Toxicol Sci* 56:165–174, 2000.

Wang W, Wine RN, Chapin RE: Rat testicular Src: Normal distribution and involvement in ethylene glycol monomethyl ether-induced apoptosis. *Toxicol Appl Pharmacol* 163:125–134, 2000.

Warren DA, Bowen SE, Jennings WB, *et al.*: Biphasic effects of 1,1,1-trichloroethane on the locomotor activity of mice: Relationship to blood and brain solvent concentrations. *Toxicol Sci* 56:365–373, 2000.

Warren DA, Graeter LJ, Channel SR, *et al.*: Trichloroethylene, trichloroacetic acid, and dichloroacetic acid: Do they affect eye development in the Sprague–Dawley rat? *Int J Toxicol* 25:279–284, 2006.

Warren DA, Reigle TG, Muralidhara S, Dallas CE: Schedule-controlled operant behavior of rats during 1,1,1-trichloroethane inhalation: Relationship to blood and brain solvent concentrations. *Neurotoxicol Teratol* 20:143–153, 1998.

Wartenberg D, Reyner D, Scott CS: Trichloroethylene and cancer: Epidemiologic evidence. *Environ Health Perspect* 108(Suppl 2):161–176, 2000.

Watanabe A, Nakano Y, Endo T, *et al.*: Collaborative work to evaluate toxicity on male reproductive organs by repeated dose studies in rats 27. Repeated toxicity study on ethylene glycol monomethyl ether for 2 and 4 weeks to detect effects on male reproductive organs in rats. *J Toxicol Sci* 25:259–266, 2000.

Watanabe M, Tanaka M, Tateishi T, *et al.*: Effects of the estrous cycle and the gender differences on hepatic drug metabolizing enzyme activities. *Pharmacol Res* 35:477–480, 1997.

Watson WA: Ethylene glycol toxicity: Closing in on rational, evidence-based treatment. *Ann Emerg Med* 36:139–141, 2000.

Watson RE, Jacobson CF, Williams AL, *et al.*: Trichloroethylene-contaminated drinking water and congenital heart defects: A critical analysis of the literature. *Reprod Toxicol* 21:117–147, 2006.

Watson WA, Litovitz TL, Rodgers GC Jr, *et al.*: 2004 Annual report of the American Association of Poison Control Centers Toxic Exposure Surveillance System. *Am J Emerg Med* 23:589–666, 2005.

Wauthier V, Verbeeck RK, Calderan PB: Age-related changes in the protein and mRNA levels of CYP2E1 and CYP3A isoforms as well as in their hepatic activities in Wistar rats. What role for oxidative stress? *Arch Toxicol* 78:131–138, 2004.

Wax PM: Elixirs, diluents, and the passage of the 1938 Federal Food, Drug and Cosmetic Act. *Ann Intern Med* 122:456–461, 1995.

Weber LWD, Boll M, Stampfl A: Hepatotoxicity and mechanisms of action of haloalkanes: Carbon tetrachloride as a toxicological model. *Crit Rev Toxicol* 33:105–136, 2003.

Weber, WW: Populations and genetic polymorphisms. *Mol Diagn* 4:299–307, 1999.

Weisel CP, Jo WK: Ingestion, inhalation, and dermal exposures to chloroform and trichloroethene from tap water. *Environ Health Perspect* 104:48–51, 1996.

Weiss NS: Cancer in relation to occupational exposure to perchloroethylene. *Cancer Causes Control* 6:257–266, 1995.

Weiss NS: Cancer in relation to occupational exposure to trichloroethylene. *Occup Environ Med* 53:1–5, 1996.

Welch LS, Schrader SM, Turner TW, Cullen MR: Effects of exposure to ethylene glycol ethers on shipyard painters: II. Male reproduction. *Am J Ind Med* 14:509–526, 1988.

Welling PG, Pool WF: Effect of liver disease on drug metabolism and pharmacokinetics, in Cameron RG, Feuer G, De la Iglesia FA (eds.): *Drug Induced Hepatotoxicity*. Berlin: Springer-Verlag, 1996, pp. 367–394.

Wenker MAM, Kerzic S, Monster AC, de Wolff FA: Metabolic capacity and interindividual variation in toxicokinetics of styrene in volunteers. *Human Exp Toxicol* 20:221–228, 2001.

WHO (World Health Organization)/Nordic Council of Ministers: *Chronic Effects of Organic Solvents on the Central Nervous System and Diagnostic Criteria*. Copenhagen, 1985.

WHO (World Health Organization of the United Nations): *Environmental Health Criteria 206: Methyl Tertiary-Butyl Ether*. Geneva, 1998.

WHO (World Health Organization): *Concise International Chemical Assessment Document 46—Carbon Disulfide*. Geneva, 2002, pp. 1–64. http://www.inchem.org/documents/cicads/cicads/cicad46.htm

Wiener HL, Richardson KE: The metabolism and toxicity of ethylene glycol. *Res Commun Subst Abuse* 9:77–87, 1988.

Wiener HL, Richardson KE: Metabolism of diethylene glycol in male rats. *Biochem Pharmacol* 38:539–541, 1989.

Wilkins-Haug L: Teratogen update: Toluene. *Teratology* 55:145–151, 1997.

Williams J, Reel JR, George JD, Lamb JC, IV: Reproductive effects of diethylene glycol and diethylene glycol monethyl ether in Swiss CD-1 mice assessed by a continuous breeding protocol. *Fundam Appl Toxicol* 14:622–635, 1990.

Williams PR, Cushing CA, Sheehan PJ: Data available for evaluating the risks and benefits of MTBE and ethanol as alternative fuel oxygenates. *Risk Anal* 23:1085–1115, 2003.

Williams PRD, Scott PK, Sheehan PJ, Paustenbach, DJ: A probabilistic assessment of household exposures to MTBE in California drinking water. *Human Ecol Risk Assess* 6:827–849, 2000a.

Williams TM, Borghoff SJ: Induction of testosterone biotransformation enzymes following oral administration of methyl *tert*-butyl ether to male Sprague–Dawley rats. *Toxicol Sci* 57:147–155, 2000.

Williams TM, Borghoff SJ: Characterization of *tert*-butyl alcohol binding to alpha2u-globulin in F-344 rats. *Toxicol Sci* 62:228–235, 2001.

Williams TM, Cattley RC, Borghoff SJ: Alterations in endocrine responses in male Sprague–Dawley rats following oral administration of methyl *tert*-butyl ether. *Toxicol Sci* 54:168–176, 2000b.

Williams WC, Riddle MM, Copeland CB, *et al.*: Immunological effects of 2-methoxyethanol administered dermally or orally to Fischer 344 rats. *Toxicology* 98:215–223, 1995.

Williams-Hill D, Spears CP, Prakash S, *et al.*: Mutagenicity studies of methyl-*tert*-butylether using the Ames tester strain TA102. *Mutat Res* 446:15–21, 1999.

Wilmarth KR, Viana ME, Abou-Donia MB: Carbon disulfide inhalation increases Ca^{2+}/calmodulin-dependent kinase phosphorylation of cytoskeletal proteins in the rat central nervous system. *Brain Res* 628:293–300, 1993.

Wilson KC, Reardon C, Farber HW: Propylene glycol toxicity in a patient receiving intravenous diazepam. *N Engl J Med* 343:815, 2000.

Wilson KC, Reardon C, Theodore AC, Farber HW: Propylene glycol toxicity: A severe iatrogenic illness in ICU patients receiving IV benzodiazepines: A case series and prospective, observational pilot study. *Chest* 128:1674–1681, 2005.

Wine RN, Ku WW, Li LH, Chapin RE: Cyclophilin A is present in rat germ cells and is associated with spermatocyte apoptosis. Reproductive Toxicology Group. *Biol Reprod* 56:439–446, 1997.

Winek CL, Shingleton DP, Shanor SP: Ethylene and diethylene glycol toxicity. *Clin Toxicol* 13:297–324, 1978.

Witzmann FA, Bauer MD, Fieno AM, *et al.*: Proteomic analysis of simulated jet fuel exposure in the lung. *Electrophoresis* 20:3659–3669, 1999.

Witzmann FA, Bauer MD, Fieno AM, *et al.*: Proteomic analysis of the renal effects of simulated occupational jet fuel exposure. *Electrophoresis* 21:976–984, 2000a.

Witzmann FA, Bobb A, Briggs GB, *et al.*: Analysis of rat testicular protein expression following 91-day exposure to JP-8 jet fuel vapor. *Proteomics* 3:1016–1027, 2003.

Witzmann FA, Carpenter RL, Ritchie GD, *et al.*: Toxicity of chemical mixtures: Proteomic analysis of persisting liver and kidney protein alterations induced by repeated exposure of rats to JP-8 jet fuel vapor. *Electrophoresis* 21:2138–2147, 2000b.

Witzmann FA, Monteiro-Riviere NA, Inman AO, *et al.*: Effect of JP-8 jet fuel exposure on protein expression in human keratinocyte cells in culture. *Toxicol Lett* 160:8–21, 2005.

Wong O: Carcinogenicity of trichloroethylene: an epidemiologic assessment. *Clin Occup Environ Med* 4:557–589, 2004.

Wong FW-Y, Chan W-Y, Lee SS-T: Resistance to carbon tetrachloride-induced hepatotoxocity in mice which lack CYP2E1 expression. *Toxicol Appl Pharmacol* 153:109–118, 1998.

Woodhouse K, Wynne HA: Age-related changes in hepatic function. Implications for drug therapy. *Drugs Aging* 2:243–255, 1992.

Wrighton SA, Stevens JC: The human cytochromes P450 involved in drug metabolism. *Crit Rev Toxicol* 22:1–21, 1992.

Wronska-Nofer T: Various disorders of cholesterol metabolism and their effect on the development of experimental arteriosclerosis in rats exposed to carbon disulfide. *Med Proc* 30:121–134, 1979.

Wronska-Nofer T, Chojnowska-Jezierska J, Nofer JR, *et al.*: Increased oxidative stress in subjects exposed to carbon disulfide (CS_2)—An occupational coronary risk factor. *Arch Toxicol* 76:152–157, 2002.

Wu L-T, Pilowsky DJ, Schlenger WE: Inhalant abuse and dependence among adolescents in the United States. *J Am Acad Child Adolesc Psych* 43:1206–1214, 2004.

Xu H, Tanphaichitr N, Forkert PG, *et al.*: Exposure to trichloroethylene and its metabolites causes impairment of sperm fertilizing ability in mice. *Toxicol Sci* 82:590–597, 2004.

Yang JH, Lee CH, Monteiro-Riviere NA, *et al.*: Toxicity of jet fuel aliphatic and aromatic hydrocarbon mixtures on human epidermal keratinocytes: Evaluation based on in vitro cytotoxicity and interleukin-8 release. *Arch Toxicol* 80:508–523, 2006.

Yin M, Ikejima K, Wheeler MD, *et al.*: Estrogen is involved in early alcohol-induced liver injury in a rat enteral feeding model. *Hepatology* 31:117–123, 2000.

Yin SJ, Han CL, Lee AI, Wu CW: Human alcohol dehydrogenase family. Functional classification, ethanol/retinol metabolism, and medical implications. *Adv Exp Med Biol* 463:265–274, 1999.

Yin S-N, Hayes RB, Linet MS, *et al.*: A cohort study of cancer among benzene-exposed workers in China: Overall results. *Am J Ind Med* 29:227–235, 1996.

Yokley K, Tran HT, Pekari K, *et al.*: Physiologically based pharmacokinetic (PBPK) modeling of benzene in humans: A Bayesian approach. *Risk Anal* 26:925–942, 2006.

Yuan R, Venitz J: Effect of chronic renal failure on the disposition of highly hepatically metabolized drugs. *Internat J Clin Pharmacol Therap* 38:245–253, 2000.

Zangar RC, Benson JM, Burnett VL, Springer DL: Cytochrome P450 2E1 is the primary enzyme responsible for low-dose carbon tetrachloride metabolism in human liver microsomes. *Chem-Biol Interact* 125:233–243, 2000.

Zhou W, Yuan D, Huang G, *et al.*: Mutagenicity of methyl tertiary butyl ether. *J Environ Pathol Toxicol Oncol* 19:35–39, 2000.

Zintzaras E, Stefanidis I, Santos M, Vidal F: Do alcohol-metabolizing enzyme gene polymorphisms increase the risk of alcoholism and alcoholic liver disease? *Hepatology* 43:352–361, 2006.

CHAPTER 25

HEALTH EFFECTS OF RADIATION AND RADIOACTIVE MATERIALS

Naomi H. Harley

INTRODUCTION

Among all the branches of toxicology, ionizing radiation provides the most quantitative estimates of health detriments for humans and animals. Five large studies provide data on the health effects of radiation on people. These effects include those due to external X-rays and gamma-ray radiation and internal alpha radioactivity. The studies encompass radium exposures, including those sustained by radium dial painters, atom bomb survivors, patients irradiated with X-rays for ankylosing spondylitis, children irradiated with X-rays for tinea capitis (ringworm), and uranium miners exposed to radon and its short-lived daughter products. The latest data on radon risk comes from over 20 domestic studies of normal radon background. The major health effect subsequent to radiation exposure seen with statistical significance to date is cancer. Some heart and digestive disease has been observed in atom bomb survivors, but only at high dose levels (>0.5 Sv). The various types and the quantitative risks are described in subsequent sections.

All the studies provide a consistent picture of the risk of exposure to ionizing radiation. There are sufficient details in the studies of atom bomb, occupational, and medical exposures to estimate the risk from lifelong low-level environmental exposure. Natural background radiation is substantial, and only within the past two decades has the extent of the radiation insult to the global population from natural radiation and radioactivity been appreciated.

BASIC RADIATION CONCEPTS

The four main types of radiation are alpha particles, electrons (negatively charged beta particles or positively charged positrons), gamma rays, and X-rays. An atom can decay to a product element through the loss of a heavy (mass = 4) charged (+2) alpha particle (He^{+2}) that consists of two protons and two neutrons. The alpha particle is ejected from the nucleus with energy depending upon the element. After it loses its energy, it is a stable helium atom. An atom can decay by loss of a negatively or positively charged electron (e^-, a beta particle or e^+, a positron). Gamma radiation results when the nucleus releases excess energy, usually after an alpha, beta, or positron transition. X-rays occur whenever an inner-shell orbital electron is removed and rearrangement of the atomic electrons results, with the release of the element's characteristic X-ray energy.

There are several excellent textbooks describing the details of radiologic physics (Evans, 1955, 1982; Andrews, 1974; Turner, 1986; Shapiro, 2002; Cember, 1996).

One of the most useful expressions relates the radioactive decay rate to the nuclide half life and the number of atoms (mass) present.

$$\text{Activity } (A) = \lambda N$$
$$\lambda = \ln(2)/T_{1/2} \tag{25-1}$$

where $T_{1/2}$ is the half-life of the radioactive element and N the number of atoms in the source.

The expression for activity may be integrated to derive the exponential radioactive decay law

$$A = A_0 e^{(-\lambda T)} \tag{25-2}$$

where A_0 is the initial decay rate at T_0 and A the decay rate at T.

Example 1. The average radon (^{222}Rn) concentration in a home is about 40 Bq m^{-3}. How many atoms exist for this concentration.

^{222}Rn $T_{1/2} = 3.8$ days
$\lambda = \ln(2)/T_{1/2} = \ln(2)/(3.8 \times 1440 \times 60) = 2.1 \times 10^{-6}$ s^{-1}
Activity (disintegrations per second) DPS = 40
$\quad = (2.1 \times 10^{-6}$ s$^{-1}) (N)$

where $N = 1.9 \times 10^7$ atoms.

There is no analytical method for a stable element that can measure a few million atoms of a substance with ease. Radioactivity provides a massless tracer in many situations.

Energy

The definition of an alpha or beta particle or a gamma ray arises from their energetic nuclear origin. Otherwise they are basically a helium atom, an electron, or a photon. Alpha particles and beta rays (or positrons) have kinetic energy as a result of their rapid motion when ejected from the nucleus. The energy is equal to

$$E = 1/2mV^2 \tag{25-3}$$

where m is the mass of the particle and V the velocity of the particle.

Alpha particles have a low velocity compared with the speed of light, and calculations of alpha particle energy do not require any corrections for relativity. Most beta particles (or positrons) have a velocity near the speed of light, and the basic expression must be corrected for their increased relativistic mass. The energy equivalent of mass is calculated from Einstein's equation $E = mc^2$. Thus, rest mass of the electron is calculated as 0.511 MeV and its total energy (increase in mass due to relativistic correction plus the rest mass) is equal to

$$E = 0.511/(1 - v^2/c^2) + 0.511 \tag{25-4}$$

where v is the velocity of the beta particle and c the speed of light.

Gamma rays and X-rays are pure electromagnetic radiation with energy equal to

$$E = hv \tag{25-5}$$

where h is the Planck's constant (6.626×10^{-34} J s) and v the frequency of radiation.

The conventional energy units for ionizing radiation are the electron volt (eV) or multiples of this basic unit, kiloelectron volts (keV), and million electron volts (MeV). The conversion to the international system of units, the Système Internationale (SI), is currently taking place in many countries, and the more fundamental energy unit of the Joule (J) is slowly replacing the older unit. The relationship is

$$1 \text{ eV} = 1.6 \times 10^{-19} \text{ J}$$

Authoritative tables of nuclear data such as those of Browne *et al.* (1986) contain the older but more widely accepted units of MeV for energy.

Alpha Particles

Alpha particles are helium nuclei (consisting of two protons and two neutrons), with a charge of +2, that are ejected from the nucleus of an atom. When an alpha particle loses energy, it slows to the velocity of a gas atom and acquires two electrons from the vast sea of free electrons present in most media, and it becomes part of the normal background helium in the environment. All helium in nature is the result of alpha particle decay. The formula for alpha decay is

$$^A_Z X \rightarrow ^{A-4}_{Z-2} Y + He^{2+} + \text{gamma} + Q_\alpha$$

where Z = atomic number and A = atomic weight.

The energy available in this decay is Q_i and is equal to the mass difference of the parent and the two products. The energy is shared among the particles and the gamma ray if one is present.

An example of the alpha decay scheme is given by the natural radionuclide radium (^{226}Ra) in Fig. 25-1. The half-lives of radioactive nuclides may be found on the web at hps.org/publicinformation/radardecaydata.cfm

The energy of alpha particles for most emitters lies in the range of 4–8 MeV. More energetic alpha particles exist but are seen only in very short-lived emitters such as those formed by reactions occurring in particle accelerators. These particles are not considered in this chapter.

Although there may be several alpha particles with very similar energy emitted by a particular element such as radium, each particular alpha particle is monoenergetic, i.e., no continuous spectrum of energies exists, only discrete energies.

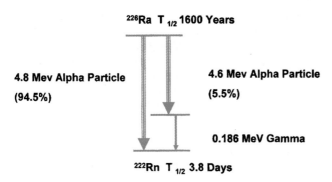

Figure 25-1. *Decay scheme for* ^{226}*Ra.*

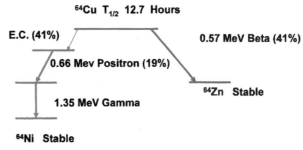

Figure 25-3. *Decay scheme for* ^{64}*Cu.*

Alpha particles are massive relative to beta particles and most alpha particles cannot penetrate a thin sheet of paper. The range of an alpha particle in air is,

$$\text{Range (air)} = 0.325\ E^{3/2}\ \text{(cm)} \qquad (25\text{-}6)$$

In tissue, the range is about 1/1000 of the range in air.

Example 2. Find the range of the ^{226}Ra alpha particle ($E = 4.8$ MeV) in air and tissue.

$$\text{Range} = 0.325(4.8^{3/2}) = 3.4\ \text{cm.}$$

In tissue, the range of the ^{226}Ra alpha particle is 3.4/1000 cm, or about 34 μm.

Beta Particles, Positrons, and Electron Capture

Beta particle decay occurs when a neutron in the nucleus of an element is effectively transformed into a proton and an electron. Subsequent ejection of the electron occurs, and the maximum energy of the beta particle equals the mass difference between the parent and the product nuclei. A gamma ray may also be present to share the energy, Q:

$$^{A}_{Z}X \rightarrow\ ^{\ A}_{Z+1}Y + \text{beta} + Q_{\beta}$$

An example of a beta decay scheme is given in Fig. 25-2 for lead 210 (^{210}Pb):

$$^{210}_{82}\text{Pb} \rightarrow\ ^{210}_{83}\text{Bi} + \text{beta (0.015 MeV)} + \text{gamma (0.046 MeV)}$$

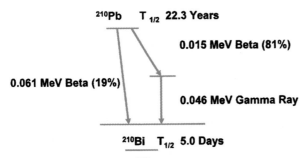

Figure 25-2. *Decay scheme for* ^{210}*Pb.*

Lead 210 emits a beta particle with energy 0.015 MeV, 80% of the time followed by the 0.046 MeV gamma ray. Twenty percent of the time it emits only a 0.061 MeV beta ray, equal to the total energy available for decay (0.015 + 0.046).

Unlike alpha decay, in which each alpha particle is monoenergetic, beta particles are emitted with a continuous spectrum of energy from zero to the maximum energy available for the transition. The reason for this is that the total available energy is shared in each decay or transition by two particles: the beta particle and an antineutrino. The total energy released in each transition is constant, but the observed beta particles then appear as a spectrum. The residual energy is carried away by the antineutrino, which is a particle with essentially zero mass and charge that cannot be observed without extraordinarily complex instrumentation. The beta particle, by contrast, is readily observed with conventional nuclear counting equipment.

Positron emission is similar to beta particle emission but results from the effective nucleon transformation of a proton to a neutron plus a positively charged electron. The atomic number decreases rather than increases, as it does in beta decay.

Figure 25-3 gives an example of positron decay for the radionuclide copper (^{64}Cu), which decays by beta emission 41% of the time, positron emission 19% of the time, and electron capture 40% of the time:

$$^{64}_{29}\text{Cu} \rightarrow\ ^{64}_{28}\text{Ni} + \text{Positron (0.66 MeV)} \quad 19\%$$

$$^{64}_{29}\text{Cu} \rightarrow\ ^{64}_{30}\text{Zn} + \text{beta (0.57 MeV)} \quad 41\%$$

$$^{64}_{29}\text{Cu} \rightarrow\ ^{64}_{28}\text{Ni}\ \text{electron capture} \quad 40\%$$

The energy of the positron appears as a continuous spectrum, similar to that in beta decay, where the total energy available for decay is again shared between the positron and a neutrino. In the case of positron emission, the maximum energy of the emitted particle is the mass difference of the parent and product nuclide minus the energy needed to create two electron masses (1.02 MeV), whereas the maximum energy of the beta particle is the mass difference itself. This happens because in beta decay, the increase in the number of orbital electrons resulting from the increase in atomic number of the product nucleus cancels the mass of the electron lost in emitting the beta particle. This does not happen in positron decay, and there is an orbital electron lost as a result of the decrease in atomic number of the product and the loss of the electron mass in positron emission. Positron emission tomography (PET) scans are a useful diagnostic tool in nuclear medicine. The positron is an unstable particle and decays immediately to two 0.511 MeV photons emitted 180° from each other. The positron emitter is typically fluorine 18 (^{18}F). The radionuclide is given in a solution that is taken up by the tissues of interest and coincidence counting of the two photons locates their tissue origin precisely.

Electron capture competes with positron decay, and the resulting product nucleus is the same nuclide. In electron capture, an orbiting electron is acquired by the nucleus, and the transformation of a proton plus the electron to form a neutron takes place. In some cases the energy available is released as a gamma-ray photon, but this is not necessary, and a monoenergetic neutrino may be emitted. If the 1.02 MeV required for positron decay is not available, positron decay is not kinetically possible and electron capture is the only mode observed.

Gamma-Ray (Photon) Emission

Gamma-ray emission is not a primary process except in rare instances, but it occurs in combination with alpha, beta, or positron emission or electron capture. Whenever the ejected particle does not utilize all the available energy for decay, the nucleus contains the excess energy and is in an excited state. The excess energy is released as photon or gamma-ray emission coincident with the ejection of the particle.

One of the rare instances of pure gamma-ray emission is technetium 99m (^{99m}Tc), which has a 6.0-hour half-life and is widely used in diagnostic nuclear medicine for various organ scans. Its decay product, ^{99}Tc, has a very long half-life (2.13×10^5 years), and as all ^{99}Tc is ultimately released to the environment, a background of this nuclide is emerging.

$$^{99m}_{43}\text{Tc} \rightarrow {}^{99}_{43}\text{Tc} + \text{gamma (0.14 MeV)}$$

Internal Conversion

In many gamma ray emitters, a photon will not actually be emitted by the nucleus but the excess excitation energy will be transferred to an orbital electron. This electron is then ejected as a monoenergetic particle with energy equal to that of the photon minus the binding energy of the orbital electron. This process is known as internal conversion. In tables of nuclear data such as those of Browne et al. (1986), the ratio of the conversion process to the photon is given as e/γ. For example, the e/γ ratio for ^{99m}Tc is 0.11, and therefore the photon is emitted 90% of the time and the conversion electron is emitted 10% of the time. The internal conversion electron is a monoenergetic particle.

INTERACTION OF RADIATION WITH MATTER

Ionizing radiation, by definition, loses energy when passing through matter by producing ion pairs (an electron and a positively charged atom residue). A fraction of the energy loss raises atomic electrons to an excited state (excitation loss). The average energy needed to produce an ion pair is given the notation W and is numerically equal to 33.85 eV in air. This energy is roughly two times the ionization potential of most gases or other elements because it includes the energy lost in the excitation process. It is not clear what role the excitation plays, for example, in damage to targets in the cellular

DNA. Ionization, by contrast, can break bonds in DNA, causing even double strand breaks.

All particles and rays interact through their charge or field with atomic or free electrons in the medium through which they are passing. There is no interaction with the atomic nucleus except at energies above about 8 MeV, which is required for interactions that break apart the nucleus (spallation). Very high-energy cosmic-ray particles, for example, produce ^{3}H, ^{7}Be, ^{14}C, and ^{22}Na in the upper atmosphere by spallation of atmospheric oxygen and nitrogen.

Alpha and beta particles and gamma rays lose energy by ionization and excitation in somewhat different ways, as described in the following sections.

Alpha Particles

The alpha particle is a heavy charged particle with a mass that is 7300 times that of the electrons with which it interacts. The massive particle interacting with a small particle (the electron) has the interesting property that it can give a maximum velocity during energy transfer to the small particle of only two times the initial velocity of the heavy particle. In terms of the maximum energy that can be transferred per interaction is

$$E_{\text{(maximum electron)}} = (4/7300)E_{\text{(alpha particle)}} \quad (25\text{-}7)$$

Although alpha particles can lose perhaps 10–20% of their energy in traveling 10 μm in tissue (1 cm in air), each interaction can impart only the small energy, given in the maximum, in Eq. (25-4). Thus, alpha particles are characterized by a high energy loss per unit path length and a high ionization density along the track length. This is called a *high linear-energy-transfer* (LET) or *high-LET* particle.

Hans Bethe (Bethe and Ashkin, 1953) derived an exact expression for the energy loss in matter per unit distance traveled, dE/dx or stopping power. Later modifications to the formula were added by Bloch and others. For alpha energies between 0.2 and 10 MeV, the Bethe–Bloch expression can be simplified to

$$dE/dx = 3.8 \times 10^{-25} C\, NZ/E\, \ln\{548E/I\}\ \text{MeV}/\mu\text{m}^{-1}$$

$$(25\text{-}8)$$

where N is the number of atoms per cm^{-3} in the medium; Z the atomic number of the medium; I the ionization potential of the medium; E the energy of alpha particle; and C the charge correction for alpha particles with energy below 1.6 MeV.

A simple rule of thumb derived by Bloch may be used to estimate the ionization potential of a compound or element.

$$I = 10(Z) \quad (25\text{-}9)$$

The Bragg additivity rule (Attix et al., 1968) may be used for compounds when the individual values of ionization potential for the elements are available. A tabulation of values of ionization potential is given in ICRU 37 (ICRU, 1984), and the stopping power in all elements has been calculated in ICRU 49 (ICRU, 1993) and by Ziegler (1977). The ionization potentials and stopping power may be found on the web at www.physics.nist.gov/PhysRefData/Star/Text/contents.html.

When alpha particles are near the end of their range, the charge is not constant at +2 but can be +1 or even zero as the particle acquires or loses electrons. A correction factor, C, is needed for energies between 0.2 and 1.5 MeV to account for this effect. Whaling

(1958) published values for the correction factor by which Eq. (25-4) should be multiplied. These factors vary from 0.24 at 0.2 MeV, 0.75 at 0.6 MeV, 0.875 at 1.0 MeV, up to 1.0 at 1.6 MeV.

For the case of tissue, Eq. (25-5) reduces to

$$dE/dx_{\text{tissue}} = [0.126C/E] \ln \{7.99E\} \text{ MeV} \mu\text{m}^{-1} \qquad (25\text{-}10)$$

Example 3. Find the energy loss (stopping power) of a 0.6 and a 5-MeV alpha particle in tissue.

For a 0.6 MeV alpha particle

$$\begin{aligned} dE/dx &= 0.126(0.75)/0.6\ln(7.99 \times 0.6) \\ &= 0.25 \text{ MeV} \mu\text{m}^{-1} \end{aligned}$$

For a 5.0 MeV alpha particle

$$\begin{aligned} &= 0.126(1.0)/5.0\ln(7.99 \times 5.0) \\ &= 0.093 \text{ MeV} \mu\text{m}^{-1} \end{aligned}$$

The slower moving (lower energy) alpha particle has more chance to interact with matter and the energy loss per unit distance is greater. The significance of this energy loss is that it requires about 33.85 eV in tissue to produce an ion pair; therefore, a 0.6 MeV alpha particle can produce $(0.25 \times 10^6 \text{ eV } \mu\text{m}^{-1})/(33.86 \text{ eV/ion pair}) = 7400$ ion pairs in 1 μm, and the 5.0 MeV alpha particle can produce 2700 ion pairs in 1 μm. The diameter of DNA is 0.002 to 0.005 μm, and the nucleosome 0.010 μm; thus, the ionization and dissociation by either a 0.6 or 5.0 MeV alpha particle can cause enough damage to cause a double-strand break (Panajotovic et al., 2006).

The alpha particle therefore disrupts DNA by direct production of ions by ejection of electrons and the electrons in turn may have enough energy to produce further ionization.

Beta Particles

The equations for beta particle energy loss in matter cannot be simplified, as in the case of alpha particles, because of three factors:

1. Even at low energies of a few tenths of a MeV, beta particles travel near the speed of light and relativistic effects (mass increase) must be considered.
2. Electrons interact with particles of the same mass in the medium (free or orbital electrons), so large energy losses per collision are possible.
3. Radiative or bremsstrahlung energy loss occurs when electrons or positrons are slowing down in matter. Such a loss also occurs with alpha particles, but the magnitude of this energy loss is negligible.

Including the effects of these three factors, the energy loss for electrons and positrons has been well quantitated. Tabulations of energy loss in various media have been prepared with the ionization energy loss and the radiative loss detailed. Tables of energy loss for electrons in tissue and many other substances as a function of electron energy can be found in ICRU 37 (1984). The stopping power for electrons may also be found on the web at physics.nist.gov/PhysRefData/Star/Text/contents.html

Gamma Rays

Photons do not have a mass or charge, as do alpha and beta particles. The interaction between a photon and matter therefore is controlled not by the electrostatic Coulomb fields but by interaction of the electric and magnetic field of the photon with the electron in the medium. There are three modes of interaction with the medium.

The Photoelectric Effect The photon interaction (energy exchange) with an orbital electron in the medium is complete, and the full energy of the photon is given to the electron minus the electron-binding energy.

The Compton Effect Part of the photon energy is transferred to an electron, and the photon scatters (usually at a small angle from its original path) (Evans, 1955) with reduced energy. The governing expressions are

$$\begin{aligned} E' &= E\, 0.511/(1 + 1/a - \cos\theta) \\ T &= E\, a(1 - \cos\theta)/[1 + a(1 - \cos\theta)] \end{aligned} \qquad (25\text{-}11)$$

where E, E' is the initial and scattered photon energy in MeV; T the kinetic energy of electron in MeV; $a = E/0.511$; and θ the angle of photon scatter from its original path.

Pair Production Pair production may occur whenever the photon energy is greater than the rest mass of two electrons, $2(0.511 \text{ MeV}) = 1.02 \text{ MeV}$. The electromagnetic energy of the photon can be converted directly to an electron–positron pair, with any excess energy above 1.02 MeV appearing as kinetic energy given to these particles.

Gamma Ray Energy Loss

The loss of photons and energy loss from a photon beam as it passes through matter are described by two coefficients. The attenuation coefficient determines the fractional loss of photons per unit distance (usually in normalized units of g/cm², which is the linear distance times the density of the medium). The mass energy absorption coefficient determines the fractional energy deposition per unit distance traveled. The loss of photons from the direct beam is given by

$$I/I_0 = \exp(\mu/\rho d) \qquad (25\text{-}12)$$

where I is the intensity of photon beam (numbers of photons); I_0 the beam intensity; μ/ρ the attenuation coefficient in medium for energy considered (in m² kg⁻²); and d the thickness of medium in superficial density units kg m⁻² (thickness in m times density in kg m⁻³).

Superficial density is convenient in that it normalizes energy absorption in different media. For example, air and tissue have approximately the same energy absorption per kg m⁻², whereas in linear dimension, the energy absorption, say, per meter, is vastly different. The energy actually deposited in the medium per unit distance is calculated using the mass energy absorption coefficient as opposed to the overall attenuation coefficient and the energy loss is given by

$$\Delta E = (\mu_{\text{en}}/\rho)E_0 \qquad (25\text{-}13)$$

Table 25-1

Mass Energy Absorption Coefficients for Air and Water

PHOTON ENERGY, MeV	AIR, μ_{en}/ρ (m² kg⁻¹)	MUSCLE, STRIATE (ICRU), μ_{en}/ρ (m² kg⁻¹)
0.01	0.46	0.49
0.015	0.13	0.14
0.02	0.052	0.055
0.03	0.015	0.016
0.04	0.0067	0.0070
0.05	0.0040	0.0043
0.06	0.0030	0.0032
0.08	0.0024	0.0026
0.10	0.0023	0.0025
0.15	0.0025	0.0027
0.20	0.0027	0.0029
0.30	0.0029	0.0032
0.40	0.0029	0.0032
0.50	0.0030	0.0033
0.60	0.0030	0.0033
0.80	0.0029	0.0032
1.00	0.0028	0.0031
1.50	0.0025	0.0028
2.00	0.0023	0.0026
3.00	0.0021	0.0023

SOURCE: Data from Hubbell, 1982.

where pE is the energy loss in medium per unit distance (in MeV m² kg⁻¹); μ_{en}/ρ the mass energy absorption coefficient (m² kg⁻²); and E_0 the initial photon energy.

The values for μ_{en}/ρ as a function of gamma-ray energy are shown in Table 25-1 for air and muscle and on the web for a variety of materials. (physics.nist.gov/PhysRefData/XrayMassCoef/cover.html). Energy loss can then be expressed per unit linear distance by multiplying by the density of the medium (kg m⁻³).

ABSORBED DOSE

Dose and Dose Rate

Absorbed dose is defined as the mean energy, e, imparted by ionizing radiation to matter of mass m (ICRU, 1993, 1998):

$$D = e/m \qquad (25\text{-}14)$$

where D is the absorbed dose; e the mean energy deposited in mass; and m the mass.

The unit for absorbed dose is gray (Gy), which is equal to 1 J kg⁻¹. The older unit of dose is rad, which is equal to 100 erg g⁻¹, a value numerically equal to 100 times the dose in gray. The conversion between the two units is 100 rad = 1 Gy.

For uncharged particles (gamma rays and neutrons), kerma (kinetic energy released in matter) is sometimes used. It is the sum of the initial kinetic energies of all the charged ionizing particles liberated in unit mass. The units of kerma are the same as those for dose.

Exposure often is confused with absorbed dose. Exposure is defined only in air for gamma rays or photons and is the charge of the ions of one sign when all electrons liberated by photons are completely stopped in air of mass m:

$$X = Q/m \qquad (25\text{-}15)$$

where X is the exposure; Q the total charge of one sign; and m the mass of air.

The unit of exposure is coulombs per kilogram of air. The older unit of exposure is roentgen, which is equal to 2.58×10^{-4} C kg⁻¹ of air.

Exposure and dose are used interchangeably in some publications, even though this is not correct. The reason is that the older numerical values of dose in rad and exposure in roentgen are similar. Although they are similar numerically, they are fundamentally different in that exposure is ionization (only in air) and dose is absorbed energy in any specified medium:

$$1 \text{ roentgen } = 0.87 \text{ rad (in air)}$$

The SI units are not numerically similar:

$$1 \text{ C kg}^{-1} = 33.85 \text{ Gy}$$

Dose Rate

Dose rate is the dose expressed per unit time interval. The dose rate delivered to the thyroid by ^{99m}Tc for a nuclear medicine scan, for example, diminishes with time because of the 6.0-hour half-life of the nuclide. The total dose is a more pertinent quantity in this case because it can be related directly to risk and compared with the benefit of the thyroid scan. The total dose over all time is expressed by

$$D = D_0 \times T_{eff}/\ln 2$$

where D_0 is the dose rate at time zero; T_{eff} the effective half-life = $\{T_r \times T_b\}/\{T_r + T_b\}$; T_r the radiologic half-life; and T_b the biological half-life.

In general, substances in the body are removed through biological processes as well as by radioactive decay; therefore, the effective half-life is shorter than the radiologic half-life.

The dose rate from natural body ^{40}K in all living cells, by contrast, is relatively constant throughout life and is usually expressed as the annual dose rate.

Equivalent Dose

Ionizing radiation creates ion pairs in a substance such as air or tissue in relatively dense or sparse distribution depending upon the particle. Alpha particles with large mass produce relatively intense ionization tracks per unit distance relative to beta particles, and beta particles produce more dense ionization than gamma rays. The ability to produce more or less ionization per unit path in a medium is expressed by the linear energy transfer (LET). The LET in a substance such as water is readily calculated from the energy loss expressions in the previous sections.

The calculated LET from alpha and beta particles is much greater than it is for gamma rays. In considering the health or cellular effects of each particle or ray, it is necessary to normalize the various

Table 25-2

Recommended Values of w_r for Various Types of Radiation

TYPE OF RADIATION	APPROXIMATE w_r
X-Rays, gamma rays, beta particles, and electrons	1
Thermal neutrons	5
Neutrons (other than thermal $\gg$ 100 keV to 2 MeV), protons, alpha particles, charged particles of unknown energy	20

SOURCE: Data from NCRP, 1993, and ICRP, 1990.

types of radiation. For a particular biological endpoint, such as cell death in an experiment with mouse fibroblasts, it is common to calculate a relative biological effectiveness (RBE). This is defined as the ratio of gamma ray dose that yields the same endpoint to the dose from the radiation under study, e.g., cell death.

Although giving the same dose to an organ from alpha particles as opposed to gamma rays would result in greater effects from the alpha particles, such refinement in the normalization of endpoints (cancer) in the human is not possible with the available data. An attempt to normalize human health effects from different types of radiation, i.e., to calculate an "equivalent" dose is made through the values for LET of the various types of radiation in water. The ratio of the LET for gamma to the radiation in question is defined as a *radiation weighting factor*, w_r (formerly Q), and the normalized (or weighted) dose is called the equivalent dose. The unit for the *equivalent dose* is sievert (Sv), and the older unit is rem:

$$H = Dw_r \qquad (25\text{-}16)$$

where H is the equivalent dose in sievert (older unit rem); D the dose in gray (older unit rad); and w_r the radiation weighting factor.

Table 25-2 gives the values of LET for different particles or rays and is reproduced from the National Council on Radiation Protection (NCRP, 1993) and the International Commission on Radiation Protection (ICRP, 1990).

Example 4. Find the equivalent dose (in sievert) for a dose to lung from an internal emitter of 0.01 Gy alpha particles and 0.01 Gy from external gamma ray radiation.

$$\text{Alpha, } H = 0.01(20) = 0.20 \text{ Sv}$$
$$\text{Gamma, } H = 0.01(1) = 0.01 \text{ Sv}$$

Effective Dose and Cancer Risk

The term *effective dose* (ED) (formerly *effective dose equivalent*) was introduced formally by the ICRP in 1977 to allow addition or direct comparison of the cancer and genetic risk from different partial-body or whole-body doses (ICRP, 1977). A partial-body gamma-ray dose of 1 Sv to the lung, for example, is thought to give 0.0064 cancers over a lifetime per sievert, whereas a whole-body dose of 1 Sv would result in 0.056 total cancers and early genetic effects over the same lifetime interval. Both values are derived from the human atom bomb follow-up data. The ratio 0.0064/0.056 was defined as a tissue weighting factor, w_t, for lung and is numerically equal to 0.12.

Table 25-3

Recommended Values of the Weighting Factors, w_t, for Calculating Effective Dose

TISSUE OR ORGAN	TISSUE WEIGHTING FACTOR, w_t
Gonads	0.20
Bone marrow (red)	0.12
Colon	0.12
Lung	0.12
Stomach	0.12
Bladder	0.05
Breast	0.05
Liver	0.05
Esophagus	0.05
Thyroid	0.05
Skin	0.01
Bone surface	0.01
Remainder	0.05*†

NOTE: The values have been developed from a reference population of equal numbers of both sexes and a wide range of ages. In the definition of effective dose, they apply to workers, to the whole population, and to either sex.

*For purposes of calculation, the remainder is composed of the following additional tissues and organs: adrenals, brain, upper large intestine, small intestine, kidney, muscle, pancreas, spleen, thymus, and uterus. The list includes organs that are likely to be selectively irradiated. Some organs in the list are known to be susceptible to cancer induction. If other tissues and organs subsequently become identified as having a significant risk of induced cancer, they will then be included either with a specific w_t or in this additional list constituting the remainder. The latter also may include other tissues or organs selectively irradiated.

†In exceptional cases in which a single one of the remainder tissues or organs receives an equivalent dose in excess of the highest dose in any of the 12 organs for which a weighting factor is specified, a weighting factor of 0.025 should be applied to that tissue or organ and a weighting factor of 0.025 should be applied to that tissue or organ and a weighting factor of 0.025 should be applied to the average dose in the rest of the remainder as defined above.

SOURCE: Data from NCRP, 1987, and ICRP, 1990.

The effective dose, H_E, is defined as a doubly weighted dose, weighted for radiation type and the tissue at risk.

$$H_E = w_t H(D)(w_r) \qquad (25\text{-}17)$$

This concept is useful in the case of occupational exposure, because H_E values from different sources to different organs can be summed to yield a direct estimate of total cancer and genetic risk.

Table 25-3 is taken from ICRP (1990) and gives the values of w_t for various organs. The occupational guideline for H_E is 20 mSv per annum (NCRP, 1987a; ICRP, 1990). This requires that the sum of all H_E be less than or equal to this value:

$$H_E = \sum w_t H \leq 20 \text{ mSv} \qquad (25\text{-}18)$$

In 1990, the ICRP revised its 1977 estimates of risk and adopted and published Publication 60. This document includes new estimates of risk for both fatal and nonfatal cancer and new guidelines for the exposure of workers to external and internal radiation. The risk estimates are based largely on the analysis of Japanese atom bomb survivors. The occupational guidelines for radiation protection developed from the 1990 document are 100 mSv in 5 years (average, 20 mSv per year) with a limit of 50 mSv in any single year. This is compared with the 1977 limit of 50 mSv per year.

Table 25-4
Nominal Probability Coefficients for Individual Tissues and Organs

TISSUE OR ORGAN	Probability of Fatal Cancer 10^{-2} Sv^{-1}		Aggregated Getriment 10^{-2} Sv^{-1}	
	WHOLE POPULATION	WORKERS	WHOLE POPULATION	WORKERS
Bladder	0.30	0.24	0.29	0.24
Bone marrow	0.50	0.40	1.04	0.83
Bone surface	0.05	0.04	0.07	0.06
Breast	0.20	0.16	0.36	0.29
Colon	0.85	0.68	1.03	0.82
Liver	0.15	0.12	0.16	0.13
Lung	0.85	0.68	0.80	0.64
Esophagus	0.30	0.24	0.24	0.19
Ovary	0.10	0.08	0.15	0.12
Skin	0.02	0.02	0.04	0.03
Stomach	1.10	0.88	1.00	0.80
Thyroid	0.08	0.06	0.15	0.12
Remainder	0.50	0.40	0.59	0.47
Total	5.00	4.00	5.92	4.74
	Probability of Severe Hereditary Disorders			
Gonads	1.00	0.6	1.33	0.80
Grand total (rounded)			7.3	5.6

NOTE: The values relate to a population of equal numbers of both sexes and a wide range of ages.
SOURCE: Data from ICRP, 1990.

The ICRP document (ICRP, 1990) is a response to the increase in lifetime cancer risk from ionizing radiation observed in atom bomb survivors. Mental retardation for those exposed in utero is a finding in the atom bomb survivor cohort and is now included in the risk estimates.

The overall risk per unit exposure for adult workers and the risk for the whole population given in the ICRP (1990) are shown in Table 25-4. The risk of fatal cancer is adopted as 0.04 per sievert [4% per sievert (100 rem)] for adult workers and 0.05 per sievert [5% per sievert (100 rem)], for the whole adult population.

The NCRP (1993) chose to limit exposure to 20 mSv per year with a lifetime limit of (age $\times$ 10 mSv). The ICRP had been criticized for excluding the effects of nonfatal cancer in previous documents. An attempt to correct this omission was made in ICRP 60 (1990). An attempt was made to calculate the total detriment and is given the notation *aggregated detriment*. The aggregated detriment is the product of four factors: the probability of attributable fatal cancer, the weighted probability of nonfatal cancer, the weighted probability of severe hereditary effects, and the relative length of life lost. The nominal probability of fatal cancer per sievert, F, and the aggregated detriment are shown in Table 25-4. The computation of the aggregated detriment proceeds as follows. A cancer lethality fraction, K (the fraction of total cancer that is lethal), is used as a weighting factor for nonfatal cancers. The total number of cancers (fatal plus nonfatal) Sv^{-1} will be F/K. The total number of nonfatal cancers is $(1 - K)F/K$. The total weighted detriment is then

$$F + K(1 - K)F/K = F(2 - K)$$

The aggregated detriment is then the product of $F(2 - K)$ times the relative length of life lost, l/l_{av}, for a particular can-

cer. The average length of life lost, l_{av}, is 15 years per cancer. The aggregated detriment is tabulated as 7.3^{-2} Sv^{-1} for the whole adult population and 5.6×10^{-2} Sv^{-1} for the working population.

In assessing radiation risk from low-dose, low-dose-rate, low-LET radiation using risk coefficients derived from high-dose, high-dose-rate exposures, a dose and rate reduction factor (DDREF) is applied. This effectively lowers the response to a linear no threshold (LNT) curve. NCRP (1980) and the United Nations Scientific Committee on the Effects of Atomic Radiation (UNSCEAR, 1988, 1993, 2000) have shown that the human data cover a range for the DDREF of 2–10. That is, the original risk coefficients derived from the high-dose data are divided by the DDREF factor to obtain the best linear estimate of effects at typical low-dose exposures. ICRP has used 2.5 as the adopted DDREF; however, in ICRP (1990) a DDREF of 2.0 was used, and this is incorporated in the nominal probability coefficients in Table 25-4. Table 25-4 is used universally to assess the effects of occupational exposure. The latest model (NAS BEIR VII, 2006) reduced the DDREF to 1.5.

The overall objective of both NCRP and ICRP dose limitation recommendations is to control the lifetime risk to maximally exposed individuals. ICRP (1990) limits the lifetime occupational effective dose to (20 mSv 50 years) = 1000 mSv. In 1993, NCRP (1993) reduced the U.S. Recommendation for Lifetime Exposure to (age $\times$ 10 mSv) or approximately 700 mSv, with an average annual limit of 20 mSv and a maximum annual limit of 50 mSv.

The dose to members of the public is also considered by ICRP and NCRP. For continuous exposure to human-made sources, i.e., other than medical or natural, it is recommended that the annual effective dose not exceed 1 mSv (100 mrem), and for infrequent exposures the annual effective dose should not exceed 5 mSv (500 mrem).

Committed Equivalent Dose

A problem arises with internal emitters in that once they are ingested, there is an irreversible dose that is committed because of the biokinetics of the particular element. The absorbed dose depends on the biological and physical half-times of the element in the body. For this reason, the concepts of committed equivalent dose and committed effective dose were derived to accommodate the potential for the dose to be delivered over long periods after incorporation in the body. The committed dose is taken over a 50-year interval after exposure and is equal to

$$H_{t,50} = \int_{t_0}^{t_0+50} H_t \, dt \qquad (25\text{-}19)$$

where $H_{t,50}$ = 50-year dose to tissue T for a single intake at time t_0, and H_t = equivalent dose rate in organ or tissue T at time t.

The NCRP (1987a,b, 1993) recognizes that for radionuclides with half-lives ranging up to about 3 months, the committed equivalent dose is equal to the annual dose for the year of intake. For longer-lived nuclides, the committed equivalent dose will be greater than the annual equivalent dose and must be calculated on an individual basis. ICRP Publication 30 (ICRP, 1978) provides the details of this calculation for all nuclides.

Negligible Individual Risk Level (Negligible Dose)

The current radiobiologic principle commonly accepted is that of linear, nonthreshold cancer induction from ionizing radiation. Thus, regardless of the magnitude of the dose, a numerical cancer risk can be calculated. For this reason, the NCRP proposed the negligible individual risk level (NIRL) and defined it as "a level of annual excess risk of fatal health effects attributable to irradiation below which further effort to reduce radiation exposure to the individual is unwarranted."

The NCRP emphasized that the NIRL is not to be confused with an acceptable risk level, a level of significance, or a limit.

The NCRP recommended an annual effective equivalent dose limit for continuous exposure of members of the public in some circumstances of 1 mSv (100 mrem). This value is in addition to that received from natural background radiation (about 2 mSv). In this context, the NIRL was taken to be 1/100th of this value or 0.01 mSv (1 mrem). In NCRP (1993) the notation used currently is negligible individual dose (NID).

MECHANISMS OF DNA DAMAGE AND MUTAGENESIS

Energy Deposition in the Cell Nucleus

DNA is a double-helical macromolecule consisting of four repeating units: the purine bases adenine (A) and guanine (G) and the pyrimidine bases thymine (T) and cytosine (C). The bases are arranged in two linear arrays (or strands) held together by hydrogen bonds centrally and linked externally by covalent bonds to sugar-phosphate residues (the DNA "backbone"). The adenine base pairs naturally with thymine (A:T base pair), while guanine pairs with cytosine (G:C base pair), so that one DNA strand has the complementary sequence of the other. The sequence of the bases defines the genetic code; each gene has a unique sequence, but certain common sequences exist in control and structural DNA elements. Damage to DNA may affect any one of its components, but it is the loss or alteration of base sequence that has genetic consequences (UNSCEAR, 2000).

Ionizing radiation loses energy and slows down by forming ion pairs (a positively charged atom and an electron). Different ionization densities result from gamma rays, beta particles, and alpha particles. Their track structure is broadly characterized as from sparsely ionizing (or low-LET), to densely ionizing (high-LET) radiation. Each track of low-LET radiation, resulting from X-rays or gamma rays, consists of a few ionizations across an average-sized cell nucleus (e.g., an electron set in motion by a gamma ray crossing an 8 μm-diameter nucleus gives an average of about 70 ionizations, equivalent to about 5 mGy (500 mrad) absorbed dose. Individual tracks vary widely about this value because of the stochastic nature of energy deposition, i.e., variability of ion pars per μm and path length through the nucleus. A high-LET alpha particle produces many thousands of ionizations and gives a relatively high dose to the cell. For example, a 4-MeV alpha-particle track yields on average, about 30,000 ionizations (3 Gy, 300 rad) in an average-sized cell nucleus. However, within the nucleus even low-LET gamma radiation will give some microregions of relatively dense ionization over the dimensions of DNA structures due to the low-energy electrons set in motion (UNSCEAR, 2000). The studies of single strand breaks (SSB) with low-energy electrons indicate that the energy threshold is practically zero (Panajotovic et al., 2006).

There was a long-standing belief that the cell nucleus must be irradiated for any biological effect to occur. In the past 15 years, research on epigenetic effects has shown this is not the case. Epigenetic (or nontargeted) effects include genomic instability (the increase in genomic alterations), bystander effects (damage that occurs in cells not traversed by radiation but close by), cytoplasmic/membrane effects (bystander effects after cytoplasm irradiation), clastogenic effects (detrimental effects from irradiated plasma), abscopal effects (partial volume irradiation induces damage in the whole organ), and transgenerational (instability passed through the germ line) effects. The new information concerning epigenetic effects (Little, 2006), although adding immensely to biological and mechanistic understanding, should not affect risk calculations which are based on observed exposure response in human and animal populations. The underlying mechanistic information should lead to better lifetime risk projection models.

Direct and Indirect Ionization

Radiation tracks may deposit energy directly in DNA (direct effect) or may ionize other molecules closely associated with DNA, hydrogen, or oxygen, to form free radicals that can damage DNA (indirect effect). Within a cell, the indirect effect occurs over very short distances, of the order of a few nanometers. The diffusion distance of radicals is limited by their reactivity. Although it is difficult to measure accurately the different contributions made by the direct and indirect effects to DNA damage caused by low-LET radiation, evidence from radical scavengers introduced into cells suggests that about 35% is exclusively direct and 65% has an indirect (scavengeable) component (Reuvers et al., 1973).

It has been argued that both direct and indirect effects cause similar early damage to DNA; this is because the ion radicals produced by direct ionization of DNA may react further to produce DNA radicals similar to those produced by water-radical attack on DNA (Ward, 1975; Cadet et al., 1999).

Douki *et al.* (2006) measured oxidized bases following irradiation of isolated DNA and human monocytes. The study used the heavy ions $^{12}C(6+)$ and $^{36}Ar(18+)$ and showed that direct ionization is a small contributor to base damage and hydroxyl radicals are major contributors. There is no consensus on the ratio of direct/indirect damage.

DNA Damage

Ionization frequently disrupts chemical bonding in cellular molecules such as DNA. If the majority of ionizations occur as single isolated events (low-LET radiation), the disruptions are readily repaired by cellular enzymes. The average density of ionization by high-LET radiations is such that several ionizations may occur as the particle traverses a DNA double helix. Therefore, much of the damage from high-LET radiations, as well as a minority of the DNA damage from low-LET radiations, will derive from localized clusters of ionizations that can severely disrupt the DNA structure (Ward, 1994). While the extent of local clustering of ionizations in DNA from single tracks of low- and high-LET radiations will overlap, high-LET radiation tracks are more efficient at inducing larger clusters and hence more complex damage. Also, high-LET radiations will induce some very large clusters of ionizations that do not occur with low-LET radiations; the resulting damage may be irreparable and may also have unique cellular consequences (Goodhead, 1994). When a cell is damaged by high-LET radiation, each track will give large numbers of ionizations, so that the cell will receive a relatively high dose, as noted in the calculation above, and there will be a greater probability of correlated damage within a single DNA molecule. As a consequence, the irradiation of a population of cells or a tissue with a "low dose" of high-LET radiation results in a few cells being hit with a relatively high dose (one track) rather than in each cell receiving a small dose. In contrast, low-LET radiation is more uniformly distributed over the cell population. At doses of low-LET radiation in excess of about 1 mGy (for an average-size cell nucleus of 8 μm in diameter), each cell nucleus is likely to be traversed by more than one sparsely ionizing track.

The interaction of ionizing radiation with DNA produces numerous types of damage; the chemical products of many of these have been identified and classified according to their structure. These products differ according to which chemical bond is attacked, which base is modified, and the extent of the damage within a given segment of DNA. Table 25-5 lists some of the main damage products that can be measured following low-LET irradiation of DNA, with a rough estimate of their abundance (UNSCEAR, 2000). Attempts have also been made to predict the frequencies of different damage types from the knowledge of radiation track structure, with certain assumptions about the minimum energy deposition (number of ionizations) required. Interactions can be classified according to the probability that they will cause a single-strand DNA alteration (e.g., a break in the backbone or base alteration) or alterations in both strands in close proximity in one DNA molecule (e.g., a double-strand break), or a more complex type of DNA damage (e.g., a double-strand break with adjacent damage). Good agreement has been obtained between these predictions and direct measurements of single-strand breaks, but there is less agreement for other categories of damage. While complex forms of damage are difficult to quantify with current experimental techniques, the use of enzymes that cut DNA at sites of base damage suggests that irradiation of DNA in solution gives complex damage sites consisting mainly of closely spaced base damage (measured as oxidized bases of aba-

Table 25-5

Estimated Yields of DNA Damage in Mammalian Cells Caused by Low-LET Radiation Exposures

TYPE OF DAMAGE	YIELD (NUMBER OF DEFECTS PER CELL Gy^{-1})
Single-strand breaks	1000
Base damage*	500
Double-strand breaks	40
DNA protein cross-links	150

*Base excision enzyme-sensitive sites or antibody detection of thymine glycol.
SOURCE: Data from UNSCEAR, 2000.

sic sites); double-strand breaks were associated with only 20% of the complex damage sites (Sutherland *et al.*, 2000). It is expected that the occurrence of more complex types of damage will increase with increasing LET, and that this category of damage will be less repairable than the simpler forms of damage. Theoretical simulations have predicted that about 30% of DNA double-strand breaks from low-LET radiation are complex because of additional breaks (Nikjoo *et al.*, 1997) and that this proportion rises to more than 70%, and the degree of complexity increases, for high-LET particles (Goodhead and Nikjoo, 1997).

Some of the DNA damage caused by ionizing radiation is chemically similar to damage that occurs naturally in the cell. This "spontaneous" damage arises from the thermal instability of DNA as well as endogenous oxidative and enzymatic processes. Several metabolic pathways produce oxidative radicals within the cell, and these radicals can attack DNA to give both DNA base damage and breakage, mostly as isolated events. The more complex types of damage caused by radiation may not occur spontaneously, because localized concentrations of endogenous radicals are less likely to be generated in the immediate vicinity of DNA (UNSCEAR, 2000).

HUMAN STUDIES OF RADIATION TOXICITY

There have been five major studies of the health detriment resulting from exposure of humans to ionizing radiation. Other studies of large worker populations exposed to very low levels of radiation and environmental populations exposed to radon are ongoing, but they are not expected to provide new data on the risk estimates from ionizing radiation. These worker or environmental populations are studied to ensure that there is no inconsistency in the radiation risk data in extrapolating from the higher exposures. The basic studies on which the quantitative risk calculations are founded include radium exposures, atom bomb survivors, underground miners exposed to radon, patients irradiated with X-rays for ankylosing spondylitis, and children irradiated with X-rays for tinea capitis (ringworm).

Radium Exposures (^{226,228}Ra)

Radium was discovered in the early part of the twentieth century. Its unique properties suggested a potential for the healing arts. It was incorporated into a wide variety of nostrums, medicines, and artifacts. The highest exposure occurred in the United States among radium dial painters who ingested from 10s to 1000s of micrograms (microcuries). These exposed groups, including patients, chemists, and dial painters, have been studied for over 60 years to determine the body retention of radium and the health effects of long-term body burdens.

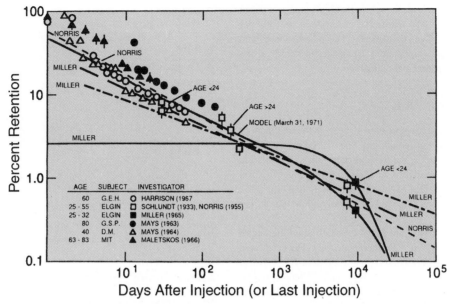

Figure 25-4. *Whole-body radium retention in humans. Summary of all available data for adult humans. (From Marshall et al., ICRP Report Number 20, 1972.)*

The only late effect of ingestion of ^{226,228}Ra seen is osteogenic sarcoma. It is significant that no study has identified a statistically significant excess of leukemia after even massive doses of radium. This implies that the target cells for leukemia residing in bone marrow are outside the short range of the radium series alpha particles (70 μm). Several thousand people were exposed to radium salts either as part of the modish therapies using radium in the era from 1900 to 1930 or occupationally in the radium dial-painting industry around 1920. Radium therapy was accepted by the American Medical Association, and in around 1915 advertisements were common for radium treatment of rheumatism and as a general tonic and in the treatment of mental disorders. Solutions were available for drinking that contained 2 μg/60 cm^3 as well as ampoules for intravenous injection containing 5–100 μg radium (Woodard, 1980). Luminous paint was developed before World War I, and in 1917 there were many plants in New England and New Jersey painting watch dials, clocks, and military instruments (Woodard, 1980).

The first large studies on osteogenic sarcoma in radium-exposed people were done by Martland (1931) and Aub *et al.* (1952), who found 30 cases of bone sarcoma; Evans *et al.* (1969) with 496 cases of sarcoma out of 1064 studied at the Massachusetts Institute of Technology; and Rowland *et al.* (1978), with 61 cases out of 1474 female dial painters (Woodard, 1980).

Radium, once ingested, is somewhat similar to calcium in its metabolism and is incorporated on bone surfaces into the mineralized portion of bone. The long half-life of ^{226}Ra (1600 years) allows distribution throughout the mineral skeleton over life. The target cells for osteogenic sarcoma reside in marrow on endosteal surfaces at about 10 μm from the bone surface. At long times after exposure, target cells are beyond the range of alpha particles from radium not on bone surfaces.

The loss of radium from the body by excretion was determined to follow a relatively simple power function (Norris *et al.*, 1958):

$$R = 0.54t^{-0.52} \tag{25-20}$$

where R is the total body retention and t the time in days.

Other models to fit the data were developed as more information became available, the most recent being that of Marshall *et al.* (1972). The entire body of radium data and the various models are shown in Fig. 25-4. It can be seen that the Norris function fits the observed data well except at very long times after exposure. A simplified form of the more complex later model of Marshall *et al.* (1972) which fits the human data over all observed times is

$$R = 0.8_t^{-0.5}(0.5e^{8t} + 0.5e - 4^{8t}) \tag{25-21}$$

where R is the whole body retention; 8 the rate of bone apposition or resorption = 0.0001 day^{-1}; and t the time in days.

For most purposes, the Norris formula is applicable. It can be seen from Fig. 25-4 for the Norris equation that even 1 year after exposure, only about 2% of the radium is retained in the body but that after 30 years, about 0.5% remains. The risk of osteogenic bone cancer after radium exposure has been summarized in the National Academy of Sciences report BEIR IV (NAS, 1988).

Equations were proposed by Rowland *et al.* (1978) for the annual risk of sarcoma (including the natural risk), and expressed as a function of either radium intake or dose from ^{226,228}Ra. Risk per unit intake is

$$I = [0.7 \times 10^{-5} + (7 \times 10^{-8})D^2] \exp[-(1.1 \times 10^{-3})D] \tag{25-22}$$

where I is the total bone sarcomas per person year at risk and D the total systemic intake of ^{226}Ra plus 2.5 times total systemic intake of ^{228}Ra (both in microcuries).

Risk per unit dose is

$$I = [10^{-5} + (9.8 \times 10^{-6})D^2] \exp(-1.5 \times 10^{-2}D) \tag{25-23}$$

where I is the total bone sarcomas per person year at risk and D the total mean skeletal dose in Gray from ^{226}Ra plus 1.5 times mean skeletal dose from ^{228}Ra.

Raabe *et al.* (1980) modeled bone sarcoma risk in the human, dog, and mouse and determined that there is a practical threshold dose and dose rate (a dose low enough so that bone cancer will not appear within the human life span). The dose rate is 0.04 Gy per day or a total dose of 0.8 Gy to the skeleton. This practical threshold for bone cancer has useful implications in considering health effects from exposures to environmental radioactivity.

Radium Exposure (^{224}Ra)

In Europe, ^{224}Ra was used for more than 40 years in the treatment of tuberculosis and ankylosing spondylitis. The treatment of children was abandoned in the 1950s, but the ability to relieve debilitating pain from ankylosing spondylitis in adults has prolonged its use. ^{224}Ra is different from ^{226}Ra in that it has a short half-life (3.62 days) and the alpha dose is delivered completely while the radium is still on bone surfaces.

Spiess and Mays (1970) and Mays (1988) studied the health of 899 German patients given ^{224}Ra therapeutically. The calculated average mean skeletal dose was 30 Gy (range, 0.06–57.5 Gy) with injection time spans ranging from 1 to 45 months. There were two groups—juveniles and adults—and the bone sarcoma response was not significantly different for the two. There were 60 patients who developed bone sarcoma (Gossner, 1999), 46 have been studied for histologic type. Further study of this group revealed other solid tumors with statistically significant excesses of male and female breast cancer, thyroid cancer, and liver cancer (Nekolla *et al.*, 1999).

In a second cohort, Wick *et al.* (1986, 1999) studied 1432 adult patients treated for ankylosing spondylitis with an average skeletal dose of 0.65 Gy. This study was originally started by Otto Hug and Fritz Schales and has been continued since their deaths. Four patients in this group have developed osteogenic sarcoma, and one in the control group.

Spiess and Mays (1973) found that the observed effectiveness of the ^{224}Ra in their cohort in producing bone sarcomas increased if the time span of the injections was long. Injections were given in 1, 10, or 50 weekly fractions. They developed an empiric expression to estimate the added risk from this protracted injection schedule:

$$I = \{0.003 + 0.014[1 - \exp(0.09m)]\}D \qquad (25\text{-}24)$$

where I is the cumulative incidence of bone sarcomas after most tumors have appeared (25 years); m the span of injections in months; and D the average skeletal dose in Gy.

Chemelevsky *et al.* (1986) analyzed the Spiess data and developed an equation for the total cumulative sarcoma risk from ^{224}Ra:

$$R = (0.0085D + 0.0017D^2)\exp(-0.025D) \qquad (25\text{-}25)$$

where R is the cumulative risk of bone sarcoma and D the average skeletal dose in Gy.

These two equations for risk predict 5.7 and 5.8 bone sarcomas in the second series of (spondylitis) patients, with two actually observed.

Chemelevsky *et al.* (1986) also showed that in the Spiess study, linearity (sarcoma response with dose) could be rejected. For example, Eq. (25-22) results in a lifetime risk of sarcoma of 0.02 Gy^{-1} at an average skeletal dose of 10 Gy but 0.01 Gy^{-1} at 1 Gy. Also, there was no difference in sarcoma response between juveniles and adults. These data are presented in Fig. 25-5. Again, no excess leukemia was found in either series of ^{224}Ra patients.

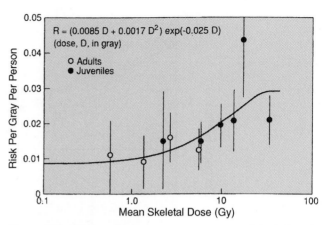

Figure 25-5. Lifetime risk per gray versus mean skeletal dose in ^{224}Ra exposed subjects. (From Chemelevsky et al., 1986, with permission.)

Atomic Bomb Survivors

The A-bomb survivor risk estimates are particularly important because the guidelines for occupational exposure are based on their experience. On August 6, 1945, the U.S. military dropped an atomic bomb on the city of Hiroshima, Japan. Three days later a second bomb was dropped on Nagasaki which effectively ended World War II. The weapons were of two different types, the first being ^{235}U and the second a ^{239}Pu device.

Within 1 km of the explosions in both cities, a total of 64,000 people were killed by the blast and the thermal effects as a result of the instantaneous gamma and neutron radiation released by the weapons. Others between 1 and 2 km from the hypocenter (the point on earth directly below the detonation point in air) received radiation doses up to several gray. Beyond 2.5 km there was no additional dose from the weapon, only natural background radiation.

Within a few years it was decided to follow the health of the people in both cities over their lifetime to determine quantitatively the effects of external ionizing radiation. The study of prospective mortality of A-bomb survivors was initiated by the Atomic Bomb Casualty Commission (ABCC) in 1950 and is ongoing by the Radiation Effects Research Foundation (RERF). The main study, called the Life Span Study (LSS), included 120,000 people, 92,228 people within 10,000 m of the hypocenter and 26,850 people who were not in either city at the time of bombing (ATB). The most recent reports of the RERF (1987, 2003) are follow-up of the cancer mortality of a subcohort (DS86 subcohort) of 75,991 persons over the periods 1950–1985, 1950–1990 (Pierce and Preston, 1993) and 1950–1997 (Preston *et al.*, 2004). The cohort includes 86,572 persons with individual dose estimates. The latest update (Preston *et al.*, 2003) report that 440 (5%) of the solid cancer deaths and 250 (0.8%) of the noncancer deaths were associated with the radiation exposure. There have been a total of 9335 cancer deaths and 31,881 noncancer deaths in 47 years of follow up.

In 1978, questions arose that the original dose estimates for persons in the LSS might be somewhat in error and that an effort should be made to improve the dose estimates. This study was published in a United States–Japan joint reassessment of dose called DS86—Dosimetry System 1986 (RERF, 1987).

Dose estimation by reconstruction of the event is always problematic, but direct computation of dose to about 18,500 persons in the LSS with detailed shielding information is complete. The remaining DS86 dose values for 57,000 individuals without detailed shielding information are also incorporated into the mortality study by various estimation techniques. Of the 75,991 persons in the DS86 subcohort, 16,207 were within 2000 m of the hypocenter, and these are the individuals who received a substantial exposure.

A new study of the A-bomb dosimetry was funded by the U.S. Department of Energy to address questions arising about the accuracy of the calculated neutron and gamma ray dose as a function of distance from the hypocenter. *The report, DS02: A new dosimetry system for A-bomb survivor studies, is available on the web www.rerf.or.jp/top/introe.htm.*

The new calculations and measurements produced during this reassessment confirmed the yield and epicenter for the Nagasaki detonation while refining these values for Hiroshima. Current measurements and calculations confirm a 21-kiloton-yield for the Nagasaki bomb and a burst point to within 2 m of previous assessments. In Hiroshima, the estimated yield has been increased from 15 kilotons to16 kilotons and the epicenter has been repositioned 20 m higher and 15 m to the west. While supercomputing technology made recalculation of the nuclear explosions possible, application of current geographic information systems technology has reconciled the exact hypocenter locations on new, more accurate maps with World War II vintage maps.

Some details from the press release concerning the new dosimetry (DS02) report, "New air over ground calculations together with newly revised fluence to dose factors resulted in recalculated estimates of the free-in-air doses from the Hiroshima weapon of about 8–10% average increase over DS86 in the total gamma-ray doses, and about 10% increase in the average neutron doses but approximately the same variation of dose with distance from the hypocenter as in DS86. Increasing the height of burst and incorporating new information on exact locations of sites relative to the epicenter did, however, improve the agreement with measurements near the hypocenter and with the slope of measurement data versus distance.

The gamma rays account for the preponderance of absorbed radiation doses to the survivors, the neutron absorbed dose at most organ depths (and distances from the hypocenter) being about 1%

of the gamma-ray absorbed dose at Hiroshima. (Note that the equivalent dose from the neutrons depends on the appropriate RBE for the neutrons, e.g., RBE of 20 would yield an equivalent dose for the neutrons of perhaps 20% of the total equivalent dose. In future risk estimations the neutron contribution at Hiroshima, about four times that at Nagasaki, should be accounted for.) Because the new DS02 fluences do not differ by much from those in DS86, one would not expect large changes in organ dose estimates for individual survivors. However, improved estimates of shielding and survivor location may result in some changes in organ dose to some survivors.

A report on the updated cancer risk using DS02 states that "For both solid cancer and leukemia, estimated age–time patterns and sex difference are virtually unchanged by the dosimetry revision. The estimates of solid-cancer radiation risk per sievert and the curvilinear dose response for leukemia are both decreased by about 8% by the dosimetry revision, due to the increase in the gamma ray dose estimates. The apparent shape of the dose response is virtually unchanged by the dosimetry revision."

The National Academy of Sciences assembled a committee (BEIR VII) to estimate the risk from low exposures to external gamma ray exposure based on the updated DS02 A-bomb dosimetry (NAS, 2006). Their estimate of lifetime excess cancer cases for an exposure of 0.1 Sv is 0.8 and 1.3% for men and women respectively. The absolute risk for men and women is similar but the excess risk differs because the baseline rate for women is much lower than for men.

Previous reports of cancer risk estimates were based on the air dose (gamma ray plus neutron tissue kerma in air) adjusted for shielding by structures or terrain. The 1987 and 1988 reports also include DS86 organ dose estimates, and these are about 80% of the shielded kerma (Shimizu *et al.*, 1988). The DS02 dosimetry improves the individual's shielding data.

The dose from fallout at Hiroshima and Nagasaki has not been included in the health effects studies. Fallout was found in certain restricted localities in Nagasaki and Hiroshima. The absorbed dose

Table 25-6

Observed and Expected Cases of Cancer in A-Bomb Survivors with DS86 Dose Estimate and Projections of Lifetime Cancer Incidence from Radiation for a Dose of 0.1 Sv

CANCER TYPE	OBSERVED CASES	EXPECTED CASES	MEAN DOSE (Sv)	Projection of Lifetime Cancer Incidence (%) for a Dose of 0.1 Sv*	
				MALES	FEMALES
Esophagus	84	77.4	0.23	0.04	0.02
Stomach	1307	1222	0.23	0.17	0.17
Colon	223	193.7	0.23	0.13	0.19
Liver	284	254.5	0.24	0.23	0.41
Lung	456	364.7	0.25	0.23	0.07
Breast	295	200	0.27	0.0	0.52
Thyroid	132	94.3	0.26	0.07	0.04
Urinary bladder	115	98.1	0.23	0.03	0.13
Other solid cancer				0.26	0.15
Solid cancer				1.16	1.70
Leukemia	141	67.4	0.25	0.05	0.05
Total				1.21	1.75

*Projection of cancer incidence based on the attained age model. Data from UNSCEAR (2000), and a whole-body exposure of 0.1 Sv at age 30. Mortality projections for total cancer 0.67 and 0.99% per 0.1 Sv, for males and females, respectively.

from gamma rays at Nagasaki for persons continuously in the fallout area from 1 hour ranged from 0.12 to 0.24 Gy. The absorbed doses at Hiroshima ranged from 0.006 to 0.02 Gy. Because the region of fallout was quite limited, the total contribution of fallout to survivor dose was probably negligible in Hiroshima but may have been significant for a limited number of survivors in Nagasaki, where an exposure of one-fifth the maximum extends over some 1000 hectares. Estimates of internal dose from ingested ^{137}Cs yield about 0.0001 Gy integrated over 40 years (Harley, 1987; RERF, 1987).

Complete mortality data and the dose estimates are reported in RERF Technical Reports 5-88 (RERF, 1987) and were updated by Pierce and Preston (1993) and in UNSCEAR (2000). The projected lifetime cancer risks as of the follow-up through 1990 are reported in UNSCEAR (2000), and these data are summarized in Table 25-6.

No statistically significant excess cancer of the gallbladder, bone, pancreas, uterus, prostate, or malignant lymphoma has been seen in the LSS to date. The latest data (Preston *et al.*, 2003) show a statistically significant excess of heart disease, stroke, digestive, and respiratory disease. The noncancer diseases were associated with exposures greater than 0.5 Sv.

It is of interest to consider the effect of smoking, as it is the most important factor in assessing lung cancer risk. The analysis performed by Shimuzu *et al.* (1988) examined the interaction of smoking and radiation in detail. The results showed no interaction indicating that smoking and the atom bomb radiation act independently rather than multiplicatively in lung cancer induction.

It is also possible to model the risk over the full life if a projection model is assumed. RERF originally preferred a constant relative risk model (radiation mortality is a constant fraction of the baseline age-specific mortality per gray) for this purpose. However, there is now evidence in the atom bomb mortality and in several other studies discussed later (ankylosing spondylitis patients, uranium miners) that the constant relative risk model is not appropriate. The excess relative risk (ERR) decreases both with time subsequent to exposure and with attained age. One model projects ERR only as a function of age at exposure because this is the stronger effect. These are biologically plausible models suggesting the loss or repair of the damaged stem cell population.

The estimates of lifetime risk of cancer may increase somewhat with time, but given the present age of the population, the final values based on risk projections from the DS02 dosimetry are unlikely to be significantly higher than the values in Table 25-6.

Tinea Capitis (Ringworm) Irradiation

During the period 1905–1960, X-ray epilation in the treatment of tinea capitis was performed regularly in children. The treatment was introduced by Sabouraud in 1904 and was standardized by Kienbock (1907) and Adamson (1909). Over the half century it was used, as many as 200,000 children worldwide may have been irradiated (Albert *et al.*, 1986).

No follow-up studies of the long-term effects of irradiation were performed until Albert and Omran (1968) reported on 2200 children irradiated at the Skin and Cancer Unit of New York University Hospital during 1940–1959. Subsequent publications on this group have appeared at regular intervals (Shore *et al.*, 1976, 1984, 2002, 2003; Shore, 1990). In the follow-up studies to 2002, there were 2224 irradiated children and 1380 in the control group. Since the New York University (NYU) study, a follow-up of 11,000 children irradiated in Israel was performed (Ron and Modan, 1984; Ron *et al.*, 1988, 1991).

Table 25-7

Average Dose to Organs in the Head and Neck from Measurements Performed with a Phantom for a Child's Head

ORGAN	AVERAGE DOSE AT 25 cm TREATMENT DISTANCE, Rad
Scalp	220–540
Brain	140
Eye	16
Internal ear	71
Cranial marrow	385
Pituitary	49
Parotid gland	39
Thyroid	6
Skin (eyelid)	16
Skin (nose)	11
Skin (midneck)	9

The mean age of children irradiated in both the New York and Israeli studies was between 7 and 8 years. The age range in the New York study was 1–15 years at the time of treatment. Dose reconstruction in the NYU series was performed using a head phantom containing the skull of a 7-year-old child covered with tissue-equivalent material (Schulz and Albert, 1963; Harley *et al.*, 1976, 1983). The doses to organs in the head and neck for a typical Adamson–Kienbock five-field treatment of the scalp are shown in Table 25-7, and the dose to the skin is shown in Fig. 25-6.

In the NYU series there were two thyroid cancers with no expected cases and 11 thyroid adenomas with 1 expected. (Shore *et al.*, 2003). In the Israeli series there were 43 thyroid cancers with 10.7 expected cases. In the NYU series there are 128 skin lesions, predominantly basal cell carcinoma, with 24 expected cases, in 41 persons. Fairness of skin is an important factor in the appearance of skin cancer (Shore *et al.*, 1984, 2002; Shore, 1990).

Skin cancer was found primarily in Caucasians even though 25% of the study population consisted of blacks. As of 2002, there were 128 cases of nonmelanoma skin cancer of the head and neck in the irradiated group and 21 in the control group. In the irradiated group 125 cases were Caucasian and 3 were African American. This and the fact that there appears to be a much lower dose response on the hair-covered scalp than on the face and neck (Harley *et al.*, 1983; Shore *et al.*, 2002) suggest that the promotional effects of UV radiation play an important role in skin cancer. The dose estimates for the thyroid in the Israeli study are 0.09 Gy and 0.06 Gy in the NYU study. The skin dose estimates range from 0.1 to 0.5 Gy on the face, but 2.5 Gy near the scalp margins.

A risk projection model was used to estimate the lifetime risk of basal cell carcinoma (BCC) for facial skin and for the hair-covered scalp after X-ray epilation in whites. The model used was a cumulative hazard plot which assumes that the BCC appearance rate in the exposed population remains constant over time (Harley *et al.*, 1983). The result of this risk projection for BCC is shown in Table 25-8.

The small numbers of tumors other than skin cancers in the NYU study make it of dubious value in estimating the lifetime risk per Gy although an excess is appearing (Shore *et al.*, 2003). There are (in 2003) 8 leukemia with 1 expected, 7 brain malignancies with none expected, and 6 salivary gland tumors with 2 expected. These are particularly important studies because children were the exposed

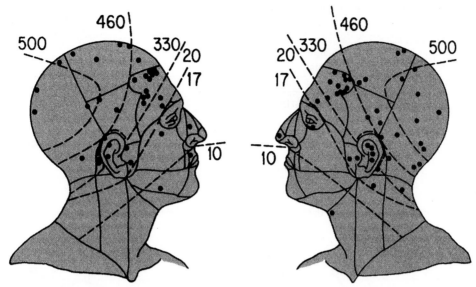

Figure 25-6. X-ray dose in rads for the Adamson–Kienbock five-field tinea capitis treatment and locations of basal cell lesions. (From Shore et al., 1984, with permission.)

Table 25-8

Estimated Lifetime Risk Estimates for Basal Cell Carcinoma (BCC) and Thyroid Cancer after X-Ray Irradiation for Tinea Capitis

	TOTAL INCIDENCE, RISK Gy^{-1}	MORTALITY, RISK Gy^{-1}
Skin malignancies (NYU study)		
BCC (facial skin)	0.32	
BCC (hair-covered scalp)	0.01	
Thyroid malignancies (Israeli study)		
Male	0.01	0.001
Female	0.04	0.004

group and because only partial body irradiation was involved. The temporal pattern of appearance of these tumors is also important. The dose was delivered over a short time interval (minutes at NYU and 5 days in Israel), and lifetime patterns are indicative of the underlying carcinogenic mechanisms.

Skin and thyroid cancers are of importance in documenting health effects from ionizing radiation. However, both types of cancer are rarely fatal. NCRP (1985) reported that about 10% of thyroid cancer is lethal. It is estimated that the fatality rate of skin cancer is 1% (NCRP, 1990). The lifetime risk per gray derived by NCRP for total thyroid cancer incidence (0.003 for females and 0.0014 for males for external X-ray or gamma radiation for persons under 18 years of age) is about a factor of 10 lower than that reported by Ron and Modan (1984; Ron *et al.*, 1991) in tinea capitis irradiations. However, the tinea irradiations were given to children with a mean age of about 7 years, also in the Israeli study there is apparently an increased sensitivity resulting from ethnicity.

The effect of ethnicity and sex is also suggested by NCRP (1985) for thyroid cancer. The incidence rates of spontaneous thyroid cancer for persons of Jewish origin in Europe and North Amer-

ica are three to four times that for other racial groups. There is an obvious susceptibility of women for thyroid cancer and adenomas in both the NYU and Israeli tinea capitis studies.

After 50 years of follow up in the New York Study, the cumulative incidence of basal cell skin cancer in the irradiated group is 16% and 4% in the control group.

Chernobyl and Radioactive Iodine (^{131}I)-Induced Thyroid Cancer

The Chernobyl accident (April 26, 1986) was the result of efforts to conduct a test on the electrical control system, which allows power to be provided in the event of a station blackout. The details of the accident have been published in reports of the International Atomic Energy Agency (IAEA, 2005) and UNSCEAR (2000). Basically, there was a rapid increase in the reactor power. Part of the fuel in the pressurized water reactor was vaporized, resulting in an explosion that blew the reactor core apart and destroyed much of the containment building. The estimates of the significant radionuclides for health effects released during the accident are 1.8 EBq (4.9×10^7 Ci) ^{131}I and 0.085 EBq (2.3×10^6 Ci) ^{137}Cs, and 0.01 EBq (2.7×10^5 Ci) ^{90}Sr and 0.003 Ebq of plutonium isotopes (UNSCEAR, 2000; IAEA, 2005). (Note 1 EBq = 10^{18} Bq, Becquerel).

The accident caused the deaths within days or weeks of 32 power plant employees and firemen (including 28 deaths that were due to radiation exposure). During 1986, 220,000 people were evacuated from areas surrounding the reactor, and, after 1986, about 250,000 people were relocated from what were at that time three constituent republics of the Soviet Union: Belarus, the Russian Federation, and Ukraine. Large areas in these three republics were contaminated, and deposition of fission product radionuclides was measurable in all countries of the northern hemisphere. In addition, about 280,000 workers, termed "liquidators," were mobilized in 1986 and 1987 to take part in major mitigation activities at the reactor and within the 30-km zone surrounding the reactor. Residual mitigation activities continued until 1990. In all, about 600,000 persons received the special status of "liquidator."

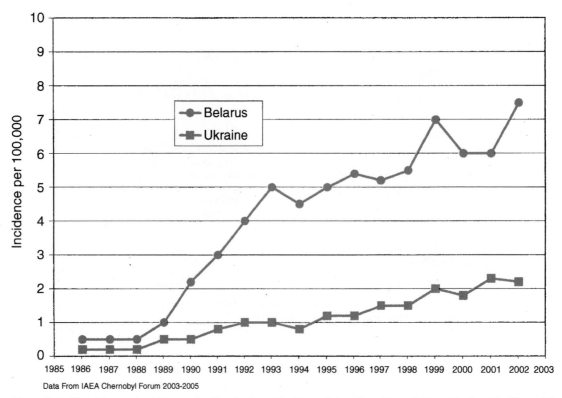

Data From IAEA Chernobyl Forum 2003-2005

Figure 25-7. *Thyroid cancer in children under 18 at the time of the Chernobyl accident. (From IAEA publication, The Chernobyl forum: 2003–2005.)*

The radiation exposures resulting from the Chernobyl accident were due initially to ^{131}I and short-lived radionuclides and subsequently to radiocesium (^{134}Cs and ^{137}Cs) from both external exposure and the consumption of foods contaminated with these radionuclides. UNSCEAR (1988) estimated that, outside the regions of Belarus, the Russian Federation, and Ukraine, thyroid doses averaged over large portions of European countries were 25 mGy for 1-year-old infants. However, the dose distribution was very heterogeneous, especially in countries near the reactor site. For example, in Poland, although the countrywide population-weighted average thyroid dose was estimated to be 8 mGy, the mean thyroid doses for the populations of particular districts ranged from 0.2 to 64 mGy. Individual dose values for about 5% of the children were 200 mGy. UNSCEAR (1988, 2000) estimates that effective dose averaged over large portions of European countries were 1 mSv or less in the first year after the accident and approximately two to five times the first-year dose over a full lifetime.

In 2002, there were 4000 cases of thyroid cancer in children from ^{131}I exposure in milk. The expected number of thyroid cancer cases is not known, but is evidently a small fraction of those observed. In 2002, there were 15 deaths related to the disease. No solid tumors other than thyroid cancer have been identified resulting from the accident. Figure 25-7 shows the sequential increase in the incidence per 100,000 of thyroid cancers in children under the age of 18 at the time of the accident. It is well established that release of ^{131}I presents the major health effect in a nuclear reactor accident. Many countries prepare for such accidents and have ready a large supply of potassium iodide (KI), which effectively blocks the thyroid uptake of radioactive iodine. Had this been available in time, and the fresh local milk supply shut down in favor of other sources, it is questionable whether the large number of tumors would have occurred.

Medical Administration of ^{131}I   Iodine-131 is given medically in three ways. Very large quantities, 3.7×10^9 Bq (100 mCi) or more are administered to ablate the thyroid in thyroid cancer, lesser quantities (about 10 mCi or 3.7×10^8 Bq) are given for hyperthyroidism, and the lowest quantity given (0.1 mCi or 3.7×10^6) is for diagnostic purposes (UNSCEAR, 1994). Individuals have also been exposed to ^{131}I as a result of nuclear weapons testing. Very few thyroid cancers have been found subsequent to these exposures, with the exception of the 243 Marshall Island inhabitants who received a large dose from a mixture of radionuclides (^{131}I, ^{132}I, ^{133}I, ^{134}I, and ^{135}I), tellurium, and gamma-ray radiation from the 1954 Bravo thermonuclear test (Conard *et al.*, 1984; Gilbert *et al.*, 2002) in the Pacific. The mean thyroid dose was estimated to be 3–52 Gy in children and 1.6–12 Gy in adults. Over a 32-year follow-up period, 7 of 130 women and 2 of 113 men developed thyroid cancer.

Attempts have been made to relate external gamma-ray radiation and ^{131}I exposure. The NCRP (1985) estimated from human data that the effectiveness ratio of ^{131}I/gamma-ray radiation is between 0.1 and 1.0. In a more recent review of the human data, Shore (1992) found 8.3 observed excess cancers derived from all ^{131}I studies and 37 cases based on risk estimates from external exposure. The ratio 8.3/37 yields an estimate for the effectiveness ratio of 0.22. The protracted dose to the thyroid during the decay of ^{131}I may explain the difference; however, the nonuniform distribution of ^{131}I in the thyroid also may be a factor (Sinclair *et al.*, 1956).

It is evident that ^{131}I can expose large populations after nuclear weapons testing or nuclear accidents. Generally, it is the ingestion pathway that is most significant. Iodine is ingested quickly either from surface deposition on edible plants or from pasture grass to the cow, to milk, and to the thyroid. A large body of data exists on the transfer coefficients, P_{24} (intake to the body per unit deposition), P_{45} (effective dose per unit intake), and P_{25} ($P_{25} = P_{24} H P_{45}$) = effective dose per unit deposition. UNSCEAR (1993) reported the transfer coefficients for ^{131}I to be

$P_{24} = 0.07$ Bq per Bq m^{-2}
$P_{45} = 61$ nSv per Bq intake (effective dose for the thyroid)
$P_{25} = P_{24}$ H $P_{45} = 4.2$ nSv per Bq m^{-2}
(effective dose for the thyroid).

Ankylosing Spondylitis

About 14,000 persons, mostly men, were treated with X-rays for ankylosing spondylitis at 87 radiotherapy centers in Great Britain and Northern Ireland between 1935 and 1954. Court Brown and Doll (1957) were the first to report that these patients had a leukemia risk substantially in excess of that for the general population. Subsequent publications have developed the time pattern of appearance not only of leukemia but also of solid tumors (Court *et al.*, 1959, 1965; Smith and Doll, 1978, 1982; Smith, 1984; Darby *et al.*, 1985, 1987; Weiss *et al.*, 1995).

A group was selected consisting of 11,776 men and 2335 women all of whom had been treated with X-rays either once or twice. About half the total group received a second X-ray treatment or treatment with thorium. The reports on the ankylosing spondylitis patients attempt to consider health effects from only the first X-ray treatment. For this reason, an individual receiving a second treatment is included in their follow-up only until 18 months after the second course (a short enough time so that any malignancies in this interval cannot be ascribed to the second X-ray treatment).

The appearance of excess leukemia is now well documented, and solid tumors are also apparent in the population. The part of the body in the direct X-ray beam (spine) received the highest dose, but it is thought that other sites received substantial radiation from scatter or from the beam itself.

The importance of this study lies in the health effects of partial body exposure and in the temporal pattern of appearance of solid tumors in irradiated adults. Smith and Doll (1978, 1982), Darby *et al.* (1985, 1987), and Weiss *et al.* (1994, 1995), in the most recent follow-up publications concerning these patients, have shown that the excess risk for solid tumors diminishes with time since exposure, with maximum appearance of 5–20 years after exposure. This has significant implications for risk projection modeling. Many projection models assume a constant rate of appearance either as an absolute number of tumors per person per unit exposure (constant absolute risk) or as a fraction of the baseline age-specific cancer mortality rate (constant relative risk). The emerging pattern is that constant risk models, either absolute or relative, are not correct for certain cancers, such as lung cancer. Thirty-five years after the first treatment, excess lung cancer had completely disappeared.

The most recent mortality study (Weiss *et al.*, 1994) included 15,577 ankylosing spondylitis (AS) patients diagnosed between 1935 and 1957 in the UK, of whom 14,556 received X-ray treatment. By January 1, 1992, over half of the cohort had died. Among the irradiated patients, cancer mortality was significantly greater than expected from the national rates for England and Wales, with a ratio of observed deaths to expected (relative risk, RR) of 1.30, and significant increases individually for leukemia, non-Hodgkin lymphoma, multiple myeloma, and cancers of the oesophagus, colon, pancreas, lung, bones, connective and soft tissue, prostate, bladder, and kidney. Among the unirradiated patients, cancer mortality was lower than expected from national rates (RR = 0.79). Among irradiated patients, the RRs for leukemia, lung cancer, and

Table 25-9

Excess Cancer in 6158 Ankylosing Spondylitis Patients Given a Single X-Ray Treatment as of the Last Follow-up

SITE	OBS	EXP	DOSE, Gy	LIFETIME RISK Gy^{-1}
Leukemia	53	17	4.8	0.0011
Lung*	563	469	2.5	0.0027
Esophagus	74	38	5.6	0.0007

*Lung cancer appearing less than 5 years after exposure is not included as less than the minimum latency for tumor expression. The doses to the pulmonary lung and main bronchi were estimated as 1.8 and 6.8 Gy, respectively. The majority of lung cancer is bronchogenic, and the dose estimates for the main bronchi are probably most pertinent Lifetime risk calculated as 30-year risk.
SOURCE: Data from UNSCEAR, 2000.

all other neoplasms all decreased significantly with increasing time since first treatment following an initial increase. By 35 years after first treatment, the radiation-related excess for lung cancer had completely disappeared, while for other neoplasms the RR remained significantly raised, although at a lower level than in earlier periods. Most irradiated patients received several courses of treatment within a 5-year period. Based on a 1 in 15 random sample, the mean total body dose received in this period was 2.64 Gy, with the heaviest dose to the vertebrae. A linear dose–response model for all neoplasms except leukemia gave an ERR of 0.18 Gy^{-1} in the period 5–24.9 years after first treatment, which decreased significantly to 0.11 Gy^{-1} in the period more than 25 years after the first treatment.

The dosimetry was redone in 1988 (Lewis *et al.*, 1988), and although better estimates of dose are now available, it is still the dose that is most uncertain for the cohort. No details about the X-ray machines used to deliver the exposures, such as output, kilovoltage, and half-value layer, are reported.

The excess cancers and the estimate of lifetime cancer risk at three sites in the ankylosing spondylitis cohort are shown in Table 25-9. For the purpose of calculating lifetime risks as of the time of follow-up, the number of persons used here as the individuals at risk is the number actually receiving only one X-ray treatment (6158). This assumes that those followed for 18 months after the second treatment do not contribute significantly to the malignancies.

The relatively low risk for leukemia (compared with atom bomb survivors) has been suggested to be due to cell sterilization at the high dose delivered. It is also possible that the low risk is due to partial irradiation of the skeletal red marrow. The volume of bone marrow irradiated in the spine, rib, and pelvis is much less than 50% of that in whole-body irradiation.

The deaths resulting from causes other than neoplasms in the total cohort are about 30% higher than expected. This higher total mortality is of significance in risk modeling as the premature deaths resulting from competing causes decrease the observed fractional cancer mortality. Thus, the lifetime risk in this population probably underestimates the risk when projecting the effects of exposure in a healthy population.

Uranium Miners

Radon is ubiquitous on earth. It is found outdoors and in all dwellings as a result of the decay of the parent ^{226}Ra, which is present in all of earth's minerals.

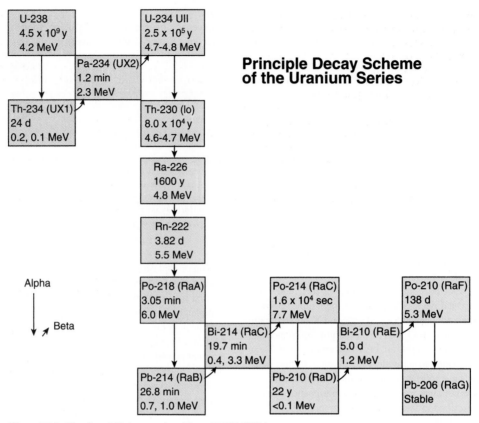

**Principle Decay Scheme
of the Uranium Series**

Figure 25-8. Uranium-238 decay series. (From NCRP, 1987.)

Although the risk of developing lung cancer from radon exposure among underground miners is firmly documented and quantitative risk estimates are available, the current interest lies in whether this risk carries over into environmental situations. Radon levels in homes that are comparable to those in mines surely confer risks to the residents. The question remains: Can the risks in mines for exposures at higher concentrations over short time periods be used to model risks at lower environmental levels over a lifetime?

The results of the domestic epidemiology have answered this question.

Radon Exposure in Underground Mines   There are 11 follow-up studies of underground miners exposed to high concentrations of radon and radon decay products. The documentation of excess lung cancer is convincing (NCRP, 1984; NAS, 1988, 1998; NIH, 1994; UNSCEAR, 2000, 2007). The carcinogen in the case of radon is actually the alpha-emitting short-lived decay products of radon, ^{218}Po, and ^{214}Po. The decay scheme for the entire uranium series, including radon and the daughter species, is shown in Fig. 25-8. The decay products or daughter products are solids and are deposited on the bronchial airways during inhalation and exhalation according to the laws of diffusion. As the airway lining (bronchial epithelium) is only about 40 μm thick, the alpha particles emitted are able to reach and transfer a significant amount of energy to all the cells implicated in lung cancer induction. Although the daughters are the carcinogen, the term *radon* is here used interchangeably for *radon decay products*, because without the parent radon, the daughters could not exist longer than a few hours. The measurements in mines were usually

of the daughter species rather than radon, and the term *working level* (WL) was adopted for occupational exposure. It indicated the total potential energy content in 1 L of air for complete decay of the short-lived daughters.[1] The exposure attributed to miners was developed in working-level months (WLMs), which is the numerical value of WL times the time exposed in multiples of a working month of 170 hours (Holaday *et al.*, 1957).

$$WLM = WL(hours\ expose/170).$$

Estimating Lung Cancer Risk from Underground Miner Epidemiology   The follow-up studies from 11 large underground mining cohorts in Australia, Canada, Czech Republic, France, Sweden, and the United States have all produced data that show that the excess lung cancer risk from exposure to radon is about 1–3 per 10,000 persons per WLM exposure (Radford and Renard, 1984; Hornung and Meinhardt, 1987; Sevc *et al.*, 1988; Muller *et al.*, 1989; Howe *et al.*, 1986, 1987; Tirmarche *et al.*, 1993; Woodward *et al.*, 1991; NCRP, 1984; NIH, 1994; NAS, 1998; UNSCEAR, 2000, 2007). Expressed another way, radon exposure increases the normal age-specific lung cancer risk by about 0.6% for each WLM exposure. This way of expressing risk leads to the concept that many epidemiologists prefer that the lung cancer risk is proportional to the normal baseline risk. The notation for this is excess relative risk (ERR). This means, e.g.,

---

[1] One working level (WL) is any combination of short-lived daughters in 1 L of air that will result in 1.3 × 10^5 MeV of alpha energy when complete decay occurs. One working level is approximately equal to 7400 Bq m^{-3} (200 pCi L^{-1}) in a home and 11,000 Bq m^{-3} (300 pCi L^{-1}) in a mine.

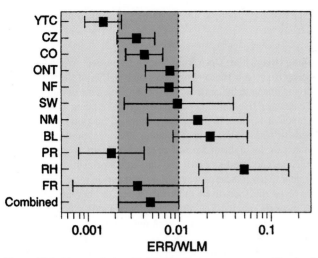

Figure 25-9. *Excess relative risk (ERR) of lung cancer per working-level month (WLM) for each of the 11 cohorts studied.*

RRs plotted per WLM exposure. YTC, Yunnan China Tin miners; CZ, Chechoslovakian uranium miners; CO, Colorado uranium miners; ONT, Ontario uranium miners; NF, Newfoundland fluorspar miners; SW, Swedish iron miners; NM, New Mexico uranium miners; BL, Beaverlodge, Canada, uranium miners; PR, Port Radium, Canada, uranium miners; RH, Radium Hill, Australia, uranium miners; FR, French uranium miners. (From NIH, 1994.)

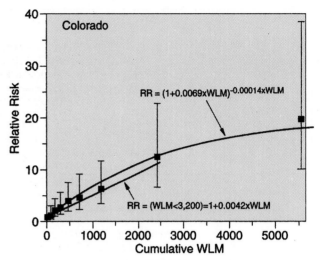

Figure 25-10. *Excess relative risk per unit exposure for the Colorado mining cohort. (From NIH, 1994.)*

1. The estimation of ERR per working level month (ERR/WLM) and the form of the exposure response.
2. The variation of ERR/WLM with attained age.
3. The variation of ERR/WLM with duration of exposure, considering total exposure as well as exposure rate.
4. The variation of ERR/WLM with age at first exposure.
5. The variation of ERR/WLM as a function of time after exposure ceased.
6. The evaluation of an optimal exposure lag interval, i.e., the interval before lung cancer death during which ^{222}Rn exposure has no effect.
7. The consistency among the 11 cohorts.
8. The joint effect of smoking and ^{222}Rn exposure.
9. The role of exposure to other airborne contaminants in mines.
10. The direct modeling of the relative risk of lung cancer with duration and rate of exposure.

that the lifetime excess lung cancer risk from radon is different for smokers and nonsmokers (NAS, 1988, 1998; NIH, 1994).

The actual data from the underground studies are not clear-cut with regard to the effect of smoking, and it is apparent from more recent analyses that radon exposure does not simply multiply the baseline risks of the population by a constant factor. This is considered in the discussion of risk, earlier in this chapter. The excess lung cancer risk in each of the exposure cohorts for the 11 major mining populations as of the date of the last published follow-up is summarized in Fig. 25-9. It can be seen in the figure that the range of risks for the same exposure varies by about a factor of 10 among the different studies. The differences are likely accounted for by errors in measuring and estimating total exposure. However, the Czech mine atmosphere contained arsenic as well as radon, and the arsenic contributed to the excess lung cancers observed. A maximum value of 50% lung cancer risk is the highest value ever observed in a mining population and was reported in mines in Saxony at the turn of the century (Muller, 1989). These mines are thought to have had about 100,000 Bq m^{-3} of radon. It is noteworthy that concentrations this high have been reported in a few homes in the United States. In Fig. 25-9, the lowest (well-documented) exposures were in the Ontario (Canadian Eldorado) mines, and in an updated study a mean exposure of 48 WLM has given an excess lung cancer risk (ERR) of about 0.5%.

To date, the most comprehensive epidemiologic analysis of underground miners exposed to high concentrations of ^{222}Rn is a joint analysis of 11 underground mining studies conducted by the National Cancer Institute (NIH, 1994), and updated by NAS (1999). The study encompasses the Chinese, Czechoslovakian, Colorado, Ontario, Newfoundland, Swedish, New Mexico, Beaverlodge, Port Radium, Radium Hill, and French mining data. The joint analysis of the 11 cohorts (NIH, 1994; NAS, 1998) focused on 10 variables:

The relative risk of lung cancer for the Colorado uranium miners is shown in Fig. 25-10 and that for all 11 cohorts—showing only the data for exposures below 400 WLM—is shown in Fig. 25-11.

The pooled cohorts included 2620 lung cancer deaths among 60,570 exposed miners, accumulating 1.2 million person-years of observation. The ERR of lung cancer is seen in Fig. 25-11 to be linearly related to the cumulative radon decay product exposure in units of WLM. The exception is at the highest exposures, where a clear reduction in ERR is evident. This is often noted as an *inverse dose rate effect*. Confusion exists concerning the inverse dose rate effect in that the relative risk is not *higher at lower dose rates* but is *lower at higher dose rates*, in agreement with cell killing and removal of damaged cells from the pool of cells that are potential sites of malignant transformation. This effect is seen in all studies of radiation damage at high doses.

Data on tobacco use were available in six of the cohorts. The lifetime domestic risk projection models based on the data estimated that the ERR/WLM was related to attained age and time since exposure. The joint effect of smoking and ^{222}Rn exposure did not show a clear pattern except that the risk was consistent with a relationship that was intermediate between additive and multiplicative.

Domestic studies now support the projected risk estimates for radon exposure in mines but the results of the domestic studies

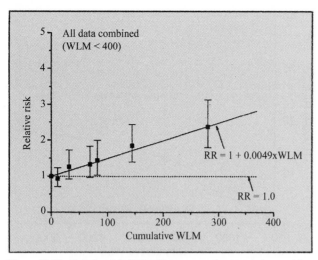

Figure 25-11. Relative risk (RR) of lung cancer by cumulative working-level month (WLM) and fitted linear excess RR model for each cohort and for all data combined (WLM <400).

RRs are plotted at mean WLM for category. When the referent category for RRs is not zero exposure, a fitted exposure-response line is adjusted to pass through the mean of the referent category. For the China, Ontario, and Beaverlodge cohorts, the excess RR model was fitted with a free intercept. (From NIH, 1994.)

should be used directly to estimate lung cancer risk. The risk projection models developed from the miner data were conservative and overestimate the domestic risk. The occupational exposure in mines is relatively short compared with that over a full life in homes and the cumulative exposure in mines is generally many times that in homes so it is possible to develop temporal risk models. The radon exposure in homes is much lower and although a value for ERR is

established it is not possible to develop models from the domestic data as yet.

Lung (Bronchial) Dose from Radon Exposure When radon gas decays to its solid decay products, some 8–15% of the ^{218}Po atoms do not attach to the normal aerosol particles. This ultrafine species (unattached fraction) is deposited with 100% efficiency on the upper bronchial airways. In mines the unattached fraction is low (4–5%) because of the normal aerosol loading. The rest of the decay products attach to the ambient aerosol of about 100-nm average diameter (George and Breslin, 1980) and only a few percent of this aerosol is deposited on these airways. Measurements in mines have mostly involved the short-lived radon daughters, as they are the easiest to measure rapidly. The alpha dose from radon gas itself is very low in comparison with that from the daughters, as the daughters deposit and accumulate on the airway surfaces. The upper airways of the bronchial tree are the region where almost all the lung cancers appear. This is true in general, not only for miners exposed to radon daughters but also for smokers.

The alpha dose from radon daughters therefore must be calculated in these airways, not in the pulmonary or gas-exchange regions. Although the dose to the pulmonary region should not be neglected, it is about 15% of that to the airways (Saccomanno *et al.*, 1996). Several calculations regarding the absorbed alpha dose exist for radon daughters (NCRP, 1984; ICRP, 1987; Harley, 1987, 1989; NRC, 1991; UNSCEAR, 2000, 2007). The authors make different assumptions about the atmospheric and biological parameters that go into the dose calculation, and this can cause discrepancies among the models. The most significant variables are the particle size of the ambient aerosol, the assumed breathing rate, and the target cells considered.

Very small particles deposit more efficiently in the airways. Therefore if small particles, such as those from open burning flame

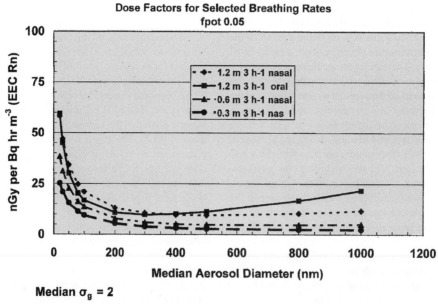

Figure 25-12. Radon decay product bronchial dose as a function of inhaled median aerosol diameter, breathing rate, for an unattached fraction (Fpot) of 0.05.

(From UNSCEAR: Sources to effects assessment for radon in homes and workplaces. Report of the United Nations Scientific Committee on the Effects of Atomic Radiation. New York: United Nations, 2007.)

(Tu and Knutson, 1988; Cohen and Asgharian, 1990), contribute to the atmosphere, the dose delivered to the bronchial epithelium can be higher per unit WLM exposure than is the dose predicted from an average particle size. Conversely, a hygroscopic particle can increase in size in the humid environment of the bronchial airways, and deposition will be diminished. The particle size of the aerosol in mines is somewhat larger than that for environmental conditions (200 to perhaps 600 nm vs. 100 nm) (George *et al.*, 1975). Figure 25-12 shows the alpha dose per unit exposure as it is related to the variables (particle size, unattached fraction, breathing rate) known to affect dose. The radon concentration in Fig. 25-12 is not the gas concentration. Because it is the decay products that deliver the dose, not the gas, the concentration is expressed in units of the equilibrium equivalent concentration (EEC). Indoors, the radon gas concentration multiplied by the equilibrium factor (Feq = 0.4) gives the EEC, i.e., the gas concentration in equilibrium with its decay products that has the same potential energy as the measured decay products. Outdoors the equilibrium factor (Feq) is 0.6 (UNSCEAR, 2000, 2006).

Example 5. Calculate the annual bronchial lung dose in nSv for a home radon concentration of 40 Bq m^{-3}. Assume 7000 hours is spent at home.
The radon EEC indoors = 0.4(40) = 16 Bq m^{-3}
The dose factor from Fig. 25-12 for a typical home environment is 15 nSv per Bq m^{-3} h (EEC).

Annual dose = 40(0.4)(15)(7000) = 1.7×10^6 nSv = 1.7 mSv

Lung cancer is related to absorbed alpha dose, and Fig. 25-12 shows that particle size is an important determinant of risk. The average dose per unit exposure for miners, shown in Fig. 25-12, is about the same as that for average environmental conditions, assuming 100 nm aerosol in homes and 200–600 nm aerosol in mines. The equilibrium factor in mines is somewhat smaller than for homes (Feq about 0.3).

Radon can deliver a greater or lesser carcinogenic potential by about a factor of 2 over the range of realistic indoor conditions (average particle size ranging from 80 to 300 nm). The allowable effective dose for continuous exposure of the population in the United States is 1 mSv/y (100 mrem/y) (NCRP, 1993). This limit would be delivered by exposure to 10 Bq m^{-3} of radon, or one-quarter the actual average measured indoor concentration in most countries where measurements have been made. Thus, the guidelines for exposure to radon cannot be set in the usual way from dosimetric considerations.

LIFETIME DOMESTIC LUNG CANCER RISK PROJECTIONS FOR RADON EXPOSURE

There are at present five sets of models based on the underground miner epidemiology that attempted to calculate risk for exposure to radon daughters in the home. The following sections describe each in detail.

National Council on Radiation Protection and Measurements

In 1984, the NCRP on Protection and Measurements (NCRP, 1984) developed a model to project the risk derived from miner studies to whole-life risk in the environment. It is a modified absolute risk

model that reduces the risk subsequent to exposure with a half-life of 20 years. Risk is not accumulated until after age 40, the time when lung cancer normally appears in the population. There is no indication that early exposure produces any significant shift to younger ages, even for young miners exposed at significantly higher concentrations. This model was the first to incorporate a time since exposure reduction in risk.

National Academy of Sciences

The National Academy of Sciences report in 1988 (BEIR IV) developed a model based on examination of the raw data from five mining cohorts (NAS, 1988). The data indicated that the highest risk appears from 5 to 15 years after exposure. After 15 years, the risk is one-half that of the 5- to 15-year risk (per unit exposure), and this risk was assumed to persist to the end of life. Again, no significant risk appears before 40, the usual age for the appearance of lung cancer. The NAS model also included a correction for attained age (at age 65, the risk is 0.4 of that for ages 55–64). The BEIR IV committee assumed a relative risk model (risk is proportional to the normal age-specific lung cancer risk per unit radon exposure), but with risk dependent on time from exposure. This was the first modified relative risk model. This means that the risk for smokers and nonsmokers differs because of their different baseline lung cancer values. Although the miners' epidemiology did not support this strictly multiplicative relationship, the NAS chose the relative risk model as a conservative one. Its analysis supported the risk reduction subsequent to exposure by using a two-step risk reduction window.

NAS 1998 (BEIR VI) expanded on the models developed in NAS (1989) using 11 underground mining cohorts rather than four. The models for the 11 cohorts were developed first by NIH (1994), see below, and updated for the NAS report.

International Commission on Radiation Protection

The ICRP (1987) developed two risk projection models: one was based on a constant relative risk and the other was a constant absolute risk model. Although neither risk model is correct because of the temporal reduction pattern of lung cancer subsequent to the cessation of exposure, the numerical values obtained for the lifetime risk of lung cancer from radon exposure are not significantly different from those in other models. Later follow-up of the Czechoslovakian underground uranium miners presented by Kunz and Sevc (1988) indicates that the excess lung cancer risk may actually be reduced to zero 35 years after exposure. If this factor was included in the NAS model (zero risk after 35 years), it would reduce those values by about a factor of 2. The risk values obtained from the various models are shown in Table 25-10. In 1993, ICRP simply adopted a lifetime lung cancer fatality coefficient of 3×10^{-4} per WLM (ICRP, 1993).

NIH Joint Analysis of 11 Underground Mining Cohorts

The pooled analysis from the 11 underground mining cohorts was used to develop two models for full-life risk projection (NIH, 1994). The models are similar to the model used by the NAS (1988), utilizing time since exposure reduction and reduction with attained age. Three time windows for reduction of risk with time since exposure

Table 25-10

Lung Cancer Risk for Continuous Whole-life Exposure to 4 pCi/L (150 Bq m^{-3} or 0.58 WLM per year at Indoor Conditions) as Predicted by Various Models of Domestic Exposure*

MODEL	LIFETIME RISK %	MODEL TYPE	COMMENT
NCRP (1984a)	0.50	Modified absolute risk. Two parameter model.	Risk decreases with time since exposure.
ICRP (1987)	0.90	Constant relative risk.	
ICRP (1987)	0.62	Constant additive risk.	
ICRP (1993)	0.56	Single-value risk per WLM.	Adopted lifetime risk per WLM exposure.
BEIR IV (NRC 1988)	1.1	Modified relative risk. Two-time windows. Two-parameter model.	Risk decreases with time since exposure.
NIH (1994)	1.8	Modified relative risk, three-time windows, age and exposure rate. Three parameter model.	Risk decreases with time since exposure and decreases with very high exposures.
BEIR VI (NRC 1998)	2.0	Modified relative risk. Three time windows, age and exposure rate. Three parameter model.	Risk decreases with time since exposure and decreases with very high exposures.
Meta-analysis of eight domestic case-control studies (Lubin and Boice, 1997)	0.7	Observed mortality.	Linear regression fit to data from eight domestic studies.

*Exposure assumes a home concentration of 148 Bq m^{-3} (4 pCi l^{-1} or 0.56 WLM), calculated with 40 percent decay product equilibrium, and actual exposure is 70 percent of the home exposure.

SOURCE: Data from NAS, 1999.

are used instead of two. Also, an additional parameter is incorporated; one model decreases the risk with increasing exposure rate, and the other decreases the risk with decreasing exposure duration. The lifetime domestic risk for lifetime exposure to unit concentration was not reported. However, the ratio of the relative risk of lung cancer for the BEIR IV and joint analysis model was given as 0.9 for continuous exposure to 4 pCi L^{-1} (1 WLM per year) for the model incorporating exposure duration as a parameter. The joint analysis estimated that there are 15,000 lung cancer deaths in the United States attributable to ^{222}Rn: 10,000 in smokers and 5000 in those who have never smoked.

BEIR VI (NAS, 1998) updated these two models and increased the calculated risk in the United States to 15,400 or 21,800 per year for ever smokers and never smokers for the two model values. The BEIR VI best annual estimate of deaths for ever smokers is stated to be 11,000 per year with 2100 or 2900 calculated deaths for never smokers, depending upon the model chosen. The results of the domestic epidemiology now indicate that the BEIR VI projected estimates of annual deaths is too large perhaps by a factor of 2.

DOMESTIC EPIDEMIOLOGY

The Domestic Studies

There is a very large body of published information on residential exposure to radon and lung cancer. A summary is given here and in the references (Neuberger, 1989, 1992; Samet *et al.*, 1991; Lubin and Boice, 1997; NAS, 1999; Pavia *et al.*, 2003; Darby *et al.*, 2005b; Krewski *et al.*, 2005; UNSCEAR, 2000, 2007).

There are at present 89 published epidemiologic studies relating radon and lung cancer. Of these, the best are 22 case control or cohort studies. One early study in the United States was performed in 1989 by the New Jersey Department of Health (NJDOH)

(Schoenberg and Klotz, 1989; Schoenberg *et al.*, 1990). This is a case-control study of women, 433 lung cancer cases and 402 controls with year long measurements of radon in the homes where the individuals lived for 10 or more years. This study devoted considerable effort to quality control concerning the exposure measurements. The results of this study are slightly positive, suggesting an association of radon and lung cancer even at concentrations of 80 Bq m^{-3}, but the results are not statistically significant. A case-control study of 538 nonsmoking women (1183 controls) in Missouri with an average exposure of 70 Bq m^{23} also showed no statistically significant increase in lung cancer (Alavanja *et al.*, 1994).

One of the largest case-control study to date concerning the effects of residential ^{222}Rn exposure was conducted nationwide in 109 municipalities in Sweden (Pershagen *et al.*, 1993). Radon was measured in 8992 homes for 3 months during the heating season. The geometric and arithmetic concentrations were 60 and 106 Bq m^{-3}. The cumulative exposure for each person from 1947 was estimated. It included all subjects 35- to 74-years old who had lived in one of the 109 municipalities at some time between January 1980 and December 31, 1984, and who had been living in Sweden on January 1, 1947. Fifty-six of the municipalities were known to have elevated ^{222}Rn concentrations on the basis of earlier measurements. There were 1360 cases and 2847 controls.

Thus, an attempt was made to study a large group of persons living in a known area of greater than average ^{222}Rn and to estimate their exposure over a large fraction of life (34 years). The primary aim of the study was to narrow the uncertainty in the estimation of lung cancer risk.

The environmental epidemiologic studies conducted before this study suffered from the small numbers of persons observed and relatively low ^{222}Rn exposures. For this reason, although the risk in underground miners was seen clearly, the outcome regarding the lung cancer risk from residential exposure had been ambiguous.

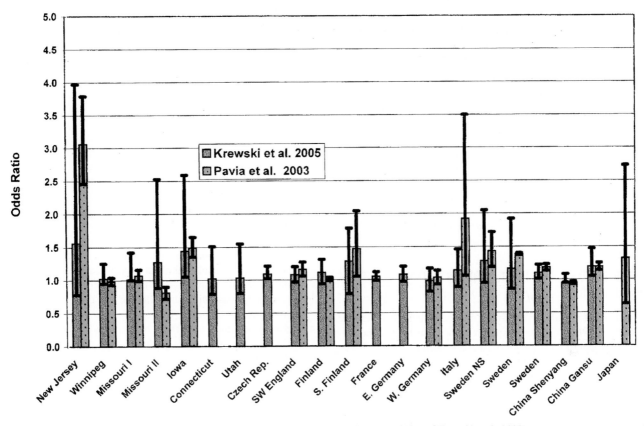

Figure 25-13. Summary data for 21 domestic case control studies. Data from Pavia et al. (2003) and Krewski et al. (2005).

All the existing domestic studies, including the measurement protocols, have been reviewed (Neuberger, 1992, 1994; Samet, 1989; Samet *et al.*, 1991; Lubin *et al.*, 1990).

The ^{222}Rn concentration in 8992 homes was measured for 3 months during the heating season. The geometric and arithmetic mean concentrations were 1.6 and 2.9 pCi L^{21} (60 and 106 Bq m^{-3}). The cumulative exposure since 1947 was estimated for each subject by the addition of the products of concentration by the length of time the subject lived in each residence.

The data were reported in terms of the relative risk (RR) of lung cancer (ratio of observed to expected lung cancer) normalized to a relative risk of 1.0 for persons who never smoked and who had radon exposure below 50 Bq m^{-3}. The excess risk due to smoking could be seen easily. Smokers smoking less than or more than 10 cigarettes per day with a radon concentration of << 50 Bq m^{-3} had RR of 6.2 (with a confidence interval from 4.2 to 9.2) and 12.6 (CI from 8.7 to 18.4), respectively.

The only statistically significant lung cancer excess resulting from ^{222}Rn was seen in those who smoked fewer than 10 cigarettes per day and had a time-weighted mean ^{222}Rn concentration >400 Bq m^{-3}. Their relative risk was 25.1 (CI 7.7 to 82.4). For those smoking more than 10 cigarettes per day, the relative risk compared with those who had never smoked and had ^{222}Rn concentrations <50 Bq m^{-3} was 32.5 (CI 10.3 to 23.7). Although this relative risk appears higher than that for those smoking <10 cigarettes per day, the result is not statistically significant. If the effect of ^{222}Rn alone is examined by comparing the risk only among smokers, i.e., those with <50 Bq m^{-3} against smokers having >400 Bq m^{-3}, the relative risk due to ^{222}Rn alone is 3.7 (CI 1.1 to 11.7) for those

smoking <10 cigarettes per day and 2.5 (CI 0.8 to 7.9) for those smoking >10 cigarettes per day (Pershagen *et al.*, 1994). Because the confidence interval includes 1.0, it cannot be stated with statistical certainty that there was increased lung cancer caused by ^{222}Rn exposure although the point estimate RR = 2.5 suggests at least an upper bound of risk.

A later study was done for a combined group of men and women (Pershagen *et al.*, 1994). There were no details given concerning lung cancer and sex difference. However, the preliminary report (Pershagen *et al.*, 1994) suggested that women may indeed have had less lung cancer than men for the same exposure conditions. Also of interest in the study of Pershagen *et al.* (1994) was the relative risk of lung cancer by histological type. In the >400 Bq m^{-3} group, only small cell carcinoma and adenocarcinoma had a statistically significant increased risk.

One of the most recent studies conducted in the United States was in Iowa and studied women only (Field *et al.*, 2000). There were 413 lung cancer cases and 614 controls. The ERR found was 0.22 (95% CI = −0.20 to 1.93).

The number of domestic case control studies is now sufficient to establish the lung cancer risk from radon exposure. The results of the studies (odds ratio or relative risk) are shown in Fig. 25-13. The domestic studies indicate that the lung cancer risk from ^{222}Rn exposure is evident at exposures of 100 Bq m^{-3}. It is interesting that the precision of the domestic studies is now better (smaller confidence intervals) than the miner studies. This is probably due to more accurate estimates of the lifetime exposure. The present studies indicate a relative risk of about 1.2 but the confidence intervals mostly include no risk.

Table 25-11

Lifetime Relative Risk (LRR) Calculated from Published Meta Analyses or Pooled Analyses of Domestic Case Control Radon and Lung Cancer Studies

STUDY	NUMBER OF STUDIES INCLUDED	LRR	95% CONFIDENCE INTERVAL
Lubin, Boice, 1997 (Meta)	8	1.14 (per 150 Bq m^{-3})	1.00–1.30
Pavia et al., 2003 (Meta)	17	1.24 (per 150 Bq m^{-3})	1.11–1.38
Lubin et al., 2004	2 China	1.33 (per 100 Bq m^{-3})	1.01–1.36
Darby et al., 2005b	13 European	1.16 (per 100 Bq m^{-3})	1.05–1.31
Krewski et al., 2005	7 North America	1.11 (per 100 Bq m^{-3})	1.00–1.28
Wichmann et al., 2005	2 Germany	1.10 (per 100 Bq m^{-3})	0.98–1.30

Unless a biological marker for radon-induced lung cancer is found, it is unlikely that further domestic epidemiology will refine the existing risk estimates.

Meta-analysis and Joint Analysis of Domestic Epidemiology

In an attempt to combine the largest domestic studies to determine whether any risk from radon exposure in the home is apparent, several meta analyses and joint analyses have been performed. Lubin and Boice (1997) were the first to perform a meta-analysis of eight domestic case control studies. A meta-analysis combines the published information from several studies into one study without actually having the raw data available. The data showed that essentially no study found statistically significant cancer deaths due to radon, but the authors state that the combined trend in the relative risk with increasing exposure was statistically significant, with an estimated RR of 1.14 (95% CI = 1.0–1.3) at an exposure of 150 Bq m^{-3} (4 pCi L^{-1}).

There are now six studies, two meta analyses, and four pooled or joint analyses to estimate the lifetime relative risk (RR) for domestic exposure to radon. The results are shown in Table 25-11.

The best estimate of relative risk (RR) at this time is probably the study of Darby et al. (2004), RR = 1.16 (95% CI 1.05–1.31) as this has the largest number of studies included. The lower confidence interval does not include any risk. This value can be used to evaluate a realistic domestic lung cancer risk from radon exposure.

Example 6. The baseline lung cancer risk in the U.S. population including smokers, nonsmokers, men, and women is about 0.05 (5%). Calculate the lifetime lung cancer risk for a continuous home concentration of 40 Bq m^{-3}.

The RR is estimated as 1.16 per 100 Bq m^{-3}. The lifetime risk is therefore increased by 0.16 above the baseline risk for 100 Bq m^{-3}.

Lifetime risk = 0.16 (0.05)(40)/(100) = 0.003 or 0.3% or 3 per 1000 persons.

What is Known about Radon Exposure

Four concepts have emerged from the radon research so far:

1. The mining epidemiology indicates that short exposure to high levels of radon and its daughters produces a clear excess of lung cancer.
2. Particle size can change the actual dose delivered by radon to bronchial tissue, with small particles giving a substantially higher dose per unit exposure. The use of open flames, electric motors, and the like indoors produces a higher dose per unit exposure.
3. Smokers are at higher risk from radon per unit exposure than nonsmokers. The domestic studies show that the relative risk for smokers and nonsmokers is about the same but their age-specific lung cancer mortality is about ten times higher than that for nonsmokers. Thus, the overall lifetime lung cancer risk is many times higher for smokers.
4. Urban areas almost universally have low radon, and apartment dwellers removed from the ground source have particularly low radon exposure at home.

The miners' data show clearly that there is a risk of lung cancer from exposure to high concentrations of radon delivered over short periods and temporal models can be derived from the data.

The results of the domestic studies are now convincing with regard to domestic radon risk. The best pooled risk estimate to date is probably that of Darby et al. (2004), who did a joint analysis of 13 European case control studies using the original data.

NATURAL RADIOACTIVITY AND RADIATION BACKGROUND

The occupational, accidental, and wartime experiences detailed in the preceding sections have provided the bases for all the current radiation risk estimates. For many years, the radioisotopes deposited internally were compared with ^{226}Ra to evaluate the maximum permissible body burden for a particular emitter. The present limits for external and internal radiation are based on dose estimates that, in turn, can be related to cancer risks. One standard of comparison has always been the exposure from natural background, and this source is assessed here.

Background radiation from all sources is described in detail in NCRP report 94 (1987b), and some of the information is summarized here.

The risk estimates in the previous sections must be placed in context with the radiation dose received by all humans from natural background radiation. A substantial dose is received annually from cosmic radiation and from external terrestrial radiation present from uranium, thorium, and potassium in the earth's crust. Internal emitters are present in the body as a consequence of dietary consumption and inhalation. For example, potassium is a necessary element in the body and is under homeostatic control. Radioactive ^{40}K constitutes a constant fraction of all natural potassium. Potassium delivers the largest internal dose from the diet of 0.15 mSv per year. However, the data are scanty on the dietary intake of other radionuclides in the U.S. population. Given the usual distribution of intakes across a

Table 25-12

Equivalent Dose Rates to Various Tissues from Natural Radionuclides Contained in the Body

RADIONUCLIDE	Equivalent Dose Rate, $mSv\ yr^{-1}$			
	BRONCHIAL EPITHELIUM	SOFT TISSUE	BONE SURFACES	BONE MARROW
^{14}C	—	0.10	0.08	0.30
^{40}K	—	1.80	1.40	2.70
^{87}Rb	—	0.03	0.14	0.07
^{238}U-^{234}Th	—	0.046	0.03	0.004
^{230}Th	—	0.001	0.06	0.001
^{226}Ra	—	0.03	0.90	0.15
^{222}Rn	—	0.07	0.14	0.14
^{222}Rn daughters	24	—	—	—
^{210}Pb-^{210}Po	—	1.40	7.00	1.40
^{232}Th	—	0.001	0.02	0.004
^{228}Ra-^{224}Ra	—	0.0015	1.20	0.22
^{220}Rn	—	0.001	—	—
Total	24	3.50	11.00	5.00

Table 25-13

Estimated Total Effective Dose Rate for a Member of the Population in the United States and Canada from Various Sources of Background Radiation

SOURCE	Total Effective Dose Rate, $mSv\ yr^{-1}$					
	LUNG	GONADS	BONE SURFACE	BONE MARROW	OTHER TISSUES	TOTAL
w_t^*	0.12	0.25	0.03	0.12	0.48	1.0
Cosmic	0.03	0.07	0.008	0.03	0.13	0.27
Cosmogenic	0.001	0.002	—	0.004	0.003	0.01
Terrestrial	0.03	0.07	0.008	0.03	0.14	0.28
Inhaled	2.0	—	—	—	—	2.0
In body	0.04	0.09	0.03	0.06	0.17	0.40
Total	2.1	0.23	0.05	0.12	0.44	3.0

*Tissue weighting factor—see Table 25.3.
SOURCE: Data from NCRP, 1987.

large population, it is probable that other emitters, notably ^{210}Pb and its decay product ^{210}Po, could deliver a significant dose to a fraction of the population. For example, ^{210}Pb is found in all tobacco products and delivers a significant lung dose.

The largest dose received by the population is from the inhaled short-lived daughters of radon. These are present in all atmospheres because radon is released rather efficiently from the ^{226}Ra in rock and soil. The short-lived daughters, ^{218}Po, ^{214}Pb, ^{214}Bi-^{214}Po, have an effective half-life of 30 minutes, but the 3.8-day parent radon supports their presence in the atmosphere. Figure 25-8 shows the entire uranium series decay.

Average outdoor concentrations in every state in the United States have been measured and summarized as 15 Bq m^{-3}, and indoors, as 40 Bq m^{-3} (NAS, 1999). A structure such as a house prevents the rapid upward distribution of radon into the atmosphere, and substantial levels can be built up indoors. The source of radon is the ground; therefore, levels in living areas above the ground are generally one-third to one-fifth the concentrations measured in basements. An effective barrier across the soil–building interface also inhibits the entry of radon to buildings. Ventilation with outdoor air reduces indoor radon. For this reason, industrial buildings with

more substantial foundations and higher ventilation rates tend to have lower radon concentrations than do single-family (or detached) houses. Apartments above ground level have radon concentrations about half the average of those in single-family dwellings.

It is of significance that an average radon concentration indoors of 40 Bq m^{-3} results in an equivalent dose to bronchial epithelium of 24 mSv per year or an effective dose of 2 mSv per year.

The equivalent doses for the major natural internal emitters are shown in Table 25-12. These are reproduced from NCRP (1987a,b).

The annual effective dose equivalents for all the external and internal emitters from natural background are summarized in NCRP Report 94 (1987a,b) and are shown in Table 25-13.

The lifetime dose from natural emitters is shown in Table 25-14, assuming an average exposure from birth to a full life of 85 years. It should be recognized that the actual dose accumulated by an individual depends on dietary habits, location (Denver, e.g., at an altitude of 1.6 km, has double the average cosmic-ray exposure), and the dwelling. An apartment dweller would accumulate approximately half the dose from inhaled radon daughters as would a person living in a single-family dwelling. Table 25-14 is informative in considering the effects of radiation exposure from other than

Table 25-14

Lifetime Effective Dose (in mSv from Birth to Age 85) from Natural Radionuclide Exposure

	LUNG	BONE MARROW	WHOLE BODY
Effective dose	180	10	260

SOURCE: Data from NCRP, 1987.

natural sources. For example, in assessing an occupational dose, which might add, say, 10 mSv effective dose equivalent, natural background would be a strong confounder. Any health detriment would have to be calculated rather than observed directly. No study would be able to detect an increase in health effects from 10 mSv above the average whole-life natural background of 260 mSv.

Figure 25-14 shows the average components of natural background in the United States, and Harley (2000) gives a detailed summary of background radiation and internal radioactivity.

Table 25-15

Estimates of Radionuclide Released and Collective Effective Dose from Human-Made Environmental Sources of Radiation

SOURCE	Release (PBq)					Collective Effective Dose* Person Sv		
	^{3}H	^{14}C	NOBLE GASES	^{90}Sr	^{131}I	^{137}Cs	LOCAL AND REGIONAL	GLOBAL
Atmospheric nuclear testing	240,000	220		604	650,000	910		2,230,000
Local								
Semipalatinsk							4600	
Nevada							500[†]	
Australia							700	
Pacific test site							160[†]	
Underground nuclear testing			50		15		200	
Nuclear weapons fabrication								
Early practice							8000[‡]	
Hanford							15,000[§]	
Chelyabinsk							1000	10,000
Later practice							30,000[¶]	
Nuclear power production							2700	
Milling and mining							3700	
Reactor operation	140	1.1	3,200		0.04		4600	
Fuel reprocessing	57	0.3	1,200	6.9	0.004	40	300,000[¶]	100,000
Fuel cycle							2000	80,000
Radioisotope production and use	2.6	1.0	52		6.0			
Accidents								
Three Mile Island			370		0.0006		40	
Chernobyl					630	70		600,000
Kyshtym				5.4		0.04	2500	
Windscale			1.2		0.7	0.02	2000	
Palomares							3	
Thule							0	
SNAP 9A								2100
Cosmos 954				0.003	0.2	0.003		20
Ciudad Juarez							150	
Mohammedia							80	
Goiania						0.05	60	
Total							380,000	23,100,000
Total collective effective dose (Person Sv)								23,500,000

*Truncated at 10,000 years.

[†] External dose only.

[‡] From release of ^{131}I to the atmosphere.

[§] From releases of radionuclides into the Techa River.

[¶] Long-term collective dose from release of ^{222}Rn from tailings.

SOURCE: Data from UNSCEAR, 1993.

Table 25-16

Lifetime Cancer Mortality per Gray from Five Major Epidemiologic Studies (in parentheses, risk per sievert for alpha emitters, $w_r = 20$)*

STUDY	ALL SITES	LEUKEMIA	LUNG	FEMALE BREAST	BONE	THYROID	SKIN
Atom bomb whole-body, gamma	0.05	0.005	0.0085	0.002	0.0005	0.0008	0.0002
Uranium miner bronchial epithelium, alpha			(0.04) 0.0020				
Ankylosing spondylitis. spincal x-ray		0.0011	0.0008 0.0028	0.0015			
Tinea capitis, head x-ray						0.0010§	0.0030‡
Radium ingestion, bone.* alpha (^{226}Ra)					0.004 (0.0002)		
Radium ingestion, bone,† alpha (^{224}Ra)					0.02 (0.0010)		

*The lifetime risk is calculated for an average skeletal dose of 10 Gy, assuming that the risk persists for 50 years and using Eq. (25-20). The risk is nonlinear and is about 0.01 Gy^{-1} at 100 Gy, for example.

†The lifetime risk is calculated for an average skeletal dose of 10 Gy using equation 25-22. The risk is nonlinear and is about 0.01 Gy^{-1} for a skeletal dose of 1 Gy.

‡The mortality for skin cancer is estimated as 1 percent of the incidence; see text.

§Thyroid mortality for males and females. Estimated as 10% of incidence.

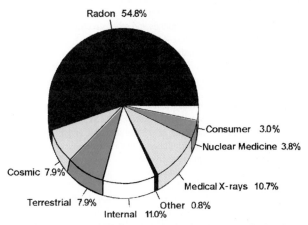

Figure 25-14. Contribution from natural background to effective dose of radiation in the U.S. population. Annual average effective dose, 3.6 mSv. (From NCRP, 1987.)

LOCAL ENVIRONMENTAL RELEASES

Large- and small-scale accidents will undoubtedly occur that release radioactivity into the environment. The accident at the Windscale nuclear power reactor in 1957 was a local incident in Great Britain. The nearby population has been studied for over 30 years without the appearance of significant health effects.

The nuclear power accident at Three Mile Island caused enormous financial damage, but the containment vessel was not breached and virtually no radioactivity escaped.

The accident at the Chernobyl nuclear power plant was another such occasion, and in this case containment did not exist and some of the radioactivity was widespread over Europe. The United

Nations Scientific Committee on the Effects of Atomic Radiation (UNSCEAR, 1988, 1993, 2000; IAEA, 2005) has summarized the committed dose from measurements made in the affected countries from various releases, and these are shown in Table 25-15. Table 25-15 includes environmental releases from most known sources.

Highly radioactive emissions from industrial or medical sources that are "lost," such as the ^{137}Cs and ^{60}Co in Goiania and Thailand, harm the persons involved, often with a few deaths due to very high radiation exposure and dose. The financial cost is usually large for cleanup and monitoring.

The criticality accident on September 30, 1999, at a fuel reprocessing facility in Tokai-Mura, Japan, resulted in the death of two workers and caused neighbors to receive a small local dose of about 2 mSv (Komura et al., 2000).

Local exposures and doses from accidents can only be anticipated to increase, as the use of radioactive materials industrially, for research and for medical diagnosis is widespread.

SUMMARY OF HUMAN CANCER RISKS FROM RADIATION

The details of the five major studies have been given in the preceding sections. The data are summarized in Table 25-16. This table shows the lifetime cancer risks that are significant. The risks are given in units of per gray (or per sievert where appropriate for alpha emitters).

Within the table, leukemia and cancers of the lung and female breast are the most critical. Osteogenic sarcoma is seen in the radium exposures. There is no clear linear dose response for ^{224,226}Ra. This has been attributed to the existence of an apparent threshold. The cancer risk to individual organs from different study groups is in general agreement regardless of radiation type or whole- or partial-body exposure.

REFERENCES

Adamson HG: A simplified method of x-ray application for the cure of ringworm of the scalp: Kienbock's method. *Lancet* 1:1378–1380, 1909.

Alavanja MCR, Brownson RC, Lubin JH, et al.: Residential radon exposure and lung cancer among nonsmoking women. *J Natl Cancer Inst* 86:1829–1837, 1994.

Albert RE, Omran A: A follow-up study of patients treated by x-ray epilation for tinea capitis: I. Population characteristics, posttreatment illnesses, and mortality experience. *Arch Environ Health* 17:899–918, 1968.

Albert RE, Shore RE, Harley NH, Omran A: Follow-up studies of patients treated by x-ray epilation for tinea capitis, in Burns F, Upton AC, Silini G (eds.): *Radiation Carcinogenesis and DNA Alterations.* New York: Plenum Press, 1986, pp. 1–25.

Andrews HL: *Radiation Biophysics.* Englewood Cliffs, NJ: Prentice-Hall, 1974.

Attix FH, Roesch WC, Tochilin E: *Radiation Dosimetry.* Vol. I. New York: Academic Press, 1968.

Aub JC, Evans RD, Hempelmann LH, Martland HS: The late effects of internally deposited radioactive materials in man. *Medicine (Baltimore)* 31:221–329, 1952.

Bethe HA, Ashkin J: Passage of radiations through matter, in Segre E (ed.): *Experimental Nuclear Physics.* New York: Wiley, 1953, pp. 166–357.

Browne E, Firestone RB, Shirley VS: *Table of Radioactive Isotopes.* New York: Wiley, 1986.

Cadet J, Delatour T, Douki T, *et al.*: Hydroxyl radicals and DNA base damage. *Mutat Res* 424:9–21, 1999.

Cember H: *Introduction to Health Physics.* New York: McGraw-Hill, 1996.

Chemelevsky D, Kellerer AM, Spiess H, Mays CW: A proportional hazards analysis of bone sarcoma rates in German radium-224 patients, in Gossner W, Gerber GB (eds.): *The Radiobiology of Radium and Thorotrast.* Munich: Urban & Schwarzenberg, 1986.

Cohen BS, Asgharian B: Deposition of ultrafine particles in the upper airways: An empirical analysis. *J Aerosol Sci* 789, 1990.

Conard RA, Boice JD, Fravwenie JF Jr (eds.): Late radiation effects in Marshall Islanders exposed to fallout 28 years ago, in Boice JD, Fraumeni JF Jr (eds.): *Radiation Carcinogenesis: Epidemiology and Biological Significance.* New York: Raven Press, 1984, pp. 57–71.

Court Brown WM, Doll R: *Leukemia and Aplastic Anemia in Patients Treated for Ankylosing Spondylitis.* London: Her Majesty's Stationery Office, 1957.

Court Brown WM, Doll R: Adult leukemia. Trends in mortality in relation to aetiology. *Br Med J* 1:1063, 1959.

Court Brown WM, Doll R: Mortality from cancer and other causes after radiotherapy for ankylosing spondylitis. *Br Med J* 2:1327, 1965.

Darby SC, Doll R, Smith PG: Long term mortality after a single treatment course with x-rays in patients treated for ankylosing spondylitis. *Br J Cancer* 55:179–190, 1987.

Darby SC, Nakashima E, Kato H: A parallel analysis of cancer mortality among atomic bomb survivors and patients with ankylosing spondylitis given x-ray therapy. *J Natl Cancer Inst* 72:1, 1985.

Darby S, Hill D, Auvinen A, *et al.*: Radon in homes and risk of lung cancer: Collaborative analysis of individual data from 13 European case-control studies. *BMJ* 330(7485):223, 2004.

Darby S, Hill D, Auvinen A, *et al.*: Radon in homes and risk of lung cancer: Collaborative analysis of individual data from 13 European case-control studies. *Br Med J* 330(7485):223, 2005a.

Darby S: Residentia radon, smoking and lung cancer. *Rad Research* 163:696, 2005b.

Douki T, Ravanat JL, Pouget JP, Testard I, Cadet J: Minor contribution of direct ionization to DNA base damage induced by heavy ions. *Int J Radiat Biol* 82:119–127, 2006.

Evans RD: *The Atomic Nucleus.* New York: McGraw-Hill, 1955, 1982.

Evans RD, Keane AT, Kolenkow RJ, *et al.*: Radiogenic tumors in the radium cases studied at M.I.T., in Mays CW, Jee WSS, Lloyd RD, *et al.* (eds.): *Delayed Effects of Bone Seeking Radionuclides.* Salt Lake City: University of Utah Press, 1969, pp. 157–194.

Field RW, Steck DJ, Smith BJ, *et al.*: Residential Radon gas exposure and lung cancer. *Am J Epidemiol* 151:1091–1102, 2000.

George AC, Breslin AJ: The distribution of ambient radon and radon daughters in residential buildings in the New Jersey–New York area, in Gesell TF, Lowder WM (eds.): *Natural Radiation Environment III CONF-780422.* Washington, DC: USDOE, 1980, pp. 1272–1292.

George AC, Hinchliffe L, Sladowski R: Size distribution of radon daughter particles in uranium mine atmospheres. *Am Ind Hyg Assoc J* 36:4884, 1975.

Gilbert ES, Land CE, Simon SL: Health effects from fallout. *Health Phys* 82:726–735, 2002.

Goodhead DT: Track structure considerations in low dose and low dose rate effects of ionizing radiation. *Adv Radiat Biol* 16:7–44, 1992.

Goodhead DT: Initial events in the cellular effects of ionizing radiations: Clustered damage in DNA. *Int J Radiat Biol* 65:7–17, 1994.

Goodhead DT, Nikjoo H: Clustered damage in DNA: Estimates from track structure simulations. *Radiat Res* 148:485–486, 1997.

Gossner W: Pathology of radium induced bone tumors. New aspects of histopathology and histogenesis. *Radiat Res* 152 (Suppl):S12–S15, 1999.

Harley JH: Dose from residual radioactivity at Hiroshima and Nagasaki, in *New Dosimetry at Hiroshima and Nagasaki and Its Implications for Risk Estimates.* Proc. Number 9. Bethesda, MD: National Council on Radiation Protection, 1987.

Harley NH: Lung Cancer Risk from Exposure to Environmental Radon. Presented at the 3rd International Conference on Anticarcinogenesis and Radiation Protection, Dubrovnik, 1989.

Harley NH: Back to background: Natural radioactivity exposed. *Health Phys* 79:121–128, 2000.

Harley NH, Albert RE, Shore RE, Pasternack BS: Follow-up study of patients treated by x-ray epilation for tinea capitis: Estimation of the dose to the thyroid and pituitary glands and other structures of the head and neck. *Phys Med Biol* 21:631–642, 1976.

Harley NH, Cohen BS: Updating radon daughter dosimetry, in Hopke PK (ed.): *American Chemical Society Symposium on Radon and Its Decay Products.* Washington, DC: American Chemical Society, 1987, pp. 419–429.

Harley NH, Cohen BS, Robbins ES: The variability in radon decay product bronchial dose. *Environment International* 22:S959–S964, 1996.

Harley NH, Kolber AB, Shore RE, *et al.*: The skin dose and response for the head and neck in patients irradiated with x-ray for tinea capitis: Implications for environmental radioactivity, in *Proceedings in Health Physics Society Mid-Year Symposium.* Albuquerque, NM: Health Physics Society, 1983, pp. 125–142.

Holaday DA, Rushing DE, Coleman RD, *et al.*: *Control of Radon and Daughters in Uranium Mines and Calculations on Biologic Effects.* U.S. PHS Report 494. Washington, DC: U.S. Public Health Service, 1957.

Hornung RW, Meinhardt TJ: Quantitative risk assessment of lung cancer in U.S. uranium miners. *Health Phys* 52:417–430, 1987.

Howe GR, Nair RC, Newcombe HB, *et al.*: Lung cancer mortality (1950–80) in relation to radon daughter exposure in a cohort of workers at the Eldorado Beaverlodge Uranium Mine. *J Natl Cancer Inst* 77:357–362, 1986.

Howe GR, Nair RC, Newcombe HB, *et al.*: Lung cancer mortality (1950–80) in relation to radon daughter exposure in a cohort of workers at the Eldorado Port Radium Mine: Possible modification of risk by exposure rate. *J Natl Cancer Inst* 79:1255–1260, 1987.

IAEA The Chernobyl Forum: 2003–2005. Chernobyl's Legacy: Health Environmental and Socio-Economic Impacts. IAEA International Atomic Energy Agency. Ed.D. Kinley III. Available at www.iaea.org/Publications/Booklets/Chernobyl/chernobyl.pdf

ICRP: *Recommendations of the International Commission on Radiological Protection.* ICRP Publication 26. New York: Pergamon Press, 1977.

ICRP: *Limits for Intakes of Radionuclides by Workers. International Commission on Radiological Protection.* ICRP Publication 30, Part I. New York: Pergamon Press, 1978.

ICRP: *Limits for Inhalation of Radon Daughters by Workers.* ICRP Publication 32. New York: Pergamon Press, 1981.

ICRP: *Lung Cancer Risk from Indoor Exposures to Radon Daughters.* ICRP Publication 50. Oxford, England: Pergamon Press, 1987.

ICRP: *1990 Recommendations of the International Commission on Radiological Protection.* ICRP Publication 60. New York: Pergamon Press, 1990.

ICRP: *Protection against Radon-222 at Home and at Work.* ICRP Publication 65. New York: Pergamon Press, 1993.

ICRU: *Stopping Powers for Electrons and Positrons.* ICRU Report Number 37. Bethesda MD: International Commission on Radiation Units and Measurements, 1984.

ICRU: *Radiation Quantities and Units in Radiation Protection.* ICRU Report Number 51 and 60. Bethesda, MD: *International Commission on Radiation Units and Measurements,* 1993, 1998.

ICRU: *Stopping Powers and Ranges for Protons and Alpha Particles.* ICRU Report Number 49. Bethesda, MD: *International Commission on Radiation Units and Measurements,* 1993.

Kienbock R: Über Radiotherapie und Harrerkrankungen. *Arch Derm Syph Wien* 83:77–111, 1907.

Komura K, Yamamoto M, Muroyama T, *et al.*: The JCO criticality accident at Tokai-Mura, Japan: An overview of the sampling campaign and preliminary results. *J Environ Radioactivity* 50:77–82, 2000.

Krewski, Daniel, Lubin, *et al.*: Residential Radon and risk of lung cancer: A combined analysis of 7 North American case-control studies. *Epidemiology* 16:137–145, 2005.

Kunz E, Sevc J: Radiation risks to underground miners in the light of Czechoslovak epidemiological studies, in Kvasnicka J (ed.): *Proceedings of the International Workshop on Radiological Protection in Mining.* Darwin, Australia, 1988.

Lewis CA, Smith PG, Stratton M, *et al.*: Estimated radiation doses to different organs among patients treated for ankylosing spondylitis with a single course of x-rays. *Br J Radiol* 61:212–220, 1988.

Little JB, Lauriston S: Taylor lecture: nontargeted effects of radiation: implications for low-does exposures. *Health Physics* 91:416–426, 2006.

Lubin JH: Studies of radon and lung cancer in North America and China. *Int J Cancer* 109:132–137, 2004.

Lubin JH, Boice JD Jr: Lung cancer in radon exposed miners and estimation of risk from indoor exposure. *J Natl Cancer Institute* 87:817–826, 1995.

Lubin JH, Boice JD: Lung cancer risk from residential radon: Meta-analysis of eight epidemiologic studies. *J Natl Cancer Institute* 89: 49–57, 1997.

Lubin JH, Samet JM, Weinberg C: Design issues in studies of indoor exposure to radon and risk of lung cancer. *Health Phys* 59:807–817, 1990.

Marshall JH, Lloyd EL, Rundo J, *et al.*: *Alkaline Earth Metabolism in Adult Man.* ICRP Report Number 20. Elmsford, NY: Pergamon Press, 1972.

Martland HS: The occurrence of malignancy in radioactive persons. *Am J Cancer* 15:2435–2516, 1931.

Mays CW: Alpha particle induced cancer in humans. *Health Phys* 55:637–652, 1988.

Muller J, Kusiak R, Ritchie AC: *Factors Modifying Lung Cancer Risk in Ontario Uranium Miners, 1955–1981.* Ontario Ministry of Labour Report. Toronto: Ministry of Labour, 1989.

NAS: *Health Risks of Radon and Other Internally Deposited Alpha Emitters Committee on the Biological Effects of Ionizing Radiation.* National Academy of Sciences Report. BEIR IV. National Research Council Washington, DC: National Academy Press, 1988.

NAS: *Health Effects of Exposure to Radon.* National Academy of Sciences Report BEIR VI. Washington, DC: National Academy Press, 1998.

NAS: *Risk Assessment of Radon in Drinking Water.* National Academy of Sciences. Washington, DC: National Academy Press, 1999.

NAS: *Health risks from exposure to Low levels radiation BEIR VII.* National Academy of Sciences. Washington, DC: National Academy Press, 2006.

NCRP: *Influence of Dose and its Distribution in Time of Dose-Response Relationships of Low-LET Radiations.* NCRP Report Number 64. Bethesda, MD: National Council on Radiation Protection and Measurements, 1980.

NCRP: *Evaluation of Occupational and Environmental Exposures to Radon and Radon Daughters in the United States.* National Council on Radiation Protection Report No. 78. Bethesda, MD: NCRP, 1984.

NCRP: *Induction of Thyroid Cancer by Ionizing Radiation.* NRCP Report Number 80. Bethesda, MD: National Council on Radiation Protection and Measurements, 1985.

NCRP: *Recommendations on Limits for Exposure to Ionizing Radiation.* National Council on Radiation Protection and Measurements, Report Number 91. Bethesda, MD: National Council on Radiation Protection and Measurements, 1987a.

NCRP: *Exposure of the Population in the United States and Canada from Natural Background Radiation.* NCRP Report Number 94, Bethesda, MD: National Council on Radiation Protection and Measurements, 1987b.

NCRP: *Recommendation on Limits of Exposure to Hot Particles on the Skin.* NRCP Report Number 106. Bethesda, MD: National Council on Radiation Protection and Measurements, 1990.

NCRP: *Limitation of Exposure to Ionizing Radiation.* Report Number 116. National Council on Radiation Protection and Measurements, Bethesda, MD: National Council on Radiation Protection and Measurements, 1993.

Nekolla EA, Kellerer AM, Kuse-Isingschulte M, *et al.*: Malignancies in patients treated with high doses of radium-224. *Radiat Res* 152(Suppl): S3–S5, 1999.

Neuberger JS: *Worldwide Studies of Household Radon Exposure and Lung Cancer.* Final Report to the U.S. Department of Energy, Office of Health and Environmental Research. Washington, DC: U.S. Department of Energy, 1989.

Neuberger JS: Residential radon exposure and lung cancer. *Health Phys* 63:503–509, 1992.

Neuberger JS: Residential radon exposure and lung cancer (letter). *N Engl J Med* 330:1685, 1994.

Neuberger JS, Gesell TF: Residential radon exposure and lung cancer: risk in nonsmokers. *Health Physics* 83:1–18, 2002.

NIH: *Radon and Lung Cancer Risk: A Joint Analysis of 11 Underground Miner Studies.* NIH Publication 94-3644. Bethesda, MD: U.S. Department of Health and Human Services, National Institutes of Health, 1994.

Nikjoo H, O'Neill P, Goodhead DT: Computational modeling of low-energy electron-induced DNA damage by early physical and chemical events. *Int J Radiat Biol* 71:467–483, 1997.

Norris WP, Speckman TW, Gustafson PF: Studies of metabolism of radium in man. *AJR* 73:785–802, 1955.

Norris WP, Tyler SA, Brues AM: Retention of radioactive bone seekers. *Science* 128:456, 1958.

NRC: *Comparative Dosimetry of Radon in Mines and Homes.* Washington, DC: National Academy Press, 1991.

Panajotovic R, Martin F, Cloutier P, Hunting D, Sanche L: Effective cross sections for production of single strand breaks in plasmid DNA by 0.1 to 4.7 eV electrons. *Rad Res* 165:452–459, 2006.

Pavia M, Bianco A, Pileggi C, Angelillio I: Meta-analysis of residential exposure to radon gas and lung cancer. *Bull WHO* 81:732–738, 2003.

Pershagen G, Ackerblow G, Axelson O, *et al.*: IMM Report 2/93—*Radon i bostader och lungcancer* (in Swedish). Stockholm: Institute for Miljomedicin, Karolinska Institute, 1993.

Pershagen G, Ackerblom G, Axelson O, *et al.*: Residential radon exposure and lung cancer in Sweden. *N Engl J Med* 330:159–164, 1994.

Pierce DA, Preston DL: Joint analysis of site specific cancer risks for the A-bomb survivors. *Radiat Res* 134:134–142, 1993.

Preston DL, Pierce DA, Shimizu Y, *et al.*: Effect of recent changes in atomic bomb survivor dosimetry on cancer mortality risk estimates. *Radiat Res* 162:377–389, 2004.

Preston DL, Shimizu Y, Pierce DA, Suyama A, Mabuchi K: Studies of mortality of atomic bomb survivors. LSS Report 13: Solid cancer and noncancer disease mortality: 1950–1997, 1998.

Raabe OG, Book SA, Parks NJ: Bone cancer from radium: Canine dose response explains data for mice and humans. *Science* 208:61–64, 1980.

Radford EP, Renard KGS: Lung cancer in Swedish iron miners exposed to low doses of radon daughters. *N Engl J Med* 310:1485–1494, 1984.

RERF: *U.S.–Japan Joint Reassessment of Atomic Bomb Radiation Dosimetry in Hiroshima and Nagasaki.* Final Report. Radiation Effects Research Foundation. Vol I. Roesch WC (ed.). Hiroshima, Japan: Radiation Effects Research Foundation, 1987.

RERF Report No. 24-02. *Radiat Res* 160(4):381–407, 2003.

Reuvers AP, Greenstock CL, Borsa J, *et al.*: Studies on the mechanism of chemical protection by dimethyl sulphoxide. *Int J Radiat Biol* 24:533–536, 1973.

Ron E, Modan B: Thyroid and other neoplasms following childhood scalp irradiation, in Boice JD, Fraumeni JF (eds.): *Radiation Carcinogenesis: Epidemiology and Biological Significance.* New York: Raven Press, 1984, pp. 139–151.

Ron E, Modan B, Boice JD Jr., *et al.*: Tumors of the brain and nervous system after radiotherapy in childhood. *N Engl J Med* 319:1033–1039, 1988.

Ron E, Modan B, Preston D: Radiation induced skin carcinomas of the head and neck. *Radiat Res* 125:318–325, 1991.

Rowland RE, Stehney AF, Lucas HF: Dose-response relationships for female radium dial painters. *Radiat Res* 76:368–383, 1978.

Saccomanno G, Auerbach O, Kuschner M, *et al.*: A comparison between the localization of lung tumors in uranium miners and in nonminers from 1947 to 1991. *Cancer* 77:1278–1283, 1996.

Samet JM: Radon and lung cancer. *J Natl Cancer Inst* 81:745–757, 1989.

Samet JM, Stolwijk J, Rose SL: Summary: International workshop on residential radon epidemiology. *Health Phys* 60:223–227, 1991.

Schoenberg J, Klotz J: *A Case-Control Study of Radon and Lung Cancer Among New Jersey Women.* NJDH Technical Report, Phase I. Trenton, NJ: New Jersey State Department of Health, 1989.

Schoenberg JB, Klotz JB, Wilcox HB, Szmaciasz SF: A case-control study of radon and lung cancer among New Jersey women, in Cross FT (ed.): 29th Hanford Symposium on Health and the Environment: *Indoor Radon and Lung Cancer: Reality or Myth.* Columbus, OH: Battelle Press, 1990, pp. 905–922.

Schulz R, Albert RE: Dose to organs of the head from the x-ray treatment of tinea capitis. *Arch Environ Health* 17:935–950, 1963.

Sevc J, Kunz E, Tomasek L, *et al.*: Cancer in man after exposure to Rn daughters. *Health Phys* 54:27–46, 1988.

Shapiro J: Radiation protection: A guide for scientists regulators and physicians, 4th edition. Cambridge MA: Harvard University Press, 2002.

Shimizu Y, Kato H, Schull WJ, *et al.*: *Life Span Study Report 11, Part 1. Comparison of Risk Coefficients for Site-Specific Cancer Mortality Based on the DS86 and T65DR Shielded Kerma and Organ Doses.* RERF Technical Report TR 12-87. Hiroshima, Japan: Radiation Effects Research Foundation, 1987a.

Shimizu Y, Kato H, Schull WJ: *Life Span Study Report 11, Part 2. Cancer Mortality in the Years 1950–85 Based on the Recently Revised Doses (DS86).* RERF Report TR-5-88. Hiroshima, Japan: Radiation Effects Research Foundation, 1988.

Shore RE: Overview of radiation-induced skin cancer in humans. *Int J Radiat Biol* 57:809–827, 1990.

Shore RE: Issues and epidemiological evidence regarding radiation-induced thyroid cancer. *Radiat Res* 131:98–111, 1992.

Shore RE, Albert RE, Pasternack BS: Follow-up of patients treated by x-ray epilation for tinea capitis. *Arch Environ Health* 31:21–28, 1976.

Shore RE, Albert RE, Reed M, *et al.*: Skin cancer incidence among children irradiated for ringworm of the scalp. *Radiat Res* 100:192–204, 1984.

Shore RA, Moseson M, Harley NH, Pasternack BS: Tumors and other diseases following childhood x-ray treatment for ringworm of the scalp (tinea capitis). *Health Phys* 85(4):404–408, 2003.

Shore RA, Moseson M, Xue X, Tse Y, Harley NH, Pasternack BS: Skin cancer after x-ray treatment for scalp ringworm. *Radiat Res* 157:410–418, 2002.

Sinclair WK, Abbatt HE, Farran HE, *et al.*: A quantitative autoradiographic study of radioactive distribution and dosage in human thyroid glands. *Br J Radiol* 29:36–41, 1956.

Smith PG: Late effects x-ray treatment of ankylosing spondylitis, in Boice JD, Fraumeni JF (eds.): *Radiation Carcinogenesis: Epidemiology and Biological Significance.* New York: Raven Press, 1984.

Smith PG, Doll R: Mortality among patients with ankylosing spondylitis after a single treatment course with x-rays. *Br Med J* 1:449, 1982.

Smith WM, Doll R: Age- and time-dependent changes in the rates of radiation-induced cancers in patients with ankylosing spondylitis following a single course of x-ray treatment, in *Late Effects of Ionizing Radiation.* Vol. 1. Vienna: International Atomic Energy Agency, 1978, p. 205.

Spiess FW, Mays CW: Bone cancers induced by Ra-224 (ThX) in children and adults. *Health Phys* 19:713–729, 1970.

Spiess H, Mays CW: Protraction effect on bone sarcoma induction of Ra-224 in children and adults, in Sanders CL, Busch RH, Ballou JE, Mahlum DD (eds.): *Radionuclide Carcinogenesis.* Springfield, VA: National Technical Information Service, 1973, pp. 437–450.

Sutherland BM, Bennett PV, Sidorkina O, *et al.*: Clustered DNA damages induced in isolated DNA and in human cells by low doses of ionizing radiation. *Proc Natl Acad Sci U S A* 97:103–108, 2000.

Tirmarche M, Raphalen A, Allin F, *et al.*: Mortality of a cohort of Rench uranium miners exposure to a relatively low radon exposure. *Br J Cancer* 67:1090–1097, 1993.

Tu KW, Knutson EO: Indoor radon progeny particle size distribution measurements made with two different methods. *Radiat Prot Dosimet* 24:251, 1988.

Turner JE: *Atoms, Radiation and Radiation Protection.* Elmsford, NY: Pergamon Press, 1986.

UNSCEAR: *Sources, Effects and Risks of Ionizing Radiation.* Report of the United Nations Scientific Committee on the Effects of Atomic Radiation. New York: United Nations, 1988.

UNSCEAR: *Sources and Effects of Ionizing Radiation.* Report of the United Nations Scientific Committee on the Effects of Atomic Radiation. New York: United Nations, 1993, pp. 125–128.

UNSCEAR: *Sources and Effects of Ionizing Radiation.* Report of the United Nations Scientific Committee on the Effects of Atomic Radiation. New York: United Nations, 1994, pp. 60–63.

UNSCEAR: *Sources and Effects of Ionizing Radiation.* Report of the United Nations Scientific Committee on the Effects of Atomic Radiation. New York: United Nations, 2000.

UNSCEAR: *Sources to Effects Assessment for Radon in Homes and Workplaces.* Report of the United Nations Scientific Committee on the Effects of Atomic Radiation. New York: United Nations, 2007.

Ward JF: Molecular mechanisms of radiation-induced damage to nucleic acids. *Adv Rad Biol* 5:181–239, 1975.

Ward JF: The complexity of DNA damage: Relevance to biological consequences. *Int J Radiat Biol* 66:427–432, 1994.

Weiss HA, Darby SC, Doll R: Cancer mortality following x-ray treatment for ankylosing spondylitis. *Int J Cancer* 59:327–338, 1994.

Weiss HA, Darby SC, Fearn T: Leukemia mortality following x-ray treatment for ankylosing spondylitis. *Int Radiat Res* 142:1–11, 1995.

Whaling W: The energy loss of charged particles in matter, in Flugge S (ed.): *Handbuch der Physik.* Berlin: Springer-Verlag, 1958, pp. 193–217.

Wick RR, Chmelevsky D, Gossner W: 224Ra risk to bone and haematopoietic tissue in ankylosing spondylitis patients, in Gossner W, Gerber GB, Hagan U, Luz A (eds.): *The Radiobiology of Radium and Thorotrast.* Munich: Urban & Schwarzenberg, 1986, pp. 38–44.

Wick RR, Nekolla EA, Gossner W, Kellerer AM: Late effects in ankylosing spondylitis patients treated with ^{224}Ra. *Radiat Res* 152(Suppl): S8–S11, 1999.

Woodward A, Roder D, McMichael AJ, *et al.*: Radon daughter exposures at the Radium Hill uranium mine and lung cancer rates among former workers 1952–1987. *Cancer Causes Control* 2:213–220, 1991.

Woodard HQ: *Radiation Carcinogenesis in Man: A Critical Review.* Environmental Measurements Laboratory Report EML-380. New York: U.S. Department of Energy, 1980.

Ziegler JF: *Helium Stopping Powers and Ranges in All Elemental Matter.* New York: Pergamon Press, 1977.

CHAPTER 26

PROPERTIES AND TOXICITIES OF ANIMAL VENOMS

John B. Watkins, III

INTRODUCTION

The animal kingdom consists of more than 100,000 species spread through major phyla including arthropods, mollusks, chordates, etc. (Mebs, 2002). Venomous animals are capable of producing a poison in a highly developed exocrine gland or group of cells and can deliver their toxin during a biting or stinging act. The venom is the sum of all natural venomous substances produced in the animal (Ménez *et al.*, 2006). Poisonous animals have no mechanism or structure for the delivery of their poisons, and poisoning usually takes place through ingestion. Venomous or poisonous animals are widely distributed throughout the animal kingdom, from the unicellular protistan *Alexandrium (Gonyaulax)* to certain mammals, including the platypus and the short-tailed shrew. At least 400 species of snakes are considered dangerous to humans. Myriad venomous and poisonous arthropods exist, and toxic marine animals are found in almost every sea and ocean (Russell and Nagabhushanam, 1996; Mebs, 2002).

Animal venom may play a role in offense, as in the capture and digestion of food, in the animal's defense, as in protection against predators or aggressors, or in both functions. In the snake, the venom provides a food-getting mechanism. Its secondary function is its defensive status. The presence of toxic venom in the snake is a superior complement to the animal's speed, size, concealment, or strength. In venomous spiders, toxin is used to paralyze the prey before the extraction of hemolymph and body fluids. The venom is not primarily designed to kill the prey, but it is only to immobilize the organism for feeding. The same can be said for the scorpions, although they do use their venom in defense. In the fishes, such as the scorpion fishes and stone fishes, and in elasmobranches, such as the stingray, the venom apparatus is generally used in the animal's defense. Venoms used in an offensive posture are generally associated with the oral pole, as in the snakes and spiders, while those used in a defensive function are usually associated with the aboral pole or with spines, as in the stingrays and scorpion fishes. Poisonous animals, on the other hand, usually derive their toxins through the food chain. As such, poison is often a metabolite produced by microorganisms, plants, or animals. Poisons are sometimes concentrated as they pass through the food chain from one animal to another.

PROPERTIES OF ANIMAL TOXINS

Venoms are very complex, containing polypeptides, high- and low-molecular-weight proteins, amines, lipids, steroids, aminopolysaccharides, quinones, glucosides, and free amino acids, as well as serotonin, histamine, and other substances. Some venoms may consist of more than a hundred proteins. The venom is a source of millions of peptides and proteins that act on myriad exogenous targets such as ion channels, receptors, and enzymes within cells and on the cell membrane (Ménez *et al.*, 2006). The venom is important for several reasons. First, the venom is a source of tools with which to study complex physiologic systems, such as the cardiovascular system, nervous system, coagulation, and homeostasis. Second, the venom is a source of potential new drugs, with at least five agents already on the market and dozens undergoing preclinical or clinical

Table 26-1

Intravenous LD$_{50}$s of Selected Toxins Determined in Mice

TOXIN SOURCE	COMMON NAME	LD$_{50}$ (μg/kg)
Clostridium botulinum	Botulinum toxin	0.0003
Crotalus viridis helleri	Southern pacific rattlesnake	1.3
Crotalus adamanteus	Eastern diamondback	1.5
Oxyuranus scutellatus	Australian taipan	2
Crotalus atrox	Western diamondback	2.2
Agkistrodon piscivorus	Eastern cottonmouth	4
Agkistrodon contortrix	Copperhead	11
Androctonus australis	North African scorpion	17
Notechis scutatus	Australian tiger snake	25
Naja siamensis	Indochinese spitting cobra	75

SOURCES: Data from Mebs (2002) and Russell (2001).

trials (Menez *et al.*, 2005). Third, additional knowledge on the composition and the function of venoms is hoped to favor development of improved protection against envenomations (Ménez *et al.*, 2006).

Novel instrument developments have permitted the greater application of mass spectrometry, coupled with various separation technologies, to tease out the complexity of natural venoms, thereby identifying the peptide and protein components of venom (Escoubas, 2006). The technology allows considerable resolution of extremely small amounts of venom. Figure 26-1 demonstrates the application of gel filtration and high-pressure liquid chromatography (HPLC), as cone snail venom was fractionated into numerous peptides with varying activities (Olivera *et al.*, 1990). Similar fractionations have been performed on many other venoms. Unfortunately, studying the chemistry, pharmacology, and toxicology of venoms requires isolating and dismantling the venoms and losing the synergy among multiple components. Nevertheless, advanced technology will permit peptide sequencing, and the characterization of post-translational modifications, such as glycosylation, and the discovery of new pharmacophores. Most venoms probably exert their effects on almost every cell and tissue, and their principal pharmacologic properties are usually determined by the amount of a fraction that accumulates at an activity site. It is clear from Table 26-1 that there is an extremely large range in the LD$_{50}$ of different toxic compounds and venoms injected intravenously into mice.

The bioavailability of a venom is determined by its composition, molecular size, amount or concentration gradient, solubility, degree of ionization, and the rate of blood flow into that tissue, as well as the properties of the engulfing surface itself. The venom can be absorbed by active or passive transport, facilitated diffusion, or pinocytosis, among other physiologic mechanisms. Besides the bloodstream, the lymph circulation not only carries surplus interstitial fluid produced by the venom, but also transports larger molecular components and other particulates back to the bloodstream. Thus, the larger toxins of snake venoms, particularly those of Viperidae, probably enter the lymphatic network preferentially and then are transported to the central venous system in the neck (Russell, 2001). Because lymphatic capillaries, unlike blood capillaries, lack a basement membrane and have fibroelastic "anchoring filaments," they can readily adjust their shape and size, facilitating absorption of excess interstitial fluid along with macromolecules of a venom.

The site of action and metabolism of venom is dependent on its diffusion and partitioning along the gradient between the plasma and the tissues where the components are deposited. Once the toxin reaches a particular site, its entry to that site is dependent on the rate of blood flow into that tissue, the mass of the structure, and the partition characteristics of the toxin between the blood and the particular tissue. Receptor sites appear to have highly variable degrees of sensitivity. In the case of complex venoms, there may be several if not many receptor sites. There is also considerable variability in the sensitivity of those sites for the different components of a venom.

A venom may also be metabolized in several or many different tissues before undergoing excretion. Some components of a venom are metabolized distant to the receptor site(s) and may never reach the primary receptor in a quantity sufficient to affect that site. The amount of a toxin that tissues can metabolize without endangering the organisms may also vary. Organs or tissues may contain enzymes that catalyze a host of reactions, including deleterious ones. Once a venom component is metabolically altered, the end substance is excreted primarily through the kidneys. The intestines play a minor role, and the contributions by the lungs and biliary system have not been determined. Excretion may be complicated by the direct action of the venom on the kidneys themselves.

ARTHROPODS

There are more than a million species of arthropods, generally divided into 25 orders, of which at least 12 are of importance to humans from an economic standpoint. Medically, however, only about 10 orders are of significant venomous or poisonous importance. These include the arachnids (scorpions, spiders, whip scorpions, solpugids, mites, and ticks); the myriapods (centipedes and millipedes); the insects (water bugs, assassin bugs, and wheel bugs); beetles (blister beetles); Lepidoptera (butterflies, moths, and caterpillars), and Hymenoptera (ants, bees, and wasps). Several texts and papers that deal with venomous and poisonous arthropods are available (Bettini, 1978; Pick, 1986; Cohen and Quistad, 1998; Russell, 2001; Kuhn-Nentwig, 2003; Isbister *et al.*, 2004).

The number of deaths from arthropod stings and bites is unknown. In Mexico, parts of Central and South America, North Africa, and India, deaths from scorpion stings, for instance, exceed several thousand a year. Spider bites probably do not account for more than 200 deaths a year worldwide. A common problem faced by physicians in suspected spider bites relates to the differential diagnosis. The arthropods most frequently involved in the misdiagnoses were ticks (including their embedded mouthparts), mites, bedbugs, fleas (infected flea bites), Lepidoptera insects, flies, vesicating beetles, water bugs, and various stinging Hymenoptera. Among the disease states that were confused with spider or arthropod bites or stings were erythema chronicum migrans, erythema nodosum, periarteritis nodosum, pyroderma gangrenosum, kerion cell-mediated response to a fungus, Stevens–Johnson syndrome, toxic epidermal necrolysis, herpes simplex, and purpura fulminans. Any arthropod may bite or sting and not eject venom. Finally, some arthropod venom poisonings accentuate the symptoms and signs of an existing undiagnosed subclinical disease.

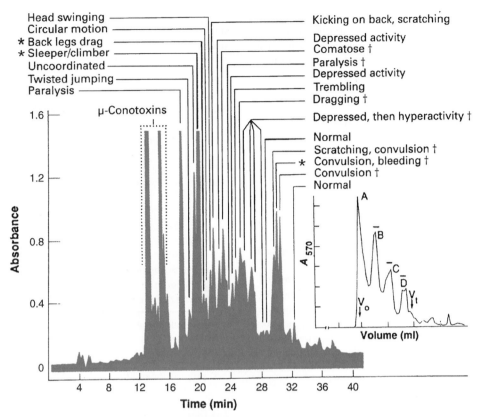

Figure 26-1. Multiple biologically active components were obtained from Conus geographus venom by first subjecting the venom to gel filtration on Sephadex G-25 into four fractions and then separation of fraction B (which contains the α-conotoxins) by high-pressure liquid chromatography on a VYDAC C18 column using a trifluoroacetic acid–acetonitrile gradient.

Various peak fractions were then injected intracerebrally into mice and different responses were noted.[†] The fraction was lethal in at least one injected animal. Reprinted with permission from Olivera BM, Rivier J, Clark C, *et al.*: Diversity of *Conus* neuropeptides. *Science* 249, 257–263, 1990.

ARACHNIDA

Scorpions

Of the more than 1000 species of scorpions, the stings of more than 75 can be considered of sufficient importance to warrant medical attention (Keegan, 1980; Polis, 1990; Russell, 2001). Scorpions spend the daylight hours under cover or in burrows. They emerge at night to ambush other arthropods or even small rodents, capture them with their pincers, sting and paralyze them, or tear them apart and digest their body fluids. Because they are carnivorous, the larger ones often feed on the smaller ones. Some of the more important ones of these species are noted in Table 26-2. In addition, members of the genera *Pandinus, Hadrurus, Vejovis, Nebo,* and some of the others are capable of inflicting painful and often erythematous lesions.

The bark scorpion, *Centruroides exilicauda*, is often found hiding under the loose bark of trees or in dead trees or logs, and may frequent human dwellings. Straw to yellowish-brown or reddish-brown in color, it is often easily distinguishable from other scorpions in the same habitat by its long, thin telson, or tail, and its thin pedipalps, or pincer-like claws. Adults of this genus show a considerable difference in length from less than 5 cm in length in *Centruroides noxius* to a length of 9 cm in *Centruroides suffuses.*

Table 26-2
Location of Some Medically Important Scorpions

GENUS	DISTRIBUTION
Androctonus species	North Africa, Middle East, Turkey
Buthus species	France and Spain to Middle East and north Africa, Mongolia, China
Buthotus species	Africa, Middle East, central Asia
Centruroides species	North, Central, South America
Heterometrus species	Central and southeast Asia
Leiurus species	North Africa, Middle East, Turkey
Mesobuthus species	Turkey, India
Parabuthus species	Southern Africa
Tityus species	Central and South America

Many scorpion venoms contain low-molecular-weight proteins, peptides, amino acids, nucleotides, and salts, among other components (Possani *et al.*, 2000; Goldin, 2001; Rodriguez de la Vega and Possani, 2004, 2005). The neurotoxic fractions are generally classified on the basis of their molecular size, the short-chain toxins being composed of 20–40 amino acid residues with three or four disulfide bonds and appear to affect potassium or chloride channels; while the long-chain toxins have 58–76 amino acid residues

(6500–8500 Da) with four disulfide bonds and affect mainly the sodium channels (Mouhat *et al.*, 2004). These particular toxins may have an effect on both voltage-dependent channels. The amino acid content is known for more than 90 species, and there appears to be a high degree of cysteines in most of these venoms. The toxins can selectively bind to a specific channel of excitable cells, thus impairing the initial depolarization of the action potential in the nerve and muscle that results in their neurotoxicity. It appears that the way some scorpion venoms differently affect mammalian, as opposed to insect tissues, is related to the structural basis of the gates in the two organisms. Not all scorpions, however, have fractions that affect neuromuscular transmission. Recently, Rodriguez de la Vega and Possani (2005) constructed a phylogenetic tree using 191 different amino acid sequences from long-chain peptides and discussed their functional divergence and extant biodiversity. The effects of scorpion venom on various potassium channels have been reviewed (Rodriguez de la Vega and Possani, 2004). More intensive research is needed to further understand scorpion toxins.

The symptoms and signs of scorpion envenomation differ considerably depending on the species (Russell, 2001). Common offenders are members of the family Vejovidae, generally found in the southwestern and western United States, Central America, and South America. Their sting gives rise to localized pain, swelling, tenderness, and mild parasthesia. Systemic reactions are rare, although weakness, fever, and muscle fasciculations have been reported. Envenomations by some members of the genus *Centruroides* are clinically the most important, particularly in the western United States, where *C. exilicauda* is found. In children, their sting may produce initial pain, although some children do not complain of pain and are unaware of the injury. The area becomes sensitive to touch, and merely pressing lightly over the injury will elicit an immediate retraction. Usually there is little or no local swelling and only mild erythema. The child becomes tense and restless and shows abnormal and random head and neck movements. Often the child will display roving eye movements. In their review of *Centruroides sculpturatus* stings, Rimsza *et al.* (1980) noted visual signs, including nystagmus roving eye and oculogyric movements, in 12 of 24 patients stung by this scorpion. Tachycardia is usually evident within 45 minutes as well as some hypertension. Although this is not seen in children as early or as severely as in adults, it is often present within an hour following the sting. Respiratory and heart rates are increased, and by 90 minutes the child may appear quite ill. Fasciculations may be seen over the face or large muscle masses, and the child may complain of generalized weakness and display some ataxia or motor weakness. Opisthotonos is not uncommon. The respiratory distress may proceed to respiratory paralysis. Excessive salivation is often present and may further impair respiratory function. Slurring of speech may be present, and convulsions may occur. If death does not occur, the child usually becomes asymptomatic within 36–48 hours.

In adults the clinical picture is somewhat similar, but there are some differences (Russell, 2001). Almost all adults complain of immediate pain after the sting, regardless of the *Centruroides* species involved. Adults do not show the restlessness that is seen in children. Instead, they are tense and anxious. They develop tachycardia and hypertension, and respirations are increased. They may complain of difficulties in focusing and swallowing. In some cases, there is some general weakness and pain on moving the injured extremity. Convulsions are very rare, but ataxia and muscle incoordination may occur. Most adults are asymptomatic within 12 hours, but may complain of generalized weakness for 24 hours or more.

Table 26-3

Some Significant Spiders, Their Toxins and the Targets of the Toxins

SPIDER	PEPTIDE	TARGET*
Acanthoscurria gomesiana	Gomesin	PLM
Agelenopsis aperta	ω-AfaI-IVA	Ca^{2+}
	μ-afatoxin 1–6	Na^+
Grammostola spatula	HaTx1,2	K^+
	GsMTx2,4	MS
	GSTxSIA	Ca^{2+}
Hadronyche versuta	ω-ACTX-Hv1a	Ca^{2+}
	ω-ACTX-Hv2a	Ca^{2+}
	δ-ACTX-Hv1a	Na^+
Heteroscodra maculate	HmTx1,2	K^+
Ornithoctonus huwena	Huwentoxin I	Ca^{2+}
	Huwentoxin IV	Na^+
Psalmopoeus cambridgei	PcTx1	ASIC
Phrixotrichus auratus	PaTx1,2	K^+
Thrixopelma pruriens	ProTxI,II	Na^+

PLM, phospholipid membranes; Ca^{2+}, K^+, and Na^+, calcium, potassium, and sodium ion channels; MS, mechano-sensitive ion channels; ASCI, acid-sensing ion channels.

Additional species, their toxins, and their targets may be obtained in the article by Corzo and Escoubas (2003).

Spiders

Of the 30,000 or so species, at least 200 have been implicated in significant bites on humans. Spiders are predaceous, polyphagous arachnids that generally feed on insects or other arthropods. Additional information of spider bites can be found elsewhere (Gertsch, 1979; Maretiĉ and Lebez, 1979; Russell, 2001). Table 26-3 provides a short list of spiders, their toxins, and the targets of their toxins.

All spiders except the Uloboridae family possess a venom apparatus that produces neurotoxins designed to paralyze or kill prey. Spider venoms are complex mixtures of low-molecular-weight components, including inorganic ions and salts, free acids, glucose-free amino acids, biogenic amines and neurotransmitters, and polypeptide toxins. The acylpolyamines, composed of a hydrophobic aromatic carboxylic acid linked to a lateral chain of one to nine aminopropyl, aminobutyl, or aminopentyl units, are voltage-dependent open-channel blockers (sodium, calcium, and potassium channels) and/or blockers of the ion channel associated with glutamate receptors. They also act on nicotinic acetylcholine receptors. The acylpolyamines possess insecticidal activity and induce fast insect paralysis via a reversible block of the insect neuromuscular junction. Polypeptide toxins include the ion channel blockers, pore-forming peptides, and enzymes. In particular, hanatoxins 1 and 2 have allowed characterization of voltage-dependent potassium channels (Swartz and MacKinnon, 1995; Yellen, 2002). The ω-agatoxins have been demonstrated to block voltage-sensitive vertebrate calcium channels (Corzo and Escoubas, 2003). The ω-atracotoxins have greater selectivity on insect voltage-sensitive calcium channels (Wang *et al.*, 2001). Many more spiders and the spider peptide toxins that have been studied to date (Fatehi *et al.*, 1997; Liu *et al.*, 1997; Corzo and Escoubas, 2003; Adams, 2004; Kuhn-Nentwig *et al.*, 2004; Rodriguez de la Vega and Possani, 2004; Ushkaryov *et al.*, 2004; Wilson and Alewood, 2006). The small spider peptide toxins are relatively easy to produce by chemical synthesis or by

Table 26-4

Comparison of Clinical Effects of Bites by Some Spiders of Australia

CLINICAL EFFECTS	*LACTRODECTUS* REDBACK SPIDERS	*STEATODA* CUPBOARD SPIDERS	LAMPONIDAE WHITE-TAIL SPIDERS	MYGALOMORPHAE FWS, MOUSE SPIDERS, TRAPDOOR SPIDERS
Severe pain (%)	62	26	27	49
Duration of pain	36 h	6 h	5 min	60 min
Fang marks (%)	6	17	17	58
Initial erythema	74	96	83	36
Swelling (%)	7	9	8	13
Itchiness (%)	38	48	44	0
Nausea, vomiting, headache, malaise (%)	35	30	9	36
Distal limb bite (%)	46	52	82	91

SOURCE: Data from Isbister and White (2004).

recombinant means. Peptide toxins from spiders have proved useful in discriminating between different cellular components of native ion channel currents and for the molecular isolation and designation of cellular receptors (Escoubas *et al.*, 2000; Corzo and Escoubas, 2003; Adams, 2004).

Poor case definition and spider identification contribute to the controversy regarding the clinical consequences and inappropriate diagnosis of spider bites worldwide. Many patients never see the spider yet many skin lesions or areas of necrosis are attributed to spider bites. The medically important spiders include the *Latrodectus* spp., *Loxosceles* spp., *Agelenopsis* spp., *Atrax* spp., *Hadronyche* spp., and *Phoneutria* spp. Table 26-4, summarized from Isbister and White (2004), lists local and systemic effects for known cases of major spider groups in Australia.

***Agelenopsis* Species (American Funnel Web Spiders)**   The American funnel web spider (*Agelenopsis aperta*) contains three classes of agatoxins that target ion channels (Adams, 2004). The α-agatoxins appear to be use-dependent, noncompetitive antagonists of the glutamate receptor channels. These are low-molecular-weight acylpolyamines that are devoid of amino acids. Mass spectrometry analysis has identified more than 33 α-agatoxins in *A. aperta* venom (Chesnov *et al.*, 2001). The μ-agatoxins are 36–37 amino acid, C-terminal amidated, peptides with four internal disulfide bridges (Skinner *et al.*, 1989). These μ-agatoxins cause increased spontaneous release of neurotransmitter from presynaptic terminals and repetitive action potentials in motor neurons. In addition, the μ-agatoxins are specific for insect sodium channels. The ω-amatoxins are a structurally diverse group of peptides that are selective for voltage-activated calcium channels. There are four types of ω-amatoxins that can be distinguished by sequence similarity and their spectrum of action against insect and vertebrate calcium channels. The action of the α-agatoxins is synergized by the μ-agatoxins causing channels to open at the normal resting potentials. It is interesting to note that the agatoxins are used as selective pharmacologic probes to characterize ion channels in organs such as brain and heart, and have been evaluated as candidate biopesticides.

***Latrodectus* Species (Widow Spiders)**   Found throughout the world in all continents with temperate or tropical climates, these spiders are commonly known as the black widow, brown widow, or red-legged spider. They, however, have many other common names

in English: hourglass, poison lady, deadly spider, red-bottom spider, T-spider, gray lady spider, and shoebutton spider. Although both male and female widow spiders are venomous, only the female has fangs that are large and strong enough to penetrate the human skin. Mature *Latrodectus mactans* females range in body length from 10 to 18 mm, whereas males range from 3 to 5 mm. These spiders have a globose abdomen varying in color from gray to brown to black, depending on the species. In the black widow, the abdomen is shiny black with a red hourglass or red spots and sometimes with white spots on the venter (Russell, 2001).

The latrotoxins, a family of high-molecular-weight proteins that are found in *Latrodectus* venoms, target different classes of animals including vertebrates, insects, and crustaceans (Grishin, 1998; 1999; Ushkaryov *et al.*, 2004). The toxins are synthesized as large precursors containing around 1000 amino acid residues (around 132–156 kDa) that undergo proteolytic processing to 110–130 kDa and activation in the lumen of the venom gland. Mature latrotoxins are structurally conserved and contain multiple ankyrin repeats. At least seven different latrotoxins have been isolated and all are large acidic proteins (pI ~ 5.0–6.0). Some are called latroinsectotoxins because they affect insects but not vertebrates, and one protein called α-latrocrustatoxin is active only in crayfish. All latrotoxins stimulate massive release of neurotransmitters after binding to specific neuronal receptors.

α-Latrotoxin is the most studied protein that is toxic only to vertebrates and not to insects or crustaceans (Ushkaryov *et al.*, 2004). α-Latrotoxin is a presynaptic toxin that is said to exert its toxic effects on the vertebrate central nervous system depolarizing neurons by increasing intracellular [Ca^{2+}] and by stimulating exocytosis of neurotransmitters from nerve terminals (Holz and Habener, 1998). The purported three-dimensional structure of α-latrotoxin consists of tetrameric complexes with a central channel that inserts into the lipid bilayer. A G-protein-coupled receptor latrophilin and a single-transmembrane receptor neurenin are high-affinity binding sites for α-latrotoxin (Ushkaryov *et al.*, 2004). The latrotoxins act by both calcium-dependent and calcium-independent mechanisms. In fact, a mutant recombinant α-latrotoxin that does not form pores has been invaluable in furthering our understanding of the multiple actions of the toxin (Volynski *et al.*, 2003). α-Latrotoxin and its mutants are versatile tools for the study of exocytosis. In particular, studies with this toxin have helped confirm the vesicular hypothesis of transmitter release (Hurlbut *et al.*, 1990), establish the requirement of calcium ion for endocytosis (Ceccarelli and Hurlbut,

1980), characterize individual neurotransmitter sites in the central nervous system (Auger and Marty, 1997), and identify two families of important neuronal cell-surface receptors (Krasnoperov *et al.*, 1997).

Bites by the black widow are described as sharp and pinprick like, followed by a dull, occasionally numbing pain in the affected extremity and by pain and cramps in one or several of the large muscle masses (Russell, 2001). Rarely is there any local skin reaction except during the first 60 minutes following the bite. Muscle fasciculations frequently can be seen within 30 minutes of the bite. Sweating is common, and the patient may complain of weakness and pain in the regional lymph nodes, which are often tender on palpation and occasionally are enlarged; lymphadenitis is frequently observed. Pain in the low back, thighs, or abdomen is a common complaint, and rigidity of the abdominal muscles is seen in most cases in which envenomation has been severe. Severe paroxysmal muscle cramps may occur, and arthralgia has been reported. Hypertension is a common finding, particularly in the elderly after moderate-to-severe envenomations. Blood studies are usually normal.

Loxosceles Species (Brown or Violin Spiders)   These primitive spiders are variously known in North America as the fiddle-back spider or the brown recluse. There are over 100 species of *Loxosceles*. The abdomen of these spiders varies in color from grayish through orange and reddish-brown to blackish and is distinct from the pale yellow to reddish-brown background of the cephalothorax. This spider has six eyes grouped in three dyads. Females average 8–12 mm in body length, whereas males average 6–10 mm. Both males and females are venomous (Russell, 2001).

The venom of *Loxosceles* spiders appears to contain phospholipase, protease, esterase, collagenase, hyaluronidase, deoxyribonuclease, ribonuclease, dipeptides, dermonecrosis factors, and sphingomyelinase D. The venom has coagulation and vasoconstriction properties and it causes selective vascular endothelial damage. There are adhesions of neutrophils to the capillary wall with sequestration and activation of passing neutrophils by the perturbed endothelial cells (Patel *et al.*, 1994). In *Loxosceles intermedia a,* the toxic effects appear to be associated with a 35-kDa protein that demonstrates a complement-dependent hemolytic activity and a dermonecrotic-inducing factor. ^{31}P-Nuclear magnetic resonance assay of the four bands representing proteins, measuring 34 kDa in the venom, produced three proteins with sphingomyelinase D activity (Merchant *et al.*, 1998). An endotoxemic-like shock, showing eosinophilic material in the proximal and distal tubules and tubular necrosis, was the most common histopathologic finding, preceded in mice by prostration, acute cachexia, hypothermia, neurological changes, and hemoglobinuria (Tambourgi *et al.*, 1998).

The bite of this spider produces about the same degree of pain as does the sting of an ant, but sometimes the patient may be unaware of the bite. In most cases, a local burning sensation, which may last for 30–60 minutes, develops around the injury. Pruritus over the area often occurs, and the area becomes red, with a small blanched area surrounding the reddened bite site. Skin temperature usually is elevated over the lesion area. With significant envenomations, the reddened area enlarges and becomes purplish during the subsequent 1–8 hours. It often becomes irregular in shape, and as time passes, hemorrhages may develop throughout the area. A small bleb or vesicle may form at the bite site, increase in size, and rupture with subsequent pustule formation. The red hemorrhagic area continues

to enlarge, as does the pustule. The whole area may become swollen and painful, and lymphadenopathy is common. During the early stages, the lesion often takes on a bull's-eye appearance, with a central white vesicle surrounded by the reddened area and ringed by a whitish or bluish border. The central pustule ruptures, and necrosis to various depths can be visualized (Russell, 2001).

In serious bites, the lesion can measure 8×10 cm^2 with severe necrosis invading muscle tissue. On the face, large lesions resulting in extensive tissue destruction and requiring subsequent plastic surgery sometimes are seen after bites by *Loxosceles laeta* in South America. Systemic symptoms and signs include fever, malaise, stomach cramps, nausea and vomiting, jaundice, spleen enlargement, hemolysis, hematuria, and thrombocytopenia. Fatal cases, while rare, usually are preceded by intravascular hemolysis, hemolytic anemia, thrombocytopenia, hemoglobinuria, and renal failure (Russell, 2001).

Steatoda Species   These spiders are variously known as the false black widow, combfooted, cobweb, or cupboard spiders. The female of *Steatoda grossa* differs from *L. mactans* and *Latrodectus hesperus* in having a purplish-brown abdomen rather than a black one. It is less shiny, and its abdomen is more oval than round. It may have pale yellow or whitish markings on the dorsum of the abdomen, and no markings on the venter. The abdomen of some species is orange, brown, or chestnut in color, and often bears a light band across the anterior dorsum (Russell, 2001).

The venom of *Steatoda paykulliana* stimulates the release of transmitter substances similar to *Latrodectus* venom (Cavalieri *et al.*, 1987). The venom is said to form ionic channels permeable for bi- and monovalent cations, and that the duration of time in the open state depends on the membrane potential (Sokolov *et al.*, 1984). *S. paykulliana* venom induces strong motor unrest, clonic cramps, exhaustion, ataxia, and then paralysis in guinea pigs. Bites by *S. grossa* or *Steatoda fulva* in the United States have been followed by local pain, often severe; induration; pruritus; and the occasional break down of tissue at the bite site (Russell, 2001).

Cheiracanthium Species (Running Spiders)   The 160 species of this genus have an almost circumglobal distribution, although only four or five species have been implicated in bites on humans (Russell, 2001). *Cheiracanthium punctorium, Cheiracanthium inclusum, Cheiracanthium mildei, Cheiracanthium diversum*, and *Cheiracanthium japonicum* are often implicated in envenomations. The abdomen is convex and egg shaped and varies in color from yellow, green, or greenish-white to reddish-brown; the cephalothorax is usually slightly darker than the abdomen. The chelicerae are strong, and the legs are long, hairy, and delicate. The spider ranges in length from 7 to 16 mm. Like *Phidippus* but even more so, *Cheiracanthium* tends to be tenacious and sometimes must be removed from the bite area. For that reason there is a high degree of identification following the bite of these spiders. The most toxic venom fraction is said to be a protein of 60 kDa, and the venom is high in norepinephrine and serotonin.

The patient usually describes the bite by *C. inclusum* as sharp and painful, with the pain increasing during the first 30–45 hours. The patient complains of dull pain over the injured part. A reddened wheal with a hyperemic border develops. Small petechiae may appear near the center of the wheal. Skin temperature over the lesion is often elevated, but body temperature is usually normal. Lymphadenitis and lymphadenopathy may develop. *C. japonicum* produces more severe manifestations, including severe local pain, nausea and vomiting, headache, chest discomfort, severe pruritus, and shock (Russell, 2001).

***Theraphosidae* Species (Tarantulas)** True tarantulas are members of the family Theraphosidae and there are around 800 species that are distributed worldwide, but especially in tropical or semitropical regions. Tarantulas are predators and they feed on various vertebrate and invertebrate preys that are captured after envenomation with venoms that act rapidly and irreversibly on the central and peripheral nervous systems. In humans, reported bites elicit mild-to-severe local pain, strong itching, and tenderness that may last for several hours. Edema, erythema, joint stiffness, swollen limbs, burning feelings, and cramps are common. In more severe cases, strong cramps and muscular spasms lasting up to several hours may be observed. *Poecilotheria* and *Stromatopelma* spp. appear to be most toxic to humans, although no fatalities have been reported (Escoubas and Rash, 2004).

Tarantula venoms have been extensively studied, and modern purification often uses orthogonal HPLC separations that combine reversed-phase and ion-exchange chromatography. Most spider peptide toxins appear to have basic pI in the 9–11 range (Escoubas *et al.*, 2000). Mass spectrometry techniques including electrospray ionization, matrix-assisted laser desorption-ionization (MALDI), and MALDI coupled to time-of-flight analysis have been extensively used for venom characterization. At least 33 peptide toxins have been described from various tarantula venoms. These have a molecular weight of 3000–5700 Da, and targets include voltage-gated potassium, sodium and calcium channels, tetrodotoxin-sensitive channels, and acid-sensing ion channels, which are sensitive to extracellular pH (reviewed by Escoubas and Rash, 2004). At least two distinct structural motifs have been characterized: the Inhibitory Cystine Knot (ICK) with a consensus sequence of $C_IX_{3-7}–C_{II}X_{3-8}–C_{III}X_{0-7}–C_{IV}X_{1-4}–C_VX_{4-13}–C_{VI}$ and disulfide bond pairing of $C_I–C_{IV}$, $C_{II}–C_V$, and $C_{III}–C_{VI}$ (Craik *et al.*, 2001), and the disulfide-directed β-hairpin (DDH) motif that comprises an antiparallel β-hairpin stabilized by two disulfide bridges (Wang *et al.*, 2000). Tarantula toxins have been classified as long-loop ICK, short-loop ICK, or DDH toxins (Escoubas and Rash, 2004).

Theraphosid spiders contain several toxins that are being evaluated for development as antiarrhythmic or as antinociceptive drugs. In particular, *Grammostola* mechanotoxin 4 from *Grammostola spatulata* has considerable promise as an antiarrhythmic. Protoxin I and II from *Thrixopelma pruriens* have promise as analgesics because they inhibit the tetrodotoxin-resistant sodium channels (Middleton *et al.*, 2002).

Future work on the toxins of tarantulas will encompass genomic and proteomic approaches. Expanding knowledge suggests trends in the association of primary and three-dimensional structures with pharmacologic activity. Continued improvement in isolation and purification technologies plus the combination of cDNA library screening with mass spectrometry will prove invaluable in characterization of toxin function and definition of toxin targets.

Ticks

Many of the approximately 900 species of ticks are associated with disease in humans and wild and domesticated animals (Rash and Hodgson, 2002; Barker and Murrell, 2004; Steen *et al.*, 2006). Tick paralysis is caused by the saliva of certain ticks of the families Ixodidae, Argasidae, and Nuttalliellidae. The tick bite involves insertion of cutting, tube-like mouthparts through the host's skin with anchoring so that the tick can feed for hours, days, or weeks. Saliva from the salivarium flows outward initially and the blood meal flows inward afterward. Ticks are known to transmit the organisms causing Lyme disease, Rocky Mountain spotted fever, babesiosis, leptospirosis, Q fever, ehrlichiosis, typhus, tick-borne encephalitis, and others. In fact, the import of immunosuppression by tick saliva in the transmission of flaviviruses has been discussed (Nuttall and Labuda, 2003).

Tick saliva contains a number of active constituents (Steen *et al.*, 2006). For example, saliva from *Ixodes scapularis* contains apyrase (ATP-diphosphohydrolase), which hydrolyzes ADP that is released at the bite site thereby inhibiting ADP-induced platelet aggregation (Mans *et al.*, 1998), kininase (ACE-like protein or angiotensin-converting enzyme-like protein), which hydrolyzes circulating kinins and reduces the host inflammatory response (Francischetti *et al.*, 2003); glutathione peroxidase (Das *et al.*, 2001); serine protease inhibitors, which inhibit coagulation enzymes (Valenzuela, 2004); an anticomplement protein that inhibits an enzyme in the alternative pathway for complement (Valenzuela *et al.*, 2000); an amine-binding protein that binds serotonin, histamine, and other biogenic amines (Sangamnetdej *et al.*, 2002); and prostanoids (PGE_2 and $PGF_{2\alpha}$ (Inokuma *et al.*, 1994). A discussion of toxins from other species may be found elsewhere (Cavassani *et al.*, 2005; Steen *et al.*, 2006).

Potentially 50 species of ticks are associated with clinical paralysis (Russell, 2001). As tick bites are often not felt; the first evidence of envenomation may not appear until several days later, when small macules 3–4 mm in diameter develop that are surrounded by erythema and swelling, often displaying a hyperemic halo. The patient often complains of difficulty with gait, followed by paresis and eventually locomotor paresis and paralysis. Problems in speech and respiration may ensue and lead to respiratory paralysis if the tick is not removed. The saliva of *Ixodes holocyclus* has yielded a peptide holocyclotoxin-1 that may cause paralysis (Masina and Broady, 1999). Peak paralytic activity was found between 60 and 100 kDa, and was a trimer of aneurotoxic protein subunit of 23 kDa (Crause *et al.*, 1993). Symptoms resolve rapidly upon removal of the tick (Russell, 2001).

CHILOPODA (CENTIPEDES)

Found worldwide, these elongated, many-segmented brownish-yellow arthropods have a pair of walking legs on most segments, and they are fast moving, secretive, and nocturnal. They feed on other arthropods and even small vertebrates and birds. The first pair of legs behind the head is modified into poison jaws. Centipedes range in length from 3 mm to almost 300 mm. In the United States, the prevalent biting genus is a *Scolopendra* species. The venom is concentrated within the intracellular granules, discharged into vacuoles of the cytoplasm of the secretory cells, and moved by exocytosis into the lumen of the gland; from thence ducts carry the venom to the jaws (Ménez *et al.*, 1990).

Centipede venoms contain high-molecular-weight proteins, proteinases, esterases, 5-hydroxytryptamine, histamine, lipids, and polysaccharides (Mebs, 2002). Such venom contains a heat-labile cardiotoxic protein of 60 kDa that produces, in humans, changes associated with acetylcholine release (Gomes *et al.*, 1983). The bite produces two tiny punctures, sharp pain, immediate bleeding, redness, and swelling often lasting for 24 hours. Localized tissue changes and necrosis have been reported, and severe envenomations may cause nausea and vomiting, changes in heart rate, vertigo, and headache. In the most severe cases, there can be mental disturbances (Bush *et al.*, 2001; Russell, 2001; Mebs, 2002).

DIPLOPODA (MILLIPEDES)

Ranging in length from 20 to 300 mm, these arthropods are cylindrical, worm-like creatures, mahogany to dark brown or black in color, and bearing two pairs of jointed legs per segment. In Australia and New Guinea particularly, the repellent secretions expelled from the sides of their bodies contain a toxin of quinone derivatives plus a variety of complex substances such as iodine and hydrocyanic acid, which the animal makes use of to produce hydrogen cyanide. Some species can spray these defensive secretions, and eye injuries are not uncommon. The lesions produced by millipedes consist of a burning or prickling sensation and development of a yellowish or brown-purple lesion; subsequently, a blister containing serosanguinous fluid forms, which may rupture. Eye contact can cause acute conjunctivitis, periorbital edema, keratosis, and much pain; such an injury must be treated immediately (Russell, 2001).

INSECTA

Heteroptera (True Bugs)

The clinically most important of the true bugs are the Reduviidae (the reduviids): the kissing bug, assassin bug, wheel bug, or cone-nose bug of the genus *Triatoma* (Russell, 2001). Generally, they are parasites of rodents and common in the nests of wood rat or in wood piles. These are elongated bugs with freely movable, cone-shaped heads, and straight beaks. The most commonly involved species appear to be *Triatoma protracta, Triatoma rubida, Triatoma magista, Reduvius personatus,* and *Arilus cristatus.* The average length of these bugs is 19 mm. The venom of these bugs appears to have apyrase activity and to lack 5-nucleotidase, inorganic pyrophosphatase, phosphatase, and adenylate kinase activities, but it is fairly rich in protease properties. It inhibits collagen-induced platelet aggregation. Three peptides isolated from the saliva of predatory reduviids are 34–36 amino acid residues in size, are calcium channel blockers similar to ω-conotoxins, and belong to the four loop disulfide bridge scaffold structural class (Corzo *et al.*, 2001). The bites of *Triatoma* species are painful and give rise to erythema, pruritus, increased temperature in the bitten part, localized swelling, and—in those allergic to the saliva–systemic reactions such as nausea and vomiting and angioedema. With some bites the wound area will slough, leaving a depression.

The water-dwelling true bugs are of at least three families, Naucordiae, Belostomatidae, and Notonectidae, which are capable of biting and envenomating humans (Russell, 2001). They are found in lakes, ponds, marshes, quiet fresh water, and swimming pools. *Lethocerus americanus,* a Belostomatidae, ranges in length from 12 to 70 mm, but some water bugs may reach 150 mm. The dorsal side is usually tan or brown, but it may be brightly colored, while the ventral side is brown. They are very strong insects and can immobilize snails, tadpoles, salamanders, and even small fish and water snakes. Water bug saliva is said to contain digestive enzymes, neurotoxic components, and hemolytic fractions. ApoLp-III isolated from the hemolymph of *Lathocerus medius* is about 19 kDa and has an amino acid composition high in methionine. If molested, water bugs will bite, and their bites give rise to immediate pain, some localized swelling, and possibly induration and formation of a small papule.

Hymenoptera (Ants, Bees, Wasps, and Hornets)

Formicidae (Ants) Most ant species sink their powerful mandibles into the flesh, providing leverage, and then drive their stings into the victim. Most ants have stings, but those that lack them can spray a defensive secretion from the tip of the gaster, which is often placed in the wound of the bite. Ants of the different species vary considerably in length, ranging from less than 1.5 mm to over 35 mm. Clinically important stinging ants are the harvesting ants (*Pagonomyrmex*), fire ants (*Solenopsis*), and little fire ants (*Ochetomyrmex*). The harvester ants are large red, dark brown, or black ranging in size from 6 to 10 mm and having fringes of long hairs on the posterior of their heads (Russell, 2001).

The venoms of the ants vary considerably. The venoms of the Ponerinae, Ecitoninae, and Pseudomyrmex are proteinaceous in character. The Myrmecinae venoms are a mixture of amines, enzymes and proteinaceous materials, histamine, hyaluronidase, phospholipase A, and hemolysins, which hemolyze erythrocytes and mast cells. Formicinae ant venom contains about 60% formic acid. Fire ant venoms are poor in polypeptides and proteins, but are rich in alkaloids such as solenopsine (Russell, 2001; Mebs, 2002). The sting of the fire ant gives rise to a painful burning sensation, after which a wheal and localized erythema develop, leading in a few hours to a clear vesicle. Within 12–24 hours, the fluid becomes purulent and the lesion turns into a pustule. It may break down or become a crust or fibrotic nodule. In multiple stings there may be nausea, vomiting, vertigo, increased perspiration, respiratory difficulties, cyanosis, coma, and even death. Cross-exposure to the venom of other species of ants is possible. Allergic reactions and fatal anaphylactic shock are seen in sensitized victims (Hoffman, 2006). Treatment of ant stings is dependent on their number, whether an allergic reaction is involved, and whether there are possible complications.

Apidae (Bees) This family includes the bumble bees, honeybees, carpenter bees, and yellow jackets. The commonest stinging bees are *Apis mellifera* and the Africanized bee, *Apis mellifer adansonii*, and the incidence of Hymenoptera poisonings is increasing. The venom of the Africanized bee is not remarkably different from that of the European bee, *A. m. mellifer.* The former bee is smaller and gives less venom, but its aggressiveness is such that attacks of fifty to hundreds of bees are not unusual (Russell, 2001).

The venom contains biologically active peptides, such as melittin, apamine, mast cell-degranulating peptide, and others, as well as phospholipases A_2 and B, hyaluronidase, histamine, dopamine, monosaccharides, and lipids (Mebs, 2002). Melittin, which is secreted as prepromelittin of 70 amino acids, consists of 26 amino acids with no cysteines that have natural detergent-like properties and causes erythrocyte lyses. Melittin also forms tetramers that form pores, thereby facilitating ion transport through membranes. In particular, melittin-tetramers cause a break down of the resting potential and rapid depolarization of nociceptors, which induces pain (Demsey, 1990; Bechinger, 1997). The compound apamine contains 18 amino acids cross-linked by two disulfide bridges. Apamine is a blocker of calcium-dependent potassium channels and is thought to be the "lethal factor" (Habermann, 1984). In addition to apamine, mast cell-degranulating peptide is also a basic peptide containing 22 amino acids with two disulfide bonds. Besides stimulating release of histamine, this peptide specifically inhibits voltage-dependent potassium channels (Dreyer, 1990; Baku, 1999).

Bee stings typically produce immediate, sharp or burning pain, slight local erythema, and edema followed by itching. The edema may vary depending on location of the sting. It is said that 50 stings can be serious and lead to respiratory dysfunction, intravascular hemolysis, hypertension, myocardial damage, hepatic changes, shock, and renal failure. With 100 or more stings, death can occur. In patients who are allergic to bee stings, immediate allergic reaction with the risk of anaphylactic shock requires urgent medical treatment (Mebs, 2002; Hoffman, 2006).

Vespidae (Wasps)   This family includes wasps and hornets. These venoms contain a high content of peptides, which include mastoparan in wasps and hornets and crabolin from hornet venom. These peptides release histamine from mast cells and consist of 13–17 amino acids with no disulfide bridges. Other peptides named waspkinins cause immediate pain, vasodilation and increased vascular permeability leading to edema. These venoms also contain phospholipases and hyaluronidases, which contribute to the break down of membranes and connective tissue to facilitate diffusion of the venom. These proteins also contribute to the allergenicity of the venoms (Mebs, 2002; Hoffman, 2006).

Lepidoptera (Caterpillars, Moths, and Butterflies)

The urticating hairs, or setae, of caterpillars are effective defensive weapons that protect some species from predators. The setae are attached to unicellular poison glands at the base of each hair. Both the larvae and the adults are capable of stinging, either by direct contact with the setae or indirectly when the creature becomes irritated. It appears that contraction of the caterpillar's abdominal muscles is sufficient to release the barbs from their sockets, allowing them to become airborne. The toxic material found in the venom glands contains aristolochic acids, cardenolides, kallikrein, and histamine among other substances. Fibrinolytic activity has been found at 16 and 18 kDa (isoelectric point of 8.5); coagulation defects such as prolonged prothrombin and partial thromboplastin times have been detected, and decreases in fibrinogen and plasminogen have been noted. It is thought that the hemorrhagic syndrome cannot be classified as being either totally fibrinolytic or a syndrome such as disseminated intravascular coagulopathy. The spicules of *Thaumetopoea pityocampa* contain a 28-kDa toxin called thaumetopoein, which is a strong dermal irritant and highly allergenic peptide (Kawamoto and Kumada, 1984; Russell, 2001; Mebs, 2002).

In some parts of the world the stings of several species of Lepidoptera give rise to a bleeding diasthesis, often severe and sometimes fatal. Envenomation by members of the family Saturniidae, the buck moths, the grapeleaf skeletonizer (family Zygaenidae), the puss moth (family Megalopygie), and the brown-tailed moth (*Euproctis* species) generally gives rise to little more than immediate localized itching and pain, usually described as burning, followed in some cases by urticaria, edema, and occasionally fever. The hemolymph and spicules contain highly active clotting enzymes, a protease with fibrinolytic activity and an enzyme that activates prothrombin. In the more severe cases—often due to *Megalopygidae, Dioptidae, Automeris,* and *Hermileucinae* species—there is localized pain as well as papules (sometimes hemorrhagic) and hematomas; on occasions there may also be headache, nausea, vomiting, hematuria, lymphadenitis, and lymphadenopathy. Contacts with larvae of the saturnid moths in South America (*Lonomia acheolus* and *Lonomia oblique*) can cause severe coagulopathy, due to inhibition of clotting Factor XIII by a venom component

called lonomine V. Severe envenomation can cause cerebral hemorrhage and death (Guerrero *et al.*, 1999).

MULLOSCA (CONE SNAILS)

Human interest in this group of mollusks has been due to the beautiful patterns on their shells. Cone snails were known to Roman scholars and natural history collectors, as the shells were often made into jewelry. The first record of fatality from cone snail sting may be found in the book of Rumphius from 1705. The genus *Conus* is a group of some 500 species of carnivorous predators found in marine habitats that use venom as a weapon for prey capture. Cone snails have a venom duct for synthesis and storage of venom and hollow harpoon-like teeth for injection of the venom (Rockel *et al.*, 1995).

Cone snails may be divided into three groups depending on preferred prey. The largest group contains worm-hunting species that feed on polychaetes (segmented marine worms in the phylum Annelida). The second group is molluscivorous and hunts other gastropods. The final group is piscivorous and has venoms that rapidly immobilize fish (Olivera, 1997, 2002; Mebs and Kauferstein, 2005).

There are probably over 100 different venom components per species (Terlau and Olivera, 2004). Components have become known as conotoxins, which may be rich in disulfide bonds, and conopeptides. Molecular targets include G-protein-coupled receptors and neuromuscular transporters, ligand- or voltage-gated ion channels. Some components have enzymatic activity.

Figure 26-2 provides an overview of peptidic *Conus* venom components, indicating gene superfamilies, disulfide bond characteristics, and general targets (McIntosh *et al.*, 1999; Olivera, 2002). The two major divisions of *Conus* toxins are the disulfide-rich conotoxins and the peptides that lack multiple disulfide cross-links. The arrangement of cysteines in the primary sequence is restricted to only a few patterns, which may be diagnostic of the gene superfamily. Most disulfide-rich conotoxins are small and consist of 12–30 amino acids. These toxins contain an unusually diverse complement of posttranslationally modified amino acids, including hydroxyproline, O-glycosylated serine or threonine, γ-carboxyl-glutamate, sulfated tyrosine, and D-amino acids (Craig *et al.*, 1999). Apparently, the posttranslational modification enzyme γ-carboxylase is present in their venom ducts (Bandyopadhyay *et al.*, 2002). The enzyme has a recognition signal in the pro region of the precursor that instructs the enzyme to modify specific amino acid residues in the mature toxin region. Thus, the pro region of conopeptide precursors provides potential anchor-binding sites for posttranslational modification enzymes (Hooper *et al.*, 2000).

Cone snails could be called sophisticated practitioners of combination drug therapy. After injection, multiple conopeptides act synergistically to affect the targeted prey. The term toxin cabal has been applied to this coordinated action of the conopeptide mixture. The fish-hunting species *Conus purpurascens* apparently has two distinct cabals whose effects differ in time and space. The "lightning-strike cabal" causes immediate immobilization of the injected prey because various venom components inhibit voltage-gated sodium channel inactivation and block potassium channels, resulting in massive depolarization of axons in the vicinity of the injection site and a tetanic state. The second physiologic cabal, the "motor cabal," acts more slowly as conotoxins must be distributed throughout the body of the prey. The overall result is total inhibition of neuromuscular transmission. Various conopeptides inhibit presynaptic calcium channels that control neurotransmitter release, the postsynaptic

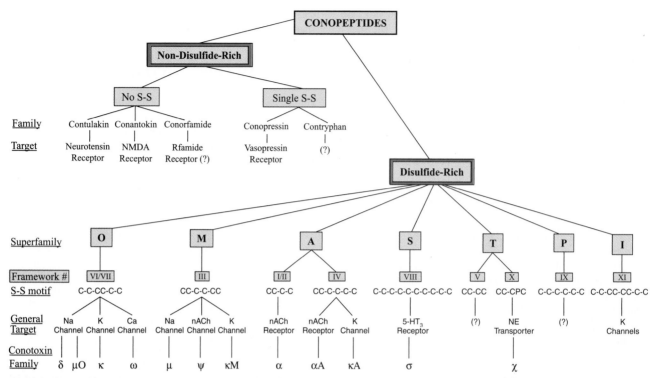

Figure 26-2. *Organizational diagram for Conus peptides, indicating gene superfamilies, disulfide patterns, and known pharmacologic targets.*

Only the superfamilies of the disulfide-rich peptides are shown. Used with permission from Terlau H, Olivera BM: *Conus* venoms: A rich source of novel ion channel-targeted peptides. *Physiol Rev* 84:41–68, 2004.

neuromuscular nicotinic receptors, and the sodium channels involved in the muscle action potential (Terlau *et al.*, 1996).

Conopeptides can affect many ion channels (Olivera *et al.*, 1994; Terlau and Olivera, 2004). For example, μ-conotoxins are peptides with 22–25 amino acids and six cysteine residues that block sodium currents by acting at a site that overlaps the tetrodotoxin-sensitive site of sodium channels. The main effect of the unusually hydrophobic δ-conotoxins, which are peptides with an inhibitory cysteine knot motif pattern of disulfide bridges, is the inhibition of the fast inactivation of sodium currents, which affects the shape and duration of the action potential. This can lead to a massive electrical hyperexcitation of the complete organism. The κ-, κA- and κM-conotoxins target potassium channels. The ω-conotoxins are peptides that target calcium channels, and these toxins have been widely used in neuroscience research. A characteristic feature of the ω-conotoxins is their high content of basic amino acids. One peptide, ω-conotoxin MVIIA from *Conus magus*, has been developed as ziconotide (Prialt®) for the treatment of intractable pain (Olivera, 2000). Other conotoxins are being studied as potential antinociceptive agents.

Conopeptides also target ligand-gated ion channels that mediate fast synaptic transmission (Kandel *et al.*, 2000). One major group of ligand-gated ion channels is activated by acetylcholine, serotonin, γ-aminobutyric acid, or glycine. These proteins differ in ligand specificity and selectivity for the permeant ion. The second family activates the glutamate receptors, *N*-methyl-D-aspartate and kainate/AMPA receptors. A third group activates synaptic transmission at certain synapses via the ATP receptors. It is evident from Fig. 26-2 that there are conopeptides that target these three different families of ligand-gated ion channels. It is clear

that our understanding of the structure and function of conopeptides is rapidly expanding and additional information regarding these toxins is available in an excellent review (Terlau and Olivera, 2004).

REPTILES

Lizards

The Gila monster (*Heloderma suspectum*) and the beaded lizards (*Heloderma horridum*) are divided into five subspecies. These large, corpulent, relatively slow moving, and largely nocturnal reptiles have few enemies other than humans. They are far less dangerous than is generally believed. Their venom is transferred from venom glands in the lower jaw through ducts that discharge their contents near the base of the larger teeth of the lower jaw. The venom is then drawn up along grooves in the teeth by capillary action (Brown and Carmony, 1991). The venom of this lizard has serotonin, amine oxidase, phospholipase A, a bradykinin-releasing substance, helodermin, gilatoxin, and low proteolytic as well as high-hyaluronidase activities, but lacks phosphomonoesterase and phosphodiesterase, acetylcholinesterase, nucleotidase, ATPase, deoxyribonuclease, ribonuclease, amino acid oxidase, and fibrinogenocoagulase activities. The clinical presentation of a helodermatid bite can include pain, edema, hypotension, nausea, vomiting, weakness, and diaphoresis. No antivenin is commercially available. Treatment is supportive (Strimple *et al.*, 1997).

The venom has been shown to contain a 25-kDa protein, helothermine, containing 223 amino acids and four pairs of disulfide bonds, which appears to inhibit Ca^{2+} flux from the sarcoplasmic reticulum (Morrissette *et al.*, 1995; Nobile *et al.*, 1996). A fraction causing hemorrhage in internal organs and the eye, a glycoprotein of 210 amino acid residues with plasma kallikrein-like properties, has also been described (Datta and Tu, 1997). A 35 amino acid residue, helodermin produces hypotension that is partially attributed to activation of glibenclamide-sensitive K$^+$ channels (Horikawa *et al.*, 1998). In fact, Helospectin I and II and helodermin are nonamidated, vasoactive intestinal peptide-like peptides, isolated from the salivary gland venom of the lizards *H. suspectum* and *H. horridum*, which have strong and potent vasodilator effects (Uddman *et al.*, 1999).

Snakes

General Information and Classification Snakes have a three-chambered heart and rely almost exclusively upon an enlarged right lung (that spans approximately half of the body length) for respiration. Of the approximately 2700 known species of snakes, about 20% are considered to be venomous (Mebs, 2002). Venomous snakes primarily belong to the following families: *Viperidae* (vipers), *Elapidae*, *Atractaspidae*, and *Colubridae*. The vipers are further divided into subfamilies, and example of which is the *Crotalinae*, or pit vipers, which possess a pit between the eyes and nostrils that serves as a heat sensor to detect warm-blooded animals. Some of the subfamilies are regarded as separate families altogether depending on the classification scheme. Overall the *Colubridae* are considered the largest venomous family, and are comprised of nearly 60% of all snakes. The *Atractaspidae* family, recently classified within the *Viperidae*, is known for burrowing into the ground and possessing the ability to expose their fangs without opening their mouth.

Another characteristic that is often used for self-defense or hunting prey is mimicry (O'Shea, 2005). Scale pattern and coloration provide distinct boundaries in the wild and often carry unspoken warnings based upon a reputation for snake venom toxicity for a given species. If a relatively harmless species is able to mimic the physical characteristics, especially color patterns, of a well-known highly toxic counterpart, then other potential predators may recognize both snakes as toxic and not pursue either.

Fang anatomy and dentition are good indicators of such factors as snake habitat and feeding habits (O'Shea, 2005). In general, the anatomical structure of fangs makes it nearly impossible for snakes to chew their prey. The distinct curvature of the fangs is not only engineered for puncturing skin and delivering venom, but also for swallowing whole prey as well. The teeth and jaw structure are relatively mobile and effectively facilitate the positioning of whole prey for swallowing. The skull and jaw possess an extremely high degree of responsiveness to stimuli. The jaw does not actually dislocate; however, it is able to rapidly reposition itself to capture, contain, and swallow prey. In addition to the capabilities of the teeth, fangs, and jaws, the classic fork-shaped tongue is another tool for identifying prey (O'Shea, 2005).

The *Viperidae* fang structure is regarded as the most developed and efficient means of venom, or toxin, delivery to prey. The venom gland is positioned at the base of a long (∼30 mm) hollow retractable fang (Mebs, 2002). Muscle pressure on the gland determines the amount of venom released. Another highly developed venom delivery apparatus is characteristic of the spitting cobras, aptly named for their ability to project venom via glands that protrude from the base of the fang opening (Mebs, 2002). Venom is carried toward the prey, or target, via forceful exhalation that is accompanied by a hissing sound. Toxin delivery via venom exposure is the primary mechanism by which snakes immobilize and kill their prey. Toxin type and specificity is dependent on the species; however, most venom comprises of complex networks of toxins that affect variable organ systems and interact with one another increasing the overall potency.

It is estimated that there are over 2.5 million snakebites annually, and that over 100,000 victims will die (White, 2005). Information resources available to physicians on management of snakebite victims may be found at the Clinical Toxinology Resources Website—www.toxinology.com or other appropriate references (Dart, 2004; Tintinalli *et al.*, 2004).

Snake Venoms These venoms are complex mixtures: proteins and peptides, consisting of both enzymatic and nonenzymatic compounds, make up over 90% of the dry weight of the venom (Phui Yee *et al.*, 2004). Snake venoms also contain inorganic cations such as sodium, calcium, potassium, magnesium, and small amounts of zinc, iron, cobalt, manganese, and nickel. The metals in snake venoms are likely catalysts for metal-based enzymatic reactions. For example, in the case of some elapid venoms, zinc ions appear to be necessary for anticholinesterase activity, and calcium may play a role in the activation of phospholipase A and the direct lytic factor. Some proteases appear to be metalloproteins. Some snake venoms also contain carbohydrates (glycoproteins), lipids, and biogenic amines, such as histamine, serotonin, and neurotransmitters (catecholamines and acetylcholine) in addition to positively charged metal ions (Russell, 2001; Mebs, 2002; Ménez, 2003; Ramos and Selistre-de-Araujo, 2006). The complexity of snake venom components is illustrated nicely in Fig. 26-3 (Ramos and Selistre-de-Araujo, 2006).

Actions of snake venoms can be said to be broad ranging in several areas (O'Shea, 2005). A simplistic approach would group toxin components as neurotoxins, coagulants, hemorrhagins, hemolytics, myotoxins, cytotoxins, and nephrotoxins. Neurotoxins produce neuromuscular paralysis ranging from dizziness to ptosis; to ophthalmoplegia, flaccid facial muscle paralysis, and inability to swallow; to paralysis of larger muscle groups; and finally to paralysis of respiratory muscles and death by asphyxiation. Coagulants may have initial procoagulant action that uses up clotting factors leading to bleeding. Coagulants may directly inhibit normal clotting at several places in the clotting cascade or via inhibition of platelet aggregation. In addition, some venom components may damage the endothelial lining of blood vessels leading to hemorrhage. Bite victims may show bleeding from nose or gums, the bite site, in saliva, urine, and stools. Myotoxins can directly impact muscle contraction leading to paralysis or cause rhabdomyolysis or the break down of skeletal muscle. Myoglobinuria, or a dark brown urine, and hyperkalemia may be noted. Cytotoxic agents have proteolytic or necrotic properties leading to the break down of tissue. Typical signs include massive swelling, pain, discoloration, blistering, bruising, and wound weeping. Sarafotoxins, which are found only in burrowing asps of Afro-Arabia, cause coronary artery constriction that can lead to reduced coronary blood flow, angina, and myocardial infarction. Finally, nephrotoxins can cause direct damage to kidney structures leading to bleeding, damage to several parts of the nephron, tissue oxygen deprivation, and renal failure.

Enzymes At least 26 different enzymes have been isolated from snake venoms, which are comprised of amino acid sequences

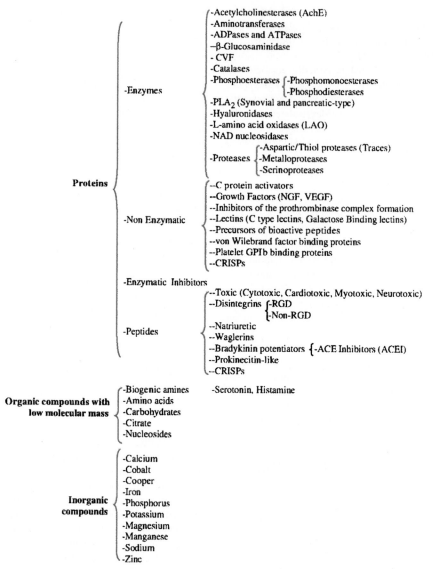

Figure 26-3. Components of snake venoms.

ACE, angiotensin-converting enzyme; CRISP, cysteine-rich secretory protein; CVF, cobra venom factor-like proteins; LAO, L-amino acid oxidase; PLA$_2$, phospholipase A$_2$; RGD, arginine–glycine–aspartate. Used with permission from Ramos OHP, Selistre-de-Araujo HS: Snake venom metalloproteases—structure and function of catalytic and disintegrin domains. *Comp Biochem Physiol, Part C* 142:328–346, Elsevier, 2006.

(150–1500) (Ménez, 2003). No single snake venom contains all of the enzymes. Some important snake venom enzymes are shown in Fig. 26-3.

Proteolytic enzymes that catalyze the break down of tissue proteins and peptides include peptide hydrolases, proteases, endopeptidases, peptidases, and proteinases. Several proteolytic enzymes may be in a single venom. The proteolytic enzymes have molecular weights between 20,000 and 95,000. Some are inactivated by ethylenediamine tetraacetic acid (EDTA) and certain reducing agents. Metals appear to be intrinsically involved in the activity of certain venom proteases and phospholipases. The crotalid venoms examined so far appear to be rich in proteolytic enzyme activity. Viperid venoms have lesser amounts, whereas elapid and sea snake venoms have minimal, if any, proteolytic activity. Venoms that are rich in proteinase activity are associated with marked tissue destruction (Russell, 2001).

Collagenase is a specific kind of proteinase that digests collagen. This activity has been demonstrated in the venoms of a number of species of crotalids and viperids. The venom of *Crotalus atrox* digests mesenteric collagen fibers but not other proteins. EDTA inhibits the collagenolytic effect, but not the argine esterase effect.

Hyaluronidase cleaves internal glycoside bonds in certain acid mucopolysaccharides resulting in a decrease in the viscosity of connective tissues. The break down in the hyaluronic barrier allows other fractions of venom to penetrate the tissues, causing hyaluronidase to be called "spreading factor." The degree to which hyaluronidase contributes to the extent of edema produced by the whole venom is not known.

Table 26-5

Miscellaneous Properties of Some α-Chain and β-Chain Fibrin(ogen)ases

PROPERTIES	α-CHAIN FIBRINOGENASE	β-CHAIN FIBRINOGENASE
Common name	Fibrolase	β-fibrinogenase
Class of enzyme	Metalloproteinase	Serine protease
Chain length	203 amino acids	232 amino acids
Molecular weight	~22.7 kDa	~26 kDa
pI	6.8	~3
Carbohydrate content	None	>30%
pH optimum	7.1–7.4	8.5–9.5

SOURCE: Data from Swenson and Markland (2005).

Phospholipase A2 (PLA$_2$s) enzymes are widely distributed throughout the tissues of animals, plants, and bacteria, and have been well studied in snake venoms (Ohno *et al.*, 2003; Soares and Giglio, 2003). Mammalian PLA$_2$ enzymes are involved in fertilization and cell proliferation, and have been implicated in respiratory ailments such as asthma, as well as skin conditions such as psoriasis (Kini, 2003; Soares and Giglio, 2003). PLA$_2$ catalyzes the Ca^{2+}-dependent hydrolysis of the 2-acyl ester bond, producing free fatty acids and lysophospholipids. However, liberation of pharmacologically active products and effects independent of enzymatic action may contribute to their overall action. In general, mammalian PLA$_2$s are considered to be nontoxic and do not elicit the same pharmacologic effects as similar enzymes in snake venoms.

As of 2003, over 280 PLA$_2$ enzymes had been classified, sharing at least 40% identify in their amino acid sequences (Kini, 2003; Soares and Giglio, 2003). Many PLA$_2$s have been sequenced. They have approximately 120 amino acids and 14 cysteine residues forming seven disulfide bonds. Surface residue recognition and covalent/non-covalent bonds stabilize complexes for receptor binding. Specific amino acid residues play an important role in the diversification and overall function of the PLA$_2$s. Of note, histidine, lysine, cysteine, and methionine have been well studied for their contribution to enzyme structure and function (Soares and Giglio, 2003). For example, alkylation of His48 diminishes the hydrolytic capabilities of certain toxins. Alkylation of amino acids has proven to effectively mitigate PLA$_2$ toxicity and has been proposed as an antivenom treatment (Soares and Giglio, 2003). PLA$_2$s interact with

other toxins in the venom as well, often resulting in synergistic reactions. Similarly, snake venom PLA$_2$ enzymes can be separated into three major groupings depending on their pharmacologic activities: low-toxicity enzymes (LD$_{50}$ > 1 mg/kg), high-toxicity enzymes (1 mg/kg > LD$_{50}$ > 0.1 mg/kg), and presynaptically acting toxins (LD$_{50}$ < 0.1 mg/kg) (Rosenberg, 1990). Although the sequences of these enzymes are homologous and their enzymatically active sites are identical, they differ widely in their pharmacologic properties. For example, taipoxin, a PLA$_2$ enzyme from the venom of the Australian elapid *Oxyuranus scutellatus*, has an intravenous LD$_{50}$ in mice of 2 μg/kg, whereas the neutral PLA$_2$ from *Naja nigricollis* has an LD$_{50}$ of 10,200 μg/kg, even though *N. nigricollis* PLA$_2$ is enzymatically more active (Russell, 2001).

Arginine ester hydrolase is one of a number of non-cholinesterases found in snake venoms. The substrate specificities are directed to the hydrolysis of the ester or peptide linkage, to which an argine residue contributes the carboxyl group. This activity is found in many crotalid and viperid venoms and some sea snake venoms but is lacking in elapid venoms with the possible exception of *Ophiophagus hannah*. Some crotalid venoms contain at least three chromatographically separable arginine ester hydrolases. The bradykinin-releasing and perhaps bradykinin-clotting activities of some crotalid venoms may be related to esterase activity.

Two distinct classes of fibrin(ogen)olytic enzymes, the metalloproteinases and the serine proteinases, have been isolated from venom of *Viperidae*, *Elapidae*, and *Crotalidae* snake families (Swenson and Markland, 2005). These two classes of proteinases differ in mechanism of action and their target in fibrin(ogen), but ultimately they break down fibrin-rich clots and help to prevent further clot formation. The properties of fibrolase, an α-chain fibrinolytic metalloproteinase from *Agkistrodon contortrix contortrix* venom, and β-fibrinogenase, a β-chain fibrinogenase from *Vipera lebetina*, are provided in Table 26-5. Properties of some newly characterized fibrin(ogen)ases are listed in Table 26-6. It is apparent that there are major differences in the properties of these enzymes from different snakes even though they have similar catalytic properties. An exciting development from the research on these enzymes is that one specific recombinant fibrinolytic enzyme derived from fibrolase called alfimeprase is progressing through clinical trials for the treatment of peripheral arterial occlusions.

The snake venom hemorrhagic metalloproteinases (SVMP) are enzymes that disrupt the hemostatic system and they are characterized by their domain structure into four primary classes, PI–PIV. SMVPs are synthesized in vivo as multimodular proteins that

Table 26-6

Miscellaneous Properties of Some α-Chain and β-Chain Fibrin(ogen)ases

PROPERTIES	α-CHAIN FIBRINOGENASE	α-CHAIN FIBRINOGENASE	α-CHAIN FIBRINOGENASE	β-CHAIN FIBRINOGENASE
Genus species	*Bothops neuwiedi*	*Agkistrodon halys*	*Lachesis stenophrys*	*Agkistrodon blomhoffi brevicadus*
Common name	Neuwiedase	Brevilysin L6	LSF	Brevinase
Chain length	198 amino acids	203 amino acids	>200 amino acids	233 amino acids
Molecular weight	22.5 kDa	22.7 kDa	24 kDa	25.7 kDa
pI	5.9	4.8	ND	5.5
Carbohydrate content	<1%	None	Glycosylated	ND
pH optimum	7.4–8.0	8.5–9.5	ND	5.5–8.5

ND, not determined.
SOURCE: Data from Swenson and Markland (2005).

Table 26-7

Comparison of Thrombin and Thrombin-like Snake Venom Enzyme Actions

ENZYMES	ACTION ON HUMAN FIBRINOGEN				
	FIBRINOPEPTIDES RELEASED	CHAIN DEGRADATION	ACTIVATION OF FACTOR XIII	PROTHROMBIN FRAGMENT CLEAVAGE	PLATELET AGGREGATION AND RELEASE
Thrombin	A - B	α(A)	Yes	Yes	Yes
Thrombin-like enzymes	A*	α(A)† or β(B)‡	No	Yes or no§	No
Agkistrodon C. contortrix Venom	B	ND	Incomplete	ND	No
Bitis gabonica Venom	A + B	ND	Yes	ND	ND

*Includes ancrod, batroxobin, crotalase, and the enzyme from *T. okinavensis*.

†Ancrod [batroxobin degrades α(A) chain of bovine but not human fibrinogen].

‡Crotalase.

§Fragment I released by crotalase and *Agkistrodon contortrix* venom, but not by ancrod or batroxobin.

ND, not determined.

SOURCE: Data from Russell (2001).

Table 26-8

Comparison of Snake Venom Thrombin-Like Enzymes

VENOM ENZYME	MOLECULAR WEIGHT	CARBOHYDRATE CONTENT (%)	ACTIVE SITE SERINE
Agkistrodon contortrix contortrix	100,000	ND	+
Bitis gabonica	32,500	ND	ND
Bothrops marajoensis	31,400	High	+
Bothrops moojeni	36,000	5.8	+
Calloselasma rhodostoma	59,000	36.0	+
Crotalus adamantus	32,700	8.3	+
Crotalus horridus horridus	19,400	Very low	ND
Deinagkistrodon acutus	33,500	13.0	+
Trimeresurus gramineus	27,000	25.0	+
Trimeresurus okinavensis	34,000	6.0	+

ND, not determined.

SOURCE: Data from Russell (2001).

comprise a signal peptide, a prodomain, and a metalloprotease domain (SVMP PI). SVMP potency tends to increase by class and those within the PIV class are larger and comprises additional disulfide bonds (Calvette *et al*., 2003, 2005). Class PII proteins exhibit a C-terminal disintegrin domain. The PII metalloproteases block the function of integrin receptors, a function that could alleviate a variety of pathological conditions such as inflammation, tumor angiogenesis and metastasis, and thrombosis. The integrin-blocking specificity of this class of metalloproteins is highly dependent on the conformation of the inhibitory loop, and thus the placement and bonding of cysteine residues. More specifically, within the inhibitory loops, RGD-containing disintegrins are specific to the class PII metalloproteases (Calvette *et al*., 2003, 2005). Class PIII SVMPs exhibit the disintegrin-like domain and the C-type lectin-like domain is present in PIV SVMPs. The metalloproteinase domain or catalytic domain is composed of about 215 amino acids and has metal-dependent endopeptidase activity (Calvette *et al*., 2005). SVMPs degrade proteins such as laminin, fibronectin, type IV collagen, and proteoglycans from the endothelial basal membrane; degrade fibrinogen and von Willebrand factor enhancing the hemorrhagic action; and inhibit platelet aggregation and stimulate release of cytokines (Ramos and Selistre-de-Araujo, 2006).

The proteolytic action of thrombin and thrombin-like snake venom enzymes is shown in Table 26-7. This table compares ancrod (from *Calloselasma rhodostoma*), batroxobin (from *Bothrops moojeni*), crotalase (from *Crotalus adamanteus*), gabonase (from *Bitis gabonica*), and venzyme (from *A. contortrix*). Table 26-8 shows the molecular size of some thrombin-like enzymes. A recent contribution on snake toxins, using mass spectrometric immunoassay and bioactive probe techniques, has been published by Ramirez *et al*. (1999). Considerable study has been given to the hemostatic properties of venoms (Markland, 1998). The hemostatically active components are summarized in Table 26-9.

Phosphomonoesterase (phosphatase) is widely distributed in the venoms of all families of snakes except the colubrids. It has the properties of an orthophosphoric monoester phosphohydrolase. There are two nonspecific phosphomonoesterases, and they have optimal pH at 5.0 and 8.5. Many types of venom contain both acid and alkaline phosphatases, whereas others contain one or the other.

Table 26-9
Snake Venom Proteins Active on the Hemostatic System

GENERAL FUNCTIONAL ACTIVITY	SPECIFIC BIOLOGICAL ACTIVITY
Procoagulant	Activates factors II, V, IX, X, and Protein C
	Fibrinogen clotting
Anticoagulant	Factor IX/factor X-binding protein
	Thrombin inhibitor
	Phospholipase A
Fibrinolytic	Fibrin(ogen) degradation
	Plasminogen activation
Vessel wall interactive	Hemorrhagic

SOURCES: Data from Markland (1998) and Russell (2001).

Phosphodiesterase has been found in the venoms of all families of poisonous snakes. It is an orthophosphoric diester phosphohydrolase that releases 5-mononucleotide from the polynucleotide chain and thus acts as an exonucleotidase, attacking DNA and RNA. More recently, it has been found that it also attacks derivatives of arabinose.

Acetylcholinesterase was first demonstrated in cobra venom and is widely distributed throughout the elapid venoms. It is also found in sea snake venoms but is totally lacking in viperid and crotalid venoms. It catalyzes the hydrolysis of acetylcholine to choline and acetic acid. The role of the enzyme in snake venoms is not clear.

RNase is present in some snake venoms in small amounts as the endopolynucleotidase RNase. It appears to have specificity toward pyrimidine-containing pyrimidyladenyl bonds in DNA. The optimum pH is 7–9 when ribosomal RNA is used as the substrate. This enzyme in Naja oxiana venom has a molecular weight of 15,900.

DNase acts on DNA to produce predominantly tri- or higher oligonucleotides that terminate in $3'$ monoesterified phosphate. C. adamanteus venom contains two DNases, with optimum pH at 5 and 9.

$5'$-Nucleotidase is a common constituent of all snake venoms; in most instances it is the most active phosphatase in snake venoms. It specifically hydrolyzes phosphate monoesters, which link with a $5'$ position of DNA and RNA. It is found in greater amounts in crotalid and viperid venoms than in elapid venoms. The molecular weight as determined from amino acid composition and gel filtration with Naja naja atra venom has been estimated at 10,000. The enzyme from N. naja venom is enhanced by Mg^{2+}, is inhibited by Zn^{2+}, is inactivated at 75°C at pH 7.0 or 8.4, and has an isoelectric point of about 8.6. That from Agkistrodon halys blomhoffi shows a pH optimum of 6.8–6.9, with activity being enhanced by Mg^{2+} and Mn^{2+} and inhibited by Zn^{2+}. The enzyme has a low order of lethality (Russell, 2001).

Nicotinamide adenine dinucleotide (NAD) nucleotidase has been found in a number of snake venoms. This enzyme catalyzes the hydrolysis of the nicotinamide N-ribosidic linkage of NAD, yielding nicotinamide and adenosine diphosphate riboside. Its optimum pH is 6.5–8.5; it is heat labile, losing activity at 60°C. Nucleotidases function as ADP scavengers thereby acting as potent inhibitors of platelet aggregation.

L-Amino acid oxidase has been found in all snake venoms examined so far. It gives a yellow color to the venom. This enzyme catalyzes the oxidation of L-α-amino and α-hydroxy acids. This activity results from a group of homologous enzymes with molec-

ular weights ranging from 85,000 to 150,000. It has a high content of acidic amino acids. The mouse intravenous LD_{50} of the enzyme from C. adamanteus venom was 9.13 mg/kg body weight, approximately four times less than the lethal value of the crude venom, and this enzyme had no effect on nerve, muscle, or neuromuscular transmission (Russell, 2001).

Polypeptides Snake venom polypeptides are low-molecular-weight proteins that do not have enzymatic activity. More than 80 polypeptides with pharmacologic activity have been isolated from snake venoms. Interested readers will find definitive reviews on these peptides in the works of Lee (1979), Eaker and Wadström (1980), and Gopalakrishnakone and Tan (1992). Most of the lethal activity of the poison of the sea snake Laticauda semifasciata was recovered as two toxins, erabutoxin-a and erabutoxin-b, using carboxymethylcellulose chromatography; 30% of the proteins were erabutoxins. More recently, erabutoxin-a, a short-chain curamimetic, has been crystallized in monomeric and dimeric forms (Nastopoulos et al., 1998). Erabutoxin-b is said to be relatively ineffective at the mammalian neuromuscular junction (Vincent et al., 1998). Another curamimetic, a long-chain polypeptide, is α-cobratoxin, while a novel "neurotoxin" from N. naja atra, having 61 amino acid residues and eight cystine residues, has been isolated by Chang et al. (1997).

Disintegrins are a family of short cysteine-rich polypeptides and are divided into five subgroups based upon the combination of length and number of disulfide bonds of polypeptides. In general, the disintegrins comprise 40–100 amino acids. Their small size coupled with a relatively dense network of disulfide bonds contributes to the tertiary structure of these compounds and high potency of such small compounds. Disintegrins are released in venoms via proteolytic processes of PII metalloproteinases, whereas structures similar in form and function to disintegrins, or disintegrin like, are subject to PIII processes (Calvette et al., 2005). Monomeric disintegrins can vary from about 50 residues and four disulfide bonds as in echistatin and obtustatin, to around 70 amino acid residues and six disulfide bridges as in albolabrin, barbourin, and halysin, to over 84 amino acids and seven disulfide bonds for bitistatin and salmosin-3. Dimeric disintegrins are about 67 amino acids long and contain four intrachain disulfide linkages and two between-chain bonds. Examples include contortrostatin and acostatin. The monomeric disintegrin-like chemicals contain around 100 amino acids and eight disulfide bonds, and include trimelysin-I, bothropasin, and jararhagin (Calvette et al., 2003; Ramos and Selistre-de-Araujo, 2006).

RGD (argine–glycine–asparagine) and non-RGD-containing disintegrins coexist in certain venoms and exhibit affinities for variable ligand receptors. In such cases, one copy of the gene encodes for the more conserved RGD function of platelet aggregation, whereas the duplicated genes have drifted toward facilitating other biological functions. Modeling and structure analysis of cyclic RGD peptides has implicated the importance of amino acid sequences on the C-terminal of the RGD sequence; furthermore, the physical features such as size of the integrin-binding loop contribute to the receptor-binding capabilities (Calvette et al., 2005). In general, the amino acid residues of this region of the RGD sequence are not well conserved and are believed to play a key role in determining integrin receptor-binding specificity. There are additional mechanisms within the C-terminal region, which include conformational epitopes that are utilized to alter receptor-binding capabilities.

The small basic polypeptide myotoxins are widely distributed in *Crotalus* snake venoms. The specific agent crotamine from *Crotalus durissus terrificus* venom induces skeletal muscle spasms and paralysis by changing the inactivation process of sodium channels, which are inhibited by tetrodotoxin and potentiated by veratridine and grayanotoxin, leading to depolarization of the neuromuscular junction. Crotamine is composed of 42 amino acid residues and three disulfide bonds. The crotamine gene contains 1.8 kbp and has three exons that are separated by a long phase-1 and a short phase-2 intron and mapped to chromosome 2. In addition, the three-dimensional structure has been published, and the structural topology is similar to that of other three disulfide bridge containing peptides such as human β-defensins and scorpion sodium channel toxin. These structural properties enable crotamine to have a unique cell penetrating ability allowing the toxin to concentrate in the nucleus by means of a probable receptor-independent mechanism. It is interesting to note that topology and diversification of functional folds are common themes in animal venom peptides acting on ion channels and other targets (Menez, 1998; Mouhat *et al.*, 2004; Oguiura *et al.*, 2006).

Toxicology   In general, the venoms of rattlesnakes and other New World crotalids produce alterations in the resistances and often in the integrity of blood vessels, changes in blood cells and blood coagulation mechanisms, direct or indirect changes in cardiac and pulmonary dynamics, and—with crotalids like *C. durrissus terrificus* and *C. scutulatus*—serious alterations in the nervous system and changes in respiration. In humans, the course of the poisoning is determined by the kind and amount of venom injected; the site where it is deposited; the general health, size, and age of the patient; the kind of treatment; and those pharmacodynamic principles noted earlier in this chapter. Death in humans may occur within less than 1 hour or after several days, with most deaths occurring between 18 and 32 hours. Hypotension or shock is the major therapeutic problem in North American crotalid bites (Russell, 2001).

Snakebite Treatment   The treatment of bites by venomous snakes is now so highly specialized that almost every envenomation requires specific recommendations. However, three general principles for every bite should be kept in mind: (1) snake venom poisoning is a medical emergency requiring immediate attention and the exercise of considerable judgment; (2) the venom is a complex mixture of substances of which the proteins contribute the major deleterious properties, and the only adequate antidote is the use of specific or polyspecific antivenom; and (3) not every bite by a venomous snake ends in an envenomation. Venom may not be injected. In almost 1000 cases of crotalid bites, 24% did not end in a poisoning. The incidence with the bites of cobras and perhaps other elapids is probably higher. The reader is referred to other appropriate texts for appropriate treatment of snakebites (Russell, 2001; Dart, 2004; Sholl *et al.*, 2004; Tintinalli *et al.*, 2004; Singletary and Holstege, 2006).

Snake Venom Evolution   Considerable efforts are being expended to examine the complex process by which snake venom components are thought to have changed over the years. This evaluation involves tracing the ancestral roots of toxins, which is made even more cumbersome due to the distinct differences in the speed at which individual components of a venom evolve. The current assemblage of snake venoms with regard to functionality and ancestral protein

Table 26-10
Basal Bioactivities of Some Toxin Types

TOXIN	ACTIVITY
3FTx	α-Neurotoxicity, blocks nicotinic acetylcholine receptor
ADAM	In Viperidae venoms, proteolytic cleavage of C-terminal domains results in direct fibrinolytic activity, liberation of disintegrins, which inhibit platelet aggregation
Cobra venom factor	Causes unregulated activation of complement cascade, hemolysis, cytolysis
Crotamine	Myonecrosis, modifies voltage-gated sodium channels
Factor V	In taipan and brown snake venom, combines with toxic form of factor X to convert prothrombin to thrombin
Kallikrein	Increases vascular permeability, stimulates inflammation, and reduces blood pressure
Kunitz	Inhibits plasmin and thrombin and other serine proteases, blocks L-type calcium channels
L-AMINO OXIDASE	Induces apoptosis, decreases platelet aggregation, inhibits blood factor IX
PLA$_2$	Releases arachadonic acid from phospholipids, resulting in inflammation and tissue destruction
VEGF	Increases permeability of vascular bed causing hypotension and shock
Whey acidic proteins	Inhibit leukoproteinases

SOURCE: Data from Fry (2005).

activity is outlined in Table 26-10 (Fry, 2005). In general, the toxins from ancestral proteins that were constructed of dense networks of cysteine cross-linkages are considered among the most diverse today in terms of toxicological insult.

Recent thinking suggests that the evolution of the PLA$_2$s appears to be directed toward modifying the molecular surface in order to maximize the diversity of the pharmacologic properties of each isozyme component (Kini and Chan, 1999; Li *et al.*, 2005). As PLA$_2$s are not crucial for snake survival, mutations in some PLA$_2$ isozymes may be ignored and allowed to progress, thereby expediting the evolution in comparison to other more critical enzymes in which mutations are monitored more closely and not allowed to progress. The functionality of PLA$_2$ isozymes can be significantly hindered by increased rates of mutations within highly conserved regions of the amino acid sequence, which could in turn displace cysteine residues and alter the tertiary protein structure. However, increased mutation of a particular subset of enzymes, such as the PLA$_2$s, may be a result of a shift in ecological niche. A recent study (Li *et al.*, 2005) reports a shift in the diet composition of the marbled sea snake as the root cause of decelerated evolution of the PLA$_2$ enzymes. The diet change from live prey to fish eggs essentially negated the need for PLA$_2$ enzymes to immobilize live prey for swallowing and digestion. Future research could focus on the declining need for PLA$_2$s, and on the altered digestive enzyme composition that has likely occurred as a result of diet shift.

ANTIVENOM

Antivenoms have been produced against most medically important snake, spider, scorpion, and marine toxins. Animals immunized with venom develop a variety of antibodies to the many antigens in the venom. Antivenom consists of venom-specific antisera or antibodies concentrated from immune serum to the venom. Antisera contain neutralizing antibodies: one antigen (monospecific) or several antigens (polyspecific). Monovalent antivenoms have a high neutralization capacity, which is desirable against the venom of a specific animal. Polyvalent antisera are typically used to cover several venoms, such as snakes from a geographic region. Polyvalent preparations usually required higher doses or volumes than monovalent antivenoms. Neutralization capacity of antivenom is highly variable as there are no enforced international standards. Antivenom may cross-react with venoms from distantly related species and may not react with venom from the intended species. Nevertheless, in general, the antibodies bind to the venom molecules, rendering them ineffective.

Antivenoms are available in several forms: intact IgG antibodies or fragments of IgG such as F(ab)$_2$ and Fab. The molecular weight of the intact IgG is about 150,000, whereas that of Fab is approximately 50,000. The molecular size of IgG prevents its renal excretion and produces a volume of distribution much smaller than that of Fab. The elimination half-life of IgG in the blood is approximately 50 hours. Its ultimate fate is not known, but most IgG is probably taken up by the reticuloendothelial system and degraded with the antigen attached. Fab fragments have an elimination half-life of about 17 hours, and are small enough to permit renal excretion.

All antivenom products may produce hypersensitivity reactions. Type I (immediate) hypersensitivity reactions are caused by antigen cross-linking of endogenous IgE bound to mast cells and basophils. Binding of antigen by a mast cell may cause the release of histamine and other mediators, producing an anaphylactic reaction. Once initiated, anaphylaxis may continue despite discontinuation of antivenom administration. Type III hypersensitivity (serum sickness) may develop several days after antivenom administration. In these cases, antigen–antibody complexes are deposited in different areas of the body, often producing inflammatory responses in the skin, joints, kidneys, and other tissues. Fortunately, these reactions are rarely serious. The risks of anaphylaxis should always be considered when one is deciding whether to administer antivenom, and thus antivenom should be given only by intravenous infusion under medical supervision (Heard *et al.*, 1999; Russell, 2001; Mebs, 2002; Dart, 2004; Tintinalli *et al.*, 2004).

POTENTIAL CLINICAL APPLICATION OF VENOMS

Animal venoms are being used as research and clinical tools based upon their high affinity for specific targets and well-studied pharmacologic properties (Menez, 1998, 2003; Dimarcq and Hunneyball, 2003; Escoubas and Rash, 2004). Toxin specificities for receptors and channels that facilitate the interface and coordination of neuromuscular activity are utilized and manipulated to study, model, diagnose, and sometimes treat acute and degenerative conditions. Upon closer examination of α-bungarotoxin and candoxin nicotinic acetylcholine receptor specificity, plans are under way to utilize the reversible and irreversible receptor binding in muscular and neuronal tissues, respectively, in Alzheimer's patients (Phui Yee *et al.*, 2004). In addition to treating neurological diseases, specific α-toxins (longer chained) are also studied for their anti-angiogenic capabilities in treating malignant tumor growth in patients suffering from small cell lung carcinoma (Tsetlin and Hucho, 2004). In cases such as this, there is an inherent trade-off between promoting some degree of neurological deficit in light of combating tumor growth. Toxins such as the snake venom thrombin-like enzymes are valuable tools in both research and therapeutic applications. Similarly, fibrin(ogen)olytic enzymes break down fibrin-rich clots preventing further clot formation may be useful as controls in blood clotting research or to treat heart attacks and strokes (Castro *et al.*, 2004; Marsh and Williams, 2005; Swenson and Markland, 2005). To facilitate research, the complement-activating cobra venom factor has been produced by recombinant techniques (Vogel *et al.*, 2004). These pharmazooticals include reptilase-R, bothrocethin, stypven, ecarin, and protac.

Other areas of active research indicate that animal venoms contain components that can reduce pain, can selectively kill specific cancers, may reduce the incidence of stroke via effects on blood coagulability, and function as antibiotics. For example, epibatidin comes from the skin of the South American frog, *Epipedobates tricolor*, and a synthetic derivative ABT-594 appears to be more effective than morphine without being addictive. TM 601 is derived from the Israeli yellow scorpion and attacks malignant brain tumors called glioma tumors responsible for two-thirds of the cases of brain cancer, without harming healthy cells. ET 743, which comes from sea squirts, is being tested for treatment of ovarian cancer and soft tissue sarcoma. Ancrod is an anticoagulant with potential to prevent cell damage and death when someone suffers a stroke. The active ingredient comes from the venom of the Malaysian pit viper. In Germany, where Ancrod has been marketed for a number of years, a specially built facility houses about 3000 snakes. Several other sources of anticoagulants are being examined. A substance called magainin 2, which comes from the skin of frogs, is an effective antibiotic to which bacteria do not appear to develop resistance. The clotting enzyme batroxobin is an ingredient in reptilase and has been used in the development of fibrin glue, which is used in surgery to stop diffuse bleeding from liver or lung by covering the surface with a thin layer of fibrin.

Another major area of investigation and success involves the venom components that act as enzyme inhibitors. In particular, venom peptides from *Bothrops jararaca* were initially called bradykinin-potentiating peptides and lowered blood pressure. After further research, it became clear that these peptides were inhibitors of angiotensin I-converting enzyme, and chemical modification lead to orally active agents such as captopril.

Venom toxins can also be used as a component of the toxin–receptor–antibody complex for diagnosis of autoimmune disorders (Ménez, 2003). In addition to providing a promising means for researching and treating muscular and neurological diseases and cancer, work is being conducted on designing methods by which to consistently reconstruct and conform the overall toxin structure to bind to a specific protein, such as HIV (Ménez, 2003).

Additional work is being conducted on animals such as the mongoose, hedgehog, and opossum, which all embody a high level of resistance to snake bites. Blood from these animals contains proteins between 400 and 700 amino acids long that inhibit hemorrhagins. The exact mechanism of the many components in animal venoms that produce toxicity or resistance to certain toxins has yet to be determined. Further research will require a multidisciplinary approach involving techniques from parasitology, chemistry, molecular biology, genomics, proteomics, physiology, pharmacology, and toxicology.

ACKNOWLEDGMENTS

The author gratefully acknowledges the assistance of Ruth A. Sanders and Ronnie L. Yeager in the preparation of this chapter.

REFERENCES

Adams ME: Agatoxins: Ion channel specific toxins from the American funnel web spider, *Agelenopsis aperta. Toxicon* 43:509–525, 2004.

Auger C, Marty A: Heterogeneity of functional synaptic parameters among single release sites. *Neuron* 19:139–150, 1997.

Baku A: Mast cell degranulating (MCD) peptide: A prototypic peptide in allergy and inflammation. *Peptides* 20:415–420, 1999.

Bandyopadhyay PK, Garrett JE, Shetty RP, *et al.*: γ-Carboxylation: An extracellular post-translational modification that antedates the divergence of molluscs, arthropods and chordates. *Proc Natl Acad Sci U S A* 99:1264–1269, 2002.

Barker SC, Murrell A: Systematics and evolution of ticks with a list of valid genus and species names. *Parasitology* 129:S15–S36, 2004.

Bechinger B: Structure and functions of channel-forming peptides: Magainins, cecropins, melittin and alamethicin. *J Membr Biol* 156:197–211, 1997.

Bettini S (ed.): *Arthropod Venoms*, Heidelberg: Springer, 1978.

Brown DE, Carmony NB: *Gila Monster.* Silver City, NM: High Lonesome Books, 1991.

Bush SP, King BO, Norris RL, *et al.*: Centipede envenomation. *Wilderness Environ Med* 12:93–99, 2001.

Calvette JJ, Marcinkiewicz C, Monleon D, *et al.*: Snake venom disintegrins: Evolution of structure and function. *Toxicon* 45:1063–1074, 2005.

Calvette JJ, Moreno-Murciano MP, Theakston RDG, *et al.*: Snake venom disintegrins: Novel dimeric disintegrins and structural diversification by disulfide bond engineering. *Biochem J* 372:725–734, 2003.

Castro HC, Zingali RB, Albuquerque MG, *et al.*: Snake venom thrombin-like enzymes: From retilase to now. *Cell Mol Life Sci* 61:843–856, 2004.

Cavalieri M, D'Urso D, Lassa A, *et al.*: Characterization and some properties of the venom gland extract of a theridiid spider (*Steatoda paykulliana*) frequently mistaken for black widow spider (*Latrodectus tredecimguttatus*). *Toxicon* 25:965–974, 1987.

Cavassani KA, Aliberti JC, Dias ARV, *et al.*: Tick saliva inhibits differentiation, maturation and function of murine bone-marrow derived dendritic cells. *Immunology* 114:235–245, 2005.

Ceccarelli B, Hurlbut WP: Ca^{2+}-dependent recycling of synaptic vesicles at the frog neuromuscular junction. *J Cell Biol* 87:297–303, 1980.

Chang LS, Chou YC, Lin SR, *et al.*: A novel neurotoxin, cobrotoxin b, from *Naja naja atra* venom: Purification, characterization and gene organization. *J Biochem* 122:1252–1259, 1997.

Chesnov S, Bigler L, Hesse M: The acylpolyamines from the venom of the spider *Agelenopsis aperta. Helv Chim Acta* 84:2178–2197, 2001.

Cohen E, Quistad GB: Cytotoxic effects of arthropod venoms on various cultured cells. *Toxicon* 36:353–358, 1998.

Corzo G, Escoubas P: Pharmacologically active spider peptide toxins. *Cell Mol Life Sci* 60:2409–2426, 2003.

Corzo G, Adachi-Akahane S, Nagao T, *et al*: Novel peptides from assassin bugs (Hemiptera: Reduviidae): Isolation, chemical and biological characterization. *FEBS Lett* 499:256–261, 2001.

Craig AG, Bandyopadhyay P, Olivera BM: Post-translationally modified peptides from *Conus* venoms. *Eur J Biochem* 264:271–275, 1999.

Craik DJ, Daly NL, Waine C: The cysteine knot motif in toxins and implications for drug design. *Toxicon* 39:43–60, 2001.

Crause JC, Vershoor JA, Coetzee J *et al.*: The localization of paralysis toxin in granules and nuclei of prefed female *Rhipicephalus evertsi evertsi* tick salivary gland cells. *Exp Appl Acarology* 17:357–363, 1993.

Dart RC (ed.): *Medical Toxicology,* 3rd ed, Philadelphia: Lippincott, 2004.

Das S, Bannerjee G, DePonte K, *et al.*: Salp25D, an *Ixodes scapularis* antioxidant, is 1 of 14 immunodominant antigens in engorged tick salivary glands. *J Infect Dis* 184:1056–1064, 2001.

Datta G, Tu AT: Structure and other chemical characterizations of gila toxin, a lethal toxin from lizard venom. *J Peptide Res* 50:443–450, 1997.

Demsey CE: The actions of melittin on membranes. *Biochim Biophys Acta* 1031:143–161, 1990.

Dimarcq J-L, Hunneyball I: Pharma-entomology: When bugs become drugs. *Drug Discovery Today* 8:107–110, 2003.

Dreyer F: Peptide toxins and potassium channels. *Rev Physiol Biochem Pharmacol* 115:93–116, 1990.

Eaker D, Wadström T (eds.):*Natural Toxins.* Elmsford, NY: Pergamon Press, 1980.

Escoubas P: Mass spectrometry in toxinology: A 21st-century technology for the study of biopolymers from venoms. *Toxicon* 47:609–613, 2006.

Escoubas P, Diochot S, Corzo G: Structure and pharmacology of spider venom neurotoxins. *Biochimie* 82:893–907, 2000.

Escoubas P, Rash L: Tarantulas: Eight-legged pharmacists and combinatorial chemists. *Toxicon* 43:555–574, 2004.

Fatehi M, Rowan EG, Harvey AL, *et al.*: Polyamine FTX-3.3 and polyamine amide sFTX-3.3 inhibit presynaptic calcium currents and acetylcholine release at mouse motor nerve terminals. *Neuropharmacology* 36:185–194, 1997.

Francischetti IBM, Mather TN, Ribeiro JMC: Cloning of a salivary gland metalloprotease and characterization of gelatinase and fibrino(gen)lytic activities in the saliva of the lyme disease tick vector *Ixodes scapularis. Biochem Biophys Res Commun* 305:869–875, 2003.

Fry BG: From genome to "venome": Molecular origin and evolution of the snake venom proteome inferred from phylogenetic analysis of toxin sequences and related body proteins. *Genome Res* 15:403–420, 2005.

Gertsch WJ: *American Spiders,* 2nd ed. New York: Van Nostrand Reinhold, 1979.

Goldin AL: Resurgence of sodium channel research. *Annu Rev Physiol* 63:871–894, 2001.

Gomes A, Datta A, Sarangi B, *et al.*: Isolation, purification and pharmacodynamics of a toxin from the venom of centipede, *Scolopendra subspinis dehaani* Brandt. *Ind J Exp Biol* 21:203–207, 1983.

Gopalakrishnakone P, Tan CK (eds.): *Recent Advances in Toxinology Research.* Singapore: National University of Singapore, 1992.

Grishin E: Polypeptide neurotoxins from spider venoms. *Eur J Biochem* 264:276–280, 1999.

Grishin EV: Black widow spider toxins: The present and the future. *Toxicon* 36:1693–1701, 1998.

Guerrero B, Perales J, Gil San Juan A, Arocha-Pinango CL: Effect on platelet FXIII and partial characterization of Lonomin V, a proteolytic enzyme from *Lonomia achelous* caterpillars. *Thrombosis Res* 93:243–252, 1999.

Habermann E: Apamin. *Pharmacol Ther* 25:255–270, 1984.

Heard K, O'Malley GF, Dart RC: Antivenom therapy in the Americas (review). *Drugs* 58:5–15, 1999.

Hoffman DR: Hymenoptera venom allergens. *Clin Rev Allergy Immunol* 30:109–128, 2006.

Holz GG, Habener JF: Black widow spider alpha-latrotoxin: A presynaptic neurotoxin that shares structural homology with the glycogen-like peptide-1 family of insulin secretagogic hormones. *Comp Biochem Physiol [B]* 121:177–184, 1998.

Hooper D, Lirazon MB, Schoenfeld R, *et al*: Post-translational modification: A two dimensional strategy for molecular diversity of *Conus* peptides, in Fields GB, Tam JP, Barany G (eds.): *Peptides for the New Millennium: Proceedings of the Sixteenth American Peptide Symposium*. Dordrecht, The Netherlands: Kluwer, 2000.

Horikawa N, Kataha K, Watanabe N, *et al*.: Glibenclamide-sensitive hypotension produced by helodermin assessed in the rat. *Biol Pharm Bull* 21:1290–1293, 1998.

Hurlbut WP, Iezzi N, Fesce R, *et al*: Correlation between quantal secretion and vesicle loss at the frog neuromuscular junction. *J Physiol* (London) 425:501–526, 1990.

Inokuma H, Kemp DH, Willadsen P: Comparison prostaglandin E2 in salivary gland of *Boophilus microplus, Haemaphysalis longicornis* and *Ixodes holocyclus* and quantification of PGE2 in saliva, hemolymph, ovary and gut of *B. microplus*. *J Vet Med Sci* 56:1217–1218, 1994.

Isbister GK, Volschenk ES, Seymour JE: Scorpion stings in Australia: Five definite stings and a review. *Int Med J* 34:427–430, 2004.

Isbister GK, White J: Clinical consequences of spider bites: Recent advances in our understanding. *Toxicon* 43:477–492, 2004.

Kandel ER, Schwartz JH, Jessel TM: *Principles of Neural Sciences,* 4th ed. New York: McGraw-Hill, 2000.

Kawamoto F, Kumada N: Biology and venoms of *Lepidoptera*, in Tu A (ed): *Insect Poisons, Allergens, and Other Invertebrate Venoms*. New York: Marcel Dekker, 1984, Vol 2, p. 292.

Keegan HL: *Scorpions of Medical Importance*. Jackson, MI: University Press of Mississippi, 1980.

Kini RM: Excitement ahead: Structure, function and mechanism of snake venom phospholipase A$_2$ enzymes. *Toxicon* 42:827–840, 2003.

Kini RM, Chan YM: Accelerated evolution and molecular surface of venom phospholipases A$_2$ enzymes. *J Mol Evol* 48:125–132, 1999.

Krasnoperov VG, Bittner MA, Beavis R, *et al*.: α-Latrotoxin stimulates exocytosis by the interaction with a neuronal G-protein-coupled receptor. *Neuron* 18:925–937, 1997.

Kuhn-Nentwig L: Antimicrobial and cytolytic peptides of venomous arthropods. *Cell Mol Life Sci* 60:2651–2668, 2003.

Kuhn-Nentwig L, Schaller J, Nentwig W: Biochemistry, toxicology and ecology of the venom of the spider *Cupiennius salei* (Ctenidae). *Toxicon* 43:534–553, 2004.

Lee C-Y (ed): Snake Venoms. New York, Springer Verlag, 1979.

Li M, Fry BG, Kini RM: Putting the brakes on snake venom evolution: The unique molecular evolutionary patterns of *Aipysurus eydouxii* (Marbled sea snake) phospholipase A$_2$ toxins. *Mol Biol Evol* 22:934–941, 2005.

Liu M, Nakazawa K, Inoue K, *et al*.: Potent and voltage-dependent block by philanthotoxin-343 of neuronal nicotinic receptor/channels in PC12 cells. *Br J Pharmacol* 122:379–385, 1997.

Mans BJ, Gaspar ARMD, Louw AI, *et al*: Purification and characterization of apyrase from the tick, *Ornithodoros savignyi*. *Comp Biochem Physiol Part B* 120:617–624, 1998.

Maretiĉ Z, Lebez D: *Araneism*. Belgrade, Yugoslavia: Nolit Belgrade, 1979.

Markland FS: Snake venoms and their hemostatic system. *Toxicon* 36:1749–1800, 1998.

Marsh N, Williams V: Practical applications of snake venom toxins in haemostasis. *Toxicon* 45:1171–1181, 2005.

Masina S, Broady KW: Tick paralysis: development of a vaccine. *Int J Parasitol* 29:535–541, 1999.

McIntosh JM, Santos AD, Olivera BM: *Conus* peptides targeted to specific nicotinic acetylcholine receptor subtypes. *Annu Rev Biochem* 68:59–88, 1999.

Mebs D: *Venomous and Poisonous Animals*. Stuttgart: Medpharm, 2002.

Mebs D, Kauferstein S: Ichthyotoxity caused by marine cone snail venoms? *Toxicon* 46:355–356, 2005.

Menez A: *The Subtle Beast: Snakes, from Myth to Medicine*. New York: Taylor & Francis, 2003.

Menez A: Functional architectures of animal toxins: A clue to drug design? *Toxicon* 36:1557–1572, 1998.

Menez A, Gillet D, Grishin E: in Gillet D, Johannes L (eds.): *Recent Research Developments on Toxins from Bacteria and Other Organisms*. Trivandrum, India: Research Signpost, 2005.

Ménez A, Stocklin R, Mebs D: "Venomics" or: The venomous systems genome project. *Toxicon* 47:255–259, 2006.

Ménez A, Zimmerman K, Zimmerman S, *et al*.: Venom apparatus and toxicity of the centipede *Ethmostigmus rubripes* (Chilopoda, Scolopendridae). *J Morphol* 206:303–312, 1990.

Merchant ML, Hinton JF, Geren CR: Sphingomyelinase D activity of brown recluse spider (*Loxosceles reclusa*) venom as studied by ^{31}P-NMR: Effects on the time-course of sphingomyelin hydrolysis. *Toxicon* 36:537–545, 1998.

Middleton RE, Warren VA, Kraus RL, *et al*.: Two tarantula peptides inhibit activation of multiple sodium channels. *Biochemistry* 41:14734–14747, 2002.

Morrissette J, Kratezschmar J, Haendler B, *et al*.: Primary structure and properties of helothermine, a peptide toxin that blocks ryanodine receptors. *Biophys J* 68:2280–2208, 1995.

Mouhat S, Jouirou B, Mosbah A, *et al*.: Diversity of folds in animal toxins acting on ion channels. *Biochem J* 378:717–726, 2004.

Nastopoulos D, Kanellopoulos PN, Tsernoglov D: Structure of dimeric and monomeric erabutoxin a refined at I.5A resolution. *Acta Crystallogr D Biol Crystallogr* 54:964–974, 1998.

Nobile M, Noceti F, Prestipino G, *et al*.: Helothermine, a lizard venom toxin, inhibits calcium current in cerebellar granules. *Exp Brain Res* 110:15–20, 1996.

Nuttall PA, Labuda M: Dynamics of infection in tick vectors and at the tick–host interface. *Adv Virus Res* 60:233–272, 2003.

Oguiura N, Boni-Mitake M, Radis-Baptista G: New view on crotamine, a small basic polypeptide myotoxin from South American rattlesnake venom. *Toxicon* 46:363–370, 2006.

Ohno M, Chijiwa T, Oda-Ueda N, *et al*.: Molecular evolution of myotoxic phospholipases A$_2$ from snake venom. *Toxicon* 42:841–854, 2003.

Olivera BM: *Conus* venom peptides, receptor and ion channel targets and drug design: 50 million years of neuropharmacology. *Mol Biol Cell* 8:2101–2109, 1997.

Olivera BM: ω-Conotoxin MVIIA: from marine snail venom to analgesic drug, in Fusetani N (ed.): *Drugs from the Sea*. Basel: Karger, 2000.

Olivera BM: *Conus* venom peptides: Reflections from the biology of clades and species. *Annu Rev Ecol Syst* 33:25–42, 2002.

Olivera BM, Miljanich G, Ramachandran J, *et al*.: Calcium channel diversity and neurotransmitter release: The ω-conotoxins and ω-agatoxins. *Ann Rev Biochem* 63:823–867, 1994.

Olivera BM, Rivier J, Clark C, *et al*.: Diversity of *Conus* neuropeptides. *Science* 249:257–263, 1990.

O'Shea M: *Venomous Snakes of the World*. Princeton: Princeton University Press, 2005.

Patel KA, Modur V, Zimmerman GA: The necrotic venom of the brown recluse spider induces dysregulated endothelial cell-dependent neutrophil activation. Differential induction of GM-CSF, IL-8, and E-selectin expression. *J Clin Invest* 94:631–642, 1994.

Phui Yee JS, Nanling G, Afifiyan F, *et al*.: Snake postsynaptic neurotoxins: Gene structure, phylogeny and applications in research and therapy. *Biochimie* 86:137–49, 2004.

Pick T (ed.): *Venoms of the Hymenoptera*. London: Academic Press, 1986.

Polis GA (ed.): *The Biology of Scorpions*. Stanford, CA: Stanford University Press, 1990, p. 482.

Possani LD, Merino E, Corona M, *et al*.: Peptides and genes encoding for scorpion toxins that affect ion-channels. *Biochimie* 82:861–868, 2000.

Ramirez MS, Sanchez EE, Garcia-Prieto C, *et al*.: Screening for fibrinolytic activity in 8 viperid venoms. *Comp Biochem Physiol Pharmacol Toxicol Endocrinol* 124:91–98, 1999.

Ramos OHP, Selistre-de-Araujo HS: Snake venom metalloproteases—structure and function of catalytic and disintegrin domains. *Comp Biochem Physiol, Part C* 142:328–346, 2006.

Rash LD, Hodgson WC: Pharmacology and biochemistry of spider venoms. *Toxicon* 40:225–254, 2002.

Rimsza ME, Zimmerman DR, Bergeson PS: Scorpion envenomation. *Pediatrics* 66:298–302, 1980.

Rockel D, Korn W, Kohn AJ: *Manual of the Living Conidae.* Weisbaden, Germany: Verlag Christa Hemmen, 1995.

Rodriguez de la Vega RC, Possani LD: Current views on scorpion toxins specific for K$^+$-channels. *Toxicon* 43:865–875, 2004.

Rodriguez de la Vega RC, Possani LD: Overview of scorpion toxins specific for Na$^+$ channels and related peptides: Biodiversity, structure–function relationships and evolution. *Toxicon* 46:831–844, 2005.

Rosenberg P: Phospholipases, in Shier WT, Mebs D (eds.): *Handbook of Toxinology.* New York: Marcel Dekker, 1990, p. 67.

Russell FE: Toxic effects of animal venoms, in Klaassen CD (ed.): *Casarett and Doull's Toxicology: The Basic Science of Poisons,* 6th ed. New York: McGraw-Hill, 2001, p. 945.

Russell FE, Nagabhushanam, R: *The Venomous and Poisonous Marine Invertebrates of the Indian Ocean.* Enfield, NH: Science Publications, 1996, p. 271.

Sangamnetdej S, Paesen GC, Slovak M, *et al.*: A high affinity serotonin- and histamine-binding lipocalin from tick saliva. *Insect Mol Biol* 11:79–86, 2002.

Sholl JM, Rathlev NK, Olshaker JS: *Wilderness Medicine.* Philadelphia: WB Saunders, 2004.

Skinner WS, Adams ME, Quistad GB, *et al.*: Purification and characterization of two classes of neurotoxins from the funnel web spider *Agelenopsis aperta. J Biol Chem* 264:2150–2155, 1989.

Singletary EM, Holstege CP: Bites and stings: Insects, marine, mammals and reptiles, in Aghababian RV (ed.): *Essentials of Emergency Medicine,* Sudbury, MA: Jones and Bartlett, 2006.

Soares AM, Giglio JR: Chemical modifications of phospholipases A$_2$ from snake venoms: Effects on catalytic and pharmacological properties. *Toxicon* 42:855–868, 2003.

Sokolov IuV, Chanturiia AN, Lishko VK: [Channel-forming properties of *Steatoda paykulliana* spider venom] [Russian]. *Biofizika* 29:620–623, 1984.

Steen NA, Barker SC, Alewood PF: Proteins in the saliva of the Ixodida (ticks): Pharmacological features and biological significance. *Toxicon* 47:1–20, 2006.

Strimple PD, Tomassoni AJ, Otten EJ, *et al*: Report on envenomation by a Gila monster (*Heloderma suspectum*) with a discussion of venom apparatus, clinical findings, and treatment. *Wilderness Environ Med* 8:111–116, 1997.

Swartz KJ, MacKinnon R: An inhibitor of the Kv2.1 potassium channel isolated from the venom of a Chilean tarantula. *Neuron* 15:35–42, 1995.

Swenson S, Markland FS, Jr: Snake venom fibrin(ogen)olytic enzymes. *Toxicon* 45:1021–1039, 2005.

Tambourgi DV, Petricevich VL, Magnoli FC, *et al.*: Endotoxemic-like shock induced by *Loxosceles* spider venoms: Pathological changes and putative cytokine mediators. *Toxicon* 36:391–403, 1998.

Terlau H, Olivera BM: *Conus* venoms: A rich source of novel ion channel-targeted peptides. *Physiol Rev* 84:41–68, 2004.

Terlau H, Shon K, Grilley M, *et al.*: Strategy for rapid immobilization of prey by a fish-hunting cone snail. *Nature* 381:148–151, 1996.

Thurn MJ, Gooley A, Broady KW: Identification of the neurotoxin from the Australian paralysis tick *Ixodes holocyclus*, in Tan P, *et al.* (eds.): *Recent Advances in Toxicological Research.* Singapore: National University of Singapore, 1992, pp. 243–256.

Tintinalli JE, Kelen GD, Stapczynski JS (Eds): *Emergency Medicine: A Comprehensive Study Guide,* 6th ed. New York: McGraw-Hill, 2004.

Tsetlin VI, Hucho F: Snake and snail toxins acting on nicotinic acetylcholine receptors: Fundamental aspects and medical applications. *FEBS Lett* 557:9–13, 2004.

Uddman R, Goadsby PJ, Jansen-Olesen I, *et al.*: Helospectin-like peptides: Immunochemical localization and effects on isolated cerebral arteries and on local cerebral blood flow in the cat. *J Cerebral Blood Flow Metabol* 19:61–67, 1999.

Ushkaryov YA, Volnski KE, Ashton AC: The multiple actions of black widow spider toxins and their selective use in neurosecretion studies. *Toxicon* 43:527–542, 2004.

Valenzuela JG: Blood-feeding arthropod salivary glands and saliva, in Marquardt, WC (ed.): *Biology of Disease Vectors.* Amsterdam: Elsevier, 2004, Chapter 28.

Valenzuela JG, Charlab R, Mather TN, *et al.*: Purification, cloning and expression of a novel salivary anticomplement protein from the tick *Ixodes scapularis. J Biol Chem* 275:18717–18723, 2000.

Vincent A, Jacobson L, Curran L: Alpha-bungarotoxin binding to human muscle acetylcholine receptor. *Neurochem Int* 332:427–433, 1998.

Vogel C-W, Fritsinger DC, Hew BE: Recombinant cobra venom factor. *Mol Immunol* 41:191–199, 2004.

Volynski KE, Capogna M, Ashton AC, *et al*: Mutant α-latrotoxin (LTX^{N4C}) does not form pores and causes secretion by receptor stimulation. This action does not require neurexins. *J Biol Chem* 278:31058–31066, 2003.

Wang X, Connor M, Smith R, *et al.*: Discovery and characterization of a family of insecticidal neurotoxins with a rare vicinal disulfide bridge. *Nat Struct Biol* 7:505–513, 2000.

Wang X, Connor M, Wilson D, *et al.*: Discovery and structure of a potent and highly specific blocker of insect calcium channels. *J Biol Chem* 276:40306–40312, 2001.

White J: Snake venoms and coagulopathy. *Toxicon* 45:951–967, 2005.

Wilson D, Alewood PF: Taxonomy of Australian Funnel-web spiders using rp-HPLC/ESI-MS profiling techniques. *Toxicon* 47:614–627, 2006.

Yellen G. The voltage-gated potassium channels and their relatives. *Nature* 419:35–42, 2002.

TOXIC EFFECTS OF PLANTS

Stata Norton

INTRODUCTION

Plants may cause toxic effects as a result of inadvertent exposure on contact or accidental ingestion of the plant. Examples are "hay fever" (rhinitis) from exposure to airborne plant pollen and oral irritation, especially in children, from biting on a leaf of a plant such as dumb cane (Diffenbachia). Another source of toxicity may be from intentional ingestion of some herbs, especially when they are taken chronically. The possibility also exists for interactions of prescribed drugs with intake of herbal remedies. For example, the chemicals in some herbs affect hepatic cytochrome enzymes (Izzo and Ernst, 2001).

In recent years, information on bioactive chemicals in plants has grown steadily, partly from increased interest in herbal remedies and from interest in identifying novel approaches to medical problems. One result of the latter interest is that toxic effects of plants are being examined for potential usefulness in cancers. This chapter will be restricted primarily to consideration of the toxic effects of plants from unintentional exposure and some intentional exposures, with only brief mention of possible value of toxic bioactive components.

In the course of evolution, plants have been attacked by viruses, bacteria, and fungi, and have been eaten by animals of many kinds. In response, plants have developed various elegant defenses, including synthesis of antimicrobial chemicals and chemicals designed to repel animals by various means. Of the many species of plants that contain toxic chemicals, only a few can be described here. Selection is based on three considerations: frequency with which exposure occurs; importance and seriousness of the exposure; and the scientific understanding of the nature of the action of the chemical.

In considering any chemical synthesized by a plant it is important to note that there may be marked variability in the amount of a toxic chemical produced by a plant. The reasons for variability in concentration of toxic chemicals are several:

1. Different portions of the plant may contain different concentrations of a chemical. An example of localization of bioactive compounds is found in the bracken fern (*Pteridium aquilinum*) in which the carcinogenic terpene, ptaquiloside, is found in high concentrations in the fronds compared with the roots (Rasmussen *et al.*, 2003).

2. The age of the plant contributes to variability. Peak concentrations of bioactive compounds often are found at different periods of growth. For example, in lettuce (*Lactuca* species) the concentration of lactucin and other sesquiterpenes increases with maturation, reaching a peak in the latex when the flower stalk is forming (Sessa *et al.*, 2000).

3. Climate and soil influence the synthesis of some chemicals. For example, lichens produce carotenoids in direct relation to the amount of sunlight, with the advantage to the plant that carotenoids protect from excessive ultraviolet light.

4. Genetic differences within a species alter the ability of plants to synthesize a chemical. Synthesis of related toxic chemicals is found in some plants as a characteristic of a genus and sometimes as a familial characteristic. For example, species of *Raunculus* (buttercup) produce an acrid juice that releases the irritating chemical, anemonin. Some other genera of the same family (Ranunculaceae) also release anemonin.

TOXIC EFFECTS BY ORGAN

Skin

Contact Dermatitis   Several plants that are common to the temperate regions worldwide contain compounds that produce irritation on contact with the intact plant. The leaves of stinging nettles (*Urtica* species, Urticaceae) bear numerous trichomes, barb-like silicified hairs that puncture skin on contact, releasing an irritating sap. The sap has been reported to contain a mixture of formic acid, histamine, acetylcholine, and serotoin (Kavalali, 2003). Although there are about 100 species of *Urtica* worldwide, *Urtica dioica* and *Urtica urens* are the most common in the United States and Europe and *Urtica ferox* is widespread in New Zealand. Exposure to *U. ferox* (poisonous tree nettle) has caused death in humans and animals. A defense by the plant against ingestion by animals, similar to that of nettles, has been developed by *Mucuna pruriens* (cowhage), a legume with pods covered with barbed trichomes that cause pain, itching, erythema, and vesication. The trichomes contain mucinain, a proteinase responsible for the pruritis (Southcott and Haegi, 1992).

Several species of *Ranunculus* (buttercup) cause contact dermatitis. These plants contain ranunculin, which releases the toxic principle protoanemonin, also present in *Anemone,* another genus of the buttercup family. Protoanemonin is readily converted to anemonin, which has marked irritant properties. In addition to contact dermatitis, ingestion of plants containing protoanemonin may result in severe irritation of the gastrointestinal tract (Kelch *et al.*, 1992).

The genus *Euphorbia* (Euphorbiaceae, spurge family) contains hundreds of species dispersed over temperate and tropical regions. Characteristically, the stems and leaves exude milky latex when damaged. The latex contains diterpene esters that are irritating to the skin. *Euphorbia marginata* (snow-on-the mountain) is a common plant in the United States, growing wild from Minnesota to Texas and cultivated for its attractive foliage. Individuals using the plant in flower arrangements may come in contact with the latex and develop skin irritation (Urushibata and Kase, 1991). Serious eye irritation has been reported (Frohn *et al.*, 1993). The latex of cultivars of *Euphorbia pulcherrima* (poinsettia) may cause contact dermatitis (Massermanian, 1998).

Allergic Dermatitis   Most people are familiar with allergic dermatitis caused by contact with some plants, such as poison ivy. These allergens tend to be located in the outer cell layers of plant organs. In allergic dermatitis to chrysanthemums (*Dendranthema* species) the allergens are sesquiterpene lactones present in small hairs (trichomes) on the stems, undersides of leaves and in flowering heads (McGovern and Barkley, 1999).

Rhus (Anacardiaceae, cashew family) and *Philodendron* (Araceae, arum family) are not closely related plants but both genera contain species causing contact dermatitis as an allergic reaction. *Philodendron scandens* is a common houseplant, while *Rhus radicans* (poison ivy) is widespread in North America. In addition to poison ivy, the toxicodendron group of plants contains *Rhus diversiloba* (poison oak) and *Rhus vernix* (poison sumac). The active chemicals in *P. scandens* are resorcinols, especially 5-*n*-heptadecatrienyl resorcinol (Knight, 1991). In *R. radicans* the allergenic component is a mixture of catechols called urushiol. The most active compound in urushiol is 3-*n*-pentadecadienyl catechol, representing about 60% of urushiol (Johnson *et al.*, 1972). As in allergies in general, there is no response to the initial exposure; even with repeated exposure, individuals show marked variation in severity of response. The allergens in usushiol will sensitize about 70% of persons exposed. Urushiol is fat soluble, penetrates the stratum corneum and binds to Langerhans cells in the epidermis. These haptenated cells then migrate to lymph nodes, where T-cells are activated (Kalish and Johnson, 1990). Ingestion of *Rhus* species has been reported to cause generalized dermatitis (Oh *et al.*, 2003). Allergic dermatitis may also develop with repeated exposure to the sap of the mango fruit. The skin of the mango (*Magnifera indica*, Anacardiaceae) contains oleoresins that cross-react with allergens of poison ivy (Tucker and Swan, 1998).

Flower growers and other individuals who handle bulbs and cut flowers of daffodils, hyacinths, and tulips sometimes develop dermatitis from contact with the sap. The rashes are due to irritation from alkaloids (masonin, lycorin, and several related alkaloids) or to needle-like crystals of calcium oxalate in the bulbs (Gude *et al.*, 1998). Most of these chemicals do not act as allergens but one, tulipalin-A, that causes "tulip fingers" from sorting and peeling tulip bulbs, has allergenic properties. Tulipalin-A, alpha-methylene-gamma-butyrolactone, is present in some cultivars in concentrations up to 2%. A safe threshold for this allergen is considered to be 0.01% (Hausen *et al.*, 1983). The advantage of the tulipalins to the plant is that they are strong antifungal agents (Christensen and Kristiansen, 1999).

An immunoglobulin-mediated hypersensitivity, called the "latex-fruit syndrome," results in cross-sensitivity in some individuals to latex in rubber gloves and some fruits. The major allergen in natural rubber latex from the tree, *Hevea brasiliensis*, is prohevein, a chitin-binding polypeptide found in several plants. Hevein, a 43-amino acid N-terminal fragment of prohevein is the major binding component. The structural analysis has been reported (Kolarich *et al.*, 2005). Individuals sensitive to rubber latex may be sensitized to fruits containing a chitinase with a hevein-like domain, including banana, kiwi, tomato, and avocado (Blanco *et al.*, 1999).

Lichens, such as species of *Usnea* and *Cladonia*, are abundant on trees in areas away from major city smog. Dermatitis from contact with lichens is known in professions where individuals are repeatedly exposed to lichens, including workers in forestry and horticulture. The allergen is usnic acid (a benzofuran) and related acids in lichens (Aalto-Korte *et al.*, 2005). Usnic acid is of current research interest as a non-genotoxic anticancer agent (Mayer *et al.*, 2005b). Usnic acid has been implicated in hepatotoxicity following use of some nonprescription weight-loss supplements (Han *et al.*, 2004).

Photosensitivity   Not all cases of dermititis from plants are due to skin contact. Poisoning of livestock from *Hypericum perforatum* (St. John's wort) has been reported from several countries. The toxic principle is hypericin (a bianthraquinone), present throughout the plant. Sheep are the most commonly affected animals, ingesting the plant in pasturage. The effect in sheep is development of edematous lesions of the skin in areas not well covered with hair, including the ears, nose, and eyes. Hypericin causes photosensitization and the lesions appear from exposure to sunlight (Sako *et al.*, 1993).

Although photosensitization in humans is a rare event after consumption of St. John's wort, enhancement of response in humans to therapeutic exposure to ultraviolet therapy has been reported (Beattie *et al.*, 2005).

Respiratory Tract

Allergic Rhinitis Rhinitis from inhalation of plant pollens, also known as "hay fever" or pollinosis, is a seasonal problem for many individuals. A chromosomal association in individuals with seasonal pollen reactivity is under investigation (Blumenthal *et al.*, 2006). Many plant species contribute to airborne pollen, especially grass pollens. *Poa* and *Festuca* species are major contributors to the allergic response. Pollen from several genera in the Asteraceae (e.g., mugwort, *Artemisia vulgaris,* in Europe, and ragweed, *Ambrosia artemisiifolia,* in North America) contains allergens causing summer rhinitis. Immunoglobulin antibodies produced by sensitized individuals from the two species cross react. The allergen has been identified as a highly conserved 14-kDa protein, profilin, found as well in birch pollen (Hirschwehr *et al.*, 1998). Pollen from pellitory (*Parietaria* species, Urticaceae) is an important cause of pollinosis in the Mediterranean region (Arilla *et al.*, 2006). Asthma and rhinitis associated with occupation are also recognized in individuals exposed to certain plants, such as cascara sagrada (*Rhamnus purshiana*) (Giavina-Bianchi *et al*, 1997), or workers in greenhouses in which bell peppers are growing (Groenewoud *et al.*, 2006).

Cough Reflex It has been found that workers who handle two types of peppers, *Capsicum annuum* (sweet pepper) and *Capsicum frutescens* (red pepper), have a significantly increased incidence of cough during exposure. The major irritants are capsaicin (*trans*-8-methyl-*N*-vanillyl-6-nonenamide) and dihydrocapsaicin (Surh *et al.*, 1998). Capsaicin-sensitive nerves in the airway are involved in the irritation and cough (Blanc *et al.*, 1991). Capsaicin activates a subtype of the vanilloid receptor found in the airway, spinal cord, dorsal root ganglion, bladder, urethra, and colon. Capsaicin can also be irritating to the skin, and individuals handling the peppers may experience irritation and vesication.

Toxin-Associated Pneumonia The formation of the pneumotoxin, 4-ipomeanol, in sweet potato roots (*Ipomea batatas*, Convolvulaceae) from the mold *Fusarium solani* has been known for some time. The toxin 4-ipomeanol is activated by human cytochrome *P*450s to a reactive intermediate that binds to DNA (Alvarez-Diez and Zheng, 2004). Differences in the pattern of organ toxicity are related to *P*450 isoforms. In cattle and rabbits, the major *P*450 activator is CYP4B1 in the lung. In the mouse, renal toxicity results from high levels of CYP4B1 in the kidney and in humans multiple subsets of liver *P*450 enzymes bioactivate 4-ipomeanol (Baer *et al.*, 2005). Fungal pneumonia from *Acremonium strictum* has been reported (Pusterla *et al.*, 2005).

Pyrrolizidine alkaloids in Boraginaceae and Asteraceae families of plants have been implicated in lung toxicity and pneumonitis in humans (Altamirano *et al.*, 2005).

Gastrointestinal System

Direct Irritant Effects The most common outcome of ingestion of a toxic plant is gastrointestinal disturbance (nausea, vomiting, and diarrhea) from irritation of the gastrointestinal tract. Many kinds of chemicals may be responsible for this. Some have found a place in medicine as mild purgatives, such as cascara sagrada. Cascara is obtained from the bark of *Rhamnus purshiana* (California buckthorn). The active ingredient is an anthraquinone, emodin.

Tung nut (*Aleurites fordii*) is grown widely in the world. The seeds, from which commercially useful oil is expressed, are the most toxic part. Ingestion of the ripe nuts causes abdominal pain, vomiting, and diarrhea. Outbreaks of poisoning are most common in children (Lin *et al.*, 1996).

Buffalo bean or buffalo pea (*Thermopsis rhombifolia*) is a legume growing wild in western United States. Loss of life in livestock has been reported from consumption of the mature plant with seeds. Children develop nausea, vomiting, dizziness, and abdominal pain from eating the beans (McGrath-Hill and Vicas, 1997). The toxic chemicals are quinolizidine alkaloids.

Aesculus hippocastanum (horse chestnut) and *Aesculus glabra* (Ohio buckeye) are common trees with attractive panicles of flowers in the spring. Nuts of both trees contain a glucoside called esculin. When eaten by humans, the main effect is gastroenteritis, which may be severe if several nuts are consumed. Esculin is poorly absorbed from the gastrointestinal tract of humans and its systemic effects are usually limited. In cattle the glucoside may be hydrolyzed in the rumen, releasing the aglycone to cause systemic effects. Cattle develop signs of nervous system stimulation—a stiff-legged gait and, in severe poisoning, tonic seizures with opisthotonus (Casteel *et al.*, 1992). While the most common poisoning of cattle occurs from ingestion of nuts, they may also be poisoned in pasture in spring from eating new leaves and buds. Beta-aescin, a triperpene saponin in horse chestnut seed extract, has been studied for use in chronic venous insufficiency in humans (Siebert *et al.*, 2002).

Antimitotic Effects *Podophyllum peltatum* (May apple, Berberidaceae) contains the toxic purgative, podophyllotoxin, especially in foliage and roots. In low doses, mild purgation predominates. Overdose results in nausea and severe paroxysmal vomiting (Frasca *et al.*, 1997). Podophyllotoxin inhibits mitosis by binding to microtubules, and this property has made the toxin of interest in treatment of cancer (Schacter, 1996).

Colchicine is best known in western medicine for its antimitotic effect, resulting from block of formation of microtubules and failure of the mitotic spindle, for which it is useful in attacks of gout. Colchicine is the major alkaloid in the bulbs of *Colchicum autumnale* (autumn crocus, Liliaceae), native to Asia Minor. Severe gastroenteritis (nausea, vomiting, diarrhea, and dehydration) follows ingestion of the bulbs that may be mistaken for wild garlic. Systemic effects (confusion, hematuria, neuropathy, and renal failure) may develop in severe poisoning. Bone marrow aplasia results from block of mitosis in bone marrow. Additional toxic effects may be due to lectins in the plant. In southern Europe, hay for cattle may contain the wild autumn crocus, and deaths occur if contamination is heavy.

Toxicity from human ingestion of tubers of *Gloriosa superba* (glory lily) similar to that from autumn crocus has been reported. This ornamental lily also contains colchicine. The plant grows wild in Sri Lanka and poisoning by *Gloriosa* tubers has been reported as the most common plant poisoning in that country. Poisoning has also been reported in India (Mendis, 1989).

Protein Synthesis Inhibition Some of the most toxic plant proteins act through inactivating protein sythesis. *Ricinus communis* (castor bean) is a member of the family Euphorbiaceae, which contains several genera that produce toxic chemicals. The castor bean is an ornamental plant introduced from India. If the attractive, mottled seeds are eaten, children and adults experience no marked symptoms of poisoning for several days. In this interval there is some loss of appetite, with nausea, vomiting, and diarrhea developing gradually. With fatal doses the gastroenteritis becomes severe, with persistent vomiting, bloody diarrhea, and icterus. Death occurs in 6–8 days. The fatal dose for a child can be five to six seeds; it may be as low as 20 seeds for an adult. However, fatality is low—less than 10% when a "fatal" dose is consumed—because the toxic protein is largely destroyed in the intestine. Death from castor beans is caused by two lectins in the beans: ricin I and ricin II. The more toxic is ricin II. Ricin II consists of two amino acid chains. The A-chain (molecular weight 30,000) inactivates the 60s ribosomal subunit of cells by catalytic depurination of an adenosine residue within the 28s rRNA (Bantel *et al.*, 1999) and blocks protein synthesis. The A-chain is endocytosed into the cell cytosol after the B-chain (molecular weight 30,000) binds to a terminal galactose residue on the cell membrane. The two chains are linked by disulfide bonds. Details of binding properties of ricin to glycoproteins have been investigated (Wu *et al.*, 2006).

Toxic lectins are found in the seeds of *Abrus precatorius* (jequirity bean, Leguminosae). They are attractive scarlet and black beans that are sometimes made into necklaces. Abrin-a, one of four isoabrins from the plant, has the highest inhibitory effect on protein synthesis and consists of an A-chain of 250 amino acids and a B-chain of 267 amino acids (Tahirov *et al.*, 1994). The LD50 of abrin injected in mice is less than 0.1 μg/kg, making abrin one of the most toxic substances known. As with ricin, the A-chain inhibits protein synthesis and the B-chain is responsible for penetration of abrin-a molecules into cells (Ohba *et al.*, 2004).

Plants that produce only A-chains offer much less risk when ingested. Young shoots of pokeweed (*Phytolacca americana,* Phytolaccaceae) are sometimes used in the spring as a salad green without toxicity. Mature leaves and berries may cause gastrointestinal irritation with nausea and diarrhea. The plant produces three isozymes of single-chain lectins (PAP, PAPII, and PAP-S; molecular weight of about 30,000) that can inhibit protein synthesis in cells by inactivating rRNA. Single-chain, ribosome-inhibiting proteins do not enter intact cells readily, but if the cell membrane has been breached by a virus, they may enter the cell (Monzingo *et al.*, 1993).

Wisteria floribunda (Leguminosae) is a common ornamental climbing vine or small tree with lilac-colored flowers from which pods with seeds develop in the fall. The seeds of wisteria cause severe gastroenteritis when ingested. A few seeds can result in headache, nausea, and diarrhea within hours, followed by dizziness, confusion, and hematemesis (Rondeau, 1993). The seeds contain a lectin with affinity for *N*-acetylglucosamine on mammalian neurons.

Cardiovascular System

Cardioactive Glycosides   Several different families of plants contain species with cardioactive glycosides, the best known of which is *Digitalis purpurea* (foxglove, Scrophulariaceae). In the lily family, squill (*Scilla maritima*) contains scillaren, and lily of the valley (*Convallaria majalis*) contains convallatoxin in the bulbs. Both glycosides have actions resembling digitalis. Milkweeds (*Asclepias* species, Asclepiadaceae) are noted for the glycosides in the plants, which are consumed by monarch butterfly caterpillars during their development. The glycosides are retained into the adult stage and

help protect the butterflies from predators. The cardiac glycoside [6'-O-(E-4-hydroxycinnamoyl) desglucouzarin] in *Asclepias asperula*, like digitalis, inhibits Na$^+$, K$^+$-ATPase (Abbott *et al.*, 1998). Other species of *Asclepias* also contain cardenolides (Roy *et al.*, 2005). Two plants in the Apocynaceae (oleander family) contain cardioactive glycosides. *Nereum oleander* (bay laurel) is native to the Mediterranean area but is grown ornamentally in many regions. The major glycosides, oleandrin and nerium, may be present in concentrations as high as 0.5 mg/g plant material. The blood level of oleandrin estimated to be toxic to humans is 1–2 ng/mL (Pietsch *et al.*, 2005). In addition to cardiac effects resembling digitalis toxicity, histopathological changes after fatal doses of *N. oleander* leaves to sheep include hemorrhages in several organs (Aslani *et al.*, 2004). A related plant, *Thevetia peruviana* (yellow oleander), is a common ornamental plant in the United States. Human poisoning has also been reported in Australia, Melanesia, Thailand, and India. The seeds are the major source of the cardiac glycosides, the most active of which is thevetin A. The fatal dose to an adult is eight to 10 seeds (Prabhasankar *et al.*, 1993).

Actions on Cardiac Nerves   *Veratrum viride* (American hellebore, Liliaceae), native to eastern North America, produces several toxic alkaloids that are distributed in all parts of the plant. European hellebore (*Veratrum album*) and *Veratrum californicum* in western North America have similar alkaloids. *V. album* was one of the medicinal drugs used for centuries to "slow and soften the pulse." These species of *Veratrum* contain a mixture of alkaloids, including protoveratrine, veratramine, and jervine. After ingestion the alkaloids cause nausea, emesis, hypotension, and bradycardia. The primary effect on the heart is to cause a repetitive response to a single stimulus resulting from prolongation of the sodium current (Jaffe *et al.*, 1990). The bulbs of the wild camas (*Zigadenus paniculatus* and other species of *Zigadenus*, Liliaceae) have been ingested by mistake as wild onions. Severe gastrointestinal toxicity may result (Peterson and Rasmussen, 2003). Cattle are also poisoned in pastures where the plants are common. Several species of *Zigadenus* contain veratrum-like alkaloids.

Aconitum   species have been used in western and eastern medicine for centuries. The European plant, *Aconitum napellus* (monkshood, Ranunculaceae) is a perennial grown in gardens for its ornamental blue flowers. The roots of *A. kusnezoffii* (chuanwu) and *A. carmichaeli* (caowu) are in the Chinese materia medica. Poisoning may occur from intentional or accidental ingestion, and the concentration of the alkaloids (aconitine, mesaconitine, and hypoaconitine) varies depending on species, place of origin, time of harvest, and processing procedures (Chan *et al.*, 1994). In addition to cardiac arrhythmias and hypotension, the alkaloids cause gastrointestinal upset and neurologic symptoms, especially numbness of the mouth and paresthesia in the extremities. The alkaloids cause a prolonged sodium current in cardiac muscle with slowed repolarization (Peper and Trautwein, 1967). The neurologic effects are due to a similar action on voltage-sensitive sodium currents in nerve fibers (Murai *et al.*, 1990).

In Greece about 2500 years ago, Xenophon described a serious condition called "mad honey poisoning" that developed in his soldiers after they had eaten honey contaminated with grayanotoxins. The poisoning resembles aconitine poisoning. In severe poisoning there is respiratory depression and loss of consciousness. Grayanotoxins bind to sodium channels in cardiac and muscle cells, increasing sodium conductance (Maejima *et al.*, 2002). Grayanotoxins are produced exclusively by several genera of Ericaceae (heath family). They have been isolated from *Rhododendron ponticum* (Onat *et al.*, 1991) and *Kalmia angustifolia* (Burke and Doskotch, 1990). The toxin gets into honey from nectar collected by bees. Grayanotoxins are present throughout the plants. The effect of the toxins is marked bradycardia, hypotension, oral paresthesia, weakness, and gastrointestinal upset, resembling aconitine poisoning. Grayanotoxins bind to sodium channels in cardiac and muscle cells, increasing sodium conductance (Maejima *et al.*, 2002). Toxicity has been reported in goats and in sheep eating leaves of *Rhododendron macrophyllum* (Casteel and Wagstaff, 1989).

Vasoactive Chemicals Mistletoe is a parasitic plant on trees and has over the centuries been considered either holy or demonic. The poisonous qualities of mistletoe were recognized by John Gerard in his herbal in 1597. He described a case of poisoning from mistletoe berries in which the tongue was inflamed and swollen, the mind dostraught, and strength of heart and wits enfeebled. The American mistletoe, *Phoradendron flavescens*, is a member of the same family as the European mistletoe (*Viscum album,* Loranthaceae). The American mistletoe contains phoratoxin, a polypeptide with a molecular weight of about 13,000. Phoratoxin and the viscotoxins cause similar effects: hypotension, bradycardia with negative inotropic actions on heart muscle, and vasoconstriction of the vessels of skin and skeletal muscle. Viscotoxins are basic polypeptides (molecular weight of about 5000). Phoratoxin is only one-fifth as active as the viscotoxins (Rosell and Samuelsson, 1988). Serious poisoning from the plants is rare, and most poisonings include gastrointestinal distress and hypotension. An instance of anaphylaxis to repeated injections of mistletoe extract has been reported (Bauer *et al.*, 2005).

Vasoconstriction is the primary toxic effect of some plant chemicals. Of the various fungi that produce toxic principles, some develop on grains that are used as food. *Claviceps purpurea* (ergot) is a fungus parasitic on grains, especially on rye. The "ergot gene cluster" of several genes is required for production of ergot alkaloids (Haarmann *et al.*, 2005). Ergot has caused outbreaks of poisonings in several European countries since the Middle Ages. The condition was called "St. Anthony's fire" from the blackened appearance of the limbs of some sufferers. The main toxic effect of ergot alkaloids is vasoconstriction, primarily in the extremities, followed by gangrene. Abortion in pregnant women is also common after ingestion of contaminated rye flower. Ergot alkaloids are derivatives of lysergic acid. Some of the alkaloids have been used in therapeutics, especially ergotamine and ergonovine. Ergot alkaloids are produced by some other fungi not closely related to *Claviceps*, such as *Aspergillus fumigatus*, a common airborne fungus (Coyle and Panaccione, 2005).

Another fungus, *Acremonium coenophialum*, grows symbiotically on the forage grass tall fescue (*Festuca arundinacea*) and produces some ergot alkaloids and other lysergic acid derivatives. The fungus causes "fescue toxicosis" in cattle grazing on infected plants (Hill *et al.*, 1994). The condition in cattle includes decreased weight gain, decreased reproductive performance, and peripheral vasoconstriction. In southwestern United States, *Stirpa robusta* (sleepy grass) also may be infected with an *Acremonium* fungus. Horses grazing on infected grass become somnolent, presumably as a result of ingesting lysergic acid amide, ergonovine, and related alkaloids produced by the fungus (Petroski *et al.*, 1992).

LIVER

Hepatocyte Damage *Senecio* (groundsel, Asteraceae) is a large genus of plants with worldwide distribution. Species containing significant concentrations of pyrrolizidine alkaloids are responsible for liver damage in the form of hepatic veno-occlusive disease associated with lipoperoxidation (Bondan *et al.*, 2005). Hepatitis in cattle grazing on *Senecio* has been reported in Africa and Asia as well as in the United States. The condition is progressive and death occurs after weeks or months of grazing on contaminated pasture. Four genera of Boraginaceae, *Echium* (bugloss), *Cynoglossum* (hound's tongue), *Heliotropium* (heliotrope), and *Symphytum* (comfrey) also contain pyrrolizidine alkaloids. Different animal species show marked differences in susceptibility to the alkaloids. Susceptible species are rats, cattle, horses, and chickens; resistant species are guinea pigs, rabbits, gerbils, hamsters, sheep, and Japanese quail. These differences are in general related to the rate of hepatic pyrrole formation, although other sources of differences must be present (Huan *et al.*, 1998). Human deaths from pyrrolizidine alkaloids have been reported in several countries, including South Africa, Jamaica, and Barbados. In Afghanistan, there was an epidemic of hepatic veno-occlusive disease from consumption of a wheat crop contaminated with seeds of a species of *Heliotropium* (Tandon *et al.*, 1978). The clinical signs associated with the liver damage resemble those of cirrhosis and some hepatic tumors may be mistaken for the hepatotoxicity (McDermott and Ridker, 1990). The clinical condition is a form of the Budd–Chiari syndrome, with portal hypertension and obliteration of small hepatic veins. Human consumption also occurs from *Symphytum* in herbal preparations, such as "comfrey tea" (Rode, 2002). In addition to veno-occlusive damage to the liver, the alkaloids in *Symphytum* have been shown to be tumorigenic and mutagenic in rats (Mei *et al.*, 2005).

Lantana camara (Verbenaceae) has been called one of the 10 most noxious weeds in the world. It is an attractive shrub, native to Jamaica and commonly cultivated in greenhouses. *L. camara* thrives outdoors in hot, dry climates. An unusual property of the plant is that it inhibits the growth of neighboring plants. In India, livestock poisoning from *L. camara* is a serious problem. Cattle grazing on the plant develop cholestasis and hyperbilirubinemia. The leaves are toxic to some nonruminants, including rabbits and guinea pigs. Several triterpenoids have been isolated from the plant. One that has been shown to induce hepatotoxicity is lantadene A (22-beta-angeloyloxy-3-oxo-olean-12-en-28-oic acid) (Sharma *et al.*, 1991).

Mushroom toxins Many of the nonedible mushrooms may cause gastrointestinal distress but most are not life threatening. Repeated consumption of the false morel, *Gyromitra esculenta*, has been reported to cause hepatitis as well as gastrointestinal disorders (Michelot and Toth, 1991). The toxic principle is gyromitrin (acetaldehyde-*N*-formylhydrazone). Several species of three genera of mushrooms are responsible for most fatal poisoning from consumption of wild mushrooms, *Amanita*, *Galerina*, and *Lepiota* (Karlson-Stiber and Persson, 2003). *Amanita phalloides*, is appropriately called "death cap." *Amanita ocreata* (death angel) is equally dangerous. *A. phalloides* contains two types of toxins, phalloidin and amatoxins. Phalloidin is a cyclic heptapeptide that may be responsible for the diarrhea that develops 10–12 hours after ingestion of *A. phalloides*. Phalloidin combines with actin in muscle cells, but is not readily absorbed from the gastrointestinal tract (Cappell and Hassan, 1992). The alpha-, beta-, and gamma-amanitins are bicyclic peptides (mw 900) and are absorbed. The most toxic, alpha-amanitin, binds strongly to RNA polymerase II in hepato-cytes, thus inhibiting protein synthesis (Jaeger *et al.*, 1993). In-testinal mucosa and kidneys are also targets. Serious clinical signs develop slowly, beginning about the third day after ingestion. Treat-ment in severe cases may require liver transplant. There is a long his-tory of use of the herb *Silybum marianum* (milk thistle, Asteraceae) for treatment of poisoning from amanitins. The active ingredient is silymarin, a flavanolignan. Silymarin and herbal preparations also have been tried in viral hepatitis and alcoholic liver disease (Ball and Kowdley, 2005; Mayer *et al.*, 2005a).

Mycotoxins   Various fungi present during harvest, or subsequent storage of food, produce toxins. Exposure to low levels of the myco-toxins by way of ingestion of the moldy foods is common, depending on geographic location and type of food. Most notable toxins are aflatoxins from *Aspergillus* species in stored grain, ochratoxin A, an immunosuppressant chemical produced by *Aspergillus* and *Penicil-lium* molds, and zearalenone, a mycotoxin produced by *Fusarium* and *Gibberella* species (Al-Anati and Petzinger, 2006; Ding *et al.*, 2006). Aflatoxin B1 from *A. flavus* and *A. parasiticus* has been asso-ciated with primary hepatocellular carcinoma in humans. The toxin forms guanine adducts and induces apoptotic cell death in human hepatocytes (Reddy *et al.*, 2006).

Fumonisins are toxins produced by the fungus *Fusarium*, pri-marily by *Fusarium moniliforme* and *Fusarium proliferatum* grow-ing on corn. Ingestion by horses of corn contaminated with *Fusarium* mold causes "moldy corn poisoning" or equine leukoencephaloma-lacia. The signs in affected horses are lethargy, ataxia, convulsions, and death (Norred, 1993). There are several target organs but the liver is a primary target in every species; in horses, it is liver and brain; in pigs, liver and lung; in rats, liver and kidney; in chickens, liver (Riley *et al.*, 1994). In humans, an association with esophageal cancer has been suggested (Yoshizawa *et al.*, 1994). Fumonisins are diesters of propane-1,2,3-tricarboxylic acid and a pentahydrox-yicosane containing a primary amino acid (Gurung *et al.*, 1999). The structure of fumonisins is similar to that of sphingosine, and their toxicity has been related to block of enzymes in sphingolipid biosynthesis (Norred, 1993).

Kidney and Bladder

Carcinogens   Bracken fern (*P. aquilinum*) grows worldwide and, in the United States, primarily east of the Rocky Mountains. It has been called one of the five most common plants on the planet and is found locally in heavy concentrations. Bracken fern is the only higher plant known to cause cancer in animals under natural condi-tions of feeding. The commonest bladder tumors in cattle are epithe-lial and mesenchymal neoplasms (Kim and Lee, 1998). The major carcinogen is ptaquiloside, a norsesquiterpene glucoside present in high concentrations in the fern, especially in crosiers and young unfolding fronds. Ptaquiloside alkylates adenines, and guanines of DNA (Shakin *et al.*, 1999). In the condition called "bovine enzootic hematuria," caused by consumption of bracken fern, the number of chromosomal aberrations is significantly increased (Lioi *et al.*, 2004). There is evidence that consumption of young bracken fern shoots by humans is associated with cancers of the upper alimentary tract (Alonso-Amelot and Avendano, 2002).

Kidney Tubular Degeneration   Species of *Xanthium* (cocklebur, Asteraceae) are annual plants found in several countries. Toxicosis

in livestock is most common in spring and early summer due to ingestion of seedlings and young plants of cocklebur. Pigs, sheep, cattle, horses, and fowl can be affected in pastures where two- and four-leaf seedlings are present. The signs are depression and dysp-nea. Pathological findings include tubular degeneration and necro-sis in the kidney and centrolobular necrosis in the liver (del Carmen Mendez *et al.*, 1998). The active ingredient is a glycoside, carboxy-atractyloside, which causes microvascular hemorrhages in multiple organs (Turgut *et al.*, 2005).

Acute renal failure is the cause of death in poisoning from *Cortinarius* species of mushroom. *Cortinarius* is a large genus of woodland fungi found especially in northern conifer forests. Species vary widely in habit and in edibility. In one series of poisonings from *Cortinarius orellanus* and related species, involving 135 cases in which the mushrooms were eaten, deaths secondary to acute renal failure occurred in almost 15% of the cases. Renal biopsy showed acute degenerative tubular lesions with inflammatory interstitial fi-brosis (Bouget *et al.*, 1990).

Blood and Bone Marrow

Anticoagulants   Fungal infections in sweet clover (*Melilotus alba*) silage and hay have caused serious toxicity and death in cattle in Cal-ifornia and in the northern plains of the United States and Canada (Puschner *et al.*, 1998). Deaths are from hemorrhages caused by dicumarol, a fungal metabolite. Dicumarol [3,3-methylene-bis(4-hydroxycoumarin)] is an effective anticoagulant, causing prothrom-bin deficiency, and is used therapeutically for this purpose.

Bone Marrow Genotoxicity   Some species of poppy, such as *Arge-mone* (Papaveraceae) produce sanguinarine, a benzophenanthridine alkaloid, that intercalates DNA. Humans may be exposed to arge-mone oil as an adulterant of mustard oil. A single low dose has been shown to increase chromosomal aberrations in bone marrow cells in mice (Ansari *et al.*, 2004). The term "epidemic dropsy" has been applied to the disease in humans and a link to gall bladder carcinoma has been suggested (Das *et al.*, 2005).

Cyanogens   Cyanogens are constituents of several different kinds of plants. One that is present in the kernels of apples, cherries, peaches, and related genera in the rose family is amygdalin, found in the highest amounts in the seeds of the bitter almond, *Prunus amygdalus*, var. *amara*. Amygdalin is not present in the seeds of the sweet al mond, the nut used for food. The amount of cyanogen in peach (*Prunus persica*) kernels is enough to cause poisoning in small children if several kernels are eaten. The seeds of apples are unlikely to present a problem. In the stomach, amygdalin releases hydrocyanic acid that combines with ferric ion in cytochrome oxi-dase or methemoglobin. The result of ingestion of several bitter al-mond seeds is classic cyanide poisoning with death from asphyxia. Amygdalin is a component of some herbal remedies for cancer in some countries and unintentional cyanide poisoning has resulted (O'Brien *et al.*, 2005). There may be an interaction with concurrent intake of large doses of vitamin C (Bromley *et al.*, 2005).

Cassava is a staple food starch from *Manihot esculenta* (Eu-phorbiaceae) grown extensively in some parts of Africa as a major food source. The untreated root contains linamarin, a cyanogenic glucoside. During processing of the root for human consumption, the cyanogen is removed. However, local processing may be inade-quate. Chronic ingestion of linamarin in cassava has been proposed as the cause of epidemics of konzo, a form of tropical myelopathy with sudden onset of spastic paralysis (Tylleskar *et al.*, 1992). Degeneration of the corticospinal motor pathway in affected individuals may be caused by production of thiocyanate from linamarin with stimulation of neuronal glutamate receptors by thiocyanate (Spencer, 1999). One important improvement in cassava as a food source is that it has been possible to produce transgenic cassava plants with marked reduction in linamarin content in the tubers (Jorgensen *et al.*, 2005). Another plant containing linamarin is flax, *Linum ustitatissumum*, the seed of which is the source of linseed oil. In some European countries, as a domestic remedy, the flax seeds are soaked overnight and the extract is used as a laxative, possibly exposing these individuals to cyanide from the linamarin (Rosling, 1993).

Nervous System

Historically, some of the most useful drugs have been plant-derived chemicals that act on the nervous system. However, some unintended serious neurotoxic syndromes may result from ingestion of certain plants.

Epileptiform Seizures The parsley family of plants (Apiaceae) contains some of the most edible (e.g., carrots) and some of the most poisonous plants in the northern hemisphere. The fleshy tubers of *Cicuta maculata* (water hemlock) may be mistaken for other edible wild tubers. A single tuber may cause fatal poisoning, characterized by tonic–clonic convulsions. The toxic principle, cicutoxin (a C17-polyacetylene), binds to GABA-gated chloride channels and this may play a role in the acute neurotoxicity (Uwai *et al.*, 2000).

Several members of the mint family (Labiatae) are noted for their essential oils, such as pennyroyal (*Hedeoma*), sage (*Salvia*), and hyssop (*Hyssopus*). These oils contain odorous monoterpenes. For example, sage contains thujone, camphor, and cineole. In high oral doses, well above amounts used for flavoring, these monoterpenes can cause tonic–clonic convulsions. Menthol is a selective modulator of inhibitory ligand-gated channels (Hall *et al.*, 2004).

Several species of *Strychnos* (Loganiaceae) contain strychnine and brucine (dimethoxystrychnine). Both indoles cause marked CNS stimulation by blocking glycine-gated chloride channels. *Strychnos nux vomixa* is a small tree native to India. Cases of unintentional poisoning from seeds of *Strychnos nux vomica* have been reported (Wang *et al.*, 2004). Seeds of *Strychnos ignatii* in the Phillipine islands have caused similar toxic effects.

Excitatory Amino Acids Widely divergent species of plants produce amino acids that mimic the action of glutamate on the central nervous system. Most fast excitatory transmission in the mammalian brain is mediated by inotropic receptors for the amino acid, glutamate, on specialized neurons. Different types of glutamate receptors respond to different excitatory amino acids from plants, acting on one or more of these glutamate receptor subtypes. The consequence of ingestion of excitatory amino acids is excessive stimulation that may result in death of neurons. One of these acids, kainic acid, is present in the marine red alga *Digenia simplex*. Under some climatic conditions the algae reproduce rapidly, causing a "red tide." Filter-feeding mussels eat the algae and humans may be poisoned by eating the mussels. A similar problem exists with the green alga *Chondria aranta* in northern oceans. The alga produces domoic acid, an analog of glutamate, as do several species of the marine diatom

Nitzschia (Kotaki *et al.*, 2005). Acute symptoms are gastrointestinal distress, headache, hemiparesis, confusion, and seizures. Prolonged effects are severe memory deficits and sensorimotor neuropathy (Teitelbaum *et al.*, 1990).

The fungus *Amanita muscaria* (fly agaric) got its name from its poisonous actions on flies. Poisoning from this woodland mushroom and from *Amanita pantherian* (panther agaric, common in western United States) is due to the content of the excitatory amino acid, ibotenic acid (isoxazole amino acid), and to its derivative, muscimol (Li and Oberlies, 2005). The effects are somewhat variable: central nervous system depression, ataxia, hysteria, and hallucinations. Myoclonic twitching and seizures sometimes develop (Benjamin, 1992). The content of ibotenic acid varies with the time of year; more has been reported in spring than in fall. Several other genera of fungi have hallucinogenic actions, notably *Psilocybe*, containing the indoles, psilocin, and psilocybin (Tsujikawa *et al.*, 2003).

Excitatory amino acids are also found in flowering plants. The pea family (Leguminosae) contains several species that produce excitatory amino acids in the seeds. Willardiine [1-(2-amino-2-carboxyethyl)pyrimidine-2,4-dione] has been isolated from *Acacia willardiana*, *Acacia lemmoni*, *Acacia millefolia*, and *Mimosa asperata* (Gmelin, 1961). Willardiine acts as an agonist on glutamate receptors. Other important excitatory amino acids are present in species of *Lathyrus*. *Lathyrus sylvestris* (flat pea) is a perennial indigenous to Europe and central Asia and naturalized in Canada and northern United States. This plant is eaten by livestock in these areas. An acute neurologic condition in sheep begins with weakness and progresses to tremors and prostration, sometimes with clonic movements and seizures (Rasmussen *et al.*, 1993). Seeds of *Lathyrus sativus* (grass pea) are used as food in several countries, including India and Ethiopia. The seeds contain the excitatory amino acid, beta-L-ODAP (beta-*N*-oxalyl-L-alpha, beta-diaminopropionic acid) (Warren *et al.*, 2004). Lathyrism develops from consumption of seeds over periods of months or longer. Affected individuals have corticospinal motor neuron degeneration with severe spastic muscle weakness and atrophy but little sensory involvement (Spencer *et al.*, 1986).

Motor Neuron Demyelination Paralysis develops from some toxins without primary excitation of neurons. *Karwinskia humboldtiana*, family Rhamnaceae, is a shrub of southwestern United States, Mexico, and Central America. Common names are buckthorn, coyotillo, and tullidora. Anthracenones are found in the seeds, the amount varying with stage of growth; green fruit may be more toxic than ripe fruit (Bermudez *et al.*, 1986). Both human and livestock poisonings occur, occasionally in epidemic proportions. The clinical syndrome that develops after a latency of several days is ascending flaccid paralysis, beginning with demyelination of large motor neurons in the legs and, in fatal cases, leading to bulbar paralysis (Martinez *et al.*, 1998). Sensory fibers are largely spared. In addition to neurotoxicity, the anthracenones in *Karwinskia*, especially peroxisomicine A$_2$, [3,39-dimethyl-3,39,8,89,9,99-hexahydroxy-3,30,4,49-tetrahydro-(7,10-bianthracene)-1,19-2*H*,29*H*-dione], causes lung atelectasis and emphysema and massive liver necrosis. Inhibition of catalase in peroxisomes has been proposed as the mechanism of cell toxicity (Martinez *et al.*, 1997).

Cerebellar Neurons Swainsonine is an indolizidine alkaloid found in the legumes *Swainsonia cansescens* (an Australian plant),

Astragalus lentiginosus (spotted locoweed) and *Oxytropis sericea* (locoweed) in western United States. Cattle consume these weeds in pasture. The common name comes from the most obvious consequence of ingestion of locoweeds: aberrant behavior with hyperexcitability and locomotor difficulty. In animals dying from locoweed poisoning, there is cytoplasmic foamy vacuolation of cerebellar neurons. The toxic ingredient, swainsonine, causes marked inhibition of liver lysosomal and cytosomal alpha-mannosidase and Golgi mannosidase II. Inhibition of the Golgi enzyme results in abnormal brain glycoproteins and accumulation of mannose-rich oligosaccharides (Tulsiani *et al.*, 1988). The pathology is not limited to the nervous system and the effects of swainsonine poisoning are found in several tissues. A major effect in animals grazing at high altitudes is congestive heart failure. The condition has been called "high mountain disease" (James *et al.*, 1991). A species of the fungus *Embellisia*, an endophyte on locoweeds, may also produce swainsonine (McLain-Romero *et al.*, 2004).

Parasympathetic Stimulation   Several plant alkaloids affect the autonomic nervous system, mimicking the transmitter acetylcholine at autonomic ganglia (nicotinic receptors) or the peripheral endings of the parasympathetic system (muscarinic receptors). The postsynaptic receptors at terminations of the parasympathetic nerve fibers are called "muscarinic" after the selective stimulation of these receptors by muscarine, a quaternary ammonium furan, that was first extracted from the mushroom *A. muscaria*. However, this mushroom contains only trace amounts of muscarine, and poisoning is due to its content of ibotenic acid. Some mushrooms of the genera *Inocybe, Clitocybe*, and *Omphalatus* contain significant amounts of muscarine, and consumption of toxic species causes diarrhea, sweating, salivation, and lacrimation, all referable to stimulation of parasympathetic receptors (de Haro *et al.*, 1999).

Parasympathetic Block   The belladonna alkaloids (atropine, L-hyoscyamine, and scopolamine), known for their block of muscarinic receptors, are found in several genera of Solanaceae, the nightshade family. The plants are widely distributed. *Datura stramonium* (jimson weed) is native to India and contains primarily scopolamine; *Hyoscyamus niger* (henbane) is native to Europe and contains primarily L-hyoscyamine; *Atropa belladonna* (deadly nightshade), also native to Europe, contains atropine; *Duboisia myoporoides* (pituri) in Australia contains L-hyoscyamine. Scopolamine has the greater action on the central nervous system. The effects of modest doses of L-hyoscyamine or atropine are referable to muscarinic receptor block: tachycardia, dry mouth, dilated pupils, and decreased gastrointestinal motility. Large doses of either or of scopolamine affect the central nervous system with confusion, bizarre behavior, hallucinations, and subsequent amnesia. In severe intoxication, tachycardia may be absent (Caksen *et al.*, 2003). Deaths are rare, although recovery may take several days.

Datura suaveolens (angel's trumpet, Solanaceae) an ornamental houseplant, contains significant quantities of atropine and scopolamine (Smith *et al.*, 1991). Seeds of *Datura ferox* contain belladonna alkaloids and are contaminants of animal feed in some parts of Europe. In areas where millet, wheat, rye, corn, and bean seeds are used for human consumption, and where *D stramonium* and *Datura metel* are common weeds, the grain sometimes has been contaminated with *Datura* seeds. Symptoms from eating bread made from contaminated flour are typical of poisoning from belladonna alkaloids (van Meurs *et al.*, 1992). The amount needed to poison an

adult is about 20 seeds. An unusual source of belladonna poisoning has been reported from eating wasp honey. *Polistes* species of wasps store honey, and atropine-like poisoning has been reported from consuming the honey when the wasps have gathered nectar from *Datura inoxia* (Ramirez *et al.*, 1999).

The seeds of *Solanum dulcamara* (bittersweet) are brilliant red-orange and are gathered in the fall for flower arrangements. The seeds contain solanine, a glycoalkaloid, responsible for the acute toxicity from ingested seeds, including tachycardia, dilated pupils, and hot, dry skin, as in atropine poisoning (Ceha *et al.*, 1997).

Sensory Neuron Block   Several plant toxins are being studied for agonist actions on sensory receptors of the vanilloid-type (VR1), especially capsaicin found in species of *Capsicum* (*C. annuum*, sweet pepper, and *C. frutescens*, red pepper, Solanaceae). Capsaicin produces a burning sensation on VR1 sensory endings, but also desensitizes the transient potential vanilloid 1 receptor (TRPV1) of sensory endings of C-fiber nociceptors to stimuli. This long-term sensory neuron blocking effect has therapeutic use in chronic pain (Szalcsany, 2002). The sensory desensitization produced by capsaicin is not due to acute cell death and long-lasting changes in mitochondria in cultured dorsal root ganglion cells have been demonstrated (Dedov *et al.*, 2001). It has recently been suggested that capsaicin may also have an action on another ion channel, the 4-aminopyridine-sensitive K^+ channel, and may inhibit contractile mechanisms by release of Ca^{2+} from intracellular storage sites (Fujimoto *et al.*, 2006).

Another plant toxin, polygodial, a sesquiterpene found in *Polygonum hydropiper*, has a capsaicin-like action on the TRPV1 (Andre *et al.*, 2006). Resiniferatoxin, a homovanillic ester from *Euphorbia resinifera* (Euphorbiaceae), is a potent agonist of TRPV1 and causes sustained depolarization of the vanilloid receptor. The long-lasting effect of resiniferatoxin on nerve terminals is related to slow activation of TRPV1 with excessive influx of Ca^{2+} without generating action potentials (Raisinghani *et al.*, 2005).

Skeletal Muscle and Neuromuscular Junction

Neuromuscular Junction   Block of the neuromuscular junction of skeletal muscle may result from either block of postsynaptic acetylcholine receptors (nicotinic receptors) by an antagonist or by an agonist causing excessive stimulation of the receptor followed by prolonged depolarization. Nicotine stimulates autonomic ganglia as well as the neuromuscular junction. An isomer of nicotine, anabasine, present in *Nicotiana glauca* (tree tobacco, Solanaceae), produces prolonged depolarization of the junction. Consumption of the leaves of the plant has caused flexor muscle spasm and gastrointestinal irritation, followed by severe, generalized weakness, and respiratory compromise (Mellick *et al.*, 1999). Curare, the South American arrow poison is a potent neuromuscular blocking agent used clinically. Curare is obtained from tropical species of *Strychnos* and *Chondrodendron*. Not all plants blocking the neuromuscular junction are tropical in origin. In warm weather, blooms of blue-green algae are not uncommon in farm ponds in temperate regions, particularly ponds enriched with fertilizer. Under these conditions, one species of alga, *Anabaena flosaquae*, produces a neurotoxin, anatoxin A, that depolarizes and blocks acetylcholine receptors, both nicotinic and muscarinic, sometimes causing death in animals that drink the pond water. The lethal effects develop rapidly, with death in minutes to hours from respiratory arrest (Short and

Edwards, 1990). Anatoxin A is 2-acetyl-9-azabicyclo(4.2.10)non-2-ene (Hyde and Carmichael, 1991).

Methyllycaconitine is a norditerpenoid present in *Delphinium barbeyi* (tall larkspur, Ranunculaceae) and in some related species. The plant contaminates western pastures in the United States and causes death of livestock. Poisoned cattle show muscle tremors and ataxia followed by prostration and respiratory arrest in fatal cases. The compound has a high affinity for the acetylcholine receptor at the neuromuscular junction like curare. Physostigmine has been used successfully as an antagonist in some cases of methyllycaconitine poisoning (Pfister *et al.*, 1994).

Skeletal Muscle Direct damage to skeletal muscle fibers has been demonstrated in some plant poisonings. Species of *Thermopsis* (Leguminosae) are common in the foothills of the Rocky Mountains. Mature seeds of these plants form in attractive pods, as in many legumes. Seeds of the poisonous species of *Thermopsis* contain quinolizidine alkaloids, principally anagyrine and thermopsine. Human poisoning from eating the seeds is rare, but cases have been reported in young children (Spoerke *et al.*, 1988). The symptoms are abdominal cramps, nausea, vomiting, and headache lasting up to 24 hours. Serious poisoning has occurred in livestock grazing on *Thermopsis montana* (false lupine). The animals develop locomotor depression and recumbancy. Microscopic areas of necrosis in skeletal muscle are found on autopsy (Keeler and Baker, 1990).

Seeds of *Cassia obtusifolia* (sicklepod, Leguminosae) have been found as a contaminant of animal feeds. Consumption of the seeds in cattle, swine, and chickens causes a degenerative myopathy in cardiac and skeletal muscle. Extracts of *C. obtusifolia* inhibit NADH-oxidoreductase in bovine and porcine mitochondria in vitro (Lewis and Shibamoto, 1989) possibly related to the anthraquinone content of the seeds.

Ingestion of white snakeroot (*Eupatorium rugosum*, Asteraceae), a common plant in central and western United States, causes tremors in cattle and "milk sickness" in humans after ingestion of milk from cows pasturing in fields infected with the plant (Beier *et al.*, 1993). The toxic effect thought to be caused by tremetone, a benzofuran, that blocks gluconeogenesis from lactate, resulting in acidosis, tremor, and death (Polya, 2003).

Bone and Tissue Calcification

Bone and Soft Tissue Worker and Carrillo (1967) proposed that a decrease in bone calcification and a wasting disease in cattle grazing along the eastern coastal plains of South America was due to the consumption of *Solanum malacoxylon* (Solanaceae). The disease, known in Argentina as "enteque seco" is characterized by calcification of the entire vascular system, especially the heart and aorta. Lungs, joint cartilage, and kidney are affected in the worst cases. Sheep and cows are both affected by ingestion of the plant. The general picture resembles vitamin D intoxication. A water-soluble vitamin D-like substance, a glycoside of 1,25-dihydroxycholecalciferol, has been isolated from the plant (Skliar *et al.*, 1992).

Cestrum diurnum (day-blooming jasmine, Solanaceae) causes hypercalcemia and extensive soft tissue calcification in grazing animals in Florida, resembling the action of *S. malacoxylon*. A dihydroxyvitamin D_3 glycoside in the leaves is the toxic agent (Durand *et al.*, 1999). *Cestrum laevigatum* causes a similar deposition of calcium in chickens (Mello and Habermehl, 1992). This species is occasionally a contaminant of hay in Europe. However, in cattle, marked hepatotoxicity occurs with centrolobular and midzonal necrosis (Peixato *et al.*, 2000).

Reproduction and Teratogenesis

Abortifacients The active alkaloid in the legumes *Astragalus* and *Oxytropus* is swainsonine. In addition to actions on the nervous system, swainsonine frequently causes abortions when locoweeds are ingested by pregnant livestock (Bunch *et al.*, 1992).

Two genera of tropical legumes, *Leucaena* and *Mimosa*, contain a toxic amino acid, mimosine [beta-*N* (3-hydroxy-4-pyridone)a-alpha-aminopropionic acid]. Mimosine is found in large amounts in foliage and seeds of *Leucaena leucocephala*, *Leucaena glauca*, and *Mimosa pudica*. In cattle the amino acid causes incoordinated gait, goiter, and reproductive disturbances including infertility and fetal death (Kulp *et al.*, 1996). Mimosine arrests the cell cycle in late G1-phase (Perry *et al.*, 2005).

Lectins that are ribosome-inactivating proteins may have many effects on reproduction when ingested, including antifertility, abortifacient, and embryotoxic actions. A lectin from bitter melon seeds (*Momordia charantia*, Curcurbitaceae) has been shown to have such effects. The lectins are alpha- and beta-momorcharins, single-chain glycoproteins with molecular weight of about 29,000. The momorcharins are known to induce midterm abortion in humans (Wang and Ng, 1998).

Caulophylline (*N*-methylcytisine) is a quinolizidine from *Caulophyllum thalictroides* (blue cohosh, Berberidaceae). The plant is widely distributed in temperate North America and eastern Asia. Caulophylline is teratogenic in rats (Kennelly *et al.*, 1999). Neonatal and maternal toxicity has been reported from maternal ingestion of herbal preparations of blue cohosh to terminate pregnancy (Jones and Lawson, 1998). The maternal signs resemble the action of an agonist to nicotinic acetylcholine receptors (Rao and Hoffman, 2002).

Many pastures of tall fescue (*Festuca arundinacea*, Poaceae) are infected by the endophytic fungus *Neotyphodium coenophialum*. The presence of the endophyte is related to production in the fescue plant of ergovaline, an ergopeptine alkaloid that acts as an agonist to dopamine D2 receptors. Ergovaline inhibits prolactin release and acts as a vasoconstrictor. Pregnant mares are most susceptible toward the end of gestation, resulting in damage to the fetus and maternal loss of milk (Blodgett, 2001). Regulation of levels of different alkaloids in grasses as a result of *Neotyphodium* infestation is closely related to plant genotype as well as the presence of the endophyte (Spiering *et al.*, 2005).

Teratogens *Veratrum californicum* (Liliaceae) is native to the mountains of North America where sheep are grazed. An incidence of teratogenesis as high as 25% has been reported in pregnant sheep in these areas, along with early embryonic death as high as 75% (Keeler, 1990). The teratogenic manifestations are dependent on the developmental stage at the time of exposure, as with many teratogens. Malformations of the offspring involve cyclopia, exencephaly, and microphthalmia. During the 4th and 5th weeks of gestation, limb defects are common; on gestational days 31–33, the result of ingestion is fetal stenosis of the trachea (Omnell *et al.*, 1990). The alkaloids in *Veratrum* that are responsible for the defects are jervine, 11-deoxyjervine and 3-*O*-glucosyl-11-deoxyjervine. Although there is species difference in sensitivity, birth defects occur in cows and goats grazing on *V. californicum*. Birth defects have been produced experimentally in chickens, rabbits, rats, and mice (Omnell *et al.*, 1990), hamsters (Gaffield and Keeler, 1993), and rainbow trout embryos

(Crawford and Kocan, 1993). The *Veratrum* alkaloids cause teratogenesis by blocking cholesterol synthesis and thus the response of fetal target tissue to the sonic hedgehog gene (Shh). The Shh locus has a role in developmental patterning of head and brain, and block of cholesterol synthesis has been shown experimentally to result in loss of midline facial structures (Cooper *et al.*, 1998).

A cluster of fetal malformations characterized by deformation of limbs and spinal cord is found after maternal ingestion of related alkaloids from different species of plants during a sensitive gestational period. The syndrome has been found in cattle grazing on *Lupinus caudatus* and *Lupinus formosus* (lupines, Luguminosae), *Nicotiana glauca* (tree tobacco, Solanaceae), and *Conium maculatum* (poison hemlock, Solanaceae). Poison hemlock is known historically as the plant that Socrates drank when condemned to death in Athens. The fatal actions of the poison have been described by Plato in his *Phaedo*. The active alkaloids in these plants are anagyrine (*L. caudatus*), ammodendrine (*L. formosus*), anabasine (*N. glauca*), and coniine (*C. maculatum*). It has been proposed that these alkaloids depress fetal movements during susceptible gestational periods and in this way cause malformations (Lopez *et al.*, 1999). Not all species are equally affected by coniine. Notably, rats and hamsters do not show teratogenesis in response to coniine, but goat and chick embryos are susceptible (Forsyth *et al.*, 1996).

SUMMARY

A great variety of toxic chemicals have been produced by plants for their own protection from the environment and from predators, including pathogenic organisms. These defensive chemicals have been both deleterious and beneficial to humans. Throughout history a select number have been incorporated into therapy against disease and to combat morbidity, often with considerable success. Morphine from the latex of the opium poppy is an ancient historical example. If fungi are included with plants (as they are in this chapter), defensive chemicals of plants are responsible for some of our more successful therapies, such as antibiotics of the penicillin type and therapy for cancer. On balance, in spite of the long list of dangerous toxic chemicals from plants, it is fair to conclude that plants have proved therapeutically more useful than harmful to humans. Finally, there is simply the pleasure of scientific inquiry into the successful adaptations of plants to their complex and often hostile environments.

REFERENCES

Aalto-Korte K, Lauerma A, Alanko K: Occupational allergic contact dermatitis from lichens in present-day Finland. *Contact Dermatitis* 52:36–38, 2005.

Abbott AJ, Holoubek CG, Martin RA: Inhibition of Na$^+$, K$^+$-ATPase by the cardenolide 6′ − *O*-(E-4-hydroxycinnamoyl) desglucouzarin. *Biochim Biophys Res Comm* 251:256–259, 1998.

Al-Anati L, Petzinger E: Immunotoxic activity of ochratoxin A. *J Vet Pharmacol Ther* 29:79–90, 2006.

Alonso-Amelot ME, Avendano M: Human carcinogenesis and bracken fern: A review of the evidence. *Curr Med Chem* 9:675–686, 2002.

Altamirano JC, Gratz SR, Wolnik KA: Investigation of pyrrolizidine alkaloids and their N-oxides in commercial comfrey-containing products and botanical materials by liquid chromatography electrospray ionization mass spectrometry. *JAOAC Int* 88:406–412, 2005.

Alvarez-Diez TM, Zheng J: Mechanism-based inactivation of cytochrome P450 3A4 by 4-ipomeanol. *Chem Res Toxicol* 17:150–157, 2004.

Andre E, Campi B, Trevisani M, *et al.*: Pharmacological characterisation of the plant sesquiterpenes polygodial and drimanial as vanilloid receptor agonists. *Biochem Pharmacology* 71:1248–1254, 2006.

Ansari KM, Chauhan LK, Dhawan A, *et al.*: Unequivocal evidence of genotoxic potential of argemone oil in mice. *Int J Cancer* 112:890–895, 2004.

Arilla MC, Gonzalez-Rioja R, Ibarrola I, *et al.*: A sensitive monoclonal antibody-based enzyme-linked immunosorbent assay to quantify *Parietaria judaica* major allergens, Par j1 and Par j2. *Clin Exp Allergy* 36:87–93, 2006.

Aslani MR, Movassaghi AR, Mhori M, *et al.*: Clinical and pathological aspects of experimental oleander (*Nerium oleander*) toxicosis in sheep. *Vet Res Commun* 28:609–616, 2004.

Baer BR, Rettie AE, Henne KR: Bioactivation of 4-ipomeanol by CYP4B1: Adduct characterization and evidence for an enedial intermediate. *Chem Res Toxicol* 18:855–864, 2005.

Ball KR, Kowdley KV: A review of *Silybum marianum* (milk thistle) as a treatment for alcoholic liver disease. *J Clin Gastroenterol* 39:520–528, 2005.

Bantel H, Engels IH, Voelter W, *et al.*: Mistletoe lectin activates caspase-8/FLICE independently of death receptor signaling and enhances anticancer drug-induced apoptosis. *Cancer Res* 59:2038–2090, 1999.

Bauer C, Oppel T, Rueff F, *et al.*: Anaphylaxis to viscotoxins of mistletoe (*Viscum album*) extracts. *Ann Allergy Asthma Immunol* 94:86–89, 2005.

Beattie PE, Dawe RS, Traynor NJ, *et al.*: Can St. John's wort (hypericin) ingestion enhance the erythremal response during high-dose ultraviolet A1 therapy? *Br J Dermatol* 153:1187–1191, 2005.

Beier RC, Norman JO, Reagor JC, *et al.*: Isolation of the major component in white snakeroot that is toxic after microsomal activation: Possible explanation of sporadic toxicity of white snakeroot plants and extracts. *Nat Toxins* 1:286–293, 1993.

Benjamin DR: Mushroom poisoning in infants and children. *J Toxicol Clin Toxicol* 30:13–22, 1992.

Bermudez MV, Gonzalez-Spencer D, Guerrero M, *et al.*: Experimental intoxication with fruit and purified toxins of buckthorn (*Karwinskia humboldtiana*). *Toxicon* 24:1091–1097, 1986.

Blanc P, Liu D, Juarez C, *et al.*: Cough in hot pepper workers. *Chest* 99:27–32, 1991.

Blanco C, Diaz-Perales A, Collada C, *et al.*: Class I chitinases as potential panallergens involved in the latex-fruit syndrome. *J Allergy Clin Immunol* 103(pt 1):507–513, 1999.

Blodgett DJ: Fescue toxicosis. *Vet Clin North Am Equine Pract* 17:567–577, 2001.

Blumenthal MN, Langefeld CD, Barnes KC, *et al.*: A genome-wide search for quantitative trait loci contributing to variations in seasonal pollen reactivity. *J Allergy Clin Immunol* 117:79–85, 2006.

Bondan C, Soares JC, Cecim M, *et al.*: Oxidative stress in the erythrocytes of cattle intoxicated with Senecio sp. *Vet Clin Pathol* 34:353–357, 2005.

Bouget J, Bousser J, Pats B, *et al.*: Acute renal failure following collective intoxication by *Cortinarius orellanus*. *Intens Care Med* 16:506–510, 1990.

Bromley J, Hughes BG, Leong DC, *et al.*: Life-threatening interaction between complementary medicines: Cyanide toxicity following ingestion of amygdalin and vitamin C. *Ann Pharmacother* 39:1566–1569, 2005.

Bunch TD, Panter KD, James LK: Ultrasound studies of the effects of certain poisonous plants on uterine function and fetal development in livestock. *J Anim Sci* 70:1639–1643, 1992.

Burke JW, Doskotch RW: High field I H- and 13 C-NMR assignments of grayanotoxins I, IV and XIV isolated from *Kalmia angustifolia*. *J Nat Prod* 53:131–137, 1990.

Caksen H, Odabas D, Akabayram S, *et al.*: Deadly nightshade (*Atropa belladonna*) intoxication: An analysis of 49 children. *Hum Exp Toxicol* 22:665–668, 2003.

Cappell MS, Hassan T: Gastrointestinal and hepatic effects of *Amanita phalloides* ingestion. *J Clin Gastroenterol* 15:225–228, 1992.

Casteel SW, Johnson GC, Wagstaff DJ: *Aesculus glabra* intoxication in cattle. *Vet Hum Toxicol* 34:55, 1992.

Casteel SW, Wagstaff DJ: *Rhododendron macrophyllum* poisoning in a group of sheep and goats. *Vet Hum Toxicol* 31:176–177, 1989.

Ceha LJ, Presperin C, Young E, *et al.*: Anticholinergic toxicity from nightshade berry poisoning responsive to physostigmine. *J Emerg Med* 15:65–69, 1997.

Chan TYF, Tomlinson B, Crichley JAJH, *et al.*: Herb-induced aconitine poisoning presenting as tetraplegia. *Vet Hum Toxicol* 36:133–134, 1994.

Christensen LP, Kristiansen K: Isolation and quantification of tuliposides and tulipalins in tulips (*Tulipa*) by high-performance liquid chromatography. *Contact Dermatitis* 40:300–309, 1999.

Cooper MK, Porter JA, Young RE, *et al.*: Teratogen-mediated inhibition of target tissue response to Shh signalling. *Science* 280:1603–1610, 1998.

Coyle CM, Panaccione DG: An ergot alkaloid biosynthesis gene and clustered hypothetical genes from *Aspergillus fumigatus*. *Appl Environ Microbiol* 71:3112–3118, 2005.

Crawford L, Kocan RM: Steroidal alkaloid toxicity to fish embryos. *Toxicol Lett* 66:175–181, 1993.

Das M, Ansari KM, Dhawan A, *et al.*: Correlation of DNA damage in epidemic dropsy patients to carcinogenic potential of argemone oil and isolated sanguinarine alkaloid in mice. *Int J Cancer* 117:709–717, 2005.

Dedov VN, Mondadi S, Armati PJ, *et al.*: Capsaicin-induced depolarisation of mitochondria in dorsal root ganglion neurons is enhanced by vanilloid receptors. *Neuroscience* 103:219–226, 2001.

de Haro L, Prost, N, David JM, *et al.*: Syndrome sudorien ou muscarinien. *Presse Med* 28:1069–1070, 1999.

del Carmen Mendez M, dos Santos RS, Riet-Correa F: Intoxication by *Xanthium cavanillesii* in cattle and sheep in southern Brazil. *Vet Hum Toxicol* 40:144–147, 1998.

Ding X, Lichti K, Staudinger JL: The mycoestrogen zearalenone induces CYP3A through activation of the pregnane X receptor. *Toxicol Sci* 91:448–455, 2006.

Durand R. Figueredo JM, Mendoza E: Intoxication in cattle from *Cestrum diurnum*. *Vet Hum Toxicol* 41:26–27, 1999.

Forsyth CS, Speth RC, Wecker L, *et al.*: Comparison of nicotinic receptor binding and biotransformation of coniine in the rat and chick. *Toxicol Lett* 89:175–183, 1996.

Frasca T, Brett AS, Yoo SD: Mandrake toxicity. *Arch Intern Med* 157:2007–2009, 1997.

Frohn A, Frohn C, Steuhl KP, *et al.*: Wolfsmilchveratzung. *Ophthalmology* 90:58–61, 1993.

Fujimoto S, Mori M, Tsushima H, *et al.*: Capsaicin-induced, capsazepine-insensitive relaxation of the guinea-pig ileum. *Eur J Pharmacol* 530:144–151, 2006.

Gaffield W, Keeler RF: Implications of C-5, C-6 unsaturation as a key structural factor in steroidal alkaloid-induced mammalian teratogenesis. *Experientia* 49:922–924, 1993.

Giavina-Bianchi, PF, Jr., Castro FF, Machado ML, *et al.*: Occupational respiratory allergic disease induced by *Passiflora alata* and *Rhamnus purshiana*. *Ann Allergy Asthma Immunol* 79:449–454, 1997.

Gmelin R: Isolierung von Willardiin [3-(1-uracyl)-L-alanin] aus den samen von *Acacia millefolia*, *Acacia lemmoni* und *Mimosa asperata*. *Acta Chem Scand* 15:1188–1189, 1961.

Groenewoud GC, de Groot H, van Wijk RG: Impact of occupational and inhalant allergy on rhinitis-specific quality of life in employees of bell pepper greenhouses in the Netherlands. *Ann Allergy Asthma Immunol* 96:92–97, 2006.

Gude M, Hausen MD, Heitsch H, *et al.*: An investigation of the irritant and allergenic properties of daffodils (*Narcissus pseudonarcissus* L., Amaryllidaceae): A review of daffodil dermatitis. *Contact Dermatitis* 19:1–10, 1988.

Gurung NK, Rankens DL, Shelby RA: In vitro ruminal disappearance of fumonisin B_1 and its effects on in vitro dry matter disappearance. *Vet Hum Toxicol* 41:196–199, 1999.

Haarmann T, Machado C, Lubbe Y, *et al.*: The ergot alkaloid gene cluster in *Claviceps purpurea*: Extension of the cluster sequence and intra species evolution. *Phytochemistry* 66:1312–1320, 2005.

Hall AC, Turcotte CM, Betts BA, *et al.*: Modulation of human GABAA and glycine receptor currents by menthol and related monoterpenoids. *Eur J Pharmacol* 506:9–16, 2004.

Han D, Matsumaru K, Rettori D, *et al.*: Usnic acid-induced necrosis of cultured mouse hepatocytes: Inhibition of mitochondrial function and oxidative stress. *Biochem Pharmacol* 67:439–451, 2004.

Hausen BM, Prater E, Shubert H: The sensitizing capacity of *Alstroemeria* cultivars in man and guinea pig. *Contact Dermatitis* 9:46–54, 1983.

Hill NS, Thompson FN, Dawe DL, *et al.*: Antibody binding by circulating ergot alkaloids in cattle grazing tall fescue. *Am J Vet Res* 55:419–424, 1994.

Hirschwehr R, Heppner C, Spitzauer S, *et al.*: Allergens, IgE mediators, inflammatory mechanisms. *J Allergy Clin Immunol* 101:196–206, 1998.

Huan J-Y, Mironda CL, Buhler DR, *et al.*: Species differences in the hepatic microsomal enzyme metabolism of the pyrrolizidine alkaloids. *Toxicol Lett* 99:127–137, 1998.

Hyde EG, Carmichael WW: Amatoxin-a(s), a naturally occurring organophosphate, is an irreversible active site-directed inhibitor of acetylcholinesterase (E.C.3.1.1.7). *J Biochem Toxicol* 6:195–201, 1991.

Izzo AA, Ernst E: Interactions between herbal medicines and prescribed drugs: A systematic review. *Drugs* 61:2163–2175, 2001.

Jaeger A, Fehl F, Flesch F, *et al.*: Kinetics of amatoxins in human poisoning: Therapeutic implications. *Clin Toxicol* 31:63–80, 1993.

Jaffe AM, Gephardt D, Courtemanche L: Poisoning due to ingestion of *Veratrum viride* (false hellebore). *J Emerg Med* 8:161–167, 1990.

James LF, Panter KE, Broquist HP, *et al.*: Swainsonine-induced high mountain disease in calves. *Vet Hum Toxicol* 33:217–219, 1991.

Johnson RA, Baer H, Kirkpatrick CH, *et al.*: Comparison of the contact allergenicity of the four pentadecylcatechols derived from poison ivy urushiol in human subjects. *J Allergy Clin Dermatol* 49:27–35, 1972.

Jones TK, Lawson BM: Profound neonotal congestive heart failure caused by maternal consumption of blue cohosh herbal medication. *J Pediatr* 132:550–552, 1998.

Jorgensen K, Bak S, Busk PK, *et al.*: Cassava plants with a depleted cyanogenic glucoside content in leaves and tubers. *Plant Physiol* 139:363–374, 2005.

Kalish RS, Johnson KL: Enrichment and function of urushiol (poison ivy)-specific T lymphocytes in lesions of allergic contact dermatitis to urushiol. *J Immunol* 145:3706–3713, 1990.

Karlson-Stiber C, Persson H: Cytotoxic fungi—an overview. *Toxicon* 42:339–349, 2003.

Kavalali G: The chemical and pharmacological aspects of *Urtica*, in Kavalali GM (ed.): *Urtica*. New York: Taylor and Francis, 2003, pp. 25–39.

Keeler RF: Early embryonic death in lambs induced by *Veratrum californicum*. *Cornell Vet* 80:203–207, 1990.

Keeler RF, Baker DC: Myopathy in cattle induced by alkaloid extracts from *Thermopsis montana*, *Laburnum anagyroides* and a *Lupinus* sp. *J Comp Pathol* 103:169–182, 1990.

Kelch WJ, Kerr LA, Adair HS, *et al.*: Suspected buttercup (*Ranunculus bulbosus*) toxicosis with secondary photosensitization in a Charolais heifer. *Vet Hum Toxicol* 34:238–239, 1992.

Kennelly EJ, Flynn TJ, Mazzola EP, *et al.*: Detecting potential teratogenic alkaloids from blue cohosh rhizomes using an in vitro rat embryo culture. *J Nat Prod* 62:1385–1389, 1999.

Kim D-Y, Lee Y-S: Ovine copper poisoning and *Pteridium aquilinum*- associated bovine urinary bladder tumor in Korea. *J Toxicol Soc* 23 (Suppl 4):645–646, 1998.

Knight TE: *Philodendron*-induced dermatitis: Report of cases and review of the literature. *Cutis* 48:375–378, 1991.

Kolarich D, Altmann F, Sunderasan E: Structural analysis of the glycoprotein allergen Hev b 4 from natural rubber latex by mass spectrometry. *Biochem Biophys Acta* 46:946–953, 2005.

Kotaki Y, Furio Ef, Satake M, *et al.*: Production of isodomoic acids A and B as major toxin components of a pennate diatom Nitzschia navis-varingica. *Toxicon* 46:946–953, 2005.

Kulp KS, Valliet PR, Richard P: Mimosine blocks cell cycle progression by chelating iron in asynchronous human breast cancer cells. *Toxicol Appl Pharmacol* 139:356–364, 1996.

Lewis DC, Shibamoto T: Effects of *Cassia obtusifolia* (sicklepod) extracts and anthraquinones on muscle mitochondrial function. *Toxicon* 27:519–529, 1989.

Li C, Oberlies NH: The most widely recognized mushroom: Chemistry of the genus Amanita. *Life Sci* 78:532–538, 2005.

Lin TJ, Hsu CI, Lee KH, *et al.*: Two outbreaks of acute Tung Nut (*Aleurites fordii*) poisoning. *J Toxicol Clin Toxicol* 34:87–92, 1996.

Lioi MB, Barbieri R, Borzacchiello G, *et al.*: Chromosome aberrations in cattle with chronic enzootic haematuria. *J Comp Pathol* 131:233–236, 2004.

Lopez TA, Cid MS, Bianchini ML: Biochemistry of hemlock (*Conium maculatum* L) alkaloids and their acute and chronic toxicity in livestock: A review. *Toxicon* 37:841–865, 1999.

Maejima H, Kinoshita E, Yuki T, *et al.*: Structural determinants for the action of grayanotoxin in D1 S4-S5 and D4 S4-S5 intracellular linkers of sodium channel alpha-subunits. *Biochem Biophys Res Commun* 295:452–457, 2002.

Martinez FJ, Duron RR, deTorres NW *et al.*: Experimental evidence for toxic damage induced by a dimeric anthracenon: Diast T-514 (peroxisome A$_2$). *Toxicol Lett* 90:155–162, 1997.

Martinez HR, Bermudez MV, Rangel-Guerra RA, *et al.*: Clinical diagnosis in *Karwinskia humboldtiana* polyneuropathy. *J Neurol Sci* 154:49–54, 1998.

Massermanian A: Contact dermatitis due to *Euphorbia pulcherrima* Willd, simulating a phototoxic reaction. *Contact Derm* 38:113–114, 1998.

Mayer KE, Myers RP, Lee SS: Silymarin treatment of viral hepatitis. *J Viral Hepat* 12:559–567, 2005a.

Mayer M, O'Neill MA, Murray KE, *et al.*: Usnic acid: A non-genotoxic compound with anti-cancer properties. *Anticancer Drugs* 16:805–809, 2005b.

McDermott WV, Ridker PM: The Budd–Chiari syndrome and hepatic veno-occlusive disease. *Arch Surg* 125:525–527, 1990.

McGovern TW, Barkley TM: Botanical briefs: Chrysanthemum—*Dendranthema* spp. *Cutis* 63:319–320, 1999.

McGrath-Hill CA, Vicas IM: Case series of *Thermopsis* exposures. *J Toxicol Clin Toxicol* 35:659–665, 1997.

McLain-Romero J, Creamer R, Zepeda H, *et al.* : The toxicosis of Embellisia fungi from locoweed (*Oxytropis lambertii*) is similar to locoweed toxicosis in rats. *J Anim Sci* 82:2169–2174, 2004.

Mei N, Guo L, Fu PP, *et al.*: Mutagenicity of comfrey (*Symphytum officinale*) in rat liver. *Br J Cancer* 92:873–875, 2005.

Mellick LB, Makowski T, Mellick GA, *et al.*: Neuromuscular blockade after ingestion of tree tobacco (*Nicotiana glauca*). *Ann Emerg Med* 34:101–104, 1999.

Mello JR, Habermehl GG: Calcinogenic plants and the incubation effect of rumen fluid. *Dtsch Tierarztl Wochenschr* 99:371–376, 1992.

Mendis S: Colchicine cardiotoxicity following ingestion of *Gloriosa superba* tubers. *Postgrad Med J* 65:752–755, 1989.

Michelot D, Toth B: Poisoning by *Gyromitra esculenta*—a review. *J Appl Toxicol* 11:235–243, 1991.

Monzingo AF, Collins EJ, Ernst SR, *et al.*: The 2.5 A structure of pokeweed antiviral protein. *J Mol Biol* 233:705–715, 1993.

Murai M, Kimura I, Kimura M: Blocking effects of hypoaconitine and aconitine on nerve action potentials in phrenic nerve-diaphragm muscles of mice. *Neuropharmacology* 29:567–572, 1990.

Norred WP: Fumonisins—mycotoxins produced by *Fusarium moniliforme*. *J Toxicol Environ Health* 38:309–328, 1993.

O'Brien B, Quigg C, Leong T: Severe cyanide toxicity from "vitamin supplements." *Eur J Emerg Med* 12:257–258, 2005.

Oh SH, Haw CR, Lee MH: Clinical and immunologic features of systemic contact dermatitis from ingestion of *Rhus* (Toxicodendron). *Contact Dermatitis* 48:251–254, 2003.

Ohba H, Moriwaki S, Bakalova R, *et al.*: Plant-derived abrin-a induces apoptosis in cultured leukemic cell lines by different mechanisms. *Toxicol Appl Pharmacol* 195:182–193, 2004.

Omnell ML, Sun FRP, Keeler RF, *et al.*: Expression of *Veratrum* alkaloid teratogenicity in the mouse. *Teratology* 42:105–119, 1990.

Onat FY, Yegen BC, Lawrence R, *et al.*: Mad honey poisoning in man and rat. *Rev Environ Health* 9:3–9, 1991.

Peixato PV, Brust LC, Duarte MD, *et al.*: *Cestrum laevigatum* poisoning in goats in southeastern Brazil. *Vet Hum Toxicol* 42:13–14, 2000.

Peper K, Trautwein W: The effect of aconitine on the membrane current in cardiac muscle. *Pflugers Arch* 296:328–336, 1967.

Perry C, Sastry R, Nasrallah IM, *et al.*: Mimosine attenuates serine hydroxymethyltransferase transcription by chelating zinc. Implications for inhibition of DNA replication. *J Biol Chem* 280:396–400, 2005.

Peterson MC, Rasmussen GJ: Intoxication with foothill camas (*Zigademus paniculatus*). *J Toxicol Clin Toxicol* 41:63–65, 2003.

Petroski RJ, Powell RG, Clay K: Alkaloids of *Stirpa robusta* (sleepy-grass) infected with an *Acremonium* endophyte. *Nat Toxins* 1:84–88, 1992.

Pfister JA, Panter KE, Manners GD: Effective dose in cattle of toxic alkaloids from tall larkspur (*Delphinium barberi*). *Vet Hum Toxicol* 36:10–11, 1994.

Pietsch J, Oertel R, Trautmann S, *et al.*: A non-fatal oleander poisoning. *Int J Legal Med* 119:236–240, 2005.

Polya G: *Biochemical Targets of Plant Bioactive Compounds.* London: Taylor & Francis, 2003, p. 583.

Prabhasankar P, Raguputhi G, Sundaravadivel B, *et al.*: Enzyme-linked immunosorbent assay for the phytotoxin thevetin. *J Immunoassay* 14:279–296, 1993.

Puschner B, Galey FD, Holstege DM, *et al.*: Sweet clover poisoning in California. *J Am Vet Med Assoc* 212:857–859, 1998.

Pusterla N, Holmberg TA, Lorenzo-Figueras M, *et al.*: *Acremonium strictum* pulmonary infection in a horse. *Vet Clin Pathol* 34:413–416, 2005.

Raisinghani M, Pabbidi RM, Premkumar LS: Activation of transient receptor potential vanilloid 1 (TRPV1) by resiniferatoxin. *J Physiol* 567 (pt 3):771–786, 2005.

Ramirez M, Rivera E, Ereu C: Fifteen cases of atropine poisoning after honey ingestion. *Vet Hum Toxicol* 41:19–20, 1999.

Rao RB, Hoffman RS: Nicotinic toxicity from tincture of blue cohosh (*Caulophyllum thalictroides*) used as an abortifacient. *Vet Hum Toxicol* 44:221–222, 2002.

Rasmussen LH, Jensen LS, Hansen HC: Distribution of the carcinogenic terpene ptaquiloside in bracken fronds, rhizomes (*Pteridium aquilinum*), and litter in Denmark. *J Chem Ecol* 29:771–778, 2003.

Rasmussen MA, Allison MJ, Foster JG: Flatpea intoxication in sheep and indications of ruminal adaptation. *Vet Hum Toxicol* 35:123–127, 1993.

Reddy L, Odhav B, Bhoola K: Aflatoxin B1-induced toxicity in HepG2 cells inhibited by carotenoids: Morphology, apoptosis and DNA damage. *Biol Chem* 387:87–93, 2006.

Riley RT, Hinton DM, Chamberlain WJ, *et al.*: Dietary fumonisin B$_1$ induces disruption of sphingolipid metabolism in Sprague–Dawley rat: A new mechanism of nephrotoxicity. *J Nutr* 124:594–603, 1994.

Rode D: Comfrey toxicity revisited. *Trends Pharmacol Sci* 23:497–499, 2002.

Rondeau ES: Wisteria toxicity. *J Toxicol* 31:107–112, 1993.

Rosell S, Samuelsson G: Effect of mistletoe viscotoxin and phoratoxin on blood circulation. *Toxicon* 26:975–987, 1988.

Rosling R: Cyanide exposure from linseed. *Lancet* 341:177, 1993.

Roy MC, Chang FR, Huang HC, *et al.* : Cytotoxic principles from the formosan milkweed, *Asclepias curassavica. J Nat Prod* 68:1494–1499, 2005.

Sako MDN, Al-Sultan II, Saleem AN: Studies on sheep experimentally poisoned with *Hypericum perforatum. Vet Hum Toxicol* 35:298–300, 1993.

Schacter L: Etopside phosphate: What, why, where and how? *Semin Oncol* 23 (suppl 13):1–7, 1996.

Sessa RA, Bennett MH, Lewis MJ, *et al.*: Metabolite profiling of sesquiterpene lactones from *Lactuca* species. *J Biol Chem* 275:26877–26884, 2000.

Shakin M, Smith BL, Prakash AS: Bracken carcinogens in the human diet. *Mutat Res* 443:69–79, 1999.

Sharma OP, Dawra RK, Pattabhi V: Molecular structure, polymorphism, and toxicity of lantadene A, the pentacyclictriterpenoid from the hepatotoxic plant *Latana camara. J Biochem Toxicol* 6:57–63, 1991.

Short SO, Edwards WC: Blue green algae toxicosis in Oklahoma. *Vet Hum Toxicol* 32:558–560, 1990.

Siebert U, Brach M, Sroczynski G, *et al.*: Efficacy, routine effectiveness, and safety of horsechestnut seed extract in the treatment of chronic venous insufficiency. A meta-analysis of randomized controlled trials and large observational studies. *Int Angiol* 21:305–315, 2002.

Skliar MI, Boland RL, Mourino A, *et al.*: Isolation and identification of vitamin D$_3$, 25-hydroxyvitamin D$_3$ 1,25-dihydroxyvitamin D$_3$ and 1,24, 25-trihydroxyvitamin D$_3$ in *Solanum malacoxylon* incubated with ruminal fluid. *J Steroid Biochem Mol Biol* 43:677–682, 1992.

Smith EA, Meloan CE, Pickell JA, *et al.*: Scopolamine poisoning from homemade "moon flower" wine. *J Anal Toxicol* 15:216–219, 1991.

Southcott RV, Haegi LAR: Plant hair dermatitis. *Med J Aust* 156:623–628, 1992.

Spencer PS: Food toxins, AMPA receptors and motor neuron diseases. *Drug Metab Rev* 31:561–587, 1999.

Spencer PS, Roy DN, Ludolph A, *et al.*: Lathyrism: Evidence for the role of the neuroexcitatory amino acid, BOAA. *Lancet* 2:1066–1067, 1986.

Spiering MJ, Lane GA, Christensen MJ, *et al.*: Distribution of the fungal endophyte *Neotyphodium lolii* is not a major determinant of the distribution of fungal alkaloids in *Lolium perenne* plants. *Phytochemistry* 66:195–202, 2005.

Spoerke DG, Murphy MM, Wruk KM, *et al.*: Five cases of Thermopsis poisoning. *J Toxicol Clin Toxicol* 26:397–406, 1988.

Surh Y-J, Lee E, Lee JM: Chemoprotective properties of some pungent ingredients present in red pepper and ginger. *Mutat Res* 404:259–267, 1998.

Szalcsany J: Capsaicin receptors as target molecules on nociceptors for development of novel analgesic agents, in Keri G and Toth I (eds.): *Molecular Pathomechanisms and New Trends in Drug Research.* London: Taylor & Francis, 2002, pp. 319–333.

Tahirov THO, Lu T-H, Liaw Y-C, *et al.*: A new crystal form of abrin-a from the seeds of *Abrus precatorius. J Mol Biol* 235:1152–1153, 1994.

Tandon HD, Tandon BN, Mattocks AR: An epidemic of veno-occlusive disease of the liver in Afghanistan. *Am J Gastroenterol* 70:607–613, 1978.

Teitelbaum JS, Zatorre RJ, Carpenter S, *et al.*: Neurologic sequelae of domoic acid intoxication due to the ingestion of contaminated mussels. *N Engl J Med* 322:1781–1787, 1990.

Tsujikawa K, Kanamori T, Iwata Y, *et al.*: Morphological and chemical analysis of magic mushrooms in Japan. *Forensic Sci Int* 138:85–90, 2003.

Tucker MO, Swan CR: The mango-poison ivy connection. *N Engl J Med* 339:235, 1998.

Tulsiani DR, Broquest HP, James LF, *et al.*: Production of hybrid glycoprotein and accumulation of oligosaccharides in the brain of sheep and pigs administered swainsonine or locoweed. *Arch Biochem Biophys* 264:607–617, 1988.

Turgut M, Alhan CC, Gurgoze M, *et al.*: Carboxyatractyloside poisoning in humans. *Ann Trop Paediatr* 25:125–134, 2005.

Tylleskar T, Banca M, Bikongi N, *et al.*: Cassava cyanogens and konzo, an upper motoneuron disease found in Africa. *Lancet* 339:208–211, 1992.

Urushibata O, Kase K: Irritant contact dermatitis from *Euphorbia marginata. Contact Dermatitis* 24:155–157, 1991.

Uwai K, Ohashi K, Takaya Y, *et al.*: Exploring the structural basis of neurotoxicity in C(17)-polyacetylenes isolated from water hemlock. *J Med Chem* 43:4508–4515, 2000.

van Meurs A, Cohen A, Edelbroek P: Atropine poisoning after eating chapattis contaminated with *Datura stramonium* (thorn apple). *Trans R Soc Trop Med Hyg* 86:221, 1992.

Wang H, Ng TB: Ribosome inactivating protein and lectin from bitter melon (*Momordica charantia*) seeds: Sequence comparison with related proteins. *Biochem Biophys Res Commun* 253:143–146, 1998.

Wang Z, Zhao J, Xing J, *et al.* : Analysis of strychnine and brucine in postmortem specimens by RP-HPLC: A case report of fatal intoxication. *J Anal Toxicol* 28:141–144, 2004.

Warren BA, Patel SA, Nunn PB, *et al.*: The Lathyrus excitotoxin beta-*N*-oxalyl-L-alpha, beta diaminopropionic acid is a substrate of the L-cystine/L-glutamate exchanger system xc-. *Toxicol Appl Pharmacol* 200:83–92, 2004.

Worker NA, Carrillo BJ: "Enteque seco," calcification and wasting in grazing animals in the Argentine. *Nature* 215:72–74, 1967.

Wu JH, Singh T, Herp A, *et al.*: Carbohydrate recognition factors of the lectin domains present in the *Ricinus communis* toxic protein (ricin). *Biochemie* 88:201–217, 2006.

Yoshizawa T, Yamashita A, Luo Y: Fumonisin occurrence in corn from high- and low-risk areas for human esophageal cancer in China. *Appl Environ Microbiol* 60:1626–1929, 1994.

UNIT 6

ENVIRONMENTAL TOXICOLOGY

CHAPTER 28

AIR POLLUTION*

Daniel L. Costa

AIR POLLUTION IN PERSPECTIVE

The second half of the twentieth century witnessed remarkable changes in environmental perspective. Until that time, national pride and prosperity were often visually depicted as an expanse of urban factories with smokestacks belching opaque clouds of industrial effluent into a seemingly neutral sky. The price of unchecked human progress through the first half of the century had led to a number of environmental catastrophes, which demonstrated the profoundly detrimental impact that such reckless prosperity could have on the natural environment. These images of "modern" prosperity gradually gave rise to public outcry for governmental action to protect environmental quality, wildlife, as well as public health.

The ensuing fifty years of regulatory legislation in the United States and Western Europe have now made such industrial scenes rare in most technologically developed nations. But, ironically, even as regulatory control measures began to reduce much of the stationary sources of air pollution, large populations have fled the cities in pursuit of a cleaner, safer lifestyle. This change in demographics post World War II altered the composition and distribution of polluted air. The commute from suburban home to city workplace back to suburban home, led to increasingly congested vehicular thoroughfares, creating a photochemical cauldron of oxidant air pollution around these newly formed, rapidly expanding metropolitan areas. More-

over, postwar population growth and rising expectations for a better (peace time) standard of living led to unrestrained consumption of inexpensive fossil fuels for energy production and recreational transportation needs. The result has been a world-wide destruction of limited environmental resources and an adverse effect on global climate, as energy-related polluted air masses drift and disperse across hundreds, even thousands of miles.

And so, air pollution remains a twenty-first-century reality, and while great legislative strides have been made to reduce emissions from both stationary and mobile sources, nonetheless, unsatisfactory air quality now plagues much broader geographic areas. More than half the U.S. population resides in counties that are not in compliance with current National Ambient Air Quality Standards (NAAQS) (Fig. 28-1). These noncompliant areas correspond well with the spread of population growth from major urban and industrial centers.

Episodes of extreme air pollution are rare in the Western world today. Occasionally, these areas experience unusual meteorological stagnations that coincide with "normal or expected" air pollution patterns that intensify the pollution over broad regions (e.g., 1995 in the United Kingdom and Western Europe). Conversely, specific locales dominated by a single, major pollutant source (e.g., Utah Valley smelter—through the 1980s and 1990s) can experience extremely poor air quality especially when exacerbated by meteorological inversions, with serious public health consequences. More typically, however, public exposures are characterized by prolonged periods of relatively low-levels of complex mixtures of photochemically transformed industrial and mobile emissions with periodic moderate excursions due to weather. This pattern of pollution now

* This article has been reviewed by the National Health and Environmental Effects Research Laboratory, U.S. Environmental Protection Agency, and approved for publication. Approval does not signify that the contents necessarily reflect the views and the policies of the Agency.

1119

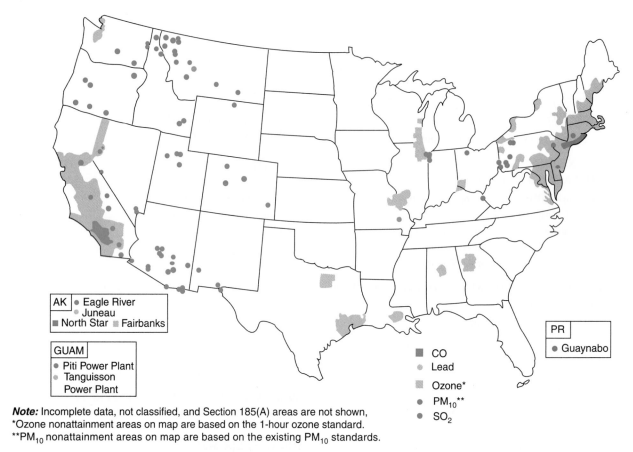

AK
- ● Eagle River
- ○ Juneau
- ■ North Star ■ Fairbanks

GUAM
- ● Piti Power Plant
- ● Tanguisson
  Power Plant

PR
- ● Guaynabo

- ■ CO
- ● Lead
- ■ Ozone*
- ● PM$_{10}$**
- ● SO$_2$

Note: Incomplete data, not classified, and Section 185(A) areas are not shown,
*Ozone nonattainment areas on map are based on the 1-hour ozone standard.
**PM$_{10}$ nonattainment areas on map are based on the existing PM$_{10}$ standards.

Figure 28-1.   Areas in the United States not in attainment for the NAAQS (September 2002) criteria pollutants: O$_3$, PM$_{10}$, SO$_2$, CO, and Pb.

No area was in violation for NO$_2$. [Note: Incomplete data, and not classified or Section 185(A) areas are not shown. Ozone nonattainment areas are based on the 1-hour NAAQS and those for PM$_{10}$ are based on the 1997 PM$_{10}$ NAAQS. *(Air Trends - Figure 4-1; http://epa.gov/airtrends/non.html).*

extends even into remote wilderness areas, where considerable damage to flora and fauna has occurred.

In contrast, many developing countries experiencing rapid population growth, industrialization, and economic expansion choose to ignore the lessons of Western industrial expansion and the consequences of inadequate air pollution control. Air pollution in some of these nations now rivals the atmospheric conditions that existed in Western Europe and America preceding the catastrophic air pollution episodes of the twentieth century. For example, two Hong Kong marathoners died in February 2006 while running during severe air pollution. In addition, industrial emissions from some developing nations and emerging economies, now contribute substantially to the global burden of many air pollutant constituents. A willingness to balance worldwide economic growth and industrialization using lessons learned from the misadventures of the Second Industrial Revolution and the Age of the Automobile will determine the impact of the "new" global economy on the health of both the earth and its inhabitants.

Previously, the scientific information regarding the impacts of air pollution on human health had largely been collected on the individual constituents that make-up air pollution's complex mixture. In turn, this knowledge was used to develop both public health standards and to establish regulatory controls. Despite the obvious complexities of urban air pollution, it was felt that single pollutant regulations were the best path to success. Indeed, great strides have been made. However, research agendas have slowly been evolving

to include the study of the interaction and transformation of individual pollutant components within atmospheric systems—a truer reflection of real-world exposure complexities.

This chapter will present an overview of the current state of knowledge regarding the production of air pollution and its subsequent impact on human health. Also, the complexities of regulatory decisions and risk assessment will be addressed. Hopefully, these topics will provide the reader with both a fundamental knowledge and appreciation of the nature of the problem, as well as a sense of the uncertainties in need of future investigation.

A Brief History of Air Pollution and Its Regulation

For most of history, air pollution has been a problem of microenvironments and domestic congestion. The smoky fires of early cave and hut dwellers choked the air inside their homes. When the emissions were vented outdoors, they combined with those of the neighbors to settle around the village on damp cold nights. With urbanization and a concomitant decrease in forest wood as a source of fuel to heat and cooking, the need for energy led to the burning of cheap coal and ambient release of sulfurous, sooty smoke. Likewise, kilns to make quicklime for construction and metal smelters pushed smoke and chemical materials into the air of active "modern" cities. Unfortunately, the city dwellers had to endure the bad air, while those with wealth frequently had country homes to which they could escape from time to time. The poor quality of urban

Table 28-1

U.S. National (Primary) Ambient Air Quality Standards*

POLLUTANT	UNIT	AVERAGING TIME	CONCENTRATION	STATISTIC
Sulfur dioxide	$\mu g/m^3$ (ppm)	Annual	80 (0.03)	Annual mean
		24 h	365 (0.14)	Maximum
Carbon monoxide	$\mu g/m^3$ (ppm)	8 h	10 (9)	Maximum
		1 h	40 (35)	Maximum
Ozone$^{\#}$	$\mu g/m^3$ (ppm)	1 h	235 (0.12)	Maximum
		8 h	157 (0.08)	Maximum
Nitrogen dioxide	$\mu g/m^3$ (ppm)	Annual	100 (0.053)	Annual mean
Particulates $PM_{10}^{\#}$	$\mu g/m^3$	Annual and 24 h	150 and 50	Annual mean
$PM_{2.5}^{\#}$	$\mu g/m^3$	Annual and 24 h	65 and 15	
Lead$^{\#}$	$\mu g/m^3$	3 months	1.5	Quarterly average

*For detailed information regarding policy and precise statistical and time-based computations to achieve attainment, contact EPA Web site: www.epa.gov/airs/criteria.html.

$^{\#}$NAAQS currently under review for potential revision in 2006. See noted Web site.

air was captured by many writers from Charles Dickens in his writings about London's fogs to the ancients: Seneca, the Roman philosopher, in AD 61 wrote: "As soon as I had gotten out of the *heavy air* of Rome, and from the *stink* of the chimneys thereof, which being stirred, poured forth whatever *pestilential vapors and soot* they had enclosed in them, I felt an *alteration to my disposition*" (emphasis added: Miller and Miller, 1993).

As in today's world efforts to regulate air pollution competed with the industrial economies and as a result, they evolved slowly. Early on, in the time of Greece and Rome, individual civil suits could be levied against local polluters, although these were of marginal success. Beginning in the thirteenth century, community-based outcries received some recognition by governing officials, one example being the banning of "sea coal" from lime kilns and domestic heaters in London by Edward I. Enforcement, however, was not effective and people largely resigned themselves to polluted air as part of urban life. By the seventeenth century, England, in the middle of several decades some refer to as "the little ice age," experienced further reductions in wood harvests, which only increased reliance on sea coal for domestic heating. Despite Percival Pott's discovery that soot was related to the incidence of scrotal cancer in chimney sweeps, the health community offered only a simple recommendation: "Fly the city, shun its turbid air; breathe not the chaos of eternal smoke . . . " (Brimblecombe, 1999)—advice hardly advanced from that of Seneca 1600 years earlier. In the late eighteenth century, the industrial revolution, which was powered by the burning of "cleaner" mined coal, added a second dimension to urban air pollution. These emissions were more acidic and hung in the air longer than the fluffy soot of the cheaper sea coal. Continued soiling of buildings and damage to nearby crops brought community boards to address sanitary reforms to cut the worse of the pollution peaks and episodes, but any gains were soon offset by growth. By the end of the nineteenth century and into the early twentieth century, power plants were being built to provide energy for factories and eventually to light homes. Steel mills and other industries proliferated along riverbanks and lakeshores, oil refineries rose in port cities and near oil fields and smelters roasted and refined metals in areas near large mineral deposits.

By 1925, air pollution was common to all industrialized nations, but people grew less tolerant of the nuisance of acidic-soot corrosion of all exposed surfaces and the general discomfort that came with smoky air—this acidic, sooty form of air pollution has been termed "reducing" air pollution. Public surveys were initiated—as in

Salt Lake City in 1926, New York City in 1937, and Leicester, Great Britain, in 1939—to bring political attention to the problem and promote the implementation of controls (Miller and Miller, 1993). However, it was not until the great air pollution disasters in the Meuse Valley, Belgium, in 1930; Donora, Pennsylvania, in 1948; and the great London fog of 1952 that air pollution was indicted primarily as a health issue. In the United States, California was already leading the way with passage of the Air Pollution Control Act of 1947 to regulate the discharge of opaque smokes. Visibility problems in Pittsburgh during the 1940s had also prompted efforts to control smoke from local industries, but it was the initiative of President Truman that provided the federal impetus to deal with air pollution. This early effort culminated in congressional passage of a series of acts starting with the Air Pollution Control Act of 1955.

The prosperity and suburban sprawl of the late 1950s provided the third and perhaps most chemically complex dimension of air pollution. The term *smog,* though originally coined to describe the mixture of smoke and fog that hung over large cities such as London, was curiously adopted for the eye-irritating photochemical reaction products of auto exhaust that blanketed cities like Los Angeles. Early federal legislation addressing stationary sources was soon expanded to include automobile-derived pollutants (the Clean Air Act of 1963, amended in 1967, and the Motor Vehicle Air Pollution Control Act of 1965). The landmark Clean Air Act (CAA) of 1970 evolved from the early legislation, and despite being only an amendment, it was revolutionary. It recognized the problem of air pollution as a national issue and set forth a plan to control it. The Act established the U.S. Environmental Protection Agency (USEPA) and charged it with the responsibility to protect the public from the hazards of polluted outdoor air. Seven "criteria" air pollutants—ozone (O_3), sulfur dioxide (SO_2), particulate matter (PM), nitrogen dioxide (NO_2), carbon monoxide (CO), lead (Pb), and total hydrocarbons; the last now dropped from the list, leaving six criteria pollutants—were specified as significant health hazards in need of *individual* National Ambient Air Quality Standards (NAAQS). These NAAQS were mandated for review every 5 years as to the adequacy of the existent standard to protect human health (Table 28-1), although in many instances adherence to this schedule has not been achieved. The explosion in the literature databases for the criteria pollutants and the extensive review process has often led to delays in completing the process on schedule. For each of the criteria pollutants, a Criteria Document or science assessment is developed, which provides a

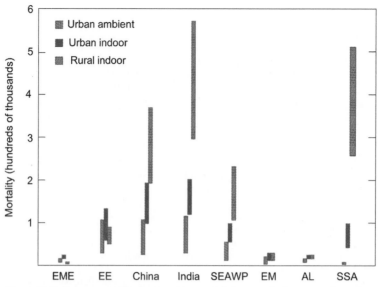

Figure 28-2. Excess mortality due to outdoor and indoor particulate matter in various international economic groupings.

Bottom and top of each bar represent the lower and upper estimates of mortality, respectively, computed using the methodology of Schwela (2000): Established Market Economics (EME); Eastern Europe (EE); China; India; South East Asia/Western Pacific (SEAWP); Eastern Mediterranean (EM); Latin America (AL); and sub-Saharan Africa (SSA). (Modified from Figure 2.6 by D. Schwela: Air Pollution in the Megacities of Asia - SEOUL WORKSHOP REPORT: Urban Air Pollution Management and Practice in Major and Megacities of Asia—*http://www.asiairnet.org/seoulreport.asp*).

detailed summary of the available literature on that pollutant. This assessment of the science is then integrated into a Staff Paper to develop a range of proposed standards based on risk analyses. The EPA Administrator considers proposals from both "evidence" and "risk" based assessments to establish policy and set the NAAQS (www.epa.gov/ttn/naaqs/naaqs_process_report_march2006.pdf). In 2006, this process was changed with the steps in the process coming to be termed: Science Assessment, Risk Assessment and Policy Assessment to replace the Criteria Document and Staff Paper. With regard to the Primary NAAQS, only health criteria can be considered in the development of the standard, including safety considerations for potentially susceptible groups. The Secondary NAAQS considers agricultural and structural welfare. Economic impacts are not to be involved in standard setting itself—only in assessing the cost of the implementation procedures. Other hazardous air pollutants (HAPs), of which there were eight listed at the time, were to undergo health assessments to establish emission controls. The CAA of 1970 was by far the most far-reaching legislation to date.

The accidental release of 30 tons of methyl isocyanate vapor into the air of the shanty village of Bhopal, India, on December 3, 1984, killed an estimated 3000 people within hours of the release, with several thousand delayed deaths, and 200,000 injured or permanently impaired. The tragedy shocked the world, and raised the issue of HAPs in the United States to a new level of concern. While such a disaster has never struck the United States, accidental industrial releases or spills of toxic chemicals are surprisingly common, with 4375 cases recorded between 1980 and 1987, inflicting 11,341 injuries and 309 deaths (Waxman, 1994). The HAPs, which had been the stepsister of the criteria pollutants for more than a decade after the passage of the 1970 CAA, have since garnered more public and policy attention. There is concern not only for accidental releases of

fugitive or secondary chemicals—such as phosgene, benzene, butadiene, and dioxin, into the air of populated industrial centers—but also for potential chronic health effects, with cancer often being the focus of attention. The slow progress of regulatory decisions on HAPs (only eight between 1970 and 1990) led to a mandated acceleration of the process under the CAA amendment of 1990. Section 112(b) currently lists 188 chemicals or classes of chemicals for which special standards and risk assessments are required. The chemicals listed are those of greatest concern on the basis of toxicity (including cancer) and estimated release volumes. Currently, there is a list of 33 HAPS from the list of 188 that are deemed to be of greatest concern, so-called a list of the "dirty thirty." Emissions are of HAPS are mandated for control to the maximal achievable control technology (MACT), and any residual health risk after MACT is to be considered in a separate quantitative risk assessment. The database for this process utilizes existing knowledge or, if necessary, mandates further research by the emitter. While many of these chemicals are now better controlled than in the past, most residual risk estimates are yet to be completed. The database from which these assessments are made is called the Integrated Risk Information System (IRIS—www.epa.gov/iris/index.html).

Emissions from motor vehicles are addressed primarily under the CAA Title II, Emission Standards for Mobile Sources. The reduction of emissions from mobile sources is complex and involves both fuel and engine/vehicle reengineering. Despite continued refinements in combustion engineering through the use of computerized ignition and timing, fuel properties have drawn recent attention for improvement. For example, to reduce wintertime CO, several oxygenates (including ethers and alcohols) have be formulated into fuels both to reduce cold-start emissions and enhance overall combustion. Perhaps the most prominent of the ethers is MTBE (methyl

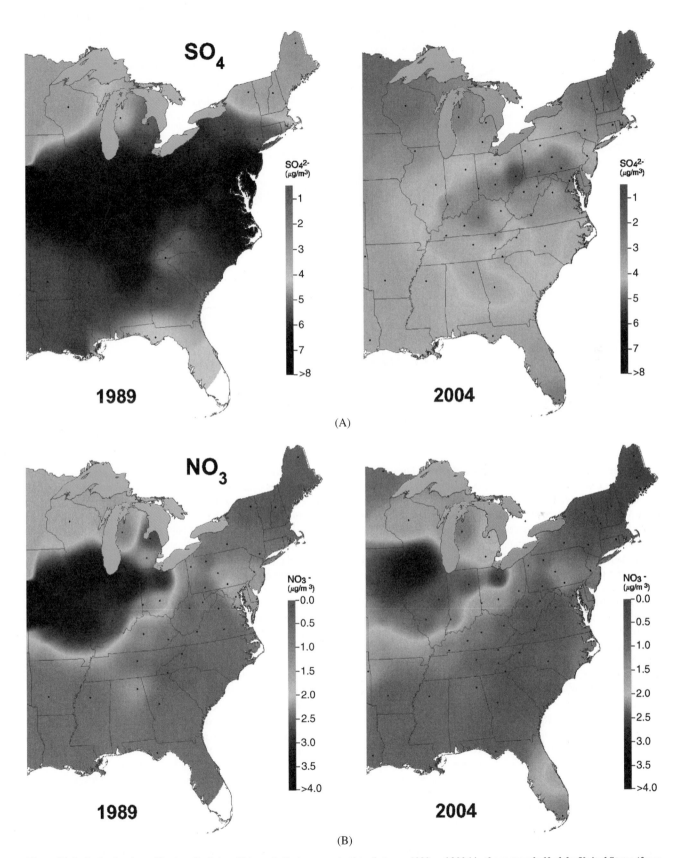

Figure 28-3. Reduction in ambient particulate sulfate and nitrate concentrations between 1989 and 2004 in the eastern half of the United States (from CASTNet monitoring data).

Sulfates and nitrates arising from industrial centers of the Midwest contribute to acid rain deposition (see Fig. 28-11). Sulfates are readily dispersed by toward the eastern half of the country. Nitrates arise from the industrial centers as well as metropolitan areas and show both a local and dispersed pattern. (Adapted from Clean Air Status and Trends Network—http://www.epa.gov/castnet/mapconc_e.html).

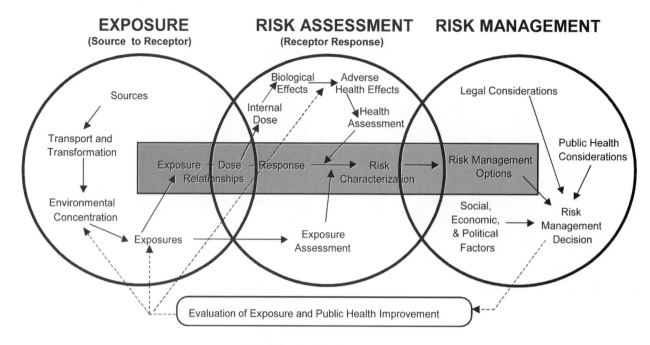

EXPOSURE
(Source to Receptor)

RISK ASSESSMENT
(Receptor Response)

RISK MANAGEMENT

ACCOUNTABILITY

Figure 28-4. NRC risk assessment paradigm.

Components of Risk Assessment within the left circle provide data to development of *Risk Management* as depicted in the right circle, modified to include an "Accountability" component as a means to address Air Quality Management impacts on the process risk reduction (National Research Council, 1983).

tertiary butyl ether), which became a controversial additive in the early 1990s, arising in part from odor and reports of asthma-like reactions by some individuals during auto refueling at service stations. Today, the controversy has taken an unexpected twist; MTBE has now been removed from fuel, not because health concerns associated with airborne exposure but rather due to leakage from service-station storage tanks into groundwater. Ironically, this prescribed remedy for an air problem has evolved into a new problem: groundwater contamination. This example illustrates the broad complexity of pollution control, measures that transcend engineering. Meanwhile, other fuel additives have been promoted or developed to boost octane ratings of fuels and/or improve engine performance and combustion (e.g., organic oxygenates, methylcyclopentadienyl manganese tricarbonyl (MMT), platinum compounds for diesel, etc.). These additives are being carefully reviewed under Title II because of concerns regarding the potential changes in combustion product reactivity or the introduction of metals into the environment, reminiscent of use lead in fuels from the 1930s to 1970s, when lead fuel additives were banned.

Internationally, the magnitude and control of air pollution sources vary considerably, especially among developing nations, which often forgo concerns for health and welfare because of cost and the desire to achieve prosperity. Figure 28-2 illustrates the international variation in air pollution related mortality (outdoor and indoor) based on economic groupings. It is clear that there are wide differences reflecting economic imbalances—particularly prominent are the indoor particulate levels in developing nations where biomass combustion is used for heating and cooking. Likewise, these regions contain many of the megacities of the world with major air pollution problems. The political upheaval in Eastern Europe since 1990 has revealed the consequences of decades of uncontrolled in-

dustrial air pollution. While vast improvements are now becoming evident in this area, as industries are being modernized and emissions controlled, many Asian, African, and South American cities have virtually unchecked air pollution. Some nations as well as the World Health Organization (WHO) have adopted air quality standards as a rational basis for guiding control measures, but the lack of binding regulations and/or economic fortune has impeded significant controls and improvements (Lipfert, 1994). In addition to local socioeconomic and political concerns, emissions of air pollutants will, in all probability, spawn problems of "international pollution" as we enter the twenty-first century, when the impact of long-range transport of polluted air masses from one country to another fully matures as a global issue (Reuther, 2000). This was the subject of some controversy between Canada and the United States in the late 1980s and into the 1990s as a result of the air mass transport of acid sulfates from industrial centers of the Midwestern United States to southern Ontario. However, reduction in SO_2 emissions has somewhat relieved the tension over the last several years (Fig. 28-3A). Improvement in NOx, also a product of stationary source fossil fuel burning, is also apparent (Fig. 28-3B).

ASSESSING RISKS ASSOCIATED WITH AIR POLLUTION

"Risk Assessment" has become a formalized process, originally described in the landmark 1983 National Research Council Report, whereby toxicity, exposure, and dose-dependent outcome data can be systematically integrated to estimate risk to a population. Figure 28-4 provides a modified version of the paradigm of the NAS incorporating recent interest in providing evidence of "accountability" that the regulations indeed did have impacts. The health database

Table 28-2
Strengths and Weaknesses of Disciplinary Approaches for Obtaining Health Information

DISCIPLINE	POPULATION	STRENGTHS	WEAKNESSES
Epidemiology	Communities	Natural exposure	Difficult to quantify exposure
			Many covariates
	Diseased groups	No extrapolation	
		Isolates susceptibility trait	Minimal dose–response data
		Long-term, low-level effects	Association vs. causation
	Field/Panel groups	Good exposure data	Usually short-term
		Fewer covariates	Volunteers
		Focus on host traits	Expensive
		Utilizes clinical evaluations	
Clinical studies	Experimental	Controlled exposures	Artificial exposures
	Diseased subjects	Few covariates	Acute effects only
		Isolates susceptibility trait	Hazards
		Cause–effect	Volunteers
Toxicology	Animals	Maximum control	Human extrapolation
		Dose-response data	Realistic models of human disease?
		Cause–effect	
	In vitro systems	Rapid data acquisition	In vivo extrapolation
		Mechanisms	

SOURCE: Data modified from Boubel *et al.*, 1994.

for any air pollutant may comprise data from animal toxicology, controlled human studies, and/or epidemiology. But, because each of these research approaches has inherent strengths and limitations, an appropriate assessment of an air pollutant requires the careful integration and interpretation of data from all three methodologies. Thus, one should be aware of the attributes of each (Table 28-2).

Epidemiologic studies reveal associations between exposure to a pollutant(s) and the health effect(s) in the *community* or *population* of interest. Because data are garnered directly under real-world exposure conditions and often involve large numbers of people, the data are of direct utility to regulators assessing pollutant impacts. With proper design and analysis, studies can explore either acute or long-term exposures and theoretically can examine trends in mortality and morbidity, accounting irreversible effects as well as responses in population subsets (i.e., sensitive groups). Why, then, is this approach to the study of air pollution not the exclusive choice of regulators in decision making? The problem is that it is difficult to control confounding personal variables in the population. Factors such as genetic diversity and lifestyle differences among individuals, and population mobility are difficult to control. Perhaps most problematic is the lack of adequate exposure data—especially on a personal basis. Exposure assessment is often one of the major weaknesses of an epidemiologic study, not only because of the difficulties of assessing exposure (as a measure of dose) to the pollutant of interest, but because it is difficult to segregate a single pollutant from correlated co-pollutants and other environmental influences, such as meteorology. Thus, only associations, and not causality, can be drawn between the broad-based exposure data and effects. Frequently, the effects are of mortality, hospitalizations, etc. Causal relationships are sometimes inferred in the presence of strong statistical significance, but such determinations are likely to be criticized. However, recent advances in exposure estimation and study design and analysis (e.g., time series) have allowed epidemiologists to examine relationships with greater confidence and specificity. These models limit the impact of covariates and longer time-based influences and thus allow epidemiologists to tease out effects

of short-term pollution not accessible formerly (Schwartz, 1991). Similarly, newer approaches that employ field studies—sometimes called *panel studies*—incorporate time-series design and multiple-regression analyses of more focused and complete exposure data (ideally personal) and targeted clinical endpoints in the exposed population under study. The endpoints often derive from empirical human and animal studies and therefore have a priori conceptual ties. The advent of new genetic approaches for characterizing polymorphisms of potentially influential traits (e.g., GSTM1—glutathione-S-transferase M1—Tujague *et al.*, 2006) opens the genomic door for assessing gene-environment interactions. These factors may well underlie much of human susceptibility to air pollution. Novel approaches such as this are evident in the most recent studies of PM air pollution (see below).

Studies that involve controlled human exposures have been used extensively to evaluate the criteria air pollutants regulated by the USEPA. Because most people are exposed to these pollutants in their daily lives, human volunteers can be ethically exposed to them in a highly controlled fashion (with the exception of Pb, which has cumulative and irreversible effects). Exposures are conducted in a controlled environment (usually in a chamber or with a mask) and are generally of short or limited repeat durations, given assurances that all responses are reversible. Clearly, data of this type are very valuable in assessing potential human risk, because they are derived from the species of concern and are rooted in well-established clinical knowledge and experience.

Suspected "susceptible or sensitive" individuals representing potential higher-risk groups can also be studied to better understand the breadth of response in the exposed public. However, clinical studies have several practical limitations. Ethical issues are involved in every aspect of a clinical test; potentially irreversible effects and carcinogenicity are also always of concern, along with the definition of an acceptable level of hyper-responsiveness in so-called sensitive individuals who volunteered to participate in the study. Likewise for any test subject, there are obvious restrictions on the invasiveness of biological procedures, although sophistication in medical technology has made accessible a large array of molecular biomarkers from peripheral blood and nasal, bronchial, and alveolar lavage fluids as well as biopsied cells from airway segments (Devlin *et al.*, 1991; Salvi *et al.*, 1999). As noted above, the advent of cutting-edge genomic and proteomic high-through-put technologies provide new tools to dissect human responses and their relationships to susceptibility. Obviously, the issue of cost, the limited numbers of subjects that can be practically evaluated, and the inability to address chronic exposure issues remain constraints on human testing. Where partnerships with animal toxicology studies have been established, studies in laboratory animal species can sometimes provide ethical justification for at least limited direct human exposure to address critical questions. Analogously, in vitro studies in both human and animal cell and tissue systems, often augmented with similar genomic tools, allow the elucidation of mechanisms of toxicity. These basic biological responses inform extrapolation models that link animal data to humans, and they support the feasibility and prescribe some of the ethical limitations of human study with some toxic air pollutants (see below).

Animal toxicology is frequently used to predict or corroborate suspected effects in humans. In the absence of human data, animal toxicology constitutes the essential first step of risk assessment: *hazard identification*. Animal toxicology is often required before any controlled human exposure can be conducted. It is particularly useful in elucidating pathogenic mechanisms involved in toxic injury or disease, providing basic knowledge that is critical to extrapolating databases across species, to estimating uncertainties, and determining the relevance of information to humans. Knowledge of the toxic mechanism(s) provides the underpinnings to the "plausibility" of findings in the human context and, under carefully defined and highly controlled circumstances, may allow *quantitative* estimates of risk to human populations. Animal toxicology studies have been used to investigate all of the criteria air pollutants and many of the HAPs as well. The strength of this discipline is that it can involve methods that are not practical in human studies and can provide more rapid turnaround of essential toxicity data under diverse exposure concentrations and durations. The minimization of uncontrolled variables (e.g., genetic and environmental) may be the greatest strength of the animal bioassay.

The clear limitation of animal studies in human risk assessment lies in the unknowns that weaken the extrapolation of findings in animals to the day-to-day human life scenario. Ideally, a test animal is selected with knowledge that it responds in a manner similar to that of the human (*homology*). *Qualitative* extrapolation of homologous effects is not unusual with many toxic inhalants, but *quantitative* extrapolation is frequently clouded by uncertainties of the relative *sensitivity* of the animal or specific target tissue compared with that of the human. Uncertainties about the target tissue dose also loom large, constituting the first obstacle to quantitative extrapolation (see below). With respect to the target tissue dose, however, most animal toxicologists make every effort to keep exposure concentrations at 5- to 10-fold that of the anticipated human exposure until appropriate dosimetric data can be ascertained. An often overlooked issue is that the dose to the target (lung region) for the test animal is less than that of the human under similar exposure conditions – especially when exposures are conducted during dormancy for the animals (Wichers *et al.*, 2006). Most human studies involve exercise exposure paradigms. Additionally, higher doses may be needed to achieve a group response among a limited pool of genetically similar animals (maybe 6–10) to represent a large population effect, where perhaps only a few of hundreds or thousands may actually be responsive if analyzed separately. Nevertheless, it must be appreciated that mechanisms may well differ at different dose levels and some responses may be misleading at the higher dose levels. Despite these limitations, however, animal studies have provided the largest database on a wide range of air toxicants and have proven utility in predicting human adverse responses to chemicals.

To be effective, any health assessment should consider the strengths and weaknesses of the approaches selected to estimate actual toxic risk. In the larger picture, other scientific disciplines can be highly valuable to a more accurate assessment of the impact of air pollution on society. The atmospheric sciences (including the chemical and physical sciences) provide insight into actual exposures by characterizing what is in the air. Better pollutant characterization, linked to exposure assessment, can only strengthen epidemiological outcome associations. Similarly, these data support toxicity evaluations based on biological test systems. In the latter case, more controlled exposures provide better insights into biological outcomes, especially with defined pollutant physicochemical attributes and interactions. Recreating realistic exposure environments to the extent possible is invaluable to developing models to estimate human risk.

Lastly, data derived from studies of botanical responses are now appreciated more than ever. Not only are commercial and native vegetation affected by pollution but some plant species are being exploited as sensitive "sentinels," warning of the impacts of pollution on both human and environmental receptors. When considered collectively, economists can inform regulators and the public at large of the cumulative impact and adversity of pollution on our quality and standard of living (Maddison and Pierce, 1999). Interestingly, some basic mechanisms (e.g., the involvement of antioxidants) between plants and animals have remarkable parallels.

Animal-to-Human Extrapolation: Issues and Mitigating Factors

The utility and value of animal toxicology is highly dependent on the ability to extrapolate or relate empirical findings to real-world scenarios. Several factors of study design play into the process of extrapolation (e.g., exposure concentration, duration, and patterns, etc.), but most important is the selection of the animal species that will serve as the toxicological model. Therefore, this selection should involve more than considerations of cost and convenience. Whenever possible, effects that are homologous and involve the same mode of action between the study species and the human should guide the decision of the most appropriate test species. For example, if upper airway irritant responses like bronchoconstriction are anticipated (e.g., SO_2 or formaldehyde), then the guinea pig, with its human-like labile and reactive airway reflexes, should be selected over the rat, which is not particularly responsive in this regard. However, if the underlying molecular events in tissue remodeling are of interest, the rat might better serve as model because of cellular mechanistic parallels with human tissue responses. In part, the availability of probes to aid in such studies would factor into the selection of the rat as well. As strains of rats differ in their neutrophilic responsiveness to deep lung inhalants (e.g., O_3), contrasting the mode of action may be more revealing and support their selection for study (Costa *et al.*, 1985). Other innate differences in sensitivity among species may also relate to differences in lung structure, specific regionality of cell metabolism, genetic polymorphisms, or antioxidant defenses (Paige and Plopper, 1999; Slade *et al.*, 1985). Thus, ideally, when such nuances are unclear or unknown, the replication of responses in multiple species builds confidence in the finding as being

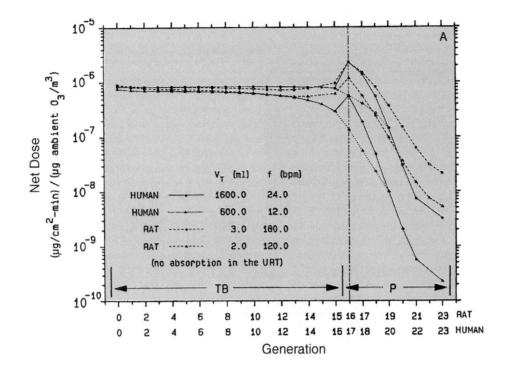

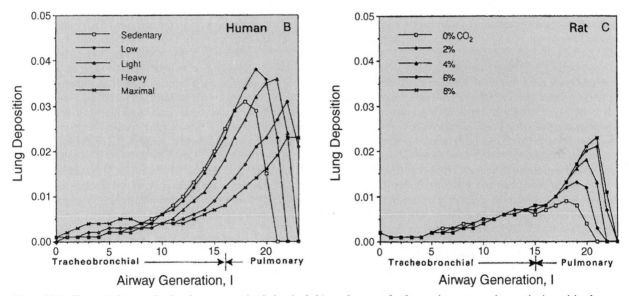

Figure 28-5. Theoretical (normalized to the concentration in inspired air) uptake curves for the reactive gas ozone in a resting/exercising human and a rat (A). Likewise, the percent deposition in the airways of a 0.6 μm insoluble particle in the respiratory tracts of a resting/exercising human (B) and rat (C).

Eight percent inspired CO_2 in the rat augments ventilation up to threefold. Airway generation refers to that airway branch numbered from the trachea (0). [Panel (A) is from Overton and Miller, 1987, and panels (B) and (C) are from Martonen *et al.*, 1992. Reproduced with permission.]

homologous or having species-conserved modes of action that are relevant to the human.

An essential, but often overlooked, part of extrapolating responses from species to species is an accurate assessment of the relative dosimetry of the pollutant along the respiratory tract. Significant advances in studies of the distribution of gaseous and particulate pollutants have been made through the use of empirical and mathematical models, the latter of which incorporate parameters of respiratory anatomy and physiology, aerodynamics, and physical chemistry into predictions of deposition and retention. Empirical

models combined with theoretical models aid in relating animal toxicity data to humans and help refine the study of injury mechanisms with better estimates of the target dose. Figures 28-5A and B illustrate the application of such an approach to the reactive gas O_3 and insoluble 0.6-μm spherical particles, respectively, as each is distributed along the respiratory tract of humans and rats. Anatomic differences between the species clearly affect the deposition of both gases and particles, but the qualitative and to a large extent quantitative similarities in deposition profiles are noticeable. This is not surprising if one argues teleologically that the lungs of each species evolved with similar functional demands (i.e., O_2–CO_2 exchange, blood acid/base balance), mechanical impediments, and environmental stresses. One needs only a cursory review of the comparative lung physiology literature to appreciate the allometric consistency of the mammalian respiratory tract to meet the challenge of breathing air. This design coherency has provided the fundamental rationale for the use of animal models for the study of air pollutants.

Susceptible subpopulations who may show exaggerated responsiveness to pollutants merit special mention. The existence of hyperresponsive individuals and groups is well accepted among those who conduct air pollution health assessments, but little is actually known about the host traits that make certain individuals responsive. This appreciation for sensitive populations is specifically noted in the CAA, where their protection is mandated in the promulgation of NAAQS. There are some definable subgroups that are considered inherently more susceptible, including children, the elderly, and those with a preexisting disease (e.g., asthma, cardiovascular disease, lung disease). The importance of susceptibility in air pollutant responses is gaining more and more attention as test subject responses that were once considered "outliers" may well be evidence of unusual responsiveness. In some cases susceptibility may simply reflect differences in dosimetry. Children who spend more time outdoors than adults, who are more active, and who have basal ventilation rates that exceed adults on a volume to body weight ratio, may experience overall greater dose to the lungs. Certainly, rapidly growing tissues may also factor in and may have contributed, perhaps with dosimetry factors, to recent findings that polluted urban air retards lung growth (Gauderman et al., 2004). Similarly, adult humans and animals with obstructive airway disease, for example, may have "hotspots" of particle deposition in the airways that exceed normal local tissue doses manyfold (Kim and Kang, 1997; Sweeney et al., 1995). Another often underappreciated aspect of susceptibility relates to the loss of functional reserve or compensation due to age or disease, perhaps altering a response threshold or impairing normal homeostasis or recovery. As already noted, there is also growing interest in gene-environment interactions where genetic differences determine responsiveness. In humans, GSTM1 polymorphisms affect ∼50% of the population and thus, may in theory undermine antioxidant defenses in some individuals (McCunney, 2005). In the end, susceptibility may be due to differences in dose, sensitivity, and/or compensation. Clearly, outcomes may be similar, but their underlying causes may be multifactoral.

Because the study of susceptibility in compromised human subjects is limited, ethically, studies must confined to subjects of only modest suspected risk (e.g., mild asthmatics). However, inroads have been made in recent years, in part because of more thorough pre-study assessments of potential risk factors, allowing researchers to design studies that need not carry undue risk. Additionally, the development of more appropriate animal models of disease or dysfunction provides a useful adjunct to explore susceptibility factors prior to study in humans and in more depth. Hence, studies in animals and human subjects are now being better coordinated, to investigate specific questions regarding the roles of diet (e.g., antioxidant content), exercise (as it relates to dosimetry), age, gender, and race, as well as disease associated frailty. The goal is to elucidate patterns or common factors that may inform potential intervention or mitigation strategies as well as basic information to reduce the uncertainties regarding risk (Kodavanti et al., 1998).

Recent advances in molecular biology have provided tools to assess traits in animal models that are under the control of identifiable genes that are homologous to humans. Natural variants in mouse genetics and specially bioengineered transgenic and knockout strains (and in some cases rats), are now widely used to address mechanistic as well as risk hypotheses regarding responses to air pollutants. These new biological tools hold great promise in better understanding responses and establishing gene-environment interactions that may underlie variation in human responsiveness. Transgenic strains can be devised to express desired traits derived from humans as well as other animals, while knockout models can be made devoid of specific traits to isolate the impact of that trait on responsivity to a toxic challenge. These animal models add to the availability of natural mutants that have been inbred historically to purify a desired genotype to achieve a specific phenotype (Ho, 1994; Glasser et al., 1994). Current technology can also target genes for specific expression in the lung (e.g., linked to surfactant protein C), and in some cases control genes can be provided with which an investigator can switch the gene of interest on or off using a pharmacologic or chemical prechallenge. Such advances allow the dissection of underlying mechanisms under very controlled scenarios and avoid the problems of having a gene be inappropriately active or inactive through all life stages (Kistner et al., 1996).

To date, the emphasis of studies using these genetically modified animal models have been on mechanisms associated with disease pathogenesis (Recio, 1995; Suga et al., 2000; Yoshida and Whitsett, 2006). Among the most popular uses of knockout and transgenic mice has been in the study of inflammatory cytokines and associated products in asthma, as the expression of many of these mediators are thought to be under the control of single genes (e.g., Kakuyama et al., 1999; Kuhn et al., 2000). Clearly these genetically modified mice are well suited for the study of mechanism of action where a specific mediator-based hypothesis can be tested as it relates to an impaired function, pathology, or altered inflammatory pattern. When these models are derived to exhibit a desired pathology or disease due to a genetic defect—for example involving lung structure or growth (e.g., emphysema or fibrosis), such that by adulthood the animal exhibits the disease—the model may serve as a surrogate of the human condition (e.g., O'Donnell et al., 1999). Analogous mouse models (e.g., ApoE $^{-/-}$) are currently being used to assess atherosclerosis and cardiac disease in long term air pollution studies (Sun et al., 2005).

The use or genetically modified animal models in air pollution research has lagged behind that of basic science and toxicology in general. The reasons for this are unclear and may relate to the difficulties in incorporating such data into conventional risk-assessment paradigms. However, with recent interest in susceptible groups, there has been a definitive upswing in the use of pharmacologically or naturally altered, as well as bioengineered animals (Kodavanti et al., 1998) to more closely link mechanistic profiles to basic human biology. Ozone has frequently been the test pollutant in these new studies, because more is known about O_3 and its effects in humans than about any other air pollutant. Frequently, these studies address aspects of inflammation and antioxidant capacity relative to challenge by O_3 and other oxidants (Johnston et al., 1999; Kleeberger et al., 2000). But with the current interest in PM health effects, these and other models are being redirected. Examples include: strain differences and acid coated PM (Ohtsuka et al., 2000); hypertransferrinemic mice and metal-rich PM (Ghio et al., 2000); and metallothionein-null mice and mercury vapor (Yoshida et al., 1999). Among rats, the Spontaneously Hypertensive Rat (SHR) has gained considerable popularity for use in studies of PM because of its resemblance to human hypertension with serum oxidant

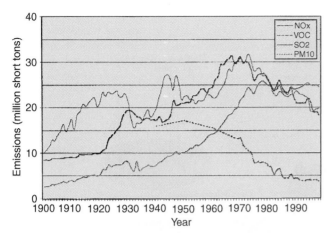

Figure 28-6. Emission trend for volatile organic compounds (VOC), nitrogen oxides (NO$_x$), sulfur dioxide (SO$_2$), and particulate matter (PM < 10 µm) from 1900 (or when records began) to 1998.

Note that since the passage of the Clean Air Act of 1970, most emissions have decreased or, in the case of nitrogen oxides, have leveled off (Reproduced from National Air Pollutant Emission Trends Report, 1998).

imbalances, heart disease, as well as its sensitivity to lung injury from inhalants (Kodavanti *et al.*, 2005). The curious are directed to the rapidly evolving literature in this area of research.

Air Pollution: Sources and Personal Exposure

In terms of tons of anthropogenic material emitted annually in the United States (as of 2002), five major air pollutants account for 98% of pollution: CO (112 thousand tons), SO$_2$ (15.3 thousand tons), volatile organic compounds (VOCs; 16.5 thousand tons), PM (6.8 thousand tons), and NO$_x$ (21.1 thousand tons). The remainder consists of Pb, which is down >98% since 1973, when phase-out from gasoline began, and a myriad of other compounds considered under the category of HAPs. On a national basis, aggregate emissions since 1970 have been cut 48%, while at the same time the U.S. Gross National Product (GNP) has increased 164%. Energy consumption has increased 42%, and vehicle miles driven have increased 155% (National Air Quality and Emissions Trends Report, 2003). The changing profile of pollutant emissions since 1900 is reflected in Fig. 28-6. Since 1993, air quality has generally continued to improve with reductions in ambient SO$_2$ being largest (−39%) but with O$_3$ changing the least, if at all. Obviously, for any specific locality, air quality can vary depending on the emission profiles of local sources, geographic topography, and meteorology. In the vicinity of a smelter for example, SO$_2$, metals, and/or PM may dominate the pollutant profile, while a refinery air shed might be dominated by VOCs and other carbonaceous products. In suburban areas, where the automobile is the main source of pollution, CO, VOCs, and NO$_2$ would prevail along with their primary photochemical product, O$_3$. NO$_x$ releases (including NO$_2$) by stationary sources also contribute to the local O$_3$ levels along with that derived secondarily from auto emissions. In all, about 146 million people in the United States live in counties that have violations of the NAAQS designed to minimize risks to the criteria pollutants.

The Evolving Profile of Air Pollution   Classically, air pollution has been distinguished on the basis of the chemical redox nature of its primary components. Dickens's eighteenth-century "London's

particular," was characterized by SO$_2$ and smoke from incomplete combustion of coal accumulated during an inversion as a chilled, acidic fog. This acidic mix reacts with surfaces, corroding metal and eroding masonry, characteristic of reductive chemistry. Historically, reducing-type atmospheres have been associated with smelting and related combustion-based industries (as along the Meuse River in 1930 and Donora, Pennsylvania, in 1948) as well as large, coal-based urban centers such as London (1952) and New York (1962). In contrast, Los Angeles has always had a characteristically "oxidant-type" pollution consisting of NO$_x$ and many secondary photochemical oxidants, such as O$_3$, aldehydes, and electron-hungry hydrocarbon radicals. Los Angeles uniquely traps auto emissions by virtue of regional topography and summer meterology, while other areas, such as Atlanta, have stagnant summer air.

The classic types of air pollution were implicitly seasonal. Reducing air pollution occurred during winter periods of oil and coal combustion and meteorological inversions, while the oxidant atmospheres occurred during the summertime, when sunlight is most intense and can catalyze reactions among the constituents of auto exhaust. Today the distinction between reducing and oxidant smogs is largely academic. Most urban areas have virtually eliminated smoky, sulfurous emissions but now have a proliferation of automobiles that contribute tons of oxidant precursors into the air. However, in the Midwest there remains heavy industry that continues to emit SO$_2$, albeit much less than decades ago. These emissions undergo complex cloud chemistry to form sulfate that disperses regionally – hence the term, regional haze. Metropolitan areas in the eastern half of the United States, now have atmospheres comprising regional reducing pollutants as well as local oxidant pollutants. Sulfates may still predominate over nitrates in the air, in contrast to the Southwest United States, but no longer is the Northeastern air pollution simply a sulfur-based problem. Not only has the composition of the haze changed, but the chemistry has affected it temporal patterns. Long extended periods of O$_3$ now prevail rather than the prototypic spike patter of Los Angeles (although challenged by Houston for the number-one spot in 1999.

Outside the U.S., however, many megacities remain plagued by the classic forms of air pollution. For example, uncontrolled industrial emissions surrounding cities like Beijing and the northern sectors of Mexico City are dominated by oil, coal, and industrial emissions, whereas southern Mexico City, Santiago, and Tokyo have substantially (but not so exclusively) automobile-derived oxidant smogs. As noted above, air pollution is a worldwide problem, where the estimate of people exposed to O$_3$ at potentially harmful levels exceeds 480 million (Schwela, 1996), with WHO estimates of PM-related mortality at 500 thousand per year.

Indoor Versus Outdoor Air Pollution   People in the United States (and in most industrialized nations) spend in excess of 80% of their time indoors at work, at school, and at home or between these places in an automobile (Robinson and Nelson, 1995). Generally, the time spent indoors is disproportionately higher for adults, who have relatively less time to participate in outdoor activities, especially during the day, when outdoor pollutants are usually at their highest levels. Children and outdoor workers, by contrast, are much more likely to encounter outdoor air pollution at its worst; in fact, because of the relatively high activity levels of these subgroups compared with inactive office workers, their lungs may incur a considerably larger dose of any given pollutant. Thus, whereas it is important to characterize and track pollution levels in outdoor air, the most

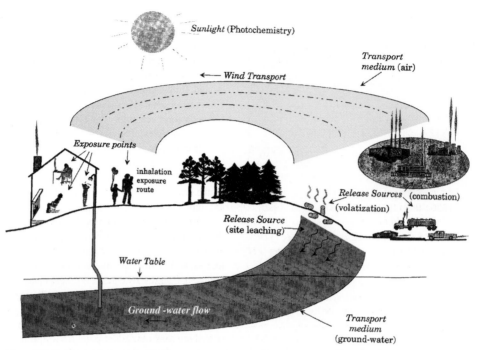

Figure 28-7. Illustration of contributors to the total personal exposure paradigm showing how these indoor and outdoor factors interact.

appropriate measure for exposure should involve a paradigm that addresses the total personal exposure of the individual or group of concern, and taken one step further, also dose to the lungs. However, defining typical paradigms of personal exposure can be extremely difficult, as personal monitoring is tedious, expensive, and complex. Outdoor pollutants can be encountered, with total exposure being influence by the personal dynamics and lifestyle of the individual. Individual monitoring is often expensive and difficult, so whenever possible, groups of people are monitored to develop models to estimate more specific exposure values.

The indoor environment has gained appreciation as a major contributor to total personal exposure. The energy crisis of the 1970s spurred efforts to increase home and building insulation, reduce infiltration of outside air, and minimize energy consumption. At the same time, indoor sources of air contaminants have been on the rise from household products and furnishings, which—when combined with poorly ventilated heating systems and overall reductions in air-exchange rates—give rise to potentially unhealthy indoor air environments. As people began to notice patterns of odors, microbiologic growth, and even ill health, measures of indoor air became a significant part of environmental assessment. Personal exposure has, therefore, come to include the myriad of potential sources, both outdoors and indoors.

It is clear now that indoor air can at times be more complex than outdoor air. The national monitoring network for the criteria pollutants has been shown to reflect human exposure reasonably well for some pollutants. Indeed, outdoor air permeates the indoor environment in spite of the reduced air exchange in most buildings. However, many variables determine how well components of the outdoor air infiltrate. The current evidence suggests that the average insulated home has about one air change per hour, resulting in indoor concentrations of pollutants that range from 30 to 80% of those outdoors. For nonreactive gases (e.g., CO), there could likely be nearly a 1:1 indoor/outdoor ratio in the absence of a "sink" for that gas;

the ratio for fine PM (<2.5 μm) could also be fairly high ($\sim$0.4–0.7), because these particles can easily penetrate through cracks and open spaces. In contrast, the indoor/outdoor ratio of O_3 would likely be low (<0.3) because of its reactivity. Obviously, household differences in the use of window ventilation and air conditioning would be important variables. Where there are independent sources of contamination indoors, the ratio of an indoor pollutant to that outdoors can even exceed 1 (e.g., NO_2). Particles and gases from tobacco smoke, unvented space heaters and poorly vented fireplaces and wood stoves as well as fresh paint and cleaning agents can be significant indoor sources. However, attention now is being directed toward the many and varied insidious sources of indoor contaminants: certain soils and construction masonry (radon), gas cooking appliances (NO_x), sidestream tobacco smoke (PM, CO, and a host of carcinogenic polyaromatics), and carpets, furnishings, dry-cleaned clothes, and household air fresheners (VOCs). Some of these chemicals can even interact with one another as has been found to occur with O_3 diffused indoors reacting with VOCs emitted from household cleaners. The complexity of these multiple sources underscores the importance of appreciating the total exposure scenario if we are to understand the nature of air pollution and its potential effects on human health (Fig. 28-7).

EPIDEMIOLOGIC EVIDENCE OF HEALTH EFFECTS

Outdoor Air Pollution

Acute and Episodic Exposures A number of air pollution incidents have been documented where concentrations of contaminants have risen to levels that are clearly hazardous to human health. When a single chemical has been accidentally released (e.g., methyl isocyanate in Bhopal, India), establishing the relationship between cause and ill effect is straightforward. However, most air pollution situations involve complex atmospheres, and establishing a specific cause other than the air pollution incident itself can be difficult. Three acute episodes of community air pollution are considered classic (Meuse Valley, Belgium; Donora, Pennsylvania; and London, United Kingdom). In each event, community inhabitants were clearly affected adversely; hospitalizations were concomitant with an elevated mortality rate. In each case, a meteorological inversion (cold air capped above by a blanket of warm air, with little or no vertical air mixing) prevailed for 3 or 5 days, during which time the concentration of pollutants rose well above the normal levels for these already heavily polluted areas. No actual measurements of pollution were made in the Meuse Valley and Donora, but crude measurements of the London fog recorded daily averages of smoke and SO_2. These were estimated at 4.5 mg/m^3 and 1.34 ppm, respectively, on the worst day. Brief (on the order of hours) peak concentrations probably reached even higher levels. During the Meuse Valley episode, 65 people died, while in Donora the number was 20. These deaths were considered "excess" deaths when compared with normal mortality rates for that time of year.

The famous "London smog" of 1952 is estimated to have resulted in 4000 excess deaths during the event itself. Hospital admissions increased dramatically, mainly among the elderly and those with preexisting cardiac and/or respiratory disease. Even otherwise healthy pedestrians, their visibility limited to as little as 3 ft, covered their noses and mouths in an attempt to minimize their exposure to the "choking" air. Many reports of sudden death were reported among workers commuting on bicycle or on foot with symptoms described as "choking." People with preexisting cardiac and lung problems were particularly affected. It is ironic that 16 years earlier, shortly after the Meuse Valley episode that 3200 deaths would occur should an analogous smog episode occur in London (Firkert, 1936). Although the London 1952 incident brought the issue of air pollution to the public consciousness, many additional episodes occurred, with the 1956 and 1962 incidents being among the most notable. Interestingly, in December 1991, London experienced a winter inversion smog-alert, but one with a very different pollutant profile: NO_2 at 423 ppb, black smoke at 148 µg/m^3, and SO_2 at 72 ppb (five, four times and twice the seasonal average, respectively). The difference between this episode and previous episodes were that the air pollution was not of the same magnitude and was largely vehicular and not the result of domestic coal burning (Anderson, 1999). Mortality and hospital admissions were difficult to discern overall, but regional comparisons suggested impacts among the elderly and cardiopulmonary-impaired (mortality: ↑14% cardiovascular and ↑22% respiratory; ↑43% for respiratory admissions). The component (and source) of the smog responsible was not clear, but overall the effects were of lesser magnitude than might have been expected.

London has not been alone among industrialized cities significantly affected by air pollution episodes in the more recent past. New York City, Steubenville, Ohio; Pittsburgh, Pennsylvania; Athens, Greece, and entire regions of Western Europe from the Netherlands to the Ruhr Valley of Germany have all had air pollution episodes of note between 1970 and 1995. While major episodes of anthropogenic air pollution continue to decrease over time in the modern world, both in their frequency and intensity, one should be aware of more "natural" events like the vegetation/forest fires of Indonesia of 1997 and 1998 can have significant impacts on air quality and health of the exposed populations. Even the forest fires of the Northwest United States in 2003 could be tracked as the plumes dispersed across the country.

So much has the air improved from the 1960s into the 1970s that many thought that the problem of sulfur-based industrial pollution was on its way to full resolution. Smokes were less visible and the air epidemiology of the times showed little health impact. However, in the late 1980s, there were revelations regarding acidic particle pollution of lakes and defoliation of forests (Calvert et al., 1985). There were also new studies showing increased emergency room visits among potentially susceptible populations—e.g., asthmatics (Bates and Sizto, 1987). A series of studies showed acute effects of regional summer haze in areas of central and Northeastern North America. These 2–3 day episodes of haze were typified by increases in O_3 and acid and neutralized (ammonium) sulfates, characteristic of the new generation of pollution in most U.S. urban areas. Interestingly, the apparent combined temporal or sequential patterns of O_3 and sulfate were associated with the health effects, but neither constituent seemed to be acting alone. Similar results were reported for the upstate New York area as well (Thurston et al., 1992), but the acidity as [H$^+$] of the haze was thought to play a more dominant role. Studies of children at summer camps, where children are active and outdoors most of the day, had reported decrements in daily measured pulmonary function on days of haze when both O_3 and acidity levels were elevated. The responses appeared to exceed those predicted by chamber studies of O_3 alone suggesting dose differences or interactions between haze components (Lippmann, 1989). Clinical studies in adolescent asthmatics and animal studies have lent further support to the belief that H$^+$ can affect airway function, particularly in the presence of O_3. Studies in the South and Southwest similarly have found effects in young asthmatics, but these appear to relate more specifically to O_3, because sulfate is less prominent in the ambient air. Early data from the Los Angeles area showed strong correlation between diminished performance among high school athletes and increased oxidant levels.

Of the many air pollution studies over the last 10–15 years, none has had more impact on the perception of pollutant risk and the direction of research today than a series of epidemiological studies that have shown association between PM and daily mortality. These studies were a novel application of time-series analyses of human health data records linked to regional air monitoring data. These studies showed significant and consistent associations between health outcomes of ambient PM at levels previously thought to be safe. Prior to this period, measurable effects of PM and SO_2 were not easily detected below the 24-hour means for smoke and SO_2—250 µg/m^3 and 0.19 ppm, respectively. In fact, the new findings showed effects, as evidenced by increases in mortality and morbidity rates at or below contemporaneous NAAQS levels [1987: 50 µg/m^3, annual mean; 150 µg/m^3 daily maximum for PM of diameter <10 µm (PM$_{10}$)]. Time-series analyses are based on Poisson regression modeling to distinguish changes in daily death counts associated with short-term changes in PM air pollution. The studies initially found effects with cruder measures of PM—total particulate material, which includes virtually all particles <35 µm in mass median aerodynamic diameter (MMAD—a median particle size normalizing the particle to unit density and spherical shape for aerodynamic comparison). These studies were followed with stronger associations with particles considered almost fully inhalable—PM$_{10}$ (an MMAD at which PM is aerodynamically separated at an initial 50% efficiency at 10 µm and increasingly at smaller sizes). Most recently, even stronger associations have been found with an analogous but fully and deeply respirable particle—PM$_{2.5}$. As the PM gets smaller, it better represents anthropogenic sources of pollution. The statistical methodology applied in these studies had an

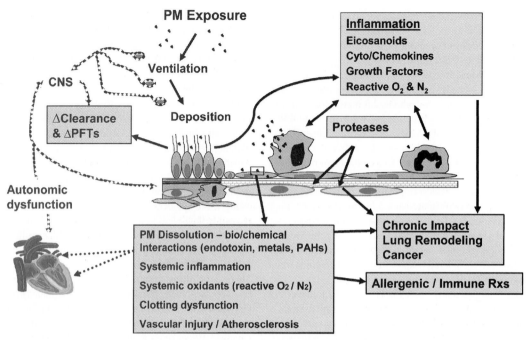

Figure 28-8. Schematic of the multiple mechanisms thought to function in cardiopulmonary response(s) to air pollutants—derived from current hypothesized mechanisms for particulate matter.

advantage over conventional regression analyses in that it could detect short-term trends and minimized the effects of other pollutants and potential confounders with longer time constants (Schwartz, 1991; reviewed by Pope and Dockery, 2006).

In contrast to the three epidemiologic studies used to develop the 1987 PM_{10} NAAQS, there were more than thirty studies for the 1997 revision and the promulgation of the new index, $PM_{2.5}$ NAAQS [15 $\mu g/m^3$, annual mean; 65 $\mu g/m^3$ daily maximum for PM of diameter <2.5 μm ($PM_{2.5}$)]. These studies showed a significant health impact of PM, linked to mass and not necessarily sulfate or any other constituent. In 2006, the PM NAAQS is again under review. More than 100 short- and long-term time-series studies have been considered, along with three major and several lesser long term cohort studies have been considered (USEPA, 2004).

The major health outcome uncovered in the study of PM is the involvement of the heart. Whereas the heart, as part of the cardiopulmonary system, has always held an indirect role in health impacts or disease from air pollution, both epidemiological and toxicological studies pointed to major cardiac involvement. Current thinking is that cardiac-mediated effects are more germane to the PM-associated mortality findings than pulmonary effects, although this concept remains under debate. Not surprisingly, effects are most apparent in subpopulations already compromised by cardiopulmonary and perhaps vascular diseases (e.g., diabetes). There exists no one generally accepted mechanism or mode of action to account for these findings (Schwartz, 1994; Costa, 2000). However, several pathways have been proposed that attempt to link exposure and cardiac effects that may or may not include pulmonary mediation. These potential mechanisms are illustrated in Fig. 28-8.

From a toxicological perspective, it has been difficult to accept that the association between particles and health outcomes is not somehow linked to PM composition rather than mass alone. The linkage to mass and not composition is counterintuitive, especially in light of the fact that all PM is not constitutively identical. The actual "biochemical lesion" caused by PM is generally thought to involve oxidant mechanisms (generation of reactive oxygen and perhaps nitrogen species) by constituents or attributes (reactive surface area) of the particles at the cell or molecular level. Initially, there was a credibility hurdle (biologically plausibility) that day-to-day fluctuations in the mass concentration of ~10 $\mu g/m^3$ airborne PM result in an increase of about 0.6–1% (excess) mortality. However, there now exist several plausible hypotheses that have some degree of empirical support: metals, organics, size difference, stable oxidants to name those most prominent. In addition to mortality, morbidity (in terms of hospital visits, inhaler use by asthmatics, and school absenteeism) has also been associated with ambient PM levels; other factors such as temperature, humidity, O_3, SO_2, and other pollutants per se do not explain the observed effects. Generally speaking, the consistency of the phenomenon from one geographic site to another and over time is remarkable (Pope and Dockery, 2006). Even revisiting the mortality data from the 1952 London incident demonstrates that PM was likely the pollutant of most prominence in terms of the adverse health consequences back almost 50 years (Schwartz and Marcus, 1990).

The direction and design of hybrid clinical-epidemiology studies today, frequently referred to as panel studies, are largely person-based, where groups of people are studied (e.g., nursing home residents, schoolchildren) in their immediate environment using non-invasive or minimally invasive clinical tools (e.g., pulmonary or cardiac function, symptoms, blood screenings, genomic profiles, etc.) to correlate effects with ambient and/or personal environmental and air pollutant measures. These studies sacrifice the power of large group numbers for more direct and individual data and controlled estimation of exposure and effect in an attempt to link biomarkers with exposure. These novel approaches have the promise of eventually offering clues as to causality, which is not possible with conventional epidemiology, and recent studies are showing increasingly more subtle changes in cardiopulmonary function with exposure to very modest air pollution.

Long-Term Exposures Epidemiologic studies of the chronic effects of air pollution are difficult to conduct by the very nature of the goal: outcomes associated with long-term exposures. Looking back in time with retrospective, cross-sectional studies is a common approach, but one frequently confounded with unknown variables and inadequate historical exposure data. A good example of the problem of confounding is cigarette smoking. Without extensive control of both active and passive smoking, the ability to discern the impact of an air pollution disease outcome, such as chronic bronchitis and emphysema, would be greatly impaired because of the high background of disease attributable to smoking and the imprecision of most indices of smoking exposure. In contrast, prospective studies have the advantage of more precise control of confounding variables, such as the tracking of urinary cotinine as an index of tobacco smoke exposure, but they can be very expensive and require substantial time and dedication on both the part of the investigators as well as the study population. Depending on the study size and design, exposure assessments can be complex, and the loss of subjects due to dropout is sometimes unpredictable.

Despite these deficiencies and problems, there are both retrospective and prospective epidemiology studies that have tackled the issue of long-term air pollution health effects. In general, these studies have suggested a positive association between urban pollution and progressive pulmonary impairments. On the one hand, cross-sectional studies in the Los Angeles Air Basin have found evidence of accelerated "aging-like" loss of lung function in people living for extended periods in regions of high oxidant pollution when compared with areas where sea air circulation lowers overall pollutant concentrations (Detels et al., 1991). Similarly, exposure to SO_2 and PM in the Netherlands over a 12-year period was shown prospectively to gradually impair lung function (Van De Lende et al., 1981). And even rural areas in western Pennsylvania, which are swept by reducing-type pollutants transported from Midwestern industrial centers, have been shown to have a higher incidence of respiratory symptoms as determined from a questionnaire-based design (Schenker et al., 1983). Whereas the role of any specific pollutant in these studies is difficult to dissect, the message that air pollution contributes to deterioration of lung health seems clear.

Among the most detailed prospective epidemiologic studies of chronic health effects across a range of levels of air pollution has been the so-called Harvard Six Cities Study begun in the early 1970s. The cities were chosen to represent a range of air quality based on SO_2 and PM. Initially, there was great dependence on routine regional air-monitoring data, but over time the investigators themselves conducted the air analyses of exposure microenvironments (local and indoor). The initial design of these studies included the gathering of parental questionnaire data (including some 20,000 people) about the prevalence of respiratory problems in schoolchildren and has continued over twenty years along with periodic assessments of pulmonary function. When compared across cities, [H$^+$] (measured in four of the six cities) was correlated (Fig. 28-9A) better than was sulfate with the prevalence of bronchitis in children age 10–12 years (Speizer, 1989). However, as the assessment program evolved, a more detailed study revealed mortality associations with PM as represented in Fig. 28-9B through D. However, the role of [H$^+$] in relation with acute mortality was less convincing than that associated with the sulfate or fine (≤ 2.5 μm) PM (sulfates co-associate with fine PM in the atmosphere) (Dockery et al., 1993). More importantly with regard to long-term health, this study showed very significant effects of PM on the life spans of people living in Steubenville, Ohio—the dirtiest of the industrial centers.

Over a 15-year period, the average human life span was reduced by about 2 years due to PM exposure. These findings were corroborated by a prospective cohort-based mortality study using a database collected on over 500 thousand people by the American Cancer Society (ACS) across 151 cities from 1982 to 1989 (Pope et al., 1995). The study showed a 15–17% increased mortality risk over 7 years due to PM, about equivalent to the risk of smoking over that period. Subsequently, Pope et al. (2002) reported results of a 10-year follow-up study of the ACS cohort. This updated analysis, which included gaseous co-pollutant and new fine-particle measurements, and more comprehensive personal information on the enrollees, confirmed the linkage of health effects, including a small risk of lung cancer, with $PM_{2.5}$ exposures. These findings reinforce the concerns for potential chronic health impacts of PM and the heightened risk of premature death from lifelong air pollution exposure. There is currently a 10-year study (results expected ~2015) to assess the impact of air pollution, with emphasis on PM, on atherosclerosis in humans as part of the MESA AIR (Multi Ethnic Study of Atherosclerosis Air Pollution—http://depts.washington.edu/mesaair/).

The role of air pollution in human lung cancer is difficult to assess because the vast majority of respiratory cancers result from cigarette smoking. The ACS study noted above for particles showed a linkage between air pollution particles and lung cancer, but in general it has been difficult to show these effects for the many HAP compounds that occur as urban air pollutants that are thought to be carcinogenic. However, most of the HAPs and even fewer (about 10%) of the more than 2800 compounds that have been identified in the air have been assayed for carcinogenic potency. Figure 28-10 gives estimates of the relative contributions of various chemicals to the lung cancer rate that is *not* associated with cigarette smoking, which, for outdoor air, is estimated to be about 2000 cases per year (Lewtas, 1993). This compares with about 2000 cases per year for passive environmental tobacco smoke and >100,000 cases per year for smokers. Volatile organic compounds (VOCs) and nitrogen-containing and halogenated organics account for most of the compounds that have been studied with animal and genetic bioassays. Most of these compounds are derived from combustion sources ranging from tobacco to power plants to incinerators. Other potential carcinogens arise from mobile sources as products of incomplete combustion and their atmospheric transformation products as well as fugitive or accidental chemical releases. This profile of carcinogens contrasts with that of indoor air, where the sources are thought to derive largely from environmental tobacco smoke and radon, with some contribution from the off-gassed organics (e.g., adhesives, carpet polymers).

The cancer risk of any individual should be some function of the carcinogenic nature of the substance, the amount of material deposited, which is itself a function of the concentration in the ambient air and the cumulative volume inhaled. Of course the innate susceptibility of the individual (including genotype and environmental factors such as diet, etc.) can also be important. A significant body of data suggests that the majority of cancer risk from ambient air pollution lies within the PM fraction. Among the many potent chemicals are the polycyclic organic chemicals, along with a group of less-volatile organics sometimes referred to as "semivolatiles" (including nitroaromatics). These persistent organics associate with the particulate matrix and thus could have a prolonged residence time at deposition sites within the respiratory tract. Genetic bioassays have revealed the potent mutagenicity, and presumably carcinogenicity, of various chemical fractions of ambient aerosols (Lewtas, 1993). Some of these compounds require metabolic transformation

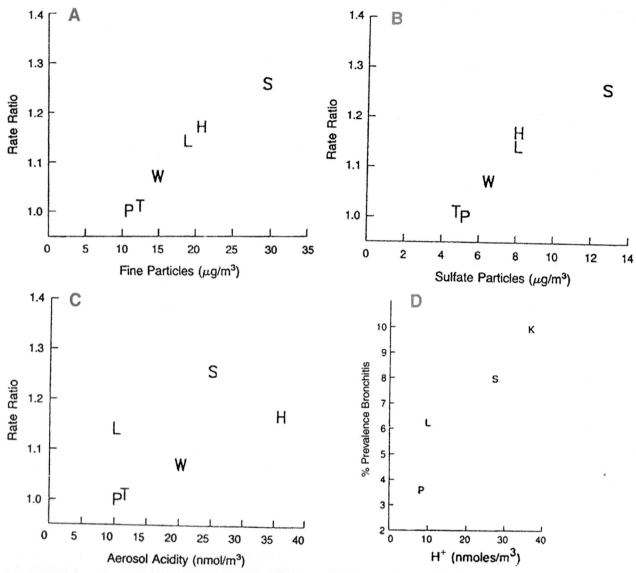

Figure 28-9. *Data from the Harvard Six Cities Study indicating the superior relationship of PM₁₀ and sulfate to mortality rates (A–C) in contrast to acidity (D), which correlates better with the prevalence of bronchitis in children [Reproduced with permission from Speizer, 1989 (D) and Dockery et al., 1993 (A–C)].*

to activate their potency whereas others may be detoxified by their metabolism.

The cells lining the respiratory tract turn over relatively quickly, because they continuously interface with the ambient environment. Conceptually, their DNA would thus be vulnerable to carcinogenic or oxidant-induced replication errors that, when fixed as mutations, could be tumorigenic. Co-pollutants, such as irritant gases, that initiate inflammation may promote carcinogenic activity by damaging cells and further enhancing their turnover. For example, there is experimental evidence that benzo(a)pyrene inhaled by rats whose respiratory tracts have been chronically exposed to SO₂ are prone to bronchogenic carcinomas. Likewise, epidermoid carcinomas were produced in mice that inhaled ozonized gasoline vapors, containing many reactive organic products, but only if these mice had been previously infected with influenza virus and presumably had inflamed lungs. Many suspect that the so-called rural–urban gradient of lung cancer, apparent even when corrected for cigarette smoking,

is a product of these complex interactions. Thus, while the phenomenon of environmental lung cancer remains poorly understood, there is general sentiment for the early opinion expressed by Kotin and Falk in 1963: "Chemical, physical and biological data unite to form a constellation that strongly implicates the atmosphere as one dominant factor in the pathogenesis of lung cancer." At the time of this statement, however, the role of tobacco smoke was not widely appreciated.

Indoor Air Pollution

As outdoor air quality has improved over the last 35 years, there has been a growing awareness of the potential for indoor air pollution to elicit adverse health effects. The concerns about indoor air that at first brought skepticism have gained an element of respectability as various attributes of the indoor environment and its effect on health and well-being have been investigated. However, the issue

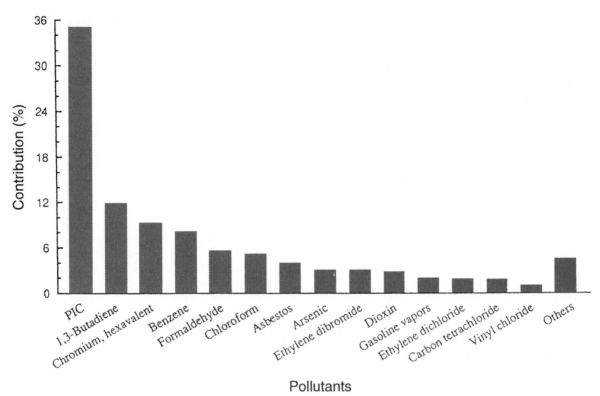

Figure 28-10. Relative contribution of individual airborne hazardous pollutants to lung cancer rates after removal of tobacco smoke cancer.

The total number of cancers from nontobacco-smoke sources is estimated to be about 2000 per year. (Reproduced with permission from Lewtas, 1993). PIC = products of incomplete combustion.

remains controversial because many of the health problems associated with indoor air pollution generally involve nonspecific symptomatology and appears to involve a wide range of potential toxicants and sources (Molhave *et al.*, 1986). The responses to indoor air pollution also appear to be affected by ambient comfort factors such as temperature and humidity. Two broadly defined illnesses that are largely unique to the indoor environment are discussed below (Brooks and Davis, 1992).

Sick-Building Syndromes   This collection of ailments, defined by a set of persistent symptoms enduring at least 2 weeks (Table 28-3), occurs in at least 20% of those exposed and is typically of unknown specific etiology, but is relieved sometime after an affected individual leaves the offending building (Hayes *et al.*, 1995). Frequently but not always, this syndrome occurs in new, poorly ventilated, or recently refurbished office buildings. The suspected causes include combustion products, household chemicals, biological materials and vapors, and emissions from furnishings; they are exacerbated by the effect of poor ventilation on comfort factors. The perception of irritancy to the eyes, nose, and throat ranks among the predominant symptoms that can become intolerable with repeated exposures. Controlled clinical studies have shown concentration- and duration-dependent worsening of sensory discomfort after exposure to a complex mixture of 22 VOCs commonly found in the indoor environment (Molhave *et al.*, 1986). The many factors contributing to such responses are poorly understood but include various host susceptibility factors, such as personal stress and fatigue, diet and alcohol use. Current biomarkers of response used in the

Table 28-3

Symptoms Commonly Associated with the Sick-Building Syndromes

Eyes, nose, and throat irritation
Headaches
Fatigue
Reduced attention span
Irritability
Nasal congestion
Difficulty in breathing
Nosebleeds
Dry skin
Nausea

SOURCE: Data modified from Brooks and Davis, 1992.

laboratory include sensory irritancy to the eyes in volunteer test subjects and sometimes in animals. However, in general, animal studies using standard measures of sensory irritation or other corporal endpoints have had limited success in assessing sick-building syndromes (SBS) and related syndromes. The biggest problem generally lies in the VOC concentrations required to achieve responses in a limited pool of animals that relate to unique human scenaios is too high to establish a plausible link to the human condition.

Building-Related Illnesses   This group of illnesses, in contrast to the SBS, consists of well-documented conditions with defined diagnostic criteria and generally recognizable etiology. These illnesses typically call for a conventional medical treatment strategies, because simply exiting the building where the illness was contracted may not readily reverse the symptoms. Several biocontaminant-related illnesses (e.g., legionnaires' disease, hypersensitivity pneumonitis, humidifier fever) fall into this group, as do allergies to animal dander, dust mites, and cockroaches. Medical treatment and mitigation of exposure (source elimination or personal protection) are generally needed to abate symptoms. Some outdoor pollutants can also be problematic indoors—most notably, CO from poorly vented heaters. Indoor exposures to NO_2 can pose problems as well, especially in people who may be sensitive—such as asthmatics. At times, however, when the concentrations of CO, NO_2, and many VOCs (passively emitted from new furniture or rugs, or from molds in the ventilation system) result in less discernible or definable signs and symptoms, the responses may be misdiagnosed as SBS, which can complicate assessment of the situation.

It should be noted that many inhalants, such as NO_2 and trichloroethylene (a VOC common to the indoor air arising from chlorinated water or dry-cleaned clothes), have been shown in animal toxicology studies to suppress immune defenses and allow opportunistic pathogens to proliferate in the lung. The involvement of immunologic suppression is a particularly controversial, yet an important attribute of indoor pollution because of its insidious nature and its implications for all building-related illnesses. This problem is further complicated in that complex indoor environments comprising of chemicals and biologicals (dust mites, fungi, molds etc.) may also lead to in unexpected interactions that remain virtually unstudied and thus are underappreciated in the assessment of indoor pollution.

POLLUTANTS OF OUTDOOR AMBIENT AIR

Classic Reducing-Type Air Pollution

The acute air pollution episodes of this century have made it clear that high concentrations of the reducing-type air pollution, characterized by SO_2 and smoke, are capable of producing dramatic human health effects. Empirical studies in human subjects and animals have long stressed the irritancy of SO_2 and its role in these incidents, while the full potential for interactions among the co-pollutants in the smoky, sulfurous mix has a mixed record of replication in the human exposure laboratory. Nevertheless, the irritancy of most S-oxidation products in the atmosphere is well documented, and there are both empirical and theoretical reasons to suspect that such products act to amplify the irritancy of fossil fuel emission atmospheres via chemical transformation. Because of its history, SO_2 is often thought of as the prototypic air pollutant of the industrial age. It is an irritant gas that has a toxicology of its own and, through atmospheric reactions, can transform into sulfites or sulfates within an irritant particle. As such it has a detailed literature base and while current levels of SO_2 in the ambient air of United States is less a threat than 30 years ago, it stands to demonstrate the role of toxicology in moving regulation to bring this contaminant under ever-increasing control.

Sulfur Dioxide

General Toxicology   Sulfur dioxide is a water-soluble irritant gas. As such, it is absorbed predominantly in the upper airways. It is a sensory irritant and can stimulate bronchoconstriction and mucus secretion in a number of species, including humans. Early studies

with relatively high exposure concentrations of SO_2 showed airway cellular injury and subsequent proliferation of mucus-secreting goblet cells. This attribute of SO_2 has led to its use (>250 ppm) in the production of laboratory animal models of bronchitis and airway injury (Kodavanti *et al.*, 2000). At much lower concentrations (<1 ppm), such as might be encountered in the polluted ambient air of industrialized areas, long-term residents experience a higher incidence of bronchitis. In fact, prior to the breakup of the Soviet block, many eastern European cities were renowned for widespread public affliction with bronchitis; now, 20 years later, the prevalence of bronchitis is greatly reduced (von Mutius *et al.*, 1994). While other factors (diet, access to health care, other pollutants) may well have been involved in this reversal, reductions in ambient smoke and SO_2 are generally thought to be most important.

The concentrations of SO_2 likely to be encountered in the United States are lower still—on average, considerably less than 0.1 ppm. Mandated use of cleaner (low-S) fossil fuels by industry as well as in diesel vehicles and emission control devices that scrub S have largely been responsible for the reductions (1970: 31,218 tons vs. 2005: 15,353 tons). Rare down-drafting of smokestack plumes due to meteorological inversions near point-sources may result in focal low-ppm levels of SO_2 that could pose a hazard to some individuals. A 2-minute exposure to 0.4–1.0 ppm can elicit bronchoconstriction in exercising asthmatics within 5–10 minutes (Gong *et al.*, 1995). However, concern remains that low-level, long-term erosion of pulmonary defenses may carry risk of reduced resistance to infection. Studies have shown that SO_2 is itself capable of impairing macrophage-dependent bacterial killing in murine models. Exposed mice have a greater frequency and severity of infection, which has been suggested to be linked to diminished ability to generate endogenous oxidants for bacterial killing. Analogously, rats exposed for 70–170 hours to 0.1, 1.0, and 20 ppm exhibited reduced clearance of inert particles, while dogs exposed to 1 ppm for a year had slowed tracheal mucocilliary transport. The fact that the low-concentration exposures showed marked effects when extended over longer periods is consistent with the epidemiologic associations between SO_2 exposure and bronchitis. The evidence is not clear, however, as some studies show no overt long-term pulmonary pathology. Guinea pigs and monkeys, for example, showed no effect on lung function or pathology after a year of continuous exposure to concentrations of 0.1–5 ppm (Alarie *et al.*, 1970, 1972).

The penetration of SO_2 into the lungs is greater during mouth as opposed to nose breathing. An increase in the airflow in deep rapid breathing augments penetration of the gas into the deeper lung. As a result, persons exercising would inhale more SO_2 and, as noted with asthmatics, are likely to experience greater irritation. Once deposited along the airway, SO_2 dissolves into surface lining fluid as sulfite or bisulfite and is readily distributed throughout the body. It is thought that the sulfite interacts with sensory receptors in the airways to initiate local and centrally mediated bronchoconstriction. Labeled $^{35}SO_2$ studies indicate, however, that some residual S (presumably as protein reaction products) persists in the respiratory system for a week or more after exposure, and is slowly excreted in the urine (Yokoyama *et al.*, 1971). In both rabbits and human subjects, sulfite that reaches the plasma has been shown to form *S*-sulfonate products of reaction with the disulfide bonds in plasma proteins (Gunnison and Palmes, 1974). The toxicological significance of *S*-sulfonate proteins is unknown, but they might serve as markers of exposure.

Pulmonary Function Effects   The basic pulmonary response to inhaled SO_2 is mild bronchoconstriction, which is reflected as a measurable increase in airflow resistance due to narrowing of the airways. Concentration-related increases in resistance have been observed in guinea pigs, dogs, and cats as well as humans. Exposure of isolated segments of the nose or airways of dogs and guinea pigs appeared to alter resistance in a manner consistent with receptor-mediated sensory stimulation. Airflow resistance increased more when the gas was introduced through a tracheal cannula than via the nose, since nasal scrubbing of the water-soluble gas was bypassed. Isolated nasal exposures increased nasal airflow resistance through the nose largely as a result of mucosal swelling, but the irritant effect appeared to signal to the more distal airways as well. Direct exposure of the trachea had a more dramatic effect on airflow resistance. Exposure of the intact nose also induced some response, consistent with the existence of a nasal neural network being involved in bronchoconstriction (Frank and Speizer, 1965; Nadel *et al.*, 1965). Intravenous injection of atropine (a parasympathetic receptor blocker) or cooling of the cervical vagosympathetic nerves abolishes bronchoconstriction in the cat model; rewarming of the nerve reestablishes the response. The rapidity of the response and its reversal emphasize the parasympathetic tonal change in airway smooth muscle. Studies in human subjects have confirmed the predominance of parasympathetic mediation, but histamine from inflammatory cells may play a secondary role in the bronchoconstrictive responses of asthmatics (Sheppard *et al.*, 1981).

Human subjects exposed to 1, 5, or 13 ppm SO_2 for just 10 minutes exhibit a rapid bronchoconstrictive response, with 1–3 ppm being a threshold for most if exercise is involved. Healthy individuals at rest seem to have a clear response at about 5 ppm, though there is considerable variation among individuals (Frank *et al.*, 1962). Even 0.25–1 ppm for a few hours can induce bronchoconstriction in adult and adolescent subjects with clinically defined mild asthma (Sheppard *et al.*, 1981; Koenig *et al.*, 1981). Findings such as these (responses <0.5 ppm) have raised concerns about potential adverse effects in this sensitive subpopulation when it is exposed to peaks of SO_2 that are known to occur near point sources.

Chronic Effects   Only a few long-term studies have been conducted with SO_2 at levels approaching those found in ambient air. Alarie *et al.* (1970) exposed guinea pigs to 0.13, 1.01, or 5.72 ppm SO_2 continuously for a year without adverse impact on lung mechanics. Similarly, monkeys exhibited no alteration in pulmonary function when exposed continuously for 78 weeks to 0.14, 0.64, and 1.28 ppm SO_2 (Alarie *et al.*, 1972). Even in the presence of 0.1 mg/m^3 sulfuric acid, dogs exposed 16 hours a day for 18 months to 0.5 ppm SO_2 showed no impairment in pulmonary function (Vaughan *et al.*, 1969). Higher levels of SO_2 for protracted periods of time [dogs to 5 ppm for 225 days (Lewis *et al.*, 1969); rats to 350 ppm for 30 days (Reid, 1963)] have been shown to alter airway mucus secretion, goblet cell topography, or lung function, but these results are of little relevance to typical SO_2 levels in ambient air.

Sulfuric Acid and Related Sulfates   The conversion of SO_2 to sulfate is favored in the environment with subsequent ammonia neutralization to ammonium sulfate [$(NH_4)_2SO_4$] or as ammonium bisulfate [NH_4HSO_4]. During oil and coal combustion or the smelting of metal ores, sulfuric acid condenses downstream of the combustion processes with available metal ions and water vapor to form submicron sulfuric acid fume and sulfated fly ash. Sulfur dioxide continues to oxidize to sulfate within dispersing smokestack plumes, which can be augmented by the presence of free soluble or partially coordinated transition metals such as iron, manganese, and vanadium within the effluent ash. When coal is burned, the acid may adsorb to the surface or solubilize in ultrafine (<0.1 μm) metal oxide particles during emission. These sulfates on the surface of coal ash may constitute as much as 9% of the emitted S—the rest is emitted as SO_2 gas. Photochemical reactions in the troposphere also promote acid sulfate formation via both metal-dependent and independent

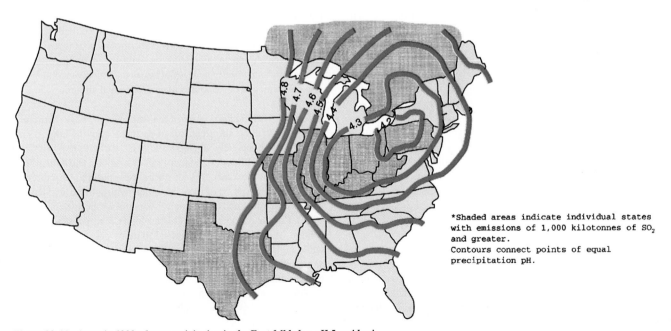

Figure 28-11.   Areas in 1988 where precipitation in the East fell below pH 5: acid rain.

*Shaded areas indicate individual states with emissions of 1,000 kilotonnes of SO_2 and greater.
Contours connect points of equal precipitation pH.

The acidity of the air in the east is thought to result from air mass transport of fine sulfated particulate matter from the industrial centers of the Midwest (National Air Pollutant Emission Trends Report, 1998).

mechanisms, but studies have shown that most of the oxidation of SO_2 occurs within plumes as they disperse in the atmosphere. Stack emissions may undergo long-range transport to areas distant from the emission source, allowing considerable time for sunlight-driven chemistry. Although the fine-particle sulfates may exist as fine sulfuric acid (the primary source of free H^+), partially or fully neutralized forms sulfate predominate, due to the abundance of natural atmospheric ammonia. As fine PM sulfates are transported long distances, they may contribute to regional summer haze and pose not only a health hazard to certain groups such as asthmatics (Koenig et al., 1989), and may also stress the general environment as acid rain (Calvert et al., 1985) (Fig. 28-11). The reduction of S emissions since the CAA and subsequent regulations (e.g., Acid Rain Program) have greatly curtailed the environmental acidification problems in North America associated with transport and deposition of acidic products formed from stack emissions. Western Europe has also made regulatory advances and similarly seen substantial recovery of acidified lakes and forest damage, although some of the Eastern Block countries continue to have problems.

General Toxicology   Sulfuric acid irritates by virtue of its ability to protonate (H^+) receptor ligands and other biomolecules. This action can either directly damage membranes or activate sensory reflexes that initiate inflammation. Ammonia, which exists in free air at about 25 ppb and in much higher concentrations within the mammalian naso-oropharynx (in the human up to 350 ppm), is capable of neutralizing most of the irritant acidic sulfates (Utell et al., 1989). The efficiency of this process is dependent on temperature, relative humidity, and air mixing and thus is a likely source of variability in biological responses. For this reason, most human test subjects rinse orally with citrus juice before a sulfuric acid study, so as to minimize this phenomenon. Neutralization can also be quite efficient in standard whole-body animal exposure-studies, in which excreta and bacteria in the chambers interact, giving rise to in-chamber ammonia concentrations up to 1100 ppb—more than enough to fully neutralize neat sulfuric acid up to several mg/m^3 (Higuchi and Davies, 1993).

Interestingly, there is considerable species variability in sensitivity to sulfuric acid, with guinea pigs being quite responsive to acid sulfates, in contrast to rats, which seem generally resistant. The reasons for this difference are not fully understood but relate to receptor type and their density in the airways, and probably not on differences in neutralization by ammonia in the airway. The sensitivity of healthy humans appears to fall somewhere in between, with asthmatic humans being perhaps best modeled by the guinea pig. Overall, however, the collective data involving animals and humans are remarkably coherent, as reviewed in an article by Amdur (1989). To illustrate this point, Table 28-4 compares the acute toxicity of SO_2 and sulfuric acid in animals and human subjects, using indices detailed below, airway resistance, and bronchial clearance. To allow direct comparisons, the concentrations are presented as μmol/m^3 of the two compounds.

Pulmonary Function Effects   Sulfuric acid produces an increase in flow resistance in guinea pigs due to reflex airway narrowing, or bronchoconstriction, which impedes the flow of air into and out of the lungs. This response might be thought of as a defensive measure to limit the inhalation of air containing noxious gases, but this explanation may be more teleological than fact. The magnitude of the response is related to both acid concentration and particle size (Amdur, 1958; Amdur et al., 1978). Early studies indicated that as particle size was reduced from 7 μm to the submicron range, the

concentration of sulfuric acid necessary to induce a response and the time to the onset of the response fell significantly. With large particles, even the sensitive guinea pig was able to withstand an exceedingly high (30 mg/m^3) challenge with little change in pulmonary resistance, in contrast to the <1 mg/m^3 challenge needed with the 0.3 μm particles (Amdur et al., 1978). Human asthmatics exposed to 2 mg/m^3 of acid fog (10 μm) for 1 hour, a very high concentration for an asthmatic, experienced variable respiratory symptoms suggesting irritation, but no changes in spirometry were elicited (Hackney et al., 1989). The apparent reason for this PM size-based differential is probably the scrubbing of large particles in the nose, while small particles are able to penetrate deep into the lung. The thicker mucus blanket of the nose may blunt (by dilution or neutralization by mucus buffers) much of the irritancy of the deposited acid, thus limiting its effects to mucous cell stimulation and a minor increase in nasal flow resistance. In contrast, the less shielded distal airway tissues, with higher receptor density, would be expected to be more sensitive to the acid particles reaching that area (Costa and Schlegele, 1998). Regional sensitivity and the longer residence times of a deposited particle relative to SO_2 gas is reflected in the relatively protracted recovery times observed in acid-exposed guinea pigs compared with animals exposed to SO_2 alone.

Asthmatics appear to be somewhat more sensitive to the bronchoconstrictive effects of sulfuric acid than are healthy individuals, but published studies have been inconsistent in this finding (Koenig et al., 1989; Utell et al., 1984). Asthma generally is characterized by hyperresponsive airways, so their tendency to constrict at low acid concentrations would be expected, just as asthmatic airways are sensitive to nonspecific airway smooth muscle agonists (e.g., carbachol, histamine, exercise) (Hanley et al., 1992). The variability may well relate to differences in the degree of impairment or underlying inflammation in the subjects, but this hypothesis remains to be confirmed. Airway hyperreactivity has been observed as an acute response in guinea pigs 2 hours after a 1 hour exposure to 200 μg/m^3 sulfuric acid, and appears to be associated with pulmonary inflammation. Likewise in rabbits, increased airway reactivity was associated with arachidonate metabolites, products of epithelial cells as well as inflammatory cells. The general correlation between airway responsiveness and inflammation that appears to be important in grading asthma severity and risk of negative clinical outcomes may also be predictive of responses to environmental stimuli.

Effects on Mucociliary Clearance and Macrophage Function Sulfuric acid alters the clearance of particles from the lung. Using insoluble, radioactively labeled ferric oxide particles as a probe, as little as a single 1 hour exposure in donkeys, rabbits, and human subjects can slow clearance. Mucus clearance appears to vary directly with the acidity ($[H^+]$) of the acid sulfate, with sulfuric acid having the greatest effect and ammonium sulfate the smallest (Schlesinger, 1984). Curiously, there appears to be a biphasic response to acid. In general, brief, single exposures of <250 μg/m^3 accelerate clearance, while high concentrations of >1000 μg/m^3 clearly depress clearance. With repeated daily exposures to low levels, there appears to be a cumulative (concentration times duration) dose-related depression of clearance. Longer-term exposure of rabbits to low-level acid also results in hyperplasia of airway mucosecretory cells (Gearhart and Schlesinger, 1989). Acidification of mucus by H^+ (i.e., a fall in pH), even if localized, is thought to have potential effects on mucus rheology and viscosity (Holma, 1989) as well as on mucus secretion and ciliary function. These effects are not unreasonable in light of

Table 28-4

Comparative Toxicity of SO$_2$ and H$_2$SO$_4$ in Acute Studies

	μmol		
	SO$_2$	H$_2$SO$_4$	REFERENCE
Guinea pigs: 1 h; 10% ↑ airway resistance	6	1	Amdur, 1974
Donkeys: 30 min; 1-h altered bronchial clearance			Spiegelman *et al.*, 1968
	8875	2	Schlesinger *et al.*, 1978
Normal subjects: 7 min; 1-h altered bronchial clearance			Lippmann and Altshuler, 1976
	520	1	Leikauf *et al.*, 1981
Normal subjects: 10 min; 5% ↓ tidal volume			
	29	1.25	Amdur, 1954
Adolescent asthmatics: 40 min; equal ↑ airway resistance			
	20	1	Koenig *et al.*, 1989

the drop in macrophage intracellular pH reported with acid exposure (Qu *et al.*, 1993).

Collectively, there seems to be coherence in the data to rank sulfate irritancy: sulfuric acid > ammonium bisulfate > ammonium sulfate. Acidity [H$^+$] appears to be the primary driver on most respiratory effects attributable to the acid sulfates even at the level of pulmonary macrophages. Lavaged rabbit macrophage phagocytosis was affected more after a single exposure to 500 μg/m^3 sulfuric acid than after 2000 μg/m^3 ammonium bisulfate (Schlesinger *et al.*, 1990). However, there is some evidence at the level of cellular activation that arachidonate metabolism might involve the anionic component of the aerosol as well. Nevertheless, in the complexity of summer haze, it remains unclear whether the bioactive form of [H$^+$] is more appropriately assayed as free ion concentration (as pH) or as total available ion concentration (titratable H$^+$).

Chronic Effects   Not surprisingly, sulfuric acid induces qualitatively similar effects in the airways as found at high concentrations of SO$_2$. As a fine aerosol, sulfuric acid deposits deeper along the respiratory tract, and its high specific acidity imparts greater effect on various cells (e.g., phagocytes and epithelial cells). Thus, a primary concern with regard to chronic inhalation of acidic aerosols is the potential for bronchitis, because this has been a problem in occupational settings in which employees are exposed to sulfuric acid mists (e.g., battery plants). Early studies in the donkey (later confirmed in a rabbit model) have provided fundamental data on this issue. The depression of clearance observed in donkeys exposed repeatedly (100 μg/m^3 1 hour per day for 6 months) raises concerns that a similar response (i.e., chronic bronchitis) can occur in humans. Studies with cigarette smoke showed parallel responses.

Studies conducted with sulfuric acid in the rabbit are in general agreement with the early findings in the donkey (Schlesinger *et al.*, 1979; Schlesinger, 1984). These studies have expanded our knowledge of the biological response and its exposure-based relationship. The initial early stimulation of clearance with subsequent depression has been shown to occur over 12 months with as little as 2 hour per day at 125 μg/m^3 sulfuric acid (Schlesinger *et al.*, 1992). Related studies also have demonstrated that the airways of exposed animals become progressively more sensitive to challenge with acetylcholine, showed a progressive decrease in diameter, and experienced an increase in the number of secretory cells, especially in the smaller airways (Gearhart and Schlesinger, 1989).

Unlike other irritants, such as O$_3$ (see below), inhaled sulfuric acid does not appear to stimulate a classic neutrophilic lung inflammation. Rather, eicosanoid homeostasis appears to be disturbed, resulting in macrophage dysfunction and altered host defense. Long-term disease attributable to connective tissue disturbances induced by sulfuric acid seems to be of lesser concern than is the impact on mucociliary function and the potential effect on ventilation and arterial oxygenation (Alarie *et al.*, 1972, 1975). Therefore, it seems reasonable to postulate that chronic daily exposure of humans to ∼100 μg/m^3 sulfuric acid may lead to impaired clearance and mild chronic bronchitis. As this is less than an order of magnitude above haze levels of sulfuric acid, the possibility that chronic irritancy may elicit bronchitis-like disease in susceptible individuals (perhaps over a lifetime or in children because of dose differences) appears to be reasonable.

Particulate Matter

Particulate matter was referred to as "soot" in the "reducing-type" air pollution of the classic episodes. The major constituents of this soot consisted of incompletely burned carbonaceous materials, acid sulfates, various metals, and silicates associated with the solid nature of the fuel. Metals were abundant, with a considerable amount of zinc in the form of zinc sulfate—as reported from post-episode analyses of the Donora PM. Soot is indicative of poorly (inefficiently) combusted fuel. Over time, combustion technology and improved fuels provided gains by increasing efficiency and minimization of gross soot emissions. Improvements in combustion methods simultaneously reduced the size of emitted particles and overall less mass. A side benefit of the smaller particles was the reduction in light diffraction through the emissions and hence a less visible plume. As such, much of the early clean-up was largely achieved through technological improvements. Carbon in fuel that is not fully oxidized to CO$_2$ persists in elemental form or as products of incomplete combustion—organic carbon. Oxidized S becomes sulfate and many of the metals appear as oxides. As noted above, sulfate was long suspected as the culprit of most health impacts associated with stationary sources, but this relationship is less discernable in contemporary particle epidemiology and toxicology.

In the last 15 years, PM has reemerged as the dominant issue in the air pollution community, overtaking O$_3$ as the pressing air pollution health issue. The reason for this shift was the emergence of epidemiology data repeatedly showing mortality, which is an adverse effect of greatest import with major impact on the cost/benefit analyses. As already noted the collective studies showed health impacts (both morbidity and mortality) at levels of PM thought to be "safe" with no apparent threshold (reviewed in Pope and Dockery, 2006). Over time, scientific advances and reanalyses have confirmed the initial mortality findings. Several hypotheses that lend "biologic plausibility" to the findings have emerged along with several "ancillary" impacts of PM on health not previously realized. Unlike any other air pollutant, PM and its demonstrable impact on mortality rates has kept this issue in the forefront of air pollution toxicology.

Particulate matter in the atmosphere can be solid, liquid, or a combination of both with a mélange of organic, inorganic, and biological compounds. The compositional matrix of PM can vary significantly depending on the emission source and secondary transformations, many of which involve gas to particle conversions. Long-range transport of emissions or transformation products can contribute significantly to the regional matrix of PM, particularly in the case of eastern sulfate of fine PM (<2.5-μm; $PM_{2.5}$). Particles of larger size tend to have more local sources being that they are formed from dispersed dust and attrition of materials. Being of larger size, they tend to "fall out" or settle from the air due to gravity (although winds can in fact carry these particles great distances—e.g., Sahara desert particles have been found on the U.S. east coast). Particles in the range of 10–2.5 μm ($PM_{10-2.5}$; coarse PM) are highly inhalable by humans. The size selection of fine and coarse particles is based on their relative respirability—those in the range of PM_{10} are inhalable into the larger thoracic airways, while the $PM_{2.5}$ is inhalable into the deeper reaches (gas exchange areas) of the lung (see Chap. 15).

The large epidemiologic database contending that PM elicits both short- and long-term health effects is largely founded on data from monitoring networks for PM regulation (Dockery and Pope, 2006). As such the PM-associated effects appear to be dependent on the gravimetric measures that these networks yield. From this, it might then be argued that the effects are not influenced by particle composition (e.g., inorganic and organic components). Further, because the findings strengthen with decreasing particle size (e.g., Total Suspended Particulate mass [pre-1978 index], PM_{10}, $PM_{2.5}$), it is the mass concentration of PM, despite compositional complexity and variation, that is the index of choice. However, toxicologists argue that a mass-based relationship contradicts the basic tenets of conventional air pollution toxicology, which is rooted in the concept of chemical-specific toxicities. A number of hypotheses that draw upon various physical and chemical attributes of PM have also been offered in search of a "biologically plausible" explanation for the reported epidemiologic observations. No one constituent has been identified as singularly determinant of health impact, although most of the suspect constituents correlate inversely with particle size, i.e., the smallest particles derive from anthropogenic combustion activities. Prominently included among the causative hypotheses that tie to particle characteristics are metals, organics, acidity, size distribution (focusing on the unique bioactivity of ultrafine PM – PM $<$ 0.1 μm), PM oxidant activity or reactivity, and the presence of potentially toxic or allergenic biologicals. However, at present, there remains insufficient understanding of the relative importance of these theories to choose one over another (especially if the spectrum of heath effects is included). As a result, there seems to be insufficient reason to unseat the PM mass-based correlation with health outcomes. Although the animal and human toxicological database is growing rapidly with regard to the issue of causation, much remains to be learned before new regulatory indices can be considered.

From research directed initially toward potential occupational hazards, it is known that several metals and silicates that make up much of the inorganic phase of PM can be cytotoxic to lung cells.

Organic constituents, as well, can induce toxicity either directly or via metabolism product—some of which are genotoxic. Other PM attributes may also come into play. Studies focusing on very small, ultrafine particles suggest that although these particles are low in mass, they are high in number and thus provide substantial reactive particle surface to interact with biological substances. Less is known about the role of biologically derived materials, such as endotoxin, other plant glycoproteins, and bioallergen fragments, which may elicit rudimentary inflammatory responses in the lung. The involvement of biologicals may be greatest in agricultural and indoor exposure environments. Finally, in the early days of air pollution toxicology, there was considerable interest in PM–co-pollutant interactions, but our knowledge in this area beyond the data derived largely from one laboratory (Amdur *et al.*, 1986) is very limited. In this regard, toxicologists need to better access the experience and knowledge of atmospheric scientists as to atmospheric interactions that are most relevant to biologic outcomes.

Metals There have been many standard acute and subchronic rodent inhalation studies with specific metal compounds, often as oxides, chlorides, or sulfates. These exposure studies relate most appropriately to occupational exposures. The varied systemic toxicities of metal compounds are presented in detail elsewhere in this text; however, it should be appreciated, that the effects of metals delivered by inhalation may differ from their impacts when administered by other routes. Metals may arise from natural as well as anthropogenic activities, and as a result metals area common constituent in ambient PM. The metal profiles differ appreciably in concentration and type and they also differ by the size mode of PM. Coarse PM (2.5–10 μm) arises largely from natural sources and thus has prominent earthen metals such as iron, sodium, silica, and magnesium – usually in oxide forms. Combustion derived metals reflect the fuel source. For example, oil may have vanadium, nickel, and perhaps zinc and iron, whereas coal may have zinc and selenium. Their chemical forms vary from water-soluble salts to oxide and phosphate forms. Other metals are emitted from vehicles burning fuels to which metal compounds were added to alter functionally (e.g., lead, manganese, platinum) or as engine wear and catalyst by-products. Similarly, metals may also derive from brake (copper, iron), tire (zinc) and dispersed road (earthen silicates) wear. As metals have many biologic properties, some essential to life while others being directly toxic to cells or act indirectly in a pro-oxidant toxic fashion. Thus metals have garnered considerable interest regarding their role in PM toxicity (Costa and Dreher, 1997).

Metal compounds can be separated nominally by physicochemical characteristics: those that are essentially water-insoluble (e.g., metal oxides and hydroxides such as those that might be released from high-temperature combustion sources or derived from the geocrustal matrix) and those that are soluble or somewhat soluble in water (often chlorides or sulfates such as those that might form under acidic conditions in a smoke plume or leach from acid-hydrated silicate particles in the atmosphere). Solubility appears to play a role in the toxicity of many inhaled metals by enhancing metal bioavailability (e.g., nickel from nickel chloride versus nickel oxide), but insolubility can also be a critical factor in determining toxicity by increasing pulmonary residence time within the lung (e.g., insoluble cadmium oxide versus soluble cadmium chloride). Moreover, some metals, either in their soluble forms or when partially coordinated on the surface of silicate or bioorganic materials, can promote electron transfer to form reactive oxidants (Ghio *et al.*,

1992). Complexes with particulate organic material in a partially hydrated form (as might be promoted by the presence of sea salt) have been shown to interact with poorly soluble metals to free coordination sites that again are pro-oxidant (Kieber *et al.*, 2005). Thus, caution is warranted in assessing inhaled PM-associated metals, as both their chemical and physical attributes as well as their interaction with co-contaminants in PM may influence their apparent toxicity. Simply measuring total metal mass to estimate effects in the lung can be misleading.

Gas-Particle Interactions   As already noted, these interactions can be extremely complex involving multiple components of the particles, gases/vapors, and sunlight. However, more than 30 years ago, generic binary interactions between particles and gases in the absence of light was shown to alter the toxicity of either the particle or the gas acting alone. The guinea pig bronchoconstriction model used for many years by Amdur and associates showed earlyon that SO_2 can interact with hydrated metal salts to potentiate particle irritancy. The mechanism(s) behind this interaction has yet to be fully discerned, but it appears to involve solubility of SO_2 in a hydrated aerosol and the ability of the metal to catalyze the oxidation of the dissolved SO_2 to sulfate. In the case of sodium chloride aerosol, potentiation appeared to be governed primarily by the solubility of SO_2 in the salt droplet and enhanced respiratory penetration. The metal salts of manganese, iron, and vanadium, on the other hand, catalyzed the formation of sulfate (Amdur and Underhill, 1968). The degree of response to the mixture was dictated by the aerosol concentration, indicating that it was the proximate irritant. Studies in humans have been less revealing about such interactions, but this database affirms the need to consider the complexity of the atmospheric challenge in estimating biological outcomes.

Complex chemistry also occurs within the effluent of the combustion source. Using a laboratory scaled furnace, the emission mix of sulfuric acid and metal oxide particles common to metal smelting and coal combustion was used to explore potential plume interactions that might impact respiratory irritancy (Amdur *et al.*, 1986). These emitted metal oxide particles, once aged and cooled, were a mixture of singlet and agglomerated ultrafine particles that would be expected to distribute throughout the lung upon inhalation. Exposures in guinea pigs of 30–60 $\mu g/m^3$ sulfuric acid combined with ultrafine zinc oxide produced progressive decreases in DL_{CO}, total lung capacity, and vital capacity and increases in cells, protein, and a variety of enzymes in lavage fluid that were not completely resolved 96 hours after exposure (Amdur, 1989). It is unclear whether the acid was on the surface of the particles or dissolved the particles, but the combination was clearly more toxic than acid alone. These effects greatly exceeded the changes in airway resistance found with relatively simple, binary mixture of SO_2 and water soluble metal salts.

Combustion studies using different coals again emphasized the significance of surface associated acidic *S*-compounds. Ultrafine combustion particles from Illinois No. 6 coal had a layer of sulfuric acid adsorbed on the surfaces resulting in greater effects in guinea pigs than the more alkaline Montana lignite. Despite the greater sulfur content of this coal, this emission ultrafine particle had adsorbed the less irritating neutralized sulfate (Chen *et al.*, 1990). Similar studies using inert carbon black appear consistent with its role as carrier for reactive gases such as O_3 and various aldehydes to enhance delivery of toxic materials to the deep lung (Jakab, 1992). The result of the latter study was enhanced infectivity when the test animals were subsequently exposed to pathologic bacteria.

Similar interactions may result from gaseous pollutants that impair the clearance of particles from the lung or otherwise alter their metabolism. Studies by Laskin at New York University in the 1960s showed an intriguing interaction of SO_2 and benzo(*a*)pyrene. It was thought that impaired clearance and greater residence time in the lung led to the enhanced the probability of carcinogenic expression of the particle. Similarly, rats exposed to an urban 8-hour daily profile of O_3 for 6 weeks, followed by a 5 hour exposure to asbestos, were found to retain three times as many fibers as did the controls 30 days postexposure. The fibers were deposited in the distal airways and penetrated more deeply into airway tissues making them less accessible to phagocytic removal (Pinkerton *et al.*, 1989). These studies, together with those focusing on irritancy and infectivity, raise the prospect that realistic exposure scenarios of gaseous and particulate pollutants can interact through either chemical or physiologic mechanisms to enhance health risks of complex polluted atmospheres.

Ultrafine Carbonaceous Matter   Ultrafine particles typically result from high temperature oxidation or as the product the atmospheric transformation involving organic vapors and sunlight. The size of these particles allow them to slip between gas molecules moving primarily by diffusion and principles of Brownian motion. Agglomeration on surfaces or other particles in the air is their primary mode of dissipation. When concentrations exceed ~million per cc, they rapidly agglomerate with each other to form larger clumps or chains of ultrafine particles. Fine PM consist in part of agglomerates of carbonaceous material which may be partially solubilized in water or coassociated organic condensate. Estimates of the carbonaceous content of ambient fine PM vary considerably, but are nominally considered to be about 30–60% of the total mass. The sources of organic carbon are varied and include the combustion products of natural smoke (e.g., forest fires), engine exhaust, and stationary sources as well as transformed condensates from VOCs in the air. Elemental carbon in diesel PM frequently combines into long ultrafine chains, with variably complex organics associated with its surface depending on the combustion conditions. It has been estimated that diesel contributes about 7% of the fine urban PM emissions, which, when expressed as an annual U.S. average, are about 2 $\mu g/m^3$ (USEPA, 1993)—but focus estimates (urban canyons) vary widely. The higher use of diesel fuel in Europe and areas of concentrated trucking in the United States has led to estimates as high as 30% of ambient fine PM mass.

As an air pollutant, elemental carbon particles generally do not exist as singlets except when emitted from high temperature sources. Elemental carbon can also be release by photocopiers and is used as a filler in some products, and as a result, some human exposure potential can occur incidentally. Elemental carbon is generally considered to be of low toxicity, although long-term, high-concentration exposure conditions in rats can lead to lung "overload" where there is evidence of lung damage and carcinogenicity (addressed below). In the environment, carbon has the potential to act as a carrier of certain irritant gases, as was noted earlier. However, carbon in the ultrafine mode (<0.1 μm) has been suggested to be more toxic than the fine-mode (2.5 μm) form, perhaps due to enhanced surface reactivity or tissue penetration (Oberdorster *et al.*, 1994, 2002; Donaldson *et al.*, 1998). Size is not the only factor as it appears that composition of the ultrafine particle also contributes to its effects and behavior (Kreyling *et al.*, 2002). Ultrafine particles in the environment exist in extremely high numbers but contribute negligibly to mass. Recent commercial introduction of "engineered" nanoparticles brings many of the same concerns as ultrafines, by virtue of their similar sizes. Additionally, being "engineered" particles they may possess design features that "natural" combustion ultrafine (or nano) particles do not.

Because diesel particulate emissions are largely ultrafine, there has been growing interest in ultrafine ambient particles. Diesel particles vary widely in the ratio of organic and elemental carbonaceous materials, which in empirical studies has been shown to influence toxic outcomes, such as to their inflammatory and carcinogenic potential (Singh *et al.*, 2004). Some diesel particles also appear to have adjuvant activity when tested with bioallergens in both animals and humans (Diaz-Sanchez *et al.*, 1999). When reacted in vitro with O_3, there appears to be an enhancement of lung inflammation relative to the diesel or O_3 alone (Madden *et al.*, 2000). However, it is important to realize that diesel particles should not be equated with whole diesel exhaust which also contains significant amounts gaseous pollutants: NO_x, CO, and SO_x as well as various VOCs and carbonyl irritants. Exposure to diluted diesel exhaust in humans reveals that the exhaust mix is very inflammogenic and to a degree cytotoxic to airway cells (Salvi *et al.*, 1999). The use of diesel particles alone in toxicology studies does not seem to display similar toxicity, thus underscoring the potential importance of interactions among air pollutants as a critical consideration in air pollution toxicity (Mauderly, 2006).

Chronic Effects and Cancer   Chronic exposure studies have been conducted with a number of particles ranging from titanium dioxide and carbon to diesel exhaust and coal fly ash aerosol. Of these substances, diesel exhaust has been the most extensively studied (reviewed by Cohen and Nikula, 1999). The primary concern with diesel has been the suspicion that it can induce lung cancer (thus its IARC classification as a Class B carcinogen). However, the evidence from over forty occupational studies (primarily railway yard, truck, and bus workers) implicating diesel exhaust as a mild carcinogen continues to be debated because of a variety of confounding issues. Taking the empirical data alone, however, carcinogenicity is suggested by several chronic exposure studies in animals and in vitro data indicating mutagenicity in *Salmonella* bacteria and enhanced sister chromatid exchange rates in Chinese hamster ovary cells. (These latter genotoxic effects have been linked to the nitroarenes associated with the diesel PM.) Rodent studies, unfortunately, have not fully resolved the question of human carcinogenic risk because of the overload need to yield positive results, and the tumors develop only in the rat. At high concentrations of diesel PM (3.5 and 7 mg/m^3), normal mucociliary clearance in the rodent models become overwhelmed, resulting in a progressive buildup of particles in the lungs. By 12 months in the rat, clearance irreversibly decreases to cessation with concomitant inflammation, oxidant generation, epithelial hyperplasia, and fibrosis. Rats seem to react more to this circumstance. Particle agglomerates within the alveolar lumen become the focus of inflammation, injury, and the eventual development of adenosarcomas and squamous cell carcinomas. At lower concentrations, where the particle buildup does not occur, tumors do not develop.

"Overload" is a common finding at the highest exposure concentrations of chronic particle inhalation bioassays. Whereas this phenomenon is not likely in humans exposed to ambient PM, it is a hypothesis worthy of consideration in a discussion of particle health effects, as it relates to the interpretation of toxicological data relevant to product use and industrial exposures. Several poorly soluble particles (PSPs) have induced lung tumors in chronic rat bioassays under conditions of overload; tumors have not developed under similar conditions in mice and hamsters. Among these particles are titanium dioxide, carbon black, toner dust, talc, and diesel emission; the potential for tumors is especially marked when the particles are in the ultrafine mode. In the rat, the time course and pattern of accumulation, chronic inflammation, epithelial hyperplasia, and tumorigenesis are essentially the same for all of the particles. In contrast, the degree of active inflammation in the mouse and hamster under similar overload conditions appears less intense, and thus is an important distinction among the species that relates to their relative sensitivities. On the one hand, such exposures do not demonstrate classic in vivo genotoxicity, but on the other, mutation of the *hprt* (hypoxanthine guanine phosphoribosyl transferase) gene was found in rat epithelial cells cultured with bronchoalveolar lavage from chronic carbon black and titanium dioxide treated rats (Driscoll *et al.*, 1997). The interpretation is that the mutation is a biomarker of genotoxicity mediated cancer, but not surprisingly, generalizing this finding to other overload cancers remains controversial. The closest analogy in humans would be coal miners who do not appear to have an enhanced risk of lung cancer, when smoking is not involved.

The issue, then, is whether rat bioassay cancer data under conditions of overload are relevant to risk assessment. A review by an expert panel (ILSI, 2000) concluded that rats, while apparently unique in this response, may represent a sensitive subgroup, and that tumorigenesis data from the rat bioassay under conditions of overload cannot be summarily dismissed as not relevant to the consideration of cancer risk in humans. However, the data should be interpreted and weighed in the context of lower concentrations and the tumor incidence and pathology found therein.

Photochemical Air Pollution

Photochemical air pollutants (notably O_3) remain the most elusive of the criteria pollutants to bring under control. It arises secondarily from a series of complex reactions in the troposphere activated by the ultraviolet (UV) spectrum of sunlight. In addition to O_3, it comprises a mixture of nitric oxides (NO_x), aldehydes, peroxyacetyl nitrates (PAN), and a myriad of aromatics and alkenes along with analog reactive radicals. If SO_2 is present, sulfates may also be formed and, collectively, they yield "summer haze." Likewise, the complex chemistry can generate organic PM, nitric acid vapor, and various condensates. Attempts to mitigate photochemical smog (especially O_3) by controlling hydrocarbon and/or NO_x emissions have proven difficult due to the complex stoichiometry of atmospheric photochemistry. Some progress has been made in controlling peak values (regulated by the 1 hour NAAQS), but the longer time frame 8 hour NAAQS has seen much smaller progress.

From the point of view of the toxicology of photochemical air pollutant gases, O_3 is by far the toxicant of greatest concern. It is highly reactive and more toxic than NO_x, and because its generation is fueled through cyclic hydrocarbon radicals, it reaches greater concentrations than the hydrocarbon radical intermediates. The gaseous hydrocarbons, so integral to the chemistry, are no longer listed collectively as a criteria pollutant because they do not have a strong health-based driver. In general, the concentrations of the hydrocarbon precursors in ambient air do not reach levels high enough to produce acute toxicity, although some individual compounds fall under the HAPs rule. Rather, the importance of these hydrocarbons stems from their role in the chain of photochemical reactions.

Although O_3 is of toxicological importance in the troposphere, in the stratosphere it plays a critical protective role. About 10 km above the earth's surface, UV light directly splits molecular O_2 into atomic $O^{\bullet}$, which then combines with O_2 to form O_3. The O_3 also dissociates back but much more slowly. The result is an accumulation of O_3 to several hundred ppm within a thin strip of the stratosphere forming an effective "permanent" barrier by absorbing the short-wavelength UV in the chemical process. This barrier had in recent years been threatened by various anthropogenic emissions (Cl_2 gas and certain chlorofluorocarbons) that enhance O_3 degradation (creation of an "O_3-hole") but recent restrictions in the use of these degrading chemicals seem to have been effective in reversing this process. The benefits are believed to be reduction of excess UV light infiltration to the earth's surface and reduced risk skin cancer risk and less risk of immune system dysfunction.

The issue is quite different in the troposphere, where accumulation of O_3 serves no known purpose and poses a threat to the respiratory tract. Near the earth's surface, NO_2 arising from combustion processes efficiently absorbs longer-wavelength UV light, from which a free O atom is cleaved, initiating the following simplified series of reactions:

$$NO_2 + hv \text{ (UV light)} \rightarrow O^{\bullet} + NO^{\bullet} \qquad (28.1)$$

$$O^{\bullet} + O_2 \rightarrow O_3 \qquad (28.2)$$

$$O_3 + NO^{\bullet} \rightarrow NO_2 \qquad (28.3)$$

This process is inherently cyclic, with NO_2 regenerated by the reaction of the $NO^{\bullet}$ and O_3. In the absence of unsaturated hydrocarbons (olefins and substituted aromatics) arising from fuel vaporization or combustion, as well as biogenic terpenes, this series of reactions would approach a steady state with little buildup of O_3. The free electrons of the double bonds of unsaturated hydrocarbons are attacked by free atomic $O^{\bullet}$, resulting in oxidized compounds and radicals that react further with $NO^{\bullet}$ to produce more NO_2. Thus, the balance of the reactions sequence shown in Eqs. 28-1 to 28-3 is tipped to the right, leading to buildup of O_3. This reaction is particularly favored when the sun's intensity is greatest at midday, utilizing the NO_2 provided by morning traffic. Carbonyl compounds (especially short-chained aldehydes) are also byproducts of these reactions. Formaldehyde and acrolein account for about 50% and 5%, respectively, of the total aldehyde in urban atmospheres. Peroxyacetyl nitrate ($CH_3COOONO_2$), often referred to as PAN, and its homologs also arise in urban air, most likely from the reaction of the peroxyacyl radicals with NO_2. In the evening when sun intensity wanes, the second rush-hour peak of NO_2 shifts the balance back by reacting with O_3 bringing the daytime peak concentration slowly down.

Short-Term Exposures to Smog

In the 1950s to 1960s, early air pollution toxicologists were challenged by the complexity of photochemical air pollution to ascertain both its potential to affect human health adversely and to determine what about these atmospheres was responsible for the effects. The focus was immediately placed on O_3 because its toxicity was found to be very high even at low ppm concentrations. Concerns that the complex atmosphere was even more hazardous led to a number of studies with actual (outdoor-derived) or synthetic (photolyzed laboratory-prepared atmospheres) smog in an attempt to assess the potency of the actual pollution mix. When human subjects were exposed to real-world photochemical air pollution (Los Angeles ambient air pumped into a laboratory exposure chamber), they experienced changes in lung function similar to those described in controlled clinical studies of O_3 alone (i.e., reduction in spirometric lung volumes; see below), thus supporting the view that this oxidant was the pollutant of primary concern. Acute animal studies using synthetic atmospheres (usually irradiated auto exhaust) provided supportive evidence indicating deep lung damage, primarily within the small airway and proximal alveolar epithelium.

While O_3 appeared to be the prime toxicant in many of these studies, there was some evidence that other co-pollutants were involved in the effects observed with smog. When guinea pigs were exposed to irradiated auto exhaust, airway resistance increased quickly, in contrast to the pattern of O_3 alone, where less effect is seen on resistance than on breathing rate. This indicated that a more soluble irritant(s) probably was active, presumably reactive aldehydes. Thus, the array of effects of a complex atmosphere may be more diverse than would be predicted if it were assumed that O_3 alone was responsible. Interestingly, the focus over time has been almost exclusively on O_3, perhaps with the emphasis coming from the regulatory perspective tied to this single pollutant.

Chronic Exposures to Smog

Epidemiological studies in human populations as well as empirical studies in animals have attempted to link degenerative lung disease with chronic exposure to photochemical air pollution. Cross-sectional and prospective field studies have suggested an accelerated loss of lung function in people living in areas of high pollution. However, as with many studies of this type, there were problems with confounding factors (meteorology, imprecise exposure assessment, and population variables). Studies have been conducted in children living in modern-day Mexico City, which has oxidant and PM levels today far in excess of any city in the United States These studies have focused on the nasal epithelium as an exposure surrogate for pulmonary tissues, using biopsy and lavage methodologies to assess damage. Dramatic effects were found in exposed children, consisting of severe epithelial damage and metaplasia as well as permanent remodeling of the nasal epithelium. When children migrated into Mexico City from cleaner, nonurban regions, even more severe damage was observed, suggesting that the tissue remodeling in the permanent residents imparted some degree of incomplete adaptation. Because the children were of middle-class origin, these observations were less likely confounded by socio-economic variables (Calderon-Garcidueñas et al., 1992). More recently, changes in lung hyperinflation as estimated by X-ray tomography and impaired lung function has been reported among similarly exposed children living in Mexico City (Calderon-Garcidueñas et al., 2003), raising further concerns of long term effects.

A now classic synthetic smog study in animals was undertaken at the Cincinnati EPA laboratory in the mid-1960s in an attempt to address the potential for long-term lung disease. Beagle dogs were exposed on a daily basis (16 hours) for 68 months, followed by a clean-air recovery period of about 3 years (Lewis et al., 1974). A series of physiologic measurements were made on the dogs after the exposure, and after their 3-year recovery. They were then moved to the College of Veterinary Medicine at the University of California at Davis. The lungs of the dogs then underwent extensive morphologic examination to correlate with the physiology. Seven groups of 12 dogs each had been studied. The dogs had been exposed to non-irradiated auto exhaust (group 1), irradiated auto exhaust (group 2), SO_2 plus sulfuric acid (group 3), the two types of exhaust plus the sulfur mixture (groups 4 and 5), and a high and a low level of NO_x (groups 6 and 7). The irradiated exhaust contained oxidant (measured as O_3) at about 0.2 ppm and NO_2 at about 0.9 ppm. The raw exhaust contained minimal concentrations of these materials and about 1.5 ppm NO. Both forms of exhaust also contained about 100 ppm CO. The controls did not show time-related lung function changes, but all the exposure groups had abnormalities, most of which persisted or worsened over the 3-year recovery period in clean air. Enlargement of airspaces and loss of interalveolar septa in proximal acinar regions were most severe in dogs that were exposed to NO_x and SO_x with irradiated exhaust (Hyde *et al.*, 1978). These studies described a morphologic lesion that was degenerative and progressive in nature, not unlike that of chronic obstructive pulmonary disease (COPD)—a condition most often associated with lifelong tobacco smoking.

Long-term "sentinel" studies in polluted cities have been attempted whereby the animals live in the same highly polluted air to which people are exposed. Such approaches have had a troubled past, but newer studies appear to have been better controlled for the problems of infection, inappropriate animal care (e.g., heat), and variable exposure atmospheres. One such study, conducted in rats exposed for 6 months to the air of São Paulo, Brazil, found considerable airway damage, lung function alterations, and altered mucus rheology (Saldiva *et al.*, 1992). The concentrations of O_3 and PM in São Paulo frequently exceed daily maximum values (in the summer months of February and March) of 0.3 ppm and 75 µg/m^3, respectively. This collage of effects is not unlike a composite of injury one might suspect from a mixed atmosphere of oxidants and acid PM in controlled laboratory animal studies. Strangely enough, however, a seven week study in rats exposed to the polluted Mexico City air, which had induced significant lesions in children, did not reveal in F-344 rats any nasal or lung histopathology (Moss *et al.*, 2001). Whereas there is no clear reason for the apparent differences in the findings, it is important to appreciate that all sentinel studies have elements of exposure that may be uncontrolled and hence at times can yield conflicting findings.

Ozone

General Toxicology   Ozone is the primary oxidant of concern in photochemical smog because of its inherent bioreactivity and its concentration relative to other reactive species. Depending on the meteorological conditions of a given year, 60–80 million Americans live in areas not in absolute compliance with the NAAQS. Los Angeles frequently attains and occasionally exceeds 1-hour levels of 0.2–0.3 ppm. Unlike SO_2 and the reducing-type pollution profile discussed above, current mitigation strategies for O_3 have been only marginally successful despite significant reductions in individual automobile emissions. These reductions have been offset by population growth, which brings with it additional vehicles and vehicle miles driven. With suburban sprawl and the downwind transport of air masses from populated areas to more rural environments, the geographic distribution of those exposed has expanded, as has the temporal profile of individual exposure. In other words, O_3 exposures are no longer stereotyped as brief 1- to 2-hour peaks. Instead, there is more typically a prolonged period of exposure of 6 hours or more at or near the NAAQS level. This recently noted change in the exposure profile to O_3 has given rise to concerns that cumulative damage over an exposure of several hours may be more significant than brief pulse-like exposures, and that as a result many more peo-

ple are at risk than was previously thought. With the revision of the O_3 NAAQS in 1997 to include an 8-hour daily average of 0.08 ppm, more cities and suburban areas find themselves in violation of the standard. If indeed the damage to the lung is cumulative over an 8-hour time period, then people in areas in compliance but near the standard may be affected. The American Lung Association estimates that nearly 50% of U.S. inhabitants live in counties that are not in O_3 compliance (State of the Air, 2006). Perhaps of greater significance is that of those who might be considered susceptible due to age and/or preexistent cardiopulmonary impairments, 80–90% live in these areas that fail to comply with the present O_3 NAAQS.

Ozone induces a variety of effects in humans and experimental animals at concentrations that occur in many urban areas (Lippmann, 1989). These effects include morphologic, functional, immunologic, and biochemical alterations. Because of its low water solubility, a substantial portion of inhaled O_3 penetrates deep into the lung, but its reactivity is such that about 17% and 40% is scrubbed by the nasopharynx of resting rats and humans, respectively (Hatch *et al.*, 1994; Gerrity *et al.*, 1988). The reason for the higher degree of scrubbing in humans is unclear, but the finding is reproducible. Moreover, the mouth appears to scrub as well as the nose. Nevertheless, regardless of species, the region of the lung that is predicted to have the greatest O_3 deposition (dose per surface area) is the centriacinar region, from the terminal bronchioles to the alveolar ducts, also referred to as the proximal alveolar ductal region (Overton and Miller, 1987). Because O_3 penetration increases with increased tidal volume and flow rate, exercise increases the dose to the target area. Using $^{18}O_3$ (a nonradioactive isotope of oxygen), Hatch and coworkers have shown that the dose to the distal lung and the degree of damage to the lung as determined by leakage of plasma protein into the alveolar space (as collected by bronchoalveolar lavage) in exercising human subjects exposed to 0.4 ppm for 2 hours with intermittent periods of 15 minutes of exercise (threefold normal ventilation on average) are similar to those in resting rats exposed for the same length of time to 2.0 ppm. Thus, it is important to consider the role of exercise in a study of O_3 or any inhalant before making cross-study comparisons, especially if that comparison is across species. With so many years invested in the study of O_3, it is surprising that only now is the nature of species differences with regard to exercise-associated dosimetry being appreciated.

Animal studies indicate that the acute morphologic responses to O_3 can involve epithelial cells along the entire respiratory tract. The pattern of injury parallels the dosimetry profile, with the majority of damage occurring in the distal lung. Along the airways, ciliated cells appear to be most sensitive to O_3, while Clara cells and mucus-secreting cells are the least sensitive. Studies in the rat nose indicate that O_3 also is an effective mucus secretagogue. In the alveolar region, type 1 epithelia are very sensitive to O_3 relative to type 2 cells, which have an active metabolic machinery. The more resistant type 2 cells serve as the stem cells for the replacement of type 1 cells. Ultrastructural damage to alveolar epithelia can be observed in rats after a few hours at 0.2 ppm, but sloughing of cells in the distal airway generally requires concentrations above 0.8 ppm. Recovery occurs within a few days, and there appears to be no residual pathology. Hence, from animal studies, it would appear that a single exposure to O_3 at a relatively low concentration is not likely to cause permanent damage. On a gross level, when a bronchoscope is used to peer into the human bronchus after O_3 exposure, the airways appear "sunburned" and, as with mild skin sunburn, recovery is typical. What is uncertain is the impact of repeated "sun-burning" of the airways and lung.

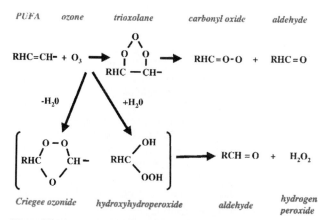

Figure 28-12. Major reactions pathways of O₃ with lipids in lung lining fluid and cell membranes. (Adapted with permission from the Air Quality Criteria Document for Ozone and Photochemical Oxidants. 600/P-93/004cF, NCEA Research Triangle Park, NC: U.S. EPA, 1996).

Studies have shown particular sensitivity to O_3-induced inflammation in neonatal rats that decreased with age into adulthood. However, enhanced sensitivity to O_3 again appears in older rats as evidenced by interstitial edema that is not seen in younger adult animals. Older rats have lower ascorbate in the lung and this diminishment of antioxidant capacity may be in part responsible. Elderly humans, however, seem less responsive to the lung function impacts of high ambient O_3. The reasons for this are unclear, but caution in linking lung function and inflammation in the O_3 response is warranted as these events appear separated in time by about 18 hours.

The mechanisms by which O_3 causes injury have been studied using cellular as well as cell-free systems. As a powerful oxidant, O_3 seeks to extract electrons from other molecules. The surface fluid lining the respiratory tract and cell membranes that underlie the lining fluid contain a significant quantity of polyunsaturated fatty acids (PUFA), either free or as part of the lipoprotein structures of the cell. The double bonds within these fatty acids have a labile, unpaired electron which is easily attacked by O_3 to form ozonides that progress through a less stable zwitterion or trioxolane (depending on the presence of water); these ultimately recombine or decompose to lipohydroperoxides, aldehydes, and hydrogen peroxide. These pathways are thought to initiate propagation of lipid radicals and autooxidation of cell membranes and macromolecules (Fig. 28-12).

Evidence of free radical-related damage in vivo includes detection of breath pentane and ethane and tissue measurements of diene conjugates. Damage to the air-blood interface disrupts its barrier function and promotes inflammation. Inflammatory cytokines (e.g., interleukins 6, 8 and others, TNF, etc.) are released from epithelial cells and macrophages that mediate early responses and initiate repair. This inflammatory process is generally transient, but it may also interact with neural irritant responses to affect lung function acutely. This latter response may have implications for those with preexistent inflammation or disease.

Pulmonary Function Effects   Exercising human subjects exposed to 0.12–0.4 ppm O_3 experience reversible concentration-related decrements in forced exhaled volumes [forced vital capacity (FVC) and forced expiratory volume in 1 second (FEV₁)] after a 2–3 hours of exposure (McDonnell *et al.*, 1983). With the recent concern that prolonged periods of exposure (6–8 hours) may lead to cumulative effects, similar protocols with lower exercise levels were ex-

tended up to 6.6 hours. In these studies, exposures to 0.12, 0.10, and 0.08 ppm induced progressive lung function impairment during the course of the exposure (Horstman *et al.*, 1989). The pattern of response was linearly cumulative as a function of exposure time such that changes not detectable at 1 or 2 hours reached significance by 4–6 hours. Decrements in FEV₁ after 6.6 hours at 0.12 ppm averaged 13.6% and were comparable to that observed after a 2 hour exposure to 0.22 ppm with much heavier exercise. It is not clear to what extent human lung dysfunction (in terms of changes in FEV₁) from O_3 is vagally mediated, but the response can be abrogated by analgesics such as ibuprofen and opiates, which also reduce pain and inflammation (see below). Thus pain reflexes involving C-fiber networks are thought to be important in the reductions in forced expiratory volumes. On the other hand, animal studies show a prominent role for vagal reflexes in altered airway reactivity and bronchconstriction. There is also evidence to implicate vagal reflexes in cardiac as well as thermal regulation, at least in rodents. Airway hyperreactivity to nonspecific agonists in humans is reported after acute 2- to 6-hour exposures to O_3 to sub-NAAQS levels of 0.08, 0.10, and 0.12 ppm (by 56, 86, and 121%, respectively, to methacholine). It is widely thought that hyperreactive airways may be a marker of predisposition to other pollutants such as sulfuric acid or aeroallergens, but such evidence is limited.

When compared with field studies, chamber exposures may underestimate responses for a given exposure to O_3. For a given concentration of O_3, greater decrements in pulmonary function have been reported in children playing outdoors at summer camps than were observed in controlled exposure studies involving exercise (Lippmann, 1989). The reasons for this difference are uncertain but might relate more to cumulative exposure in the children at camp, as they were outside all day, or to the fact that the ambient exposures probably involve other haze co-pollutants, such as H⁺. The responses to the ambient exposures also have slightly altered temporal patterns and pre-exposure histories (Kinney *et al.*, 1988). Animal studies are consistent with the fact that both duration and concentration are important in assessing the response to O_3 exposure (Costa *et al.*, 1989). Pulmonary function decrements increased with $C \times T$ (concentration times time) in rats exposed for 2, 4, or 8 hours to O_3 at 0.2, 0.4, and 0.8 ppm. Rats exposed for 7 hours to 0.5 ppm with 8% CO_2 added to increase ventilation, produced functional decrements similar to those observed in human chamber studies of 6.6 hours at 0.12 ppm when ventilation-adjusted $C \times T$ products were factored in. This would imply that rats and humans respond with about the same sensitivity and opens the door to the study of various scenarios of exposure to predict human responses. It should be cautioned, however, that it is unknown whether CO_2-stimulated breathing in the rat might alter response thresholds beyond mere incrementing of the dose. However, in related studies without stimulated breathing, lavage fluid protein content (an index of permeability) 24-hours postexposure was also nearly linearly cumulative, with exaggerated responses at the higher concentrations suggestive of an exponential pattern (Highfill *et al.*, 1992) common to other biological functions.

Inflammation of the Lung and Host Defense   The mechanism by which O_3 produces decrements in pulmonary function is not fully understood. In contrast to sulfuric acid and SO_2, O_3-induced lung dysfunction does not appear correlate with nonspecific hyperreactivity, and appears not to be enhanced in asthmatics (the distress may be due to less functional reserve), as appears to be the case with sulfated acids. It was hypothesized that lung inflammation might reflect parallel sensitivity to lung dysfunction suggesting mechanistic linkages. Koren *et al.* (1989) found an eightfold increase in *neutrophils* in bronchoalveolar lavage fluid recovered from human subjects 18 hours after a 2-hour exposure to 0.40 ppm with intermittent exercise. There was also evidence of increased epithelial permeability (a twofold increase in serum proteins and albumin). However, when compared to lung function the inflammatory markers did not correlate. Arachidonate metabolites, including the prostaglandins PGE_2 and PGF_{2a} and the leukotriene thromboxane B_2, have also been seen to increase in human bronchoalveolar lavage fluid after 0.4 ppm O_3 for 2 hours (Seltzer *et al.*, 1986). Pretreatment with the anti-inflammatory agents, indomethacin and ibuprofen (both cyclooxygenase inhibitors), decreased the pulmonary function deficit and PGE_2, but other indicators of cell injury and vascular leak in lavage fluid (neutrophils, extravasated protein, and lactate dehydrogenase) were not attenuated after exposure (Hazucha *et al.*, 1996). Because PGE_2 can have either pro- or anti-inflammatory functions under certain conditions as well as bronchodilatory action on constricted airways, it remains unclear what if any causal relationship exists between arachidonate metabolites and changes in FEV_1. Studies in animal models suggests a role for C-fiber mediated responses that might tie to pain on inspiration in the human as the limit to full inhalation for the forced expiratory maneuvers.

Sensitivity to O_3 appears to have a genetic component as well. Studies in inbred stains of mice have shown that O_3-induced pulmonary neutrophilia and permeability are governed by a single gene linked to the Toll4 locus that has been associated with endotoxin sensitivity (Kleeberger *et al.*, 2000). The growth of genomic and proteomic technologies has made it possible to begin studies in humans to define genetic linkages to O_3 sensitivity. Again using Mexico City as a backdrop, it has been found that polymorphism in GSTM1 (as noted above with regard to PM) appears to convey O_3 sensitivity as well (Romieu *et al.*, 2004). More detailed controlled O_3 exposures may identify even more genes associated with responsiveness.

The potential for O_3 to influence allergic sensitization or challenge-responses has received limited investigation in either humans or animals. In general, animal studies have shown the ability of O_3 to enhance the sensitization process under certain conditions (Osebold *et al.*, 1980), but evidence of this in humans is lacking. Controlled studies of heightened antigen responsiveness in allergic subjects have only been suggestive, with enhancement of allergic rhinitis after 0.5 ppm for 4 hours providing the only credible data to date. However, diary studies of asthmatic nurses reported worsened allergy symptoms, as well as durations thereof, at concentrations of O_3 near the NAAQS (Schwartz, 1992).

Exposure to O_3 before a challenge with aerosols of infectious agents produces a higher incidence of infection than is seen in control animals (Coffin and Blommer, 1967). Studies have demonstrated that this effect in a mouse model using an aerosol of *Streptococcus* (group C) bacteria is a direct result of altered phagocytosis by macrophages in the O_3-exposed animals (Gilmour *et al.*, 1993), allowing the bacteria to develop a thickened capsule that reduces their attractiveness to phagocytes and enhances their virulence. This host resistance model has shown responsiveness to an exposure as low as 0.08 ppm for 3 hours. The susceptibility of mice and hamsters to *Klebsiella pneumoniae* aerosol is also increased by prior exposure to O_3. In the rat, altered microbe-killing may relate to membrane damage in macrophages, thus impairing the production of bactericidal superoxide anions. The rat appears less susceptible than mice because it has a more vigorous PMN response to bacteria than do mice, which seems to compensate for macrophage impairments. This is yet another example of where susceptibility lies more in the inability to compensate than in the initial responsiveness to a given challenge.

Chronic Effects Morphometric studies of the centriacinar region of rats exposed for 12 hours per day for 6 weeks to 0.12 or 0.25 ppm O_3 have shown hyperplasia and hypertrophy of type 1 alveolar cells (smaller and thicker cells) coupled with damage and alterations in ciliated and Clara cell populations in small airways (Barry *et al.*, 1988). A collective cross-protocol analysis of type 1 cell hypertrophy was conducted, type 1 cell thickness appeared to be linearly related to the O_3 $C \times T$ (Chang *et al.*, 1991, 1992). This finding suggested that over a season, the impact of O_3 in the distal lung may be cumulative and perhaps more importantly may be without threshold. The biological significance of this change is unclear—it may be part of a compensatory response to "thicken" that part of the alveolar duct junction that receives the greatest dose and is most affected. This response may be protective as the thickened cells were also smaller, offering therefore a smaller exposure-surface to the incoming O_3. This changed morphology could limit membrane damage. When returned to clean air, most of the epithelial morphologic changes regressed, but there was evidence of residual interstitial remodeling below the epithelium in the alveolar duct region. Examination of autopsied lung specimens from young smokers shows many analogous tissue lesions that come to be described as the "smoldering" precursor of emphysema.

Studies involving episodic exposures of rats and monkeys using a pattern of alternating months of O_3 (0.25 ppm) for 18 months indicate that there may be carry-over effects, notably thickening of interstitial fibrous matrix (Tyler *et al.*, 1988, 1991). These interstitial changes were quantitatively similar regardless of the twofold difference in the cumulative exposure dose (i.e., $C \times T$). This would imply that a pattern of exposure resembling seasonal O_3 patterns might result in more serious lesions than predicted by dose alone—indeed more than would have occurred had the exposure been continuous. Hence, the concept of "more dose . . . more effect" may not hold in chronic episodic scenarios, as it appears to do with uninterrupted exposures. The number of episodes experienced may well be more significant to long-term outcomes than total dose—a phenomenon not unlike that of repeated sun-burning and deterioration of the skin.

Studies of lung function in rodents exposed chronically to O_3 have been conducted, but have yielded mixed results. Generally, the dysfunction is reflective of stiffened or fibrotic lungs, particularly at higher concentrations. There have been two prominent chronic O_3 studies—the EPA 18-month chronic study fashioned after a realistic urban exposure profile with a peak exposure of 0.25 ppm (Chang *et al.*, 1992; Costa *et al.*, 1995) and the National Toxicology Program (NTP)—Health Effects Institute (HEI Report, 1994/1995) study of 0.125–1 ppm for 20 months (square wave; 6 h/d; 5d/week). From an environmental relevance perspective, the $C \times T$ doses for these studies were similar, but the urban profile study produced evidence for centriacinar interstitial fibrosis suggesting a possible influence of the exposure pattern. There was no general biochemical evidence for fibrosis (Last *et al.*, 1994), as reported in monkey and rat studies that had been conducted at higher O_3 concentrations. If one attempts to compare these results with the Cincinnati beagle study, one finds that the synthetic smog atmosphere showed degenerative and not fibrotic lung lesions. However, it should be noted that the air pollutant mixture used in the beagle study was both more complex and involved considerably higher concentrations than more recent studies.

The ability of O_3 to induce tolerance to itself is a curious phenomenon that has implications for both episodic and chronic exposures. Classic O_3 tolerance takes the form of protection against a lethal dose in animals that received a very low initial challenge 7 days before. This term, *tolerance*, is sometimes used to describe "adaptation" or acclimatization over time to near-ambient levels of O_3, and as such, has led to some confusion. However, with regard to "adaptation" to O_3, the process begins during and immediately after the initial exposure and progresses to completion in at most 2–4 days. This adaptive phenomenon has been well established in humans with regard to lung function and recently has been correlated with several inflammatory endpoints (Devlin *et al.*, 1993). Lavage lactate dehydrogenase (LDH; a marker of cell injury) and elastase (enzymatically active against lung matrix), interestingly, do not appear to adapt in humans based on the Devlin study. An analogous pattern of adaptation of functional and biochemical endpoints (including LDH and elastase) in rodents also takes place with repeated exposures up to a week. But to date, the linkages between acute, adaptive, and long-term process remain unclear, because over longer periods of exposure both morphologic and functional effects do appear to develop. The precise mechanism for O_3 adaptation is not known and several theories abound, including changes in cell profiles, lung surface fluids, and induced antioxidants. Few studies have tackled the problem but in rats the adaptation of the neurtophilic response appears to be related to the induction of an endogenous acute-phase response (McKinney *et al.*, 1998). On the other hand, adaptation to lung function changes in rats after chronic exposure appears linked to lung antioxidants (Wiester *et al.*, 2000) such as ascorbic acid. The significance of this finding in humans is uncertain because ascorbic acid is not endogenously synthesized as it is in the rat. However, self-administration of ascorbate has been shown to reduce O_3-induced lung function decrements in adults (Samet *et al.*, 2001; Mudway *et al.*, 1999), and in children, supplementation with ascorbate and α-tocopherol lessened nasal inflammatory responses to O_3 in Mexico City (Sienra-Monge *et al.*, 2004). Despite these interesting findings, it remains unclear if antioxidant supplements can protect humans from long-term O_3 effects given the many mechanisms that may be involved in the various responses. How these interplay with long-term adaptation and the likelihood of degenerative disease is unclear.

Ozone Interactions with Copollutants   An approach simplifying the complexity of synthetic smog studies, yet addressing the issue of pollutant interactions involves the exposure of animals or humans to binary or more complex synthetic mixtures of pollutants that occur together in ambient air. The most frequent combination involves interactions of O_3 and NO_2 or O_3 and sulfuric acid. Not surprisingly, study design adds a level of complexity in interpretation such that evidence exists supporting either augmentation or antagonism of lung function impairments, lung pathology, and other indices of injury (Kleinman *et al.*, 1985). This apparent conflict in the findings only emphasizes the need to carefully consider the myriad of factors than might affect studies involving multiple determinants and the nature of the exposure that is most relevant to reality.

When O_3 and NO_2 (1 ppm and 14 ppm, respectively) were administered to rats from a premixed retention chamber, the resulting damage evident in bronchoalveolar lavage exceeded that of either toxicant alone, regardless of the temporal sequence of exposure (Gelzleichter *et al.*, 1992). Biochemical and histological indices of fibrogenesis also were increased in related studies (Last *et al.*, 1994). In retrospect, it was hypothesized that the two oxidants formed rela-tively stable intermediate nitrogen radicals that were more toxic than either gas alone. At lower, more realistic concentrations (0.3 ppm O_3 and 3.0 ppm NO_2), where this reaction would not be favored, the impact of these irritants on rabbits was only additive (Schlesinger *et al.*, 1991). This contrast in response serves to illustrate that the tenets of dose-dependency that hold for any single-toxicant response may be of equal or more importance when two or more pollutants coexist and have the potential to interact.

Studies of O_3 mixed with acid aerosols also have shown enhanced or antagonistic responses that were time dependent during the period of exposure. On the one hand, as noted above, field studies of children in camps and studies of asthma admissions in the Northeast and in Canada, suggested an interaction of acid and O_3 underlying responses to summer haze. Yet, in an experimental setting with rabbits exposed over an extended period, there was exposure duration-specific evidence of enhanced as well as antagonized secretory cell responses with combined O_3 (0.1 ppm) and sulfuric acid (125 $\mu g/m^3$) over the course of the 1-year exposure (Schlesinger *et al.*, 1992). As the number of interacting variables increases, so does the difficulty in interpretation. Studies of complex atmospheres involving acid-coated carbon combined with O_3 at near-ambient levels also show varied evidence of interaction on lung function and macrophage receptor activity (Kleinman *et al.*, 1999). As such, the platform of any multicomponent study is its statistical design and the ability to either separate or determine the nature of the interacting variables. However, it is indeed the complex mixture to which people are exposed that we wish to evaluate. Creative approaches to understanding mixture responses are a likely part of the new agenda that toxicologists will need to address in the next decade (Mauderly, 1993, 2006).

Nitrogen Dioxide

General Toxicology   Nitrogen dioxide, like O_3, is a deep lung irritant that can produce pulmonary edema if it is inhaled at high concentrations. It is a much less potent irritant and oxidant than O_3, but NO_2 can pose clear toxicological problems. Potential life-threatening exposure is a real-world problem for farmers, as near-lethal high levels of NO_2 can be liberated from fermenting fresh silage. Being heavier than air, the generated NO_2 and CO_2 displace air and oxygen at the base of silo and diffuse into closed spaces where workers can inadvertently get exposed to very high concentrations perhaps with depleted oxygen. Typically, shortness of breath rapidly ensues with exposures nearing 75 to 100 ppm NO_2, with delayed edema and symptoms of pulmonary damage. Not surprisingly, the symptoms are collectively termed "silo-filler's disease." Nitrogen dioxide is also an important indoor pollutant, especially in homes with unventilated gas stoves or kerosene heaters (Spengler and Sexton, 1983). Under such circumstances, very young children and their mothers who spend considerable time indoors may be especially at risk. Sidestream tobacco smoke is yet another source of indoor NO_2, although the levels from this source are not likely to generate NO_2 levels of acute concern. In general, indoor environments with NO_2 sources achieve concentrations far in excess those observed outdoors. However, protocols that simulate an urban (rush-hour) or household (cooking) patterns of two daily peaks superimposed on a low continuous background concentration have elicited effects in experimental animals that continuous exposure to NO_2 did not evoke, suggesting an important dependency on exposure profile. Among the common air pollutants, empirical studies of NO_2 have frequently shown greater effects with higher peak concentrations at equivalent $C \times T$ steady-state concentrations.

Although the distal lung lesions produced by acute NO$_2$ are similar among species, there exist differences in species sensitivity. Where direct comparison is possible, guinea pigs, hamsters, and monkeys appear more sensitive than rats, although comparative dosimetry information might explain some of this difference. As in the case of O$_3$, theoretical dosimetry studies indicate that NO$_2$ is deposited along the length of the respiratory tree, with preferential deposition being in the distal airways. Not surprisingly, the pattern of damage to the respiratory tract reflects this profile: damage is most apparent in the terminal bronchioles, just a bit more proximal in the airway than is seen with O$_3$. At high concentrations, the alveolar ducts and alveoli are also affected, with type 1 cells again showing their sensitivity to oxidant challenge. In the airways of these animals there is also damage to epithelial cells in the bronchioles, notably with loss of ciliated cells, as well as a loss of secretory granules in Clara cells. The pattern of injury of NO$_2$ is quite similar to that of O$_3$, but its potency is about an order of magnitude lower.

Pulmonary Function Effects   Exposure of normal human subjects to concentrations of ≤ 4 ppm NO$_2$ for up to 3 hours produces no consistent effects on spirometry. However, a study has shown slightly enhanced airway reactivity with 1.5–2.0 ppm. Interestingly, ascorbic acid pretreatment of human subjects appeared to protect them from this hyperreactivity (Mohsenin, 1987). Whether asthmatics have a particular sensitivity to NO$_2$ is a controversial issue. A number of factors appear to be involved (e.g., exercise, inherent sensitivity of the asthmatic subject, exposure method). Some studies have reported effects in some individuals at 0.2 ppm, which approximates an ambient level in a household with an unvented gas stove. Recent meta-analyses, which have incorporated the findings of many studies to achieve a weight-of-evidence perspective, support an effect of NO$_2$ on asthmatics. As for an appropriate animal model, only very high concentrations (10 ppm NO$_2$) invoke an irritancy response in guinea pigs (tachypnea); these levels are well above those a person probably would encounter in everyday life. However, recently, NO$_2$ has been found to be associated with mortality in some time-series studies of air pollution attempting to tease out specific pollutant effects (focusing mainly on PM) (Gold et al., 2000). NO$_2$ in these studies is thought to be a marker for vehicular traffic rather than as an indication of a specific NO$_2$ effect. These studies have found correlates with cardiovascular deaths, which have raised new questions of the mechanisms by which pollutants might affect health in susceptible subgroups (Rosenlund et al., 2006).

Inflammation of the Lung and Host Defense   Unlike O$_3$, NO$_2$ does not induce significant neutrophilic inflammation in humans at exposure concentrations encountered in the ambient outdoor environment. There is some evidence for bronchial inflammation after 4–6 hours at 2.0 ppm, which approximates the highest transient peak indoor levels of this oxidant. Exposures at 2.0–5.0 ppm have been shown to affect T lymphocytes, particularly CD8$^+$ cells and natural killer cells that function in host defenses against viruses. Although these concentrations may be high, epidemiologic studies variably show effects of NO$_2$ on respiratory infection rates in children, especially in indoor environments. Animal models, by contrast, have for years shown associations between NO$_2$ and bacterial infection (Gardner, 1984). As noted for other effects, the incidence of infection in exposed models appears to be governed more by the peak exposure concentration than by exposure duration. The effects are ascribed to suppression of macrophage function and clearance from the lung, in the form of suppressed bactericidal and/or motility functions of macrophages from rabbits exposed to 0.3 ppm for 3 days (Schlesinger, 1987). Similar effects have been reported in humans exposed to 0.10 ppm for 6.6 hours (Devlin et al., 1991).

Toxicological studies of the interaction of NO$_2$ with viruses also suggest enhanced infectivity. Squirrel monkeys infected with nonlethal levels of A/PR-8 influenza virus and then exposed continuously to 5 or 10 ppm NO$_2$ suffered high mortality rates; 6/6 monkeys exposed to 10 ppm died within 3 days, while only 1/3 exposed to 5 ppm died (Henry et al., 1970). Other experiments suggest that exposure of squirrel monkeys for 5 months to 5 ppm NO$_2$ depresses the formation of protective antibodies against the A/PR-8 influenza virus. Controlled human studies with virus challenges, however, have been inconclusive, perhaps because of low subject numbers. One study showed decreased virus inactivation by alveolar macrophages recovered from 4 of 9 subjects when cultured and exposed for 3.5 hours to 0.6 ppm NO$_2$ in vitro. The responsive macrophages produced interleukin-1, a known cytokine modulator of immune cell function (Frampton et al., 1989). Thus, the potential for augmented risk of viral infection associated with NO$_2$ exposure remains unclear and suggests a role for underlying host susceptibility. This concern would be greatest for children who have less mature pulmonary immune function, especially during seasonal use of unvented gas-heaters.

Chronic Effects   Concern about the chronic effects of NO$_2$ stem from observations that a continuous 30 day, 30-ppm exposure produces emphysema in hamsters. Whether the result of this exposure scenario relates to cyclic human exposures at 1/100th that level is unclear. On the one hand, an 18-month study in rats exposed to an urban pattern of NO$_2$ in which a background of 0.5 ppm for 23 hours per day peaked at 1.5 ppm for 4 hours each day showed little ultrastructural damage to the distal lung (Chang et al., 1988). On the other hand, mice exposed for a year to a base level of 0.2 ppm NO$_2$ with a 1-hour spike of 0.8 ppm twice a day 5 days per week (Miller et al., 1987) displayed effects that differed between the base-only and peak-only exposure groups. The base level produced no effects, while the overlaid peaks induced slight functional impairment and augmented susceptibility to bacterial infection. Early studies (Ehrlich and Henry, 1968) showed that clearance of bacteria from the lungs is suppressed with 0.5 ppm NO$_2$ through 12 months of exposure. Interestingly, studies with a similar double diurnal peak design for NO$_2$, with NO used as a negative control, showed more pronounced effects of NO on alveolar septal remodeling than did NO$_2$ (Mercer et al., 1995). Apparently, NO acts intercellularly to interrupt collagen metabolism; the potential for NO$_2$ to act in this manner is not known. These and similar studies utilizing varied peak-plus-baseline NO$_x$ exposures indicate the importance of exposure profile for at least this pollutant.

Other Oxidants   A number of other reactive oxidants have been identified in photochemical smog, however most are short-lived because of their reaction with copollutants. Peroxyacetyl nitrate (PAN), which is thought to be responsible for much of the eye-stinging activity of smog, is known to exist in smog situations. It is more soluble and reactive than O$_3$, and hence rapidly decomposes in mucous membranes before it can penetrate into the respiratory tract. The cornea is a sensitive target and is prominent in the burning/stinging discomfort often associated with oxidant smogs. A few studies with high levels of PAN have shown that it can cause lung damage and have mutagenic activity in bacteria, but it is not likely that these scenarios are relevant to ambient levels of PAN.

Aldehydes   Carbonyl compounds, notably short-chained (2–4 C) aldehydes, are common photo-oxidation products of unsaturated hydrocarbons. Two aldehydes are of major interest by virtue of their concentrations and irritancy: formaldehyde (HCHO) and acrolein (H_2C=CHCHO). They contribute to the odor as well as eye and sensory effects of smog. Formaldehyde accounts for about 50% of the estimated total aldehydes in polluted air, while acrolein, the more irritating of the two, accounts for about 5% of the total. Acetaldehyde (C_3HCHO) and many other longer chain aldehydes make up the remainder, but they are not as intrinsically irritating, exist at low concentrations, and have less solubility in airway fluids. Formaldehyde and particularly acrolein are also found in mainstream tobacco smoke (~90 and ~8 ppm, respectively, per puff) and are likely to be found at lower levels in sidestream smoke as well. Formaldehyde is also an important indoor air pollutant and can often achieve higher concentrations indoors than outdoors due to out-gassing by new upholstery or other furnishings.

Empirical studies have shown that formaldehyde and acrolein are competitive agonists for similar irritant receptors in the airways. Thus, irritation may be related not to "total aldehyde" concentration but to specific ratios of acrolein and formaldehyde. Their relative difference in solubility, with formaldehyde being somewhat more water-soluble and thus having more nasopharyngeal uptake, may distort this relationship under certain exposure conditions (e.g., exercise). On the other hand, acrolein is very reactive and may interact easily with many tissue macromolecules.

Formaldehyde   Formaldehyde is a primary sensory irritant. Because it is very soluble in water, it is absorbed in mucous membranes in the nose, upper respiratory tract, and eyes. The dose–response curve for formaldehyde is steep: 0.5–1 ppm yields a detectable odor; 2–3 ppm produces mild irritation; and 4–5 ppm is intolerable to most people. Formaldehyde is thought to act via sensory C-fibers that signal locally as well as through the trigeminal nerve to reflexively induce broncheoconstriction through the vagus nerve. In guinea pigs, a 1 hour exposure to about 0.3 ppm of formaldehyde induces an increase in airflow resistance accompanied by a smaller decrease in compliance (Amdur, 1960). Respiratory frequency and minute volume also decreased, but these changes were not statistically significant until >10 ppm. The no observed effect level (NOEL) using these lung function criteria is about 0.05 ppm. The general pattern of the irritant response and its rapid recovery is similar to that produced by higher concentrations of SO_2. Like SO_2, breathing through a tracheal cannula to bypass nasal scrubbing greatly augments the irritant response, indicating that deep lung irritant receptors can also be activated by this vapor.

The irritancy of inhaled formaldehyde vapor, again like SO_2, has been shown to be potentiated by water-soluble salt aerosols. Irritancy appears to be augmented in proportion to the aerosol concentration, but the potentiation could not be accounted for by a simple aerosol "carrier" effect (Amdur, 1960). Moreover, reversal of bronchoconstriction was slower than had been observed with SO_2. Thus it appeared that the vapor-aerosol itself constituted a new irritant species, the product of a chemical transformation of formaldehyde—perhaps methylene hydroxide (Underhill, 2000). In addition to interactions with water-soluble particles, formaldehyde has been shown to interact with carbon-based particles (Jakab, 1992) to augment bacterial infectivity in a murine model. In this case, the potentiation appears to correlate with the surface carrying capacity of the inhaled particle.

Two aspects of formaldehyde toxicology have brought it from relative obscurity to the forefront of attention in recent years. One is its near ubiquitous presence in indoor atmospheres as an off-gassed product of construction materials such as plywood, furniture, or improperly polymerized urea-formaldehyde foam insulation (Spengler and Sexton, 1983). Complaints of formaldehyde irritation in industry have been reported at 50 ppb (Horvath *et al.*, 1988). In studies relating household formaldehyde to chronic effects, children were found to have significantly lower peak expiratory flow rates (about 22% in homes with 60 ppb) than did unexposed children, and asthmatic children were affected below 50 ppb. Thus, this irritant vapor can cause respiratory effects, and perhaps act as an allergen, at commonly experienced exposure levels (Krzyzanowski *et al.*, 1990).

A longtime concern regarding formaldehyde has been its potential carcinogenicity. In 2004, IARC concluded, based on a through review of the published data, that formaldehyde was a probable carcinogen; IARC deemed that there was "sufficient" epidemiologic evidence that formaldehyde causes nasopharyngeal cancer, "strong but not sufficient" evidence of leukemia, and limited evidence of sinonasal cancer, along with "sufficient" evidence that formaldehyde causes nasal cancer in animals (Cogliano, 2005). Nasal cancer had been induced empirically with formaldehyde vapor in a 2-year study where rats were exposed to 2, 6, or 14 ppm 6 hours per day, 5 days per week. The incidence of nasal squamous cell carcinomas was zero in the control and 2-ppm groups, 1% in the 6-ppm group, and 44% in the 14-ppm group. Exposure-related induction of squamous metaplasia occurred in the respiratory epithelium of the anterior nasal passages in all exposed groups. A 20-fold increase in cell proliferation in the nasal epithelium occurred after 5 days to 14 ppm. Mice were much less sensitive; only one carcinoma was seen at 14 ppm. The detection of DNA adducts in the two species paralleled the difference in the incidence of tumors as well as regional dosimetry. Formaldehyde, with its large and diverse database and potential public health impact, has remained the focus of considerable debate among modelers and risk assessors. The arguments behind this debate crosses both cancer and noncancer considerations and is beyond that which can be discussed in this chapter. The reader is encouraged to sample the recent literature (e.g., Connolly *et al.*, 2004).

Acrolein   Because acrolein is an unsaturated aldehyde, it is more reactive than formaldehyde. It penetrates a bit deeper into the airways and may not have the same degree of sensory irritancy but it may cause more damage. Concentrations below 1 ppm cause irritation of the eyes and the mucous membranes of the respiratory tract. Exposure of guinea pigs to ≥0.6 ppm reversibly increased pulmonary flow resistance and tidal volume and decreased respiratory frequency (Murphy *et al.*, 1963). With irritants of this type, flow resistance is increased by concentrations below those that cause the classic decrease in frequency seen with sensory irritants. This suggests that increases in flow resistance would be produced by far lower concentrations of acrolein than were tested. The mechanism of increased resistance appears to be mediated through both local C-fiber and centrally mediated cholinergic reflexes. Ablation of the C-fiber network and atropine (muscarinic blocker) block this response. On the other hand, aminophylline, isoproterenol, and epinephrine (sympathetic agonists) partially or completely reversed the changes, whereas the antihistamines pyrilamine and tripelennamine had no effect.

Exposures of rats to 0.4, 1.4, or 4.0 ppm for 6 hours per day, 5 days per week for 13 weeks resulted in paradoxical effects on lung function (Costa *et al.*, 1986). The lowest concentration resulted in hyperinflation of the lung with an apparent reduction in small-airway flow resistance, while the highest concentration resulted in airway injury and peribronchial inflammation and fibrosis. The intermediate concentration was functionally not different from the control, although airway pathology was evident. It appears that the high-concentration response reflected the cumulative irritant injury and remodeling as a result of the repeated acrolein, while the low-concentration group had little overt damage and appeared to have slightly stiffened airways, perhaps a result of the protein cross-linking action of acrolein. The pathology in these rats contrasts with that found in formaldehyde studies of similar duration, where more upper airway involvement was observed. Ambient exposure to acrolein probably would be about 10–20% the low concentration used in the subchronic study discussed above. However, these concentrations of acrolein are well below those found in mainstream tobacco smoke and the occupational Threshold Limit Value.

Thus, as a class the aldehydes can be very irritating and may constitute a significant fraction of the discomfort and sensation experienced during an oxidant pollution episode, especially in mixed atmospheres containing particles.

Carbon Monoxide   Carbon monoxide is classed toxicologically as a chemical asphyxiant because its toxic action stems from its formation of carboxyhemoglobin, preventing oxygenation of the blood for systemic transport. The fundamental toxicology of CO and the physiologic factors that determine the level of carboxyhemoglobin attained in the blood at various atmospheric concentrations of carbon monoxide are detailed in Chap. 11.

The normal concentration of carboxyhemoglobin (COHb) in the blood of nonsmokers is about 0.5%. This is attributed to endogenous production of CO from heme catabolism. Blood COHb is a function of the concentration in air, the length of exposure, and the ventilation of the exposed individual. Uptake is said to be ventilation-limited, implying that virtually all the CO inspired in a breath is absorbed and bound to the available hemoglobin. Thus, continuous exposure of human subjects to 30 ppm CO leads to an equilibrium value of 5% COHb. The Haldane equation is used to compute the COHb equilibrium under a given exposure situation. The equilibrium values generally are reached after 8 hours or more of exposure. The time required to reach equilibrium can be shortened by physical activity.

Analysis of data from air-monitoring programs in California indicates that 8 hour average values can range from 10 to 40 ppm CO. Depending on the location in a community, CO concentrations can vary widely. Vehicle emissions are the major source of CO outside accidental domestic exposures and tobacco smoke. Concentrations predicted inside passenger compartments of motor vehicles in downtown traffic were almost 3 times those for central urban areas and 5 times those expected in residential areas. Occupants of vehicles traveling on expressways had CO exposures somewhere between those in central urban areas and those in downtown traffic. Concentrations above 87 ppm have been measured in underground garages, tunnels, and buildings over highways.

No overt human health effects have been demonstrated for COHb levels below 2%, while levels above 40% cause fatal asphyxiation. A 90-minute exposure to about 50 ppm CO would likely result in COHb levels of ~2.5%, with a resultant impairment of time-interval discrimination; at approximately 5% COHb, there is an impairment of other psychomotor faculties. At 5% COHb in nonsmokers (the median COHb value for smokers is about 5%), however, maximal exercise duration and maximal oxygen consumption are reduced (Aronow, 1981). Cardiovascular changes also may be produced by exposures sufficient to yield COHb in excess of 5%. These include increased cardiac output, arteriovenous oxygen difference, and coronary blood flow in patients without coronary disease. Decreased coronary sinus blood PO$_2$ occurs in patients with coronary heart disease, and this would impair oxidative metabolism of the myocardium. In the early 1990s, a series of studies in subjects with cardiovascular disease were conducted in several laboratories under the sponsorship of the Health Effects Institute (HEI) to determine the potential for angina pectoris when they exercised moderately with COHb levels in the range of 2–6% (Allred *et al.*, 1989). The results of these studies indicate that premature angina can occur under these conditions but that the potential for the induction of ventricular arrhythmias remains uncertain. Thus, the reduction in ambient CO brought about by newer controls should reduce the risk of myocardial infarct in predisposed persons.

The recent introduction of gasoline oxygenates like MTBE and other ether derivatives was an attempt to enhance fuel combustion and reduce CO emissions. The ensuing problems with MTBE have been discussed earlier, but the goal of achieving lower CO was only partially successful. This finding reinforces the need to carefully consider whether resolution of one problem has the potential for generating others.

Hazardous Air Pollutants   Hazardous air pollutants (so-called air toxics or HAPs) represent an inclusive classification for air pollutants that are of anthropogenic origin that are generally of measurable quantity in the air, and are not covered in the Criteria Pollutant list. They are covered under Section 112 of the Clean Air Act. Selected regulatory issues of the HAPs were discussed above. Most exposure estimates for these pollutants are derived from emission inventories that are modeled into the National Air Toxics Assessment (www.epa.gov/ttn/atw/nata/sitemap.html). The most recent NATA assessment (2002) used 1999 data on the 33 HAPs (so-called "dirty 30" noted above), plus diesel emissions. The diverse nature of even 33 of the 188 HAPs complicates a general discussion of their toxicology because the group includes various classes of organic chemicals (by structure, e.g., acrolein, benzene), minerals (e.g., asbestos), polycyclic hydrocarbon particulate material [e.g., benzo(a)pyrene], and various metals and metal compounds (e.g., mercury, beryllium compounds) and pesticides (e.g., carbaryl, parathion).

The focus to date on the HAPs has been on their potential carcinogenicity, as shown in chronic bioassays, mutagenicity tests in bacterial systems, structure-activity relationships, or—in a few special cases (e.g., benzene, asbestos)—their known carcinogenicity in humans. These cancers need not be, and generally are not, pulmonary. Noncancer issues frequently relate to direct lung toxicants that, upon fugitive emissions or accidental release, which might risk those with preexisting diseases (e.g., asthma) or which might lead to chronic lung disease. The assessment of noncancer risk by air toxics to any organ system is based on the computation of long-term risk reference exposure concentrations (RfCs) to which individuals may be exposed over a lifetime without adverse, irreversible injury. This approach to hazardous air pollutant assessment is discussed in detail by Jarabek and Segal (1994). An analogous short-term RfC method has been developed for exposures up to 30 days. Of the noncancer risks deemed highest in this analysis, acrolein ranks at the top based on emission inventories, the potential for exposure, and its inherent irritancy. Discussion of this topic and an approach to mixed exposures to noncancer HAPs has been reviewed (Costa, 2004).

Accidental versus "Fence-Line" Exposures The relationship between the effects associated with an accidental release of a large quantity of a volatile chemical into the air from a point source such as a chemical plant and the effects associated with a chronic low-level exposure over many years or a lifetime is not clear. With regard to cancer, which defaults to a linearized model of dose and effect (through some alternative models can be used if there is some data), the issue is fairly straightforward. Any exposure must be minimized if not eliminated if cancer risk is to be kept as close to zero as possible. With noncancer risks, the roles of nonspecific or specific host defenses, thresholds of response, and repair and recovery after exposure complicate the assessment of risk. In large part the issue here relates to $C \times T$. Can we better relate disease or injury to *cumulative dose* or *peak* concentration for protracted exposures? Is there an exposure peak beyond which a cumulative approach fails (i.e., the effect is concentration-driven), or is concentration always the dominant determinant? Many of these questions have yet to be answered, not to mention their specificity with regard to individual compounds and tissues affected.

Methyl isocyanate provides a contrast between the effects of a large accidental release versus those produced by cyclic or continuous small fugitive vapor releases. The reactive nature of methyl isocyanate with aqueous environments is of such magnitude that upon inspiration, almost immediate mucous tissue corrosion can be perceived. The vapor undergoes hydrolysis within the mucous lining of the airways to generate hydrocyanic acid, which destroys the airway epithelium and causes acute bronchoconstriction and edema. The damage is immediately life-threatening at concentrations above 50 ppm; at 10 ppm, it is damaging in minutes. These concentrations are in the range of the dense vapor cloud that for several hours enshrouded the village of Bhopal bordering the Union Carbide pesticide plant. Studies in guinea pigs showed the immediate irritancy of this isocyanate, which in just a few minutes also resulted in significant pathology (Alarie *et al.*, 1987). Rats exposed to 10 or 30 ppm for 2 hours also showed severe airway and parenchymal damage, which did not resolve in surviving rats; transient effects were seen at 3 ppm. Even 6 months after exposure, the airway and lung damage remained, having evolved into patchy, mostly peribronchial fibrosis with associated functional impairments (Stevens *et al.*, 1987). There was also cardiac involvement secondary to the damage to the pulmonary parenchyma and arterial bed. As a result, there was pulmonary hypertension and right-sided heart hypertrophy. This same spectrum of health effects has resulted in disability and deaths of thousands of initial survivors since the incident.

In the United States, methyl isocyanate has been measured in Katawba Valley, Texas, as a result of small but virtually continual fugitive releases of the vapor into the community air ("fence-line") from an adjoining region with several chemical plants. While these levels of methyl isocyanate are not sufficient to cause the damage seen in Bhopal, there is concern that low-level exposure over many years may have more diffuse, chronic effects. Residents complain of odors and a higher frequency of respiratory disorders, but clear evidence of injury or disease is lacking.

Phosgene is best known for its use as a war gas, but it is also one of the most common intermediate reactants used in the chemical industry, particularly in pesticide formulation. It is also a constituent of photochemical smog. Because of its direct pulmonary reactivity, it lends itself to use as a model pulmonary toxicant for studies addressing $C \times T$ relationships. These studies suggest that there may be a threshold below which compensatory and other bodily defenses (e.g., antioxidants) may be able to cope with long-term low-level exposure (tolerance). For phosgene, this appears to be at or below the current threshold limit value of 0.1 ppm for 8 hours. At higher concentrations, however, concentration appears to be the primary determinant of injury or disease regardless of duration. Thus, even though there is some adaptation with time, there continues to be a concentration-driven response that exceeds that predicted by $C \times T$. This relationship appears to be different from that of O_3 at ambient levels, which can be approximated acutely by the $C \times T$ paradigm.

WHAT IS AN ADVERSE HEALTH EFFECT?

Any attempt to establish criteria to define an "adverse effect" of air pollution is likely to be questioned. Some effects would pass uncontested as adverse, e.g., death, acute life-threatening dysfunction or disease, irreversible impairments, and pain. Other effects that may reflect minor and temporary dysfunctions or discomfort could be argued by some as not warranting significant or costly concern, especially if effects are minor or transient. The goal of air-quality management is clearly to avoid or, at worst, limit negative impacts of air pollution on public health. However, one must appreciate the distinction between risk to the individual and to a population. Clearly, risk to an individual can be beyond an acceptable limit and can put that person's health in jeopardy, but this response may be lost in a population index. On the other hand, risk to a population is the summation of individual risks such that there is a shift in the normal distribution putting unspecified individuals at risk. These two forms of risk are clearly related, but most often in practice, the population risk is considered most appropriate and most reasonably quantifiable. This population-based risk or susceptibility is that identified in the CAA.

In 1985, the American Thoracic Society issued a position paper that attempted to define an adverse effect related to air pollution. This definition has recently been revised because of the many advances in clinical medicine and empirical health sciences (ATS, 2000). This statement considers seven broad areas: biomarkers, quality of life, physiologic impacts, symptoms, clinical outcomes, mortality, and population health versus individual risk. The summary conclusion states that caution should be exercised in evaluating the many new biomarkers of effect (especially cell and molecular markers), as there is need for validation that *small* changes in these markers represent a progression along a course to disease or permanent impairment. Admittedly, in the clinical environment many of these markers may appear as salient features of a disease or injury, but the health implications of minor changes in these biomarkers remains uncertain. Significant alterations of standard clinical measures of health due to pollution are clearly adverse. However, a shift from the 1985 ATS statement is that transient pulmonary function deficits (where a 10% or more drop in FVC was defined as adverse) may not necessarily be adverse. On the other hand, any irreversible reduction in pulmonary function would be adverse either for an individual or

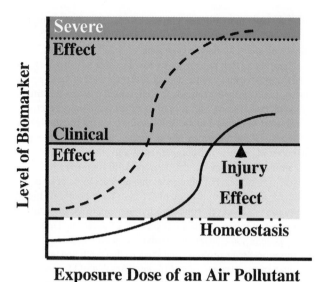

Figure 28-13. *Schematic illustration of the elements of the dose response to an air pollutant(s) of a susceptible versus a healthy individual.*

The hypothetical susceptible individual may be more sensitive or may have a *loss of reserve*, either of which results in an *inability to maintain homeostasis*. The *leftward shift or increased slope* in the dose–response curve suggests an increase in responsiveness. Either situation may contribute to sensitivity and the likelihood of enhanced progression from subtle to severe outcomes.

across a population. Any population for which a significant mortality risk can be detected must be considered adverse. Of course, a common thread through all these subject areas is the influential role of susceptibility, which can take the form of hyper-responsiveness or loss of reserve. What was a minor reversible effect may now be a dysfunction that cannot be reversed or compensated (Fig. 28-13). Obvious examples would be cardiopulmonary compromised individuals who function with little or no reserve. In the end, however, the ATS statement realizes the limits of definitions and the importance of value judgment in the final assessment. Implied in this

position is that a loss of quality of life due to air pollution as well as enduring its associated effects may also be designated as adverse. As science continues to advance, especially in the realm of molecular biology where small signals can be detected that may forecast an adverse effect or otherwise may identify individuals or groups at risk, the definition of adverse will certainly need re-examination. That same sensitivity in measurement that serves to predict an adverse effect must be separated from signals that are essential for homeostasis and the maintenance of life. Clearly, dissecting and defining these phenomena will have implications not only for assessing clinical adversity but will have implications for predictive toxicology.

CONCLUSIONS

In writing this textbook chapter on air pollution toxicology, the author's goal has been to relate empirical studies in animals to phenomena known to occur in humans through epidemiologic or controlled clinical study. The breadth and complexity of the problem of air pollution—from the development of credible databases to supporting regulatory action and decision making—has been the theme throughout. The classic and still most important air pollutants provide a foundation for understanding and appreciating the nuances of the issues and strategies for air pollution control and protection of public health. The key role of the toxicologist is to develop sensitive methods to assay responses to low pollutant concentrations, apply these methods to relevant exposure scenarios and test species, and develop paradigms to relate empiric toxicological data to real life through an understanding of mechanism. Last, the toxicologist must continually integrate laboratory data with those of epidemiology and clinical study to ensure their maximum utility.

ACKNOWLEDGMENT

The author would like to thank Mr. James R. Lehmann of the USEPA for his constructive comments on the chapter, and Dr. Urmila Kodavanti and Mr. William Russo, also of the USEPA, for their critical reviews.

REFERENCES

Alarie Y, Ferguson JS, Stock MF, *et al.*: Sensory and pulmonary irritation of methyl isocyanate in mice and pulmonary irritation and possible cyanide-like effects of methyl isocyanate in guinea pigs. *Environ Health Perspect* 72:159–168, 1987.

Alarie YC, Krumm AA, Busey WM, *et al.*: Long-term exposure to sulfur dioxide, sulfuric acid mist, fly ash, and their mixtures: Results of studies in monkeys and guinea pigs. *Arch Environ Health* 30:254–262, 1975.

Alarie YC, Ulrich CE, Busey WM, *et al.*: Long-term continuous exposure of guinea pigs to sulfur dioxide. *Arch Environ Health* 21:769–777, 1970.

Alarie YC, Ulrich CE, Busey WM, *et al.*: Long-term continuous exposure to sulfur dioxide in cynomolgus monkeys. *Arch Environ Health* 24:115–128, 1972.

Allred EN, Bleeker ER, Chaitman BR, *et al.*: Short-term effects of carbon monoxide exposure on individuals with coronary heart disease. *N Engl J Med* 321:1426–1432, 1989.

Amdur MO: Toxicological studies of air pollutants. *US Public Health Reports* 69:724–726, 1954.

Amdur MO: The respiratory response of guinea pigs to sulfuric acid mist. *AMA Arch Ind Health* 18:407–414, 1958.

Amdur MO: The response of guinea pigs to inhalation of formaldehyde and formic acid alone and with a sodium chloride aerosol. *Int J Air Pollut* 3:201–220, 1960.

Amdur MO: 1974 Cummings memorial lecture: The long road from Donora. *Am Ind Hyg Assoc J* 35:589–597, 1974.

Amdur MO: Sulfuric acid: The animals tried to tell us: 1989 Herbert E. Stokinger Lecture. *Appl Ind Hyg Assoc J* 4:189–197, 1989.

Amdur MO, Dubriel M, Creasia DA: Respiratory response of guinea pigs to low levels of sulfuric acid. *Environ Res* 15:418–423, 1978.

Amdur MO, Sarofim AF, Neville M, *et al.*: Coal combustion aerosols and SO_2: An interdisciplinary analysis. *Environ Sci Tech* 20:139–145, 1986.

Amdur MO, Underhill DW: The effect of various aerosols on the response of guinea pigs to sulfur dioxide. *Arch Environ Health* 16:460–468, 1968.

American Thoracic Society: What constitutes an adverse health effect of air pollution? *Am J Respir Crit Care Med* 161:665–673, 2000.

Anderson HR: Health effects of air pollution episodes, in: Holgate ST, Samet JM, Koren H, Maynard RL (eds): *Air Pollution and Health.* London: Academic Press, 1999, pp. 461–484.

Aronow WS: Aggravation of angina pectoris by two percent carboxyhemoglobin. *Am Heart J* 101:154–157, 1981.

Barry BE, Mercer RR, Miller FJ, et al.: Effects of inhalation of 0.25 ppm O₃ on the terminal bronchioles of juvenile and adult rats. *Exp Lung Res* 14:225–245, 1988.

Bates DV, Sizto R: Air pollution and hospital admissions in southern Ontario: The acid summer haze effect. *Environ Res* 65:172–194, 1987.

Boubel RW, Fox DL, Turner DB et al.: *Fundamentals of Air Pollution,* 3rd edn. New York: Academic Press, 1994, pp. 107.

Brimblecombe P: Air pollution and health history, in Holgate ST, Samet JM, Koren H, Maynard RL (eds): *Air Pollution and Health.* London: Academic Press, 1999, pp. 10.

Brooks BO, Davis WF: *Understanding Indoor Air Quality.* Boca Raton, FL: CRC Press, 1992.

Calderon-Garciduenas L, Mora-Tiscareno A, Fordham LA, et al.: Respiratory damage in children exposed to urban pollution. *Pediatr Pulmonol* 36(2):148–161, 2003.

Calderon-Garcidueñas L, Osorno-Velazquez A, Bravo-Alvarez H, et al.: Histopathological changes of the nasal mucosa in southwest metropolitan Mexico City inhabitants. *Am J Pathol* 140:225–232, 1992.

Calvert JG, Lazrus A, Kok GL, et al.: Chemical mechanisms of acid generation in the troposphere. *Nature* 317:27–35, 1985.

Chang L, Huang Y, Stockstill BL, et al.: Epithelial injury and interstitial fibrosis in the proximal alveolar regions of rats chronically exposed to a simulated pattern of urban ambient ozone. *Toxicol Appl Pharmacol* 115:241–252, 1992.

Chang L, Miller FJ, Ultman J, et al.: Alveolar epithelial cell injuries by subacute exposure to low concentrations of ozone correlate with cumulative exposure. *Toxicol Appl Pharmacol* 109:219–234, 1991.

Chang LY, Mercer RR, Stockstill BL, et al.: Effects of low levels of NO₂ on terminal bronchiolar cells and its relative toxicity compared to O₃. *Toxicol Appl Pharmacol* 96:451–464, 1988.

Chen LC, Lam HF, Kim EJ, et al.: Pulmonary effects of ultrafine coal fly ash inhaled by guinea pigs. *J Toxicol Environ Health* 29:169–184, 1990.

Coffin DL, Blommer EJ: Acute toxicity of irradiated auto exhaust: Its indication by enhancement of mortality from streptococcal pneumonia. *Arch Environ Health* 15:36–38, 1967.

Cogliano VJ: IARC Monographs, leukemia, nasopharyngeal cancer, sinonasal cancer. *Environ Health Perspect* 113:1205–1208, 2005.

Cohen AJ, Nikula, KJ: The health effects of diesel exhaust: Laboratory and epidemiology studies, in Holgate ST, Samet JM, Koren HS, Maynard RL (eds): *Air Pollution and Health.* San Diego, CA: Academic Press, 1999, pp. 707–745.

Conolly RB, Kimbel JS, Janszen D, et al.: Human respiratory tract cancer risks of inhaled formaldehyde: Dose-Response predictions derived from biologically motivated computational modeling of a combined rodent and human dataset. *Toxicol Sci* 82: 279–296, 2004.

Costa DL: Particulate matter and cardiopulmonary health: A toxicologic perspective. *Inhal Toxicol* 12(Suppl 3):35–44, 2000.

Costa DL: Issues that must be addressed for risk assessment of mixed exposures: The U.S. EPA experience with air quality. *J Toxicol Environ Health A* 67(3):195–207, 2004.

Costa DL, Dreher KL: Bioavailable transition metals in particulate matter mediate cardiopulmonary injury in healthy and compromised animal models. *Environ Health Perspect* 105 (Suppl 5):1053–1060, 1997.

Costa DL, Hatch GE, Highfill J, et al.: Pulmonary function studies in the rat addressing concentration vs. time relationships for ozone, in Schneider T, Lee SD, Wolters GJR, Grant LD (eds): *Atmospheric Ozone Research and Its Policy Implications.* Amsterdam: Elsevier, 1989, pp. 733–743.

Costa DL, Kutzman RS, Lehmann JR, et al.: Altered lung function and structure in the rat after subchronic exposure to acrolein. *Am Rev Respir Dis* 133:286–291, 1986.

Costa DL, Schafrank SN, Wehner RW, et al.: Alveolar permeability to protein in rats differentially susceptible to ozone. *J Appl Toxicol* 5(3):182–186, 1985.

Costa DL, Schlegele E: Irritant air pollutants, in Swift DL, Foster WM (eds): *Air Pollutants and the Respiratory Tract.* New York: Marcel Dekker, 1998, pp. 119–145.

Costa DL, Tepper JS, Stevens MA, et al.: Restrictive lung disease in rats chronically exposed to an urban profile of ozone. *Am J Respir Crit Care Med* 151:1512–1518, 1995.

Detels R, Tashkin DP, Sayre JW, et al.: The UCLA population studies of CORD: X. A cohort study of changes in respiratory function associated with chronic exposure to SOₓ, NOₓ, and hydrocarbons. *Am J Public Health* 81:350–359, 1991.

Devlin RB, Folinsbee LJ, Biscardi F, et al.: Attenuation of cellular and biochemical changes in the lungs of humans exposed to ozone for five consecutive days. *Am Rev Respir Dis* 147:A71, 1993.

Devlin RB, McDonnell WF, Mann R, et al.: Exposure of humans to ambient levels of ozone for 6.6 hours causes cellular and biochemical changes in the lung. *Am J Respir Cell Mol Biol* 4:72–81, 1991.

Diaz-Sanchez D, Garcia MP, Wang M, et al.: Nasal challenge with diesel exhaust particles can induce sensitization to a neoallergen in the human mucosa. *J Allergy Clin Immunol* 104(6):1183–1188, 1999.

Dockery DW, Pope CA, Xu X, et al.: An association between air pollution and mortality in six U.S. cities. *N Engl J Med* 329(24):1753–1759, 1993.

Dockery D, Pope III CA: Health effects of fine particulate air pollution: Lines that connect. *J Air Waste Manag Assoc* 56(6):709–742, 2006.

Donaldson K, Li XY, MacNee W: Ultrafine (nanometre) particle mediated lung injury. *J Aerosol Sci* 29:553–560, 1998.

Driscoll KE, Deyo LC, Carter JM, et al.: Effects of particle exposure and particle-elicited inflammatory cells on mutation in rat alveolar epithelial cells. *Carcinogenesis* 18(2):423–430, 1997.

Ehrlich R, Henry MC: Chronic toxicity of nitrogen dioxide: I. Effect on resistance to bacterial pneumonia. *Arch Environ Health* 17:860–865, 1968.

Environmental Progress and Challenges: EPA's Update. U.S. EPA, Office of Policy Planning and Evaluation (PM-219), EPA-230-07-88-033. Washington, DC: EPA, 1988, p. 29.

Firkert M: Fog along the Meuse Valley. *Trans Faraday Soc* 32:1192–1197, 1936.

Frampton MW, Smeglin AM, Roberts NJJ, et al.: Nitrogen dioxide exposure *in vivo* and human macrophage inactivation of influenza virus *in vitro.* *Environ Res* 48:179–192, 1989.

Frank NR, Amdur MO, Worchester J, et al.: Effects of acute controlled exposure to SO₂ on respiratory mechanics in healthy male adults. *J Appl Physiol* 17:252–258, 1962.

Frank NR, Speizer FE: SO₂ effects on the respiratory system in dogs: Changes in mechanical behavior at different levels of the respiratory system during acute exposure to the gas. *Arch Environ Health* 11:624–634, 1965.

Gardner DE: Oxidant induced enhanced sensitivity to infection in animal models and their extrapolation to man. *J Toxicol Environ Health* 13:423–439, 1984.

Gauderman WJ, Avol E, Gilliland F, et al.: The effect of air pollution on lung development from 10 to 18 years of age. *N Engl J Med* 351(11):1057–1067, 2004.

Gearhart JM, Schlesinger RB: Sulfuric acid-induced changes in the physiology and structure of the tracheobronchial airways. *Environ Health Perspect* 79:127–136, 1989.

Gelzleichter TR, Witschi H, Last JA: Synergistic interaction of nitrogen dioxide and ozone on rat lungs: Acute responses. *Toxicol Appl Pharmacol* 116:1–9, 1992.

Gerrity TR, Weaver RA, Bernsten J, et al.: Extrathoracic and intrathoracic removal of ozone in tidal breathing humans. *J Appl Physiol* 65:393–400, 1988.

Ghio AJ, Carter JD, Richards JH, et al.: Diminished injury in hypertranferrinemic mice after exposure to a metal-rich particle. *Am J Physiol Lung Cell Mol Physiol* 278(5):L1051–L1061, 2000.

Ghio AJ, Kennedy TP, Whorton AR, et al.: Role of surface complexed iron in oxidant generation and lung inflammation induced by silicates. *Am J Physiol Lung Cell Mol Physiol* 263(7):L511–L518, 1992.

Gilmour MI, Park P, Doerfler D, Selgrade MK: Ozone-enhanced pulmonary infection with *Streptococcus zooepidemicus* in mice: The role of alveolar macrophage function and capsular virulence factors. *Am Rev Respir Dis* 147:753–760, 1993.

Glasser SW, Korfhagen TR, Wert S, et al.: Transgenic models for study of pulmonary development and disease. *Am J Physiol: Lung Cell Mol Physiol* 267(11):L489–L497, 1994.

Gold DR, Litonjua A, Schwartz J, *et al.*: Ambient pollution and heart rate variability. *Circulation* 101(11):1267–1273, 2000.

Gong Jr H, Lachenbruch PA, Haber P, *et al.*: Comparative short term health responses to sulfur dioxide exposure and other common stressors in a panel of asthmatics. *Toxicol Ind Health* 11:467–487, 1995.

Gunnison AF, Palmes ED: S-Sulfonates in human plasma following inhalation of sulfur dioxide. *Am Ind Hyg Assoc J* 35:288–291, 1974.

Hackney JD, Linn WS, Avol EL: Acid fog: Effects on respiratory function and symptoms in healthy asthmatic volunteers. *Environ Health Perspect* 79:159–162, 1989.

Hanley QS, Koenig JQ, Larson TV, *et al.*: Response of young asthmatic patients to inhaled sulfuric acid. *Am Rev Respir Dis* 145:326–331, 1992.

Hatch GE, Boykin E, Graham JA, *et al.*: Inhalable particles and pulmonary host defense: *In vivo* and *in vitro* effects of ambient air and combustion particles. *Environ Res* 36:67–80, 1985.

Hatch GE, Slade R, Harris LP, *et al.*: Ozone dose and effect in humans and rats: A comparison using oxygen-18 labeling and bronchoalveolar lavage. *Am J Respir Crit Care Med* 150:676–683, 1994.

Hayes SM, Gobbell RV, Ganick NR (eds): *Indoor Air Quality: Solutions and Strategies.* New York: McGraw-Hill, 1995.

Hazucha M, Madden M, Pape G, *et al.*: Effect of cycloxygenase inhibition on ozone induced respiratory inflammation and lung function changes. *Environ J Appl Physiol Occup Health* 73(1–2):17–27, 1996.

Health Effects Report: Consequences of Prolonged Inhalation of Ozone on F344 Rats: Collaborative Studies. Studies I–XIII, Report #65. Boston: Health Effects Institute, 1994–1995.

Henry MC, Findlay J, Spengler J, Ehrlich R: Chronic toxicity of NO_2 in squirrel monkeys: III. Effect on resistance to bacterial and viral infection. *Am Ind Hyg Assoc J* 20:566–570, 1970.

Highfill JH, Hatch GE, Slade R, *et al.*: Concentration time models for the effects of ozone on bronchoalveolar lavage fluid protein in rats and guinea pigs. *Inhal Toxicol* 4:1–16, 1992.

Higuchi MA, Davies DW: An ammonia abatement system for whole-body animal inhalation exposures to acid aerosols. *Inhal Toxicol* 5:323–333, 1993.

Ho YS: Transgenic models for the study of lung biology and disease. *Am J Physiol Lung Cell Mol Physiol* 266(10):L319–L353, 1994.

Holma B: Effects of inhaled acids on airway mucus and its consequences for health. *Environ Health Perspect* 79:109–114, 1989.

Horstman DH, Folinsbee LJ, Ives PJ, *et al.*: Ozone concentration and pulmonary response relationships for 6.6 hours with five hours of moderate exercise to 0.08, 0.10, and 0.12 ppm. *Am Rev Respir Dis* 142:1158–1162, 1989.

Horvath E, Anderson H, Pierce W, *et al.*: Effects of formaldehyde on mucous membranes and lungs: A study of an industrial population. *JAMA* 259:701–707, 1988.

Hyde D, Orthoefer J, Dungworth D, *et al.*: Morphometric and morphologic pulmonary lesions in beagle dogs chronically exposed to high ambient levels of air pollutants. *Lab Invest* 38(4):455–469, 1978.

ILSI Report: The relevance of the rat lung response to particle overload for human risk assessment: A workshop consensus report. ILSI Sponsored Workshop, March, 1998, *Inhal Toxicol* 12:101–117, 2000.

Jakab GJ: Relationship between carbon black particulate-bound formaldehyde, pulmonary antibacterial defenses and alveolar macrophage phagocytosis. *Inhal Toxicol* 4:325–342, 1992.

Jarabek AM, Segal SA: Noncancer toxicity of inhaled toxic air pollutants: Available approaches for risk assessment and risk management, in Patrick DR (ed): *Toxic Air Pollution Handbook.* New York: Van Nostrand Reinhold, 1994, pp. 100–132.

Johnston CJ, Finkelstein JN, Oberdorster G, *et al.*: Clara cell secretory protein-deficient mice differ from wild-type mice in inflammatory chemokine expression to oxygen and ozone, but not to endotoxin. *Exp Lung Res* 25(1):7–21, 1999.

Kakuyama M, Ahluwalia A, Rodrigo J, *et al.*: Cholinergic contraction is altered in nNOS knockouts: Cooperative modulation of neural bronchoconstriction by NOS and COX. *Am J Respir Crit Care Med* 160:2072–2078, 1999.

Kieber RJ, Skrabal SA, Smith BJ, Willey JD: Organic complexation of Fe(II) and its impact on the redox cycling of iron in rain. *Environ Sci Technol* 39(6):1576–1583, 2005.

Kim CS, Kang TC: Comparative measurement of lung deposition of inhaled fine particles in normal subjects and patients with obstructive airway disease. *Am J Respir Crit Care Med* 155(3):899–905, 1997.

Kinney PJ, Ware JH, Spengler JD: A critical evaluation of acute epidemiology results. *Arch Environ Health* 43:168–173, 1988.

Kistner A, Gossen M, Zimmermann F, Jerecic J, *et al.*: Doxycycline mediated quantitative and tissue specific control of gene expression in transgenic mice. *Pro Natl Acad Sci U S A* 93:10933–10938, 1996.

Kleeberger SR, Reddy S, Zhang LY, *et al.*: Genetic susceptibility to ozone-induced lung hyperpermeability. Role of toll-like receptor 4. *Am J Respir Cell Mol Biol* 22(5):620–627, 2000.

Kleinman MT, Bailey RM, Whynot JD *et al.*: Controlled exposure to a mixture of SO_2, NO_2, and particulate air pollutants: Effects on human pulmonary function and respiratory symptoms. *Arch Environ Health* 40:197–201, 1985.

Kleinman MT, Mautz WJ, Bjarnason S: Adaptive and non-adaptive responses in rats exposed to ozone, alone and in mixtures, with acidic aerosols. *Inhal Toxicol* 11(3):249–264, 1999.

Kodavanti UP, Costa DL, Bromberg P: Rodent models of cardiopulmonary disease: Their potential applicability in studies of air pollutant susceptibility. *Environ Health Perspect* 106 (Suppl 1):111–130, 1998.

Kodavanti UP, Mebane R, Ledbetter A, *et al.*: Variable pulmonary responses from exposure to concentrated ambient air particles in a rat model of bronchitis. *Toxicol Sci* 54(2):441–451, 2000.

Kodavanti UP, Schladweiler MC, Ledbetter AD, *et al.*: Consistent pulmonary and systemic responses from inhalation of fine concentrated ambient particles: Roles of rat strains used and physicochemical properties. *Environ Health Perspect* 113(11):1561–1568, 2005.

Koenig JQ, Covert DS, Pierson WE: Effects of inhalation of acidic compounds on pulmonary function in allergic adolescent subjects. *Environ Health Perspect* 79:127–137, 173–178, 1989.

Koenig JQ, Pierson WE, Horike M, Frank R: Effects of SO_2 plus NaCl aerosol combined with moderate exercise on pulmonary function in asthmatic adolescents. *Environ Res* 25:340–348, 1981.

Koren HS, Devlin RB, Graham DE, *et al.*: Ozone-induced inflammation in the lower airways of human subjects. *Am Rev Respir Dis* 139:407–415, 1989.

Kotin P, Falk HF: Atmospheric factors in pathogenesis of lung cancer. *Cancer Res* 7:475–514, 1963.

Kreyling WG, Semmler M, Erbe F, *et al.*: Translocation of ultrafine insoluble iridium particles from lung epithelium to extrapulmonary organs is size dependent but very low. *J Toxicol Environ Health A* 65(20):1513–1530, 2002.

Krzyzanowski M, Quackenboss JJ, Lebowitz MD: Chronic respiratory effects of indoor formaldehyde exposure. *Environ Res* 52:117–125, 1990.

Kuhn III C, Homer RJ, Zhu Z, *et al.*: Airway hyperresponsiveness and air obstruction in transgenic mice: Morphologic correlates in mice over-expressing IL-11 and IL-6 in the lung. *Am J Respir Cell Mol Biol* 22:289–295, 2000.

Last JA, Gelzleichter TR, Harkema J, Hawk S: *Consequences of Prolonged Inhalation of Ozone on Fischer-344/N Rats: Collaborative Studies.* Part I: *Content and Cross-Linking of Lung Collagen*: Res. Report No. 65. Cambridge, MA: Health Effects Institute, April 1994.

Leikauf G, Yeates DB, Wales KA, *et al.*: Effects of sulfuric acid aerosol on respiratory mechanics and mucociliary particle clearance in healthy nonsmoking adults. *Am Ind Hyg Assoc J* 42:273–282, 1981.

Lewis TR, Campbell KI, Vaughan Jr TR: Effects on canine pulmonary function: Via induced NO_2 impairment, particulate interaction, and subsequent SO_x. *Arch Environ Health* 18:596–601, 1969.

Lewis TR, Moorman WJ, Yang YY, Stara JF: Long-term exposure to auto exhaust and other pollutant mixtures. *Arch Environ Health* 21:102–106, 1974.

Lewtas J: Airborne carcinogens. *Pharmacol Toxicol* 72(Suppl 1):S55–S63, 1993.

Lipfert FW: *Air Pollution and Community Health: A Critical Review and Data Sourcebook.* New York: Van Nostrand Reinhold, 1994, pp. 10–57.

Lippmann M: Health effects of ozone: A critical review. *J Air Pollut Control Assoc* 39:67–96, 1989.

Lippmann M, Altshuler B: Regional deposition of aerosols, in Aharonson EF, Ben-David A, Klingberg MA (eds): *Air Pollution and the Lung.* Jerusalem: Halsted Press - John Wiley, 1976, pp. 25–48.

Madden MC, Richards J, Daily LA, *et al.*: Effect of ozone on diesel exhaust particle toxicity in the rat lung. *Toxicol Appl Pharmacol* 168:140–148, 2000.

Maddison D, Pierce D: Costing the health effects of poor air quality, in Holgate ST, Samet JM, Koren H, Maynard RL (eds): *Air Pollution and Health.* London: Academic Press, 1999, pp. 917–930.

Martonen TB, Zhang Z, Yang Y: Interspecies modeling of inhaled particle deposition patterns. *J Aerosol Sci* 23(4):389–406, 1992.

Mauderly JL: Toxicological approaches to complex mixtures. *Environ Health Perspect* 101(Suppl 4):155–165, 1993.

Mauderly JL: Health hazards of complex environmental exposures: A difficult challenge to inhalation toxicology. *Inhal Toxicol* 18:137–141, 2006.

McCunney RJ: Asthma, genes, and air pollution. *J Occup Environ Med* 47(12):1285–1291, 2005.

McDonnell WF, Horstman DH, Hazucha MJ, *et al.*: Pulmonary effects of ozone exposure during exercise: Dose-response characteristics. *J Appl Physiol* 5:1345–1352, 1983.

McKinney WJ, Jaskot RH, Richards JH, *et al.*: Cytokine mediation of ozone-induced pulmonary adaptation. *Am J Respir Cell Mol Biol* 18:696–705, 1998.

Mercer RR, Costa DL, Crapo JD: Effects of prolonged exposure to low doses of nitric oxide on the alveolar septa of the adult rat lung. *Lab Invest* 73(1):1–9, 1995.

Miller FJ, Graham JA, Raub JA, *et al.*: Evaluating the toxicity of urban patterns of oxidant gases: II. Effects in mice from chronic exposure to nitrogen dioxide. *J Toxicol Environ Health* 21:99–112, 1987.

Miller FW, Miller RM: *Environmental Hazards: Air Pollution—A Reference Handbook. Contemporary World Issues.* Santa Barbara, CA: ABC-CLIO, Inc., 1993, pp. 1–18.

Mohsenin V: Effect of vitamin C on NO_2-induced airway hyperresponsiveness in normal subjects. *Am Rev Respir Dis* 136:1408–1411, 1987.

Molhave LB, Bach B, Pederson O: Human reactions to low concentrations of volatile organic compounds. *Environ Int* 12:165–167, 1986.

Moss OR, Gross EA, James RA, *et al.*: Respiratory tract toxicity in rats exposed to Mexico City air. *Res Rep Health Eff Inst* (100):1–24, 2001.

Motor vehicle-related air toxics study, U.S.EPA, EPA 420-R-93-005, Ann Arbor, MI: Office of Mobile Sources, 1993.

Mudway IS, Krishna MT, Frew AJ, *et al.*: Compromised concentrations of ascorbate in fluid lining the respiratory tract in human subjects after exposure to ozone. *Occup Environ Med* 56(7):473–481, 1999.

Murphy SD, Klingshirn DA, Ulrich CE: Respiratory response of guinea pigs during acrolein inhalation and its modification by drugs. *J Pharmacol Exp Ther* 141:79–83, 1963.

Nadel JA, Salem H, Tamplin B, Tokiwa Y: Mechanism of bronchoconstriction during inhalation of sulfur dioxide. *J Appl Physiol* 20:164–167, 1965.

National Air Pollutant Emission Trends Reports, 1998. EPA 454/R-00-002. Research Triangle Park, NC: U.S. EPA Office of Air Quality Planning and Standards, Mar. 2000, pp. 21.

National Air Quality & Emission Trends Report, 1998. EPA 454/R-00-003. Research Triangle Park, NC: U.S. EPA Office of Air Quality Planning and Standards, Mar. 2000, pp. 2, 5.

National Air Quality & Emission Trends Report, 2003. EPA 454/R-03-005. Research Triangle Park, NC: U.S. EPA Office of Air Quality Planning and Standards, Sept. 2003, pp. 2, 5.

National Research Council (NRC) and Committee on the Institutional Means for Assessment of Risks to Public Health: *Risk Assessment in the Federal Government: Managing the Means.* Washington, DC: National Academy Press, 1983.

O'Donnell MD, O'Conner CM, FitzGeral d MX, *et al.*: Ultrastructure of lung elastin and collagen in mouse models of spontaneous emphysema. *Matrix Biol* 18(4):357–360, 1999.

Oberdorster G, Ferin J, Lehnert BE: correlation between particle size, *in vivo* particle persistence, and lung injury. *Environ Health Perspect* 102 (Suppl 5):173–179, 1994.

Oberdorster G, Sharp Z, Atudorei V, *et al.*: Extrapulmonary translocation of ultrafine carbon particles following whole-body inhalation exposure of rats. *J Toxicol Environ Health A* 65(20):1531–1543, 2002.

Ohtsuka Y, Clarke RW, Mitzner W, *et al.*: Interstrain variation in murine susceptibility to inhaled acid-coated particles. *Am J Physiol Lung Cell Mol Physiol* 278(3): L469–L476, 2000.

Osebold JW, Gershwin LJ, Zee YC: Studies on the enhancement of allergic lung sensitization by inhalation of ozone and sulfuric acid aerosol. *J Environ Pathol Toxicol* 3:221–234, 1980.

Overton JH, Miller FJ: Modeling ozone absorption in the respiratory tract. 80th Annual Meeting of the Air Pollution Control Association, paper no. 87–99.4, 1987.

Paige RC, Plopper CG: Acute and chronic effects of ozone in animal models, in Holgate ST, Samet JM, Koren H, Maynard RL (eds): *Air Pollution and Health.* London: Academic Press, 1999, pp. 531–557.

Pinkerton KE, Brody AR, Miller FJ, Crapo JD: Exposure to low levels of ozone results in enhanced pulmonary retention of inhaled asbestos fibers. *Am Rev Respir Dis* 140(4):1075–1081, 1989.

Pope III CA, Burnett RT, Thun MJ, *et al.*: Lung cancer, cardiopulmonary mortality, and long-term exposure to fine particulate air pollution. *JAMA* 287(9):1132–1141, 2002.

Pope III CA, Thun MJ, Namboodiri MM, *et al.*: Particulate air pollution as a predictor of mortality in a prospective study of U.S. adults. *Am J Respir Crit Care Med* 151(3 Pt 1):669–674, 1995.

Pope III CA, Dockery DW: 2006 critical review – Health effects of fine particulate air pollution: Lines that connect. *JAWMA* 56:709–748, 2006.

Qu QS, Chen LC, Gordon T, Amdur M, Fine JM: Alteration of pulmonary macrophage intracellular pH regulation by sulfuric acid aerosol exposures. *Toxicol Appl Pharmacol* 121(1):138–143, 1993.

Recio L: Transgeneic animal models and their application in mechanistically based toxicology research. *CIIT Activities* 15(10):1–7, 1995.

Reid L: An experimental study of hypersecretion of mucus in the bronchial tree. *Br J Exp Pathol* 44:437–440, 1963.

Reuther CG: *FOCUS—Winds of change: Reducing transboundary air pollutants. *Environ Health Perspect* 108(4):A170–A175, 2000.

Robinson J, Nelson WC: *National Human Activity Pattern Survey Data Base.* Research Triangle, Park, NC: U.S. Environmental Protection Agency, 1995.

Romieu I, Sienra-Monge JJ, Ramirez-Aguilar M, *et al.*: Genetic polymorphism of GSTM1 and antioxidant supplementation influence lung function in relation to ozone exposure in asthmatic children in Mexico City. *Thorax* 59(1):8–10, 2004.

Rosenlund M, Berglind N, Pershagen G, *et al.*: Long-term exposure to urban air pollution and myocardial infarction. *Epidemiology* 17(4):383–390, 2006.

Saldiva PHN, King M, Delmonte VLC, *et al.*: Respiratory alterations due to urban air pollution: An experimental study in rats. *Environ Res* 57:19–33, 1992.

Salvi S, Blomberg A, Rudell B, *et al.*: Acute inflammatory responses in the airways and peripheral blood after short-term exposure to diesel exhaust in healthy human volunteers. *Am J Respir Crit Care Med* 159:702–709, 1999.

Samet JM, Hatch GE, Horstman D, Steck-Scott S, *et al.*: Effect of antioxidant supplementation on ozone-induced lung injury in human subjects. *Am J Respir Crit Care Med* 164(5):819–825, 2001.

Schenker MB, Samet JM, Speizer FE, *et al.*: Health effects of air pollution due to coal combustion in the Chestnut Ridge region of Pennsylvania: Results of cross-sectional analysis in adults. *Arch Environ Health* 38:325–330, 1983.

Schlesinger RB: Comparative irritant potency of inhaled sulfate aerosol: Effects on bronchial mucociliary clearance. *Environ Res* 34:268–279, 1984.

Schlesinger RB: Intermittent inhalation of nitrogen dioxide: Effects on rabbit alveolar macrophages. *J Toxicol Environ Health* 21:127–139, 1987.

Schlesinger RB, Chen LC, Finkelstein I, Zelikoff JT: Comparative potency of inhaled acidic sulfates: Speciation and the role of hydrogen ion. *Environ Res* 52:210–224, 1990.

Schlesinger RB, Gorczynski JE, Dennison J, *et al.*: Long-term intermittent exposure to sulfuric acid aerosol, ozone, and their combination: Alterations in tracheobronchial mucociliary clearance and epithelial secretory cells. *Exp Lung Res* 18:505–534, 1992.

Schlesinger RB, Halpern M, Albert RE, Lippmann M: Effects of chronic inhalation of sulfuric acid mist upon mucociliary clearance from the lungs of donkeys. *J Environ Pathol Toxicol* 2:1351–1367, 1979.

Schlesinger RB, Lippmann M, Albert RE: Effects of short-term exposures to sulfuric acid and ammonium sulfate aerosols upon bronchial airway function in the donkey. *Am Ind Hyg Assoc J* 39:275–286, 1978.

Schlesinger RB, Weidman PA, Zelikoff JT: Effects of repeated exposures to ozone and nitrogen dioxide on respiratory tract prostanoids. *Inhal Toxicol* 3:27–36, 1991.

Schwartz J: Particulate air pollution and daily mortality in Detroit. *Environ Res* 56:204–213, 1991.

Schwartz J: Air pollution and the duration of acute respiratory symptoms. *Arch Environ Health* 47(2):116–22, 1992.

Schwartz J: Air pollution and daily mortality: A review and meta analysis. *Environ Res* 64:36–52, 1994.

Schwartz J, Marcus A: Mortality and air pollution in London. *Am J Epidemiol* 131:185–194, 1990.

Schwela DH: Exposure to environmental chemicals relevant for respiratory hypersensitivity: Global aspects. *Toxicol Lett* 86:131–142, 1996.

Schwela DH: The World Health Organization Guidelines for Air Quality. Part 1: Exposure-response relationships and air quality guidelines. *EM* pp. 29–34, 2000.

Seltzer J, Bigby BG, Stulbarg M, *et al.*: O$_3$-induced change in bronchial reactivity to methacholine and airway inflammation in humans. *J Appl Physiol* 60:1321–1326, 1986.

Sheppard DA, Saisho A, Nadel JA, Boushey HA: Exercise increases sulfur dioxide induced bronchoconstriction in asthmatic subjects. *Am Rev Respir Dis* 123:486–491, 1981.

Sienra-Monge JJ, Ramirez-Aguilar M, Moreno-Macias H.: Antioxidant supplementation and nasal inflammatory responses among young asthmatics exposed to high levels of ozone. *Clin Exp Immunol* 138(2):317–322, 2004.

Singh P, DeMarini DM, Dick CA, *et al.*: Sample characterization of automobile and forklift diesel exhaust particles and comparative pulmonary toxicity in mice. *Environ Health Perspect* 112(8):820–825, 2004.

Slade R, Stead AG, Graham JA, Hatch GE: Comparison of lung antioxidant levels in humans and laboratory animals. *Am Rev Respir Dis* 131:742–746, 1985.

Speigelman JR, Hanson GD, Lazurus A, *et al.*: Effect of acute sulfur dioxide exposure on bronchial clearance in the donkey. *Arch Environ Health* 17:321, 1968.

Speizer FE: Studies of acid aerosols in six cities and in a new multi-city investigation: Design issues. *Environ Health Perspect* 79:61–68, 1989.

Spengler JD, Sexton K: Indoor air pollution: A public health perspective. *Science* 221:9–17, 1983.

State of the Air: 2006. American Lung Association. Available: at http://lungaction.org/reports/stateoftheair2006.html

Stevens MA, Fitzgerald S, Menache MG, *et al.*: Functional evidence of persistent airway obstruction in rats following a two-hour inhalation exposure to methyl isocyanate. *Environ Health Perspect* 72:89–94, 1987.

Suga T, Kurabayashi M, Sando Y, *et al.*: Disruption of the klotho gene causes pulmonary emphysema in mice. *Am J Respir Cell Mol Biol* 22:26–33, 2000.

Sun Q, Wang A, Jin X, *et al.*: Long-term air pollution exposure and acceleration of atherosclerosis and vascular inflammation in an animal model. *JAMA* 294(23):3003–3010, 2005.

Sweeney TD, Skornik WA, Brain JD, *et al.*: Chronic bronchitis alters the pattern of aerosol deposition in the lung. *Am J Respir Crit Care Med* 151(2 Pt 1):482–488, 1995.

Thurston GD, Ito K, Kinney PL, Lippmann M: A multi-year study of air pollution and respiratory hospital admissions in three New York state metropolitan areas: Results for 1988 and 1989 summers. *J Expos Anal Environ Epidemiol* 2:429–450, 1992.

Tujague J, Bastaki M, Holland N, *et al.*: Antioxidant intake, GSTM1 polymorphism and pulmonary function in healthy young adults. *Eur Respir J* 27:282–288, 2006.

Tyler WS, Tyler NK, Hinds D, *et al.*: Influence of exposure regimen on effects of experimental ozone studies: Effects of daily and episodic and seasonal cycles of exposure and post-exposure. Presented at the 84th annual meeting of the Air Waste Management Association, Vancouver, BC, Canada. Paper No. 91–141.5, 1991.

Tyler WS, Tyler NK, Last JA, *et al.*: Comparison of daily and seasonal exposures of young monkeys to ozone. *Toxicology* 50:131–144, 1988.

USEPA: Air Quality Criteria for Ozone and Related Photochemical Oxidants (1996). U.S. Environmental Protection Agency, Office of Research and Development, National Center for Environmental Assessment, Washington Office, Washington, DC, 1996.

USEPA: Air Quality Criteria for Particulate Matter (October 2004). U.S. Environmental Protection Agency, Washington, DC, EPA 600/P-99/002aF-bF, 2004.

Underhill DW: Aerosol synergism and hydrate formation—A possible connection. *Inhal Toxicol* 12 (Suppl 1):189–198, 2000.

Utell MJ, Mariglio JA, Morrow PE, *et al.*: Effects of inhaled acid aerosols on respiratory function: The role of endogenous ammonia. *J Aerosol Med* 2:141–147, 1989.

Utell MJ, Morrow PE, Hyde RW: Airway reactivity to sulfate and sulfuric acid aerosols in normal and asthmatic subjects. *J Air Pollut Control Assoc* 34:931–935, 1984.

Van De Lende R, Kok TJ, Reig RP, *et al.*: Decreases in VC and FEV$_1$ with time: Indicators for effects of smoking and air pollution. *Bull Eur Physiopathol Respir* 17:775–792, 1981.

Vaughan TR, Jennelle LF, Lewis TR: Long-term exposure to low levels of air pollutants: Effects on pulmonary function in the beagle. *Arch Environ Health* 19:45–50, 1969.

von Mutius E, Martinez FD, Fritzsch C, *et al.*: Prevalence of asthma and atopy in two areas of West and East Germany. *Am J Respir Crit Care Med* 149(2 Pt 1):358–364, 1994.

Waxman HA: Title III of the 1990 Clean Air Act amendments, in Patrick DR (ed): *Toxic Air Pollution Handbook.* New York: Van Nostrand Reinhold, 1994, pp. 25–32.

Wichers LB, Rowan WH, Nolan JP, *et al.* : Particle deposition in spontaneously hypertensive rats exposed via whole-body inhalation: Measured and estimated dose. *Tox Sci* 93(2):400–410, 2006.

Wiester MJ, Winsett DW, Richards JE, *et al.*: Ozone adaptation in mice and its association with ascorbic acid in the lung. *Inhal Toxicol* 12:577–590, 2000.

Yokoyama E, Toder RE, Frank NR: Distribution of ^{35}SO$_2$ in the blood and its excretion in dogs exposed to ^{35}SO$_2$. *Arch Environ Health* 22:389–395, 1971.

Yoshida M, Satoh M, Shimada A, *et al.*: Pulmonary toxicity caused by acute exposure to mercury vapor is enhanced in metallothionein-null mice. *Life Sci* 64(20):1861–1867, 1999.

Yoshida M, Whitsett JA: Alveolar macrophages and emphysema in surfactant protein-D-deficient mice. *Respir* 11:S37–S40, 2006.

CHAPTER 29

ECOTOXICOLOGY

Richard T. Di Giulio and Michael C. Newman

INTRODUCTION

Ecotoxicology is the science of contaminants in the biosphere and their effects on constituents of the biosphere (Newman and Unger, 2003). It follows from this definition that ecotoxicologists examine large-scale ecological phenomenon (Preston, 2002) in addition to those normally addressed in toxicology: ecotoxicology has an overarching goal of explaining and predicting effect or exposure phenomena at several levels of biological organization (Fig. 29-1). Essential explanations and models include those applied in conventional toxicology and a range of environmental sciences.

Although Truhaut's original definition of this new science encompassed effects to humans (Truhaut, 1977), most recent definitions of ecotoxicology do not. Relevant effects to nonhuman targets range from biomolecular to global. Taking on the classic toxicology vantage initially, suborganismal and organismal effects were emphasized during ecotoxicology's nascent stage; however, studies of higher level effects and interactions are becoming increasingly commonplace as the science matures. Such indirect effects[1] were initially considered problematic and reluctantly relegated to secondary importance (Fleeger *et al.*, 2003) relative to direct effects to individuals. Indirect effects are now known to be as important as direct effects to nonhuman targets (Fleeger *et al.*, 2003; Chapman, 2004). As the need to predict major effects to populations, communities, ecosystems, and other higher level entities has become increasingly apparent, more cause–effect models relevant to these higher levels of biological organization are added to the conventional set of toxicology models applied by pioneering ecotoxicologists.

Contaminant chemical form, phase association, and movement among components of the biosphere are also central issues in ecotoxicology because they determine exposure, bioavailability, and realized dose. The context of these biogeochemical studies has expanded in the last several decades to encompass issues of larger and larger scale such as global movement of persistent organic pollutants (Wania and Mackay, 1996).

From a practical vantage, ecotoxicology informs decision makers about ecological risks associated with contamination. Risk to ecological entities are estimated or predicted by combining exposure and effect information. Risk might involve diminished fitness of individuals, increased risk of local population extinction, a drop in species diversity, or reduced nutrient cycling or primary productivity. Because potential ecological endpoints are so diverse, the ecological risk framework tends to be more flexible than that of the conventional human health risk assessment (Fig. 29-2). This important role of ecotoxicology in ecological risk assessment will be discussed in more detail below.

SOME DISTINCT ASPECTS OF EXPOSURE

Predicting exposure and effect is difficult for all relevant ecological entities. In contrast to human toxicology in which information about a few species might be used to predict harm to one (humans), ecotoxicology commonly uses sparse information for a few species to predict effects to many species and their interactions. Exposure pathways, bioavailability, bioaccumulation, and toxicant transfer for all relevant ecological entities are also difficult issues requiring considerable effort to adequately understand.

Relevant exposure routes are the conventional ingestion, inhalation, and dermal absorption. But, unique features of exposure

---

[1] Indirect effects are effects of toxicants mediated by another ecosystem component (Krivtsov 2004) such as those that might occur to a flowering plant if a pesticide were to eliminate its primary insect pollinator.

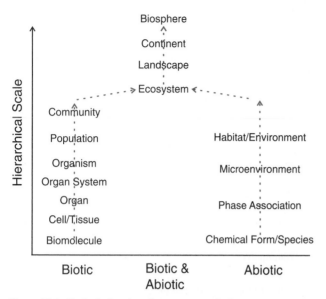

Figure 29-1. Ecological scales relevant to ecotoxicology.

Solely biological scales relevant to ecotoxicology range from the molecular to the community levels: solely abiotic scales range from the chemical to the entire habitat. Biotic and abiotic components are usually combined at levels above the ecological community and habitat. The ecological community and physicochemical habitat combined to form the ecosystem. Ecological systems can be considered at the landscape scale, i.e., the combination of marine, freshwater, and terrestrial systems at a river's mouth. Recently, the continental and biospheric scales have become relevant as in the cases of ozone depletion, acid precipitation, and global warming.

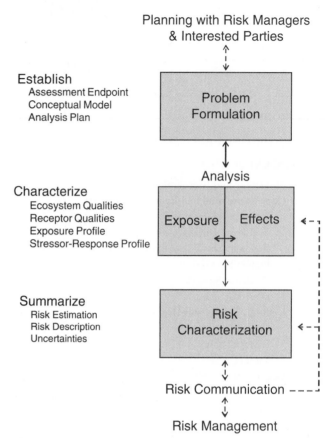

Figure 29-2. The general form of an ecological risk assessment including problem formulation, analysis, and risk characterization stages.

Problem formulation is done in dialog with risk managers and stakeholders, and involves a clear statement of the ecological entity to be assessed, a conceptual model for the process, and a plan for conducting the assessment. The analysis stage involves exposure and effects characterizations. Using the context developed during problem formulation and information organized together in the analysis stage, a statement of risk and associated uncertainties are made in the risk characterization stage.

pathways must be accommodated for species that ingest a wide range of materials using distinct feeding mechanisms, breathe gaseous or liquid media using different structures, and come into dermal contact with a variety of gaseous, liquid, and solid media.

Prediction of oral exposure can be limited because species feed on different materials; however, conventional principles regarding oral bioavailability remain relevant. As an example, some birds are uniquely at high risk of lead poisoning because they ingest and then use lead shot as grit. Shot are ground together in their gizzards under acidic conditions, releasing significant amounts of dissolved lead (Kendall *et al.*, 1996). As true with humans (i.e., the ionic hypothesis of Mathews, 1904), the dissolved form of lead is more available to do harm than solid lead shot. Similar high risk of lead poisoning is present for some raptors feeding on game birds whose tissues can contain lead shot (Wayland and Bollinger, 1999). Complex sorting of filtered materials on the gills of bivalve molluscs strongly influences the metal content and bioavailability of the material that eventually passes into their guts (Allison *et al.*, 1998). Some invertebrate species have elaborate feeding structures that are also involved in respiration (e.g., lugworms and bivalve molluscs) or locomotion (copepods and other zooplankton species). Some zooplankton species feed and digest algal cells in such a way that only metals soluble in the algal cytosol are bioavailable (Reinfelder and Fisher, 1991). Unlike mammalian species, many invertebrate species are capable of sequestering large amounts of metals in intracellular granules (Mason and Nott, 1981). Incorporation of metals into granules by prey species reduces metal bioavailability to predators (Nott and Nicolaidou, 1993). Just as noted with 5-fluoruracil administration or chronic ethanol consumption, some pollutant exposures cause malabsorption by damaging the intestine wall. A relevant sit-

uation would be intestinal damage to otters caused by ingestion during grooming of oiled fur (Lipscomb *et al.*, 1996; Ormseth and Ben-David, 2000). The principles remain the same in all of these cases but critical exposure pathway details are different.

Many techniques applied to determining human oral bioavailability are available to the ecotoxicologist; however, as just illustrated, modifications are needed for the many pathways for nonhuman species exposure. Typical are those associated with estimating contaminant bioavailability in aquatic environments. As an example, biomimetic and related extraction methods used to predict human oral bioavailability can be modified to predict sediment-bound contaminant bioavailabilities. Sediments are placed into contact with biomimetic solutions (Chen and Mayer, 1998; Leslie *et al.*, 2002) or digestive fluids taken from organisms (Mayer *et al.*, 1996; Weston and Maruya, 2002), and the amount of extracted contaminant used to estimate bioavailability.

Estimation of chemical speciation is central to predicting bioavailability of water-associated contaminants. Speciation can determine the bioavailability of dissolved metals. Movements of nonionic and ionizable organic compounds across the gut or gills are strongly influenced by lipid solubility and the pH partition theory, respectively. Consequently, determination of a compounds lipophilicity or calculation of pH- and pK_a-dependent ionization facilitates some predictive capability for bioavailability. A common application of this approach would be estimation of water pH effects on ammonia toxicity as the consequence of the ease with which unionized ammonia passes through gills relative to ionized ammonia (Lloyd and Herbert, 1960). The Free Ion Activity Model (FIAM) states that uptake and toxicity of cationic trace metals are best predicted from their free ion activity or concentration (Campbell and Tessier, 1996) although exceptions exist to this extension of the ionic hypothesis. Consequently, dissolved metal exposure assessments often begin by estimating the amount of a metal present as the free ion. Normally, such calculations require only thermodynamic modeling based on measured concentrations of dissolved cations and anions. Lipid partitioning is often used to predict dissolved, nonionizing organic compound accumulation in and effects to aquatic biota. The propensity for an organic compound to accumulate in aquatic organisms increases with lipid solubility as often described with a simple Quantitative Structure Activity Relationship (QSAR) (Neely et al., 1974; Mckay, 1982; Chiou, 1985; Connell, 1990). The log of the octanol–water partition coefficient (log K_{ow}) is used to predict measures such as the bioconcentration factor (the quotient of the concentration in the organism and that in the water from which the organic compound is being accumulated):

$$Bioconcentration\ Factor\ (BCF) = \frac{C_{Organism}}{C_{Water}}$$

Bioavailability, bioaccumulation, or exposure concentrations for sediment-associated toxicants are also approached by considering chemical speciation and phase partitioning. Metals in sediments are either incorporated into one of many solid phases or dissolved in the interstitial waters surrounding the sediment particles. Bioavailabilities of metals in these different forms are difficult to predict (Luoma, 1989) but, nonetheless, various schemes have been applied to that end. Bioavailable metals have been estimated by normalizing sediment metal concentrations to easily extracted iron and manganese concentrations because solid iron and manganese oxides sequester metals in poorly bioavailable solid forms (Luoma and Bryan, 1978). Other chemical extraction methods have been applied with some success (Tessier et al., 1984). A pragmatic method for predicting sediment metal bioavailability has emerged that is based on the assumption that the sediment metal form of most concern is the dissolved metal. Further, for many metals and sediments, the dissolved interstitial metal concentrations are determined by equilibrium between solid (iron and manganese) sulfides and the interstitial water.

$$Cd^{2+} + FeS_{Solid} \longleftrightarrow CdS_{Solid} + Fe^{2+}$$

Because the equilibrium so favors formation of metal sulfide (CdS in this case) at the expense of FeS, insignificant amounts of dissolved metal will be present in the interstitial waters if enough FeS is present. This premise has given rise to a standard technique for determining if sediments might contain enough metal to warrant concern (Di Toro et al., 1990). First, a sediment aliquot is extracted with cold hydrochloric acid. Then the amounts of sulfide (acid volatile sulfides, AVS) and simultaneously extracted metals (SEM) are measured in that extract. The difference between the SEM and AVS suggests whether or not enough metal will be dissolved in the interstitial waters to warrant concern. This method has enjoyed wide application and was recently refined by Di Toro et al.

(2005) by including metal partitioning to sediment organic matter. Some ecotoxicologists such as Lee et al. (2000) suggest that further refinement remains to be done because metal exposure of organisms that ingest sediment particulates is not fully defined by interstitial water concentrations alone.

Bioavailability and accumulation of sediment-associated organic compounds are predicted with tools similar to those described for waters. The bioavailability of ionizable organic compounds can be approximated with the pH-partition hypothesis that relates the availability of an ionizable compound to the diffusion of its unionized form through membranes as determined by pH and pK_a. Availability of nonionizing organic compounds for accumulation can often be estimated with its log K_{ow} and equilibrium partitioning theory as described already for accumulation from waters. The challenge with nonionizing organic compounds becomes adequately defining the phases between which the compound is partitioning. This might be done by estimating the partitioning of the compound between sediment solid phases and the interstitial water as done by Di Toro et al. (1991). Descriptions of nonionizing organic compound bioaccumulation from sediments can also entail normalization of concentrations to phases thought to be dictating partitioning:

$$Biota\ Sediment\ Accumulation\ Factor\ (BSAF)$$

$$= \frac{\mu g/kg\ lipid}{\mu g/kg\ organic\ carbon}$$

where the mass of compound in the organisms is divided by kg of organism-associated lipid and the mass of compound in the sediment is divided by kg of sediment-associated organic carbon.

Another issue of importance to the ecotoxicologist is the possibility of biomagnification, the increase in contaminant concentration as it moves through a food web. As will be described below, biomagnification can result in harmful exposures to species situated high in the food web such as birds of prey.

TOXICANT EFFECTS

While determining *exposure* comprises one-half of the risk assessment paradigm, the other half, understanding chemical effects, lies at the heart of toxicology and hence, comprises the focus of this chapter. The effects, or deleterious consequences of chemical exposures, can be enormously diverse as demonstrated by previous chapters, and investigated by numerous techniques. One approach to this complex topic of ecotoxicological effects, which we employ here, is to organize effects according to biological levels of organization. Thus, one may consider effects, in ascending order, at the subcellular (molecular and biochemical), cellular, organismal, population, community, and ecosystem levels of organization. As noted earlier, an important distinction between traditional biomedical, or human health-oriented, toxicology and ecotoxicology is the emphasis by the latter on higher levels of biological organization, specifically populations, communities, and ecosystems, while biomedical toxicology focuses on lower levels, from organismal and below. This difference arises from the focus of biomedical toxicology on one species and concerns for protecting the health of individuals of that species. Ecotoxicology, in contrast, deals with, theoretically at least, all species; and in line with other aspects of natural resource management, the primary concern is one of sustainability. That is, policies and regulations surrounding chemical effects in natural ecosystems are designed to protect ecological features such as population dynamics,

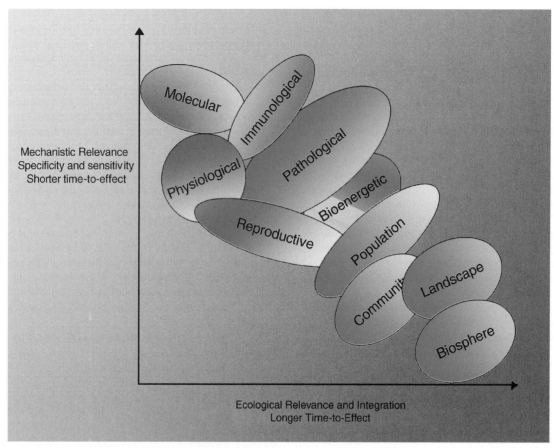

Figure 29-3. Hierarchical types of effects considered in ecotoxicology, indicating relative attributes such mechanistic vs. ecological relevance and time lags between exposure and observable effect.

Based on artwork kindly provided by S.Marshall Adams, Oak Ridge National Laboratory.

community structures, and ecosystem functions. In this light, the individual organism is essentially viewed as expendable, as long as these higher level variables are protected. An exception here is that of endangered or threatened species, where the loss of an individual may have unacceptable legal or ecological consequences.

While higher levels of organization comprise the ultimate focus of those concerned with chemical pollution of natural systems, the science of ecotoxicology includes studies across the entire range. Studies at lower levels (cellular and below) provide insights into mechanisms of toxicity that can be valuable for making predictions among related compounds or species, and establishing cause–effect relationships in field studies, for generating useful "biomarkers" of chemical exposure and effect, and for providing insights into higher level, particularly population level, effects. Studies at the organism level have historically played a dominant role in regulatory ecotoxicology; many traditional bioassays, described later, can be viewed as organismal level queries. Again, understanding effects at the population and higher levels can be viewed as the "gold standard" in ecotoxicology. However, because these effects can require a relatively long time beyond the initial exposure of a system to emerge, their quantification is often difficult, and they generally do not serve to identify the nature of the stressor. Thus, the elucidation of effects of chemical pollutants, as well as other stressors, in natural systems draws upon multiple approaches and conclusions are generally based on the weight of evidence available. Examples of effects, or endpoints, that can be measured spanning levels of organization and

their relative sensitivities and ecological relevancies are illustrated in Fig. 29-3. The originator of this figure, S.M. Adams (Oak Ridge National Laboratory) has discussed the importance of integrating studies across levels of organization and mathematical approaches for accomplishing this (Adams *et al.*, 2000).

In the following sections, we describe important chemical effects that have been addressed at different levels of biological organization in ecotoxicological contexts, including illustrative examples. It is beyond the scope of this chapter to provide discussions of all chemicals that have received ecotoxicological attention. Other chapters in this text, particularly those in Unit 5 (Toxic Agents) provide detailed information for most classes of chemicals of concern as pollutants of natural systems, albeit in a primarily mammalian context. Many of the effects described are relevant to other animals, and of course mammals do occur in natural systems! Some plant-specific effects will be addressed herein. It should be noted that, while we have employed a biological level of organization approach as a meaningful way to organize and convey a complex array of information, the phenomena we have categorized into various levels are ultimately interwoven, as will become apparent.

Molecular and Biochemical Effects

This lowest level of organization includes fundamental processes associated with the regulation of gene transcription and translation, biotransformation of xenobiotics, and the deleterious

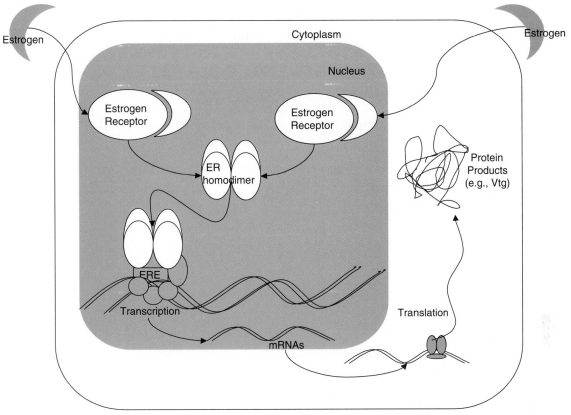

Figure 29-4. A simplified model of estrogen receptor signaling including the estrogen receptor (ER), which upon binding to native hormone ligand (estrogen) or xenoestrogen (see Fig. 29–5) forms the transcriptionally active ER homodimer complex that binds to genes containing estrogen response elements (ERE) and thereby upregulates transcription and translation of genes/proteins regulated by the system, such as vitellogenin (Vtg). Kindly provided by Carla Rosenfeld, Duke University.

biochemical effects of xenobiotics on cellular constituents including proteins, lipids, and DNA. These effects have been described elsewhere throughout this book in various contexts related to human health. Here we will highlight some aspects of subcellular effects that have received particular attention in the context of ecotoxicology. Research in this area has been performed for a variety of reasons, including the elucidation of mechanisms of adaptation and toxicity, understanding species similarities and differences (e.g., to compare selected wildlife species with standard mammalian models, and to identify particularly sensitive species), and to develop useful biomarkers of chemical exposure and toxicity for environmental assessments. More in depth discussions are provided in monographs such as Hoffman *et al.* (2003), Newman and Unger (2003), Mommsen and Moon (2005), and Di Giulio and Hinton (in press).

Gene Expression and Ecotoxicogenomics

A long-standing mechanistic issue in toxicology concerns chemical effects on gene and protein expression. Xenobiotics can affect gene transcription through interactions with transcription factors and/or the promoter regions of genes that bind transcription factors in the process of activating transcription. In the context of environmental toxicology, perhaps the most studied xenobiotic effects involve ligand-activated transcription factors. These intracellular receptor proteins recognize and bind specific compounds, thus forming a complex that binds to specific promoter regions of genes, thereby activating transcription of mRNAs, and ultimately translation of

the associated protein. Two examples of substantial importance in ecotoxicology that illustrate these interactions involve the estrogen receptor (ER) and the aryl hydrocarbon receptor (AHR).

Estrogen Receptor   A number of chemicals have been shown to perturb various components of the endocrine system, and the identification and elucidation of "endocrine disruptors" has been a subject of much research and regulatory action in recent years, in the contexts of both human and wildlife health (see Chap. 10; Rotchell and Ostrander, 2003). Perhaps the most studied component of the vertebrate endocrine system in this context is the estrogen receptor, particularly estrogen receptor α (ER), and responses associated with it. The dominant natural ligand for this nuclear receptor is estradiol (E2); binding of E2 with ER produces a complex that can then bind to estrogen response elements (ERE) of specific genes that contain one or more EREs, thereby causing gene transcription (see Fig. 29-4). Genes regulated in this manner by E2–ER play various important roles in, for example, sexual organ development, behavior, fertility, and bone integrity (Deroo and Korach, 2006).

A number of chemicals including certain drugs and environmental pollutants can serve as ligands for ER; in most cases these "xenoestrogens" activate gene transcription, i.e., similar to estradiol, acting as receptor agonists. The first xenoestrogen identified was diethylstilbestrol (DES), a drug used to prevent miscarriage in the 1940s to the 1970s until it was discovered to have profound developmental effects in some offspring of women receiving the treatment (Trimble, 2001). In recent years, a number of environmental

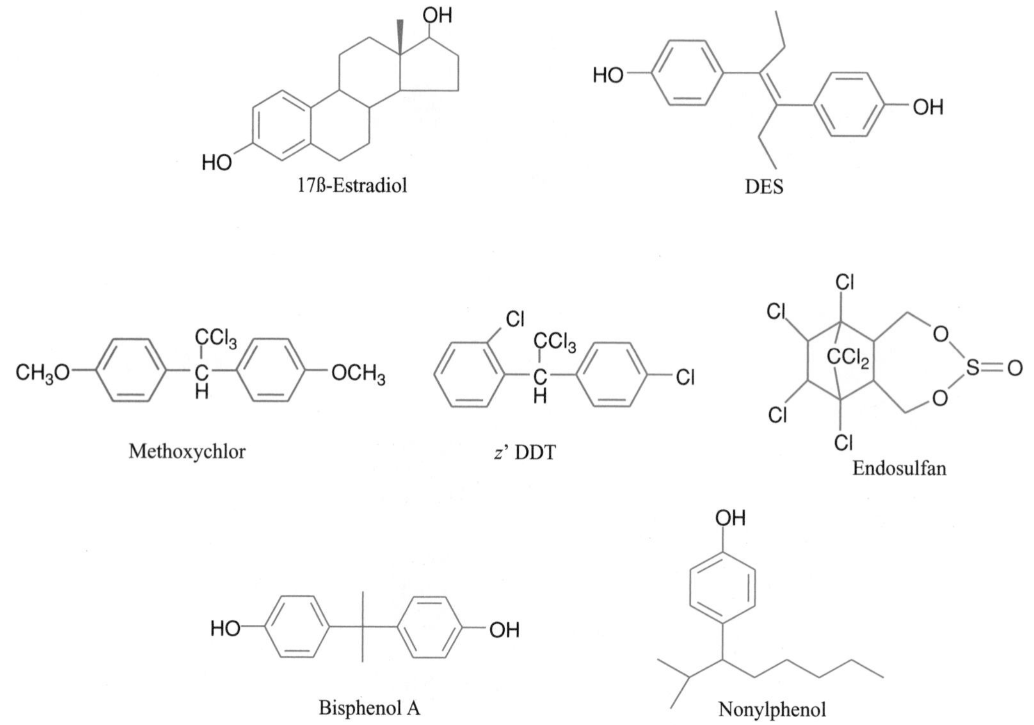

Figure 29-5. Estrogen receptor agonists, including a native estrogen (17β-estradiol), the drug diethylstilbestrol (DES), a surfactant component (nonylphenol), an industrial intermediate (bisphenol A), and several pesticides (remainder).

pollutants with estrogenic activity have been identified, including certain chlorinated hydrocarbon insecticides (e.g., DDT, methoxychlor, endosulfan), surfactants (nonyl-phenol), some PCBs, bisphenol A (used in plastics manufacturing), and ethinyl estradiol, a synthetic estrogen used in birth control pills and observed in municipal effluents and surface waters (Shelby *et al.*, 1996; Larsson *et al.*, 1999; van der Oost *et al.*, 2003; see Fig. 29-5). With the exception of ethinyl estradiol, these pollutants exhibit relatively low binding affinities to ER, as compared to E2 or DES (Shelby *et al.*, 1996); however, environmental exposures may be sufficient to perturb reproduction or development.

Evidence for such "endocrine disruptions" by environmental xenoestrogens appears to be overall stronger for wildlife than for humans, likely due to instances of elevated exposures that are less prone to confounding factors than is typically the case for human exposures. Also, egg-laying vertebrates provide a unique biomarker of estrogen exposure that has contributed to ecotoxicological studies in this area. Vitellogenin (Vtg) is a protein that is normally produced by the liver of females and transported via the bloodstream to the ovary where, as a key component of yolk, it provides nourishment to the developing embryo. The production of Vtg is regulated by the estrogen–estrogen receptor system. Interestingly, males of egg-laying vertebrate species contain the molecular machinery to produce Vtg, but production and circulating levels are normally very low, due to low titers of estrogen. However, exposures of males to estrogen and xenoestrogens upregulate Vtg production, which can be readily measured in blood samples. Consequently, elevated Vtg in males of these species is a useful biomarker of estrogenic chemical exposures (Sumpter and Jobling, 1995; see **Biomarker** discussion below). Examples include rainbow trout (*Oncorhynchus mykiss*) caged in surface waters below industrial or municipal effluent sources enriched in alkylphenolic surfactants in the UK (Harries

et al., 1997) or natural and synthetic estrogens in Sweden (Larsson *et al.*, 1999), and whitefish (*Coregonus lavaretus*) caged near paper mill effluents in Finland (Mellanen *et al.*, 1999). While the bulk of research related to estrogenic compounds in natural systems have focused on fish, this approach has merit for other egg-laying vertebrates (Lorenzen *et al.*, 2003; Huang *et al.*, 2005), and for some invertebrates that produce Vtg-like proteins (Porte *et al.*, 2006).

Aryl Hydrocarbon Receptor The aryl hydrocarbon receptor (AHR) is a member of the basic helix–loop–helix Per ARNT Sim (bHLH-PAS) family of receptors/transcription factors that play roles in development, as sensors of the internal and external environment in order to maintain homeostasis, and in establishment and maintenance of circadian clocks (Denison and Nagy, 2003; Hahn *et al.*, 2005). The AHR is among the most intensively studied receptors in toxicology due to its role in regulating a number of genes coding for proteins involved in xenobiotic metabolism, and its responsiveness to a number of widespread environmental contaminants, as well as some drugs and endogenous compounds. The AHR is a ligand-activated cytosolic receptor that upon binding to a ligand traverses to the nucleus where it complexes with another transcription factor, the AHR nuclear translocator (ARNT) protein (Fig. 29-6) to form a transcriptionally active dimer. This AHR–ARNT complex binds to promoter sequences of genes regulated by the AHR system; these promoters are most often referred to as "xenobiotic response elements" (XRE) or "dioxin response elements" (DRE).

Characterized genes that are upregulated by the AHR system in large part code for enzymes involved in the metabolism of lipophilic chemicals, including organic xenobiotics and some endogenous substrates such as steroid hormones. These enzymes include specific cytochrome P450s (mammalian CYP1A1, 1A2, and 1B1 and

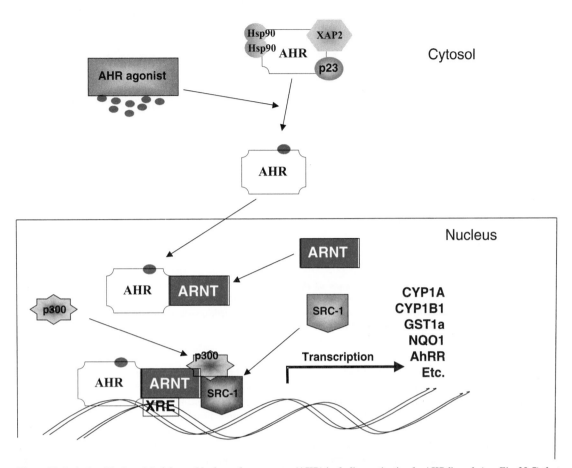

Figure 29-6. *A simplified model of the aryl hydrocarbon receptor (AHR) including activation by AHR ligands (see Fig. 29-7) that allows for dimerization with the AHR nuclear transporter (ARNT) that forms the transcriptionally active complex that binds to xenobiotic response elements (XRE) and thereby upregulates a number of genes, including several involved in biotransformation, indicated here, as well as the AHR repressor (AHRR) that provides negative feedback control of the system.*

Hsp 90, XAP2, and p23 are chaperone proteins; SRC-1 and p300 are examples of coregulator proteins involved in transcription. Kindly provided by Carrie Fleming and Carla Rosenfeld, Duke University.

their counterparts in other vertebrates), a glutathione transferase (GST), a glucuronosyl transferase (UDPGT), an alcohol dehydrogenase (ALD), and a quinone oxidoreductase (NQO). In addition to these enzymes, AHR–ARNT upregulates the AHR repressor protein (AHRR), which then competes with AHR for ARNT. This results in a transcriptionally inactive complex and effectively provides a negative feedback loop for controlling AHR-mediated gene transcription (Hahn *et al.*, 2005). The biotransformation enzymes regulated by the AHR system are described in detail in Chap. 6. Briefly, they play key roles for transforming many lipophilic chemicals, including numerous common organic contaminants, into more water soluble, and hence excretable, products. However, this biotransformation activity can result in production of highly reactive products that are more toxic than their parent compounds, i.e., "activation."

Of particular relevance to the present discussion, however, is the ability of some ubiquitous pollutants to act as AHR ligands and markedly upregulate gene transcription via the AHR–ARNT signaling pathway described above (Denison and Nagy, 2003). In some cases, this can be interpreted as an adaptive response—the organism is reacting to exposure to a lipophilic xenobiotic in order to enhance its elimination. However, as noted above, biotransformation can also lead to enhanced toxicity of some substrates. The two

major classes of pollutants that have members that act as ligands for the AHR and upregulate gene expression (and thereby "induce" biotransformation enzymes), and have received the greatest attention in ecotoxicology are the polycyclic aromatic hydrocarbons (PAHs) and the polyhalogenated aromatic hydrocarbons (pHAHs); examples of both are provided in Fig. 29-7. The most studied pHAHs are particular "coplanar" polychlorinated biphenyls (PCBs) and chlorinated dioxins. Whereas some PAHs and pHAHs share the ability to activate the AHR, important differences between these classes exist. PAHs, whether they are ligands for the AHR or not, are overall very good substrates for the biotransformation systems upregulated via the AHR, which can act to both detoxify and enhance the toxicity of some PAHs (discussed below under section "Cancer"). In general, pHAH-type AHR ligands are more potent AHR ligands and enzyme inducers than PAHs, but due to extensive halogenation are much poorer substrates for biotransformation. One of the most potent ligands for the AHR is the dioxin, 2,3,7,8-tetrachlorodibenzodioxin (TCDD), which is highly recalcitrant to biotransformation (Denison and Nagy, 2003).

In similarity with xenoestrogen-mediated inductions of Vtg via the ER, the inducibility of biotransformation enzymes via the AHR by xenobiotics has been used for biomonitoring. In this

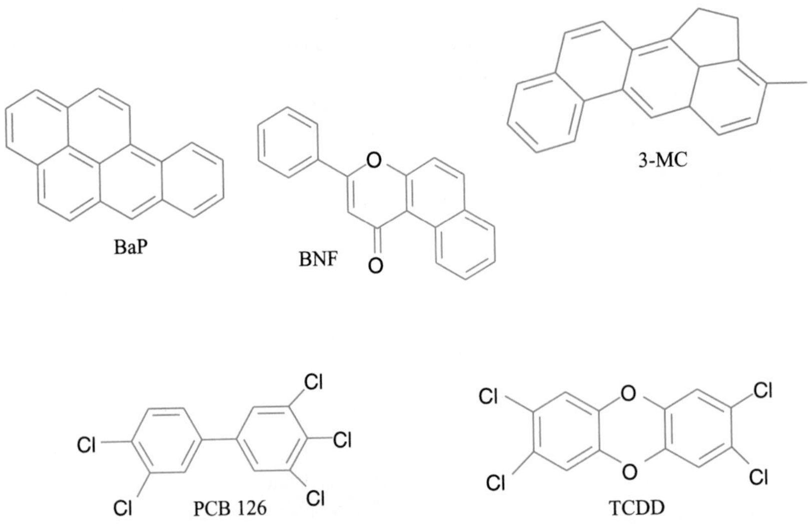

Figure 29-7. Representative ligands of the aryl hydrocarbon receptor, including 2,3,7,8-tetrachlorodibenzodioxin (TCDD), a co-planar polychlorinated biphenyl (PCB 126), two polycyclic aromatic hydrocarbons (benzo(a)pyrene—BaP, and 3-methlycholanthrene—3-MC), and a flavone (β-naphthoflavone—BNF).

regard, enzymatic activities associated with the CYP1As have been the most widely used AHR-related biomarker, particularly an activity that appears highly specific for these CYPs, ethoxyresorufin *O*-deethylase (EROD), which is most often measured in liver tissue of vertebrates. Elevated activities of EROD in various vertebrates have been associated with exposures to PCBs, dioxins, PAHs, and complex mixtures of these associated with, for example, harbor sediments, municipal effluents, paper mill effluents, refinery effluents, and crude oil spills (Custer *et al.*, 2001; van der Oost, 2003; Miller *et al.*, 2005). Invertebrate AHR homologues examined do not bind to ligands similarly to vertebrate AHRs and do not demonstrate protein inductions analogous to those observed in vertebrates (Butler *et al.*, 2001; Hahn, 2002; Chaty *et al.*, 2004). Polycyclic aromatic hydrocarbon and pHAH toxicities and the potential roles played by their interactions with the AHR will be discussed at various points in subsequent sections of this chapter, and related discussions from a human health standpoint appear in other chapters.

Genomics and Ecotoxicogenomics   Recent advances in gene sequencing and associated techniques for investigating mechanism underlying gene expression have revolutionized molecular biology. These advances are rapidly permeating many areas of biological research, including toxicology and environmental science. Underlying these advances are very large projects to sequence the entire genomes of various species, such as the highly publicized Human Genome Project that was completed in 2003 (Little, 2005). Other species that have been completely or largely sequenced include the mouse, rat, cow, dog, chimpanzee, chicken, zebrafish (*Danio rerio*), puffer fish (*Fugu rubripes*), medaka (*Oryzias latipes*), fruit fly (*Drosophila melanogaster*), a sea urchin (*Strongylocentrotus purpuratus*), a soil nematode (*Caenorhabditis elegans*), a yeast (*Saccharomyces cerevisiae*), and rice (*Oryza sativa*), and the number of species sequenced is anticipated to expand rapidly (see www.genome.gov; Crollius and Weissenbach, 2005). Genome sequencing set the stage for genome-wide analysis of gene expression ("transcriptomics"); cDNAs for known genes can be spotted on glass slides, or chips, resulting in "microarrays" that can be employed to quantify relative levels, i.e., expression, of mRNAs for those genes in samples of interest. The study of changes in gene expression arising from chemical exposures is a key component of "toxicogenomics" (Schmidt, 2002). Microarrays for genomes or genome components of interest (such as genes associated with stress responses, carcinogenesis, and development) are commercially available for many species, and rapidly expanding. Also advancing rapidly are related analyses of global changes in proteins (the translation products of mRNAs), refereed to as "proteomics," and resulting metabolite profiles (amounts of sugars, lipids, amino acids, etc. in various tissues that are controlled in part by enzyme activities), referred to as "metabolomics." A major complexity in these global analyses is the extremely large data sets that arise, for example, when one examines the responses of thousands of genes from organisms exposed to one or more concentrations of a chemical at one or more time points. This has led to the development of the field of "bioinformatics" that includes the application of sophisticated statistical and computing approaches for revealing biologically meaningful patterns of gene expression such as relationships to cellular signaling pathways. "Omics" is a term used to refer collectively to these interrelated approaches (i.e., transcriptomics, proteomics, metabolomics, and bioinformatics).

Omics have spread into the science and applications of ecotoxicology, collectively termed ecotoxicogenomics. As is the case for human health-oriented toxicogenomics, ecotoxicogenomics has great potential for elucidating impacts of chemicals of ecological concern and ultimately for playing an important role in ecological risk assessments and regulatory ecotoxicology (Snape *et al.*, 2004; Ankley *et al.*, 2006; Watanabe and Iguchi, 2006). Specific areas to which this emerging field can contribute include prioritization of chemicals investigated in ecological risk assessments, identification of modes of action of pollutants, identification of particularly sensitive species, and effect prediction at higher levels of organization. As in other areas of ecotoxicology, a major complexity faced is the vast array of species of potential concern. This is a particularly problematic issue in ecotoxicogenomics which requires substantial species-specific molecular information. However, as mentioned earlier, the number of ecologically relevant species for which this information is becoming available is expanding rapidly, and is likely to accelerate as tools are refined. Moreover, as information grows, genomic approaches hold great promise for identifying appropriate surrogate species for laboratory studies used in basic ecotoxicological research and in support of regulatory ecotoxicology (Benson and Di Giulio, 2006).

Protein Damage The study of chemical effects on proteins, particularly enzymes, has a long history in toxicology. Of particular interest within ecotoxicology are the inhibitions of acetylcholinesterase (AChE) by certain pesticides and of delta-aminolevulinic acid dehydratase (ALAD) by lead. AChE degrades the neurotransmitter acetylcholine, and in so doing, controls nerve transmission in cholinergic nerve tracts. The widely used organophosphate and carbamate classes of insecticides kill by inhibiting AChE, and this mechanism is operative for "non-target" organisms including invertebrates, wildlife, and humans. (See Chap. 22 for a detailed discussion of these pesticides and AChE inhibition.) Of particular ecological concern have been the ingestions of AChE-inhibiting insecticides with food items or granular formulations (mistaken as seed or grit) by birds and exposures to aquatic animals from agricultural run-off (Mineau, 1991; Carr *et al.*, 1997; Wilson *et al.*, 2001). In many field studies, effects of these insecticides on mortality, and relationships between AChE inhibition and mortality, have been of primary concern. However, relationships between AChE inhibition and important sublethal impacts such as behavior have also been observed (Sandhal *et al.*, 2005). ALAD catalyzes the rate-limiting step of heme synthesis, a key component of cytochromes, hemoglobin, and myoglobin, and ALAD activity is very sensitive to inhibition by lead (ATSDR, 1999). This sensitivity has been exploited widely as a biomarker for lead exposure in humans and wildlife. In wildlife, concerns for lead exposure have included ingestion by birds of spent lead shot used in hunting (Kendall *et al.*, 1996), accumulation of lead by wildlife living near highways (Birdsall *et al.*, 1986), and aquatic organisms inhabiting surface waters contaminated by lead from mine run-off and other industrial activities (Schmitt *et al.*, 2005). In addition to enzyme inhibition, chemicals can damage proteins in other ways, including oxidative damage as described below, and by forming stable adducts similar to those formed with DNA, also discussed below.

Oxidative Stress The classic depiction of aerobic respiration shows molecular oxygen (O_2) as the terminal electron acceptor, with its reduction resulting ultimately in water as high-energy intermediates (NADH, $FADH_2$) are oxidized and cellular energy is captured as ATP. This reduction of O_2 to H_2O requires four electrons that are sequentially added; this process is tightly coupled so that the one, two, and three electron intermediates are released at low amounts (less than 0.1% of O_2 inspired; Fridovich, 2004). These intermediates are, in sequence, the superoxide anion radical (O_2^-), hydrogen peroxide (H_2O_2), and the hydroxyl radical ($\cdot OH$). This tight coupling is fortunate because these intermediates, produced during aerobic respiration and other O_2 consuming or producing processes (such as photosynthesis and CYP-mediated biotransformations) are potentially deleterious products that can indiscriminately damage cellular components; hence they are referred to as "reactive oxygen species" (ROS). Some ROS, including O_2^- and $\cdot OH$, are free radicals, i.e., they possess an unpaired electron; among ROS, $\cdot OH$ is particularly reactive and toxic. In order to defend themselves from the damag-

ing effects of ROS, all aerobic organisms have evolved complex antioxidant defense systems that include enzymatic and nonenzymatic components (Halliwell and Gutteridge, 1999). Antioxidant enzymes include superoxide dismutases that convert O_2^- to H_2O_2, catalases and peroxidases that detoxify peroxides including H_2O_2, and enzymes involved in the production and maintenance of reduced glutathione (GSH) such as glutamate–cysteine ligase (GCL) and glutathione reductase (GR). Low molecular weight, nonenzymatic antioxidants include vitamins A, C, and E, and GSH.

Oxidative stress has been defined as "a disturbance in the prooxidant-antioxidant balance in favor of the former, leading to potential damage" (Sies and Cadenas, 1985)—i.e., the point at which the production of ROS exceeds the capacity of antioxidants to prevent damage. Numerous environmental contaminants can act as prooxidants and enhance the production of ROS. The resulting oxidative damage can account wholly or partially for toxicity (Halliwell and Gutteridge, 1999). Mechanisms by which chemicals can enhance ROS production include redox cycling, interactions with electron transport chains (notably in mitochondria, microsomes, or chloroplasts), and photosensitization.

Redox cycling is perhaps the most common mechanism by which a diverse array of chemicals including many environmental pollutants generates intracellular ROS. Redox cycling chemicals include diphenols and quinones, nitroaromatics and azo compounds, aromatic hydroxylamines, bipyridyliums, and certain metal chelates, particularly of copper and iron (Di Giulio *et al.*, 1989; Halliwell and Gutteridge, 1999). These include compounds of broad industrial use, many pesticides, ubiquitous elements, and metabolic products of numerous pollutants. In the redox cycle, the parent compound accepts an electron from a reduced cofactor, such as NADH or NADPH; this reaction is typically catalyzed by a reductase such as xanthine oxidase or cytochrome P450 reductase (Kappus, 1986). In the presence of O_2, the unpaired electron of the radical metabolite is donated to O_2, yielding O_2^- and regenerating the parent compound; importantly, the parent compound can repeat this cycle until it is cleared or metabolized to an inactive product. In the course of each redox cycle, two potentially deleterious events occur—a high-energy reducing equivalent is expended (the oxidation of NADPH to $NADP^+$, for example), and an oxygen radical is produced. A generalized redox cycle that includes associations with cellular toxicities and antioxidant defenses comprises Fig. 29-8.

Additionally, pHAH AHR ligands such as coplanar PCBs and TCDD can enhance ROS production, possibly by inducing CYP1A activity and concomitantly interfering with electron flow mediated by these enzymes (Schlezinger and Stegeman, 2001). Polycyclic aromatic hydrocarbons can also upregulate CYP1A and can enhance the production of ROS-generating redox-active quinone metabolites, in contrast to uncoupling mechanisms proposed for pHAHs; Nebert *et al.* (2000) discuss potential mechanisms by which AHR agonists can produce oxidative stress. The herbicide paraquat is phytotoxic due to interference with chloroplast electron transport. Interestingly, it is a very potent lung toxicant because of its specific uptake by this tissue and subsequent redox cycling (Halliwell and Gutteridge, 1999). Another important mechanism particularly significant in aquatic systems is photosensitization. Ultraviolet (UV) radiation (specifically UVB and UVA) radiation can penetrate surface waters to depths dependent on the wavelength of the radiation and the clarity of the water. The ultraviolet radiation generates ROS and other free radicals either via excitation of photosensitizing chemicals, including common pollutants of aquatic systems (Larson and Weber, 1994). For example, due to photosensitization, many

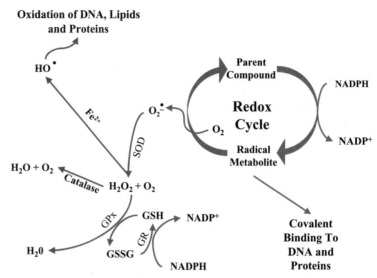

Figure 29-8. Overview of oxidative stress, including reactive oxygen species stimulation initially by redox cycling, key antioxidant defenses, and potential deleterious biochemical effects.

"Parent compound" in redox cycle could include a number of chemicals such as quinones, nitroaromatics, azo dyes, paraquat and diquat, and transition metal chelates.

PAHs are orders of magnitude more acutely toxic to aquatic organisms in the presence of UV radiation than in its absence (Arfsten *et al.*, 1996; Ankley *et al.*, 1997). The ecological relevance of photosensitization, however, is controversial (McDonald and Chapman, 2002).

As noted, ROS are generally indiscriminant molecules and can potentially damage any cellular component. Well-characterized biochemical impacts of ROS include oxidations of unsaturated lipid components of membranes ("lipid peroxidation"), oxidations of amino acids and proteins (resulting in, for example, the addition of carbonyl groups), and DNA oxidations resulting in products such as 8-hydroxy-guanosine and thyme glycol (Halliwell and Gutteridge, 1999). Another important impact is perturbed redox status (Schafer and Buettner, 2001). Healthy cells typically maintain high ratios of cofactors in their reduced, high-energy state relative to their oxidized state (e.g., NADH/NAD$^+$, NADPH/NADP$^+$, and GSH/GSSG), as the reduced forms are those most employed for energy production, biosynthesis, and antioxidant defense, for example. The ROS can drive redox status to a more oxidized state by several direct and indirect mechanisms, potentially reducing cell viability. These ROS-mediated impacts and others have been associated with a number of human diseases including atherosclerosis, arthritis, cancer, and neurodegenerative diseases such as Alzheimer's disease, Parkinson's disease, and amyotrophic lateral sclerosis (Halliwell and Gutteridge, 1999). With the exception of cancer (see below), the role of ROS in specific diseases in wildlife has received little attention. However, numerous studies have documented oxidative stress-mediated biochemical and cellular effects in wildlife associated with environmental contamination (Bainy *et al.*, 1996; Livingstone, 2001; van der Oost, 2003; Dorval *et al.*, 2005). As with humans and various animal models for human disease, it is reasonable to assume that oxidative stress comprises an important mechanism accounting in part for the toxicity of diverse pollutants to free-living organisms. Also, oxidative stress is involved in the effects of air pollutants on plants and likely plays a role in forest die-backs observed downwind

of industrialized areas (Richardson *et al.*, 1989; Hippeli and Elstner, 1996).

DNA Damage The importance of DNA as a molecular target in toxicology is indicated by the devotion of Chapter 9 of this text to genetic toxicology. As indicated, perhaps the most pressing human health issue associated with xenobiotic–DNA interactions is cancer. Cancer is also an important health outcome associated with chemical exposures in wildlife, particularly for bottom-dwelling fishes, as discussed under section "Cancer" below. Of greater concern in ecotoxicology versus human health are other, multi-generational effects of pollutants on genetic structures and resulting phenotypes of populations and communities, through both direct effects on DNA (mutations) and indirect effects (selection); this topic is discussed under **Population** effects below.

Chemical contaminants can damage DNA through several mechanisms, including the formation of DNA–xenobiotic adducts, by causing strand breaks, and by oxidations of DNA bases. In the context of ecotoxicology, the most widely studied form of damage has been the formation of stable DNA adducts, particularly by PAHs. In order to form these adducts, PAHs must first be activated to reactive metabolites by enzyme systems such as the cytochrome P450s. The bulk of PAHs metabolized to various oxidized products (such as phenols, diols, and epoxides) is subsequently conjugated by phase II enzymes (such as glutathione, sulfate, and glucuronosyl transferases; see Chapter 6); however, some fraction can react with DNA, mainly through covalent bonding with DNA bases. The most studied example of this is benzo(*a*)pyrene (BaP) which can be metabolized to the highly reactive benzo(*a*)pyrene diol epoxide (BPDE) that can bond to DNA. In field studies, the resulting large adducts of DNA with BPDE and other activated PAHs and related compounds can be measured with the highly sensitive ^{32}P-postlabeling assay (Phillips, 1997). This technique has been used extensively to monitor DNA adducts in benthic fish and bivalves inhabiting systems contaminated with hydrocarbons, particularly PAHs (Maccubbin, 1994; Reichert *et al.*, 1998; Shugart, 2000; Amat *et al.*, 2004). Other forms of DNA damage that have been investigated in ecotoxicological studies include DNA strand breaks and oxidized DNA bases (Shugart, 2000; Malins *et al.*, 2006).

Once DNA damage has occurred, whether from chemical exposures or other causes (respiration, UV radiation, viral interactions, normal wear and tear), several subsequent outcomes can occur, including: the damage can be properly repaired, the damage can lead to cell death, or a resulting change in DNA structure (base sequence) can become fixed and passed on to daughter cells, i.e., mutation occurs. Complex DNA repair systems have been elucidated in prokaryotic and eukaryotic organisms (see Chapters 8 and 9), and while these systems have received relatively little attention in species of ecological relevance, it is a safe assumption that these conserved systems are qualitatively similar across diverse phyla. Overall, these systems exhibit a remarkable capacity for surveying the cellular genome, detecting damage such as oxidations, adducts, and strand breaks, and repairing the damage by, for example, removing a damaged base and replacing it with the correct base. However, misrepair does sometime occur, with the result that an incorrect base is incorporated. Depending on the gene involved and the site within the gene, this change may lead to cell death, or may result in a mutation that may have no effect (occurs at noncritical base sequence) or one that leads to functional change in the protein coded by the gene. Some chemicals cause cancer by mutating genes that play pivotal roles in cellular growth and differentiation, particularly oncogenes and tumor suppressor genes. Examples of discoveries of activated genes (in liver tumors) in field studies include the *K-ras* oncogene in tomcod (*Microgadus tomcod*) from the Hudson River, NY (Wirgin *et al.*, 1989) and in winter flounder (*Pseudopleuronectes americanus*) collected from Boston Harbor (McMahon *et al.*, 1990), and the retinoblastoma (*Rb*) tumor suppressor gene in the marine flatfish, dab (*Limanda limanda*) from the UK (du Corbier *et al.*, 2005).

Cellular, Tissue, and Organ Effects

Cells Cellular organelles that have received attention as targets in species of ecological interest include mitochondria, lysosomes, and nuclei. Most free-living organisms routinely experience energy deficits. For example, food resources are often highly depleted during the winter for many animals, which adapt by conserving energy (by hibernating or lowering metabolism) or by storing energy beforehand (as the case for many migratory birds). Thus, effects of pollutants on mitochondrial energy metabolism can be of particular importance to wildlife. For example, Sokolova and coworkers (Sokolova, 2004; Cherkasov *et al.*, 2006) have elegantly described the effects of cadmium on several aspects of mitochondrial function in isolated gill and hepatopancreas cells from the eastern oyster (*Crassostrea virginica*), and noted a marked synergy between the metal and increasing environmental temperatures. Lysosomes are involved in the degradation of damaged organelles and proteins, and also sequester a wide variety of environmental contaminants, including metals, PAHs, and nanoparticles (Moore *et al.*, 2005). The accumulation of xenobiotics by lysosomes can elicit membrane damage, or "membrane instability," that has been used as an early warning measure of pathological chemical effects in both invertebrates and vertebrates (Hwang *et al.*, 2002; Kohler *et al.*, 2002; Moore *et al.*, 2006).

In addition to specific damage to DNA bases described above, chemical effects on nuclei have been examined in ecological

contexts with additional techniques. Micronuclei are chromosomal fragments that are not incorporated into the nucleus at cell division, and chemical exposures can markedly increase their frequency. Elevated micronuclei numbers have been observed, for example, in fish erythrocytes from polluted coastal sites in California (Hose *et al.*, 1987) and in hemocytes in clams from a PCB-polluted harbor in Massachusetts (Dopp *et al.*, 1996). Also, a standardized higher plant (*Tradescantia*) assay for micronuclei has been used for monitoring air pollution (Solenska *et al.*, 2006). A cell-based assay that has been used widely in environmental applications is the Comet assay. In this assay, cells are imbedded in agarose, lysed and subjected to gel electrophoresis, and the features of the resulting "comets tail" on the gel used to assess DNA damage. With appropriate manipulations, the comet assay can be employed to detect and distinguish among a variety of genotoxicities including strand breaks, oxidative damage, and adducts (Moller, 2006). It has been used in a variety of field applications, particularly with bivalves (Steinert, 1996; Nigro *et al.*, 2006), fish (Heuser *et al.*, 2004), and mice (Husby and McBee, 1999).

Histopathology The detailed microscopic analysis of the structure of cells and tissues can provide important links among chemical exposures, cellular targets and mechanisms, and effects at the organismal level (Hinton, 1994). Moreover, the determination that tissue damage has occurred as demonstrated by histopathological analysis is extremely useful for inferring that a significant deleterious effect has occurred. However, the substantial expertise required for proper histopathological analyses of this nature and the oftentimes time- and labor-intensive nature of these analyses has perhaps limited the application of this powerful approach in ecotoxicological contexts. Nevertheless, histopathological analysis has played an important role in confirming chemically mediated tissue damage in numerous laboratory and field studies. For example, Pacheco and Santos (2002) integrated histopathological analysis with biochemical studies of the effects of various environmental contaminants on the European eel (*Anguilla anguilla*), and Devlin (2006) similarly incorporated this approach in studies of the effects of methylmercury in fathead minnows (*Pimephales promelas*). Handy *et al.* (2002) relied upon histopathology in a study of fish health in rivers in southern England. Wester *et al.* (2002) reviewed the application and potential contributions of histopathology in aquatic toxicology, particularly in the context of small fish models. In subsequent sections concerning organismal-level impacts, other examples of the use of histopathology will be provided.

Target Organs Descriptions of chemical impacts on all organ systems of the myriad species relevant to ecotoxicology are beyond the scope of this chapter. Other chapters in this volume address key target organs in the mammalian context, and much of this is relevant to other vertebrates. Target organ toxicology is also the subject of comprehensive reviews by Schlenk and Benson (2001) concerning marine and freshwater fishes, and by Gardner and Oberdorster (2005) concerning reptiles. Relevant information in marine mammals was reviewed in Vos *et al.* (2002). We are unaware of similar reviews for birds or invertebrates. The unique properties of the avian respiratory system and its utility for investigating respiratory system toxicity and air pollution were reviewed by Brown *et al.* (1997).

Another important target organ in ecotoxicology that is not covered elsewhere in this text is the respiratory organ of nonmammalian aquatic vertebrates and many invertebrates, the gill; gills of fishes have received the most attention as targets of toxicants. The gill epithelium is the major site of gas exchange, ionic regulation, acid–base balance, and nitrogenous waste excretions for fishes and other aquatic animals (Evans, 1987). Gills are immersed in a major exposure medium for these animals (surface water) so metabolically active epithelial cells are in direct contact with this medium. They also receive blood supply directly from the heart, through the ventral aorta. Thus, it is not surprising that gills comprise a very important target for many environmental pollutants, due to their critical physiological functions, central position in blood circulation pathways, and intimate relationship with the environment. The basic structure of fish gills is comprised by branchial arches from which extend numerous filaments; from the filaments extend the lamellae (Wendelaar Bonga and Lock, in press). The lamellae are covered by a layer of epithelial cells that function in gas exchange, whereas the filament epithelium is dominated by other cell types, including pavement cells, mucous cells, and chloride cells; chloride cells are the primary location for ATPase activity and ion channels involved in ion transport.

Common structural lesions in gills caused by a diverse array of chemicals include cell death (via necrosis and apoptosis), rupture of the epithelium, hyperplasia and hypotrophy of various cell populations that can lead to lamellar fusion, epithelial swelling, and lifting of the respiratory epithelium from the underlying tissue (Wendelaar Bonga and Lock, in press). Chloride cells have received particular attention due to their key role in ionic homeostasis. For example, metals such as cadmium, copper, lead, silver, and zinc have been shown to interfere with their function in ion transport. In some cases, this may be due to inhibition of ATPase activities and/or increased membrane permeability (Spry and Wood, 1985; Wendelaar Bonga and Lock, 1992; Li et al., 1998; Rogers et al., 2003; Bury, 2005). The stress response, which results in elevated blood concentrations of epinephrine and cortisol, and associated responses such as increased cardiac output and elevated blood pressure, can also perturb ionic balance by promoting passive loss of ions such as Na^+ and Cl^- (McDonald and Milligan, 1997). A variety of contaminants have been shown to evoke the stress response in fish, sometimes concomitantly with perturbations in ionic balance (Hontela, 1997; Webb and Wood, 1998; Chowdhury et al., 2004). Also, gill damage appears to be the primary cause of the acute toxicity of PAH-mediated phototoxicity in fish (see section "Oxidative Stress", above). Weinstein et al. (1997) reported histopathological impacts of UV + fluoranthene in gills of fathead minnows including severe damage to mucosal cells, inflammation, and apparent accumulation of lipid peroxidation products; these effects likely resulted in respiratory stress, and lethality. This study elegantly demonstrates a progression from biochemical mechanism (oxidative stress) to target organ damage (gill respiration) to an important organismal impact (death). Mortality and important sublethal organismal impacts that have received substantial attention among ecotoxicologists comprise the following section.

Organismal Effects

Mortality   In similarity with impacts on human health, chemical pollution of the environment does not in most cases attain levels sufficient to outright kill wildlife. Concern in the ecotoxicological context is overall more for long-term, chronic impacts on organismal variables such as reproduction and development, behavior, and disease susceptibility, and how such impacts parlay into impacts at population and higher levels of organization. However, numerous cases of wildlife mortalities (particularly birds) due to exposures to chemical pollution have been observed, including cases associated with chronic oil discharges (Wiese and Robertson, 2004) and major oil releases from events such as the Exxon Valdez tanker wreck in Alaska (Peterson et al., 2003) and the 1991 Gulf War (Evans et al., 1993), lead from spent shot (Clark and Scheuhammer, 2003) and mines (Henny, 2003), and pesticide exposures (Mineau et al., 1999). While not a direct toxic chemical effect, hypoxia can be an important cause of fish and invertebrate mortality in aquatic systems; anthropogenic inputs of nutrients associated with sewage or fertilizers that enhance the growth of phytoplankton can cause or exacerbate hypoxia (Paerl et al., 1998; Wu, 1999). While direct mortality may not be a commonplace effect of toxic chemicals in natural systems, mortality comprises a major endpoint in toxicity testing, discussed later.

Reproduction and Development   Impacts on reproduction and development comprise perhaps the greatest concern among potential sublethal effects of xenobiotics on animals inhabiting natural systems. This is due to sensitivities of the physiological processes involved that have been described for a number of pollutants, and the importance of reproduction and development to population dynamics, a key ecological concern. Moreover, the discovery of the effects of some organochlorine insecticides on avian reproduction (particularly eggshell thinning) and resulting population crashes of several predatory bird species, and the public's awareness through the publication of Rachel Carson's Silent Spring in 1962, can be associated with the birth of ecotoxicology. Concern for reproductive and developmental effects has blossomed in recent years, with the widespread detection of endocrine disruptors in the environment.

A variety of environmental contaminants have been associated with reproductive and/or developmental effects in wildlife populations, with this association supported by controlled laboratory studies. Chlorinated hydrocarbons have continued to generate concerns although many (DDT and other insecticides, and PCBs) have had their production and use sharply curtailed. For example, DDT, its major metabolite in birds (DDE), and PCBs have been associated with reproductive and developmental impacts in bird populations in the Great Lakes, southern California, the Puget Sound and the Arctic (Fry, 1995; Custer et al., 1999; Bustnes et al., 2005). Also, alligators (Alligator mississippiensis) inhabiting a DDT-polluted lake in Florida have exhibited reproductive and developmental perturbations (Guillette et al., 2000). Evidence also indicates that PCBs impact marine mammal reproduction, including that of bottlenose dolphins (Tursiops truncates) (Schwacke et al., 2002; Wells et al., 2005).

Deleterious impacts on fish reproduction have been associated with environmental exposures to a number of contaminants. Case studies include PAHs (and other chemicals) accumulated in sediments in urban areas and harbors in the Puget Sound (Johnson et al., 1993) and northeastern United States (Johnson et al., 1994) or associated with oil spills such as the Exxon Valdez (Sol et al., 2000). Other examples include effluents from bleached paper mills in various locations, including Canada (Munkittrick et al., 1991), and selenium, for example, emanating from coal-fired power plant fly ash stored near freshwater lakes (Lemly, 2002) or in streams due to coal mine run-off (Holm et al., 2005). Notably, selenium produced severe developmental effects in water birds feeding in a created wetland in central California (Kesterson National Wildlife Refuge) that concentrated naturally occurring selenium (Ohlendorf, 2002). Additionally, severe developmental anomalies have also been observed in natural populations of marine gastropods exposed to tributyltin (TBT), which has been used extensively as an anti-fouling paint on ship hulls (Ruiz *et al.*, 2005).

The developmental effects of dioxins (TCDD) and coplanar PCBs on vertebrate development have received substantial attention. To some extent, this work was motivated by analyses that indicated that these compounds were responsible for population crashes of Great Lakes' fisheries (particularly lake trout, *Salvelinus namaycush*, in Lake Ontario) in the 1950s and 1960s, as well as for developmental impacts on other wildlife, particularly piscivorous birds and mammals in the region (Gilbertson *et al.*, 1991; Cook *et al.*, 2003). Laboratory investigations, largely with fish and bird models, have shown that embryo development is very sensitive to these compounds, and such effects likely underlaid the population crashes (Fairbrother *et al.*, 1999; Cook *et al.*, 2003). These investigations have included elegant mechanistic studies that revealed cardiac development was particularly sensitive to these chemicals, and concluded that developmental perturbations are largely receptor mediated, that is, they are dependent upon binding of the chemical (such as TCDD) with the aryl hydrocarbon receptor (AHR) described above (Hankinson, 1995; Heid *et al.*, 2001; Tanguay *et al.*, 2003; Antkiewicz *et al.*, 2005). Much of the more recent work in this area has been done with zebrafish (*Danio rerio*), a powerful model for molecular and developmental toxicology due to ease of visually examining development through a clear chorion, rapid development (~4 days from fertilization to hatch), and abundant genetic information, including gene sequences (Carney *et al.*, 2006). For example, with a known gene sequence, one can design morpholinos to block translation of specific mRNAs; morpholinos are oligonucleotides with a modified "backbone" that renders them stable (resistant to DNA/RNA-ase activities) and thus able to transiently block translation of specific protein targets. Carney *et al.* (2004) employed morpholinos to knock down AHR translation in zebrafish embryos, which greatly reduced the developmental toxicity of TCDD, confirming the role of the AHR in dioxin toxicity. Morpholinos were also employed to investigate the role of CYP1A; for example, its upregulation via TCDD activation of the AHR could enhance oxidative stress. Teraoka *et al.* (2003) observed marked reductions of TCDD toxicity with either AHR or CYP1A morpholinos, while Carney *et al.* (2004) observed protection with the AHR but not the CYP1A morpholino. While the role of CYP1A in dioxin effects on development remain unclear, pathways downstream of the AHR other than CYP1A are likely involved.

Similar concerns have emerged for the developmental effects of PAHs, particularly in fish. Hydrocarbons, in large part PAHs, associated with oil spills, contaminated sediments, paper mill effluents, and creosote used for wood treatment have profound developmental effects in fish embryos (Billiard *et al.*, 1999; Carls *et al.*, 1999; Meyer *et al.*, 2002). In many cases, the effects observed visually appear similar to those observed in fish embryos exposed to dioxins and co-planar PCBs, and include malformed hearts ("tube heart"), craniofacial deformities, hemorrhaging, and edema of the pericardium and yolk sac, the latter resulting in a distended, faintly blue yolk sac and hence a name given this syndrome—"blue sac disease" (Spitsbergen *et al.*, 1991). The mechanisms by which PAHs produce this effect are unresolved, and likely include more than a single mechanism—not surprising in light of the myriad of chemicals comprising hydrocarbon/PAH mixtures in the environment. In some cases, effects appear to be AHR-independent. Incardona *et al.* (2005) concluded in studies with zebrafish and employing morpholinos, that in weathered crude oil, tricyclic PAHs (such as phenanthrene

and dibenzothiophene—DBT, the latter a sulfur-substituted PAH) accounted for the bulk of cardiovascular teratogenesis, and rather than mediating toxicity, the AHR-CYP1A pathway afforded some protection. Wassenberg and Di Giulio (2004a) and Wassenberg *et al.* (2005) observed marked synergies in the developmental toxicity to killifish (*Fundulus heteroclitus*) embryos between higher molecular weight PAHs that are AHR agonists (BaP and BNF) and PAHs that inhibit CYP1A (α-naphthoflavone—ANF, fluoranthene, DBT, and carbazole—a nitrogen-substituted PAH). Also, ANF enhanced the toxicity of a water-based extract of sediments contaminated with weathered creosote (Wassenberg and Di Giulio, 2004b). In subsequent studies with zebrafish embryos investigating the synergistic toxicity of BNF and ANF, the AHR morpholino provided protection, while the CYP1A morpholino enhanced toxicity (Billiard *et al.*, 2006). Collectively, these PAH studies suggest that in the context of embryo toxicity, CYP1A plays a protective role, presumably by mediating metabolism and clearance of these metabolically labile compounds. This is in contrast to the metabolism-resistant dioxin-like compounds, where CYP1A appears to either play a role in mediating toxicity, or has no effect. For some PAHs, such as lower molecular weight (tricyclic) PAHs that have little or no activity as AHR ligands, developmental toxicity appears AHR-independent, while the developmental toxicity of some higher molecular weight PAHs that are AHR agonists appears in part AHR-mediated. In addition, oxidative stress may play a role in the developmental toxicity of some PAHs to fish embryos (Bauder *et al.*, 2005). Polycyclic aromatic hydrocarbons comprise a ubiquitous class of contaminants that appear to be generally increasing in the environment, reflecting urbanization, population growth, and use of fossil fuels (Van Metre and Mahler, 2005).

Contaminant effects on development are often difficult to discern in field studies, due to the small size of embryos and the fact that developmental impacts are generally either lethal or greatly reduced survival. However, early life stages of most organisms are generally more sensitive to xenobiotics than other life stages; thus developmental impacts merit careful attention by ecotoxicologists.

Disease Susceptibility Disease plays an important role in regulating and sometimes seriously impacting populations of free-living organisms. Of great concern are interactions between disease organisms and environmental contaminants, particularly potential impacts of chemicals on immune systems that render organisms more susceptible to disease. The question is often raised about how chemical pollution elevates the role of disease in population viability and dynamics.

Both field observational and laboratory experimental studies motivate this concern. For example, forensic evidence suggested that pHAHs such as dioxins and PCBs may have played a role in mass mortalities of seals and other marine mammals in the Baltic Sea that were directly attributed to viral infections (Ross *et al.*, 1996). Captive harbor seals (*Phoca vitulina*) fed fish from the Baltic Sea displayed a number of immune system deficits relative to seals fed fish from uncontaminated Atlantic Ocean sites, including impaired natural killer (NK) cell activity, in vitro T-lymphocyte function, antigen-specific in vitro lymphocyte proliferative responses, and in vivo delayed-type hypersensitivity and antibody responses to ovalbumin. These effects were correlated with greater concentrations of TCDD equivalents in fish from the Baltic Sea. In a case-control study using long-term data from studies of marine mammal strandings in the UK, Hall *et al.* (2006) concluded that each 1 mg/kg increase in total PCB concentrations in blubber resulted in an average increase in mortality due to infectious disease of 2% in harbor porpoises (*Phocoena phocoena*). In a study of free-ranging loggerhead sea turtles (*Caretta caretta*) collected in North Carolina, Keller *et al.* (2006) observed significant correlations between selected immune responses (lysozyme activity and lymphocyte proliferation) and concentrations of PCBs and chlorinated insecticides (DDE and chlordanes); these correlations were supported by in vitro studies with these chemicals in isolated turtle leukocytes. Similarly, Auffret *et al.* (2006) observed responses associated with immunosuppression in mussels (*Mytilus galloprovincialis*) that generally tracked chemical pollution gradients in the western Mediterranean Sea. Using available laboratory and field data, Loge *et al.* (2005) developed a model to assess the effects of environmental stressors, including chemicals, on disease susceptibility in migrant juvenile salmon in the Columbia River Basin, Washington. They concluded that chemical and nonchemical stressors contributed equally to disease-induced mortalities that were predicted to range from 3% to 18% of the population, depending on residence time.

Numerous laboratory studies have demonstrated chemical impacts on immune systems in animals of ecological relevance. These include effects of pesticides in amphibians (Christen *et al.*, 2004), PCBs in channel catfish (*Ictalurus punctatus*) (Rice and Schlenk, 1995), heavy metals in rainbow trout (Sanchez-Dardon *et al.*, 1999), PAHs in bivalves (Wootten *et al.*, 2003), and flame retardants (polybrominated diphenyl ethers, PBDEs) in American kestrels (*Falco sparverius*) (Fernie *et al.*, 2005). Fairbrother *et al.* (2004) reviewed the literature concerning effects of chemicals on immune systems of birds, emphasizing potential impacts on wildlife species, and Zelikoff *et al.* (2002) performed a similar review for fish. The potential effects of chemicals on immune function and disease susceptibility in wildlife is clearly a very important subject in ecotoxicology and one likely to see significant advances in the near future as powerful genomic tools become more available for representative species.

Behavior   The impacts of chemicals on animal behavior have received significant attention among ecotoxicologists. Relatively subtle effects on behaviors associated with, for example, mating and reproduction, foraging, predator–prey interactions, preference/avoidance of contaminated areas, and migration have potentially important ramifications for population dynamics. However, difficulties in objective quantifications of behaviors and laboratory to field extrapolations appear to have limited the application of this area to ecological risk assessments, and by extension, perhaps to funds available for basic research. In some cases, however, biochemical mechanisms underlying behavioral effects have been elucidated that may assist with these issues and provide useful biomarkers for behavioral toxicants in field studies.

As noted by Rand (1985), chemicals causing behavioral effects in wildlife are often known from mammalian studies to be neurotoxicants. For example, in an early study, Grue *et al.* (1982) noted reduced nest attentiveness in female starlings dosed with the AChE-inhibiting organophosphate insecticide dicrotophos; this study took advantage of the relative ease of attracting wild starlings to artificial nest boxes that is advantageous for detailed studies, a phenomenon that has been employed in subsequent avian ecotoxicological studies (Parker and Goldstein, 2000). Grue *et al.* (1997) and Walker (2003) reviewed the behavioral effects in birds of these and other neurotoxic insecticides.

Behavioral effects of insecticides have also been observed in fish. For example, Scholz *et al.* (2000) reported adverse impacts of the organophosphate diazinon on olfactory mediated behaviors such as the alarm response and homing in the Chinook salmon (*Oncorhynchus tshawytscha*), and Sandhal *et al.* (2005) observed similar thresholds for the effects of another organophosphate (chlorpyrifos) on swimming and feeding behaviors and on AChE inhibition in coho salmon (*O. kistich*). The effects of pollutants, including pesticides, on fish behavior were reviewed by Scott and Sloman (2004).

Mercury, particularly as methylmercury, comprises another potent neurotoxin that has been shown to perturb behavior in wildlife. For example, golden shiners (*Notemigonus crysoleucas*) fed diets containing methylmercury that resulted in tissue mercury concentrations consistent with those observed in this species in northern U.S. lakes exhibited perturbed predator avoidance behaviors (Webber and Haines, 2003). In a study employing fish captured in the field and brought into the laboratory for behavioral analysis, Smith and Weis (1997) observed that killifish captured from a mercury-polluted tidal creek in New Jersey exhibited reduced feeding activity and greater mortality due to predation than killifish from an uncontaminated site. Using mercury concentrations in feathers as a marker for exposure, Heath and Frederick (2005) observed a negative correlation between mercury exposure and nesting activity among White Ibises (*Eudocimus albus*) in the Florida Everglades that may be related to behavioral effects. In studies with wild mink (*Mustela vision*) collected in Canada, Basu *et al.* (2005) observed significant correlations between mercury concentrations in brains and densities of neurochemical receptors (cholinergic and dopaminergic) associated with animal behavior. The effects of mercury on wildlife, including behavioral impacts, were reviewed by Wolfe *et al.* (1998).

Environmental contaminants not generally thought of as neurotoxicants have also been shown to perturb behavior. For example, cadmium and copper have been shown to impact olfactory neurons and associated behaviors (preference/avoidance to chemicals, including pheromones) in several fish species (Saucier *et al.*, 1991; Baker and Montgomery, 2001; Baldwin *et al.*, 2003). Copper exposure in zebrafish also led to loss of neurons in the peripheral mechanosensory system ("lateral line"), which could lead to altered behaviors associated with schooling, predator avoidance, and rheotaxis (physical alignment of fish in a current) (Linbo *et al.*, 2006). Carvalho and Tillitt (2004) reported loss of retinal ganglion cells in rainbow trout exposed to TCDD; these cells link the eye with the brain, and in this study deficits in visual acuity and prey capture rates were noted in TCDD-exposed fish. Clearly, numerous mechanisms of chemical toxicity can result in behavioral impacts, including direct toxicity to neurons, alterations in hormones that modulate behaviors, and impaired energy metabolism. In some cases, impaired behavior may comprise a sublethal impact with substantive ecological consequence (Scott and Sloman, 2004).

Cancer   Beginning in the 1960s, numerous cases of cancer epizootics in wildlife that are associated with chemical pollution, particularly in specific fish populations, have been reported in North America and northern Europe (Harshbarger and Clark; 1990; Vethaak, 1992). As in humans, cancer in these animals occurs largely in relatively older age classes and therefore is oftentimes considered a disease unlikely to directly impact population dynamics or other ecological parameters. However, this may not always be the case, particularly in species that require many years to attain sexual maturity and/or have low reproductive rates. In any event, the occurrence of high incidences of cancer in wildlife populations raises serious concerns for environmental quality at those locations experiencing these epizootics. For these reasons, as well as for concerns for human health in these areas, and the advantages of alternative models such as fish for understanding chemical carcinogenesis, these epizootics have motivated substantial research in several areas relevant to human health and ecotoxicology.

In field studies of cancer outbreaks in aquatic and marine systems, typically only selected species exhibit elevated cancer rates associated with chemical contamination. A major contributor to this differential cancer susceptibility in wild fish populations is clearly lifestyle; benthic (bottom-dwelling) species such as brown bullhead (*Ameriurus nebulosus*) and white sucker (*Catostomus commersoni*) in freshwater systems, and English sole (*Parophrys vetulus*) and winter flounder (*Pseudopleuronectes americanus*) in marine systems generally exhibit the highest cancer rates in polluted systems (Baumann, 1998). The bulk of chemicals in these systems associated with cancer epizootics, such as PAHs, PCBs, and other halogenated compounds, reside in sediments; benthic fish live in contact with these sediments and prey in large measure on other benthic organisms. Thus benthic fish experience greater exposures to carcinogens than other species in these systems. Inherent biological differences may also play a role in species susceptibilities to chemical carcinogenesis; for example, laboratory studies have revealed marked differences among fish species in their abilities to activate PAH procarcinogens to DNA adduct-forming metabolite as well as to detoxify them through phase II metabolism (Collier *et al.*, 1992; Hasspieler *et al.*, 1994; Ploch *et al.*, 1998).

In their analysis of cancer epizootics in fish, Harshbarger and Clark (1990) concluded that cancers of the liver (hepatocellular neoplasms) had the strongest associations with chemical pollution, although cancers have been observed in other tissues in wild fish as well (Ostrander and Rotchell, 2005). Polycyclic aromatic hydrocarbons appear to be the most implicated class of carcinogens associated with liver neoplasms in fish cancer epizootics. Studies implicating a key role for PAHs (and key PAH sources) include English sole in the Puget Sound (various urban and industrial sources; Malins *et al.*, 1987), brown bullhead in the Black River, Ohio (a coal-coking facility; Baumann and Harshbarger, 1998) and in the Potomac River watershed near Washington, DC (various point and nonpoint discharges; Pinkney *et al.*, 2001), and killifish in the Elizabeth River, Virginia (a wood treatment plant using creosote; Vogelbein *et al.*, 1990). As stated earlier, PAHs appear to comprise a class of contaminant generally increasing in the environment. The metabolism of PAHs such as BaP to reactive metabolites that form DNA adducts that initiates carcinogenesis, or conversely to excretable conjugates, was described earlier. It is noteworthy that the molecular and biochemical pathways underlying chemical carcinogenesis, such as PAH metabolism, DNA damage, and effects on oncogenes, are qualitatively similar between most fish and mammalian species examined.

This recognition of shared pathways has in part contributed to the use of various fish models for studying chemical carcinogenesis from a human health as well as from a broader environmental standpoint. An important historical event was the identification in Italy, France, and the U.S. during the 1950s and 1960s of aflatoxin as a potent liver carcinogen in farm-raised rainbow trout (Sinnhuber *et al.*, 1977). Subsequently aflatoxin, a fungal toxin produced by *Aspergillus flavus* that is of concern where grains and nuts are stored in wet conditions, was found to be carcinogenic to

mammals including humans. Thus, the rainbow trout observations led to the discovery of a new and important class of chemical carcinogens, and the recognition that fish can be very sensitive to chemical carcinogenesis. Since that time, other fish species have been employed for laboratory studies related to chemical carcinogenesis, particularly medaka (*Oryzias latipes*) and platyfish/swordtails hybrids (*Xiphophorus* spp.); zebrafish also show promise as a laboratory model (Ostrander and Rotchell, 2005). Compared to rodent models, fish models have advantages of reduced costs for propagation and housing, briefer time intervals between exposures and the expression of tissue changes indicative of carcinogenesis, and greater feasibility of performing large-scale studies with many animals to quantify dose–response relationships.

It is noteworthy that the great bulk of reports of elevated cancer rates in free-living animals occur in fish, with few reports of potentially chemically related cancers to our knowledge in other vertebrates. California sea lions (*Zalophus californianus*) stranded along the central California coast were found to have elevated cancer rates (18%), and concentrations of DDT and PCBs were greater in animals with cancer versus those determined to die of other causes (Ylitalo *et al.*, 2005). Martineau *et al.* (2002) reported elevated cancer rates (also 18%) in carcasses of beluga whales (*Delphinapterus leucas*) stranded along the shores of the St. Lawrence River estuary in Quebec, a system with elevated levels of PAHs. The authors noted that beluga was the only species of marine mammal among 20 inhabiting this system that exhibited elevated cancer rates, and that cancers are rare worldwide in marine mammals. It is likely that elevated exposures play an important role in the relatively high frequency of reports of cancers in benthic fishes; relative inherent sensitivities among mammals, birds, reptiles, and amphibians, and fishes are unclear.

Population

A population is a collection of individuals of the same species that occupy the same space and within which genetic information can be exchanged. The study of populations is a central theme in ecological sciences and ecotoxicology is no exception. Assessment of toxicant effects upon populations has been important in ecotoxicology since its inception (Newman, 2001). A well-known, early instance is the sharp drop and then slow recovery of coastal populations of osprey (Spitzer *et al.*, 1978) and brown pelican (Anderson *et al.*, 1975) that occurred as a consequence of widespread DDT and DDE spraying and eventual banning. Another was the enhanced, genetically based tolerance of pest insect populations chronically sprayed with pesticides (Mallet, 1989). Industrial melanism, the premier example in biology textbooks of natural selection in wild populations, is another example of population ecotoxicology (Newman, 2001). Population ecotoxicology covers a wide range of topics with core research themes being (1) epidemiology of chemical-related disease, (2) effects on general population qualities including demographics and persistence, and (3) population genetics.

The level of belief warranted for possible contaminant-related effects in nonhuman populations is assessed by applying routine epidemiological methods. Many methods described in epidemiology textbooks (Anders, 1993; Woodward, 2005) are applied to nonhuman populations although with a slightly different balance because much more experimental exposure data are potentially available for nonhuman populations than for human populations. Rules of thumb for gauging the level of belief warranted by evidence that emerged from human epidemiology are also applied in population

Table 29-1

A Summary of One Popular Set of Rules of Thumb (Data from Fox, 1991) for Assessing Plausibility of a Causal Association in an Ecological Epidemiology

RULE	DESCRIPTION
1. Strength of association	How strong the association is between the possible cause and the effect, e.g., a very large relative risk
2. Consistency of association	How consistently is there an association between the possible cause and the effect, e.g., consistent among several studies with different circumstances
3. Predictive performance	How good is the prediction of effect made from the presence/level of the possible cause
4. Monotonic trend	How consistent is the association between possible cause and effect to a monotonic trend (i.e., either a consistent increase or decrease in effect level/prevalence with an increase in exposure)
5. Inconsistent temporal sequence	The effect, or elevated level of effect, occurs before exposure to the hypothesized cause
6. Factual implausibility	The hypothesized association is implausible given existing knowledge
7. Inconsistency with replication	Very poor reproducibility of association during repeated field assessments encompassing different circumstances or repeated formal laboratory testing

NOTE: According to Fox, the first four rules are most useful in supporting a causal hypothesis if found to be true (i.e., very strong, consistent, predictive, or monotonic association). The others are most useful for lessening belief in the causal hypothesis if true.

ecotoxicology. Hill's nine aspects of human disease association (Hill, 1965) might be used directly or after minor modification. As an example, Fox (1991) (Table 29-1) modified such rules of thumb to accommodate slight differences in the subject matter and approaches in population ecotoxicology. Conventional epidemiological descriptors and models are also applied. For example, Horness et al. (1998) quantified prevalence and relative risks for neoplastic liver lesions in English sole inhabiting areas with different sediment concentrations of polycyclic aromatic hydrocarbons. Logistic regression models were also used to identify relationships between these lesions and chemical and biological risk factors (Myers et al., 1994).

Defining and predicting alterations in population size, dynamics, and demographic composition due to toxicant exposure has always been central in ecotoxicology and has become increasingly so in the last 15 years as regulatory agencies such as the U.S. Environmental Protection Agency clearly reinforced their long-standing commitment to understanding chemical exposure effects on natural population viability.

Protecting populations is an explicitly stated goal of several Congressional and Agency mandates and regulations. Thus it is important that ecological risk assessment guidelines focus upon protection and management at the population, community, and ecosystem levels . . .

EPA (1991)

Ecological theory and research (e.g., Forbes and Calow, 1999) also indicate that metrics of effect to individuals are not especially good metrics of toxicant exposure effects to populations.

Models of exposed population dynamics suggest that reductions on population densities are not the only important changes brought about by chemical exposure. Some species populations fluctuate within a range of densities. These fluctuations are characteristic of the species strategy for maintaining itself in various types of habitats and toxicant exposure could potentially change this range (Simkiss et al., 1993). Combined with decreases in population densities driven by external forces such as weather events, these toxicant-induced modifications of the average population densities and dynamics can increase the risk of a population's

density falling so low that local extinction occurs (Newman, 1995).

Demographic qualities can change with toxicant exposure in ways that influence the risk of local population extinction. Toxicants can change a species population's vital rates, i.e., age- and sex-dependent death, birth, maturation, and migration rates, in complex ways. These changes in combination determine the population density and distribution of individuals among ages and sexes during exposure. The population's ability to resist external forces that reduce its size is determined by these demographic features (Gard, 1992; Sherratt et al., 1999; Kammenga and Lawkowski, 2000; Aubone, 2004). Consequently, considerable research effort is being spent on demographic methods for predicting exposed population changes and risks of extinction.

Demography explores vital rates of populations composed of individuals that differ in age and sex. Individuals in field populations can also differ in their spatial distribution and this influences the impact of toxicants (Newman, 2001). Individuals of the same species often are grouped into subpopulations within a habitat and all of these subpopulations together comprise a metapopulation (Fig. 29-9). Subpopulations in the metapopulation have different levels of exchange and different vital rates that depend on the nature of their habitat. Spatial distances and obstacles or corridors for migration influence migration among patches: habitat quality determines vital rates. An inferior habitat, such as a grossly contaminated one, can act as a sink into which individuals migrate from nearby superior (source) habitat. Migration can rescue a subpopulation or reduce its risk of local extinction. An individual migrating from the contaminated habitat to an uncontaminated one can express an adverse effect despite its present distance from the contamination, i.e., the action-at-distance hypothesis of ecotoxicology (Spromberg et al., 1998). The viability of the metapopulation can also be as strongly influenced by maintaining important migration corridors among subpopulations and protecting high-quality habitats (i.e., keystone habitats) as by the general level of contamination within the metapopulation's habitat (Maurer and Holt, 1996; O'Connor, 1996; Spromberg et al., 1998; Newman, 2001).

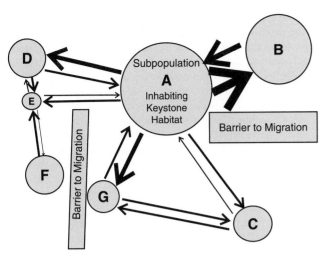

Figure 29-9. Metapopulations are composed of subpopulations that differ in their vital rates and tendency to exchange individuals.

In this illustration, subpopulation A occupies a keystone habitat. The loss of subpopulation A would devastate the metapopulation. Also, loss of the migration corridor between subpopulations A, B, and D would devastate the metapopulation. In contrast, the loss of subpopulation F would not influence the metapopulation to the same degree.

The genetics of exposed populations are studied to understand changes in tolerance to toxicants and to document toxicant influence on field populations. The capacity of some populations to become more tolerant of toxicants via selection is well documented. A few examples include increased tolerance of pine mice to endrin (Webb and Horsfall, 1967) and rats to warfarin (Partridge, 1979) after years of application of these agents for rodent control. More recently, Ownby *et al.* (2002) documented enhanced tolerance in populations of an estuarine fish chronically exposed to PAHs. Although genetically based increases in tolerance are well documented in wild populations, many exposed populations probably find themselves in situations in which they cannot adapt adequately because of their genetic resources, nature of the toxicant, or spatial/temporal context within which the enhanced tolerance must evolve are inadequate. Also, in an ecotoxicological sense, all cases of increased tolerance do not fit the conventional context manifested in the examples just given. Some do not involve suborganismal changes to biochemical or anatomical features resulting in enhanced tolerance. For example, industrial melanism increases a peppered moth's fitness in the presence of soot by reducing its likelihood of being taken by a predator. The dominant light form of this moth has a lowered fitness in the presence of dark soot, and genetically based changes in color increases its fitness. The selective mechanism here is ecological, i.e., fitness relative to avoiding visual predators.

Genetic qualities are also used to infer past toxicant influence in an exposed population. For example, Mulvey *et al.* (2002, 2003) showed distinct genetic qualities in estuarine fish populations exposed to high concentrations of PAHs. Another piece of evidence demonstrating past toxicant influence on populations can be a change in genetic diversity. A drop in genetic diversity in populations is thought to be an adverse effect because genetic diversity is required in populations to evolutionarily adapt to environmental changes. Toxicants can influence genetic diversity by purely stochastic means. Genes can be lost in the population if the population is so drastically reduced in size that the chance of a rare gene being lost between generations becomes very high. Also, the

average rate at which the frequency of a rare gene decreases through time due to genetic drift increases as the effective population size decreases. The effective population is the number of individuals contributing genes to the next generation so toxicant-related changes in demographic qualities can also accelerate genetic drift.

Community

An ecological community is an interacting assemblage of species populations occupying a defined habitat at a particular time. Populations in a community interact in many ways and, because these many interactions are complex, a community has properties that are not predictable from those of its component populations. Some species have such a crucial role (keystone species) or numerical dominance (dominants) that they are essential to maintaining community structure.[2] Other species contribute to the nature of the community in more subtle ways.

Ambiguity exists about the importance of all the species in a community relative to maintaining overall structure and balancing essential functions such as nutrient cycling, primary productivity, community respiration, and detritus processing. The redundant species hypothesis suggests that species function redundantly: if a species were lost, another with a similar function would increase in numbers to compensate. Only certain critical species such as dominant or keystone species are essential to the community. The rivet popper hypothesis suggests otherwise. Each species in a community is similar to one of the many rivets holding an airplane fuselage together. Each lost rivet contributes to a gradual weakening of the fuselage that will lead eventually to a failure in function. By analogy, each species disappearance diminishes a community's functioning.

Ecotoxicologists remain divided about which hypothesis is most relevant. Pratt and Cairns (1996) argue from evidence and a conservative stance that the rivet popper is the most appropriate. Ecotoxicologists and regulators who pragmatically set standards based on concentrations that will not harm more than a specified percentage of species in a community (e.g., Stephan *et al.*, 1985) assume that the redundant species hypothesis is more pertinent. Although the redundant species hypothesis is assumed to be correct in many ecological risk assessments (Solomon and Sibley, 2002), recent theory (Loreau 2004), modeling (Naeem *et al.*, 1994), and experimental evidence (Tilman, 1996; Tilman *et al.*, 1996; Salminen *et al.*, 2001) seem to support the rivet popper hypothesis. Biodiversity tends to foster community stability and function.

Communities take on characteristic structures as predicted by the Law of Frequencies: the number of individual organisms in a community is related by some function to the number of species in the community (Fig. 29-10). Ecotoxicants[3] can alter the resulting community structure in predictable ways by either directly impact-

---

[2] In its most rudimentary context, community structure refers to the number of species present and the numbers of individuals present in each of these species. It can also refer to the distribution of species among different functional groups such as decomposers, detritivores, primary producers, primary consumers such as herbivores, secondary consumers such as carnivores that consume herbivores, etc.

[3] The conventional context for the term toxicant becomes difficult to retain without some qualification when dealing with populations, communities, and other higher level entities because an agent does not necessarily have to directly interact with the individual in order to harm it. As an example, an agent might eliminate a prey species, leading indirectly to the disappearance of a predator species that depended on it for sustenance. The "toxicant" did not poison the predator yet it caused its demise nonetheless. A distinct term, ecotoxicant, is often applied to avoid confusion in such cases.

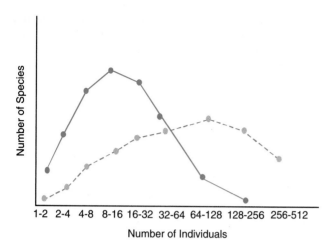

Figure 29-10. Log-normal model of species abundance for an unexposed (solid line and black points) and toxicant-exposed community (dashed line and open points).

Communities have distinct structure as shown here with the typical log-normal species abundance model. As first described by data from Patrick (1973), ecotoxicants tend to lower the mode of the species abundance curve and stretch the right tail outward. Ecotoxicants result in fewer intermediate abundance species and more extremely abundant species.

ing the fitness of individuals in populations that make up the community or by altering population interactions. Community ecotoxicologists spend considerable effort trying to understand and predict ecotoxicant influences on community structure and essential functions.

Direct effects involve removal of a population or metapopulation from the community by reducing the Darwinian fitness of individuals enough that the population falls below some critical minimum size. Indirect effects can involve interference with interspecies competition, predator–prey interactions, host–disease/parasite interactions, or symbiotic relationships such as pollination. The simplest competition model (Lotka–Volterra Model) can be used to illustrate the potential for both direct and indirect effects on populations:

$$\frac{dN_1}{dt} = r_1 N_1 \left[1 - \frac{N_1}{K_1} - \frac{\alpha_{12} N_2}{K_1}\right]$$

$$\frac{dN_2}{dt} = r_2 N_2 \left[1 - \frac{N_2}{K_2} - \frac{\alpha_{21} N_1}{K_2}\right]$$

where N_1 and N_2 = population size of competitors 1 and 2, K_1 and K_2 = carrying capacities of the environment for competitors 1 and 2, r_1 and r_2 = intrinsic rate of population increase (i.e., birth rate—death rate) for competitors 1 and 2, α_{12} = competition coefficient quantifying the impact of the presence of competitor 2 on competitor 1, and α_{21} = impact of competitor 1 on competitor 2. Not only can exposure directly impact birth rates, death rates, and carrying capacity of each species, it can influence species persistence by shifting competition coefficients in favor of another species. Mathematically, it can be shown that the two competitors depicted in the Lotka-Volterra Model can co-exist only if two conditions are met, $K_1 < K_2/\alpha_{21}$ and $K_2 < K_1/\alpha_{12}$. So, a population can be lost from a community as readily by changing its competitive interactions as by directly changing its death and reproductive rates. Similar statements can be made about changes in predator–prey, host–disease, and various symbiotic interactions. As an example,

concern expressed recently about unintended pesticide reductions in the number and diversity of pollinators in European farmlands (Newman *et al.*, 2006) could be partially responsible for the recently reported decline in insect-pollinated plant species in Britain and The Netherlands (Biesmeijer *et al.*, 2006). In another instance, reduced habitat cover and insect densities in European farmlands has had a significant impact on grey partridge populations (Rands, 1985; Chiverton, 1999). As another and final example involving predator–prey interactions, amphibian tadpole exposure to endosulfan increases the risk of predation by dragonfly larvae (Broomhall, 2002). None of these examples involves a direct poisoning by a toxicant, but instead, involves an ecotoxicant that adversely modifies species interactions.

Structural changes to communities can be detected in species abundance plots (see Fig. 29-10) or shifts in conventional community metrics calculated from community samples taken in the proximity of contaminated sites. Common metrics for species richness, diversity, and evenness are used to express changes in biodiversity. Richness is simply the number of species in the sampled community, or if a relative number of species in different communities is all that is needed, the number of species expected in a specified sample size such as a rarefaction richness estimate of 12 species in a sample of 100 individuals from a community. Evenness is a measure of how equitably the individuals in a community are spread among the species. Finally, diversity (heterogeneity) indices combine the elements of richness and evenness into one number. Generally, but not always, ecotoxicants lower species richness, evenness, and overall diversity. The regulatory premise is that these changes reflect a diminished community.

Recently, structural and functional qualities in communities have been combined to generate multimetric indices such as the Biotic Index of Integrity (IBI) (Karr, 1991). Ecological insight is used to select and then numerically combine community qualities such as species richness, health of individual animals in a sample, and the number of individuals in a sample belonging to a particular functional group, such as number of piscivorous fish. The IBI score for a study site is calculated and compared to that expected for an unimpacted site in order to estimate its biological integrity.

Another central theme in community ecotoxicology is toxicant transfer during trophic interactions. Toxicant concentrations can decrease (biodiminution), remain constant, or increase (biomagnification) with each trophic transfer within a food web. Persistent organic pollutants with moderately high lipid solubility ($5 < \log K_{ow} < 7$ or 8; Thomann, 1989; Connell, 1990) and minimal metabolic breakdown in an organism can biomagnify to harmful concentrations. Metals that biomagnify are mercury and the alkali metals, cesium and rubidium. Zinc, an essential metal that is actively regulated in individuals, can exhibit biomagnification or biominification depending on whether ambient levels are below or above those required by the organism to function properly. Biominification is facilitated in a marine food web after sequestration in intracellular phosphate granules of molluscan prey species (Nott and Nicolaidou, 1993) and biomagnification by active regulation in zinc-deficient terrestrial communities (Beyer, 1986). The biomagnification of mercury is enhanced by its microbial transformation to methylmercury. Biomagnification of the potassium analogs, cesium and rubidium, is facilitated by the differences in their influxes and effluxes that favor retention in organisms (Rowan and Rasmussen, 1994; Campbell *et al.*, 2005).

Quantifying the trophic position of a species in a community is essential to modeling biomagnification. Most trophic systems are

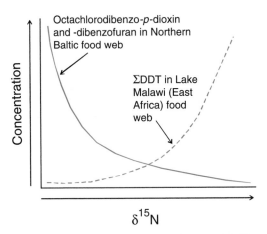

Figure 29-11. Modeling ecotoxicant concentration versus trophic position as quantified with $\delta^{15}N$.

Power models were applied to octachlorodibenzo-*p*-dioxin/dibenzofuran concentrations in a North Baltic food chain (Data from Broman *et al.*, 1992) and the ΣDDT (sum of primarily the *p, p'* isomers of DDD, DDE, and DDT) in food webs of Lake Malawi (Data from Kidd *et al.*, 2001). Biomagnification and minification were evident for ΣDDT and octachlorodibenzo-*p*-dioxin/dibenzofuran, respectively.

not simple "food chains." Most individuals in a community can feed on different species depending on their life stage, seasons, and relative abundances of prey species. These trophic interactions are best described as occurring in a trophic web, not a trophic chain.

Conveniently, trophic position of an individual within a complex food web can be quantified with nitrogen isotopes. Generally, ^{14}N passes through biochemical pathways faster than ^{15}N, resulting in excretion of waste with a slightly higher $^{14}N/^{15}N$ ratio than in ingested food. The relative amounts of ^{14}N and ^{15}N will be slightly biased toward the heavy isotope in tissues of a species relative to those of its foodsource(s). This discrimination between the heavy and light N isotopes continues through food webs, allowing the trophic position of each participating species to be estimated. The metric used for this purpose, the $\delta^{15}N$, expresses the quotient of these two isotopes in the biological tissue of interest relative to the quotient expected in the atmosphere.

$$\delta^{15}N = 1000\left[\frac{[^{15}N_{Tissue}]/[^{14}N_{Tissue}]}{[^{15}N_{Air}][^{14}N_{Air}]} - 1\right]$$

The change in toxicant concentrations within food webs is modeled using the $\delta^{15}N$ which quantifies trophic position of the species from which the tissue sample was taken (Fig. 29-11). Linear and exponential models are commonly applied.

$$Concentration = a + b\delta^{15}N$$
$$Concentration = 10^{a+b\delta^{15}N} \quad or \quad e^{a+b\delta^{15}N}$$

Ecosystem to Biosphere

Ecosystems are the functional unit of ecology composed of the ecological community and its abiotic habitat. Systems ecologists try to describe and predict energy and mass cycling in and flow from ecosystems. The ecotoxicologist's interest in ecosystems includes understanding how toxicants diminish an ecosystem's capacity to

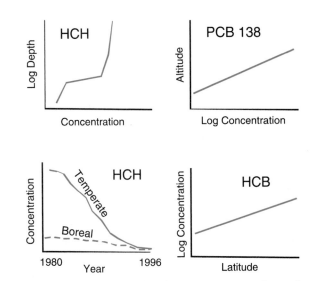

Figure 29-12. Examples of scales relevant to assessments of ecotoxicant distributions.

The smallest scale example (top left) is the vertical distribution of α-hexachlorocyclohexane (HCH) in a stratified region of the Sea of Japan (Data from Chernyak *et al.*, 1995). A slightly larger scale is reflected in the change in the polychlorinated biphenyl congener PCB-138 in tissues of fish inhabiting European lakes at different altitudes (top right panel, Data from Fernandez and Gromalt, 2003). Representing a subcontinental scale study is the temporal change in atmospheric α-hexachlorocyclohexane concentrations in temperate and boreal regions of central northern Europe (bottom left panel, Data from Wania *et al.*, 1999). The largest scale encompasses the entire Earth, showing the influence of latitude on hexachlorobenzene (HCB) concentration in tree bark (bottom right panel, Data from Simonich and Hites 1995).

perform essential functions and to understand toxicant movement enough to assess exposure within different ecosystem components.

Many of the effects described above for exposed communities are relevant here. As an example, Allred and Giesy (1988) demonstrated that elevating cadmium concentrations in an artificial stream reduced decomposition rates of dead leaves. Odum (1985) suggested that other changes to be expected with increased ecosystem stress include an increased loss of nutrients, increased community respiration, and an imbalance of primary production and respiration.

Studies of toxicant movement within ecological systems are conducted at extremely different scales (Fig. 29-12). Conventional ecosystem studies involve descriptions of contaminant concentrations and movements in easily defined ecosystems such as lakes, forests, or fields. Some toxicants, especially those subject to wide dispersal by air or water, cannot be completely understood in this framework so a landscape scale might be chosen instead. As an example, acid precipitation might be examined in the context of an entire watershed, mountain range, or even a continental region. As another example (see Fig. 29-12, top right panel), the fish tissue concentrations of a PCB congener and other persistent organic pollutants (POPs) were measured in high mountain region lakes of Europe. Concentrations for several were related to the altitude at which a lake sat. The relationships between altitude and concentrations of the various POPs was interpreted based on atmospheric movement of the POPs and each POP's propensity to either volatilize or condense at a particular altitude-dependent temperature regime. Still other ecotoxicants require a global context in order to fully understand their movements and accumulation. As an example, hexachlorobenzene concentration in tree bark collected worldwide showed a clear latitudinal gradient. Its global distribution and those of other sampled POPs were a function of their relative volatilities. The volatile hexachlorobenzene moved more readily toward the poles than less volatile POPs such as endosulfan and DDT. The differential global movement of POPs due to differences in volatility and partitioning behavior was called global distillation (Wania and Mackay, 1996). The balance between a POP's tendency to condense or evaporate at different latitude-related temperatures determines its atmospheric mobility and its ultimate global deposition pattern (Wania and Mackay, 1996).

APPROACHES

Many approaches have been developed to detect and quantify contaminant effects. These span the levels of organization described above. Approaches widely applied in ecotoxicology include standardized toxicity tests deigned to meet regulatory needs and biomarkers for organismal exposure and effects. For higher levels, a range of ecological methods exists for population, community, and ecosystem effects. Other techniques such as Geographic Information System (GIS) analysis of impacts allow the ecotoxicologist to assess impact encompassing large spatial scales. These approaches and examples of their applications are described in this section.

Toxicity Tests

Toxicity testing encompassing representative animals and plants at different levels of organization offers a practical approach to characterize chemical effects on biological systems. While it is widely known that toxicity tests cannot mimic the complex interactions and variable conditions of natural ecosystems, they address the potential direct effects of toxic substances on individual ecosystem components in a controlled and reproducible manner. A number of testing guidelines have been put forth by regulatory bodies and organizations worldwide to meet requirements for chemical registration or authorization (OECD, 1981; MAFF, 1985; US EPA OPPTS, 1996a; ASTM International, 2006), with numerous subsequent revisions. Different sets of guidelines apply to specific countries, regions, or products, and can differ significantly in their requirements. The harmonized guidelines put forth by the U.S. EPA Office of Prevention, Pesticides and Toxic Substances (U.S. EPA OPPTS, 1996a) were created in an attempt to lessen variations in testing requirements, and bring together requirements from the Organisation for Economic Co-Operation and Development (OECD), the U.S. EPA Office of Pollution Prevention and Toxics (OPPT) and the Office of Pesticide Programs (OPP).

Ecotoxicology tests feature a wide variety of aquatic (including algae, invertebrates, tadpoles, bivalves, shrimp, fish), avian (quail, duck), and terrestrial species (soil microorganisms, crops, honey bees, earthworms, wild mammals). Species are selected based on their traditional use as laboratory animals, but also on ecological relevance, which further complicates global harmonization of ecological testing. In addition, special considerations apply to testing of aquatic species due to the unmistakable differences in the way aquatic species are exposed to toxicants (U.S. EPA OPPTS, 1996b). For instance, water quality monitoring, investigation of the solubility and stability of the test substance under the conditions of testing, along with determination of nominal versus measured concentrations are common practices in aquatic toxicology. Testing can be conducted in aqueous systems without renewal of the test substance (static), renewal at predetermined time intervals (static-renewal), or continuous flow of test substance through the test compartment (flow-through).

Acute toxicity testing consists of single species exposed to various concentrations of the test substance. The most common endpoint in acute tests is death, although abnormal behavioral or other gross observations are commonly noted, and nonlethal endpoints occasionally apply (e.g., immobilization for daphnids, shell deposition in oysters). Variations in acute toxicity studies comprise testing of different species (such as fresh versus saltwater fish, bobwhite quail versus mallard duck), life-stages (embryo, larva, juvenile), environmental influences (e.g., presence of organic material), or sediment exposures. Data from different test concentrations and time points are used to derive concentration–response curves and predicted values such as the LC_{50} (median lethal concentration), EC_{50} (median effective concentration), or IC_{50} (median inhibition concentration). The LC_{50} represents the concentration of test substance killing 50% of the tested animals and EC_{50} the concentration of test substance affecting 50% of the test population during a specified period of time, such as growth; the IC_{50} is the concentration causing a 50% reduction in a nonquantal measurement (such as movement) for the test population. More quantitative values derived from acute tests are the lowest observed effect concentration (LOEC), i.e., the lowest concentration where an effect is observed, and the no-observed-effect-concentration (NOEC), the highest concentration resulting in no adverse effects.

Short-term laboratory studies conducted with single species are useful for rapid screening, provide information on thresholds for effects, selective and comparative toxicity, and can be used as range finders to guide subsequent, often more involved studies. Long-term and reproductive studies evaluate the effects of substances on organisms over extended periods of time and/or sequential generations (chronic toxicity, life cycle, reproduction). Endpoints include both quantal (such as mortality) and nonquantal (reproduction, growth) measurements, and can be used to derive additional values, other than previously mentioned in acute toxicity tests. These include the calculation of threshold values, such as the MATC (maximum acceptable toxicant concentration) which is the maximum chemical concentration not toxic to test organisms, and the BCF (bioconcentration factor) which estimates the tissue concentration in relation to the average exposure concentration in the test medium (e.g., water).

Unique to ecotoxicology are the more elaborate microcosm, mesocosm, and field studies. Microcosms are representative aquatic or terrestrial ecosystems created under laboratory conditions that include a number of relevant species (such as protozoa, plankton, algae, plants, invertebrates). Simulated field studies or mesocosms can be created in the laboratory or in the field (e.g., artificial streams, ponds) or consist of enclosures of existing habitats, containing representative soil, water, and biota. Lastly, full-scale field studies (aquatic organisms, terrestrial wildlife, pollinators) evaluate the effects of a substance on wildlife under real-life scenarios of actual use conditions of a product (e.g., pesticide field usage rate), and thus, are more complicated, subject to considerable variability, and require extensive background knowledge of the local population and community dynamics.

As a final point, plant studies are a significant component of ecological toxicity testing, particularly for pesticide registration, and involve tiered testing of both target area and nontarget terrestrial and aquatic plants. Target area plants are those that are present in the area where the substance will be routinely used (application area), but which are not anticipated to be affected. Nontarget plants are those outside of the intended use area. Endpoints of phytotoxicity include seedling emergence and growth, vegetative vigor, and rhizobium-legume toxicity, among others, and central to the toxicity testing with plants are the substrate and environmental conditions, which greatly influence plant health.

Biomarkers

The National Academy of Sciences (1987) defined a biomarker as "a xenobiotically induced variation in cellular or biochemical components or processes, structures, or function that is measurable in a biological system or sample." In the context of ecotoxicology, this definition has been modified slightly to refer to biochemical physiological or histological indicators of either exposure to, or effects of, xenobiotic chemicals at the suborganismal or organismal level (Huggett *et al.*, 1992). The term is most often employed to refer to molecular, physiological, and organismal responses to contaminant exposure that can be quantified in organisms inhabiting or captured from natural systems. A response that is limited to laboratory studies falls outside the generally held concept of a biomarker.

By definition, biomarkers do not directly provide information concerning impacts on the higher levels of organization that ecotoxicology ultimately endeavors to discern. Nevertheless, biomarkers often provide important ancillary tools for discerning contaminant exposures and potential impacts of ecological importance. The development and use of biomarkers in ecotoxicology is motivated by several factors. These include the inherent instabilities of many contaminants (such as PAHs and many pesticides) that make measures of exposure by direct tissue residue analysis difficult, the relative biological sensitivity of many biomarkers, the chemical specificity of some biomarkers that serve to contribute to the identification of chemicals having biological effects, and relatedly, the linkage of some biomarkers to underlying mechanisms of toxic action. Additionally, while populations and higher level effects are of greatest concern, variables associated with these levels are oftentimes relatively insensitive to chemicals and other stressors, take long periods of time to become manifest, and/or methods for their analysis are difficult or imprecise. Thus, biomarkers can provide sensitive early warning signals of incipient ecological damage (van der Oost *et al.*, 2003), in essence an ecological counterpart to the "canary in the coal mine" approach for preventing harm to coal miners. However, biomarkers do not provide adequate standalone data in the context of ecological assessments of contaminant effects. At this time and for the foreseeable future, such assessments generally involve a "weight of evidence approach," coalescing information obtained from chemical analyses, toxicity tests, biomarkers, and ecological indicators (sometimes referred to as "bioindicators").

In earlier discussions, a number of contaminant effects at the organismal level and below that have been utilized as biomarkers were pointed out. These include effects with some degree of chemical specificity and relationship to a mechanism of toxicity (AChE inhibition by organophosphate and carbamate insecticides, ALAD inhibition by lead, DNA-PAH adducts), responses associated with exposures to chemicals acting through a common receptor (Vtg induction by estrogen receptor agonists such as natural and synthetic estrogens, some surfactants, plasticizers, and pesticides; CYP1A induction by aryl hydrocarbon receptor agonists such as certain pHAHs and PAHs), and broader indices of cellular stress or tissue damage, such as markers of oxidative stress, lysosomal membrane stability, and histopathology. Numerous other identified

mechanisms of toxicity, indices of chemical exposure, and cellular and organismal impacts have been exploited, with varying degree of success, as biomarkers (see reviews by Huggett *et al.*, 1992; Peakall, 1992; Adams, 2002; van der Oost *et al.*, 2003). In addition, new biomarkers continue to emerge; for example, considerable attention is now being given to biomarkers arising from advances in genomic technologies, discussed above.

In considering the development or use of a selected biomarker, several issues and limitations warrant consideration. For example, while sensitivity is overall an advantage of many biomarkers, it can sometimes raise important questions surrounding interpretation. For example, some molecular and biochemical measures are very sensitive to chemical exposures, but their ramifications for organismal health are unclear. For this reason, some distinguish between biomarkers of exposure and biomarkers of effect (see reviews cited above). However, this distinction is often blurred and is subject to an individual's view of what constitutes a significant biological chemical effect; some may say the formation of DNA adduct is a significant effect, while others will argue that such adducts only indicate exposure and will require tumor formation to occur before denoting an effect. Certainly most would agree that the tumor is a clearer marker of effect than the adducts, and something more readily grasped by policy makers and the general public. On the other hand, tumors are far less sensitive as a biomarker, a key *raison d'etre*; such trade-offs merit consideration.

Chemical specificity among biomarkers is also highly variable and is imbued with trade-offs. In some cases, such as where one has a good idea of the nature of contaminants likely to occur at a site, chemical-specific biomarkers will likely be most informative. In contrast, if such information is lacking, or mixtures encompassing several classes of chemicals likely occur, nonspecific markers may be superior. In most cases, suites of biomarkers prove to be most effective, although the larger the suite, the more time-intensive and costly the analysis will be, another trade-off. Another important consideration is the influence of the biomarker to variables other than those of concern (chemical contamination). Effects of environmental variables such as temperature, time of day or year, salinity and dissolved oxygen, and physiological variables such as sex, age, reproductive status, and nutritional status need to be controlled for or at least understood and accounted for. Many biomarkers are invasive and require sacrifice of the organism in order to obtain needed tissues. This can be problematic, particularly in cases involving rare species or charismatic species such as marine mammals. In such cases, and in others where feasible, the use of noninvasive biomarkers is either preferred or required (Fossi and Marsili, 1997). In summary, biomarkers can provide powerful tools as early warning signals of ecological damage, to assist in assessments of environmental contamination, and in determining the effectiveness of various environmental management decisions such as clean-ups. However, careful case-specific thought must go into the selection of biomarkers, and they rarely are efficacious alone.

Population

Population-level effects are quantified with both field and laboratory approaches (see Newman, 1995, 2001). Population density is the most common of field population qualities measured in surveys of contaminated habitats. Quadrat, mark-recapture, and removal-based methods are applied. The density of individuals in a series of random quadrats within the area of interest is used to estimate densities in quadrat methods. The total population size can be estimated with knowledge of the total number of quadrats in the area of interest. In cases in which individuals are mobile and capable of avoiding being counted in a quadrat, a mark-recapture method might be applied instead. This involves marking a subset of individuals from the population, allowing them to randomly mix back into the population, and resampling the population. The number of marked and unmarked individuals taken, and the total number originally marked, can be used to estimate population size. Removal-based methods involve repeated sampling of the population without replacement, noting how the number collected per unit of effort declines through the sequence of samplings, and extrapolating this trend down to the point (total number caught previous to a sampling) at which no more individuals will be taken. This point is an estimate of the population size. Obviously, this approach is useful only if sampling decreases the catch noticeably between sampling episodes.

As noted earlier in discussions of metapopulations, the spatial distribution of individuals in a habitat is important to understand. Fortunately, well-established methods are available for this task. Methods vary depending on whether the sampling units are discrete or arbitrary. An arbitrary unit might be the number of razor clam per square meter of beach or number of a zooplankton species per cubic meter of water. A discrete sampling unit might be the number of mallard ducks per pond or squirrels per oak tree. Some methods associated with discrete sampling units attempt to fit the spatial pattern to a specific distribution. Methods for arbitrary sampling units include quadrat-based or distance-to-nearest neighbor approaches as described by Krebs (1998).

Demographic surveys or experiments can be conducted for exposed populations. Some studies explore age-specific vital rates but others are designed to explore vital rates for different life ages such as nestling, fledgling, juvenile, and adult. Most result in data sets that can be analyzed profitably using either a simple life table or more involved matrix analysis. The matrix method allows one to describe the population state and also to understand the sensitivity of the population to effects occurring to vital rates for various ages or stages (Caswell, 2001). The value of such studies lies in the ability to integrate effects to several effects into a projection of population consequences. Demographic studies are becoming more common in ecotoxicology, especially with species amenable to laboratory manipulation (Jensen et al., 2001; Tanaka and Nakanishi, 2001; Chandler et al., 2004).

Conventional studies of increased tolerance after generations of exposure and molecular genetic surveys of exposed populations are the primary approaches by which genetic consequences are assessed. Increased tolerance is usually detected by subjecting individuals from the chronically exposed population and a naïve population to toxicant challenge and formally testing for tolerance differences. A recent example is the study by Ownby et al. (2002) of enhanced tolerance for a PAH-exposed population of killifish from Elizabeth River (Virginia). Alternatively, a change associated with a tolerance mechanism might be examined in chronically exposed and naïve populations. As an example, Meyer et al. (2003) found upregulated antioxidant defenses in the same populations of exposed Elizabeth River killifish studied by Ownby et al. (2002). Close examinations of population genetics associated with contaminated habitats are also used to infer consequences of multi-generational exposure. Continuing with the Elizabeth River killifish example, Mulvey et al. (2002, 2003) examined the genetic qualities of fish sampled within the Elizabeth River estuary using allozymes and mDNA. Clear evidence was found using both tools for the influence of contamination on the population genetics of killifish subpopulations within the estuary.

Community and Ecosystem

Most community and ecosystem effects studies by ecotoxicologists use modified methods developed in community and systems ecology (see Magurran, 1988, for method descriptions). Recent books such as Newman (1995) and Clements and Newman (2002) provide some details of ecotoxicological applications of these methods. Several general approaches are taken. The approach affording the most control and ability to replicate treatments involves laboratory microcosms. A microcosm is a simplified system that is thought to possess the community or ecosystem qualities of interest. The experimental control and reproducibility associated with microcosms come at the cost of losing ecological realism. Is the laboratory microcosm actually responding in a way that provides insight about how the actual community or ecosystem would respond? Microcosm studies are so common throughout the ecotoxicological literature that standard methods have been proposed for their execution (Taub, 1997). As a microcosm example, Clarke (1999) established invertebrate communities in the laboratory to determine the influence of oil drilling muds on offshore benthic communities. Relative to the issue of community redundancy discussed above, zinc-amended soil microcosms was used in another case by Salminen et al. (2001) and provided minimal evidence to support the current reliance on the redundant species theory by ecological risk assessors. Gaining back some realism by giving up some degree of tractability, outdoor mesocosms are also applied to community and ecosystem ecotoxicology. Mesocosms are larger experimental systems, usually constructed outdoors that also attempt to simulate some aspect of an ecosystem such as community species composition. Often, terrestrial ecotoxicologists apply the term enclosure instead of mesocosm for such experimental units. Aquatic mesocosms can be artificial ponds such as those developed by Woin (1998), streams such as those used by Kreutzweiser et al. (2000), or river segments such as those used by Culp et al. (2000). Terrestrial mesocosms can be pens, enclosures, or large soil plots depending on the effects being quantified. An example of a terrestrial mesocosm study is that conducted by Korthals et al. (1996) of the effects of long-term copper exposure to soil nematode communities. Field studies are the third means of exploring effects at the community or ecosystem level. The high realism of associated findings from field studies is balanced against the difficulty of achieving true replication and sufficient control of other factors influencing the system's response. Field studies can involve manipulations such as introducing toxicant into replicate water bodies; however, the majority of field studies involve biomonitoring of an existing, notionally impacted, community or ecosystem. This might involve close examination of species composition and comparison to that expected or measured in a similar, but uncontaminated, system. Most biomonitoring efforts focus on community structure instead of function because it is generally believed that changes in community structure will be seen before those to functions. As examples, metal effects on invertebrate and plant community structure were studied by Peeters et al. (2000) and Strandberg et al. (2006), respectively. Despite the tendency to study community structure, study of functions can provide valuable insights as in the case of Day (1993), who found changes in photosynthesis in periphytic algae in response to herbicide exposure. Because mesocosm and field studies involve data generation in the presence of many uncontrolled variables and poor replication or pseudoreplication, multivariate statistical techniques for recognizing patterns among locations or through time are commonly applied, for example, Landis *et al.* (1997) and Kedwards *et al.* (1999).

Landscape to Biosphere

The creation and eventual convergence of several key technologies facilitate ecotoxicological study at the landscape to biosphere vantages. These same technologies have also allowed the emergence of large context, environmental disciplines such as landscape[4] ecology (Forman and Godron, 1986), global ecology (Rambler *et al.*, 1989), and global biogeochemistry (Butcher *et al.*, 1992) that contribute concepts to large-scale ecotoxicology efforts.

Technologies for acquiring, processing, and analyzing large amounts of information have been essential. Archived and new imagery from satellites and high-altitude platforms are now integrated with off-the-shelf Geographic Information Systems (GIS) software with affordable computers. Much of this imagery is gathered with remote sensing technologies, i.e., technologies that do not require physical contact with the feature being measured. However, arrays of sensors are rapidly coming together such as the network coastal observing systems that are quickly linking to form a readily accessible real-time data stream for all of our oceans. Remote sensing data from satellites or aircraft provide information for wide spatial areas and the rapidly emerging, ground- or water-based observing system networks have begun to produce extremely rich data streams. Such technologies facilitate ecotoxicological explorations at spatial scales that were impossible to consider only a few decades ago.

ECOLOGICAL RISK ASSESSMENT

Ecological risk assessment (ERA) applies ecotoxicological knowledge in support of environmental decision making. The ERA approach is an adaptation of human risk assessment methods, notably those articulated in the National Academy of Sciences paradigm (National Research Council, 1983). Adaptations are needed to accommodate differences in exposure pathways and the entities for which risk is to be estimated. Risk might be to an endangered or threatened species, or to a damaged natural resource for which remuneration might be required from a responsible party. In such cases, the ERA might estimate risk to individuals. Alternatively, as emphasized in the above EPA quote, the risk might be to a local species population or to the integrity of an ecological community. A widely dispersed ecotoxicant such as acid precipitation or widely used product such as the herbicide, atrazine, might require assessment of risk at a landscape or subcontinental scale. A recent example of such a risk assessment is that for atrazine, an herbicide used throughout North America (Solomon *et al.*, 1996). Ecotoxicants requiring a global ERA might include greenhouse gases contributing to global warming, hydrofluorocarbons depleting the ozone layer, and POPs that accumulate to harmful concentrations in polar regions far from their point of release at highly industrialized latitudes.

Adaptations are based on the context of an ERA. Some ERAs address existing situations. Considerable field information might be available for such a retroactive ERA and epidemiological methods might be applied advantageously. In contrast, predictive ERA assess possible risk associated with a future or proposed toxicant

exposure. In this case, the ERA might rely more heavily on exposure modeling and laboratory-derived effects data. A special case of predictive risk assessment is a life cycle assessment in which "cradle-to-grave" predictions are done for a product that includes all aspects of its raw material extraction, manufacture, distribution, use, and final disposal. Finally, an ERA will be structured slightly differently if it compares the ecological risk of one or more options. An example would be the comparative risk associated with a spill of Bunker oil versus Orimulsion® (a bitumen-based fossil fuel). Such a comparative risk assessment might draw insight and data from existing spill sites, laboratory tests, and exposure models. Despite adaptations and differing contexts, most ERA have the same general form (see Fig. 29-2).

Risk assessors, risk managers, and key stakeholders engage in initial planning together with the intention of formulating a clear statement of the problem. What valued ecological entity or quality is being assessed (assessment endpoint) is defined. A conceptual model is created that links the assessment endpoint and the toxicant, including descriptions of exposure pathways and possible effects. A clear statement of possible or predicted effects (risk hypothesis) is formulated. A clear formulation of the problem with concurrence of key stakeholders is critical to the ERA because of the diversity of possible assessment endpoints and exposure pathways.

Exposure characterization describes or predicts contact between the toxicant and the assessment endpoint. Depending on the ERA context, this could involve a simple calculation of average exposure, or a temporally and spatially explicit description of amounts present in relevant media. Toxicant sources, transport pathways, kinds of contact, and potential co-stressors are also defined.

Ecological effects characterization describes the qualities of any potential effects of concern, describes the connection between the potential effects and the assessment endpoint, and describes how changes in the level of exposure might influence the effects manifesting in the assessment endpoint. Normally, a statement about the strength of evidence associated with the descriptions is presented in the ecological effects characterization. As a common example of evidentiary uncertainty often requiring explanation is the measurement endpoint. It is not always desirable to derive effects information directly from an assessment endpoint such as an endangered species so uncertainty is introduced by gauging effects to a surrogate (measurement endpoint). Ecological effects characterizations must describe the justifiable confidence in extrapolating from measurement to assessment endpoints.

Risk characterization uses the analysis of exposure and ecological effects to address the risk question(s) posed in the problem formulation. This can involve an explicit statement of risk, that is, the probability of a specified intensity of an adverse effect occurring to the assessment endpoint. Often, the information needed to make such an explicit statement is absent and a qualitative statement of the likelihood of an adverse effect is made instead. Regardless of whether a quantitative or qualitative statement of risk is produced, the risk characterization must provide details surrounding the statement, including important uncertainties.

INTERCONNECTIONS BETWEEN ECOSYSTEM INTEGRITY AND HUMAN HEALTH

As noted at the beginning of this chapter, while the original definition of ecotoxicology included effects on humans, most subsequent treatments exclude discussions of humans except as a source of

---

[4] A landscape is formally defined by Forman and Godron (1986) as a heterogeneous landscape that is "composed of a cluster of interacting ecosystems that is repeated in a similar form throughout." Each ecosystem is a part of a whole landscape much as a tessera is part of a mosaic or a subpopulation is part of a metapopulation.

contaminants, with some notable exceptions (e.g., Newman and Unger, 2003). This ecotoxicology chapter, imbedded in a book focused on human or biomedical toxicology, describes the younger science of elucidating chemical effects in natural systems. While ecotoxicology has features distinct from biomedical toxicology, it is important to consider parallelisms in the two fields and more broadly, interconnections between human health and ecological integrity, or health. While obviously related, biomedical and ecological toxicology have historically exhibited relatively little coordination or collaboration among scientists across these fields. This is likely due to a number of reasons, including the different levels of biological organization considered, as well as different academic cultures populating the two fields. However, it is questionable if this gulf has been in the best interest of understanding chemical effects, and ultimately protecting both human and ecological health. This concern has prompted several broad discussions intended to bridge this divide and enhance interdisciplinary natural and social scientific research in these areas (see reviews by Costanza *et al.*, 1992; Di Giulio and Monosson, 1996; Di Giulio and Benson, 2002).

This gulf has resulted in two fields that, while largely disconnected, parallel one another and share common paradigms such as dose–response, toxicokinetics, mechanisms of action, and risk assessment frameworks. However, by generally ignoring how chemicals and other anthropogenic stressors that degrade ecosystems can ultimately impact human health and well-being, and vice versa, an opportunity to holistically understand the results of environmental contamination is lost. Miranda *et al.* (2002) developed a conceptual model for elucidating the interconnections paradigm that links natural and social systems in a circular manner with continuous feedbacks, as opposed to parallel linear models (exposure to response, either in humans or ecosystems) that dominate toxicology currently. In this conceptual model, the natural system produces both positive outputs (such as natural resources, raw materials) and negative outputs (e.g., hurricanes, disease vectors) to the social system. The culture and institution of the social system in turn transforms the natural system outputs in various ways and subsequently delivers various positive outputs (consumer goods, conservation efforts) and negative outputs (pollution, deforestation) to the natural system. These outputs influence the quantity and quality of life (human and nonhuman) of the natural system, and the circular flow of resources continually creates conditions that influence the well-being of individuals, societies, and ecosystems, now and in the future.

This rather abstract model formalizes the interconnections between human and ecological health that most of us intuitively sense. Some of these connections, in the context of environmental pollution, are obvious. Chemical contamination of seafoods valued by humans is one example. Others are less clear but potentially very significant, such as human impacts on aquatic systems that foster the propagation of human disease vectors, or human impacts on global climate that may concomitantly impact humans and ecosystems in varied and complex ways. Also important to consider is the matter of human perceptions of their environment; people's sense of the health of the environment in which they live (whether their perception is correct or not) can have substantial impacts on their mental and physical health (O'Keefe and Baum, 1996). As noted by Kendall *et al.* (2001), "the indirect effects of environmental pollution may, in the end, be more important than the direct effects for human health."

There are significant indications that these fields are converging and meaningful interactions are increasing. The inclusion of an ecotoxicology chapter in this text is favorable evidence. This trend is motivated in part by the genomics revolution which provides powerful methods for evaluating fundamental biological similarities across species, including those employed in biomedical and ecotoxicological research. Research in this area has revealed genetic similarities, or conservation, in many genes and the proteins they code for that are important to organismal adaptations and impacts due to environmental stressors, including chemicals (Eaton *et al.*, 2006). Certainly many important species differences also exist that contribute to the great complexity of understanding human-ecological interconnections, but as pointed out by Winston *et al.* (2002), "in the final analysis, the biological similarities across living systems are probably more impressive than the differences." Discussions among diverse scientists of the promises, limitations, and potential applications of genomics for elucidating cross-species extrapolations are provided by Benson and Di Giulio (2006). Such cross-fertilizations among biomedical and environmental scientists, as well as social scientists and policy-makers, are likely to enhance all areas, and catalyze the integrated protection of human and ecosystem health.

ACKNOWLEDGMENT

A special thanks to Dr. Adriana M. Doi for her expert assistace.

REFERENCES

Adams SM: Evaluating effects of contaminants on fish health at multiple levels of biological organization: Extrapolating from lower to higher levels. *Human Ecol Risk Assess* 6:15–27, 2000.

Adams SM, Shepard KL, Greeley MS, Jimenez BD, Ryon MG, Shugart LR: The use of bioindicators for assessing the effects of pollutant stress on fish. *Mar Environ Res* 28:459–464, 1989.

Allison N, Millward GE, Jones MB: Particle processing by *Mytilus edulis*: Effects on bioavailability of metals. *J Exp Mar Biol Ecol* 22:149, 1998.

Allred PM, Giesy JP: Use of in situ microcosms to study mass loss and chemical composition of leaf litter being processed in a blackwater stream. *Arch Hydrobiol* 114:231, 1988.

Amat A, Pfol-Leskowicz A, Burgeot T, Castegnaro M: DNA adducts as a biomarker of pollution: Field study on the genotoxic impact evolution of the *Erika* oil spills on mussels (*Mytilus edulis*) over a period of eleven months. *Polycyclic Aromatic Cmpds* 24:713–732, 2004.

Anders A: *Biostatistics for Epidemiologists*. Boca Raton, FL: CRC Press, 1993.

Anderson DW, Jehl JR, Risebrough RW, Woods LA, Deweese LR, Edgecomb WG: Brown pelicans: Improved reproduction off the Southern California Coast. *Science* 190:806, 1975.

Ankley GT, Daston GP, Degitz SJ *et al.*: Toxicogenomics in regulatory ecotoxicology. *Environ Sci Technol* 40: 4055–4065, 2006.

Ankley GT, Erickson RJ, Sheedy BR, *et al.*: Evaluation of models for predicting the phototoxic potency of polycyclic aromatic hydrocarbons. *Aquatic Toxicol* 37:37–50, 1997.

Antkiewicz DS, Burns CG, Carney SA, Peterson RE, Heideman W: Heart malformation is an early response to TCDD in embryonic zebrafish. *Toxicol Sci* 84:368–377, 2005.

Arfsten DP, Schaeffer DJ, Mulveny DC: The effects of near ultraviolet radiation on the toxic effects of polycyclic aromatic hydrocarbons in animals and plants: A review. *Ecotoxicol Environ Saf* 33:1–24, 1996.

ASTM International, 2006. Annual Book of ASTM Standards Volume 11.05, Pesticides; Environmental Assessment; Hazardous Substances and Oil Spill Responses. ASTM International, West Conshohocken, PA.

ATSDR: *Toxicological Profile for Lead*, Washington DC: U.S. Department of Health and Human Services, Agency for Toxic Substances and Disease Registry, 1999.

Aubone A: Loss of stability owing to a stable age structure skewed toward juveniles. *Ecol Modelling* 175:55, 2004.

Auffret M, Rousseau S, Boutet I, *et al.*: A multiparametric approach for monitoring immunotoxic responses in mussels from contaminated sites in Western Mediterranean, *Ecotoxicol Environ Saf* 63:393–405, 2006.

Bainy ACD, Saito E, Carvalho PSM, Junqueira VBC: Oxidative stress in gill, erythrocytes, liver and kidney of Nile Tilapia (*Oreochromis niloticus*) from a polluted site. *Aquatic Toxicol* 34:151–162, 1996.

Baker CF, Montgomery JC: Sensory deficits induced by cadmium in banded kokopu, *Galaxias fasciatus*, juveniles. *Environ Biol Fishes* 62:455–464, 2001.

Baldwin DH, Sandahl JF, Labenia JS, Scholz NL: Sublethal effects of copper on coho salmon: Impacts on nonoverlapping receptor pathways in the peripheral olfactory nervous system. *Environ Toxicol Chem* 22:2266–2274, 2003.

Basu N, Klenavic K, Gamberg M, *et al.*: Effects of mercury on neurochemical receptor-binding characteristics in wild mink. *Environ Toxicol Chem* 24:1444–1450, 2005.

Bauder MB, Palace VP, Hodson PV: Is oxidative stress the mechanism of blue sac disease in retene-exposed trout larvae? *Environ Toxicol Chem* 24:694–702, 2005.

Baumann PC: Epizootics of cancer in fish associated with genotoxins in sediment and water. *Mutat Res Rev Mutat Res* 411:227–233, 1998.

Baumann PC, Harshbarger JC: Long term trends in liver neoplasm epizootics of brown bullhead in the Black River, Ohio. *Environ Monitor Assess* 53:213–223, 1998.

Benson WH, Di Giulio RT (eds.): *Emerging Molecular and Computational Approaches for Cross-Species Extrapolations*. New York, Taylor & Francis, 2006.

Biesmeijer JC, Roberts SPM, Reemer M, *et al.*: Parallel declines in pollinators and insect-pollinated plants in Britain and the Netherlands. *Science* 313:351, 2006.

Billiard SM, Querbach K, Hodson PV: Toxicity of retene to early life stages of two freshwater fish species. *Environ Toxicol Chem* 18:2070–2077, 1999.

Billiard SM, Timme-Laragy AR, Wassenberg DM, Cockman C, Di Giulio RT: The role of the aryl hydrocarbon receptor pathway in mediating synergistic developmental toxicity of polycyclic aromatic hydrocarbons to zebrafish. *Toxicol Sci* 92:526–536, 2006.

Birdsall CW, Grue CE, Anderson A: Lead concentrations in bullfrog (*Rana catesbeiana*) and green frog (*Rana clamitans*) tadpoles inhabiting highway drainages. *Environ Pollut* 40A:233–247, 1986.

Broman D, Naf C, Rolff C, Zebuhr Y, Fry B, Hobbie J: Using ratios of stable nitrogen isotopes to estimate bioaccumulation and flux of polychlorinated dibenzo-*p*-dioxins (PCDDs) and dibenzofurans (PCDFs) in two food chains from the Northern Baltic. *Environ Toxicol Chem* 11:331, 1992.

Broomhall S: The effects of endosulfan and variable water temperature on survivorship and subsequent vulnerability to predation in *Litoria citropa* tadpoles. *Aquatic Toxicol* 61:243, 2002.

Brown RE, Brain JD, Wang N: The avian respiratory system: A unique model for studies of respiratory toxicosis and for monitoring air quality. *Environ Health Perspect* 105:188–200, 1997.

Bury NR: The changes to apical silver membrane uptake, and basolateral membrane silver export in the gills of rainbow trout (*Oncorhynchus mykiss*) on exposure to sublethal silver concentrations. *Aquatic Toxicol* 72:135–145, 2005.

Bustnes JO, Miland O, Fjeld M, *et al.*: Relationships between ecological variables and four organochlorine pollutants in an artic glaucous gull (*Larus hyperboreus*) population. *Environ Pollut* 136:175–185, 2005.

Butcher SS, Charlson RJ, Orians GH, Wolfe GV: *Global Biogeochemical Cycles*. London, Academic Press, 1992.

Butler RA, Kelley ML, Powell WH, Hahn ME, Van Beneden RJ: An aryl hydrocarbon receptor (AHR) homologue from the soft-shell clam, *Mya arenaria*: Evidence that invertebrate AHR homologues lack 2,3,7,8-tetrachlorodibenzo-*p*-dioxin and beta-naphthoflavone binding. *Gene* 278:223–234, 2001.

Campbell PGC, Tessier A: Ecotoxicology of metals in the aquatic environment: Geochemical aspects, in Newman MC, Jagoe CH (eds.): *Ecotoxicology. A Hierarchical Treatment*. Boca Raton, FL: CRC Press, 1996, p. 11.

Carls MG, Rice SD, Hose JE: Sensitivity of fish embryos to weathered crude oil: Part I. Low-level exposure during incubation causes malformations, genetic damage, and mortality in larval Pacific herring (*Clupea pallasi*). *Environ Toxicol Chem* 18:481–493, 1999.

Carney SA, Peterson RE, Heideman W: 2,3,7,8-Tetrachlorodibenzo-*p*-dioxin activation of the aryl hydrocarbon receptor/aryl hydrocarbon receptor nuclear translocator pathway causes developmental toxicity through a CYP1A-independent mechanism in zebrafish. *Mol Pharmacol* 66:512–521, 2004.

Carney SA, Prasch AL, Heideman W, Peterson RE: Understanding dioxin developmental toxicity using the zebrafish model. *Birth Defects Res A* 76:7–18, 2006.

Carr RL, Ho LL, Chambers JE: Selective toxicity of chlorpyrifos to several species of fish during an environmental exposure: Biochemical mechanisms. *Environ Toxicol Chem* 16:2369–2374, 1997.

Carson R: *Silent Spring*, Houghton Mifflin, Boston, 1962.

Carvalho PSM, Tillitt DE: 2,3,7,8-TCDD effects on visual structure and function in swim-up rainbow trout. *Environ Sci Technol* 38:6300–6306, 2004.

Caswell H: *Matrix Population Models. Construction, Analysis, and Interpretation,* Sunderland. MA: Sinauer Associates, 2001.

Chandler GT, Cary TL, Bejarano AC, Pender J, Ferry JL: Population consequences of Fipronil and degradates to copepods at field concentrations: An integration of life cycle testing with Leslie matrix population modeling. *Environ Sci Technol* 38:6407, 2004.

Chapman PM: Indirect effects of contaminants. *Mar Pollut Bull* 48:411, 2004.

Chaty S, Rodius F, Vasseur P: A comparative study of the expression of CYP1A and CYP4 genes in aquatic invertebrate (freshwater mussel, *Unio tumidus*) and vertebrate (rainbow trout, *Oncorhynchus mykiss*). *Aquatic Toxicol* 69:81–93, 2004.

Chen Z, Mayer LM: Mechanisms of Cu solubilization during deposit feeding. *Environ Sci Technol* 32:770, 1998.

Cherkasov AS, Biswas PK, Ridings DM, Ringwood AH, Sokolova IM: Effects of acclimation temperature and cadmium exposure on cellular energy budgets in the marine mollusk *Crassostrea virginica*: Linking cellular and mitochondrial responses. *J Expt Biol* 209:1274–1284, 2006.

Chernyak SM, McConnell LL, Rice CP: Fate of some chlorinated hydrocarbons in arctic and far eastern ecosystems in the Russian Federation. *Sci Total Environ* 75:160–161, 1995.

Chiou CT: Partition coefficients of organic compounds in lipid-water systems and correlations with fish bioconcentration factor. *Environ Sci Technol* 19:57, 1985.

Chiverton PA: The benefits of unsprayed cereal crop margins to grey partridge *Perdix perdix* and pheasants *Phasianu colchicus* in Sweden. *Wildl Biol* 5:8, 1999.

Chowdhury MJ, Pane EF, Wood CM: Physiological effects of dietary cadmium acclimation and waterborne cadmium challenge in rainbow trout: Respiratory, ionoregulatory, and stress parameters. *Comp Biochem Physiol* 139C:163–173, 2004.

Clark AJ, Scheuhammer AM: Lead poisoning in upland-foraging birds of prey in Canada. *Ecotoxicology* 12:23–30, 2003.

Collier TK, Singh SV, Awasthi YC, Varanasi U: Hepatic xenobiotic metabolizing enzymes in 2 species of benthic fish showing different prevalences of contaminant-associated liver neoplasms. *Toxicol Appl Pharmacol* 113:319–324, 1992.

Connell DW: *Bioaccumulation of Xenobiotic Compounds*. Boca Raton, FL: CRC Press, 1990.

Cook PM, Robbins JA, Endicott DD, *et al.*: Effects of aryl hydrocarbon receptor-mediated early life stage toxicity on lake trout populations in Lake Ontario during the 20th century. *Environ Sci Technol* 37:3864–3877, 2003.

Costanza R, Norton BG, Haskell BD (eds.): *Ecosystem Health. New Goals for Environmental Management*, Island Press, Washington DC, 1992.

Crollius HR, Weissenbach J: Fish genomics and biology. *Genome Res* 15:1675–1682.

Culp JM, Lowell RB, Cash KJ: Integrating mesocosm experiments with field and laboratory studies to generate weight-of-evidence risk assessments for large rivers. *Environ Toxicol Chem* 19:1167, 2000.

Custer TW, Custer CM, Dickerson K, Allen K, Melancon MJ, Schmidt LJ: Polycyclic aromatic hydrocarbons, aliphatic hydrocarbons, trace elements, and monooxygenase activity in birds nesting on the North Platte River, Casper, Wyoming, USA. *Environ Toxicol Chem* 20:624–631, 2001.

Custer TW, Custer CM, Hines RK, *et al.*: Organochlorine contaminants and reproductive success of double-crested cormorants from Green Bay, Wisconsin, USA. *Environ Toxicol Chem* 18:1209–1217, 1999.

Day KE: Short-term effects of herbicides on primary productivity of periphyton in lotic environments. *Ecotoxicol* 2:123, 1993.

de Andrade VM, da Silva J, Heuser VD, Dias JF, Yoneama ML, de Freitas TRO: Fish as bioinclicators to assess the effects of pollution in two Southern Brazilian rivers using the comet assay and micronucleus test. *Environ Mol Mutagen* 44:459–468, 2004.

Denison MS, Nagy SR: Activation of the aryl hydrocarbon receptor by structurally diverse exogenous and endogenous chemicals. *Ann Rev Pharmacol Toxicol* 43:309–334, 2003.

Deroo BJ, Korach KS: Estrogen receptors and human disease. *J Clin Invest* 116:561–570, 2006.

Devlin EW: Acute toxicity, uptake and histopathology of aqueous methyl mercury to fathead minnow embryos. *Ecotoxicology* 15:97–110, 2006.

Di Giulio RT, Hinton DE, eds.: *The Toxicology of Fishes*, CRC Press, in press.

Di Giulio RT, Monosson E, (eds.): *Interconnections Between Human and Ecosystem Health*. London: Chapman and Hall, 1996.

Di Giulio RT, Washburn PC, Wenning RJ, Winston GW, Jewell CS: Biochemical responses in aquatic animals: A review of determinants of oxidative stress. *Environ Toxicol Chem* 8:1103–1123, 1989.

Di Toro DM, Mahony JD, Hansen DJ, *et al.*: Toxicity of cadmium in sediments: The role of acid volatile sulfide. *Environ Toxicol Chem* 9:1487, 1990.

Di Toro DM, McGrath JA, Hansen DJ, Barry WJ, *et al.*: Predicting sediment metal toxicity using a sediment biotic ligand model: Methodology and initial application *Environ Toxicol Chem* 24:2410–2427, 2005.

Dopp E, Barker CM, Schiffmann D, Reinisch CL: Detection of micronuclei in hemocytes of *Mya arenaria*: Association with leukemia and induction with an alkylating agent. *Aquatic Toxicol* 34:31–45, 1996.

Dorval J, Leblond V, Deblois C, Hontela A: Oxidative stress and endocrine endpoints in white sucker (*Catostomus commersoni*) from a river impacted by agricultural chemicals. *Environl Toxicol Chem* 24:1273–1280, 2005.

du Corbier FA, Lyons BP, Stentiford GA, Rotchell JM: The role of the retinoblastoma gene in liver tumor development in fish. *Environ Sci Technol* 39:9785–9790, 2005.

Eaton D, Gallagher E, Hooper M, Schlenk D, *et al.*: Species differences in response to toxic substances: Shared pathways of toxicity—values and limitations of omic technologies to elucidate mechanism or mode of action. In: Benson WH, Di Giulio RT, (eds.): *Emerging Molecular and Computational Approaches for Cross-Species Extrapolations*. New York: Taylor & Francis, 2006.

Environmental Protection Agency: *Summary Report on Issues in Ecological Risk Assessment*, EPA/625/3-91/018, Springfield, VA, NTIS, 1991.

Evans DH: The fish gill: Site of action and model for toxic effects of environmental pollutants. *Environ Health Perspect* 71:47–58, 1987.

Evans MI, Syemens P, Pilcher CWT: Short-term damage to coastal bird populations in Saudi-Arabia and Kuwait following the 1991 Gulf War marine pollution. *Mar Pollut Bull* 27:157–161, 1993.

Fairbrother A, Ankley GT, Birnbaum LS, *et al.*: Reproductive and developmental toxicology of contaminants in oviparous animals, in: Di Giulio RT, Tillitt DE (eds.): *Reproductive and Developmental Effects of Contaminants in Oviparous Vertebrates*. SETAC Press, 1999, pp. 283–361.

Fairbrother A, Smits J, Grasman KA: Avian immunotoxicology. *J Toxicol Environ Health Crit Rev* 7B:105–137, 2004.

Fernandez P, Grimait JO: On the global distribution of persistent organic pollutants. *CHIMIA* 57:514, 2003.

Fernie KJ, Mayne G, Shutt JL, *et al.*: Evidence of immunomodulation in nestling American kestrels (*Falco sparverius*) exposed to environmentally relevant PBDEs. *Environ Pollut* 138:485–493, 2005.

Fleeger JW, Carman KR, Nisbet RM: Indirect effects of contaminants in aquatic ecosystems. *Sci Total Environ* 317:207, 2003.

Forbes VE, Calow P: Is per capita rate of increase a good measure of population-level effects in ecotoxicology? *Environ Toxicol Chem* 18:1544, 1999.

Forman RTT, Godron M: *Landscape Ecology*. New York: Wiley, 1986.

Fossi MC, Marsili L: The use of non-destructive biomarkers in the study of marine mammals. *Biomarkers* 2:205–216, 1997.

Fox G: Practical causal inference for ecoepidemiologists. *J Toxicol Environ Health* 33:359, 1991.

Fridovich I: Mitochondria: Are they the seat of senescence? *Aging Cell* 3:13–16, 2004.

Fry DM: Reproductive effects in birds exposed to pesticides and industrial chemicals. *Environ Health Perspect* 103 (Suppl 7):165–171, 1995.

Gard TC: Stochastic models for toxicant-stressed populations. *Bull Math Biol* 54:827, 1992.

Gardner SC, Oberdorster E: *Toxicology of Reptiles*. Taylor and Francis, 2005.

Gilbertson M, Kubiak T, Ludwig J, *et al.*: Great Lakes embryo mortality, edema, and deformities syndrome (GLEMEDS) in colonial fish-eating birds—similarity to chick edema disease. *J Toxicol Environ Health* 33:455–520, 1991.

Grue CE, Gilbert PL, Seeley ME: Neurophysiological and behavioral changes in non-target wildlife exposed to organophosphate and carbamate pesticides: Thermoregulation, food consumption, and reproduction. *Amer Zool* 37:369–388, 1997.

Grue CE, Powell GVN, McChesney MJ: Care of nestlings by wild female starlings exposed to an organo-phosphate pesticide. *J Appl Ecol* 19:327–335, 1982.

Guillette LJ, Crain DA, Gunderson MP, *et al.*: Alligators and endocrine disrupting contaminants: A current perspective. *Amer Zool* 40:438–452, 2000.

Hahn ME: Aryl hydrocarbon receptors: Diversity and evolution. *Chem Biol Interact* 141:131–160, 2002.

Hahn ME, Merson RR, Karchner SI: Xenobiotic receptors in fish: Structural and functional diversity and evolutionary insights, in Mommsen TP, Moon TW (eds.): *Environmental Toxicology, Vol 6, Biochemistry and Molecular Biology of Fishes*, Elsevier, 2005.

Hall AJ, Hugunin K, Deaville R, *et al.*: The risk of infection from polychlorinated biphenyl exposure in the *harbor porpoise* (*Phocoena phocoena*): A case-control approach. *Environ Health Perspect* 114:704–711, 2006.

Halliwell B, Gutteridge JMC: *Free Radicals in Biology and Medicine*. 3rd edn. Oxford University Press, 1999.

Handy RD, Runnalls T, Russell PM: Histopathologic biomarkers in three spined sticklebacks, *Gasterosteus aculeatus*, from several rivers in Southern England that meet the freshwater fisheries directive. *Ecotoxicology* 11:467–479, 2002.

Hankinson O: The aryl hydrocarbon receptor complex. *Ann Rev Pharmicol Toxicol* 35:307–340, 1995.

Harries JE, Sheahan DA, Jobling S *et al.*: Estrogenic activity in five United Kingdom rivers detected by measurement of vitellogenesis in caged male trout. *Environ Toxicol Chem* 16:534–543, 1997.

Harshbarger JC, Clark JB: Epizootiology of neoplasms of bony fish of North America. *Sci Total Environ* 94:1–32, 1990.

Hasspieler BM, Behar JV, Di Giulio RT: Glutathione-dependent defense in channel catfish (*Ictalurus punctatus*) and brown bullhead (*Ameriurus nebulosus*). *Ecotoxicol Environ Saf* 28:82–90, 1994.

Heath JA, Frederick PC: Relationships among mercury concentrations, hormones, and nesting effort of White Ibises (*Eudocimus albus*) in the Florida Everglades. *Auk* 122:255–267, 2005.

Heid SE, Walker MK, Swanson HI: Correlation of cardiotoxicity mediated by halogenated aromatic hydrocarbons to aryl hydrocarbon receptor activation. *Toxicol Sci* 61:187–196, 2001.

Henny CJ: Effects of mining lead on birds: A case history at Coeur d'Alene Basin, Idaho, in Hoffman DJ, Rattner BA, Burton GA Jr, Cairns J Jr (eds.): *Handbook of Ecotoxicology*. 2nd edn, Lewis, 2003.

Hill AB: The environment and disease: Association or causation? *Proc R Soc Med* 59:295, 1965.

Hinton DE: Cells, cellular responses, and their markers in chronic toxicity, Malins DC, Ostrander GK: *Aquatic Toxicology: Molecular, Biochemical, and Cellular Perspectives*, Lewis, 1994, pp. 207–239.

Hippeli S, Elstner EF: Mechanisms of oxygen activation during plant stress: Biochemical effects of air pollutants. *J Plant Physiol* 148:249–257, 1996.

Hoffman DJ, Marn CM, Marois KC: Sublethal effects in avocet and stilt hatchlings from selenium-contaminated sites. *Environ Toxicol Chem* 21:561–566, 2002.

Hoffman DJ, Rattner BA, Burton GA, Cairns J (eds.): *Handbook of Ecotoxicology*. Lewis/CRC Publishers, 2003.

Holm J, Palace V, Siwik P, et al.: Developmental effects of bioaccumulated selenium in eggs and larvae of two salmonid species. *Environ Toxicol Chem* 24:2373–1381, 2005.

Hontela A: Endocrine and physiological responses to xenobiotics in fish: Role of glucocorticoid hormones. *Rev Toxicol* 1:1–46, 1997.

Horness BH, Lomax DP, Johnson LL, Myers MS, Pierce SM, Collier TK: Sediment quality thresholds: Estimates from hockey stick regression of liver prevalence in English sole (*Pleuronectes vetulus*). *Environ Toxicol Chem* 17:872, 1998.

Hose JE, Cross JN, Smith SG, Diehl DL: Elevated circulating erythrocyte micronuclei in fishes from contaminated sites off southern California. *Mar Environ Res* 22:167–176, 1987.

Huang YW, Matthews JB, Fertuck KC, Zacharewski TR: Use of *Xenopus laevis* as a model for investigating in vitro and in vivo endocrine disruption in amphibians. *Environ Toxicol Chem* 24:2002–2009, 2005.

Huggett RJ, Kimerle RA, Mehrle PM Jr, Bergman HL (eds.): *Biomarkers. Biochemical, Physiological, and Histological Markers of Anthropogenic Stress*. Boca Raton, FL: Lewis, 1992.

Husby MP, McBee K: Nuclear DNA content variation and double-strand DNA breakage in white-footed mice (*Peromyscus leucopus*) collected from abandoned strip mines. Oklahoma, USA. *Environ Toxicol Chem* 18:926–931, 1999.

Hwang HM, Wade TL, Sericano JL: Relationship between lysosomal membrane destabilization and chemical body burden in eastern oysters (*Crassostrea virginica*) from Galveston Bay, Texas, USA. *Environ Toxicol Chem* 21:1268–1271, 2002.

Jansen A, Forbes VE, Parker Jr ED: Variation in cadmium uptake, feeding rate, and life-history effects in the gastropod *Potamopyrgus antipodarum*: Linking toxicant effects on individuals to the population level. *Environ Toxicol Chem* 20:2503, 2001.

Keller JM, McClellan-Green PD, Kucklick JR, Keil DE, Peden-Adams MM: Effects of organochlorine contaminants on loggerhead sea turtle immunity: Comparison of a correlative field study and in vitro exposure experiments. *Environ Health Perspect* 114:70–76, 2006.

Incardona JP, Carls MG, Teraoka H, et al.: Aryl hydrocarbon receptor-independent toxicity of weathered crude oil during fish development. *Environ Health Perspect* 113:1755–1762, 2005.

Johnson L, Casillas E, Sol S, Collier T, Stein J, Varanasi U: Contaminant effects on reproductive success in selected benthic fish. *Mar Environ Res* 35:165–170, 1993.

Johnson LL, Stein JE, Collier TK, Casillas E, Varanasi U: Indicators of reproductive development in prespawning female winter flounder (*Pleuronectes americanus*) from urban and nonurban estuaries in the northeast United States. *Sci Total Environ* 141:241–260, 1994.

Kammenga J, Laskowski R: *Demography in Ecotoxicology*. Chichester, UK: Wiley, 2000.

Kappus H: Overview of enzyme systems involved in bio-reduction of drugs and in redox cycling. *Biochem Pharmacol* 35:1–6, 1986.

Karr JR: Biological integrity: A long-neglected aspect of water resource management. *Ecol Appl* 1:66, 1991.

Kedwards TJ, Maund SJ, Chapman PF: Community level analysis of ecotoxicological field studies: I. Biological monitoring. *Environ Toxicol Chem* 18:149, 1999.

Kendall RJ, Anderson TA, Baker RJ, et al.: Ecotoxicology, in Klaassen CD (ed.): *Casarett and Doull's Toxicology, the Basic Science of Poisons*. 6th edn, New York: McGraw-Hill, 2001.

Kendall RJ, Lacher TE Jr, Bunck C, et al.: An ecological risk assessment of lead shot exposure in non-waterfowl avian species: Upland game birds and raptors. *Environ Toxicol Chem* 15:4–20, 1996.

Kidd KA, Bootsma HA, Hesslein RH, Muir DCG, Hecky RE: Biomagnification of DDT through the benthic and pelagic food webs of Lake Malawi, East Africa: Importance of trophic level and carbon source. *Environ Sci Technol* 35:14–20, 2001.

Kohler A, Wahl E, Soffker K: Functional and morphological changes of lysosomes as prognostic biomarkers of toxic liver injury in a marine flatfish (*Platichthys flesus* (L.)). *Environ Toxicol Chem* 21:2434–2444, 2002.

Korthals GW, Alexiev AD, Lexmond TM, Kammenga JE, Bongers T: Long-term effects of copper and pH on the nematode community in an agroecosystem. *Environ Toxicol Chem* 15:979, 1996.

Krebs CJ: *Ecological Methodology*. 2nd edn. New York: Benjamin Cummings, 1998.

Kreutzweiser DP, Capell SS, Scarr TA: Community-level responses by stream insects to NEEM products containing azadirachtin. *Environ Toxicol Chem* 19:855, 2000.

Krivtsov V: Investigations of indirect relationships in ecology and environmental science: A review and the implications for comparative theoretical ecosystem analysis. *Ecol Model* 174:37, 2004.

Landis WG, Matthews RA, Matthews GB: Design and analysis of multispecies toxicity tests for pesticide registration. *Ecol Appl* 7:1111, 1997.

Larsson DGJ, Adolfsson-Erici M, Parkkonen J, et al.: Ethinyloestradiol—an undesired fish contraceptive? *Aquatic Toxicol* 45:91–97, 1999.

Larson RA, Weber EJ: *Reaction Mechanisms in Environmental Organic Chemistry*. Lewis Publishers, 1994.

Lee B-G, Griscom SB, Lee J-K, et al.: Influences of dietary uptake and reactive sulfides on metal bioavailability from aquatic sediments. *Science* 287:282, 2000.

Lemly AD: Symptoms and implications of selenium toxicity in fish: The Belews Lake case example. *Aquatic Toxicol* 57:39–49, 2002.

Leslie HA, Oosthoek AJP, Busser FJM, Kraak MHS, Hermens JLM: Biomimetic solid-phase microextraction to predict body residues and toxicity of chemicals that act by narcosis. *Environ Toxicol Chem* 21:229, 2002.

Linbo TL, Stehr CM, Incardona JP, Scholz NL: Dissolved copper triggers cell death in the peripheral mechanosensory system of larval fish. *Environ Toxicol Chem* 25:597–603, 2006.

Lipscomb TP, Harris RK, Rebar AH, Ballachey BE, Haebler RJ: Exxon Valdez oil spill state/federal natural resource damage assessment, Final report. *Pathological Studies of Sea Otters (Marine Mammal Study 6–11)*, US FWS, Anchorage, AK, June 1996.

Li J, Quabius ES, Wendelaar Bonga SE, Flik G, Lock RAC: Effects of water-borne copper on branchial chloride cells and Na+/K+-ATPase activities in Mozambique tilapia (*Oreochromis mossambicus*). *Aquatic Toxicol* 43:1–11, 1998.

Little PFR: Structure and function of the human genome. *Genome Res* 15:1759–1766, 2005.

Livingstone DR: Contaminant-stimulated reactive oxygen species production and oxidative damage in aquatic organisms. *Mar Pollut Bull* 42:656–666, 2001.

Lloyd R, Herbert DWM: The influence of carbon dioxide on the toxicity of un-ionized ammonia to rainbow trout (*Salmo gairdneri* Richardson). *Ann Appl Biol* 48:399, 1960.

Loge FJ, Arkoosh MR, Ginn TR, Johnson LL, Collier TK: Impact of environmental stressors on the dynamics of disease transmission. *Environ Sci Technol* 39:7329–7336, 2005.

Loreau M: Does functional redundancy exist? *OIKOS* 104:606, 2004.

Lorenzen A, Williams KL, Moon TW: Determination of the estrogenic and antiestrogenic effects of environmental contaminants in chicken embryo hepatocyte cultures by quantitative-polymerase chain reaction. *Environ Toxicol Chem* 22:2329–2336, 2003.

Luoma SN: Can we determine the biological availability of sediment-bound trace elements? *Hydrobiologia* 379:176–177, 1989.

Luoma SN, Bryan GW: factors controlling the availability of sediment-bound lead to the estuarine bivalve *Scrobicularia plana. J Mar Biol Ass UK* 58:793, 1978.

Maccubbin AE: DNA adduct analysis in fish: Laboratory and field studies, in Malins DC, Ostrander GK (eds.): *Aquatic Toxicology: Molecular, Biochemical, and Cellular Perspectives.* Boca Raton, FL: Lewis Publishers, 1994, pp. 267–294.

Mackay D: Correlation of bioconcentration factors. *Environ Sci Technol* 16:274, 1982.

MAFF (Ministry of Agriculture, Forestry and Fisheries): Guidance on toxicological study data for application of pesticide registration, No.59-Nousan-4200, Ministry of Agriculture, Forestry and Fisheries, Japan, 1985.

Magurran AE: *Ecological Diversity and its Measurement.* Princeton, NJ: Princeton University Press, 1988.

Malins DC, Anderson KM, Stegeman JJ, et al.: Biomarkers signal contaminant effects on the organs of English sole (*Parophrys vetulus*) from Puget Sound. *Environ Health Perspect* 114:823–829, 2006.

Malins DC, Krahn MM, Brown DW, et al.: Toxic chemicals in marine sediment and biota from Mukilteo, Washington: Relationships with hepatic neoplasms and other hepatic lesions in English sole (*Parophrys vetulus*). *J Natl Cancer Inst Monogr* 74:487–494, 1987.

Mallet J: The evolution of insecticide resistance: Have the insects won?, *Trends Ecol Evol* 14:336, 1989.

Martineau D, Lemberger K, Dallaire A, et al.: Cancer in wildlife, a case study: Beluga from the St. Lawrence estuary, Quebec,Canada. *Environ Health Perspect* 110:285–292, 2002.

Mason AZ, Nott JA: The role of intracellular biomineralized granules in the regulation and detoxification of metals in gastropods with special reference to the marine prosobranch *Littorina littorea. Aquatic Toxicol* 1:239, 1981.

Mathews AP: The relation between solution tension, atomic volume, and the physiological action of elements. *Am J Physiol* 10:290, 1904.

Mauer BA, Holt RD: Effects of chronic pesticide stress on wildlife populations in complex landscapes: processes at multiple scales. *Environ Toxicol Chem* 15:420, 1996.

Mayer LM, Chen Z, Findlay RH et al.: Bioavailability of sedimentary contaminants subject to deposit-feder digestion. *Environ Sci Technol* 30:2641, 1996.

McMahon G, Huber LJ, Moore MJ, Stegeman JJ, Wogan GN: Mutations in c-Ki-ras oncogenes in diseased livers of winter flounder from Boston Harbor. *Proc Natl Acad Sci U S A* 87:841–845, 1990.

McDonald BG, Chapman PM: PAH phototoxicity—An environmentally irrelevant phenomenon? *Mar Pollut Bull* 44:1321–1326, 2002.

Mellanen P, Soimasuo M, Holmbloom B, Oikari A, Santti R: Expression of the Vitellogenin gene in the liver of juvenile whitefish (*Coregonus lavaletus* L. s.l.) exposed to effluents from pulp and paper mills. *Ecotoxicol Environ Saf* 43:133–137, 1999.

Meyer JN, Smith JD, Winston GW, Di Giulio RT: Antioxidant defenses in killifish (*Fundulus heteroclitus*) exposed to contaminated sediments and model prooxidants: Short-term and heritable responses. *Aquatic Toxicol* 65:377, 2003.

Meyer JN, Nacci D, Di Giulio RT: Cytochrome P4501A (CYP1A) in killifish (*Fundulus heteroclitus*): Heritability of altered expression and relationship to survival in contaminated sediments. *Toxicol Sci* 68:69–81, 2002.

Miller KA, Assuncao MGL, Dangerfield NJ, Bandiera SM, Ross PS: Assessment of cytochrome P450 1A in harbour seals (Phoca vitulina) using a minimally-invasive biopsy approach. *Mar Environ Res* 60:153–169, 2005.

Mineau P (ed.): *Cholinesterase-Inhibiting Insecticides: Their Impact on Wildlife and the Environment.* Amsterdam, The Netherlands: Elsevier, 1991.

Mineau P, Fletcher MR, Glaser LC, Thomas NJ, et al.: Poisoning of raptors with organophosphorus and carbamate pesticides with emphasis on Canada, US and UK. *J Raptor Res* 33:1–37, 1999.

Miranda ML, Mohai P, Bus J, Charnley G, et al.: Policy concepts and applications, in Di Giulio RT, Benson WH (eds.): *Interconnections Between Human Health and Ecological Integrity.* Pensacola FL: SETAC Press, 2002,

Moller P: The alkaline comet assay: Towards validation in biomonitoring of DNA damaging exposures. *Basic Clin Pharmacol Toxicol* 98:336–345, 2006.

Mommsen TP, Moon TW: Environmental toxicology. *Biochemistry and Molecular Biology of Fishes*, vol. 6. Amsterdam, The Netherlands: Elsevier, 2005.

Moore MN, Allen JI, McVeigh A: Environmental prognostics: An integrated model supporting lysosomal stress responses as predictive biomarkers of animal health status. *Mar Env Res* 61:278–304, 2006.

Mulvey M, Newman MC, Vogelbein W, Unger MA, Ownby, DR: Genetic structure and mtDNA diversity of *Fundulus heteroclitus* populations from PAH-contaminated and neighboring sites. *Environ Toxicol Chem* 22:671, 2003.

Mulvey M, Newman MC, Vogelbein W, Unger MA: Genetic structure of *Fundulus heteroclitus* from PAH-contaminated and neighboring sites in the Elizabeth and York Rivers. *Aquatic Toxicol* 61:195, 2002.

Munkittrick KR, Portt CB, van der Kraak GJ, et al.: Impact of bleached kraft mill effluent on population characteristics, liver MFO activity, and serum steroid levels of a Lake Superior white sucker (*Catostomus commersoni*) population. *Can J Fish Aquat Sci* 48:1371–1380, 1991.

Myers MS, Stehr CM, Olson OP, et al.: Relationships between toxicopathic hepatic lesions and exposure to chemical contaminants in English sole (*Pleuronectes vetulus*), starry flounder (*Platichthys stellatus*), and white croaker (*Genyonemus lineatus*) from selected marine sites on the Pacific coast, USA. *Environ Health Perspects* 102: 200, 1994.

National Research Council: *Risk Assessment in the Federal Government: Managing the Process.* Washington, DC: National Academy of Sciences, 1983.

Nebert DW, Roe AL, Dieter MZ, Solis WA, Yang Y, Dalton TP: Role of the aromatic hydrocarbon receptor and [*Ah*] gene battery in the oxidative stress response, cell cycle control, and apoptosis. *Biochem Pharmacol* 59:65–85, 2000.

Neely WK, Branson DR, Blau GE: Partition coefficient to measure bioconcentration potential of organic chemicals in fish. *Environ Sci Technol* 8:1113, 1974.

Newman MC, Crane M, Holloway G: Does pesticide risk assessment in the European Union assess long-term effects? *Rev Environ Toxicol* 187:1, 2006.

Newman MC, Unger MA: *Fundamentals of Ecotoxicology*, 2nd edn. Boca Raton: Lewis/CRC Publishers, 2003.

Newman MC: *Population Ecotoxicology*. Chichester, UK: Wiley, 2001.

Newman MC: *Quantitative Methods in Aquatic Ecotoxicology*. Boca Raton, FL: CRC/Lewis Press, 1995.

Nigro M, Falleni A, Del Barga I et al.: Cellular biomarkers for monitoring estuarine environments: Transplanted versus native mussels. *Aquatic Toxicol* 77:339–347, 2006.

Nott JA, Nicolaidou A: Bioreduction of zinc and manganese along a molluscan food chain. *Comp Biochem Physiol* 104A:235, 1993.

O'Connor RJ: Toward the incorporation of spatiotemporal dynamics into ecotoxicology, in Rhodes Jr OE, Chesser RK, Smith MH (eds.): *Population Dynamics in Ecological Space and Time.* Chicago IL: The University of Chicago Press, 1996, p. 281.

Odum EP: Trends expected in stressed ecosystems. *Bioscience* 35:419, 1985.

OECD (Organisation for Economic Co-operation and Development). *OECD Guidelines for the Testing of Chemicals.* Paris, France: OECD Publishing, 1981.

Ohlendorf HM: The birds of Kesterson Reservoir: a historical perspective. *Aquatic Toxicol* 57:1–10, 2002.

O'Keefe MK, Baum A: Perceptions of ecosystem health, stress and human well-being, in Di Giulio RT, Monosson E (eds.): *Interconnections Between Human and Ecosystem Health.* London: Chapman and Hall, 1996.

Ormseth OA, Ben-david M: Ingestion of crude oil: Effects on digesta retention times and nutrient uptake in captive river otters. *J Comp Physiol B* 170:419, 2000.

Ostrander GK, Rotchell JM: Fish models of carcinogenesis, in Mommsen TP, Moon TW (eds.): *Environmental Toxicology, Biochemistry and Molecular Biology of Fishes,* vol. 6. Amsterdam, The Netherlands: Elsevier, 2005.

Ownby D, Newman MC, Mulvey M, Unger M, Vogelbein W: Fish (*Fundulus heteroclitus*) populations with different exposure histories differ in tolerance of creosote-contaminated sediments. *Environ Toxicol Chem* 21:1897, 2002.

Pacheco M, Santos MA: Biotransformation, genotoxic, and histopathological effects of environmental contaminants in European eel (*Anguilla anguilla* L.). *Ecotoxicol Environ Saf* 53:331–347, 2002.

Paerl HW, Pinckney JL, Fear JM, Peierls BL: Ecosystem responses to internal and watershed organic matter loading: Consequences for hypoxia in the eutrophying Neuse river estuary, North Carolina, USA. *Mar Ecol Prog Ser* 166:17–25, 1999.

Parker ML, Goldstein MI: Differential toxicities of organophosphate and carbamate insecticides in the nestling European starling (*Sturnus vulgaris*). *Arch Environ Contam Toxicol* 39:233–242, 2000.

Partridge GG: Relative fitness of genotypes in a population of *Rattus norvegicus* polymorphic for Warfarin resistance. *Heredity* 43:239, 1979.

Patrick R: Use of algae, especially diatoms in the assessment of water quality. *ASTM Spec Tech Bull* 528:76, 1973.

Peakall D: *Animal Biomarkers as Pollution Indicators.* New York: Chapman and Hall, 1992.

Peeters ETHM, Gardeniers JJP, Koelmans AA: Contribution of trace metals in structuring *in situ* macroinvertebrate community composition along a salinity gradient. *Environ Toxicol Chem* 19:1002, 2000.

Peterson CH, Rice SD, Short JW, Esler D, Bodkin BE, Irons DB: Long-term ecosystem response to the Exxon Valdez oil spill. *Science* 302:2082–2086, 2003.

Phillips DH: Detection of DNA modifications by the ^{32}P-postlabelling assay. *Mutat Res* 178:1–12, 1997.

Pinkney AE, Harshbarger JC, May EB, Melancon MJ: Tumor prevalence and biomarkers of exposure in brown bullheads (*Ameiurus nebulosus*) from the tidal Potomac River, USA, watershed. *Environ Toxicol Chem* 20:1196–1205, 2001.

Ploch SA, King LC, Kohan MJ, Di Giulio RT: Comparative *in vitro* and *in vivo* benzo(a)pyrene-DNA adduct formation and its relationship to CYP1A activity in two species of Ictalurid catfish. *Toxicol Appl Pharmacol* 149:90–98, 1998.

Porte C, Janer G, Lorusso LC, *et al.*: Endocrine disruptors in marine organisms: Approaches and perspectives. *Comp Biochem Physiol* 143C:303–315, 2006.

Pratt JR, Cairns Jr J: Ecotoxicology and the redundancy problem: Understanding effects on community structure and function, in Newman MC, Jagoe CH (eds.): *Ecotoxicology. A Hierarchical Treatment.* Boca Raton, FL: CRC/Lewis, 1996, p. 347.

Preston BL: Indirect effects in aquatic ecotoxicology: Implications for ecological risk assessment. *Environ Manage* 29:311, 2002.

Rambler MB, Margulis L, Fester R: *Global Ecology. Towards a Science of the Biosphere.* Boston: Academic Press, 1989.

Rand GM: Behavior, in Rand GM, Petrocelli AR (eds.): *Fundamentals of Aquatic Toxicology.* Hemisphere, 1985, pp. 221–263.

Rands MRW: Pesticide use on cereals and the survival of grey partridge *Perdix perdix* chicks in a field experiment. *J Appl Ecol* 22:49, 1985.

Reichert WL, Myers MS, Peck-Miller K, *et al.*: Molecular epizootiology of genotoxic events in marine fish: Linking contaminant exposure, DNA damage, and tissue-level alterations. *Mutat Res, Rev Mutat Res* 411:215–225, 1998.

Reinfelder JR, Fisher NS: The assimilation of elements ingested by marine copepods. *Science* 251:794, 1991.

Rice CD, Schlenk D: Immune function and cytochrome P4501A activity after acute exposure to 3,3′,4,4′,5-pentachlorobiphenyl (PCB 126) in channel catfish. *J Aquatic Animal Health* 7:195–204, 1995.

Richardson CJ, Di Giulio RT, Tandy NE: Free radical mediated processes as markers of air pollution stress in trees. *Biologic Markers of Air-pollution Stress and Damage in Forests.* Washington, DC: National Academy Press, 1989, pp. 251–260.

Rogers JT, Richards JG, Wood CM: Ionoregulatory disruption as the acute toxic mechanism for lead in the rainbow trout (*Oncorhynchus mykiss*). *Aquatic Toxicol* 64:215–234, 2003.

Ross P, DeSwart R, Addison R, *et al.*: Contaminant-induced immunotoxicity in harbour seals: Wildlife at risk? *Toxicology* 112:157–169, 1996.

Rotchell JM, Ostrander GK: Molecular markers of endocrine disruption in aquatic organisms. *J Toxicol Environ Health B* 6:453–495, 2003.

Ruiz JM, Barreiro R, Gonzalez JJ: Biomonitoring organotin pollution with gastropods and mussels. *Mar Ecol Progr Ser* 287:169–176, 2005.

Salminen J, Van Gestel CAM, Oksanen J: Pollution-induced community tolerance and functional redundancy in a decomposer food web in metal-stressed soil. *Environ Toxicol Chem* 20:2287, 2001.

Sanchez-Dardon J, Voccia I, Hontela A, *et al.*: Immunomodulation by heavy metals tested individually or in mixtures in rainbow trout (*Oncorhynchus mykiss*) exposed *in vivo*. *Environ Toxicol Chem* 18:1492–1497, 1999.

Sandahl JF, Baldwin DH, Jenkins JJ, Scholtz NL: Comparative thresholds for acetylcholinesterase inhibition and behavioral impairment in coho salmon exposed to chlorpyrifos. *Environ Toxicol Chem* 24:136–145, 2005.

Saucier D, Astic L, Rioux P: The effects of early chronic exposure to sublethal copper on the olfactory discrimination of rainbow trout, *Oncorhynchus mykiss*. *Environ Biol Fishes* 30:345–351, 1991.

Schafer FQ, Buettner GR: Redox environment of the cell as viewed through the redox state of the glutathione disulfide/glutathione couple. *Free Radic Biol Med* 30:1191–1212, 2001.

Schlezinger JJ, Stegeman JJ: Induction and suppression of cytochrome P450 1A by 3,3′,4,4′,5-pentachlorobiphenyl and its relationship to oxidative stress in the marine fish scup (*Stenotomus chrysops*). *Aquatic Toxicol* 52:101–115, 2001.

Schmidt CW: Toxicogenomics. *Environ Health Perspect* 110:A750–A755, 2002.

Schmitt CJ, Whyte JJ, Brumbaugh WG, Tillitt DE: Biochemical effects of lead, zinc, and cadmium from mining on fish in the Tri-States District of northeastern Oklahoma, USA. *Environ Toxicol Chem* 24:1483–1495, 2005.

Schlenk D, Benson W: *Target Organ Toxicity in Marine and Freshwater Teleosts.*Taylor and Francis, 2001.

Scholz NL, Truelove NK, French BL, *et al.*: Diazinon disrupts antipredator and homing behaviors in chinook salmon (*Oncorhynchus tshawytscha*). *Can J Fish Aquat Sci* 57:1911–1918, 2000.

Schwacke LH, Voit EO, Hansen LJ, *et al.*: Probabilistic risk assessment of reproductive effects of polychlorinated biphenyls on bottlenose dolphins (*Tursiops truncatus*) from the southeast United States coast. *Environ Toxicol Chem* 21:2752–2764, 2002.

Scott GR, Sloman KA: The effects of environmental pollutants on complex fish behaviour: Integrating behavioural and physiological indicators of toxicity. *Aquatic Toxicol* 68:369–392, 2004.

Shelby MD, Newbold RR, Tully DB, Chae K, Davis VL: Assessing environmental chemicals for estrogenicity using a combination of in vitro and in vivo assays. *Environ Health Perspect* 104:1296–1300, 1996.

Sherratt TN, Roberts G, Williams P, *et al.*: A life-history approach to predicting the recovery of aquatic invertebrate populations after exposure to xenobiotic chemical. *Environ Toxicol Chem* 18:2512, 1999.

Shugart L: DNA damage as a biomarker of exposure. *Ecotoxicology* 9:329–340, 2000.

Sies H, Cadenas E: Oxidative stress: Damage to intact cells and organs. *Philosoph Trans Royal Soc London, Ser B, Biol Sci* 311:617–631, 1985.

Simkiss K, Daniels S, Smith RH: Effects of population density and cadmium toxicity on growth and survival of blowflies. *Environ Pollut* 81:41, 1993.

Simonich SL, Hites RA: Global distribution of persistent organochlorine compounds. *Science* 269, 1861, 1995.

Sinnhuber RO, Hendricks JD, Wales JH, Putnam GB: Neoplasms in rainbow trout, a sensitive animal model for environmental carcinogenesis. *Ann NY Acad Sci* 298:389–408, 1977.

Smith GM, Weis JS: Predator-prey relationships in mummichogs (*Fundulus heteroclitus* (L)): Effects of living in a polluted environment. *J Exper Mar Biol Ecol* 209:75–87, 1997.

Snape JR, Maund SJ, Pickford DB, Hutchinson TH: Ecotoxicogenomics: The challenge of integrating genomics into aquatic and terrestrial ecotoxicology. *Aquatic Toxicol* 67:143–154, 2004.

Sokolova IM: Cadmium effects on mitochondrial function are enhanced by elevated temperatures in a marine poikilotherm, *Crassostrea virginica* Gmelin (Bivalvia: Ostreidae). *J Expt Biol* 207:2639–2684, 2004.

Solomon KR, Baker DB, Richards RP, et al.: Ecological risk assessment of atrazine in North America surface waters. *Environ Toxicol Chem* 15:31–76, 1996.

Solomon KR, Sibley P: New concepts in ecological risk assessment: Where do we go from here? *Mar Pollut Bull* 44:279, 2002.

Sol SY, Johnson LL, Horness BH, Collier TK: Relationship between oil exposure and reproductive parameters in fish collected following the Exxon Valdez oil spill. *Mar Pollut Bull* 40:1139–1147, 2000.

Solenska M, Micieta K, Misik M: Plant bioassays for an in situ monitoring of air near an industrial area and a municipal solid waste—Zilina (Slovakia). *Environ Monitor Assess* 115:499–508, 2006.

Spitsbergen JM, Walker MK, Olson JR, Peterson RE: Pathological alterations in early life stages of lake trout, *Salvelinus namaycush*, exposed to 2,3,7,8-tetrachloro-para-dioxin as fertilized eggs. *Aquatic Toxicol* 19:41–71, 1991.

Spitzer PR, Risebrough RW, Walker W II, et al.: Productivity of ospreys in Connecticut-Long Island increases as DDE residues decline. *Science* 202:333, 1978.

Spromberg JA, John BM, Landis WG: Metapopulation dynamics: Indirect effects and multiple distinct outcomes in ecological risk assessment. *Environ Toxicol Chem* 17:1640, 1998.

Spry DJ, Wood CM: Ion flux rates, acid-base status, and blood gases in rainbow trout, *Salmo gairdneri*, exposed to toxic zinc in natural soft water. *Can J Fish Aquat Sci* 42:1332–1341, 1985.

Steinert SA: DNA damage as a bivalve biomarker. *Biomarkers* 4:492–496, 1999.

Stephan CE, Mount DI, Hansen DJ, Gentile JH, Chapman GA, Brungs WA: *Guidelines for Deriving Numerical National Water Quality Criteria for the Protection of Aquatic Organisms and Their Uses.* Duluth, MN: US EPA, 1985.

Strandberg B, Axelsen JA, Pedersen MB, Jensen J, Attrill MJ: Effect of a copper gradient on plant community structure. *Environ Toxicol Chem* 25:743, 2006.

Sumpter JP, Jobling S: Vitellogenesis as a biomarker for estrogenic contamination of the aquatic environment. *Environ Health Perspect* 103 (Suppl 7):173–178, 1995.

Tanaka Y, Nakanishi J: Life history elasticity and the population-level effect of *p*-nonylphenol on *Daphnia galeata*. *Ecol Res* 16:41, 2001.

Tanguay RL, Andreasen EA, Walker MK, Peterson RE: Dioxin toxicity and aryl hydrocarbon receptor signaling in fish, in Schecter A, Gasiewicz TA (eds.): *Dioxins and Health*. Wiley, 2003, pp. 603–628.

Teraoka H, Dong W, Tsujimoto Y, et al.: Induction of cytochrome P450 1A is required for circulation failure and edema by 2,3,7,8-tetrachlorodibenzo-*p*-dioxin in zebrafish. *Biochem Biophys Res Commun* 304:223–228, 2003.

Tessier A, Campbell PGC, Auclair JC, Bisson M: Relationships between partitioning of trace metals in sediments and their accumulation in the tissues of the freshwater mollusc *Elliptio complanata* in a mining area. *Can J Fish Aquatic Sci* 41:1463, 1984.

Thomann RV: Bioaccumulation model of organic chemical distribution in aquatic food chains. *Environ Sci Technol* 23:699, 1989.

Tilman D: Biodiversity: Population versus ecosystem stability. *Ecol* 77:350, 1996.

Tilman D, Wedin D, Knops J: Productivity and sustainability influenced by biodiversity in grassland ecosystems. *Nature* 379:718, 1996.

Trimble EL: A guest editorial: Update on diethylstilbestrol. *Obstret Gynecol Surv* 56:187–189, 2001.

Truhaut R: Ecotoxicology: Objectives, principles and perspectives. *Ecotoxicol Environ Saf* 1:151, 1977.

US EPA OPPTS, OPPTS harmonized guidelines, Series 850—Ecological Effects Test Guidelines. Office of Prevention, Pesticides, and Toxic Substances, U.S. Environmental Protection Agency, Washington, DC, 1996a.

US EPA OPPTS, Ecological Effects Test Guidelines, OPPTS 850.1000. Special Considerations for Conducting Aquatic Laboratory Studies. EPA 712–C–96–113. Office of Prevention, Pesticides, and Toxic Substances, U.S. Environmental Protection Agency, Washington, DC, 1996b.

van der Oost R, Beyer J, Vermeulen NPE: Fish bioaccumulation and biomarkers in environmental risk assessment. *Environ Toxicol Pharmacol* 13:57–149, 2003.

Van Metre PC, Mahler BJ: Trends in hydrophobic organic contaminants in urban and reference lake sediments across the United States, 1970–2001. *Environ Sci Technol* 39:5567–5574, 2005.

Vethaak ADT: Fish disease as a monitor for marine pollution: The case of the North Sea. *Rev Fish Biol Fish* 2:1–32, 1992.

Vogelbein WK, Fournie JW, Van Veld PA, Huggett RJ: Hepatic neoplasms in the mummichog *Fundulus heteroclitus* from a creosote-contaminated site. *Cancer Res* 50:5978–5986, 1990.

Vos JG, Bossart G, Fournier M, O'Shea T: *Toxicology of Marine Mammals*. Taylor and Francis, 2002.

Walker CH: Neurotoxic pesticides and behavioural effects upon birds. *Ecotoxicology* 12:307–316, 2003.

Wania DM, Mackay D: Tracking the distribution of persistent organic pollutants. *Environ Sci Technol* 30:390A, 1996.

Wania DM, Mckay D, Li Y-F, Bidleman TF, Strand A: Global chemical fate of ∀-hexachlorocyclohexane. 1. Evaluation of a global distribution model. *Environ Toxicol Chem* 18:1390, 1999.

Wassenberg DM, Di Giulio RT: Synergistic embryotoxicity of polycyclic aromatic hydrocarbon aryl hydrocarbon receptor agonists with cytochrome P4501A inhibitors in *Fundulus heteroclitus*. *Environ Health Perspect* 112:1658–1664, 2004a.

Wassenberg, DM, Di Giulio RT: Teratogenesis in *Fundulus heteroclitus* embryos exposed to a creosote-contaminated sediment extract and CYP1A inhibitors. *Mar Environ Res* 58:163–168, 2004b.

Wassenberg D, Nerlinger A, Battle L, Di Giulio R: Effects of the PAH-heterocycles, carbazole and dibenzothiophene, on *in vivo* and *in vitro* CYP1A activity and PAH-derived embryotoxicity. *Envirol Toxicol Chem* 24:2526–2532, 2005.

Watanabe H, Iguchi T: Using ecotoxicogenomics to evaluate the impact of chemicals on aquatic organisms. *Mar Biol* 149:107–115, 2006.

Wayland M, Bollinger T: Lead exposure and poisoning in bald eagles and golden eagles in the Canadian prairie provinces. *Environ Pollut* 104:341, 1999.

Webb NA, Wood CM: Physiological analysis of the stress response associated with acute silver nitrate exposure in freshwater rainbow trout (*Oncorhynchus mykiss*). *Environ Toxicol Chem* 17:679–588, 1998.

Webb RE, Horsfall Jr F: Endrin resistance in pine mouse. *Science* 156:1762, 1967.

Webber HM, Haines TA: Mercury effects on predator avoidance behavior of a forage fish, golden shiner (*Notemigonus crysoleucas*). *Environ Toxicol Chem* 22:1556–1561.

Weinstein JE, Oris JT, Taylor DH: An ultrastructural examination of the mode of UV-induced toxic action of fluoranthene in the fathead minnow, *Pimephales promelas*. *Aquat Toxicol* 39:1–22, 1997.

Wells RS, Tornero V, Borrell A, *et al.*: Integrating potential life-history and reproductive success data to examine relationships with organochlorine compounds for bottlenose dolphins (*Tursiops truncatus*) in Sarasota Bay, Florida. *Sci Total Environ* 349:106–119, 2005.

Wendelaar Bonga SE, Lock RAC: Toxicants and osmoregulation in fish. *Netherlands J Zool* 42:478–493, 1992.

Wendelaar Bonga SE, Lock RAC: The osmoregulatory system, in Di Giulio RT, Hinton DE (eds.): *The Toxicology of Fishes*, CRC Press, in press.

Wester PW, van der Ven LTM, Vethaak AD, Girnwis GCM, Vos JG: Aquatic toxicology: Opportunities for enhancement through histopathology. *Environ Toxicol Pharmacol* 11:289–295, 2002.

Weston DP, Maruya KA: Predicting bioavailability and bioaccumulation with in vitro digestive fluid extraction. *Environ Toxicol Chem* 21:962, 2002.

Wiese FK, Robertson GJ: Assessing seabird mortality from chronic oil discharges at sea. *J Wildl Manage* 68:627–638, 2004.

Wilson L, Martin PA, Elliot JE, Mineau P, Cheng KM: Exposure of California quail to organophosphorus insecticides in apple orchards in the Okanagan Valley, British Columbia. *Ecotoxicology* 10:79–90, 2001.

Winston GW, Adams SM, Benson WH, Gray LE Jr, *et al.*: Biological bases of similarities and differences, in Di Giulio RT, Benson WH (eds.): *Interconnections Between Human Health and Ecological Integrity*. Pensacola, FL: SETAC Press, 2002.

Winston GW, Di Giulio RT: Prooxidant and antioxidant mechanisms in aquatic organisms. *Aquatic Toxicol* 19:137–161, 1991.

Wirgin I, Currie D, Garte SJ: Activation of the K-ras oncogene in liver tumors of Hudson River tomcod. *Carcinogenesis* 10:2311–2315, 1989.

Woin P: Short- and long-term effects of the pyrethroid insecticide fenvalerate on an invertebrate pond community. *Ecotox Environ Saf* 41:137, 1998.

Wolfe MF, Schwarzbach S, Sulaiman RA: Effects of mercury on wildlife: A comprehensive review. *Environ Toxicol Chem* 17:146–160, 1998.

Woodward M: *Epidemiology. Study Design and Data Analysis*, 2nd edn. Boca Raton, FL: Chapman & Hall/CRC, 2005.

Wootton EC, Dyrynda EA, Ratcliffe NA: Comparisons of PAH-induced immunomodulation in three bivalve mollusks. *Aquatic Toxicol* 65:13–25, 2003.

Wu RSS: Hypoxia: From molecular responses to ecosystem response. *Mar Pollut Bull* 45:35–45, 2002.

Ylitalo GM, Sten JE, Hom T, *et al.*: The role of organochlorines in cancer-associated mortality in California sea lions (*Zalophus californianus*). *Mar Pollut Bull* 50:30–39, 2005.

Zelikoff JT, Carlson E, Li Y, *et al.*: Immunotoxicity biomarkers in fish: Development, validation and application for field studies and risk assessment. *Human Ecol Risk Assess* 8:253–263, 2002.

UNIT 7

APPLICATIONS OF TOXICOLOGY

CHAPTER 30

FOOD TOXICOLOGY

Frank N. Kotsonis and George A. Burdock

INTRODUCTION TO FOOD TOXICOLOGY

The typical Western diet contains hundreds of thousands of substances naturally present in food and many more which form in situ when food is cooked or prepared. Many of these substances affect the nutritional and esthetic qualities of food including appearance and organoleptic properties (i.e., conferring flavor, texture, or aroma) that determine whether or not we will even try the food or take a second bite, respectively. Whereas substances present in food may be nutritional and/or gratifying, they may not necessarily be "safe" in *any* amount or for *any* intended use. The Federal Food, Drug and Cosmetic (FD&C) Act gives the federal government the authority to ensure that all food involved in interstate commerce is safe. Congress, in writing the Act (and its subsequent amendments), understood that safety cannot be proved absolutely and indicated instead that the safety standard for substances added to food can be no more than a *reasonable certainty of no harm*. As will be pointed out in other sections of this chapter, the language of the FD&C Act effectively provides for practical and workable approaches to the assessment of safety for food, food ingredients, and food contaminants. Because food is highly complex, the legal framework provided by Congress for the regulation of food and substances in food was kept simple so that it would work.

The basic element of the framework is that food, which is defined as articles or components of articles used for food or drink for humans or animals, bears the presumption of safety [Sections 201(f) and 402(a)(1) of the FD&C Act]. This means that a steak or a potato is presumed to be safe unless it contains a poisonous or deleterious substance in an amount, which is shown to make it *ordinarily injurious* to health. In essence, this presumption of safety was born of necessity. If the hundreds of thousands of substances naturally present in food were subject to the same strictures and limitations that apply to added substances, virtually all food would be suspect and food shortages could easily result. To avoid such crises, Congress developed a safety standard that would not force regulatory authorities to ban common, traditional foods. In cases where the substance is not naturally present in food but is a contaminant or added ingredient, the safety standard is quite different. This standard decrees a food to be adulterated if it contains any poisonous or deleterious substance that *may render it injurious*.

Thus, for additives and contaminants, Congress recognized that these substances are not as complex as food and should therefore meet a higher standard of safety. However, because neither the law nor Food and Drug Administration (FDA) or U.S. Department of Agriculture (USDA) regulations explicitly define the term "safety" for substances added to food, scientists and their legal and regulatory counterparts have worked out operational definitions for the safety of such substances.

As with food, a practical and workable approach must be found for the contaminants of added ingredients, because all substances contain a myriad of contaminants at trace or even undetectable amounts with current technology. In this case, the approach involves setting specification limits on contaminants that are intended to exclude the possibility that the level present in an additive *may render* the food to which the substance is added, *unsafe*. It should be emphasized that specifications can serve their purpose of assuring suitable purity only if the manufacturing processes used are adequately controlled to assure consistency in the quality and purity of the product. The philosophy by which specifications are established for substances added to food embodies the belief that not all risks are worthy of regulatory concern and control (i.e., the concept of *de minimis*).[1] Implicit in this philosophy is the important unifying concept of *threshold of regulation* in food safety assessment (Flamm *et al.*, 1994, 2002).

Food, as stated earlier, contains hundreds of thousands of substances, most of which have not been fully characterized or tested. The presumption that a food is safe is based on a history of common use and that the consumption of certain foods is deeply rooted in tradition. When the uncertainty about the risk of the added substance is

small compared with the uncertainties attending food itself, the standard of "reasonable certainty of no harm" for the added substance has been satisfied. Thus, for food-like substances, the presumption is that the substance resembles food, is digested and metabolized as food, and consequently raises fewer toxicological and safety-related questions than do non-food-like substances. Moreover, when non-food-like substances are added in only very small or trace amounts, the low levels of exposure aid in demonstrating that the intended conditions of use of these substances are safe. These broad generalizations, however, do not suffice to exempt these food ingredients from the requirements of thorough safety evaluation.

Over the past decade, there has been increasing interest on the part of consumers about the health-enhancing properties of foods and the components they contain. Substances such as phytosterols from vegetable oils and isoflavones from soy have been isolated and added to other foods at elevated levels to impart cholesterol-lowering abilities. Such products have raised regulatory questions about whether these substances are functioning as drugs, and should be regulated as such, or whether they should be viewed as new nutrients and allowed in foods, as are vitamin C and iron. Recently, experts in nutritional science concluded that the concept of nutrients should be expanded to include a growing number of desirable food constituents that produce quantifiable health benefits related to disease prevention (Sansalone, 1999). This isolation of, and fortification with, new food components will necessitate a thorough evaluation of safety at the intended level of intake and for the population at large (Mackey and Kotsonis, 2002).

Finally, it should be recognized that in most of the world, microbiological contamination of food represents by far the greatest food-borne risk facing consumers. Thus, while vigilance in assuring the safety of substances added to food under their intended conditions of use is appropriate, we should not lose sight of the major concern of food safety.

Uniqueness of Food Toxicology

The nature of food is responsible for the uniqueness of food toxicology. Food occupies a position of central importance in virtually all cultures, and because most food cannot be commercially produced in a definable environment under strict quality controls, food generally cannot meet the rigorous standards of chemical identity, purity, and good manufacturing practice met by most consumer products. The fact that food is harvested from the soil, the sea, inland waters, or is derived from land animals, which are subject to the unpredictable forces of nature, makes the constancy of raw food unreliable. Experience has supported the safety of commonly consumed foods, and the good agricultural practices (GAP) under which food is produced mandates the need for quality controls (i.e., current Good Manufacturing Practice, cGMP). Nevertheless, it is clear that food is held to a different standard as a practical matter dictated by necessity.

Food also acquires uniqueness from its essential nutrients, which, like Vitamin A, may be toxic at levels only 10-fold above those required to prevent deficiencies. The evaluation of food ingredients often must rely on reasoning unique to food science in the sense that such substances may be normal constituents of food or modified constituents of food as opposed to the types of substances ordinarily addressed in the fields of occupational, environmental, and medical toxicology. Assessing the safety of such substances, which are added to food for their technical effects, often focuses on digestion and metabolism occurring in the gastrointestinal (GI) tract. The reason for this focus is that in many cases an ingested

---

[1] *de minimis non curat praetor* or *de minimis non curat lex*, in the sense that law is not interested in trivial matters. In this sense, a risk so small it is not worthy of concern.

Table 30-1

Food as a Complex Mixture

NUTRIENTS	NON-NUTRIENTS
Carbohydrates	Naturally occurring substances
Proteins	Food additives
Lipids	Contaminants
Minerals	Products of food processing
Vitamins	

SOURCE: Smith RL: Does one man's meat become another man's poison? *Transactions of the Medical Society of London* Nov. 11, 1991, p. 6. With permission from Medical Society of London.

Table 30-2

Non-nutrient Substances in Food

FOOD	NUMBER OF IDENTIFIED NON-NUTRIENT CHEMICALS
Cheddar cheese	160
Orange juice	250
Banana	325
Tomato	350
Wine	475
Coffee	625
Beef (cooked)	625

SOURCE: Smith RL: Does one man's meat become another man's poison? *Trans Medl Soc Lond* Nov. 11:6, 1991. With permission from Medical Society of London.

substance is not absorbed through the GI tract; only products of its digestion are absorbed, and these products may be identical to those derived from natural food.

Nature and Complexity of Food

Food is an exceedingly complex mixture of nutrient and non-nutrient substances whether it is consumed in the "natural" (unprocessed) form or as a highly processed ready-to-eat meal such as a "Meal Ready to Eat" (MRE) (Table 30-1). Among the "nutrient" substances, the Western diet consists of items of caloric and noncaloric value; that is, carbohydrates supply 47% of caloric intake, fats supply 37%, and protein supplies 16% (all three of which would be considered "macronutrients"), whereas minerals and vitamins, the "micronutrients," obviously have no caloric value but are no less essential for life.

Non-nutrient substances are often characterized in the popular literature as being contributed by food processing, but nature provides the vast majority of non-nutrient constituents. For instance, in Table 30-2 one can see that even among "natural" (or minimally processed) foods, there are far more non-nutrient than nutrient constituents. Many of these non-nutrient substances are vital for the growth and survival of the plant, including hormones and naturally occurring pesticides (estimated at approximately 10,000 by Gold *et al.* (1992)). Some of these substances may be antinutrient (e.g., lectins, saponins, trypsin, and/or chymotrypsin inhibitors in soybeans, phytates that may bind minerals (present in soybeans) and anti-thiamines in fish and plants) or even toxic (e.g., tomatine, cycasin) to humans. An idea of the large number of substances present in food is given in the series *Database of Volatile Compounds in Food* (BACIS, 1999), in which approximately 5500 volatile substances are noted as occurring in one or more of the 246 different foods. However, this is only the tip of the iceberg, as the number of unidentified natural chemicals in food vastly exceeds the number that has been identified (Miller, 1991).

Non-nutrient substances are also added as a result of processing, and in fact, 21 CFR 170.3(o) lists 32 categories of direct additives, of which there are about 3000 individual substances. Approximately 2000 of these are flavor ingredients, most of which already occur naturally in food and are non-nutritive (Burdock, 2002). Of the 2000 flavoring ingredients that may be added to food, approximately one-third are used at concentrations below 10 ppm (Hall and Oser, 1968), about the same concentration as is found naturally.

Importance of the Gastrointestinal Tract

It is essential to appreciate the fact that the gut is a large, complex, and dynamic organ with several layers of organization and a vast absorptive surface that has been estimated to be from 200 to 4500 m^2 (Concon, 1988). The GI transit time provides for adequate exposure of ingesta to a variety of environmental conditions (i.e., variable pH), digestive acids and enzymes (trypsin, chymotrypsin, etc., from the pancreas and carbohydrases, lipases, and proteases from the enterocytes), saponification agents (in bile), and a luxuriant bacterial flora providing a repertoire of metabolic capability not shared by the host (e.g., fermentation of "nondigestible" sugars such as xylitol and sorbitol) (Drasar and Hill, 1974). The enterocytes (intestinal epithelium) possess an extensive capacity for the metabolism of xenobiotics that may be second only to the liver, with a full complement of phase (type) I and phase (type) II reactions present. The enteric monooxygenase system is analogous to the liver, as both systems are located in the endoplasmic reticulum of cells, require NADPH and O$_2$ for maximum activity, are inhibited by many of the same substances, and are qualitatively similar in their response to enzyme induction (Hassing *et al.*, 1989). Induction and inhibition of xenobiotic metabolism and effects on transporter *P*-glycoprotein are discussed in another section (see section Food–drug interactions).

The constituents of food and other ingesta (e.g., drugs, contaminants, inhaled pollutants dissolved in saliva and swallowed) are a physicochemically heterogeneous lot, and because the intestine has evolved into a relatively impermeable membrane, mechanisms of absorption have developed that allow substances to gain access to the body from the intestinal lumen. The four primary mechanisms for absorption are passive or simple diffusion, active transport, facilitated diffusion, and pinocytosis. Each of these mechanisms characteristically transfers a defined group of constituents from the lumen into the body (Table 30-3). As is noted in the table, xenobiotics and other substances may compete for passage into the body.

Aiding this absorption is the rich vascularization of the intestine, with a normal rate of blood flow in the portal vein of approximately 1.2 L/h/kg. However, after a meal, there is a 30% increase in blood flow through the splanchnic area (Concon, 1988). It follows then, that substances, which affect blood flow, also tend to affect the absorption of compounds; an example is alcohol, which tends to increase blood flow to the stomach and thus enhances its own absorption. Few stimuli tend to decrease flow to this area, with the possible exception of energetic muscular activity and hypovolemic shock.

Lymph circulation is important in the transfer of fats, large molecules (such as botulinum toxin), benzo[*a*]pyrene, 3-methylcholanthrene, and *cis*-dimethylaminostilbene (Chhabra and

Table 30-3
Systems Transporting Enteric Constituents

SYSTEM	ENTERIC CONSTITUENT
Passive diffusion	Sugars (e.g., fructose, mannose, and xylose, which may also be transported by facilitated diffusion), lipid-soluble compounds, water
Facilitated diffusion	D-xylose, 6-deoxy-1,5-anhydro-D-glucitol, glutamic acid, aspartic acid, short-chain fatty acids, xenobiotics with carboxy groups, sulfates, glucuronide esters, lead, cadmium, zinc
Active transport	Cations, anions, sugars, vitamins, nucleosides (pyrimidines, uracil, and thymine, which may be in competition with 5-fluorouracil and 5-bromouracil), cobalt, manganese (which competes for the iron transportation system)
Pinocytosis	Long-chain lipids, vitamin B_{12} complex, azo dyes, maternal antibodies, botulinum toxin, hemagglutinins, phalloidins, *E. coli* endotoxins, virus particles

Eastin, 1984). Lymph has a flow rate of about 1–2 mL/h/kg in humans, and few factors are known to influence its flow, with the exception of tripalmitin, which has been shown to double the flow and therefore double the absorption of *p*-aminosalicylic acid and tetracycline (Chhabra and Eastin, 1984). Another factor that lends importance to lymph is the fact that the lymph empties via the thoracic duct into the point of junction of the left internal jugular and subclavian veins, preventing "first-pass" metabolism by the liver, unlike substances transported by the blood.

Many food ingredients are modified proteins, carbohydrates, fats, or components of such substances. Thus, understanding the changes these substances undergo in the GI tract, their possible effect on the GI tract, and whether they are absorbed or affect the absorption of other substances is critical to an understanding of food toxicology and safety assessment. Some of the factors that may affect GI absorption and the rate of absorption are listed in Table 30-4.

SAFETY STANDARDS FOR FOODS, FOOD INGREDIENTS, AND CONTAMINANTS

The FD&C Act Provides for a Practicable Approach

The FD&C Act presumes that traditionally consumed foods are safe if they are free of contaminants. For the FDA to ban such foods, it must have clear evidence that death or illness can be traced to consumption of a particular food. The fact that foods contain many natural substances, some of which are toxic at a high concentration, is in itself an insufficient basis under the Act for declaring a food as being unfit for human consumption. Examples of this concept include acceptance of Generally Recognized As Safe (GRAS) status and the implementation of tolerances.

The Application of Experience: Generally Recognized as Safe (GRAS)   The FD&C Act permits the addition of substances to food to accomplish a specific technical effect if the substance is determined to be GRAS. The Act does not require the FDA to make this determination, though it does not exclude the agency from making such decisions. The Act instead requires that scientific experts base a GRAS determination on the adequacy of safety, as shown through scientific procedures or through experience based on common use in food before January 1, 1958, under the intended conditions of use of the substance [FD&C Act, section 201(s)].

In addition to allowing GRAS substances to be added to food, the Act provides for a class of substances that are regulated food additives, which are defined as "any substances the intended use of which results in its becoming a component...of any food...if such substance is not generally recognized...to be safe." Hence,

Table 30-4
Factors Affecting Intestinal Absorption and Rate of Absorption

FACTOR	EXAMPLE
Gastric emptying rate	Increased fat content
Gastric pH	Antacids, stress, H_2-receptor blockers
Intestinal motility	Diarrhea due to intercurrent disease, laxatives, dietary fiber, disaccharide intolerance, amaranth
Food content	Lectins of *Phaseolus vulgaris* (inhibition of glucose absorption and transport)
Surface area of small intestine	Short-bowel syndrome
Intestinal blood flow	Alcohol
Intestinal lymph flow	Tripalmitin
Enterohepatic circulation	Chlordecanone (prevented by cholestyramine)
Permeability of mucosa	Inflammatory bowel disease, celiac disease
Inhibition of digestive processes	Catechins of tea which inhibit sucrase and therefore glucose absorption
Concomitant drug therapy	Iron salts/tetracycline

SOURCE: Modified from Hoensch HP, Schwenk M: Intestinal absorption and metabolism of xenobiotics in humans, in Schiller CM (ed): *Intestinal Toxicology*. New York: Raven Press, 1984, pp. 169–192. With permission from Lippincott Williams & Wilkins.

a legal distinction is drawn between regulated food additives and GRAS substances. Regulated food additives must be approved and regulated for their intended conditions of use by the FDA under 21 CFR 172–179 before they can be marketed. Under section 409 of the Act, the requirements for data to support the safe use of a food additive are described in general terms. The requirements or recommended methods for establishing safe conditions of use for an additive are available in the form of guidelines issued by the FDA. These guidelines, referred to as the Redbook, provide substance and definition to the safety standard applicable to regulated food additives: "reasonable certainty of no harm under conditions of intended use" (Burdock and Carabin, 2004).

Use of Tolerances If a food contains an *unavoidable* contaminant even with the use of current good manufacturing practice (cGMP), it may be declared unfit as food if the contaminant may render the food injurious to health. Thus, for a food itself to be declared unfit, it must be ordinarily injurious, while an unavoidable contaminant in food need only pose the risk of harm for the food to be found unfit, and subject to FDA action. The reason for the dichotomy is practicality. Congress recognized that if authority were granted to ban traditional foods for reasons that go beyond clear evidence of harm to health, the agency would be subject to pressure to ban certain foods.

Foods containing unavoidable contaminants are not automatically banned because such foods are subject to the provisions of section 406 of the FD&C Act, which indicates that the quantity of unavoidable contaminants in food may be limited by regulation for the protection of public health and that any quantity of a contaminant which exceeds the fixed limit shall be deemed unsafe. This authority has been used by the FDA to set limits on the quantity of unavoidable contaminants in food by regulation (tolerances) or by informal action levels which do not have the force of law. Such action levels have been set for aflatoxins, fumonisins, and patulin (Table 30-5). Action levels have the advantage of offering greater flexibility than is provided by tolerances established by regulation. Whether tolerances or action levels are applied to unavoidable contaminants of food, the FDA attempts to balance the health risk posed by unavoidable contaminants against the loss of a portion of the food supply. In contrast, contaminants in food that are *avoidable* by cGMP are deemed to be unsafe under section 406 if they are consid-

ered poisonous or deleterious. Under such circumstances, the food is typically declared *adulterated* and unfit for human consumption. The extent to which consumers who are already in possession of such food must be alerted depends on the health risk posed by the contaminated food. If there is a reasonable probability that the use of or exposure to such a food will cause serious adverse health consequences or death, the FDA will seek a Class I recall which provides the maximum public warning, the greatest depth of recall, and the most follow-up. Classes II and III represent progressively less health risk and require less public warning, less depth of recall, and less follow-up (21 CFR 7.3).

Food and Color Additives

An intentionally added ingredient, not considered GRAS, is either a direct food additive or color additive. As with all ingredients intentionally added to food, there must be a specific and justifiable functionality. While a color additive has only one function, a food additive may have any one of 32 functionalities (Table 30-6).

The term "color additive" refers to a material which is a dye, pigment, or other substance made by a process of synthesis or extracted and isolated from a vegetable, animal, or mineral source [FD&C Act 201(t)]. Blacks, whites, and intermediate grays also are included in this definition. When such additives are added or applied to a food, drug, or cosmetic or to the human body, they are capable of imparting color. Color additives are not eligible for GRAS status.

There are two distinct types of color additives that have been approved for food use: those requiring certification by FDA chemists and those exempt from certification. Certification, which is based on chemical analysis, is required for each batch of most organic synthesized colors because they may contain impurities that may vary from batch to batch. Most certified colors approved for food use bear the prefix FD&C. Certification involves in-depth chemical analysis of major and trace components of each individual batch of color additives by FDA chemists and is required before any batch can be released for commercial use. Such color additives consist of aromatic amines or aromatic azo structures (FD&C Blue No. 1, Blue No. 2, Green No. 3, Red No. 3, Red No. 40, Yellow No. 5, and Yellow No. 6) that cannot be synthesized without a variety of impurities. Orange B and Citrus Red No. 2 are the only certified food colors that lack the FD&C designation (21 CFR 74 Subpart A).

Despite the fact that aromatic amines are generally considered relatively toxic substances, the FD&C colors are notably nontoxic. Table 30-7, which is adopted from a publication of the National Academy of Sciences (NAS) (Committee on Food Protection, 1971), shows that certified food colors have a low order of toxicity. The principal reason involves sulfonation of the aromatic amine or azo compound that constitutes a color additive. Such sulfonic acid groups are highly polar, which, combined with their high molecular weight, prevents them from being absorbed by the GI tract or entering cells. All the FD&C food colors have been extensively tested in all Concern Level (CL) III tests (Table 30-8) and have been found to be 'remarkably' nontoxic.

Food colors that are exempt from certification typically have not been subjected to such extensive testing requirements. The exempt food colors are derived primarily from natural sources. Whereas synthetic food colors have received the majority of public, scientific, and regulatory attention, natural color agents are also an important class. Currently, 26 color additives have been given exemption from certification in 21 CFR 73. These agents consist

Table 30-5

FDA Action Levels for Mycotoxins

COMMODITY	LEVEL, ng/g
Aflatoxins	
All products, except milk, designated for humans	20
Aflatoxins: Milk	0.5
Patulin: Apple juice	50
Deoxynivalenol (DON or vomitoxin): All finished wheat products that may be consumed by humans	1000
Fumonisins, Total ($FB_1 + FB_2 + FB_3$)	
Degermed dry milled corn product	2000
Cleaned corn intended for popcorn	3000
Cleaned corn for masa production	4000

SOURCE: Mycotoxins in Domestic Foods (http://www.cfsan.fda.gov/~comm/cp07001.html)

Table 30-6
Direct Food Additives by Functionality

NUMBER	DESIGNATION	DESCRIPTION	EXAMPLES
170.3(o) (1)	Anticaking agents and free-flow agents	Substances added to finely powdered or crystalline food products to prevent caking, lumping, or agglomeration	Glucitol, sodium ferrocyanide, silicon dioxide
(2)	Antimicrobial agents	Substances used to preserve food by preventing growth of microorganisms and subsequent spoilage, including fungistats, mold, and rope inhibitors and the effects listed by the NAS/NRC under "preservatives"	Nisin; methyl-, ethyl-, propyl-, or butyl-ester of p-hydroxybenozoic acid; sodium benzoate; sorbic acid and its salts
(3)	Antioxidants	Substances used to preserve food by retarding deterioration, rancidity, or discoloration due to oxidation.	Butylated hydroxyanisole (BHA), butylated hydroxytoluene (BHT), propyl gallate
(4)	Colors and coloring adjuncts	Substances used to impart, preserve, or enhance the color or shading of a food, including color stabilizers, color fixatives, color-retention agents	FD&C Yellow No. 5 (tartrazine), FD&C Red No. 4, β-carotene, annatto, turmeric
(5)	Curing and pickling agents	Substances imparting a unique flavor and/or color to a food, usually producing an increase in shelf life	Calcium chloride, glucitol
(6)	Dough strengtheners	Substances used to modify starch and gluten, producing a more stable dough, including the applicable effects listed by the NAS/NRC under "dough conditioners"	Calcium bromate, baker's yeast extract, calcium carbonate
(7)	Drying agents	Substances with moisture-absorbing ability used to maintain an environment of low moisture	Calcium stearate, cobalt caprylate, cobalt tallate
(8)	Emulsifiers and emulsifier salts	Substances that modify surface tension in the component phase of an emulsion to establish a uniform dispersion or emulsion	Phosphate esters of mono- and diglycerides, acetylated monoglycerides, calcium stearate
(9)	Enzymes	Enzymes used to improve food processing and the quality of the finished food	Papain, rennet, pepsin
(10)	Firming agents	Substances added to precipitate residual pectin, strengthening the supporting tissue and preventing its collapse during processing	Calcium acetate, calcium carbonate
(11)	Flavor enhancers	Substances added to supplement, enhance, or modify the original taste and/or aroma of a food without imparting a characteristic taste or aroma of their own	Monosodium glutamate, inositol
(12)	Flavor agents and adjuvants	Substances added to impart or help impart a taste or aroma in food	Cinnamon, citral, p-cresol, thymol, zingerone

(Continued)

Table 30-6
(Continued)

NUMBER	DESIGNATION	DESCRIPTION	EXAMPLES
(13)	Flour-treating agents	Substances added to milled flour at the mill to improve its color an/or baking qualities, including bleaching and maturing agents	Calcium bromate
(14)	Formulation aids	Substances used to promote or produce a desired physical state or texture in food, including carriers, binders, fillers, plasticizers, film formers, and tableting aids	Palm kernel oil, tallow
(15)	Fumigants	Volatile substances used for controlling insects or pests	Aluminum phosphide, potassium bromide
(16)	Humectants	Hygroscopic substances incorporated in food to promote retention of moisture, including moisture-retention agents and antidusting agents	Arabic gum, calcium chloride
(17)	Leavening agents	Substances used to produce or stimulate production of carbon dioxide in baked goods to impart a light texture, including yeast, yeast foods, and calcium salts listed by the NAS/NRC under "dough conditioners"	Carbon dioxide, adipic acid
(18)	Lubricants and release agents	Substances added to food contact surfaces to prevent ingredients and finished products from sticking to them	Mineral oil, acetylated monoglycerides
(19)	Nonnutritive sweeteners	Substances having less than 2% of the caloric value of sucrose per equivalent unit of sweetening capacity	Acesulfame, aspartame, saccharin
(20)	Nutrient supplements	Substances that are necessary for the body's nutritional and metabolic processes	Calcium carbonate
(21)	Nutritive sweeteners	Substances that have greater than 2% of the caloric value of sucrose per equivalent unit of sweetening capacity	Lactitol, hydrogenated starch hydrolysate
(22)	Oxidizing and reducing agents	Substances that chemically oxidize or reduce another food ingredient, producing a more stable product, including the applicable effects listed by the NAS/NRC under "dough conditioners"	Calcium peroxide, chloride, hydrogen peroxide
(23)	pH control agents	Substances added to change or maintain active acidity or basicity, including buffers, acids, alkalis, and neutralizing agents	Acetic acid, propionic acid, calcium acetate, calcium carbonate, carbon dioxide
(24)	Processing aids	Substances used as manufacturing aids to enhance the appeal or utility of a food or food component, including clarifying agents, clouding agents, catalysts, flocculents, filler aids, and crystallization inhibitors	Carbon dioxide, ammonium carbonate, ammonium sulfate, potassium bromide

(Continued)

Table 30-6
(Continued)

NUMBER	DESIGNATION	DESCRIPTION	EXAMPLES
(25)	Propellants, aerating agents, and gases	Gases used to supply force to expel a product or reduce the amount of oxygen in contact with the food in packaging	Carbon dioxide, nitrous oxide
(26)	Sequestrants	Substances that combine with polyvalent metal ions to form a soluble metal complex to improve the quality and stability of products	Acetate salts, citrate salts, gluconate salt, metaphosphate, edetic acid, calcium acetate
(27)	Solvents and vehicles	Substances used to extract or dissolve another substance	Acetic acid, acetylated monoglycerides
(28)	Stabilizers and thickeners	Substances used to produce viscous solutions or dispersions, to impart body, improve consistency, or stabilize emulsions, including suspending and bodying agents, setting agents, jellying agents, and bulking agents	Calcium acetate, calcium carbonate
(29)	Surface-active agents	Substances used to modify surface properties of liquid food components for a variety of effects other than emulsifiers but including solubilizing agents, dispersants, detergents, wetting agents, rehydration enhancers, whipping agents, foaming agents, and defoaming agents	Sorbitan monostearate, mono- and diglycerides, polysorbate 60, acetostearin
(30)	Surface-finishing agents	Substances used to increase palatability, preserve gloss, and inhibit discoloration of foods, including glazes, polishes, waxes, and protective coatings	Ammonium hydroxide, arabic gum
(31)	Synergists	Substances used to act or react with another food ingredient to produce a total effect different from or greater than the sum of the effects produced by the individual ingredients	Acetic acid, propionic acid
(32)	Texturizers	Substances that affect the appearance or feel of food	Calcium acetate

of a variety of natural compounds generally obtained by various extraction and treatment technologies. Included in this group of colors are preparations such as dried algae meal, beet powder, grape skin extract, fruit juice, paprika, caramel, carrot oil, cochineal extract, ferrous gluconate, and iron oxide. A problem encountered in attempts to regulate these additives is the lack of a precise chemical definition of many of these preparations. With a few exceptions such as caramel, which is the most widely used color, the natural colors have not been heavily used. In part, this may be due to economic reasons, but these colors generally do not have the uniformity and

intensity characteristic of the synthetic colors, therefore necessitating higher concentrations to obtain a specific color intensity. They also lack the chemical and color stability of the synthetic colors and have a tendency to fade with time.

Intake of color additives varies among individuals. The maximal intake of food colors is estimated to be ~53.5 mg/d, whereas the average intake per day is ~15 mg (Committee on Food Protection, 1971). Only about 10% of the food consumed in the United States contains food colors. The foods that utilize food colors in order of the quantity of color utilized are (1) beverages, (2) candy and

Table 30-7

Data on Certified Food Colors Permanently Listed in the United States

COLOR	NO ADVERSE EFFECT DIETARY LEVELS AND ANIMALSTUDIES	SAFE LEVEL FOR HUMANS (mg/day)	ESTIMATED MAXIMUM INGESTION (mg/day/person)
FD&C Blue No.1	5.0% rats 2.0% dogs	363	1.23
FD&C Blue No. 2	1.0% rats, dogs	181	0.29
FD&C Green No. 3	5.0% rats 1.0% dogs 2.0% mice	181	0.07
Orange B	5.0% rats 1.0% dogs 5.0% mice	181	0.31
Citrus Red No. 2	0.1% rats	18	Not applicable
FD&C Red No. 3	0.5% rats 2.0% dogs 2.0% mice	91	1.88
FD&C Yellow No. 5	2.0% rats 2.0% dogs	363	16.3
FD&C Yellow No. 6	2.0% rats 2.0% dogs 2.0% mice	363	15.5

SOURCE: Committee on Food Protection (1971). Reprinted with permission from (**Food Colors**) © (**1971**) by the National Academy of Sciences, Courtesy of the National Academies Press, Washington, D.C.

Table 30-8

Summary of the Toxicity Tests Recommended for Different Levels of Concern[1]

TOXICITY STUDIES [2]	CONCERN LEVELS		
	I	II	III
Short-term tests for genetic toxicity	X	X	X
Metabolism and pharmacokinetic studies		X	X
Short-term (28-day) toxicity studies with rodents	X[3]		
Subchronic (90-day) toxicity studies with rodents		X[3]	X[3]
Subchronic (90-day) toxicity studies with nonrodents		X[3]	
Reproduction studies with teratology phase		X[3]	X[3]
One-year toxicity studies with nonrodents			X
Carcinogenicity studies with rodents			X[4]
Chronic toxicity/carcinogenicity studies with rodents			X[4,5]

[1]http://www.cfsan.fda.gov/~redbook/redtoc93.html.

[2] Not including dose range-finding studies, if appropriate.

[3]Including neurotoxicity and immunotoxicity screens.

[4]An in utero phase is recommended for one of the two recommended carcinogenicity studies with rodents, preferably the study with rats.

[5]Combined study may be performed as separate studies.

confections, (3) dessert powders, (4) bakery goods, (5) sausages (casing only), (6) cereals, (7) ice cream, (8) snack foods, and (9) gravies, jams, jellies, and so forth (Committee on Food Protection, 1971).

Methods Used to Evaluate the Safety of Foods, Ingredients, and Contaminants

Safety Evaluation of Direct Food and Color Additives The basic concept that forms the foundation for the safety evaluation of direct food and color additives is the recognition that the safety of any added substance to food must be established on the basis of the intended conditions of use in food. Factors that need to be taken into account include (1) the purpose for use of the substance, (2) the food to which the substance is added, (3) the concentration level used in the proposed foods, and (4) the population expected to consume the substance.

The evaluation of a new food additive is a complicated and expensive undertaking, especially when the additive will be widely used in many foods. Each additive can pose unique safety questions depending on its chemistry, stability in use, metabolism, toxicity study results, and estimated human exposure. Integral to a discussion of exposure is the concept of the "whole food additive." This refers to the additive, the degradation or conversion products arising from the use of the additive in foods, and the impurities found in the manufactured additive itself (Kotsonis and Hjelle, 1991, 1996).

Exposure: The Estimated Daily Intake Prior to 1958, the FDA held to the philosophy that food additives (and potential contaminants) should not be harmful at any level. This is impractical, as many substances critical to life are toxic at high doses. For example, distilled water is harmless if consumed at low amounts, but if enough is ingested to cause electrolyte imbalance, fatalities may occur. Other substances that may be toxic at high concentrations, such as acids or bases, are used at low concentrations to control pH or inhibit bacterial growth during the processing of meats and cheeses,

Table 30-9
Food Categories

NUMBER	DESIGNATION	DESCRIPTION	EXAMPLES
170.3(n)			
(1)	Baked goods and baking mixes	Includes all ready-to-eat and ready-to bake products, flours, and mixes requiring preparation before serving	Doughnuts, bread, croissants, cake mix, cookie dough
(2)	Beverages, alcoholic	Includes malt beverages, wines, distilled liquors, and cocktail mix	Beer, malt liquor, whiskey, liqueurs, wine coolers
(3)	Beverages and beverage bases, nonalcoholic	Includes only special or spiced teas, soft drinks, coffee substitutes, and fruit- and vegetable-flavored gelatin drinks	Herbal tea (non-tea-containing "teas"), soda pop, chicory
(4)	Breakfast cereals	Includes ready-to-eat and instant and regular hot cereals	Oatmeal (both regular and instant), farina, corn flakes, wheat flakes

are considered GRAS by the FDA. These examples underscore the fact that exposure level is a major factor in a safety evaluation, and is reflected in the FDA's *Toxicological Principles for the Safety Assessment of Direct Food Additives and Color Additives Used in Food* (FDA, 1982a),[2] a source used to determine which testing methods should be conducted to determine safety levels of a substance.

In food additive safety determinations, exposure is usually referred to an estimated daily intake (EDI) and is based on the daily intake (I) of the food in which the substance will be used, and the concentration (C) of the substance when it is in the food. Many food ingredients are used in several different food categories, but as an example, we will assume that an additive is used only in breakfast cereals. If the substance is added at a concentration that does not exceed 20 μg/g (ppm), and the mean daily intake of breakfast cereals is 175 g/person/day, the EDI is calculated at 3500 μg/person/day. As most food additives are used in many foods, the total exposure is the sum of the exposures from each of the food categories. The formula for exposure to food additive B is

$$\text{EDI}_B = (C_B f \times I_f) + (C_B g \times I_g) + (C \ldots)$$

where $C_B f$ and $C_B g$ are the concentration of B in food category f and g, respectively. I_f and I_g are the daily intake of food category f and g, respectively. Therefore, the EDI is the sum of the individual contributions of B in each of the food categories.

The same principles may be applied to the estimation of the consumption of residue from secondary direct additives (substances not intended to remain in a food after the technical effect has been accomplished; examples include solvents, sanitizers, and defoaming agents), and contaminants. Additional information on the estimation of exposure to direct food additives and contaminants has been made available by the agency's Center for Food Safety and Applied Nutrition.[3]

Calculating the EDI raises several basic questions: (1) How does one determine the amount of a food additive that is added to

each food category? and (2) How are food categories determined? To determine the amount of food additive added to each food category, the highest end of the range of use levels for the new substance is used. These food group maximums are not to be exceeded by a food manufacturer, based on the current Good Manufacturing Practice regulation (cGMPs; 21 CFR 110), which binds a manufacturer not to add more of an additive than is reasonably required to achieve the specific technical effect of the food additive (additional information on cGMPs may be found in the Food Chemicals Codex (FCC, 2003).

General food categories have been specified by the FDA. A sample of the categories is presented in Table 30-9. These categories were derived from a survey of food additives conducted by the National Academy of Sciences/National Research Council and published in 1972 (NRC/NAS, 1979). This survey pioneered the use of categorizing foods, but changes in the consumption patterns of the U.S. population, in addition to changes in the types of foods available, have necessitated the generation of additional, more current data.

More contemporary data on food intake has been calculated through the use of food consumption surveys (Table 30-10). Food consumption databases have specific characteristics and are based on particular assumptions. Methods commonly used by regulatory agencies, manufacturers, nutritionists, and general researchers for assessing food consumption by individuals include 24-hour dietary recalls, dietary records, food frequency records, and dietary history accounts (Matulka, 2005). For example, one database may be based on an individual's food intake from the past 24 hours, while another may utilize dietary records taken over a three-day period of time, and yet another may cover average consumption over 14 days. Some databases may provide only general population consumption values, while others may provide a detailed breakout of particular subpopulations (e.g., the elderly, women, teenagers).

In safety assessments, one must consider other sources of consumption for the proposed intended use of the food additive, such as whether it is already used in food for another purpose, is used in nonfood products (e.g., toothpaste, lipstick, drugs), or the additive occurs naturally in foods. In summary, to estimate human consumption of a particular food substance, it is necessary to know (1) the levels of the substance in food, (2) the daily intake of each food containing the substance, (3) the distribution of food intake within the population, and (4) the potential exposure to the substance from nonfood sources (Tennant, 2002).

---

[2] The Agency is in the process of updating the Redbook and is now making Redbook 2000 chapters available electronically (http://www.cfsan.fda.gov/~redbook/red-toca.html). The Redbook 2000 chapters now substitute for, or supplement, guidance available in the 1982 Redbook I and in the 1993 Draft Redbook II, which can be obtained from the Office of Food Additive Safety. As additional chapters of Redbook 2000 are completed they will become available electronically.

[3] U.S. FDA, Center for Food Safety and Applied Nutrition, Office of Premarket Approval, September, 1995, available online at http://www.cfsan.fda.gov/~dms/opa-cg8.html.

Table 30-10

Databases for Estimating Food Intake

Continuing Survey of Food Intakes by Individuals, USDA, 1985, 1986, 1989, 1990, 1991

The Nationwide Food Consumption Survey, USDA, 1987–1988*

Estimates of Daily Intake (NRC/NAS), 1979 (Abrams, 1992)

The FDA Total Diet Study (Pennington and Gunderson, 1987)

Foods Commonly Consumed by Individuals, USDA (Pay *et al.*, 1984)

USDA Economic Research Service Reports Continuing Survey of Food Intakes by Individuals, USDA, 1985, 1986, 1989*, 1990, 1991

National Health and Nutrition Examination Survey I, II, III, 2001–2002, 2003–2004

What We Eat In America, USDA 2001–2002

*Indicates current use by FDA.

SOURCE: (R. Matulka, personal communication). Reprinted with permission from (**The 1977 Survey of the Industry on the Use of Food Additives**) © (**1979**) by the National Academy of Sciences, Courtesy of the National Academies Press, Washington, D.C.

Before a food additive is approved, evidence is required by regulatory agencies that indicate the additive is safe for its intended use(s) and that the EDI for the additive is less than its acceptable daily intake (ADI) (Butchko and Kotsonis, 1996). Regulatory agencies may impose restrictions on certain uses of food additives if the EDI exceeds the ADI, or restrict future approvals for new categories of use. Chronic, long-term rodent toxicity studies are usually used in determining the ADI. These studies are used to determine the no-observed-adverse-effect level (NOAEL) for the additive. To provide an adequate level of safety from animal to human extrapolation, a 100-fold safety factor is usually employed to account for species differences and the inter-individual variation among humans, to determine the ADI for a food additive. This factor provides a reasonable certainty in estimating safe doses in humans from animal studies (Lehman and Fitzhugh, 1954).[4]

Assignment of Concern Level (CL) and Required Testing

Structure–activity (SA) relationships are now the basis for developing many therapeutic drugs, pesticides, and food additives. These relationships are put to good use in the Toxicological Principles for the Safety Assessment of Direct Food Additives and Color Additives Used in Foods (FDA, 1982a), which describes a qualitative "decision tree" that assigns categories to substances on the basis of the structural and functional groups in the molecule. Additives with functional groups with a high order of toxicity are assigned to category C, those of unknown or intermediate toxicity are assigned to category B, and those with a low potential for toxicity are assigned to category A. For example, a simple saturated hydrocarbon alcohol such as pentanol would be assigned to category A. Similarly, a substance containing an α,β-unsaturated carbonyl function, epoxide, thiazole, or imidazole group would be assigned to category C. Thus, based on structure assignment and calculated exposure, the Concern Levels (CLs) are assigned (Table 30–11). For example, 0.03 ppm of a substance in Structure Category B would be assigned

to CL II. In contrast, the same dose (i.e., 0.03 ppm) of a substance in Structure Category A would be assigned to the lesser CL I.

Once the CL is established, a specific test battery is prescribed, as shown in Table 30-8. The tests for CL III are the most demanding and provide the greatest breadth for the determination of adverse biological effects, including effects on reproduction. The tests are comprehensive enough to detect nearly all types of observable toxicity, including malignant and benign tumors, preneoplastic lesions, and other forms of chronic toxicity. The tests for CL II are of intermediate breadth. These tests are designed to detect the most toxic phenomena other than late-developing histopathological changes. The short-term (genotoxicity) tests are intended to identify substances for which chronic testing becomes critical. The CL I test battery is the least broad, as is appropriate for the level of hazard which substances in this category may pose. However, if untoward effects are noted, additional assessment becomes necessary. Studies of the absorption, distribution, metabolism, and elimination characteristics of a test substance are recommended before the initiation of toxicity studies longer than 90 days' duration. Of particular importance for many proposed food ingredients is data on their processing and metabolism in the GI tract.

Unique to food additive carcinogenicity testing is the controversial use of protocols that include an in utero phase. Under such protocols, parents of test animals are exposed to the test substance for 4 weeks before mating and throughout mating, gestation, and lactation. Most countries and international bodies do not subscribe to the combining of an in utero phase with a rat carcinogenicity study, as this presents a series of logistical and operational problems and substantially increases the cost of conducting a rat carcinogenicity study. The FDA began requesting in utero studies of the food industry in the early 1970s, when it was discovered from lifetime feeding studies that the artificial sweetener saccharin produced bladder tumors in male rats when in utero exposure was introduced. Subsequently, the FDA required the food, drug, and cosmetic color industries to conduct lifetime carcinogenicity feeding studies of 18 color additives in rats using an in utero exposure phase.

Special note should also be made of genetic toxicity testing. Genetic toxicity tests are performed for two reasons: (1) to test chemicals for potential carcinogenicity and (2) to assess whether a chemical may induce heritable genetic damage. Currently, genetic toxicity assays can be divided into three major groups: (1) forward and reverse mutation assays (e.g., point mutations, deletions), (2) clastogenicity assays detecting structural and numerical changes in chromosomes (e.g., chromosome aberrations, micronuclei), and (3) assays that identify DNA damage (e.g., DNA strand breaks, unscheduled DNA synthesis).

Because the correlation between carcinogens and mutagens has proved to be less than desirable, as has been demonstrated by false–positive and false–negative findings when carcinogens and noncarcinogens have been examined in genetic toxicity tests, it is recommended that several tests be selected from a battery of tests. It should be kept in mind that as the number of tests employed increases, the possibility of false-negative results increases as well. Consequently, the National Toxicology Program (NTP) has advised that only a single gene mutational assay be used (*Salmonella typhimurium*) to optimize the prediction of carcinogenicity (Tennant and Zeiger, 1993).

Safety Determination of Indirect Food Additives   Indirect food additives are food additives that are not added directly to food but

---

[4] This is the source of the 100 safety factor.

Table 30-11
Assignment of Concern Level

STRUCTURE CATEGORY A	STRUCTURE CATEGORY B	STRUCTURE CATEGORY C	CONCERN LEVEL
<0.05 ppm in the total diet (<0.0012 mg/kg/day) or	<0.025 ppm in the total diet (<0.00063 mg/kg/day) or	<0.0125 ppm in the total diet (<0.00031 mg/kg/day) or	I
≥0.05 ppm in the total diet (≥0.0012 mg/kg/day) or	≥0.025 ppm in the total diet (≥0.00063 mg/kg/day) or	≥0.0125 ppm in the total diet (≥0.00031 mg/kg/day) or	II
≥1 ppm in the total diet (≥0.025 mg/kg/day)	≥0.5 ppm in the total diet (≥0.0125 mg/kg/day)	≥0.25 ppm in the total diet (≥0.0063 mg/kg/day)	III

enter food by migrating from surfaces that contact food. These surfaces may be from packaging material (e.g., cans, paper, plastic) or the coating of packaging materials or surfaces used in processing, holding, or transporting food.

Essential to demonstrating the safety of an indirect additive are extraction studies with food-simulating solvents. The FDA recommends the use of three food-simulating solvents—10% ethanol, 50% ethanol, and corn oil or a synthetic triglyceride—for aqueous and acidic, alcoholic, and fatty foods, respectively (FDA, 2002a). The conditions of extraction depend in part on the intended conditions of use. Extraction studies are used to assess the level or quantity of a substance that might migrate and become a component of food, leading to consumer exposure.

To convert extraction data from packaging material into anticipated consumer exposure, the FDA has determined the fraction of the U.S. diet which comes into contact with different classes of material: glass, metal (coated and uncoated), paper (coated and uncoated), and polymers. For each class, the FDA has assigned a "consumption factor" (CF), which is the fraction of the total diet that comes into contact with an individual class of material.

The fraction of individual food types (aqueous, acidic, alcoholic, fatty) for which such packaging material is used is referred to as the food-type-distribution factor (f_T). To calculate cumulative estimated daily intake (CEDI), the following equation is used:

$$CEDI = CF \times [(f_{T\,aqueous} + f_{T\,acidic}) \times (\text{ppm of migrating substance}$$
$$\text{in 10\% ethanol}) + (f_{T\,alcoholic} \times \text{ppm of migrating}$$
$$\text{substance in 50\% ethanol}) + (f_{T\,fatty} \times \text{ppm of}$$
$$\text{migrating substance in corn oil})] \times 3\,kg/person/day$$
$$= mg/person/day[5].$$

For additives with virtually no migration (<0.5 ppb), in which the CEDIs correspond to 1.5 μg/person/day, no safety studies are recommended. Migration levels, as determined by extraction studies, that are greater than 0.5 ppb to 50 ppb (150 μg/person/day), in vitro genotoxicity tests should include bacterial mutagenicity and cytogenetic evaluation of chromosomal damage using mammalian cells or an in vitro mouse lymphoma assay. Where there is significant migration, i.e., 50 ppb to 1 ppm (3 mg/person/day), genetic toxicity tests should be conducted and the substance should be further evaluated by two subchronic oral toxicity studies (one in a rodent species

and one in a nonrodent species). The studies should provide an adequate basis for determining an acceptable daily intake (ADI) for the indirect additive or a constituent in the indicated range of CEDIs. In addition, the results of these studies will help determine whether longer-term or specialized safety tests (e.g., metabolism studies, teratogenicity studies, reproductive toxicity studies, neurotoxicity studies, and immunotoxicity studies) should be conducted to assess the safety of these substances. For cumulative exposure greater than 1 ppm, FDA recommends submission of a food additive petition (FDA, 2002a).

Safety Requirements for GRAS Substances   In spite of the fact that the FD&C Act and the relevant regulations scrupulously avoid defining food except in a functional sense—"food means articles used for food or drink for man or other animals... [and includes] chewing gum, and... articles used for components of any such article"—it regards foods as GRAS when they are added to other food, for example, green beans in vegetable soup (Kokoski *et al.*, 1990; Burdock and Carabin, 2004). It also regards a number of food ingredients as GRAS, and these ingredients are listed under 21 CFR 182, 184, and 186. However, the language used acknowledges that there are substances the FDA considers to be GRAS which are not listed. This accomplishes two things: (1) It leaves the door open for additional nonlisted substances to be affirmed as GRAS by the agency and (2) reinforces the concept that substances can be deemed GRAS whether or not they are listed by the FDA or on a publicly available list. A list of examples of substances regarded as GRAS is given in Table 30-12. It is important to re-emphasize that GRAS substances, though used like food additives, are not food additives. Although the distinction may seem to be one of semantics, it allows GRAS substances to be exempt from the premarket clearance restrictions enforced by the FDA and exempt from the Delaney carcinogens clause, because that clause of the Act pertains only to food additives.[6]

While the courts have ruled that GRAS substances must be supported by the same quantity and quality of safety data that support food additives, this does not mean that the data must be identical in nature and character to those for a food additive. For uses of substances to be eligible for classification as GRAS, there must be common knowledge throughout the scientific community about the safety of substances directly or indirectly added to food (21 CFR

---

[5] The 3 kg is FDA's value for daily food consumption which, when multiplied by mg/kg (ppm) and the weighting factors, reduces to milligrams of the additive *per* day.

[6] See Assessment of Carcinogens.

Table 30-12
Examples of GRAS Substances and Their Functionality

CFR NUMBER	SUBSTANCE	FUNCTIONALITY
Substances Generally Recognized as Safe 21 CFR 182		
182.2122	Aluminum calcium silicate	Anticaking agent
182.8985	Zinc chloride	Nutrient supplement
Direct Food Substances Affirmed as Generally Recognized as Safe 21 CFR 184		
184.1005	Acetic acid	Several
184.1355	Helium	Processing aid
Indirect Food Substances Affirmed as Generally Recognized as Safe 21 CFR 186		
186.1025	Caprylic acid	Antimicrobial
186.1374	Iron oxides	Ingredient of paper and paperboard

170.30); this is termed the "common knowledge standard" by FDA.[7] The studies relied on for concluding that a given use of a substance is GRAS ordinarily are based on generally available data and information published in the scientific literature. Such data are unlikely to be conducted in accordance with FDA-recommended protocols, as these studies often are conducted for reasons unrelated to FDA approval. Thus, the first basis for a GRAS determination is by "scientific procedures" (i.e., test data). GRAS status also can be based on experience with common use in food before January 1, 1958,[8] which further distinguishes GRAS data requirements from those demanded of food additives. Such experience need not be limited to the United States, but if it comes from outside the United States, it must be published or corroborated by an independent source. The FDA has made it clear, that while an ingredient may have an extensive history of use prior to 1958, this does not place it beyond regulatory reach, as new data generated must be taken into account—new data trumps history of use.[9]

Importance of the GRAS Concept

The importance of the GRAS provision is obvious from its many applications. Many substances, for example, that are used in food processing have never received formal FDA approval. The use of these substances in the manufacture of food products is considered appropriate under cGMPs, while the substance itself is considered GRAS for such purposes. Similarly, certain substances are permitted as optional ingredients in standardized foods [foods with standards of identity specified by regulation (21 CFR 130-169)] even though they are not approved food additives and are not on any of the GRAS lists.

The GRAS concept as traditionally applied in the United States also has applicability to certain novel foods which may differ only slightly from traditional foods or which, after careful consideration, can be regarded as raising no issues or questions of safety beyond that raised by the traditional foods they are intended to replace. The GRAS approach may therefore permit the introduction of novel foods that contain less saturated fat and/or cholesterol or more fiber or are in other ways modified.

Transgenic Plant (and New Plant Varieties) Policy Crops have been genetically modified using conventional breeding methods for more than a hundred years to produce new plant varieties with improved characteristics. Methods such as wide crosses of distantly related species that normally would not interbreed and mutagenesis of developing seeds using radiation or chemical mutagens have been successfully employed to produce genetic variation for selection of improved plant varieties. Over the past decade, scientists have employed biotechnology to add one or more specific genes into crops like soybean, corn, cotton, and canola, to improve pest and disease management, resulting in agronomic, economic, environmental, health, and social benefits for farmers (Brooker and Barfoot, 2005; James, 2006). For example, much of the corn crop planted in the United States contains a gene from the bacterium Bacillus thuringiensis that produces a Bt insecticidal protein (James, 1999). Bt is a protein toxic to certain caterpillar insect pests that destroy corn plants (EPA, 1988; McClintock et al., 1995). By enabling the corn plant to protect itself from this insect pest, the use of this product can reduce the need for and use of conventional insecticides (Gianessi and Carpenter, 1999).

Irrespective of the breeding method used to produce a new plant variety, tests must be done to ensure that the levels of nutrients or toxins in the plants have not changed and that the food is still safe to consume. For food/feed from biotechnology-derived crops, compositional analyses are done to ensure that the levels of key nutrients or toxins are comparable to food from conventional varieties. This is also done for a few conventionally bred crops where levels of important toxins such as glyoalkaloids in potatoes and erucic acid in rapeseed oil have been monitored. The International Life Sciences Institutes (ILSI, 2006) supports a large crop composition database that provides information on the natural variability in composition for conventional corn, soybean, and cotton crops. This database provides a reference for comparing the nutrient composition of new crop varieties (Taylor et al., 1999; George et al., 2004; Herman et al., 2004; Oberdoerfer et al., 2005). Animal feeding studies are also done with biotechnology-derived crops fed over several weeks to months to a variety of farm animal species

---

[7] http://www.cfsan.fda.gov/~rdb/opa-g092.html (site visited 10 April 2006).

[8] There are some exceptions to this rule. In at least one case, FDA has indicated that use before 1958 was not sufficient to demonstrate safety. (See GRAS Notice No. GRN 00040 on mineral oil). http://www.cfsan.fda.gov/~rdb/opa-g040.html, site visited 9 April 2006).

[9] http://www.cfsan.fda.gov/~rdb/opa-g071.html (site visited 10 April 2006).

to ensure that the performance (feed efficiency, milk production, etc.) is comparable to that of conventional controls (Flachowsky *et al.*, 2005). Food safety studies have also been done with various biotechnology-derived crops to ensure that there are no treatment-related adverse findings (Brake and Evenson, 2004; Hammond *et al.*, 2005; MacKenzie *et al.*, 2005). Clearly, new proteins produced in plant varieties must be nontoxic and not have the characteristics of proteins known to cause allergies. Thus, the proteins produced in genetically modified crops are evaluated for toxicity (Sjoblad *et al.*, 1992; Harrison *et al.*, 1996; Betz *et al.*, 2000; Pariza and Johnson, 2001) and allergenicity (Metcalf *et al.*, 1996; Astwood *et al.*, 2003). The DNA that is introduced into genetically modified plants to direct the production of such new proteins has been determined to be Generally Recognized As Safe (FDA, 1992).

The safety of new plant varieties (transgenic plants, genetically modified plants) is regulated primarily under the FDA's postmarket authority [section 402(a)(1) of the FD&C Act]. This section, previously applied to occurrences of unsafe levels of toxicants in food, is now applied to new plant varieties whose composition has been altered by an added substance. The new policy has been applied to plants containing substances that are GRAS [Federal Register 57(104): 22984–23005]. The *Federal Register* notice (May 29, 1992) indicates that "[i]n most cases, the substances expected to become components of food as a result of genetic modification of a plant will be the same as or substantially similar to substances commonly found in food, such as proteins, fats and oils, and carbohydrates." The notice also indicates the responsibility of the FDA to exercise the premarket review process when the "objective characteristics of the substance raise questions of safety." In regard to substances within the new variety that are not similar to substances commonly found in food, a food additive petition may have to be filed.

The *Federal Register* notice offers points of consideration for the safety assessment of new plant varieties (Table 30-13). Accompanying these points of consideration are a decision flowchart and advice that the FDA be consulted on certain findings, for example, transference of allergens from one plant to another, a change in the concentration or bioavailability of nutrients, and the introduction of a new macroingredient.

In the United States new plant varieties are regulated not only by the FDA, but also by the Environmental Protection Agency (EPA) and U.S. Department of Agriculture (USDA). The FDA is responsible for the safety and labeling of foods and feeds derived from crops, irrespective of the method used to produce the new plant variety. The EPA is responsible for assuring the safety of pesticides, thus in the example cited above whereby a pesticide is produced in a new plant variety, this product would also fall under EPA's jurisdiction. The USDA's Animal and Plant Health Inspection Service has responsibility for the environmental safety of field-testing and commercial planting of new plant varieties.

The developer of a biotechnology-derived crop variety must obtain registration from not only the country of origin but from importing countries as well (OECD, 1993). A variety of European/Global Scientific authorities (WHO, 1995; FAO, 1996; OECD, 1997; Codex, 2003; EFSA, 2004) have provided guidance on the safety assessment process for food and feed derived from biotechnology-derived crops. The process considers two main categories of potential risks: those related to the properties and function of the introduced protein(s), and those related to the whole food crop since insertion of the introduced gene(s) into the plant genome theoretically could cause unintended environmental effects. As in conventional crop breeding, agronomic studies carried out under diverse environmental conditions are used to screen for varieties that exhibit unintended changes so they can be eliminated from development.

Methods for Establishing Safe Conditions of Use for Novel Foods

Novel foods, including those derived from new plant varieties and macroingredient substitutes, present new challenges and may require new methods of determining safety. For example, with each new additive, it has been traditional (and rooted in a regulation such as 21 CFR 170.22) to establish an ADI, which is usually based on 1/100 of the NOEL established in animal testing. This works well for additives projected to be consumed at a level of 1.5 g/d or less (which is equal to or less than 25 mg/kg), for this extrapolates at a 100-fold safety factor to consumption by a rat at a level of 2500 mg/kg/d (about 5% of the rat's diet). The problem arises when a new food or macroingredient substitute becomes a substantive part of the diet (estimated to constitute as much as 15–20%). For example, a macroingredient substitute or food projected to be consumed at a level of just 5% of the diet (150 g/d) would require the test animal (rat) to consume 250 g/kg/d, or slightly more than the rat's body weight. This is an untenable test requirement, for at those levels, the investigator would establish an effect level only for malnutrition, not for the toxicity of the macroingredient. The converse is true for some essential nutrients, such as vitamins A and D and iron, which at doses 100 times the nutritional use level would be toxic (Kokoski *et al.*, 1990). The answer therefore lies in careful interpretation of toxicological data and the conduct, where appropriate, of special studies to assess drug interactions, nutrient interactions changes in gut flora, changes in gut activity, and the like (Munro, 1990; Borzelleca, 1992a,b). Also, it may be appropriate to consider what effect, if any, macroingredients may have on individuals with compromised digestive tracts, those dependent on laxatives, and those on high-fiber diets.

The regulatory approval of a new food additive is generally based on traditional toxicology studies. The rationale is that data from such studies will adequately predict adverse effects that could occur in humans. However, such studies, especially for novel foods, may not be adequate. Therefore, although human studies are not generally required for food additives, in the case of novel foods, human studies are likely essential in evaluating their safety (Stargel *et al.*, 1996).

Another useful tool in ensuring the safety of a food additive is monitoring it after its approval, or postmarketing surveillance. With widespread use of a food additive, *monitoring for consumption* can determine whether actual consumption exceeds the EDI and

Table 30-13

Points of Consideration in the Safety Assessment of New Plant Varieties

Toxicants known to be characteristic of the host and donor species

The potential that food allergens will be transferred from one food source to another

The concentration and bioavailability of important nutrients for which a food crop is ordinarily consumed

The safety and nutritional value of newly introduced proteins

The identity, composition, and nutritional value of modified carbohydrates or fats and oils *monitoring for anecdotal complaints* may identify adverse health effects that escaped detection in earlier studies. This could be especially important for novel foods when traditional toxicology studies are not done at large multiples of the EDI (Butchko *et al.*, 1994, 1996a). Thus, the combination of traditional toxicity studies, special animal and human studies, and possibly postmarketing surveillance will ensure the safety of consumers and provide evidence to justify a safety factor different from 100.

Nanotechnology Nanotechnology offers some distinct advantages in delivery systems using micelles and liposomes and other technological advantages as nanoemulsions (emulsion stability), biopolymeric nanoparticles (encapsulation technology), and cubosomes (solubilize hydrophobic, hydrophilic, and amphiphilic molecules, among other uses), thus allowing new and more efficient uses of old products. Nanotechnology can enhance solubility, facilitate controlled release, improve bioavailability, and protect labile substances (including micronutrients and bioactive substances) during processing, storage, and distribution (Chen *et al.*, 2006).

Although the GI tract is an organ for absorption, it is also the first barrier to substances that we do not wish to absorb (e.g., large molecules such as colors) or serve their function best by not being absorbed (e.g., fiber). The question then arises as to what impact nanotechnology might have on this balance. Size has always mattered and in the range of what has been accepted as "nano",[10] many of the principles of absorption (as well as distribution, metabolism, and excretion) may be affected (EPA, 2005). Further, a striking observation regarding particle health effects is the ability of particles to generate toxic effects at the site of initial deposition as well as significant systemic toxic responses (EPA, 2004). Another observation that "size does matter" is that degraded carrageenan (MW 30,000) may have carcinogenic properties,[11] while undergraded carrageenan (MW 100,000) apparently does not. Also, food packaging can incorporate the ultraviolet-blocking material, TiO_2, but because titanium dioxide's safety is predicated upon its lack of absorption (IFST, 2006b), the use of nanotechnology may ultimately mandate a new safety review. Presently, the FDA has taken no action on nanotechnology, as it prefers to regulate on a product-by-product basis and does not regulate a technology.[12]

Safety Requirements for Dietary Supplements

Dietary supplements have a special status within the law and the regulations—supplements are regarded as foods or food constituents and not food additives, nor drugs. There is also a different standard of safety, the concept of *reasonable expectation of no harm*, although articulated in the Federal Food Drug and Cosmetic Act (FFDCA) definition of adulterated food (Section 402) as [no] "significant or unreasonable risk of illness or injury."[13] This is a lesser safety standard than the *reasonable certainty* standard for substances *added to foods*. The basis for this rationale is that consumption of a dietary supplement is by choice, not involuntary as for a food (i.e., food must have a presumption of safety and therefore, the higher standard of safety). Therefore, because there is (1) a deliberate choice involved in consuming a dietary supplement and (2) because the daily recommended intake is clearly stated on the label, there is an implied assumption of some risk on the part of the consumer.

In many respects, passage of the Dietary Supplement Health and Education Act (DSHEA) in October, 1994, was a safety valve, venting consumer discontent with the high degree of restriction placed upon health claims and the narrowing of the window of availability of dietary supplements as the result of actions by the FDA. In response to these pressures, a tacit bargain between Congress and the consumers was struck, whereby Congress granted continued access by the public to dietary supplements by (1) providing for this lower threshold of evidence for safety, (2) changing the role of the FDA from gate-keeper to policeman (i.e., abandoning pre-market approval),[14] and (3) allowing a type of claim (i.e., structure function claims, not health claims). The consumer's concessions were that (1) supplements could not be added to food (because of the lower threshold for safety), (2) consumption will always remain the product of an overt, voluntary act on the part of the consumer (a dietary supplement can never be represented as a food or meal replacement), and (3) because the recommended daily dose is presented on the supplement, the consumer will assume at least some risk[15] from consumption (articulated by the standard of reasonable *expectation* of no harm (21 CFR 190.6(a)[16]). As a final safeguard, Congress empowered the *Secretary* of Health and Human Services HHS (not the *Commissioner* of FDA), to take action through the "imminent hazard" clause of the regulation if a supplement is determined to have an unexpected consequence (Burdock, 2000; Mackey and Kotsonis, 2002; Burdock *et al.*, 2006).

Assessment of Carcinogens

Carcinogenicity as a Special Problem Congress provided the FDA with wide latitude in assessing safety and assuring a safe food supply with one exception. That exception is a provision of the FD&C Act known as the Delaney clause, which prohibits the approval of regulated food additives "found to induce cancer when ingested by man or animals" [sections 409(c)(3)(A), 706(b)(5)(B), and 512(d)(1)(H)].

The Delaney prohibition applies only to the approval of food additives, color additives, and animal drugs; it does not apply to unavoidable contaminants or GRAS substances or ingredients sanctioned by the FDA or USDA before 1958. The clause also does not apply to constituents that are present in food or color additives or animal drugs, provided that the level of such contaminants can be demonstrated to be safe and the whole additive, including its contaminants, is not found to induce cancer in humans or animals.

---

[10] A nonometer is one billionth of a meter (10^{-9} m)—about one ten-thousandth of the diameter of a human hair, a thousand times smaller than a red blood cell, or about half the size of the diameter of DNA (EPA, 2005).

[11] Degraded carrageenan is classified by the International Agency for Research on Cancer (IARC) as 2B, a possible human carcinogen, based on animal study data. Native carrageenan has been classified by IARC as 3, unclassifiable with respect to carcinogenicity in humans.

[12] FDA Regulation of Nanotechnology Products (http://www.fda.gov/nanotechnology/regulation.html) (site visited 9 April 2006).

[13] Also articulated in the FFDCA (§413) as "reasonably be expected to be safe".

[14] FFDCA§402(f)(1) "In any proceeding under this subparagraph, *the United States shall bear the burden of proof* on each element to show that a dietary supplement is adulterated."

[15] FDA has stated that it would use a "reasonable consumer" standard in determining whether a claim is misleading. The reasonable consumer standard replaced the standard of "the ignorant, the unthinking, and the credulous" consumer, used by courts at the request of FDA in the past (Walsh *et al.*, 2005).

[16] Referred in the FFDCA (§402(f)(1)(A)) as "significant or unreasonable risk of illness or injury."

Table 30-14

Uncertainty Parameters and Their Associated Range of Risk Factors

UNCERTAINTY PARAMETERS	ESTIMATED RANGE (FACTOR)
Extrapolation model	1–10,000
Total dose vs. dose rate	30–45
Most sensitive sex/strain vs. average sensitivity	1–100
Sensitivity of human vs. test animal	1–1000
Potential synergism or antagonism with other carcinogens or promoters	1–1000?
Total population vs. target population, potential vs. actual market penetration	1–1000
Absorptive rate (gut, skin, lung) for animals at high dose vs. humans at low dose	1–10
Dose scaling: mg/kg body weight, ppm (diet, water, feed) surface area	1–15
Upper confidence on users or exposed	1–10
Specifications or tolerances	1–10
Limits of detection vs. actual levels	1–1000
Additivity vs. nonadditivity of multiple sites	1–3
Survival or interim sacrifice adjustments	1–2
Knowledge of only high-end plateau dose response	1–10
Error or variation in detection methods	1–10
Adjustments for less than lifetime bioassays	1–100
Adjustments for intermittent and less than lifetime human exposure	1–100
Use vs. nonuse of historical data	1–2
Upper confidence and lower confidence limits vs. expected values in extrapolation level of acceptable risk	1–1000
Level of acceptable risk	1–1000
Adding or not adding theoretical risks from many substances	1–100

SOURCE: Flamm WG, Lorentzen RJ: Quantitative risk assessment (qra): A special problem in the approval of new products, in Cothern CR, Mehlman MA, Marcus WL (eds.): *Risk Assessment and Risk Management of Industrial and Environmental Chemicals*. Princeton Scientific Publishing Co., Inc., Princeton, NJ, 1988.

This interpretation of the Delaney clause was set forth by the FDA in its so-called "constituent policy" published on April 2, 1982, as an Advanced Notice of Proposed Rulemaking (ANPR). The policy mandates the development and use of animal carcinogenicity data and probabilistic risk assessment to establish a safe level for the contaminant in the additive under its intended conditions of use.

The constituent policy and, as will be discussed later, the implementation of the so-called DES (diethylstilbestrol) proviso for animal drugs under the Delaney clause have forced the FDA to develop a means for establishing safe levels for carcinogenic substances. The DES proviso allows the addition of carcinogenic animal drugs to animal feed if they leave no residue in edible tissue as determined by an approved analytic procedure. To do this, the FDA has turned to the use of probabilistic risk assessment in which tumor data in animals are mathematically extrapolated to an upper bound risk in humans exposed to particular use levels of the additive. The FDA takes the position that considering the many conservative assumptions inherent in the procedure, an upper bound lifetime risk of one cancer in a million individuals is the biological equivalent of zero.

Much controversy surrounds the use of risk assessment procedures, in part because estimates of risk are highly dependent on the many assumptions that must be made. The common practice of testing at a maximum tolerated dose (MTD) (Williams and Weisburger, 1991) raises the question of appropriateness to human exposure. Do high test doses cause physiological changes unlike those from human exposure? The basic assumption in quantitative risk assessment (QRA) that the dose–response curve is linear beneath the lowest observable effect may result in the calculation of relatively high risks even at doses that are much lower than the lowest dose that produces cancer in experimental animals. QRA is more a process than a science; many steps in the process are based on assumptions, not proven scientific facts. If only the most conservative assumptions are made throughout the process, many will represent overestimates of human risk by 10- or 100-fold, leading to a combined overestimate of perhaps a million-fold or more. Table 30-14 provides some rough estimates of potential ranges of uncertainty that might lead to large overestimates (Flamm and Lorentzen, 1988).

Historically, the FDA has employed a high threshold for establishing that a food or color additive has been found to induce cancer when ingested by humans or animals. If these additives are found to induce cancer, they cannot be approved for foods or colors no matter how small the estimated risk. In the end, very few substances have been disapproved or banned because of the Delaney clause. Two indirect food additives (Flectol H and mercaptoimidazoline) that migrate from packaging material were banned. Among direct additives, safrole, cinnamyl anthranilate, thiourea, and diethylpyrocarbonate were banned because of the Delaney clause, diethylpyrocarbonate because it forms urethane.

A number of substances (e.g., butylated hydroxyanisole (BHA), xylitol, methylene chloride, sorbitol, trichloroethylene, nitrilotriacetic acid (NTA), diethylhexyl phthalate, melamine, formaldehyde, bentonite) listed in the Code of Federal Regulation as food additives are also listed as carcinogens by National Toxicology Program (NTP), the International Agency for Research on Cancer (IARC), or the state of California (under the Safe Drinking Water and Toxic Enforcement Act of 1986, also known as Proposition 65). How is this possible, and on what basis do these food additive listings continue?

Despite the fact that tests and conditions exist under which each of these substances will produce cancer in animals, the FDA has found it possible to continue listing these substances as food additives. The reasoning applied in almost every case is based on secondary carcinogenesis. The one exception is formaldehyde, which is carcinogenic only on inhalation, and there are compelling reasons to believe that inhalation is not an appropriate test in this case (Flamm and Frankos, 1985). Therefore, formaldehyde is not treated as a carcinogen prohibited by the Delaney clause.

For BHA, which induces forestomach cancer, the concept has been advanced that its carcinogenicity is attributable primarily to a cycle of irritation and restorative hyperplasia (Clayson *et al.*, 1986). For xylitol, a sugar alcohol, an increase in bladder tumors and adrenal pheochromocytomas is considered secondary to calcium imbalance resulting from the indigestibility of sugar alcohols and their fermentation in the lower GI tract. Sorbitol, another sugar alcohol, behaves in a similar manner. For NTA, the argument is secondary carcinogenesis, and although specific explanations vary, the mechanism involving zinc imbalance has considerable scientific support.

Thus, the FDA has generally interpreted the phrase "found to induce cancer when ingested by man or animals" as excluding cancers that arise through many secondary means. Therefore, to be a carcinogen under the Delaney clause, a food or color additive must be demonstrated to induce cancer by primary means when ingested by humans or animals or to induce cancer by other routes of administration that are found to be appropriate. This is interpreted to mean that the findings of cancer must be clearly reproducible and that the cancers found are not secondary to nutritional, hormonal, or physiological imbalances. This position allows the agency to argue that changing the level of protein or fat in the diet does not induce cancer but simply modulates tumor incidence (Kritschevsky, 1994).

Biological *vs.* Statistical Significance   Much can be learned about the proper means of assessing carcinogenicity data by studying large databases for substances that have been tested for carcinogenicity many times. The artificial sweetener cyclamate is an example. The existence of more than a dozen studies on cyclamate and the testing of multiple hypotheses at dozens of different organ and tissue sites in all these studies led to the awareness that the overall false-positive error rate could be inflated if individual findings were viewed out of context (FDA, 1984). Therefore, very careful attention must be paid to the totality of the evidence.

The possibility of false–negative error is always of concern because of the need to protect public health. However, it should be recognized that any attempt to prove absolutely that a substance is not carcinogenic is futile. Therefore, an unrelenting effort to minimize false-negative errors can produce an unacceptably high probability of a false-positive. Further, demanding certainty (i.e., a zero or implicitly an extremely low probability of false-negative error) has negative consequences for an accurate decision-making process. This is the case because it severely limits the ability to discriminate between carcinogens and noncarcinogens on the basis of bioassays (FDA, 1984).

In addition to the false–positive/false–negative trap, which is a statistical matter, there are many potential biological traps. The test substance, typically administered at high MTDs, may affect one or more of the many biological processes known to modulate tumor incidence at a specific organ site without causing an induction of tumors at that or any other site. Nutritional imbalances such as choline deficiency are known to lead to a high incidence of liver cancer in rats and mice. Simple milk sugar (lactose) is known to increase the incidence of Leydig cell tumors in rats. Caloric intake has been shown to be a significant modifying factor in carcinogenesis. Im-

pairment of immune surveillance by a specific or nonspecific means (stress) affecting immune responsiveness and hormonal imbalance can result in higher incidences of tumors at specific organ sites. Hormonal imbalance, which can be caused by hormonally active agents (e.g., estradiol) or by other substances that act indirectly, such as vitamin D, may result in an increased tumor incidence. Chronic cell injury and restorative hyperplasia resulting from treatment with lemon flavor (D-limonene) probably are responsible for renal tumor development in male rats by mechanisms that are of questionable relevance to humans (Flamm and Lehman-McKeeman, 1991). In these examples, the increases in tumor incidence at specific organ sites probably are secondary to significant changes in normal physiological balance and homeostasis. Moreover, the increases in tumor incidence, and hence the increases in the risk of cancer, probably would not occur except at toxic doses (Ames and Gold, 1997).

To preserve the ability of a bioassay to discriminate between carcinogens and noncarcinogens, the possibility of false–positive or false–negative results and the possibility of secondary effects must be considered. To be meaningful, evaluations must be based on the weight of evidence. Particular attention must be given to the many factors that are used in deciding whether tumor incidences are biologically as well as statistically significant. These factors include (1) the historical rate of the tumor in question (is it a rare tumor, or does it occur frequently in the controls?); (2) the survival histories of dosed and test animals (did dosed animals survive long enough to be considered "at risk" and what effect did chemical toxicity and reduced survival have in the interpretation of the data?); (3) the patterns of tumor incidence (was the response dose-related?); (4) the biological meaningfulness of the effect (was it experimentally consistent with the evidence from related studies and did it occur in a target organ?); (5) the reproducibility of the effect with other doses, sexes, or species; (6) evidence of hyperplasia, metaplasia, or other signs of an ongoing carcinogenic process (is the effect supported by a pattern of related non-neoplastic lesions, particularly at lower doses?); (7) evidence of tumor multiplicity or progression; and (8) the strength of the evidence of an increased tumor incidence (what is the magnitude of the p value, for pairwise comparison and for trend?).

A good discussion of the use of these factors by scientists in deciding whether a substance induces cancer in animals is contained in the notice of a final rule permanently listing FD&C Yellow No. 6 (51 *Federal Register* 41765–41783, 1988). An elevation of tumor incidence in rats was identified at two organ and/or tissue sites: (1) medullary tumors of the adrenal glands in female rats only and (2) renal cortical tumors in female rats only. Scientists at the FDA concluded that the increase in medullary tumors of the adrenal glands in female rats did not suffice to establish that FD&C Yellow No. 6 is a carcinogen. The basis for the decision was (1) a lack of dose response, (2) the likelihood of false positives, (3) the lack of precancerous lesions, (4) morphological similarity of adrenal medullary lesions in treated and control rats, (5) an unaffected latency period, (6) a lack of effect in male rats, and (7) a comparison with other studies in which there was no association between exposure to FD&C Yellow No. 6 and the occurrence of adrenal medullary tumors.

A similar judgment was made with respect to the cortical renal lesions in female rats, which were not found to provide a basis for concluding that FD&C Yellow No. 6 can induce cancer of the kidneys. The main reasons leading to this conclusion were (1) the relatively common occurrence of proliferative renal lesions in aged male control rats (28 months or older), (2) the lack of renal tumors in treated males despite their usually greater sensitivity to renal carcinogens, (3) the lack of malignant tumors indicating no progression of adenomas to a malignant state, (4) the lack of a decreased latency period compared with controls, (5) the coincidence of renal proliferative lesions and chronic renal disease, (6) the lack of genotoxicity, and (7) a lack of corroborative evidence from other studies that suggests a treatment-related carcinogenic effect of FD&C Yellow No. 6 on the kidney. Both these examples emphasize the importance of considering all the evidence in attempting to decide the significance of any subset of data.

As essential elements, vitamins, sugars, and calories by themselves can increase tumor incidence in test animals; the mechanism by which tumors arise as the result of exposure to food or food ingredients is critically important to assessing the relevance of the finding to the safety of the substance under its intended conditions of use in food. McClain (2002) provides an excellent discussion of mechanistic considerations in the regulation and classification of chemical carcinogens.

Carcinogenic Contaminants   The Delaney clause, which prohibits the addition of carcinogens to food, could ban many food additives and color additives if strictly interpreted to include contaminants of additives within its definition. Clearly, this was not Congress's intent, and just as clearly, the FDA needed to develop a common sense policy for addressing the problem that all substances, including food and color additives, may contain carcinogenic contaminants at some trace level.

Toward this end, the agency argued (FDA, 1982b) that banning food and color additives simply because they have been found or are known to contain a trace level of a known carcinogen does not make sense because all substances may contain carcinogenic contaminants. The agency asserted in its constituent policy that the mere fact an additive contains a contaminant known to be carcinogenic should not automatically lead the agency to ban that food additive but should instead cause the agency to consider the health risks it poses based on its level of contamination and the conditions of its use (FDA, 1977).

SAFETY OF FOOD

Adverse Reactions to Food or Food Ingredients

In a survey of Americans, 30% indicated that they or someone in their immediate families has a food sensitivity of one type or another. Although this number is likely too high, as much as 7.5% of the population may be allergic (i.e., their body's immune system is activated due to exposure to food ingredient) to some food or component thereof, such as a peanut allergy (Taylor *et al.*, 1989). Lactose intolerance (a deficiency of the disaccharide enzyme, lactase) is high among some groups; for example, there is an incidence of 27% in black children age 12–24 months, which may increase to 33% by age six years (Juambeltz *et al.*, 1993). The percentage of young northern European children allegedly intolerant to food additives ranges from 0.03 to 0.23% (Wuthrich, 1993) to 1–2% (Fuglsang *et al.*, 1993). Further, there are certain drug–food incompatibilities about which physicians and pharmacists are obligated to warn patients, such as monoamine oxidase (MAO) inhibitors and tyramine in cheese or benzodiazapenes and naringenin in grapefruit juice. People who are prescribed tetracycline also must be alerted not to take milk with this antibiotic. By any standard, there are large numbers of real and perceived adverse reactions to or incompatibilities with food (Thomas and Cotter, 2002). The first step in understanding

these reactions is to define the nomenclature, a task undertaken by the American Academy of Allergy and Immunology (Committee on Adverse Reactions to Foods) and the National Institute of Allergy and Infectious Diseases (Anderson and Sogn, 1984). An adaptation of their definitions and classification is represented in Table 30-15. In the table, the definitions proceed from general to more specific. Obviously, there is little to distinguish the terms "adverse reaction" and "sensitivity" to a food or a food "intolerance," except perhaps in the lexicon of the individual, colored by his or her own experience. That is, an "adverse reaction" may indicate something as simple as an unpleasing esthetic or hedonic quality such as an unpleasant taste, which may in fact have a genetic basis as in the ability to taste phenylthiocarbamide (Guyton, 1971), or may indicate a fatal outcome resulting from an immune or toxic reaction.

Clinical descriptions of adverse reactions to food are not new. Hippocrates (460–370 B.C.) first recorded adverse reactions to cow's milk that caused gastric upset and urticaria, and Galen (AD 131–210) described allergic symptoms to goat milk. However, the immunologic basis of many adverse reactions to food was not established until the passive transfer of sensitivity to fish was described in the early 1960s (Frankland, 1987; Taylor *et al.*, 1989; Taylor and Hefle, 2002). This test, which evolved into the (skin) prick test and later the Radioallergosorbent (RAST) test, allowed a distinction to be made between immunologically based adverse reactions (true allergies) and adverse reactions with other causation.

Food Allergy

Description   Food hypersensitivity (allergy) refers to a reaction involving an immune-mediated response. Such a response is generally IgE-mediated, although IgG_4- and cell-mediated immunity also may play a role in some instances (Fukutomi *et al.*, 1994). What generally distinguishes food allergy from other reactions is the involvement of immunoglobulins, basophils, or mast cells (the latter being a source of mediating substances including histamine and bradykinin for immediate reactions and prostaglandins and leukotrienes for slower-developing reactions) and a need for a prior exposure to the allergen or a cross-reactive allergen. An allergic reaction may be manifested by one or more of the symptoms listed in Table 30-16. The list of foods known to provoke allergies is long and is probably limited only by what people are willing to eat. Although cutaneous reactions and anaphylaxis (i.e., severe allergic reaction, resulting in a drop of blood pressure, and may be fatal) are the most common symptoms associated with food allergy, the body is replete with a repertoire of responses that are rarely confined to only a few foods.

A curious type of food allergy, the so-called exercise-induced food allergy, is apparently provoked by exercise which has been immediately preceded or followed by the ingestion of certain foods (Kivity *et al.*, 1994), including shellfish, peach, wheat, celery, and "solid" food (Taylor *et al.*, 1989; Taylor and Hefle, 2002). The exact mechanism is unknown, but it may involve enhanced mast cell responsiveness to physical stimuli and/or diminished metabolism of histamine similar to red wine allergy (Taylor *et al.*, 1989). Meanwhile, food intolerance in patients with chronic fatigue may have less to do with allergic response and has been shown to be a somatization trait of patients with depressive symptoms and anxiety disorders (Manu *et al.*, 1993).

Chemistry of Food Allergens   Most allergens (antigens) in food are protein in nature, and although almost all foods contain one

Table 30-15
Adverse Reaction to Food: Definition of Terms

TERM	DEFINITION	CHARACTERISTICS/EXAMPLES
Adverse reaction (sensitivity) to a food	General term that can be applied to a clinically abnormal response attributed to an ingested food or food additive	Any untoward pathological reaction resulting from ingestion of a food or food additive. May be immune-mediated
Food hypersensitivity (allergy)	An immunologic reaction and may occur only in some patients, may occur after only a small amount of the substance is ingested, and is unrelated to any physiological effect of the food or food additive	Immune-mediated (cellular or humoral response), requires prior exposure to antigen or cross-reacting antigen. First exposure may have been asymptomatic
Food anaphylaxis	A classic allergic hypersensitivity reaction to food or food additives	A humoral immune response most often involving IgE antibody and release of chemical mediators. Mortality may result
Food intolerance	A general term describing an abnormal physiological response to an ingested food or food additive; this reaction may be an immunologic, idiosyncratic, metabolic, pharmacological, or toxic response	Any untoward pathological reaction resulting from ingestion of a food or food additive. May be immune-mediated. Celiac disease (intolerance to wheat, rye, barley, oats)
Food toxicity (poisoning)	A term use to imply an adverse effect caused by the direct action of a food or food additive on the host recipient without the involvement of immune mechanisms. This type of reaction may involve nonimmune release of chemical mediators. Toxins may be contained within food or released by microorganisms or parasites contaminating food products	Not immune-mediated. May be caused by bacterial endo- or exotoxin (e.g., hemorrhagic *E. coli*) fungal toxin (e.g., aflatoxin), tetrodo-toxin from pufferfish, domoic acid from mollusks, histamine poisoning from fish (scombroid poisoning), nitrate poisoning (i.e., methemoglobinuria)
Food idiosyncrasy	A quantitatively abnormal response to a food substance or additive; this reaction differs from its physiological or pharma-cological effect and resembles hypersensitivity but does not involve immune mechanisms. Food idiosyncratic reactions include those which occur in specific groups of individuals who may be genetically predisposed	Not immune-mediated, Favism (hemolytic anemia related to deficiency of erythrocytic glucose-6-phosphate dehydrogenase), fish odor syndrome, beetanuria, lactose intolerance, fructose, intolerance, asparagus urine, red wine intolerance
Anaphylactoid reaction to a food	An anaphylaxis-like reaction to a food or food additive as a result of nonimmune release of chemical mediators. This reaction mimics the symptoms of food hypersensitivity (allergy)	Not immune-mediated. Scombroid poisoning, sulfite poisoning, red wine sensitivity
Food–drug interaction	A change in the pharmacokinetic or pharmacodynamic action of a drug as the result of ingestion of a food	Not immune-mediated. Ingestion of fats, phytates, or fiber to change absorption; upregulation of genes by *Brassica*, polyunsaturated fats; unregulation of polypeptide transporters by St. Johns wort
Metabolic food reaction	Toxic effects of a food when eaten in excess or improperly prepared	Cycasin, vitamin A toxicity, goiterogens, licorice

SOURCE: Adapted from Anderson JA, Sogn DD (eds.): *Adverse Reactions to Foods*. Washington, DC, U.S. Department of Health and Human Services, 1984.

or more proteins, a few foods are associated more with allergic reactions than are others. For example, anaphylaxis to peanuts is more common than is anaphylaxis to other legumes (e.g., peas, soybeans). Similarly, although allergies may occur from bony fishes, there is no basis for cross-reactivity to other types of seafood (e.g., mollusks and crustaceans), although dual (and independent) sensitivities may exist (Anderson and Sogn, 1984). Interestingly, patients who are allergic to milk usually can tolerate beef and inhaled cattle dander, and patients allergic to eggs usually can tolerate ingestion of chicken and feather-derived particles (Anderson and Sogn, 1984), although in the "bird–egg" syndrome patients can

be allergic to bird feathers, egg yolk, egg white, or any combination of the three (DeBlay *et al.*, 1994; Szepfalusi *et al.*, 1994).

Some of the allergenic components of common food allergens are listed in Table 30-17. Although food avoidance is usually the best means of protection, it is not always possible because (1) the content of some prepared foods may be unknown (e.g., the presence of eggs or cottonseed oil); (2) there is the possibility of contamination of food from unsuspected sources (e.g., *Penicillium* in cheeses or meat, *Candida albicans* (Dayan, 1993; Dorion *et al.*, 1994), and cow's milk antigens in the breast milk of mothers who

Table 30-16

Symptoms of IgE-Mediated Food Allergies

Cutaneous	Urticaria (hives), eczema, dermatitis, pruritus, rash
Gastrointestinal	Nausea, vomiting, diarrhea, abdominal cramps
Respiratory	Asthma, wheezing, rhinitis, bronchospasm
Other	Anaphylactic shock, hypotension, palatal itching, swelling including tongue and larynx, methemoglobinemia*

*An unusual manifestation of allergy reported to occur in response to soy or cow milk protein intolerance in infants.
SOURCE: Murray KF, Christie, DL: Dietary protein intolerance in infants with transient methemoglobinemia and diarrhea. *J Pediatr* 122:90, 1993, with permission from Elsevier.
SOURCE: Adapted from Taylor SL, Scanlan RA (eds.): *Food Toxicology: A Perspective on the Relative Risks.* New York, Marcel Dekker, 1989. With permission from Copyright Clearance Center.

Table 30-17

Known Allergenic Food Proteins

FOOD	ALLERGIC PROTEINS
Cow's milk	Casein (Dorion *et al.*, 1994; Stoger and Wuthrich, 1993)
	β-Lactoglobulin (Piastra *et al.*, 1994; Stoger and Wuthrich, 1993)
	a-Lactalbumin (Bernaola *et al.*, 1994; Stoger and Wuthrich, 1993)
Egg whites	Ovomucoid (Bernhisel-Broadbent *et al.*, 1994)
	Ovalbumin (Fukotomi *et al.*, 1994; Bernhiesel-Broadbent *et al.*, 1994)
Egg yolks	Livetin (de Blay *et al.*, 1994; Szepfalusi *et al.*, 1994)
Peanuts	Ara h II (Dorion *et al.*, 1994)
	Peanut I (Sachs *et al.*, 1981)
Soybeans	β-Conglycinin (7S fraction) (Rumsey *et al.*, 1994)
	Glycinin (11S fraction) (Rumsey *et al.*, 1994)
	Gly mIA (Gonzalez *et al.*, 1992)
	Gly mIB (Gonzalez *et al.*, 1992)
	Kunitz trypsin inhibitor (Brandon *et al.*, 1986)
Codfish	Gad cI (O'Neil *et al.*, 1993)
Shrimp	Antigen II (Taylor *et al.*, 1989)
Green peas	Albumin fraction (Taylor *et al.*, 1989)
Rice	Glutelin fraction (Taylor *et al.*, 1989)
	Globulin fraction (Taylor *et al.*, 1989)
Cottonseed	Glycoprotein fraction (Taylor *et al.*, 1989)
Peach guava, banana, mandarin, strawberry	30 kD protein (Wadee *et al.*, 1990)
Tomato	Several glycoproteins (Taylor *et al.*, 1989)
Wheat	Gluten (Stewart-Tull and Jones, 1992)
	Gliadin (O'Hallaren, 1992)
	Globulin (O'Hallaren, 1992)
	Albumin (O'Hallaren, 1992)
Okra	Fraction I (Manda *et al.*, 1992)

SOURCE: Modified from Taylor SL, Scanlan RA (eds.): *Food Toxicology: A Perspective on the Relative Risks.* New York, Marcel Dekker, 1989, p. 265. With permission from Copyright Clearance Center.

have consumed cow's milk (Halken *et al.*, 1993)); (3) the presence of an allergen in a previously unknown place (the insertion of Brazil nut DNA into soybeans and subsequent appearance of the allergic 2S protein in soybean products (Nordlee *et al.*, 1996)); and (4) there is a lack of knowledge about the phylogenetic relationships between food sources (legumes include peas, soybeans, and peanuts).

Demographics of Food Allergy and Intolerance   Although children appear to be the most susceptible to food allergy, with adverse reactions occurring in 4–6% of infants, the incidence appears to taper off with maturation of the digestive tract, with only 1–2% of

young children (4–15 years) susceptible (Fuglsang *et al.*, 1993). The increase in the number of adults exhibiting food allergy may be due in part to an expanded food universe, that is, an increased willingness to try different foods. In one study, allergies among young children were most commonly to milk and eggs, whereas allergies that developed later in life tended to be to fruit and vegetables (Kivity *et al.*, 1994).

Familial relationships also play a role. Schrander and colleagues (1993) noted that among infants with cow's milk protein intolerance, 65% had a positive family history (first- or second-degree relatives) for atopy compared with 35% of healthy controls.

Table 30-18
Idiosyncratic Reactions to Foods

FOOD	REACTION	MECHANISM	REFERENCE
Fava beans	Hemolysis, sometimes accompanied by jaundice and hemoglobinuria; also, pallor, fatigue, nausea, dyspnea, fever and chills, abdominal and dorsal pain	Pyramidene aglycones in fava bean cause irreversible oxidation of GSH in G-6-PD-deficient erythrocytes by blocking NADPH supply, resulting in oxidative stress of the erythrocyte and eventual hemolysis	Chevion *et al.*, 1985
Chocolate	Migraine headache	Phenylethylamine-related (?)	Gibb *et al.*, 1991; Settipane, 1987
Beets	Beetanuria: passage of red urine (often mistaken for hematuria)	Excretion of beetanin in urine after consumption of beets	Smith, 1991
Asparagus	Odorous, sulfurous-smelling urine	Autosomal dominant inability to metabolize methanthiol of asparagus and consequent passage of methanthiol in urine	Smith, 1991
Red Wine	Sneezing, flush, headache, diarrhea, skin itch, shortness of breath	Diminished histamine degradation: deficiency of diamine oxidase (?) Histamines present in wine	Wantke *et al.*, 1994
Choline- and carnitine-containing foods	Fish odor syndrome: foul odor of body secretions	Choline and carnitine metabolized to trimethylamine in gut by bacteria, followed by absorption but inability to metabolize to odorless trimethylamine *N*-oxide	Ayesh *et al.*, 1993
Milk	Abdominal pain, bloating, diarrhea	Lactase deficiency	Mallinson, 1987
Fructose-containing foods	Abdominal pain, vomiting, diarrhea, hypoglycemia	Reduced activity of hepatic aldolase B toward fructose-1-phosphate	Frankland, 1987; Catto-Smith and Adams, 1993

Food Toxicity (Poisoning)   See "**Substances for which tolerances may not be set.**"

Food Idiosyncrasy   Food idiosyncrasies are generally defined as *quantitatively* abnormal responses to a food substance or additive; this reaction differs from the physiological effect, and although it may resemble hypersensitivity, it does not involve immune mechanisms. Food idiosyncratic reactions include those that occur in specific groups of individuals who may be genetically predisposed. Examples of such reactions and the foods that probably are responsible are given in Table 30-18.

Probably the most common idiosyncratic reaction is lactose intolerance, a deficiency of the lactase enzyme needed for the metabolism of the lactose in cow's milk. A lack of this enzyme results in fermentation of lactose to lactic acid and an osmotic effect in the bowel, with resultant symptoms of malabsorption and diarrhea. Lactose intolerance is lowest in northern Europe at 3–8% of the population; it reaches 70% in southern Italy and Turkey and nearly 100% in southeast Asia (Anderson and Sogn, 1984; Gudmand-Hoyer, 1994).

Anaphylactoid Reactions   Anaphylactoid reactions are historically thought of as reactions mimicking anaphylaxis through direct application of the primary mediator of anaphylactic reactions: histamine. Ingestion of scombroid fish (e.g., tuna, mackerel, bonito) as well as some nonscombroid fish (mahimahi and bluefish) that have been acted upon by microorganisms to produce histamine may

result in an anaphylactoid reaction also called "scombrotoxicosis" (Table 30-19) (Clark *et al.*, 1999). The condition was reported to be mimicked by the direct ingestion of 90 mg of histamine in unspoiled fish (Van Geldern *et al.*, 1992), but according to Taylor (1986), the effect of simply ingesting histamine does not produce the equivalent effect. Instead, Taylor claims that histamine ingested with spoiled fish appears to be much more toxic than is histamine ingested in an aqueous solution as a result of the presence of histamine potentiators in fish flesh. The apparent mechanism of potentiation involves the inhibition of intestinal histamine-metabolizing enzymes (diamine oxidase), which causes increased histamine uptake. Melnik *et al.* (1997) proposed that anaphylactoid responses may be the sum of several mechanisms: (1) an increased intake of biogenic amines (including histamine) with food, (2) an increased synthesis by the intestinal flora, (3) a diminished catabolism of biogenic amines by the intestinal mucosa, and (4) an increased release of endogenous histamine from mast cells and basophils by histamine-releasing food. Scombrotoxicosis in the absence of high histamine levels (less than the FDA action level for tuna of 50 mg histamine/100 g fish) was reported by Gessner *et al.*, 1996. Ijomah *et al.* (1991) claimed that dietary histamine is not a major determinant of scombrotoxicosis, because potency is not positively correlated with the dose and volunteers tend to fall into susceptible and nonsusceptible subgroups. Ijomah *et al.* (1991) suggested that endogenous histamine released by mast cells plays a significant role in the etiology of scombrotoxicosis, whereas the role of dietary histamine is minor. An exception to this endogenous histamine theory was described by Morrow *et al.* (1991), who found the

Table 30-19
Anaphylactoid Reactions to Food

FOOD	REACTION	MECHANISM	REFERENCE
Western Australian salmon (*Arripis truttaceus*)	Erythema and urticaria of the skin, facial flushing and sweating, palpitations, hot flushes of the body, headache, nausea, vomiting, and dizziness	Scombroid poisoning; high histamine levels demonstrated in the fish	Smart, 1992
Fish (spiked with histamine)	Facial flushing, headache	Histamine poisoning; histamine concentration in plasma correlated closely with histamine dose ingested	Van Gelderen *et al.*, 1992
Cape yellow tail (fish) (*Seriola lalandii*)	Skin rash, diarrhea, palpitations, headache, nausea and abdominal cramps, paraesthesia, unusual taste sensation, and breathing difficulties	Scombroid poisoning, treated with antihistamines.	Muller *et al.*, 1992
Sulfite sensitivity	Bronchospasm, asthma	Sulfite oxidase deficiency to meta-bisulfites in foods and wine	Smith, 1991
Tuna, albacore, mackerel, bonito, mahimahi, and bluefish	Reaction resembling an acute allergic reaction	Scombroid poisoning treated with antihistamines and cimetidine	Lange, 1988
Cheese	Symptoms resembling acute allergic reaction	Responds to antihistamines; histamine poisoning?	Taylor, 1986

expected increase in urinary histamine in scombroid-poisoned individuals but did not find an increase in urinary 9α,11β-dihydroxy-15-oxo-2,3,18,19-tetranorprost-5-ene-1,20-dioic acid, the principal metabolite of prostaglandin D$_2$, a mast cell secretory product; thus, no mast cell involvement was indicated.

Smith (1991) described sulfite-induced bronchospasm (sometimes leading to asthma), which was first noticed as an acute sensitivity to meta-bisulfites sprayed on restaurant salads and in wine. Sulfite normally is detoxicated rapidly to inorganic sulfate by the enzyme sulfite oxidase. In sensitive individuals, there is apparently a deficiency in this enzyme, making them supersensitive to sulfites. Thus, the addition of sulfite to food is considered safe only when properly disclosed on the food label.

Food–Drug Interactions Once known as pharmacological food reactions or as "false food allergies" (Moneret-Vautrin, 1987), these adverse reactions were once thought to be exaggerated responses to pharmacological agents in food and possibly due to receptor sensitization. However, the majority of food and drug interactions are actually the result of food-induced changes in drug bioavailability or metabolism (i.e., *pharmacokinetic* interactions), although some are the result of *pharmacodynamic* interactions. For drugs with a narrow therapeutic index and the need for dose titration, even small changes in the dose–response effects can have great consequences (Schmidt and Dalhoff, 2002). The potential to alter therapeutic effect can be great and in recognition of the role that food plays, test meals are now given to determine their effect on drug therapeutic effect (FDA, 2002b).

Pharmacokinetic effects on absorption (e.g., gastric pH, gastric emptying, lymphatic flow) were described earlier. Examples of foods affecting a number of cytochromes, Phase II enzymes, and transporters are provided in Table 30-20, although the effects on CYP3A4 and P-glycoprotein may be the clinically most important (Harris *et al.*, 2003). Other dietary ingredients that may produce an

effect on the overall pharmacokinetics of drugs would include substances that would change the pH of urine or simply the presence of fiber in the intestine. Examples of pharmacodynamic interactions might include the effect of unsaturated fatty acids in the diet on anticoagulants or membrane potentials of the membranes in which they become incorporated; or high potassium intake from potassium-rich foods and the risk of hyperkalemia during therapy with angiotensin enzyme converting enzyme inhibitors or spironolactone (Schmidt and Dalhof, 2002). Other pharmacodynamic interactions might include phytoestrogens and other estrogen-stimulating substances during treatment for hormonally sensitive cancers (e.g., breast and prostate) and; caffeine or other stimulatory methylxanthines from coffee, chocolate, and soft drinks flavored with guarana, during treatment for hypertension.

Metabolic Food Reactions Metabolic food reactions are distinct from other categories of adverse reactions in that the foods are more or less commonly eaten and demonstrate toxic effects only when eaten to excess or improperly processed (Table 30-21). The susceptible population exists as a result of its own behavior, that is, the "voluntary" consumption of food as a result of a limited food supply or an abnormal craving for a specific food. Such an abnormal craving was reported by Bannister *et al.* (1977), who noted hypokalemia leading to cardiac arrest in a 58-year-old woman who had been eating about 1.8 kg of licorice per week. In "glycyrrhizism," or licorice intoxication, glycyrrhizic acid is the active component, with an effect resembling that of aldosterone, which suppresses the renin–angiotensin–aldosterone axis, resulting in the loss of potassium. Clinically, hypokalemia with alkalosis, cardiac arrhythmias, muscular symptoms together with sodium retention and edema, and severe hypertension are observed. The syndrome may develop at a level of 100 g licorice/day but gradually abates upon withdrawal of the licorice (Isbrucker and Burdock, 2006).

Table 30-20
Food–Drug Interactions (Activity may be Enhanced or Inhibited)

ENZYME OR TRANSPORTER	FOOD	DRUG
CYP1A2	Caffeine, theophylline, grapefruit juice (naringen and furanocoumarins bergamottin and dihydroxybergamotin), grape juice, cruciferous vegetables, apiaceous vegetables, cooked meat	Clozapine, fluvoxamine, imipramine
CYP2E1	Watercress and possibly other isothiocyanate-containing cruciferous vegetables; polyunsaturated fatty acids (corn oil, menhaden oil)	Ethanol, halothane, enflurane
CYP3A4	Grapefruit juice, orange juice, red wine, possibly other polyphenol-containing substances, St. Johns wort, garlic	Ketoconazole, cyclosporin, erythromycin, protease inhibitors, HMG-CoA reductase inhibitors
UGT &GST	Brussel sprouts, cabbage, watercress, broccoli	Acetominophen, oxazepam, morphine, ibuprofen
P-glycopeptide &OATP	Vegetables, fruit juice, St. Johns wort	Digoxin, cyclosporine, pravastatin

UGT, uridine diphosphate glycuronosyltransferases; GST, glutathione-*S*-transferases; OATP, organic anion transporting polypeptides.

Table 30-21
Metabolic Food Reactions

FOOD	REACTION	MECHANISM	REFERENCE
Lima beans, Cassava roots, millet (sorghum) sprouts, bitter almonds, apricot, and peach pits	Cyanosis	Cyanogenic glycosides releasing hydrogen cyanide on contact with stomach acid	Anderson and Sogn, 1984
Cabbage family, turnips, soybeans, radishes, rapeseed, and mustard	Goiter (enlarged thyroid)	Isothiocyanates, goitrin, or *S*-5-viny-thiooxazolidone interferes with utilization of iodine	Anderson and Sogn, 1984; van Etten and Tookey, 1985
Unripe fruit of the tropical tree *Blighia sapida,* common in Caribbean and Nigeria	Severe vomiting, coma, and acute hypoglycemia sometimes resulting in death, especially among the malnourished	Hypoglycin A, isolated from the fruit, may interfere with oxidation of fatty acids, so that glycogen stores have to be metabolized for energy, with depletion of carbohydrates, resulting in hypoglycemia	Evans, 1985
Leguminosae, Cruciferae	Lathyritic symptoms: neurological symptoms of weakness, leg paralysis, and sometimes death	L-2-4-Diaminobutyric acid inhibition of ornithine transcarbamylase of the urea cycle, inducing ammonia toxicity	Evans, 1985
Licorice (glycyrrhizic acid)	Hypertension, cardiac enlargement, sodium retention	Glycyrrhizic acid mimicking Mineralocorticoids.	Farese *et al.,* 1991
Polar bear and Chicken liver	Irritability, vomiting, increased intracranial pressure, death	Vitamin A toxicity	Bryan, 1984
Cycads (cycad flour)	Amyotrophic lateral sclerosis (humans), hepatocarcinogenicity (rats and nonhuman primates)	Cycasin (methylazoxymethanol); primary action is methylation, resulting in a broad range of effects from membrane destruction to inactivation of enzyme systems	Matsumoto, 1985; Sieber *et al.,* 1980

Isothiocyanates are present in a number of foods, especially cruciferous vegetables; in mustard and horseradish (as allyl isothiocyanate), providing the 'bite' associated with these foods and in watercress (as methyl isothiocyanate), which confers a slight zaniness to the taste. In mustard seed, the glycoside, sinigrin, is acted upon by myrosin in the presence of water and when the seed is injured, liberating the (allyl)-isothiocyanate, a potent antimicrobial (especially antifungal). Other members of the *Brassica* family, including broccoli, kale, and cabbage, release thiocyanate ion. Once ingested, both the iso- and thiocyanates bind iodine in the body, preventing its organification, leading to *diffuse hyperplastic (iodine-deficient) goiter.* Although the degree to which I$^-$ is bound by the thiocyanates is not comparable to say, percholorate anion (ClO$_4^-$), nevertheless, in areas of low iodine and high *Brassica* consumption, pathology could result (Capen *et al.*, 2002; Farwell and Braverman, 2006). Ermans *et al.* (1972) indicate that chronic consumption of thiocyanate may play a role in endemic cretinism. Paradoxically, excess iodine may also cause goiter (i.e., *iodine-excess goiter*). Excess iodine appears primarily to block the release of T_3 and T_4 from thyroglobulin and interferes with peroxidation of $2I^-$ to I_2 and disrupts the conversion of monoiodothyronine to diiodothyronine (Capen *et al.*, 2002). The FDA is aware of the possibility of iodine toxicity and has placed limits on iodine in kelp, the products of which have extensive use in food.[17]

This category also includes the ingestion of improperly prepared food such as cassava or cycad, which if prepared properly will result in a toxin-free food. Exposure to cycad seed kernel is an etiologic factor for the western Pacific amyotrophic lateral sclerosis (ALS) and parkinsonism-dementia complex (PDC); present also are mutagenic and carcinogenic substances. The neurotoxins found in cycad are *beta-N*-methylamino-L-alanine (BMAA) and methylazoxymethanol *beta-D*-glucoside (cycasin). Cyanogenic glycosides are also found in cassava (as they are in lima beans). The cycad (*Cacaos circinalis*) is a particularly hardy tree in tropical to subtropical habitats around the world. Cycads often survive when other crops have been destroyed (e.g., a natural disaster such as a typhoon or drought) and therefore may serve as an alternative source of food. Among people who have used cycads for food, the method of detoxification is remarkably similar despite the wide range of this plant: The seeds and stems are cut into small pieces and soaked in water for several days and then are dried and ground into flour. The effectiveness of leaching the toxin (cycasin) from the bits of flesh is most directly dependent on the size of the pieces, the duration of soaking, and the number of water changes (Matsumoto, 1985). Shortcuts in processing may have grave consequences.

Fiddleheads (crosiers) of the ostrich fern (*Matteuccia struthiopteris*) are a seasonal delicacy harvested commercially in the northeastern United States and in coastal provinces of Canada. The ostrich fern was a spring vegetable for American Indians of eastern North America and became part of the regular diet of settlers to New Brunswick in the late 1700s. Until recently, it was consumed primarily in the Maritime Provinces of Canada and in the northeastern United States. The ferns are available commercially either canned or frozen, but since the early 1980s, farmers' markets and supermarket chains have sold fresh ferns in season. None of the fiddlehead ferns of eastern and central North America previously have been reported to be poisonous. Although some ferns may be carcinogenic, the ostrich fern has been considered to be safe to eat either raw or cooked. However, in May 1994, outbreaks of food poisoning were associated with eating raw or lightly cooked fiddlehead ferns in New York and western Canada. Approximately 60% of restaurant patrons consuming raw or minimally processed ferns (e.g., light sauté ing) experienced nausea, vomiting, abdominal cramps, and/or diarrhea within hours. Those consuming ferns subjected to more rigorous processing (e.g., boiling for at least 6 minutes) did not experience symptoms. The authors speculated the ferns contained a heat-labile toxin and recommended that ferns be boiled for 10 minutes prior to eating (MMWR, 1994).

Importance of Labeling

The importance of labeling was first realized in its ability to protect consumers from economic fraud by requiring that the weight and exact contents of the product be stated; otherwise, the product was *mislabeled*. Later, it became obvious that labels could also serve a purpose in assuring the safety of the consumer by including safety warnings for particularly susceptible groups.

Food allergies have a considerable impact on modern society. There is no known cure for food allergies and although accidental exposure is common, avoidance of the offending foods is the only successful noninterventional approach. Food allergy is the leading cause of anaphylaxis, a severe type of allergic reaction requiring hospitalization. It is estimated that 2% of adults and about 5% of infants and young children in the United States suffer from food allergies. Approximately 30,000 individuals require emergency room treatment, 2000 are hospitalized, and 150 die because of allergic reactions to food.[18]

Effective January 1, 2006, as a result of the Food Allergen Labeling and Consumer Protection Act of 2004 (FALCPA), manufacturers are required to identify the presence of ingredients that contain protein derived from milk, eggs, fish, crustacean shellfish, tree nuts, peanuts, wheat, or soybeans. These eight major food allergens account for 90% of food allergic reactions. In addition, FALCPA labeling regulations require declaration of the specific type of tree nut (e.g., almonds, pecans, or walnuts), the species of fish (e.g., bass, flounder, or cod), and the kind of crustacean shellfish (e.g., crab, lobster, or shrimp). FALCPA requires with a few exceptions the label on a food product (conventional foods, dietary supplements, infant formula, and medical foods) that is or contains an ingredient (spice, flavoring, coloring, or incidental additive) that includes a "major food allergen" (Carabin and Magnuson, 2006).

Labeling requirements for nonallergens include those for intolerance (e.g., lactose or gluten intolerance) or the presence of phenylalanine for PKU patients, are especially important when these substances may be present in foods where their presence may not be expected. Label warnings also include those warning of a threshold for a laxative effect (e.g., polydextrose, mannitol, sorbitol). The FDA has indicated that, at this time, they are not aware of any information that foods developed through genetic engineering differ as a class in any attribute from foods developed through conventional means that would warrant a special label (Thompson, 2000). The FDA allows companies to include on the label of a product any statement as long as the statement is truthful and not misleading.

TOLERANCE SETTING FOR SUBSTANCES IN FOODS

Pesticide Residues

A pesticide is defined under the Federal Insecticide, Fungicide and Rodenticide Act (FIFRA), as any substance used to control or mitigate pests (such as insects, rodents, weeds, or fungi), or intended for use as a plant growth regulator, defoliant, or dessicant. In the United States, the regulation of pesticides is the responsibility of the Environmental Protection Agency (EPA) and is accomplished under both FIFRA and the FD&C Act. FIFRA governs the registration, sale, and use of all pesticides. It is illegal to use a pesticide unless it is specifically registered and labeled for the intended use. In order to obtain registration, an applicant must supply EPA with data on pesticide composition, mammalian and ecological toxicity, environmental fate, and potential human and environmental exposures.

---

[17] 21 CFR §172.365.

[18] http://www.cfsan.fda.gov/~dms/alrgact.html (site visited 8 April 2006).

A major part of the registration process for most pesticides involves the establishment of tolerances. The EPA must establish tolerances, or exemptions from tolerances, for all pesticides that may come into contact with food or feed, i.e., those intended for use during the production, storage, transportation, or processing of food or feed crops, on livestock, or in food-handling establishments. The tolerances are intended to represent the highest expected residue levels from legal uses of the pesticide. All pesticide tolerances are now established under Section 408 of the FD&C Act. Prior to 1996, if pesticide residues in processed foods exceeded those in raw agricultural commodities, they were considered to be intentional food additives and were required to be assigned "Food Additive Tolerances" under Section 409 of the Act. If the pesticide chemical in question had been classified by the EPA as a human or animal carcinogen, the Delaney clause would be invoked and the Section 409 food additive tolerance(s) could be denied on that basis. However, the Food Quality Protection Act (FQPA) of 1996 revised Section 201(s) of the FD&C Act to exclude pesticides from the definition of *food additive*—even in the case of concentration residues in processed fractions. Although an additional tolerance for a processed fraction is still required if the pesticide residue in the fraction exceeds the tolerance for the raw agricultural commodity (RAC), that tolerance is now established under Section 408 rather than Section 409. Consequently, although the Delaney clause has *not* been repealed from Section 409, and continues to apply to intentional food additives *other than pesticides*, it is no longer applicable for *pesticides*.

Prior to 1996, the EPA used 100× as a default safety factor when conducting risk assessments to ensure that the necessary food and feed tolerances would be safe for human health. However, FQPA also requires that an additional 10× safety factor "shall be applied for infants and children to take into account potential pre- and postnatal toxicity and completeness of the data with respect to exposure and toxicity to infants and children." It further states, however, that "the Administrator may use a different margin of safety for the pesticide chemical residue only if, on the basis of reliable data, such margin will be safe for infants and children."

Drugs Used in Food-Producing Animals

An animal drug "means any drug intended for use for animals other than man" [section 201(w) of the FD&C Act]. Animal drugs, which typically are used for growth promotion and increased food production, present a complex problem in the safety assessment of animal drug residues in human food. Determination of the potential human health hazards associated with animal drug residues is complicated by the metabolism of an animal drug, which results in residues of many potential metabolites.

The primary factors which must be considered in the evaluation of animal drugs are (1) consumption and absorption by the target animal, (2) metabolism of the drug by the target food animal, (3) excretion and tissue distribution of the drug and its metabolites in food animal products and tissues, (4) consumption of food animal products and tissues by humans, (5) potential absorption of the drug and its metabolites by humans, (6) potential metabolism of the drug and its metabolites by humans, and (7) potential excretion and tissue distribution in humans of the drug, its metabolites, and the secondary human metabolites derived from the drug and its metabolites. Thus, the pharmacokinetic and biotransformation characteristics of both the animal and the human must be considered in an assessment of the potential human health hazard of an animal drug.

When an animal drug is considered GRAS, the safety assessment of the drug is handled as described under the section on GRAS. With respect to new animal drugs, safety assessment is concerned primarily with residues that occur in animal food products (milk, cheese, etc.) and edible tissues (muscle, liver, etc.). Toxicity studies in the target species (chicken, cow, pig, etc.) should provide data on metabolism and the nature of metabolites, along with data on the drug's pharmacokinetics. During this phase, the parent drug and its metabolites are evaluated both qualitatively and quantitatively in the animal products of concern (eggs, milk, meat, etc.). This may involve the development of sophisticated analytic methodologies. Once these data are obtained, it is necessary to undertake an assessment to determine potential human exposure to these compounds from the diet and other sources, pursuant to the establishment of a tolerance.

To comply with the Congressional intent regarding the use of animal drugs in food-producing animals as required in the no residue provision of the Delaney clause, the FDA began to build a system for conducting risk assessment of carcinogens in the early 1970s (FDA, 1977). In the course of developing a policy and/or regulatory definition for "no residue," the FDA was compelled to address the issue of residues of metabolites of animal drugs known to induce cancer in humans or animals. As the number of metabolites may range into the hundreds, it became apparent that as a practical matter, not every metabolite could be tested with the same thoroughness as the parent animal drug. This forced the FDA to consider threshold assessment for the first time. Threshold assessment combines information on the structure and in vitro biological activity of a metabolite for the purpose of determining whether carcinogenicity testing is necessary (Flamm *et al.*, 1994, 2002). If testing is necessary and if the substance is found to induce cancer, the FDA's definition states that a lifetime risk of one in a million is equivalent to the meaning of "no residue" as intended by Congress.

Unavoidable Contamination during Growth, Storage, or Processing

Certain substances, such as polyhalogenated aromatic hydrocarbons (PHAHs), including dioxins, dibenzofurans, and biphenyls, or heavy metals, are unavoidable in food because of their widespread use, presence in the earth's crust which has resulted in their becoming a persistent and/or ubiquitous contaminant in the environment or presence as a product of normal food processing. As a result, foods and animal feeds, principally those of animal (e.g., PHAHs accumulate in dairy/meat products due to lipophilicity of these compounds) and marine origin, contain unavoidable contaminants at some level. Tolerances for residues of unavoidable contaminants are established for foods and food ingredients to ensure that they are safe under expected or intended conditions of use.

Heavy Metals   There are 92 natural elements; approximately 22 are known to be essential nutrients of the mammalian body and are referred to as micronutrients (Concon, 1988). Among the micronutrients are iron, zinc, copper, manganese, molybdenum, selenium, iodine, cobalt, and even aluminum and arsenic. However, among the 92 elements, lead, mercury, and cadmium are familiar as contaminants or at least have more specifications setting their limits in food ingredients (e.g., Food Chemicals Codex (FCC, 2003)). The prevalence of these elements as contaminants is due to their ubiquity in nature but also to their use by humans.

Lead   Although the toxicity of lead is well known, lead may be an essential trace mineral. A lead deficiency induced by feeding rats <50 ppb (vs. 1000 ppb in controls) over one or more generations, produced effects on the hematopoietic system, decreased iron stores in the liver and spleen, and caused decreased growth (Kirchgessner and Reichmayer-Lais, 1981), but apparently not as a result of an effect on iron absorption. Although the toxic effects of lead are discussed elsewhere in this text, it is important to note that the effects are profound (especially in children) and appear to be long-lasting, because mechanisms for excretion appear to be inadequate in comparison to those for uptake (Linder, 1991). Foods may become contaminated with lead if they are grown, stored, or processed under conditions that could introduce larger amounts of lead into the food, such as when a root crop is grown in soil that has been contaminated from the past use of leaded pesticides. Under such conditions, the resulting contamination of the food may pose a health risk to consumers.

Over the years, recognition of the serious nature of lead poisoning in children has caused the World Health Organization (WHO) and FDA to adjust the recommended tolerable total lead intake from all sources of not more than 100 μg/d for infants up to 6 months old and not more than 150 μg/d for children from 6 months to 2 years of age to the considerably lower range of 6–18 μg/d as a provisional tolerable range for lead intake in a 10-kg child. As the result of recent publicity, the FDA is recommending that lead levels in candy products likely to be consumed frequently by small children not exceed 0.1 ppm because such levels are achievable under good manufacturing practices and would not pose a significant risk to small children for adverse effects. This recommended maximum level is consistent with the FDA's longstanding goal of reducing lead levels in the food supply (FDA, 2005).

Initiatives to reduce the level of lead in foods, such as the move to eliminate lead-soldered seams in soldered food cans that was begun in the 1970s, and efforts to eliminate leachable lead from ceramic ware glazes, have resulted in a steady decline in dietary lead intake. Although food and water still contribute lead to the diet, data from the FDA's Total Diet Study indicated a reduction in mean dietary lead intake for adult males from 95 μg/d in 1978 to 9 μg/d in the period 1986–1988 (Shank and Carson, 1992).

Some lead sources are difficult to curtail as lead often survives food processing; for example, lead in wheat remains in the finished flour (Linder, 1991). Therefore, reducing the contribution from dietary sources remains a challenge, but elimination of lead-soldered cans, lead-soldered plumbing, and especially the use of tetraethyl lead as a gasoline additive has produced substantial reductions in lead ingestion. What is needed now is continued vigilance of largely imported lead-based ceramic ware, lead-containing calcium supplements, and lead leaching into groundwater (Shank and Carson, 1992).

Arsenic   Arsenic is a ubiquitous element in the environment; it ranks 20th in relative abundance among the elements of the earth's crust and twelfth in the human body (Concon, 1988). (Because arsenic is discussed in detail elsewhere in this text, the discussion here is limited to its relationship to foods.) There is some competition for arsenic absorption with selenium, which is known to reduce arsenic toxicity; arsenic is also known to antagonize iodine metabolism and inhibit various metabolic processes, as a result affecting a number of organ systems. There are a number of sources of arsenic, including drinking water, air, and pesticides (Newberne, 1987), but arsenic consumed via food is largely in proportion to the amount of seafood eaten (74% of the arsenic in a market-basket survey came from the meat-poultry-fish group, of which seafood has the consistently highest concentration) (Johnson *et al.*, 1981). Although arsenic is used as an animal feed additive, this source does not contribute much to the body burden, as 0.1% arsanilic acid or docecylamine-p-chlorophenylarsonate fed to turkeys resulted in tissue residues of only 0.31 and 0.24 ppm in fresh muscle (Underwood, 1973).

At a time when arsenic use was common as a pesticide, acute poisoning with arsenic often resulted from mistaking arsenic for sugar or baking soda and adding it to food. The time between exposure and symptoms ranged from 10 minutes to several days, and the symptoms include burning of the mouth or throat, a metallic taste, vomiting, diarrhea (watery and bloody), borborigmi (rumbling of the bowels caused by movement of gas in the GI tract), painful tenesmus (spasm of the anal or vesical sphincter), hematuria, dehydration, jaundice, oliguria, collapse, and shock. Headache, vertigo, muscle spasm, stupor, and delirium may occur (Bryan, 1984). Episodes of acute arsenic poisoning are now rare.

Cadmium   Cadmium is a relatively rare commodity in nature and usually is associated with shale and sedimentary deposits. It is often found in association with zinc ores and in lesser amounts in fossil fuel. Although rare in nature, it is a nearly ubiquitous element in American society because of its industrial uses in plating, paint pigments, plastics, and textiles. Exposure to humans often occurs through secondary routes as a result of dumping at smelters and refining plants, disintegration of automobile tires (which contain cadmium-laden rubber), subsequent seepage into the soil and groundwater, and inhalation of combustion of cadmium-containing materials. The estimated yearly release of cadmium from automobile tires ranges from 5.2 to 6.0 metric tons (Davis, 1970; Lagerwerff and Specht, 1971).

Although like mercury, cadmium can form alkyl compounds, unlike mercury, the alkyl derivatives are relatively unstable and consumption almost always involves the inorganic salt. Of two historical incidents of cadmium poisoning, one involved the use of cadmium-plated containers to hold acidic fruit slushes before freezing. Up to 13–15 ppm cadmium was found in the frozen confection, 300 ppm in lemonade, and 450 in raspberry gelatin. Several deaths resulted. A more recent incident of a chronic poisoning involved the dumping of mining wastes into rice paddies in Japan. Middle-aged women who were deficient in calcium and had had multiple pregnancies seemed to be the most susceptible. Symptoms included hypercalciuria; extreme bone pain from osteomalacia; lumbago; pain in the back, shoulders, and joints; a waddling gait; frequent fractures; proteinuria; and glycosuria. The disease was called *itai itai* (ouch-ouch disease) as a result of the pain with walking. The victims had a reported intake of 1000 μg/d, approximately 200 times the normal intake in unexposed populations (Yamagata and Shigematsu, 1970). Cadmium exposure has also been associated with cancer of the breast, lung, large intestine, and urinary bladder (Newberne, 1987).

Chlorinated Organics   Chlorinated organics have been with us for some time, and given their stability in water and resistance to oxidation, ultraviolet light, microbial degradation, and other sources of natural destruction, chlorinated organics will continue to reside in the environment for some time to come, albeit in minute amounts. However, with the introduction of chlorinated hydrocarbons as pesticides in the 1930s, diseases associated with an insect vector such

Table 30-22
Examples of Levels of Chlorinated Hydrocarbons in British Food

FOOD	CHLORINATED HYDROCARBONS μg/kg								
	$CHCl_3$	CCl_4	TCE	TCEY	TTCE	PCE	HCB	HCBD	PerCE
Milk	5.0	0.2		0.3	—	—	1.0	0.08	0.3
Cheese	33.0	5.0		3.0	0.0	0.0	0.0	0.0	2.0
Butter	22.0	14.0		10.0	—	—	—	2.0	13.0
Chicken eggs	1.4	0.5		0.6	0.0	0.0	0.0	0.0	0.0
Beef steak	4.0	7.0	3.0	16.0	0.0	0.0	0.0	0.0	0.9
Beef fat	3.0	8.0	6.0	12.0					1.0
Pork liver	1.0	9.0	4.0	22.0	0.5	0.4			5.0
Margarine	3.0	6.0	—		0.8				7.0
Tomatoes	2.0	4.5	—	1.7	1.0		70.1	0.8	1.2
Bread (fresh)	2.0	5.0	2.0	7.0	—	—	—	—	1.0
Fruit drink (canned)	2.0	0.5	—	5.0		0.8			2.0

$CHCl_3$, chloroform; CCl_4, carbon tetrachloride; TCE, trichloroethane; TCEY, trichloroethylene; TTCE, tetrachloroethane;
PCE, pentachloroethane; HCB, hexachlorobenzene; HCBD, hexachlorobutadiene; PerCE, perchloroethylene.
SOURCE: Modified from McConnell, G. Gerguson, GM Pearson CR: Chlorinated hydrocarbons and the environment.
Endeavour 34:14, 1975, with kind permission from Elsevier Science.

as malaria were nearly eliminated. In the industrialized world, chlorinated organics brought the promise of nearly universal solvents, and their extraordinary resistance to degradation made them suitable for use as heat transfer agents, carbonless copy paper, and fire retardants (Table 30-22).

As persistent as these substances are in the environment and despite the degree of toxicity that might be implied, the possible hazard from chlorinated substances is relatively low. Ames *et al.* (1987) described a method for interpreting the differing potencies of carcinogens and human exposures: the percentage HERP (human exposure dose/rodent potency dose). Using this method, they demonstrated that the hazard from trichloroethylene-contaminated water in Silicon Valley or Woburn, Massachusetts, or the daily dietary intake from DDT (or its product, DDE) at a HERP of 0.0003–0.004% is considerably less than the hazard presented by the consumption of symphytine in a single cup of comfrey herb tea (0.03%) or the hazard presented by aflatoxin in a peanut butter sandwich (0.03%). The FDA's authority to set tolerances has been used only once in establishing levels for polychlorinated biphenyls (21 CFR 109.15 and 109.30).

There have been only a few incidents of mass poisonings via food, three of which involved contaminated cooking oil. The first became known as *yusho*, or rice oil disease, from rice oil contamination by polychlorinated biphenyls (PCBs). This occurred in 1968 in Japan and affected approximately 2000 individuals. The most vulnerable were newborns of poisoned mothers. The liver and skin were the most severely affected. Symptoms included dark brown pigmentation of nails; acne-like eruptions; increased eye discharge; visual disturbances; pigmentation of the skin, lips, and gingiva; swelling of the upper eyelids; hyperemia of the conjunctiva; enlargement and elevation of hair follicles; itching; increased sweating of the palms; hyperkeratotic plaques on the soles and palms; and generalized malaise. Recovery requires several years (Anderson and Sogn, 1984; Guo *et al.*, 2003). The second incident occurred in 1979 in Yucheng, Taiwan, which also involved PCB-contaminated cooking oil and exposed a similar number of people as the earlier incident in Japan (Guo *et al.*, 2003). The third incident has become known as "Spanish toxic oil syndrome" and although details are still not

fully known, occurred when aniline-contaminated rapeseed oil was distributed as cooking oil in Spain in 1981. Approximately 20,000 people were affected and several deaths occurred. Because symptoms were unique and included respiratory effects, eosinophilia and muscle wasting, but not typical of aniline poisoning, the exact etiologic agent is still unknown. Because the source of the aniline may have been improperly cleaned tank trucks that had imported industrial chemicals, three hypotheses have been offered: the etiologic agent may have been (1) a contaminant in the aniline, (2) a contaminant introduced during transportation or, (3) a reaction product of normal oil components and the potential contaminants (the fraction of the oil most commonly associated with toxicity contained $C_{18:3}$—anilide, also called oleyl anilide and "fatty acid anilide") (Wood *et al.*, 1994; Posada de la Paz *et al.*, 1996; Borda *et al.*, 1998).

Nitrosamines, Nitrosamides, and *N*-Nitroso Substances Nitrogenous compounds such as amines, amides, guanidines, and ureas can react with oxides of nitrogen (NO_x) to form *N*-nitroso compounds (NOCs) (Hotchkiss *et al.*, 1992). The NOCs may be divided into two classes: the nitrosamines, which are *N*-nitroso derivatives of secondary amines, and nitrosamides, which are *N*-nitroso derivatives of substituted ureas, amides, carbamates, guanidines, and similar compounds (Mirvish, 1975).

Nitrosamines are stable compounds, while many nitrosamides have half-lives on the order of minutes, particularly at pH ≫ 6.5. Both classes have members which are potent animal carcinogens, but by different mechanisms. In general, the biological activity of an NOC is thought to be related to alkylation of genetic macromolecules. *N*-nitrosamines are metabolically activated by hydroxylation at an α-carbon. The resulting hydroxyalkyl moiety is eliminated as an aldehyde, and an unstable primary nitrosamine is formed. The nitrosamine tautomerizes to a diazonium hydroxide and ultimately to a carbonium ion. Nitrosamides spontaneously decompose to a carbonium ion at physiological pH by a similar mechanism (Hotchkiss *et al.*, 1992). This is consistent with in vitro laboratory findings because nitrosamines require S9 for activity and nitrosamides are mutagenic de novo.

Table 30-23
Sources of Dietary NOCs

The use of nitrate and/or nitrite as intentional food additives, both of which are added to fix the color of meats, inhibit oxidation, and prevent toxigenesis.

Drying processes in which the drying air is heated by an open flame source. NO_x is generated in small amounts through the oxidation of N_2, which nitrosates amines in the foods. This is the mechanism for contamination of malted barley products.

NOCs can migrate from food contact materials such as rubber bottle nipples.

NOCs can inhabit spices which may be added to food.

Cooking over open flames (e.g., natural gas flame) can result in NOC formation in foods by the same mechanism as drying.

SOURCE: Adapted with permission from Hotchkiss JH, Helser MA, Maragos CM, *et al.*: Nitrate, nitrite, and *N*-nitroso compounds: Food safety and biological implications, in Finley JW, Robinson SF, Armstrong DJ (eds.): *Food Safety Assessment*. Washington, DC, American Chemical Society, 1992, pp. 400–418.

NOCs originate from two sources: environmental formation and endogenous formation (Table 30-23). Environmental sources have declined over the last several years but still include foods (e.g., nitrate-cured meats) and beverages (e.g., malt beverages), cosmetics, occupational exposure, and rubber products (Hotchkiss, 1989). NOCs formed in vivo may actually constitute the greatest exposure and are formed from nitrosation of amines and amides in several areas, including the stomach, where the most favorable conditions exist (pH 2 to 4), although consumption of H_2-receptor blockers or antacids decreases the formation of NOCs.

Environmentally, nitrite is formed from nitrate or ammonium ions by certain microorganisms in soil, water, and sewage. In vivo, nitrite is formed from nitrate by microorganisms in the mouth and stomach, followed by nitrosation of secondary amines and amides in the diet. Sources of nitrate and nitrite in the diet are given in Table 30-24. Many sources of nitrate are also sources of vitamin C. Another possibly significant source of nitrate is well water; although the levels are generally in the range of 21 μM, average levels of 1600 μM (100 mg/L) have been reported (Hotchkiss *et al.*, 1992). However, on the average, Western diets contain 1–2 mmol nitrate/person/day (Hotchkiss *et al.*, 1992). Nitrosation reactions can be inhibited by preferential, competitive neutralization of nitrite with naturally occurring and synthetic materials such as vitamin C, vitamin E, sulfamate, and antioxidants such as BHT, BHA, gallic acid, and even amino acids or proteins (Hotchkiss, 1989; Hotchkiss *et al.*, 1992).

N-nitrosoproline is the most common nitrosoamine present in humans and is excreted virtually unchanged in the urine. The basal rate of urinary excretion of nitrosoproline, which is claimed to be noncarcinogenic, is 2–7 g/d in subjects on a low nitrate diet (Oshima and Bartsch, 1981). Epidemiological studies have not provided evidence of a causal association between nitrate exposure and human cancer nor has a causal link been shown between *N*-nitroso compounds, pre-formed in the diet or endogenously synthesized, and the incidence of human cancer (Gangolli, 1999).

Food-borne Molds and Mycotoxins Molds have served humans for centuries in the production of foods (e.g., ripening cheese) and have provided various fungal metabolites with important medicinal uses; they also may produce secondary metabolites with the potential to produce severe adverse health effects, including behavioral changes (Cousins *et al.*, 2005). It is possible the ergot mycotoxins may have exerted a major role in restricting population expansion and only the reduced dependency on rye cereal as the staple food in

the sixteenth and seventeenth centuries, arising from the introduction of wheat and potatoes, allowed the steady upward movement in population growth (CAST, 2003; IFST, 2006a).

Mycotoxins are secondary fungal metabolites (i.e., not essential for survival of the mold) secreted into the microenvironment around the mold. Mycotoxins represent a diverse group of chemicals that can occur in a variety of plants used as food, including commodities such as cereal grains (barley, corn, rye, wheat), coffee, dairy products, fruits, nuts, peanuts, and spices. A few mycotoxins also can occur in animal products derived from animals that consume contaminated feeds (e.g., milk). However, because commodities are eaten in the greatest amounts, the mycotoxins present in these foods represent the greatest risk (Cousins *et al.*, 2005).

The current interest in mycotoxicosis was generated by a series of reports in 1960–1963 that associated the death of turkeys in England (so-called turkey X disease) and ducklings in Uganda with the consumption of peanut meal feeds containing mold products produced by *Aspergillus flavus* (Stoloff, 1977). The additional discovery of aflatoxin metabolites (e.g., aflatoxin M_1 in milk) led to more intensive studies of mycotoxins and to the identification of a variety of these compounds associated with adverse human health effects, both retrospectively and prospectively.

Moldy foods are consumed throughout the world during times of famine, as a matter of taste, and through ignorance of their adverse health effects. Epidemiological studies designed to ascertain the acute or chronic effects of such consumption are few. Data from animal studies indicate that the consumption of food contaminated with mycotoxins has the potential to contribute to a variety of human diseases (Miller, 1991). Reports of acute intoxications are few; however, prolonged exposure to small quantities of mycotoxin may lead to more insidious effects including growth retardation, birth defects, impaired immunity, decreased disease resistance, and tumor formation in humans and decreased production in farm animals (CAST, 2003).

With some exceptions, molds can be divided into two main groups: "field fungi" and "storage fungi." The former group contains species that proliferate in and under field conditions and do not multiply readily once grain is in storage. Field fungi may be superseded and overrun by storage fungi if conditions of moisture and oxygen allow.

Importantly, the presence of a toxigenic mold does not guarantee the presence of a mycotoxin, which is elaborated only under certain conditions. Further, more than one mold can produce the same mycotoxin (e.g., both *Aspergillus flavus* and several *Penicillium*

Table 30-24
Nitrate and Nitrite Content of Food

VEGETABLES	NITRATE (ppm)	NITRITE (ppm)	MEAT	NITRATE (ppm)	NITRITE (ppm)
Artichoke	12	0.4	Unsmoked side bacon	134	12
Asparagus	44	0.6	Unsmoked back bacon	160	8
Green beans	340	0.6	Peameal bacon	16	21
Lima beans	54	1.1	Smoked bacon	52	7
Beets	2400	4	Corned beef	141	19
Broccoli	740	1	Cured corned beef	852	9
Brussel sprouts	120	1	Corned beef brisket	90	3
Cabbage	520	0.5	Pickled beef	70	23
Carrots	200	0.8	Canned corn beef	77	24
Cauliflower	480	1.1	Ham	105	17
Celery	2300	0.5	Smoked ham	138	50
Corn	45	2	Cured ham	767	35
Radish	1900	0.2	Belitalia (garlic)	247	5
Rhubarb	2100	NR	Pepperoni (beef)	149	23
Spinach	1800	2.5	Summer sausage	135	7
Tomatoes	58	NR	Ukranian sausage (Polish)	77	15
Turnip	390	NR	German sausage	71	17
Turnip greens	6600	2.3			

NR = not reported.
SOURCE: Adapted with permission from Hotchkiss JH, Helser MA, Maragos CM, *et al.*: Nitrate, nitrite, and *N*-nitroso
   compounds: Food safety and biological implications, in Finley JW, Robinson SF, Armstrong DJ (eds.): *Food Safety
   Assessment*. Washington, DC, American Chemical Society, 1992, pp. 400–418.

species produce the mycotoxin cyclopiazonic acid) (El-Banna *et al.*, 1987; Truckness *et al.*, 1987). Also, more than one mycotoxin may be present in an intoxication; that is, as in the outbreak of turkey X disease, there is speculation that aflatoxin and cyclopiazonic acid both exerted an effect, but the profound effects of aflatoxin would have overshadowed those of cyclopiazonic acid (Miller, 1989). Although there are many different mycotoxins and subgroups (Table 30-25), this discussion will be confined largely to six of the more toxicologically and economically important: aflatoxins, trichothecenes, fumonisins, zearalenone, ochratoxin A, and ergot alkaloids.

Organic foods, produced without the use of insecticides and fungicides, may be more susceptible to mycotoxin contamination than foods produced using conventional agricultural practices. The UK Food Standards Agency found several organic maize meal products highly contaminated with fumonisin mycotoxins whereas conventional produced maize meal products analyzed concurrently had levels below recommended limits (UK Food Standards Agency, 2003). Because European agriculture faces a growing demand by consumers for organic produce, the European Union has established a project called "safe organic vegetables and vegetable products by reducing risk factors and sources of fungal contaminants throughout the production chain" focusing on organic carrots and reduction of alternaria toxins (EU, 2002).

Aflatoxins Among the various mycotoxins, the aflatoxins have been the subject of the most intensive research because of the extremely potent hepatocarcinogenicity and toxicity of aflatoxin B_1 in rats. Epidemiological studies conducted in Africa and Asia suggest that it is a human hepatocarcinogen, and various other reports have implicated the aflatoxins in incidences of human toxicity (Krishnamachari *et al.*, 1975; Peers *et al.*, 1976).

Generally, aflatoxins occur in susceptible crops as mixtures of aflatoxins $B_1, B_2, G_1,$ and G_2, with only aflatoxins B_1 and G_1 demonstrating carcinogenicity. A carcinogenic hydroxylated metabolite of aflatoxin B_1 (termed aflatoxin M_1) can occur in the milk from dairy cows that consume contaminated feed. Aflatoxins may occur in a number of susceptible commodities and products derived from them, including edible nuts (peanuts, pistachios, almonds, walnuts, pecans, Brazil nuts), oil seeds (cottonseed, copra), and grains (corn, grain sorghum, millet) (Stoloff, 1977). In tropical regions, aflatoxin can be produced in unrefrigerated prepared foods. The two major sources of aflatoxin contamination of commodities are field contamination, especially during times of drought and other stresses, which allow insect damage that opens the plant to mold attack, and inadequate storage conditions. Since the discovery of their potential threat to human health, progress has been made in decreasing the level of aflatoxins in specific commodities in developed countries. For example, in the United States and Western European countries, control measures include ensuring adequate storage conditions and careful monitoring of susceptible commodities for aflatoxin level and the banning of lots that exceed the action level for aflatoxin B_1.

Aflatoxin B_1 is acutely toxic in all species studied, with an LD_{50} ranging from 0.5 mg/kg for the duckling to 60 mg/kg for the mouse (Wogan, 1973). Death typically results from hepatotoxicity. Aflatoxin B_1 is also highly mutagenic, hepatocarcinogenic, and possibly teratogenic. A problem in extrapolating animal data to humans is the extremely wide range of species susceptibility to aflatoxin B_1. For instance, whereas aflatoxin B_1 appears to be the most hepatocarcinogenic compound known for the rat, the adult mouse is essentially totally resistant to its hepatocarcinogenicity.

Aflatoxin B_1 is an extremely reactive compound biologically, altering a number of biochemical systems. The hepatocarcinogenicity of aflatoxin B_1 is associated with its biotransformation to a highly

Table 30-25

Examples of Selected Mycotoxins Produced by Various Molds and Some of Their Effects and Commodities and Foods that are Potentially Contaminated

MYCOTOXIN	SOURCE	EFFECT	COMMODITIES CONTAMINATED
Aflatoxins B_1, B_2, G_1, G_2	*Aspergillus flavus, A. parasiticus*	Acute aflatoxicosis, carcinogenesis	Corn, peanuts, and others
Aflatoxin M_1	Metabolite of AFB_1	Hepatotoxicity	Milk
Fumonisins B_1, B_2, B_3, B_4, A_1, A_2	*Fusarium verticillioides*	Renal and liver carcinogenesis	Corn
Trichothecenes (for example, T-2, deoxynivalenol, diacetoxyscirpenol)	*Fusarium, myrothecium*	Hematopoietic toxicity, meningeal hemorrhage of brain, "nervous" disorder, necrosis of skin, hemorrhage in mucosal epithelia of stomach and intestine, emesis, feed refusal, immune suppression	Cereal grains, corn
Zearalenones	*Fusarium*	Estrogenic effect	Corn, grain
Cyclopiazonic acid	*Aspergillus, Penicillium*	Muscle, liver, and splenic toxicity	Cheese, grains, peanuts
Kojic acid	*Aspergillus*	Hepatotoxic?	Grain, animal feed
3-Nitropropionic acid	*Arthrinium sacchari, A. saccharicola, A. phaeospermum*	Central nervous system impairment	Sugarcane
Citreoviridin	*Penicillium citreoviride, P. toxicarium*	Cardiac beriberi	Rice
Cytochalasins E, B, F, H	*Aspergillus* and *Penicillium*	Cytotoxicity	Corn, cereal grain
Sterigmatocystin	*Aspergillus versiolar*	Carcinogenesis	Corn
Penicillinic acid	*Penicillium cyclopium*	Nephrotoxicity, abortifacient	Corn, dried beans, grains
Rubratoxins A, B	*Penicillium rubrum*	Hepatotoxicity, teratogenic	Corn
Patulin	*Penicillium patulatum*	Carcinogenesis, liver damage	Apple and apple products
Ochratoxin	*Aspergillus ochraceus, A. carbonarius, Penicillium verrucosum*	Endemic nephropathy, carcinogenesis	Grains, peanuts, grapes, green coffee
Citrinin	*Aspergillus* and *Penicillium*	Nephrotoxicity	Cereal grains
Penitrem(s)		Tremors, incoordination, bloody diarrhea, death	Moldy cream cheese, English walnuts, hamburger bun, beer
Ergot alkaloids	*Clavicepts purpurea*	Ergotism	Grains

reactive electrophilic epoxide, which forms covalent adducts with DNA, RNA, and protein. Damage to DNA is thought to be the initial biochemical lesion resulting in the expression of the pathological tumor growth (IARC, 2002). Species differences in the response to aflatoxin may be due in part to differences in biotransformation and susceptibility to the initial biochemical lesion (Monroe and Eaton, 1987).

Trichothecenes Trichothecenes represent a group of toxic substances in which it is likely that several forms may be consumed concomitantly. They represent many different chemical entities, all containing the trichothecene nucleus, and are produced primarily by *Fusarium*, but also by a number of commonly occurring molds, including *Myrothecium*, *Trichothecium*, *Stachybotrys*, and *Cephalosporium*. The trichothecenes were first discovered during attempts to isolate antibiotics, and although some show antibiotic activity, their toxicity has precluded their use as therapeutic agents. Trichothecenes most often occur in moldy cereal grains. There have been many reported cases of trichothecene toxicity in

farm animals and a few in humans. One of the more famous cases of presumed human toxicity associated with the consumption of trichothecenes occurred in Russia during 1944 around Orenburg, Siberia. Disruption of agriculture caused by World War II resulted in millet, wheat, and barley being overwintered in the field. Consumption of these commodities resulted in vomiting, skin inflammation, diarrhea, and multiple hemorrhages, among other symptoms. About 10% of the population was affected and mortality rates were as high as 60% in some counties (Ueno, 1977; Beardall and Miller, 1994), and was subsequently identified as alimentary toxic aleukia (ATA) (CAST, 2003). Trichothecenes are protein synthesis inhibitors known to bind to ribosomes. The extent of toxicity associated with the trichothecenes in humans and farm animals is poorly understood, owing in part to the number of entities in this group and the difficulty of assaying for these compounds (JECFA, 2001). The acute LD_{50}s of the trichothecenes range from 0.5 to 70 mg/kg, and though there have been reports of possible chronic toxicity associated with certain members of this group, more research will be needed before the magnitude of their potential to produce adverse human health effects is understood (Sato and Ueno, 1977).

Fumonisins Fumonisins are mycotoxins produced by *Fusarium verticillioides* (formerly known as *F. moniliforme*) and several other *Fusarium* species. Corn products contaminated with *F. verticilliodes* are responsible for agriculturally important diseases in horses and swine (ICPS, 2000) and are actively being evaluated to determine how great a threat they pose to public health. Initial evidence of the involvement of *F. verticilliodes* produced toxins in human disease, was reported by Marasas *et al.* (1988), who found that an increased incidence of esophageal cancer was associated with the consumption of contaminated corn (maize) by humans in a region in South Africa. Fumonisins have been associated with cancer, reproductive toxicity (neutral tube defects), and acute disease outbreaks where low-quality corn is consumed on a regular basis (Cousins *et al.*, 2005). Fumonisins target different organs in different species, but the underlying mechanism is a disruption of lipid metabolism by inhibition of ceramide synthetase, an enzyme integral to the formation of complex lipids for use in membranes (ICPS, 2000; IARC, 2002).

Corn borer insect pests cause damage to the developing grain, which enables spores of the toxin-producing fungi, *Fusarium*, to germinate. The fungus then proliferates, which leads to ear and kernel rot and the production of potentially hazardous levels of fumonisins. Corn varieties which express the Bt insecticidal protein recently have been shown to contain significantly reduced levels of fumonisin because the Bt protein significantly reduces corn borer-induced tissue damage in corn products (Munkvold *et al.*, 1997, 1999; Masoero *et al.*, 1999; Hammond *et al.*, 2004; Papst *et al.*, 2005).

Zearalenone Another mycotoxin produced by some *Fusarium* species is zearalenone. It was first discovered during attempts to isolate a chemical from feeds that produced a hyperestrogenic syndrome in swine that was characterized by a swollen and edematous vulva and vaginal prolapse in severe cases (Stob *et al.*, 1962). Zearalenone can occur in corn, barley, wheat, hay, and oats as well as other agricultural commodities (Mirocha *et al.*, 1977). Zearalenone consumption can decrease the reproductive potential of farm animals, especially swine.

Ochratoxin A This mycotoxin is primarily produced by *Aspergillus ochraceous*, *A. carbonarius*, and *Penicillium verrucosum* and human exposure occurs as the result of contamination of small grains (barley, wheat, corn), coffee beans and grapes. The effects of ochratoxin A were discovered as the result of feeding the mycotoxin to pigs, who subsequently drank copious amounts of water, urinated near continuously, and exhibited pain in the area of the kidney. Ochratoxin A is nephrotoxic and carcinogenic in mice and rats. Ochratoxin A is absorbed from the gastrointestinal tract and enters the enterohepatic circulation; it is also absorbed by the proximal and distal tubules of the kidney. It binds tightly to albumin in the blood and can therefore have a very long serum half-life. Epidemiologic evidence indicates nearly half the European population is exposed to ochratoxin A and there is an association of endemic nephropathy and renal tumors in humans in parts of Eastern Europe (CAST, 2003).

Ergot Alkaloids Produced by several species of *Claviceps*, these mycotoxins are divided into four major groups based on chemical structure: (1) clavines, (2) lysergic acids, (3) lysergic acid amides, and (4) ergopeptines. There are two primary types of ergotism of humans, convulsive and gangrenous. Convulsive ergotism is typified by muscle twitching and spasms, changes in mental state, hallucinations, sweating, and fever lasting for several weeks, all suggestive of serotonergic overstimulation of the CNS (Eadie, 2003). Postmortem findings include bleeding and softening of the brain and lesions in the posterior horns of the spinal cord. Full mental recovery from a nonfatal case is rare (Beardall and Miller, 1994). The gangrenous form of ergotism is characterized by edema, pruritis, necrotic extremities, prickling sensations, and severe muscular pain (CAST, 2003), all of which are likely the result of peripheral vasoconstriction.

Solanine and Chaconine The humble potato, *Solanum tuberosum*, may produce toxic steroidal glycoalkaloids if exposed to light in the field or during storage or otherwise stressed by mechanical damage or improper storage or sprouting. Previously known only as "solanine" or now, (total) solanaceous glycoalkaloids (SGA), the major players are α-solanine and α-chaconine and are normally present in amounts of <5 mg/100 g of tuber fresh weight although a normal toxin load in the potatoes of 20–100 mg/kg tuber, is considered safe. The toxins are not affected by baking, frying, or microwave cooking. SGAs inhibit cholinesterases and can alter the effects of neuromuscular blocking drugs and anesthetics (Sorensen, 2002). Low doses of these glycoalkaloids can produce gastrointestinal upset with diarrhea, vomiting, and severe abdominal pain. At higher doses, neurological symptoms are evident with drowsiness and apathy, confusion, weakness, and vision disturbances, followed by loss of consciousness and sometimes, death.

Rodents do not absorb solanines well and the LD_{50} is >1000 mg/kg in mice and 590 in the rat; values that are 300–500 times more than the toxic dose of 2 mg/kg in humans and, in which, the estimated lethal dose may be as little as 3–6 mg/kg. There was thought to be an association of potato (and SGA) consumption with neural tube defects in children, although prospective studies have not borne out this hypothesis, nor has this effect been seen in animal testing (ICPS, 1993).

In the 1960s, a scientist bred a new variety of potato, crossing a Delta Gold with a wild type from Peru. The new variety called "Lenape" was excellent for making potato chips and was tested as a "new potato" for roasting with meats and vegetables. Upon eating the potato however, the grower was sickened and upon analysis, the potato was found to have high levels of glycoalkaloids. As a product of the breeding process, the gene for glycoalkaloids was stimulated to produce a high level of SGA. Immediately, all the seed potato growers were contacted and stocks were recalled or destroyed (Fedoroff and Brown, 2004).

Ethyl Carbamate Ethyl carbamate or urethane, the ethyl ester of carbamic acid, was used for many years as an intravenous anesthetic until its mutagenic and carcinogenic properties became known. It has since been classified by the International Agency for Research on Cancer (IARC) as "possibly carcinogenic to humans" (Group 2B) and "reasonably anticipated to be a human carcinogen" by the National Toxicology Program (NTP, 2004a). The primary use of urethane is as a chemical intermediate in the preparation of amino resins, with lesser uses as a solubilizer in the manufacture of pesticides, fumigants, and cosmetics and as an intermediate for pharmaceuticals and biochemical research. It is allowed in some anticonvulsant drugs at a level of 1 ppm and is still used as a veterinary anesthetic. Urethane has been found in fermented foods and beverages including liquor, wine, beer, bread, soy sauce, and yogurt. Diethylpyrocarbonate, an inhibitor of fermentation, can form ethyl carbamate.

Ethyl carbamate is easily absorbed and undergoes CYP2E1-mediated metabolic activation to vinyl carbamate epoxide, which binds covalently to nucleic acids and proteins, producing adducts. Ethyl carbamate is a multisite carcinogen with a short latency period. Single doses or short-term oral dosing at 100–200 mg/kg BW/d has been shown to induce tumors in mice, rats, and hamsters. Intake estimates from food and alcoholic beverages range from a mean of 0.015 µg/kg BW/d to 0.080 µg/kg BW/d for high-end users. The BMDL (benchmark dose lower confidence limit) as set by JECFA is 0.3 mg/kg BW/d, which yields a margin of safety of 20,000 (JECFA, 2005).

Trans Fatty Acids *Trans* fatty acids, also known as *trans* fat, are made through the process of hydrogenation of unsaturated bonds that solidifies (liquid) oils. Hydrogenation increases the melting point, shelf life, and flavor stability of these oils and foods that contain them. The hydrogenation process was developed in the 1930s and has been in widespread commercial use since the 1940s. Dietary fats containing hydrogenated fatty acids, such as those used in margarine, have gradually displaced animal fats, such as butter and lard. *Trans* fat is found in vegetable shortenings, and in some margarines, crackers, cookies, snack foods, and other foods. The scientific literature is replete with studies indicating that consumption of *trans* fatty acids contributes to increased blood LDL-cholesterol ("bad" cholesterol) levels, which increase the risk of coronary heart disease (CHD). Recent information from the American Heart Association indicates that CHD causes about 500,000 deaths annually, making it the number one cause of death in the United States (FDA, 1999a,b). To remedy this problem, it is now required to label foods indicating the amount of *trans* fat present.

Furan Furan was once known only as an industrial chemical intermediate in the synthesis of polymers used to prepare temperature-resistant structural laminates and to prepare copolymers used in machine dishwashing products. Furan has recently been found to occur in a number of foods that undergo heat treatment, such as canned and jarred foods, including baby food. It is considered by IARC (1995) to be possibly carcinogenic to humans. According to the NTP, furan is hepatotoxic and shows clear evidence of carcinogenicity to both sexes and both species of mice and rats (NTP, 1993). Furan is produced in a variety of experimental systems, including heating of sugars (e.g. glucose, lactose, fructose, xylose, rhamnose), heating sugars in the presence of amino acids or protein (e.g., alanine, cysteine, casein), and thermal degradation of vitamins (ascorbic acid, dehydroascorbic acid, thiamin) (FDA, 2004).

Furan has been found in a small number of heat-treated foods, including coffee, canned meat, baked bread, cooked chicken, sodium caseinate, filberts (hazelnuts), soy protein isolate, hydrolyzed soy protein, rapeseed protein, fish protein concentrate, and caramel (FDA, 2004). Very little information has been developed on furan levels in food.

Dinoflagellate Poisoning (Paralytic Shellfish Poisoning or PSP; Saxitoxin) In contrast to other seafood toxins, there is a tolerance set for PSP. The etiologic agent in this type of poisoning is saxitoxin or related compounds and is found in mussels, cockles, clams, soft shell clams, butter clams, scallops, and shellfish broth. Bivalve mussels are the most common vehicles. Saxitoxin, originally isolated from toxic Alaskan butter clams (*Saxidomus giganticus*) is actually a family of neurotoxins and includes neosaxitin and gonyautoxins 1 through 4. All block neural transmission at the neuromuscular junction by binding to the surface of the sodium channels and interrupting the flow of Na^+ ions; AV nodal conduction may be suppressed, there may be direct suppression of the respiratory center and progressive reduction of peripheral nerve excitability. The toxin produces parathesia and neuromuscular weakness without hypotension and lacks the emetic and hypothermic action of tetrodotoxin. Moderate symptoms are produced by 120–180 µg/person and are reversible within hours or days, whereas 80 µg of purified toxin per 100 g of tissue (0.5–2 mg/person) may be lethal, due to asphyxiation, usually within 12 hours of ingestion. The toxin is an alkaloid and is relatively heat stable. The toxin is produced by several genera of plankton (*Gonyaulax* (now known as *Alexandrium*) *catenella*, *G. acatenella*, and *G. tamarensis*, *Pyrodinium* spp., *Ptychodiscus brevis*, *Gymnodinium catenaturm* and others), and during red tide blooms may reach 20 million to 40 million per milliliter. Toxic materials are stored in various parts of the body of shellfish. Digestive organs, liver, gills, and siphons contain the greatest concentrations of poison during the warmer months. Distribution is worldwide (Bryan, 1984; Clark *et al.*, 1999; Liston, 2000). The tolerance for PSP for clams, mussels, and oysters is 80 µg/100 g of meat (Compliance Policy Guideline, 540.250).

Added Substances—Fluoride Fluorine, in the form of fluoride, is nearly ubiquitous in nature. Primary human exposure is via drinking water, although it is also present in some foods, notably some teas, vegetables, and marine fish. Exposure also occurs via processed food made with fluoridated water or produce washed with fluoridated water (the so-called 'halo' effect). The greatest nondietary source is fluoridated toothpaste (NRC, 2006). Fluoride taken in water has a high degree of bioavailability with an absorption of 90% and with food, approximately 50%. Consumption of fluoride results in uptake by bone and in teeth, where enamel crystallites form fluorhydroxyapatite in place the naturally formed hydroxyapatite; the former being stronger and more acid resistant than the latter, resisting and even reversing the initiation and progression of dental caries. Ionic fluoride rarely exists in blood, most is trapped by bone tissue, where new bone growth is stimulated and this mechanism has served as the basis of some treatments for osteoporosis (WHO, 1996).

Fluorosis occurs as the result of high fluoride intake and may be complicated by low calcium intake; it is cumulative and endemic to some areas of the world (e.g., China and India). Fluorosis is dose responsive, producing a range of effects from cosmetic (mottling of teeth) to adverse functionality (skeletal fluorosis). Enamel fluorosis occurs as the result of high fluoride consumption prior to tooth eruption (i.e., in children up to the age of eight years, exposed to water with a fluoride content of ≥ 4 mg/L) and can range from a mild discoloration of the tooth surface to severe (brown) staining and pitting of the teeth to the point of enamel loss (NRC, 2006). In skeletal fluorosis, in the asymptomatic, preclinical stage, patients have an increased bone density. Stage 1 skeletal fluorosis is characterized by occasional stiffness, pain in joints or some osteosclerosis of the pelvis and vertebra. Stage 2 skeletal fluorosis is characterized by sporadic pain, stiffness of joints and osteosclerosis of the pelvis and spine, although mobility is not severely affected. In Stage 3 (rarely seen in the U.S.), there may be crippling, dose-related calcification of ligaments, osteosclerosis, exotoses, osteoporosis of long bones, muscle wasting, and neurological effects due to hypercalcification of vertebrae (at this point, bone ash fluoride may be 2–3 times that of the bones of normal subjects). While it is agreed that skeletal fluorosis is the result of prolonged exposure to increased amounts of fluoride, because the incidence of crippling skeletal fibrosis continues to be rare even in geographic areas of high exposure, unidentified intervening metabolic or dietary factors may have rendered skeletons more or less susceptible. Other effects attributed to excess fluoride include lower IQ's and decreased thyroid function, increased calcitonin activity, increased parathyroid hormone activity, secondary hyperparathyroidism, impaired glucose tolerance and possible effects on timing of sexual activity (NRC, 2006). The reports of possible carcinogenic effects of fluoride are mixed and inconclusive.

Guidelines for fluoridation of the public water supply recommend addition at levels of 0.7–1.2 mg/L, to achieve target Adequate Intake levels based on a 2 L water/day intake by adults; with adjustments in warmer regions where water intake is high in the summer months, or where fluoride occurs naturally at high levels (e.g., some areas of Colorado, 11.2 mg/L; Oklahoma, 12.0 mg/L; New Mexico, 13.0 mg/L; and Idaho, 15.9 mg/L). Although the essentiality of fluorine has not been described, an Adequate Intake (AI) has been established for various age groups as a balance between caries resistance and possible fluorosis of teeth. For example, the AI for infants at 0.01 mg/d, for adult females and males at 3 and 4 mg/d, respectively and, a range of graduated AI's for intervening age groups (IOM, 1997).

SUBSTANCES FOR WHICH TOLERANCES MAY NOT BE SET

All the contaminants of food described to this point are those associated with synthesis, growth, production, or storage and are regarded by FDA as *unavoidable*. Because they are unavoidable, the FDA sets limits rather than bans them, as described earlier. The substances in this section are regarded as (1) *avoidable* or of such hazard that a safe level cannot be set and as such, FDA has determined that food containing such substances is banned or; (2) are beyond the control of FDA and cannot be regulated (e.g., substances produced in the home).

Toxins in Fish, Shellfish, and Turtles

There are a number of seafood toxins (to be distinguished from marine venoms), many of which are not confined to a single species (over 400 species have been incriminated in ciguatera toxicity) and are therefore most likely to be influenced by the environment. However, some seafood toxins are specific to a single species or genus. A complicating factor in the study of seafood toxins is the sporadic frequency and nonpredictability of the presence of the toxin.

Seafood toxins generally can be classified according to the location of the poison. For example, (1) ichthyosarcotoxin is concentrated in the muscles, skin, liver, or intestines or is otherwise not associated with the reproductive system or circulatory system, (2) ichthyootoxin is associated with reproductive tissue, (3) ichthyohemotoxin is confined to the circulatory system, and (4) ichthyohepatotoxin is confined to the liver. In general, seafood toxins under FDA

policy have a zero tolerance, with any detectable level considered cause for regulatory action.

Neurotoxic Shellfish Poisoning (NSP)   Traditionally limited to the coast of Florida, *Gymnodinium breve* form red tide blooms containing polycyclic ether toxins called brevetoxins (based on the backbone structure of the molecule generally divided into Type 1 or Type 2), with Type 2 the most often found. Brevetoxins bind to voltage-dependent sodium channels and strength of binding varies with the specific affinity of the toxin and thus the relative potency. Symptoms of NSP include nausea, tingling, and numbness of the oral area, loss of motor control and severe muscular ache; all of which resolve in a few days and no deaths have been reported, unlike PSP. An additional route of entry for mammals may result from inhalation of aerosolized toxin as the result of the relative ease of lysis of the unarmored *G. breve* organism during the breaking of waves on the shore. Symptoms of this type of exposure are seen as irritation of the throat and upper respiratory tract. A "kill" of nearly 150 manatees was reported during an unprecedented large outbreak of the toxin, although the specific mode of transmission is uncertain. Human exposure is primarily via consumption of filter-feeding organisms, which may concentrate the toxin (Van Dolah, 2000).

Amnesic Shellfish Poisoning (Domoic Acid)   Consumption of mussels harvested from the area off Prince Edward Island in 1987 resulted in gastroenteritis and many older consumers or those with underlying chronic diseases, experienced neurologic symptoms including memory loss. Despite treatment, three patients (71–84 years old) died within 11–24 days. The poisoning was attributed to domoic acid produced by the diatom *Nitzschia pungens* f. *multiseries* (now called *Pseudonitzschia multiseries*) which had been ingested by the mussels during the normal course of feeding. Occurrence of domoic acid has also been reported in California shellfish and produced by *N. pseudodelicatissima* and in anchovies (resulting in pelican deaths) produced by *N. pseudoseriata* (now called *Pseudonitzchia australis*). Domoic acid has been reported in shellfish in other provinces of Canada, Alaska, Washington, and Oregon and may be as frequent as PSP toxins. Domoic acid has also been reported in seaweed. Domoic acid was reported in Japan in 1958 and was isolated from the red algae *Chondria armata*.

In the Canadian outbreak, mice injected with extracts (as in the PSP assay) died within 3.5 hours. The mice exhibited a scratching syndrome uniquely characteristic of domoic acid that was followed by increasingly uncoordinated movements and seizures until the mice died. Levels of domoic acid >40 μg/g wet weight of mussel meat caused the mouse symptoms (Canadian authorities require cessation of harvesting when levels approach 20 μg/g). Mice and rats can generally tolerate 30–50 mg/kg. Domoic acid is dose-responsive in humans: with no effect at 0.2–0.3 mg/kg, mild gastrointestinal symptoms at 0.9–2.0 mg/kg, and the most serious symptoms at 1.9–4.2 mg/kg with gastrointestinal effects and neurological effects, including dizziness, disorientation, lethargy, seizures, and permanent loss of short-term memory. Although rodents appear to be more tolerant, the fatalities in humans were likely associated with underlying illness. Domoic acid is an analog of glutamine, a neurotransmitter and of kainic acid; the toxicity of all three are similar as they are excitatory and act on three types of receptors in the CNS with the hippocampus being the most sensitive. Domoic acid may be a more potent activator of kainic acid receptors than kainic acid itself.

The stimulatory action may lead to extensive damage of the hip-pocampus, but less severe injury to the thalamic and forebrain regions (Todd, 1993; Clark *et al.*, 1999; Van Dolah, 2000).

Ciguatera Poisoning The "cigua" in ciguatera toxin is derived from the Spanish name for the sea snail *Turbo pica* in which the symptoms were first reported. Ciguatera and related toxins (scaritoxin and maitotoxin) are ichthyosarcotoxic neurotoxins (anticholinesterase) and are found in 11 orders, 57 families, and over 400 species of fish as well as in oysters and clams. The penultimate toxin (gambiertoxin) is produced by the dinoflagellate *Gambierdiscus toxicus*, commonly isolated from microalgae growing on or near coral reefs that have ingested the dinoflagellate. The pre-toxin appears to pass through the food chain and is biotransformed upon transfer to or by the ingesting fish to the active, which is consumed by mammals. Other toxins, including palytoxin and okadaic acid, unrelated to gambiertoxin, may be present in ciguarteric fish and may contribute to toxicity. The asymptomatic period is 3–5 hours after consumption but may last up to 24 hours. The onset is sudden, and symptoms may include abdominal pain, nausea, vomiting, and watery diarrhea; muscular aches; tingling and numbness of the lips, tongue, and throat; a metallic taste; temporary blindness; and paralysis. Deaths have occurred. Recovery usually occurs within 24 hours, but tingling may continue for a week or more. The intraperitoneal (i.p.) LD_{50} of maitotoxin in mice is 50 ng/kg (Bryan, 1984; Liston, 2000).

Palytoxin Poisoning Palytoxin is produced by the zoanthind soft coral of the genus *Palythoa*, and fish, crabs, and polychaete worms living in close association with or eating this mass, may become contaminated with palytoxin. The toxin is not part of the stinging nematocyst of the coral, but may be produced by female polyps and mature eggs of the organism, possibly requiring the presence of an unidentified symbiotic algae (possibly the dinoflagellate *Ostreopsis siamensis*). Palytoxin, in various forms, is produced by any number of species, including *P. tuberculosa* in the tropical waters in the Pacific and Japan, *P. mammilosa* and *P. caribaeorum* in the West Indies, Puerto Rico, and the Bahamas, *P. vestitus* and other *Palythoa* spp. On occasion, the coral becomes detached from its anchorage and becomes a soft floating mass with a seaweed or moss-like appearance, a very attractive feeding ground for fish. Indigenous peoples of Hawaii knew this as *limu-make-o-Hana* (the deadly seaweed of Hana) and some are said to have smeared the moss on spear points to enhance their utility as a weapon (Onuma *et al.*, 1999; Tan and Lau, 2000; Tosteson, 2000).

The toxin has been reported in mackerel, parrotfish, and several species of crabs. Victims report a bitter, metallic taste from the meat (most often muscle, liver, ovary, and digestive tract), followed immediately by nausea, vomiting, and diarrhea. Within several hours, symptoms include myoglobinuria, a burning sensation around the mouth and extremities, muscle spasms, dyspnea, and dysphonia. Cause of death may be the result of mycocardial injury, although it is known in vitro to be a powerful hemolysin.

Although there are several isoforms and possibly minor toxins associated with palytoxin (depending on the producing species), the predominant action is as a oubain-sensitive Na^+K^+-ATPase inhibitor. Unlike oubain, palytoxin has no effect on H^+-, Ca^{2+}-, or H^+/K^+-transporting ATPases. The toxin is quite effective with intravenous LD_{50}s of 0.078, 0.45, 0.033, and 0.089 µg/kg for monkeys, mice, dogs, and rats, respectively. The standard assay is measured in mouse units (MU), the time taken to kill a mouse weighing 20 grams in 4 hours following intraperitoneal (i.p.) injection of 0.25 mL (Tan and Lau, 2000; Tosteson, 2000).

Puffer Fish Poisoning (Tetrodotoxin) *Tetrodon* or puffer fish poisoning is caused by the improper preparation and consumption of any of about 90 species of puffer fish (fugu, blowfish, globefish, porcupine fish, molas, burrfish, balloonfish, toadfish, etc.); although the toxin has also been reported present in newts, frogs, octopus, starfish, flatworms, various crabs, and gastropods. Pufferfish are found in subtropical and tropical marine waters in the Atlantic (including off the coast of Florida), Pacific, and Indian Oceans. Some puffers live in brackish and fresh water. The toxin (tetrodotoxin) is located in nearly all the tissues, but the ovaries, roe, liver, intestines, and skin are the most toxic. Toxicity is highest during the spawning period, although a species may be toxic in one location but not in another. Tetrodotoxin is associated with the presence of several bacteria on and in fish and shellfish and is an evolutionary advantage providing protection against predators (i.e., they are *endosymbiotic* bacteria). A total of 21 species can produce tetrodotoxins including *Vibros*, *Pseudomonas*, and *E. coli*, and at least two strains of red algae.

Tetrodotoxin is a neurotoxin and causes paralysis of the central nervous system and peripheral nerves by blocking the movement of all monovalent cations. The toxin is water-soluble and is stable to boiling except in an alkaline solution. A fatal dose may be as little as 1–4 mg/person. The victim is asymptomatic for 10–45 minutes but may have a reprieve for as long as 3 or more hours. Toxicity is manifested as a tingling or prickly sensation of the fingers and toes; malaise; dizziness; pallor; numbness of the lips, tongue, and extremities; ataxia; nausea, vomiting, and diarrhea; epigastric pain; dryness of the skin; subcutaneous hemorrhage and desquamation; respiratory distress; muscular twitching, tremor, incoordination, and muscular paralysis; and intense cyanosis. Fatality rates are high (Bryan, 1984; Liston, 2000).

Moray Eel Poisoning Although the moray eel (*Gymnothorax javanicus*) and other carnivorous fishes may accumulate ciguatoxin as the result of eating other contaminated fish, the Indo-Pacific moray eel (*Lycodontis nudivomer*) has been shown to possess a mucous skin secretion with hemolytic, toxic and hemagglutinating properties, unrelated to ciguatoxin. The hemolytic properties can be separated from the hemagglutinating properties. The hemolytic property is lost upon treatment with trypsin and is unstable in the presence of heat, acidic or alkaline media (Randall *et al.*, 1981). The skin mucous of other species of eels, the common European eel (*Anguilla anguilla*) and pike eel (*Muraenesox cinereus*) were found to have proteinaceous toxins, immunologically similar to that of the skin mucous toxin from the Japanese eel (*Anguilla japonica*) (Shiomi *et al.*, 1994).

Abalone Poisoning (Pyropheophorbide) Abalone poisoning is caused by abalone viscera poison (located in the liver and digestive gland) and is unusual in that it causes photosensitization. The toxin, pyropheophorbide a, is stable to boiling, freezing, and salting. It is found in Japanese abalone, *Haliotis discus* and *H. sieboldi*. The development of symptoms is contingent on exposure to sunlight. The symptoms are of sudden onset and include a burning and stinging sensation over the entire body, a prickling sensation, itching, erythema, edema, and skin ulceration on parts of the body exposed to sunlight (Bryan, 1984; Shiomi, 1999). Paralytic shellfish toxin

(PST) has been detected in abalone, probably through consumption of the mossworm, a plankton feeder that also clings to seaweed and some shellfish (Takatani *et al.*, 1997).

Sea Urchin Poisoning The etiologic agent forms during the reproductive season and is confined to the gonads. The sea urchins involved include *Paracentrotus lividus*, *Tripneustes ventricosus*, and *Centrechinus antillarum*. The symptoms include abdominal pain, nausea, vomiting, diarrhea, and migraine-like attacks (Bryan, 1984). The toxin has been shown to interfere with calcium uptake in nerve preparations (Zhang *et al.*, 1998).

Sea Turtle Poisoning (Chelonitoxin) The etiologic agent here is chelonitoxin, which is found in the liver (greatest concentration) but also in the flesh, fat, viscera, and blood. Toxicity is described as sporadic or even seasonal, indicating the poison may be derived from toxic marine algae. Most outbreaks occur in the Indo-Pacific region. The turtles involved include the green sea turtle, the hawksbill and leatherback turtles. Local custom in Sri Lanka is to first offer the liver to crows and if the birds eat it, the flesh is regarded as safe, but because the symptoms appear over a few hours to several days, this bioassay requires patience. Symptoms of intoxication in humans include vomiting; diarrhea; sore lips, tongue, and throat; foul breath, difficulty in swallowing; a white coating on the tongue, which may become covered with pin-sized, pustular papules; tightness of the chest; coma; and death. The toxin has been reported transferred to nursing infants from intoxicated mothers. Post-mortem examinations reveal congestion of internal organs, interstitial pulmonary edema, and necrosis of myocardial fibers. Fatality rates of 7% and 25% have been reported (Bryan, 1984; Ariyananda and Fernando, 1987; Chandrasiri *et al.*, 1988; Champetier De Ribes *et al.*, 1997).

Haff Disease Haff disease is a syndrome of unknown etiology following consumption of certain types of fish found in both salt and fresh water. The syndrome consists of rhabdomyolysis with a release of muscle cell contents into the blood. Patients are often rigid, sensitive to touch and unable to move; urine may have a dark brown color. Symptoms appear 18 hours (with a range of 6–21 hours) after consumption; symptoms resolve within 2–3 days and the fatality rate is approximately 1% (Frenzen, 2004). "Haff disease" was first reported in the 1920s along the Koenigsberg Haff, a brackish inlet on the Baltic sea, although outbreaks have been reported in Sweden, the former Soviet Union and in the United States beginning in 1984. U.S. poisonings have been associated with buffalo fish (*Ictiobus cyprnellus*) caught in California, Missouri, and Louisiana. No etiologic agent has been identified (Anonymous, 1998).

Microbiological Agents—Preformed Bacterial Toxins

Although the United States likely has the safest and cleanest food supply in the world, most food-related illness in the United States results from microbial contamination. Food-borne disease outbreaks are tracked by the Centers for Disease Control and Prevention (CDC) in Atlanta, Georgia. The CDC reports that there are approximately 400 outbreaks of food-borne disease per year involving 10,000–20,000 people. However, the actual frequency may be as much as 10–200 times as high because (1) an outbreak is classified as such only when the source can be identified as affecting two or more people and (2) most home poisonings are mild or have a long incubation time

and are therefore not connected to the ingested food, go unreported and are often felt to be only a "24-hour bug." Naturally, because of differences in virulence and opportunity, some species are more likely than others to cause outbreaks.

If all the microbiological food-borne health concerns could be divided into two categories—*poisonings* and *infections*—the former would include chemical poisonings and intoxications, which may have a plant, animal, or microbial origin. In the infections category, food acts as a vector for organisms that exhibit their pathogenicity once they have multiplied inside the body. Infections include the two subcategories: enterotoxigenic infections (with the release of toxins following colonization of the GI tract) and invasive infections in which the GI tract is penetrated and the body is invaded by organisms.

There are a number of food toxins of microbial origin; however, discussion in this chapter will be limited to pre-formed bacterial toxins—that is, those toxins elaborated by bacteria concomitant to their residence and growth in or on the food *prior* to ingestion. Importantly, the bacteria need not be present for the intoxication to take place because the bacteria may have been killed by heat while the toxin survives. Bacterial toxins may be divided on the basis of activity: *emetic toxins* (i.e., *Bacillus cereus*), which produce their effect by binding to specific receptors in the duodenum, *neurotoxins* (whose action is self explanatory) and, *enterotoxins*, which are protein toxins having action on the *enteric* cells of the intestine. Enterotoxins can be subdivided into cytotoxic enterotoxins which disrupt the cell membrane or other vital functions of the cell and cytotonic enterotoxins, which enter the epithelial cell and cause diarrhea without direct membrane disruption or cell death (Granum, 2006). Bacterial toxins may also be divided on the basis of their origin: an *endotoxin* is generally a lipopolysaccharide membrane constituent released from a dead or dying Gram-negative bacteria, these toxins are nonspecific and stimulate inflammatory responses from macrophages including, but not limited to prostaglandins, thromboxanes, interleukins, and other mediators of immunity; *exotoxins* which are synthesized and released (usually by Gram-positive bacteria) and are not an integral part of the organism, but may enhance its virulence. Some bacteria, such as *Shigella* spp., *Staphylococcus aureus*, or *Escherichia coli* (which releases the shiga-like vero toxin), can elaborate both endotoxin and exotoxin.

Clostridium Botulinum, C. butyricum and C. baratti Food botulism rarely causes illness because the confluence of conditions required for its germination and toxin production—low acidity, high water activity, absence of preservatives, ambient temperature, and anaerobic environment—such a combination rarely occurs in foods, but botulinum poisoning remains important, the result of its potency (Sobel *et al.*, 2004). All *Clostridia* are Gram-positive, spore-forming anaerobes. Botulism is a product of the toxins: A (the predominant form in the U.S.), B (the predominant form in Europe), E (the predominant form in Northern latitudes), and F that may be produced by one or more strains of *C. botulinum*, *C. butyricum* (Type E only) and *C. baratti*; toxins C and D cause botulism in animals. Type G has not caused any human cases. *C. botulinum* toxins are categorized as Group I to IV on the basis of toxin produced; additionally, Group I is proteolytic in culture (liquefying egg white, gelatin, and other solid proteins). The toxin is elaborated in foods, wounds, and infant gut and is neurotoxic, interfering with acetylcholine at peripheral nerve endings. Botulinum neurotoxins induce blockage of voluntary motor and autonomic cholinergic neuromuscular junctions, which prevents motor fiber stimulation. Clinical illness is characterized by cranial nerve palsies, followed by descending flaccid muscle paralysis, which can involve the muscles of respiration. Although ptosis and dysarthria may be mistaken for signs of encephalopathy, patients are fully alert, and the results of a sensory examination are normal. Recovery often takes weeks to months (Sobel *et al.*, 2004). Although the spores are among the most heat-resistant, the toxins are heat-labile (the toxin may be rendered harmless at 80–100°C for 5–10 minutes). Botulinum toxins are large zinc-metalloproteins of ~150,000 Da, composed of two parts, a 50,000 Da piece, the catalytic subunit and the 100,000 Da piece containing an N-terminal translocation domain and a C-terminal binding domain. The structural features are similar to tetanus toxin. For Types B, D, F, and G (and tetanus toxin), the target protein is VAMP/synaptobrevin, a protein associated with the synaptic vesicle. Types A and E cleave a protein associated with the presynaptic membrane, ANAP25. Botulinum toxin C cleaves SNAP25 and syntaxin, another protein involved in exocytosis. Although intracellular mechanisms of botulinum and tetanus toxins are similar, symptoms are different because different populations of neurons are targeted. The symptoms may include respiratory distress and respiratory paralysis that may persist for 6–8 months. The case fatality rate in the United States is 4% (Sobel *et al.*, 2004) and the poison is fatal in 3–10 days; a lethal dose is approximately one nanogram.

Current methods for detecting botulinum toxin include a mouse bioassay and an enzyme-linked immunosorbent assay (ELISA). The mouse bioassay is the accepted standard, where the mouse is injected with a lethal dose, the signs of which should develop in 8 hours and, if not, the mouse is observed for 4 days. The mouse bioassay can also be used to differentiate between the toxin types by mixing neutralizing antibodies with the sample, prior to injection. Determining which mice survive following which combination of toxin and antisera, determines the specific toxin type. The absolute amount of toxin detected in the mouse bioassay is not well defined but is thought to be 10–20 pg/mL for type A (Barr *et al.*, 2005).

Sources and reservoirs for *Clostridia* include soil, mud, water, and the intestinal tracts of animals. Foods associated with botulinum toxin include improperly canned low-acid foods (green beans, corn, beets, asparagus, chili peppers, mushrooms, spinach, figs, baked potato, cheese sauce, beef stew, olives, and tuna). The toxin also may occur in smoked fish, fermented food (seal flippers, salmon eggs) and improperly home-cured hams. An increasing source of poisonings is from the use of flavored oils or oil infusion, most typically in garlic-in-oil preparations; in 1993, FDA required acidification of such preparations to prevent the growth of *Clostridia*. Whereas a proteolytic strain of *C. botulinum* (Group I) may cause the food to appear and smell "spoiled" (by-products include isobutyric acid, isovaleric acid, and phenylpropionic acid), this is not the case with nonproteolytic strains, many of which can flourish and elaborate toxin at temperatures as low as 3°C (Loving, 1998; Belitz and Grosch, 1999; Crane, 1999; Lund and Peck, 2000).

The successful use of nitrates in meat to prevent spoilage by *C. botulinum* resulted in the petitioning of FDA by the USDA to have sodium and potassium nitrate approved for addition by "prior sanction" (21 CFR 181.33). The mechanism of nitrates is believed to be due to an inactivation by nitric oxide of iron–sulfur proteins such as ferrodoxin and pyruvate oxidoreductase within the germinated cells. The activity is dependent on the pH and is proportional to the level of free HNO_2; 100 mg nitrate/kg of meat is necessary for the antimicrobial effect, although this effect can be enhanced with ascorbates and chelating agents. Other antibacterials that prevent *C. botulinum* include nisin (used in cheese spreads), parabens, phenolic antioxidants, polyphosphates, and carbon dioxide (Belitz and Grosch, 1999; Lund and Peck, 2000).

Clostridium perfringens Unlike *C. botulinum*, the primary reservoir for *C. perfringens* is the intestinal tract of warm-blooded animals (including humans). Most incidences of *C. perfringens* food poisoning are associated with the consumption of roasted meat that has been contaminated with intestinal contents at slaughter, followed by roasting and inadequate storage, allowing *C. perfringens* growth and enterotoxin (CPE) to be elaborated (although some CPE may actually be released during a "second sporulation" process in the stomach of the victim). Virtually all food poisoning is produced by type A strain, although a particularly severe form (a necrotic enteritis called "pig-bel" among indigenous peoples of the New Guinea highlands or in Germany known as "Darmbrand") and is produced by type C strain, which has a mortality rate of 15–25% even with treatment. The toxin is normally trypsin sensitive, but people with low intakes of protein or who consume trypsin-inactivating foods (e.g., sweet potatoes) are more at risk than carnivorous people with normal trypsin levels (Granum and Brynestad, 1999; Granum, 2006).

CPE is enterotoxic and follows an ordered series of events, first causing cellular ion permeability, followed by macromolecular (DNA, RNA) synthesis inhibition, morphologic alteration, cell lysis, and villi tip desquamation and severe fluid loss. This is manifested by abdominal cramping and diarrhea occurs within 8–16 hours, although symptoms are of short duration, one day or less. Foods associated with *C. perfringens* poisoning include cooked meat or poultry, gravy, stew, and meat pies. *C. perfringens* is also associated with the production of another 11 toxins, including those associated with gas gangrene (Hobbs *et al.*, 1953; Hauschild, 1971; Walker, 1975; Hobbs, 1976; Crane, 1999; Labbe, 2000).

Bacillus cereus *Bacillus cereus* is also a Gram-positive, spore-forming rod, but is an aerobe. *Bacillus cereus* is a causative agent of emetic or diarrheagenic exo- and enterotoxins elaborated in food. The emetic thermostable toxin (surviving 259°F for 90 minutes) is called cerulide (a small cyclic peptide, 1.2 kDa that acts on 5-HT$_3$ receptors stimulating the vagus afferent nerve) and is produced by serotypes 1, 3, and 8; it is also resistant to pH and proteolysis, but is not antigenic. The diarrheagenic thermolabile toxin (133°F for 20 minutes), is produced by serotypes 1, 2, 6, 8, 10, and 19; and may also be produced in situ in the lower intestine of the host. The diarrheal form may actually consist of three toxins, one of which is hemolytic (Granum, 2006). Reservoirs are soil and dust. Foods associated with this organism and its toxic properties, include boiled and fried rice (principally the emetic form), while the diarrheal form has a wider occurrence and may be found in meats, stews, pudding, sauces, dairy products, vegetable dishes, soups, and meat loaf (Goepfert *et al.*, 1972; Gilbert, 1979; Bryan, 1984; Crane, 1999; Granum and Lund, 1997). The foods associated with the two types somewhat reflect the geographic distribution of the types, as the emetic type predominates in Japan, while in North America and Europe, the diarrhea type is most often seen.

Evidence is accumulating that other species of *Bacillus* may elaborate food toxins, including *Bacillus thurigensis*, *B. subtilis*, *B. licheniformis*, and *B. pumilis* (Crane, 1999; Granum and Baird-Parker, 2000; Granum, 2006).

Staphylococcus aureus Staphylococcal intoxication includes staphyloenterotoxicosis and staphylococcus food poisoning. *S. aureus* produces a wide variety of exoproteins, including toxic shock syndrome toxin-1 (TSST-1), the exfoliative toxins ETA and ETB, leukociden and the staphylococcal enterotoxins (SEA, SEB, SECn,[19] SED, SEE, SEG, SHE, and SEI). TSST-1 and the staphylococcal enterotoxins (SE) are also known as pyrogenic toxin superantigens (PTSAgs) on the basis of their biological characteristics. There is a relatively wide degree of molecular diversity among SE toxins and this is thought to be the result of adaptation to allow for a broad range of potential hosts (Monday and Bohach, 1999). Some, but not all, SE require Zn^{++} for superantigen activity. Although enterotoxemia only develops from ingestion of large amounts of SE, emesis is produced as the result of stimulation of the putative SE receptors in the abdominal viscera, following which is a cascade of inflammatory mediator release. All the SE toxins share a number of properties: an ability to cause emesis and gastroenteritis in primates, superantigenicity, intermediate resistance to heat and pepsin digestion, and tertiary structural similarity, including an intramolecular disulfide bond. Induction of emesis separates the SE toxins from TSST-1, but the induction of emesis is not directly correlated to superantigen activity (Granum, 2006). The exact link between superantigenicity and lethality by the SE toxins and TSST-1 is not known, but may be dependent upon cytotoxicity for certain cells, possibly in the kidneys, liver, or vascular endothelium (Monday and Bohach, 1999). Sources of *Staphylococcus* include nose and throat discharges, hands and skin, infected cuts, wounds, burns, boils, pimples, acne, and feces. The anterior nares of humans are the primary reservoirs. Other reservoirs include mastitic udders of cows and ewes (responsible for contamination of unpasteurized milk); and arthritic and bruised tissues of poultry. Foods usually are contaminated after cooking by persons cutting, slicing, chopping, or otherwise handling them and then keeping them at room temperature for several hours or storing them in large containers. Foods associated with staphylococcal poisoning include cooked ham; meat products, including poultry and dressing; sauces and gravy; cream-filled pastry; potatoes; ham; poultry; fish salads; milk; cheese; bread pudding; and generally high protein leftover foods (Cohen, 1972; Bryan, 1976, 1984; Minor and Marth, 1976; Crane, 1999; Dinges *et al.*, 2000).

Escherichia coli Although *E. coli* does not produce a pre-formed toxin, it deserves mention because of the overwhelming publicity the emergent strain O157:H7 has received (H and O refer to flagellar antigens and virulence markers). There are four categories of *E. coli* associated with diarrheal disease: enteropathogenic (EPEC), enterotoxigenic (ETEC), enteroinvasive (EIEC), and Vero cytotoxin-producing *E. coli* (VTEC). The classification VTEC also includes "shiga-like toxin"-producing *E. coli* (or SLTEC) and "shiga toxin"-producing *E. coli* (STEC). Enterohemorrhagic *E. coli* (EHEC) refers to those strains producing bloody diarrhea and are a subset of VTEC. The reference to shiga toxin is the result of the clinical similarity of the bloody diarrhea caused by EHEC to that caused by *Shigellae*. Each of the diseases presented by the four categories is also associated with one or more toxins (Willshaw *et al.*, 2000).

Because cattle are a significant reservoir of *E. coli*, it is logical that most outbreaks in the United States have been associated with hamburgers and other beef products although raw vegetables (often fertilized with manure) and unpasteurized apple cider and juice have been reported as sources of outbreaks. Outbreaks in Europe are more often associated with contamination of recreational waters (swimming pools, lakes, etc.). Other sources of contamination include person-to-person contact (especially in families and among institutionalized persons) and contact with farm animals especially following educational farm visits (Karch *et al.*, 1999).

The subject of organic food has increasingly captured the public interest. Within this issue, is a debate concerning the use of organic fertilizers (e.g., cow manure) in organic and conventional farming, which may contain *E. coli* O157:H7 (Stephenson, 1997). Data reported to the U.S. Centers for Disease Control and Prevention (CDC) in 1996, and tabulated in a CDC document entitled "Clusters/Outbreaks of *E. coli* O157:H7 reported to CDC in 1996," show that approximately 10% of all *E. coli* O157:H7 infections reported that year were from organically grown lettuce, although organic foods apparently account for less than 1% of the total food supply.

At the basis of the potential problem is the use of inadequately treated manure for fertilizer. Human cases of *E. coli* O157:H7 infection have been reported from consumption of contaminated lettuce, potatoes, radish sprouts, alfalfa sprouts, cantaloupe, and unpasteurized apple cider and juice (Karch *et al.*, 1999). Adequate treatment of manure requires composting the manure for a minimum of 3 months during which, the heap must reach a temperature of 60°C and although this may be adequate to kill vegetative pathogens, it will not destroy spore-formers such as *Clostridium perfringens* or *C. botulinum*. Survival of viruses and protozoa during composting is not known (Anonymous, 1999).

Bovine Spongiform Encephalopathy

Bovine spongiform encephalopathy (BSE) was first identified in Great Britain in 1986. BSE is a neurological disease classified as a transmissible spongiform encephalopathy (TSE) and is similar to TSEs in other species including scrapie (sheep and goats), transmissible mink encephalopathy (ranch-bred mink), chronic wasting disease (mule deer and elk), exotic ungulate encephalopathy (captive exotic bovoids such as bison, oryx, kudu) and feline spongiform encephalopathy (domestic cats and zoo Felidae). TSEs among humans include kuru, Creutzfeldt-Jakob Disease (CJD), and "new variant" CJD (nvCJD) and Gerstmann–Sträussler–Scheinker syndrome (to be distinguished from CJD by an earlier onset and tends to run in families).

Clinically, all these diseases present neurological deterioration and wasting, with the incubation period and interval from clinical onset to inexorable death determined by the dose of infective agent, its virulence and genetic makeup of the victim. The incubation of BSE in cattle is generally 4–5 years (range of 20 months to 18 years) and an interval of 1–12 months from presentation of clinical signs to death. Characteristic histologic lesions in the brain and spinal cord are vacuolation and "spongiform" changes. BSE fibrils (long strands of host glycoprotein called prion protein or PrP) in spinal cord preparations may be seen with electron microscopy following detergent extraction and proteinase K digestion. BSE/scrapie tissues with highest infectivity are brain and spinal cord, followed by retina, spleen, tonsil lymph nodes, distal ileum, and proximal colon. The infective agent can be transferred using preparations of neural tissue from infected animals across species barriers. The most effective method of transfer is direct injection into the brain or spinal cord, but transfer has been reported with intraperitoneal injection and oral

---

[19] "n" indicating seven subtypes.

Table 30-26
Amounts of Heterocyclic Amines in Cooked Foods

SAMPLE	AMOUNT (ng/g) IN COOKED FOOD				
	IQ	MEIQX	4,8-DIMEIQX	TRP-P-1	TRP-P-2
Broiled beef	0.19	2.11		0.21	0.25
Fried ground beef	0.70	0.64	0.12	0.19	0.21
Broiled chicken		2.33	0.81	0.12	0.18
Broiled mutton		1.01	0.67		0.15
Food-grade beef extract		3.10			

SOURCES: Sugimura T, Wakabayashi K, Nagao M, *et al.*: Heterocyclic amines in cooked food, in Taylor SL, Scanlan RA (eds.): *Food Toxicology: A Perspective on the Relative Risks.* New York, Marcel Dekker, 1989, p. 45. With permission from Copyright Clearance Center.

Adamson RH: Mutagens and carcinogens formed during cooking of foods and methods to minimize their formation. *Cancer Prevention Vol 1(November)*: 1–7 (1990). With permission from Lippincott Williams &Wilkins.

IQ = 2-amino-3-methylimidazo[4,5-f]quinoline; MeIQx = 2-amino-3,8-dimethylimidazo[4,5-f]quinoxaline; 4,8-DiMeIQx = 2-amino-3,4,8-trimethyl-3H-imidazo[4,8-f]quinoxaline; Trp-P-1 = 3-amino-1,4-dimethyl-5h-pyrido[4,3-*b*]indole; Trp-P-2 = 3-amino-1-methyl-5h-pyrido[4,3-*b*]indole.

dosing. Vertical transfer (mother to offspring) has been reported among domestic cattle and lateral transfer through biting or injury (especially among mink) has also been reported. Indirect transmission of chronic wasting disease (CWD) has been reported recently (Miller *et al.*, 2004); CWD of mule deer (*Odocoileus hemionus*) can be transmitted from environments contaminated by excreta 2.2 years earlier or decomposed carcasses ~1.8 years earlier.

It is generally agreed that the infective agent is likely a variant of scrapie (endemic to sheep) and was transferred to cattle from rendered sheep via inadequately processed meat and bone meal protein supplement. There is strong evidence and general agreement that the outbreak was amplified and spread throughout the UK cattle industry by feeding rendered (contaminated) bovine meat- and-bone meal to young calves. Disputes have arisen about other details of BSE and its relationship to other TSEs and effects in man because of an expectation of conformation by BSE to historical principles of disease transmission. Based on the BSE controversy, the FDA has published a proposed rule (Federal Register 70:58569-58601, 2005), which lists so-called high-risk tissues not allowed in animal or pet food due to potential BSE risk to livestock or pets and ultimately, humans.

The currently most accepted theory is that the infective agent is a modified form of a normal cell surface component known as prion protein PrP^c (*alpha*-helix form), which when introduced into an organism causes a conversion of PrP^c into a likeness of itself (i.e., the isoform), but then designated as the pathogenic form, PrP* or PrP^{sc} for scrapie; or PrP^{res} for protease resistant (beta-pleated sheet form) (Flechsig and Wissmann, 2004; Frosch *et al.*, 2005). The agent does not possess nucleic acid. The pathogenic form of the protein, PrP*, is both less soluble and more resistant to enzyme degradation than the normal form. The protein is resistant to heat, antimicrobials, ultraviolet or ionizing radiation, and is not consistently inactivated with alcohol, formaldehyde, glutaraldehyde, or sodium hydroxide. Phenol and sodium hypochlorite disinfection have had variable success.

Investigators have concluded that the agent in nvCJD and BSE is the same strain and may be the same agent in feline spongiform encephalopathy and exotic ungulate encephalopathy. While this information might indicate a simple mode of transmission, workers with the highest potential incidence of exposure to BSE or TSE (sheep farmers, butchers, veterinarians, cooks, and abattoir workers) do not have an unusually high incidence of nvCJD (Prusiner, 1991; Collee, 2000). Likewise, hemophilic patients have not reflected an increased incidence of nvCJD, although CJD transmission has been documented as the result of injections of human growth hormone or gonadotrophin (derived from human pituitary gland), implantation of dura mater and corneas and even infected EEG electrodes and neurosurgical instruments (Prusiner, 1994; Lee *et al.*, 1998; Collee, 2000).

Substances Produced by Cooking

Heterocyclic Amines Tolerances cannot be set for contaminants that are produced as a result of an action taken by the consumer. An example of this type of contaminant is heterocyclic amines, which are generated during cooking. Heterocyclic amines (HCAs) were discovered serendipitously by Japanese investigators who, while examining the mutagenicity of smoke generated by charred foods, found that the extracts of the charred surfaces of the meat and fish were quantitatively more mutagenic than could be accounted for by the presence of polycyclic aromatic hydrocarbons (Sugimura *et al.*, 1989). Collectively, there are more than 20 HCAs. They are formed as a result of high-temperature cooking of proteins (especially those containing high levels of creatinine) and carbohydrates. Normally, as a result of such heating, desirable flavor components are formed, for example, pyrazines, pyridines, and thiazoles. Intermediates in the formation of these substances are dihydropyrazines and dihydropyridines, which in the presence of oxygen form the flavor components; however, in the presence of creatinine, HCAs are formed (Table 30-26) (Chen and Chiu, 1998; Schut and Snyderwine, 1999).

These substances are rapidly absorbed by the GI tract, are distributed to all organs, and decline to undetectable levels within 72 hours. HCAs behave as electrophilic carcinogens (Table 30-27). They are metabolized first by *N*-hydroxylation followed by further activation by *O*-acetylation or *O*-sulfonation to react with DNA. DNA adducts are formed with guanosine in various organs, including the liver, heart, kidney, colon, small intestine, forestomach, pancreas, and lung. Unreacted substances are subject to phase II detoxication reactions and are excreted via the urine and feces. In vitro, HCAs require metabolic activation, with some requiring *O*-acetyltransferase and others not. Although much of the mutagenicity testing has been carried out in TA98 and TA100, these substances are mutagenic in mammalian cells both in vitro and in vivo, *Drosophila*, and other strains of *Salmonella* (Munro *et al.*, 1993; Skog *et al.*, 1998; Sugimura and Wakahayashi, 1999).

Table 30-27

Mutagenicity and Carcinogenicity of Heterocyclic Amines

| HCA | NUMBER OF REVERTANTS u/g (STRAIN TA98) | CARCINOGENICITY | |
		SPECIES	STATISTICALLY SIGNIFICANT TUMORS
MeIQ	47,000,000	Mouse	Liver, forestomach
		Rat	Zymbal gland, oral cavity, colon, skin, mammary gland
IQ	898,000	Mouse	Liver, forestomach, lung
		Rat	Liver, mammary gland, Zymbal gland
		Monkey	Liver, metastasis to lungs
MeIQx	417,000	Mouse	Liver, lung, lymphoma, leukemia
		Rat	Liver, Zymbal gland, clitoral gland, skin
Glu-P-1	183,000	Mouse	Liver, blood vessels
		Rat	Liver, small and large intestine, brain, clitoral gland, Zymbal gland
DiMeIQx	126,000	No data	
Trp-P-2	92,700	Mouse	Liver, lung
		Rat	Liver, clitoral gland
Trp-P-1	8,990	Mouse	Liver
		Rat	Liver, metastasis to lungs
PhIP	1,800	Mouse	Liver, lung, lymphoma
		Rat	Colon, mammary gland
Glu-P-2	930	Mouse	Liver, blood vessels
		Rat	Liver, small and large intestine, Zymbal gland, brain, clitoral gland

SOURCE: Adapted from Sugimura T, Wakabayashi K, Nagao M, *et al*.: Heterocyclic amines in cooked food, in Taylor SL, Scanlan RA (eds.): *Food Toxicology: A Perspective on the Relative Risks*. New York, Marcel Dekker, 1989, pp. 36–43. With permission from Copyright Clearance Center. MeIQ = 2-amino-3,4-dimethylimidazo[4,5-f]quinoline; IQ = 2-amino-3-methylimidazo[4,5-f]quinoline; MeIQx = 2-amino-3,8-dimethyl-limidazo[4,5-f]quinoxaline; Glu-P-1 = 2-amino-6-methyldipyrido[1,2-*a*:3′,2′-*d*]imidazole; 4,8-DiMeIQx = 2-amino-3,4,8-trimethyl-3H-imidazo[4,8-f]quinoxaline; Trp-P-1 = 3-amino-1,4-dimethyl-5*h*−pyrido[4,3-*b*]indole; Trp-P-2 = 3-amino-1-methyl-5*h*−pyrido[4,3-*b*]indole; PhIP = 2-amino-1-methyl-6-phenylimidazo[4,5-*b*]pyridine; glu-p-2 = 2-aminodipyrido[1,2-*a*:3′,2′-*d*]imidazole.

Acrylamide Prior to 2002, when Swedish investigators detected acrylamide in food (Table 30-28), it was of interest only to specialists in worker safety, as this chemical is an important intermediate in the manufacture of polyacrylamides. Although there are many industrial and manufacturing uses of polyacrylamides, the bulk of production are used as chemical flocculants for water treatment, oil recovery and, in construction of dam foundations, tunnels and sewers—consumer exposure is largely incidental (NTP, 2004b). End users are exposed to polyacrylamide, which is not toxic as long as the monomer is not present. Acrylamide (the monomer) was known to be a neurotoxin, creating morphological changes in peripheral nerves at doses as low as 1 mg/kg BW/d. Much more is now known about acrylamide and its primary metabolite, glycidamide, which is produced from acrylamide by the enzyme CYP2E1; both acrylamide and glycidamide will form adducts with hemoglobin. Acrylamide is absorbed rapidly and extensively (23–48% of the administered dose to rodents) from the gastrointestinal tract. Both acrylamide and glycidamide are largely eliminated as mercapturic acid conjugates. Repeated dosing of acrylamide (in drinking water at 21 mg/kg BW/d for 40 days) produces morphological changes in the brain areas critical for learning, memory, and other cognitive functions (i.e., cerebral cortex, thalamus, and hippocampus) (JECFA, 2005). Acrylamide was classified as "probably carcinogenic to humans" (IARC Group 2A) by the International Agency for Research on Cancer (IARC, 1994) and "reasonably anticipated to be a human carcinogen" by the National Toxicology Program (NTP, 2004b).

Acrylamide is formed in foods that are high in carbohydrate, but low in protein, which are subjected to processing temperatures of at least 120°C. These high-temperature processing conditions are largely the same as required for the Maillard reaction which imparts a toasted, or baked (i.e., "crust") flavor to breads, toast, and other baked goods and, breaded meats and vegetables for sauté ing or frying and, most critical in production of French fries and potato chips. Most acrylamide is formed in the final stages of baking, grilling, or frying as the moisture content of the food falls and the surface temperature rises (JECFA, 2005). The presence of ammonium bicarbonate as a leavening agent increases the formation of acrylamide.

A critical element is the presence of asparagine, and amino acids competing with asparagine in the Maillard reaction, which reduce the levels of acrylamide in the final product. Strategies for mitigation focus on reduction of asparagine through use of asparaginase, breeding and selection of low asparagine plants and prolonged yeast fermentation; alternatively, processing temperature could be lowered (JECFA, 2005).

Acrylamide intake estimates range from 0.3 to 2.0 μg/kg BW/d for the average population, with the 90th to 97th percentile at 0.6 to 3.5 μg/kg BW/d at the 99th percentile at 5.1 μg/kg BW/d. Primary sources include French fries (1–30%), potato chips (6–46%), coffee (13–39%), pastry and cookies (10–20%), and bread and rolls/toasts (10–30%). The national average and "high intake users" are 1 and 4 μg/kg BW/d, respectively. The NOEL for morphological change in nerves and for reproductive effects is 200 and 2000 μg/kg BW/d, respectively (JECFA, 2005).

Table 30-28

Representative Concentrations of Acrylamide in Several Foods

FOOD	MEAN CONC. (μg/kg)	REPORTED MAXIMUM (μg/kg)
Cereal-based products		
Breads and rolls	446	3436
Pastry and cookies	350	7834
Breakfast cereals	96	1346
Roots and tubers		
Baked potato	169	1270
Potato chips	752	4080
French fries	334	5312
Coffee		
Coffee, brewed, ready to drink	13	116
Coffee extracts	1100	4948
Coffee, decaffeinated	668	5399
Coffee substitutes	845	7300
Vegetables		
Raw, boiled and canned	4.2	25
Processed (toasted, baked, fried, grilled)	59	202
Infant formula	<5	15
Baby food (biscuits)	181	1217

JECFA (2006) Evaluation of Certain Food Additives and Contaminants. Sixty-fourth report of the Joint FAO/WHO Expert Committee on Food Additives (JECFA). WHO Technical Report Series 930. World Health Organization (WHO), Geneva, pp. 20–21. (http://whqlibdoc.who.int/trs/WHO_TRS_930_eng.pdf) (accessed on 17 May 2007).

Miscellaneous Contaminants in Food

Sometimes the items under the miscellaneous heading are the most interesting. For example, Rodricks and Pohland (1981) pointed out an interesting historical case of the possible transfer of a toxic botanic chemical from an animal to humans, which was first identified by Hall (1979). It is found in the Bible, Book of Numbers, 11:31–33, which describes hungry Israelites inundated with quail blown in from the sea; those who ate the quail quickly died. Hall speculated that the quail had consumed various poisonous berries, including hemlock, while they overwintered in Africa. The hemlock berry contains coniine, a neurotoxic alkaloid to which quail are resistant and which can accumulate in their tissue. Humans are not resistant to coniine, and consumption of large quantities of quail tissue containing the neurotoxin could result in death as described in the biblical text.

Mountain laurel, rhododendron, and azaleas all possess andromedotoxin (now called acetylandromedol) and grayanotoxins (I, II, and II) in their shoots, leaves, twigs, and flowers. Honey made from flowers of these plants is toxic to humans, and after an asymptomatic period of 4–6 hours, salivation, malaise, vomiting, diarrhea, tingling of the skin, muscular weakness, headache, visual difficulties, coma, and convulsions occur. Life-threatening bradycardia and arterial hypotension may occur. Needless to say, beekeepers maintain apiaries well away from these species of plants. A similar poisoning occurs with oleander (*Nerium oleander* and *N. indicum*), where honey made from the flowers, meat roasted on oleander sticks, or milk from a cow that eats the foliage can produce prostrating symptoms. The oleander toxin consists of a series of cardiac glycosides: thevetin, convallarin, steroidal, helleborein, ouabain, and digitoxin. Sympathetic nerves are paralyzed; the cardiotoxin stimulates the heart muscles similar to the action of digitalis, and gastric distress ensues (Anderson and Sogn, 1984; VonMalottki and Weichmann, 1996).

Other contaminations include contamination of milk with pyrrolizidine and other alkaloids after a cow has fed on tansy ragwort (*Senecio jacobaea*) and tremetol contamination of milk from white snakeroot (*Eupatorium rugusum*).

CONCLUSION

Food toxicology differs in many respects from other subspecialties of toxicology largely because of the nature and chemical complexity of food. Food consists of hundreds of thousands of chemical substances in addition to the macro- and micronutrients that are essential to life. The federal law defining food safety in the United States, the FD&C Act, provides a scheme for establishing the safety of foods, food ingredients, and contaminants. Whereas the act does not specify how the safety of food and its components and ingredients is to be demonstrated, it emphasizes the need for reasonable approaches in both the application of tests and their interpretation. New policies, consistent with the safety provisions of the Act, are being developed to provide guidance for determination of the safety-in-use of novel foods and those foods derived from new plant varieties.

Contaminants found in food may be divided into two large classes: those that are unavoidable by current good manufacturing practice and those that are not. The former class is represented by substances such as certain chlorinated organic compounds, heavy metals, and mycotoxins which have been determined to be unavoidable by current food-manufacturing practice and for which tolerances or action levels may be established. Additionally, pesticide residues and residues of drugs used in food-producing animals may have tolerances established when necessary to protect public health. For avoidable class of contaminants, tolerances are not set either because public health concerns dictates that the mere presence of the substance or agent demands immediate regulatory action or because contamination results from food preparation in the home, which is beyond FDA control.

It is important to emphasize that the vast majority of food-borne illnesses in developed countries is attributable to microbiological contamination of food arising from the pathogenicity and/or toxigenicity of the contaminating organism. Thus, the overwhelming concern for food safety in the United States remains directed toward preserving the microbiological integrity of food.

REFERENCES

Abrams IJ: Using the menu census survey to estimate dietary intake-Post-market surveillance of aspartame, in Finley JW, Robinson SF, Armstrong DJ (eds.): *Food Safety Assessment*. Washington, DC: American Chemical Society, 1992, p. 201.

Ames BN, Gold LS: Environmental pollution, pesticides, and the prevention of cancer: Misconceptions. *FASEB J* 11:1041, 1997.

Ames BN, Magaw R, Gold LS: Ranking possible carcinogenic hazards. *Science* 236:271, 1987.

Anderson JA, Sogn DD (eds.): *Adverse Reactions to Foods*. Washington, DC: US Department of Health and Human Services, 1984.

Anonymous: Haff disease associated with eating buffalo fish—United States, 1997. *MMWR Morb Mortal Wkly Rep* 47:1091, 1998.

Anonymous: Organic food. *Food Sci Technol Today* 13:108, 1999.

Ariyananda OL, Fernando SSD: Turtle flesh poisoning. *Ceylon Med J* 32:213, 1987.

Astwood JD, Bannon GA, Dobert RL, et al.: Food biotechnology and genetic engineering, in Metcalf DD, Sampson HA, Simon RA (eds.): *Food Allergy,* 3rd edn. Maiden, MA: Blackwell Scientific Inc, 2003.

Ayesh R, Mitchell SC, Zhang A, et al.: The fish odour syndrome: Biochemical, familial and clinical aspects. *Br Med J* 307:655, 1993.

BACIS: *Database of Volatile Compounds in Food*. TNO Nutrition and Food Research, Boelens Aroma Chemical Information Service, The Netherlands. CD-ROM, 1999.

Bannister B, Gibsburg G, Shneerson T: Cardiac arrest due to licorice induced hypokalemia. *BMJ* 2:738, 1977.

Barr JR, Moura H, Boyer AE, et al.: Botulinum neurotoxin detection and differentiation by mass spectrometry. *Emerg Infect Dis* 2005. http://www.cdc.gov/ncidod/EID/vol11no10/04-1279.htm (site visited 22 March 2006).

Beardall JM, Miller JD: Diseases in humans with mycotoxins as possible causes, in Miller JD, Trenhold HL (eds.): *Mycotoxins in Grain. Compounds Other than Aflatoxin*. St. Paul, MN: JEagan Press, 1994, p. 487.

Belitz H-D, Grosch W: *Food Chemistry*. Berlin: Springer-Verlag, 1999, p. 992.

Bemaola G, Echechipia S, Urrutia I, et al.: Occupational asthma and rhinoconjunctivitis from inhalation of dried cow's milk caused by sensitization to alpha-lactalbumin. *Allergy* 49:189, 1994.

Bernhisel-Broadbent J, Dintzis HM, Dintzis RZ, et al.: Allergenicity and antigenicity of chicken egg ovomucoid (Gal d III) compared with ovalbumin (Gal d I) in children with egg allergy and in mice. *J Allergy Clin Immunol* 93:1047, 1994.

Betz FS, Hammond BG, Fuchs RL: Safety and advantages of *Bacillus thuringiensis*-protected plants to control insect pests. *Regul Toxicol Pharmacol* 32(2):156, 2000.

Borda IA, Philen RM, Posada de la Paz M, et al.: Toxic oil syndrome mortality: The first 13 years. *Int J Epidemiol* 27:1057, 1998.

Borzelleca JF: Macronutrient substitutes: Safety evaluation. *Regul Toxicol Pharmacol* 16:253, 1992a.

Borzelleca JF: The safety evaluation of macronutrient substitutes. *Crit Rev Food Sci Nutr* 32:127, 1992b.

Brake D, Evenson DP: A generational study of glyphosate-tolerant soybeans on mouse fetal, postnatal, pubertal and adult testicular development. *Food Chem Toxicol* 42(1):29, 2004.

Brandon DL, Haque S, Friedman M: Antigenicity of native and modified Kunitz soybean trypsin inhibitors. *Adv Exp Med Biol* 199:449, 1986.

Brooker G, Barfoot P: GM Crops—The global economic and environmental impact—the first nine years 1996–2004. *AgBioForum* 8(2–3):187, 2005.

Bryan FL: *Staphylococcus aureus*, in Defigueiredo MP, Splittstoesser DF (eds.): *Food Microbiology: Public Health and Spoilage Aspects*. Westport, CT: AVI, 1976.

Bryan FL: Diseases transmitted by foods—A classification and summary, in Anderson JA, Sogn DN (eds.): *Adverse Reactions to Foods*, Appendix. Washington, DC: US Department of Health and Human Services, 1984, pp. 1–101.

Burdock GA: Dietary supplements and lessons to be learned from GRAS. *Regul Toxicol Pharmacol* 31:68, 2000.

Burdock, GA: Regulation of flavor ingredients, in Kotsonis FN, Mackey M (eds.): *Nutritional Toxicology*. New York: Taylor & Francis, 2002, p. 316.

Burdock GA, Carabin IC: Generally recognized as safe (GRAS): History and description. *Toxicol Lett* 150(1):3, 2004.

Burdock GA, Carabin IC, Griffiths JC: The importance of GRAS to the functional food and nutraceutical industries. *Toxicology* 221:17, 2006.

Butchko H, Kotsonis F: Acceptable daily intake and estimation of consumption, in Tschanz C, Butchko HH, Stargel WW, Kotsonis FN (eds.): *The Clinical Evaluation of a Food Additive, Assessment of Aspartame*. Boca Raton, FL: CRC Press, 1996, p. 43.

Butchko HH, Tschanz C, Kotsonis FN: Postmarketing surveillance of anecdotal medical complaints, in Tschanz C, Butchko HH, Stargel WW, Kotsonis FN (eds.): *The Clinical Evaluation of a Food Additive, Assessment of Aspartame*. Boca Raton, FL: CRC Press, 1996, p. 183.

Butchko HH, Tschanz C, Kotsonis FN: Postmarketing surveillance of food additives. *Regul Toxicol Pharmacol* 20:105, 1994.

Capen CC, DeLellis RA, Yarrington JT: Endocrine system, in Haschek WM, Rousseaux CG, Wallig MA (eds.): *Handbook of Toxicologic Pathology*, 2nd edn. San Diego, CA: Academic Press, 2002, p. 681.

Carabin IC, Magnuson BA: New labeling requirements for food allergens. *Nutr Outlook* 9:28, 2006.

CAST (Council for Agricultural Science and Technology): *Mycotoxins: Risks in Plant, Animal, and Human Systems*, Task Force Report No. 139. Ames, Iowa, 2003, p. 199.

Catto-Smith AG, Adams A: A possible case of transient hereditary fructose intolerance. *J Inherit Metab Dis* 16:73, 1993.

Champetier De Ribes G, Rasolofonirina RN, Ranaivoson G, et al.: [Intoxication by marine animal venoms in Madagascar (ichthyosarcotoxism and chelonitoxism): Recent epidemiological data.] *Bull Soc Pathol Exot* 90:286, 1997.

Chandrasiri N, Ariyananda PL, Fernando SSD: Autopsy findings in turtle flesh poisoning. *Med Sci Law* 28:142, 1988.

Chen BH, Chiu CP: Analysis, formation and inhibition of heterocyclic amines in foods: An overview. *J Food Drug Anal* 6:625, 1998.

Chen H, Weiss J, Shahidi F: Nanotechnology in nutraceuticals and function foods. *Food Technol* 3:30, 2006.

Chevion M, Mager J, Glaser G: Naturally occurring food toxicants: Favism-producing agents, in Rechcigl M, Jr. (ed.): *CRC Handbook of Naturally Occurring Food Toxicants*. Boca Raton, FL: CRC Press, 1985, p. 63.

Chhabra RS, Eastin WC Jr: Intestinal absorption and metabolism of xenobiotics in laboratory animals, in Schiller CM (ed.): *Intestinal Toxicology*. New York: Raven Press, 1984, p. 145.

Clark RF, Williams SR, Nordt SP, *et al.*: A review of selected seafood poisonings. *Undersea Hyperb Med* 26:175, 1999.

Clayson DB, Iverson F, Nera F, *et al.*: Histopathological and radioautographical studies on the forestomach of F344 rats treated with butylated hydroxyanisole and related chemicals. *Food Chem Toxicol* 24:1171, 1986.

Codex: Joint FAO/WHO Food Standards Programme. Codex Alimentarius Commission. Report of the fourth session of the Codex *Ad Hoc* Intergovernmental Task Force on Foods Derived from Biotechnology, Alinorm 03/34A, 2003.

Cohen JO (ed.): *The Staphylococci*. New York: Wiley-Interscience, 1972.

Collee JG: Transmissible spongiform encephalopathies. *The Microbiological Safety and Quality of Food*. Gaithersburg, MD: Aspen, 2000, p. 1589.

Committee on Food Protection: *Food Colors*. Washington, DC: National Academy of Sciences, 1971.

Concon J: *Food Toxicology*. New York: Marcel Dekker, 1988.

Cousins MA, Riley RT, Pestka JJ: Foodborne mycotoxins: Chemistry, biology, ecology, and toxicology, in Fratamico PM, Bhunia AK (eds.): *Foodborne Pathogens: Microbiology and Molecular Biology*. Norfok, UK: Horizon Scientific Press, 2005, p. 164.

Crane JK: Preformed bacterial toxins. *Clin Lab Med* 19:583, 1999.

Davis WE: *National Inventory of Sources and Emissions of Cadmium, Nickel, and Asbestos. Cadmium*, Section 1. Report PB 192250. Springfield, VA: National Technical Information Service, 1970.

Dayan AD: Allergy to antimicrobial residues in food: Assessment of the risk to man. *Vet Microbiol* 35:213, 1993.

DeBlay F, Hoyet C, Candolfi E, *et al.*: Identification of *alpha* livetin as a cross reacting allergen in bird-egg syndrome. *Allergy Proc* 15:77, 1994.

Dinges MM, Orwin PM, Schlievert PM: Exotoxins of *Staphylococcus aureus*. *Microbiol Rev* 13:16, 2000.

Dorion BJ, Burks AW, Harbeck R, *et al.*: The production of interferon-*gamma* in response to a major peanut allergy, Arh h II, correlates with serum levels of IgE anti-Ara h II. *J Allergy Clin Immunol* 93:93, 1994.

Drasar BS, Hill MJ: *Human Intestinal Flora*. New York: Academic Press, 1974.

Eadie MJ. Convulsive ergotism: Epidemics of the serotonin syndrome. *Lancet Neurol* 2(7):429, 2003.

EFSA: Guidance document of the scientific panel on genetically modified organisms for the risk assessment of genetically modified plants and derived food and feed, 8 November, 2004.

El-Banna AA, Pitt JI, Leistner L: Production of mycotoxins by *Penicillium* species. *Syst Appl Microbiol* 10(1):42, 1987.

EPA (Environmental Protection Agency): Guidance for the re-registration of pesticide products containing *Bacillus thuringiensis* as the active ingredient. *Re-registration Stand* 540:RS-89-023, 1988.

EPA (Environmental Protection Agency): Air quality criteria for particulate matter. Report Number EPA/600/P-99/002a,bF. USEPA, Washington, DC, October, 2004. (http://cfpub.epa.gov/ncea), (site visited 9 April 2006).

EPA (Environmental Protection Agency): Nanotechnology White Paper (external review draft). Science Policy Council, USEPA, Washington, DC, December 2, 2005.

Ermans AM, Delange F, Van der Velden M, *et al.*: Possible role of cyanide and thiocyanate in the etiology of endemic cretinism. *Adv Exp Med Biol* 30:455, 1972.

EU: Safe organic vegetables: The development of strategies to ensure a safe organic food supply by minimizing mycotoxin risks: The carrot—Alternaria model. (http://www.seedcentre.nl/Projects/EU_SafeOrganicVegetables/safe_ organic_ vegetables.htm), 2002.

Evans CS: Naturally occurring food toxicants: Toxic amino acids, in Rechcigl M, Jr. (ed.): *CRC Handbook of Naturally Occurring Food Toxicants*. Boca Raton, FL: CRC Press, 1985, p. 3.

FAO: Biotechnology and food safety. Report of a Joint FAO/WHO Consultation, Rome, Italy, 30 September–4 October 1996. FAO Food and Nutrition Paper 61, 1996.

Farese RV, Biglieri EG, Shackleton CHL, *et al.*: Licorice-induced hypermineralocorticoidism. *N Engl J Med* 325:1223, 1991.

Farwell AP, Braverman LE: Thyroid and antithyroid drugs, in Brunton LL, Lazo JS, Parker KL (eds.): *Goodman and Gilmans, The Pharmacological Basis of Therapeutics,* 11th edn. New York: McGraw-Hill, 2006, p. 1511.

FCC: *Food Chemicals Codex*, 5th edn. Washington, DC: National Academy Press, 2003.

FDA: Food producing animals: Criteria and procedures for evaluating assays for carcinogenic residues. *Fed Regist* 42:1977.

FDA: *Toxicological Principles for the Safety Assessment of Direct Food Additives and Color Additives used in Food*. Washington, DC: U.S. Food and Drug Administration, Bureau of Foods, 1982a.

FDA: Policy for regulating carcinogenic chemicals in food and color additives. *Fed Regist* 47:14464, 1982b.

FDA: Scientific review of the long-term carcinogen bioassays performed on the artificial sweetener, cyclamate. *Report of the Cancer Assessment Committee for Food Safety and Applied Nutrition*. Washington, DC: Food and Drug Administration, 1984.

FDA: Statement of policy: Foods derived from new plant varieties. *Fed Regist* 57:104, 22984, 1992.

FDA: FDA proposes new rules for *trans* fatty acids in nutrition labeling, nutrient content claims, and health claims. *HHS NEWS*. US Department of Health and Human Services, 1999a. (http://www.cfsan.fda.gov/~lrd/hhtfacid.html) (site visited 16 April 2006.)

FDA: Food labeling: Trans fatty acids in nutrition labeling, nutrient content claims, and health claims, proposed rule. *Federal Register* 64:62745, 1999b.

FDA: Guidance for industry: Preparation of food contact notifications and food additive petitions for food contact substances—Chemistry recommendations. *CFSAN/Office of Food Additive Safety*. Washington, DC: Food and Drug Administration, 2002a. (http://www.cfsan.fda.gov/~dms/opa2pmnc.html) (site visited 16 April 2006.)

FDA: Guidance for industry. Feed-effect bioavailablity and fed bioequivalence studies. Rockville, MD: Food and Drug Administration, 2002b. (http://www.fda.gov/cder/guidance/5194fnl.pdf) (site visited 16 April 2006.)

FDA: Furan in food, thermal treatment: Request for data and information. *Fed Regist* 69:25911, 2004.

FDA: Lead in candy likely to be consumed frequently by small children: Recommended maximum level and enforcement policy (draft guidance). December, 2005 (http://www.cfsan.fda.gov/~dms/pbguid2.html) (site visited 8 April 2006).

Fedoroff NV, Brown NM: *Mendel in the Kitchen*. Washington, DC: Joseph Henry Press, 2004, p. 171.

Flachowsky G, Chesson A, Aulrich K: Animal nutrition with feeds from genetically modified plants. *Arch Anim Nutr* 59(1):1, 2005.

Flamm WG, Frankos V: Nitrates: Laboratory evidence, in Walk NJ, Doll R (eds.): *Interpretation of Negative Epidemiological Evidence for Carcinogenicity*. Lyons, France: IARC Scientific Publications No. 65, 1985, p. 85.

Flamm WG, Kotsonis FN, Hjelle JJ: Threshold of regulation: A unifying concept in food safety assessment, in Kotsonis F, Mackey M, Hjelle J (eds.): *Nutritional Toxicology*. New York: Raven Press, 1994, p. 223.

Flamm WG, Kotsonis FN, Hjelle JJ: Threshold of regulation: A unifying concept in food safety assessment, in Kotsonis F, Mackey M, Hjelle J (eds.): *Nutritional Toxicology,* 2nd edn. New York: Taylor & Francis, 2002, p. 190.

Flamm WG, Lehman-McKeeman LD: The human relevance of the renal tumor-inducing potential of *d*-limonene in male rats: Implications for risk assessment. *Regul Toxicol Pharmacol* 13:70, 1991.

Flamm WG, Lorentzen RL: Quantitative risk assessment (QRA): A special problem in approval of new products, in Mehlman M (ed.): *Risk Assessment and Risk Management*. Princeton, New Jersey: Princeton Scientific Publishing, 1988, p. 91.

Flechsig E, Weissmann C: The role of PrP in health and disease. *Curr Mol Med* 4:337, 2004.

Frankland AW: Anaphylaxis in relation to food allergy, in Brostoff J, Challacombe SJ (eds.): *Food Allergy and Intolerance*. Philadelphia: Bailliere and Tindall, 1987, p. 456.

Frenzen PD: Deaths due to unknown foodborne agents. *Emerging Infectious Diseases*, [serial on the Internet] 2004. http://www.cdc.gov/ncidod/EID/vol10no9/03-0403.htm (site visited 22 March 2006).

Frosch MP, Anthony DC, DeGirolami U: The central nervous system, in Kumar V, Abbas AK, Fausto N (eds.): *Robbins and Cotran Pathologic Basis of Disease*. Philadelphia: Elsevier Saunders, 2005, p. 1380.

Fuglsang G, Madsen C, Saval P, *et al*.: Prevalence of intolerance to food additives among Danish school children. *Pediatr Allergy Immunol* 4(3):123, 1993.

Fukutomi O, Kondo N, Agata H, *et al*.: Timing of onset of allergic symptoms as a response to a double-blind, placebo-controlled food challenge in patients with food allergy combined with a radioallergosorbent test and the evaluation of proliferative lymphocyte responses. *Int Arch Allergy Immunol* 104(4):352, 1994.

Gangolli SD: Nitrate, nitrite and *n*-nitroso compounds, in Ballantyne B, Marrs T, Turner P (eds.): *General and Applied Toxicology*. New York: Stockton Press, 1999, p. 2111.

George C, Ridley WP, Obert JC, *et al*.: Composition of grain and forage from corn rootworm-protected corn event MON 863 is equivalent to that of conventional corn (*Zea mays* L.). *J Agric Food Chem* 52(13):4149, 2004.

Gessner BD, Hokama Y, Isto S: Scombrotoxicosis-like illness following the ingestion of smoked salmon that demonstrated low histamine levels and high toxicity on mouse bioassay. *Clin Infect Dis* 23:1316, 1996.

Gianessi LP, Carpenter JE: Agricultural Biotechnology: Insect control benefits. National Center for Food and Agricultural Policy, 1999.

Gibb CM, Davies PT, Glover V, *et al*.: Chocolate is a migraine-provoking agent. *Cephalalgia* 11(2):93, 1991.

Gilbert R: *Bacillus cereus* gastroenteritis, in Reimann H, Bryan FL (eds.): *Food-Borne Infections and Intoxications*, 2nd edn. New York: Academic Press, 1979.

Goepfert JM, Spira WM, Kim HU: *Bacillus cereus*: Food poisoning organism: A review. *Journal of Milk and Food Technology* 35:213, 1972.

Gold LS, Slone TH, Stern BR, *et al*.: Rodent carcinogens: Setting priorities. *Science* 258:261, 1992.

Gonzalez R, Polo F, Zapatero L, *et al*.: Purification and characterization of major inhalant allergens from soybean hulls. *Clin Exp Allergy* 22(8):748, 1992.

Granum PE: Bacterial toxins as food poisons, in Alouf JE, Popoff MR (eds.): *The Comprehensive Sourcebook of Bacterial Protein Toxins*, 3rd edn. New York: Elsevier/Academic Press, 2006, p. 949.

Granum PE, Baird-Parker TC: *Bacillus* species, in Lund BM, Baird-Parker TC, Gould GW (eds.): *The Microbiological Safety and Quality of Food*. Gaithersburg, MD: Aspen, 2000, p. 1029.

Granum PE, Brynestad S: Bacterial toxins as food poisons, in Alouf JE, Freer JH (eds.): *The Comprehensive Sourcebook of Bacterial Protein Toxins*, 2nd edn. New York: Academic Press, 1999, p. 669.

Granum PE, Lund T: *Bacillus cereus* and its food poisoning toxins. *FEMS Microbiol Lett* 157:223, 1997.

Gudmann-Hoyer E: The clinical significance of disaccharide maldigestion. *Am J Clin Nutr* 59(Suppl 3):735S, 1994.

Guo YL, Yu ML, Hsu CC: The Yucheng rice oil poisoning incident. *Dioxins and Health*. Hoboken, NJ: Hoboken Press, 2003, p. 893.

Guyton AC: The chemical senses—Taste and smell. *Textbook of Medical Physiology*, 4th edn. Philadelphia: WB Saunders, 1971, p. 639.

Halken S, Host A, Hansen LG, *et al*.: Preventive effect of feeding high-risk infants a casein hydrolysate formula or an ultrafiltrated whey hydrolysate formula. A prospective, randomized, comparative clinical study. *Pediatr Allergy Immunol* 4(4):173, 1993.

Hall R, Oser B: The safety of flavoring substances. *Residue Rev* 24:1, 1968.

Hall RL: *Proceedings of Marabou Symposium on Foods and Cancer*. Stockholm: Caslan Press, 1979.

Hammond BG, Campbell KW, Pilcher CD, *et al*.: Lower fumonisin mycotoxin levels in the grain of Bt corn grown in the United States in 2000–2002. *J Agric Food Chem* 52(5):1390, 2004.

Harris RZ, Jang GR, Tsunoda S: Dietary effects on drug metabolism and transport. *Clin Pharmacokinet* 42:1071, 2003.

Harrison LA, Bailey MR, Naylor MW, *et al*.: The expressed protein in glyphosate-tolerant soybean, 5-enolpyruvylshikimate-3-phosphate synthase from Agrobacterium sp. strain CP4, is rapidly digested *in vitro* and is not toxic to acutely gavaged mice. *J Nutr* 126(3):728, 1996.

Hassing JM, Al-Turk WA, Stohs SJ: Induction of intestinal microsomal enzymes by polycyclic aromatic hydrocarbons. *Gen Pharmacol* 20(5):695, 1989.

Hauschild AHW: *Clostridium perfringens* enterotoxin. *J Milk Food Technol* 34:596, 1971.

Herman RA, Phillips AM, Collins RA, *et al*.: Compositional equivalency of Cry1F corn event TC6275 and conventional corn (*Zea mays* L.). *J Agric Food Chem* 52(9):2726, 2004.

Hobbs G: *Clostridium botulinum* and its importance in fishery products. *Adv Food Res* 22:135, 1976.

Hobbs BC, Smith ME, Oakley CL, *et al*.: *Clostridium welchii* food poisoning. *J Hyg (Lond)* 51:75, 1953.

Hotchkiss JH: Relative exposure to nitrite, nitrate, and *N*-nitroso compounds from endogenous and exogenous sources, in Taylor SL, Scanlan RA (eds.): *Food Toxicology: A Perspective on the Relative Risks*. New York: Marcel Dekker, 1989, p. 57.

Hotchkiss JH, Helser MA, Maragos CM, *et al*.: Nitrate, nitrite, and *N*-nitroso compounds: Food safety and biological implications, in Finley JW, Robinson SF, Armstrong DJ (eds.): *Food Safety Assessment*. Washington, DC: American Chemical Society, 1992, p. 400.

IARC: Acrylamide. *Some Industrial Chemicals*, vol. 60. International Agency for Research on Cancer (IARC) Working Group on the Evaluation of Carcinogenic Risk to Humans. Lyon, France: IARC Press, 1994, p. 389.

IARC (International Agency for Research on Cancer): Dry cleaning, some chlorinated solvents and other industrial chemicals. *IARC Monographs on the Evaluation of Carcinogenic Risks to Humans*, vol 63. Lyon, France: IARC Press, 1995, p. 394.

IARC (International Agency for Research on Cancer): Some traditional herbal medicines, some mycotoxins, naphthalene and styrene. IARC Working Group on the Evaluation of Carcinogenic Risk to Humans. Lyon, France: IARC Press, 2002, p. 171.

ICPS (International Chemical Safety Programme): Solanine and chaconine, Environmental Health Criteria 764 (WHO Food Additives Series 30), 1993. http://www.inchem.org/documents/jecfa/jecmono/v30je19.htm (site visited 15 April 2006).

ICPS (International Chemical Safety Programme): Fumonisin B1, environmental health criteria 219, United Nations Environmental Programme, the International Labour Organization and the World Health Organization International Programme on Chemical Safety, Geneva, 2000, p. 153.

IFST (Institute of Food Science and Technology Trust Fund): Mycotoxins: Information statement, 2006a. http://www.ifst.org/myco.pdf (site visited 12 March 2006).

IFST (Institute of Food Science and Technology Trust Fund): Nanotechology: Information statement, 2006b. http://www.ifst.org/nano.pdf (site visited 12 March 2006).

Ijomah P, Clifford MN, Walker R, *et al*.: The importance of endogenous histamine relative to dietary histamine in the aetiology of scombrotoxicosis. *Food Addit Contam* 8(4):531, 1991.

ILSI: ILSI Crop Composition Database, version 3 (www.crop-composition.org). International Life Sciences Institute (ILSI), 2006.

IOM (Institute of Medicine). Fluoride. *Dietary Reference Intakes for Calcium, Phosphorus, Magnesium, Vitamin D and Fluoride*, Chap. 8. Washington, DC: National Academy Press, 1997, p. 288.

Isbrucker RA, Burdock GA: Risk and safety assessment on the consumption of licorice root (*Glycyrrhiza* sp.), its extract and powder as a food ingredient, with emphasis on the pharmacology and toxicology of glycyrrhizin. *Regul Toxicol Pharmacol* 46(3):167, 2006.

James C: Preview: Global review of commercialized transgenic crops. *ISAA Briefs* No. 12. Ithaca, NY: ISAAA, 1999.

James C: Global status of commercialized biotech/GM crops—2005. Executive summary in *ISAA Briefs* No. 34. International Service for the Acquisition of Agri-Biotech Applications, (ISAA), 2006, p. 1.

JECFA (Joint FAO/SHO Expert Committee on Food Additives): *Safety Evaluation of Certain Mycotoxins in Food.* WHO Food Additives Series 47. WHO, Geneva, 2001, p 419.

JECFA (Joint FAO/WHO Expert Committee on Food Additives): Sixty-fourth meeting. Rome, 8–17 February 2005, pp. 1–47, http://www.who.int/ipcs/food/jecfa/summaries/summary_report_64_final.pdf (site visited 13 April 2006).

Johnson RD, Manske DD, New DH, et al.: Food and feed pesticides, heavy metal and other chemical residues in infant and toddler total diet samples. *Pestic Monit J* 15:39, 1981.

Juambeltz JC, Kula K, Perman J: Nursing caries and lactose intolerance. *ASDC J Dent Child* 60(4):377, 1993.

Karch H, Bielaszewska M, Bitzan M, et al.: Epidemiology and diagnosis of Shiga toxin-producing *Escherichia coli* infections. *Diagn Microbiol Infect Dis* 34:229, 1999.

Kirchgessner M, Reichlmayer-Lais AM: *Trace Element Metabolism in Man and Animals (TEMA-4).* Canberra: Australian Academy of Science, 1981.

Kivity S, Sunner K, Marian Y: The pattern of food hypersensitivity in patients with onset after 10 years of age. *Clin Exp Allergy* 24:1, 1994.

Kokoski CJ, Henry SH, Lin CS, et al.: Methods used in safety evaluation, in Branen AL, Davidson PM, Salminen S (eds.): *Food Additives.* New York: Marcel Dekker, 1990.

Kotsonis FN, Hjelle JJ: The safety assessment of aspartame: Scientific, and regulatory considerations, in Tschanz C, Butchko HH, Stargel W, Kotsonis FH (eds.): *The Clinical Evaluation of a Food Additive. Assessment of Aspartame.* Boca Raton, FL: CRC Press, 1996, p. 23.

Krishnamachari KAVR, Bhat RV, Nagarajan V, et al.: Hepatitis due to aflatoxicosis. *Lancet* 1(7915):1061, 1975.

Kritschevsky D: The role of fat, calories and fiber in disease, in Kotsonis F, Mackey M, Hjelle J (eds.): *Nutritional Toxicology.* New York: Raven Press, 1994, p. 67.

Labbe RG: *Clostridium perfringens*, in Lund BM, Baird-Parker TC, Gould GW (eds.): *The Microbiological Safety and Quality of Food.* Gaithersburg, MD: Aspen, 2000, p. 1110.

Lagerwerff JV, Sprecht AW: Occurrence of environmental cadmium and zinc and their uptake by plants, in Hemphill DD (ed.): *Proceedings of the University of Missouri 4th Annual Conference on Trace Substances in Environmental Health.* Columbia: University of Missouri, 1971, p. 85.

Lange WR: Scombroid poisoning. *Am Fam Physician* 37:163, 1988.

Lee CA, Ironside JW, Bell JE, et al.: Retrospective neuropathological review of prion disease in UK haemophilic patients. *Thromb Haemost* 80:909, 1998.

Lehman AJ, Fitzhugh OG: 100-Fold margin of safety. *Quarterly Bulletin of the Association of Food and Drug Officials of the United States*, January:33, 1954.

Linder MC: *Nutritional Biochemistry and Metabolism*, 2nd edn. Norwalk, CT: Appleton and Lange, 1991.

Liston J: Fish and shellfish poisoning, in Lund BM, Baird-Parker TC, Gould GW (eds.): *The Microbiological Safety and Quality of Food.* Gaithersburg, MD: Aspen, 2000, p. 1518.

Loving AL: Botulism in flavored oils—A review. *Dairy, Food and Environmental Sanitation* 18:438, 1998.

Lund BM, Peck MW: Clostridium botulinum, in Lund BM, Baird-Parker TC, Gould GW (eds.): *The Microbiological Safety and Quality of Food.* Gaithersburg, MD: Aspen, 2000, p. 1057.

MacKenzie SA, Pavely C, Malley LA, et al.: Evaluation of the subchronic toxicity of 1507XNK603 transgenic maize. *Toxicologist* 84(S-1):14105, 2005.

Mackey M, Kotsonis FN: Functional foods: Regulatory and scientific considerations, in Kotsonis F, Mackey M, Hjelle J (eds.): *Nutritional Toxicology*, 2nd edn. New York: Taylor & Francis, 2002, p. 243.

Mallinson CN: Basic functions of the gut, in Brostoff J, Challacombe SJ (eds.): *Food Allergy and Intolerance.* Philadelphia: Bailtiere and Tindalf, 1987, p. 27.

Manda F, Tadera K, Aoyama K: Skin lesions due to Okra (*Hibiscus esculenius* L.): Proteolytic activity and allergenicity of okra. *Contact Dermatitis* 26(2):95, 1992.

Manu P, Matthews DA, Lane TJ: Food intolerance in patients with chronic fatigue. *Int J Eat Disord* 13:203, 1993.

Marasas WFO, Jaskiewicz K, Venter FS, et al.: Fusarium moniliforme contamination of maize in oesophageal cancer areas in the transkei. *S Afr Med J* 74:110, 1988.

Masoero F, Moschini M, Rossi F, et al.: Nutritive value, mycotoxin contamination and *in vitro* rumen fermentation of normal and genetically modified corn (CryIA(B)) grown in northern Italy. *Maydica* 44:205, 1999.

Matsumoto H: Cycasin, in Rechcigl M Jr (ed.): *CRC Handbook of Naturally Occurring Food Toxicants.* Boca Raton, FL: CRC Press, 1985, p. 43.

Matulka RH: Understanding ingredient consumption analysis. *Nat Prod Ind Insid* 10:46, 2005.

McClain RM: Mechanistic considerations in the regulation and classification of chemical carcinogens, in Kotsonis FN, Mackey M, Hjelle JJ (eds.): *Nutritional Toxicology,* 2nd edn. New York: Taylor & Francis, 2002, p. 387.

McClintock JT, Schaffer CR, Sjoblad RD: A comparative review of the mammalian toxicity of *Bacillus thuringiensis*-based pesticides. *Pestic. Sci* 45:95, 1995.

Melnik B, Szliska C, Noehle M, et al.: Food intolerance: Pseudoallergic reactions induced by biogenic amines. *Allergo J* 20:163, 1997.

Metcalfe DD, Astwood JD, Townsend R, et al.: Assessment of the allergenic potential of foods derived from genetically engineered crop plants. *Crit Rev Food Sci Nutr* 36(S):S165, 1996.

Miller CD: *Selected Toxicological Studies of the Mycotoxin Cyclopiazonic Acid in Turkeys.* (dissertation). Ann Arbor, MI: University of Michigan Dissertation Services, 1989.

Miller MW, Williams ES, Hobbs NT, et al.: Environmental sources of prion transmission in mule deer. *Emerg Infect Dis* 10:1003, 2004.

Miller SA: Food additives and contaminants, in Amdur MO, Doull J, Klaassen CD (eds.): *Toxicology: The Basic Science of Poisons.* New York: Taylor & Francis, 1991, p. 819.

Minor TE, Marth EH: *Staphylococci and their Significance in Foods.* Amsterdam: Elsevier, 1976.

Mirocha CJ, Pathre SV, Christensen CM: Zearalenone, in Rodericks ^EJV, Hesseltine CW, Mehlman MA (eds.): *Mycotoxins in Human and Animal Health.* Park Forest South, IL: Pathtox, 1977, p. 345.

Mirvish SS: Formation of *N*-nitroso compounds: Chemistry kinetics, and *in vivo* occurrence. *Toxicol Appl Pharmacol* 31:325, 1975.

MMWR: Ostrich fern poisoning—New York and Western Canada. *MMWR Morb Mortal Wkly Rep* 43:677, 1994.

Monday SR, Bohach GA: Properties of *Staphylococcus aureus* enterotoxins and toxic shock syndrome toxin-1, in Alouf JE, Freer JH (eds.): *The Comprehensive Sourcebook of Bacterial Protein Toxins*, 2nd edn. New York: Academic Press Limited, 1999, p. 589.

Moneret-Vautrin DA: Food intolerance masquerading as food allergy: False food allergy, in Brostoff J, Challacombe SJ (eds.): *Food Allergy and Intolerance.* Philadelphia: Balliere Tindall, 1987, p. 836.

Monroe DH, Eaton DL: Comparative effects of butylated hydroxyanisole on hepatic *in vivo* DNA binding and *in vitro* biotransformation of aflatoxin B$_1$ in the rat and mouse. *Toxicol Appl Pharmacol* 90:401, 1987.

Morrow JD, Margiolies GR, Rowland J, et al.: Evidence that histamine is the causative toxin of scombroid-fish poisoning. *N Engl J Med* 324(11):716, 1991.

Muller GJ, Lamprechi JH, Barnes JM, et al.: Scombroid poisoning: Case series of 10 incidents involving 22 patients. *S African Med J* 81(8):427, 1992.

Munkvold GP, Hellmich RL, Rice LR: Comparison of fumonisin concentrations in kernels of transgenic Bt maize hybrids and nontransgenic hybrids. *Plant Dis* 83:130, 1999.

Munkvold GP, Hellmich RL, Showers WB: Reduced fusarium ear rot and symptomless infection in kernels of maize genetically engineered for European corn borer resistance. *Phytopathology* 87:1071, 1997.

Munro IC: Issues to be considered in the safety evaluation of fat substitutes. *Food Chem Toxicol* 28:751, 1990.

Munro IC, Kennepohl E, Erickson RE, *et al.*: Safety assessment of ingested heterocyclic amines: Initial report. *Regul Toxicol Pharmacol* 17:S1, 1993.

Newberne PM: Mechanisms of interaction and modulation of response, in Vouk VB, Butler GC, Upton AC, *et al.* (eds.): *Methods for Assessing the Effects of Mixtures of Chemicals*. New York: Wiley, 1987, p. 555.

Nordlee JA, Taylor SL, Townsend JA, *et al.*: Transgenic soybeans containing Brazil nut 2S storage protein issues regarding allergenicity, in: Eisenbrand G, *et al.* (eds.): *Food Allergies and Intolerances*. New York: VCH Publishers, 1996, p. 196.

NRC (National Research Council): *Fluoride in Drinking Water: A Scientific Review of EPA's Standards*. Washington, DC: National Academy Press, 2006, p. 576.

NRC/NAS (National Research Council/National Academy of Science): *The 1977 Survey of Industry on the Use of Food Additives by the NRC/NAS*. October 1979, U.S. Department of Commerce, NTIS PB 80-113418. Volume III: *Estimates of Daily Intake*. Committee on GRAS list survey—Phase III Food and Nutrition Committee, National Research Council, 1979.

NTP (National Toxicology Program): *Toxicology and Carcinogenesis Studies of Furan (CAS No. 110-00-9) in F344/N Rats and B6C3F1 Mice (gavage studies)*, NTP Technical Report No. 402. Research Triangle Park, NC: U.S. Department of Health and Human Services, Public Health Service, National Institutes of Health, 1993.

NTP: Urethane. *Report on Carcinogens*, 11th edn. Washington, DC: U.S. Department of Health and Human Services, Public Health Service, National Toxicology Program (NTP), 2004a. http://ntp-server.niehs.nih.gov/index.cfm?objectid=32BA9724-F1F6-975E-7FCE50709CB4C932 (site visited 15 April 2006).

NTP: Acrylamide. *Report on Carcinogens*, 11th edn. Washington, DC: U.S. Department of Health and Human Services, Public Health Service, National Toxicology Program (NTP), 2004b. http://ntp-server.niehs.nih.gov/index.cfm?objectid=32BA9724-F1F6-975E-7FCE50709CB4C932 (site visited 15 April 2006).

Oberdoerfer RB, Shillito RD, de Beuckeleer M, *et al.*: Rice (*Oryza sativa* L.) containing the bar gene is compositionally equivalent to the non-transgenic counterpart. *J Agric Food Chem* 53(5):1457, 2005.

OECD: *Safety Evaluation of Foods Derived by Modern Biotechnology: Concepts and Principles*. Organization for the Economic Co-operation and Development (OECD). Paris: OECD Press, 1993.

OECD: *Report of the Workshop on the Toxicological and Nutritional Testing of Novel Foods*, SG/ICGB(98)1. Organization for the Economic Co-operation and Development (OECD). Paris: OECD Press, 1997.

O'Hallaren MT: Baker's asthma and reactions secondary to soybean and grain dust, in Bardana EJ, Jr, Montanaro A, O'Hallaren MT (eds.): *Occupational Asthma*. Philadelphia: Hanley and Belfus, 1992, p. 107.

O'Neil C, Helbling AA, Lehrer SB: Allergic reactions to fish. *Clin Rev Allergy* 11(2):183, 1993.

Onuma Y, Satake M, Ukena T, *et al.*: Identification of putative palytoxin as the cause of clupeotoxism. *Toxicon* 37(1):55, 1999.

Oshima H, Bartsch H: Quantitative estimation of endogenous nitrosation in humans by monitoring *N*-nitrosoproline excreted in the urine. *Cancer Res* 41:3658, 1981.

Papst C, Utz HF, Melchinger AE, *et al.*: Mycotoxins produced by *Fusarium* spp. In isogenic Bt *vs.* non-Bt maize hybrids under European corn borer pressure. *Agron J* 97:219, 2005.

Pariza MW, Johnson EA: Evaluating the safety of microbial enzyme preparations used in food processing: Update for a new century. *Regul Toxicol Pharmacol* 33(2):173, 2001.

Pay EM, Fleming KH, Guenther PM, *et al.*: *Foods Commonly Eaten by Individuals: Amount per Day and per Eating Occasion*. Washington, DC: USDA (HERR No. 44), 1984.

Peers FG, Gilman GA, Linsell CA: Dietary aflatoxins and human liver cancer: A study in Swaziland. *Int J Cancer* 17:167, 1976.

Pennington JAP, Gunderson EL: History of the Food Drug Administration total diet study-1961–1987. *J Assoc Off Anal Chem* 70:772, 1987.

Piastra M, Stabile A, Fioravanti G, *et al.*: Cord blood mononuclear cell responsiveness to beta-lactoglobulin: T-cell activity in "atopy-prone" and "non-atopy-prone" newborns. *Int Arch Allergy Immunol* 104:358, 1994.

Posada de la Paz M, Philen RM, Borda IA, *et al.*: Toxic oil syndrome: Traceback of the toxic oil and evidence for a point source epidemic. *Food Chem Toxicol* 34:251, 1996.

Prusiner SB: *Prion Diseases of Animals and Humans*. Washington, DC: Toxicology Forum, 1991, p. 203.

Prusiner SB: Prion diseases of humans and animals. *J R Coll Physicians* 28:1, 1994.

Randall JE, Aida K, Oshima Y, *et al.*: Occurrence of a crinotoxin and hemagglutinin in the skin mucus of the moray eel *Lycodontis nudivomer*. *Mar. Biol.* 62:179, 1981.

Rodricks JV, Pohland AE: Food hazards of animal origin, in Roberts HR (ed.): *Food Safety*. New York: Wiley, 1981, p. 181.

Rumsey GL, Siwicki AK, Anderson DP, *et al.*: Effect of soybean protein on serological response, non-specific defense mechnisms, growth, and protein utilization in rainbow trout. *Vet Immunol Immunopathol* 41:323, 1994.

Sachs MI, Jones RT, Yunginger JW: Isolation and partial characterization of a major peanut allergen. *J Allergy Clin Immunol* 67:27, 1981.

Sansalone W (ed.): *What is a Nutrient: Defining the Food-Drug Continuum*. Proceedings, Georgetown University, Center for Food and Nutritional Policy, Washington, DC, 1999, p. 82.

Sato N, Ueno Y: Comparative toxicities of trichothecenes, in Rodericks JV, Hesseltine CW, Mehlman MA (eds.): *Mycotoxins in Human and Animal Health*. Park Forest South, IL: Pathtox Publishers, 1977, p. 295.

Schmidt LE, Dalhoff K: Food-drug interactions. *Drugs* 62:1481, 2002.

Schrander JJ, van den Bogart JP, Forget PP, *et al.*: Cow's milk protein intolerance in infants under 1 year of age: A prospective epidemiological study. *Eur J Pediatr* 52(8):640, 1993.

Schut HAJ, Snyderwine EG: DNA adducts of heterocyclic amine food mutagens: Implications for mutagenesis and carcinogenesis. *Carcinogenesis* 20:353, 1999.

Settipane GA: The restaurant syndromes. *N Engl Reg Allergy Proc* 8:39, 1987.

Shank FR, Carson KL: What is safe food? in Finley JW, Robinson SF, Armstrong DJ (eds.): *Food Safety Assessment*. Washington, DC: American Chemical Society, 1992, p. 26.

Shiomi K, Utsumi K, Tsuchiya S, *et al.*: Comparison of proteinaceous toxins in the skin mucous from three species of eels. *Comp Biochem Physiol Biochem Mol Biol* 107:389, 1994.

Shiomi K: Toxins in marine animals. *J Jpn Assn Acute Med* 10:4, 1999.

Sieber SM, Correa P, Dalgard DW, *et al.*: Carcinogenicity and hepatotoxicity of cycasin and its aglycone methylazoxymethanol acetate in nonhuman primates. *JNCI* 65:177, 1980.

Sjoblad RD, McClintock JT, Engler R: Toxicological considerations for protein components of biological pesticide products. *Regul Toxicol Pharmacol* 15(1):3, 1992.

Skog KI, Johannsson MAE, Jagerstad MI: Carcinogenic heterocyclic amines in model systems and cooked foods: A review on formation, occurrence and intake. *Food Chem Toxicol* 36:879, 1998.

Smart DR: Scombroid poisoning: A report of seven cases involving the Western Australian salmon, *Arripis truttaceus*. *Med J Aust* 157:748, 1992.

Smith RL: Does one man's meat become another man's poison? *Trans Med Soc Lond* Nov. 11:6, 1991.

Sobel J, Tucker N, Sulka A, *et al.*: Foodborne botulism in the United States, 1990–2000. *Emerg Infect Dis* 10:1606, 2004.

Sorensen JM: Herb-drug, food-drug, nutrient-drug, and drug-drug interactions: Mechanisms involved and their medical implications. *J Altern Complement Med* 8:293, 2002.

Stargel WW, Sanders PG, Tschanz C, *et al.*: Clinical Studies with Food Additives, in Tschanz C, Butchko HH, Stargel WW, Kotsonis FN (eds.): *The Clinical Evaluation of a Food Additive. Assessment of Aspartame.* Boca Raton, Florida: CRC Press, 1996, p. 11.

Stephenson J: Public health experts take aim at a moving target: Foodborne infections. *JAMA* 277:97, 1997.

Stewart-Tull DE, Jones AC: Adjuvanted oral vaccines should not induce allergic responses to dietary antigens. *FEMS Microbiol Lett* 79:489, 1992.

Stob M, Baldwin RS, Tuite J, *et al.*: Isolation of an anabolic, uterotropic compound from corn infected with *Gibberella zeae*. *Nature* 196:1318, 1962.

Stoger P, Wuthrich B: Type I allergy to cow milk proteins in adults: A retrospective study of 34 adult milk- and cheese-allergic patients. *Int Arch Allergy Immunol* 102:399, 1993.

Stoloff L: Aflatoxins—An overview, in Rodericks JV, Hesseltine CW, Mehlman MA (eds.): *Mycotoxins in Human and Animal Health*. Park Forest South, IL: Pathtox, 1977.

Sugimura T, Wakabayashi K: Carcinogens in foods, in Shils ME (ed.): *Modern Nutrition in Health and Disease*. Baltimore: Williams and Wilkins, 1999, p. 1255.

Sugimura T, Wakabayashi K, Nagao M, *et al.*: Heterocyclic amines in cooked food, in Taylor SL, Scanlan RA (eds.): *Food Toxicology: A Perspective on the Relative Risks*. New York: Marcel Dekker, 1989, p. 31.

Szepfalusi Z, Ebner C, Pandjaitan R, *et al.*: Egg yolk *alpha*-livetin (chicken serum albumin) is a cross-reactive allergen in the bird-egg syndrome. *J Allergy Clin Immunol* 93:932, 1994.

Takatani T, Akaeda H, Arakawa O, *et al.*: Occurrence of paralytic shellfish poison (PSP) in bivalves, along with mossworm adherent to their shells, collected from Fukue Island, Nagasaki, Japan during 1995 and 1996. *J Food Hygienic Soc Jpn* 38:430, 1997.

Tan CH, Lau CO: Chemistry and detection, in Botana LM (ed): *Seafood and Freshwater Toxins. Pharmacology, Physiology and Detection*. New York: Marcel Dekker, 2000, p. 533.

Taylor NB, Fuchs RL, MacDonald J, *et al.*: Compositional analysis of glyphosate-tolerant soybeans treated with glyphosate. *J Agric Food Chem* 47(10):4469, 1999.

Taylor SL: Histamine food poisoning: Toxicology and clinical aspects. *Crit Rev Toxicol* 17(2):91, 1986.

Taylor SL, Hefle SL: Allergic reactions and food intolerances, in Kotsonis F, Mackey M, Hjelle J (eds.): *Nutritional Toxicology*, 2nd edn. New York: Taylor & Francis, 2002, p. 93.

Taylor SL, Nordlee JA, Rupnow JH: Food allergies and sensitivities, in Taylor SL, Scanlan RA (eds.): *Food Toxicology: A Perspective on the Relative Risks*. New York: Marcel Dekker, 1989, p. 255.

Tennant D: Estimation of food chemical intake, in Kotsonis F, Mackey M, Hjelle J (eds.): *Nutritional Toxicology*, 2nd edn. New York: Taylor & Francis, 2002, p. 263.

Tennant R, Zeiger E: Genetic toxicology: Current status of methods of carcinogen identification. *Environ Health Perspect* 100:307, 1993.

Thomas JA, Cotter R: Interactions between foods, nutritional supplements and drugs, in Kotsonis FN, Mackey M, HjelleJ J (eds.): *Nutritional Toxicology*, 2nd edn. New York: Taylor & Francis, 2002, p. 155.

Thompson L: Are Bioengineered foods safe. *FDA Consum* 34:18, 2000.

Todd ECD: Domoic acid and amnesic shellfish poisoning: A review.*J Food Prot* 56:69, 1993.

Tosteson MT: Mechanism of action, pharmacology and toxicology, in Botana LM (ed.): *Seafood and Freshwater Toxins. Pharmacology, Physiology and Detection*. New York: Marcel Dekker, 2000, p. 549.

Truckness MW, Mislivec PB, Young K, *et al.*: Cyclopiazonic acid production by cultures of *Aspergillus* and *Penicillium* species isolated from dried beans, corn meal, macaroni, and pecans. *J Assoc Off Anal Chem* 70:123, 1987.

Ueno Y: Trichothecenes: Overview address, in Rodericks JV, Hesseltine CW, Mehlman MA (eds.): *Mycotoxins in Human and Animal Health*. Park Forest South, IL: Pathtox, 1977, p. 189.

UK Food Standards Agency: www.food.gov.uk/news/newsarchive/maize (site visited 10 September 2003).

Underwood JE: Trace elements. *Toxicants Occurring Naturally in Foods*, 2nd ed. Washington, DC: National Academy of Sciences, 1973, p. 178.

Van Dolah FM: Diversity of marine and freshwater algal toxins, in Botana LM (ed.): *Seafood and Freshwater Toxins. Pharmacology, Physiology and Detection*. New York: Marcel Dekker, 2000, p. 19.

Van Etten CH, Tookey HL: Glucosinotates, in Rechcigl J, Jr (ed.): *CRC Handbook of Naturally Occurring Food Toxicants*. Boca Raton, FL: CRC Press, 1985, p. 15.

Van Gelderen CE, Savelkoul TJ, van Ginkel LA, *et al.*: The effects of histamine administered in fish samples to healthy volunteers. *J Toxicol Clin Toxicol* 30(4):585, 1992.

VonMalottki K, Wiechmann HW: Acute life threatening bradycardia: Food poisoning by Turkish wild honey. *Dtsch Med Wochenschr* 121:936, 1996.

Wadee AA, Boting L2Da, Rabson AR: Fruit allergy: Demonstration of IgE antibodies to a 302Dkd protein present in several fruits. *J Allergy Clin Immunol* 85:801, 1990.

Walker HW: Foodborne illness from *Clostridium perfringens*. *CRC Crit Rev Food Sci Nutr* 7:71, 1975.

Walsh EM, Leitzan EK, Hutt PB: The importance of the court decision in *Pearson v. Shalala* to the marketing of conventional food and dietary supplements in the United States, in Hasler C (ed.): *Regulation of Functional Foods and Nutraceuticals*. New York: IFT Blaikestone, 2005, p. 109.

Wantke F, Gotz M, Jarisch R: The red wine provocation test: Intolerance to histamine as a model for food intolerance. *Allergy Proc* 15(1):27, 1994.

WHO: *Application of the Principles of Substantial Equivalence to the Safety Evaluation of Foods or Food Components from Plants Derived by Modern Biotechnology*. Report WHO/FNU/FOS/95.1. Geneva: World Health Organization (WHO), 1995.

WHO: Fluoride. *Trace Elements in Human Nutrition and Health*, Chap 15. Geneva: World Health Organization (WHO), 1996, p. 187.

Williams GM, Weisburger JH: Chemical carcinogenesis, in Amdur MO, Doull J, Klaassen CD (eds.): *Toxicology: The Basic Science of Poisons*. New York: Raven Press, 1991, p. 127.

Willshaw GA, Cheasty T, Smith HR: *Escherichia coli*, in Lund BM, Baird-Parker TC, Gould GW (eds.): *The Microbiological Safety and Quality of Food*. Gaithersburg, MD: Aspen, 2000, p. 1136.

Wogan GN: Aflatoxin carcinogenesis, in Busch H (ed.): *Methods in Cancer Research*. New York: Academic Press, 1973, p. 309.

Wood GM, Slack PT, Rossell JB, *et al.*: Spanish toxic oil syndrome (1981): Progress in the identification of suspected toxic components in simulated oils. *J Agric Food Chem* 42:2525, 1994. [Correction published in *J Agric Food Chem* 43:854, 1995.]

Wuthrich B: Adverse reactions to food additives. *Ann Allergy* 71(4):379, 1993.

Yamagata N, Shigematsu I: Cadmium pollution in perspective. *Inst Public Health Tokyo Bull* 19:1, 1970.

Zhang YA, Wada T, Ichida S, *et al.*: Partially purified sea urchin toxin inhibits $^{45}Ca^{2+}$ uptake in P2 fraction from chick brain under physiological ionic conditions. *Bull Pharm Res Technol Inst* 7:67, 1998.

CHAPTER 31

ANALYTIC/FORENSIC TOXICOLOGY

Alphonse Poklis

It is impossible to consider the topic of forensic toxicology without discussing analytic toxicology in detail. However, analytic toxicology has its roots in forensic applications. Therefore, it is logical to discuss these mutually dependent areas together. Analytic toxicology involves the application of the tools of analytic chemistry to the qualitative and/or quantitative estimation of chemicals that may exert adverse effects on living organisms. Generally, the chemical that is to be measured (the analyte) is a xenobiotic that may have been altered or transformed by metabolic actions of the organism. Frequently, the specimen that is to be analyzed presents a matrix consisting of body fluids or solid tissues from the organism. Both the identity of the analyte and the nature of the matrix present formidable problems to an analytic toxicologist.

Forensic toxicology involves the use of toxicology for the purposes of the law (Cravey and Baselt, 1981). Although this broad definition includes a wide range of applications, such as regulatory toxicology and urine testing to detect drug use, by far the most common application is to identify any chemical that may serve as a causative agent in inflicting death or injury on humans or in causing damage to property. Frequently, as a result of such unfortunate incidents, charges of liability or criminal intent are brought that must be resolved by the judicial system. At times, indirect or circumstantial evidence is presented in an attempt to prove cause and effect. However, there is no substitute for an unequivocal identification of a specific chemical substance that is demonstrated to be present in tissues from the victim at a sufficient concentration to explain the injury with a reasonable degree of scientific probability or certainty. For this reason, forensic toxicology and analytic toxicology have long shared a mutually supportive partnership.

Some forensic toxicologic activities have been deemed so important by society that a great effort is expended to initiate and implement analytic procedures in a forensically credible manner as an aid in deciding whether adverse effects have been produced by certain chemicals. Attempts to control drivers whose driving ability may be impaired by ethanol or certain drugs are evidenced by laws prescribing punishment to individuals who are so impaired. The measurement of ethanol in blood or breath at specific concentrations is generally required to prove impairment by this agent (Fisher *et al.*, 1968). Similarly, the decade of the 1980s saw a growing response by society to the threat of drug abuse. Attempts to identify drug users by testing urine for the presence of drugs or their metabolites, using methods and safeguards developed by forensic toxicologists, have become required by law (Department of Health and Human Services, 1988).

The diagnosis and treatment of health problems induced by chemical substances (Blanke and Decker, 1986) and the closely allied field of therapeutic drug monitoring (Moyer *et al.*, 1986) also rely greatly on analytic toxicology. Although the analytes are present in matrices similar to those seen in forensic toxicology, the results must be reported rapidly to be of use to clinicians in treating patients. This requirement of a rapid turnaround time limits the number of chemicals that can be measured because methods, equipment, and personnel must all be available for an instant response to toxicologic emergencies.

Occupational toxicology (see Chap. 33) and regulatory toxicology require analytic procedures for their implementation or monitoring. In occupational toxicology, the analytic methods used to monitor threshold limit values (TLVs) and other means of estimating the exposure of workers to toxic hazards may utilize simple, nonspecific, but economical screening devices. However, to determine the actual exposure of a worker, it is necessary to analyze blood, urine, breath, or another specimen by employing methods similar to those used in clinical or forensic toxicology. For regulatory purposes, a variety of matrices (food, water, air, etc.) must be examined for extremely small quantities of analytes. Frequently, this requires the use of sophisticated methodology with extreme sensitivity. Both of these applications of analytic toxicology impinge on forensic toxicology because an injury or occupational disease in a worker can result in a legal proceeding, just as a violation of a regulatory law may.

Other applications of analytic toxicology occur frequently during the course of experimental studies. Confirmation of the concentration of dosing solutions and monitoring of their stability often can be accomplished with the use of simple analytic techniques. The bioavailability of a dose may vary with the route of administration and the vehicle used. Blood concentrations can be monitored as a means of establishing this important parameter. In addition, an important feature in the study of any toxic substance is the characterization of its metabolites as well as the distribution of the parent drug, together with its metabolites, to various tissues. This requires sensitive, specific, and valid analytic procedures. Similar analytic studies can be conducted within a temporal framework to gain an understanding of the dynamics of the absorption, distribution, metabolism, and excretion of toxic chemicals.

It is evident that analytic toxicology is intimately involved in many aspects of experimental and applied toxicology. Because toxic substances include all chemical types and because the measurement of toxic chemicals may require the examination of biological or nonbiological matrices, the scope of analytic toxicology is broad. Nevertheless, a systematic approach and a reliance on the practical experience of generations of forensic toxicologists can be used in conjunction with the sophisticated tools of analytic chemistry to provide the data needed to understand the hazards of toxic substances more completely. These concepts are described in detail in the rest of this chapter.

ANALYTIC TOXICOLOGY

In light of the statement by Paracelsus five centuries ago, "All substances are poisons: there is none which is not a poison," analytic toxicology potentially encompasses all chemical substances. Forensic toxicologists learned long ago that when the nature of a suspected poison is unknown, a systematic, standardized approach must be used to identify the presence of most common toxic substances. An approach that has stood the test of time was first suggested by Chapuis in 1873 in *Elements de Toxicologie*. It is based on the origin or nature of the toxic agent (Peterson *et al.*, 1923). Such a system can be characterized as follows:

1. Gases
2. Volatile substances
3. Corrosive agents
4. Metals
5. Anions and nonmetals
6. Nonvolatile organic substances
7. Miscellaneous

Closely related to this descriptive classification is the method for separating a toxic agent from the matrix in which it is embedded. The matrix is generally a biological specimen such as a body fluid or a solid tissue. The agent of interest may exist in the matrix in a simple solution or may be bound to protein and other cellular constituents. The challenge is to separate the toxic agent in sufficient purity and quantity to permit it to be characterized and quantified. At times, the parent compound is no longer present in large enough amounts to be separated. In this case, known metabolites may indirectly provide a measure of the parent substance (Hawks and Chiang, 1986). With other substances, interaction of the poison with tissue components may require the isolation or characterization of a protein adduct (SanGeorge and Hoberman, 1986). Methods for separation have long provided a great challenge to analytic toxicologists. Only recently have methods become available that permit direct measurement of some analytes without prior separation from the matrix.

Gases are most simply measured by means of gas chromatography. Some gases are extremely labile, and the specimen must be collected and preserved at temperatures as low as that of liquid nitrogen. Generally, the gas is carefully liberated by incubating the specimen at a predetermined temperature in a closed container. The gas, freed from the matrix, collects over the specimen's "headspace," where it can be sampled and injected into the gas chromatograph. Other gases, such as carbon monoxide, interact with proteins. These

gases can be carefully released from the protein, or the adduct can be measured independently, as in the case of carboxyhemoglobin.

Volatile substances are generally liquids of a variety of chemical types. The temperature at which they boil is sufficiently low that older methods of separation utilized microdistillation or diffusion techniques. Gas–liquid chromatography is the simplest approach for simultaneous separation and quantitation in favorable cases. The simple alcohols can be measured by injecting a diluted body fluid directly onto the column of the chromatograph. A more common approach is to use the headspace technique, as is done for gases, after incubating the specimen at an elevated temperature.

Corrosives include mineral acids and bases. Many corrosives consist of ions that are normal tissue constituents. Clinical chemical techniques can be applied to detect these ions when they are in great excess over normal concentrations. Because these ions are normal constituents, the corrosive effects at the site of contact of the chemical, together with other changes in blood chemistry values, can confirm the ingestion of a corrosive substance.

Metals are encountered frequently as occupational and environmental hazards. Elegant analytic methods are available for most metals even when they are present at extremely low concentrations. Classic separation procedures involve destruction of the organic matrix by chemical or thermal oxidation. This leaves the metal to be identified and quantified in the inorganic residue. Unfortunately, this prevents the determination of the metal in the oxidation state or in combination with other elements, as it existed when the metal compound was absorbed. For example, the toxic effects of metallic mercury, mercurous ion, mercuric ion, and dimethylmercury are all different. Analytic methods must be selected that determine the relative amount of each form present to yield optimal analytic results. The analytic difficulty in doing this has lent support to the unfortunate practice of discussing the toxicity of metals as if each metal existed as a single entity.

Toxic anions and nonmetals are a difficult group for analysis. Some anions can be trapped in combination with a stable cation, after which the organic matrix can be destroyed, as with metals. Others can be separated from the bulk of the matrix by dialysis, after which they are detected by colorimetric or chromatographic procedures. Still others are detected and measured by ion-specific electrodes. There are no standard approaches for this group, and other than phosphorus, they are rarely encountered in an uncombined form.

The *nonvolatile organic substances* constitute the largest group of substances that must be considered by analytic toxicologists. This group includes drugs, both prescribed and illegal, pesticides, natural products, pollutants, and industrial compounds. These substances are solids or liquids with high boiling points. Thus, separation procedures generally rely on differential extractions of tissue specimens (Fig. 31-1). These extractions often are not efficient, and recovery of the toxic substance from the matrix may be poor. When the nature of the toxic substance is known, immunoassay procedures are useful because they allow a toxicologist to avoid using separation procedures. These compounds can be classified as

1. organic strong acids
2. organic weak acids
3. organic bases
4. organic neutral compounds
5. organic amphoteric compounds

Separation generally is achieved by adjusting the acidity of the aqueous matrix and extracting with a water-immiscible solvent or a solid-phase absorbent material. Finally, a *miscellaneous* category

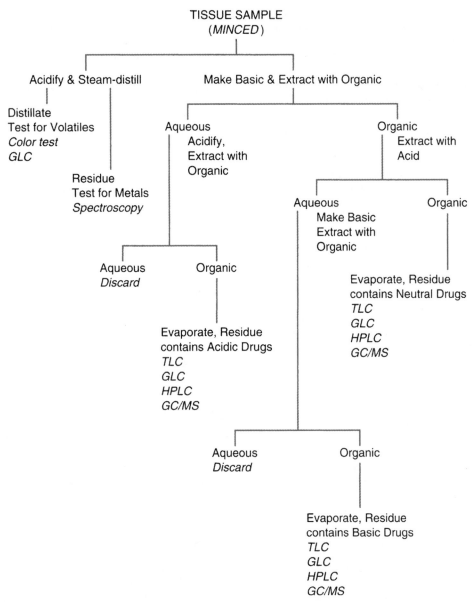

Figure 31-1. A scheme of separation for poisons from tissues by steam distillation and differential solvent extraction.

Abbreviations: GC/MS, gas chromatography/mass spectrometry; GLC, gas-liquid chromatography; HPLC, high-pressure liquid chromatography; TLC, thin-layer chromatography.

must be included to cover the large number of toxic agents that cannot be detected by the routine application of the methods described above. Venoms and other toxic mixtures of proteins or uncharacterized constituents fall into this class. Frequently, if antibodies can be grown against the active constituent, immunoassay may be the most practical means of detecting and measuring these highly potent and difficult-to-isolate substances. Unfortunately, unless highly specific monoclonal antibodies are used, the analytic procedure may not be acceptable for forensic purposes. Most frequently, specific analytic procedures must be developed for each analyte of this type. At times, biological endpoints are utilized to semiquantify the concentration of the isolated product.

After this brief description of the scope of analytic toxicology, we shall now show how it is applied to a variety of aspects of toxicology.

ANALYTIC ROLE IN GENERAL TOXICOLOGY

In almost all experimental studies in toxicology, an agent, generally a single chemical substance, is administered in known amounts to an organism. It is universally acknowledged that the chemical under study must be pure or the nature of any contaminant must be known to interpret the experimental results with validity. However, it is a common practice to proceed with the experimental study without verifying the purity of the compound. Not only does this practice lead to errors in establishing an accurate dose, but, depending on the nature of the study, other erroneous conclusions may be drawn. For example, the presence of related compounds in the dosage form of a tricyclic antidepressant led to erroneous conclusions about the metabolic products of the drug when it was administered together with the unidentified contaminants (Saady *et al.*, 1981). An even greater error may result when a small amount of a contaminant may be supertoxic. A well-publicized example of this error involved the presence of dioxin in mixtures of the defoliants 2,4-D and 2,4,5-T (Panel on Herbicides, 1971) used during the Vietnam War as Agent Orange. Some of the adverse effects of Agent Orange may have been due to the low concentration of dioxin in those mixtures. Other researchers have reported that the toxicity of mixtures of polybrominated biphenyls may be due to the high toxicity of specific components, while other brominated biphenyls are relatively nontoxic (Mills *et al.*, 1985).

A related application of analytic toxicology is in monitoring dosage forms or solutions for stability throughout the course of an experimental study. Chemicals may degrade in contact with air, by exposure to ultraviolet or other radiation, by interaction with constituents of the vehicle or dosing solution, and by other means. Developing an analytic procedure by which these changes can be recognized and corrected is essential in achieving consistent results throughout a study (Blanke, 1989).

Finally, analytic methods are important in establishing the bioavailability of a compound that is under study. Some substances with low water solubility are difficult to introduce into an animal, and a variety of vehicles may be tried. However, measuring blood concentrations of the compound under study provides a simple means of comparing the effectiveness of vehicles. Introducing a compound into the stomach in an oil vehicle may not be the most effective means of enhancing the absorption of that compound (Granger *et al.*, 1987). Rather than observing dose–effect relationships, it may be more accurate to describe blood (serum) concentration–effect relationships.

ANALYTIC ROLE IN FORENSIC TOXICOLOGY

The duties of a forensic toxicologist in postmortem investigations include the qualitative and quantitative analysis of drugs or poisons in biological specimens collected at autopsy and the interpretation of the analytic findings in regard to the physiologic and behavioral effects of the detected chemicals on the deceased at the time of death.

The complete investigation of the cause or causes of sudden death is an important civic responsibility. Establishing the cause of death rests with the medical examiner, coroner, or pathologist, but success in arriving at the correct conclusion often depends on the combined efforts of the pathologist and the toxicologist. The cause of death in cases of poisoning cannot be proved beyond contention without a toxicologic analysis that establishes the presence of the toxicant in the tissues and body fluids of the deceased.

Many drugs or poisons do not produce characteristic pathologic lesions; their presence in the body can be demonstrated only by chemical methods of isolation and identification. If toxicologic analyses are avoided, deaths resulting from poisoning may be erroneously ascribed to an entirely different cause or poisoning may be designated as the cause of death without definite proof. Such erroneous diagnoses may have significant legal and social consequences.

Additionally, a toxicologist can furnish valuable evidence concerning the circumstances surrounding a death. Such cases commonly involve demonstrating the presence of intoxicating concentrations of ethanol in victims of automotive or industrial accidents or such concentrations of carbon monoxide in fire victims. The degree of carbon monoxide saturation of the blood may indicate whether the deceased died as a result of the fire or was dead before the fire started. Arson is commonly used to conceal homicide. Also, licit or illicit psychoactive drugs often play a significant role in the circumstances associated with sudden or violent death. The behavioral toxicity of many illicit drugs may explain the bizarre or "risk-taking" behavior of the deceased that led to his or her demise. At times, a negative toxicologic finding is of particular importance in assessing the cause of death. For example, toxicology studies may demonstrate that a person with a seizure disorder was not taking the prescribed medication and that this contributed to the fatal event.

Additionally, the results of postmortem toxicologic testing provide valuable epidemiologic and statistical data. Forensic toxicologists are often among the first to alert the medical community to new epidemics of substance abuse (Poklis, 1982) and the dangers of abusing over-the-counter drugs (Garriott *et al.*, 1985). Similarly, they often determine the chemical identity and toxicity of novel analogs of psychoactive agents that are subject to abuse, including "designer drugs" such as "china white" (methylfentanyl) (Henderson, 1988) and "ecstasy" (methylenedioxymethamphetamine) (Dowling *et al.*, 1987).

Today, there are numerous specialized areas of study in the field of toxicology; however, it is the forensic toxicologist who is obliged to assist in the determination of the cause of death for a court of law and who has been historically recognized by the title "toxicologist."

Until the nineteenth century, physicians, lawyers, and law enforcement officials harbored extremely faulty notions about the signs and symptoms of poisoning (Thorwald, 1965). Unless a poisoner was literally caught in the act, there was no way to establish the fact that the victim died from poison. In the early eighteenth century, a Dutch physician, Hermann Boerhoave, theorized that various poisons in a hot, vaporous condition yield characteristic odors. He placed substances suspected of containing poisons on hot coals and tested their smells. While Boerhoave was not successful in applying his method, he was the first to suggest a chemical method for proving the presence of poison.

White arsenic (arsenic trioxide) has been widely used with murderous intent for over a thousand years. Therefore, it is not surprising that the first milestones in the chemical isolation and identification of a poison in body tissues and fluids centered on arsenic. In 1775, Karl Wilhelm Scheele, a Swedish chemist, discovered that white arsenic is converted to arsenous acid by chlorine water. The addition of metallic zinc reduced the arsenous acid to poisonous arsine gas. If gently heated, the evolving gas would deposit metallic arsenic on the surface of a cold vessel. In 1821, Serullas utilized the decomposition of arsine for the detection of small quantities of arsenic in stomach contents and urine in poisoning cases. In 1836, James M. Marsh, a chemist at the Royal British Arsenal in Woolwich, applied Serullas' observations in developing the first reliable method to determine the presence of an absorbed poison in body tissues and fluids such as liver, kidney, and blood. After acid digestion of the tissues, Marsh generated arsine gas, which was drawn through a heated capillary tube. The arsine decomposed, leaving a dark deposit of metallic arsenic. Quantitative measures were performed by comparing the length of the deposit from known concentrations of arsenic with those of the test specimens.

The 1800s witnessed the development of forensic toxicology as a scientific discipline. In 1814, Mathieiv J. B. Orfila (1787–1853), the "father of toxicology," published *Traité des Poisons,* the first systematic approach to the study of the chemical and physiological nature of poisons (Gettler, 1977). Orfila's role as an expert witness in many famous murder trails, particularly his application of the Marsh test for arsenic in the trial of the poisoner Marie Lafarge, aroused both popular and scholarly interest in the new science. As dean of the medical faculty at the University of Paris, Orfila trained numerous students in forensic toxicology.

The first successful isolation of an alkaloidal poison was done in 1850 by Jean Servials Stas, a Belgian chemist, using a solution of acetic acid in warm ethanol to extract nicotine from the tissues of the murdered Gustave Fougnie. As modified by the German chemist Fredrick Otto, the Stas–Otto method was quickly applied to the isolation of numerous alkaloidal poisons, including colchicine, coniine, morphine, narcotine, and strychnine. In the latter half of the nineteenth century, European toxicologists were in the forefront of the development and application of forensic sciences, providing valuable evidence of poisoning. A number of these trials became "causes célèbres" and the testimony of forensic toxicologists captured the imagination of the public and increased awareness of the development and application of toxicology. Murderers could no longer poison with impunity.

In the United States, Rudolph A. Witthaus, professor of chemistry at Cornell University Medical School, made many contributions to toxicology and called attention to the new science by performing analyses for the city of New York in several famous morphine poisoning cases, including the murder of Helen Potts by Carlyle Harris and that of Annie Sutherland by Dr. Robert W. Buchanan. In 1911, Witthaus and Tracy C. Becker edited a four-volume work on medical jurisprudence, forensic medicine, and toxicology—the first standard forensic textbook published in the United States. In 1918, the city of New York established a medical examiner's system, and the appointment of Dr. Alexander O. Gettler as toxicologist marked the beginning of modern forensic toxicology in this country. Although Dr. Gettler made numerous contributions to the science, perhaps his greatest was the training and direction he gave to future leaders in forensic toxicology. Many of his associates went on to direct laboratories within coroners' and medical examiners' systems in major urban centers throughout the country.

In 1949, the American Academy of Forensic Sciences was established to support and further the practice of all phases of legal medicine in the United States. The members of the toxicology section represent the vast majority of forensic toxicologists working in coroners' or medical examiners' offices. Several other international, national, and local forensic science organizations, such as the Society of Forensic Toxicologists and the California Association of Toxicologists, offer a forum for the exchange of scientific data pertaining to analytic techniques and case reports involving new or infrequently used drugs and poisons. The International Association of Forensic Toxicologists, founded in 1963, with over 750 members in 45 countries, permits worldwide cooperation in resolving the technical problems confronting toxicology.

In 1975, the American Board of Forensic Toxicology (ABFT) was created to examine and certify forensic toxicologists. One of the stated objectives of the board is "to make available to the judicial system, and other publics, a practical and equitable system for readily identifying those persons professing to be specialists in forensic toxicology who possess the requisite qualifications and competence." Those certified as diplomats of the board must have a doctor of philosophy or doctor of science degree, have at least 3 years of full-time professional experience, and pass a written examination. In 2000, the board began certifying "forensic toxicology specialists." Specialists must have a master's or bachelor's degree

and 3 years of full-time professional experience and must pass a written examination. At present, there are approximately 225 diplomats and 20 specialists certified by the board. In 1998, the board began an accreditation program for forensic toxicology laboratories. ABFT accredited laboratories must meet standards of qualified, experienced personnel and forensically sound procedures for the handling of evidence, analysis of specimens, and reporting of results. Laboratories must pass periodic on-site inspections involving a review of laboratory procedures and previous casework since the last inspection in order to maintain their continuous accreditation.

TOXICOLOGIC INVESTIGATION OF A POISON DEATH

The toxicologic investigation of a poison death may be divided into three steps: (1) obtaining the case history and suitable specimens, (2) the toxicologic analyses, and (3) the interpretation of the analytic findings.

Case History and Specimens

Today, thousands of compounds are readily available that are lethal if ingested, injected, or inhaled. Usually, a limited amount of specimen is available on which to perform analyses; therefore it is imperative that, before the analyses are initiated, as much information as possible concerning the facts of the case be collected. The age, sex, weight, medical history, and occupation of the decedent as well as any treatment administered before death, the gross autopsy findings, the drugs available to the decedent, and the interval between the onset of symptoms and death should be noted. In a typical year, a postmortem toxicology laboratory will perform analyses for such diverse poisons as prescription drugs (analgesics, antidepressants, hypnotics, tranquilizers), drugs of abuse (hallucinogens, narcotics, stimulants), commercial products (antifreeze, aerosol products, insecticides, rodenticides, rubbing compound, weed killers), and gases (carbon monoxide, cyanide). Obviously, thorough investigation of the death scene including a tentative identification of the administered poison is helpful prior to beginning the analysis (Ernst *et al.*, 1982).

The pathologist at autopsy usually performs the collection of postmortem specimens for analysis. Specimens of many different body fluids and organs are necessary, as drugs and poisons display varying affinities for body tissues (Fig. 31-2). Therefore, detection of a poison is more likely in a tissue in which it accumulates. A large quantity of each specimen is needed for thorough toxicologic analysis because a procedure that extracts and identifies one compound or class of compounds may be ineffective in extracting and identifying others (Table 31-1).

In collecting the specimens, the pathologist labels each container with the date and time of autopsy, the name of the decedent, the identity of the sample, an appropriate case identification number, and his or her signature or initials. It is paramount that the handling of all specimens, their analysis, and the resultant reports be authenticated and documented. A form developed at the collection site that identifies each specimen is submitted to the laboratory with the specimens. The form is signed and dated by the pathologist and subsequently by any individual handling, transferring, or transporting the specimens from one individual or place to another. In legal terms, this form constitutes a "chain of custody" of specimens, documenting by time, date, name, and signature of all persons transferring or receiving the specimens. The chain of custody enables a toxicologist

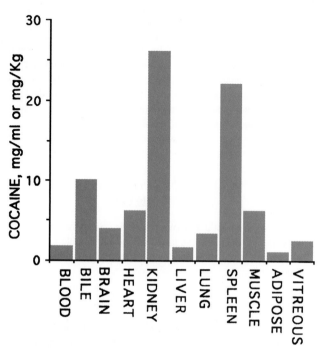

Figure 31-2. Cocaine tissue distribution in a fatal poisoning. (Data drawn from Poklis A, Mackell MA, Graham M: Disposition of cocaine in a fatal poisoning in man. J Anal Toxicol 9:227–229, 1985.)

to introduce his or her results into legal proceedings, having established that the specimens analyzed came from the decedent.

Specimens should be collected before embalming, as this process may destroy or dilute the poisons present, rendering their detection impossible. Conversely, methyl or ethyl alcohol may be a constituent of embalming fluid, giving a false indication of the decedent's drinking before death.

On occasion, toxicologic analysis is requested for cases of burned, exhumed, and skeletal remains. In such instances, it is necessary to analyze unusual specimens such as bone marrow, hair, skeletal muscle, vitreous humor, and even maggots (Inoue, 1992). Numerous drugs have been successfully identified in bone marrow and bone washings from skeletal remains even after decomposition and burial (Benko, 1985). Similarly, the vitreous humor of the eye is isolated and sequestered from putrefaction, charring, and trauma;

Table 31-1

Suggested List of Specimens and Amounts to be Collected at Autopsy

SPECIMEN	QUANTITY (g)
Brain	100
Liver	100
Kidney	50
Heart blood	25
Peripheral blood	10
Vitreous humor	All available
Bile	All available
Urine	All available
Gastric contents	All available

SOURCE: Appendix, Report of the Laboratory Guidelines Committee, Society of Forensic Toxicologist and Toxicology Section, American Academy of Forensic Sciences. *J Anal Toxicol* 14:18(A), 1990, with permission.

thus, it is a useful specimen for the detection of most drugs, anions, and even volatile poisons such as alcohols, ketones, and glycols (Coe, 1993). Hair analysis is a rapidly growing technique in forensic toxicology. Recently, numerous therapeutic agents such as antibiotics and antipsychotic drugs as well as drugs subject to abuse (morphine, phencyclidine, and cocaine) have been identified in hair (Tagliro, 1993). Limited data are available to support a direct correlation between hair values and drug doses or between physiologic and behavioral effects; however, qualitative results have been accepted as indicators of drug use. In severely decomposed bodies, the absence of blood and/or the scarcity of solid tissues suitable for analysis have led to the collection and testing of maggots (fly larvae) feeding on the body (Pounder, 1991). The fundamental premise underlying maggot analysis is that if drugs or intoxicants are detected, they could only have originated from the decedents' tissues on which the larvae were feeding. Surprisingly, analysis of maggots is rather straightforward, requiring no special methodology beyond that routinely applied in toxicology laboratories. Case reports have documented the detection of numerous drugs and intoxicants in maggots collected from decomposed bodies. The compounds detected include barbiturates, benzodiazepines, phenothiazines, morphine, and malathion. Controlled studies in which maggots were allowed to feed on tissues to which drugs had been added have demonstrated the accumulation of propoxphene and amitriptyline in the larvae (Goff *et al.*, 1993).

Toxicologic Analysis

Before the analysis begins, several factors must be considered, the amount of specimen available, the nature of the poison sought, and the possible biotransformation of the poison. In cases involving oral administration of the poison, the gastrointestinal (GI) contents are analyzed first because large amounts of residual unabsorbed poison may be present. The urine may be analyzed next, as the kidney is the major organ of excretion for most poisons and high concentrations of toxicants and/or their metabolites often are present in urine. After absorption from the GI tract, drugs or poisons are carried to the liver before entering the general systemic circulation; therefore, the first analysis of an internal organ is conducted on the liver. If a specific poison is suspected to have caused or contributed to a death, the toxicologist may first analyze the tissues and fluids in which the poison concentrates.

A knowledge of drug biotransformation is often essential before an analysis is performed. The parent compound and any major physiologically active metabolites should be isolated and identified. In some instances, the metabolites provide the only evidence that a drug or poison has been administered. Many screening tests, such as immunoassays, are specifically designed to detect not the parent drug but its major urinary metabolite. An example of the relationship of pharmacokinetic and analytic factors is provided by cocaine. The major metabolites of cocaine biotransformation are benzoylecgonine and ecgonine methylester (Fig. 31-3). The ingestion of alcohol combined with the administration of cocaine results in the hepatic transesterification of cocaine to form cocaethylene (Hime *et al.*, 1991) (Fig. 31-3). The disposition of these compounds in various body fluids and hair is shown in Fig. 31-4. Thus, the initial testing of urine to determine cocaine use is performed with immunoassays specifically designed to detect the presence of benzoylecgonine, the major urinary metabolite. If saliva or hair is tested, parent cocaine is the analyte sought. To determine a cocaine profile of each compound present in a specimen, chromatographic procedures such as

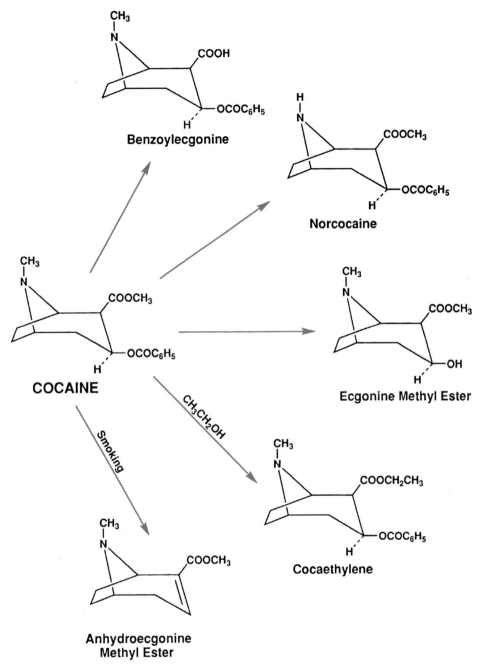

Figure 31-3. Biotransformation and pyrolysis products of cocaine.

gas chromatography/mass spectrometry (GC/MS), that allow the simultaneous separation and quantification of each compound, are used.

The analysis may be complicated by the normal chemical changes that occur during the decomposition of a cadaver. The autopsy and toxicologic analysis should be started as soon after death as possible. The natural enzymatic and nonenzymatic processes of decomposition and microbial metabolism may destroy a poison that was present at death or produce substances or compounds with chemical and physical properties similar to those of commonly encountered poisons. As early as the 1870s, the so-called cadaveric alkaloids isolated from the organs of putrefied bodies were known to produce color test reactions similar to those produced

by morphine and other drugs. These cadaveric alkaloids resulted from the bacterial decarboxylation of the amino acids ornithine and lysine, producing putrescine and cadaverine, respectively (Evans, 1963). Similarly, during decomposition, phenylalanine is converted to phenylethylamine, which has chemical and physical properties very similar to those of amphetamine. The hydrolysis, oxidation, or reduction of proteins, nucleic acids, and lipids may generate numerous compounds, such as hydroxylated aliphatic and aromatic carboxylic acids, pyridine and piperidine derivatives, and aromatic heterocyclics such as tryptamine and norharmane (Kaempe, 1969). All these substances may interfere with the isolation and identification of the toxicants being sought. The concentration of cyanide and ethyl alcohol and the carbon monoxide saturation of the blood

PERCENT

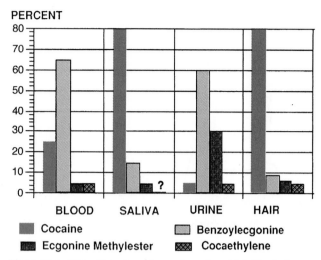

Figure 31-4. Disposition of cocaine and cocaine metabolites in human fluids and hair. (Data redrawn from Spiehler V: Society of Forensic Toxicology Conference on Drug Testing in Hair, Tampa, FL, October 29, 1994.)

may be decreased or increased, depending on the degree of putrefaction and microbial activity. However, many poisons—such as arsenic, barbiturates, mercury, and strychnine—are extremely stable and may be detectable many years after death.

Before analysis, the purity of all chemicals should be established. The primary reference material used to prepare calibrators and controls should be checked for purity, and the salt form or degree of hydration should be determined (Blanke, 1989). All reagents and solvents should be of the highest grade possible and should be free of contaminants that may interfere with or distort analytic findings. For example, the chloroform contaminants phosgene and ethyl chloroformate may react with primary or secondary amine drugs to form carbamyl chloride and ethyl carbamate derivatives (Cone *et al.*, 1982). Specimen containers, lids, and stoppers should be free of

contaminants such as plasticizers, which often interfere with chromatographic or GC/MS determinations. Care should be exercised to ensure a clean laboratory environment. This is of particular concern in the analysis of metals, as aluminum, arsenic, lead, and mercury are ubiquitous environmental and reagent contaminants.

Forensic toxicology laboratories analyze specimens by using a variety of analytic procedures. Initially, nonspecific tests designed to determine the presence or absence of a class or group of analytes may be performed directly on the specimens. Examples of tests used to rapidly screen urine are the FPN (ferric chloride, perchloric, and nitric acid) color test for phenothiazine drugs and immunoassays for the detection of amphetamines, benzodiazepines, and opiate derivatives. Positive results obtained with these tests must be confirmed by a second analytic procedure that identifies the particular drug. The detection limit of the confirmatory test should be lower than that of the initial nonspecific test. Some analytic procedures identify specific compounds. Even in such instances, a second test should be performed to identify the analyte. The second test should be based on a chemical or physical principle different from that of the first test. Such additional testing is performed to establish an unequivocal identification of the drugs or poisons present. Whenever possible, the most specific test for the compound of interest should be performed. Today, GC/MS or high-performance liquid chromatography (HPLC)/MS is the most widely applied methodology in toxicology and is generally accepted as unequivocal identification for most drugs. Analyte identification is based upon the retention time in the chromatographic system coupled with the ion fragmentation spectrum in the mass spectrometer. The analyte mass spectrum is the pattern of mass to charge ion fragments and their relative abundance. Even drugs such as amitriptyline and cyclobenzaprine that display similar chromatographic behavior and differ in their chemical structure by only a double bond may be readily identified by GC/MS (Fig. 31-5).

The lower limit of detection, the smallest concentration of analyte reliably identified by the assay, and the specificity of all qualitative methods should be well documented. The laboratory must

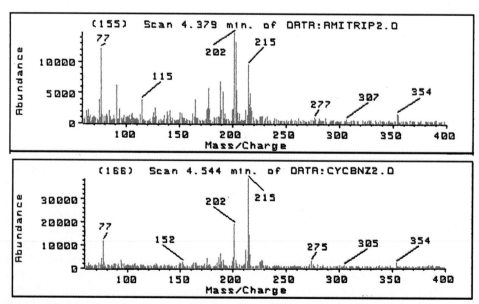

Figure 31-5. Electron impact mass spectra of amitriptyline and cyclobenzaprine, scanning ion mass from 60 to 400 m/e. (From Poklis A: Cyclobenzaprine in emergency toxicology. Clin Chem CC96-3:43–57, 1996. American Society of Clinical Pathologists, with permission.)

demonstrate that the assay response to blank or negative calibrators does not overlap with the response of the lowest-positive calibrator. In certain instances, qualitative identification of a poison or drug is sufficient to resolve forensic toxicology issues. However, most cases require reliable estimates of poison concentrations for forensic interpretation. For quantitative analysis, the linearity, precision, and specificity of the procedure must be established. Linearity should be determined by using at least a drug free and three drug added calibrators whose concentrations bracket the anticipated concentrations in the specimen. Precision, which statistically demonstrates the variance in the value obtained, is determined by replicate analyses of a specimen of a known concentration. For a variety of reasons, a quantitative result occasionally will deviate spuriously from the true value. Therefore, replicate quantitative determinations should be performed on all specimens, at least in duplicate (Blanke, 1987).

When unusual samples such as bone marrow, hair, and maggots are analyzed, the extraction efficiency of a procedure may vary greatly, depending on the nature of the specimens. Therefore, all calibrators and controls should be prepared in the same matrix as the specimens and analyzed concurrently with the specimens. Often the matrix is "unique" or impossible to match, such as decomposed or embalmed tissue. In these instances, the method of "standard additions" may be used. Known amounts of the drug or poison of interest are added to specimen aliquots and these are analyzed. The concentration of poison in the test specimen is determined by comparing the proportional response of the "poison added" specimens to that of the test specimens. When comparable results are obtained from analysis of specimens by both direct extraction methods and standard addition, not only is the efficacy of the extraction method validated, but also the accuracy of the results is assured (Poklis *et al.*, 1998).

Interpretation of Analytic Results

Once the analysis of the specimens is complete, the toxicologist must interpret his or her findings in regard to the physiologic or behavioral effects of the toxicants on the decedent at the concentrations found. Specific questions may be answered, such as the route of administration, the dose administered, and whether the concentration of the toxicant present was sufficient to cause death or alter the decedent's actions enough to cause his or her death. Assessing the physiologic or behavioral meanings of analytic results is often the most difficult problem faced by the forensic toxicologist.

In determining the route of administration, the toxicologist notes the results of the analysis of the various specimens. As a general rule, the highest concentrations of a poison are found at the site of administration. Therefore, the presence of large amounts of drugs and/or poisons in the GI tract and liver indicates oral ingestion, while higher concentrations in the lungs than in other visceral organs can indicate inhalation or intravenous injection. The ratio or relative distribution of drugs in different tissues may also differentiate oral from parenteral administration (Fig. 31-6). Drugs may also be detected in the tissue surrounding an injection site following intramuscular or intravenous injection. Smoking is a popular route of administration for abusers of controlled substances such as cocaine, heroin, and phencyclidine. Pyrolysis of these drugs leads to the inhalation not only of the parent drug but also of characteristic breakdown products of combustion. For example, a major pyrolysis product of "crack" cocaine smoking is anhydroecgonine methylester (Martin *et al.*, 1989) (Fig. 31-3). Thus, identification of relatively high concentrations of this compound along with cocaine

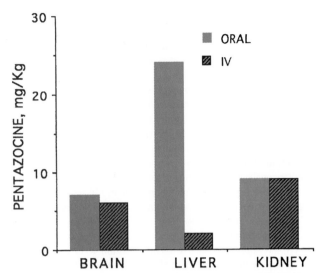

Figure 31-6. Comparison of pentazocine distribution in fatal poisonings due to intravenous injection and oral administration. (Data from Baselt RC: Disposition of Toxic Drugs and Chemicals in Man, 2nd ed. Davis, CA: Biomedical Publications, 1982, pp. 603–606, and Poklis A, MacKell MA: Toxicological findings in deaths due to pentazocine: A report of two cases. Forensic Sci Int 20:89–95, 1982.)

or cocaine metabolites in urine or other body fluids or tissues indicates smoking as the route of cocaine administration (Jacob *et al.*, 1990).

The presence of a toxic material in the GI tract, regardless of the quantity, does not provide sufficient evidence to establish that agent as the cause of death. It is necessary to demonstrate that absorption of the toxicant has occurred and that it has been transported by the general circulation to the target organ in order to exert its lethal effect. This is established by blood and tissue analysis. An exception to the rule is provided by strong, corrosive chemicals such as sulfuric acid, lye, and phenol, which exert their deleterious effects by directly digesting tissue, causing hemorrhage and shock. The results of urinalysis are often of little benefit in determining the physiologic effects of a toxic agent. Urine results establish only that the poison was present in the body at some time before death. Correlation of urine values with physiologic effects is poor because of various factors that influence the rate of excretion of specific compounds and the urine volume.

The physiologic effects of most drugs and poisons are correlated with their concentrations in blood or blood fractions such as plasma and serum. Indeed, in living persons, this association is the basis of therapeutic drug monitoring. However, postmortem blood has been described as a fluid resembling blood that is obtained from the vasculature after death. Therefore, interpretation of postmortem blood results requires careful consideration of the case history, the site of collection, and postmortem changes. The survival time between the administration of a poison and death may be sufficiently long to permit biotransformation and excretion of the agent. Blood values may appear to be nontoxic or consistent with therapeutic administration. Death from hepatic failure after an acetaminophen overdose usually occurs at least 3 to 4 days after ingestion. Postmortem acetaminophen concentrations in blood may be consistent with the ingestion of therapeutic doses. Therefore, fatal acetaminophen overdose is established by case history, central lobular necrosis of the liver, and, if available, analysis of serum specimens collected from the decedent when he or she was admitted to the emergency department (Price *et al.*, 1991). Emergency medical treatment—such as the administration of fluids, plasma extenders, diuretics, and blood transfusions—may dilute or remove toxic agents. Similarly, prolonged survival on a mechanical respirator, hemodialysis, or hemoperfusion may significantly reduce initially lethal blood concentrations of poisons.

Until recently, it was generally assumed that postmortem blood drug concentrations were more or less uniform throughout the body. However, in the 1970s, several investigators noted that postmortem concentrations of digoxin in heart blood greatly exceeded those in simultaneously collected femoral blood. They also observed that postmortem blood concentrations, particularly in heart blood, exceeded the expected values at the time of death (Vorpahl and Coe, 1978; Aderjan *et al.*, 1979). This postmortem increase in blood digoxin concentrations was apparently due to release of the drug from tissue stores, particularly the myocardium. Recently, other researchers have demonstrated that for many drugs, blood concentrations in the same body vary greatly depending on the site from which the specimen is collected—subclavian vein, thoracic aorta, inferior vena cava, femoral vein, and so forth. For example, in a case of fatal multiple drug ingestion, analysis of postmortem blood collected from 10 different sites demonstrated imipramine concentrations that differed by as much as 760% (2.1–16.0 mg/L) (Jones and Pounder, 1987). In an extensive investigation, Prouty and Anderson (1990) demonstrated that postmortem blood drug concentrations were not only site-dependent but also increased greatly over the interval between death and specimen collection, particularly in heart blood. This increase over the postmortem interval was most pronounced for basic drugs with large apparent volumes of distribution, such as tricyclic antidepressants.

In an overt drug overdose, postmortem blood concentrations are elevated sufficiently to render an unmistakable interpretation of fatal intoxication. However, in many cases, the postmortem redistribution of drugs may significantly affect the interpretation of analytic findings. For drugs whose volume of distribution, plasma half-life, and renal clearance vary widely from person to person or that undergo postmortem redistribution, tissue concentrations readily distinguish therapeutic administration from drug overdose (Apple, 1989). Therefore, to provide a foundation of reasonable medical certainty in regard to the role of a drug in the death of an individual, it is recommended that, in addition to heart blood, a peripheral blood specimen and tissues be analyzed.

The analysis of tissue specimens is important for the estimation of a "minimal administered dose" or body burden of a drug or poison. In order to calculate a minimum body burden, it is necessary to analyze as many different body tissues and fluids as possible to determine the concentrations of the drug present. The concentration of drug in each separate specimen is then multiplied by the total weight or volume of that particular tissue or fluid. In this manner, the total amount of drug in each different tissue or fluid is determined. The amounts of drug in each separate tissue and fluid are then added together to give the total body burden or minimal administered dose. This simple approach has often proven extremely effective in resolving legal medical issues. For example, lidocaine is commonly administered in 50- to 100-mg bolus injections as an antiarrythmic agent for ventricular arrhythmia during resuscitation efforts. Because of poor circulation and tissue perfusion during arrhythmias, lidocaine is not well distributed in the body of the victim of a fatal heart attack. Postmortem bloods often exceed 50 mg/L in such cases, while values for effective antiarrythmic prophylaxis do

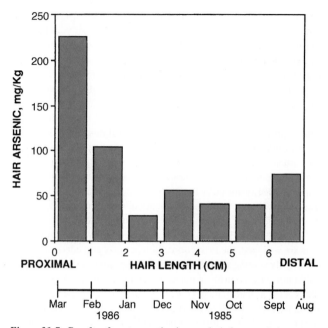

Figure 31-7. Results of neutron activation analysis for arsenic in sequential sections of hair, demonstrating chronic arsenic poisoning. Increased exposure in the first two sections is consistent with fatal events. Lower values in section 3 are consistent with 2 weeks of hospitalization. (Data from Poklis A, Saady JJ: Arsenic poisoning: Acute or chronic? Suicide or murder? Am J Forensic Med Pathol 11:226–232, 1990.)

not exceed 5 mg/L. Therefore, a blood lidocaine value of 50 mg/L may be an artifact of resuscitation efforts or might represent a fatal overdose. Tissue distribution studies have resolved this issue in both accidental and homicidal poisoning with lidocaine (Poklis *et al.*, 1984).

Postmortem toxicology results are often used to corroborate investigative findings. For example, the analysis of sequential sections of hair provides a reliable correlation with the pattern of arsenic exposure. Significant increases in the arsenic content of the root and the first 5 mm of the hair occur within hours after the ingestion of arsenic (Smith, 1964). The germinal cells are in relativity close equilibrium with circulating arsenic; thus, as arsenic concentrations in blood rise or fall, so does arsenic deposition in growing hair. Normal arsenic content in hair varies with nutritional, environmental, and physiologic factors; however, the maximum upper limit of normal with a 99% confidence limit in persons not exposed to arsenic is 5 mg/kg (Shapiro, 1967). Hair grows at a rate of approximately 12.5 mm (in.) per month. Therefore, analysis of 1.0-cm segments provides a monthly pattern of exposure (Fig. 31-7). Such analyses are often performed in cases of homicidal poisoning to demonstrate that increases in arsenic deposition in the victim's hair correlate with times when a poisoner had an opportunity to administer the poison. Continuously, elevated hair arsenic values indicate chronic rather than acute poisoning as the cause of death.

A new extension of forensic toxicology is the analysis of impurities of illicit drug synthesis in biological specimens. Many drugs of abuse are illicitly manufactured in clandestine laboratories, particularly methamphetamine. There are several popular methods of methamphetamine synthesis; when these are applied in clandestine laboratories, side reactions or incomplete conversion of the reactants yield an impure mixture of methamphetamine and synthetic impurities. These impurities can be characteristic of a particular synthetic method and their detection in biological specimens can indicate use of an illicitly produced drug that is not a legal pharmaceutical product; suggest the synthetic method that was used to produce the drug; point to a possible common source of illicit production; and provide a link between manufacturers, dealers, and users. An example of impurity analysis was the detection of metabolites of α-benzyl-N-methylphenethylamine (BNMPA) in the urine of abusers of methamphetamine (Moore *et al.*, 1996) and in a case of fatal drug overdose involving methamphetamine (Moore *et al.*, 1996). BNMPA is an impurity arising from the synthesis of methamphetamine via the Leukart reaction using phenyl-2-propanone (P2P) synthesized from phenylacetic acid. Clandestine laboratories often must synthesize the P2P starting material, as its sale and distribution is regulated by the Federal Drug Enforcement Agency.

CRIMINAL POISONING OF THE LIVING

Over the past few decades, forensic toxicologists have become more and more involved in the analysis of specimens obtained from living victims of criminal poisonings. Generally, this increase in testing has arisen from two types of cases: (1) administration of drugs to incapacitate victims of kidnapping, robbery, or sexual assault and (2) poisoning as a form of child abuse.

For centuries, those severely intoxicated from alcohol often became victims of kidnapping, robbery, or sexual assault. In the days of sail, the kidnapping of drunks in seaports was a common way of obtaining sailors for long commercial voyages such as those involved in whaling. Late in the nineteenth century, the mixing of the powerful hypnotic chloral hydrate with alcohol produced the legendary "Mickey Finn." While alcohol is still often a primary factor in cases of alleged sexual assault, common drugs of abuse or other psychoactive drugs are often involved (Table 31-2). Of particular concern are the many potent inductive agents medically administered prior to general anesthesia. Many of these drugs, such as benzodiazepines and phenothiazines, are available today through illicit sources or legal purchase in foreign countries. When administered surreptitiously, they cause sedation and incapacitate the victim while also producing amnesia in the victim as to the events while drugged without causing severe central nervous system depression. These cases often present a difficult analytic challenge to the toxicologist.

Table 31-2

Distribution of Drugs of Abuse Encountered Urine Specimens in 578 Cases of Alleged Sexual Assault

RANK	DRUG/DRUG GROUP	INCIDENCE	PERCENT OF CASES* (%)
1.	No drugs found	167	29
2.	Ethanol	148	26
3.	Benzodiazepines	70	12
4.	Marijuana	67	12
5.	Amphetamines	41	7
6.	Gamma-hydroxybutyrate	24	4
7.	Opiate (morphine/codeine)	20	4
8.	Other drugs	13	3

*Percentages do not add to 100% due to rounding.

SOURCE: Data from ElSohly MA, *et al.*: Analysis of flunitrazepam metabolites and other substances in alleged cases of sexual assault. Presentation at the 50th Anniversary Meeting of the American Academy of Forensic Sciences; San Francisco, CA, February 13, 1997.

Usually, the victim does not bring forth an allegation of assault until 24 hours to several days after the attack. Thus, the intoxicating drug may have been largely eliminated or extensively metabolized such that extremely low concentrations of drug or metabolites are present in the victim's blood, urine, and/or hair specimens. Sophisticated, highly sensitive analytic methods such as GC/MS or HPLC/MS may be required to accurately identify drugs in such specimens. To provide guidance in the choice of analytic approaches to such cases, recommendations for the toxicologic investigation of sexual assaults have recently been formulated by the Toxicology Section of the American Academy of Forensic Sciences (LeBeau *et al.*, 1999).

Poisoning as a form of child abuse involves the deliberate administration of toxic or injurious substances to a child, usually by a parent or other caregiver. The victims of such poisonings range in age from a few months to the teens. Common agents used to intentionally poison children have included syrup of ipecac, table salt, laxatives, diuretics, antidepressants, sedative-hypnotics, and narcotics (Dine and McGovern, 1982). The motivation for such heinous behavior is in the province of psychiatry, not toxicology. However, toxicologists must have some understanding of the nature of these poisonings to aid in the investigation of such cases. In some instances, it is a form of child battering committed by persons with low tolerance to the child's upsetting behaviors. The poison may be given to an infant to stop its crying or be force-fed to older children as a form of punishment. Such behavior is characteristic of persons with a cultural background where violence toward children is common or who have severe personality disorders or other mental illnesses. "Munchausen syndrome by proxy" is another form of child poisoning (Murray, 1997). The term *Munchausen syndrome* (MS) is used to describe patients who seek admission to hospitals with apparent illness along with plausible, dramatic, albeit fictitious medical histories. Such people seek medical treatment solely to assume the role of a patient and receive the attention derived from this deception. "MS by proxy" refers to the situation in which an individual, usually a parent, presents not himself or herself but a child with a fictitious illness often induced by physical or chemical means. The purpose of the poisoning is not to kill the child but to induce signs and symptoms of illness that will assure medical attention. Thereby, the parent as caregiver gains the craved attention. Given a fictitious case history and the obvious illness of the child, these cases are almost always and understandably misdiagnosed. Often, the child may be chronically poisoned at home and in the hospital for as long as a year before suspicion leads to the collection of specimens for extensive toxicologic testing. Although the parent may not have intended such an outcome, some children have died from fatal poisoning in these situations. As in the case of sexual assault, sophisticated GC/MS testing methods may be required to detect such agents as emetine and cephaeline, the emetic alkaloids in syrup of ipecac. Testing in these cases is best performed in a laboratory with forensic experience, as positive drug findings will usually result in some form of legal proceeding.

FORENSIC URINE DRUG TESTING

Concerns about the potentially adverse consequences of substance abuse both for the individual and for society have led to widespread urine analysis for the detection of controlled or illicit drugs (Gust and Walsh, 1989). Currently, such testing is conducted routinely by the military services, regulated transportation and nuclear industries, many federal and state agencies, public utilities, federal and state criminal justice systems, and numerous private businesses and

Table 31-3

Forensic Urine Drug-Testing Analytes and Cutoff Concentrations

	CONCENTRATION (ng/mL)	
	INITIAL TEST	CONFIRMATORY TEST
Marijuana metabolite(s)	50	15[†]
Cocaine metabolite(s)	300	150[‡]
Opiate(s)	2000*	—
Morphine	—	300
Codeine	—	300
6-Monoacetylmorphine	—	15
Phencyclidine	25	25
Amphetamines	1000	—
Amphetamine	—	500
Methamphetamine	—	500

*25 ng/mL if immunoassay is specific for free morphine; [†] *D*-9-tetrahydrocannabinol-9-carboxylic acid; [‡] Benzoylecgonine.

SOURCE: Department of Health and Human Services: Mandatory guidelines for federal workplace drug testing programs. *Fed Reg* 53(69), 11983, April 11, 1988; revised: *Fed Reg* 58(14), 6063, January 25, 1993.

industries. Significant ethical and legal ramifications are associated with such testing. Those having positive test results may not receive employment, be dismissed from a job, be court-martialed, or suffer a loss of reputation.

To assure the integrity of workplace urine testing, two certification programs currently accredit forensic urine-testing laboratories. Laboratories conducting testing of federal employees are required to be certified under the Department of Health and Human Services Mandatory Guidelines for Workplace Drug Testing as published in the April 11, 1988, *Federal Register* (Department of Health and Human Services, 1988). The College of American Pathologists (CAP) also conducts a certification program for urine-testing laboratories. The federal program regulates a specific program from specimen collection through testing to the reporting of results, whereas the CAP program allows flexibility in the construction of programs servicing a broad range of clients. Both programs involve periodic on-site inspection of laboratories and proficiency testing.

Forensic urine drug testing (FUDT) differs from other areas of forensic toxicology in that urine is the only specimen analyzed and testing is performed for a limited number of drugs. At present, under the federal certification program, analyses are performed for only five drug classes or drugs of abuse (Table 31-3). While FUDT laboratories typically analyze 100–1000 urine specimens daily, only a relatively small number of those specimens are positive for drugs. To handle this large workload, initial testing is performed by immunoassays on high-speed, large-throughput analyzers. A confirmation analysis in FUDT-certified laboratories is performed by GC/MS.

Proper FUDT is a challenge to good laboratory management. As with all forensic activities, every aspect of the laboratory operation must be thoroughly documented—specimen collection, chain of custody, quality control procedures, testing, qualifications of personnel, and the reporting of results. The facility must be constructed and operated to assure total security of specimens and documents. Confidentiality of all testing results is paramount; only specifically authorized persons should receive the results. The presence of a controlled or illicit drug in a single random urine specimen is gen-

erally accepted as proof of recent or past substance abuse. However, positive urine drug findings are only evidence that, at some time before the collection of the sample, the individual was administered the drug, self-administered it, or was exposed to it. Positive urine tests do not prove impairment from the drug abuse or addiction.

FUDT results are reported only as positive or negative for the drugs sought. Cutoff values are established for both the initial and confirmation assays (Table 31-2). The cutoff value is a concentration at or above which the assay is considered positive. Below the cutoff value, the assay is negative. Obviously, drugs may be present below the cutoff concentration. However, the use of cutoff values allows uniformity in the drug testing and reporting of results. All test reports indicate the drug tested and its cutoff value. FUDT laboratories must be thoroughly familiar with all regulatory and analytic issues related to urine testing and devise strategies to resolve uncertainties. Many individuals who are subject to regulated urine testing have devised techniques to mask their drug use either by physiologic means such as the ingestion of diuretics or by attempting to adulterate the specimen directly with bleach, vinegar, or other products that interfere with the initial immunoassay tests (Warren, 1989). Thus, specimens are routinely tested for adulteration by checking urinary pH, creatinine, and specific gravity and noting any unusual color or smell. Recently, a mini-industry has developed to sell various products that are alleged to "fool drug testers." These products often have colorful trade names such as UrinAid, Instant Clean ADD-IT-ive, and Klear. They contain chemicals that, when added to a urine specimen, interfere with either the initial or confirmatory drug test. For example, several of these products contain glutaraldehyde, which will react with the nitrogen atoms of the antibody proteins of the immunoassay screening test, thereby cross-linking the antibodies and inactivating the assay. However, this destruction of the test is so complete that the immunoassay analyzer records almost no signal, thus indicating possible adulteration of the specimen. Another adulterant, for the marijuana metabolite urine test, contains sodium nitrite. In acidic urine, the nitrite salt is converted to nitrous acid, which then converts the marijuana metabolites to nitroso derivatives, rendering them undetectable by routine GC/MS analysis (Lewis *et al.*, 1999). Often, the pH of the urine is insufficiently acidic for complete nitroso conversion of the tetrahydrocannabinol (THC) metabolite, THC–carboxylic acid. Thus, the urine will be screen positive by the initial immunoassay. When urine is acidified to extract the THC acid metabolite for MS confirmation testing, the metabolite is completely oxidized and undetectable. However, the deuterated THC–carboxylic acid added to the sample as the internal standard of the confirmation test is also completely destroyed. Failure to detect the internal standard readily alerts the analyst that an oxidant adulterant had been added to the urine. In such cases, a quantitative test for nitrite is performed. Nitrite may be present in urine from numerous internal and external sources such as foods, drugs, pathologic conditions, and infection from nitrate-reducing microorganisms. However, none of these sources produces urinary nitrite concentrations that even begin to approach those obtained by the addition of adulterant amounts of potassium nitrite = 1000 mg/L (Urey *et al.*, 1998). Most chemical adulterants can be detected in urine by specific colorimetric tests that can be readily adapted to high-volume autoanalyzers (Table 31-4). Thus, FUDT laboratories now routinely test not only for drugs of abuse but also for a wide variety of chemical adulterants. In most instances, a positive test result for adulteration has as serious a consequence as a positive drug test.

Table 31-4

Urine Adulterants Detected by Chemical Test

ADULTERANT	DETECTION METHOD
Acids, baking soda	pH
Bleach	Smell, color test (substituted benzene complex)
Detergents, diuretics, salt	Specific gravity
Diuretics	Creatinine
Glutaraldehyde	Altered immunoassay, GC
Nitrite	Color test (azo dye formation)
Pyridium chromate	Color, AAS (chromate), GC (pyridine)

NOTE: GC, gas chromatography; AAS, atomic absorption spectrophotometry.

There may be valid reasons other than substance abuse for positive drug findings, such as therapeutic use of controlled substances, inadvertent intake of drugs via food, and passive inhalation. For example, the seed of *Papaver somniferum,* poppy seed, is a common ingredient in many pastries and breads. Depending on their botanical source, poppy seeds may contain significant amounts of morphine. Several studies have demonstrated that the ingestion of certain poppy-seed foods results in the urinary excretion of readily detectable concentrations of morphine (ElSohly and Jones, 1989). Morphine is a major urinary metabolite of heroin. Therefore, to readily differentiate heroin abuse from poppy-seed ingestion, analysis may be performed for 6-monoacetylmorphine, a unique heroin metabolite (Fehn and Megges, 1985).

Even over-the-counter medications may present potential problems for laboratories conducting urine drug testing. Methamphetamine may occur as a racemic mixture of D and L optical isomers. D-Methamphetamine, a Schedule II controlled substance, is a potent central nervous system stimulant subject to illicit drug abuse, while L-methamphetamine (L-desoxyephedrine) is an alpha-adrenergic stimulant available in over-the-counter Vicks inhalers as a nasal decongestant. Cross-reactivity of L-desoxyephedrine with the initial immunoassay screening test may occur after excessive use of the Vicks inhaler (Poklis and Moore, 1995). Additionally, the most popular confirmational GC/MS products for amphetamines are achiral. Therefore, if such analyses are performed, a "false-positive" result for D-methamphetamine may be reported. This dilemma is easily resolved if confirmational testing is done with a *chiral* GC/MS procedure, which can readily resolve the stereoisomers of methamphetamine (Fitzgerald *et al.,* 1988).

HUMAN PERFORMANCE TESTING

Forensic toxicology activities also include the determination of the presence of ethanol and other drugs and chemicals in blood, breath, or other specimens and the evaluation of their role in modifying human performance and behavior. The most common application of human performance testing is to determine driving under the influence of ethanol (DUI) or drugs (DUID). While operation of a motor vehicle is a common experience to most people, few appreciate the complexity of mental and physical functioning involved. A driver must simultaneously coordinate fine motor skills in tracking the road course and applying pressure to accelerator or brake—with visual attention immediately in front, to the horizon, and to the periphery of the vehicle—while continuously judging distance, speed, and appropriateness of response to signals, traffic, and unexpected events. The threshold blood ethanol concentration (BAC) for diminished driving performance of these complex functions in many individuals is as low as 0.04 g/dL, the equivalent of ingestion of two beers within an hour's time. The statutory definition of DUI in the United States is a BAC of either 0.08 or 0.10 g/dL, depending on the particular state law. These concentrations are consistent with diminished performance of complex driving skills in the vast majority of individuals. Over the past half century, an enormous amount of data has been developed correlating blood ethanol concentrations with intellectual and physiologic impairment, particularly of the skills associated with the proper operation of motor vehicles. Numerous studies have demonstrated a direct relationship between an increased BAC in drivers and an increased risk of involvement in road accidents (Council on Scientific Affairs, 1986). Alcohol-impaired drivers are responsible for 25–35% of all crashes causing serious injury in single-vehicle accidents, and 55–65% percent of fatally injured drivers have a BAC of 0.10 g/dL or greater.

During the past decade, there has been growing concern about the deleterious effects of drugs other than ethanol on driving performance. Several studies have demonstrated a relatively high occurrence of drugs in impaired or fatally injured drivers (White *et al.,* 1981; Mason and McBay, 1984). These studies tend to report that the highest drug-use accident rates are associated with the use of such illicit or controlled drugs as cocaine, benzodiazepines, marijuana, and phencyclidine. However, most studies test for only a few drugs or drug classes, and the repeated reporting of the same drugs may be a function of limited testing. Before "driving under the influence of drugs" testing is as readily accepted by the courts as ethanol testing, many legal and scientific problems concerning drug concentrations and driving impairment must be resolved (Consensus Report, 1985). The ability of analytic methodology to routinely measure minute concentrations of drug in blood must be established. Also, drug-induced driving impairment at specific blood concentrations in controlled tests and/or actual highway experience must be demonstrated.

COURTROOM TESTIMONY

The forensic toxicologist often is called upon to testify in legal proceedings. As a general rule of evidence, a witness may testify only to facts known to him or her. The witness may offer opinions solely on the basis of what he or she has observed (Moenssens *et al.,* 1973). Such a witness is called a "lay witness." However, the toxicologist is referred to as an "expert witness." A court recognizes a witness as an expert if that witness possesses knowledge or experience in a subject that is beyond the range of ordinary or common knowledge or observation. An expert witness may provide two types of testimony: objective testimony and "opinion." Objective testimony by a toxicologist usually involves a description of his or her analytic methods and findings. When a toxicologist testifies as to the interpretation of his or her analytic results or those of others, that toxicologist is offering an "opinion." Lay witnesses cannot offer such opinion testimony, as it exceeds their ordinary experience.

Before a court permits opinion testimony, the witness must be "qualified" as an expert in his or her particular field. In qualifying someone as an expert witness, the court considers the witness's education, on-the-job training, work experience, teaching or academic appointments, and professional memberships and publications as well as the acceptance of the witness as an expert by other courts. Qualification of a witness takes place in front of the jury members, who consider the expert's qualifications in determining how much weight to give his or her opinions during their deliberations.

Whether a toxicologist appears in criminal or civil court, workers' compensation, or parole hearings, the procedure for testifying is the same: direct examination, cross-examination, and redirect examination. The attorney who has summoned the witness to testify conducts direct examination. Testimony is presented in a question-and-answer format. The witness is asked a series of questions that allow him or her to present all facts or opinions relevant to the successful presentation of the attorney's case. During direct examination, an expert witness has the opportunity to explain to the jury the scientific bases of his or her opinions. Regardless of which side has called the toxicologist to court, the toxicologist should testify with scientific objectivity. Bias toward his or her client and prejudgments should be avoided. An expert witness is called to provide informed assistance to the jury. The jury, not the expert witness, determines the guilt or innocence of the defendant.

After direct testimony, the opposing attorney questions the expert. During this cross-examination, the witness is challenged as to his or her findings and/or opinions. The toxicologist will be asked to defend his or her analytic methods, results, and opinions. The opposing attorney may imply that the expert's testimony is biased because of financial compensation, association with an agency involved in the litigation, or personal feelings regarding the case. The best way to prepare for such challenges before testimony is to anticipate the questions the opposing attorney may ask.

After cross-examination, the attorney who called the witness may ask additional questions to clarify any issues raised during cross-examination. This allows the expert to explain apparent discrepancies in his or her testimony raised by the opposing attorney. Often an expert witness is asked to answer a special type of question, the "hypothetical question." A hypothetical question contains only facts that have been presented in evidence. The expert is then asked for his or her conclusion or opinion based solely on this hypothetical situation. This type of question serves as a means by which appropriate facts leading to the expert's opinion are identified. Often these questions are extremely long and convoluted. The witness should be sure he or she understands all the facts and implications in the question. Like all questions, this type should be answered as objectively as possible.

ANALYTIC ROLE IN CLINICAL TOXICOLOGY

Analytic toxicology in a clinical setting plays a role very similar to its role in forensic toxicology. As an aid in the diagnosis and treatment of toxic incidents as well as in monitoring the effectiveness of treatment regimens, it is useful to clearly identify the nature of the toxic exposure and measure the amount of the toxic substance that has been absorbed. Frequently, this information, together with the clinical state of the patient, permits a clinician to relate the signs and symptoms observed to the anticipated effects of the toxic agent. This may permit a clinical judgment as to whether the treatment must be vigorous and aggressive or whether simple observation and symptomatic treatment of the patient are sufficient.

A cardinal rule in the treatment of poisoning cases is to remove any unabsorbed material, limit the absorption of additional poison, and hasten its elimination. The clinical toxicology laboratory serves an additional purpose in this phase of the treatment by monitoring the amount of the toxic agent remaining in circulation or measuring what is excreted. In addition, the laboratory can provide the data needed to permit estimations of the total dosage or the effectiveness of treatment by changes in known pharmacokinetic parameters of the drug or agent ingested.

While the instrumentation and the methodology used in a clinical toxicology laboratory are similar to those utilized by a forensic toxicologist, a major difference between these two applications is responsiveness. In emergency toxicology testing, results must be communicated to the clinician within hours to be meaningful for therapy. A forensic toxicologist may carefully choose the best method for a particular test and conduct replicate procedures to assure maximum accuracy. A clinical laboratory cannot afford this luxury and frequently sacrifices accuracy for a rapid turnaround time. Additionally, because it is impossible to predict when toxicologic emergencies will occur, a clinical laboratory must provide rapid testing 24 hours a day every day of the year. The most commonly encountered intoxicants in emergency toxicology testing and the rapid methodologies to detect their presence in serum and/or urine specimens are presented in Table 31-5.

Primary examples of the usefulness of emergency toxicology testing are the rapid quantitative determination of acetaminophen,

Table 31-5

Most Commonly Encountered Drugs and Methods for Analysis in Emergency Toxicology

RANK	DRUG/DRUG GROUP	SPECIMEN	ANALYTICAL METHOD
1.	Drugs of Abuse (amphetamines, cocaine, opiates, phencyclidine)	Urine	Immunoassays
2.	Ethanol	Serum	GC
3.	Benzodiazepines	Urine/serum	Immunoassay/GC/MS
4.	Acetaminophen, salicylates	Serum	Immunoassay/HPLC
5.	Tricyclic antidepressants	Serum	Immunoassay/HPLC
6.	Ibuprofen	Urine/serum	TLC/HPLC
7.	Dextropropoxyphene	Urine	Immunoassay
8.	Fluoxetine	Urine/serum	TLC/HPLC
9.	Barbiturates (50% phenobarbital)	Urine/serum	Immunoassay/GC
10.	Diphenhydramine	Urine	TLC

NOTE: GC, gas chromatography; GC/MS, gas chromatography/mass spectrometry; HPLC, high-pressure liquid chromatography; TLC, thin-layer chromatography.

SOURCE: Data from Year-End 1998 Emergency Department Data from the Drug Abuse Warning Network, Department of Health and Human Services, December 1999.

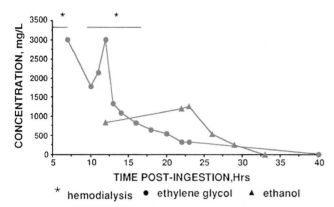

Figure 31-8. Serum ethylene glycol and ethanol concentrations monitored during dialysis and ethanol infusion therapy. (Data from the Toxicology Laboratory, Medical College of Virginia Hospital, Richmond, VA.)

salicylate, alcohols, and glycol serum concentrations in instances of suspected overdose. Acetaminophen serum values related to the time after ingestion (see Chap. 32) not only indicate an overdose, but provide a prognosis for possible delayed hepatotoxicity and the need to continue administration of *N*-acetylcystine antidote. In addition, continuous monitoring of serum values permits an accurate pharmacokinetic calculation of the ingested dose (Melethil *et al.*, 1981). Similarly, salicylate serum values related to the time after ingestion may indicate an overdose, providing a prognosis for possible delayed severe metabolic acidosis and the need for lifesaving dialysis treatment. Continuous monitoring of serum salicylate values permits an accurate assessment of the efficacy of dialysis.

Ethanol is the most common agent encountered in emergency toxicology. While little fatal intoxications occur with ethanol, serum values are important in the assessment of behavioral and neurologic function, particularly in trauma cases where the patient is unable to communicate and surgery with the administration of anesthetic or analgesic agents is indicated. Intoxications from accidental or deliberate ingestion of other alcohols or glycols—such as methanol from windshield deicer or paint thinner, isopropanol from rubbing alcohol, and ethylene glycol from antifreeze—are often encountered in emergency departments. Following ingestion of methanol or ethylene glycol, patients often present with similar neurologic symptoms and severe metabolic acidosis due to the formation of toxic aldehyde and acid metabolites. A rapid quantitative serum determination for these intoxicants will indicate the severity of intoxication and the possible need for dialysis therapy. Alcohol infusion, in order to saturate the enzyme alcohol dehydrogenase, blocks the conversion of methanol and ethylene glycol to their toxic metabolites. Continuous monitoring of serum values not only permits an assessment of the clearance of the intoxicant by dialysis but also assures a proper infusion rate of alcohol for effective antidotal concentrations (Fig. 31-8). To provide effective service to the emergency department, laboratories should have available chromatographic methods for the rapid separation and detection of alcohols and glycols (Edinboro *et al.*, 1993).

The utilization of the analytic capabilities of a clinical toxicology laboratory has increased enormously in recent years. Typically, the laboratory performs testing not only for the emergency department but also for a wide variety of other medical departments, as drugs and toxic agents may be a consideration in diagnosis. Urine is analyzed from substance abuse treatment facilities to monitor the administration of methadone or other therapeutic agents and/or to

assure that patients do not continue to abuse drugs. Similarly, psychiatrists, neurologists, and physicians treating patients for chronic pain need to know whether patients are self-administering drugs before such patients undergo psychiatric or neurologic examinations. Analysis for drugs of abuse in meconium and urine obtained from neonates is used to corroborate the diagnosis of withdrawal symptoms in newborns and document fetal exposure to controlled substances. Toxic metal determinations, such as blood lead concentration, are often performed to assess possible toxic metal exposure or severity of toxicity (see Chap. 23). Analysis of heavy metals in 24-hour urine specimens is often used to rule out toxic metal exposure as a cause of symmetrical peripheral neuropathy prior to the diagnosis of neurologic disorders such as Guillian–Barré syndrome. The clinical toxicology laboratory may often perform unique diagnostic tests that require sophisticated analytic capabilities such as GC/MS and HPLC analysis for organic acids and amino acids to detect inborn errors of metabolism in infants and children. Methods for the analysis of abnormal organic acids will also detect acidic drugs and other intoxicants such as salicylates, ethylene glycol, gamma-hydroxybutyric acid, and valproic acid. Another such diagnostic test requiring sensitive chromatography is the timed metabolism of lidocaine to its monoethylglycinexylidide (MEGX) metabolite (O'Neal and Poklis, 1996). The rate of this conversion is a sensitive indicator of hepatic dysfunction and is often used to assess hepatic viability in donor livers prior to transplantation. MEGX formation may also be useful in monitoring the severity of the histologic condition of patients with chronic hepatitis and cirrhosis (Shiffman *et al.*, 1994).

ANALYTIC ROLE IN THERAPEUTIC MONITORING

Historically, the administration of drugs for long-term therapy was based largely on experience. A dosage amount was selected and administered at appropriate intervals based on what the clinician had learned was generally tolerated by most patients. If the drug seemed ineffective, the dose was increased; if toxicity developed, the dose was decreased or the frequency of dosing was altered. At times, a different dosage form might be substituted. Establishing an effective dosage regimen was particularly difficult in children and the elderly.

The factors responsible for individual variability in responses to drug therapy include the rate and extent of drug absorption, distribution, and binding in body tissues and fluids, rate of metabolism and excretion, pathologic conditions, and interaction with other drugs (Blaschke *et al.*, 1985). Monitoring of the plasma or serum concentration at regular intervals will detect deviations from the average serum concentration, which, in turn, may suggest that one or more of these variables need to be identified and corrected.

In a given patient, when the various factors are assumed to be constant, the administration of the same dose of a drug at regular intervals eventually produces a steady-state condition (Fig. 31-9) (Moyer *et al.*, 1986). Monitoring of steady-state drug concentrations assures that an effective concentration is present. For drugs that have a defined correlation between serum values and undesired toxic effects, the lowest serum value immediately prior to dosing (trough) and the highest expected serum concentration (peak) are monitored to assure efficacy and minimize toxicity. Appropriate situations for therapeutic drug monitoring are presented in Table 31-6.

Because the drug being administered is known, qualitative characterization of the analyte generally is not required. Quantitative accuracy is required, however. Frequently, the methodology

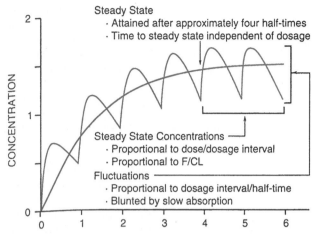

Figure 31-9. Fundamental pharmacokinetic relationships for the repeated administration of drugs.

The blue line is the pattern of drug accumulation during the repeated administration of a drug at intervals equal to its elimination half-time, when drug absorption is 10 times as rapid as elimination. As the relative rate of absorption increases, the concentration maxima approach 2 and minima approach 1 during steady state. The black line depicts the pattern during administration of equivalent dosage by continuous intravenous infusion. Curves are based upon the one-compartment model. Average concentration (C_{SS}) when steady state is attained during intermittent drug administration is $C_{SS} = F \times dose/Cl \times T$, where F = fractional bioavailability of the dose and T = dosage interval (time). By substitution of infusion rate for $F \times dose/T$, the formula is equivalent to Eq. (1) and provides the concentration maintained at steady state during continuous intravenous infusion. [From Hardman JG, Limbird LE, Molinoff PB, *et al.* (eds.): *Goodman & Gilman's The Pharmacological Basis of Therapeutics,* 9th edn. New York: McGraw-Hill, 1995, p 23.]

applied is important, particularly in regard to its selectivity. For example, methods that measure the parent drug and its metabolites are not ideal unless the individual analytes can be quantified separately. Depending on the drug, metabolites may or may not be active to a different degree than the parent drug. The cardiac antiarrythmic drug procainamide is acetylated during metabolism to form *N*-acetylprocainamide (NAPA). This metabolite has antiarrythmic activity of almost equal potency to that of the parent drug, procainamide. There is bimodal genetic variation in the activity of the *N*-acetyltransferase for procainamide, so that, in "fast acetylators," the concentration of NAPA in the serum may exceed that of the parent drug. For optimal patient management, information should be available about the concentrations of both procainamide and NAPA in serum (Bigger and Hoffman, 1985).

Because absolute characterization of the analyte is not necessary for many drugs, immunoassay procedures are commonly used. This is particularly true of drugs with extremely low serum concentrations, such as cardiac glycosides, and drugs that are difficult to extract because of a high degree of polarity, such as the aminoglycoside antibiotics. In these cases, serum can be conveniently assayed directly by using commercially available kits for immunoassays.

The chromatographic methods in which an appropriate internal standard is added are favored when more than one analyte is to be measured or if metabolites with structures similar to those of the parent drugs must be distinguished. Because the nature of drugs is varied, many different analytic techniques may be applied, including atomic absorption spectrophotometry for measuring lithium used to treat manic disorders. Virtually, all the tools of the analyst may be used for specific applications of analytic toxicology. Drugs that are commonly monitored during therapy, their usual effective therapeutic serum concentrations, "panic values," and typical analytic methodologies applied to serum measurements are presented in Table 31-7. The term *panic value* denotes a serum drug concentration associated with the development of potentially serious toxicity. In clinical laboratories, the panic value alerts the toxicologist that the treating physician must be *immediately* contacted and notified of the test result.

ANALYTIC ROLE IN BIOLOGICAL MONITORING

In the workplace, good industrial hygiene practices require monitoring of the environment to which workers are exposed in order to identify potentially harmful amounts of hazardous chemicals. Despite

Table 31-6
Appropriate Use of Therapeutic Drug Monitoring

USE	EXAMPLES
Optimize efficacy while minimizing toxicity	
Optimal SDC for clinical effect	
Routine, prophylactic peak serum	Aminoglycosides
Poor patient response	Antiarrhythmics, antidepressants
Suspected toxicity	
Resolve complicating factors	
Patient characteristics	Age, smoking, noncompliance
Disease	Renal failure, hepatic disorders
Drug interactions	Induction or inhibition of drug metabolism
Sudden change in physiologic state	Improved cardiac function on lidocaine therapy increases clearance
Dosage regimen design	
Individualize future dosing (single SDC)	
Pharmacokinetic profiling (multiple SDC)	Ideal dosage for aminoglycosides
Follow-up SDC	Single steady-state lidocaine
Verify therapy	Medicolegal lithium

NOTE: SCD, serum drug concentration.

Table 31-7
Drugs Commonly Indicated for Therapeutic Monitoring

THERAPEUTIC USE DRUG	EFFECTIVE SERUM RANGE (mg/L)	PANIC VALUE = OR = (mg/L)	ANALYTIC METHODOLOGY
Antiarrythmic			
Digoxin	0.0005–0.002	0.0024	Immunoassay
Procainamide	4–10	12	Immunoassay
NAPA	5–30	40	Immunoassay
Anticonvulsant			
Carbamazepine	4–12	15	Immunoassay
Gabapentin	2–15	20	GC
Lamotrigine	0.5–8	10	HPLC
Phenobarbital	15–30	50	Immunoassay
Phenytoin	10–20	40	Immunoassay
Tropiramate	2–10	Undetermined	GC
Valproic acid	50–100	200	GC
Antidepressants			
Amitriptyline	0.08–0.250	0.5	HPLC
Desipramine	0.125–0.30	0.4	HPLC
Nortriptyline	0.08–0.250	0.5	HPLC
Antimicrobials			
Tobramycin	0.5–1.5 (trough)	2	Immunoassay
	5–10 (peak)	12	
Vancomycin	5–10 (trough)		Immunoassay
	30–40 (peak)	90	
Immunosuppressant			
Cyclosporine	0.1 (trough, whole blood)		HPLC
Neonatal apnea			
Caffeine	8–20	50	HPLC

NOTE: GLC, gas chromatography; HPLC, high-pressure liquid chromatography.

these precautions, it has become apparent that monitoring a worker directly can be a better indicator of exposure because it can show what has actually been absorbed. This is biological monitoring, and it can take a variety of forms. Often, environmental exposures are to a mixture of compounds and/or to compounds that are converted to physiologically important metabolites. Thus, analytic methods must be capable of separating a family of chemical agents and their major metabolites (Fig. 31-10). Additionally, methods must be sufficiently specific and sensitive to measure minute concentrations of the compounds in complex biological matrices.

An example of biological monitoring is presented in Table 31-8, which shows data relating to benzene exposure of chemists engaged in pesticide residue analysis in a state regulatory laboratory. Air-monitoring devices in this laboratory indicated that the ambient benzene concentration never exceeded the time-weighted average (TWA) of 32 mg/m^3 (10 ppm). Monitoring of the breathing zones at different locations around the laboratory where benzene was in use showed other concentrations of this material. When expired air was monitored, one worker showed a significantly greater amount of benzene exposure than did others. Upon questioning, she recalled spilling some of the solvent on a laboratory bench, in the process saturating a portion of her laboratory coat. Presumably, her exposure by inhalation and skin absorption was considerably greater than was indicated by the air monitor.

In addition to the measurement of the chemical or its metabolites in the body fluids, hair, or breath of the worker, other, more indirect methods may be employed. Substances that interact with macromolecules may form adducts that persist for long periods.

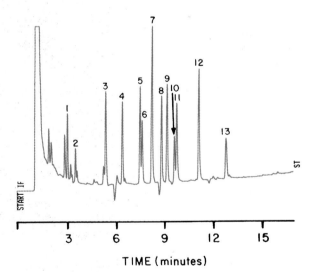

Figure 31-10. Capillary gas chromatographic separation of chlorinated hydrocarbon pesticides added to human serum at concentrations ranging from 1 to 4 ng/mL.

Peak number 1, a-lindane; 2, c-lindane; 3, heptachlor; 4, internal standard; 5, heptachlor epoxide; 6, oxychlordane; 7, c-chlordane; 8, a-chlordane; 9, *trans*-nonachlor; 10, dieldrin; 11, *p,p'*-DDE; 12, *p,p*-DDD; 13, *p,p'*-DDT. (Separation based on the method of Saady JJ, Poklis A: Determination of chlorinated hydrocarbon pesticides by solid phase extraction and capillary GC with electron capture detection. *J Anal Toxicol* 14:301–304, 1990. Reproduced from the Journal of Analytical Toxicology, by permission of Preston Publications, a Division of Preston Industries, Inc.)

Table 31-8

Benzene Exposure of Chemists Performing Pesticide Residue Analysis

SOURCE	BREATH BENZENE (ppm)	AIR BENZENE (ppm)
Chemist A	0.45	—
Chemist B	0.13	—
Chemist C	0.41	—
Chemist D	0.48	—
Chemist E	0.34	—
Chemist F	0.37	—
Chemist G	2.50	—
Chemist H	0.56	—
Fume hood breathing zone	—	14.2
Fume hood breathing zone	—	51.2

These adducts can be sampled periodically and potentially can serve as a means of integrating exposure to certain substances over long periods. For example, adducts of ethylene oxide with DNA or hemoglobin have been studied in workers. This technique may also be applicable in other situations that are not necessarily related to occupational hazards. Acetaldehyde, a metabolite of ethanol, forms adducts with hemoglobin. This marker may be of use in forensic cases (Stockham and Blanke, 1988).

Another approach that is useful in biological monitoring is to measure changes of normal metabolites induced by xenobiotics. The profile of glucuronic acid metabolites excreted in urine can be altered after exposure to substances that induce monooxygenase activity. Although monitoring the alteration of the urinary excretion of these metabolites may not indicate exposure to specific substances, this technique can be used in a generic fashion to flag a potentially harmful exposure to a hepatotoxic agent (Saady and Blanke, 1990). The early recognition of a toxicologic problem may permit the protection of a worker before irreversible effects occur.

SUMMARY

The analytic techniques initiated by forensic toxicologists have continued to expand in complexity and improve in reliability. Many new analytic tools have been applied to toxicologic problems in almost all areas of the field, and the technology continues to open new areas of research. Forensic toxicologists continue to be concerned about conducting unequivocal identification of toxic substances in such a manner that the results can withstand a legal challenge. The problems of substance abuse, designer drugs, increased potency of therapeutic agents, and widespread concern about pollution and the safety and health of workers present challenges to the analyst's skills. As these challenges are met, analytic toxicologists continue to play a significant role in the expansion of the discipline of toxicology.

REFERENCES

Aderjan R, Bahr H, Schmidt G: Investigation of cardiac glycoside levels in human postmortem blood and tissues determined by a special RIA procedure. *Arch Toxicol* 42:107–114, 1979.

Apple FS: Postmortem tricyclic antidepressant concentrations: Assessing cause of death using parent drug to metabolite ratio. *J Anal Toxicol* 13:197–198, 1989.

Benko A: Toxicological analysis of amobarbital and glutethimide from bone tissue. *J Forensic Sci* 30:708–714, 1985.

Bigger JT Jr, Hoffman BF: Antiarrhythmic drugs, in Gilman AG, Goodman LS, Rall TW, Murad F (eds): *The Pharmacological Basis of Therapeutics,* 7th edn. New York: Macmillan, 1985, p 763.

Blanke RV: Quality assurance in drug-use testing. *Clin Chem* 33:41B–45B, 1987.

Blanke RV: *Validation of the Purity of Standards.* Irving, TX: Abbott Laboratories, Diagnostic Division, 1989.

Blanke RV, Decker WJ: Analysis of toxic substances, in Tietz NW (ed): *Textbook of Clinical Chemistry.* Philadelphia, PA: WB Saunders, 1986, pp. 1670–1744.

Blaschke TF, Nies AS, Mamelock RD: Principles of therapeutics, in Gilman AG, Goodman LS, Rall TW, Murad F (eds): *The Pharmacological Basis of Therapeutics,* 7th ed., New York: Macmillan, 1985, p 52.

Chapuis E: *Elements de toxicologie,* 1873, cited in Peterson F, Haines WS, Webster RW: *Legal Medicine and Toxicology.* 2nd ed. Vol 2. Philadelphia, PA: WB Saunders, 1923.

Coe JI: Postmortem chemistry update: Emphasis on forensic applications. *Am J Forensic Med Pathol* 14:91–117, 1993.

Cone EJ, Buchwald WF, Darwin WD: Analytical controls in drug metabolism studies: 11. Artifact formation during chloroform extraction of drugs and metabolites with amine substitutes. *Drug Metab Dispos* 10:561–567, 1982.

Consensus Report: Drug concentrations and driving impairment. *JAMA* 254:2618–2621, 1985.

Council on Scientific Affairs: Alcohol and the driver. *JAMA* 255:522–527, 1986.

Cravey RH, Baselt RC: The science of forensic toxicology, in Cravey RH, Baselt RC (eds): *Introduction to Forensic Toxicology.* Davis, CA: Biomedical Publications, 1981, pp. 3–6.

Department of Health and Human Services, ADAMHA: Mandatory guidelines for federal workplace drug testing: Final guidelines: Notice. *Fed Reg* 53(69):11970–11989, 1988.

Dowling GP, McDonough ET, Bost RO: "Eve" and "ecstasy": A report of five deaths associated with the use of MDEA and MDMA. *JAMA* 257:1615–1617, 1987.

Edinboro LE, Nanco CR, Soghoian DM, Poklis A: Determination of ethylene glycol in serum utilizing direct injection on a wide bore capillary column. *Ther Drug Monit* 15:220–223, 1993.

ElSohly MA, Jones AB: Morphine and codeine in biological fluids: Approaches to source differentiation. *Forensic Sci Rev* 1:13–22, 1989.

Ernst MF, Poklis A, Gantner, GE: Evaluation of medicolegal investigators' suspicious and positive toxicology findings in 100 drug deaths. *J Forensic Sci* 27:61–65, 1982.

Evans WED: *The Chemistry of Death.* Springfield, IL: Charles C Thomas, 1963.

Fehn J, Megges G: Detection of O6-monoacetylmorphine in urine samples by GC/MS as evidence for heroin use. *J Anal Toxicol* 9:134–138, 1985.

Fisher RS, Hine CH, Stetler CJ (Committee on Medicolegal Problems): *Alcohol and the Impaired Driver: A Manual on the Medicolegal Aspects of Chemical Tests for Intoxication.* Chicago: American Medical Association, 1968.

Fitzgerald RL, Ramos JM, Bogema SC, Poklis A: Resolution of methamphetamine stereoisomers in urine drug testing: Urinary excretion of R(-)-methamphetamine following use of nasal inhalers. *J Anal Toxicol* 12:255–259, 1988.

Garriott JS, Simmons LM, Poklis A, Mackell MS: Five cases of fatal overdose from caffeine-containing "look-alike" drugs. *J Anal Toxicol* 9:141–143, 1985.

Gettler AD: Poisoning and toxicology, forensic aspects: Part 1: Historical aspects. *Inform* 9:3–7, 1977.

Goff ML, Brown WA, Omori AI, LaPointe DA: Preliminary observations of the effects of amitriptyline in decomposing tissue on the development of parasarcophaga ruficornis (Diptera: Sarcophagidae) and implications of this effect to estimation of postmortem interval. *J Forensic Sci* 38:316–322, 1993.

Granger RH, Condie LW, Borzelleca JF: Effect of vehicle on the relative uptake of haloalkanes administered by gavage. *Toxicologist* 40:1, 1987.

Gust SW, Walsh JM: *Drugs in the Workplace: Research and Evaluation Data.* NIDA Research Monograph 91. Washington, DC: U.S. Government Printing Office, 1989.

Hawks RL, Chiang CN: Examples of specific drug assays, in Hawks RL, Chiang CN (eds): *Urine Testing for Drugs of Abuse.* NIDA Research Monograph 73. Rockville, MD: U.S. Department Health and Human Services, PHS, ADAMHA, 1986, p 93.

Henderson GL: Designer drugs: Past history and future prospects. *J Forensic Sci* 33:569–575, 1988.

Hime GW, Hearn WL, Rose S, Cofino J: Analysis of cocaine and cocaethylene in blood and tissues by GC-NPD and GC-Ion Trap mass spectrometry. *J Anal Toxicol* 15:241, 1991.

Inoue T, Seta S: Analysis of drugs in unconventional samples. *Forensic Sci Rev* 4:89–107, 1992.

Jacob P, Lewis ER, Elias-Baker BA, Jones RT: A pyrolysis product, anhydroecgonine methyl ester (methylecgonidine), is in the urine of cocaine smokers. *J Anal Toxicol* 14:353, 1990.

Jones GR, Pounder DJ: Site-dependence of drug concentrations in postmortem blood—A case study. *J Anal Toxicol* 11:186–190, 1987.

Kaempe B: Interfering compounds and artifacts in the identification of drugs in autopsy material, in Stolman A (ed): *Progress in Chemical Toxicology.* Vol 4. New York: Academic Press, 1969, pp. 1–57.

Klaassen CD, Amdur MO, Doull J: *Casarett and Doull's Toxicology: The Basic Science of Poisons,* 3rd ed. New York: Macmillan, 1986.

LeBeau M, Andollo W, Hearn WL, et al.: Recommendations for toxicological investigation of drug-facilitated sexual assaults. *J Forensic Sci* 44:227–230, 1999.

Lewis SA, Lewis LA, Tuinman A: Potassium nitrite reaction with 11-nor-delta-9-tetrahydrocannabinol-9-carboxylic acid in urine in relation to drug screening analysis. *J Forensic Sci* 44:951–955, 1999.

Martin BR, Lue LP, Boni JP: Pyrolysis and volatization of cocaine. *J Anal Toxicol* 13:158, 1989.

Mason AP, McBay AJ: Ethanol, marijuana, and other drug use in 600 drivers killed in single-vehicle crashes in North Carolina. *J Forensic Sci* 29:987–1026, 1984.

Melethil S, Poklis, A, Schwartz HS: Estimation of the amount of drug absorbed in acetaminophen poisoning: A case report. *Vet Hum Toxicol* 23:421–423, 1981.

Mills RA, Millis CD, Dannan GA, et al.: Studies on the structure-activity relationships for the metabolism of polybrominated biphenyls by rat liver microsomes. *Toxicol Appl Pharmacol* 78:96–104, 1985.

Moenssens AA, Moses RE, Inbau FE: *Scientific Evidence in Criminal Cases.* Mineola, NY: Foundation Press, 1973.

Moore KA, Daniel J, Fierro M, et al.: Detection of a metabolite of α-benzyl-N-methylphenylamine synthesis in a mixed drug fatality involving methamphetamine. *J Forensic Sci* 41:524–526, 1996.

Moore KA, Ismaiel A, Poklis A: α-Benzyl-N-methylphenylamine (BN-MPA) an impurity of illict methamphetamine synthesis: lll. Detection of BNMPA and metabolites in urine from methamphetamine users. *J Anal Toxicol* 20:89–92, 1996.

Moyer TP, Pippenger CE, Blanke RV: Therapeutic drug monitoring, in Tietz NW (ed): *Textbook of Clinical Chemistry.* Philadelphia, PA: WB Saunders, 1986, pp. 1615–1669.

Murray JB: Munchausen syndrome/Munchausen syndrome by proxy. *J Psychol* 131:343–352, 1997.

O'Neal CL, Poklis A: A sensitive HPLC assay for the simultaneous quantitation of lidocaine and its metabolites; monoethylglcinexylididie and glycinexylidide in serum. *Clin Chem* 42:330–331, 1996.

Panel on Herbicides: Report on 2,4,5-T, in *A Report of the Panel on Herbicides of the President's Science Advisory Committee.* Executive Office of the President, Office of Science and Technology. Washington, DC: U.S. Government Printing Office, 1971.

Petersen F, Haines WS, Webster RW: *Legal Medicine and Toxicology,* 2nd ed. Vol 2. Philadelphia, PA: WB Saunders, 1923.

Poklis A: Pentazocine/tripelennamine (T's and blues) abuse: A five year survey of St. Louis, Missouri. *Drug Alcohol Depend* 10:257–267, 1982.

Poklis A, Mackell MA, Tucker E: Tissue distribution of lidocaine after fatal accidental injection. *J Forensic Sci* 29:1229–1236, 1984.

Poklis A, Moore KA: Response of Emit amphetamine immunoassays to urinary desoxyephedrine following Vicks inhaler use. *Ther Drug Monit* 17:89–94, 1995.

Poklis A, Poklis, JL, Trautman D, et al.: Disposition of valproic acid in a case of fatal intoxication. *J Anal Toxicol* 22:537–540, 1998.

Pounder DJ: Forensic entomo-toxicology. *J Forensic Sci Soc* 31:469–472, 1991.

Price LM, Poklis A, Johnson DE: Fatal acetaminophen poisoning with evidence of subendocardial necrosis of the heart. *J Forensic Sci* 36:930–935, 1991.

Prouty BS, Anderson WH: The forensic science implications of site and tempered influences on postmortem blood-drug concentrations. *J Forensic Sci* 35:243–270, 1990.

Saady JJ, Blanke RV: Measurement of glucuronic acid metabolites by high resolution gas chromatography. *J Chromatogr Sci* 28:282–287, 1990.

Saady JJ, Narasimhachari N, Friedel RO: Unsuspected impurities in imipramine and desipramine standards and pharmaceutical formulations. *Clin Chem* 27:343–344, 1981.

SanGeorge RC, Hoberman RD: Reaction of acetaldehyde with hemoglobin. *J Biol Chem* 262:6811–6821, 1986.

Shapiro HA: Arsenic content of human hair and nails: Its interpretation. *J Forensic Med* 14:65–71, 1967.

Shiffman ML, Luketic VA, Sanyal AJ, et al.: Hepatic lidocaine metabolism and liver histology in patients with chronic hepatitis and cirrhosis. *Hepatology* 31:933–940, 1994.

Smith H: The interpretation of the arsenic content of human hair. *J Forensic Sci Soc* 4:192–199, 1964.

Stockham TL, Blanke RV: Investigation of an acetaldehyde-hemoglobin adduct in alcoholics: Alcoholism. *Clin Exp Res* 12:748–754, 1988.

Tagliro F (ed): Hair analysis as a diagnostic tool for drugs of abuse investigation. *Proceeding of the 1st International Meeting,* Genoa, Italy, December 10–11, 1992. Special Issue. *Forensic Sci Int* 63:1–316, 1993.

Thorwald J: *The Century of the Detective.* New York: Harcourt, 1965.

Urey FM, Komaromy-Hiller G, Staley B, et al.: Nitrite adulteration of workplace urine drug-testing specimens: Part 1: Sources and associated concentrations of nitrite in urine and distinction between natural sources and adulteration. *J Anal Toxicol* 22:8995, 1998.

Vorpahl TE, Coe JI: Correlation of antemortem and postmortem digoxin levels. *J Forensic Sci* 23:329–334, 1978.

Warren A: Interference of common household chemicals in immunoassay methods for drugs of abuse. *Clin Chem* 35:648–651, 1989.

White JM, Clardy MS, Groves MH, et al.: Testing for sedative-hypnotic drugs in the impaired driver: A survey of 72,000 arrests. *Clin Toxicol* 18:945–957, 1981.

CHAPTER 32

CLINICAL TOXICOLOGY

Louis R. Cantilena Jr.

HISTORY OF CLINICAL TOXICOLOGY

Historical Aspects of the Treatment of Poisoning

The history of poisons and poisoners dates back to ancient times. The *Odyssey* and *Shastras* from approximately 600 BC contained references to antidotes. The first documentation of use of a specific antidote may be found in Homer's *Odyssey* where it is suggested to Ulysses that he take moli to protect himself from poisoning. Moli may actually be *Galanthus nivalis*, a plant derived cholinesterase inhibitor that might counteract the effects of the anticholinergic plant *Datura stramonium* (Plaitakis and Duvoisin, 1983).

Galen (AD 129–200) wrote three books called *De Antidotis I, De Antidotis II,* and *De Theriaca ad Pisonem* that described the development of a universal antidote known as a alexipharmic or theriac by King Methridates VI of Pontus who lived from 132–63 BC (Wax, 1997). The antidote reportedly contained 36 or more ingredients and was ingested every day conferring protection against a broad spectrum of poisons such as venomous stings and bites from vipers, spiders, and scorpions (Jarcho, 1972).

The refinement of theriac (antidote) formulations is documented for nearly 2000 years. Andromachus (first century AD) was a physician to Nero and improved the Methridates' theriac by modifying the formula to include up to 73 ingredients (Wax, 1997). The use of these ancient antidotes included treatment of acute poisoning and prophylactic treatment to make one "poison proof." The Methridates' theriac with subsequent modifications remained in use until the early twentieth century. William Heberden wrote *Antitheriaka: An Essay on Mithridatium and Theriaca* in 1745 in which he questioned the effectiveness of these products (Jarcho, 1972). Despite the skepticism concerning these antidote formulations, their use continued for two millenniums.

One of the earliest writings on the prevention of the gastrointestinal absorption of poisons was by Nicander (Major, 1934). In this ancient writing, the induction of emesis by ingestion of an emetic agent or mechanical stimulation of the hypopharynx was described as a method to prevent poison absorption. It was not until the 1600s when the use of ipecacuanha for induction of emesis was recommended by William Piso (Reid, 1970).

The use of oral charcoal, now a mainstay in the treatment of many human poisonings, can be dated to early Greek and Roman civilizations when wood charcoal was used for the treatment of maladies such as anthrax and epilepsy (Cooney, 1995). The antidotal properties of charcoal were demonstrated in the 1800s by the French with dramatic demonstrations of a reduction in lethality when charcoal was ingested with potentially lethal dosages of arsenic trioxide by Bertrand and strychnine by Touery (Holt and Holz, 1963). One of the earliest reported human studies examining the efficacy of charcoal in poisoning was in 1948 by the American physician Rand (Holt and Holz, 1963). The use of superheated steam to treat the charcoal to enhance its absorption capacity was reported by Ostrejko, a Russian scientist in 1900 (Greensher *et al.*, 1987). By the 1960s, the use of activated charcoal was routinely recommended for the treatment of patients poisoned with substances thought to be adsorbed to charcoal.

Introduction of the Poison Control Center

Advances in the field of clinical toxicology have paralleled the evolution of poison control centers. One of the earliest local efforts to systematically collect, analyze and distribute to physicians, clinical information about poisoning was led by Jay Arena, a Duke University pediatrician. In 1939 he published a case series detailing the clinical outcome of 50 cases of lye poisoning (Martin and Arena, 1939). Interest in clinical information regarding the treatment of poisoned patients and resultant patient outcomes was also growing in Europe during approximately the same time. During the 1940s, several European communities developed hospital-based treatment facilities for poisoning (Manoguerra and Temple, 1984). This local, poison information effort continued for several years as further realization of the growing importance of the problem of poisoning occurred. A study by the American Academy of Pediatrics completed in 1952 reported that more than half of childhood accidents involved unintentional poisoning in the United States. Possibly in response to this study, Edward Press and Louis Gdalman started the first United States poison control center in Chicago, Illinois. Mr. Gdalman had collected toxicological information on more than 9,000 commercial and noncommercial products throughout the 1940s and early 1950s. Their Chicago poison center provided telephone advice to health care professionals as well as collected poisoning data systematically during the information sharing process. These centers became valuable resources for information about product ingredients, potential toxicity, and recommendations for the treatment of poisoned patients. Poison control centers proliferated over the next two decades and peaked at 661 centers in 1978 (Scherz and Robertson, 1978). Most of these centers served small areas; each state had a least one poison center; several states had more than 20 poison centers active at the same time; and there was little standardization throughout the specialty. Through regionalization, consolidation and certification, the number of poison control centers have significantly decreased to 63 centers in 2004 (IOM, 2004).

Staffing of a poison control center usually consists of a medical director (medical toxicologist), administrator or managing director, specialists in poison information, and educators for poison prevention programs. The medical toxicologist, managing director, and specialists in poison information are health care professionals who are credentialed by their respective boards. The American Board of Medical Subspecialties offers a subspecialty certificate in medical toxicology to physicians who successfully complete the certifying examination. The American Board of Applied Toxicology (ABAT) offers a certification examination for nonphysicians and the American Association of Poison Control Centers (AAPCC) provides a certification of the specialists in poison information who are usually nurses or pharmacists. The managing director is usually either the same person as the medical director or a nonphysician certified by the ABAT.

The public health services provided by poison control centers have been well documented. These services include direct information to patients with recommendations for needed treatment, critical diagnostic and treatment information for health care professionals, education for health care personnel and poison prevention activities through public education. Several studies have shown that poison information centers are cost effective. An often cited example of the economic benefit from access to a poison control center comes from a one year forced closure of the Louisiana State Poison Center. When there was no poison center to call, the community was left with the alternative of an emergency room or doctor's office visit for information and possible treatment of their exposure. It was estimated that the increased costs to the state for emergency medical services was $1.4 million for that year (King, 1991). Studies have shown that for each dollar spent to operate a poison control center a saving of approximately $3–6.50 can be realized for the health care system (Miller and Lestina, 1997).

Recently, the Institute of Medicine commissioned an in-depth study of poison prevention and control services in the United States. The resulting report affirmed the need for, and the value of, the poison control centers and recommended several changes in the interest of public safety, standardization, and process improvement including: regional centers continue to serve the population; federal funding be provided to stabilize core functions of each center; and integration of poison control centers with public health agencies at the federal, state, and local level including integration with the Centers for Disease Control and Prevention for chemical and biological terrorism preparedness (IOM, 2004).

CLINICAL STRATEGY FOR TREATMENT OF THE POISONED PATIENT

The initial phases of treatment of a seriously poisoned patient usually occur in the setting of a hospital emergency room but initial treatment in other, less ideal settings such as the battlefield, workplace, home or street setting can be required as well. Most clinical toxicologists agree that a methodically executed, stepwise approach to the treatment of the poisoned patient is recommended for optimal care (Goldfrank, 2006; Ellenhorn, 1997). This section will refer primarily to the treatment of poisoned patients in the Emergency Department (ED) setting. In that setting, the following general steps represent important elements of the initial clinical encounter for a poisoned patient:

1. Stabilization of the patient
2. Clinical evaluation (history, physical, laboratory, radiology)
3. Prevention of further toxin absorption
4. Enhancement of toxin elimination
5. Administration of antidote
6. Supportive care and clinical follow-up

Clinical Stabilization

The first priority in the treatment of the poisoned patient is clinical stabilization. This is the so-called ABCs (Airway, Breathing, Circulation) of initial emergency treatment. Assessment of the vital signs and the effectiveness of respiration and circulation are the primary objectives of this initial encounter. Early in the course of some poisonings there is a varying range of severity of demonstrated toxic effects by patients poisoned with even lethal dosages of toxins. Some chemicals, such as a benzodiazepine can cause pronounced clinical effects early such as sedation but can have a comparatively mild clinical course; while other chemicals, such as camphor, show little clinical effects initially but can produce a fatal outcome. Some chemicals can cause seizures early in the course of their presentation. Control of chemical-induced seizures can be an important component of the initial stabilization of the poisoned patient. The degree of initial clinical stabilization required for a poisoned patient therefore is highly variable. The clinical procedures available to stabilize a critically ill poisoned patient include the initial and ongoing assessment and, if indicated, support of ventilation, circulation, and oxygenation. A detailed description of the various clinical methods available to treat abnormalities in these parameters is beyond the scope of this chapter. The reader is referred to textbooks of emergency medicine and critical care medicine for further information on this subject. Once the poisoned patient is clinically stabilized, the remainder of the assessment and treatment steps can proceed. In critically ill patients, sometimes treatment interventions must be initiated before a patient is truly stable.

Clinical History in the Poisoned Patient

The primary goal of taking a medical history in poisoned patients is to determine, whenever possible, what substance the poisoned patient has been exposed to and to determine the extent and time of exposure. Unfortunately, in contrast to most specialties of medicine, the clinical history available during the initial clinical encounter in the treatment of poisoned patients is sometimes not helpful because it may be either unreliable or unobtainable. In the setting of a suicide attempt, the patient often is not willing to provide a history or may give incorrect information to increase the possibility of success of their attempt to bring harm to themselves. For these reasons, additional sources for the clinical history are often incorporated to aid the clinical team in determining what substances the patient has been exposed to. Examples of possible sources sometimes employed

Table 32-1
Clinical Features of Toxic Syndromes

	BLOOD PRESSURE	PULSE	TEMPERATURE	PUPILS	LUNGS	ABDOMEN	NEUROLOGIC
Sympathomimetic	Incr.	Incr.	Slight Incr.	Mydriasis	NC	NC	Hyperalert, incr. reflexes
Anticholinergic	Slight incr. or NC	Incr.	Incr.	Mydirasis	NC	Decr. Bowel sounds	Altered mental status
Cholinergic	Slight decr. or NC	Decr.	NC	Miosis	Incr. bronchial sounds	Incr. bowel sounds	Altered mental status
Opioid	Decr.	Decr.	Decr.	Miosis	NC or rales (late)	Decr. Bowel sounds	Decr. level of consciousness

to obtain an accurate history include family members, emergency medical technicians who were at the scene, a pharmacist who can sometimes provide a listing of prescriptions recently filled or an employer who can provide a list of chemicals that are in the work environment.

In estimating the exposure level to the poison, generally one should maximize the possible dose received. That is, one should assume that the entire prescription bottle contents were ingested, that the entire bottle of liquid was consumed or that the highest possible concentration of airborne contaminant was present for a patient poisoned by inhalation unless definite evidence exists to the contrary. Maximizing the potential dose or exposure level reduces the probability of encountering an unexpected clinical outcome in a poisoned patient.

With an estimate of dose, the toxicologist can refer to various information resources to determine what the range of expected clinical effects might be from the estimated exposure. The estimation of expected toxicity greatly assists with the triage of poisoned patients. Poison information specialists working in Poison Information Centers routinely give telephone recommendations regarding the level of medical care required for a given ingestion based on the expected clinical effects from the reported ingestion. The vast majority of in-the-home accidental pediatric exposures are treated with at-home observation, home-administered activated charcoal, or the induction of emesis. In the hospital setting, ED staff use the estimation of expected clinical effects to effectively triage the poisoned patient. For example, a three-year-old patient who accidentally ingested 25 children's chewable multivitamins without iron would likely be triaged to a non-critical care area of the ED, whereas another three-year-old who drank a mouthful of caustic alkali drain cleaner would be triaged to a high intensity of care section of the ED.

Estimating the timing of the exposure to the poison is frequently the most difficult aspect of the clinical history when treating the poisoned patient. Often the toxicologist must turn detective to determine the most likely window of time that the exposure occurred. For example, if a pediatric patient was being watched by the babysitter at all times except for a 20-minute period that preceded the onset of symptoms and the discovery of an open prescription bottle for digoxin, then one would estimate that the ingestion occurred in that 20-minute window. Other situations require estimation of a far broader window for exposure. A person found with a suicide note could have taken the contents of the empty prescription bottle (or anything else available) at any time from when they were last seen by someone to a short time before they were discovered.

Due to these and other limitations, obtaining an accurate history of the poisoned patient can be very challenging and in some cases the treating personnel are not successful. When the history is unobtainable the clinical toxicologist is left without a clear picture of the exposure history in the poisoned patient. When this occurs, treatment proceeds empirically as an "unknown ingestion" poisoning. This type of treatment will be discussed later in this chapter.

Physical Examination

One of the most important aspects of the initial clinical encounter in the treatment of the poisoned patient is the physical examination. A thorough examination of the patient is required to assess the patient's condition, categorize the patient's mental status and, if altered, determine possible additional explanations for the abnormal mental status such as trauma or central nervous system infection. One very helpful tool for the clinical toxicologist is to categorize the patient's physical examination parameters into broad classes referred to as toxic syndromes. These toxic syndromes have been called toxidromes (Mofenson and Greensher, 1970). A toxidrome is a constellation of clinical signs and symptoms that, when taken together, are likely associated with exposure from certain toxicologic classes of chemicals. The major toxic syndromes include narcotic, cholinergic, sympathomimetic, and anticholinergic. Table 32-1 lists the clinical features of these major toxic syndromes.

In certain treatment settings, the chemicals responsible for the poisoning are not known during the critically important phase of initial treatment of the poisoned patient. Categorization of the patient presentation into toxic syndromes allows for the initiation of rationale treatment based on the most likely category of toxin responsible. For example, if a patient presents in a coma, with miosis (pinpoint pupils), hypotension, bradycardia, a markedly reduced respiratory rate, and slight hypothermia with an otherwise non-localizing neurological examination, the clinical toxicologist can characterize the patient's presentation as consistent with the narcotic toxic syndrome. The presence of needle tracks on the skin would support this categorization. The treatment would then be directed at support of respiration and pharmacological reversal with a mu-receptor opioid antagonist such as naloxone. In this example, lifesaving treatment can be administered in a timely manner, even in the absence of definitive identification of the ingested poison.

Occasionally a characteristic odor can be detected on the poisoned patient's breath or clothing which may point toward exposure or poisoning by a specific agent. Table 32-2 lists some of the better recognized odors and the substance associated with the odor. Detection of one of these odors may provide an important historical clue as to the agent responsible for the poisoning.

Table 32-2
Characteristic Odors Associated with Poisonings

ODOR	POTENTIAL POISON
Bitter almonds	Cyanide
Eggs	Hydrogen sulfide, mercaptans
Garlic	As, organophosphates, DMSO, Thallium
Mothballs	Naphthalene, camphor
Vinyl	Ethchlorvynol
Wintergreen	Methylsalicylate

Periodic reexamination of the patient is a very important aspect of clinical toxicology treatment procedures. Follow-up clinical examinations can help gauge the progression of the clinical course of poisoning as well as determine the effectiveness of treatment interventions and gauge the need for additional treatment procedures.

Laboratory Evaluation

A common misconception concerning the initial treatment of poisoned patients is that a definitive diagnosis of the specific agent or poison responsible for the patient's clinical presentation is frequently made by the clinical laboratory during the initial patient evaluation. Unfortunately, the repertoire of specific assays for toxins available in clinical laboratories on a rapid turnaround basis (STAT, e.g., within 1 hour) is very limited. Table 32-3 lists drugs or other chemical substances that are typically available for STAT measurement in a medical center type hospital facility. As one can see, the number of chemicals for which quantitative detection is possible in the rapid turnaround clinical setting is extremely limited compared to the number of possible chemicals that can poison patients. This further emphasizes the importance of recognizing clinical syndromes for poisoning and for the clinical toxicologist to be able to initiate general treatment and supportive care for the patient with poisoning from an unknown substance.

For the relatively few substances that can be measured on a rapid turnaround basis in an ED setting, the quantitative measurement can often provide both prognostic and therapeutic guidance. Several authors have suggested certain "action levels" for specific therapeutic drugs and chemicals which when met or exceeded during the measurement in patient plasma, should trigger specific interventions or predict likely clinical outcomes. In some cases, measurement of an indicator of the biologic effect of a poison provides sufficient information to render definitive treatment to the patient. Measurement of methemoglobin concentration in a patient poisoned by one of many chemicals that can cause this chemical transformation of the hemoglobin molecule is sufficient to initiate treatment for methemoglobinemia without identification of the specific toxin that caused the condition. Similarly, most hospital laboratories have the capability for rapid measurement of carboxyhemoglobin concentrations, which permits treatment of carbon monoxide poisoning based on the laboratory test measuring a surrogate marker for carbon monoxide exposure.

For some commonly ingested drugs, a nomogram has been established to predict the severity of the poisoning and is important in some cases to guide therapeutic intervention based on the measured plasma concentration of the drug and the time elapsed from the exposure. Proper use of such nomograms is necessary for the clinical management of poisoning cases.

Table 32-3
Drugs Commonly Measured in a Hospital Setting on a STAT Basis

Acetaminophen
Acetone
Carbamazepine
Carboxyhemoglobin
Digoxin
Ethanol
Ethyl alcohol
Gentamycin
Iron
Lithium
Methemoglobin
Osmolality
Phenobarbital
Phenytoin
Procainamide/NAPA
Quinidine
Salicylates
Theophylline
Tobramycin
Valproic acid

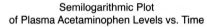

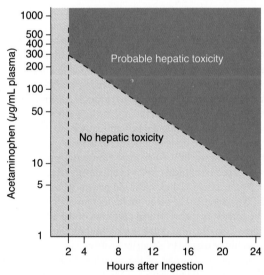

Figure 32-1. Rumack-Mathew nomogram for acetaminophen poisoning. (From Rumack and Mathew, 1975, with permission. Copyright American Academy of Pediatrics, 1975.)

The clinical usefulness of a drug plasma concentration measured by the clinical laboratory was suggested for salicylates approximately 40 years ago. In 1960, Done published a nomogram to predict the clinical outcome from poisoning with salicylates (Done, 1960).

In 1975, Rumack and Mathews published a nomogram for acetaminophen poisoning shown in Figure 32-1 (Rumack and Mathew, 1975). This nomogram predicts clinical outcome and is also valuable to guide the clinician in the decision as to whether or not to administer N-acetyl cysteine (NAC), an antidote for significant acetaminophen ingestion. Laboratory evaluation of a patient potentially poisoned with acetaminophen is crucial to assess what hepatic injury may have already occurred and to determine plasma concentrations of acetaminophen for prognostic purposes. Accurate estimation of acetaminophen in the plasma should be done on samples drawn at least 4 hours after ingestion, when or past the time that peak plasma levels can be expected. Once an accurate plasma concentration of acetaminophen has been obtained, it should be plotted on the Rumack-Matthew nomogram (Fig. 32-1) to determine whether NAC therapy is indicated. This nomogram is based on a series of patients with and without hepatotoxicity and their corresponding acetaminophen plasma concentrations at presentation.

In the appropriate patient, the decision to treat an acetaminophen-poisoned patient is based on the plasma concentration of parent acetaminophen plotted on the nomogram. Although some authors recommend that NAC treatment only be administered to a patient with an acetaminophen plasma concentration in the "definite toxic" range, most clinical toxicologists agree that NAC should be given at or above the "probably toxic" action level. It should be noted however that proper use of this nomogram is required, namely that certain conditions should be met to apply the nomogram to a specific clinical case. The nomogram was validated for a single acetaminophen ingestion, the time of ingestion is critically important to establish the X-axis coordinate for the data point and the plasma concentration should have been obtained at least 4 hours after ingestion to assure that the peak plasma concentration of parent acetaminophen has occurred.

Similar, though perhaps less well established, predictive relationships of drug plasma concentration and clinical outcome and/or suggested concentrations that require therapeutic interventions are available for several other chemicals including lithium, salicylates, digoxin, iron, phenobarbital, and theophylline. Some authors have identified "action levels" or toxic threshold values for the measured plasma concentrations of various drugs or chemicals (Ellenhorn, 1997). Generally, these values represent mean concentrations of the respective substance that have been retrospectively shown to produce a significant harmful effect. The pharmaco- (or toxico-) dynamic variability for a given toxin or for a combination of toxins is significant, however. For example, a patient with a "normal" or "nontoxic" digoxin level may display significant toxic effects and conversely a patient with an elevated or "toxic" plasma concentration of digoxin may not show any sign of harmful effects. The clinical toxicologist must critically evaluate the laboratory data and treat the patient and not just the laboratory value.

Because of the limited clinical availability of "diagnostic" laboratory tests for poisons, toxicologists utilize specific, routinely obtained, clinical laboratory data to establish a differential diagnosis of what poisons may have been ingested. There are two calculations that toxicologists can perform using clinical laboratory values routinely obtained in an acute clinical setting. The calculations performed on routine clinical labs are the anion gap and the osmol gap. An abnormal anion gap or osmol gap suggests a differential diagnosis for significant exposure of a poisoned patient. Both calculations are used as diagnostic aids when the clinical history suggests poisoning and the patient's condition is consistent with exposure to agents known to cause elevations of these parameters (i.e., metabolic acidosis, altered mental status, etc.).

The anion gap is calculated as the difference between the serum Na ion concentration and the sum of the serum Cl and HCO_3 ion

Table 32-4

Differential Diagnosis of Metabolic Acidosis with Elevated Anion Gap: "AT MUD PILES"

A	Alcohol (Ethanol ketoacidosis)
T	Toluene
M	Methanol
U	Uremia
D	Diabetic ketoacidosis
P	Paraldehyde
I	Iron, Isoniazid
L	Lactic Acid
E	Ethylene Glycol
S	Salicylate

concentrations.

$$Anion\,Gap = [Na\,mEq/L - (Cl\,mEq/L + HCO_3\,mEq/L)]$$

$$Normal\,Anion\,Gap \leq 12$$

When there is laboratory evidence of metabolic acidosis in a poisoned patient, the finding of an elevated anion gap would suggest systemic toxicity from a relatively limited number of agents. A popular clinical pneumonic (AT MUD PILES) is commonly employed as a memory aid for this differential diagnosis. Table 32-4 lists the more common agents that have metabolic acidosis with an elevated anion gap as part of the clinical presentation that are included in this pneumonic.

The second calculated parameter from clinical chemistry values is the osmol gap. The osmol gap is calculated as the numerical difference between the measured serum osmolality and the serum osmolarity calculated from the clinical chemistry measurements of the serum sodium ion, glucose, and blood urea nitrogen (BUN) concentrations (Smithline and Gardner, 1976).

$$OsmoGap = Measured\,Serum\,Osmolality\,(mOsm)$$

$$- Calculated\,Serum\,Osmolarity$$

where calculated serum osmolarity $= 2 \times Na\,mEq/L + Glucose\,mg/dL/18 + BUN\,mg/dL/2.8$,

$$Normal\,osmol\,gap < 10\,mOsm.$$

Note that the serum osmolality must be measured by freezing point depression and not boiling point elevation as the later method can fail to detect the osmolality contribution of volatile, low-molecular-weight substances due to vaporization of the substance during measurement.

An elevated osmol gap in the setting of a poisoned patient suggests the presence of an osmotically active substance in the plasma that is not accounted for by the Na, glucose or BUN concentrations. Table 32-5 lists several substances that when ingested can be associated with an elevated osmol gap in humans.

While calculation of both the anion gap and the osmol gap can provide very useful information from readily available clinical chemistry measurements, these determinations must be interpreted cautiously in certain clinical settings. For example, even though a patient may have ingested a large, significantly toxic amount of

Table 32-5
Differential Diagnosis for Elevated Osmol Gap

Methanol
Ethanol
Ethylene glycol
Isopropanol

methanol, if measured late in the clinical course of the exposure, the osmol gap may not be significantly elevated as most of the osmotically active methanol has left the plasma and has been biotransformed or cleared but still producing serious clinical effects.

Radiographic Examination

The utility of the radiographic examination to diagnose specific poisonings is relatively limited. The use of clinical radiographs to visualize drug overdose or poison ingestions is also relatively limited. This is due primarily to the lack of radiopacity of many oral forms of medication. Early radiographic surveys of the radiopacity of oral medications revealed that the vast majority of commercially available tablets and capsules surveyed were essentially undetectable by radiograph (Handy, 1971; O'Brien et al., 1986). These and other studies have shown that relatively few formulations of drugs are radiopaque and would likely be detectable by plain X-ray of the abdomen. Generally, plain radiographs can detect a significant amount of ingested oral medication containing ferrous or potassium salts. However, a study of the in vitro and in vivo visualization of chewable oral formulations of iron supplements showed that once the chewable iron was ingested it was no longer detectable by plain abdominal radiograph (Everson et al., 1989). However, certain formulations that have an enteric coating or certain types of sustained release products are radiopaque and can be visualized (Savitt et al., 1987; Nelson et al., 1993).

The most useful radiographs ordered in an overdose or poisoned patient include the chest and abdominal radiographs and the computed head tomography study. The abdominal radiograph has been used to detect recent lead paint ingestion in children due to pica for many years. Although the presence of radiographic evidence of lead based paint chips probably underrepresented the proportion of children with moderate to severe lead poisoning in one study, an abdominal radiograph showing pica was associated with significantly elevated blood lead concentrations (McElvaine et al., 1992). Another situation in which an abdominal radiograph may be helpful is the setting of a halogenated hydrocarbon such as carbon tetrachloride or chloroform. If a sufficient amount of either liquid is ingested it is likely that these organic solvents will be visualized as a radiopaque liquid in the gut lumen on the abdominal film relatively recently after ingestion (Dally et al., 1987). Finally, abdominal plain radiographs have been helpful in the setting where foreign bodies are detected in the gastrointestinal tract. An example of this is in the situation where an international traveler coming to the United States, becomes acutely ill with signs of severe sympathomimetic excess and numerous foreign bodies are visualized throughout the gastrointestinal tract. This patient would be known as a body packer who smuggles illegal substances by swallowing latex or plastic storage vesicles filled with cocaine or some other substance (Beerman et al., 1986; McCarron and wood, 1983; Sporer and Firestone, 1997). Occasionally these storage devices rupture and the drug is released into the gastrointestinal tract with serious and sometimes fatal results.

Aside from these relatively uncommon situations, the overall clinical utility for detection and diagnosis of poisons by radiography is limited.

In contrast to the limited clinical utility of plain radiography for the identification of a specific poison or to diagnose poisoning, plain radiography and other types of diagnostic imaging in clinical toxicology can be extremely valuable for the diagnosis of toxin-induced pathology and to aid the clinical toxicologist in the ongoing treatment and patient management phases of the drug overdose. Detection of drug-induced noncardiac pulmonary edema is associated with serious intoxication with salicylates and opioid agonists (Stern et al., 1968; Heffner et al., 1990). Plain chest radiography can detect this abnormality, which would likely correlate with the findings observed during physical examination of the lungs. This radiographic finding would increase the severity classification of the poisoning and potentially alter the planned therapeutic strategy for the patient.

Another example of the use of radiological imaging in clinical toxicology is with computed tomography (CT) of the brain. Significant exposure to carbon monoxide (CO) has been associated with CT lesions of the brain consisting of low-density areas in the cerebral white matter and in the basal ganglia, especially the globus pallidus. Although not clinically employed for diagnostic purposes in the acute phases of a carbon monoxide poisoning, these CT findings of the brain have been useful for estimating the clinical prognosis of a patient who survives the initial phase of CO poisoning (Miura et al., 1985; Jones et al., 1994). Finally, concurrent intracranial pathology, such as trauma or hemorrhage can be detected by CT or MRI of the brain to aid in the diagnosis of additional injury or pathology previously not appreciated during the treatment of a poisoned patient.

The initial clinical evaluation of the poisoned patient is a critically important phase of the therapeutic process to treat poisoned individuals. The physical, laboratory and radiological examination all contribute to the initial diagnostic steps for poison treatment. The physical and laboratory examinations are generally utilized more from a diagnostic and acute management standpoint, whereas the radiological examination tends to be more useful for detection and management of toxicant-induced pathology.

Prevention of Further Poison Absorption

During the early phases of poison treatment or intervention for a toxic exposure via the oral, inhalation or the topical route, the treatment team may have an opportunity to prevent further absorption of the poison to minimize the total amount that reaches the systemic circulation. For chemicals presented by the inhalation route, the main intervention to prevent further absorption is removal of the patient from the environment where the chemical is found and to provide adequate ventilation and oxygenation for the patient. For topical exposures, patient clothing containing the toxin must be removed and properly disposed in airtight wrappings or containers to ensure that the rescuers and health care providers are adequately protected from secondary exposure. Most topical exposures require gentle washing of the skin with water and mild soap taking care not to cause cutaneous abrasions of the skin that may enhance dermal absorption.

The optimal time to intervene to prevent continued absorption of an oral poison is as soon as possible after the ingestion. The four primary methods currently available for this purpose are: induction of emesis with syrup of ipecac, gastric lavage, oral administration of activated charcoal and whole bowel irrigation. Historically, induction of emesis with a variety of agents was the sole modality employed to treat poisoning by seeking to reduce the gastrointestinal absorption of poisons. Tartar emetic was an antimony salt used for induction of emesis and other medicinal purposes. Other emetic agents used later on included mustard mixed in water, concentrated solutions of copper and zinc salts and various botanical substances. In hospitals, apomorphine injection was given even into the 1980s to cause emesis in patients with a history of potentially toxic ingestion.

Currently syrup of ipecac is the only agent available for induction of emesis in the treatment of a potentially toxic ingestion. Previously poison center directed, home use of syrup of ipecac was the most widely used poison treatment intervention. Syrup of ipecac has been available in the United States since the early 1960s. Typically, 15–20 ml of syrup of ipecac is given orally with water and vomiting (usually more than a single episode) can be expected within the ensuing 30 minutes. However, recently the efficacy and potential abuse liability of syrup of Ipecac have significantly impacted on the product's use in the management of poisoning. Controlled studies have demonstrated significant variability in the amount of drug or test markers removed by administration of syrup of ipecac. In addition, the efficacy to remove gastric contents and therefore subsequent absorption of the toxin declines with increase in the time interval between poison ingestion and syrup of ipecac administration (Neuvonen *et al.*, 1983). Despite being available as an over-the-counter drug product in the United States since 1965, a citizen's petition was filed with the Food and Drug Administration to request removal of syrup of ipecac from the OTC market in 2002 based on limited efficacy data and published reports of increasing abuse liability for the product. In June, 2003 the FDA's advisory committee for nonprescription drugs met to review the pros and cons of continued OTC availability for this product. Due to a nuance in regulations and FDA policy, if removed from the OTC market, because no prescription "sponsor" is available for the product, syrup of ipecac would effectively be removed from the entire US market (prescription and nonprescription) and unavailable for sale. At the present time, the FDA has yet to decide the fate of the OTC availability for syrup of ipecac. The American Academy of Clinical Toxicology and the European Association of Poisons Centres and Clinical Toxicologists issued a position paper regarding the use of syrup of ipecac in 2004, which stated that the product should not be used routinely in the management of the poisoned patient and that there was insufficient data to either support or exclude ipecac administration soon after poison ingestion (Krenzelok *et al.*, 2004). Many clinical toxicologists believe that there remains a limited role for the clinical use of syrup of ipecac, mainly is rural areas where the length of time before a poisoned patient can reach medical care is significant. The accepted contraindications for use of syrup of ipecac are: (1) children less than 6 months of age; (2) in the ingestion of a caustic agent (acid or alkali); (3) in a patient with a depressed level of consciousness or gag reflex or when the toxin ingested is expected to cause either condition within a short period of time; or (4) when there is a significant risk of aspiration of gastric contents such as for ingestion of a liquid hydrocarbon with high aspiration potential.

The use of gastric lavage, the technique of placing an orogastric tube into the stomach and aspirating fluid then cyclically instilling fluid and aspirating until the effluent is clear, has diminished significantly in recent years. The reasons for the decline in use of this technique include a growing appreciation of the risk of aspiration during the lavage procedure and growing evidence that the effectiveness of gastric lavage may be more limited than originally thought. Careful attention to the patient's gag reflex prior to initiation of this procedure is important. If the patient does not exhibit a gag reflex, then endotracheal intubation must be performed to adequately protect the airway and prevent aspiration. Most clinical toxicologists would agree that the current role of gastric lavage, if there is a role at all, would be in the initial treatment of the overdose patient who had a recent (within 1 hour) oral ingestion. It is essential that the orogastric tube be of sufficient size (40–44 French for an adult) to be useful. Even with a large bore orogastric tube some tablets or capsules may not be able to pass through the tube. In the pediatric patient, there are practical limitations to the use of large bore tubes. In this case, orogastric lavage may only be useful to attempt removal of liquid toxins or possibly dissolved tablets or capsules. Due to recent questioning of the effectiveness of the technique and the availability of data showing that other modalities for prevention of further toxin absorption (e.g., oral activated charcoal) are possibly as or more effective, the use of gastric lavage has greatly diminished.

As described earlier, the medicinal use of charcoal dates back more than 150 years. The first reported medicinal use of oral charcoal to adsorb an ingested toxin is credited to the American physician, Hort, who, in 1834, used large amounts of powdered charcoal to successfully treat a patient poisoned with a chloride salt of mercury. A dramatic demonstration of the adsorptive effect of oral charcoal was that by Tourey, a French pharmacist who reportedly mixed a lethal dose of strychnine with charcoal and consumed the combination before his colleagues at the French Academy in 1930 (Andersen, 1946). Early in vitro investigations of the adsorptive properties of activated charcoal demonstrated the effect of charcoal on various chemical substances in aqueous solutions (Andersen, 1946), the effect of pH on charcoal adsorption properties (Andersen, 1947) and the effect of activated charcoal on the adsorption of strychnine from gastric contents (Andersen, 1948).

During the last 20–30 years there has been growing use of oral charcoal as a therapeutic intervention for oral poisoning. For many years, orally administered activated charcoal has been routinely incorporated into the initial treatment of a patient poisoned by the oral route. The term "activated" refers to the substantially increased adsorptive capacity that results from the processing of charcoal obtained from the burning of carbonaceous substances such as wood pulp, sugars, organic material and industrial wastes. The processing involves extensive treatment with steam, carbon dioxide, oxygen, zinc chloride, sulfuric acid, or phosphoric acid at temperatures of 500–900 degrees Fahrenheit "activate" the residue oxidation which leads to a significant increase in surface area through creation of small pores in the material. Many organic molecules are significantly bound to activated charcoal. Generally low-molecular-weight, and polar compounds, such as ethanol, tend to be less well bound to activated charcoal. Substances such as lithium, iron and certain inorganic salts are also not appreciably bound. In acute oral overdose, activated charcoal is typically administered at a dosage of 1.0–1.5 g/kg. When the patient is unable to safely drink the charcoal it is placed into the stomach via orogastric or nasogastric tube.

The usefulness of whole bowel irrigation for the treatment of the poisoned patient is very limited. Whole bowel irrigation is a procedure that in essence "washes" the lumen of the gastrointestinal tract clear of unabsorbed material. The procedure is accomplished with a poorly absorbed, osmotically neutral polyethylene glycol electrolyte solution that is administered orally to expel the contents of the intestines via the rectal route. This procedure is used to prepare the lower intestine for endoscopic medical procedures of the large intestine. The primary role of this technique is for removal of ingested packets of illegal drugs that may or may not be causing toxic effects due to leakage. Other potential roles for this gastrointestinal technique are to treat ingestion of sustained release formulations of drugs and ingestions of substantial amounts of iron preparations (Tenebein *et al.*, 2004).

Most clinical toxicologists agree that, for the prevention of further absorption following oral ingestion of most toxins, the administration of oral activated charcoal provides the most consistent efficacy and best safety profile (Goldfrank, 2006). The other modalities described above have more limited roles (whole bowel irrigation, syrup of ipecac) or only rare circumstances when their use should be considered at all (gastric lavage). Most treatment centers favor the use of activated charcoal without gastric decontamination (lavage or ipecac) for treatment of oral poisoning and drug overdose. Many poison control centers recommend home use of a premixed slurry of activated charcoal for immediate treatment of potentially significant poisonings. The use of ipecac syrup is largely limited to individual patients in whom it is likely to make a difference in outcome, who are in rural environments, hours away from more definitive medical treatment, in whom it appears to be the most effective method available in that particular set of circumstances, or in whom it is the only method available to attempt gastric emptying.

Enhancement of Poison Elimination

There are several methods available to enhance the elimination of specific poisons or drugs once they have been absorbed into the systemic circulation. The primary methods employed for this use today include: alkalinization of the urine, hemodialysis, hemoperfusion, hemofiltration, plasma exchange or exchange transfusion, and serial oral activated charcoal.

The use of urinary alkalinization results in the enhancement of the renal clearance of certain weak acids. The basic principle is to increase urinary filtrate pH to a level sufficient to ionize the weak acid and prevent renal tubule reabsorption of the molecule. This is also referred to as ion trapping. The ion-trapping phenomenon occurs when the pK_a of the agent is such that after glomerular filtration into the renal tubules, alteration of the pH of the urinary filtrate can ionize and "trap" the agent in the urinary filtrate. Once the toxin is ionized, reabsorption from the renal tubules is impaired, and as a result, more of the drug remains in the urinary filtrate and is excreted in the urine.

Clinical use of this alkalinization procedure requires adequate urine flow and close clinical monitoring including that of the pH of the urine. The procedure is accomplished by adding sterile sodium bicarbonate to sterile water with 5% dextrose for intravenous infusion and titrating the urine pH to 7.5 to 8.5. The drugs for which this procedure has been shown clinically efficacious include salicylate compounds and phenobarbital which have pK_a's of 3.2 and 7.4, respectively. The increase in total body clearance for salicylate for example, by increasing urinary pH from 5.0 to 8.0 can be substantial. The American Association of Poison Control Centers and the European Association of Poisions Centres and Clinical Toxicologists 2004 Position Paper on Urinary Alkalinization recommends this procedure for moderately severe salicylate poisoning for patient not meeting criteria for hemodialysis (Proudfoot *et al.*, 2004).

Theoretically there are similar advantages to be gained from acidification of the urine regarding enhancement of clearance of drugs such as amphetamine and phencyclidine, however there are significant adverse events associated with acidification such as acute renal failure and acid-base and electrolyte disturbances. For this reason, acidification of the urine is not recommended as a therapeutic intervention in the treatment of poisoning.

The dialysis technique, either hemodialysis or peritoneal dialysis, relies on passage of the toxic agent through a semipermeable dialysis membrane (or the peritoneal membrane) so that it can equilibrate with the dialysate and subsequently be removed. Hemodialysis incorporates a blood pump to pass blood next to a dialysis membrane to allow agents permeable to the membrane to pass through and reach equilibrium. In order for this method to be clinically beneficial the chemcial must have a relatively low volume of distribution, low protein binding, a relatively high degree of water solubility and low molecular weight. Use of hemodialysis to attempt to remove a chemical with the later three characteristics but with a high volume of distribution, such as digoxin, would not be clinically beneficial because the vast majority of the drug is not in the physiologic compartment (blood) accessible to the dialysis membrane. Therefore, despite hemodialysis being able to effectively clear the digoxin in plasma during the dialysis run, most of the body burden of digoxin is located outside of the blood compartment and is not appreciably affected by the procedure. Similarly, if a drug is highly protein-bound, only a small percentage (the free fraction) would be available to pass through the dialysis membrane and be cleared from the body. Some drugs, such as phenobarbital, can readily cross these membranes and go from a high concentration in plasma to a lower concentration in the dialysate. Phenobarbital has a relatively low volume of distribution (0.5–0.7 L/kg) and protein binding (30–50%) so there is a reasonable opportunity for enough drug to be removed from the total body burden to make the technique valuable in serious cases of overdose (Brown *et al.*, 1985; Cutler *et al.*, 1987). Drugs and toxins for which hemodialysis has been shown to be clinically effective in the treatment of poisoning by these agents is shown in Table 32-6.

The technique of hemoperfusion is similar to hemodialysis except there is no dialysis membrane or dialysate involved in the procedure. The patient's blood is pumped through a perfusion cartridge where it is in direct contact with adsorptive material (usually

Table 32-6

Agents for which Hemodialysis Has Been Shown Effective as a Treatment Modality for Poisoning

Alcohols
Antibiotics
Boric acid
Bromide
Calcium
Chloral hydrate
Fluorides
Iodides
Isoniazid
Lithium
Meprobamate
Metformin
Paraldehyde
Phenobarbital
Potassium
Salicylates
Strychnine
Theophylline
Thiocynates
Valproic acid

activated charcoal) that has a coating of material such as cellulose or a heparin-containing gel to prevent the adsorptive material from being carried back to the patient's circulation. The principle characteristics for a drug or toxin to be successfully removed by this technique are low volume of distribution and adsorption by activated charcoal. This method can be used successfully with lipid soluble compounds and with higher molecular weight compounds than for hemodialysis. Protein binding does not significantly interfere with removal by hemoperfusion. Because of the more direct contact of the patient's blood with the adsorptive material, the medical risks of this procedure include thrombocytopenia, hypocalcemia and leukopenia. This technique is primarily used for the treatment of serious theophylline overdose, and possibly amanita toxin exposure, paraquat and meprobamate poisoning. The technique is seldom used currently and it is possible that access to the sterile hemoperfusion cartridge necessary for the procedure may be limited, even at major medical centers.

The use of the technique of hemofiltration for the treatment of poisoning is relatively new and consequently there is much less experience with the modality for enhancement of chemical elimination. During this procedure, the patient's blood is delivered through hollow fiber tubes and an ultrafiltrate of plasma is removed by hydrostatic pressure from the blood side of the membrane. Different membrane pore sizes are available for use so the size of the filtered molecules can be controlled during the procedure. The perfusion pressure for the technique is either generated by the patient's blood pressure (for arteriovenous hemofiltration) or by a blood pump (for venovenous hemofiltration). Needed fluid and electrolytes removed in the ultrafiltrate are replaced intravenously with sterile solutions. The procedure has the advantage of continuous use compared to the 4–6 hour limitation for a hemodialysis run. One theoretical advantage of continuous filtration versus intermittent hemodialysis is that the rebound phenomenon is not seen with hemofiltration as it is with certain poisons after hemodialysis. The rebound of serum concentrations occurs when there is redistribution of the dialyzed poison to the blood when dialysis is interrupted. This rebound is commonly seen during hemodialysis for lithium overdose (Bosinski et al., 1998). Whether or not hemofiltration becomes a routine technique employed in poisoning treatment is unclear at this time.

The use of either plasma exchange or exchange transfusions has been relatively limited in the field of clinical toxicology. While the techniques afford the potential advantage of being able to remove high molecular weight and/or plasma protein bound toxins, the clinical utility in poison treatment has been limited. Plasma exchange, or pheresis involves removal of plasma and replacement with frozen donor plasma, albumin or both with intravenous fluid. The risks and complications of this technique include allergic type reactions, infectious complications and hypotension (Mokrzycki and Kaplan, 1994). Exchange transfusion involves replacement of a patient's blood volume with donor blood. The use of this technique in poison treatment is relatively uncommon and mostly confined to the setting of inadvertent drug overdose in a neonate or premature infant in the setting of a neonatal intensive care unit.

Serial oral administration of activated charcoal, also referred to as multiple-dose activated charcoal (MDAC), has been shown to increase the systemic clearance of various drug substances. The mechanism for the observed augmentation of non-renal clearance caused by repeated doses of oral charcoal is thought to be translumenal efflux of drug from blood to be adsorbed to the charcoal passing through the gastrointestinal tract (Berg et al., 1982). In addition, MDAC is thought to produce its beneficial effect by interrupting the enteroenteric-enterohepatic circulation of drugs. After systemic absorption, a drug may reenter the gut lumen by passive diffusion if the intraluminal drug concentration is lower than that in blood. The rate of this passive diffusion depends on the concentration gradient and the intestinal surface area, permeability, and blood flow. The activated charcoal in the gut lumen serves as a "sink" for toxin. A concentration gradient is maintained and the toxin passes continuously into the gut lumen, where it is adsorbed to charcoal. The characteristics of toxins that favor enhanced elimination by MDAC include (1) significant enteroenteric-enterohepatic circulation, including the formation of active recirculating metabolites, (2) prolonged plasma half-life after an overdose, (3) small (<1.0 L/kg) volume of distribution, (4) limited (<60%) plasma protein binding, (5) a pK_a that maximizes transport of drug across cell membranes, (6) sustained-release/resin-form tablets and/or capsules, and (7) onset of organ failure (e.g., kidney) that results in reduced capacity of the major route of elimination of the toxin so that MDAC may make a considerable contribution to total body clearance.

The technique involves continuing oral administration of activated charcoal beyond the initial dosage (described above) every 2–4 hours with approximately one-half the initial dose, or 0.5 g/kg. The charcoal is generally mixed as an aqueous slurry and a cathartic substance is not incorporated due to the potential for electrolyte abnormalities with repeated administration of cathartic agents. An alternative technique for MDAC is to give the activated charcoal via an orogastric tube or nasogastric tube a loading dose of 1.0 g/kg of an aqueous slurry or activated charcoal (not the combination product that contains the cathartic sorbitol) followed by a continuous infusion intragastrically of 0.2 g/kg/h. The duration of gastric infusion depends on the clinical status of the patient and repeated monitoring of plasma drug levels where indicated (Ilkhanipour et al., 1992; Ohning et al., 1986; Chyka, 1995; Goulbourne et al., 1994; Mofenson et al., 1985; Park et al., 1983, 1986; Pollack et al., 1981; Van de Graaff et al., 1982).

Studies in animals and human volunteers have shown that MDAC increases drug elimination significantly, but few prospective randomized controlled clinical studies in poisoned patients have been published demonstrating a significant reduction in patient morbidity or mortality when MDAC is employed. One recent study however does provide a striking example of clinical benefit from the use of MDAC (de Silva et al., 2003). The study showed that patients who intentionally poisoned themselves with yellow oleander seeds (a cardiac poison) and were randomized to MDAC (after all patients received an adequate initial single dose of activated charcoal) had a statistically improved outcome in both mortality and cardiac morbidity. The early use of MDAC is an attractive alternative to more complex methods of enhancing toxin elimination, such

Table 32-7

Agents for which activated charcoal has been shown as an effective means of enhanced body clearance

Carbamazepine
Dapsone
Digoxin
Digitoxin
Nadolol
Phenobarbital
Salicylates
Theophylline

as hemodialysis and hemoperfusion, although only in a relatively small subset of patients. The decision to use MDAC depends on the clinical situation including the specific chemical involved, the presence of contraindications (e.g., intestinal obstruction) to the use of MDAC, and the likely effectiveness of alternative methods of therapy. A list of chemicals for which MDAC has been shown as an effective means of enhanced body clearance is shown in Table 32-7.

Use of Antidotes in Poisoning

A relatively small number of specific antidotes are available for clinical use in the treatment of poisoning. This is partially due to a paucity of effort in drug development for antidotes as drugs. Significant barriers exist for poison antidote drug development including the small projected market for antidotes and the practical difficulties in performing clinical trials in overdose patients, an important component of an application for drug approval. The typical standard for clinical proof of drug safety and efficacy is the prospective, randomized, double-blinded, placebo controlled clinical trial. Practical considerations make it very difficult to perform this type of clinical trial for rare conditions such as specific poisonings. The United States Food and Drug Administration (FDA) placed incentives for sponsors to develop drugs for rare diseases or conditions through the Orphan Drug Act. Via the Orphan Drug pathway, an antidote for a fairly common poisoning was approved using the orphan drug pathway in December, 1997. Fomepizole (4-methylpyrazole), a chemical inhibitor of alcohol dehydrogenase, was approved as an antidote for ethylene glycol (and later methanol) poisoning. Despite that early success there have not been a large number of antidote products approved to this point in time as a result of this regulatory incentive. Another potential stimulus for antidote drug development has been the "post 9/11" federal funding increase for antiterrorism efforts including research for prevention and treatment of chemical, biological and radiologic poisons. Hopefully this large increase in federal spending will result in the development and approval of new antidotes.

The mechanism of action of various antidotes is quite different. For example, a chelating agent or Fab fragments specific to digoxin work by physically binding the toxin, preventing the toxin from exerting a deleterious effect in vivo and in some cases, facilitating body clearance of the toxin. Other antidotes pharmacologically antagonize the effects of the toxin. Atropine, an antimuscarinic, anticholinergic agent is used to pharmacologically antagonize at the receptor level, the effects of organophosphate insecticides or acetylcholinesterase inhibiting nerve gases, which produce cholinergic, muscarinic effects, which if sufficient, can be lethal. Certain chemicals exert their antidote effects by chemically reacting with biological systems to increase detoxifying capacity for the toxin. For example, sodium nitrite is given to patients poisoned with cyanide to cause formation of methemoglobin, which serves as an alternative binding site for the cyanide ion thereby making it less toxic to the body.

The time course for antidote onset of action is highly variable across currently available antidotes. Intravenous naloxone can have a dramatic effect on the level of consciousness of an opiate-poisoned patient within minutes. Chelating agents such as desferoxamine may require multiple dosages over many days before a clinically detectable effect is seen.

The skillful therapeutic use of antidotes is essential to optimize the treatment of the poisoned patient. Many antidotes have a relatively narrow safety margin or low therapeutic index. Excessive dosing with an antidote can in some instances be more harmful than the expected effects of the toxin itself. Some antidotes require an adjustment of their dosage based on a measured blood concentration of the toxin (for example, digoxin Fab fragments) or based on the clinical assessment of the patient such as with sodium bicarbonate usage in a tricyclic antidepressant overdose. A significant part of the clinical training in the field of medical toxicology is devoted to learning how to use antidotes skillfully.

An important area of research in clinical toxicology has been in the study of prognostic indicators of poisoning severity and predictors for the level of treatment required. For practical reasons much of this work has been retrospective in nature but has resulted in significant aids to guide the treatment rendered by clinical toxicologists. Several authors have proposed "action levels" that are a threshold for a certain level of clinical intervention based upon a measured plasma concentration of the toxin or a clinical manifestation of the poisoning. For example, a patient with a measured plasma theophylline concentration of 90 mg/L after a single oral exposure would be expected to exhibit significant toxicity. If the patient's clinical condition correlated with the measured laboratory plasma concentration (i.e., laboratory error was unlikely), the patient would likely require aggressive treatment measures. Another way that prognostic information is studied is when a constellation of clinical signs and symptoms is proven to correlate with a clinical outcome following exposure to a specific poison. An example of this would be a worker with a significant topical methanol exposure who demonstrates a metabolic acidosis with an elevated anion gap, an osmol gap and visual symptoms. Based on clinical signs and symptoms, this patient would likely undergo hemodialysis even in the absence of a confirmatory measurement of the methanol concentration in serum. These relationships, the correlation of serious clinical effects with a theophylline level above 90 mg/L (Weisman, 1998) or visual symptoms in a methanol poisoned patient (Ellenhorn, 1997) have come from years of observational study by investigators in the field of clinical toxicology. Early on in the field, the majority of publications were primarily case reports making it difficult to determine the relative effectiveness of various treatments being assessed. The case series or meta-analysis type of scientific analysis was an important step to advance the study of clinical outcomes and assess the quality of treatment provided to poisoned patients. An example of the case series study includes the publication that described the relationship of the QRS interval on the patient's 12-lead ECG to the severity of poisoning by tricyclic antidepressant drugs (Boehnert and Lovejoy, 1985). This important observational study helped to stratify patients poisoned with an overdose of first generation tricyclic antidepressants into risk categories for development of seizures or cardiac arrhythmias. The field now tries to incorporate the prospective, controlled clinical trials, whenever possible which better enables clinicians to validate (or dismiss) new therapeutic modalities and treatment strategies.

Supportive Care of the Poisoned Patient

Once the initial treatment phase in the clinical management of the poisoned patient has been completed, the care of the patient is generally shifted to an inpatient hospital setting for those patients who will require admission. This supportive care phase of poison treatment is very important. Poisoned patients who are unstable or at risk for significant clinical instability are generally admitted to a medical intensive care unit for close monitoring. In addition, patients who are excessively sedated from their poisoning or those who require mechanical ventilation or invasive hemodynamic monitoring are usually candidates for an intensive care stay. Not only are there certain poisonings that have delayed toxicity such as acetaminophen, paraquat and diphenoxylate, but there are also toxins that exhibit multiple phases of toxicity that include delayed effects (i.e., ethylene glycol, salicylate).

Similar to other ill, hospitalized patients, patients admitted for continued treatment of poisoning are at risk for nosocomial infections, iatrogenic fluid and electrolyte disturbances as well as potential harmful effects from the initial therapies that they received for treatment of their poisoning. For example, induction of emesis, gastric lavage or orogastric infusion of activated charcoal can cause aspiration and lead to pneumonitis. Any drug that severely alters a patient's mental status causing obtundation can allow aspiration of gastric contents associated with a loss of the gag reflex. Close clinical monitoring can detect these later phase poisoning complications and allow for prompt medical intervention to minimize patient morbidity and mortality. These are but a few of the reasons that close vigilance is a very important component of the support phase of poison treatment.

Another important component of the supportive care phase of poison treatment is the psychiatric assessment. For intentional self poisonings, a formal psychiatric evaluation of the patient should be performed prior to patient discharge. In many cases, it is not possible to perform a psychiatric interview of the patient during the early phases of treatment and evaluation. Once the patient has been stabilized and is able to communicate, the psychiatric evaluation should be obtained in this setting. Generally a patient who has attempted suicide should be constantly monitored until they have been evaluated by the psychiatric consultant and judged to be "safe" to remove from constant surveillance.

CASE EXAMPLES OF SPECIFIC POISONINGS

Acetaminophen

A thirty-six-year-old male patient comes to the ED and reports taking an "overdose" earlier that day in an attempt to commit suicide. Apparently he was discharged from his job one day prior and had "given up." He reports some abdominal pain approximately and two episodes of emesis 3–4 hours prior to arrival in the ED. Initially he refused to identify what substance he ingested during the suicide attempt. He denied regular or recent use of prescription or over-the-counter medications or dietary supplements as well as regular consumption of alcoholic beverages. No other medical history is available.

On physical examination the vital signs were: blood pressure 138/88, pulse 92/min and regular, respiratory rate 20/min, and temperature 37.2 Celsius. He was awake, alert and oriented and responded to questions appropriately. The remainder of the physical examination was significant for normal bowel sounds, mild epigastric tenderness without guarding or rebound, the rectal examination was normal, the stool was without detectable occult blood. The neurologic examination was within normal limits.

Routine clinical laboratory studies were ordered STAT (electrolytes, creatinine, blood urea nitrogen, glucose, complete blood count with differential, coagulation studies, urine analysis and urine toxicology screen) and a plasma acetaminophen level. Chest and abdominal radiography were normal.

The patient was given 1.5 g/kg oral activated charcoal prepackaged with a sorbitol cathartic. The patient was closely monitored in the ED while the laboratory tests were being performed. Within one hour the laboratory results returned significant for a slight increase in white blood cell count, liver transaminase values were slightly elevated but <3 times the upper limit of normal and an acetaminophen concentration of 290 ug/mL. When confronted with the acetaminophen lab data, the patient admitted ingesting an entire bottle of 500 mg acetaminophen capsules. The estimate of the maximum amount of acetaminophen consumed was 25 g, well above what is considered a highly toxic dosage.

The patient did not recall seeing capsule fragments in the emesis material. He denied taking any other medications or substances with the acetaminophen. Based on the Rumack-Mathew nomogram (Fig. 32-1), a plasma acetaminophen concentration of 290 ug/kg at approximately 6 hours after ingestion is well within the "probable hepatic toxicity" range and therefore treatment with N-acetylcysteine (NAC) was required.

The patient received his first dose of intravenous (IV) NAC in the ED and was admitted to the medical ward to complete the treatment course of NAC. Only mild (<4 times the upper limit of normal) elevation of hepatic transaminases was measured on follow-up assessments. The patient was seen by the Psychiatry Consultation service and judged not to be actively suicidal. He was discharged from the hospital 2 days after admission with scheduled psychiatric and medical follow-up appointments.

Acetaminophen has been used as an analgesic and antipyretic since the mid-1950s and has become more prominently recognized as a potential hepatotoxin in the overdose situation since the original British reports in the late 1960s (Proudfoot and Wright, 1970). Work on the mechanisms of the liver toxicity of this drug has provided a theoretical basis for therapy (Mitchell et al., 1973).

The clinical presentation of patients poisoned with acetaminophen is sufficiently confusing in some cases it is difficult to estimate the time of ingestion. Due to the paucity of clinical symptoms with acute overdose, waiting for the appearance of symptoms is an inadequate strategy for the clinical decision making process regarding institution of treatment.

Acetaminophen in normal individuals is inactivated by sulfation (approximately 52%) and glucuronide conjugation (42%). About 2% of the drug is excreted unchanged. The remaining 4% is biotransformed by the cytochrome P-450 mixed-function oxidase system. The P-450 isozyme responsible for acetaminophen biotransformation is CYP2E1. Metabolism by CYP2E1 results in a potentially toxic metabolite that is normally detoxified by conjugation with glutathione and excreted as the mercapturate. Evidence extrapolated from animals estimates that when 70% of endogenous hepatic glutathione is consumed, the toxic metabolite becomes available for covalent binding to hepatic cellular components. However, patients who are concurrently using, or have recently used, agents that induce CYP2E1, such as in the case of chronic ethanol exposure or phenobarbital use, may produce more than 4% of the toxic metabolite. It is therefore important to determine, whenever possible, whether or not the patient's CYP2E1 system may be induced when determining the risk of hepatic necrosis in any given individual. When there is evidence (medical history) of concurrent agents that induce CYP2E1, the treatment nomogram from acetaminophen should be modified to a lower threshold for treatment with NAC (Rumack et al., 1981).

Follow-up liver biopsy studies of patients who have recovered 3 months to a year after hepatotoxicity have demonstrated no long-term sequelae or chronic toxicity (Clark et al., 1973). A very small percentage (0.25%) of patients in the national multiclinic study conducted in Denver may progress to hepatic encephalopathy with subsequent death. The clinical nature of the overdose is one of a sharp peak of serum glutamic-oxalocaetic transaminase (SGOT) by day 3, with recovery to less than 100 IU/L by day 7 or 8. Patients with SGOT levels as high as 20,000 IU/L have shown complete recovery and no sequelae 1 week after ingestion (Arena *et al.*, 1978).

Laboratory evaluation of a potentially poisoned patient is crucial in terms of both hepatic measures of toxicity and plasma levels of acetaminophen. Accurate estimation of acetaminophen in the plasma should be done on samples drawn at least 4 hours after ingestion, when peak plasma levels can be expected.

Once an accurate plasma level has been obtained, it should be plotted on the Rumack-Matthew nomogram to determine if NAC therapy is indicated (Fig. 32-1). This nomogram is based on a series of patients with and without hepatotoxicity and their corresponding measured plasma acetaminophen concentrations.

Treatment should be instituted in any patient with a plasma concentration in the potentially toxic range. Some clinical toxicologists recommend withholding NAC treatment unless the plasma concentration is at or above the "probably toxic" demarcation but most often the more conservative approach is recommended. Standard support with administration of activated charcoal, or gastric lavage (a seldom used option for very recent acetaminophen ingestions) should be followed by administration of N-acetylcysteine. The protective effect of NAC in oral acetaminophen poisoning was demonstrated when contrasted with controls not receiving antidotal therapy (Rumack *et al.*, 1981; Smilkstein *et al.*, 1988). Because NAC is most effective if it is given within 8–12 hours of acetaminophen ingestion, patients in whom blood levels cannot be obtained should have NAC treatment instituted and therapy terminated only if levels are nontoxic. The dosing regimen for oral NAC is a loading dose of 140 mg/kg orally, followed by 70 mg/kg orally for 17 additional doses (Peterson and Rumack, 1977). The dosage regimen for IV NAC is 150 mg/kg loading dose over 15 minutes, followed by 50 mg/kg over the next 4 hours then 100 mg/kg over 16 hours for a total dose of 300 mg/kg in 20 hours. Anaphylactoid reactions are a significant concern surrounding the use of IV NAC. The decision to use IV instead of oral NAC is not straightforward. Most authors recommend IV NAC for adults without asthma or other contraindications to IV NAC (Howland, 2006). Children can receive IV NAC but the volume required for the dilution can cause electrolyte abnormalities. The potential advantage from using the IV form is that the complete dosage regimen is completed in 20 hours in contrast to the 72 hour oral regimen. Children less than 9–12 years of age have a lower incidence of hepatotoxicity after an overdose than do adults but are still treated with NAC according to the same nomogram. Oral NAC is more frequently given to poisoned pediatric patients. Patients with trivial or "nontoxic" acetaminophen ingestions should not be given NAC therapy because the antidote can produce clinical significant adverse events.

Methanol

A twenty-seven-year-old male was brought to the ED after being found unresponsive in a chemical storage tank at an electrical components manufacturing plant where he worked. The patient was obtunded, responsive to pain and without obvious signs of trauma. At the scene, emergency medical personnel learned that he was last seen entering the 1200 gallon tank with a cleaning solvent 35 minutes prior to a coworker's discovery that he was unconscious. The plant supervisor was not certain as to what the tank had previously con-

tained as it had not been used for approximately 2 years. Coworkers stated that the patient would occasionally talk about drinking some of the chemicals found in the workplace. The emergency medical personnel brought the cleaning solvent container with them to the ED. The solvent listed "methyl alcohol" as its primary active ingredient. All patient clothing was removed, placed in sealed plastic bags and removed from the ED area.

Physical exam was significant for a blood pressure of 105/56, the pulse was 74/min, the respiratory rate was 28/min, and the body temperature 37.0°C. The skin on the patient's distal upper and lower extremities was slightly erythematous. The pupils were 3 mm and reactive to light. The lung and heart examinations were normal. Abdominal examination revealed diminished but present bowel sounds, no tenderness was noted and no organomegaly or masses were detected. The rectal examination was normal; the stool was without detectable occult blood. Neuro exam was nonfocal with a diminished gag reflex.

The patient was placed on a cardiac monitor, an intravenous line was started, clinical laboratory specimens were obtained and he was placed on oxygen, given naloxone, thiamine, and dextrose, intravenously. These four treatments are standard for patients presenting with an altered mental status to an ED. Chest and abdominal radiography was without abnormality. A 12 lead electrocardiogram was also normal. Faced with the uncertainty of oral ingestion versus topical and inhalation exposure a decision was made to proceed with gastric decontamination. Because no direct history from the patient was available, a mixed ingestion could not be ruled out as well. Because of the diminished gag reflex, the patient was endotracheally intubated to protect his airway before an orogastric tube was placed. Gastric lavage was performed and no blood or detectable foreign substances were removed. Activated charcoal (2.0 g/kg) was placed via the orogastric tube into the stomach with a cathartic.

Clinical laboratory results returned showing the following:

Serum Chemistries:

Na = 140 mEq/L	K = 3.0 mEq/L
Cl = 94 mEq/L	HCO_3 = 8 mEq/L
BUN = 12 mg/dl	Glucose = 100 mg/dl

Arterial blood gas (ABG):

pH = 7.20; pCO_2 = 20 mm Hg; pO_2 = 98 mm Hg

The complete blood count was normal, the urine analysis was normal, measured serum osmolarity was 330 mOsm/kg, acetaminophen and salicylate levels were below the limits of detection, and the urine toxicology screen was negative.

The laboratory results were interpreted as follows: a metabolic acidosis with elevated anion gap (AG = 38) and an elevated osmol gap (40 mOsm). These findings are consistent with methanol poisoning as well as ethylene glycol (note cross reference Tables 32-4 and 32-5). A blood sample for measurement of methanol and ethylene glycol was sent for analysis but based on the solvent container; the working diagnosis of methanol poisoning was established. The patient was treated with intravenous (sterile) ethanol infusion while fomepizole (4-methylperazole) was requested from the nearby regional hospital. Sodium bicarbonate was given intravenously for the profound metabolic acidosis and the patient was prepared for hemodialysis. After 4 hours of hemodialysis, his acid-base and electrolyte abnormalities corrected. Approximately 9 hours after the blood specimen was sent, the laboratory reported a "toxic" serum methanol concentration of 67 mg/dL. The patient underwent a second 4-hour course of hemodialysis 8 hours later when his metabolic acidosis recurred. He regained normal consciousness within 12 hours and recovered completely. Subsequently the patient admitted that he spilled the solvent on him after becoming lightheaded in the storage tank and that he drank some of the solvent as well while cleaning the tank. A past medical history of alcoholism was later obtained and a psychiatric consultation recommended inpatient detoxification for what turned out to be an active alcohol dependency problem after he was medically stabilized.

This case demonstrates the importance of utilizing the anion and osmol gap calculations in overdose patients. Although not considered diagnostic (Walker *et al.*, 1986), the presence of both a metabolic acidosis with an anion gap and an osmol gap is highly suggestive of either methanol or ethylene glycol given the patient's presentation despite a scant history. Known access to a methanol containing product clearly made that substance the most likely poison in this case but consideration of alternate substances should always be held open. Initiation of antidote therapy and hemodialysis to increase removal of the poison prior to receipt of the confirmatory laboratory test was also required in this case. It is quite possible that if the clinicians had not instituted therapy until the confirmatory laboratory test (i.e., the methanol level) had returned, the patient may have had a fatal or significantly morbid outcome. It is quite common for hospital clinical laboratories to have to "send out" blood specimens for ethylene glycol and methanol analysis becasuse these are not routinely performed on-site. A turnaround time of 6–12 hours for this test result to be available is not uncommon.

Methanol exerts is primary toxicity after undergoing biotransformation by alcohol dehydrogenase to formaldehyde and then to formic acid by the action of aldehyde dehydrogenase. The formic acid is thought to be responsible for both the ocular (blindness) and the acid-base toxicity of methanol (Swartz *et al.*, 1981). If untreated or treated too late, methanol poisoning can result in fatal cerebral edema with seizures as a preterminal event. Hemodialysis can remove the unmetabolized methanol, eliminating the substrate for production of the toxic metabolite. Administration of an inhibitor or competing substrate for alcohol dehydrogenase can be instituted while transporting the patient to a health care facility where hemodialysis is available. Ethanol (sterile, for intravenous administration) can be given to effectively inhibit the metabolism of methanol and prevent the potentially devastating effects of the poisoning. 4-methylperazole is a commercially available inhibitor of alcohol dehydrogenase that is FDA approved for the treatment of methanol and ethylene glycol poisoning. Finally, the administration of folic acid in animal models has been shown to enhance the in vivo clearance of formate, the toxic metabolite of methanol (McMartin *et al.*, 1977). Folate or folinic acid has been given to methanol poisoned patients and is suggested to hasten formic acid metabolism thereby accelerating its clearance. Many clinical toxicologists will include folic or folinic acid in their therapeutic regimen for methanol poisoned patients.

Tricyclic Antidepressants

An thirty-six-year-old female nurse is brought to the ED by her spouse who tells the desk nurse that she has just taken a drug overdose with a tricyclic antidepressant. The patient was driven to the hospital by her husband and walked into the ED. The patient was immediately taken to the acute or intensive care section of the ED. The husband reports that she took her entire prescription of amitriptyline approximately 40 minutes prior to arrival in the ED in an apparent suicide attempt. The patient denied any other ingestion, which was confirmed by her husband who witnessed the ingestion. The patient's initial vital signs were: blood pressure 125/70, pulse 94/min, respiratory rate 20/min, and temperature 37.2°C. The unit clerk called the patient's pharmacy to confirm a recent prescription of thirty 50 mg tablets of imipramine. Within 15 minutes the patient becomes unresponsive. The vital signs at that time are: blood pressure of 80/55, pulse 135/min, respiratory rate of 8/min and temperature unchanged. Intravenous lines are started, and intravenous fluids are administered as rapidly as possible, the cardiac monitor reveals sinus tachycardia.

The remainder of the physical examination shows the patient to be well dressed without obvious signs of trauma; the skin is warm and dry, without track marks. The pupils are 7 mm and poorly reactive to light. Other significant findings include the examination of the abdomen, which shows markedly diminished bowel sounds. The rectal examination is negative for occult blood. The neurological examination reveals coma without focal motor abnormalities and an absent gag reflex.

Initial laboratories show no significant acid base disturbance, no elevated anion or osmol gaps, normal glucose, liver function tests and renal function tests. The chest and abdominal radiographs are normal. The 12-lead ECG reveals sinus tachycardia, a right axis deviation, 1st degree heart block and a prolonged QRS duration of 125 ms.

A Foley catheter was inserted and 600 ml of urine was obtained. The patient has a generalized seizure lasting approximately 20 seconds. Endotracheal intubation, followed by gastric lavage was performed and only a several pill fragments were seen in the lavage fluid. The patient was placed on a ventilator to support her respiration. Activated charcoal (2.0 g/kg) was administered via the orogastric tube immediately following the lavage procedure. The blood pressure continued to remain low despite intravenous fluid administration. The patient developed intermittent (non-sustained) ventricular tachycardia. Sodium bicarbonate was administered intravenously and an arterial monitor was instituted to closely track the arterial pH. The patient clinically stabilized, with return of normal blood pressure and cardiac rhythm, then transferred to the medical intensive care unit and closely monitored. Alkaline intravenous fluid was continued for 8 hours to maintain the arterial pH at 7.50. MDAC was employed via the gastric tube for approximately 18 hours. The patient regained consciousness and was evaluated by the psychiatry service which recommended transfer to the inpatient psychiatric ward for continued care when medically stable.

Tricyclic antidepressant (TCA) agents can be very deadly in overdose situations. During the 1980s the TCAs were consistently ranked at or near the top of the list of most frequently fatal drug overdose cases reported to the American Association of Poison Control Centers. No diagnostic laboratory tests are available to acutely aid the clinician treating a patient poisoned with a TCA. Clinically, anticholinergic effects appear early. The TCAs are the most deadly cause of the anticholinergic toxic syndrome. The clinical presentation of the TCA overdose is complex, with CNS, cardiovascular, and respiratory components most prominent. Usually, serious toxicity from TCAs appears within 2–3 hours of ingestion. The prognostic value of the QRS duration from the 12-lead ECG was discussed above (Boehnert and Lovejoy, 1985). In this case the prolonged QRS duration predicted the observed systemic toxicity of the reported overdose and specifically, an increased likelihood of seizures.

The TCAs are available in a wide variety of brands, including amitriptyline, doxepin, and imipramine, and also in combination with phenothiazine drugs. TCAs have three primary pharmacological actions: anticholinergic effects, reuptake blockade of catecholamines at the adrenergic neuronal site, and quinidine like (fast sodium channel) effects on cardiac tissue. The latter cardiac effect is responsible for the changes seen in the QRS interval on the ECG. The newer TCAs, such as amoxapine, have a significantly higher incidence of seizures and a lower incidence of cardiac arrhythmia than do the older TCAs. TCA overdose represents a life-threatening episode (Crome, 1986; Frommer *et al.*, 1987). The initial symptoms seen are CNS depression with manifestations of lethargy, disorientation, ataxia, respiratory depression, hypothermia, and agitation. Severe toxicity may be associated with hallucinations, loss of deep tendon reflexes, muscle twitching, coma, and convulsions. The anticholinergic effects of these drugs include dry mouth, hyperpyrexia, dilated pupils, urinary retention, tachycardia, and reduced GI motility, which may result in marked delay of the onset of symptoms. Life-threatening sequelae of the tricyclic antidepressants are the cardiovascular effects, resulting in cardiac arrhythmias such as supraventricular tachycardia, premature ventricular contractions, ventricular tachycardia, ventricular flutter, and ventricular fibrillation that progresses to hypotension and shock. The ECG characteristically demonstrates a prolonged PR interval, widening of the QRS complex, QT prolongation, T-wave flattening or inversion, ST segment depression, and varying degrees of heart block progressing to asystole. Widening of the QRS complex has been reported to correlate well with the severity of the toxicity after acute overdose ingestions (Bigger, 1977). Widening of the QRS complex past 100 ms or greater within the first 24 hours is an indication of severe toxicity (Boehnert and Lovejoy, 1985; Liebelt *et al.*, 1995).

Gastric lavage may be indicated if the oral ingestion was very recent (within one hour), followed by the administration of activated charcoal. Activated charcoal may be beneficial even hours after ingestion due to delayed gastric emptying from the anticholinergic effects of TCA drugs. Patients admitted with TCA overdose but without symptoms should be monitored in the hospital setting for a minimum of 6–8 hours to detect any possible delayed onset of symptoms. Vital signs and the ECG should be monitored in symptomatic patients, as fatal cardiac arrhythmias have occurred late in the course. Hypotension should be treated with fluids and may respond to sodium bicarbonate as well as vasopressors such as dopamine or norepinephrine. Adjustment of blood pH with bicarbonate to pH greater than 7.45, coupled with antiarrhythmia drugs that do not prolong the QRS interval (such as lidocaine) is the primary approach to therapy for cardiac arrhythmias. Seizures may also be responsive to benzodiazepines, barbiturates or propofol.

SUMMARY

The practice of clinical toxicology encompasses the expertise of the specialties of medical toxicology, applied toxicology, and clinical poison information specialists. Basic and clinical science has significantly contributed to the present state of the discipline over the past 50 years. The evolution of the poison control (information) center has paralleled that of the discipline. The incorporation of evidence based, outcome driven practice recommendations has significantly improved the critical evaluation of treatment modalities and methods for poison treatment. Application of a stepwise approach to the poisoned patient as described above is a useful method for the evaluation and treatment of the poisoned patient. A methodically performed, clinical diagnostic approach to a poisoned patient is essential as the important medical history is often absent or unreliable. Skillful use of antidotes is an important component of the practice of Medical Toxicology. Continued research will increase the repertoire of effective treatments for poisoning and ultimately improve patient outcomes.

REFERENCES

Anderson AH: Adsorption power of charcoal in aqueous solution. Experimental studies on the pharmacology of activated charcoal. *Acta Pharm* 2:69–78, 1946.

Anderson AH: The Effect of pH on the adsorption by charcoal from aqueous solutions. Experimental studies on the pharmacology of activated charcoal. *Acta Pharm* 3:199–218, 1947.

Anderson AH: Adsorption from gastro-intestinal contents. Experiemntal studies on the pharmacology of activated charcoal. *Acta Pharm* 4:275–284, 1948.

Arena JM, Rourk MHJ, Sibrack CD: Acetaminophen: Report of an unusual poisoning. *Pediatrics* 61:68–72, 1978.

Beerman R, Nunez D, Wetli C: Radiographic evaluation of the cocaine smuggler. *Gastrointest Radiol* 11:351–354, 1986.

Berg MJ, Berlinger WG, Goldberg MJ, *et al.*: Acceleration of the body clearance of phenobarbital by oral activated charcoal. *N Eng J Med* 307:642–644, 1982.

Bigger JT: Tricyclic antidepressant overdose: Incidence of symptoms. *JAMA* 238:135–138, 1977.

Boehnert MT, Lovejoy FH: Value of the QRS duration versus the serum drug level in predicting seizures and ventricular arrhythmias after an acute overdose of tricyclic antidepressants. *N Eng J Med* 313:474–479,1985.

Bosinski T, Bailie GR, Eisele G: Massive and extended rebound of serum lithium concentrations following hemodialysis in two chronic overdose cases. *Am J Emerg Med* 16:98–100, 1998.

Brown TR, Evans JE, Szabo GK, *et al.*: Studies with stable isotopes II: Phenobarbital pharmacokinetics during monotherapy. *J Clin Pharmacol* 25:51–58, 1985.

Chyka PA: Mutiple-dose activated charcoal enhancement of systematic drug clearance: Summary of studies in animals and human volunteers. *J Toxicol Clin Toxicol* 33:399–405, 1995.

Clark R, Borirakchanyavat V, Davidson AR, *et al.*: Hepatic damage and death from overdose of paracetamol. *Lancet* 1:66, 1973.

Cooney DO: *Activated Charcoal in Medical Applications.* New York: Dekker, 1995.

Crome P: Poisoning due to tricyclic antidepressant overdose. *Med Tox* 1:261–285, 1986.

Cutler RE, Forland SC, Hammond PGSJ, *et al.*: Extracorporeal removal of drugs and poisons by hemodialysis and hemoperfusion. *Annu Rev Pharmacol Toxicol* 27:169–191, 1987.

Dally SL, Garneir R, Bismuth C: Diagnosis of chlorinated hydrocarbon poisoning by x-ray examination. *Br J Ind Med* 44:424–425, 1987.

de Silva HA, Foneska M, Pathmeswaran A, *et al.*: Multiple dose activated charcoal for treatment of yellow oleander poisoning: A single-blind, randomized, placebo controlled trial. *Lancet* 361:1935–1938, 2003.

Done AK: Salicylate intoxication: Significance of measurements of salicylate in blood in cases of acute ingestion. *Pediatrics* 26:800–807, 1960.

Ellenhorn MJ: Alcohols and glycols, in Ellenhorn, MJ (ed): *Ellenhorn's Medical Toxicology, Diagnosis and Treatment of Poisoning,* 2nd edn.Philadelphia: Williams and Wilkins, 1997.

Ellenhorn MJ: *Ellenhorn's Medical Toxicology, Diagnosis and Treatment of Poisoning,* 2nd edn. Philadelphia: Williams and Wilkins, 1997.

Everson GW, Oudjhane K, Young LW, *et al.*: Effectiveness of abdominal radiographs in visualizing chewable iron supplements following overdose. *Am J Emerg Med* 7:459–463, 1989.

Frommer DA, Kulig KW, Marx JA, Rumack B: Tricyclic antidepressant overdose: A review. *JAMA* 257:521–526, 1987.

Goldfrank LR: Chapter 3, in Goldfrank NR, Flomenbaum NE, Lewin NA, *et al.* (eds): *Goldfrank's Toxicologic Emergencies,* 8th edn. New York: The McGraw-Hill Companies, Inc., 2006.

Goulbourne KB, *et al.*: Small-bowel obstruction secondary to activated charcoal and adhesions. *Ann Emerg Med* 24:108–109, 1994.

Greensher J, Mofenson HC, Caraccio TR: Ascendency of the black bottle (activated charcoal). *Ped* 80:949–950, 1987.

Handy CA: Radiopacity of oral non-liquid medications. *Radiology* 98:522–533, 1971.

Heffner JE, Harley RA, Schabel SI: Pulmonary reactions from illicit substance abuse. *Clin Chest Med* 11:151–162, 1990.

Holt LE, Holz PH: The black bottle: A consideration in the role of charcoal in the treatment of poisoning in children. *J Pediatr* 63:306–314, 1963.

Howland MA: Antidotes in depth: N-Acetylcysteine, in Goldfrank LR, Flomenbaum NE, Lewin NA, *et al.* (eds). *Goldfrank's Toxicologic Emergencies,* 8th edn. New York: McGraw-Hill, 2006.

Ilkhanipour K, *et al.*: The comparative efficacy of various multiple-dose activated charcoal regimens. *Am J Emerg Med* 10:298–300, 1992.

Institute of Medicine: *Forging a Poison Prevention and Control System.* Washington D.C.: National Academy Press, 2004.

Jarcho S: Medical numismatic notes VII: Mithridates IV. *Bull NY Cad Med* 48:1059–1064, 1972.

Jones JS, Lagasse J, Zimmerman G: Computed tomographic findings after acute carbon monoxide poisoning. *Am J Emerg Med* 12:448–451, 1994.

King WD, Palmisano PA: Poison control centers: Can their value be measured? *South Med J* 84:722–726, 1991.

Krenzelok EP, McGuigan M, Lheureuz P, The American Academy of Clinical Toxicology, European Association of Poisions Centres and Clinical Toxicologists: Position paper: Ipecac syrup. *J Toxicol Clin Toxicol* 42(2):133–143, 2004.

Liebelt EL, Francis PD, Woolf AD: ECG lead aVR versus QRS in predicting seizures and arrhythmias in acute tricyclic antidepressant toxicity. *Ann Emerg Med* 26:195–201, 1995.

Major RH: History of the stomach tube. *Ann Med Hist* 6:500–509, 1934.

Martin JM, Arena JM: Lye poisoning and stricture of the esophagus: A report of 50 cases. *South Med J* 32:286–290, 1939.

Manoguerra AS, Temple AR: Observations on the current status of poison control centers in the United States. *Emerg Med Clin North Am* 2:185–197, 1984.

McCarron MM, Wood JD: The cocaine "body packer" syndrome. *JAMA* 250:1417–1420, 1983.

McElvaine MD, DeUngria EG, Matte TD, *et al.*: Prevalence of radiographic evidence of paint chip ingestion among children with moderate to severe lead poisoning, St. Louis, Missouri, 1989 through 1990. *Pediatrics* 89:740–742, 1992.

McMartin KE, Martin-Amat G, Makar AT, *et al.*: Methanol poisoning V: Role of formate metabolism in the monkey. *J Pharmacol Exp Ther* 201:564–572, 1977.

Miller TR, Lestina DC: Costs of poisoning in the united states and savings from poison control centers: A benefit-cost analysis. *Ann Emerg Med* 29(2):239–245, 1997.

Mitchell JR, Jollow DJ, Potter WZ, *et al.*: Acetaminophen induced hepatic necrosis. *J Pharmacol Exp Ther* 187:185–194, 1973.

Miura T, Mitomo M, Kawai R, Harada K: CT of the brain in acute carbon monoxide intoxication: Characteristic features and prognosis. *AJNR* 6:739–742, 1985.

Mofenson HC, Caraccio TR, Greensher J, D'Agustino R, Rossi A: Gastrointestinal dialysis with activated charcoal and cathartic in the treatment of adolescent intoxications. *Clin Pediatrics* 24:678–684, 1985.

Mokrzycki MH, Kaplan AA: Therapeutic plasma exhange: Complications and management. *Am J Kidney Dis* 23:817–827, 1994.

Nelson JC, Liu D, Olson KR: Radiopacity of modified release medications. *Vet Hum Toxicol* 35:317, 1993.

Neuvonen P, Vartiainen M, Tokola O: Comparison of activated charcoal and ipecac syrup in prevention of drug absorption. *Eur J Clin Pharmacol* 24:557–562, 1983.

O'Brien RP, McGeehan PA, Helmeczi AW, *et al.*: Detectability of drug tablets and capsules by plain radiography. *Am J Emerg Med* 4:302–312, 1986.

Ohning BL, *et al.*: Continuous nasogastric administration of activated charcoal for the treatment of theophylline intoxication. *Pediatr Pharm* 5:241–245, 1986.

Park GD, Radomski L, Goldberg MJ, *et al.*: Effects of size and frequency of oral doses of charcoal on theophylline clearance. *Clin Pharm Ther* 34:663–666, 1983.

Peterson RG, Rumack BH: Treatment of acute acetaminophen poisoning with acetylcysteine. *JAMA* 237:2406–2407, 1977.

Plaitakis A, Duvoisin RC: Homer's moly identified as galanthus nivalis: Physiologic antidote to stramonium poisoning. *Clin Neuropharmacol* 6:1–5, 1983.

Pollack MM, *et al.*: Aspiration of activated charcoal and gastric contents. *Ann Emerg Med* 10:528–529, 1981.

Proudfoot AT, Wright N: Acute paracetamol poisoning. *Br Med J* 2:557, 1970.

Proudfoot AT, Krenzelok EP, Vale JA: Position paper on urine alkalinization. *J Toxicol Clin Toxicol* 42:1–26, 2004.

Reid DHS: Treatment of the poisoned child. *Arch Dis Child* 45:428–433, 1970.

Rumack BH, Matthew H: Acetaminophen poisoning and toxicity. *Pediatrics* 55:871, 1975.

Rumack BH, Peterson RC, Koch GG, *et al.*: Acetaminophen overdose: 662 cases with evaluation of oral acetylcysteine treatment. *Arch Intern Med* 141:380–385, 1981.

Savitt DL, Hawkins HH, Roberts JR: The radiopacity of ingested medications. *Ann Emerg Med* 16:331–339, 1987.

Scherz RG, Robertson WO: The history of poison control centers in the United States. *Clin Toxicol* 12(3):291–296, 1978.

Smilkstein MJ, Knapp GL, Kulig KW, *et al.*: Efficacy of oral N-acetylcysteine in the treatment of acetaminophen overdose. *N Engl J Med* 319:1557–1562, 1988.

Smithline N, Gardner KD: Gaps: Anionic and osmolal. *JAMA* 236:1594–1597, 1976.

Sporer KA, Firestone J: Clinical Course of crack cocaine body stuffers. *Ann Emerg Med* 29:596–601, 1997.

Stern WZ, Spear PW, Jacobson HG: The roentgen findings in acute heroin intoxication. *AJR* 103:522–532, 1968.

Swartz RD, Millman RP, Billi JE, *et al.*: Epidemic methanol poisoing: Clinical and biochemical analysis of a recent episode. *Medicine* 60:373–382, 1981.

Tenebein M, Lheureuz P, The American Academy of Clinical Toxicology, European Association of Poisions Centres and Clinical Toxicologists: Position Paper: Whole Bowel Irrigation. *J Toxicol Clin Toxicol* 42(6):843–854, 2004.

Van de Graaff WB, Thompson WL, Sunshine I, *et al.*: Adsorbent and cathartic inhibition of enteral drug absorption. *J Pharmacol Exp Ther* 221:656–663, 1982.

Walker JA, Schwartzbard A, Krauss EA, *et al.*: The missing gap: A pitfall in the diagnosis of alcohol intoxication by osmometry. *Arch Intern Med* 146:1843–1844, 1986.

Wax PM: Analeptic use in clinical toxicology: A historical appraisal. *Clin Toxicol* 35:203–209, 1997.

Weisman RS: Theophylline, in Goldfrank (ed.): *Goldfrank's Toxicologic Emergencies,* 6th edn. Stanford, Connecticut: Appleton and Lange, 1998.

CHAPTER 33

OCCUPATIONAL TOXICOLOGY

Peter S. Thorne

INTRODUCTION

For centuries the work environment has played a significant role in the occurrence of adverse human health effects due to chemical and biological hazards. Early writings by Agricola (1494–1555) and Paracelsus (1492–1541) revealed the toxic nature of exposures in mining, smelting, and metallurgy. A systematic treatise by Ramazzini (1633–1714) described the hazards as they applied to miners, chemists, metal workers, tanners, pharmacists, grain sifters, stonecutters, sewage workers, and even corpse bearers. Today we continue to be concerned with occupational health and safety in these and other work environments. Although occupational settings are safer now than in the past, the levels of risk deemed acceptable have decreased while the recognition of the causal link of exposures to chronic diseases or diseases with long latencies has increased. As new hazards arise with the emergence of new technologies, we must be prepared to assess the risks and protect the health of workers.

Occupational toxicology is the application of the principles and methodology of toxicology toward understanding and managing chemical and biological hazards encountered at work. The objective of the occupational toxicologist is to prevent adverse health effects in workers that arise from exposures in their work environment. Because nonoccupational exposures can act as confounders or can increase the susceptibility of individual workers, occupational toxicologists must evaluate the entire spectrum of exposures experienced by the work force under consideration. Occupational toxicology is a discipline that draws on occupational hygiene, epidemiology, occupational medicine, and regulatory toxicology. The occupational toxicologist must have an intimate knowledge of the work environment and be able to recognize and prioritize exposure hazards. Because the work environment can present exposures to complex mixtures, the occupational toxicologist must also recognize those that are particularly hazardous when occurring in combination.

It is often difficult to establish a causal link between a worker's illness and job. First, the clinical expressions of occupationally induced diseases are often indistinguishable from those arising from nonoccupational causes. Second, there may be a protracted but biologically predictable latent interval between exposure and the expression of disease. Third, diseases of occupational origin may be multifactorial with personal or other environmental factors contributing to the disease process. Nevertheless, studies have repeatedly shown that the dose of toxicant is a strong predictor of the likelihood, severity, and type of health effect.

WORKPLACES, EXPOSURES, AND STANDARDS

The Nature of the Work Force

The demographics and distribution of the work force in industrialized nations has undergone a progressive shift over the past three decades, moving away from jobs in heavy industry and toward jobs in the service sector and high-technology industries. In some instances, these manufacturing jobs have moved to less developed countries with less stringent worker health protection. There are currently 144.9 million people in the United States in the civilian, paid work force (seasonally adjusted data). The civilian labor force participation rate is 66.2% (USDL, 2006b), a figure that has grown steadily over the past 50 years owing to the increased entry of women into the labor force (Fullerton, 1999). The 25 countries of the EU have an estimated 201.7 million workers (Employment in Europe, 2006), and Japan has about 66.4 million (Japan Statistical Yearbook, 2006). Table 33-1 shows the breakdown of employment in the United States. This illustrates that there are about 24.6 million workers (17%) engaged in manufacturing, construction, natural resources and mining, and agriculture—occupations that have the potential for significant exposure to chemical and biological agents. Furthermore, there are occupations in the service sector, such as

Table 33-1

The U.S. Seasonally Adjusted Civilian Labor Market

SECTOR	NUMBER EMPLOYED	AVERAGE WORK WEEK, HOURS
Nonfarm*	135,613,000	
Goods-producing	22,427,000	40.3
Manufacturing	14,210,000	45.4
Construction	7,535,000	38.4
Natural resources and mining	682,000	45.1
Service-providing	113,185,600	33.5
Retail trade	15,196,700	30.4
Wholesale trade	5,865,600	38.0
Transportation, warehousing, utilities	4,997,300	37.3
Information	3,058,000	36.9
Finance, insurance, real estate	8,347,000	35.7
Professional and business services	17,413,000	34.4
Education and health services	17,817,000	32.5
Leisure and hospitality services	13,092,000	25.6
Other services	5,411,000	30.7
Government	21,988,000	N.A.[†]
Farm[‡]	2,143,000	42.2[§]
Self-employed	932,000	43.3[§]
Wage and salary workers	1,196,000	40.6[§]
Unpaid family workers[¶]	13,000	36.2[§]
Total[‡]	144,900,000	—

*SOURCE: Current Employment Statistics Survey (Establishment Survey), U.S. Bureau of Labor Statistics. Data as of September 2006.

[†] Not available but has averaged ~38 h in earlier surveys.

[‡] SOURCE: Current Population Survey (Household Survey), U.S. Bureau of Labor Statistics. Data as of September 2006.

[§] Data from 1998.

[¶] Data so marked are not seasonally adjusted.

automobile repair; other repair and maintenance; work in gasoline stations, pipeline transportation, truck and rail transportation; waste management and remediation services; and employment in botanical gardens that can also include exposures to hazardous chemicals. Service-producing occupations account for the majority (83.5%) of U.S. nonfarm jobs. On average, employees in the service sector work 6.8 fewer hours per week than in the goods-producing sector. Farm work employs an estimated 2.14 million workers 16 years of age and older, and the U.S. Bureau of Labor Statistics has documented an average of 42.2 hours worked per week. Work in agriculture is markedly different from most other occupations in four fundamental ways. First, 44% of those employed in agriculture are self-employed or unpaid family members. Second, the overwhelming majority of farm establishments (90%) have fewer than 20 employees and these work sites represent 35% of the agricultural work force (USDL, 2006a). Third, although the annual national average hours worked per week is slightly over 42, many farmers, ranchers, and farm workers have periods when they work as many as 20 hours per day, 7 days per week. Fourth, according to the U.S. Bureau of the Census there are in excess of 290,000 children who identify agricultural work as their major employment (GAO/HEHS, 1998). Department of Labor data indicate that, on average, 128,500 hired farm workers between the ages of 14 and 17 were working annually in crop production (GAO/HEHS, 1998). The presence of children in the work force has important ramifications for body burdens, disease latency, toxicokinetics, and biotransformation of toxicants.

Determinants of Dose

Dose is defined as the amount of toxicant that reaches the target tissue over a defined time span. In occupational environments, *exposure* is often used as a surrogate for *dose*. The response to a chemical is dependent upon both host factors and dose. Figure 33-1 illustrates the pathway from exposure to subclinical disease or to adverse health effect and suggests that there are important modifying factors: contemporaneous exposures, genetic susceptibility, age, gender, nutritional status, and behavioral factors. These modifying factors can influence whether a worker remains healthy, develops subclinical disease that is repaired, or progresses to illness. Workplace health protection and surveillance programs (shown in blue) can reduce exposures, disrupt the exposure-dose pathway, or identify internalized dose and early effects before irreparable disease develops. These programs help to ensure a safe workplace and a healthy work force.

As illustrated in Fig. 33-1, dose is a function of exposure concentration, exposure duration, and exposure frequency. Individual and environmental characteristics can also affect dose. Exposure assessment is the process of quantifying the intensity, frequency, and duration of exposures and their determinants in order to better estimate dose. Table 33-2 indicates determinants of dose for exposure via the inhalation and dermal routes. For determining inhalation exposures, environmental conditions such as concentration, particle size distribution, and properties of the chemical are important. However, respiratory rate and breathing volume as well as other

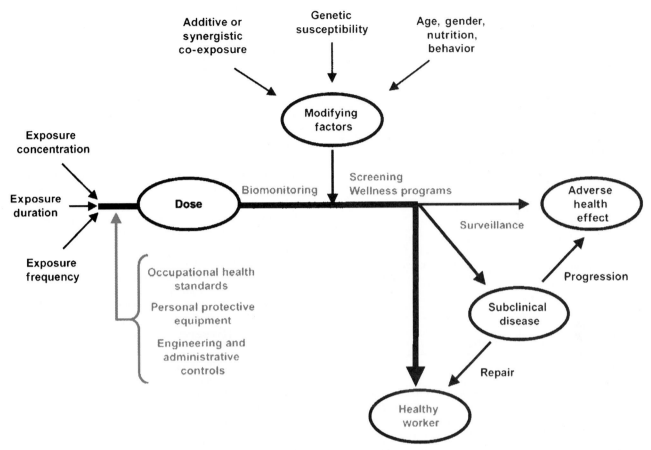

Figure 33-1. *Pathway from exposure to disease, showing modifying factors and opportunities for intervention.*

host factors contribute. Protection afforded by personal protective equipment (especially respirators) will reduce but not eliminate exposure. The degree of exposure reduction for a particular respirator (the workplace protection factor) varies with respirator design, fit, maintenance, manner of use, and environmental conditions from less than 5 to 10,000. Thus, for a respirator with a workplace protection factor of 10, when used properly, particulate matter concentrations inside the mask will be one-tenth that outside the mask. A commonly used two-strap fiber respirator for lowering particulate matter exposure, the N95, should reduce exposures by 95% but may fail to meet this criterion for submicron aerosols (Balazy *et al.*, 2006).

Dermal exposures depend upon toxicant concentration; work conditions, including the degree and duration of wetness; and the ambient conditions at the work site (Table 33-2). Some determinants of dermal dosing relate to the physicochemical properties of the chemical as they affect the percutaneous absorption rate. These include solubility, temperature, pH, molecular size, and chemical characteristics of the vehicle. Host factors also influence dermal absorption and distribution. Important factors include the surface area of the skin that is exposed, the integrity of the skin, blood flow, and biotransformation. Because the stratum corneum, the outer layer of the epidermis, is the principal barrier to dermal uptake, the thickness of this layer in the exposed area has great significance. As an example, the absorption of hydrocortisone through the plantar foot arch is 1/25 less than through the back and 1/300 less than through scrotal skin (Bason *et al.*, 1991). The use of protective gloves and clothing or aprons and the application of barrier creams can greatly reduce

exposure. For maximal protection, it is important that the glove be constructed of material tailored to the toxicant(s) of concern.

Occupational Exposure Limits

One of the roles of the occupational toxicologist is to contribute data to the process of establishing standards or determining the appropriateness of those standards. Workplace exposure limits exist for chemical, biological, and physical agents and are recommended as guidelines or promulgated as standards in order to promote worker health and safety. For chemical and biological agents, exposure limits are expressed as acceptable ambient concentration levels (occupational exposure limits) or as concentrations of a toxicant, its metabolites, or a specific marker of its effects in biological systems (biological exposure indices).

Occupational exposure limits (OELs) are established as standards by regulatory agencies or as guidelines by research groups or trade organizations. In the United States, the Occupational Safety and Health Administration (OSHA) under the Department of Labor promulgates legally enforceable standards known as permissible exposure limits (PELs). These standards are determined and supported by the best scientific evidence available and assure "to the extent feasible. . . that no employee will suffer material impairment of health or functional capacity" with regular exposure "for the period of his working life." OSHA has defined an 8-hour time-weighted average (TWA) PEL (Federal Register, 1992) as the "employee's average airborne exposure in any 8-hour work shift of a 40-hour

Table 33-2
Determinants of Toxicant Dose

Inhalation exposure
   Airborne concentration
   Particle size distribution
   Respiratory rate
   Tidal volume
   Other host factors
   Duration of exposure
   Chemical, physical, or biological properties of the hazardous
      agent
   Effectiveness of personal protective devices
Dermal exposure
   Concentration in air, droplets, or solutions
   Degree and duration of wetness
   Integrity of skin
   Percutaneous absorption rate
   Region of skin exposed
   Surface area exposed
   Preexisting skin disease
   Temperature in the workplace
   Vehicle for the toxicant
   Presence of other chemicals on skin

work week which shall not be exceeded." The TWA PEL is established as the highest level of exposure to which an employee may be exposed without incurring the risk of adverse health effects (OSHA, 1995). Although approximately 500 PELs have been promulgated, there are not enough to regulate exposures to the vast number of compounds to which workers are exposed, and some of the existing PELs do not reflect current knowledge.

The National Institute for Occupational Safety and Health (NIOSH), under the Centers for Disease Control and Prevention, publishes recommended exposure limits (RELs) that are more frequently updated and are generally more stringent than PELs. NIOSH also performs research and disseminates information on workplace hazards and their prevention. Most developed countries have governmental inspectorate agencies analogous to OSHA that are responsible for establishing and enforcing OELs. In some countries, the insurance system also plays a significant role.

The European Commission has established legally enforceable binding occupational exposure limit values (BOELV) and biological limit values (BLV) for the protection of health and safety in the workplace. Socioeconomic and technical feasibility factors are also considered in setting these values. The OELs are established based on recommendations of the Scientific Committee on Occupational Exposure Limits (SCOEL), which evaluates published scientific data on hazardous compounds for regulation and provides assessment of exposure limits that "it believes will protect workers from chemical risks"(European Commission, 1995; European Commission, 1998). EU member countries may not promulgate OELs less stringent than these values.

The American Conference of Governmental Industrial Hygienists (ACGIH) is a trade organization that publishes OELs for chemicals and for physical agents. These take the form of threshold limit values (TLVs) and biological exposure indices (BEIs). They are frequently revisited and generally reflect current knowledge in occupational toxicology and industrial hygiene. They are developed as guidelines and are not enforceable standards; however, many industries adopt TLVs and BEIs as internal OELs. As stated by the ACGIH, "The TLVs and BEIs represent conditions under which ACGIH believes that nearly all workers may be repeatedly exposed without adverse health effects." (ACGIH, 2006 TLV and BEI Book).

Three types of TLVs are suggested, depending on the time scale of adverse effects inducible by the toxicants. The time-weighted average TLV (TLV-TWA) is an OEL for exposures averaged over an 8-hour day, 5-day work week regimen. These are generally applied to toxicants that exert their effects over long periods. The short-term exposure limit (TLV-STEL) is an OEL for a 15-minute measurement period. The TLV-STEL should not be exceeded in any 15-minute sampling window and there should be 60 minutes or more between exposures in this range. The ceiling limit (TLV-C) represents a concentration that should never be exceeded. These are usually applied to toxicants that cause acute effects (such as asphyxia or potent sensory irritation) and for which real-time monitoring devices are available. BEIs are guidelines for biological monitoring and represent levels "most likely to be observed in specimens collected from healthy workers who have been exposed to chemicals to the same extent as workers with inhalation exposure at the Threshold Limit Value" (ACGIH, 2006). BEIs are recommended for analysis of urine, blood, and exhaled air. While hair, fingernails, and other specimens are used in research and forensic toxicology, there are no BEIs for these.

It is important to recognize that OELs do not correspond to exposure conditions devoid of health risk. The concept of acceptable exposure level must be understood as the level of exposure below which the probability of impairing the health of the exposed workers is acceptable. The process of deciding what is an acceptable risk to occupational or environmental hazards blends the scientific disciplines of exposure assessment and toxicology with often vexing policy issues. Historically, acceptable risk in a society is related to the general health of the population and to a host of factors that influence how risks are perceived. To determine that the risks from an occupational hazard are acceptable, it is necessary to characterize the hazard, identify the potential diseases or adverse outcomes, and establish the relationship between exposure intensity or dose and the adverse health effects. If biological markers of exposure or early reversible effects are identified, this can aid in the risk-assessment process.

OCCUPATIONAL DISEASES

Routes of Exposure

Diseases arising in occupational environments involve exposure primarily through inhalation, ingestion, or dermal absorption. In the vast majority of work environments, inhalation of toxicants is a primary concern. Inhalation exposures can occur with gases, vapors, liquid aerosols, particulate aerosols, fumes, and mixtures of these. Dermal exposures are also important and can arise from airborne materials as well as liquids splashed onto the skin, immersion exposures, or from material handling.

Additional exposure hazards exist for infectious agents. Exposures leading to occupational infections may arise through inhalation or ingestion of microorganisms but can also arise from needlesticks in health-care workers or through insect bites among farmers, natural resource workers, and others employed out of doors. Additionally, poisonings from toxic plants or venomous animals can occur through skin inoculation (e.g. zookeepers, horticulturists, or commercial divers).

Table 33-3
Examples of Occupational Diseases and the Toxicants That Cause Them

ORGAN SYSTEM OR DISEASE GROUP	DISEASE	CAUSATIVE AGENT
Lung and airways	Acute pulmonary edema, bronchiolitis obliterans	Nitrogen oxides, phosgene
Allergic rhinitis		Pollens, fungal spores
	Asphyxiation	Carbon monoxide, hydrogen cyanide, inert gas dilution
	Asthma	Toluene diisocyanate, α-amylase, animal urine proteins
	Asthma-like syndrome	Swine barn environments, cotton dust, bioaerosols
	Bronchitis, pneumonitis	Arsenic, chlorine
	Chronic bronchitis	Cotton dust, grain dust, welding fumes
	Emphysema	Coal dust, cigarette smoke
	Fibrotic lung disease	Silica, asbestos
	Hypersensitivity pneumonitis	Thermophilic bacteria, avian proteins, pyrethrum, *Penicillium, Aspergillus*
	Metal fume fever	Zinc, copper, magnesium
	Mucous membrane irritation	Hydrogen chloride, swine barn environments
	Organic dust toxic syndrome	"Moldy" silage, endotoxin
	Upper respiratory tract inflammation	Endotoxin, peptidoglycan, glucans, viruses
Cancer	Acute myelogenous leukemia	Benzene, ethylene oxide
	Bladder cancer	Benzidine, 2-naphthylamine, 4-biphenylamine
	Gastrointestinal cancers	Asbestos
	Hepatic hemangiosarcoma	Vinyl chloride
	Hepatocellular carcinoma	Aflatoxin, hepatitis B virus
	Mesothelioma, lung carcinoma	Asbestos, arsenic, radon, bis-chloro methyl ether
	Skin cancer	Polycyclic aromatic hydrocarbons, ultraviolet irradiation
Skin	Allergic contact dermatitis	Natural rubber latex, isothiazolins, poison ivy, nickel
	Chemical burns	Sodium hydroxide, hydrogen fluoride
	Chloracne	TCDD[†], polychlorinated biphenyls
	Irritant dermatitis	Sodium dodecyl sulfate
Nervous system	Cholinesterase inhibition	Organophosphate insecticides
	Neuronopathy	Methyl mercury
	Parkinsonism	Carbon monoxide, carbon disulfide
	Peripheral neuropathy	N-hexane, trichloroethylene, acrylamide
Immune system	Autoimmune disease	Vinyl chloride, silica
	Hypersensitivity	See entries for allergic rhinitis, asthma, hypersensitivity pneumonitis, allergic contact dermatitis
	Immunosuppression	TCDD[†], lead, mercury, pesticides
Renal disease	Indirect renal failure	Arsine, phosphine, trinitrophenol
	Nephropathy	Paraquat, 1,4-dichlorobenzene, mercuric chloride
Cardiovascular disease	Arrhythmias	Acetone, toluene, methylene chloride, trichloroethylene
	Atherosclerosis	Dinitrotoluene, carbon monoxide
	Coronary artery disease	Carbon disulfide
	Cor pulmonale	Beryllium
	Systemic hypotension	Nitroglycerine, ethylene glycol dinitrate
Liver disease	Fatty liver (steatosis)	Carbon tetrachloride, toluene
	Cirrhosis	Arsenic, trichloroethylene
	Hepatocellular death	dimethylformamide, TCDD[†]
Reproductive system	Male	Chlordecone (Kepone), dibromochloropropane, hexane
	Female	Aniline, styrene
	Both sexes	Carbon disulfide, lead, vinyl chloride

(Continued.)

Agents Associated with Diseases

There are a myriad of agents responsible for occupational diseases. While some act on a particular organ such as the liver or kidney, others can affect multiple organ systems. Table 33-3 presents a list of the major occupational diseases and examples of agents that cause them. This is not intended to be all-inclusive. Rather it is meant to highlight what are historically the most prevalent and widely recognized occupational diseases plus those that continue to be prevalent in the workplace. The toxicants listed are those for which there is

Table 33-3
Examples of Occupational Diseases and the Toxicants That Cause Them

ORGAN SYSTEM OR DISEASE GROUP	DISEASE	CAUSATIVE AGENT
Infectious diseases*	Arboviral encephalitides	Alphavirus, Bunyavirus, Flavivirus
	Aspergillosis	*Aspergillus niger, A. fumigatus, A. flavus*
	Cryptosporidiosis	*Cryptosporidium parvum*
	Hepatitis B	Hepatitis B virus
	Histoplasmosis	*Histoplasma capsulatum*
	Legionellosis	*Legionella pneumophila*
	Lyme disease	*Borrelia burgdorferi*
	Psittacosis	*Chlamydia psittaci*
	Tuberculosis	*Mycobacterium tuberculosis hominis*

*For more on occupational infectious diseases, see Douwes *et al.*, 2003.
†TCDD = 2,3,7,8-tetrachlorodibenzo-*para*-dioxin.

a strong association with the disease or the most conclusive data to support causality. Examples are shown for cancer and for diseases of the lung and airways, heart, liver, kidney, skin, nervous system, immune system, and reproductive system. Several examples of occupational infectious diseases are also listed to highlight the fact that, in many work settings, infectious agents may constitute the major hazard and may coexist with chemical hazards. Most of the occupational diseases listed in Table 33-3 are associated with industrial chemicals. These are discussed in other chapters throughout this book.

Table 33-4 lists the agents that are known by the International Agency for Research on Cancer (IARC) to be carcinogens in humans (Group 1) and for which there is extensive occupational exposure. This list includes agents such as asbestos, arsenic, benzene, vinyl chloride, and coal tars. IARC Group 1 refers to agents or mixtures that are known to be carcinogenic to humans based on sufficient epidemiologic evidence usually accompanied by limited or sufficient animal evidence.

Occupational Respiratory Diseases

Because inhalation generally represents the most significant route of exposure, many of the major occupational diseases affect the lung and airways. These diseases have been studied extensively and are largely responsible for the creation of the occupational regulatory framework. Deaths due to occupational lung diseases such as coal workers' pneumoconiosis, silicosis, asbestosis, byssinosis, and occupational asthma led to important legislation such as the U.S. Occupational Safety and Health Act (1970). These occupational lung diseases continue to have significant associations with morbidity. Table 33-5 lists the crude U.S. death rate and annual deaths and illustrates that while the death rates are fairly low, there are still about 2780 deaths per year attributable to asbestos, silica, coal dust, and other pneumoconiotic dusts; 2485 malignant mesothelioma deaths; and 57 deaths from hypersensitivity pneumonitis. However, fatalities are just the tip of the iceberg as some resulting diseases are rarely fatal yet may still be debilitating. Every year in the U.S., there are 20,000 hospital discharges related to cases of asbestosis and 188,000 coal workers receive federal Black Lung benefits (NIOSH, 2006). The U.S. Mine Safety and Health Administration has compiled data on inspector- and mine operator-collected samples in coal mining operations and found that 29.3% of these exceeded the PEL for

respirable quartz and 7.5% were over the PEL for respirable coal dust.

Many of the diseases listed in Table 33-3 are known by other names that refer to a particular occupation or agent. One example is hypersensitivity pneumonitis, an allergic lung disease marked by interstitial lymphocytic pneumonitis and granulomatous lesions. Hypersensitivity pneumonitis is also known as extrinsic allergic alveolitis, farmer's lung disease, bagassosis (sugar cane), humidifier fever, Japanese summer house fever, pigeon breeder's lung, and maple bark stripper's lung, depending upon the occupational setting in which it arises. Although we often think of these as the same disease, it is important to recognize that the exposures and physiologic responses they induce are complex and may differ in the manifestation of the disease.

The U.S. Bureau of Labor Statistics tracks data for respiratory conditions arising from exposure to toxic agents and dust diseases of the lung. The former category includes pneumonitis, pharyngitis, rhinitis, and acute lung congestion. Table 33-6 shows data for rates and cases in 2001 by industry division. These data indicate 14,500 cases per year of respiratory conditions attributed to toxic agents and 1300 dust diseases of the lung. These represent a decrease of 10,000 cases per year since 1995. The manufacturing and services industries contributed 69% of the toxic agent exposure cases. Ten manufacturing industries exceed a nonfatal incidence rate of 10 per 10,000 full-time workers for this type of exposure. These are: secondary nonferrous metals; metal plating and polishing; engine electrical equipment; ship building and repairing; motorcycles, bicycles and parts; laboratory apparatus and furniture; photographic equipment and supplies; chocolate and cocoa products; weft knit fabric mills; and plastic bottle manufacturing. The two other industries that exceed 10 per 10,000 are public water supply utilities and recreational vehicle dealers.

Toxic gas injuries are often characterized by leakage of both fluid and osmotically active proteins from the vascular tissue into the interstitium and airways. Important determinants of the severity and location of injury are the concentration and water solubility of the toxic gas or vapor. Anhydrous ammonia, with its extremely high solubility, primarily damages the eyes, sinuses, and upper airways. The vapors combine with water in the tissue and form ammonium hydroxide, quickly producing liquefaction necrosis. Chemicals with lower solubility, such as nitrogen dioxide, act more on the distal airways and alveoli and take longer to induce tissue damage.

Table 33-4

Occupational Exposure Agents Classified by IARC as Definite Human Carcinogens

AGENT	INDUSTRIES AND OCCUPATIONS WHERE SOME WORKERS MAY BE EXPOSED
Particulate matter	
Asbestos	Miners, abatement workers, construction workers, sheet metal workers, steam fitters, shipyard workers
Crystalline silica	Stone and ceramics industry, foundries, construction, abrasives manufacturing
Talc containing asbestiform fibers	Ceramics industry
Erionite	Waste treatment workers, building materials manufacturing
Wood dust	Wood and wood-products industries, pulp and paper industry, wood working trades
Metals	
Arsenic and arsenic compounds	Miners, nonferrous metal smelting, arsenical pesticide manufacturers and applicators
Beryllium	Specialty metallurgy workers, avionics, electronics, nuclear industry
Cadmium and cadmium compounds	Cadmium smelting, battery production, dyes and pigment making, electroplating
Hexavalent chromium compounds	Chromate production plants, dye and pigment making, welders, tanners,
Nickel compounds*	Nickel smelting, welding
Organic chemicals	
Benzene	Refineries, shoe industry, chemical, pharmaceutical and rubber industry, printing industry
Coal tars and pitches	Coke production, coal gasification, refineries, foundries, road paving, hot tar roofing
Mineral oils, untreated and mildly treated	Metal machining and honing, roll steel production, printing
Shale oils or shale-derived lubricants	Mining and processing, cotton textile industry
Soots	Chimney sweeps, heating and ventilation contractors, firefighters, metallurgical workers
Vinyl chloride	Plastics industry, production of polyvinyl chloride products and copolymers
Bis(chloromethyl) ether and Chloromethyl ether (technical grade)	Chemical industry, laboratory reagent, plastic manufacturing
4-Aminobiphenyl	Chemical industry, dyestuffs and pigment manufacturing
Benzidine	Chemical industry, dyestuffs and pigment manufacturing
2-Naphthylamine	Chemical industry, dyestuffs and pigment manufacturing
Ethylene oxide	Chemical industry, dry vegetable fumigation, hospital sterilizing
2,3,7,8-Tetrachlorobibenzo-*para*-dioxin (TCDD)	Hazardous waste processing, chlorophenoxy herbicide production and use, pulp and paper industry
Aflatoxin	Animal feed industry, grain handling and processing
Other agents with occupational exposure	
Environmental tobacco smoke	Restaurant, bar and entertainment industry; other smoke-exposed workers
Mustard gas	Production, soldiers, some research laboratories
Strong inorganic acid mists containing sulfuric acid	Steel industry, petrochemical industry, fertilizer industry, pickling industry
Physical Agents	
Ionizing radiation[†]	Radiology and nuclear medicine staff, nuclear workers, miners, hazardous waste workers
Solar radiation	Farmers, gardeners and landscapers, lifeguards, construction workers

*Certain combinations of nickel oxides and sulfides.

[†]Includes x-rays, γ-rays, neutrons and radon gas.

SOURCE: Siemiatycki *et al. Environ Health Perspect* 112:1447–1459, 2004.

Occupational asthma may be defined as a "disease characterized by variable airflow limitation and/or airway hyperresponsiveness and/or inflammation due to causes and conditions attributable to a particular occupational environment and not to stimuli encountered outside the workplace" (Bernstein IL *et al.*, 2006). The U.S. National Health Interview Survey has provided data on the prevalence of asthma based upon usual industry and smoking status (Table 33-7). These data indicate that asthma prevalence is highest in general merchandise stores; food, bakery, and dairy stores; furniture, lumber and wood products industries; trucking and ware-

housing; health services; and the primary metals industry. Interestingly, in some industries current smokers demonstrate the higher prevalence while in other industries the higher prevalence is seen among nonsmokers. This may reflect that many people diagnosed with these conditions quit smoking.

There are a variety of industries in which there is increased risk of developing work-related asthma. In chemical-based industries, plastic and rubber polymer precursors, diisocyanates, reactive dyes, and acid anhydrides are recognized low-molecular-weight sensitizing compounds. Biocides and fungicides used in metal fabrication

Table 33-5

U.S. Deaths and Crude Death Rates Attributed to Selected Occupational Lung Diseases

DISEASE	NUMBER OF DEATHS	DEATH RATE PER MILLION WORKING AGE PEOPLE
Asbestosis	1265	6.0
Coal workers pneumoconiosis	1003	4.7
Silicosis	187	0.9
Byssinosis	7	0.03
Other pneumoconioses*	318	1.5
Malignant Mesothelioma	2485	11.7
Hypersensitivity pneumonitis	57	0.3

*This includes aluminosis, berylliosis, stannosis, siderosis, and fibrosis from bauxite, graphite fibers, wollastonite, cadmium, portland cement, emery, kaolin, antimony, and mica.
SOURCE: NIOSH Worker Health Chartbook 2004, U.S. Bureau of Labor Statistics.

and machining, custodial services, lawn and turf growing, and agriculture are also chemicals associated with occupational asthma. A number of metals can induce sensitization and asthma, including chromium, cobalt, nickel, platinum, and zinc. Enzymes pose significant risks for occupational asthma (Heederik et al., 2002). Examples include α-amylase among bakery workers and subtilisin, a protease used in laundry detergents (Houba et al., 1998). The enzyme production industry has had to adopt strict environmental and process controls to reduce the incidence of occupational asthma in their production facilities.

Those working with animals or animal products are at increased risk of developing allergy (Elliott et al., 2005) and occupational asthma (Pacheco et al., 2003). Animal handlers, processors, and laboratory technicians who work with animals can become immunologically sensitized to urine or salivary proteins in many

vertebrates; proteins in bat guano and bird droppings; animal dander; serum proteins in blood products; dust from horns, antlers, and tusks; or the shells of crustaceans. Very high rates of sensitization can occur in shellfish processors (Glass et al., 1998). Arthropods such as insect larvae, cockroaches, mites, or weevils are recognized inducers of work-related asthma. Plants and plant products (e.g., soy flour, spices, and coffee beans) can also cause asthma among workers. In a variety of occupations, exposure to fungi, especially of the genera Aspergillus, Penicillium, Rhizopus, Mucor, and Paecilomyces, are associated with allergic rhinitis and asthma. These are especially present in sawmills, woodchip handling, and composting facilities (Duchaine et al., 2000; Eduard et al., 1992; Halpin et al., 1994). Apart from the contaminating microorganisms, certain woods themselves produce chemical sensitizing agents. Examples include western red cedar, redwood, and some tropical hardwoods.

Asthma emerged in the 1980s as a major occupational health concern among health-care workers. In order to reduce the risk of hepatitis B and other infectious diseases, health-care workers adopted the use of natural rubber latex gloves for barrier protection. Proteins from the latex of the rubber tree, Hevea braziliensis, led to immunologic sensitization. Thirteen of these high-molecular-weight proteins have now been characterized as allergens (Bernstein et al., 2003). Many other plants of less commercial value produce a similar milky fluid when cut and have similar sensitizing properties. A shift to powder-free and nonlatex examination gloves has reduced the incidence of latex allergy among health-care workers and patients.

Studies of asthma prevalence in occupational settings with exposure to low-molecular-weight agents have suggested prevalence rates of 5–10% for toluene diisocyanate (Baur, 1996; Becklake et al., 2006), 3.2–18% for anhydrides (Venables et al., 1985; Wernfors et al., 1986), 4% for plicatic acid from western red cedar (Chan-Yeung et al., 1984), and 54% in a platinum refinery (Venables et al., 1989). For high-molecular-weight allergens, prevalence

Table 33-6

Rate of Nonfatal Occupational Illnesses 2001. Rate Per 10,000 Workers.

INDUSTRY DIVISION	RESPIRATORY CONDITIONS DUE TO TOXIC AGENTS*	DUST DISEASES OF THE LUNG	POISONING	SKIN DISEASES OR DISORDERS†
Manufacturing	2.4	0.2	0.8	9.3
Durable goods	2.7	0.3	1.2	10.1
Nondurable goods	1.8	0.2	0.3	8.1
Construction	0.8	0.1	0.2	2.3
Mining	0.3	1.7	0.1	0.2
Agricultural production‡	0.9	0.2	0.2	12.5
Forestry services	1.3	<0.05	<0.05	42.2
Transportation, public utilities	2.1	0.2	0.2	2.4
Services§	2.1	0.1	0.2	4.8
Wholesale and retail trade	0.8	0.1	0.2	1.4
Finance, insurance, real estate	1.0	<0.05	0.2	0.9
Total, all private industry	1.6	0.1	0.3	4.3
Number of reported cases	14,500	1300	2800	38,900

*These conditions are pneumonitis, pharyngitis, rhinitis, and acute congestions due to chemicals, dusts, gases, or fumes.
†These conditions are contact dermatitis, eczema, or rash caused by primary irritants and sensitizers or poisonous plants; oil acne; friction blisters, chrome ulcers; and inflammation.
‡Excludes farms with fewer than 11 employees.
§Includes auto repair, other repair, health care, hotel, personal, business, entertainment, educational, social, and engineering services.
SOURCE: Bureau of Labor Statistics, U.S. Department of Labor, 2006.

Table 33-7

U.S. Asthma Prevalence by Usual Industry and Smoking Status for Selected Industry Codes*

	ASTHMA PREVALENCE, %	
INDUSTRY	NONSMOKERS	CURRENT SMOKERS
General merchandise stores	13.0	14.7
Food, bakery and dairy stores	12.8	11.7
Furniture, lumber and wood products	12.5	5.7
Trucking service and warehousing	10.7	10.1
Health services except hospitals	10.2	12.1
Primary metal industries	10.1	10.5
Transportation equipment	10.0	9.9
Fabricated metal industries	9.7	11.1
Hospitals	8.8	9.1
Wholesale trade	7.4	8.9
Printing, publishing and allied industries	7.2	5.9
Textile mill and finished textile products	6.2	3.5
Construction	5.7	4.7
Repair services	5.0	10.9
Agriculture	4.4	5.0
Chemicals and allied products	3.7	2.8

*The U.S. adult self-reported lifetime asthma prevalence rate is 11.6% for males and 14.9% for females and the prevalence rate for current asthma is 6.1% for males and 10.0% for females (BRFSS, 2004).
SOURCE: National Health Interview Survey, Work-related Lung Diseases Surveillance Report 2003.

among shellfish processors was estimated at 21–26% (Desjardin et al., 1995; Glass et al., 1998), 11–44% among lab animal workers (Cullinan et al., 1994; Fuortes et al., 1996, 1997; Hollander et al., 1997), and 5–7% among bakers exposed to wheat and alpha-amylase (Houba et al., 1998). Surveillance through the NIOSH SENSOR program in California, Massachusetts, Michigan, and New Jersey indicates that of over 2500 cases reported in 1993–1999, 20% were for work-aggravated asthma and 80% for new-onset asthma (NIOSH, 2003).

Agricultural workers exposed to grain dust, cotton dust, or atmospheres in swine or poultry confinement barns are at risk for the development of an asthma-like syndrome. This syndrome is an acute nonallergic airway response characterized by self-limited inflammation with neutrophilic infiltrates and increased proinflammatory cytokines and chemokines (e.g,. TNFα, IL-6, and IL-8) but it does not include persistent airway hyperreactivity, as in occupational asthma (Schenker et al., 1998). Asthma-like syndrome includes cough, mild dyspnea, fever, malaise, and cross-shift declines in lung function. Endotoxin in combination with other inflammatory bioaerosols is the likely etiologic agent (Douwes et al., 2003; Schwartz et al., 1994; Schwartz et al., 1995).

Other Occupational Diseases

Occupational diseases of the skin are common but less often fatal that those of the respiratory system. Irritant dermatitis and allergic contact dermatitis have the highest incidence of reported skin conditions. Table 33-6 shows data for rates of skin diseases or disorders in 2001 by industry division. These data indicate that forestry services, agricultural production, and manufacturing carrying the highest risks. However, three-quarters (29,500) of the 38,900 cases reported in 2001 were among workers in the manufacturing and service industries.

Occupational toxicants may induce diseases in a variety of body sites distant from the lung or skin. These include tumors arising in the liver, bladder, gastrointestinal tract, or hematopoietic system and are attributable to a variety of chemical classes. Further discussion of other occupational diseases and the toxicants listed in Table 33-3 can be found in the relevant chapters in Units 4 and 5 of this text.

Nervous system damage can be central, peripheral, or both. It may be acute, as with some organophosphate exposures, or chronic, as with organomercury poisoning or acrylamide-induced neuropathy. Injury affecting the immune system may arise from the immunosuppressive effects of chemicals such as dioxins or toxic metals. Many occupational diseases of the immune system occur due to hypersensitivity leading to respiratory or dermal allergy or systemic hypersensitivity reactions. Autoimmune syndromes have been associated with occupational exposures to crystalline silica and vinyl chloride.

Occupational diseases of the cardiovascular system include atherosclerosis, a variety of arrhythmias, problems with coronary blood supply, systemic hypotension, and cor pulmonale (right ventricular hypertrophy usually due to pulmonary hypertension as with chronic obstructive pulmonary disease). Liver diseases such as carbon tetrachloride-induced fatty liver and hepatocellular death due to toxic concentrations of acetaminophen have classically been used to illustrate chemical mechanisms of cellular injury leading to organ failure. These are thoroughly discussed in Chap. 13. Occupational diseases of the reproductive system can be gender- and organ-specific; but several toxicants—including carbon disulfide, lead, and vinyl chloride—may affect both sexes.

Exposures to infectious agents are a part of a variety of occupations (Thorne and Duchaine, 2007. Veterinarians, health-care workers, and biomedical researchers studying infectious agents have exposures that are largely known and infection control strategies can limit their risks. For others, such as farmers and foresters, specific risks may be less obvious. Zoonotic diseases such as Q-fever, rabies, leptospirosis, and brucellosis may affect abattoir workers, zookeepers, animal handlers, and veterinarians. Foresters, field biologists, and natural resource workers who spend time in wooded areas experience tick- and mosquito-borne illnesses at a higher frequency than that of the general population. These illnesses include the arboviral encephalitides, Rocky Mountain spotted fever, Lyme disease, and ehrlichiosis. Occupational infections may arise as a result of work settings bringing people into close proximity with other people or animals, thus facilitating the transmission of microorganisms. Occupational infectious diseases attributable to the clustering of people affect workers in such facilities as day care centers, schools, healthcare settings, correctional facilities, dormitories, military barracks, or shelters for the homeless, among others. Industrial settings can place large numbers of workers in a shared space, leading to increased transmission of diseases. This is especially true for diseases with annual outbreaks, such as influenza and Norwalk-like viruses. Exposures to chemicals may increase the susceptibility of workers to infection through irritation of mucosa or the pulmonary epithelium or through immunosuppression leading to impaired host defense.

Both industrial and nonindustrial occupational environments may pose occupational hazards due to the presence of chemical or biological agents. Reports of work environments with ineffective ventilation or decreased ventilation rates and increased utilization of synthetic building materials have demonstrated a rise in complaints associated with occupancy in buildings. In some cases, service sector workers in a problem building develop specific clinical conditions with recognized etiology. This is defined as building-related illness. In other cases, symptoms are nonspecific and disappear when the worker leaves the problem building. When this occurs with sufficient prevalence, it is termed *sick building syndrome*. This can arise from volatile and semivolatile chemicals released from office materials, building materials, floor coverings, furniture, cleaning products, and microorganisms. Office buildings and residential settings comprise a complex ecology consisting of people, molds, mites, volatile organic compounds of microbial and nonmicrobial origin, and sometimes plants, pets, cockroaches, and other vermin (Thorne and Heederik, 1999b). Molds, house dust mites, and animal proteins are potent human allergens that can lead to allergy and asthma. Exposure to chemicals and biomolecules such as endotoxin may enhance this process (Douwes *et al.*, 2003). Workers in laboratory animal facilities exhibit a high prevalence of allergy to rodent urinary proteins. In some cases, the occupied space of a building may be clean and dry, but local amplification sites for molds may develop. These may arise in ventilation systems, utility closets, subfloors or basements that serve as return air plenums, or in local sites of water damage. Such sites can become sources of microorganisms and aeroallergens of sufficient volume to generate significant bioaerosol exposures throughout the environment. Airborne viruses, bacteria, and fungi are responsible for a variety of building-related illnesses arising from organisms that are pathogenic to humans. Nonpathogenic microorganisms may induce symptoms or diseases through inflammatory processes, by stimulating the immune response, or by releasing noxious odors, allergenic compounds, or bioactive macromolecules. These may combine with industrial chemicals released into the air to create complex exposure environments.

TOXICOLOGIC EVALUATION OF OCCUPATIONAL AGENTS

Evaluation of Occupational Risks

In most instances of prolonged exposure to low levels of chemicals, there is a continuum between being healthy and being ill. The exposures may impart biochemical or functional changes that are without signs or symptoms, subclinical changes, or in cases of more significant toxicity, manifest as clinical disease. The health significance of the identified changes resulting from exposure to a particular agent must be assessed in order to determine which effects are adverse. Following this assessment, one must consider the interindividual variability or susceptibility factors that influence the risks. There is no one single dose-effect relationship but a distribution of responses. Therefore, in order to recommend an acceptable exposure level to an industrial chemical, one must attempt to define the risk associated with adverse effects in the most sensitive populations exposed. It then remains to be determined what proportion of exposed subjects may still develop an adverse effect at the proposed acceptable exposure level. This acceptable risk level will vary according to a value judgment of the severity, permanence, and equality of the potential adverse effects and the characteristics of the most susceptible population. Clearly, inhibition of an enzyme without functional consequences will be viewed as more acceptable than a more serious toxic effect, such as teratogenicity leading to a congenital malformation in the offspring of the exposed individual.

Establishing Causality   In complex occupational environments, it may be difficult to establish a causal relationship between a toxic substance and a disease. For this reason a number of systematic approaches have been devised to help define causation. In 1890, Robert Koch proposed postulates for "proving" that a specific organism caused a specific disease. T. M. Rivers extended this approach to viruses in 1937. Sir Austin Bradford Hill suggested epidemiologic criteria for assessing causality in 1965 considering strength, specificity, consistency, temporality, exposure period, exposure gradients, and biological plausibility of the associations. These schema and modern weight-of-evidence determination criteria were later combined to suggest a set of postulates for the evaluation of evidence for disease agents in organic dust (Donham and Thorne, 1994). A matrix was developed and is extended here to evaluate the weight of evidence for a causal association between a toxicant and an occupational disease (Fig. 33-2). Evidence from well-conducted in vitro studies, animal studies, human challenge studies, case reports, and epidemiologic investigations are evaluated with regard to data quality and clarity of evidence in support of the establishment of causality. This evaluation is guided by seven criteria (shown in blue). If a chemical were thoroughly studied in animals, humans, and in vitro studies and produced clear and convincing evidence of an exposure–response relationship in controlled studies that used appropriate models and relevant endpoints, that would constitute compelling evidence of a causal relationship between that chemical and that disease. Figure 33-2 reminds us that a consortium of study types contributes data used for the evaluation of occupational hazards. These are discussed below.

To evaluate with some degree of confidence the level of exposure at which the risk of health impairment is acceptable, a body of toxicologic information is required. Five sources of data may be available to inform the occupational risk-assessment process.

	Assessment of Exposure to Specific Agents	Consideration or Control of Confounders	Evidence of a Dose-Response Relationship	Consistent Results From Different Studies	Objective Clinical Data	Endpoints Related to Human Pathology	Appropriate Subjects or Models
In Vitro Studies	▓▓				▓▓		
Animal Studies					▓▓		
Human Challenge Studies						▓▓	
Case Studies						▓▓	▓▓
Epidemiology Studies						▓▓	

For each type of study listed in the first column weight the quality of data from existing studies based on the criteria listed in the column headings as follows:

0	No evidence or condition is not met
1	Equivocal evidence or condition is partially met
2	Some evidence or condition is mostly met
3	Clear evidence or condition is convincingly met

Figure 33-2. Matrix for assessing the strength of an association between a toxicant and an occupational disease.

- In vitro assays
- Animal toxicology studies
- Human challenge studies
- Case reports
- Epidemiology studies

In Vitro Assays A number of useful in vitro assays have been developed over the past several decades in order to provide screening data and, in some cases, mechanistic insight without the need or expense of exposing animal or human subjects. While at this time there are few validated methods to determine complex toxicologic responses such as immune hypersensitivity or peripheral neuropathy, there are validated and very useful screening assays. Notable examples are the *Salmonella typhimurium* reverse mutation assay, or Ames test, the Corrositex assay for dermal corrosivity potential of chemicals (ICCVAM, 2003; NIH-99-4495, 1999), and the in vitro ocular toxicity test for identifying severe irritants and corrosives (ICCVAM, 2006). In addition, quantitative structure–activity relationships can help suggest potential toxicologic effects for an unstudied compound if structurally similar compounds have been evaluated.

Animal Toxicology Studies Animal toxicology studies serve an important function in terms of identifying adverse effects, providing mechanistic data, establishing dose-response relationships, and aiding the process of establishing standards. Because animal studies can be conducted before there is any human exposure, these studies play an important role in hazard identification and prevention of human disease. There are numerous animal models for occupational injury and illness; these are described throughout this textbook in the context of the affected organ system and the classes of toxicants. Generation of animal toxicology data to predict health effects in workers is a central function of experimental toxicologists.

Toxicologic investigations using animals often serve to establish a tentative acceptable exposure level. Other important information that may also be derived from these investigations concerns the relationships between the metabolic handling of the chemical and its interactions with target molecules (mechanism of action), identification of methods for biological monitoring of exposure and early health effects, and identification of preexisting pathologic states that may increase susceptibility to the chemical. However, animal testing can provide only an estimate of the toxicity of a chemical for humans. Animals do not always respond to a chemical exposure in the same way as humans. For instance, there are very significant species and strain differences in responsiveness to aryl hydrocarbon receptor agonists such as polychlorinated dibenzo-p-dioxins (Abnet *et al.*, 1999; Boverhof *et al.*, 2006). In some instances, interspecies differences in metabolism or mechanism of action cause certain chemicals to induce cancer in rodents but not in humans. One such example is kidney cancer, attributable to the accumulation of a rat-specific protein (α_{2u}-globulin) in proximal tubular cells, and produced in male rats chronically exposed to unleaded gasoline (Hard *et al.*, 1993). There are a few compounds for which predictive animal models have not been found. As discussed further, skin and internal cancers caused in humans by excessive oral exposure to inorganic arsenic were not reproduced during classic carcinogenicity studies in animals (ATSDR, 2005).

Human Challenge Studies Human challenge studies, or clinical exposure studies, are a useful approach for verifying findings from animal toxicology studies in humans and for establishing whether biotransformation pathways in the animal models represent those in exposed humans. Human challenge studies with occupational toxicants are usually designed to answer very specific questions regarding rates of uptake, biotransformation pathways, the time course of metabolite excretion during and after exposure, evaluation of the threshold concentration for sensory responses (odor, irritation of the nasal mucosa, etc.), and acute effects of toxicant exposure on perception, vigilance, and function. Human challenge studies help to establish biomarkers of exposure. For reversible conditions, they can be useful for testing therapeutic options. They may also be useful for investigating bronchial hyperresponsiveness to inhaled agents. Extreme caution must be exercised to ensure the safety of research subjects. Idiosyncratic responses can cause a subject to be exceptionally sensitive. For inhalation studies, equipment malfunction can result in overexposure, so real-time exposure monitoring is a necessity. In the past 25 years, there have been several serious injuries and fatalities associated with human challenge studies. These have been attributed to hypersensitivity reactions and generally used mock workplace simulations without rigorous control and monitoring of exposures, as is the current standard of practice. Thus, such studies should be undertaken only when the same results cannot be obtained through other means and under circumstances in which the risk for volunteers can reasonably be estimated as negligible.

Case Reports When new toxicants, new combinations of toxicants, or changes in process conditions occur in the workplace, a case or outbreak of cases can occur. These may be identified through workplace surveillance systems or through workers associating their disease with workplace exposures. In some cases, the problem is identified quickly and resolved, while others take years to resolve. These are often published as case reports and may give rise to animal or epidemiologic studies. Cases of hypersensitivity pneumonitis among machinists exposed to metalworking fluids contaminated with mycobacteria is but one recent example (Thorne *et al.*, 2006, Weiss *et al.*, 2002). NIOSH has a Health Hazard Evaluation (HHE) program in place in which employees or their authorized representatives or employers at a job site can request an investigation to evaluate a potentially hazardous situation. This program issues HHE Reports to disseminate information regarding the hazard. NIOSH also publishes NIOSH Alerts, Criteria Documents, Special Occupational Hazard Reviews, Occupational Hazard Assessments, and Current Intelligence Bulletins. While useful for hazard identification, case reports and HHE Reports do not establish incidence or prevalence of diseases associated with an occupational hazard.

Epidemiology Studies Epidemiology studies help to unravel the associations between occupational diseases, exposures, and personal risk factors. Exposure may be characterized using a surrogate measure such as job classification or via questionnaire, or more directly through exposure monitoring or biomonitoring. Adverse effects may be expressed in terms of mortality, incidence or prevalence of clinical disease, irreversible or reversible functional changes, or critical biological changes.

Several types of epidemiologic studies are used to gather data on the association of workplace exposures with human disease. Cross-sectional studies compare disease prevalence or health status between groups of workers classified according to job title, work site, or exposure status. Cohort studies compare exposed workers versus unexposed or less exposed workers either prospectively or retrospectively in order to associate the occurrence of disease with exposure. Because many occupational diseases have a long induction period or occur only rarely, prospective cohort studies may require a long time and need a large number of subjects to establish significant findings. Retrospective cohort studies can resolve the latency problem but require that relevant exposure data have been collected over time. In the absence of measured exposures, job titles, tasks routinely performed, and years of employment may allow exposure categorization (e.g., low, medium, high). Exposure misclassification is frequently a problem in retrospective studies.

Case-control studies are useful for investigating rare diseases or diseases with long induction periods. As the name suggests, case-control studies compare workers with disease to workers without disease with regard to their past exposure intensity, frequency, and duration, plus other postulated risk factors. In some instances where the exposure–disease relationship is not understood, it may be difficult to identify an appropriate control group. Case-control studies are strongest when accompanied by a rich data set of measured exposures to the candidate causative agents spanning the relevant exposure period. If exposure history is assessed by questionnaire after workers have developed adverse health effects, there arises the potential for recall bias in which those with disease may recall past exposures differently than those who are free of disease. Error can also arise due to selection bias if those who agree to participate in the study are not representative of the population of interest.

Characteristics of observational epidemiology studies are listed in Table 33-8. Occupational epidemiology studies assess relationships between exposures and human health outcomes and, therefore, are particularly useful for risk assessment. Confounding may arise due to exposures of risk factors not associated with the work environment.

Because measures of effect may be subtle and may overlay a background level of incidence, results generally require sophisticated statistical comparisons between a group of exposed workers and a similar group of workers without the exposure of interest. Ideally, the group of unexposed workers should be matched on variables such as age, race, gender, socioeconomic status, and smoking habits. They should also undergo the same standardized clinical, biological, or physiologic evaluation at the same time as the exposed group. Comparison with the general population is ill-advised because an employed population is a highly selected group and may have a higher degree of physical fitness. Because occupational epidemiologic studies often last for several years, all methods of investigation—such as questionnaires, measurement instruments, and analytic techniques—must be validated and standardized before the start of the study. The number of subjects under study should be chosen based on a sample size calculation to be able to detect a difference between exposed and unexposed subjects (should there be a difference) and should take into account labor turnover and those declining participation in any aspects of the study. If exposures are high enough to induce an adverse effect, it is expected that these studies may permit establishment of the relationship between integrated exposure (intensity × time) and frequency of abnormal results and, consequently, a redefinition of the OEL.

In most cases, occupational epidemiologic studies encompass the collection of samples from the subjects or data obtained through interaction with the subjects. Because this often includes identifiable private information, the confidentiality of the data must be protected. U.S., EU, and international laws require that subjects must always have the right to refuse participation and investigators must have written consent from a duly informed volunteer obtained without coercion.

Table 33-8
Comparison of Epidemiologic Studies and Experimental Exposure Studies

	OBSERVATIONAL EPIDEMIOLOGIC STUDIES	EXPERIMENTAL ANIMAL EXPOSURE STUDIES
Toxicant exposure Character	Reflects true exposure among population at risk Complex and variable in space and time May include nonoccupational exposures to toxicant or related compounds	Controlled to represent major toxicant of interest Usually 1 or 2 test compounds May not reflect complexity of human exposures
Frequency and duration	Work day, work week, and years in that job May be task specific	Acute, sub-acute, sub-chronic, chronic
Exposure route	Inhalation, ingestion, percutaneous, or a combination	Injection, inhalation, oral, or dermal. Rarely a combination by design
Appropriateness of dose	Reflect the actual range of exposure	Often doses studied are far higher than human exposures
Assessment	Environmental sampling or measurement of biomarkers May be retrospective and based on employer records, group-based approaches or questionnaires	Measurement of administered dose with or without measurement of biomarkers Sampling of exposure chamber air for inhalation studies
Species considerations	Humans—cohorts or cases and controls Must protect the safety and confidentiality of subjects	Laboratory animals, usually inbred strains of mice or rats Must ensure proper care and use of animals
Representativeness	May exist a selection bias such that the study population may not represent the occupational work force	Experimental animal species may not represent humans
Relevance to human health	Directly relevant if appropriate outcomes are studied	Relevant if species differences are known Of limited relevance if species or strain effects on absorption, distribution, metabolism, and disease are unknown
Analytical challenges	Selection bias, misclassification, and confounding in characterization of outcomes Within- and between-subject variance may be high	Control of genetics, feeding and housing between exposed and control groups Low variance in outcomes

Animal Toxicology Testing for Establishing Acceptable Levels of Exposure

It is evident that certainty as to the complete safety of a chemical can never be obtained, regardless of the extent of toxicologic investigations performed on animals. Nevertheless, animal studies provide valuable data from which to estimate the level of exposure at which the risk of health impairment is acceptable. Table 33-8 compares the information gained from animal studies to epidemiology studies. To the extent possible, animal studies should employ species for which the metabolic pathways and disease processes reflect those of humans. Guidelines and protocols for assessing experimentally the toxicologic hazards of chemicals have been formulated by various national and international agencies. These tests include local and systemic acute toxicity tests, tests of toxicity following repeated exposure, investigations of metabolism and mechanism of action, short-term tests for detecting potential mutagens and carcinogens, studies of effect on reproduction and of teratogenic activity, chronic studies to detect carcinogenesis and other long-term effects, interaction studies, tests for immunosuppression, and dermal and pulmonary hypersensitivity tests. The need for performing these testing protocols should be carefully evaluated for the inclusion of any occupational toxicant to which workers will be exposed. In selecting the studies most appropriate for safety evaluation, the toxicologist should be guided by an understanding of the following:

- physicochemical properties of the chemical
- potential for the generation of toxic derivatives when the chemical is submitted to heat, pH changes, and UV light
- conditions of use and route of exposure
- type of exposure (continuous, intermittent, or incidental)
- degree of exposure

Toxicologic information already available on other chemicals with similar chemical structure and reactive chemical groups can suggest potential hazards and reactivity.

Conclusions drawn from any toxicologic investigation are useful only if the composition and physical state of the tested preparation is known. This would include the nature and concentration of impurities or degradation products, speciation of inorganic compounds, characterization of physical properties for inhaled materials, and characterization of the vehicle (if any). Sensitive and specific methods of analysis of the chemical in solution, air, and biological material should also be available. The assessment of the toxicity of malathion conducted in the 1970s illustrates this point. Malathion is an organophosphate insecticide that normally has relatively low human toxicity. This pesticide was responsible for a 1976 episode of mass poisoning among malaria workers in Pakistan because the specific product contained impurities (mainly isomalathion) capable of inhibiting tissue and plasma carboxyesterases (Baker *et al.*,

1978; Aldridge *et al.*, 1979). The toxicity evaluation for malathion had not anticipated isomalathion coexposure.

The duration of tests necessary to establish an acceptable level for occupational exposure is primarily a function of the type of toxic action suspected. It is generally recognized that for systemically acting chemicals, subacute and short-term toxicity studies are usually insufficient for proposing OELs. Subacute and short-term toxicity tests are usually performed to find out whether the compound exhibits immunotoxic properties and cumulative characteristics. They also aid in selection of the doses for long-term-exposure studies and the kind of tests that may be most informative when applied during long-term exposures. A number of studies have drawn attention to the fact that the reproductive system may also be the target organ of industrial chemicals (e.g., glycol ethers, styrene, lead, dibromochloropropane). Thus, studies designed to evaluate reproductive effects and teratogenicity should also be considered during routine toxicologic testing of occupational toxicants.

Information derived from exposure routes similar to those experienced by workers is clearly the most relevant. For airborne pollutants, inhalation exposure studies provide the basic data on which provisional OELs are based. Experimental methodology is much more complicated for inhalation studies than for oral administration experiments and requires more specialized equipment and expertise (Thorne, 2000). For example, in the case of exposure to an aerosol, particle size distribution must be evaluated and the degree of retention in the respiratory tract of the animal species under study should be established. Ideally, particle size should be selected according to the deposition pattern of dry or liquid aerosols in the particular animal species used in order to represent human lung deposition with occupational exposures. Particle deposition and retention curves have been published for human, monkey, dog, guinea pig, rat, and mouse (Asgharian *et al.*, 2003; Hsieh *et al.*, 1999; Schlesinger, 1985). Recent research coupling asymmetric multiple-path models of the bronchial tree and ventilation parameters can provide more accurate prediction of site-specific particle deposition (Asgharian and Price, 2006). It should also be kept in mind that the concentration of the material in the air and the duration of exposure do not give a direct estimate of the dose, because retained dose is also dependent on the minute volume and the proportion of inhaled particles retained. Measurement of pulmonary dust retention following exposure to a radiolabeled or fluorescently tagged test aerosol should be performed prior to conducting acute, subchronic, or chronic studies. This allows one to assess deposition and determine whether the selected levels of exposure may overwhelm pulmonary clearance mechanisms (ILSI, 2000; Oberdörster, 2002).

The choice of studies to perform and their routes of administration must be evaluated scientifically for each toxicant. Important considerations include its target sites and mechanism of action, metabolism, the nature of its adverse effects, and how workers are exposed to the toxicant. The morphologic, physiologic, and biological parameters that are usually evaluated, either at regular intervals in the course of the exposure period or at its termination, are described in Units 4 and 5 of this text. Investigations that can make use of specific physiologic or biochemical tests, based on knowledge of the principal target organ or function, produce highly valuable information and increase confidence in the OEL derived from them.

Worker Health Surveillance

The primary objective of worker health surveillance programs is to provide both periodic screening of general health and wellness plus health and exposure monitoring tailored to recognized hazards of the workplace. The monitoring of exposures to toxicants in the workplace may play an important role in detecting excessive exposures before the occurrence of significant biological disturbances and health impairment. A scheme for biological monitoring of exposure and of early biological effects is possible only when sufficient toxicologic information has been gathered from animal or human studies on the mechanism of action and the metabolism of xenobiotics to which workers are exposed. When a new chemical is being used on a large scale, the careful clinical surveillance of workers and monitoring of workplaces should be instituted in order to address three aims: (1) to identify overexposure or adverse effects on the health of the workers and quickly intervene, (2) to evaluate the validity of an existing or proposed OEL, and (3) to test the validity of a proposed method for biological monitoring.

Evaluation of the validity of the proposed OEL derived from animal experiments through workplace surveillance is the major aim because studies and observations on humans are the final basis for deciding whether an OEL set originally on the basis of animal toxicity testing is truly acceptable as one that will not produce excess health risks. This means that sensitive clinical, biochemical, physiologic, or behavioral tests for detecting an adverse effect of a toxicant should ideally be performed on the workers concurrent with exposure assessment. It is helpful if health surveillance programs can include the same biomarkers as used in prior animal or human exposure studies. Occupational toxicologists and occupational physicians cannot rely solely on the standard diagnostic tools used in clinical medicine, as they were established primarily to reveal advanced pathologic states and not to detect early adverse effects at a stage when they are still reversible. For example, the measurement of serum creatinine is still a widely used clinical test for assessing renal integrity; yet it is known that the glomerular filtration rate of the kidney must be reduced by more than 50% before serum creatinine rises significantly.

The main limitation of current OELs or BEIs is that some are based on limited experimental data or clinical studies in which only late effects have been investigated and correlated with past exposure. Furthermore, several BEIs are derived from the study of external-internal exposure relationships and not from relationships between internal dose and early adverse effects. The validity of an OEL is much stronger if it is based on the study of dose-response relationships in which the dose is expressed in terms of the cumulative target dose and the monitored effect reflects a critical biological event. However, for some chemicals and some adverse effects (e.g., induction of hypersensitivity and possibly genotoxic effects), the frequency of peak exposure may be more important for health risk assessment than the integrated dose. For example, long-term low-level exposures to commercial enzymes rarely induce sensitization. However, a single exposure to a high concentration can produce hypersensitivity and occupational asthma.

In cases where a surveillance program was not instituted before the introduction of a new chemical, it is more difficult to establish the efficacy of the OEL. In this situation, evaluation depends on retrospective cohort studies or case-control studies on workers who have already sustained exposure. Evaluation of a "no observed adverse effect level" (NOAEL) is difficult because information on past exposures is often incomplete and frank effects are generally the focus of retrospective or case-control studies. Provided that a satisfactory assessment of past exposure is possible, cross-sectional studies that rely on preclinical signs of toxicity may, to a certain extent, overcome these difficulties. Whether or not clinical investigations are planned from the introduction of a new chemical or process, it is essential to keep standardized records of occupational histories and exposure. The need may arise for mortality or case history studies in order to answer an urgent question on a suspected risk.

Careful investigation of overexposures resulting from specific incidents such as containment breaches, chemical spills, or vessel or pipe ruptures can provide useful information. Although such observations are usually not helpful for determining the NOAEL in humans, they may indicate whether human symptomatology is similar to that found in animals and may suggest functional or biological tests that might prove useful for routine monitoring of exposed workers.

Linkage of Animal Studies and Epidemiologic Studies

In the field of occupational toxicology, perhaps more than in other areas of toxicology, close cooperation between those conducting animal studies and studies of workers is essential for examining risks associated with overexposure to chemicals and other toxicants. A few examples will serve to illustrate the complementarity of these disciplines.

Several occupational carcinogens have been identified clearly through combined epidemiologic and experimental approaches (IARC, 1987). For example, the carcinogenicity of vinyl chloride was first demonstrated in rats (Viola et al., 1971), and a few years later, epidemiologic studies confirmed the same carcinogenic risk for humans (Creech and Johnson, 1974; Monson et al., 1974). This observation stimulated several investigations on the metabolism of vinyl chloride in animals and on its mutagenic activity in in vitro systems. Identification of vinyl chloride metabolites led to the conclusion that there is microsomal oxidation leading to the formation of an epoxide derivative, which acts as a proximate carcinogen (ATSDR, 2006). This finding triggered further studies on the biotransformation of structurally related halogenated ethylenes, such as vinyl bromide, vinylidene chloride, 1,2-dichloroethene, trichloroethylene, and perchloroethylene (Bonse et al., 1975; Uehleke et al., 1977; Dekant et al., 1987). Comparison of their oncogenic activity in relation to their metabolism suggested that an interplay between the stability and reactivity in reaching the DNA target and reacting with it after being formed would determine their genotoxic risk. It is now recognized that vinyl chloride produces promutagenic etheno-DNA adducts including etheno-guanine, etheno-cytosine, and lesser amounts of etheno-adenine (Bolt, 2005; NTP, 2005).

1,3-Butadiene is a known human carcinogen that is used in the manufacture of synthetic rubber products. Experimental studies in rats and mice demonstrated carcinogenicity, with mice being particularly sensitive (NTP, 2005). Subsequent to these findings, 1,3-butadiene was shown to follow the same metabolic pathway in humans as in rats and mice, forming mutagenic and carcinogenic epoxides. That led to cohort and case-control studies establishing 1,3-butadiene as a human carcinogen (NTP, 2005). Recent studies have considered the relative importance of the metabolic pathway leading to formation of the reactive metabolite 1,2-epoxy-3-butene, which reacts with hemoglobin to form 1- and 2-hydroxy-3-butenyl valine adducts (MHBVal) and with DNA to form guanine adducts. Under the assumption of a genotoxic mechanism and cross-species comparisons of hemoglobin and DNA binding, these data facilitate a more informed cancer risk assessment. This analysis suggests that for exposures to 1,3-butadiene, the cancer risk is lower for humans than rats or mice on an equivalent dose basis (Van Sittert et al., 2000).

Furthermore, this work illustrates that the measurement of the MH-BVal adducts is a sensitive method for monitoring 1,3-butadiene metabolism via the epoxide-forming pathway in workers.

In 1973, an outbreak of peripheral neuropathy occurred in workers exposed to the solvent methyl butyl ketone (MBK) (McDonough, 1974; Allen et al., 1975). The same lesion was reproduced in animals (Mendell et al., 1974; Spencer et al., 1975). Biotransformation studies were then undertaken in rats and guinea pigs and some MBK metabolites (2,5-hexanedione, 5-hydroxy-2-hexanone) were also found to possess neurotoxic activity (Spencer and Schaumburg, 1975; DiVincenzo et al., 1976; DiVincenzo et al., 1977). Similar oxidation products are formed from n-hexane, the neurotoxicity of which is probably due to the same active metabolite as that produced from MBK. Because methyl isobutyl ketone and methyl ethyl ketone cannot give rise to 2,5-hexanedione, they were suggested as replacement solvents.

These examples demonstrate that studies of the metabolic handling of occupational toxicants in animals are instrumental in the characterization of reactive intermediates and may suggest unsuspected risks or indicate new methods of biological monitoring. Conversely, clinical observations of workers may stimulate studies of the metabolism or the mechanism of toxicity of a toxicant in animals, thereby revealing the health significance of a biological disturbance.

Arsenic is one of the very few compounds for which there are limited data of predictive value from animal studies to human health effects. Arsenic has been used as a medicine since the time of Hippocrates. Initially used to treat ulcers, arsenicals achieved notoriety as medicinals for a wide variety of ailments, and then, in the first half of the twentieth century, for the treatment of syphilis and parasites. Many foods and beverages contaminated with arsenic have been associated with accidental and intentional poisonings. Inorganic pentavalent arsenic (arsenate) is readily absorbed across tissues and converted to the trivalent form (arsenite). This is then methylated to form monomethyl arsenic acid and dimethyl arsenic acid (ATSDR, 2005). These are primarily transported in the blood bound to sulfhydryl groups in proteins. The half-life in humans for arsenic compounds is 2–4 days and the major excretion is via the urine (Nriagu, 1994).

Inorganic arsenic was first noted as a human carcinogen by Hutchinson in 1887 (Hutchinson, 1887). Epidemiologic studies led to classification of arsenic by the IARC as a skin and lung carcinogen in 1980 (IARC, 1980). Since then studies among occupationally exposed populations and populations with high arsenic in their drinking water have shown conclusively that arsenic causes human cancers of the skin, lung, bladder, kidney, liver, nasal tissue, and prostate. There is also evidence for arsenic-associated cutaneous effects, cardiovascular and cerebrovascular disease, diabetes mellitus, and adverse reproductive outcomes (EPA, 2000; WHO, 2001).

A large number of carefully executed cancer bioassays in mice, rats, beagles, and monkeys have been performed using sodium arsenate, sodium arsenite, lead arsenite, arsenic trioxide, and dimethylarsinic acid. These studies have been uniformly negative for cancer. A number of subsequent studies that tested for tumor-promotion activity following dosing with recognized tumor initiators also yielded negative results. Recent studies using transgenic mice, high-dose in utero exposures, or administration of a cocarcinogen have yielded tumors in mice (Hughes, 2006). However, negative results in standard animal carcinogenicity screens have been problematic in the face of unquestionable oncogenic activity in humans.

The examples above demonstrate that the occupational toxicologist cannot rely solely on animal or epidemiologic studies.

A combined approach is necessary in order to identify, elucidate, and prioritize risks and to develop interventions and techniques for worker health surveillance.

EXPOSURE MONITORING

Two important applications of occupational toxicologic investigations are compared below: environmental monitoring and biological monitoring. As described above under "Occupational Health Standards," both are important in worker health surveillance and are essential elements of toxicology studies with dosing via the inhalation or dermal routes.

Environmental Monitoring for Exposure Assessment

An important objective of experimental and clinical investigations in occupational toxicology is the proposal of safe levels of exposure. OELs must be reevaluated at regular intervals as new information on the toxicity of industrial chemicals develops. Adherence to OELs may not protect everyone and, therefore, cannot supplant close medical surveillance of workers. Various private and official institutions regularly review the toxicologic information on chemicals in order to propose or update permissible levels of exposure. These include governmental organizations worldwide and trade organizations such as the ACGIH. A critical element of establishing OELs is the accurate and uniform assessment of exposure. Methodology for exposure assessment must be specifically tailored to the agent under study and the environment in which it appears. To assess airborne exposures for compliance purposes, personal samples taken in the breathing zone are generally used. In a few specific environments, area samples form the basis of an exposure standard (e.g., the OSHA standard for exposure to raw cotton dust specifies use of the vertical elutriator or an equivalent method). Occupational environmental surveys may employ area sampling to determine areas with higher or lower toxicant concentrations. However, concentrations determined from personal samples typically exceed area concentrations, depending on the work practices and environmental controls. For example, geometric mean concentrations of inhalable dust assessed from 159 personal samples in dairy barns were 1.78 mg/m^3, compared with 0.74 mg/m^3 for 252 area samples collected simultaneously in two locations in the same barns (Kullman *et al.*, 1998). Thus, in this environment, area sampling alone would underestimate personal exposures by a factor of 2.4.

Repeated random sampling is theoretically the best approach to developing unbiased measures of exposure. However, this is rarely the approach that is taken. Variability in exposure, especially variability over time, is often large; therefore, a considerable number of repeated measurements are needed to obtain an accurate proxy of the true exposure. When the number of repeats is insufficient, the slope of the exposure–response relationship will be biased, usually leading to considerable underestimation of the relationship (Heederik and Attfield, 2000). Recent studies have demonstrated that group-based approaches, assessing exposures to groups rather than to individuals, are more efficient in terms of measurement effort for obtaining a desired level of accuracy (Vermeulen and Kromhout, 2005). In a group-based approach, workers are grouped by job title, task performed, or through exposure modeling studies to elucidate determinants of exposure, and the group mean is used as the average exposure for each worker (Kromhout *et al.*, 1996). Further statistical modeling of the exposure data can reduce problems of bias and large

temporal and spatial variability (Preller *et al.*, 1995; Tielemans *et al.*, 1998). Whereas this approach is gaining acceptance among occupational epidemiologists for evaluating exposure–response data and assessing risks, it is not accepted for compliance monitoring.

Although one cannot assess dose directly through exposure monitoring, it does have several distinct advantages over biomonitoring. Exposure monitoring allows one to quantify workplace exposure by route through selective air monitoring in the breathing zone of the worker and dermal dosimetry using absorptive material affixed to the workers' skin or clothing. Biomonitoring cannot provide route-specific exposure data. Environmental monitoring techniques are generally less expensive and less invasive than techniques involving the collection and analysis of biological samples such as blood or urine. Thus, a larger population of workers can be studied for the same amount of money. Workers are accustomed to wearing personal samplers for exposure assessment and are generally quite willing to do so. However, they are often unwilling to give a blood or urine sample, fearing that the sample will be surreptitiously used for drug testing, DNA testing, or experimentation. Another benefit of air sampling in the workplace is that spatial, temporal, and work practice associations can be established and can suggest better interventions and engineering controls to reduce exposures. Finally, analytic interferences and variabilities are generally lower with environmental samples than with biological samples.

A fully validated sampling and analysis method requires specification of the sampling methods; sample duration, handling, and storage procedures; the analytic method and measurement technique; the range, precision, accuracy, bias, and limits of detection; quality assurance issues; and known interferences. It is also important to document intralaboratory and interlaboratory variability. Once a standard method is established, it must be closely followed in every detail in order to assure consistency of results.

The development of accurate and precise analytic methods for environmental assessment is an ongoing effort. NIOSH publishes the extensive *NIOSH Manual of Analytical Methods* (NIOSH-NMAM, 2006) and these are widely used. The American Society for Testing Materials (ASTM) has also developed a rigorous system for the establishment of methods. It generally requires 5 or more years to establish a new ASTM method for exposure assessment. The International Organization for Standardization (ISO) is a global federation of national standards bodies with over 150 member countries. The subcommittee on workplace atmospheres is administered by the American National Standards Institute (ANSI). ISO has completed harmonization on a number of air sampling methods—for example, the determination of the number concentration of airborne inorganic fibers by phase contrast optical microscopy. The American Industrial Hygiene Association (AIHA) and the ACGIH publish compilations with descriptions of analytic devices and methodology (Cohen and McCammon, 2001; DiNardi, 2003). Methods have also been developed for bioaerosol exposure assessment and these have been reviewed (Heederik *et al.*, 2003; Thorne and Heederik, 1999a; Willeke and Macher, 1999).

Biological Monitoring for Exposure Assessment

Biomonitoring consists of the measurement of toxicants, their metabolites, or molecular signatures of effect in specimens from humans or animals, including urine, blood, feces, exhaled breath, hair, finger or toenails, bronchial lavage, breast milk, and adipose tissue. These may serve as biomarkers of exposure, biological effect, or susceptibility. New technologies are emerging that will allow measurement and monitoring of chemicals in the body and transmission of the data from indwelling biosensors. Biomonitoring data provide a measurement of exposure based upon internalized dose and, thus, account for all exposures by all routes for the assessed analyte.

Depending on the chemical and the analyzed biological material, the term *internalized dose* may have different meanings. The measured biomarker may reflect the amount of chemical absorbed shortly before sample collection, as with the concentration of a solvent in exhaled air or in a blood sample obtained during the work shift. It may reflect exposure during the preceding day, as with the measurement of a metabolite in blood or urine collected after the end of exposure. For toxicants with a long biological half-life, the measured parameter may reflect exposure accumulated over a period of weeks or months as with arsenic in toenails. *Internal dose* may refer to the amount of chemical stored in one or in several body compartments or in the whole body (*the body burden*).

When biological measurements are available to assess the internal dose, they offer important advantages over monitoring the air of the workplace. The greatest advantage is that the biological measure of exposure is more directly related to the adverse health effects than environmental measurements because it reflects the amount of toxicant absorbed. Therefore, it may offer a better estimate of the risk than can be determined from ambient monitoring. Biological monitoring accounts for uptake by all exposure routes. Many industrial chemicals can enter the organism by absorption through the skin or the gastrointestinal tract as well as the lung. For example, some solvents (e.g., dimethylformamide) and many pesticide formulations exhibit substantial exposure via the dermal route. In these situations, exposures determined through monitoring airborne concentrations underestimate true exposure. Monitoring of an early biomarker of effect is useful when the subjects are exposed to a complex mixture and the agents responsible for the effect are unknown or several agents are working in synergy.

Several factors can influence uptake. Personal hygiene habits vary from one person to another, and there is some degree of individual variation in the absorption rate of a chemical through the lungs, skin, or gastrointestinal tract. Use of size-selective air sampling to determine the inhalable or respirable fraction can strengthen the exposure estimate. However, biological factors such as ventilatory parameters can affect the strength of such a correlation. For example, increased workload can markedly increase the respiratory uptake of an airborne toxicant. Because of its ability to encompass and evaluate the overall exposure (whatever the route of entry), biological monitoring can also be used to test the overall efficacy of personal protective equipment such as respirators, gloves, or barrier creams. Another consideration with biological monitoring is the fact that nonoccupational exposures (through hobbies, residential exposures, dietary habits, smoking, second jobs) may also be expressed in the biological sample. The organism integrates the total external (environmental and occupational) exposure into one internal load. Whereas this is beneficial for worker health and safety, it may be confounding in epidemiologic studies or compliance monitoring. Thus, while biomonitoring is an important exposure measurement tool for health risk assessment, it generally does not allow one to relate sources and levels of exposure to adverse health effects (Albertini *et al.*, 2006).

The value of biological monitoring is heightened when the relationships between external exposure, internal dose, and adverse effects are established. Normally, biological monitoring of exposure cannot be used for assessing exposure to substances that exhibit their toxic effects at the sites of first contact and are poorly absorbed. Examples include dermally corrosive compounds and primary lung irritants. In this situation, the only useful relationship is that between external exposure and the intensity of the local effects.

Relationships between air monitoring and biological monitoring may be modified by genetic or external factors that influence the fate of an occupational toxicant in vivo. Metabolic interactions can occur when workers are exposed simultaneously to chemicals that are biotransformed through identical pathways. Exposure to chemicals that modify the activity of the biotransformation enzymes (e.g., microsomal enzyme inducers or inhibitors) may also influence the fate of another compound. Furthermore, metabolic interferences may occur between occupational toxicants and alcohol, tobacco, food additives, prescription drugs, natural product remedies, or recreational drugs. Changes in any of several biological variables (weight, body mass, pregnancy, diseases, immune status, etc.) may modify the metabolism of an occupational chemical. These factors have to be taken into consideration when the results of biomonitoring are interpreted. Whatever the parameter measured, whether it is the substance itself, its metabolite, or an early biomarker of effect, the test must be sufficiently sensitive and specific to provide meaningful data in the range of workplace exposures.

Some chemicals have a long biological half-life in various body compartments (e.g., hydrophobic persistent organic pollutants) and the time of sampling may not be critical. For other chemicals, the time of sampling is critical because, following exposure, the compounds or their metabolites may be rapidly eliminated from the body. In these cases, the biological sample is usually collected during exposure, at the end of the exposure period, or sometimes just before the next work shift. When biological monitoring consists of the sampling and analysis of urine, it is usually performed on "spot" urine specimens or on the first morning void. It is a standard practice for most organic compounds to adjust the results for urine output by expressing the results per gram of creatinine in the urine. Analyses performed on very dilute urine samples are not reliable. The WHO has specified acceptable limits for urine specimens of between 0.3 and 3.0 g/L creatinine or 1.010–1.030 specific gravity (ACGIH, 2006). When samples exhibit large interindividual variability or high "background" levels the interpretation of a single measurement may be difficult. In such cases, it may be useful to analyze biological material collected before and after the exposure period and gauge exposure based upon the cross-shift change.

The majority of BEIs listed by the ACGIH refer to analysis of the parent compound or its phase I metabolite. Analytical advances over the past decade have yielded methods for detecting reactive intermediates of metabolism and macromolecular adducts that may induce mutations or cell cycle disruption. These methods are important for comparing human and animal toxicity data for risk assessment and may help to explain differential responses in animal models and susceptibility in human populations. These methods are also useful for occupational health surveillance programs.

Environmental monitoring plays an important role in the evaluation and prevention of excessive exposure to toxicants in the workplace. However, the prevention of acute toxic effects on the respiratory tract, skin, or eye mucosa can only be achieved by keeping the concentration of the irritant substance below a certain level or by eliminating the exposure. Local acute effects of chemicals do not lend themselves to a biological surveillance program. Likewise, biological monitoring is usually not indicated for detecting peak exposure to dangerous chemicals such as arsine (AsH_3), carbon monoxide, or prussic acid (HCN). Furthermore, identification

Table 33-9

Control Approaches for Occupational Inhalation Hazards

Change the process to use or produce less hazardous compounds.
Automate and enclose the process to isolate the compounds.
Incorporate administrative and work practice controls to reduce duration or intensity of exposure.
Install or upgrade local exhaust systems and dilution exhaust.
Institute a comprehensive program for personal protective equipment use where necessary.

of emission sources and the evaluation of the efficiency of engineering control measures are usually best performed by ambient air analysis. Table 33-9 lists the approaches most useful for controlling inhalation exposures in the workplace. It should be emphasized that process changes and application of engineering controls are preferable to reliance on personal protective equipment.

In summary, environmental and biological monitoring should not be regarded as opposites but as complementary elements of an occupational health and safety program. They should be integrated as much as possible to ensure low levels of contaminants and optimal health for workers.

CONCLUSION

The working environment will always have the potential to overexpose workers to various toxicants. Recognition of these risks should not wait until epidemiologic studies have uncovered hazardous levels. A combined experimental, clinical, and epidemiologic approach is most effective for evaluating and managing the potential risks. One can then promulgate scientifically based occupational health standards, apply effective workplace controls to ensure adherence to those standards, and institute worker health surveillance programs to identify unexpected effects in susceptible individuals.

REFERENCES

Abnet CC, Tanguay RL, Heideman W, Peterson RE: Transactivation activity of human, zebrafish, and rainbow trout aryl hydrocarbon receptors expressed in COS-7 cells: Greater insight into species differences in toxic potency of polychlorinated dibenzo-*p*-dioxin, dibenzofuran, and biphenyl congeners. *Toxicol Appl Pharmacol* 159(1):41–51, 1999.

ACGIH: *2006 TLVs and BEIs: Threshold Limit Values for Chemical Substances and Physical Agents and Biological Exposure Indices.* Cincinnati, OH: American Conference of Governmental Industrial Hygienists, 2006.

Albertini R, Bird M, Doerrer N, et al: The use of biomonitoring data in exposure and human health risk assessments. *Environ Health Perspect* 114:1755–1762, 2006.

Aldridge WN, Miles JM, Mount DL, Verschoyle RD: The toxicological properties of impurities in malathion. *Arch Toxicol* 42:95–106, 1979.

Allen N, Mendell JR, Billmaier DJ, et al: Toxic polyneuropathy due to methyl n-butylketone. *Arch Neurol* 32:209–218, 1975.

Asgharian B, Kelly JT, Tewksbury EW: Respiratory deposition and inhalability of monodisperse aerosols in Long-Evans rats. *Toxicol Sci* 71:104–111, 2003.

Asgharian B, Price OT: Airflow distribution in the human lung and its influence on particle deposition. *Inhal Toxicol* 18:795–801, 2006.

ATSDR (Agency for Toxic Substances and Disease Registry): *Draft Toxicological Profile for Arsenic.* Atlanta: Department of Health and Human Services, 2005. Available at http://atsdr.cdc.gov/toxprofiles/tp2.pdf.

ATSDR (Agency for Toxic Substances and Disease Registry): *Toxicological Profile for Vinyl Chloride.* Atlanta: Department of Health and Human Services, 2006. Available at http://atsdr.cdc.gov/toxprofiles/tp20.pdf.

Baker EL, Zack M, Miles JV, et al.: Epidemic malathion poisoning in Pakistan malaria workers. *Lancet* 1:31–33, 1978.

Balazy A, Toivola M, Adhikari A, et al.: Do N95 respirators provide 95% protection level against airborne viruses, and how adequate are surgical masks? *Am J Infection Control* 34:51–57, 2006.

Bason M, Lammintausta K, Maibach HI: Irritant dermatitis (irritation), in Marzulli FN, Maibach HI (eds.): *Dermatotoxicology,* 4th ed. New York: Hemisphere, 1991, pp. 223–252.

Baur X. Occupational asthma due to isocyanates. *Lung* 174:23–30, 1996.

Becklake MR, Malo JL, Chan-Yeung M: Epidemiological approaches in occupational asthma, in Bernstein IL et al. (eds.) *Asthma in the Workplace,* 3d ed. New York: Taylor & Francis Group, 2006, pp. 37–77.

Bernstein DA, Biagini RE, Karnani R, et al.: In vivo sensitization to purified Hevea brasiliensis proteins in health care workers sensitized ti natural rubber latex. *J Allergy Clin Immunol* 111:610–616, 2003.

Bernstein IL, Bernstein DI, Chan-Yeung M, Malo JL: Definition and classification of asthma in the workplace, in Bernstein IL et al. (eds): *Asthma in the Workplace, 3d* ed. New York: Taylor & Francis Group, 2006, pp. 1–4.

Bolt HM Vinyl chloride - a classical industrial toxicant of new interest. *Crit Rev Toxicol* 35:301–323, 2005.

Bonse G, Urban T, Reichert D, Henschler D: Chemical reactivity, metabolic oxirane formation and biological reactivity of chlorinated ethylenes in the isolated perfused rat liver preparation. *Biochem Pharmacol* 24:1829–1834, 1975.

Boverhof DR, Burgoon LD, Tashiro C, et al.: Comparative toxicogenomic analysis of the hepatotoxic effects of TCDD in Sprague Dawley rats and C57BL/6 mice. *Tox Sic* 94:398–416, 2006.

Chan-Yeung M, Vedal S, Kus J, et al.: Symptoms, pulmonary function and bronchial hyperactivity in western red cedar workers compared with those in office workers. *Am Rev Respir Dis* 130:1038–1041, 1984.

Cohen BS, McCammon CS, Jr. (eds): *Air Sampling Instruments for Evaluation of Atmospheric Contaminants,* 9th ed. Cincinnati, OH: American Conference of Governmental Industrial Hygienists, 2001.

Creech JL, Johnson HM: Angiosarcoma of the liver in the manufacture of polyvinylchloride. *J Occup Med* 16:150–151, 1974.

Cullinan P, Lowson D, Nieuwenhuijsen MJ, et al.: Work related symptoms, sensitisation, and estimated exposure in workers not previously exposed to laboratory rats. *Occup Environ Med* 51:589–592, 1994.

Dekant W, Martens G, Vamvakas S, et al.: Bioactivation of tetrachloroethylene. *Drug Metab Dispos* 15:702–709, 1987.

Desjardins A, Malo JL, L'Archevçque J, et al.: Occupational IgE-mediated sensitization and asthma due to clam and shrimp. *J Allergy Clin Immunol* 96:608–617, 1995.

DiNardi SR (ed.): *The Occupational Environment—Its Evaluation and Control.* Fairfax, VA: American Industrial Hygiene Association, 2003.

DiVincenzo GD, Hamilton ML, Kaplan CJ, Dedinas J: Metabolic fate and disposition of ^{14}C-labeled methyl n-butyl ketone in the rat. *Toxicol Appl Pharmacol* 41:547–560, 1977.

DiVincenzo GD, Kaplan CJ, Dedinas J: Characterization of the metabolites of methyl-n-butyl ketone, methyl iso-butyl ketone, and methyl ethyl ketone in guinea pig serum and their clearance. *Toxicol Appl Pharmacol* 36:511–522, 1976.

Donham KJ, Thorne PS: Agents in organic dusts: Criteria for a causal relationship. *Am J Ind Med* 25:33–39, 1994.

Douwes J, Thorne PS, Pearce N, Heederik D: Biological agents—recognition, in Perkins JL (ed): *Modern Industrial Hygiene:* Vol II. *Biological Aspects.* Cincinnati, OH: American Conference of Governmental Industrial Hygienists, pp. 219–292, 2003.

Duchaine C, Meriaux A, Thorne PS, Cormier Y: Assessment of particulates and bioaerosols in Eastern Canadian sawmills. *Am Ind Hyg Assoc J* 61:727–732, 2000.

Eduard W, Sandven P, Levy F: Relationships between exposure to spores from *Rhizopus microsporus* and *Paecilomyces variotii* and serum IgG antibodies in wood trimmers. *Int Arch Allergy Immunol* 97:274–282, 1992.

Elliott L, Heederik D, Marshall S, Peden D, Loomis D: Incidence of allergy and allergy symptoms among workers exposed to laboratory animals. *Occup Environ Med* 62:766–771, 2005.

Employment in Europe 2006. European Commission Directorate General for Employment, Social Affairs, and Equal opportunities, October 2006. Available at http://ec.europa.eu/employment_social/news/2006/nov/employment_europe_en.pdf.

EPA. 40 CFR Parts 141 and 142, National primary drinking water regulations; arsenic and clarifications to compliance and new source contaminants monitoring; proposed rule. *Fed Reg* 65(121):38888–38983, 2000.

European Commission. European Commission Directive 95/320/EC, 1995. Available at http://ec.europa.eu/employment_social/health_safety/scoel_en.htm.

European Commission. European Commission Directive 98/24/EC, 1998. Available at http://ec.europa.eu/employment_social/health_safety/scoel_en.htm.

European Union: Employment rates report 1998 Employment performance in the member states. http://europa.eu.int/comm/employment social/empl&est/empL99/rates en.pd f, pp. 1–31, 1998.

Fullerton HN, Jr.: Labor force participation: 75 years of change, 1950–98 and 1998–2025. *Monthly Labor Review* Dec:3–12, 1999.

Fuortes LJ, Weih LA, Jones M, et al.: Epidemiologic assessment of laboratory animal allergy among university employees. *Am J Ind Med* 29:67–74, 1996.

Fuortes LJ, Weih L, Pomrehn P, et al.: Prospective epidemiologic evaluation of laboratory animal allergy among university employees. *Am J Ind Med* 32:665–669, 1997.

GAO/HEHS: Child *Labor in Agriculture—Changes Needed to Better Protect Health and Educational Opportunities.* GAO/HEHS-98-193. Washington, DC: U.S. Government Accountability Office, 1998, pp. 1–90.

Glass WI, Power P, Burt R, et al.: Work-related respiratory symptoms and lung function in New Zealand mussel openers. *Am J Ind Med* 34:163–168, 1998.

Halpin DM, Graneek BJ, Lacey J, et al.: Respiratory symptoms, immunological responses, and aeroallergen concentrations at a sawmill. *Occup Environ Med* 51:165–172, 1994.

Hard GC, Rodgers IS, Baetcke KP, et al.: Hazard evaluation of chemicals that cause accumulation of α_{2u}-globulin, hyaline droplet nephropathy, and tubule neoplasia in the kidneys of male rats. *Environ Health Perspect* 99:313–349, 1993.

Heederik D, Attfield M: Characterization of dust exposure for the study of chronic occupational lung disease: A comparison of different exposure assessment strategies. *Am J Epidemiol* 151(10):982–990, 2000.

Heederik D, Thorne PS, Doekes G: Health-based occupational exposure limits for high molecular weight sensitizers: how long is the road we must travel? *Ann Occup Hyg* 46(5):439–446, 2002.

Heederik D, Thorne PS, Douwes J: Biological agents - monitoring and evaluation of bioaerosol exposure, in Perkins JL (ed): *Modern Industrial Hygiene:* Vol II. *Biological Aspects.* Cincinnati, OH: American Conference of Governmental Industrial Hygienists, pp. 293–327, 2003.

Hollander A, Heederik D, Doekes G: Respiratory allergy to rats: Exposure-response relationships in laboratory animal workers. *Am J Respir Crit Care Med* 155:562–567, 1997.

Houba R, Doekes G, Heederik D: Occupational respiratory allergy in bakery workers: A review of the literature. *Am J Ind Med* 34:529–546, 1998.

Hsieh TH, Yu CP, Oberdorster G: Deposition and clearance models of Ni compounds in the mouse lung and comparisons with the rat models. *Aerosol Sci Technol* 31:358–372, 1999.

Hughes MF: Biomarkers of exposure: a case study with inorganic arsenic. *Environ Health Perspect* 114:1790–1796, 2006.

Hutchinson J: Arsenic cancer. *Br Med J* 2:1280–1281, 1887.

IARC (International Agency for Research on Cancer): *IARC Monographs on the Evaluation of Carcinogenic Risks to Humans.* Suppl 7. Lyons, France: IARC, 1987.

IARC: *Metals and metallic compounds. IARC Monographs on the Evaluation of Carcinogenic Risks to Humans,* Vol 23. Lyon, France: International Agency for Research on Cancer, 1980.

ICCVAM (Interagency Coordinating Committee on the Validation of Alternative Methods). 2003. http://iccvam.niehs.nih.gov/methods/ corrode.htm

ICCVAM (Interagency Coordinating Committee on the Validation of Alternative Methods). 2006. http://iccvam.niehs.nih.gov/methods/ocudocs/otmer102706.pdf

ILSI Risk Science Institute Workshop Participants. The relevance of the rat lung response to particle overload for human health risk assessment: A workshop consensus report. *Inhal Toxicol* 12:1-17: 2000.

Japan Statistical Yearbook 2006. 2006. Statistics Bureau and Statistical Research and Training Institute, Chap. 16. Japanese Ministry of Internal Affairs and Communications. Available at http://www.stat.go.jp.

Kromhout H, Tielemans E, Preller L, Heederik D: Estimates of individual dose from current measurements of exposure. *Occup Hyg* 3:23–39, 1996.

Kullman GJ, Thorne PS, Waldron PF, et al.: Organic dust exposures from work in dairy barns. *Am Ind Hyg Assoc J* 59:403–413, 1998.

McDonough JR: Possible neuropathy from methyl-*n*-butyl ketone. *N Engl J Med* 290:695, 1974.

Mendell JR, Saida K, Ganasia MF, et al.: Toxic polyneuropathy produced by methyl-*n*-butyl ketone. *Science* 185:787–789, 1974.

Monson RR, Peters JM, Johnson MN: Proportional mortality among vinylchloride workers. *Lancet* 2(7877):397–398, 1974.

NIH-99-4495: *Corrositex: An in Vitro Test Method for Assessing Dermal Corrosivity Potential of Chemicals.* NIH-99-4495. Washington, DC: National Toxicology Program, 1999, pp 1–236. Available at http://iccvam.niehs.nih.gov/docs/reports/corprrep.pdf.

NIOSH: *Work-Related Lung Disease Surveillance Report,* 2002. Number 2003-111. Washington, DC: Department of Health and Human Services (NIOSH), 2003. Available at: http://www.cdc.gov/niosh/docs/2003-111/pdfs/2003-111j.pdf.

NIOSH: *Work-Related Lung Disease (eWoRLD) Surveillance System,* 2006. Available at: http://www2a.cdc.gov/drds/WorldReportData/.

NIOSH_NMAM 2006. Available at http://www.cdc.gov/NIOSH/NMAM.

Nriagu JO: *Arsenic in the Environment:* Part II: *Human Health Effects and Ecosystem Effects.* New York: Wiley. 1994, pp 1–91.

NTP (National Toxicology Program): *11th Report on Carcinogens.* Research Triangle Park, NC: National Toxicology Program, U.S. Department of Health and Human Services, 2005. Available at http://ntp.niehs.nih.gov/ntp/roc/roc11.zip.

Oberdörster G.: Toxicokinetics and effects of fibrous and nonfibrous particles Regul. *Toxicol Pharmacol* 27:123–135, 2002.

OSHA. Standard Interpretations: 10/06/1995—8-hour total weight average (TWA) permissible exposure limit (PEL). 1995. Available at http://www.osha.gov/pls/oshaweb/owadisp.show_document?p_table= INTERPRETATIONS&p_id=24470.

Pacheco KA, McCammon C, Liu AH, et al.. Airborne endotoxin predicts symptoms in non-mouse-sensitized technicians and research scientists exposed to laboratory mice. *Am J Respir Crit Care Med* 167:983–990, 2003.

Preller L, Kromhout H, Heederik D, Tielen MJM: Modeling long-term average exposure in occupational exposure-response analysis. *Scand J Work Environ Health* 21:504–512, 1995.

Schenker MB, Christiani D, Cormier Y, et al.: Respiratory health hazards in agriculture. *Am J Respir Crit Care Med* Suppl 158(pt 2):S1–S76, 1998.

Schlesinger RB: Comparative deposition of inhaled aerosols in experimental animals and humans: A review. *J Toxicol Environ Health* 15:197–214, 1985.

Schwartz DA, Thorne PS, Jagielo PJ, *et al.*: Endotoxin responsiveness and grain dust–induced inflammation in the lower respiratory tract. *Am J Physiol* 267:L609–L617, 1994.

Schwartz DA, Thorne PS, Yagla SJ, *et al.*: The role of endotoxin in grain dust–induced lung disease. *Am J Respir Crit Care Med* 152:603–608, 1995.

Spencer PS, Schaumburg HH: Experimental neuropathy produced by 2,5-hexanedione A major metabolite of the neurotoxic industrial solvent methyl-*n*-butyl ketone. *J Neurol Neurosurg Psychiatry* 38:771–775, 1975.

Spencer PS, Schaumburg HH, Raleigh RL, Terhaar CJ: Nervous system degeneration produced by the industrial solvent methyl-n-butyl ketone. *Arch Neurol* 32:219–222, 1975.

Thorne PA, Adamcakova-Dodd A, Kelley KM *et al.*. Metalworking fluid with mycobacteria and endotoxin induces hypersensitivity pneumonitis in mice. *Am J Respir Crit Care Med* 173:759–768; 2006.

Thorne PS, Duchaine C. Airborne bacteria and endotoxin, in Hurst CT, Crawford RL, Garland JL, Lipson DA, Mills AL, Stetzenbach LD (eds): *Manual of Environmental Microbiology*, 3rd Ed., Washington DC: ASM Press, 2007, pp. 989–1004.

Thorne PS, Heederik D: Assessment methods for bioaerosols, in Salthammer T (ed): *Organic Indoor Air Pollutants—Occurrence, Measurement, Evaluation.* Weinheim, Germany: Wiley/VCH, 1999a; pp. 85–103.

Thorne PS, Heederik D: Indoor bioaerosols—Sources and characteristics, in Salthammer T (ed): *Organic Indoor Air Pollutants—Occurrence, Measurement, Evaluation.* Weinheim, Germany: Wiley/VCH, 1999b; pp 275–288.

Thorne PS: Inhalation toxicology models of endotoxin- and bioaerosol-induced inflammation. *Toxicology* 152:13–23, 2000.

Tielemans E, Kupper LL, Kromhout H, *et al.*: Individual-based and group-based occupational exposure assessment: Some equations to evaluate different strategies. *Ann Occup Hyg* 42(2):115–119, 1998.

Uehleke H, Tabarelli-Poplawski S, Bonse G, Henschler D: Spectral evidence for 2,2,3-trichloro-oxirane formation during microsomal trichloroethylene oxidation. *Arch Toxicol* 37:95–105, 1977.

USDL (United States Department of Labor): *The Employment Situation: September 2006 USDL 06–1770.* U.S. Department of Labor, Bureau of Labor Statistics 2000b, pp. 1–26. Available at http://www.bls.gov/news.release/archives/empsit_10062006.pdf.

USDL (United States Department of Labor): *Career Guide to Industries: Agricultural Production.* 2006–07 ed. Washington, DC: U.S. Department of Labor, Bureau of Labor Statistics, http://www.bls.gov/oco/cg/cgs001.htm, 2006a.

U.S. Federal Register. Vol 57, No. 114, June 12, 1992, pp.26539-26590.

van Sittert NJ, Megens HJJJ, Watson WP, Boogaard PJ: Biomarkers of exposure to 1,3-butadiene as a basis for cancer risk assessment. *Toxicol Sci* 56:189–202, 2000.

Venables KM, Dally MB, Nunn AJ, *et al.*: Smoking and occupational allergy in workers in a platinum refinery. *Br Med J* 299:939–942, 1989.

Venables KM, Topping MD, Howe W, *et al.*: Interaction of smoking and atopy in producing specific IgE antibody against a hapten protein conjugate. *Br Med J* 290:201–204, 1985.

Vermeulen R, Kromhout H: Historical limitations of determinant based exposure groupings in the rubber manufacturing industry. *Occup Envir Med* 62:793–799, 2005.

Viola PL, Bigotti A, Caputo A: Oncogenic response of rat skin, lungs, and bones to vinyl chloride. *Cancer Res* 31:516–522, 1971.

Weiss LPC, Lewis R, Rossmoore H, *et al.*: Respiratory illness in workers exposed to metal working fluid contaminated with nontuberculous mycobacteria – Ohio, 2001. *Morb Mortal Wkly Rer* 51:349–352, 2002.

Wernfors M, Nielsen J, Schültz A, Skerfving S: Phthalic anhydride-induced occupational asthma. *Int Arch Allergy Appl Immunol* 79:77–82, 1986.

WHO. *Arsenic and Arsenic Compounds,* 2nd ed. Environmental Health Criteria 224. Geneva, World Health Organization, 2001. Available at http://www.who.int/ipcs/publications/ehc/ehc_224/en/.

Willeke K, Macher J: Air sampling, in Macher J (ed): *Bioaerosols—Assessment and Control.* Cincinnati, OH: American Conference of Governmental Industrial Hygienists, 1999, pp. 11-1–11-25.

INDEX

NOTE: Page numbers followed by a *t* refer to tables and page numbers followed by an *f* indicate figures.